DISEASES OF THE LIVER

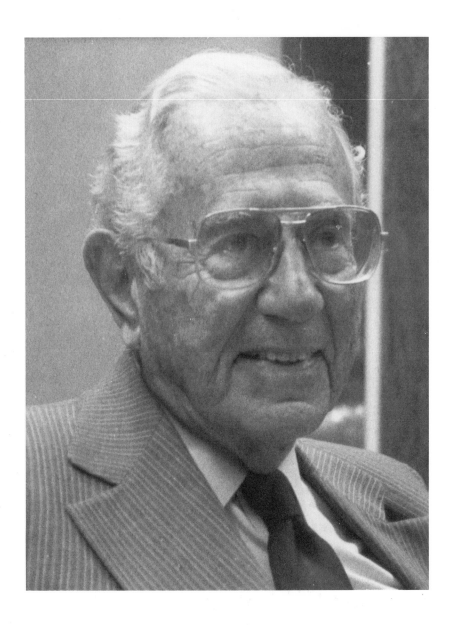

Leon Schiff

SIXTH EDITION

DISEASES OF THE LIVER

Edited by

LEON SCHIFF, M.D., Ph.D.
Emeritus Professor of Medicine
University of Cincinnati
College of Medicine
Cincinnati, Ohio;
Clinical Professor of Medicine
University of Miami Medical School
Miami, Florida

EUGENE R. SCHIFF, M.D.
Chief, Division of Hepatology
University of Miami School of Medicine;
Chief, Hepatology Section
Veterans Administration Medical Center
Miami, Florida

79 Contributors

J. B. LIPPINCOTT COMPANY

Philadelphia

London • Mexico City • New York
St. Louis • São Paulo • Sydney

Sponsoring Editor: Delois Patterson
Manuscript Editor: Leslie E. Hoeltzel
Indexer: Alexandra Weir
Design Coordinator: Susan Hess Blaker
Production Manager: Kathleen P. Dunn
Production Coordinator: Ken Neimeister
Compositor: Tapsco, Inc.
Printer/Binder: Maple Press Company, Inc.

Sixth Edition

6   5   4   3   2

Library of Congress Cataloging-in-Publication Data

Diseases of the liver.

Includes bibliographies and index.
1. Liver—Diseases.   I. Schiff, Leon, 1901–
II. Schiff, Eugene R. [DNLM: 1. Liver Diseases.
W1 700 D615]
RC845.D53   1987   616.3'62   86-21410
ISBN 0-397-50747-X

The authors and publisher have exerted every effort to ensure that drug selection and dosage set forth in this text are in accord with current recommendations and practice at the time of publication. However, in view of ongoing research, changes in government regulations, and the constant flow of information relating to drug therapy and drug reactions, the reader is urged to check the package insert for each drug for any change in indications and dosage and for added warnings and precautions. This is particularly important when the recommended agent is a new or infrequently employed drug.

Dedicated to the memory of Edward A. Gall,
distinguished physician, pathologist, teacher, and devoted colleague,
for his invaluable contributions to the field of liver disease.

Contributors

DAVID H. ALPERS, M.D.

Chief, Gastroenterology Division
Washington University School of Medicine
Washington University Medical Center
St. Louis, Missouri

COLIN E. ATTERBURY, M.D.

Associate Professor of Medicine
Yale University School of Medicine
New Haven, Connecticut
Chief, Intermediate Care Section
West Haven Veterans Administration Medical
  Center
West Haven, Connecticut

WILLIAM F. BALISTRERI, M.D.

Director, Division of Pediatric Gastroenterology
  and Nutrition
Children's Hospital Medical Center
Associate Professor of Pediatrics
University of Cincinnati College of Medicine
Cincinnati, Ohio

JEAN-PIERRE BENHAMOU, M.D.

Professor, Université de Paris
Unité de Recherches de Physiopathologie
  Hépatique (INSERM)
Hôpital Beaujon
Clichy, France

GEORGE BERCI, M.D., F.A.C.S.

Associate Director of Surgery
Cedars-Sinai Medical Center
Clinical Professor of Surgery
University of California School of Medicine
Los Angeles, California

**BARBARA H. BILLING, M.D., Ph.D.,
  F.R.C.Path.**

Professor of Biochemistry Applied to Medicine
  (Emeritus)
Department of Medicine
Royal Free Hospital
London, England

D. MONTGOMERY BISSELL, M.D.

Associate Professor
Department of Medicine
Liver Center Laboratory
University of California
San Francisco, California

**THOMAS H. BOTHWELL, D.Sc., M.D.,
  F.R.C.P., F.R.S.(S.A.), F.A.C.P.(Hon.)**

Professor and Head, Department of Medicine
University of the Witwatersrand Medical School
Chief Physician
Johannesburg Hospital
Director, South African Medical Research Council
Iron and Red Cell Metabolism Unit
Johannesburg, Republic of South Africa

H. WORTH BOYCE, JR., M.D.

Professor of Medicine
Director, Division of Digestive Diseases and
  Nutrition
University of South Florida College of Medicine
Tampa, Florida

JAMES L. BOYER, M.D.

Professor of Medicine
Director, Liver Study Unit
Chief, Division of Digestive Diseases
Yale University School of Medicine
New Haven, Connecticut

ROBERT W. CHARLTON, M.D., F.R.C.P.E.

Vice Principal
University of the Witwatersrand
Senior Physician
Johannesburg Hospital
Johannesburg, Republic of South Africa

ALAN S. COHEN, M.D.

Chief, Department of Medicine
Boston City Hospital
Director, Arthritis Section of Boston University
    School of Medicine
Conrad Wesselhoeft Professor of Medicine
Boston University School of Medicine
Boston, Massachusetts

HAROLD O. CONN, M.D.

Professor of Medicine
Yale University School of Medicine
New Haven, Connecticut
Chief, Liver Research Laboratory
West Haven Veterans Administration Medical
    Center
West Haven, Connecticut

JOHN R. CRAIG, M.D., Ph.D.

Assistant Clinical Professor
University of Southern California School of
    Medicine
Los Angeles, California

JOHN DALY, M.D.

Associate Attending in Surgery
Department of Surgery
Memorial Sloan–Kettering Cancer Center
Assistant Professor of Surgery
Cornell University Medical College
New York, New York

MICHAEL E. DeBAKEY, M.D.

Chancellor
The Olga Keith Wiess Professor of Surgery and
    Chairman
Cora and Webb Mading Department of Surgery
Director, National Heart and Blood Vessel
    Research and Demonstration Center
Baylor College of Medicine
Houston, Texas

KEVIN M. De COCK, M.D., M.R.C.P.(U.K.), DTM&H

Assistant Professor of Medicine
University of Southern California School of
    Medicine
Los Angeles, California

HUGH A. EDMONDSON, M.D.†

Emeritus Professor of Pathology
University of Southern California School of
    Medicine
Los Angeles, California

MURRAY EPSTEIN, M.D.

Professor of Medicine
University of Miami School of Medicine
Associate Director
Nephrology Section
Veterans Administration Medical Center
Miami, Florida

SERGE ERLINGER, M.D.

Professeur à la Faculté de Médecine Xavier-Bichat
Service d'Hépatologie et Unité de Recherches de
    Physiopathologie Hépatique
Hôpital Beaujon
Clichy, France

CARLOS O. ESQUIVEL, M.D., Ph.D.

Assistant Professor of Surgery
University of Pittsburgh School of Medicine
Attending Surgeon
Presbyterian–University Hospital of Pittsburgh
Children's Hospital of Pittsburgh
Pittsburgh, Pennsylvania

JOHN T. GALAMBOS, M.D.

Professor of Medicine
Director, Division of Digestive Diseases
Emory University School of Medicine
Atlanta, Georgia

JOSEPH E. GEENAN, M.D.

Clinical Professor of Medicine
Medical College of Wisconsin
Milwaukee, Wisconsin

† Deceased.

ROBERT D. GORDON, M.D.

Assistant Professor of Surgery
University of Pittsburgh School of Medicine
Attending Surgeon
Presbyterian–University Hospital of Pittsburgh
Children's Hospital of Pittsburgh
Pittsburgh, Pennsylvania

KAMAL G. ISHAK, M.D., Ph.D.

Chairman, Department of Hepatic Pathology
Armed Forces Institute of Pathology
Washington, D.C.
Clinical Professor of Pathology
Uniformed Services University of the Health
    Sciences
Medical Care Consultant
Clinical Center
National Institutes of Health
Bethesda, Maryland
Professorial Lecturer
Mount Sinai School of Medicine
Consultant, Department of Pathology
College of Physicians and Surgeons
Columbia University
New York, New York

SHUNZABURO IWATSUKI, M.D.

Associate Professor of Surgery
University of Pittsburgh School of Medicine
Attending Surgeon
Presbyterian–University Hospital of Pittsburgh
Children's Hospital of Pittsburgh
Pittsburgh, Pennsylvania

GEORGE L. JORDAN, JR., M.D.

Distinguished Service Professor of Surgery
Baylor College of Medicine
Chief of Staff
Harris County Hospital District
Attending in Surgery
The Methodist Hospital
Consultant in Surgery
Veterans Administration Medical Center, St.
    Luke's Episcopal Hospital, and Texas
    Children's Hospital
Houston, Texas

MARSHALL M. KAPLAN, M.D.

Chief, Gastroenterology Section
New England Medical Center
Professor of Medicine
Tufts University School of Medicine
Boston, Massachusetts

FRED KERN, JR., M.D.

Professor of Medicine
Head, Division of Gastroenterology
University of Colorado School of Medicine
Denver, Colorado

RAYMOND S. KOFF, M.D.

Professor of Medicine
Boston University School of Medicine
Chief, Hepatology Section
Boston University Medical Center
Boston, Massachusetts
Chief of Medicine
Framingham Union Hospital
Framingham, Massachusetts

PATRICIA S. LATHAM, M.D.

Assistant Professor of Medicine and Pathology
University of Maryland School of Medicine and
    Baltimore Veterans Administration Hospital
Baltimore, Maryland

ERIC G. LeVEEN, M.D.

Research Associate
Department of Surgery
Medical University of South Carolina
Charleston, South Carolina

HARRY H. LeVEEN, M.D.

Professor of Surgery
Department of Surgery
Medical University of South Carolina
Charleston, South Carolina

CHARLES J. LIGHTDALE, M.D.

Associate Attending Physician
Department of Medicine
Memorial Sloan–Kettering Cancer Center
Associate Professor of Clinical Medicine
Cornell University Medical College
New York, New York

WILLIS C. MADDREY, M.D.

Magee Professor of Medicine and Chairman of the
    Department
Jefferson Medical College of Thomas Jefferson
    University
Philadelphia, Pennsylvania

MANUEL A. MARCIAL, M.D.

Research Fellow in Gastrointestinal Pathology
Brigham and Women's Hospital and Harvard
    Medical School
Boston, Massachusetts

RAÚL A. MARCIAL–ROJAS, M.D., J.D.,
    M.P.H., M.P.A., F.A.C.P.

Professor of Pathology and Dean
School of Medicine
Universidad Central del Caribe
Cayey, Puerto Rico
Former Chairman
Department of Pathology
Universidad de Puerto Rico
School of Medicine
San Juan, Puerto Rico

JAY W. MARKS, M.D.

Associate Director, Gastroenterology
Cedars-Sinai Medical Center
Adjunct Associate Professor of Medicine
University of California, Los Angeles
Los Angeles, California

SHIRLEY McCARTHY, Ph.D., M.D.

Assistant Professor
Diagnostic Radiology
Yale University School of Medicine
New Haven, Connecticut

CHARLES L. MENDENHALL, M.D., Ph.D.

Chief, Digestive Diseases
Cincinnati Veterans Administration Medical
    Center
Professor of Medicine
University of Cincinnati College of Medicine
Cincinnati, Ohio

DENIS J. MILLER, M.D.

Associate Clinical Professor of Medicine
Liver Study Unit
Department of Medicine
Yale University School of Medicine
New Haven, Connecticut

FRANK G. MOODY, M.D.

Professor and Chairman
Department of Surgery
The University of Texas Medical School at
    Houston
Houston, Texas

RONALD D. NEUMANN, M.D.

Associate Chief
Nuclear Medicine Clinical Center
National Institutes of Health
Bethesda, Maryland

RAOUL V. PEREIRAS, M.D.

Clinical Assistant Professor of Medicine
Assistant Professor of Radiology
University of Miami School of Medicine
Miami, Florida

M. JAMES PHILLIPS, M.D.

Professor
Department of Pathology
University of Toronto
Pathologist-in-Chief
Hospital for Sick Children
Toronto, Ontario, Canada

SIRIA POUCELL, M.D.

Department of Pathology
Hospital for Sick Children and University of
    Toronto
Toronto, Ontario, Canada

P. R. RAJAGOPALAN, M.D.

Associate Professor of Surgery
Department of Surgery
Medical University of South Carolina
Charleston, South Carolina

ARON M. RAPPAPORT, M.D., Ph.D.

Professor Emeritus, Department of Physiology
University of Toronto
Toronto, Ontario, Canada

OSCAR D. RATNOFF, M.D.

Professor of Medicine
Case Western Reserve University
Career Investigator, American Heart Association
Physician, University Hospitals of Cleveland
Cleveland, Ohio

TELFER B. REYNOLDS, M.D.

Clayton Loosli Professor of Medicine
University of Southern California
Chief, Hepatology Division, Los Angeles County–
    University of Southern California Medical
    Center
Los Angeles, California

CAROLINE A. RIELY, M.D.

Associate Professor of Medicine and Pediatrics
Liver Study Unit
Yale University School of Medicine
New Haven, Connecticut

SEYMOUR M. SABESIN, M.D.

Chairman, Section of Digestive Diseases
Director, Senior Attending Physician
Rush Presbyterian–Saint Luke's Hospital
Chicago, Illinois

PHILIP SANDBLOM, M.D., Ph.D.(H.C.)

Professor Emeritus of Surgery
Past President, University of Lund
Lund, Sweden

JAY P. SANFORD, M.D.

Uniformed Services University of the Health
    Sciences
F. Edward Hebert School of Medicine
Bethesda, Maryland

ROBERT R. SCHADE, M.D.

Assistant Professor of Medicine
University of Pittsburgh School of Medicine
Pittsburgh, Pennsylvania

EUGENE R. SCHIFF, M.D., F.A.C.P.

Chief, Division of Hepatology
University of Miami School of Medicine
Chief, Hepatology Section
Veterans Administration Medical Center
Miami, Florida

GILBERT M. SCHIFF, M.D.

President
James N. Gamble Institute of Medical Research
Professor of Medicine
University of Cincinnati College of Medicine
Cincinnati, Ohio

LEON SCHIFF, M.D., Ph.D., M.A.C.P.

Clinical Professor of Medicine
Division of Hepatology
University of Miami School of Medicine
Miami, Florida

RUDI SCHMID, M.D., Ph.D.

Professor of Medicine
Dean
University of California at San Francisco
San Francisco, California

LESLIE J. SCHOENFIELD, M.D., Ph.D.

Director, Gastroenterology
Cedars-Sinai Medical Center
Professor of Medicine
University of California, Los Angeles
School of Medicine
Los Angeles, California

WILLIAM K. SCHUBERT, M.D.

Professor and Chairman
Department of Pediatrics
Attending Gastroenterologist
Children's Hospital Medical Center
Cincinnati, Ohio

SHEILA SHERLOCK, D.B.E., M.D.

Professor and Chairman Emeritus
Department of Medicine
The Royal Free Hospital
School of Medicine
University of London
London, England

MARTHA SKINNER, M.D.

Professor of Medicine
Research Program Director
Arthritis Section
Boston University School of Medicine
Boston, Massachusetts

THOMAS E. STARZL, M.D., Ph.D.

Professor of Surgery
University of Pittsburgh School of Medicine
Attending Surgeon, Presbyterian–University
    Hospital of Pittsburgh
Children's Hospital of Pittsburgh
Oakland Veterans Administration Hospital
Pittsburgh, Pennsylvania

BRADFORD G. STONE, M.D.

Assistant Professor of Medicine
University of Pittsburgh School of Medicine
Pittsburgh, Pennsylvania

ERIC G. C. TAN, F.R.A.C.S.

Senior Lecturer in Surgery
University of Western Australia
Nedlands, Western Australia, Australia

**KENNETH J. W. TAYLOR, M.D., Ph.D.,
    F.A.C.P.**

Professor, Diagnostic Imaging
Yale University School of Medicine
Director, Diagnostic Ultrasound
Yale–New Haven Hospital
New Haven, Connecticut

**HOWARD C. THOMAS, M.D., Ph.D.,
    M.R.C.Path., F.R.C.P.(Lond.),
    F.R.C.P.(Glas.)**

Professor of Medicine
The Royal Free Hospital
London, England

DAVID A. THOMPSON, M.D.

Assistant Professor
Department of Surgery
The University of Texas Medical School at
    Houston
Houston, Texas

DAVID H. VAN THIEL, M.D.

Professor of Medicine
Chief of Gastroenterology
University of Pittsburgh School of Medicine
Pittsburgh, Pennsylvania

RAMA P. VENU, M.D.

Associate Professor of Medicine
Medical College of Wisconsin
Milwaukee, Wisconsin

J. M. WALSHE, Sc.D., F.R.C.P.

Reader in Metabolic Diseases
University of Cambridge Clinical School
Physician to Addenbrooke's Hospital
Cambridge, England

KENNETH W. WARREN, M.D.

Surgeon, New England Baptist Hospital
Former Chairman, Department of Surgery
Lahey Clinic Foundation
Former Surgeon-in-Chief
New England Baptist Hospital
Boston, Massachusetts

CAROL I. WILLIAMS, M.D.

Staff Surgeon
New England Baptist Hospital
Boston, Massachusetts

SHELDON M. WOLFF, M.D.

Endicott Professor and Chairman
Department of Medicine
Tufts University School of Medicine
Physician-in-Chief
New England Medical Center
Boston, Massachusetts

DAVID J. WYLER, M.D.

Professor of Medicine
Tufts University School of Medicine
Physician
New England Medical Center
Boston, Massachusetts

LESLIE ZIEVE, M.D.

Professor of Medicine
University of Minnesota Medical School
Section of Gastroenterology
Hennepin County Medical Center
Minneapolis, Minnesota

HYMAN J. ZIMMERMAN, M.D.

Distinguished Physician
Veterans Administration Medical Center
Professor of Medicine
George Washington University School of
    Medicine
Washington, D.C.

DAVID S. ZIMMON, M.D., F.A.C.P.

Professor of Clinical Medicine
New York University School of Medicine
Gastroenterologist
St. Vincent's Hospital and Beth Israel Hospital
New York, New York

Preface

There is no doubt that the method of collaboration [in a multiple author textbook] invites overlapping and presentation of various or even divergent points of view. It is perhaps less likely to favor dogma or the ultra-authoritarian attitude.

C. J. Watson, in foreword to First Edition (1956) of *Diseases of the Liver*

The field of liver disease continues its rapid growth. This is evidenced not only by the increase in the number and size of societies devoted to the study of liver disease both in this country and abroad, but also by the number of new textbooks dealing with the subject and the establishment of multiple liver transplant centers. Further attesting to the growth is the steady increase in the size of *Diseases of the Liver* from the First Edition to the Sixth Edition, both in the number of contributors (from 28 to 79) and pages (from 738 to 1477).

A panoramic view of changes occurring in the field of liver disease over the three decades since the First Edition appeared would include those procedures or data that are obsolete or are becoming so and those that represent advances. Among the former are the cephalin flocculation test, thymol turbidity, zinc turbidity, galactose tolerance, urinary and fecal urobilinogen, BSP excretion, intravenous cholangiography, transduodenal biliary drainage, oral cholecystography, and exploratory laparotomy to establish the cause of jaundice, most notably in cases of primary biliary cirrhosis.

Among the advances—primarily clinical—the following may be included:

1. Discovery of the Australia and delta antigens
2. Classification of viral hepatitis
3. Conjugation of serum bilirubin (1956)
4. Determination of serum transaminases
5. Development of the hepatitis B vaccine
6. Relationship of chronic B viral hepatitis to hepatocellular carcinoma
7. Increasing incidence and recognition of primary sclerosing cholangitis
8. Earlier detection of primary biliary cirrhosis in the form of elevated serum alkaline phosphatase, the more favorable outlook, and the diagnostic value of the mitochondrial antibody test
9. Hepatobiliary imagery—its various aspects—and, among other categories, its diagnostic value in jaundiced states
10. Endoscopic sphincterotomy and extraction of common duct stones
11. ERCP and biliary manometry in elucidating postcholescystectomy syndromes
12. Medical dissolution of gallstones
13. Oral contraceptives and tumors of the liver
14. Alpha₁-antitrypsin deficiency and cirrhosis
15. Newer diuretics in the management of ascites
16. Peritoneal jugular shunt for ascites
17. Detection and treatment of spontaneous bacterial peritonitis
18. Sclerotherapy for bleeding esophageal varices
19. Advances in selective portacaval shunting
20. Management of portosystemic encephalopathy
21. Treatment of chronic active autoimmune hepatitis
22. Medical treatment of pyogenic liver abscess
23. Alpha-fetoprotein and hepatocellular carcinoma
24. Greater survival in hepatic transplantation

Ed Gall, to whose memory this Sixth Edition is affectionately dedicated, was indeed a man of distinction. He was one of the most literate individuals with whom it was the Senior Editor's good fortune to be associated. In the opinion of Dr. Henry Winkler, former President of the University of Cincinnati, Ed could readily have qualified for chairmanship of a department of English. He possessed a brilliant mind, a sharp tongue, and a keen sense of humor. Much of the Senior Editor's accomplishments he would attribute to his close association with Ed through the years, and, as noted in the Fifth Edition of *Diseases of the Liver,* he still sorely misses Ed's wise counsel, which was readily forthcoming, whenever it was sought.

The Editors extend a warm welcome to the new contributors and deeply appreciate their cooperation.

We deeply regret the passing of William Altemeier, Robert L. Peters, Hugh Edmondson, and Cecil Watson since the appearance of the Fifth Edition, all of them truly giants in the field of liver disease.

And finally, we wish to express our thanks to Vivian Gonzalez and Mrs. Patricia Villacorta for their invaluable secretarial assistance, and the staff of J. B. Lippincott, especially Delois Patterson, Les Hoeltzel, and Karen Joseph, for their editorial assistance.

Leon Schiff, M.D., Ph.D.
Eugene R. Schiff, M.D.

Preface to the First Edition

In the recent words of Himsworth, the present time seems to be particularly opportune for reviewing our knowledge of liver disease. A partial list of reasons would include the advances made in the fundamental sciences as they pertain to liver structure and function; the advances in the experimental approach to liver disease; the increased knowledge in the field of viral hepatitis; the newer clinical criteria and concept of hepatic coma, with attention focused on disturbance in the metabolism of ammonia; a better understanding of the pathogenesis and the treatment of cirrhosis; a clearer concept of the metabolic defect in hemochromatosis and the apparent effectiveness of depleting iron stores in the treatment of this disorder; the implication of disturbed copper metabolism in hepatolenticular degeneration; the increasing experience with needle biopsy of the liver; and the surgical attack on portal hypertension.

This book is not intended to be encyclopedic in nature but rather the expression of present-day information pertaining to various aspects of liver disease by a group of authors particularly qualified by their experience, interest and scientific contributions. The reader may discover certain omissions; but he usually will find these to be matters of lesser importance. They will be more than compensated by the quality of the information contained, which deals with those aspects of hepatic disease that are much more apt to concern him, including the description of the principles of treatment, both medical and surgical, by experts in the field. Furthermore, he will frequently find it unnecessary to consult other books, particularly on points dealing with basic concepts.

To various contributors the editor expresses his deep gratitude for their excellent and willing cooperation. He has considered it good fortune indeed to have been associated with them in this undertaking. He wishes to express his thanks to Cecil J. Watson, Arthur J. Patek, Jr., and to his colleague, Edward A. Gall, for their helpful suggestions. He is particularly indebted to Miss Olive Mills, without whose tireless and able secretarial and editorial assistance he would not have been able to accomplish his task.

In some instances individual authors have appended acknowledgements of assistance to their respective chapters. To those concerned the editor wishes to express his apologies for not having included these expressions of gratitude for the sake of uniformity of composition and conservation of space.

Leon Schiff

Contents

† Deceased.

chapter 1
Physioanatomic Considerations

ARON M. RAPPAPORT

The time when anatomy consisted of tabulated data from the dissecting rooms has passed. Today the work of anatomists and physiologists interlaces continuously. Indeed, the concepts of the morphology of the liver have changed with the advances in hepatic electron microscopy, physiology, and pathology. Experimentalists and clinicians too have added to the knowledge of normal and abnormal morphology. Functional anatomy is thus on the march, and we shall strive to follow it in our presentation.

In the following pages the development of the liver, its lobes, surface, peritoneal connections (ligaments), its microanatomy, vessels, and nerves are considered. Also, the bile ducts and gallbladder and general topography are discussed.

GROSS ANATOMY

The liver is covered by the fibrous capsule of Glisson, which, in turn, is invested with serosa. At the porta hepatis this capsule turns deep into the liver substance along the vessels and the biliary ducts, following them to their finest ramifications.

The liver of an adult weighs from 1400 g to 1600 g, accounting for one fiftieth of the body weight. In the newborn, the greater comparative size of the liver (one twentieth of the body weight) is due to its blood-forming activity during fetal life.

Although it is the largest gland of the body, the liver is believed to yield a relatively small amount of secretion (600–800 ml of bile daily). The daily output of canalicular bile has not yet been determined by microcannulation of the bile capillaries. However, in view of the large secretory surface of the bile canaliculi and of the rich hepatic blood supply, one may expect it to be much higher than the daily amount collected from the choledochus or calculated by indirect methods.

The hardened adult specimen *in situ* has the appearance of a wedge with the base to the right. The normal liver extends from the right fifth intercostal space in the midclavicular line down to the right costal margin. The lower margin of a normal liver usually transgresses the costal border; its greatest thickness (12–15 cm) is at the level of the upper pole of the right kidney, and its greatest transverse diameter is 15 cm to 20 cm. A convenient site of transthoracic puncture for liver biopsy is in the anterior axillary line at the seventh, eighth, or ninth interspace,

always one interspace below the upper limit of liver dullness. The morphologic and topographic variations of the normal liver were studied by Villemin and associates.[341]

EMBRYOLOGY

The liver arises from the entodermal lining of the foregut during the fourth week of gestation. The hepatic diverticulum is situated at the ventral side of the foregut, cranial to its opening into the yolk sac. In embryos of 5 mm to 6 mm in length, the original hepatic diverticulum can be distinguished as differentiating cranially into proliferating hepatic cords and bile ducts, caudally into the gallbladder. The tip of the hepatic diverticulum sheds hepatoblasts arranged in tubules to interdigitate with the developing sinusoids. The hepatic tubular cords sprout tridimensionally (cranially, ventrally, and laterally), penetrating the septum transversum and passing between the two layers of splanchnic mesoderm. The latter envelop the sprouting lobules, provide their interstitial connective tissue, and form the liver capsule.

The formation of the vascular spaces is self-differentiating. The vitelline veins become completely incorporated into the hepatic sinusoidal bed; the sinusoids act as templates for the growth of the hepatic cords.

The earliest intrahepatic portal vein (PV) branches are afferent vitelline veins. Mesenchyma migrates around them, and the earliest bile ducts form by conversion of adjacent hepatic cords that already contain bile canaliculi. There are no arterioles in the early portal spaces. There are two hepatic veins to one PV. The umbilical vein develops from the left umbilical vein, and the ductus venosus is established in a 6-mm embryo to permit direct flow from the umbilical vein to the inferior vena cava. The umbilical vein develops a sphincter at the junction with the ductus venosus to regulate flow to the fetal heart.[124] As development of bile ducts in portal spaces increases, they become highly vascularized by arterioles that spiral around the bile ducts. The development of the bile ducts continues into the neonatal period. The human liver, initially a simple gland, changes into a "composite labyrinthine gland."[36] Although the differentiation of the liver anlage is conditioned by the interrelation of both entodermal and mesenchymal elements, the primary factor remains the proliferation of the epithelium in tubular cords that communicate with the bile ductules.[23] Similar observations have been made by Wilson and co-workers in the liver of the mouse embryo.[350]

A chemomorphological study of the development of the liver in the golden hamster indicates the formation of primary lobules as evidenced by the high periportal activity of the glycogen-forming enzyme. The glycogen storage around the hepatic end venules is a secondary phenomenon and occurs after birth.[292] In rats, during the postnatal period, the acini widen and formation of new acini continues. The cells most active in protein synthesis are located now mainly in zone 1 (Z_1); their periportal prevalence is due to predominance of arterial flow in this zone.[175]

Recent studies of the liver in human fetuses[11] demonstrate that the earliest organized structures formed by the association of hepatocytes and cholangiolar cells are situated around the small portal branches (*i.e.,* Zone$_1$); they represent the anlage of the liver acinus.[257]

The primordium of the gallbladder is a diverticular dilation of the original outgrowth from the gut, situated caudal to the confluence of the hepatic ducts. Since it elongates quickly and becomes saccular, developmental disturbance in this region can produce malformations of the gallbladder in the presence of a normal liver. Aberrant biliary ducts, vasa aberrantia, are considered by most authors to be proliferating branches of primitive tubular liver cords that were arrested in their development.

Anomalies in the blood supply of the liver are due to anomalies of the vascular anlage rather than of the liver anlage.

In summary, the liver is an entodermal outgrowth of the foregut into mesodermal surroundings increasing the metabolic and digestive activities of the gut. The liver

grows by tridimensional budding of the hepatoblasts, the primary bile ductules around the smallest portal spaces. Thus small parenchymal masses (liver acini) are formed around a central biliovascular axis. The final shape of the liver and its attached excretory apparatus is an expression of the developmental case history of the organ.

LOBES

As distinguished from the multilobulated liver of many mammals, the human liver is one compact and continuous mass. It is divided conventionally into two lobes by the line of insertion of the falciform ligament. The right lobe is larger and shows on its posterior-inferior surface two smaller lobes—the caudate and the quadrate lobes (Fig. 1-1). The former with its caudate process is wedged between the groove of the inferior vena cava and the porta hepatis. The quadrate lobe lies between the round ligament and the gallbladder. Cantlie[47] and Sérégé[313] considered the gallbladder–caval line as the true dividing line of the liver.

Hjortsjö injected the hepatic ducts *in situ* with red lead in celloidin and took stereoscopic cholangiograms.[137] Then he filled the portal vessels with colored celloidin, corroded them, and described their course in relation to the stereogram. In his corrosion specimen he saw a fissure running toward the caval area from the right septal fissure, which is situated to the right of the gallbladder fundus. Occasionally there were other fissures subdividing the left lobe. These fissures harbor major branches of the hepatic vein and are bridged *in vivo* by sinusoids.

With a view to operations on the parenchyma, Couinaud[57] and Junès[152] have studied the segmental distri-

Fig. 1-1. Posterior view of the liver. The marks impressed upon the liver surface by neighboring organs mirror its intricate topographic relation with the surroundings. (Anson BJ, McVay CB: Callander's Surgical Anatomy, 5th ed. Philadelphia, WB Saunders, 1971)

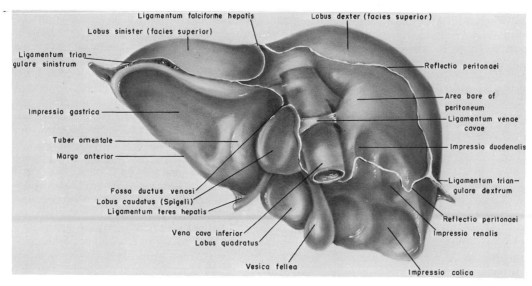

Ligamentum falciforme hepatis
Lobus dexter (facies superior)
Lobus sinister (facies superior)
Ligamentum trian-
gulare sinistrum
Reflectio peritonaei
Area bare of
peritoneum
Impressio gastrica
Ligamentum venae
cavae
Tuber omentale
Impressio duodenalis
Margo anterior
Ligamentum trian-
gulare dextrum
Fossa ductus venosi
Lobus caudatus (Spigeli)
Ligamentum teres hepatis
Reflectio peritonaei
Impressio renalis
Vena cava inferior
Lobus quadratus
Vesica fellea
Impressio colica

bution of the vascular and biliary tree within the liver. The lobes of the liver cannot be compared with the pulmonary lobes; the liver is one parenchymal mass and the lobes are not delimited by any fibrous septum traversing the liver substance. Each conventional hepatic lobe has its own vascular and biliary systems, but there are intercommunications between the respective systems. Surgical anastomosis of a major intrahepatic bile duct of one lobe with an intestinal loop drains the entire liver.[157,184]

There is no preferential blood flow to the right or the left liver lobe[56], but there is sufficient mixture in the questionable streamlined flow to guarantee unity of function of the organ. Splenic portography shadows the entire liver at once. Furthermore, of all the liver functions, none ever has been attributed to any lobe. However, from a developmental and microstructural viewpoint, the liver is to be considered as lobulated not only on its surface but also into its innermost parts. The accessory lobes scattered in various organs (mesentery, suspensory ligaments, spleen, adrenals) are the remainders of parenchymal clusters around the sprouting bile ductules that have split off from the entire liver mass.[341] Riedel's lobe is a downward prolongation of the right liver lobe often caused by an adhesion to the mesocolon.

In summary, the liver consists of a uniform mass of parenchyma that conventionally appears to be divided into lobes by deep vascular or avascular grooves. In spite of the demonstrated bilateral portal blood flow when the intestines are exposed, there is not enough evidence to prove that under normal circumstances the named lobes of the adult liver receive their blood each from a different intestinal area, nor that they have distinct functions. On the microscopic level, however, the liver is lobulated throughout.

SURFACE OF THE LIVER

Of the five surfaces of the liver (superior, anterior, right lateral, posterior, and inferior), the posterior and inferior show more structural features.

The superior, anterior, and lateral surfaces are smooth and convex to fit into the dome of the diaphragm. They are completely covered by peritoneum except for a small triangular area where the two layers of the upper part of the falciform ligament diverge.

In the marks of the posterior and the inferior surfaces of the liver (see Fig. 1-1) we can read the glorious past, when the liver represented one fifth of the entire body weight. The groove of the venous ligament separating conventionally the left liver lobe from the rest of the organ is the site at which the gastrohepatic omentum is inserted. Once in this furrow lay a main afferent channel that brought oxygenated blood from the umbilical vein into the hepatic sinusoids. Some of the blood in this channel also passed through the venous duct (duct of Arantius) directly into the inferior vena cava and so to the right atrium. The umbilical vein, an arterial channel now obliterated and transformed into the round hepatic ligament, runs in the lower half of its groove. It delimits the quadrate lobe from the left liver lobe. Thus from the beginning, the liver, especially its left lobe, has had arterial blood of first quality.

The inferior vena cava runs through the posterior surface of the liver at the base of its bare area. In some livers the vein passes under a bridge of liver substance. Here the hepatic veins, arranged in a superior group of three (left, right, and median hepatic) with a variable inferior group, empty into the inferior vena cava. Thus the coronary ligament attaching the triangular bare area of the right liver lobe to the diaphragm by areolar tissue encloses the above large veins.

The fossa of the gallbladder delimits the quadrate from the right liver lobe. The horizontal portal fissure, which joins the upper ends of the gallbladder fossa and the groove of the round ligament, contains the branches of the hepatic artery and of the PV, the hepatic nerve plexus, the hepatic ducts, and the lymph vessels. In the portal fissure the arterial branches lie between the bile ducts in front and the portal branches behind.

The diaphragmatic, renal, suprarenal, colic, duodenal, pyloric, gastric, and esophageal areas that we see on a posterior view of the liver are the impressions made by neighboring organs. These imprints should remind us also of a variety of pathologic processes that can involve the liver, together with any of these organs. Generally speaking the surface mirrors what is close to it and is exposed to injury from its surroundings.

PERITONEAL CONNECTIONS: LIGAMENTS

The liver is connected to the diaphragm, abdominal wall, stomach, and duodenum by bands of connective tissue in peritoneal folds. These have the function of conveying afferent, efferent, and collateral blood vessels, lymphatics, and nerve plexuses to the liver and of helping to maintain the organ in position.

Falciform Ligament. This peritoneal fold connects the liver to the diaphragm and the anterior abdominal wall. It ascends from the umbilicus, from which during fetal life it conducted the umbilical vein to the liver. The obliterated vessel forms the free edge of the sickle-shaped peritoneal fold. It carries between its peritoneal layers the paraumbilical veins, the clinically important collaterals of the PV. These veins are often exposed surgically and used as a route for catheterization and radiography of the PV, permitting collection of blood samples for metabolic studies.[172] When dilated in cirrhosis and in Cruveilhier–Baumgarten syndrome, blood sampling and visualization of the portal system become possible without recourse to catheterization.[317]

Coronary Ligament. The "bare area" of the posterior surface of the liver, connected by areolar tissue with the diaphragm, is enclosed by an upper and a lower layer of peritoneum. The inferior vena cava and the hepatic veins are contained within the coronary ligament.

Hepatorenal Ligament. The lower layer of the coronary ligament, passing along the lower limit of the right posterior hepatic surface, may be reflected on the upper part of the anterior surface of the right kidney, thus forming the hepatorenal ligament. It often contains collateral vessels of the liver.

Right Triangular Ligament. This is the free margin of the coronary ligament.

Left Triangular Ligament. This consists of two closely applied layers of peritoneum that continue with the falciform ligament in front and the lesser omentum behind. Both triangular ligaments, besides attaching the liver lobes to the diaphragm, convey collateral branches from the phrenic and the musculophrenic vessels to the liver.[279]

Ligaments are ties that connect the organ with the rest of the organism. Through them, nutrients, hormones, raw materials for function, and stimuli are carried in and out by blood and lymph vessels, bile ducts, and nerves.

MICROANATOMY

Hepatic Cytology

See Chapter 2.

Hepatic Histology

Even in its early stage of development, the liver shows the close association of entodermal and mesodermal elements that characterizes this organ. The rows of epithelial cells radiating from the terminal portal vessels (TPVs) to the terminal hepatic ("central") veins (THVs or ThVs) are sustained by fine reticulin fibers and sinusoidal capillaries of mesodermal origin. However, the amount of fibrous tissue around the afferent and the efferent channels is in proportion to their size. They are the continuation of Glisson's capsule, a remainder of the septum transversum.

We may well think of the liver as a tree that has grown out from the virgin land of the foregut to increase its metabolic and digestive functions. It has spread its crown of parenchyma into the space of the septum transversum but continues to draw its nutrients through the portal capillary roots from the daily enriched soil of the intestines. As the liver anlage develops by tridimensional budding of the hepatoblasts and the bile ducts to the final shape of the organ, small parenchymal clusters remain centered around the spread-out terminal branches of the duct. Here the zonal arrangement of the cells with respect to circulation, function, and pathology proves to us that lobulation is an essential structural feature of the hepatic parenchyma.

Hepatic lobules were described by Malpighi[191] in 1666, and Mascagni[194] represented them as grapelike bunches attached to the extremities of the PV. A more descriptive concept of hepatic lobulation was introduced by Francis Kiernan in 1833.[163] He envisaged a hexagonal lobule centered around the radicles of the hepatic veins. This lobule is still presented in some textbooks of histology as the ultimate unit of the liver. However, the idea of a parenchymal mass filling a hexagonal space around the central vein would not integrate functional unity, either normal or abnormal. Therefore, the existence of a hexagonal lobule has been questioned by many authors.[8,38,188,230,251,268,288] In spite of its arrangement within an incomplete hexagonal framework of vessels, the hexagonal lobule is not conspicuous under *in vivo* microscopic observation of the hepatic circulation.[254] The blood flowing through the pairs of terminal afferent vessels streams into sinusoids of an area extending into sectors only of adjacent hexagonal fields. Thus these terminal afferent vessels accompanied by a terminal bile ductule are the orientating landmarks around which the parenchymal tissue is arranged in clumps or small clusters; they can be well delimited under suitable conditions.

Two differently colored gelatin masses of the same viscosity, injected simultaneously and under the same pressure into the two main branches of the PV of a dog or a rabbit, sharply delimit parts of the liver. Microscopically, differently colored areas are found to be situated around terminal portal branches, to occupy adjacent parts of neighboring hexagonal fields, and to extend from the "central vein" of one hexagon to the "central vein" of another (Fig. 1-2). The same arrangement is observed when the colored masses are injected into the two branches of the hepatic artery or bile duct. Thus the hexagonal fields are broken down into distinct areas that are the cross sections of berrylike *irregular* parenchymal masses surrounding a trio of axial channels. Of these, the hepatic arteriole and the portal venule bring in the materials for metabolism, whereas the accompanying terminal bile ductule carries away the product of secretion. Each outlined parenchymal mass represents the structural, microcirculatory, and functional unit of the liver, which we named the *liver acinus.*[250]

Simple Liver Acinus

The simple liver acinus is a small parenchymal mass, irregular in size and shape, arranged around an axis consisting of a terminal hepatic arteriole, portal venule, bile ductule, lymph vessels, and nerves that grow out together from a small triangular portal field. The simple liver acinus lies between two (or more) THVs with which its vascular and biliary axis interdigitates. In a two-dimensional view it occupies sectors only of two adjacent hexagonal fields.

If one injects simultaneously the main (lobar) branches of the PV and the entire hepatic venous system of the human liver, each with differently colored vinylite acetate, and, after the injection mass has hardened, removes the

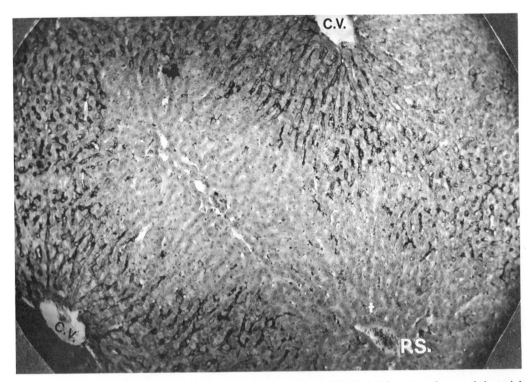

Fig. 1-2. Acinar unit in a rabbit liver. The area clear of India ink is centered around the axial channels that grow out from a small portal space (*P.S.*). It extends into two adjacent hexagonal fields, the "central veins" (*C.V.*) of which are seen in the lower left and upper right corners. (× 100, approx.) (Rappaport AM et al: Anat Rec 119:11, 1954)

parenchyma by acid digestion, a three-colored cast is obtained.[20] The cast clearly shows that the area around each THV ("central vein") is supplied with blood derived from different sources, remote from one another.[261] Hence there is *no* microcirculatory unity in the tissue around a THV (*i.e.,* "central vein" of Kiernan).

Similar casts were obtained also of the liver of the dog, rabbit, pig, and monkey. The terminal branches of the visualized afferent vessels and bile ducts represent the axes around which the hepatic parenchyma is organized. Because of their variety in length, course, and capillary ramification, the parenchymal masses supplied and drained by them vary likewise.

The width of an acinus is twice the length of a radial sinusoid and measures about .25 mm in the *in vivo* transilluminated liver of weanling rats. Measurements in serial sections of human liver acini[260] with their peripheries outlined by bands of ischemic necrosis revealed that the average length and width of the acini are 1480 μm and 1070 μm, respectively. The plates and cords of the simple acini, although definitely oriented upon their axial channels, *are in cellular and capillary continuity with adjacent or overlapping acini.* There is no capsular investment around these irregularly shaped microscopic clumps that separates them from one another. Nevertheless, the terminal afferent and draining channels pervade the entire liver mass in a definite way, subdividing it into small functional clumps. These clumps, although matted together, hang berrylike on their axial stalks; the dividing line between the acini is the watershed of biliary drainage. Each acinus empties its biliary secretion into the bile ductule with which it originated and to which it stays linked. Since the terminal vascular branches, which bring the materials for nutrition and metabolism into the acinus, run along the terminal bile ductule draining the secretory product of the same acinus, structural, circulatory, and functional unity is established in this small clump of parenchyma. In spite of extensive intersinusoidal communication, blood and nutrients are preferentially carried into the sinusoids of each acinus by its parent vessels. An injection of the portal system with India ink (Fig. 1-3) indicates also the course of the other channel systems and nerves; they are included in our description, although not always mentioned specifically. The dependence of the parenchyma on the preferential supply lines is also evidenced under circulatory (*e.g.,* ischemia) or nutritional (*e.g.,* choline deficiency) stress.*

* For a better illustration of this strict relationship between nutrient vessels, bile duct, and parenchymal clump, I would give the following analogy: Imagine a mat glass wall evenly illuminated from behind by a multitude of small bulbs. Because of the fusion

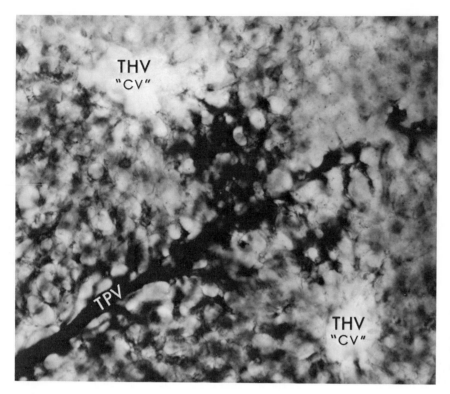

Fig. 1-3. Liver acinus in a human. The acinus occupies sectors only of two adjacent hexagonal fields and reaches their "central veins" (*"CV"*). The axial terminal portal branch (*TPV*) of the structural unit is injected with India ink and runs perpendicular to the two terminal hepatic ("central") venules (*THV*) with which it interdigitates. It is visualized by a fortunate cut parallel to almost its entire length. The THVs lie close to each other in this section. (Thick cleared section × 300)

Acinar Circulatory Zones. There is a zonal relationship between the cells constituting the acini and their blood supply. The hepatocytes situated close to the axial terminal vascular branches in zone 1 (Fig. 1-4) are the first to be supplied with fresh blood, rich in oxygen and substrate. They form the most active and resistant core of the acinus in circulatory or nutritional deficiency: they are the last to die and the first to regenerate.[113,296] The more distant the cells are, in any plane, from the site where the terminal portal and arterial branches empty into the sinusoids, the poorer is the quality of blood that bathes them, and the less is their resistance to damage. The greater distance from the supply lines is indicated by the higher order of zones (zones 2 and 3). The circulatory zones run concentrically around the *terminal* afferent vessels (*i.e.,* around the *smallest nontriangular* portal spaces).

Periportal location is generally assumed to be close to the supply of fresh blood, but it is evident that cells around differently sized and shaped portal spaces do not share such supply equally. Some cells in area B or C (Fig. 1-4), farther from the triangular portal space, have an excellent blood supply from the terminal afferent vessels branching

out from the preterminal vessels of this triangular space. *In vivo* transillumination of a rat liver and microscopic observation of the blood flow pattern during circulatory stress also reveal a darkening of the portion of the sinusoid that is remote from the TPVs and hepatic arterioles.

Enzymic and Metabolic Areas in the Acini: Heterogeneity of Liver Cells. *Morphologic.* All cells within the liver lobule have always been considered to be structurally homogeneous with some differences "in cells immediately surrounding the central veins."[185] Karyometric investigations have demonstrated higher nuclear volumes in zone 3 (Z_3) close to the THV.[303]

Although no particular function can as yet be ascribed exclusively to one group of hepatocytes, their lack of uniformity is now evident in electron microscopic and histochemical studies.[154] Porter[241] noticed an even intermingling of large mitochondria and ergastoplasmic reticulum (ER) in the hepatocytes of Z_1 and ER clusters in the parenchymal cells of Z_3. Morphometric studies using stereologic methods bring evidence of quantitative differences between the vast and highly reactive surface areas (measured in square meters!) of the mitochondria of Z_1 and Z_3.[347] The secretory poles of the hepatocytes[119] in Z_1 are rich in Golgi apparatus, which is large in size and volume. Periportal cells contain two times the volume of Golgi apparatus as hepatocytes in Z_3. The canalicular ectoplasm has a larger diameter and volume in Z_1 than in Z_3 after a bile-salt load.[150] There are more lysosomes and less

---

of light one could hardly indicate which small area of the wall is lighted primarily by which bulb. However, if one or several bulbs suddenly emit only a dim light, the specific area they illuminate becomes manifest. Similarly, in the liver, the individual simple, complex, or agglomerated acini become sharply outlined when physiopathologic changes occur in them.

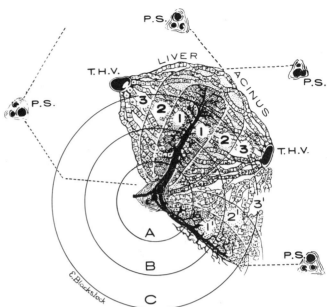

Fig. 1-4. Blood supply of the simple liver acinus and the zonal arrangement of cells. The acinus occupies adjacent sectors of neighboring hexagonal fields. Zones 1, 2, and 3, respectively, represent areas supplied with blood of first, second, and third quality with regard to substrate, oxygen, and nutrients. These zones center around the terminal afferent vascular branches, terminal bile ductules, lymph vessels, and nerves and extend into the triangular portal field from which these branches crop out. Zones 1', 2', and 3' designate corresponding areas in a portion of an adjacent acinar unit. In zones 1 and 1', the afferent vascular twigs empty into the sinusoids. Circles B and C indicate peripheral circulatory areas as commonly described around a "periportal" area A; P.S. = portal space; T.H.V. = terminal hepatic venules ("central veins").

smooth endoplasmic reticulum (SER) in Z_1 than in Z_3. The endothelial cells show a higher surface to volume ratio in the richly anastomotic sinusoids of Z_1 than in Z_3.[203] Also, the endothelia of Z_1 are endowed with large fenestrae that are contractile as a result of microfilaments (50–70 nm) surrounding them and taking part in the regulation of sinusoidal blood flow.[226] All these anatomic peculiarities allow a regulated solute–sinusoidal and hepatocytic wall interaction that is greater at the acinar inlet than at its outlet.[203]

Enzymic–Metabolic. It is obvious that the microenvironment of the cells in the three zones shows some difference with regard to pressure, dynamics of flow, and supply of oxygen and substrates.[102] Thus conditions are favorable for the presence of some enzymes in one zone while in other zones different enzymic activities are predominant. The topography of hepatic enzymes in relation to the microcirculation[253] and as a part of an integrated metabolic system is a frequent topic of research.[304] Figure 1-5 illustrates and summarizes the distribution of common hepatic enzymes in the microcirculatory zones. Thus, the integration of the enzyme pattern into metabolic systems enables us to identify the circulatory zones as metabolic areas. A certain metabolic activity is promoted in these areas under normal conditions; as these conditions change, so does the distribution of enzymes.[77,294]

Immediately after birth there is an increase in enzyme activities (*e.g.,* glucose 6-phosphatase); the great change in the intrahepatic circulation due to the occlusion of the umbilical vein, the ductus Arantii, and the increase in hepatic arterial flow suddenly create a new environment different for the cells in Z_1 than for those in Z_3. It is as if a branch of the Gulf Stream suddenly changed its course;

areas of luxurious growth become barren, whereas in other areas new vegetation develops.[253] Localization of enzyme activity in close dependence to the partial pressure of oxygen (PO_2) is illustrated best by changes in the γ-glutamyl transpeptidase activity. The fetal hepatic circulation in the rat delivering blood of uniform PO_2 to all hepatocytes is instrumental in the equal distribution of γ-glutamyl transpeptidase activity over *all* zones of the acinus. In the adult rat liver such activity is limited to the highly arterialized Z_1. Arterialization of the liver by diverting portal blood through a portacaval anastomosis distributes again the activity of γ-glutamyl transpeptidase over all acinar zones.[211]

The arterioles deliver their blood exclusively[205,356] into the beginning of the sinusoids (*i.e.,* Z_1); hence the tissue PO_2 in this area is closer to arterial tension than in Z_3, where the PO_2 in the proximity of the THV is closer to venous tension. Direct measurements of the tissue PO_2 gradient have been carried out recently by Ji and co-workers.[146] They found an oxygen gradient of 350 mmHg across the lobule. Quistorff and Chance[246] reported a periportal–perivenous redox potential in the normoxic rat liver. Different physiological oxygen tensions can modulate the induction of liver enzymes and contribute to heterogeneity of hepatocytes.[153]

Activity of respiratory enzymes such as succinic dehydrogenase and cytochrome oxidase in horse and pig livers has been shown to be particularly concentrated in Z_1.[304] In this zone the hepatocytes, with their numerous large mitochondria, are exposed first to arterial blood entering the acinus; oxidative processes by way of the Krebs cycle operate at high level (see Fig. 5). In addition, the abundance in Z_1 of large lysosomes rich in acid phospha-

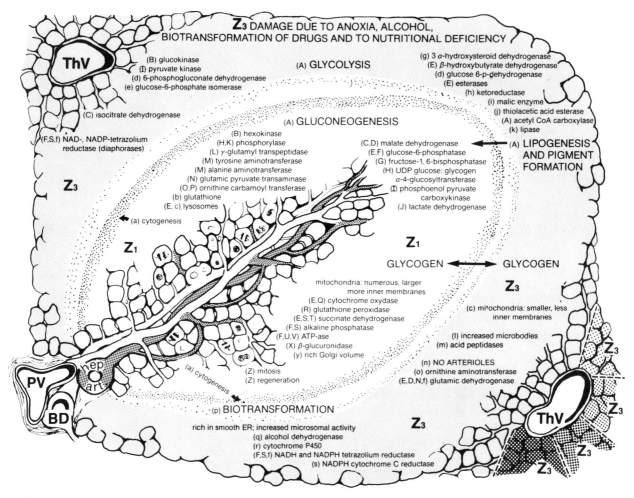

Fig. 1-5. Metabolic areas and their enzymatic pattern (for description, see text). The letters indicate corresponding references: **A,** Jungermann and Sasse[154]; **B,** Fisher et al[87]; **C,** Novikoff et al[225]; **D,** Wimmer and Pette[351]; **E,** Novikoff and Essner[223]; **F,** Wachstein[342]; **G,** Schmidt et al[300]; **H,** Sasse[292]; **I,** Guder and Schmidt[117]; **J,** Rutenburg and Seligman[287]; **K,** Sasse and Köhler[294]; **L,** Albert et al[1]; **M,** Welsh[348]; **N,** Shank et al[314]; **O,** Cohen and Marshall[54]; **P,** Mizutani[206]; **Q,** Burstone[45]; **R,** Yoshimura[358]; **S,** Schumacher[304]; **T,** Nolte and Pette[219]; **U,** Padykula and Herman[233]; **V,** Novikoff et al[224]; **X,** Hayashi[130]; **Y,** Jones et al[150]; **Z,** Grisham[112]; **a,** Schepers[296]; **b,** Smith et al[323]; **c,** Reith et al[280]; **d,** Hildebrand[133]; **e,** Gearhart and Oster-Granite[95]; **f,** Pette and Brandau[236]; **g,** Balogh[12]; **h,** Johnson[147]; **i,** Teutsche[335]; **j,** Wachstein et al[343]; **k,** Klein et al[165]; **l,** Loud[185]; **m,** Rutenburg and Seligman[287]; **n,** Mitra[205]; **o,** Swick et al[330], **p,** Axelrod et al[9]; **q,** Greenberg et al[108]; **r,** Gooding et al[100]; **s,** Taira et al[332]; PV = portal vein; ThV = terminal hepatic venule; BD = bile ductule; hep. art. = hepatic arteriole; Z_1 = periportal area; Z_3 = periacinar and perivenular area.

tase may facilitate a higher rate of pinocytosis and entrance of proteins and other material from the nutrient-laden portal blood into the hepatocytes.

Enzymic activity necessary for *protein metabolism* is preferentially located in Z_1. LeBouton[174] demonstrated with radioautographic studies using ^{3}H leucine that the prime area of protein metabolism and new formation of plasma proteins, presumably albumin, is found in Z_1. The formation of albumin has been questioned recently by

the finding that all liver cells normally synthesize and secrete albumin at any time.[177] Synthesis of acute-phase proteins (fibrinogen, α-macroglobulin, haptoglobulin) takes place first in Z_1 but later uniformly through the acinus.[58]

Cytogenesis, particularly after hepatectomy or toxic injury, is closely connected with DNA metabolism; it occurs mainly in Z_1. However, each zone is capable of regenerating cells that lie close to areas of toxic damage. Schepers,[296] studying cellular gigantism after toxic injury, calls the areas close to the afferent vessels the "cytogenic zones" because there the newborn cells are smallest. While the cells are moving toward the "cytoclastic locus" around the THV, they fulfill their physiologic tasks, become polyploidic, age, die, and are then eliminated into the hepatic veins. Such movements toward Z_3 have been confirmed by Grisham[113] in rats after partial hepatectomy. Liver cells regenerate rapidly, a fact known since ancient times, when it led to the legend of Prometheus, renowned for stealing fire from the gods and giving it to man. Zeus punished him by chaining him to a mountain, where everyday an eagle plucked at his liver, which regenerated every night.

Z_1 *is the gluconeogenic compartment,*[154] and glycogen synthesis, glycogenolysis, and transport of glucose along the glycogen-laden cells depend in the end on the quality of blood offered to the cells by the afferent vessels and on the predominance of a number of enzymes, including hexokinase, glucose 6-phosphatase, lactate dehydrogenase, phosphoenolpyruvate carboxykinase, and fructose 1-6 bisphosphatase 300 (see also Fig. 5); the activity of the latter two are the rate-limiting factors in gluconeogenesis.[117] The entrance of lactate and alanine into the glucogenic pathway is mediated in Z_1 by lactate dehydrogenase and alanine aminotransferase.[348] The gluconeogenesis from amino acids is handled primarily by the hepatocytes in Z_1, which are stimulated by glucagon, while insulin has its glycolytic effect on all hepatocytes. The presence of alanine aminotransferase, tyrosine transferase, and ornithine carbamoyl-transferase is an indication that urea formation from amino acids is taking place here. In the end, gluconeogenesis is an endergonic process[154] that is driven by oxidative catabolism, which is facilitated in cells exposed directly to the activity of the arterioles and their oxygen-rich blood.

Glycolysis and liponeogenesis occur primarily in acinar Z_3, the tips of which form the "perivenous" area (see Fig. 5, right lower corner); its cells are most remote from arteriolar supply.[86] These are the enzymes instrumental in glycolysis of Z_3 hepatocytes: glucokinase,[8] pyruvate kinase,[117] as well as the nicotinamide-adenine dinucleotide phosphate (NADPH)-generating enzymes: glucose 6-phosphate dehydrogenase[133] and malic enzyme,[335] which are necessary for fatty acid synthesis. Glycolysis and lipogenesis are exergonic processes that can take place in the absence of oxygen; they are well at home near the sinusoids of Z_3 carrying blood that has already exchanged its oxygen with cells in Z_1 and Z_2.

Ammonia is produced by the colon and kidney, and is transformed into urea in the liver. The distribution of glutamate dehydrogenase and NADPH-generating isocitrate dehydrogenase in the hepatocytes of Z_3 points to the localization of ureagenesis from ammonia in this zone.

Z_3 is indeed the site of general detoxification as well as of *biotransformation of drugs,* which is also dependent on NADPH production. The zonal distribution of drug-induced toxic lesions in Z_3 is due to the topography of the enzymes involved in the biotransformation of these substances, which are detoxified by oxidation, reduction, or hydrolysis. The SER is rich in NADPH-dependent hydroxylases. Glucose 6-phosphatase, glucose 6-phosphate dehydrogenase,[133] isocitrate dehydrogenase, and malic enzyme are all predominant in the hepatocytes of Z_3 and generate NADPH, which is used by cytochrome C reductase in the process of metabolizing our "daily drugs." Finally, alcohol dehydrogenase, the key enzyme for metabolic degradation of alcohol, is active mainly in Z_3. This is one of the reasons that alcohol damage to the liver cells is first noted around the THV.[179] An additional reason is given by Smith and co-workers,[323] who refer to the reciprocal gradient of glutathione and cytochrome P450. The Z_3 hepatocytes are exposed to a higher risk of damage as a result of the higher activity of their detoxifying enzymes and their lower content of the protective glutathione.

The heterogeneity of the hepatocytes is also manifest in the *excretion of bile salts and bile pigments.* There is an intracellular concentration gradient of endogenous bile salts from Z_1 to Z_3.[151] Selective destruction of the hepatocytes in Z_3 by bromobenzene has demonstrated that the remaining cells of Z_1 still excrete 85% of the injected taurocholate.[120] This area is rich in Golgi apparatus,[150] which is involved in the excretion of bile salts and bile pigments.[101] However, Z_3 cells also have the reserve capacity to excrete bile salts in a liver whose bile excretion has been partially blocked.[150] It is concluded that the bile salt–dependent portion of canalicular bile is predominantly the excretory product of the periportal cells (Z_1); the nondependent fraction is excreted by the hepatocytes of Z_3.[115]

Thus, we note that the concept of metabolic heterogeneity[118,174,295] in the various zones is still evolving and will probably undergo various modifications; nevertheless, it has already permitted selective microchemical studies on cells from different circulatory zones isolated by microdissection and less invasive methods.[146] Similarly, metabolic heterogeneity of cells must be implicated in some way in the selective toxic injury of tissue in different circulatory zones of the liver acinus.[259,327,349] This susceptibility to different degrees of damage by anoxia or malnutrition, characteristic of each acinar zone, enabled us to delimit these zones before their enzymatic pattern was known. Thus, histopathologic changes in the injured liver of the dog, rat, rabbit, monkey, and human and the work done independently by histochemists[66] and enzymologists[223,342] confirm the subdivision of the simple acinus into zones. *However, the enzymic activity in the liver of different species outlined here should not be regarded as a fixed map.* Each hepatic cell is capable of multiple metabolic functions; a *prevalent enzymic activity is the result of an adaptation to the microenvironment regulated by the hepatic microcirculation.* Pathologic changes in structure and circulation may cause an enzymic shift from one acinar zone to another.[294] Thus the lines delimiting the dynamic zones[153] should not be regarded as fixed frontiers. The metabolic activity changes in a gradient from one zone to another.[294] The dividing Z_2 is to be viewed as a fence that one tends to shift to the neighbor's property. With increase in arteriolar activity, Z_2 is moved toward Z_3 as a result of enlargement of Z_1. In ischemia or anoxia, Z_3 enlarges at the expense of Z_2 and Z_1.

Deductions made from experimental reversal of intrahepatic blood flow in dogs to disprove the dependence of the enzymic topography on the direction of intra-acinar blood flow are not valid. The "reversed liver" does *not* receive portal blood at all, and the venous (caval) blood flows in a direction opposing the arterial stream. Severe hepatic congestion and ascites occurred in the few animals surviving the experiments.[52,320] Some authors, by comparing the metabolic effects of anteroperfusion of the liver (with hemoglobin-free solutes) to those of retroperfused ones attempt to disprove acinar zonation. Paradoxically they end up demonstrating that metabolic zonation is due to the *direction of blood flow,* which is indeed the foundation on which the tridimensional organization of the parenchyma into acini rests. The reliance on the two-dimensional hexagons, cleaving the tissue into "periportal" and "pericentral" ("perivenous"), disrupts the reality of a continuum of parenchyma, consisting of interconnected microcirculatory units (acini); in them there is a natural blood flow gradient from terminal afferent to terminal efferent channels.

As long as our liver tissue remains anteroperfused by the hepatic arterioles and portal venules, the gradients of PO_2, substrates, and enzymic activity in dynamic acinar zones will persist.

Complex Acinus

A complex acinus is a microscopic clump of tissue composed of at least three simple acini and a sleeve of parenchyma around the preterminal arterial, portal, and biliary branches, lymph vessels, and nerves that give origin to the terminal axial channels of the simple acini constituting this larger unit.

Figure 1-6 represents a longitudinal cut through a complex liver acinus. A preterminal portal branch ramifies in three directions. Each of its terminal branches forms the axis of a simple acinus. Each acinus has a well-delimited periphery that extends toward the pertaining portal space. It drains into two areas about THVs (these areas in the upper half of the picture are poorly injected). Also a distinct clump of tissue surrounds the preterminal channels as a sleeve. This sleeve of parenchyma consists of tiny clumps—acinuli—that are nourished by small axial venules and hepatic arterioles branching off from the preterminal vessels. Such vascular twigs have been demonstrated radiologically by Daniel and Pritchard[61]: they arborize into a thicket of sinusoids.

A cross section through this complex acinus at the level at which the preterminal vessel divides into its terminal branches would have to be inclined toward the left in order to lay bare the origin of all three branches by the same plane of section. The preterminal parent vessels and biliary channel supply and drain this complex parenchymal unit (Fig. 1-6). The subdivision of the complex acinus into circulatory zones is difficult to illustrate. Z_3 continues from one simple acinus into the neighboring one, thus generating a three-vaulted structure that tops as a cupola the cores of the three acini (see also Fig. 1-20). As usual Z_3, is prone to ischemic, toxic, or nutritional damage, and the localization of these injuries serves indeed to outline the irregular size and shape of the complex acini in the rat, dog, monkey, and human. Studies of serial sections of such lesions in the human liver demonstrate the interconnections of Z_3 of neighboring acini. Data on the function of the normal complex acinus as a whole are yet to be established.

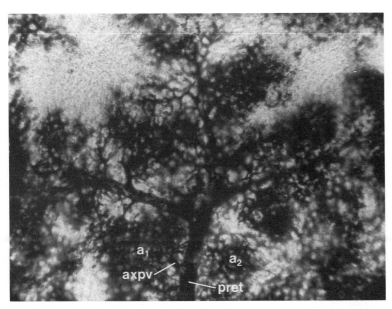

Fig. 1-6. Human complex acinus. The sinusoids injected with India ink are supplied by three terminal portal branches and their parent preterminal vessel (*pret*). These portal venules help form the axial channels of a complex acinus cut longitudinally. The sleeve of parenchyma around pret is formed by acinuli (*a₁, a₂*); axpv = axial portal venule supplying the sinusoids of a_1. The poorly injected white areas (in the upper corners) are parts of zone 3 around terminal hepatic venules (not shown): (150 μm thick section × 88).

Structural and functional unity in these clumps is also demonstrated by the three-color injection technique.[19] The specimens show that the axial vessels of the simple acini are always of the same color as the parent stems of the complex acini. The complex acini are, of course, parts of greater microscopic clumps of tissue, the acinar agglomerates.

Acinar Agglomerate

The acinar agglomerate is a microscopic parenchymal clump, composed of three or four complex acini and the acini forming the sleeve of parenchyma around the large portal space, containing the supplying and draining channels and nerves of the agglomerate.

Figure 1-7 illustrates acinar agglomerates in the human liver. A large portal branch runs diagonally through the field and divides into its preterminal (1) and terminal branches (2). The tissue organized around this vascular structure is an acinar agglomerate. It has unity because the main route of vascular supply and the biliary drainage are common to the whole clump as well as to its subdi-

visions. Furthermore, the handle of the catapult-like vascular structure originates from a large macroscopic vascular branch from which other vessels also ramify; they are of appropriate size to form the axis of other acinar agglomerates. The lumina of portal venous branches supplying acinar agglomerates in the human liver are usually oval shaped on cut, with the long diameter averaging 200 μm and the short diameter 100 μm.[260] The field in Figure 1-7 comprises a group of acinar agglomerates. Vessels and bile ducts in the portal space that form the axis of a group of acinar agglomerates have passed the microscopic threshold and become visible to the naked eye. They should not be included in the microscopic study of liver structure, but it is easy to imagine that a number of groups of acinar agglomerates may form a small liver lobe in an animal with a multilobulated liver.

Architectural Framework in the Liver

The vessels and bile ducts form the architectural framework of the acini of various orders; they run in irregular curved lines as shown in Fig. 1–8. Consequently, the acini

Fig. 1-7. Group of acinar agglomerates. Human liver injected with India ink. Three large portal branches grow out in different directions from a portal space (*PS* in right upper corner). One of these runs diagonally through the field and represents the axis of an acinar agglomerate. From this portal branch, preterminal (1) and terminal (2) branches grow out and form the axes of the outcropping complex and simple acini, respectively. (100-μm-thick cleared section $\times$ 18)

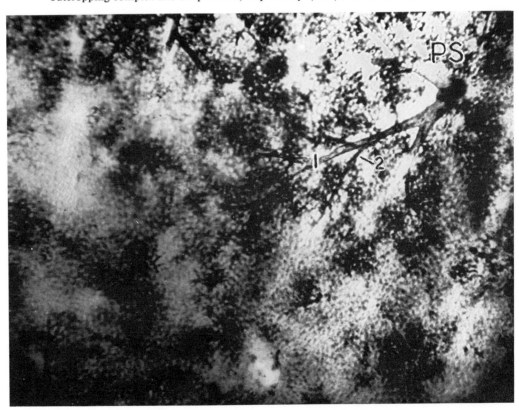

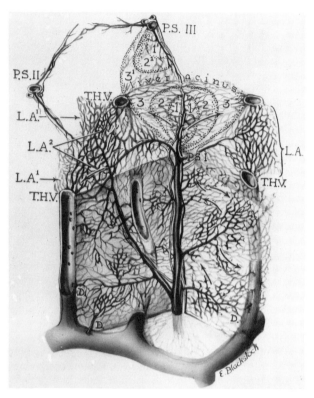

Fig. 1-8. Vascular and biliary architecture of an acinar agglomerate and the relation of the acini to the assumed hexagonal framework of the liver. For explanation, see text. P.S. I, P.S. II, P.S. III = portal spaces; L.A., L.A.[1] = simple liver acinus; L.A.[2] = simple acinus penetrating a hexagonal field situated well above the level of origin of the acinus; T.H.V. = terminal hepatic venule; D = channels of Deysach; 1, 2, 3 = circulatory zones of the simple liver acinus. Note the arcuate courses of the terminal portal branches, the irregularly arranged simple acini, and the short portal vessels that form the axes of tiny acini (acinuli) constituting the mantle of parenchyma around the longitudinally cut portal space. Arrows indicate intercommunicating paths of acini and acinuli.

have no rigid geometric arrangement around the THVs (Fig. 1-8). The blood coming up through the portal spaces with the respiratory tides in the portal branches and with pulsating jets in the arterial channels disperses like a fountain through the terminal afferent twigs and sinusoids, waters and nourishes the parenchyma of the acini, each of them extending into several adjacent hexagonal fields. The bile secreted by the hepatocytes is collected in the bile canaliculi and drained into ductules and ducts accompanying the afferent vascular channels. These course mainly perpendicularly to the THVs with which they interdigitate (Fig. 1-9).

The regular interdigitation of the terminal radicles of the hepatic veins (the "central veins") with the tridimensionally arranged terminal afferent channels brings about a hexagonal pattern in the parenchyma at microscopic

level. The distance between two such THVs is equal to the width of one liver acinus. This distance is halved by the perpendicularly running pair of afferent axial vessels of the acinus (see Fig. 1-3). The veins are situated at the periphery of the structure they drain, an arrangement that corresponds to the rule in vascular anatomy. Interdigitation of the gross afferent and efferent hepatic channels is equally conspicuous in their corrosion casts.[20]

The portal spaces can be classified according to their function. The smallest *triangular* portal spaces in a microscopic field contain the *preterminal* branches of PV, hepatic artery and bile duct, lymph vessels, and nerves. The triangular shape of the portal space is due to the tridimensional outcropping of terminal branches from the channels of the triad and their sheath of connective tissue.[252] In proximity to the triangular spaces and deriving from them are a number of small, *round, or oval* portal spaces representing the multiple cross sections of the *terminal* channels that supply and drain the simple acini. *These smallest portal spaces are the most important functional landmarks in the hepatic parenchyma* (see section on Anatomic Pattern of Pathologic Processes). Larger portal spaces, either triangular with rounded edges or roughly oval, are the cross sections of the trio of channels servicing acinar agglomerates or groups of acinar agglomerates. In contradiction to the geometric lobulation taught by the classicists, we must state that the liver acini are irregular in size and shape and depend very much on the configuration of the axial channels and their ramifying twigs.

The hexagonal pattern in the hepatic parenchyma that has fascinated the histologists for (about) 150 years is seen to be the result of tridimensional budding of the terminal bile ducts and accumulation of connective tissue around them.[251,268]

Although earlier authors[79,188,288] denied the existence of the hexagonal lobule, one still finds it presented in the literature as a means of quick orientation in the light microscopic field. However, visually caging the hepatic parenchyma within an imaginary hexagonal space disregards the path of gradual exchange of substrate[102] between blood and hepatocytes along the continuum of the differently organized microcirculation of the liver and its units (see pages 26–29).

Structural Elements of the Acinar Units. The following elements are present in all acini:

Hepatic Cords and Plates. The oversimplified description of a test tube–like hepatic epithelium arranged in cords, two cells thick with a bile canaliculus between has been revised by Elias' tridimensional studies of the mammalian liver.[78,79] The parenchyma of the human liver is fashioned in cribriform sheets or plates one cell thick. Each cell is surrounded by a polygonal network of bile canaliculi that unite to empty into the bile ductules. This concept leans on earlier observations of Hering (1872),[131] Braus,[36] and Pfuhl.[237] Perhaps it can be challenged by the observations made with intravital fluorescence micros-

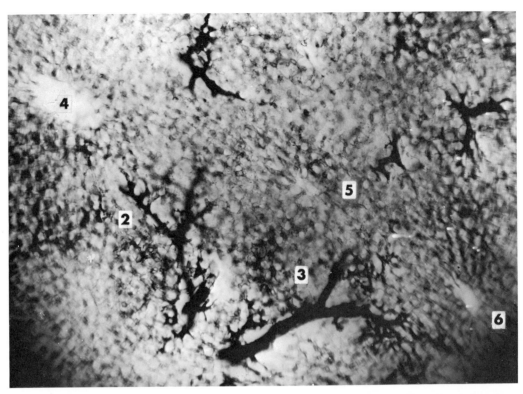

Fig. 1-9. Human liver injected with India ink. Interdigitation of portal and hepatic vein branches. Two horizontal terminal portal branches (*2, 3*), forming the axes of acini, interdigitate with three cross-sectioned vertical terminal hepatic venules (*4, 5, 6*), around which they arch. (Cleared thick section × 110)

copy.[127] Also, in random sections hepatic cells in sheet arrangement are observed rarely.

    Bile Canaliculi, Intermediate Canals of Hering,[131] and (Axial) Terminal Bile Duct Branches. The study of the bile canaliculi has reached safer ground since Hanzon[127] proved *in vivo* that a bile capillary plexus surrounds each liver cell in a lamina except for the side exposed to the sinusoids. Bile canaliculi in their zigzag course reach the intermediate canal of Hering (Fig. 1-10). As confirmed by electron microscopy,[35] the walls of the canaliculi are formed by the modified membranes of the surrounding hepatic cells. The canaliculi are wider in Z_1 than in Z_3 of the acini.[173]

    The intermediate canal, Zwischenstück of Hering, was reinvestigated with the electron microscope.[326] Its wall, endowed with microvilli, is formed by the cell membranes of hepatocytes and of cuboidal epithelial cells lining the smallest bile ductules; the cells are poor in mitochondria and contain a dark-staining argentophilic nucleus. The intermediate canal of Hering is only 2 to 4 cells long;[326] it is richly vascularized and is the site of parenchymal repair and perhaps of fluid secretion and absorption. Several intermediate canals join the axial terminal branch of the bile duct (see Fig. 1-10).

Fig. 1-10. SEM view of the rat bile canaliculi, casted by monomeric methacrylate injection medium after perfusion fixation (a well-injected area, × 860) coated with gold. B = terminal twig of the bile duct, part of the biliovascular axis of a simple liver acinus; b = canal of Hering; c = bile canaliculi emptying into canals of Hering. (Courtesy of Murakami T, Itoshima T et al [Department of Anatomy, Okayama University]: Arch Histol Jpn 47:223, 1984)[214]

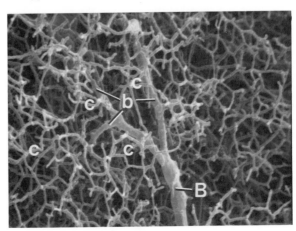

Blood Vessels, Lymph Vessels, and Nerves will be discussed in following sections.

In summary, the essential feature of the hepatic parenchyma is its lobulation. It is not a matter of conjecture but a biologic principle that secreting cells have a definite arrangement around the very small afferent vessels on which their nutrition and function depend. They also have an intimate connection with the very small excretory channels through which their products are discharged. This principle is depicted in the liver acinus, the hepatic structural and functional unit. It is clearly visible in the *in vivo* transilluminated liver; it can be demonstrated by special injection techniques[261] and is also revealed in the pattern of certain pathologic processes.

VESSELS OF THE LIVER

Extrahepatic Distribution of the Hepatic Vessels

The liver receives blood through the PV and through the hepatic artery, a branch of the celiac axis. Since the PV drains the blood of an area supplied by the other branches of the celiac axis and by the superior and the inferior mesenteric arteries, the amount of blood flowing into the liver depends in fact on the flow in these arteries.

Common Hepatic Artery. This artery, the second major branch of the celiac axis, courses to the right along the upper border of the pancreas in the right gastropancreatic fold, which conducts the artery to the medial border of the hepatoduodenal part of the lesser omentum. It ascends in front of the PV in 91% of humans and to the left of and behind the bile duct in 64% of cases. It divides into the left and the right hepatic arteries to supply the corresponding lobes of the liver. Michels[202] sees the hepatic artery dividing into three terminal branches: right, middle (for quadrate lobe), and left. There is an extensive and continuously growing literature[162] on the anomalies of the hepatic artery and its branches.

Cystic Artery. The cystic artery arises in about a third of cases from the right hepatic artery in the upper part of Calot's triangle formed by the cystic and the hepatic ducts. The cystic artery divides into a superficial branch that is distributed to the peritoneal surface of the gallbladder and a deep branch that supplies the attached wall of the gallbladder and its bed. The artery is single in 75% of cases and double in 25%. In the latter, the deep and the superficial branches each have a separate origin.

Because the cystic artery arises in about 35% of cases from the right hepatic branch only or from a right hepatic artery, the variations and the topographic relationship of these arteries with the bile duct and the PV are important. They were described by Daseler and co-workers.[63]

Anomalies of the Hepatic Artery. In about 50% of cases there are aberrant hepatic arteries. The right hepatic artery springs from the superior mesenteric artery, whereas the left aberrant hepatic artery derives frequently from the left gastric artery. Each of these arteries is often the single hepatic artery, and its injury can damage the liver severely. Knowledge of the anomalies of the hepatic artery is important for any surgery in the hepatic and duodenal area and for an effective chemotherapeutic infusion of a cancerous liver.[162]

Portal Vein. The valveless PV is an afferent nutrient vessel of the liver and in this sense is an arterial channel. Analogy between the PV and the pulmonary artery has been based on studies by Reeves and associates.[277] They compare the lung lobule with its central pulmonary arterial inflow to the liver acinus with its portal venular axis. It carries blood from the entire capillary system of the digestive tract, spleen, pancreas, and gallbladder.

The PV derives from the omphalomesenteric veins, which bring blood from the yolk sac and the intestines to the liver. The omphalic portion of the veins regresses with the disappearance of the yolk sac. With the growth of the intestines the mesenteric portions persist and become the tributaries of the PV. Its stem is formed by the omphalomesenteric trunks arranged in a figure eight around the first and third portions of the duodenum. Its spiral course is formed by dropping out the posterior (right) limb of the "8" below and the anterior (left) limb of the "8" above.

In recent years, more frequent operations on the PV have led to new investigations of its anatomy.[97] It has been found constant in its length but extremely variable in its tributaries.

Splenic Vein. This vein (0.94 cm diam) commences with five to six branches that return the blood from the spleen and unite to form a single nontortuous vessel. In its course across the posterior abdominal wall, it grooves the upper part of the pancreas, from which it collects numerous short tributaries. It can be visualized preoperatively by splenoportography (see Chap 14). It runs close to the hilum of the left kidney and terminates behind the neck of the pancreas, where it joins at a right angle the superior mesenteric vein. Because of its nearness to the vessels of the left kidney, the splenic vein can be anastomosed to the renal vein. Its tributaries are the short gastric veins, the pancreatic veins, the left gastroepiploic vein, and the inferior mesenteric vein. In the Warren[346] operation the short gastric veins are used for collateral drainage of the gastroesophageal varices; portal blood flow to the liver is diminished but not curtailed.

Inferior Mesenteric Vein. This vein (0.24 cm diam) returns blood from the area drained by the superior and the inferior left colic and the superior rectal veins.

Superior Mesenteric Vein. This vein (0.78 cm diam) is second in diameter to the PV itself and well suited for anastomosis with the caval system. It carries blood from the veins of the small intestine, the cecum, and the ascending and the transverse colon. The portal trunk (about 2 cm diam) is formed behind the neck of the pancreas by the confluence of its roots, that is, the splenic and the superior mesenteric veins. The length of the portal trunk is approximately 5.5 cm to 8 cm (Fig. 1-11). The portal trunk receives also the rootlets of the superior pancreaticoduodenal vein, some accessory pancreatic veins, the pyloric vein, the left gastric (coronary) vein, and the cystic vein. Usually there is an upper segment of the portal trunk, averaging 5 cm in length, which is devoid of major branches.[97] Here surgical dissection can be started without danger of hemorrhage.

The most troublesome tributary of the portal trunk is the left gastric (coronary) vein. It runs upward along the lesser curvature of the stomach, where it receives some esophageal veins. With progressing cirrhosis of the liver, these enlarge to form varices that are apt to produce fatal hemorrhage. The portal trunk runs in the hepatoduodenal ligament in a plane dorsal to the bile duct and the hepatic artery and divides into two lobar branches before entering the portal fissure. The right lobar branch, short and thick, receives the cystic vein. The left lobar branch, longer and smaller, is joined by the umbilical vein (ligamentum teres) and the associated paraumbilical veins. It connects by the venous ligament (ductus Arantii) with the inferior vena cava. The left lobar branch gives branches to the quadrate lobe and also to the caudate lobe before entering the liver at the left end of the porta hepatis.

Anomalies of the Portal Vein. These are relatively rare. The cavernomatous transformation of the PV is considered by some authors as an acquired anatomic anomaly due to early thrombosis and recanalization of the portal system.[321] Others consider it an atypical development of the plexus of veins between the omphalomesenteric and the hepatic veins during the second month of fetal life.[88] Leger and associates have thoroughly discussed the anatomy and pathogenesis of the portal cavernoma.[176] They stress the viewpoint that the postnatal obliterative process in the umbilical vein and the duct of Arantius may spread to the portal stem and its tributaries. A number of small cavernomatous veins form in the process of bypassing the obliterated vascular area.

Intrahepatic Distribution of the Hepatic Vessels

The topography of the vascular and biliary structures within the liver has been studied by Segall[309] and Hjortsjö[137]; Couinaud,[57] Junès,[152] and Bilbey[19] have rein-

Fig. 1-11. Mensuration of the portal vein and its main branches. Figures are in centimeters. (Gilfillan RS: Arch Surg 61:449, 1950)

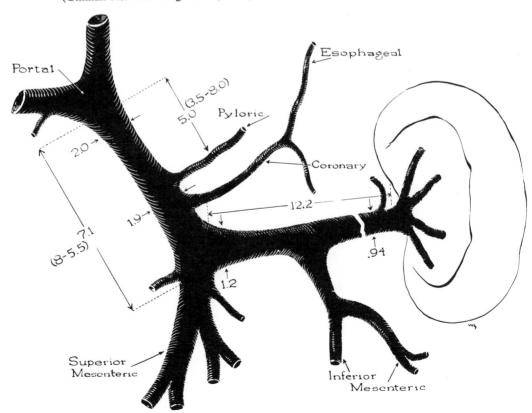

vestigated the gross intrahepatic distribution of the PV, the hepatic artery, and the hepatic vein. We shall follow their description (Fig. 1-12).

Portal Vein. The portal trunk divides in the portal fissure into the left and right hepatic lobar branches, which form an angle of 90° with each other. The left branch is longer than the right and consists of transverse and umbilical parts. The latter is the remainder of the umbilical vein. It has a longitudinal course and continues into the round hepatic ligament. Thus, a bend is formed between transverse and umbilical parts of the left lobar branch. The paraumbilical veins, important hepatofugal collaterals within the falciform ligament, spring from the umbilical part of the left portal branch.

The injection of multicolored vinylite acetate into the vascular branches and the biliary ducts accessible in the porta hepatis has demonstrated that the liver can be divided into segments according to the distribution of the major supplying and efferent vascular or biliary branches (Fig. 1-12). These branches have been named by Bilbey[19] after the segments of the liver they service. The outline in Figure 1-12 summarizes his nomenclature for the intrahepatic branches of the PV, the hepatic artery, and the bile duct. Superior, inferior, medial, and lateral branches of the (right) anterior segment radiate from a common, deeply situated central vessel and are difficult to isolate surgically. The surgical topography of the liver segments has been well presented by Reifferscheid.[278]

Each segment depends on its major vessel for blood supply. There is no anastomosis between the macroscopic branches but large intercommunication at the level of the sinusoids.

Hepatic Artery. Segall[309] likened the straight intrahepatic arterial branches in the younger person to those of a maple tree and the tortuous branches of the older person (over 40 years) to those of a bare apple tree. Left and right arterial lobar branches anastomose rarely outside the portal fissure but intercommunicate by small twigs present in the deeper folds of the capsule of Glisson within the groove of the round ligament.[99] This explains why, after ligation of one branch of the hepatic artery in the autopsy specimen, the entire liver still can be injected with a barium mass through the other arterial branch.[309] Inside the liver substance, the terminal branches of the hepatic artery communicate with each other and the PV only through capillaries and sinusoids.

Fig. 1-12. Intrahepatic distribution of portal venous and hepatic venous branches; portal and hepatic venous segments of the liver overlap. For explanation, see text.

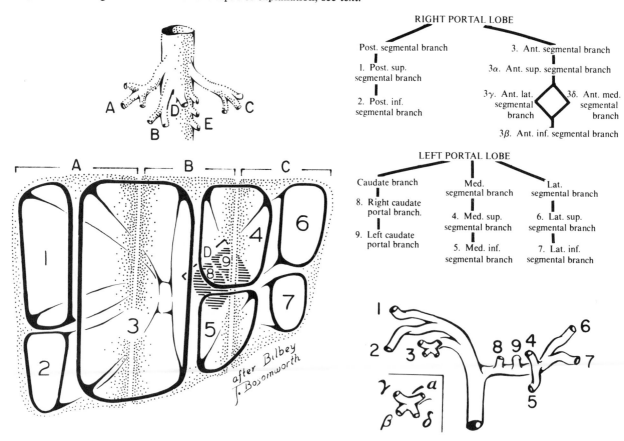

The intrahepatic arterial branches follow the smaller portal branches closely, "climbing along them like a vine on a tree." This feature can be observed *in vivo* at microscopic level.[166] There is commonly an irregularity in the branching of the arterial trunks and the major rami. They do not run close and parallel to the corresponding portal channels or the major intrahepatic bile ducts. Coordination of the courses of the branches of PV, hepatic artery, and bile duct is accomplished in the peripheral parts of the liver, at the level where tridimensional branching is the major law for the housing of a maximum of parenchyma in a limited space. Also, the dome-shaped diaphragm may determine the hemispheric shape of the hepatic surfaces underneath which tridimensional growth is favored by ideal conditions.

Hepatic Veins. The hepatic veins empty into the inferior vena cava where it lies in the groove of the posterior surface of the liver. They are enveloped by the coronary ligament. Since catheterization of the hepatic veins for the determination of hepatic blood flow and sinusoidal pressure has become a frequently used procedure[30,116,315] and guided catheterization of the hepatic veins has permitted their roentgenography,[217,248,270,336] a brief outline of the intrahepatic branches of these veins may be useful.

An upper group of three major hepatic veins (right, middle and left) empties into the inferior vena cava. They drain three hepatic venous segments (Fig. 1-12*A, B, C*) that interdigitate and overlap the outlined portal segments.

Left Hepatic Vein. This vessel (Fig. 1-12*C* and 1-13*C*) drains the left lobe. It is composed of two major radicles: an upper one coming from the upper half and a lower one from the lower half of the territory they drain.

Middle Hepatic Vein. This vein carries blood from the central parts of the liver from areas irrigated by the right and the left lobar portal branches (Fig. 1-12*B* and 1-13*B*). The middle vein sometimes unites with the left hepatic vein to form a short common trunk before emptying into the vena cava.

Right Hepatic Vein. This vessel (Fig. 1-12*A* and 1-13*A*) is the remainder of the cardiac portion of the right omphalomesenteric vein. It drains the territory to the right of the Sérégé gallbladder-caval line.

Several smaller veins (Fig. 1-12*D* and *E* and 1-13*D* and *E*) empty below the group of the major three or two veins into the vena cava. They drain blood from around the gallbladder, from the caudate process, and from the posterior portal segment and the lateral portion of the anterior portal segment in the right liver lobe.

The intrahepatic course of the valveless hepatic veins is straight and simple. Their smaller branches are in direct contact with the hepatic parenchyma. There are frequent anastomoses among the various branches of the hepatic veins.

There is a definite spatial relationship between the branches of the hepatic veins and those of the PV and hepatic artery. The branches of the hepatic vein interdigitate with the afferent vessels (Fig. 1-13); this architectural

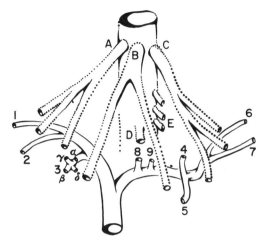

Fig. 1-13. Scheme of interdigitation of hepatic and portal venous trees.

arrangement is maintained up to their finest ramifications. A uniform and quick drainage from all parts of the liver is thus accomplished.

Terminal (Axial) Branches of Afferent Vessels, Sinusoids, Radicles of Hepatic Veins

These vessels lead into and out of the exchange vessels of the liver, the sinusoids, together forming the hepatic microcirculation.

Portal Vein. Elias[80] introduced a distinctive nomenclature for the finer intrahepatic ramifications of the PV. His differentiation into "conducting" and "axial distributing veins," although possible only when these vessels happen to be cut longitudinally, is very suitable for practical purposes. However, serial sections of conducting veins reveal the regular branching out of venules to supply the acinuli in the periportal cuff of tissue. Thus the "conducting veins" distribute blood too. Similar observations were made by Daniel and Pritchard.[61] Conversely, the "axial distributing vein"[80] is a terminal branch of the PV and is the axis of an acinar unit, the sinusoidal glomus of which it supplies with its arborizing inlet venules. These venules show *in vivo* sphincter-like activity that finely adjusts the amount of portal blood in the sinusoids.[166,255,271]

TPVs are easily recognized in the microscopic slide; their cross section is found in the *smallest round or oval portal spaces;* in a longitudinal section one can see the sinusoids branching off the TPV. Preterminal portal branches, the axial vessels of complex acini, lie in small *triangular* portal spaces.

Hepatic Artery. The branches of this vessel supply all the structures in the portal tracts and also the parenchyma. There is now general agreement that the arterioles and arterial capillaries join the terminal portal venules and the sinusoids in Z_1 only; *no arteriole enters Z_3*. Thus two bloodstreams flow into a firmly encapsulated organ under quite different pressures. The question as to how the portal blood streams uphill against arterial pressure is not answered fully. It is believed that sluice mechanisms raise one stream to the level of the other by means of sphincters at the junction of arterioles and arterial capillaries with portal venules and sinusoids.[167] There is also sphincter-like activity at the outlets of the sinusoids into the peripheral veins, which has been observed by several workers.[166,271,345] The information about the histologic features of these sphincters is recent.[43,80] McCuskey describes the sphincters as consisting of reticuloendothelial cells.[197] These cells contain contractile protein, that is, actin and myosin filaments[226,353]; when contracted, they bulge with their nuclear region into the vascular lumen and occlude it.

According to Hale's clear review,[123] the distribution of the terminal (axial) branches of the hepatic artery may be divided into a general plexus within the portal tract, a special capillary plexus surrounding the bile ducts (peribiliary plexus), and the arterial capillaries emptying directly into the sinusoids (Fig. 1-14).

General plexus supplies the structures within the portal tract, except for the terminal branches of the bile duct. These capillaries have a more open network woven around the contents of the portal space and send branches into the radial or peripheral sinusoids.[227]

Peribiliary Arteriolar Plexus. Figure 1-15 illustrates the close network of arterioles and arterial capillaries forming an outer and inner layer around the bile ducts up to their terminal branches; it supplies their walls. Alcohol injected into the hepatic artery perfuses also the peribiliary plexus and produces scarring of the bile ducts, yielding a cholangiographic picture of sclerosing cholangitis.[72] The capillaries of the plexus play an important role in the regulation of hepatic arterial flow, in secretion, absorption, and concentration of primary bile. The arteriolar network is a known route for collaterals instrumental in the regeneration of hepatic parenchyma.[269] The collaterals are derived from the left gastric artery and the superior mesenteric artery through the gastroduodenal and pancreatic arcades. They can become so prominent as to be angiographically demonstrated,[53] especially in hepatic tumors close to the porta hepatis. Branches of the peribiliary plexus pass into radial[10,227] and peripheral[4,80] sinusoids and through capillary connections join the PV, forming "internal roots of the PV."[4,10,163] Murakami has studied injection specimens of the plexus in rodents and monkeys with scanning electron microscopy (SEM).[213] Grooves in the casts, suggestive of sphincters, have been noted in the efferent vessels of the plexus (Fig. 1-15). Random sphincter activity has been confirmed through microscopic observation of the intrahepatic circulation *in vivo*.[166,271,345]

Arterioles Emptying Directly into Sinusoids. The intralobular arterioles running freely through the hepatic parenchyma have been described by both early[44] and recent investigators.[80] We have repeatedly observed *in vivo* the activity of hepatic arterioles in Z_1 only.[271] One also notes *in vivo* selective arterialization and dilatation of transa-

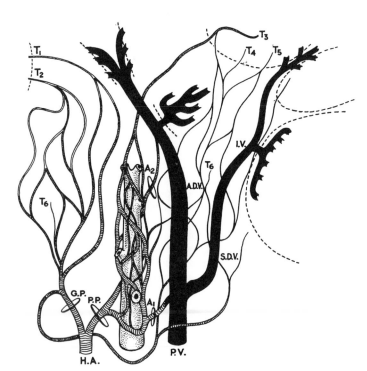

Fig. 1-14. A_1 = arteriolar–venular anastomosis between hepatic artery and portal vein; A_2 = capillary anastomosis between hepatic artery and portal vein; A.D.V. = axial distributing vein; H.A. = hepatic artery; G.P. = general plexus of hepatic artery; I.V. = inlet venule; P.P. = peribiliary plexus of hepatic artery; P.V. = portal vein; S.D.V. = small distributing vein. Branches from general plexus: T_1 = emptying into a radial sinusoid; T_2, emptying into the peripheral sinusoid; T_3, intralobular capillary. Branches from peribiliary plexus: T_4 = emptying into a radial sinusoid; T_5 = emptying into a peripheral sinusoid. Stippled area represents bile ducts. Interrupted lines represent the limits of hexagonal fields. (Hale AJ: Glasgow Med J 32:283, 1951)

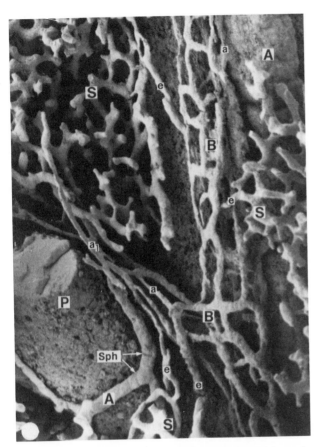

Fig. 1-15. Scanning electron micrograph of cast blood vessels in the liver of Rhesus monkey. Peribiliary plexus (*B*) receives blood from arterial branches (*A*) by means of afferent arterioles (*a*); it supplies the sinusoids (*S*) through efferent arterioles (*e*). Note the grooves indicating arteriolar sphincters (*Sph*). Arterioles (*a₁*) bypass the plexus and empty directly into sinusoids. P = portal venous branch. (Methyl methacrylate cast × 135) (Courtesy of Dr. T. Murakami, Department of Anatomy, Okayama University, Okayama, Japan)[213]

cinar sinusoids receiving arterial blood under higher pressure.[258] In methacrylate casts these sinusoids may be seen running through all the lobule.[156] No arteriolar wall structures have ever been demonstrated histologically in the "translobular arterioles." A clear and detailed electron microscopic study at low magnification of the various anastomotic ways of the hepatic arterioles with the sinusoids and portal venules in the rat has been published by Burkel[42] and recently confirmed in casts by Yamamoto[356]; for similar distribution in the monkey see Figure 1-15.

The structural complexity of the arterioportal junctions indicates multiple possibilities for the hepatic artery to regulate the flow of arterial and portal blood in the acini.

Sinusoids. These hepatic capillaries are unique in their thin endothelial syncytial lining as they are in their large

Kupffer cells.[166] The latter are, in fact, a self-proliferating population of mobile macrophages[352] attached mainly to the endothelial plasmodium and spreading their stellate processes through the capillary lumen toward various points of the wall, where they anchor.[354] In addition to their role in the production of bilirubin, they are the scavengers of this complex canal system, clearing it of particulate matter, old erythrocytes, bacteria,[193] and debris that they engulf.

The littoral cells are seen under the electron microscope as a discontinuous layer[83,125,223] of endothelium composed of cells of various types.[299] Some are very thin, 0.8 μm, and extend over three or four parenchymal cells; some are thicker, up to 5 μm to 6 μm. Their overlapping cytoplasmic lamellae are separated from each other by narrow passages (fenestrae) that provide access for the plasma to Disse's space, which continues into an extensive labyrinth of narrower spaces between the hepatocytes and the spaces at both ends of the sinusoids.[210] The large Kupffer cells have an oval nucleus and cytoplasmic projections on their undersurface for interlacing contact with the microvilli of the parenchymatous cells. These Kupffer cells have a few round mitochondria; their endoplasmic reticulum and Golgi apparatus are not prominent; their large lysosomes are rich in acid phosphatase. Kupffer cells metabolize phagocytized material (pigments, fat, cholesterol, colloids), and they produce reticular fibers; their nuclei also synthesize protein.[84] For other littoral cells, see Chapter 2. The fenestrations of the endothelium can change their size[91] and may selectively permit easy passage of the various macromolecules of the blood plasma into Disse's spaces; their functional role has been recently stressed by Oda[226] and by Fraser.[92]

Evidence has been presented that the surface-to-volume ratio of the sinusoids in Z_1 is significantly larger than that of Z_3. This structural organization favors solute-membrane interactions in Z_1.[203] The width of the sinusoids can vary from 6 μm to 30 μm and can increase to 180 μm when necessary. The change in caliber is due to contractility, an exquisite feature of these capillaries, the structural elements of which are microtubules and microfilaments; recently actin and myosin have been found in endothelial cells.[353] There is also tonic contractility[166] that helps to regulate the amount of flow through a vascular area. Groups of sinusoids shift their work asynchronously. The circulatory activity spreads simultaneously to those sectors of neighboring hexagonal fields that are adjacent to the active axial vessel. This phenomenon explains itself as circulatory activity of single acini. Thus is disclosed the microscopic feature of the function of the liver as a "venesector and blood giver of the circulatory system."[158]

Radicles of the Hepatic Veins. Abrupt transition from capillaries to such large vessels as the "central veins" is unusual in vascular anatomy. The majority of the sinusoids, as seen *in vivo,*[254] empty individually, some through collecting venules into the radicles of the hepatic veins, the THV. Hanzon's microphotos of the various phases of uranin secretion *in vivo* (his Figs. 16 and 39) demonstrated that different acini around a THV empty into collecting venules, which they border.[127] The central veins (THVs) are the *drainage centers* of collecting venules as well as of individual sinusoids from several acini (see Fig. 1-8). The sluice channels of Deysach[68,254] are collecting venules surrounded by sphincters at their site of junction with the preterminal hepatic venules into which they short-circuit a certain amount of sinusoidal blood when needed. The absence of a limiting plate around the THV also indicates that the surrounding tissue is not bound together but belongs to different acini.

The walls of the hepatic venous branches also have contractile sphincters. In dogs, the smooth muscles in the wall of the hepatic veins contract during shock.[196] The presence of these muscle fibers in dogs and humans was described by early workers[38,239] and demonstrated later by Popper,[240] who found that an inversely proportional rate of flow is possible in the hepatic veins and in their mural lymphatics.

The interdigitating relationship between the branches of the hepatic vein and the PV, observed in the gross specimen, is maintained in the microscopic field between terminal branches of these veins. The terminal (axial) branches of the PV and of the hepatic artery in the simple acini run mainly perpendicular to the radicles of the hepatic veins that they surround.

Hepatic Collateral Circulation

Arterial Channels. The frequent fatal outcome after severance of the hepatic artery in humans and in laboratory animals has led for a long time to the belief that the hepatic artery is a terminal vessel. A review of this problem[193] has shown that Haberer[121] in 1905 was the first to prove experimentally that ligation of the hepatic artery proximal to its gastroduodenal branch is not fatal. However, the study of the collateral hepatic circulation did not advance until it was demonstrated that in the dog all branches of the hepatic artery can be ligated with impunity when the animal is treated with antibiotics postoperatively. The liver deprived of the hepatic arterial channels develops a rich collateral arterial supply on which it survives.[90,250] The literature on this subject has grown at a rapid pace since the hepatic artery was ligated in human patients for the treatment of the sequelae of portal hypertension.[16,169]

Extrahepatic Collaterals. The hepatic artery is provided with collateral flow through its anastomoses with adjacent arteries arising from the celiac axis and the superior mesenteric artery. Good collateral circulation becomes manifest in cases of gradual occlusion of the artery. The liver as an outgrowth of the gut shares one of its architectural features, the vascular arcade. The supramesocolic organs are provided with blood by their own vessels and by collaterals that run in modified arcades. In fact, collateral circulation is due to the persistence of modified pathways of fetal circulation.

During the fetal period of life the organs lie closer together, and their vascular interrelationship is more intimate. Growth, increasing the distance between the organs, weakens their vascular interconnections. Thus the gastroepiploic, the pancreaticoduodenal, and the primary branches of the colic arteries represent the *dorsal* anastomosis of the embryonic ventral splanchnic arteries, whereas the left and the right gastric and hepatic arteries are the equivalent of the *ventral* anastomosis of the fetal ventral splanchnic arteries.

The many aberrant hepatic arteries described in about 50% of human cases and their anastomosis with the regular vessels are similarly modified vascular arcades. The frequent and extensive communication between the ultimate and the penultimate branches of the right, the middle, and the left hepatic arteries[201] that takes place in the capsular folds within the fossa for the umbilical vein, and in the region around the caudate lobe,[99] denotes the same arching principle that the splanchnic vessels follow before sending their terminals into the organ. Of course, sudden interruption of the hepatic arterial supply through the celiac axis[16] always means putting all hope in collaterals, if any.

Interruption of arterial flow to the cirrhotic liver is absolutely unphysiological[266] and often induces hepatic failure. This operation has now become obsolete. However, the effects of ligation of the hepatic artery or one of its branches in humans are not necessarily fatal in patients with relatively normal hepatic function; adequate perfusion can be provided by portal and remaining arterial flow until arterial collaterals have developed fully.[39]

Michels[202] has listed 26 potential collateral pathways that may develop to supply the human liver deprived of its arterial blood flow: 10 of these are anatomic variations of the hepatic artery. However, only seven provide sufficient communication between hepatic and nonhepatic vessels to guarantee an immediate collateral supply after occlusion of the hepatic artery. Any deductions about functions (metabolism) made after experimental ligation of the common or proper hepatic artery or some of its branches should be met with grave doubt, since blood from many collateral sources enters the hepatic arterial circuit immediately, especially via the peribiliary plexus.

The main collaterals of the common hepatic artery are right and left gastrics; right and left gastroepiploics; gastroduodenal, supraduodenal, retroduodenal, superior, and inferior pancreaticoduodenals; aberrant hepatic arteries; and inferior phrenic arteries.[250,279]

In the liver of the rat and the dog, after interruption of the arterial supply, revascularization is provided also by the increasing pericholedochal arterial network and its microscopic extension, the peribiliary arterial plexus.[64,269] We wonder how much the rich ramifications of the supraduodenal and the inferior pancreaticoduodenal arteries, around the supraduodenal and the retroduodenal parts of the common bile duct, are capable of such a task in humans. The lack of a similar collateral supply in the transplanted liver may be one of the causes of the frequent biliary postoperative complications.

The role of the hepatic arterial collaterals in the relief of experimentally induced hepatic coma was stressed by Rappaport and associates[267]; they further investigated the metabolic role of the hepatic artery[267] and the part it plays in prolonging the survival of totally depancreatized dogs at no time treated with insulin.[272]

Intrahepatic Collaterals. They develop in the cirrhotic liver as it becomes gradually deprived of portal blood. As the normal flow of portal blood through the sinusoids is blocked by fibrosis in Z_3, an arterial network of collateral vessels develops into a perinodular plexus (see Fig. 1-21).

Portal Channels. Pick has divided the portal collaterals into *hepatopetal* and *hepatofugal*.[238] The hepatopetal pathways develop in patients with unimpeded intrahepatic circulation but with extrahepatic blockage of the PV. The blood bypasses this obstruction by using normal and anomalous channels that enlarge and accommodate the increasing flow through them.

The number and size of hepatopetal collaterals depend on the site of portal obstruction. They usually consist of deep cystic veins, epiploic veins of the lesser omentum and of the hepatocolic and the hepatorenal ligaments, veins in the wall of the common bile duct, diaphragmatic veins, veins of the suspensory ligament of the liver, and the paraumbilical veins.

We found in dogs in which an Eck[76] fistula had been formed by the classic technique, not comprising the complete ligation of the smallest tributaries of the portal stem, that hepatopetal collaterals developed in spite of the portacaval anastomosis. Thus intestinal blood bypassed the wide-open portacaval shunt and continued to flow through the narrow pathways in the porta hepatis.

The hepatofugal collaterals shunt the blood from the abdominal viscera round the intrahepatic obstacle. McIndoe classified these collaterals embryologically into three groups[198]:

1. Veins located in the gastrointestinal tract at the junction of absorbing epithelium with protective epithelium. In portal hypertension, varices are formed in the "stomachoesophageal and hemorrhoidal plexuses." The former shunts blood from the left gastric (coronary) veins by way of the inferior hemiazygos and through the diphragmatic and the azygos veins into the superior vena cava. The hemorrhoidal plexus transfers blood from the superior rectal (inferior mesenteric) vein through the middle and the inferior rectal veins into the inferior vena cava. Both plexuses are vulnerable, but the esophageal plexus mainly gives rise to prolonged bleeding in patients suffering from portal hypertension.
2. Veins occurring at the site of the obliterated fetal circulation, the so-called accessory portal system of Sappey. These are the paraumbilical veins in the falciform and the round ligaments. They unite with the epigastric and internal mammary veins as well as with the azygos vein through the diaphragmatic veins. Veins may pass along the round ligament to the umbilicus and there develop prominent varicosities known as the "caput medusae." A large vein over which a loud murmur can be heard is present in patients with Cruveilhier–Baumgarten syndrome. Its superficial tortuous course was displayed by phlebography.[270,317] Other varieties of collaterals can be observed in the many ramifications of the venous channels in the thoracicoabdominal wall.
3. Veins in the abdomen found at all sites where the gastrointestinal tract and the glands derived from it become retroperitoneal in their development or adhere to the abdominal wall because of pathologic processes. These veins of Retzius can arise from the duodenum, omentum, spleen, pancreas, small intestine, and colon. They establish connections between the portal bed and the ascending lumbar azygos and renal veins. Of clinical importance is the "portorenal plexus," consisting of anastomoses between the left renal vein and the portal beds in the pancreas, spleen, and descending colon. Had its function been understood earlier, the possibility of alleviating portal hypertension by splenorenal anastomosis[181] might have been recognized sooner. Simonds gives a classic description of such a naturally occurring anastomosis that was disturbed during splenectomy with fatal consequences.[321] Other rare portacaval shunts pass by way of the adrenal vein.[88]

Within the hepatic parenchyma collateral channels are formed by anastomoses between smaller branches of the portal and the hepatic veins, the tributaries of the caval system. Moschcowitz[209] made an extensive study of their genesis and considered them "intrahepatic Eck fistulae." Their presence was demonstrated by multicolored injection of cirrhotic liver specimens.[240]

LYMPH VESSELS OF THE LIVER

In the human liver a well-developed subserous hepatic network communicates with the lymph vessels of the gallbladder. The deep lymphatic channels run in the portal tracts where they are visible as the spaces of Mall,[188] especially when serous exudation is present.[134] The lymphatics surround the branches of the hepatic artery and the PV up to their finest ramifications in the simple liver acini. Also the biliary tree and hepatic lymph vessels are connected intimately. The injection of Chicago blue into the clamped choledochus against the direction of bile flow under 310 mm H_2O pressure makes the dye appear immediately in the hepatic lymph vessels.[190]

The lymph from these vessels is drained toward the lymph nodes of the hilum of the liver. Frequently, the lymphatics surrounding the tributaries of the hepatic veins are overlooked. They run along the walls of the tributaries of the hepatic veins and drain into the nodes around the inferior vena cava. The wall of the lymphatic capillaries is formed of spindle- and scallop-shaped and of irregular endothelial cells; there is no basement membrane, no pericytes. Slits between the endothelial cells can narrow or dilate.[145]

Lymph capillaries have not been detected between the parenchymal cells. Disse[69] in 1890 put forward the theory that lymph spaces exist around the hepatic sinusoids. Electron microscopy has revealed a continuous tissue space along the sinusoidal linings that terminates at the limiting plates. The connection between the Disse spaces and the lymph vessels in the terminal portal fields has not yet been demonstrated. Lymph capillaries exist in the walls of the portal and the hepatic veins and extend to their endothelial lining. Therefore, one may assume that some lymph percolates from these veins into the lymph vessels of the surrounding connective tissue. All hepatic lymph vessels drain into lymph nodes: those from the convex part of the liver drain into nodes of the falciform ligament, celiac and esophageal nodes, and xiphosternal nodes; from the under surface of the liver into nodes of the common bile duct and inferior vena cava. Lymph vessels along the PV drain into nodes at the left side of the porta hepatis.

HEPATIC BLOOD FLOW

The preceding detailed description of the vascular system of the liver, of its structural variety and differentiation, will help us in the interpretation of unexpected and anticipated complexities of hepatic circulation. The vascular network of the liver is interposed between the gastrointestinal and systemic circulation. It has often been called the "antechamber of the heart" because it collects all gastrointestinal and splenic blood through the PV and delivers it to the right side of the heart. A fifth of the cardiac output of blood passes each minute by way of the hepatic artery and PV, through the huge sinusoidal network of the liver.

Arterial Flow

The role of the hepatic arterial circulation has been considered for centuries to be of minor importance to the function of the hepatic parenchyma; it was supposed to supply only the connective tissue and gallbladder. Generations of surgeons in the preantibiotic era, however, dreaded accidental injury to the hepatic artery during operations because it was followed by death in at least 50% of the cases.[103] Following the successful experimental ligation of all branches of the hepatic artery in which the animal survived,[250,269] a preparation became available for determining the hepatic functions exerted by this vessel, as they were missing after its ligation.

Arterial Pressure and Volume Flow. The mean pressure in the hepatic artery under anesthesia is around 100 mm Hg. The resistance in the hepatic artery bed is 30 to 40 times that in the portal venous one. The arterial blood passes through a long path of fine, muscular resistance vessels before joining the wide sinusoids. The hepatic arterial bed shows pressure-induced autoregulation.[126,338] The basal tone of the resistance vessels is minimal at 80 mm Hg and increases as arterial pressure rises.[110]

Interactions Between Hepatic Artery and Portal Vein. There is physiologic evidence of intrahepatic mixing of portal and arterial blood[55] and of a one-way hepatic artery–to-PV flow.[247] Hepatic arterial flow increases with reduced PV flow,[244,270,289] for example, during hemorrhage, in which the hepatic artery would deliver 65% of total liver blood flow[62,129,140]; also, hepatic arterial flow doubles after the formation of a side-to-side portacaval shunt.[183] Materials present in the portal stream can modulate flow in the hepatic artery. Vasoactive substances, originating from the gastrointestinal tract, when in sufficient concentrations, will influence vascular resistance in the arterial circuit.[285]

Increased PV pressure in the liver results in increased constriction of the hepatic arterioles. The effects are most marked at portal pressure below 10 mm Hg.[189] Occlusion of the hepatic artery causes small and transient decreases in portal pressure, but the results are not uniform.[46,106,338] The injudicious clinical application of these observations led to the surgical treatment of portal hypertension by ligation of the hepatic artery with unfortunate results.[266,267] In the dog the hepatic arterioles react with vasoconstriction to increases in hepatic venous pressure,[136] and arteriolar resistance may double when the pressure in the hepatic veins rises to 10 mm Hg.[186] However, arterial flow still manages to pass through the experimentally congested vascular network of the rabbit liver.[242] In perfusion experiments[192] one finds that *during nonpulsatile perfusion the vascular resistance is increased by 115%* compared with pulsatile perfusion, a fact to be taken into consideration because in the majority of experimental liver perfusions nonpulsatile perfusion pumps are used. Resistance rises progressively with increases in perfusion rate.

The arteriolar constriction following a rise in arterial, portal, or hepatic venous pressure is considered to be a myogenic reaction to a rise in transmural pressure across the arteriolar wall,[89,170] and this rise enhances the rhythmic activity of the smooth muscle cells in the vessel wall.

Studies of the hemodynamic role of arterioles in the hepatic microcirculation have been made using the transillumination technique (see Hemodynamics of Microcirculation). The hepatic arterioles are constricted effectively by smooth muscle elements.[43,271] The angle at which arterioles and arterial capillaries join the sinusoids determines the direction of blood flow through the sinusoids,[197,277,325] the mixture of portal and arterial blood, and thus the O_2 saturation.[264,271] Our own *in vivo* observations show a marked slowing of flow after the hepatic artery has been occluded. With PV occlusion there is an incomplete circulatory block because the hepatic arterioles continue to deliver blood.[48]

Control of Hepatic Arterial Flow. Hepatic arterial flow is controlled by the following factors.

Neural. The hepatic plexus receives fibers from the celiac plexus, the vagi, and the right phrenic nerves and forms a thick coat around the hepatic artery. The origin and distribution of these fibers have been investigated by Ungváry and co-workers.[339] The splanchnic arteries have an outer nerve plexus in the adventitia, a plexus between adventitia and media, and a plexus within the muscular media. Nerve fibers have been demonstrated histochemically and by transmission electron microscopy (TEM) in association with endothelial cells of the terminal vessels in the portal spaces.[226] Neither dorsal root fibers nor sympathetic vasodilator nerve fibers are present in splanchnic vessels. Dilatation of these vessels is due to diminished vasoconstrictor tone. Stimulation of vagal fibers produces no obvious change in intrahepatic resistance.[7]

Reflex responses occur within the hepatic vasculature. Stimulation of the hepatic nerves decreases liver volume, and 50% of the blood in the liver is maximally expelled. This again proves the role of the liver as a blood reservoir.[111] Stimulation of the plexus in dogs causes an increase in pressure in the hepatic artery and a marked reduction in flow.[107] Following the flow reduction there is reactive hyperemia; α-adrenergic receptors[107,318] mediate these effects; phenoxybenzamine blocks the receptors. Reactive hyperemia involves a combination of metabolic and myogenic mechanisms, an increase of metabolites (CO_2, lactate, pyruvate, adenosine) and of osmolarity (H^+, K^+ ions) in the stagnant blood during occlusion of the vessel. The repayment of flow debt is inversely proportional to the duration of vascular occlusion. Myogenic and metabolic factors are less active with venous than with arterial occlusion.[148] In the cat there is an autoregulatory escape and return to control levels within 4 minutes in spite of maintained stimulation.[82,110] Accumulation of vasodilator metabolites may be the cause of this escape. After sinoaortic denervation in dogs, there is a *transient* increase in hepatic arterial resistance indicating that the hepatic artery takes only a minor part in the adjustment of systemic blood pressure changes.[212] There is a definite reduction in hepatic blood flow and splanchnic blood volume in the human during muscular exercise.[21,28]

Arterioles are richly supplied with unmyelinated nerve fibers and respond to sympathetic stimulation with transient constriction. The regulation of intrahepatic flow takes place at the arteriolar level, whereas the rate of flow in the PV is determined by the state of constriction or dilatation of the mesenteric, splenic, and gastric arterioles. Caliber changes in the TPV are adjustments to decreased volume flow due to arteriolar constriction or to changes in shape and volume of the large endothelial cells at both ends of the sinusoids. Expansion of the portal venous lumen elicits a "venomotor" reflex,[355] that is, arteriolar constriction proximal to the site of venous distention; a similar response occurs to an elevation of portal pressure.[311] Traction on the mesenteric vessels produces in humans and in experimental animals a *fall* in arterial pressure, provided that the nerve supply is intact.[235,337] Heating or chilling the skin, a rise in carotid sinus pressure, and stimulation of the central end of the cut sciatic nerve all elicit changes in the splanchnic and hepatic vasculature.[2]

Metabolic. Although metabolism and circulation of an organ are interdependent, little is known about the relationship between hepatic arterial flow and hepatic metabolic rate.[29] However, metabolites flowing into the sinusoidal network through the PV can have a "transhepatic" effect on the arterioles opening into these channels.[284] In dogs, an 87% increase in hepatic arterial flow is noted after an infusion of amino acids.[301] Glucose infusion dilates the arterioles and renders their jets conspicuous during microscopic observation *in vivo*.[325] Adenosine and potassium seem to be metabolic dilators of the hepatic arterioles.[197]

Changes in the composition of blood gases affect the hepatic circulation. In severe hypoxia with an O_2 saturation 50% less than normal, there is a fall in estimated hepatic blood flow (EHBF), and the intrahepatic arterioles are constricted.[85] No "reactive hyperemia" develops in the liver.[337]

Hypercapnia always causes an increase in splanchnic vasoconstriction of arterioles and venous channels.[207] Contraction of the spleen occurs by neural and neurohumoral factors.

Secretory. The fact that the arterioles of the excretory bile channels are situated upstream and deliver the arterial blood to the sinusoids (see Fig. 1-16*A*) indicates a certain dependence of sinusoidal flow on the prepositioned and filtering periductular vascular glomus. The earlier observation by Schwiegk[307] that an injection of Na-dehydrocholate produces an increase in hepatic artery blood flow together with choleresis has been confirmed[204,243,302]; the choleretic dilates the arterioles.[75] Increased amounts of thin watery bile are also produced by infusion or injection of Na-taurocholate.[115,275] There is increased secretion by the ductular epithelium that is supplied by the periductular arterioles. Na-taurocholate is a part of the reabsorbed bile salt pool; its reabsorption increases hepatic artery flow and O_2 supply during the heightened postabsorptive metabolic activity of the liver.

Hormonal. Regulation of flow occurs in the microcirculatory units mainly by the glycogenolytic hormones, glucagon, epinephrine, and possibly also by secretin[197]; the latter two dilate the arterioles and relax the precapillary sphincters. Glucagon causes an arterial pressure reduction in the pig; the hepatic artery flow increases by 80% 2 minutes after administration and by 58% in 10 minutes.[180] The arteriolar smooth muscles and precapillary sphincters are extremely sensitive to stimulation by vasoactive substances circulating in the blood.[122] Norepinephrine is released from the nerve endings supplying the splanchnic vessels. The arterioles are *constricted* by norepinephrine and dopamine. The hepatic arterioles are *dilated* by ace-

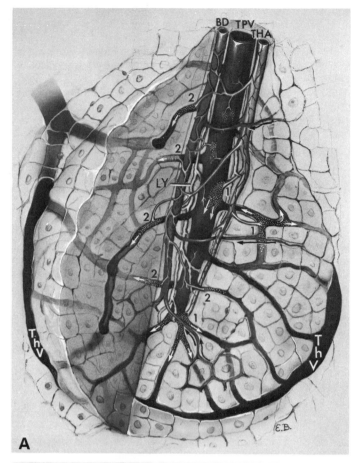

A

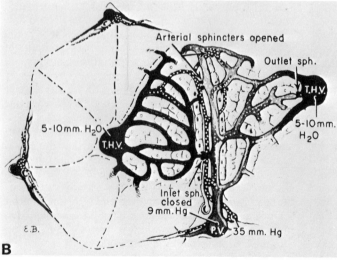

B

Fig. 1-16. A. Microcirculatory hepatic unit, comprising the terminal portal venule (*TPV*) with the sinusoids branching off it and forming a glomus; the hepatic arteriole (*THA*) lacing with its branches a plexus around the terminal bile ductule (*BD*). The arterioles empty either directly (*1*) or through the peribiliary plexus (*2*) into the TPV and sinusoids. The sinusoids run along the outside of cell plates and cords, inside of which are the capillaries of the hepatic secretory and excretory system. The glomus of sinusoids is drained by at least two terminal hepatic venules (*ThV*); LY = lymphatics. (Rappaport AM: Microvasc Res 6:222, 1973) **B.** Microcirculation in a liver acinus. The pressure in the terminal portal, arterial, and hepatic venous branches is indicated. In the left half of the figure note an opened arteriolar inlet sphincter that admits arterial (*white dotted*) blood into the sinusoidal area primarily filled with portal (*black*) blood; the outlet sphincters around the left terminal hepatic venules (*T.H.V.*) are open. In the right half of the figure, arteriolar–portal and arteriolar–sinusoidal sphincters have opened, admitting blood and thus raising velocity and pressure in all the sinusoids. One outlet sphincter at the junction of a sinusoid with the THV is closed. P.V. = portal venule.

tylcholine (1–5 μg into hepatic artery)[6] and by histamine, secretin, pituitrin,[305] and decholine[75,204] and by bile salts given intravenously.[275]

The role of the hepatic artery has been reviewed[265]; its part in protein, fat, and carbohydrate metabolism[264,272,274]

awaits further elucidation. Lautt sees the purpose of the hepatic artery in maintenance of the clearance of blood-borne substances, hormones, and other endogenous products; fluctuations in the clearance of these substances are eliminated.[170] Alteration in hepatic clearance results in changed plasma levels liable to produce serious toxic reactions. The hepatic artery alters parameters affecting O_2 uptake, but the O_2 delivery to the hepatocyte is not controlled by the artery. Oxygen extraction by the hepatic parenchyma is at a maximum because the structure of the normal microcirculatory pathways does not permit short-circuiting of O_2 from arterial or portal blood into the hepatic venules.

Portal Circulation

The portal circulation carries blood from the gastrointestinal and splenic vascular beds. Portal flow depends upon the pressure in the arterioles of these vascular beds; pressure may vary as the smooth muscles of the microvessels display myogenic autoregulation. Increase in intra-abdominal pressure above 40 cm H_2O will decrease portal flow by 90%[228]; this has been demonstrated by angiography.

Rhythmic segmental and tonic contractions of the intestinal wall greatly influence blood flow within the bowel loops.[319] The minute volume of portal flow increases with the rate of rhythmic intestinal contraction but decreases with the duration of the tonic contraction. As the bowel distention increases, intestinal circulation decreases to complete cessation in the overextended obstructed loop; this may eventually lead to necrosis of the bowel wall. Food intake and the quality of food (*e.g.,* protein and carbohydrate) increase portal circulation.[32,93]

It is estimated that two thirds of total hepatic blood flow is of portal origin. The osmolarity, hormones, and metabolites in the portal blood determine to a great extent the inner environment of the hepatocytes. The O_2 content and PO_2 in the hepatic blood are greatly influenced by the corresponding values in the arterial blood. Because portal blood is venous and 70% saturated, with a PO_2 of around 50 mm Hg, the "inner milieu" and PO_2 of the hepatocytes will depend on the interplay and reciprocity of flow between hepatic artery and PV.[15,24,96]

Portal Pressure. Portal pressure depends primarily on the state of constriction or dilatation of the mesenteric and splenic arterioles and on the intrahepatic resistance, be it at the site of inflow or outflow from the liver. Normal hepatic arterial pressure is already greatly reduced within the sinusoids and has little influence on the portal pressure.[334] Hormones, for example, epinephrine, dilate the mesenteric arterioles, thereby increasing portal pressure; vasopressin constricts the mesenteric arterioles and causes a drop in pressure , a dilatation of the PV vascular bed, and reduction in circulating blood volume.[285,305] In cirrhosis, the pressure is increased because of augmented *postsinusoidal* resistance, due mainly to fibrosis in Z_3 of the acini, where the outflow portion of all sinusoids is situated. In addition, the entire hepatic venous bed is significantly diminished. There is also *presinusoidal* and *sinusoidal* portal hypertension depending on the site of the increased hindrance factor.[273] There is also a strong cor-

relation between hepatocyte enlargement and raised portal and intrahepatic pressure.[22]

Regulation of Portal Flow. The intrahepatic portal vessels do not show pressure-induced autoregulation of flow.[109,285] The PV does not differ in this respect from other venous vessels.[200] The absence of smooth muscle fibers in the TPV wall eliminates autoregulation at the microscopic level. The muscular elements of the macroscopic portal venous branches, however, respond to stretch with myogenic activity.[138]

Stimulation of the hepatic nerves or administration of adrenalin produces in the rat, rabbit, guinea pig, and cat blanching of the peripheral parts of the liver, indicating restricted flow[60]; portal flow is diverted toward the portions of the liver lobes that lie closer to the hilum. Thus, in states of circulatory distress, the short-circuited portal blood returns faster through the hepatic veins into the systemic circulation. There is as yet no angiographic proof that similar shunting is present in the human liver.

Streamlined flow as noted in the PV of restrained, anesthetized and laparotomized rabbits is not present in the human liver. During splenoportography, opacification of the liver is not segmental but occurs in all lobes at once. Iodine-labeled rose bengal was uniformly distributed in the liver of the dog following injection into spleen, small intestine, cecum, and colon.[56]

Physical Forces Modifying Hepatic Blood Flow

The liver moves with the diaphragm and is influenced also by the motion of the neighboring organs, intestines, and lungs. These mechanical factors produce shifts in the position of the hepatic vessels as well as in their filling. The blood content of the intraperitoneal organs influences the intra-abdominal pressure; experimental increase in intra-abdominal pressure causes a decrease in hepatic blood flow.[31,228] Gravity too affects hepatic blood flow, and orthostasis decreases EHBF.[59] Exercise causes changes in circulating blood volumes at the expense of the splanchnic circulation; consequently hepatic blood flow decreases because of splanchnic vasoconstriction.[44,344] These observations have initiated the introduction of prolonged rest in the therapy of patients with acute hepatitis.

It was commonly assumed that the phases of the respiratory cycle have their definite effects on emptying and filling the great splanchnic venous reservoir, thus increasing venous return during inspiration.[37,229] Deep inspiration may reduce the luminal cross section of the veins and impede the outflow of splanchnic blood.[139,220] The modifying effects of respiration on splanchnic blood flow will depend on the forces (position, rate, and depth of respiratory excursions; tone of diaphragm, and abdominal wall muscles; intestinal filling) active in the respiratory cycle.

As the "antechamber of the heart," the hepatic circulation is in close relationship with the systemic circulation. This is most evident in pathologic circulatory states, for example, hemorrhagic hypotension[340] and congestive heart failure.

In hemorrhagic shock, splanchnic blood volume decreases to a greater extent than the total blood volume.[281] There is mesenteric arteriolar constriction together with general vasoconstriction, but the hepatic arterioles have a tendency to dilate moderately and assure the O_2 supply of the hepatic parenchyma unless severe hypotension (<80 mm Hg) occurs.

In congestive heart failure there is passive distention of the splanchnic veins, and the hepatic veins and venules are engorged. The trapping of blood in the venous reservoir may reduce the load on the failing heart. However, the large volume of blood in the abdominal veins can be easily displaced by increases in intra-abdominal pressure (forceful respiration, cough, defecation) and thrown as a dangerous load on the heart at any time.

Experimental alteration of hepatic blood flow such as portacaval anastomosis,[76,181] ligation of the hepatic artery,[269] total devascularization of the liver followed by hepatic coma,[87,231,266] occlusion of the hepatic veins,[26] and portacaval transposition[51] have added to the understanding and therapy of liver diseases caused primarily by derangements of the hepatic circulation.

Lymph Flow

The movement of lymph in mammals is part of the continuous circulation of the extracellular body fluids[218]; it is caused by the *vis a tergo* of tissue turgor and by the position and motion of body and limbs. Muscular activity, stretching, breathing, and variations in thoracic pressure are additional sources of energy for driving the lymph. The main function of the lymph is the collection and transport of large molecules, that is, plasma proteins, particulate matter, tissue debris, bacteria, foreign substances, and tissue fluids. The liver lymph originates from the interstitial fluid in the intercellular crevices and in the spaces of Disse. These extend toward the limiting liver plates, and thus lymph fluid finds its way into the initial lymph clefts of Mall[188] situated in the portal spaces. Owing to the permeability of the hepatic sinusoids to large molecules, the hepatic lymph contains 3% to 5% of protein, mainly albumin, thus approximating the protein content of blood plasma. Quantitative studies of hepatic lymph flow have been carried out by the Mayo Group.[25] They indicate that 80% of the hepatic lymph flow passes through the hilar lymphatics and cysterna chyli into the thoracic duct. Hilar lymph flow is greatly increased in glycogenosis of the liver,[286] in cirrhosis, and in veno-occlusive disease. Lymph flow increases when hepatic venous pressure is raised 1 cm to 5 cm H_2O above hilar interstitial pressure. The augmented flow parallels the rise in hepatic venous pressure.[34] At the highest venous pressure induced, the protein composition of the lymph was almost identical to that of plasma. This is easily explained by the many communications (fenestrations) of various and changing sizes[91]

between the sinusoids and the space of Disse. Histamine in low doses increases hepatic lymph flow, its protein content, and its specific gravity by changing the permeability of the endothelial cells lining the sinusoids.[226,359]

There is a close connection between lymph flow and hepatic blood flow. Ligation of the thoracic duct and of the lymphatics at the hilum of the liver leads to a 30% decrease in total hepatic blood flow due to stasis in the portal vessels and in the Disse spaces.[331] The stasis in the lymph leads to increased resistance in the arterial and portal vessels all situated in Z_1 of the acinus. Ligation of the bile duct also increases the intrahepatic vascular resistance, but the maximal increase in tissue pressure occurs in Z_3; there results an increased hepatic artery flow that overcomes the tissue pressure. Experimental production of ascites by constriction of the inferior vena cava above the hepatic veins blocks the efferent lymph vessels in the wall of the great vein in addition to raising hepatic venous pressure.[199] Experimental hepatic venous congestion or carbon tetrachloride poisoning in dogs and rats[71,144] as well as liver cirrhosis in humans leads to an increase in number, widening, and increased permeability of the superficial and deep lymphatic vessels.

Measurement of Hepatic Blood Flow

Methods for quantitation of blood flow have been classified by Bradley.[29]

Direct methods. Older invasive techniques,[98,310] of which the "collection" method became possible in humans with the use of a double balloon catheter,[270] have been supplanted by the use of the electromagnetic flowmeter. The measurement of regional microcirculatory flow in the liver of small animals[141] requires microcannulation of the terminal hepatic vessels.[216,257] Radiologic evaluation of hepatic blood flow is still uncertain.[14] Determination of hepatic blood volume, greatly influenced by the metabolically active microcirculatory "storage phase," has not yet been attempted in humans.[345]

Indirect methods. These have grown in number and complexity and are presented with a slant toward clinical application by Mathie[195] in his clear monograph, to which the reader is referred.

HEPATIC MICROCIRCULATION: THE MICROCIRCULATORY HEPATIC UNIT

The microcirculation is the most active part of the hepatic circulation because it regulates nutrition and function of the parenchyma and its supporting tissues. It is the result of the total merging of the hepatic arterial and portal streams in a common delta. However, the arterial blood with its high pressure does *not* drop like a waterfall into the sinusoidal bed with its low pressure level; it does not dissipate its energy at once. The stream in the hepatic artery breaks up into uncounted rivulets, each of them passing through an arteriole. The arteriole becomes the center of a microvascular glomus around which the acinar parenchyma is organized (Fig. 1-16A). Thus the microcirculation of the liver is organized in units in which pressure and flow are primarily under arteriolar control.

Ultrastructure and Dimensions of the Microvessels. Electron microscopy has confirmed the philosophical dictum that the world is infinite not only upward but also downward.[40,41] The ultrastructural studies of hepatocytes and of the terminal vascular bed have opened new vistas for further investigations. Knowledge of the electron microscopic structure and of the exact dimensions of these vessels in humans is still scant. Burkel and associates[42,43] have provided data on the rat's liver; they facilitate the understanding of the dynamics of the hepatic microcirculation.

The Arterioles. The average inner diameter of the human hepatic arteriole is 25 μm. In the rat, arterioles of the largest size (100 μm diam) have an elastica interna, a double layer of smooth muscle cells (media), and a thin adventitia containing unmyelinated nerve fibers. The terminal arterioles (50 to 20 μm diam) have *no* elastica interna, only a single layer of smooth muscle cells richly supplied with unmyelinated nerve fibers. The arterioles branch into capillaries that form the peribiliary (periductular) arterial plexus and eventually join the sinusoids. The capillaries originate at right angles to the axis of the arterioles; here, for a distance of 30 μm, their wall is surrounded by strong smooth muscle cells forming "precapillary sphincters."[283] The capillaries are lined by a nonfenestrated endothelium.

The Terminal Portal Venule. The TPV in the rat is 50 μm to 70 μm long with an inner diameter of 15 μm to 35 μm; its wall is formed by an endothelial lining and a basement membrane but has no smooth muscle cells. In the human liver the TPV is larger (av. 45 μm) and longer (av. 720 μm).[260] Regulation of blood flow through TPV is not efficient; it is possible only through contractile swelling and shrinking of large endothelial cells at the entry into the sinusoids.[197,226]

Sinusoids. Sinusoids are the venous capillaries of the liver. The length of a human sinusoid varies between 223 μm and 477 μm; the sinusoids of the rat are 250 μm long and 7μm to 15 μm wide; 90% of their length is lined by a fenestrated endothelium that has no basement membrane. This porosity is chiefly of hemodynamic importance because the low hydrostatic pressure (2 mm to 3 mm Hg) is not appropriate for a quick exchange between blood plasma and hepatic cells.[255] There are numerous large pores in the sinusoidal endothelium at Z_1; they are small and more numerous in Z_3.[114] Pores can narrow or widen to become gaps.[353]

Terminal Hepatic Venules. The structure of these radicles of the hepatic venous system is different from that of the TPV. The average inner diameter of a THV in the human liver is 66 μm. The THV has no structured wall; it is an endothelial tube surrounded by few pericytes, fibroblasts, and reticular fibers and by a small tissue space; the hepatocytes lie close to the venule.

In summary, the microcirculatory hepatic unit (Fig. 1-16A) is structured around the terminal hepatic arteriole, which eventually twines itself as a plexus of arterial capillaries around the terminal bile ductule. The arterial capillaries empty into the sinusoids at the site at which they branch off from the TPV. The sinusoids form a glomus around the axis of arterial and portal terminal vessels and empty at their peripheral end into at least two THVs, which interdigitate with the axial afferent vessels.

The anatomic features important for the dynamics of the hepatic microcirculation are the smooth muscle cells around the larger arterioles, the precapillary sphincters, the variable size of the endothelial fenestrae and, to a lesser degree, the actin-like microfilaments in the large endothelial cells at the entry and exit of the sinusoids and arterial capillaries.

Hemodynamics in the Microcirculatory Unit. There are scant data on direct measurements of pressure in the microvessels.[216,257] Orientation in the hepatic microcirculation is lacking in clarity because it was based for a long time on the concept of a hexagonal lobule.

Cannulation of the arterioles and determination of the pressure in them has not been accomplished as yet; the arterioles lie deep to the liver surface. Arteriolar openings into sinusoids and TPVs can be seen in the transilluminated liver; however, one would have to distinguish between the direct end branches of the axial arterioles and vessels coming from the periductular capillary plexus (Fig. 1-16A; 1, 2). There is now general agreement that *no* arteriolar activity can be observed outside Z_1.[155,197,215] The outward movement of plasma fluid into the tissue spaces is greatest in this area. Plasma fluid lowers the extracellular protein concentration and provides the stimulus for increased DNA synthesis and mitosis in Z_1, the most active site for growth and regeneration in the acini.[175]

Because there are no structural differences between the hepatic arterioles and any other arterioles (*e.g.,* the mesenteric), one is justified in assuming that the hepatic arteriolar pressure is 30 mm to 35 mm Hg, the same as in any other terminal vessel of the arterial system.

The question arises: How can low-pressured portal blood pass into sinusoids that are filled with arterial blood under pressure eight times as high? This is possible for the following reasons:

Reduction of arteriolar pressure in the periductular arterial plexus: the capillaries arising from this plexus do not gush their blood forcefully into the sinusoids.

There is an immediate drop to sinusoidal or to terminal portal pressure at the opening of the arterial capillaries into the sinusoids or the TPV; the energy of pressure is transformed into velocity and the flow of portal blood is speeded up.

Intermittent closure of the arterioles facilitates the entry of portal blood into microcirculatory areas shielded from arteriolar pressure by closed sphincters.[254,264]

The sinusoidal area (Fig. 1-16*B:* black in left half of acinus) has been filled with portal blood when the arterioles were closed. The sphincters guarding the arteriolar-portal anastomoses and the inlets of the arterioles into the sinusoids open, the arterial jets (*white dotted*) increase the *vis a tergo* and sweep the portal blood ahead through open outlet sphincters into the THVs.[264] During this event flow is speeded up and exerts through intersinusoidal connections a siphoning effect on neighboring sinusoids.[254] When, however, the outlet sphincters are closed, the rich mixture of arterial and portal blood, appropriate for specific metabolic activities, undergoes a thorough chemical exchange with the liver cell. At a later phase when the sphincters of the arterioles and of the arteriolar-portal anastomoses have closed again, the portal inlet sphincters open and venous blood may flow into the same area following the pressure gradient between the terminal portal and terminal hepatic venules (approximately 50 mm H_2O). A comparison with a sluice mechanism is suggestive, since with the reopening of the arteriolar sphincters the low pressure level of the portal stream will be raised to a higher level.

Micropuncture of the TPV established a pressure about half of that in the portal stem. Flow in the TPV is continuous but is modified by the intermittent activity of the hepatic arterioles and by the pressure gradient between afferent and efferent venules during the phases of respiration. Cannulation of a TPV with the tip of the microcannula positioned close to an arteriolar opening showed pulsatile pressure changes from 50 mm to 250 mm saline.[257]

The sinusoids have not been micropunctured to date. Wedged hepatic venous pressure readings transmit arterial rather than sinusoidal pressure.[290] One notices a puzzling substantial pressure drop (40%) in the wide and multibranching sinusoids between TPV and THV, for which we offer their porosity as an explanation.[255]

The sinusoidal endothelium has been recently studied with SEM and TEM under high magnification; studies revealed the presence of actin filaments (50–70 nm in diameter) that respond to adrenergic and cholinergic stimulations. They mediate constriction and dilatation of the sinusoidal endothelium, the fenestrae, and the venular inlets and outlets.[226]

Sinusoidal pressure and flow are modified by the interplay of the large endothelial cells at the inlet and outlet of the sinusoids. Constriction of the endothelial cells at the inlet causes a drop in sinusoidal pressure and the return of plasma and tissue fluid into the sinusoids. Relaxation of the endothelial cells at the inlet and/or their constriction at the outlet as well as any rise in hepatic venous pressure will cause a pouring out of the plasma into the parenchyma.

Flow in single sinusoids, as recorded on film in the *in vivo* transilluminated mammalian liver,* is definitely pulsatile.[316] The overall impression of continuous sinusoidal flow is due to random intermittent activity of innumerable sphincters in a given time.

Regulation of Blood Flow in the Hepatic Microvessels. The regulation of portal flow by the TPV is practically nil because its wall has no smooth muscles. Still, it can adjust its width to the volume flow that is determined by constriction or dilatation of the splanchnic arterioles. McCuskey[197] has observed *in vivo* the dilation of the arterioles and of the precapillary sphincters by glycogenolytic substances, intermediaries, and metabolites. Glucagon thus yields a swift current of arterial blood for moving the glucose out of the liver quickly; it also provides oxygenated blood to increase gluconeogenesis. The hepatic arterioles are highly responsive to metabolites, electrolytes, and vasoactive substances, all adjusting the arterial microcirculation to local requirements. Tight myoendothelial junctions[283] in the endothelial lining of the arterioles facilitate the stimulation of the muscular elements in their wall by substances contained in the blood. The rich supply of the smooth muscles of the arterioles and precapillary sphincters with unmyelinated nerve fibers permits transmission of impulses from the autonomic nervous system. Thus the merging of the hepatic arterial stream with the portal stream occurs in the uncounted well-controlled microcirculatory hepatic units.

Finally, there is adjustment of flow in these units through bile secretion. The excretory arrangement in the acini is comparable to that in the kidneys.[5] The afferent arterioles enter the wall of the bile ductules and form the peribiliary arterial plexuses from which arise the efferent arterioles; the latter empty into the straight sinusoids that run along the outside of the liver cell plates containing the canaliculi, the finest channels of the excretory system. It will be difficult to micropuncture the afferent and efferent arterioles of the peribiliary arterial plexus to determine the pressure in these microvessels. However, the observation *in vivo* of the arteriolar openings in Z_1 shows a distinct difference in circulatory activity between arterial capillaries of the peribiliary plexus that empty into the sinusoids (Fig. 1-16*A: 2*) and those that bypass the plexus and deliver their blood in strong pulsating jets directly into the TPVs and their sinusoids (Fig. 1-16*A: 1*). The location of the arterial peribiliary plexus upstream to the sinusoids, parenchyma, and its bile canaliculi indicates that the importance of the plexus lies in (1) the modification of the primary bile as it arrives from the bile capillaries and percolates down in the ductular system , the

---

* The color films with sound entitled "Normal Microcirculation of the Mammalian Liver" and "Pathologic Microcirculation in the Mammalian Liver" are available through the Division of Instructional Media Services, Medical Sciences Building, Faculty of Medicine, University of Toronto, Toronto, Ontario, Canada.

result of a countercurrent ionic exchange between blood and bile, and (2) the regulation of arteriolar flow to the sinusoids. Arteriolar dilatation depends in part on the level of bile salts present in portal and systemic blood. Arteriolar activity increases within minutes after raising experimentally the bile salt level in the systemic or portal circulation.[275] On the other hand, increase in secretion is favored by raised plasma flow.[333]

We may thus perceive a direct link between food digestion, absorption, and increased hepatic arterial flow mediated by the dilated arterioles of the peribiliary plexus. Increase in arterial supply further aids in maintaining the proportion between arterial and portal flow that is augmented during digestion. On the other hand, the intimate connection between hepatic microcirculation and biliary secretion in the same microscopic clump of parenchyma demonstrates again the structural, microcirculatory, and secretory unity of the acinus.

In summary, the microcirculatory hepatic unit represents the junction between the hepatic arterial and portal microcirculation, which is artfully modified into a glomus of sinusoids with its afferent and efferent vessels, all within a parenchymal, structural, metabolic, and secretory unit, namely, the simple liver acinus.

Pathways of Hepatic Circulation

The circulation of the liver is characterized by its dual blood supply. As in the similarly supplied lungs, vital metabolic changes of the blood are effected in the liver. From these organs the blood is sent almost directly to the heart for distribution. However, the dynamics in the pulmonary and in the portal circuits differ. Whereas the venous pulmonary stream is driven through its capillary bed by the muscle of the right ventricle and the pulsatile flow is conditioned by the respiratory phases, the flow in the PV could be likened to that of a swampy river. Having its sources in the capillary network of the large splanchnic marsh, the movement of the blood is nonpulsatile and subjected to many fluctuations. The velocity and pressure of the portal stream are very much determined by the flow through the hepatic venous delta, which, in turn, changes with the phases of respiration. If one observes the exposed PV of a dog, one is amazed by the sudden gains in speed of the portal bloodstream; the latter becomes turbulent during inspiration. Indeed, the hepatic veins within the parenchyma do not collapse during inspiration, and the aspirating force of the thorax has its full effect on the entire sinusoidal network.

The vascular branches of the portal and hepatic veins interdigitate and run close to each other. They are separated only by small parenchymal masses, the length of a sinusoid or half the width of an acinus, that is, the distance between its axial vessels and THV. After ingestion of food, the muddy bed of the intestinal capillaries is flooded, and the tide in the portal stream rises. During exercise, the circulation in the musculocutaneous areas is increased at the expense of that in the splanchnic area, and the hepatic minute volume drops. Thus, inflow into the splanchnic area and outflow from the hepatic sinusoidal network determine the volume of flow and the pressure level in the PV. Other factors influencing inflow and outflow are the number and width of irrigated collateral venous channels and the amount of arterial blood flowing through the liver.

There is a reciprocal relationship between arterial and portal blood passing through the liver. Competition of inflow is controlled where the hepatic artery meets the PV. This junction is arteriolar, capillary, or sinusoidal.[197,245,271] Thus, as in other vascular areas, the regulation takes place at the terminal vascular branches, which, in the liver, we defined as the afferent axial channels of the acinar structural and functional units. The blood coming up in a tidal flow through the portal branch and in pulsating jets through the companion arterial twig disperses like a fountain. It runs through the sinusoids down into the radicles of the hepatic veins and waters and nourishes the parenchyma of liver acini. The various ways of branching and anastomosing of the terminal afferent vessels with vascular areas situated above and below a hexagonal field (see Fig. 1-8) indicate that the structural units are intimately connected with each other by the blood channels and form *one* parenchymal mass.

Inflow and outflow from the sinusoidal delta are regulated by an intricate sluice mechanism, the morphology[42] and the nervous control of which have been investigated recently.[226] Thanks to the marvelous play of sphincters at the arterioles, of the endothelium at the inlet and outlet venules[166,271], the variability of the endothelial fenestrae and the pre-capillaries, the arterial and the portal streams, coming into the same compartment under a remarkable pressure difference, further each other's flow instead of inhibiting it. The arterial jets break up the sluggish portal flow in the sinusoids and send it on. The rushing blood column may exert a siphoning effect on communicating lateral sinusoids and empty them. The opening and closing of adjacent blood channels by sphincters has a valvular effect similar to that in the heart cavities, where low-pressured blood is passed intermittently to a chamber that is under high pressure in its active phase.

Under stress conditions, the portal stream, which keeps the sinusoidal system filled (sometimes one third of the entire blood volume is stored in it) may detour its blood from the peripheral sinusoidal and hepatic venous delta and short-circuit it by direct channels into the large hepatic veins. Also, extrahepatic collateral venous channels are used to transfer the blood rapidly into the inferior vena cava.[61] Thus portal circulation time is reduced, and the blood returns more quickly to the heart.

Collateral arterial circulation also plays a definite role in the liver. This becomes manifest under pathologic and experimental conditions. After all branches of the hepatic artery *and* the PV in a dog have been ligated in a stepwise procedure, the liver, this huge vascular organ, can still survive on collateral arterial circulation alone.[269]

From the related data, much of which has been gathered since the observation of the intrahepatic circulation *in vivo*,[136,197,271,345] one might be inclined to believe that we know a great deal about the hepatic circuit interposed between the splanchnic capillaries and the heart. However, most of the data concern only the changing circulatory phenomena. We still lack sufficient quantitative data on pressure and flow rate within the microcirculatory hepatic units. Further investigations of the physiology and pharmacology of the hepatic microcirculation and the integration of the findings into the regulatory mechanisms of splanchnic blood flow will advance our knowledge of the pathology and therapy of the liver.

In summary, the study of the morphology of the hepatic circulation shows that the liver consists of a large vascular delta formed by the confluence of the portal and arterial streams. Their arms, which subdivide the delta into lobar areas, start to run parallel and close to each other when they are still visible to the naked eye; dwindled down to microscopic size, the vessels become the scaffold for the parenchymal cell masses nestling between them. The arterioles as they merge with the sinusoidal and portal channels assume the role of organizing the microcirculation into units. These units are the *vascular core* of the structural and functional liver acini. It is now demonstrated beyond doubt that there exists a PO_2 gradient in the hepatic vessels and tissues decreasing from the site of the arteriolar rivulets joining the portal venous stream in Z_1 only toward the site of their common egress through the THVs. The gradient permits the subdivision of the microscopic vascular units into three microcirculatory zones, each of them creating an appropriate microenvironment for specific enzymic and metabolic activity. The microcirculatory shifts in arterial flow from tide to ebb due to digestion or neurohumoral causes will cause change in the activity of the zones. These are *essentially dynamic* subdivisions of the metabolic activity in the hot liver swamp. Here also start the tiny rivulets forming a green river, the bile stream, that runs in the opposite direction to the portal and hepatic arterial flow. It is to be expected that the quantity and quality of bile carrying important products back to the gastrointestinal area for digestion and absorption of fat are influenced by the tides in portal and arterial flow. All in all, it is evident that vascular morphology is the visual aspect of the dynamic blood flow permitting us to perceive its functional orderliness and to study the circulatory physiology in the hepatic delta; the relationship between hepatic blood flow and metabolism is not yet clearly established.

The role of the arterial and portal components of the hepatic circulation has been analyzed. There is a reciprocal relationship between arterial and portal volume flow; it is effected by the state of constriction or dilation of the mesenteric and hepatic arterioles, both under myogenic control. The portal blood secures the nutrition of the hepatocytes and the delivery of the greater part of the absorbed products of digestion to the liver. The hepatic artery maintains an appropriate PO_2 gradient between the acinar zones and the flow of blood against increased tissue resistance; it ensures a steady clearance of blood-borne substances, for example, hormones and endogenous products. Regulation of arterial flow is less neural than neurohumoral; metabolites and bile salts exert additional effects on blood flow. Phases of respiration, intra-abdominal pressure, intestinal contraction and relaxation, as well as gravity and exercise, are forces that modify the hepatic circulation.

Lymph flow is intimately connected with the circulation because it provides an additional way of egress from the liver of protein-rich plasma and tissue fluids. Lymph flow is greatly increased in states of impeded blood flow through the liver.

NERVE SUPPLY OF THE LIVER

Sympathetic fibers deriving from bilateral ganglia T7 to T10 and synapsing in the semilunar ganglion of the celiac plexus intermingle with fibers from the right and the left vagus and the right phrenic nerve to form the hepatic arterial nerve plexus.[105] It is known also as the anterior nerve plexus, and it surrounds the hepatic artery as a thick coat. Other nerve bundles ramify around the PV and bile ducts and form a posterior hepatic plexus[143]; both plexuses intercommunicate. Other nerve bundles travel freely in the peritoneal folds linked with the porta hepatis. Some nerve fibers from the plexus around the gallbladder enter the hepatic parenchyma. The arteries are innervated mainly by the sympathetic fibers, whereas the bile ducts are innervated by both sympathetic and parasympathetic fibers. Some fibers follow the vessels and bile ducts into their finest ramifications and send off branches supplying the structural elements of the portal tracts.[3,171] Histochemical investigations have demonstrated the extension of cholinergic nerve fibers into hepatocytes of the limiting plate. TEMs reveal the presence of unmyelinated nerve endings in the vicinity of the smooth muscle fibers, close to portal endothelium in the portal space.[226] The nerve fibers also join the nerve plexus around the hepatic venous branches.[329] Others pass into the parenchyma and form the parenchymal plexus around the cell cords, and some end in small knobs around single cells.[329]

Resection of the anterior nervous plexus[189] changes the quality of bile secretion: the concentration of bile salts and pigments increases. Interruption of the anterior nerve plexus prevents the accumulation of fat in the liver. Degeneration of the nerve fibers around the hepatic veins has been observed in the human cirrhotic liver.[140]

STROMA OF THE LIVER

The connective tissue of the liver, *stroma,* shows a varying degree of cellularity: fixed histiocytes, monocytes, plasma cells, and lymphocytes. It forms the capsule of Glisson, which is attached to the parenchyma by radial processes. The capsule is thick around the inferior vena cava and at the porta hepatis. The intrahepatic spread of connective tissue follows the vascular and biliary branches through the porta into the segments of the liver, ramifying in them, and almost joining up at their surface with the capsule. The sparse connective tissue around the hepatic veins merges with the fibrous tissue around the inferior vena cava. The connective tissue carries the lymphatics and the nerve fibers. There is also the mesh of *reticulum* fibers suspended among the bundles of connective tissue fibers around the portal and hepatic venous tree. The argentaffin reticulum framework, probably a product of the reticular cells lining the sinusoids, sustains the liver cords and plates. When this framework survives hepatic injury, the hepatocytes can regenerate more rapidly and fill the empty spaces in an orderly fashion. Under the electron microscope the reticulum fibers show a characteristic segmentation that distinguishes them from the collagenous and elastic fibers.

ANATOMIC PATTERN OF PATHOLOGIC PROCESSES

The concept of a hexagonal lobule that is situated around a THV offers the pathologist only two or three landmarks for the orientation of lesions he observes:[262,263] the "central vein," the "periphery," and, rarely, the "midzone."[135] On the other hand, in the acinar concept attention is focused on the dynamic lines along which adequate or deficient nutrients and oxygen are moved into the parenchyma and along which the produced bile is carried away (Fig. 1-17A). Noxious agents, ascending infections of bile ducts, and lymph vessels all enter the liver along the same lines. In severe injury, large areas of parenchyma are wiped out, and lobular orientation becomes impossible, but in cases of less damage the pathologic change is patterned on the anatomy of the acini and their circulatory zones:[256] The lesions are often well delimited; their sharp borders have been tentatively explained by an interplay in disturbed specific enzymic activity.[293]

A *"paracentral" lesion*—necrotic, fatty, or fibrous—is a *focal* lesion occupying about one triangular sector of the hexagon, with the base toward one of its sides.[322] It represents the tangential cut of the damaged periphery of an acinus that lies above or below the plane of section (Fig. 1-17A: 1).[74] Similar lesions were produced experimentally by Kettler and called *Gruppennekrosen.*[161] "Midzonal" lesions have been explained by Rappaport and co-workers[268] as tangential cuts of the damaged periphery of acini. Cheng[50] demonstrated by serial histologic sections that the "midzonal" necrosis produced by experimental intoxication with beryllium sulfate represents the tangential cut of a necrotic area near a terminal afferent vascular branch. If one ceases to consider as a unit the tissue contained within the imaginary hexagonal field and sees it composed of parts of simple acini surrounding a THV, "focal" and "midzonal" lesions are easily recognized as sectioned lesions of acinar zones.

A periportal lesion unfolding toward two adjacent central veins (Fig. 1-17A: 2) represents the transverse section of an acinus entirely diseased (*e.g.,* the necrosis in phosphorus poisoning).

The *perivenular ("pericentral") lesions* seen in ischemic necrosis (Fig. 1-17B), in fatty change,[35,312] in chronic active hepatitis[298] ("Kollapsstrassen," "confluent necrosis" *i.e.,* "bridging"),[18,67,297] in early dietary fibrosis,[128] alcoholic liver disease,[232] and cirrhosis[94,182,282] demonstrate by their stellate processes extending into adjacent hexagonal fields (Fig. 1-17B) that in reality the progressing damage skirts the tissue in Z_1 and Z_2 that surrounds the supplying vessels. Thus a triangle-shaped area is outlined (Fig. 1-17B: II; N_1) with a THV in its center. These less severe lesions are located at the periphery of parenchymal clumps representing complex acini. As the injury progresses, the stellate processes increase and widen to form a starfish-shaped lesion around the THV (Fig. 1-17B: III, N_2 and Fig. 1-18). In advanced lesions, the line of damage follows the periacinar course, creating within adjacent acini venovenous necrotic or fibrotic bands that are known as "bridging" (Fig. 1-17: III and Fig. 1-18). The peripheries of the simple acini surrounding a THV are *not* bound together by a limiting plate[80]; this facilitates the cleavage of the individual acini by any damage that spreads in a stellate fashion along the acinar peripheries.[308,327] Necrotic, fatty, or fibrotic lesions, as they progress, broaden and form *periacinar* bands,[256] tridimensionally interwoven septa, like baskets, containing only the surviving Z_1, the core of the simple acini (see Fig. 1-17B: RSA).[128]

Scanning a wider microscopic area, one can find in the same slide small periportal rims, islets, and clumps of surviving parenchyma in the midst of necrotic, fatty, or fibrotic tissue (Fig. 1-19A). It is easily recognized that the surviving cells are oriented around terminal (Fig. 1-19A: 1) and preterminal (Fig. 1-19A: 2) afferent axial vessels and bile ductules. The THVs have become separated from the normal tissue. A band of damaged tissue connecting several THVs to one another and to portal fields may arch as the broken line in Figure 1-19A over many hexagonal fields to surround an area of healthy tissue that represents the cross section of acinar agglomerates (Fig. 1-19A: 3). Within this area the contiguity of the parenchyma is maintained because the pathologic change is not severe enough to injure the peripheries of complex or simple acini. The lesser degree of damage may be due to the fact that the parenchyma has been spared massive invasion of the area under study. The cleavage of the uniform hepatic parenchyma into regenerating nodules and nodes (Fig. 1-19B) by fatty change or diffuse fibrosis[17] occurs along the peripheries of simple acini or portions thereof,[276] complex acini, and acinar agglomerates, where the radicles of the hepatic veins are normally situated.

This peculiar position of "central veins" at the periphery of the regenerating nodules has been reemphasized.[160] However, no adequate explanation has been given for this "move" of the radicles of hepatic veins from a central to a peripheral position in the tissue. The anatomic expla-

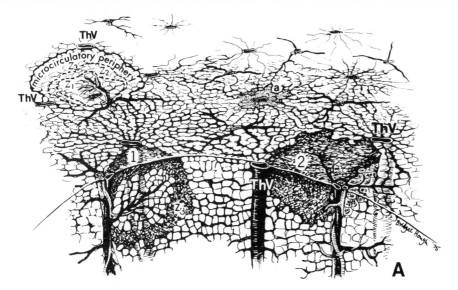

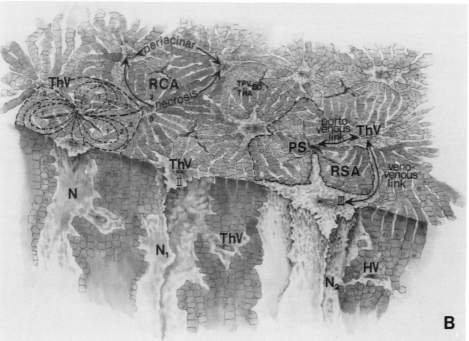

Fig. 1-17. A. Hepatic lesions limited to single acini. *Crosshatched area 1* = "paracentral" necrosis revealed by a tangential cut of a lesion in the peripheral part, zone 3, of an acinus beneath the plane of section. *Area 2* = transverse section of an entirely diseased acinus close to its axial vessels; the injury therefore extends into two sections of neighboring hexagonal fields and reaches their ThV. *Perivenular* ("pericentral") necrosis and fatty or fibrous change (*a*) result from mild damage to the parts of zone 3 most remote from the terminal afferent vessels of the complex acini occupying parts of at least three adjacent hexagonal fields. **B.** Diagram illustrating tridimensionally the chief patterns of necrosis (*N, N₁, N₂*). A complex acinus comprising three simple acini, their microcirculatory zones, and the terminal hepatic venule (*ThV*) is shown (*far left*). There is perivenular necrosis around the ThV and at I(*N*), cut here vertically. The lesion around II, N₁, is triangular as the perivenular injury has progressed along zone 3 of adjacent complex acini. The spreading processes of the triangular necrosis link ThV to ThV (*periacinar arrows, upper left*) and surround the remnant of a complex acinus (*RCA*). Necrosis may progress further and assume the shape of a *starfish* (*III, N₂*) by extending its processes along Z_3 of simple acini; the confluent necrosis then reaches a ThV and a portal space (*PS*). These venovenous and portovenous necrotic links follow also the periacinar course ("bridging"); they have isolated the remnant of a simple acinus (*RSA*). HV = hepatic venule; TPV = terminal portal venule; THA = terminal hepatic arteriole; BD = terminal bile duct.

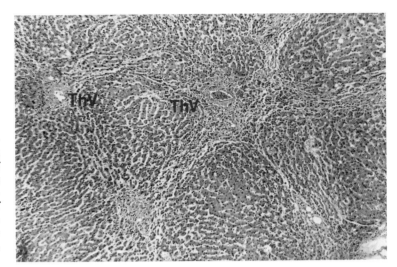

Fig. 1-18. Starfish-shaped fibrosis around terminal hepatic venules (ThV) in the liver of a cirrhotic patient. This design is the result of partial fibrosis of zone 3 of several acini; the fibrous bands link ThV to ThV. Tridimensionally seen, the bands are cross-sections of fibrous septa that envelop the nodular remnants of the acini. (Trichrome × 68). (Rappaport AM et al: Virchows Arch Pathol [A], 1983. Courtesy of Springer Verlag, NY)

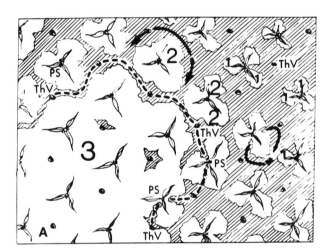

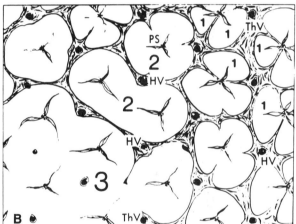

Fig. 1-19. A. Hepatic damage affecting simple acini (*1*), complex acini (*2*), and acinar agglomerates (*3*). The lesion is severest in the right half of the diagram where the simple acini have lost most of their parenchyma and have been reduced to small "periportal" rims of tissue (*1*) around the nutrient vessels. The injury is less in the center of the figure where complex acini (*2*) have survived; however, they are already separated from each other and from the bulk of well-preserved acinar agglomerates (*3*) by strands of damaged tissue (*broken line*) linking the portal spaces (*PS*) to terminal hepatic venules (*ThV*) situated at the microcirculatory periphery of the acinar agglomerates. **B.** Regeneration of the acinar remnants. Regeneration and hyperplasia, starting from the surviving remnants of the acini, have created a nodular pattern of the hepatic parenchyma. The monoacinar nodules (*1*) developed from the remnants of simple acini can be distinguished easily from small nodules (*2*) formed from surviving remnants of complex acini. The large node (*3*) is the result of hyperplasia in preserved acinar agglomerates. Note that the hepatic veins are in their normal position, that is, at the periphery of the acini and their regenerated remnants. HV = hepatic vein. (Modified from Rappaport AM, Hiraki GY: Acta Anat 32:126, 1958)

nation is now possible on the basis of the acinar concept, which presents the THVs as drainage centers at the outskirts of several acini; these veins do not "move"; they just retain their original position.

Irregularity of Nodes and Nodules

The irregularity of nodes and nodules is usually attributed to the varying degree of regenerating power that the organ has preserved. However, the established irregularity in size and shape of normal simple and complex acini and acinar agglomerates makes clear how nodules deriving from their remnants will likewise show a great variety in size and form. Also, when certain parts of the liver suffer either from a mild injury or from occasional noxious agents and deficiencies, the lesions will affect only the circulatory periphery of an acinar agglomerate or of a group of acinar agglomerates (Fig. 1-19*A: 3*). The lesions will delimit in a wide sweep an area that is serviced by one major trio of axial channels. Within this area the circulation is still coherent, and the intrahepatic flow of nutrients is not arrested at the monoacinar peripheries, as in Figure 1-19*A* and *B: 1;* they continue to intercommunicate largely, ensure the resistance of the hepatic parenchyma, and preserve an apparent polygonal pattern. Regeneration in a region, favored by good supply, is active and produces large nodes (Fig. 1-19*B: 3*) that have hypertrophied in an "orderly" fashion. However, tissue that by the pathologic processes has undergone subdivision into a complex or monoacinar pattern will regenerate and form nodes and nodules that are divorced from their THVs and give the impression of pseudolobulation (Fig. 1-19*B*). On the basis of our structural and functional concept we can now understand "pseudolobulation"; it reveals, although in a dis-

torted way, the true acinar lobulation of the liver. However, the classification of cirrhosis based on the variety of nodules is confusing. Also, the study of the intrahepatic microcirculatory changes, so important for the nutrition of the nodular parenchyma, has been neglected. These changes induce vascular sequelae that lead to the death of the patients.

In a recent paper[276], we have defined cirrhosis as follows: *the scarring of the liver acini in Z_3 or Z_1 or in both.* By serial sectioning of a variety of cirrhotic livers, we confirmed that nodules are scarred and modified remnants of various acini. Since blood supply is essential for function and survival of the tissues, we have classified the nodules according to the way they are supplied by their nutrient vessels into *triadal, paratriadal,* and *atriadal* nodules. The classification of nodules into "micronodules" and "macronodules" is difficult to justify, since their two-dimensional appearance changes at different planes of section (Fig. 1-20). Early scar formation precedes the change in microcirculatory dynamics. Sprouting of vascular branches, especially of arterioles, takes the leading role in the development of mature scars, that is, fibrovascular membranes. The fibrous repair is at the same time the road builder for collateral flow. The pathophysiology of the *intrahepatic* collateral circulation is the *basic deter-*

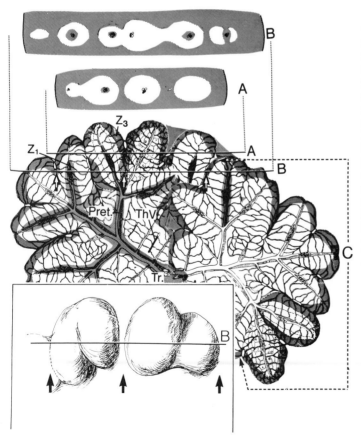

Fig. 1-20. Diagram of changing appearance of paratriadal nodules. Paratriadal nodules result from the maintained interconnection of parenchymal remnants of acini sclerosed at zone 1 (Z_1) and zone 3 (Z_3). The cross-hatched areas indicate fibrosed zonal portions of the acini of various order. The shaded area at the periphery of the entire clump of tissue marks the microcirculatory periphery of the group of acinar agglomerates fed by the triad TR. The cross-hatched zone 3 of one agglomerate is outlined by C; it contains peripheries of complex and of simple acini. (Cross-sections at a superficial (*A*) and deeper (*B*) level of the same scarred acini show nodules of different size and shape. The tridimensional aspect of the nodules situated between the arrows is shown in the lower inset. Z_3 includes the microcirculatory periphery. Pret. = preterminal arterial and portal branches; ThV = terminal hepatic venule. (Rappaport AM et al: Virchows Arch Pathol [A], 1983. Courtesy of Springer Verlag, NY)

minant in the formation of the cirrhotic patterns. These patterns are illustrated in Figure 1-21. The arteriolar flow in an acinar agglomerate decreases progressively from the normal triadal trichotomy in the left complex acinus toward the right complex acinus. In the latter, periacinar fibrosis with its collateral vascular network has dissected out the simple acini. The sinusoidal route has become blocked at its egress into the THV by the perivenular fibrosis, and the triadal arterioles, unable to overcome the resistance to flow, have progressively fibrosed.

Collateral vessels develop from the patent preterminal arteriole with pressure that is higher than that in the terminal arterioles. Neogenesis of collateral arterioles starts at capillary level, that is, in the capillaries of the granulation tissue instrumental in the scar formation. Capillaries in which flow predominates gradually develop into arterioles and arterial branches[221]; they lengthen and follow a spiral course. Flow in the periacinar arterial and venous plexus meanders to find its way into still patent hepatic

venules and veins where perivenous fibrosis is less pronounced. In the end (Fig. 1-21; right *CA*) there are no axial vessels in the acinar remnants, which have become transformed into nodules with perinodular plexuses of vessels, lymphatics, bile ductules, and nerves.

Three microcirculatory phases in the cirrhotic process nodules can be delimited; they are due to a changeover of the intrahepatic circulatory path from normal trichotomy of the preterminal vascular branches to convoluted collateral channels. The three phases of the cirrhotic process are described below:

1. *The triadal nodule.* It receives blood from the stunted TPVs and terminal hepatic artery and partly from the perinodular plexus evolving in Z_3 along the periacinar path (see 1-17*B*). The nodular parenchyma may thus become segregated from the THV, a situation that leads to portal hypertension.

2. *The paratriadal nodule.* It is a conglomerate of nodules

Fig. 1-21. Diagram illustrating the evolution of the arteriolar bypass of the sinusoidal route within the scarring acini in an agglomerate. The left complex acinus (*CA*) is irrigated by terminal arterioles derived from the trichotomy of the preterminal (*Pret*) arterial branch. The light arrows indicate the normal sinusoidal path toward the terminal hepatic venules (*ThV*). In the middle CA, fibrosis (cross-hatched) following damage at the microcirculatory periphery of the simple acinus (SA) surrounded the ThVs and created dams around them (increasing from left to right). The axial arterioles are partially fibrosed, while there is concomitant increase in collateral vessels. The right CA consists of three acinar remnants of parenchyma, that is, nodules without axial supplying vessels but with a very rich plexus of arterioles spiraling in the thick fibrous membranes around the nodules. This perinodular plexus is supplied by the larger preterminal arteriole (*black arrows*); the number of ThVs has decreased. ThV_1 and ThV_2 = venules narrowed by fibrosis.

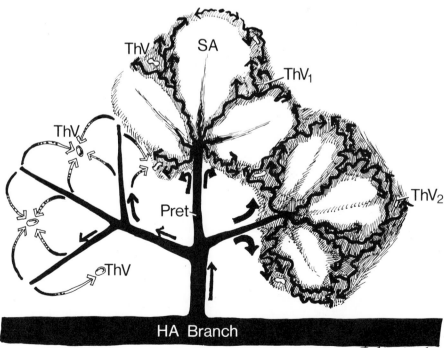

not completely separated from one another; they are derived from neighboring acini of various orders that receive blood from large triads contained in the perinodular scar. The blood arrives into the sinusoids primarily via a plexus surrounding the conglomerate of nodules. Some sinusoids may receive additional blood through sclerosing remnants of terminal afferent branches and through irregular vascular twigs, which, along with septa, enter the nodules at various sites (see Fig. 1-20).

3. *The atriadal nodule.* It is completely separated from neighboring nodules by thick scars; its parenchyma is totally segregated from afferent and efferent vascular branches. The nodules receive blood only from a dense perinodular capillary plexus. Atriadal nodules are seen rarely at autopsy, since most patients die of vascular accidents and hepatic failure during the paratriadal phase.

BILIARY SYSTEM

Ducts

Bile excretion starts in the intercellular bile canaliculi that empty into the smallest bile ductules (see Fig. 1-10); the entire biliary tree participates in the formation of the final product, the bile.[49] The uniting bile canals form the terminal "interlobular" ductules. The latter are lined by tall cuboidal epithelium and follow the course of the terminal (axial) branches of the PV surrounding them in a plexiform way. From the confluence of the terminal bile ductules, ducts arise. Their epithelium is taller and contains mitochondria; their walls are thicker; also, they are surrounded by the larger amount of connective tissue present in the portal tracts. The peribiliary arterial plexus is woven around these ducts and is in intimate connection with the outpocketings of their walls described by Beale (1889).[13] They were recently demonstrated with SEM by Yamamoto[357] in the portal spaces of rat and human liver. There is a dense plexus of ductules especially in the rat[132] that communicates with the ductal branches and provides collateral safeguards for bile flow.

Plexus and parietal sacculi help concentrate the bile by the absorption of water.[132] Considering the weight of the gland and the volume of hepatic blood flow (1,500 ml/min), a larger bile secretion than the daily outflow from the bile duct is to be expected. An absorptive mechanism in the ductules and smaller ducts similar to that in the renal tubules was suggested.[250] Brauer, in his studies of bile secretion of the removed and perfused liver, demonstrated that the bile secreted by the hepatic cells in passing down the biliary tree is afforded an opportunity to reach electrolyte equilibrium with the blood plasma.[33] He further concurred that the peribiliary plexus is an excellent anatomic device for effecting the exchange between blood and bile constituents. Finally, more recent studies[81,291] as well as observations with the electron microscope of mi-crovilli protruding into the lumen of the bile canaliculi[234] and of the striated border of the isoprismatic epithelium lining the bile ductules[35] have corroborated this suggestion.

Intrahepatic Ducts. The wall of the microscopic intrahepatic bile ducts has dense fibrous tissue that contains many elastic fibers. The mucosa formed by tall to columnar epithelium tends to be folded. The localized occurrence of smooth muscle fibers in the wall of the ducts[324] near the hilum of the liver forms the morphologic basis for the narrowing of the bile ducts seen in the cholangiograms. Topographic studies of the intrahepatic distribution of the bile ducts have been carried out to enable a correct interpretation of the cholangiograms.[137,324] Exact knowledge of the intrahepatic topography of the major bile channels is required when anastomosis between them and the intestinal lumen must be established in order to bypass a heavily scarred bile duct, especially in biliary atresia.[157]

In the hilar region there is no fixed coordination between the major ducts and the major branches of the PV. In the peripheral parts of the liver, branches of the PV, the hepatic artery, and bile ducts run together. Of all the major intrahepatic bile ducts, the most constant in its course is the lateral superior segmental duct. It runs straight toward the suspensory ligament and is found when the liver is approached from its upper left corner. On the right side the inferior branch is easily accessible.

Extrahepatic Ducts. The anatomy of the extrahepatic ducts has been well researched, since they are in the domain of surgical activity.

Common Hepatic Duct. This duct arises from the confluence of the right and left lobar ducts, which leave the liver in the right end of the portal fissure to become the right and left hepatic ducts. The common hepatic duct is 3 cm long and is situated to the right of the hepatic artery and in front of the PV. It is joined by the cystic duct at its right side and in an acute angle to form the bile duct (ductus choledochus).[149] This manner of junction is considered normal. Anatomic variations in the types of anastomosis between the cystic and hepatic ducts are of surgical importance.

Bile Duct (Ductus Choledochus). The length of the bile duct depends on the site of junction of the cystic duct with the common hepatic duct.[104] If this junction is very low, the choledochus is short. Its average length is quoted as 7 cm, its diameter, the size of a goose quill. The free or supraduodenal part of the choledochus runs downward and slightly to the left and lies in the right border of the lesser omentum, anterior to the aditus to the lesser sac. Usually, surgical revision of the common bile duct is carried out at this free part; also, it is the most common site of strictures.[222]

The *pancreatic part* of the bile duct passes retroperitoneally behind the first portion of the duodenum. It then runs in a groove on the posterior surface of the head of the pancreas, where it is situated in front of the inferior vena cava. At the left side of the duodenum it is joined in 89% of cases by the pancreatic duct (Wirsung) and forms the ampulla of Vater, 3 mm to 5 mm long.

Studies of the *duodenal or intramural part* of the choledochus have been made to clarify the intricate sphincter mechanism present here.[27,306] It is destined to regulate a one-way flow of biliary and pancreatic secretion into the intestine. In their passage through the duodenal wall, the united bile and pancreatic ducts form a wartlike elevation of the mucosa called the papilla of Vater. A shallow dilation inside the papilla, averaging 3 mm deep and as some believe inconstant, is called the ampulla of Vater. Cholangiography reveals in about one fourth of the cases a reflux from the bile duct into the pancreatic duct. In these cases the openings of both ducts lead into a common cavity; thus biliary disease can easily reflect upon the pancreas.

The circular smooth muscle fibers surrounding these structures are defined as the *sphincter of Oddi*. It is composed of the following parts:

1. *Choledochus sphincter.* This consists of circular muscle fibers that surround the intramural portion of the common bile duct in its course through the intestinal submucosa. The sphincter, which is always present, constricts the lumen of the bile duct.
2. *Pancreatic sphincter.* This is present in only 33% of persons and is not a real muscle ring.[168] Thus the reflux of bile from the bile duct into the lumen of the pancreatic duct is possible.
3. *Sphincter ampullae.* This consists of longitudinal fibers surrounding a weak layer of sparse circular fibers.[164] The longitudinal fibers in contracting shorten the ampulla and raise mucosal folds to prevent reflux of intestinal content into the lumina of the ducts.

Endoscopic partial sphincterotomy does not abolish the motor characteristics of the proximal parts of the sphincter of Oddi.[65]

Gallbladder

The gallbladder is a receptacle for bile (30–50 ml). In the form of a pear-shaped sac 3 cm wide and 7 cm long, it lies on the undersurface of the right liver lobe. Its parts are designated as fundus, body, and neck. The fundus projects beyond the inferior border of the liver at the site at which the lateral margin of the rectus crosses the costal margin. The body is directed upward and to the left. Posteriorly, fundus and body are in close relation with transverse colon and duodenum, respectively. Gallstones can perforate into these viscera.

The cystic artery reaches the neck of the gallbladder at the site of its attachment to the liver by areolar tissue. The neck is curved anteriorly in an S-shape and when enlarged forms the so-called Hartmann's pouch. The mucous membrane of the neck forms a spiral valve of Heister that continues into the cystic duct. The latter arises from the left upper corner of the pouch and has a proximal

valvular and a distal smooth portion. The spiral valve has the function of regulating bile flow both ways—into and out of the gallbladder. During the fasting state the gallbladder receives bile from the hepatic duct through the cystic duct. When stimulated by food or cholecystokinin, the gallbladder delivers the concentrated bile through the cystic duct into the common bile duct and the intestine.[142] Some consider the mucosal folds of Heister's valve as an architectural device to prevent distention and collapse of the cystic duct when sudden change of pressure occurs in the gallbladder or the common duct.[178]

Histology of Extrahepatic Ducts and Gallbladder. The cystic, the hepatic, and the common bile ducts all possess a mucosa, a submucosa, and a muscularis. The mucosa consists of a single layer of columnar epithelium and a tunica propria that contains mucous glands. These are of the type of utricular glands, and their openings are visible to the naked eye. They are lined by simple cylindrical epithelium and are surrounded by a wall of connective tissue rich in capillary network. Some believe that they represent small receptacles in which the bile is concentrated as in the gallbladder. In the dog these sacculi dilate and increase in number after cholecystectomy.

The wall of the extrahepatic ducts is formed by a strong layer of connective tissue fibers into which sparse muscle elements are interspersed,[187] except for the region of the neck of the gallbladder and at the lower end of the common duct where muscle rings are conspicuous. Taking into consideration the absorptive and the sphincter mechanisms, it is to be emphasized that the extrahepatic bile ducts are not passive conducting tubes; they are involved in the secretin-mediated production and absorption[291] of bile. They take part in the concentration and intermittent discharge of bile.

The gallbladder is lined by a mucosa thrown into multiple folds, which serve to increase the absorptive capacity of the organ. The epithelial lining of the mucosa is columnar; the cells are provided with a striated border (for absorption). At TEM the cells show microvilli, a well-developed Golgi apparatus, and numerous but small mitochondria.[149] Glands of the tubuloalveolar type are found in the region of the neck. They are the only glands to produce mucus in the gallbladder. The Rokitansky–Aschoff sinuses are only outpouchings of the mucosa into defects of the muscularis that favor bacterial retention and inflammation. However, the ducts of Luschka are lined with mucosa of the bile duct type. They are situated in the areolar tissues of the hepatic surface of the gallbladder and communicate with intrahepatic bile ducts rather than with the gallbladder cavity. Their presence is an indication for drainage of the gallbladder bed following cholecystectomy. A small amount of areolar tissue separates the mucosa from a skimpy layer of decussated smooth muscle bands well developed only in the fundus and the neck of the organ. Their arrangement is similar to that of the urinary bladder. There are many elastic fibers in the body of the gallbladder. The serosa is attached to the muscularis by a subserous layer of connective tissue that contains the vessels, nerves, and lymphatics.

Blood Supply of Bile Ducts and Gallbladder. The arterial supply of the bile ducts comes mainly from the right hepatic artery. The gallbladder may be supplied by one, two, or three arteries. Its venous network does not accompany the arteries but empties directly into hepatic areas connecting with right and left portal venous branches.[159] Branches of the posterior, superior, and posteroinferior pancreaticoduodenal arteries forming abundant anastomotic loops contribute also to the formation of Zuckerkandel's plexus around the common bile duct.[73]

A continuation of this plexus within the liver along the intrahepatic bile ducts forms the peribiliary plexus. In the dog whose hepatic artery has been ligated, these vascular networks become pathways by which the hepatic parenchyma connects with collateral arterial vessels, mainly from the phrenicoabdominal and inferior pancreaticoduodenal arteries. The periductal plexus in such animals has been demonstrated by catheterization and roentgenography of the celiac axis *in vivo*.[249,269]

The cystic artery usually arises from the right hepatic arterial branch, joins the gallbladder at its neck, divides into two branches that run under the serosa of the gallbladder, supplying this organ as a terminal artery. Injury to this vessel or its parent artery is followed by gangrene of the gallbladder. In some cases, in which the gallbladder is buried more deeply into the liver substance, collateral blood supply from the hepatic parenchyma may prevent this cataclysm. The anomalies of its arterial supply have been described by Michels.[201] The veins of the gallbladder empty into the PV or form a vein at the neck of the gallbladder that passes directly into the hepatic parenchyma joining the sinusoids.

Lymph Vessels of Bile Ducts and Gallbladder. The lymph vessels of the hepatic, cystic, and upper parts of the common bile duct empty into glands of the hilum. Those of the lower part of the common bile duct drain into glands around the head of the pancreas.

The lymph vessels of the gallbladder investigated by Sudler are connected intimately with the lymph vessels of Glisson's capsule.[328] The gallbladder, although an outgrowth of the intestine, has no lymph follicles. However, there is a superficial subserous network of lymphatics and a submucous one that does not penetrate the mucosal folds. They empty into the "lymph gland of the neck" of the gallbladder.

Nerves. Nerve fibers supplying the extrahepatic ducts derive mainly from the sympathetic hepatic plexus laced around the hepatic artery. These also receive filaments from the right and left vagus nerves. Some nerve fibers deriving from the plexus can be seen running along the common bile duct. Sparse ganglion cells are present in the muscularis and the mucosa of the gallbladder. Most nerve cells are found in the fibromuscular layer of the cystic duct. Nervous connection with the spinal system is brought about by fibers from the right phrenic and the musculophrenic nerves. Since these nerves derive from the third or fourth cervical nerve, the anatomic basis for shoulder pain in gallbladder disease is seen readily.

Anatomic Variations of Bile Ducts and Gallbladder. These anomalies are much less frequent than those in the vascular supply of the liver and its bile receptacle. The absence or the obliteration of the bile duct is noticed early in the newborn. It is fatal when not corrected in time.[157] Absence of the gallbladder is normal for the rat,[132] horse, and deer. It is rare in humans (1 in 4000 cases), and in two-thirds of cases it shows some symptoms.[70] Usually it is associated with absence of the cystic duct.

Accessory hepatic ducts, low junction of the branches of the hepatic duct, anomalies in the anastomoses between cystic duct and hepatic duct, and congenital cystic dilatation of the common bile duct are the most common malformations of the duct system.

The common hepatic duct can receive accessory hepatic ducts, or it may be completely absent. In the latter case two hepatic ducts run separately and join close to the duodenum. Then the right duct anastomoses with the cystic duct.

Double gallbladder usually produces symptoms of biliary disease and sometimes can be discovered by cholecystogram or during operation.[208] This anomaly is due to nonconfluent cavitation of the solid gallbladder anlage. Bilobed, hourglass-constricted gallbladders and those with folded fundus (phrygian cap) or persistent septum favor retention and inflammation. The gallbladder can be completely buried in liver substance or attached loosely to it by a mesenterium (floating gallbladder). The latter variety is preferred by the surgeon.

SUMMARY

Although the liver occupies a shielded corner of the abdominal cavity, because of its size, topography, and vascular, biliary, and nervous connections, it maintains an intricate relationship with almost all abdominal organs. In the end, morphology is a snapshot of the immensity of physicochemical events as they appear to our senses in the *nunc stans,* be it in the natural gross range or in grandiose magnifications. The functional anatomy of the liver is a fine illustration of the fact that structure and function are only different aspects of the same package of atomar change.[41]

REFERENCES

1. Albert Z et al: Histochemical and biochemical investigation of gammaglutamyltranspeptidase in the tissues of man and laboratory rodents. Acta Histochem 18:78, 1964
2. Alexander RS: The participation of the venomotor system in pressor reflexes. Circ Res 2:405, 1954

3. Alexander WF: Innervation of biliary system. J Comp Neurol 72:357, 1940

4. Andrews WHH et al: Studies on the liver circulation: II. The micro-anatomy of the hepatic circulation. Ann Trop Med Parasitol 43:229, 1949

5. Andrews WHH et al: Excretory function of the liver: A reassessment. Lancet 2:116, 1955

6. Andrews WHH et al: The action of adrenaline, noradrenaline, acetylcholine and histamine on the perfused liver of the monkey, cat and rabbit. J Physiol 132:509, 1956

7. Andrews WHH et al: Observations on the innervation of hepatic blood vessels. Ann Trop Med Parasitol 52:200, 1958

8. Arey LB: On the presence of the so-called portal lobules in the seal's liver. Anat Rec 51:315, 1932

9. Axelrod J et al: Mechanism of the potentiating action of B-diethyl aminoethyl diphenylpropylacetate. J Pharmacol Exp Ther 112:49, 1954

10. Bailey FR: Bailey's Textbook of Histology, 16th ed. Baltimore, Williams & Wilkins, 1971

11. Balis JU et al: Electron microscopy study of the developing human liver. In Vandenbroucke J, DeGrote J, Standaert LO (eds): Advances in Hepatology, Trans. Symp. I.A.S.L., Brussels and Leuven, 1964, p 133. Baltimore, Williams & Wilkins, 1965

12. Balogh K Jr: Histochemical demonstration of 3-α-hydroxysteroid dehydrogenase activity. J Histochem Cytochem 14:77, 1966

13. Beale LS: The Liver, p 30. London, J & A Churchill, 1889

14. Bengmark S, Rosengren K: Angiographic study of the collateral circulation to the liver after ligation of the hepatic artery in man. Am J Surg 119:620, 1970

15. Benyó I et al: The mechanism of the changes in splanchnic blood flow after feeding. Res Exp Med 171:255, 1977

16. Berman JK, Hull JE: Hepatic, splenic and left gastric arterial ligations in advanced portal cirrhosis. Arch Surg 65:37, 1952

17. Best CH et al: Liver damage produced by feeding alcohol or sugar and its prevention by choline. Br Med J 2:1001, 1949

18. Bianchi L et al: Acute and chronic hepatitis revisited. Lancet 2:914, 1977

19. Bilbey DLJ, Rappaport AM: The segmental anatomy of the human liver. Anat Rec 136:165, 1960

20. Bilbey DLJ, Rappaport AM: Segmental anatomy of human liver. Anat Rec 136:330, 1960

21. Bishop JM et al: Changes in arterial-hepatic venous oxygen content difference during and after supine leg exercise. J Physiol 137:319, 1957

22. Blendis LM et al: The role of hepatocyte enlargement in hepatic pressure in cirrhotic and noncirrhotic alcoholic liver disease. Hepatology 2:539, 1982

23. Bloom W: The embryogenesis of human bile capillaries and ducts. Am J Anat 36:451, 1925/26

24. Bollman JL, Grindley JH: Hepatic function modified by alteration of hepatic blood flow. Gastroenterology 25:532, 1953

25. Bollman JL et al: Technique for the collection of lymph from the liver, small intestine or thoracic duct of the rat. J Lab Clin Med 33:1349, 1948

26. Bolton C, Barnard WG: The pathological occurrences in the liver in experimental venous stagnation. J Pathol Bacteriol 34:701, 1931

27. Boyden EA: The sphincter of Oddi. Surgery 1:25, 1937

28. Bradley SE: Variations in hepatic blood flow in man during health and disease. N Engl J Med 240:456, 1949

29. Bradley SE: The hepatic circulation. In Hamilton WF, Dow PH (eds): Circulation, Handbook of Physiology, vol II, section 2, p 1387. Washington, DC, Am Physiol Soc 1966

30. Bradley SE et al: Estimation of hepatic blood flow in man. J Clin Invest 24:890, 1945

31. Bradley SE et al: Determinants of hepatic hemodynamics. In Ciba Foundation Symposium, Visceral Circulation, p 219, 1953

32. Brandt JL et al: The effect of oral protein and glucose feeding on splanchnic blood flow and oxygen utilization in normal cirrhotic subjects. J Clin Invest 34:1017, 1955

33. Brauer RW: Mechanisms of bile secretion. Gastroenterology 34:1021, 1958

34. Brauer RW et al: Changes in liver function and structure due to experimental passive congestion under controlled hepatic vein pressures. Am J Physiol 197:681, 1959

35. Braunsteiner H et al: Elektronenmikroskopische Beobachtungen an normalen Leberschnitten sowie nach Gallenstauung, Histamin und Allylformiatvergiftung. Z Ges Exp Med 121:254, 1953

36. Braus H: Anatomie des Menschen, 2nd ed, pp 14, 324. Berlin, Springer–Verlag, 1924

37. Brecher GA: Venous Return, p 149. New York, Grune & Stratton, 1956

38. Brissaud E, Sabourin C: Sur la constitution lobulaire du foie et les voies de la circulation sanguine intrahépatique. CR Soc Biol 40:757, 1888

39. Brittain RS et al: Accidental hepatic artery ligation in humans. Am J Surg 107:82, 1964

40. Brunner C: Die Lehre von den Geistigen und vom Volke, pp 244–555. Stuttgart, Cotta, 1962

41. Brunner C: Science, Spirit, Superstition: A New Enquiry into Human Thought, pp 43–44. Toronto, Toronto University Press, 1968

42. Burkel WE, Low FN: The fine structure of rat liver sinusoids, space of Disse, and associated tissue space. Am J Anat 118:769, 1966

43. Burkel WE: The fine structure of the hepatic arterial system of the rat. Anat Rec 167:329, 1970

44. Burns GP, Schenk WG Jr: Effect of digestion and exercise on intestinal blood flow and cardiac output: An experimental study in the conscious dog. Arch Surg 98:790, 1969

45. Burstone MS: New histochemical techniques for the demonstration of tissue oxidase (cytochrome oxidase). J Histochem Cytochem 7:112, 1959

46. Caldwell RS et al: Observations on portal venous pressure following hepatic artery ligation in experimental animals. Surgery 36:1068, 1954

47. Cantlie J: On a new arrangement of the right and left lobe of the liver. J Anat Physiol 32:4, 1897

48. Chenderovitch J: La circulation hépatique. Étude micro-cinématographique 1: Le foie normal du rat blanc. Pathol Biol 10:629, 1962

49. Chenderovitch J: Les conceptions actuelles des mécanismes de la sécrétion biliaire. Presse Med 71:2645, 1963

50. Cheng K–K: Experimental studies on the mechanisms of the zonal distribution of beryllium liver necrosis. J Pathol Bacteriol 71:265, 1956

51. Child CG III et al: Liver regeneration following porta-caval transposition in dogs. Ann Surg 138:600, 1953

52. Child CG III et al: Reversal of hepatic venous circulation in dogs. Ann Surg 150:445, 1959

53. Cho KJ, Lunderquist A: The peribiliary vascular plexus:

The microvascular architecture of the bile duct in the rabbit and in clinical cases. Radiology 147:357, 1983

54. Cohen PP, Marshall M: Carbamyl group transfer. In Boyer D (ed): The Enzymes, vol 6. New York, Academic Press, 1972

55. Cohn JN, Pinkerson AL: Intrahepatic distribution of hepatic arterial and portal venous flows in the dog. Am J Physiol 216:285, 1969

56. Cole JW et al: An experimental study of intrahepatic distribution of portal blood. Surg Gynecol Obstet 102:543, 1956

57. Couinaud C: Les enveloppes vasculobiliaires du foie ou capsule de Glisson. Leur intérêt dans la chirurgie vésiculaire, les résections hépatiques et l'abord du hile du foie. Lyon Chir 49:589, 1954

58. Courtoy PJ et al: Synchronous increase of four acute phase proteins synthesized by the same hepatocytes during the inflammatory reaction. Lab Invest 44:105, 1981

59. Culbertson JW et al: The effect of the upright posture upon hepatic blood flow in normotensive and hypertensive subjects. J Clin Invest 30:305, 1951

60. Daniel PM, Pritchard MML: Effects of stimulation of the hepatic nerves and of adrenaline upon the circulation of the portal venous blood within the liver. J Physiol 114:538, 1951

61. Daniel PM, Pritchard MML: Variations in the circulation of the portal venous blood within the liver. J Physiol 114:521, 1951

62. Darle N, Lim C Jr: Hepatic arterial and portal venous flows during hemorrhage. Eur Surg Res 7:259, 1975

63. Daseler EH et al: The cystic artery and constituents of the hepatic pedicle: Study of 500 specimens. Surg Gynecol Obstet 85:47, 1947

64. DeLong RP: Revascularization of the rat liver following interruption of its arterial supply. Surg Forum 4:388, 1953

65. De Masi E et al: Motor activity in the sphincter of Oddi (SO) after distal partial sphincterotomy. Gastroenterology 86:1060, 1984

66. Desmet VJ: Experimentelle levercarcinogenese, histochemisetic studie, pp 80, 317. Brussels, Presses Académiques Européenes SC, 1963

67. Desmet VJ: Die Morphogenese der chronischen Hepatitis. Münich Med Wochschr 120:1523, 1978

68. Deysach LJ: The nature and location of the "sphincter mechanism" in the liver as determined by drug actions and vascular injections. Am J Physiol 132:713, 1941

69. Disse J: Über die Lymphbahnen der Säugetierleber. Arch Mikr Anat 36:203, 1890

70. Dixon CF, Lichtman AL: Congenital absence of gallbladder. Surgery 17:11, 1945

71. Dolgova MA: 1962, as quoted by Jdanov DA (1964). (See Reference 144.)

72. Doppman JL, Girton ME: Bile duct scarring following ethanol embolization of the hepatic artery: An experimental study in monkeys. Radiology 152:621, 1984

73. Douglass TC, Cutter WW: Arterial blood supply of the common bile duct. Arch Surg 57:599, 1948

74. Dubin IN: Anoxic necrosis of liver in man. Am J Pathol 33:589, 1957

75. Duffin J et al: Simultaneous blood flow measurements with square wave electromagnetic flowmeters. Preconference Digest, pp 32–33. Canadian Electronics Conference, Oct. 4–6, 1965, Toronto, Ontario

76. Eck N: Ligature of the portal vein. Voenno—Meditsinskiy Jurnal (St Petersburg), 130, No. 2:1, 1877

77. Eger W: Zur Struktur und Funktion des Lebergewebes. Ärztl Sammelblätter 50:1, 1961

78. Elias H: The liver cord concept after one hundred years. Science 110:470, 1949

79. Elias H: A re-examination of the structure of the mammalian liver: I. Parenchymal architecture. Am J Anat 84:311, 1949

80. Elias H: A re-examination of the structure of the mammalian liver: II. The hepatic lobule and its relation to the vascular and biliary systems. Am J Anat 85:379, 1949

81. Erlinger S: Secretion of bile. In Schiff L, Schiff ER (eds): Diseases of the Liver, 5th ed, p 93–118, Philadelphia, JB Lippincott, 1982

82. Fara JW, Ross G: Escape from drug-induced constriction of isolated arterial segments from various vascular beds. Angiologica 9:27, 1972

83. Fawcett DW: Observations on the cytology and electron microscopy of hepatic cells. J Natl Cancer Inst 15:1475, 1955

84. Ficq A: Radioautographic studies on nuclear activity in the liver. J Histochem Cytochem 7:215, 1959

85. Fischer A: Dynamics of the circulation in the liver. In Rouiller CH (ed): The Liver, vol 1, pp 330–371. New York, Academic Press, 1963

86. Fischer W et al: Reciprocal distribution of hexokinase and glucokinase in the periportal and perivenous zone of the rat liver acinus. Hoppe Seylers Z Physiol Chem 363:375, 1982

87. Fisher JE, Baldassarini RJ: False neurotransmitters and hepatic failure. Lancet 2:75, 1971

88. Fleischhauer H: Über den chronischen Pfortaderverschluss. Virchows Arch Pathol Anat 286:747, 1932

89. Folkow B: Transmural pressure and vascular tone—Some aspects of an old controversy. Arch Int Pharmacodyn Ther 139:455, 1962

90. Fraser D Jr et al: Effects of the ligation of the hepatic artery in dogs. Surgery 30:624, 1951

91. Fraser R: Thoughts on the liver sieve. Bull Kupffer Cells Foundation 1:46, 1978

92. Fraser R et al: High perfusion pressure damages the sieving ability of the sinusoidal endothelium in rat livers. Br J Exp Pathol 61:222, 1980

93. Fronek K, Stahlgren LH: Systemic and regional hemodynamic changes during food intake and digestion in nonanesthetized dogs. Circ Res 23:687, 1968

94. Galambos JT: Natural history of alcoholic hepatitis: III. Histological changes. Gastroenterology 63:1026, 1972

95. Gearhart J, Oster-Granite ML: An immunofluorescence procedure for the tissue localization of glucosephosphate isomerase. Histochem Cytochem 28:245, 1980

96. Gelman S, Ernst EA: Role of pH, P_{CO_2} and O_2 content of portal blood in hepatic circulatory autoregulation. Am J Physiol 233:E255, 1977

97. Gilfillan RS: Anatomic study of the portal vein and its main branches. Arch Surg 61:449, 1950

98. Ginsburg M, Grayson J: Factors controlling liver blood flow in the rat. J Physiol 123:574, 1954

99. Glauser F: Studies of intrahepatic arterial circulation. Surgery 33:333, 1953

100. Gooding PE et al: Cytochrome P-450 distribution in rat liver and the effect of sodium phenobarbitone administration. Chem Biol Interac 20:299, 1978

101. Goresky CA: The hepatic uptake process: Its implications for bilirubin transport. In Goresky CA, Fisher MM (eds): Jaundice, pp 159–174. Plenum Press, New York, 1975

102. Goresky CA et al: On the uptake of materials by the intact liver: The transport and net removal of galactose. J Clin Invest 52:991, 1973

103. Graham RR, Cannel D: Accidental ligation of hepatic artery: Report of one case with review of cases in the literature. Br J Surg 20:566, 1932

104. Grant JCB: Atlas of Anatomy, 6th ed, Fig. 144. Baltimore, Williams & Wilkins, 1972

105. Gray H: Anatomy of the Human Body, 29th ed. Philadelphia, Lea & Febiger, 1973

106. Grayson J, Mendel D: Observations on the intrahepatic flow, interactions of the hepatic artery and portal vein. J Physiol 139:167, 1957

107. Green HD et al: Autonomic vasomotor responses in the canine hepatic arterial and venous beds. Am J Physiol 196:196, 1959

108. Greenberger NJ et al: The effect of chronic ethanol administration on liver alcohol dehydrogenase activity in the rat. Lab Invest 14:264, 1965

109. Greenway CV, Stark RD: Hepatic vascular bed. Physiol Rev 51:23, 1971

110. Greenway CV et al: The effects of stimulation of the hepatic nerves, infusions of noradrenaline and occlusion of the carotid arteries on liver blood flow in the anesthetized cat. J Physiol 192:21, 1967

111. Greenway CV et al: Capacitance responses and fluid exchange in the cat liver during stimulation of the hepatic nerves. Circ Res 25:277, 1969

112. Grisham JW: Lobular distribution of hepatic nuclei labeled with tritiated-thymidine in partially hepatectomized rats. Fed Proc 18:478, 1959

113. Grisham JW: Deoxyribose nucleic acid synthesis and cell renewal in regenerating rat liver. J Histochem Cytochem 8:330, 1960

114. Grisham JW et al: Scanning electronmicroscopy of normal rat liver: The surface structure of its cells and tissue components. Am J Anat 144:295, 1975

115. Grodins FS et al: The effect of bile acids on hepatic blood flow. Am J Physiol 132:375, 1941

116. Groszman RJ et al: Wedged and free hepatic venous pressure measured with a balloon catheter. Gastroenterology 76:253, 1979

117. Guder WG, Schmidt U: Liver cell heterogeneity: The distribution of pyruvate kinase and phosphoenolpyruvate carboxykinase (GTP) in the liver lobule of fed and starved rats. Hoppe Seylers Z Physiol Chem 357:1793, 1976

118. Gumucio JJ, Miller DL: Functional implications of liver cell heterogeneity. Gastroenterology 80:393, 1981

119. Gumucio JJ, Miller DL: Liver cell heterogeneity. In Arias IM, Popper H, Schachter D et al (eds): The Liver: Biology and Pathobiology, pp 647–661. New York, Raven Press, 1982

120. Gumucio JJ et al: Bile salt transport after selective damage to acinar zone 3 hepatocytes by bromobenzene in the rat. Toxicol Appl Pharmacol 50:77, 1979

121. Haberer H: Experimentelle Unterbindung der Leberarterie. Arch Klin Chir 78:557, 1905

122. Haddy FJ, Scott JB: Metabolically linked vasoactive chemicals in local regulation of blood flow. Physiol Rev 48:688, 1968

123. Hale AJ: The minute structure of the liver: A review. Glasgow Med J 32:283, 1951

124. Hamilton WJ, Mossman HW: Human Embryology, 4th ed, chap 11, pp 339–349. Baltimore, Williams & Wilkins, 1972

125. Hampton JC: A re-evaluation of the submicroscopic structure of the liver. Tex Rep Biol Med 18:602, 1960

126. Hanson KM, Johnson PC: Local control of hepatic arterial and portal venous flow in the dog. Am J Physiol 211:712, 1966

127. Hanzon V: Liver cell secretion under normal and pathologic conditions studied by fluorescence microscopy on living rats. Acta Physiol Scand (suppl 101, Fig 14), 28:93, 1952

128. Hartroft WS: The trabecular anatomy of late stages of experimental dietary cirrhosis. Anat Rec 119:71, 1954

129. Hay EB, Webb JK: The effect of increased arterial blood flow to the liver on the mortality rate following hemorrhagic shock. Surgery 29:826, 1951

130. Hayashi M: Distribution of β-glucuronidase activity in rat tissues employing the Naphthol AS-Bi glucuronide hexazonium pararosanilin method. J Histochem Cytochem 12:659, 1964

131. Hering E: Manual of Human and Comparative Histology, vol 2. Power N (trans): Berlin, Stricer, 1872

132. Higgins GM: The biliary tract of certain rodents with and those without a gallbladder. Anat Rec 32:89, 1926

133. Hildebrand R: Nuclear volume and cellular metabolism. Adv Anat Embryol Cell Biol 60:1, 1980

134. Hill KR: Liver disease in Jamaican children. In Hoffbauer FW (ed): Trans 10th Liver Injury Conf, p 263. New York, Macy, 1951

135. Himsworth HP: Lectures on the Liver and its Diseases. pp 40–42 (Fig. 23A). Cambridge, Harvard University Press, 1948

136. Hinshaw LB et al: Venous–arteriolar response in the canine liver. Proc Soc Exp Biol Med 118:979, 1965

137. Hjortsjö CH: The topography of the intrahepatic duct system. Acta Anat 11:599, 1951

138. Holman ME: Electrophysiology of vascular smooth muscle. Ergeb Physiol 61:137, 1969

139. Holt JP: The collapse factor in the measurement of venous pressure: The flow of fluid through collapsible tubes. Am J Physiol 134:292, 1941

140. Honjo I, Hasebe S: Studies on the intrahepatic nerves in the cirrhotic liver. Rev Int Hepat 15:595, 1965

141. Intaglietta M: The measurement of pressure and flow in the microcirculation. Microvasc Res 5:357, 1973

142. Ivy AC: Factors concerned in the evacuation of the gallbladder. Medicine 11:345, 1932

143. Jayle GE: Les nerfs du foie, étude anatomique et histologique. Nutrition 7:57, 1937

144. Jdanov DA: Nouvelles données sur l'anatomie fonctionnelle des vaisseaux sanguins et lymphatiques du foie et leur rôle dans la pathogénie des malades du foie. Ann Anat Pathol (Paris) 9:411, 1964

145. Jdanov DA: Anatomy and function of the lymphatic capillaries. Lancet 2:895, 1969

146. Ji S et al: Periportal and pericentral pyridine nucleotide fluorescence from the surface of the perfused liver: Evaluation of the hypothesis that chronic treatment with ethanol produces pericentral hypoxia. Proc Natl Acad Sci USA 79:5415, 1982

147. Johnson AB: The use of phenazine methosulphate for improving the histochemical localization of ketose reductase (L-iditol: NAD oxidoreductase or sorbitol dehydrogenase). J Histochem Cytochem 15:207, 1967

148. Johnson PC: The microcirculation and local and humoral control of the circulation. In Guyton AC, Jones EC (eds): Cardiovascular Physiology, vol 1, p 163. London, Butterworth & Co, 1974

149. Jones AL, Spring-Mills E: The liver and gallbladder. In Weiss L, Greep RO (eds): Histology, 4th ed, pp 701–746. New York, McGraw-Hill, 1977

150. Jones AL et al: A quantitative analysis of hepatic ultrastructure in rats during enhanced bile secretion. Anat Rec 192:277, 1978

151. Jones AL et al: Autoradiographic evidence for hepatic lobular concentration gradient of bile acid derivative. Am J Physiol 238:G233, 1980

152. Junès MP: Les arborisations biliovasculaires intrahépatiques: (étude anatomo-chirurgicale en vue des hépatectomies) d'après 50 moulages hépatiques en matières plastiques. Bordeaux Chir 1:5, 1954

153. Jungermann K, Katz N: Functional hepatocellular heterogeneity. Hepatology 2:385, 1982

154. Jungermann K, Sasse D: Heterogeneity of liver parenchymal cells. TIBS, Sept 1978, p 198

155. Kaman J: Zur terminalen Ramifikation der Arteria hepatica des Schweines. Mikroskopie 20:129, 1965

156. Kardon RH, Kessel RG: Three dimensional organization of the hepatic microcirculation in the rodent as observed by scanning electron microscopy of corrosion casts. Gastroenterol 79:72, 1980

157. Kasai M et al: Surgical treatment of biliary atresia. J Pediatr Surg 3:665, 1968

158. Katz LN, Rodbard S: The integration of the vasomotor responses in the liver with those in other systemic vessels. J Pharmacol Exp Ther 67:407, 1939

159. Kedzior E, Kus J: The blood vessels of the gallbladder. Folia Morphol (Warsz) 24:393, 1965

160. Kelty RH et al: Relation of the regenerated liver nodule to the vascular bed in cirrhosis. Gastroenterology 15:285, 1950

161. Kettler LH: Untersuchungen über die Genese von Lebernekrosen auf Grund experimenteller Kreislaufstörungen. Virchows Arch Pathol Anat 316:525, 1949

162. Khazei AM, Watkins E Jr: Hepatic artery anomalies or deformities managed during infusion chemotherapy of liver cancer. Surg Clin North Am 45:639, 1965

163. Kiernan F: The anatomy and physiology of the liver. Philos Trans R Soc Lond 123:711, 1833

164. Kirk J: The sphincter papillae. J Anat 78:118, 1944

165. Klein H et al: Die histochemische Bestimmung der Lipaseaktivität der Leber. Zentralbl Allg Pathol Anat 88:295, 1952

166. Knisely MH et al: Selective phagocytosis: I. Microscopic observations concerning the regulation of blood flow through the liver and other organs and the mechanism and rate of phagocytic removal of particles from the blood. Det Kong Dans Videnskab Selskab Biol Skri IV: No. 7, 1, 1948

167. Knisely MH et al: Hepatic sphincters. Science 125:1023, 1957

168. Kreilkamp BL, Boyden EA: Variability in the composition of the sphincter of Oddi: A possible factor in the pathologic physiology of the biliary tract. Anat Rec 76:485, 1940

169. Laufman H et al: Graded hepatic arterial ligations in experimental ascites. Surg Gynecol Obstet 96:409, 1953

170. Lautt WW: The hepatic artery subservient to hepatic metabolism or guardian of normal hepatic clearance rates of humoral substances. Gen Pharmacol 8:73, 1977

171. Lautt WW: Hepatic nerves: A review of their functions and effects. Can J Physiol Pharmacol 58:105, 1980

172. Lavoie P et al: The umbilico-portal approach for the study of splanchnic circulation: Technical, radiological, and hemodynamic consideration. Can J Surg 9:338, 1966

173. Layden TJ, Boyer JL: Influence of bile acids on bile canalicular membrane morphology and the lobular gradient in canalicular size. Lab Invest 39:110, 1978

174. LeBouton AV: Heterogeneity of protein metabolism between liver cells as studied by radioautography. Curr Mod Biol 2:111, 1968

175. LeBouton AV, Marchand R: Changes in the distribution of thymidine-^{3}H labeled cells in the growing liver acinus of neonatal rats. Dev Biol 23:524, 1970

176. Leger L et al: Les cavernômes de la veine porte; étude anatomique, physio-patho-génique. J Chir 84:145, 1962

177. Le Rumeur E et al: All normal rat hepatocytes produce albumin at a rate related to their degree of ploidy. Biochem Biophys Res Commun 101:1038, 1981

178. Lichtenstein ME, Ivy AC: The function of the "valves" of Heister. Surgery 1:38, 1937

179. Lieber ChS et al: Choline fails to prevent liver fibrosis in ethanol-fed baboons but causes toxicity. Hepatology 5:561, 1985

180. Lindberg B, Darle N: Effect of glucagon on hepatic circulation in the pig. Arch Surg 111:1379, 1976

181. Linton RR: The selection of patients for portacaval shunts with a summary of results in 61 cases. Ann Surg 134:433, 1951

182. Lischner MW et al: Natural history of alcoholic hepatitis: I. The acute disease. Am J Dig Dis 16:481, 1971

183. Loisance DY et al: Hepatic circulation after side-to-side portacaval shunt in dogs: Velocity pattern and flow rate changes studied by an ultrasonic velocimeter. Surgery 73:43, 1973

184. Longmire WP Jr, Sanford MC: Intrahepatic cholangiojejunostomy with partial hepatectomy for biliary obstruction. Surgery 24:264, 1948

185. Loud AV: A quantitative stereological description of the ultrastructure of normal rat liver parenchymal cells. J Cell Biol 37:27, 1968

186. Lutz J et al: Appearance and size of venovasomotoric reactions in the liver circulation. Pflügers Arch Ges Physiol 299:311, 1968

187. Mahour GH et al: Structure of the common bile duct in man: Presence or absence of smooth muscle. Ann Surg 166:91, 1967

188. Mall FP: A study of the structural unit of the liver. Am J Anat 5:227, 1906

189. Mallet–Guy P et al: Étude expérimentale de la neuréctomie périartère hépatique. I. Effects de la résection du "pédicule nerveux antérieure" sur le foie normal. Lyon Chir 51:45, 1956

190. Mallet–Guy P et al: Recherches expérimentales sur la circulation lymphatique du foie. I. Donnés immédiates sur la perméabilité biliolymphatique. Lyon Chir 58:847, 1962

191. Malpighi M: De viscerum structura exercitatio anatomica. London, 1666

192. Mandelbaum I et al: Regional blood flow during pulsatile and nonpulsatile perfusion. Arch Surg 91:771, 1965

193. Markowitz J, Rappaport AM: The hepatic artery. Physiol Rev 31:188, 1951

194. Mascagni P: Prodromo della grande Anatomia. Firenze, 1819

195. Mathie RT (ed): Blood Flow Measurement in Man. London, Castle House Publications, 1982

196. Mautner H, Pick EP: Über die durch Schockgifte erzeugten Zirkulationsstörungen: II. Das Verhalten der überlebenden Leber. Biochem Z 127:72, 1922

197. McCuskey RS: A dynamic and static study of hepatic arterioles and hepatic sphincters. Am J Anat 119:455, 1966

198. McIndoe AH: Vascular lesions of portal cirrhosis. Arch Pathol Lab Med 5:23, 1928

199. McKee FW et al: Protein metabolism and exchange as influenced by constriction of the vena cava: Experimental ascites and internal plasmapheresis. J Exp Med 87:457, 1948

200. Mellander S, Johansson B: Control of resistance, exchange and capacitance functions in the peripheral circulation. Pharmacol Rev 20:117, 1968

201. Michels NA: The hepatic, cystic and retroduodenal arteries and their relation to the biliary ducts. Ann Surg 133:503, 1951

202. Michels NA: Collateral arterial pathways to liver after ligation of hepatic artery and removal of celiac axis. Cancer 6:708, 1953

203. Miller DL et al: Quantitative morphology of sinusoids of the hepatic acinus. Gastroenterology 76:965, 1979

204. Mitchell GG, Torrance HB: The effects of a bile-salt: Sodium dehydrocholate upon liver blood-flow in man. Br J Surg 53:807, 1966

205. Mitra SK: The terminal distribution of the hepatic artery with special reference to arterio-portal anastomosis. J Anat 100:651, 1966

206. Mizutani A: Cytochemical demonstration of ornithine carbamoyl transferase activity in liver mitochondria of rat and mouse. J Histochem Cytochem 16:172, 1968

207. Mohamed MS, Beau JW: Local and general alterations of blood CO_2 and influence of intestinal motility in regulation of intestinal bloodflow. Am J Physiol 167:413, 1951

208. Moore TC, Hurley AG: Congenital duplication of the gallbladder, review of the literature and report of an unusual symptomatic case. Surgery 35:283, 1954

209. Moschcowitz E: Laennec's cirrhosis: Its histogenesis with special reference to the role of angiogenesis. Arch Pathol 45:187, 1948

210. Motta P, Porter KR: Structure of rat liver sinusoids and associated tissue spaces as revealed by scanning electron-microscopy. Cell Tissue Res 148:111, 1974

211. Müller E et al: Histochemical demonstration of γ-glutamyltranspeptidase in rat liver after portacaval anastomosis. Experientia 30:1128, 1974

212. Mundschau GA et al: Hepatic and mesenteric artery resistances after sino-aortic denervation and hemorrhage. Am J Physiol 211:77, 1966

213. Murakami T et al: Peribiliary portal system in the monkey liver as evidenced by the injection replica scanning electronmicroscope method. Arch Histol Jpn 37:254, 1979

214. Murakami T et al: A monomeric methyl and hydroxypropyl methacrylate injection medium and its utility in casting blood capillaries and liver bile canaliculi for scanning electron microscopy. Arch Histol Jpn 47:223, 1984

215. Nakata K, Kanbe A: The terminal distribution of the hepatic artery and its relationship to the development of focal liver necrosis following interruption of the portal blood supply. Acta Pathol Jpn 16:313, 1966

216. Nakata K et al: Direct measurement of blood pressures in minute vessels of the liver. Am J Physiol 199:1181, 1960

217. Ney HR: Die Kontrastdarstellung der Lebervenen im Röntgenbild. Fortschr Röntgenstr 86:302, 1957

218. Nisimara Y: Concept of body fluid circulation. Hiroshima J Med Sci 31:199, 1982

219. Nolte J, Pette D: Microphotometric determination of enzyme activity in single cells in cryostat sections: I. Application of the gel film technique to microphotometry and studies on the intralobar distribution of succinate dehydrogenase and lactate dehydrogenase activities in the rat liver. J Histochem Cytochem 20:567, 1972

220. Norhagen A: Selective angiography of the hepatic veins. Experimental investigations of basal circulatory dynamics. Acta Radiol (suppl) 221:30, 1963

221. North KAK et al: The development of anastomotic circulation to transplanted tissue. Br J Exp Pathol 41:520, 1960

222. Northoven JMA, Terblanche J: A new look at the arterial supply of the bile duct in man and its surgical implications. Br J Surg 65:379, 1979

223. Novikoff AB, Essner E: The liver cell: Some new approaches to its study. Am J Med 29:102, 1960

224. Novikoff AB et al: The localization of adenosine triphosphate in liver: In situ staining and cell fractionation studies. J Histochem Cytochem 6:61, 1958

225. Novikoff AB et al: Cold acetone fixation for enzyme localization in frozen sections. J Histochem Cytochem 8:37, 1960

226. Oda M et al: Some dynamic aspects of the hepatic microcirculation: Demonstration of sinusoidal endothelial fenestrae as a possible regulatory factor. Excerpta Medica 625:105, 1983

227. Olds JM, Stafford ES: On the manner of anastomosis of the hepatic and portal circulation. Bull Johns Hopkins Hosp 47:176, 1930

228. Olerud S: Experimental studies on portal circulation at increased intra-abdominal pressure. Acta Physiol Scand (Suppl 109) 30:1, 1953

229. Opdyke DF et al: Further evidence that inspiration increases right atrial inflow. Am J Physiol 162:259, 1950

230. Opie EL: The pathogenesis of tumours of the liver produced by butter yellow. J Exp Med 80:231, 1944

231. Opolon P et al: Coma hépatique expérimental par necrose ischémique aigue du foie chez le porc. Tentatives de prevention et de traitement par hémodialyse croisée. Ann Med Interne 122:819, 1971

232. Orrego H et al: Effect of short term therapy with propylthiouracyl in patients with alcoholic liver disease. Gastroenterology 76:105, 1979

233. Padykula HA, Herman E: The specificity of the histochemical method for adenosine triphosphatase. J Histochem Cytochem 3:170, 1955

234. Palade GE: The fine structure of mitochondria. Anat Rec 114:427, 1952

235. Peterson LH: Some characteristics of certain reflexes which modify the circulation in man. Circulation 2:351, 1950

236. Pette D, Brandau H: Enzymehistiogramme und Enzymaktivitätsmuster der Rattenleber. Nachweis Pyridinnukleotidspezifischer Dehydrogenasen im Gelschicht-Verfahren. Enzyme Biol Clin 6:79, 1966

237. Pfuhl W: Handbuch der Mikroskopischen Anatomie des Menschen, vol 5, part 2, p 226. Berlin, Springer–Verlag, 1932

238. Pick L: Über totale hämangiomatöse Obliteration des Pfortaderstammes. Arch Pathol Anat 197:490, 1909

239. Pollister AW, Pollister PF: Über Drosselvorrichtungen an Lebervenen. Klin Wochenschr 10:2129, 1931

240. Popper H et al: Vascular pattern of the cirrhotic liver. Am J Clin Pathol 22:717, 1952

241. Porter KR: Personal communication, 1962

242. Potvin P: Les effets de modifications de la pression sushépatique sur la circulation du foie chez le lapin. Agressologie 10:45, 1969

243. Preisig R et al: The relationship between taurocholate se-

cretion rate and bile production in the unanesthetized dog during cholinergic blockade and during secretin administration. J Clin Invest 41:1152, 1962

244. Price JB et al: The validity of chronic hepatic blood flow measurements obtained by electromagnetic flowmeter. J Surg Res 5:313, 1965

245. Prinzmetal M et al: Arteriovenous anastomoses in liver, spleen, and lungs. Am J Physiol 152:48, 1948

246. Quistorff B et al: Two and three dimensional redox heterogeneity of rat liver: Effects of anoxia and alcohol on the lobular redox pattern. In Dutton PL et al (eds): Frontiers of Biological Energetics: From Electrons to Tissues, vol 2, p 1487. New York, Academic Press, 1978

247. Rabinovici N, Vardi J: The intrahepatic portal vein-hepatic artery relationship. Surg Gynecol Obstet 120:38, 1965

248. Rappaport AM: Hepatic venography. Acta Radiol 36:165, 1951

249. Rappaport AM: The guided catheterization and radiography of the abdominal vessels. Can Med Assoc J 67:93, 1952

250. Rappaport AM: Circulatory aspects of liver physiology. PhD Thesis, University of Toronto, 1952

251. Rappaport AM: In discussion of Elias H: Morphology of the liver, p 196. Trans 11th Liver Injury Conf New York, Macy, 1953

252. Rappaport AM: The structural and functional unit in the human liver (liver acinus). Anat Rec 130:673, 1958

253. Rappaport AM: Liver morphology, Discussion Workshop. Ann NY Acad Sci 111:527, 1963

254. Rappaport AM: "The normal microcirculation of the mammalian liver." 16 mm color film, sound, 19 min. Division of Instructional Media Services, Faculty of Medicine, University of Toronto (1972). Toronto, Canada.

255. Rappaport AM: The microcirculatory hepatic unit. Microvasc Res 6:212, 1973

256. Rappaport AM: The microcirculatory acinar concept of normal and pathological hepatic structure. Beitr Pathol 157: 215, 1976

257. Rappaport AM: Microcirculatory units in the mammalian liver; their arterial and portal components. Bibl Anat 16: 116, 1977

258. Rappaport AM: "The pathologic microcirculation of the mammalian liver." 16 mm color film, sound, 25 min. Division of Instructional Media Services, Faculty of Medicine, University of Toronto (1979). Toronto, Canada.

259. Rappaport AM: Physioanatomical basis of toxic liver injury. In Farber E, Fisher MM (eds): Toxic Injury to the Liver, chap 1. New York, Dekker, 1979

260. Rappaport AM: The acinus—Microvascular unit of the liver. In Lautt WW (ed): Hepatic Circulation in Health and Disease, pp 175–192. New York, Raven Press, 1981

261. Rappaport AM, Bilbey DLJ: Segmentation of the liver at microscopic level. Anat Rec 136:262, 1960

262. Rappaport AM, Hiraki GY: Histopathological changes in the structural and functional unit of the human liver. Acta Anat 32:240, 1958

263. Rappaport AM, Hiraki GY: The anatomical pattern of lesions in the liver. Acta Anat 32:126, 1958

264. Rappaport AM, Knoblauch M: The hepatic artery, its structural, circulatory and metabolic functions. In Vanderbroucke J, DeGrote J, Standaert LO (eds): Liver Research. 3rd Int Symp Int Assoc Study of Liver, Kyoto, 1966. Tijdschrift voor Gastroenterologie, p 116. Antwerpen, Belgium, 1967

265. Rappaport AM, Schneiderman JH: The function of the hepatic artery. Rev Physiol Biochem Pharmacol 76:130, 1976

266. Rappaport AM et al: Experimental hepatic coma. Surg Forum 4:504, 1952

267. Rappaport AM et al: Hepatic coma following ischemia of the liver. Surg Gynecol Obstet 97:748, 1953

268. Rappaport AM et al: Subdivision of hexagonal liver lobules into a structural and functional unit: Role in hepatic physiology and pathology. Anat Rec 119:11, 1954

269. Rappaport AM et al: Experimental hepatic ischemia collateral circulation of the liver. Ann Surg 140:695, 1954

270. Rappaport AM et al: Hepatic venography. Gastroenterology 46:115, 1964

271. Rappaport AM et al: Normal and pathologic microcirculation of the living mammalian liver. Rev Int Hépat 16: 813, 1966

272. Rappaport AM et al: Effects of hepatic artery ligation on survival and metabolism of depancreatized dogs. Am J Physiol 215:898, 1968

273. Rappaport AM et al: Hepatic microcirculatory changes leading to portal hypertension. Ann NY Acad Sci 170:48, 1970

274. Rappaport AM et al: Effects of arterial and portal ischemia on survival and metabolism of partially and totally depancreatized dogs. Z Exper Chir 8:326, 1975

275. Rappaport AM et al: The effect of injected Na-taurocholate on the microcirculation of the rat liver. Gastroenterology 79:1047, 1980

276. Rappaport AM et al: The scarring of the liver acini (cirrhosis): Tridimensional and microcirculatory considerations. Virchows Arch Pathol Anat. A, 402:107, 1983

277. Reeves JT et al: Microradiography of the rabbit's hepatic microcirculation: The similarity of the hepatic portal and pulmonary arterial circulations. Anat Rec 154:103, 1966

278. Reifferscheid M: Chirurgie der Leber. Stuttgart, Thieme, 1957

279. Reinmann B et al: Anastomosen zwischen Segmentarterien der Leber und phrenico-hepatische arterio-arterielle Anastomosen. Langenbecks Arch Chir 359:81, 1983

280. Reith A et al: Quantitative und qualitative elektronenmikroskopische Untersuchungen zur Struktur des Leberläppchens normaler Ratten. Z Mikrosk Anat Forsch 89: 225, 1968

281. Reynell PC et al: Changes in splanchnic blood volume and splanchnic blood flow in dogs after hemorrhage. Clin Sci 14:407, 1955

282. Reynolds TB, Edmondson HA: Editorial: Alcoholic hepatitis. Ann Intern Med 74:440, 1971

283. Rhodin JAG: The ultrastructure of mammalian arterioles and precapillary sphincters. J Ultrastruc Res 18:181, 1967

284. Richardson PDI, Withrington PG: Pressure flow relationships and effects of noradrenaline and isoprenaline on the hepatic arterial and portal venous vascular beds in the dog. J Physiol 282:451, 1978

285. Richardson PDI, Withrington PG: Physiological regulation of the hepatic circulation. Ann Rev Physiol 44:57, 1982

286. Riddell AG et al: Portacaval transposition in the treatment of glycogen-storage disease. Lancet 2:1146, 1966

287. Rutenburg AM, Seligman AM: The histochemical demonstration of acid phosphatase by a post-incubation coupling technique. J Histochem Cytochem 3:455, 1955

288. Sabourin C: Recherches sur l'anatomie normale et pathologique de la glande biliaire de l'homme. Paris, Alcan, 1888

289. Sancetta SM: Dynamic and neurogenic factors determining the hepatic arterial flow after portal occlusion. Circ Res 1: 414, 1953

290. Sapirstein LA: Indicator dilution methods in the measurement of the splanchnic blood flow of normal dogs. In Brauer RW (ed): Liver Function, pp 93–105. Washington, DC, American Institute of Biological Sciences, 1958

291. Sasaki H et al: Bile ductules in cholestasis: Morphologic evidence for secretion and absorption in man. Lab Invest 16:84, 1967

292. Sasse D: Chemomorphologie der Glykogensynthese und des Glykogengehalts während der Histogenese der Leber. Histochemie 20:159, 1969

293. Sasse D, Germer M: Zonation of hepatocellular injury. In Keppler D, Popper H, Bianchi L et al (eds): Mechanisms of Hepatocyte Injury and Death, pp 31–36. Lancaster, MTP-Press, 1984

294. Sasse D, Köhler J: Die topochemische Verlagerung von Funktionseinheiten des Glykogenstoffwechsels in der Leber durch Allylformiat. Histochemie 18:325, 1969

295. Sasse D et al: Functional heterogeneity of rat liver parenchyma and of isolated hepatocytes. FEBS Lett 57:83, 1975

296. Schepers GWH: Hepatic cellular gigantism as a manifestation of chemical toxicity, p 785. Proc 13th Int Cong Occupational Health, 1961

297. Scheuer PJ: Liver biopsy in chronic hepatitis: 1968–78. Gut 19:544, 1978

298. Schmid M: Die chronische Hepatitis. Habilitationsschrift der Medizinischen Fakultät, Univ Zürich, pp 59–61. Berlin, Springer–Verlag, 1966

299. Schmidt FG: Electronmikroskopische Untersuchungen an den Sinusoid Wandzellen (Kupfferschen Sternzellen) der weissen Maus. Anat Anz 108:376, 1960

300. Schmidt U et al: Liver cell heterogeneity: the distribution of fructose-bisphosphatase in fed and fasted rats and in man. Hoppe Seylers Z Physiol Chem 359:193, 1978

301. Scholtholt J: Das Verhalten der Durchblutung der Leber bei Steigerung des Sauerstoffverbrauches der Leber. Pflügers Arch 318:202, 1969

302. Scholtholt J, Siraishi T: The effect of sodium dehydrocholate on blood flow and oxygen consumption of the liver in the anesthetized dog. Arzneim Forsch 18:197, 1968

303. Schultz M, Hildebrand R: Karyometric investigation on circadian rhythmic changes in the periportal and perivenous zones of the acinus of the rat liver. Cell Tissue Res 231: 643, 1983

304. Schumacher HH: Histochemical distribution pattern of respiratory enzymes in the liver lobule. Science 125:501, 1957

305. Schwartz SI: Influence of vasoactive drugs on portal circulation. Ann NY Acad Sci 170:296, 1970

306. Schwegler RA Jr, Boyden EA: The development of the pars intestinalis of the common bile duct in the human fetus, with special reference to the origin of the ampulla of Vater and the sphincter of Oddi. Anat Rec 68:17, 1937

307. Schwiegk H: Untersuchungen über die Leberdurchblutung und den Pfortaderkreislauf. Arch Exper Pathol Pharmakol 168:693, 1932

308. Seawright AA, Hrdlicka J: The effect of prior dosing with phenobarbitone and β-diethylaminoethyl diphenylpropyl acetate (SKF525A) on the toxicity and liver lesion caused by Ngaione in the mouse. Br J Exp Pathol 53:242, 1972

309. Segall HN: An experimental anatomical investigation of the blood and bile channels of the liver. Surg Gynecol Obstet 37:152, 1923

310. Selkurt EE: Comparison of the bromsulphalein method with simultaneous direct hepatic blood flow. Circ Res 2:155, 1954

311. Selkurt EE, Johnson PC: Effect of acute elevation of portal venous pressure on mesenteric blood volume, interstitial fluid volume, and hemodynamics. Circ Res 6:592, 1958

312. Sellers EA, You RW: Propylthiouracyl, thyroid and dietary liver injury. J Nutr 44:513, 1951

313. Sérégé H: Sur la teneur en urée de chaque lobe du foie en rapport avec les phases de la digestion. CR Soc Biol 54: 200, 1902

314. Shank RE et al: Cell heterogeneity within the hepatic lobule (quantitative histochemistry). J Histochem Cytochem 7: 237, 1959

315. Sherlock S: Hepatic vein catheterization in clinical research. Proc Inst Med Chic 18:335, 1951

316. Sherlock S: Estimation of hepatic blood flow. In Diseases of the Liver and Biliary System, 3rd rev ed, pp 192–196. Oxford/Edinburgh, Blackwell Scientific Publications, 1971

317. Sherlock S, Walshe V: The use of portal anastomotic vein for absorption studies in man. Clin Sci 6:113, 1946

318. Shoemaker CP: A study of hepatic hemodynamics in the dog. Circ Res 15:216, 1964

319. Sidky M, Bean JW: Influence of rhythmic and tonic contractions of intestinal muscle on blood flow and on blood reservoir capacity in dog intestine. Am J Physiol 193:386, 1958

320. Sigel B et al: Effect of blood flow reversal in liver autotransplants upon the site of hepatocyte regeneration. J Clin Invest 47:1231, 1968

321. Simonds JP: Chronic occlusion of the portal vein. Arch Surg 33:397, 1936

322. Smetana HF et al: Symposium on diseases of the liver: Histologic criteria for differential diagnosis of liver diseases in needle biopsies. Rev Gastroenterol 20:227, 1953

323. Smith MT et al: The distribution of glutathione in the rat liver lobule. Biochem J 182:103, 1979

324. Stahle J: Studies on the bile ducts, and the blood vessels in Glisson's capsule: A histological investigation of the incidence of smooth muscle in the intrahepatic bile ducts. Acta Soc Med Upsalien 57:455, 1952

325. Stefenelli N: Die terminale Strombahn der Mikrozirkulation der Rattenleber im Intravitalmikroskop. Wien Klin Wochenschr 82:575, 1970

326. Steiner JW, Carruthers JS: Studies on the fine structure of the terminal branches of the biliary tree. Am J Pathol 38: 639, 1961

327. Stoner HB: The mechanism of toxic hepatic necrosis. Br J Exp Pathol 37:176, 1956

328. Sudler MT: The architecture of the gallbladder. Bull Johns Hopkins Hosp 12:126, 1901

329. Sutherland SD: The intrinsic innervation of the liver. Rev Int Hepat 15:569, 1965

330. Swick RW et al: The unique distribution of Ornithine aminotransferase in rat liver mitochondria. Arch Biochem Biophys 136:212, 1970

331. Szabo G et al: The effect of occlusion of liver lymphatics on hepatic blood flow. Res Exp Med 169:1, 1976

332. Taira Y et al: Immunohistochemical studies on NADPH-cytochrome c reductase in rat liver. Fed Proc 37:425, 1978

333. Tanturi CA, Ivy AC: A study of the effect of vascular changes in the liver and the excitation of its nerve supply on the formation of bile. Am J Physiol 121:61, 1938

334. Taylor FW, Rosenbaum D: The case against hepatic arterial ligation in portal hypertension. JAMA 151:1066, 1953

335. Teutsch HF: Chemomorphology of liver parenchyma. Progr Histochem Cytochem 14:1, 1981

336. Tori G, Scott WG: Experimental method for visualization of the hepatic vein: Venous hepatography. AJR 70:242, 1953

337. Torrance HB: Liver blood flow during operations on the upper abdomen. JR Coll Surg 2:216, 1957

338. Torrance HB: The control of the hepatic arterial circulation. J Physiol 158:39, 1961

339. Ungváry G et al: Die Innervation der A. hepatica und V. portae. Experimentell-histologische und histochemische Studien. Anat Anz Ergänzungsheft 130:187, 1971

340. Vanecko RM et al: Microcirculatory changes in primate liver during shock. Surg Gynecol Obstet 129:995, 1969

341. Villemin F et al: Variations morphologiques et topographiques du foie. Arch Mal Appar Dig 40:63, 1951

342. Wachstein M: Enzymatic histochemistry of the liver. Gastroenterology 37:525, 1959

343. Wachstein M et al: Histochemistry of thiolacetic acid esterase: A comparison with non-specific esterase with special regard to the effect of fixatives and inhibitors on intracellular localization. J Histochem Cytochem 9:325, 1961

344. Wade OL et al: The effect of exercise on the splanchnic blood flow and splanchnic blood volume in normal man. Clin Sci 15:457, 1956

345. Wakim KG, Mann FC: The intrahepatic circulation of the blood. Anat Rec 82:233, 1942

346. Warren WD et al: Selective trans-splenic decompression of gastroesophageal varices by distal splenorenal shunt. Ann Surg 166:437, 1967

347. Weibel ER et al: Correlated morphometric and biochemical studies on the liver cell. J Cell Biol 42:68, 1969

348. Welsh FA: Changes in distribution of enzymes within the liver lobule during adaptive increases. J Histochem Cytochem 20:107, 1972

349. Wilson JW: Hepatic structure. In Brauer RW (ed): Liver Function, No. 4, p 175. Washington, DC, Am Inst Biol Sci Pub, 1958

350. Wilson JW et al: Histogenesis of the liver. Ann NY Acad Sci 111:8, 1963

351. Wimmer M, Pette D: Microphotometric studies on intra-acinar enzyme distribution. Histochemistry 64:23, 1979

352. Wisse E: Ultrastructure and function of Kupffer cells and other sinusoidal cells in the liver. Med Chir Dig 6:409, 1977

353. Wisse E et al: The liver sieve: Considerations concerning the structure and function of endothelial fenestrae, the sinusoidal wall and the space of Disse. Hepatology 5:683, 1985

354. Wolf–Heidegger G, Beydl W: Zur Morphologie und Topographie d. Kupfferschen Sternzellen. Acta Anat 19:15, 1953

355. Yamada S, Burton AC: Effect of reduced tissue pressure on blood flow of the fingers: The veni-vasomotor reflex. J Appl Physiol 6:501, 1954

356. Yamamoto K et al: Three dimensional observations of the hepatic arterial terminations in rat, hamster and human liver by scanning electron microscopy of microvascular casts. Hepatology 5:452, 1985

357. Yamamoto K et al: Hilar biliary plexus in human liver. Lab Invest 52:103, 1985

358. Yoshimura S et al: Purification and immunohistochemical localization of rat liver glutathione perioxidase. Biochim Biophys Acta 621:130, 1980

359. Zeppa R, Womack NA: Humoral control of hepatic lymph flow. Surgery 54:37, 1963

chapter **2**

Electron Microscopy of Human Liver Diseases

M. JAMES PHILLIPS, PATRICIA S. LATHAM, and SIRIA POUCELL

Electron microscopic examination of the liver has contributed greatly to a better understanding of the structure and function of the liver in both health and disease.[23,41,94,105,114,125,153,188,189,197,202] The two main instruments used in ultrastructural studies are the transmission electron microscope, which permits two-dimensional examination of ultrathin sections of the liver, and the scanning electron microscope, which allows the visualization of surface structures in three dimensions. Technical advances have been made in recent years that make the application of electron microscopy practical. One such advance is the "universal fixative."[116] This glutaraldehyde paraformaldehyde fixative is a stable compound in which the tissue can be placed and retained for days or even months, if desired, while maintaining excellent preservation of fine structural details. In addition, many histochemical procedures have been developed that have extended the usefulness of electron microscopy in the analysis of subcellular structures.

Because of the small sample size taken for electron microscopy, it is important to preselect the appropriate blocks for ultrathin sections. These should include representative areas from zone 1 and zone 3. This selection is accomplished by cutting 1-μm toluidine blue–stained plastic embedded sections followed by light microscopic examination. Traditionally, human liver disease has been diagnosed by correlation of light microscopy with other clinical and laboratory findings. However, diagnostic accuracy can now be greatly refined by incorporation of electron microscopy as a routine procedure.

NORMAL LIVER

Normal hepatocytes maintain their familiar light microscopic angular polyhedral shape in electron microscopic sections (Fig. 2-1). Nevertheless, there are subtle ultrastructural differences between hepatocytes in acinar zones 1 and 3. For example, the smooth endoplasmic reticulum is more prevalent in zone 3 (centrilobular), which correlates well with more intense activity of cytochrome P450 in this region. In contrast, mitochondria in zone 1 (periportal) are larger and more pleomorphic, reflecting the

increased activity of succinic dehydrogenase. The sinusoidal surface of the hepatocyte is separated from the cellular elements of the blood by the sinusoidal lining cells, of which there are four types; the endothelial, Kupffer, fat-storing, and pit cells.[23,98,215,216] In transmission electron micrographs, the endothelial cells are thin and have numerous processes. The endothelium is seen by the scanning electron microscope to form a thin sinusoidal lining, in which perforations or fenestrae exist. This sievelike structure permits exchange between the blood plasma and the space of Disse (Fig. 2-2).[215] The Kupffer cells that are intermingled with the endothelial cells are highly phagocytic and contain many lysosomes. The fat-storing cell, also known as the lipocyte, vitamin A–storing cell, perisinusoidal cell, stellate cell, or Ito cell, is located beneath the endothelium in the perisinusoidal recesses between neighboring hepatocytes.[90] Pit cells are characterized by the presence of neurosecretory-type dense core and rod-shaped granules and are presently thought to represent specialized lymphocytes.[98,216] The space of Disse lies between the liver cells and the endothelium and is known to be a zone of rapid transcellular exchange. It contains mainly plasma, occasional strands of collagen, and the microvilli of hepatocytes; a basement membrane is lacking (see Fig. 2-1).

The liver cell is highly polarized, with approximately 50% of its surface facing the sinusoids and 15% forming the bile canaliculus.[41] The plasma membrane of hepatocytes has several specialized zones: the sinusoidal region and the biliary regions, both of which are rich in microvilli; the lateral cell membranes, which run parallel to adjacent cells, lack microvilli, and are 100 nm apart; and the specialized areas comprising the cell junctions. The cell junctions are of four main types: the desmosome (macula adherens), a button-like plaque that serves as the site of attachment of tonofilaments to maintain cell shape[183]; the intermediate junction (zonula adherens), the site of insertion of actin filaments (4–7 nm) and intermediate filaments (10 nm), which serve as strong adhesive structures between liver cells[131]; the gap junction (macula communicans, nexus), which allows intimate cell-to-cell communication[57,68] and acts as a site of electrical coupling[113]; and the tight junction (zonula occludens), which is composed

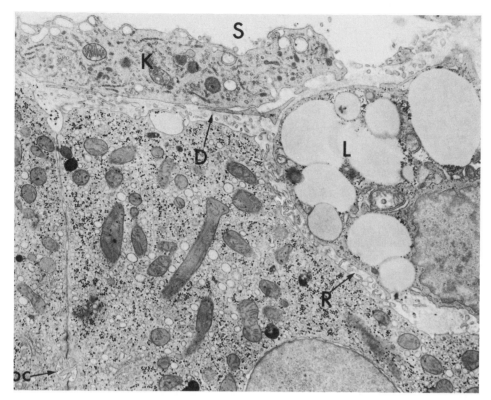

Fig. 2-1. Normal human liver. A portion of two hepatocytes, a Kupffer cell (*K*), processes of an endothelial cell, and a lipocyte (*L*) or Ito cell bordering a sinusoid (*S*) are shown. Note that microvilli on the sinusoidal border of the hepatocytes project into the space of Disse (*D*) and the perisinusoidal recess (*R*). Note the absence of collagen (reticulin) fibers. A normal bile canaliculus (*bc*) is shown on the lower left, its lumen filled with microvilli. (× 8775; transmission electron micrograph by V. Edwards)

of rows of contact points between adjacent membranes. The tight junctions of hepatocytes are situated at the margins of the bile canaliculi. It was initially thought that they were impermeable barriers. There is now experimental evidence to suggest that they may provide a potential passageway for the paracellular movement of fluid between the sinusoids and the bile canaliculi.[108] The complexity of the weave of fibers extending between the cells at the tight junctions is seen to be intermediate in degree (Figs. 2-3 and 2-4) compared with that of the compact weave of impermeable tight junctions and the very loose weave of permeable tight junctions.[58,68] The junctions may be capable of transmitting fluids and electrolytes. The concept of a paracellular pathway for the movement of materials between the hepatic sinusoids and the bile canaliculi is supported by recent electron-cytochemical findings of hepatic membrane–bound Na$^+$,K$^+$-adenosine triphosphatase (ATPase) on the lateral and sinusoidal membrane surfaces.[18,106,107] *

The cytoplasm of the hepatocyte is replete with organelles. It is estimated that the average hepatocyte contains

* Phillips MJ et al: Mechanisms of cholestasis. Lab Invest 54: 593, 1986.

over 2000 mitochondria.[197] Other organelles include peroxisomes, Golgi apparatus, rough endoplasmic reticulum (RER) and smooth endoplasmic reticulum (SER), primary and secondary lysosomes including lipofuscin type of secondary lysosomes and residual bodies, coated and smooth vesicles, and multivesicular bodies. Other normal cytoplasmic components in hepatocytes are glycogen rosettes (alpha particles), free ribosomes and polysomes, and small amounts of lipid, especially triglyceride and very low density lipoproteins (VLDL). In addition, cytoskeletal elements may be seen, including abundant microfilaments, intermediate filaments, and microtubules. Nuclei are large (8 μm), round to oval, and centrally placed and most commonly have a prominent single nucleolus. The nucleus is enveloped by a double membrane, which is periodically interrupted by nuclear pores formed at the sites of inner and outer membrane fusion, thus allowing for nuclear–cytoplasmic exchange. The outer nuclear membrane is studded with ribosomes and is in continuity with the RER in the cytoplasm.

There are two types of nuclear inclusions that may be found in the normal liver: true inclusions and pseudoinclusions. Nuclear glycogenoses or "glycogen nuclei" represent true non–membrane-bound nuclear inclusions;

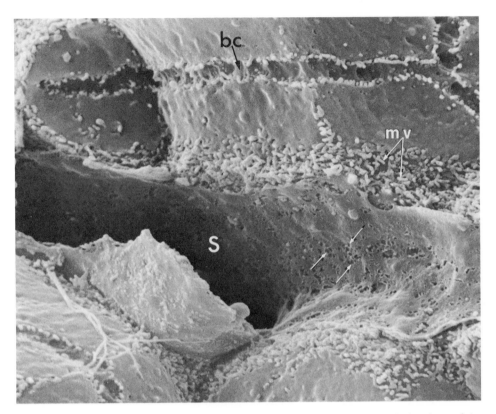

Fig. 2-2. Normal rat liver. A portion of several hepatocytes fractured through the plane of the bile canaliculus (*bc*) is shown. Microvilli (*mv*) can be seen in the canalicular lumen and on the sinusoidal surfaces of the hepatocytes. The endothelial lining of a sinusoid (*S*) is shown. Perforations (fenestrae) in the endothelium are marked by the unlabeled arrows. The thin strands seen on the lower left are type III collagen fibrils. (× 4500; scanning electron micrograph by M. Teitelbaum)

Fig. 2-3. Close-up view of freeze-fractured bile canaliculus from normal rat liver. The tight junction is recognizable as more or less parallel strands or ridges in the P face. The ridges are interrupted at one point by a small gap junction. Bile canalicular microvilli can also be seen (*v*). (× 37,550) (DeVos R, Desmet VJ: Br J Exp Pathol 59:220, 1978)

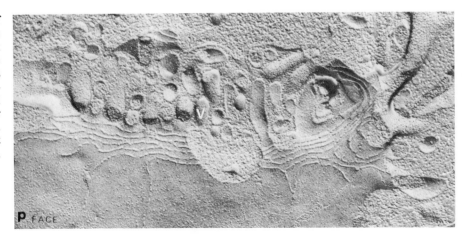

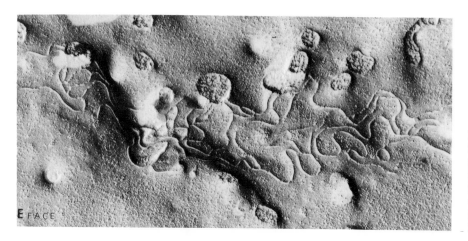

Fig. 2-4. Close-up view of freeze-fractured bile canaliculus from rat liver after 21 days of bile duct obstruction. Note the irregular tight junctional network (P face). ($\times$ 37,550) (DeVos R, Desmet VJ: Br J Exp Pathol 59:220, 1978)

glycogen particles are usually of the monoparticulate type (beta particles). Interestingly, the nuclear glycogen is sometimes arranged in rosettes (alpha particles) that have diameters greatly exceeding the size of the nuclear pores and suggesting that the glycogen is formed or aggregated within the nucleus. Pseudoinclusions are cytoplasmic invaginations and are commonly seen in the elderly. The mitochondria of hepatocytes measure 0.5 μm to 1 μm; they are elongated and are enveloped by a double membrane. Each mitochondrion contains three to five intramatrical granules per ultrathin section and is known to contain calcium and magnesium. The matrix is protein rich and also contains mitochondrial DNA.

The endoplasmic reticulum occurs in two forms, rough and smooth. The RER is composed of membranes that are disposed as cisternae, often arranged in stacks. The outer surface of the RER cisternae is covered by ribosomes that produce proteins for export, for example, plasma proteins. The SER, or agranular endoplasmic reticulum, is ribosome free and appears as smooth-surfaced vesicles or tubules. It contains heme proteins, for example, cytochrome P450, which is important in lipid synthesis, inactivation of hormones, and drug detoxification. It also contains glucose 6-phosphatase, which is important in the formation of free glucose for the blood. The SER is a labile organelle that increases dramatically following treatment with many drugs used in clinical medicine, such as phenobarbital. In such circumstances, there is a concomitant increase in drug-metabolizing enzymes that can greatly alter the expected response from subsequently administered drugs. There are also occasions during which an increase in SER is associated with decreased enzyme activity. The term hypertrophic hypoactive endoplasmic reticulum has been used for such a reticulum. Free ribosomes and polysomes unattached to membranes are also found in the cytoplasm and synthesize proteins for use by the hepatocyte.

Peroxisomes (microbodies) are membrane-bound organelles that are, slightly smaller than mitochondria, measuring 0.4 μm to 1.3 μm. In human liver, peroxisomes lack the crystalline uricase-dense body, characteristic of the organelle in many species. The number of peroxisomes increases greatly following the administration of certain drugs that reduce serum lipid levels (*e.g.,* clofibrate).[75,159] Peroxisomes are also increased in many human liver diseases. They have been found to be abnormal and drastically reduced in number in Refsum's disease and completely absent in the familial and fatal cerebrohepatorenal syndrome of Zellweger.[148,156] Peroxisomes play an important role in the beta oxidation of fatty acids and possibly a role in cholic acid synthesis.[124,162] The Golgi apparatus of the hepatocyte is interposed between the RER and the biliary aspect of the cell and consists of stacked, smooth-faced cisternae whose lateral rims are dilated. The structure is directional and has two distinct faces; the convex, or CIS, face, which is adjacent to the RER, and the more distal concave, or TRANS, face. The Golgi apparatus processes and packages products received via vesicles from the RER into end-product vesicles; the Golgi apparatus then sorts the vesicles and directs them to their proper intracellular or extracellular destinations. Lysosomes are commonly situated in the biliary region, are recognized as electron-dense structures limited by a single membrane, and contain numerous enzymes capable of degrading most biologic materials. Because digestive processes are found at various stages of maturation and because the lysosomal contents are variable, marked pleomorphism of lysosomes is the main characteristic of these organelles.

Microfilaments of actin (4–7 nm), intermediate (keratin) filaments (10 nm in diameter), thick filaments of myosin (15 nm in diameter), and microtubules (20–26 nm) represent the major components of the cytoskeleton. In hepatocytes, actin filaments are distributed throughout the cell; higher concentrations of these filaments are associated with the plasma membrane, especially in the canalicular region. The contractile system of hepatocytes is formed by actin and myosin, which influence bile flow through active contractions of the canalicular system.[57,131,139]

Isolated and cultured hepatocytes (Figs. 2-5 and 2-6) are excellent models for experimental metabolic and pharmacologic studies, since hormonal, nervous, and vascular influences are completely eliminated.[12,45,91–93,119,144,184] Incompletely separated cell groups, particularly

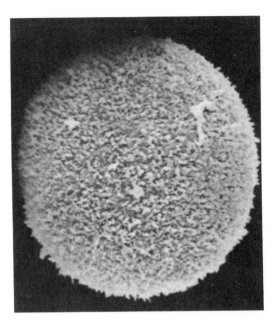

Fig. 2-5. Isolated hepatocyte from normal liver in spinner culture. The exterior surface is covered by microvilli. ($\times$ 5000; scanning electron micrograph by Dr. M. Oda)

Fig. 2-6. Isolated hepatocyte from normal liver sectioned through its center. The nucleus is central. Cytoplasmic organelles are normally disposed. Note microvilli on plasma membrane (compare with Fig. 2-5). ($\times$ 5750; transmission electron micrograph by Dr. M. Oda)

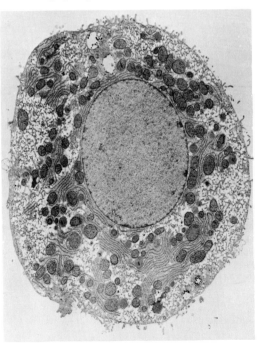

couplets and triplets, can be made in which polarity of the cells is maintained; such cells constitute the smallest secretory units of the liver. Under special conditions the hepatocytes maintain a morphologic appearance very similar to that *in vivo* for up to 24 hours or longer. They become a suitable model system to test the effects of drugs on canalicular contractions as well as the effects of hormones and carcinogenic compounds. The ability of the pericanalicular filaments to produce movement was first demonstrated in this model.

Biliary epithelial cells contain few organelles and have a round to oval nucleus located near the basal lamina. A small, eccentric nucleolus may be observed. The biliary cell is smaller than the hepatocyte, and its nucleus occupies half of the cell. Its mitochondria are also smaller and more elongated, and the mitochondrial matrix is less electron dense than that of hepatocytes; furthermore, biliary epithelial cells contain fewer dense granules and have transverse cristae, which produce a striped appearance. The RER is not prominent. Vesicles from the SER are scattered throughout the cytoplasm but predominate at the periphery of the cells. The Golgi apparatus is inconspicuous and is generally found in the apical region of biliary cells. Free ribosomes are numerous, and cytokeratin filaments are found in the cytosol; the latter are organized in randomly oriented bundles. The apical region is provided with abundant microvilli. The presence of numerous periluminal pinocytic vacuoles reflects the highly active processes that take place between the biliary cells and the luminal contents. Cilia are infrequent. Biliary epithelial cells show interdigitations of their adjoining lateral membranes toward the apical region. Occasionally, slitlike openings between the lateral cell membranes give rise to secondary lumina. The biliary epithelium is always enclosed by a basement membrane.[96,148,197]

VIRAL HEPATITIS

The identification of the hepatitis B virus is a landmark among the contributions of electron microscopy to the diagnosis of liver disease.[10] Immunoelectron microscopy has been particularly valuable in localizing antigen-specific viral particles for visualization.[63] The hepatitis B virus has been recently classified as a hepatotropic DNA virus, or hepadna virus. The hepatitis B virus consists of two distinct antigenic subunits, the viral coat and the core. The assemblage of subunits gives rise to the complete virus, also known as the Dane particle, which measures approximately 42 nm. The outer component of the hepatitis B virus, the surface antigen (HBsAg), comprises spherical or elongated tubular structures, which on transverse section measure 22 nm and may or may not appear to be hollow. On longitudinal sections, the surface antigen particles are found either singly or in tightly packed groups that distend the endoplasmic reticulum cisternae (Fig. 2-7). The inner component, or core particle (HBcAg), is a spherule that in section appears ring shaped and measures 28 nm. It is known to contain "e" antigen, partially double-stranded DNA, and DNA polymerase. Core particles

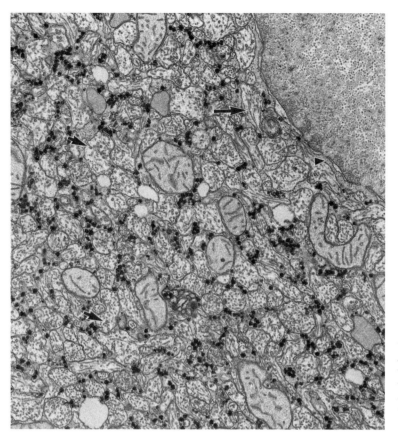

Fig. 2-7. Ground-glass hepatocyte from a hepatitis B carrier. A portion of the nucleus and the cytoplasm of one cell is shown. The endoplasmic reticulum is increased in amount and dilated. It contains spherical and tubular structures corresponding to hepatitis B surface antigen (*long arrow*). The larger spherical particles are Dane particles (*short arrows*). Note also the numerous core antigen particles within the nucleus (*sanded nucleus*); some viral core particles are present in the hyaloplasm as well (*arrowhead*), near the nuclear pores. (Original magnification × 30,000; transmission electron micrograph by J. Patterson)

are found in the nucleus and less frequently in the cytosol, bile canaliculi, and the extracellular space. The core particles migrate from the nucleus and enter the endoplasmic reticulum, where assembly of the two components, core (HBcAg) and surface (HBsAg), results in the formation of the complete virion.[5,35,62–64,78,83,128,136,148,175,189]

Characteristically, in patients with chronic hepatitis B infection and in carriers, cells known as aldehyde-fuchsin (orcein)–positive ground-glass hepatocytes are seen. The peculiar light microscopic appearance of ground-glass hepatocytes correlates ultrastructurally with the presence of HBsAg particles within the proliferated endoplasmic reticulum.[128,129,178,196,214]

These particles react specifically with anti-HBsAg to produce a diffuse cytoplasmic pattern by immunofluorescence or immunoperoxidase. This immunohistochemical finding is in contrast to that seen when the core particle is treated with anti-HBcAg. In this instance, the sanded nuclear appearance by light microscopy of infected hepatocytes results from the presence of HBcAg. When stained histochemically with anti-HBcAg, positive nuclei are homogeneously stained, and a less striking dotted pattern may be observed in the cytoplasm.

Ultrastructurally, in immunosuppressed patients, in whom HBcAg is abundant, nuclear details can be completely obscured by the massive presence of core

particles[74,78,80,83–85,148] (see Fig. 2-7). Core antigen can be observed in the nuclei of hepatocytes in the acute phase, whereas HBsAg cytoplasmic inclusions are rarely seen. However, the occurrence of demonstrable HBsAg in the acute phase is an ominous finding that usually indicates that transition to chronicity may ensue.[140,148] The presence of ground-glass hepatocytes is inversely related to the activity of the inflammation in chronic disease.[62,214] A similar relationship between chronicity, inflammation, and viral particles has also been observed for immune complexes of viral antigen and antibody.[1,46,129]

Hepatitis A virus measures 27 nm and is a nonenveloped single-stranded RNA enterovirus from the family of Picornaviridae.[34,109,111,148] Cytoplasmic granular accumulations of these particles have been demonstrated by immunofluorescence, but nuclei have been persistently negative. In hepatocytes of experimentally infected animals, electron microscopy has revealed viral particles within the cisternae of the endoplasmic reticulum, in cytoplasmic vesicles, and within the lumina of bile canaliculi. Lysosomes of Kupffer cells have also been found to harbor clusters of hepatitis A viral particles. In a study of 11 patients with infectious hepatitis, viral-like particles were reported to be seen within cytoplasmic saccules.[4,34]

The subcellular changes observed in acute hepatitis A are indistinguishable from those in hepatitis B. Chronic hepatitis, carrier state, cirrhosis, and hepatocellular carcinoma have not been documented as a sequelae of hepatitis A.[109,148]

Non-A, non-B (NANB) hepatitis is a relatively newly described type of viral hepatitis, that shares some similarities with both hepatitis A and hepatitis B. Studies carried out in chimpanzees and marmosets infected experimentally with NANB virus,[51,138] as well as—albeit less convincingly—studies of clinical NANB hepatitis in humans,[5,27] have demonstrated nuclear particles of 20 nm to 27 nm and a range of cytoplasmic alterations affecting primarily the endoplasmic reticulum. Curved membranes, peculiar tubular or cylindrical structures that measure 150 nm to 330 nm in width, spongelike networks, and tubuloreticular inclusions represent some of the most common ultrastructural findings in NANB hepatitis. Of these cytoplasmic changes, tubuloreticular inclusions are the most frequent type found in human acute and chronic NANB hepatitis; fibrillar or tubular reticular inclusions closely resemble the morphologic appearance of the viroplasmic aggregates seen in other viral infections. The cytoplasmic changes observed in hepatocytes in NANB hepatitis do not represent the NANB virus *per se,* since they have also been documented in delta superinfection. The above-mentioned nuclear and cytoplasmic findings have been mutually exclusive in experimental studies, suggesting that NANB hepatitis represents more than one viral strain.[2,5,22,50,51,115,138,179] Interestingly, cytochemical studies performed on the fibrillar reticular inclusions suggest that one of their components may be RNA. On the other hand, there is current evidence to support the view that one of the NANB agents may be a DNA virus that shares many similarities with hepatitis B virus.[2,4,22,27,50,51,179]

The delta agent is an incomplete, hepatotropic, and transmissible RNA virus whose infectivity is restricted to patients in whom HBsAg is present.[148,160,161,173] The delta agent viral particle measures 35 nm to 37 nm in diameter. The inner component corresponds to the delta antigen in which a single-stranded linear RNA represents the genome of the virion. The outer component is acquired by the delta agent from the HBsAg-infected hepatocytes. Therefore, replication and virulence of the delta agent depends on HBsAg accessibility. Furthermore, delta superinfection may obscure the natural history of hepatitis B. The coinfection of hepatitis B virus and hepatitis "D" or delta virus has been reported to greatly increase the severity of the illness and the frequency in which acute B hepatitis evolves to chronicity.[148,150,160,161,173]

Immunohistochemical studies for the delta agent have revealed patterns similar to those depicted in HBcAg-harboring hepatocytes. However, all attempts to characterize the ultrastructure of the delta agent in human liver have thus far been unsuccessful.

In viral hepatitis, the degree of cellular damage seen by electron microscopy roughly parallels that seen by light microscopy. Not infrequently, however, the damage to subcellular organelles is far more profound than simple loss of hepatocytes would suggest.[140,196] Aside from the specific findings pertaining to the viral particles *per se,* the changes in hepatocyte ultrastructure in viral hepatitis are nonspecific. The characteristic swollen hepatocyte or ballooned cell is one in which there is extensive dilation and vesiculation of the RER and SER. This may be a reversible condition in mild degrees but when widespread may lead to a critical failure of metabolism in the hepatocytes.[136,166,203] Ribosomes fail to become attached to the endoplasmic reticulum. Glycogen may appear to be decreased in the cell, and lysosomes are increased. Bile canaliculi may be normal or dilated with swollen or reduced microvilli. Mitochondria may be swollen. It has been suggested that this latter change may correlate with the increased AST (serum glutamic-oxaloacetic transaminase [SGOT]) seen in acute hepatitis.[200] Another important finding in viral hepatitis, but not specific for this disease, is "focal cytoplasmic necrosis" or "focal cytoplasmic degradation," a process whereby part of the cell dies but the total cell continues to survive.[140,164] The cell remains viable by sequestering the damaged organelles into cytophagocytic vacuoles. These vacuoles fuse with primary lysosomes to become autophagic vacuoles, a prominent feature of the ultrastructural pathology of acute viral hepatitis. The cell will continue to maintain its intact appearance on routine histology until the autophagocytic vacuoles can no longer cope with the degree of damage. Imbalance of electrolytes (sodium, potassium, and calcium) may cause the cell to swell. Eventually integrity of the plasma membrane is lost, resulting in single-cell necrosis. Hepatocellular necrosis may also occur by progressive dehydration and condensation of the cytoplasm with nuclear pyknosis. In this type of necrosis, the liver cell takes on a deeply eosinophilic appearance on light microscopy and forms the typical acidophilic or Councilman-like body.[13,15,96,140] By electron microscopy, organelles of acidophilic bodies show a remarkable preservation of morphology, but a generalized deeply osmiophilic appearance is classic. When the acidophilic body becomes extruded from the liver cell plate into the space of Disse or the sinusoid, it is engulfed by Kupffer cells. At later stages, the cytoplasmic organelles undergo degeneration, and the plasma membrane may be absent.[15,136,148,203]

Concomitant with hepatocellular necrosis and regeneration, mesenchymal cells proliferate. The Kupffer cells are hypertrophied, extensions of cytoplasm contain increased RER and show evidence of active phagocytosis of cellular remnants.[200,203,212] Inflammatory cells, including lymphocytes, polymorphonuclear leukocytes, plasma cells, and some eosinophils migrate into the space of Disse or wedge between the closely apposed neighboring hepatocytes.[96,140,148,197] It has been suggested that the relationship of the mononuclear inflammatory cells to the hepatocytes may be in reaction to an altered immune status of the liver cells and may contribute to their eventual necrosis.

In acute viral hepatitis, features of regeneration are also evident. There is an early increase in autophagocytosis along with restoration to normal of the organelle changes described above. There is an increase in polyribosomes,[166] an increase in nuclear size, and an increase in RER compatible with the increased demand for protein synthesis. The appearance of intracellular glycogen in regeneration occasionally takes the form of "glycogen bodies," which are parallel arrays of SER alternating with rows of multiparticulate glycogen.[15,212] Many of the patterns of subcellular injury and regeneration described above in liver cells are similar to those seen experimentally.[6]

Biliary epithelial cells of interlobular ducts may show a widened intercellular space, cytoplasmic condensation, and increased osmiophilia. Shrinkage and retraction of the biliary cells also occur. Additionally, polymorphonuclear cells and lymphocytes may surround the bile duct and invade the epithelium. An occasional inflammatory cell may be seen in the lumen. However, unlike hepatocellular damage, injury to bile ducts may or may not be present in viral hepatitis.[30,170] A secondary narrowing of the lumen may be caused by the development of cytoplasmic blebs along the apical surface of these cells, with an associated decrease in true microvilli. An occasional inflammatory cell may be seen in the lumen. Proliferation of ductules, cholangioles, and neocholangioles occurs as the inflammation becomes more severe or chronic. The phenomenon of ductular proliferation has been linked to the appearance of fibrosis and is discussed below.

DRUG EFFECTS

Many drugs and chemical agents cause liver damage; examination of the liver by light and electron microscopy has disclosed several underlying patterns of cellular injury[95,108,148,149,159,162,182,184,222–224] (Figs. 2-8 through 2-12). In both drug-induced cholestasis and hepatitis, such studies provide some clues to the possible pathogenesis or the primary site of cell damage. In this chapter two examples of drug-induced hepatitis, are discussed briefly, halothane-induced and galactosamine-induced, since they may serve as prototypes and both have been the subject of many studies.[44,96,104,148,207] Halothane is thought to induce inflammation in the liver as an unpredictable hypersensitivity reaction. Galactosamine, on the other hand, is used experimentally as a model of direct hepatotoxicity associated with liver cell necrosis. The inflammation and necrosis that result are predictable and dose related. The drug effects on ultrastructure in both cases frequently include pronounced mitochondrial swelling, alterations of the outer mitochondrial membrane and cristae, and crystalloid inclusions. Hypertrophy of the SER, glycogen and ribosomal depletion, liposome accumulation, and the presence of protein-containing vacuoles have been described in galactosamine hepatitis.[118,207,213] These changes occur to varying degrees in viral hepatitis, but some features are more commonly associated with drug effects and may suggest that drugs cause alterations and injury in some way different than that of the hepatitis viruses. For example, the hypertrophy of SER which is one of the hallmarks of adverse drug reactions, may be related to increased utilization of cytochrome P450 and other microsomal enzymes.[202] An increase in lipids may be due to many factors, including a decreased ability to transport lipoprotein out of the cell or an inhibition of lipoprotein synthesis for transport.[200]

Fig. 2-8. Drug-induced mitochondrial changes: The markedly enlarged mitochondrion shown (∗) contains numerous paracrystalline inclusions and increased numbers of matrical granules. Some of the neighboring mitochondria are also pleomorphic. Lipid droplets (*L*) and lipofuscin granules are present. The patient is on methotrexate therapy. (Original magnification × 11,000; transmission electron micrograph by J. Patterson)

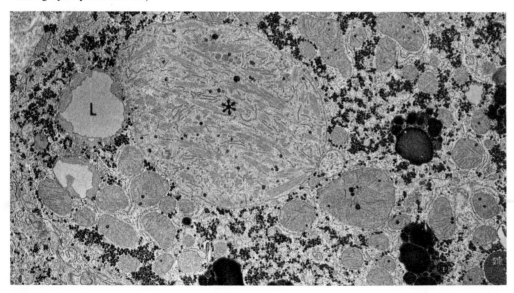

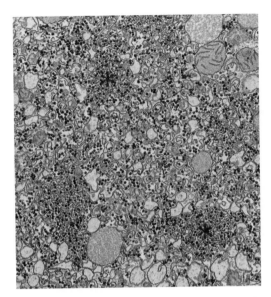

Fig. 2-9. Drug-induced proliferation of the smooth endoplasmic reticulum is shown (∗). The patient is on phenobarbital therapy. (Original magnification × 11,000; transmission electron micrograph by J. Patterson)

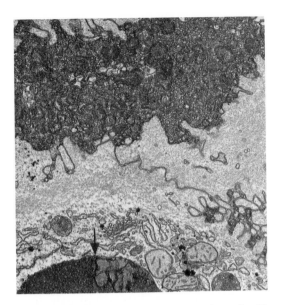

Fig. 2-11. Drug-induced cholestasis. A portion of a dilated canaliculus that contains a deeply osmiophilic bile plug is shown; a lysosome (*arrow*) has similar contents. The patient is on amiodarone therapy. (Original magnification × 15,500; electron micrograph by J. Patterson)

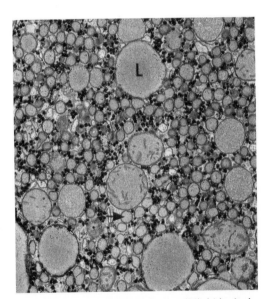

Fig. 2-10. Drug-induced steatosis. Small lipid inclusions (*L*) alternate with membrane-bound microvesicular lipid droplets (*arrow*). The patient is on 6-mercaptopurine therapy. (Original magnification × 15,000; transmission electron micrograph by J. Patterson)

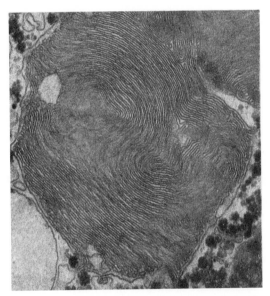

Fig. 2-12. Drug (amiodarone)-induced phospholipidosis. An enlarged lysosome contains tightly packed, parallel membranes. (× 60,000; transmission electron micrograph by J. Patterson)

Not all drug reactions are similar, nor do they share common pathways of cell injury. Many drugs can produce characteristic electron microscopic changes. For instance, phenobarbital produces a marked hypertrophy of the SER, actinomycin D causes striking nuclear and nucleolar abnormalities, certain antilipidemic agents cause a great increase in peroxisomes, norethandrolone affects the bile canaliculus, glucagon causes cytolysosome formation, colchicine damages microtubules, amiodarone produces osmiophilic lamellar inclusions identical to those seen in the primary phospholipidoses, whereas tetracycline can cause severe mitochondrial damage and fatty

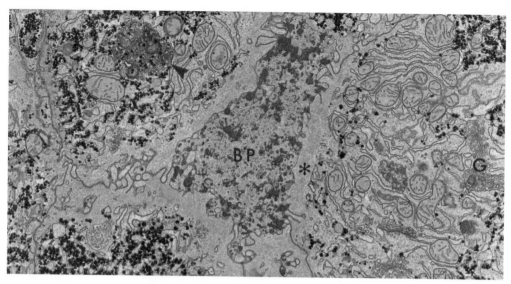

Fig. 2-13. Extrahepatic biliary tract obstruction. The bile secretory apparatus of two neighboring hepatocytes is shown. The ectoplasmic zone (∗) around the bile canaliculus is widened, and the dilated lumen is filled with a bile plug (*BP*); there is a reduction in microvilli. Note also the presence of retained biliary material within a lysosome (*arrowhead*). The Golgi apparatus (*G*) is prominent. (Original magnification × 12,000; transmission electron micrograph by J. Patterson)

liver.[94,97,134,146,148,155,159,182] Drug-induced cholestasis is discussed in the next part of this chapter. Some experimental drugs have specific subcellular cytopharmacologic effects also; for example, phalloidin causes actin filaments to accumulate in hepatocytes,[60] whereas cytochalasin B causes them to break down.[130]

Ultrastructural patterns of drug and toxic injury to the liver can simulate those seen in a wide range of other hepatic diseases. However, with careful evaluation of clinical, histologic, and ultrastructural studies, a diagnosis of liver damage secondary to drugs or chemicals can often be made. Undoubtedly, further investigations and documentation in this important area are necessary to fully elucidate the pathogenetic mechanisms reflected in abnormal organelle function and structure.

CHOLESTASIS

The ultrastructure of the liver in intrahepatic and extrahepatic cholestasis has been the subject of a number of recent reviews.[40,141,146,148,151] Enhanced interest in this subject has arisen partly because of the increased awareness of drug-induced liver disease, of which intrahepatic cholestasis is a common type,[141,145,146,148,149,203] ∗ and because of interest in the relationship of bile acids to gallstone disease and possibly to cholestasis.[20,52,59,121,122,147,199,220] The

∗ Phillips MJ et al: Mechanisms of cholestasis. Lab Invest 54: 593, 1986.

ultrastructural hallmark of cholestasis in humans is the presence of biliary material in dilated bile canaliculi (Fig. 2-13 and 2-14). Bile canalicular microvilli are also usually altered, showing swelling and a reduction in number or even a total absence. It has been noted that the microvilli immediately adjacent to the tight junctions tend to be preserved, and this may have special functional significance.[141,208] In scanning electron micrographs, the canaliculi appear not only dilated but tortuous, saccular, and associated with diverticula.[33] No communications with the space of Disse, however, have been found. Other findings include hypertrophy of the Golgi apparatus, increased numbers of vesicles, increased numbers of lysosomes and cytolysosomes, dilation and vesiculation of the RER, variation in size and shape of mitochondria, often with curled cristae or paracrystalline inclusions, and hypertrophy of the SER. Some of the vesicles contain biliary pigment, and similar material can be found in intercellular locations and in the space of Disse. The biliary material in the cytoplasm and in bile canaliculi is of two major morphologic types: it is partly granular and partly membranous or lamellar. The precise chemical nature of these components is not known, but they presumably represent bile pigment and phospholipid liquid crystals or phospholipid–bile salt complexes. In some instances, the cytoplasm of the hepatocytes contains a great deal of this material, and in such conditions the liver cells show feathery degeneration by light microscopy.

It is significant that the bile canaliculi do not rupture even in the face of prolonged biliary obstruction; the regurgitation appears transcellular and occurs by way of

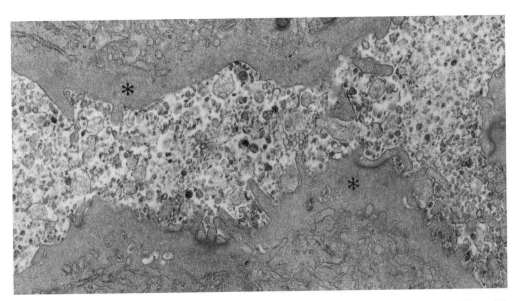

Fig. 2-14. Intrahepatic cholestasis (Byler's disease). A large, dilated bile canaliculus is shown. Microvilli are greatly reduced in number, but some are near normal. The lumen contains coarse particulate biliary material, and the pericanalicular ectoplasmic zone (∗) is greatly widened. (Original magnification × 19,000; transmission electron micrograph by Dr. D. Yu)

vesicles that transport biliary materials from the canalicular pole to the sinusoidal region of the liver cell where the biliary material is released by reversed pinocytosis. The tight junctions bordering the bile canaliculi have been examined in rat liver following experimental bile duct ligation using the freeze-fracture technique.[42] It was found that the normal parallel strands became reduced and had an irregular pattern, a conformation suggesting altered permeability. In addition, gap junctions disappeared, resulting in a lack of intercellular communication and uncoupling of liver cells. This might help to explain the variation in bile canalicular changes found ultrastructurally in cholestasis. Bile ducts show a variety of fine-structural changes similar to those described in hepatocytes, including increased vesicular activity, evidence of reversed pinocytosis, biliary pigment in the duct lumen and in vesicles, reduction in microvilli, shedding and bleb formation, prominence of the Golgi apparatus, and, less frequently, curling of mitochondrial cristae. Reduplication of the basement membrane and increased numbers of ducts of Hering are also features.[165] In primary biliary cirrhosis (Fig. 2-15), duct epithelial cells show a wide range of changes including an increase in cytoplasmic filaments, swollen mitochondria, large cytophagosomes, marked blebbing and shedding of the luminal surface of the cell membrane, vesiculation of the RER, apoptotic bodies, and lymphocytes wedged between biliary epithelial cells; a deeply electron-dense granular or laminated material alternates with layers of duplicated basement membrane.[11,148,168] Essentially similar findings are seen in sclerosing cholangitis; however, in this condition bile ducts are reduced in size and compressed by concentric bun-

dles of collagen fibers and fibroblastic processes[29,148] (Fig. 2-16).

In many clinical conditions associated with jaundice, such as alcoholic liver disease, viral hepatitis, cirrhosis, and several types of drug-induced jaundice, there is nothing distinctive about the ultrastructural pathology associated with the cholestasis aside from canalicular and pericanalicular changes as are seen in other forms of cholestasis.[8,32,79,103,169] Moreover, the ultrastructural changes in the liver in intrahepatic cholestasis are virtually identical to those found in mechanical obstruction.[33,79,103] However, there are a number of cholestatic conditions in which the electron microscopic findings might be specific or at least are distinctive. Copper-containing granules are frequently found in hepatocytes in the late stages of primary biliary cirrhosis; in sclerosing cholangitis copper deposits appear to be less common. They are found mainly in hepatocytes at the periphery of the cirrhotic nodules and are presumably a reflection of prolonged cholestasis, with interference of copper excretion in the bile. In Byler's disease, a familial fatal form of intrahepatic cholestasis thought to be due to a primary defect in bile acid metabolism, the ultrastructural appearance of bile pigment is unusual.[148] Bile canaliculi are dilated and contain coarsely particulate biliary material (see Fig. 2-14). Moreover, the filamentous pericanalicular ectoplasmic zone is generally greatly widened. Biliary epithelial cells in Byler's disease may show intense cytolysosome formation and bile necrosis; in later stages there is extensive deposition of collagen fibers, and cirrhosis may develop.[148] Microfilament dysfunction has been suggested as a possible cause of intrahepatic cholestasis in some forms of drug-induced experimental cho-

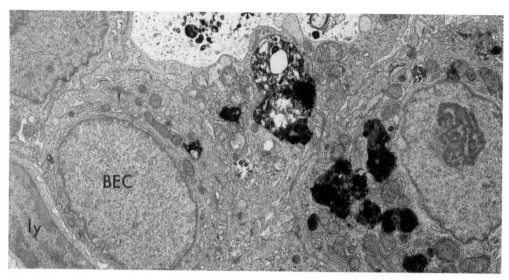

Fig. 2-15. Primary biliary cirrhosis. Detail of part of a bile duct is shown. Two types of lysosomes are present within the biliary epithelial cells (*BEC*): A large electron lucent cytolysosome contains a sparse amount of electron dense material (∗); other secondary lysosomes with electron dense material stained positively for copper by light microscopy. A lymphocyte (*Ly*) is in close contact with two of the biliary cells. (Original magnification × 8500; transmission electron micrograph by Dr. P. Valencia)

lestasis such as that produced by cytochalasin B, phalloidin, and norethandrolone.[60,145,146] ∗ Decrease in bile flow in some instances may be explained by an effect on Na^+,K^+-ATPase, which is thought to influence bile salt–independent bile blow, or on altered fluidity of the liver cell membranes with altered membrane permeability and secretory activity.[180] ∗

ALCOHOLIC LIVER DISEASE

Mallory bodies, or alcoholic hyalin, have interested electron microscopists for many years. They are one of the hallmarks of acute alcoholic hepatitis, but histologically and ultrastructurally identical structures have been observed in more than 30 conditions involving the liver, including Wilson's disease, primary biliary cirrhosis, chronic and acute hepatitis, jejunoileal bypass for obesity, extrahepatic biliary obstruction, Indian childhood cirrhosis, and hepatomas.[148] In early reports, Mallory bodies were considered to be megamitochondria or regions of focal cytoplasmic degradation. Studies of Biava,[14] Yokoo,[219] and French and Davies[56] have shown convincingly that Mallory bodies are filamentous in nature. There is now growing evidence that they are made up of 10-nm filaments that correspond in size to intermediate filaments. As the Mallory body evolves, the cytoskeleton of liver cells appears to retract into the Mallory body. These cells, when decorated with keratin antibody, reveal a positively

∗ Phillips MJ et al: Mechanisms of cholestasis. Lab Invest 54: 593, 1986.

stained inclusion surrounded by a swollen, empty-looking cytoplasm in which the cytoskeletal components are severely deranged; keratin filaments appear greatly diminished or completely absent. These observations are substantial evidence that intermediate filaments of the cytokeratin subtype constitute the major element of Mallory bodies.[54,55,127,211] Denk and associates have been successful in producing an experimental model of Mallory bodies using griseofulvin and colchicine, two well-known antimicrotubular agents.[37–39,54] The interference with assembly of microtubules in treated animals followed by a pathologic increase in numbers of intermediate filaments could theoretically lead to the formation of Mallory bodies. In other studies it has been demonstrated that an inverse relationship exists between the accumulation of intermediate filaments and the reduction of the number of microtubules.[37–39,56] Further, the preneoplasia hypothesis attempts to explain Mallory body formation on the basis of their association with the development of oncofetal markers in experimental hepatic carcinogenesis. However, most of the conditions in which Mallory bodies are present are not neoplastic or preneoplastic. Recently, vitamin A deficiency followed by squamous metaplasia of hepatocytes has also been postulated as a possible mechanism in the pathogenesis of the Mallory body. It is important to note here that ethanol has been implicated in the inhibition of microtubule assembly and function. Alcohol has also been shown to cause enlargement of hepatic cells and delayed secretion of albumin and transferrin by the liver, which is explained on the basis of decreased liver microtubules. Hence, an effect of ethanol on microtubules may help to explain a number of the findings in acute

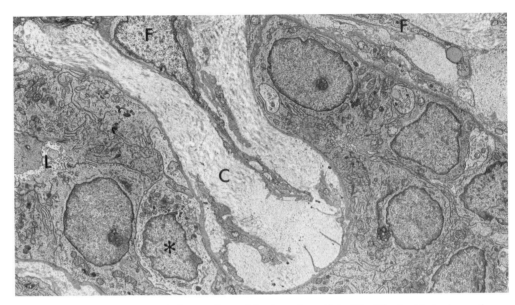

Fig. 2-16. Sclerosing cholangitis in a patient with ulcerative colitis. The bile duct is tortuous, has a narrow lumen (*L*), and the whole biliary structure is encroached upon by dense collagen bundles (*C*). The basement membrane is thickened. A mononuclear cell is wedged between two of the biliary cells (∗). Note also the presence of fibroblasts (*F*) and fibroblastic processes around the bile duct. (Original magnification × 5000; transmission electron micrograph by J. Patterson)

ethanol-induced liver injury, including swelling of the hepatocytes, possibly the Mallory body, and the low levels of serum proteins, which may result in part from functional impairment.

Ultrastructural aspects of Mallory bodies in alcoholic liver disease as classified by Yokoo and colleagues fall into three categories: type I is composed of filaments running parallel to one another; Type II is characterized by filaments that have a random orientation (Fig. 2-17); and Type III, formed by a granular or homogeneous electron-dense mass, represents structural degeneration of the Mallory body.[219]

Fig. 2-17. Alcoholic liver disease. Part of a Mallory body is shown; it comprises parallel arrays (*arrow*) and randomly oriented intermediate filaments (∗) (types I and II of Yokoo; see text). (Original magnification × 51,000; transmission electron micrograph by J. Patterson)

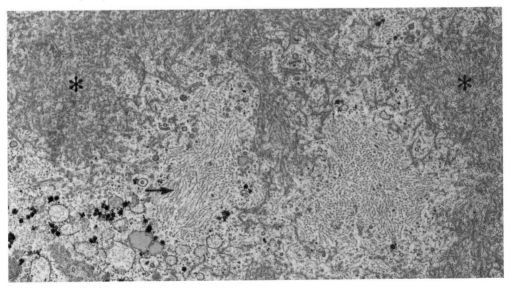

Other frequent ultrastructural findings in acute alcoholic liver injury include cytoplasmic lipid accumulation, predominantly triglyceride, which can displace other organelles. When microvesicular lipid accumulation is extensive in the cytoplasm of zone 3 hepatocytes, the hepatocytes become markedly enlarged and have a foamy appearance on light microscopy. By electron microscopy, the cytoplasm is densely packed with lipid droplets, glycogen is depleted, and the RER may be dilated. The term "alcoholic foamy degeneration" refers to this type of steatosis.[206] Significant alterations are found in mitochondria, including enlargement with variability in size and shape, rearrangement of cristae into longitudinal stacks, increase in the number and size of dense granules and crystalline inclusions. Giant forms are also common and may even be visible by light microscopy.[24] The morphologic changes in mitochondria relate to disturbed energy production and may explain hepatic insufficiency and instances of sudden death.[168] Fat accumulation and mitochondrial enlargement are the earliest changes found and have been produced in normal human volunteers fed ethanol as isocaloric substitution for carbohydrates.[163] The SER is increased. The amount of RER tends to be reduced, and stacks of cisternae are usually absent. The reduction in the RER may be partly responsible for the low serum albumin levels seen in chronic alcoholic liver disease. Bile canaliculi are usually normal, but some are dilated, lack microvilli, and contain biliary pigment. At the sinusoidal border, microvilli may be reduced in number. The space of Disse may harbor a basement membrane and is often filled and blocked by collagen fibers, Kupffer cells, lipocytes (fat-storing cells), myofibroblastic processes, fibroblasts, and transitional cells. The latter represent an intermediate cell between lipocytes and fibroblasts and have been reported to be numerous in alcoholic liver disease.[110] Myofibroblasts presently are implicated in the process of fibrogenesis. These cells are more common in zone 3 (perivenular area) and are recognized by the presence of patchy accumulations of microfilaments at the periphery of the cell and a surrounding basement membrane. Myofibroblasts have been shown to synthesize collagen types I, III, IV and laminin. The scarring process and mesenchymal cell reaction progress down the sinusoids from zone 3, resulting eventually in both intralobular perisinusoidal and pericellular fibrosis.[110,142,172] These changes may impair diffusion of substances between the hepatocellular and sinusoidal interface.

HEPATIC FIBROSIS AND CIRRHOSIS

The final common denominator in many forms of chronic liver injury, as a result of necrosis, regeneration, altered vasculature, and a changing architectural scaffold, is the formation of nodules of liver cells surrounded by collagenous fibrous tissue. This section discusses general aspects of the cirrhotic and fibrotic processes.

One of the earliest and initially puzzling contributions

of electron microscopy in this field was the failure to find a continuous linear reticulin deposit along the margins of the sinusoids. This reticulin framework is one of the hallmarks of the light microscopic examination of the liver. By electron microscopy, however, the space of Disse has been clearly defined and shows no basement membrane or continuous network of reticulin fibers (see Fig. 2-1). Reticulin fibers are now known to be type III collagen.[191] In the electron micrographs, they appear as a focal deposit of what seems to be a few randomly oriented fibrils. It should be remembered, however, that these sections are extremely thin. If serial sections with three-dimensional reconstructions were made, it is most likely that the original notion of a fibril-formed architectural scaffold would be confirmed. In any event, in the lobule there normally are no collagen bundles at all and at best only a few single collagen strands; the presence of more than this constitutes fibrosis at the ultrastructural level (Fig. 2-18).

Of the major types of collagen described, most of the collagen in the portal tracts and surrounding central veins is in bundles and is type I.[61] Type III is located in small amounts in the triads and in the parenchyma. Collagen type IV is found in basement membranes such as those around portal bile ducts and blood vessels. A small amount of basement membrane–like material is occasionally found in the space of Disse, but a true basement membrane in chronic liver disease is found only in periportal areas. It is noteworthy that basement membrane material in the sinusoids—so called capillarization of the sinusoids—is mainly a feature of actively developing cirrhosis. Basement membranes are usually not present in the nodules of advanced cirrhosis.[171] In actively developing cirrhosis, the hepatic sinusoid may be encroached upon by layers of collagen, basement membranes, fibroblasts, and other mesenchymal cells, all of which serve to obliterate Disse's space as a plasma-filled compartment and to separate the hepatic cell plasma membrane from the blood in the sinusoids. In cirrhotic nodules with thickened liver cell plates, the normal disposition of hepatocytes in relation to the sinusoids is deranged. Instead of approximately 50% of the surface area facing the sinusoids, this figure is greatly reduced. Indeed, as a result of regeneration, rearrangement of liver cell cords takes place, and numerous hepatocytes are trapped amidst other hepatocytes, isolating them from the sinusoids.[6,142] In these instances, the intercellular space between hepatocytes is widened and the contiguous plasma membrane surfaces are provided by anomalous microvilli. These intercellular spaces or canals communicate eventually with perisinusoidal recesses and the space of Disse. The formation of pericellular canals has been deemed an adaptive change whereby the liver cells return to a more fetal type.[6,142]

Ductular proliferation is seen in many forms of liver disease. It is important because it may serve as a scaffold for the deposition of fibrous tissue.[29,152,170,185,187] The proliferated ductules are of two main types: those lined only by biliary cells and those lined by a combination of biliary cells, hepatocytes, and intermediate cells. The former are

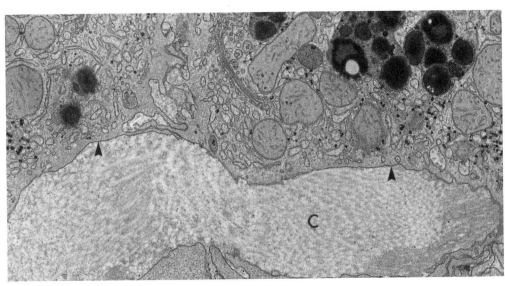

Fig. 2-18. Advanced inactive cirrhosis. The space of Disse is filled with densely packed collagen fibers (*C*). Note also that the sinusoidal surface of the plasma membrane (*arrowheads*) of the hepatocytes is devoid of microvilli. (Original magnification × 20,000; transmission electron micrograph by J. Patterson)

completely enclosed by a basement membrane. The latter group has two subtypes: cholangioles and neocholangioles. Neocholangioles, unlike cholangioles, are present only in pathologic states and are seen to best advantage in active cirrhosis, chronic active hepatitis, massive or submassive necrosis, and alcoholic liver disease. In cholangioles, the basement membrane is seen only around the bile duct epithelium, whereas in neocholangioles it encloses both biliary epithelial cells and hepatocytes. Furthermore, neocholangioles frequently contain "biliary hepatocytes," which represent an intermediate cell form. Cholangioles and neocholangioles are long anastomosing biliary channels with irregular lumina.[140,148,154] In addition, ultrastructural studies have shown that the "oval" cells seen in the cellular fibrous tissue by light microscopy are in fact biliary epithelium.[71,171,187] In the phase of proliferation, the endoplasmic reticulum and ribosomal content of biliary epithelial cells may increase, and microfilaments in the cell may become conspicuous.[71,152,186] The luminal surface of the cell membrane may show prominent blebs. The smooth plasma membranes, usually closely apposed between neighboring cells, may become separated, but the smooth basilar plasma membrane remains unchanged. The enclosing basement membrane of proliferated ductules is frequently thickened or reduplicated and surrounded by a cuff of inflammatory cells and mesenchymal cells.[170] The inflammatory cells may migrate through the basement membrane and enter the intercellular space. Many of these ductules have been found to maintain continuity with bile ducts despite extension of their growth well into the lobular parenchyma, whereas others end blindly. The stimulus to the growth of these ductules and to the relationship of the associated fibrosis has been the

subject of conjecture and controversy. They have been implicated in regeneration and in the persistence of active inflammation,[152] but their role in fibrogenesis is the most widely discussed.[71,148,152,170,185,187]

There is evidence that with piecemeal necrosis the area of the necrosis and ductular proliferation at the terminal plate of the lobule is also the area in which active fibrosis occurs. It has been suggested, therefore, that ductular proliferation is a reaction to a stimulus such as inflammation that will inevitably result in an increased basement membrane along with the ductular cell growth. The basement membrane then will provide the stimulus and scaffold for the collagen deposition that follows.[152] The correlation of collagen deposition with inflammation, ductular proliferation, or basement membrane, however, is not invariable.[163]

The source of collagen formation in the liver has always been presumed to be the fibroblast. However, evidence obtained *in vitro* suggests that the hepatocyte also forms collagen and may play a significant role in some types of collagen synthesis *in vivo*.[204] The hepatocyte *in vitro* appears to produce a predominance of collagen types III and V, whereas the fibroblast produces a predominance of collagen type I. In recent studies, the lipocyte, or Ito cell, has also been noted *in vivo* to be a conspicuous cell type in regions of active fibrosis.[81,82] This is the perisinusoidal fat-storing cell described earlier in this chapter (see Fig. 2-1). Fibrils have been seen in vacuoles in its cytoplasm. Its number has been noted to increase when collagen fibers are being synthesized,[29,81,82,102,152] and it has been observed surrounding proliferating ductules in portal triads. It may have the capacity to differentiate into a fibroblast-like or transitional cell with collagen-forming capacity.[82,102] In experimental fibrosis, consequent to necrosis and inflammation, it is the lipocyte or fat-storing cell that increases in number.[81,82,102] As the lesion matures, however, lipocytes are no longer increased in number, but fibroblasts are seen in association with collagen deposition.[190] This observation has been considered to be evidence that fibroblasts and transitional cells in the liver are derived from the lipocytes.[110,148,190,215]

METABOLIC LIVER DISEASES

Electron microscopic observations have proved to be helpful in the diagnosis of metabolic diseases involving the liver. The discussion that follows highlights some of the metabolic conditions in which the contribution of electron microscopy has been significant.

α_1-Antitrypsin Deficiency

α_1-antitrypsin enzyme has been found to be deficient in a population of adults and children with emphysema and/or liver disease.[53,123] The liver disease seen can range from no apparent pathologic changes, through mild inflammation and cholestasis, to fatal cirrhosis.[47,53,69,73,123,176,221] By light microscopy, hyaline globules may be seen in hepatocytes predominantly from the periportal area. The finding of these globules does not correlate invariably with symptoms or histologic evidence of disease, but analysis of the globules by immune staining does reveal them to be composed of α_1-antitrypsin.[53,69] Special staining on light microscopy with periodic acid-Schiff (PAS) has shown the globules to be positive and diastase resistant. On electron microscopy, the globules correspond to dilated cisternae of SER or RER with a content of homogeneous, finely granular, moderately electron-dense material that often displays a clear peripheral halo (Fig. 2-19). These ultrastructural features are virtually diagnostic of α_1-antitrypsin deficiency.[148] On the contrary, light microscopy may at times be misleading in the diagnosis of α_1-antitrypsin deficiency because hyaline globules in sections stained with hematoxylin and eosin may be the result of alcoholic hyalin deposits, giant mitochondria, or autophagic vacuoles, and PAS-diastase–resistant globules may occur with lipofuscin and intracellular bile. However, if the tissue sections are decorated with appropriate fluorescein- or peroxidase-labeled antibodies, the diagnosis of α_1-antitrypsin deficiency can be confirmed. It has been suggested that the subcellular localization of the abnormal α_1-antitrypsin may indicate difficulty in transport or secretion of the abnormally formed glycoprotein through the endoplasmic reticulum. One theory states that this failure of transport prevents the protein from arriving at the site of sialic acid addition, which is required for export of the protein.[221] The specificity of liver tissue in the expression of the defect is confirmed by the failure to acquire the deposits in transplant livers and a serologic conversion of phenotype in the recipient to that of the donor.[148]

Fig. 2-19. Adult patient with alpha-1-antitrypsin deficiency. The cisternae of the endoplasmic reticulum are widely dilated and contain homogeneous material (∗). This corresponds to the PAS-positive diastase-resistant cytoplasmic inclusions seen on light microscopy. (Original magnification × 8500; transmission electron micrograph by J. Patterson)

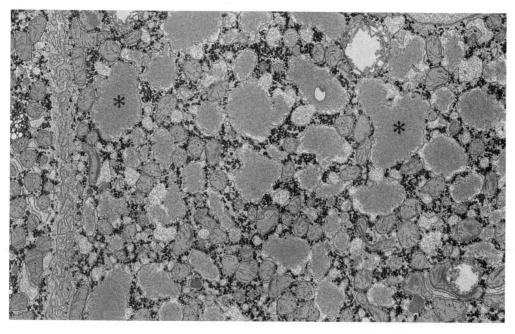

Amyloidosis

The light microscopic changes of amyloid deposition at the sinusoidal margins along liver cell plates are clarified by electron microscopy.[148,181,197] Amyloid is composed of 10-nm filaments that have a hollow core around which are globules of protein. The amyloid fibril is characterized by a periodicity of 4 nm. A similar appearance of the ultrastructure of the fibrils is seen whether the deposit is of the primary or secondary type. The amyloid deposits lie in the space of Disse and extend into the intracellular recesses between hepatocytes. The hepatocytes are compressed and appear atrophic with a loss of microvilli and occasional blebs at the sinusoidal surface.[137] A globular presentation of hepatic amyloidosis has also been reported. The amyloid globules measure 5 μm to 40 μm in diameter and are found in the space of Disse and portal tracts. These globules lack a limiting membrane and are formed of fibrils that are arranged in a disorderly fashion. The fibrils of globular amyloid share characteristics identical to those of the diffuse form.[99]

Wilson's Disease

In Wilson's disease, excretion of hepatic copper along its normal pathway from liver to bile is deficient; however, the basic defect remains unknown.[148,195] The site of greatest injury due to the toxic effect of copper is the liver, although copper accumulates in many other tissues.[148,192] The light microscopic changes of early steatosis, progressing to chronic act hepatitis and finally cirrhosis, are

paralleled by ultrastructural findings of subcellular injury.[193] In the early stages, when the disease is often asymptomatic, the hepatocytes demonstrate a copper content that is diffusely distributed in the cytoplasm of periportal hepatocytes by staining with rubeanic acid or silver sulfide.[66] By electron microscopy, hepatocytes show a spectrum of changes, which together make the ultrastructure of Wilson's disease very typical (Figs. 2-20 and 2-21). A major feature is the presence of copper granules, which are found in two main forms: partially or entirely surrounded by a single membrane, or lying free in the hyaloplasm. The latter accumulations of copper are found as electron-dense, finely granular material, resembling iron deposition, whereas the former electron-dense homogeneous masses represent copper-containing lysosomes.[148,195] The sequestration of copper into lysosomes has been considered an attempt to protect the cell from the toxicity of copper.[66,112,193] The mitochondria may show a number of alterations, including increased mitochondrial size with varied shapes; giant forms are often seen, as are paracrystalline inclusions, and an increase in the size and number of dense granules is also common. The dilation of the intramembranous space of cristae has been considered a hallmark of the disease; however, this aberration may also be observed in other conditions, especially those associated with copper overload.[148,192,194] Copper has been noted to inhibit mitochondrial enzymes and may produce a condensation of mitochondrial matrix and increased intracristal space in vitro.[25]

Glycogen nuclei in Wilson's disease are also similar to glycogen nuclei of other diseases such as diabetes and gly-

Fig. 2-20. Wilson's disease. Neocholangiole from a periportal area comprising of biliary cells (*BEC*) and hepatocytes (*H*) surrounded by a basement membrane (*bm*). Note the dilated tips of the hepatocyte mitochondrial cristae (*arrowheads*); some mitochondria have enlarged matrical granules, whereas others are devoid of granules. Note also numerous lysosomes. C = collagen, F = fibroblast. (Original magnification $\times$ 10,000; transmission electron micrograph by J. Patterson)

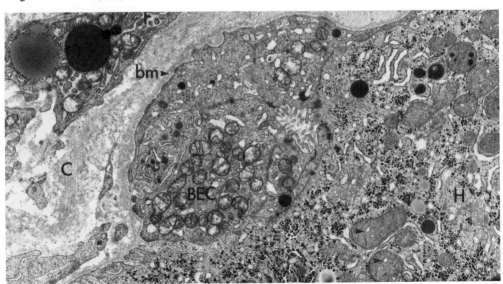

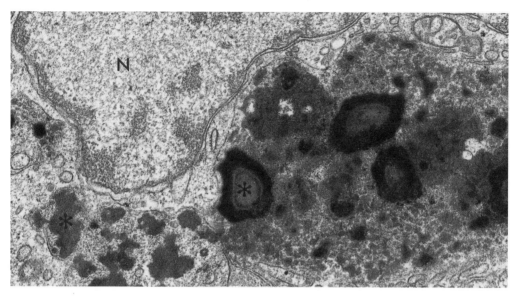

Fig. 2-21. Wilson's disease. Typical copper containing lysosomes (coppersomes, *). Note also severe cytoplasmic and nuclear damage; the nucleus (N) has segregated and clumped chromatin. (Original magnification × 39,000; transmission electron micrograph by J. Patterson)

cogen storage diseases. In glycogen nuclei of any etiology, the nucleus usually, but not invariably, contains monoparticulate glycogen. The mechanism by which glycogenosis of the nucleus occurs is unknown. Other features of this disorder include membrane-bound and microvesicular steatosis, an increase in the number of lipofuscin granules in the pericanalicular region, numerous lipolysosomes, glycogen bodies, and atypical bile canaliculi lined by elongated, metaplastic brush border–like microvilli[148] As the activity of the liver inflammation wanes with the progression of fibrosis, the copper levels in liver tissue begin to fall. The distribution of copper in the hepatocytes of Wilson's disease also changes over time as measured by radionucleotide-labeled copper. There is a decrease in the diffuse cytoplasmic distribution of the metal in favor of an increased sequestration in lysosomal vacuoles.[195] A finding of particular interest in Wilson's disease is the presence of Mallory bodies in zone 1 hepatocytes structurally identical in every respect to those seen in alcoholic liver disease.[148,193]

The Porphyrias

The degree of liver damage due to porphyria alone has most frequently been noted in erythropoietic protoporphyria (defective ferrochelatase) in which acute inflammation and fatal cirrhosis have been reported.[19] The inflammation and fibrosis are believed to be changes in reaction to the toxicity of the pigment accumulated in hepatocytes and Kupffer cells.[19,72,217] There may also be an obstructive component caused by its inspissation in bile ducts and canaliculi. The pigment itself on electron

microscopy may show a range of presentations. In its most dramatic form, it is seen as a "star burst" of fine needle-like electron-dense crystals[19,72,217] 0.4 μm to 0.5 μm in length and 7 nm to 13 nm in width. Such crystals have been confirmed to be protoporphyrin by specific fluorescence and birefringent characteristics.[72,217] The crystals occur free or membrane bound in the cytoplasm of hepatocytes or free in the canalicular space. The largest aggregates tend to occur where concentrations of the pigment is great and liver damage is severe. In milder form, the crystalline aggregates may not be well seen in hepatocytes by conventional light microscopy, but electron microscopy or polarization will reveal crystals in hepatocytes and Kupffer cells. In Kupffer cells (Fig. 2-22) they may form large aggregates that are always contained in lysosomes.[217] Hepatocytes may also show another inclusion, the "paracrystalline body." These crystals are found free in the cytoplasm of hepatocytes and have been seen as well in extracellular sites and within mitochondria. The deposits have been observed in mice following griseofulvin administration.[72] They have also been observed in patients with porphyria cutanea tarda (defective uroporphyrinogen decarboxylase).[210] The characteristics of accumulation in hepatic tissue are similar by electron microscopy to the diffuse deposits seen in eyrthropoietic protoporphyria. When followed sequentially, the crystalline aggregations are at first membrane bound in hepatocytes. As the crystals grow, however, the membrane ruptures, and organelle changes are seen that include vesiculation of the endoplasmic reticulum and autophagocytosis, swelling of mitochondria, and finally cell necrosis.[72] The electron microscopic observations in this experimental model support

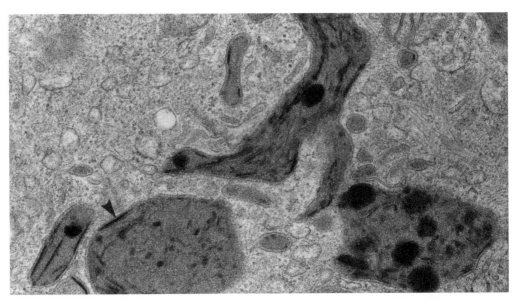

Fig. 2-22. Hepatic protoporphyria. Protoporphyria pigment is seen within enlarged, pleomorphic lysosomes in a Kupffer cell. A granular appearing matrix contains variable electrondense masses and some needle-shaped crystals (*arrowhead*). (Original magnification × 45,000; transmission electron micrograph).

biochemical data suggesting that the occurrence of protoporphyrin pigment in the liver is primary.[174]

The only other porphyria in which porphyrin pigment has been described is porphyria cutanea tarda.[210] It is seen to be a needle-like inclusion in hepatocytes of approximately 4 μm to 5 μm in length. It is frequently surrounded by lysosomal-like contents but without a clear delimiting membrane. The mitochondria may be enlarged with giant transformation and decreased matrical density containing myelin figures or paracrystalline inclusions.[17,205,210] In a few cells, the SER and RER may be dilated. Other changes of increased autophagic vacuoles, lipofuscin granules, and associated ferritin and hemosiderin have also been described. In fact, iron deposition has been frequently noted in association with this condition. Improvement of symptoms and of pathologic changes has occurred with phlebotomy. The mechanisms of these interrelationships are not clear.[16,17,77,205,210]

Disorders of Bile Pigment

In the Dubin–Johnson syndrome the characteristic cytoplasmic pigment in hepatocytes is found to be contained in enlarged pericanalicular lysosomes, whereas other organelles appear normal (Fig. 2-23). The pigment in Dubin–Johnson syndrome is a melanin-like substance as demonstrated by histochemical and physiochemical studies.[3,48,120,148] In Rotor's syndrome, the liver is normal by light microscopy, but there are fine structural changes including enlarged mitochondria with paracrystalline rearrangement of their cristae, immature-looking bile

canaliculi that have decreased microvilli, prominent Golgi apparatus, lysosomes containing a deeply osmiophilic pigment, and frequent glycogen nuclei. In addition, anomalous intercellular microvilli and fibers in the space of Disse have been reported.[120,148] In Gilbert's syndrome, the commonly described finding is hypertrophy of the SER, but in other cases altered sinusoidal plasma membranes or increased pericanalicular pigment granules have been observed.[7,117,120,148]

Iron Overload

The defect in iron-overload syndromes may be an inborn error of metabolism as in primary hemochromatosis, or it may be toxic. Both types may result in liver injury and lead to cirrhosis.[67]

The effects of excessive iron on the liver seem to depend in part on the route of its administration. Some degree of iron storage in the liver is common; according to one study it occurs in 28% of normal livers. Dietary intake favors direct entry of ferritin into the hepatocytes and Kupffer cells.[101] In normal metabolism with oral iron intake, the iron is stored in the hepatocyte as fine 10-nm granules with a dense 6-nm central core bounded by apoferritin. These particles are organized in clusters free in the hyaloplasm of the hepatocyte. The other storage form is hemosiderin. The hemosiderin granules comprise iron-containing particles stored in lysosomes or siderosomes. Lysosomal storage is favored when iron is administered by the intravenous route.[101,157] In lysosomes, iron particles measuring 5 nm to 13 nm in diameter may occur in a

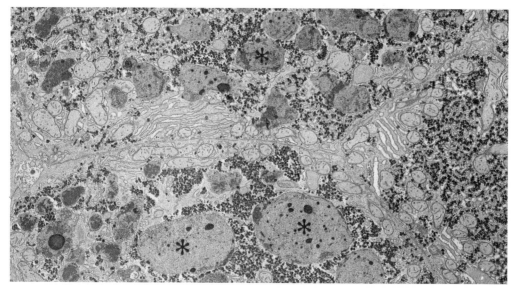

Fig. 2-23. Dubin–Johnson syndrome. Lysosomal pigment granules are numerous and of variable size (∗). They have a finely granular, moderately electron dense matrix that alternates with denser areas and osmiophilic droplets. (Original magnification × 9000; transmission electron micrograph by J. Patterson)

diffuse form or in paracrystalline or lamellar arrays.[87] Ferritin is a water-soluble form of iron in the cell. It is increased in all conditions of enhanced hepatic iron deposition.[158] It is probably the form of iron storage that is most readily mobilized on demand for iron in hemoglobin synthesis.[70,157] The amount of iron stored as ferritin at any one time seems to be predetermined, evidenced by the observation that the number of ferritin granules will increase under stress of iron loading only to a finite amount, beyond which the iron may be directly deposited in the more stable form, hemosiderin.[89] When iron loading overwhelms the lysosomal storage compartment of the cell, it is then seen to be deposited in the hyaloplasm and in mitochondria.[101,198,201] Deposits of iron in these sites may be toxic to the cell; as the hepatocytes become overloaded, a greater share of iron is given to reticuloendothelial cells and bile duct epithelium.

The tendency for the early iron accumulation to be in hepatocytes is an important diagnostic observation in idiopathic hemochromatosis. As is true in light microscopy, however, there are no specific electron microscopic features that allow one to differentiate iron overload of the secondary type from familial idiopathic hemochromatosis. The most important clinical feature continues to be the discovery of other family members with iron excess.[67] The susceptibility locus for primary hemochromatosis has been located in the short arm of chromosome 6, close to the HLA-A locus, whereas the ferritin gene has been assigned to chromosome 19. Furthermore, hemochromatosis may present with variable biochemical and clinical manifestations, which may explain the genetic heterogeneity observed.[126,157] It is not clearly understood in what way the accumulated iron causes liver cell damage or cirrhosis, however, circumstantial evidence does suggest an association.[70] It has also been suggested that iron may affect membrane lipid peroxidation as a mode of injury.[201] Although a precise correlation has not been established, it is possible that the resultant injury to the cell with necrosis and inflammation is sufficient to induce collagen deposition, as has been observed in rats fed a diet high in iron.[198]

Reye's Syndrome

By electron microscopy, diffuse microvesicular steatosis, together with the typical mitochondrial abnormalities, is virtually diagnostic of Reye's syndrome. On light microscopy, aside from small droplet fat, the histologic appearance of the liver is normal.[21,88,135] Mitochondria are characteristically swollen, pale, and frequently "ameboid" (Fig. 2-24). Less pleomorphic mitochondria are crescent shaped and are closely apposed to the lipid inclusions. Disoriented cristae, which often appear to be floating in the matrix, absence of dense granules, narrowing of the intercristae space, as well as collapse of the mitochondria-enveloping membranes, are constant findings in the ameboid mitochondria of Reye's syndrome. Glycogen content of hepatocytes varies from cell to cell and tends to diminish as the disease progresses. Peroxisomes may be increased. All of the changes described are transient and reversible in the early course of the disease and rapidly return to normal in successfully treated patients.

The clinical and histologic findings in Reye's syndrome are often compared in the literature with those of fatty liver of pregnancy. However, they can usually be differ-

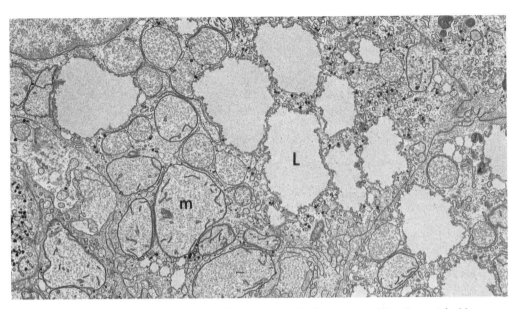

Fig. 2-24. Reye's syndrome. Large "ameboid" mitochondria (*m*) are seen. Note the matrical lucency, absence of dense granules, and altered cristae of the mitochondria. These changes, along with the presence of lipid droplets (*L*) and marked diminution in the amount of glycogen particles, constitute the classic ultrastructural findings in hepatocytes in this condition. (Original magnification × 9000; transmission electron micrograph by J. Patterson)

entiated ultrastructurally. In fatty liver of pregnancy, mitochondria can be swollen and pleomorphic but not ameboid in shape. They frequently bear paracrystalline inclusions, which are not seen in Reye's syndrome, and cholestasis, which may accompany fatty liver of pregnancy, is not a feature of Reye's syndrome.[148]

Glycogen Storage Diseases

Most of the glycogenoses involve the liver except for types V and VII. In many instances, the organelles of the liver are crowded by an increased number of multiparticulate (rosette form) glycogen particles[86] (Fig. 2-25). There is

Fig. 2-25. Glycogen storage disease. Low-power view of hepatocytes; their abundant cytoplasm is occupied mostly by glycogen particles. In some hepatocytes the organelles are displaced to the cell margins. Lipid droplets (*L*) are also present. N = nucleus. (Original magnification × 2300; transmission electron micrograph by J. Patterson)

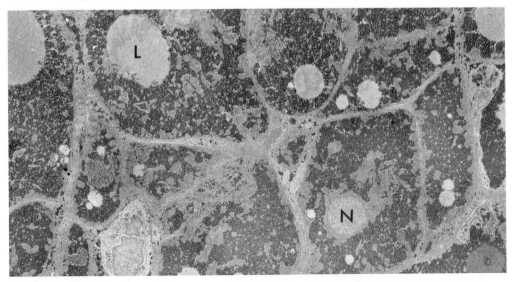

also an increased tendency for lipid droplets to accumulate.[197] Type I, glucose 6-phosphatase deficiency, has a particular tendency for the appearance of glycogen in nuclei.[177] Type II, acid alpha-1,4-glucosidase deficiency, is characterized by the accumulation of monoparticulate and multiparticulate glycogen within lysosomes.[9] The surrounding cytoplasm has normal or slightly increased glycogen particles, and the remaining organelles show no conspicuous abnormalities. Partial or total absence of pericanalicular primary lysosomes has been noted. The accumulation of glycogen in lysosomes is also seen in Kupffer cells. In Kupffer cells, however, the particles are described as smaller with occasional dense aggregates of particles considered to be phagocytosed glycogen.[9] Lysosomes morphologically similar to those in type II glycogenosis have also been described in type IX, phosphorylase kinase deficiency, but to a significantly less degree.[86] Type IV glycogenosis, alpha-1,4-glucan alpha-1-4 glucan 6-alpha glycosyltransferase deficiency, is always associated with cirrhosis. The abnormal glycogen appears on electron microscopy as a fibrillar material seen as small or large aggregates in the cytoplasm of hepatocytes. The fibrillar glycogen is usually randomly oriented, admixed with tubular structures, and surrounded by enlarged glycogen rosettes. Hepatocytes may disclose one mass of fibrillar glycogen that occupies most of the cytoplasm or several small aggregates. Mitochondria frequently display enlarged matrical-dense granules.[148] Glycogen storage disease type IX, or phosphorylase kinase deficiency, is characterized ultrastructurally by large pools of densely packed monoparticulate and multiparticulate glycogen that alternate with scattered areas of finely granular or-

ganelle-free cytosol, which accounts for the distinctive "starry sky" appearance.[148] This pattern of glycogen accumulation may be seen occasionally in other glycogenoses; however, in glycogen storage disease type IX it is striking and present in every cell. The other glycogenoses show no specific hepatic ultrastructural abnormalities to date.[86,148]

Lipidoses

Examination of the ultrastructure in conjunction with biochemical analysis of liver tissue has been diagnostically helpful for several of the storage diseases and, in particular, the lipidoses. The unique morphology associated with several of the lipidoses has been reviewed.[65,86,96,209] Neimann–Pick disease is due to a deficiency of a sphingomyelinase resulting in an accumulation of sphingomyelin. On light microscopy, foamy Kupffer cells accumulate in the sinusoidal spaces and are seen ultrastructurally to contain finely laminated, osmiophilic membranous material that alternates with electron-lucent areas[31,148,209] (Fig. 2-26). Hepatocytes may also contain these lipid membranous inclusions, which are found near the biliary pole. Endothelial cells, lipocytes, fibroblasts, and macrophages may also show similar cytoplasmic changes.[65,148] Gaucher's disease is due to a deficiency of glucocerebroside-cleaving enzyme and results in an accumulation of glycosyl ceramide in Kupffer cells in the liver and in other reticuloendothelial cells. These cells have a characteristic appearance caused by large lysosomes filled with parallel tubular structures (Fig. 2-27) that are responsible for the

Fig. 2-26. Niemann–Pick disease. Sphingomyelin is stored within lysosomes as laminated inclusions of variable size, shape, and electron density. Note their typical pericanalicular location. bc = bile canaliculus. (Original magnification × 14,000; transmission electron micrograph by J. Patterson)

Fig. 2-27. Gaucher's disease. Close-up of the enlarged pleomorphic lysosomes found in Gaucher's cells. The stored cerebroside appears typically as long, tightly packed, tubular structures (*arrowhead*). (Original magnification × 25,500; transmission electron micrograph by J. Patterson)

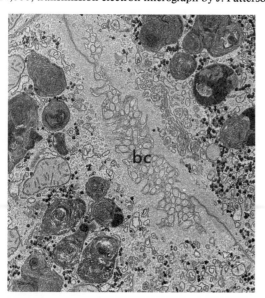

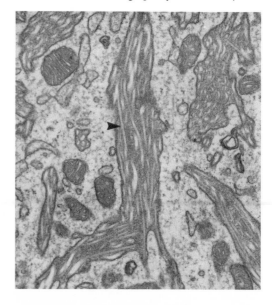

peculiar striations seen in the cytoplasm of Gaucher cells by light microscopy.[43,148,209] The hepatocytes are not directly involved by accumulating glucocerebroside. In chronic myelocytic leukemia, Gaucher cells are due to an acquired deficiency.[100] Hurler's syndrome (defective α_1-iduronidase) is one of many conditions resulting from abnormal accumulations of acid mucopolysaccharides.[28,76] Hepatocytes and Kupffer's cells show numerous vacuoles, which are pale and contain sparse finely granular or reticular material.[28,148,209] Tay–Sachs disease is the result of hexosaminidase deficiency resulting in GM2 ganglioside accumulation. In the liver, this is manifested by the presence of prominent lysosomes in pericanalicular areas containing tightly laminated concentric membranes. These peculiar osmiophilic lysosomal inclusions have been termed zebra-like bodies and are highly characteristic of the disease.[65,148,209,218] Wolman's disease is a deficiency of acid lipase that results in cholesterol accumulation and electron-lucent angular crystals in lysosomes of Kupffer cells. The hepatocytes are filled with lipid, and necrosis results from cell injury.[26] In a more benign form of cholesterol ester–storage disease, electron microscopy demonstrates the cholesterol crystals to be in hepatocyte lysosomes as well.[148,197]

Liver Tumors and Tumor-like Conditions

Two benign proliferative lesions of current interest are focal nodular hyperplasia and liver cell adenoma. Focal nodular hyperplasia is a localized, conspicuously nodular lesion composed of hepatocytes, ductules, Kupffer cells, and blood vessels. Electron microscopy has shown important differences between this tumor-like lesion and liver cell adenoma. Ultrastructurally, the parenchymal liver cells in focal nodular hyperplasia are almost indistinguishable from the hepatocytes seen in the nodules of inactive cirrhosis, including the presence of anomalous microvilli between neighboring cells.[142,143,148] An excess of cytoplasmic glycogen is a common finding. In the central scars, which are characteristic of the light microscopic appearance of focal nodular hyperplasia, there are numerous structurally abnormal blood vessels and myofibroblasts rather than fibroblasts. In sharp contrast are the ultrastructural findings in liver cell adenoma. In this condition, the liver cells ultrastructurally are clearly neoplastic. Even in the most differentiated liver cell adenoma there is an overall reduction in cellular organelles, especially of the RER. Gross dilation of the RER is often seen, frequently with regions devoid of membranes. Free ribosomes are increased, as are cytoplasmic filaments. A striking finding is the marked variation of fine structure from one cell to the next within the same tumor. Glycogen and lipid, especially triglyceride, are variable and often increased. Bile canaliculi are reduced in number and may be malformed. Tight junctions are often small, reduced in number, and frequently appear rudimentary. Hence, by electron microscopy, it is easy to distinguish the hepatocytes of focal nodular hyperplasia from those of liver cell adenoma. The latter condition is obviously neoplastic; the former is not.

Well-differentiated hepatocellular carcinoma closely resembles liver cell adenoma, and it is doubtful whether well-differentiated hepatocellular carcinoma cells can be distinguished ultrastructurally from those seen in the adenoma. However, in progressively less well-differentiated tumors there is parallel reduction in the number and size of mitochondria, reduction in the RER and SER, reduction of cell junctions, reduction or absence of bile canaliculi, and nuclear pleomorphism frequently associated with pseudoinclusions due to cytoplasmic invaginations (Fig. 2-28). In contrast there is an inverse increase in free ribosomes and also in cytoplasmic filaments, particularly 10-nm intermediate filaments, which may form Mallory bodies that are identical to those seen in alcoholic liver disease. Other common intracytoplasmic inclusions frequently found in well- and moderately differentiated tumors are the PAS-positive diastase-resistant α_1-antitrypsin globules seen by light microscopy. The α_1-antitrypsin material is contained within cisternae of the endoplasmic reticulum, and its ultrastructural characteristics are identical to those described in the metabolic section. Inclusions of α-fetoprotein may also be encountered.[134,148] Structures not ordinarily seen in hepatocytes such as cilia and annulate lamellae are occasionally found. In the extreme, anaplastic liver cell carcinoma may be composed of cells having none of the ultracytologic features of hepatocytes. In a sequential, experimental study of chemically induced hepatic carcinogenesis,[132] a similar progression of ultrastructural changes, from putative preneoplastic cells to frankly malignant cells has been seen. Although there is a growing association between primary liver cell carcinoma and the hepatitis B virus, no virus particles have been reported as yet in tumor cells. However, orcein or Shikata-positive (HBsAg) cells have been found in up to 25% of patients in the surrounding "normal" or cirrhotic liver tissue.[133,134] It is possible that the increased SER present in these cells may reflect a capacity for enhanced microsomal biotransformation. This capability may render these hepatocytes more susceptible to normal metabolites, drugs, or toxins, perhaps by excessive formation or reduced degradation of a biologically active metabolite. In other words, the effect of the HBsAg may be to select these hepatocytes as the precursor cells for malignant transformation. This concept of cellular selection is completely in keeping with the current theory of chemical carcinogenesis proposed by Farber.[49]

Angiosarcoma of the liver is rare but is of interest because of its association with vinyl chloride, a monomer used extensively in the plastics industry. It has been suggested that angiosarcomas may be derived from lipocytes (perisinusoidal cells or Ito cells).[167] It is beyond the scope of this chapter to discuss the role of electron microscopy in the differential diagnosis of metastatic tumors of the liver. Suffice it to say that tumor cells in needle biopsies of the liver are usually well preserved and are eminently suitable for electron microscopic study.

Fibrolamellar carcinoma is a recently described primary liver tumor that warrants a special comment on its ultrastructural aspects (Figs. 2-29 and 2-30). The tumor cells

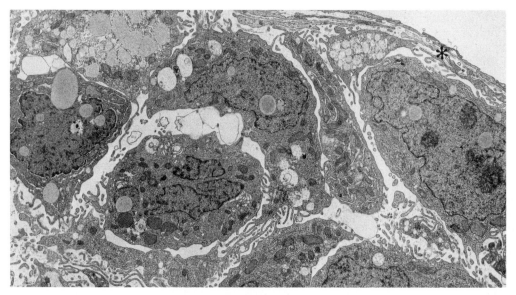

Fig. 2-28. Hepatocellular carcinoma, moderately differentiated. The nuclei of the neoplastic hepatocytes are highly convoluted and have prominent nucleoli and occasional lipid inclusions. Note the large nuclear/cytoplasmic ratio and abundance of microvilli. The tumor cells tend to form a liver cell cord with a space of Disse and with layered endothelium (*). (Original magnification × 6700; transmission electron micrograph by J. Patterson)

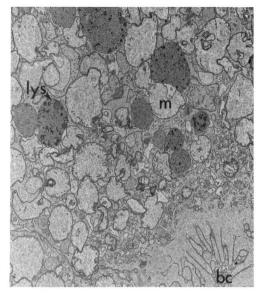

Fig. 2-29. Fibrolamellar carcinoma. Swollen mitochondria (*m*) devoid of dense granules, conspicuous lysosomes (*lys*) containing round, dense inclusions, and a bile canaliculus (*bc*) with long, pleomorphic microvilli are classic findings. (Original magnification × 9000; transmission electron micrograph by J. Patterson)

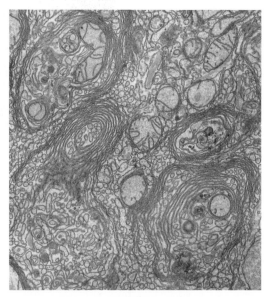

Fig. 2-30. Fibrolamellar carcinoma. Complex membranous arrays derived from the endoplasmic reticulum are another frequent finding. (Original magnification × 7500; transmission electron micrograph by J. Patterson)

are arranged in groups or cords and are embedded within bands of fibrous tissue. The finding of myofibroblasts and fibroblasts immersed in collagen fibers accounts for the spindle-shaped cell component of this tumor. The neo-

plastic cells in fibrolamellar carcinoma have a giant cytoplasm with a single nucleus whose nucleolus has a striking target-like appearance. The tumor cells are filled with mitochondria to the extent that other organelles are frequently inconspicuous. The mitochondria are large, swollen, and rounded with a pale matrix that may have focal condensations. Dense granules are usually absent. The membrane bilayers of the mitochondrial envelope and the cristae are collapsed on one another, making it difficult to visualize the intracristal space. The cristae are disoriented, and occasional whorls of membranes may be found. The mitochondrial membrane changes in fibrolamellar carcinoma resemble those seen in Reye's syndrome and have not been seen in other liver conditions.[148] Large membrane-bound cytoplasmic inclusions are a prominent feature both by light microscopy and electron microscopy. Ultrastructurally, they are formed by a single membrane and are often occupied by bundles of fibrin with its characteristic periodicity. Glycogen is very sparse or absent, giving the cell a very pale, monotonous appearance. The lysosomes are osmiophilic and therefore contrast with the remaining organelles. The lysosomal contents vary in electron density, giving it a spotted appearance. Characteristically, the endoplasmic reticulum forms geometric, complex membranous whorls; frequently the membranes are devoid of ribosomes. Individual cells may form pleomorphic hemicanaliculi. Internalized bile canaliculi, surrounded by a cuff of filaments may show numerous long and slender microvilli, which frequently fill the lumen.[148]

Fibrolamellar carcinoma is an excellent example to illustrate the key role electron microscopy plays in diagnostic pathology. Although the light microscopic features of this tumor are characteristic, its ultrastructural aspects are unique such that it cannot be mistaken for any other primary liver cell tumor.[148]

REFERENCES

1. Almeida JD, Waterston AP: Immune complexes in hepatitis. Lancet 2:933, 1969
2. Alter HJ, Dienstag, JL: The evolving spectrum of non-A, non-B hepatitis. In Chisari FV (ed): Advances in Hepatitis Research, p 281. New York, Masson Publishing, 1984
3. Baba N, Ruppert RD: The Dubin-Johnson syndrome: Electron microscopy observation of hepatic pigment: A case study. Am J Clin Pathol 57:306, 1972
4. Babudieri B et al: Presence of virus-like bodies in liver cells of patients with infectious hepatitis. J Clin Pathol 19:577, 1966
5. Bamber M et al: Ultrastructural features in chronic non-A, non-B hepatitis: A controlled blind study. J Med Virol 8:267, 1981
6. Bartel H et al: Ultrastructure of hepatocytes in the regenerating liver. Acta Med Pathol 18:279, 1977
7. Barth RF et al: Excess lipofuscin accumulation in constitutional hepatic dysfunction (Gilbert's syndrome): Light and electron microscopic observations. Arch Pathol 91:41, 1971
8. Bateson MC et al: Effect of gallstones dissolution therapy on human liver structure. Dig Dis 22:293, 1977
9. Baudhuin P et al: An electron microscopic and biochemical study of type II glycogenosis. Lab Invest 13:1139, 1964
10. Bayer ME et al: Particles associated with Australia antigen in the sera of patients with leukemia, Down's syndrome, and hepatitis. Nature 218:1057, 1968
11. Bernuau D et al: Ultrastructural lesions of bile ducts in primary biliary cirrhosis: A comparison with the lesions observed in graft versus host disease. Hum Pathol 12:782, 1981
12. Berry MN, Friend DS: High yield preparations of isolated rat liver parenchymal cells. J Cell Biol 43:506, 1969
13. Bianchi L: Morphologic features in biopsy diagnosis of acute viral hepatitis. In Popper H, Schaffner F (eds): Progress in Liver Disease, vol 3, p 236. New York, Grune & Stratton, 1970
14. Biava C: Mallory alcoholic hyalin: A heretofore unique lesion of hepatocellular ergastoplasm. Lab Invest 13:301, 1964
15. Biava C, Mukhlova–Montiel M: Electron microscopic observations on Councilman-like acidophilic bodies and other forms of acidophilic changes in human liver cells. Am J Pathol 46:775, 1965
16. Biempica L et al: Hepatic porphyria, cytochemistry and ultrastructure of liver in acute intermittent porphyria and porphyria cutanea tarda. Arch Pathol 98:336, 1974
17. Blekkenharst, GH et al: Hepatic haem metabolism in porphyria cutanea tarda (PCT): Enzymatic studies and their relation to liver ultrastructure. Ann Clin Res, 8:108, 1976
18. Blitzer BL, Boyer JL: Cytochemical localization of Na^+,K^+-ATPase in the rat hepatocyte. J Clin Invest 62:1104, 1978
19. Bloomer J et al: Hepatic disease in erythropoietic protoporphyria. Am J Med 58:869, 1975
20. Bonvicini F et al: Cholesterol in acute cholestasis induced by taurolithocholic acid: A cytochemical study in transmission and scanning electron microscopy. Lab Invest 38:487, 1978
21. Bove K et al: The hepatic lesion in Reye's syndrome. Gastroenterology 69:685, 1975
22. Bradley DW: Transmission, etiology and pathogenesis of viral hepatitis non-A, non-B in non-human primates. In Chisari, FV (ed): Advances in hepatitis research, chap 31, p 268. New York, Masson Publishing 1984
23. Bronjenmajor S et al: Fat storing cells (lipocytes) in human liver. Arch Pathol 82:447, 1966
24. Bruguera M et al: Giant mitochondria in hepatocytes: A diagnostic hint for alcoholic liver disease. Gastroenterology 73:1383, 1977
25. Burka T et al: Structure changes of liver cells in copper intoxication. Arch Pathol 78:331, 1964
26. Burke JA, Schubert WK: Deficient activity of hepatic acid lipase in cholesterol ester storage disease. Science 176:309, 1972
27. Busachi CA et al: Ultrastructural changes in the liver of patients with chronic non-A, non-B hepatitis. J Med Virol 7:205, 1981
28. Callahan W, Lowricz A: Hepatic ultrastructure in the Hurler syndrome. Am J Pathol 48:277, 1966
29. Carruthers JS et al: The ductular cell reaction of rat liver in extrahepatic cholestasis: II. The proliferation of connective tissue. Exp Mol Pathol 1:377, 1962
30. Cavalli G et al: Ultrastructural studies of bile ductules in the course of acute hepatitis. Acta Hepatospleno 18:355, 1971
31. Chan EC et al: Adult Niemann-Pick disease: A case report. J Pathol 121:177, 1977
32. Chedid A et al: Ultrastructural aspects of primary biliary cirrhosis and other types of cholestatic liver disease. Gastroenterology 67:858, 1974

33. Compagno J, Grisham JW: Scanning electron microscopy of extrahepatic biliary obstruction. Arch Pathol 97:348, 1974

34. Cook EH et al: Ultrastructural studies of hepatitis A virus by electron microscopy. J Virol 20:687, 1976

35. Dane DS et al: Virus-like particles in serum of patients with Australia antigen associated hepatitis. Lancet 1:695, 1970

36. De Brabander N et al: Effects of antimicrotubular compounds on monolayer cultures of adult rat hepatocytes. J Biol Cell 31:127, 1978

37. Denk H, Eckerstorfer R: Colchicine-induced Mallory body formation in the mouse. Lab Invest 36:563, 1977

38. Denk H et al: Experimental Mallory bodies ("alcoholic hyalin"): New findings on evolution, structure and pathology significance. In Preisig R, Paumgartner G, Bircher J (eds): The Liver: Quantitative Aspects of Structure and Function, p 43. Basel, Karger, 1979

39. Denk HG et al: Hepatocellular hyalin (Mallory bodies) in long term griseofulvin-treated mice: A new experimental model for the study of hyalin formation. Lab Invest 32:773, 1975

40. Desmet VJ: Morphologic and histochemical aspects of cholestasis. In Popper H, Schaffner F (eds): Progress in Liver Disease, vol 4, p 97. New York, Grune & Stratton, 1972

41. Desmet VJ: Anatomy: I. Hepatocyte-canaliculus. In Bianchi L et al (eds): Liver and Bile, p 3. Lancaster, MTP Press, 1977

42. De Vos R, Desmet VJ: Morphologic changes of the junctional complex of the hepatocytes in rat liver after bile duct ligation. Br J Exp Pathol 59:220, 1978

43. Djaldert M et al: The surface ultrastructure of Gaucher cells. Am J Clin Pathol 71:146, 1979

44. Dragier M et al: Quantitative electron microscopic studies of the changes in rat hepatocytes following halothane induced anesthesia. Folia Med 19:32, 1977

45. Drochmans P et al: Isolation and subfractionation of Ficoll gradient of adult rat hepatocytes: Size, morphology and biochemical characteristics of cell fractions. J Cell Biol 66:1, 1975

46. Edgington TS: Immunologic aspects of viral hepatitis, pp 12–21. Postgraduate Symposium on Viral Hepatitis, AASLD, Chicago, Nov. 3–4, 1976

47. Eriksson S, Larsson C: Purification and partial characterization of PAS-positive inclusion bodies from the liver in alpha-1-antitrypsin deficiency. N Engl J Med 292:176, 1975

48. Essner E, Novikoff A: Human hepatocellular pigments and lysosomes. J Ultrastruct Res 3:374, 1960

49. Farber E et al: Newer insights into the pathogenesis of liver cancer. Am J Pathol 89:477, 1977

50. Feinstone SM, Hoofnagle JH: Non-A, maybe-B hepatitis. N Engl J Med 311:185, 1984

51. Feinstone SM et al: Non-A, non-B hepatitis in chimpanzees and marmosets. J Infect Dis 144:588, 1981

52. Fisher MM et al: Bile acid metabolism in mammals: IV. Sex differences in chenodeoxycholic acid metabolism in the rat. Lab Invest 27:254, 1972

53. Fisher R et al: Alpha-1-antitrypsin deficiency in liver disease: The extent of the problem. Gastroenterology 71:646, 1976

54. Franke WW et al: Ultrastructural biochemical and immunologic characterization of Mallory bodies in livers of griseofulvin-treated mice: Fimbriated rods of filaments containing prekeratin-like polypeptides. Lab Invest 40:207, 1979

55. Franke WW et al: Characterization of the intermediate-sized filaments in liver cells by immunofluorescence and electron microscopy. Biol Cellulaire 34:99, 1979

56. French SW: The Mallory body: Structure, composition and pathogenesis. Hepatology 1:76, 1981

57. French SW, Davies PL: Ultrastructural localization of actin like filaments in rat hepatocytes. Gastroenterology 68:765, 1975

58. Friend DS, Gilula NB: Variations in tight and gap junctions in mammalian tissue. J Cell Biol 53:758, 1972

59. Fromm H et al: Studies of liver function and structure in patients with gallstones before and during treatment with chenodeoxycholic acid. Acta Hepatogastroenterol 22:359, 1975

60. Gabbiani G et al: Phalloidin-induced hyperplasia of actin filaments. Lab Invest 33:562, 1975

61. Gay S et al: Liver cirrhosis: Immunofluorescence and biochemical studies demonstrate two types of collagen. Klin Wochenschr 53:205, 1975

62. Gerber MA, Paronetto F: Hepatitis B antigen in human tissues. In Schaffner F et al (ed): The Liver and its Diseases. p 54. New York, Intercontinent Medical Books, 1974

63. Gerber MA et al: Immuno-electron microscopy of hepatitis B antigen in liver. Proc Soc Exp Biol Med 140:1334, 1972

64. Gerber MS et al: Incidence and nature of cytoplasmic hepatitis B antigen in hepatocytes. Lab Invest 32:251, 1975

65. Glew RH et al: Lysosomal storage diseases. Lab Invest 53:250, 1985

66. Goldfischer S, Sternlieb I: Changes in the distribution of hepatic copper in relation to the progression of Wilson's disease. Am J Pathol 53:883, 1968

67. Gollan J et al: Diagnosis of hemochromatosis. Gastroenterology 84:418, 1983

68. Goodenough DA, Revel JP: A fine structural analysis of intercellular junctions in mouse liver. J Cell Biol 45:272, 1970

69. Gordon HW et al: Alpha-1-antitrypsin (A_1AT) accumulation in livers of emphysematous patients with A_1AT deficiency. Hum Pathol 3:361, 1972

70. Grace ND, Powell LW: Iron storage disorders of the liver. Gastroenterology 64:1257, 1974

71. Grisham JW, Hartroft WS: Morphologic identification by electron microscopy of "oval" cells in experimental hepatic degeneration. Lab Invest 10;317, 1961

72. Gschnatt, F et al: Mouse model for protoporphyria: I. Liver and hepatic protoporphyrin crystals. J Invest Dermatol 65:290, 1975

73. Hadchouel M, Gautier M: Histopathologic study of the liver in the early cholestatic phase of alpha-1-antitrypsin deficiency. J Pediatr 89:211, 1976

74. Hadziyannis SJ: The ground-glass hepatocyte: An aid to diagnosis, a challenge to pathophysiology. In Berk PD, Chalmers TC (eds): Frontiers in Liver Disease, p 106. New York, Thieme–Straton, 1981

75. Hanefeld M et al: Der effeckt der regardin (CPIB)-therapy von hyerlipoproteinaneum (HIP) auf die Leber. Dtsch Gesundh-Wesen 32:2267, 1977

76. Haust MD et al: The fine structure of liver in children with Hurler's syndrome. Exp Mol Pathol 10:141, 1969

77. Heilmann E et al: Special clinical, light and electron microscopic aspects of acute intermittent porphyria. Ann Clin Res 8:213, 1976

78. Hirschman SZ et al: Purification of naked intranuclear

particles from human liver infected by hepatitis B virus. Proc Natl Acad Sci 71:3345, 1974

79. Hollander M, Schaffner F: Electron microscopic studies in biliary atresia: I. Bile ductular proliferation. Am J Dis Child 116:49, 1968

80. Hoofnagle JH et al: Antibody to hepatitis B virus core in man. Lancet 2:869, 1973

81. Hopwood D, Nylars A: Effect of methotrexate therapy in psoriasis on the Ito cells in liver biopsies, assessed by point-counting. J Clin Pathol 29:698, 1976

82. Hruban Z et al: Ultrastructural changes in livers of two patients with hypervitaminosis A. Am J Pathol 76:451, 1974

83. Huang SN: Hepatitis-associated antigen hepatitis: An electron microscopic study of virus-like particles in liver cells. Am J Pathol 64:483, 1971

84. Huang SN et al: Virus-like particles in Australia antigen-associated hepatitis. Am J Pathol 67:453, 1972

85. Huang SN et al: A study of the relationship of virus-like particles and Australia antigen in liver. Hum Pathol 5:209, 1974

86. Hug G: Non-bilirubin genetic disorders. In Gall EA, Mostofi FK (eds): The Liver, p 21. Baltimore, Williams & Wilkins, 1973

87. Iancu TC, Neustein HB: Ferritin in human liver cells of homozygous beta-thalassaemia: Ultrastructural observations. Br J Haematol 37:527, 1977

88. Iancu TC et al: Ultrastructural abnormalities of liver cells in Reye's syndrome. Hum Pathol 8:421, 1977

89. Iancu TC et al: Pathogenetic mechanisms in hepatic cirrhosis of thalassemia major: Light and electron microscopy. Pathol Annu 1:171, 1977

90. Ito T: Recent advances in the study of the fine structure of the hepatic sinusoidal wall: A review. Gumma Rep Med Sci 6:119, 1973

91. Jeejeebhoy KN, Phillips JJ: Isolated mammalian hepatocytes in culture. Gastroenterology 71:1087, 1976

92. Jeejeebhoy KN, Phillips MJ: Unpublished observations.

93. Jeejeebhoy KN et al: Effects of hormones on the synthesis of (acute phase) glycoprotein in isolated rat hepatocytes. Biochem J 168:347, 1977

94. Jezequel AM et al: A morphometric study of the endoplasmic reticulum in human hepatocytes. Gut 15:737, 1974

95. Jezequel AM et al: Early structural and functional changes in liver of rats treated with a single dose of valproic acid. Hepatology 4:1159, 1984

96. Johannessen JV: Electron microscopy in human medicine. In The Liver, the Gallbladder and Biliary Ducts, vol 8. New York, McGraw-Hill, 1979

97. Jones AL, Fawcett DW: Hypertrophy of the agranular endoplasmic reticulum in hamster liver induced by phenobarbital. J Histochem Cytochem 14:215, 1966

98. Kaneda K et al: Distribution and morphological characteristics of the pit cell in the liver of the rat. Cell Tissue Res 233:485, 1983

99. Kanel GC et al: Globular hepatic amyloid: An unusual morphologic presentation. Hepatology, 1:647, 1981

100. Katlove HE et al: Gaucher cells in chronic myelocytic leukemia: An acquired abnormality. Blood 233:279, 1969

101. Kent G, Schneider KA: Cirrhosis and iron overload. In Schaffner F et al (eds): The Liver and Its Disorders. p 314. New York, International Medical Book Corporation, 1974

102. Kent G et al: Role of lipocytes (perisinusoidal cells) in fibrogenesis. In Wisse E, Knook DL (eds): Kupffer Cells and Other Sinusoidal Cells, p 73. Amsterdam, Elsevier Holland Biomedical Press, 1977

103. Klion FM, Schaffner F: Electron microscopic observations in primary biliary cirrhosis. Arch Pathol 81:151, 1966

104. Klion FM et al: Hepatitis after exposure to halothane. Ann Intern Med 81:467, 1969

105. Koch MM et al: A stereological and biochemical study of the human liver in uncomplicated cholelithiasis. Digestion 18:162, 1978

106. Latham PS, Kashgarian M: The ultrastructural localization of transport ATPase in the rat liver at non-bile canalicular plasma membranes. Gastroenterology 76:988, 1979

107. Layden TJ et al: Bile formation in the rat: The role of the paracellular "shunt" pathway. J Clin Invest 62:1375, 1978

108. Lefkowitch JH et al: Oxyphilic granular hepatocytes: Mitochondrion-rich liver cells in hepatic disease. Am J Clin Pathol 74:432, 1980

109. Lemon SM: Type A viral hepatitis: New developments in an old disease. N Engl J Med 313:1054, 1985

110. Lieber CS: Metabolism of alcohol and associated hepatic effects. In Berk, JE (ed): Bockus Gastroenterology, Vol 5, Liver, p. 2957. Philadelphia, WB Saunders, 1985

111. Locarnini SA et al: The relationship between a 27 nm virus-like particle and hepatitis A as demonstrated by immune electron microscopy. Intervirology 4:110, 1974

112. Lough J, Wiglesworth FW: Wilson's disease: Comparative ultrastructure in a subship of nine. Arch Pathol Lab Med 100:659, 1976

113. Lowenstein WL: Membrane junctions in growth and differentiation. Fed Proc 32:60, 1971

114. Ma MH, Biempica L: The normal human liver cell. Am J Pathol 63:353, 1971

115. Mc Caul TF et al: Application of electron microscopy to the study of structural changes in the liver in non-A, non-B hepatitis. J Virol Methods 4:87, 1982

116. Mc Dowell EM, Trump BF: Histologic fixatives suitable for diagnostic light and electron microscopy. Arch Pathol Lab Med 100:405, 1976

117. Mc Gee JOD et al: Liver ultrastructure in Gilbert's syndrome. Gut 16:220, 1975

118. Medline A et al: Ultrastructural features in galactosamine-induced hepatitis. Exp Mol Pathol 12:201, 1970

119. Michalopoulos G et al: Hormonal regulation and the effects of glucose on tyrosine aminotransferase activity in adult rat hepatocytes cultured on floating collagen membranes. Cancer Res 39:1550, 1978

120. Minio F et al: L'ultrastructure du foie humain lors d'icterus idiopathiques chronic: III. Inclusions pigmentaires dans les syndromes de Gilbert, de Rotor, et de Dubin Johnson. Z Mikrosk Anat Forsch 72:168, 1966

121. Miyai K et al: Bile acid metabolism in mammals: Ultrastructural studies on the intrahepatic cholestasis induced by lithocholic and chenodeoxycholic acids in the rat. Lab Invest 24:292, 1971

122. Miyai K et al: Freeze fracture study of bile canalicular changes induced by lithocholic acid. Lab Invest 30:384, 1974

123. Morse JO: Alpha-1-antitrypsin deficiency: A review. N Engl J Med 299:1045, 1978

124. Moser HW, Goldfischer SL: The peroxisomal disorders. Hospital Prac 20:61, 1985

125. Mota PM: The three-dimensional microanatomy of the liver. Arch Histol Jpn 47:1, 1984

126. Muir WA et al: Evidence for heterogeneity in hereditary hemochromatosis: Evaluation of 174 persons in nine families. Am J Med 76:806, 1984

127. Nenci I: Identification of actin-like proteins in alcoholic hyaline by immunofluorescence. Lab Invest 32:256, 1975

128. Nowoslanski A et al: Cellular localization of Australia antigen in the liver of patients with lympho-proliferative disorders. Lancet 1:494, 1970

129. Nowoslanski A et al: Tissue localization of Australia-antigen immune complexes in acute and chronic hepatitis and liver cirrhosis. Am J Pathol 68:31, 1972

130. Oda M, Phillips MJ: Bile canalicular membrane pathology in cytochalsin B-induced cholestasis. Lab Invest 37:350, 1977

131. Oda M et al: Ultrastructure of bile canaliculi with special reference to the surface coat and the pericanalicular web. Lab Invest 31:314, 1974

132. Ogawa K et al: Sequential analysis of hepatic carcinogenesis: A comparative study of the ultrastructure of preneoplastic, malignant, prenatal, postnatal and regenerating liver. Lab Invest 41:22, 1979

133. Okuda K, Nakashima T: Hepatocellular carcinoma: A review of the recent studies and developments. In Popper H, Schaffner F (eds): Progress in Liver Disease, vol 6, p 639. New York, Grune & Stratton, 1979

134. Ordonez NG, Mackay B: Ultrastructure of liver cell and bile duct carcinomas. Ultrastruct Pathol 5:201, 1983

135. Partin J: Liver ultrastructure in Reye's syndrome. In Pollack J (ed): Reye's syndrome, p 117. New York, Grune & Stratton, 1975

136. Pavel I et al: Ultrastructural aspects of the liver in the viral hepatitis. Digestion 2:221, 1969

137. Pfeifer U, Aterman K: Shedding of peripheral cytoplasm: A mechanism of liver cell atrophy in human amyloidosis. Virchows Arch Cell Pathol 29:229, 1979

138. Pfeifer U et al: Experimental non-A, non-B hepatitis: Four types of cytoplasmic alterations in the hepatocytes of infected chimpanzees. Virchows Arch Cell Pathol 33:233, 1980

139. Phillips MJ, Oda M: The bile canalicular web. Fed Proc 33:626, 1974

140. Phillips MJ Poucell S: Modern aspects of the morphology of viral hepatitis. Hum Pathol 12:1060, 1981

141. Phillips MJ, Poucell S: Cholestasis: Surgical pathology, mechanisms and new concepts. In Farber E, Phillips MJ (eds): Pathogenesis of Liver Diseases. International Academy of Pathology Monograph. Baltimore, Williams & Wilkins, 1986

142. Phillips MJ, Steiner JW: Electron microscopy of liver cell in cirrhotic nodules: I. The lateral cell membrane. Am J Pathol 45:985, 1965

143. Phillips MJ et al: Benign liver cell tumours: Classification and ultrastructural pathology. Cancer 32:463, 1973

144. Phillips MJ et al: Ultrastructural and functional studies of isolated hepatocytes. Lab Invest 31:533, 1974

145. Phillips MJ et al: Microfilament dysfunction as a possible cause of intrahepatic cholestasis. Gastroenterology 68:48, 1975

146. Phillips MJ et al: Evidence of microfilament involvement in norethandrolone induced intrahepatic cholestasis. Am J Pathol 93:729, 1978

147. Phillips MJ et al: Ultrastructural evidence of intrahepatic cholestasis before and after chenodeoxycholic acid therapy in patients with cholelithiasis: The National Cooperative Gallstone study. Hepatology 3:209, 1983

148. Phillips MJ et al: The liver: An atlas of ultrastructural pathology with emphasis on metabolic and drug-induced disorders. New York, Raven Press (in press)

149. Plaa GL et al: Intrahepatic cholestasis induced by drugs and chemicals. Pharmacol Rev 28:207, 1977

150. Ponzetto A et al: Hepatitis B markers in United States addicts with special emphasis on the delta hepatitis virus. Hepatology 6:1111, 1984

151. Popper H, Schaffner F: The organelle pathology of cholestasis. In Gentilini P et al (ed): Intrahepatic Cholestasis, p 35. New York, Raven Press, 1979

152. Popper H et al: Has proliferation of bile ductules clinical significance? Acta Hepatospleno 9:129, 1962

153. Popper H et al: Environmental hepatic injury in man. In Popper H, Schaffner E (eds): Progress in Liver Disease, vol 6, p 605. New York, Grune & Stratton, 1979

154. Poucell S et al: Neocholangiole. Lab Invest 46:65, 1982

155. Poucell S et al: Amiodarone associated phospholipidosis and fibrosis of the liver: Light, immunohistochemical and electron microscopic studies. Gastroenterology 86:926, 1984

156. Poulos A, Sharp P, Whiting M: Infantile Refsum's disease (phytanic acid storage disease): A variant of Zellweger's syndrome? Clin Genet 26:579 1984

157. Powell LW, Halliday JW: Hemochromatosis. In Berk JE (ed): Bockus Gastroenterology, Vol 5, Liver, p 3203. Philadelphia, WB Saunders, 1985

158. Rager R, Finegold MJ: Cholestasis in immature newborn infants: Is parenteral alimentation responsible? J Pediatr 86:264, 1975

159. Reddy JK: Possible properties of microbodies (peroxisomes), microbody proliferation and hypolipidemic drugs. J Histochem Cytochem 21:967, 1973

160. Rizzetto M: The delta agent. Hepatology 5:729, 1983

161. Rizzetto M et al: Biological, clinical and epidemiologic aspects of the delta system. In Chisari FV (ed): Advances in Hepatitis Research, p 258. New York, Masson, 1984

162. Roels F et al: Peroxisomes (microbodies) in human liver: Cytochemical and quantitative studies of 85 biopsies. J Histochem Cytochem 31:235, 1983

163. Rubin E et al: Experimental hepatic fibrosis without hepatocellular regeneration: A kinetic study. Am J Pathol 52:111, 1968

164. Sandritter W, Riede UN: Morphology of liver cell necrosis. In Keppler D (ed): Pathogenesis and mechanism of liver cell necrosis, p 1. Lancaster, MTP Press, 1975

165. Sasaki H et al: Bile ductules in cholestasis: Morphologic evidence of secretion and absorption in man. Lab Invest 16:84, 1967

166. Schaffner F: Intralobular changes in hepatocytes and the electron microscopic mesenchymal response in acute viral hepatitis. Medicine 45:547, 1966

167. Schaffner F: Personal communication.

168. Schaffner F: Primary biliary cirrhosis. In Berk JE (ed): Bockus Gastroenterology, Vol 5, The Liver, p 3150. Philadelphia, WB Saunders, 1985

169. Schaffner F, Popper H: Morphologic studies in cholestasis. Gastroenterology 37:565, 1959

170. Schaffner F, Popper H: Electron microscopic studies of

normal and proliferated bile ductules. Am J Pathol 39:393, 1961

171. Schaffner F, Popper H: Capillarization of hepatic sinusoids in man. Gastroenterology 44:239, 1963

172. Schaffner F et al: Hepatocellular cytoplasmic changes in acute alcoholic hepatitis. JAMA 183:343, 1963

173. Schiff ER, De Medina MD: Delta agent: Another hepatitis virus. Diag Med 8:17, 1985

174. Scholonick P et al: Erythropoietic protoporphyria: Evidence for multiple sites of excess protoporphyrin formation. J Clin Invest 50:203, 1971

175. Scotto J et al: Electron microscopic studies of severe hepatitis. Am J Dis Child 123:311, 1972

176. Sharp HL: Alpha-1-antitrypsin deficiency. Hosp Pract 6: 83, 1971

177. Sheldon H et al: On the differing appearance of intranuclear and cytoplasmic glycogen in liver cells in glycogen storage disease. J Cell Biol 13:468, 1962

178. Shikata T et al: Staining methods of Australia antigen in paraffin section-detection of cytoplasmic inclusion bodies. Jpn J Exp Med 44:25, 1974

179. Shimizu YK et al: Non-A, non-B hepatitis: Ultrastructural evidence for two agents in experimentally infected chimpanzees. Science 205:13, 1979

180. Simon FR et al: Studies on drug induced cholestasis: Effect of ethinyl estradiol on hepatic bile acid receptors and (Na+-K+)-ATPase. In Paumgartner G, Stiehl A (eds): Bile acid metabolism in health and disease, p 133. Lancaster, MTP Press, 1977

181. Skinner MS et al: Electron microscopic observation of early amyloidosis in human liver. Gastroenterology 50:243, 1966

182. Smuckler EA, Barker EA: Effect of drugs on amino acid incorporation in the liver. Excerpta Med (Int Cong Ser) 15: 83, 1966

183. Staehelin LA: Structure and function of intercellular junctions. Int Rev Cytol 30:121, 1974

184. Stein O et al: Colchicine-induced inhibition of lipoprotein and protein secretion into the serum and lack of interference with secretion of biliary phospholipids and cholesterol by rat liver in vivo. J Cell Biol 62:90, 1974

185. Steiner JW, Carruthers JS: Studies on the fine structure of proliferated bile ductules: II. Changes of the ductule-connective tissue envelope relationship. Can Med Assoc J 85: 1275, 1961

186. Steiner JW, Carruthers JS: Experimental extrahepatic obstruction: Some aspects of the fine structural changes of bile ductules and preductules (ducts of Hering). Am J Pathol 40:253, 1962

187. Steiner JW et al: The ductular reaction of rat liver in extrahepatic cholestasis: I. Proliferated biliary epithelial cells. Exp Mol Pathol 1:162, 1962

188. Steiner JW et al: Ultrastructural and subcellular pathology of the liver. Int Rev Exp Pathol 3:65, 1964

189. Steiner JW et al: Some aspects of the ultrastructural pathology of the liver. In Popper H, Schaffner F (eds): Progress in Liver Disease. vol 2, chap 21, p 303. New York, Grune & Stratton, 1965

190. Stenger RJ: Hepatic sinusoids in carbon tetrachloride induced cirrhosis: An electron microscopic study. Arch Pathol 81:439, 1966

191. Stern R: Experimental aspects of hepatic fibrosis. In Popper H, Schaffner, F (eds): Progress in Liver Disease, vol 6, p 173. New York, Grune & Stratton, 1979

192. Sternlieb I: Mitochondrial and fatty changes in hepatocytes of patients with Wilson's disease. Gastroenterology 55:354, 1968

193. Sternlieb I: Evolution of the hepatic lesion in Wilson's disease (hepatolenticular degeneration). In Popper H, Schaffner F (eds): Progress in Liver Disease, vol 4, p 511. New York, Grune & Stratton, 1972

194. Sternlieb I, Scheinberg JH: Wilson's disease. In Schaffner F, Sherlock S, Leevy CM (eds): The Liver and its Diseases, p 328. Int Med Biol Co 1974

195. Sternlieb I et al: Lysosomal defect of hepatic copper excretion in Wilson's disease (hepatolenticular degeneration). Gastroenterology 64:99, 1973

196. Sun SC et al: Hepatocellular ultrastructure in asymptomatic hepatitis B antigenemia. Arch Pathol 97:373, 1974

197. Tanikawa K: Ultrastructural aspects of the liver and its disorders, 2nd ed. Tokyo, Igaku-Shoin, 1979

198. Theron JJ et al: The pathogenesis of experimental dietary siderosis of the liver. Am J Pathol 43:73, 1963

199. Thistle JL, Hofmann A: Efficacy and specificity of chenodeoxycholic acid therapy for dissolving gallstones. N Engl J Med 289:655, 1973

200. Trump BF et al: The ultrastructure of the human liver cell and its common patterns of reaction to injury. In Gall EA, Mostoffi FK (eds): The Liver, p 80. Baltimore, Williams & Wilkins, 1973

201. Trump BF et al: The relationship of intracellular pathways of iron metabolism to cellular iron overload and the iron storage diseases: Cell sap and cytocavitary network pathways in relation to lysosomal storage and turnover of iron macromolecules. Am J Pathol, 72:295, 1973

202. Trump BF et al: The application of electron microscopy and cellular biochemistry to the autopsy. Hum Pathol 6: 499, 1975

203. Trump BF et al: Cellular pathophysiology of hepatitis. Am J Clin Pathol 65:828, 1976

204. Tseng SCG et al: Types of collagen synthesized by normal rat liver hepatocytes in primary culture. Hepatology 3:955, 1983

205. Tumme A et al: Symptomatic porphyria. S Afr Med J 8: 1803, 1974

206. Uchida T et al: Alcoholic foamy degeneration: A pattern of acute alcoholic injury of the liver. Gastroenterology 84: 683, 1983

207. Uzunalimoglu B et al: The liver in mild halothane hepatitis: Light and electron microscopic findings with special reference to the mononuclear cell infiltrate. Am J Pathol 61: 457, 1970

208. Vial JD et al: Effect of bile duct ligation on the ultrastructural morphology of hepatocytes. Gastroenterology 70:85, 1976

209. Volk B, Wallace B: The liver in lipidosis. Am J Pathol 49;203, 1966

210. Waldo ED, Tobias H: Needle-like cytoplasmic inclusions in the liver in porphyria cutanea tarda. Arch Pathol 96: 368, 1973

211. Wiggers KD et al: The ultrastructure of Mallory body filaments. Lab Invest 29:652, 1973

212. Wills EJ: Acute infective hepatitis. Arch Pathol 36:184, 1968

213. Wills EJ, Walton B: A morphological study of unexplained hepatitis following halothane anaesthesia. Am J Pathol 91: 11, 1978

214. Winckler K et al: Ground-glass hepatocytes in unselected

liver biopsies. Ultrastructure and relationship to hepatitis B surface antigen. Scand J Gastroenterol 11:167, 1976

215. Wisse E, Knook DL: Sinusoidal liver cells. Amsterdam, Elsevier Biomedical Press, 1982

216. Wisse E et al: The pit cell: Description of a new type of cell occurring in rat liver sinusoids and peripheral blood. Cell Tissue Res 173:423, 1976

217. Wolfe K et al: Liver inclusions in erythropoietic protoporphyria. Eur J Clin Invest 5:21, 1975

218. Yamamoto A et al: Localized B-galactosidase deficiency occurrence in cerebellar ataxia with myoclonus epilepsy and macular cherry-red spot: A new variant of GM_1-gangliosidosis? Arch Invest Med 134:627, 1974

219. Yokoo H et al: Morphologic variants of alcoholic hyaline. Am J Pathol 69:25, 1972

220. Yousef IM et al: Lithocholate induced intrahepatic cholestasis. Gastroenterology 70:996, 1976

221. Yunis EK et al: Fine structural observation of the liver in alpha-1-antitrypsin deficiency. Am J Pathol 82:265, 1976

222. Zimmerman HJ: Drug induced chronic liver disease. In Farber E, Fisher, MM (ed): Toxic Injury of the Liver, part B, p 687. New York, Marcel Dekker, 1980

223. Zimmerman HJ: Drug induced liver disease: An overview. Sem Liver Dis 1:93, 1981

224. Zimmerman HJ, Ishak KG: Valproate-induced hepatic injury: Analysis of 23 fatal cases. Hepatology 2:591, 1982

chapter **3**

Secretion of Bile

SERGE ERLINGER

Bile, the exocrine secretion of the liver, is a complex aqueous solution of organic and inorganic compounds. The organic compounds include bile acids, bile pigments, cholesterol, and phospholipids, and the inorganic compounds are mainly the plasma electrolytes. Bile also contains small amounts of proteins. Bile is secreted by the liver cells into the bile canaliculi, transported and modified by the intrahepatic and extrahepatic biliary system, and delivered to the duodenum through the ampulla of Vater. After entry into the duodenum, some bile constituents, such as bile pigments, are irreversibly excreted into the feces, whereas others, mainly the bile acids, are reabsorbed by the intestine, return to the liver, and are reexcreted into bile. This enterohepatic circulation is therefore essential to normal biliary physiology. This chapter is concerned primarily with the mechanisms of bile flow and their possible alterations and with the enterohepatic circulation of bile acids. Several reviews are available.[26,104,108,211,306]

STRUCTURAL BASIS OF BILE SECRETION

Morphology

A schematic view of the biliary system is shown in Figure 3-1. Bile is formed by the hepatocytes (parenchymal liver cells) and secreted by them into the bile canaliculi. The bile canaliculi are channels about 1 μm in diameter grooving the 1-cell thick hepatocyte plates. They branch and communicate with one another to form a continuous three-dimensional network. They are closed at one end (situated near the central part of the hepatic lobule); at their other end, situated near the portal space at the periphery of the lobule, they drain into larger channels, the bile ductules, which in turn join to form bile ducts. A bile canaliculus consists of a localized separation between the limiting (plasma) membranes of two, sometimes three, adjoining hepatocytes. The canaliculi have no walls of their own; however, the hepatocyte plasma membrane that bounds them is often called, for convenience, the canalicular membrane. The canalicular membrane has an extensive surface area because numerous microvilli project into the lumen of the canaliculi. The canaliculus is surrounded by a narrow zone of organelle-poor cytoplasm, known as pericanalicular ectoplasm. In this region, the presence of actin microfilaments (about 7 nm in di-

ameter) has been demonstrated by several techniques, including biochemical analysis.[72] Although microfilaments are also seen beneath the sinusoidal membrane (which bounds the sinusoidal face of the hepatocyte), they occur mainly in the pericanalicular area, where they form a web. They insert in the part of the intercellular junction called the intermediate junction (see below), form a network around the canaliculus, and extend into the canalicular microvilli, where they appear to insert on the inner part of the membrane. Microfilaments probably have a role in the maintenance of the shape of the microvilli and of the canaliculus itself.

Microtubules, another element of the cytoskeleton, about 24 nm in diameter, are more randomly distributed within the cytoplasm but are also present in the pericanalicular area. They may interact with plasma-membrane components.[20]

On each side of the canaliculus, the cell membranes of adjacent cells form structures known as intercellular junctions. They consist of three main elements encountered in the following order from the canaliculus to the perisinusoidal space: tight junction, intermediate junction, and desmosome. A fourth element, the gap junction, may be found as small patches in the tight junction or as larger areas on the intercellular surface. The desmosome appears to protect the membranes from deformation and damage due to distention. The intermediate junction is thought to serve as an adhesive structure to the cells; it also provides sites for attachment of actin microfilaments. The gap junction includes channels that appear to establish a cell-to-cell communication system. The tight junction is generally regarded as a sealing structure between the lumen of the bile canaliculus and the intercellular space and, hence, the sinusoidal blood.

The ductules and ducts, unlike the canaliculi, are lined with true epithelial cells forming the biliary epithelium. These cells have a prominent Golgi apparatus, and microvilli project from their luminal face. They are separated from one another by intercellular spaces. The ducts in the portal tracts possess a rich blood supply, mainly arterial.[96,98] The ductules are arranged in a complex anastomosing network.[367]

Relation of Morphology to Function

Among functional implications emerging from structural studies, several merit special attention.

77

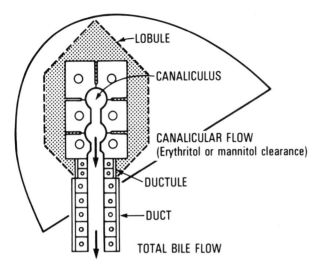

Fig. 3-1. Schematic view of the biliary system.

The bile canaliculus is a long, narrow channel open at one end and closed at the other. It has a high surface volume ratio and is well adapted to the creation of local osmotic water flow.[79,81] The canalicular surface area (not including the microvilli) available for movement of water and solutes through the canalicular membrane has been estimated at about 7000 cm²/100 g of liver,[356] or some 10.5 m² for a human liver. Alternatively, or in addition, the microvilli and the spaces between them may also serve as structures for osmotic water flow as proposed for other secretory epithelia.[257]

The permeability of the tight junction is of particular importance for the process of bile formation. It was formerly believed that all tight junctions were impermeable.[122] However, more recent studies have revealed that tight junctions differ among epithelia.[57,78,135] In impermeable epithelia, such as in the toad bladder, which has a high transepithelial electrical resistance, the tight junctions are deep and are made of a complex network of continuous contact lines between adjacent plasma membranes. These epithelia are referred to as "tight" epithelia. In contrast, in relatively permeable epithelia, such as the proximal kidney tubule, with a low transepithelial resistance, the tight junctions are made of a few discontinuous contact lines. These epithelia, which allow for paracellular fluid flux, are referred to as "leaky" epithelia. The liver seems to be of an intermediate type,[135] with relatively numerous contact lines; it is considered to be a potential pathway for transjunctional fluid or solute movement, as postulated by Ashworth and Sanders.[7]

The microcirculation within the hepatic lobule allows many compounds absorbed by the alimentary tract (into the portal blood) to gain access to the hepatocytes for eventual metabolism before entry into the systemic blood or excretion into bile. Blood, flowing from the portal space through the sinusoids, is then drained by a branch of the hepatic vein. Provided there is a unidirectional plasma flow, the hepatocytes adjacent to portal spaces are first exposed to afferent blood and hence should receive blood with the highest solute concentrations. The amount of solute then removed by the hepatocyte as blood flows in the sinusoids toward the hepatic vein depends on the extraction efficiency for each solute. This results in a translobular concentration gradient (Fig. 3-2) and, hence, in a nonuniform exposure of hepatocytes to the solute. This has been clearly illustrated by an autoradiographic study of D-galactose uptake[151] and of uptake of labeled bile acid analogues.[192,339] A similar view may well apply to secretion into bile. For instance, measurements of the diameter of canaliculi around the portal areas and around hepatic vein areas have suggested that at physiologic loads, bile acids are secreted mostly into periportal bile canaliculi.[223] At higher doses, recruitment of more distal hepatocytes seems to occur. However, it appears that blood flow through the sinusoids is not always unidirectional because of the complexity of the sinusoidal network and the variation of resistances within it. Pulsatile pressure changes within the sinusoids probably allow for mixing of solutes before hepatocyte uptake and reduce the steepness of the translobular gradient. This probably exposes the hepatocytes to plasma of a more uniform composition.

Canalicular bile within the lobule flows in a direction opposite to that of sinusoidal plasma flow. In this way, hepatocytes at the portal venous end of the sinusoid can elaborate bile containing solutes at a concentration higher than those at the hepatic venous end. This bile does not come into contact with hepatocytes that may contain lesser amounts of the same solute, a pattern that reduces back-diffusion of solutes from bile to hepatocytes and sinusoidal blood. This arrangement favors formation of bile with a high concentration of organic solutes.[189]

Finally, some structural characteristics of the biliary epithelial cells are usually associated with fluid trans-

Fig. 3-2. The concept of translobular gradient. A solute enters the sinusoid (*S*) at its portal end. Solute concentration (*dots*) decreases as it is progressively taken up (*arrows*) by the hepatocytes (*H*). Bile flows opposite to the direction of blood flow, so that bile in the periportal canaliculi is more concentrated than in canaliculi in the hepatic vein area. PS = perisinusoidal space; BC = bile canaliculus.

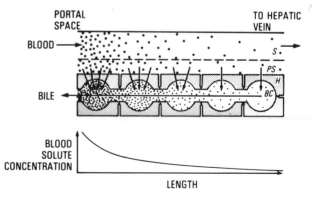

port.[329-331] This fact, together with the abundant arterial vascularity of the portal bile ducts, suggests that the bile elaborated by the hepatocytes may be modified on its way through the ductules or ducts.

BILE COMPOSITION

Water and Electrolytes

In general, inorganic electrolytes are present in bile at concentrations closely reflecting those in plasma.[38] The range of reported values is shown in Table 3-1. However, concentrations in bile of sodium, potassium, calcium, and bicarbonate may be appreciably higher than in plasma, whereas the chloride level may be lower. Hypothetically, these differences may be due to one or more of the following phenomena: the formation by the bile acids of polymolecular aggregates (or micelles),[50] which have low osmotic activity; differences in electrical potential between the biliary lumen and the extracellular fluid; variable repartition of different electrolytes due to the Donnan distribution; or possible active transport of inorganic ions.

The predominant biliary cation is sodium, which is present in normal human bile in concentrations ranging between 145 mEq and 165 mEq/liter.[124,345,353] Lower concentrations prevail when substances such as dehydrocholate, phenol red, or polyethylene glycol 1500, whose micelle-forming capacity is inferior to that of the natural bile acids, are excreted in the bile.[327] Micelle formation probably also explains why, under physiologic conditions, fluctuations in biliary bile acid concentration are accompanied by equivalent fluctuations in biliary sodium concentration.[274,360] Sodium concentrations of up to 340 mEq/liter have been observed in concentrated gallbladder bile of rabbits,[83,243] and concentrations of up to 240 mEq/liter have been observed in the hepatic bile of cholecys-

tectomized dogs.[271,360] Variations of bile potassium levels usually parallel those of sodium.

The concentration of calcium in bile, especially gallbladder bile, may be even higher, in comparison with its plasma concentration, than is the case with sodium and potassium.[42,44] This may also be due to binding to bile acids and micelle formation.[63] In addition, the electronegativity of the gallbladder lumen[83] may predispose to higher concentrations of divalent than of monovalent cations.

The concentration of bicarbonate in bile is often higher that its concentration in plasma,[124,271,345] especially in rabbits[314] and guinea pigs,[128] whereas the concentration of chloride is generally similar to, or even lower than, that prevailing in plasma.[124,274,345] The reason for these observations is not known, but a bicarbonate-transporting mechanism has been suggested (see below). One result of these variations is that the pH of bile, although generally alkaline, also varies.[271,360]

In dogs and in humans, bicarbonate concentration in bile is higher than in plasma after administration of the hormone secretin (see Ductular–Ductal Secretion).

Organic Solutes

The main organic compounds of bile are the conjugated bile acids, phospholipids, cholesterol, and the bile pigments. Proteins are present in bile at low concentrations. Metabolites of various endogenous compounds (chiefly hormones) may also be found in bile.

Bile acid concentration in human hepatic bile ranges from 2 mM to 45 mM.[345] Bile acids are mostly present as glycine and taurine conjugates, with a pK well below the physiologic range of biliary pH, and are therefore present as anions (referred to as bile salts) rather than as undissociated bile acids.

TABLE 3-1.   Flow and Electrolyte Concentrations of Hepatic Bile*

SPECIES	FLOW	Na^+	K^+	Ca^{++}	Mg^{++}	Cl^-	HCO_3^-	BILE ACIDS	REFERENCES
	$\mu l \cdot min^{-1} \cdot kg^{-1}$	←			mEq/liter			→ mM	
Man	1.5–15.4	132–165	4.2–5.6	1.2–4.8	1.4–3.0	96–126	17–55	3–45	124, 270, 345, 353
Dog	10	141–230	4.5–11.9	3.1–13.8	2.2–5.5	31–107	14–61	16–187	60, 271, 274, 280, 360
Sheep	9.4	159.6	5.3	–	–	95	21.2	42.5	317
Rabbit	90	148–156	3.6–6.7	2.7–6.7	0.3–0.7	77–99	40–63	6–24	110, 120, 314, 336
Rat	30–150	157–166	5.8–6.4	–	–	94–98	22–26	8–25	23, 208
Guinea pig	115.9	175	6.3	–	–	69	49–65	–	317
Turkey	10	161–223	4.4–6.8	–	–	85–110	18–54	74	176
Dogfish shark	1.2	227	5.0	18.0	9.0	224	5.8	21	36

* Numbers indicate range or means of published values.

Bile acids and salts are amphipathic molecules that form micelles (or polymolecular aggregates) above a critical micellar concentration.[50,182] The concentration of bile acids in human hepatic and gallbladder bile is usually well above the critical micellar concentration; hence bile acids are mostly in the micellar form in normal bile, as well as in the duodenal and jejunal lumen. The major bile acids of humans are conjugates of the primary (cholic and chenodeoxycholic) and secondary (deoxycholic and, to a lesser extent, lithocholic) bile acids. Phospholipid and cholesterol concentrations of human hepatic bile range, respectively, from 25 mg/dl to 810 mg/dl and from 60 mg/dl to 320 mg/dl or from 0.3 mM to 11 mM and 1.6 mM to 8.3 mM.[345] In gallbladder bile, the concentrations of nonabsorbable constituents (bile acids, phospholipids, cholesterol) are appreciably higher, owing to reabsorption of water (and inorganic electrolytes) by the gallbladder. However, theoretically, the molar percentage of each of these compounds in gallbladder bile relative to the total biliary lipid concentration should remain unchanged compared with hepatic bile, although deviations may be observed.[322] The secretion into bile of cholesterol and phospholipid is intimately dependent on bile acid secretion in animals[89,165,201,352,357] and in humans.[178,308,352] It is also well recognized that bile acids are a major determinant of phospholipid and cholesterol solubilization in bile. This process probably occurs through mixed micellar formation, a phenomenon that explains why biliary phospholipid and cholesterol concentrations far exceed the maximal solubility of these compounds in a simple aqueous solution. Solubilization of cholesterol into a liquid crystalline phase may also occur. However, cholesterol concentration in human bile frequently exceeds the maximal cholesterol solubilizing capacity; this may lead to cholesterol precipitation and cholesterol gallstone formation.

Bile pigments are present in human hepatic and gallbladder biles at a concentration averaging, respectively, 0.3 mM and 3.2 mM (0.5 g/liter and 2 g/liter).[325] The solubility of the various bile pigments and its relationship to pigment gallstone formation have been discussed by Soloway and co-workers.[325]

Protein concentrations in bile are extremely low, of the order of 60 mg/liter to 400 mg/liter in canine bile, and 300 mg/liter to 3000 mg/liter in human bile.[170,288,294,345] Serum albumin is the most abundant and is derived from the plasma pool.[85,86,288] Other bile proteins probably also originate from plasma, and their concentrations appear to be inversely related to their molecular weights.[85,86] Some, like immunoglobulin A, are transported into bile by a vesicular pathway after receptor-mediated endocytosis.[69,148,218] Bile also contains a variety of lysosomal enzymes, probably excreted by hepatocyte exocytosis independently of bile acid secretion.[219]

Osmolality

Bile osmolality, as measured by freezing-point depression, is usually approximately 300 mosm/kg.[54,143,323,360] It varies in parallel to plasma osmolality.[143] Slight deviation from isotonicity has been observed in dogs: during high bile acid infusions, bile tends to be hypotonic, whereas during secretin administration, it tends to be hypertonic.[168,271] The significance of these deviations has not been fully elucidated but may be related, in part, to the nonideal osmotic behavior of the bile acids.[168]

Total ion concentration (especially cation concentration), however, may be much higher in bile than in plasma,[360] in spite of the isotonicity of bile. Total osmotic activity has been found empirically to be accounted for only by the inorganic electrolytes, ignoring the bile salt anions.[360] It is therefore generally assumed that bile acids, because they are in micellar form, have little or no osmotic activity and that the osmolality of bile is attributable mostly to the osmotic activity of the inorganic ions.

FLUID MOVEMENT IN THE BILIARY SYSTEM: MECHANISMS AND SITES

Absorption and secretion of fluid in living organisms result from net movement of water. Active transport of water has never been observed in a living organism, and the water potential is identical inside and outside the living mammalian cell.[233] Therefore, the driving force for water transport across epithelia must come from hydrostatic pressure or osmotic pressure.

Hydrostatic filtration is unlikely to be the initiating event in bile flow: in the isolated perfused rat liver, bile can be secreted at pressures exceeding the perfusion pressure[39,41]; in the intact animal, maximum biliary pressure (or maximum secretory pressure) is invariably greater than sinusoidal (or portal) pressure.[12,13,66,101,284,318,337] However, under experimental or pathologic conditions, variations in hydrostatic pressure may affect bile formation. Excessive output of bile has been observed in cirrhosis and attributed, at least in part, to increased hepatic venous pressure.[226] Acute increase in hepatic venous pressure in dogs may, on the other hand, reduce bile flow.[269] Partial obstruction of the suprahepatic portion of the inferior vena cava has been reported both to increase bile flow[87] or to have no effect.[297]

Osmotic filtration is widely assumed to be the major bile flow–generating mechanism. The mechanisms of osmotic water flow across epithelia have been studied extensively in absorptive epithelia, such as the gallbladder and the intestine. Current concepts of osmotic absorption of water are derived from the models of Curran[64] and Diamond,[77,79–81] in which the active transport of a solute is coupled to water transport until osmotic equilibration is achieved. Such models have been postulated to apply also to secretory epithelia.[257] Prerequisites are a lumen closed at one end and provided with a high surface/volume ratio, and active (energy-dependent) transport of one or several solutes. The bile canalicular network, as we have seen, satisfies the first of these conditions. As for the second, the solutes in question may be either non-reabsorb-able solutes that induce choleresis analogous to osmotic diuresis or solutes of lower molecular weight that induce choleresis by establishing a local osmotic gradient. Appropriate solutes are considered in a later section.

The anatomic sites of fluid movement in the biliary system are the bile canaliculi, the ductules, the ducts, and the gallbladder. Water movement of canalicular origin can be distinguished from movement of water of ductal or ductular origin by measurement of biliary clearance of inert solutes (see next section). More detailed analysis must await the development of more refined techniques, such as micropuncture. Water transport in the gallbladder has been fully studied elsewhere.[75,76,363]

EXPERIMENTAL SYSTEMS AND METHODS

Systems for the Study of Bile Secretion

The simplest experimental preparation for studying bile formation is the total biliary fistula. Its major disadvantage is the total interruption of the enterohepatic circulation and the consequent depletion of the natural bile acids. This is usually overcome by constant intravenous or intraduodenal administration of exogenous bile acids at controlled rates. The partial biliary fistula allows interruption of the enterohepatic circulation: after collection of a known quantity of bile, bile is returned to the stomach or duodenum, thus replenishing the pool of natural bile acids.[88] The isolated perfused liver preparation[29,40,203] is useful for observing the effects of single factors or of drugs with a toxic systemic action. Isolated[22,315] and cultured liver cells are used for transport studies.[4,140,305,312,313] For an accurate characterization of transport systems, membrane vesicle preparations derived from the basolateral[27] or canalicular[186] membrane are being used with increased frequency. This variety of techniques indicates that, in interpreting the results of an experiment, it is necessary to take into account the species of animal and the experimental preparation used.

Estimation of Canalicular Bile Flow

Canalicular bile flow may be estimated by measuring the biliary clearance of nonmetabolized solutes that enter the canalicular bile by passive processes[302] and that are neither secreted nor reabsorbed by the ductules or the ducts. This method is analogous to measurement of the glomerular filtration rate by urinary clearance of substances that do not cross the renal tubular epithelium. The theoretic basis of the method and some of its limitations have been discussed by Forker[128,129,131,134] and Wheeler and co-workers.[361] In brief, when such a solute is administered in the systemic circulation, its excretion rate in bile during a steady state should depend on the permeability of the epithelium and on bile flow. The biliary clearance (C) is calculated as

$$C = F \times \frac{[B]}{[P]}$$

where F is bile flow, and [B] and [P] are the biliary and plasma concentrations of the solute. The technique implies that the selected solute is unable to cross the ductular epithelium and that its permeability in the canaliculi is high enough that diffusion equilibrium is achieved at the highest rates of canalicular bile flow. Neither of these assumptions is presently accessible to direct experimental testing. However, an operational test of adequate canalicular permeability is the finding that increments in bile flow produced by bile acid infusions (which are presumably of canalicular origin) are accompanied by parallel increases in clearance. Erythritol (Mol wt: 122) meets this requirement in dogs,[361] hamsters,[299] rats,[29] rabbits,[110] monkeys,[338] and humans.[268] Mannitol (Mol wt: 182) appears to equilibrate in canalicular bile in dogs[361] but not in hamsters,[299] rabbits,[110] or humans.[31] In guinea pigs, passage of both solutes in the canaliculi is restricted.[128]

The assumption that these solutes are unable to cross the bile ductular or ductal epithelium is tested, again operationally, by the finding that their clearance is unaltered by secretin choleresis.[128,361] The reasonable conclusion is that secretin acts at a site distal to the canaliculus and impermeable to the solutes, supposedly the bile ductules or ducts. It should be pointed out, however, that secretin does not enhance choleresis in rabbits or rats; hence, the assumption cannot be tested in these species. Moreover, experiments in dogs have shown an increase in the biliary clearances of erythritol and mannitol during secretin choleresis.[18,249] This observation can be explained either by stimulation of canalicular secretion by the hormone or by permeability of the bile ductules or ducts to erythritol and mannitol. Finally, it is impossible, with this method, to determine whether secretin choleresis originates in the small periportal bile ductules or in the larger bile ducts.

How do erythritol and mannitol pass from the sinusoids into the canalicular bile? The predominant mode of transit is thought, conventionally, to be by osmotic filtration through, successively, the sinusoidal membrane, the hepatocyte, and the canalicular membrane (Fig. 3-3). The findings that (1) the equilibrium between plasma and hepatic concentrations of five- or six-carbon sugars and polyalcohols is rapidly established in the steady state[46,296,302] and (2) the hepatic venous dilution curve of erythritol after a single intraportal injection is superimposable upon that of water[146] suggest that the sinusoidal membrane is permeable to those solutes and that they rapidly penetrate the totality of the hepatocyte. If this is so, their entry into bile depends mainly upon their passing through the canalicular membrane. However, several observations suggest the possibility of a paracellular pathway (Fig. 3-3). The bile-to-plasma concentration ratios of relatively larger solutes, such as insulin (Mol wt: 5000), sucrose (Mol wt: 342), or polyethylene glycol 4000, stabilize well before the hepatocyte-to-plasma concentration ratios.[131,190]

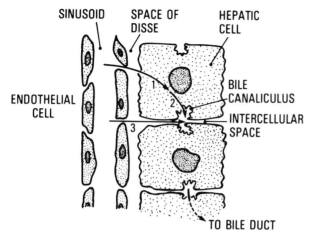

Fig. 3-3. Schematic diagram of the possible anatomic pathways for solute transport into bile. Materials may enter bile after hepatocellular uptake (*1*) and secretion into the bile canaliculi (*2*) (transcellular pathway), or through the intercellular space (*3*) (paracellular pathway). (After Ashworth CT, Sanders E: Am J Pathol 37:343, 1960)

Consistent with the view of a paracellular pathway is the rapid appearance in bile (approximately 10 minutes) of ferrocyanide (Mol wt: 484, hydrated form).[37] This alternate route of entry should not preclude the use of such solutes as indicators of canalicular flow, provided that a parallel increase in bile flow and solute clearance is clearly demonstrated during bile acid–induced choleresis. Finally, it has been shown that the biliary clearances of charged solutes (such as ferrocyanide and carboxylinulin) are consistently lower than those of uncharged solutes of similar molecular size, an observation suggesting that the pathway of entry into bile includes a barrier that selectively restricts passive anionic movement.[37]

Solutes such as sucrose and inulin also enter canalicular bile; however, their bile-to-plasma concentration ratio in the rat is approximately 0.15 to 0.20 and 0.05 to 0.10, respectively.[131,302] This is due to restriction to movement across the pathway that permits their entry into canalicular bile. Consequently their biliary clearance does not estimate canalicular bile flow. They may be used, however, to estimate qualitatively changes in the permeability of the biliary system.[130]

CANALICULAR (HEPATOCYTIC) BILE FORMATION

Canalicular bile formation is regarded as an osmotic water flow in response to "active" solute transport. Because of the excellent correlation between bile flow and bile acid output in bile, bile acids are considered one of the solutes that generate bile flow: the term *bile acid–dependent flow* is used to describe this fraction of bile flow. In contrast, flow that may be generated at low bile acid outputs, in the absence of bile acids, or in addition to bile acid–dependent flow is described as *bile acid–independent flow.*[108,132,189,211]

Bile Acid–Dependent Flow

Uptake, Transport, and Secretion of Bile Acids

The mechanisms for the uptake of bile acids into the hepatocytes, their intracellular transport, and their secretion into bile are incompletely understood.[116] The liver has a high extraction efficiency for bile acids.[256] The uptake of bile acids by the liver cells meets the criteria of a carrier-mediated process. As illustrated in Figure 3-4, it appears to be saturable, as shown by an indicator dilution technique in the intact dog,[144,145] in the *in-situ* perfused rat liver,[277,278] and by studies with isolated and cultured liver cells.[4,305,312] Competitive inhibition may be shown when two bile acids are administered simultaneously,[145] but not with other organic anions, such as indocyanine green.[259]

A marked dependence of bile acid uptake on extracellular sodium has been clearly demonstrated in the isolated perfused liver,[278] in isolated[312] and cultured[305] hepatocytes, and in plasma membrane vesicles.[27,92,185,293] This strongly suggests that bile acid uptake is a secondary active transport energized by the transmembrane sodium gradient. The carrier probably moves the bile acid and sodium across the membrane (symport or cotransport) simultaneously. The sodium gradient is continuously maintained by the sodium-potassium–activated adenosine triphos-

Fig. 3-4. Hepatic uptake of taurocholate in the dog. Uptake was measured by the indicator dilution technique. The initial velocity of uptake increased in a nonlinear way with the dose, indicating saturation. (Glasinovíc JC et al: J Clin Invest 55: 419, 1975. Copyright by The American Society for Clinical Investigation)

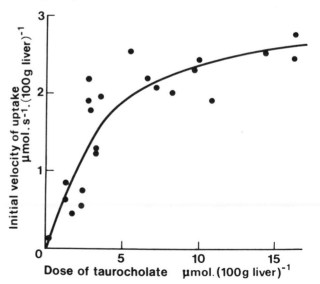

phatase (Na^+,K^+-ATPase), the enzymatic basis of the sodium pump.[61] This system is analogous to the intestinal and kidney tubule transport systems of bile acids.[82,364,365]

The exact nature of the postulated carrier system is not known. However, a bile acid–binding protein has been characterized in the plasma membrane of the liver cell.[1,149] It is not known whether this protein is actually on the sinusoidal membrane (and available for uptake) or on the canalicular membrane.

The maximal capacity for uptake (about 4.5 $\mu mol \cdot s^{-1} \cdot 100$ g liver^{-1}) is approximately ten times greater than the maximal capacity for sodium sulfobromophthalein (Bromsulphalein [BSP]) uptake.[150] It also greatly exceeds the maximal capacity for biliary excretion (see below).

Little is known about the intracellular transport from the sinusoidal to the canalicular pole of the hepatocyte. Bile acids appear to have little affinity for the Y (ligandin) or Z proteins[5,227,283] that bind a variety of other organic anions, including BSP and iodinated contrast agents. However, cytoplasmic bile acid–binding proteins have been detected and partially purified[334,335] and may play a role in transport. One of them exhibits glutathione-transferase activity and may actually be identical to ligandin.[335] Bile acid–binding proteins different from ligandin have also been identified.[333,340] During this phase of hepatic transport, unconjugated bile acids are conjugated to taurine and glycine. Conjugation may be a limiting step in overall hepatic transport for certain bile acids: the maximal biliary transport capacity (transport maximum [Tm] or maximal secretory rate [SRm]) of some conjugated bile acids administered intravenously is far greater than that of the unconjugated compounds.[115,349,369] Keto bile acids can also be hydroxylated.[71,164,324]

The secretion of bile acids into bile probably takes place through another carrier-mediated process. Secretion into bile is saturable, with a Tm of 8 μmol to 8.5 $\mu mol \cdot min^{-1} \cdot kg^{-1}$ in dogs,[254] 14 $\mu mol \cdot min^{-1} \cdot kg^{-1}$ in sheep,[3] and 10 μmol to 12 $\mu mol \cdot min^{-1} \cdot kg^{-1}$ in rats.[2] Three lines of evidence suggest that the hepatic secretory mechanism for bile acids is not the same as that for other organic anions excreted in the bile, in particular bilirubin, BSP, and iodinated contrast agents: (1) The Tm for bile acids is five to ten times higher than that for BSP.[359] (2) Bile acids and BSP do not compete for biliary excretion; on the contrary, administration of bile acids increases the apparent Tm for BSP[35,74,157,255] (the mechanism of which is examined below). (3) In mutant Corriedale sheep, which have an inherited defect in biliary excretion of organic anions that is closely related to the Dubin–Johnson syndrome in humans, maximal biliary excretion of BSP was low, whereas that of bile acids was normal.[3]

The canalicular carrier system appears to be independent of sodium, as demonstrated in canalicular membrane vesicles.[186] There is no evidence that it requires a source of energy, and it may be a carrier-mediated system (facilitated diffusion). It has also been suggested that transport may be driven by the membrane potential.[238] A schematic

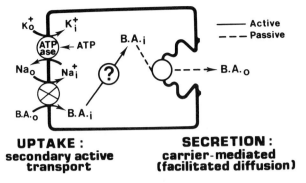

Fig. 3-5. Schematic representation of bile acid transport by hepatocytes. Uptake is mediated by a bile acid/sodium co-transport (symport) system energized by the transmembrane sodium gradient maintained by Na^+,K^+-ATPase. Canalicular secretion is probably a carrier-mediated, energy-independent process driven by the membrane potential. The mechanisms of intracellular transport are largely unknown.

view of the steps of hepatocellular transport of bile acids is shown on Figure 3-5. It can be noted that the active step is probably the uptake, which allows concentration in the hepatocyte. This is probably responsible, in part, for the concentration gradient between blood and bile: the biliary concentration (10–100 mM) is about 100 to 1000 times higher than the plasma concentration in systemic or portal blood. Part of this concentration gradient, however, is probably best explained by micelle formation, which prevents reabsorption from bile.

Because of their efficient hepatic transport and their enterohepatic circulation,[49,179,180,181,211,236] bile acids are secreted into bile in considerable amounts: with a synthetic rate of approximately 600 mg/day, the liver is able to maintain a bile acid pool of 2 g to 3 g and to secrete into bile 20 g to 30 g of bile acids per day.

Effect of Bile Acid Secretion on Canalicular Bile Flow

Bile acids stimulate bile production in many animal species. An apparently linear relation between bile acid secretion rates and bile flow has been demonstrated in the dog,[271] the rabbit,[109,110] the rat, and the isolated rat liver,[23,29,32] the rhesus monkey,[88,338] and in humans.[268,270,308] This relation is illustrated in Figure 3-6. Bile acid–induced choleresis is presumably of canalicular origin, for it is accompanied by a parallel increase in erythritol clearance.[128,129,361] A linear relation is also found between bile acid secretion rate and erythritol or mannitol clearance, both in animals[29,361] and in humans.[31,231,268] This relation is shown in Figure 3-7.

The hypothesis that bile acids increase bile flow because they provide an osmotic driving force for filtration of water and electrolytes was first proposed by Sperber.[326,327] The reduction in bile flow and electrolyte excretion without reduction in bile acid secretion that has been recorded

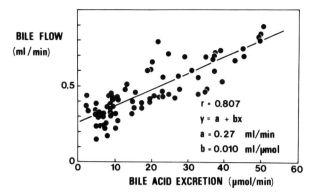

Fig. 3-6. Relation between bile flow and bile acid secretion rate in humans. Data obtained from patients with T-tubes in common bile duct after cholecystectomy. There is a linear relation between bile flow and bile acid secretion, with a slope of 0.010 ml/μmol (10 μl of bile being formed per each μmol of bile acid secreted) (bile acid-dependent flow) and an intercept for a zero bile acid secretion of 0.27 ml/min, indicating a total (canalicular + ductal/ductular) bile acid-independent flow of 0.27 ml/min. (Prandi D et al: Eur J Clin Invest 5:1, 1975)

after intravenous injections of hypertonic solutions[54] may be due to a fall in this osmotic gradient. The observation that other osmotically active compounds—organic anions other than bile acids and nonanionic substances—that also appear in bile at high concentrations also have a choleretic action proportional to the osmotic load is an additional point in favor of this hypothesis. Finally, bile acids that do not form micelles (such as dehydrocholate) or bile acids that have a high critical micellar concentration, such as norcholate,[252] have a greater choleretic effect than that of physiologic bile acids.

Fig. 3-7. Relation between canalicular flow and bile acid secretion rate in humans. Data obtained from the same patients as in Figure 3-6. Canalicular flow is estimated by erythritol clearance. There is a linear relation between canalicular bile flow and bile acid secretion rate, with a slope of 11 μl of bile per μmol of bile acid and an intercept of 0.157 ml/min (canalicular bile acid-independent flow). (Prandi D et al: Eur J Clin Invest 5:1, 1975)

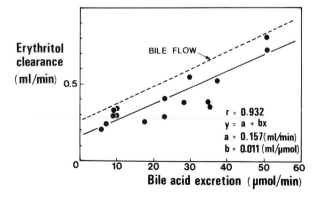

Because bile acids are in the micellar form, as noted above, most of the osmotic activity must be accounted for by their accompanying counterions. The slope of the line that relates bile flow to bile acid secretion, which is an operational estimate of the osmotic effect of bile acids, varies from species to species. Expressed in microliters of bile per micromole of bile acid secreted, it is approximately 8 in the dog,[271,361] 13 in the rhesus monkey,[88] 15 in the rat,[23] and 30 in the rabbit.[109] The smallest of these volumes is far larger than the amount of water that would be expected if bile acids alone were secreted in an isotonic solution. The reasonable conclusion is that bile acid–dependent bile flow includes substantial amounts of other osmotically active solutes, probably driven by passive diffusion and solvent drag. The magnitude of these processes depends on the permeability characteristics of the canaliculus and may differ, therefore, from species to species.

An alternative hypothesis to explain bile acid–dependent bile flow is that the choleretic effect of bile acids may be due, at least in part, to their regulating the activity of other solute pumps.[108,324] This hypothesis is supported by several pieces of suggestive evidence:

In some species, dehydrocholate produces a higher bile flow than do other bile acids.[71,327] This difference is traditionally regarded as being due to this compound and its metabolites having less tendency to micelle formation than the natural bile acids.[253,326,327] However, it has been noted that, during dehydrocholate choleresis, bile flow reached a maximum well after the bulk of the bile acid load had been secreted into bile,[324] an observation not easily explained by the osmotic theory, which predicts simultaneity between the secretion of the osmotic load and the choleresis.

Experiments in rats with ursodeoxycholate and 7-ketolithocholate (its precursor during synthesis from chenodeoxycholic acid) have shown that the choleretic effect of these compounds was again much greater than that of taurocholate and deviated from the expected linearity.[94] This hypercholeresis was associated with a marked increase in bicarbonate biliary secretion.

In the rhesus monkey, erythritol clearance was greater per mole of secreted taurocholate when the bile acid was infused at a high rate than when infused at a low rate.[9]

In the dog, bile flow associated with unconjugated cholate secretion is much higher than that associated with taurocholate secretion at the same rate[254]; the "extra" bile flow does not appear to be related to a higher osmotic activity of the unconjugated bile acid.[254] It could again be due to stimulation of fluid secretion other than by the osmotic effect of cholate. Alternatively, it could be due to a change in permeability at the site of bile acid–dependent bile formation.

In rats with selective biliary obstruction, an increase in bile acid flux through the nonobstructed liver together with a disproportionate increase in bile flow has been reported.[354] All these observations suggest that bile acids may stimulate inorganic ion transport. Sodium transport mediated by the Na[+],K[+]-ATPase, the role of which is discussed later in this chapter, might be one of the candidates for such an activation. In rats with selective biliary obstruction,[354] the activity of this enzyme in liver plasma membranes was increased. In other cases, bicarbonate transport may be stimulated, as observed with ursodeoxycholate, 7-keto-lithocholate and several other compounds.[94]

Pathway of Fluid Movement

The pathway of fluid transport during bile acid–induced choleresis is unclear. Because bile acids are transported through the canalicular membrane of the hepatocyte, it is often stated that the osmotic water flow in response to this transport also occurs through the canalicular membrane. However, the ionic composition of bile closely resembles that of the extracellular fluid. It is therefore necessary to postulate either an ionic equilibration downstream along the biliary channels or a paracellular fluid pathway from the intercellular space into the bile canaliculi. Evidence that solutes such as inulin, sucrose, polyethylene glycol, or ferrocyanide may gain access to canalicular bile through this pathway has already been presented. Experiments with dehydrocholate and taurodehydrocholate have demonstrated a progressive increase in the bile-to-plasma concentration ratio of sucrose, a penetration of ionic lanthanum into the tight junctions, and an increase in the number of intercellular "blisters".[224] These observations have suggested that the paracellular pathway may be an important site for bile acid–induced water and solute movement into bile.

In summary, bile acid–dependent canalicular bile flow is probably related to the osmotic activity of bile acids or of their associated counterions. In addition, evidence suggests that some bile acids, such as dehydrocholate, ursodeoxycholate, or others, may, in certain species, increase canalicular bile flow by stimulating inorganic ion transport. Bile acid–induced water and solute movement into bile may take place, at least in part, through the paracellular (tight junction) pathway.

Bile Acid–like Choleretic Effect of Exogenous Substances

Organic Anions

Organic anions include BSP, fluorescein, indocyanine green, ioglycamide, iodipamide, phenol red, phloridzin, and rose bengal, all of which are secreted into the bile. In general, they increase bile flow in proportion to their secretion rate into bile, and the choleresis is thought to depend upon an osmotic mechanism similar to that of bile acid choleresis.[102,177,327] However, marked differences among species are observed in the effect of these compounds on bile flow.

In a study in dogs, the choleretic response to infusions of BSP, ioglycamide, and taurocholate was proportional to biliary output, and the volume of water secreted per micromole of the three compounds was, respectively, 9.2 μl, 11.9 μl, and 7.3 μl.[177] The greater choleretic potency of BSP and ioglycamide compared with taurocholate may be explained by a higher osmotic activity. This is even more marked with iodipamide, which "obligates" 22 μl of bile/μmol[123]; however, its osmotic activity in bile (1.5 mosm/mmol) is only twice as great as that of taurocholate (0.8 mosm/mmol). The reason for the apparent "extra" water is not clear: it could be due to stimulation of an inorganic solute pump, modifications of canalicular permeability, generation of an electrical potential with subsequent passive movement of ions, or a combination of these mechanisms.

Increased bile flow has been induced by fluorescein in the rat, by phenol red in the chicken, and by phloridzin in the chicken and in the dog.[327] Rose bengal increased bile flow in dogs but reduced it in rabbits.[73] In contrast to its choleretic action in the dog, BSP has been shown to reduce bile flow in the rat.[74,159,272,309] Anticholeresis in the rat by indocyanine green has also been reported.[159,183] The mechanism of action is examined below.

Bilirubin in physiologic doses does not seem to cause choleresis[341]; this is possibly due to the fact that the osmotic load is low and to the incorporation of bilirubin into micelles, with loss of osmotic activity. Choleresis after infusion of bilirubin in quantities close to its Tm has been recorded.[362] Reproduction of this experiment in our laboratory showed the choleretic response to be transitory and followed by a decrease in flow.

Organic Cations

Organic cations are also excreted into bile.[184,303] Their transport process appears to be different from that which secretes organic anions. Their effect on choleresis, if any, has not been documented.

Neutral Substances

Many substances other than organic anions or cations are excreted into bile and increase choleresis. Although they include compounds as chemically disparate as polyethylene glycol 1500,[327] ferrioxamine derivatives,[240] and ouabain,[154] they may be grouped into two categories: neutral substances excreted into bile in the form of metabolites, chiefly glucuronides, including 4-methylumbelliferone,[126,127,215] dihydroxy-dibutyl-ether,[60] and probably many of the commercial choleretics; and neutral substances excreted into bile unconverted into anionic compounds. For some of them, such as dihydroxy-dibutyl-ether,[60] a correlation has been found between bile flow and the biliary output of the substance. This suggests that these compounds also increase bile flow by an osmotic mechanism.

Effect of Bile Acids on the Biliary Secretion of Organic Anions

Bile acid administration is usually associated with an increase in the Tm into bile of organic anions such as

BSP,[3,35,74,157,255,285] indocyanine green,[351] iopanoic acid,[21,248] bilirubin,[152] and ampicillin.[234] Four explanations may be considered to explain such an effect: a role of bile flow, a sequestration of the agent in micelles formed by the bile acid, a direct effect of the bile acid on the organic anion carrier, or a recruitment of transporting hepatocytes under the influence of the bile acid. There is evidence that the increase in Tm is not related to the increase in flow: canalicular choleresis induced by agents other than bile acids, such as theophylline,[15,112] 4-methyl-umbelliferone,[112] and the bicyclic organic anion SC 2644,[21,142] has no influence on the Tm of BSP or iopanoic acid. Incorporation into mixed micelles has been shown to occur *in vitro*[304,351] and may serve as a micellar "sink"[304]; however, no correlation has been found *in vivo* between incorporation into micelles and the effect of several bile acids on the Tm of various compounds.[351] Moreover, dehydrocholate and its metabolites, which have no or little micelle-forming capacity, increase BSP Tm to the same extent as micelle-forming bile acids.[24,74,285,350] In contrast, glycodihydrofusidate, a steroid compound that forms mixed micelles *in vitro* and is excreted into bile, did not increase BSP Tm in the hamster.[70] Therefore, it seems more likely that bile acids increase the biliary Tm of other organic anions by a direct action on the transport system of these agents. The theoretic possibilities are that (1) the active transport of bile acids provides the driving force for other organic anions by a cotransport system; (2) bile acids modify, possibly in an allosteric way, the carrier of the other organic anions[133]; (3) bile acids increase, by a recruitment process, the number of hepatocytes available for transport. Available kinetic data do not allow us to distinguish among these possibilities at the present time.

Anticholeretic Effect of Organic Anions

Administration of taurolithocholate or taurocholenate to rats and hamsters decreases bile flow and bile acid secretion and leads to the electron microscopic changes of cholestasis.[191,301] The diminution of bile flow can be prevented or corrected by administration of taurocholate or taurochenodeoxycholate. A similar effect has been observed with the water-soluble conjugates tauro-3β-hydroxy-5-cholenoate-3-sulfate[237] and lithocholate glucuronide.[250] The mechanism is poorly understood. Several possibilities have been proposed: precipitation of taurolithocholate in the canaliculi (because of its low water solubility) with resultant canalicular obstruction[188]; decrease in bile acid–independent flow, as suggested in the hamster[204]; toxic effect of the bile acid on membrane structure, as suggested by scanning electron microscopic observations[225]; and intracellular calcium binding[251] with alteration of cellular transport processes. Cholestasis may be induced by other bile acids, such as chenodeoxycholic acid in the rat,[241,242] or even taurocholate when given at rates above its biliary Tm.[311]

Some of the anionic dyes used for investigation of liver function are anticholeretic when given in high doses. Bile flow in rabbits is lowered by the phthalein dye rose bengal[73]; BSP and indocyanine green have been shown to reduce bile flow in the rat.[74,159,183,272,309] These effects have been attributed, at least in part, to inhibition of bile acid–independent bile formation.[78,183]

Bile Acid–Independent Flow

Evidence and Estimation

In all animal species studied, plots of bile acid secretion rates against bile flow[23,29,32,88,109,268,270,271,308] and against erythritol or mannitol clearance[29,31,32,110,231,268,338,361] yield a positive intercept upon extrapolation to the flow axis (Fig. 3-7). The extrapolated value of erythritol clearance at zero bile acid secretion is generally regarded as estimating the bile acid–independent fraction of canalicular bile. Its actual amount differs from species to species: in microliters min$^1 \cdot$ kg b. wt.$^{-1}$, it was about 5 in dogs,[361] 70 in rats,[23] 60 in rabbits,[110] 7 in rhesus monkeys,[338] and 1.5 to 2 in humans.[31,231,268]

This procedure, however, rests on the assumption that the osmotic activity of bile acids does not increase when their concentration falls below the critical micellar concentration. Testing this assumption requires examination of the relation between bile flow and bile acid secretion at low bile acid concentrations and secretion rates. In the isolated perfused rat liver, linearity seems to extend into the critical range,[29,32] and the intercept measured in this preparation correlates well with the value calculated by extrapolation. In the rat *in vivo*, however, careful analysis of this relation has revealed a variation of the slope with bile acid concentration[10]: the slope, expressed in microliters of bile per micromole of bile acid, decreased from 90 at concentrations below 10 mM, to 12 at concentrations between 30 to 45 mM. This suggests that quantitation of the bile acid–independent flow by the extrapolation procedure may be subject to error.

More convincing evidence for canalicular flow-generating mechanisms independent of bile acid secretion comes from the study of drugs that increase in parallel bile flow and erythritol clearance, without modifying bile acid secretion rate. These include phenobarbital and other barbiturates,[23,207,259] theophylline[111] and glucagon,[202] hydrocortisone,[93,232] and SC 2644[357] (see below). With the possible exception of hydrocortisone, neither these drugs themselves nor their metabolites are excreted into bile in sufficient amounts to provide an osmotic driving force. They do not seem to increase the osmotic activity of the bile acids, as estimated by the slope of the bile flow–bile acid secretion plot,[23,207,259] or the permeability of the canalicular membrane or tight junction to water and ions, as estimated by the bile-to-plasma concentration ratio of sucrose.[357] The most reasonable hypothesis to explain the effect of these compounds on bile flow is that they stimulate the transport into bile of some other solute (or solutes), probably inorganic electrolytes. Sodium transport linked to Na^+,K^+-ATPase[29,105,110,113,114,153] and, more recently, bicarbonate transport[169] have been implicated as possible mediators and are now examined in light of how certain drugs affect bile formation. The mechanisms of electrolyte transport by the liver and their possible role in bile acid–independent bile formation have been discussed in several reviews.[104,153,306]

Role of Sodium Transport

Active sodium transport occurs through most cell plasma membranes; it is associated with a membrane-bound enzyme, Na^+,K^+-ATPase.[310,321] In isolated cells, extrusion of sodium is coupled with entry of potassium and does not generate osmotic water flow. However, in transporting epithelia, Na^+,K^+-ATPase has been implicated in various secretions and is thought to generate water flow by local osmosis. Plasma membranes of hepatocytes[33,99] have been shown to contain Na^+,K^+-ATPase. The localization of the enzyme on the membrane is discussed below. Several lines of indirect evidence suggest that it is implicated in the generation of bile flow.

Inhibitors of Sodium Transport. Three inhibitors of sodium transport, ouabain, ethacrynic acid, and amiloride, diminished or suppressed the bile acid–independent flow when injected into the portal vein of anesthetized rabbits.[110,113,114] Scillaren had the same effect in the isolated perfused liver.[29] Interpretation of *in vivo* experiments with these agents may be difficult, however, because ouabain[216] and ethacrynic acid metabolites[55,209] are excreted into bile by concentrative processes and may produce an osmotic choleresis. This choleresis may mask, in part or in totality, their possible inhibitory effects. Indeed, in subsequent experiments, both ouabain and ethacrynic acid have been reported to induce choleresis in various species[55,154,209,317] and, with ethacrynic acid, a linear relation between drug excretion and erythritol clearance has been observed.[55] Thus, the effect of these agents in any given experimental situation will probably depend on the relative contribution of the inhibitory and osmotic stimulatory effects.

Estrogen. Cholestasis has been observed in both rats and humans after treatment with estrogens.[138,171,174,214,246] The mechanism is not fully understood. It has been shown with ethinyl estradiol in rats that the decrease in bile flow was due mainly to a decrease in the bile acid–independent flow,[162] although a diminution of the bile acid Tm and a moderate diminution of bile acid secretion were also observed. Inhibition of Na^+,K^+-ATPase activity in liver plasma membranes *in vitro* has been reported,[173] whereas steroids having no effect on Na^+,K^+-ATPase had no effect on bile flow.[173] Subsequent experiments *in vivo* with estrogen-treated rats have shown a parallel decrease in Na^+,K^+-ATPase activity in liver cell plasma membranes and in bile acid–independent bile flow.[65,279] It is noteworthy that a decrease in bile acid–independent bile flow and Na^+,K^+-ATPase activity has also been reported during

pregnancy.[282] The mechanism of the decrease in enzyme activity may be an alteration of the lipid composition of the membrane.[65] These observations suggest that estrogen-induced cholestasis may be initiated by a failure of the sodium pump. In estrone-treated rats, increases in the bile-to-plasma concentration ratio of sucrose and in sucrose biliary clearance have been reported.[130] This suggests that the decreased flow may be due, at least in part, to increased permeability of the biliary system, leading to an increased "back-diffusion" of bile. These two proposed mechanisms are not necessarily mutually exclusive. It should be noted, however, that increased permeability may also be observed during bile acid–induced choleresis,[224] and its contribution to cholestasis, although still a possibility, requires further evaluation.

Phenobarbital. Phenobarbital, when given to rats for 3 or 4 days, results in an increase in bile flow[172,205,229,286] due solely to an increase in the bile acid–independent flow, with no change in bile acid secretion[23,207,260] or in the relative outputs of individual bile acids.[260] When given to rats for 7 days[160] or to rhesus monkeys for 14 days,[276] it also stimulates bile acid secretion. Again, studies *in vivo* in phenobarbital-treated rats have shown parallel increases in bile flow and Na^+,K^+-ATPase activity in liver cell plasma membranes,[279,319] although two previous experiments did not detect any effect of phenobarbital on the activity of the enzyme.[34,217] The increase in activity is suppressed by inhibitors of protein synthesis, suggesting that it is due to enhanced synthesis.[321]

Phenobarbital has a number of other effects on the liver and on biliary function.[47] It decreases serum bilirubin concentration in patients with familial nonhemolytic hyperbilirubinemia[62,366]; it may improve cholestasis, especially in children[316,332,344]; and it enhances the biliary clearance and elimination of certain dyes.[206,210] The relation of these effects to the stimulation of bile flow is, at present, unclear. It is apparent, however, that the effect on bile flow is not related to the induction of microsomal drug-metabolizing enzymes because (1) other microsomal enzyme inducers do not affect bile flow[205]; (2) pentobarbital may increase bile flow without producing any detectable microsomal enzyme induction[48]; and (3) inhibition of microsomal enzyme induction by SKF-525A or cobaltous chloride does not suppress the effect of phenobarbital on bile flow.[56]

Thyroid Hormones. Bile flow is reduced in hypothyroid rats[139] because of a decrease in bile acid–independent bile flow[222]; a parallel decrease in Na^+,K^+-ATPase activity in liver plasma membranes is observed.[222] Administration of L-thyroxine restores both bile flow and Na^+,K^+-ATPase levels to normal. Animals made hyperthyroid by administration of L-3,5,3'-triiodothyronine have an increased bile acid–independent flow (as well as an increase in bile acid secretion) and a parallel increase in plasma membrane Na^+,K^+-ATPase activity.[222]

Chlorpromazine. In the rhesus monkey, chlorpromazine hydrochloride infused intravenously in pharmacologic doses results in a dose-dependent inhibition of the bile acid–independent flow.[287] It also inhibits both Mg^{2+} and Na^+,K^+-ATPase in liver plasma membranes in a dose-dependent fashion.[298] The inhibition is reduced by glutathione and enhanced when chlorpromazine semiquinone free-radical formation is increased, observations that may explain in part the irregular appearance of chlorpromazine-induced cholestasis in humans.

Location of Sodium Transport. The localization of transport Na^+,K^+-ATPase on the hepatocyte plasma membrane is not firmly established. A simple view of sodium pumping into the canalicular lumen would require the enzyme to be located on the canalicular ("mucosal") site of the membrane, facing secretion. However, in most epithelia, the enzyme appears to be situated on the basolateral ("serosal") site of the epithelial cell.[118,119,273] Cytochemical[25,220] and biochemical[239,266] studies have also supported a basolateral site (i.e., sinusoidal and intercellular) of the hepatocyte Na^+,K^+-ATPase. This localization appears paradoxical because the enzyme is oriented in the wrong direction to transport sodium into the canalicular lumen. This apparent paradox, however, extends to many secretory organs, in particular osmoregulatory organs with high Na^+,K^+-ATPase activity.[118,119,121,200,273] A Na^+,K^+-ATPase orientation opposite the direction of net electrolyte and water secretion is therefore consistent with a role of this enzyme in bile formation. Moreover, experiments using labeled monoclonal[307] or polyclonal[342] antibodies have suggested that the enzyme was also present on the canalicular membrane. It should be clear, however, that the mechanism of coupling of enzyme to net electrolyte and water transport into bile remains to be elucidated. Among the theoretic possibilities are secondary transport of other electrolytes along the electrical gradient created by sodium extrusion; establishment of a standing gradient within the intercellular space, followed by an osmotic flow through the relatively leaky junctional complexes; and direct pumping of sodium across the canalicular membrane. None of these possibilities has yet been tested, although a paracellular sodium movement from the sinusoids to the canalicular lumen has been suggested.[155]

Attempts have also been made to localize sites of origin of the bile acid–independent flow within the hepatic lobule. After selective destruction of centrilobular hepatocytes by bromobenzene, canalicular bile flow decreased, with no change in bile acid secretion.[161] This suggests that centrilobular hepatocytes contribute predominantly to the secretion of the bile acid–independent fraction at physiologic bile acid loads.

Other Possible Mechanisms

Bicarbonate Transport. In the isolated perfused rat liver, perfusion with a bicarbonate-free solution reduced the bile acid–independent flow by 50%.[169] Under this condition, bicarbonate secretion was nearly eliminated, whereas sodium secretion was markedly reduced. In contrast, administration of SC-2644 to dogs increased canalicular bile flow and bicarbonate concentration in bile.[17] These observations led to the suggestion that a bicarbonate transport mechanism may have a role in the elaboration of the bile acid–independent flow. As noted above, ursodeoxycholate and 7-ketolithocholate increase bicarbonate secretion as well as canalicular bile flow, an effect possibly related to stimulation of the bicarbonate transport system by these bile acids. The cellular mechanism remains to be elucidated. In other epithelia, such as the kidney tubule or the pancreas, bicarbonate transport has been attributed to the activity of a Na^+/H^+ exchange system (antiport) on the opposite membrane. An amiloride hydrochloride-sensitive Na^+/H^+ antiport, again energized by the sodium gradient, has been found on the sinusoidal membrane of rat hepatocytes.[6] Its role in bicarbonate transport remains to be established. An alternative mechanism could be a canalicular bicarbonate-sensitive ATPase. Attempts to demonstrate a bicarbonate-sensitive ATPase in liver cell plasma membranes have thus far been unsuccessful,[169,187] although a bicarbonate-stimulated ATPase activity of bovine liver alkaline phosphatase has been demonstrated.[59]

Effect of Other Pharmacologic Agents. Cyclic 3',5'-adenosine monophosphate (cAMP) is known to increase sodium transport. It stimulates choleresis in dogs by increasing the bile acid–independent flow.[244] Theophylline and glucagon, which increase the intracellular concentration of cAMP, also increase bile flow in dogs and in humans.[16,95,111,194,202,244,245] This has led to the suggestion that cAMP may play a role in bile formation, perhaps by regulating electrolyte transport. In a systematic study of liver cAMP in rats and dogs, however, no correlation could be found between cAMP content and choleresis during administration of theophylline, methyl isobutylxanthine, dibutyryl cAMP, or glucagon.[265] Therefore the role of the cAMP system in bile formation is still uncertain. It is also claimed to have a role in secretin-induced choleresis.[228] Prostaglandins A_1, E_1, and E_2 increase bile flow in dogs, rats, and cats.[199,213,221] In the rat this effect appears to be due to stimulation of bile acid–independent bile formation,[199,221] whereas in the cat, available data suggest an inhibition of fluid reabsorption by the bile ducts.[213] The cellular mechanisms are not known. Somatostatin decreases bile flow in the dog,[163,281] probably mostly by enhanced ductular reabsorption, an effect opposite to that of secretin.[281] *Salicylates* are choleretics in dogs and rats,[43,45,107,295] also by stimulation of bile acid–independent flow.[107] Choleresis is due, in part, to their secretion into bile and osmotic activity.

In summary, flow-generating mechanisms that cannot be attributed to the active transport of bile acids are present in the canaliculi. Flow due to these mechanisms is generally referred to as bile acid–independent canalicular bile flow. Suggestive evidence has accumulated in favor of a role of Na^+,K^+-ATPase–mediated ion transport. Bicarbonate transport, although as yet less clearly characterized, may also play a role.

A schematic representation of transport systems that probably participate in the generation of bile flow is shown in Figure 3-8.

Role of Microfilaments and Microtubules

There is circumstantial evidence that microfilament dysfunction may alter bile formation. Cytochalasin B, an agent that destroys microfilaments, causes cholestasis in the isolated rat liver preparation.[261] Phalloidin, a cyclic peptide isolated from the mushroom *Amanita phalloides,* which accelerates the polymerization of actin into microfilaments, induces a decrease in bile flow in rats.[90,346] At the same time, a proliferation of the microfilamentous network is seen.[90,137] The decrease in bile flow is parallel to the increase in microfilaments,[90] suggesting a causal relationship between the cholestasis and the changes in microfilaments. The morphologic appearance of the canaliculi in this model, with dilatation of the lumen, loss of microvilli, and increased thickness of the pericanalicular microfilamentous network,[90] resembles that observed in human cholestasis. The mechanism of phalloidin-induced cholestasis is not known. It has been proposed that cholestasis may be related to the loss of the normal canalicular architecture needed for the generation of local osmotic fluid flow.[103]

Alternatively, microfilaments may be responsible for canalicular "contractions," as suggested by experiments on hepatocyte cultures[262,263,355] and, to some extent, *in vivo.* Paralysis of these contractions may result in cholestasis. Finally, it has also been shown that phalloidin increases biliary permeability to sucrose and inulin,[90,97] suggesting a microfilament-mediated change in junctional permeability.

Agents interfering with microtubules have variable effects on bile formation. In the rat *in vivo,* colchicine has been reported to have no effect on basal bile flow[91,328] and

to decrease bile acid–stimulated bile flow.[91] In the isolated rat liver preparation, antimicrotubular agents have been reported to decrease bile flow and biliary phospholipid secretion.[156] The role of microtubules in bile formation, if any, remains to be established.

SECRETION AND ABSORPTION IN THE BILE DUCTS

Secretion (Ductular/Ductal Bile Acid–Independent Flow)

The earliest indication that secretion may occur in the bile ductules and ducts was obtained in isolated segments of canine bile duct[289]; it has been confirmed by studies using the hormone secretin, which has long been known to possess choleretic activity,[19] and by observing secretion in isolated segments of bile duct.[52,53,247]

The choleretic action of secretin has been demonstrated in cats,[314] dogs,[194,195,271,360] guinea pigs,[128] rhesus monkeys,[338] baboons,[228] humans,[158,275,353] and in the isolated perfused pig liver.[166] It appears not to occur in the rabbit[314] or the rat,[67] although increased bile flow rates have been reported after infusion of secretin into the hepatic arterial circulation of the rat[8] and after intravenous injections in rabbits.[120]

Secretin choleresis is generally accompanied by changes in bile composition, chiefly a rise in bicarbonate (and *p*H) and a fall in bile acids.[271,314,360] Bicarbonate and chloride concentrations of about 120 mEq and 50 mEq/liter, respectively, were found in the secretin-stimulated bile fraction from the perfused pig liver.[167] Intraduodenal infusion of hydrochloric acid in dogs induces the same choleretic response as exogenous secretin,[271] an effect probably due to endogenous secretin release. Endogenous secretin release is thought to be responsible for spontaneous variations of "basal" bile flow in dogs and is blocked by

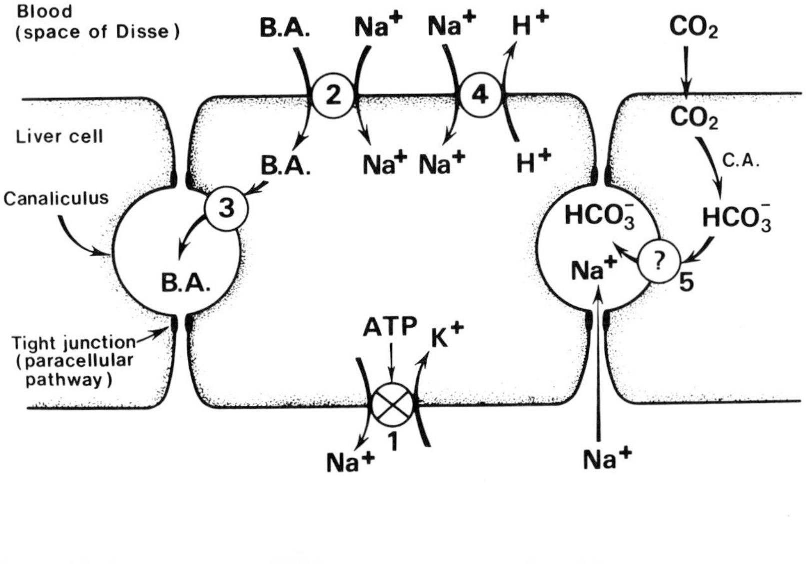

Fig. 3-8. Transport systems of hepatocytes important for bile flow: (*1*) the Na^+,K^+-ATPase, or sodium pump; (*2*) the bile acid/sodium symport system; (*3*) the canalicular bile acid carrier system; (*4*) the Na^+/H^+ antiport; (*5*) the bicarbonate transport system (not precisely characterized), possibly a Cl^-/HCO_3 antiport.

administration of pipenzolate methylbromide, an anticholinergic drug.[360]

Several lines of evidence support the view that secretin acts chiefly on the duct system and not on the hepatocyte. (1) The choleretic response to secretin was greater when it was infused into the hepatic artery (which provides the main blood supply to the bile ducts) than when it was infused into the portal system.[358] (2) The biliary "wash-out volume" during constant-rate BSP infusion was less during secretin choleresis than during bile acid choleresis, a finding that suggests that secretin acts distal to the canaliculi.[358] (3) Biliary clearances of erythritol and mannitol are increased during bile acid choleresis and not during secretin choleresis, as discussed above.[128,361] In the rabbit, isolated segments of bile duct secreted electrolyte solutions isotonic with plasma, in vivo[52] and in vitro[53]: the secretion was inhibited by 2,4-dinitrophenol.[53] An isolated segment of canine bile duct likewise secreted 0.55 ml to 0.81 ml of an electrolyte solution per hour.[247]

Secretin is the only hormone or agent known thus far to stimulate bile duct secretory activity. Gastrin also increased choleresis in dogs,[196,368] although pentagastrin had no effect.[198] Gastrin choleresis was associated with an increase in concentration and output of bicarbonate.[368] Study of an isolated segment of dog bile duct after intravenous administration of synthetic gastrin suggested that the site of action of gastrin on bile flow may be the bile ducts.[247]

The secretory activity of the bile ductules and ducts explains the choleresis that occurs in certain diseases. Elevated bile flows have been recorded in patients with cirrhosis or other chronic liver diseases associated with ductular proliferation.[51,226] An increased response to secretin in these patients suggests a ductular/ductal origin for the increased bile flow.[28] High bile flows have also been reported in patients with congenital dilatation of the intrahepatic biliary tree.[117,348] An augmented surface of the biliary epithelium is common to these conditions. Ductular cell proliferation induced experimentally by α-naphthylisothiocyanate and by ethionine is also associated with increased bile flow and increased capacity of the biliary tree.[14,147,264]

Reabsorption

The bile ductules and/or ducts appear also to be capable of a reabsorptive function. This was suggested by study of bile composition in cholecystectomized dogs[360]; bile stored in the common bile duct of fasting animals was similar in composition to typical gallbladder bile. Bile-to-plasma concentration ratios above unity in the steady state, which were found for mannitol in the dog,[361] for erythritol in the rabbit,[110] occasionally for mannitol or erythritol in the rat,[222,302] and for erythritol in the rhesus monkey,[338] strongly suggest water reabsorption in the ductal/ductular system, since neither of these solutes is thought to be transported by active concentrative processes. As indicated above, somatostatin is apparently ca-

pable of enhancing reabsorption by the bile ducts or ductules, an effect opposite that of secretin.[163,281] Structural evidence that absorption can take place in human bile ductules has been obtained in cholestasis from various causes.[300] The relative importance of these two processes—secretion and absorption—probably varies during the day in the normal person but has not been quantitated precisely.

OTHER FACTORS

Insulin and Vagal Stimulation

Insulin increases bile flow and, more specifically, the canalicular bile acid–independent fraction.[11,136,193,292] The mechanism is unknown. It does not seem to be mediated by hypoglycemia and vagus nerve stimulation: in the dog, truncal vagotomy has variable effects on insulin-induced choleresis,[136,141,197] whereas in the rat, 2-deoxy-D-glucose and acetylcholine, two vagal stimulants, have no effect on bile flow.[68]

Vascular Factors

Bile flow was largely unaffected by variations in blood flow rates in the isolated perfused rat liver.[39,41] However, a small decrease in bile acid–independent bile formation has been recorded in the isolated rat liver perfused at a low rate,[343] possibly as a consequence of regional alterations of perfusion. End-to-side portacaval anastomosis and arterialization of the portal circulation were without effect on bile flow in dogs[125]; in rats, an end-to-side portacaval shunt caused a reduction of the canalicular bile acid–independent bile flow,[175,267] together with a reduction in liver weight. Pronounced decrease in bile flow has been recorded to result from acute hepatic ischemia[39,100] and from acute increase in hepatic venous pressure.[269]

Ethanol

Acute ethanol administration in the isolated rat liver impaired bile flow and excretion of BSP and indocyanine green.[212] In contrast, the long-term feeding of ethanol to rats was associated with a moderate increase in canalicular bile flow and bile acid excretion.[30]

Other Drugs

Diuretics other than amiloride and ethacrynic acid have variable effects on bile flow. Spironolactone increases canalicular bile acid–independent bile formation,[370] an effect that resembles that of phenobarbital and is likewise associated with an increase in liver weight. Furosemide may decrease or increase bile flow.[84,320]

Various hypolipidemic drugs[230,290,291] have been shown to increase bile flow; the choleresis is bile acid–independent and associated with increased liver weight.

Carbonic anhydrase inhibitors cause a rise in biliary chloride concentration in dogs and humans.[235,258,353,360] Their effect on bile flow is controversial.

BILIARY SECRETION IN HUMANS

The existence of the processes described above is inferred largely from studies of various animal species. However, available data suggest that similar processes may operate in humans. As noted above, there is a linear relationship between bile flow and bile acid secretion and between erythritol (or mannitol) clearance and bile acid secretion.[31,231,268] The mean rate of secretion of canalicular bile is 11 μl/μmol bile acid. In the presence of an intact enterohepatic circulation, a mean of approximately 15 μmol of bile acid is secreted per minute, giving a mean bile acid–dependent flow of 0.15 ml to 0.16 ml/minute. The estimated canalicular bile acid–independent flow is 0.16 ml to 0.17 ml/minute, and the estimated ductular/ductal secretion is about 0.11 ml/minute. These studies point to a daily production of bile of approximately 600 ml. The contribution of each fraction of bile flow (canalicular bile acid–dependent, canalicular bile acid–independent, ductal/ductular) is shown in Figure 3-9. Similar values have been obtained in patients with T-tubes in the common bile duct.[345,353] However, under physiologic conditions, the volume of bile reaching the duodenum depends on the production of hepatocyte bile, which itself depends in part on the rate at which the bile acid pool circulates within the enterohepatic circulation; reabsorption in the gallbladder and bile ducts; and secretion in the ductules or ducts, which depends on endogenous secretin.

FUNCTIONS OF BILE AND ALTERATIONS OF BILE SECRETION

The major function of bile is the efficient absorption of dietary fat from the gut lumen. Bile salt molecules, with lecithin and cholesterol, first adsorb to the surface of fat (triglyceride) globules and provide stable emulsification. This is followed by micellar solubilization. The micelle is composed of bile salt, lecithin, and cholesterol; upon action of pancreatic lipases, triglycerides are transformed into fatty acids and monoglycerides, and the micelles change their composition into bile salt, cholesterol, fatty acid, monoglyceride, lecithin, lysolecithin, and diglyceride. Micellar solubilization serves essentially to facilitate diffusion of these products (as well as liposoluble vitamins or drugs) through the unstirred water layer at the intestinal surface. After passive absorption into the enterocyte, triglycerides and lecithin are resynthesized, and chylomicrons and very low density lipoproteins are formed (with specific apoproteins). These are transported into the lymphatics by exocytosis. It has been estimated that, by these processes, the bile salt pool is able to transport 25 times its weight of fat from intestinal lumen to lymph each day.

In addition, as seen above, bile salts are one of the major driving forces for bile formation. Bile serves as an important excretory pathway for degradation products, such as bilirubin, drug and hormone metabolites, and other organic compounds.

In the large intestine, the dihydroxy bile acids induce fluid secretion and probably increase motility. Altered bile acid metabolism may have clinical significance in syndromes of diarrhea[179] and constipation.

Finally, bile acids have an important role in sterol, particularly cholesterol, homeostasis.[347] Cholesterol is an essential constituent of living tissues, as a structural component of most biologic membranes and as a precursor of vitamins and hormones. Cholesterol can be acquired from the environment by the diet and by *de novo* synthesis from acetylcoenzyme A. Usually more cholesterol enters the body through these two mechanisms than is used during normal metabolism. The excess must be metabolized or excreted to prevent a potentially harmful accumulation. Transformation of cholesterol into bile acids is a major pathway of cholesterol catabolism. Thus bile acids are the principal water-soluble excretory products of cholesterol, and they serve to disperse and transport their precursor.

Altered bile secretion is observed in two major clinical situations: cholestasis and gallstones. Cholestasis, or bile secretory failure, is the result of obstruction of extrahepatic bile ducts (extrahepatic cholestasis), obstruction of intrahepatic bile ducts, or failure of the hepatocyte to secrete bile (intrahepatic cholestasis), the mechanisms of which are incompletely understood. The proposed mechanisms, which have been discussed above, include[106]: inhibition of Na^+,K^+-ATPase; increased permeability of the paracellular pathway with back-diffusion (leakage) of bile constituents into plasma; altered microfilament function with possibly decreased canalicular "contractions"; and de-

Fig. 3-9. Components of bile flow in humans. Values are derived from measurements in patients with T-tubes after cholecystectomy.

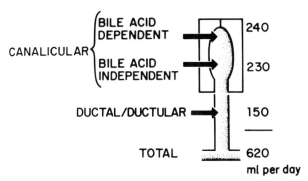

creased intracellular calcium concentration. Gallstone formation results from precipitation of cholesterol (cholesterol gallstones) or bile pigment (pigment stones) into bile. Cholesterol gallstones are the most prevalent in western countries. Many are due to excessive cholesterol secretion into bile, which may be related, in part, to increased cholesterol synthesis by the liver. This results in supersaturation of bile with cholesterol, followed by precipitation and nucleation of cholesterol crystals. Stone growth is promoted by continuous further aggregation of cholesterol crystals.

SUMMARY OF PROCESSES IN BILE FLOW

Bile is an osmotic aqueous solution of bile acids, cholesterol, phospholipids, bile pigments, and inorganic electrolytes. It is secreted by the hepatocytes into the bile canaliculi and modified in the bile ductules or ducts. The three main processes identified in bile flow are shown in Figure 3-10. They are defined as follows:

1. *Concentrative secretion of bile acids* by the hepatocytes, responsible for the bile acid–dependent fraction of canalicular bile flow. Coupling between water flow and bile acid secretion is probably effected mainly through an osmotic mechanism. Because the osmotic activity of the bile acid anions is reduced by their aggregation into micelles, the major component of the osmotic gradient is probably provided by counterions. There is suggestive evidence that water flows through the intercellular junctions. The bile acid–dependent fraction accounts for 30% to 60% of spontaneous basal bile flow.

2. *A canalicular bile acid–independent secretion,* probably driven by Na^+,K^+-ATPase–mediated ion transport (and possibly other inorganic ion pumps) and stimulated by phenobarbital. It has been suggested that bile acids may also have some influence on this fraction of bile flow. It represents 30% to 60% of basal bile flow.

   Normal canalicular bile flow may also depend on the integrity of intracellular organelles, mainly pericanalicular microfilaments.

3. *Reabsorption and secretion* of fluid and inorganic electrolytes by the ductules or ducts. Secretion occurs chiefly in response to secretin and represents 30% of basal bile flow in humans.

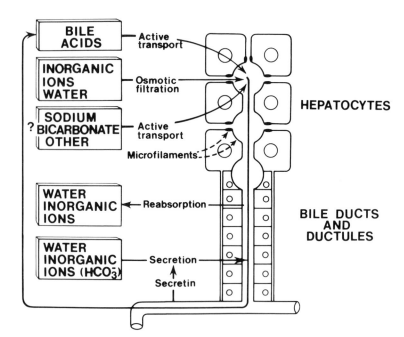

Fig. 3-10. Schematic view of bile secretion. Canalicular bile flow includes bile formed in response to active bile acid transport (bile acid-dependent flow) and in response, probably, to active secretion of inorganic electrolytes. Water and inorganic ions enter into the canalicular lumen by osmotic filtration, probably through the paracellular pathway. Microfilaments are important for normal canalicular flow. Canalicular bile is modified in the ductules or ducts, or both, by net reabsorption and secretion of water and inorganic ions.

REFERENCES

1. Accatino L, Simon FR: Identification and characterization of a bile acid receptor in isolated liver surface membranes. J Clin Invest 57:496, 1976

2. Adler RD, Wannagat FJ, Ockner RK: Bile secretion in selective biliary obstruction: Adaptation of taurocholate transport maximum to increased secretory load in the rat. Gastroenterology 73:129, 1977

3. Alpert S, Mosher M, Shanske A et al: Multiplicity of hepatic excretory mechanisms for organic anions. J Gen Physiol 53:238, 1969

4. Anwer MS, Kroker R, Hegner D: Cholic acid uptake into isolated rat hepatocytes. Hoppe-Seyler's Z Physiol Chem 357:1477, 1976

5. Arias IM, Fleischner G, Listowski I et al: Ligandin structure and function. In Bianchi L, Gerok W, Sickinger K (eds): Liver and Bile, pp 157–166. Lancaster, MTP Press, 1977

6. Arias IM, Forgeac M: The sinusoidal domain of the plasma membrane of rat hepatocytes contains an amiloride-sensitive Na^+/H^+ antiport. J Biol Chem 259:5406, 1984

7. Ashworth CT, Sanders E: Anatomic pathway of bile formation. Am J Pathol 37:343, 1960

8. Back DJ, Calvey TN: Infusion of secretin into the hepatic arterial circulation of the rat. J Physiol 219:14, 1971

9. Baker AL, Wood RAB, Moossa AR et al: Sodium taurocholate modifies the bile acid–independent fraction of canalicular bile flow in the rhesus monkey. J Clin Invest 64:312, 1979

10. Balabaud C, Kron KA, Gumucio JJ: The assessment of the bile salt–nondependent fraction of canalicular bile water in the rat. J Lab Clin Med 89:393, 1977

11. Baldwin J, Heer FW, Albo R et al: Effect of vagus nerve stimulation on hepatic secretion of bile in human subjects. Am J Surg 11:66, 1966

12. Barber–Riley G: Rat biliary tree during short periods of obstruction of common duct. Am J Physiol 205:1127, 1963

13. Barber–Riley G: The rate of biliary secretion during flow up vertical cannulas of different bore. Experientia 20:639, 1964

14. Barber–Riley G: Biliary capacity in rats following ethionine ingestion. Am J Physiol 214:133, 1968

15. Barnhart JL, Combes B: Effect of theophylline on hepatic excretory function. Am J Physiol 227:194, 1974

16. Barnhart JL, Combes B: Characteristics common to choleretic increments of bile induced by theophylline, glucagon and SQ-20009 in the dog. Proc Soc Exp Biol Med 150:591, 1975

17. Barnhart JL, Combes B: Characterization of SC 2644-induced choleresis in the dog: Evidence for canalicular bicarbonate secretion. J Pharmacol Exp Ther 206:190, 1978

18. Barnhart JL, Combes B: Erythritol and mannitol clearances with taurocholate and secretin-induced choleresis. Am J Physiol 234:E146, 1978

19. Bayliss WM, Starling EH: The mechanism of pancreatic secretion. J Physiol 28:325, 1902

20. Becker JS, Oliver JM, Berlin RD: Fluorescence techniques for following interactions of microtubules subunits and membranes. Nature 254:152, 1975

21. Berk RN, Golberger LE, Loeb PM: The role of bile salts in the hepatic excretion of iopanoic acid. Invest Radiol 9:7, 1974

22. Berry MN, Friend DS: High-yield preparation of isolated rat liver parenchymal cells: A biochemical and fine structural study. J Cell Biol 43:506, 1969

23. Berthelot P, Erlinger S, Dhumeaux D et al: Mechanism of phenobarbital-induced hypercholeresis in the rat. Am J Physiol 219:809, 1970

24. Binet S, Delage Y, Erlinger S: Influence of taurocholate, taurochenodeoxycholate, and taurodehydrocholate on sulfobromophthalein transport into bile. Am J Physiol 236:E10, 1979

25. Blitzer BL, Boyer JL: Cytochemical localization of Na^+,K^+-ATPase in the rat hepatocyte. J Clin Invest 62:1104, 1978

26. Blitzer BL, Boyer JL: Cellular mechanisms of bile formation. Gastroenterology 82:346, 1982

27. Blitzer BL, Donovan CB: A new method for the rapid isolation of basolateral plasma membrane vesicles from rat liver: Characterization, validation, and bile acid transport studies. J Biol Chem 259:9295, 1984

28. Bode C, Zelder O, Goebell H et al: Choleresis induced by secretin: Distinctly increased response in cirrhotics. Scand J Gastroenterol 7:697, 1972

29. Boyer JL: Bile formation in the isolated perfused rat liver. Am J Physiol 221:1156, 1971

30. Boyer JL: Effect of chronic ethanol feeding on bile formation and secretion of lipids in the rat. Gastroenterology 62:294, 1972

31. Boyer JL, Bloomer JR: Canalicular bile secretion in man: Studies utilizing the biliary clearance of [^{14}C]mannitol. J Clin Invest 54:773, 1974

32. Boyer JL, Klatskin G: Canalicular bile flow and bile secretory pressure: Evidence for a non–bile salt dependent fraction in the isolated perfused rat liver. Gastroenterology 59:853, 1970

33. Boyer JL, Reno D: Properties of $(Na^+ + K^+)$-activated ATPase in rat liver plasma membranes enriched with bile canaliculi. Biochim Biophys Acta 401:59, 1975

34. Boyer JL, Reno D, Layden T: Bile canalicular membrane Na^+,K^+-ATPase: The relationship of enzyme activity to the secretion of bile salt independent canalicular flow. In Leevy CM (ed): Diseases of the Liver and Biliary Tract, pp 198–212. Basel, Karger, 1976

35. Boyer JL, Scheig RL, Klatskin G: The effect of sodium taurocholate on the hepatic metabolism of sulfobromophthalein sodium (BSP): The role of bile flow. J Clin Invest 49:206, 1970

36. Boyer JL, Schwarz J, Smith N: Biliary secretion in elasmobranchs: I. Bile collection and composition. Am J Physiol 230:970, 1976

37. Bradley SE, Herz R: Permselectivity of biliary canalicular membrane in rats: Clearance probe analysis. Am J Physiol 235:E570, 1978

38. Brauer RW: Mechanisms of bile secretion. JAMA 169:1462, 1959

39. Brauer RW: Hepatic blood supply and the secretion of bile. In Taylor W (ed): The Biliary System, pp 41–67. Oxford, Blackwell, 1965

40. Brauer RW, Leong GF, Holloway RJ: Mechanics of bile secretion: Effect of perfusion pressure and temperature on bile flow and bile secretion pressure. Am J Physiol 177:103, 1954

41. Brauer RW, Pessotti RL, Pizzolato P: Isolated rat liver preparation: Bile production and other basic properties. Proc Soc Exp Biol Med 78:174, 1951

42. Briscoe AM, Ragan C: Bile and endogenous fecal calcium in man. Am J Clin Nutr 16:281, 1965

43. Bullock GR, Delaney VB, Sawyer BC et al: Biochemical and structural changes in rat liver resulting from the parenteral administration of a large dose of sodium salicylate. Biochem Pharmacol 19:245, 1970

44. Burnett W: The pathogenesis of gall stones. In Taylor W (ed): The Biliary System, pp 601–618. Oxford, Blackwell, 1965

45. Buttar HS, Coldwell BB, Thomas BH: The effect of salicylate on the biliary excretion of ^{14}C-bishydroxy-coumarin in rat. Br J Pharmacol 48:278, 1973

46. Cahill GF Jr, Ashmore J, Earle AS: Glucose penetration into liver. Am J Physiol 192:491, 1958

47. Capron JP, Dumont M, Feldmann G et al: Barbiturate-induced choleresis: Possible independence from microsomal enzyme induction. Digestion 15:556, 1977

48. Capron JP, Erlinger S: Barbiturates and biliary function. Digestion 12:43, 1975

49. Carey MC: The enterohepatic circulation. In Arias I, Popper H, Schachter D et al (eds): The Liver: Biology and Pathobiology, pp 429–465. New York, Raven Press, 1982

50. Carey MC, Small DM: Micelle formation by bile salts: Physical-chemical and thermodynamic considerations. Arch Intern Med 130:506, 1972

51. Caroli J, Tanasoglu Y: Le temps d'apparition de la bromesulfonephtaléine dans la bile: Nouveau test pour le diagnostic des ictères incomplets par rétention et des blocages anictériques de la voie biliaire principale. Sem Hôp Paris 29:591, 1953

52. Chenderovitch J: Transport d'eau et d'électrolytes dans le cholédoque du lapin "in vivo." Rev Eur Etud Clin Biol 16:591, 1971

53. Chenderovitch J: Secretory function of the rabbit common bile duct. Am J Physiol 223:695, 1972

54. Chenderovitch J, Phocas E, Rautureau M: Effects of hypertonic solutions on bile formation. Am J Physiol 205:863, 1963

55. Chenderovitch J, Raizman A, Infante R: Mechanism of ethacrynic acid–induced choleresis in the rat. Am J Physiol 229:1180, 1975

56. Chivrac D, Dumont M, Erlinger S: Lack of parallelism between microsomal enzyme induction and phenobarbital-induced hypercholeresis in the rat. Digestion 17:516, 1978

57. Claude P, Goodenough DA: Fracture faces of zonulae occludentes from "tight" and "leaky" epithelia. J Cell Biol 58:390, 1973

58. Cook DL, Beach DA, Bianchi RG et al: Factors influencing bile flow in the dog and rat. Am J Physiol 163:688, 1950

59. Corbic M, de Couët G, Bertrand O et al: Bicarbonate-stimulated ATPase activity of bovine liver alkaline phosphatase. J Hepatol 1:167, 1985

60. Corbic M, Dumont M, de Couët G et al: Choleretic and diuretic properties of dihydroxydibutyl ether in the rat. J Pharmacol Exp Ther 221:769, 1982

61. Crane RK: The gradient hypothesis and other models of carrier-mediated active transport. Rev Physiol Biochem Pharmacol 78:99, 1977

62. Crigler JF Jr, Gold NI: Sodium phenobarbital-induced decrease in serum bilirubin in an infant with congenital nonhemolytic jaundice and kernicterus. J Clin Invest 45:998, 1966

63. Cummings SA, Hofmann AF: Physiologic determinants of biliary calcium secretion in the dog. Gastroenterology 87:664, 1984

64. Curran PF, McIntosh JR: A model system for biological water transport. Nature 193:347, 1962

65. Davis RA, Kern F Jr, Showalter R et al: Alterations of hepatic Na^+,K^+-ATPase and bile flow by estrogen: Effects on liver surface membrane lipid structure and function. Proc Natl Acad Sci USA 75:4130, 1978

66. Debray C, Besançon F: Le débit et la pression au cours de l'obstruction biliaire graduée chez le rat. Rev Int Hepat 11:49, 1961

67. Debray C, de la Tour J, Rozé C et al: Independence from vagal control of biliary secretion in the rat. Digestion 10:413, 1974

68. Debray C, Vaille C, de la Tour J et al: Action des sécrétines du commerce sur la sécrétion pancréatique externe du rat. J Physiol 54:549, 1962

69. Delacroix DL, Hodgson HJF, McPherson A et al: Selective transport of polymeric immunoglobulin A in bile: Quantitative relationships of monomeric and polymeric immunoglobulin A, immunoglobulin M, and other proteins in serum, bile, and saliva. J Clin Invest 70:230, 1982

70. Delage Y, Dumont M, Erlinger S: Effect of glycodihydrofusidate on sulfobromophthalein transport maximum in the hamster. Am J Physiol 231:1875, 1976

71. Desjeux JF, Dumont M, Erlinger S: Métabolisme et influence sur la sécrétion biliaire du dehydrocholate chez le chien. Biol Gastroentérol 6:9, 1973

72. Desmet VJ. Anatomy I: Hepatocyte-canaliculus. In Bianchi L, Gerok W, Sickinger K (eds): Liver and Bile, pp 3–31. London, MTP Press, 1977

73. Dhumeaux D, Berthelot P, Préaux AM et al: A critical study of the concept of maximal biliary transport of sulfobromophthalein (BSP) in the Wistar rat. Rev Europ Etud Clin Biol 15:279, 1970

74. Dhumeaux D, Erlinger S, Benhamou JP et al: Effects of rose bengal on bile secretion in the rabbit: Inhibition of a bile salt–independent fraction. Gut 11:134, 1970

75. Diamond JM: The reabsorptive function of the gallbladder. J Physiol 161:442, 1962

76. Diamond JM: The mechanism of water transport by the gallbladder. J Physiol 161:503, 1962

77. Diamond JM: The mechanisms of isotonic water transport. J Gen Physiol 48:15, 1964

78. Diamond JM: Tight and leaky junctions of epithelia: A perspective on kisses in the dark. Fed Proc 33:2220, 1974

79. Diamond JM, Bossert WH: Standing-gradient osmotic flow: A mechanism for coupling of water and solute transport in epithelia. J Gen Physiol 60:2061, 1967

80. Diamond JM, Tormey JM: Studies on the structural basis of water transport across epithelial membranes. Fed Proc 25:1458, 1966

81. Diamond JM, Tormey JM: Role of long extracellular channels in fluid transport across epithelia. Nature 210:817, 1966

82. Dietschy JM: Mechanisms for the intestinal absorption of bile acids. J Lipid Res 9:297, 1968

83. Dietschy JM, Moore EW: Diffusion potentials and potassium distribution across the gallbladder wall. J Clin Invest 43:1551, 1964

84. Di Padova C, Zuin M, Bellomi M et al: Choleretic and anticholeretic effects of furosemide in the rat. Ital J Gastroenterol 10:92, 1978

85. Dive C, Heremans JF: Nature and origin of the proteins of bile: I. A comparative analysis of serum and bile proteins in man. Eur J Clin Invest 4:235, 1974

86. Dive C, Nadalini RA, Vaerman JP et al: Origin and nature of the proteins of bile: II. A comparative analysis of serum, hepatic lymph and bile proteins in the dog. Eur J Clin Invest 4:241, 1974

87. Donovan AJ, Child MA, Masto AS: The effect of hepatic venous obstruction on the rate of flow of bile. Surg Gynecol Obstet 134:89, 1972

88. Dowling RH, Mack E, Picott J et al: Experimental model for the study of the enterohepatic circulation of bile in rhesus monkeys. J Lab Clin Med 72:169, 1968

89. Dowling RH, Mack E, Small DM: Biliary lipid secretion and bile composition after acute and chronic interruption of the entero-hepatic circulation in the rhesus monkey: IV. Primate biliary physiology. J Clin Invest 50:1917, 1971

90. Dubin M, Maurice M, Feldmann G et al: Phalloidin-induced cholestasis in the rat: Relation to changes in microfilaments. Gastroenterology 75:450, 1978

91. Dubin M, Maurice M, Feldmann G et al: Influence of colchicine and phalloidin on bile secretion and hepatic ultrastructure in the rat: Possible interaction between microtubules and microfilaments. Gastroenterology 79:646, 1980

92. Duffy MC, Blitzer BL, Boyer JL: Direct determination of the driving forces for taurocholate uptake into rat liver plasma membrane vesicles. J Clin Invest 72:1470, 1983

93. Dumont M, Erlinger S: Influence of hydrocortisone on bile formation in the rat. Biol Gastroenterol 6:197, 1973

94. Dumont M, Uchman S, Erlinger S: Hypercholeresis induced by ursodeoxycholic acid and 7-ketolithocholic acid in the rat: Possible role of bicarbonate transport. Gastroenterology 79:82, 1980

95. Dyck WP, Janowitz HD: Effect of glucagon on hepatic bile secretion in man. Gastroenterology 60:400, 1971

96. Elias H: A re-examination of the structure of the mammalian liver: II. The hepatic lobule and its relation to the vascular and biliary systems. Am J Anat 85:379, 1949

97. Elias E, Hruban Z, Wade JB et al: Phalloidin-induced cholestasis: A microfilament-mediated change in junctional complex permeability. Proc Natl Acad Sci USA 77:2229, 1980

98. Elias H, Petty D: Terminal distribution of the hepatic artery. Anat Rec 116:9, 1953

99. Emmelot P, Bos CJ, Benedetti EL et al: Studies on plasma membranes: I. Chemical composition and enzyme content of plasma membranes isolated from rat liver. Biochim Biophys Acta 90:126, 1964

100. Engstrand L: Bile secretion and hepatic nitrogen metabolism in relation to variations of blood and oxygen supply to the liver. Acta Chir Scand 146(suppl):1, 1949

101. Erlinger S: Les mecanismes de la sécrétion biliaire. Rev Int Hepat 18:1, 1968

102. Erlinger S: Influence of drugs on bile flow. Isr J Med Sci 10:354, 1974

103. Erlinger S: Cholestasis: Pump failure, microvilli defect of both? Lancet 1:533, 1978

104. Erlinger S: Hepatocyte bile secretion: Current views and controversies. Hepatology 1:352, 1981

105. Erlinger S: Does Na$^+$-K$^+$-ATPase have any role in bile secretion? Am J Physiol 243:G243, 1982

106. Erlinger S: What is cholestasis in 1985? J Hepatol 1:687, 1985

107. Erlinger S, Bienfait D, Poupon R et al: Effect of lysine acetylsalicylate on biliary lipid secretion in dogs. Clin Sci Mol Med 49:253, 1975

108. Erlinger S, Dhumeaux D: Mechanisms and control of secretion of bile water and electrolytes. Gastroenterology 66:281, 1974

109. Erlinger S, Dhumeaux D, Benhamou JP et al: La sécrétion biliaire du lapin: Preuves en faveur d'une importante fraction indépendante des sels biliaires. Rev Fr Etud Clin Biol 14:144, 1969

110. Erlinger S, Dhumeaux D, Berthelot P et al: Effect of inhibitors of sodium transport on bile formation in the rabbit. Am J Physiol 219:416, 1970

111. Erlinger S, Dumont M: Influence of theophylline on bile formation in the dog. Biomedicine 19:27, 1973

112. Erlinger S, Dumont M: Influence of canalicular bile flow on sulfobromophthalein transport maximum in bile in the dog. In Paumgartner G, Preisig R (eds): The Liver: Quantitative Aspects of Structure and Function, pp 306–313. Basel, Karger, 1973

113. Erlinger S, Dumont M, Benhamou JP: Effets de l'ouabaine sur la sécrétion biliaire du lapin. Rev Fr Etud Clin Biol 14:1007, 1969

114. Erlinger S, Dumont M, Benhamou JP: Effect of inhibitors of sodium transport on bile formation in the rabbit. Nature 223:1276, 1969

115. Erlinger S, Dumont M, Zouboulis-Vafiadis I et al: The importance of conjugation in biliary secretion of ursodeoxycholate and 7-ketolithocholate in the rat. Clin Sci 487, 1984

116. Erlinger S, Glasinovic JC, Poupon R et al: Hepatic transport of bile acids. In Taylor W (ed): The Hepatobiliary System, pp 433–447. New York, Plenum Press, 1976

117. Erlinger S, Sakellaridis D, Maillard JN et al: Les formes angiocholitiques de la fibrose hépatique congénitale. Press Med 77:1189, 1969

118. Ernst SA: Transport adenosine triphosphatase cytochemistry: II. Cytochemical localization of ouabain-sensitive, potassium-dependent phosphatase activity in the secretory epithelium of the avian salt gland. J Histochem Cytochem 20:23, 1972

119. Ernst SA, Mills JW: Basolateral plasma membrane localization of ouabain-sensitive transport sites in the secretory epithelium of the avian salt gland. J Cell Biol 75:74, 1977

120. Esteller A, Lopez MA, Murillo A: The effect of secretin and cholecystokinin-pancreozymin on the secretion of bile in the anaesthetized rabbit. Q J Exp Physiol 62:363, 1977

121. Eveloff J, Karnaky KJ Jr, Silva P et al: Elasmobranch rectal gland cell: Autoradiographic localization of [^{3}H]ouabain-sensitive Na,K-ATPase in rectal gland of dogfish, *squalus acanthias.* J Cell Biol 83:16, 1979

122. Farquhar M, Palade G: Junctional complexes in various epithelia. J Cell Biol 17:375, 1963

123. Feld GK, Loeb PM, Berk RN et al: The choleretic effect of iodipamide. J Clin Invest 55:528, 1975

124. Fink S: Studies on hepatic bile obtained from a patient with an external biliary fistula: Its composition and changes after diamox administration. N Engl J Med 254:258, 1956

125. Fisher B, Lee SH, Fedor EJ: Effect of permanent alteration of hepatic blood flow upon biliary secretion. Arch Surg 76:41, 1958

126. Fontaine L, Belleville M, Lechevin JC et al: Etude du métabolisme de la méthyl-4-ombelliferone sur l'animal et chez l'homme. Thérapie 23:373, 1968

127. Fontaine L, Grand M, Molho D et al: Activités cholérétiques et spasmolytique: Pharmacologie générale de la méthyl-4-ombelliférone. Thérapie 23:51, 1968

128. Forker EL: Two sites of bile formation as determined by

mannitol and erythritol clearance in the guinea-pig. J Clin Invest 46:1189, 1967

129. Forker EL: Bile formation in guinea-pigs: Analysis with inert solutes of graded molecular radius. Am J Physiol 215: 56, 1968

130. Forker EL: The effect of estrogen on bile formation in the rat. J Clin Invest 48:654, 1969

131. Forker EL: Hepatocellular uptake of inulin, sucrose and mannitol in rats. Am J Physiol 219:1568, 1970

132. Forker EL: Mechanisms of hepatic bile formation. Annu Rev Physiol 39:323, 1977

133. Forker EL, Gibson G: Interaction between sulfobromophthalein (BSP) and taurocholate: The kinetics of transport from liver cells to bile in rats. In Paumgartner G, Preisig R (eds): The Liver: Quantitative Aspects of Structure and Function, pp 326–335. Basel, S Karger, 1973

134. Forker EL, Hicklin T, Sornson H: The clearance of mannitol and erythritol in rat bile. Proc Soc Exp Biol Med 126: 115, 1967

135. Friend DS, Gilula NB: Variations in tight and gap junctions in mammalian tissues. J Cell Biol 53:758, 1972

136. Fritz ME, Brooks FP: Control of bile flow in the cholecystectomized dog. Am J Physiol 204:825, 1963

137. Gabbiani G, Montesano R, Tuchweber B et al: Phalloidin-induced hyperplasia of actin filaments in rat hepatocytes. Lab Invest 33:562, 1975

138. Gallagher TF, Mueller MN, Kappas A: Estrogen pharmacology: IV. Studies on the structural basis for estrogen-induced impairment of liver function. Medicine 45:471, 1966

139. Gartner LM, Arias IM: Hormonal control of hepatic bilirubin transport and conjugation. Am J Physiol 222:1091, 1972

140. Gebhardt R, Jung W: Biliary secretion of sodium fluorescein in primary monolayer cultures of adult rat hepatocytes and its stimulation by nicotinamide. J Cell Sci 56:233, 1982

141. Geist RE, Jones RS: Effect of selective and truncal vagotomy on insulin-stimulated bile secretion in dogs. Gastroenterology 60:566, 1971

142. Gibson GE, Forker EL: Canalicular bile flow and bromosulfophthalein transport maximum: The effect of a bile salt independent choleretic, SC 2644. Gastroenterology 66: 1046, 1974

143. Gilman A, Cowgill GR: Osmotic relations between blood and body fluids: IV. Pancreatic juice, bile and lymph. Am J Physiol 104:476, 1933

144. Glasinovic JC, Dumont M, Duval M et al: Hepatocellular uptake of taurocholate in the dog. J Clin Invest 55:419, 1975

145. Glasinovic JC, Dumont M, Duval M et al: Hepatocellular uptake of bile acids in the dog: Evidence for a common carrier-mediated transport system: An indicator dilution study. Gastroenterology 69:973, 1975

146. Glasinovic JC, Dumont M, Duval M et al: Hepatocellular uptake of erythritol, mannitol and sucrose in the dog. Am J Physiol 229:1455, 1975

147. Goldfarb S, Singer EJ, Popper H: Biliary ductules and bile secretion. J Lab Clin Med 62:608, 1963

148. Goldman IS, Jones AL, Hradek GT et al: Hepatocyte handling of immunoglobulin A in the rat: The role of microtubules. Gastroenterology 85:130, 1983

149. Gonzalez MC, Sutherland E, Simon FR: Regulation of hepatic transport of bile salts: Effect of protein synthesis inhibition on excretion of bile salts and their binding to liver surface membrane fractions. J Clin Invest 63:684, 1969

150. Goresky CA: The hepatic uptake and excretion of sulfobromophthalein and bilirubin. Can Med Assoc J 92:851, 1965

151. Goresky CA, Bach GB, Nadeau BE: On the uptake of materials by the intact liver: The transport and net removal of galactose. J Clin Invest 52:991, 1973

152. Goresky CA, Haddad HH, Kluger WS et al: The enhancement of maximal bilirubin excretion with taurocholate-induced increments in bile flow. Can J Physiol Pharmacol 52:389, 1974

153. Graf J: Canalicular bile salt–independent bile formation: Concepts and clues from electrolyte transport in rat liver. Am J Physiol 244:G233, 1983

154. Graf J, Korn P, Peterlik M: Choleretic effect of ouabain and ethacrynic acid in the isolated perfused rat liver. Naunyn-Schmiedebergs Arch Pharmacol 272:230, 1972

155. Graf J, Peterlik M: Ouabain-mediated sodium uptake and bile formation by isolated perfused rat liver. Am J Physiol 230:876, 1976

156. Gregory DH, Vlahcevic ZR, Prugh MF et al: Mechanism of secretion of biliary lipids. Role of a microtubular system in hepatocellular transport of biliary lipids in the rat. Gastroenterology 74:93, 1978

157. Gronwall R, Cornelius CE: Maximal biliary excretion of sulfobromophthalein sodium in sheep. Am J Dig Dis 15: 37, 1970

158. Grossman MI, Janowitz HD, Ralston H: The effect of secretin on bile formation in man. Gastroenterology 12:133, 1949

159. Groszmann RJ, Kotelanski B, Kendler J et al: Effect of sulfobromophthalein and indocyanine green on bile excretion. Proc Soc Exp Biol Med 132:712, 1969

160. Gumucio JJ, Accatino L, Macho AM et al: Effect of phenobarbital on the ethynyl estradiol–induced cholestasis in the rat. Gastroenterology 65:651, 1973

161. Gumucio JJ, Balabaud C, Miller DL et al: Bile secretion and liver cell heterogeneity in the rat. J Lab Clin Med 91: 350, 1978

162. Gumucio JJ, Valdivieso VD: Studies on the mechanism of ethynylestradiol impairment of bile flow in the rat. Gastroenterology 61:339, 1971

163. Hanks JB, Kortz WJ, Andersen DK et al: Somatostatin suppression of canine fasting bile secretion. Gastroenterology 84:130, 1983

164. Hardison WGM: Metabolism of sodium dehydrocholate by the rat liver: Its effect on micelle formation in bile. J Lab Clin Med 77:811, 1971

165. Hardison WGM, Apter JT: Micellar theory of biliary cholesterol excretion. Am J Physiol 222:61, 1972

166. Hardison WGM, Norman JC: Effect of bile salt and secretin upon bile flow from the isolated perfused pig liver. Gastroenterology 53:412, 1967

167. Hardison WGM, Norman JC: Electrolyte composition of the secretin fraction of bile from the perfused pig liver. Am J Physiol 214:758, 1968

168. Hardison WGM, Norman JC: Effect of secretin on bile osmolality. J Lab Clin Med 73:34, 1969

169. Hardison WGM, Wood CA: Importance of bicarbonate in bile salt independent fraction of bile flow. Am J Physiol 235:E158, 1978

170. Hardwicke J, Rankin JG, Baker KJ et al: The loss of protein in human and canine hepatic bile. Clin Sci 26:509, 1964

171. Harkavy M, Javitt NB: Effect of ethynyl estradiol on hepatic excretory function of the rat. In Salhanic HA, Kipnis DM, Van de Wielde RL (eds): Metabolic Effects of Gonadal

Hormones and Contraceptive Steroids, pp 11–18. New York, Plenum Press, 1960

172. Hart LG, Guarino AM, Adamson RH: Effects of phenobarbital on biliary excretion of organic acids in male and female rats. Am J Physiol 217:46, 1969

173. Heikel TAJ, Lathe GH: The effect of 17-ethinyl-substituted steroids on adenosine triphosphatases of rat liver plasma membrane. Biochem J 118:187, 1970

174. Heikel TAJ, Lathe GH: The effect of oral contraceptive steroids on bile secretion and bilirubin Tm in rats. Br J Pharmacol 38:593, 1970

175. Herz R, Paumgartner G, Preisig R: Bile salt metabolism and bile formation in the rat with a portacaval shunt. Eur J Clin Invest 4:223, 1974

176. Himes JA, Bruss ML, Simpson CF et al: Hypercholeresis in turkeys following the ingestion of crotolaria spectabilis seeds. Cornell Vet 66:551, 1976

177. Hoenig V, Preisig R: Organic-anionic choleresis in the dog: Comparative effects of bromsulfalein, ioglycamide and taurocholate. Biomedicine 18:23, 1973

178. Hofmann AF: Biliary lipid secretion in man. In Bianchi L, Gerok W, Sickinger K (eds): Liver and Bile, pp 101–118. Lancaster, MTP Press, 1977

179. Hofmann AF: The enterohepatic circulation of bile acids in man. Clin Gastroenterol 6:3, 1977

180. Hofmann AF: Chemistry and enterohepatic circulation of bile acids. Hepatology 4:4S, 1984

181. Hofmann AF, Molino G, Milanese M et al: Description and simulation of a physiological pharmacokinetic model for the metabolism and enterohepatic circulation of bile acids in man: Cholic acid in healthy man. J Clin Invest 71:1003, 1983

182. Hofmann AF, Small DM: Detergent properties of bile salts: Correlation with physiological function. Annu Rev Med 18:333, 1967

183. Horak W, Grabner G, Paumgartner G: Inhibition of bile salt–independent bile formation by indocyanine green. Gastroenterology 64:1005, 1973

184. Hunter A, Klaassen CD: Species differences in the plasma disappearance and biliary excretion of procaine amide ethobromide. Proc Soc Exp Biol Med 139:1445, 1972

185. Inoue M, Kinne R, Tran T et al: Taurocholate transport by rat liver sinusoidal membrane vesicles: Evidence of sodium cotransport. Hepatology 2:572, 1982

186. Inoue M, Kinne R, Tran T et al: Taurocholate transport by rat liver canalicular membrane vesicles: Evidence for the presence of an Na^+-independent transport system. J Clin Invest 73:659, 1984

187. Izutsu KT, Siegel IA, Smuckler EA: HCO_3-ATPase activity distribution in rat liver cell fractions prepared by zonal centrifugation. Experientia 34:731, 1978

188. Javitt NB: Current status of cholestasis induced by monohydroxylated bile acids. In Goresky CA, Fisher MM (eds): Jaundice, pp 401–509. New York, Plenum Press, 1975

189. Javitt NB: Hepatic bile formation. N Engl J Med 295:1464, 1469, 1511, 1976

190. Javitt NB, Dillon D, Kok E et al: Mechanisms of bile formation: Transcellular and paracellular pathways. In Preisig R, Bircher J (eds): The Liver: Quantitative Aspects of Structure and Function, pp 197–202. Aulendorf, Editio Cantor, 1979

191. Javitt NB, Emerman S: Effect of sodium taurolithocholate on bile flow and bile acid excretion. J Clin Invest 47:1002, 1968

192. Jones AL, Hradek GT, Renston RH et al: Autoradiographic evidence for hepatic lobular concentration gradient of bile acid derivative. Am J Physiol 238:G233, 1980

193. Jones RS: Effect of insulin on canalicular bile formation. Am J Physiol 231:4043, 1976

194. Jones RS, Geist RE, Hall AD: The choleretic effects of glucagon and secretin in the dog. Gastroenterology 60:64, 1971

195. Jones RS, Grossman MI: Choleretic effects of secretin and histamine in the dog. Am J Physiol 217:532, 1969

196. Jones RS, Grossman MI: Choleretic effects of cholecystokinin, gastrin II and caerulein in the dog. Am J Physiol 219:1014, 1970

197. Jones RS, Smith BM: The effect of truncal vagotomy on taurocholate choleresis and secretin choleresis. J Surg Res 23:149, 1977

198. Kaminski DL, Rose RC, Nahrwold DL: Effect of pentagastrin on canine bile flow. Gastroenterology 64:630, 1973

199. Kaminski DL, Ruwart M, Willman VL: The effect of prostaglandin A_1 and E_1 on canine hepatic bile flow. J Surg Res 18:391, 1975

200. Karnaky KJ Jr, Kinter LB, Kinter WB et al: Teleost chloride cell: II. Autoradiographic localization of gill Na,K-ATPase in killifish *Fundulus heteroclitus* adapted to low and high salinity environments. J Cell Biol 70:157, 1976

201. Kay RE, Entenman C: Stimulation of taurocholic acid synthesis and biliary excretion of lipids. Am J Physiol 200:855, 1961

202. Khedis A, Dumont M, Duval M et al: Influence of glucagon on canalicular bile production in the dog. Biomedicine 21:176, 1974

203. King JE, Oshiba S, Schoenfield LJ: Bile secretion in isolated hamster liver. J Appl Physiol 28:495, 1970

204. King JE, Schoenfield LJ: Cholestasis induced by sodium taurolithocholate in isolated hamster liver. J Clin Invest 50:2305, 1971

205. Klaassen CD. Biliary flow after microsomal enzyme induction. J Pharmacol Exp Ther 168:218, 1969

206. Klaassen CD: Plasma disappearance and biliary excretion of sulfobromophthalein and phenol-3,6-dibromphthalein disulfonate after microsomal enzyme induction. Biochem Pharmacol 19:1241, 1970

207. Klaassen CD: Studies on the increased biliary flow produced by phenobarbital in rats. J Pharmacol Exp Ther 176:743, 1971

208. Klaassen CD: Bile flow and composition during bile acid depletion and administration. Can J Physiol Pharmacol 52:334, 1974

209. Klaassen CD, Fitzgerald TJ: Metabolism and biliary excretion of ethacrynic acid. J Pharmacol Exp Ther 191:548, 1974

210. Klaassen CD, Plaa GL: Studies on the mechanism of phenobarbital-enhanced sulfobromophthalein disappearance. J Pharmacol Exp Ther 161:361, 1968

211. Klaassen CD, Watkins JB III: Mechanisms of bile formation, hepatic uptake, and biliary excretion. Pharmacol Rev 36:1, 1984

212. Kotelanski B, Groszmann RJ, Kendler J: Effect of ethanol on sulfobromophthalein and indocyanine green metabolism in isolated perfused rat liver. Proc Soc Exp Biol Med 132:715, 1969

213. Krarup N, Larsen JA, Munck A: Secretin-like choleretic effect of prostaglandins E_1 and E_2 in cats. J Physiol 254:813, 1976

214. Kreek MJ, Peterson RE, Sleisenger MH et al: Influence of ethinyl estradiol-induced cholestasis on bile flow and biliary

excretion of estradiol and bromosulfophthalein by the rat. (abstr). J Clin Invest 46:1080 1967

215. Kroker R, Anwer MS, Hegner D: Characterization of methylumbelliferone (Mendiaxon®)-induced choleresis in the isolated perfused rat liver. Acta Hepatogastroenterol 24:348, 1977

216. Kupferberg HJ, Schanker LS: Biliary secretion of ouabain-^{3}H and its uptake by liver slices in the rat. Am J Physiol 214:1048, 1968

217. Laperche Y, Launay A, Oudea P et al: Effects of phenobarbital and rose bengal on the ATPases of plasma membranes of rat and rabbit liver. Gut 13:920, 1972

218. LaRusso NF: Proteins in bile: How they get there and what they do. Am J Physiol 247:G199, 1984

219. LaRusso NF, Fowler S: Coordinate secretion of acid hydrolases in rat bile: Hepatocyte exocytosis of lysosomal protein? J Clin Invest 64:948, 1979

220. Latham PS, Kashgarian M: The ultrastructural localization of transport ATPase in the rat liver at non-bile canalicular plasma membranes. Gastroenterology 76:988, 1979

221. Lauterburg B, Paumgartner G, Preisig R: Prostaglandin-induced choleresis in the rat. Experientia 31:1191, 1975

222. Layden TJ, Boyer JL: The effect of thyroid hormone on bile salt–independent bile flow and Na$^+$,K$^+$-ATPase activity in liver plasma membranes enriched in bile canaliculi. J Clin Invest 57:1009, 1976

223. Layden TJ, Boyer JL: Influence of bile acids on bile canalicular membrane morphology and the lobular gradient in canalicular size. Lab Invest 39:110, 1978

224. Layden TJ, Elias E, Boyer JL: Bile formation in the rat: The role of the paracellular shunt pathway. J Clin Invest 62:1375, 1978

225. Layden TJ, Schwarz J, Boyer JL: Scanning electron microscopy of the rat liver: Studies of the effect of taurolithocholate and other models of cholestasis. Gastroenterology 69:724, 1975

226. Lenthall J, Reynolds TB, Donovan AJ: Excessive output of bile in chronic hepatic disease. Surg Gynecol Obstet 130:243, 1970

227. Levi AJ, Gatmaitan Z, Arias IM: Two hepatic cytoplasmic protein fractions, Y and Z, and their possible role in the hepatic uptake of bilirubin, sulfobromophthalein, and other anions. J Clin Invest 48:2156, 1969

228. Levine RA, Hall RC: Cyclic AMP in secretin choleresis: Evidence for a regulatory role in man and baboons but not in dogs. Gastroenterology 70:537, 1976

229. Levine WG, Braunstein IR, Meijer DKF: Effect of nafenopin (SU-13,437) on liver function: Mechanism of choleretic effect. Naunyn Schmiedebergs Arch Pharmacol 290:221, 1975

230. Levine WG, Millburn P, Smith RL et al: The role of the hepatic endoplasmic reticulum in the biliary excretion of foreign compounds by the rat: The effect of phenobarbitone and SKF 525-A (diethylaminoethyldiphenylpropylacetate). Biochem Pharmacol 19:235, 1970

231. Lindblad L, Scherstén T: Influence of cholic and chenodeoxycholic acid on canalicular bile flow in man. Gastroenterology 70:1121, 1976

232. Macarol V, Morris TQ, Baker KJ et al: Hydrocortisone choleresis in the dog. J Clin Invest 49:1714, 1970

233. Maffly RH, Leaf A: The potential of water in mammalian tissues. J Gen Physiol 42:1257, 1959

234. Mandiola S, Johnson BL, Winters RE et al: Biliary excretion of ampicillin in the anesthetized dog: I. Effect of serum ampicillin concentration, taurocholate infusion rate, biliary secretion pressure, and secretin infusion. Surgery 71:664, 1972

235. Maren TH, Ellison AC, Fellner SK et al: A study of hepatic carbonic anhydrase. Mol Pharmacol 2:144, 1966

236. Matern S, Gerok W: Pathophysiology of the enterohepatic circulation of bile acids. Rev Physiol Biochem Pharmacol 85:126, 1979

237. Mathis U, Karlaganis G, Preisig R: Monohydroxy bile salt sulfates: Tauro-3β-hydroxy-5-cholenoate-3-sulfate induced intrahepatic cholestasis in rats. Gastroenterology 85:674, 1983

238. Meier PJ, St. Meier–Abt A, Barrett C et al: Mechanisms of taurocholate transport in canalicular and basolateral rat liver plasma membrane vesicles. J Biol Chem 259:10614, 1984

239. Meier PJ, Sztul ES, Reuben A et al: Structural and functional polarity of canalicular and basolateral plasma membrane vesicles isolated in high yield from rat liver. J Cell Biol 98:991, 1984

240. Meyer–Brunot HG, Keberle H: Biliary excretion of ferrioxamines of varying liposolubility in perfused rat liver. Am J Physiol 214:1193, 1968

241. Miyai K, Fisher MM: The hepatotoxicity of chenodeoxycholic acid. Gastroenterology (abstr) 60:189, 1971

242. Miyai K, Price VM, Fisher MM: Bile acid metabolism in mammals: Ultrastructural studies on the intrahepatic cholestasis induced by lithocholic and chenodeoxycholic acids in the rat. Lab Invest 24:292, 1971

243. Moore EW, Dietschy JM: Na and K activity coefficients in bile and bile salts determined by glass electrodes. Am J Physiol 206:1111, 1964

244. Morris TQ: Choleretic responses to cyclic AMP and theophylline in the dog (abstr.). Gastroenterology 62:187, 1972

245. Morris TQ, Sardi GF, Bradley SE: Character of glucagon-induced choleresis (abstr). Fed Proc 26:774, 1967

246. Mueller MN, Kappas A: Estrogen pharmacology: I. The influence of estradiol and estriol on hepatic disposal on sulfobromophthalein (BSP) in man. J Clin Invest 43:1905, 1964

247. Nahrwold DL, Shariatzedeh AN: Role of the common bile duct in formation of bile and in gastrin-induced choleresis. Surgery 70:147, 1971

248. Nelson JA, Staubus AE, Riegelman S: Saturation kinetics of iopanoate in the dog. Invest Radiol 10:371, 1975

249. Nicholls RJ: Biliary mannitol clearance and bile salt output before and during secretin choleresis in the dog. Gastroenterology 76:983, 1979

250. Oelberg DG, Chari MV, Little JM et al: Lithocholate glucuronide is a cholestatic agent. J Clin Invest 73:1507, 1984

251. Oelberg DG, Dubinsky WP, Adcock EW et al: Calcium binding by lithocholic acid derivatives. Am J Physiol 247:G112, 1984

252. O'Maille ERL, Kozmary SV, Hofmann AF et al: Differing effects of norcholate and cholate on bile flow and biliary lipid secretion in the rat. Am J Physiol 246:G67, 1984

253. O'Maille ERL, Richards TG: The secretory characteristics of dehydrocholate in the dog: Comparison with the natural bile salts. J Physiol 261:337, 1976

254. O'Maille ERL, Richards TG, Short AH: Acute taurine depletion and maximal rates of hepatic conjugation and secretion of cholic acid in the dog. J Physiol 180:67, 1965

255. O'Maille ERL, Richards TG, Short AH: Factors determining the maximal rate of organic anion secretion by the liver

and further evidence on the hepatic site of action of the hormone secretin. J Physiol 186:424, 1966

256. O'Maille ERL, Richards TG, Short AH: The influence of conjugation of cholic acid on its uptake and secretion: Hepatic extraction of taurocholate and cholate in the dog. J Physiol 189:337, 1967

257. Oschman JL, Berridge MJ: The structural basis of fluid secretion. Fed Proc 30:49, 1971

258. Pak BH, Hong SS, Pak HK et al: Effect of acetazolamide and acid-base changes on biliary and pancreatic secretion. Am J Physiol 210:624, 1966

259. Paumgartner G, Horak W, Probst P et al: Effect of phenobarbital on bile flow and bile salt excretion in the rat. Naunyn-Schmiedebergs Arch Pharmacol 270:98, 1971

260. Paumgartner G, Reichen J: Different pathways for hepatic uptake of taurocholate and indocyanine green. Experientia 31:306, 1975

261. Phillips MJ, Oda M, Mak E et al: Microfilament dysfunction as a possible cause of intrahepatic cholestasis. Gastroenterology 69:48, 1975

262. Phillips MJ, Oshio C, Miyairi M et al: A study of bile canalicular contractions in isolated hepatocytes. Hepatology 2:763, 1982

263. Phillips MJ, Oshio C, Miyairi M et al: Intrahepatic cholestasis as a canalicular motility disorder: Evidence using cytochalasin. Lab Invest 48:205, 1983

264. Popper H: Roles of the bile ductules in bile formation. Am J Med Sci 242:519, 1961

265. Poupon RE, Dol ML, Dumont M et al: Evidence against a physiological role of cAMP in choleresis in dogs and rats. Biochem Pharmacol 27:2413, 1978

266. Poupon RE, Evans WH: Biochemical evidence that Na$^+$,K$^+$-ATPase is located at the lateral region of the hepatocyte surface membrane. FEBS Lett 108:374, 1979

267. Prandi D, Dumont M, Erlinger S: Influence of portacaval shunt on bile formation in the rat. Eur J Clin Invest 4:197, 1974

268. Prandi D, Erlinger S, Glasinovic JC et al: Canalicular bile production in man. Eur J Clin Invest 5:1, 1975

269. Preisig R, Bircher H, Paumgartner G: Physiologic and pathophysiologic aspects of the hepatic hemodynamics. In Popper H, Schaffner F (eds): Progress in Liver Diseases, vol 4, pp 201–216. New York, Grune & Stratton, 1972

270. Preisig R, Bucher H, Stirnemann H et al: Postoperative choleresis follow bile duct obstruction in man. Rev Fr Etud Clin Biol 14:151, 1969

271. Preisig R, Cooper HL, Wheeler HO: The relationship between taurocholate secretion rate and bile production in the unanesthetized dog during cholinergic blockade and during secretin administration. J Clin Invest 41:1152, 1962

272. Priestly BG, Plaa GL: Reduced bile flow after sulfobromophthalein administration in the rat. Proc Soc Exp Biol Med 135:373, 1970

273. Quinton PM, Tormey JM: Localization of Na$^+$,K$^+$-ATPase sites in the secretory and reabsorptive epithelia of perfused eccrine sweat glands: A question of the role of the enzyme in secretion. J Membr Biol 29:383, 1976

274. Ravdin IS, Johnston CG, Riegel C: Studies of gall-bladder function: VII. The anion-cation content of hepatic and gall-bladder bile. Am J Physiol 100:317, 1932

275. Razin E, Feldman MG, Dreiling DA: Studies on biliary flow and composition in man and dog. J Mt Sinai Hosp NY 32:42, 1965

276. Redinger RN, Small DM: Primate biliary physiology: VIII. The effect of phenobarbital upon bile salt synthesis and pool size, biliary lipid secretion and bile composition. J Clin Invest 52:161, 1973

277. Reichen J, Paumgartner G: Kinetics of taurocholate uptake by the perfused rat liver. Gastroenterology 68:132, 1975

278. Reichen J, Paumgartner G: Uptake of bile acids by the perfused rat liver. Am J Physiol 231:734, 1976

279. Reichen J, Paumgartner G: Relationship between bile flow and Na$^+$,K$^+$ adenosine triphosphatase in liver plasma membranes enriched in bile canaliculi. J Clin Invest 60:429, 1977

280. Reinhold JG, Wilson DW: The acid-base composition of hepatic bile. Am J Physiol 107:378, 1934

281. René E, Danzinger RG, Hofmann AF et al: Pharmacologic effect of somatostatin on bile formation in the dog: Enhanced ductular reabsorption as the major mechanism of anticholeresis. Gastroenterology 84:120, 1983

282. Reyes H, Kern F Jr: Effect of pregnancy on bile flow and biliary lipids in the hamster. Gastroenterology 76:144, 1979

283. Reyes H, Levi AJ, Gatmaitan Z et al: Studies of Y and Z, two hepatic cytoplasmic organic anion-binding proteins: Effect of drugs, chemicals, hormones, and cholestasis. J Clin Invest 50:2242, 1971

284. Richards TG, Thomson JY: The secretion of bile against pressure. Gastroenterology 40:705, 1961

285. Ritt DJ, Combes B: Enhancement of apparent excretory maximum of sulfobromophthalein sodium (BSP) by taurocholate and dehydrocholate. J Clin Invest 46:1108, 1967

286. Roberts RJ, Plaa GL: Effect of drug on the excretion of an exogenous bilirubin load. Biochem Pharmacol 16:827, 1967

287. Ros E, Small DM, Carey MC: Effects of chlorpromazine hydrochloride on bile salt synthesis, bile formation, and biliary lipid secretion in the Rhesus monkey: A model for chlorpromazine-induced cholestasis. Eur J Clin Invest 9:29, 1979

288. Rosenthal WS, Kubo K, Dolinski M et al: The passage of serum albumin into bile in man. Am J Dig Dis 10:271, 1965

289. Rous P, McMaster PD: Physiological causes for the varied character of stasis bile. J Exp Med 34:75, 1921

290. Rozé C, Cuchet P, Souchard M et al: The effects of tiadenol, clofibrate and clofibride on bile composition in the rat. Eur J Pharmacol 43:57, 1977

291. Rozé C, Debray C, Vaille C et al: Hypercholérèse induite et excrétion des sels biliaires après traitement par le clofibrate. CR Acad Sci 274:3472, 1972

292. Rozé C, Feldmann D: Stimulation par l'insuline d'une fraction de la cholérèse indépendante des sels biliaires chez le rat. CR Acad Sci 273:887–890, 1971

293. Ruifrok PG, Meijer DKF: Sodium ion-coupled uptake of taurocholate by rat-liver plasma membrane vesicles. Liver 2:28, 1982

294. Russel IS, Fleck A, Burnett W: The protein content of human bile. Clin Chim Acta 10:210, 1964

295. Rutishauser SCB, Stone SL: The effect of sodium salicylate on bile secretion in the dog. J Physiol 245:549, 1975

296. Sacks J, Bakshy S: Insulin and tissue distribution of pentose in nephrectomized cats. Am J Physiol 189:339, 1957

297. Sadiq S, Rao SP, Enquist IF: Hepatic congestion and bile secretion. Arch Surg 105:749, 1972

298. Samuels AM, Carey MC: Effects of chlorpromazine hydrochloride and its metabolites on Mg^{2+}- and Na$^+$,K$^+$-ATPase activities of canalicular-enriched liver plasma membranes. Gastroenterology 74:1183, 1978

299. Sarfeh IJ, Beeler DA, Treble DH et al: Studies of the hepatic excretory defects in essential fatty acid deficiency: Their possible relationship to the genesis of cholesterol gallstones. J Clin Invest 53:423, 1974

300. Sasaki H, Schaffner F, Popper H: Bile ductules in cholestasis: Morphologic evidence for secretion and absorption in man. Lab Invest 16:84, 1967

301. Schaffner F, Javitt NB: Morphologic changes in hamster liver during intrahepatic cholestasis induced by taurolithocholate. Lab Invest 15:1783, 1966

302. Schanker LS, Hogben CAM: Biliary excretion on inulin, sucrose, and mannitol: Analysis of bile formation. Am J Physiol 200:1087, 1961

303. Schanker LS, Solomon AM: Active transport of quaternary ammonium compounds into bile. Am J Physiol 204:829, 1963

304. Scharschmidt BF, Schmid R: The micellar sink. A quantitative assessment of the association of organic anions with mixed micelles and other macromolecular aggregates in rat bile. J Clin Invest 62:1122, 1978

305. Scharschmidt BF, Stephens JE: Transport of sodium, chloride, and taurocholate by cultured rat hepatocytes. Proc Natl Acad Sci USA 78:986, 1981

306. Scharschmidt BF, Van Dyke RW: Mechanisms of hepatic electrolyte transport. Gastroenterology 85:1199, 1983

307. Schenk DB, Leffert HL: Monoclonal antibodies to rat Na$^+$,K$^+$-ATPase block enzymatic activity. Proc Natl Acad Sci USA 80:5281, 1983

308. Scherstén T, Nilson S, Cahlin E et al: Relationship between the biliary excretion of bile acids and the excretion of water, lecithin and cholesterol in man. Eur J Clin Invest 1:242, 1971

309. Schulze PJ, Czok G: Reduced bile flow in rats during sulfobromophthalein infusion. Toxicol Appl Pharmacol 32:213, 1975

310. Schwartz A, Lindenmayer GE, Allen JC: The sodium-potassium adenosine triphosphatase: Pharmacological, physiological and biochemical aspects. Pharmacol Rev 27:3, 1975

311. Schwarz HP, Herz R, Sauter K et al: Taurocholate induced anticholeresis in the rat (abstr). Eur J Clin Invest 3:268, 1973

312. Schwarz LR, Burr R, Schwenk M et al: Uptake of taurocholic acid into isolated rat-liver cells. Eur J Biochem 55:617, 1975

313. Schwenk M, Burr R, Schwarz L et al: Uptake of bromosulfophthalein by isolated liver cells. Eur J Biochem 64:189, 1976

314. Scratcherd T: Electrolyte composition and control of biliary secretion in the cat and rabbit. In Taylor W (ed): The Biliary System, pp 515–529. Oxford, Blackwell, 1965

315. Seglen PO: Preparation of rat liver cells: I. Effect of Ca^{2+} on enzymatic dispersion of isolated, perfused liver. Exp Cell Res 74:450, 1972

316. Sharp HL, Mirkin BL: Effect of phenobarbital on hyperbilirubinemia, bile acid metabolism, and microsomal enzyme activity in chronic intrahepatic cholestasis of childhood. J Pediatr 81:116, 1972

317. Shaw H, Caple I, Heath T: Effect of ethacrynic acid on bile formation in sheep, dogs, rats, guinea-pigs and rabbits. J Pharmacol Exp Ther 182:27, 1972

318. Shorter RG, Bollman JL, Baggenstoss AH: Pressures in the common hepatic duct of the rat. Proc Soc Exp Biol Med 102:682, 1959

319. Simon FR, Sutherland E, Accatino L: Stimulation of hepatic sodium and potassium-activated adenosine triphosphatase activity by phenobarbital: Its possible role in regulation of bile flow. J Clin Invest 59:849, 1977

320. Siro–Brigiani G, Campese VM, Antoncecci E: Azione coleretica del furosemide e della teofillina nel ratto. Boll Soc Ital Biol Sper 46:607, 1970

321. Skou JC: Enzymatic basis for active transport of Na$^+$ and K$^+$ across cell membrane. Physiol Rev 45:596, 1965

322. Small DM, Rapo S: Source of abnormal bile in patients with cholesterol gallstones. N Engl J Med 283:53, 1970

323. Sobotka H: Physiological Chemistry of the Bile. Baltimore, Williams & Wilkins, 1937

324. Soloway RD, Hofmann AF, Thomas PJ et al: Triketocholanoic (dehydrocholic) acid: Hepatic metabolism and effect on bile flow and biliary lipid secretion in man. J Clin Invest 52:715, 1973

325. Soloway RD, Trotman BW, Ostrow JD: Pigment gallstones. Gastroenterology 72:167, 1977

326. Sperber I: Secretion of organic anions in the formation of urine and bile. Pharmacol Rev 11:109, 1959

327. Sperber I: Biliary secretion of organic anions and its influence on bile flow. In Taylor W (ed): The Biliary System, pp 457–467. Oxford, Blackwell, 1965

328. Stein O, Sanger L, Stein Y: Colchicine-induced inhibition of lipoprotein and protein secretion into the serum and lack of interference with secretion of biliary phospholipids and cholesterol by rat liver in vivo. J Cell Biol 62:90, 1974

329. Steiner JW, Carruthers JS: Studies on the fine structure of the terminal branches of the biliary tree: I. The morphology of normal bile canaliculi, bile preductules (ducts of Hering) and bile ductules. Am J Pathol 38:639, 1961

330. Sternlieb I: Electron microscopic study of intrahepatic biliary ductules. J Microscopie 4:71, 1965

331. Sternlieb I: Functional implications of human portal and bile ductular ultrastructure. Gastroenterology 63:321, 1972

332. Stiehl A, Thaler MM, Admirand WH: The effects of phenobarbital on bile salts and bilirubin in patients with intrahepatic and extrahepatic cholestasis. N Engl J Med 286:858, 1972

333. Stolz A, Sugiyama Y, Kuhlenkamp J et al: Identification and purification of a 36kDa bile acid binder in human hepatic cytosol. FEBS Lett 177:31, 1984

334. Strange RC, Cramb R, Hayes JD et al: Partial purification of two lithocholic acid–binding proteins from rat liver 100,000 g supernatants. Biochem J 165:425, 1977

335. Strange RC, Nimmo IA, Percy-Robb IW: Binding of bile acids by 100,000 g supernatants of rat liver. Biochem J 162:659, 1977

336. Stransky E: Untersuchungen über die Pharmakologie der Gallensekretion: IV. Mitteilung. Mitgteilung. Ausssheidung von Stoffen durch die Galle. Z Ges Exp Med 77:807, 1931

337. Strasberg SM, Dorn BC, Redinger RN et al: Effects of alterations of biliary pressure on bile composition: A method for study: Primate biliary physiology V. Gastroenterology 61:357, 1971

338. Strasberg SM, Ilson RG, Siminovitch KA et al: Analysis of the components of bile flow in the rhesus monkey. Am J Physiol 228:115, 1975

339. Suchy FJ, Balistreri WF, Hung J et al: Intracellular bile acid transport in rat liver as visualized by electron microscope autoradiography using a bile acid analogue. Am J Physiol 245:G681–G689, 1983

340. Sugiyama U, Yamada T, Kaplowitz N: Newly identified

bile acid binders in rat liver cytosol: Purification and comparison with glutathione S-transferases. J Biol Chem 258:3602, 1983

341. Takane S: Uber den einfluss verschiedener narkosemittel auf die Leberfunktion: Experimentelle untersuchungen mit bilirubin unt Kongorot. Arch Klin Chir 170:672, 1932

342. Takemura S, Omori K, Tanaka K et al: Quantitative immunoferritin localization of (Na⁺,K⁺)ATPase on canine hepatocyte cell surface. J Cell Biol 99:1502, 1984

343. Tavoloni N, Reed JS, Boyer JL: Hemodynamic effects on determinants of bile secretion in isolated rat liver. Am J Physiol 234:E584, 1978

344. Thompson RPH, Williams R: Treatment of chronic intrahepatic cholestasis with phenobarbitone. Lancet 2:646, 1967

345. Thureborn E: Human hepatic bile: Composition changes due to altered enterohepatic circulation. Acta Chir Scand 303(suppl):1, 1962

346. Tuchweber B, Gabbiani G: Phalloidin-induced hyperplasia of actin microfilaments in rat hepatocytes. In Preisig R, Bircher J (eds): The Liver: Quantitative Aspects of Structure and Function, pp 84–90. Aulendorf, Editio Cantor, 1976

347. Turley SD, Dietschy JM: Cholesterol metabolism and excretion. In Arias I, Popper H, Schachter D et al (eds): The Liver: Biology and Pathobiology, pp 467–492. New York, Raven Press, 1982

348. Turnberg LA, Jones EA, Sherlock S: Biliary secretion in a patient with cystic duct dilatation of the intrahepatic biliary tree. Gastroenterology 54:1155, 1968

349. Vessey DA, Whitney J, Gollan JL: The role of conjugation reactions in enhancing biliary secretion of bile acids. Biochem J 214:923, 1983

350. Vonk RJ, Jekel P, Meijer DKF: Choleresis and hepatic transport mechanisms: II. Influence of bile salt choleresis and biliary micelle binding on biliary excretion of various organic anions. Naunyn Schmiedebergs Arch Pharmacol 290:375, 1975

351. Vonk RJ, van der Veen H, Prop G et al: The influence of taurocholate and dehydrocholate choleresis on plasma disappearance and biliary excretion of indocyanine green in the rat. Naunyn Schmiedebergs Arch Pharmacol 282:401, 1974

352. Wagner CI, Trotman BW, Soloway RD: Kinetic analysis of biliary lipid excretion in man and dog. J Clin Invest 57:473, 1976

353. Waitman AM, Dyck WP, Janowitz HD: Effect of secretin and acetazolamide on the volume and electrolyte composition of hepatic bile in man. Gastroenterology 56:286, 1969

354. Wannagat FJ, Adler RD, Ockner RK: Bile acid–induced increase in bile acid–independent flow and plasma membrane NaK-ATPase activity in rat liver. J Clin Invest 61:297, 1978

355. Watanabe S, Miyairi M, Oshio C et al: Phalloidin alters bile canalicular contractility in primary monolayer cultures of rat liver. Gastroenterology 85:245, 1983

356. Wheeler HO: Water and electrolytes in bile. In Code CF (ed): Handbook of Physiology, vol 5, Section 6, Alimentary Canal, pp 2409–2431. Washington, DC, American Physiological Society, 1968

357. Wheeler HO, King KK: Biliary excretion of lecithin and cholesterol in the dog. J Clin Invest 51:1337, 1973

358. Wheeler HO, Mancusi-Ungaro PL: Role of bile ducts during secretin choleresis in dogs. Am J Physiol 210:1153, 1966

359. Wheeler HO, Meltzer JI, Bradley SE: Biliary transport and hepatic storage of sulfobromophthalein sodium in the unanesthetized dog, in normal man, and in patients with hepatic disease. J Clin Invest 39:1131, 1960

360. Wheeler HO, Ramos OL: Determinants of the flow and composition of bile in the unanesthetized dog during constant infusions of sodium taurocholate. J Clin Invest 39:161, 1960

361. Wheeler HO, Ross ED, Bradley SE: Canalicular bile production in dogs. Am J Physiol 214:866, 1968

362. Whelan G, Combes B: Depression of biliary excretion of infused bilirubin in rats and guinea-pigs by bile. Am J Physiol 220:683, 1971

363. Whitlock RT, Wheeler HO: Coupled transport of solute and water across rabbit gallbladder epithelium. J Clin Invest 43:2249, 1964

364. Wilson FA: Intestinal transport of bile acids. Am J Physiol 241:G83, 1981

365. Wilson FA, Burckhardt G, Murer H et al: Sodium-coupled taurocholate transport in the proximal convolution of the rat kidney in vivo and in vitro. J Clin Invest 67:1141, 1981

366. Yaffe SJ, Levy G, Matsuzawa T et al: Enhancement of glucuronide-conjugating-capacity in a hyperbilirubinemic infant due to apparent enzyme induction by phenobarbital. N Engl J Med 275:1461, 1966

367. Yamamoto K, Phillips MJ: A hitherto unrecognized bile ductular plexus in normal rat liver. Hepatology 4:381, 1984

368. Zaterka S, Grossman MI: The effect of gastrin and histamine on secretion of bile. Gastroenterology 50:500, 1966

369. Zouboulis–Vafiadis I, Dumont M, Erlinger S: Conjugation is rate limiting in hepatic transport of ursodeoxycholate in the rat. Am J Physiol 243:G208, 1982

370. Zsigmond G, Solymoss B: Effect of spironolactone, pregnenolone-16-carbonitrile and cortisol on the metabolism and biliary excretion of sulfo bromophthalein and phenol-3,6-dibromphthalein disulfonate in rats. J Pharmacol Exp Ther 183:499, 1972

chapter 4

Bilirubin Metabolism

BARBARA H. BILLING

Although bilirubin can be regarded as a waste product of metabolism, its formation is essential for mammalian life because it is the main means by which heme is eliminated from the body. Unless the accumulation of heme liberated from senescent erythrocytes is prevented, then new heme will not be synthesized and many important compounds such as the cytochromes as well as hemoglobin will not be formed.

An appreciation of the manner in which bilirubin is transported by the liver will help in our understanding of the etiology of jaundice, whether it is congenital or pathologic. It will also increase our knowledge of the hepatic transport of many organic anions that share similar pathways and have important biological functions.

In this chapter the chemistry, biosynthesis, and metabolism of bile pigments as well as the various congenital types of adult hyperbilirubinemia that result from disorders of bilirubin metabolism will be discussed.

STRUCTURE OF BILE PIGMENTS

Bile pigments may be defined as compounds that consist of a chain of four substituted pyrrole rings linked together at their α positions by three methene ($-CH_2$) or methyne ($-CH=$) groups. The naturally occurring pigments are derived from ferroprotoporphyrin IX (heme) as the result of oxidative scission at the α linkage (*i.e.,* between the two pyrrole rings bearing the vinyl groups) and therefore possess a IX$_\alpha$ structure (Fig. 4-1). Biliverdin is the pigment whose structure is most closely related to protoporphyrin since its four pyrrole rings are joined through three of the original methyne bridges and the side-chains are unaltered; its central methyne bridge is readily reduced so that it is converted from a green pigment to the yellow pigment bilirubin.

X-ray crystallographic analysis[55] supports the view that, both in solution and in the solid state, the two terminal pyrroles of bilirubin occur predominantly in the lactam form ($-NH-C=O$)[158] and that the molecule is stabilized by six intramolecular hydrogen bonds between the $-COOH$ and $-NH$ groups (Fig. 4-2). This provides an explanation for the insolubility of bilirubin at a physiologic *p*H and probably acounts for its behavior in the Van den Bergh reaction in the presence of accelerators such as ethanol, caffeine, and urea, all of which are capable of

disrupting intramolecular hydrogen bonds. The bilirubin IX$_\alpha$ molecule is constrained to a Z,Z configuration (see Fig. 4-2). Since it has an unsymmetrical structure, rotation of either of the outer pyrrole rings A and D will produce the geometric isomers E,E, Z,E, and E,Z, thereby decreasing intramolecular bonding so that the solubility of the molecule is increased.[55]

In acid solution, naturally occurring bilirubin IX$_\alpha$ is cleaved at the central $-CH_2$ bridge and the two dissimilar halves will reunite at random (dipyrrole exchange) so that bilirubin III$_\alpha$ and bilirubin XIII$_\alpha$ are formed.[198] Small quantities of these isomers are found in commercial preparations of bilirubin and have also been identified in the early labeled bilirubin of bile.[230] In mammals, very small amounts of heme may be cleaved at carbon bridge positions other than α so that β, γ, and δ isomers of bilirubin IX (which do not form intramolecular hydrogen bonds) appear in trace amounts in bile. Bilirubin IX$_\beta$ has been found in fetal bile and meconium of newborns.[54]

Reduction of bilirubin either by chemical or bacterial hydrogenation results in the formation of a heterogeneous group of compounds known collectively as urobilinogens and urobilins. The relationships between some of the more common urobilinoids is shown schematically in Figure 4-3.

Only a few of the large number of urobilinoid stereoisomers that have been demonstrated by modern physicochemical techniques have been isolated and characterized.[276] It is not easy to determine these pigments individually but a semiquantitative estimate of the sum of the urobilinoids can be obtained using Erlich's aldehyde reaction provided they are first converted to their fully hydrogenated precursors, the urobilinogens.

Phototherapy

Bilirubin acts as a photoreceptor, thus enabling treatment with blue light to cause bilirubin to undergo photo-oxidation so that several colorless polar products are formed that can be excreted in urine.[190] In addition it has become apparent that the main photochemical event associated with phototherapy is photoisomerization; this results in changes in the shape of the molecule so that it becomes a polar compound without being fragmented.[200] The fastest photochemical reaction is configurational (geometric) isomerization so that the normal (4Z, 15Z) bilirubin is

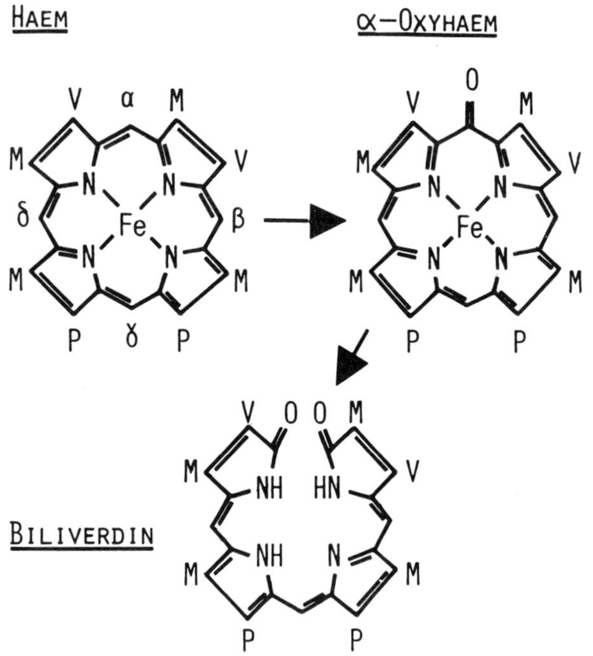

Fig. 4-1. Pathway of heme catabolism (M_1—CH_3: V, —CH=CH_2: P, —CH_2 CH_2COOH). (Brown SB, King RFGJ: Biochemistry 170:297, 1978)

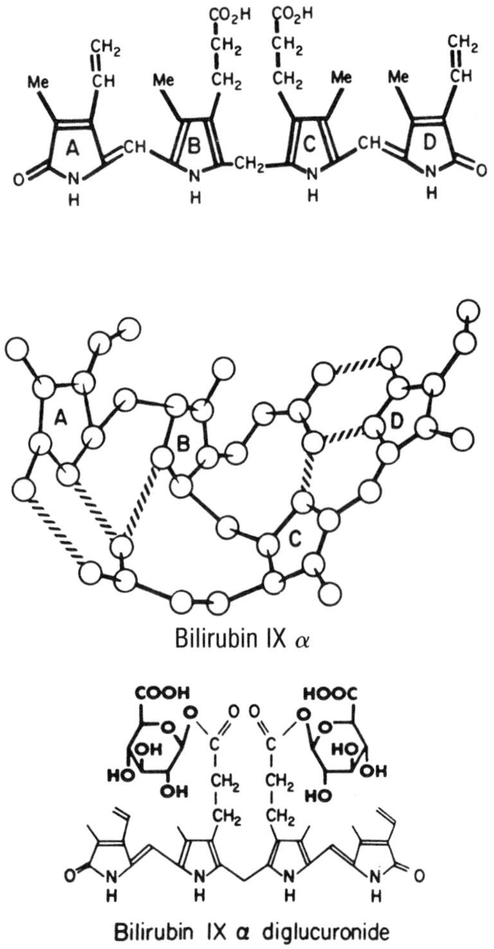

Bilirubin IX α

Bilirubin IX α diglucuronide

Fig. 4-2. Structures of I unconjugated bilirubin. Rings A and B lie in one plane and rings C and D in another. Dotted lines indicate intramolecular hydrogen bonds. (Bonnett R et al: Nature 262:326, 1976) II Bilirubin diglucuronide.

converted to (4Z, 15E) bilirubin (photobilirubin I). This reaction is reversible so that during therapy some of the bilirubin formed in the skin and subsequently excreted in the bile will revert to (4Z, 15Z) bilirubin and be reabsorbed in the intestine. The formation of lumirubin (photobilirubin II), a "structural" isomer of bilirubin containing a seven member ring, is a slower reaction, which is irreversible. It is, therefore, cleared more rapidly from the plasma than the "configurational" isomer (half-life; 2 hours vs. 15 hours) and is probably the most important pathway for bilirubin elimination in the newborn during phototherapy.[102,175] In the presence of impaired liver function lumirubin may undergo polymerization and form the pigment responsible for the bronze baby syndrome.[221]

ORIGIN OF BILIRUBIN

It has been known for over 100 years that bilirubin formation is dependent on red cell destruction. The senescent cells are mainly removed from the circulation by sequestration in the reticuloendothelial cells of the spleen, liver, and bone marrow where they undergo lysis and the liberated hemoglobin is immediately degraded.[172] In hemolytic states, or after splenectomy, the hepatic sinusoidal cells play an important role.[35] Under conditions of intravascular hemolysis the conversion of hemoglobin heme to bilirubin occurs in the hepatic parenchymal cells, which

take up free hemoglobin as well as haptoglobin-bound hemoglobin, methemoglobin, methemalbumin, hemin, and heme-hemopexin.[155] When the haptoglobin-binding capacity is exceeded, free hemoglobin may be filtered by the renal glomeruli and be partially taken up by the epithelial cells of the proximal convoluted tubules in the kidney and converted to bilirubin.[234]

Although the heme moiety of hemoglobin is responsible for approximately 80% of the circulating bilirubin, the remainder comes from other sources. It was shown that when an isotopic precursor of heme such as ^{15}N- or ^{14}C-glycine was administered to human subjects, the majority of the labeled bile pigment formed was excreted in the feces as urobilin (or stercobilin) between 90 and 150 days after the administration of the isotope, corresponding to the end of the life span of the average erythrocyte.[148,191] In addition, there was a significant excretion of early labeled bilirubin (ELB) in the feces within 10 days of the

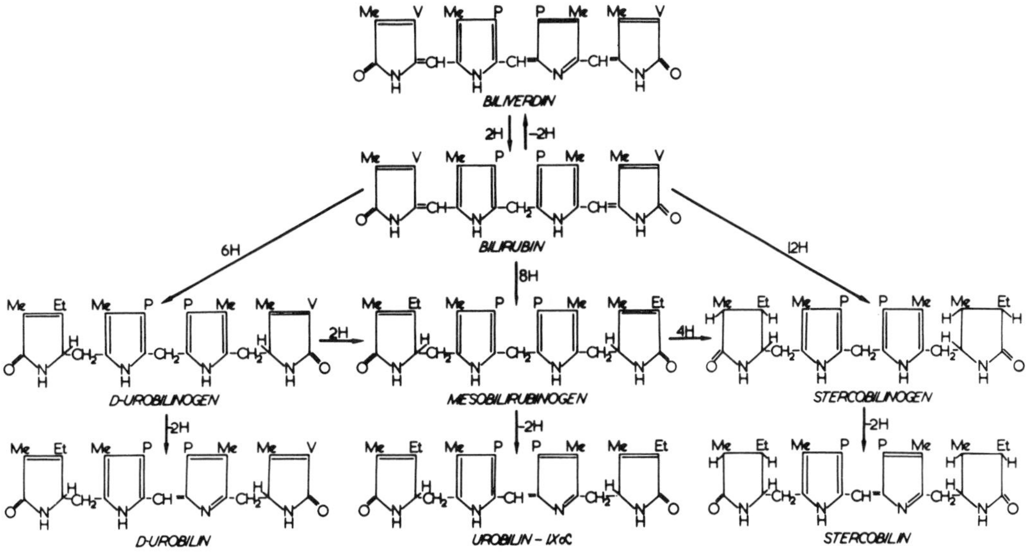

Fig. 4-3. Structural relation between bilirubin and urobilinoids (M_1—CH_3: Et, —C_2H_5: V, —CH=CH_2: P, —CH_2CH_2COOH).

administration of the isotopic precursor that accounted for 10% to 20% of the total labeled pigment excretion. Part of the ELB was shown to arise from a nonerythroid source when it was observed that there was increased early labeling of fecal urobilin in a patient with erythroid aplasia.[164] This has since been confirmed by the administration of isotopic δ-aminolevulinic acid (ALA), which preferentially labels heme from nonerythroid sources.[159,160,242,249,310] Studies in patients with ineffective erythropoiesis established that there was also an erythroid component of ELB[15] (see section on Diseases Associated with Early Labeled Bilirubin Production).

The presence of both nonerythroid and erythroid ELB has been demonstrated in plasma following the administration of isotopic heme precursors.[228,309] With ^{14}C-glycine, labeled ELB is detected within 90 minutes due to the rapid turnover of free heme pools in the liver and marrow erythroid cells.[135,187,242] Two peaks of radioactivity at 12 to 24 hours and another at 3 to 5 days also occur. The latter plasma component is believed to be derived almost exclusively from erythropoietic sources,[228,242] and to be responsible for the exaggerated fecal urobilin peak observed in patients with ineffective erythropoiesis (see section on hemolytic disease). The liver appears to be the main organ responsible for the first plasma component of ELB[187,264] and the microsomal heme enzymes, which have a fast turnover, have been considered to be the most likely precursors, although catalase and tryptophan pyrrolase may also be involved.[261] There is also good evidence from animal experiments that substantial quantities of hepatic heme may be degraded to compounds other than bilirubin and carbon monoxide.[37]

It is now possible to quantitate the rate of synthesis of ELB either by determining the total bilirubin turnover

$(3.89 \pm 0.67$ mg/kg/day)[19] and bilirubin production from senescent erythrocytes[28] or by measuring the incorporation of labeled glycine and ALA into bile pigments.[249] It appears that, in the normal subject, 21% of the daily bilirubin turnover is independent of erythropoiesis and that for every 100 mg of bilirubin derived from the breakdown of hemoglobin an additional 8.9 mg is produced as the result of ineffective erythropoiesis.[28] Compartmental models using tracer doses of ^{14}C bilirubin and ^{3}H-ALA have been designed in order to investigate the handling of bilirubin formed in the liver.[169,173] It would appear that approximately two thirds of the hepatic bilirubin formed passes into the plasma as unconjugated bilirubin and is then taken up by the liver and subsequently excreted in the bile; only a small proportion of the hepatic bilirubin is excreted directly in the bile. Animal experiments have indicated that hepatic ELB can be increased by anesthesia, sham operation, bile duct ligation, and administration of phenobarbital.[159,160] It may, therefore, contribute to the rise in serum bilirubin frequently observed in the immediate postoperative period, but this has not been proved.

FORMATION OF BILIRUBIN FROM HEME

There has been considerable controversy as to whether *in vivo* heme catabolism is an enzymatic or a nonenzymatic process. Current thinking[261] indicates that the two mechanisms are not mutually exclusive but favors the microsomal heme oxygenase system, whose specific activity is highest in the spleen, bone marrow, and liver[156,283,285] where heme degradation is known to occur. This microsomal enzyme has an absolute and stoichiometric requirement for reduced nicotinamide adenine dinucleotide phosphate (NADPH) and requires 3 mol of oxygen for the conversion of heme to equimolar amounts of biliverdin IX_α and carbon monoxide. Heme oxygenase reacts preferentially with free heme and only attacks bound heme (*e.g.*, metalbumin) if it is easily dissociated from its parent apoprotein.[285] Hemoglobin and many hemoproteins are not good substrates for this reaction *in vitro* so that it seems likely that *in vivo* the protein moiety is first degraded and then the heme becomes bound to heme oxygenase in the membrane of the endoplasmic reticulum.[62,312] The ferric iron of the bound heme is reduced by NADPH, which is generated by cytochrome c reductase and a reactive oxygen radical is generated that binds to the complex and selectively attacks the heme at its α bridge to form α-oxyheme.[62] Two more molecules of oxygen are required to cleave the α-oxyheme ring[61] so that 1 mol of carbon monoxide is liberated and an iron biliverdin complex is formed. Ferrous iron is detached from the complex and returns to the iron pool, and active heme oxygenase is regenerated. Biliverdin IX_α is released and then reduced to bilirubin IX_α by biliverdin reductase,[284] a cystosolic enzyme that has a stereochemical preference for the α isomer.[77] Experiments with purified preparations of NADPH cytochrome-c-reductase, heme oxygenase, and biliverdin reductase have raised the possibility that *in vivo* a ternary enzyme complex is formed at the cytosol-endoplasmic reticulum boundary that is responsible for the enzymatic conversion of heme to bilirubin.[313]

These findings are in agreement with the *in vivo* observations that bilirubin turnover is related to carbon monoxide production[25] and that intravenously administered biliverdin can be recovered in bile as bilirubin. The newly formed bilirubin appears to reflux with the plasma bilirubin pool before it is excreted, thereby providing further evidence that elimination of bilirubin from the plasma compartment occurs by hepatic channels that do not communicate with those responsible for endogenously formed pigment.[169,173] Somewhat surprisingly, an injection of heme in humans did not cause a rise in plasma bilirubin concentration until 12 hours after the injection; this observation warrants further investigation.[197]

Although the heme oxygenase system utilizes the electron transport mechanism of the microsomal drug-oxidizing mixed function oxidase system it is distinct from the cytochrome P450 system. Thus, cobalt and other heavy metals will simultaneously induce hepatic heme oxygenase and decrease the hepatic cytochrome P450.[194] Heme oxygenase activity is dependent on the presence of a central iron or cobalt atom in the porphyrin ring; otherwise the porphyrin will be excreted unchanged in the bile.[194] Activity of the enzyme in the liver, spleen, bone marrow,[285] macrophages,[233] and renal tubules[234] can be significantly increased by heme or hemoglobin so that the human body readily adapts to the increased loads of heme requiring catabolism in hemolytic disorders[285] and intravascular hemolysis.[234]

Hemoglobin is not the only naturally occurring substrate for heme oxygenase. It has been shown that bilirubin can also be formed from the catabolism of hemoproteins such as myoglobin, catalase, peroxidase, and cytochrome P450 and b_5 but not cytochrome c, since in this molecule heme forms two covalent bonds with the apoprotein and cannot, therefore, be cleaved by heme oxygenase. Both the microsomal cytochromes P450 and b_5, which catalyze the biotransformation of many hormones, drugs, and toxins have a short biologic half-life, and it has been postulated that they are the probable precursors for ELB (see section on origin of bilirubin).[262]

It has been demonstrated that some synthetic metalloporphyrins, in which the central iron atom of heme is replaced by other elements, can be competitive inhibitors in the heme oxygenase reaction, although they are not themselves degraded to bile pigments. Tin protoporphyrin is the most potent inhibitor tested, and it has been used experimentally to prevent the development of hyperbilirubinemia in neonatal rats[97] and rhesus monkeys[82] by diminishing the production of bilirubin. It has also been used therapeutically in a few patients with Gilbert's syndrome and primary biliary cirrhosis, but only small reductions in serum bilirubin levels have been achieved.[171]

Although the formation of bilirubin and carbon monoxide in equimolar amounts has been demonstrated *in vitro*, it is usually somewhat less than would be expected on the basis of heme disappearance. This observation is in keeping with *in vivo* studies, which showed that the intravenous administration of hematin and hemoglobin or damaged red cells[222,271] did not result in the recovery of the expected amount of bilirubin. Moreover, under certain conditions, carbon monoxide production may exceed bilirubin production[21,25,75,182] so the possibility that alternate pathways of heme catabolism exist has to be considered. Studies in normal rat liver and primary hepatocyte culture[37] have established that endogenous hepatic heme, in contrast to exogenous heme, is degraded predominantly by pathways which probably do not involve bile pigment or carbon monoxide formation. It has been postulated that microsomal lipid peroxidation may be involved since the heme moiety of cytochrome P450 is known to be susceptible to peroxidative attack yielding hematinic acid, methylvinylmaleimide and propentdypents but not carbon monoxide.[253] Support for this hypothesis comes from a study with purified NADPH–cytochrome-P450 reductase, which will degrade heme in the absence of heme oxygenase in a similar manner to hydrogen peroxide.[95]

BILIRUBIN METABOLISM

Transport in Blood

Unconjugated bilirubin has a very limited solubility in aqueous solutions at a physiologic *p*H (7 mM at *p*H 7.4, temperature 37° C); its solubility in apolar solvents is also low so that theoretically it should not be regarded as a lipophilic substance although interaction with lipids can occur and the pigment is soluble in solvents such as chloroform and dimethylsulfoxide.[59] A small fraction of the bilirubin in circulating blood may be bound to erythrocytes,[14] but the majority is reversibly bound to plasma albumin; in the newborn binding to α-fetoprotein may be important.[293] If the molar ratio of bilirubin to albumin is 1:1 or less, then the bilirubin is very tightly bound to a single high-affinity site with a binding constant of 6.4×10^7 M^{-1}. Histidine residues of albumin play an important role in the covalent binding of bilirubin; arginine, tyrosine, and tryptophan may also be involved.[162] There are also two low affinity sites, with a dissociation constant of 4.4×10^6 M^{-1} that are important when the molar ratio of bilirubin to albumin is greater than 1.[162]

The distribution of bilirubin between plasma and tissues is dependent on the presence of a very small fraction of bilirubin that exists in the plasma as a protein-free, diffusible anion; the amount present is related to the concentration of albumin available to bind bilirubin, as well as pH, ionic strength, and the presence of other organic anions.[208] The administration to pregnant women or newborns of anionic drugs such as sulfonamides and salicylates, which compete with bilirubin for protein binding, may increase the risk of kernicterus in the jaundiced infant since only "unbound bilirubin" can cross the blood–brain barrier (which is more permeable in the newborn than in the adult.)[58,161,168] Some food additives, radiographic contrast media, and diuretics also have the ability to displace bilirubin from its binding site on albumin, and there is the possibility that the high plasma concentration of free fatty acids in breast milk–fed infants may act in this way and cause jaundice.[314] In addition, asphyxia, hypoxia, and acidosis may interfere with bilirubin–albumin binding, as well as increase the permeability of the brain for unconjugated bilirubin.[94]

In spite of the strong affinity of unconjugated bilirubin for plasma albumin, the pigment can cross biologic membranes by nonionic diffusion or carrier-mediated transport. This has been shown for the placenta, liver,[4] intestine,[185] gallbladder,[223] and kidney.[208]

Conjugated bilirubin is also transported in the plasma bound to albumin, although its affinity for the protein is not as great as that of unconjugated bilirubin and a small fraction is dialyzable (see section on renal excretion). It may also bind to other plasma proteins and appears to be distributed in the tissues in a different manner from unconjugated bilirubin.[4]

Hepatic Uptake

Under normal circumstances newly formed bilirubin is removed from the circulation very rapidly by the liver[4] so that the plasma bilirubin concentration remains less than 1 mg/dl (17 μmol/liter). Blood flow carries the bilirubin–albumin complex through the hepatic sinusoids where it tranverses the space of Disse and reaches the plasma membrane of the hepatocyte. Dissociation of the bilirubin–albumin complex occurs more rapidly in vivo than would be predicted from physiochemical studies in vitro. This suggests that there may be some form of interaction with the cell membrane so that the albumin molecule undergoes a conformational change that enables the bilirubin to be rapidly transferred into the hepatocyte and the albumin molecule to be detached from the binding site and returned to the circulation.[297] This hypothesis remains to be validated since specific albumin receptors have not been identified on liver sinusoidal membranes. Moreover, there is good evidence that bilirubin uptake is not facilitated by albumin binding.[277] It has, however, been possible for two separate groups of investigators to isolate a binding protein for bilirubin that acts as a receptor.[278,301]

Current evidence supports the view that hepatic uptake is a carrier-mediated saturable process that obeys Michaelis-Menten kinetics. The pathway appears to be shared by other organic anions (e.g., sulfobromophthalein and indocyanine green), which show competitive inhibition, but not by bile acids.[143,144,227,255] The hepatic uptake system normally operates well below saturation, and its maximum capacity greatly exceeds that of the excretory transport so that uptake is not the rate-limiting factor in bilirubin excretion.[255] Studies in Gunn rats[255] and patients with congenital nonhemolytic jaundice[50] indicate that the initial rate of uptake of a tracer dose of bilirubin is independent of subsequent conjugation and biliary excretion, although they do influence net transport. The bi-directional flux of bilirubin across the plasma membrane has been demonstrated experimentally[144,255] and has also been deduced from compartmental analysis of plasma bilirubin disappearance curves.[19,33] It has been calculated that in normal subjects approximately 40% of bilirubin removed by the liver in a single pass refluxes unchanged into the plasma; this may be increased in unconjugated hyperbilirubinemia.[20,33,173]

In the hepatocyte, bilirubin binds primarily to the cytosolic proteins, ligandin (glutathione S-transferase B) and Z protein, which play an important role in the intrahepatic transport and detoxification of many molecules including fatty acids, cortisol, and carcinogens.[9] There has been considerable debate as to whether these proteins are mainly concerned with the storage of bilirubin in a nontoxic form or whether they play a role in the uptake process. Multiple indicator dilution studies, performed in an isolated perfused rat liver with variable ligandin concentrations, support the hypothesis that ligandin has an intracellular binding function similar to that of albumin in plasma so that when it is increased the reflux of bilirubin into the plasma is decreased.[304] Although ligandin appears to play a regulatory role in controlling the net hepatic uptake of bilirubin, this function is not shared by Z protein.[286]

Little is known about the mechanism underlying the transfer of unconjugated bilirubin from the cytoplasmic binding proteins to the membranes of the endoplasmic reticulum, where bilirubin glucuronide is formed, or of the transfer of the latter pigment to the bile canaliculus. There is indirect evidence that bilirubin transport within the hepatocyte is compartmentalized since bilirubin produced from the turnover of hepatic heme appears to use different channels from those taken by bilirubin that is present in the plasma before it is conjugated and enters the bile.[173]

An alternative mechanism for the intracellular transport of bilirubin is being considered based on the fact that the pigment is hydrophobic. It could, therefore, partition into phospholipid bilayers in the plasma membrane and undergo rapid diffusion into the intracellular membranes. It might even be possible for bilirubin to be transferred by direct, membrane-to-membrane contact to the endoplasmic reticulum as has been proposed for the heme oxygenase system.

Biosynthesis of Bilirubin Conjugates: Structure

Conjugation is essential for the elimination of bilirubin IX_α from the body. It involves esterification of one or both of the propionic side-chains (Fig. 4-2) usually with a glycosidic moiety, such as glucuronic acid; intracellular hydrogen bonding is thereby reduced and in a less constrained conformation bilirubin becomes more hydrophilic and can be excreted in the bile and urine; its reabsorption from the gut[185] and gallbladder[223] is also impaired. All conjugates give a "direct" reaction in the Van den Bergh test. Because of the asymmetrical nature of the pigment, monoconjugated bilirubin occurs in two isomeric forms; one is esterified at the propionic acid side-chain attached to C-8 (C-8 isomer) and the other attached to C-12 (C-12 isomer). With appropriate chromatographic systems,[71,79,118,140,220,272] it is possible with bile to separate and quantitate both these monoconjugates, which are predominantly glucuronides, from the diconjugates, which may comprise mixed diconjugates, containing one glucuronosyl moiety and either one xylosyl or glucosyl group in addition to the diglucuronide. The instability of bile pigments in cholestasis and the lack of a suitable reference compound have limited the use of high-pressure liquid chromatography for the analysis of tetrapyrroles in serum.[165] Provided the composition of the individual conjugates is not required, some of these difficulties can be overcome by first converting the conjugates to stable methyl derivatives. The results obtained by high-pressure liquid chromatography will then provide estimates of the monoconjugates and diconjugates on a group basis, as well as unconjugated bilirubin.[42,45,202]

In human bile, about 80% of the total pigments occur as bilirubin diglucuronide while bilirubin monoglucuronide accounts for less than 20%; small amounts of glucose and xylose conjugates may also be present.[114] Other conjugates such as sulfates[207] have been postulated but have not been confirmed when very sensitive analytical techniques were used.[178] The pigment composition of bile varies considerably in different species[83,116] and may be altered in obstructive jaundice[79,114] and familial hyperbilirubinemia.[115,141]

In cholestatic serum there is a fourth bile pigment fraction, in addition to unconjugated bilirubin, bilirubin monoconjugates, and bilirubin diconjugates, which is tightly bound to protein. This fraction was first described in 1960[179] but was not characterized until 1982[183] when a reverse-phase high-pressure liquid chromatographic technique was devised for its estimation.[184] The δ-bilirubin, which has been denoted as biliprotein, bilirubin-protein conjugate, and albumin-bound bilirubin, is predominantly "direct reacting" in the Van den Bergh test and binds more strongly to protein than the other three fractions. The binding is resistant to physical (e.g., urea, guanidine), chemical (e.g., HCl, NaOH, and boiling MeOH), or enzymatic treatments[183] and appears to involve a covalent amide linkage between one of the propionic acid side-chains of the tetrapyrrole and a functional lysine group on plasma albumin.[307] The formation of bilirubin protein conjugate is probably nonenzymatic and may involve acyl migration of bilirubin from a bilirubin glucuronic acid ester to a nucleophilic site on albumin.[128,199]

Biosynthesis of Bilirubin Conjugates: Mechanism

The enzyme responsible for the formation of bilirubin IX_α monoglucuronide is bilirubin UDP-glucuronyl transferase, which transfers the glucuronic acid moiety of uridine diphosphate glucuronic acid (UDPGA) to bilirubin so that a mixture of C-8 and C-12 isomers of bilirubin monoglucuronide is formed.[44,71,73,142] Bilirubin UDP-glucuronyl transferase is a membrane-bound enzyme whose activity is modulated by the phospholipid composition and physicochemical properties of the membrane.[315] It is widely distributed in the liver, the majority being found in the rough and smooth endoplasmic reticulum but has not been detected in plasma membranes or cytosol.[153] Since the rough membranes comprise 60% of the endoplasmic reticulum of the hepatocyte, it is likely that this organelle is the major site of bilirubin glucuronidation in the liver.

Bilirubin UDP-glucuronyl transferase activity has also been demonstrated in other organs. Immunocytochemical techniques have shown that it occurs in the rat in the epithelial cells of the jejunum while in the kidneys the highest concentration is in the epithelial cells of the proximal convoluted tubules.[72] Extrahepatic conjugation of bilirubin in vivo has been demonstrated in hepatectomized animals,[122] and when kidneys were grafted from normal Wistar rats into Gunn rats, a marked reduction in hyperbilirubinemia occurred.[119] Similar results were observed when a clonal strain of rat hepatoma cells, which have glucuronyl transferase activity, were transplanted into homozygous Gunn rats.[248] It is not known, however, whether renal conjugation plays a role in the disposition of bilirubin IX_α in the normal rat.

The proposal that the conversion of bilirubin monoglucuronide to bilirubin diglucuronide, which has been demonstrated in vivo,[46] is due to the activity of a transmutase in the canalicular membrane[71] is no longer tenable since there is now good evidence that the reported mechanism was a nonenzymatic phenomenon.[111,142,269] It has been clearly established from studies with rat microsomes and primary monolayer culture of hepatocytes[36] that the formation of bilirubin diglucuronide is a two-step reaction involving bilirubin glucuronyl transferase, in which the monoglucuronide is formed first and is then converted to the diglucuronide. Both steps require UDPGA as co-substrate and probably have similar pH optima.[44,63] Diglucuronide formation *in vitro* is favored by a low bilirubin concentration, a relatively high UDPGA concentration, the removal of glucuronyl transferase latency by digitonin or lubrol, the presence of the allosteric effector uridine 5′-diphospho-*N*-acetyl glucosamine, and treatment with trypsin under anaerobic conditions.[87,142]

Studies with a highly purified bilirubin UDP-glucuronyl transferase preparation support the hypothesis that the formation of both bilirubin monoglucuronide and diglucuronide is catalyzed by a single microsomal enzyme, which may also be responsible for the formation of bilirubin monoglucosides and diglucosides.[63] It has been postulated that bilirubin UDP-glucuronyl transferase consists of four subunits, the complete tetrameric enzyme being required for the formation of the diglucuronide while the biosynthesis of the monoglucuronide can be mediated by a single subunit.[229] Bilirubin UDP-glucuronyl transferase appears to have a different molecular mass from that of the enzymes responsible for the glucuronidation of such substrates as estrone, testosterone, *p*-nitrophenol, and phenolphthalein.[229,265] With the use of immunoblot analysis it has been possible to obtain convincing evidence that bilirubin UDP-glucuronyl transferase activity is completely absent from the congenitally jaundiced Gunn rat.[265]

Kinetic studies in a perfused rat liver have established that hepatic deconjugation of a small fraction of bilirubin glucuronides is probably a physiologic event.[139] This could occur as the result of hepatic β-glucuronidase activity (although its specificity with respect to bilirubin glucuronides has not been adequately studied) or as the reverse reaction of UDP-glucuronyl transferase catalyzed glucuronidation, which has an optimum pH of 5.1 compared with 7.8 for the forward reaction.[88] If the reverse reaction occurs this could explain why some patients with parenchymatous liver disease, who tend to have a reduction in intracellular pH, have increased levels of unconjugated bilirubin in their plasma. Deconjugation could also explain the accumulation of bilirubin monoglucuronide and unconjugated bilirubin in the cholestatic rat liver.[2]

In vivo administration of microsomal enzyme inducers such as phenobarbital, glutethimide, antipyrine, and clofibrate[120] will cause induction of bilirubin glucuronyl transferase activity in experimental animals[33] and decrease the plasma bilirubin concentration in patients with familial unconjugated hyperbilirubinemia (see Gilbert's syndrome). It appears that induction causes a similar proportional increase in enzyme activity regardless of whether native, detergent-activated, or allosterically activated enzyme preparations are used.[282] The activity of the enzyme is greater in female than in male rats and can be modified by pregnancy or by the administration of steroid hormones.[203,205,206] The temporary induction caused by glucagon appears to be mediated by adenosine 3′5′-monophosphate.[80]

Biliary Excretion

Although normal human bile does contain small amounts of unconjugated bilirubin (1.2% of total bilirubin in gallbladder[56,272]), conjugation is virtually essential for the excretion of the pigment. This could be due to the glucuronide moiety binding to a specific carrier or to conjugation disrupting the internal hydrogen bonding so that the pigment can be transported by a carrier system that has a broad specificity for hydrophilic anions. Little is known about the transport of bilirubin from the endoplasmic reticulum to the canalicular membrane and whether ligandin and an intracellular vesicular pathway are involved. Secretion appears to occur against a concentration gradient and to involve a carrier-mediated transport system that is shared by many other organic anions (*e.g.*, sulfobromophthalein, indocyanine green, and cholecystographic agents) but not by bile acids.[6] Studies with sulfobromophthalein suggest that there may be two canalicular carriers responsible for its secretion,[193] one of which appears to be shared by bilirubin glucuronide.[74] In common with other substances excreted in bile at high concentrations relative to plasma, maximal bilirubin excretion can be enhanced by taurocholate[145] in spite of the fact that it has a separate excretory mechanism. It has been postulated that the bile salts form a "micellar sink" in the bile canaliculus so that the conjugated bilirubin is removed from the nonmicellar phase and a net concentration gradient is formed, which enhances the passive diffusion of pigment from the liver cell into the bile. Support for this concept comes from the observation that bilirubin conjugates, which may be in the form of aggregates, are excreted in bile incorporated into mixed lipid micelles.[240,257] This interpretation is controversial since the infusion of taurocholate during bilirubin-decreased phospholipid secretion does not increase maximal biliary bilirubin secretion although phospholipid secretion is restored to normal.[127] Another possible explanation for the increased bilirubin excretion with taurocholate is that the bile acid infusion causes centrilobular hepatocytes, as well as periportal cells, to be recruited for secretion.[145]

In addition to the organic anions mentioned previously, anabolic steroids, particularly C-17 alkyl derivatives, will compete with bilirubin for excretion and may cause jaundice.[7] Although the normal subject has a large functional reserve for bilirubin excretion,[238] the capacity of the excretory system is less than that of uptake. It appears from experimental studies that conjugation rather than secretion is probably the rate-limiting step for the hepatic transport of bilirubin.[204,205,291]

Intestinal Metabolism

In the intestine the bilirubin glucuronides excreted in the bile are first deconjugated by bacterial or intestinal βglucuronidases. They are then reduced by bacteria to form colorless urobilinogens, which subsequently undergo dehydrogenation to give orange-yellow urobilins (see Fig. 4-3). The structure of the urobilinoid formed will depend on the nature of the bacterial flora and does not appear to be of diagnostic value.[296] In the presence of broad-spectrum antibiotics, and in the newborn, bilirubin is excreted directly in the feces and urobilinogen is not formed, so that it seems likely that reduction of bile pigments only occurs if bilirubin is in the conjugated form. Enterohepatic circulations for both unconjugated bilirubin[134,185] and urobilinogen[186] have been demonstrated, but they are of minor importance in the disposition of bilirubin in the normal adult. It is, however, possible that in the newborn reabsorption of bilirubin from the intestine may be a cause of "physiologic" jaundice.

Estimations of fecal urobilinogen in the normal subject may vary between 47 and 276 mg/day and are slightly higher (on a body weight basis) in men than women.[49] A poor relationship has been found between bilirubin production, determined by the analysis of ^{14}C plasma disappearance curves and fecal urobilinogen excretion.[49] This discrepancy has been attributed to catabolism of bilirubin in the gastrointestinal tract, as well as difficulties inherent in the chemical estimation. Fecal urobilinogen estimations may, therefore, give false-negative results in patients with hemolytic disease; a significantly raised excretion will, however, be of diagnostic value in indicating an overproduction of bilirubin. Very low results will indicate complete biliary obstruction or a significant defect in hepatic bilirubin glucuronyl transferase. The color of normal feces is not due to urobilinoids but may be dependent on fuscins, which are derived from dipyrromethane polymers and probably originate from early labeled hemes.[133,231]

The intestine has the potential to contribute to the elimination of bilirubin from the body in a similar manner to the liver. Isolated mucosal cells from the intestine can synthesize radioactive heme from δ-amino-(^3H)-levulinic acid and then convert the heme to both monoglucuronide and diglucuronide conjugates of bilirubin[152]; they can also degrade bilirubin to dipyrroles.[311] The role, if any, of the intestine in the metabolism of bilirubin in the normal subject remains to be established, but it could be important in the hepatectomized animal.[122]

Renal Excretion

Bilirubin

Bilirubin is only excreted by the kidney in significant amounts when there is a raised level of conjugated bilirubin in the plasma. It cannot, therefore, be detected in the urine of normal subjects or patients with an unconjugated hyperbilirubinemia. The excretion of conjugated bilirubin is dependent on the small fraction in the plasma that is not protein bound[125] and is therefore available for glomerular filtration.[3,113,124,295] Compounds such as salicylate, sulfisoxazole, and bile salts, which compete with conjugated bilirubin for protein binding, and thus increase the amount of diffusible conjugated bilirubin, will augment the renal excretion of bilirubin in experimental animals when given in high doses.[5,125]

The histochemical demonstration of conjugated bilirubin in proximal tubular cells in obstructive jaundice supports the view that, in addition to glomerular filtration, either tubular absorption and/or tubular secretion are involved. The administration of inhibitors of tubular secretion such as probenecid and p-aminohippurate to jaundiced dogs[124] and rats[5] did not cause an increase in bilirubin clearance or influence the fractional reabsorption of bilirubin in the isolated perfused rat kidney.[138] Apart from the results of stop flow studies in bile duct ligated in dogs, there is, therefore, no good evidence that tubular secretion of conjugated bilirubin occurs.

Although it was not possible to demonstrate the presence of a major reabsorption process[125] in dogs, indirect evidence of this mechanism was obtained in rats when it was observed that conjugated bilirubin excretion increased after the administration of alkali, probably due to diminished reabsorption of the pigment.[3] In the isolated rat kidney, perfused with a protein-free medium, it was shown that tubular reabsorption exceeded 70% of the filtered conjugated bilirubin load, but it was not possible to establish whether this process involved active as well as passive diffusion.[138] In vivo studies[3,124] do not, however, support the view that nonionic diffusion is an important factor in the renal excretion of bile pigments. There are some preliminary studies that indicate that bile acids compete with conjugated bilirubin for reabsorption.[13]

The threshold level of serum conjugated bilirubin at which bilirubinuria occurs appears to vary greatly and to alter during the course of the disease. This is due in part to the formation of a fraction of conjugated bilirubin that becomes covalently bound to plasma albumin[183] and is, therefore, not available for renal excretion (see section on cholestatic jaundice). Compared with biliary excretion, the renal excretion of conjugated bilirubin is a relatively inefficient method of disposing of bilirubin. Values ranging from 0.07 ml to 0.82 ml/min for the "apparent" renal clearance of conjugated bilirubin have been recorded· these measurements have little diagnostic value.[113] The diversity in the results reported in the literature is probably due to the use of nonspecific analytical methods for the urinary estimation of bilirubin, which is very unstable, as well as the lack of a suitable method for determining unbound (or diffusible) plasma bilirubin.

Urobilinogen

The appearance of urobilinogen in the urine will depend on the amount of conjugated bilirubin appearing in the bile and the site of the urobilinogen forming bacteria, since urobilinogen is more efficiently absorbed from the intestine than from the colon. In the normal subject the small amount of urobilinogen that is reabsorbed will be almost entirely re-excreted by the liver so that values for the daily renal excretion of urobilinoids (expressed as urobilinogen) only range from 0 to 4 mg/day.[57] In hemolytic disease greater amounts of urobilinogen will presumably be formed and reabsorbed into the systemic circulation, and in hepatocellular disease there may be a failure to re-excrete the absorbed urobilinogen into the bile.[30] In these circumstances increased renal excretion of urobilinoids may, therefore, occur.

Urobilinogen is approximately 80% bound to plasma protein so that only a small fraction of that in the plasma is filtered by the glomerulus. There are preliminary data indicating that urobilinogen is secreted by the proximal tubules and that pH-dependent nonionic diffusion occurs in the distal nephron.[57,189]

Since urobilinoids are unstable, the collection of urine is often made over a 2- to 4-hour period, and in order to take account of the fact that there is a diurnal variation in urobilinogen excretion, it has been recommended that the urine specimen be collected between noon and 4 PM.[296] Urinary determinations of urobilinogen do not appear, however, to be of diagnostic value, except to demonstrate that biliary excretion has recommenced following relief of obstruction or during recovery from hepatitis.

PIGMENT GALLSTONES

There are two major types of pigment stones that are morphologically and clinically distinctive.[288] The typical brown laminated stones obtained mainly from Asians are qualitatively similar in composition to recurrent common bile duct stones found in Western patients associated with bacterial infection. This raises the possibility that the hydrolysis of bilirubin conjugates by bacterial β-glucuronidase may be a causative factor. The brown stones are composed of calcium salts from bilirubin and palmitate and cholesterol in a glycoprotein matrix.

The black amorphous pigment stone, which predominates in Western subjects, is also composed of calcium bilirubinate in addition to calcium carbonate and phosphate but rarely contains fatty acids or cholesterol. The major qualitative difference between the two types of stones is that in the black stones the calcium bilirubinate is polymerized to a greater degree. There is an increased incidence of black stones in patients with hemolysis due to the increased biliary bilirubin concentration, while in cirrhosis decreased concentrations of bile salts may play an etiologic role.

ALTERNATE PATHWAYS OF BILIRUBIN METABOLISM

Studies with radioactive bilirubin in patients and rats with prolonged cholestasis[66,67] and defective bilirubin conjugation[260] have established that catabolism of bilirubin can be an important mechanism for disposal of the pigment. The enzymes responsible for these alternate pathways of bilirubin metabolism have not yet been identified. It has been postulated that a microsomal P448–dependent mono-oxygenase may be involved since inducers of this enzyme, such as the toxic drug 2,3,7,8 tetrachloro-dibenzo-p-dioxin (TCDD)[170] and β-naphthoflavone[68] will increase the turnover of bilirubin in the Gunn rat and thus reduce its plasma bilirubin level. The existence of a mitochondrial bilirubin oxygenase that in vitro will degrade bilirubin to a variety of catabolites, including propentdyopents, has been demonstrated in rat brain,[60] intestine,[311] kidney,[311] and liver.[68] The role of this enzyme in vivo has still to be defined.

NORMAL PLASMA BILIRUBIN CONCENTRATION

The concentration of bilirubin in the plasma represents a balance between the rate of entry of the pigment into the plasma and the hepatic clearance of bilirubin. Studies in which the plasma disappearance rate of radioactive bilirubin was determined in 57 normal individuals[51] have established that the plasma unconjugated bilirubin concentration (Br) is related to the bilirubin production rate (BRP) and hepatic bilirubin clearance (C_{BR}) by the following equation:

$$Br = BRP \div C_{BR}$$

The results obtained from this study for the distribution for Br in the normal population are in agreement with those obtained by standard diazo techniques[11,224,237] and indicate that anyone with a Br exceeding 1.0 mg/dl (17 μmol/liter) should be suspected of having either abnormal hepatic function or bilirubin overproduction, or both. In a study of 18,454 men and 5,471 women attending a screening center, the median total bilirubin value for men was 0.56 mg/dl (9.6 μmol/liter), which was significantly higher ($p < .001$) than that for women (0.45 mg/dl, 7.6 μmol/liter).[11] These findings are in agreement with earlier observations[224,237,258] and probably reflect the higher activities of hepatic bilirubin UDP-glucuronyl transferase in females than males, as has been shown in rats.[203,204]

In normal subjects almost all the bilirubin in the plasma appears to be in the unconjugated form,[45] although with a very sensitive high-pressure liquid chromatographic assay it is possible to show that approximately 4% of the pigment is present as bilirubin conjugates with equal amounts of monoglucuronides and diglucuronides.[202] Routine diazo procedures tend to give artifactually high values for "direct" (conjugated) bilirubin at low levels of total bilirubin so that calculated values of "indirect" (unconjugated) bilirubin, obtained by subtracting conjugated bilirubin from total bilirubin, are not meaningful without knowledge of the limitations of the method employed in a particular laboratory.[112]

ABNORMALITIES IN BILIRUBIN METABOLISM ASSOCIATED WITH JAUNDICE

If there is either a marked increase in the rate of formation of bilirubin or a defect in any of the processes underlying the hepatic clearance of unconjugated bilirubin (*i.e.,* hepatic uptake, intracellular binding, and conjugation), then unconjugated bilirubin will accumulate in the plasma. In contrast, impairment to biliary flow either at a canalicular or bile ductular level will cause reflux of conjugated bilirubin into the plasma. In the presence of diffuse liver injury there will often be a combination of bilirubin overproduction and impairment in one or more of the different hepatic transport mechanisms; however, the overall effect will be to cause a conjugated hyperbilirubinemia.

Unconjugated Hyperbilirubinemia

Hemolytic Disease

Hemolysis causes an increased production of bilirubin and a raised fecal and urinary urobilinogen excretion. The ability of the liver to excrete bilirubin is greatly in excess of that normally required so that a 50% reduction in red cell survival in a patient with normal liver function will not necessarily result in a plasma bilirubin concentration outside the normal range.[236] In severe cases of hemolytic disease the excretory capacity of the liver will be exceeded and an unconjugated hyperbilirubinemia will result. However, even if the rate of red cell destruction is increased sixfold, the plasma bile pigment excretion is unlikely to rise above 5 mg/dl.

Although the plasma bilirubin in hemolytic jaundice is predominantly unconjugated, with only 4% in the conjugated form,[112] significant increases in conjugated bilirubin are not infrequently reported from the routine laboratory; if these exceed 15% of the total bilirubin, then this is probably the result of concomitant hepatic dysfunction.[287] In acute massive hemolytic episodes, such as may occur after multiple transfusions during surgery,[181] in Wilson's disease,[201] in acute infections[101,105] or after drug administration,[254] then a mixed hyperbilirubinemia will result due to excessive production of bilirubin associated with hepatic dysfunction.

Some patients with hemolytic disease have higher plasma bilirubin concentrations than would be expected from their red cell survival.[22,236] Their pattern of radiobilirubin clearance is, however, similar to that in patients with classic Gilbert's syndrome.[20] Studies in patients undergoing splenectomy for hereditary spherocytosis[29] have shown that those who, preoperatively, had reduced values for hepatic bilirubin clearance (C_{BR}) and bilirubin glucuronyl transferase activity, tended to normalize their C_{BR} postoperatively. These findings were interpreted as indicating that a hemolytic stress can unmask a latent state for Gilbert's syndrome. There have been several other re-

ports of reduced bilirubin glucuronyl transferase activity in chronic hemolytic anemia, but not in aplastic anemia.[10] In a series of 37 patients with clinically overt hemolytic disease, 41% had defects in bilirubin conjugation and 51% had pigment stones in the gallbladder.[117] Although the two abnormalities did not appear to exhibit a direct causal relationship,[117] the solubility of bilirubin in the bile would be impaired so that it is not surprising that pigment stones are more common in hemolytic disease than in any other pathologic condition in the Western Hemisphere. It is possible that unconjugated bilirubin may play a role in the initiation of cholesterol stones since these patients may also have a defect in hepatic bilirubin glucuronidation.[99]

Diseases Associated with Early Labeled Bilirubin Production

Marked increases in early labeled bilirubin (ELB) formation have been noted in diseases associated with ineffective erythropoiesis, such as iron deficiency anemia,[243] pernicious anemia,[252] thalassemia,[151,241] dyserythropoietic jaundice (shunt hyperbilirubinemia),[18,159] erythropoietic porphyria,[149,192] and lead poisoning.[21] Patients with these conditions, which are characterized by abnormalities in heme biosynthesis within the developing normoblast, have significant increases in total bile pigment turnover but do not show evidence of increased red cell destruction. In contrast, in paroxysmal nocturnal hemoglobinuria and sickle cell anemia,[163] or following hemorrhage,[147] there is an absolute but not a relative increase in erythroid ELB production together with increased red cell destruction. This source of bilirubin is often reduced in aplastic or hypoplastic anemia[15] but can be increased if there is a favorable response to treatment with vitamin B_{12}.[252]

Quantitative studies have shown that the hepatic component of ELB is not changed in megaloblastic anemia, thalassemia, or sideroblastic anemia.[250] There is, however, evidence that some of the increased bilirubin production in patients with erythropoietic porphyria[149] and pernicious anemia[250,309] may be hepatic in origin. There have also been reports in cirrhosis and acute hepatitis[251,281] of increased turnover of hepatic heme proteins that require confirmation.

The term primary shunt hyperbilirubinemia has been used to describe a rare heterogeneous group of patients with mild unconjugated hyperbilirubinemia and increased ELB production.[159,160] Dyserythropoietic jaundice,[18] would, however, probably be a more appropriate description since there is no evidence that porphyrins can be converted to bile pigments without heme as an intermediate. Israels[159] has reviewed 11 such cases in which there was evidence of rapid turnover of heme and hemoglobin within the bone marrow, possibly due to premature destruction of red cell precursors. These patients also had erythroid hyperplasia of the bone marrow, increased iron turnover, hemosiderosis of hepatic parenchymal and Kupffer cells, marked increases in urobilinogen excretion, and a normal peripheral red cell survival time.[174] Spleno-

TABLE 4-1. Classification of Nonhemolytic Unconjugated Hyperbilirubinemia

| | CRIGLER-NAJJAR SYNDROME | | GILBERT'S SYNDROME |
	Type I	Type II	
Plasma bilirubin (mg/dl)	25–48	6–25	1–6
Bile	Pale yellow (trace bilirubin and monoglucuronide)	Yellow; mainly bilirubin monoglucuronide	Normal appearance; relative increase in bilirubin monoglucuronide
Fecal urobilinogen (mg/day)	<10	20–80	Lower limit of normal range
Hepatic bilirubin glucuronyl transferase	None	Trace (?)	Significantly reduced
Kernicterus	Usual	Rare	Never
Prognosis	Poor	Good	Good
Effect of phenobarbital on plasma bilirubin	None	Marked reduction to 4–8 mg/dl	Reduction to normal levels
Routine liver function tests cholecystography, hematology, liver histology	Normal	Normal	Normal
Inheritance	Autosomal recessive	? Autosomal dominant	? Autosomal dominant

megaly has been described in 50% of patients, but hepatomegaly was not present and tests of liver function were normal. Reticulocytes tend to be raised, which may be a useful diagnostic feature of this condition. The prognosis appears to be excellent, although, like hemolytic jaundice, it predisposes to cholelithiasis.

Chronic Nonhemolytic Unconjugated Hyperbilirubinemia

Compartmental analysis of plasma disappearance curves[20] has suggested that alterations in the hepatic uptake process, either at the cell membrane or cytoplasmic binding level, could be responsible for the development of unconjugated hyperbilirubinemia. As yet there are no firm data to substantiate this hypothesis. It has, however, been well established that the deficiency of hepatic bilirubin UDP-glucuronyl transferase seen in the newborn may persist into adult life so that the patient has a chronic unconjugated hyperbilirubinemia, in the absence of overt hemolysis and coexistent hepatic or systemic disease associated with reduced hepatic blood flow. Results of liver function tests and histology on light microscopy are normal. The extent of the deficiency of glucuronyl transferase and the degree of jaundice attained are variable, and for convenience the patients have been arbitrarily divided into three main groups, that is, Crigler-Najjar type I, Crigler-Najjar type II, and Gilbert's syndromes (Table 4-1), as suggested by Arias and co-workers.[8]

Crigler-Najjar Type I Syndrome. Crigler-Najjar type I syndrome (congenital nonhemolytic jaundice) is an extremely rare condition that appears early in life.[86] The hyperbilirubinemia, which may range from 25 mg to 45 mg/dl (428 μmol to 796 μmol/liter) has been shown to be due to an absolute deficiency of bilirubin glucuronyl transferase, when bilirubin or bilirubin monoglucuronide is used as a substrate in a new sensitive assay.[106] It is associated with kernicterus, which causes severe cerebral damage and mental retardation. Death usually occurs within 18 months of life. Some affected patients have survived until puberty and then developed bilirubin encephalopathy.[26,47,53] Treatment with phlebotomy,[27] plasmapheresis,[26] and phototherapy[47,106,209] has been attempted, and reduced levels of serum bilirubin have been attained; the condition has only been temporarily alleviated, however, and the plasma bilirubin concentration has never been reduced by more than 50%. Enzyme replacement is a potential means of treatment, but this has not yet been successful in the Gunn rat,[248] which is an excellent animal model for this condition, with its absolute deficiency of bilirubin glucuronyl transferase. Now that clones for glucuronyl transferase have been isolated,[64] genetic engineering has become a possibility. Transplantation could also be considered; this would probably have to involve the liver because, although renal transplantation has been shown to be successful in the Gunn rat,[119] bilirubin UDP-glucuronyl transferase has not been detected in the human kidney.[116] Further prolonged testing in nonhuman primates is necessary before therapy with tin protoporphyrin, which would limit bilirubin production, could be advocated.[171]

Bilirubin production in patients with the Crigler-Najjar syndrome is essentially normal whether determined by standard techniques or radiobilirubin kinetics. The hepatic bilirubin clearance is greatly diminished, giving a biologic half-life of the pigment in excess of 156 hours.[27,47,260] This appears to be mainly due to a lack of bilirubin UDP-glucuronyl transferase activity.[8,47] As a result, only minimal amounts of bilirubin appear in the bile and fecal urobilinogen excretion is very low. Analysis of the pale yellow bile has shown that 30% to 57% of the bilirubin pigments exist as unconjugated bilirubin and that trace amounts of bilirubin monoglucuronide can be detected.[115] By definition the administration of microsomal enzyme inducers such as phenobarbital or glutethimide[47,106] do not influence bilirubin metabolism in these patients.

The exact mechanism whereby the plasma bilirubin level in these patients remains relatively constant, in spite of their inability to excrete bilirubin into bile or urine, is a matter for conjecture. The classic studies of Schmid and Hammaker[260] in which ^{14}C bilirubin was administered to a child with the Crigler-Najjar syndrome and to Gunn rats have indicated that the main means of disposal of the pigment is in the form of catabolites in the urine and feces. These include hydroxyl derivatives of bilirubin in addition to significant amounts of diazo-negative compounds, some of which give a propentdyopent reaction and may be dipyrroles (see section on alternate pathways of bilirubin metabolism).

Examination of the literature in which 60 or more cases of the type I syndrome have been reported indicates that it is probably inherited as an autosomal recessive trait. Support for this mode of inheritance comes mainly from excretion studies with aglycones such as menthol, which are also excreted as glucuronides[8] but whose formation involves a different glucuronyl transferase.

Crigler-Najjar Type II Syndrome. Patients with the Crigler-Najjar type II syndrome have plasma bilirubin concentrations ranging from 6 mg to 25 mg/dl (103 μmol to 428 μmol/liter), virtually all in the unconjugated form, and are less severely affected than those with the type I syndrome. When they are treated with phenobarbital[8,38,48,136,270] or other microsomal enzyme inducers such as glutethimide[41,48] their plasma bilirubin concentration drops dramatically. This suggests that these patients have bilirubin UDP-glucuronyl transferase activity in their tissues in reduced amounts, although our present techniques are often not sufficiently sensitive to detect it.[136] (See section on Gilbert's syndrome.) Bilirubin monoglucuronide is the predominant pigment in bile,[115,141] so there may also be a defect in the conversion of the monoglucuronide to the diglucuronide. This impairment in the diglucuronide to monoglucuronide ratio in bile is still apparent in the presence of acquired cholestasis when phenobarbital does not reduce the serum bilirubin level but will increase the biliary bilirubin excretion.[289]

The high level of circulating unconjugated bilirubin does not appear to cause neurologic damage in the adult. Indeed, three brothers over 50 years of age were reported who had serum bilirubin levels greater than 20 mg/dl and who did not appear to have suffered any ill effects from their jaundice, which had been present since birth.[136] In common with most other sufferers of this condition they were delighted to be "white washed" by treatment with phenobarbital (Fig. 4-4). Their serum bilirubin concentration fell to 4 mg to 5 mg/dl and has remained at this level for 10 years. In common with patients with Gilbert's syndrome their hyperbilirubinemia increased with fasting or removal of lipid from their diet.[137]

The exact mode of inheritance of the type II syndrome is in doubt, but from data obtained with the menthol glucuronide test, it is generally accepted that it is transmitted as an autosomal dominant trait with incomplete penetrance; tests with bilirubin as the substrate for glucuronidation are needed to establish this point. Individuals with Gilbert's syndrome often occur in families of patients with the Crigler-Najjar syndrome.[8,136,157] It has been suggested that two allelic genes may be involved in the Crigler-

Fig. 4-4. Effect of a 400-calorie diet and treatment with phenobarbitone (t.d.s.) on the plasma bilirubin concentration of a 53-year-old man with the Crigler–Najjar syndrome, type II. During the 5-day control period on a ward diet, his plasma bilirubin concentration varied from 21 to 23 mg/dl. (Gollan JL et al: Gastroenterology 68:1543, 1975)

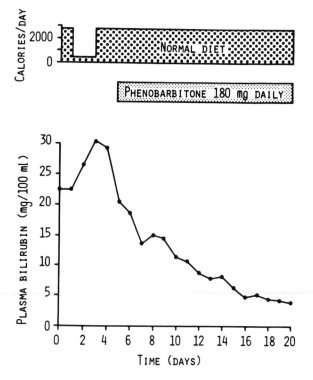

Najjar syndrome and that Gilbert's syndrome results when only one of these genes is present,[157] but this hypothesis requires testing with molecular biologic techniques.

Gilbert's Syndrome. It is now generally believed that Gilbert's syndrome (constitutional hepatic dysfunction, idiopathic unconjugated hyperbilirubinemia)[121,132] and the Crigler-Najjar syndrome have a similar pathogenesis and differ only in the severity of the condition. The analysis of plasma disappearance curves following the administration of isotopically labeled bilirubin to patients with both the Crigler-Najjar syndrome type II[41,85,260] and Gilbert's syndrome[20,41] has confirmed studies with nonisotopic bilirubin (2 mg/kg),[34,215] in showing that all these patients have a characteristic reduction in hepatic bilirubin clearance that is responsible for their hyperbilirubinemia. These findings have been interpreted by most investigators as indicating defects in both the hepatic uptake and the conjugation of bilirubin, although a study with varying loads of nonradioactive bilirubin has failed to confirm the occurrence of defective hepatic uptake.[146] The bilirubin transport maximum appears to be low in patients with Gilbert's syndrome, whereas the relative storage capacity is normal.[215,238] Reduced values for hepatic bilirubin glucuronyl transferase activity in needle biopsy specimens (measured after digitonin activation) have been found in all patients who have been clinically diagnosed as having Gilbert's syndrome (Fig. 4-5).[39,109] The observation that the bile of these patients contains proportionally less bil-

irubin diglucuronide than the normal subject, in addition to a decrease in the total bile pigments, has been interpreted as indicating that there are defects in the formation of both the monoglucuronide and the diglucuronide.[115] It has been postulated that the reduction in glucuronyl transferase activity might be due to alterations in the microenvironment in the microsomal membrane rather than to a specific protein defect,[239] but there are no data to support this hypothesis. Preliminary studies with needle biopsy specimens provide indirect evidence for the presence of reduced amounts of the normal enzyme rather than the existence of an abnormal enzyme.[31,84]

Reductions in enzyme activity have also been reported in chronic persistent hepatitis,[107] hemolytic disorders,[10,117] noncirrhotic portal fibrosis, portal vein thrombosis, and granulomatous liver disease.[89] The differential diagnosis of these conditions, however, is unlikely to be confused with Gilbert's syndrome. There is no good correlation between the raised plasma unconjugated bilirubin concentration and the reduced enzyme activity in Gilbert's syndrome. This is probably because 40% to 50% of these patients (who do not have congenital spherocytosis or glucose-6-phosphate dehydrogenase deficiency) also have an increased bilirubin turnover owing to a slight reduction in red cell survival in addition to a decrease in hepatic bilirubin clearance.[20,22,236] Recognition of this group of patients can be achieved from analysis of plasma disappearance curves of radioactive bilirubin[20,24] or a knowledge of the patients' red cell volume, chromium-51 red cell half-life, and plasma bilirubin concentration.[22] Kinetic studies with nonradioactive bilirubin and radioactive heme precursors have established that these patients with Gilbert's syndrome, who have an increased bilirubin turnover, comprise both patients with an increased erythroid heme turnover and patients with increased metabolism of hepatic heme.[316]

The heterogeneity of patients classified as having Gilbert's syndrome is further demonstrated by the fact that some of them have mild defects in their ability to clear sulfobromophthalein[23]; a proportion, but not all, of these patients also exhibit defective plasma clearance of indocyanine green.[196] Further variants of Gilbert's syndrome, which are characterized by defective indocyanine green uptake in the presence of normal sulfobromophthalein metabolism have been reported from Japan.[213,218] Abnormalities in the hepatic transport of drugs, including tolbutamide,[69] rifamycin SV,[130,131] and nicotinic acid[130,131] have also been detected in Gilbert's syndrome. There is, therefore, increasing evidence of the existence of subgroups of patients with Gilbert's syndrome whose hepatic defects are not limited to bilirubin glucuronidation but also involve hepatic uptake of organic anions, excluding bile acids other than ursodeoxycholate.[212] The possibility that morphologic heterogeneity exists has also been postulated[90] but has not been confirmed.[167]

Effects of Drugs. Treatment of patients with Gilbert's syndrome with phenobarbital,[9,41,110] glutethimide,[41,48] and clofibrate[180] has been shown to cause a significant drop

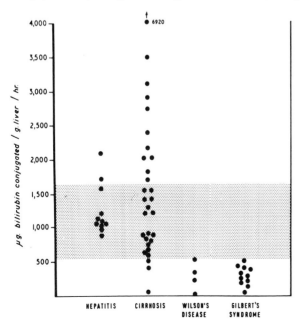

Fig. 4-5. Hepatic bilirubin UDP-glucuronyl transferase activity in patients with hepatocellular disease and Gilbert's disease. Hatched area indicates the normal range (mean ± SD). (Black M, Billing BH: N Engl J Med 280:1266, 1971)

in plasma bilirubin concentration due mainly to an increase in hepatic bilirubin clearance, which becomes almost indistinguishable from that of a normal subject; in addition, there may be a slight reduction in plasma bilirubin turnover. Since studies in surgical patients[40] and patients with hepatitis[109] have demonstrated that chronic phenobarbital administration will increase hepatic bilirubin glucuronyl transferase activity, it is somewhat surprising that two groups of investigators[41,109] have been unable to demonstrate more convincing changes in enzyme activity following treatment in Gilbert's disease. Moreover, in patients with the Crigler-Najjar syndrome type II it has not been possible to demonstrate hepatic glucuronyl transferase activity either before or after phenobarbital treatment despite impressive decreases in plasma bilirubin levels, a rapid clearance of isotopic bilirubin from the plasma, and enhanced excretion of isotope in the feces. This failure has been attributed to insufficient sensitivity of the enzyme assay or the possibility that an *in vitro* assay gives only an approximation of the activity of the enzyme *in vivo*[41,136] Corticosteroids can also cause a reduction in plasma bilirubin, probably by enhancing hepatic uptake or storage of bilirubin rather than biliary excretion.[214] Treatment does not, however, influence the parameters of the nicotinic acid test.[210]

Incidence and Prognosis. Mild icterus is the only abnormal physical finding in Gilbert's syndrome, and this may not always be apparent in the majority of cases with mild hyperbilirubinemia. Serum unconjugated bilirubin levels tend to fluctuate, and approximately one third of patients may at some time have a normal value. Transient rises have been associated with intercurrent infections, fatty foods, caloric deprivation, alcohol ingestion, and physical exercise[121] as well as with premenstrual tension.[308] A high proportion of patients appear to present with gastrointestinal complaints[121,237] and complain of nonspecific symptoms such as fatigue, weakness, and abdominal pain. There is no evidence that these symptoms are related to the hyperbilirubinemia per se, although they did persist in one third of 17 patients who had been followed for 7 to 20 years but did not involve loss of time from work. The hyperbilirubinemia of the patients in this study remained relatively constant during the entire period of observation (Makinen, Billing BH, Sherlock S: Unpublished observations).

Gilbert's syndrome is most often diagnosed in the late teens or early 20s; there is, however, no reliable data to indicate whether the symptoms occur before puberty, although isolated cases have been reported. Males predominate in a ratio of approximately 4:1 in most series.[11,121,224,237] This sex difference probably reflects the lower distribution of bilirubin concentrations in normal women than in men[11,224,237,258] rather than sex-linked inheritance. The incidence of Gilbert's syndrome, based on an abnormal serum bilirubin value, may be as high as 5% of the male population.[11,224] Although there is no doubt that there is a familial incidence[121,224,237] in this syndrome (Fig. 4-6), its heterogeneity makes it difficult to establish the mode of inheritance. Studies based on plasma bilirubin

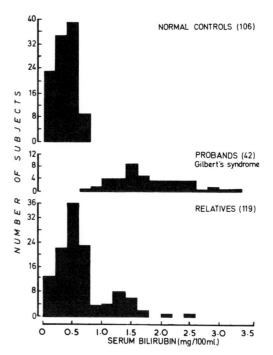

Fig. 4-6. Distribution of values for serum total bilirubin concentration in normal controls, patients with Gilbert's syndrome, and healthy first-degree relatives. The results for the relatives showed a bimodal distribution; 17 of the 42 families (40%) had one or more affected relatives. (Powell LW et al: N Engl J Med 277:1108, 1967)

concentrations suggest that it is probably inherited as an autosomal dominant trait with incomplete penetrance.[237]

Invasive Tests. Fasting (or a low lipid 400 caloric diet)[108,137,225] will cause a twofold to threefold rise in plasma bilirubin concentration in patients with Gilbert's syndrome, even if the serum bilirubin is initially normal. Modest rises in plasma bilirubin may also be seen in patients with hemolysis, acute viral hepatitis, and biliary cirrhosis so that a positive response to fasting can only be considered to be diagnostic if other liver functions tests are normal and overt hemolysis has been excluded. Moreover, not all patients with Gilbert's syndrome respond to this test,[137] which is less sensitive and less specific for females than males.[219] The mechanism of fasting hyperbilirubinemia is still incompletely understood.[110,216,299] It appears that there is an increase in bilirubin production, but perhaps more important is a reduction in hepatic bilirubin clearance.

Nicotinic acid increases the osmotic fragility of human erythrocytes so that there is a greater load of bilirubin available for disposal.[211] In the presence of a defect in bilirubin glucuronyl transferase an injection of nicotinic acid (50 mg) will cause a significant rise in plasma bilirubin.[123] It is claimed that the nicotinic acid test will differentiate Gilbert's syndrome from chronic liver disease but not from hemolytic anemia.[210] The sensitivity of the test can be improved if the area under the bilirubin concentration time curve is measured rather than the maximal increment of unconjugated serum bilirubin or the retention at 4 hours.[246]

The use of plasma bilirubin disappearance curves (4-hour retention), bilirubin UDP-glucuronyl transferase determinations in liver biopsy, and reduced ratio of bilirubin diglucuronide to monoglucuronide in bile have already been discussed.[217]

Diagnosis. When making the diagnosis of Gilbert's syndrome caution must be exercised to eliminate the possibility that the chronic unconjugated hyperbilirubinemia is not due to some acquired diseased state such as cardiac disease, fatty liver and alcoholism, cirrhosis, biliary tract disease, chronic persistent hepatitis, malignant tumors, and infarctions.[188] Unconjugated hyperbilirubinemia may follow viral hepatitis and appear in patients who have undergone portacaval shunt due to hemolysis.[92] It can also occur in thyrotoxicosis[150] and may be present in people living at high altitudes.[17]

Since Gilbert's disease is a benign condition and the only obvious abnormality is a fluctuating plasma bilirubin level due to a decreased ability to clear bilirubin from the plasma, the establishment of the diagnosis is largely a matter of exclusion. The tests listed in the previous section do not enable the clinician to make a firm diagnosis of Gilbert's syndrome since abnormal results may be seen in other types of disease. Liver biopsy permits the immediate exclusion of structural liver disease but is not considered by some physicians to be a justifiable risk except in special circumstances. A report from seven different centers in Europe and the United States[217] has adopted a pragmatic approach to the problem and has recommended that a presumptive diagnosis of Gilbert's syndrome can be made after a careful history and physical examination, if the individual, who is essentially asymptomatic, has (1) an unconjugated hyperbilirubinemia on several occasions; (2) normal results of complete blood cell count, examination of blood smear, and reticulocyte count; and (3) normal values for serum glutamic oxaloacetic/pyruvic transaminases, alkaline phosphatase, γ-glutamyl transpeptidase, and fasting/postprandial serum bile acid determination.[96,244,294] If no further laboratory abnormalities develop on two to three follow-up visits during the next 12 to 18 months, then the presumptive diagnosis becomes definitive. Once the diagnosis has been established, then the patient can be reassured that he has a benign condition with an excellent prognosis. An unnecessary operation may be avoided, and any difficulties with regard to insurance or employment resulting from the patient's hyperbilirubinemia can be overcome by a suitable report from the physician.

Conjugated Hyperbilirubinemia

Cholestasis

In the majority of patients with liver disease red cell survival is reduced[232] so that there may be more bilirubin for disposal than in the normal subject unless the patient becomes severely anemic. In the presence of bile duct obstruction, whether intrahepatic or extrahepatic in origin, the concentration of bilirubin in the plasma gradually rises and then, if the obstruction is complete, plateaus at a value ranging between 10 mg and 30 mg/dl.[126,305] Concentrations greater than 30 mg/dl are more likely to be found in patients with hepatocellular disease than in those with extrahepatic obstruction. A survey of 11 patients with alcoholic nutritional cirrhosis and 8 patients with acute viral hepatitis revealed that the development of "extreme hyperbilirubinemia" (33 mg to 75 mg/dl) was often due to impaired renal function or excessive hemolysis resulting from sickle cell anemia or a deficiency of erythrocyte glucose-6-phosphate dehydrogenase.[126]

Radioisotopic studies in biliary atresia[66] and in experimental animals with bile duct ligation[1,4,67] indicate that urinary excretion is the main means of controlling bilirubin homeostasis in obstructive jaundice. Catabolism of a proportion of the pigments to unknown compounds, some of which give a propentdyopent reaction and are probably dipyrroles, also occurs. The rise in plasma bile pigment concentration in hepatitis, cirrhosis, and cholestasis is due to a mixture of monoconjugates and diconjugates of bilirubin that are refluxed into the plasma as the result of impaired biliary excretion. In patients with hepatocellular disease the dominant pigments in plasma tend to be the monoconjugates, whereas in obstructive jaundice the diconjugates are the major group of pigments.[256,290] There is, however, a considerable overlap in the results so that the relative amounts of monoconjugates and diconjugates do not appear to be of diagnostic significance.

Bile retention results in the nonenzymatic formation of positional glucuronide isomers due to sequestral migration of the bilirubin acyl group from C-1 to C-2, C-3, and C-4 of the sugar residue.[43,78] These non–C-1 glucuronides, which accumulate in bile and plasma, are resistent to β-glucuronidase and thus will not be hydrolyzed in the gallbladder or gut lumen. It has been postulated that they may play a protective role in preventing pigment cholelithiasis and excessive reabsorption of unconjugated bilirubin.

In hepatitis, bilirubinuria is often the first abnormality to be detected. In contrast, during recovery, bilirubinuria may be absent.[235] These apparent alterations in the threshold level of plasma conjugated bilirubin are due to the nonenzymatic formation of a tightly bound bilirubin protein conjugate (see section on bile pigments) that cannot be filtered by the glomerulus. The life span of this bilirubin complex, is therefore, dependent on the half-life of albumin, and not on urinary excretion, so that the jaundice resolves slowly in spite of improvement in other tests of liver function.[290] Raised levels of plasma bilirubin–protein conjugates have been reported in almost all cases of obstructive jaundice (intrahepatic or extrahepatic) and in the Dubin-Johnson syndrome.[298] They are dependent on the duration of the cholestasis but do not have any recognizable diagnostic meaning. In hepatobiliary disease there is a discrepancy between the sum of the unconjugated bilirubin and monoesterified and diesterified bilirubins determined by the alkaline methanolysis–high-pressure liquid chromatography method[45] and the total bilirubin values obtained by diazo methods[257,290]; this is due to the loss of the bilirubin complex on the protein precipitate.

Since bilirubin conjugation occurs only in the liver, it has been postulated that in anicteric patients, with normal serum total bilirubin values, determination of esterified bilirubin values might provide a more sensitive marker of hepatobiliary disease than standard liver function tests including serum bile acids.[112,166,290]

Analytical problems have prevented the satisfactory determination of pool sizes and turnover rates of unconjugated and conjugated bilirubin in obstructive jaundice. However, the results of investigations in which ^{14}C bilirubin has been given to animals, whose bile ducts have been ligated, do suggest that the extravascular pool of conjugated bilirubin is considerably greater than that of unconjugated bilirubin, probably due to differences in protein binding.[1,4]

The hepatic clearance of unconjugated ^{14}C bilirubin from the plasma of patients with cholestatic liver disease appears to be normal.[52] In cirrhosis the efficiency of the liver in extracting unconjugated bilirubin from the plasma is, however, impaired even though the liver's capacity to conjugate bilirubin may be normal.[226]

In most types of cholestatic liver disease the pattern of serum bilirubin concentrations follows that of serum bile acids. In benign recurrent intrahepatic cholestasis there is a marked dissociation between bilirubin and bile acid levels,[279] so that whereas at the beginning of an attack serum bile acid concentrations are often extremely high, the serum bilirubin concentrations may be normal. Subsequently the bile acid concentration falls while the serum bilirubin value rises and a maximum value is attained after a month when the bile acid concentration has significantly decreased. It remains to be determined whether this distinctive pattern in benign recurrent intrahepatic cholestasis is of diagnostic value.

Dubin-Johnson Syndrome (Chronic Idiopathic Jaundice)

Dubin-Johnson syndrome is a benign chronic or intermittent form of jaundice with both unconjugated and conjugated bilirubin in the plasma[65,98,274]; bilirubin–protein conjugates have also been detected.[298] Plasma total bilirubin concentrations as high as 27 mg/dl have been reported, but on most occasions the patient is only mildly jaundiced. Physical examination is normal apart from vague abdominal pains, and pruritus is not a problem.[300] The syndrome is characterized by the presence of large amounts of a yellow–brown-black pigment in the lysosomes of centrilobular hepatocytes,[266] which are otherwise histologically normal (Fig. 4-7). The black pigment can be easily detected on visual examination in a needle biopsy

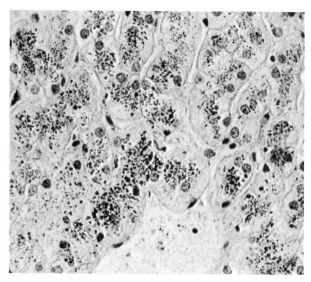

Fig. 4-7. Dubin–Johnson syndrome. Photomicrograph showing pigmentation in liver cells. (Courtesy of the Armed Forces Institute of Pathology)

specimen and probably has a melanin-like structure,[280] but it tends to disappear during an attack of hepatitis.[292] The pigment has also been found in Corriedale sheep,[81] which have proved to be a useful model for studying the condition. There is a poor correlation between the amount of pigment in the liver and the degree of jaundice.

Results of liver function tests are usually normal in patients with the Dubin-Johnson syndrome,[98] although the urine urobilinogen value may be raised. The gallbladder is not usually visualized on oral cholecytography, and indeed acute renal failure has been reported in one patient with the Dubin-Johnson syndrome[273] who was sensitive to biligrafin. However, with ^{99m}Tc-HIDA, visualization of the liver and gallbladder, but not the intrahepatic biliary tree, can be achieved after 90 minutes, and the isotope can be detected in the intestine.[12] Loading studies with bilirubin[34] and sulfobromophthalein[263] have clearly demonstrated that the principal defect in this syndrome is a reduced ability to transport organic anions from the liver cell into the bile. Retention of rose bengal, methylene blue, and indocyanine green has also been reported, but the excretion of bile acids is normal, except for the β-hydroxy bile acid ursodeoxycholate.[212] An extended sulfobromophthalein[70,195] (2 mg/kg) test has been found to be of diagnostic value since in the majority of patients studied the plasma sulfobromophthalein concentration 90 to 120 minutes after the injection is greater than that at 45 minutes, regardless of whether the 45-minute value is normal or increased; appreciable quantities of the injected dye can also be recovered from the urine. This abnormal response in the test is due to the reflux of dye (mainly as its glutathione conjugate) from the liver cell into the plasma. A delayed rise in the plasma level of sulfobromophthalein after 75 minutes has also been reported for extrahepatic jaundice and amyloidosis.[245] No reflux is seen when dyes such as disulfobromophthalein or indocyanine green, which are not conjugated by the liver, are administered.[103] The Dubin-Johnson syndrome is the only hepatic disorder in which the transport maximum for sulfobromophthalein is almost nil while the relative storage capacity of the liver is normal.[76]

It has been shown that the urinary coproporphyrin I excretion is increased in the Dubin-Johnson syndrome to a greater extent than in patients with other hepatic and biliary tract disorders (90% total), while that of the coproporphyrin III isomer tends to be decreased.[16,177,302] These changes are diagnostic and are also reflected in the feces and bile.[176] Family studies have shown that with respect to urinary coproporphyrin excretion[16,302] and abnormal sulfobromophthalein metabolism[100,268] the Dubin-Johnson syndrome is probably inherited as an autosomal recessive characteristic.

Cases of the Dubin-Johnson syndrome have been reported from all over the world and in particular in Israel amongst the Ashkenazi and Sephardic Jews, as well as Arabs.[16,267,268] Many patients are asymptomatic at the time of diagnosis, and the disease is detected for the first time during family studies for the evaluation of a relative with jaundice. Pregnancy and the use of oral contraceptives, which reduce hepatic excretory function, may unmask the presence of the Dubin-Johnson syndrome by temporarily converting a mild conjugated hyperbilirubinemia into overt jaundice.[76]

Rotor's Syndrome

Rotor's syndrome is another rare type of benign, familial chronic conjugated hyperbilirubinemia. It differs in many respects from the Dubin-Johnson syndrome.[154,247,259] The jaundice may fluctuate in intensity and increase in the presence of intercurrent infections; the plasma bilirubin concentration is usually less than 10 mg/dl and consists of approximately equal amounts of unconjugated and conjugated bilirubin; results of other liver function tests are normal, and there is no evidence of hemolysis. In contrast to the Dubin-Johnson syndrome the oral cholecystogram is reported to be normal; nevertheless it has been reported that ^{99m}Tc-HIDA administration does not result in visualization of the liver, gallbladder, or biliary tract and that the isotope, instead of accumulating in the intestine, is excreted by the kidneys.[12] There is no pigment in the liver cells. Changes seen on electron microscopy appear to be relatively nonspecific and include multiple phagolysosomal pigment bodies, mitochondria of variable size and matrix density, abnormal peroxisomes, and focal bile canalicular abnormalities.[104,275]

The kinetics of the cholephilic dyes are very different in Rotor's syndrome from those in the Dubin-Johnson syndrome. In particular, the initial slope of the plasma disappearance curve for both indocyanine green[91,206] and sulfobromophthalein[206,306] is impaired, suggesting a defect in hepatic uptake, and there is no secondary rise. The 45-minute plasma sulfobromophthalein retention is elevated by 30% to 50%. The sulfobromophthalein transport maximum is modestly reduced, whereas the relative storage capacity may be reduced by as much as 90%, which is in contrast to the findings in the Dubin-Johnson syndrome in which the transport maximum is almost zero and the storage capacity is normal.[306] Similar findings have been reported for patients with hepatic storage disease,[93] and it now seems likely that these two conditions are identical. The hepatic uptake of bilirubin is also diminished in Rotor's syndrome.[259] The total urinary coproporphyrin excretion is usually greater than normal in Rotor's syndrome and has a pattern similar to that seen in other hepatobiliary disorders.[303] The increase in coproporphyrin I is proportionately greater than that of coproporphyrin III, but when expressed as a percentage of total coproporphyrin it is significantly less than that seen in the Dubin-Johnson syndrome (i.e., mean 64.8 ± 2.5 [SEM] vs. 88.9 ± 1.3).[303]

Family studies of abnormalities in urinary coproporphyrin[303] excretion and sulfobromophthalein[91,306] metabolism have confirmed that Rotor's syndrome is inherited as an autosomal recessive trait (Fig. 4-8). It appears that the main defects in this condition are in hepatic uptake and storage. Since the hyperbilirubinemia is due to both conjugated and unconjugated bilirubin, one has to postulate that there is either an additional excretory defect

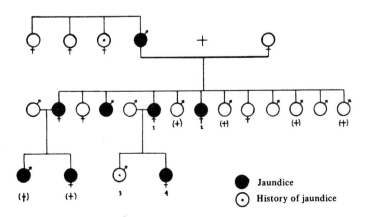

Fig. 4-8. Genealogy of a family with Rotor's syndrome. (Rotor AB et al: Acta Med Philipp 5:37, 1948)

● Jaundice

⊙ History of jaundice

or a diminution in the intraheptic binding of bilirubin so that the conjugated bilirubin refluxes into the plasma.[32]

REFERENCES

1. Abei T et al: The distribution and kinetics of removal of carbon-14 labeled bilirubin in the dog with ligation of the common bile duct. Johns Hopkins Med J 122:112, 1968

2. Acocella G et al: Does deconjugation of bilirubin glucuronide occur in obstructive jaundice? Lancet 1:68, 1968

3. Ali MAM, Billing BH: Effect of acid–base changes in renal clearance of bile pigments. Clin Sci 30:543, 1966

4. Ali MAM, Billing BH: Plasma disappearance of conjugated and unconjugated bilirubin C^{14} in the rat with obstructive jaundice. Proc Soc Exp Biol Med 124:339, 1967

5. Ali MAM, Billing BH: Renal excretion of bilirubin by the rat. Am J Physiol 214:1340, 1968

6. Alpert S et al: Multiplicity of hepatic excretory mechanisms for organic anions. J Gen Physiol 53:238, 1969

7. Arias IM: Effect of a plant acid (icterogenin) and certain anabolic steroids on the hepatic metabolism of bilirubin and sulfobromophthalein (B.S.P.). Ann NY Acad Sci 104:1014, 1963

8. Arias IM et al: Chronic non-hemolytic unconjugated hyperbilirubinemia with glucuronyl transferase deficiency: Clinical, biochemical, pharmacologic and genetic evidence for heterogenicity. Am J Med 47:395, 1969

9. Arias IM et al: On the structure, regulation and function of ligandin. In Arias IM, Jakoby WB (eds): Glutathione Metabolism and Function, p. 175. New York, Raven Press, 1976

10. Auclair C et al: Bilirubin and paranitrophenol glucuronyl transferase activities and ultrastructural aspects of the liver in patients with chronic hemolytic anemias. Biomedicine 25:61, 1976

11. Bailey A et al: Does Gilbert's disease exist? Lancet 1:931, 1977

12. Bar-Meir S et al: ^{99m}Tc-HIDA cholescintigraphy in Dubin-Johnson and Rotor syndromes. Radiology 142:743, 1982

13. Barnes S et al: The role of tubular reabsorption in the renal excretion of bile acids. Biochem J 166:65, 1977

14. Barnhart JL, Clarenburg R: Binding of bilirubin to erythrocytes. Proc Soc Exp Biol Med 142:1101, 1973

15. Barrett PVD et al: The association of urobilin "early peak" and erythropoiesis in man. J Clin Invest 45:1657, 1966

16. Ben-Ezzer J et al: Abnormal excretion of the isomers of urinary coproporphyrin by patients with the Dubin-Johnson syndrome in Israel. Clin Sci 40:17, 1971

17. Berendsohn S: Hepatic function at high altitudes. Arch Intern Med 109:256, 1962

18. Berendsohn S et al: Idiopathic dyserythropoietic jaundice. Blood 24:1, 1964

19. Berk PD et al: Studies of bilirubin kinetics in normal adults. J Clin Invest 48:2176, 1969

20. Berk PD et al: Constitutional hepatic dysfunction (Gilbert's syndrome): A new definition based on kinetic studies with unconjugated radiobilirubin. Am J Med 49:296, 1970

21. Berk PD et al: Haematologic and biochemical studies in a case of lead poisoning, Am J Med 48:137, 1970

22. Berk PD, Blaschke TF: Detection of Gilbert's syndrome in patients with hemolysis: A method using radioactive chromium. Ann Intern Med 77:527, 1972

23. Berk PD et al: Defective bromosulfophthalein clearance in patients with constitutional hepatic dysfunction (Gilbert's syndrome). Gastroenterology 63:472, 1972

24. Berk PD et al: Bilirubin production as a measure of red cell life span. J Lab Clin Med 79:364, 1972

25. Berk PD et al: Comparison of plasma bilirubin turnover and carbon monoxide production in man. J Lab Clin Med 83:29, 1974

26. Berk PD et al: Unconjugated hyperbilirubinemia: Physiologic evaluation and experimental approaches to therapy. Ann Intern Med 82:552, 1975

27. Berk PD et al: The effect of repeated phlebotomy on bilirubin turnover, bilirubin clearance and unconjugated hyperbilirubinemia in the Crigler-Najjar syndrome and the jaundiced Gunn rat: Application of computers to experimental design. Clin Sci Mol Med 50:333, 1976

28. Berk PD et al: A new approach to quantitation of the various sources of bilirubin in man. J Lab Clin Med 87:767, 1976

29. Berk PD et al: Effect of splenectomy on hepatic bilirubin clearance in patients with hereditary spherocytosis: Implications for the diagnosis of Gilbert's syndrome. J Lab Clin Med 98:37, 1981

30. Bernstein RB et al: The effect of hepatobiliary disease on urobilinogen excretion. Gastroenterology 54:150, 1968

31. Berry CS et al: Kinetics of hepatic bilirubin monoglucuronide formation in needle biopsy specimens from patients with hyperbilirubinemia. In Preisig R, Bircher J (eds): The Liver: Quantitative Aspects of Structure and Function, p 226. Aulendorf, Edition Cantor, 1979

32. Berthelot P, Dhumeaux D: New insights into the classification and mechanisms of hereditary, chronic, nonhaemolytic hyperbilirubinaemias. Gut 19:474, 1978

33. Billing BH: Role of conjugating enzymes in the biliary excretion of bilirubin. In Heirwegh KPM, Brown SB (eds): Bilirubin, Vol II, Metabolism, p 85. Boca Raton, FL, CRC Press, 1982

34. Billing BH et al: Defects in hepatic transport of bilirubin in congenital hyperbilirubinemia: An analysis of plasma disappearance curves. Clin Sci 27:245, 1964

35. Bissell DM et al: Hemoglobin and erythrocyte catabolism in rat liver: THe separate roles of parenchymal and sinusoidal cells. Blood 40:812, 1972

36. Bissell DM, Billing BH: Bilirubin metabolism in primary hepatocyte culture.: In Preisig R, Bircher J (eds): The Liver: Quantitative Aspects of Structure and Function, p 110. Aulendorf, Edition Cantor, 1979

37. Bissell DM, Guzelian PS: Degradation of endogenous hepatic heme by pathways not yielding carbon monoxide. J Clin Invest 65:1135, 1980

38. Black M, Sherlock S: Treatment of Gilbert's syndrome with phenobarbitone. Lancet 1:1359, 1970

39. Black M, Billing BH: Hepatic bilirubin UDP-glucuronyl transferase activity in liver disease and Gilbert's syndrome. N Engl J Med 280:1266, 1971

40. Black M et al: Hepatic bilirubin UDP-glucuronyl transferase activity and cytochrome P450 content in a surgical population and the effects of preoperative drug therapy. J Lab Clin Med 81:704, 1973

41. Black M et al: Effect of phenobarbitone in plasma(^{14}C) bilirubin clearance in patients with unconjugated hyperbilirubinaemia. Clin Sci Mol Med 45:517, 1973

42. Blanckhaert N: Analysis of bilirubin and bilirubin mono- and diconjugates. Biochem J 185:115, 1980

43. Blanckhaert N et al: The fate of bilirubin IX glucuronide

in cholestasis and during storage *in vitro*. Biochem J 171: 203, 1978

44. Blanckhaert N et al: Bilirubin diglucuronide synthesis by a UDP-glucuronic acid–dependent system in rat liver microsomes. Proc Natl Acad Sci USA 76:2037, 1979

45. Blanckhaert N et al: Measurement of bilirubin and its monoconjugates and diconjugates in human serum by alkaline methanolysis and high-pressure liquid chromatography. J Lab Clin Med 96:198, 1980

46. Blanckhaert N et al: Mechanism of bilirubin diglucuronide formation in intact rats. J Clin Invest 65:1332, 1980

47. Blaschke TF et al: Crigler-Najjar syndrome: An unusual course with development of neurologic damage at age eighteen. Pediatr Res 8:573, 1974

48. Blaschke TF et al: Drugs and the liver: I. Effects of glutethimide and phenobarbital on hepatic bilirubin clearance, plasma bilirubin turnover and carbon monoxide production in man. Biochem Pharmacol 23:2795, 1974

49. Bloomer JR et al: Comparison of fecal urobilinogen excretion with bilirubin production in normal volunteers and patients with increased bilirubin production. Clin Chim Acta 29:463, 1970

50. Bloomer JR et al: Bilirubin metabolism in congenital nonhemolytic jaundice. Pediatr Res 5:256, 1971

51. Bloomer JR et al: Interpretation of plasma bilirubin levels based on studies with radioactive bilirubin. JAMA 218: 216, 1971

52. Bloomer JR et al: Hepatic clearance of unconjugated bilirubin in cholestatic liver diseases. Am J Dig Dis 19:9, 1974

53. Blumenschein SD et al: Familial nonhemolytic jaundice with late onset of neurological damage. Pediatrics 42:786, 1968

54. Blumenthal SG et al: Changes in bilirubin in human prenatal development. Biochem J 186:693, 1980

55. Bonnett R et al: Structure of bilirubin. Nature 262:326, 1976

56. Boonyapisit ST et al: Unconjugated bilirubin and the hydrolysis of conjugated bilirubin in gallbladder bile of patients with cholelithiasis. Gastroenterology 74:70, 1978

57. Bourke E et al: Mechanisms of renal excretion of urobilinogen. Br Med J 2:1510, 1965

58. Brodersen R: Competitive binding of bilirubin and drugs to human serum albumin, studied by enzymatic oxidation. J Clin Invest 54:1353, 1974

59. Brodersen R: Bilirubin: Solubility and interaction with albumin and phospholipid. J Biol Chem 254:2364, 1979

60. Brodersen R, Bartels P: Enzymic oxidation of bilirubin. Eur J Biochem 10:468, 1969

61. Brown SB, King RFGJ: The mechanism of haem catabolism: A study of bile pigment formation in living rats by (^{18}O) oxygen labelling. Biochem J 170:297, 1978

62. Brown SB, Troxler RF: Heme degradation and bilirubin formation. In Heirwegh KPM, Brown SB (eds): Bilirubin, vol 2, p 1. Boca Raton, FL, CRC Press, 1982

63. Burchell B, Blanckhaert N: Bilirubin mono- and diglucuronide formation by purified rat liver microsomal bilirubin UDP-glucuronyl transferase. Biochem J 223:461, 1984

64. Burchell B et al: Isolation of cloned cDNA coding for UDP-glucuronyl transferases (UDPGT). Falk Symposium 40, Advances in glucuronide conjugation, p. 119. Falcon House, Lancaster, United Kingdom, MTP Press, 1985

65. Butt HR et al: Studies of chronic jaundice (Dubin-Johnson syndrome): Evaluation of a large family with the trait. Gastroenterology 51:619, 1966

66. Cameron JL et al: Metabolism and excretion of ^{14}C-labelled bilirubin in children with biliary atresia. N Engl J Med 274: 231, 1966

67. Cameron JL et al: Metabolism and excretion of bilirubin ^{14}C in experimental obstructive jaundice. Ann Surg 163: 330, 1966

68. Cardenas-Vazquez R et al: Enzymatic oxidation of unconjugated bilirubin by rat liver. Biochem J 236:625, 1986

69. Carulli N et al: Alteration of drug metabolism in Gilbert's syndrome. Gut 17:581, 1976

70. Charbonnier A, Brisbois P: Note sur l'epuration de la bromesulfonephtaleine dans cet ictère de Dubin-Johnson. Rev Med Mal Foie 35:75, 1960

71. Chowdhury JR et al: Bilirubin monoglucuronide and diglucuronide formation by human liver *in vitro*: Assay by high-pressure liquid chromatography. Hepatology 1:622, 1981

72. Chowdhury JR et al: Distribution of UDP-glucuronosyl transferase in rat tissue. Proc Natl Acad Sci USA 82:2990, 1985

73. Chowdhury JR et al: Bilirubin diglucuronide formation in intact rats and in isolated Gunn rat liver. J Clin Invest 69: 595, 1982

74. Clarenberg R, Kao C-C: Shared and separate pathways for biliary excretion of bilirubin and BSP in rats. Am J Physiol 225:192, 1973

75. Coburn RF et al: Effect of erythrocyte destruction on carbon monoxide production in man. J Clin Invest 43:1098, 1964

76. Cohen L et al: Pregnancy, oral contraceptives and chronic familial jaundice with predominantly conjugated hyperbilirubinemia (Dubin-Johnson syndrome). Gastroenterology 62:1182, 1972

77. Colleran E, O'Carra P: Enzymology and comparative physiology of biliverdin reduction. In Berk PD, Berlin NI (eds): Chemistry and Physiology of Bile Pigments, p. 69, Fogarty International Center Proceedings, No. 35. Washington, DC, US Government Printing Office, 1977

78. Compernolle F et al: Glucuronic acid conjugates of bilirubin IX in normal bile compared with postobstructive bile. Biochem J 171:185, 1978

79. Compernolle F: Bilirubin conjugates: Isolation, structure analysis and synthesis. In Heirwegh KPM, Brown SB (eds): Bilirubin, vol 1. p. 59. Boca Raton, FL, CRC Press, 1982

80. Constantopoulos A, Matsaniotis N: Augmentation of uridine diphosphate glucuronyl transferase activity in rat liver by adenosine 3',5'-monophosphate. Gastroenterology 75: 486, 1978

81. Cornelius CE, Arias IM: Hepatic pigmentation with photosensitivity: A syndrome in Corriedale sheep resembling Dubin-Johnson syndrome in man. J Am Vet Assoc 146: 709, 1965

82. Cornelius CE, Rodgers PA: Prevention of neonatal hyperbilirubinemia in rhesus monkeys by tin protoporphyrin. Pediatr Res 18:728, 1984

83. Cornelius CE et al: Heterogeneity of bilirubin conjugates in several animal species. Cornell Vet 65:90, 1975

84. Cowlishaw J et al: Kinetics of bilirubin monoglucuronide formation in Gilbert's syndrome (abstr.) Gastroenterology 79:1010, 1980

85. Crigler JF, Gold NI: Effect of sodium phenobarbital on bilirubin metabolism in an infant with congenital, nonhemolytic unconjugated hyperbilirubinemia. J Clin Invest 48:42, 1969

86. Crigler JF, Najjar VA: Congenital familial nonhemolytic jaundice with kernicterus. Pediatrics 10:169, 1952

87. Cuypers HTM et al: Microsomal conjugation and oxidation of bilirubin. Biochim Biophys Acta 758:135, 1983

88. Cuypers HTM et al: UDP-glucuronyl transferase catalysed deconjugation of bilirubin monoglucuronide. Hepatology 4:918, 1984

89. Datta DV et al: Estimation of hepatic bilirubin UDP-glucuronyl transferase in patients with noncirrhotic portal fibrosis and liver disease: Significance and limitations. Dig Dis 20:961, 1975

90. Dawson J et al: Gilbert's syndrome: Evidence of morphological heterogeneity. Gut 20:848, 1979

91. Delage Y et al: Rotor's syndrome: Evidence for an impairment of hepatic uptake and storage of cholephilic organic anions. Digestion 15:228, 1977

92. De Silva LC et al: Pathogenesis of indirect reacting hyperbilirubinemia after portacaval anastomosis. Gastroenterology 44:117, 1963

93. Dhumeaux D, Berthelot P: Chronic hyperbilirubinaemia associated with hepatic uptake and storage impairment: A new syndrome resembling that of the mutant Southdown sheep. Gastroenterology 69:998, 1975

94. Diamond I, Schmid R: Experimental bilirubin encephalopathy: The mode of entry of bilirubin ^{14}C in the central nervous system. J Clin Invest 45:678, 1966

95. Docherty JC et al: Methene bridge carbon atom elimination in oxidative heme degradation catalysed by heme oxygenase and NADPH-cytochrome P450 reductase. Arch Biochem Biophys 235:657, 1984

96. Douglas JG et al: Bile salt measurements in Gilbert's syndrome. Eur J Clin Invest 11:421, 1981

97. Drummond GS, Kappas A: Prevention of neonatal hyperbilirubinaemia by tin protoporphyrin IX, a potent competitive inhibitor of heme oxidation. Proc Natl Acad Sci USA 78:6466, 1981

98. Dubin IN: Chronic idiopathic jaundice: A review of 50 cases. Am J Med 24:268, 1958

99. Duvaldestin P et al: Possible role of a defect in hepatic bilirubin glucuronidation in the initiation of cholesterol gallstones. Gut 21:650, 1980

100. Edwards RH: Inheritance of the Dubin-Johnson-Sprinz syndrome. Gastroenterology 68:734, 1975

101. Eley A et al: Jaundice in severe infections. Br Med J 2:75, 1965

102. Ennever JF et al: Phototherapy for neonatal jaundice: In vivo clearance of bilirubin photoproducts. Pediatr Res 19:205, 1985

103. Erlinger S et al: Hepatic handling of unconjugated dyes in the Dubin-Johnson syndrome. Gastroenterology 64:106, 1973

104. Evans J et al: Fecal porphyrin abnormalities in a patient with features of Rotor's syndrome. Gastroenterology 81:1125, 1981

105. Fahrlander H et al: Intrahepatic retention of bile in severe bacterial infections. Gastroenterology 47:590, 1964

106. Farrell GC et al: Crigler-Najjar type I syndrome: Absence of hepatic bilirubin UDP glucuronyl transferase activity and therapeutic response to light. Aust NZ J Med 28:280, 1982

107. Felsher BE, Carpio NM: Chronic persistent hepatitis and unconjugated hyperbilirubinemia. Gastroenterology 76:248, 1979

108. Felsher BF et al: The reciprocal relation between caloric intake and the degree of hyperbilirubinemia in Gilbert's syndrome. N Engl J Med 283:170, 1970

109. Felsher BF et al: Hepatic bilirubin glucuronidation in Gilbert's syndrome. J Lab Clin Med 81:829, 1973

110. Felsher BF et al: Effect of fasting and phenobarbital on hepatic UDP-glucuronic acid formation in the rat. J Lab Clin Med 93:414, 1979

111. Fevery J: The bilirubin diglucuronide controversy. J Hepatol 1:437, 1985

112. Fevery J, Blanckhaert N: What can we learn from analysis of serum bilirubin? J Hepatol 2:113, 1986

113. Fevery J et al: Renal bilirubin clearance in liver patients. Clin Chim Acta 17:63, 1967

114. Fevery J et al: Bilirubin conjugates in bile of man and rat in the normal state and in liver disease. J Clin Invest 51:2482, 1972

115. Fevery J et al: Unconjugated bilirubin and an increased proportion of bilirubin monoconjugates in the bile of patients with Gilbert's syndrome and Crigler-Najjar disease. J Clin Invest 60:970, 1977

116. Fevery J et al: Comparison in different species of biliary bilirubin IX_α conjugates with the activities of hepatic and renal bilirubin IX_α-uridine diphosphate glycosyl transferases. Biochem J 164:737, 1977

117. Fevery J et al: Glucuronidation of bilirubin and the occurrence of pigment gallstones in patients with chronic hemolytic disease. Eur J Clin Invest 10:210, 1980

118. Fevery J et al: Analysis of bilirubins in biological fluids by extraction and thin layer chromatography of the intact tetrapyrroles: Application to bile of patients with Gilbert's syndrome, hemolysis or cholelithiasis. Hepatology 3:177, 1983

119. Foliot A et al: Bilirubin UDP-glucuronyl transferase activity of Wistar rat kidney. Am J Physiol 229:340, 1975

120. Foliot A et al: Increase in the hepatic glucuronidation and clearance of bilirubin in clofibrate-treated rats. Biochem Pharmacol 26:547, 1977

121. Foulk WOT et al: Constitutional hepatic dysfunction (Gilbert's disease): Its natural history and related syndromes. Medicine 38:25, 1959

122. Franco D et al: Extrahepatic formation of bilirubin glucuronides in the rat. Biochim Biophys Acta 286:55, 1972

123. Fromke VL, Miller D: Constitutional hepatic dysfunction: A review with special reference to a characteristic increase and prolongation of the hyperbilirubinemic response to nicotinic acid. Medicine 51:451, 1972

124. Fulop M, Brazeau P: The renal excretion of bilirubin in dogs with obstructive jaundice. J Clin Invest 43:1192, 1964

125. Fulop M et al: Dialysability, protein binding and renal excretion of plasma conjugated bilirubin. J Clin Invest 44:666, 1965

126. Fulop M et al: Extreme hyperbilirubinemia. Arch Intern Med 127:254, 1971

127. Garcia-Marin JJ, Esteller A: Biliary inter-relationship between phospholipid, bilirubin and taurocholate in the anaesthetised rat. Clin Sci 67:499, 1984

128. Gautam A et al: Irreversible binding of conjugated bilirubin to albumin in cholestatic rats. J Clin Invest 73:873, 1984

129. Gentile S et al: The implication of bilitranslocase function in the impaired rifamycin-SV metabolism in Gilbert's syndrome. Clin Sci 68:675, 1985

130. Gentile S et al: Gilbert's syndrome: Heterogeneity in hepatic uptake of nicotinic acid and rifamycin-SV. Ital J Gastroenterol 17:73, 1985

131. Gentile S et al: Sex differences of nicotinate-induced hyperbilirubinaemia in Gilbert's syndrome. J Hepatol 1:417, 1985

132. Gilbert A et al: Les trois cholémies congenitales. Bull Mem Soc Med Hop Paris 24:1203, 1907

133. Gilbertsen AS et al: Studies of the dipyrryl-methene ("fuscin") pigments. J Clin Invest 38:1166, 1959

134. Gilbertsen AS et al: Enterohepatic circulation of unconjugated bilirubin in man. Nature 196:141, 1962

135. Glass J et al: Rapidly synthesized heme: Relationship to erythropoiesis and haemoglobin production. Blood Cells 1:557, 1975

136. Gollan JL, et al: Prolonged survival in three brothers with severe type 2 Crigler-Najjar syndrome: Ultrastructural and metabolic studies. Gastroenterology 68:1543, 1975

137. Gollan JL et al: Effect of dietary composition on the unconjugated hyperbilirubinaemia of Gilbert's syndrome. Gut 17:335, 1976

138. Gollan JL et al: Excretion of conjugated bilirubin in the isolated perfused rat kidney. Clin Sci Mol Med 54:381, 1978

139. Gollan JL et al: Bilirubin kinetics in intact rats and isolated perfused liver: Evidence for hepatic deconjugation of bilirubin glucuronides. J Clin Invest 67:1003, 1981

140. Gordon ER, Goresky CA: A rapid and quantitative high performance liquid chromatographic method for assaying bilirubin and its conjugates in bile. Can J Biochem 60:1050, 1982

141. Gordon ER et al: Bilirubin secretion and conjugation in the Crigler-Najjar syndrome type II. Gastroenterology 70:761, 1976

142. Gordon ER et al: Mechanism and subcellular site of bilirubin diglucuronide formation in rat liver. J Biol Chem 259:5500, 1984

143. Goresky CA: The hepatic uptake and excretion of sulfobromophthalein and bilirubin. Can Med Assoc J 92:851, 1965

144. Goresky CA: Hepatic membrane carrier transport processes: their involvement in bilirubin uptake. In Berk PD, Berlin NI (eds): The Chemistry and Physiology of Bile Pigments, p 265. Washington DC, US Government Printing Office, 1977

145. Goresky CA et al: Enhancement of maximal bilirubin excretion with taurocholate-induced increments in bile flow. Can J Physiol Pharmacol 52:389, 1974

146. Goresky CA et al: Definition of a conjugation dysfunction in Gilbert's syndrome: studies of the handling of bilirubin loads and of the pattern of bilirubin conjugates secreted in bile. Clin Sci Mol Med 55:63, 1978

147. Gray CH, Scott JJ: The effect of hemorrhage on the incorporation of $(\alpha\text{-}^{14}C)$-glycine into stercobilin. Biochem J 71:38, 1959

148. Gray CH et al: Studies in congenital porphyria: II. Incorporation of ^{15}N in the stercobilin in the normal and in the porphyric. Biochem J 47:87, 1950

149. Gray CH et al: Isotope studies in a case of erythropoietic protoporphyria. Clin Sci 26:7, 1964

150. Greenberger NJ et al: Jaundice and thyrotoxicosis in the absence of congestive heart failure. Am J Med 36:840, 1964

151. Grinstein M et al: Hemoglobin metabolism in thalassemia: *In vivo* studies. Am J Med 29:18, 1960

152. Hartman F et al: Metabolism of heme and bilirubin in rat and human small intestinal mucosa. J Clin Invest 70:23, 1982

153. Hauser SC et al: Subcellular distribution and regulation of hepatic bilirubin UDP-glucuronyl transferase. J Biol Chem 259:4257, 1984

154. Haverback BJ, Wortschafter SK: Familial nonhemolytic jaundice with normal liver histology and conjugated bilirubin. N Engl J Med 262:113, 1960

155. Hershko C et al: Storage iron kinetics: II. The uptake of haemoglobin iron by hepatic parenchymal cells. J Lab Clin Med 80:624, 1972

156. Hughes-Jones NC, Cheney B: The use of ^{51}Cr and ^{39}Fe as red cell labels to determine the fate of normal erythrocytes in the rat. Clin Sci 20:323, 1961

157. Hunter JO et al: Inheritance of type 2 Crigler-Najjar hyperbilirubinaemia. Gut 14:16, 1973

158. Hutchinson DW et al: Tautomerism and hydrogen bonding in bilirubin. Biochem J 123:483, 1971

159. Israels LG: The bilirubin shunt and shunt hyperbilirubinaemia. In Popper H, Schaffner F (eds): Progress in Liver Disease, vol 3, p 1. London, William Heineman, 1970

160. Israels LG et al: The early bilirubin. Medicine 45:517, 1966

161. Iwatsuru M et al: The classification of drugs on the basis of the drug-binding site on human serum albumin. Chem Pharm Bull 30:4489, 1982

162. Jacobsen C, Jacobsen J: Dansylation of human serum albumin in the study of the primary binding sites of bilirubin and L-tryptophan. Biochem J 181:251, 1979

163. James GW III, Abbott LD Jr: Erythrocyte destruction in sickle cell anaemia: Simultaneous N^{15} hemin and N^{15} stercobilin studies. Proc Soc Exp Biol Med 88:398, 1955

164. James GW III, Abbott LD Jr: N^{15}-glycine labelling of stercobilin in refractory anemia. J Clin Invest 40:1051, 1961

165. Jansen PLM: β-Glucuronidase–resistant glucuronide isomers in cholestatic liver disease: Determination of bilirubin metabolites in serum by means of high-pressure liquid chromatography. Clin Chem Acta 110:309, 1981

166. Jansen PLM et al: Quantitation of bilirubin conjugates with high-performance liquid chromatography in patients with low total serum bilirubin levels. Eur J Clin Invest 14:295, 1984

167. Jezequel AM: Gilbert's syndrome: New acquisitions from ultrastructural morphometry. Gastroenterology 79:1111, 1980

168. Johnson L et al: Kernicterus in rats with an inherited deficiency of glucuronyl transferase. Am J Dis Child 97:591, 1959

169. Jones EA et al: Quantitative studies of the delivery of hepatic synthesized bilirubins to plasma utilizing δ-amino levulinic acid-4-^{14}C and bilirubin H^3 in man. J Clin Invest 51:2450, 1972

170. Kapitulnik J, Ostrow JD: Stimulation of bilirubin catabolism in jaundiced Gunn rats by an inducer of microsomal mixed-function mono-oxygenases. Proc Natl Acad Sci USA 75:682, 1978

171. Kappas A et al: Control of heme oxygenase and plasma levels of bilirubin by a synthetic heme analogue, tin-protoporphyrin. Hepatology 4:336, 1984

172. Keene WR, Jandl JH: The sites of hemoglobin catabolism. Blood 26:705, 1965

173. Kirshenbaum G et al: An expanded model of bilirubin kinetics: Effect of feeding, fasting and phenobarbital in Gilbert's syndrome. J Pharmacokinet Biopharm 4:115, 1976

174. Klaus D, Feine U: Primary shunt hyperbilirubinaemia. Germ Med Month 10:89, 1965

175. Knox I et al: Urinary excretion of an isomer of bilirubin during phototherapy. Pediatr Res 19:198, 1985

176. Kondo T et al: Coproporphyrin isomers in Dubin-Johnson syndrome. Gastroenterology 70:1117, 1976

177. Koskelo P et al: Urinary coproporphyrin isomer distribution in the Dubin-Johnson syndrome. Clin Chem 11:1006, 1976

178. Kuenzle CC: Bilirubin conjugates of human bile: Nuclear-magnetic-resonance, infra-red and optical spectra of model compounds. Biochem J 119:395, 1970

179. Kuenzle CC et al: The nature of four bilirubin fractions from serum and of three bilirubin fractions from bile. J Lab Clin Med 67:294, 1966

180. Kutz K et al: Effect of clofibrate on the metabolism of bilirubin, bromosulphthalein and indocyanine green and on the biliary lipid composition in Gilbert's syndrome. Clin Sci 66:389, 1984

181. LaMont JT, Isselbacher KJ: Postoperative jaundice. N Engl J Med 288:305, 1973

182. Landaw SA et al: Catabolism of heme in vivo: Comparison of the simultaneous production of bilirubin and carbon monoxide. J Clin Invest 49:914, 1970

183. Lauff JJ et al: Isolation and preliminary characterization of a fraction of bilirubin in serum that is firmly bound to protein. Clin Chem 28:629, 1982

184. Lauff JJ et al: Quantitative liquid chromatographic estimation of bilirubin species in pathological serum. Clin Chem 29:800, 1983

185. Lester R, Schmid R: Intestinal absorption of bile pigments: II. Bilirubin absorption in man. N Engl J Med 269:178, 1963

186. Lester R et al: Intestinal absorption of bile pigments: IV. Urobilinogen absorption in man. N Engl J Med 272:939, 1965

187. Levitt M et al: The non-erythropoietic component of early bilirubin. J Clin Invest 47:1281, 1968

188. Levine RA, Klatskin G: Unconjugated hyperbilirubinemia in absence of overt hemolysis. Am J Med 36:541, 1964

189. Levy M et al: Renal excretion of urobilinogen in the dog. J Clin Invest 47:2117, 1968

190. Lightner DA, Linane WP, Ahlfors CE: Photo-oxidation products in the urine of jaundiced neonates receiving phototherapy. Pediatr Res 18:696, 1984

191. London IM et al: On the origin of bile pigment in normal men. J Biol Chem 184:351, 1950

192. London IM et al: Porphyrin formation and hemoglobin metabolism in congenital porphyria. J Biol Chem 184:365, 1950

193. Mahu JL et al: Biliary transport of cholephilic dyes: Evidence for 2 different pathways. Am J Physiol 232:E445, 1977

194. Maines MD, Kappas A: Enzymatic oxidation of cobalt protoporphyrin IX: Observations on the mechanism of heme oxygenase action. Biochemistry 16:419, 1977

195. Mandema E et al: Familial chronic idiopathic jaundice. (Dubin-Sprinz disease) with a note on bromsulphthalein metabolism in this disease. Am J Med 28:42, 1960

196. Martin JF et al: Abnormal hepatic transport of indocyanine green in Gilbert's syndrome. Gastroenterology 70:385, 1976

197. McCormack LR et al: Effect of haem infusion on biliary secretion of porphyrins, haem and bilirubin in man. Eur J Clin Invest 12:257, 1982

198. McDonagh AF: Bile pigments: Bilatrienes and 5,15-biladienes. In Dolphin D (ed): Porphyrins, vol VI, p 293. New York, Academic Press, 1979

199. McDonagh AF et al: Origin of mammalian biliprotein and rearrangement of bilirubin glucuronides in vivo in the rat. J Clin Invest 74:763, 1984

200. McDonagh AF, Lightner DA: Like a shrivelled blood orange—bilirubin, jaundice and phototherapy. Pediatrics 75:443, 1985

201. McIntyre N et al: Hemolytic anemia in Wilson's disease. N Engl J Med 276:439, 1967

202. Muraca M, Blanckhaert N: Liquid chromatographic assay and identification of mono- and diester conjugates of bilirubin in normal serum. Clin Chem 29:1767, 1983

203. Muraca M, Fevery J: Influence of sex and sex steroids on bilirubin uridine diphosphate glucuronyl transferase activity in rat liver. Gastroenterology 87:308, 1984

204. Muraca M et al: Sex differences of hepatic conjugation of bilirubin determine its maximal biliary excretion in non-anaesthetised male and female rats. Clin Sci 64:85, 1983

205. Muraca M et al: Conjugation and maximal biliary excretion of bilirubin in the rat during pregnancy and lactation and during estroprogestogen treatment. Hepatology 4:633, 1984

206. Namihisa T et al: The constitutional conjugated hyperbilirubinemia (Dubin-Johnson syndrome and Rotor's type of hyperbilirubinemia): New definitions based on transport with indocyanine green and bromosulfophthalein. Gastroenterol Jpn 8:217, 1973

207. Noir BA: Bilirubin conjugates in bile of man, rat and dog. Biochem J 155:365, 1976

208. Odell GB: The distribution and toxicity of bilirubin. Pediatrics 46:16, 1970

209. Odievrez M et al: Case of congenital non-obstructive, non-haemolytic, jaundice: Successful long-term phototherapy at home. Arch Dis Child 53:81, 1978

210. Ohkubo H, Okuda K: The nicotinic acid test in constitutional conjugated hyperbilirubinemias and effects of corticosteroid. Hepatology 4:1206, 1984

211. Ohkubo H et al: Studies on nicotinic acid interaction with bilirubin metabolism. Dig Dis Sci 24:700, 1979

212. Ohkubo H et al: Ursodeoxycholic acid oral tolerance test in patients with constitutional hyperbilirubinemias and effect of phenobarbital. Gastroenterology 81:126, 1981

213. Ohkubo H et al: A constitutional unconjugated hyperbilirubinemia with indocyanine green intolerance: A new functional disorder? Hepatology 1:319, 1981

214. Ohkubo H et al: Effects of corticosteroids on bilirubin metabolism in patients with Gilbert's syndrome. Hepatology 1:168, 1981

215. Okolicsanyi L et al: An evaluation of bilirubin kinetics with respect to the diagnosis of Gilbert's syndrome. Clin Sci Mol Med 54:539, 1978

216. Okolicsanyi L et al: A modeling study of the effect of fasting on bilirubin kinetics in Gilbert's syndrome. Am J Physiol 240:R266, 1981

217. Okolicsanyi L et al: How should mild, isolated unconjugated hyperbilirubinemia be investigated? Semin Liver Dis 3:36, 1983

218. Okuda K et al: Marked delay in indocyanine green plasma clearance with a near-normal bromosulphophthalein retention test: A constitutional abnormality? Gut 17:588, 1976

219. Olsson R, Lindstedt G: Evaluation of tests for Gilbert's syndrome. Acta Med Scand 207:425, 1980

220. Onishi S et al: An accurate and sensitive analysis by high-pressure liquid chromatography of conjugated bilirubin IX_α in various biological fluids. Biochem J 185:281, 1980

221. Onishi S et al: Mechanism of development of bronze baby syndrome in neonates treated with phototherapy. Pediatrics 69:273, 1982

222. Ostrow JD et al: The formation of bilirubin from hemoglobin *in vivo.* J Clin Invest 41:1628, 1962

223. Ostrow JD: Absorption of bile pigments by the gallbladder. J Clin Invest 46:2035, 1967

224. Owens D, Evans J: Population studies on Gilbert's syndrome. J Med Genet 12:152, 1975

225. Owens D, Sherlock S: Diagnosis of Gilbert's syndrome: Role of reduced caloric test. Br Med J 3:559, 1973

226. Owens D et al: Studies on the kinetics of unconjugated [^{14}C] bilirubin metabolism in normal subjects and patients with compensated cirrhosis. Clin Sci Mol Med 52:555, 1977

227. Paumgartner G, Reichen J: Kinetics of hepatic uptake of unconjugated bilirubin. Clin Sci Mol Med 51:169, 1976

228. Perugini S et al: Ricerche sulla bilirubina precocemente marcata. I. Incorporazione della glicina-2-^{14}C e del Δ-ALA-3,5-^{3}H, nella bilirubina del plasma, nell'emina e nella globina degli eritrociti in condizioni di eritropoiesi normale e stimolata. Haematologica 56:21, 1971

229. Peters WHM et al: The molecular weights of UDP-glucuronyl transferase determined with radiation-inactivation analysis: A molecular model of bilirubin UDP-glucuronyl transferase. J Biol Chem 259:11701, 1984

230. Petryka ZJ: The identification of isomers differing from 9,α in the early labelled bilirubin of the bile. Proc Soc Exp Biol Med 123:464, 1966

231. Petryka ZJ: Dipyrroles in urine and feces. In Chemistry and Physiology of Bile Pigments, p 77. Washington, DC, DHEW Publication No. (NH1), 1977

232. Pitcher CS, Williams R: Reduced red cell survival in jaundice and its relation to abnormal glutathione metabolism. Clin Sci 24:239, 1963

233. Plimstone NR et al: The enzymatic degradation of haemoglobin to bile pigments by macrophages. J Exp Med 133:1264, 1971

234. Plimstone NR et al: Inducible heme oxygenase in the kidney: A model for the homeostatic control of hemoglobin catabolism. J Clin Invest 50:2042, 1971

235. Pollock MR: Preicteric stage of infective hepatitis: Value of biochemical findings in diagnosis. Lancet 2: 626, 1945

236. Powell LW et al: The assessment of red cell survival in idiopathic unconjugated hyperbilirubinaemia (Gilbert's syndrome) by the use of radioactive diisopropylfluorophosphate and chromium. Aust Ann Med 16:221, 1967

237. Powell LW et al: Idiopathic unconjugated hyperbilirubinemia (Gilbert's syndrome). N Engl J Med 277:1108, 1967

238. Raymond GD, Galambos JT: Hepatic storage and transport of bilirubin in man. Am J Gastroenterol 55:135, 1971

239. Reichen J: Familial unconjugated hyperbilirubinaemia syndromes. Semin Liver Dis 3:1, 1983

240. Reuben A et al: Physical state of bilirubin and organic anions in bile. Hepatology 4:212S, 1984

241. Robinson S et al: Jaundice in thalassemia minor: A minor consequence of "ineffective erythropoiesis." N Engl J Med 267:523, 1962

242. Robinson SH: The origins of bilirubin. N Engl J Med 279: 143, 1968

243. Robinson SH, Koeppel E: Preferential hemolysis of immature erythrocytes in experimental iron deficiency anemia: Source of erythropoietic bilirubin formation. J Clin Invest 50:1847, 1971

244. Roda A et al: Serum primary bile acids in Gilbert's syndrome. Gastroenterology 82:71, 1978

245. Rodes J et al: Metabolism of bromsulphalein in Dubin-Johnson syndrome: Diagnostic value of the paradoxical increase in plasma levels of BSP. Am J Dig Dis 17:545, 1972

246. Rollinghoff W et al: Nicotinic acid test in the diagnosis of Gilbert's syndrome: correlation with bilirubin clearance. Gut 22:663, 1981

247. Rotor AB et al: Familial non-hemolytic jaundice with direct van den Bergh reaction. Acta Med Philipp 5:37, 1948

248. Rugstad HE et al: Transfer of bilirubin uridine diphosphate-glucuronyl transferase to enzyme-deficient rats. Science 170: 553, 1970

249. Samson D et al: Quantitation of ineffective erythropoiesis from the incorporation of (^{15}N)delta-aminolaevulinic acid and (^{15}N)glycine into early labelled bilirubin: I. Normal subjects. Br J Haematol 34:33, 1976

250. Samson D et al: Quantitation of ineffective erythropoiesis from the incorporation of (^{15}N)delta-aminolaevulinic acid and (^{15}N)glycine into early labelled bilirubin: II. Anaemic patients. Br J Haematol 34:45, 1976

251. Samson D et al: Enhancement of bilirubin clearance and hepatic haem turnover by ethanol. Lancet 2:256, 1976

252. Samson D et al: Reversal of ineffective erythropoiesis in pernicious anemia following B$_{12}$ therapy. Br J Haematol 35:217, 1977

253. Schaefer WH et al: Characterization of the enzymatic and nonenzymatic peroxidetixe degradation of iron porphyrins and cytochrome P450 heme. Biochemistry 24:3254, 1985

254. Schalm L, Weber AP: Jaundice with conjugated bilirubin in hyperhaemolysis. Acta Med Scand 176:549, 1964

255. Scharschmidt BF et al: Hepatic organic anion uptake in the rat. J Clin Invest 56:1280, 1975

256. Scharschmidt BF et al: Measurement of serum bilirubin and its mono- and diconjugates: Application to patients with hepatobiliary disease. Gut 23:643, 1982

257. Scharschmidt BF, Schmid R: The micellar sink: A quantitative assessment of the association of organic anions with mixed micelles and other macromolecular aggregates in rat bile. J Clin Invest 62:1122, 1978

258. Schiff L: Serum bilirubin in health and in disease. Arch Intern Med 40:800, 1927

259. Schiff L et al: Familial nonhemolytic jaundice with conjugated bilirubin in the serum: A case study. N Engl J Med 260:1315, 1959

260. Schmid R, Hammaker L: Metabolism and disposition of C^{14} bilirubin in congenital nonhemolytic jaundice. J Clin Invest 42:1720, 1963

261. Schmid R, McDonagh AF: The enzymatic formation of bilirubin. Ann NY Acad Sci 244:533, 1975

262. Schmid R et al: Enhanced formation of rapidly labelled bilirubin by phenobarbital: Hepatic microsomal cytochromes as possible source. Biochem Biophys Res Commun 24:319, 1966

263. Schoenfield LJ et al: Studies of chronic idiopathic jaundice (Dubin-Johnson syndrome): I. Demonstration of hepatic excretory defect. Gastroenterology 44:101, 1963

264. Schwartz S, Cardinal R: Nonhemoglobin heme intermediates in the biosynthesis of bile pigments. Medicine 46: 73, 1967

265. Scragg I et al: Congenital jaundice in rats due to the absence of hepatic bilirubin UDP glucuronyl transferase enzyme protein. FEBS Lett 183:37, 1985

266. Seymour CA et al: Lysosomal changes in liver tissue from

patients with the Dubin-Johnson-Sprinz syndrome. Clin Sci Mol Med 52:241, 1977

267. Shani M et al: Dubin-Johnson syndrome in Israel: I. Clinical, laboratory and genetic aspects of 101 cases. QJ Med 39:549, 1970

268. Shani M et al: Sulfobromophthalein tolerance test in patients with the Dubin-Johnson syndrome and their relatives. Gastroenterology 59:842, 1970

269. Sieg A et al: Uridine diphosphate-glucuronic acid–dependent conversion of bilirubin monoglucuronides to diglucuronide in presence of plasma membranes from rat liver is nonenzymatic. J Clin Invest 69:347, 1982

270. Sleisenger MH et al: Nonhemolytic unconjugated hyperbilirubinemia with hepatic glucuronyl transferase deficiency: A genetic study in four generations. Trans Assoc Am Physicians 80:259, 1967

271. Snyder AL, Schmid R: The conversion of hematin to bile pigment. J Lab Clin Med 65:817, 1965

272. Spivak W, Carey MC: Reverse phase h.p.l.c. separation, quantification and preparation of bilirubin and its conjugates from native bile. Biochem J 225:787, 1985

273. Sprent J et al: Acute renal failure complicating intravenous cholangiography in a patient with Dubin-Johnson syndrome. Med J Aust 2:446, 1969

274. Sprinz H, Nelson RS: Persistent nonhemolytic hyperbilirubinemia associated with lipochrome-like pigment. Ann Intern Med 41:952, 1954

275. Sternlieb I: Electron microscopy of mitochondria and peroxisomes in human hepatocytes. In Popper H, Schaffner F (eds): Progress In Liver Disease, vol VI, p 81. New York Grune & Stratton, 1979

276. Stoll MS, Gray CH: The oxidation products of crude mesobilirubinogen. Biochem J 117:271, 1970

277. Stollman YR et al: Hepatic bilirubin uptake in the isolated perfused rat liver is not facilitated by albumin binding. J Clin Invest 72:718, 1983

278. Stremmel W et al: Physiochemical and immunological studies of a sulphobromophthalein and bilirubin binding protein from rat liver plasma membranes. J Clin Invest 71:1976, 1983

279. Summerfield JA et al: A distinctive pattern of serum bile acid and bilirubin concentrations in benign recurrent intrahepatic cholestasis. Hepatogastroenterology 28:139, 1981

280. Swartz HM et al: On the nature and excretion of the hepatic pigment in the Dubin-Johnson syndrome. Gastroenterology 76:958, 1979

281. Tarao K et al: The effects of acute infectious hepatitis and cirrhosis of the liver on the non-erythropoietic component of early bilirubin. J Lab Clin Med 87:240, 1976

282. Tavaloni N et al: Effect of low dose phenobarbital on hepatic microsomal UDP-glucuronyl transferase activity. Biochem Pharm 32:2143, 1983

283. Tenhunen R et al: Microsomal heme oxygenase. Characterisation of the enzyme. J Biol Chem 244:6388, 1969

284. Tenhunen R et al: Reduced nicotinamide-adenine dinucleotide phosphate–dependent biliverdin reductase: Partial purification and characterisation. Biochemistry 9:298, 1970

285. Tenhunen R et al: The enzymatic catabolism of haemoglobin: Stimulation of microsomal heme oxygenase by hemin. J Lab Clin Med 75:410, 1970

286. Theilman L et al: Does Z-protein have a role in transport of bilirubin and bromosulfophthalein in isolated perfused rat liver? Hepatology 4:923, 1984

287. Tisdale WA et al: The significance of direct reacting fraction of serum bilirubin in hemolytic jaundice. Am J Med 26:214, 1959

288. Trotman BW, Soloway RD: Pigment gallstone disease: Summary of the National Institutes of Health—International Workshop. Hepatology 2:879, 1982

289. Trotman BW et al: Effect of phenobarbital on serum and biliary parameters in a patient with Crigler-Najjar syndrome type II and acquired cholestasis. Dig Dis Sci 28:753, 1983

290. Van Hootegem P et al: Serum bilirubins in hepatobiliary disease: Comparison with other liver function tests and changes in the postobstructive period. Hepatology 5:112, 1985

291. Van Steenbergen W, Fevery J: Maximal biliary secretion of bilirubin in the anaesthetised rat: dependence on UDP-glucuronosyl transferase activity. Clin Sci 62:521, 1982

292. Varma RR et al: A case of the Dubin-Johnson syndrome complicated by acute hepatitis. Gut 11:817, 1970

293. Versée V, Barel AO: Interaction of rat foetoprotein with bilirubin. Biochem J 179:705, 1979

294. Vierling JM et al: Normal fasting-state levels of serum cholyl-conjugated bile acids in Gilbert's syndrome: an aid to the diagnosis. Hepatology 2:340, 1982

295. Wallace DK, Owen EE: An evaluation of the mechanism of bilirubin excretion by the human kidney. J Lab Clin Med 64:741, 1964

296. Watson CJ: Composition of the urobilin group in urine, bile and feces and the significance of variations in health and disease. J Lab Clin Med 54:1, 1959

297. Weisiger RA et al: The role of albumin in hepatic uptake processes. Prog Liver Dis 7:71, 1982

298. Weiss JS et al: The clinical importance of a protein-bound fraction of serum bilirubin in patients with hyperbilirubinemia. N Engl J Med 309:147, 1983

299. Whitmer DI, Gollan JL: Mechanism and significance of fasting and dietary hyperbilirubinaemia. Semin Liver Dis 3:42, 1983

300. Wolkoff AW: Inherited disorders manifested by conjugated hyperbilirubinemia. Semin Liver Dis 3:65, 1983

301. Wolkoff AW, Chung CT: Identification, purification and partial characterization of an organic anion binding protein from rat liver cell plasma membranes. J Clin Invest 65:1152, 1980

302. Wolkoff AW et al: Inheritance of the Dubin-Johnson syndrome. N Engl J Med 288:113, 1973

303. Wolkoff AW et al: Rotor's syndrome: A distinct inheritable pathophysiologic entity. Am J Med 60:173, 1976

304. Wolkoff AW et al: Role of ligandin in transfer of bilirubin from plasma into liver. Am J Physiol 236:E638, 1979

305. Wollaeger EE, Gross JB: Complete obstruction of the extrahepatic biliary tract due to carcinoma as determined by the fecal urobilinogen test: Incidence and effect on serum bilirubin concentrations. Medicine 45:529, 1966

306. Wolpert E et al: Abnormal sulfobromophthalein metabolism in Rotor's syndrome and obligate heterozygotes. N Engl J Med 296:1099, 1977

307. Wu TW: Delta bilirubin: The fourth fraction of bile pigments in human serum. Isr J Chem 23:341, 1983

308. Yamaguchi K et al: Cyclic premenstrual unconjugated hyperbilirubinaemia. Ann Intern Med 83:514, 1975

309. Yamamoto T et al: The early appearing bilirubin: Evidence for 2 components. J Clin Invest 44:31, 1965

310. Yanomoni CZ, Robinson SH: Early labelled haem in erythroid and hepatic cells. Nature 258:330, 1975

311. Yokosuka O, Billing BH: Catabolism of bilirubin by intestinal mucosa. Clin Sci 58:138, 1980

312. Yoshida T, Kikuchi G: Features of the reaction of heme degradation catalysed by the reconstituted microsomal heme oxygenase system. J Biol Chem 253:4230, 1978

313. Yoshinaga T et al: The occurrence of molecular interactions among NADPH, cytochrome c reductase, heme oxygenase and biliverdin reductase in heme degradation. J Biol Chem 257:7786, 1982

314. Young FC, Cheah SS: Breast milk jaundice: An *in vitro* study of the effect of free fatty acids on the bilirubin-serum albumin complex. Res Commun Chem Pathol Pharmacol 17:679, 1977

315. Zakim D, Vessey DA Regulation of microsomal enzymes by phospholipid IX. Production of uniquely modified forms of microsomal UDP-glucuronyl transferase by treatment with phospholipase A and detergents. Biochem Biophys Acta 410:61, 1975

316. Zeneroli ML et al: Sources of bile pigment overproduction in Gilbert's syndrome: Studies with non-radioactive bilirubin kinetics and with δ-(3,5-^{3}H)aminolaevulinic acid and (2-^{14}C)glycine. Clin Sci 62:643, 1982

chapter **5**

The Liver and Its Effect
on Endocrine Function
in Health and Diseases

DAVID H. VAN THIEL, BRADFORD G. STONE,
and ROBERT R. SCHADE

MECHANISM OF ACTION
OF HORMONES

The liver is perhaps the most biochemically complex organ within the body. It possesses the enzymes and cofactors necessary for an unparalleled number of metabolic reactions. Regulation of these reactions is a function of all three broad cases of hormones: the polypeptides, steroids, and tyrosine derivatives.

In the last two decades it has been shown that hormones exert their effects on the liver as well as on other tissues following their interaction with specific receptors either on the cell surface or within the cytosol. Table 5-1 lists some of the hormones known to have specific receptors in the liver. In addition to classic hormones, the liver has specific receptors for an impressive number of physiologically active compounds and drugs, including low-density lipoproteins, haptoglobin-hemoglobin, transferrin, the bile acids, bilirubin, albumin, benzodiazepines, trifluoperazine, chlorpromazine, phenytoin, and cimetidine.

Before discussing the way in which hormones function, we shall first provide a brief overview of the historical aspects of receptor physiology. A quantitative basis for receptor theory was established in 1926 by Clark[66] and Gaddum,[128] who formulated the occupancy theory, which states that the intensity of a pharmacologic (or hormonal) effect is directly proportional to the number of receptors occupied by a specific drug (or hormone) known to produce the effect. This theory further states that the drug or hormonal effect increases proportionately to the number of receptors occupied, becoming maximal when all or nearly all receptors are occupied.

Using this concept, and on the basis of potency comparisons, Ahlqvist[2] defined two principal types of catecholamine receptors, which he identified as alpha and beta. He recognized the agonists or ligands for alpha receptors in order of their potency as being norepinephrine > epinephrine > isoproterenol, whereas beta-adrenergic receptors recognize isoproterenol > epinephrine > norepinephrine.

As noted previously, there are three broad classes of hormones: polypeptides, steroids, and tyrosine derivatives. The polypeptide hormones, typified by insulin, glucagon, thyroid-stimulating hormone (TSH), adrenocorticotropic hormone (ACTH), and a very large number of small peptides, such as hypothalamic-releasing factors, all of which are water soluble, have their receptors located on the hepatocyte cell surface. In contrast, lipophilic hormones, like steroid hormones such as estradiol, progesterone, and cortisol, have their receptors located within the interior of the cell within the cytoplasm and/or nucleus. Tyrosine-like derivatives present a mixed pattern, with acetylcholine receptors, alpha-adrenergic receptors, and beta-adrenergic receptors located on the cell surface, whereas thyroid hormone receptors are located within the cell on mitochondria and the nucleus.

Polypeptide hormones and catecholamines, being water soluble, are not bound to serum proteins and circulate free in plasma. Therefore, they have relatively short half-lives and at their target tissues bind to specific receptors located on the external surface of the target cell. The cell-surface receptors for this group of hormones vary in size from large symmetric glycoproteins having molecular weights of several hundred thousand daltons (*e.g.,* the insulin receptor, 350,000 d)[224,261] to small proteins (*e.g.,* catecholamine beta-adrenergic receptor 64,000 d).[48] The binding reaction between the receptor and hormone is both specific for the particular hormone and reversible. The high degree of specificity of a given hormonal effect of a given cell is conferred by the presence of the specific receptors for the hormone involved. The presence of such specific receptors determines both the high degree of tissue selectivity of hormone action and the multiplicity of biologic effects produced by a given hormone at different target cells.

TABLE 5-1.   Hormones Having Specific Receptors in the Liver

POLYPEPTIDES

Insulin	Human chorionic gonadotropin
Glucagon	
Growth hormone	Angiotension II
Prolactin	Cholecystokinin
Epidermal growth factors	Vasoactive intestinal peptide

STEROIDS

Cortisol	Estrogens
Progesterone	Vitamin D
Dihydrotestosterone	

AMINO ACID DERIVATIVES

Thyroxine	Triiodothyronine
Epinephrine	Norepinephrine
Acetylcholine	

The response of any tissue such as the liver to a given hormone depends upon the concentration of the hormone in the plasma about the cell, the number of receptors for the particular hormone in question, and the binding characteristics of the receptor on the cell for its ligand. Thus, administration of a small amount of hormone may activate only those receptors that have a high affinity for the hormone, even though their number may be limited. Administration of larger amounts of hormone may saturate other receptors that are present on the cell and cross react with the hormone in question, thereby producing an entirely different response to the administered hormone. Different types of receptors differ in their primary and secondary structure. Thus, they have different affinities for their various cross-reacting hormones. Differences between receptors can be demonstrated by use of either hormonal analogues or antagonists or both, each of which will have a different effect on the various types of receptors for a given hormone.

For the polypeptide hormones, with the notable exceptions of insulin, growth hormone, prolactin, and the various somatomedins, the effector within the cell is the membrane-bound enzyme adenylate cyclase. This enzyme converts adenosine triphosphate (ATP) to cyclic AMP, the actual intracellular mediator for hormone action within the cell (Fig. 5-1).[318] The mechanism of activation of adenylate cyclase by the hormone is complicated and requires three major components: the hormone-receptor complex; a membrane protein known as N-protein that serves as a coupler and whose activity is regulated by the guanine nucleotide, GTP; and the catalytic unit of adenylate cyclase. The activation sequence consists of the binding of specific hormone to its receptor, which leads to a conformational change in the receptor; subsequent

Fig. 5-1. Schematic representation of the mechanism of action of hormones that interact with membrane receptors.

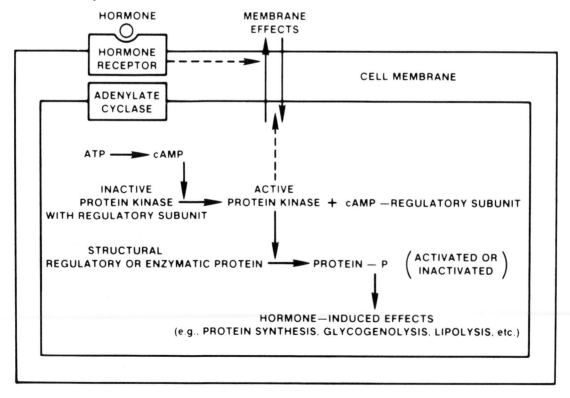

movement of the receptor within the membrane, which permits it to interact with the N-protein, which then binds GTP and, as a result, undergoes a conformational change that allows it to activate the catalytic unit of adenylate cyclase. A GTPase inherent in the N-protein terminates the activation of the receptor and adenyl cyclase by converting GTP to GDP.[47,178] The resultant cyclic AMP generated exerts its effects within the cell through a complex series of reactions that involve its binding to a regulatory subunit on the enzyme protein kinase. In turn, protein kinase phosphorylates specific serine and threonine residues of specific proteins within the cell that are responsible for producing the response characteristic of the cell in question to the specific hormone in question (Fig. 5-1).

Mechanism of Action of Sex Steroids

A general scheme for the mechanism of action for steroid hormones is shown in Figure 5-2. Steroid hormones, such as estradiol, progesterone, and cortisol travel via the bloodstream to their specific target tissues bound by plasma-binding protein and albumin. Only a small fraction of these lipophilic hormones exists free in plasma. It is only the free hormone that is available for diffusion into the target cell and that is responsible for the hormone action at the level of the target cell. Because of their lipophilic nature, steroid hormones enter both target and nontarget cells via passive diffusion. Once within the cell of a target tissue, however, it binds to a specific cytoplasmic receptor for the hormone. Following binding, an apparently temperature-dependent activation process of the hormone-receptor complex occurs that results in the translocation of the hormone receptor complex to the nucleus.[210] The exact nature of the interaction between the steroid hormone-receptor complex and the nucleus has not been completely defined. However, it is clear that the hormone-receptor complex interacts with nuclear DNA via an acceptor protein, which exerts some influence on DNA expression. The net effect is the generation of new messenger RNA specific for the hormone. The new messenger RNA then moves to the cytoplasm, where the translational process results in the synthesis of hormone-specific structural and enzymatic proteins that actually produce the hormone "action."

DIABETES MELLITUS AND THE LIVER

Diabetes mellitus is a chronic disease of pancreatic origin characterized by hyperglycemia and, in the more severe cases, ketosis and protein wasting. It has significant impact in terms of morbidity and mortality as well as an increased

Fig. 5-2. Schematic representation of steroid hormone action.

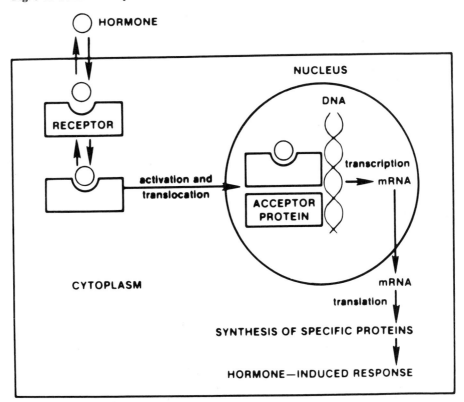

risk of certain associated diseases, including those involving the liver. Table 5-2 shows the four-part classification of diabetes mellitus. This classification, proposed by the National Diabetes Data Group,[245] dispenses with previous age distinctions and defines the syndrome of diabetes mellitus based on the following criteria: (1) classic symptoms of diabetes and hyperglycemia; (2) a fasting glucose level greater than 140 mg/dl; or (3) a serum glucose level greater than 200 mg/dl after an oral glucose load.

The Liver and Energy Metabolism

The liver occupies a unique role in carbohydrate homeostasis. After feeding, the liver actively takes up glucose and either uses it for fuel or stores it as glycogen. During fasting, the liver synthesizes glucose from amino acids. As a result of these two opposite functions of storage and synthesis, the liver maintains a relatively stable plasma-glucose concentration in the fasting as well as the fed state. We shall explain how the liver accomplishes this task before discussing the abnormalities of glucose regulation found in diabetes mellitus.

With ingestion of a meal, a large bolus of glucose is delivered to the liver via the portal vein (Fig. 5-3). The fact that the peripheral glucose concentration rises only slightly (50% above baseline) after a meal compared with the very high levels observed when the same load of glucose is given intravenously implies that the liver is the principal site of glucoregulation after a meal.[330] This supposition was substantiated by the studies of Felig and associates,[119] who used splanchnic vein catheterization techniques to trace the fate of an administered glucose load. Based on their data, only 40% of an ingested glucose load escapes the splanchnic circulation to reach the peripheral circulation as glucose, amino acids, and fat (Fig. 5-3).

With fasting or hypoglycemia due to any cause, these peripherally stored materials are broken down and made available to the liver to reform glucose so that the crucial energy needs of the body can be maintained.[391]

The tight homeostatic control of peripheral glucose levels is maintained by hepatic glucose uptake in response to increases in portal venous glucose. This process does not appear to be an insulin-dependent one. Rather, it is the result of the enzyme kinetics of the initial step in glucose handling by the hepatocyte. This initial step is regulated by the enzyme glucokinase, which irreversibly phosphorylates glucose, trapping it within the hepatocyte. The kinetics of this reaction are such that they allow for the modulation of large or small changes in portal glucose concentrations. Specifically, glucose is taken up by the liver via facilitated diffusion, and, within the range of glucose concentrations seen by the liver, this mechanism is saturated.[391] Once glucose is present within the hepatocyte, it is rapidly phosphorylated to glucose-6-phosphate by the enzyme glucokinase. This enzyme, as distinguished from the nonhepatic enzymes in the hexokinase family, has a relatively low affinity for glucose, and saturation occurs only at a concentration of glucose much greater than that seen under physiologic conditions.[383] As a result, this enzyme is never saturated, and its reaction rate is dependent on only the intracellular substrate concentration. Thus, greater intrahepatic substrate concentrations increase the rate of phosphorylation and produce in effect a "glucose sink" within the hepatocyte.[205,391]

Although hepatic glucokinase in the normal situation is in relative excess compared with its substrate concentration, the amount of this enzyme within the liver is under glucose as well as insulin control. In the fasting state or with acute insulin deficiency, the enzyme level declines. In contrast, during the fed state, the intrahepatic level of the enzyme increases, as does the glucose level.[383]

TABLE 5-2.   Classification of Diabetes Mellitus

1. Spontaneous diabetes mellitus, or primary diabetes mellitus
   Type I, or insulin-dependent diabetes (formerly called juvenile-onset diabetes)
   Type II, or insulin-independent diabetes (formerly called maturity-onset diabetes)
2. Secondary diabetes associated with certain syndromes or conditions
   Pancreatic disease (pancreoprivic diabetes, e.g., pancreatectomy, pancreatic insufficiency, hemochromatosis)
   Hormonal: excess secretion of contrainsulin hormones (e.g., acromegaly, Cushing's syndrome, pheochromocytoma)
   Drug-induced (e.g., potassium-losing diuretics, contrainsulin hormones, psychoactive agents, diphenylhydantoin)
   Associated with complex genetic syndromes (e.g., ataxia telangiectasia, Laurence-Moon-Biedl syndrome, myotonic dystrophy, Friedreich's ataxia
3. Impaired glucose tolerance (formerly called chemical diabetes, latent diabetes, and subclinical diabetes): normal fasting plasma glucose, and 2-hour value on glucose tolerance test >140 mg/dl but <200 mg/dl
4. Gestational diabetes: glucose intolerance that has its onset in pregnancy

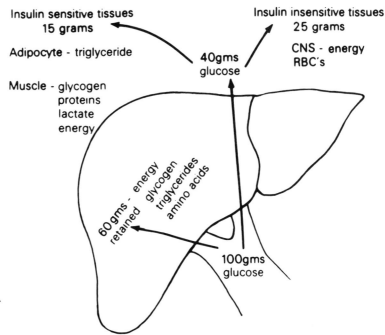

Fig. 5-3. The fate of an oral glucose load. The liver regulates the serum glucose concentration, avoiding a large rise in serum glucose after an oral glucose ingestion by retaining most of the glucose load within the liver. Only 15% of the glucose load escapes to the peripheral circulation above the 25 g delivered to the obligate glucose metabolizing tissues. Fifteen grams of glucose is stored in insulin-sensitive tissues to be released when needed.

Once glucose has been phosphorylated, it can either be stored as glycogen or broken down to acetyl coenzyme A (CoA) and further converted to either an amino acid, fatty acid, or energy. In the fed state, glycogen synthesis predominates. The major regulators of glycogen production are the concentrations of glucose and its product, glucose-6-phosphate. This regulation is mediated through a phosphorylation-dephosphorylation mechanism that modulates the activity of the enzymes involved.[313] This sequence is initiated by glucose binding to phosphorylase A, leading to its inactivation.[313] In turn, this inactivation of phosphorylase A leads to a decrease in glycogenolysis, and, as the concentration of active phosphorylase drops further, a derepression of glycogen synthetase and glycogen synthesis occurs. This enhancement of glycogen synthesis appears to respond within minutes to changes in the systemic concentration of glucose present in blood.[89] Therefore, although insulin appears to increase the levels of the enzymes involved in glycogen synthesis, the intrahepatic glucose concentration and not a hormonal change is the more important of the two in regulating the rapid changes in glycogen metabolism that occur in the postabsorptive state in response to a meal and during fasting.[27,89]

Insulin also appears to have an important effect on he-

Fig. 5-4. Interrelation of glucose and its metabolites within the hepatocytes. Glucose enters the hepatocyte by facilitative diffusion, with the rate-limiting step being the formation of glucose-6-phosphate by glucokinase. The product of this reaction can then be formed into glycogen or pyruvate, depending on the cellular influence at the time. Alanine can also be metabolized to pyruvate for subsequent glucose or energy formation.

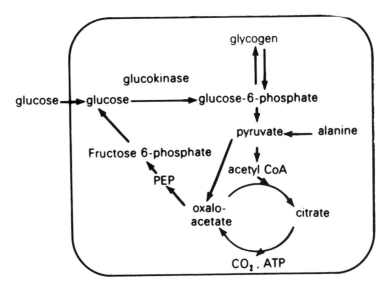

patic glucose production. Low doses of insulin inhibit glycogen breakdown, and, at higher doses, it inhibits glucose synthesis from amino acid precursors.[58] Thus, low doses of insulin lead to hepatic glycogen accumulation, not by augmenting glycogen synthesis, but rather by inhibiting its breakdown. At higher levels of insulin, both glycogenolysis and gluconeogenesis are inhibited.[58] The net result is a smaller increase in the hepatic venous glucose concentration than would be expected, with storage of most of the ingested glucose as glycogen within the liver.

The inhibition of hepatic glucose production with high insulin levels is a direct effect of insulin on the liver rather than a consequence of some peripheral effect of insulin, such as a reduction of the availability of various potential gluconeogenic precursors.[118] High insulin levels actually lead to a decrease in the hepatic extraction of potential gluconeogenic substances and a resultant diminished formation of glucose, Thus, when there are high splanchnic glucose concentrations, insulin stimulates a net hepatic glucose uptake.[56,118] Neither the ratio of insulin to glucagon nor the absolute amount of glucagon appears to be important in this process.[56,314]

The difference between portal venous and systemic insulin levels suggests that the liver is not only the major site of glucose regulation but also the main site of insulin degradation. This occurs as a consequence of binding of insulin to specific insulin receptors found on the hepatocyte surface. This is followed by internalization of the receptor and its bound hormone, with the subsequent breakdown of the bound insulin by cytosolic proteases.[131] The receptor is recycled to the cell surface.[112] Thus, the amount of insulin degraded by the liver is determined by the amount bound to hepatocyte receptors, which is, in turn, dependent on a variety of stimuli that control insulin receptor number or affinity or both.[110,130,324] Recently, it has been suggested that the amount of insulin required for maximal expression of its hormonal effect represents only a small portion of the total insulin bound to receptor. The excess bound insulin is thought to be directed solely for insulin degradation.[131,187]

With a prolonged fast, the noninsulin-dependent organs adapt to ketone body metabolism, and gluconeogenesis is decreased significantly as a result of depletion of the glucose precursor pool.[44,115] Because this is a nonphysiologic situation, no further discussion of glucoregulation by the liver in this state will be undertaken here.

The following comments pertain to glucoregulation as it occurs in a more "physiologic" overnight fast. Following an overnight fast, plasma insulin levels decline to a level that is approximately one fifth that observed after feeding. This, coupled with a lower portal venous glucose concentration, results in essentially no hepatic uptake of glucose. The maintenance of plasma glucose under these conditions is accomplished by the hepatic glucose production and release into the systemic circulation. Under such circumstances, hepatic glucose production is necessary to supply the obligate glucose metabolizing tissues with an adequate energy source for their needs, which necessitates

the production of 150 g to 200 g of glucose per day.[117] Initially, 75% of this glucose produced by the liver is derived from the breakdown of hepatic glycogen stores.[114] The remainder is derived from gluconeogenesis. Lactate derived from red blood cells, muscles, and brain metabolism contributes 10% to 15% of the precursor substrate necessary for this hepatic gluconeogenesis, whereas glycerol derived from fat breakdown in adipose tissue contributes a very small percentage.[44,202,276] A large contribution of the precursors required for hepatic gluconeogenesis is derived from amino acids that are released as a result of peripheral protein breakdown. The most important amino acid precursor is alanine.[115] Because the liver normally contains only 70 g of glycogen, existing hepatic glycogen stores are utilized within 24 hours of initiating a fast.[171] As the fast continues, a progressively greater contribution of total hepatic glucose production must come from gluconeogenesis in order for the liver to supply the total amount of glucose required for the maintenance of the glucose-dependent tissues of the rest of the body.[44]

The signals that initiate glycogenolysis appear to be multifactorial. A decrease in the portal venous glucose inhibits glycogen synthesis and stimulates glycogen degradation as a result of a derepression of the phosphorylase enzyme.[391] This derepression of phosphorylase also inhibits glycogen synthetase. The net result is a breakdown of glycogen to glucose. However, glycogenolysis is also under hormonal control. Plasma glucagon levels, derived from increased pancreatic release, rise during the first 24 to 48 hours of fasting and initiate glycogen breakdown via a cycle adenosine monophosphate (cAMP)-mediated process.[219,313] Moreover, the decline in insulin levels that occurs with fasting also derepresses glycogenolysis.[55] As glycogen stores in the liver are depleted, hepatic gluconeogenesis increases to maintain peripheral blood glucose concentrations.

Gluconeogenesis appears to be regulated by the peripheral release and hepatic uptake of gluconeogenic precursors as well as a stimulation of the hepatic enzymes responsible for their assembly into glucose.[116,217] This process is under hormonal regulation and is enhanced by a reduction in insulin levels as well as a relative excess of glucagon.[44,55,107] The most important gluconeogenic amino acids released by such breakdown of muscle protein are alanine, serine, glycine, and threonine, with alanine constituting almost half of all the amino acids taken up by the liver for gluconeogenesis.[115] Formation of glucose from pyruvate is favored by the overabundance of acetyl CoA groups, which are derived from the obligate hepatic fatty acid oxidation that occurs with fasting. The free fatty acids oxidized are derived principally from adipose cells, which promptly increase their lipolytic activity with fasting. This lipolysis by adipose cells is stimulated by the increased glucagon levels seen and the resultant accumulation of cAMP within the adipocyte.[391] The liver responds to the increased plasma levels of free fatty acids by a passive increase in their hepatic clearance.[19]

Two pathways exist for disposal of these fatty acids in

the liver: esterification to triglycerides, and oxidation to energy and acetyl CoA. The fate of fatty acids within the liver primarily depends on the feeding state. In the fed state, oxidation of fatty acids is inhibited by increased levels of malonyl CoA, which accompany carbohydrate ingestion. During fasting, intrahepatic levels of malonyl CoA decrease and the constraint they exert on fatty acid oxidation is removed.[228] Another factor that regulates the rate of fatty acid oxidation is the rate of hepatic esterification of fatty acids to triglycerides.[226] An increased rate of esterification results in a decreased amount of fatty acid available for oxidation. In the fed state, esterification of fatty acids is favored as a result of the greater availability of the glycerol backbone needed to form triglycerides. However, high intrahepatic concentrations of fatty acids inhibit esterification.[391] The rate of fatty acid esterification and, therefore, the amount of fatty acid available for oxidation is also related to the length of the available fatty acid carbon chains.[197] Fatty acids with chain lengths greater than 12 carbons are esterified more readily.

The acetyl CoA formed from the oxidation of fatty acids can either be further metabolized to energy through the tricarboxylic acid (TCA) cycle or, alternatively, can yield ketone bodies that are released into the plasma. Ketone body production is favored when the amount of acetyl CoA present in the liver is in excess of that which can be utilized via the TCA cycle. Moreover, inadequate insulin levels also enhance ketone body formation.[391]

Type I Diabetes Mellitus

Central to the pathogenesis of the hyperglycemia seen in the insulin-deficient diabetic is the obvious lack of sufficient insulin levels.[226] Glucose production by the liver is doubled in patients with an acute deficiency of insulin and reverts to normal when sufficient insulin is made available to the liver.[116,374] This increase in hepatic glucose production with insulin deficiency is accompanied by an increase in the hepatic vein urea concentration, demonstrating that the glucose synthesized and released by the liver under these circumstances is derived from amino acids.[38] The fact that continued hepatic glucose production occurs in the presence of hyperglycemia demonstrates that a loss of the normal feedback inhibition on gluconeogenesis by plasma glucose levels has occurred.[38]

This fact, coupled with the observation that peripheral glucose extraction does not differ between the decompensated diabetic patient and the normal individual, underscores the role of the liver in the production of hyperglycemia seen in insulin-dependent diabetes mellitus.[38] Not only is the overproduction of glucose by the liver a characteristic finding in the syndrome of insulin-deficient diabetes, but, in addition, there is a marked underutilization of glucose by the liver.

The hyperglycemia seen early in the course of uncontrolled diabetes mellitus may be due to not only insufficient insulin levels *per se* but also, at least in part, a relative glucagon excess. The initial effect of a relative hyperglu-

cagonemia is stimulation of glycogen breakdown.[55] After 4 hours, this effect is no longer present. However, even after this time, a basal level of glucagon is required to exert a "permissive" effect on the continued hepatic glucose production seen with insulin deficiency. However, concentrations of glucagon above basal levels do not appear to be an important modulator of the hyperglycemia associated with insulin deficiency.

In severe and prolonged insulin deficiency, ketosis develops. Insulin normally inhibits adipocyte lipolysis. Thus, the ketosis associated with insulin deficiency has been attributed to an increase in adipose triglyceride breakdown and the release of free fatty acids into the circulation.[108] Recently, the suppression of glucagon levels present in insulin-dependent diabetics has been shown to prevent the development of ketoacidosis.[138] This effect is associated with a reduction in plasma free fatty acid, glycerol, and ketone levels. Thus, in the decompensated diabetic patient, the presence of glucagon enhances the release of free fatty acids from peripheral adipose tissue.

The resultant increased plasma free fatty acids are taken up by the liver, where fatty acetyl CoA derivatives are formed. These fatty acyl CoAs can either be oxidized or esterified to phospholipids or triglycerides. Adequate levels of insulin inhibit fatty acid oxidation; a deficiency of insulin allows oxidation to proceed at a maximal rate.[391] In experimentally induced diabetes mellitus, the mitochondria of hepatocytes develop an increase in their capacity to oxidize fatty acids to acetyl CoA. This increase in fatty acid oxidation is reversed by insulin treatment.[157] The resulting elevation of the intracellular acetyl CoA concentration that occurs with insulin deficiency exceeds the ability of the liver to metabolize fatty acids to carbon dioxide and energy. As a result, the excess acetyl CoA is metabolized to ketone bodies. Thus, the ketone body formation that accompanies decompensated diabetes mellitus appears to be primarily a result of insulin deficiency.

Type II Diabetes Mellitus

In the insulin-independent diabetic, the pathogenesis of the observed hyperglycemia is not as clear. At least four separate mechanisms have been proposed to explain the observed carbohydrate intolerance. These mechanisms are (1) loss of the initial increase in insulin in response to a postprandial increase in plasma glucose levels, (2) a decrease in the absolute amount of insulin released in response to a given glucose load, (3) insulin resistance as seen in obesity, and (4) elevated glucagon levels.[262,375] It is not known why ketosis does not develop in such patients as it does in patients with insulin-dependent diabetes.

Finally, the liver of patients with insulin resistance appears to lack the ability to respond to a normal or even an elevated level of insulin. In such patients, hepatic insulin resistance occurs in the basal state and appears to correlate with their degree of obesity.[262,375] Therefore, the hepatocyte sees a relative lack of insulin, although ambient serum levels are elevated. This apparent hepatic insulin deficiency results in carbohydrate intolerance despite the presence of adequate or elevated insulin levels.

Disorders of Fat Metabolism Occurring in Diabetes Mellitus

The syndrome of diabetes mellitus includes both an enhanced breakdown of fat for hepatic oxidation and profound disturbances in intrahepatic triglyceride and cholesterol metabolism. The alarming rate of atherosclerosis present in diabetic patients and the alleged increase in cholesterol gallstone disease seen in such individuals suggest that disturbances in intrahepatic lipid metabolism are important untoward consequences of the diabetes mellitus syndrome.[211,255]

Hyperlipidemia is an extremely common problem in patients with poorly controlled diabetes mellitus. The frequency of elevated plasma lipids runs between 20% and 90%, depending on the type of diabetes and the degree of control.[91] Hypertriglyceridemia appears to be the most common lipid abnormality observed in diabetic populations and results from an accumulation of very low-density lipoproteins (VLDL) in the plasma of such patients.[91] It is important to remember that the liver is the major site of VLDL production as well as VLDL remnant and low-density lipoprotein (LDL) clearance from plasma. Thus, disorders in triglyceride metabolism are not unexpected in patients with diabetes mellitus.

The pathogenesis of the observed hypertriglyceridemia that accompanies clinical diabetes mellitus is related to the type of diabetes.[91] In the insulin-dependent diabetic, the mechanism appears to be a combination of an increased production of VLDL triglyceride and decreased removal. With acute insulin deficiency, the mobilization of peripheral free fatty acids and their increased hepatic uptake enhance triglyceride synthesis and VLDL output.[15] This effect appears to be short-lived because the increasing levels of hepatic fatty acids ultimately inhibit triglyceride synthesis and the coexistent elevated glucagon levels inhibit hepatic VLDL output.[108,161] Therefore, in the type I diabetic, there is an initial but nonsustained increase in VLDL secretion by the liver, which is followed by a decreased VLDL removal. In the normal individual, triglycerides carried on VLDL particles are hydrolyzed peripherally by the enzyme lipoprotein lipase. The action of this enzyme on VLDL produces a remnant particle that is relatively triglyceride depleted. The triglyceride remaining in the remnant particle can either be further hydrolyzed with formation of a LDL particle or be cleared by the liver through a remnant receptor pathway. In the insulin-dependent diabetic, the activity of lipoprotein lipase, the enzyme responsible for VLDL hydrolysis, is reduced compared with that found in normal people.[247] Insulin therapy in the insulin-dependent diabetic restores the level of this enzyme and thereby reduces the plasma VLDL triglyceride level.[25,270] The decrease in VLDL clearance seen in type I diabetes is thought to be the major cause of the hypertriglyceridemia associated with type I diabetes mellitus.

In contrast, in the type II diabetic, lipoprotein lipase activity is usually normal. This suggests that the cause of the observed hyperlipidemia present in this disorder is VLDL overproduction.[247] In a series of nonketotic patients with diabetes mellitus, an increase in VLDL production with no significant defect in VLDL hydrolysis has been confirmed.[1] These data suggest that one of three possible mechanisms may be responsible for the findings: (1) an excessive caloric intake associated with obesity, (2) an elevated free fatty acid level seen in the nonketotic diabetic, or (3) the associated hyperglycemia that results in an increased hepatic triglyceride production.[1] Whether any or all three of these mechanisms are responsible for the hyperlipidemia of type II diabetes is difficult to ascertain. At present, however, the excess production of VLDL in the nonketotic diabetic appears to be multifactorial.

Cholesterol Metabolism in Diabetes Mellitus

Cholesterol metabolism is thought to be disturbed universally in the diabetic patient. Hypercholesterolemia has been well documented in the poorly controlled diabetic and improves with insulin therapy.[25,310] Early studies demonstrated an increase in total body cholesterol synthesis in diabetics compared with normal individuals, which decreases with the initiation of insulin therapy.[1,25] More recent research has challenged these observations by demonstrating an increased total body cholesterol synthesis with the institution of insulin therapy in diabetics.[125] Until more definitive data are available, however, it appears that diabetic patients have an increased rate of cholesterol synthesis.

Animal data, however, demonstrate a decreased hepatic cholesterol synthesis in uncontrolled diabetes mellitus.[143,244] This decrease in hepatic synthesis is difficult to explain when there is an increased total body cholesterol synthesis because the liver normally contributes more than half the total body synthesis of cholesterol.[328] This discrepancy may be rectified by the fact that intestinal cholesterol synthesis is markedly increased in animals with experimentally induced diabetes mellitus.[143,244] Cholesterol formed in the intestine is carried by chylomicrons to the liver where it contributes to regulation of hepatic cholesterol synthesis by negative feedback.[329] Thus, the following sequence of events is suggested in experimentally induced diabetes mellitus. The observed increase in total body cholesterol synthesis is due predominantly to an increased intestinal cholesterol synthesis, which is offset partially by a diminished hepatic cholesterol synthesis. Institution of insulin therapy reestablishes a more normal rate of intestinal cholesterol synthesis and decreases the amount of cholesterol delivered to the liver from the intestine. This allows a derepression of hepatic cholesterol formation to occur, which accounts for the observed increase in hepatic cholesterol synthesis that accompanies the institution of insulin therapy.

Not only is the liver an important site of cholesterol synthesis, but also it is a major site of lipoprotein uptake and metabolism. Thus, altered lipoprotein metabolism may contribute importantly to the hypercholesterolemia observed in diabetics. Specifically, two defects in lipoprotein metabolism have been identified in diabetics. First, increased hepatic VLDL output and a decreased hepatic VLDL uptake occurs. Because 20% of the VLDL particle is made up by cholesterol, the resultant cholesterol concentration in plasma must increase. Second, the cholesterol carried in LDL, a particle that has a significant positive correlation with the development of atherosclerosis, is elevated in patients with insulin-dependent diabetes mellitus.[310] The LDL particle in man is almost exclusively formed from the hydrolysis of VLDL.[12] LDL particles are cleared from the plasma by an LDL receptor-mediated mechanism found on most tissues.[12] However, the liver is thought to be quantitatively the most important site of LDL cholesterol uptake.[12]

Protein Metabolism and Diabetes Mellitus

The liver plays a unique role in protein metabolism. Not only does it utilize endogenous and peripherally supplied amino acids, but also it is exposed to the high levels of portal venous amino acids absorbed from the intestinal tract. Fifty percent of the amino acids metabolized in the liver are derived from hepatic protein degradation. The other half are derived from extrahepatic sources, either peripheral tissue sites or dietary sources.[322] In the fed state, the majority of the amino acids delivered to the liver are derived from dietary proteins (90 g).[322] In addition, 50 g of amino acids is derived from exfoliated cell proteins that have been digested and are absorbed by the intestine; 16 g is derived from secreted gastrointestinal enzymes; and 1 g to 2 g arises from exuded plasma proteins.[322] In the fasting state, the total amount of amino acids that influx through the portal vein to the liver is reduced to about one sixth of that found in the fed state and is derived almost exclusively from exfoliated intestinal cell protein. The liver adapts to this reduction in amino acids delivered to it by the portal vein by metabolizing endogenous and peripheral amino acids to supply its needs.

Hepatic protein synthesis appears to be under hormonal control. This is true for proteins retained within the hepatocyte as well as for those manufactured in the liver but secreted into the systemic circulation. Adequate levels of insulin and glucagon are necessary for intrinsic hepatic protein synthesis observed during hepatic regeneration after injury.[208] In this situation, these two hormones stimulate hepatic DNA synthesis, hepatic protein synthesis, and subsequent cell division.

Secretory protein synthesis by the liver is modulated by fasting and protein ingestion. Fasting promptly decreases albumin synthesis. This reduction in albumin synthesis is associated with a decreased hepatic RNA concentration, a decreased hepatic protein concentration, and, finally, a reduced state of aggregation of the endoplasmic reticulum (ER)-bound polysomes.[282] In this condition, the free polysomes do not appear to be affected to any significant degree. These changes are quickly reversed with feeding or amino acid delivery to the liver. It is of interest that fasting affects the hepatic level of ER–bound polysomes, which are thought to be important in secretory protein synthesis, without affecting hepatic levels of free polysomes, which are thought to be responsible for endogenous protein synthesis.[164] A basal insulin level is necessary to maintain the state of aggregation of the ER–bound polysomes for secretory protein synthesis.[183,241] In insulin-deficient animals, a loss of rough ER, smooth ER proliferation, decreased amino acid incorporation, and a decreased amount of rough ER–bound ribosomes existing as polyribosomes are seen.[273] The relative sparing of the smooth ER suggests that patients with diabetes mellitus have a defect in secretory protein synthesis predominantly while they maintain adequate endogenous protein synthesis.

DIABETES MELLITUS AND LIVER DISEASE

Up to this point, this discussion of diabetes mellitus and the liver has centered on the role of the liver in the clinical syndrome of diabetes mellitus. However, it should also be noted that a variety of hepatic disorders are associated with diabetes mellitus (Table 5-3).

A variety of hepatic histopathologic lesions are observed with increased frequency in diabetic populations.[336] The most common lesion seen is an increase in liver glycogen demonstrated both at autopsy and in biopsy material.[59,81,333] The incidence of increased hepatic glycogen in diabetes has been reported to be as high as 80%.[81] Initially, this would appear to be a rather surprising finding in that under the influence of a lack of sufficient insulin, the liver should have little or no glycogen. Interestingly, increased glycogen deposits are observed with increased frequency in brittle diabetics who are prone to hypoglycemia.[106,218] In addition, insulin therapy in such patients has been shown to increase hepatic glycogen deposition further.[39] Together, these findings suggest that an intermittent excess in insulin levels associated with exogenous insulin therapy is the cause of the lesion and the associated hypoglycemia. The hepatocyte responds to the transient influence of the excess exogenous insulin by an overac-

TABLE 5-3.   Liver Disease Associated With Diabetes Mellitus

Hepatic disease caused by diabetes mellitus
  Glycogen deposition
  Fatty liver
  Cirrhosis
  Biliary tract disease
Liver disease associated with therapy of diabetes mellitus
  Viral hepatitis (? needle stick)
  Lesions associated with oral hypoglycemic drugs
Liver diseases associated with diabetes mellitus
  Hemochromatosis
  Autoimmune chronic active liver disease
Hepatogenic diabetes

cumulation of hepatic glycogen. The increased liver glycogen and accompanying hepatomegaly can be reversed quickly when more appropriate insulin therapy is instituted.[41]

Fatty liver is defined as the accumulation of lipid, usually in the form of triglyceride, that exceeds 5% of the liver weight.[168] Recently, an increase in lipolysosomes was documented in diabetics with fatty liver; such increases appear to correlate with increased serum cholesterol levels.[159] Diabetic patients commonly have elevated serum cholesterol levels, suggesting that cholesterol may be an important contributing factor in the pathogenesis of the fatty liver associated with diabetes (see preceding sections).

The prevalence of fatty liver in diabetic populations varies but, in general, 50% of diabetics will have excess fat in their livers, as shown by a biopsy.[81] There are several potential etiologies of this fatty liver, and, in any given series of patients with fatty liver, diabetes has been reported to be the cause, with a frequency of between 4% and 46%.[81] This wide range may be explained by the concurrent obesity seen in many patients with noninsulin-dependent diabetes.[52] Because obesity in and of itself appears to be a major cause of fatty liver and because the incidence of fatty liver in patients with diabetes mellitus without concurrent obesity is not known, it is difficult to isolate diabetes *per se* as a specific etiologic factor responsible for the finding of a fatty liver.[168]

Nonetheless, it has been demonstrated that the presence of fatty liver in diabetics correlates with age, the relative mildness of the carbohydrate abnormality, and the duration of the diabetes but does not correlate with the degree of diabetic control.[81,398] Rarely does the insulin-dependent diabetic develop fatty liver. In the type II diabetic population, fatty liver can be demonstrated in more than 50% of the patients examined. Insulin insensitivity rather than the degree of glucose intolerance is predictive of the occurrence of fatty liver in this population.[381,398]

Although patients with fatty livers often present with hepatomegaly, this finding is not invariable.[156,397] No abnormality of liver enzymes reliably predicts the presence or absence of excess hepatic fat in diabetics (or nondiabetics).

Histologically, the fat appears as either large or small droplets within the hepatic cytosol.[156] With intensive fatty infiltration, there is a coalescing of the cytoplasmic fat into large droplets that eccentrically relocate the nucleus and that can cause hepatocyte destruction. In dense areas of fatty infiltration, an increase in connective tissue is occasionally seen. Inflammation is characteristically absent.[156] Because of the lack of good correlation among the various laboratory tests of hepatic injury and function and because of the presence or absence of fat in liver cells, it appears that liver biopsy is the only reliable way to diagnose fatty liver in diabetics and in nondiabetics, although the CT scan is quite accurate in this regard.

The pathophysiologic mechanism(s) responsible for the development of a diabetic fatty liver is (are) not completely understood. However, recent knowledge of hepatic lipoprotein formation has helped to elucidate the potential mechanisms. In diabetes mellitus, free fatty acids, released from adipocytes, are taken up by the liver in a concentration-dependent manner. The fate of these fatty acids is either oxidation to ketone bodies or esterification to phospholipids and triglycerides with subsequent excretion in VLDL particles. It appears that fatty liver occurs when the rate of hepatic triglyceride synthesis exceeds the rate of hepatic secretion of VLDL. This situation can occur as a result of four potential mechanisms: (1) increased hepatic free fatty acid concentrations derived from synthesis, dietary intake, or peripheral lipolysis; (2) increased triglyceride synthesis; (3) decreased oxidation of fatty acids to ketone bodies; and (4) decreased output of triglycerides in VLDL particles.[168] The mechanism responsible for the development of fatty liver in a given subject depends on the type of diabetes mellitus and the degree of diabetic control achieved.

Fatty liver seen in insulin-dependent diabetics occurs only when diabetic control is inadequate. In the presence of reduced serum insulin levels, there is a marked increase in hepatic free fatty acid concentrations that stimulate ketone body production and hepatic triglyceride synthesis. Also, glucagon inhibits triglyceride secretion as VLDL but does not inhibit triglyceride synthesis.[161] Together, these data suggest that the fatty liver seen in the poorly controlled insulin-dependent diabetic is due to an increased influx of free fatty acids that forces triglyceride synthesis.

In type II diabetics, the imbalance between hepatic triglyceride synthesis and VLDL secretion occurs for different reasons. Hepatic free fatty acid concentrations are increased in these patients as a result of a greater intake of dietary fat and carbohydrate and the resultant elevated plasma-free fatty acid concentrations.[3,312] Triglyceride synthesis is stimulated as a result of the increased hepatic free fatty acid content of both endogenus and exogenous sources.[42,386] Because, as yet, there is no evidence that suggests that triglyceride secretion in the type II diabetic is impaired, intracellular lipid accumulation in these patients presumably occurs solely because the rate of triglyceride synthesis exceeds the liver's capacity to secrete newly formed triglyceride as VLDL.

The clinical significance of fatty liver in patients with diabetes mellitus is subject to debate. It is generally believed that fatty liver does not progress to more severe disease. However, some evidence to the contrary has been presented. In pancreatectomized dogs, the progression of fatty liver to fibrosis and ultimately cirrhosis has been documented.[168] Similarly, serial liver biopsies in two diabetic patients with fatty liver have demonstrated progression to cirrhosis.[206] More recently, fatty steatosis, pericentral fibrosis, and intracellular hyalin have been described in the livers of a small series of poorly controlled female diabetics.[109] Such steatonecrosis is more commonly seen in the alcoholic population, in whom the presence of this lesion associated with polymorphonuclear leukocytic inflammation, not seen in diabetics, suggests the subsequent development of Laennec's cirrhosis.[369]

Despite the prevailing opinion that fatty liver *per se* does not lead to cirrhosis, many researchers report an increased prevalence of cirrhosis in diabetic patients.[81,156,181,397] The data can be summarized as follows. There appears to be an approximately fourfold increase of cirrhosis in diabetics, with no special type of cirrhosis prevailing. The ability to draw conclusions from the available data is problematic because the definition of what constitutes diabetes varies considerably from study to study.

The consequences of diabetes mellitus on biliary lipid secretion are seen most often in the type II diabetic who tends to be overweight and secretes a lithogenic bile. Haber and Heaton[154] have addressed this issue by comparing mature-onset diabetics with obesity-matched controls. Using these more appropriate controls, they found that duodenal bile from both groups was supersaturated and therefore lithogenic. This suggests that obesity *per se* and not the diabetes is the etiologic factor common to patients with lithogenic bile and type II diabetes mellitus. In conflict with this suggestion, Bennion and Grundy[25] studied nonobese type II diabetic Pima Indians and found that they secreted a supersaturated bile. However, this group of patients is not a representative population because this unique American Indian population tends to secrete a supersaturated bile even without diabetes mellitus.[150] Finally, a study of nonobese, non-Indian patients with significant fasting hyperglycemia, who did not develop ketoacidosis, demonstrated that these patients had an increase in bile acid and hepatic cholesterol synthesis without an increase in bile acid pool size or cholesterol saturation.[1] Therefore, in the insulin-independent diabetic, it appears that the secretion of a lithogenic bile is related more to obesity or an associated genetic predisposition than to the diabetes *per se*.

The insulin-dependent diabetic has not been investigated as carefully. Meinders and associates[230] studied a group of 12 insulin-dependent diabetics who were not overweight and found no increase in biliary cholesterol saturation compared with that present in 28 control subjects. Moreover, they found that the total biliary lipid concentration was lower in the diabetic group.

In conclusion, both in the insulin-dependent and non-insulin-dependent diabetic, there is no evidence that suggests that diabetic patients secrete bile with a composition different from that present in appropriately matched controls.

It is of interest that the institution of insulin therapy changes the biliary saturation index in a given patient. Specifically, a study by Bennion and Grundy[25] demonstrates that a lack of diabetic control is associated with an increased bile salt synthesis and pool size and that the institution of insulin therapy decreased the bile salt secretion rate and reduced the bile acid pool size toward normal. This resulted in a net increase in the cholesterol saturation of the bile. This increase in cholesterol saturation index has been confirmed in a second study.[1] With experimentally induced diabetes, a decrease in hepatic cholesterol synthesis that can be reversed with institution

of insulin therapy is observed.[143] In man, cholesterol synthesis appears to be an important determinant of biliary cholesterol secretion.[190] Biliary cholesterol secretion has been documented to be higher in the uncontrolled and insulin-treated diabetic than in normal control subjects.[1] A decrease in the bile acid pool size associated with an increased biliary cholesterol secretion results in the formation of a supersaturated bile, a necessary prerequisite for gallstone formation. Therefore, by decreasing bile salt secretion and increasing biliary cholesterol secretion, insulin therapy would appear to increase the risk for gallstone formation.[105]

However, many normal people secrete a supersaturated bile. Thus, the mere presence of a lithogenic bile *per se* does not completely explain the increased frequency of gallstones reported to occur in the diabetic population. The diabetic also has an additional risk factor for gallstone formation—that of decreased gallbladder contractility.[24,291] This decreased contractility results in incomplete emptying of the gallbladder, which promotes cholesterol nucleation. Once nucleation occurs, stone formation and growth are favored.[105]

Earlier research suggested that patients with diabetes and cholelithiasis have a higher mortality rate than does the normal population if emergent surgical intervention is required.[190] In diabetics, emergency surgery for acute cholecystitis has been associated with a 10% to 20% mortality rate compared with a 1% to 4% mortality in nondiabetics.[336] This has led to the suggestion that screening to identify silent gallstones should be considered in diabetic populations, so that elective surgical intervention could be instituted in these patients before acute cholecystitis occurs. It appears that the increased surgical risk in the diabetic with cholecystitis is related primarily to the coexistent presence of vascular or renal disease.[377] In the diabetic patient without vascular or renal disease, surgical intervention for acute cholecystitis has not been associated with an increased mortality over that observed in the general population. Importantly, it is not certain that elective surgery for silent gallstones in the subpopulation of diabetics with vascular or renal disease will decrease the mortality from cholelithiasis. At this point, however, it appears that an elective cholecystectomy might reasonably be considered in such patients who have abdominal complaints.

LIVER DISEASE ASSOCIATED WITH DIABETES MELLITUS

Various hepatobiliary diseases are seen with increased frequency in patients with diabetes mellitus. Unfortunately, therapy for diabetes entails an increased risk of liver disease. Insulin therapy, presumably through needle exposure, is thought to increase the risk of viral hepatitis. These data are derived from early series when insulin treatment of diabetes was just being developed. With our increased understanding of the transmission of hepatitis and the use of disposable needles and syringes for insulin administration, this is probably no longer true. Nevertheless, viral hepatitis is thought to be more common in diabetics than in nondiabetics.[81]

Treatment of diabetes with oral hypoglycemic agents also appears to increase the risk of liver disease. The most commonly used group of oral hypoglycemics consists of the sulfonylurea agents (chlorpropamide, tolazamide, tolbutamide, and acetohexamide). Each of these agents has been shown to produce jaundice, although the frequency of reported hepatic toxic reactions varies with the particular agent used. The reported incidence of such toxicity is greatest with chlorpropamide, occurring at a rate of 0.5% to 1%.[297] Sulfonylurea hepatic toxicity usually consists of a cholestatic reaction, although a picture of hepatocellular injury or a mixed picture can be seen.[297] Rarely, oral hypoglycemic agents are implicated as a cause of granulomatous liver disease.[33] The occasional hepatocellular necrosis seen with administration of these agents appears to be most common with acetohexamide.[142]

THYROID HORMONE HOMEOSTASIS AND THE LIVER

Thyroid hormone synthesis and secretion is regulated by a classic feedback loop system. The hypothalamus, through the release of thyrotropin-releasing hormone (TRH), stimulates production of thyroid-stimulating hormone (TSH) by the anterior pituitary. TSH in turn stimulates various parameters of thyroid gland function, increasing the rates of synthesis as well as the rates of release of both tetraiodothyronine (T_4) and triiodothyronine (T_3). This feedback loop system is then completed by the ability of T_4 and T_3 to inhibit the subsequent secretion of TSH and probably that of TRH.

Thyroid hormones circulate in blood attached primarily to three proteins that are synthesized in the liver: thyroxine-binding globulin (TBG), thyroxine-binding prealbumin, and albumin. After release from the thyroid gland, the majority of both T_4 and T_3 is protein bound, the primary carrier protein being TBG. Only a small percentage of thyroid hormones circulate free or unbound (0.05% of T_4, and 0.5% of T_3). It is important to recognize that the bound fraction serves as a large reserve of thyroid hormone; only the free fraction is available to diffuse into target cells and exert biologic activity.

Recently, attention has focused on the importance of the metabolism of thyroid hormones after they have been secreted by the thyroid gland. These studies have established that hepatic metabolism of T_4 plays a major role in the regulation of thyroid function and have opened up a new area for which we must examine the changes in thyroid hormone economy that occur in both health and disease.[61,294,380]

The liver is one of the main sites for extra thyroidal thyroid hormone metabolism. It is also the source for synthesis of the three major thyroid hormone carrier proteins in human serum.[163] Of the total thyroid hormone released from the thyroid gland, approximately 85% is in the form of T_4, and 15% is in the form of T_3. Current theories on the cellular action of thyroid hormone suggest that T_3 is significantly more potent than T_4, giving rise to the concept that T_4 represents a prohormone that must be metabolically converted to T_3 in the course of normal hormone metabolism. This occurs by the monodeiodination of the outer ring of T_4 by the enzyme 5'-monodeiodinase to yield 3,5,3'-triiodothyronine (T_3). It has been estimated that approximately 40% of the total amount of T_4 secreted by the thyroid is eventually converted to T_3. This, in turn, represents approximately 85% of the total T_3 produced in the body.

The remainder of T_4 available for deiodination undergoes inner ring deiodination by 5'-monodeiodinase to form 3,3',5'-triiodothyronine, also known as reverse T_3 (rT_3), a biologically inactive form of thyroid hormone that is less highly bound to carrier proteins and more rapidly cleared than T_3. The extra thyroidal deiodination of T_4 to T_3 and to rT_3 occurs in many tissues, including skeletal muscle, but the main sites of conversion are the liver and kidneys.[163] The remainder of the T_4 metabolized by the liver occurs by sulphation, glucuronidation, and other phase II reactions.

Many recent reports have documented alterations in thyroid hormone levels in patients with a wide variety of nonthyroidal illnesses. These illnesses include starvation, diabetes mellitus, chronic renal disease, systemic infection, psychiatric disease, and the many different forms of liver disease. In general, these conditions are characterized by a decreased formation of T_3 from T_4 and an increase in serum levels of rT_3.[61,186,294,380] The entire process probably occurs secondarily to a decrease in 5'-monodeiodinase activity that has the dual effect of decreasing T_3 production and decreasing the clearance of rT_3.

Acute Liver Disease and Thyroid Hormone Homeostasis

Several studies have shown that patients with acute hepatitis have elevated serum levels of T_4 without clinical signs of hyperthyroidism.[132,281,335] The increased T_4 could be secondary to increased T_4 secretion from the thyroid gland or increased circulating TBG concentration during the acute illness, or both, both of which resolve with clinical recovery. It has been suggested that the increase in TBG concentration observed occurs as a result of increased release of TBG from injured hepatocytes, because a significant correlation has been found between the changes in serum TBG levels and aspartate aminotransferase levels.[132] This rise in T_4 coincides with a rise in serum TBG, and the continued euthyroid state of the patient is reflected by a lowered T_3 resin uptake and normal free thyroxine index. If the diagnosis of hyperthyroidism is mistakenly considered in such cases, a normal TSH response to TRH will exclude the possibility.

The T_3 levels measured in acute hepatitis have been reported to be lower, unchanged, or increased.[281] Much research must be undertaken to explain these discrepancies. Reverse T_3 levels are increased during acute illness and return to normal with recovery.[132] TSH concentrations are generally reported to be normal in patients with acute hepatitis.[132]

Chronic Liver Disease and Thyroid Hormone Homeostasis

Both chronic active liver disease (CAH) and primary biliary cirrhosis (PBC) can alter thyroid function test results.[102,299,300] Similar to acute hepatitis, some patients with these diseases exhibit an increase in total T_4 secondary to an increase in TBG levels.[299,300] In this group of patients, there is the expected decrease in T_3 resin uptake; however, the free T_4 index is usually normal. Schussler and associates[299] measured T_3 resin-binding ratios in patients with CAH and PBC and found that the ratio was approximately 50% higher in patients with such diseases than in control subjects. There is a group of patients with either CAH or PBC who have normal serum T_4 and T_3 levels. Schussler and co-workers[299] and others have reported a high incidence of antithyroglobulin antibodies in this population.[82,102] Elta and associates[102] report positive antimicrosomal antibodies in 34% of patients with PBC, whereas Crowe and co-workers[82] report positive antithyroid antibodies in 26% of PBC patients.

Since both CAH and PBC appear to have an autoimmune etiology, it would not be surprising to find coexistent autoimmune Hashimoto's thyroid disease in this setting; in fact, the incidence of hypothyroidism presumed to be due to Hashimoto's disease in PBC patients is reported to be 18% to 22%. The latter can be diagnosed in all cases with appropriate measurements of TSH levels either with or without TRH testing. HLA antigens, A1, B8, and Dr3 are commonly found in patients with Hashimoto's thyroiditis and chronic liver disease, regardless of whether it is CAH, PBC, or primary sclerosing cholangitis (PSC).

Chronic liver disease is associated with important changes in almost all aspects of thyroid hormone metabolism and is associated as a result with clinically important alterations in most standard thyroid function tests. Thyroxine levels in chronic liver disease have been reported to be normal or low.[62,148,163,172,248] Low thyroxine levels are often due to reduced circulating levels of thyroid hormone binding proteins, which occur as a result of the decreased synthetic capacity of the diseased liver.[172] They may also occur in some cases as a result of decreased binding affinity of T_4 for TBG.[61] When directly measured, free T_4 has been found to be normal or slightly elevated.[62,172,248] One of the most consistent findings in chronic liver disease is a decline in T_3 levels.[62,148,248] This finding has been attributed to a decreased extrathyroidal T_4 to T_3 conversion, rather than to a limitation in thyroidal secretion of T_3. By noncompartmental analysis, Nomura and colleagues[248] have shown that there is a decrease in the percentage of T_4 converted to T_3 from 35.7% in normal persons to 15.6% in cirrhotic patients. In addition to the low T_3 levels reported in patients with liver disease, rT_3

levels in patients with chronic liver disease have been reported to be elevated.[60,63] Such elevated rT_3 levels are thought to be due to a decreased clearance rate, which presumably occurs as a result of the reduced activity of 5'-monodeiodinase present in such patients. The levels of rT_3 have been used as prognostic indicators for survival while waiting for orthotopic liver transplantation (OLTx) and/or recovery in patients with alcoholic hepatitis.[177,253,354,376]

Basal levels of TSH are either normal or mildly elevated in patients with cirrhosis.[158,177] None of the patients studied in these series has been clinically hypothyroid, and there have been no findings consistent with Hashimoto's thyroiditis. The clinical impression of euthyroidism in such patients is strengthened by the finding of a normal TSH response to TRH stimulation, normal Achilles reflex time, and a normal index of myocardial contractility when such studies have been performed.[62] In contrast Green and associates[148] and Van Thiel and colleagues[368] have reported elevated basal TSH levels and a delayed response to TRH stimulation in chronic alcoholics with liver disease. These authors have suggested that some patients with cirrhosis, particularly those with chronic alcoholism, have a defect in their hypothalamic regulation of TSH secretion.

It has been suggested by several other investigators that the derangements of thyroid metabolism seen in patients with advanced liver disease have prognostic importance for the short-term outcome of chronic liver disease.[163,177,180,354] Hepner and Chopra[163] have evaluated a combination of prothrombin time, aminopyrine breath test, and T_3 and rT_3 formation in patients with liver disease. They found that both T_3 and rT_3 provide a sensitive index for the severity and prognosis of chronic liver disease. Those patients with cirrhosis who died within 3 months of study had significantly lower T_3 levels than did patients who survived at least 6 months.[163]

Hegedus[160] recently reported that chronic alcoholic patients with histologically proven cirrhosis have a significant decrease in the size of their thyroid glands compared with control subjects. Interestingly, however, he did not find any significant correlations between the thyroid gland volume and biochemical indices of liver function or thyroid function tests.

A recent experimental study in animals has shown that animals chronically fed ethanol have a hypermetabolic state with an increased rate of hepatic oxygen consumption similar to that observed in hyperthyroidism.[176] This alcohol-induced hypermetabolic state can be abolished by administration of propylthiouracil (PTU).[175] These animals studies led directly to an evaluation of the effects of PTU in patients with alcoholic hepatitis and cirrhosis by these same authors.[177,253] Interestingly, it was observed that PTU exerted a beneficial effect on both the rate and magnitude of improvement in patients with alcoholic hepatitis and that the greatest benefit was obtained in those patients with the most severe liver disease.[177,253] Unfortunately, not all investigators have found PTU to be beneficial. Thus, further clinical studies must be carried out either to confirm or to refute these findings before the use of PTU in acute alcoholic hepatitis can be considered appropriate therapy.

Thyroid Hormone Homeostasis and Hepatic Cancer

Many authors have reported finding increased levels of TBG and therefore T_4 levels in patients with hepatocellular carcinoma. Moreover, some of these authors have suggested that serial monitoring of the serum level of TBG may be an effective method of early identification of those cirrhotic patients who have undergone malignant transformation within their diseased liver. Prospective studies evaluating this point are currently in progress. The mechanism thought to be responsible for the increased TBG levels in such patients is a derepression of the TBG gene that occurs as part of the malignant transformation of the hepatocyte in such cases.

Not only can TBG levels be used to monitor patients for the development of hepatic cancer, but also TBG can be used as a relative guide as to the amount of cancer present and the response to either chemotherapy or surgery in patients with recognized hepatic cancer and elevated levels of TBG.

Drug-Induced Alterations of Thyroid Hormone Levels

Several drugs have been shown to inhibit the hepatic enzymatic monodeiodination of T_4 to T_3 and, as a result, potentially, to cause hyperthyroxinemia. Most important among these to the hepatologist are glucocorticoids, propranolol, and iodinated contrast reagents used in hepatobiliary scanning procedures as well as other such studies. There are two distinct monodeiodinase enzymes within microsomes: Type I occurs in the liver and the kidney, and type II is found in the pituitary gland. Drugs that have been reported to cause hyperthyroxinemia by inhibiting these enzymes can be divided into either of two categories, depending on whether they inhibit the type I enzyme alone or both enzymes.

Drugs that inhibit only the 5′deiodinase type I activity include PTU (at a dose greater than 600 mg/day),[304] dexamethasone,[64] and propranolol at high doses (usually greater than 160 mg/day).[78] Interestingly, propranolol is the only beta blocker reported to be capable of inhibiting the conversion of T_4 to T_3. The second group of drugs that inhibit both types I and II enzymes includes amiodarone (a new oral antiarrhythmic agent that resembles T_4) and the radiographic contrast agents iopanoic acid and ipodate, which are used for oral cholecystograms.[113] All these drugs have iodine in their chemical structure and, in part, have a structure that resembles the clinical structure of thyroxine. The observed changes in thyroid function studies seen after use of these drugs include an increased serum T_4 level and decreased serum T_3 level secondary to impaired peripheral conversion and clearance, a rise in serum rT_3, and a rise in serum TSH secondary to impaired T_4 conversion to T_3 by the pituitary. Cholecystographic agents may also elevate T_4 levels by inhibiting the hepatic uptake and binding of T_4.[113] Moreover, failure of a patient treated with amiodarone to develop hyperthyroxinemia may suggest the presence of hypothyroidism.[4,221]

Liver Function in Diseases of the Thyroid Gland

Abnormal liver function tests have been reported to occur in hyperthyroidism. The reported incidence of abnormal liver function tests in such cases varies from 15% to 76%.[221,326] The abnormalities include mild increases in serum glutamic oxaloacetic transaminase (SGOT), alkaline phosphatase, and bilirubin concentrations. The most common abnormality is an elevated alkaline phosphatase.[326] Studies of alkaline phosphatase isoenzymes have indicated that the elevations can originate from liver, bone, or both.[326] Usually, however, it reflects enhanced T_4 bone tumor rather than primary hepatobiliary disease. Liver function test abnormalities in hyperthyroidism show a slow, steady improvement over a period of months to a year as patients are treated and return to a euthyroid state.

Although elevated serum levels of bilirubin have been reported in hyperthyroidism, clinical jaundice develops infrequently. When the pathogenesis of hepatic dysfunction occurs in hyperthyroidism, it is unclear but may be related to tissue hypoxemia.

No consistent or specific abnormalities of hepatic function are seen in patients with hypothyroidism. However, serum levels of SGOT may be abnormal in as many as 50% of such patients, suggesting the presence of coexistent hepatocellular disease. When the source of the transaminase elevation is investigated, however, the findings of a concomitant increase in creatinine kinase (MM isoenzyme) and aldolase levels usually indicate a skeletal muscle site of origin. In myxedema, both an increased release of these enzymes as a result of myxedema as well as a decreased clearance of these muscle enzymes explain the finding of increased muscle enzymes in such patients.

THE HYPOTHALAMIC-PITUITARY-GONADAL AXIS

Normal Physiology

The hypothalamic-pituitary-gonadal axis consists of the gonads, hypothalamus, and pituitary gland. The hypothalamus receives a variety of sensory inputs that regulate noradrenergic neurons in the hypothalamus and the locus ceruleus of the midbrain. These brain regions have axonal connections with neurons in the median eminence that secrete gonadotropin-releasing hormone (GnRH). GnRH is responsible for stimulating the gonadotrophs of the anterior pituitary to secrete the two gonadotropins, follicle-stimulating hormone (FSH), and luteinizing hormone (LH).

Under basal conditions, pituitary secretion of the two gonadotropins is episodic, with secretory bursts occurring approximately once per hour. The amplitude of individual secretory bursts varies and is affected by circulating levels of the sex steroid. Thus, the bursts are greater in castrate or hypogonadal subjects than in normal subjects. Factors other than noradrenergic neurotransmitters that affect GnRH secretion include visual and olfactory stimuli, stress, pineal gland function, enkephalins, and possibly other peptidergic neurotransmitters that act to inhibit or free amino acid-bound copper, which stimulates GnRH secretion.

The principal inhibitors of GnRH secretion are estrogens (mainly estradiol) in women and testosterone in men. These steroids act primarily at the hypothalamic level, but some data suggest that estradiol can also act as a potent inhibitor of gonadotropin secretion at the pituitary level. The principal neurotransmitter agents that inhibit GnRH secretion are the endogenous opioids (met- and leuenkephalin).

Effects of Liver Disease on the Hypothalamic-Pituitary-Gonadal Axis

A disease such as hemochromatosis, which involves the abnormal accumulation of iron in the hypothalamus, pituitary, and gonads, disturbs the functioning of the entire hypothalamic-pituitary-gonadal complex at a variety of sites, which varies from person to person depending on the site within the person that is most involved. Thus, in some persons with hemochromatosis, gonadotropin levels are low despite advanced gonadal failure.[28,51,229,378] In such cases, the toxic effect of the accumulated iron appears to be manifest either at the level of the hypothalamus or at the level of the pituitary. In the former situation, GnRH secretion is reduced and the administration of exogenous GnRH would be expected to increase gonadotropin secretion if the pituitary were not also involved. If the anterior pituitary gland is the principal site of the toxic injury, exogenous GnRH would not be effective at inducing gonadotropin secretion.

Infiltrative Diseases of the Liver That Also Involve the Hypothalamic-Pituitary-Gonadal Axis

Sarcoidosis, amyloidosis, histiocytosis X, and other infiltrative diseases of the liver can involve the hypothalamus and/or pituitary as well as the liver and can be associated with gonadal failure. Such diseases are unusual, however, and, in the absence of coexistent hypothalamic-pituitary involvement, the functioning of the hypothalamic-pituitary-gonadal axis is normal. In contrast, when hypothalamic and/or pituitary dysfunction is the major finding, the injury to the hypothalamic-pituitary-gonadal axis reflects this primary central neuroendocrine injury rather than a primary gonadal injury.

In contrast to the situation with hemochromatosis, Wilson's disease, another hepatic disease resulting from an abnormal hepatic accumulation of a metal, in this case copper, is rarely, if ever, associated with gonadal failure. The reason for this remarkable difference between these two hepatic disorders of metal metabolism is that the copper that accumulates in the brain in Wilson's disease does not involve the hypothalamus and pituitary but, instead, occurs principally in the basal ganglia, a site that does not affect the integrity of the hypothalamic-pituitary-gonadal axis. Moreover, circulating copper bond to amino acids acts as a stimulant for GnRH secretion and guarantees adequate gonadal functioning at a time when other hepatic diseases, with similar degrees of advanced injury characterized by hepatic high-grade encephalopathy and portosystemic shunting, usually manifest evidence of gonadal failure.[18,43]

Hepatic encephalopathy and advanced portosystemic shunting due to any hepatic disease can adversely affect the hypothalamic-pituitary-gonadal axis by altering central neurotransmitter synthesis, secretion, and turnover. Moreover, portosystemic shunting also allows relatively weak sex steroids (androstenedione, dehydroepiandrosterone, and estrone) and other substances such as dietary phytoestrogens as well as other as yet unrecognized substances to escape the normal enterohepatic circuit (Fig. 5-5) and thereby disturb the normal functioning of the hypothalamic-pituitary-gonadal axis.[343,351] Thus, for example, in advanced cases of hepatic encephalopathy, alterations in the dopaminergic activity of the hypothalamus could adversely affect GnRH secretion directly by altering dopaminergic control of GnRH secretion or indirectly by altering prolactin secretion, which suppresses GnRH release. Both dopamine and norepinephrine normally act to enhance GnRH secretion. Any reduction in their levels in or replacement by false neurotransmitters within the median eminence would be expected to reduce the frequency of GnRH secretory bursts and lead to central (secondary) hypogonadism. Moreover, a reduction in dopamine levels in these same areas results in enhanced prolactin secretion, which acts to inhibit GnRH secretion centrally and thereby contribute to the development of secondary hypogonadism.[387]

In contrast, excessive levels of dopamine and norepinephrine at sites such as the median eminence would be expected to result in unrestrained GnRH secretion. When there is excessive GnRH secretion, the pituitary receptors for GnRH down-regulate, and gonadotropin secretion either ceases or declines remarkably, and hypogonadism results. This sequence of events is used clinically in the management of precocious puberty with GnRH analogues.[80,86]

Alcoholic Liver Disease and the Hypothalamic-Pituitary-Gonadal Axis

Alcoholic liver disease, unlike the hepatic diseases discussed thus far, is commonly associated with failure of the hypothalamic-pituitary-gonadal axis even before the liver disease is clinically or pathologically advanced.[346,363]

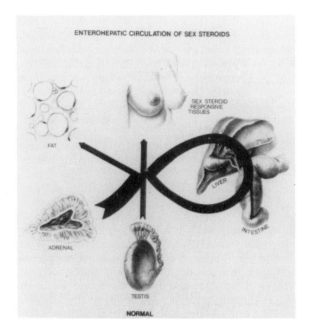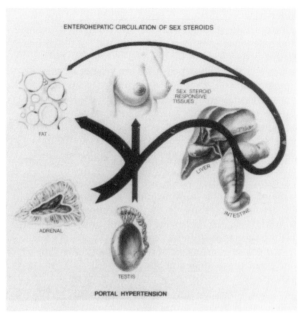

Fig. 5-5. Enterohepatic circulation of sex steroids under normal circumstances (*left*) and as occurs with portosystemic shunting due to portal hypertension (*right*).

Furthermore, alcohol abuse, even in the absence of any detectable alcoholic liver disease, can result in severe gonadal failure in both men and women.[337] Such gonadal failure occurs principally as a consequence of ethanol's intrinsic toxicity, which can be manifest at several sites in the hypothalamic-pituitary-gonadal axis. A discussion follows of the various mechanisms by which ethanol abuse and alcoholic liver disease alone and together can adversely affect gonadal function.

The Alcoholic Man. Hypoandrogenization is commonly seen in chronic alcoholic men; 70% to 80% of such men experience reduced libido and/or impotence.[334,338] Reproductive as well as Leydig cell failure is common in such men, with 70% to 80% of them demonstrating gross testicular atrophy and infertility after years of alcohol abuse.[338,340,344,356,360] Histologic studies of the testicular tissue obtained from chronic alcoholic men usually demonstrate marked seminiferous tubular atrophy and loss of mature germ cells.[341] Many of the residual, less mature germ cells present in such testes have an abnormal morphology.

Evidence for hyperestrogenization is also present in such men but occurs less often than does hypoandrogenization. Thus, a female escutcheon and palmar erythema are seen in 50%, spider angiomata in 40%, and gynecomastia in 20%.[209,212,341,357] These "estrogenic" signs of chronic alcoholism, unlike the transient impotence experienced with an acute alcoholic bout, persist in the absence of intoxication and are due, in large measure, to alcohol-induced permanent tissue injury.

Until recently, the alcoholic liver disease present in many such men was considered to be of primary impor-

tance in the pathogenesis of these evidences of endocrine dysfunction.[212,382] However, during the past 15 years, this concept has been challenged and a diametrically opposite point of view has gained favor. This change in thinking has occurred as a result of the demonstration that endocrine dysfunction can be present in alcoholic men with a broad spectrum of morphologic alcohol-associated hepatic injuries, varying from essentially normal liver to that of severe alcoholic hepatitis and/or cirrhosis.[363] Moreover, testosterone concentrations can be shown to fall in normal male volunteers within hours of their ingesting sufficient amounts of alcohol to produce a hangover.[338,364] In addition, many features of the syndrome of alcohol-induced endocrine dysfunction can be produced in experimental animals and appear in such animals at a time when hepatic biochemical function and morphologic appearance are altered only minimally.[13,136,345,349] Thus, the concept that the endocrine changes observed in chronic alcoholic men are the result of alcohol abuse *per se,* rather than the indirect consequence of alcohol-induced liver disease, has gained considerable credence.

The most direct evidence that alcohol, and possibly acetaldehyde (the first metabolic product of the metabolism of ethanol), may disturb testicular function has been developed in studies using isolated perfused rat testes and isolated Leydig's cells maintained in culture.[70,71,76,342] In these studies, testes are perfused with a defined tissue culture medium that contains gonadotropin. When alcohol or acetaldehyde is added to either the perfusion medium or the culture medium at concentrations comparable to those found in the blood of chronic alcoholic or acutely intoxicated persons, testosterone production and secretion by Leydig's cells is markedly reduced.

The specific mechanisms by which alcohol adversely affects testicular function are slowly being discovered.[362] Alcohol interferes with testicular vitamin A activation, which is essential for normal spermatogenesis.[101,348,361] In addition, alcohol metabolism shifts the testicular balance between NAD and NADH as it does in the liver, thereby secondarily inhibiting testosterone biosynthesis.[57,146,184,362] Similarly, acetaldehyde, either produced directly in the testes as a result of testicular metabolism of ethanol or entering the testes from the plasma as a result of ethanol metabolism by the liver, has a deleterious effect upon testicular mitochondria, organelles critical for normal steroidogenesis. Thus, the conversion of cholesterol to pregnenolone, a reaction that occurs in the mitochondria, is inhibited as a result of mitochondrial exposure to either ethanol or acetaldehyde. In addition, several investigators have demonstrated reduced activity of several microsomal enzymes essential for testosteronogenesis, particularly 17-α-hydroxylase, 3-β-hydroxysteroid dehydrogenase/isomerase and desmolase.[57,146,184] Not only is testicular testosterone production inhibited as a result of alcohol exposure, but recent studies have demonstrated that ethanol interferes with gonadotropin (LH) binding to testicular tissue and that chronic alcohol exposure is associated with a hypothalamic-pituitary defect in gonadotropin secretion.[29,30,135,359,364] Thus, alcoholics not only have inappropriately low plasma gonadotropin concentrations for the degree of their gonadal failure but also demonstrate inadequate responses to exogenous stimuli that normally provoke gonadotropin release such as clomiphene and GnRH.[338,341,363,364] Similarly, inadequate gonadotropin responses can be demonstrated in chronic alcohol-fed rats and in normal rats following alcohol administration.[13,136,345]

As noted previously, in addition to being hypogonadal, chronic alcoholic men are often feminized.[338,340,344,356,360] Thus, palmar erythema, spider angiomata, female escutcheon, and gynecomastia are common physical findings in such men. Biochemical evidence of "hyperestrogenization" in such men is documented by reported increases in estrogen responsive proteins, such as sex steroid-binding globulin and estrogen responsive neurophysin.[350,366] It is probable that the observed increase in prolactin levels seen in cirrhosis are related, at least in part, to increased estrogen levels or estrogen responsiveness.[358,360,365-367] Moreover, because testicular atrophy can be produced by estrogen administration, the testicular damage in alcoholic men with cirrhosis can, at least in part, be ascribed to a "hyperestrogenemic" state. However, when plasma estradiol levels are actually measured in such men, they are found to be either normal or only slightly increased.[338,340,344,356,360] In contrast, plasma estrone levels are increased moderately.[144,360,366]

This finding of normal to near-normal estrogen levels in the presence of androgen deficiency is paradoxical in that estrogens can be produced only by conversion from preformed androgens. Thus, the mechanism of normal or moderately increased plasma estrogen levels in the presence of markedly reduced plasma androgen levels requires further explanation. Preliminary results suggest that the "hyperestrogenemic" state is a result of both the direct effects of alcohol and the indirect effects of alcohol mediated through the development of liver disease.[209,341,357] Unlike what was expected initially, the metabolic clearance rate for estradiol in men with Laennec's cirrhosis is normal, not reduced.[251] Most recently, phytoestrogens (nonsteroidal estrogenic materials of plant origin) have been found in alcoholic beverages. Whether such materials accumulate in the plasma of chronic alcoholic men, however, has not yet been determined.

Evidence suggests that the adrenal overproduction of weak androgens and estrogen precursors regularly occurs in chronic alcoholic men.[72-75,275,306,307,339] Moreover, signs and symptoms of adrenocorticoid hyperresponsiveness resembling Cushing's syndrome have been described in such men.[275,306,307] Thus, these patients not infrequently develop loss of peripheral muscle mass, truncal obesity, hypertension, facial erythema, increased plasma cortisol and androstenedione levels, loss of the normal diurnal variation of plasma cortisol, and failure to demonstrate dexamethasone suppression. The mechanism responsible for this overproduction of adrenocortical precursors of estrone remains uncertain. Recent studies suggest, however, that ethanol and acetaldehyde directly stimulate the adrenal cortex by activating adenyl cyclase.[72-75,339] In addition, in clinical studies, weakly androgenic steroids, such as androstenedione and dehydroepiandrosterone sulfate, have been shown to undergo aromatization to estrogens in various tissues, including skin, fat, muscle, bone, and brain.[1,12,25,125,143,244,247,270,310,322,328,329] Such peripheral aromatization has been shown to be enhanced in men with Laennec's cirrhosis.[251,306] In addition, aromatase activity in the liver, and presumably other tissues, is enhanced in experimental animals as a result of ethanol administration.[352] Thus, a normal metabolic clearance rate and an increased production rate of androstenedione and estrone account for the observed increases in the plasma concentrations of these two steroids seen in alcoholics.[145,209,341,352]

Compounding this overproduction of adrenal androgens, which can be converted to estrogens, portosystemic shunting, which occurs as a consequence of alcoholic liver disease, has been shown to allow steroidal estrogen precursors such as androstenedione and dehydroepiandrosterone, which are secreted into the systemic circulation, to escape the confines of the enterohepatic circulation. As a result, these steroids are converted to estrogens at peripheral sites where aromatase activity is increased.[145,209,341,352] Therefore, the slight increase in plasma estrogen levels observed in alcoholics reflects the levels that reflux back into the plasma from these peripheral sites after aromatization has occurred rather than gonadal production per se.[145,209,341,352]

Compounding the effect of this increased peripheral aromatization of androgens to estrogens is the observation that at least in the liver, cytosolic estrogen receptor activity is enhanced in chronic alcohol-fed animals and also, presumably, in alcoholic men.[92-94,97] Normal male rat liver contains one third the amount of cytoplasmic estrogen receptor present in normal female liver. After castration of the male rat, cytoplasmic estrogen receptor activity increases toward the level found in female rats. Treatment of the castrated rat with dehydrotestosterone (DHT) prevents the castration-induced change toward the female level. Moreover, chronic alcohol feeding of otherwise normal male rats is associated with a decline in the hepatic cytosolic content of a male-specific estrogen-binding protein and an increase in the classic estrogen receptor, thus, in effect, converting the male alcohol-fed rat liver to that which is more similar to that of a female in terms of its cytosolic estrogen-binding characteristics. Such increased estrogen receptor activity and reduced levels of the non-receptor male-specific estrogen-binding protein allow the male liver obtained from alcohol-fed animals to hyperrespond to the normal or only moderately increased plasma estrogen levels present in such male rats.

The Alcoholic Woman. In contrast to the alcoholic man, the alcoholic woman is not superfeminized (hyperestrogenized) but instead shows severe gonadal failure commonly manifested as oligoamenorrhea, loss of secondary sex characteristics (such as breast and pelvic fat accumulation), and infertility.[340,356] Histologic studies of the ovaries obtained at autopsy from chronic alcoholic women who died of cirrhosis while still in their reproductive years (20–40 years of age) have shown a paucity of developing follicles and few or no corpora lutea, thus documenting reproductive failure.[185,353] Moreover, these findings have recently been reproduced in animal models with alcohol administration in the absence of alcoholic liver histologic or biochemical injury.[136,353] Endocrine failure of the ovary of alcoholic women is manifested by reduced plasma levels of estradiol and progesterone, loss of secondary sex characteristics, and ovulatory failure.[338,340,356] The biochemical mechanisms for such endocrine failure are probably the same as those occurring within the testes of the male, because the pathways for steroidogenesis are the same in the gonads of the two sexes, and an alcohol dehydrogenase has been reported to be present within the ovary as well as within the testes.

Since 1958, nine studies by seven different investigative groups have examined the effect of alcohol exposure in female mice, rats, rabbits, and monkeys on the estrus cycle of animals.[6,35,104,179,191,231,345,347,353] In general, as the alcohol exposure either increases in dose or is prolonged over time, the number of female animals demonstrating a total loss of estrus cyclicity or a disruption of the existing cycles (usually with irregular prolongations of the cycle) increases. Similarly, in female rabbits, mice, rats, and monkeys, an increased incidence of ovulatory failure documented by a failure to conceive, absence of expected ova in the fallopian tubes following the time of expected ovulation, absence of ovarian corpus hemorrhagicum and corpora lutea, a loss of the midcycle ovulatory gonadotropin surge, and a failure of plasma estradiol and progesterone levels to increase in the latter half of the cycle have been seen following ethanol exposure to female animals.[32,35,49,134,191,231,347,353] Not unexpectedly, as a result

of this increased prevalance of ovulatory failure with increasing alcohol exposure, the fertility of alcohol-exposed female animals is affected adversely.[49,92,179]

In contrast to the considerable amount of data available concerning the adverse effects of ethanol exposure on endocrine and reproductive function in female animals, few data exist regarding humans.[170,232,233,242,288,332] In contrast to the generally negative *acute* studies that have been performed in human female subjects, *chronic* ethanol abuse by human female subjects has been shown to disturb hypothalamic-pituitary-gonadal function by most investigators studying the problem.[170,232,233]

SOMATOMEDINS AND THE LIVER

Normal Physiology

Initially, three substances in human serum appeared to qualify as somatomedins and were named somatomedins A, B, and C. Somatomedin C has been extensively characterized and is now known to be identical to insulin-like growth factor I (IGF-I).[192] Somatomedin B never met all the criteria for a somatomedin and was subsequently shown to derive its mitogenicity from contaminating epidermal growth factor.[162] The status of somatomedin A remains unclear, although recent amino acid sequence data suggest that it may not be different from SmC/IGF-I.[103]

Significant support for the somatomedin hypothesis that many of the effects of pituitary growth hormone on somatic growth are mediated by somatomedins has been obtained from the demonstration that SmC/IGF-I stimulates the growth of hypophysectomized rats in the absence of growth hormone.[298] In addition, SmC/IGF-I has been shown to participate in a classic negative feedback loop on growth hormone secretion. When injected into the ventricles of intact rats, it inhibits the release of growth hormone from the pituitary. This action occurs because SmC/IGF-I induces the secretion from the hypothalamus of somatostatin, a powerful inhibitor of growth hormone release, and also blocks the action of growth hormone-releasing factor (GRF) on growth hormone release at the level of the pituitary.[26,40]

Although not apparent initially, the growth hormone-dependent mitogens in serum have insulin-like properties and are the same as the insulin-like growth factors (IGFs) of serum. Originally termed *nonsuppressible insulin-like activity,* this residual insulin activity of serum was found by Rinderknecht and Humbel[279,280] to reside in two peptides having a strong structural homology to proinsulin. They were later designated IGF-I and IGF-II.

The insulin-like properties of the somatomedins are demonstrable in typical insulin target tissues both *in vivo* and *in vitro;* they differ from insulin only in their potency.[393] They require concentrations of IGFs 10 to 100 times the insulin concentration required for the same effect.[394]

The third characteristic of the somatomedins is their mitogenic effect on cultured cells. Pierson and Temin[260] initially proposed the term *multiplication stimulating activity* (MSA) for such serum factors, but it was soon learned that they were similar, if not identical, to the somatomedins and that a variety of cultured cells elaborate mitogenic substances into their medium and presumably also into serum.

Two major somatomedins predominate in the serum of most species studied: an electrically basic molecule, SmC/IGF-I; and an electrically neutral molecule, IGF-II/MSA. The concentrations of SmC/IGF-I in serum are highly dependent on growth hormone, whereas those of IGF-II/MSA are much less so. The nature of the two somatomedins are contrasted in Table 5-4. The structural homology of the two somatomedins with proinsulin strongly suggests that a common ancestral gene gave rise to both insulin and the somatomedins.[34]

In contrast to insulin and other peptide hormones, the somatomedins circulate in the plasma bound entirely to larger serum proteins. In human serum, 75% to 90% of the total SmC/IGF-I is associated with a binding protein complex having an estimated molecular weight of about 140,000, and the remainder is associated with various protein complexes ranging down to molecular weights of 35,000.[79] The larger binding protein is composed of two subunits, at least one of which, like the somatomedins, appears to be growth hormone dependent.[126] The presence of these serum-binding proteins probably serves to maintain the somatomedins in an inactive form, because the total circulating concentrations of SmC/IGF-I are about tenfold higher than those required for maximum mitogenic potency in culture.

The quantitation of somatomedins in serum and tissue extracts has been accomplished using a variety of biologic assays, radioreceptor assays, and specific radioimmunoassays. Bioassays utilize the insulin-like or mitogenic characteristics of somatomedins.[274,395] The advantage of these assays is that they measure the total serum somatomedin activity, but they are also tedious and sensitive to nonspecific inhibitors that may independently influence the target tissue. Radio receptor assays, using placenta or other tissues with somatomedin receptors, greatly reduce the interference experienced by nonsomatomedins, but their use is limited by their inability to distinguish SmC/

IGF-I from IGF-II/MSA.[220] Many studies in the current literature on the physiology of the somatomedins have used specific radioimmunoassays performed on whole plasma or on plasma that has been acid extracted to displace the somatomedins from their binding proteins.[127,396] Acid extraction permits measurement of the total somatomedin content of the plasma. Both measurements, however, accurately reflect changes in somatomedin concentrations within the physiologic range.[69,83]

Somatomedin biologic assays have revealed the existence in serum of physiologically important somatomedin inhibitors that are not binding proteins for the somatomedins. These substances inhibit somatomedin action at target tissues and result in a low bioassay of somatomedin activity when there are normal concentrations determined by radioimmunoassay. A number of compounds, including fatty acids, glucocorticoids, and a variety of small peptides have been shown to be somatomedin inhibitors.[37,290,370] The liver appears to be an important source of these substances in situations such as malnutrition, hypopituitarism, and diabetes.[259,334,370,372]

Like other peptide hormones, somatomedins initiate responses in their target cells by interacting with plasma membrane receptors. Two distinct tissue somatomedin receptors have been identified, each with a specificity for one of the two major somatomedins found in serum. Type I receptors have the highest affinity for SmC/IGF-I, although they also bind IGF-II/MSA/ and insulin at supraphysiologic concentrations.[223] Type I receptors show strong homology with the insulin receptor, with each consisting of two subunits linked by interchain disulfide bridges in a heterotetrameric configuration.[54] Type II somatomedin receptors have a preferential affinity for IGF-II/MSA and do not bind insulin. Moreover, they show no homology with either the type I somatomedin or the insulin receptor and exist as a monomeric structure with an internal disulfide bridge.[223]

No biologic effects have been linked to type II somatomedin receptors, although they have been shown to cycle more rapidly from the cell surface to the cytoplasm in response to insulin than do type I receptors.[252] Although somatomedin receptors are widely distributed throughout the body, hepatocytes as well as some other cells of epi-

TABLE 5-4.   Comparison of the Two Major Somatomedins With Regard to Biologic and Physical Characteristics

	SmC/IGF-I	IGF-II/MSA
In vitro insulin-like activity	+	+++
Mitogenicity	+++	+
Isoelectric point	8.3	Neutral
Molecular weight	7649	7471
Serum concentration in humans	193 ± 58 ng/ml	647 ± 126 ng/ml
Growth hormone dependence of serum concentration	+++	+

thelial origin appear to lack significant numbers of the mitogenic type I receptor.[223] In contrast, these cells are rich in insulin and type II somatomedin receptors, and insulin appears to stimulate their growth through its own receptor.[198,222,272,317]

Growth Hormone and the Liver

Growth hormone effects on the liver are initiated by an interaction between growth hormone and specific growth hormone membrane receptors on hepatocytes. A somatogenic class of liver receptors probably initiates the growth-promoting effects, whereas a class of lactogenic receptors probably mediates the effects of the closely related hormone, prolactin. Human growth hormone binds to both somatogenic and lactogenic receptors and has both somatotropic and lactogenic effects clinically.[272] In contrast, bovine growth hormone binds only to somatogenic receptors, whereas human prolactin binds only to lactogenic receptors.

The number of growth hormone receptors in liver is controlled by growth hormone and by other hormones, such as prolactin, with the two receptor classes apparently being regulated independently. Somatogenic receptors are found in equal numbers in the liver of men and women. In contrast, the lactogenic receptors are present only in the liver of women and occur in roughly equal numbers to those of the somatogenic receptors.[272] Metabolic influences are also important modulators of somatogenic growth hormone receptors in liver. Somatogenic, but not lactogenic, receptors are depressed in fasted animals and return to normal with refeeding.[21,216,265] These effects may result in part from the diminished insulin concentrations of fasting. Somatogenic receptors are selectively reduced in hepatic membranes from diabetic animals and are restored with adequate insulin treatment.[22,215]

Growth hormone regulation of hepatic somatomedin production is postulated to be mediated largely by somatogenic receptors, although prolactin can stimulate somatomedin production in hypophysectomized animals and in vitro.[14,123,166] Humans with prolactin-secreting tumors do not have elevated somatomedin levels, but in those instances in which a prolactin-secreting tumor has been associated with growth hormone deficiency, somatomedin levels are found in the normal range.[68] This suggests a physiologic role for prolactin and, presumably, lactogenic receptors in somatomedin regulation.

Growth hormone has long been known to stimulate protein synthesis in the liver.[53] It stimulates amino acid uptake into the livers of intact rats and the incorporation of labeled amino acids into protein within 30 minutes of perfusion into isolated rat livers.[182,278] In addition, growth hormone rapidly stimulates the synthesis of RNA in perfused livers and also increases the number of ribosomes involved in protein synthesis.[199,201,385] Although it has been shown that growth hormone stimulates the hepatic synthesis of mRNA for specific plasma proteins, such as albumin, and alpha-2u globulin, it is as yet unclear whether these substances are preferentially synthesized over other

substances.[149,188,283] A recent report by Seelig and associates[302] indicates that growth hormone acts at a pretranslational level in cultured hepatocytes to increase the concentration of three separate mRNAs.[302]

Growth hormone treatment has also been shown to induce hepatic enzymes regulating the flow of substrates into a number of important metabolic pathways. Both in hypophysectomized animals and in cultured hepatocytes, growth hormone induces the enzyme glutamine synthetase.[137,388] Growth hormone also causes the induction of tryptophan oxygenase, ornithine decarboxylase, and tyrosine aminotransferase.[200,254,271]

Growth hormone also has complex influences on hepatic carbohydrate and lipid metabolism that include both insulin-like and insulin-antagonistic effects.[11,214] In addition, as discussed earlier, growth hormone is thought to be the pituitary factor that permits the development of the sexually dimorphic patterns of drug metabolism that can be well documented in rat liver and that also occurs, but to a lesser extent, in human liver.[151]

The liver plays a critical role in growth hormone metabolism in that it is the chief site of growth hormone degradation. Growth hormone clearance is generally reduced in conditions of hepatic failure, and growth hormone concentrations are elevated in patients with chronic liver disease.[45] In addition to reduced clearance, there appears to be an enhanced pituitary secretion of growth hormone in response to a wider variety of stimuli, such as thyrotropin-releasing hormone (TRH) and oral glucose.[45,289,355] This pattern is also typical in patients with malnutrition and a variety of chronic diseases. There is little evidence to suggest that either growth hormone or the somatomedins are important regulators of liver growth.

Regulation of Hepatic Somatomedin Production

Studies in vivo and in vitro document the regulation of hepatic somatomedin production by growth hormone. Treatment of hypophysectomized rats with growth hormone increases the immunoreactive and bioassayable somatomedin content of their livers.[85,371] Perfusion of the isolated rat liver with growth hormone results in an increase in the perfusate content of bioassayable and immunoreactive somatomedins, as does growth hormone treatment of liver explants and cultured hepatocytes.[31,196,225,227,257,293,295,301,311] Interpretation of the data derived from cultured tissue and cells must, however, be made with some caution. Putative regulators of hormone synthesis in cultured tissues and cells may have effects that are not specific for somatomedin production but that influence other factors, such as cell viability or general protein synthesis and degradation. Furthermore, cells in culture often lose sensitivity to substances to which they respond in vivo, or, in the process of adaptation to culture conditions, they elaborate substances that are not normally elaborated in vivo.

The issue of whether somatomedins are synthesized de novo or released from storage sites in the liver before release by growth hormone remains unresolved, but available data suggest a minimal hepatic storage of somatomedins. In response to a bolus injection of growth hormone, there is a lag of 6 hours before a significant increase in plasma concentrations of SmC/IGF-I is observed in hypopituitary patients.[79] Similarly, Mayer and Schalch[225] found that MSA release from BRL cells in culture was blocked by inhibitors of protein synthesis, a fact that suggests *de novo* synthesis prior to release.

Malnutrition is a potent depressor of somatomedin; it overrides the influence of growth hormone. Somatomedin concentrations in plasma are low in protein-calorie malnutrition and in experimentally fasted adult humans and animals.[67,147,165,174,235,258,268,269,303,308] Moreover, somatomedin levels do not respond to additional exogenous growth hormone in cases with these conditions.[235]

The mechanisms by which nutritional variables modulate hepatic somatomedin production remain to be explained. Nutritional factors can influence the liver by altering the concentrations of key substrates available to the liver from the portal vein, as well as by altering the hormonal milieu that bathe the liver.

Somatomedin Levels in Liver Disease

Somatomedin concentrations are reduced in patients with chronic liver diseases, generally alcohol-induced cirrhosis or other fibrotic disorders, and tumors. Wu and associates[390] have shown depressed somatomedin bioactivity in 21 such patients. They found the depression of somatomedin activity to correlate with the severity of the liver disease and with a wide variety of biochemical indices such as serum albumin, alkaline phosphatase, and bilirubin. Similar results have been reported in a group of patients studied by Schimpff and colleagues,[296] who also showed a significant somatomedin depression from normal in patients with cirrhosis and a further depression in patients with hepatitis associated with cirrhosis. Zapf and co-workers[392] confirmed these results in 20 cirrhotic patients with an IGF radioimmunoassay, and Takano and associates[321] found similar depression with a receptor assay for somatomedin A. Although these studies have been interpreted to confirm the role of liver mass in the determination of plasma somatomedin concentrations, they have failed to take into consideration the nutritional status of the subjects studied. Generally, only acutely ill patients or chronic alcoholics have been studied, and the authors of these reports have focused on hepatocellular failure as the cause of the observed somatomedin depression.

ESTROGEN AND ANDROGEN RECEPTORS IN THE LIVER AND THEIR ROLE IN HEPATIC FUNCTION

Historically, the description and characterization of sex hormone receptors has been limited to only target tissues for such hormones, such as the ovary, testes, uterus, and prostate, sites where the levels of these somewhat labile proteins are maximal. In the mid-1970s, however, several laboratories began to publish reports that female rat liver contained estrogen-binding activity with characteristics similar, if not identical, to those of classic estrogen receptors (ERs) found in target tissues.[50,100,373] Since then, hepatic ERs have been described in both male and female liver.[8,92,97,250,267] Like ER in classic sex steroid–dependent tissues, the ER of liver of both sexes binds estradiol with high affinity. It also binds a variety of other estrogenic compounds, such as estrogen metabolites, phytoestrogens, antiestrogens, and xenobiotics such as the insecticide chlorophenothane (DDT).[92,195,203,250,266] As noted earlier in this chapter, male liver contains about one fourth the amount of ER as that found in female liver.[92] The ER content in male liver appears to be lower because testosterone represses the level of ER in the liver. Castration of the male results in an increase in hepatic ER. Similarly, estrogen treatment of males increases hepatic ER activity.[92] In females, the liver contains about 25% as much cytosolic receptor as does the uterus. Moreover, hepatic ER appears to have many of the same physical and chemical properties that are present in ER in classic hormonally dependent target tissues, such as the uterus. It also differs from the ER of such organs in two major regulatory aspects. First, much higher doses of estrogen are required to translocate the ER to the nucleus of the liver cell. Presumably, this occurs because metabolism of the estrogen by the liver cell limits the availability of the steroid for the receptor.[90] Because of this metabolism, both the liver and the ER are exposed to a wide variety of estrogenic metabolites and other xenobiotics that may potentially interact with the receptor.

Consistent with the animal work described above, recent work has demonstrated the presence of cytosolic ER in the liver of men and women.[9,10,264] The hepatic ER in humans is an estrogen binder of high affinity and low capacity and is specific for both steroidal and nonsteroidal estrogens.[264] In addition, studies have demonstrated that, in addition to the cytosolic ER, human liver also contains ER in its nuclear fraction.[263] This suggests that ER within liver is in fact a functional entity, because it appears to interact with the nucleus, a requirement for sex hormone expression.

These findings were not to be unexpected, however, because of the well-known responses of human liver to estrogens, such as enhanced synthesis of several plasma transport proteins. Specifically, estrogen administration increases the synthesis of sex steroid-binding globulin, thyroxine-binding globulin, transcortin, ceruloplasmin, and so on.[139,140,240,309] A variety of other hepatic proteins and enzymes are also enhanced by estrogens. Animal studies have shown that estrogen administration results in an increase in hepatocyte low-density lipoprotein (LDL) receptor, thus increasing uptake of LDL-associated cholesterol from the blood.[384] In addition, ovariectomized female rats given estrogen display a significant increase in VLDL-associated triglycerides, but not cholesterol, compared with a group of animals not treated with hormone.[325]

The Sexual Dimorphism of Hepatic Function

The sexual dimorphism of liver function in mammals is well recognized.[16,77,151,152,284] Many observations in humans clearly demonstrate that men and women differ markedly in their ability to metabolize different classes of xenobiotics. In general, men exhibit a higher hepatic content of microsomal oxidative enzymes, whereas women have a greater capacity for reductive activity. Androgens appear to be the major steroids that determine the "masculine" pattern of hepatic metabolic function. In fact, most of the metabolic functions that are elevated in men require androgen imprinting, that is, a brief surge of testicular androgen synthesis early in life, in order to achieve and maintain adult levels of these "masculine" activities.[99] The imprinting process most likely occurs at the level of the hypothalamus or pituitary. However, it is unclear whether or not there is an additional direct effect of imprinting on the liver *per se*. Some imprinted functions require the constant presence of androgen after puberty, whereas others retain partial activity even after castration. Certain enzyme activities, such as 5-α-reductase, an androgen-metabolizing enzyme, are low in adult men but are high in the liver of women, presumably as a result of a putative "feminizing factor" that permits the greater expression of certain proteins in the liver of women while it represses others.

Androgen Receptors in Liver

Although androgenic hormones have been shown to exert powerful effects on the liver, whether directly or indirectly through their effects on the hypothalamus and pituitary, no one has yet shown convincingly the presence of a hepatic androgen receptor (AR) within the liver. Roy and associates[285,286] have described an AR present in liver cytosol that binds both androgen and estrogen and is male specific; however, these same authors have since reconsidered their findings because of the inability of their androgen-binding protein to interact with the nucleus. Several reports describe the presence of an androgen-binding protein in the liver, but the reported affinities for the androgen ligand (Kd values of 10–100 nM) or the specificity of binding demonstrated have not been consistent with those of a receptor.[207,292] Nonetheless, Barrack[17] has described the presence of sites on liver nuclear matrix that are capable of binding activated prostate cytosolic AR. Moreover, Eagon and colleagues[95,96] have described the partial characterization of a high-affinity androgen-binding protein in both cytosolic and nuclear fractions of male rat liver that appears to be an AR.[95,96] These latter studies have characterized both the nuclear and cytosolic fractions of male liver as having high affinity and specificity for androgen's characteristics that are compatible with and essential for its identity as an AR.[95,96]

Hepatic Imprinting

The pituitary plays an important role in the development of the sexually dimorphic "masculine" and "feminine" patterns of hepatic steroid and drug-metabolizing enzyme systems. Developmentally, male and female rats have similar male-like hepatic enzyme patterns until about 30 days of age, at which time the pituitary matures, presumably under the influence of the hypothalamus, and in females secretes a "feminizing factor" that gives rise to the female pattern of hepatic steroid metabolism.[151,152] Gustafsson and colleagues[151] have since purified this "feminizing" factor and have presented evidence of its identity with that of growth hormone. Eden[98] reported a sexual difference in the pattern of growth hormone release. The male pattern of growth hormone secretion is programmed by the action of neonatal androgens at the level of the hypothalamus, as are those for LH and FSH. Relevant to this issue, Rumbauch and Colby[287] have reported feminization of hepatic steroid metabolism in rats in response to the administration of growth hormone twice daily to hypophysectomized male animals also given ACTH and T_4.[287] Recently, Gustafsson and colleagues[151,152] have presented evidence that the putative "feminizing factor" is growth hormone. The continuous administration of growth hormone by minipumps to mimic the female pattern of growth hormone secretion results in the feminization of hepatic steroid metabolism in normal and hypophysectomized males and "refeminization" of the hypophysectomized and ovariectomized females. The same effect has been achieved with injections of growth hormone every 3 to 6 hours, but not when it is given every 12 hours. Apparently the 12-hour schedule permits plasma growth hormone levels to decrease to undetectable levels between surges, a characteristic of the male pattern of growth hormone secretion.[249] When males are castrated or treated with estrogen, a change to the female pattern of growth hormone secretion is observed, concomitant with a change to the feminine pattern of hepatic steroid metabolism.[236] Norstedt and Palmiter[249] monitored two sex-specific liver activities as a function of the administration of growth hormone, given either continuously or as pulses. Their results suggest that "feminine" hepatic function, as monitored by high hepatic-prolactin receptor levels is the result of continuous growth hormone receptor occupancy, whereas the "masculine" pattern is the result of pulsatile growth hormone receptor occupancy separated by periods of low-receptor occupancy and undetectable levels of growth hormone in the plasma.

Although the presence of hepatic sex steroid receptors has been elucidated or at least postulated, the role of these receptors in the regulation of hepatic steroid metabolism is as yet unclear. Thus, it is difficult to determine what role these steroid receptors play in the regulation of hepatic steroid metabolism. The same factors that have primary control over hepatic steroid metabolism also appear to control the level of the sex hormone receptors in the liver.

Sex Hormone-Related Liver Disease

Numerous examples of liver-estrogen interactions have been associated with human liver disease. Women exposed to oral contraceptive steroids (OCS) are at increased risk for hepatic neoplasms, jaundice and cholestatis hepatitis, gallstones, and hepatic vein thrombosis (Budd-Chiari syndrome).[20,23,65,84,111,129,141,169,189,193,204,246,256,316,331] Pregnant women exposed to gestational levels of both estrogenic and progestational hormones develop liver abnormalities, which include fatty liver of pregnancy, intrahepatic cholestasis of pregnancy, and gallstones.[46,155,277,319] Not only does the liver respond to estrogen exposure, but it also plays a major role in the metabolism of sex steroid hormones, converting them to less potent compounds.[167] Many of these metabolites have the potential to alter the rate of metabolism and excretion of other hormones and drugs, thus further influencing the interaction between these compounds and the hepatocyte (e.g., catechol estrogens, although weak estrogens are noncompetitive inhibitors of the demethylation of mestranol, a 17-α-ethinyl estrogen found in OCS).[36] Such a decrease in catabolism could theoretically expose the hepatocyte to higher levels of a potential hepatotoxin for longer periods of time, increasing the likelihood of estrogen-hepatocyte interactions.

Anabolic-androgenic steroids (AAS) are also associated with significant liver disease. The most common manifestation that occurs in patients treated with androgens is mild hepatic dysfunction without jaundice that resolves without sequelae upon discontinuation of the drug.[194,327] Cholestasis with jaundice is unusual but may take weeks to months to resolve.[320] Such cholestasis is caused by a direct hepatotoxic effect of the drug and is particularly related to the presence of an alkyl group on the steroid's nucleus at the C-17 position. Androgens interfere with exertion of conjugated bilirubin into the canaliculus. Other problems reported to occur with androgen treatment include peliosis hepatitis and hepatic neoplasia. However, some reported cases of hepatocellular carcinoma (HCC) have been disputed on pathologic grounds and have suggested that the tumors are hepatic adenomas.[5,153,243,320] Because many of the patients treated with AAS also have Fanconi's anemia, which is associated with malignancy independent of androgen exposure, some investigators suggest that the occurrence of HCC in such androgen-treated patients may be a complication of the underlying Fanconi's syndrome rather than that of the administered androgen.[153]

Nonetheless, it is of interest that several groups have reported the presence of ER in HCC as well as in adjacent normal human liver. Molteni and associates[239] reported finding cytosolic ER in one HCC specimen. Similarly, Friedman and colleagues[124] assayed five human HCC specimens and the normal liver obtained with three of the cancers. All contained cytosolic ER. The data presented in this report suggest that the ER levels were lower in HCC than in normal liver, but the differences reported between the two types of tissue were not significant. Based on these preliminary data, these investigators treated another group of five patients with HCC with progestins and noted tumor regression in two of the patients at 6 and 10 months of therapy. The other three patients died at 1, 2, and 4 months. Unfortunately, none in the treatment group had their tumors assayed for ER or AR, either before or after treatment. The same laboratory also assayed one hepatoblastoma and found cytosolic ER in it, as did Iqbal and co-workers[173] in a similar tumor. This latter group assayed normal male and female liver, fetal tissue, and four HCC. All had cytosolic and nuclear ER–binding capacity except for the fetal tissue, which had only cytosolic receptor demonstrable. There was a wide range of values with no distinguishable pattern between tissues either by sex, tissue type, or localization of the measured binding to either the cytosolic or nuclear compartments. In contrast to these studies, Wong and associates[389] assayed 10 HCC specimens for ER using an immunocytochemical localization technique and found only one tumor to be positive for ER. It is difficult to correlate or compare the data present in these reports because of the small numbers of tumors examined, the marked variability in assay conditions used, the lack of documentation that ER was in fact the protein being measured, and the wide range of binding values obtained.

Data on AR in HCC, as in normal hepatic tissue, are sparse. Iqbal and colleagues[173] reported finding cytosolic and nuclear AR levels in four HCC, but they could not detect AR in normal human liver, in contrast to the reports of Aten and Eisenfeld.[9,10]

Other investigators have looked for ER in human hepatic adenomas.[133,213] Christopherson and Mays[65] assayed six hepatic adenoma specimens removed from young women who had been exposed to OCS. They found insignificant levels of cytosolic ER in five of the specimens. In the one ER-positive hepatic adenoma studied, they found that the ER-binding capacity in the tumor was less than that found in the adjacent normal liver and less than that in liver from normal control subjects who were not exposed to exogenous steroids. This finding of greater ER content in normal liver tissue adjacent to tumor was also reported by Friedman and colleagues[124] and in the studies of hepatic adenomas reported by Porter and co-workers.[263,264]

Porter and colleagues[263] assayed hepatic adenomas and associated normal liver tissue resected from three menstruatng young women for cytosolic and nuclear ER activity. One of these women was treated with pharmacologic doses of the antiestrogen tamoxifen in an unsuccessful attempt to reduce tumor size before her surgery. The two hepatic adenomas not treated with tamoxifen had measurable cytosolic ER, but the binding capacity was significantly less than that demonstrated in the normal liver adjacent to the adenomas, and also less than that demonstrated in normal liver obtained from female control subjects. However, the hepatic adenomas contained significantly more nuclear ER-binding capacity than did the normal liver. This increase in nuclear ER-binding capacity suggests that these adenomas may be more responsive to estrogenic hormones than is the normal liver. Such increased responsiveness to estrogen may explain the association between certain hepatic adenomas and OCS. In contrast, Porter and associates[263] were unable to demonstrate cytosolic ER in the tamoxifen-treated hepatic adenomas. The nuclear ER capacity present in the adenoma exposed to tamoxifen was significantly less than that found in other hepatic adenomas not exposed to the drug, despite the fact that the tumor increased in size during drug treatment. This finding suggests that tamoxifen was acting as an estrogen, or as a growth promoter, early in the course of the disease. It is possible that as the tumor progressed, it dedifferentiated and may have lost both its cytosolic and nuclear receptors.

It has clearly been shown in experimental studies that estrogens promote the development of hepatic neoplasms associated with increased hepatocyte activity. For example, Wanless and Medline[379] reported estrogens promote diethylnitrosamine-induced liver tumors. As described above, Porter and colleagues[263] found changes in the content and distribution of ER in the liver of persons with oral contraceptive-associated focal nodular hyperplasia and hepatic adenomas. In addition, Francavilla and colleagues[122] reported a very low level of cytosolic ER in a transplantable rat hepatoma, Morris 7777, compared with normal rat liver. All these data indicate that there is a possible interaction between estrogen and its receptor and the process of hepatocyte proliferation and possibly regeneration.

Despite this evidence, only two studies have reported on the effect of estrogen in liver regeneration after partial hepatectomy.[120,121] In order to establish a link between estrogen and hepatic regeneration, Francavilla and colleagues[121] monitored the temporal relationship between ER redistribution in the liver cell, the mitotic index, and the DNA synthesis rate in regenerating liver. At 3 hours after potential hepatectomy, ER levels were unchanged; however, a significant decrease in cytosolic ER was evident at 12, 24, and 48 hours. At 72 hours and thereafter, the level of ER had returned to the normal level prior to partial hepatectomy. A parallel increase in the amount of nuclear ER represents a clear demonstration of translocation of the cytosolic receptor to the nucleus as a sequela of the partial hepatectomy. Moreover, the authors of this study demonstrated that the binding of estrogen to both the cytosolic and nuclear ER was highly specific for estrogens, indicating that the receptor had not undergone unexpected alterations in specificity after partial hepatectomy or as a consequence of the regenerative process. Furthermore, no alterations in the affinity of the receptor for estrogen had occurred. The redistribution of the cytosolic ER started at the same time as the measured stimulation of DNA synthesis and reached its maximum at 48 hours, a point that coincides with the highest value of the mitotic index. The interrelationships of these phenomena with hepatocyte division is further demonstrated by the fact that a normal distribution of receptor was found in the cytosol and nucleus 72 hours after partial hepatectomy when few mitoses were observed. Thus, the active translocation of the ER into the nucleus correlated temporally with the other markers of hepatocyte regeneration, including several biochemical activities, such as DNA polymerase, protein synthesis, and deoxythymidine kinase activity.

The effect of ER translocation after partial hepatectomy may be related to either an increase in serum estradiol or an increase in hepatic intracellular estradiol resulting from a decrease in the estrogen metabolizing capacity of the liver remnant or both. The experimental data demonstrating that estrogen administration to nonhepatectomized rats results in a translocation of ER to the nucleus, as well as increased liver weight and DNA synthesis, support this view.

This work was supported in part from grants from the NIAAA #AA04425 and #AA06601 and NIAMDKD #AM32556, as well as grants from the Gastroenterology Medical Research Foundation of Southwestern Pennsylvania.

REFERENCES

1. Abrams JJ, Ginsberg H, Grundy SM: Metabolism of cholesterol and plasma triglycerides in nonketotic diabetes mellitus. Diabetes 31:903, 1982
2. Ahlqvist RP: Study of adrenotropic receptors. Am J Physiol 153:586, 1948
3. Alpers DH, Sabesin SM: Fatty liver: Biochemical and clinical aspects. In Schiff L, Schiff ER (eds): Diseases of the Liver. Philadelphia, JB Lippincott, 1982
4. Amico JA, Richardson V, Alpert B et al: Clinical and chemical assessment of thyroid function during therapy with amiodarone. Arch Intern Med 144:487, 1984
5. Anthony AP: Hepatoma associated with androgenic steroids. Lancet 1:485, 1975
6. Aron E, Glanzy M, Combescot C et al: L'alcool, est-il dans le vin l'element qui perturbe, chez la ratte, le cycle vaginal? Bull Acad Natl Med 149:112, 1965
7. Ashkar FS, Miller R, Smoak WM et al: Liver disease in hyperthyroidism. South Med J 64:462, 1971
8. Aten RF, Dickson RB, Eisenfeld AJ: Estrogen receptor in adult male rat liver. Endocrinology 103:1629, 1978
9. Aten RF, Eisenfeld AJ: Androgen and estrogen receptors in human liver (Abstr 245A) Presented at the 7th International Congress of Endocrinology, Quebec City, Quebec, 1984
10. Aten RF, Eisenfeld AJ: Human liver contains androgen and estrogen receptors (Abstr 373A) Presented at the Annual Meeting of the Endocrine Society, San Antonio, 1983
11. Atszuler N: Actions of growth hormone on carbohydrate metabolism. In Handbook of Physiology: Endocrinology IV, Part 2, Bethesda MD. American Physiological Society, 1972, p 233
12. Attie AD, Pittman RC, Steinberg D: Hepatic catabolism of low-density lipoprotein: Mechanisms and metabolic consequences. Hepatology 2:269, 1982
13. Badr FM, Bartke A: Effect of ethyl alcohol on plasma testosterone levels in mice. Steroids 23:921, 1974
14. Bala RM, Bohnet HG, Carber JW et al: Effect of ovine prolactin on serum somatomedin bioactivity in hypophysectomized female rats. Can J Physiol Pharmacol 56:984, 1978
15. Balasse EO, Bier DM, Havel RJ: Early effects of anti-insulin serum on hepatic metabolism of plasma free fatty acids in dogs. Diabetes 21:280, 1972
16. Bardin CW, Catteral JS: Testosterone: A major determinant of extragenital sexual dimorphism. Science 211:1285, 1981

17. Barrack ER: The nuclear matrix of the prostate contains acceptor sites for androgen receptors. Endocrinology 113: 430, 1983

18. Barrea A, Cho G: Evidence that copper-amino acid complexes are potent stimulators of the release of luteinizing hormone–releasing hormone from isolated hypothalamic granulae. Endocrinology 115:936, 1984

19. Basso LV, Havel RJ: Hepatic metabolism of free fatty acids in normal and diabetic dogs. J Clin Invest 49:537, 1970

20. Baum JK, Holtz F, Bookstein JJ et al: Possible association between benign hepatomas and oral contraceptives. Lancet 2:926, 1973

21. Baxter RC, Bryson JM, Turtle JR: The effect of fasting on liver receptors for prolactin and growth hormone. Metabolism 30:1086, 1981

22. Baxter RC, Bryson JM, Turtle JR: Somatogenic receptors of rat liver: Regulation by insulin. Endocrinology 107:1176, 1980

23. Bennion LJ, Ginsbert RL, Garnick BM et al: Effects of oral contraceptives on the gallbladder bile of normal women. N Engl J Med 294:189, 1976

24. Bennion LJ, Grundy SM: Risk factors for the development of cholelithiasis. N Engl J Med 299:1161, 1978

25. Bennion LJ, Grundy SM: Effects of diabetes mellitus on cholesterol metabolism in man. N Engl J Med 296:1365, 1977

26. Berelowitz M, Szabo M, Frohman LA et al: Somatomedin-C mediates growth hormone negative feedback by effects on both the hypothalamus and the pituitary. Science 212: 1279, 1981

27. Bergman RN: Integrated control of hepatic glucose metabolism. Fed Proc 36:265, 1977

28. Bezwoda WR, Bothwell TH, Vander Wait LA et al: An investigation into gonadal dysfunction in patients with idiopathic haemochromatosis. Clin Endocrinol 6:377, 1977

29. Bhalla VK, Chen CJH, Gramnaprakasam MS: Effects of in vivo administration of human chorionic gonadotropin and ethanol on the process of testicular receptor depletion and replenishment. Life Sci 24:1315, 1979

30. Bhalla VK, Haskell J, Grier H et al: Gonadotropin binding factors. J Biol Chem 251:4947, 1976

31. Binoux M, Hossenlopp P, Lasarre C et al: Somatomedin production by rat liver in organ culture. I. Validity of the technique. Influence of the released material on cartilage sulphation. Effects of growth hormone and insulin. Acta Endocrinol 93:73, 1980

32. Blake CA: Paradoxical effects of drugs acting on the central nervous system on the pro-ovulatory release of pituitary luteinizing hormone in prooestrous rats. J Endocrinol 79: 319, 1978

33. Bloodworth JMB, Hamwi GJ: Histopathologic lesions associated with sulfonylurea administration. Diabetes 10:90, 1959

34. Blundell TL, Humbel RE: Hormone families: Pancreatic hormones and homologous growth factors. Nature 287:781, 1980

35. Bo WJ, Krueger WA, Rudeen PK et al: Ethanol-induced alterations in the morphology and function of the rat ovary. Anat Rec 202:255, 1982

36. Bolt HM, Kappus H: Interaction by 2-hydroxyestrogens with enzymes of drug metabolism. J Steroid Biochem 7: 311, 1976

37. Bomboy JD Jr, Burkhalter VJ, Nicholson WE et al: Similarity of somatomedin inhibitor in sera from starved, hy-pophysectomized, and diabetic rats: Distinction from a heat-stable inhibitor of rat cartilage metabolism. Endocrinology 112:371, 1983

38. Bondy PK, Bloom WL, Whitner VS et al: Studies of the role of the liver in human carbohydrate metabolism by the venous catheter technic. II. Patients with diabetic ketosis, before and after the administration of insulin. J Clin Invest 78:1126, 1948

39. Bondy PK, Sheldon WH, Evans LD: Changes in liver glycogen studied by the needle aspiration technic in patients with diabetic ketosis. With a method for the estimation of glycogen from histologic preparations. J Clin Invest 28: 1216, 1949

40. Brazeau P, Guillemen R, Ling N et al: Inhibition by somatomedin of growth hormone secretion stimulated by hypothalamic growth hormone-releasing factor (somatocrinin, GRF) or the synthetic peptide hpGRF. CR Acad Sci Paris 295:651, 1982

41. Bronstein HD, Kantrowitz PA, Schaffner F: Marked enlargement of the liver and transient ascites associated with the treatment of diabetic acidosis. N Engl J Med 261:1314, 1959

42. Brunengraber H, Boutry M, Lowenstein JM: Fatty acid and 3-β-hydroxysterol synthesis in the perfused rat liver. J Biol Chem 248:2656, 1973

43. Burrows GH, Barrea A: Copper stimulates the release of luteinizing hormone-releasing hormone from isolated hypothalamic granulae. Endocrinology 115:1456, 1982

44. Cahil GF, Herrera MG, Morgan AP et al: Hormone-fuel interrelationships during fasting. J Clin Invest 48:584, 1968

45. Cameron DP, Burger HG, Catt KJ et al: Metabolic clearance of human growth hormone in patients with hepatic and renal failure, and in the isolated perfused pig liver. Metabolism 21:895, 1972

46. Cano R, Delman R, Pitchemoni CS et al: Acute fatty liver of pregnancy. JAMA 231:159, 1975

47. Cassel D, Pfeuffer T: Mechanism of cholera toxin action: Covalent modification of the guanyl nucleotide-binding protein of the adenylate cyclase system. Proc Natl Acad Sci USA 75:2669, 1978

48. Cerione RA, Strulovici B, Benovic JL et al: Pure β-adrenergic receptor: The single polypeptide confers catecholamine responsiveness to adenylate cyclase. Nature 306:562, 1983

49. Chadhury RR, Matthews M: Effect of alcohol on the fertility of female rabbits. J Endocrinol 34:275, 1966

50. Chamness GC, Costlow ME, McGuire WL: Estrogen receptor in rat liver and its dependence on prolactin. Steroids 26:363, 1975

51. Charbonnel B, Chupin M, LeGrand A et al: Pituitary function in idiopathic haemochromatosis. Acta Endocrinol 98: 178, 1981

52. Cheah JS, Tan BY: Diabetes among different races in a similar environment. In Waldhausl WK (ed): Diabetes. Amsterdam, Excerpta Medica, 1979

53. Cheek DB, Graystone JE: The action of insulin, growth hormone, and epinephrine on cell growth in the liver, muscle, and brain of the hypophysectomized rat. Pediatr Res 3:77, 1969

54. Chernausek SD, Jacobs S, Van Wyk JJ: Structural similarities between human receptors for somatomedin C and insulin: Analysis by affinity labeling. Biochemistry 20:7345, 1981

55. Cherrington AD, Lacy WW, Chiasson JL: Effect of glucagon

on glucose production during insulin deficiency in the dog. J Clin Invest 62:664, 1978

56. Cherrington AD, Steiner KE: The effects of insulin on carbohydrate metabolism *in vivo*. Clin Endocrinol Metab 11: 307, 1982

57. Chiao Y-B, Johnston AB, Gavaler JS et al: Effect of chronic ethanol feeding on testicular content of enzymes required for testosteronogenesis. Alcoholism 5:230, 1981

58. Chiasson JL, Atkinson RL, Cherrington AD et al: Effects of insulin at two-dose levels on gluconeogenesis from alanine in fasting man. Metabolism 29:810, 1980

59. Chipps HD, Duff GL: Glycogen infiltration of the liver cell nuclei. Am J Pathol 18:645, 1942

60. Chopra IJ, Chopra U, Smith SR et al: Reciprocal change in serum concentrations of 3,5′,3′-triiodothyronine (T3) and 3,3′,5′-triiodothyronine (rT3) in systemic illness. J Clin Endocrinol Metab 41:1043, 1975

61. Chopra IJ, Hershman JM, Pardridge WM et al: Thyroid function in nonthyroidal illness. Ann Intern Med 98:946, 1983

62. Chopra IJ, Solomon DH, Chopra U et al: Alterations in circulating thyroid hormones and thyrotropin in hepatic cirrhosis: Evidence for euthyroidism despite subnormal serum triiodothyronine. J Clin Endocrinol Metab 39:501, 1974

63. Chopra IJ, Solomon DH, Hepner GW et al: Misleadingly low free thyroxine index and usefulness of reverse triiodothyronine measurement in nonthyroidal illnesses. Ann Intern Med 90:905, 1979

64. Chopra IJ, Williams DE, Orgiazzi J et al: Opposite effects of dexamethasone on serum concentrations of 3,3′,5-triiodothyronine (T3). J Clin Endocrinol Metab 41:911, 1975

65. Christopherson WM, Mays ET, Barrows GH: Liver tumors in women on contraceptive steroids. Obstet Gynecol 46: 221, 1975

66. Clark AJ: The antagonism of acetylcholine by atripine. J Physiol 61:547, 1926

67. Clemmons DR, Klibanski A, Underwood LE et al: Reduction of plasma immunoreactive somatomedin C during fasting in humans. J Clin Endocrinol Metab 53:1247, 1981

68. Clemmons DR, Underwood LE, Ridgway EC et al: Hyperprolactinemia is associated with increased immunoreactive somatomedin C in hypopituitarism. J Clin Endocrinol Metab 52:731, 1981

69. Clemmons DR, Van Wyk JJ: Factors controlling blood concentration of somatomedin C. Clin Endocrinol Metab 13:113, 1984

70. Cobb CF, Ennis MF, Van Thiel DH et al: Acetaldehyde and ethanol are direct testicular toxins. Clin Toxicol 29: 921, 1978

71. Cobb CF, Gavaler JS, Van Thiel DH: Is ethanol a testicular toxin? Clin Toxicol 32:149, 1981

72. Cobb CF, Van Thiel DH: Mechanism of ethanol-induced adrenal stimulation. Alcoholism 6:202, 1982

73. Cobb CF, Van Thiel DH, Ennis MF et al: Is acetaldehyde an adrenal stimulant? Curr Surg 36:431, 1979

74. Cobb CF, Van Thiel DH, Gavaler JS: Isolated rat adrenal perfusion: A new method to study adrenal function. Metabolism 31:347, 1981

75. Cobb CF, Van Thiel DH, Gavaler JS et al: Effects of ethanol and acetaldehyde on the rat adrenal. Metabolism 30:537, 1981

76. Cobb CF, Ennis MF, Van Thiel DH et al: Isolated testes perfusion: A method using a cell- and protein-free perfusate

useful for the evaluation of potential drug and/or metabolic injury. Metabolism 29:71, 1980

77. Colby HD: Regulation of hepatic drug and steroid metabolism by androgens and estrogens. In Thomas JA, Singal RL (eds): Advances in Sex Hormone Research. Baltimore, Urban and Schwartzenberg, 1980

78. Cooper DS, Daniels GH, Ladenson PW et al: Hyperthyroxinemia in patients treated with high-dose propranolol. Am J Med 73:867, 1982

79. Copeland KC, Underwood LE, Van Wyk JJ: Induction of immunoreactive somatomedin in human serum by growth hormone: Dose response relationships and effects on chromatographic profiles. J Clin Endocrinol Metab 50:690, 1980

80. Corbin A, Bex FJ: Physiology and contraceptive effects of LHRH and agonistic analogues in female animals. In Zatuchni GJ, Smelton JD, Sciarra JJ (eds): LHRH Peptides as Female and Male Contraceptives. Philadelphia, Harper & Row, 1981

81. Creutzfeldt W, Frerichs H, Sickinger K: Liver diseases and diabetes mellitus. Prog Liver Dis 13:371, 1970

82. Crowe JP, Christensen E, Butler J et al: Primary biliary cirrhosis: The prevalence of hypothyroidism and its relationship to thyroid autoantibodies and sicca syndrome. Gastroenterology 78:1437, 1980

83. Daughaday WH, Mariz IK, Blethen SL: Inhibition of access of bound somatomedin to membrane receptor and immunobinding sites: A comparison of radioreceptor and radioimmunoassay of somatomedin in native and acid-ethanol-extracted serum. J Clin Endocrinol Metab 51:781, 1980

84. David RA, Kern F Jr: Effects of ethinyl estradiol and phenobarbital on bile acid synthesis and biliary bile acid and cholesterol excretion. Gastroenterology 70:1130, 1976

85. D'Ercole AJ, Stiles AD, Underwood LE: Tissue concentrations of somatomedin C: Further evidence for multiple sites of synthesis and paracrine or autocrine mechanisms of action. Proc Natl Acad Sci USA 81:935, 1984

86. DeFazio J, Lu JKH, Vale W et al: Effects of the (lm Bzl) D-His⁶, Desgly analog of GnRH on gonadotropin and estradiol secretion in normal women. Endocr Rev 10:163, 1984

87. Demanes DJ, Friedman MA, McKerrow JH et al: Hormone receptors in hepatoblastoma: A demonstration of both estrogen and progesterone receptors. Cancer 50:1828, 1981

88. DeMeyts P: Cooperative properties of hormone receptors in cell membranes. J Supramol Struc 4:241, 1976

89. DeWulf H, Hers HG: The stimulation of glycogen synthesis and of glycogen synthetase in the liver by administration of glucose. Eur J Biochem 2:50, 1967

90. Dickson RB, Eisenfeld AJ: 17-ethinyl estradiol is more potent than estradiol in receptor interactions with isolated hepatic parenchymal cells. Endocrinology 108:1551, 1981

91. Dunn FL: Hyperlipidemia and diabetes. Med Clin North Am 77:1347, 1982

92. Eagon PK, Fisher SE, Imhoff AF et al: Estrogen binding proteins of male rat liver: Influences of hormonal changes. Arch Biochem Biophys 201:486, 1980

93. Eagon PK, Porter LE, Gavaler JS et al: Effect of ethanol feeding upon levels of a male-specific hepatic estrogen binding protein: A possible mechanism for feminization. Alcoholism 5:183, 1981

94. Eagon PK, Van Thiel DH: E2T/ratio: An update. In Langer M, Chiandussi L, Chopra IJ, Martini L (eds): The Endocrines and the Liver. New York, Academic Press, 1982

95. Eagon PK, Willett JE, Rogerson BJ: Androgen receptor in male rat liver; separation from male-specific estrogen binder. (Abstr. 650) Presented at the 7th Annual Meeting of the Endocrine Society, San Antonio, 1983

96. Eagon PK, Willett JE, Seguiti SM et al: Androgen receptor in male rat liver. (Abstr. 777) Presented at the 7th International Congress of Endocrinology, Quebec City, Quebec, Canada, 1984

97. Eagon PK, Zdunek JR, Van Thiel DH et al: Alcohol-induced changes in hepatic estrogen binding proteins: A mechanism explaining feminization in alcoholics. Arch Biochem Biophys 211:48, 1981

98. Eden S: Age and sex-related differences in episodic growth hormone secretion in the rat. Endocrinology 105:555, 1979

99. Einarsson K, Gustafsson JA, Stenberg A: Neonatal imprinting of liver microsomal hydroxylation and reduction of steroids. J Biol Chem 248:4987, 1973

100. Eisenfeld AJ, Aten R, Weinberger MJ et al: Estrogen receptor in the mammalian liver. Science 191:862, 1976

101. Ellingboe J, Vananelli CC: Ethanol inhibits testosterone biosynthesis by direct action on Leydig cells. Res Commun Chem Pathol Pharmacol 24:87, 1979

102. Elta GH, Sepersky RA, Goldberg MJ et al: Increased incidence of hypothyroidism in primary biliary cirrhosis. Dig Dis Sci 28:971, 1982

103. Engberg B, Carlqvist M, Jornvall H et al: Isolation and characterization of somatomedin A from human plasma. Abstracts of the 7th International Congress of Endocrinology, p 588. Quebec City, Quebec, Canada, Amsterdam, Excerpta Medica International Congress Series 652, 1984

104. Eskay RL, Ryback RS, Goldman M et al: Effect of chronic ethanol administration on plasma levels of LH and the estrous cycle in the female rat. Alcoholism 5:204, 1981

105. Evans DF, Cussler EL: Physiochemical considerations in gallstone pathogenesis. Hosp Pract 9:133, 1974

106. Evans RW, Littler TR, Pemberton HS: Glycogen storage in the liver in diabetes mellitus. J Clin Pathol 8:110, 1955

107. Exton JH: Gluconeogenesis. Metabolism 21:945, 1972

108. Fain JN, Kovacev VP, Scow RO: Antilipolytic effect of insulin in isolated fat cells of the rat. Endocrinology 78:773, 1966

109. Falchuk KR, Fiske SC, Haggitt RC et al: Pericentral hepatic fibrosis and intracellular hyalin in diabetes mellitus. Gastroenterology 78:535, 1980

110. Fantus GI, Saviolakis GA, Hedo JA et al: Mechanism of glucocorticoid-induced increase in insulin receptors of cultured human lymphocytes. J Biol Chem 257:8277, 1982

111. Fechner RE: Benign hepatic lesions and orally administered contraceptives. Hum Pathol 8:255, 1977

112. Fehlmann M, Carpenter JL, Van Obberghen E et al: Internalized insulin receptors are recycled to the cell surface in rat hepatocytes. Proc Natl Acad Sci USA 79:5921, 1982

113. Felicetta JV, Green WL, Melp WB: Inhibition of hepatic binding of thyroxine by cholecystographic agents. J Clin Invest 65:1032, 1980

114. Felig P: The glucose-alanine cycle. Metabolism 22:179, 1973

115. Felig P, Owan OE, Wahren J et al: Amino acid metabolism during prolonged starvation. J Clin Invest 48:584, 1969

116. Felig P, Pozefsky T, Marliss E et al: Alanine: Key role in gluconeogenesis. Science 167:1003, 1970

117. Felig P, Sherwin R: Carbohydrate homeostasis, liver and diabetes. Prog Liver Dis 5:149, 1976

118. Felig P, Wahren J: Influence of endogenous insulin secretion on splanchnic glucose and amino acid metabolism in man. J Clin Invest 50:1702, 1971

119. Felig P, Wahren J, Hendler R: Influence of oral glucose ingestion on splanchnic glucose and gluconeogenesis substrate metabolism in man. Diabetes 24:468, 1975

120. Fisher B, Gundes M, Saffer EA et al: Relation of estrogen and its receptors to rat liver growth and regeneration. Cancer Res 64:2410, 1984

121. Francavilla A, DiLeo A, Eagon PK et al: Regenerating rat liver: Correlation between estrogen receptor localization and deoxyribonucleic acid synthesis. Gastroenterology 86:562, 1984

122. Francavilla A, Eagon PK, DiLeo A et al: Estrogen binding protein activity in Morris hepatoma 7777 compared to normal rat liver. Gastroenterology 86:1410, 1984

123. Francis MJO, Hill DJ: Prolactin-stimulated production of somatomedin by rat liver. Nature 255:167, 1975

124. Friedman MA, Demanes DJ, Hoffman PG: Hepatomas: Hormone receptors and therapy. Am J Med 73:263, 1982

125. Frier BM, Saudek CD: Cholesterol metabolism in diabetes: The effect of insulin on the kinetics of plasma squalene. J Clin Endocrinol Metab 49:824, 1979

126. Furlanetto RW: Somatomedin C binding protein: Evidence for a heterologous subunit structure. J Clin Endocrinol Metab 51:12, 1980

127. Furlanetto RW, Underwood LE, Van Wyk JJ et al: Estimation of somatomedin C levels in normals and patients with pituitary disease by radioimmunoassay. J Clin Invest 60:648, 1977

128. Gaddum JH: The action of adrenalin and ergotamine on the uterus of the rabbit. J Physiol 61:141, 1926

129. Gallagher TF, Meuller NW, Kappas A: Estrogen pharmacology. IV. Studies on structural basis for estrogen-induced impairment of liver function. Medicine 45:471, 1966

130. Gammeltoft S, Keiding S, Tygstrup N: Carbohydrate metabolism in relation to liver physiology and disease. In Arias IM, Frenkel M, Wilson JHP (eds): The Liver Annual 4. Amsterdam, Elsevier, 1984

131. Gammeltoft S, Tygstrup N: Carbohydrate metabolism in relation to liver physiology and disease. In Arias IM, Frenkel M, Wilson JHP (eds): The Liver Annual 3. Amsterdam, Elsevier, 1983

132. Gardner DF, Carithers RL, Utiger RD: Thyroid function tests in patients with acute and resolved hepatitis B virus infection. Ann Intern Med 96:450, 1982

133. Gastard J, Gasselin M, Bretagne JF et al: Dosage des recepteurs de l'oestradiol dans un adenome hepatique observe apres prise d'oestroprogestatifs. Nouv Press Med 9:43, 1980

134. Gavaler JS: Sex-related differences in ethanol-induced hypogonadism and sex steroid responsive tissue atrophy: Analysis of the weaning ethanol-fed rat model using epidemiologic methods. In Cicero TJ (ed): Ethanol Tolerance and Dependence: Endocrinologic Aspects. Alcohol and Health Monograph Series No. 13. Bethesda, Maryland, National Institutes on Alcohol Abuse and Alcoholism, 1983

135. Gavaler JS, Gay V, Egler KM et al: Evaluation of the differential in vivo toxic effects of ethanol and acetaldehyde on the hypothalamic-pituitary-gonadal axis using 4-methylpyrazole. Alcoholism 7:332, 1983

136. Gavaler JS, Van Thiel DH, Lester R: Ethanol, a gonadal toxin in the mature rat of both sexes: Similarities and differences. Alcoholism 4:271, 1980

137. Gebhardt R, Mecke D: The role of growth hormone, dexamethasone, and triiodothyronine in the regulation of glu-

tamine synthetase in primary cultures of rat hepatocytes. Eur J Biochem 100:519, 1979

138. Gerich JE, Lorenzi M, Bier DM et al: Prevention of human diabetic ketoacidosis by somatostatin. N Engl J Med 292:985, 1975

139. Gilnoer DM, Gershengorn MC, DuBois A et al: Stimulation of thyroxin binding globulin synthesis by isolated rhesus monkey hepatocytes after *in vitro* β-estradiol administration. Endocrinology 100:807, 1977

140. Gilnoer DM, McGuire RA, Gershengorn MC et al: Effects of estrogen on thyrotropin-binding globulin metabolism in rhesus monkeys. Endocrinology 100:9, 1977

141. Goldfarb S: Sex hormones and hepatic neoplasia. Cancer Res 36:2584, 1976

142. Goldstein MJ, Rothenberg AJ: Jaundice in a patient receiving acetohexamide. N Engl J Med 275:97, 1966

143. Goodman MW, Michels LD, Keane WF: Intestinal and hepatic cholesterol synthesis in the alloxan diabetic rat. Proc Soc Exp Biol Med 170:286, 1982

144. Gordon GG, Olivo J, Rafii F et al: Conversion of androgens to estrogens in cirrhosis of the liver. J Clin Endocrinol Metab 40:1018, 1975

145. Gordon GG, Southren AL, Vittek J et al: The effect of alcohol ingestion on hepatic aromatase activity and plasma steroid hormones in the rat. Metabolism 28:20, 1979

146. Gordon GG, Vittek J, Southren AL: Effects of chronic alcohol ingestion on the biosynthesis of steroids in rat testicular homogenate *in vitro*. Endocrinology 106:1880, 1980

147. Grant DB, Hambley J, Becker D et al: Reduced sulphation factor in undernourished children. Arch Dis Child 48:596, 1973

148. Green JC, Snitcher EJ, Mowat NA et al: Thyroid function and thyroid regulation in euthroid men with chronic liver disease. Clin Endocrinol 7:453, 1977

149. Griffin EE, Miller LL: Effects of hypophysectomy of liver donor on net synthesis of specific plasma proteins by the isolated rat liver. J Biol Chem 249:5062, 1974

150. Grundy SM, Metzger AL, Adler RD: Mechanisms of lithogenic bile formation in American Indian women with cholesterol gallstones. J Clin Invest 51:3026, 1972

151. Gustafsson JA, Mode A, Norstedt G et al: Sex steroid–induced changes in hepatic enzymes. Annu Rev Physiol 45:51, 1983

152. Gustafsson JA, Mode A, Norstedt G et al: The hypothalamo-pituitary-liver axis: A new hormonal system in control of hepatic steroid and drug metabolism. Biochem Action Horm 7:47, 1980

153. Guy JT, Auslander MO: Androgenic steroids and hepatocellular carcinoma. Lancet 1:148, 1973

154. Haber GB, Heaton KW: Lipid composition of bile in diabetics and obesity-matched controls. Gut 20:518, 1979

155. Haemmerli UP: Jaundice during pregnancy. Acta Med Scand 444:1, 1975

156. Hano T: Pathohistological study on the liver cirrhosis in diabetes mellitus. Kobe J Med Sci 14:87, 1968

157. Harano Y, DePalma RG, Lavine L et al: Fatty acid oxidation, oxidative phosphorylation, and ultrastructure of mitochondria in the diabetic rat liver. Diabetes 21:257, 1972

158. Hasselbach HC, Bech K, Eskildsen PC: Serum prolactin and TSH responses to TRH in men with alcoholic cirrhosis. Acta Med Scand 209:37, 1981

159. Hayashi H, Hotta Y, Sakamoto N: Electron microscopic study on the floating lipids of human liver. Acta Pathol Jpn 33:923, 1983

160. Hegedus L: Decreased thyroid gland volume in alcoholic cirrhosis of the liver. J Clin Endocrinol Metab 58:930, 1984

161. Heimberg M, Weinstein I, Kohout M: The effects of glucagon, dibutyryl cyclic adenosine 3′,5′-monophosphate, and concentration of free fatty acid on hepatic lipid metabolism. J Biol Chem 244:5131, 1969

162. Heldin C-H, Wasteson A, Fryklund L et al: Somatomedin B: Mitogenic activity derived from contaminant epidermal growth factor. Science 213:1122, 1981

163. Hepner GW, Chopra IJ: Serum thyroid hormone levels in patients with liver disease. Arch Intern Med 139:1117, 1979

164. Hicks SJ, Drysdale JW, Munro HN: Preferential synthesis of ferritin and albumin by different populations of liver polysomes. Science 164:584, 1969

165. Hintz RL, Suskind R, Amatyakul K et al: Plasma somatomedin and growth hormone values in children with protein-calorie malnutrition. J Pediatr 92:153, 1978

166. Holder AT, Wallis M: Actions of growth hormone, prolactin, and thyroxine on serum somatomedin-like activity and growth in hypopituitary dwarf mice. J Endocrinol 74:223, 1977

167. Hoffman AR, Paul SM, Axelrod J: Estrogen-ehydroxylase in the rat: Distribution and response to hormone manipulation. Biochem Pharmacol 29:83, 1980

168. Hoyumpa AM, Greene HL, Dunn GD et al: Fatty liver: Biochemical and clinical considerations. Dig Dis 20:1142, 1975

169. Hoyumpa AM, Schiff L, Helfman EL: Budd-Chiari syndrome in women taking oral contraceptives. Am J Med 50:137, 1971

170. Hughes ND, Perret G, Adessi G et al: Effects of chronic alcoholism on the pituitary-gonadal function of women during menopausal transition and in the postmenopausal period. Biomedicine 29:279, 1978

171. Hultman E, Nilsson LH: Liver glycogen in man. Effect of different diets and muscular exercise. In Pernow B (ed): Muscle Metabolism During Exercise. New York, Plenum Press, 1971

172. Inada M, Sterling M: Thyroxine turnover and transport in Laennec's cirrhosis of the liver. J Clin Invest 46:1275, 1967

173. Iqbal MJ, Wilkinson ML, Johnson PJ et al: Sex steroid receptor proteins in foetal, adult, and malignant liver tissue. Br J Cancer 48:791, 1983

174. Isley WL, Underwood LE, Clemmons DR: Dietary components that regulate serum somatomedin C concentrations in humans. J Clin Invest 71:175, 183

175. Israel Y, Kalant H, Orrego H et al: Experimental alcohol-induced hepatic necrosis: Suppression by propylthiouracil. Proc Natl Acad Sci USA 72:1137, 1975

176. Israel Y, Videla L, Bernstein J: Liver hypermetabolic state after chronic ethanol consumption: Hormonal interrelationships and pathogenic implications. Fed Proc 34:2052, 1975

177. Israel Y, Walfish PB, Orrego H et al: Thyroid hormones in alcoholic liver disease; effect of treatment with 6-n-propylthiouracil. Gastroenterology 76:116, 1979

178. Iyengar R, Swartz TL, Birnbaumer L: Coupling of glucagon receptor to adenyl cyclase: Requirement of a receptor guanyl nucleotide binding site for coupling of receptor to the enzyme. J Biol Chem 254:119, 1979

179. James VHT, Green JRB, Walker JG et al: The endocrine status of postmenopausal cirrhotic women. In Langer L, Chiandussi I, Chopra J, et al (eds): The Endocrines and the Liver. New York, Academic Press, 1982

180. Janni A, D'Azzo G, Pinzello GB et al: The prognostic value of thyroid function tests in liver cirrhosis. In Langer M, Chiandussi L, Chopra IJ, et al (eds): The Endocrines and the Liver. Academic Press, London, 1982

181. Jaques WE: The incidence of portal cirrhosis and fatty metamorphosis in patients dying with diabetes mellitus. N Engl J Med 249:442, 1953

182. Jefferson LS, Korner A: A direct effect of growth hormone on the incorporation of precursors into proteins and nucleic acids of perfused rat liver. Biochem J 104:826, 1967

183. John DW, Miller LL: Regulation of net biosynthesis of serum albumin and acute phase plasma proteins. J Biol Chem 244:6134, 1969

184. Johnston DE, Chiao Y-B, Gavaler JS et al: Inhibition of testosterone synthesis by ethanol and acetaldehyde. Biochem Pharmacol 30:1827, 1981

185. Jung Y, Russfield AB: Prolactin cells in the hypophysis of cirrhotic patients. Arch Pathol 94:265, 1972

186. Kaptein EM, Grieb DA, Spencer CA et al: Thyroxine metabolism in the low thyroxine state of critical nonthyroidal illnesses. J Clin Endocrinol Metab 53:764, 1981

187. Kasuga M, Kahn RC, Hedo JA et al: Insulin-induced receptor loss in cultured human lymphocytes is due to accelerated receptor degradation. Proc Natl Acad Sci USA 78:6917, 1981

188. Keller GH, Taylor JM: Effect of hypophysectomy and growth hormone treatment on albumin mRNA levels in the rat liver. J Biol Chem 254:276, 1979

189. Kern F Jr: Effect of estrogens on the liver. Gastroenterology 75:512, 1978

190. Key PH, Bonorris GG, Coyne MJ et al: Hepatic cholesterol synthesis: A determinant of cholesterol secretion in gallstone patients. Gastroenterology 72:1182, 1977

191. Kieffer JD, Ketchel M: Blockade of ovulation in the rat by ethanol. Acta Endocrinol 65:117, 1979

192. Klapper DG, Svoboda ME, Van Wyk JJ: Sequence analysis of somatomedin C: Confirmation of identity with insulin-like growth factor I. Endocrinology 112:2215, 1983

193. Klatskin G: Hepatic tumors: Possible relationship to use of oral contraceptives. Gastroenterology 73:386, 1977

194. Klatskin G: Toxic and drug-induced hepatitis. In Schiff L (ed): Diseases of the Liver, 4th ed. Philadelphia, JB Lippincott, 1975

195. Kneifel R, Katzenellenbogen BS: Comparative effects of estrogen and antiestrogen on plasma renin substrate levels and hepatic estrogen receptors in rats. Endocrinology 108:545, 1981

196. Kogawa M, Takano K, Hizuka N et al: Effect of GH and insulin on the generation of somatomedin by perfused rat liver. Endocrinol Jpn 29:141, 1982

197. Kohout M, Kohoutova B, Heimberg M: The regulation of hepatic triglyceride metabolism by free fatty acids. J Biol Chem 246:5067, 1971

198. Koontz JW, Iwahashi M: Insulin as a potent, specific growth factor in a rat hepatoma cell line. Science 211:947, 1981

199. Korner A: The effect of hypophysectomy and growth hormone treatment of the rat on the incorporation of amino acids into isolated liver ribosomes. Biochem J 81:292, 1961

200. Korner A, Hogan BLM: III. The effect of growth hormone on inducible liver enzymes. In Pecile A, Muller EE (eds): Growth and Growth Hormone, p 98. Amsterdam, Excerpta Medica, 1972

201. Kostyo JL, Nutting DF: Growth hormone and protein metabolism. In Handbook of Physiology: Endocrinology IV, Part 2, p 187. Bethesda, Maryland, American Physiological Society, 1974

202. Kreisberg RA: Glucose-lactate interrelations in man. N Engl J Med 287:132, 1972

203. Kupfer D, Bulger WH: Estrogenic properties of DDT and its analogs. In McLaughlin JA (ed): Estrogens in the Environment. New York, Elsevier/North Holland, 1980

204. Langer B, Stone RM, Colapinto RF et al: Clinical spectrum of the Budd-Chiari syndrome and its surgical management. Am J Surg 129:137, 1975

205. Lea MA, Walker DG: Factors affecting hepatic glycolysis and some changes that occur during development. Biochem J 94:655, 1965

206. Leevy CM: Fatty liver: A study of 270 patients with biopsy proven fatty liver and a review of the literature. Medicine 41:249, 1962

207. Lefebvre YA, Morante SJ: Binding of dihydrotestosterone to a nuclear-envelope fraction from the male rat liver. Biochem J 202:225, 1982

208. Lefferte HL, Koch KS, Lad PJ et al: Hepatocyte growth factors. In Zakim D, Boyer TD (eds): Hepatology. Philadelphia, WB Saunders, 1982

209. Lester R, Eagon PK, Van Thiel DH: Feminization of the alcoholic: The estrogen/testosterone ratio (E/T). Gastroenterology 76:415, 1979

210. Levey GS, Robinson AG: Introduction to the general principles of hormone-receptor interactions. Metabolism 31:639, 1982

211. Lieber MM: The incidence of gallstones and their correlation with other diseases. Ann Surg 135:394, 1952

212. Lloyd CW, Williams RH: Endocrine changes associated with Laennec's cirrhosis of the liver. Am J Med 4:315, 1948

213. MacDonald JS, Lippman ME, Wooley PV et al: Hepatic estrogen and progesterone receptors in an estrogen-associated neoplasm. Cancer Chemother Pharmacol 1:135, 1978

214. MacGorman LR, Rizza RA, Gerich JE: Physiological concentrations of growth hormone exert insulin-like and insulin antagonistic effects on both hepatic and extrahepatic tissues in man. J Clin Endocrinol Metab 53:556, 1981

215. Maes M, Ketelslegers J-M, Underwood LE: Low plasma somatomedin C in streptozotocin-induced diabetes mellitus. Diabetes 32:1060, 1983

216. Maes M, Underwood LE, Ketelslegers J-M: Plasma somatomedin C in fasted and refed rats; close relationship with changes in liver somatogenic but not lactogenic binding sites. J Endocrinol 97:243, 1983

217. Mallette LE, Exton JH, Park CR: Effects of glucagon on amino acid transport and utilization in the perfused rat liver. J Biol Chem 244:5724, 1969

218. Manderson WG, McKiddie MT, Manners DJ et al: Liver glycogen accumulation in unstable diabetes. Diabetes 17:13, 1968

219. Marliss EB, Aoki TT, Unger RH et al: Glucagon levels and metabolic effects in fasting man. J Clin Invest 49:2256, 1970

220. Marshall RN, Underwood LE, Voina SJ et al: Characterization of the insulin and somatomedin C receptors in human placental cell membranes. J Clin Endocrinol Metab 39:283, 1974

221. Martino E, Safran M, Aghini SP et al: Environmental iodine intake and thyroid dysfunction during chronic amiodarone therapy. Ann Intern Med 101:28, 1984

222. Massague J, Blinderman LA, Czech MP: The high affinity

insulin receptor mediates growth stimulation in rat hepatoma cells. J Biol Chem 257:958, 1982

223. Massague J, Czech MP: The subunit structures of two distinct receptors for insulin-like growth factors I and II and their relationship to the insulin receptor. J Biol Chem 257: 5036, 1982

224. Massague J, Pilch PF, Czech MP: Electrophoretic resolution of three major insulin receptor structures with subunit stoichiometries. Proc Natl Acad Sci USA 77:7137, 1980

225. Mayer PW, Schalch DS: Somatomedin synthesis by a subclone of Buffalo rat liver cells: Characterization and evidence for immediate secretion of *de novo* synthesized hormone. Endocrinology 113:588, 1983

226. Mayes PA, Felts JM: Regulation of fat metabolism in the liver. Nature 215:716, 1967

227. McConaghey P, Sledge CB: Production of "sulphation factor" by the perfused liver. Nature 225:1249, 1970

228. McGarry JD, Foster DW: Regulation of hepatic fatty acid oxidation and ketone body production. Annu Rev Biochem 49:395, 1980

229. McNeil LW, McKee LC Jr, Lorber D et al: The endocrine manifestations of hemochromatosis. Am J Med Sci 285:7, 1983

230. Meinders AE, Van Berge Henegouwen GP, Willekens FLA et al: Biliary lipid and bile acid composition in insulin-dependent diabetes mellitus. Dig Dis Sci 26:402, 1981

231. Mello NK, Bree MP, Mendelson JH et al: Alcohol self-administration disrupts reproductive function in female Macaque monkeys. Science 222:677, 1983

232. Mendelson JH, Mello NK, Bauli S et al: Alcohol effects on female reproductive hormones. In Cicero TJ (ed): Ethanol Tolerance and Dependence: Endocrine Aspects. NIAAA Research Monograph No. 13, DHHS Publication #(ADM) 83–1285, p 146. Washington DC, US Government Printing Office, 1983

233. Mendelson JH, Mello NK, Ellingboe J: Acute alcohol intake and pituitary gonadal hormones in normal human females. J Pharmacol Exp Ther 218:23, 1981

234. Merari A, Ginton A, Heifez T et al: Effects of alcohol on the mating behavior of the female rat. Q J Stud Alcohol 34:1095, 1973

235. Merimee TJ, Zapf J, Froesch ER: Insulin-like growth factors in the fed and fasted states. J Clin Endocrinol Metab 55: 999, 1982

236. Mode A, Gustafsson JA, Jansson JD et al: Association between plasma levels of growth hormone and sex differentiation of hepatic steroid metabolism in the rat. Endocrinology 111:1692, 1982

237. Mode A, Norstedt G, Eneroth P et al: Purification of liver feminizing factor from rat pituitaries and demonstration of its identity with growth hormone. Endocrinology 113: 1250, 1983

238. Mode A, Norstedt G, Simic B et al: Continuous infusion of growth hormone feminizes hepatic steroid metabolism in the rat. Endocrinology 108:2103, 1981

239. Molteni A, Baher RM, Battifora HA et al: Estradiol receptor assays in normal and neoplastic tissues. Ann Clin Lab Med 9:103, 1979

240. Moore DE, Kawagoe S, Davajan V et al: An *in vivo* system in man for quantitation of estrogenicity. II. Pharmacologic in binding capacity of serum corticosteroid-binding globulin induced by conjugated estrogens, menstranol, and ethinyl estradiol. Am J Obstet Gynecol 130:482, 1978

241. Moore DH, Kowlessar OD: Hepatic synthesis and degradation of plasma proteins. In Zakim D, Boyer TD (eds): Hepatology. Philadelphia, WB Saunders, 1982

242. Moskovic S: Effect of chronic alcohol intoxication on ovarian dysfunction. Stiar 20:2, 1975

243. Mulvihill JJ, Ridolfi RL, Schultz FR et al: Hepatic adenoma in Fanconi anemia treated with oxymethylone. J Pediatr 87:122, 1975

244. Nakayama H, Nakagawa S: Influence of streptozotocin diabetes on intestinal 3-hydroxy-3-methylglutaryl coenzyme A reductase activity in the rat. Diabetes 26:439, 1977

245. National Diabetes Data Group: Classification and diagnosis of diabetes mellitus and other categories of glucose intolerance. Diabetes 28:1039, 1979

246. Neuberger J, Portmann B, Nunnerley HB et al: Oral contraceptive-associated liver tumors: Occurrence of malignancy and difficulties in diagnosis. Lancet i:273:1980

247. Nikkila EA, Huttunen JK, Ehnholm C: Postheparin plasma lipoprotein lipase and hepatic lipase in diabetes mellitus. Diabetes 26:11, 1977

248. Nomura S, Pittmen CS, Chambers JB et al: Reduced peripheral conversion of thyroxine to triiodothyronine in patients with hepatic cirrhosis. J Clin Invest 56:643, 1975

249. Norstedt G, Palmiter R: Secretory rhythm of growth hormone regulates sexual differentiation of mouse liver. Cell 36:805, 1984

250. Norstedt G, Wrange O, Gustafsson JA: Multihormonal regulation of the estrogen receptor in rat liver. Endocrinology 108:1190, 1981

251. Olivo J, Gordon GG, Rafii F et al: Estrogen metabolism in hyperthyroidism and in cirrhosis of the liver. Steroids 26:47, 1975

252. Oppenheimer CL, Pessin JE, Massague J et al: Insulin action rapidly modulates the apparent affinity of the insulin-like growth factor II receptor. J Biol Chem 258:4824, 1983

253. Orrego H, Kalant H, Israel Y et al: Effect of short-term therapy with propylthiouracil in patients with alcoholic liver disease. Gastroenterology 76:105, 1979

254. Paleckar AG, Collipp PJ, Maddaiah VI: Growth hormone and rat liver mitochondria: Effects on urea cycle enzymes. Biochem Biophys Res Commun 100:1604, 1981

255. Palumbo PJ, Elveback LR, Chu C et al: Diabetes mellitus: Incidence, prevalence, survivorship, and causes of death in Rochester, MN, 1945–1970. Diabetes 25:566, 1976

256. Pertsemlidis D, Panveliwalla D, Ahrens EH: Effects of clofibrate and of an estrogen-progestin combination on fasting biliary lipids and cholic acid kinetics in man. Gastroenterology 66:565, 1974

257. Phillips LS, Herington AC, Karl IE et al: Comparison of somatomedin activity in perfusates of normal and hypophysectomized rat livers with and without added growth hormone. Endocrinology 98:606, 1975

258. Phillips LS, Young HS: Nutrition and somatomedin. I. Effect of fasting and refeeding on serum somatomedin activity and cartilage growth activity in rats. Endocrinology 99:304, 1976

259. Phillips LS, Young HS: Nutrition and somatomedin II. Serum somatomedin activity and cartilage growth activity in streptozotocin-diabetic rats. Diabetes 25:516, 1976

260. Pierson RW Jr, Temin HM: The partial purification from calf serum of a fraction with multiplication stimulating activity for chicken fibroblasts in cell culture and with non-suppressible insulin-like activity. J Cell Physiol 79:319, 1972

261. Pollet RJ, Kempner ES, Standaert ML: Structure of the

insulin receptor: Evidence suggesting that two subunits are required for insulin binding. J Biol Chem 257: 894, 1982

262. Porte D, Halter JB: The endocrine pancreas and diabetes mellitus. In Williams RH (ed): Textbook of Endocrinology. Philadelphia, WB Saunders, 1981

263. Porter LE, Elm MS, Van Thiel DH et al: Estrogen receptor in human liver nuclei. Hepatology 4:1085, 1984

264. Porter LE, Elm MS, Van Thiel DH et al: Characterization and quantitation of human hepatic estrogen receptor. Gastroenterology 81:704, 1983

265. Postel-Vinay MC, Cohen-Tanugi E, Charrier J: Growth hormone receptors in rat liver membranes: Effects of fasting and refeeding, and correlation with plasma somatomedin activity. Mol Cell Endocrinol 28:657, 1982

266. Powell-Jones W, Raeford S, Lucier GW: Binding properties of zearalenone mycotoxins to hepatic estrogen receptors. Mol Pharmacol 20:35, 1981

267. Powell-Jones W, Thompson C, Nayfeh SN et al: Sex differences in estrogen binding by cytosolic and nuclear components of rat liver. J Steroid Biochem 13:219, 1980

268. Prewitt TE, D'Ercole AJ, Switzer BR et al: Relationship of serum immunoreactive somatomedin C to dietary protein and energy in growing rats. J Nutr 112:114, 1982

269. Price DA, Wit JM, van Bull-Offers S et al: Serum somatomedin activity and cartilage metabolism in acutely fasted, chronically malnourished and refed rats. Endocrinology 105:851, 1979

270. Pykalisto OJ, Smith PH, Brunzell JD: Determinants of human adipose tissue lipoprotein lipase: Effect of diabetes and obesity on basal and diet-induced activity. J Clin Invest 56:1108, 1975

271. Raina A, Holtta E: The effect of growth hormone on the synthesis and accumulation of polyamines in mammalian tissues. In Pecile A, Muller EE (eds): Growth and Growth Hormone, p 143. Amsterdam, Excerpta Medica, 1972

272. Ranke MB, Stanley CA, Tenore A et al: Characterization of somatogenic and lactogenic binding sites in isolated hepatocytes. Endocrinology 99:1033, 1976

273. Reaven EP, Peterson DT, Reaven GM: The effect of experimental diabetes mellitus and insulin replacement on hepatic ultrastructure and protein synthesis. J Clin Invest 52:248, 1973

274. Rechler MM, Fryklund L, Nissley SP et al: Purified human somatomedin A and rat multiplication stimulating activity: Mitogens for cultured fibroblasts that crossreact with the same growth peptide receptors. Eur J Biochem 82:5, 1978

275. Rees LH, Besser GM, Jeffcoate WJ: Alcohol-induced pseudo Cushing's syndrome. Lancet 1:726, 1977

276. Reichard GA, Moury NF, Hochella NJ et al: Quantitative estimation of the Cori cycle in the human. J Biol Chem 238:495, 1963

277. Reyes H: Prevalence of intrahepatic cholestasis of pregnancy in Chile. Ann Intern Med 88:487, 1978

278. Riggs TR, Walker LM: Growth hormone stimulation of amino acid transport into rat tissues *in vivo*. J Biol Chem 235:3603, 1960

279. Rinderknecht E, Humbel RE: The amino acid sequence of human insulin-like growth factor I and its structural homology with proinsulin. J Biol Chem 253:2769, 1978

280. Rinderknecht E, Humbel RE: Primary structure of human insulin-like growth factor II. FEBS Lett 89:283, 1978

281. Ross DS, Daniels GH, Dienstag JL et al: Elevated thyroxine levels due to increased thyroxine binding globulin in acute hepatitis. Am J Med 74:564, 1983

282. Rothschild MA, Oratz M, Schreiber SS: Alcohol, amino acids, and albumin synthesis. Gastroenterology 67:1200, 1974

283. Roy AK, Arun K: Hormonal regulation of alpha 2u globulin. In Litwack G (ed): Biochemical actions of hormones, Vol VI, p 481. New York, Academic Press, 1979

284. Roy AK, Chatterjee B: Sexual dimorphism in the liver. Annu Rev Physiol 45:37, 1983

285. Roy AK, Chatterjee B, Demyan WF et al: Hormone and age-dependent regulation of alpha 2u globulin gene expression. Recent Prog Horm Res 39:425, 1983

286. Roy AK, Milan BS, McMinn DM: Androgen receptor in rat liver: Hormonal and developmental regulation of the cytoplasmic receptor and its correlation with the androgen-dependent synthesis of alpha 2u globulin. Biochim Biophys Acta 354:213, 1974

287. Rumbaugh RC, Colby HD: Is growth hormone the pituitary feminizing factor mediating the actions of estradiol on hepatic drug and steroid metabolism? Endocrinology 107:719, 1984

288. Ryback RS: Chronic alcohol consumption and menstruation. JAMA 238:2143, 1977

289. Salerno F, Cocchi D, Lampertico M et al: Effects of hypophysiotropic stimuli and neuroactive drugs on growth hormone secretion in cirrhotic patients. In Langer M, Chiandussi L, Chopra IJ et al (eds): The Endocrines and the Liver, p 289. London, Academic Press, 1982

290. Salmon WD, Holladay LA, Burkhalter VJ: Inibitors of somatomedin activity. In Giordano G, Van Wyk JJ, Minuto F (eds): Somatomedins and Growth, p 197. London, Academic Press, 1974

291. Sarva RP, Shreiner DP, Van Thiel DH et al: Gallbladder function: Methods for measuring filling and emptying. J Nucl Med 26:140, 144, 1985

292. Sato N, Ota M, Obara K: Presence of binding components for testosterone in rat liver cytosol. Endocrinol Jpn 27:315, 1980

293. Schalch DS, Heinrich UE, Drazin B et al: Role of the liver in regulating somatomedin activity: Hormonal effects on the synthesis and release of insulin-like growth factor and its carrier protein by the isolated perfused rat liver. Endocrinology 104:1143, 1979

294. Schimmel M, Utiger RD: Thyroidal and peripheral production of thyroid hormones. Review of recent findings and their clinical implications. Ann Intern Med 878:760, 1977

295. Schimpff RM, Donnadieu M, Gautier M: Somatomedin activity measured as sulphation factor in culture media from normal human liver and connective tissue explants. Effects of human growth hormone. Acta Endocrinol 98:24, 1981

296. Schimpff RM, Lebrec D, Donnadiu M: Serum somatomedin activity measured as sulphation factor in peripheral, hepatic, and renal veins of patients with alcoholic cirrhosis. Acta Endocrinol 88:729, 1978

297. Schneider HL, Hornback KD, Kniaz JL et al: Chlorpropamide hepatotoxicity: Report of a case and review of the literature. Am J Gastroenterol 79:721, 1984

298. Schoenle E, Zapf J, Humbel RE et al: Insulin-like growth factor I stimulates growth in hypophysectomized rats. Nature 296:252, 1982

299. Schussler GC, Schaffner F, Henley J et al: Thyroid function in primary biliary cirrhosis. Clin Res 27:259A, 1979

300. Schussler GC, Schaffner F, Korn F: Increased serum thyroid

hormone binding and decreased free hormone in chronic active liver disease. N Engl J Med 299:510, 1978

301. Schwander JC, Hauri C, Zapf J et al: Synthesis and secretion of insulin-like growth factor and its binding protein by the perfused rat liver: Dependence on growth hormone status. Endocrinology 113:197, 1983

302. Seelig S, Mariash CN, Topliss DJ et al: Growth hormone acts at a pretranslational level in hepatocyte cultures. Biochem Biophys Res Commun 115:882, 1983

303. Shapiro B, Pimstone BL: Sulphation factor (somatomedin activity) in experimental protein malnutrition in the rat. J Endocrinol 77:233, 1978

304. Silva JE, Larsen PR: Contributions of plasma triiodothyronine and local thyroxine monodeiodination to triiodothyronine to nuclear triiodothyronine receptor saturation in pituitary liver, and kidney of hypothyroid rats. J Clin Invest 61:1247, 1978

305. Small DM, Rapo S: Source of abnormal bile in patients with cholesterol gallstones. N Engl J Med 283:53, 1977

306. Smals AG, Kloppenborg PW: Alcohol-induced Cushingoid syndrome. (Letter) Lancet 1:1369, 1977

307. Smals AG, Njo KT, Knoben JM et al: Alcohol-induced Cushingoid syndrome. J R Coll Physicians Lond 12:36, 1977

308. Smith IF, Latham MC, Azubuike JA et al: Blood plasma levels of cortisol, insulin, growth hormone, and somatomedin in children with marasmus, kwashiorkor and intermediate forms of protein-energy malnutrition. Proc Soc Exp Biol Med 167:607, 1981

309. Song CS, Kappas A: Hormones and hepatic function. In Schiff L (ed): Diseases of the Liver, 4th ed. Philadelphia, JB Lippincott, 1975

310. Sosenko JM, Breslow JL, Miettinen OS et al: Hyperglycemia and plasma lipid levels: A prospective study on young insulin-dependent diabetic patients. N Engl J Med 302:650, 1980

311. Spencer EM: Synthesis by cultured hepatocytes of somatomedin and its binding protein. FEBS Lett 99:157, 1979

312. Stacpoole PW, Harwood JH, Varnado CE: Dietary carbohydrate decreases 3-hydroxy-3-methylglutaryl coenzyme A reductase activity and cholesterol synthesis in rat liver. Biochem Biophys Res Commun 113:888, 1983

313. Stalmans W: The role of the liver in the homeostasis of blood glucose. In Horecker BL, Stadtman ER (eds): Current Topics in Cellular Regulations. New York, Academic Press, 1976

314. Steiner KE, Williams PE, Lacy WW et al: Effects of the insulin/glucagon molar ratio on glucose production in the dog. Fed Proc 40:843, 1981

315. Stephenson RP: A modification of receptor theory. Br J Pharmacol Chemother 11:379, 1956

316. Stoll BA, Andrews JT, Matterum R: Liver damage from oral contraceptives. Br Med J 1:960, 1966

317. Strauss DS: Growth-stimulatory actions of insulin *in vitro* and *in vivo*. Endocr Rev 5:356, 1984

318. Sutherland EW, Robinson GA, Butcher RW: Some aspects of the biological role of adenosine 3,5-monophosphate (cyclic AMP). Circulation 37:279, 1968

319. Svanborg A, Ohlsson S: Recurrent jaundice of pregnancy. Acta Obstet Gynecol Scand 33:134, 1954

320. Sweeney EC, Evans DJ: Liver lesions and androgenic steroid therapy. Lancet 2:1042, 1975

321. Takano K, Hizuka N, Shizume K et al: Serum somatomedin peptides measured by somatomedin. A radioreceptor

assay in chronic liver disease. J Clin Endocrinol Metab 45: 828, 832, 1977

322. Tavill AS: Protein metabolism and the liver. In Wright R, Alberti KGMM, Karan S et al (eds): Liver and Biliary Disease. London, WB Saunders, 1979

323. Tell GP, Haour F, Saez JM: Hormonal regulation of membrane receptors and cell responsiveness: A review. Metabolism 27:1566, 1978

324. Terris S, Steiner DF: Binding and degradation of ^{125}I-insulin by rat hepatocytes. J Biol Chem 250:8389, 1975

325. Thompson C, Hudson PM, Lucier GW: Correlation of hepatic estrogen receptor concentrations and estrogen-mediated elevation of very low-density lipoproteins. Endocrinology 112:1389, 1983

326. Thompson P, Stru O: Abnormalities of liver function tests in thyrotoxicosis. Milit Med 143:548, 1978

327. Ticktin HE, Zimmerman HJ: Effects of a synthetic anabolic agent on hepatic function. Am J Med Sci 251:674, 1966

328. Turley SD, Dietschy JM: Cholesterol metabolism and excretion. In Arias I, Popper H, Schachter D et al (eds): The Liver: Biology and Pathobiology. New York, Raven Press, 1982

329. Turley SD, Dietschy JM: Regulation of biliary cholesterol output in the rat: Dissociation from the rate of hepatic cholesterol synthesis, the size of the hepatic cholesteryl ester pool, and the hepatic uptake of chylomicron cholesterol. J Lipid Res 20:923, 1979

330. Tygstrup N, Iverson J: Carbohydrate metabolism in relation to liver physiology and disease. In Arias IM, Frenkel M, Wilson JHP (eds): The Liver Annual 1. Amsterdam, Elsevier, 1981

331. Urban E, Frank BW, Kern J Jr: Liver dysfunction with menstranol but not with norethynodrel in a patient with Enovid-induced jaundice. Ann Intern Med 68:598, 1968

332. Valimaki H, Harkonen M, Yilkahri R: Acute effects of alcohol on female sex hormones. Alcoholism 7:289, 1983

333. Vallance-Owen J: Liver glycogen in diabetes mellitus. J Clin Pathol 5:42, 1952

334. Van den Brande JL, Van Buul S, Heinrich U et al: Further observations on plasma somatomedin activity in children. Adv Metab Disord 8:171, 1974

335. Vannotti A, Beraud T: Functional relationships between the liver, the thyroxine binding protein of serum, and the thyroid. J Clin Endocrinol Metab 19:466, 1959

336. Van Thiel DH: Diabetes mellitus and hepatobiliary disease. Acta Med Port 5:59, 1984

337. Van Thiel DH: Effects of ethanol upon organ systems other than the central nervous system. In Tabakoff B, Sutker PB, Randall CL (eds): Medical and Social Aspects of Alcohol Abuse. New York, Plenum, 1983

338. Van Thiel DH: Ethanol: Its adverse effects upon the hypothalamic-pituitary-gonadal axis. J Lab Clin Med 101:21, 1983

339. Van Thiel DH: Adrenal response to ethanol: A stress response? In Pohorecky LA, Brick J (eds): Stress and Alcohol Use. New York, Elsevier, 1983

340. Van Thiel DH: Disorders of the hypothalamic-pituitary-gonadal axis in patients with liver disease. In Zakim D, Boyer TD (eds): Hepatology, a Textbook of Liver Diseases. Philadelphia, WB Saunders, 1982

341. Van Thiel DH: Feminization of chronic alcoholic men: A formulation. Yale J Biol Med 52:219, 1979

342. Van Thiel DH, Cobb CF, Herman GB et al: An examination of various mechanisms for ethanol-induced testicular injury

studies utilizing the isolated perfused rat testes. Endocrinology 109:2009, 1981

343. Van Thiel DH, Gavaler JS, Cobb CF et al: An evaluation of the respective roles of portosystemic shunting and portal hypertension in rats upon the production of gonadal dysfunction in cirrhosis. Gastroenterology 85:199, 1983

344. Van Thiel DH, Gavaler JS, Cobb CF et al: Effects of ethanol upon the hypothalamic-pituitary-gonadal axis. In Langer M, Chiandussi L, Chopra IJ et al (eds): The Endocrines and the Liver. New York, Academic Press, 1982

345. Van Thiel DH, Gavaler JS, Cobb CF et al: Alcohol-induced testicular atrophy in the adult male rat. Endocrinology 105:888, 1979

346. Van Thiel DH, Gavaler JS, Eagon P et al: Hypogonadism and feminization in alcoholic men: The past, present, and future. In Galanter M (ed): Currents in Alcoholism VII. New York, Grune & Stratton, 1981

347. Van Thiel DH, Gavaler JS, Lester R: Ethanol: A gonadal toxin in the female. Drug Alcohol Depend 2:373, 1977

348. Van Thiel DH, Gavaler JS, Lester R: Ethanol inhibition of vitamin A metabolism in the testes: Possible mechanism for sterility in alcoholics. Science 186:941, 1974

349. Van Thiel DH, Gavaler JS, Lester R et al: Alcohol-induced testicular atrophy: An experimental model for hypogonadism occurring in chronic alcoholic men. Gastroenterology 69:326, 1975

350. Van Thiel DH, Gavaler JS, Lester R et al: Plasma estrone, prolactin, neurophysin, and sex steroid binding globulin in chronic alcoholic men. Metabolism 24:1015, 1975

351. Van Thiel DH, Gavaler JS, Sanghvi A: Lack of dissociation of prolactin responses to thyrotropin-releasing hormone and metoclopramide in chronic alcoholic men. J Endocrinol Invest 5:281, 1982

352. Van Thiel DH, Gavaler JS, Slone FL et al: Is feminization in alcoholic men due in part to portal hypertension: A rat model. Gastroenterology 78:81, 1980

353. Van Thiel DH, Gavaler JS, Sherins RJ et al: Alcohol-induced ovarian failure in the rat. J Clin Invest 61:624, 1978

354. Van Thiel DH, Gavaler JS, Tarter RE et al: Pituitary and thyroid hormone levels before and after orthotopic hepatic transplantation and their responses to thyrotropin-releasing hormone. J Clin Endocrinol Metab 60:569, 1985

355. Van Thiel DH, Gavaler JS, Wight C et al: Thyrotropin-releasing hormone (TRH)–induced growth hormone responses in cirrhotic men. Gastroenterology 75:66, 1978

356. Van Thiel DH, Lester R: Hypothalamic-pituitary-gonadal function in liver disease. Viewpoints Dig Dis 12:13, 1980

357. Van Thiel DH, Lester R: The effect of chronic alcohol abuse on sexual function. Clin Endocrinol Metab 8:499, 1979

358. Van Thiel DH, Lester R: Further evidence for hypothalamic-pituitary dysfunction in alcoholic men. Alcoholism 2:265, 1978

359. Van Thiel DH, Lester R: Hypothalamic-pituitary-gonadal dysfunction in patients with alcoholic liver disease. In Davidson CS (ed): Problems in Liver Disease. New York, Stratton Intercontinental Medical Book Corp, 1977

360. Van Thiel DH, Lester R: Alcoholism: Its effect on hypothalamic-pituitary-gonadal function. Gastroenterology 71:318, 1976

361. Van Thiel DH, Lester R: Sex and alcohol: A second peek. N Engl J Med 295:835, 1976

362. Van Thiel DH, Lester R: Sex and alcohol. N Engl J Med 291:251, 1974

363. Van Thiel DH, Lester R, Sherins RJ: Hypogonadism in alcoholic liver disease: Evidence for multiple defect. Gastroenterology 67:1188, 1974

364. Van Thiel DH, Lester R, Vaitukaitis J: Evidence for a defect in pituitary secretion of luteinizing hormone in chronic alcoholic men. J Clin Endocrinol Metab 47:499, 1978

365. Van Thiel DH, Loriaux DL: Evidence for an adrenal origin of plasma estrogens in alcoholic men. Metabolism 28:536, 1979

366. Van Thiel DH, McClain CJ, Elson MK et al: Hyperprolactinemia and thyrotropin-releasing factor (TRH) responses in men with alcoholic liver disease. Alcoholism 2:344, 1978

367. Van Thiel DH, Smith WI, McClain CJ et al: Abnormal prolactin and growth hormone responses to thyrotropin-releasing hormone in chronic alcoholic men. Curr Alcohol 5:71, 1979

368. Van Thiel DH, Smith WI, Wight C et al: Elevated basal and abnormal thyrotropin-releasing hormone–induced thyroid stimulating hormone secretion in chronic alcoholic men with liver disease. Alcoholism 3:302, 1979

369. Van Waes L, Lieber CS: Early perivenular sclerosis in alcoholic fatty liver: An index of progressive liver injury. Gastroenterology 73:646, 1977

370. Vassilopoulou-Sellin R, Oyedeji CO, Samaan NA: Extraction of cartilage sulfation inhibitors and somatomedins from rat liver. Endocrinology 114:576, 1984

371. Vassilopoulou-Sellin R, Phillips LS: Extraction of somatomedin activity from rat liver. Endocrinology 110:582, 1982

372. Vassilopoulou-Sellin R, Phillips LS, Reichard LA: Nutrition and somatomedin. VII. Regulation of somatomedin activity by the perfused rat liver. Endocrinology 106:260, 1980

373. Viladiu P, Delgado C, Pensky J et al: Estrogen binding protein of rat liver. Endocr Res Commun 2:273, 1975

374. Wahren J, Felig P, Cerasi E et al: Splanchnic and peripheral glucose and amino acid metabolism in diabetes mellitus. J Clin Invest 51:1870, 1972

375. Waldhausl WK: Treatment of diabetes mellitus: Pathophysiological aspects and state of the art. In Walhausl WK (ed): Diabetes 1979. Amsterdam, Excerpta Medica, 1980

376. Walfish PG, Orrego H, Israel Y et al: Serum triiodothyronine and other clinical and laboratory indices of alcoholic liver disease. Ann Intern Med 91:13, 1979

377. Walsh DB, Eckhauser FE, Ramsburgh SR et al: Risk associated with diabetes mellitus in patients undergoing gallbladder surgery. Surgery 91:254, 1982

378. Walton C, Kelly WF, Laing I et al: Endocrine abnormalities in idiopathic haemochromatosis. Q J Med 52:99, 1983

379. Wanless IR, Medline A: Role of estrogens as promoters of hepatic neoplasia. Lab Invest 46:313, 1982

380. Wartofsky L, Burman KD: Alterations in thyroid function in patients with systemic illness: The "euthroid sick syndrome." Endocr Rev 3:164, 1982

381. Wasantjerna C, Reissel P, Karjalainen J et al: Fatty liver in diabetes. Acta Med Scand 19:225, 1972

382. Weichsilbaum A: Ueber veranderungen der hoden bei chronichen alcoholismus. Berh Dtsch Pathol Ges 14:234, 1910

383. Weinhouse S: Regulation of glucokinase in liver. In Horecker BL, Stadtman ER (eds): Current Topics in Cellular Regulation. New York, Academic Press, 1976

384. Windler EET, Kovaner PT, Chao Y-S et al: The estradiol-stimulated lipoprotein receptor of rat liver. A binding site

that mediates the uptake of rat lipoproteins containing aproproteins B and E. J Biol Chem 255:464, 1980

385. Windnell CC, Tata JR: Additive effects of thyroid hormone, growth hormone, and testosterone on deoxyribonucleic acid–dependent acid polymerase in rat liver nuclei. Biochem J 98:621, 1966

386. Windmueller HG, Spaeth AE: *De novo* synthesis of fatty acid in perfused rat liver as a determinant of plasma lipoprotein production. Arch Biochem Biophys 122:363, 1967

387. Winters SJ, Troen P: Altered pulsatile secretion of luteinizing hormone in hypogonadal men with hyperprolactinemia. Clin Endocrinol 21:257, 1984

388. Wong BS, Chenoweth ME, Dunn A: Possible growth hormone control of liver glutamine synthetase activity in rats. Endocrinology 106:268, 1980

389. Wong LY, Chan SH, Oon CJ et al: Immunocytochemical localization of testosterone in human hepatocellular carcinoma. Histochem J 16:687, 1984

390. Wu A, Grand DB, Hambley J et al: Reduced serum somatomedin activity in patients with chronic liver disease. Clin Sci 47:359, 1974

391. Zakim D: Metabolism of glucose and fatty acids by the liver. In Zakim D, Boyer TD (eds): Hepatology. Philadelphia, WB Saunders, 1982

392. Zapf J, Morell B, Walter H et al: Serum levels of insulin-like growth factor (IGF) and its carrier protein in various metabolic disorders. Acta Endocrinol 95:505, 1980

393. Zapf J, Schmidt CH, Froesch ER: Biological and immunological properties of insulin-like growth factors (IGF) I and II. Clin Endocrinol Metab 13:3, 1984

394. Zapf J, Schoenle E, Froesch ER: Insulin-like growth factors I and II: Some biological actions and receptor binding characteristics of two purified constituents of nonsuppressible insulin-like activity of human serum. Eur J Biochem 87:285, 1978

395. Zapf J, Schoenle E, Jagars G et al: Inhibition of the action of nonsuppressible insulin-like activity in isolated rat fat cells by binding to its carrier protein. J Clin Invest 63:1077, 1979

396. Zapf J, Walter H, Froesch ER: Radioimmunological determination of insulin-like growth factors I and II in normal subjects and in patients with growth disorders and extra pancreatic tumor hypoglycemia. J Clin Invest 68:1321, 1981

397. Zimmerman HJ, MacMurray FG, Rappaport H et al: Studies of the liver in diabetes mellitus. J Lab Clin Med 36:912, 1950

398. Zimmerman HJ, MacMurray FG, Rappaport H et al: Studies of the liver in diabetes mellitus, II. J Lab Clin Med 36:922, 1950

chapter 6

Immunologic Aspects of Liver Disease

HOWARD C. THOMAS

Many of the immunologic phenomena associated with both acute and chronic liver disease are secondary to liver damage and have no primary pathogenetic significance. Changes of diagnostic and possibly pathogenetic significance in each disease state will be emphasized.

HEPATITIS A VIRUS INFECTION

This virus is a picornavirus that replicates within the liver, is excreted in the stool,[45] and evokes a strong antibody response. A rapid rise in IgM antibody titer occurs at onset and is of diagnostic use (Fig. 6-1). This antibody lasts for 3 to 6 months.[23] IgG antibodies are present in high titer from the clinical onset and remain for life, conferring protective immunity. The virus neutralizing antibody is directed to a conformational determinant, including sequences from the VP1 structural capsid peptide.[89] The majority of the antibody is directed to a limited number of epitopes.[41,126] In North America and Western Europe, by middle age, approximately 40% of people have immunity.[64] The prevalence of infection increases by 10% per decade of life.[64] The infection rate is greater in developing countries. In most tropical areas of Africa, more than 90% of the population will have immunity by 10 years of age.[249]

It is suspected that hepatitis A virus (HAV) replicates initially in the intestinal mucosa and then subsequently in the hepatocytes. This is supported by the observation that in marmosets immunosuppressed with prednisolone, HAV antigens can be detected in the enterocytes of the upper jejunum and ileum.[102] There is an IgA class antibody response within the intestinal mucosa,[102] and it is likely that this is important in conferring protective immunity against enteric challenge.

Cell-mediated immunity to the virus capsid antigens has been demonstrated.[58] Whether the liver damage is caused by a cytopathic effect of the virus or by cell-mediated immune responses directed to viral determinants on the infected hepatocytes has not been established.

During the acute phase of the infection, serum IgM concentrations increase,[218] and large amounts of circulating immune complexes are present.[221] The composition of these complexes is unknown. Low-titer smooth muscle antibody is often present.[1] Low-titer IgM class liver membrane antibodies (LMA) are found in most sera[261] and may be causatively related to the piecemeal necrosis that is seen in most of these patients.[216] It should be emphasized, however, that chronic infection and chronic hepatitis are not seen.

Prevention

Household contacts can be protected by administering immune serum globulin, 0.02 ml/kg IM, within 10 days. The development of a vaccine has been problematic. The virus has been grown in tissue culture,[178] and progress has been made in developing attenuated strains. An enteric attenuated live vaccine would seem to be the logical approach.

HEPATITIS B VIRUS INFECTION

Hepatitis B virus (HBV) infection is parenterally transmitted, usually during therapeutic use of blood or blood products, sexual contact, or sharing of needles during drug abuse. The incubation period is 3 to 6 months.

When infection occurs in adult life, it may result in acute hepatitis of varying severity, fulminant hepatitis, or, in 10% of cases, in chronic infection with the development of chronic hepatitis[163] (Fig. 6-2). More rarely, extrahepatic syndromes, including polyarteritis nodosum, membranoproliferative glomerulonephritis, polyneuropathy, papular acrodermatitis (Gionotti disease), and mixed cryoglobulinemia, may occur.

In Japan and China, infection usually occurs at birth. The child born to a chronic carrier mother who has viremia at the time of birth will almost certainly be infected, and more than 95% of these patients develop chronic infection[9] (Fig. 6-2). In these communities, between 10% and 20% of the population is chronically infected.

The delta agent is an RNA virus that replicates only in patients with HBV infection.[182,183] Both HDV and HBV

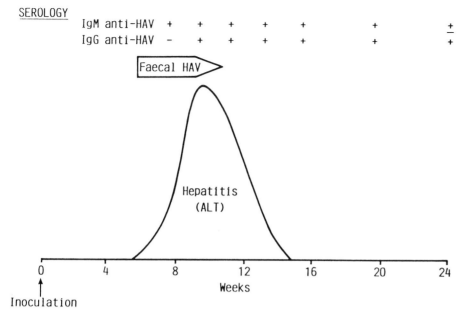

SEROLOGY

| IgM anti-HAV | + | + | + | + | + | | + | | + |
| IgG anti-HAV | − | + | + | + | + | | + | | + |

Faecal HAV

Hepatitis
(ALT)

0   4   8   12   16   20   24
Weeks

Inoculation

Fig. 6-1. HAV virus is shed into the feces before the development of humoral immunity (IgM anti-HAV) and before the hepatitis.

may be introduced in the same inoculum (coinfection) (Fig. 6-3) and give rise to acute hepatitis with a 5% to 10% chance of chronicity. In other cases, delta virus superinfects an established chronic HBV carrier and causes an acceleration of the course of the chronic hepatitis, so that the patient rapidly progresses to cirrhosis.[185,187] Both coinfection and superinfection can, in the acute phase, be diagnosed by the demonstration of delta antigen[183] or IgM anti-delta[195] in the serum. In coinfection, but not in superinfection, high-titer IgM anti-HBc is also present. In chronic delta virus infection, higher-titer IgG antibody is found, and continuing IgM antibody responses are observed.[195]

Mechanisms of Liver Damage

Acute Hepatitis

HBV itself is not directly cytopathic,[124] and the diversity of lesions described in infected patients has been attributed to variation in the capacity of the host's immune response to eliminate or suppress the infective agent.[48] The virus is first detected in the blood 6 to 8 weeks after the exposure. At this stage, before there is a detectable humoral immune response to the virus, alpha interferon can be detected in the serum.[173] This is probably responsible for the prodromal symptoms of fever and malaise that are often seen in

CLINICAL MANIFESTATIONS OF HBV INFECTION

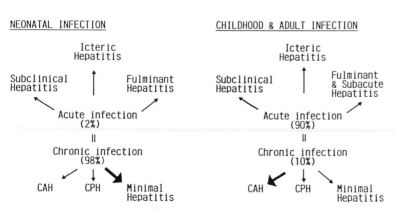

NEONATAL INFECTION

Icteric
Hepatitis

Subclinical   Fulminant
Hepatitis   Hepatitis

Acute infection
(2%)

∥

Chronic infection
(98%)

CAH   CPH   Minimal
              Hepatitis

CHILDHOOD & ADULT INFECTION

Icteric
Hepatitis

Subclinical   Fulminant
Hepatitis   & Subacute
                         Hepatitis

Acute infection
(90%)

∥

Chronic infection
(10%)

CAH   CPH   Minimal
              Hepatitis

Fig. 6-2. Syndromes occurring after HBV infection in neonatal and later life.

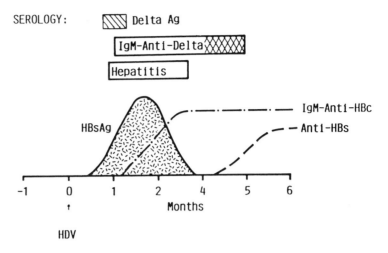

CO-INFECTION WITH HBV AND DELTA

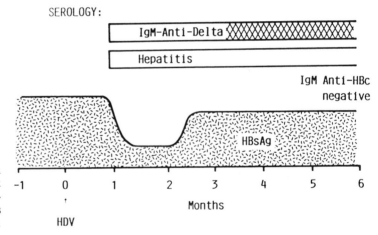

SUPERINFECTION WITH DELTA VIRUS IN CHRONIC HBV CARRIER

Fig. 6-3. Coinfection and superinfection with HDV. **Top.** Coinfection results in development of IgM anti-HBc and IgM anti-HDV. **Bottom.** Superinfection of an HBV carrier with HDV results in IgM anti-HDV in the absence of IgM anti-HBc.

these patients. This interferon induces an antiviral state in both infected and uninfected hepatocytes and stimulates an increased display of HLA class 1 protein on the hepatocyte membrane. At this time, there is an accumulation of natural killer (NK) and cytotoxic T cells in the hepatic parenchyma.[52] The cytotoxic T cells recognize the nucleocapsid proteins of the virus (HBc[243] and HBe[172]) in association with HLA class 1 proteins displayed in the hepatocyte membrane, and lysis of infected cells occurs[173] (Fig. 6-4).

The humoral immune response during the acute phase has been studied in detail and is summarized in Figure 6-5. The appearance of anti-HBe[124] and anti-HBV reactive antibody[2] is associated with the disappearance of HBe antigen and of HBV particles from the serum. The antibody conferring protective immunity is anti-HBs. This develops late in the illness, sometimes 1 to 2 months after the disappearance of HBs antigen from the serum. The antigenic determinants recognized by these virus-neutralizing antibodies are conformational[251] and involve the pre-S and S peptides.[92] IgM anti-HBc is present from the first 2 weeks after onset of HBs antigenemia and for 6 months thereafter.[28] It is absent or in low titer during chronic infection. This antibody is of diagnostic importance, and its presence in high-titer differentiates the acute from the chronic infection.

Chronic Infection

A major enigma in this field is the mechanism by which the virus persists and why chronically infected subjects develop hepatic lesions varying from severe chronic active hepatitis to minimal hepatitis and, in some cases, extrahepatic syndromes. It has been postulated that defects in

INTERFERON : ENHANCEMENT OF CLEARANCE OF HBV INFECTED HEPATOCYTES IN ACUTE HEPATITIS

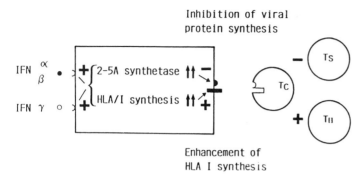

Fig. 6-4. Effect of interferon on virus-infected cells. Alpha (α)- and beta (β)-IFN acting through a common receptor and γ-IFN acting through a separate receptor activate several enzyme systems, including a 2-5A synthetase. This catalyzes production of oligoadenylates, which activate an endogenous ribonuclease, leading to clearage of viral RNA. IFN also causes enhanced expression of HLA class I proteins on the hepatocyte surface, facilitating recognition of virus-infected cells by the cellular immune mechanisms of the host.

the mechanism of elimination of infected hepatocytes[225] and in neutralization of infectious virus particles[51] underlie the chronic infection. It is now clear that, at the pathogenetic level, there is heterogeneity of the carrier state.

Infection at birth from an HBe antigen–positive carrier mother, virtually always results in chronic infection,[9] and it now seems probable that maternal IgG anti-HBc, passively transferred across the placenta, is involved in modulating or suppressing cell-mediated responses to nucleocapsid proteins,[172,223] thereby preventing effective clearance of infected cells (Fig. 6-6).

Infection in adults results in chronic infection in 5% to 10% of cases.[140] In many cases, there is a deficiency of alpha and, in some cases, also gamma interferon production.[91] This deficiency impedes the process of control of

viral protein synthesis and prevents adequate recognition and lysis of infected cells by sensitized lymphocytes (Fig. 6-7). It seems likely that the heterogeneity of hepatic and extrahepatic lesions is dependent upon variation in the effectiveness of the immune response in eliminating infected hepatocytes and neutralizing extracellular virus. A useful analogy can be drawn to the tuberculoid and lepromatoid responses to *Mycobacterium leprae* infection: Chronic active hepatitis (CAH) may be the result of a dominant cell-mediated (tuberculoid) response to the virus, whereas the extrahepatic diseases (polyarteritis nodosum and membranoproliferative glomerulonephritis) may represent a dominant humoral (lepromatoid) response.[219] The carrier state associated with only minimal hepatitis, which is most often seen after neonatal infection,

Fig. 6-5. Humoral immune response to HBV. The anti-HBc response is initially of IgM and IgG class.

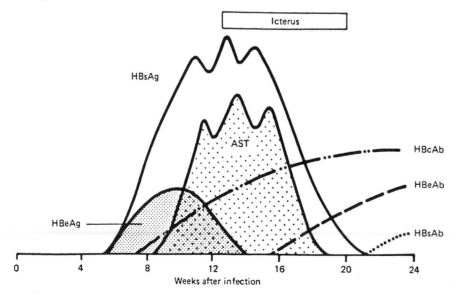

POSTULATED MECHANISM OF NEONATAL CARRIER STATE

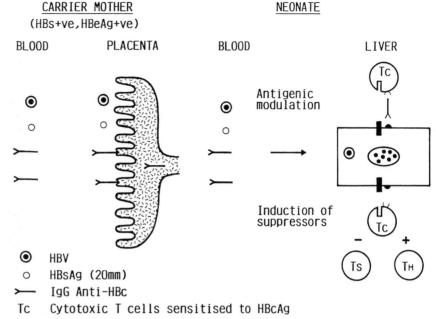

CARRIER MOTHER
(HBs+ve, HBeAg+ve)

NEONATE

BLOOD   PLACENTA   BLOOD   LIVER

Antigenic modulation

Induction of suppressors

⊙   HBV
○   HBsAg (20mm)
>—   IgG Anti-HBc
Tc   Cytotoxic T cells sensitised to HBcAg

Fig. 6-6. Postulated mechanism of neonatal carrier state. Material IgG anti-HBc crosses the placenta into the neonatal circulation. HBV infection of the neonatal liver is thus facilitated as maternal IgG blocks recognition of virus-infected cells by cytotoxic T-cells. Early exposure to soluble-virus proteins may induce a state of antigenic tolerance to the virus with specific suppressor cells inhibiting host defense mechanisms.

has been postulated to represent a state of partial or split tolerance to the virus,[223] perhaps occurring because of immaturity of the host's immune system at birth.

Natural History of Chronic HBV Infection

The presence in the serum of HBe antigen, a low–molecular weight component of the nucleocapsid of the virus, usually indicates the presence of virus particles in the circulation and therefore a state of relatively high infectivity.[202] Patients at this stage of the infection readily transmit infection to sexual contacts, and inoculation of even small amounts of their blood during needle-stick injury will cause infection.

After several years of chronic infection, HBeAg disappears from the serum and HBeAb appears (Fig. 6-8). Although no virus particles are visible by electron-microscopy in the serum of most of these patients and they are therefore rendering these patients to be of low or "zero" infectivity, when hybridization techniques are used to look for viral DNA, small numbers of viral particles can be detected in some (5%–60%) cases.[33,75,106] These cases are presumably, under some circumstances, infectious. Clearance of HBV particles from the blood is usually marked by a period of lobular hepatitis and elevated transaminases.[33,85] This transient exacerbation of the disease during HBe antigen–to-antibody conversion represents immune lysis of hepatocytes supporting HBV replication.

Fig. 6-7. Postulated defects occurring in childhood- and adult-acquired carrier state. Reduced IFN production leads to failure of HLA protein display and reduced 2-5A synthetase production.

POSTULATED MECHANISM OF CHILDHOOD & ADULT CARRIER STATE

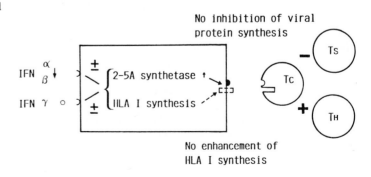

No inhibition of viral protein synthesis

IFN α/β ↓

IFN γ ○

2-5A synthetase ↑
HLA I synthesis

No enhancement of HLA I synthesis

NATURAL HISTORY OF HBV - INFECTION

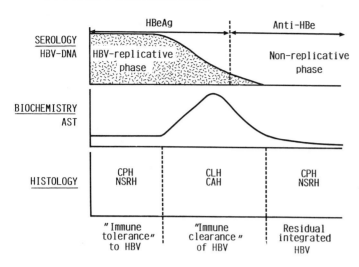

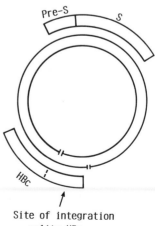

Fig. 6-8. Natural history of chronic HBV infection. During the period of viral replication, HBeAg is present in the patient's serum. Continued production of HBs antigen after cessation of HBV replication indicates the presence of hepatocytes that contain integrated HBV sequences.

Cytolytic T cells probably sensitized to HBc[146,243] or HBe[172] antigen contribute to this elimination process.

The continued secretion of the viral coat protein (HBsAg) in the absence of active viral replication probably represents a phase of infection in which the viral DNA has become integrated into the host DNA, so that some of the viral genes are transcribed and translated as though they were hepatocyte DNA. This integration event may be involved, late in the infection, in the malignant transformation of hepatocytes.[187,198] In order for this to result in a clinical hepatocellular tumor, these cells containing integrated sequences must evade the immune elimination processes. This may occur because the HBc and HBe antigens, the putative targets on the hepatocytes for cytolytic T cells, are absent on the cells containing integrated sequences.[225] Since the preferred site of integration on the viral genome is in the promoter region of the HBc gene[43] (Fig. 6-9), this transcription unit is therefore destroyed during the integration process. HBsAg continues to be expressed in these cells because this gene is intact in the integrated viral sequence.[43] Why the immune system fails to recognize this protein remains to be determined (Fig. 6-10).

The site of integration in the host genome is variable. However, the recent identification of a sequence within the DR2 region of HBV, which is homologous to a sequence within the host genome that determines the responsiveness to interferon of host genes encoding for several proteins responsible for the antiviral state,[220] would result in integration of HBV selectively within these sites (Fig. 6-11). Thus, integration may render the infected cell unable to respond to interferon and would allow a focus of HBV infection to persist. This process may reduce the chance of success when treating these patients with interferon.[220]

Low-titer antibodies to smooth muscle (actin) are present[81] as a reflection of the immune response to partially denatured antigens released from necrotic liver cells. Antibodies to single-stranded and double-stranded DNA are present for similar reasons.[95]

Fig. 6-9. Preferred site, within the HBV genome, at which integration with genomic DNA occurs. Integration results in disruption of the transcription unit for HBc.

SITE OF HBV INTEGRATION

Site of integration splits HBc

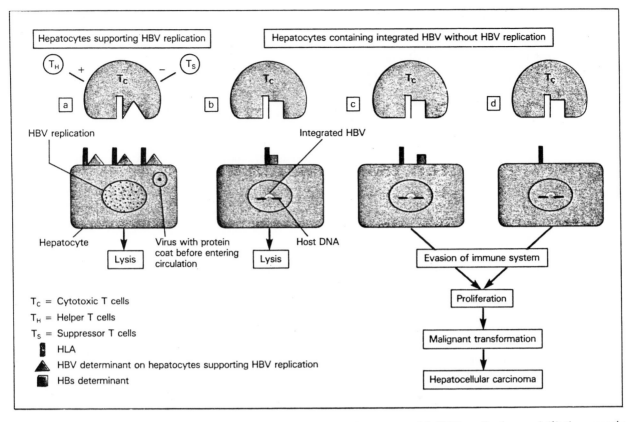

Fig. 6-10. Clearance of hepatocytes that support (*a*) HBV replication and (*b*) that contain integrated HBV sequences requires recognition of viral proteins associated with HLA protein by cytotoxic T-cells. Failure of this system may occur because of (*c*) nondisplay of HBs antigen or (*d*) nonassociation of viral proteins with HLA molecules.

HLA–DR	A G A G T T T C T C C T C T - C A
HLA–A3	G C A G T T T C T T T T C T - C T
HLA*	G C A G T T T C T C T T C T T C T
MT II	G C A G T T T C T C C T C T - C T
HBV	C A A C T T T T T C A C C T - C T

Fig. 6-11. A. A sequence of HBV (1821-1834 bases in subtype adw) is partially homologous to interferon-sensitive nucleotide sequences in the liver cell genome 220. Episomal or integrated virus may render the hepatocyte unable to respond to interferon.

Antibodies to liver-specific lipoprotein, an extract of liver cell antigens, are present in acute and chronic HBV-induced liver disease,[98] and the titer appears to be proportional to the degree of liver cell damage.[98] These antibodies are distinct from liver membrane antibodies[86] and are probably the consequence of liver damage rather than the cause.

Immunologic Aspects of the Treatment of Chronic HBV Infection

Carriers resulting from neonatal infection are resistant to all present attempts at treatment. Interferons are probably of no value in this group.[229] Procedures to modify the immune response to the virus will be required to treat this subgroup.

Patients who contract the infection later in life and who are actively replicating the virus (HBeAg positive) may be treated with either alpha-interferon or adenine arabinoside monophosphate.[229,253] Both of these agents will reproducibly inhibit viral replication, and, in cases with continuing immune competence, during the period of inhibition of viral replication, lysis of residual infected cells will occur. Lymphoblastoid interferon is effective in approximately 60% of patients, including homosexual as well as heterosexual cases.[229] Adenine arabinoside monophosphate is effective only in the heterosexual group; the homosexual patients respond less frequently,[165] probably because of secondary immunodeficiency.[171]

Attempts at immunotherapy have largely been unsuccessful, but immunotherapy has the theoretic advantage of perhaps destroying clones of cells that contain integrated as well as replicating HBV.[225]

NON-A, NON-B HEPATITIS VIRUS INFECTION

The non-A, non-B viruses are an important cause of sporadic (presumably enterally transmitted) and post-transfusion (parenterally transmitted) hepatitis. The diagnosis depends upon the exclusion of HAV and HBV infection by demonstrating the absence of IgM anti-HAV and IgM anti-HBc, respectively. Epstein-Barr virus and cytomegalovirus infection must also be excluded by IgM antibody tests.

Sporadic enterally transmitted non-A, non-B virus infection causes a mild illness; many persons are asymptomatic. A putative virus particle has been identified in the stools of these patients, and a serum antibody of IgG class has been identified.[5,105] These patients recover and do not develop chronic infection.[6]

An epidemic form of enterally transmitted non-A, non-B hepatitis has been described in Kasmir[110] and North Africa.[10] This form of the disease is similar to acute HAV infection. Whether the virus is the same as that causing sporadic non-A, non-B virus has not been established. The epidemic form is particularly severe in pregnant women. No diagnostic serologic tests are available.

Post-transfusion (parenterally transmitted) non-A, non-B hepatitis is important in that although the acute illness is mild, 20% to 80% of patients develop chronic infection,[4,11] ultimately leading, in some cases, to cirrhosis. There are at least two parenterally transmitted viruses that can be characterized by the duration of their incubation periods (2 to 4 and 6 to 10 weeks) and that commonly cause chronic hepatitis.

Pathogenic Mechanisms

The sporadic form of non-A, non-B hepatitis is associated with an increase in serum IgG levels.[269] The cause of this is unknown. This IgG increase allowed non-A, non-B hepatitis to be differentiated from acute HAV and HBV infections.[269]

The parenterally transmitted viruses are probably cytopathic. Low-titer smooth muscle antibody occurs, but hyperglobulinemia is not evident until cirrhosis is present. Serologic methods for the positive identification of this group of viruses are not yet available.

Treatment and Prevention

There is no proven method of therapy. Immune serum globulin may confer protection if given before blood transfusion[113] or with clotting factor concentrates (preexposure prophylaxis).[110] Its value in preventing infection in needle-stick victims (postexposure prophylaxis) has not been proved. The dosage and use of immune serum globulin are currently under investigation; therefore, no definitive recommendations can be made.

AUTOIMMUNE CHRONIC HEPATITIS

General Considerations

Chronic hepatitis is defined as chronic hepatic inflammation continuing without improvement for longer than 6 months. Inflammation of the intrahepatic biliary tree is usually excluded from this group of diseases. Several etiologic factors may initiate chronic hepatitis. These include a primary defect in regulation of the immune response (autoimmune), persistent viral infection (type B and non-A, non-B hepatitis viruses), prolonged administration of drugs (oxyphenisatin, methyldopa, isoniazid, nitrofurantoin), alcohol, and Wilson's disease. In a substantial number of cases, no etiologic factor can be identified.

The distribution of the inflammatory infiltrate in the portal tracts and hepatic lobules, established by hepatic biopsy, allows a further classification into chronic persistent, chronic active, and chronic lobular hepatitis; this is justifiable on prognostic grounds. These lesions may be seen with any of the etiologic factors.

In autoimmune CAH, there is mononuclear and plasma cell infiltration of the portal and periportal areas of the liver. Groups of mononuclear cells surround hepatocytes, some of which appear to be damaged, in a lesion called *piecemeal necrosis.* The lymphoid cells are predominantly T cells of the helper phenotype (OKT4 positive).[148] Cytotoxic-suppressor cells are less frequent than in the virus-induced forms of chronic hepatitis.[148] The disease has an insidious onset in most cases but occasionally presents abruptly with features suggestive of acute viral hepatitis. In these cases, the acute symptoms that call attention to chronic hepatitis probably represent intercurrent (new) infections with type A, B, or non-A, non-B viruses.

About half the patients have other immunologic disorders, including arthralgia or arthritis, vasculitis, ulcerative colitis,[73] glomerulonephritis,[67] fibrosing alveolitis,[241]

Hashimoto's thyroiditis,[179] autoantibody-positive hemolytic anemia,[122] leukopenia,[22] thrombocytopenia, and diabetes mellitus.

There is often hematologic evidence of hypersplenism secondary to portal hypertension. Serum IgG is usually markedly elevated, with smaller changes in IgM and IgA levels.[60,217] Antinuclear antibodies,[86,101] antibodies to double-stranded DNA[40,95] and to smooth muscle (actin),[100,257] are present in high titer, usually greater than 1:40 by immunofluorescence. The term *lupoid chronic active hepatitis* was given this syndrome because of the presence of antinuclear factor. More recently, additional autoantibodies have been described in these patients, including the liver-kidney microsomal[188] and mitochondrial antibodies.[15] Whether these antibodies define separate subgroups with different etiologies has not been determined. The liver-kidney microsomal antibody also binds to the hepatocyte membrane.[228]

Autoantibodies

Liver-Specific Lipoprotein

Meyer zum Buschenfelde and colleagues extracted and characterized two proteins from supernatants of liver cell homogenates, a stable protein and an unstable lipoprotein.[143] Immunization of rabbits with these proteins in Freund's complete adjuvant induced the production of specific antisera, and repetitive immunization induced chronic hepatitis resembling human CAH.[141] Initially three peaks were obtained when the supernatants were fractionated by column chromatography. The first contained liver-specific antigenic material; further fractionation yielded two proteins, a low-density macromolecular liver membrane lipoprotein—then termed *LPI*—and a cytoplasmic protein termed *LPII*. LPI was subsequently identified by immunofluorescence on isolated hepatocytes as a membrane antigen that had organ specificity but appeared to lack species specificity.[143] This membrane protein was later extracted in purer form and became known as liver-specific protein (LSP) (Fig. 6-12).[134] LSP is structurally very complex, and the molecular weight of the apoprotein is 4 million daltons to 20 million daltons. The lability of LSP made it difficult to study this material until stabilization with EDTA was used in the extraction procedure, and improved yields resulted.[134] Recent studies indicate that human LSP has species-specific and non-species-specific determinants.[263]

LSP is a candidate liver autoantigen because of its capacity to (1) induce chronic hepatitis in rabbits,[141] (2) act as reactant in migration inhibition tests with blood lymphocytes from patients with chronic hepatitis,[140] (3) inhibit the cytotoxic activity of blood mononuclear cells of patients with CAH for isolated hepatocytes,[70] and (4) have antigenic activity in radioimmunoassays with sera of pa-

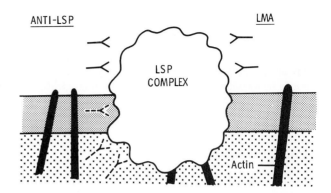

Fig. 6-12. Liver-specific lipoprotein (*LSP*) and liver membrane antigen (*LMA*).

tients with chronic hepatitis.[98] Although most investigators consider LSP to be truly liver-specific,[29] some disagree.[8a] Given the extraction problems, some preparations of LSP could contain non–organ-specific components.[263]

Immune reactivity to LSP, whether humoral or cellular, may not be specific for any one type of liver disease. Thus, humoral antibody to LSP, demonstrable by radioimmunoassays, can be transiently detected in acute viral hepatitis, in CAH of the autoimmune or HBsAg-associated type, and in alcoholic cirrhosis and primary biliary cirrhosis.[98] Thus, in some circumstances, an immune response to LSP may occur as a consequence of liver cell injury. Still at issue is the question of whether an ongoing immune response to LSP as an organ-specific target antigen provides an explanation for the self-perpetuation of autoimmune CAH.

Liver Membrane Antigen

In studies on the organ specificity of LSP, Hopf and coworkers, in 1976, found that heterologous (rat and rabbit) antisera to their two preparations of liver-specific proteins LPI and LPII reacted by immunofluorescence with a liver cell membrane.[86] Later it was shown that 30% to 85% of hepatocytes isolated from biopsies of patients with CAH were coated *in vivo* with an autoantibody reactive with the hepatocyte membrane.[85] This was called *liver membrane autoantibody* (LMAb). Moreover, serum of patients reacted *in vitro* with the membrane of isolated rabbit hepatocytes in a linear type of staining. These reactions were found to characterize cases of autoimmune CAH and contrasted with a different granular pattern of fluorescence observed on the liver cell membrane in cases of HBsAg-associated CAH.[86] LMAb can also be detected by radioimmunoassay techniques, using rat hepatocytes as target, in various liver diseases, with a high frequency in

HBsAg-negative cases of cirrhosis (61%) and CAH (38%), and in acute viral hepatitis (18%).[261] It seldom occurs in all other categories of liver disease. The antigen reactive with LMAb has been separated by affinity chromatography using insolubilized LMAb-positive sera and appears not to be a constituent of LSP.[142] Accordingly, LMAb is claimed to be a specific marker for autoimmune-type CAH and to be reactive with the antigen that evokes this disease.

Antinuclear Antibodies

Antinuclear antibodies (ANA) were first recognized in CAH by positivity in the lupus erythematosus (LE) cell test.[101] ANA reactions in CAH are now recognized by immunofluorescence.[258] The conventional nuclear substrate for detection of ANA is provided by frozen sections of rat liver. A suggested "cut-off" dilution of serum for positivity is 1/10. Human blood smears are also diagnostically useful as substrates. These provide nuclei of lymphocytes and granulocytes as substrate; thus, they enable recognition of a granulocyte-specific ANA that is characteristic of autoimmune CAH.[258] The "patterns" of ANA reactivity seen with immunofluorescence include (1) "homogenous" indicating reactivity with the nucleoprotein histone complex and characterizing autoimmune CAH; (2) "rim" or "peripheral," indicating reactivity with DNA; (3) "speckled," specifying reactivity with extractable nuclear antigens (Sm and ribonucleoprotein); and (4) nucleolar.

Antibodies to native double-stranded DNA, detected by radioimmunoassay, do occur in CAH, although infrequently.[40,95] There is a high incidence of reactivity to denatured single-stranded DNA.[95]

Smooth Muscle Antibody

Demonstrated in 1965 in CAH by immunofluorescence,[100] smooth muscle antibody (SMA) is not entirely specific for CAH. It is also found in patients with alcoholic hepatitis,[257] rheumatoid arthritis,[257] multiple sclerosis,[135] cancer,[259] and particularly acute viral disease.[237] Curiously, however, the reaction for SMA seems uniformly lacking in systemic lupus erythematosus (SLE).[257] SMA is found in 70% of cases of CAH and in only 3% to 14% of the normal population. Smooth muscle from any source in the body and from all species down to amphibia is reactive with SMA, and positive sera react with smooth muscle of autologous origin.

Actin was recognized as one important determinant for SMA reactivity. The description of three different immunofluorescent-staining patterns on frozen sections of rat kidney—namely, SMA-T (tubules), SMA-G (glomeruli), and SMA-V (vessels) and the finding that the reactivity of SMA-T and some SMA-G was neutralized by actin but that of SMA-V was not—indicated that SMA might have "actin" or "non-actin" specificity.[21] Studies

on acetone-fixed cultured fibroblasts[237] established that SMA could be reactive with different ultrastructural components of the cellular cytoskeleton—namely, microfilaments (6 nm), which form actin "cables," microtubules (25 nm); and intermediate filaments (10 nm). The main protein subunits are, respectively, actin, tubulin, and vimentin. Immunofluorescence studies using antibodies raised in rabbits to pure proteins suggest the presence of various proteins among each of these cytoplasmic filaments.[237]

Immunologic Aspects of Pathogenesis

Both the number[146,218] and function of nonspecific suppressor cells[80,97] are diminished in these patients. A defect in antigen-specific suppressor cell functions may be responsible for the development of autoantibodies reacting with liver membrane antigens.[242] These antibodies are found in high titer in autoimmune CAH and are thought to mediate the lesion of periportal piecemeal necrosis.[98,261] The nature of the hepatocyte membrane antigen that is the target is unknown. Some investigators suggest involvement of LSP, but more recent data favor a major role for LMA. Mice immunized with the latter develop florid chronic hepatitis,[8] whereas rabbits immunized with LSP develop minimal disease,[141] which is also found in animals given adjuvant alone.[25] These antibodies are also found in patients with primary biliary cirrhosis who exhibit piecemeal necrosis.[261] A reflection of the diminished activity of nonspecific suppressor cells is the high serum immunoglobulin concentrations, particularly IgG.[60] The fact that this defect may be genetically determined is suggested by the finding of an increased incidence of autoantibodies and raised globulin levels in the relatives of these patients[65] and a state of linkage disequilibrium of the disease with the human leukocyte antigens HLA-B8[127] and -Dw3.[128] The latter association suggests that the inheritance of a gene or genes close to the B and D loci of the major histocompatibility complex (MHC) on chromosome 6 predisposes to the development of the disease, either spontaneously or in response to some environmental trigger factor.

Immunologic Aspects of Treatment

Until we are able to correct the defect in the immunoregulatory system, immunosuppression represents the mainstay of therapy. Controlled trials have demonstrated that corticosteroids produce a prolongation of survival over a period of 10 years.[111] Azathioprine may occasionally be added to allow maintenance with lower doses of steroids. The defect in immunoregulatory function returns to normal during steroid therapy.[164,218] In most cases, relapse will occur on cessation of therapy[47] and may be predicted by the continuing presence of anti-LSP.[125] It seems probable that therapy must be continued for life.

PRIMARY BILIARY CIRRHOSIS

General Considerations

In this disease, a chronic granulomatous inflammatory process results in destruction of the intrahepatic biliary tree.[160,192,201] Patients with this disease also exhibit lesions of the salivary, lacrimal, and pancreatic glands, scleroderma, rheumatoid arthritis, and thyroid disease.[67,68] The finding of mitochondrial antibody in the serum of these patients led to the conclusion that the disease was probably of autoimmune origin.[227]

The disease occurs commonly in middle-aged women, who present with symptoms of cholestasis. Liver function tests show an elevated alkaline phosphatase level, often with normal transaminases and bilirubin. The most prominent symptom is pruritus. The rate of progression is variable. Many patients remain anicteric for 10 to 20 years. Once jaundice develops, life expectancy is considerably reduced.[199]

Immunologic Aspects of Pathogenesis

Recently, evidence of an abnormality in the immunoregulatory system in these patients has been obtained. Both the concentrations[218] and functions of suppressor T cells[97] are markedly reduced. It is hypothesized that this abnormality allows the expansion of a clone of autoreactive lymphocytes with the potential to mount an immune response to both hepatic and nonhepatic ductular antigens.[54] Similarity of the syndrome to chronic graft-versus-host disease,[71,72] in which transplanted bone marrow cells attack the tissues of the body that have a high density of HLA antigens, has led to the suggestion that the target antigen in primary biliary cirrhosis (PBC) may be either a native or an altered HLA protein.[54]

One result of the reduced suppressor cell activity is an increased rate of synthesis of IgM[97] with failure of polymerization, leading to release of monomeric IgM.[56] An additional abnormality of the humoral immune system is failure to convert from IgM to IgG antibody production.[222] The protracted IgM response may be the result of failure of feedback inhibition because of the poor IgG antibody response (Fig. 6-13).

Mitochondrial Antibody

Mitochondrial antibody (MA) was first described in 1966 by Doniach and associates.[46] The pattern by immunofluorescence is coarsely granular, and mitochondria of all tissues are reactive; however, renal tubular cells rich in mitochondria are the usual substrate. MA exist in the three main immunoglobulin classes, but mostly IgM.[169] Tests for MA have high sensitivity and specificity for PBC; the antibody is present in more than 95% of cases.[154] It is detectable in only a few other diseases, including Sjögren's disease.[255] MA is notably not demonstrable in jaundice because of extrahepatic biliary obstruction.[256]

The specific reactivity of MA with mitochondria has been established using subcellular fractions and marker enzymes.[14] The antigen has been localized to the inner membrane of mitochondria and is a lipoprotein of molecular weight 180,000 to 200,000 daltons. The "classical" MA of PBC is one of four types:[15] (1) anticardiolipin (M1); (2) antibody of PBC (M2); (3) antibody of the pseudolupus syndrome (M3); and (4) antibody of the CAH-PBC "overlap" disease (M4). Labro and co-workers[114] described another type (M5) seen in patients with SLE.

Immune Complexes and Complement Activation

These patients have large amounts of "immune complex-like" factors in their serum[221,248] that result in activation of the classical[175] and alternative pathways[248] of complement. These "complexes" are cleared abnormally slowly[99] because of antibodies to the C3B receptor.[145] The complexes may be responsible for some of the extrahepatic manifestations of the disease, including, in some cases, arthritis, arteritis, and glomerulonephritis.[230] Their role in the genesis of hepatic granulomas is unknown.

Fig. 6-13. Abnormal regulation of the humoral immune response in primary biliary cirrhosis.

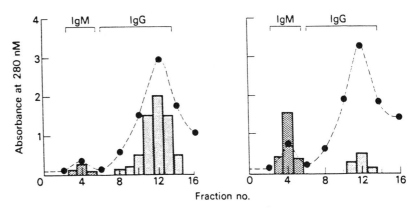

Abnormalities of Cell-Mediated Immunity

Patients with PBC are severely anergic in delayed hypersensitivity skin tests.[62] Serum factors appear to be important,[137] and, recently, evidence has focused on the role of abnormal high- and low-density lipoproteins in the anergic state.[166,167]

Immunologic Aspects of Treatment

Penicillamine, a copper chelating and anti-inflammatory compound, has been shown in some studies to produce biochemical and histologic improvement,[55,94] but its effect on survival has not been proved. This drug has been shown to reduce the ratio of helper to suppressor T cells,[218] and this may be one factor responsible for improvement. Cyclosporin produces similar changes in the T-cell subsets and a marked improvement in liver biochemistry.[189] Clinical trials are currently being carried out.

ALCOHOL-INDUCED LIVER DISEASE

Several factors contribute to the liver damage that occurs in persons who consume large amounts of alcohol. The alcohol or its metabolites are undoubtedly directly hepatotoxic, producing ultrastructural changes within a few hours after ingestion.

Since persons with similar exposure histories may respond with widely different degrees of liver damage, it is suspected that factors other than the amount of alcohol consumed influence susceptibility.[116,117] It seems likely that alcohol ingestion induces steatosis in all persons, but progression to hepatitis and cirrhosis does not always occur. Some investigators suggest that all patients with alcohol-induced cirrhosis have gone through a stage of hepatitis, but in other studies, this suggestion is less clear. The factors that determine the rate of development of the disease are not yet understood.

Recent studies have revealed an increased incidence of HLA-B8 in a group of patients with alcohol-induced hepatitis.[4,150] The incidence in patients with steatosis is similar to that found in the normal population, and persons who have established cirrhosis without obvious hepatitis exhibit a low incidence of this phenotype. The authors suggest that in persons who have progressed to cirrhosis with or without hepatitis, the mechanism of liver damage may be similar but the presence of the gene or genes linked to HLA-B8 predisposes the patient to a more florid hepatitic component of the disease. Other investigators have found linkage with other HLA phenotypes[11,12,139] or no linkage at all.[194,206]

Immunologic Aspects of Pathogenesis

Immune Response to Liver Cell Antigens

The liver biopsy specimen in alcohol-induced liver disease has some features that may be compatible with an immunologically mediated component to the disease process. Although a major feature is central necrosis and polymorphonuclear cell infiltration, in some cases the portal zones reveal a mononuclear cell infiltrate and stellate fibrosis. This periportal infiltrate is similar to that seen in CAH and may represent an immunologic reaction to hepatocytes at the point of entry of lymphocytes to the hepatic lobule. This possibility is supported by the observation that lymphocytes from patients with alcohol-induced hepatitis are sensitized to liver cell antigens[144] and are cytotoxic for rabbit hepatocytes.[103] More recently, antibodies to alcohol-altered hepatocytes have been found in sera of patients with alcohol-induced hepatitis.[3]

The involvement of immune mechanisms in alcohol-induced liver disease is further supported by studies of the hepatic cellular infiltrate. Eighty percent of the cells in the liver of patients with alcoholic hepatitis are T-lymphocytes, and 20% are B-lymphocytes.[191] This contrasts with other forms of liver disease, in which the ratio of T- to B-lymphocytes is nearer 50:50. These findings are consistent with the suggestion that T-lymphocytes have become sensitized to liver antigens[144] and are mediating a tissue-damaging reaction.

The role of an immune response to Mallory's hyalin in the pathogenesis of alcohol-induced hepatitis is more difficult to determine. Hyalin is found in about 50% of cirrhotic patients with a history of alcohol abuse, but it is also found in Indian childhood cirrhosis, Wilson's disease, and PBC. The material is a highly refractile, eosinophilic, cytoplasmic inclusion that probably represents a condensation of intracellular contractile filaments. Interest in this material has increased following the demonstration that patients with alcohol-induced hepatitis and cirrhosis are sensitized to the purified material.[267] These patients also exhibit low-titer antibodies to smooth muscle[63] and aggregated albumin,[76] and it seems probable that all are a reflection of an immune response to intracellular proteins released from denatured and degenerating hepatocytes.

Altered Humoral Immunity

Although many of the immunologic features of alcohol-induced disease are common to other types of liver injury and presumably result from changes in hepatic phagocyte function,[224] some features are peculiar to the disease. In alcohol-induced disease, one of the earliest changes is an increase in serum IgA concentration.[150] This occurs at a stage when the liver is either normal or exhibits only a mild degree of steatosis. Since this class of antibody is produced in the intestinal wall, one explanation of this increase would be that alcohol exposure results in an increase in permeability of the mucosa, thereby allowing increased access of intestinal antigens to the IgA immunocytes of the lamina propria and mesenteric lymph nodes. This change may represent merely an epiphenomenon, but it also seems possible that the change in permeability allows absorption of factors that contribute to the induction of hepatic damage. Increased titers of antibody to *Escherichia coli* occur at this early stage,[205] indicating that endotoxin is absorbed and may be one of the intestine-derived factors contributing to the ongoing liver damage.[190]

Altered Cell-Mediated Immunity

Cell-mediated immunity is altered in patients with alcohol-induced liver disease.[13] Since many of the changes are also found in other types of liver disease[88] and in animal models of cirrhosis,[234] it seems probable that they are the result of liver damage rather than the chemical effect of alcohol.

Eighty percent of patients with alcohol-induced liver disease fail to develop a delayed hypersensitivity reaction to a challenge with dinitrochlorobenzene and exhibit a significant decrease in responsiveness to streptokinase and to mumps, antigens to which the subjects are likely to have been sensitized previously.[13] This demonstrates a defect in the efferent part of the delayed hypersensitivity response but does not exclude a coexisting defect in the afferent limb. The normal response to croton oil rules out a defect in the inflammatory response.[13] A normal *in vitro* response to T-cell mitogens excludes an intrinsic T-cell defect,[13] but serum inhibitors of this response can be demonstrated.[88]

Immunologic Aspects of Treatment

Withdrawal of alcohol is the main goal of therapy. In florid alcohol-induced hepatitis, corticosteroid therapy has been tried without significant beneficial effect.[18,27,78,129,180,193,203] In poorly nourished alcoholics, some of the immunologic abnormalities may respond to improved diet.

The response to abstinence is variable and partly dependent upon the degree of damage and consequent hepatic cirrhosis.

DRUG-INDUCED LIVER DISEASE

An increasing number of widely used and generally well-tolerated drugs can cause hepatic injury, ranging from a transient asymptomatic elevation of serum transaminases to clinically overt acute or chronic liver disease. These drug-induced states are often clinically, biochemically, and histologically indistinguishable from virally induced forms of liver injury; this makes it difficult to establish a causal relationship between the drug and the disease. For this reason, the list of drugs suspected of inducing liver injury is much longer than that of drugs that have been proved to play a role in inducing liver injury.

Most drugs that injure the liver do so by one of two mechanisms. Some drugs or their metabolites are hepatotoxic by a chemical interaction with an essential structural component or metabolic enzyme system of the liver cell, whereas others involve a hypersensitivity reaction. In both cases, host factors may influence the probability of a significant adverse reaction. The rate of generation and de-

toxification of a toxic metabolite will influence both types of reactions, and immune response genes may be involved in determining whether or not a patient manifests an idiosyncratic hypersensitivity response.

Direct Hepatotoxins

Drugs toxic to the liver usually cause acute hepatic necrosis. Prolonged administration causes protracted or repeated episodes of necrosis and may ultimately lead to the development of chronic liver disease. Salicylates and acetaminophen are two such drugs.

The onset of liver damage is immediate in all subjects exposed to sufficient dosage if direct toxicity is the mechanism. Such drugs also produce liver damage in animals and are usually identified as hepatotoxic in preliminary animal toxicology studies. A causal relationship between the drug and the adverse reaction is readily established in a patient by studying the effect of drug withdrawal on recovery.

Drugs Inducing Hypersensitivity Responses

A drug or its metabolite may induce liver damage by immunologic mechanism (Fig. 6-14). The drug may alter either the regulatory system of the immune response, so that reactions to self-antigens are no longer suppressed, or they may alter hepatocyte antigens, so that they are no longer recognized as self-components. In the former case, the ensuing disease may be multisystemic, whereas the alteration of liver antigens would be expected to produce an autoaggressive assault solely on the liver.

The problem can be approached in two ways: (1) define the host factors that determine susceptibility, and (2) define the mechanism by which the drug produces liver damage.

The involvement of host factors is suggested by the observation that only a small minority of exposed persons develop hepatic injury. This is in contrast to the high susceptibility rates to hepatotoxins. The factors involved are poorly understood. The increased incidence in atopic subjects and the occurrence of identical reactions in several generations of a family suggest that hereditary factors exist. Genetic factors may influence the rate and form of metabolism of the drug, thereby influencing the rate of formation of immunogenic complexes of drug metabolite with cellular macromolecules. The demonstration that microsomal enzyme activity is genetically determined shows that some progress has been made. In the field of immunology, evidence suggests that HLA phenotypes may be linked to immune response genotypes.

The mechanism by which the drug initiates an autoaggressive immune response is unknown. The drug may act as a hapten and combine with a membrane component of the hepatocyte, or it may denature a self-antigen (Fig. 6-14). This will result in a response to either the drug or a native or denatured liver cell antigen. Successful attempts to demonstrate these humoral and cellular responses are rare. When responses have been found, they are usually

a

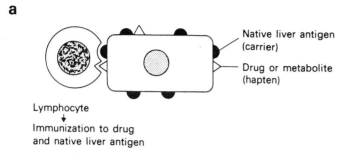

Lymphocyte
↓
Immunization to drug
and native liver antigen

b

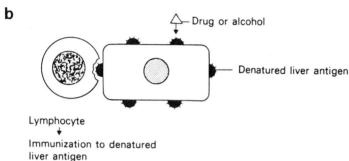

Lymphocyte
↓
Immunization to denatured
liver antigen

Fig. 6-14. Drugs (*a*) associated with carrier proteins or (*b*) denaturing liver membrane proteins cause an immune response to the hepatocyte.

of the delayed hypersensitivity type. The paucity of positive data may in part be attributed to the insensitivity of the test systems but also probably is a result of failure to test with both the drug and its metabolites complexed to the appropriate carrier molecule.

Although it is theoretically possible that the autoimmune reaction may continue after removal of the offending drug, this does not usually occur. Thus, for chronic liver disease to develop, prolonged exposure over several months would be necessary. Establishing a causal relationship between the drug and the liver lesion is a major problem. Withdrawal of the suspected drug usually results in clinical and biochemical improvement, and, in a clinical setting, this is all that can be done. Rechallenge carries the risk of a severe exacerbation and is not permissible. Very little help can be derived from biochemical, histologic, or serologic studies. For example, CAH induced by methyldopa,[130] oxyphenisatin,[181] or isoniazid,[250] and nitrofurantoin[200] is indistinguishable on biochemical and histologic grounds from other forms of the disease, and, in many cases, the autoimmune markers (antinuclear antibody, LE cells[130]) are also present. The type of liver injury may be classified on histologic and biochemical grounds as hepatocellular or cholestatic and, in some cases, as a mixture of the two. There are no specific features that incriminate one drug rather than another. The history usually points to exposure to a specific drug.

Hepatic Reactions

Hepatic reactions have been reported with monoamine oxidase inhibitors,[130] oxyphenisatin,[181] methyldopa,[130] and halothane.[152,247] If exposure is prolonged, the patient may develop chronic liver disease.

Monoamine Oxidase Inhibitors. These drugs produce a predominantly hepatitis-like picture. Iproniazid was the first recorded example, which was followed by phenelzine, pheniparzine, and isocarboxazid—all hydrazine derivatives. The reaction may be severe, and fulminant cases have been reported.

Isoniazid is a member of this group. Ten percent of patients show increased transaminase levels during the first 2 months of therapy, and liver biopsy shows a mild hepatitis. Only a minority of patients (less than 1%) develop symptomatic liver disease, and fatalities are rare. The reaction is usually mild, and the transaminases return to normal when the drug is stopped. It is possible, however, that continued administration may occasionally induce CAH associated with positive ANF and SMA, and hyperglobulinemia. Sensitization of T cells can be demonstrated using the drug conjugated to albumen.[250]

Oxyphenisatin. A constituent of many laxatives, oxyphenisatin has been associated with hepatocellular damage.[81] Only a minority of exposed persons react adversely, usually after at least 6 months of continual use. Most patients develop an acute hepatic illness, but some present with CAH indistinguishable from the lupoid variety.[181] The LE test and antinuclear factor are often positive, and hyperglobulinemia develops. The illness subsides when the drug is stopped, and the challenge leads rapidly to worsening liver function as disclosed by appropriate tests.

Methyldopa. Methyldopa produces mild subclinical abnormalities in transaminases in 5% of patients. The frequency of this reaction and its occurrence early after ingestion suggests a direct toxic mechanism.[130] In a minority of patients, a more severe hepatic reaction occurs

3 to 16 weeks after starting treatment. The prodromal symptoms are similar to those of acute viral hepatitis, and the patient becomes jaundiced. The Coombs' test and tests for antinuclear factor and smooth muscle antibody may be positive. The patient usually recovers uneventfully when the drug is stopped, but occasionally the course is fulminant or a stage of subacute hepatic necrosis proceeds to CAH and then cirrhosis.

Halothane. Halothane is now established in controlled trials as a cause of postoperative jaundice.[266] Many of the features of the hepatitis strongly suggest a hypersensitivity mechanism. The reaction occurs 8 to 13 days after the first operation, and earlier after subsequent exposures. Pyrexia usually precedes the development of jaundice by 2 to 3 days and may be accompanied by eosinophilia.[152] The outcome is good in most cases. However, if the patient becomes icteric, the mortality rate is very high—up to 20%.

Early reports of mitochondrial antibodies in these patients' sera have not been confirmed,[186] but a recent study did demonstrate that 40% of cases were positive for liver-kidney microsomal antibody.[247] Demonstrations of cell-mediated immunity to the drug by lymphocyte transformation or leucocyte migration inhibition are also conflicting.[153,169,246]

It seems likely that the reaction occurs to a metabolite of the native drug, and, therefore, the rate of metabolism and the degree of sensitization will determine the severity of the reaction. Antibodies that react with halothane-altered hepatocytes have been associated with the severe hepatic reaction. The antigen is in greatest density during anoxic metabolism of the hepatocyte.[162] The drug may produce damage as a result of both direct toxicity and hypersensitization.

Aminosalicylate. Aminosalicylate (PAS) reactions involving the liver are common and are usually part of a generalized reaction. Pyrexia, rashes, and arthralgias accompany the hepatitis. Cholestatic features are common.

Cholestatic Reactions

A cholestatic reaction occurs in association with phenothiazines, oral hypoglycemics (chlorpropamide), and antithyroid drugs (thiouracil). Only chlorpromazine will be discussed here.

Chlorpromazine-induced reactions are often of a mixed hepatitic-cholestatic type. The reaction occurs 1 to 3 weeks after starting treatment in approximately 0.5% of patients who receive the drug. The reaction is unrelated to the dose and may occur several weeks after the patient has stopped taking the drug. If chlorpromazine is given a second time, approximately 40% of patients suffer a relapse; it is postulated that the remaining patients, who do not respond to challenge, are desensitized by subsequent doses.

Prodromal symptoms of fever and rash and blood and tissue eosinophilia all support a hypersensitivity mecha-

nism as the cause of the syndrome. Liver biopsy shows cholestasis and marked portal mononuclear and eosinophilic infiltrate. There is variable hepatitis. The prognosis is good. There have been two reports of progression to biliary cirrhosis.

Granulomatous Reactions

Granulomatous reactions are seen in patients treated with phenylbutazone and sulfonamides. Although clinical and histologic features suggest an immunologic basis for the lesion, serologic tests and tests for lymphocyte sensitization have been unrewarding.

INFLUENCE OF LIVER DISEASE ON THE IMMUNE RESPONSE

Hyperglobulinemia[60,217,239] and depressed cell-mediated immunity[217,234] are common to most forms of chronic liver disease, and it seems probable that these changes are a result of liver damage. This is supported by the observation that similar changes can be induced in rats when they are rendered cirrhotic.[224,234]

Phagocytic Function

Phagocytic function is markedly altered in patients with hepatic cirrhosis.[224,235,239] This results in changes in antigen distribution,[224] which is a major factor in determining the characteristics of the ensuing humoral and cellular immune responses.[224]

Antigens enter the circulation from the gastrointestinal tract, the larger ones via the mesenteric lymphatics and the smaller ones via the mesenteric venous circulation.[217] The liver, which is an important phagocytic organ, may therefore receive intestinally derived antigen either directly, via the portal circulation when it acts as a filter interposed in series with the rest of the body, or it may receive antigen from the systemic circulation via its arterial supply and in this situation acts as a filter in parallel (Fig. 6-3). The hepatic phagocytes render antigens nonimmunogenic, whereas splenic and lymph node–derived macrophages serve to enhance immunogenicity.[224] The distribution of antigen between liver and spleen (and other lymphoid organs) will therefore influence the magnitude of the immune response.[224] Diversion of antigen from the liver to the spleen will enhance the immune response.[224] Changes in the phagocytic function of the liver have an effect on both portal and systemic routes of immunization.[217]

Immune complexes are cleared from the portal and systemic blood by the hepatic sinusoidal phagocytes. Large complexes that fix complement are avidly cleared by the liver, whereas smaller complexes which do not fix complement, are cleared by the spleen.[133] In hepatic cirrhosis, these functions are impaired, and complexes accumulate in the plasma.[235] In most cases, these complexes do not result in significant activation of C3 and do not cause tissue damage. The composition of such complexes is unknown, but it seems probable that many will contain food and bacterial antigens derived from the gut.

Endotoxins are phagocytosed and detoxified by the liver: They can be demonstrated in portal blood but not in systemic blood in normal subjects.[24] Endotoxinemia has been demonstrated during fulminant hepatic failure[263] and in some subjects with established cirrhosis,[121] presumably as a result of impaired hepatic clearance of this substance. It is suggested that it plays a significant role in the renal malfunction that often accompanies these diseases.[263]

Humoral Immunity

The altered handling of antigen in subjects with hepatic cirrhosis has a significant effect on the humoral immune response.[208,224,239] This is seen most clearly in the response to putative thymus-independent antigens,[20,205,239] which are not influenced by changes in cell-mediated immunity that accompany the development of chronic liver disease. It seems probable that the increased *E. coli* titers found in patients with alcohol-induced cirrhosis,[20] chronic active liver disease,[240] and PBC[205] are the result of this phenomenon.

The response to thymus-dependent antigens is more complex, involving the cooperation not only of antigen-presenting cells and B-lymphocytes but also of T-lymphocytes. When patients with alcohol-induced cirrhosis, chronic active liver disease, and PBC were immunized intravenously with the bacteriphage ϕX174, a thymus-dependent antigen, the primary and secondary responses were significantly decreased when compared with the responses of normal subjects.[222] In the presence of increased responses to thymus-independent antigens, this implies that the cooperating functions of T cells are reduced, so that B cells challenged with thymus-dependent antigens cannot respond to the increased antigenic stimulus.

In addition to the quantitative changes in the humoral response of subjects with hepatic cirrhosis, there are also qualitative changes. In normal subjects, during a secondary response, more than 90% of the antibody is IgG, whereas in patients with PBC, CAH, and alcohol-induced cirrhosis, the percentage of IgM antibody is much increased.[222] This relative failure to change from IgM to IgG antibody production during the evolution of the immune response is also compatible with a defect in helper T-cell function.

The relationship of the increased viral antibody titers, which have been described in chronic liver disease,[34,35,39,231,238] to altered mononuclear phagocytic function is more vexed. Small increases in titer to lipoprotein-coated viruses such as herpes simplex, cytomegalovirus, influenza A, rubella, and measles are seen in HBsAg-positive, and HBsAg-negative CAH,[39] alcohol-induced cirrhosis,[39] and PBC,[39] but the sixfold increase in titer to measles and rubella viruses seen in lupoid chronic active

liver disease[39] is peculiar to this disease. It seems probable that the one- to twofold increase in titer to several viruses, which is common to all types of chronic liver disease, is a reflection of the altered immune function that occurs in any type of chronic liver injury but that the specific association of a high-titer response to measles and rubella with lupoid chronic active liver disease is an indication of the presence of an additional diathesis in the immune system of these patients.[155]

The cumulative effect of these increased humoral responses is readily seen in the hypergammaglobulinemia that accompanies any form of experimental[12,117] or natural chronic liver disease.[19,60] The fact that this change is probably secondary to alterations in the mononuclear phagocytic system of the liver should not be allowed to direct attention away from the increased IgM of PBC and IgA of alcohol-related disease (Fig. 6-15)—changes specific to these diseases that may therefore give further clues to their pathogenesis.

Cell-Mediated Immunity

The incidence of positive delayed hypersensitivity skin tests to common bacterial and viral antigens is decreased in alcohol-related liver disease, CAH, and PBC. This occurrence in all types of liver disease suggests that this is in part secondary to the chronic liver disease.

The delayed hypersensitivity response involves the cooperation of macrophages and T cells in the presence of various serum factors that may enhance or inhibit the response. The afferent limb of the system, whereby cells become sensitized to the antigens concerned, has not been

Fig. 6-15. Immunoglobulin levels in chronic liver disease. Note the high IgM in PBC, high IgG in lupoid CAH, and high IgA in alcohol-related disease.

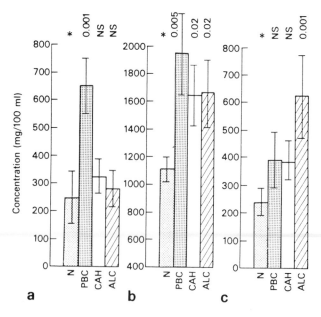

evaluated in patients with chronic liver disease because of the limitations of the test systems.

The efferent limb requires that T-lymphocytes be present in adequate concentrations, that they be sensitized to and recognize the antigen under test, and that they be capable of producing the lymphokine mediators of the delayed hypersensitivity reaction. The concentrations of peripheral blood T-lymphocytes measured by rosetting techniques is diminished in HBsAg-positive and HBsAg-negative chronic active liver disease,[37,42] alcohol-related disease,[13,17] and PBC.[226] The presence of plasma or serum inhibitors of T-lymphocyte function may also contribute to the anergy seen in patients with chronic liver disease. Serum factors that inhibit mitogen transformation of lymphocytes have been demonstrated in PBC,[137,167] and alcohol-induced liver disease,[88] as well as in an animal model of hepatic cirrhosis.[234] Increased macrophage suppressor cell activity, which is dependent upon the level of antigenic stimulation, has also been described in animals[234] and in patients with hepatic cirrhosis. Although the humoral and cellular inhibitors of T-lymphocyte function are readily demonstrated *in vitro,* their functional importance *in vivo* remains uncertain. Many of the inhibitors appear to be common to several types of liver disease and are therefore probably a reflection of the altered metabolic state in these conditions.

Immunologically Active Plasma Proteins

The liver is the major site of synthesis for many plasma proteins, some of which have either a regulator or effector role in the immune response.

Alpha-Fetoprotein. Alpha-fetoprotein (AFP) is produced by the entodermal cells of the foregut, particularly the liver. It is present in high concentration in the plasma of the fetus and mother. Within a few hours after birth, the concentration starts to fall, and by 1 year of age, adult levels are attained (10 ng/ml to 20 ng/ml).

Increased concentrations of AFP have been demonstrated in 90% to 95% of primary hepatocellular carcinomas. Smaller increases (500 ng/ml) are seen following acute hepatic necrosis and acute viral hepatitis and in patients with chronic liver disease, particularly those with macronodular cirrhosis. In these circumstances, the increase is believed to be a reflection of an increased rate of liver cell division (*i.e.,* regeneration). Thus, this protein is synthesized at an increased rate during hyperplastic and neoplastic growth.

The immunosuppressant properties of AFP were shown to be dependent upon the induction of a suppressor cell.[156-158] The presence of sialic acid residues on the protein appears to be essential for these biologic effects. More recently, however, other investigators have failed to confirm these observations.[123]

Alpha Globulins. A complex group of proteins, alpha globulins are produced by the liver and have immuno-regulatory properties.[26,38] Pregnancy-associated globulin inhibits T-cell functions.[210,211] It is increased mainly in pregnancy but also in patients with chronic liver disease and in cancer. Alpha$_2$ macroglobulin is an important inhibitor of both the complement and coagulation systems.[209] It has recently been suggested that it has immunoregulatory properties in relation to K-cell function.[26] Increased concentrations are found in PBC and HBsAg-negative CAH.[136]

Complement Components. Complement components are produced by either the mononuclear phagocytes or hepatocytes and are often reduced in acute and chronic liver disease.[176]

REFERENCES

1. Adjukiewicz AB et al: Immunological studies in an epidemic of infective short incubation hepatitis. Lancet 2:380, 1972
2. Alberti A et al: Detection of a new antibody system reacting with Dane particles in HBV infection. Br Med J 2:1056–1058, 1978
3. Anthony RS et al: Liver antibodies in alcohol-related liver disease and antibodies to alcohol-altered hepatocytes. In press.
4. Bailey RJ et al: Histocompatibility antigens, autoantibodies, and immunoglobulins in alcoholic liver disease. Br Med J ii:727–731, 1976
5. Balayan MS et al: Evidence for a virus in Non-A, Non-B hepatitis transmitted via the fecal-oral route. Intervirology 20:23–31, 1983
6. Bamber M et al: Short incubation non-A, non-B hepatitis transmitted by factor VIII concentrates in patients with congenital coagulation disorders. Gut 22:854–859, 1981
7. Bamber M et al: Clinical and histological features of patients with sporadic non-A, non-B hepatitis. J Clin Pathol 34:1175–1180, 1981
8. Bartholomaeus WN, Reed WD, Joske RA, and Shilkin KB: Autoantibody responses to liver-specific lipoprotein in mice. Immunology 43:219–226, 1981
8a. Behrens UJ, Paronetto F: Studies on "liver-specific" antigens. I. Evaluation of the liver specificity of "LSP" and "LP-2." Gastroenterology 77:1045, 1979
9. Beasley RP et al: Hepatitis B immune globulin (HBIG) efficacy in the interruption of perinatal transmission of hepatitis B carrier state. Lancet 2:388–393, 1981
10. Belabbes H et al: Non-A, non-B epidemic viral hepatitis in Algeria: Strong evidence for its water spread. In Vyas GN, Dienstag JC, Hoffnagle JH (eds): Viral Hepatitis and Liver Disease. New York, Grune and Stratton Inc, 1984
11. Bell H, Nordhagen R: Association between HLA-BW40 and alcoholic liver disease with cirrhosis. Br Med J 1:822–829, 1978
12. Bell H, Nordhagen R: HLA antigens in alcoholics with special reference to alcoholic cirrhosis. Scand J Gastroenterol 15:453–459, 1980
13. Berenyi MR et al: *In vitro* and *in vivo* studies of cellular immunity in alcoholic cirrhosis. Dig Dis 19:199, 1974
14. Berg PA et al: Mitochondrial antibodies in primary biliary cirrhosis: I. Localization of the antigen to mitochondrial membranes. J Exp Med 126:277, 1967

15. Berg PA et al: Serological classification of chronic cholestatic liver disease by the use of two different types of antimitochondrial antibodies. Lancet 1:1329, 1980
16. Berman M: The chronic sequelae of NANB hepatitis. Ann Intern Med 91:1–6, 1979
17. Bernstein IM et al: Reduction in T lymphocytes in alcoholic liver disease. Lancet ii:488, 1974
18. Blitzer BL et al: Adrenocorticosteroid therapy in alcoholic hepatitis: A prospective, double-blind randomized study. Dig Dis 22:477, 1977
19. Bjorneboe M et al: Tetanus anti-toxin production and gamma globulin levels in patients with cirrhosis of the liver. Acta Med Scand 188:541, 1970
20. Bjorneboe M et al: Antibodies to intestinal microbes in serum of patients with cirrhosis of the liver. Lancet i:58, 1972
21. Bottazzo GF et al: Classification of smooth muscle autoantibodies detected by immunofluorescence. J Clin Pathol 29:403, 1976
22. Boxer LA et al: Autoimmune neutropenia associated with chronic active hepatitis. Am J Med 52:280, 1972
23. Bradley DW et al: Serodiagnosis of viral hepatitis A by a modified competitive binding radioimmunoassay for IgM anti-HAV. J Clin Microbiol 9:120–127, 1979
24. Braude AI et al: Studies with radioactive endotoxin ii. Correlation of physiological effects with distribution of radioactivity in rabbits injected with lethal doses of E. coli endotoxin labeled with radioactive sodium chromate. J Clin Invest 34:858, 1955
25. Butler RC et al: Studies on experimental chronic active hepatitis in the rabbit: Induction of the disease by immunization with muscle as well as liver proteins. Br J Exp Pathol 65:499–510, 1984
26. Calder EA et al: The effect of anti-$_2$ macroglobulin on K-cell cytolysis and T- and B-cell formation. Immunology 22:112, 1975
27. Campra JL et al: Prednisone therapy of acute alcoholic hepatitis. Ann Intern Med 79:625, 1973
28. Chau KH et al: Serodiagnosis of recent hepatitis B virus infection by IgM class anti-HBc. Hepatology 3:142–149, 1983
29. Chisari FV: Liver-specific protein in perspective. Gastroenterology 78:168, 1980
30. Cherrick GR et al: Immunologic response to tetanus toxoid inoculation in patients with hepatic cirrhosis. N Engl J Med 261:340, 1959
31. Chisari FV, Edginton TS: Lymphocyte E-rosette inhibitory factor: A regulatory serum lipoprotein. J Exp Med 142:1092, 1975
32. Chisari FV, Edginton TS: Human T-lymphocyte E-rosette function 1. A process modulated by intracellular cyclic AMP. J Exp Med 140:1122, 1974
33. Chu CM et al: Natural history of chronic hepatitis B virus infection in Taiwan: Studies of hepatitis B virus DNA in serum. Hepatology 5:431–434, 1985
34. Closs O et al: High titres of antibodies against rubella and morbilli virus in patients with chronic hepatitis. Scand J Gastroenterol 8:523, 1973
35. Closs O: Raised antibody titres in chronic liver disease. Lancet ii:1202, 1971
36. Colombo M et al: Long-term delta superinfection in hepatitis B surface antigen carriers and its relationship to the course of chronic hepatitis. Gastroenterology 85:235–239, 1983
37. Colombo M et al: T and B lymphocytes in patients with chronic active hepatitis. Clin Exp Immunol 30:4, 1977
38. Cooperband SR et al: The effect of immunoregulatory globulin (IRA) upon lymphocytes in vitro. J Immunol 109:154, 1972
39. Crimmins FB et al: Viral antibody titres in HBs antigen positive and negative chronic active hepatitis. Scand J Gastroenterol 15:107–112, 1980
40. Davis P, Read AE: Antibodies to double-stranded (native) DNA in active chronic hepatitis. Gut 16:41, 1975
41. Dawson GJ et al: Monoclonal antibodies to hepatitis A virus. J Med Virol 14:1–8, 1984
42. De Horatius RJ et al: T and B lymphocytes in acute and chronic hepatitis. Clin Immunol Immunopathol 2:353, 1974
43. Dejean A et al: Specific hepatitis B virus integration in hepatocellular carcinoma DNA through a viral 11-base-pair chart repeat. Proceedings of the National Academy of Science (USA) 81:5350, 1985
44. De Meo AN, Anderson BR: Defective chemotaxis associated with a serum inhibitor in cirrhotic patients. J Lab Clin Med 78:980, 1971
45. Dienstag JL et al: Hepatitis A antigen isolated from liver and stool: Immunologic comparison of antigen prepared in guinea pigs. J Immunol 117:876–881, 1976
46. Doniach D et al: Tissue antibodies in primary biliary cirrhosis, active chronic (lupoid) hepatitis, cytogenic cirrhosis, and other liver diseases and their clinical implications. Clin Exp Immunol 1:237, 1966
47. Dooley JS et al: Prediction of relapse following withdrawal of treatment in hepatitis B surface antigen negative chronic active liver disease. Gut 20:A954, 1978
48. Dudley FJ et al: Cellular immunity and hepatitis-associated (Australia) antigen liver disease. Lancet i:743, 1972
49. Dudley FJ et al: Serum autoantibodies and immunoglobulins in hepatitis-associated antigen (HAA)–positive and –negative liver disease. Gut 14:360, 1973
50. Eddleston ALWF et al: Cell-mediated immune response in primary biliary cirrhosis to a protein fraction from human bile. Br Med J 4:274–275, 1973
51. Eddleston ALWF, Williams R: Inadequate antibody response to HBsAg or suppressor T-cell defect in development of active chronic hepatitis. Lancet ii:1543, 1974
52. Eggink HF et al: Cellular and humoral immune reactions in chronic active liver disease: Lymphocyte subsets and viral antigen in acute and chronic hepatitis B. Clin Exp Immunol 56:121–128, 1984
53. Eleftheriou N et al: Serum alpha-fetoprotein levels in patients with acute and chronic liver disease. J Clin Pathol 30:704, 1977
54. Epstein O et al: Primary biliary cirrhosis is a dry gland syndrome with features of chronic graft-versus-host disease. Lancet 1:1166–1168, 1980
55. Epstein O et al: D-penicillamine treatment improves survival in primary biliary cirrhosis. Lancet 1:1275, 1984
56. Fakunle YM et al: Monometric (7S) IgM in chronic liver disease. Clin Exp Immunol 38:204, 1979
57. Farci P et al: The effect of acute and chronic HDV infection on HBV replication: Are anti–HBe-positive HBV carriers without HBV replication more susceptible to HDV superinfection. Hepatology (in press)
58. Fasel-Felley J et al: A specific immune response to purified HA antigen demonstrated by leukocyte migration inhibition

in patients recovering from viral hepatitis A. J Hepatology (in press)

59. Fehér J et al: Inhibition of autoimmune hepatitis with hot labeled liver specific antigen. Clin Exp Immunol 55:360–368, 1984

60. Feizi T: Immunoglobulins in chronic liver disease. Gut 9:193, 1968

61. Fox RA et al: The primary immune response to haemocyanin in patients with primary biliary cirrhosis. Clin Exp Immunol 14:480, 1973

62. Fox RA et al: Impaired delayed hypersensitivity in primary biliary cirrhosis. Lancet 1:959–962, 1969

63. French SW et al: Alcoholic hepatitis. In Fisher MM, Rankin JG (eds): Alcohol and the Liver. New York, Plenum, 1974

64. Frosner GG et al: Antibody against hepatitis A in seven European countries. Comparison of prevalence data in different age groups. Am J Epidemiol 110:563–569, 1979

65. Galbraith RM et al: High prevalence of sero-immunologic abnormalities in relatives of patients with active chronic hepatitis or primary biliary cirrhosis. N Engl J Med 290:63, 1974

66. Gerber MA et al: Antibodies to ribosomes in chronic active hepatitis. Gastroenterology 76:138, 1979

67. Golding PL et al: Multisystem involvement in chronic liver disease. Am J Med 55:772–782, 1973

68. Golding PL et al: Sicca complex in liver disease. Br Med J IV:340, 1970

69. Goldstein A et al: The role of thymosin and the endocrine thymus on the mitogenesis and function of T-cells. In Molecular Approaches to Immunology, p 243. New York, Academic Press, 1975

70. Gonzales C et al: Mechanisms responsible for antibody-dependent cell-mediated cytotoxicity to isolated hepatocytes in chronic active hepatitis. Gut 20:1979

71. Gratwhol AA et al: Sjogren-type syndrome after allogeneic bone marrow transplantation. Ann Intern Med 87:703–706, 1977

72. Graze PR, Gales RP: Chronic graft-versus-host disease: A syndrome of disordered immunity. Am J Med 66:611–620, 1979

73. Gray N et al: Hepatitis, colitis, and lupus manifestations. Am J Dig Dis 3:481, 1958

74. Hadden JW et al: Effect of levamisole and imidazole on lymphocyte proliferation and cyclic nucleotide levels. Cell Immunol 20:98, 1975

75. Hadziyannis SJ et al: Analysis of liver disease, nuclear HBcAg viral replication, and hepatitis B virus DNA in liver and serum of HBcAg virus anti–HBe-positive carriers. Hepatology 3:656–662, 1983

76. Hauptman S, Tomasi TB: Antibodies to human albumin in cirrhosis sera. J Clin Invest 54:122–127, 1974

77. Havens P et al: Production of antibody by patients with chronic hepatic disease. J Immunol 67:347, 1951

78. Helman RA et al: Alcoholic hepatitis: Natural history and evaluation of prednisolone therapy. Ann Intern Med 74:311, 1971

79. Hochwald GM et al: Site of formation of immunoglobulins and of a component of C3. (i) A new technique for the demonstration of syntheses of individual serum proteins by tissues in vitro. J Exp Med 114:459, 1961

80. Hodgson HJF et al: Alteration in suppressor cell activity in chronic active hepatitis. Proc Natl Acad Sci USA 75:1549, 1978

81. Holborow EJ: Immunological aspects of viral hepatitis. Br Med Bull 28:142, 1972

82. Holborow EJ et al: Smooth muscle autoantibodies in infectious mononucleosis. Br Med J 3:323, 1973

83. Holdsworth CD et al: Ulcerative colitis in chronic liver disease. Q J Med 34:211, 1965

84. Hooper B et al: Autoimmunity in a rural community. Clin Exp Immunol 12:79, 1972

85. Hopf U, Meyer zum Buschenfelde KH: Studies on the pathogenesis of experimental chronic active hepatitis in rabbits. II. Demonstration of immunoglobulin on isolated hepatocytes. Br J Exp Pathol 55:509, 1974

36. Hopf U et al: Detection of a liver-membrane autoantibody in HBsAg-negative chronic active hepatitis. N Engl J Med 194:578, 1976

87. Horne CHW et al: Studies in pregnancy-associated globulin. Clin Exp Immunol 13:603, 1973

88. Hsu CCS, Leevy CM: Inhibition of PHA-stimulated lymphocyte transformation by plasma from patients with advanced cirrhosis. Clin Exp Immunol 8:749, 1971

89. Hughes JV et al: Neutralizing monoclonal antibodies to hepatitis A virus: Partial localization of a neutralizing antigen site. J Virol 52:465, 1984

90. Husby G et al: Localization of T and B cells and alpha-fetoprotein in hepatic biopsies from patients with liver disease. J Clin Invest 56:1198, 1975

91. Ikeda T et al: A deficiency of alpha interferon production in patients with chronic hepatitis B infection. Hepatology (in press)

92. Iwarsen S et al: Neutralization of hepatitis B virus infectivity by a murine monoclonal antibody: An experimental study in the chimpanzee. J Med Virol 16:89–95, 1985

93. Jacob AI et al: Endotoxin and bacteria in portal blood. Gastroenterology 72:1268, 1977

94. Jain S et al: A controlled trial of D-penicillamine in primary biliary cirrhosis. Lancet 1:831, 1977

95. Jain S et al: Double-stranded DNA binding capacity of serum in acute and chronic disease. Clin Exp Immunol 26:35, 1976

96. James O et al: Primary biliary cirrhosis—a revised clinical spectrum. Lancet 1:1278, 1981

97. James SP et al: Abnormal regulation of immunoglobulin synthesis in vitro in primary cirrhosis. Gastroenterology 76:1268, 1979

98. Jensen DM et al: Detection of antibodies directed against a liver specific membrane lipoprotein in patients with acute and chronic active hepatitis. N Engl J Med 299:1, 1978

99. Jones EA et al: Primary biliary cirrhosis and the complement system. Ann Intern Med 90:72, 1979

100. Johnson GD et al: Antibody to smooth muscle in patients with liver disease. Lancet 2:878, 1965

101. Joske RA, King WE: The LE cell phenomenon in active chronic viral hepatitis. Lancet 2:477, 1955

102. Karayannis P et al: Studies of hepatitis A virus replication and the host immune response to HAV in relation to the pathogenesis of liver cell damage. J Med Virol 18:261, 1986

103. Kakumu S, Leevy CM: Lymphocyte cytotoxicity in alcoholic hepatitis. Gastroenterology 72:594, 1977

104. Kanagasundaram N et al: Alcoholic hyaline antigen (AHAg) and antibody (AHaB) in alcoholic hepatitis. Gastroenterology 73:1368, 1977

105. Kane MA et al: Epidemic non-A, non-B hepatitis in Nepal: Recovery of a possible etiological agent and transmission studies in marmosets. JAMA (in press)

106. Karayannis P et al: Detection of serum HBV-DNA by molecular hybridization. Correlation with HBeAg/anti-HBe status, racial origin, liver histology, and hepatocellular carcinoma. J Hepatol 1:99, 1985

107. Kawai K et al: Experimental chronic nonsuppurative destructive cholangitis in rabbits following immunization with bile duct antigen. Gastroenterology 15:345, 1980

108. Keraan M et al: Increased serum immunoglobulin following portacaval shunt in the normal rat. Gut 15:468, 1974

109. Kernoff PBA et al: High risk of NANB hepatitis after a first exposure to volunteer or commercial clotting factor concentrates: Effects of prophylactic immune serum globulin. Br J Haematol 60:469–479, 1985

110. Khuroo MS: Study of an epidemic of non-A, non-B hepatitis: Possibility of another human hepatitis virus distinct from post-transfusion. Am J Med 68:818, 1980

111. Kirk AP et al: Late results of Royal Free Hospital controlled trial of prednisolone therapy in hepatitis B surface antigen–negative chronic active hepatitis. Gut 21:78, 1980

112. Koffler D et al: Antibodies to polynucleotides. Distribution in human serums. Science 166:1648, 1969

113. Knodell RG et al: Development of chronic liver disease after acute non-A, non-B post-transfusion hepatitis: Role of gamma-globulin prophylaxis in its prevention. Gastroenterology 72:902–909, 1977

114. Labro MT et al: A new pattern of non-organ and non-species-specific anti-organelle immunofluorescence: The mitochondrial antibody number 5. Clin Exp Immunol 31:357, 1978

115. Lee RG et al: Granulomas in primary biliary cirrhosis: A prognostic feature. Gastroenterology 81:983, 1981

116. Leevy CM et al: Liver disease of the alcoholic: The role of immunologic abnormalities in pathogenesis, recognition, and treatment. Prog Liver Dis 5:515, 1976

117. Leevy CM et al: Alcoholic hepatitis, cirrhosis, and immunologic reactivity. Ann NY Acad Sci 252:106, 1975

118. Liaw Y-F et al: Clinical and histological events preceding hepatitis e antigen seroconversion in chronic-type B hepatitis. Gastroenterology 84:216, 1983

119. Lidman K et al: Antiactin specificity of human smooth muscle antibodies in chronic active hepatitis. Clin Exp Immunol 24:266, 1976

120. Lieberman HM et al: Detection of HBV-DNA in human serum by a simplified molecular hybridization test: Comparison to HBeAg/anti-HBe status in HBsAg carriers. Hepatology 3:285, 1983

121. Liehr H et al: Endotoxaemia in liver cirrhosis, treatment with polymyxin D. Lancet ii:810, 1975

122. Lightwood AM et al: Autoimmune haemolytic anaemia due to red cell antibodies of different specificities in a patient with chronic hepatitis. Vox Sang 24:331, 1973

123. Littman BM et al: The effect of purified alpha-fetoprotein on in vitro assays of cell-mediated immunity. Cell Immunol 30:35, 1977

124. Lok ASF et al: Studies of HBV replication during acute hepatitis followed by recovery and acute hepatitis progressing to chronic liver disease. J Hepatol 5:671, 1985

125. McFarlane IG et al: Antibodies to liver specific protein predict outcome of treatment withdrawal in autoimmune chronic active hepatitis. Lancet ii:964, 1984

126. MacGregor A et al: Monoclonal antibodies against hepatitis A virus. J Clin Microbiol 18:1237, 1983

127. MacKay IR, Morris PJ: Association of autoimmune active chronic hepatitis with HLA1, B8. Lancet ii:793, 1972

128. MacKay IR, Tait BD: HLA associations with autoimmune-type chronic active hepatitis: identification of B8-DRW3 haplotype by family studies. Gastroenterology 79:95, 1980

129. Maddrey WC et al: Corticosteroid therapy of alcoholic hepatitis. Gastroenterology 75:193, 1978

130. Maddrey WC, Boitnott JK: Drug-induced chronic liver disease. Gastroenterology 72:1348, 1977

131. Manns M et al: The liver specific protein: Evidence for species-specific and non–species-specific determinants. J Clin Lab Immunol 3:9, 1980

132. Manns M et al: Autoantibodies against liver-specific membrane lipoprotein in acute and chronic liver disease: Studies on organ-, species-, and disease specificity. Gut 21:955, 1980

133. Mannik M, Arend WP: Fate of preformed immune complexes in rabbits and rhesus monkey. J Exp Med 134:195, 1971

134. McFarlane IG et al: Purification and characterization of human liver-specific membrane lipoprotein (LSP). Clin Exp Immunol 27:381, 1977

135. McMillan SA et al: Antibodies to lymphocytes and smooth muscle in the sera of patients with multiple sclerosis. Clin Immunol Immunopathol 16:374, 1980

136. MacSween RNM: Serum protein levels in primary biliary cirrhosis. J Clin Pathol 25:789, 1972

137. MacSween RNM, Thomas MA: Lymphocyte transformation by phytohaemagglutinin (PHA) and purified protein derivative (PPD) in primary biliary cirrhosis: Evidence of serum inhibitory factors. Clin Exp Immunol 15:523, 1973

138. MacSween RNM et al: In Leevy CM (ed): Diseases of the Liver and Biliary Tract, p 23. Basel, Switzerland, S. Karger, 1976

139. Melenderc M et al: Distribution of HLA compatibility antigens, ABO groups, and Rh antigens in alcoholic liver disease. Gut 20:288–292, 1979

140. Meyer zum Büschenfelde KH et al: Celluläre Immunoreaktionen gegenüber homologen leberspezifischen Antigenen (HLP) bei chronischen Leberentzündungen. Klin Wochenschr 52:246, 1974

141. Meyer zum Büschenfelde KH, Hoff U: Studies on the pathogenesis of experimental chronic active hepatitis in rabbits: Induction of the disease and protective effect of allogenic liver specific protein. Br J Exp Pathol 55:498, 1974

142. Meyer zum Büschenfelde KH et al: LM-Ag and LSP—two different target antigens involved in the immunopathogenesis of chronic active hepatitis. Clin Exp Immunol 37:205, 1979

143. Meyer zum Büschenfelde KH, Miescher PA: Liver specific antigens. Purification and characterization. Clin Exp Immunol 10:89, 1972

144. Mihas AA et al: Cell-mediated immunity to liver in patients with alcoholic hepatitis. Lancet 1:951, 1975

145. Minuti GY et al: IgM anti-complement receptor antibodies in serum of patients with primary biliary cirrhosis. Abstract No. 212, AASLD, 1982

146. Mondelli M, Eddleston ALWF: Mechanisms of liver cell injury in acute and chronic hepatitis B virus infection. Semin Liver Dis 4:47, 1984

147. Thomas L et al: Inducer and suppressor T cells in hepatitis B virus–induced liver disease. Hepatology 2:202, 1982

148. Montano L et al: An analysis of the composition of the inflammatory infiltrate in autoimmune and hepatitis B virus–induced chronic liver disease. Hepatology 3:292, 1983

149. Montano L et al: Hepatitis B virus and HLA antigen display

in the liver during chronic hepatitis B virus infection. Hepatology 2:557, 1982

150. Morgan MY et al: HLA-B8 viral antibodies, immunoglobulins and autoantibodies in alcohol-related liver disease. J Clin Pathol 33:488, 1980

151. Mowbray J, Cooperband SR: Alpha globulins affecting the immune response. In Brent and Holborrow (eds): Progress in Immunology II, Vol 5, p 383. Amsterdam, North-Holland, 1974

152. Moult PJA, Sherlock S: Halothane-related hepatitis: A clinical study of 26 cases. Q J Med 44:99, 1975

153. Moult PJA et al: Lymphocyte transformation in halothane-related hepatitis. Br Med J 2:69–75, 1975

154. Munoz LE et al: Is mitochondrial antibody diagnostic of primary biliary cirrhosis? Gut 22:136, 1981

155. Munoz LE et al: Complement activation in chronic liver disease. Clin Exp Immunol 47:548, 1982

156. Murgita RA, Tomas TB: Suppression of the immune response by alpha-fetoprotein. ii. The effect of mouse alpha-fetoprotein on mixed lymphocyte reactivity and mitogen-induced lymphocyte transformation. J Exp Med 141:440, 1975

157. Murgita RA, Tomas TB: Suppression of the immune response by alpha-fetoprotein. (i). The effect of mouse alpha-fetoprotein on the primary and secondary antibody response. J Exp Med 141:269, 1975

158. Murgita RA et al: Alpha-fetoprotein induces suppressor T cells in vitro. Nature 267:257, 1977

159. Murray K et al: Hepatitis B virus antigens made in microbial cells immunize against viral infection. EMBO J 3:645, 1984

160. Nakanuma Y, Ohta G: Histometric and serial section observations of the intrahepatic bile ducts in primary biliary cirrhosis. Gastroenterology 76:1326, 1979

161. Neurath AR et al: Hepatitis B virus contains pre-S gene–encoded domains. Nature 315:154, 1985

162. Neuberger JM et al: Oxidative metabolism of halothane in the production of altered hepatocyte membrane antigen in acute halothane–induced hepatic necrosis. Gut 22:669, 1981

163. Nielsen JO et al: Incidence and meaning of persistence of Australia antigen in patients with acute viral hepatitis: Development of chronic hepatitis. N Engl J Med 285:1157, 1971

164. Nouri-Aria UJ et al: Effect of corticosteroids on suppressor cell activity in autoimmune and chronic active hepatitis. N Engl J Med 307:1301, 1982

165. Novick DM et al: Diminished responsiveness of homosexual men to antiviral therapy for HBsAg-positive chronic liver disease. J Hepatol 1:29, 1984

166. Owen JS: Plasma lipoproteins and the regulation of cellular function. In Reid E, Cook GMW, Moore DJ (eds): Investigation of Membrane-Located Receptors, Chapter 6. New York, Plenum, 1984

167. Owen JS et al: The effect of high-density lipoprotein from patients with liver disease on erythrocyte morphology and lymphocyte transformation. Gastroenterology 79:1119, 1980

168. Paronetto F et al: Antibodies to cytoplasmic antigens in primary biliary cirrhosis and chronic active hepatitis. J Lab Clin Med 69:979, 1967

169. Paronetto F, Popper H: Lymphocyte stimulation induced by halothane in patients with hepatitis following exposure to halothane. N Engl J Med 283:277–285, 1980

170. Parr EL: Diversity of expression of H-2 antigens on mouse liver cells demonstrated by immunoferritin labeling. Transplanation 27:45, 1979

171. Perrillo RP et al: Comparative efficacy of adenine arabinoside 5′monophosphate and prednisolone followed by adenine arabinoside 5′monophosphate in treatment of type B CAH. Gastroenterology 88:780, 1985

172. Pignatelli M et al: Evidence that cytotoxic T-cells sensitive to HBe are responsible for hepatocyte lysis in chronic hepatitis B virus infection. J Hepatol (in press)

173. Pignatelli M et al: HLA Class I antigens on the hepatocyte membrane during recovery from acute hepatitis B virus infection and during interferon therapy on chronic HBV infection. Hepatology 6:349–353, 1986

174. Porter HP et al: Corticosteroid therapy in severe alcoholic hepatitis: A double-blind drug trial. N Engl J Med 284:1350, 1971

175. Potter BJ et al: Hypercatabolism of the third component of complement in patients with primary biliary cirrhosis. J Lab Clin Med 88:427, 1976

176. Potter BJ et al: Profiles of serum complement in patients with hepatobiliary diseases. Digestion 18:371, 1978

177. Potter BJ et al: Complement metabolism in chronic liver disease: Catabolism of Clq in chronic active liver disease and primary biliary cirrhosis. Gastroenterology 78:1034, 1981

178. Provost PJ, Hilleman MR: Propagation of human hepatitis A virus in cell culture in vitro. Proc Soc Exp Biol Med 160:213, 1979

179. Read AE et al: 'Juvenile cirrhosis': Part of a systemic disease. The effect of corticosteroid therapy. Gut 4:378, 1963

180. Rennick RH, Iber FL: Progress report: Treatment of acute alcoholic hepatitis. Gut 13:68, 1972

181. Reynolds JB et al: Chronic active and lupoid hepatitis caused by a laxative oxyphenisatin. N Engl J Med 280:813, 1971

182. Rizzetto M et al: Immunofluorescence detection of a new antigen/antibody system (delta/anti-delta) associated with hepatitis B virus in liver and serum of HBsAg carriers. Gut 18:997, 1977

183. Rizzetto M et al: Delta antigen: The association of delta antigen with hepatitis B surface antigen and ribonucleic acid in the serum of delta-infected chimpanzees. Proc Natl Acad Sci USA 77:6124, 1980

184. Rizzetto M et al: The hepatitis B virus–associated delta antigen: Isolation from liver, development of solid-phase radioimmunoassays for delta antigen and anti-delta and partial characterization of delta antigen. J Immunol 125:318, 1980

185. Rizzetto M et al: Chronic hepatitis in carriers of hepatitis B surface antigen, with intrahepatic expression of the delta antigen: An active and progressive disease unresponsive to immunosuppressive treatment. Ann Intern Med 98:437, 1983

186. Rodriguez M et al: Antimitochondrial antibodies in jaundice following drug administration. J Am Med Assoc 208:148–153, 1969

187. Weller IVD et al: Significance of delta antigen infection in chronic hepatitis B virus infection: A study in British carriers. Gut 24:1061, 1983

188. Rizzetto M et al: Microsomal antibodies in active chronic hepatitis and other disorders. Clin Exp Immunol 15:331, 1973

189. Routhier G et al: Effects of cyclosporin A on suppressor

and inducer T-lymphocytes in primary biliary cirrhosis. Lancet 2:1223, 1980

190. Rutenberg AM et al: The role of intestinal bacteria in the development of dietary cirrhosis in rats. J Exp Med 106:1, 1957

191. Sanchez-Tapias J et al: Lymphocyte populations in liver biopsy specimens from patients with chronic liver disease. Gut 18:472, 1977

192. Scheuer PJ: Biliary disease and cholestasis. Chronic hepatitis. In Liver Biopsy Interpretation, 3rd ed. London, Bailiere Tindall, 1985

193. Schlichting P et al: Alcoholic hepatitis superimposed on cirrhosis: Clinical significance and effect of long-term prednisone treatment. Scand J Gastroenterol 11:305, 1976

194. Scott BB et al: Histocompatibility antigens in chronic liver disease. Gastroenterology 72:122–129, 1972

195. Smedile A et al: Radioimmunoassay detection of IgM antibodies to the HBV-associated delta antigen, clinical significance in infection. J Med Virol 9:131, 1982

196. Szmuness W et al: On the role of sexual behavior in the spread of hepatitis B infection. Ann Intern Med 83:489, 1975

197. Shafritz DA et al: Integration of hepatitis B virus DNA into the genome of liver cells in chronic liver disease and hepatocellular carcinoma. N Engl J Med 305:1067, 1981

198. Shafritz DA, Kew HC: Identification of integrated hepatitis B virus DNA sequences in human hepatocellular carcinomas. Hepatology 1:1, 1981

199. Shapiro JM et al: Serum bilirubin: A prognostic factor in primary biliary cirrhosis. Gut 20:137, 1979

200. Sharp JR et al: Chronic active hepatitis and severe hepatic necrosis associated with nitrofurantoin. Ann Intern Med 92:14, 1980

201. Sherlock S, Scheuer PJ: The presentation and diagnosis of 100 patients with primary biliary cirrhosis. N Engl J Med 289:674, 1973

202. Shikata T et al: Hepatitis B e antigen and infectivity of hepatitis B virus. J Infect Dis 136:571, 1977

203. Shumaker JB et al: A controlled trial of 6-methyl-prednisolone in acute alcoholic hepatitis. Gastroenterology 69:443, 1978

204. Silva H et al: Renal involvement in active juvenile cirrhosis. J Clin Pathol 18:157, 1965

205. Simjee AE et al: Antibodies to Escherichia coli in chronic liver disease. Gut 16:871, 1975

206. Simon M et al: Idiopathic hemochromatics and iron overload in alcoholic liver disease: Differentiation by HCA phenotype. Gastroenterology 73:655–662, 1977

207. Smalley MJ et al: Antinuclear factor and human leucocytes: Reaction with granulocytes and lymphocytes. Aust Ann Med 17:28, 1968

208. Souhami RL: The effect of colloidal carbon on the organ distribution of sheep red blood cells and the immune response. Immunology 22:685, 1972

209. Steinbach M et al: Biology and pathology of plasma proteinase inhibitors. In Bayer Symposium V. Proteinase Inhibitors, p 78. Berlin, Springer-Verlag, 1974

210. Stimson WH: Studies on the immunosuppressive properties of a pregnancy-associated macroglobulin. Clin Exp Immunol 25:199, 1976

211. Stimson WH: Variations in the level of a pregnancy-associated macroglobulin in patients with cancer. J Clin Pathol 28:868, 1975

212. Strickland RG, Miller JV: The pathogenesis of alcoholic hepatitis and cirrhosis. Aust NZ J Med 6:78, 1976

213. Svec KH et al: Immunologic studies of systemic lupus erythematosus (SLE). Tissue-bound immunoglobulin in relation to serum anti-nuclear immunoglobulins in systemic lupus and in chronic liver disease with LE cell factor. J Clin Invest 46:558, 1967

214. Szmuness W et al: Hepatitis B vaccine. Demonstration of efficacy in a controlled clinical trial in a high-risk population in the United States. N Engl J Med 303:833–841, 1980

215. Tage-Jensen U et al: Liver-cell membrane autoantibody specific for inflammatory liver disease. Br Med J 1:206, 1977

216. Teixeira MR et al: The pathology of hepatitis A in man. Liver 2:53, 1982

217. Thomas HC: The role of the liver in immunological disease. Proc R Soc Med 70:521, 1977

218. Thomas HC: T-cell subsets in patients with acute and chronic HBV infection, primary biliary cirrhosis, and alcohol-induced liver disease. In J Immunopharmacol 3:301, 1981

219. Thomas HC: The relationship of cell-mediated and humoral immunity to the hepatic and renal injury following HBV infection. In Bertoli, Chiandussi, Sherlock (eds): Systemic Effects of HBsAg Immune Complexes. Padua, Piccin Medical Books, 1981

220. Thomas HC, Pignatelli M, Lever A: Homology between HBV-DNA and a sequence regulating the interferon-induced antiviral system: A possible mechanism of persistent infection. J Med Virol 19:63–69, 1986

221. Thomas HC et al: Immune complexes in acute and chronic liver disease. Clin Exp Immunol 31:150, 1978

222. Thomas HC et al: Immune response to X174 in man. 5. Primary and secondary antibody production in primary biliary cirrhosis. Gut 17:844, 1976

223. Thomas HC, Lever A: Immunology for hepatologists. Prog Liver Dis 8:179–190, 1985

224. Thomas HC et al: The role of the liver in controlling the immunogenicity of commensal bacteria in the gut. Lancet i:1288, 1973

225. Thomas HC et al: Immunological mechanisms in chronic hepatitis B virus infection. Hepatology 2:116S, 1982

226. Thomas HC et al: Peripheral blood lymphocyte populations in chronic liver disease. Clin Exp Immunol 26:222, 1976

228. Thomas HC: Potential pathogenic mechanisms in primary biliary cirrhosis. Semin Liver Dis 1:344–388, 1981

229. Thomas HC et al: Interferon in the management of chronic HBV infection. Br Med Bull 41:374–380, 1985

230. Thomas HC et al: Is primary biliary cirrhosis an immune complex disease? Lancet 2:1251, 1977

231. Thomas HC et al: Measles, rubella, and lymphocyte antibodies in chronic active hepatitis. Clin Sci Med 49:27, 1975

232. Thomas HC et al: The HLA system: Its relevance to the pathogenesis of liver disease. In Popper H, Schaffner F (eds): Progress in Liver Diseases, Vol VII, p 517. New York, Grune & Stratton, 1982

233. Thomas WG, Hart IR: Chronic active hepatitis and Crohn's disease. Am J Dig Dis 18:111, 1973

234. Thomas HC et al: The immune response in cirrhotic rats: Antigen distribution, humoral immunity, cell-mediated immunity, and splenic suppressor cell activity. Clin Exp Immunol 26:574, 1976

235. Thomas HC, Vaez-Zadeh F: A homeostatic mechanism for the removal of antigen from the portal circulation. Immunology 26:375, 1974

236. Tindall, Schwartz RS: Trojan horse lymphocytes. N Engl J Med 290:397, 1974

237. Toh BH: Smooth muscle antibodies and autoantigens. Clin Exp Immunol 38:621, 1979

238. Triger DR et al: Raised antibody titres to measles and rubella viruses in chronic active hepatitis. Lancet i:665, 1972

239. Triger D et al: Bacterial and dietary antibodies in liver diseases. Lancet i:60, 1972

240. Triger DR: Bacterial, viral, and autoantibodies in acute and chronic liver disease. Ann Clin Res 8:174, 1976

241. Turner-Warwick M: Fibrosing alveolitis and chronic liver disease. Q J Med 37:133, 1968

242. Vento S et al: Antigen-specific suppressor cell function in autoimmune chronic active hepatitis. Lancet 1:1200, 1984

243. Vento S et al: T-lymphocyte sensitization to HBcAg and T–cell-mediated unresponsiveness to HBsAg in hepatitis B virus–related chronic liver disease. Hepatology 5:192, 1985

244. Vergani D et al: Antibodies to the surface of halothane-altered rabbit hepatocytes in patients with severe halothane-associated hepatitis. N Engl J Med 303:66, 1980

245. Walker JG et al: Serological tests in diagnosis of primary biliary cirrhosis. Lancet 1:827, 1965

246. Walton B et al: Lymphocyte transformation. Absence of increased responses to alleged halothane jaundice. JAMA 225:494–498, 1973

247. Walton B et al: Unexplained hepatitis following halothane. Br Med J 1:1171, 1976

248. Wands JR et al: Circulating immune complexes and complement activation in primary biliary cirrhosis. N Engl J Med 298:233, 1978

249. Wankya BM et al: Seroepidemiology of hepatitis A and B in Kenya. A rural population survey in Machakos district. East Afr Med J 56:134, 1979

250. Warrington RJ et al: Evaluation of isoniazid-associated hepatitis by immunological tests. Clin Exp Immunol 32: 97, 1978

251. Waters J et al: Virus neutralizing antibodies to hepatitis B virus: The nature of an immunogenic epitope on the "S" gene peptide. J Gen Virol (in press)

252. Waters J et al: Identification of a dominant immunogenic epitope of the nucleocapsid (HBc) of the hepatitis B virus. J Med Virol 19:79–86, 1986

253. Weller IVD et al: A randomized controlled trial of ARAMP for chronic type B hepatitis. Gut 26:745–751, 1985

254. Wells R: Prednisolone and testosterone propionate in cirrhosis of the liver: A controlled trial. Lancet 2:1416, 1960

255. Whaley K et al: Sjögren's syndrome. 2. Clinical associations and immunological phenomena. Q J Med 42:513, 1973

256. Whittingham S: Immunofluorescence reactions in patients with prolonged extrahepatic biliary obstruction. Gastroenterology 66:169, 1974

257. Whittingham S et al: Smooth muscle autoantibody (SMA) in "autoimmune" hepatitis. Gastroenterology 51:499, 1966

258. Whittingham S et al: An autoantibody reactive with nuclei of polymorphonuclear neutrophils: A cell differentiation marker. Blood 58:768–771, 1981

259. Whitehouse et al: Smooth male antibody in malignant disease. Br Med J 4:511, 1971

260. Wiedmann K et al: Identification of shared epitope on liver/kidney microsomal and liver plasma membranes. J Hepatol (submitted)

261. Wiedmann KH et al: Liver membrane antibodies detected by immunoradiometric assay in acute and chronic virus–induced and autoimmune liver disease. Hepatology 4:199, 1984

262. Wiedmann KH et al: Analysis of the antigenic composition of liver-specific lipoprotein using murine monoclonal antibodies. Gut 26:510, 1985

263. Wiedmann KH et al: Analysis of the antigen composition of liver-specific lipoprotein using murine monoclonal antibodies. Gut 26:510–517, 1985

264. Wilkinson SP et al: Relation of renal impairment and hemorrhagic diathesis to endotoxemia in fulminant hepatic failure. Lancet i:521, 1974

265. Willems TH et al: Viral inhibition of the phytohemagglutinin response of human lymphocytes and applications to viral hepatitis. Proc Soc Exp Biol (NZ) 130:652, 1969

266. Wright R et al: Controlled prospective study of the effect on liver function of multiple exposure to halothane. Lancet i:817, 1975

267. Zetterman RK et al: Alcoholic hepatitis. Cell-mediated immunological response to alcoholic hyaline. Gastroenterology 70:382, 1976

268. Zetterman EF et al: Immunosuppression by mouse sialylated fetoprotein. Nature 265:354, 1977

269. Zhuang et al: Serum immunoglobulin levels in acute A, B, and non-A, non-B hepatitis. Gastroenterology 82:549–553, 1982

chapter **7**

Disordered Hemostasis
in Hepatic Disease

OSCAR D. RATNOFF

A characteristic and troublesome feature of many disorders of the liver or biliary tree is the appearance of generalized hemorrhagic phenomena. The association was recognized early. In 1846, Budd wrote: "There is . . . a tendency to hemorrhage from the nose and other parts in which there is no particular stress on the vessels. Small purpuric spots often appear on the face or forehead, sometimes on the distended belly; and, if the patient be cupped, ecchymosis is apt to take place about the puncture."[32] Since Budd's day, innumerable careful clinical descriptions of the hemorrhagic phenomena associated with hepatic or biliary tract disease have been published. Although the usual case of viral hepatitis is not complicated by a bleeding tendency, severely affected patients may bleed from the skin and mucous membranes, an event that may presage a fatal outcome;[76] as many as half or more of patients with fulminant hepatic failure may have hemorrhagic symptoms, and these may provide the lethal event.[2] Other acute disorders that involve the liver, as diverse as leptospirosis and mushroom poisoning, may be complicated by cutaneous or mucosal bleeding, but these symptoms are not necessarily related to hepatic dysfunction. Patients with chronic hepatic disease are more likely to have clinical evidence of a bleeding tendency. In one series, one fourth of patients with Laennec's cirrhosis had epistaxis, cutaneous purpura, gingival bleeding, or menometrorrhagia;[201] similar phenomena are common in postnecrotic cirrhosis or chronic active hepatitis.[2,202] Hemorrhage from the upper gastrointestinal tract is most often from esophageal varices, an event that complicates about one fourth of cases of Laennec's cirrhosis and one third of cases of postnecrotic cirrhosis,[201,202] but bleeding may also arise from superficial mucosal erosions or peptic ulcer.[280] Bleeding into the skin or from the mucous membranes is also a concomitant finding of untreated chronic obstruction of the biliary tree, and the danger of surgery under these conditions was commented upon as early as 1878.[234]

As one might expect from the central metabolic role of the liver, the pathogenesis of bleeding is often complex. In hepatic disorders, clotting factors may be deficient in plasma or qualitatively defective, the platelets may be qualitatively or quantitatively defective, endogenous anticoagulant substances may be present, the plasma fibrinolytic systems may behave abnormally, and tests for intravascular coagulation may be positive. Among patients with cirrhosis, those who sustain episodes of gastrointestinal, vaginal, or postoperative hemorrhage severe enough to require transfusion are more likely to have laboratory evidences of a bleeding tendency than those who do not bleed.[239] Admittedly, it is difficult to prove that the prognosis after bleeding from esophageal varices is related to hemostatic function. Nonetheless, patients in whom the normal mechanisms of hemostasis are impaired may bleed excessively at surgery, and, in such individuals, biopsy of the liver may be dangerous. The care of patients with hepatic disease is often influenced by the physician's assessment of the degree to which the hemostatic mechanisms are deranged and by his awareness of the measures that can be used to treat or prevent hemorrhage.

PHYSIOLOGY OF HEMOSTASIS

Several interrelated mechanisms stanch the flow of blood from injured blood vessels. In the smallest vessels, the earliest discernible event is the rapid accumulation of platelets at the site of the damage. Vasodilatation, which may follow injury to small vessels, slows the flow of blood, diverting platelets from the center of the stream to the periphery. There, platelets adhere to the vascular wall, probably at sites of endothelial damage that expose the underlying collagen-like proteins. Other platelets then adhere to those adherent to the vascular wall and to each other, forming aggregates of these cells at the site of vascular injury. Aggregation is brought about by adenosine diphosphate (ADP) released by damaged endothelial cells and, perhaps stimulated by the collagen-like proteins, by the platelets themselves. Platelet aggregation may also be brought about by stimulation by collagen of the formation of prostaglandin endoperoxides, particularly thromboxane A2, within these cells. After a brief interval, thrombin forms in the vicinity of the platelet mass, and, under its influence, the platelets undergo gross morphologic changes, fibrin fibers appear, and a more stable plug forms that can seal the gap in the blood vessel.

Although platelets undoubtedly participate in the control of bleeding from defects in larger blood vessels, hemostasis under these conditions is largely a function of the clotting mechanism. The final stage in the events leading to blood coagulation is the formation of a network of insoluble fibrin in the meshes of which serum and the cellular elements of blood are trapped. The clot almost always plugs the hole in the vessel. If this is unsuccessful, exsanguination ensues, or, if bleeding has occurred in a confined area, the pressure of the extravasated blood may slow hemorrhage until treatment is possible. The exposed anatomic situation of esophageal varices is unopposed by the back pressure of distended tissues.

Fibrin is formed through the action of a proteolytic enzyme, thrombin, which splits off four small fragments, the fibrinopeptides, from each molecule of fibrinogen, the precursor of fibrin. The molecules of fibrinogen from which the fibrinopeptides have been separated, now called *fibrin monomers,* polymerize to form insoluble threads of fibrin, a process accelerated by calcium ions at physiologic concentrations. In purified systems, this fibrin is held together loosely and can be dissolved by agents such as 5 M urea or 1% monochloroacetic acid. In normal blood, on the other hand, the fibrin molecules are bound by firm chemical bonds induced by a second enzyme, fibrin-stabilizing factor (factor XIII, fibrinoligase), a tetramer of two alpha and two beta chains. This enzyme is inactive in circulating blood but is activated by thrombin during clotting. If calcium ions are present, it unites adjacent fibrin monomers by transamidation. Factor XIII also binds fibronectin (cold-insoluble globulin) to fibrin.

Thrombin, the agent responsible for the formation of fibrin, cannot be detected in freshly drawn blood but evolves during coagulation from its precursor, prothrombin. At least two mechanisms have been discerned. In one, clotting is initiated by contact of blood with injured tissue; this process is therefore described as the *extrinsic pathway.* The active principle of injured tissue, tissue thromboplastin, interacts with a plasma protein, factor VII, to form a complex which, in the presence of calcium ions, activates another plasma protein, Stuart factor (factor X). The enzyme responsible for activation of Stuart factor is factor VII. Activated Stuart factor then releases thrombin from its parent molecule, prothrombin (factor II) by an enzymatic process. Thrombin formation is at first slow, but, as this enzyme forms, it alters another plasma protein proaccelerin (factor V). Once this has occurred, proaccelerin, in association with phospholipids and calcium ions, greatly potentiates the conversion of prothrombin to thrombin by activated Stuart factor. The phospholipid for this reaction is furnished by the injured tissue, by the plasma itself, and by platelets.

The second sequence through which thrombin generates in shed blood does not involve the intervention of tissue thromboplastin and has therefore been called the *intrinsic pathway.* The waterfall[56] or cascade[145] hypothesis of blood coagulation envisions the successive participation of a number of plasma proteins. When blood comes into contact with glass or similar insoluble agents, Hageman factor (factor XII), a plasma protein, is changed to an activated form that brings about reactions leading not only to clotting but, additionally, to fibrinolysis, increased vascular permeability and, through the transformation of plasma prekallikrein (Fletcher factor) to the proteolytic enzyme, plasma kallikrein, the liberation of biologically active peptide kinins from plasma kininogens. There are two groups of kininogens in plasma, differing in molecular weight, and it is primarily upon those of high molecular weight that plasma kallikrein acts. The kinins induce some of the phenomena of inflammation. The biologic counterpart of glass is not known, although collagen, sebum, and disrupted endothelial cells have been implicated in the activation of the intrinsic pathway. Activated Hageman factor changes plasma thromboplastin antecedent (PTA, factor XI) to a hydrolytic enzyme, which, in the presence of calcium ions, activates Christmas factor (factor IX). Plasma prekallikrein, functionally deficient in plasma in asymptomatic persons with Fletcher trait, potentiates the action of activated Hageman factor upon its substrates, including PTA, whereas high-molecular–weight kininogen, deficient in the plasmas of asymptomatic persons with Fitzgerald, Williams, Flaujeac, Reid, or Fujiwara trait, is apparently an absolute requirement for these reactions.

The activated form of Christmas factor (factor IXa) interacts with antihemophilic factor (AHF, factor VIII) to generate clot-promoting activity. Both are bound to phospholipid micelles, a process requiring the presence of calcium ions; the phospholipid is furnished by platelets and by the plasma itself. The complex of activated Christmas factor, AHF, phospholipid, and calcium ions then activates Stuart factor (factor X). The enzymatic groups responsible for the coagulant properties of the complex are on the Christmas factor moiety, but clot-promoting activity also requires an alteration in AHF brought about by thrombin. The subsequent steps of the intrinsic and extrinsic pathways are apparently identical. This formulation is undoubtedly simplistic; evidence has accrued that agents of the intrinsic pathway augment the reactions of the extrinsic pathway and vice versa. Thus, the enzymatic activity of factor VII is enhanced if it is first altered by thrombin, plasmin, or the activated forms of Hageman factor, Christmas factor, or Stuart factor, and the factor VII–tissue thromboplastin complex activates not only Stuart factor but also Christmas factor.

Platelets, essential for normal hemostasis, are derived from the cytoplasm of megakaryocytes, located principally, in the normal adult, in the bone marrow. Besides their capacity to plug small vascular defects and to furnish phospholipids for clotting, platelets promote clot retraction, a process in which the clot shrinks, expelling the serum contained within. Retraction is initiated by thrombin and depends upon the presence in platelets of a contractile protein, thrombasthenin, or platelet actomyosin, which, like muscle actomyosin, is an adenosine triphosphatase. Perhaps this enzyme helps to provide the energy required for retraction. Although the utility of retraction is not known, persons in whom this function is impaired have a bleeding tendency. Platelets also contain proteins identical with or closely similar to plasma proaccelerin (factor V), AHF (factor VIII), PTA (factor XI), fibrinogen, and the α chain of fibrin-stabilizing factor (factor XIII). During the clotting process, proaccelerin on the surface of platelets is activated by thrombin and, in turn, binds activated Stuart factor (factor Xa) that has generated in plasma. In this situation, the conversion of prothrombin to thrombin by activated Stuart factor is greatly enhanced. The role of platelet AHF, PTA, and fibrinogen is less clear, although platelet aggregation is dependent upon the presence of fibrinogen in plasma and probably of platelet fibrinogen as well.

Plasma has the potential capacity not only to form fibrin but also to dissolve clots, as though to protect against inadvertent intravascular coagulation. Plasma's potential for digesting fibrin resides in the plasma protease, plasmin. Not surprisingly, in normal individuals, plasmin is largely or completely in the form of an inert precursor, plasminogen, which is synthesized in the liver.[217] Plasminogen can be activated in the test tube in many ways, for example, by incubation of plasma with streptokinase (a product of certain β-hemolytic streptococci), urokinase (a proteolytic enzyme in urine), or activators derived from various tissues. The tissue activators appear to be separable into two classes, those that adhere readily to fibrin and those that, like urokinase, adhere poorly to this protein. Blood drawn distal to a vein that has been occluded by a tourniquet has enhanced fibrinolytic activity; a similar response can be elicited by exercise, emotional stress, or the injection of epinephrine, vasopressin, or pyrogens. The plasminogen activator derived from vascular endothelium seems unrelated to urokinase. Plasminogen can also be converted to plasmin by enzymes that participate in the early, surface-mediated steps of the intrinsic pathway, namely, kallikrein, activated PTA (factor XIa), and, to a lesser extent, activated Hageman factor (factor XIIa). *In vivo,* plasmin generation can also be brought about by the activated form of protein C (*vide infra*). The frequency with which fibrinolysis accompanies diffuse intravascular coagulation emphasizes the importance of the relationship between the clotting and fibrinolytic mechanisms.

The transformation of plasminogen to plasmin is greatly enhanced by its adsorption to fibrin. Activation is modulated by plasma inhibitors of the activation of plasminogen, including histidine-rich glycoprotein, which reduces binding of plasminogen to fibrin.[8,20,138,175] Plasmin is a protease of broad specificity. In addition to digesting fibrin, it hydrolyzes fibrinogen; inactivates the coagulant properties of proaccelerin (factor V), antihemophilic factor (factor VIII:C), Christmas factor, and prothrombin;[63,134] and digests gamma globulin, adrenocorticotropic hormone (ACTH), glucagon, and somatotropin. Plasmin also con-

verts the first component of complement to its active form, $C\bar{1}$ or C1 esterase, and releases biologically active kinins from their precursors in plasma, thus contributing to the events of inflammation. In addition to substrates that it might meet in nature, plasmin hydrolyzes casein, gelatin, denatured hemoglobin and other proteins, and various synthetic amino acid esters and amides.

The digestion of fibrinogen by plasmin takes place through a series of steps. First, it separates fragments from the carboxy-terminal ends of the α chains and the amino-terminal ends of the β chains. The principal residue, fragment X, can still be clotted by thrombin. Fragment X is further digested by plasmin, yielding fragments Y, D, and E. The degradation of fibrin proceeds in a similar manner, but fragment X is incoagulable. Products of the digestion of fibrinogen or fibrin impede clotting by interfering with the generation of thrombin and its action upon fibrinogen and with the normal polymerization of fibrin monomers. The digestive products of the fibrinolytic process can be demonstrated immunologically in the sera of patients who have spontaneous fibrinolytic states or who have been treated with such activators of plasminogen as urokinase,[70,158] but the usual laboratory tests for these fibrin(ogen)-split products do not distinguish them from soluble fibrin complexes.

Not unexpectedly, plasma contains inhibitory substances that may limit the processes of coagulation and fibrinolysis. The principal inhibitor of thrombin is antithrombin III, a protein synthesized by hepatic and vascular endothelial cells. Antithrombin III also blocks the enzymatic activity of activated Stuart factor (factor Xa) and, less effectively, plasmin, plasma kallikrein, and the activated forms of Hageman factor (factor XIIa), PTA (factor XIa), and Christmas factor (factor IXa). Heterozygotes for hereditary antithrombin III deficiency have a partial functional deficiency of this protein and have recurrent episodes of thromboembolism in both arteries and veins.

α_2-Plasmin inhibitor serves to block the enzymatic properties of plasmin rapidly and is the major inhibitor of this enzyme.[8,143] It is bound to fibrin by fibrin-stabilizing factor (factor XIII), and, in this way α_2-plasmin inhibitor interferes with the binding of plasminogen to fibrin. This property of α_2-plasmin inhibitor probably accounts for the increased resistance to fibrinolysis of clots formed in the presence of fibrin-stabilizing factor. A hereditary deficiency of α_2-plasmin inhibitor is associated with a hemophilia-like bleeding tendency, presumably because of the rapid dissolution of clots.[10]

α_2-Macroglobulin is a slower acting inhibitor of plasmin than α_2-antiplasmin and also blocks the actions of thrombin and plasma kallikrein.[79] α_1-Antitrypsin (α_1-antiproteinase) inhibits activated PTA (factor XIa) and plasmin; its importance in hemostasis is not clear. Its functional deficiency is associated with pulmonary emphysema and hepatic disease. $C\bar{1}$ inactivator (C1 esterase inhibitor) is a plasma protein that blocks the enzymatic properties of the first component of complement (C1), as well as plasmin, plasma kallikrein, and the activated forms of Hageman factor and PTA. The basic biochemical lesion in hereditary angioneurotic edema is a functional deficiency of C$\bar{1}$ inhibitor.

Protein C and protein S are vitamin K–dependent plasma proteins that serve to modulate the clotting and fibrinolytic systems. Protein C is converted by thrombin to an activated form that inactivates the coagulant properties of antihemophilic factor and proaccelerin; inactivation is more rapid if these clotting factors are in the thrombin-altered form. *In vivo,* activated protein C also enhances fibrinolysis in animal models. *In vitro* studies suggest that this effect is indirect, through the release of an intermediary that increases circulating plasminogen activator activity. Activation of protein C *in vivo* appears to take place preferentially on the vascular endothelial surface where its activator, thrombin, is bound to a specific receptor, thrombomodulin. Activation of protein C is also accelerated by thrombin-altered proaccelerin. Complicating matters further, protein S forms a complex with activated protein C and serves as a cofactor that enhances its activity; protein S also binds to the C4b-binding protein of complement. Plasma contains an inhibitor of activated protein C that may limit its inhibitory properties. Hereditary deficiencies of protein C have been described. Heterozygotes for protein C deficiency have a thrombotic tendency and are susceptible to the development of the severe local cutaneous necrosis that rarely complicates oral anticoagulant therapy. Several instances of neonatal purpura fulminans have been ascribed to homozygous deficiency of protein C.

Current evidence suggests that except for a part of the molecule of antihemophilic factor all the plasma protein clotting and fibrinolytic factors and their inhibitors are synthesized exclusively or for the most part by the liver. For example, cultured human hepatoma cells synthesize fibrinogen, prothrombin, Stuart factor, antithrombin III, and α_2-plasmin inhibitor.[67,219] As will be discussed subsequently, completion of the synthesis of prothrombin, Christmas factor, Stuart factor, factor VII, and proteins C and S are dependent upon the presence of vitamin K.

Antihemophilic factor (AHF, factor VIII) is a complex molecule comprised of two unequal parts held together by noncovalent bonds. The smaller subcomponent, factor VIII:C, provides the clot-promoting activity of the molecule; its synthesis has been localized to the liver and possibly the kidney and takes place under the direction of a gene on the X chromosome. The larger part, sometimes designated von Willebrand's factor (factor VIII:VWF), fosters the adhesion of platelets to exposed subendothelial vascular tissues. This portion of antihemophilic factor forms precipitates with heterologous antiserum against the whole antihemophilic factor molecule and has therefore been designated as factor VIIIR:Ag, that is, factor VIII-related antigen. It is required for agglutination of platelets by the antibiotic ristocetin, a property described as factor VIII:RCo, that is, factor VIII cofactor for ristocetin-induced agglutination; the biologic significance of this phenomenon is not clear. Synthesis of the larger subcom-

ponent of antihemophilic factor has been localized to vascular endothelial cells and to megakaryocytes and is under the direction of an autosomal gene. In classic hemophilia, factor VIII:C is functionally deficient, whereas the concentrations of factor VIIIR:Ag and factor VIII:RCo are both normal. The abnormally long bleeding time in von Willebrand's disease has been ascribed to factor VIIIR:Co.

Proaccelerin (factor V) has long been thought to be synthesized in the liver, but recent studies indicate that endothelial cells may also synthesize this molecule.

TESTS OF HEMOSTATIC FUNCTION

For the most part, defects in hemostasis are diagnosed in the laboratory. Certain tests are particularly helpful in the clinical care of patients with hepatic disease.

The *clotting time* of whole blood is a function of the concentration of factors that participate in the intrinsic pathway of blood clotting. Measured in glass tubes, the clotting time is prolonged only when the deficiency of these factors is profound; it is unaltered by thrombocytopenia or by deficiencies of factor VII or fibrin-stabilizing factor. Its insensitivity to minor deficiencies of clotting factors and its technical difficulty have made measurement of the clotting time much less useful than that of the partial thromboplastin time. An abnormally long clotting time may also reflect the presence of intrinsic or extrinsic inhibitors of blood clotting, of which heparin, administered therapeutically, is the most common. In patients with catastrophic fibrinolytic purpura, whole blood may seem to be incoagulable because the fibrin strands dissolve as rapidly as they form. The sensitivity of the clotting time may be enhanced by use of silicone-coated or polystyrene tubes, but the tedium of this modification makes it impractical for routine use.

Both in obstructive jaundice and in parenchymal hepatic disease, particularly cirrhosis of the liver, the clotting time is occasionally prolonged when measured in glass tubes and, more often, when tested in silicone-coated or plastic tubes.

Because of its insensitivity, the whole blood clotting time has been replaced for almost all purposes by the *partial thromboplastin time.* This test is performed by measuring the clotting time of a mixture of citrated plasma, calcium ions, and crude phospholipid derived from brain tissue or soybeans; the test is usually modified by the addition of kaolin, Celite, or ellagic acid to activate Hageman factor as completely as possible. Like the clotting time of whole blood, the partial thromboplastin time is prolonged if factors of the intrinsic pathway are deficient or qualitatively abnormal or if inhibitors are present. Although more sensitive than the clotting time of whole blood, the partial thromboplastin time may be normal in mild coagulative disorders. In hepatic disease or obstructive jaundice, the partial thromboplastin time is often moderately prolonged.

Several simple tests help to localize the clotting defects of patients with hepatic disease. The *thrombin time,* that is, the clotting time of a mixture of citrated plasma and bovine thrombin, measures the rate of formation of fibrin from fibrinogen. The thrombin time may be prolonged if the concentration of fibrinogen is excessively low or high or if this protein is qualitatively abnormal. It is also long if intrinsic or extrinsic inhibitors of fibrin formation, such as the proteolytic digestion products of fibrinogen or fibrin or therapeutically administered heparin, are present. The thrombin time is not affected by the concentration of fibrin-stabilizing factor, a deficiency of which is detected by noting the solubility in 5 M urea or in 1% monochloroacetic acid of clots formed by the addition of calcium ions to citrated plasma.

The *prothrombin time* assesses the extrinsic pathway of thrombin formation. The test is performed by measuring the clotting time of a mixture of citrated plasma, tissue thromboplastin, and calcium ions. A long prothrombin time, a common finding in obstructive jaundice or hepatic disease, may reflect deficiencies or qualitative abnormalities of factor VII, Stuart factor, proaccelerin, prothrombin, or fibrinogen or the presence of inhibitors of the formation of activated Stuart factor, thrombin, or fibrin. A pronounced increase in the prothrombin time is an indicator of poor prognosis in severe viral hepatitis or paracetamol poisoning.[125] Among patients with cirrhosis, those who have had a major episode of bleeding are more likely to have a prolonged prothrombin time than those who have escaped this complication.[239]

When the prothrombin time is normal, an abnormally long partial thromboplastin time suggests qualitative or quantitative deficiencies of Hageman factor, plasma prekallikrein, high-molecular-weight kininogen, PTA, Christmas factor, or antihemophilic factor or the presence of inhibitors of these substances.

The *platelets* may be counted by a variety of means, but mechanized platelet counters are least accurate in severe thrombocytopenia; the normal range is 150,000/μl to 350,000/μl. Platelet function may be tested by observing *clot retraction* grossly or by measuring it semiquantitatively. Clot retraction is usually reduced only if the count is less than about 100,000/μl; retraction may also be impaired if the platelets are qualitatively abnormal. Qualitative defects of platelets may also be identified because these cells do not aggregate normally upon addition of ADP, collagen, or epinephrine. Agglutination upon addition of the antibiotic ristocetin may also be impaired, a defect said to be due in hepatic disease to an abnormality of platelets. The release of clot-promoting substances (PF3) upon incubation of platelet-rich plasma with kaolin is another useful but rarely used measure of qualitative defects of platelets.

Thrombocytopenia and qualitative abnormalities of platelets are usually accompanied by prolongation of the bleeding time. I prefer to measure the bleeding time by a modification of Duke's method, in which the tip of the finger is punctured with a scalpel blade. Other investigators use variations of the Ivy technique, in which bleeding is measured from incised wounds of the forearm, distal to an occlusive tourniquet, using a template to standardize the length and depth of the incision, but this may leave permanent scarring. In thrombocytopenic states, the bleeding time gives abnormal results only when the platelet count is less than 100,000/μl, a level not often reached in hepatic disease. A long bleeding time is also found in thrombocythemia, in which the platelet count is above about 800,000/μl; in von Willebrand's disease, a hereditary disorder classically characterized by a decreased titer of antihemophilic factor in clotting assays, a decreased concentration of antigens related to this factor as measured by heterologous antiserum, and decreased ristocetin-induced platelet agglutination; in disorders in which the platelets are qualitatively defective; and in one or another of the dysproteinemias. In some patients with abnormal bleeding, no obvious cause for a prolonged bleeding time can be found.

Further investigation of the hemostatic mechanisms requires procedures not always readily available. Quantitative or semiquantitative assays can be performed for each plasma clotting factor, as well as tests that detect and localize circulating anticoagulants in plasma, that is, abnormal inhibitory substances. Abnormal fibrinolytic activity can be measured, with increasing sensitivity, in clots of whole blood, plasma, or the euglobulin fraction of plasma. The detection of fibrin(ogen)-related antigens in serum, which is normally devoid of fibrinogen, suggests that disseminated intravascular coagulation (DIC) or intravascular fibrinolysis has occurred. A widely used procedure, the Thrombo-Wellco test (Burroughs Wellcome Co.) depends upon the aggregation of latex particles coated with antiserum against fibrinogen fragments D and E. This reagent reacts with fibrinogen monomers, with soluble, incompletely aggregated complexes of fibrin monomers, and with complexes of fibrin monomers with fibrinogen or with the fibrin(ogen) split or degradation products generated during fibrinolysis (FSP or FDP). Thus, a positive result should not be interpreted as proof that a fibrinolytic process has taken place. The components of the fibrinolytic system can be assayed with some confidence. Other tests provide information concerning the possibility that intravascular clotting has occurred. The tourniquet test, widely used to demonstrate increased capillary fragility, is unreliable and provides little useful information.

DISORDERS OF VITAMIN K-DEPENDENT CLOTTING FACTORS

Four clotting factors in mammalian plasma—Christmas factor (factor IX), factor VII, Stuart factor (factor X), and prothrombin—and proteins C and S are synthesized only if vitamin K is available. The properties of these agents are extraordinarily similar, as though they were derived phylogenetically from a single ancestor protein. Their synthesis is impaired in obstructive jaundice or hepatic disease, contributing in an important way to the bleeding tendency in these conditions. Vitamin K is also needed for the synthesis of proteins in bone, lung, kidney, and placenta. Functional deficiencies of prothrombin, Stuart factor, and factor VII are recognized by the presence of an abnormally long prothrombin time, and deficiency of Christmas factor is recognized by an abnormally long partial thromboplastin time.

A wide variety of compounds, all derivatives of naphthoquinone, exhibit vitamin K–like activity. These agents cannot be synthesized by mammals but are furnished by the ingestion of plant foods, particularly leafy green vegetables, and by intestinal flora. In adults, deprivation of vitamin K for 4 or 5 weeks does not result in depletion of this vitamin unless oral antibiotic therapy is given concomitantly.[77] Naturally occurring compounds with vitamin K–like activity are lipid-soluble, and, as a consequence, their optimal absorption from the gastrointestinal tract requires a normal capacity to absorb lipids, as well as the presence of bile salts and, probably, pancreatic lipase.[109,235]

Once absorbed, vitamin K is used by the parenchymal cells of the liver to synthesize the proteins that depend upon this agent.[18,177,186] The role of the liver in synthesis, well established experimentally, has been demonstrated by clinical observation that the plasma concentration of the vitamin K–dependent clotting factors is reduced by partial hepatectomy[4,174] or interruption of the hepatic arterial circulation.[5] The vitamin is not incorporated into the structure of the clotting factors. Olson and associates[177] and Suttie[251] have demonstrated that puromycin, which blocks the protein synthetic function of ribosomes, inhibits the formation of vitamin K–dependent clotting factors. Olson and colleagues'[177] experiments suggest that vitamin K acts only after the formation of a protein precursor of the clotting factors. Thus, the first step in synthesis of the vitamin K–dependent clotting factors is the synthesis of polypeptide chains that lack clot-promoting properties.[193,252] In liver disease, synthesis of these polypeptides is deficient.[89] In contrast, a deficiency of vitamin K or administration of coumarin-like agents prevents the formation of functionally active molecules, but not of the protein precursors, whose presence can be detected immunologically or by measurement of their clot-inhibitory properties.[15,89,178]

The role of vitamin K in the synthesis of Christmas factor, factor VII, Stuart factor, and prothrombin, long obscure, has been clarified through studies by Magnuson and colleagues,[146] Stenflo and associates,[245] and others. Vitamin K is a necessary cofactor for a carboxylase that inserts carbon dioxide into the gamma carbon of certain glutamic acid residues of the precursors of these proteins. The unique tricarboxylic glutamic acids thus created are essential for the functional activity of these clotting factors. Vitamin K is oxidized in the process and is salvaged by a vitamin K reductase that is inhibited by warfarin-like "anticoagulants." Calcium ions, needed for the action of the vitamin K–dependent factors, are apparently joined to these proteins at the unique tricarboxylic acids, where they serve as points of attachment of the phospholipids, which are also needed for their optimal function.

The physiologic role of vitamin K in the synthesis of clotting factors is put to practical use in the care of patients with obstructive jaundice or hepatic disease. In obstructive jaundice, vitamin K is absorbed poorly because bile salts are prevented from entering the duodenum. During the first few days after biliary duct obstruction by stone, the titers of the vitamin K–dependent factors are normal or even elevated.[38] Shortly, however, the exclusion of bile salts from the gastrointestinal tract prevents the normal absorption of vitamin K, so that the carboxylation of the precursors of the vitamin K–dependent factors is impeded. As a result, patients with obstructive jaundice may be functionally deficient in each vitamin K–dependent factor, a change reflected by an abnormally long prothrombin time.[190] The critical need for bile salts for absorption of vitamin K is clearly seen in patients with biliary fistulas in whom therapy with *oral* vitamin K is ineffective unless bile salts are also administered.[288] Similarly, the administration of cholestyramine, used in the treatment of pruritus in patients with hepatic or biliary tract disease, may, by binding bile salts, impede the absorption of lipids and *pari passu* of vitamin K.[94]

The deficiencies of the vitamin K–dependent clotting factors that result from malabsorption of the vitamin are apparently responsible for the susceptibility to hemorrhage of patients with obstructive jaundice. Bleeding, once a common and dangerous complication of surgery in obstructive jaundice, can usually be prevented by daily parenteral administration of vitamin K;[34] small amounts of vitamin K_1 or a water-soluble analogue such as menadione sulfate, for example, 5 mg/day, are usually sufficient. The effects of therapy can be assessed by measuring the prothrombin time. If this is abnormally long because the absorption of vitamin K is impaired, it will shorten within a few days after therapy is instituted. A more rapid response follows the intramuscular injection of 25 mg of vitamin K_1. Intravenous injections are seldom indicated and best avoided because they may be followed by severe reactions. The response to vitamin K is useful not only therapeutically but also diagnostically,[143] because, as will be noted shortly, patients with hepatic disease usually do not benefit from the injection of small amounts of this substance. The revolution in the care of patients with obstructive jaundice brought about by therapy with vitamin K is epitomized by one writer's statement that "in patients with calculus obstruction of the common duct, the defect in hemostasis is rarely so severe as to cause spontaneous bruising and bleeding."[128]

Vitamin K–dependent clotting factors may be deficient in both acute and chronic parenchymal hepatic disease. Deficiencies of prothrombin, factor VII, Stuart factor (factor X), and Christmas factor (factor IX) are usually found together.[56,151,195,222,239] In general, the functional titer of factor VII shows the greatest decline and that of Christmas factor the least.[125,264] Rarely, deficiency of a single factor, for example, Christmas factor, may dominate the picture.[127] The decrease in the titer of the vitamin K–

dependent factors detected in clotting assays is paralleled by decreased concentrations of these proteins, as measured immunologically.[51,87,125,180] Additionally, in most patients with hepatitis or cirrhosis, the titer of incompletely carboxylated prothrombin (and presumably other vitamin K–dependent proteins) is increased, as though the precursor proteins were prematurely liberated into the plasma or the carboxylase responsible for the formation of tricarboxylic glutamic acid residues were functionally deficient.[25,50,51]

At least in hepatic failure, the degree of deficiency of factor VII may be related to prognosis; in 12 such cases, the 6 patients in whom the titer of factor VII was more than 8% of the average normal survived, whereas the others died.[65] Other abnormalities in hepatic disease, notably, a deficiency of proaccelerin (factor V) or, much less commonly, a deficiency or qualitative abnormality of fibrinogen, also prolong the prothrombin time. As noted above, an abnormally low concentration of Christmas factor is not detected by the prothrombin time.[145]

In some patients with parenchymal hepatic disease, particularly those with severe jaundice, the prothrombin time is shortened by the administration of vitamin K (for example, the intramuscular injection of vitamin K_1).[231,243] In such cases, this response to vitamin K may suggest a component of intrahepatic obstruction of the biliary tree, indistinguishable physiologically from extrahepatic obstruction. This explanation is probably too simple, however, because the dose of vitamin K needed to shorten the prothrombin time in parenchymal hepatic disease is often much larger than that needed in obstructive jaundice; patients with parenchymal disease may respond only to doses of 25 mg to 50 mg of vitamin K_1.

In most patients in whom an abnormally long prothrombin time is associated with parenchymal hepatic disease, the administration of vitamin K is without obvious benefit. Spector and Corn[239] found that patients who had had a major hemorrhage never responded to therapy with this vitamin. Presumably, vitamin K cannot be used in these patients because the precursor proteins cannot be carboxylated. As a result, in hepatic disease, therapy of the hemorrhagic state associated with a deficiency of the vitamin K–dependent factors is difficult. If the patient does not respond to vitamin K, for example, 25 mg of vitamin K_1 given intramuscularly daily for 3 days, its use should not be continued. Transfusion of normal plasma may get the patient through an acute crisis. Since the vitamin K–dependent factors are stable during storage at 4° C or frozen, there is no particular necessity to use fresh blood or plasma, but pooled plasma should be avoided because of the risk of hepatitis. Other defects in the plasma of patients with hepatic disease, such as proaccelerin deficiency, are not corrected by the use of ordinary stored plasma. Thus, the use of fresh frozen plasma, which contains adequate amounts of proaccelerin (factor V), or fresh blood, which also contains viable platelets, is preferable.[14,240]

When an adult with hepatic disease is thought to be bleeding because of a deficiency of the vitamin K–dependent clotting factors, the infusion of 1000 ml of fresh frozen plasma may improve hemostasis, although normal titers of the deficient factors will not be achieved; proportionately smaller amounts are used in children. Unfortunately, the transfused factors, particularly factor VII, disappear rapidly from the circulation, so that the patients must be transfused repeatedly; 200 ml of plasma every 4 hours is a minimal amount. Greater volumes may so overload the circulation as to pose the danger of rupture of esophageal varices unless, at the same time, blood is being lost through active hemorrhage. Concentrates of the vitamin K–dependent factors, such as Proplex (Hyland) or Konȳne (Cutter) may help to sustain the level of these agents without overloading the circulation,[24] but such preparations may induce thrombotic complications, including postoperative portal vein thrombosis, pulmonary embolism, DIC, fatal infectious hepatitis, or acquired immune deficiency syndrome (AIDS).[17,118,153,284] If bleeding is sufficient to reduce the hematocrit, as in esophageal variceal hemorrhage, transfusion of blood cells will be needed to sustain blood volume. Fresh whole blood, if available, is probably the treatment of choice.

A peculiar association of factor VII deficiency with Dubin-Johnson syndrome, Gilbert's syndrome, and its variant, Rotor's syndrome, has been described.[225,226] Paradoxically, the titers of prothrombin, factor VII, and Stuart factor may be elevated in primary biliary cirrhosis or obstruction of the common duct by biliary stone,[38] a change that has been attributed to a generalized increase in protein synthesis by the liver.

Anticoagulant therapy is seldom indicated in hepatocellular disease. If the need arises, however, treatment with coumarin-like anticoagulants should be approached with caution. Experimentally, hepatic damage prolongs the effect of these drugs, and the response of patients with hepatic disease to the administration of coumarin-like compounds is exaggerated compared to that in persons with no hepatic damage.[203,230] Heparin therapy, too, has its dangers, because patients with thrombocytopenia may be peculiarly sensitive to this agent, and heparin itself may induce thrombocytopenia.

PROACCELERIN (FACTOR V) DEFICIENCY

In addition to deficiencies of the vitamin K–dependent clotting factors, the most common coagulative defect in acute and chronic hepatic disease is probably a decrease in the concentration of proaccelerin (factor V) in plasma.[182,195,264] This defect is unusual in uncomplicated obstructive jaundice, primary biliary cirrhosis, or metastatic disease in the liver, in which the titer of proaccelerin may be normal or increased.[36,61,195] In infants with biliary atresia, the level of proaccelerin in plasma is decreased in those in whom hepatic damage is prominent, but normal in those in whom vitamin K deficiency is still present after hepatic portoenterostomy.[285]

Proaccelerin is probably synthesized largely or exclusively in the liver, where it has been localized to parenchymal cells, but the cell specifically responsible for synthesis has not been definitively determined.[83,84,230] Recent studies indicate that endothelial cells elaborate this protein.[39] Proaccelerin is elaborated by the perfused liver, and synthesis is suppressed by the administration of puromycin.[177] Further, the concentration of proaccelerin is depressed in experimental animals subjected to hepatectomy[150,167] or chloroform intoxication[253] and in humans after partial hepatectomy.[4] Therefore, probably, in hepatic disease, the concentration of proaccelerin is the result of impaired synthesis of the protein. Alternatively, a decreased titer of proaccelerin may reflect its utilization in the formation of thrombin during DIC, its destruction by the excessive plasma proteolytic activity that is common in chronic liver disease or by activated protein C.[1,63,134] It is, however, doubtful that this abnormality can be attributed to plasma proteolytic activity in most cases, because, in other situations, similar degrees of proteolytic activity do not affect the concentration of proaccelerin.[99] Perhaps, in the rare cirrhotic with fibrinolytic purpura, plasmin contributes to the deficiency of proaccelerin.[19] An isolated deficiency of proaccelerin is reflected by an abnormally long prothrombin time. Because this test is sensitive to deficiencies of other factors, specific procedures are needed for the measurement of proaccelerin, but these are rarely indicated clinically. That a deficiency of proaccelerin contributes to the bleeding tendency of patients with hepatic disease is known only by analogy; patients with hereditary deficiencies of proaccelerin, similar in degree to those of patients with cirrhosis, may have a slight tendency to bleed, usually after injury. Still, severe depression of proaccelerin has been correlated with a poor prognosis in hepatic disease.[154]

In hepatic disease, an isolated deficiency of proaccelerin does not usually need to be corrected. The only available measure is the transfusion of fresh blood or fresh frozen plasma. Proaccelerin survives storage at 4° C in the blood bank only erratically. Since its half-disappearance time after transfusion is 15 to 30 hours, such therapy is suitable only for an acute episode of bleeding. The schedule for transfusion is similar to that used for the vitamin K–dependent clotting factors. Vitamin K therapy is useless, because this vitamin is not used in the synthesis of proaccelerin.

FIBRINOGEN AND FIBRIN FORMATION

A commonly mentioned but relatively unusual defect in hepatic disorders is a decrease in the concentration of fibrinogen in circulating plasma. This protein is synthesized largely or exclusively in the liver. Direct evidence of hepatic synthesis was first obtained by Miller and associates,[161,162] who demonstrated that the isolated liver, unlike the liverless animal, incorporated radioactive amino acids into fibrinogen. This observation has been confirmed repeatedly in the perfused liver,[177] in hepatic slices,[246] and in cultured human embryonal liver cells[88] and hepatoma

cells.[120] Fluorescent antibody techniques have localized the site of synthesis to the parenchymal cells.[72]

The concentration of fibrinogen in normal plasma averages about 280 mg/dl, ranging in one series from 165 mg/dl to 485 mg/dl. Its half-disappearance time from plasma is 3 to 4 days. Hypofibrinogenemia may result from decreased synthesis of fibrinogen, from its consumption during intravascular coagulation, from unreplaced loss during massive hemorrhage, or from its destruction by abnormal plasma fibrinolytic activity.

Hypofibrinogenemia, usually of moderate degree, is occasionally found in patients with severe acute or chronic hepatic disease, in whom it suggests a poor prognosis.[69,82,136] More often, the concentration of fibrinogen is normal or even elevated.[99,125,262,264] Patients with cirrhosis may not respond to stimuli such as infection that in other persons would induce an increased concentration of fibrinogen in plasma.[100]

The rate of synthesis of fibrinogen in hepatic disease is usually normal[270] or even increased,[97] but decreased synthesis is probably an important element in the rare case of hypofibrinogenemia accompanying severe acute hepatitis of whatever cause. In clinical situations in which hypofibrinogenemia is an isolated finding, abnormal bleeding does not occur if the concentration of fibrinogen is above about 100 mg/dl plasma. Below this point, bleeding is excessive from the sites of injury or surgical procedures, but spontaneous bleeding is uncommon. In liver disease, hypofibrinogenemia is invariably only one of many hemostatic defects and can therefore be expected to be of greater moment. If hypofibrinogenemia is thought to contribute to a bleeding tendency and is unaccompanied by signs of significant DIC, attempts should be made to correct this defect, at least temporarily. A ready source of fibrinogen is the cryoprecipitate fraction of normal plasma used in the treatment of classic hemophilia (factor VIII "deficiency"). Each bag, prepared from one unit of blood, contains 200 mg to 250 mg of fibrinogen, on the average, but the amount in any one bag varies widely.[170] An adequate initial dose is 1 bag of cryoprecipitate for every 3 kg of body weight; subsequently, 1 bag for every 15 kg should be given daily to sustain the patient's level of fibrinogen.[233] Needless to say, the transfusion of cryoprecipitate, prepared as it is from the blood of many donors, bears the risk of inducing hepatitis.

Within the last few years, increasing attention has been paid to the possible role of DIC in the pathogenesis of bleeding in some patients with both acute and chronic hepatic disease of various types.[21,36,115,247,269] Conceivably, in such patients, clot-promoting agents gain access to circulating blood, where they induce slow formation of fibrin throughout the vasculature. Several biologic consequences result. The titer of clotting factors is diminished, as these are consumed in the process of coagulation or are inactivated by thrombin that forms *pari passu*. Decreases in the coagulant titer of antihemophilic factor (factor VIII) and proaccelerin (factor V) may also result from their digestion by thrombin or activated protein C; perhaps reflecting the latter, the plasma inhibitor of protein C may be decreased by DIC.[74] The titer of antithrombin III is also significantly reduced during DIC,[23] but whether this is due to its utilization during the clotting process or impaired hepatic synthesis is uncertain.[3] The concentration of platelets is also decreased, possibly because these cells, clumped by thrombin, are removed prematurely from the circulation. Curiously, few intravascular fibrin deposits are found upon pathologic examination either in animals or patients with DIC; sometimes small thrombi are seen in the liver, lungs, or kidney. The dearth of thrombi may be related to several phenomena that are not mutually exclusive. Conceivably, fibrin polymerization is incomplete, and soluble fibrin polymers or polymers of fibrinogen and fibrin may be removed from the circulation, or particulate fibrin is rapidly removed from the blood vessels by cells of the reticuloendothelial system that, in experimental animals, contain material antigenically related to fibrinogen.[126] Alternatively, the clots are dissolved either by plasmin that has generated as a consequence of stress or of the activation of Hageman factor or by proteases liberated from leukocytes.

Patients thought to have undergone DIC may have multiple clotting factor deficiencies and thrombocytopenia. Their serum, which normally would be devoid of fibrinogen, contains antigenic material recognized by antiserum against fibrinogen or fibrin. The fibrinogen-related antigens, often misnamed fibrin(ogen) degradation or split products, are usually ascribed to degradation of fibrin by plasmin (*vide supra*) but may represent circulating, incompletely polymerized fibrin or complexes of fibrin monomers with fibrinogen or with fibrinogen- or fibrin degradation products.[141,172,229] The abnormally low titer of antithrombin III found in some patients with hepatic disease has been ascribed to DIC, as noted above, but another plausible explanation is its decreased synthesis by the diseased liver.[3,99,106,273] Hiller and associates[108] reported that after the onset of severe esophageal hemorrhage, a decreased titer of antithrombin III and an increased concentration of fibrin(ogen)-related antigens were signs of a poor prognosis.

As Minna and colleagues[163] and Straub[247] have emphasized, recognition of DIC is difficult in patients with hepatic disease, who may have thrombocytopenia and impaired blood coagulation from a variety of causes. Although DIC is nowadays much overdiagnosed in liver disease,[176] this process, nonetheless, appears to be of considerable importance. Accelerated catabolism of fibrinogen, possibly the consequence of DIC, has been observed in some, but not all patients with hepatic disease and is said to be reversed by the administration of heparin or by correcting the concomitant deficiency of antithrombin III by tranfusion of a purified preparation of this inhibitor.[7,26,42,223,224,262] Inhibition of fibrinolysis by administration of tranexamic acid[262] or ε-aminocaproic acid[7] has given erratic results in patients with cirrhosis, but one can conclude that fibrinolysis is only a minor factor in accelerated catabolism of fibrinogen in this disease. Increased rates of catabolism have also been reported in severe acute hepatic necrosis of diverse etiologies,[191,247] biliary tract obstruction, cholangitis, and contusion of the liver.[276] Support for the theory that DIC may be responsible for the increased rate of catabolism of fibrinogen comes from the demonstration of fibrinogen-related antigens or soluble fibrin monomer complexes in some patients with cirrhosis,[70,159,173,224,257] primary hepatocellular carcinoma,[264] or acute hepatic necrosis.[65,191] Further, the titer of fibrinopeptide A, presumably released from the Aα chain of fibrinogen by the action of thrombin, may be modestly increased in patients with cirrhosis, as though some degree of DIC were present.[165] Additional support for a possible role of DIC comes from the observation that the titer of coagulant antihemophilic factor (factor VIII:C) is relatively lower than the concentration of antihemophilic factor–like antigens detected by heterologous antiserum (factor VIIIR:Ag) in patients bleeding from esophageal varices, as though the coagulant antihemophilic factor had been inhibited by thrombin or by activated protein C.[22] Rarely, the red blood cells may be fragmented, an abnormality associated with experimental intravascular coagulation.[33] Alternative possibilities to be considered are that accelerated catabolism is due to fibrinogenolysis by plasmin (*vide infra*) or other proteases or that the supposed shortening of the half-life of fibrinogen in hepatic disease may be the artefactual result of its loss into extravascular spaces or of unrecognized bleeding.[247]

The pathogenesis of intravascular coagulation in hepatic disease is obscure. Verstraete and associates[269] have suggested that necrotic hepatocytes may activate clotting factors within circulating plasma and that defective clearance of activated factors by the liver and reticuloendothelial system, combined with depressed levels of inhibitors of coagulation of plasma, may enhance the effects of these activated factors so as to allow intravascular coagulation to occur. Another possibility, proposed by Collen,[45] is that in portal hypertension, the endothelial cells of the expanded collateral circulation and spleen may be damaged, perhaps by hypoxia resulting from the abnormally slow blood flow, and that these alterations may predispose to local clotting. Still another view is that the source of activators of clotting is the gastrointestinal tract. Experimental extirpation of the bowel prevents defibrination after hepatectomy.[212] Perhaps endotoxins, liberated into the blood stream from the gastrointestinal tract, may induce intravascular coagulation in patients with hepatic disorders.[276,279] In agreement with this, endotoxemia has been observed in some patients with hepatic disease, particularly those with concomitant renal failure. This interpretation of the pathogenesis of DIC is appealing, since evidences of this syndrome are rare in otherwise uncomplicated cirrhosis,[92,247] whereas many patients with liver disease and DIC have concomitant septicemia,[163] albeit controversy exists concerning the frequency with which endotoxemia can be found.[78,266]

In recent years, treatment of ascites in patients with hepatic cirrhosis by autotransfusion of ascitic fluid and peritoneovenous (LeVeen) shunts has gained popularity. These procedures have almost always resulted in transient or sustained alterations of the patient's circulating plasma, resembling those of DIC, or, more rarely, dramatic fibrinolysis.[85,183,225,244] Occasionally, life-threatening or lethal hemorrhagic symptoms ensue.[130,156] These changes have variously been related to the presence in ascitic fluid of thromboplastin, to a direct activator of Stuart factor (factor X), or to endotoxin.[129,184,255] Additionally, concentrates of cell-free ascitic fluid aggregate platelets, but the significance of this observation is lessened by the absence of this property in unconcentrated ascitic fluid.[221] In patients with minor DIC, this complication is usually self-limited, but the presence of clinical symptoms is an indication for interruption of the shunt. Therapy with heparin or purified antithrombin III has yielded disappointing results.[75]

DIC may explain at least some instances of severe bleeding during or immediately after liver transplantation.[27,265] Beyond transfusion to replace blood loss, other measures, such as the administration of plasma, cryoprecipitates, platelets, or antifibrinolytic agents may produce disappointing results.[265]

When intravascular coagulation is suspected, the use of fibrinogen therapy is limited by the accelerated catabolism of this protein. Further, the possibility that the infused fibrinogen will induce further thrombosis cannot be ignored. In this situation, treatment with heparin has been proposed.[42,115,192,268,286] Evidence for its value is currently insecure, and this anticoagulant is, of course, potentially dangerous, particularly when thrombocytopenia is present. Therapy with heparin should be avoided when active bleeding is present. The proposed beneficial effects of infusions of antithrombin III for repair of a deficiency of this inhibitor during DIC have not yet been established.[23,105,224]

A different anomaly of the final stages of clotting is common in hepatic disease. When citrated plasma of some patients with cirrhosis or metastatic disease of the liver is mixed with thrombin, the clotting time of the mixture, that is, the thrombin time, is often prolonged.[114,198,240,257] In contrast, the thrombin time is usually normal in primary hepatocellular carcinoma.[264] Many different changes may contribute to the delay in the formation of a clot. Excessively high or low concentrations of plasma fibrinogen lengthen the thrombin time.[99] Sometimes the fibrinogen molecule itself is abnormal, so that it reacts more slowly than normal to the addition of thrombin.[198,267,271] The basic nature of the alterations that are responsible is not clear, although abnormalities of the carbohydrate content of these abnormal fibrinogens have been described.[91,159,238] Among these alterations is an increase in the sialic acid content of fibrinogen, which has been correlated with an increased thrombin time.[155,237] The functional defect of the abnormal fibrinogens is delayed aggregation of fibrin monomers that are formed by the action of thrombin.[60,93,123] Poller[185] made the disturbing observation that, among patients with cirrhosis who had bled from esophageal varices, this complication was more likely to be lethal if indirect evidence of impaired fibrin aggregation was found than in those in whom this defect was not detected. Whether there was a causal relationship between the presence of an abnormal fibrinogen and the lethal event was not clear. In severe viral hepatitis, the presence of an abnormal fibrinogen has not been related to a poor prognosis.[237]

In most patients in whom qualitatively abnormal fibrinogens have been found, the thrombin time is usually increased two to four times above that of control plasma. A much less impressive increase in the thrombin time is found in other patients with cirrhosis or biliary tract obstruction.[16,114,198] The pathogenesis of the long thrombin time in these circumstances is uncertain and may be different from patient to patient. In some patients, aggregation of fibrin monomers may be impeded, perhaps by an agent or agents in plasma; in one recent case of cytomegalovirus hepatitis, this defect was ascribed to the presence of β_2-microglobulin in plasma.[101,277] In other patients, the plasma may be qualitatively or quantitatively deficient in an agent that accelerates the conversion of fibrinogen to fibrin by thrombin.[114,198] In support of this possibility, Spector and colleagues[240] noted that the transfusion of fresh frozen plasma shortened the abnormally long thrombin time in patients with cirrhosis. I am unfamiliar with more recent studies concerning this phenomenon. In other cases, circulating anticoagulants, whose nature is not always clear, may be present.[48] Perhaps, in some instances, these anticoagulants are soluble intermediates of the transformation of fibrinogen to fibrin or are the products of digestion of fibrinogen or fibrin by plasmin. In one series of patients with cirrhosis, however, the long thrombin time did not correlate with the presence of fibrin(ogen)-related antigens in plasma.[30] Further, treatment of cirrhosis patients with ε-aminocaproic acid, a potent antifibrinolytic agent, does not shorten an abnormally long thrombin time.[21] A related theory suggests that the long thrombin time reflects the presence in plasma of degraded forms of fibrinogen.[142]

The abnormally long thrombin time of plasma obtained from patients with hepatic disease cannot be attributed to an alteration in its antithrombic properties. Normally, plasma inactivates thrombin, but at a rate too slow to affect the thrombin time. The concentration of the principal inhibitor of thrombin, antithrombin III, is often diminished in patients with either chronic hepatic disease or acute yellow atrophy.[12,99,106,110,264,274] In hepatitis, on the other hand, plasma antithrombic activity is ordinarily normal,[99] and, in obstructive jaundice, it may be increased.[106]

The degree to which prolongation of the thrombin time contributes to a bleeding tendency is uncertain. The modest prolongation usually found in cirrhosis is of the same order of magnitude as that observed in preeclampsia, which is unassociated with evidences of a hemorrhagic tendency. Possibly, abnormalities in fibrin formation augment defective hemostasis when other defects are present.

In normal blood clotting, the fibrin strands are bound covalently by fibrin-stabilizing factor (factor XIII), which is probably synthesized in the liver. Individuals with a hereditary deficiency of fibrin-stabilizing factor have a severe bleeding diathesis, and wounds may break down, delaying healing. In hepatic disorders, particularly severe cirrhosis or primary or metastatic neoplasms, the plasma occasionally behaves as though it were deficient in fibrin-stabilizing factor;[61,125,148] fibrin-stabilizing factor activity is normal in obstructive jaundice.[274] Whether the deficiency of fibrin-stabilizing factor in hepatic disease is due to decreased synthesis or to the effect of DIC is uncertain. Fibrin formed in the absence of fibrin-stabilizing factor is more readily lysed by plasmin than normal, covalently bound fibrin, presumably because the binding of α_2-antiplasmin to fibrin is impaired under these conditions, exaggerating the effect of plasmin. Conceivably, in some cases of fibrin-stabilizing-factor deficiency, this susceptibility renders fibrin clots more susceptible to fibrinolysis. Perhaps, when the defect is sufficiently severe, it contributes to the bleeding tendency of patients with hepatic disease.

ABNORMAL PLASMA FIBRINOLYTIC ACTIVITY

In 1914, Goodpasture[90] described an extraordinary phenomenon in patients with cirrhosis of the liver: their clotted blood reliquified upon incubation at 37°C. He ascribed the liquefaction to the digestion of fibrin by the plasma's intrinsic proteolytic activity. Goodpasture's studies have been confirmed many times.[19,58,68,122,197] When normal plasma is clotted by the addition of calcium or thrombin, the fibrin that forms may not lyse for many days, if at all; clots formed from the euglobulin (water-insoluble) fraction of normal plasma may dissolve within 6 to 8 hours. In contrast, in cirrhosis, fibrinolysis of clotted plasma may take place within a day or two and, of the clotted euglobulin fraction of plasma, much more rapidly than in normal euglobulin clots.

The pathogenesis of the increased rate of fibrinolysis in cirrhotic plasma is not clear. Fibrinolysis is mediated by the plasma proteolytic enzyme, plasmin, although it is possible that in whole blood, proteases released by blood cells may contribute to the dissolution of fibrin. Whatever the mechanism, it does not seem to be operative in most forms of acute hepatic disease, carcinoma of the liver, biliary cirrhosis, or obstructive jaundice, in which the rate of fibrinolysis of clotted plasma or its euglobulin fraction is not increased.[58,113,197,264] Indeed, total hepatectomy in experimental animals does not have to be associated with increased fibrinolytic activity,[40,64] although this observation is not universally accepted,[80,272] and, in the totally hepatectomized human subject, fibrinolysis is greatly accelerated.[272]

A variety of influences may be responsible for the enhanced rate of fibrinolysis in cirrhosis, none mutually exclusive. As Goodpasture[90] knew, the proteolytic enzyme responsible for the lysis of a clot, now called *plasmin,* is relatively inert in unclotted plasma. The formation of

plasmin from its precursor, plasminogen, is brought about by activators derived from tissues or intrinsic to the plasma itself. Activation of plasminogen appears to take place preferentially upon the surface of fibrin, to which this enzyme precursor is readily adsorbed. Activation is impeded by inhibitory agents in plasma and by the clearance of plasminogen activators by the liver. Once formed, plasmin is subject to inhibition by a congerie of plasma inhibitory agents, limiting the process of fibrinolysis.

Presumably, alterations of any of the components of this fibrinolytic system may be responsible for the rapid fibrinolysis characteristic of cirrhosis. Thus, fibrinolysis might be due to entrance into the bloodstream of excessive amounts of plasminogen activators. It is known, for example, that rapid fibrinolysis, as measured *in vitro,* may follow the parenteral injection of nicotinic acid, epinephrine, or vasopressin, as though these vasoactive agents released plasminogen activator from vascular endothelium and perhaps from other tissues. Perhaps the same mechanisms are responsible for the rapid fibrinolysis seen after a variety of stresses such as exercise, anxiety, childbirth, or surgical procedures.

Conceivably, too, the rapid fibrinolysis of cirrhotics may be due to ready access of tissue plasminogen activators into the bloodstream. Thus, tissue plasminogen activators of hepatic origin may contribute to fibrinolysis. Although Beaumont and colleagues[19] reported that extracts of normal liver prevent fibrinolysis, the cirrhotic liver is rich in an activator of plasminogen.[13a] If this agent were to enter the bloodstream, it might contribute to plasma fibrinolytic activity.

Another activator of plasminogen that has been described is protein C, a vitamin K–dependent protein. The importance of this agent in the pathogenesis of the increased rate of fibrinolysis observed *in vitro* in cirrhosis is not clear; its concentration in this disorder is decreased.[28,152] Further, the titer of the plasma inhibitor of protein C is only occasionally decreased in cirrhosis, as though a deficiency of this inhibitor did not contribute to accelerated fibrinolysis.[74]

Rapid fibrinolysis might also be the result of impaired clearance of plasminogen activators from the circulation by the diseased liver.[47,71] This may help to explain the fibrinolytic state noted in human subjects after total hepatectomy.[272]

Rapid fibrinolysis in cirrhosis does not appear to be due to the presence in plasma of excessive amounts of plasminogen, which, indeed, is usually found in decreased concentrations in hepatic disease.[9,189,200,257,264,281] The decreased concentration of plasminogen has been ascribed to decreased synthesis by the liver as well as to a shortening of its survival in the circulation.[244] The titer of plasminogen may be elevated in patients with primary biliary cirrhosis or obstruction of the common duct by stone, conditions in which rapid fibrinolysis is unusual.[38]

Rapid fibrinolysis might also ensue if there were impairment of the normal inhibition of the activation[8,20,104,175] or activity of plasmin. The chief inhibitor of plasmin in plasma, α_2-plasmin inhibitor, is reduced in titer in hepatic disease, at least in part because its synthesis is impaired.[11,12,119] Such a deficiency might contribute to enhanced fibrinolysis. Patients with a hereditary deficiency of α_2-plasmin inhibitor have a severe bleeding tendency, supporting this view.[10] Further, histidine-rich glycoprotein, which may normally interfere with the binding of plasminogen to fibrin and thus inhibit the formation of plasmin on the fibrin meshwork, is significantly reduced in cirrhosis, an alteration that may contribute to enhanced fibrinolysis.[138,218] As noted earlier, the concentration of antithrombin III, which contributes to the inhibition of plasmin in plasma, may be normal or diminished in liver disease. In contrast, the concentrations of α_2-macroglobulin[11,12,160] and α_1-antitrypsin[11,160] may be increased. Antithrombin III levels are peculiarly severely decreased in DIC seen in women with fatty liver of pregnancy.[137,166] In obstruction of the common duct by stone and in primary biliary cirrhosis, increased titers of α_1-antitrypsin, α_2-macroglobulin, and possibly antithrombin III have also been reported, whereas the concentration of α_2-plasmin inhibitor is normal.[12,38]

In the test tube, plasma inhibitors of plasmin appear to be less stable in cirrhotics than in normal individuals, their potency decreasing sharply at the same time that fibrinolysis occurs.[196] This early observation seems to be explained by Collen's[44] demonstration that the emergence of fibrinolysis is correlated with the disappearance of α_2-plasmin inhibitor, which is presumably neutralized by its inhibition of the first plasmin that forms.

Thus, the enhanced rate of fibrinolysis in cirrhosis appears to be the result of a series of biochemical changes. In the clinic, the determination that the "clot lysis time" is shortened in cirrhosis is interesting as a laboratory oddity, but its role in the pathogenesis of bleeding in affected patients is uncertain. Poller[185] has proposed its association with a common complication of cirrhosis, peptic ulceration. It is doubtful whether the observation of fibrinolytic phenomena serves either as a diagnostic aid or as an explanation for the hemorrhagic tendency of most patients with cirrhosis of the liver. A short clot-lysis time of the degree found in cirrhosis is found after many stresses, unaccompanied by a bleeding tendency. If the fibrinolysis were to occur in vivo in cirrhosis, the impairment of coagulation by the products of digestion might aggravate a pre-existing bleeding tendency. Such products have been demonstrated in the plasma or serum of some but not all cirrhotics.[70,158,173,257,258]

The question must be raised whether bleeding from esophageal varices is exaggerated by lysis of clots that form within the ruptured vessels. Data concerning this possibility are not yet available. If fibrinolysis were of importance in this situation, therapy with ϵ-aminocaproic acid, which inhibits the activation and action of plasmin, might seem in order. But Lewis and Doyle[133] noted no improvement in hemostatic function in patients treated with 10 g of this drug daily, and one of their patients died of gastrointestinal hemorrhage after a day of therapy. Similarly, therapy of patients with cirrhosis with tranexamic acid, another inhibitor of the activation of plasminogen, was unimpressive.[262]

Fibrinolytic purpura, that is, a bleeding state induced by excessive fibrinolysis, has been described in a few patients with hepatic disease,[19,254,263] but it is rare and, when it occurs, may be secondary to intravascular coagulation.[19] If fibrinolysis is thought to be the primary process, ϵ-aminocaproic acid may be beneficial, but, if fibrinolysis is secondary to intravascular coagulation, attempts to inhibit it are probably contraindicated.

Grossi, Rousselot, and Panke[95] were impressed with the frequency with which portasystemic shunts led to increased fibrinolytic activity in patients with cirrhosis. Excessive fibrinolysis was usually detectable more readily in portal than systemic venous blood. These investigators believed that the intravenous injection of 4 g of ϵ-aminocaproic acid reduced capillary bleeding during surgery and that this agent also helped to control systemic hemorrhage in the weeks after surgery.[96] The dosage used suggests that little benefit derived from this therapy.

OTHER COAGULATIVE PROBLEMS IN HEPATIC DISEASE

Each of the four clotting factors that are involved in the surface-mediated generation of activated PTA—Hageman factor, plasma prekallikrein, high-molecular–weight kininogen, and PTA—is probably synthesized in the liver, given that the concentrations are reduced in patients with cirrhosis.[62,102,168,214–216] Hageman factor synthesis has been demonstrated in isolated rat liver preparations.[220] Hereditary solitary deficiencies of Hageman factor, prekallikrein, and high-molecular–weight kininogen are not usually accompanied by a significant bleeding tendency, whereas PTA deficiency is associated with hemorrhagic symptoms that vary from patient to patient but are usually mild. To what extent the additional burden of deficiencies of these factors contributes to the hemostatic problems of patients with hepatic disease is not known. Presumably, these would be corrected by transfusion of blood or plasma.

Antihemophilic factor activity, as measured in clotting assays (factor VIII:C) is usually normal or even elevated in patients with hepatitis, cirrhosis, primary hepatocellular carcinoma, or metastatic hepatic disease.[69,157,195,248,264,287] In decompensated cirrhosis, the coagulant titer of antihemophilic factor may be greatly elevated; the concentration of antigens detected by heterologous antiserum against this factor (factor VIIIR:Ag) is also strikingly increased, often disproportionately more than coagulant activity.[92] On cross-immunoelectrophoresis, the antihemophilic factor–like antigens appear to be more heterogeneous than normal, and the capacity of plasma to enhance ristocetin-induced platelet agglutination (factor VIIIR:Co) may be increased.[147] Agglutination of platelets by ristocetin is said to be impaired in some cases of hepatic disease, a defect localized to the platelets and attributed to deficiency of glycoprotein I.[179,205] The mechanisms responsible for the rise in antihemophilic factor titer in hepatic disease are not known beyond the vague view that this complex protein is an acute phase reactant. Alternatively, perhaps the increased titer is due to decreased catabolism of this protein by the liver.[236] The high titer of antihemophilic factor may account for the reported increase in platelet adhesiveness to glass in hepatic diseases.[124]

Little attention has been paid to defects in blood coagulation in patients with metastatic liver disease. In one series, no striking abnormalities were found; the concentration of fibrinogen was invariably elevated, and antithrombin III levels were moderately depressed in those with extensive hepatic involvement.[211]

PLATELET ABNORMALITIES

Portal hypertension is a common result of cirrhosis of the liver and may sometimes accompany other forms of hepatic disease. Patients in whom the portal pressure is elevated may bleed as the result of rupture of distended collateral veins, particularly esophageal varices. In these individuals, the immediate cause of bleeding is the mechanical break in the vascular wall. The extent to which defects in hemostatic mechanisms contribute to bleeding has not been clarified, but, presumably, it varies from patient to patient.

Portal hypertension may result in thrombocytopenia, an association emphasized by Rosenthal in 1928.[207] A significantly low platelet count is common in cirrhosis and in primary hepatocellular carcinoma. In one series, for example, 53 of 119 patients with alcoholic cirrhosis had platelet counts below 100,000/μl.[132] On the average, however, the decline in platelet count in severe but stable cirrhosis is modest.[244] Gastrointestinal hemorrhage is probably more the result of increased portal pressure than of coincident thrombocytopenia. In none of the cirrhotic patients studied by Desforges, Bigelow, and Chalmers[59] did thrombocytopenia appear to be responsible for the continuation of massive gastrointestinal bleeding.

The pathogenesis of thrombocytopenia in portal hypertension has been disputed. Megakaryocytes are in the marrow in normal or increased numbers.[144] One hypothesis proposed suggests that the diseased spleen removes platelets from the circulation at an excessive rate or so alters them that they are removed from the circulation prematurely. This view is in accord with data suggesting that the life span of platelets in congestive splenomegaly is sometimes shortened,[41] a change not corrected by treatment with heparin.[244] Thrombocytopenia is more likely the direct consequence of the congestive splenomegaly associated with portal hypertension. Normally, about one third of platelets are sequestered within the spleen. When the spleen is enlarged, as in portal hypertension, a larger proportion of platelets may be found within the spleen, reducing the number present in the peripheral circulation.[13,155] In agreement with this view, the life span of platelets in patients with congestive splenomegaly may be normal,[13,49,81,204] and the proportion of platelets sequestered within the spleen but returned to the circulation upon stimulation by epinephrine is increased.[29] Cohen, Gardner, and Barnett[41] reported that platelet production may also be diminished, but more recent studies suggest that in severe but stable cirrhosis, platelet production may be significantly increased.[41] Agglutinins directed against platelets have been described in patients with cirrhosis, whether or not thrombocytopenia is present. There is no evidence that these agglutinins are antibodies directed against platelets or that the agglutinins contribute to the development of thrombocytopenia. Techniques other than agglutination for the demonstration of antiplatelet antibodies have given negative results in patients with portal hypertension.[117]

The thrombocytopenia of portal hypertension is seldom severe enough to be the sole cause of a generalized bleeding tendency. When, however, the platelet count is less than 100,000/μl, the question of whether splenectomy should be performed is certain to arise.[259] Unquestionably, splenectomy is often followed by a rise in the platelet count and amelioration of hemorrhagic phenomena. A proper concern, however, is whether such a procedure should not be combined with splenorenal anastomosis in an attempt to relieve the underlying portal hypertension. Interestingly, portacaval anastomosis without splenectomy is sometimes followed by a rise in the platelet count.[249] If surgery is contemplated in patients with severe thrombocytopenia, the transfusion of platelet concentrates just before and during the operation may help to minimize bleeding.

A rare complication of splenectomy in portal hypertension is worth noting because of its perplexing nature. I have observed the development of thrombocythemia, that is, platelet counts above 800,000/μl, after splenectomy in two patients and once in a patient with extrahepatic portal hypertension. Somewhat similar cases have been described.[37,73] The pathogenesis of the thrombocythemia is unknown, and even more puzzling is the fact that serious bleeding phenomena, notably epistaxes, may occur. The proper course of treatment in the thrombocythemia observed in this situation is not clear; in other situations, marrow depressants have been given. A more modest thrombocytosis, of no apparent significance, is seen in some patients with hepatocellular carcinoma or juvenile hepatoblastoma.[171,228,264]

Other causes of thrombocytopenia in cirrhosis of the liver must be considered. Treatment of severe bleeding from esophageal varices may entail the transfusion of many liters of blood over a short period of time. Under these circumstances, a generalized bleeding tendency may supervene. Although the pathogenesis of this complication is complex, a major element is the appearance of thrombocytopenia.[121] Presumably, in such cases, platelets lost through bleeding are not restored by the transfused blood, which, under ordinary conditions of storage, is depleted of viable platelets. Antihemophilic factor and proaccelerin are also deficient in stored blood, compounding the difficulty. The only known prophylaxis for the hemorrhagic state that arises from massive transfusion is the use of blood drawn with minimal trauma and transfused as soon as possible.[66,69] Unfortunately, the volume needed too often necessitates the use of stored blood. One pragmatic solution is the transfusion of packed cells, platelet concentrates, and fresh frozen plasma.

In some patients with Laennec's cirrhosis, thrombocytopenia may be due to a concomitant deficiency of folic acid rather than to portal hypertension.[107] In such persons, the thrombocytopenia may respond to folic acid therapy. A dosage as small as 0.2 mg/day administered orally or intramuscularly is probably adequate to correct the deficiency. Whether the deficiency of folic acid is due to an inadequate dietary supply of this substance or to a defect in its metabolism is not certain.

Another cause of thrombocytopenia in patients with cirrhosis is alcoholism. Heavy ingestion of alcoholic beverages often results in a sharp decrease in the platelet count, which may be severe enough to induce hemorrhagic phenomena.[139,181] The thrombocytopenia is not associated with either folic acid or vitamin B_{12} deficiency, from which it must be distinguished. The syndrome can be reproduced by the ingestion[140] or intravenous infusion[188] of ethanol. Thrombocytopenia appears to be due both to suppression of platelet formation by megakaryocytes and to a decrease in the life span of platelets, for which new formation of platelets cannot compensate adequately.[53,54,213,250] Those platelets that reach the peripheral circulation may display multiple anatomic and functional abnormalities including impaired aggregation by collagen, thrombin, adenosine diphosphate, and epinephrine.[54,103]

Thrombocytopenia is occasionally seen in acute infectious hepatitis.[6,282] in which its pathogenesis is obscure. Perhaps, in some instances, thrombocytopenia is a manifestation of DIC[191] and, in other cases, reflects the presence of antiplatelet antibodies.[117] Rarely, congestive splenomegaly may be a factor,[164] whereas in other cases, particularly those of non-A, non-B hepatitis, thrombocytopenia is part of a pancytopenia or frank aplastic anemia.[208,209] No therapy is available for correcting the thrombocytopenia of infectious hepatitis; the efficacy of steroids is uncertain.[35,98]

An instance of lethal acute thrombotic thrombocytopenic purpura has been reported in a patient with alcoholic Laennec's cirrhosis.[169]

The suggestion has been made that platelets are qualitatively defective in hepatic disease.[31,52,57,149,179,181] Qualitative platelet abnormalities are said to be particularly prominent in fulminant hepatic failure and are thought to contribute in this condition to the development of hypotension during hemoperfusion through activated charcoal, a complication that may be averted by concomitant infusion of prostacyclin (PGI_2).[86,210,278] One biochemical defect that has been described in hepatic disease is a deficiency of glycoprotein I in the platelet membrane.[179] In

patients with "hypersplenism," most of whom had chronic active hepatitis or Laennec's cirrhosis, the volume of individual platelets was often significantly below normal.[116] Thomas and colleagues[258] found that in patients with Laennec's cirrhosis, the aggregation of platelets, normally induced *in vitro* by the addition of ADP or thrombin, was delayed in those patients in whom the thrombin time was prolonged. These investigators attributed the delay to the presence in plasma of abnormal fibrinogen breakdown products, secondary to excessive fibrinolysis. Although this may be true, it must be recalled that the long thrombin time in cirrhosis has many possible causes. Further, the significance of this observation is lessened by a recent report that platelet aggregation by ADP, collagen, and epinephrine was normal in a large group of patients with severe but stable cirrhosis.[244] Thomas[256] has also delineated a group of cirrhotics whose platelet-poor plasma accelerated aggregation of normal platelets, an action ascribed to the presence of fibrin monomers in the abnormal plasma. Whether this observation has pragmatic significance remains to be determined; impaired aggregation of platelets of cirrhotic patients by ADP has been related to a lengthening of the bleeding time, suggesting that this phenomenon may enhance their hemorrhagic tendency.[16]

NEEDLE BIOPSY OF THE LIVER

A frequent question asked concerns the safety of needle biopsy of the liver when there are the hemostatic defects so common in patients with hepatic disease. Sherlock's[232] cautions seem sound. She suggests that needle puncture not be performed if the prothrombin time is more than 3 seconds longer than that of control plasma or if the platelet count is less than 80,000/μl. If examination of liver tissue is imperative, transient correction of the hemostatic defect by the transfusion of 1 liter of fresh frozen plasma and, if indicated, by the transfusion of platelets may be attempted. The use of concentrates of the vitamin K–dependent factors should be avoided for the reason stated previously. Better still, if at all feasible, open biopsy, perhaps through a peritoneoscope, may make possible local control of abnormal bleeding.

LIVER TRANSPLANTATION

During hepatic transplantation, pronounced changes in the clotting and fibrinolytic systems take place. The titers of the plasma clotting factors fall, particularly during the anhepatic phase of the procedure, and may reach levels that impair hemostasis. The fall in the titer of coagulant antihemophilic factor (factor VIII:C) may be especially impressive.[135] Additionally, the platelet count may fall, and there is a transient increase in plasma fibrinolytic activity that is believed to contribute to the bleeding tendency.[27,135] The changes described have been ascribed to DIC induced, perhaps, by activation of clotting factors during the operative procedure, combined with impaired clearance of activated clotting factors in the absence of the liver.[27] Enhanced fibrinolysis may be secondary to DIC, but it is also likely to be the result of the release of tissue plasminogen activators during surgery that cannot be cleared until the new liver is in place. In earlier days, the bleeding tendency during the anhepatic phase was exacerbated by heparin that was used to prevent clotting in the donor liver before transplantation, but this is now avoided.[241] Attempts to control fibrinolysis by the administration of such antifibrinolytic agents as ε-aminocaproic acid are best avoided, because their use has led to severe thrombotic complications.[241] Once the circulation to the donor liver is established, excessive fibrinolysis is no longer detected.[112,135]

Hemorrhagic complications were originally a major problem during the first week after liver transplantation, but current experience suggests that this is now rarely a critical problem.[111,206,242] Among 100 consecutive patients in whom liver transplantation was performed, 3 who had abnormally small portal veins died of hemorrhage during attempts to obtain adequate portal flow from the confluence of the splenic and superior mesenteric veins.[112] Another patient developed a leak from choledochojejunostomy and bled fatally during an attempt to drain an abscess at the hepatic hilum and to reconstruct the biliary system. A fifth patient developed hematobilia from a mycotic aneurysm of the hepatic artery; the artery was repaired with a homograft that subsequently ruptured, resulting in lethal hemorrhage. Reviewing these cases, one is impressed that bleeding was mechanical in each instance rather than the result of failure of hemostatic mechanisms.

This chapter has stressed the complex origin of the hemorrhagic tendency seen in some patients with hepatic disease. Not all the defects described are susceptible to treatment, but effective therapy, to the extent that it is available, is based on a rational analysis of the pathogenesis of bleeding in each individual patient.

REFERENCES

1. Alagille D, Soulier JP: Action des enzymes protéolytiques sur le sang total "in vitro"; modifications des facteurs de coagulation et du complément. Sem Hôp Paris 32:355, 1956
2. Aledort LM: Blood clotting abnormalities in liver disease. In Popper VH, Schaffner F (eds): Progress in Liver Diseases, p 350. New York, Grune & Stratton, 1976
3. Anker E et al: Low antithrombin in severe disease: Consumption or decreased synthesis? Scand J Haematol 30: Suppl 39:59, 1983
4. Almersjö O et al: The coagulation defect after extensive liver resection in man. Scand J Gastroenterol 2:204, 1967
5. Almersjö O et al: Changes in coagulation factors after hepatic dearteriolization in man. Am J Surg 116:414, 1968
6. Alt HL, Swank RL: Thrombocytopenic purpura associated with catarrhal jaundice: Report of a case. Ann Intern Med 10:1049, 1937
7. Amris A, Amris CJ: Turnover and distribution of [131]iodine-labeled human fibrinogen. Thromb Diath Haemorrh 11:404, 1964
8. Aoki N, von Kaulla KN: Human serum plasminogen antiactivator: Its distinction from antiplasmin. Am J Physiol 220:1137,1971
9. Aoki N et al: Abnormal plasminogen. A hereditary molecular abnormality found in a patient with recurrent thrombosis. J Clin Invest 61:1186, 1978
10. Aoki N et al: Congenital deficiency of α₂-plasmin inhibitor associated with severe hemorrhagic tendency. J Clin Invest 63:877, 1979
11. Aoki N, Yamanaka T: The α₂-plasmin inhibitor levels in liver disease. Clin Chim Acta 84:99, 1978
12. Arman R et al: Natural protease inhibitors to fibrinolysis in liver diseases. Hepatogastroenterology 27:254, 1980
13. Aster RH: Pooling of platelets in the spleen: Role in the pathogenesis of "hypersplenic" thrombocytopenia. J Clin Invest 45:645, 1966
13a. Astrup T et al: Fibrinolytic activity of cirrhotic liver. Nature 185:619, 1960
14. Auslander MO, Gitnick GL: Vigorous medical treatment of acute fulminant hepatitis. Arch Intern Med 137:599, 1977
15. Babior BM: The role of vitamin K in clotting factor synthesis. I. Evidence for the participation of vitamin K in the conversion of a polypeptide precursor to factor VII. Biochim Biophys Acta 123:606, 1966
16. Ballard HS, Marcus AJ: Platelet aggregation in portal cirrhosis. Arch Intern Med 136:316, 1976
17. Blatt P, Roberts HR: Letter: Prothrombin-complex concentrates in liver disease. Lancet 2:189, 1975
18. Barnhart MI: Cellular site for prothrombin synthesis. Am J Physiol 199:360, 1960
19. Beaumont JL et al: Research on the spontaneous fibrinolytic activity of the plasma in liver cirrhosis. Rev Franc Etud Clin Biol 1:667, 1956
20. Bennett NB: A method for the quantitative assay of inhibitor of plasminogen activation in human serum. Thromb Diath Haemorrh 17:12, 1967
21. Bergström K et al: Studies on the plasma fibrinolytic activity in a case of liver cirrhosis. Acta Med Scand 168:291, 1960
22. Bertaglia E et al: Bleeding in cirrhotic patients: A precipitating factor due to intravascular coagulation or to hepatic failure? Haemostasis 13:328, 1983
23. Bick RL: Clinical relevance of antithrombin III. Semin Thromb Hemost 8:276, 1982
24. Bidwell E et al: The preparation for therapeutic use of a concentrate of Factor IX containing also Factors II, VII, and X. Br J Hematol 13:568, 1967
25. Blanchard RA et al: Acquired vitamin K–dependent carboxylation deficiency in liver disease. N Engl J Med 305:242, 1981
26. Blombäck B et al: Turnover of ^{131}I-labeled fibrinogen in man. Acta Med Scand 179:557, 1966
27. Bohmig HJ: The coagulation disorder in orthoptic hepatic transplantation. Thromb Haemost (abstr) 4:57, 1977
28. Boyer C et al: Dosage immunologique de la protein C. Variations en pathologie. Nouv Rev Fr Hématol 26:120, 1984
29. Branehög I et al: The exchangeable splenic platelet pool studied with epinephrine infusion in idiopathic thrombocytopenic purpura and in patients with splenomegaly. Br J Hematol 25:239, 1973

30. Braunstein KM et al: Regulation of the thrombin time in cirrhosis. Thromb Res 9:309, 1976

31. Breddin K: Hämorrhagische Diathesen bei Lebererkrankungen unter besonderer Berücksichtigung der Thrombocytenfunktion. Acta Haematol 27:1, 1962

32. Budd G: On Diseases of the Liver. Philadelphia, Lea & Blanchard, 1846

33. Bull BS et al: Microangiopathic haemolytic anaemia: Mechanisms of red-cell fragmentation. In vitro studies. Br J Hematol 14:643, 1968

34. Butt HR et al: The use of vitamin K and bile in treatment of the hemorrhagic diathesis in cases of jaundice. Proc Staff Mayo Clin 13:74, 1938

35. Camitta BM et al: Posthepatic severe aplastic anemia: An indication for early marrow transplantation. Blood 43:473, 1974

36. Cano RI et al: Acute fatty liver of pregnancy. Complication by disseminated intravascular coagulation. JAMA 231:159, 1975

37. Case Reports Massachusetts General Hospital. N Engl J Med 280:1113, 1969

38. Cederblad G et al: Observations of increased levels of blood coagulation factors and other plasma proteins in obstructive jaundice. Scand J Gastroenterol 11:391, 1976

39. Cerveny TJ et al: Synthesis of coagulation factor V by cultured aortic endothelium. Blood 63:1467, 1984

40. Clay RC, Ratnoff OD: Modified one-stage hepatectomy in the dog, with some notes on the effect of hepatectomy on the coagulability and proteolytic activity of the blood. Bull Johns Hopkins Hosp 88:457, 1951

41. Cohen P et al: Reclassification of the thrombocytopenias by the Cr^{51}-labeling method for measuring platelet life span. N Engl J Med 264:1294, 1961

42. Coleman M et al: Fibrinogen survival in cirrhosis: Improvement by "low-dose" heparin. Ann Intern Med 83:79, 1975

43. Collen D: Identification and some properties of a new fast-reacting plasmin inhibitor in human plasma. Eur J Biochem 69:209, 1976

44. Collen D: On the regulation and control of fibrinolysis. Thromb Haemost 43:77, 1980

45. Collen D: Intravascular coagulation in liver disease. In Fondu P, Thijs O (eds): Haemostatic Failure in Liver Disease, pp 44–51. Boston, Martinus Nijhoff, 1984

46. Collen D et al: Turnover of radiolabeled plasminogen and prothrombin in cirrhosis of the liver. Eur J Clin Invest 8:185, 1978

47. Comp PC et al: A lysine-adsorbable plasminogen activator is elevated in conditions associated with increased fibrinolytic activity. J Lab Clin Med 97:637, 1981

48. Conley CL et al: Circulating anticoagulants: Technique for their detection and clinical studies. Bull Johns Hopkins Hosp 84:255, 1949

49. Cooney DP, Smith BA: The pathophysiology of hypersplenic thrombocytopenia. Arch Intern Med 121:332, 1968

50. Corrigan JJ Jr, Earnest DL: Factor II antigen in liver disease and warfarin-induced vitamin K deficiency. Correlation with coagulant activity using Echis venom. Am J Hematol 8:249, 1980

51. Corrigan JJ et al: Prothrombin antigens and coagulant activity in patients with liver disease. JAMA 248:1736, 1982

52. Cortet P et al: Le facteur plaquettaire au cours des cirrhoses alcooliques. Étude de l'adhésivité in vivo par le test de Borchgrevink. Arch Mal Appar Dig 53:1041, 1964

53. Cowan DH: Thrombokinetic studies in alcohol-related thrombocytopenia. J Lab Clin Med 81:64, 1973

54. Cowan DH: Effect of alcoholism on hemostasis. Semin Hematol 17:137, 1980

55. Davey MG: The Survival and Destruction of Human Platelets. Basel, Switzerland S Karger, 1966

56. Davie EW, Ratnoff OD: Waterfall sequence for intrinsic blood clotting. Science 145:1310, 1964

57. De Nicola P: Liver and blood coagulation. Changes in blood coagulation factors in experimental liver injuries and hepatopathies. Acta Hepatosplen (Stuttg) 7:86, 1960

58. De Nicola P, Soardi F: Fibrinolysis in liver diseases: Study of 109 cases by means of the fibrin plate method. Thromb Diath Haemorrh (Stuttg) 2:290, 1958

59. Desforges JF et al: The effects of massive gastrointestinal hemorrhage on hemostasis. I. The blood platelets. J Lab Clin Med 43:501, 1954

60. Dettori AG et al: Impaired fibrin formation in advanced cirrhosis. Haemostasis 6:137, 1977

61. Deutsch E: Blood coagulative changes in liver diseases. In Popper H, Schaffner F (eds): Progress in Liver Diseases, pp 69–83. Grune & Stratton, New York, 1965

62. Deutsch E et al: Prekallikrein, HMW-kininogen, and factor XII in various disease states. Thromb Res 31:351, 1983

63. Donaldson VH: Effect of plasmin in vitro on clotting factors in plasma. J Lab Clin Med 56:644, 1960

64. Drapanas T et al: Studies of fibrinolytic activity after hepatectomy. Arch Surg 87:64, 1963

65. Dymock IW et al: Coagulation studies as a prognostic index in acute hepatic failure. Br J Hematol 29:385, 1975

66. Ebeling WC et al: Management of patients with portal hypertension undergoing venous-shunt surgery. N Engl J Med 254:141, 1956

67. Fair DS, Bahnak BL: Human hepatoma cells secrete single chain factor X, prothrombin, and antithrombin III. Blood 64:194, 1984

68. Fearnley R: Fibrinolysis. London, Edward Arnold & Co., 1965

69. Finkbiner RB et al: Coagulation defects in liver disease and response to transfusion during surgery. Am J Med 26:199, 1959

70. Fisher S et al: Immunoelectrophoretic characterization of plasma fibrinogen derivatives in patients with pathological plasma proteolysis. J Lab Clin Med 70:903, 1967

71. Fletcher AP et al: Abnormal plasminogen-plasmin system activity (fibrinolysis) in patients with hepatic cirrhosis: Its cause and consequences. J Clin Invest 43:681, 1964

72. Forman WB, Barnhart MI: Cellular site for fibrinogen synthesis. JAMA 187:128, 1964

73. Fountain JR, Losowsky MS: Haemorrhagic thrombocythaemia and its treatment with radioactive phosphorus. Q J Med 31:207, 1962

74. Francis RB Jr, Thomas W: Behavior of protein C inhibitor in intravascular coagulation and liver disease. Thromb Haemost 52:71, 1984

75. Franco D et al: Coagulation defects following peritoneovenous shunts. In Fondu P, Thijs O (eds): Haemostatic Failure in Liver Disease, pp 108–120. Boston, Martinus Nijhoff, 1984

76. Frerichs FT: Murchison C (trans): A Clinical Treatise on Diseases of the Liver. Baltimore, Wood, 1860

77. Frick PG et al: Dose response and minimal daily requirement for vitamin K in man. J Appl Physiol 23:387, 1967

78. Fulenwider JT et al: Endotoxemia of cirrhosis: An observation not substantiated. Gastroenterology 78:1001, 1980

79. Ganrot PO, Miléhn JE: Competition between plasmin and thrombin for α_2-macroglobulin. Clin Chim Acta 17:511, 1967

80. Gans H: Study of fibrinogen turnover rates after total hepatectomy in dogs. Surgery 55:544, 1964

81. Gehrmann G, Elbers C: Thrombopenisches Hyperspleniesyndrom bei splenomegaler Leberzirrhose. Dtsch Med Wochenschr 95:1429, 1970

82. Geill T: Die differentialdiagnostische Bedeutung des Fibringehaltes im Blut bei Leber und Gallenwegsleiden. Acta Med Scand (Suppl) 78:243, 1936

83. Giddings JC: Coagulation factors synthesis by the liver, with special reference to factor VIII and V. In Fondu P, Thijs O (eds): Haemostatic Failure in Liver Disease, pp 5–23. Boston, Martinus Nijhoff, 1984

84. Giddings JC et al: The immunological localization of factor V in human tissue. Br J Haematol 29:57, 1975

85. Giles AR et al: Changes in the coagulation status of patients undergoing autotransfusion of concentrated ascitic fluid as treatment of refractory ascites. (abstr) Blood (Suppl) 50:1, 267, 1977

86. Gimson AES et al: Prostacyclin to prevent platelet activation during charcoal hemoperfusion in fulminant hepatic failure. Lancet 1:173, 1980

87. Girolami A, Patrassi G, Capellato G, Quiano V: An immunological study of prothrombin in liver cirrhosis. Blut 41:61, 1980

88. Gitlin D, Biasucci A: Development of γ G, γ A, γ M, β IC/β IA, C'1 esterase inhibitor, ceruloplasmin, transferrin, hemopexin, haptoglobin, fibrinogen, plasminogen, alpha$_1$-antitrypsin, orosomucoid, beta-lipoprotein, alpha$_2$-macroglobulin, and prealbumin in the human conceptus. J Clin Invest 48:1433, 1969

89. Goodnight SH Jr et al: Factor VII antibody–neutralizing material in hereditary and acquired Factor VII deficiency. Blood 38:1, 1971

90. Goodpasture EW: Fibrinolysis in chronic hepatic insufficiency. Bull Johns Hopkins Hosp 25:330, 1914

91. Gralnick HR et al: Dysfibrinogenemia associated with hepatoma. Increased carbohydrate content of the fibrinogen molecule. N Engl J Med 299:221, 1978

92. Green A, Ratnoff OD: Elevated antihemophilic factor (AHF, Factor VIII) procoagulant activity and AHF-like antigen in alcoholic cirrhosis of the liver. J Lab Clin Med 83:189, 1974

93. Green G et al: Association of abnormal fibrin polymerization with severe liver disease. Gut 18:909, 1977

94. Gross L, Brotman M: Hypoprothrombinemia and hemorrhage associated with cholestyramine therapy. Ann Intern Med 72:95, 1970

95. Grossi CE et al: Coagulation defects in patients with cirrhosis of the liver undergoing portasystemic shunts. Am J Surg 104:512, 1962

96. Grossi CE et al: Hemorrhagic diatheses during and after portacaval shunts in patients with cirrhosis of the liver; their recognition and management. Am J Gastroenterol 41:117, 1964

97. Grün M et al: Regulation of fibrinogen synthesis in portal hypertension. Thromb Diath Haemorrh 32:292, 1974

98. Hagler L et al: Aplastic anemia following viral hepatitis: Report of two fatal cases and literature review. Medicine 54:139, 1975

99. Hallén A, Nilsson IM: Coagulation studies in liver disease. Thromb Diath Haemorrh (Stuttg) 11:51, 1964

100. Ham TH, Curtis FC: Plasma fibrinogen response in man. Influence of the nutritional state, induced hyperpyrexia, infectious disease, and liver damage. Medicine 17:413, 1938

101. Hammerschmidt DE, Moldow CF: Impaired fibrin polymerization in viral hepatitis. Report of a case. Probable identity of the inhibitor with β_2-microglobulin. J Lab Clin Med 92:1002, 1978

102. Hathaway WE, Alsever J: The relation of "Fletcher factor" to factors XI and XII. Br J Haematol 18:161, 1970

103. Haut MJ, Cowan DH: The effect of ethanol on hemostatic properties of human platelets. Am J Med 56:22, 1974

104. Hedner U: Studies on an inhibitor of plasminogen activation in human serum. Thromb Diath Haemorrh 30:414, 1973

105. Hellgren M et al: Antithrombin-III concentrate as adjuvant in DIC treatment. A pilot study in 9 severely ill patients. Thromb Rev 35:459, 1984

106. Hensen A, Loeliger EA: Antithrombin III: Its metabolism and its function in blood coagulation. Thromb Diath Haemorrh (Stuttg) (Suppl) 9:1, 1963

107. Herbert V: Hematopoietic factors in liver diseases. In Popper H, Schaffner F (eds): Progress in Liver Disease, p 257. New York, Grune & Stratton, 1965

108. Hiller EJ et al: Hypercoagulability in acute variceal bleeding. Thromb Res 22:243, 1981

109. Hollander D: Intestinal absorption of vitamins A, E, D, and K. J Lab Clin Med 97:449, 1981

110. Innerfield I et al: Plasma antithrombin titer in incipient and advanced liver failure. Gastroenterology 20:417, 1952

111. Iwatsuki S et al: Experience with 150 liver resections. Ann Surg 197:247, 1983

112. Iwatsuki S et al: Current status of hepatic transplantation. Semin Liver Dis 3:173, 1983

113. Jedrychowski A et al: Fibrinolysis in cholestatic jaundice. Br Med J 1:640, 1973

114. Jim RTS: A study of the plasma thrombin time. J Lab Clin Med 50:45, 1957

115. Johannson SA: Studies on blood coagulation factors in a case of liver cirrhosis; remission of the hemorrhagic tendency on treatment with heparin. Acta Med Scand 175:177, 1964

116. Karpatkin S, Freedman ML: Hypersplenic thrombocytopenia differentiated from increased peripheral destruction by platelet volume. Ann Intern Med 89:200, 1978

117. Karpatkin S et al: Cumulative experience in the detection of antiplatelet antibody in 234 patients with idiopathic thrombocytopenic purpura, systemic lupus erythematosus, and other clinical disorders. Am J Med 52:776, 1972

118. Kasper CK: Clinical use of factor IX concentrates: Thromboembolic complications. Thromb Diath Hemorrh 33:640, 1975

119. Knot EAR: α_2-Plasmin inhibitor metabolism in patients with liver cirrhosis. J Lab Clin Med 105, 353, 1985

120. Knowles, BB et al: Human hepatocellular carcinoma cell lines secrete the major plasma proteins and hepatitis B surface antigen. Science 209:497, 1980

121. Krevans JR, Jackson DP: Hemorrhagic disorder following massive whole blood transfusions. JAMA 159:171, 1955

122. Kwaan HC et al: Plasma fibrinolytic activity in cirrhosis of the liver. Lancet 1:132, 1956

123. Lane DA et al: Acquired dysfibrinogenemia in acute and chronic liver disease. Br J Hematol 35:301, 1977

124. Langley P et al: Platelet adhesiveness to glass in liver disease. Acta Haematol 67:124, 1982

125. Lechner K et al: Coagulation abnormalities in liver disease. Semin Thromb Haemost 4:40, 1977

126. Lee L, McCluskey RT: Immunohistochemical demonstration of the reticuloendothelial clearance of circulating fibrin aggregates. J Exp Med 116:611, 1962

127. Lee S et al: Factor IX deficiency in liver disease. JAMA 221:1410, 1972

128. LeQuesne LP: Choledocholithiasis. In Smith R, Sherlock S (eds): Surgery of the Gall Bladder and Bile Ducts. London, Butterworth & Co, 1964

129. Lerner RG et al: Intravascular coagulation complicating peritoneal-atrial shunts (abstr) Blood (Suppl) 50:1, 274, 1977

130. Lerner RG et al: Disseminated intravascular coagulation. Complication of LeVeen peritoneovenous shunts. JAMA 240:2064, 1978

131. Levin J, Conley CL: Thrombocytosis associated with malignant disease. Arch Intern Med 114:497, 1964

132. Levrat M, Truchot R: Le role de la thrombopénie dans les hémorragies des cirrhoses du foie. Arch Mal Appar Dig 51: 1394, 1962

133. Lewis JH, Doyle AP: Effects of epsilon aminocaproic acid on coagulation and fibrinolytic mechanisms. JAMA 188: 56, 1964

134. Lewis JH et al: Thrombin formation. II. Effects of lysin (fibrinolysin, plasmin) on prothrombin, Ac-globulin and tissue thromboplastin. J Clin Invest 28:1507, 1949

135. Lewis JH et al: Liver transplantation: Intraoperative coagulation findings. Blood 62:276a, 1983

136. Lian C et al: Valeur séméiologique du dosage pondéral de la fibrinémie dans les affections hépatiques. Bull Soc Med Paris 52:603, 1936

137. Liebman JA et al: Severe depression of antithrombin III associated with disseminated intravascular coagulation in women with fatty liver of pregnancy. Ann Intern Med 98: 330, 1983

138. Lijnen HR et al: Histidine-rich glycoprotein in a normal and a clinical population. Thromb Res 22:519, 1981

139. Lindenbaum J, Hargrove RL: Thrombocytopenia in alcoholics. Ann Intern Med 68:526, 1968

140. Lindenbaum J, Lieber CS: Hematologic effects of alcohol in man in the absence of nutritional deficiency. N Engl J Med 281:333, 1969

141. Lipinski B et al: Soluble unclottable complexes formed in the presence of fibrinogen degradation products (FDP) during the fibrinogen–fibrin conversion and their potential significance in pathology. Thromb Diath Haemorrh (Stuttg) 17:65, 1967

142. Lipinski B et al: Abnormal fibrinogen heterogeneity and fibrinolytic activity in advanced liver disease. J Lab Clin Med 90:187, 1977

143. Lord JW Jr, Andrus W deW: Differentiation of intrahepatic and extrahepatic jaundice. Response of the plasma prothrombin to intramuscular injection of menadione (2-methyl-1,4-naphthoquinone) as a diagnostic aid. Arch Intern Med 68:199, 1941

144. Lozner EL: Differential diagnosis, pathogenesis, and treatment of thrombocytopenic purpuras. Am J Med 14:459, 1953

145. Macfarlane RG: An enzyme cascade in the blood clotting mechanism, and its function as a biochemical amplifier. Nature 202:498, 1964

146. Magnuson S et al: Primary structure of the vitamin K–dependent part of prothrombin. FEBS Lett 44:189, 1974

147. Maisonneuve P, Sultan Y: Modification of factor VIII complex properties in patients with liver disease. J Clin Pathol 30:221, 1977

148. Mandel EE, Gerhold WM: Plasma fibrin-stabilizing factor: Acquired deficiency in various disorders. Am J Clin Pathol 52:547, 1969

149. Mandel EE, Lazerson J: Thrombasthenia in liver disease. N Engl J Med 265:56, 1961

150. Mann FD et al: Effect of removal of the liver on blood coagulation. Am J Physiol 164:111, 1951

151. Mann JD: Plasma prothrombin in viral hepatitis and hepatic cirrhosis; evaluation of the two-stage method in 75 cases. Gastroenterology 21:263, 1952

152. Mannucci PM, Vigano S: Deficiencies of protein C, an inhibitor of blood coagulation. Lancet 2:463, 1982

153. Marassi A et al: Letter: Thromboembolism following prothrombin complex concentrates and major surgery in severe liver disease. Thromb Haemost 39:787, 1978

154. Martinez J, Palascak JE: Hemostatic alterations in liver disease. In Zakim D, Boyer TD (eds): Hepatology. A Textbook of Liver Disease, pp 546–580. Philadelphia, WB Saunders, 1982

155. Martinez J et al: Abnormal sialic acid content of the dysfibrinogenemia associated with liver disease. J Clin Invest 61:535, 1978

156. Matsche JW et al: Fatal disseminated intravascular coagulation after peritoneovenous shunt for intractable ascites. Mayo Clin Proc 53:526, 1978

157. Meili EO, Straub PW: Elevation of factor VIII in acute fatal liver necrosis. Thromb Diath Haemorrh (Stuttg) 24: 161, 1966

158. Merskey C et al: Quantitative estimation of split products of fibrinogen in human serum, relation to diagnosis and treatment. Blood 28:1, 1966

159. Mester L, Szabados L: Structure défectuese et biosynthèse des fractions glucidiques dans les variantes pathologique du fibrinogène. Nouv Rev Fr Hématol 10:679, 1970

160. Miesch F et al: The α_2-antitrypsin and α_2-macroglobulin content and the protease-inhibitory capacity of normal and pathological sera. Clin Chim Acta 31:231, 1971

161. Miller LL, Bale WF: Synthesis of all plasma protein fractions except gamma globulins by the liver. The use of zone electrophoresis and lysine-ϵ-C^{14} to define the plasma proteins synthesized by the isolated perfused liver. J Exp Med 99: 125, 1954

162. Miller LL et al: The dominant role of the liver in plasma protein synthesis. A direct study of the isolated perfused rat liver with the aid of lysine-ϵ-C^{14}. J Exp Med 94:431, 1951

163. Minna JD et al: Disseminated Intravascular Coagulation in Man, p 160. Springfield, Charles C Thomas, 1974

164. Monteil R et al: Purpura thrombocytopénique au cours d'une hépatite virale. Hémostase 1:267, 1961

165. Morongiu F et al: α_2-Antiplasmin and fibrinopeptide A in liver cirrhosis. Haemostasis (abstr) 14:110, 1984

166. Mosvold J et al: Low antithrombin III in acute hepatic failure at term. Scand J Haematol 29:48, 1982

167. Munro FL et al: Changes in components A and B of prothrombin in dog following hepatectomy. Am J Physiol 145: 206, 1945

168. Naeye RL: Hemophilioid factors: Acquired deficiencies in several hemorrhagic states. Proc Soc Biol Med 94:623, 1957

169. Nally JV, Metz EN: Acute thrombotic thrombocytopenic purpura. Another cause for hemolytic anemia and thrombocytopenia in cirrhosis. Arch Intern Med 139:711, 1979

170. Ness PM, Perkins HA: Cryoprecipitate as a reliable source of fibrinogen replacement. JAMA 241:1690, 1979

171. Nickerson HJ et al: Hepatoblastoma, thrombocytosis, and increased thrombopoetin. Cancer 45:35, 1980

172. Niewiarowski S et al: Formation of highly ordered polymers from fibrinogen and fibrin degradation products. Biochim Biophys Acta 221:326, 1970

173. Niléhn JE, Nilsson IM: Demonstration of fibrinolytic split products in human serum by an immunologic method in spontaneous and induced fibrinolytic states. Scand J Haematol 1:313, 1964

174. Niléhn JE et al: Studies on blood clotting factors in man after massive liver resection. Acta Chir Scand 133:189, 1967

175. Nilsson IM et al: Severe thrombotic disease in a young man with bone marrow and skeletal changes and with a high content of an inhibitor in the fibrinolytic system. Acta Med Scand 169:323, 1961

176. Oka K, Tanaka K: Intravascular coagulation in autopsy cases with liver disease. Thromb Haemost 42:564, 1979

177. Olson JP et al: Synthesis of clotting factors by the isolated perfused rat liver. J Clin Invest 45:690, 1966

178. Olson RE: The mode of action of vitamin K. Nutr Rev 28: 171, 1970

179. Ordinas A et al: A glycoprotein defect in the platelets of three patients with severe cirrhosis of the liver. Thomb Res 13:297, 1978

180. Orlando M et al: Factor VII in liver cirrhosis. Haemostasis 11:73, 1982

181. Owen CA Jr et al: Platelet function and coagulation in patients with Wilson's disease. Arch Intern Med 136:148, 1976

182. Owren PA: Diagnostic and prognostic significance of plasma prothrombin and Factor V levels in parenchymatous hepatitic and obstructive jaundice. Scand J. Clin Invest 1: 131, 1949

183. Parbhoo SP et al: Treatment of ascites by continuous ultrafiltration and reinfusion of protein concentrate. Lancet 1:949, 1974

184. Phillips LL, Rodgers JB: Procoagulant activity of ascitic fluid in hepatic cirrhosis: In vivo and in vitro. Surgery 86: 714, 1979

185. Poller L: Coagulation abnormalities in liver disease. In Poller L (ed): Recent Advances in Blood Coagulation, No. 2, p 267. Edinburgh, Churchill Livingstone, 1977

186. Pool JG, Robinson J: In vitro synthesis of coagulation factors by rat liver slices. Am J Physiol 196:423, 1959

187. Post RM, Desforges JF: Thrombocytopenia and alcoholism. Ann Intern Med 68:1230, 1968

188. Post RH, Desforges JF: Thrombocytopenic effect of ethanol infusion. Blood 31:344, 1968

189. Purcell G Jr, Phillips LL: Fibrinolytic activity in cirrhosis of the liver. Surg Gynecol Obstet 117:1963

190. Quick AJ et al: Study of the coagulation defect in hemophilia and in jaundice. Am J Med Sci 190:501, 1935

191. Rake MO et al: Intravascular coagulation in acute hepatic necrosis. Lancet 1:533, 1970

192. Rake MO et al: Early and intensive therapy of intravascular coagulation in acute liver failure. Lancet 2:1215 1971

193. Ranhotra GS, Johnson BC: Vitamin K and the synthesis of factor VII–X by isolated rat liver cells. Proc Soc Exp Biol Med 132:509, 1969

194. Rapaport SI: Plasma thromboplastin antecedent levels in

195. Rapaport SI et al: Plasma clotting factors in chronic hepatocellular disease. N Engl J Med 263:278, 1960

196. Ratnoff OD: Studies on proteolytic enzyme in human plasma. III. Some factors controlling rate of fibrinolysis. J Exp Med 88:401, 1948

197. Ratnoff OD: Studies on proteolytic enzyme in human plasma. IV. The rate of lysis of plasma clots in normal and diseased individuals, with particular reference to hepatic disease. Bull Johns Hopkins Hosp 84:29, 1949

198. Ratnoff OD: An accelerating property of plasma for the coagulation of fibrinogen by thrombin. J Clin Invest 33: 1175, 1954

199. Ratnoff OD: The liver; three aspects of hepatic failure: Cholemia, ascites, and hemorrhagic phenomena. In Mellors RC (ed): Analytic Pathology, p 245. New York, McGraw-Hill, 1957

200. Ratnoff OD, Donaldson VH: Physiologic and pathologic effects of increased fibrinolytic activity in man: With notes on the effects of exercise and certain inhibitors of fibrinolysis. Am J Cardiol 6:378, 1960

201. Ratnoff OD, Patek AJ Jr: The natural history of Laennec's cirrhosis of the liver: An analysis of 386 cases. Medicine 21:207, 1942

202. Ratnoff OD, Patek AJ Jr: Postnecrotic cirrhosis of the liver. J Chron Dis 1:266, 1955

203. Reisner EH Jr et al: The effect of liver dysfunction on the response to Dicumarol. Am J Med Sci 217:445, 1949

204. Ries CA, Price DC: Platelet kinetics in thrombocytopenia. Correlation between splenic sequestration of platelets and response to splenectomy. Ann Intern Med 80:702, 1974

205. Rodés, J et al: Increased factor VIII complex and defective platelet aggregation in liver disease. Thromb Res 11:899, 1977

206. Rolles K et al: The Cambridge and King's College Hospital experience of liver transplantation, 1968–1983. Hepatology 4:505, 1984

207. Rosenthal N: The blood picture in purpura. J Lab Clin Med 13:303, 1927–28

208. Rosner F: Aplastic anemia and viral hepatitis. Lancet 2: 1080, 1970

209. Rubin E et al: Syndrome of hepatitis and aplastic anemia. Am J Med 45:88, 1968

210. Rubin MH et al: Abnormal platelet function and ultrastructure in fulminant hepatic failure. QJ Med NS 46:339, 1977

211. Rubin RN et al: Coagulation profiles in patients with metastatic liver disease (abstr). Blood 52:(Suppl 1) 193, 1978

212. Rutherford RB, Hardaway RM III: Significance of the rate of decrease in fibrinogen level after total hepatectomy in dogs. Ann Surg 163:51, 1966

213. Sahud MA: Platelet size and number in alcoholic thrombocytopenia. N Engl J Med 286:355, 1972

214. Saito H et al: Fitzgerald factor (high molecular weight kininogen) clotting activity in human plasma in health and disease in various animal plasmas. Blood 48:941, 1976

215. Saito H et al: Radioimmunoassay of human Hageman factor (factor XII). J Lab Clin Med 88:506, 1976

216. Saito H et al: Human plasma prekallikrein (Fletcher factor) clotting activity and antigen in health and disease. J Lab Clin Med 92:84, 1978

217. Saito H et al: Production and release of plasminogen by

patients receiving coumarin anticoagulants and in patients with Laennec's cirrhosis. Proc Soc Exp Biol Med 108:115, 1961

isolated perfused rat liver. Proc Natl Acad Sci USA 77: 6837, 1980

218. Saito H et al: Reduced histidine-rich glycoprotein levels in plasmas of patients with advanced liver cirrhosis. Possible implications for enhanced fibrinolysis. Am J Med 73:179, 1982

219. Saito H et al: Synthesis and secretion of α_2-plasmin inhibitor by established human cell lines. Proc Natl Acad Sci USA 79:5684, 1982

220. Saito H et al: Synthesis and release of Hageman factor (factor XII) by the isolated perfused rat liver. J Clin Invest 72:948, 1983

221. Salem HH et al: The aggregation of platelets by ascitic fluid: A possible mechanism for disseminated intravascular coagulation complicating LeVeen shunts. Am J Hematol 11: 153, 1981

222. Scanlon GH et al: Plasma prothrombin and the bleeding tendency; with special reference to jaundiced patients and vitamin K therapy. JAMA 112:1898, 1939

223. Schipper HG et al: Antithrombin-III transfusion in disseminated intravascular coagulation. Lancet 2:854, 1978

224. Schipper HG, ten Cate JW: Antithrombin III transfusion in patients with hepatic cirrhosis. Br J Hematol 52:25, 1982

225. Schwarts ML et al: Coagulopathy following peritoneous venous shunting. Surgery 85:671, 1979

226. Seligsohn U et al: Dubin-Johnson syndrome in Israel. II. Association with Factor-VII deficiency. Q J Med 39:569, 1970

227. Seligsohn U et al: Gilbert's syndrome and factor VII deficiency. Lancet 1:1398, 1970

228. Selroos O: Thrombocytosis. Acta Med Scand 193:431, 1973

229. Shainoff JR, Page IH: Significance of cryoprofibrin in fibrinogen–fibrin conversion. J Exp Med 116:687, 1962

230. Shaw E et al: Synthesis of procoagulant factor VIII, factor–VIII related antigen, and other coagulation factors by the isolated perfused rat liver. Br J Haematol 41:585, 1979

231. Sherlock SPV et al: Anticoagulants and the liver. In Pickering GW (ed): Proc Symp Anticoagulants. London, Harvey, 1960

232. Sherlock S: Diseases of the Liver and Biliary System, 6th ed, p 28. Oxford, Blackwell Scientific Publications, 1981

233. Shulman NR: Surgical care of patients with hereditary disorders of blood coagulation. In Ratnoff OD (ed): Treatment of Hemorrhagic Disorders, p 61. New York, Harper & Row, 1968

234. Sims JM: Remarks on cholecystotomy in dropsy of the gallbladder. Br Med J 1:811, 1878

235. Smith HP et al: Bleeding tendency and prothrombin deficiency in biliary fistula dogs: Effect of feeding bile and vitamin K. J Exp Med 67:911, 1938

236. Sodetz JM et al: Relation of sialic acid to function and *in vivo* survival of human factor VIII/von Willebrand factor protein. J Biol Chem 252:5538, 1977

237. Soria J, Soria C: Abnormalities of fibrin formation in severe hepatic disease. In Fondu P, Thijs O (eds): Haemostatic Failure in Liver Disease, pp 52–68. Boston, Martinus Nijhoff, 1984

238. Soria J et al: Dysfibrinogènémies acquise dans les atteintes hépatique sévères. Coagulation 3:37, 1970

239. Spector I, Corn M: Laboratory tests of hemostasis; the relation to hemorrhage in liver disease. Arch Intern Med 119: 577, 1967

240. Spector I et al: Effect of plasma transfusions on the pro-

thrombin time and clotting factors in liver disease. N Engl J Med 275:1032, 1966

241. Starzl TE et al: Analysis of liver transplantation. Hepatology, 4:475, 1984

242. Starzl TE et al: Fifteen years of clinical liver transplantation. Gastroenterology 77:375, 1979

243. Steigmann F et al: Vitamin K therapy in liver disease: Need for a reevaluation. Am J Gastroenterol 31:369, 1959

244. Stein SF, Harker LA: Kinetic and functional studies of platelets, fibrinogen, and plasminogen in patients with hepatic cirrhosis. J Lab Clin Med 99:217, 1982

245. Stenflo J et al: Vitamin K–dependent modification of glutamic acid residues in prothrombin. Proc Natl Acad Sci USA 71:2730, 1974

246. Straub PW: A study of fibrinogen production by human liver slices *in vitro* by an immunoprecipitin method. J Clin Invest 42:130, 1963

247. Straub PW: Diffuse intravascular coagulation in liver disease? Semin Thromb Haemost 4:29, 1977

248. Straub PW et al: Erhöhung des antihämophilen γ-globulins (Factor VIII) bei letaler Lebernekrose. Schweiz Med Wochenschr 96:1199, 1968

249. Sullivan BH Jr, Tumen HJ: Effect of portacaval shunt on thrombocytopenia associated with portal hypertension. Ann Intern Med 55:598, 1961

250. Sullivan LW et al: Induction of thrombocytopenia by thrombophoresis in man: Patterns of recovery in normal subjects during ethanol ingestion and abstinence. Blood 49:197, 1977

251. Suttie JW: Control of prothrombin and factor VII biosynthesis by vitamin K. Arch Biochem 118:166, 1967

252. Suttie JW: Mechanism of action of vitamin K: Demonstration of a liver precursor of prothrombin. Science 179: 192, 1973

253. Sykes EM Jr et al: Effect of acute liver damage on ac-globulin activity of plasma. Proc Soc Exp Biol Med 67:506, 1948

254. Tagnon TJ et al: Occurrence of fibrinolysis in shock, with observations on prothrombin time and plasma fibrinogen during hemorrhagic shock. Am J Med Sci 211:88, 1946

255. Tarao K et al: Detection of endotoxin in plasma and ascites fluid of patients with cirrhosis: Its clinical significance. Gastroenterology 73:539, 1977

256. Thomas DP: Abnormalities of platelet aggregation in patients with alcoholic cirrhosis. Ann NY Acad Sci 201:243, 1972

257. Thomas DP et al: A comparative study of four methods for detecting fibrinogen degradation products in patients with various diseases. N Engl J Med 283:663, 1970

258. Thomas DP et al: Platelet aggregation in patients with Laennec's cirrhosis of the liver. N Engl J Med 276:1344, 1967

259. Tocantins LM: The hemorrhagic tendency in congestive splenomegaly (Banti's syndrome); its mechanism and management. JAMA 136:616, 1948

260. Triantaphyllopoulos DC: Anticoagulant effect of incubated fibrinogen. Can J Biochem Physiol 36:249, 1958

261. Tytgat G et al: Investigations on the fibrinolytic system in liver cirrhosis. Acta Haematol 40:265, 1968

262. Tytgat GN et al: Metabolism of fibrinogen in cirrhosis of the liver. J Clin Invest 50:1690, 1971

263. Vachon A et al: Fibrinolyse hémorragique mortelle au cours d'une cirrhose avec ictère. Lyon Med 187:165, 1952

264. van der Walt JA et al: Hemostatic factors in primary hepatocellular carcinoma. Cancer 40:1593, 1977

265. van Imhoff GW et al: Bleeding during orthoptic liver transplantation in man. In Fondu P, Thijs O (eds): Haemostatic Failure in Liver Disease, pp 121–126. Boston, Martinus Nijhoff, 1984

266. van Vliet ACM et al: Plasma prekallikrein and endotoxemia in liver cirrhosis. Thromb Haemost 45:65, 1981

267. Verhaeghe R et al: Dysfibrinogenaemia associated with primary hepatoma. Scand J Haematol 9:451, 1972

268. Verstraete M et al: Excessive consumption of blood coagulation components as cause of hemorrhagic diathesis. Am J Med 38:899, 1965

269. Verstraete M et al: Intravascular coagulation in liver disease. Ann Rev Med 25:447, 1974

270. Volwiler W et al: Biosynthetic determination with radioactive sulfur of turn-over rates of various plasma proteins in normal and cirrhotic man. J Clin Invest 34:1126, 1955

271. von Felten A et al: Dysfibrinogenemia in a patient with primary hepatoma. N Engl J Med 280:405, 1969

272. von Kaulla KN et al: Changes in blood coagulation before and after hepatectomy or transplantation in dogs and man. Arch Surg 92:71, 1966

273. von Kaulla E, von Kaulla KN: Antithrombin III and its disorders. Am J Clin Pathol 48:69, 1967

274. Walls WD, Losowsky MS: The hemostatic defect of liver disease. Gastroenterology 60:108, 1971

275. Walls WD, Losowsky MS: Plasma fibrin stabilizing factor (FSF) activity in normal subjects and patients with chronic liver disease. Thromb Diath Haemorrh (Stuttg) 21:134, 1969

276. Wardle EN: Fibrinogen in liver disease. Arch Surg 109:741, 1974

277. Weinstein MJ, Deykin D: Quantitative abnormality of an Aα chain molecular weight form in the fibrinogen of cirrhotic patients. Br J Hematol 40:617, 1979

278. Weston MJ et al: Platelet function in fulminant hepatic failure and effect of charcoal hemoperfusion. Gut 18:897, 1979

279. Wilkinson SP et al: Relation of renal impairment and haemorrhagic diathesis to endotoxaemia in fulminant hepatic failure. Lancet 1:521 1974

280. Williams R, Crossley IR: Clinical manifestations of the hemostatic failure in acute and chronic liver disease. In Fondu P, Thijs O (eds): Haemostatic Failure in Liver Disease, pp 94–107. Boston, Martinus Nijhoff, 1984

281. Witte S, Dirnberger P: Über die Verlängerung der Profibrinolysinzeit bei Leberkrankheiten. Klin Wochenschr 33:931, 1955

282. Woodward TE: Thrombocytopenic purpura complicating acute catarrhal jaundice: Report of a case, review of the literature, and review of 48 cases of purpura at University Hospital. Ann Intern Med 19:799, 1943

283. Wu FC, Laskowski M: Crystalline acid-labile trypsin inhibitor from bovine blood plasma. J Biol Chem 235:1680, 1969

284. Wyke RJ et al: Transmission of non-A, non-B hepatitis to chimpanzees by factor-IX concentrates after fatal complications in patients with chronic liver disease. Lancet 1:520, 1979

285. Yanofsky RA et al: The multiple coagulopathies of biliary atresia. Am J Hematol 16:171, 1984

286. Zetterqvist E, von Francken I: Coagulation disturbances with manifest bleeding in extrahepatic portal hypertension and in liver cirrhosis. Preliminary results of heparin treatment. Acta Med Scand 173:753, 1963

287. Zetterqvist E, von Francken I: Koagulationsfaktoren vid levers-jukdom. Nord Med 69:81, 1963

288. Zuckerman IC et al: Studies in human biliary physiology. III. The effect of bile and vitamin K on experimentally produced hemorrhagic diathesis in a human with a total external biliary fistula. Am J Dig Dis 6:332, 1939

chapter 8
Jaundice: A Clinical Approach

LEON SCHIFF

Jaundice is indeed a mere symptom and, as we have seen, may occur in most diseases of the liver, but it is a symptom that is so striking and is such an important element in any case in which it may happen that a separate consideration of it is almost requisite.[10]

Jaundice, or icterus, is the condition recognized clinically by a yellowish discoloration of the plasma, the skin, and the mucous membranes caused by staining by bile pigment. It is often the first and sometimes the sole manifestation of liver disease. Frequently, it is detected best in the peripheral portions of the ocular conjunctivae; it can also be observed in the mucous membrane of the hard palate or in the lips when compressed with a glass slide. It may be overlooked in poor or artificial light. It may be preceded for a day or more by the passage of dark urine or light-colored stools. Its presence is usually first recognized by a family member or friend. Occasionally, attention is first directed to it by a laboratory report of "serum icteric." Icterus may be detected when the concentration of serum bilirubin exceeds 2 mg/100 ml.

The physician still faces the diagnostic challenge of whether jaundice in a given patient is "medical" or "surgical" in order to determine whether to use medical or surgical treatment. Surgery may prove hazardous in intrahepatic jaundice but curative or palliative when icterus is due to mechanical biliary obstruction.

In the differentiation of the various causes of jaundice, the physician should stress the clinical examination and laboratory tests and, if necessary, select one or more of such diagnostic procedures as abdominal ultrasonography, HIDA scan, percutaneous transhepatic cholangiography (PTC), endoscopic retrograde cholangiopancreatography (ERCP), and less frequently, computed tomography (CT). In cases in which a definitive diagnosis is not reached, the physician has recourse to needle biopsy of the liver with or without guidance by ultrasonography or CT, and in selected instances, guided fine needle aspiration or exploratory laparotomy.

In 1962, Steven Schenker, John Balint, and I[58] reported that a careful history, physical examination, and review of the standard liver chemistries in a group of jaundiced patients yielded a diagnostic accuracy of approximately 85%. Years later, a report by Lumeng and colleagues[42] not only confirmed these observations but also pointed out that the clinical examination was as efficient as individual diagnostic procedures in current use.[48,49,50,56-59,70]

ETIOLOGY AND PATHOGENESIS

"Listen to the patient; he will tell you what is wrong."
David Segal

The familial occurrence of icterus should suggest the possibilities of congenital hemolytic jaundice, Gilbert's syndrome, the Dubin-Johnson syndrome, Rotor's syndrome, or benign recurrent intrahepatic cholestasis. A history of consanguinity of parents should arouse suspicion of Wilson's disease. A history of allergic disorders may predispose to drug-induced liver injury.

Recent foreign travel with particular reference to areas of endemic hepatitis and to contact with jaundiced persons should arouse suspicion of viral hepatitis. A high index of suspicion of hepatitis should be held in homosexuals, drug addicts, patients undergoing hemodialysis and attendants in such units, and in clinical laboratory personnel. All medications that the patient has been taking should be brought in and listed, particularly anabolic steroids, oral contraceptives, thorazine, erythromycin estolate 30 isoniazid, methyldopa,[43] acetaminophen in doses of 4 g/day, and aspirin in doses sufficient to produce blood salicylate levels of greater than 15 mg/dl in patients with rheumatic fever, systemic lupus erythematosus, and juvenile rheumatoid arthritis.[73] Liver injury resulting from drugs may be indistinguishable from viral hepatitis, especially when caused by isoniazid or methyldopa, or it may present as cholestasis, especially following use of anabolic steroids, thorazine, or oral contraceptives. The clinician must guard against mistaking drug-induced cholestasis for extrahepatic obstructive jaundice.

Blood transfusions administered 2 weeks to 6 months prior to the onset of jaundice should lead to suspicion of post-transfusion hepatitis; the more blood used, the stronger the suspicion. The incidence is said to be six or seven times higher in recipients of commercial blood than volunteer blood. Hepatitis A is rarely transmitted by transfusion. As many as 90% of cases of post-transfusion hepatitis are of the non-A, non-B types, outbreaks of which have also been reported after the administration of blood clotting factors VIII and IX.

A history of alcoholism should always be sought, and in doubtful situations, an interview should be arranged with spouse, mistress, minister, golfing partner, or bartender. The importance of determining the alcoholic content of the urine has been advocated in assessing the patient's estimate of the quantity of alcohol consumption.[51] In young people, a history of alcoholism may detract from consideration of viral hepatitis. In older patients, the symptoms of anorexia, weakness, and weight loss (and the presence of hepatomegaly) may wrongly suggest a malignant tumor of the liver. On the other hand, a bout of alcoholic hepatitis with its acute abdominal pain, nausea and vomiting, fever, right upper abdominal tenderness, and leukocytosis may be mistaken for an acute surgical abdominal disorder. It is important to remember that nonalcoholic liver disease may simulate alcoholic hepatitis and cirrhosis.[44]

The physician should adopt a conservative attitude in cases of postoperative jaundice. If much blood accumulated in the peritoneal or pleural cavities and resulted in shock, anorexia, and liver damage and if much blood was transfused, the damaged liver is unable to excrete the increased bilirubin load, although it is able to conjugate it. The resulting cholestasis is not harmful *per se* and does not require specific therapy. In case of a cholecystectomy, accidental injury to the common bile duct should be suspected. If the duct has been ligated, jaundice will appear early; if it has been severed or incised, prolonged drainage of bile from the operative area will ensue, to be followed later by icterus and evidences of associated cholangitis.

Jaundice occurred in 23.4% of 154 adult patients having cardiac surgery. The jaundice was usually mild. The severity of right heart failure before operation and hypoxia, hypotension, and amount of blood used during and shortly after operation are factors contributing to the development of jaundice.[14]

If halothane was the anesthetic used and, particularly, if it had been administered in the past and was followed by unexplained fever, toxic hepatitis as a result of halothane must be strongly considered. The first exposure is likely to trigger symptoms after 7 days, whereas following multiple exposures, symptoms tend to appear in 3 days. It is of interest that children are relatively resistant to halothane hepatotoxicity.

Careful inquiry should be made regarding abdominal pain. It is usually improminent—more of a heavy or dragging sensation—in viral hepatitis, although occasionally it is severe enough to simulate gallstone colic.[54] In approximately 10% of elderly patients, common duct stone may be painless and may manifest itself many years after cholecystectomy for calculous cholecystitis. The stone may be residual or may have formed *de novo* in the bile duct. Glenn[29] believed that any calculus recognized within the biliary ductal system during a period of 1 year or less following surgery for calculous biliary tract disease is indeed a retained stone. A case of common duct stone has been reported with neither pain nor icterus, presenting itself as a fever of undetermined origin.[67] Jaundice may occur in acute cholecystitis in the absence of common duct stones.[20] It is believed to be primarily due to reduced excretion of bile, which may be caused by pressure on the ducts by the distended gallbladder.

The pain caused by pancreatic cancer is quite characteristic, as originally pointed out by Chauffard.[13] It is usually located in the upper abdomen or right upper quadrant and radiates to the back. It is worse in the recumbent position and is lessened by turning on either side, by assuming the prone position, or by sitting up and flexing the spine. It is usually severe and often requires an opiate, although aspirin at frequent intervals may provide relief. The pain, when accompanied by weakness, weight loss, pruritus, jaundice, and frequently hyperglycemia, warrants the strongest suspicion of pancreatic cancer and may provide the prime basis for diagnosis.

Tumors of the liver, both primary and metastatic, may present with abdominal pain, which may be dull or boring or sharp and usually localized to the right hypochondrium. The pain may radiate to the back, right infrascapular area, or right flank and may be increased by deep breathing, cough, exertion, or changes in posture. The pain is presumably due to invasion or stretching of the liver capsule by the neoplasm. Hemorrhage into a tumor may result in sudden severe pain. Rupture of the tumor may produce an acute catastrophic hemoperitoneum.

Although a history of chronic jaundice—recurrent or continuous—with chills, fever, and usually abdominal pain is generally indicative of common duct stones, it nevertheless warrants inspection for sclerosing carcinoma of the bile ducts, sclerosing cholangitis, especially in the presence of ulcerative colitis, and, much less commonly, congenital malformation of bile ducts, especially choledochal cyst and Caroli's disease. In patients with previous biliary tract surgery, iatrogenic stenosis (stricture) or a residual stone should be suspected. It is of interest that recurrent obstructive jaundice has been reported in cases of fibrolamellar hepatocellular carcinoma.[3]

Chills and fever do not usually occur in extrahepatic obstruction resulting from pancreatic tumor because the bile is not infected, in contrast to common duct stones. Chills and fever may be present during the preicteric phase of viral hepatitis and may occur in thorazine or other drug-induced liver injury, leptospirosis, and chronic active hepatitis. In the experience of the author, chills and fever after the onset of jaundice would be unusual in uncomplicated acute viral hepatitis.

More than one hundred years ago, Budd[10] pointed out that pruritus is most pronounced in cases of occlusion of the common bile duct, particularly by tumor. According to Schoenfield,[62] pruritus occurs with extrahepatic obstruction in 75% of patients with malignant lesions and in 50% of those with benign conditions. He believes that the itching that occurs in 20% of patients with hepatitis and 10% of those with cirrhosis is often associated with clinical and laboratory evidence of intrahepatic cholestasis, and he has found that approximately 75% of patients with bile duct stricture or primary biliary cirrhosis have pruritus. Itching is prominent in recurrent intrahepatic cholestasis and in the recurrent jaundice of pregnancy.

Although an increase in serum bile acids has long been suspected as the cause of the pruritus, itching of the skin not infrequently precedes or follows the appearance or disappearance of icterus. It is not surprising, therefore, that pruritus may occur with low serum bile acid concentrations or may not occur with very high serum bile acid values, and relief of itching may follow the use of norethandrolone without concomitant decrease in serum bile acids.

According to Javitt,[34,35] the pruritis occurring in cholestatic syndromes can be distinguished from that occurring in other diseases by its diurnal variation; it is worse at bedtime and gone by morning. He points out that serum bile acids are highest in the evening after dinner and can become normal by morning. He believes that the absence of pruritus in some persons regardless of the height of the serum bile acid concentration implies "some variation in the perception of pruritus as a sensory phenomenon, or variation in the type of bile acid and the moderating effects of bilirubin and other components that are also retained in the skin and other tissues."[34,35]

The appearance of dark urine—"looking like tea or Coca-cola"—is the most reliable criterion of the onset of jaundice and is likely to precede the yellowish discoloration of the skin or sclerae by days. Occasionally, a seemingly acholic stool may be due to admixture of barium ingested during an upper gastrointestinal x-ray study. The occurrence of brown stools in the presence of deep jaundice is usually indicative of hepatocellular disease but may occur rarely in carcinoma of the head of the pancreas. Although it may prove to be caused by a bleeding peptic ulcer or ruptured esophageal varices, the passage of tarry stools by an icteric patient should also arouse suspicion of hemobilia or carcinoma of the ampulla of Vater or pancreas eroding the duodenum or stomach.

PHYSICAL EXAMINATION

Age and Sex

"The time honored skill of physical examination should be revived especially where the physician is confronted with a jaundiced patient" Okuda[49,50]

The age and sex of the patient may prove to be of diagnostic significance. Viral hepatitis type A is seen most commonly in children of school age, whereas common duct stone and neoplastic jaundice usually occur in middle-aged or older patients. Leptospirosis is primarily a disease of children and young adults and occurs predominantly in males. Portal cirrhosis, chronic type B hepatitis, hepatoma, pancreatic cancer, sclerosing cholangitis, and primary hemochromatosis predominate in males, whereas common duct stone, primary biliary cirrhosis, and carcinoma of the gallbladder are more prevalent in females.

Eyes

Mild degrees of icterus may be detectable only in the scleral periphery and may be overlooked in artificial light. Kayser-Fleischer rings should be looked for in all patients younger than 30 years of age with chronic active hepatitis, because Wilson's disease may present in this form.[66] Pigmented corneal rings have also been described in non-Wilsonian liver disease, notably primary biliary cirrhosis.[24] Conjunctival suffusion, occasionally accompanied by conjuctival hemorrhage, should suggest leptospirosis.

Vascular Spiders

Vascular spiders should be searched for carefully with the aid of good light. Inspection with a hand-lens may be necessary to distinguish them from small papular lesions. Vascular spiders may pulsate and can be obliterated by pressing on their central point with the point of a pencil. They usually indicate the presence of hepatic cirrhosis and have been linked to the presence of esophageal varices.[9] They seldom appear in patients with jaundice owing to neoplasm or common duct stone. They may be seen in acute hepatitis, chronic active hepatitis, pregnancy, and, occasionally, in normal persons, in whom they are likely to be solitary. They usually occur on the face, neck, arms, fingers, and upper part of the trunk and, exceptionally, on the lower trunk and lower extremities.[5]

Breath

A peculiar, sickly sweetish breath (hepatic foetor) is characteristic of severe hepatic disease with necrosis, but it may be encountered in cases of extensive collateral circulation. The foetor is probably due to a mixture of the three related volatile compounds: methethiol, dimethyl sulfide, and dimethyl disulfide. Detection of the peculiar foetor in a patient in coma should arouse suspicion of hepatic encephalopathy.

Abdominal Examination

I cannot overemphasize the importance of Olser's advice: "*Don't* touch the patient—state first what you see; cultivate your powers of observation."[4]

Prominent superficial abdominal veins are most often observed in patients with hepatic cirrhosis but may occur in the presence of peritoneal tumor implants, obstruction of the portal vein by tumor, or inferior caval obstruction. Normal veins may be made more prominent by stretching and thinning of the overlying skin as a result of abdominal distention in the absence of portal hypertension. In portal hypertension, the blood flow in the abdominal veins is radially away from the umbilicus, whereas in inferior or caval obstruction, it is upward over the abdominal wall.[63]

Liver

F. M. Hanger noted: "One good feel of the liver is worth any two liver function tests."[60] I have been so much impressed with the truth of this dictum that I would strongly emphasize the necessity for painstaking palpation of the liver in the detection of hepatic disease. To obtain a good "feel" of the liver, the examiner's hand should be warm, and the patient should lie on his or her back, with the head slightly raised, arms at his or her sides, and knees flexed. Having the patient think of something pleasant may promote abdominal relaxation. It is best to first place the examining hand over the lower right abdomen and proceed upward while asking the patient to breathe deeply. The first "feel" is often the best, because flipping the liver edge at the end of the inspiration may be painful and cause the patient to restrict subsequent inspirations. Yet, two good feels may be better than one. The normal liver is soft, smooth, and frequently tender. It has a sharp edge that usually is not palpable but may extend one to two fingerbreadths below the right costal margin.

Although it has been shown that a direct relationship between the position of lower liver borders and liver weight does not exist,[23] it is safe to assume that a liver that extends three fingerbreadths or more below the right costal margin is probably enlarged (and hence the seat of the disease), provided that one may exclude downward displacement by right pleural cavity fluid or pulmonary emphysema or the presence of marked visceroptosis. Variations in the shape and position of the liver appear to be in relation to body types. In a stocky person, the liver may often extend to the left lateral abdominal wall, with its lower edge lying relatively high; it may not be palpable beneath the costal margin. In a lanky person, the normal liver, including the left lobe, may lie entirely in the right abdomen and may extend five fingerbreadths below the costal margin.[23] Here, the slant of the liver edge may be steep enough and may approach an angle of 60°, according to Fleischner and Sayegh.[23] I recall a patient with a marked hyposthenic habitus whose liver extended down to the level of the navel over the years and was found to be normal at laparotomy and surgical biopsy.

The liver should be palpated on more than one visit, because variations in the degree of abdominal relaxation, in the examiner's own perceptivity, and in the time the examiner devotes to the examination will explain the ability to palpate the organ on one day and failure to do so on another. Before concluding that the liver is impalpable, it is good to feel the abdomen in the lateral decubitus position.

A liver that is unduly firm is likely to be diseased, as is one with a blunted edge or an irregular contour. Lesser degrees of surface irregularity may not be detectable clinically. A very irregular, firm, nodular liver is most commonly indicative of intrahepatic malignant neoplasm. However, the large regenerating nodules of postnecrotic cirrhosis may produce an irregularity of contour that may closely simulate that produced by tumor. The same may be true in congenital cystic disease of the liver.

The examiner should palpate and listen for a friction rub over the liver. Occasionally, the rub may be detected in the right lower chest, anteriorly or anterolaterally. It may come and go like a pericardial rub. A hepatic friction rub is most commonly indicative of malignant tumor (invading or breaking through the liver capsule).[27] It may

also be found in hepatic syphilis and hepatic abscess. It may follow percutaneous needle biopsy of the liver. Rarely, a friction rub produced by fibrinous exudate localized to an area of pericolic extension of a neoplasm of the ascending colon proves confusing.

The examiner should auscultate the abdomen for the presence of a bruit. The detection of a harsh (arterial) murmur over the liver either with systolic accentuation or purely systolic in character should suggest the presence of hepatoma or alcoholic hepatitis.[15] This type of murmur is not affected by posture, respiration, or local pressure with the stethoscope. It is apparently due to locally increased arterial blood flow and should be contrasted with the venous hum of portal hypertension, which arises from collateral venous channels.[63] The venous hum is lower in pitch than the arterial murmur, is altered by posture and by respiration, and is frequently obliterated by pressure with the stethoscope. A systolic murmur over the liver has been described in cases of anemia and may decrease after appropriate blood transfusion.[38] In a case of multiple liver abscesses observed by the author, a loud bruit was audible over the liver and resembled that described in cases of hepatoma.

The liver may not extend below the right costal margin in cases of hepatitis or cirrhosis. Usually it is found 1 to 2 (or 2 to 3) fingerbreadths below the right costal margin in viral hepatitis and is frequently tender in this disease. A very large liver (one extending four to five fingerbreadths or more below the right costal margin) is usually indicative of fatty vacuolization, cirrhosis, tumor, amyloidosis, cystic disease, or congestive failure.

The absence of a palpable liver in a patient who has had jaundice for 2 to 3 weeks or more would, in my experience, tend to exclude obstruction of the bile ducts by pancreatic cancer, because sufficient bile stasis should result, by this time, to produce detectable hepatic enlargement.[61] A nonpalpable liver is rarely the seat of a neoplasm.

Gallbladder

The presence of a smooth, nontender, distended gallbladder in a patient with jaundice, once considered to be indicative of neoplastic obstruction of the common bile duct in accordance with Courvoisier's law, occurred in 25% of cases of common duct stone reported by Flood and associates.[25] It is such a reliable indicator of obstructive jaundice as to warrant limiting the choice of diagnostic maneuvers to establish biliary tract obstruction. A distended gallbladder is found much more frequently at operation or necropsy than at the bedside due to concealment of the overlying right lobe of the liver or, less frequently, by a thick abdominal wall. Painless distention of the gallbladder may be encountered in patients who have been vomiting and not ingesting fats.[36]

Rarely, a distended gallbladder may be more visible than palpable. At times, it may be found in the right lower abdominal quadrant and may be mimicked by a tumor of the colonic flexure or right kidney. Lateral mobility, descent on inspiration, and lack of forward displacement by pressure over the right lumbar region may prove helpful in identification of the gallbladder. As in the case of a palpable liver, and for the same reasons, a distended gallbladder may be detected on one examination and not on another.

Spleen

The spleen is usually palpated best with the patient on his or her right side, knees bent, and left arm extended over the head. The patient is instructed to breathe deeply, because the spleen is felt best at the end of inspiration. Palpation of the spleen should be gentle, as Galambos has emphasized,[28] because the organ is quite superficial and may be overlooked with very deep palpation. In some instances, it may be more readily palpated with the patient lying supine with or without the left arm extending across the back. As in the case of the liver, palpation should proceed upward from well below the left costal margin. In obstructive jaundice of long standing, splenomegaly may be a manifestation of secondary biliary cirrhosis; in cancer of the body and tail of the pancreas, it may result from encroachment of the tumor on the splenic vein.[19]

Increase in splenic size may also be determined by percussion. Nixon[47] advises that the patient be placed in the right lateral recumbent position with the left arm extended forward and upward and that percussion be initiated at the lower level of pulmonary resonance in approximately the posterior axillary line and carried downward obliquely toward the lower midanterior costal margin. He finds that the upper border of dullness extends 6 cm to 8 cm above the costal margin and that dullness over 8 cm is indicative of an enlarged spleen in the adult.

Ascites

The presence of ascites in a jaundiced patient is usually indicative of hepatic cirrhosis but may also be observed in massive or submassive hepatic necrosis, the presence of peritoneal tumor implants, or in invasion of the portal vein by tumor. Because of its occurrence in alcoholics, pancreatic ascites may at times be mistaken for cirrhotic ascites.[12] Marked elevation of amylase and higher protein values characterize pancreatic ascites. A high protein content (over 3 gm/ml) and a lactic dehydrogenase level of over 400 sigma units are strongly suggestive of peritoneal carcinoma.[8] Relatively small quantities of ascitic fluid may escape clinical detection but may be revealed by abdominal ultrasonography in amounts as little as 300 ml.[30] An enlarged spleen may obscure shifting dullness when the patient turns on his or her right side.[28]

A cell count of more than 500/cu mm of ascitic fluid with more than 50% polymorphonuclear leukocytes is very much in keeping with spontaneous bacterial peritonitis[16] but may also occur in peritonitis secondary to perforated peptic ulcer or gallbladder, as may a positive culture for enteric organisms. When the ascitic fluid white cell count is greater than 500/cu mm and mononuclear cells are predominant, tuberculosis, malignant neoplasm, and pancreatic ascites should be considered. Hoefs[32] has pointed out that ascitic fluid protein and cell counts may rise during diuresis.

Ascitic fluid may conceal an enlarged liver even on palpation by dipping or ballotting. It is not unusual to be unable to palpate an enlarged tumorous liver following development of ascites, only to readily feel it again after abdominal paracentesis. Hemorrhagic ascitic fluid should suggest hepatoma, peritoneal tumor implants, or tuberculous peritonitis. Palpation of the umbilicus, especially in patients with ascites, may at times reveal small metastatic nodules.

Miscellaneous findings include the presence of an abdominal mass, usually indicative of intra-abdominal tumor. Absence of axillary or pectoral hair is suggestive of cirrhosis of the liver, as are testicular atrophy and gynecomastia, although the last two conditions have been reported in hepatitis. Parotid enlargement, Dupuytren's contracture, and palmar erythema may also be noted in cases of cirrhosis. The presence of multiple venous thrombi in a jaundiced patient should suggest cancer of the body or the tail of the pancreas[37] and calf tenderness leptospirosis.

ROUTINE TESTS

Blood Count

The white blood cell count is usually reduced during the preicteric phase and normal during the icteric phase of viral hepatitis. The chief value of a white blood cell count in a patient with jaundice is in ruling out uncomplicated viral hepatitis by the presence of leukocytosis, which is frequently found in toxic hepatitis, alcoholic hepatitis, metastatic hepatic neoplasm, common duct stone (with cholangitis), leptospirosis, and fulminant hepatitis. The presence of eosinophilia should suggest toxic hepatitis.

Blood Urea Nitrogen

Elevation in the blood urea nitrogen (BUN) level in a patient with jaundice should suggest the possibility of leptospirosis or exposure to an hepatotoxic agent that is also injurious to the kidney, such as carbon tetrachloride. Renal failure complicating liver disease—the hepatorenal syndrome—must also be considered. Depression of BUN below 5 mg/dl is said to be characteristic of alcoholic cirrhosis.[28]

Urine Analysis

The presence of albuminuria should suggest the possibility of leptospirosis or carbon tetrachloride hepatotoxicity, although it may occur in the preicteric and the early icteric phases of viral hepatitis. Given the fact that jaundice may occur in amyloidosis, the simultaneous occurrence of marked albuminuria should also arouse suspicion of this disorder.

Liver Profile

Among the so-called liver function tests, the serum bilirubin determination possesses diagnostic value that is not fully appreciated. Watson[71] emphasized the value of the ratio of conjugated to total serum bilirubin in subdividing cases of jaundice. A ratio of less than 15% would indicate unconjugated hyperbilirubinemia constituting hemolytic disease, Gilbert's syndrome, and Crigler-Najjar syndrome whereas a value between 15% and 40%, which Watson designated as semiconjugated, characterizes liver disease with a hemolytic component or hypersplenism and hemolytic disease with liver injury. Ratios exceeding 40% are to be found in cholestasis as a result of biliary obstruction or liver disease.

A total serum bilirubin value of less than 10 mg/dl is usually encountered in common duct stone, largely because of intermittent and incomplete obstruction; whereas greater concentrations favor the persistent and often complete obstruction resulting from neoplasm. The peak concentration of total serum bilirubin in acute viral hepatitis is usually 15 mg/dl but may reach higher levels. A concentration above 25 mg/dl is unusual in extrahepatic obstruction unless complicated by oliguria and/or hemolysis. Billing[6] has recently assessed the value of bile pigment determination in the diagnosis of jaundice.

A daily increase of 1.5 mg/dl to 2 mg/dl in the total serum bilirubin is characteristic of extrahepatic biliary obstruction. I recall a consultation in which I rightfully suspected extrahepatic obstruction (which was proved to be due to a pancreatic tumor) because of a reported daily increase in the serum bilirubin of approximately 1.5 mg/dl. A diagnosis of viral hepatitis had been based on serum transaminase values exceeding 1000 units.

During my examination of another patient with very high serum transaminases attributed to viral hepatitis, the patient cried out with upper abdominal pain and bent forward in bed and asked for a hypodermic injection to relieve his pain. This behavior led to a suspicion of obstructive jaundice, which proved to be due to a pancreatic cancer.

Although obstructive jaundice is almost always accompanied by an increase in the serum alkaline phosphatase, this increase may be of moderate degree, even in cases of biliary obstruction resulting from neoplasm. A steadily rising concentration of both serum alkaline phosphatase and serum bilirubin in the absence of corresponding increases in the serum transaminases constitutes a most reliable index of obstructive jaundice. One may exclude increases in the enzyme concentration attributable to bone disease by determining the level of serum 5-nucleotidase, or gamma glutamyl transpeptidase, which are not influenced by osseous factors. It is increasingly being realized that elevation of the serum alkaline phosphatase may prove to be the forerunner of pruritus and jaundice by years in primary biliary cirrhosis.

Patients with alcoholic fatty liver show a significant increase in gamma glutamyl transferase activity both in the liver and serum, which has been attributed to hepatic enzyme induction rather than to liver cell injury.[68]

Determination of the serum glutamic oxaloacetic transaminase (SGOT) and serum glutamic pyruvic transaminase (SGPT) levels has proved to be of great value in the distinction between hepatocellular and obstructive jaundice. In obstructive jaundice, the concentration of these enzymes is usually not greater than 300 units to 400 units, whereas in the very early stages of hepatitis, an increase of 1000 or more units is frequent. The diagnostic value of these enzyme determinations varies with the duration of jaundice, because the most marked increases occur in the very early stages of hepatitis. Thus, in patients first seen 2 or 3 weeks after the onset of hepatitis, the enzyme level may have fallen to that ordinarily observed in obstructive jaundice. The degree of elevation of serum transaminases is of no prognostic significance. A progressive decrease is usually a favorable omen, but in fulminant hepatitis very low values may be obtained due to failure of the liver to produce the enzymes normally. In cirrhosis, the SGOT is usually greater than the SGPT, which may even be normal; whereas the reverse is usually true in viral hepatitis.

Although serum transaminases exceeding 500 Karmen units are unusual in extrahepatic obstructive jaundice, exceptions do occur that may lead to erroneous diagnosis of viral hepatitis[1,11] as noted above. Such elevations are likely to be more transient than those occurring in viral hepatitis, and there is evidence suggesting that they may follow a hypodermic injection of morphine with resultant spasm of the sphincter of Oddi.

Tests should be made for HBsAg in all cases of jaundice that appear to be of hepatocellular origin, and, if indicated, determinations should be made of HBs antibody, HBc antibody, E antigen and antibody, and IgM A antibody. The mitochondrial antibody test, although not specific for primary biliary cirrhosis, has proved to be of inestimable value in differentiating this disorder from extrahepatic obstructive jaundice,[18] thus virtually eliminating the need for exploratory laparotomy for diagnostic purposes.

PROTHROMBIN RESPONSE

It is well known that an abnormally long prothrombin time may be due to the exclusion of bile from the intestine as well as severe liver injury. If the prothrombin time of the blood of an icteric patient is markedly prolonged (i.e., if prothrombin activity is under 40% of normal) but returns to normal within 24 hours after parenteral administration of vitamin K, it is probable that liver-cell function is reasonably good and that jaundice is due to extrahepatic obstruction. The failure of the prothrombin time to shorten under these circumstances indicates the presence of parenchymal liver disease.[41] An adequate amount of vitamin K is provided by 10 mg of phytonadione (AquaMEPHYTON) given subcutaneously. In order to exclude intrinsic errors in the test itself, it is best to determine the blood prothrombin time on two separate days, both before and after the administration of vitamin K.

HEPATOBILIARY IMAGERY

Following the clinical examination and laboratory tests, the clinician should utilize hepatobiliary imaging beginning with abdominal real-time ultrasonography.[17] If dilated ducts are displayed—an indication of obstructive jaundice—the clinician should invoke either percutaneous transhepatic cholangiography (PTC) or endoscopic retrograde cholangiopancreatography (ERCP), depending largely upon local expertise. In suspected common duct stone, ERCP is preferred because of the approach it affords for simultaneous removal of the stones.[55] As a specific diagnostic aid in bile duct cancer, PTC is more effective. Niederou and associates[46] compared extrahepatic bile duct size measured by ultrasound and by different radiographic methods. (Failure to demonstrate dilated ducts does not necessarily rule out biliary tract obstruction.)

The usefulness of abdominal ultrasonography is limited by the presence of marked abdominal distention or obesity. Recourse may be had to use an abdominal CT scan, which, although helpful, is usually not required in the study of a jaundiced patient. The CT-scan has the advantage of greater resolution of pancreatic mass enlargement, periportal tumor infiltration, and depicting common duct stones. For example, because of an overlying duodenal shadow or gas in the colon, ultrasonography is said to reveal common duct stones in only about 15% of cases in contrast to a positive incidence of 50% or more with abdominal CT-scan.[22,59]

Radionuclide scanning with ^{99m}Tc HIDA[31,52] or ^{99m}Tc DISIDA plays a limited but useful role. The primary indication for either is in the diagnosis of acute cholecystitis by failing to show gallbladder filling because of obstruction of the cystic duct. Both are useful in evaluating the patency of a postoperative biliary tract reconstruction or the presence of extravasated bile in the right upper abdominal quadrant.

The accuracy of the test is greatest when the serum bilirubin is less than 5 mg/dl and tends to diminish the higher the serum bilirubin level. The accuracy of the test is also said to be diminished when extrahepatic obstruction is only partial. In a preliminary study, Kuni and associates[39] found the test useful in differentiating intrahepatic cholestasis from other hepatobiliary disorders in which the parenchymal transit time was increased disproportionately to any decrease in hepatocyte clearance.

NEEDLE BIOPSY OF THE LIVER

When the diagnosis as to the cause of jaundice is still in doubt, recourse should be to needle biopsy of the liver. This procedure is being used more sparingly in the differential diagnosis of jaundice largely as a result of the contributions of hepatobiliary tract imagery. Although its risk in obstructive jaundice has been exaggerated, it should not be used in the presence of a Courvoisier gallbladder because of the reliability of this finding as a sign of extrahepatic obstructive jaundice and because the great increase in intrabiliary pressure it reflects would predispose to bile peritonitis on liver puncture. Another reason for the decline in the use of liver biopsy in the jaundiced patient is the frequent difficulty in distinguishing intrahepatic from extrahepatic cholestasis histologically. Nevertheless, the procedure retains its value in the diagnosis of alcoholic and chronic hepatitis and primary biliary cirrhosis. The changes in alcoholic hepatitis, once considered pathognomonic, have been described following jejunoileal bypass[53] and in nonalcoholics.[2]

Sampling errors in needle specimens of the liver are most likely to occur in cases of cirrhosis, chronic hepatitis, and in one third or more cases of neoplastic invasion. A sample obtained from one area may be interpreted as normal, from a second area as questionable cirrhosis, and from a third area as micronodular cirrhosis.[69] Soloway and associates[65] observed five instances in which a biopsy specimen that did not show cirrhosis was preceded and followed by specimens that did; Edmondson[21] had a similar experience.

LAPAROSCOPY

Experience in the Liver Unit of the Los Angeles County Hospital has shown that hepatocellular carcinoma can be diagnosed at laparoscopy in approximately 65% of cases.[54a] Since "liver function tests" and needle biopsy specimens can be normal in cirrhosis, laparoscopy may prove very rewarding in demonstrating cirrhosis in the presence—or even absence—of suspicion of this diagnosis. In experienced hands the risk from liver biopsies under laparoscopic control is the same or less than the risk of blind liver biopsy. In a recent alcoholic patient, with icterus and ascites, suspected of having cirrhosis, laparoscopy revealed a congested liver which, in turn, led to detection of constructive pericardites.

CONCLUSION

Clinical examination of the jaundiced patient retains its importance in providing valuable clues to accurate diagnosis and to selection of the more helpful laboratory procedures to the exclusion of the unnecessary or least helpful. Not only is appropriate therapy thus expedited, but the cost and hazards of medical care are reduced concomitantly.

Repeated abdominal examination may detect abnormalities overlooked because of a previously hurried and less perceptive examination or poor abdominal relaxation.

Although advances in the radiologic imaging of the liver and biliary tract have contributed so importantly to the diagnostic approach in the jaundiced patient, they should not be permitted to replace or lessen the importance of the clinical examination.

When diagnosis of the cause of jaundice still remains in doubt, recourse may be had to exploratory laparotomy, which was performed in 23 of 144 consecutive cases of jaundice.[14] Four of these were unnecessary. The accuracy of the clinician's decision on this procedure was 83%.[14]

"The most brilliant discoveries in therapeutics and the most skillful surgery avail nothing if the patient's disease is not correctly diagnosed."[26] N. B. Foster

REFERENCES

1. Abbruzzese A, Jeffrey RL: Marked elevation of serum glutamic oxaloacetic transaminase and lactic dehydrogenase activity in chronic extrahepatic biliary disease. Am J Dig Dis 14:332, 1969
2. Adler M, Schaffner F: Fatty liver, hepatitis, and cirrhosis in obese patients. Am J Med 67:811, 1979
3. Albaugh JS et al: Recurrent obstructive jaundice caused by fibrolamellar hepatocellular carcinoma. Dig Dis Sci 29:762, 1984
4. Bean NB: Osler Aphorisms. New York, Henry Schuman, 1950
5. Bean WB: Vascular spiders and related lesions of the skin. Springfield, IL, Charles C Thomas, 1958
6. Billing BH: A 1983 assessment of the value of bile pigment determination in the diagnosis of jaundice. Postgrad Med J 89 (Suppl):19, 1983
7. Black M et al: Isoniazid-associated hepatitis in 114 patients. Gastroenterology 69:289, 1979
8. Boyer TD et al: Diagnostic value of ascitic fluid, lactic dehydrogenase, protein, and WBC levels. Arch Intern Med 138:1103, 1978
9. Brick IB, Palmer ED: Esophageal varices and vascular spiders (nevi araneosi) in cirrhosis of the liver. JAMA 155:8, 1954
10. Budd G: Diseases of the Liver. Philadelphia, Lee & Blanchard, 1946
11. Burckhardt D, Ladue JS: Provocation of serum enzyme activity in cholecystectomized patients given opiates. Am J Gastroenterol 46:43, 1966
12. Cameron JL et al: Pancreatic ascites. Surg Gynecol Obstet 125:328, 1967
13. Chauffard MA: Le cancer de corps de pancreas. Bull Acad Natl Med 60:242, 1908
14. Chio-Ming-Chu et al: Jaundice after open heart surgery: A prospective study. Thorax 39:52, 1984
15. Clain H et al: Abdominal arterial murmurs in liver disease. Lancet 2:516, 1966
16. Conn H, Fessel JM: Spontaneous bacterial peritonitis in cirrhosis: Variations on a theme. Medicine 50:161, 1971
17. Cooperberg P: High resolution real-time ultrasound in the evaluation of the normal and obstructed biliary tract. Radiology 129:477, 1978
18. Doniach D, Walker G: Progress report mitochondrial antibodies (AMA). Gut 15:664, 1974
19. Duff GL: The clinical and pathological features of carcinoma of the body and tail of the pancreas. Bull Johns Hopkins Hosp 65:69, 1939
20. Edlund G et al: Jaundice in acute cholecystitis without common duct stones. Acta Chir Scand 149:597, 1983
21. Edmondson H: Personal communication.
22. Ferruci JI: Imaging in obstructive jaundice. In Moody FG (ed): Advances in diagnosis and surgical treatment of biliary tract disease. New York, Masson Publishing USA Inc, 1983
23. Fleischner FG, Sayegh V: Assessment of the size of the liver; roentgenologic considerations. N Engl J Med 249:271, 1958
24. Fleming CR et al: Pigmented corneal rings in non-Wilsonian liver disease. Ann Intern Med 86:285, 1977
25. Flood CA et al: The differential diagnosis of jaundice. A study of 235 cases of nonhemolytic jaundice due to carcinoma, calculus in the common bile duct, and liver degeneration. Am J Med Sci 185:358, 1933
26. Foster NB: The Examination of Patients. Philadelphia, WB Saunders, 1923
27. Fred HL, Brown GR: The hepatic friction rub. N Engl J Med 266:554, 1962
28. Galambos J: Cirrhosis. Philadelphia, WB Saunders, 1979
29. Glenn F: Common Duct Stones. Springfield, IL, Charles C Thomas, 1975
30. Goldberg BB: Ultrasonic evaluation of intraperitoneal fluid. JAMA 235:2427, 1976
31. Harvey E et al: Tc 99m hida: A new radiopharmaceutical for hepatobiliary imaging. J Nucl Med 16:533, 1975
32. Hoefs JC: Increase in ascites white blood cell and protein concentrations during diuresis in patients with chronic liver disease. Hepatology 1:249, 1981
33. Inman HW, Rawson NSB: Erythromycin estolate and jaundice. Br Med J 286:1954, 1983
34. Javitt NB: Cholestatic liver disease: Mechanisms, diagnosis, and therapy. Adv Intern Med 25:146, 1980
35. Javitt NB: Bile acids and hepatobiliary disease. In Schiff L, Schiff ER (eds): Diseases of the Liver, 5th ed. Philadelphia, JB Lippincott, 1982
36. Jones CM: Personal communication.
37. Kenney WE: The association of carcinoma of the body and tail of the pancreas with multiple venous thrombi. Surgery 14:600, 1943
38. Konar MR et al: Murmur over liver in cases of severe anemia. Br Med J 4:154, 1967
39. Kuni CC et al: Evaluation of intrahepatic cholestasis with radionuclide hepatobiliary imaging. Gastrointest Radiol 9: 163, 1984
40. Lindberg et al: A description of diagnostic strategies in jaundice. Scand J Gastroenterol 18:257, 1983
41. Lord JW Jr, Andrus W deW: Differentiation of intrahepatic and extrahepatic jaundice: Response of the plasma prothrombin to intramuscular injection of menadione (2 methyl-1,4-naphthoquinone) as a diagnostic aid. Arch Intern Med 68:199, 1941
42. Lumeng L et al: Final report of a blinded prospective study comparing current noninvasive approaches in the differential diagnosis of jaundice (abstr). Gastroenterology 78:1313, 1980
43. Maddrey WC, Boinott JK: Severe hepatitis from methyldopa. Gastroenterology 68:351, 1975
44. Miller DJ et al: Nonalcoholic liver disease mimicking alcoholic hepatitis and cirrhosis. Gastroenterology 77:A27, 1979
45. Morgenstern L: Postoperative jaundice. In Schiff L, Schiff ER (eds): Diseases of the Liver, 5th ed. Philadelphia, JB Lippincott, 1982
46. Niederou C et al: Comparison of the extrahepatic bile duct size measured by ultrasound and by different radiographic methods. Gastroenterology 87:615, 1984
47. Nixon RK Jr: Detection of splenomegaly by percussion. N Engl J Med 250:166, 1954

48. O'Connor KW et al: A blinded prospective study comparing four current noninvasive approaches in the differential diagnosis of medical versus surgical jaundice. Gastroenterology 84:1498, 1983

49. Okuda K et al: How to investigate cholestasis: Utility of ultrasound as the first imaging study. Semin Liver Dis 3: 308, 1983

50. Okuda K, Tsuchiya Y: Ultrasonic anatomy of the biliary system. Clin Gastroenterol 12:49, 1983

51. Orrego H et al: Reliability of assessment of alcohol intake based on personal interviews in a liver clinic. Lancet 22 (29): 1354, 1979

52. Pelot D et al: Pipida excretory scintigraphy in the diagnosis of hepatobiliary disorders. Am J Gastroenterol 75:22, 1981

53. Peters R et al: Post-jejunoileal-bypass hepatic disease. Am J Clin Pathol 63:318, 1975

54. Pickles WN: Epidemiology in Country Practice. Baltimore, Williams & Wilkins, 1939

54a. Reynolds TB: Diagnostic methods for hepatocellular carcinoma. In Okuda K, Peters RL (eds): Hepatocellular Carcinoma. New York, John Wiley & Sons, 1976

55. Safrany L, Cotton PB: Endoscopic Management of Cholelithiasis. Surg Clin North Am 62:825, 1982

56. Sampluer RE: Evaluation of the patient with jaundice. Ariz Med 41:302, 1984

57. Scharshmidt BF et al: Approach to the patient with cholestatic jaundice. N Engl J Med 308:1515, 1983

58. Schenker S et al: Differential diagnosis of jaundice: A report of a prospective study of 61 proved cases. Am J Dig Dis 7: 449, 1962

59. Schiff L: Jaundice. In Blacklow RS (ed): Signs and Symptoms, 6th ed. Philadelphia, JB Lippincott, 1983

60. Schiff L: One feel of the liver. Gastroenterology 26:506, 1954

61. Schiff L: Absence of a palpable liver: A sign of value in excluding obstructive jaundice due to pancreatic cancer. Gastroenterology 32:1143, 1957

62. Schoenfield LJ: The relationship of bile acids to pruritus in hepatobiliary disease. In Schiff L et al (eds): Bile salt metabolism. Springfield IL, Charles C Thomas, 1969

63. Sherlock S: Cirrhosis of the liver. Postgrad Med J 26:472, 1960

64. Simone JF, Ferruci JT: New trends in gallbladder imaging. JAMA 246:381, 1981

65. Soloway et al: Observer error and sampling variability tested in evaluation of hepatitis and cirrhosis by liver biopsy. Am J Dig Dis 17:1082, 1971

66. Sternlieb I, Scheinberg IH: Chronic hepatitis as a first manifestation of Wilson's disease. Ann Intern Med 76:59, 1972

67. Taub S, Schiff L: Common duct stone and cholangitis simulating fever of unknown origin. South Med J 74:230, 1981

68. Teschle R et al: Hepatic gamma glutamyl transferase activity in alcoholic fatty liver. Comparison with other liver enzymes in man and rats. Gut 24:625, 1983

69. Thaler H: Leberbiopsie. Berlin, Springer-Verlag, 1969

70. Vennes JA, Bond JH: Approach to the jaundiced patient. Gastroenterology 84:1615, 1983

71. Watson CJ: The prognosis and treatment of hepatic insufficiency. Ann Intern Med 31:405, 1959

72. Weisman HS et al: Cholescintigraphy, ultrasonography, and computerized tomography in the evaluation of biliary tract disorders. Semin Nucl Med 9:22, 1979

73. Zimmerman HJ: Effects of aspirin and acetaminophen on the liver. Arch Intern Med 141:333, 1981

chapter 9
Laboratory Tests

MARSHALL M. KAPLAN

Laboratory tests, often referred to as liver function tests, or LFTs, are useful in the evaluation and management of patients with hepatic dysfunction. First, they provide a sensitive, noninvasive method of screening for the presence of liver dysfunction. This is particularly important in anicteric patients who may have unsuspected disorders such as viral hepatitis, chronic active hepatitis, cirrhosis, or partial bile duct obstruction. Second, once the presence of hepatic dysfunction is recognized, the pattern of laboratory test abnormalities may allow one to recognize the general type of liver disorder. For example, laboratory tests will usually allow one to distinguish hepatocellular disorders such as viral hepatitis from cholestatic syndromes such as primary biliary cirrhosis and bile duct obstruction. Third, laboratory tests allow one to assess the severity of liver dysfunction and occasionally permit one to predict outcome early in the course of disease. Finally, liver function tests allow the physician to follow the course of liver disease, to evaluate accurately the response to treatment, and to adjust treatment when necessary. This is particularly true in patients with steroid-responsive autoimmune chronic hepatitis.

Although laboratory tests are indispensable in the management of patients with liver disease, they have certain limitations. First, they lack sensitivity. Normal results may be obtained in patients with serious liver disorders such as cirrhosis or hepatocellular carcinoma. Second, these tests are not specific for liver dysfunction. For example, the serum albumin may be decreased in inflammatory bowel disease and the aminotransferases may be elevated in musculoskeletal or cardiac diseases. Finally, liver function tests rarely provide a specific diagnosis; rather, they suggest a general category of liver disorder. They will not distinguish viral hepatitis from drug hepatitis or intrahepatic cholestasis from extrahepatic bile duct obstruction.

It is important to recognize that no one liver function test enables the clinician to assess accurately the total functional capacity of the liver. The liver carries out thousands of biochemical functions, most of which cannot be easily measured by blood tests. The laboratory tests in current use measure only a limited number of these functions. In fact, many tests, such as the aminotransferases or alkaline phosphatase, do not measure liver function at all. Rather, they detect liver cell damage or interference with bile flow. In order to increase both the sensitivity and specificity of laboratory tests in the detection of liver disease, it is helpful to use them as a battery. When more than one of these tests provides abnormal findings, the probability of liver disease is high. When all test results are normal, the possibility of missing occult liver disease is low.

When evaluating patients with liver disorders, it is helpful to group these tests into general categories. The classification that the author has found most useful is given below:

1. Tests of the liver's capacity to transport organic anions and metabolize drugs. Included in this group are the serum bilirubin, the bromosulfphthalein and indocyanine green tests, serum bile acids, and breath tests. Each of these tests measures the liver's ability to clear endogenous or exogenous substances from the circulation, so they are grouped together.
2. Tests that detect injury to hepatocytes. These include all the enzyme tests, of which the aminotransferases and alkaline phosphatase are still the most useful.
3. Tests of the liver's biosynthetic capacity. Included in this group are the serum albumin, ceruloplasmin, ferritin, α_1-antitrypsin, lipoproteins, and blood clotting factors. These are substances synthesized in the liver for transport into the circulation.
4. Tests that detect chronic inflammation in the liver, altered immunoregulation, or viral hepatitis. These include the immunoglobulins, hepatitis serologies, and specific autoantibodies. These are not truly liver function tests, because most of these are proteins made by B-lymphocytes, not by hepatocytes. Nevertheless, some are quite specific for certain liver diseases.

In this chapter, those tests that the author believes to be most useful in evaluating liver diseases will be discussed. Other tests, which are of less value in the author's opinion but are still used, will be discussed briefly. Whenever possible, the pathophysiologic basis of each test will be reviewed together with the test's sensitivity and specificity for detecting the nature and severity of liver dysfunction.

TESTS OF THE LIVER'S CAPACITY TO TRANSPORT ORGANIC ANIONS AND METABOLIZE DRUGS

Bilirubin (see Chapter 10 for complete coverage)

Bilirubin Metabolism

Bilirubin, a tetrapyrrole pigment, is a breakdown product of ferroprotoporphyrin IX (heme), an integral part of

219

heme-containing proteins.[57,312] Approximately 70% to 80% of the 250 mg to 300 mg of bilirubin produced each day is derived from the breakdown of hemoglobin in senescent red blood cells.[123,172,189] The remainder comes from prematurely destroyed erythroid cells in bone marrow and from the turnover of hemoproteins in tissues throughout the body.[257,346] The liver is the major source of the latter because of its high concentration of hemoproteins with relatively high turnover rates such as cytochrome p-450.[203,283] Initial steps leading to the formation of bilirubin occur in reticuloendothelial cells, primarily in the spleen and liver.[310] The first reaction, catalyzed by the microsomal enzyme heme oxygenase, oxidatively cleaves the α bridge of the porphyrin group, opens the heme ring, and produces equimolar amounts of biliverdin and carbon monoxide (Fig. 9-1).[180] The second reaction, catalyzed by the cytosolic enzyme, biliverdin reductase, reduces the central methylene bridge of biliverdin converting it to bilirubin (Fig. 9-1).[311] Bilirubin formed in the reticuloendothelial cells is lipid soluble and virtually insoluble in water. In order to be transported in blood, it must be solubilized. This is accomplished by its reversible, noncovalent binding to albumin.[172,189] Bilirubin is then transported to the liver, where it, but not the albumin, is taken up by hepatocytes by a process that appears to involve carrier-mediated membrane transport (Fig. 9-2).[278] In the hepatocyte, bilirubin is coupled to the cytosolic protein, ligandin, (formerly called the Y protein).[12,190] A small fraction may be bound to a second cytosolic protein, the Z protein,[12] although its role in bilirubin metabolism is currently in doubt.[313] Bilirubin is then solubilized by conjugation to glucuronic acid, forming bilirubin monoglucuronide and diglucuronide, both referred to as direct-

acting bilirubins.[31,38] The conjugation of glucuronic acid to bilirubin is catalyzed by an enzyme system in the endoplasmic reticulum of the hepatocyte that transfers glucuronic acid from UDP-glucuronic acid to the acyl groups of the proprionic acid side chains of bilirubin (Fig. 9-3).[31,123,172] The bilirubin conjugates are then transported from the hepatocyte into canalicular bile by a process that appears to involve saturable, carrier-mediated membrane transport. This is assumed to be the rate-limiting step in hepatic bilirubin excretion.[247] The conjugated bilirubins drain from the bile duct into the duodenum and are carried distally through the intestine. In the distal ileum and colon, the conjugated bilirubins are hydrolyzed to unconjugated bilirubin by bacterial β-glucuronidases.[98a,327] The unconjugated bilirubin is reduced by normal gut bacteria to form a group of colorless tetrapyrroles called *urobilinogens*.[327] Approximately 80% to 90% of these products are excreted in feces, either unchanged or oxidized to orange derivatives called *urobilins*. The remaining 10% to 20% of the urobilinogens are passively absorbed, enter the portal venous blood, and are re-excreted by the liver. A small fraction escapes hepatic uptake, filters across the renal glomerulus, and is excreted in urine; usually less than 3 mg/dl.[47] The renal excretion of urobilinogen is complicated, in part because urobilinogen is a weak acid that passively diffuses across the renal tubule when in its undissociated form. Its appearance in urine depends upon many factors, including urine pH and the rate of urine flow.

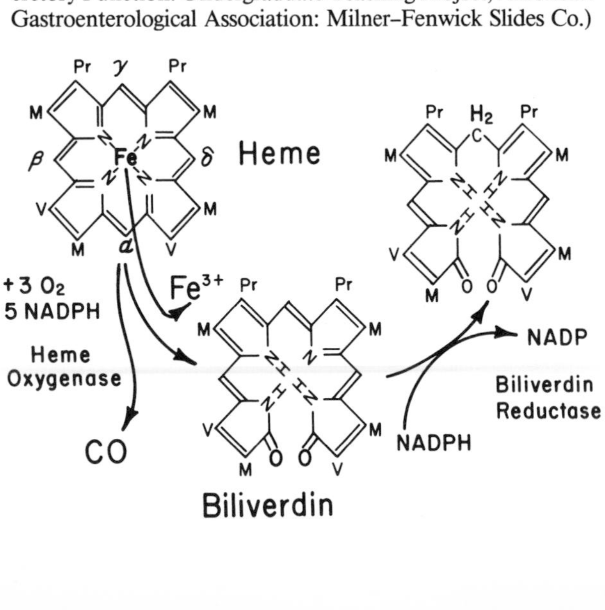

That unconjugated bilirubin was insoluble in aqueous solution was an enigma for many years because of the chemical structure of bilirubin (Fig. 9-4). It is an openchain tetrapyrrole with two proprionic acid groups. These carboxylic acids would be expected to ionize almost completely in aqueous solution at physiologic pH and confer polar properties on bilirubin. However, bilirubin behaves as a nonpolar molecule. In fact, the insolubility of bilirubin in aqueous media may contribute to the requirement that bilirubin be conjugated before it can be excreted in bile. An explanation for the nonpolar properties and water insolubility of bilirubin has been provided by recent studies using infrared spectroscopy and x-ray diffraction.[46,110,284] These studies demonstrate that intramolecular hydrogen bonds tightly link the acyl groups of the proprionic acid side chains to the nitrogens and oxygen of opposite pyrrole rings in the physiologically occurring bilirubin IX α (Fig. 9-4). These intramolecular hydrogen bonds render the bilirubin molecule rigid, bury the polar parts of the molecule within the nonpolar shell of the molecule, and prevent the proprionic acid carboxylic acid groups from ionizing and becoming hydrated. These intramolecular hydrogen bonds confer nonpolar properties on a seemingly polar molecule.[284] This hydrogen bonding occurs only in the naturally occurring isomer IX α. Exposure to visible light will disrupt these hydrogen bonds and allow changes in the configuration around the double bonds of the methene bridges. These altered configurations lead to the formation of a mixture of geometrical isomers, which, for

Fig. 9-1. Formation of bilirubin from heme by the sequential actions of the enzymes heme oxygenase and biliverdin reductase. M = methyl; V = vinyl; Pr = proprionic acid sidechains. (Adapted from Ostrow JD et al: Unit 1, Hepatic Excretory Function. Undergraduate Teaching Project, American Gastroenterological Association: Milner–Fenwick Slides Co.)

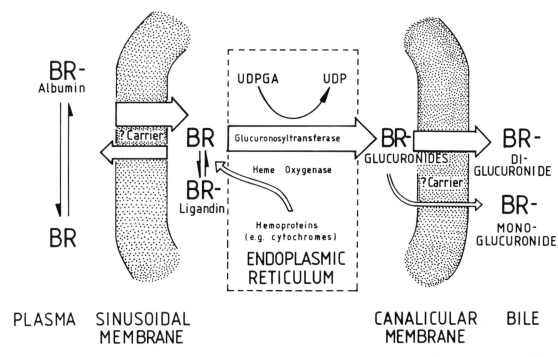

Fig. 9-2. Bilirubin transport and conjugation in the hepatocyte. Bilirubin is taken up from plasma into the hepatocyte of the plasma membrane and bound to ligandin. It is then carried to the endoplasmic reticulum where it is conjugated to glucuronic acid, forming bilirubin monoglucuronide and diglucuronide. Conjugated bilirubin is transported across the canalicular membrane and excreted in bile (Blanckaert N, Schmid R: Physiology and pathophysiology of bilirubin metabolism. In Zakim T, Boyer TA [eds]: Hepatology. A Textbook of Liver Disease, p 247. Philadelphia, WB Saunders, 1982)

Fig. 9-3. Structure of bilirubin IX α and bilirubin IX α diglucuronide. In the latter, the glucuronides prevent intramolecular hydrogen bonding between the proprionic acid groups and the pyrrole ring nitrogens. (Schmid R: Gastroenterology 74:1307, 1978)

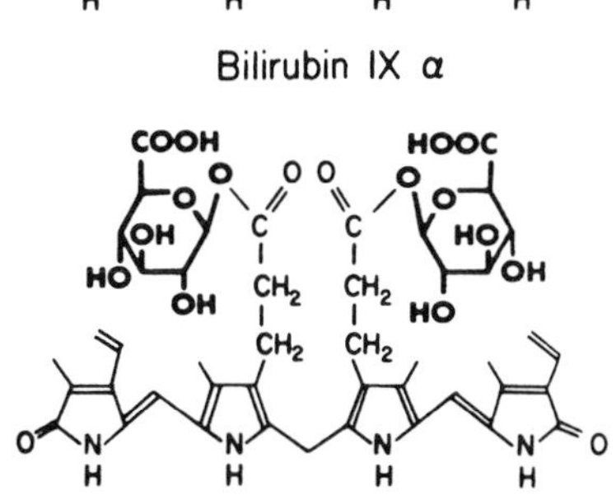

Bilirubin IX α

Bilirubin IX α diglucuronide

steric reasons, cannot form tight intramolecular hydrogen bonds.[37] These isomers are water soluble, can be excreted in bile without conjugation, and account for the effectiveness of phototherapy in treating neonatal unconjugated hyperbilirubinemia.[68] Conjugation of bilirubin to glucuronic acid also disrupts these internal hydrogen bonds and solubilizes bilirubin.[148]

Measurement of Serum Bilirubin

The terms direct- and indirect-reacting bilirubin are based on the original van den Bergh method, which is still used in most clinical chemistry laboratories to determine the serum bilirubin.[351] In this assay, bilirubin reacts with diazotized sulfanilic acid and splits into two relatively stable dipyrryl azopigments that absorb maximally at 540 nm. The direct fraction is that which reacts with diazotized sulfanilic acid in 1 minute in the absence of alcohol.[351] This fraction provides an approximate determination of the conjugated bilirubin in serum. The total serum bilirubin is that amount that reacts in 30 minutes after the addition of alcohol. The indirect fraction is the difference between the total and direct bilirubin and provides an estimate of the unconjugated bilirubin in serum. With the

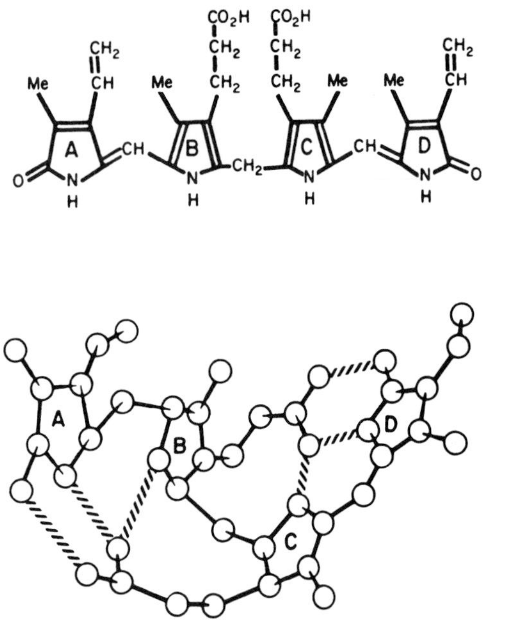

Fig. 9-4. Structure of bilirubin IX α: conventionally written structure (*top*) and internally hydrogen-bonded structure (*bottom*). In the latter, the proprionic acid groups of pyrrole rings B and C are linked to the nitrogen of the opposite pyrrole rings (*broken lines*). (Schmid R: Gastroenterology 74:1307, 1978)

van den Bergh method, the normal serum bilirubin concentration is usually less than 1.0 mg/dl. Up to 20% to 30% or 0.3 mg/dl of the total is direct-reacting bilirubin.[107,317,351] Total serum bilirubin concentrations are between 0.2 mg/dl and 0.9 mg/dl in 95% of a normal population and below 1.0 in 99%.[329,351] Some differences in

the properties of unconjugated and conjugated bilirubin are listed in Table 9-1.

Recent advances in methodology indicate that the diazo method does not accurately reflect the true values of the indirect- and direct-reacting fractions of bilirubin, particularly at low total serum bilirubin concentrations.[39,40] Although these new, more accurate methods provide information that resolves many of the enigmas of bilirubin metabolism, they are less convenient to perform. In most clinical situations, they do not provide enough clinical advantages to replace the older, familiar diazo methods. One new, more precise method involves alkaline methanolysis of bilirubin followed by chloroform extraction of the bilirubin methyl esters, separation of these esters with high performance liquid chromatography (HPLC) and spectrophotometric determination at 430 nm.[39,40] There are, in addition, other HPLC methods that do not require alkaline methanolysis, although globulins and other high molecular–weight proteins must be precipitated from serum prior to chromatography.[82,185] Other assays, based on dry reagent chemistry, have recently been reviewed.[82] One method, which is used in increasing numbers of clinical chemistry laboratories, is based on photographic film technology.[82] It can be automated and appears able to accurately measure conjugated and unconjugated bilirubin as well as to detect a newly recognized bilirubin fraction, bilirubin delta. Bilirubin delta is conjugated bilirubin that is tightly linked to albumin, probably by covalent bonding.[328]

These new techniques add considerably to our understanding of bilirubin metabolism. First, they demonstrate that almost 100% of the serum bilirubin in normal persons or those with Gilbert's syndrome is unconjugated. (Fig. 9-5). Less than 3% is monoconjugated bilirubin. Second, in jaundiced patients with hepatobiliary disease, the total serum bilirubin concentration measured by these new, more accurate methods is lower than the values found

TABLE 9-1.   Differences Between Unconjugated and Conjugated Bile Pigments

PROPERTY	UNCONJUGATED BILIRUBIN	CONJUGATED BILIRUBIN
van den Bergh reaction	Indirect (+ alcohol)	Direct
Solubility in aqueous solution	—	+
Solubility in lipid solvents	+	—
Attachment to plasma albumin	+	+
Presence in icteric urine	—	+
Presence in bile	—*	+
Affinity for brain tissue	+	—
Association with hemolytic jaundice	++	±
Association with obstructive and hepatocellular jaundice	+	+++

* A small quantity of unconjugated bilirubin may be present in common duct bile. There is a relative increase in unconjugated bilirubin in bile in conditions associated with severe unconjugated hyperbilirubinemia such as Crigler–Najjar syndrome.[78]

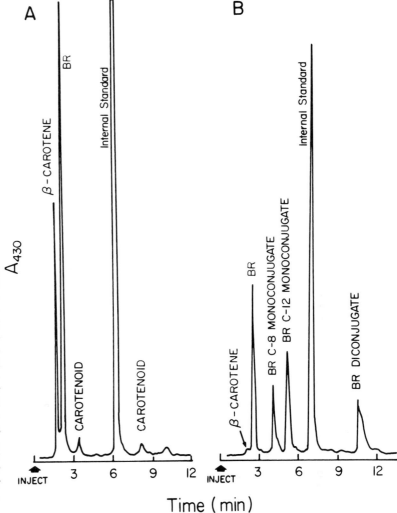

Fig. 9-5. Chromatograms of bilirubin in plasma of a healthy adult (*A*) and a patient with obstructive jaundice (*B*). BR = unconjugated bilirubin. There are no detectable bilirubin glucuronides in the healthy adult. In the patient with obstructive jaundice there is a mixture of unconjugated bilirubin, bilirubin monoglucuronides, and bilirubin diglucuronide. Bilirubin conjugates in plasma were converted to their methyl ester derivatives, then extracted and separated by high-pressure liquid chromatography. Xanthobilirubic acid was used as an internal standard. (Blanckaert N, Schmid R: Physiology and pathophysiology of bilirubin metabolism. In Zakim D, Boyer TA [eds]: Hepatology. A Textbook of Liver Disease, p 261. Philadelphia, WB Saunders, 1982)

with diazo methods.[40] This suggests that there are diazo-positive compounds distinct from bilirubin in the serum of patients with hepatobiliary disease. Third, these studies indicate that in jaundiced patients with hepatobiliary disease, monoglucuronides of bilirubin predominate over the diglucuronides (Fig. 9-5). Fourth, part of the direct-reacting bilirubin fraction includes conjugated bilirubin that is covalently linked to albumin (Fig. 9-6).[328] This albumin-linked bilirubin fraction represents an important fraction of total serum bilirubin in patients with cholestasis and hepatobiliary disorders (Fig. 9-7).[328] Albumin-bound bilirubin is formed in serum when hepatic excretion of bilirubin glucuronides is impaired and the glucuronides are present in serum in increasing amounts. By virtue of its tight binding to albumin, the clearance rate of albumin-bound bilirubin from serum approximates the half-life of albumin, 12 to 14 days, rather than the short half-life of bilirubin, approximately 4 hours.[43] The prolonged half-life of albumin-bound bilirubin explains two previously

unexplained enigmas in jaundiced patients with liver disease: (1) that some patients with conjugated hyperbilirubinemia do not exhibit bilirubinuria during the recovery phase of their disease, and (2) that the elevated serum bilirubin declines more slowly than expected in some patients who otherwise appear to be recovering quite satisfactorily. Late in the recovery phase of hepatobiliary disorders, all the conjugated bilirubin may be in the albumin-linked form. It is therefore not filtered by the renal glomerulus and does not appear in urine, although the serum bilirubin concentration is high. Its value in serum falls slowly because of the long half-life of albumin. The slow decline is unrelated to the actual hepatic status.

Diagnostic Value of Serum Bilirubin

The bilirubin normally present in serum represents a balance between input from production and hepatic removal of the pigment. Hyperbilirubinemia, therefore, may result

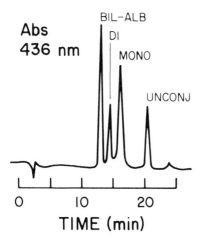

Fig. 9-6. Chromatogram of serum bilirubin from a patient with obstructive jaundice demonstrating the presence of a bilirubin fraction that is bound to albumin, BIL-ALB. DI = bilirubin diglucuronide; MONO = bilirubin monoglucuronide; UNCONJ = conjugated bilirubin. Serum bilirubin was separated by reversed-phase high-performance liquid chromatography. (Reprinted by permission of the New England Journal of Medicine, vol 309, p 147, 1983)

from (1) overproduction of bilirubin; (2) impaired uptake, conjugation, or excretion of bilirubin; or (3) regurgitation of unconjugated or conjugated bilirubin from damaged hepatocytes or bile ducts. One may anticipate that an increase in unconjugated bilirubin in serum results from overproduction or impairment of uptake or conjugation, whereas an increase in the conjugated moiety is due to decreased excretion or backward leakage of the pigment.

Total serum bilirubin is not a sensitive indicator of hepatic dysfunction and may not accurately reflect the degree of liver damage. Hyperbilirubinemia may not be detected in instances of moderate or severe hepatic parenchymal damage or of a partially or briefly obstructed common bile duct. This lack of sensitivity is partly explained by observations obtained in normal persons given infusions of unconjugated bilirubin[315] and in patients with uncomplicated hemolysis,[238] suggesting that the capacity of the human liver to remove bilirubin from serum before hyperbilirubinemia occurs is at least twofold greater than the daily pigment load (250 mg to 300 mg) normally presented to this organ. The capacity may be even higher based on the maximal rate of excretion of bilirubin in bile, approximately 55.2 mg/kg/day,[248] and the average amount of bilirubin formed from the destruction of senescent red blood cells, 3.9 mg/kg/day.[27] In a steady state, the height of the serum bilirubin usually reflects the intensity of jaundice and the increase in total body bile pigment. However, occasionally the serum bilirubin concentration may be lowered transiently by the presence in serum of substances such as salicylates, sulfonamides, or free fatty acids that displace bilirubin from its attachment to plasma albumin and enhance transfer of the pigment

Fig. 9-7. Albumin-bound bilirubin (*BIL-ALB*) as a percentage of total bilirubin (*T BILI*). The number of subjects is indicated for each diagnostic category. Each solid circle represents a serum sample from a patient with a clinically deteriorating condition and increasing total bilirubin. Each open circle represents a sample from a patient with clinical improvement and falling total bilirubin. The bars indicate means ± 1 SD. Serial measurements were not obtained in subjects with unconjugated hyperbilirubinemia and Dubin–Johnson syndrome. (Reprinted by permission of the New England Journal of Medicine, vol 309, 147, 1983)

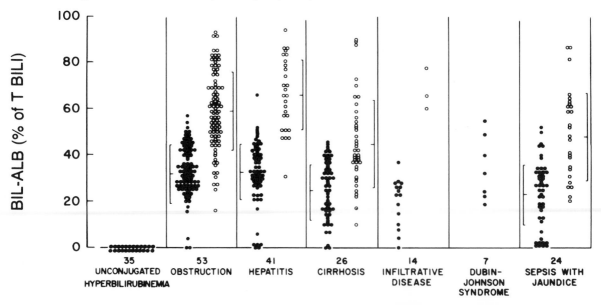

into tissues.[282] Conversely, an increase in serum albumin concentration may induce a temporary shift of bilirubin from tissue sites into the circulation.[93,157]

The height of the total serum bilirubin is seldom of value in specifying the cause of jaundice in the individual patient because values among the various types of jaundice overlap considerably.[144] On the average, however, uncomplicated hemolysis seldom causes a serum bilirubin in excess of 5 mg/dl,[172] and parenchymal liver disease or incomplete extrahepatic obstruction due to biliary calculi gives lower serum bilirubin values than those seen with malignant obstruction of the common bile duct.

Few controlled studies have critically assessed the prognostic value of height and duration of hyperbilirubinemia in liver disease. In general, the higher the serum bilirubin concentration in viral hepatitis, the greater the histologic evidence of hepatocellular damage and the longer the course of the disease.[293] Nevertheless, patients may die of fulminant hepatitis with only modest elevation of serum bilirubin. The presence of concomitant hemolysis with overproduction of bilirubin and diminished glomerular filtration rate causing decreased excretion of the pigment may also confuse the issue by causing higher serum bilirubin values than would be expected for any degree of hepatocellular damage present. In acute alcoholic hepatitis, hyperbilirubinemia in excess of 5 mg/dl is one of the findings that connotes a poor prognosis.[132,133]

The major value of fractionating total serum bilirubin into unconjugated and direct-reacting moieties is in the detection of states characterized by unconjugated hyperbilirubinemia (Table 9-2). Such a diagnosis appears warranted when the serum indirect-reacting bilirubin is in excess of 1.2 mg/dl and the direct-reacting fraction constitutes less than 20% of the total serum bilirubin. Unfortunately, when the total serum bilirubin is minimally elevated, it may be difficult to distinguish the nature of the bilirubin elevation. This is due to the inaccuracy of the diazo methods in distinguishing conjugated from unconjugated bilirubin at low total serum bilirubin concentrations. This is one of the instances in which the new, more precise HPLC methods of bilirubin determination

will provide clinically useful information not attainable with the older diazo methods. This is particularly true in the detection of early or mild liver injury. Total bilirubin may initially be normal in some patients with cirrhosis, hepatitis, congestive heart failure, and other disorders.[115,276,326] However, an increase in the direct fraction above 0.3 mg/dl should alert one to the possibility of mild liver injury. If the newer, more accurate techniques are used, conjugated bilirubin concentrations above 0.1 mg/dl should accurately detect patients with early liver injury, since, normally, bilirubin glucuronides are undetectable in serum except in hepatobiliary disorders.[40]

At present, measurement and fractionation of the serum bilirubin in jaundiced patients does not allow one to distinguish accurately between parenchymal (hepatocellular) and cholestatic (obstructive) jaundice. The accurate HPLC methods for measuring serum bilirubin demonstrate that unconjugated and conjugated bilirubins are both increased in hepatobiliary disease. There is no consistent pattern of elevation of these fractions that distinguishes hepatocellular from cholestatic liver disease.[40] Both bilirubin monoglucuronide and diglucuronide are elevated, with the monoglucuronides predominating. This is true in both hepatocellular and cholestatic liver disease.

Urine Bilirubin

The presence of bilirubin in the urine indicates hepatobiliary disease. Unconjugated bilirubin is tightly bound to albumin, is not filtered by the glomerulus, and is not present in urine. Only conjugated bilirubin is found in urine. This occurs only when there is conjugated bilirubin in serum, that is, when there is hepatobiliary disease. The newer, more precise methods for measuring serum bilirubin indicate that virtually 100% of the serum bilirubin in normal persons and those with Gilbert's syndrome is unconjugated bilirubin. Measureable amounts of conjugated bilirubin in serum are found only in hepatobiliary disease. Because the renal threshold for conjugated bilirubin is low and methods currently in use can detect bilirubin concentrations as low as 0.05 mg/dl of urine,[173]

TABLE 9-2. Causes of Unconjugated Hyperbilirubinemia

PATIENT GROUP	MECHANISM
PEDIATRIC	
Physiologic	Immaturity or inborn or acquired
Crigler–Najjar syndrome[78]	impairment of hepatic
Breast milk[10]	glucuronide-conjugating system
Lucey–Driscoll syndrome[11]	
PEDIATRIC AND ADULT	
Intravascular hemolysis	Overproduction of bilirubin
"Shunt" hyperbilirubinemia	Overproduction of bilirubin
Gilbert's syndrome	Impaired uptake and/or conjugation
Posthepatic[103]	Impaired uptake and/or conjugation
Miscellaneous (e.g., cardiac, hepatobiliary)[191]	Unspecified

conjugated bilirubin may be found in urine when the total serum bilirubin is normal and the patient is not clinically jaundiced. This may occur early in the course of viral hepatitis or other hepatobiliary disease when conjugated bilirubin first appears in serum. Conversely, the urine may become free of bilirubin long before the conjugated serum bilirubin falls to normal values in patients recovering from hepatobiliary diseases.[328] When this occurs, all the conjugated bilirubin is in the albumin-bound form and is not filtered by the glomerulus.

Dye Tests

Because it has long been recognized that the serum bilirubin is an insensitive test of hepatic dysfunction and that at low serum levels measurement of the total and direct bilirubin lacks biochemical precision, an effort was made to develop other tests of hepatic excretory capacity that were more sensitive and specific. The aim was to develop tests that would more critically and specifically evaluate the excretory and/or detoxification capacity of the liver. Although all these tests are clearly more sensitive than the serum bilirubin, they have limited value at present because of their nonspecificity, that is, the extent of the abnormality is, in general, comparable in all types of hepatobiliary disorders. These tests include the dye tests, the breath tests, and the serum bile acid tests.

Sulfobromophthalein Sodium

Sulfobromophthalein sodium (BSP) (Fig. 9-8) was introduced in 1924[264] and used as a sensitive indicator of liver

Fig. 9-8. Structural formula from BSP, sulfobromophthalein sodium (sodium phenoltetrabromophthalein disulfonate).

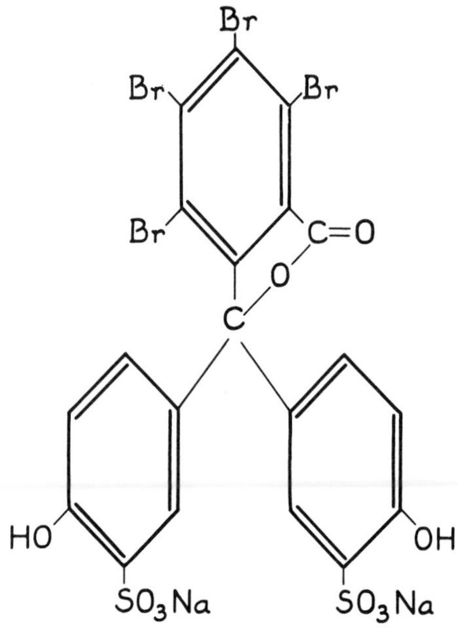

dysfunction until the 1970s when its use as a liver function test greatly decreased. It is rarely used now except in research laboratories and in specific situations such as the diagnosis of the Dubin–Johnson syndrome.[59,94,200,290,291] The following discussion is included as much for historical interest as for practical use by the hepatologist and clinical investigator.

BSP is completely soluble in water but binds rapidly to albumin and α_1-lipoprotein when it is injected intravenously.[16] BSP or the BSP–albumin complex binds to the hepatocyte plasma membrane,[305,327a] and BSP is avidly taken up by the hepatocyte where it binds to ligandin (the Y protein) but probably not to the Z protein as was formerly believed.[313] Hepatic uptake of BSP appears saturable,[122] and there is competition for uptake with bilirubin, indocyanine green, rose bengal, and bunamiodyl.[147] BSP has a high first-pass clearance by the liver, 50% to 80%, and its removal from the circulation is closely related to hepatic blood flow.[62,130] Much of the BSP within hepatocytes is conjugated to glutathione in a thioether linkage.[73,154,155] The reaction is catalyzed by ligandin, the same protein that binds BSP and bilirubin within hepatocytes (Fig. 9-9).[73,124,155] A number of other conjugates, including BSP-cysteinyl glycine and BSP-cysteine, are also formed, presumably by cleavage of glutamic acid and glycine from the glutathione moiety. Both conjugated and free BSP are then excreted across canalicular membranes into the biliary tract. Conjugation is not required for uptake[72,233] nor for biliary excretion of the dye. However, it does appear to be advantageous for the latter process in some species in which conjugated BSP compounds are preferentially excreted into bile.[72,233,324,325,336]

BSP compounds are transported into bile in high concentration and, when compared to intracellular concentration, against large concentration gradients. There is also evidence that other organic anions compete with BSP for biliary excretion and thus, presumably, for a common canalicular transport system.[71] Finally, biliary excretion appears to have many of the characteristics of a rate-limited transport process,[74,333,334] although several studies indicate that the apparent maximal rate of biliary excretion of BSP can be enhanced by infusion of taurocholate.[125,224,254]

Prolonged infusions of BSP have been used to quantify the liver's excretory capacity by measuring BSP's hepatic uptake, storage, and maximal biliary excretion rate.[333,334] BSP will accumulate in liver in proportion to the serum concentration, up to a maximal capacity, the hepatic storage capacity, S.[333,334] If BSP is infused at two different rates that are each greater than the liver's maximum capacity to excrete BSP into bile, the maximum excretion rate for BSP, Tm, can be calculated.[333,334]

More recently, similar types of data have been generated by simply determining the plasma disappearance following a standard intravenous injection of BSP.[130] By use of a semilogarithmic clearance curve, two rate constants can be measured (Fig. 9-10). K_1, the rapid, initial clearance rate, correlates closely with estimated hepatic blood flow,

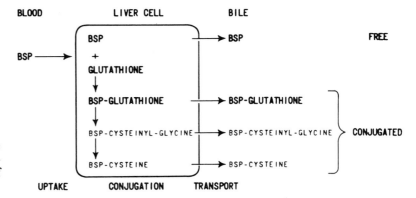

Fig. 9-9. Conjugation of BSP to glutathione in hepatocytes, metabolism of BSP-glutathione within hepatocytes, and excretion of BSP conjugates into bile.

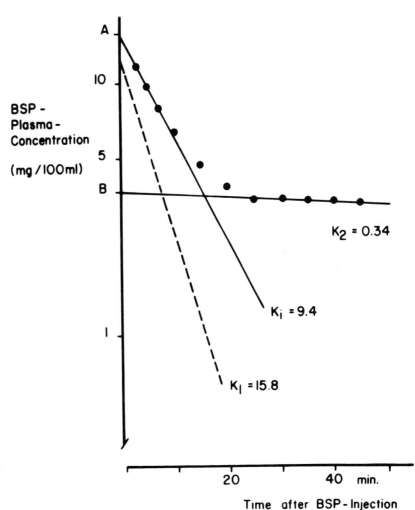

Fig. 9-10. Representative BSP-plasma disappearance curve in a patient with primary biliary cirrhosis after injection of 5 mg/kg of BSP. The lines for K_1 and K_2 were fitted graphically. K_i was calculated from K_1 and K_2. A and B are extrapolated zero-time intercepts. The disappearance rate constants are expressed in percent per minute. (Hacki W et al: J Lab Clin Med 88:1019, 1976)

(Fig. 9-11) whereas K_2, the second slower experimental component, correlates closely with the Tm for BSP (Fig. 9-12).[130] Serial determinations of BSP-Tm may prove useful in the management of certain chronic cholestatic syndromes such as primary biliary cirrhosis. In this disease, the earliest changes involve damage to the small bile ductules and result in diminished bile flow. The BSP-Tm may be a sensitive way to measure this function and to evaluate the response to drugs being used to treat primary biliary cirrhosis.

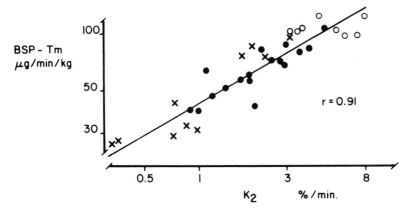

Fig. 9-11. Double logarithmic correlation between BSP-Tm and the second exponential component, K_2. Control subjects are shown by open circles, patients with cirrhosis by closed circles, and patients with miscellaneous liver diseases by X's. (Hacki W et al: J Lab Clin Med 88:1019, 1976)

Observations in mutant sheep with congenital transport defects, in Corriedale sheep with a hepatic excretory defect,[9] and in Southdown sheep with a hepatic uptake defect[77] for many organic anions, including BSP, indicate that carrier activity may be determined genetically. This further suggests that the functioning of the sinusoidal and canalicular carrier mechanisms depends in some way upon genetically determined proteins. Such genetic factors may also determine the sensitivity of carriers to other compounds, for example, the probable sensitivity of the canalicular transport system in cholestatic jaundice of pregnancy to various steroids, including oral contraceptive agents.[218]

The standard test involves the intravenous injection of a fixed dose of BSP, usually 5 mg/kg body weight, followed

Fig. 9-12. Double logarithmic correlation between estimated hepatic plasma flow (EHPF) and the first experimental component, K_1, in patients with cirrhosis. The normal range ± 1 SD is given by the rectangle. (Hacki W et al: J Lab Clin Med 88:1019, 1976)

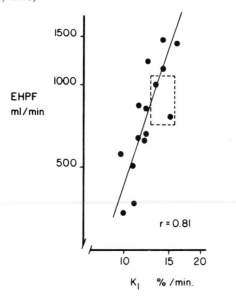

by sampling of blood from the noninjected arm at various times after injection. Serum is separated and alkalinized, and the BSP is read at 580 nm in a spectrophotometer. The purpose is to determine the percentage of dye remaining in plasma at a given time after injection. The zero-time concentration is assumed to be 10 mg/dl.[350] Normal values at 30 minutes and 45 minutes are 10% and 5%, respectively, although these values may exclude up to 30% of normal persons.[350] Values in men and women are the same if the dose is adjusted to lean body weight, although both Tm and S are greater in men.[239]

Local tissue damage may occur if dye is injected into the perivascular tissues. Anaphylactic reactions, sometimes fatal, have been reported but are rare.[149] Care should be taken to ensure that the dye is administered intravenously and slowly over a period of a few minutes. Toxic reactions have also resulted from injection of cold solutions of BSP that contain crystals of the dye.[159]

Because the BSP retention test is dependent upon so many factors, including hepatic blood flow, hepatic mass, functional capacity of hepatocytes, and bile flow, the test is abnormal in all types of liver disease. As would be expected, it is also nonspecific. In addition, results are affected by fever[42] and the concomitant use of drugs that either displace BSP from its plasma-binding proteins or inhibit its uptake or excretion by the liver.[153] There is one clinical situation in which the BSP test is useful, the diagnosis of Dubin–Johnson syndrome and its differentiation from Rotor's syndrome. In Dubin–Johnson syndrome, there is an initial rapid fall in the plasma BSP concentration followed by a secondary rise 45 minutes to 90 minutes later.[59,94,200,290,291] This is due to regurgitation of conjugated BSP. In Rotor's syndrome, there is a slower clearance of BSP from serum but no secondary rise.[77,255] Tm is nearly zero in Dubin–Johnson syndrome, whereas S is low in Rotor's syndrome. The BSP test is still useful in clinical research and in the elucidation of hepatobiliary transport disorders.

Indocyanine Green

Indocyanine green (ICG) (Fig. 9-13), another dye used to evaluate liver function,[188,229] is bound to albumin and α_1-

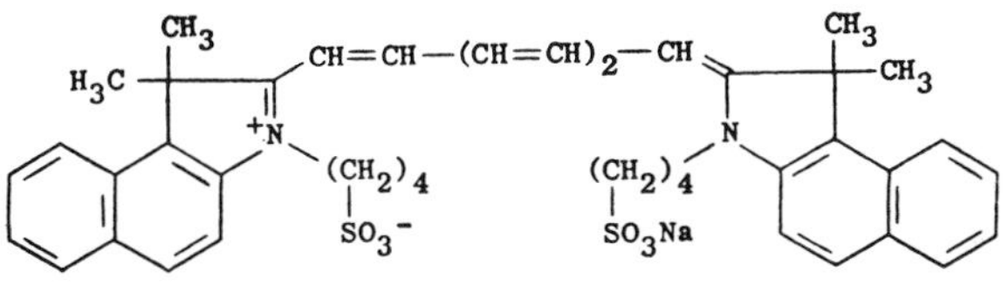

Fig. 9-13. Structural formula for indocyanine green.

lipoprotein more avidly than BSP.[16] It has a higher hepatic extraction ratio than BSP, 70% to 96%.[62] Ninety-seven percent of an administered dose is excreted unchanged in bile,[332] and the liver appears to be the only site of clearance of ICG in humans.[229] ICG and BSP appear to share the same sinusoidal and canalicular transport systems,[147,332] but ICG has no enterohepatic circulation. ICG can be measured directly by spectrophotometry. Theoretically, ICG disappearance curves can be measured without repeated blood samplings by dichromatic ear lobe densitometry,[188] but this method is not always reliable and the ear lobe readings do not correlate closely with simultaneously obtained plasma values.[126] ICG is used primarily to estimate hepatic blood flow.[33,229,353] If ICG is infused intravenously at a rate well below the liver's capacity to clear it, a steady state is reached within 1 hour. At this time, the rate of hepatic clearance is equal to the infusion rate. Since this is known and ICG concentration in peripheral venous blood is easily measured, hepatic blood flow can be estimated by use of the Fick equation:

$$F = \frac{R}{(ICG)_a - (ICG)_{hv}}$$

F is the estimated hepatic blood flow, R is the hepatic removal rate of ICG, $(ICG)_a$ is the concentration of ICG in the hepatic artery and portal vein blood, and $(ICG)_{hv}$ is the concentration of ICG in hepatic vein blood. $(ICG)_a$ is the same as the concentration of ICG in peripheral venous blood. Measurement of $(ICG)_{hv}$ would require catheterization of the hepatic vein and is impractical in most clinical settings. Because first pass extraction of ICG by the liver is very high, 70% to 96%, the clearance rate is assumed to be 100%, and $(ICG)_{hv}$ is accordingly set at zero. This method can be performed at the bedside but will always underestimate hepatic blood flow,[33] because $(ICG)_{hv}$ is always more than zero.

ICG clearance is not as sensitive an indicator of hepatic dysfunction as BSP because at doses of ICG that are safe to administer, the liver's excretory capacity for ICG is far below its maximum.[229] In order to estimate the maximal ICG capacity, one would have to use four or five different doses of ICG at different times and then use Michaelis–Menton-type data analysis. This is time consuming and impractical except in a research setting. Those who have used ICG in the evaluation of liver disease recommend single intravenous injections ranging from 0.64 μmol/kg to 6.4 μmol/kg[229] and determination of a single blood level 20 minutes later. Both doses are well below the dose needed to saturate the liver's excretory capacity for ICG, more than 72 μmol/kg. In contrast to the BSP test, ICG

clearance is not affected by fever[188] and is normal in the Dubin–Johnson syndrome[83] and in newborns.[188] ICG is rarely used in the evaluation of patients with liver disease but is useful in clinical research.

Bile Acid Tests

Although sensitive tests to measure serum bile acid concentration (see Chap. 3) have been available for more than 10 years,[295] physicians are still searching for a role for these tests in the evaluation of patients with suspected liver disease. Bile acids are synthesized from cholesterol in hepatocytes, conjugated to glycine or taurine, and then secreted into bile. Approximately 80% to 90% of the bile acids are stored in the gallbladder between meals while the remaining fraction is secreted continuously into the duodenum. This fraction accounts for the bile acids normally present in serum after a long fast, the concentration of which is 5 μmol/L to 10 μmol/L.[2] Cholic acid conjugates constitute less than 20% of this amount, and dihydroxy bile acids constitute the remainder.[2] During a meal, the gallbladder contracts and discharges its pool of bile acids into the duodenum. Bile acids move rapidly down the intestinal tract, where some are absorbed throughout the whole intestine by nonionic passive diffusion and most are actively reabsorbed by carrier-mediated transport in the terminal ileum and carried back to the liver via the portal vein.[29] The liver efficiently extracts bile acids from portal blood; approximately 70% to 80% of dihydroxy bile acids undergo first pass extraction, whereas 90% of trihydroxy bile acids are extracted.[2,8] This difference in extraction rates is probably due to the tighter binding of dihydroxy bile acids to albumin. The fractional extraction rates of bile acids are relatively constant in health.[240] Since a larger quantity of bile acids reach the liver following a meal and the proportion extracted is constant, a larger quantity of bile acids escapes into the circulation postprandially. This produces the normal postprandial rise in serum bile acid concentration, to a level approximately two- to fivefold greater than fasting levels.[181] In health, all the serum bile acids are from intestinal input; none comes directly from the liver.[183] Maintenance of normal serum bile acid concentrations is dependent upon hepatic blood flow, hepatic uptake, secretion of bile acids, and intestinal motility.[29] A disease that affects any of these functions should theoretically affect serum bile acid levels. This has proved to be true in practice. Serum bile acids are very sensitive but nonspecific indicators of hepatic dysfunction. They do allow some quantification of functional hepatic reserve.

There are now several accurate ways to measure serum bile acid concentration.[101] These include enzymatic assays in which the bacterial enzyme 3-α-hydroxysteroid dehydrogenase is coupled either to fluorimetric[20] or biluminescence techniques,[259] gas–liquid chromatography,[231] radioimmunoassay,[84,258,277] and a highly specific assay combining gas–liquid chromatography and mass spectrometry.[7] Only the enzyme and radioimmunoassays are easily adapted to the clinical chemistry laboratory. Although the radioimmunoassays can be automated, a variety of individual radioimmunoassays that detect cholic and chenodeoxycholic acids and their conjugates would have to be used in order to measure the total amount of bile acids in serum. This is probably not necessary if the purpose of the assay is to detect liver disease.

To date, the serum bile acid tests appear to have contributed little to the differential diagnosis of liver disease. There appears to be no consistent advantage to the postprandial test compared to the fasting test.[105,195,231,318] As might be expected, the bile acid tests are more sensitive than the serum bilirubin in all types of hepatobiliary disorders[144,212,296] and correlate moderately well with results of the aminopyrine breath test (Fig. 9-14).[215] Serum bile acid levels are normal in patients with Gilbert's syndrome[55,258] and Dubin–Johnson syndrome.[4] Serum bile acid tests are as sensitive as the aminotransferases in detecting acute viral hepatitis but less so than the aminotransferases in detecting post-transfusion hepatitis.[213] They are also less sensitive than the aminotransferases as screening tests for detecting subclinical liver disease.[105,252] Serum bile acids are invariably abnormal in cirrhosis of any etiology[106,296,314,321] and are equal to or more sensitive than tests such as the serum albumin or prothrombin time.

This is not unexpected and is due to the decreased functioning liver cell mass, decreased bile excretion, and portasystemic shunting usually present in chronic liver diseases, all of which will affect serum bile acid levels. It has been suggested that serum bile acid tests can predict histologic severity[215] and might replace percutaneous liver biopsy, but there are insufficient data to comfortably support this hypothesis. Some investigators have found a poor correlation between serum bile acids and histologic severity in chronic hepatitis and alcoholic liver disease (Fig. 9-15).[98,158,212] The observation that a twofold increase in serum bile acid concentration will accurately predict impending relapse in patients with chronic hepatitis who are in remission[174] also has not been confirmed. There is, in fact, too much overlap between serum bile acid levels in patients with persistent hepatitis and chronic active hepatitis with bridging necrosis or cirrhosis to obviate liver biopsy.[212,215,296] The attempt to improve the sensitivity and/or specificity of the serum bile acid tests by intravenous or oral tolerance tests has not proved successful.[8,118,182]

In summary, serum bile acid tests offer the advantage that they are highly specific indicators of liver dysfunction. However, they are less sensitive than they were originally hoped to be and nonspecific in distinguishing among the various types of liver disease. In this respect, they appear similar to the BSP and ICG clearance tests, sensitive liver function tests that are rarely used. They may have usefulness in ruling out liver disease in patients with suspected Gilbert's syndrome and Dubin–Johnson syndrome.

Breath Tests

The introduction of breath tests in man using ^{14}C-aminopyrine,[139] ^{14}C-phenacetin,[51] ^{14}C-diazepam,[142] and [14]C-

Fig. 9-14. Correlation between the aminopyrine breath test and the logarithm of 2-hour postprandial serum cholylglycine levels in 44 patients who underwent both tests. Closed circles indicate chronic active hepatitis with bridging necrosis or cirrhosis; open circles indicate chronic persistent hepatitis and chronic active hepatitis. Cholylglycine levels were determined by radioimmunoassay. (Monroe PS et al: Hepatology 2:317, 1982)

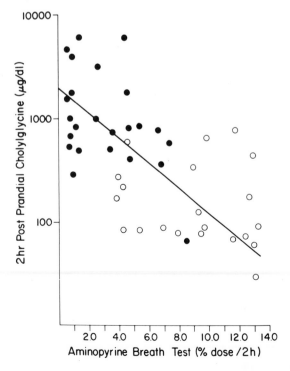

Fig. 9-15. Serum bile acids in normal subjects and in patients with alcohol-induced fatty liver and alcoholic cirrhosis. Note the overlap in individual values among the three groups. Serum bile acids, shown on the ordinate, were determined by combined gas–liquid chromatography and mass spectrometry using deuterium-labeled internal standards. (Einarsson K et al: Hepatology 5:108, 1985)

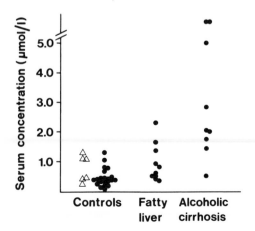

or ^{13}C-galactose[294] represents an attempt to develop a practical test of hepatic functional reserve. The principle and methodology of breath tests are simple. A substance labeled with ^{14}C, which is converted primarily in the liver to [14]CO_2, is given orally or parenterally. As long as absorption is complete or reproducible, the oral route is more convenient. The [14]CO_2 exhaled in the breath is collected at various intervals in an alkaline medium that serves as a CO_2 trap. Metabolism of the labeled agent by the liver can be determined semiquantitatively by multiplication of the specific activity of exhaled [14]CO_2 over a given time interval by a value for endogenous CO_2 output of 9 mm/kg/hr.[342]

An ideal drug for use in a breath test of hepatic drug-metabolizing capacity would have the following characteristics: (1) Metabolism of the test drug should be primarily hepatic. This important parameter is often difficult to validate in humans. (2) When the drug is given orally, its absorption must be rapid and complete or at least predictable. (3) The generated [14]CO_2 should be evenly distributed in the body and not sequestered in an unavailable compartment. (4) For ease of collection of [14]CO_2, the drug should have a short elimination half-life. (5) The drug must be safe. In general, these characteristics seem to have been met for the drugs currently in use as breath tests, although some points have not been worked out completely.

Most experience has been obtained with the ^{14}C-aminopyrine breath test. The radioactive methyl groups of aminopyrine undergo demethylation and eventual conversion through formaldehyde and formate to bicarbonate-CO_2 with exhalation of [14]CO_2 in breath (Fig. 9-16). Studies in rats demonstrate that the rate of [14]CO_2 appearance in breath correlates with the hepatic mixed function oxidase system mass.[186] Studies in humans also suggest that the aminopyrine breath test is a measure of mixed function oxidase mass, because in control subjects, the rate of appearance of [14]CO_2 in breath correlates with clearance of aminopyrine from blood[32,114a,139,140]; furthermore, the rate of [14]CO_2 appearance increases following pretreatment with phenobarbital, a known microsomal

inducer, whereas it decreases after treatment with disulfiram, an inhibitor of the microsomal mixed function oxidase system.[139] The decreased rate of [14]CO_2 appearance in breath also correlates well with decreased clearance of aminopyrine from blood in patients with cirrhosis, a state in which mixed function oxidase mass is likely to be decreased. The concept that the breath test is a measure of functioning hepatic microsomal mass is further supported by observations that low results of the aminopyrine breath test in patients with hepatocellular disease correlate well with the tests that reflect functional mass: the degree of prothrombin time prolongation,[61] with the extent of decrease in serum albumin[139,140]; serum bile acid levels,[215] Figure 9-14; galactose elimination capacity[32]; and impaired BSP removal from blood.[32,140] Low aminopyrine breath test results also correlate well with the degree of necrosis and inflammation in liver biopsies in patients with alcohol-related cirrhosis (Fig. 9-17).[61] Although only 30% of the administered label is recovered in 48 hours and only 60% of the administered aminopyrine is recovered as demethylated metabolites in urine,[56,117] a recent detailed analysis of the pharmacokinetics of the aminopyrine breath test supports its validity as a measurement of hepatic microsomal enzyme function.[151] However, one must be aware that factors such as diet, folate deficiency, and use of other drugs may alter the results of this test.

The test is usually performed after an overnight fast. A known dose of ^{14}C-aminopyrine, 1.0 μCi to 2.0 μCi, is administered orally and breath samples are collected at 30-minute intervals for up to 4 hours. The expired CO_2 is trapped in alkali and counted. There is an excellent correlation between the percentage of administered ^{14}C expired in 2 hours, the plasma clearance rate of aminopyrine, and the fractional disappearance rate of [14]CO_2.[141] Because of this, most investigators have found it satisfactory to rely upon a single sample collected at 2 hours. Normal persons excrete 6.6% ± 1.3% of the administered dose in the breath in 2 hours. Patients with hepatocellular injury excrete significantly less (Fig. 9-17). A single measurement at 60 minutes is more convenient for patients, yields similar data, and has recently been recommended.[15]

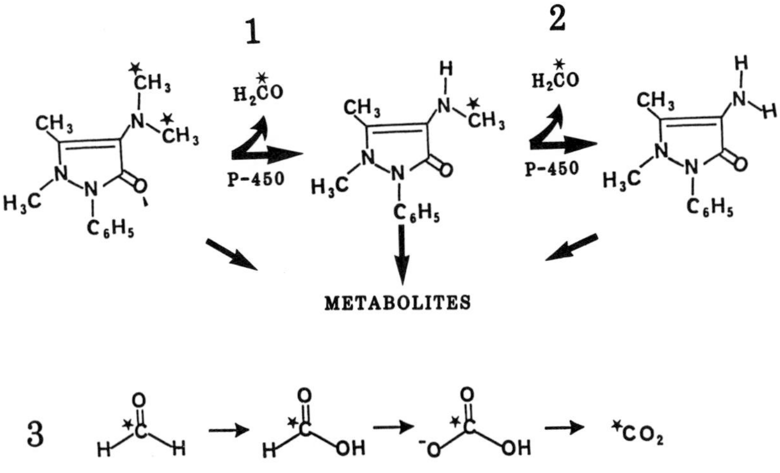

Fig. 9-16. Metabolism of [^{14}C]-aminopyrine. (Baker AL et al: Semin Liver Dis 3:318, 1983)

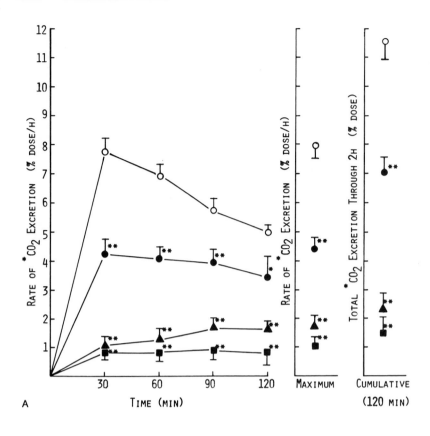

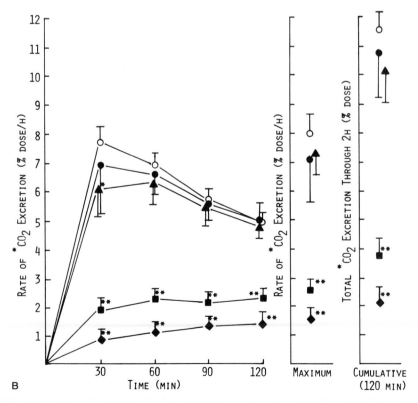

Fig. 9-17. Average excretion rate of labeled CO_2 from aminopyrine in normal subjects and in patients with alcoholic liver disease and chronic active liver disease. **A.** Open circles indicate normal subjects; closed circles, mild alcoholic hepatitis; triangles, moderate alcoholic liver disease; and squares, severe alcoholic liver disease. Bars indicate SEM Statistical difference from normal controls: *p ≤ 0.05; **p ≤ 0.01. **B.** Open circles indicate normal subjects; closed circles, chronic persistent hepatitis; triangles, chronic active hepatitis; squares, chronic active hepatitis with bridging necrosis; diamonds, chronic active hepatitis with cirrhosis. Other symbols are the same as those in *A*. (Schoeller DA et al: Hepatology 2:455, 1982)

The data are clear that a single breath result cannot distinguish among the different types of liver disease. Levels are equally depressed in patients with alcoholic cirrhosis, postnecrotic cirrhosis, advanced primary biliary cirrhosis, and severe hepatitis.[15] The test may have clinical value in quantifying residual functioning liver cell mass and in establishing prognosis in diseases such as alcoholic hepatitis.[15] The aminopyrine breath test appears to be as sensitive as the aminotransferases in detecting hepatocellular diseases and more sensitive than the serum bilirubin, prothrombin, and albumin.[114a,145] It may be more specific for detecting histologic severity in chronic hepatitis[214,219] and alcoholic liver disease[61,216,230,275,286] than conventional liver tests (Fig. 9-17). The breath test appears to be as sensitive as a 2-hour postprandial bile acid test, and there is a moderately good correlation between the two.[114a,215] The test is abnormal more frequently in hepatocellular than in obstructive liver disease.[114a,140] However, the degree of depression of breath test results overlaps considerably in all types of severe liver disease, including cirrhosis, hepatitis, hepatic malignancy, and various histologic forms of alcohol-related disease (Fig. 9-18).[114a,138,140] In one study, the aminopyrine breath test predicted short-term survival and clinical improvement of patients with alcoholic hepatitis more reliably than conventional liver tests.[286] This important observation must be confirmed in other studies involving more patients.

Although breath tests have been available for almost 10 years in the United States, they are still used infrequently. There are several reasons for this. They are less convenient to perform than simple blood tests and use the radioisotope ^{14}C, which has a long half-life and is not widely used by departments of nuclear medicine.[145] Although identical testing can be done with the stable isotope ^{13}C, its use requires sophisticated and expensive mass spectrometers, which are not widely available, and there is still little evidence that breath tests are significantly more sensitive or specific than the currently used liver function tests. Breath tests have been suggested as substitutes for liver biopsy in patients with chronic hepatitis and alcoholic hepatitis. However, there is little evidence that they will replace the liver biopsy, which permits a specific diagnosis and an assessment of the extent of liver damage. Breath tests are useful in measuring residual functional microsomal mass and may prove helpful for establishing the prognosis and response to therapy of certain types of liver disease.

TESTS THAT DETECT INJURY TO HEPATOCYTES (SERUM ENZYMES)

The liver contains thousands of enzymes, some of which are also present in serum in very low concentrations. These enzymes have no known function in serum and behave like other serum proteins. They are distributed in plasma and in interstitial fluid and have characteristic half-lives of disappearance, usually measured in days. Little is known about their catabolism or clearance. The elevation of a given enzyme activity in serum is thought to primarily reflect its increased rate of entrance into serum from damaged liver cells. Serum enzyme tests can be grouped into two categories: (1) enzymes whose elevation in serum reflects generalized damage to hepatocytes, and (2) enzymes whose elevation in serum primarily reflects cholestasis.

Fig. 9-18. The percentage of administered [^{14}C] excreted as [^{14}C]O_2 in breath 2 hours after oral administration of [^{14}C]-aminopyrine. Transverse lines represent ± SEM; hatched areas represent SD. (Hepner GW, Vesell ES: Ann Intern Med 83:632, 1975)

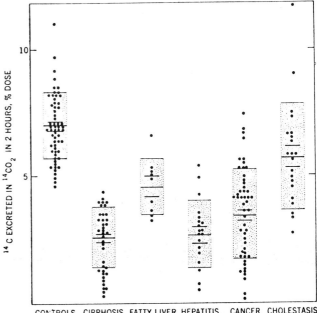

ENZYMES THAT DETECT HEPATOCELLULAR NECROSIS

Aminotransferases

The serum aminotransferases (formerly called transaminases) are sensitive indicators of liver cell injury[80,89,99,340,345,352] and are most helpful in recognizing acute hepatocellular diseases such as hepatitis. Alanine aminotransferase (ALT, serum glutamic-pyruvic transaminase [SGPT]) and aspartate aminotransferase (AST, serum glutamic-oxaloacetic transaminase [SGOT]) activities in serum are the most frequently measured indicators of liver disease. These enzymes catalyze the transfer of the alpha amino groups of alanine and aspartic acid, respectively, to the alpha keto group of ketoglutaric acid. This results in the formation of pyruvic acid and oxalacetic acid (Fig. 9-19). Of the numerous methods developed for measuring ALT and AST activity in serum, the most specific method couples the formation of pyruvate and oxalacetate, the products of the aminotransferase reactions, to their enzymatic reduction to lactate and malate.[250] NADH, the cofactor in this reduction, is oxidized to NAD. Since NADH, but not NAD, absorbs light at 340 nm, the event can be followed spectrophotometrically by the loss of absorptivity at 340 nm.

Both aminotransferases are normally present in serum in low concentrations, less than 30 units/L to 40 units/L. The organ source of these enzymes in serum has never been firmly identified, although they most likely originate in tissues rich in ALT and AST. AST is found in liver, cardiac muscle, skeletal muscle, kidney, brain, pancreas, lung, leukocytes, and erythrocytes, in decreasing order of concentration, whereas ALT is present in highest concentration in liver.[49,249] The increase in ALT and AST serum values is related to damage to or destruction of tissue rich in the aminotransferases or to changes in cell membrane permeability that allow ALT and AST to leak into serum. Their activity in serum at any moment reflects the relative rate at which they enter and leave the circulation. Injected aminotransferases are distributed in interstitial fluid as well as in plasma. From there, they are gradually cleared like other serum proteins, AST being cleared more rapidly than ALT.[97] They are presumably catabolized by cells in the reticuloendothelial system. Hepatic sinusoidal cells appear to be the major site for AST clearance.[160] Virtually no aminotransferases are present in urine and only very small amounts in bile.[97,112] It is, therefore, unlikely that biliary or urinary excretion plays a role in the clearance of ALT or AST.

ALT and AST both require pyridoxal 5'-phosphate as cofactors and both may be present in serum in apoenzyme as well as in holoenzyme form.[85,249] In tissues, ALT is found in the cytosol, whereas AST occurs in two locations, the cytosol and mitochondria.[249] The cytosolic and mitochondrial forms of AST are true isoenzymes and are immunologically distinct.[217] They can be separated from one another by a number of techniques, including immunoprecipitation, chromatography, and electrophoresis. Approximately 80% of AST activity in human liver is

Fig. 9-19. Enzymatic assay of aspartate aminotransferase (*AST*) and alanine aminotransferase (*ALT*). MDH = malic dehydrogenase; LDH = lactic dehydrogenase; NADH = reduced nicotinamide-adenine dinucleotide; NAD = nicotinamide-adenine dinucleotide.

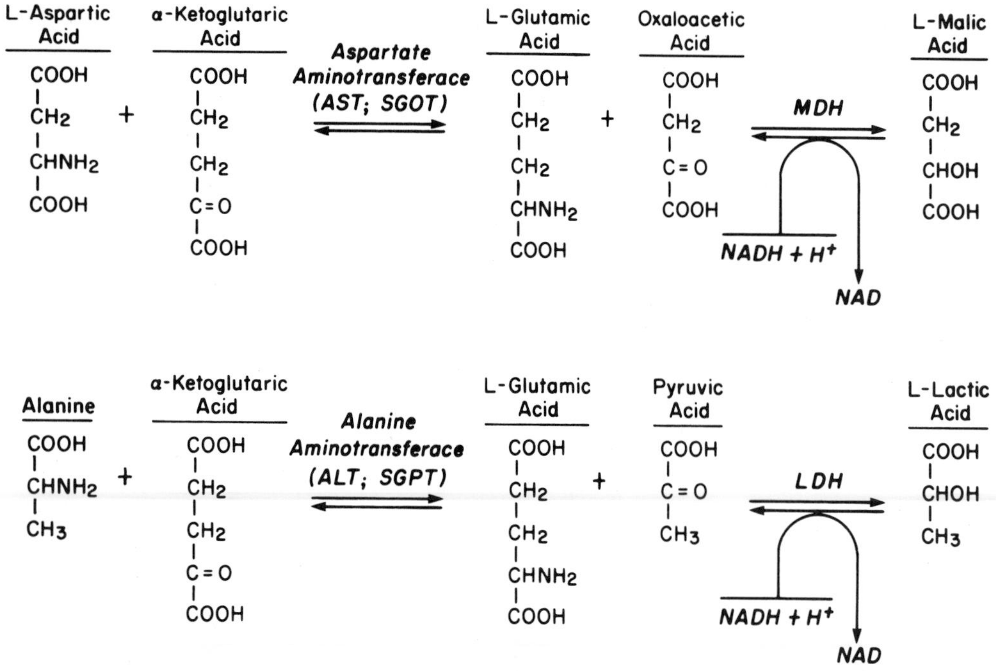

contributed by the mitochondrial isoenzyme,[249] whereas most of the circulating AST activity in normal persons is derived from the cytosolic isoenzyme.[49] Neither ALT nor AST have isoenzymes that are tissue specific. Hence, isoenzyme analysis of serum ALT or AST is rarely useful. Patients with acute myocardial infarction may be an exception. Large increases in mitochondrial AST in serum occur following extensive tissue necrosis. Because of this, assay of mitochondrial AST has been advocated as an accurate test for the detection of myocardial infarction.[250]

Aminotransferases are usually elevated in all liver disorders. These include all types of acute and chronic hepatitis, cirrhosis, infectious mononucleosis, acute and chronic heart failure, various infections, metastatic carcinoma, and granulomatous and alcoholic liver diseases (Fig. 9-20).[87,89,99,340,345,352] Elevations up to eight times the upper limit of normal are nonspecific and may be found in any of the above disorders. The highest elevations occur in disorders associated with extensive hepatocellular injury, such as drug and viral hepatitis, acute heart failure, and exposure to hepatotoxins such as carbon tetrachloride and phalloidin.[66,96,345] Values are often in the low thousands, although values in the 10,000 to 15,000 range may occur in rare persons with viral hepatitis who make uneventful recoveries. The aminotransferases are rarely elevated above 500 units in obstructive jaundice and cir-

Fig. 9-20. Activities of SGOT (*AST*) and SGPT (*ALT*) in patients with various types of hepatobiliary diseases. G STONES = gallstone; Ca HP = carcinoma of head of pancreas; MALIG OB = carcinoma of bile duct; Int CHOL = intrahepatic cholestasis; CIRRHOSIS = portal cirrhosis; PBC = primary biliary cirrhosis; EARLY IH = early infectious hepatitis; LATE IH = late infectious hepatitis; CAH = chronic active hepatitis; ALC = alcoholic hepatic disease; CHOLEC = cholecystitis; CHOLANG = cholangitis; MET = hepatic metastases. Upper limit of normal is shown by dotted lines. (Ellis G et al: Am J Clin Pathol 70:248, 1978)

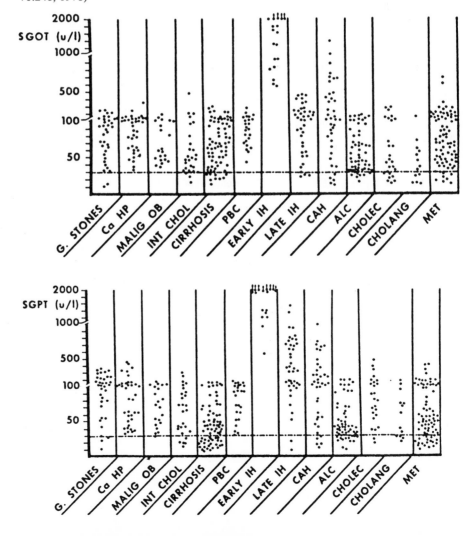

TABLE 9-3. Aminotransferase Values in Patients with Infectious Hepatitis and Obstructive Jaundice*

| UNITS | AST (SGOT) | | ALT (SGPT) | |
| | Infectious Hepatitis | Obstructive Jaundice | Infectious Hepatitis | Obstructive Jaundice |
	(Cumulative percent)		(Cumulative percent)	
Normal	1	10	1	20
34:46†–200	27	81	27	60
201–400	43	98	39	93
401–600	50	99	43	97
601–800	64	99	48	99
801–1000	72	100	53	100
1001–2000	95	—	83	—
2001–3000	99	—	91	—
3000	100	—	100	—
Total pts	274	181	177	97

(Clermont, RJ, Chalmers TC: Medicine 46:197, 1967)

* These aminotransferase values were reported in 28 papers with data on patients with infectious hepatitis and in 14 papers with data on patients with obstructive jaundice.

† Upper limit of normal 33 units for AST and 45 units for ALT.

rhosis (Tables 9-3 and 9-4)[66,119,204] and usually less than 300 units in alcoholic liver disease.[70,133] One exception is in acute bile duct obstruction owing to a common duct stone.[1] AST and ALT values may reach the thousands within 24 to 48 hours following acute bile duct obstruction but then rapidly decline to lower values. The AST and ALT are equally elevated in most hepatobiliary disorders, with the ALT usually somewhat higher than the AST.[88,89] ALT appears to be a more sensitive and specific test of acute hepatocellular damage than AST and is often used to document the incidence of viral hepatitis in epidemiologic studies.[88,89]

There is a poor correlation between the extent of liver cell necrosis and the elevation of serum aminotransferases. Likewise, the absolute elevation of aminotransferases is of little prognostic value in predicting the outcome of acute hepatocellular disorders. Rapid decreases in the aminotransferase levels in serum are usually a sign of recovery

TABLE 9-4. Ratio of AST to ALT in Patients with High and Low Values (<500 or ≥500 Units)

| HIGHEST VALUE OF EITHER TEST | <500 Ratio | | ≥500 Ratio | | TOTAL PTS |
	<1.0	≥1.0	<1.0	≥1.0	
Infectious hepatitis					
No. pts	66	37	61	7	171
Percent	64	36	90	10	
Infectious mononucleosis					
No. pts	43	7	4	0	54
Percent	86	14			
Obstructive jaundice					
No. pts	33	22	6	1	62
Percent	60	40	86	14	
Cirrhosis					
No. pts	4	64	1	1	70
Percent	6	94			
Total pts	146	130	72	9	337

(Clermont RJ, Chalmers TC: Medicine 46:197, 1967)

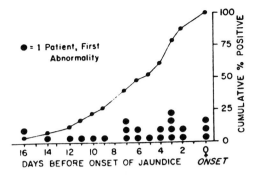

Fig. 9-21. Elevation of AST (*SGOT*) in the early stages of acute viral hepatitis. Relation of the first abnormality is compared to the onset of jaundice in 23 patients or volunteers followed closely during the incubation period of viral hepatitis. (Clermont RJ, Chalmers TC: Medicine 46:197, 1967)

from disease. However, this may be a poor prognostic sign in fulminant hepatitis, where decreasing serum values may reflect the massive destruction and loss of viable hepatocytes.

Elevated aminotransferase activities are among the first laboratory abnormalities detected in the early phases of viral hepatitis (Fig. 9-21).[66,174] In patients with jaundice due to hepatitis, elevation of the serum bilirubin usually lags behind the rise in aminotransferases by about 1 week. Thus, the aminotransferases are frequently declining as the bilirubin is increasing. There is typically a steady decline in the aminotransferases during recovery from viral hepatitis. Secondary increases of the aminotransferases or their persistent elevation may indicate recrudescence of acute hepatitis or the development of chronic active hepatitis. Non-A, non-B hepatitis is often associated with fluctuations in ALT and AST that may continue for many months or even years.[116] Many persons with persistently elevated aminotransferase will have liver biopsy evidence of chronic hepatitis. The aminotransferases are one of the important means of following the clinical activity of viral hepatitis and of evaluating the response to immunosuppressive therapy in chronic hepatitis.[297]

The AST to ALT ratio is usually of little value in distinguishing among various hepatobiliary disorders. There is one important exception, the recognition of alcoholic liver disease. If the ALT is less than 300, an AST to ALT ratio more than 2 is suggestive of alcoholic liver disease, and a ratio greater than 3 is highly suggestive of alcoholic liver disease (Figs. 9-22 and 9-23).[70,113] The increased ratio primarily reflects the low serum activity of ALT in patients with alcoholic liver disease (Fig. 9-24).[204] This is secondary to a deficiency of pyridoxal 5'-phosphate in persons with

Fig. 9-22. AST/ALT ratio in patients with biopsy-proven liver disease. The ratio was calculated from the serum sample that had the highest individual aminotransferase values, be it AST or ALT. (Adapted from Cohen JA, Kaplan MM: Dig Dis Sci 24:835, 1979)

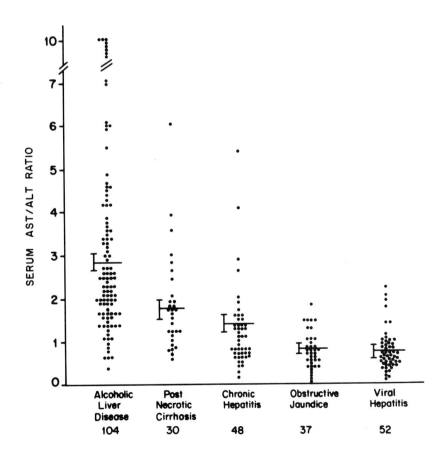

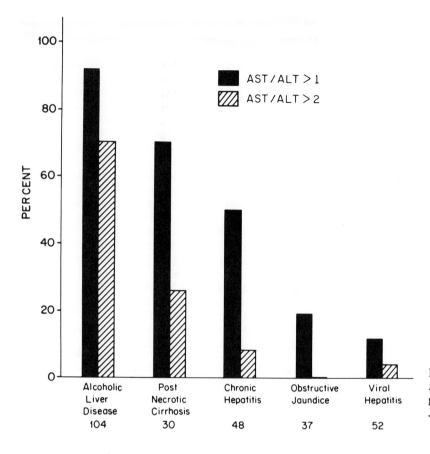

Fig. 9-23. Percentage of patients with AST/ALT ratios greater than one and greater than two. (Adapted from Cohen JA, Kaplan MM: Dig Dis Sci 24:835, 1979)

Fig. 9-24. Alanine aminotransferase (*ALT*) and aspartate aminotransferase (*AST*) activities in human liver. NL = normal liver; FL = fatty liver in the absence of alcoholism; ALD = alcoholic hepatitis or cirrhosis, or both; PBC = primary biliary cirrhosis; CAH = chronic active hepatitis; CPH = chronic persistent hepatitis. The activity of GPT is selectively decreased in livers of patients with alcoholic hepatitis or cirrhosis, or both. (Adapted from Matloff DS et al: Gastroenterology 78:1389, 1980)

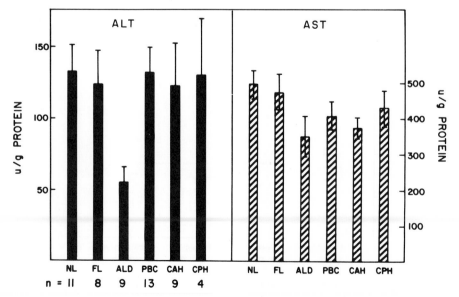

alcoholic liver disease.[85] ALT synthesis in liver requires pyridoxal phosphate more than does AST synthesis.[85] The altered AST to ALT ratio in serum appears to reflect the altered ratios in the liver (Fig. 9-24). However, the less-than-expected increase in the serum ALT and AST values in alcoholic liver disease, usually less than 200 units and 300 units, respectively, cannot be explained simply by the decreased hepatic concentrations. This becomes evident whenever a patient with alcoholic liver disease develops concomitant heart failure or viral hepatitis. When this occurs, the serum AST and ALT may soar to the thousands. Note, however, that despite their striking elevations, the AST to ALT ratio will remain increased and typical of alcoholic liver disease.[164,166]

Elevated serum aminotransferase values are not specific for hepatobiliary disorders. They may also be found in patients with severe cardiac and skeletal muscle damage.[345,352] AST is more often increased in patients with myocardial infarction than is ALT and is undoubtedly of cardiac origin. Large increases in ALT in cardiac disease are probably of hepatic origin, because they are frequently seen in the setting of large hemodynamically significant infarcts, associated with congestive heart failure and circulatory collapse, in which hepatic ischemia and central hepatocellular necrosis are likely to occur.

Increased AST and ALT values in muscle disease are probably derived from muscle.[96,345] The extent of enzyme elevation in muscle disease is almost invariably less than 300 units. Except in instances of acute rhabdomyolysis, values rarely reach the range observed in acute hepatocellular disorders. Serum AST and occasionally ALT activities may also increase slightly following vigorous exercise.[251,281] They then rapidly return to normal. This may account for the slight, usually unexplained increases in aminotransferase values observed in joggers.

The aminotransferases may be falsely elevated or diminished under certain circumstances. Drugs such as erythromycin and para-aminosalicylic acid may yield falsely elevated aminotransferase values if older colorometric tests are used.[272,295a,348] Conversely, low values of AST may be seen in uremia.[325] These low values increase after dialysis, suggesting that a dialyzable inhibitor of the aminotransferase reaction is present in the serum of uremic patients.[325]

Other Enzyme Tests Indicative of Hepatocellular Necrosis

There are a number of other serum enzyme tests that have been promulgated as being either more specific or more sensitive in detecting hepatocellular necrosis than the aminotransferases. Some of these enzymes are found only in liver tissues and theoretically should be more specific for liver disease than the aminotransferases. However, none of them has proved more useful in practice than the aminotransferase and none are widely used. A brief description of some of these enzyme tests follows.

Glutamate Dehydrogenase

Glutamate dehydrogenase, a mitochondrial enzyme, is found primarily in liver, heart, muscle, and kidneys.[285] In the liver, it is present in highest concentration in centrilobular hepatocytes.[127] Because of this location and the fact that it is particularly elevated after acute right-sided heart failure, serum glutamate dehydrogenase was investigated as a specific marker for liver disorders that affect primarily centrilobular hepatocytes, such as alcoholic hepatitis.[322] An initial report that glutamate dehydrogenase may be a sensitive and relatively specific marker for alcoholic hepatitis was not confirmed by others.[99,166] Glutamate dehydrogenase is rarely used as a liver function test.

Isocitrate Dehydrogenase

Isocitrate dehydrogenase, a cytoplasmic enzyme, is found in liver, heart, kidney, and skeletal muscle.[263] Its activity in serum parallels that of the aminotransferases in acute and chronic hepatitis, but it is less sensitive.[26,304] Although elevations of the serum isocitrate dehydrogenase are relatively specific for liver disorders, increased levels have been reported in disseminated malignancy without detectable hepatic involvement.[330] It offers no diagnostic advantage over the aminotransferases.

Lactate Dehydrogenase

Lactate dehydrogenase is a cytoplasmic enzyme present in tissues throughout the body. Five isoenzyme forms of lactate dehydrogenase are present in serum and are readily separated by a variety of electrophoretic techniques. The slowest migrating band predominates in the liver. This test is not as sensitive as the aminotransferases in liver disease and has poor diagnostic specificity, even when isoenzyme analysis is used. It is more useful as a marker of myocardial infarction and hemolysis.[84]

Sorbitol Dehydrogenase

Sorbitol dehydrogenase is a cytoplasmic enzyme found predominantly in the liver with only relatively low concentrations in the prostate and kidney.[263] Its activity in serum parallels that of the aminotransferases in hepatobiliary disorders. However, it appears to be less sensitive, and values may be normal in cirrhosis and other chronic liver disorders. Its instability in serum further limits its diagnostic usefulness.[263]

ENZYMES THAT DETECT CHOLESTASIS

Alkaline Phosphatase

Alkaline phosphatase is the name given to a group of enzymes that catalyze the hydrolysis of a large number of organic phosphate esters at an alkaline *p*H optimum. Inorganic phosphate and the organic radical are generated by the reaction.[129,235] The alkaline phosphatases of different tissues are true isoenzymes because they catalyze the same reaction but differ in certain physicochemical properties.[163] The precise function of alkaline phosphatase is unknown. Alkaline phosphatases are found in many locations throughout the body, including bone osteoblasts, the canalicular membranes of hepatocytes, the brush border of the mucosal cells of the small intestine, the proximal convoluted tubules of the kidney, the placenta, and white blood cells.[163] In bone, the enzyme appears to be concerned with calcification, although its precise function is unknown. At other sites, it may participate in transport processes, but its actual physiologic functions are also largely unknown.[79] Alkaline phosphatase activity is normally demonstrable in serum. There is good evidence that serum enzyme in the normal adult is derived primarily from three sources: liver, bone, and, in some instances, the intestinal tract (Fig. 9-25). Liver and bone are the major sources.[163] Contribution from the intestine (about 10% to 20%) is of importance primarily in persons with blood groups 0 and B who are secretors of the ABH red blood cell antigen and is enhanced by prior consumption of a fatty meal.[17,235,236,256] Based on studies with infused placental alkaline phosphatase, circulating enzyme appears to behave like other serum proteins.[67] Its half-life is 7 days, and its clearance from serum is independent of the functional capacity of the liver or of the patency of the bile ducts.[67] Its sites of degradation are not known.[235]

Some details of the more popular procedures used to measure alkaline phosphatase activity, including substrates used, end products measured, and the usual range of normal values for adults aged 17 to 55 years, are contained in Table 9-5.[91,163,344] Currently, the most widely used procedure utilizes p-nitrophenyl phosphate as substrate and an amino alcohol such as 2-amino-2-methyl-1-propanol as buffer. It measures the rate of release of p-nitrophenol or of phosphate from the substrate under specified incubation conditions. The results are expressed in international units (units/L), which is the activity of alkaline phosphatase that releases 1 μmol of chromogen or Pi per minute. Results obtained with these methods appear to be equally effective in detecting a wide variety of clinical diseases.[91] Conversion factors permit interchange of values obtained by the different methods. However, these factors are based on average values and correlate poorly in individual patients.[91,316] This is not surprising, because serum alkaline phosphatase consists of isoenzymes that differ in their reactivity in various assay systems.[163] A simple way of comparing results of different methods is to express the results as multiples of the upper limit of normal. A number of analytic sources of error exist. Factors such as the concentrations of phosphate, citrate, and magnesium and the type and concentration of the buffer may be important.[129,196,235,344]

In the 15-year to 50-year age group, mean serum alkaline phosphatase activity is somewhat higher in men than in women (Fig. 9-26).[65,90,233] By contrast, for persons over 60 years of age, the enzyme activity of women equals or exceeds that of men, and both sexes tend to have somewhat higher values than younger adults.[137a,171,233] The reasons for these differences are not known. In children, serum alkaline phosphatase activity is considerably elevated in both sexes, correlates well with the rate of bone growth, and appears to be accounted for by influx of enzyme from osteoid tissue.[65,169] Serum alkaline phosphatase in normal adolescent males may reach mean levels three times greater than in normal adults without implying the presence of hepatobiliary disease.[65,274] Enzyme activity in serum may double late in normal pregnancy, primarily because of influx of placental phosphatase.[34,206]

Although elevation of serum alkaline phosphatase ac-

Fig. 9-25. Alkaline phosphatase isoenzymes separated in 7½% polyacrylamide gel slabs at *p*H 7.5. **Lane A.** Liver isoenzyme from a patient with obstructive jaundice. **Lane B.** Bone isoenzyme from a patient with Paget's disease of bone. **Lane C.** Liver and intestinal isoenzymes from a patient with alcoholic cirrhosis. **Lane D.** Liver and bone isoenzymes from a patient with celiac sprue and osteomalacia. (Kaplan MM: Gastroenterology 62:452, 1972)

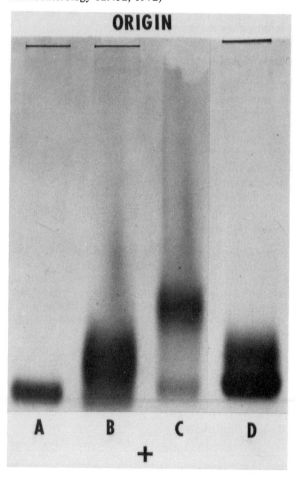

TABLE 9-5. Clinical Methods of Serum Alkaline Phosphatase Determination

METHOD	SUBSTRATE (μmol/ml)	TEMPER-ATURE (°C)	pH	BUFFER	UNIT	NORMAL RANGE
Bessey–Lowry–Brock	p-Nitrophenylphospate (5.4)	39	10.5	Glycine	1 μmol p-nitrophenol/ L/60 min	0.8–3.0
Bodansky	β-Glycerophosphate (14.5)	37	8.6	Diethyl barbiturate	1 mg pi/100 ml/60 min	1.5–4.0
International	p-Nitrophenylphosphate (2.8)	37	10.5	2-amino-2-methyl-1-propanol	1 μmol p-nitrophenol/ L/min	21.0–85.0
International	Phenylphosphate (9.2)	37	10.0	Sodium carbonate	1 mg phenol/100 ml/ 30 min	3.0–13.0
King–Armstrong	Phenylphosphate (4.75)	37	9.3	Diethyl barbiturate	1 mg phenol/100 ml/ 30 min	3.0–13.0
Klein–Read–Babson	Phenolphthalein diphosphate (2.5)	37	9.3	Tris	1 mg phenolphthalein/ 100 ml/30 min	1.0–4.0
Shinowara–Jones Reinhart	β-Glycerophosphate (3.2)	37	9.3	Diethyl barbiturate	1 mg phenol/100 ml/ 60 min	2.2–8.6

(Kaplan M: Gastroenterology 62:452, 1972)

tivity is observed frequently in various hepatobiliary diseases, similar elevations are observed in disorders of bone characterized by increased osteoblastic activity and, as indicated, occur normally during growth and pregnancy. Occasionally, the intestinal tract and rarely the kidney may be the sources of an elevated serum enzyme value.[163]

If an elevated serum alkaline phosphatase is the only abnormal finding in an apparently healthy person or if the degree of elevation is higher than expected in the clinical setting, identification of the source of elevated isoenzyme is helpful. There are several different ways to approach this problem. First, and most precise, is the fractionation of the alkaline phosphatase by electrophoresis.[161] Alkaline phosphatases derived from liver, bone, intestine, and placenta have differing electrophoretic mobilities. In most clinical situations, this amounts to separating liver from bone alkaline phosphatase.[52] In a study of 317 patients in a university hospital, selected because of elevated serum alkaline phosphatase activities, the liver isoenzyme was the source of the elevation in 253 patients, bone in 58 patients, a mixture of bone and liver in 4 patients and intestine in only 2 patients.[52] Unfortunately, the bone and liver isoenzymes differ only slightly in electrophoretic mobility. These isoenzymes often overlap if

Fig. 9-26. Normal serum alkaline phosphatase values at various ages in men (*open circles*) and women (*closed circles*). (Data derived from Clarke LC, Beck EJ: J Pediatr 36:335, 1950; and Wolf PL: Arch Pathol Lab Med 102:497, 1978)

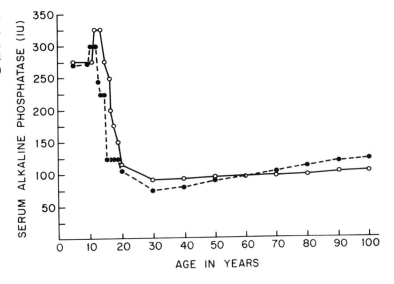

run on the electrophoretic systems used in most routine clinical laboratories. Separation on polyacrylamide gel slabs is the most reliable method and produces clear-cut separations of the liver, bone, intestinal, and placental isoenzymes (Fig. 9-25). However, this method is not always available. Electrophoresis on cellulose acetate with the addition of heat inactivation[237] may accomplish the same purpose.

The second approach is based on the observation that alkaline phosphatases from individual tissues differ in susceptibility to inactivation by heat or by 2 M urea.[14,163,206,237] Placental alkaline phosphatase and an isoenzyme found in certain cancers, the Regan isoenzyme, are fully "heat-stable" after exposure to a temperature of 56° C for 15 minutes.[109] The enzymes derived from bone, intestine, and liver are partly inactivated. Accordingly, the finding of an elevated serum alkaline phosphatase in a patient with all the excess activity in a "heat-stable" fraction strongly suggests that the placenta or a tumor is the source of the elevated enzyme in serum. Susceptibility to inactivation by heat and urea increases, respectively, for intestine, liver, and bone alkaline phosphatases, bone being by far the most sensitive.[14,163,237]

Unfortunately, in assessments of nonselected patients, both heat inactivation and 2 M urea were not found to be diagnostically useful.[164,343] A confounding factor in the use of heat inactivation is the fact that slight changes in temperature, as little as 0.2° C, will alter the rates of inactivation substantially.[163] The presence of more than one alkaline phosphatase isoenzyme in serum, each with its own rate of heat denaturation, may also yield uninterpretable results. The author has not found these methods useful and does not recommend them.

In the third, and, at present, the best substantiated approach, serum leucine aminopeptidase, 5'-nucleotidase, and gamma glutamyl transpeptidase activity are measured (Fig. 9-27). These enzymes, discussed below, are not elevated by bone disorders but only with liver dysfunction or, in the case of leucine aminopeptidase and possibly 5'-nucleotidase, in pregnancy. An increase of these enzymes in serum in nonpregnant patients indicates, therefore, that an elevated serum alkaline phosphatase is due at least in part to hepatobiliary disease. In contrast, lack of increased 5'-nucleotidase in serum in the presence of elevated alkaline phosphatase does not rule out liver disease, because these enzymes do not necessarily increase in a parallel manner in early or modest hepatic injury.[76]

In all patients studied, the elevated levels of alkaline phosphatase in serum originate in the tissues whose metabolism is either functionally disturbed (the obstructed liver) or greatly stimulated (placenta in the third trimester of pregnancy and bone in growing children). There is general agreement regarding the skeletal origin of the elevated serum alkaline phosphatase in patients with bone disorder and in growing children and the placental origin in women during the third trimester of pregnancy.[79] Only in patients with hepatobiliary disorders has there been any question regarding the mechanism of the increased serum alkaline

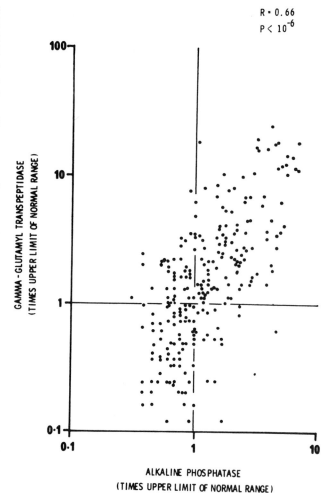

Fig. 9-27. Correlation between serum γ-glutamyl transpeptidase and serum alkaline phosphatase in 245 healthy subjects and patients with hepatobiliary diseases. The units on the abscissa and ordinate are the logarithms of the multiples of the upper limits of normal for each test. Each point represents one patient. Although there is good correlation between the logarithmic values of the population (r = 0.66), there is considerable variation between the percent γ-glutamyl transpeptidase and alkaline phosphatase elevations in individual patients. (Whitfield JB et al: Gut 13:702, 1972)

phosphatase.[129] The following two theories have been proposed: (1) The damaged liver regurgitates hepatic alkaline phosphatase back into serum; and (2) the damaged liver, particularly if due to obstructive jaundice, fails to excrete alkaline phosphatases made in bone, intestine, and liver.

This long-standing debate has been resolved in favor of the former, the regurgitation of liver alkaline phosphatase into serum. There are compelling data that support this theory. First, as noted above, only hepatic alkaline phosphatase is found in the serum of patients with liver disease, particularly cholestasis.[52,63,161,221] Second, the clearance rates of infused placental alkaline phosphatase are the same in patients with bile duct obstruction and in normal persons.[67] Third, in experimental models of bile duct obstruction in rats, the entire increase in serum alkaline phosphatase activity is due to the leakage of hepatic alkaline phosphatase into serum.[45,162] The increased serum activity is paralleled by a striking increase in hepatic alkaline phosphatase activity. The increased hepatic activity cannot be accounted for by biliary retention of alkaline phosphatase.[162]

The mechanism by which hepatobiliary disease leads to an elevation of serum alkaline phosphatase has been greatly clarified. Most evidence suggests that this elevation occurs primarily because of *de novo* synthesis of the enzyme in the liver and release of the phosphatase into the circulation.[45,162,165] This appears to be mediated by the action of bile acids, which induce the synthesis of the enzyme and may cause it to leak into the circulation, perhaps by disruption of hepatic organelles and solubilization of phosphatase bound to such membranes.[135,136,280] The precise manner in which the phosphatase reaches the circulation is not clear. However, in some persons with cholestasis, small vesicles that contain many basolateral (sinusoidal) membrane enzymes, including alkaline phosphatase, still bound to these membranes, have been found in serum.[80,81]

The major value of the serum alkaline phosphatase in the diagnosis of liver disorders is in the recognition of cholestatic disorders. Approximately 75% of patients with prolonged cholestasis will have alkaline phosphatase values increased fourfold or greater. Such elevations occur in both extrahepatic and intrahepatic obstruction, and the extent of the elevation does not distinguish between the two. There is essentially no difference among the values found in obstructive jaundice due to malignancy, common duct stone, sclerosing cholangitis, or bile duct stricture.[79] Values are similarly increased in patients with intrahepatic cholestasis due to drug-induced hepatitis, primary biliary cirrhosis, rejection of transplanted livers, and, rarely, in alcohol-induced steatonecrosis.[232] Lesser increases in alkaline phosphatase activity, up to three times the upper limit of normal, are nonspecific and may occur in all types of liver disorders, including viral hepatitis, chronic hepatitis, cirrhosis, infiltrative diseases of the liver, and congestive heart failure.[52,129,235]

Isolated elevations of hepatic alkaline phosphatase, or disproportionate elevation compared to other tests, such as the aminotransferases and serum bilirubin, may occur in partial bile duct obstruction owing to gallstones or tumor, as well as in infiltrative diseases such as sarcoidosis, hepatic abscesses, tuberculosis, and metastatic carcinoma.[163,235] The mechanism is unknown but probably represents local areas of bile duct obstruction with induction and leakage into serum of hepatic alkaline phosphatase from these obstructed areas. However, elevated serum alkaline phosphatase in patients with primary extrahepatic malignancy does not necessarily imply metastasis to liver

or bone.[3] Some cancers may secrete their own alkaline phosphatase into serum[109] or may cause leakage of hepatic alkaline phosphatase into serum by some unknown mechanism.[52]

Finally, it should be recognized that moderate elevations of alkaline phosphatase of hepatic origin may occur in disorders that do not directly involve the liver. These may occur in patients with stage I and II Hodgkin's disease, myeloid metaplasia, congestive heart failure, intra-abdominal infections, and osteomyelitis.[52] In addition, certain families may have increased serum alkaline phosphatase that is genetic in origin.[341]

5'-Nucleotidase

This phosphatase specifically catalyzes hydrolysis of nucleotides such as adenosine 5'-phosphate and inosine 5'-phosphate, in which the phosphate is attached to the 5 position of the pentose moiety. 5'-nucleotidase is found in the liver, intestines, brain, heart, blood vessels, and endocrine pancreas.[120] In the liver, the enzyme is associated primarily with canalicular and sinusoidal plasma membranes.[298] Its physiologic function is unknown. In most laboratories, 5'-nucleotidase activity is assayed by using adenosine 5'-phosphate as substrate and measuring either the released inorganic phosphate[60] or the free adenosine. The presence of alkaline phosphatase in serum complicates the assay, because it will also hydrolyze the 5'-nucleotide substrates. Corrections must be made for its activity. This can be done in two ways: (1) by preliminary incubation of serum with appropriate concentrations of EDTA, which will selectively inactivate only alkaline phosphatase,[143] or (2) by assaying in the presence and absence of Ni^{++}, a heavy metal that specifically inhibits 5'-nucleotidase.[60] In most clinical laboratories, free inorganic phosphate is measured. A unit of 5'-nucleotidase activity is designated as equivalent to that amount of enzyme that liberates 1 mg of phosphate per hour per 100 ml of serum. These units are analogous to the old Bodansky units of alkaline phosphatase activity and are expressed as such.[347] In most series of normal adult patients, the serum 5'-nucleotidase ranges from 0.3 Bodansky units to 3.2 Bodansky units and is not clearly influenced by sex or race.[19,143,175,347] Values are substantially lower in children than in adults, rise gradually with adolescence, and reach a plateau after the age of 50 years.[24]

Serum values of this enzyme are elevated primarily in hepatobiliary diseases with a spectrum of abnormality similar to that found for alkaline phosphatase. The parallel behavior of these two enzymes in hepatobiliary diseases probably reflects their similar subcellular location in hepatocytes.[253,280,298] Both are bound to bile canalicular and sinusoidal membranes and must be solubilized in order to gain access to the circulation. Bile acids may act as detergents and solubilize them. In experimental bile duct obstruction in rats, bile acid concentrations rapidly reach levels sufficient to disrupt plasma membranes and solubilize both these enzymes.[280] The same situation may occur in hepatobiliary disorders in which there is any degree of cholestasis.[253]

Most studies indicate that alkaline phosphatase and 5'-nucleotidase are equally valuable in demonstrating biliary obstruction or hepatic infiltrative and space-occupying lesions.[143,175,278a,347] In selected patients, however, one enzyme may be elevated and the other may be normal.[19,109,143,320] Although the coefficient of correlation between the two enzymes is high,[278a] the values may not rise proportionately in individual patients.[19,100]

Most data suggest that the 5'-nucleotidase and serum alkaline phosphatase are of equal value in differentiating obstructive from parenchymal liver disease.[99] All investigators have shown some overlap in 5'-nucleotidase values in obstructive and hepatocellular jaundice.[99] Some investigators have found this overlap to be small and have concluded that this assay is equal to or better than the measurement of serum alkaline phosphatase for differentiating between these two types of jaundice,[19,347] whereas others reported that the alkaline phosphatase had greater selective value.[100]

Conflicting data have been reported for values of 5'-nucleotidase activity in serum during normal pregnancy. Some investigators have found an increase in enzyme activity in the third trimester,[168,177] and others report no change during pregnancy.[288] It is not clear whether or not these different experiences are accounted for by differences in methodology used to measure 5'-nucleotidase activity. The major advantage of 5'-nucleotidase over the nonspecific alkaline phosphatase measurement in serum is enhancement of specificity. Most studies show that serum 5'-nucleotidase does not rise in bone disease,[147,175,347] and, in the few instances in which an increase was observed, it was of low magnitude.[100,143] This is in striking contrast to alkaline phosphatase.

The major value of the 5'-nucleotidase assay is its specificity for hepatobiliary disease. An increased serum 5'-nucleotidase level in a nonpregnant person suggests that a concomitantly increased serum alkaline phosphatase is of hepatic origin. A normal nucleotidase in the presence of an elevated serum alkaline phosphatase, however, does not rule out the liver as the source of elevated phosphatase. As noted above, occasionally one enzyme may be normal and the other elevated in liver disease.[143]

γ-Glutamyl Transpeptidase

γ-Glutamyl transpeptidase (GGT) catalyzes the transfer of the γ-glutamyl group from γ-glutamyl peptides such as glutathione to other peptides and to L-amino acids. γ-L-glutamyl-p-nitroanilide is most commonly used as a substrate in its assay with glycylglycine as the acceptor.[307,308] The enzyme catalyzes the transfer of the γ-glutamyl moiety from the substrate to glycylglycine and so liberates the chromogen p-nitroaniline, which can be measured spectrophotometrically. GGT is present in cell membranes in many tissues, including kidney, pancreas, liver, spleen, heart, brain, and seminal vesicles.[121] It is

thought to play a role in amino acid transport across membranes as part of the γ-glutamyl cycle.[207-209] More recent data suggest that hydrolysis of glutathione rather than transpeptidation may be its true physiologic function.[292] The enzyme is present in normal human serum, where values are usually comparable in men and women,[13,198,309,349] although some investigators have found higher values in men.[270,307] Children older than 4 years of age have normal adult values in serum.[169,323] Serum enzyme activity does not rise during the course of normal pregnancy.[198,323]

Elevated serum activity of this enzyme is found predominantly and in high frequency in diseases of the liver, biliary tract, and pancreas.[13,30,150,198,270,309,349] Abnormal values appear in approximately the same spectrum of hepatobiliary diseases as for alkaline phosphatase, leucine aminopeptidase, and 5'-nucleotidase. Some investigators find GGT to be more sensitive than alkaline phosphatase[198,270] and leucine aminopeptidase[198] in detecting liver disease. Others find little difference in sensitivity between GGT and alkaline phosphatase.[30] There is a reasonably good, albeit far from perfect, correlation between GGT levels and those of 5'-nucleotidase and alkaline phosphatase in liver disease (Figs. 9-27 and 9-28).

The major clinical value of GGT lies in its use in conferring organ specificity to an elevated value for alkaline phosphatase, since GGT activity is not elevated in patients with diseases of bone.[30,198] In addition, high GGT values are found in people who take medicines such as barbiturates or dilantin[261,295a,338,339] or ingest large quantities of alcohol,[179,260,262,331,337] even when values for other serum enzyme tests and serum bilirubin are normal. When the elevated GGT is associated with the use of anticonvulsant drugs or alcohol abuse, there is no correlation between the serum GGT and alkaline phosphatase.[121] Some investigators have found an isolated elevation of GGT or a GGT elevation out of proportion to that of other enzymes such as the alkaline phosphatase or ALT to be an indicator of alcohol abuse or alcoholic liver disease (Fig. 9-29).[166] Induction of hepatic microsomal GGT by alcohol and other drugs may account for some of the observations.[22,121] However, this is not the only explanation, since neither elevated serum GGT levels nor a history of recent alcohol ingestion correlates with hepatic GGT activity in patients with biopsy proven alcoholic liver disease.[152,289] In addition, the activities of alkaline phosphatase and GGT in liver tissue are increased similarly in patients with alcoholic hepatitis; yet, GGT levels in serum were 1300% of normal, whereas those of alkaline phosphatase were only slightly above normal (Fig. 9-29).[152,166,289] Recent in vitro studies suggest that alcohol may also cause the leakage of GGT from hepatocytes.[22]

Normal values for GGT in childhood and in pregnancy offer additional diagnostic possibilities for this test, but there is little published clinical experience with GGT determinations in liver disease occurring during these states. The extent of rise of GGT activity in serum may be depressed by female sex hormones.[75] This was inferred from

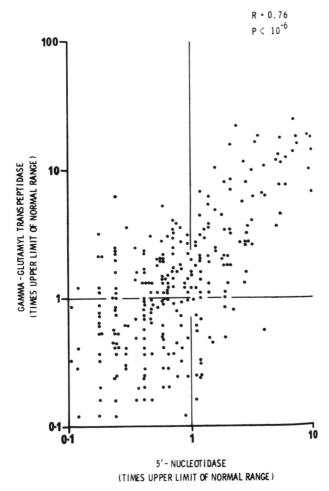

$R = 0.76$
$P < 10^{-6}$

GAMMA - GLUTAMYL TRANSPEPTIDASE (TIMES UPPER LIMIT OF NORMAL RANGE)

5' - NUCLEOTIDASE
(TIMES UPPER LIMIT OF NORMAL RANGE)

Fig. 9-28. Correlation between serum γ-glutamyl transpeptidase and serum 5'-nucleotidase in 245 healthy subjects and patients with hepatobiliary diseases. The units on the abscissa and ordinate are logarithms of the multiples of the upper limits of normal for each test. Although there is good correlation between the logarithmic values of the population (r = 0.76), there is considerable variation between the percent γ-glutamyl transpeptidase and 5'-nucleotidase elevations in individual patients. (Whitfield JB et al: Gut 13:702, 1972)

reports that GGT activity was increased less frequently and to a lesser degree in women who developed viral hepatitis during the last half of pregnancy or while taking birth control pills.[75] In the latter study, it was also demonstrated that hyperbilirubinemia interfered with measured activity of GGT *in vitro*.[75] Both these factors seem to operate in other disorders of the liver and undoubtedly contribute to impaired differential diagnostic usefulness of the GGT enzyme test. Aside from its value in conferring liver specificity to an elevated alkaline phosphatase and its possible use in identifying patients with alcohol abuse, GGT offers no advantage over the aminotransferase and alkaline phosphatase. In one prospective study of 1040

nonselected inpatients, 139 (13.4%) had elevated serum GGT activity. However, only 32% of these patients had hepatobiliary diseases, and the remaining 68% had other diseases not involving the liver.[58]

Leucine Aminopeptidase

Leucine aminopeptidase, a proteolytic enzyme, hydrolyzes amino acids found in tissues throughout the body from the N-terminal end of proteins and polypeptides. It has highest activity when leucine is the N-terminal residue, hence its name. Leucine aminopeptidase is found in all human tissues assayed, with high activity in the liver, where it is localized primarily in biliary epithelium.[175] The function of this enzyme is not known but possibly involves hydrolysis of a peptide bond near an L-leucine residue or the transfer of L-leucine from one peptide to another.[269] The leucine aminopeptidase of normal serum as a rule is electrophoretically homogeneous and probably originates in liver. In hepatobiliary disease, several peaks of activity are detected.[176] They probably represent isoenzymes.

The prevalent method for measuring serum leucine aminopeptidase involves α-leucyl-β-naphthylamide hydrochloride as a substrate with the liberated β-naphthylamine assayed colorimetrically.[119a] There is some evidence that the peptidase responsible for this reaction differs from those that hydrolyze other leucine compounds.[228] Accordingly, in extrapolating data from one study to another, one should carefully consider the substrate used. Normal values when α-leucyl-β-naphthylamide is used usually range from 50 units to 220 units without significant difference owing to sex, age (from 18 to 75 years), or fasting.[18,241]

Leucine aminopeptidase elevation, like that of 5'-nucleotidase and, to a lesser degree, GGT, appears to be specific for liver disorders. Leucine aminopeptidase is not elevated in patients with bone disease,[18,175,268] and values of the enzyme in children, although based on a small number of determinations, are comparable to those of adults.[271] The only condition other than hepatobiliary disease known to result in an increase in this enzyme is pregnancy.[53,54,323] Serum leucine aminopeptidase rises progressively during gestation and reaches a peak at term. After delivery, the enzyme level falls, decreasing by about 35% in 4 days. Electrophoresis of serum leucine aminopeptidase from pregnant women and people with liver disease shows much overlap between the various isoenzymes. This procedure is probably of no practical value in differentiating between these two sources of the enzyme.[23]

Serum leucine aminopeptidase is as sensitive as alkaline phosphatase and 5'-nucleotidase in detecting obstructive, infiltrative, or space-occupying lesions of the liver.[18,19,54,175] Indeed, some investigators consider leucine aminopeptidase a more sensitive indicator of infiltrative diseases than alkaline phosphatase in the nonjaundiced patient.[268] Contrary to original reports, pancreatic malignancy without hepatobiliary disease does not cause an elevation in serum leucine aminopeptidase.[54,209]

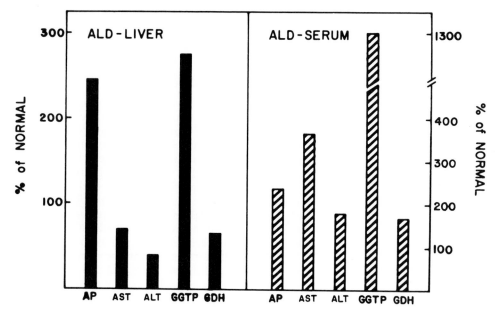

Fig. 9-29. Enzyme values in liver tissue and serum of patients with biopsy-proven alcoholic hepatitis and cirrhosis (*ALD*). Values are expressed as a percentage of the values in normal subjects. AP = alkaline phosphatase; AST = aspartate aminotransferase; ALT = alanine aminotransferase; GGTP = γ-glutamyltranspeptidase; GDH = glutamate dehydrogenase. Note that AP and GGTP activities are similarly elevated in the liver tissue of patients with ALD but that serum GGTP is 1300% of normal whereas serum AP is only 240% of normal. The data suggest that induction of hepatic GGTP by alcohol is not the sole or major cause of the serum GGTP elevation. (Kaplan MM: Biochemical basis of serum enzyme abnormalities in alcoholic liver disease. In Chang NC, Chao HM (eds): Early Identification of Alcohol Abuse, p 186. NIAAA, Research Monograph 17, 1985)

Leucine aminopeptidase activity is elevated in most types of liver disease,[54,175] but values are highest in biliary obstruction. Some have promulgated it as a reliable test to distinguish obstructive from hepatocellular liver disease.[262] Others observed a considerable overlap in values among the various patient groups and found the serum alkaline phosphatase to be at least as selective.[54,175] The controversy regarding the specificity of leucine aminopeptidase as a test of biliary obstruction has never been resolved. Because of the availability of other equally sensitive, convenient, and specific tests, leucine aminopeptidase is not widely used. Its only possible value is its specificity for liver disease. In this regard, it, the 5'-nucleotidase, and GGT seem to have comparable merit.

TESTS OF THE LIVER'S BIOSYNTHETIC CAPACITY

Serum Proteins

Serum contains a complex mixture of proteins that have been studied extensively by a variety of techniques.[242] A schematic representation of the results of some of the methods in current use is shown in Figure 9-30. The liver is the major source of most of these serum proteins; the parenchymal cells are responsible for synthesis of albumin, fibrinogen, and other coagulation factors and most of the alpha and beta globulins.[111,178,202,210] Gamma globulins are an important exception, being synthesized by B-lymphocytes.[319]

In this section, we will discuss only those proteins used in the diagnosis of liver disease, albumin and prothrombin, both of which are synthesized exclusively by hepatocytes, and the immunoglobulins that are synthesized by B-lymphocytes. Lipoproteins are discussed in Chapter 23. Ceruloplasmin, the blue copper–containing protein, is discussed in Chapter 28, ferritin in Chapter 27, and α_1-antitrypsin in Chapter 40.

Total serum protein is usually determined by a variation of the biuret reaction. Its fractionation into its major constituents, albumin and globulins, is done by automated dye binding methods[95] or by paper or cellulose acetate electrophoresis.[226] Older salting out techniques do not quantitatively remove all the alpha and beta globulins from albumin and are less commonly used.[106,128,145]

Albumin

Albumin, quantitatively the most important plasma protein, is synthesized exclusively by the liver. Normal serum values range from 3.5 g/dl to 4.5 g/dl. The average adult

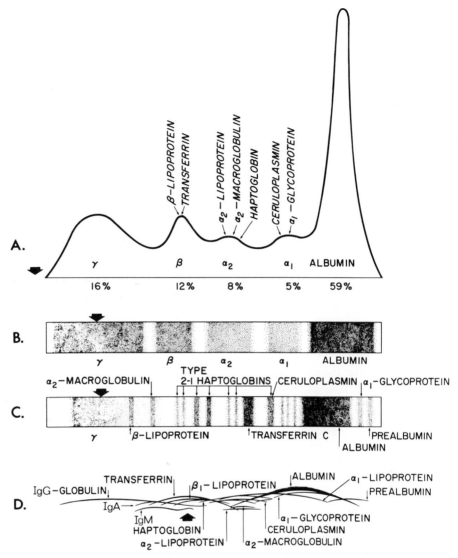

Fig. 9-30. Schematic representation of the electrophoretic pattern of normal human serum in *p*H 8.6 buffer as obtained by four methods. **A.** Tiselius or free boundary electrophoresis. **B.** Paper electrophoresis. **C.** Starch-gel electrophoresis. **D.** Immunoelectrophoresis. The broad, vertical arrow indicates the starting point with each method. Beta-2 M-globulin remains at the origin in starch-gel electrophoresis but moves in the γ- to β-range with other methods. (Putnam FW: The Proteins, vol I, 2nd ed, p 18. Orlando, Academic Press, 1975)

has approximately 300 g to 500 g of albumin distributed in body fluids and synthesizes about 12 g/day. The synthesis rate may double in situations in which there is rapid albumin loss or a fall in the serum albumin concentration owing to dilution such as occurs during the rapid accumulation of ascitic fluid.[265] Albumin has a long half-life, 15 to 20 days. Approximately 4% is degraded per day, but little is known about its site of degradation. The serum level at any time reflects the rate of synthesis, the degradation rate, and the volume of distribution. Albumin synthesis is regulated by changes in nutritional status, osmotic pressure, systemic inflammation, and hormones.[265,267] The

precise mechanism is not totally known but appears to be related to the formation of albumin-mRNA polysomes within the liver.[267] Substances that stimulate albumin synthesis cause individual ribosomes to bind to the albumin-mRNA to form polysomes that will more efficiently synthesize albumin.[266,267] Amino acids such as tryptophan, phenylalanine, glutamine, and lysine, for example, function in this way and increase albumin synthesis in *in vitro* systems.[266,267] Albumin synthesis is also stimulated by those amino acids that increase urea synthesis, ornithine and arginine.[225] Ornithine serves as precursor of the polyamine spermine, a compound that promotes polysome formation.[225] Corticosteroids stimulate albumin synthesis by increasing the concentration of albumin-mRNA in hepatocytes, either by increasing its synthesis or decreasing its degradation.[156] In *in vitro* models, alcohol decreases albumin synthesis by inhibiting the formation of polysomes,[267] whereas inflammation decreases albumin synthesis[28] perhaps through the effects of interleukin-1.[86]

Serum albumin levels tend to be normal in liver diseases such as acute viral hepatitis, drug-related hepatotoxicity, and obstructive jaundice. Albumin levels below 3 g/dl in hepatitis should raise the possibility of chronic hepatitis. Hypoalbuminemia is more common in chronic liver disorders such as cirrhosis and usually reflects severe liver damage and decreased albumin synthesis. One exception is the patient with ascites in whom synthesis may be normal or even increased, but levels are low because of the increased volume of distribution.[134,265] Heavy alcohol ingestion, chronic inflammation, and protein malnutrition may inhibit albumin synthesis.[266,272] Hypoalbuminemia is not specific for liver disease and may occur in protein malnutrition of any cause, protein-losing enteropathies, chronic infections, and nephrotic syndrome.

PROTHROMBIN TIME

Clotting is the end result of a complex series of enzymatic reactions involving at least 13 factors.[243] The liver is the major site of synthesis of 11 blood coagulation proteins: factor I—fibrinogen[111,131,211,223,306]; factor II—prothrombin[5,6,21,170,205,223a]; factor V—proaccelerin, labile factor[205,223a]; factor VII—serum prothrombin conversion accelerator (SPCA), stable factor[170,205,223,223a,234]; factor IX—Christmas factor, plasma thromboplastin component[170,246]; factor X—Stuart–Prower factor[170,205,223,223a]; factors XII and XIII—prekallikrein and high molecular-weight kininogen.[201] The liver is also involved in clearing some of the clotting factors from serum.[255] Components of the clotting mechanism are frequently abnormal in the course of hepatic diseases.[92,108,222,244,246,255,295a] These abnormalities can be assessed by tests that measure one factor or the interplay of a number of factors. The one-stage prothrombin time of Quick[243] is one of the most useful tests available (see Chap. 6). It measures the rate at which available prothrombin is converted to thrombin in the presence of a tissue extract (thromboplastin), calcium ions, and a series of activated coagulation factors, followed by the polymerization of fibrinogen by thrombin to fibrin (Fig. 9-31). It is influenced by factors I, II, V, VII, and X. The results may be expressed in time in seconds or as a ratio of the plasma prothrombin time to a control plasma time.[287] A normal control is usually in the range of 9 to 11 seconds. In general, a prolongation of 2 seconds or more is considered abnormal, and values more than 4 seconds prolonged indicate a group at risk from bleeding.[299] The prothrombin time is prolonged if any of the involved factors is deficient, either singly or in combination.

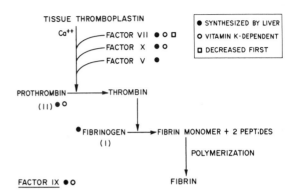

Fig. 9-31. Factors involved in Quick one-stage prothrombin time.

The hepatic synthesis of biologically active forms of factors II, VII, IX, and X requires vitamin K for the addition of carboxylic acid moieties to the gamma positions of glutamic acid residues in these proteins.[220,300,303] The gamma carboxylation step is a post-translational process[192] that allows these proteins to bind Ca^{++} avidly, a necessity for them to function as clotting factors.[300] The absence of vitamin K, the ingestion of vitamin K antagonists, or the presence of certain hepatic disorders (hepatocellular carcinoma) inhibits this vitamin K–dependent carboxylation and allows the release of des-γ-carboxy prothrombin (abnormal prothrombin) into serum.[192] This can be detected by a specific radioimmunoassay.[35] Normal subjects have no abnormal prothrombin in serum. Its presence in serum is a more sensitive indicator of vitamin K deficiency than measurement of the prothrombin time, and abnormal prothrombin may be present in high concentration despite a normal prothrombin time.[36] It is present in high concentration in 91% of patients with biopsy-confirmed hepatocellular carcinoma.[193] Measurement of the abnormal prothrombin in serum shows great promise as a diagnostic test for the detection of vitamin K deficiency and liver disorders but is not yet widely available.

A prolonged prothrombin time is not specific for liver disease, being observed in various congenital deficiencies of coagulation factors[245,246] and in acquired conditions, including consumption of clotting factors and ingestion of drugs that affect the prothrombin complex.[243,246,255] In these instances, the underlying cause can usually be elucidated. When the above are excluded, a prolonged prothrombin time may be the consequence of either (1) hypovitaminosis K, as observed with prolonged obstructive jaundice, steatorrhea,[48] or, much less commonly, dietary deficiency[114,167] or intake of antibiotics that alter the gut flora[114]; or (2) poor utilization of vitamin K due to parenchymal liver disease. These two situations can usually be differentiated by parenteral administration of vitamin K_1.[48,92,197,301,302] If the prothrombin time returns to normal or improves by at least 30% within 24 hours after a single parenteral injection of vitamin K_1 (doses of 5 mg to 10 mg are usually used), one may surmise that parenchymal function is good and that hypovitaminosis K was responsible for the original prothrombin time. By contrast, slight if any improvement is observed in most patients with parenchymal liver disease. Most patients with extrahepatic obstruction respond promptly to vitamin K, and one would hesitate to make such a diagnosis if the prothrombin time did not respond. In jaundice, the type of response to vitamin K_1 is therefore of some value in differential diagnosis. However, observations of sluggish responses to vitamin K_1, with prolonged values still recorded 24 hours before normalization at 48 to 72 hours in some patients with obstructive jaundice, and of good responses in some patients with hepatocellular disease have been reported and complicate interpretation.

The prothrombin test is not a sensitive index of liver disease, because, even in severe cirrhosis, results may be normal or the prothrombin time may be prolonged only slightly. On the other hand, the test has high prognostic value, particularly in acute hepatocellular disease. An abnormal prothrombin time with confirmed prolongation more than 5 to 6 seconds above control is the single laboratory test that draws attention to the possibility of fulminant hepatic necrosis developing in the course of acute viral hepatitis. Such a prolonged prothrombin time often precedes by days the manifestations of liver failure. Nevertheless, not all patients with abnormal prothrombin times of this extent develop evidence of fulminant hepatic necrosis.[104] Progressive shortening of the prothrombin time to normal usually precedes or accompanies other evidence of clinical improvement in this latter group. The degree of prolongation of the prothrombin time is also prognostic in alcoholic steatonecrosis. A prothrombin time greater than 4 seconds above control values occurred six times as often in a group of patients who died (60%) than in a group who survived (10%).[133] In chronic hepatocellular disease, an abnormal prothrombin time, particularly one prolonged more than 4 to 5 seconds that does not respond to parenteral vitamin K_1, indicates extensive parenchymal damage and carries a poor long-term prognosis.[169,299] The test is also used as an early predictor of outcome in acetaminophen overdose.[64]

The prothrombin test is particularly important in the management of patients with liver disease. It permits an assessment of the tendency to bleed before any contemplated surgical or diagnostic procedure such as closed liver biopsy, splenic puncture, or transhepatic cholangiography. When the prothrombin time is prolonged, vitamin K_1 should be administered routinely in doses of 5 mg/day to 10 mg/day parenterally for up to 3 doses. It is difficult to indicate at what level of prothrombin time diagnostic procedures such as a needle biopsy of the liver are contraindicated, because the risks of bleeding have not been well correlated with the values of this test. Furthermore, vascular reactivity and coagulation factors such as platelets exert an important contributory role. Closed needle biopsies are rarely done in my hospital if the prothrombin time is more than 4 seconds prolonged. For patients with prothrombin times prolonged at least 4 seconds who do not respond to vitamin K_1, mortality is high after surgery such as portacaval shunt.[194] Obviously the performance of any open surgical procedure is determined by the urgency of the situation. The more pressing the need, the more prolonged the prothrombin time that is accepted. It can often be corrected by infusions of fresh frozen plasma with careful monitoring of the prothrombin time.

TESTS THAT DETECT CHRONIC INFLAMMATION OR ALTERED IMMUNOREGULATION

Immunoglobulins

Serum immunoglobulins are produced by stimulated B-lymphocytes and so do not directly test liver function. Their elevation in many patients with chronic liver disease is believed to be indicative of impaired function of reticuloendothelial cells in hepatic sinusoids or to shunting of portal venous blood around the liver.[319] Data indicate that antibodies directed against antigens of the normal colonic flora account for much of the increased serum immunoglobulins in patients with cirrhosis.[319] In cirrhosis, these antigens are not taken up and degraded by hepatic reticuloendothelial cells as they normally are and reach lymphoid tissue outside the liver where they elicit an antibody response.

In most cases of acute hepatitis, immunoglobulins are normal or minimally increased.[137] Persistent hypergammaglobulinemia of a moderate degree is suggestive of chronic active hepatitis,[187,297] whereas striking increases are suggestive of autoimmune chronic hepatitis.[187,199] Immunoglobulins are also increased in most types of cirrhosis, although the values tend to be lower than in autoimmune chronic active hepatitis. Diffuse polyclonal increases in IgG and IgM are found in most types of cirrhosis and are nonspecific.[199] Specific increases in IgM are suggestive of primary biliary cirrhosis,[227] whereas increases in IgA may be seen in alcoholic cirrhosis.[102] Immunoglobulin levels are usually normal in obstructive jaundice. The major value of measuring the immunoglobulins is in detecting patients who might have cirrhosis or chronic hepatitis. It is also useful in monitoring the response to immunosuppressive therapy in patients with autoimmune chronic hepatitis.[297] Hypergammaglobulinemia, with or without hypoalbuminemia, is not specific for liver disease and may be found in other chronic inflammatory and malignant diseases.

A more detailed description of immunologic aspects of liver disease is provided in Chapters 21 and 22. A discussion of antimitochondrial antibody, a marker of primary biliary cirrhosis, is provided in Chapter 26.

USE OF LIVER FUNCTION TESTS

The author has found it useful to obtain the tests listed in Table 9-6 during the initial encounter with a patient

TABLE 9-6. Liver Function Test Patterns in Hepatobiliary Disorders and Jaundice

TYPE OF DISORDER	BILIRUBIN	AMINOTRANS-FERASES	ALKALINE PHOSPHATASE	ALBUMIN	GLOBULIN	PROTHROMBIN TIME
Hemolysis Gilbert's syndrome	Normal to 5 mg/dl >85 % due to indirect fraction No bilirubinuria	Normal	Normal	Normal	Normal	Normal
Acute hepatocellular necrosis (viral and drug hepatitis, hepatotoxins, acute heart failure)	Both fractions may be elevated; peak usually follows aminotransferases Bilirubinuria	Elevated, often >500 units: ALT ≥ AST	Normal to <3× elevation	Normal	Normal	Usually normal; if >5 sec above control and not corrected by parenteral vitamin K, suggests massive necrosis and poor prognosis
Chronic hepatocellular disorders Alcoholic hepatitis Cirrhosis	Both fractions may be elevated Bilirubinuria	Elevated, but usually <300 units AST/ ALT > 2 suggests alcoholic hepatitis or cirrhosis	Normal to <3× elevated	Often decreased	Increased gamma globulin	Often prolonged; fails to correct with parenteral vitamin K
Intrahepatic cholestasis Obstructive jaundice	Both fractions may be elevated Bilirubinuria	Normal to moderate elevations Rarely >500 units	Elevated, often >4× normal	Normal, unless chronic	Gamma globulin normal Beta globulin may be increased	Normal; if prolonged will correct with parenteral vitamin K
Infiltrative diseases (tumor, granulomata) Partial bile duct obstruction	Usually normal	Normal to slight elevation	Elevated, often >4× normal Fractionate, or confirm liver origin with 5'-nucleotidase, gamma glutamyl transpeptidase	Normal	Usually normal Gamma may be increased in granulomatous disease	Normal

(Kaplan M: Evaluation of hepatobiliary diseases. In Stein JH (ed): Internal Medicine, p 58. Boston, Little, Brown and Co, 1983)

with jaundice or suspected liver disease. These include the total and direct bilirubin, urine for bilirubin, the aminotransferases, alkaline phosphatase, albumin, globulin, and prothrombin time. The use of these tests as a battery increases their specificity and sensitivity in the diagnosis of liver disease and renders it unlikely that any person with clinically important liver disease will not be identified.

Conceptually, it is helpful to divide the various causes of jaundice and liver dysfunction into the broad categories shown in Table 9-6. These include disorders of bilirubin metabolism, acute parenchymal or hepatocellular disease, chronic hepatocellular diseases such as cirrhosis, cholestasis, and infiltrative diseases. Because the pattern of liver function test abnormalities is often similar in patients with infiltrative diseases and those with partial bile duct obstruction, these two types of disorders are listed together.

A patient with hemolysis or Gilbert's syndrome may have total serum bilirubins elevated to as much as 5 mg/dl. If the standard van den Bergh bilirubin fractionation is performed, more than 85% of the bilirubin will be in the indirect fraction. There is no bilirubinuria. If HPLC were used to fractionate the bilirubin, all the bilirubin would be in the indirect fraction. All the other screening tests of liver function listed in Table 9-5 would be normal. Compensated hemolysis can be detected by measuring the reticulocyte count, serum hemoglobin, or haptoglobin. If there is bilirubinuria and if more than 15% to 20% of the elevated bilirubin is due to the direct fraction, one must consider disorders of bilirubin metabolism such as the Dubin–Johnson syndrome and Rotor's syndrome, in which other tests of liver function will also be normal. Since Dubin–Johnson syndrome and Rotor's syndrome are both benign conditions, one could argue cogently that no further investigation is required except to repeat these tests and verify them. For those who are not satisfied with uncertainty, the BSP test with blood sampling at 45 and 90 minutes would be an option in order to diagnose the Dubin–Johnson syndrome and distinguish it from Rotor's syndrome. A serum bile acid test might also be obtained since it will be normal in the Dubin–Johnson syndrome.[4]

The aminotransferases are clearly the most sensitive test in the detection of acute hepatocellular disorders such as viral or drug-induced hepatitis. Aminotransferase levels greater than 500 make such a diagnosis probable. Depending upon the severity of the underlying hepatocellular disorder, bilirubin may be normal or elevated. If bilirubin is elevated, there should be bilirubinuria and increases in both the direct and indirect bilirubin fractions. Alkaline phosphatase elevations as high as three times the upper limit of normal are common in acute hepatocellular disorders, but values greater than three times normal are unusual except in some drug-induced hepatitis. Serum albumin is usually normal, and immunoglobulins are normal or minimally elevated. The prothrombin time is typically normal in most patients with viral or drug-induced hepatitis. Prolongation of the prothrombin time to more than 5 seconds above control and its failure to correct within 24 to 48 hours with the parenteral administration of vitamin K suggests a poor prognosis and should alert one to the possibility of massive hepatic necrosis. If the liver function tests are typical of acute hepatitis, a careful medication history must be obtained together with serologic tests for hepatitis A and hepatitis B. The possibility of hepatic ischemia should also be considered.[69]

Liver function tests are less precise in the diagnosis of chronic hepatocellular disorders such as cirrhosis. The activity of the disease and the degree of hepatic reserve are variable and the results of liver function tests will vary with the activity of the process and the amount of hepatic reserve. Liver function tests may be highly insensitive in cirrhosis. Patients with end-stage postnecrotic or alcoholic cirrhosis may have shrunken livers and striking portal hypertension and yet have liver function tests that are almost normal. The author has seen such patients and been surprised by the normal or nearly normal serum bilirubin, aminotransferases, alkaline phosphatase, prothrombin time, albumin, and globulin in some of them. Breath tests, serum bile acid tests, and measurements of the undercarboxylated form of prothrombin[35,192] would all be useful tests in such patients. On the other hand, liver function tests may be strikingly abnormal in patients with chronic hepatic disorders. A serum albumin below 3 g/dl, increased immunoglobulins, a prothrombin time three or more seconds above control that fails to correct with parenteral vitamin K, and aminotransferases that are elevated but less than 300 units make the diagnosis of cirrhosis likely. An AST/ALT ratio greater than two raises the possibility of alcoholic liver disease, and an AST/ALT ratio greater than three is highly suggestive of this possibility. The alkaline phosphatase is rarely helpful in the diagnosis of cirrhosis. However, threefold or greater elevations should suggest the possibility of primary biliary cirrhosis in the setting of cirrhosis or portal hypertension.

There is a characteristic pattern of the liver function tests in cholestasis, although the routine laboratory tests in Table 9-6 do not distinguish between intrahepatic and extrahepatic cholestasis. The alkaline phosphatase is usually elevated out of proportion to other tests. Values four times or greater than normal suggest some type of cholestasis. Depending upon the severity of the underlying condition, the bilirubin will be normal or elevated. If elevated, the direct fraction will be increased and there will be bilirubinuria. Aminotransferases are usually elevated, but values greater than 500 units are rare. Aminotransferases are usually less than 300 unless tests are done within 24 hours of the development of acute bile duct obstruction, for example, that due to the passage of a common duct stone.[1] Albumin and globulin are usually normal. Increased immunoglobulins suggest cirrhosis in the patient with cholestasis; an increased IgM fraction suggests primary biliary cirrhosis. The antimitochondrial antibody test is helpful in this situation. It is positive in 90% to 95% of patients with primary biliary cirrhosis and negative in extrahepatic bile duct obstruction or sclerosing cholangitis.

The prothrombin time is usually normal. If elevated, it is usually due to vitamin K deficiency and should correct with parenteral vitamin K.

Infiltrative liver diseases produce similar liver function test abnormalities as partial bile duct obstruction. Often the earliest and only abnormal test is the alkaline phosphatase. If this is the case or if the serum alkaline phosphatase is elevated out of proportion to the other tests, it is helpful to identify the origin of the alkaline phosphatase. This can be done with electrophoretic techniques or by measuring the 5′-nucleotidase or GGT. The bilirubin is often normal early in infiltrative diseases and usually normal in patients with partial bile duct obstruction. If the total serum bilirubin is elevated, the direct fraction is certain to be elevated and there will be bilirubinuria. Aminotransferases are normal or minimally elevated in patients with infiltrative diseases and partial bile duct obstruction as are the serum albumin, immunoglobulins, and prothrombin time.

It is important to recognize that these laboratory tests *suggest* but rarely make a specific diagnosis. However, once this information is obtained, the results will facilitate the efficient use of other diagnostic tests such as the hepatitis serologies, echography, CT scanning, percutaneous liver biopsy, and cholangiography.

It is possible that with increasing experience, the breath tests and serum bile acid tests may be added to the routinely used tests listed in Table 9-6 or replace some of them. For example, serum bile acid tests may someday replace the direct bilirubin test as a general screening test for detecting hepatic dysfunction.[145] This has not yet occurred. However, any conveniently performed inexpensive test that will increase the diagnostic power of the standard liver function battery will be welcomed.

REFERENCES

1. Abbruzzese A, Jeffrey RL: Marked elevation of serum glutamic oxalacetic transaminase and lactic dehydrogenase activity in chronic extrahepatic biliary disease. Am J Dig Dis 14:332, 1969
2. Ahlberg J et al: Individual bile acids in portal venous and systemic blood serum in fasting man. Gastroenterology 73:1377, 1977
3. Aisenberg AC et al: Serum alkaline phosphatase at the onset of Hodgkin's disease. Cancer 26:318, 1970
4. Albert S et al: Multiplicity of hepatic excreting mechanisms for organic anions. J Gen Physiol 53:238, 1969
5. Anderson GF, Barnhart MI: Intracellular localization of prothrombin. Proc Soc Exp Biol Med 116:1, 1964
6. Anderson GF, Barnhart MI: Prothrombin synthesis in the dog. Am J Physiol 206:929, 1964
7. Angelin B et al: Individual serum bile acid concentrations in normo- and hyperlipoproteinemia as determined by mass fragmentography: Relation to bile acid pool size. J Lipid Res 19:527, 1978
8. Angelin B et al: Hepatic uptake of bile acids in man. Fasting and postprandial concentrations of individual bile acids in portal venous and systemic blood venous. J Clin Invest 70:724, 1982
9. Arias I et al: Black liver disease in Corriedale sheep; a new mutation affecting hepatic excretory function (abstr). J Clin Invest 43:1249, 1964
10. Arias IM et al: Prolonged neonatal unconjugated hyperbilirubinemia associated with breast feeding and a steroid pregnane-2(α),20(β)-diol, in maternal milk that inhibits glucuronide formation *in vitro*. J Clin Invest 43:2037, 1964
11. Arias IM et al: Transient familial neonatal hyperbilirubinemia. J Clin Invest 44:1442, 1965
12. Arias IM et al: On the structure, regulation, and function of ligandin. In Arias IM, Jakoby WB (eds): Glutathione: Metabolism and Function, p 175. New York, Raven Press, 1976
13. Aronsen KF et al: The value of γ-glutamyl transpeptidase in differentiating viral hepatitis from obstructive jaundice. Acta Chir Scand 130:92, 1965
14. Bahr M, Wilkinson JH: Urea as a selective inhibitor of human tissue alkaline phosphatases. Clin Chim Acta 17:367, 1967
15. Baker AL et al: Clinical utility of breath tests for the assessment of hepatic function. Semin Liver Dis 3:318, 1983
16. Baker KJ: Binding of sulfobromophthalein (BSP) sodium and indocyanine green (ICG) by plasma α_1 lipoproteins. Proc Soc Exp Biol Med 122:957, 1966
17. Bamford KF et al: Serum-alkaline-phosphatase and the ABO blood groups. Lancet 1:530, 1965
18. Banks BM et al: Clinical value of serum leucine aminopeptidase determinations. N Engl J Med 263:1277, 1960
19. Bardawill C, Chang G: Serum lactic dehydrogenase, leucine aminopeptidase, and 5′-nucleotidase activities: Observations in patients with carcinoma of the pancreas and hepatobiliary disease. Can Med Assoc J 89:755, 1963
20. Barnes S, Spenney JG: Improved enzymatic assays for bile acids using resazarin and NADH oxidoreductase from *Clostridium kluyveri*. Clin Chim Acta 102:241, 1980
21. Barnhart MJ: Prothrombin synthesis: An example of hepatic function. J Histochem Cytochem 13:740, 1965
22. Barouki R et al: Ethanol effects in a rat hepatoma cell line: Induction of γ-glutamyl transferase. Hepatology 3:323, 1983
23. Bechman L: Monographs in Human Genetics. I. Isozyme Variations in Man. Basel, Switzerland, S Karger, 1966
24. Belfield A, Goldberg A: Normal ranges and diagnostic value of serum 5′-nucleotidase and alkaline phosphatase activities in infancy. Arch Dis Child 46:842, 1971
25. Belfield A et al: A specific colorimetric 5′-nucleotidase assay utilizing the Berthelot reaction. Clin Chem 16:396, 1970
26. Bell JL et al: Serum isocitrate dehydrogenase in liver disease and some other conditions. Clin Chem 23:57, 1962
27. Berk PD et al: Studies of bilirubin kinetics in normal adults. J Clin Invest 48;2176, 1969
28. Bernau D et al: Decreased albumin and increased fibrinogen secretion by single hepatocytes from rats with acute inflammatory reaction. Hepatology 3:29, 1983
29. Berry W, Reichen J: Bile acid metabolism: Its relation to clinical disease. Semin Liver Dis 3:330, 1983
30. Betro MG et al: Gamma-glutamyl transpeptidase in diseases of the liver and bone. Am J Clin Pathol 60:672, 1973
31. Billing BH et al: The excretion of bilirubin as a diglucuronide giving the direct van den Bergh reaction. Biochem J 65:774, 1957
32. Bircher J et al: Aminopyrine demethylation measured by

breath analysis in cirrhosis. Clin Pharmacol Ther 20:484, 1976

33. Bircher J: Quantitative assessment of deranged hepatic function: A missed opportunity. Semin Liver Dis 3:275, 1983

34. Birkett DJ et al: Serum alkaline phosphatase in pregnancy: An immunological study. Br Med J 1:1210, 1966

35. Blanchard RA et al: Acquired vitamin K–dependent carboxylation deficiency in liver disease. N Engl J Med 305:242, 1981

36. Blanchard RA et al: Immunoassays of human prothrombin species which correlate with functional coagulant activities. J Lab Clin Med 101:242, 1983

37. Blanckaert N et al: Comparison of the biliary excretion of the four isomers of bilirubin-IX in wistar and homozygous Gunn rats. Biochem J 164:237, 1977

38. Blanckaert N et al: Bilirubin diglucuronide synthesis by a UDP-glucuronic acid–dependent enzyme system in the rat liver microsomes. Proc Natl Acad Sci 76:2037, 1979

39. Blanckaert N: Analysis of bilirubin and bilirubin mono- and di-conjugates. Biochem J 185:115, 1980

40. Blanckaert N et al: Measurement of bilirubin and its monoconjugates and diconjugates in human serum by alkaline methanolysis and high-performance liquid chromatography. J Lab Clin Med 96:198, 1980

41. Blanckaert N, Schmid R: Physiology and pathophysiology of bilirubin metabolism. In Zakim D, Boyer TD (eds): Hepatology—A Textbook of Liver Disease, p 278. Philadelphia, WB Saunders, 1982

42. Blaschke TF et al: Effects of induced fever on sulfobromophthalein kinetics in man. Ann Intern Med 78:221, 1971

43. Bloomer JR et al: Interpretation of plasma bilirubin levels based on studies of radioactive bilirubin. JAMA 218:216, 1971

44. Bloomer JR et al: Serum bile acids in primary biliary cirrhosis. Arch Intern Med 136:57, 1976

45. Boernig H et al: Zum mechanismus der aktivitat sanderung der alkalinischen phosphatase in leber und darm der ratte. Acta Biol Med Germ 22:537, 1969

46. Bonnett R et al: Structure of bilirubin. Nature 262:326, 1976

47. Bourke E et al: Mechanisms of renal excretion of urobilinogen. Br Med J 2:1510, 1965

48. Bouvier CA, Maurice PA: Liver and blood coagulation. In Rouiller C (ed): The Liver, Vol II, pp 177–213. New York, Academic Press, 1964

49. Boyde TRC, Latner AL: Starch gel electrophoresis of transaminase in human tissue extracts and serum. Biochem J 82:52, 1961

50. Boyde TRC: Detection and assay of mitochondrial aspartate aminotransferase in serum. Z Klin Chem 6:431, 1968

51. Breen KJ et al: ^{14}C-phenacetin breath test in the assessment of hepatic function. Gastroenterology 72:1033, 1977

52. Brensilver HL, Kaplan MM: Significance of elevated liver alkaline phosphatase in serum. Gastroenterology 68:1556, 1975

53. Bressler R, Forsyth BR: Serum leucine aminopeptidase activity in normal pregnancy and in patients with hydatidiform mole. N Engl J Med 261:746, 1959

54. Bressler R et al: Serum leucine aminopeptidase activity in hepatobiliary and pancreatic disease. J Lab Clin Med 56:417, 1960

55. Briheim G et al: Serum bile acids in Gilbert's syndrome before and after reduced caloric intake. Scand J Gastroenterol 17:877, 1982

56. Brodie BB, Axelrod J: The fate of aminopyrine (pyramidon) in man and methods for the estimation of aminopyrine and its metabolites in biological material. J Pharmacol Exp Ther 99:171, 1950

57. Brown SB, King RFGJ: The mechanism of haem catabolism. Bilirubin formation in living rats by ^{18}O oxygen labeling. Biochim J 170:297, 1978

58. Burrows S et al: Serum gamma-glutamyl transpeptidase. Evaluation in screening of hospitalized patients. Am J Clin Pathol 64:311, 1975

59. Caesar J et al: The use of indocyanine green in the measurement of hepatic blood flow and as a test of hepatic function. Clin Sci 21:43, 1961

60. Campbell DM: Determination of 5'-nucleotidase in blood serum. Biochem J 82:348, 1962

61. Carlisle R et al: The relationship between conventional liver tests, quantitative function tests, and histopathology in cirrhosis. Dig Dis Sci 24:358, 1979

62. Cherrick GR et al: Indocyanine green: Observations on its physical properties, plasma decay, and hepatic extraction. J Clin Invest 39:592, 1960

63. Chiandussi L et al: Serum alkaline phosphatase fractions in hepatobiliary and bone diseases. Clin Sci 22:425, 1962

64. Clarke E et al: Coagulation abnormalities in acute liver failure: Pathogenetic and therapeutic implications. Scand J Gastroenterol 8(Suppl 19):63, 1973

65. Clarke LC, Beck E: Plasma "alkaline" phosphatase activity. I. Normative data for growing children. J Pediatr 36:335, 1950

66. Clermont RJ, Chalmers TC: The transaminase tests in liver disease. Medicine 46:197, 1967

67. Clubb JS et al: The behavior of infused human placental alkaline phosphatase in human subjects. J Lab Clin Med 66:493, 1965

68. Cohen AN, Ostrow JD: New concepts in phototherapy: Photoisomerization of bilirubin IXα and potential toxic effects of light. Pediatrics 65:740, 1980

69. Cohen JA, Kaplan MM: Left-sided heart failure presenting as hepatitis. Gastroenterology 74:583, 1978

70. Cohen JA, Kaplan MM: The SGOT/SGPT ratio—an indicator of alcoholic liver disease. Dig Dis Sci 24:835, 1979

71. Combes B: Excretory function of the liver. In Rouiller C (ed): The Liver Vol. II, Chap 12. New York, Academic Press, 1964

72. Combes B: The importance of conjugation with glutathione for sulfobromophthalein sodium (BSP) transfer from blood to bile. J Clin Invest 44:1214, 1965

73. Combes B, Stakelum GS: Conjugation of sulfobromophthalein sodium with glutathione in thioether linkage by the rat. J Clin Invest 39:1214, 1960

74. Combes B et al: The mechanisms of Bromsulphalein removal from the blood. Trans Assoc Am Phys 69:276, 1956

75. Combes B et al: Serum gamma-glutamyl transpeptidase activity in viral hepatitis: Suppression in pregnancy and by birth control pills. Gastroenterology 72:271, 1977

76. Connell MD, Dinwoodie AJ: Diagnostic use of serum alkaline phosphatase isoenzymes and 5-nucleotidase. Clin Chim Acta 30:235, 1970

77. Cornelius CE, Gronwall RR: A mutation in Southdown sheep affecting the hepatic uptake of sulfobromophthalein (BSP), indocyanine green, rose bengal, sodium cholate, and phylloerythrin from blood (abstr). Fed Proc 24;144, 1963

78. Crigler JF, Najjar VA: Congenital familial nonhemolytic jaundice with kernicterus. Pediatrics 10:169, 1952

79. Crofton PM: Biochemistry of alkaline phosphatase isoenzymes. CRC Crit Rev Clin Lab Sci 16;161, 1982

80. Debroe ME et al: The separation and characterization of liver plasma membrane fragments circulating in the blood of patients with cholestasis. Clin Chim Acta 59:369, 1975

81. Debroe ME et al: Liver plasma membrane is the source of high molecular–weight alkaline phosphatase in human serum. Hepatology 5:118, 1985

82. Defreese JD, Wang TSC: Properties and determinations of serum bilirubin. CRC Crit Rev Clin Lab Sci 19:267, 1984

83. Dejeux JF et al: Hepatic clearance and biliary excretion of unconjugated dyes in the Dubin–Johnson syndrome. Gut 12:758, 1971

84. Demers LM, Hepner G: Radioimmunoassay of bile acids in serum. Clin Chem 22:602, 1976

85. Diehl AM et al: Relationship between pyridoxal 5'-phosphate deficiency and aminotransferase levels in alcoholic hepatitis. Gastroenterology 86:632, 1984

86. Dinarello C: Interleukin-I and the pathogenesis of the acute phase response. N Engl J Med 311:1413, 1984

87. De Ritis F et al: Transaminase activity in liver disease. Lancet II:214, 1958

88. De Ritis F et al: Serum transaminase activities in liver disease. Lancet I:685, 1972

89. De Ritis F et al: Biochemical laboratory tests in viral hepatitis and other hepatic diseases. Bull WHO 32:59, 1965

90. Dent CE, Harper CM: Plasma-alkaline-phosphatase in normal adults and in patients with primary hyperparathyroidism. Lancet I:559, 1962

91. Deren JJ et al: Comparative study of four methods of determining alkaline phosphatase. N Engl J Med 270:1277, 1964

92. Deutsch E: Blood coagulation changes in liver diseases. In Popper H, Schaffner F (eds): Progress in Liver Diseases, Vol 2, pp 69–83. New York, Grune & Stratton, 1965

93. Diamond I, Schmid R: Experimental bilirubin encephalopathy; the mode of entry of bilirubin-^{14}C into the central nervous system. J Clin Invest 45:678, 1966

94. Dollinger MR, Brandborg LL: Late elevation in serum Bromsulphalein in Dubin–Johnson Syndrome. Am J Digest Dis 72:413, 1967

95. Doumas BT et al: Albumin standards and the measurement of serum albumin with bromcresol green. Clin Chim Acta 31:87, 1971

96. Dreyfus JC et al: Serum enzymes in the physiopathology of muscle. Ann NY Acad Sci 75:235, 1959

97. Dunn M et al: The disappearance rate of glutamic oxaloacetic transaminase from the circulation and its distribution in the body's fluid compartments and secretions. J Lab Clin Med 51:259, 1958

98. Einarsson K et al: The diagnostic value of fasting individual serum bile acids in anicteric alcoholic liver disease: Relation to liver morphology. Hepatology 5:108, 1985

98a. Elder G et al: Bile pigment fate in gastrointestinal tract. Semin Hematol 9:71, 1972

99. Ellis G et al: Serum enzyme tests in diseases of the liver and biliary tree. Am J Clin Pathol 70:248, 1978

100. Eshchar J et al: Serum levels of 5'-nucleotidase in disease. Am J Clin Pathol 47:598, 1967

101. Everson GT, Kern F Jr: Bile acid metabolism. In MacSween T (ed): Advances in Hepatology. London, Churchill Livingstone, 1983

102. Feizi T: Immunoglobulins in chronic liver disease. Gut 9: 193, 1968

103. Felsher BF, Carpio NM: Chronic persistent hepatitis and unconjugated hyperbilirubinemia. Gastroenterology 76: 248, 1979

104. Fenster LF: Viral hepatitis in the elderly; an analysis of 23 patients over 65 years of age. Gastroenterology 49:262, 1965

105. Ferraris R et al: Diagnostic value of serum bile acids and routine liver function tests in hepatobiliary disease. Sensitivity, specificity, and predictive value. Dig Dis Sci 28: 129, 1983

106. Festi D et al: Diagnostic effectiveness of serum bile acids in liver disease as evaluated by multivariate statistical methods. Hepatology 3:707, 1983

107. Fevery J et al: Hyperbilirubinemia: Significance of the ratio between direct-reacting and total bilirubin. Clin Chim Acta 17:73, 1967

108. Finkbiner RB et al: Coagulation defects in liver disease and response to transfusion during surgery. Am J Med 26:199, 1959

109. Fishman WH: Immunologic and biochemical approaches to alkaline phosphatase isoenzyme analysis: The Regan isoenzyme. Ann NY Acad Sci 116:745, 1969

110. Fog J, Jellum E: Structure of bilirubin. Nature 198:88, 1963

111. Forman WB, Barnhart MI: Cellular site for fibrinogen synthesis. JAMA 187:168, 1964

112. Frankl HD, Merritt JH: Enzyme activity in the serum and common duct bile of dogs. Am J Gastroenterol 31:166, 1959

113. Franklin M et al: Electrophoretic studies in liver disease. II. Gamma globulin in chronic liver disease. J Clin Invest 30:729, 1951

114. Frick PG et al: Dose response and minimal daily requirement for vitamin K in man. J Appl Physiol 23:387, 1967

114a. Galizzi J et al: Assessment of the ^{14}C aminopyrine breath test in occult liver disease. Gut 19:40, 1978

115. Gambino SR et al: Direct serum bilirubin and sulfobromophthalein test in occult liver disease. JAMA 201:1047, 1967

116. Gerety RJ (ed): Non-A, Non-B Hepatitis. New York, Academic Press, 1981

117. Gikalov I, Bircher J: Dose dependence of the ^{14}C-aminopyrine breath tests. Intrasubject comparison of tracer and pharmacologic doses. Eur J Clin Pharmacol 12:229, 1977

118. Gilmore IT, Thompson RPH: Plasma clearance of oral and intravenous cholic acid in subjects with and without chronic liver disease. Gut 21:123, 1980

119. Ginsberg AL: Very high levels of SGOT and LDH in patients with extrahepatic biliary tract obstruction. Am J Dig Dis 15:803, 1970

119a. Goldberg JA, Rutenburg AM: Colorimetric determination of leucine aminopeptidase in urine and serum of normal subjects and patients with cancer and other diseases. Cancer 11:283, 1958

120. Goldberg DM: 5'-Nucleotidase: Recent advances in cell biology, methodology, and clinical significance. Digestion 8: 87, 1973

121. Goldberg DM: Structural, functional, and clinical aspects of γ-glutamyl transferase. CRC Crit Rev Clin Lab Sci 12: 58, 1981

122. Goresky CA: Initial distribution and rate of uptake of sulfobromophthalein in the liver. Am J Physiol 207:13, 1964

123. Gray CH: Bile Pigments in Health and Disease. Springfield, IL, Charles C Thomas, 1961

124. Grodsky GM et al: Biosynthesis of a sulfobromophthalein mercaptide with glutathione. Proc Soc Exp Biol Med 106:526, 1961

125. Gronwall R, Cornelius CE: Biliary excretion of sulfobromophthalein in sheep (abstr). Fed Proc 25:576, 1966

126. Groszman R, Kaplan MM: Personal communication.

127. Guker WG et al: The diagnostic significance of liver cell inhomogeneity: Serum enzymes in patients with central liver necrosis and the distribution of glutamatic dehydrogenase in normal human liver. Z Klin Chem Klin Biochem 13:311, 1975

128. Gutman AB: The plasma proteins in disease. In Anson ML, Edsall JT (eds): Advances in Protein Chemistry, Vol IV, p 155. New York, Academic Press, 1948

129. Gutman AB: Serum alkaline phosphatase activity in diseases of the skeletal and hepatobiliary systems. Am J Med 27:875, 1959

130. Hacki W et al: A new look at the plasma disappearance of sulfobromophthalein (BSP): Correlation with the BSP transport maximum and the hepatic plasma flow in man. J Lab Clin Med 88:1019, 1976

131. Hamashima Y et al: The localization of albumin and fibrinogen in human liver cells. J Cell Biol 20:271, 1964

132. Hardison WG, Lee FI: Prognosis in acute liver disease of the alcoholic patient. N Engl J Med 275:61, 1966

133. Harinasuta U et al: Steatonecrosis-Mallory body type. Medicine 46:141, 1967

134. Hasch E et al: Albumin synthesis rate as a measure of liver function in patients with cirrhosis. Arch Intern Med 182:38, 1967

135. Hatoff DE, Hardison WGM: Induced synthesis of alkaline phosphatase by bile acids in rat liver cell culture. Gastroenterology 77:1062, 1979

136. Hatoff DE, Hardison WG: Hepatic bile acid content controls alkaline phosphatase increase during cholestasis. Gastroenterology 78:1307, 1980

137. Havens WP Jr: Viral hepatitis, clinical pattern and diagnosis. Am J Med 32:665, 1972

137a. Heino AE, Jokipii SG: Serum alkaline phosphatase levels in the aged. Ann Med Intern Fenn 51:105, 1962

138. Hepner GW et al: Abnormal aminopyrine metabolism in patients with hepatic neoplasm: Detection by breath test. JAMA 236:1587, 1976

139. Hepner GW, Vesell ES: Assessment of aminopyrine metabolism in man by breath analysis after oral administration of ^{14}C-aminopyrine. Effects of phenobarbital, disulfiram, and portal cirrhosis. N Engl J Med 291:1384, 1974

140. Hepner GW, Vessell ES: Quantitative assessment of hepatic function by breath analysis after oral administration of (^{14}C)aminopyrine. Ann Intern Med 83:632, 1975

141. Hepner GW, Vessell ES: Aminopyrine disposition: Studies on breath, saliva, and urine of normal subjects and patients with liver disease. Clin Pharmacol Ther 20:654, 1976

142. Hepner GW et al: Disposition of aminopyrine, antipyrine, diazepam, and indocyanine greens in patient with liver disease or on anticonvulsant drug therapy: Diazepam breath test and correlations in drug elimination. J Lab Clin Med 90:440, 1977

143. Hill PG, Sammons HG: An assessment of 5′-nucleotidase as a liver-function test. Q J Med 36:457, 1967

144. Hoffbauer FW et al: Limitations and merits of a single serum sample analysis in differential diagnosis of jaundice. J Lab Clin Med 34:1259, 1949

145. Hofman A: The aminopyrine demethylation breath test and the serum bile acid level: Nominated but not yet elected to join the common liver tests. Hepatology 4:512, 1982

146. Howe PE: The determination of proteins in blood—a micro method. J Biol Chem 49:109, 1921

147. Hunton DB et al: The plasma removal of indocyanine green and sulfobromophthalein: Effect of dosage and blocking agents. J Clin Invest 40:1648, 1961

148. Hutchinson DW et al: The reaction between bilirubin and aromatic diazo compounds. Biochem J 127:907, 1972

149. Iber FL: Reactions to sulfobromophthalein sodium injection. USP Bull Johns Hopkins Hosp 116:132, 1965

150. Ideo G et al: γ-Glutamyl transpeptidase: A clinical and experimental study. Digestion 5:326, 1972

151. Irving CJ et al: The aminopyrine breath test as a measure of liver function. J Lab Clin Med 100:356, 1982

152. Ivanov E et al: Elevated liver gamma-glutamyl transferase in chronic alcoholics. Enzyme 25:304, 1980

153. Jablonski P, Owens JA: The clinical chemistry of bromosulfophthalein and other cholephilic dyes. Adv Clin Chem 12:309, 1969

154. Javitt NB: Phenol 3,6-dibromphthalein disulfonate, a new compound for the study of liver disease. Proc Soc Exp Biol Med 117:254, 1964

155. Javitt NB et al: The intrahepatic conjugation of sulfobromophthalein and glutathione in the dog. J Clin Invest 39:1570, 1960

156. Jefferson DM et al: Effects of dexamethasone on albumin and collagen gene expression in primary cultures of adult rat hepatocytes. Hepatology 5:14, 1985

157. Johnson LM: The effect of certain substances on bilirubin levels and occurrence of kernicterus in genetically jaundiced rats. In Sass-Kortsak A (ed): Kernicterus, pp 208–218. Toronto, University of Toronto Press, 1961

158. Jones MB et al: Clinical values of serum bile acid levels in chronic hepatitis. Dig Dis Sci 26:978, 1981

159. Juhl E et al: Atypical reactions to bromosulphthalein (BSP). Lancet 2:424, 1970

160. Kamimoto Y et al: Plasma clearance of intravenously injected aspartate aminotransferase isozymes: Evidence for preferential uptake by sinusoidal liver cells. Hepatology 5:367, 1985

161. Kaplan MM, Rogers L: Separation of serum alkaline phosphatase isoenzymes by polyacrylamide gel electrophoresis. Lancet 2:102, 1968

162. Kaplan MM, Righetti A: Induction of rat liver alkaline phosphatase: The mechanism of the serum elevation in bile duct obstruction. J Clin Invest 49:508, 1970

163. Kaplan M: Alkaline phosphatase. Gastroenterology 62:452, 1972

164. Kaplan MM: Understanding serum enzyme tests in clinical liver disease. In Davidson CS (ed): Problems in Liver Diseases, pp 79–85. New York, Stratton Intercontinental Medical Book Corp, 1979

165. Kaplan MM et al: Increased synthesis of rat liver alkaline phosphatase by bile duct ligation. Hepatology 3:368, 1983

166. Kaplan MM et al: Biochemical basis for serum enzyme abnormalities in alcoholic liver disease. In Chang NC, Chan NM (eds): Early Identification of Alcohol Abuse. Research Monograph, No. 17, NIAAA, p 186, 1985

167. Kark R, Lozner EL: Nutritional deficiency of vitamin K in man: Study of 4 nonjaundiced patients with dietary deficiency. Lancet 2:1162, 1939

168. Kater RMH, Mistilis SP: Obstetric cholestasis and pruritus of pregnancy. Med J Aust 1:638, 1967

169. Kattwinkel J et al: The effects of age on alkaline phosphatase and other serologic liver function tests in normal subjects and patients with cystic fibrosis. J Pediatr 82:234, 1973

170. Kazmier FJ et al: Release of vitamin K–dependent coagulation factors by isolated perfused rat liver. Am J Physiol 214:919, 1968

171. Klaassen CHL: Age and serum-alkaline-phosphatase. Lancet 11:1361, 1966

172. Klatskin G: Bile pigment metabolism. Annu Rev Med 12:211, 1961

173. Klatskin G, Bungards L: An improved test for bilirubin in urine. N Engl J Med 248:712, 1953

174. Korman MG et al: Assessment of activity in chronic active liver disease. Serum bile acids compared with conventional tests and histology. N Engl J Med 290:1399, 1974

175. Kowlessar OD et al: Comparative study of serum leucine aminopeptidase, 5'-nucleotidase and nonspecific alkaline phosphatase in diseases affecting the pancreas, hepatobiliary tree, and bone. Am J Med 31:231, 1961

176. Kowlessar OD et al: Localization of leucine aminopeptidase in serum and body fluids by starch gel electrophoresis. J Clin Invest 39:671, 1960

177. Kreek MJ: Cholestasis of pregnancy and during ethinyl estradiol administration in the human and rat. In Salhanick HA, Kipnis DM, Vande Wiele RL (eds): Metabolic Effects of Gonadal Hormones and Contraceptive Steroids, pp 40–58. New York, Plenum Press, 1969

178. Kukral JC et al: Synthesis of α- and β-globulins in normal and liverless dog. Am J Physiol 204:262, 1963

179. Lamy J et al: Determination de la γ-glutamyl transpeptidase senque des ethyliques a la suite du sevrage. Clin Chim Acta 56:169, 1974

180. Landow SA et al: Catabolism of heme in vivo: Comparison of the simultaneous production of bilirubin and carbon monoxide. J Clin Invest 49:914, 1970

181. La Russo NF et al: Diagnosis of the enterohepatic circulation of bile acids—postprandial serum concentration of conjugates of cholic acid in healthy cholecystectomized patients and patients with bile acid malabsorption. N Engl J Med 291:689, 1974

182. La Russo NF et al: Validity and sensitivity of an intravenous bile acid tolerance test in patients with liver disease. N Engl J Med 292:1209, 1975

183. La Russo NF et al: Determinations of fasting and postprandial serum bile acid levels in healthy man. Am J Dig Dis 23:385, 1978

184. Latner AL, Skillen AW: Isoenzymes in Biology and Medicine, pp 146–157, London and New York, Academic Press, 1968

185. Lauff JL et al: Quantitative liquid chromatographic estimation of bilirubin species in pathological serum. Clin Chem 29:800, 1983

186. Lauterburg BH, Bircher J: Expiratory measurement of maximal aminopyrine demethylation in vivo. Effects of phenobarbital, partial hepatectomy, portocaval shunt, and bile duct ligation in the rat. J Pharmacol Exp Ther 196:501, 1976

187. Lee FI: Immunoglobulins in viral hepatitis and active alcoholic liver disease. Lancet 2:1034, 1965

188. Leevy CM et al: Physiology of dye extraction by the liver: Comparative studies of sulfobromophthalein and indocyanine green. Ann NY Acad Sci 111:161, 1963

189. Lester R, Schmid R: Bilirubin metabolism. N Engl J Med 270:779, 1964

190. Levi AJ et al: Two hepatic cytoplasmic protein fractions, Y and Z, and their possible role in the hepatic uptake of bilirubin, sulfobromophthalein, and other anions. J Clin Invest 48:2156, 1969

191. Levine RA, Klatskin G: Unconjugated hyperbilirubinemia in the absence of overt hemolysis; importance of acquired disease as an etiologic factor in 366 adolescent and adult subjects. Am J Med 36:541, 1964

192. Liebman HA et al: Hepatic vitamin K–dependent carboxylation of blood-clotting proteins. Hepatology 2:488, 1982

193. Liebman HA et al: Des-γ-carboxy (abnormal) prothrombin as a serum marker of primary hepatocellular carcinoma. N Engl J Med 310:1427, 1984

194. Liebowitz HR, Rousselot LM: Bleeding Esophagel Varices; Portal Hypertension. Springfield, IL, Charles C Thomas, 1959

195. Linnet K et al: Diagnostic values of fasting and postprandial concentrations in serum of 3 alpha-hydroxy bile acids and gamma glutamyl transferase in hepatobiliary disease. Scand J Gastroenterol 18:49, 1983

196. Long CH et al: Serum alkaline phosphatase in the postnatal pig and effect of serum storage on enzyme activity. Proc Soc Exp Biol Med 119:412, 1965

197. Lord JW Jr, Andrus W deW: Differentiation of intrahepatic and extrahepatic jaundice. Response of the plasma prothrombin to intramuscular injection of menadione (2-methyl-1,4 naphthaquinone) as a diagnostic aid. Arch Intern Med 68:199, 1941

198. Lum G, Gambino SR: Serum gamma-glutamyl transpeptidase activity as an indicator of disease of liver, pancreas, or bone. Clin Chem 18:358, 1972

199. Maclachlan MJ et al: Chronic active (lupoid) hepatitis. Ann Intern Med 62:425, 1965

200. Mandema E et al: Familial chronic idiopathic jaudice (Dubin–Sprinz disease), with a note on Bromsulphalein metabolism in this disease. Am J Med 28:42, 1960

201. Mannucci PM, Forman SP: Hemostasis and liver disease. In Colman RM et al (eds): Hemostasis and Thrombosis: Basic Principles and Clinical Practice, pp 595–601. Philadelphia, JB Lippincott, 1982

202. Marsh JB, Whereat AF: The synthesis of plasma lipoprotein by rat liver. J Biol Chem 234:3196, 1959

203. Marver HS, Schmid R: The porphyrias. In Stanbury JB, Wyngaarden JB, Frederickson DS (eds): The Metabolic Basis of Inherited Disease, p 1087. New York, McGraw-Hill, 1972

204. Matloff DS et al: Hepatic transaminase activity in alcoholic liver disease. Gastroenterology 78:1389, 1980

205. Mattii R et al: Production of members of the blood coagulation and fibrinolysin systems by the isolated perfused liver. Proc Soc Exp Biol Med 116:69, 1964

206. McMaster Y et al: The mechanism of the elevation of serum alkaline phosphatase in pregnancy. J Obstet Gynaecol Br Emp 71:735, 1964

207. Meister A: The γ-glutamyl cycle. Diseases associated with specific enzyme deficiencies. Ann Intern Med 81:247, 1974

208. Meister A: Glutathione and the γ-glutamyl cycle. In Arias JM, Jakoby WB (eds): Glutathione: Metabolism and Function, p 35. New York, Raven Press, 1976

209. Meister A, Tate SS: Glutathione and related γ-glutamyl compounds: Biosynthesis and utilization. Annu Rev Biochem 45:559, 1976

210. Miller LL, Bale WE: Synthesis of all plasma protein fractions

except gamma globulin by the liver. J Exp Med 99:125, 1954

211. Miller LL et al: The dominant role of the liver in plasma protein synthesis; a direct study of isolated perfused rat liver with the aid of lysine-ε-C^{14}. J Exp Med 94:431, 1951

212. Milstein HJ et al: Serum bile acids in alcoholic liver disease. Comparison with histological features of the disease. Am J Dig Dis 21:281, 1976

213. Mishler JM et al: Serum bile acids and alanine aminotransferase concentrations. JAMA 246:2340, 1981

214. Monroe P et al: The aminopyrine breath test (CABT) predicts histology and correlates with course in patients with chronic hepatitis. Gastroenterology 78:1314, 1980

215. Monroe PS et al: The aminopyrine breath test and serum bile acids reflect histologic severity in chronic hepatitis. Hepatology 2:317, 1982

216. Morelli A et al: The relationship between aminopyrine breath test and severity of liver disease in cirrhosis. Am J Gastroenterol 76:110, 1981

217. Morino Y et al: Immunochemical distinction between glutamic-oxalacetic transaminases from soluble and mitochondrial fractions of mammalian tissues. J Biol Chem 239:943, 1964

218. Mueller MH, Kappas A: Estrogen pharmacology. I. The influence of estradiol and estriol on hepatic disposal of sulfobromophthalein (BSP) in man. J Clin Invest 43:1905, 1964

219. Narducci F, Morelli A: Usefulness of aminopyrine breath test in chronic hepatitis. IRCS Med Sci 9:493, 1981

220. Nelsestuen GL et al: The mode of action of vitamin K: Identification of γ-carboxyglutamic acid as a component of prothrombin. J Biol Chem 249:6347, 1974

221. Newton MA: The clinical application of alkaline phosphatase electrophoresis. Q J Med 36:17, 1967

222. Norcross JW: The anemia of liver disease. Med Clin North Am 50:543, 1966

223. Olson JP et al: Synthesis of coagulation factors by the in vitro perfused liver. Blood 22:828, 1963

223a. Olson JP et al: Synthesis of clotting factors by the isolated perfused rat liver. J Clin Invest 45:690, 1966

224. O'Maille ERL et al: Factors determining the maximal rate of organic anion secretion by the liver and further evidence on the hepatic site of action of the hormone secretin. J Physiol 186:424, 1966

225. Oratz M et al: The role of the urea cycle and polyamines in albumin synthesis. Hepatology 3:567, 1983

226. Owen JA: Paper electrophoresis of proteins and protein-bound substances in clinical investigations. In Sobotka H, Stewart CP (eds): Advances in Clinical Chemistry, Vol I, p 237. New York, Academic Press, 1958

227. Paronetto F et al: Immunocytochemical and serologic observations in primary biliary cirrhosis. N Engl J Med 271:1123, 1964

228. Patterson EK et al: Evidence from purification procedures that the enzyme that hydrolyzes L-leucyl-β-naphthylamide is not the classical leucine aminopeptidase (abstr). J Histochem Cytochem 9:609, 1961

229. Paumgartner G: The handling of indocyanine green by the liver. Schweiz Med Wochenschr (Suppl) 105:1, 1975

230. Pauwels S et al: Breath $^{14}CO_2$ after intravenous administration of [^{14}C]aminopyrine in liver diseases. Dig Dis Sci 27:49, 1982

231. Pennington CR et al: Serum bile acids in the diagnosis of hepatobiliary disease. Gut 18:903, 1977

232. Perrillo RP et al: Alcoholic liver disease presenting with marked elevation of serum alkaline phosphatase: A combined clinical and pathological study. Dig Dis Sci 23:1061, 1978

233. Philip JR et al: Mercaptide conjugation in the uptake and secretion of sulfobromophthalein. Am J Physiol 200:545, 1961

234. Pool JG, Robinson J: In vitro synthesis of coagulation fraction by rat liver slices. Am J Physiol 196:423, 1959

235. Posen S et al: Alkaline phosphatase. Ann Intern Med 67:183, 1967

236. Posen S et al: Intestinal alkaline phosphatase in human serum. Am J Clin Pathol 48:81, 1967

237. Posen S et al: Heat inactivation in the study of human alkaline phosphatase. Ann Intern Med 62:1234, 1965

238. Powell LW et al: An assessment of red cell survival in idiopathic unconjugated hyperbilirubinemia (Gilbert's syndrome) by the use of radioactive diisopropylfluorophosphate and chromium. Aust Ann Med 16:221, 1967

239. Presig R et al: Changes in sulfobromophthalein transport and storage by the liver during viral hepatitis in man. Am J Med 40:170, 1966

240. Pries JM et al: Hepatic extraction of bile salts in conscious dog. Am J Physiol 226:E191, 1979

241. Pruzanski W, Fischl J: The evaluation of serum leucine aminopeptidase estimation; the influence of the administration of steroids on S-LAP activity in obstructive disease of the biliary tract (preliminary report). Am J Med Sci 248:581, 1964

242. Putnam FW: The Plasma Proteins, Vol I, 2nd ed, p 18. Orlando, Florida, Academic Press, 1975

243. Quick AJ: Hemorrhagic Diseases and Thrombosis, 2nd ed, p 391. Philadelphia, Lea & Febiger, 1966

244. Rapaport SI et al: Plasma clotting factors in chronic hepatocellular disease. N Engl J Med 263:278, 1960

245. Ratnoff OD: Bleeding Syndromes: A Clinical Manual. Springfield, IL, Charles C Thomas, 1960

246. Ratnoff OD: Hemostatic mechanisms in liver disease. Med Clin North Am 47:721, 1963

247. Raymond GD, Galambos JT: Hepatic storage and excretion of bilirubin in the dog. Am J Gastroenterol 55:119, 1971

248. Raymond GD, Galambos JT: Hepatic storage and excretion of bilirubin in man. Am J Gastroenterol 55:135, 1971

249. Rej R: Aspartate aminotransferase activity and isoenzyme proportions in human liver tissues. Clin Chem 24:1971, 1978

250. Rej R: Measurement of aminotransferase: Part 1: Aspartate aminotransferase. CRC Crit Rev Clin Lab Sci 21:99, 1985

251. Remmers AR Jr, Kaljot V: Serum transaminase levels. Effects of strenuous and prolonged physical exercise on healthy young subjects. JAMA 185:968, 1963

252. Rickers H et al: The diagnostic value of fasting serum total bile acid concentration in patients with suspected liver disease. A prospective consecutive study. Scand J Gastroenterol 17:565, 1982

253. Righetti ABB, Kaplan MM: Disparate responses of serum and hepatic alkaline phosphatase and 5'-nucleotidase to bile duct obstruction in the rat. Gastroenterology 62:1034, 1972

254. Ritt DJ, Combes B: Enhancement of apparent excretory maximum of sulfobromophthalein sodium (BSP) by taurocholate and dehydrocholate (abstr). J Clin Invest 46:1108, 1967

255. Roberts HR, Cederbaum AI: The liver and blood coagu-

lation: Physiology and pathology. Gastroenterology 63:297, 1972

256. Robinson JC, Goldsmith LA: Genetically determined variants of serum alkaline phosphatase: A review. Vox Sang 13:289, 1967

257. Robinson S et al: Early-labeled peak of bile pigment in man. Studies with glycine-^{14}C and delta aminolevulinic acid-^{3}H. N Engl J Med 277:1323, 1967

258. Roda A et al: Serum primary bile acids in Gilbert's syndrome. Gastroenterology 82:77, 1982

259. Roda A et al: Bioluminescent measurement of bile acids using immobilized 7 α-hydroxysteroid dehydrogenase: Application to serum bile acids. J Lipid Res 23:1354, 1982

260. Rollason JG et al: Serum gamma glutamyl transpeptidase in relation to alcohol consumption. Clin Chim Acta 39:75, 1972

261. Rosalki SB et al: Plasma gamma-glutamyl transpeptidase elevation in patients receiving enzyme-inducing drugs. Lancet 2:376, 1971

262. Rosalki S, Rau D: Serum gamma-glutamyl transpeptidase activity in alcoholism. Clin Chim Acta 39:41, 1972

263. Rosalki SB: Enzyme tests in disease of the liver and hepatobiliary tract. In Wilkinson JH (ed): The Principles and Practice of Diagnostic Enzymology, pp 303–360. London, Edward Arnold, 1973

264. Rosenthal SM, White EC: Studies in hepatic function. VI. A. The pharmacological behavior of certain phthalein dyes; B. The value of selected phthalein compounds in the estimation of hepatic function. J Pharmacol Exp Ther 24:265, 1924

265. Rothschild MA et al: Albumin synthesis in cirrhotic subjects studied with carbonate ^{14}C. J Clin Invest 48:344, 1969

266. Rothschild MA et al: Effect of tryptophan on the hepatotoxic effects of alcohol and CCl_4. Trans Assoc Am Phys 84:313, 1971

267. Rothschild MA et al: Alcohol, amino acids, and albumin synthesis. Gastroenterology 67:1200, 1974

268. Rutenberg AM et al: A comparison of serum aminopeptidase and alkaline phosphatase in the detection of hepatobiliary disease in anicteric patients. Ann Intern Med 61:50, 1964

269. Rutenberg AM et al: Leucine aminopeptidase activity; observations in patients with cancer of the pancreas and other diseases. N Engl J Med 259:469, 1958

270. Rutenberg AM et al: Serum γ-glutamyl transpeptidase activity in hepatobiliary pancreatic disease. Gastroenterology 45:43, 1963

271. Rutenberg AM et al: Serum leucine aminopeptidase activity: In normal infants, in biliary atresia, and in other diseases. Am J Dis Child 103:47, 1962

272. Sabath LD et al: Serum glutamic oxalacetic transaminase. False elevation during administration of erythromycin. N Engl J Med 279:1137, 1968

273. Salispuro MP, Maenpaa PH: Influence of ethanol on the metabolism of perfused normal, fatty and cirrhotic rat livers. Biochem J 100:769, 1966

274. Salz JL et al: Serum alkaline phosphatase activity during adolescence. J Pediatr 82:536, 1973

275. Saunders JB et al: Early diagnosis of alcoholic cirrhosis by aminopyrine breath test. Gastroenterology 79:112, 1980

276. Schaefer J, Schiff L: Liver function tests in metastatic tumor of the liver: Study of 100 cases. Gastroenterology 49:360, 1965

277. Schalm SW et al: Radioimmunoassay of bile acids; development, validation, and a preliminary application of an assay for conjugates of chenodeoxycholic acid. Gastroenterology 73:285, 1977

278. Scharschmidt BF et al: Hepatic organic anion uptake in the rat. J Clin Invest 56;1280, 1975

278a. Schenker S et al: Differential diagnosis of jaundice: Report of a prospective study of 61 proved cases. Am J Dig Dis 7:449, 1962

279. Schiff L et al: Familial nonhemolytic jaundice with conjugated bilirubin in the serum; a case study. N Engl J Med 260:1315, 1959

280. Schlaeger R et al: Studies on the mechanism of the increase in serum alkaline phosphatase activity in cholestasis: Significance of the hepatic bile acid concentration for the leakage of alkaline phosphatase from rat liver. Enzyme 28:3, 1982

281. Schlang HA, Kirkpatrick CA: The effect of physical exercise on serum transaminase. Am J Med Sci 242:338, 1961

282. Schmid R et al: Interaction of bilirubin with albumin. Nature (London) 204:1041, 1965

283. Schmid R et al: Enhanced formation of rapidly labeled bilirubin by phenobarbital: Hepatic microsomal cytochromes as possible source. Biochem Biophys Res Commun 24;319, 1966

284. Schmid R: Bilirubin metabolism: State of the art. Gastroenterology 74:1307, 1978

285. Schmidt E, Schmidt FW: Methode and wert der bestimmung der glutaminsaure—dehydrogenase-aktivitat in serum. Klin Wochenschr 40:962, 1962

286. Schneider JF et al: Aminopyrine N-demethylation: A prognostic test of liver function in patients with alcoholic liver disease. Gastroenterology 79:1145, 1980

287. Seide MJ: Laboratory control of coumarin therapy: The clinician's dilemma. Ann Intern Med 57:572, 1962

288. Seitanidis B, Moss DW: Serum alkaline phosphatase and 5'-nucleotidase levels during normal pregnancy. Clin Chim Acta 25:183, 1969

289. Selinger MJ et al: γ-Glutamyl transpeptidase activity in liver disease: Serum elevation is independent of hepatic GGTP activity. Clin Chim Acta 125:283, 1982

290. Shani M et al: Sulfobromophthalein tolerance test in patients with Dubin–Johnson syndrome and their relatives. Gastroenterology 59:842, 1970

291. Shani M et al: Dubin–Johnson syndrome in Israel. Q J Med 39:549, 1970

292. Shaw LM, Neuman DA: Hydrolysis of glutathione by human liver γ-glutamyl transferase. Clin Chem 27:75, 1979

293. Sherlock S: Biochemical investigations in liver disease; some correlations with hepatic histology. J Pathol Bacteriol 58:523, 1946

294. Shreeve WW et al: Test for alcoholic cirrhosis by conversion of ^{14}C- or ^{13}C-galactose to expired CO_2. Gastroenterology 71:98, 1976

295. Simmonds WJ et al: Radioimmunoassay of conjugated cholyl bile acids in serum. Gastroenterology 65:705, 1973

295a. Singh HP et al: Effect of some drugs on clinical laboratory values as determined by the Technicon SMA 12/60. Clin Chem 18:137, 1972

296. Skrede S et al: Bile acids measured in serum during fasting as a test for liver disease. Clin Chem 24:1095, 1978

297. Soloway R et al: Clinical, biochemical, and histological remission of severe chronic active liver disease: A controlled study of treatments and early prognosis. Gastroenterology 63:820, 1972

298. Song CS et al: 5'-Nucleotidase of plasma membranes of the rat liver: Studies on subcellular distribution. Ann NY Acad Sci 161:565, 1969

299. Spector I, Corn M: Laboratory tests of hemostasis. The relation to hemorrhage in liver disease. Arch Intern Med 119:577, 1967

300. Sperling R et al: Metal binding properties of γ-carboxyglutamic acid: Implications for the vitamin K–dependent blood coagulation proteins. J Biol Chem 253:3898, 1978

301. Stein HB: Effect of 2-methyl-1,4-naphtoquinone on clotting factors of blood of jaundiced patients with hypoprothrombinemia. S Afr J Med Sci 7:72, 1942

302. Stein HB: "Prothrombin response to vitamin K test" in the differentiation between intra- and extrahepatic jaundice. S Afr J Med Sci 9:111, 1944

303. Stenflo J et al: Vitamin K–dependent modifications of glutamic acid residues in prothrombin. Proc Natl Acad Sci USA 71:2730, 1974

304. Sterkel RL et al: Serum isocitric dehydrogenase activity with particular reference to liver disease. J Lab Clin Med 52:176, 1958

305. Stollman YR et al: Hepatic bilirubin uptake in the isolated perfused rat liver is not facilitated by albumin binding. J Clin Invest 72:718, 1983

306. Straub PW: A study of fibrinogen production by human liver slices in vitro by an immunoprecipitin method. J Clin Invest 42:130, 1963

307. Szasz G: A kinetic photometric method for serum γ-glutamyl transpeptidase. Clin Chem 15:124, 1969

308. Szasz G: Reaction rate method for γ-glutamyl transferase activity in serum. Clin Chem 22:2051, 1976

309. Szezeklik E et al: Serum γ-glutamyl transpeptidase activity in liver disease. Gastroenterology 41:353, 1961

310. Tenhunen R et al: Microsomal heme oxygenase: Characterization of the enzymes. J Biol Chem 244:6388, 1969

311. Tenhunen R et al: Reduced nicotinamide-adenine dinucleotide phosphate–dependent biliverdin reductase: Partial purification and characterization. Biochemistry 9:288, 1970

312. Tenhunen R et al: Enzymatic degradation of heme: Oxygenative cleavage requiring cytochrome P-450. Biochemistry 11:1716, 1972

313. Theilmann L et al: Does Z-protein have a role in the transport of bilirubin and bromosulfophthalein by isolated perfused rat liver? Hepatology 4:923, 1984

314. Thjodleifsson B et al: Assessment of the plasma disappearance of choly-1^{14}C-glycine as a test of hepatocellular disease. Gut 18:697, 1977

315. Thompson HE, Wyatt BL: Experimentally induced jaundice (hyperbilirubinemia); report of animal experimentation and of physiologic effect of jaundice in patients with atrophic arthritis. Arch Intern Med 61:481, 1938

316. Tietz NW et al: A comparative study of the Bodansky and the Bessey–Lowry and Brock methods for alkaline phosphatase in serum. Clin Chim Acta 15:365, 1967

317. Tisdale WA et al: The significance of the direct-reacting fraction of serum bilirubin in hemolytic jaundice. Am J Med 26:214, 1959

318. Tobiasson P, Boeryd B: Serum cholic acid and chenodeoxycholic acid conjugates and standard liver function test in various morphological stages of alcoholic liver disease. Scand J Gastroenterol 15:657, 1980

319. Triger DR, Wright R: Hypergammaglobulinemia in liver disease. Lancet 1:1494, 1973

320. Vinnik IE et al: Serum 5'-nucleotidase and pericholangitis in patients with chronic ulcerative colitis. Gastroenterology 45:492, 1963

321. Van Blankenstein M et al: The endogenous bile acid tolerance test. Neth J Med 20:235, 1977

322. Van Waes L, Lieber S: Glutamate dehydrogenase: A reliable marker of liver cell necrosis in the alcoholic. Br Med J ii:1508, 1977

323. Walker FB et al: Gamma glutamyl transpeptidase in normal pregnancy. Obstet Gynecol 43:745, 1974

324. Ware AJ, Combes B: Influence of diet on the metabolism and excretion of bromosulphthalein sodium (BSP). Am J Physiol 225:1260, 1973

325. Warnock LE et al: Decreased aspartate aminotransferase ("SGOT") activity in serum of uremic patients. Clin Chem 20:1213, 1974

326. Watson CJ: The importance of the fractional serum bilirubin determination in clinical medicine. Ann Intern Med 45:351, 1956

327. Watson CJ: Gold from dross: The first century of the urobilinoids. Ann Intern Med 70:839, 1969

327a. Weisiger R et al: Receptor for albumin on the liver cell surface may mediate uptake of fatty acids and other albumin-bound substances. Science 211:1048, 1981

328. Weiss JS et al: The clinical importance of a protein-bound fraction of serum bilirubin in patients with hyperbilirubinemia. N Engl J Med 309:147, 1983

329. Werner M et al: Influence of sex and age on the normal range of eleven serum constituents. Z Klin Chem Klin Biochem 8:105, 1970

330. West M et al: Glycolytic and oxidative enzymes and transaminases in patients with carcinoma of the kidney, prostate, and urinary bladder. Cancer 17:432, 1964

331. Westwood M et al: Serum gamma-glutamyl transpeptidase activity: A chemical determinant of alcohol consumption during adolescence. Pediatrics 62:560, 1978

332. Wheeler HO et al: Hepatic uptake and biliary excretion of indocyanine green in the dog. Proc Soc Exp Biol Med 99:11, 1958

333. Wheeler HO et al: Hepatic storage and excretion of sulfobromophthalein sodium in the dog. J Clin Invest 39:236, 1960

334. Wheeler HO et al: Biliary transport and hepatic storage of sulfobromophthalein sodium in unanesthetized dog, in normal man, and in patients with hepatic disease. J Clin Invest 39;1131, 1960

335. Whelan G, Combes B: Competition by unconjugated and conjugated sulfobromophthalein sodium (BSP) for transport into bile. Evidence for a single excretory system. J Lab Clin Med 78:230, 1971

336. Whelan G et al: A direct assessment of the importance of conjugation for biliary transport of sulfobromophthalein sodium. J Lab Clin Med 75:542, 1970

337. Whitehead TP et al: Biochemical and haematological markers of alcohol intake. Lancet 1:978, 1978

338. Whitefield JB et al: Serum γ-glutamyl transpeptidase activity in liver disease. Gut 13:702, 1972

339. Whitefield JB et al: Changes in plasma γ-glutamyl transferase activity associated with alterations in drug metabolism in man. Br Med J 1:316, 1973

340. Wilkinson JH: Blood enzymes in diagnosis. In London University (Br Post Grad Med Fed): Lectures on the Scientific Basis of Medicine. London, Athlone Press, 1958

341. Wilson JW: Inherited elevation of alkaline phosphatase ac-

tivity in the absence of disease. N Engl J Med 301:983, 1979

342. Winchell HS, Wiley K: Considerations in analysis of breath $^{14}CO_2$ data. J Nucl Med 11:708, 1970

343. Winkelman J et al: The clinical usefulness of alkaline phosphatase isoenzyme determinations. Am J Clin Pathol 57:625, 1972

344. Wolf PL: Clinical significance of an increased or decreased serum alkaline phosphatase level. Arch Pathol Lab Med 102:497, 1978

345. Wroblewski F: The clinical significance of transaminase activities of serum. Am J Med 27:911, 1959

346. Yamamoto T et al: The early appearing bilirubin: Evidence for two components. J Clin Invest 44:31, 1965

347. Young II: Serum 5'-nucleotidase: Characterization and evaluation in disease states. Ann NY Acad Sci 75:357, 1958

348. Young DS et al: Effects of drugs on clinical laboratory tests. Clin Chem 18:1041, 1972

349. Zein M, Discombe G: Serum gamma-glutamyl transpeptidase as a diagnostic aid. Lancet 2:748, 1970

350. Zieve L, Hill E: An evaluation of factors influencing the discriminative effectiveness of a group of liver function tests. II. Normal limits of 11 representative hepatic tests. Gastroenterology 28:766, 1955

351. Zieve L et al: Normal and abnormal variations and clinical significance of the one-minute and total serum bilirubin determinations. J Lab Clin Med 38:446, 1951

352. Zimmerman HJ, West M: Serum enzyme levels in the diagnosis of hepatic disease. Am J Gastroenterol 40:387, 1963

353. Zito RA, Reid PA: Lidocaine kinetics predicted by indocyanine green clearance. N Engl J Med 298:1160, 1978

chapter 10

Noninvasive Imaging of the Hepatobiliary System

KENNETH J. W. TAYLOR, SHIRLEY McCARTHY,
and RONALD D. NEUMANN

There are few better examples of the progress of medical technology than the changes in the field of noninvasive hepatobiliary imaging that have taken place during the past 2 decades. Despite these advances, the traditional radionuclide liver–spleen scan has retained some value as an initial screening procedure, although it is limited in sensitivity and specificity. Both computed tomography (CT) and ultrasonography produce high-resolution tomograms of the liver that are invaluable for disclosing the specific nature of space-occupying masses.[12,19,23] These newer imaging techniques can be used to guide aspiration or biopsy of liver lesions for definitive diagnosis.[60,104] The recent advent of magnetic resonance imaging (MRI) adds a further exciting modality that provides functional data relating to flow in addition to tomographic imaging in any plane.[30]

It is important to appreciate the different physical mechanisms on which imaging depends. Ultrasound imaging depends primarily on the rigidity of tissues, with the collagen and fat contents probably being important determinants. Thus, there is an ability to image soft tissues without the use of contrast agents and highly accurate differentiation between solid and cystic natures. Scintigraphy is largely dependent on the functional integrity of the tissue, relying on phagocytosis of Technetium-99m (^{99m}Tc)-labeled sulfur colloid, the excretion of biliary imaging agents, or the uptake of gallium citrate-67 (^{67}Ga) in tumors or inflammatory lesions.

CT imaging is dependent on tissue differences in radiographic attenuation. Thus, water, fat, air, and calcium are clearly differentiated, whereas discrimination among soft tissues of subtle density differences may necessitate the use of contrast media. The differential enhancement between normal and abnormal tissues improves sensitivity.

MRI of the body depends on four tissue parameters: hydrogen density, two magnetic relaxation times (T_1 and T_2), and blood flow. Differences in hydrogen density among fat, muscle, blood, and bone are major determinants of contrast in the MR image. These differences are greater than the equivalent determinant of radiographic contrast—electron density. Hence there is inherently more contrast in the MR image than in its radiographic counterpart (CT). Furthermore, the observed intensity of hydrogen density is strongly modulated by local physical and chemical factors that affect the rate at which nuclei align within the magnetic field (T_1) and the rate at which nuclear energy emission decays (T_2). Varying the time between successive excitations (TR) and the time of listening (TE) selectively enhances tissue contrast via T_1 and T_2, respectively. Since rapidly flowing blood does not generate a signal, patent vessels are readily identified without administration of contrast medium.[128]

Owing to these differences in the physical basis for imaging, a pathologic process missed by one modality is usually detected by another. Thus, although a sensitivity in excess of 85% can be achieved by any of these methods, their use is often complementary, and the use of a further modality usually improves accuracy.[1,29,96,110,164] In view of the similarity in results, the choice of modality must be based on local availability of equipment and expertise, as well as on the cost to the patient both in money and ionizing radiation. The relative costs of examinations in 1985 dollars are given in Table 10-1.

CLINICAL INDICATIONS FOR HEPATOBILIARY IMAGING

It is now popular to present algorithms for organ imaging. An algorithm for liver imaging usually begins with the radionuclide liver–spleen scan and proceeds to ultrasound or CT for more specific identification of observed lesions. We believe that there are certain indications for proceeding directly to the newer tomographic modalities and that rigid adherence to an imaging algorithm may not be cost effective for any particular patient. There are a number of occasions when the liver–spleen scan is unlikely to produce the required information and a tomographic technique with greater specificity may be indicated as the initial investigation. Such indications include the following:

TABLE 10-1.   Relative Cost of Modalities for Liver Imaging

MODALITY	COST (1985 DOLLARS)
Abdominal sonogram	250
^{99m}Tc-HIDA scintigram	268
[99m]Tc liver–spleen scan	350
[67]Ga scintigram	450
Liver CT with contrast	450
Magnetic resonance imaging	800

Obstructive jaundice. Ultrasound is the most economic and highly sensitive technique for detecting dilated biliary vessels and is appropriate for the initial investigative modality.[170] In many patients, ultrasound not only permits accurate differentiation between extrahepatic and intrahepatic causes for jaundice but also delineates the precise anatomic site and pathologic cause of the obstruction.[170] If the site is not localized, CT scanning is usually most helpful especially in the region of the head of the pancreas, where bowel gas may limit ultrasound penetration. Hepatobiliary scintigraphy using agents such as ^{99m}Tc-HIDA provides a useful assessment of biliary function and patency of the biliary vessels.[180]

Palpable mass. When a mass is palpated in the right upper quadrant, it is almost invariably cold on radionuclide scanning. Under these conditions, ultrasound or CT can demonstrate the anatomic location and nature of the mass and its relation to the surrounding organs, thereby allowing a more specific provisional diagnosis to be made.

Guidance of biopsy and aspiration procedures.[60,104,188] (See pp. 272, 286.)

Nonspecific symptoms. To investigate nonspecific symptoms and signs, an imaging modality is preferred that allows examination of the entire anatomy of the upper abdomen rather than one isolated organ. Either ultrasound or CT can display the pathology, whether it be in the liver, kidneys, adrenals, pancreas, great vessels, or biliary system.

Fever of unknown origin. When time is not at a premium, ^{67}Ga or indium-111 (^{111}In) autologous leukocyte scintigraphy is a very sensitive, albeit expensive, screening procedure for an inflammatory focus.[43,59]

Although conventional liver scintigraphy may reveal a defect from an intrahepatic or subphrenic abscess, CT and to a lesser extent ultrasound permit a more extensive evaluation of the entire abdomen, pelvis, and retroperitoneum in a search for an abscess, and also permit guided aspiration and catheter drainage (see p. 272). Experience has shown that CT is the most sensitive technique for the detection of abscesses, but it is more expensive than ultrasound and the availability of equipment becomes important in the choice of one modality over another in a particular institution.

The accuracy of CT in detecting abscesses is reported to be 90% to 100%.[51] The inherent advantage of CT includes exquisite anatomic detail of the site and extent of the abscess, including detection of minute amounts of gas, a capability not shared by other modalities. Unlike sonography, body habitus, wounds, and dressings do not hinder the examination. However, artifacts due to surgical hardware or poor bowel opacification can cause interpretation problems. Similarly, localized ascites cannot be differentiated from an abscess unless air is present. Intramesenteric and retroperitoneal abscesses are best evaluated with CT since bowel gas hinders ultrasound examination.

Liver–spleen scintigraphy as the primary procedure is still indicated in some patients, although these indications may decrease with further improvements of the other modalities. However, at present, radionuclide scintigraphy is available in a large number of hospitals at modest expense and is largely independent of operator skills. It also provides an overview of the entire liver, as opposed to tomograms through it. Liver scintigraphy is indicated as an initial procedure in the following patients:

In patients presenting with primary tumors, the low prevalence of liver involvement at the time of initial presentation makes a standarized screening procedure for hepatic metastases desirable, and liver scintigraphy fulfills this requirement. Equivocal results, usually due to anatomic variation, can be further investigated by ultrasound or CT.[29,108,148,164]

In patients with cirrhosis, liver scintigraphy is useful to provide a functional overview of the entire liver. This overview may be valuable to the clinician who is attempting to assess the entire liver on the basis of a limited biopsy sample with well-recognized inherent sampling errors.

Liver scintigraphy can be combined with ^{67}Ga to help diagnose a hepatoma,[59] but it is often faster and more economic to proceed directly and biopsy a focal defect under ultrasound or CT guidance to provide definitive cytology.[104,171]

Ultrasound and CT are also indicated after scintigraphy in a substantial number of patients when a liver–spleen scan is equivocal and reasonable doubt exists between anatomic variations and significant pathology.[164] Ultrasound or CT can help resolve such issues.[100,164] Furthermore, in the presence of a definitely abnormal liver–spleen scan, CT or ultrasound can add specificity by disclosing the nature of the mass.[1,168]

PHYSICAL PRINCIPLES AND INSTRUMENTATION

Ultrasound

Ultrasound imaging depends on the small differences that exist in the acoustic properties of soft tissue. A very short pulse of ultrasound approximately 1 microsecond in duration is transmitted into the patient. At each interface between tissues of different acoustic properties, a small portion of the energy is reflected back to the transducer. The presence of soft tissue interfaces is thereby detected and imaged (Fig. 10-1*A*). If the transducer is moved while up to 3000 short pulses per second are emitted, 3000 lines of reflection can be built up each second.

To appreciate the following information on ultrasound physics and instrumentation, it is important to be familiar with the following terms:

A-scan or A-mode. The A-scan is a single line of ultrasound data. With the transducer in any fixed position passing through the liver substance, an entire line of echoes is returned from the passage of each short pulse of ultrasound (Fig. 10-1*B*). When the beam passes through a medium without any interfaces, such as water, no echoes return. Thus, the absence of echoes on the A-scan very reliably indicates the presence of a cyst (Fig. 10-1*C*).

B-mode or B-scan. The B-scan is composed of a large number of A-scans that are redisplayed so that large interfaces are shown as bright dots rather than as big deflections from the baseline. A B-scan tomogram can be produced in any plane. In the transverse plane, these tomograms are similar to those conventionally produced by CT. However, tomograms in the longitudinal, oblique, or any other plane can be produced by the operator by orientation of the transducer. This flexibility of scanning planes is a major advantage because it allows the plane of the tomogram to be adjusted for viewing of the entire structure such as the portal vein or bile duct. However, for those who are inexperienced in the interpretation of ultrasonograms, the final images are in unfamiliar planes and present confusing anatomy as well as unfamiliar pathology.

It is important to understand that, at the frequencies used (2–5 MHz), ultrasound cannot penetrate air or bone to any appreciable extent. Therefore, scanning planes may be dictated by availability of access. For example, a patient

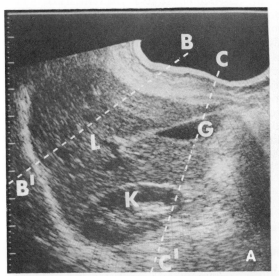

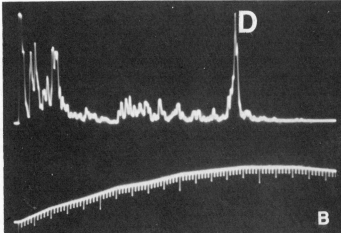

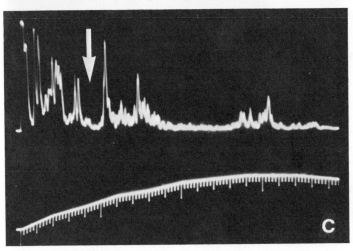

Fig. 10-1. A. Longitudinal ultrasonogram through the right lobe of the liver, showing the liver (*L*), gallbladder (*G*), and right kidney (*K*). **B.** A-scan through the line B-B′ shown in *A*, demonstrating the small echoes that originate in the parenchyma of the liver and the large echo from the diaphragm (*D*) that limits the liver posteriorly. **C.** A-scan through the gallbladder and liver along the line C-C′ shown in (*A*). Note that the cystic contents of the gallbladder return no echoes (*arrow*); this allows reliable differentiation of solid from cystic masses.

with a high subcostal liver may have to be scanned entirely through intercostal spaces, yielding many cone-shaped sections, rather than by a complete transverse tomogram. Multiple samplings allow the ultrasonographer to examine most, if not all, of the liver parenchyma. Entire transverse sections are seldom obtained as they are with CT.

Real-time Ultrasound Instrumentation

Real-time ultrasound refers to the rapid acquisition and display of multiple tomograms to form a movie of the scanned anatomy and pathology. Real-time ultrasound is useful for imaging the abdomen because it allows recognition of certain structures by their characteristic movement. It also makes it possible to trace the course of a structure in a process similar to fluoroscopy. A further advantage of real-time ultrasound is the automatic acquisition of ultrasound images independent of the skill of the operator. Movement of the ultrasound beam is achieved either mechanically by rotating transducers on a wheel or by moving the beam through a sector electronically. Both techniques result in a triangular scan with its apex at the skin line and usually a 90°C sector. Linear arrays can also be used in which the beam is moved electronically along a plane face that is up to 10 cm in length. Such equipment is popular in Japan where the thin population is especially well suited to excellent ultrasonic imaging. In the more obese American population, sector scanners are usually required and there is serious degradation of the image quality by scattering of the ultrasound beam by fat. More detailed consideration of the physics of ultrasound image formation and instrumentation is beyond the scope of this chapter, and the reader is referred elsewhere.[140,165]

Doppler Ultrasound

The Doppler effect is the change in frequency of backscattered ultrasound due to the movement of scattering particles. In moving blood, ultrasound energy is scattered from red cells and their movement causes a change in frequency that can be detected and displayed. Conveniently, this Doppler-shifted frequency lies in the audible range, which allows Doppler ultrasound to be used most simply as a supersensitive stethoscope. Detection of the Doppler-shifted frequency allows confirmation of the presence and direction of flow. A more sophisticated way to display hemodynamic data is achieved by subjecting the returned Doppler signal to fast Fourier transform (FFT), which results in a time–velocity spectrum. Examples of Doppler waveform spectra are shown for all the hepatic vessels in Figure 10-2. The vertical axis of the waveform is proportional to the velocity of blood while the horizontal axis is time.

Pulsed Doppler ultrasound refers to a development that allows precise anatomic localization of the sample volume. A short train of ultrasound pulses is emitted, and its receipt is timed to allow sampling at any given distance from the transducer face. In addition, the size of the sample volume can be adjusted by the operator to sample the maximal axial velocities or to encompass the entire vessel, thereby providing an estimate of average velocity.

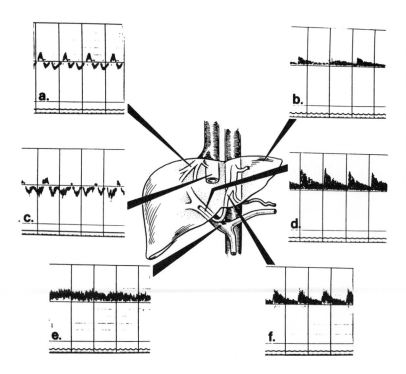

Fig. 10-2. Montage to show Doppler waveform spectra in blood vessels around the liver. The vertical axis of each waveform is velocity, and the horizontal axis is time. **a, c.** Waveforms in hepatic vein and inferior vena cava, respectively, showing both respiratory and cardiac oscillatory variations. **b.** Intrahepatic branch of hepatic artery. Note the damped flow with little variation between systole and diastole. **d.** Waveform in proper hepatic artery. **f.** Waveform in common hepatic artery. **e.** Waveform in portal vein. Note continuous flow with slight respiratory variation. (Courtesy of the editors of Radiology)

The ability to measure the average velocity allows the possibility of estimation of absolute portal vein volume flow, and this is considered later (see p. 290). After 2 years of clinical evaluation of a pulse Doppler device (ATL 600), we believe that the main use of pulse Doppler is the noninvasive means to demonstrate patency of the hepatic vessels, as demonstrated in Figure 10-2. Doppler ultrasound can also be used to help in the diagnosis of unusual vascular structures, as demonstrated in cavernous transformation of the portal vein (see p. 291). It provides an inexpensive portable alternative to MRI to demonstrate patency of various vessels without the use of contrast media. We have shown this to be invaluable for the assessment of hepatic transplant perfusion using mobile equipment in the intensive care unit.[172]

Scintigraphy

Instrumentation

For hepatic imaging, the appropriate radiopharmaceutical is injected into a peripheral vein and allowed to localize in the liver. Images are then made with the gamma camera positioned to provide several anatomic projections of the liver.

A scintillation camera produces an image by detecting the photons produced during the radioactive decay of radionuclide atoms administered in the radiopharmaceutical. Radioactive decay is a random process, and the photons produced leave the patient's body in all directions. In order for an image of an organ to be produced, the desired photons are passively focused; the photons must pass through septa in a lead collimator that is attached to the camera face much like the lens in a conventional camera. The collimated photons then interact with a thallium-activated sodium iodide crystal that produces scintillation light each time a photon is detected. Each scintillation within this crystal is proportional in intensity and corresponds in position to the photon that was detected. Attached to the back surface of the crystal is an array of photomultiplier tubes. These tubes "see" the very faint blue scintillation light and produce an amplified electrical output to signal that a photon was detected. The electronic pulse from the array of photomultiplier tubes is subsequently modified to produce a visible light image on a cathode ray tube. This image accurately reproduces the distribution of the radiopharmaceutical within the liver. The final image or "scintigram" of the liver may be photographed on Polaroid or x-ray film. The same signals may also be fed into a computer for image processing and analysis, as desired.[123]

The development of commercially available tomographic nuclear medicine instruments has made possible cross-sectional nuclear computed tomography (SPECT), which permits visualization of the three-dimensional distribution of a radionuclide. Preliminary results from SPECT studies of the liver report greater sensitivity than planar scintigraphy in detection of intrahepatic lesions.[32,66,73]

Radiopharmaceuticals

The particular radiopharmaceutical used for an individual hepatic examination is chosen according to the information desired, such as anatomic structure evaluation, detection of metastases, or biliary system function. Both the parenchymal cells (hepatocytes) and the reticuloendothelial cells (Kupffer cells) may be used for radionuclide imaging of the liver. The gross anatomic configuration of the organ may be demonstrated by labeling a compound that will demonstrate either of these cell populations.

^{99m}Tc-Sulfur Colloid. The most commonly used radiopharmaceutical for anatomic evaluation of the liver is ^{99m}Tc-labeled colloid, which is taken up by the reticuloendothelial (RE) cells. The method assumes a relatively uniform distribution of the RE cell population in a normal liver.[21] Thus, the phagocytosis of this radiopharmaceutical produces a uniform image of the normal organ. Any disease process that causes replacement of RE cells, including metastases, primary tumors, cysts, or abscesses, produces a "cold" area in the hepatic scintigram. Other conditions such as hepatitis, which may produce functional disturbances in the Kupffer cells, change the relative distribution pattern of the radiolabeled colloid. This occurs because colloidal radionuclide preparations do not selectively go to the liver alone. Such radiopharmaceuticals are phagocytosed by RE cells in the spleen and bone marrow as well. Abnormal RE cell function in the liver produces a shift in the amount of material that localizes in the spleen and bone marrow. Such changes in relative distribution are indirect evidence of hepatic disease, particularly in conditions such as acute hepatitis or cirrhosis. In a normal person, about 90% of the injected colloid localizes in the liver and the remaining 10% is distributed between the spleen and bone marrow. The radiopharmaceutical in the RE cells of the spleen allows evaluation of the spleen as well as the liver during the imaging procedure.

Hepatic parenchymal cells may potentially be imaged by labeling any of the multitude of substances metabolized by these cells. Unlike the colloidal radiopharmaceutical, most metabolized compounds offer the additional advantage of imaging the biliary system as the radioactive label is excreted into the bile. Thus, over a suitable period of time, one can obtain, first, blood pool images of the liver, next, images of the parenchymal cells as they process the radiopharmaceutical, and, finally, the biliary system as the radioactive label is excreted into the bile.

Radiopharmaceuticals for Biliary Scintigraphy. The earliest conventional agent for biliary imaging was iodine-131-rose bengal. Its primary use is to obtain information analogous to that provided by the intravenous cholangiogram, with secondary importance given to any information about liver parenchyma *per se*. Several chemical compounds have replaced ^{131}I-rose bengal for hepatobiliary imaging. These materials may be labeled with ^{99m}Tc, which is more suitable for imaging than [131]I. The amount of ^{131}I-rose bengal that can be administered to patients is very small because ^{131}I produces a significant radiation exposure. Small doses mean fewer photons for producing images and therefore usually poorer images. In addition, most nuclear medicine instrument systems are now designed to produce optimum images using the 140-KeV photon produced by [99m]Tc. Much effort has been expended to develop compounds that produce hepatic images when labeled with [99m]Tc. A number of ^{99m}Tc-labeled hepatobiliary radiopharmaceuticals have been produced thus far, including penicillamine, pyriodoxylidine glutamate, dihydrothioctic acid, and several iminodiacetic acid derivatives.[157,180] Firnau described the essential chemical structural characteristics necessary for compounds to undergo hepatobiliary uptake and excretion. These are a molecular weight between 300 and 10,000 daltons, strong polar groups, two or more ring systems in different geometric planes, and a strong affinity for albumin.[35]

^{99m}Tc-HIDA (N-N[1]-[2,6-dimethyl-phenyl] carbamoylmethyl iminodiacetic acid) initially was one of the most popular hepatobiliary agents. This radiopharmaceutical has been evaluated in a large number of clinical protocols and has been shown to be useful for the diagnosis of acute cholecystitis as well as of other hepatobiliary disorders. Other derivatives of iminodiacetic acid are being evaluated for clinical efficacy; these include the parabutyl, diisobutyl, diisopropyl, and other variants.

The compounds tested thus far with the highest extraction into hepatocytes and rapid intracellular transport are ^{99m}Tc-diisopropyl-IDA and ^{99m}Tc-trimethyl bromo-IDA. These two agents have hepatocyte extraction efficiencies of about 65% and are secondarily excreted by the kidneys.[42,82] The aim of these studies is to find a radiopharmaceutical that will give optimum images of the biliary system even in patients whose bilirubin levels prohibit conventional radiographic contrast medium studies. It must be emphasized that these hepatobiliary agents are intended to assess the functional status of the liver and biliary system rather than to produce detailed anatomic images. Investigators initially thought that these ^{99m}Tc-labeled compounds were cleared by the liver as was bromosulfophthalein (BSP). Competition studies using BSP have shown a decrease in clearance of these compounds as the administered amount of BSP increased.[42] Hepatobiliary studies in patients with Gilbert's disease have not shown any decrease in hepatocyte clearance.[82,89]

When patients are referred for hepatobiliary imaging, a 2-hour fast immediately before the study is suggested. The patient then lies supine under a gamma camera and receives an intravenous injection of the hepatobiliary radiopharmaceutical. If desired, a flow study can be started immediately to follow the distribution of the radionuclide during its intravascular phase. Approximately 1 minute after the injection an initial static image is made to record the equilibrium blood pool phase. Subsequent images are made at 5-minute intervals for 30 to 60 minutes. In a normal patient, the liver, gallbladder, and segments of the biliary tree are visualized. Once radionuclide excreted into the bile passes through the ampulla of Vater, segments of the intestine are also seen by virtue of the activity now present in the lumen. If these structures are not apparent, delayed scintigrams are obtained as required over the next several hours. The procedure may include an assessment of the contractile response of the visualized gallbladder through either a natural or a drug-stimulation test. Given that images of the entire liver are produced while the radiopharmaceutical is in the hepatocyte phase, examination of the gross morphology of the liver is also possible. When serum bilirubin levels exceed the upper limit for these radiopharmaceuticals (presently 5 mg to 30 mg/dl, depending on which compound is used), the main route of excretion shifts to the kidneys and these studies become less reliable in visualizing the biliary system.

[67]Ga. Gallium citrate-67 is also an important radiopharmaceutical in evaluating hepatic disease. Successful imaging of certain human tumors by gallium was noted in 1969.[31] Several years later investigators began using the isotope to detect inflammatory lesions as well.[94,97] Since these early reports, a large body of information has accumulated concerning the use of gallium for tumor and abscess detection.[59]

Scintigraphy is started 6 to 24 hours after the patient receives an intravenous injection of the agent. Appropriate areas of the body are imaged with a large-field Anger scintillation camera or tomographic camera.[55]

During the first 24 hours after injection, 10% to 25% of the isotope dose is excreted into the urine. Subsequent elimination of the drug from the body is slower and occurs primarily through the intestine. Because activity of ^{67}Ga within the intestine may cause difficulties in the interpretation of abdominal images, some form of bowel cleansing before imaging is usually necessary. Much of the drug that is retained in the body normally localizes in the liver and skeletal system. When disease is present, a portion of the isotope concentrates in the tumor or inflammatory lesion. This alters the normal distribution and frequently causes decreased hepatic uptake. A persistent focal area of increased activity, that is, a "hot spot," is the usual criterion of abnormality in a gallium scintigram. Leukocytes, histiocytes, and the bacteria themselves appear to play a role in concentrating the isotope in inflammatory lesions. The mechanism for tumor localization of ^{67}Ga is not completely understood, but imaging with this agent has been shown to be particularly useful in detecting Hodgkin's disease, some non-Hodgkin's lymphomas, melanomas, and hepatomas.[59]

Gallium citrate-67 is not an ideal tracer for the detection of inflammation because it accumulates not only in some tumors but normally also concentrates in liver, bone marrow, and the gastrointestinal tract. Leukocytes labeled with ^{111}In have an increased specificity but similar sensitivity. However, for chronic low-grade infections, these leukocytes are not as sensitive as ^{67}Ga citrate scintigraphy. When symptoms can be localized to a well-defined body region such as the abdomen or pelvis, ultrasound or CT should be the first choice.[19,169]

Computed Tomography

Subsequent to the discovery of x-rays, it became apparent that transmission images of the human body could yield an immense amount of anatomic information. However, projection of a three-dimensional object onto a two-dimensional display resulted in masking of specific internal tissues by the shadows of overlying and underlying structures. Tomographic techniques were developed to eliminate the unwanted structures in the final image. In conventional linear tomography, the plane of interest is held in focus while the overlying and underlying structures are blurred due to the relative motion of the x-ray source and film. The radiation exposure is relatively high for a complete examination since the planes above and below the focal plane are also exposed to the full x-ray beam for each exposure. The advent of axial tomography resolved this problem. In axial tomography a fan x-ray beam rotates around the body, exposing only a single cross section. A film on the opposite side of the x-ray source is rotated with the source.

CT produces a two-dimensional representation of the linear x-ray attenuation coefficients distributed in a narrow plane of the human body.[17] The final image is the electron density distribution of the tissues within the scan section. Computers subtract the blurring that results, and hence the technique is called computed axial tomography. Because tissues of different structures within the body have different elemental compositions, they have different x-ray attenuation. Computers reconstruct these attenuation coefficients into a gray scale to form the CT image. The linear attenuation coefficients for air and water serve as reference values to transform the measured attenuation coefficients of tissues into a relative unit called the CT number. Water is assigned the CT number of 0, and currently, air has the value -1000, dense bone, $+1000$–2000, and soft tissue, $+40$–60. The gray scale is called the Hounsfield scale and its units (CT number) are termed Hounsfield units (HU). A change of 1 HU corresponds to a change of 0.1% in linear attenuation coefficient relative to water. The entire scale is not displayed because subtle differences in tissue density would be obscured. The window (range of CT numbers) is set around a level (CT numbers of the tissue of interest). For the liver, the window is usually 0 to 100 HU.

The reconstructed CT image is a two-dimensional matrix of CT numbers. The technique of filtered back projection, which is the reconstruction of a two-dimensional object from many angles of view, is the image reconstruction process used by all modern CT scanners. The number of individual projection measurements varies between 25,000 and 1 million. The final reconstruction matrix is between 160×160 and 1000×1000. The matrix size of most CT scanners is 160×160 to 512×512 picture elements. Picture elements are referred to as pixels. The volume element, voxel, refers to the fact that there is a finite section thickness that is generally between 2 mm and 20 mm.

A typical CT scanner contains a scanning gantry that holds the collimated x-ray source and detectors, a motorized patient handling table, a computer for data acquisition and reconstruction, and a viewing console. Commercial differences in scanners primarily relate to differences in the gantry design, particularly the number and type of x-ray detectors and their relative motion with the x-ray source. The complexity of the computer depends on the size of the detector arrays, the speed of scanning, and image reconstruction. CT scanners with a slow scan time (1 to 5 minutes) usually have the CT image reconstructed while scanning occurs. With faster scanners (2 to 20 seconds), image reconstruction occurs after scanning. The larger the number of detectors that are simultaneously recording transmitted x-ray attenuations, the faster is the scanning sequence. Spatial resolution is also increased with larger detector arrays since the individual detector element can be minimized. Four categories of scanners have been classified according to their sequence of development (generation). The most significant factor relates to the data gathering method via movements of the x-ray source and detector (Fig. 10-3). For detector arrays of up to about 90 elements, the translate-rotate scan sequence (first generation) is used similar to the original EMI brain scanner. If multiple detectors are used, simultaneous readings from a fan beam of radiation can be obtained (second generation). Historically, this system allowed body scan times less than the breath-holding time of the patient. Third- and fourth-generation scanners use a pure rotary motion. A rotating fan of x-rays greatly reduces the scan time.

Typical CT examination radiation doses are in the range of 0.5 to 5 rad. CT scanning results in approximately the same marrow dose as do chest radiographs but much less than upper gastrointestinal series, barium enemas, or excretory urograms.[33] Dosage can be reduced by decreasing the scan time, increasing the slice thickness, and increasing the pixel size. The scanner geometry also affects patient dosage.

Magnetic Resonance Imaging

Magnetic resonance imaging (MRI) is the current major advance in medical imaging. Although nuclear magnetic resonance spectroscopy has been used in analytical chemistry for at least 30 years, its use in diagnostic radiology has only become apparent in the past few years. MRI creates multiplanar images by interaction between static magnetic fields, radio waves, and atomic nuclei. The energy changes in MRI are enormously different from x-ray CT. One x-ray photon has almost a billion times the energy of an electromagnetic photon concerned in nuclear magnetic resonance. Hence, MRI appears to be a very safe technique. Unlike CT, which detects tissue electron den-

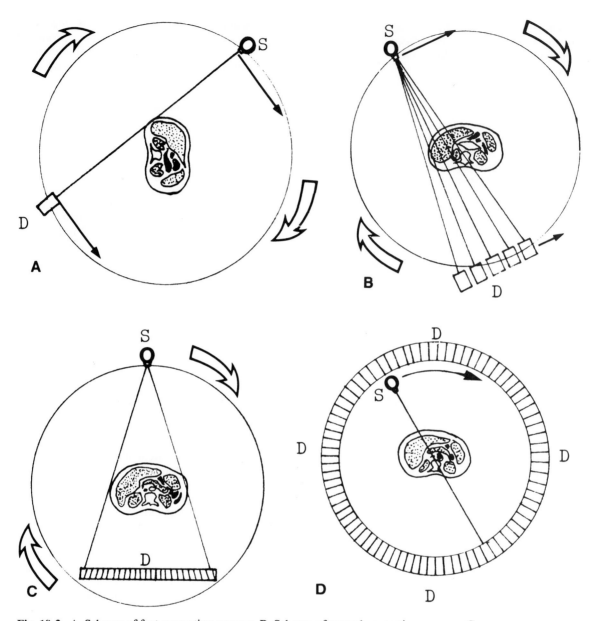

Fig. 10-3. A. Schema of first-generation scanner. **B.** Schema of second-generation scanner. **C.** Schema of third-generation scanner. **D.** Schema of fourth-generation scanner. (Courtesy of Dr. Caroline R. Taylor)

sity, MR images are basically density maps of water or lipid protons and their relaxation times. These time constants, T_1 and T_2, reflect the local molecular environment. T_1 is the rate at which nuclei align themselves within the external magnetic field, whereas T_2 represents the rate at which nuclear energy emission decays.

Since protons have an odd number of particles, they behave like magnets when placed in a strong magnetic field. If weak radio waves of a resonant frequency (RF pulses) are applied, the nuclei will change their direction of spin and reorient in the static magnetic field. As the nuclei return to their original alignment, they emit radio waves with the same frequency as those absorbed. In a given magnetic field, the frequency of the radio waves causing resonance is specific for each nucleus. Thus, superimposition of a nonuniform small-field gradient enables spatial encoding of the signal such that a proton map (image) is produced.[128]

Imaging consists of a period of tissue excitation followed by a period of listening for the emission of the absorbed excitation. Manipulation of the timing of the 90° or 180° RF pulses changes the relative contribution of hydrogen density, T_1, and T_2. The resultant images can therefore be "weighted." Changing the interval between successive excitations (TR) will selectively enhance tissues according to their T_1. A short interval results in tissues having a long T_1 to yield less signal than those with a short T_1, since the former have less time to realign with the magnetic field. Varying the interval between excitation and observation of the signal (TE) selectively enhances tissues via their T_2. Tissues with a long T_2 generate larger signals, appearing brighter on the MR gray scale. If hydrogen nuclei move through the imaged volume before data acquisition is complete, their signal is lost. Thus, rapidly flowing blood is signal free. The choice of technique used for data acquisition is determined by the contrast resolution necessary for a particular tissue and its pathology. The spin echo technique of data acquisition is most commonly used today. Inversion recovery and saturation recovery sequences have fewer applications.

An MRI system consists of a large magnet to create the static magnetic field, gradient coils for spatial encoding, a radiofrequency coil to apply and receive the resonant frequency, and computers for data acquisition, processing, and display. The static field can be created by iron-core, resistive air-core, or superconducting magnets. The latter type is currently the most useful.

In the future, multinuclear MR spectroscopy will prove useful as a clinical biochemical tool. Currently, MRI is based on hydrogen because it is the most sensitive of the stable nuclei to MR and also is the most abundant nucleus in the body. In proton imaging, the individual voxel is characterized by a single intensity value, whereas the spectroscopic voxel (which may be part of the anatomic image) contains spectral (biochemical) information. Phosphorus-31 spectroscopy of tumors, *in vitro* and *in vivo,* may prove useful not only to distinguish malignant from benign tissue but also to differentiate well-vascularized anaerobic tumors from poorly vascularized hypoxic tumors. The latter information may provide a rationale for the timing of radiation and chemotherapy in response to the tumor.

ANATOMY OF THE LIVER

Every reader is familiar with the normal liver–spleen scintigram (Fig. 10-4). Since both ultrasound and CT are tomographic techniques, only sample tomograms can be shown here. Figure 10-1*A* shows a B-scan ultrasonogram through the right lobe of the liver, which is limited by the right hemidiaphragm on the left, the anterior abdominal wall above, and the right kidney below. The gallbladder is seen in its most common position. An A-scan is shown taken in the plane B-B' in Figure 10-1*A*. The size of the parenchymal echoes is small compared with the large dia-phragmatic echo (Fig. 10-1*B*). This relationship demonstrates normal echogenicity through the liver substance. Figure 10-1*C* shows an A-scan in the plane of C-C'. There are no echoes from within the gallbladder lumen because of the absence of interfaces. Fluid-filled areas are completely anechoic on ultrasound, making for a high degree of confidence in the diagnosis of cysts. It should be recalled that ultrasound tomograms, although shown mainly in the longitudinal and transverse planes, can be taken in any plane.

A normal CT scan of the liver is shown in Figure 10-5. Note that the fissures of the liver are well demonstrated and that the normal liver parenchyma has a homogeneous appearance, owing to a uniform x-ray attenuation. Figures 10-6 and 10-7 are illustrations of the somewhat variant normal hepatic anatomy. Figure 10-6 shows an unusual configuration of the lateral division of the left lobe with extension across the abdomen into the left flank. Figure 10-7 shows a prominent caudate lobe. Its inferior and lateral extension can mimic a mass in the porta hepatis or the head of the pancreas. Analysis of serial sections shows continuity, thus differentiating the normal papillary and caudate processes from extrahepatic lesions.[5]

Knowledge of the segmental anatomy of the liver enables localization of masses so that resectability can be determined. Since the vascular anatomy best defines the location of the segments, angiography, contrast-enhanced CT, and sonography have been used to localize lesions.[103,127,131] MRI displays vasculature without the need for any contrast media, since rapidly flowing blood is signal free. The vessels are easily distinguished from liver parenchyma, the latter having a homogeneous moderate signal intensity. Furthermore, hepatic vasculature can be directly depicted in any plane (Fig. 10-8).[36] Angiography, once the gold standard for evaluation of hepatic surgical anatomy, is no longer routinely necessary.

The main lobar fissure divides the liver into its right and left lobes. This fissure can be identified by a line drawn between the gallbladder fossa and the inferior vena cava. On more cephalic scans, the right and left lobes are separable by locating the middle hepatic vein.

The most obvious fissure is the left intersegmental fissure, which divides the medial and lateral segments of the left lobe.[103] For ease of identification, the left intersegmental fissure can be subdivided into cranial, middle, and caudal portions.[103] The left hepatic vein courses within the cranial portion, thus dividing the most cephalic portions of the medial and lateral segments of the left lobe. The falciform ligament, a remnant of the fetal ventral mesentery, extends between the left portal vein and the anterior abdominal wall. Dividing the caudal part of the medial and lateral segments, it is not routinely seen on sonography or CT unless fibrofatty tissue or ascites is present. The ligamentum teres, the obliterated umbilical vein, lies in the inferior edge of the falciform ligament. The ascending or vertical segment of the left portal vein identifies the middle third of the left intersegmental fissure.

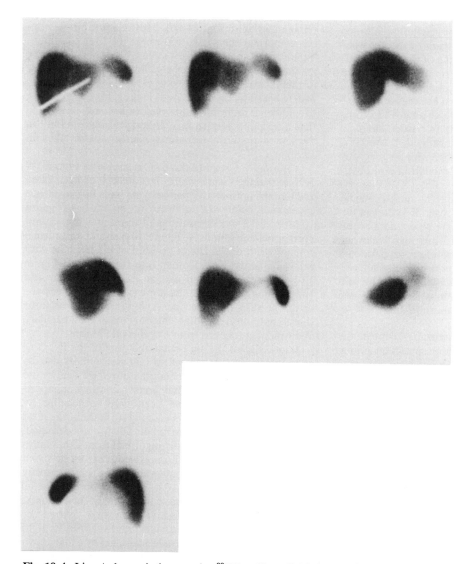

Fig. 10-4. Liver/spleen scintigram using ^{99m}Tc sulfur colloid. Conventional multiple views are shown.

The right intersegmental fissure can be ascertained by locating the right portal and right hepatic veins. The latter courses within the right intersegmental fissure, dividing it into anterior and posterior segments. The anterior and posterior divisions of the right portal vein course centrally in their corresponding segments. On transaxial scans, the right hepatic vein in cross section bisects the anterior and posterior divisions.

The caudate lobe is a separate anatomic lobe since it receives branches from both the right and left portal veins and hepatic arterial vessels. This lobe lies between the inferior vena cava and the fissure for the ligamentum venosum. The latter structure and the transverse portion of the left portal vein define the anterior surface of this lobe.

FOCAL DISEASE OF THE LIVER

Liver Cysts

Small hepatic cysts are common incidental findings. They are seldom of clinical significance but do lead to confusing liver scintigrams in patients who are being investigated for metastatic disease. Occasionally, these liver cysts attain huge dimensions (Fig. 10-9B and C) Liver cysts are usually very easily detected by liver scintigraphy as cold areas (Fig. 10-9A), but ultrasound and CT have two great advantages: First, they allow recognition that a mass is a cyst with regular walls and therefore an incidental finding of no clinical significance. In addition, the kidneys and

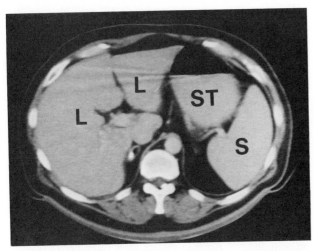

Fig. 10-5. CT scan at midhepatic level showing normal liver (*L*) with fissures. The stomach (*ST*) and the spleen (*S*) are shown.

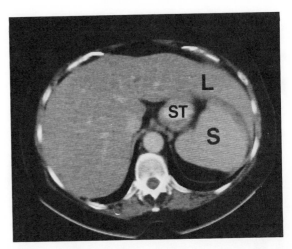

Fig. 10-6. CT scan of normal variant anatomy showing large left lobe of the liver (*L*) extending around the lateral aspect of the spleen (*S*). A section of stomach (*ST*) is seen.

other abdominal organs are imaged, so that, when liver cysts are due to polycystic disease, the kidneys and other possible sites for the disease are imaged.[142] CT and ultrasound offer not only a more specific diagnosis but also the ability to survey the adjacent organs for concomitant disease.

Figure 10-10 demonstrates the value of this ability to survey the entire abdomen. An elderly patient with a known oat-cell carcinoma of the lung presented with a rapidly enlarging liver and falling hematocrit. The liver–spleen scintigram (Fig. 10-10*A*) shows a huge cold area in the right lobe of the liver that could be tumor, abscess, or cyst. Ultrasound (Fig. 10-10*B*) and CT (Fig. 10-10*C*) show that the liver lesion is a huge fluid-filled mass and dem-

onstrate, in addition, a tumor in the upper pole of the right kidney. A longitudinal ultrasound scan allowed both lesions to be imaged in one view, so that the tumor is seen posterior to the liver lesion and there is obvious invasion of the perirenal tissues, producing a large intrahepatic hematoma.

CT may be more highly specific owing to quantitation of a precise CT number characteristic of blood. The value of CT is further illustrated by Figure 10-11. A large incidental cyst is seen in the left lobe of the liver. This displaces the stomach to the left and is clearly benign, whereas the additional lower slice shows marked deformity of the right lobe of the liver by the patient's retroperitoneal sarcoma.

Fig. 10-7. **A.** CT scan showing prominent caudate lobe (*C*) that is clearly part of the liver. **B.** CT scan of the liver at a lower level than that shown in *A*. Extension of the caudate lobe mimics a mass in the head of the pancreas (*P*).

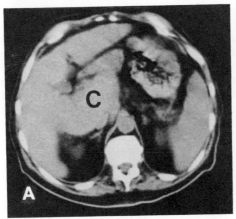
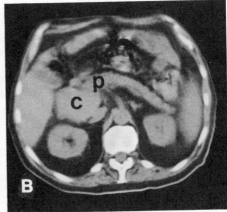

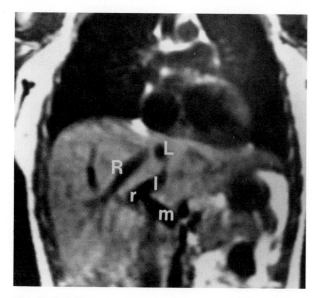

Fig. 10-8. MR scan (coronal spin echo TR2000, TE40) of liver demonstrating the main (*m*), left (*l*), and right (*r*) portal veins and the left (*L*) and right (*R*) hepatic veins.

The majority of cystic lesions within the liver have attenuation values on the Hounsfield scale from −5 to +15. Lesions with values above and below these numbers should not be considered to be simple cysts.[8]

On MRI, simple cysts have a characteristic intensity. Like other body fluids (*e.g.,* urine, hepatic bile, and cerebrospinal fluid), hepatic cysts are low intensity on T_1-weighted images and high intensity on T_2-weighted sequences.[159]

Liver Abscesses

Liver abscesses still cause significant morbidity and mortality, and since the modern imaging modalities described here are capable of detecting virtually every abscess, mortality is often related to inappropriate usage and delay in therapy.

Scanning with ^{67}Ga is a sensitive technique for demonstrating inflammatory change in the liver but is nonspecific and time consuming. In practice, therefore, ultrasound and CT are preferred initial modalities for the evaluation of intrahepatic and subphrenic abscesses.[2,19,23,169]

On ultrasound scanning, a liver abscess characteristically presents as a fluid-filled lesion (Fig. 10-12), often with thick and irregular edges and debris within the fluid collection.[169] However, the finding of any perihepatic fluid collection in a patient with clinical suspicion of an abscess should stimulate a diagnostic aspiration[60,161] rather than a request for numerous confirmatory studies that waste time and money.

When gas is present within a lesion, CT is highly specific for abscess. In general, gas is present less often in hepatic abscesses than other intra-abdominal abscesses (19% vs 30% to 50%). If no air is present, then the CT appearance is nonspecific. Abscesses can vary from well-defined rounded cavities near water density (resembling cysts) to higher-density ill-defined areas indistinguishable from neoplasms.[51,132] Nonetheless, CT is highly sensitive. Thus, if the CT scan is completely normal, an abscess is ruled out. Intravenous contrast media are used routinely since the contents of abscesses do not enhance whereas the normal surrounding liver does.[106,113]

Nonpyogenic infections can have a fairly specific appearance. If calcium is present in the wall of the cyst, hydatid disease should be included in the differential diagnosis. If calcium is contained within a hypodense heterogeneous lesion, an alveolar echinococcal cyst should be excluded.[22,27] Amebic abscess most often presents as a solitary low density area in the right lobe.

Intrahepatic abscesses have no characteristic appearance on MRI since the relaxation characteristics depend on the contents of the abscess. The amount of protein related to pus or blood alters the relaxation characteristics. Thus, T_1 and T_2 values are not specific enough to obviate the need for aspiration to establish the diagnosis. Currently, interventional procedures are cheaper and easier to perform with ultrasound or CT.

Liver–lung scanning has been described as a useful diagnostic procedure, but we have become disillusioned with this technique. In the case of a pleural effusion, there is an apparent false-positive result; and pus in Morison's pouch is too low to lead to a separation between liver and lung, so, in this case, the technique results in a false-negative result (Fig. 10-13).

The value of a ^{67}Ga scan is illustrated in the patient with Reye's syndrome. Figure 10-14*A* shows abnormal uptake of gallium in the subhepatic region and in the left subphrenic region. A liver sulfur colloid scintigram was normal (Fig. 10-14*B*). Plain radiography demonstrated abnormal air collections in the subhepatic region and left subphrenic region (Fig. 10-14*C*). On ultrasound examination, a left subphrenic abscess was found but the subhepatic appearances were confusing (Fig. 10-14*D*). The air could easily be dismissed as being in the colon or stomach. However, further examination of the scan shows that the air collection is between the medial and lateral segments of the left lobe of the liver and definitely anterior to the plane of the duodenum. These appearances are perfectly consistent with the presence of a subhepatic abscess, as demonstrated by plain radiography and gallium scanning. When air is present in a lesion, plain film radiography may be useful to confirm the ultrasound findings.

Abscess Drainage

Diagnostic aspiration under ultrasound or CT guidance is the procedure of choice in any patients with a fluid

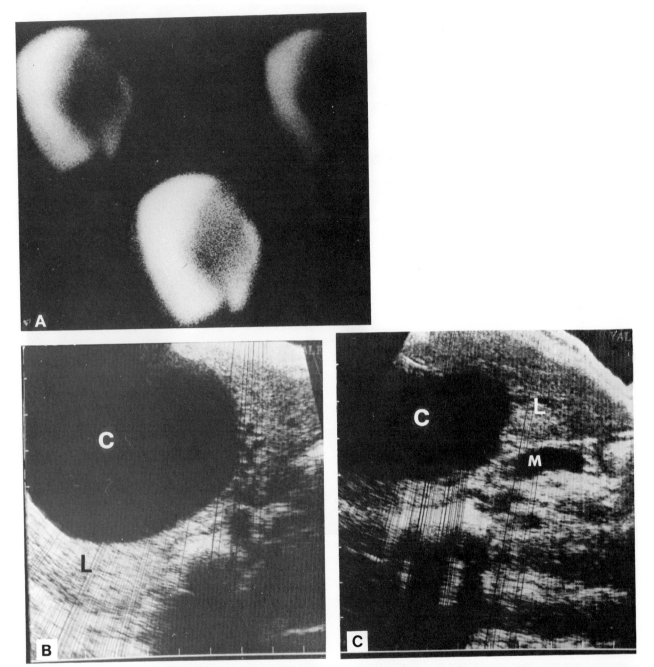

Fig. 10-9. A. Liver sulfur colloid scintigram showing a large cold area that could be due to a cyst, abscess, or tumor. Right anterior oblique view with three different intensities is shown. **B.** Transverse ultrasonogram showing a huge cystic mass (*C*) 12 cm in diameter surrounded by compressed liver tissue (*L*). **C.** Longitudinal ultrasonogram of a cystic mass (*C*) within the liver (*L*). M, superior mesenteric vein.

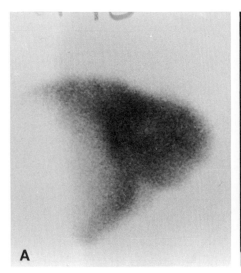

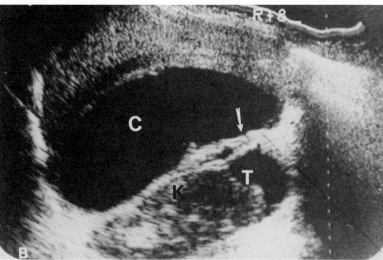

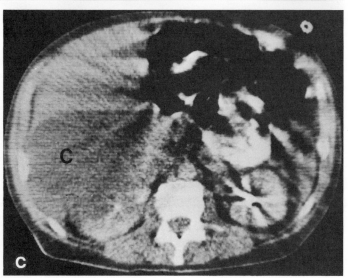

Fig. 10-10. A. Liver sulfur colloid scintigram. A right anterior oblique view shows a huge cold area in the right lobe of the liver. **B.** Longitudinal ultrasonogram through the right lobe of the liver and the right kidney. The kidney (*K*) is disorganized and partially necrotic; its appearance is consistent with the presence of a tumor (*T*). The liver shows a huge cystic mass (*C*), and there is evidence of rupture of the tumor through Gerota's fascia (*arrow*). Appearances are consistent with hemorrhage into the liver from a renal tumor. **C.** CT scan confirming the presence of a large cystic mass in the right lobe of the liver. Lower sections demonstrate the renal mass. Note that this is a second-generation CT scan and of poor quality.

collection of unknown nature, especially if they have a fever of unknown origin and leukocytosis. Incidental liver and renal cysts are very common and need not be aspirated unless there is clinical suspicion of infection or tumor.[138] If calcium is detected in the wall of a cyst or the patient is from an area where echinococcus is endemic, aspiration should be deferred until immunologic tests are performed. Cyst puncture can cause anaphylaxis or dissemination.

Perihepatic and intrahepatic fluid collections, especially if they are increasing in size in a patient with symptoms and signs of sepsis, should be aspirated. In the upper abdomen, this is usually most rapidly achieved using real-time ultrasound guidance. A biopsy guide can be used to provide continuous monitoring of the position of the needle, but more frequently the surface projection of the fluid collection can be marked and the ultrasound equipment discarded, making it easier to sterilize the field and aspirate the collection. When the abscess is obviously infected,

diagnostic aspiration should be followed by catheter drainage.[77] Abscesses should not merely be subjected to diagnostic aspiration since subsequent leakage may occur along the needle track and cause septic shock. The abscess should be decompressed and left to drain by a catheter (Fig. 10-15). Numerous different catheters have been used and different techniques described.[77,161] For most perihepatic and intrahepatic abscesses, a direct approach suffices, usually after ultrasound localization. For deeper collections near bowel, CT localization is required and use of the Seldinger technique under fluoroscopic control is mandatory. Similarly, lesions near the dome of the diaphragm necessitate fluoroscopic monitoring to avoid pleura.[122,124]

Diagnostic needle puncture is very safe, but long-term drainage catheters must be strategically positioned to prevent contamination of subphrenic, perihepatic, and/or pleural spaces. The results of aspiration and catheter

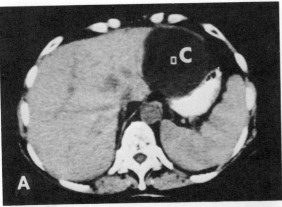

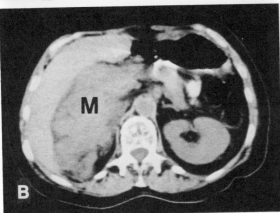

Fig. 10-11. A. CT scan showing a large cyst (*C*) in the left lobe of the liver. A cursor has been placed in the cyst to provide the Hounsfield number, which is within the cystic range. This disease was incidental to a huge retroperitoneal sarcoma (*M*), shown in *B*. A metastasis was suspected on the basis of a nonspecific defect seen on the liver scintigram.

drainage are excellent, with morbidity and mortality lower than that of conventional surgical drainage. Although the use of small catheters is contrary to conventional surgical wisdom there are very few failures and the low morbidity and mortality is probably related to closed drainage, which prevents superimposed infection (see Fig. 10-15).[77]

There is usually dramatic improvement in the clinical condition of a patient within a few hours of catheter drainage with greatly improved sense of well-being, and resolution of fever and toxicity. This is in contrast to the continuing toxicity when abscesses are treated by purely medical therapy, which, while eventually successful, causes prolonged debility and hospitalization.

Metastatic Liver Disease

The most frequent indication for liver imaging is the exclusion of metastatic disease. For these purposes, liver scintigraphy serves well, provided that equivocal scans

can be further investigated by ultrasound or CT. Unfortunately, to date there are no reliable published figures for the negative predicative value of a completely normal liver–spleen scan after exclusion of all equivocal results, but our anecdotal experience is that such scans should command a high level of confidence.

On scintigraphy with ^{99m}Tc-sulfur colloid, all metastatic lesions appear as cold areas and are indistinguishable from those due to cysts or abscesses. On ultrasound examination, a wide spectrum of appearances is seen, from hypoechoic to echogenic lesions, and there are considerable differences of opinion in the published data.[50,111,151,166] Figure 10-16*A* shows minimal metastatic disease from breast carcinoma, also well demonstrated by liver scintigraphy (Figure 10-16*B*). Of echogenic tumors seen at Yale–New Haven Hospital, 50% are from primary tumors in the colon (Fig. 10-17), and a further 25% are hepatomas.[166]

We have investigated the value of ultrasound to improve the sensitivity and specificity of equivocal liver scintigrams. One hundred patients with equivocal liver–spleen scans were subjected to ultrasound examination.[164] For review purposes, the liver scintigrams were classified as (1) equivocal but probably normal, (2) definitely equivocal, or (3) equivocal but probably abnormal. The corresponding sensitivities and specificities for ultrasound and scintigraphy are presented in Tables 10-2 and 10-3. Most important, the study showed that the overall accuracy could be elevated from 74% to 93% by the use of the two modalities in this complementary fashion.

This study on the value of ultrasound to enhance the utility of equivocal scintigrams led to the identification of "high risk" areas on the scintigram. These include edge defects, the region of the porta hepatis, the impression of the gallbladder, and the right renal fossa. Figure 10-18*A* shows a possible edge defect in the left lobe of the liver, although such a defect may occur as a normal variant. The ultrasound scan (Fig. 10-18*B*) in the longitudinal plane shows a partially necrotic but highly irregular mass replacing the left lobe; this finding was subsequently confirmed at autopsy (Fig. 10-18*C*).

The region of the porta hepatis has long been known to produce both false-negative and false-positive results on scintigraphy. In a follow-up study of a large number of patients, McClelland found that portal defects were due to pathology in only 40% of patients and to anatomic variation in 60%.[108] Thus, defects in the region of the porta hepatis need further investigation by either ultrasound or CT. False-positive radionuclide scans due to anatomic variation in liver configuration or adjacent extrahepatic structures are easily recognized and explained with CT.[29] One group has also reported on the value of tomographic scintigraphy for further delineation of this area.[148]

Studies comparing CT to sonography or radionuclide scanning have shown CT to be the best single method to detect metastases.[1,83] The most recent prospective study using 2- and 10-second CT scanners found CT to have the highest sensitivity (93%). CT had the highest true pos-

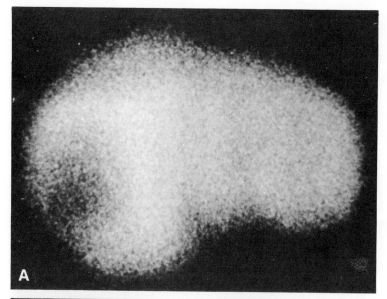

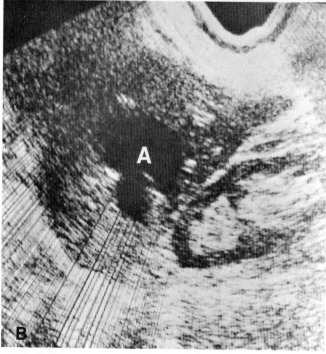

Fig. 10-12. A. Liver sulfur colloid scintigram. Right anterior oblique view shows a cold area in the lateral aspect of the right lobe of the liver. **B.** Longitudinal ultrasonogram through the right lobe of the liver shows good transmission and few echoes in this lesion, indicating a fluid-filled mass (*A*). At surgery, an intrahepatic abscess was drained.

itive ratio at every false-positive ratio.[1,41] CT can detect lesions 1 mm to 2 mm in size whereas radionuclide scanning does not routinely find lesions less than 2 cm in size. Due to the high sensitivity of CT for detecting focal lesions, there is greater confidence in a negative result. Therefore, a normal CT scan in a patient with biochemical disease is strong evidence for diffuse liver disease. Although all diagnostic tests depend on diagnostic performance and interpretation, sonography is particularly vulnerable since it is highly dependent on the operator's maneuvers and

observations that must be made during the study. Retrospective analysis of images rarely provides more information. With CT, the examination is standardized and subsequent interpretation can occur in consultation with others. Furthermore, the information is permanently on tape and can be reviewed at leisure with selection of numerous levels and windows to bring out density differences. The advantages of mobility and real-time scanning in sonography, however, focus attention on suspicious areas identified on CT. For example, cystic hepatic neo-

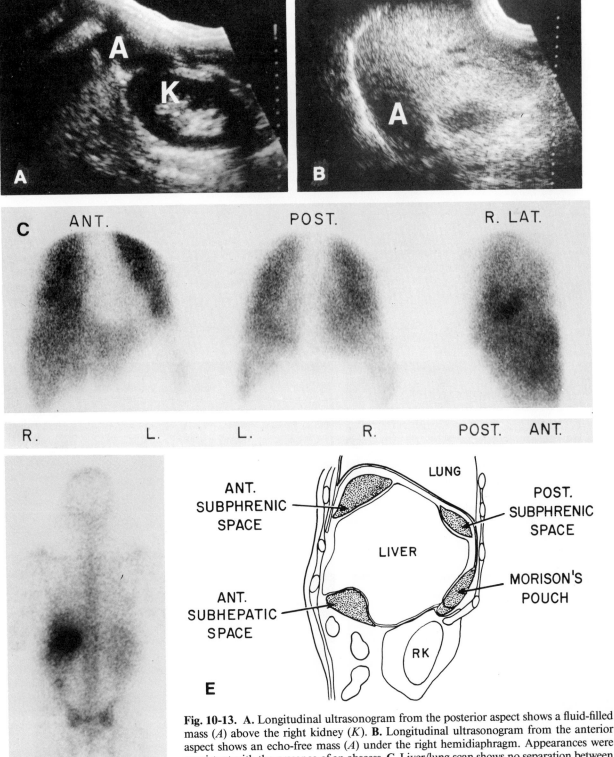

Fig. 10-13. **A.** Longitudinal ultrasonogram from the posterior aspect shows a fluid-filled mass (*A*) above the right kidney (*K*). **B.** Longitudinal ultrasonogram from the anterior aspect shows an echo-free mass (*A*) under the right hemidiaphragm. Appearances were consistent with the presence of an abscess. **C.** Liver/lung scan shows no separation between the liver and lung, a finding in apparent conflict with those demonstrated in *A* and *B*. **D.** Gallium-67 scan showing marked uptake of isotope in the right upper quadrant. Single posterior view. (Searle Pho/Con) **E.** Schema of the perihepatic spaces in which abscesses are commonly found. An abscess located in the posterior subphrenic space produces separation between the liver and lung and is apparent on a liver/lung scan. In this patient, the abscess was immediately above the right kidney in Morison's pouch and did not produce separation between liver and lung. Pus was aspirated from this area under ultrasound localization. (Berger H: Subhepatic intraperitoneal abscess. JAMA 242:657–659, 1979) (Courtesy of the Editors of JAMA)

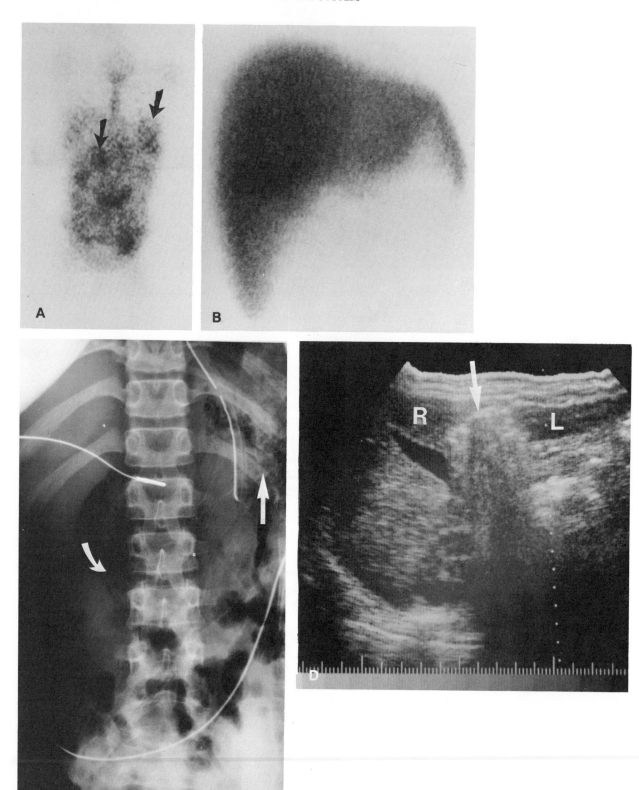

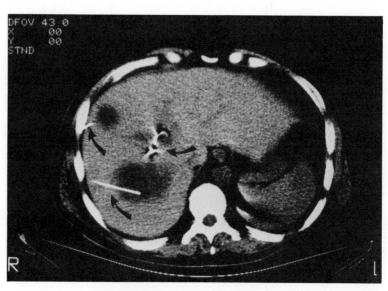

Fig. 10-15. CT scan demonstrating three intrahepatic abscesses diagnosed and treated by a CT-guided aspiration and drainage. Note that the location and the course of the catheters (*arrows*) are easily identified.

plasms such as metastatic ovarian cancer can sometimes look like benign cysts on CT. Sonography can differentiate a simple cyst from a cystic neoplasm by identifying wall thickness, mural nodules, septations, and/or fluid levels.

Bolus injection with incremental dynamic scanning is the most commonly employed technique for the detection of primary metastatic disease.[38] Usually, a 50-g iodine load is administered within 2 minutes. Most metastases are hypodense; thus liver to tumor contrast is maximized by rapid scanning following high-dose (bolus) delivery of contrast medium. The equilibrium phase in contrast enhancement is reached approximately 2 minutes after termination of a bolus and immediately after termination of an infusion.[18] Scanning during the equilibrium phase does not significantly improve visualization of hepatic tumors when compared with the precontrast or bolus examination and actually carries a risk of obscuring tumors since they may be isodense with normal parenchyma. For similar reasons, tumors also may be concealed when intravenous contrast material has been used for other radiologic studies preceding the CT examination. In the equilibrium phase, contrast concentration gradients between the vascular and interstitial water spaces are relatively small. Therefore, to optimize density differences created by bolus injections, dynamic incremental scanning is usually employed. The latter necessitates a scanner with fast scanning times and rapid table movement.

The following protocol is suggested in the CT workup of a patient with possible hepatic malignancy. The initial examination can be a precontrast study. If diffuse liver lesions are identified, no further scans are necessary. If the study demonstrates a potentially resectable lesion (*i.e.*, isolated to one segment or lobe), a postcontrast study should be obtained to exclude the possibility of lesions elsewhere in the liver, which would make the disease unresectable. In departments where throughout is important due to time constraints and scheduling, only a direct contrast study can be obtained. Postcontrast survey dynamic scans are more informative than precontrast examinations.

Although intravenous contrast improves lesion detectability, there is no characteristic appearance to a particular

Fig. 10-14. A. Gallium-67 scan showing abnormal uptake of gallium in the left subphrenic region and the right subhepatic region (*arrows*). Other abdominal activity is represented by gallium in the intestines. Single anterior image. (Searle Pho/Con) **B.** Liver sulfur colloid scintigram is normal because the lesion is subhepatic. Anterior view. **C.** A plain abdominal film showing an air collection in the left subphrenic region (*straight arrow*) and a further collection in the right subhepatic region (*curved arrow*). Both appearances are suggestive of air-containing abscesses. **D.** Transverse ultrasonogram. Ultrasound reflection characteristic of air is seen (*arrow*) between the medial (*R*) and lateral (*L*) segments of the liver but could be dismissed as air in the colon or duodenum; however, given that this air was visualized within the liver, it was concluded that this was an air-containing abscess. A CT scan or MR scan would show this clearly. At surgery, a subhepatic abscess was found that extended inferiorly anterior to the duodenum. This demonstrates the value of plain films and ^{67}Ga in the interpretation of ultrasonograms.

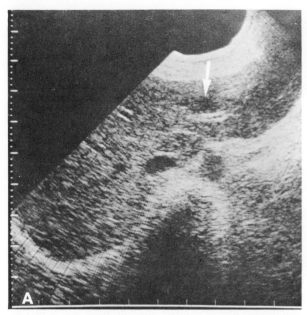

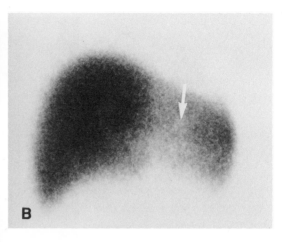

Fig. 10-16. A. Transverse ultrasonogram of the liver showing subtle defect (*arrow*) in the left lobe of the liver. This defect is approximately 2 cm in diameter. **B.** Liver sulfur colloid scintigram. The anterior view shows a defect (*arrow*) in the left lobe of the liver corresponding to the metastasis demonstrated in *A*.

Fig. 10-17. Longitudinal ultrasonogram showing an echogenic mass (*arrow*) under the right hemidiaphragm (*D*). At the Yale–New Haven Hospital, 50% of echogenic metastases have proved to originate from colonic primaries.

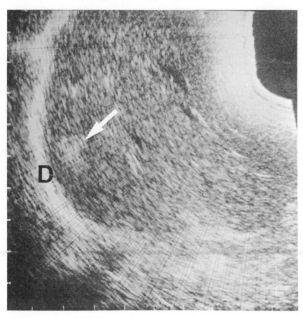

tumor type. A spectrum of contrast enhancement patterns can be found in multiple lesions of similar pathology in any one liver, and changes in contrast enhancement can occur rapidly within the same lesion. Most metastases are hypovascular with the exception of metastatic carcinoid, islet cell, and renal cell.

Intra-arterial delivery of contrast during dynamic hepatic scanning does create the greatest enhancement of lesions and thus the highest detectability. However, this is not practical in most instances since an intra-arterial catheter has to be placed prior to the study.[118]

Figure 10-19 shows large metastatic deposits within the liver appearing as low-density lesions. Within the lesions

TABLE 10-2. Accuracy of Ultrasound and Scintigraphy at Initial Reading

SCINTIGRAPHY READING	SCINTIGRAPHY ACCURACY	ULTRASOUND ACCURACY
Probably normal	95%	95%
Indeterminate	?	94%
Probably abnormal	47%	91%

(Sullivan DC et al: The use of ultrasound to enhance the diagnostic utility of the equivocal liver scintigraph. Radiology 128:727–732, 1978)

TABLE 10-3.   Correlation of Ultrasound and Scintigraphy with Final Diagnosis

	SCINTIGRAPHY	ULTRASOUND
Sensitivity	89%	83%
Specificity	69%	97%
Accuracy	74%	93%

(Sullivan DC et al: The use of ultrasound to enhance the diagnostic utility of the equivocal liver scintigraph. Radiology 128:727–732, 1978)

themselves, speckled calcifications can be demonstrated, suggesting a diagnosis of a colonic primary lesion.[13]

The superior contrast resolution of MRI offers theoretic advantages in the detection of metastases.[58] Proper choice of pulse sequence is critical in MRI to optimize liver to lesion contrast. Although it seems unlikely that a specific T_1 and T_2 can be ascribed to a particular tumor, in general, malignancy has a sufficiently prolonged T_1 and T_2 to make it readily identifiable (Figure 10-20). In one study of 28 tumors the mean T_1 was 40% longer and the mean T_2 was 20% longer than normal parenchyma.[119] The relaxation times are prolonged, probably due to increased free water content. T_2 values of metastasis have been correlated with the degree of cancer cellularity.[126]

Benign Liver Lesions

Benign hepatic masses have no pathognomonic appearance on ultrasound or CT.[37] Occasionally, hepatic scintigraphy can be definitive.[76] Focal nodular hyperplasia (FNH) can be echogenic or echopenic on ultrasound, while on CT the lesion commonly appears as a hypodense area that variably enhances with intravenous contrast. Detection of a central fibrous scar is highly suggestive of FNH (Fig. 10-21). The scar corresponds to the central fibrous core and radiating septa described pathologically. Since FNH contains Kupffer cells, ^{99m}Tc colloid scintigraphy may demonstrate uptake in the tumor (40%–50% of cases).[20,26,139,150]

Similarly, hepatic adenoma has no characteristic appearance on sonography. On CT, identification of a calcific focus with a focal lesion is suggestive of adenoma. The calcification represents prior hemorrhage, while a hyperdense area suggests recent hemorrhage. In a young patient with right upper quadrant pain and a history of oral contraceptive use, a hemorrhagic lesion should be considered hepatic adenoma until proven otherwise.[56] Since adenomas do not contain Kupffer cells, they are cold on ^{99m}Tc-sulfur colloid radionuclide scans. Hepatic adenomas do not demonstrate any characteristic contrast medium enhancement.[37] The presence of a low-density peripheral ring, due to an excess of lipid-laden hepatocytes, may enable a more specific diagnosis of adenoma.[3]

Hemangiomas have a characteristic appearance on CT if contrast material is administered with single-level dynamic and delayed scans (Fig. 10-22).[71,72] Hemangiomas characteristically enhance from peripherally to centrally. Delayed scans are essential to demonstrate that the lesion fills in with contrast medium.[71,86] Hemangiomas smaller than 2 cm may be too small to follow the temporal phases of contrast medium enhancement; nonetheless larger hemangiomas have CT features sufficiently characteristic to obviate arteriography or biopsy.[39,156]

MRI is extremely sensitive in the detection of hemangiomas.[159] They have a consistent appearance on MR images (Fig. 10-23), and their T_2 is greater than 80 msec,[126] which enables differentiation from hepatic malignancy, which usually has a T_2 of less than 80 msec. In one study, MRI identified more hemangiomas than CT, ultrasound, or selective arteriography.[46]

CT has significant advantages over other modalities in the diagnosis of hepatic injury from upper abdominal trauma.[54,117] The size of the hepatic laceration, hematoma and/or hemoperitoneum can be readily identified. An acute hemoperitoneum is characteristically hyperdense on CT (approximately 45 HU). A large hemoperitoneum indicates the need for surgery. Parenchymal hemorrhage is initially hyperdense due to clot and then becomes water density in 2 to 3 weeks. Hemobilia can be recognized as a dependent density within the gallbladder. The progress of healing or recurrent bleeding is easily monitored with CT.[54]

Radiation can be injurious to the liver. However, radiation hepatitis is usually not observed in patients receiving less than 3500 rad. Radiation injury is seen as a low-density bandlike lesion corresponding to the radiation port. Both noncontrast and contrast scans show a region of low attenuation that gradually resolves with time.[75,84]

Hepatoma

There is no general agreement as to the ultrasound appearances of hepatomas. In one report on a small series of hepatomas, these tumors were always echogenic on ultrasound examination,[78] but our experience is that hepatomas present a very wide spectrum of appearances from malignant necrotic cysts to homogeneous tumors and echogenic masses. In Figure 10-24A and B a predominantly solid mass is shown that protrudes from the lower border of the right lobe of the liver. The mass shows quite marked central necrosis, and the lesion is seen on the liver scintigram as an edge defect (Fig. 10-24C). Biopsy revealed a hepatoma; however, these appearances are nonspecific and could be due to any partially necrotic primary or metastatic tumor. One of the most useful attributes of ultrasound is its ability to define focal lesions in the presence of a cirrhotic liver and, thereby, to detect hepatomas.[171]

Technetium-99m-sulfur colloid scintigrams are usually abnormal in the presence of hepatoma. The finding of a

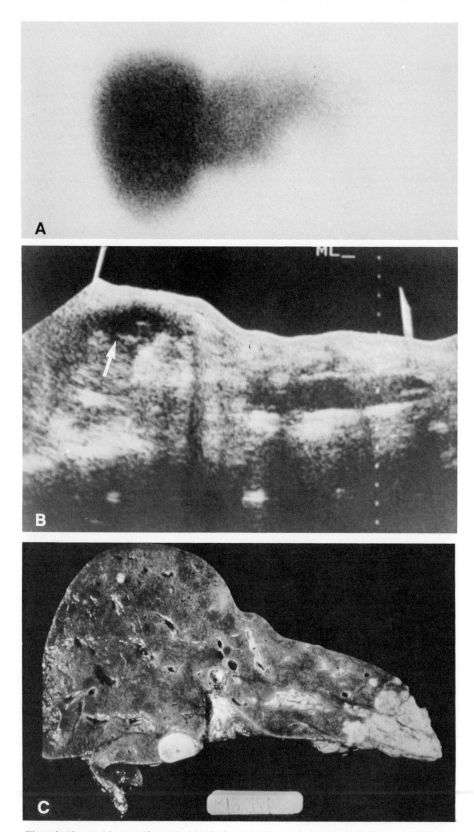

Fig. 10-18. A. Liver sulfur colloid scintigram. The anterior view shows possible edge defect in the left lobe of the liver. **B.** Longitudinal ultrasonogram showing a partially necrotic, irregular mass (*arrow*) on the anterior part of the left lobe of the liver. **C.** Pathologic specimen confirming the presence of a metastasis amputating the tip of the left lobe of the liver.

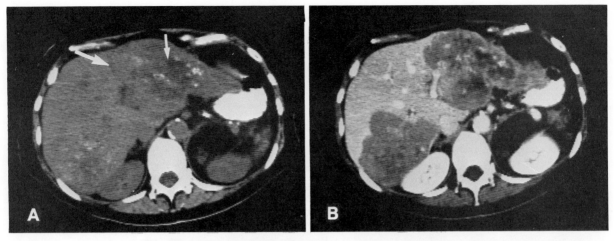

Fig. 10-19. A. CT scan without contrast medium showing metastatic disease to the liver as areas of low attenuation (*arrow*). There are also scattered areas of high attenuation, indicating calcification, that were not apparent on plain film radiography. Such calcifications suggest colonic metastases. **B.** CT scan with contrast enhancement of the liver. This improves differentiation between normal liver and metastatic lesions.

"cold" lesion due to a hepatoma is nonspecific and cannot be distinguished from other causes of "cold" zones such as fibrous tissue or regenerative nodules occurring in cirrhotic livers. Since the clinical problem is most often to diagnose a hepatoma in the presence of cirrhosis, the ^{99m}Tc-sulfur colloid images alone are not sufficient. Lomas and co-workers explored the use of ^{67}Ga imaging for detecting hepatomas.[98] These investigators found that virtually all hepatomas have uptake of this agent that equals or exceeds its concentration in normal liver tissue. Pseudotumors in cirrhotic livers do not concentrate gallium. This differential gallium uptake between hepatomas and

pseudotumors is the basis of the clinical usefulness of this radiopharmaceutical for detecting hepatomas in patients with cirrhosis. However, ^{67}Ga uptake is also increased in abscesses and some tumor metastases. In addition, because gallium concentration in hepatomas may not exceed normal hepatic tissue concentration, it is the "filling in" on the ^{67}Ga scan of "cold spots" detected by the conventional ^{99m}Tc-sulfur colloid images that is often the clue to the correct diagnosis of hepatomas. Most investigators have reported sensitivities of 90% or greater for the detection of hepatoma by ^{67}Ga.[59] Cornelius and Atterbury reviewed the literature on ^{67}Ga scintigraphy of hepatomas.[24] They

(*Text continues on p. 286*)

Fig. 10-20. MR scan (coronal spin echo TR2000 TE28) showing tumor (*T*) in right lobe as high signal area compressive IVC (*arrow*). Note that normal liver (*L*) is lower intensity.

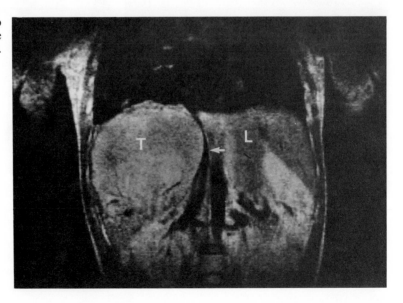

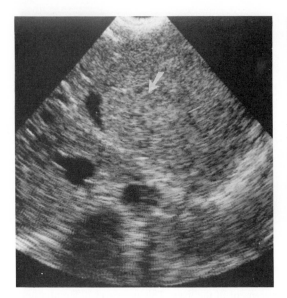

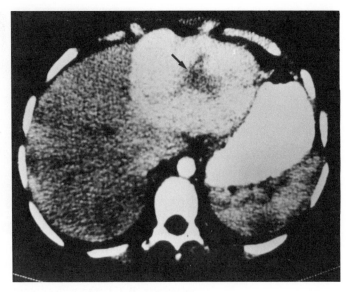

Fig. 10-21. Left. Transverse sonogram through left lobe showing an echogenic lesion (*arrow*). **Right.** Contrast-enhanced CT demonstrates central fibrous scar (*arrow*) typical of focal nodular hyperplasia.

Fig. 10-22. Left. Ultrasonogram showing an echogenic mass (*H*) in the right lobe of the liver. The appearance is identical to that of a large metastasis; however, the mass proved to be a hemangioma. **Right.** CT scan conducted with single-level dynamic bolus enhancement. Note early peripheral opacification 12 seconds after contrast (second image) to complete filling in of lesion 27 seconds after contrast (sixth image). This sequence of opacification from the periphery to the center is diagnostic of a hemangioma.

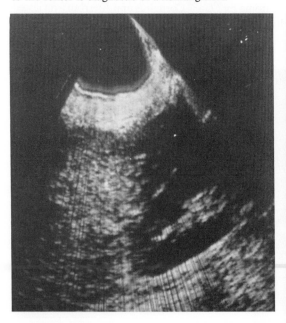

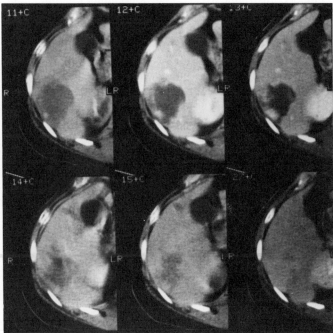

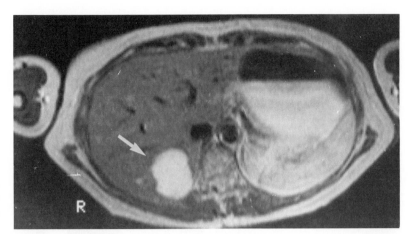

Fig. 10-23. MR scan (axial spin echo TR2000 TE60) showing typical high-intensity hemangioma (*arrow*). (Courtesy of Dr. David Stark)

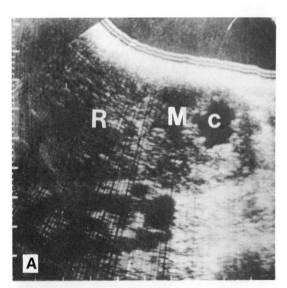

Fig. 10-24. A. Longitudinal ultrasonogram through the right lobe of the liver (*R*) and right kidney. A predominantly solid mass (*M*) with an irregular, necrotic mass center (*c*). **B.** Transverse ultrasonogram showing a partially necrotic mass (*arrow*). Biopsy of this area under ultrasound guidance disclosed a hepatoma. **C.** Liver sulfur colloid scintigram, anterior view, showing a defect in the lower border of the right lobe of the liver.

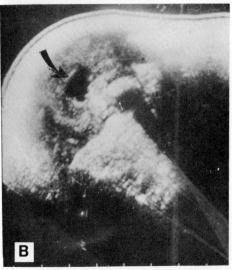

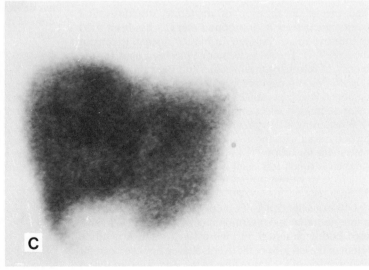

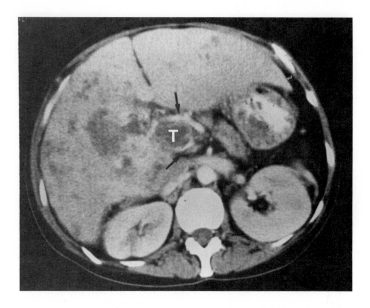

Fig. 10-25. Contrast-enhanced CT scan demonstrating portal vein thrombosis from hepatoma (hypodense areas in liver). Note splaying of left and replaced right hepatic arteries (*arrows*) by thrombus (*T*) in portal vein.

found that in studies of 164 patients reported in nine separate articles, 63% of hepatomas concentrated more of the agent than the host liver tissue, 25% of hepatomas had uptake of the radiopharmaceutical roughly equal to the surrounding liver tissue, and 12% of hepatomas had uptake that was less than the host liver.[24]

Figure 10-25 shows a patient with a biopsy-proved hepatoma that had no specific CT characteristics. Hepatomas have CT numbers suggesting solid tumors and, because of their vascularity, very often show contrast medium enhancement.[62,65,67] With the use of bolus contrast medium administration, portal vein thrombosis and cavernous transformation are demonstrable, improving the specificity for hepatoma.[65,90,105]

Ultrasonic or CT Guidance of Liver Biopsy

The precise localization of anatomic structures and pathologic defects by ultrasound and CT has been used to improve the success rate of biopsy of small lesions in the liver.[60,188] The same technique has been used for the biopsy of retroperitoneal lesions and pancreatic tumors (Fig. 10-26). A preference for CT over ultrasound by some authors is largely personal, although variations in available instrumentation affect this choice.

When using CT to guide biopsy, it is customary to perform the scan with the needle *in situ* to ensure the correct placement for biopsy.[188] In practice, however, such reassurance is much less helpful than the pathology report, which, in most institutions, can now be obtained within 30 minutes.

Ultrasonic guidance of a biopsy can be done with either a fine needle or a conventional cutting needle. We have used both techniques. In Figure 10-27*A* and *B* a subtle lesion in the left lobe of the liver is shown; however, careful examination of the entire lobe of the liver failed to reveal

any evidence of metastatic tumor. Routine biopsy of the right lobe of the liver would therefore be almost certainly unsuccessful. Thus, in fixed respiration, the position, angle, and depth of attack were noted, and a Klatskin needle biopsy was taken with those parameters. Histology revealed adenocarcinoma. The pancreatic primary tumor was also visualized by ultrasound (Fig. 10-27*C*).

The use of the fine-needle biopsy (22 gauge) attains most importance for the biopsy of retroperitoneal lesions, in which the needle can perforate the stomach and allow outpatient biopsy. The biopsy specimen obtained may be less satisfactory than that obtained by a cutting needle, but it may well suffice to confirm the presence of meta-

Fig. 10-26. CT scan showing a large tumor mass (*m*) that has deflected the pancreas (*p*) toward the left and extended upward to involve the liver. Biopsy revealed a lymphosarcoma. Note calcification in the wall of the aorta.

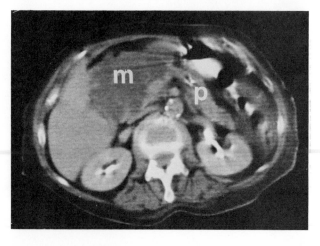

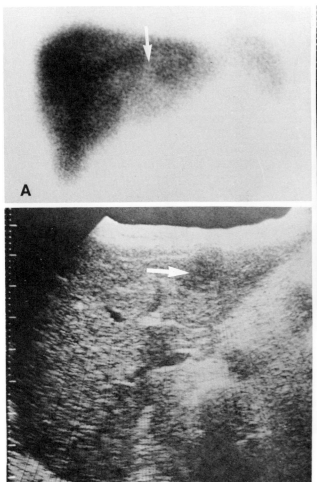

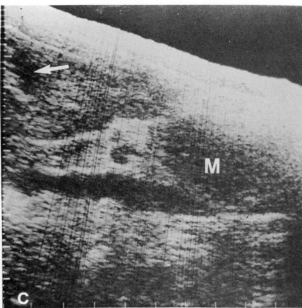

Fig. 10-27. A. Liver sulfur colloid scintigram, anterior view, showing cold defect (*arrow*) in the left lobe of the liver. **B.** Transverse ultrasonogram showing a relatively hypoechoic area (*arrow*) in the left lobe of the liver, consistent with the presence of a solid liver tumor. A biopsy guided by ultrasound revealed adenocarcinoma. **C.** Longitudinal ultrasonogram in the plane of the inferior vena cava. The left lobe of the liver shows a hypoechoic area (*arrow*) consistent with the presence of a liver metastasis. A pancreatic mass (*M*) is seen encroaching upon the lumen of the inferior vena cava. Appearances are consistent with the presence of a pancreatic mass and a liver metastasis.

static disease in a patient with a known primary lesion. This technique is of particular value when a patient with a carcinoma of the lung or pancreas, for example, presents with subtle lesions in the liver and an equivocal liver–spleen scan. Ultrasound or CT may detect these lesions quite clearly, and their malignant nature may be confirmed by fine-needle biopsy. Such patient management radically alters patient treatment.

DIFFUSE DISEASE OF THE LIVER

Scintigraphy, ultrasonography, and CT all contribute toward the diagnosis of fatty infiltration and established cirrhosis (Fig. 10-28).[61,99,121] For sensitivity, they obviously cannot compete with the results of biopsy; however, they are valuable for solving some of the problems of clinical management; they allow exclusion of focal abnormality in patients with hepatomegaly, and they provide a functional and anatomic overview of the liver in cirrhotics.

Scintigraphy in diffuse liver disease can present a wide spectrum of appearances, including alteration in the size of the liver, heterogeneous uptake of ^{99m}Tc-sulfur colloid, shift of colloid to the spleen, and uptake of colloid in the bone marrow. This functional overview of the liver is valuable for the clinician. Relatively minor histologic changes in the presence of a grossly abnormal liver scintigram also suggest a sampling error.

The ability to display the liver parenchyma by ultrasound introduces the possibility of a more precise diagnosis of diffuse liver disease. A cirrhotic or fatty liver gives rise to bigger amplitude echoes.[11,16,120] In a retrospective review of 22 alcoholic patients who underwent ultrasound and liver biopsy during a period of 18 months at the Yale–New Haven Hospital, ultrasound was found to be sensitive in detection of fatty infiltration and cirrhosis of moderate severity.[171] On a scale of 0 to IV, grade I fat, connective tissue, and necrosis were not detected. Grades II, III, and IV were successfully detected with a sensitivity of 95%, although fat and fibrosis could not be differentiated.

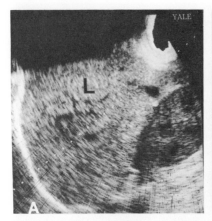

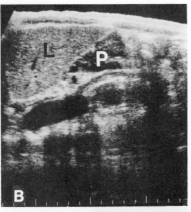

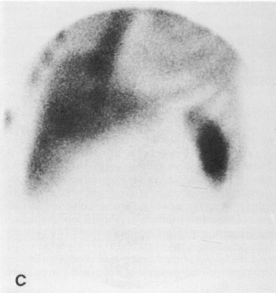

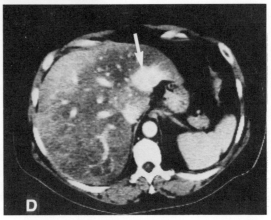

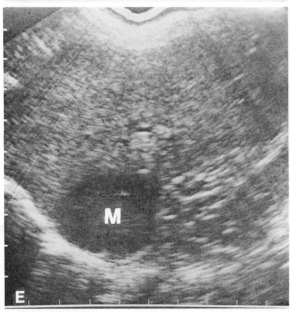

Fig. 10-28. A. Longitudinal ultrasonogram of a patient with alcoholic liver disease. The liver (*L*) is echogenic with high-amplitude parenchymal echoes almost as high as those of the diaphragm and higher than those of the kidney. These appearances are consistent with the presence of fatty infiltration or cirrhosis. **B.** Longitudinal ultrasonogram showing an echogenic liver (*L*) and an enlarged, hypoechoic pancreas (*P*). Appearances are consistent with the presence of pancreatitis or a tumor. Ultrasound cannot differentiate between the changes of pancreatitis and those due to a tumor. **C.** Liver sulfur colloid scintigram showing patchy uptake of isotope by an enlarged liver with a shift of colloid to the spleen and bone marrow. Appearances are consistent with the presence of diffuse hepatocellular liver disease. Right anterior oblique view. **D.** CT scan with contrast enhancement. Note low attenuation areas in the parenchyma of the liver, consistent with the presence of fatty infiltration. In the medial aspect of the liver, a mass is seen (*arrow*) that shows good contrast enhancement due to either a regenerating nodule or a hepatoma. **E.** Longitudinal ultrasonogram showing an enlarged liver with a diffusely abnormal parenchymal pattern. On the posterior aspect, there is a hypoechoic focal lesion (*M*). Such a lesion must be regarded as a probable hepatoma and biopsied. Biopsy in this patient revealed hepatoma. Regenerating nodules are seldom apparent as focal defects on an ultrasound scan; all focal defects must be regarded with suspicion.

There have been numerous efforts to diagnose cirrhosis by measuring attenuation through the liver. Our work has demonstrated that when liver ultrasonic attenuation is compared with liver biopsies, any increased attenuation is due to the concomitant presence of fat.[173] Thus, it appears at present that all imaging methods can detect the presence of fat, but none of them are sensitive to the presence of fibrosis.

In Figure 10-28D there is a CT scan of a patient who was on long-term hyperalimentation and showed diffuse fatty infiltration of the liver. The heterogeneous nature of the attenuation values can easily be appreciated. Closer observation yielded evidence for a dense lesion in the lateral division of the left lobe. At surgery, this proved to be a regenerating nodule. The liver had attenuation values similar to or slightly higher than those of the spleen.[137] In diffuse hepatocellular disorders, the CT findings can vary from normal to grossly abnormal with alterations in size, shape, or density. Normal scans are typically found in patients with amyloidosis, sarcoidosis, hepatitis, Hodgkin's disease, and early cirrhosis. However, a variety of specific CT findings can be found in such processes as fatty infiltration, advanced cirrhosis, and hemochromatosis, which permit quantification of the extent of the disease process.

Increase in hepatic fat content causes a decrease in the hepatic attenuation value. Experimental work in animals has demonstrated that for each milligram of triglyceride deposited in a gram of liver there is a decrease in attenuation of 1.6 HU.[47] A qualitative estimation of hepatic fat is based on the relative attenuation of liver compared with spleen. The attenuation value of the spleen does not change in fatty infiltration of the liver. The mean normal liver CT number is greater than the spleen. Higher than normal hepatic CT values are associated with higher than normal spleen CT values. Therefore, if the hepatic CT number is less than the spleen, then fatty infiltration is present.[130] Additionally, on noncontrast scans of diffuse fatty liver, the portal venous structures stand out as dense structures surrounded by a background of low density, a reversal of the norm. Nonuniform fatty infiltration or focal collections of fat can produce disconcerting ultrasound or CT appearances.[10,52] It is difficult to distinguish metastases from normal parenchyma when extensive fatty infiltration is present. If the portal vessels traverse these areas without mass effect, then fatty infiltration is likely. If necessary, percutaneous aspiration biopsy can provide definitive proof.

Early cirrhosis is not detectable by CT since density changes are usually not present. In advanced cirrhosis, however, changes in the liver contour, size, and/or homogeneity in CT number are often present. A small liver with a nodular contour is indicative of focal atrophy, fibrosis, and/or regenerating nodules. Often seen is prominence of the caudate lobe associated with a decreased size of the right lobe.[176] Ancillary findings are the presence of ascites and liver masses. The latter may indicate regenerating nodules or hepatomas. Portal hypertension is suggested by serpiginous densities occurring in the porta he-

patis, perigastric, umbilical, and splenic regions. Use of intravenous bolus contrast media demonstrates that these enhance, a finding that is diagnostic of varices. Regenerating nodules are usually of normal hepatic density, whereas hepatomas are not commonly hypodense.

Hemochromatosis is identified on CT as a marked increase in the density of the hepatic parenchyma.[115] The high atomic number of iron increases the CT number. At 120 kVp, the average number ranges between 75 HU and 132 HU. Dual energy techniques enable quantitation of the amount of iron present; thus the progress of therapy can be noninvasively followed.[48] Amiodarone, an iodinated compound used in the treatment of refractory ventricular arrythmias causes increased hepatic density on CT, probably secondary to the increased iodine content. The accumulation of the drug in hepatic liposomes causes a secondary phospholipidosis.[49] Thoratrast also increases hepatic density. Glycogen storage disease can increase or decrease hepatic attenuation values.[145] Dual energy CT can be helpful in distinguishing hemochromatosis from glycogen deposition and quantitating either disease.[145]

MRI can also serve as a noninvasive method for the diagnosis and monitoring of storage diseases. Iron and copper when present in sufficient amount cause a decrease in the T_1. This enhancement of relaxation occurs because of the interaction between the magnetic moment of the paramagnetic ion and that of the hydrogen proton. On conventional imaging sequences the liver appears black (see Fig. 10-29).[16,146,158]

With conventional pulse sequences MRI has thus far not proved extremely sensitive to fatty infiltration of the liver.[187] However, a simple proton spectroscopic imaging strategy has the potential to be useful clinically.[95] Since it exploits differences in the rate of precession of the protons in water and fat molecules, this method has achieved unequaled precision in quantifying fat.[141] On CT scans irregular fatty infiltration of the liver can occasionally present a diagnostic dilemma when it coexists with focal abnormalities. It is particularly difficult to distinguish metastases from normal parenchyma when extensive fatty infiltration is present. Ability to separate fat and water images would resolve this ambiguity since metastases contain no fat and thus stand out on subtracted (opposed) MR images.

MRI has demonstrated prolongation of the T_1 and the T_2 in patients with hepatitis. On spin echo images the involved liver appears more intense than normal parenchyma. Focal hepatitis can be distinguished.[160] Experience with cirrhosis is limited.

DUPLEX SONOGRAPHY OF THE LIVER

Normal Liver

All the major vessels of the liver can be sampled by pulsed Doppler ultrasound and their waveform recorded (see Fig. 10-2).[167] The right hepatic artery can always be sampled

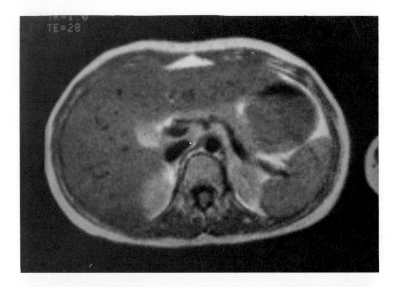

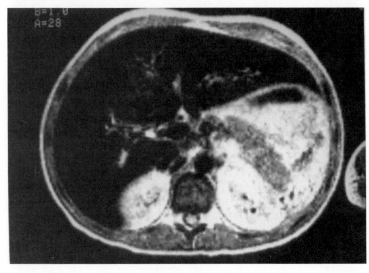

Fig. 10-29. Top. MR scan of normal liver containing 0.15 mg/g iron. **Bottom.** Loss of signal low intensity from liver containing 12.5 mg/g iron in a patient with hemochromatosis.

as it passes anterior to the portal vein. More deeply, the main portal vein can be sampled as well as the right and left branches. The portal vein exhibits almost continuous flow with some respiratory variation (see Fig. 10-2e), but this may be lost in severe portal hypertension. Bolondi and co-workers reported a sensitivity of 80% and a specificity of 100% for the recognition of portal hypertension based on diminished response of the portal vessels to the respiratory cycle.[15] The pressure changes in the inferior vena cava are freely transmitted to the hepatic veins (see Fig. 10-2a). Thus, the patency of all the major vessels to and from the liver can be noninvasively evaluated. In addition, the direction of flow in the portal vein can be established since flow away from the probe is below the zero line whereas flow toward the probe appears above the zero line. Thus, pulsed Doppler ultrasound allows recognition

of reversal of flow in the portal vein. It is important to note that some current duplex machines are extremely sensitive and are capable of detecting flow in small vessels throughout the liver that are not apparent on the ultrasound image (see Fig. 10-2b). Therefore, if the main vessels cannot be imaged for any reason, the sample volume can be moved throughout the liver parenchyma and liver viability can be confirmed by the demonstration of typical arterial and portal venous waveforms.

Attempts have been made to measure portal vein flow by Doppler techniques. The method is simple. The average velocity of blood in the portal vein is estimated and multiplied by the diameter. However, there are many sources of error in this computation that generally have not been sufficiently considered.[45] Considerable variations in the range of portal venous flow have been estimated, especially in cirrhosis. There are numerous sources of error, one of the most serious of which is the large angle that usually occurs between the beam and the vessel. Angles in excess of 60° lead to unacceptable errors. Further errors arise from the oval shape of the portal vein and its variations with respiration.

Intuitively, portal venous volume flow is unlikely to be a useful parameter in cirrhotics since it is unlikely to be related directly to pressure. The lack of respiratory variation in the portal vein in portal hypertension may be helpful.[15] However, the hepatologist is more interested in the flow that bypasses the portal vein into life-threatening varices.

Portal Vein Thrombosis

Portal vein thrombosis can be diagnosed by duplex ultrasound. On the ultrasound image, an occluded portal vein contains echoes after recent thrombosis and the lumen is replaced by an echogenic line in due time. Doppler examination reveals no portal flow. Conversely, detection of normal portal venous signal (see Fig. 10-2e) excludes portal vein thrombosis.

Cavernous Transformation of the Portal Vein

Following portal vein thrombosis, approximately 30% of patients eventually develop collateral channels, resulting in the so-called cavernous transformation of the portal vein. This pathologic entity can be diagnosed by duplex

Doppler ultrasound.[186] These channels can have confusing appearances and indeed may be misinterpreted as an abscess unless the vascular nature is demonstrated by pulsed Doppler technique (Fig. 10-30). The absence of respiratory variation in these collaterals indicates the presence of portal hypertension.[15]

Evaluation of Liver Transplants

The ability to obtain all the vascular signals illustrated in Figure 10-2 is invaluable for a transplant surgeon to evaluate patency of vessels prior to transplantation, and also on longitudinal studies following transplantation to exclude vascular compromise. On our first 18 liver transplants, we have detected hepatic arterial occlusion on one occasion, portal vein thrombosis on three occasions, and portal vein stenosis on two occasions (Fig. 10-31)[172] In the pretransplant evaluation of the liver, the presence of the inferior vena cava can be confirmed, and this is important since infants with biliary atresia may have congenital absence of this vessel. It is also important to be able to ascertain patency and direction of flow in the portal vein so that the surgeon is prepared for any difficulties during surgery.

Scintigraphic techniques, such as quantitative evaluation of hepatic transit time and excretion of ^{99m}Tc-di-iso-propyl iminodiacetic acid (DISIDA), may provide early detection of hepatic graft rejection since this results in a significant increase in the half-time excretion of ^{99m}Tc-DISIDA.[136]

Fig. 10-30. Cavernous transformation of the portal vein. **Left.** Transverse scan of liver shows multiloculated region of the porta hepatis (*arrow*). **Right.** Doppler examination of this area shows continuous flow characteristic of hypertensive portal venous flow. (Weltin G. et al: Duplex Doppler: Identification of cavernous transformation of the portal vein. AJR 144: 99–1001, 1985)

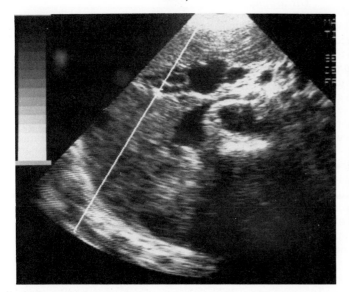
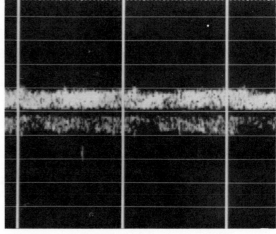

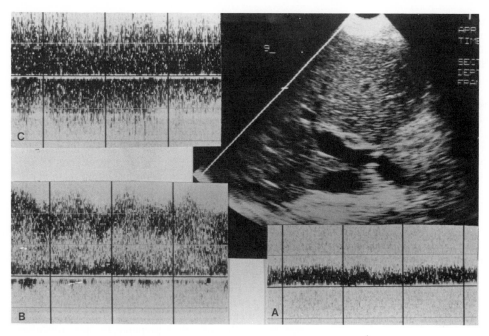

Fig. 10-31. Portal vein stenosis. **A.** Normal portal vein flow is seen before the stenosis. **B.** A high-velocity jet occurs at the stenosis. **C.** There is distal turbulence owing to eddy currents. (Taylor K et al: Liver transplant recipients: Portable duplex US with correlative angiography. Radiology 159: 357–363, 1986)

THE BILIARY SYSTEM

Imaging of the Gallbladder

In view of the acknowledged accuracy of approximately 97% of oral cholecystography (OCG) in the diagnosis of gallstones,[6] it is surprising that ultrasound has made such an impact on this field. However, in reality, the sensitivity and specificity of OCG is unknown. Many patients with symptoms of acute biliary tract disease such as nausea, vomiting, and jaundice are not suitable candidates for OCG, whereas many more patients with nonvisualized gallbladders on OCG do not have sufficient symptoms to prompt surgery. The accuracy of 97% for OCG is therefore based on the follow-up of those patients who come to surgery and those are mainly selected by their clinical symptoms. Thus, although OCG still remains a simple, inexpensive, and well-standardized screen for investigation of the gallbladder, in practice ultrasound and the new iminodiacetic acid agents have largely replaced it.

Proponents of the two techniques have discussed the relative value of them in the literature,[91,179] but the clinician is still left with the final decision of the order in which to use them or which one alone should be ordered. It must be recalled that in many patients the diagnosis of acute cholecystitis can be made with great accuracy on clinical grounds alone. If a surgeon merely requires one test to confirm a strong clinical suspicion, then the iminodiacetic acid scintigram is adequate. If acute cholecys-

titis is but one of several possible differential diagnoses, then ultrasound should be requested since many organs can be examined at the same time, and the point of maximum tenderness can be accurately localized to a specific organ. This "ultrasonic Murphy's sign" is very helpful in making the diagnosis of acute cholecystitis in the presence of gallstones.[134,135]

Ultrasound

We now recognize several different ultrasound appearances for gallbladder pathology, and each of these has a different level of clinical confidence.[25] The classic appearances of gallstones include an opacity within the dilated gallbladder lumen, its free movement with gravity, and distal shadowing because of the high attenuation of the sound beam by the stone (Fig. 10-32A). In such cases, the level of diagnostic confidence is virtually 100%. Shadowing from the edges of the gallbladder may occur, owing to refraction at the tissue–fluid interface (Fig. 10-32B), so that shadowing from the neck of the gallbladder must be interpreted with caution. We now recognize a further group of patients in whom the diagnosis of gallbladder pathology may be made with a high degree of confidence. In these patients, there is no obvious lumen to the gallbladder despite fasting, because the gallbladder is shrunken and fibrosed. Such gallbladders almost invariably contain gallstones and exhibit distal shadowing (Fig. 10-33A). These are the ultrasonic appearances of chronic chole-

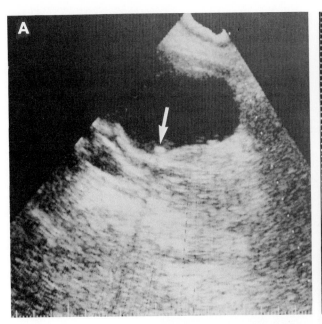
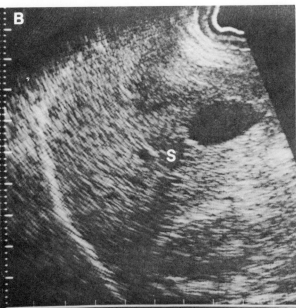

Fig. 10-32. A. Gallbladder lumen with a clearly visible opacity about 3 mm in diameter (*arrow*). Note the shadow distal to the opacity. Free movement of the opacity was demonstrated. The appearances are diagnostic of gallstones. **B.** Ultrasonogram of a gallbladder. Shadowing (*S*) from the neck of the gallbladder may be due to refraction of the beam at the bile–liver interface or may occur from the valves of Heister. Shadowing from a suspected stone in the neck of the gallbladder should be further investigated by attempts to dislodge the stone into the body of the gallbladder, where shadowing can be elicited from the stone alone.

cystitis and cholelithiasis in whom the gallbladder is incapable of physiologic distention. It should be noted, however, that such organs may be capable of iatrogenic distention (Fig. 10-33B). Although these appearances could also be due to congenital absence, the incidence of this anomaly is so low (0.03%) that the appearances are most commonly an indicator of gallbladder pathology.[116]

The third group of appearances, present in approximately 12% of the population scanned for gallbladder symptoms, consists of nonshadowing opacities within the gallbladder (Fig. 10-34).[25] Unfortunately, these are nonspecific appearances, and they are seen in normal patients who have calcium bilirubinate crystals due to biliary stasis and in the presence of sludge or empyema of the gallbladder. Thus, these appearances are truly equivocal and other imaging methods are required. Ultrasound also has extreme limitations in the diagnosis of acalculous cholecystitis. In such cases, the demonstration of a coincidence between the maximum site of tenderness and the underlying gallbladder may be of some clinical value. There may also be some thickening of the gallbladder wall, although we have found poor correlation between the thickness documented by ultrasound and that consequently displayed at surgery, unless the thickening is quite gross and exceeds 5 mm. The so-called rim sign, that is, an echo-free halo around the gallbladder, may be due to surrounding edema but may also be mimicked by fat or

ascites. Thus, we believe that the diagnosis of acalculous cholecystitis should be made by scintigraphic techniques.

Scintigraphy

Functional hepatobiliary scintigraphy using the various technetium ^{99m}Tc-labeled iminodiacetic acid conjugates can provide useful information in a number of clinical conditions. Hepatobiliary scans are requested most often to evaluate patients suspected of having acute cholecystitis. These studies can also be used in evaluating patients with chronic cholecystitis, intrahepatic cholestasis and hepatocellular disease, congenital abnormalities of the biliary system, bile leaks, and postoperative biliary tract abnormalities.[80]

A normal ^{99m}Tc-HIDA hepatobiliary study is shown in Figure 10-35. The radiolabeled compound is given intravenously and imaging is started within 5 minutes. The activity is seen first in the hepatic parenchymal cells, then is excreted into the intrahepatic biliary ducts, permitting visualization of at least the major intrahepatic ducts. The extrahepatic duct system, gallbladder, and finally, the small intestine are seen in images as the radioactive material follows the flow of bile. Several normal variants of this pattern can be seen. The first occurs in patients on prolonged fasts, which can result in nonvisualization of the gallbladder or the intestine by 1 to 2 hours after ra-

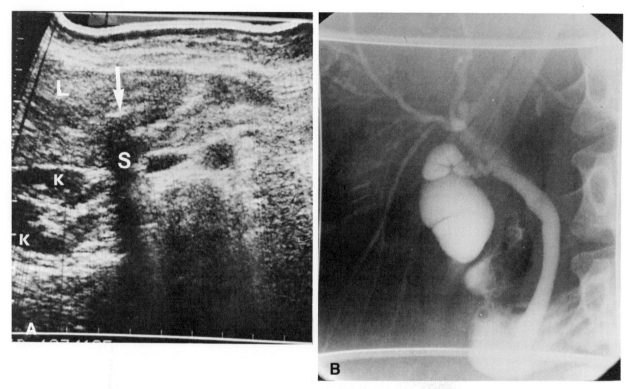

Fig. 10-33. A. Transverse ultrasonogram of the liver (*L*) and right kidney (*K*). Despite fasting, there is no evidence of physiologic dilatation of the gallbladder, and the gallbladder fossa appears as an echogenic area (*arrow*) with distal shadowing (*S*). These appearances are consistent with the existence of a small gallbladder contracted by chronic cholecystitis and almost invariably containing gallstones. **B.** Endoscopic retrograde cholangiography of the same patient as shown in *A.* Note that iatrogenic distension of the gallbladder has occurred, although not physiologically. (Courtesy of Drs. John Dobbins and Morton Burrell)

diopharmaceutical administration. Similarly, hospitalized patients receiving parenteral nutrition may not have a normal gallbladder image during a hepatobiliary study, presumably as the result of extreme concentration of the bile by the gallbladder.[154] Reflux of bile into the stomach can be seen in studies of apparently normal individuals as well as in patients with bile reflux gastritis.[175]

Those patients with acute cholecystitis typically have cystic duct obstruction so that the gallbladder is not visualized during the hepatobiliary study (Fig. 10-36).[143] A pattern of persistent nonvisualization of the gallbladder on images extending to several hours after radiopharmaceutical administration when there is normal demonstration of the liver, bile ducts, and intestine is nearly 95% accurate for the diagnosis of acute cholecystitis.[181] However, the interpretation of hepatobiliary studies must be done with full knowledge of the patient's nutritional status, current medications (narcotics can interfere), alcohol-use history, and other clinical information.

Radionuclide hepatobiliary studies are less accurate in patients with chronic cholecystitis. These studies do not have sufficient anatomic resolution to demonstrate gall-

stones or delineate enlarged intrahepatic ducts. Images obtained in patients with chronic cholecystitis will vary depending on whether the gallbladder, cystic duct, or common duct contains bile stones or "sludge." In a large percentage of patients with chronic cholecystitis, the hepatobiliary scan will be normal.[40,182] Delayed gallbladder visualization is the most common abnormal pattern in cholescintigraphy of chronic cholecystitis (Fig. 10-37). This delayed visualization must not be misinterpreted as acute cholecystitis; delayed images are needed to detect the gallbladder visualization, which can occur as long as 24 hours after radiopharmaceutical administration.[143] Delayed biliary tract to bowel transit times for the radiolabeled iminodiacetic acid compounds are sometimes seen in chronic cholecystitis. This transit delay, however, is not a specific finding since it can also be found in forms of common bile duct obstruction produced by ampullary stenosis, pancreatitis, narcotic administration, and so on.

Intrahepatic cholestasis can be studied with ^{99m}Tc-IDA cholescintigraphy. Depending on the cause of the bile stasis, studies in these patients can show normal or decreased hepatocyte uptake, prolonged parenchymal transit

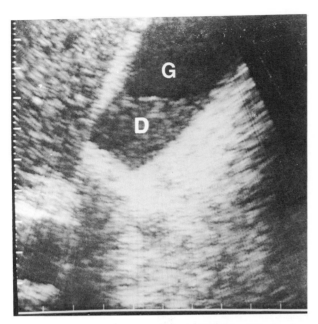

Fig. 10-34. Ultrasonogram of the gallbladder (*G*) showing nonshadowing debris (*D*) layered in the neck of the gallbladder. This debris is seen when there is inspissated bile secondary to stasis, sludge, which commonly occurs in alcoholics, or an empyema of the gallbladder. Therefore this appearance is not diagnostic of disease; if seen in a patient with suspected acute cholecystitis, the condition should be confirmed by technetium–HIDA study.

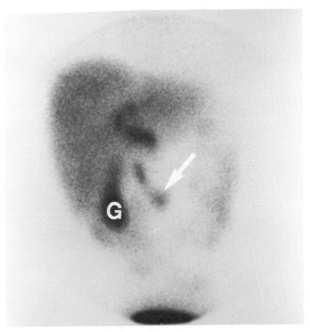

Fig. 10-35. Technetium–HIDA cholescintigram at 60 minutes showing normal uptake of the isotope by parenchymal cells and concentration of the isotope in the intrahepatic and extrahepatic bile ducts and within the gallbladder (*G*). Activity is seen within the duodenum (*arrow*), confirming the patency of the biliary tree.

Fig. 10-36. Technetium–HIDA cholescintigram 60 minutes after injection showing parenchymal activity of the isotope and concentration in the bile ducts without visualization of the gallbladder. These appearances are consistent with those of acute cholecystitis.

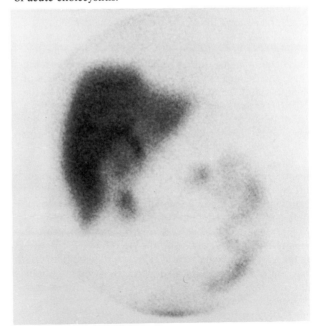

times, and variable visualization times of the extrahepatic ducts and intestine. If the hepatic clearance of the radiopharmaceutical is decreased, there will be prominent renal excretion. The scan patterns seen in the various types of cholestasis differ from acute obstructive diseases in which the hepatic parenchymal cell uptake is usually initially preserved and hepatic excretion is prolonged or absent. If the extrahepatic biliary tract is not demonstrated in a hepatobiliary study, it is not possible to distinguish accurately between intrahepatic cholestasis and chronic forms of obstructive biliary tract disease. The utility of cholescintigraphy also varies with the serum bilirubin level. With ^{99m}Tc-HIDA, best results are obtained at bilirubin levels less than 5 mg to 8 mg/dl. Other iminodiacetic acid–type radiopharmaceuticals can be used successfully in patients with bilirubin levels in the range of 20 mg to 30 mg/dl.

Anatomic biliary tract obstruction (so-called surgical jaundice) is well suited for study by ^{99m}Tc-IDA cholescintigraphy. The scintigraphic study is in fact capable of diagnosing early or partial biliary obstruction prior to sonographic evidence of ductular dilatation and occasionally before the bilirubin or other liver function tests have reached abnormal levels.[81,183,191] Cholescintigraphy has thus proved useful for evaluating the acutely obstructed patient, the cholestatic patient with hepatic parenchymal cell dysfunction or obstructive disease, patients with lo-

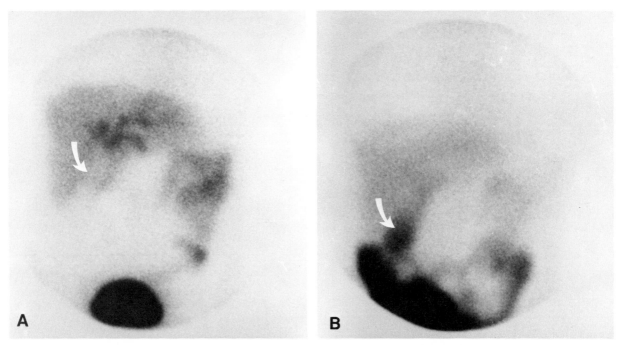

Fig. 10-37. A. Technetium–HIDA cholescintigram after 60 minutes shows activity in the bile ducts but not in the gallbladder (*arrow*). **B.** At 90 minutes, there is delayed concentration of isotope in the gallbladder (*arrow*). These appearances exclude acute cholecystitis but may be found in chronic cholecystitis. Ultrasound examination of the gallbladder should be performed to search for possible stones.

calized intrahepatic biliary duct obstruction, and patients with air or gas in the biliary tree, which can interfere with sonographic studies.[179]

Hepatobiliary studies are done in infants and children to differentiate forms of neonatal jaundice and to diagnose congenital abnormalities. Cholescintigraphy can aid in the difficult diagnosis of biliary atresia since even a small amount of radionuclide activity seen in the intestine during a hepatobiliary study excludes the diagnosis of atresia. These infants are often studied following 3 to 7 days of phenobarbital therapy, which enhances excretion of the ^{99m}Tc-IDA radiopharmaceutical in those infants with a patent biliary tree.[101] Other diseases such as choledochal cysts,[53,64,162] Caroli's disease, and Rotor's syndrome[7] can be identified using hepatobiliary scintigraphy.

Hepatic injury is common following both blunt and penetrating abdominal trauma. Penetrating hepatic injuries usually require surgical exploration, but blunt trauma to the liver can be managed conservatively unless there are specific indications for surgical exploration. Although extrahepatic bile duct or gallbladder rupture is usually readily detected with bile staining of the peritoneum, other intrahepatic, partial, or sequestered bile leaks may not be detected clinically. Hepatobiliary scintigraphy can provide useful information in cases of blunt or penetrating trauma; it is extremely sensitive for detecting a bile leak regardless of cause (Fig. 10-38).[163,184,192]

Cholescintigraphy can also be of great benefit for evaluating the postoperative patient. In the postcholecystectomy patient the ^{99m}Tc-IDA scans can be used to evaluate duct patency, detect cystic duct remnants, find sites of bile leakage, and evaluate hepatic parenchymal function.[185,193] ^{99m}Tc-IDA scintigraphy can provide information about the integrity and patency of surgical anastomoses of biliary tract structures and biliary gastrointestinal tract anastomoses (Fig. 10-39).[144,194]

Computed Tomography

CT scanning is not the primary modality for investigation of gallbladder disease, but it has been useful in several instances for carcinoma and in demonstrating morphologic problems or equivocal results.[57] Cholecystitis can be suggested on CT where there is a thickening of the gallbladder wall, fluid around the gallbladder, and/or infiltration of the pericholecystic fat.[155] Calcified gallstones are readily apparent on CT. However, the number of stones visible depends on the slice thickness and interslice gap. Emphysematous cholecystitis and porcelain gallbladder have a pathognomonic appearance on CT. Carcinoma of the gallbladder presents as a mass lesion within the gallbladder or a gallbladder fossa usually with gallstones and often with biliary dilatation.[69,70]

With MRI, gallbladder intensity varies depending on

the fasting state of the patient.[63] In the fasting subject, its intensity is higher than liver, whereas in the nonfasting person, the intensity can be lower than liver since dilute intrahepatic bile is present. Layering of dilute over concentrated bile is often seen. Within 4 hours of gallbladder emptying, 90% of the water content is absorbed by the gallbladder wall. Concentrated bile has a high intensity due to this change in water content. By 8 hours of fasting, the gallbladder should be hyperintense. In a preliminary study of fasting patients with cholecystitis, the gallbladder was abnormally hypointense or isointense.[107]

Specific Diseases of the Gallbladder

Hydrops. Hydrops of the gallbladder gives rise to a cold area of variable size on the liver–spleen scan and to non-filling of the gallbladder with normal demonstration of the extrahepatic ducts on ^{99m}Tc-HIDA cholescintigraphy. On ultrasound examination (Fig. 10-40) there is distention of the gallbladder, which tends to become spherical in contour. Sometimes the gallbladder also becomes very large; however, more frequently, its size is within normal limits. On CT scans, a dilated gallbladder is easily identified (Fig. 10-41A), and any accompanying dilation of the biliary tree can also be appreciated (Fig. 10-41B).

Polyps. Polyps of the gallbladder appear on ultrasound as small projections from the walls that do not shadow and do not move with gravity. These criteria allow them to be differentiated from gallstones. However, few patients with polyps come to surgery, so that the sensitivity and specificity of these observations is unknown.

Thickening of the Gallbladder Wall. Several articles have appeared on the use of ultrasound to detect thickening of the gallbladder wall,[34,102,112] but we remain unconvinced of its usefulness. There is general agreement that the gallbladder wall appears abnormally thick in the presence of ascites and that this may be due to edema of the gallbladder wall associated with hypoalbuminemia. It is commonly seen in patients with hepatitis. Thus, we regard thickening of the gallbladder wall as a nonspecific change. The presence of a fluid collection around the gallbladder should raise the possibility of a pericholecystitic abscess (Fig. 10-42), although ascites must be differentiated. Diffuse gallbladder wall thickening on CT may represent cholecystitis, whereas focal gallbladder wall thickening is more suggestive of a carcinoma.

Carcinoma. Carcinoma of the gallbladder tends to occur in patients with gallstones and may be found fortuitously at cholecystectomy (Fig. 10-43A). More frequently, it presents as a large, palpable mass in the right costal margin, with extensive spread into the right lobe of the liver and to the periportal nodes, often producing obstructive jaundice. Liver–spleen scanning and iminodiacetic acid scanning have limited value since they lack specificity in the diagnosis of such advanced tumors. Ultrasound and CT

demonstrate no more than a nonspecific solid tumor with irregular contours in the region of the gallbladder fossa; such a mass could be a primary tumor of the biliary tree, a hepatoma, or metastatic disease (Fig. 10-43B). Nonetheless, the visualization of a focal soft tissue mass, biliary obstruction at the level of the porta hepatis, direct hepatic invasion or metastases, and/or lymphadenopathy at the distal common bile duct and pancreatic head are highly suggestive of gallbladder carcinoma.[174,177] Guided percutaneous biopsy usually provides a definitive diagnosis of a disease that is so virulent that surgery is contraindicated.[14] Thus, a percutaneous biopsy for diagnosis and a percutaneous stent for internal biliary drainage when necessary may replace surgery.

Imaging of the Bile Ducts

Ultrasound

Although we believe that the normal intrahepatic bile ductules can be visualized by ultrasound, they are at the limits of our resolution, and, for practical purposes, we regard them as normal unless the lumen is visible.[170] However, the common hepatic duct and common bile duct can be visualized, and the portal vein is used as an important landmark. The common hepatic duct and common bile duct pass down the hepatoduodenal ligament anterior to the portal vein. The lower part of the common bile duct in the noncholecystectomized patient by ultrasound should be less than 6 mm, with 95% being less than 4 mm.[125] The common duct may be larger in patients post cholecystectomy, although it is probable that this is due to present or past biliary obstruction. Intrahepatic bile ducts usually appear larger on cholangiography than they do on ultrasonography, even allowing for a small magnification factor. Thus, the presence of contrast medium within the bile ducts may be responsible for some dilation, or there may be iatrogenic distention.

Many studies have been published on the accuracy of ultrasound in differentiating between extrahepatic and intrahepatic causes of jaundice on the basis of dilatation of the biliary tree. Our series, the largest of these, was based on 275 jaundiced patients coming to follow-up. Using dilated ducts as a criterion of extrahepatic obstruction, a sensitivity of 94% was achieved.[170] In the remaining 6% of the patients, no dilatation was detected by any modality, and the obstruction was usually due to gallstones. We therefore suggested that there might be intermittent obstruction due to a ball-valve effect by the gallstone. Whatever the mechanism, the study implies that either ultrasonic or CT demonstration of normal ducts does not exclude the possibility of a surgically correctable obstructing lesion. The specificity of 100% in this series suggests that false-positive results are very unusual. In the practical management of the jaundiced patient and where experience in ultrasound exists, ultrasound can be used as the initial test. The demonstration of dilated ducts indicates

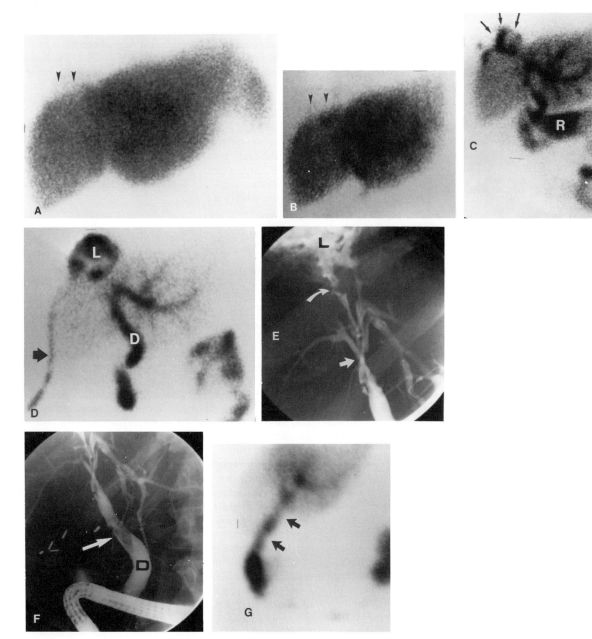

Fig. 10-38. A 59-year-old man was involved in a motor vehicle accident. Because of hemo-dynamic instability, laparotomy was performed, resulting in ligation of the right hepatic artery to control bleeding. Eight weeks later, fever and right upper quadrant pain developed. **A.** Tech-netium-99m sulfur colloid scan obtained 8 weeks after injury shows mild atrophy of the right hepatic lobe. The superior surface of the right lobe appears flattened (*arrowheads*). **B.** Technetium-99m disofenin scan obtained 20 minutes after administration of the radionuclide shows a similar appearance to the right lobe (*arrowheads*). **C.** Technetium-99m disofenin scan (as in *B* above) obtained 1 hour after administration of the radionuclide shows the presence of extensive biliary leakage (*arrows*) and pooling of activity in the left hepatic ducts and common duct. Note the gastric reflux of tracer (*R*). **D.** Technetium-99m disofenin scan, 2-hour image, obtained 1 week later, after dilatation of the patient's previous surgical drain site with percutaneous catheter insertion. Leakage (*L*) is again noted with activity accumulating in the patient's drainage catheter (*arrow*). Pooling of tracer is also noted in the left hepatic duct and common bile duct (*D*).

(*Continued on facing page*)

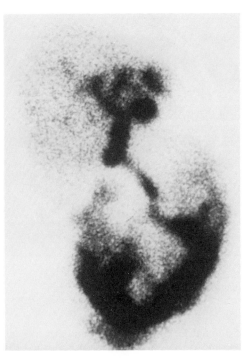

Fig. 10-39. Technetium–HIDA cholescintigraphy demonstrates patency of an anastomosis between the hepatic duct and the jejunal loop.

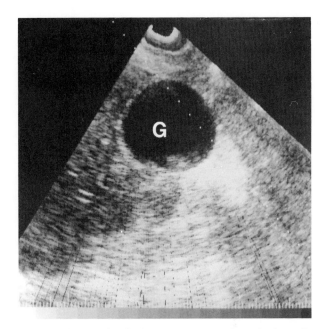

Fig. 10-40. Longitudinal ultrasonogram through the gallbladder (*G*). This patient had a tender ballotable mass easily palpated in the right subcostal region. The size of the gallbladder was not increased, but distension produced a more spherical organ. Appearances are consistent with the presence of a hydrops of the gallbladder.

a very high probability of extrahepatic obstruction. In 50% of these patients, the level and cause of the obstruction can be predicted.[170] The patient can then be scheduled for surgery, and the level and extent of obstruction can be further investigated by transhepatic cholangiography (THC) immediately before surgery. In the presence of dilated ducts, THC is successful in virtually all patients. When the obstructing lesion is obscured by gas, CT is an excellent alternative modality for the investigation of jaundice,[28] although confusion between dilated bile ducts and the portal venous system requires the use of contrast medium.[88] Figure 10-41*B* shows dilatation of the entire biliary tree due to a carcinoma at the head of the pancreas. Either CT or ultrasound can be used to guide a fine-needle biopsy of a liver or a pancreatic mass.

Two further phenomena must be considered. First, obstruction to the biliary tree may be manifest only by dilatation of the extrahepatic ducts.[190] Although, in our experience, it is very unusual for there not to be minimal dilatation of some of the intrahepatic ducts, in some series, the intrahepatic ductules have been normal in up to 30% of the patients (Fig. 10-44).[149] These differences probably result from the strict criteria that we use to recognize such dilatation.

A similar phenomenon by CT scanning is shown in Figure 10-44*B*. The amount of dilatation of the common bile duct is out of proportion to that of the intrahepatic biliary tree.[152] We have observed that the degree of dilatation of the biliary ducts appears to bear no relation to the duration of jaundice and may be more affected by the compliance of the vessels and the surrounding structures.

The second important phenomenon is the fact that

Fig. 10-38. (*Continued*) **E.** ERCP, oblique view, centered at the bifurcation confirms biliary leakage (*L*), as evidenced by contrast material extravasation. The right system partially drains normally into the common duct (*arrow*). Other more posterior ducts are draining directly into the biloma (*curved arrow*). The left system appears also to be disrupted at the bifurcation and is peripherally dilated. **F.** ERCP, anterior view, demonstrates a flame-shaped bile cast (*arrow*) that at fluoroscopy acted as a ball-valve obstruction within the dilated common duct (*D*). **G.** Technetium-99m disofenin scan, 1-hour image, 1 week after cholangiojejunostomy reveals dramatic resolution of leakage once normal biliary drainage and egress have been restored. The Roux-en-Y portion of the anastomosis (*arrows*) is well demonstrated. (Zeman RK: Radiology 151:771–777, 1984)

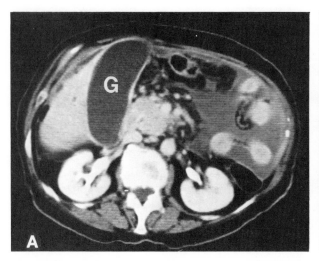 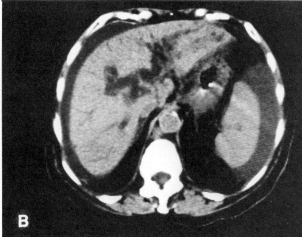

Fig. 10-41. A. CT scan shows distension of the gallbladder (*G*). **B.** CT scan shows gross dilatation of the intrahepatic bile ducts due to a carcinoma of the head of the pancreas. Ascites may be seen around the liver.

subtotal obstruction may produce biliary dilatation without jaundice. Two series of such patients have been reported in the radiologic literature.[178,189] In our series, biliary dilatation in the presence of normal serum bilirubin was due to three conditions:

1. To unilateral biliary obstruction due to a Klatskin type of tumor, for example, in which there is dilatation

Fig. 10-42. Transverse ultrasonogram showing the gallbladder lumen (*G*). Note the fluid collection (*arrow*) around the gallbladder. The presence of fluid raises the possibility of pericholecystitic abscess. At surgery, a perforated empyema of the gallbladder was found.

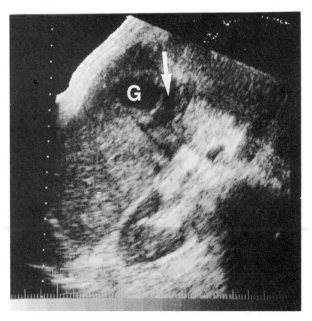

of one half of the biliary tree while the other half is normal, so that serum bilirubin is normal (Fig. 10-45). Such patients usually have elevation of serum alkaline phosphatase levels. In Klatskin's original series, one such patient with preicteric biliary dilatation was noted.[79] Figure 10-45*A* shows a CT scan through the upper portion of the left lobe of the liver of a patient with a known cholangiocarcinoma. Obstruction of the biliary tree distal to the lesion can easily be identified. Note the normal appearance of the remainder of the liver substance.

2. To subtotal obstruction due to tumor
3. To surgical relief of biliary obstruction after long-standing biliary dilatation

The intrahepatic biliary system is not seen on CT unless there is biliary obstruction, an enterobiliary anastomosis, or biliary contrast administration. The small size of the intrahepatic ducts and their oblique course relative to the axial CT cut results in volume averaging of adjacent hepatic parenchyma. The normal common bile duct is discernable. When there is a biliary dilatation, the ducts are readily discerned. Differentiation of veins from dilated ducts is easiest on contrast medium–enhanced scans since the density of the hepatic venous structures becomes greater than the hepatic parenchyma whereas the biliary system remains hypodense.

Sonography and CT are advocated as the initial procedures in the evaluation of the jaundiced patient. Ultrasound is preferred as the initial screening procedure because of its low cost, lack of ionizing radiation, and high accuracy in detecting gallstones. CT is used whenever the sonographic findings are in question, when a mass lesion is suspected, when the distal common duct is not clearly shown, when a segmental obstruction is suspected, or when any hepatic parenchymal abnormality is identified. Reported accuracy of CT in distinguishing obstructive or

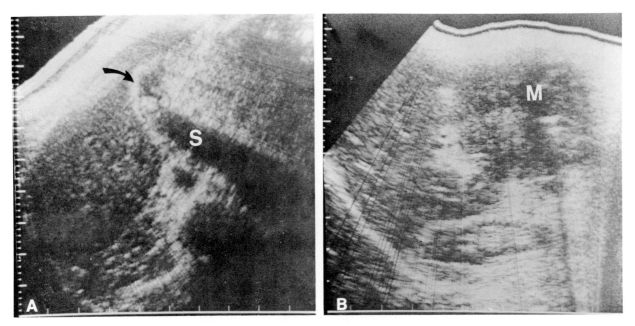

Fig. 10-43. A. Transverse scan of the gallbladder showing a small, contracted organ (*arrow*). Obvious gallstones are seen within the lumen, and there is distal shadowing (*S*). These appearances are consistent with the existence of chronic cholelithiasis and cholecystitis; in addition, a small carcinoma of the gallbladder was found at surgery. **B.** Longitudinal ultrasonogram shows an irregular mass (*M*) occupying the gallbladder fossa. These appearances are not specific for either an inflammatory mass or a neoplastic mass, but they raise the possibility of an advanced carcinoma of the gallbladder. Obstruction to the pancreatic duct as well as to the common bile duct was due to a small tumor in the ampulla of Vater.

Fig. 10-44. A. Longitudinal ultrasonogram showing marked dilatation of the common bile duct, which has a diameter of 1.5 cm. There is little evidence for peripheral ductular dilatation. Note the presence of multiple stones (*arrow*) in the common bile duct. **B.** CT scan shows disparate dilatation between the common bile duct (*arrow*) and the intrahepatic bile ducts. Common bile duct dilatation is due to cholelithiasis.

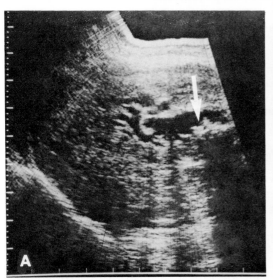
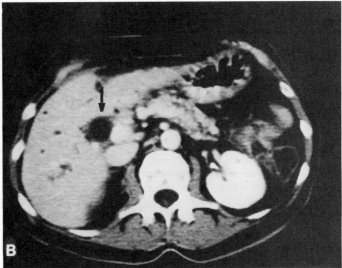

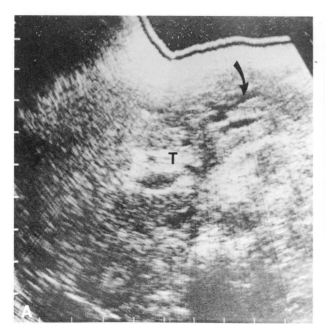
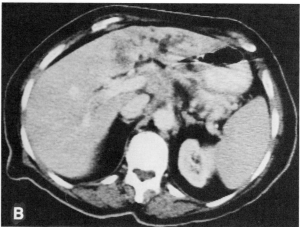

Fig. 10-45. A. Transverse ultrasound scan showing an echogenic tumor (*T*) in the region of the porta hepatis. The left lobe of the liver clearly shows dilatation of the distal bile ducts (*curved arrow*). **B.** CT scan showing metastasis from a cholangiocarcinoma (Klatskin tumor) in the region of the porta hepatis producing distal biliary duct dilatation.

nonobstructive jaundice ranges from 87% to 98%.[4,129,153] The level of obstruction is readily ascertained with CT. Demonstration of an enlarged gallbladder greater than 5 cm in diameter usually indicates obstruction distal to the cystic duct. Lack of gallbladder dilatation in patients with intrahepatic ductal dilatation indicates a level of obstruction above the cystic duct.[68] Demonstration of biliary calculi, the size of the dilated bile duct, the shape of the distal end of the obstructed duct, and the level of obstruction all aid in determining the cause of obstruction (which can be ascertained in 75% to 94% of cases). Pancreatitis usually produces a mild to moderately dilated common bile duct that smoothly tapers. In 50% of cases there is evidence of calcific pancreatitis. An abrupt change in the size of the dilated duct to one that is undetectable is usually due to a malignant lesion. The distal bile duct may be rounded, irregular, or nipple shaped. Associated diagnostic findings are lymphadenopathy in the porta hepatis and/or a peripancreatic mass. Ancillary findings include gallbladder dilatation and marked dilatation of the common hepatic or common bile duct such that it courses in a horizontal plane for part of its length.[9]

Common duct calculi are visible in 82% to 90% of cases by CT but only in about 30% by ultrasound.[114] Identification of calcific foci at the level of the obstruction is diagnostic. Pure cholesterol calculi have a lower attenuation than bile and are not as readily seen.[74] The dilatation of the bile duct is usually mild to moderate, with the duct tapering slightly. Sclerosing cholangitis appears as focal discontinuous areas of minimal intrahepatic bil-

iary dilatation without an associated mass lesion. The only differential diagnosis for this finding would be the rare diffuse form of cholangiocarcinoma.[133]

To assess the biliary tree, CT scans should be performed with 5-mm sections and collimation, therefore increasing the likelihood of finding small masses or stones. Intravenous contrast medium is necessary to opacify the vascular system to better differentiate vessels from the biliary tree. Although the sensitivity for CT in the identification of dilated ducts is greater than 95%, bile duct evaluation is more difficult in the presence of a fatty liver. Fatty liver can have the same attenuation value as bile within the dilated biliary system, making the bile ducts indistinguishable. In this setting, both precontrast and postcontrast scans may be necessary for optimal evaluation of the intrahepatic ducts. On one of these two scans, the attenuation value will be different. Furthermore, on the contrast medium–enhanced scans the peribiliary venous plexus may enhance, enabling identification of biliary structures.

Scintigraphy

The extrahepatic bile ducts are also well seen on ^{99m}Tc-HIDA scanning (see section on scintigraphy earlier in this chapter).

Specific Diseases of the Bile Ducts

Tumors. Tumors of the extrahepatic biliary tree are relatively rare. McDermott summarized 15 years of experience and found a total of only 34 patients with such pathology.[109] After an extensive review of the literature, Sako and co-workers concluded that malignant disease of the biliary tract occurs in less than 0.5% of autopsy examination.[147] Most frequently on ultrasound, CT, or scintigraphy using ^{99m}Tc-HIDA, tumors of the lower part of the biliary tract are manifest as biliary obstruction by a mass of unknown etiology. Only histologic examination can differentiate between a primary tumor of the bile duct, gallbladder, retroperitoneal lymphoma, or sarcoma, or metastatic disease to the region of the porta hepatis. The Klatskin tumor has been considered previously.

Congenital Cystic Dilatation of the Biliary Tract. Cystic dilatation of the biliary tract comprises the various types of choledochal cysts and Caroli's syndrome and may be associated with congenital hepatic fibrosis. A choledochal cyst can easily be demonstrated by ultrasound, CT, or ^{99m}Tc-HIDA. A typical choledochal cyst is shown in Figure 10-46A. Bile ducts are seen opening into the cystic mass,

thereby allowing it to be differentiated from a distended gallbladder. It was also differentiated from a compressed gallbladder, which was seen more laterally. These findings are diagnostic of a choledochal cyst. The same findings were demonstrated by ^{99m}Tc-HIDA scintigraphy, which showed a cold area initially corresponding to the cyst as visualized by ultrasound (Fig. 10-46B). Subsequently, activity appeared in the lesion, showing that it communicated with the biliary tree.

Cavernous dilatation of the intrahepatic biliary tree is also easily apparent on ultrasound examination (Fig. 10-47A and B). This constitutes Caroli's syndrome, which is also very well demonstrated by ^{99m}Tc-HIDA scanning (Fig. 10-47C), as confirmed by percutaneous transhepatic cholangiography (Fig. 10-47D).

CONCLUSIONS

In the past 5 years we have seen a dramatic increase in the methods available for imaging of the liver. The ad-

Fig. 10-46. A. Longitudinal ultrasonogram through the right lobe of the liver. A large cystic lesion is seen (*C*). Multiple bile ducts are seen opening into this lesion. These characteristics are diagnostic of a choledochal cyst. **B.** Technetium–HIDA cholescintigram. A large cold area (*arrow*) corresponds to the cystic mass demonstrated on ultrasound. Delayed films showed activity in this area, confirming the biliary origin of this cystic mass.

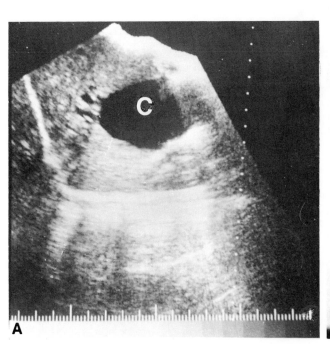

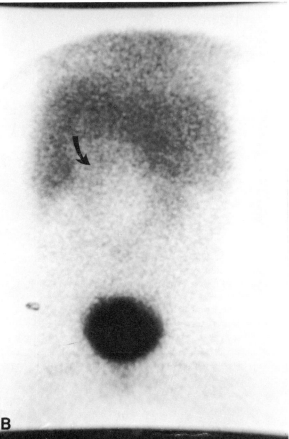

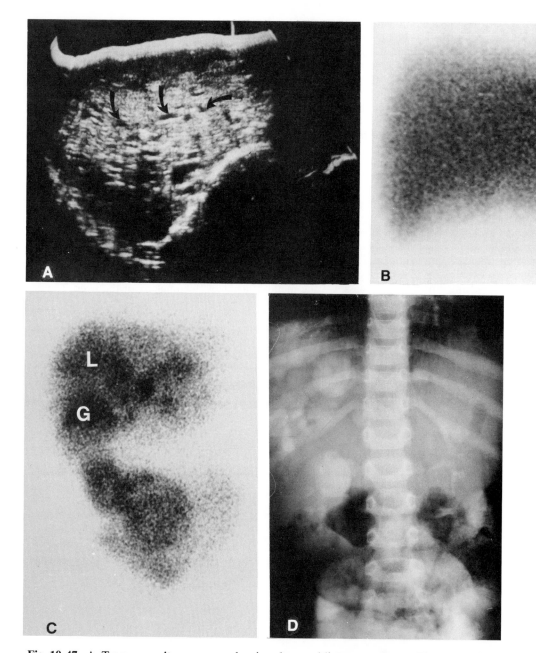

Fig. 10-47. **A.** Transverse ultrasonogram showing abnormal liver parenchyma. The echogenic liver is consistent with the presence of congenital hepatic fibrosis. There are multiple defects throughout the liver substance (*arrows*), consistent with cavernous dilatation of the biliary tree. **B.** Liver sulfur colloid scintigram showing nonspecific enlargement of the liver, with more uptake of the isotope in the spleen (*S*) than in the liver. **C.** Technetium–HIDA scintigram of entire abdomen showing cystic dilatation of biliary vessels of the liver (*L*), a subhepatic concentration, probably in the gallbladder (*G*), and bile activity in the lower abdomen. **D.** Percutaneous transhepatic cholangiography showing cystic dilatation of the biliary tree. All these appearances are consistent with the presence of Caroli's syndrome and congenital hepatic fibrosis. (Courtesy of Dr. Morton Burrell)

vantages of the fine spatial resolution produced by both ultrasound and CT scanning are probably offset by the limitations of a tomographic technique, so that liver–spleen scintigraphy remains valuable for an overview of the anatomy and function of the liver. The introduction of the new biliary imaging agents is welcome. These agents are valuable for investigation of biliary tract function and patency in jaundiced patients. Many studies have been published comparing the values of ultrasound and CT and demonstrating the superiority of one technique over another.[8,20,25,48] However, many variations are due to differences in instrumentation and expertise. There is no doubt that ultrasound is much more operator dependent than CT, and the presence of the rib cage and intestinal air challenge the technologist and may preclude obtaining a complete tomograph. However, real-time (automated) machines are now available that cost less than 5% of a CT scanner and require no contrast medium or ionizing radiation. These are good reasons to use ultrasound as an initial imaging procedure, requiring further training of technologists, radiologists, and hepatologists in the interpretation of these scans.

The next decade is unlikely to produce such dramatic changes as the 1970s. We can expect further modest improvement in image quality, but the major thrust may be toward more measurement of pathologic processes by ultrasound and CT and further development of isotope techniques to study the pathophysiology of the liver while MRI may constitute the next major impact on liver imaging.

REFERENCES

1. Alderson P et al: Computed tomography, ultrasound and scintigraphy of the liver in patients with colon or breast carcinoma: A prospective comparison. Radiology 149:225–230, 1983
2. Alexander E et al: CT differentiation of the subphrenic abscess and pleural effusion. AJR 140:47–51, 1983
3. Angres G et al: Unusual ring in liver cell adenoma. AJR 135:172, 1980
4. Araki T et al: Computed tomography of localized dilatation of the intrahepatic bile ducts. Radiology 141:733–736, 1981
5. Auh Y et al: CT of the papillary process of the caudate lobe of the liver. AJR 142:535–538, 1984
6. Baker HL: Further studies on the accuracy of oral cholecystography. Radiology 74:239–245, 1960
7. Bar-Meir S et al: ^{99m}Tc HIDA cholescintigraphy in Dubin-Johnson and Rotor's syndromes. Radiology 142:743, 1982
8. Barnes P et al: Pitfalls in the diagnosis of hepatic cysts by computed tomography. Radiology 141:129–133, 1981
9. Baron R et al: Computed tomographic features of biliary obstruction. AJR 140:1173–1178, 1983
10. Bashist B et al: Computed tomographic demonstration of rapid changes in fatty infiltration of the liver. Radiology 142:691–692, 1982
11. Behan M, Kazam E: The echographic characteristics of fatty tissues and tumors. Radiology 129:143–151, 1978
12. Berland L: Screening for diffuse and focal liver disease: The case for hepatic computed tomography. J Clin Ultrasound 12:83–89, 1984
13. Bernardino ME: Computed tomography of calcified liver metastases. J Comput Assist Tomogr 3:32–35, 1979
14. Bismuth H, Malt RA: Current concepts in cancer: Carcinoma of the biliary tract. N Engl J Med 301:704–706, 1979
15. Bolondi L et al: Ultrasonography in the diagnosis of portal hypertension: Diminished response of portal vessels to respiration. Radiology 142:167–172, 1982
16. Brasch R: Magnetic resonance imaging of transfusional hemosiderosis complicating thalassemia major. Radiology 150:767–771, 1984
17. Brooks RA, DiChiro G: Theory of image reconstruction in computed tomography. Radiology 117:561–572, 1975
18. Burgener F, Hamlin D: Contrast enhancement of hepatic tumors in CT: Comparison between bolus and infusion techniques. AJR 140:291–295, 1983
19. Callen PW: Computed tomographic evaluation of abdominal and pelvic abscesses. Radiology 131:171–175, 1979
20. Casarella WJ et al: Focal nodular hyperplasia and liver cell adenoma: Radiologic and pathologic differentiation. AJR 131:393–402, 1978
21. Chaudhuri T et al: Autoradiographic studies of distribution in the liver of ^{198}Au and ^{99m}Tc-sulfur colloids. Radiology 109:633–637, 1973
22. Choliz J et al: Computed tomography in hepatic echinococcosis. AJR 139:699–702, 1982
23. Cooperman AM et al: Computed tomography and abdominal abscesses: A valuable diagnostic aid. Am J Gastroenterol 69:579–581, 1978
24. Cornelius EA, Atterbury CE: Problems in the imaging diagnosis of hepatoma. Clin Nucl Med 9:30–38, 1984
25. Crade M et al: Surgical and pathologic correlation of cholecystosonography and cholecystography. AJR 131:227–229, 1978
26. Diament M et al: Technetium sulphur colloid uptake simulating focal nodular hyperplasia. AJR 139:168–171, 1982
27. Didier D et al: Hepatic alveolar echinococcosis: Correlative US and CT study. Radiology 154:179–186, 1985
28. DiGiacomo PJ et al: Evaluation of cholestatic jaundice by computed tomography. Surg Gynecol Obstet 145:570–572, 1977
29. Djang W et al: Computed tomography of the liver: Evaluating focal defects on radionuclide liver spleen scans. AJR 141:937–940, 1984
30. Doyle F et al: Nuclear magnetic resonance imaging of the liver: Initial experience. AJR 138:193–200, 1982
31. Edwards CL, Haynes RL: Tumor scanning with gallium citrate. J Nucl Med 10:103–105, 1969
32. Ell PJ, Khan O: Emission computerized tomography: Clinical applications. Semin Nucl Med 11:50–60, 1981
33. Evens R, Mettler F: National CT use and radiation exposure: United States 1983. AJR 144:1077–1081, 1985
34. Finberg HJ, Birnholz J: Ultrasound evaluation of the gallbladder wall. Radiology 133:693–698, 1979
35. Firnau G: Why do ^{99m}Tc cholates work for cholescintigraphy? Eur J Nucl Med 1:137, 1976
36. Fisher M et al: Hepatic vascular anatomy on magnetic resonance imaging. AJR 144:739–746, 1985
37. Fishman E et al: Computed tomography of benign hepatic tumors. J Comput Assist Tomogr 6:472–481, 1982
38. Foley W et al: Contrast enhancement technique for dynamic hepatic computed tomographic scanning. Radiology 147:797–803, 1983

39. Freeny PC et al: Cavernous hemangioma of the liver: Ultrasonography, arteriography, and computed tomography. Radiology 132:143–148, 1979

40. Freitas JE, Fink-Bennett DM: Asymptomatic cystic duct obstruction in chronic cholecystitis. J Nucl Med 21:17, 1980

41. Frick MP et al: Computed tomography, radionuclide imaging and ultrasonography in hepatic mass lesions. Comput Tomogr 3:49–55, 1979

42. Fritzberg AR, Bloedow DC: Animal models in the study of hepatobiliary radiotracers. In Lambrecht RM, Eckelman WC (eds): Animal Models in Radiotracer Design, pp 179–209. New York, Springer-Verlag, 1983

43. Froelich J, Swanson D: Imaging of inflammatory processes with labeled cells. Semin Nucl Med 14:128–140, 1984

44. Giannotta SL et al: Computerized tomography of the liver. AJR 128:579–590, 1977

45. Gill RW: Measurement of blood flow by ultrasound: Accuracy and sources of error. Ultrasound Med Biol 11:625–641, 1985

46. Glazer G et al: Hepatic cavernous hemangioma: Magnetic resonance imaging. Radiology 155:417–420, 1985

47. Goldberg HI: CT scanning of diffuse parenchymal liver disease. In Moss AI, Goldberg HI (eds): Computerized Tomography, Ultrasound and X-ray: An Integrated Approach. San Francisco, University of California, 1980

48. Goldberg HI et al: Non-invasive quantitation of liver iron in dogs with hemochromatosis using dual energy CT scanning. Invest Radiol 17:375, 1982

49. Goldman I et al: Increased hepatic density and phospholipidosis due to amiodarone. AJR 144:541–546, 1985

50. Green RL et al: Gray scale ultrasound evaluation of hepatic neoplasms: Patterns and correlations. Radiology 124:203–208, 1977

51. Halvorsen R et al: The variable CT appearance of hepatic abscesses. AJR 141:941–946, 1984

52. Halvorsen R et al: CT appearance of focal fatty infiltration of the liver. AJR 139:277–281, 1982

53. Han BK et al: Choledochal cyst with bile duct dilatation: Sonography and ^{99m}Tc-IDA cholescintigraphy. AJR 136:1075, 1981

54. Haney P et al: Liver injury and complications in the postoperative trauma patient: CT evaluation. AJR 139:271–275, 1982

55. Hauser MR, Gottschalk A: Comparison of Anger tomographic scanner and the 15-inch scintillation camera in gallium imaging. J Nucl Med 18:603, 1977

56. Havrilla T et al: Benign hepatic tumors and cysts in women using oral contraceptive agents: Computed tomography as a diagnostic aid. Cleve Clin Q 44:41–47, 1977

57. Havrilla T et al: Computed tomography of the gallbladder. AJR 130:1059–1067, 1978

58. Heiken J et al: Hepatic metastases studied with MR and CT. Radiology 156:423–427, 1985

59. Hoffer PB et al: Gallium-67 Imaging, Part I. New York, John Wiley & Sons, 1978

60. Holm HH, Kristensen JK: Interventional Ultrasound. Copenhagen, Munksgaard, 1985

61. Holmes JH: Ultrasonic diagnosis of liver disease. Am J Dig Dis 8:249–263, 1963

62. Hosoki T et al: Dynamic computed tomography of hepatocellular carcinoma. AJR 139:1099–1106, 1982

63. Hricak H et al: Work in progress: Nuclear magnetic resonance imaging of the gall bladder. Radiology 147:481–484, 1983

64. Huang MJ, Liau YF: Intravenous cholescintigraphy using ^{99m}Tc-labeled agents in the diagnosis of choledochal cyst. J Nucl Med 23:113, 1982

65. Inamoto K et al: CT of hepatoma: Effects of portal vein obstruction. AJR 136:349–353, 1981

66. Israelson A et al: Detection of space occupying lesions of the liver and spleen: A comparison of emission computed reconstructive tomography and conventional gamma camera scintigraphy. In Emission Computed Tomography: The Single Photon Approach, Publication No. FDA 171–176. Washington, DC, Bureau of Radiological Health, 1981

67. Itai Y et al: Computed tomography in the evaluation of hepatocellular carcinoma. Radiology 131:165–170, 1979

68. Itai Y et al: Computed tomography and ultrasound in the diagnosis of intrahepatic calculi. Radiology 136:399–405, 1980

69. Itai Y et al: Computed tomography of primary intrahepatic biliary malignancy. Radiology 147:485–490, 1983

70. Itai Y et al: Computed tomography of gallbladder carcinoma. Radiology 137:713–718, 1980

71. Itai Y et al: Computed tomography of cavernous hemangioma of the liver. Radiology 137:149–155, 1980

72. Itai Y et al: Computed tomography and sonography of cavernous hemangioma of the liver. AJR 141:315–320, 1983

73. Jaszczak RJ et al: Lesion detection with single-photon emission computed imaging (SPECT) compared with conventional imaging. J Nucl Med 23:97–102, 1982

74. Jeffrey R et al: Computed tomography of choledocholithiasis. AJR 140:1179–1183, 1983

75. Jeffrey R et al: CT of radiation-induced hepatic injury. AJR 135:445–448, 1980

76. Jhingran SG et al: Hepatic adenomas and focal nodular hyperplasia of the liver in young women on oral contraceptives: Case reports. J Nucl Med 18:263–266, 1977

77. Johnson R et al: Percutaneous drainage of pyogenic liver abscesses. AJR 144:463–467, 1985

78. Kamin PD et al: Ultrasound manifestations of hepatocellular carcinoma. Radiology 131:459–461, 1979

79. Klatskin G: Adenocarcinoma of the hepatic duct at its bifurcation within the porta hepatis—an unusual tumor with distinctive clinical and pathological features. Am J Med 38:241–256, 1965

80. Klingensmith WC: Radionuclide assessment of hepatic function with emphasis on cholestasis. In Freeman LM, Weissman HS (eds): Nuclear Medicine Annual, 1984. New York, Raven Press, 1984

81. Klingensmith WC et al: Effect of complete biliary tract obstruction on serial hepatobiliary imaging in an experimental model. J Nucl Med 22:866–868, 1981

82. Klingensmith WC et al: Clinical evaluation of ^{99m}Tc-trimethylbromo-IDA and ^{99m}Tc-diisopropyl-IDA for hepatobiliary imaging. Radiology 146:181–184, 1983

83. Knopf D et al: Liver lesions: Comparative accuracy of scintigraphy and computer tomography. AJR 138:623–627, 1982

84. Kolbenstvedt A et al: Post-irradiation change in the liver demonstrated by computed tomography. Radiology 135:391, 1980

85. Kormano M, Dean PO: Extravascular contrast material: The major component of contrast enhancement. Radiology 121:379–382, 1976

86. Kreel L: Computerised tomography and the liver. Clin Radiol 28:571–581, 1977

87. Kressel HY, Filly RA: Ultrasonic appearance of gas-containing abscesses in the abdomen. AJR 130:71–73, 1978

88. Kressel HY, Korobkin M: The portal venous tree simulating dilated biliary ducts on computed tomography of the liver. J Comput Assist Tomogr 1:169–175, 1977

89. Kuni CC, Klingensmith WC: Hepatocyte dysfunction. In Kuni CC, Klingensmith III WC (eds.): Atlas of Radionuclide Hepatobiliary Imaging, pp 31–36. GK Hall, Boston, 1983

90. LaBerge J et al: Hepatocellular carcinoma: Assessment of resectability by computed tomography and ultrasound. Radiology 152:485–490, 1984

91. Laing FC et al: Ultrasonic evaluation of patients with acute right upper quadrant pain. Radiology 140:449, 1981

92. Larsen MJ et al: Nonvisualization of the gallbladder secondary to a prolonged fast in radionuclide hepatobiliary imaging. J Nucl Med 23:1003–1005, 1982

93. Larsen SM: Mechanism of localization of gallium-67 in tumors. Semin Nucl Med 8:193–203, 1978

94. Lavender JP et al: Gallium 67 citrate scanning in neoplastic and inflammatory lesions. Br J Radiol 44:361–366, 1971

95. Lee J et al: Fatty infiltration of the liver: Demonstration by proton spectroscopic imaging. Radiology 153:195–201, 1984

96. Lee J et al: Detection of hepatic metastases by proton magnetic spectroscopic imaging. Radiology 156:429–433, 1985

97. Littenberg RL et al: Gallium-67 for localization of septic lesions. Ann Intern Med 79:403–406, 1973

98. Lomas F et al: Increased specificity of liver scanning with the use of gallium-67 citrate. N Engl J Med 286:1323, 1972

99. Luthra M et al: Scintiphotography in cirrhosis. Arch Intern Med 122:207–213, 1968

100. MacCarty RL et al: Retrospective comparison of radionuclide scans and computed tomography of the liver and pancreas. AJR 129:23–28, 1977

101. Majd M et al: Effect of phenobarbital on ^{99m}Tc-IDA scintigraphy in the evaluation of neonatal jaundice. Semin Nucl Med 11:194, 1981

102. Marchal G et al: Gallbladder wall thickening: A new sign of gallbladder disease visualized by gray scale cholecystosonography. J Clin Ultrasound 6:177–179, 1978

103. Marks W et al: Ultrasonic anatomy of the liver: A review with new applications. J Clin Ultrasound 7:137–146, 1979

104. Martino C et al: CT guided liver biopsies: Eight years' experience. Radiology 152:755–757, 1984

105. Mathieu D et al: Portal vein involvement in hepatocellular carcinoma: Dynamic CT features. Radiology 152:127–132, 1984

106. Mathieu D et al: Dynamic CT features of hepatic abscesses. Radiology 154:749–752, 1985

107. McCarthy S et al: Cholecystitis: Detection with MR imaging. Radiology 158:333–336, 1986

108. McClelland RR: Focal porta hepatis scintiscan defects: What is their significance? J Nucl Med 16:1007–1012, 1975

109. McDermott WV, Peinert RA: Carcinoma in the supra-ampullary portion of the bile ducts. Surg Gynecol Obstet 149:681–686, 1979

110. McClees E, Gedgaudas-McClees R: Screening for diffuse and focal liver disease: The case for hepatic scintigraphy. J Clin Ultrasound 12:75–81, 1984

111. Meire H: Gray scale echographic appearances of liver metastases. In White DN, Brown RE (eds): Ultrasound in Medicine, vol 3A, pp 315–319. New York, Plenum Press, 1977

112. Mindell HJ, Ring BA: Gallbladder wall thickening: Ultrasonic findings. Radiology 133:699–701, 1979

113. Mintz M et al: An algorithmic approach to the radiologic evaluation of a suspected abdominal abscess. Semin Ultrasound 4:80–90, 1983

114. Mitchell S, Clark R: A comparison of computed tomography and sonography in choledocholithiasis. AJR 142:729–733, 1984

115. Mitnick J et al: CT in β-thalassemia: Iron deposition in the liver, spleen, and lymph nodes. AJR 136:1191–1194, 1981

116. Monroe SE, Ragen FJ: Congenital absence of the gallbladder. Calif Med 85:422–423, 1956

117. Moon K, Federle M: Computed tomography in hepatic trauma. AJR 141:309–314, 1983

118. Moss A et al: Dynamic CT of hepatic masses with intravenous and intra-arterial contrast material. AJR 138:847–852, 1982

119. Moss A et al: Hepatic tumors: Magnetic resonance and CT appearance. Radiology 150:141–147, 1984

120. Mountford RA, Wells PNT: Ultrasonic liver scanning: The A-scan in the normal and cirrhosis. Phys Med Biol 17:261–269, 1972

121. Mulhern CB et al: Nonuniform attenuation in computed tomography study of the cirrhotic liver. Radiology 132:399–402, 1979

122. Neff C et al: Serious complications following transgression of the pleural space in drainage procedures. Radiology 152:335–341, 1984

123. Neumann RD, Gottschalk A: Diagnostic techniques in nuclear medicine. Annu Rev Nucl Particle Sci 29:285–288, 1979

124. Nichols D et al: The safe intercostal approach? Pleural complications in abdominal interventional radiology. AJR 141:1013–1018, 1984

125. Niderau C et al: Extra-hepatic bile ducts in healthy subjects, in patients with cholelithiasis and in postcholecystectomy patients: A prospective ultrasonic study. J Clin Ultrasound 11:23–27, 1983

126. Ohtomo K et al: Hepatic tumors: Differentiation by transverse relaxation time (T2) of magnetic resonance imaging. Radiology 155:421–423, 1985

127. Pagani J: Intrahepatic vascular territories shown by computed tomography. Radiology 147:173–178, 1983

128. Partain C et al: Nuclear magnetic resonance and computed tomography. Radiology 136:767–770, 1980

129. Pedrosa C et al: Computed tomography in obstructive jaundice. Radiology 139:635–645, 1981

130. Piekarski J et al: Difference between liver and spleen CT numbers in the normal adult: Its usefulness in predicting the presence of diffuse liver disease. Radiology 137:727–729, 1980

131. Prando A et al: Computed tomographic arteriography of the liver. Radiology 130:697–701, 1979

132. Quinn M et al: Computed tomography of the abdomen in evaluation of patients with fever of unknown origin. Radiology 136:407–411, 1980

133. Rahn N et al: CT appearance of sclerosing cholangitis. AJR 141:549–552, 1983

134. Ralls PW et al: Prospective evaluation of ^{99m}Tc-IDA cholescintigraphy and gray-scale ultrasound in the diagnosis of acute cholecystitis. Radiology 144:369, 1982

135. Ralls PW et al: Prospective evaluation of the sonographic Murphy's sign in suspected acute cholecystitis (abstr). Radiology 145:282, 1982

136. Reuben A et al: The value of hepatobiliary scanning in assessing graft function after liver transplantation (abstr). Hepatology 5:943, 1985

137. Ritchings RT et al: An analysis of the spatial distribution of attenuation values in computed tomographic scans of liver and spleen. J Comput Assist Tomogr 1:36–39, 1979

138. Roemer C et al: Hepatic cysts: Diagnosis and therapy by sonographic needle aspiration. AJR 136:1065–1070, 1981

139. Rogers J et al: Hepatic focal nodular hyperplasia: Angiography, CT, sonography and scintigraphy. AJR 137:983–990, 1981

140. Rose JL, Goldberg BB: Basic Physics in Diagnostic Ultrasound. New York, Wiley Medical, 1979

141. Rosen B et al: Proton chemical shift imaging: An evaluation of the clinical potential using an in vivo fatty liver model. Radiology 154:469–472, 1985

142. Rosenfield AT et al: Gray scale ultrasonography, computerized tomography in the evaluation of polycystic kidney and liver disease. Urology 9:436–438, 1977

143. Rosenthall L et al: Diagnosis of hepatobiliary disease by ^{99m}Tc-HIDA cholescintigraphy. Radiology 126:467–474, 1978

144. Rosenthall L et al: ^{99m}Tc-IDA hepatobiliary imaging following upper abdominal surgery. Radiology 130:735, 1979

145. Royal S et al: Detection and estimation of iron, glycogen and fat in the liver of children with hepatomegaly using CT. Pediatr Res 13:408, 1979

146. Runge VM et al: Nuclear magnetic resonance of iron and copper disease states. AJR 141:943–948, 1983

147. Sako S et al: Carcinoma of the extrahepatic bile ducts: Review of the literature and report of six cases. Surgery 41:416, 1957

148. Sample WF et al: Nuclear imaging, tomographic nuclear imaging and gray scale ultrasound in the evaluation of the porta hepatis. Radiology 122:773–779, 1977

149. Sample WF et al: Gray-scale ultrasonography of the jaundiced patient. Radiology 128:719–725, 1978

150. Sandler M et al: Ultrasonic features and radionuclide correlation in liver cell adenoma and focal nodular hyperplasia. Radiology 135:393–397, 1980

151. Scheible W et al: Gray scale echographic patterns of hepatic metastatic disease. AJR 129:983–987, 1977

152. Shanser JD et al: Computed tomographic diagnosis of obstructive jaundice in the absence of intrahepatic ductal dilatation. AJR 131:389–392, 1978

153. Shimizu H et al: The diagnostic accuracy of computed tomography in obstructive biliary disease: A comparative evaluation with direct cholangiography. Radiology 138:411–416, 1981

154. Shuman WP et al: PIPIDA scintigraphy for cholecystitis: False positives in alcoholism and total parenteral nutrition. AJR 138:1–5, 1982

155. Smathers R et al: Differentiation of complicated cholecystitis from gallbladder carcinoma by computed tomography. AJR 143:255–259, 1984

156. Solbiati L et al: Fine-needle biopsy of hepatic hemangioma with sonographic guidance. AJR 144:471–474, 1985

157. Stadalnik RC et al: Technetium-99m pyridoxylidene glutamate cholescintigraphy. Radiology 121:657–661, 1976

158. Stark D et al: Magnetic resonance imaging and spectroscopy of hepatic iron overload. Radiology 154:137–142, 1985

159. Stark D et al: Magnetic resonance imaging of cavernous hemangioma of the liver: Tissue specific characterization. AJR 145:213–222, 1985

160. Stark D et al: Chronic liver disease: Evaluation by magnetic resonance. Radiology 150:149–151, 1984

161. Stephenson TF et al: CT-guided Seldinger catheter drainage of a hepatic abscess. AJR 131:323–324, 1978

162. Sty JR et al: Technetium ^{99m} biliary imaging in pediatric surgical problems. J Pediatr Surg 16:686, 1981

163. Sty JR et al: Radionuclide hepatobiliary imaging in the detection of traumatic biliary tract disease in children. Pediatr Radiol 12:115, 1982

164. Sullivan DC et al: The use of ultrasound to enhance the diagnostic utility of the equivocal liver scintigraph. Radiology 128:727–732, 1978

165. Taylor KJW, Kremkau FW: Basic principles of diagnostic ultrasound. In Taylor KJW (ed): Atlas of Gray Scale Ultrasonography, 2nd ed, pp 1–22. Edinburgh, Churchill Livingstone, 1985

166. Taylor KJW, Viscomi GN: Spectrum of ultrasonic appearances of liver metastases and accuracy of the technique. Proceedings of EORTC Conference, Brussels, Belgium, 1978

167. Taylor KJW et al: Blood flow in deep abdominal and pelvic vessels: Ultrasonic pulsed Doppler analysis. Radiology 154:487–493, 1985

168. Taylor KJW et al: Gray scale ultrasound and isotope scanning: Complementary techniques for imaging the liver. AJR 128:277–281, 1977

169. Taylor KJW et al: Accuracy of grey-scale ultrasound diagnosis of abdominal and pelvic abscesses in 220 patients. Lancet 1:83–84, 1978

170. Taylor KJW et al: Diagnostic accuracy of gray scale ultrasonography for the jaundiced patient: A report of 275 cases. Arch Intern Med 139:60–63, 1979

171. Taylor KJW et al: Ultrasonography of alcoholic liver disease with a histological correlation. Radiology 141:157–161, 1981

172. Taylor KJW et al: Liver transplant recipients: Portable duplex US with correlative angiography. Radiology 159:357–363, 1986

173. Taylor KJW et al: Quantitative US attenuation in normal liver and in patients with diffuse liver disease: Importance of fat. Radiology 160:65–71, 1986

174. Thorsen M et al: Primary biliary carcinoma: CT evaluation. Radiology 152:479–483, 1984

175. Tolin RD et al: Enterogastric reflux in normal subjects and patients with Billroth II gastroenterostomy. Gastroenterology 77:1027, 1979

176. Waller R et al: Computed tomography and sonography of hepatic cirrhosis and portal hypertension. Radiographics 4:715, 1984

177. Weiner S et al: Sonography and computed tomography in the diagnosis of carcinoma of the gallbladder. AJR 142:735–739, 1984

178. Weinstein DP et al: Ultrasonography of biliary tract dilatation without jaundice. AJR 132:729–734, 1979

179. Weissmann HS, Freeman LM: The Biliary Tract. In Freeman LM, Johnson PM (eds): Clinical Radionuclide Imaging. New York, Grune & Stratton, 1984

180. Weissmann HS et al: Cholescintigraphy, ultrasonography and computerized tomography in the evaluation of biliary tract disorders. Semin Nucl Med 9:22–35, 1979

181. Weissmann HS et al: Spectrum of ^{99m}-Tc-IDA cholescintigraphic patterns in acute cholecystitis. Radiology 138:167, 1981

182. Weissmann HS et al: The clinical role of technetium 99m iminodiacetic acid cholescintigraphy. Nucl Med Annu 1981

183. Weissmann HS et al: Early diagnosis of acute common duct obstruction by ^{99m}Tc-IDA cholescintigraphy. J Nucl Med 21:41, 1980

184. Weissmann HS et al: Role of ^{99m}Tc-IDA scintigraphy in the evaluation of hepatobiliary trauma. Semin Nucl Med 13:199, 1983

185. Weissmann HS et al: Evaluation of the post-operative patient with ^{99m}Tc-IDA cholescintigraphy. Semin Nucl Med 12:27–51, 1982

186. Weltin G et al: Duplex Doppler—an aid in the diagnosis of cavernous transformation of the portal vein. AJR 144:999–1001, 1984

187. Wenker J et al: Focal fatty infiltration of the liver: Demonstration by magnetic resonance imaging. AJR 143:573–574, 1984

188. Wittenberg J, Ferrucci JT: Radiographically guided needle biopsy of abdominal neoplasms—who—where—why? J Clin Gastroenterol 1:273–284, 1979

189. Zeman RK et al: Ultrasound demonstration of anicteric dilatation of the biliary tree. Radiology 134:689–692, 1980

190. Zeman RK et al: Hepatobiliary scintigraphy and sonography in early biliary obstruction. Radiology 153:793–798, 1984

191. Zeman RK et al: Acute experimental biliary obstruction in the dog: Sonographic findings and clinical implications. AJR 136:965–967, 1981

192. Zeman RK et al: Strategy for the use of biliary scintigraphy in non-iatrogenic biliary trauma. Radiology 151:771–777, 1984

193. Zeman RK et al: Postcholecystectomy syndrome: Evaluation using biliary scintigraphy and endoscopic retrograde cholangiopancreatography. Radiology 156:787–792, 1985

194. Zeman RK et al: Ultrasonography and hepatobiliary scintigraphy in the assessment of biliary-enteric anastomoses. Radiology 145:109–115, 1982

chapter **11**

Gastrointestinal Endoscopy in the Diagnosis and Management of Hepatobiliary Disease

DAVID S. ZIMMON

The increased clinical skill and technical sophistication that the endoscopist has developed in the past few years is now supported by a vast array of new or improved techniques and devices that make previously difficult or impossible maneuvers simple and safe. Disillusionment with the accuracy of noninvasive investigation such as ultrasound, computed tomography, and isotopic hepatobiliary scanning[46,55] and appreciation of the risk and expense of the prolonged algorithmic diagnostic approach[73,106] has emphasized the value of prompt definitive diagnostic investigations in hepatobiliary diseases.[45] The virtue of a definitive endoscopic diagnosis in a patient with jaundice or gastrointestinal hemorrhage is amplified by the low risk and "noninvasive" character of diagnostic endoscopy and the proven efficacy of therapeutic endoscopy for numerous diseases.[11,105]

The close linkage between endoscopic diagnosis and therapy in the management of obstructive jaundice and gastrointestinal bleeding limit the value of noninvasive radiologic approaches since therapy is the ultimate goal. Exploratory surgery has receded with the development of palliative or definitive nonsurgical therapy. Endoscopic sclerosis replaces balloon tamponade[24,59] and surgical portacaval shunt[90] as the primary therapy for bleeding esophageal varices. Endoscopic sphincterotomy is the procedure of choice for postcholecystectomy choledocholithiases, papilla of Vater stenosis, and sphincter of Oddi dysfunction and for high-risk patients who have bile duct disease with gallbladder *in situ*. Endoscopic stents are used for palliation of the unfortunate majority of patients with malignant bile duct obstruction and yield results equal to surgical or radiologic techniques with less morbidity.[40,77]

Implied judgments as to the applicability of specific techniques to individual clinical situations must remain generalities. The constant competition among techniques (endoscopic, radiologic, and surgical) gives rise to productive tension that can only be resolved by careful clinical judgment in each individual patient. The senior field—surgery—is rapidly losing ground to the low-risk, shorter hospital stay, shorter convalescence, less painful, nonsurgical procedures.[14] The junior field—endoscopy—is rapidly gaining due to the low risk of diagnostic[4,34] and therapeutic maneuvers that do not traverse mucosal boundaries and therefore are noninvasive compared with percutaneous transhepatic puncture for cholangiography and stent placement[50] or varix sclerosis via retrograde portal catheterization.[5]

The endoscopist has the further advantage of withholding therapeutic commitment until after completion of a precise diagnostic survey. Therapy may be impossible in the jaundiced patient with multiple intrahepatic metastasis or hepatoma invading the proximal bile duct or unnecessary in gallstone pancreatitis if the stone has passed. Often temporizing procedures such as placement of a nasobiliary or nasopancreatic drain will relieve sepsis or pancreatitis. Definitive therapy may be delayed until the patient has been resuscitated. The excess risk of emergency intervention is obviated, and a low-risk procedure can replace high-risk emergent intervention. These concepts are important particularly when treating patients at high risk because of age or complicating cardiac, pulmonary, renal, or other disease or when the clinical circumstance increases risk, as in cholangitis with systemic sepsis.

Important in this litigious era is the precise preoperative documentation of indications and hazards if abdominal surgery is entertained. This can only be achieved by direct cholangiography. Intraoperative radiography often fails technically[29,96] or documents the fruitlessness of abdominal surgery after a laparotomy is underway.[14]

Preoperative biliary or pancreatic decompression particularly in high-risk patients is valuable even when surgical indications appear to be present.[8,104] For example, in periampullary cancer only a trial of biliary decompression will identify the one third of the patients in whom jaundice does not respond to relief of bile duct obstruction and who have an 88%, 30-day mortality.[9,52] The need for patient stratification by nonoperative biliary decompression in periampullary cancer testifies to the limitations of computed tomography and ultrasound in identifying patients who will not respond to surgical measures and should be spared this trauma in the last few weeks of their life.[40]

The ability to provide a precise diagnosis at low risk even in emergent clinical circumstances combined with numerous therapeutic alternative options to emergent abdominal surgery has advanced gastrointestinal endoscopy and endoscopic retrograde cholangiopancreatography to the forefront of diagnosis and management in hepatobiliary diseases. Close cooperation among the referring primary physician, endoscopists, radiologists, and surgeon is essential nevertheless if the benefits of these recent advances are to be translated into improved patient care.

ENDOSCOPIC RETROGRADE CHOLANGIOPANCREATOGRAPHY

Endoscopic retrograde cholangiopancreatography (ERCP) is a combined endoscopic and radiologic procedure that uses a specialized lateral viewing fiberoptic endoscope of 1 cm in diameter to visualize the upper gastrointestinal tract, identify the papilla of Vater, and, under visual control, cannulate the pancreatic or biliary duct system for the retrograde injection of radiopaque contrast media. This complex and highly sophisticated procedure has evolved rapidly over the past 15 years. The flexible endoscope contains fiberoptic bundles that transmit a bright light to the mucosal surface as well as a high-quality lens system coupled with a coherent fiberoptic bundle to return a detailed image of the mucosal surface to the endoscopist. A small channel allows the introduction of air under pressure to distend the intestine and inject small quantities of fluid to wash the lens and blow it dry. An instrument channel 4.2 mm in diameter courses the length of the endoscope to permit the passage of biopsy instruments, cannulating catheters, electrosurgical devices, and baskets or balloons for endoscopic manipulations. The distal tip of the endoscope is controlled by the operator, who adjusts the tension of cables within the endoscope wall with a series of concentric knobs in the handle.

Initially, attempts to cannulate the papilla of Vater were made with curved devices that were fashioned to fit the anatomy of the second duodenum and that used only radiologic control. Almost simultaneously, endoscopists appreciated the fact that the duodenum and papilla of Vater could be visualized with endoscopes primarily designed for examination of the upper gastrointestinal tract, particularly the stomach. These two lines of investigation rapidly converged. In 1970, Japanese investigators published preliminary experience with fiberoptic cannulation of the papilla of Vater for the performance of retrograde pancreatography and cholangiography.[56] The procedures were performed under general anesthesia, because they both were time consuming and required control of patient movement and peristalsis in the duodenum. From 1970

to the present, rapid technical advances in operator skill and appreciation of the pharmacology, radiology, and physiology of the duodenum, pancreas, and biliary tree have made ERCP a brief procedure. In expert hands, it requires only 10 to 15 minutes for the average patient. Therefore, the short-acting intravenous sedation employed for standard gastrointestinal fiberoptic endoscopy is adequate. As a result, ERCP is now commonly performed on an ambulatory basis. From the patient's viewpoint, ERCP is similar to a routine endoscopic examination.[34]

Diagnostic Spectrum

Since ERCP is a brief, atraumatic procedure, its use is limited only by the time and effort required to master its technical complexities. The diagnostic spectrum of this technique includes all the mucosal and submucosal diseases of the upper gastrointestinal tract from the esophagus to the jejunum that are elucidated by fiberoptic endoscopy. In addition, the proximal jejunum and periampullary area including the papilla of Vater may be examined in meticulous detail. Target biopsies of mucosal lesions, cytologic brush or fluid sampling, bile analysis or culture, and the collection of pancreatic secretion for biochemical or cytologic study may precede or follow radiologic examination of the pancreatic duct or biliary tree (Table 11-1).

ERCP is a remarkable advance in the diagnosis and management of pancreatic diseases. The pancreas had been an elusive organ because of its inaccessible retroperitoneal position and the substantial hazard associated with surgical exploration and biopsy. Fortunately, the pathologic changes associated with both chronic pancreatitis[108] and pancreatic neoplasia[101] are reflected in anatomic alterations of the duct system. Therefore, pancreatography provides a reliable and objective diagnostic tool for the definition of pancreatic disease (Fig. 11-1). This is in contrast to arteriography, with which pathologic change is seen late in pancreatic disease. Furthermore, after definition of a pancreatic ductal lesion, percutaneous biopsy under radiologic control has a high diagnostic yield with minimal risk in patients with neoplasia.[58] The pancreatogram defines the extent of pancreatic inflammatory disease as well as duct obstruction and the presence of intraductal calculi and yields a road map for the surgeon undertaking remedial pancreatic surgery (Fig. 11-2). Although percutaneous pancreatography using standard radiologic landmarks has been used successfully when ERCP has failed,[113] it must be considered a higher-risk, secondary procedure at least until more experience has been gathered. These general considerations can only hint at the revolutionary impact of endoscopic pancreatography on the diagnosis and management of pancreatic diseases.

Endoscopic cholangiography had its initial emphasis in the diagnosis of frankly jaundiced patients suspected of having extrahepatic bile duct obstruction when other more familiar techniques such as laparoscopy or percutaneous cholangiography were contraindicated. With the development of expertise, ERCP supplanted these techniques.

TABLE 11-1.   Diagnostic and Therapeutic Spectrum of Endoscopy with ERCP

FIBEROPTIC ENDOSCOPY (ESOPHAGUS TO JEJUNUM)
Mucosal diseases
  Inflammation (esophagitis, gastritis, duodenitis)
  Neoplasia
Submucosal diseases
  Esophagogastric varices
  Neoplasia
  Inflammation (pancreatitis)
Papilla of Vater
  Location
  Lumen
  Pathology (inflammation, neoplasia)
Diagnostic Aids
  Documentation and measurement (film, videotape)
  Cytologic, brush, or fluid samples
  Bile analysis and culture
  Bile duct biopsy with or without sphincterotomy
  Pancreatic secretion analysis, cytology, and culture
  Transduodenal endoscopic or percutaneous pancreatic biopsy guided by pancreatography
  Sphincter of Oddi manometry
  Trial of decompression by biliary or pancreatic stent or drain (pain, pancreatitis, or cholestasis)

ENDOSCOPIC RETROGRADE PANCREATOGRAPHY
Pancreatic inflammatory disease
Pancreatic neoplasia
Preoperative and postoperative pancreatic duct anatomy (plan surgery, avoid duodenotomy and pancreatography, progress of disease, confirm success of drainage)

ENDOSCOPIC RETROGRADE CHOLANGIOGRAPHY
Extrahepatic biliary tree (lithiasis, neoplasia, stricture, variant anatomy)

Cystic duct and gallbladder (lithiasis, neoplasia)
Intrahepatic biliary tree (infiltration, cirrhosis, abscess, neoplasia)

THERAPEUTIC ENDOSCOPY
Lithiasis: balloon or basket extraction/aided by balloon spincter dilatation or mechanical stone fragmentation-lithotripsy, endoscopic papillotomy, or sphincteroplasty
Papilla of Vater stenosis: endoscopic sphincteroplasty
Benign bile duct stenosis
  Distal: endoscopic sphincteroplasty and/or stents
  Proximal: stent(s) and/or balloon dilatation
Choledochocele: endoscopic excision
Neoplastic stenosis
  Papilla of Vater: infundibulotomy with stent(s) or stent(s)
  Distal and proximal bile duct: endoscopic papillotomy with stent(s)
Cholecystitis: retrograde irrigation with antibiotic, cystic duct disimpaction
Cholangitis
  Decompression: stone disimpaction and removal
  Irrigation: nasobiliary drain or stent(s)
Pancreatitis: sphincterotomy, stent or drain
Gallstone pancreatitis: urgent endoscopic sphincterotomy and stent
Pancreas divisum: pain or pancreatitis, duct of Santorini (minor papilla) stent
Anomolous biliary-pancreatic junction: sphincterotomy
Long common channel: sphincterotomy
Idiopathic pancreatitis: sphincterotomy
Pancreatitis with prepapillary stenosis or lithiasis: sphincterotomy, stone extraction, stent

It was then appreciated that the intrahepatic biliary tree provided important diagnostic information that could be gained with little hazard by a simple increase in the volume of contrast material injected.[22] Furthermore, ERCP allows the forceful injection of radiopaque contrast medium into the cystic duct and gallbladder as well as into the intrahepatic biliary tree beyond sites of obstruction. This permits therapeutic endoscopic options and the diagnosis of cystic duct obstruction.

The broad diagnostic spectrum of endoscopy combined with endoscopic retrograde pancreatography and cholangiography yields a positive diagnosis or excludes a wide spectrum of diseases when such diseases are clinically manifest or in their early stages, when symptoms are not typical or are transient.[34] In this sense, a negative ERCP carries great weight and generally terminates the diagnostic workup. Furthermore, access to the gastrointestinal tract through the natural orifices of the mouth and the papilla

of Vater allows these procedures to be performed with a minimum of risk. Although retrograde cholangiopancreatography was approached with great trepidation, it early became apparent that, in experienced hands, complications rarely if ever occur in patients without obstructed duct systems.[68,109] Because of this, ERCP approaches the ideal for an "invasive" diagnostic procedure, since any hazard is appropriate to the diagnostic yield with little risk incurred in the absence of mechanical duct obstruction. In patients with intrahepatic cholestasis, for example, ERCP carries little or no risk, even if severe hepatic dysfunction is present. Suspected sepsis or hemorrhagic disorders are not contraindications.

With these concepts in mind, endoscopy combined with ERCP became an important primary diagnostic procedure for seriously ill patients suspected of disease of the biliary tract or pancreas.[110] After our initial experience in developing technical skill, my colleagues and I studied a con-

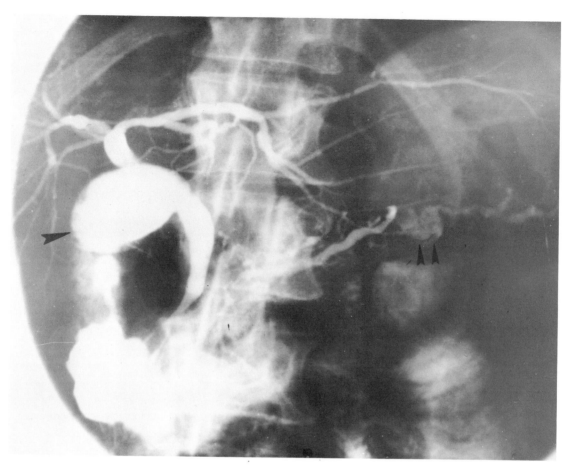

Fig. 11-1. Endoscopic cholangiogram and pancreatogram from a patient who had recurrent attacks of pancreatitis. The cholangiogram demonstrates a small shrunken gallbladder with multiple radiolucent stones (*single large arrow*). The common duct is slightly dilated and tapers within the pancreas, indicating extrinsic compression. The pancreatic duct is irregular with dilated and clubbed secondary pancreatic radicles, suggesting the presence of acute or early chronic pancreatitis. An area of ductal disruption and pseudocyst formation is seen in the midportion of the pancreas (*two small arrows*). This is an example of pancreatitis associated with gallstones in which disruption of the pancreatic duct and pseudocyst formation have taken place.

secutive series of 91 patients, aged 23 to 70, with a tentative diagnosis on admission of rapidly evolving serious pancreatic or biliary tract disease that might require prompt abdominal surgery. Endoscopic visualization of the entire upper gastrointestinal tract and identification of the papilla of Vater was successful in all but one patient, who had an active duodenal ulcer with pyloric stenosis. Chronic pancreatitis in exacerbation was confirmed at laparotomy. A positive diagnosis was established in the remaining patients by either endoscopy or cholangiopancreatography in 77 of 91 (85%). Endoscopy yielded the diagnosis in 13 (17%), cholangiography in 39 (51%), and pancreatography in 25 (32%). In 53 jaundiced patients, the etiology of the jaundice was established by endoscopy in 11 and by retrograde radiographic studies in 33, for a diagnostic success rate of 83%. Distal common bile duct obstruction demonstrated by subsequent percutaneous transhepatic cholangiography (PTC) prevented collection of bile or retrograde cholangiography in two patients with choledocholithiasis. A normal extrahepatic biliary tree was found by retrograde cholangiography in 25 of 29 patients (86%) with intrahepatic cholestasis.

The diagnosis of pancreatitis with a precipitating cause (gallstones) or complication (pseudocyst) was established in 27 patients. Of 51 patients with acute pancreatitis, alcohol abuse was a factor in 11, and gallstones were present in 4. Of 12 patients with chronic pancreatitis, pseudocyst was found in 2.

This integrated approach to the diagnosis of rapidly evolving intra-abdominal disease narrows the diagnostic

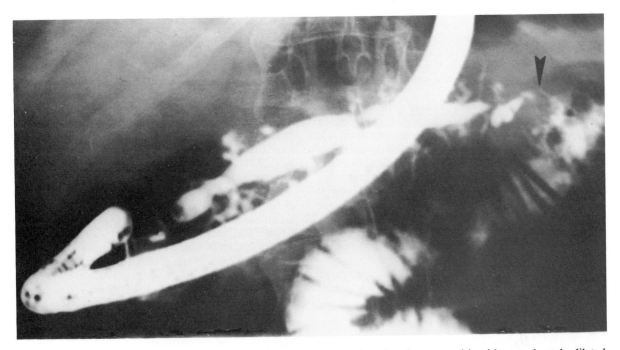

Fig. 11-2. Retrograde pancreatogram showing chronic pancreatitis with a moderately dilated main pancreatic duct and dilated secondary radicles extending laterally from it. An area of ductal stricture is seen in the head of the pancreas adjacent to the tip of the endoscope (*small arrow*). Contrast medium has been forced through this blocked segment. The terminal pancreatic duct is narrowed, with two areas of stricture. The black arrow on the right marks the site of a pancreaticojejunostomy performed at the time of a previous pancreatic resection. The pancreaticojejunostomy was performed because an earlier pancreatogram had shown the obstruction in the head of the pancreas demonstrated here. This anastomosis is not considered adequate for drainage of the pancreas, because a stricture has formed at the anastomosis. Delayed films prepared after withdrawal of the endoscope demonstrated extremely slow emptying of contrast from the pancreatic duct system. This surgical attempt to relieve pancreatic duct obstruction and preserve the function of the gland must be considered a technical failure.

field and yet leaves little residual. It may be preceded by an ultrasound examination and followed immediately by laparotomy, liver biopsy, percutaneous cholangiography, angiography, intravenous pyelography, or evaluation of the colon. If a team is available to perform ERCP on an emergency basis for patients who may require immediate abdominal surgery, it seems reasonable to follow this same rapid advantageous route in the evaluation of less seriously ill individuals rather than following proposed algorithms that emphasize noninvasive procedures, require numerous intervals for gut cleansing after barium or other radiopaque contrast agents, and ultimately require a procedure that yields a definitive anatomic diagnosis.[73,106]

Indications

After analysis of the procedure records of our first 1089 attempts at ERCP, we defined groups of indications in retrospect.[34] Only one third of the patients studied were investigated for cholestasis. In jaundiced patients, ERCP immediately displaced intravenous cholangiography, be-

cause, even when bilirubin levels are below 3 mg/dl, intravenous cholangiography fails to visualize the bile duct adequately in 45% of patients and yields a high incidence (40%) of both false-positive and false-negative interpretive errors.[26]

ERCP is unique in visualizing the pancreatic duct for the diagnosis of neoplasm or inflammatory disease. Approximately 20% of the patients were studied for the evaluation of the pancreatic duct system to confirm a clinical suspicion of pancreatic neoplasia when initial studies were negative or to differentiate inflammatory from neoplastic masses and estimate resectability before laparotomy.

Patients with gallbladder disease were either evaluated during active illness or presented as diagnostic problems in which ultrasound, oral cholecystography, or intravenous cholangiography had failed to adequately visualize the gallbladder or indicate a cause for pain. In this 10% of the patients, ERCP was used to document the presence of gallstones, prove the presence of cystic duct obstruction, or demonstrate a rigid nondistensible gallbladder as an indication for cholecystectomy.[89]

Ten percent of the patients were studied for postcholecystectomy syndromes in which high-resolution cholangiography was essential to rule out the presence of small stones retained in the common bile duct or in the cystic duct stump as well as to rule out other gastrointestinal tract or pancreatic diseases.

Twenty percent of the patients were evaluated for abdominal pain.[67] This group yielded a wide spectrum of diagnoses and often multiple pathologic processes that made it difficult to determine the origin of the pain precipitating evaluation. Particularly in populations in which alcohol abuse is frequent and biliary lithiasis is commonplace, peptic ulcer, duodenitis, cholelithiasis, and pancreatitis often coexist and make determination of the source of pain or signs of inflammation difficult (Fig. 11-3).

Diagnostic Value

Methods for quantitating diagnostic value have received considerable attention. Narrowly focused studies such as oral cholecystography, radionuclide biliary scanning, or PTC may be considered diagnostically successful if they visualize the gallbladder, demonstrate cystic duct patency, or visualize the biliary tree. A broad diagnostic test such as endoscopy with ERCP may establish or rule out numerous diagnoses. As has been emphasized, incidental pathologic processes such as cholelithiasis often coexist with other causes of jaundice or abdominal pain. The ideal diagnostic test must either identify the only pathologic process producing the patient's signs and symptoms or exclude all pathologic processes by examination of the entire upper gastrointestinal tract, biliary tree, and pancreatic duct. Although no single diagnostic test can exclude all forms of upper gastrointestinal tract disease, endoscopy combined with ERCP most closely approaches this ideal when the upper gastrointestinal tract from the esophagus to the jejunum is visualized endoscopically and both pancreatic and biliary duct systems are radiologically opacified.

The diagnostic value of ERCP in 1089 patients was

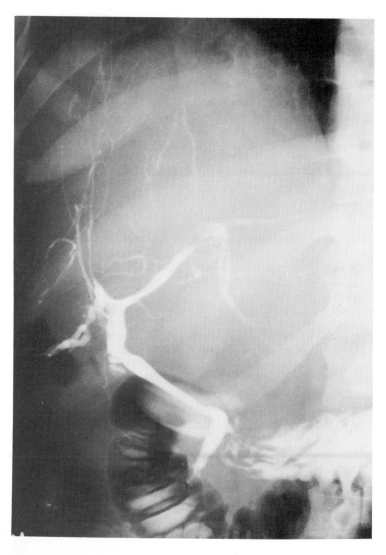

Fig. 11-3. ERCP in a jaundiced patient with chronic active hepatitis following cholecystectomy. Laboratory data suggested extrahepatic obstruction. The intrahepatic bile ducts are compressed and distorted by regeneration and fibrosis. Caudate lobe hypertrophy splays and displaces the right and left hepatic ducts inferiorly. Shrinkage of the right lobe with massive hypertrophy of the left lobe has shifted the porta hepatis to the right and angulated the common bile duct. A short cystic duct stump is visible. The possibility of extrahepatic bile duct obstruction was ruled out by this examination. The compression with narrowing of the intrahepatic bile ducts and distorted anatomy, along with the presence of severe fibrosis and portal hypertension, would make a percutaneous transhepatic examination in this patient both likely to fail and hazardous.

estimated on this basis. Diagnostic studies were carried out in 75.2% of these patients. Endoscopic findings alone established a diagnosis in 4.4%. Endoscopy with cannulation and opacification of both pancreatic and biliary ducts was carried out in 45.4%. Endoscopy with opacification of a single duct demonstrating a diagnostic pattern was done in 25.4%. Diagnostic studies were done in 83.5% of 201 consecutive patients studied at St. Vincent's Hospital in New York. In this subgroup, endoscopic findings were positive in 7.5%. Both pancreatic and bile ducts were visualized in 54%. A single diagnostic duct was visualized in 21.8%. A nondiagnostic duct was cannulated in 9.5%. In only 7% of the patients was the papilla of Vater not cannulated and the diagnostic value therefore limited to the endoscopic examination. Therefore, in this subgroup, diagnostic studies were done in 83.5% and the entire diagnostic spectrum of endoscopy and ERCP was covered in 54%.

Complications

This initial experience with 1000 cases studied before 1975 has been vastly improved on.[34] With greater experience, improved radiologic equipment, and a better understanding of the physiology, pharmacology, and pathology of the biliary tree and pancreas, the diagnostic success rate increases, and complications decrease. Failure to cannulate a specific duct by an experienced operator indicates an unusual anatomic condition or disease within the duct system. During the years from 1970 to 1975, the Erlangen group, under the direction of Demling, performed 2507 examinations.[4] They increased their success rate from 88.3% to 94.5%. At the same time, the incidence of complication fell from 7.4% in the years 1970 to 1973 to 1.3% in 1975.

Complications have been further reduced by recent advances in the management of bile obstruction with the use of endoscopic retrograde biliary drains and stents and percutaneous biliary drainage.[114] The two deaths after ERCP in our first 1089 cases (0.18%) would both have been managed by these newer methods. One of the patients died of cholangitis after ERCP for bile duct obstruction secondary to carcinoma of the pancreas. At the time, the patient's condition was considered inoperable. Today, she would have managed with either an endoscopic retrograde stent or a percutaneous transhepatic biliary drain or stent.

The second patient with choledocholithiasis died after surgery for biliary tract and pancreatic sepsis. Today, she would have been managed by an endoscopic sphincterotomy (Fig. 11-4).

Failure

The identification of the papilla of Vater and cannulation of its 2-mm potential orifice requires precise control of endoscope, cannula, duodenal peristasis, and patient movement. This is achieved by the meticulous intravenous use of sedatives combined with glucagon, a potent agent for producing duodenal aperistalsis and relaxation of the papilla of Vater with minimal systemic effects. Glucagon is a major advance over atropine. In our initial report of ERCP complications,[109] atropine toxicity played a major role and limited our approach to patients with severe cardiac or pulmonary disease. This problem has been completely overcome with glucagon, with which systemic effects on the heart, lungs, and urinary bladder are rarely observed. During the course of endoscopy and ERCP, instrumental manipulation and the passage of time evoke peristalsis in the duodenum. Instrumentation of the papilla of Vater produces sphincter spasm. After successful cannulation of the duct of prime clinical interest, the time required for careful injection of radiopaque contrast medium, patient positioning, and radiography may force termination of the procedure when aperistalsis and relaxation of the periampullary musculature is lost. Cannulation of the insignificant duct may result from pathologic obstruction in the duct of prime clinical interest that lies immediately adjacent or from the technical problem of passing a small catheter into the relatively collapsed distal part of the other duct system after the injection of contrast medium into the insignificant system. Periampullary cancer may infiltrate the duct system to produce obstruction without evidence of mucosal disease. The cannulating catheter may enter a papilla with a normal configuration but not pass beyond 6 mm, and contrast medium cannot be injected into the ducts. These cases appear to be pharmacologic failures of sphincter relaxation, given that no anatomic cause for failure to cannulate is evident endoscopically. With increasing experience, it is frequently possible to position the cannulation catheter directly within the orifice of the duct and, by force, to inject contrast material through the obstructed segment or demonstrate a short obstructed segment of normal duct (Fig. 11-5). Initial publications emphasize the limitation of ERCP in visualizing the duct system proximal to an obstruction. This problem has been overcome with appreciation of the technical problems and improved radiographic technique. It is generally feasible to inject contrast retrograde through obstructing lesions in the pancreatic duct or biliary tree when clinically indicated.[12,82,104] Furthermore, techniques for endoscopic dilatation of stenotic segments, passage of stents or drains, and electrosurgical incision and drainage are well established.

Anatomic causes for failure to cannulate include pyloric obstruction, a Bilroth II gastrectomy, a papilla within a diverticulum, and severe narrowing of the duodenum associated with pancreatitis or neoplastic infiltration.

COMPARISON OF ENDOSCOPIC RETROGRADE CHOLANGIOPANCREATOGRAPHY AND PERCUTANEOUS TRANSHEPATIC CHOLANGIOGRAPHY

It should be apparent that the precision of diagnosis required for the appropriate management of bile duct obstruction cannot be achieved by any method but direct

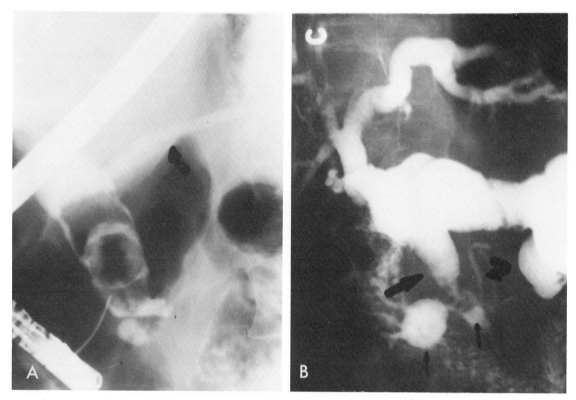

Fig. 11-4. A. The common bile duct after ERCP in a 76-year-old man who presented with fever and jaundice. The pancreatic duct is normal (*curved arrow*). Three common-duct stones measuring 2 cm in diameter are impacted in the distal common bile duct. The size of the stones was determined by comparison with the endoscope, which is 1 cm in diameter. After the biliary tree had been opacified and the diagnosis established, an endoscopic sphincterotomy was performed. The sphincterotomy catheter containing an opaque wire is seen at the upper margin of the sphincterotomy, which is about 3 cm in length. This produced a lateral choledochoduodenostomy that allowed extraction of the three stones. **B.** A gastrointestinal series was performed 2 days after passage of the stones. The curved arrow shows the pancreatic duct outlined by barium. The large straight arrow indicates the distal common bile duct. The two small vertical arrows show barium in periampullary diverticula on either side of the common bile duct. Dilatation of the intrahepatic bile ducts testifies to this patient's long-standing high-grade bile duct obstruction.

cholangiography or pancreatography.[45,55] The endoscopic portion of ERCP completes the diagnostic workup of the upper gastrointestinal tract and is used to avoid barium contrast studies that impede sophisticated tests. On the other hand, PTC generally requires a preliminary evaluation of the upper gastrointestinal tract. In this sense, ERCP is a primary diagnostic procedure that may be performed after the initial history, physical examination, and minimal laboratory evaluations if clinically indicated. PTC has a diagnostic spectrum limited to visualization of the biliary tree and, occasionally, the pancreatic duct by reflux.[103] When the Chiba "fine" (0.7 mm) technique is used, the duct system is often filled by injection of contrast material into the needle track. Contrast medium streams through the track into the punctured duct and simulta-

neously through the punctured vascular spaces. Bile also refluxes from the punctured duct into the vascular spaces. This bile duct to blood vessel fistula[38] limits the volume and pressure of contrast medium entering the gallbladder and bile duct, and inadequate radiographs may result. Even though bile duct dilatation and mechanical obstruction is confirmed, sufficient information for a precise diagnosis may be lacking. Failure to visualize the distal biliary tree and pancreatic duct beyond the obstruction prevents a definitive differential diagnosis of periampullary cancer when carcinoma of the pancreas must be differentiated from more favorable, operable lesions (Fig. 11-6).[14]

The complications of ERCP[4,34] are much less frequent than those of PTC[39,103] and are rare in the absence of duct

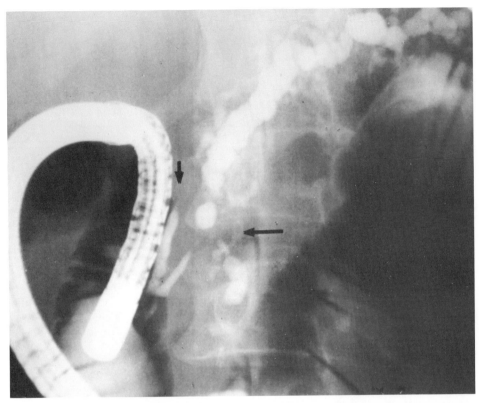

Fig. 11-5. Both the common bile duct and the pancreatic duct are opacified on this ERCP film. The common bile duct on the left (*short arrow*) is obstructed 2 cm above the papilla of Vater. The pancreatic duct on the right (*long arrow*) shows an area of no ducts 1 cm above the papilla of Vater (field defect) and markedly dilated proximal ducts and ducts extending inferiorly into the uncinate process. The mass (approximately 2 cm in diameter) that blocks both the pancreatic and the biliary ducts represents the "double duct sign" characteristic of pancreatic carcinoma.

obstruction. In particular, ERCP is the procedure of choice in patients with relative or absolute contraindications to PTC. This includes patients with known or suspected liver disease, patients who are poor operative risks when obstructive jaundice must be ruled out, patients with a bleeding diathesis, and patients suspected of having diseases in which PTC is risky or unlikely to succeed, such as sclerosing cholangitis or metastatic liver disease.[22] When there is no intrahepatic bile duct dilatation, the success rate of PTC is 70% at best, whereas ERCP visualizes the bile duct in 85% to 95% of patients, depending on the experience of the endoscopist.

A large category of patients in whom ERCP is superior to PTC consists of those in whom a pancreatogram is required. This includes patients with known or suspected pancreatic inflammatory disease and patients with suspected gallstone pancreatitis. Cholecystectomy is unlikely to help patients with chronic pancreatitis, a diagnosis easily established with pancreatography.

The largest group of patients in whom ERCP is vital consists of suspected cases of periampullary neoplasia.

Although it is possible to be suspicious of carcinoma of the pancreas from the appearance of a percutaneous cholangiogram, it is difficult to differentiate carcinoma of the pancreas from cancer of the terminal bile duct or of the papilla of Vater or from a neoplastic process invading the porta hepatis. Pancreatography, on the other hand, gives a definitive diagnosis of carcinoma of the pancreas.[14] Atlthough percutaneous aspiration biopsy of obstructing ductal lesions is extremely useful (Fig. 11-7) for histologic documentation of cancer, it does not differentiate adenocarcinoma of the bile duct or papilla, a resectable and curable lesion, from carcinoma of the head of the pancreas, a rarely resectable and even more rarely curable lesion that may be managed with biliary stents to avoid the risk and disability of laparotomy when life expectancy is short (Fig. 11-8).[40,77] Similarly, pancreatography allows separation of adenocarcinoma rising from the duct system from the rare endocrine tumors that arise in the parenchyma of the gland.

The removal of common duct stones by endoscopic techniques has been raised to a high art (Figs. 11-4, 11-

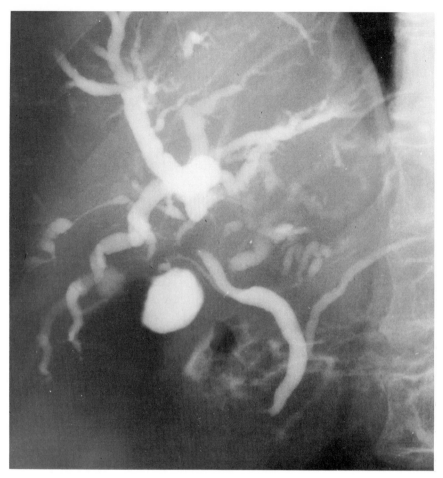

Fig. 11-6. A deeply jaundiced patient, who had had a colon carcinoma resected several years earlier, presented with intense cholestasis, suggesting extrahepatic bile duct obstruction. ERCP showed the distal common bile duct to be normal. There is compression of the hepatic duct with amputation of the cystic duct and an irregular collection of contrast within the gallbladder (*small arrowhead*). The intrahepatic ducts are alternately dilated and compressed. A typical segment of compressed proximal bile duct can be seen with a markedly dilated distal portion extending to the left (*large arrowhead*). This finding is characteristic of intrahepatic metastatic cancer producing intrahepatic bile duct obstruction and dilatation. Puncture of the liver may produce marked leakage of bile.

9). This is the procedure of choice in patients who have undergone cholecystectomy and in high-risk patients with the gallbladder *in situ.*[21,31,53,71] If ERCP is to be the definitive therapeutic mode, little is to be gained by accepting the risk of a diagnostic PTC. Therefore, the above categories of patients should be submitted to ERCP for diagnosis and therapy. PTC is a secondary procedure and ERCP primary in terms of point of application in the diagnostic work up, diagnostic yield, and relative risk (Table 11-2).

Access to the Biliary Tree

To appreciate the complications of PTC and ERCP, it is necessary to understand the concepts of direct cholangiography[13] and the therapy of bile duct disease that these techniques afford.[114] Both ERCP and PTC provide access to the biliary tree without laparotomy, but they do so by different routes. In PTC, the skin, peritoneum, hepatic capsule, and hepatic parenchyma are penetrated to enter the biliary tree. It is often necessary to puncture the liver numerous times to position a needle in the bile ducts and inject contrast material. Once the contrast medium is introduced into the liver, a second puncture may be required with a larger-bore catheter needle in order that a drain or stent may be placed in the main biliary tree.[114]

During the performance of this series of hepatic punctures and manipulations, the complications of PTC arise. The puncture of dilated bile ducts or blood vessels on the hepatic surface results in bile leakage into the peritoneal cavity[33] or intra-abdominal hemorrhage.[49] Laceration of vessels within the hepatic parenchyma produces intrahepatic hematomas similar to those seen at liver biopsy.[27] The track of the needle produces a fistula between the vascular system and the bile duct that risks the passage of bile into the blood.[38] In patients with bile duct obstruction, the pressure in the biliary tree exceeds that in the hepatic veins and the intra-abdominal cavity. In patients with cholangitis, either clinically apparent or occult, this bile to blood fistula may produce gram-negative shock or sepsis when a large volume of infected bile passes directly into the bloodstream. The leakage of bile into the peritoneal cavity may produce bile peritonitis or, in the antibiotic-treated patient, appear in the postoperative period as a subphrenic or subhepatic abscess. These complications accrue to the surgeon. In addition, hemobilia is occasion-

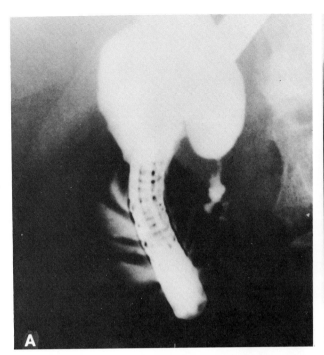
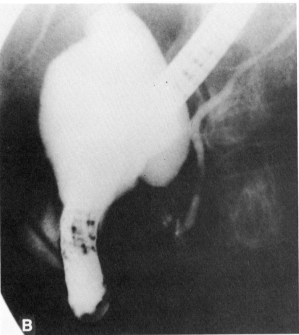

Fig. 11-7. A. On this ERCP film, the endoscope (1 cm in diameter) is seen in the duodenum. The large arrow marks an irregular stenotic segment of the distal bile duct just adjacent to the papilla of Vater. Radiopaque contrast material has been instilled through the strictured segment to delineate the dilated bile duct above it. The short, irregular stenotic segment (<1 cm in length) is typical of primary bile duct carcinoma. This patient had resection for cure. **B.** Additional information gained from retrograde pancreatography: The pancreatic duct adjacent to the distal bile duct carcinoma shows compression (*arrow*) from infiltration by the surrounding tumor. The remainder of the proximal duct is normal. This confirms the presence of a primary bile duct carcinoma less than 2 cm in diameter.

ally precipitated by PTC. These potentially serious complications require meticulous follow-up after the procedure, as does liver biopsy. Their relatively frequent occurrence make it advisable that laparotomy follow PTC promptly when duct obstruction is present if some other decompressive maneuver is not performed. Similarly, the intrinsic risks of the percutaneous transhepatic technique account for the need for prophylactic antibiotic therapy, which should be initiated at least 24 hours before PTC. Shock may follow the creation of a bile to blood fistula when endotoxin is released, even though the bacteria are not viable. We follow the contraindications described by Okuda, including bleeding tendency, sensitivity to iodine, high or continuous fever, poor general condition, extreme jaundice, ascites, moderate to severe anemia, and recent severe pain.[57]

ERCP has the virtue of approaching the biliary tree through the duodenum and papilla of Vater. This avoids the problems associated with the PTC techniques. There is no risk of hemorrhage, bile duct to blood vessel fistula, or bile leakage into the peritoneal cavity. Because the duodenal route is not sterile, bacteria contamination of

the obstructed biliary tree or pancreatic duct was anticipated when ERCP was first initiated; however, this early concern appears to have been unwarranted. The initial septic complications reported with the use of ERCP were traced to inadequate disinfection of the endoscope.[20] Many early complications of ERCP were the result of poor techniques and drugs that are no longer in use.[109] It was common to fill ductal systems until adequate radiographic detail was obtained. This high pressure provoked both disruption of biliary epithelium with fever and pancreatitis.[27] Furthermore, it did not yield superior radiographs. Subsequently, we learned to inject relatively small amounts of radiopaque contrast and to manipulate the patient's position to fill all the ducts. The simultaneous use of prophylactic antibiotics may also be of value, but attempts to study the efficacy of a prophylactic antibiotic after ERCP have been thwarted by the infrequency of septic complications.

Initially, there was great concern that pancreatography would initiate pancreatitis in a normal duct system or aggravate it in patients with pancreatitis. This has not proved true. With proper technique, only a small amount

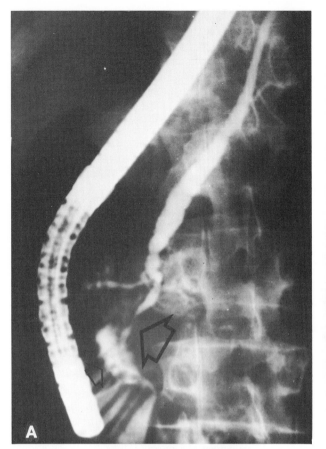

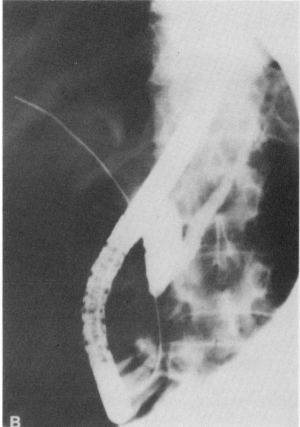

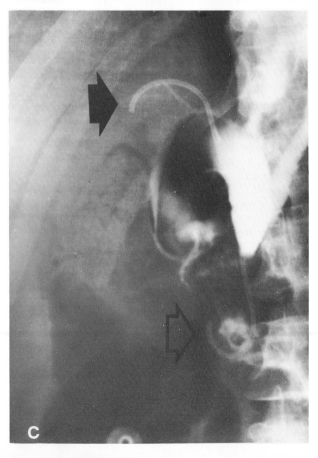

Fig. 11-8. A. Retrograde pancreatogram showing the endoscope in the position of cannulation. The small open arrow is placed just above the cannulating catheter, which can be seen passing into the papilla of Vater. A short normal segment of the pancreatic duct is visible in front of a minute stenotic area (*large arrowhead*). The more proximal pancreatic duct is normal and drains effectively through the duct of Santorini. This stenotic area is a constricting carcinoma of the pancreas. **B.** After repositioning of the endoscopic catheter in the common bile duct, the dilated distal common bile duct in this jaundiced patient is visible. A stenting wire guide was passed through the cannulating catheter above the contrast-filled distal common bile duct into the hepatic duct. The common bile duct measures about 12 mm in diameter when compared to the endoscope. **C.** The double pigtail multihole endoscopic biliary stent is positioned with its upper pigtail in the hepatic duct above the stenosis (*closed arrowhead*). The lower pigtail (*open arrowhead*) is seen in the duodenum. Contrast and bile enter the pigtail in the hepatic duct to traverse the stenosis within the stent and exit into the duodenum. In this patient, the diagnostic ERCP and therapeutic biliary stent were combined as a single procedure.

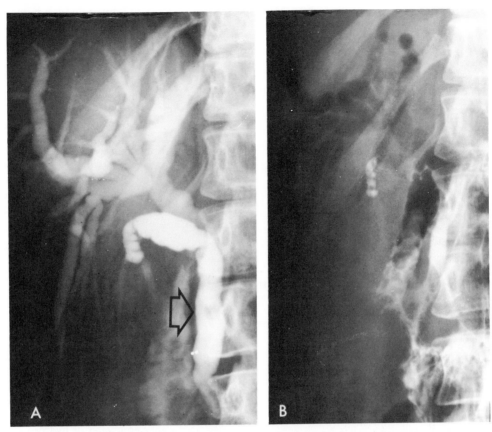

Fig. 11-9. A. Diagnostic ERCP showing a 7-mm stone in the midcommon bile duct that was forced upward from its site of impaction in the distal bile duct by the injection of radiopaque contrast and gentamicin. The dilated cystic duct stump and intrahepatic ducts result from high-grade bile duct obstruction and cholangitis. **B.** After endoscopic sphincterotomy, the stone and contrast have passed into the duodenum, and the biliary tree is filled with air. Biliary decompression was achieved without the risk of peritoneal soilage.

of contrast is injected, and its position is followed fluoroscopically so that the ducts are not distended. This is in contrast to operative or percutaneous pancreatography,[20] with which it is much more difficult to monitor the quantity and pressure of contrast material injected.

Obviously, if there is no therapeutic benefit for the patient, no procedures should be performed. We do not advocate the performance of pancreatography in patients with exacerbation of chronic pancreatitis unless an unfavorable course indicates a likely remedial complication.[7] In patients suspected of gallstone pancreatitis, ERCP remains the diagnostic procedure of choice, and pancreatography can be performed with impunity, providing that proper technique is followed (see Fig. 11-11).[25,66,70,87]

Sphincter of Oddi Manometry

Sphincter of Oddi manometry is an interesting investigational technique that has been proposed as a method for identifying patients with presumed biliary pain who do not have objective evidence of duct obstruction. Although a number of functional abnormalities of the sphincter mechanism have been identified,[2] the correlation between response of pain to endoscopic sphincterotomy and sphincter of Oddi manometry is disputed.[54,65] Clearly, an initial period of temporizing drug therapy should be undertaken in the absence of objective signs of biliary tract disease. In a patient who is disabled by abdominal pain thought to be of biliary origin, an endoscopic sphincterotomy is probably justified as an alternative to the transabdominal sphincteroplasty. In a group of carefully selected patients in whom objective evidence of disease has been excluded by careful cholangiopancreatography, approximately one half of the patients achieve substantial relief of their symptoms.[65] This is a taxing group of patients to manage either by use of drugs or endoscopic sphincterotomy. To date there has been little satisfaction from provocative or manometric investigations.

TABLE 11-2.   Diagnostic and Therapeutic Spectrum of Endoscopy

DIAGNOSIS IN ESOPHAGEAL VARICES

Documentation (color film, videotape)
Measurement (size, extent)
Direct measurement of portal pressure by transesophageal puncture
Direction of variceal blood flow (Doppler ultrasound probe)
Identification of subepithelial vascular channels on varices
Detection of variceal bleeding site
Identification of alternative potential or actual bleeding site (gastritis, ulcer)

THERAPY

Endoscopic injection varix sclerosis
   Intravariceal sclerosis
   Paravariceal sclerosis
Endoscopic laser varix sclerosis
Endoscopic therapy of associated nonvariceal hemorrhage (gastritis, ulcer, Mallory-Weiss esophageal laceration) with electrocoagulation, injection sclerosis, or laser

Pancreas Divisum

Pancreas divisum is the most common anomaly of the pancreatic duct system, occurring in 7% to 9% of the surveyed population.[18] It is thought to rarely be associated with pancreatitis either as a result of hypoplasia or acquired stenosis of the duct system as it enters the duodenum or of the unique, separate blood supply, acinar structure, and hormonal character of the dorsal and ventral segments.[35,80] Endoscopic and surgical therapy directed at either dorsal or ventral pancreas has met with varied success[91] and must be applied on a highly individualized basis.[16]

Sclerosing Cholangitis

Sclerosing cholangitis is a subtle inflammatory disease of the biliary tree associated with a high incidence of potentially curable bile duct neoplasms and remedial intrahepatic and extrahepatic bile duct strictures.[92] Liver biopsy may be suggestive, but only cholangiography gives a definitive diagnosis and identifies threatening lesions.[19] ERCP is the diagnostic procedure of choice and may be useful for biopsy, balloon dilatation, or stenting of obstructing lesions of the main duct system.

ENDOSCOPIC RETROGRADE CHOLANGIOPANCREATOGRAPHY AS A THERAPEUTIC PROCEDURE

In the past, only abdominal surgery could approach the biliary tree. The surgeon drained and irrigated an infected bile duct. If he could not remove the obstruction, he placed a stent (T-tube) through it or performed a biliodigestive anastomosis. Similar technical and therapeutic goals may be achieved without laparotomy by ERCP or PTC.[7,40,65,66,105]

Local Injection of Antibiotics

Systemically administered antibiotics do not penetrate closed spaces such as an obstructed bile duct during an episode of cholangitis or an acute empyema of the gallbladder. If percutaneous cholangiography is performed on a patient with cholangitis, an attempt should be made to decompress the biliary tree, and antibiotics should be injected. When the distal bile duct is patent, the flow of bile into the duodenum may prevent the filling of a diseased gallbladder with radiopaque contrast material or antibiotics.

ERCP uses the retrograde route for the injection of radiopaque contrast medium under pressure. This forces antibiotics into obstructed areas, including the gallbladder and the common bile duct proximal to obstructing stones or tumors. Failure to fill the gallbladder at ERCP indicates cystic duct obstruction and either empyema or hydrops when acute gallbladder disease is present. The forceful injection of antibiotics into the biliary tree at ERCP may open an occluded cystic duct and visualize the gallbladder. When acute empyema is present, 80 mg of gentamicin mixed with contrast medium is injected. In this way, the acute empyema is sterilized and drained, and elective surgery with its lesser hazards can be performed. Cystic duct obstruction in the presence of acute symptoms indicates either empyema or hydrops. This is an important indication for emergency surgery in patients with acute empyema of the gallbladder, because, on conservative management, resolution is unlikely, and perforation is frequent. These findings are particularly valuable in diabetic patients, who often present with little more than fever and slight right upper quadrant discomfort. Exclusion of gallbladder disease is essential in these patients, because perforation is common if surgery is not performed.

Irrigation of the Biliary Tree and Gallbladder

In cholecystitis or cholangitis, pus and biliary sludge may obstruct the flow of bile, preventing drainage and recovery. Irrigation of the common bile duct or the gallbladder by ERCP washes the obstructing material into the duodenum. Small stones may be forced into the duodenum by the injection of contrast material. Retrograde irrigation combined with balloons or ureteral-type baskets may be used to extract small stones from the common bile duct. When, as in 20% of patients with choledocholithiasis, the previous passage of common duct stones has created a biliary fistula or the papilla has been enlarged surgically by sphincterotomy or sphincteroplasty, stones larger than 1 cm in diameter may be extracted by ERCP.[112] A similar approach is used to remove obstructing food or stones in patients after choledochoduodenostomy.

Drainage

Spontaneous drainage of the gallbladder or bile duct occurs after antibiotic therapy in the majority of patients with cholecystitis or cholangitis. This favorable outcome may be accelerated by the local injection of antibiotics and irrigation. Reimpaction of common duct stones can be prevented and continued drainage ensured by the use of drains placed in the common bile duct at ERCP through the papilla of Vater (Fig. 11-10). The retrograde endoscopic methods avoid all the complications inherent in the percutaneous transhepatic technique when it is used in a patient with infected bile. ERCP is particularly advantageous, because patients with choledocholithiasis often do not have dilated intrahepatic bile ducts, and PTC therefore succeeds in only 70%. Furthermore, it is technically demanding to place a percutaneous drain in a biliary tree that is not dilated.

Preoperative biliary drainage is used to reduce operative mortality in patients with periampullary cancer. Nakayama and co-workers[51] have demonstrated a reduction in operative mortality from 28% to 8% ($p < .05$) when preoperative bilirubin was reduced to less than 5 mg/dl by drainage in patients with periampullary cancer resected for cure.[61] Presumably, similar benefits would accrue to patients with benign disease. Obviously, the resolution of acute cholecystitis and cholangitis reduces the hazard of intra-abdominal and wound infection. Many errors of

Fig. 11-10. ERCP film from a 35-year-old man who had undergone a cholecystectomy several years earlier (note clips in the right upper quadrant). The man was referred from another hospital because of cholangitis and gram-negative sepsis not controllable by parenteral antibiotics. Emergency diagnostic ERCP demonstrated a 7-mm common duct stone (*open arrowhead*) impacted in the distal common bile duct. The intrahepatic ducts were dilated. After proximal displacement of the stone and injection of 80 mg of gentamicin, a nasobiliary drain (*closed arrowhead*) was placed in the common bile duct. The 1.6-mm diameter drain is seen after removal of the endoscope passing through the duodenum and stomach. With continued antibiotic therapy, cholangitis and sepsis rapidly resolved. An endoscopic papillotomy was performed and the stone removed.

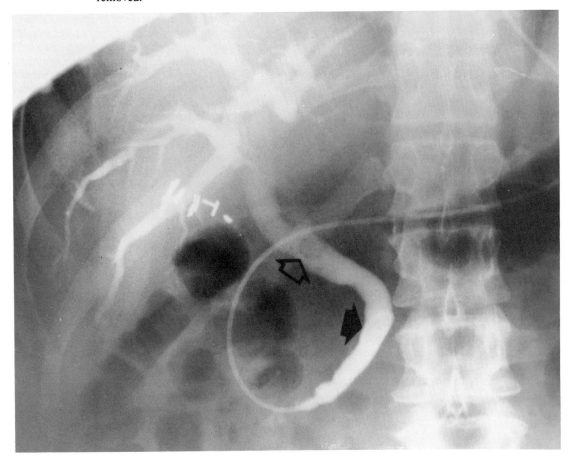

technique that occur during abdominal surgery arise with difficult dissection of inflamed tissue. Unavoidable complications such as suture failure and anastomotic disruption also result from operation during periods of acute infection.

Endoscopic Retrograde Stents and Drains

A biliary stent or drain is a tube placed within the bile duct to maintain drainage and an adequate lumen. The traditional T-tube is a stent that allows the choledochotomy incision to heal without stenosis. In patients with bile duct strictures who undergo remedial bile duct repair, it is common surgical practice to leave stents in the bile ducts for years.[7] A biliary stent placed by ERCP follows the same surgical principle. The stent may remain in place for the duration of the patient's life or may be removed.[51,64] An endoscopic drain is a tube of small diameter (No. 5 or 7 F) that is passed through the endoscope by way of the papilla of Vater into the proximal biliary tree above an obstruction. The endoscope is then removed, leaving the biliary drain in place. This device maintains the free flow of bile from the liver into the duodenum or serves as a partial or complete external biliary fistula. Since the biliary drain is brought out through the patient's nose, serial cholangiograms may be obtained by simple injection of contrast medium into the drain catheter (see Fig. 11-10).

Decompression of the obstructed biliary tree with the resumption of bile flow encourages the rapid resolution of cholangitis and cholestasis. Definitive therapy may then be undertaken in the most favorable circumstances. If abdominal surgery is necessary, the excess risk posed by infection and cholestasis may be substantially reduced by drainage. Even when endoscopic biliary surgery is to be used, it is wise first to gain control of systemic sepsis secondary to cholangitis with its associated hemorrhagic diathesis and to reduce the edema associated with severe cholangitis before the performance of endoscopic biliary surgery. Anatomic landmarks may be obscured by edema, and severely infected tissue may be prone to bleed. With decompression, the apparently obstructed cystic duct often regains patency. Serial cholangiograms obtained by injection of contrast through the nasobiliary drain allow the objective assessment of progress and may reveal intrahepatic abscesses or metastasis.

Endoscopic stents and drains have substantial advantages over the percutaneous techniques. By approaching the biliary tree through the papilla of Vater, they avoid all the risks of bleeding, bile leaks, and sepsis associated with puncture of the liver. This is particularly important in patients with cholangitis, because the intrahepatic biliary tree is commonly not dilated. In this case, the diagnostic yield of PTC is substantially less and the hazard much greater than for ERCP. In neoplastic bile duct obstruction, the endoscopic approach has the advantage of defining biliary tract geography before a hazardous hepatic puncture is made (see Fig. 11-6). With percutaneous techniques, it may not be possible to reestablish bile flow into the duodenum. The patient may be left with a total external biliary fistula or with drainage of a segmental hepatic duct that is separated from the main biliary tree by intrahepatic tumor. On the other hand, endoscopic stents and drains require considerable skill and experience for their use and may be unsuccessful in patients for whom percutaneous drainage is possible. Our approach is to define biliary anatomy by ERCP and place an endoscopic drain or stent as appropriate. If these techniques fail, we then approach the liver percutaneously, with biliary geography defined (Fig. 11-11).

Techniques of Biliary Decompression

Preoperative biliary decompression by percutaneous transhepatic methods was first proposed by Nakayama to reduce the high operative mortality (28%) of patients undergoing "curative" surgery for periampullary and bile duct cancer. Endoscopic methods immediately found a role in providing a reliable differentiation of periampullary cancers. Carcinoma of the duodenum and papilla of Vater are obvious on endoscopic inspection of the duodenum, and the pancreatogram identifies the small 1 cm to 2 cm adenocarcinoma of the pancreas invading the bile duct or metastatic to the porta hepatis that is invisible to ultrasound and computed tomography.[14] Placement of an endoscopic stent or drain carries less risk than the percutaneous procedures and always returns bile to the gut.[40,77,82] Without the percutaneous wound the patient is free of pain as well as the pulmonary, hepatic, and peritoneal complications. Endoscopic sphincterotomy or infundibulotomy, a puncture of a portion of the intraduodenal bile duct above the tumor, provides long-term palliation for slow-growing papilla of Vater or terminal bile duct neoplasms. Most important is the fact that the endoscopic prosthesis cannot be pulled out accidentally and does not provide a continuous reminder to the patient of the incurable disease process.

Subsequent trials have shown that only 5% to 10% of patients with malignant jaundice are suitable for surgical resection.[23,28,61] Since the operative mortality of 10% is similiar to the 5-year survival, the value of surgery is seriously questioned, particularly in patients with carcinoma of the pancreas.[14,23]

The need for careful selection is further emphasized by the fact that two thirds of the patients with malignant jaundice fail to respond satisfactorily to any form of biliary decompression.[9,53,102] These patients have tumor dissemination that is not apparent to noninvasive imaging procedures. Therefore the response to biliary decompression is vital to differentiate patients with malignant jaundice who are unresponsive to therapy and are a very high-risk group[9,52] (88% operative mortality) from a favorable group who are relieved of jaundice and may be considered for resective surgery or other types of palliation in an attempt to prolong the 6-month average survival.[40] A trade of nonsurgical for surgical decompression is of little value

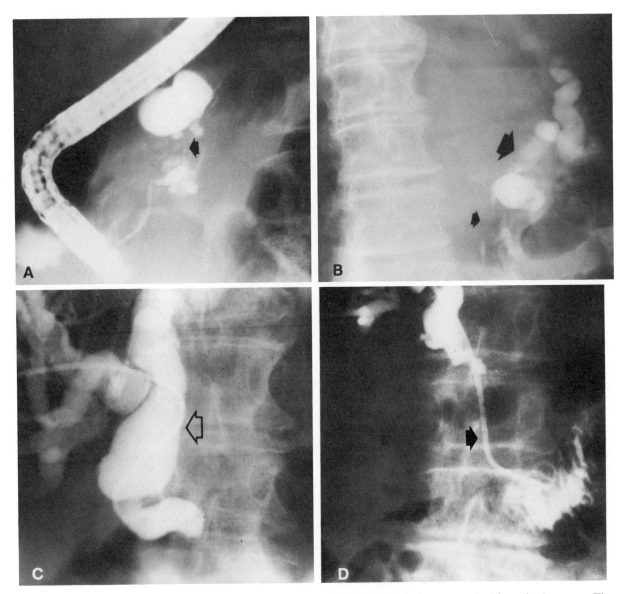

Fig. 11-11. A. ERCP performed in a 72-year-old cholecystectomized jaundiced woman. The endoscope is seen in the position of cannulation. A normal 1-cm segment of pancreatic duct is followed by a stenotic area (*arrowhead*) with dilatation of the proximal duct. On the basis of the fluoroscopic impression gained from this volume of contrast, the procedure was terminated. **B.** Film obtained after withdrawal of the endoscope gives a good lateral view of the area of pancreatic duct stenosis (*small arrowhead*), with marked proximal dilatation visible as the contrast diffuses proximally in the dilated duct system (*large arrowhead*). Findings from this study were considered diagnostic of carcinoma of the pancreas. **C.** Percutaneous biliary drain was put in place after percutaneous cholangiography (*open arrowhead*). There is marked dilatation of the proximal common bile duct and intrahepatic ducts. The distal hepatic duct is obstructed. No contrast passed beyond the obstruction. This illustrates the nonspecific percutaneous cholangiographic findings in carcinoma of the pancreas. A percutaneous cholangiogram alone would not give adequate diagnostic information. **D.** Percutaneous biliary stent was placed through the obstructing carcinoma of the pancreas. The approximate position of the papilla of Vater is marked by the arrowhead. Jaundice was palliated in this patient, who survived 7 months.

unless a specific indication is present because the survival is similar for all 3 methods.[40]

The issues of stent size and shape are not yet settled. Physically a 5 F stent with a 1-mm lumen 10 cm in length will pass 1 ml/min of bile (1440 ml/day) at 10 cm H_2O pressure. Measured human bile production is approximately 900 ml/day. Therefore a single stent with a lumen of 1 to 1.5 mm is adequate and was initially used successfully both endoscopically and percutaneously.[9,97] Stents are slowly occluded by deposition of biliary sludge. Rapid occlusion occurs from infection or bleeding because bile secretory pressure is low (maximum 30 cm H_2O). Early and late stent occlusion are related to the quantity and quality of bile flow and the contamination of bile from reflux of duodenal contents when the 10 cm pressure gradient between duodenum and bile duct is breeched by the stent. Attempts to prolong stent function have used different materials, increased stent bore, or used multiple small stents. Large-bore stents are rigid and promote duodenal reflux. Multiple small-lumen stents may occlude with sludge but provide an extraluminal space between the two or three No. 5 or 7 F stents. Experience with percutaneous stents ranging from No. 8 to 10 F suggest that stent changes are required every 3 to 4 months in favorable cases and more frequently in patients in whom bleeding, infection, tumor detritus, or low bile flow rates complicate management.[50] Similar service requirements are found for endoscopic stents. The massively dilated intrahepatic duct system with infection is poorly drained by any technique. When this situation is complicated by aggressive infection in a debilitated patient only external drainage to gravity will control cholangitis. The issue of stent size and type is dwarfed by the varied pathology, presenting circumstances, and course in this diverse group of patients.

Early Complications

Failure of endoscopic stent placement occurs in 10% to 20% of the cases even in experienced hands.[12] The difficult case with duodenal invasion or a long irregular stenosis may best be handled by initial placement of a nasobiliary drain followed at a later sitting by a large single or multiple smaller stents. Nasobiliary drainage establishes the quality and quantity of bile flow. Continued external drainage until adequate volumes (700 ml to 900 ml) of clear, sterile bile return is the best assurance that the stent will function and that hepatic function is adequate.[9] Bleeding from manipulation and erosion by pressure from the stent may cause immediate stent occlusion. If bile flow is maintained by irrigation or stent replacement, satisfactory drainage may be established. Early stent occlusion occurs in approximately 10% of patients. Repeated hemobilia is difficult to manage. Infection is controlled by maintaining bile flow and appropriate antibiotic therapy.

Cystic duct or left hepatic duct obstruction may occur following stent placement, particularly when large stents are used. The initial concerns over the production of pan-creatitis were unfounded. This is a rare occurrence after placement of percutaneous stents without the benefits of endoscopic papillotomy to relieve pressure within the sphincter. Bleeding from an endoscopic sphincterotomy through tumor tissue is difficult to control and therefore should be avoided.

After successful resolution of jaundice a period of 3 to 6 months of satisfactory stent function is anticipated. Since average survival in palliated patients is 6 months, the recurrence of jaundice or a rising alkaline phosphatase level is often the result of disease progression with hepatic metastasis or portal vein or duodenal obstruction.[8,40] Duodenal ulceration with bleeding or hemobilia may occlude stents repeatedly. A shift to a percutaneous stent that can be irrigated, drained, or changed frequently may be useful, but the risks are great and the benefits small late in the course of these diseases.[50] We advise a prophylactic ambulatory stent change at 3 months to evaluate disease progression and avoid stent occlusion in patients who achieve good palliation. The examination of the stent and duodenum as well as the intrahepatic biliary tree allows a fair estimate of the future course and timing of stent service in the future if necessary.

This complex area cannot be summarized briefly. Our approach is to initiate nasobiliary drainage in patients with cholangitis, dense jaundice, evidence of hepatic failure, advanced age, probable dissemination of malignancy, or other risk factors suggesting that the prognosis is guarded. Bile flow and decrease in the serum bilirubin value are observed. Repeated cholangiography through the drain ensures duct decompression. If hepatic failure is confirmed, therapy may be stopped or endoscopic stent placed and the patient dismissed. A good response to external drainage allows stent placement with confidence that cholestasis will resolve. The choice of stent is based on anatomic measurements with the duct system well decompressed and clear radiographic visualization of the biliary tree. In good-risk patients a definitive stent(s) may be placed during the initial diagnostic ERCP using a No. 7 F or larger single stent or two No. 5 F stents. In patients who are candidates for palliative or curative surgery it should be anticipated that 4 to 6 weeks of preoperative biliary decompression with return of bile to the gut will be required to correct hepatic, immune, and metabolic dysfunctions.[61] If cholestasis does not resolve completely, tumor dissemination is probable and should be sought. The initial goal of a bilirubin value less than 5 mg/dl set by Nakayama for preoperative biliary decompression appears inadequate both for resolution of functional deficits and to identify patients with subtle dissemination.

There are no trials to date that meet these criteria.[61] Furthermore, most operations performed in trials of biliary decompression have been relatively low-risk bypass procedures rather than the higher-risk resections.[61] In adenocarcinoma of the pancreas only 10% of the patients reaching abdominal exploration have a localized disease that might be considered for palliative resection.[23] Only this small group would benefit from preoperative decompression followed by a resection. A type II statistical error is highly probable unless patients are stratified carefully.

Endoscopic Biliary Surgery

Extraction of Common Duct Stones with Balloon or Basket

Stones slightly larger than the opening of the papilla (4 mm in diameter) may be extracted by grasping with a basket or by the passing of the basket or balloon beyond the stone and withdrawal of the device to force the stone through the orifice of the papilla. Our current experience suggests that, if the papilla of Vater is intact, this procedure is effective only when stones are less than 4 mm in diameter or when they are of the pigment type and can be deformed during extraction.[112]

In patients who have had sphincterotomy or papillotomy, instrumentation of the biliary tree is facilitated. Extraction of stones may be difficult if the diameter of the stones is larger than the fibrotic orifice. The baskets used for this technique are easily deformed during passage through the endoscope and by the manipulations required during stone extraction. A stone too firm to be crushed by compression between the basket and the catheter and too large to pass through the papilla will trap the basket within the bile duct.

Lithotripsy

Mechanical fragmentation of pigment stones with balloons or loops is used to avoid the hazard of the larger endoscopic sphincterotomy incision.[83] A metal oversleeve can be passed over the shaft of a wire basket to crush the trapped stone within the bile duct.[63] This is similar to the techniques used percutaneously or through the T-tube tract to fragment stones. An extension of this method proposes stone fragmentation and extraction through an intact papilla to further reduce the risk of the procedure. Capture of the stone within the wire basket can be difficult. After lithotripsy, numerous troublesome, smaller fragments may remain in the bile duct. Most importantly the availability of the lithotripsy basket and sleeve reduces the hazard of basket impaction when attempting to remove a large stone through a relatively small incision in the terminal bile duct. These techniques will undoubtedly be developed further. It will require considerable experience to determine whether a modest endoscopic papillotomy with a low risk of bleeding and other complications of the incision will be displaced by extraction of stones through an intact papilla with the risk of pancreatitis and trauma to the biliary sphincter mechanism.[81,88]

Endoscopic Electrosurgical Papillotomy

Endoscopic electrosurgical papillotomy permits the controlled enlargement of the orifice of a normal papilla of Vater or the extension of a previous sphincterotomy to allow the extraction or passage of stones up to 1 cm in diameter. Experience suggests that the submucosal and inferior sphincters of the papilla of Vater retain stones of up to approximately 1 cm in diameter. After the endoscopic papillotomy, stones may be extracted at the same sitting, or a period of time may be allowed for spontaneous passage of the stones. The endoscopic papillotomy heals in 3 to 5 days, with formation of a terminal biliary fistula. Follow-up examination after endoscopic papillotomy reveals an intact distal biliary sphincter mechanism. Reflux of air or intestinal contents into the bile duct does not occur (Fig. 11-12).

Endoscopic Electrosurgical Sphincterotomy

In endoscopic electrosurgical sphincterotomy, the endoscopist attempts to incise the full length of the intraduodenal bile duct, including submucosal, inferior, and superior sphincters of the distal bile duct. The hazard is greater than with endoscopic electrosurgical papillotomy, and this procedure should be reserved for patients with stones greater than 10 mm in diameter that require a large incision for spontaneous passage or extraction (see Fig. 11-4). After endoscopic electrosurgical sphincterotomy, there may be reflux of intestinal contents into the common bile duct. The physiologic effect is identical to that of surgical sphincteroplasty. The lateral choledochoduodenal fistula allows the endoscopic retrograde passage of instruments into the bile duct for extraction or fragmentation of residual stones. We have fragmented and removed stones 20 mm in diameter through an endoscopic sphincterotomy incision (see Fig. 11-12).

Advantages

The endoscopic retrograde biliary tract approach uses a new field to enter the distal bile duct and is not impeded by prior abdominal surgery. Precise anatomic and pathologic definition of pancreatic, biliary, and periampullary areas is obtained before the procedure. The endoscopist is uncommitted until the actual performance of the electrosurgical procedure. He may terminate the endoscopy at any point, if circumstances are unfavorable, and resume it on another occasion. In the presence of severe edema, sepsis, or pancreatitis, he may decide to identify the pathologic findings and await resolution of the inflammatory process by injection of antibiotics into the biliary tree and initiation of systemic antibiotic therapy. Stone extraction alone or a small initial incision (endoscopic papillotomy) may be performed with little hazard for drainage of the biliary tree or dislodgement of an impacted stone responsible for pancreatitis. At that point, the procedure may be terminated and several days allowed for resolution of periampullary edema or associated pancreatitis. Sepsis is controlled by retrograde injection of antibiotics, papillotomy, and a biliary drain to convert the obstructed bile duct into a freely draining system.

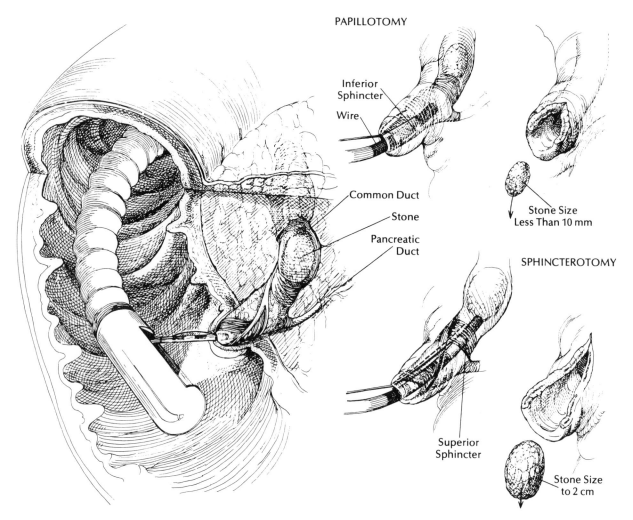

Fig. 11-12. Cannulation of the papilla of Vater by an endoscope catheter (*left*) sets the stage for endoscopic papillotomy or sphincterotomy. In papillotomy, the catheter is usually advanced no more than 15 mm and then flexed by tautening of the cautery wire, through which electric current passes for simultaneous cutting and coagulation; the resulting incision, which is usually 6 to 9 mm long, cuts into the inferior sphincter and allows stones of up to 10 mm in diameter and sometimes larger to pass or be extracted (*upper right*). In sphincterotomy, the catheter probes more deeply, and the incision extends for 1.5 to 3.5 cm; this cuts the sphincter completely, allowing spontaneous passage or extraction of stones up to 2 cm in diameter (*lower right*). (Zimmon DS: Hosp Pract 13[12], 1978. Reprinted with permission)

The procedure may be staged. Two to 5 days after an initial papillotomy, a full sphincterotomy may be performed. Stone extraction may be undertaken at this point, after an in-hospital delay, or the patient may be discharged from the hospital to return for stone extraction after resolution of inflammation and edema.

In benign stenosis of the papilla or with distal biliary tumors, a similar fractional procedure may be performed using endoscopic biopsy sampling after incision of the papilla to establish or exclude the presence of a submucosal periampullary tumor. The adequacy of biliary drainage and passage of stones is determined by follow-up retrograde cholangiography and manometric studies comparing the pressure within the bile duct to that in the duodenum. A normal pressure gradient should be less than 20 cm H_2O.

Endoscopic biliary surgery is ideal for elderly patients either before cholecystectomy or without cholecystectomy, if unnecessary.[21,31,53,71] It may be used to facilitate clearance of the bile duct of stones at the time of cholecystectomy if the common bile duct contains impacted stones that might otherwise require duodenotomy or choledochoduodenostomy.

If there are no complications, the procedure is brief. No anesthesia is required. There is no abdominal incision or postoperative recovery. The patient is immediately ambulatory, and the cardiovascular complications associated with major abdominal surgery are obviated (Fig. 11-13).

Disadvantages

When stones cannot be removed by extraction or flushing, the performance of ERCP and endoscopic electrosurgery requires a high degree of technical skill. Complications such as hemorrhage, pancreatitis, cholangitis, or duode-

nal perforation require skilled surgical intervention (Fig. 11-14).

Indications

Endoscopic biliary surgery is indicated in postcholecystectomy choledocholithiasis when there is no T-tube or when stone extraction through the T-tube tract fails. In choledocholithiasis with the gallbladder *in situ,* endoscopic electrosurgery may be lifesaving as a temporizing procedure to control infection and relieve biliary obstruction before cholecystectomy. Successful endoscopic management of choledochlithiasis may allow a delay before cholecystectomy and avoid common duct exploration in high-risk patients. In selected patients, endoscopic management of choledocholithiasis may be coupled with stone dissolution therapy for cholelithiasis. Endoscopic biliary surgery is ideal for patients requiring relief of terminal bile duct

Fig. 11-13. A. Common bile duct of an elderly man who underwent a cholecystostomy for cholangitis and cholecystitis. Unremitting cholangitis resulted from a 7-mm triangular stone in the distal common bile duct. **B.** After an endoscopic sphincterotomy, the stone passed into the duodenum. The probable sequence of events was impaction of the common duct stone followed by cholangitis and cholecystitis.

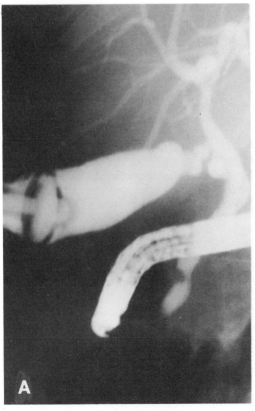 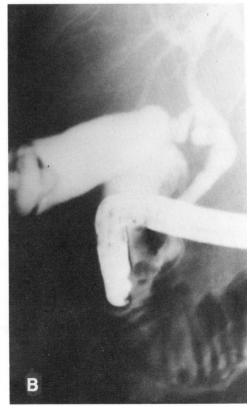

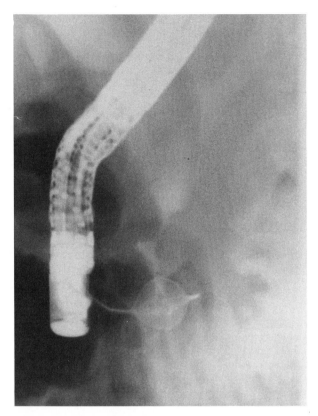

Fig. 11-14. After an endoscopic papillotomy this 14-mm stone was extracted without difficulty in a 4-wire basket. If the stone had been trapped in the bile duct a lithotripsy sleeve could have been used for fragmentation.

obstruction, as in papilla of Vater stenosis, the sump syndrome after choledochoduodenostomy, and anomalies such as choledochocele (Table 11-3).

Stone Dissolution

The use of nasobiliary drains for solvent perfusion of common duct stones is a prolonged and often unsuccessful therapy presumably due to the presence of insoluble pig-

ment stones or a pigment coating on cholesterol stones.[88] Until more effective, less toxic methods of perfusion are found, extraction and lithotripsy techniques are to be preferred. After placement of a biliary bridge stent with an endoscopic papillotomy, spontaneous stone fragmentation and passage due to mechanical abrasion and dissolution from refluxed intestinal contents usually occurs within 3 to 6 months. During this interval the bridging stent prevents stone impaction. Often both stone and stent pass spontaneously. If this is unsuccessful, lithotripsy is easily performed in an interval period after cholestasis, infection, and duodenal edema have resolved.

Results

Ten centers in West Germany have collaborated in reporting the results of endoscopic biliary surgery.[1] Over the past 6 years, endoscopic techniques have been the preferred procedures in West Germany for the management of choledocholithiasis after cholecystectomy, in high-risk patients with the gallbladder *in situ,* for the management of stenosis of the papilla of Vater, and in selected patients with distal papillary carcinoma (see Table 11-3).

It should be emphasized that these results arise from ten collaborating centers in which the procedure is performed by experts. Of 1554 attempts, endoscopic electrosurgical procedures were performed in 1458 instances. Sixty-nine percent of these patients were older than 60 years of age, and 39% were older than 70. Spontaneous stone passage occurred in 54% of patients. Endoscopic stone extraction after endoscopic electrosurgery was perfomed in 32%. Fourteen percent of the patients had incomplete procedure or failure of the procedure or were lost to follow-up. The overall success rate in patients operated on for choledocholithiasis was 93.8% (Table 11-4). The incidence of complications (7.7%) was remarkably low for this large group of aged, high-risk patients. The number of deaths, 16 (1.1%), was approximately ten times smaller than that expected for traditional abdominal surgery.[55] On the basis of these results, endoscopic biliary surgery is considered to be the preferred procedure for the indications listed, if an expert endoscopist is available.

Our experience with endoscopic management of biliary tract disease has been similar to the German reports: only

TABLE 11-3. Indications for Endoscopic Biliary Surgery in 1458 Patients

INDICATION	NUMBER OF PATIENTS	%
Choledocholithiasis	1223	83.9
After cholecystectomy	968	79.2
Gallbladder *in situ* (high-risk)	255	20.8
Papillary stenosis	194	13.3
Papillary carcinoma	25	1.7
Other	16	1.1

TABLE 11-4. Results of Endoscopic Biliary Surgery for Choledocholithiasis in 1459 Patients

RESULT	NUMBER OF PATIENTS	%
Spontaneous stone passage	663	54.2
Stone extraction	394	32.2
No follow-up	30	2.5
Overall success	1223	93.8

11 of our patients required laparotomy, and there were only six postoperative deaths in a series of more than 900 patients. The age distribution of our patients is similar to that of the German experience: more than half the patients were older than 70 years of age, and eight were older than 90.

Our initial approach was to refuse technically difficult cases, such as patients with liver disease and those not considered candidates for conventional surgical approaches. We frequently have patients referred to us who are not likely to survive surgical intervention if a complication of endoscopic biliary surgery requiring open surgical management should occur. In cases in which endoscopic biliary surgery is the last resort, the favorable experience to date suggests that the use of these procedures is warranted. In particular, the combination of endoscopic papillotomy with an endoscopic biliary stent achieves complete biliary decompression with little risk. This is an ideal approach for aging high-risk patients with a huge common duct stone and serious complicating diseases (Fig. 11-15).[98,115]

An important aspect of the preoperative preparation of a patient for abdominal surgery or use of endoscopic biliary surgery, when feasible, is the reduction in morbidity and convalescence. However, this is difficult to measure. Median hospital stay for 900 patients undergoing endoscopic biliary surgery was 3 days. Uncomplicated patients required only 36 hours of hospitalization. Survival after abdominal surgery may still leave aged patients disabled, unable to regain prior life-style, or with a prolonged uphill convalescent course lasting for months. A substantial number of aging patients are demented after abdominal surgery, although they survive.[31,48,62]

Modern surgery needs a precise data base to meet the demands for speed, accuracy, and a successful outcome. The sequential approach to the differential diagnosis of

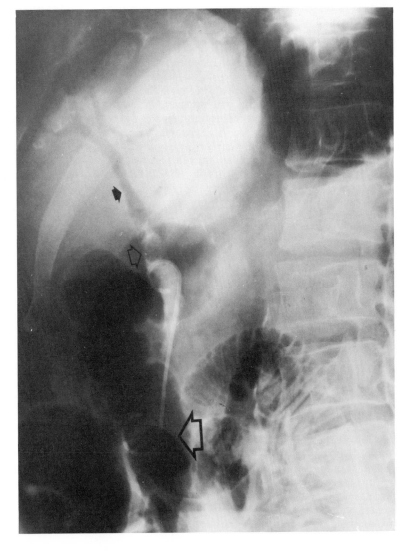

Fig. 11-15. ERCP of an 80-year-old man who was referred for management of cholangitis and choledocholithiasis after a cardiac arrest. An 8-mm stone in the common bile duct could not be extracted through the narrow intrapancreatic portion of the common bile duct by endoscopic papillotomy. A double pigtail biliary stent was therefore placed in the bile duct. The upper pigtail maintains the proximal position of the stone and allows free flow of bile (*small open arrow*). The distal pigtail is seen in the duodenum (*large open arrow*). The combination stent and endoscopic papillotomy produced reflux of air into the biliary tree with complete biliary decompression (*closed arrowhead*). The patient has maintained excellent health for the subsequent 2 years.

jaundice, with its emphasis on noninvasive diagnostic tests[73,106] and lengthy evaluation[46,55] has been preempted by precise positive diagnostic studies. Our approach to patients suspected of having pancreatic or biliary tract disease has been revolutionized by developments in fiberoptic endoscopy and radiology, culminating in the techniques of ERCP, endoscopic biliary surgery, PTC, and the removal of common duct stones through the T-tube tract. The therapeutic value of endoscopic biliary surgery and T-tube tract extraction of retained common duct stones as alternatives to secondary biliary tract surgery is clearly established. Preoperative diagnosis of periampullary cancer permits the patient's referral to a specialized center that promises a lower operative mortality and the best chance for cure. The frustrations and disappointments of operations for pancreatic cancer can be reduced by accurate preoperative diagnosis.[3]

There is close link between diagnostic and therapeutic approaches in patients with disease of the biliary tract and pancreas. Unnecessary complications may arise by virtue of delay in coordinating diagnosis and therapy. The therapeutic techniques of local antibiotic injection, biliary tract irrigation, and biliary tract drainage by PTC or ERCP reduce the incidence of complications after diagnostic procedures and provide important avenues for therapy.[100,102,105] A substantial group of patients who are at high risk for abdominal surgery should have these techniques applied. These include patients over 60 years of age, patients with serious complicating hepatic, cardiovascular, pulmonary, or renal diseases, patients who have previously undergone biliary tract surgery, and patients with severe infection of the biliary tract or pancreas. Because the hazard of emergency surgery is substantially greater than that of elective surgery, temporizing therapeutic maneuvers are important, even when abdominal surgery is necessary. Such maneuvers gain time and allow an elective operation (Fig. 11-16).

The new and varied diagnostic and therapeutic techniques that are available for diseases of the biliary tract and pancreas must be integrated with traditional abdominal surgery. Patients with these diseases will benefit substantially from being the focus of sophisticated techniques at the interface of endoscopy, radiology, and surgery.

UPPER GASTROINTESTINAL FIBEROPTIC ESOPHAGOGASTRODUODENOSCOPY WITH ENDOSCOPIC VARIX SCLEROSIS

Gastrointestinal bleeding in liver disease is a complex clinical problem. The cirrhotic patient, occult or obvious, is subject to all the causes of gastrointestinal bleeding. Portal hypertension may be incidental, a complicating factor, or primary in variceal hemorrhagic or hemorrhagic gastritis.[47] The exact pathogenesis of these individual clinical entities is poorly understood. Only fiberoptic esophagogastroduodenoscopy can visualize the entire upper gastrointestinal tract and identify the bleeding site(s) that are active or potential. In liver disease, particularly when associated with ethanol abuse, multiple potential or actual sources of upper gastrointestinal tract bleeding are common. Conversely, variceal hemorrhage often can be deduced only from the presence of esophagogastric varices visualized on endoscopy and the absence of other lesions in the visualized stomach and duodenum. Therefore early endoscopy is essential to solving the questions of differential diagnosis and activity (rate of bleeding) in a patient with suspected or proven upper gastrointestinal hemorrhage.

Dagradi[17] first recognized the increased frequency of variceal hemorrhage in patients with "varices on varices." Beppu and co-workers[6] identified red wale marks (minute linear blood vessels) and cherry-red spots, the equivalent of Dagradi's varices on varices, and also confirmed the association of these endoscopic findings with bleeding. Why these endoscopically visible lesions are associated with variceal hemorrhage was not known until the Belfast group examined the excised rings of esophageal mucosa from cirrhotic patients undergoing esophageal transection for recurrent variceal hemorrhage. Intraepithelial vascular channels with markedly attenuated vascular epithelium were identified just below the squamous mucosal surface.[78,79] The intraepithelial channels undoubtedly correspond to the endoscopically visable varices on varices (red wale marks) seen in linear profile and to cherry-red spots when seen en face. The mechanism of this unique lesion's formation is unknown,[47] but it is the hallmark of esophageal bleeding in cirrhosis with portal hypertension. It thus appears that an increased portohepatic pressure gradient of greater than 10 mm Hg in cirrhotic patients combined with a mucosal defect of intraepithelial vascular channels in the distal esophageal squamous mucosa leads to recurrent variceal hemorrhage from this site.

Rationale

Theoretically and technically the endoscopist may aim to inject and sclerose the varices[32] or the paravariceal mucosa.[60,76] The practical facts of technique require paravariceal submucosal spread of sclerosant in all patients. Therefore, mucosal and submucosal fibrosis (sclerosis)[30] is the inevitable result of endoscopic varix sclerosis with a variable thrombosis of esophageal and paraesophageal portosystemic collateral veins.[74] Control of variceal hemorrhage probably results from mucosal and submucosal fibrosis that obliterates intraepithelial vascular channels and separates the varices from the lumen.

The complex esophageal venous drainage in the cirrhotic patient with portal hypertension makes it unlikely that all varices could be obliterated without severe mucosal injury and esophageal stenosis. Clinically, bleeding is usually controlled by endoscopic sclerosis of the distal 5 cm of esophageal mucosa just above the cardioesophageal junction.[60] This is the area where intraepithelial vascular channels were found by Spence and his colleagues.[32,78,79] Taken together, this evidence suggests that paravariceal

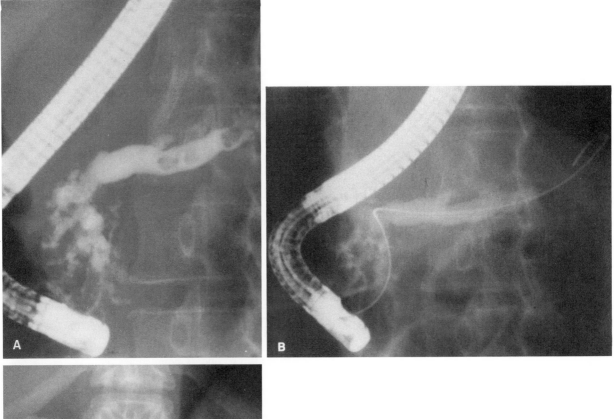

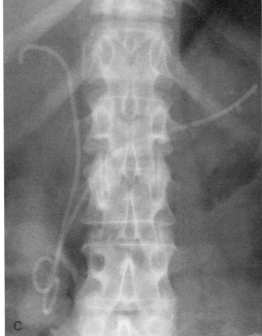

Fig. 11-16. A. This patient suffers from alcohol-associated pancreatitis and intractable abdominal pain. ERCP demonstrates severe pancreatic duct injury in the head of the pancreas with duct stenosis adjacent to the papilla of Vater. Multiple pancreatic duct stones were present. An adjacent bile duct stenosis produced an elevated alkaline phosphatase (not shown). **B.** After an endoscopic sphincterotomy has been performed and the pancreatic duct stones extracted with a balloon, the stent wire guide is passed to the tail of the pancreas. **C.** Pancreatic and biliary stents are in place. Pancreatic calcification is noted to the left of the spine adjacent to the stent. This follow-up film was obtained to assure that the stents remained in position. The patient was not relieved of abdominal pain, indicating the source of the pain to be related to inflammation, probably in the head of the pancreas, and not related to duct obstruction or the intraductal calculi. These findings strongly suggest that a pancreatic surgical procedure to achieve only duct drainage would not relieve the patient's symptoms.

sclerosis of the distal 5 cm of the esophagus as proposed by Paquet is appropriate to control variceal hemorrhage. It seems likely that the various trials and controlled trials of varix sclerosis, although claiming to use specific paravariceal or variceal injection in fact all use to a greater or lesser extent paravariceal sclerosis.[11,15,43,84,99]

Soderlund and associates[74] examined the effects of intravariceal sclerosis on paraesophageal portosystemic collateral vessels. They showed extensive occlusive thrombosis of paravariceal vessels by transhepatic portography. This raises the additional therapeutic possibility of returning portosystemic collateral flow to the liver by intentional intravariceal sclerosis. This is a therapeutic effect similar to that sought by transhepatic angiographic or surgical obliteration of collateral vessels.[5] A theoretic base[107] has been established for these maneuvers, but clinical efficacy cannot yet be demonstrated. The value of endoscopic varix sclerosis in controlling hemorrhage,[75,94] reducing the incidence of recurrent hemorrhage, and prolonging life after varix hemorrhage is well documented.[43,60,84,85,94] Controlled comparisons of endoscopic varix sclerosis versus propranolol therapy[95] and endoscopic varix sclerosis versus distal splenorenal shunt[90] favor endoscopic varix sclerosis. Prophylactic therapy is under consideration.[99]

Technique

Emergent control of variceal hemorrhage by endoscopic varix sclerosis is vastly superior to the previously used alternatives, balloon tamponade[24,59] or portacaval anastomosis,[90] in both morbidity and mortality. Nevertheless, all techniques have limitations and may fail. Endoscopic expertise is vitally important. Occasionally, endotracheal intubation and general anesthesia are required when the patient cannot be sedated safely or hemorrhage is massive. A brief period of balloon tamponade with resuscitation may be necessary prior to endoscopic varix sclerosis. Most emergent patients are treated at routine diagnostic endoscopy for bleeding. Follow-up treatments may be performed on an ambulatory basis if the patient's general condition and extramural support is available.[72]

Sclerosants seem essentially similiar. In Europe polidocanol is preferred. In the United States tetradecylsulfate and sodium morrhuate are available. My preference is for 10 to 30 injections of 1% tetradecylsulfate to a total volume of 20 ml using the paravariceal technique of Paquet.[60] Injections are begun at the cardioesophageal junction and advance proximally. The initial injections are made on either side of the bleeding site. Successful sclerosis raises a linear epithelial bleb that compresses the bleeding site (Fig. 11-17).

Complications

The risks of endoscopy include oversedation and aspiration and are more common and severe in emergency circumstances.[72] Acute complications specifically related to endoscopic varix sclerosis include laceration of the varix with the injection needle or puncture with both the needle and shaft, which is 1.7 mm to 2.2 mm in diameter. Although these complications are to be feared, they may also be controlled by circumferential sclerosis, as is true of most bleeding sites in the upper gastrointestinal tract.[76]

The aim of varix sclerosis is mucosal and submucosal inflammation, fibrosis, and varix thrombosis.[74] Ulceration should be considered a complication because it is variable in occurrence. Esophageal ulcers and inflammatory polyps can lead to secondary hemorrhage requiring endoscopic or surgical therapy (esophageal transection or portacaval anastomosis).[90] The 4 to 6 weeks encompassing three to six endoscopic sittings required for the sclerosing injections followed by esophageal healing and protective fibrosis and thrombosis are a high-risk period during which bleeding may recur. After the course is completed, hemorrhage becomes much less frequent and probably less severe. The desire to get through this danger period encourages the use of more sclerosant and more frequent injections. This may lead to esophageal ulceration, hemorrhage, and sepsis, requiring bouginage.

Long-Term Results

Endoscopic surveillance at 6-month intervals has been proposed. In contrast to many new therapies the early

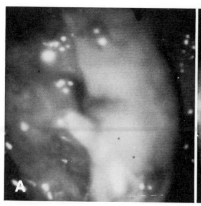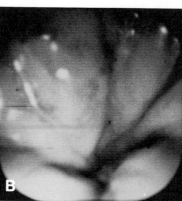

Fig. 11-17. A. Endoscopic photograph demonstrates typical "cherry red spots" or "varices on varices." Note the marked distension of the varix compared to the adjacent esophageal wall. B. After three sittings of paravariceal sclerosis, the same site is compressed and covered with a layer of fibrous tissue. There is no longer the sharp demarcation between the dilated varix and the esophageal wall. A few residual "cherry red spots" are visible through an opaque layer of fibrosis.

results of endoscopic varix sclerosis were confirmed repeatedly by controlled trials. The start-up costs of learning a demanding technique apparently were overcome by the clinical efficacy of varix sclerosis. Despite the unresolved issues of sclerosant, intravariceal versus paravariceal injections, and mucosal versus collateral vessel effect, the clinical efficacy of endoscopic varix sclerosis is well established as the preferred therapy for bleeding esophageal varices. The presence of what appears to be a specific anatomic lesion (intraepithelial vascular channels) that should be controlled by an appropriate technique (paravariceal varix sclerosis) suggests that at last a rational therapy for the group of cirrhotic patients who suffer from variceal hemorrhage is available.

REFERENCES

1. Alendt R et al: Experience with endoscopic sphincterotomy: A collective study of six centres. Endoscopy 15:173–174, 1983
2. Bar-Meir S et al: Biliary and pancreatic duct pressures measured by ERCP manometry in patients with suspected papillary stenosis. Dig Dis Sci 24:209–213, 1979
3. Beall MS et al: Disappointments in the management of patients with malignancy of pancreas, duodenum and common bile duct. Arch Surg 101:461, 1970
4. Belohlavek D et al: Five years experience in endoscopic retrograde cholangiopancreaticography (ERCP). Endoscopy 8:115–118, 1976
5. Bengmark B et al: Obliteration of esophageal varices by percutaneous transhepatic portography. Ann Surg 190:549–554, 1979
6. Beppo K et al: Prediction of variceal hemorrhage by esophageal endoscopy. Gastrointest Endosc 27:213–218, 1981
7. Braasch JW et al: Progress in biliary structure repair. Am J Surg 129:34–37, 1975
8. Burcharth F: Nonsurgical drainage of the biliary tract. Semin Liver Dis 2:75–84, 1982
9. Burcharth F et al: A new endoprosthesis for nonoperative intubation of the biliary tract in malignant obstructive jaundice. Surg Gynecol Obstet 146:76–78, 1978
10. Case records of the Massachusetts General Hospital. N Engl J Med 297:1054, 1977
11. Cello P et al: Endoscopic sclerotherapy versus portacaval shunt in patients with severe cirrhosis and variceal hemorrhage. N Engl J Med 311:1589–1594, 1984
12. Classen M, Hagenmuller F: Biliary drainage. Endoscopy 15:221–229, 1983
13. Clemett AR: Percutaneous transhepatic cholangiography. In Berk RN, Clemett AR (eds): Radiology of the Gallbladder and Bile Ducts, p 241. Philadelphia, WB Saunders, 1977
14. Cooperman A et al: Periampullary cancer, 1983. Semin Liver Dis 3:181–192, 1983
15. Copenhagen Group: Sclerotherapy after first variceal hemorrhage in cirrhosis. N Engl J Med 311:1594–1600, 1984
16. Cotton PB et al: Pancreas divisum: Curiosity or culprit? Gastroenterology 89:1431–1435, 1985
17. Dagradi AE et al: Bleeding esophageal varices. Arch Surg 92:944–947, 1966
18. Delhaye M et al: Pancreas divisum. Gastroenterology 89: 951–958, 1985
19. Elias E et al: Endoscopic retrograde cholangiopancreatography in the diagnosis of jaundice associated with ulcerative colitis. Gastroenterology 67:107–111, 1974
20. Elson CO et al: Polymicrobial sepsis following endoscopic retrograde cholangiopancreatography. Gastroenterology 69: 507–510, 1975
21. Escourrou J et al: Early and late complications after endoscopic sphincterotomy for biliary lithiasis with and without the gallbladder in situ. Gut 25:598–602, 1984
22. Falkenstein DB et al: The endoscopic intrahepatic cholangiogram: Clinco-pathological correlation with post-mortem cholangiograms. Invest Radiol 10:358–365, 1975
23. Feduska NJ et al: Results of palliative operations for carcinoma of the pancreas. Arch Surg 103:330–334, 1971
24. Fleig WE et al: Emergency endoscopic sclerotherapy for bleeding esophageal varices: A prospective study of patients not responding to balloon tamponade. Gastrointest Endosc 29:8–14, 1983
25. Gebhardt CL et al: The importance of ERCP for the surgical tactic in haemorrhagic necrotizing pancreatitis. Endoscopy 15:558, 1983
26. Goodman MW et al: Is intravenous cholangiography still useful? Gastroenterology 79:642–645, 1980
27. Gothlin J, Tranberg KG: Complications of percutaneous transhepatic cholangiography (PTC). AJR 117:426–431, 1973
28. Gudry SR et al: Efficacy of preoperative biliary tract decompression in patients with obstructive jaundice. Arch Surg 119:703–708, 1984
29. Hall RC, Sckiyakk P, Kim SK: Failure of operative cholangiography to prevent retained common duct stones. Am J Surg 125:51–63, 1973
30. Helpap B, Bollweg L: Morphological changes in the terminal esophagus with varices, following sclerosis of the wall. Endoscopy 6:229, 1981
31. Huber DF et al: Cholecystectomy in elderly patients. Am J Surg 146:719, 1983
32. Johnston GW, Rogers HW: A review of 15 years experience in the use of sclerotherapy in the control of acute hemorrhage from esophageal varices. Br J Surg 60:797, 1973
33. Juler GL et al: Bile leakage following percutaneous transhepatic cholangiography with the Chiba needle. Arch Surg 112:954–958, 1977
34. Kessler RE, Falkenstein DB, Clemett AR et al: Indications, clinical value and complications of endoscopic retrograde cholangiopancreatography. Surg Gynecol Obstet 142:865–870, 1976
35. Kleitsch WP et al: Anatomy of the pancreas. Arch Surg 71: 795, 1955
36. Koch H: Operative endoscopy. Gastrointest Endosc 24:65–68, 1977
37. Koch H et al: Endoscopic papillotomy. Gastroenterology 73:1393, 1977
38. Koch RL, Gorder JL: Bile-blood fistula: A complication of percutaneous transhepatic cholangiography. Radiology 93: 67, 1969
39. Kreek M, Balint JA: "Skinny needle" cholangiography. Gastroenterology 78:598–604, 1980
40. Leung JWC et al: Management of malignant obstructive jaundice at the Middlesex Hospital. Br J Surg 70:584–586, 1983
41. Luft HS et al: Should operations be regionalized? The empirical relation between volume and mortality. N Engl J Med 301:1364–1369, 1979

42. Lumeng L et al: Final report of a blinded prospective study comparing current noninvasive approaches in the differential diagnosis of medical and surgical jaundice (abstr). Gastroenterology 78:1312, 1980

43. MacDougall BRD et al: Increased long-term survival in variceal hemorrhage using injection sclerotherapy. Lancet 1:124–127, 1982

44. Margulis AR: Cholestasis in ulcerative colitis: Radiologic evaluation. Gastroenterology 73:362, 1977

45. Matzen P, Haubek A, Holst-Christensen J et al: Accuracy of direct cholangiography by endoscopic or transhepatic route in jaundice: A prospective study. Gastroenterology 81:234–241, 1981

46. Matzen P, Malchow-Moller A, Brun B et al: Ultrasonography, computed tomography, and cholescintography in suspected obstructive jaundice: A prospective comparative study. Gastroenterology 84: 1492–1497, 1983

47. McCormack TT et al: Gastric lesions in portal hypertension: Inflammatory gastritis or congestive gastropathy? Gut 26: 1226–1232, 1985

48. McSherry CK, Glenn F: The incidence and causes of death following surgery for nonmalignant biliary tract disease. Ann Surg 191:271–275, 1980

49. Mori W, Mukawa K: Wound healing and complications to the liver after percutaneous transhepatic cholangiography. Acta Hepatogastroenterol 24:86–92, 1977

50. Mueller PR et al: Percutaneous biliary drainage: Technical and catheter related problems in 200 procedures. Am J Radiol 135:17–23, 1982

51. Nakayama T et al: Percutaneous transhepatic drainage of the biliary tract. Gastroenterology 74:554–559, 1978

52. Neff RA et al: The radiologic management of malignant biliary obstruction. Clin Radiol 34:143–146, 1983

53. Neptolemos JP et al: The management of common bile duct calculi by endoscopic sphincterotomy with gallbladders in situ. Br J Surg 71:69–71, 1984

54. Novis BH et al: Endoscopic manometry of the pancreatic duct and sphincter zone in patients with chronic pancreatitis Dig Dis Sci 30:225–228, 1985

55. O'Connor KW, Sondgrass PJ, Swonder JE et al: A blinded prospective study comparing four current noninvasive approaches in the differential diagnosis of medical versus surgical jaundice. Gastroenterology 84:1498–1504, 1983

56. Oi I et al: Endoscopic pancreatocholangiography. Endoscopy 2:103–106, 1970

57. Okuda K et al: Nonsurgical, percutaneous transhepatic cholangiography—diagnostic significance in medical problems of the liver. Am J Dig Dis 19:21–36, 1974

58. Oscarson J et al: Selective angiography and fine-needle aspiration cytodiagnosis of gastric and pancreatic tumors. Acta Radiol 12:737–749, 1972

59. Paquet KJ, Feussner H: Endoscopic sclerosis and esophageal balloon tamponade in acute hemorrhage from esophagogastric varices: A prospective controlled randomized trial. Hepatology 5:580–583, 1985

60. Paquet KJ et al: Endoscopic paravariceal injection sclerotherapy of the esophagus—indications, technique, complications: Results of a period of 14 years. Gastrointest Endosc 29:310–315, 1983

61. Pitt HA et al: Does preoperative percutaneous biliary drainage reduce operative risk or increase hospital cost? Ann Surg 201:545–553, 1985

62. Ratner JT, Rosenberg GM: Management of gallstones in the aged. J Am Geriatr Soc 23:258, 1975

63. Riemann JF, Demling L: Lithotripsy of bile duct stones. Endoscopy 15:191–196, 1983

64. Ring EJ et al: Therapeutic applications of catheter cholangiography. Radiology 128:333–338, 1978

65. Roberts-Thomson IC, Toouli J: Is endoscopic sphincterotomy for disabling biliary-type pain after cholecystectomy effective? Gastrointest Endosc 6:370–373, 1985

66. Rosseland AR, Solhaug JH: Early or delayed endoscopic papillotomy in gallstone pancreatitis. Ann Surg 199:165–167, 1984

67. Ruddell WSJ et al: The diagnostic yield of ERCP in the investigation of unexplained abdominal pain. Br J Surg 70: 74–75, 1983

68. Ruppin H et al: Acute pancreatitis after endoscopic/radiological pancreatography. Endoscopy 6:94, 1974

69. Safrany L: Duodenoscopic sphincterotomy and gallstone removal. Gastroenterology 72:338, 1977

70. Safrany L, Cotton PB: A preliminary report: Urgent duodenoscopic sphincterotomy for gallstone pancreatitis. Surgery 89:424–428, 1981

71. Safrany L, Cotton PB: Endoscopic management of choledocholithiasis. Surg Clin North Am 62:825–836, 1982

72. Sauerbruch T et al: Bacteraemia associated with endoscopic sclerotherapy of esophageal varices. Endoscopy 17:170–172, 1985

73. Scharschmidt BF, Goldberg HI, Schmid R: Approach to the patient with jaundice. N Engl J Med 308:1515–1519, 1983

74. Soderlund C et al: Sclerotherapy of esophageal varices: An endoscopic and portographic study. Hepatology 5:877–884, 1984

75. Sohendra N et al: Sclerotherapy of esophageal varices: Acute arrest of gastrointestinal hemorrhage or long term therapy? Endoscopy 15:136–140, 1983

76. Sohendra N et al: Injection of nonvariceal bleeding lesions of the upper gastrointestinal tract. Endoscopy 4:129–132, 1985

77. Speer AG et al: Randomized trial comparing endoscopic and percutaneous prostheses in poor risk patients with malignant obstructive jaundice. Gut 26:A1135, 1985

78. Spence RAJ et al: Esophageal mucosal changes in patients with varices. Gut 24:1024–1029, 1983

79. Spence RAJ et al: Histologic factors of the esophageal transection ring as clues to the pathogenesis of bleeding varices. Surg Gynecol Obstet 159:253–259, 1984

80. Spooner BS et al: The developement of the dorsal and ventral mammalian pancreas in vivo and in vitro. J Cell Biol 47:235, 1970

81. Starlitz M et al: Endoscopic removal of common duct stones through the intact papilla after medical sphincter dilation. Gastroenterology 88:1807–1811, 1985

82. Stoker J et al: Results of endoscopic stenting in malignant stricture of the biliary tract. Gut 26:A1135, 1985

83. Stolte M et al: Vaskularisation der Papilla Vater; und Blutungsgefahybe, der Papillotomie. Leber Magen Darm 10: 293–301, 1980

84. Terblanche J et al: A prospective controlled trial of sclerotherapy in the long-term management of patients after variceal bleeding. Surg Gynecol Obstet 148:322, 1979

85. Terblanche J et al: Long-term management of patients after an esophageal variceal bleed: The role of sclerotherapy. Br J Surg 72:88–90, 1985

86. Titchener JL: The psychology of the aged surgical patient.

In Powers JH (ed): Surgery of the Aged and Debilitated Patient, p 254. Philadelphia, WB Saunders, 1968

87. Vander Spuys S: Endoscopic sphincterotomy in the management of gallstone pancreatitis. Endoscopy 13:25–26, 1981

88. Velasco N et al: Treatment of retained common bile duct stones: A prospective controlled study comparing monoctanon and heparin. World J Surg 7:266–270, 1983

89. Veno RP et al: ERCP: Diagnosis of cholelithiasis in patients with normal gallbladder x-ray and ultrasound studies. JAMA 249:74–75, 1983

90. Warren WD et al: Distal splenorenal shunt versus endoscopic sclerotherapy in management of variceal bleeding: Early results of a randomized trial. Hepatology 5:984A, 1985

91. Warshaw AL et al: The cause and treatment of pancreatitis associated with pancreas divisum. Ann Surg 198:443–452, 1983

92. Weiserner RH, La Russo NF: Clincopathologic features of the syndrome of primary sclerosing cholangitis. Gastroenterology 79:200–206, 1980

93. Westaby D, Williams R: The history of injection sclerotherapy for esophageal varices. Gastrointest Endosc 29:303–307, 1983

94. Westaby D, Williams R: Followup study after sclerotherapy. Scand J Gastroenterol 19:(suppl 102):71–75, 1984

95. Westaby D et al: By selective adrenoreceptor blockade for the long-term management of variceal bleeding: A prospective randomized trial comparing metoprolol with injection sclerotherapy in cirrhosis. Gut 26:421–425, 1985

96. White TT, Hart MJ: Cholangiography and small duct injury. Am J Surg 149:640–643, 1985

97. Wiechel KL et al: Percutaneous transhepatic cholangiography. Acta Chir Scand Suppl 330:1, 1964

98. Winstanley PA et al: Medium term complications of endoscopic biliary sphincterotomy. Gut 26:730–733, 1985

99. Witzel L et al: Prophylactic endoscopic sclerotherapy of esophageal varices: A prospective controlled study. Lancet 1:773–776, 1985

100. Zimmon DS: Endoscopic biliary surgery: The American experience. In Demling L, Rösch W (eds): Operative Endoskopie 1979, pp 117–124. Berlin, Acron Verlag, 1979

101. Zimmon DS: Endoscopic diagnosis and management of biliary and pancreatic disease. Curr Probl Surg 16:1–46, 1979

102. Zimmon DS: New uses of ERCP in the management of biliary and pancreatic disease. In Progress in Gastroenterology, vol 4, pp 477–504. New York, Grune & Stratton, 1983

103. Zimmon DS, Clemett AR: Visualization of the bile ducts. In Popper H, Schaffner F (eds): Progress in Liver Diseases, vol VI, pp 503–518. New York, Grune & Stratton, 1979

104. Zimmon DS, Clemett AR: Endoscopic stents and drains in the managment of pancreatic and bile duct obstruction. Surg Clin North Am 62:837–844, 1982

105. Zimmon DS, Clemett AR: Nonsurgical biliary drainage in cancer. In DeCosse JJ, Sherlock P (eds): Clinical Management of Gastrointestinal Cancer, pp 275–302, Boston, M Nijhoff, 1984

106. Zimmon DS, Clemett AR, Cooperman A: Letter: Cholestatic jaundice. N Engl J Med 309:1192, 1983

107. Zimmon DS, Kessler RE: The effect of portal venous blood flow diversion on portal pressure. J Clin Invest 65:1388–1397, 1980

108. Zimmon DS et al: Endoscopic retrograde cholangiopancreatography (ERCP) in the diagnosis of pancreatic inflammatory disease. Radiology 3:287–292, 1974

109. Zimmon DS et al: Complications of endoscopic retrograde cholangiopancreatography: Analysis of 300 consecutive cases. Gastroenterology 69:303–309, 1975

110. Zimmon DS et al: Endoscopy with endoscopic cholangiopancreatography: The combination as a primary diagnostic procedure. JAMA 233:447–449, 1975

111. Zimmon DS et al: Endoscopic papillotomy for choledocholithiasis. N Engl J Med 293:1181–1182, 1975

112. Zimmon DS et al: Management of biliary calculi by retrograde endoscopic instrumentation (lithocenosis). Gastrointest Endosc 23:82–86, 1976

113. Zimmon DS et al: Percutaneous pancreatography. Gastroenterology 77:1101–1104, 1979

114. Zimmon DS et al: Advances in the management of bile duct obstruction: Percutaneous transhepatic cholangiography and endoscopic retrograde cholangiopancreatography. Med Clin North Am 63:593–609, 1979

115. Zimmon DS et al: Endoscopic biliary surgery: The American Experience. In Deming L, Rösch W (eds): Operative Endoskopic 1979, p 117. Berlin, Acron Verlag, 1979

chapter 12
Special Radiologic Procedures in Liver Diseases

RAOUL PEREIRAS

PERCUTANEOUS TRANSHEPATIC CHOLANGIOGRAPHY

One of the most common and difficult problems that the internist must confront in his regular practice is the differential diagnosis of cholestasis. This syndrome results from a decrease in bile flow and encompasses a wide array of conditions that affect the biliary tree anywhere from the hepatocyte to the duodenum. The difficulty arises in defining the site of biliary pathology. The effect may be an intra- or extraphepatic lesion, the latter being amenable to surgery and the former not. Clinical, biochemical, and pathologic studies often fail to differentiate hepatocellular causes from mechanically obstructive ones, making visualization of the biliary tree highly desirable. From the therapeutic point of view, one must decide whether or not to operate. Surgery in a patient with intrahepatic cholestasis is at least a relative, if not an absolute, contraindication because of the deleterious effect of surgery upon a damaged liver, particularly if significant hepatic obstruction requires a palliative or curative solution. Surgical intervention precludes the complications of cholangitis and cirrhosis.

The first report of a percutaneous transhepatic cholangiography came from Huart and Do-Xuan-Hop in 1937. However, because of the high incidence of complications such as bile peritonitis and bleeding observed with the large needle originally used, surgical intervention had to be arranged immediately after the procedure. In many cases, dilated biliary trees were undetected, and rarely was the nondilated biliary tree visualized. This technique was improved with the advent of the image intensifier first reported by Arnel and Glenn in 1962. Weichel, in 1964, published a very comprehensive review with various measures to improve its safety, the most important being a change from a rigid needle to a catheter needle combination.[132] After the report by Okuda and co-workers in 1974 of the so-called Chiba method, in which a sharp, thin, flexible 23-gauge needle is used, this technique was rapidly accepted as the preferred approach for direct opacification of the biliary ducts in the evaluation of cholestatic jaundice.[28,83,85,87,88,105]

Technique

After confirmation of a cholestatic syndrome by clinical and biochemical parameters, prothrombin time (PT), partial thromboplastin time (PTT), and a platelet count are obtained. The PT should be within 4 seconds of control, the PTT less than 40 seconds, and the platelet count greater than $40,000/mm^3$. The patient is fasted overnight, and no sedation is used. Patients with clinical cholangitis receive I.V. antibiotics whenever possible for 24 hours before the examination.

After adequate sterilization of the skin, local anesthesia is administered, and the needle is introduced in a site slightly anterior to the midaxillary line and as high as possible, avoiding the right costophrenic angle. The needle is aimed at a lead landmark placed over the abdomen equidistant between the dome of the diaphragm and the duodenal bulb, which is outlined by air.[85,87,88] With this approach, one attempts to enter a duct slightly above the confluence of the hepatic ducts (Fig. 12-1). The highest entry point below the costophrenic angle avoids going through the gallbladder. The stylet is then removed, and normal respiration is permitted. Contrast material (Renografin, 60%) is injected through a polyethylene tube attached to the needle, which is slowly withdrawn under fluoroscopic monitoring. If a nondilated biliary tree is entered, several quick exposures are obtained. Enough contrast media is then injected to fill the biliary tree and the gallbladder, and the needle is removed. It is important to obtain multiple films in different positions, even if the ducts are not dilated, in order not to overlook small calculi. If a dilated biliary tree is encountered, 20 ml to 50 ml of bile are withdrawn, and similar amounts of contrast material are injected. Aspiration of bile alternating with the injection of contrast meterial is repeatedly performed until there is complete filling of the biliary tree without over-

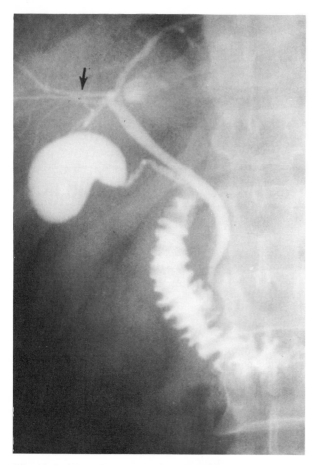

Fig. 12-1. Normal transhepatic cholangiogram. The patient has alcoholic hepatitis. Arrow shows the entry point of the needle just above the confluence of the hepatic ducts.

distention. Overdistention of the bile ducts in a patient with cholangitis frequently leads to bacteremia with fever and sometimes shock.

After multiple films are obtained at all possible projections, the ducts are completely decompressed, the needle is removed, and the entry point is covered with a small Band-Aid. Contrast material in blood vessels is easily recognized by the direction of the flow and by its rapid disappearance (Fig. 12-2). Liver lymphatics are differentiated from normal ducts by their tortuosity, increased number, and drainage toward the midline into the cisterna chyli (Fig. 12-3). Perivascular injection can be a problem, because contrast material here can simulate the appearance of intraluminal contrast in a dilated system (Fig. 12-4). Fluoroscopically, the slower flow of contrast permits the differentiation of contrast material within the lumen from that in the biliary system, where centrifugal flow is more rapid. If no biliary ducts can be entered after six or seven passes of the needle, we can only assume that the bile

ducts are of normal size or are minimally dilated. However, a false sense of security may result if one does not attempt to visualize the nondilated biliary tree, which may still be the site of surgically correctable pathology. The most common type of pathology in this group of patients is choledocholithiasis (Fig. 12-5).[113] In these patients, a rapid fluctuation in biliary tree size occurs because of a ball–valve phenomenon (Fig. 12-6). Patients with long-standing postoperative benign strictures of the extrahepatic bile ducts usually do not get a marked distention of the intrahepatic radicles because of secondary biliary cirrhosis caused by long-standing ascending cholangitis (Fig. 12-7).

We have encountered a surgically correctable jaundice in 4% of patients studied in whom the bile ducts were not dilated. We believe that the success rate in nondilated ducts is significantly improved by an increase in the number of passes made with the Chiba needle. If no biliary ducts can be entered before discontinuation of the procedure, we always make an attempt to puncture the gallbladder. This has further increased the success rate in patients with nondilated ducts, and we believe that we have not significantly affected the morbidity rate. Illescas and co-workers reported on ultrasound-guided percutaneous transcholecystal cholangiography for visualization of the biliary tree on five patients following failed endoscopic retrograde cholangiography. In all cases, the visualization was excellent, and there were no complications.[47]

Although some investigators report that it is almost always impossible to aspirate bile through a Chiba needle,[22,48] we have not encountered this problem in more than 1400 examinations. If the ducts are dilated and bile cannot be aspirated in spite of rotation of the needle, a small peripheral duct has probably been entered. Reposition of the needle into a more central branch will solve the problem.

In patients with severe obstruction of the distal common duct, a high pseudo-obstruction at the level of the hilum of the liver is very commonly encountered (Fig. 12-8A). This pseudo-obstruction is due to incomplete filling of the biliary tree and demonstrates the importance of aspirating bile and injecting contrast media. Complete replacement of the existing bile together with a change in the position of the patient will delineate the real level of obstruction (Fig. 12-8B).

Indications and Contraindications

We can simplify the indications for this procedure to include any situation in which surgery is contemplated for possible obstructive jaundice. An absolute exclusion of surgical intervention is probably the only contraindication.[9] Severe bleeding disorders can usually be corrected by administering platelets or fresh frozen plasma before the procedure, but, in many of these patients, it is probably safer to use ERCP.[123]

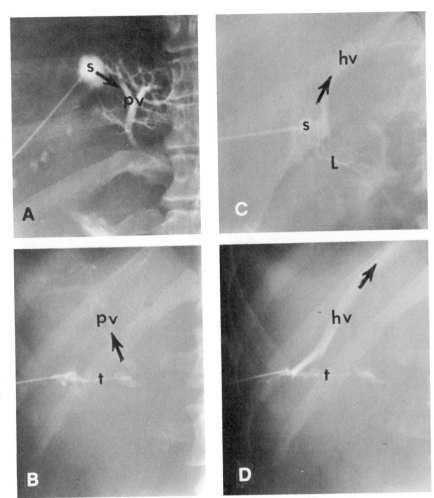

Fig. 12-2. A. Injection into a sinusoid in a patient with portal hypertension shows reversal of flow (*arrow*) into portal vein **B.** Demonstration of normal direction of flow (*arrow*) of portal vein (*pv*). t, needle tract. **C.** Injection into a sinusoid with normal flow (*arrow*) in the hepatic vein (*hv*). Note the filling of the small lymphatic (*L*). **D.** Direct injection into a hepatic vein (*hv*) showing normal flow (*arrow*). t, needle tract.

Interpretation

With good radiologic technique, stones in the bile ducts rarely represent a diagnostic problem. At fluoroscopy, stones are seen to move about freely in the dilated portion of the duct system. Impacted stones are easily diagnosed when it is possible to inject contrast media past the stone and visualize its proximal and distal margins (Fig. 12-9). Stone impaction with complete obstruction sometimes has an appearance that is nonspecific in character; an irregular calculus may simulate a polypoid tumor. In cases in which calculi are suspected, it is very important that some early radiographs be obtained in which only a few of the contrast media have been injected. Even if the ducts are not very dilated, a small calculus can be obscured by large amounts of contrast media when the ducts are completely filled (Fig. 12-10). Dilution of contrast material with saline is also used routinely when calculi are sus-

pected. The diagnostic problem arises when we have failed to demonstrate the biliary tree. In our experience, most patients with failure to visualize the biliary tree but with surgically correctable pathology were later found to have a nondilated system with biliary calculi.

Parasites usually do not present a problem in diagnosis. Ascaris lumbricoides are easily recognized because of the size and shape of the adult worms, even when coiled in the duct. Children with choledocholithiasis or any patient with intrahepatic calculi or hepatic duct stones without cholelithiasis should be investigated for parasitic infestation, particularly ascaris. The liver flukes are flat leaflike worms that have an oval or elliptic shape when viewed *en face* and measure at most 1 cm to 2 cm in diameter.

Recurrent chronic cholangitis causes changes in the bile duct that can be recognized radiographically. The extrahepatic ducts and larger intrahepatic ducts are dilated. The smaller intrahepatic ducts are straightened and taper abruptly. Areas of stricture and ill-defined margins are

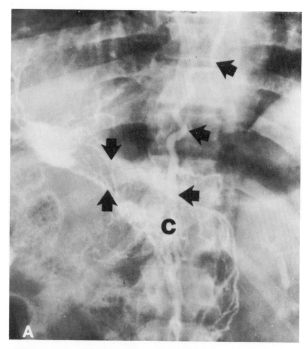

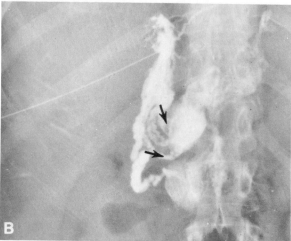

Fig. 12-3. A. Skinny needle transhepatic cholangiogram showing filling of multiple liver lymphatics, which drain into the cisterna chyli (*C*) and into the thoracic duct (*arrows*). B. Filling of engorged and tortuous liver lymphatics, which drain into enlarged hilar nodes (*arrows*) in a patient with primary biliary cirrhosis.

also present. If these are complicated with multiple small liver abscesses that communicate with the bile ducts, the diagnosis is even easier (Fig. 12-11).

Sclerosing cholangitis is a nonspecific, chronic, low-grade fibrosing inflammatory reaction of the biliary system of unknown etiology. Not infrequently, it is associated with ulcerative colitis.[129] Differentiation from certain slow-growing scirrhous carcinomas of the bile ducts may not be possible, even at surgery. An association between long-standing ulcerative colitis and bile duct tumor has also been suggested.[36] Stricture is the characteristic radiologic feature. The length of the stricture can vary, ranging from uniform involvement of the extrahepatic bile ducts to short focal strictures of the hepatic ducts. The alternation of short focal strictures with focal areas of minimal dilatation may result in a beaded appearance of the hepatic ducts (Fig. 12-12). A decreased arborization of the intrahepatic radicles is also very common, resulting in what has been described as a "pruned tree" appearance (Fig. 12-13.).[129] One important finding that is very useful in differential diagnosis is the absence of marked dilatation of the intrahepatic ducts proximal to a stricture. This is explained by the histologic finding of a subepithelial inflammatory fibrosis of the walls of the bile duct. Another important x-ray finding is that, although obstructive jaundice is present, the contrast material usually passes through the stenotic duct into the duodenum.

Choledochal cyst is a segmental dilatation of the common bile duct that may also involve the adjacent cystic and common hepatic ducts. In Caroli's disease, there is a segmental saccular dilatation of the intrahepatic bile ducts. The usual complications are intrahepatic stone formation with recurrent cholangitis and liver abscesses.

In chronic pancreatitis, there is usually a long stricture of the distal common bile duct, which is quite smooth. There is moderate dilatation of the extrahepatic bile ducts and normal or only slight dilatation of the intrahepatic radicles (Fig. 12-14). Complete common duct obstruction is rarely seen. Marked displacement of the strictured portion of the duct occurs when an associated pseudocyst is located in the head of the pancreas (Fig. 12-15).

Papillary stenosis is a controversial subject. The surgical criterion for diagnosis is failure to pass a dilator larger than a Bakes No. 3 from the common duct into the duodenum.[118] The diagnosis can be suspected if a stenosis of the terminal bile duct with a retention of contrast media in dilated proximal bile ducts is demonstrated. Radiographically, it is impossible to make a differential diagnosis of the tumor.

Obstruction of the Bile Ducts by Tumor

Total obstruction of the common duct at the superior margin of the pancreas is almost always due to pancreatic carcinoma.[9] We rarely encounter a complete obstruction of the common bile duct using good cholangiographic technique. Usually, there is more dilatation of proximal radicles than with a primary bile duct carcinoma. Because there is almost always a large mass associated with pancreatic carcinoma, a frequent finding is a median upward displacement of the obstructed duct.[71] If, indeed, a complete obstruction is encountered, the configuration of the duct at the point of obstruction may show a rat-tail deformity or may be blunt or rounded (Fig. 12-16*A,B*). Car-

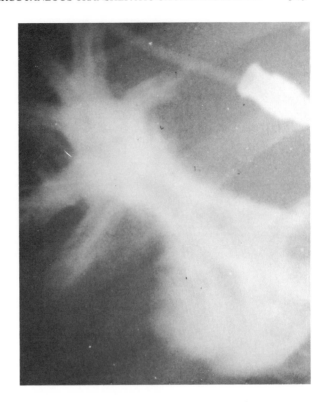

Fig. 12-4. Branching pattern of perivascular injection at time of transhepatic cholangiography may, at time of fluoroscopy, simulate contrast media in a dilated system.

Fig. 12-5. Normal-sized biliary tree with multiple small calculi in the distal portion of the common duct (*CD*) and in the gallbladder. The common duct measures less than 4 mm. E, area of extravasation.

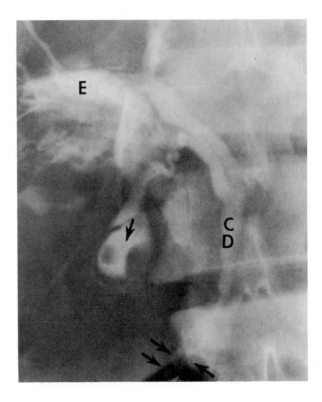

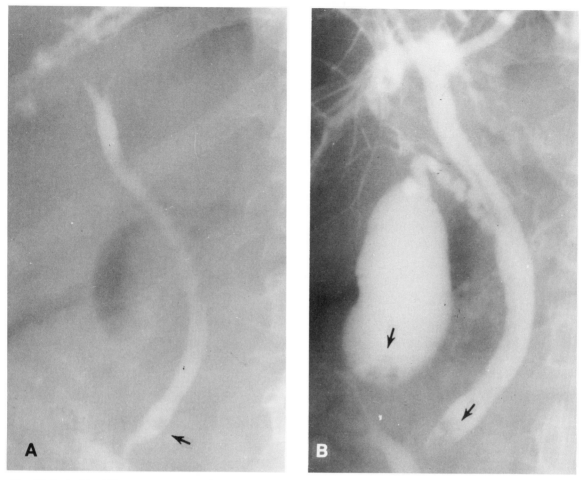

Fig. 12-6. A. The biliary tree may experience fluctuations in size among patients with chole-docholithiasis. Transhepatic cholangiogram shows normal-sized ducts with a small distal filling defect (*arrow*). **B.** The same study repeated 20 minutes later. During that time, the patient experienced right upper quadrant pain. The new study shows that several calculi have migrated from the cystic duct and are impacted in the distal common duct (*arrow*), which is larger in size. Also note other calculi within the gallbladder.

cinomas of the papilla are usually very small tumors that cause a very severe or complete obstruction of the distal end of the common duct. If a tumor is polypoid, the radiographic findings are characteristic (Fig. 12-17).

Bile Duct Carcinoma. Primary carcinoma of the bile ducts is no longer considered rare. Several large series have been reported.[15,48] Most of these tumors are small nodular or annular scirrhous infiltrating lesions. Less than 5% are papillary or polypoid lesions. They can arise anywhere in the biliary tree, although the two anatomical sites of preference are the common hepatic duct, including the bifurcation (37%), and the common bile duct (28%). In the past, most of these tumors were undetected at the time

of an exploratory laparotomy in patients presenting with obstructive jaundice.

Small sclerosing lesions, especially those located high in the porta hepatis, were frequently overlooked by both the surgeon and the radiologist, because operative cholangiograms are usually of poor quality (Fig. 12-18). The infrequent polypoid intraluminal tumors are easily recognized (Fig. 12-19). The small scirrhous carcinoma presents with a short area of stenosis and a variable degree of dilatation of the proximal ducts (Fig. 12-20). Cases with extensive axial spread present with a long stenosis that cannot be differentiated from metastatic carcinoma (Fig. 12-21). Primary tumor of the bile duct and hepatocellular carcinoma can cause similar changes.[13]. Extrahepatic duct

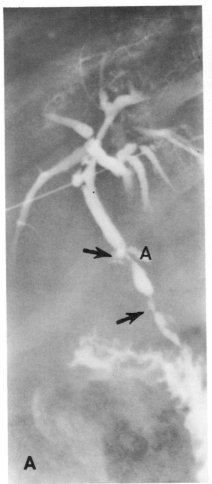

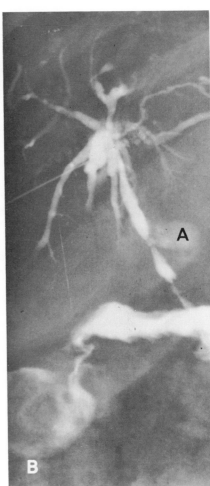

Fig. 12-7. A nondilated biliary tree with surgical jaundice. Multiple postoperative strictures of the common duct (*arrows*) with an area of extravasation into a small abscess (*A*) resulted in secondary biliary cirrhosis. Note beading of the intrahepatic radicles, which are crowded together. These changes are secondary to long-standing ascending cholangitis. This patient benefited from resection of the common duct and abscess and from a high hepaticojejunostomy.

obstruction, although rare, has also been reported with hepatocellular carcinoma. (Fig. 12-22). The location of primary biliary carcinoma can be a problem for differential diagnosis. Those lesions occurring at the level of the porta hepatis at times cannot be differentiated from metastatic disease to the lymph nodes of the hilum of the liver, Hodgkin's disease, carcinoma of the gallbladder, or primary hepatocellular carcinoma. There is usually a longer stenosis in metastatic carcinoma than in primary bile duct carcinoma. In carcinoma of the gallbladder, besides the stenosis or complete obstruction of the common hepatic and cystic ducts, there is usually a large massive lesion in the region of the gallbladder.

Metastatic carcinoma of the liver may cause distortion and displacement of the intrahepatic ducts with areas of segmental stenosis or occlusion (Fig. 12-23). This is best seen when the ducts are not fully distended with contrast media. Polycystic disease may cause compression of intrahepatic ducts, which can simulate metastatic carci-

noma, and the hepatic ducts, especially the small branches, may be straightened and narrowed in diffuse lymphoma.[9] In cirrhosis, the ducts are usually tortuous and irregular in caliber (Fig. 12-24.)[121]

Complications

The most important complications of percutaneous transhepatic cholangiography that are seen especially in patients with partially obstructing biliary calculi are fever and sepsis. In a recently published multi-institutional survey based on more than 2000 procedures, fever not accompanied by hypotension or a positive blood culture occurred in 3.4%.[39] In the same study, sepsis, which was defined as fever and chills accompanied by hypotension, positive blood culture, or severe prostration, occurred in 1.4%. Our personal experience with more than 1400 examinations shows similar results except for fewer complications resulting from sepsis (0.8%). It is advised that

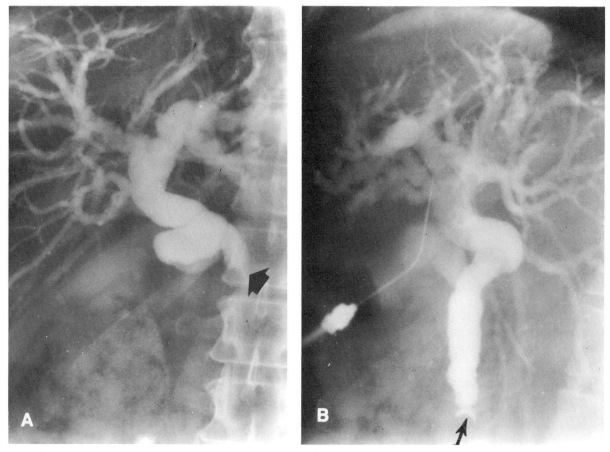

Fig. 12-8. A. A pseudo-obstruction high in the common hepatic duct (*arrow*) is a common finding when the ducts are not completely filled. **B.** After aspiration of bile alternating with injection of contrast media, the true level of obstruction was pinpointed. Note the small stone impacted at the ampulla (*arrow*).

any patient referred for percutaneous cholangiography with clinical signs of cholangitis be placed on high doses of systemic antibiotics for 1 to 2 days before the examination. We use a combination of ampicillin and gentamicin. An immediate surgical or nonsurgical decompression is recommended in those patients with mechanical obstructive jaundice complicated by clinical or radiographic evidence of cholangitis. Needle puncture of the liver may be painless, but most patients note a dull pain in the epigastrium. Severe pain can occur if bile cannot be aspirated and the ducts are overdistended with contrast media.

Clinical peritonitis caused by intraperitoneal bile leakage occurred in 0.6% of the patients in the abovementioned study.[39] We believe that a significant intraperitoneal leakage of sterile bile occurs in a good percentage of patients without causing any peritoneal signs. We have personal experience with three patients, two of whom had traumatic rupture of the gallbladder and one of whom had postsurgical leak of bile diagnosed 2 to 3 months after surgery; the only clinical complaint of the latter patient was an increase in the size of the abdomen resulting from the accumulation of several liters of bile (Fig. 12-25.). Intraperitoneal hemorrhage is an uncommon complication. We encountered our first significant postprocedure hemorrhage when we had more than 800 examinations. The patient was treated conservatively with blood transfusions, and the bleeding stopped within 24 hours; however, the patient died from a coronary thrombosis 4 days postprocedure. Harbin reported intraperitoneal hemorrhage in 0.35% of his cases and death in 0.2%.[39] Ariyama, in 1983, published the complications in 2745 procedures. Sepsis occurred in 1.7%, bile leakage in 0.9%, bleeding in 0.2%, and death in 0.1%.[6] Hepatic arteriovenous fistulas, almost always arterioportal, are of no clinical significance and usually close spontaneously.[131]

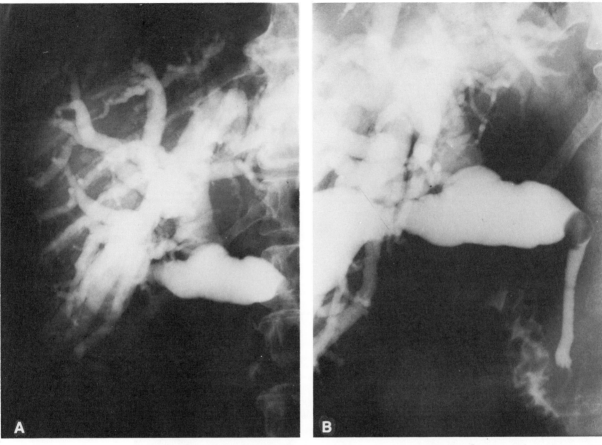

Fig. 12-9. **A.** Complete obstruction at the proximal portion of the common duct is shown with marked dilatation of the biliary tree. The configuration of the duct at the point of obstruction is not diagnostic. Clinically, carcinoma of the pancreas was suspected, given that the patient's jaundice was painless. **B.** Once contrast media flows distal to the obstruction, the diagnosis of an impacted calculi is obvious.

Important Features

The success of percutaneous cholangiography in opacifying the biliary system is directly related to the presence of ductal dilatation and the number of attempts made.[50] The use of multiple passes when necessary (average 12–14) brings the success rate to 99%.[4,39,88] Ariyama, in 1983, reviewing 2515 cases, found a success rate of 98% in the dilated and 82% in the nondilated group.[6] A comparison of groups that limit their number of passes to fewer than six with others that routinely use more than six shows no difference in the incidence of serious complications.[39]

Contrast media should be continuously injected during withdrawal of the thin-gauge flexible needle. This permits demonstration of normal-sized ducts in a high percentage of patients.[28,41,85,87,88,105]

Aspiration of bile alternating with the injection of contrast material prevents overdistention in dilated ducts.[41,87,88]

Dilated ducts should be completely decompressed before removal of the needle.[41,99]

A right flank approach should be used. This is superior to the anterior subcostal approach, because it produces less of a likelihood of bile leakage into the peritoneal cavity.[85]

Prophylactic antibiotic therapy should be used.[31,39,88]

Under no circumstances is it appropriate to draw a conclusion if the biliary tree is not entered and visualized successfully, because patients with nondilated ducts can harbor a surgical jaundice.[73,88] Percutaneous transhepatic cholangiography with the Chiba needle is the procedure of choice in resolving the differential diagnosis of obstructive jaundice. This is the simplest, cheapest, and most

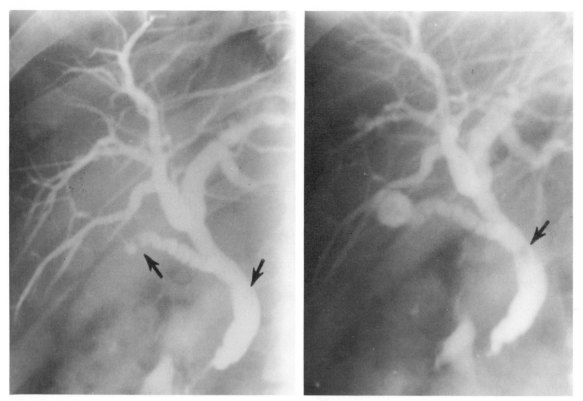

Fig. 12-10. Common duct and cystic duct calculi (*arrows*) partially obscured by contrast media.

Fig. 12-11. A. Recurring cholangitis showing ill-defined markings of the intrahepatic radicles. **B.** Multiple liver abscesses (*A*) that communicate with the biliary tree.

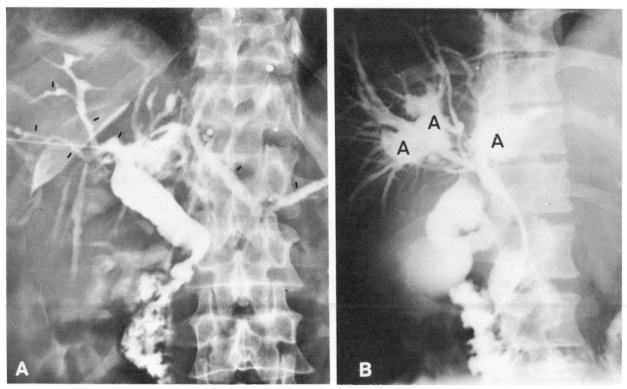

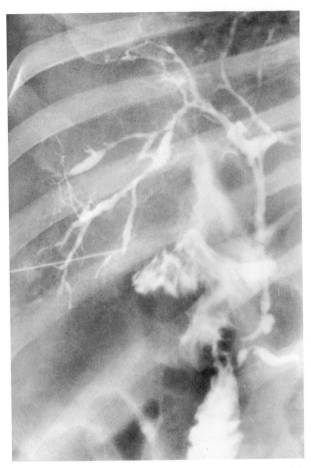

Fig. 12-12. Classic example of primary sclerosing cholangitis with the hepatic ducts having a beaded appearance.

widely available single examination capable of preventing unnecessary exploration of the jaundiced patient with primary liver parenchymal disease. It is also the most useful potential source of practical information if laparotomy is necessary to correct biliary tract obstruction.

ANGIOGRAPHY OF LIVER MASSES

Selective arteriography is the best method currently available for detecting the presence and nature of hepatic masses.[80a] Furthermore, in spite of advances with computerized tomography (CT) and ultrasound of the liver, angiography remains the most critical examination for determining the extent of disease and potential surgical cure in patients with hepatic malignancy.

Technique

With the Seldinger technique[116]—from a femoral artery approach—the arteries supplying the liver are selectively catheterized. Both celiac and superior mesenteric arteries are routinely catheterized, because, in one fourth of the cases, a portion or all of the arterial blood supply of the liver arises from the superior mesenteric artery.[76] Also, in 18% of cases, the hepatic artery arises from the left gastric artery.[76] Whenever technically possible, we routinely inject each hepatic artery selectively, even if it arises from the superior mesenteric or left gastric artery. We do this in order to obtain greater detail of the intrahepatic circulation and, more important, to produce a high-density hepatogram, which is the key to detecting small avascular or hypovascular masses. Difficulty arises in evaluation of the left lobe of the liver, where details are usually obscured by the spine and superimposed gastric and splenic vessels. Here, a superselective left hepatic arteriogram has great value (Fig. 12-26).

If the tip of the catheter is placed in the hepatic artery beyond the origin of the gastroduodenal, 70 ml of Renografin 76% is injected at the fastest rate possible without allowing reflux into the celiac trunk. The best indirect portogram is obtained from a superior mesenteric artery injection. Renografin 76% (80 ml) is injected 45 seconds after intra-arterial Priscoline (50 mg). During injection into the hepatic artery, rapid serial filming at the rate of two films/second for 4 seconds, one film/second for 4 seconds, and one film/2 seconds for 15 seconds is obtained.

Space-Occupying Lesions

Space-occupying lesions of the liver include tumors, cystic liver diseases, and abscesses.

Neoplastic lesions
1. Malignant
   A. Hepatocellular carcinoma
   B. Metastatic carcinoma
   C. Cholangiocarcinoma
   D. Miscellaneous
2. Benign
   A. Adenoma
   B. Nodular hyperplasia
   C. Regenerating nodules
   D. Hemangioma

Non-neoplastic lesions
1. Abscesses (pyogenic, amebic, tuberculoma, gumma)
2. Hematoma
3. Cysts (solitary, polycystic, hydatid)

Malignant Liver Tumors. The angiographic findings of hepatocellular carcinoma have been well described by Boysen and Abrams[13] and by Nebessar and co-workers.[77] They usually are multinodular with 20% to 40% presenting as unicentric lesions.[11] At the time of diagnosis, these so-called unicentric tumors usually have daughter lesions, which can easily be overlooked if high-quality angiograms are not performed with large doses of contrast media injected selectively into the hepatic arteries (Fig. 12-27). These tumors usually have a rich arterial supply,[80a] and

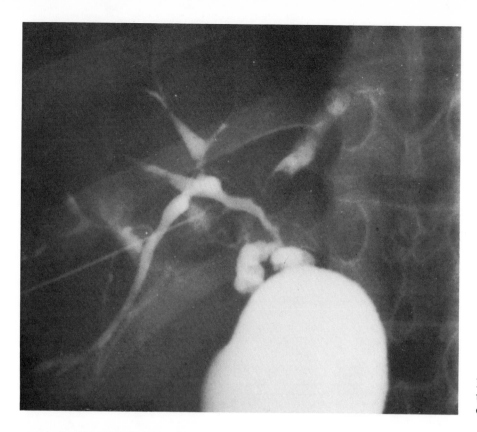

Fig. 12-13. Classic "pruned tree" appearance of sclerosing cholangitis.

Fig. 12-14. Chronic pancreatitis with a long, smooth common duct stricture and minimal dilatation of the intrahepatic radicles.

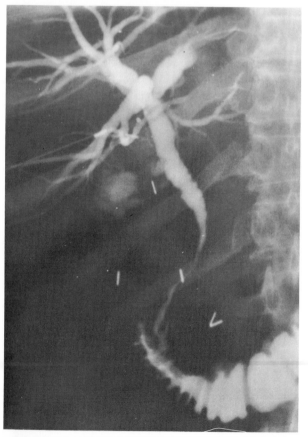

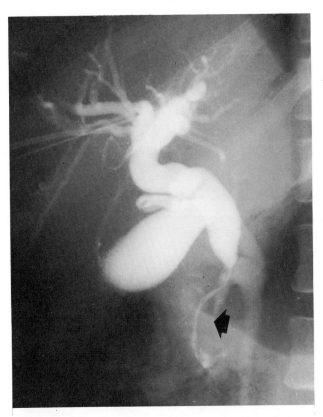

Fig. 12-15. Chronic pancreatitis with compression of a long stricture of the common duct from a pseudocyst in the head of the pancreas (*arrow*).

the degree of vascularity varies according to the gross anatomic type. Dilatation of the common hepatic duct and the branches of the hepatic artery feeding the tumor reflect the increases in arterial blood supply (Fig. 12-28). There is widening, displacement, and stretching of intrahepatic arteries, with a lack of normal peripheral tapering. Bizarre tumor vessels are clustered within a large single area or are scattered in small nodules (see Fig. 12-27). A dense tumor stain is usually also present. The tumor vessels remain filled with contrast media for several seconds after the material has disappeared from the uninvolved branches of the hepatic artery.

The tumor stain has usually begun to fade 10 seconds after the end of the injection.[102] Arteriovenous anastomoses[2] (Fig. 12-29) are characteristic of hepatocellular carcinoma; they are seldom seen in metastatic liver carcinoma. Nakashima and associates have shown that the portal vein branches are often sharply severed by tumor growth, and their periphery may be opacified during the arterial phase. Portal vein thrombosis with esophageal varices caused by intravenous tumor growth is another angiographic feature of hepatocellular carcinoma. This can be demonstrated by superior mesenteric indirect por-

tography (Fig. 12-30). The so-called thread-and-streaks sign[84] is a reliable sign of hepatocellular carcinoma thrombus growing within veins. It is seen in from 8% to 27% of patients with hepatocellular carcinoma,[62,84] and we have not seen it in patients with cholangiocarcinoma or hepatic metastases. The thread-and-streaks sign corresponds to the longitudinal spaces between the thrombus and the venous wall as well as to the vessels that form in the thrombus. These vessels receive arterial blood and are usually visualized in a retrograde fashion before the venous phase. They can also be visualized in an antegrade fashion by contrast medium carried by portal blood delineating the streaks. This angiographic sign has great value in the determination of which patients should undergo hepatic surgery for tumor resection.

In spite of all these signs that have been described in hepatocellular carcinoma, differential diagnosis from other primary liver tumors and from metastatic disease may at times be impossible.[86] We have seen cases of metastatic disease with every characteristic, with the exception of the thread-and-streak sign, that has been described in hepatocellular carcinoma. Differential diagnosis from leiomyosarcoma of the inferior vena cava can also be very difficult. A large filling defect shown by an inferior vena-cavogram with neovascularity confined to this area aids in the determination of this rare tumor.

Cholangiocarcinomas are poorly vascularized tumors. Their neoplastic vessels are usually thin and irregular and confined to the liver hilum (Fig. 12-31).[51] Encasement or obstruction rather than displacement of hepatic arteries also occurs commonly (Fig. 12-32).[13,51]

Neoplastic vasculature in hepatocellular carcinoma varies with the different types, but tumor vessels are almost always present and are much richer than in cholangiocarcinoma. In some forms of poorly vascularized necrotic or mixed types, the angiographic differential diagnosis of cholangiocarcinoma may be impossible.[106] Portal vein obstruction has been reported to be low in cholangiocarcinoma. Kaude has reported it in 13% of cases, whereas it occurs in 45% of all cases of hepatocellular carcinoma.[51] Studies, including microangiography in experimental hepatocellular and cholangiocarcinoma,[46,79] explain the observation of frequent hepatic artery involvement in cholangiocarcinoma and portal vein obstruction in hepatocellular carcinoma.

Hepatic metastases are the most common cause of hepatic mass lesions in the United States. There is a wide variance in the degree of angiographic vascularity of metastatic tumors in the liver, depending upon the site of origin and the cell type. This makes it at times impossible to differentiate angiographically hepatocellular carcinoma from a metastatic tumor. The most common vascular hepatic metastatic deposits are carcinoid, malignant islet cell tumor, choriocarcinoma, renal tumors, leiomyosarcoma, angiosarcoma, and thyroid carcinoma. They are easily detected by angiography, and tumors of just a few millimeters can be pinpointed (Fig. 12-33). Moderate neovascularity is seen in metastatic adenocarcinoma of the colon,

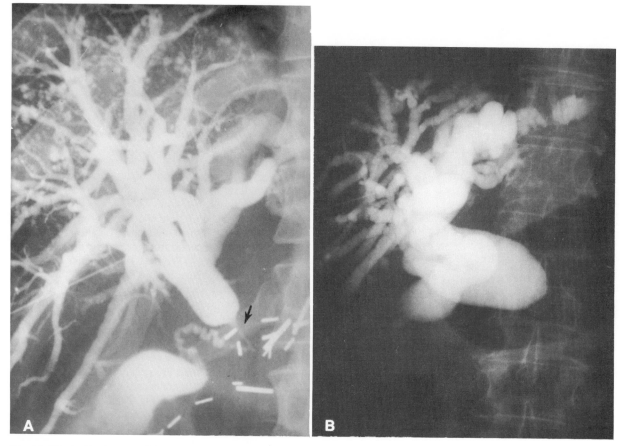

Fig. 12-16. A. Carcinoma of the head of the pancreas with complete obstruction of the common hepatic duct showing a rat-tail configuration (*arrows*). Also note marked dilatation of the intrahepatic radicles with multiple small liver abscesses. **B.** Carcinoma of the head of the pancreas with complete obstruction and marked dilatation of the intrahepatic radicles. Note rounded configuration of the duct at the point of obstruction.

stomach, and breast, and hypovascular lesions occur with lung or esophageal metastases (Fig. 12-34).

Angiographic findings that at times are helpful in the differentiation of secondary liver carcinoma from primary carcinoma are as follows:

1. Space-occupying lesions are usually multiple and round in shape.
2. Angiographically, metastatic lesions are less vascular than hepatocellular carcinoma.
3. The halo effect is commonly seen in late angiograms (Fig. 12-35).
4. Arteriovenous shunts and and portal thrombosis occur rarely in metastatic disease.
5. Signs of portal hypertension are absent or minimal.

In spite of the angiographic signs mentioned in the discussion of hepatocellular carcinoma, differential diagnosis between primary and metastatic liver tumors may be im-

possible. Most primary tumors are multicentric and show a variable degree of vascularity, including the halo sign (Fig. 12-36). Hypervascular metastases may present arteriovenous shunting (Fig. 12-37), and portal vein thrombosis, although reported to be rare, was found in 18% of our cases with metastatic liver tumors.

Hepatic angiosarcoma has been seen with increasing frequency in vinyl chloride workers, who exhibit a central hypovascularity with puddling surrounded by a peripheral stain.[133]

Benign Liver Tumors. Cavernous hemangiomas of the liver usually yield definite angiographic findings that enable us to differentiate them from hepatocellular carcinoma.[1,102] In contrast to hepatocellular carcinoma, the common hepatic artery is not enlarged. The smaller feeding vessels may be dilated and crowded together.[1] They fill large, irregular, well-defined sinusoidal spaces, which

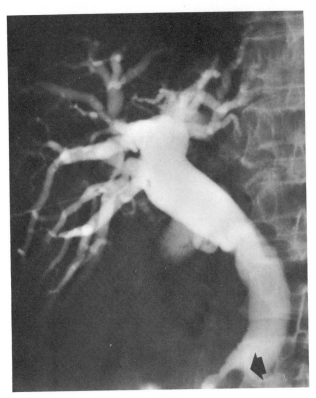

Fig. 12-17. Polypoid ampullary carcinoma (*arrow*) with complete obstruction and marked biliary tree dilatation.

retain contrast medium for as long as 20 seconds (Fig. 12-38A,B);[102] in contrast, hepatocellular carcinomas retain a diffuse tumor stain for a very short time.[101,102] The portal venous system is not involved. In hepatocellular carcinoma, portal vein displacement or thrombosis is very common.

Adenomas and focal nodular hyperplasia present similar angiographic features.[34] These are usually well-defined hypervascular lesions with less bizarre vessels than those seen in hepatocellular carcinoma. The arterial supply characteristically originates at the periphery of the mass, with multiple parallel feeding vessels coursing toward the the center (Fig. 12-39). A prolonged stain is usually present (Fig. 12-40), but laking, portal vein thrombosis or arteriovenous shunting does not occur. We also believe that the circumferential branches are due to displacement of feeding arteries, which are a reflection of slow growth (Fig. 12-41).[64] We have seen this sign in slow-growing hepatocellular carcinomas and liver metastases in which no arteriovenous shunting or portal vein invasion has occurred. In these cases, differential diagnosis is impossible. However, we have seen two cases of liver adenoma that occurred with the use of contraceptives and in which the tumors were hypovascular, probably because of internal

bleeding. The few vessels that were demonstrated resembled malignant tumor vessels.

In regenerating nodules, the angiographic findings are those of a cirrhotic liver with corkscrewing and crowded vessels. If the nodules are large, stretched and displaced vessels are also present. The arterial hepatogram is heterogeneous, with alternating areas of increased stain and lucency.[104] The nodules with increased stain are usually distinguishable from hepatocellular carcinoma arising in a cirrhotic liver because they are supplied by tiny vessels that show no arteriovenous shunting or laking and no portal vein invasion (Fig. 12-42).

The extreme hypervascularity seen in the so-called arterialization of the liver in cases with long-standing portal vein occlusion or reversal of flow should pose no problem to the experienced angiographer (Fig. 12-43).

Liver cysts and abscesses are avascular lesions that may cause displacement and stretching of hepatic arteries. Chronic, large abscesses usually have a thick hypervascular wall (Fig. 12-44).

TRANSHEPATIC OBLITERATION OF BLEEDING GASTROESOPHAGEAL VARICES

Transhepatic obliteration of gastroesophageal varices is an effective method for control of variceal bleeding.[56,90,91,93,127] It is the technique of choice in patients who have not responded to intensive medical therapy, especially those with severe decompensated cirrhosis.[90,91,93] After control of bleeding, the patient can be evaluated for the ultimate therapy to prevent rebleeding; such therapy consists of elective surgical decompression of the varices and the portal system. An elective shunt is preferable to emergency shunt surgery, because it carries a much lower mortality.

Technique

The entry point for this procedure is the highest possible point in the midaxillary line; attention should be directed toward the lateral inferior projection of the right costal diaphragmatic sulcus during fluoroscopy. The skin, subcutaneous planes, intercostal space, and liver capsule should be infiltrated with a local anesthetic. A stab incision is then made in the skin with a No. 11 blade, and the skin and subcutaneous tissues are separated with a straight forceps. A trochar assembly measuring 25 cm in length with a No. 5 French sleeve is advanced close to the upper edge of the lower rib and parallel to the plane of the x-ray table. It is directed toward the intervertebral space between T-11 and T-12, which has been marked on the skin with a lead marker. The tip of the trochar is introduced to a point about 4 cm from the lateral border of the vertebrae, and the stylet is removed.

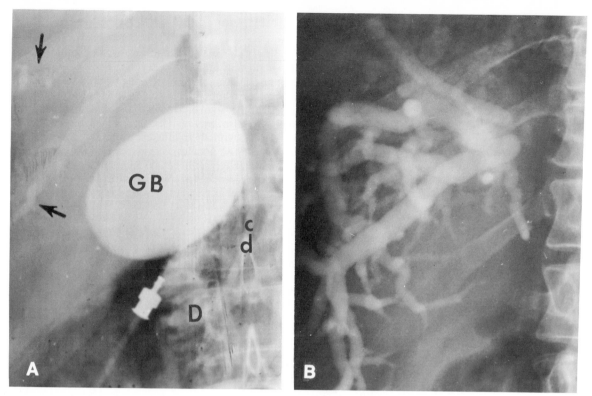

Fig. 12-18. Klatskin tumor. **A.** The tumor was missed at the time of exploratory laparotomy, and this operative cholangiogram injecting through the gallbladder (*GB*) was interpreted as normal. Arrows point to very faint demonstration of dilated intraphepatic radicles. The common duct (*cd*) is of normal size and empties into the duodenum (*D*). **B.** Skinny needle transhepatic cholangiogram shows complete obstruction high at the bifurcation with no communication with the left hepatic ducts.

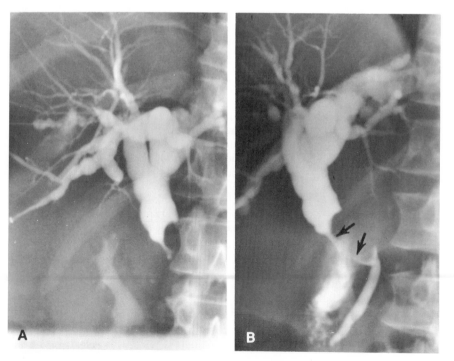

Fig. 12-19. Polypoid cholangiocarcinoma at the junction of the common ducts causing marked dilatation of the biliary tree. **A.** Large calculi make differential diagnosis impossible. **B.** Lobulated contour of the tumor can be identified (*arrows*).

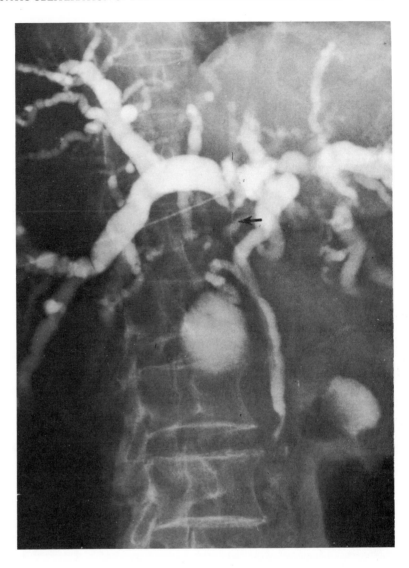

Fig. 12-20. Small scirrhous carcinoma, the so-called Klatskin tumor, at the common hepatic bifurcation (*arrow*).

The No. 5 French sleeve is then slowly withdrawn until good venous return is obtained. With the aid of a small, curved guidewire with an outside diameter of 0.25 mm, the portal vein is selectively catheterized, and the catheter is advanced into the splenic vein, close to the splenic hilum. A transhepatic splenoportogram is obtained by injection of 60 ml of Renografin 76% within a period of 5 seconds. It is unnecessary and costly to use ultrasonic or CT guidance for routine catheterization of the portal vein. In over 80% of our studies, we were able to cannulate the portal vein merely by feel, using fewer than three passes of the trochar. The other 20% of the studies required more than three punctures. After a good venous return is obtained, the curved guidewire is manipulated blindly until the wire can be felt entering a vessel. Its position is then checked by fluoroscopy before the sleeve is advanced further, because it is not uncommon to cannulate a hepatic

vein and the inferior vena cava. This technique reduces the dose of radiation to the hands of the operator.

Frequently, the advancement of the catheter over the wire is difficult or unsuccessful in cirrhotic patients, despite the use of guidewires with larger diameters, because of the catheter friction that results from the fibrotic nature of the liver and the presence of ascites (Fig. 12-45). In these patients, the liver tract is dilated to a No. 6 French caliber with a dilator that encompasses a translumbar aortagram set without a stylet (Fig. 12-46).[96]

After the preliminary splenoportogram, the coronary and short gastric veins are selectively catheterized as peripherally as possible (Fig. 12-47) with a preshaped Kifa guidewire or a deflector system. These vessels are then embolized with very small particles of Gelfoam soaked with 3% Sotradecol.[91,93] The resulting gel-like suspension is injected very slowly by hand with a 1-mm tuberculin

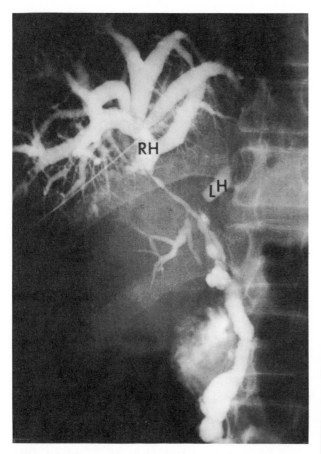

Fig. 12-21. Long stricture in the common hepatic duct. Note the bifurcation and central extension of the stricture into the right hepatic duct (*RH*) from the cholangiocarcinoma. LH, left hepatic duct.

Following completion of the study, obliteration of the juxtacapsular portion of the needle tract is recommended in order for leakage of blood into the peritoneal cavity to be avoided in patients with low platelet levels and abnormal prothrombin time.

Discussion

Since the original publication by Dr. Lunderquist in 1974,[58] we have used the technique of transhepatic portal vein catheterization and variceal obliteration in 300 patients. The technique has been applied to active as well as to stabilized bleeders under circumstances in which surgical treatment is refused or highly risky.

Due to the high frequency of recanalization of obliterated veins, we abandoned early in our series the use of hypertonic glucose, intimal damage plus thrombin, bal-

Fig. 12-22. Extrahepatic duct obstruction by a hepatocellular carcinoma. Note stricture at the bifurcation (*arrow*) with complete occlusion of the left hepatic duct. RH, right hepatic duct.

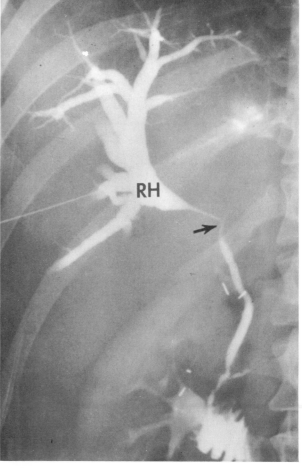

syringe; increments of no more than 0.3 mm for the largest coronary veins and smaller increments for the smaller vessels are used. A small amount of contrast medium is administered under fluoroscopic control after each embolization. When blood flow starts to slow down, a 3- to 5-minute interval is allowed between each embolization. By this technique, one tries to achieve a peripheral obliteration of the varices (Fig. 12-47*C*), producing a cast of Gelfoam over a long segment of vein (Fig. 12-47*D*). Embolization with a large amount of Gelfoam at one time usually produces a proximal occlusion of a short segment of vein (Fig. 12-48). This occlusion usually disintegrates, migrating peripherally in a short period of time. In some patients, a peripheral occlusion interrupts the flow in other collateral vessels that have not been embolized, thereby reducing the procedure time (Fig. 12-49). Other patients may require several days of embolization before total obliteration of the gastroesophageal flow is achieved (Fig. 12-50).

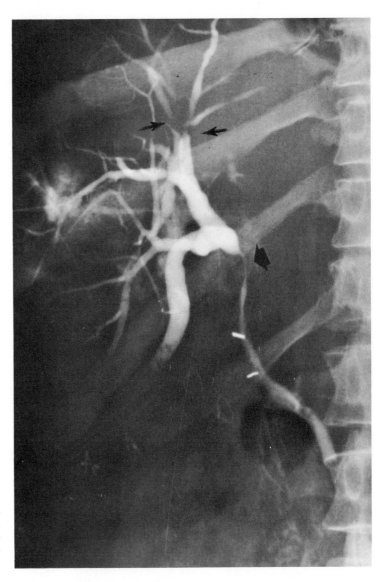

Fig. 12-23. Extrahepatic obstruction caused by a metastatic carcinoma of the colon to the hilum of the liver (*large arrow*). Note distortion and stenosis of intrahepatic ducts (*arrows*) from parenchymal liver metastases.

loon occlusion, and embolization with modified autogenous clot.[58,59,91,134] Lunderquist also reported that isobutyl 2-cyanoacrylate did not produce permanent occlusion, with six of eight patients showing recanalized veins in follow-up studies.[60] We have had good results embolizing with Gelfoam soaked with Sotradecol using the technique described above. Only two recanalized veins have been detected in 30 follow-up studies. In contrast, Lunderquist reported a high frequency of recanalization with the use of Gelfoam and a similar sclerosing agent (Etolin).[59] We believe that the key is to embolize (Fig. 12-50) with small increments to achieve a peripheral obliteration, producing a cast of Gelfoam over a long segment of a vein. We have also used fine particles of Ivalon, also with good results, but it is more cumbersome to use than Gelfoam; we have

had problems with obstruction of the catheter. Absolute ethanol is readily available and inexpensive. It also has the advantage over particulate material or acrylic polymers that it will not cause complications by passages through the variceal system into the pulmonary circulation owing to the dilution with large amounts of flowing blood.[52,139] Yune also postulated that ethanol causes permanent occlusion at the variceal plexus itself rather than at the feeding veins alone.

After a short trial, we abandoned the use of ethanol because of a great increase in the amount of ascites that occurred following variceal embolization. Other disadvantages include the marked increase in the time required to produce occlusion. The incidence of portal vein thrombosis also greatly increased. This is produced by

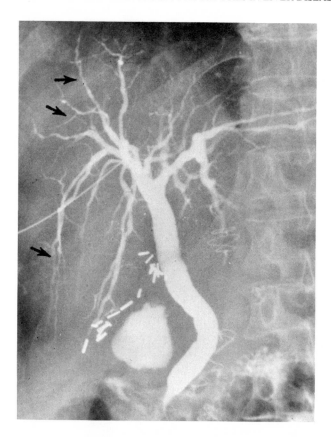

Fig. 12-24. Tortuosity and irregularity of intrahepatic ducts (*arrows*) secondary to liver cirrhosis.

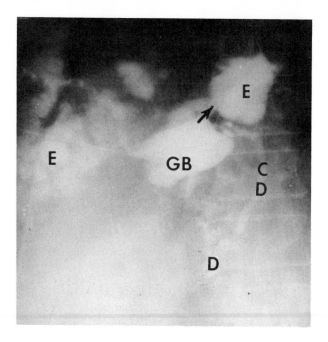

Fig. 12-25. Traumatic rupture of the gallbladder. Arrow points to area of laceration with extravasation. (*E*) into the lesser sac and the peritoneal cavity. GB, gallbladder; CD, common duct; D, duodenum.

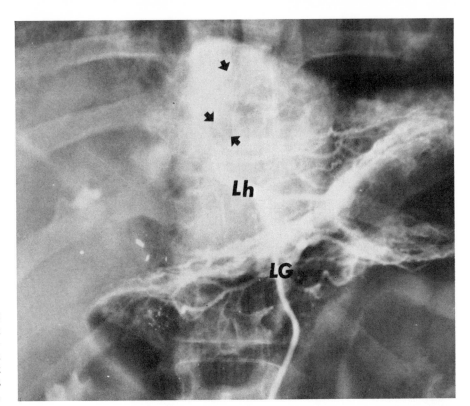

Fig. 12-26. Highly selective left hepatic arteriogram showing large avascular metastatic lesions coming from a carcinoma of the colon (*arrows*). Note that the left hepatic artery (*Lh*) arises from the left gastric artery (*LG*).

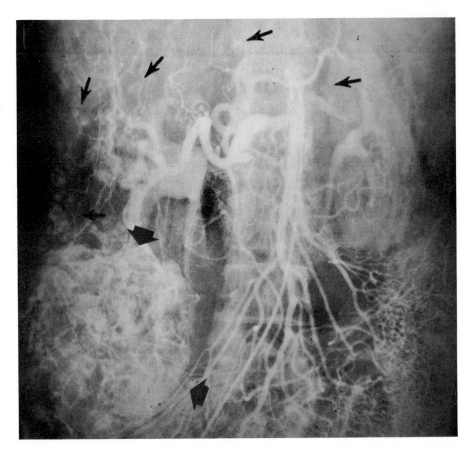

Fig. 12-27. Hepatocellular carcinoma. Note the bizarre tumor vessels clustered in a large area (*large arrows*) in which a dense tumor stain may also be observed. Multiple, very small vascular daughter lesions are visible throughout the rest of the liver.

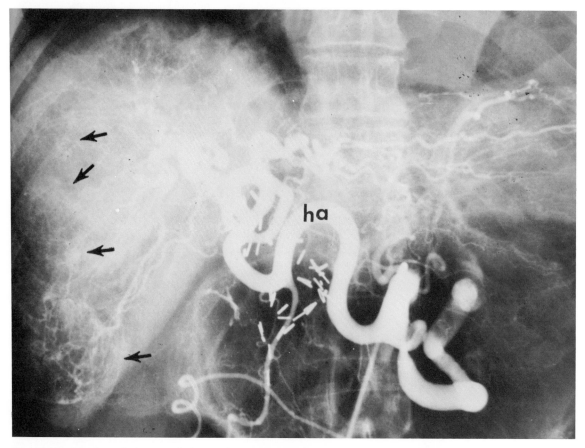

Fig. 12-28. Multicentric hepatocellular carcinoma (*arrows*) in a cirrhotic liver in a patient with hemochromatosis. Note the rich supply to the tumor nodules and the marked dilatation of the common hepatic artery (*ha*).

reflux of ethanol in patients with severe portal hypertension in which the portal blood flow is virtually stagnant.[52,139] Ohnishi has obtained excellent results embolizing with a combination of stainless coils with hypertonic glucose and Gelfoam.[82] We use only large stainless coils to embolize gastric varices in patients with spontaneous portal systemic shunts such as the gastrorenal. This type of connection cannot be embolized with small particles, because they will pass into the lung.

We have had experience with ten patients with large bleeding gastric varices. Four patients had spontaneous gastrorenal shunts and the other six had had a distal splenorenal shunt from 1 to 5 years. After several months, this type of shunt will become like a central shunt owing to large collaterals that draw blood from the portal system into the surgical shunt. Part of this collateral pathway may be by means of submucosal veins, such as gastric varices, which have a tendency to bleed. All of these patients were embolized with a combination of very large coils followed by Gelfoam to prevent pulmonary embolization.

Mendez and colleagues reported that patients with hepatofugal portal vein flow are associated with a continued hemorrhage following percutaneous transhepatic obliteration; they recommended that this procedure be denied in this type of patient.[66] We strongly disagree. A total reversal of the portal flow indicates only that there is a very large spontaneous portal systemic shunt. This condition makes the procedure technically more difficult, because the branches of the portal vein are very small and are difficult to enter. We have performed embolization in 22 patients with total reversal of the portal flow, many of them with partial portal vein thrombosis. Seven of these patients were massively bleeding; the rest were elected procedures. We found no significant difference in controlling of the bleeding episode. Benner and associates[8] also found different results than did Mendez and colleagues and recommended not to deny this procedure on the basis of complete hepatofugal portal flow.

Control of massive hemorrhage was achieved in 95% of patients successfully embolized (Fig. 12-51), with less

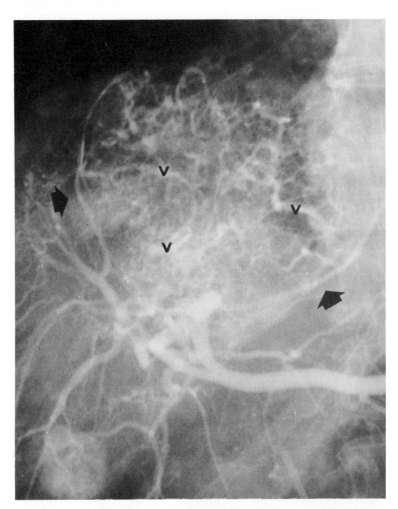

Fig. 12-29. Solitary hepatocellular carcinoma with multiple areas of arteriovenous anastomosis (*V*). Note the rich supply of bizarre tumor vessels with large feeding arteries displaced along the mass surface.

Fig. 12-30. Complete occlusion of the portal vein by hepatocellular carcinoma. Indirect portography shows complete occlusion of the portal vein (*PV*), with reversal of flow (*arrows*) into the coronary vein (*CV*) and the inferior mesenteric vein (*IMV*).

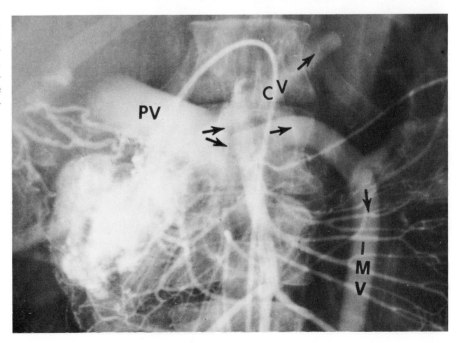

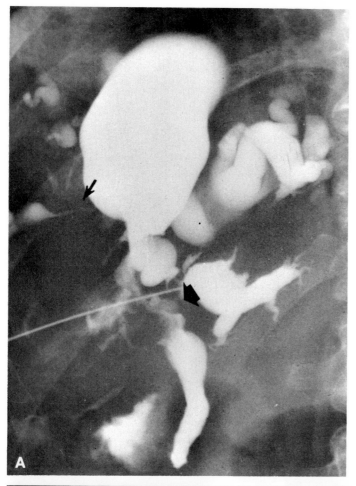

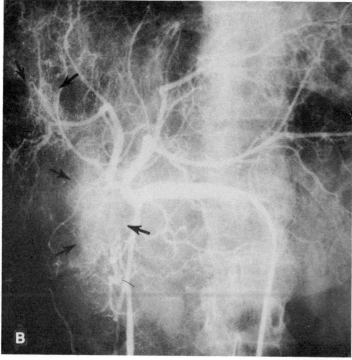

Fig. 12-31. Extensive cholangiocarcinoma. **A.** Transhepatic cholangiography shows large polypoid cholangiocarcinoma at the hepatic bifurcation (*large arrow*) causing tremendous dilatation of the biliary tree. Also note intrahepatic extension of the tumor (*small arrow*). **B.** Hepatic arteriogram shows areas of neovascularity with thin and irregular vessels and a mild stain (*arrows*). These areas correlate well with the findings in the transhepatic cholangiocarcinoma of *A*.

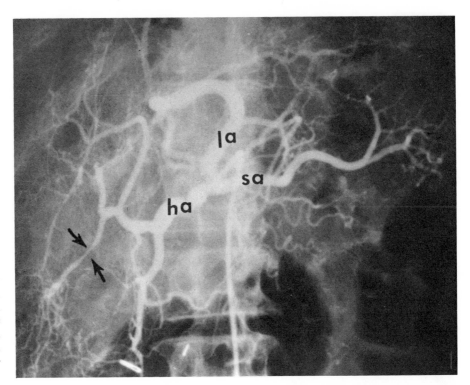

Fig. 12-32. Celiac arteriography showing encasement of a branch of the hepatic artery (*arrows*) in the region of the hilum of the liver in a patient with a Klatskin tumor. ha, hepatic artery; sa, splenic artery; la, left gastric artery.

than 7% rebleeding in the first 2 weeks. However, long-term follow-up (1–2 years) showed recurrence of bleeding in 30% of our patients who did not undergo surgery. Similar results were obtained by Widrich.[136] He also reported that 60% of his patients, where bleeding was inadequately controlled with Pitressin, had no recurrent variceal bleed within 30 days of the transhepatic obliteration.[136] Of those patients treated electively, 95% had no recurrent variceal bleeding within the first 30 days. Before the advent of transhepatic obliteration, the in-hospital, 1-month mortality of patients whose variceal bleeding was not controlled with Pitressin was 88%. The mortality of this subgroup decreases to 37% with transhepatic obliteration.[132]

Smith-Laing and associates[119] have reported the highest rebleeding rate—65% at a mean interval of 4.6 months. The mean interval to rebleed among the 65% of patients in this study who suffered recurrent hemorrhage was 8 months, with varices documented as the bleeding source in over 75% of the cases. The study of Smith-Laing[119] failed to show improved survival in a small prospective randomized trial of transhepatic embolization versus standard medical therapy.

Benner reported that half of his patients who were at risk of rebleeding did so by 30 weeks and 80% had rebled at 2 years.[8]

Ohnishi and associates[82] reported in 27 emergency cases in which transhepatic obliteration was performed first that the variceal rebleeding rate at 1, 2, and 12 months after complete or incomplete variceal obliteration was 16%, 29%, and 56%, respectively. In 17 elective cases in which transhepatic obliteration was performed with success, the variceal rebleeding rate at 1, 2, and 12 months was 0%, 0%, and 39%, respectively. In 18 conservatively treated controlled cases, the rebleeding rate at 1, 2, and 12 months after cessation of initial variceal hemorrhage was 22%, 28%, and 89%, respectively. The rebleeding rate was significantly greater in the conservative cases than in the elective cases.

There have been several reports discussing the possible efficacy of spontaneous portosplenic shunts, which have appeared after variceal embolization, in decompressing the portal system.[59,90,93,127] In reality, most spontaneous portosystemic shunts are inadequate to decompress the portal system; thus, most of the patients embolized should be re-evaluated for shunt surgery. In our experience, after variceal obliteration, only those patients with large spontaneous splenorenal shunts (Fig. 12-52) may be spared shunt surgery.

Complications

The most frequent complications were pain and low-grade fever, which occurred in about 50% of our patients. Intra-abdominal bleeding resulted in the death of two of our patients and five in Widrich's series.[136] Other rare com-

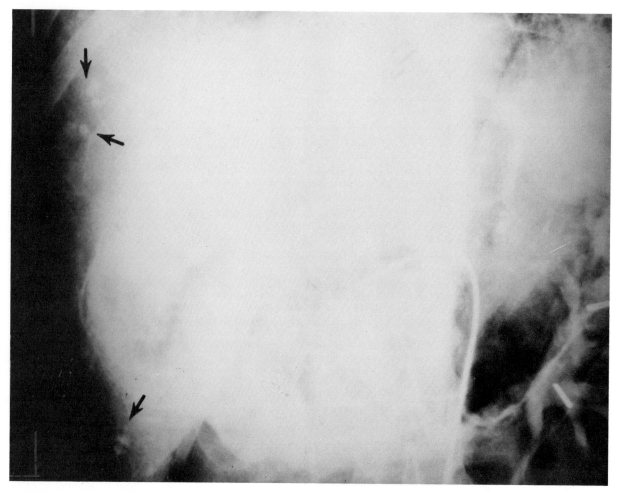

Fig. 12-33. Renal cell carcinoma metastatic to liver. When metastatic deposits are vascular, even tiny ones can be pinpointed by hepatic arteriography (*arrows*).

plications included bleeding from an intercostal artery, right pleural effusions, right hemothorax, and leak of ascitic fluid. Pulmonary embolism should not occur if one does not embolize a vein that leads to a spontaneous portal systemic shunt.[93]

Reported complications range between 20% and 52%.[8,119,127,134,136] Portal vein thrombosis is reported to be between 3% and 22%. We believe that this complication can be greatly reduced with experience because it is related to prolonged procedure time and reflux of embolizing material or sclerosing agents into the portal vein. Death has been reported in 0% to 14% of the patients in the series.[59,65]

Transhepatic obliteration of gastroesophageal varices is a relatively safe, palliative procedure that can successfully control bleeding varices. It is indicated when intensive medical therapy of bleeding varices fails. It may delay or prevent rebleeding in poor surgical candidates, thus pro-

viding time for reversibility of liver damage and reconsideration for definitive surgery.

PERCUTANEOUS TRANSHEPATIC BILIARY DECOMPRESSION

Primary malignancies of the extrahepatic bile ducts often remain unsuspected until very late in the course of the disease. Secondary spread to adjacent structures has occurred in about 90% of the cases when the diagnosis is made.[27] Radical surgery in such advanced stages is not possible, but the establishment of a permanent bile drainage is mandatory. Palliation in obstructive jaundice due to malignancy can be performed by nonsurgically placed—external, internal–external, or internal—biliary drains.[12,69,93,95,100,107,118,120,122,139] Temporary percutaneous biliary drainage has also been advocated to decrease op-

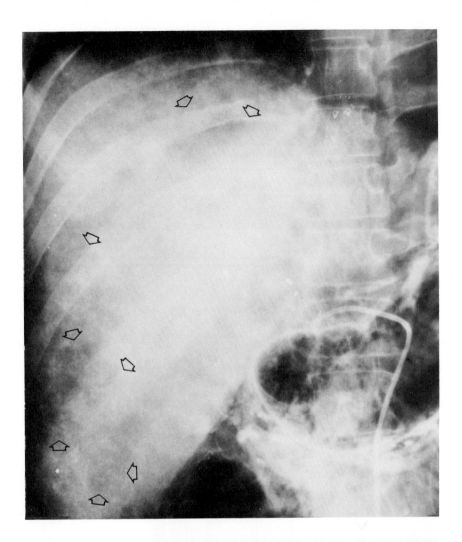

Fig. 12-34. Hepatic arteriogram showing multiple avascular filling defects (*arrows*) from the late parenchymal phase of a metastatic adenocarcinoma of the colon.

Fig. 12-35. Adenocarcinoma of the stomach metastatic to liver. In the parenchymal phase, hepatic arteriography discloses multiple large necrotic metastases, with thick vascular walls, showing the so-called halo sign.

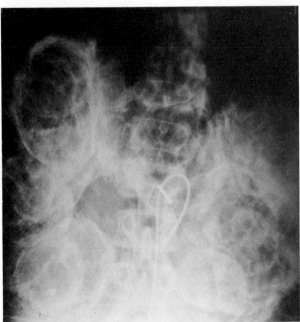

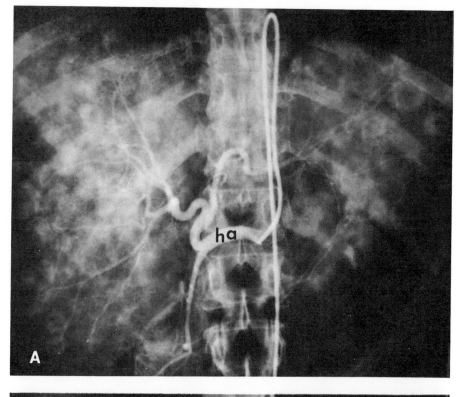

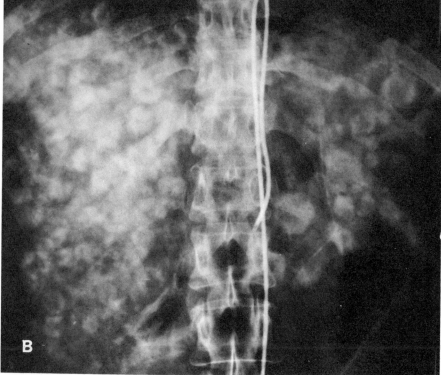

Fig. 12-36. Selective injection into the hepatic artery (*ha*) shows involvement of the entire liver by a multicentric hepatocellular carcinoma. Most of these tumors are small and show evidence of central necrosis, giving the appearance of a halo sign, which is characteristic of metastatic lesions. (Courtesy of Dr. Tieslich, Augusta, GA)

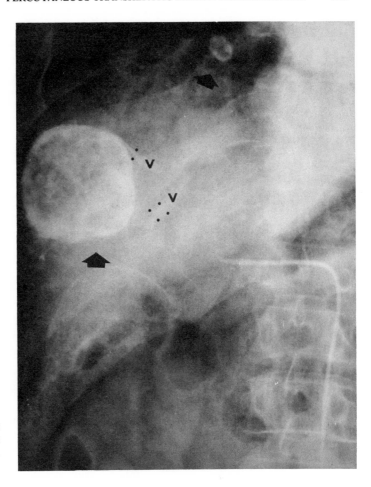

Fig. 12-37. Metastatic renal cell carcinoma to the liver. Late-phase hepatic arteriogram shows multiple vascular masses with a necrotic center (*arrow*) and evidence of AV shunting (*V*).

erative mortality in patients with serum bilirubin levels of about 10 mg/dl.[22,23,35,40,75,80,100] It has also been used for emergency management of severe biliary tract infections.[53,122] Benign biliary strictures can be dilated percutaneously with balloon catheters.[70,97,98,100,113,123]

Balloon Dilatation of Benign Biliary Strictures

It is generally believed that correction of obstructive jaundice secondary to benign strictures should be accomplished by surgery, although the stricture recurs in 25% to 35% of patients reoperated.[14,32,129,130] Transhepatic balloon dilatation of benign choledochoenterostomy strictures was first reported by Molnar and co-workers. This technique provides a simple and promising alternative. In patients with a benign bile duct stricture in whom an attempted surgical repair fails to prevent the recurrence of obstructive jaundice, transhepatic dilatation and drainage may be lifesaving. Molnar reported that eight of nine patients treated by this method became asymptomatic, with normal serum bilirubin values and no recurrence of jaundice

or ascending cholangitis for seven years.[70] Burhenne reported successful dilatation of high hepatojejunostomies in three patients.[20] Hudson and associates[45,111] described a new technique of balloon dilatation of biliary strictures through a choledochojejuno-cutaneous fistula. They demonstrated that biliary strictures can be repeatedly and safely dilated through the stomatized jejunal limb. Management of sclerosing cholangitis is extremely difficult and frequently requires combined medical, surgical, and radiologic techniques.[55,63,66] For example, a T-tube can be surgically inserted below an obstruction. After the tract matures, catheters can be inserted through the T-tube tract for balloon dilatation and drainage.

We have had excellent results with balloon dilatation of 21 benign biliary strictures related to prior surgery. Forty percent of our patients needed a second dilatation at approximately 1 year's time. We have long-term follow-ups of 7 years in three patients who remain almost asymptomatic, with only an occasional bout of cholangitis and minimal fluctuations in the alkaline phosphatase level. We have also been successful in dilating primary benign

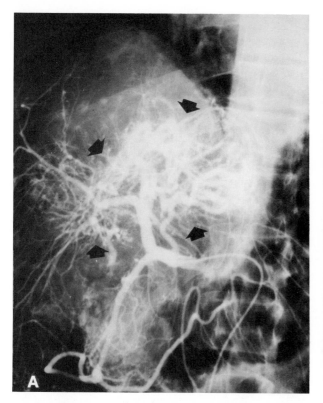
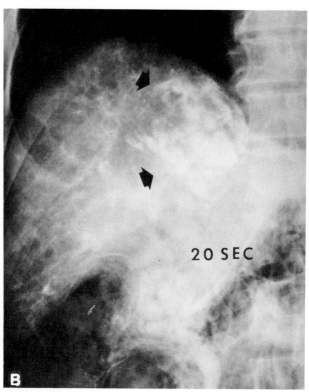

Fig. 12-38. Characteristic findings of cavernous hemangioma of the liver with dilated and crowded feeding vessels (*arrows in A*) and irregular, well-defined sinusoidal spaces with contrast media retained for as long as 20 seconds (*arrows in B*).

Fig. 12-39. Hepatic arteriography shows multiple liver adenomas with the characteristic arterial supply that originates at the periphery of the mass, with multiple parallel feeding vessels coursing toward the center of the lesion.

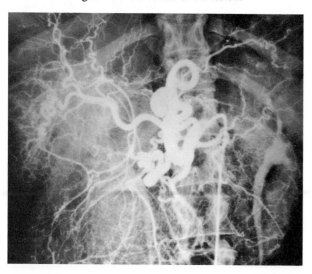

strictures of the distal common duct. The patient in Figure 12-54 remained asymptomatic following his original dilatation.

Technique

Transhepatic cholangiography with the Chiba needle is performed first for determination of the nature and location of the obstructing lesion. Also, as the ducts remain filled with contrast material, puncture with the Chiba needle facilitates subsequent puncture with a large-sheathed trochar. If a T-tube is in the biliary tree, dilatation can be performed by use of the T-tube tract (see Fig. 12-2).

With a right-flank approach, the trochar assembly with an outer No. 5 French sheath is introduced into the liver and directed under fluoroscopic guidance into a branch of the right hepatic duct that appears to have a straight course into the common hepatic duct. After removal of the needle, the sheath is slowly withdrawn until a free flow of bile is observed. If the desired duct is missed, the needle is reinserted into the sheath and the whole assembly is

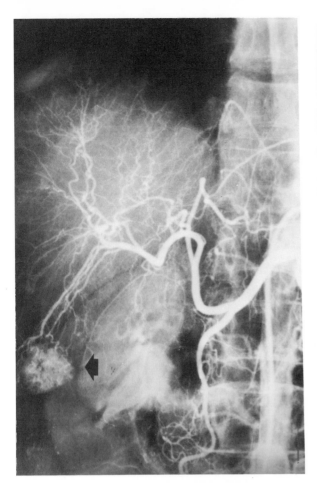

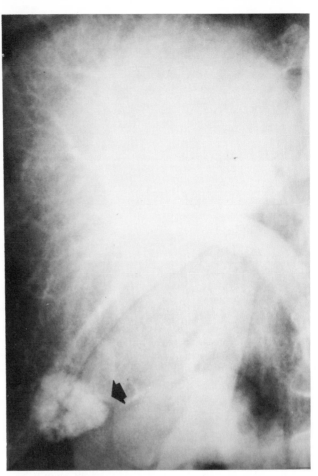

Fig. 12-40. Focal nodular hyperplasia. Hepatic arteriograms show a small hypervascular lesion with circumferential feeding vessels and a prolonged, well-defined stain characteristic of focal nodular hyperplasia (*arrows*).

Fig. 12-41. Extensive carcinoid liver metastases. Selective hepatic arteriograms show multiple large and small vascular metastases with circumferential feeding vessels and well-defined, prolonged stain.

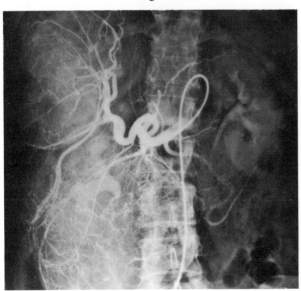

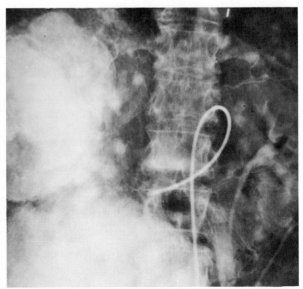

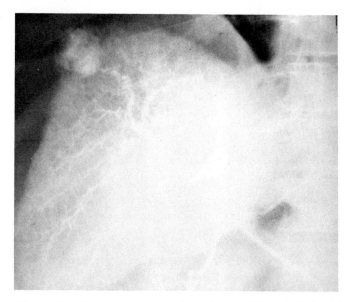 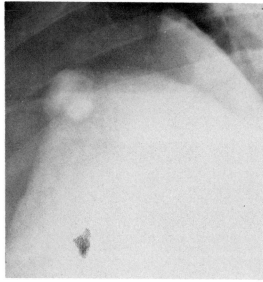

Fig. 12-42. Hepatic arteriograms show changes of liver cirrhosis with corkscrewing of the hepatic arteries and a small area of neovascularity supplied by tiny vessels with a mild stain. No AV shunting was demonstrated. This lesion represented a small regenerating nodule.

redirected more dorsally or ventrally. Complete removal of the sheath from the liver after a miss is not advisable; only a single capsular puncture should be required. Once the sheath is intraductal, it can be advanced with a 0.025-in. curved guidewire. If the stenotic segment cannot be cannulated, we recommend the use of a 0.038-in. IFA guidewire, which has excellent torque. Its tip can be curved according to the anatomy of the ducts for a successful cannulation.[56] Once the wire is placed distal to the stenosis, the sheath is exchanged for a Gruntzig type of double-lumen balloon catheter. Then the stricture is dilated by the pulling of the inflated balloon across the stenosis (Figs. 12-53, 12-54). This maneuver is repeated 10 or 15 times, at the end of which the balloon catheter is exchanged for a No. 7 French internal–external biliary drainage catheter with multiple side holes. The tip of this catheter lies distal to the stenosis in the duodenum or jejunum (Figs. 12-53, 12-54). Under fluoroscopic control, contrast medium is injected to ensure that the side holes are positioned above and below the stenosis. No side holes should be left outside the duct in the liver parenchyma. Daily balloon dilatations are recommended for 7 to 14 days. The degree of stenosis can be assessed from movement of the inflated balloon across the site of the stenosis. As the dilatation progresses, the pressure needed to keep the inflated balloon in its original shape across the stenosis gradually decreases. Satisfactory dilatation is reached when an 8-mm balloon readily passes through the site of the stenosis. We use a Gruntzig type of balloon designed for dilatation of arterial stenosis. The balloon diameter ranges from 4 mm to 8 mm. The main advantages of this type of balloon are the

following: first, rupture, which was a serious problem with latex balloons, even with the protection of a cage, rarely occurs; second, and probably more important, the elongated shape of this balloon permits maintenance of the equator of the balloon at the level of the stricture, something that was almost impossible with the old spherical type of balloon.

External Biliary Drainage

External biliary drainage is provided by percutaneous transhepatic insertion into the biliary tree of a catheter with multiple side holes with its tip resting just proximal to the point of obstruction (Fig. 12-55). This modality of percutaneous biliary drainage should be used only if one is not technically able to place a catheter distal to the obstruction. Even for temporary external biliary drainage, an internal–external type of catheter, which causes dislodgement with very low frequency, is recommended. Percutaneous external transhepatic biliary drainage offers an alternative to surgery purely for decompressive purposes.[72,122,124]

Technique

After visualization of the biliary tree by percutaneous cholangiography performed with a Chiba needle by way of a right-flank approach, a trochar assembly with an outer No. 5 French sheath is introduced into the liver and directed under fluoroscopic guidance into a branch of the right hepatic duct that appears to have a straight course

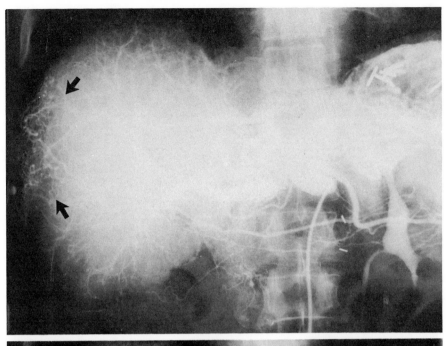

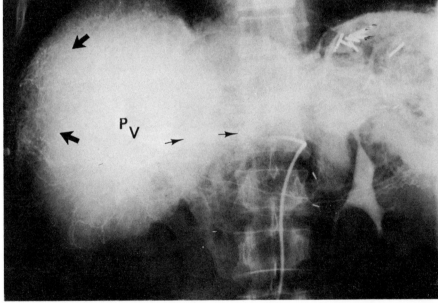

Fig. 12-43. Arterialization of the liver secondary to reversal of portal flow (*small arrows*). Note extreme neovascularity with increasing size and number of small hepatic arteries (*large arrows*). These vessels are not as bizarre as those seen in hepatocellular carcinoma. PV, portal vein.

into the common hepatic duct. The needle is removed at this point, and the sheath is slowly withdrawn until a free flow of bile is observed. The No. 5 French catheter is advanced with the help of a 0.025-in. curved guidewire. A guide-wire 0.38 in. in diameter is then substituted for the thinner one, and a No. 7 or No. 8 French Teflon or polyethylene catheter is exchanged for the No. 5 French sheath. The tip of this catheter is tapered to facilitate in-

troduction. It also has four to six large side holes arranged in spiral fashion in the distal 5 cm to ensure adequate external drainage (Figs. 12-55, 12-56). The introduction of the catheter over the guidewire is greatly facilitated by the use of a metallic cannula, which is inserted over the guidewire and through the catheter.[93] Similar results can be obtained with a hard guidewire with a flexible tip.[57] Once introduced, the catheter is advanced to the point of

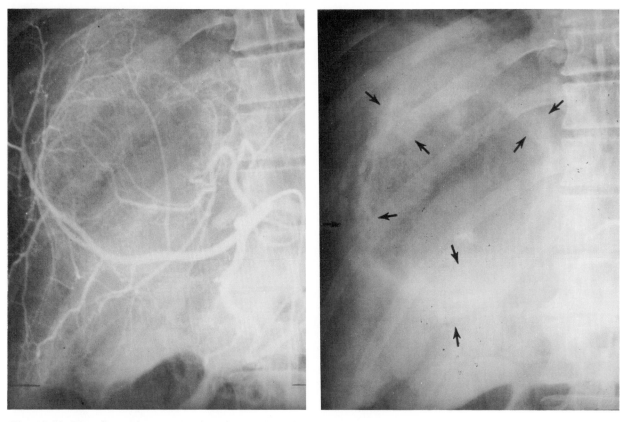

Fig. 12-44. Hepatic arteriogram showing characteristic signs in a large chronic liver abscess with a thick hypervascular wall (*arrows*). These findings are undistinguishable from those in a large necrotic primary or metastatic carcinoma of the liver.

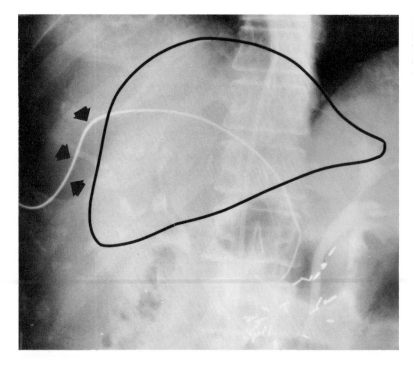

Fig. 12-45. The catheter and wire are coiled in the peritoneal space (*arrows*) of this patient. The catheter could not be advanced over the guidewire beyond the main portal vein (*arrow*).

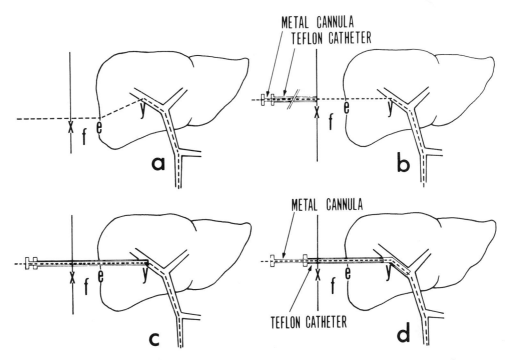

Fig. 12-46. Procedure for dilatation. **a.** Although the guidewire is in place, the path from x to y is not straight because the respiratory phase is not appropriate for dilatation. **b.** The respiratory phase has been corrected, and the patient is apneic. The path of the dilator (x-y) should be relatively straight to accommodate the stiff cannula. **c.** The catheter and cannula are advanced through the parenchyma of the liver to point y. **d.** The No. 6 French Teflon catheter is advanced into the portal vein. x, skin incision; y, junction of the parenchyma of the liver, the portal system, and the point at which the wire usually curves; f, ascitic fluid space; e, margin of the liver.

obstruction. The bile that drains externally through the catheter is collected in a plastic bag. To prevent dislocation of the catheter from the liver, a certain degree of consistency of the catheter is required. However, a very stiff catheter may break because of constant respiratory movement and bending. It is important to secure fixation of the drainage catheter; for this purpose, we use the Molnar disk, which is applied over the catheter and sutured to the skin. Tissue adhesives are used to provide a permanent bond between the disk and the outer catheter (Fig. 12-57). The sutures can be removed after several weeks, and the disk is then secured to the skin by adhesive tape. By this time, a fibrous bridging sheath has formed between the liver and the parietal peritoneum; this facilitates reinsertion of the catheter if it becomes dislocated.

Internal–External Biliary Drainage

At present, internal–external drainage is the most popular type of percutaneous transhepatic biliary drainage. A catheter with multiple side holes is placed transhepatically into the biliary tree through the area of obstruction and into the duodenum or jejunum (Fig. 12-58). This tech-nique has great advantages over external drainage alone;[44,69,107] the drainage tube is less easily displaced, and, with properly functioning side holes, it returns the bile to the gastrointestinal tract so that the patient's nutrition is maintained.

Technique

The initial steps are the same as for external drainage. After cannulation of the biliary tree, the No. 5 French sheath is advanced through the stenotic segment into the duodenum with the aid of a 0.025-in. or a 0.038-in. Kifa guidewire. Even when dealing with what appeared to be a complete obstruction, we have successfully placed the catheter through the lesion and into the duodenum on the first attempt in over 90% of our cases. If the guidewire cannot be advanced across the obstruction, an external drainage catheter is left in place (Fig. 12-59A). After several days of external drainage, it is usually possible to advance the guidewire through the obstruction. Once the tip of the sheath is in the duodenum, it is changed for internal–external catheter drainage with a thicker guidewire. The catheter used is No. 7 or No. 8 French and is constructed

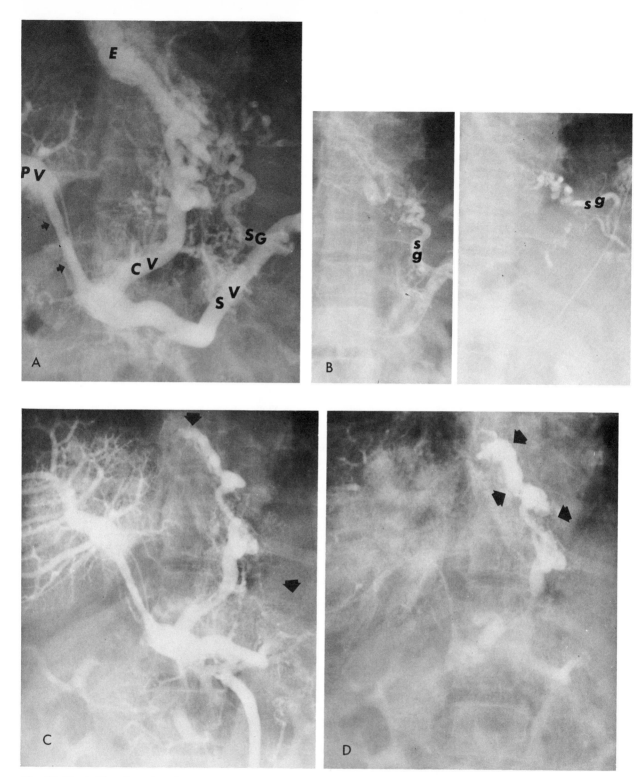

Fig. 12-47. A. Transhepatic splenoportogram shows huge gastroesophageal varices. Note the mural thrombus involving the portal vein (*arrows*). **B.** Selective catheterization of the two short gastric veins and of the coronary vein (not shown) was performed before embolization. **C, D.** Postembolization splenoportogram demonstrates complete obliteration of the gastroesophageal varices. Note the long segment of embolic material within the varices (*short arrows in D*). PV, portal vein; CV, coronary vein: SV splenic vein; SG, short gastric veins; E, esophageal varices.

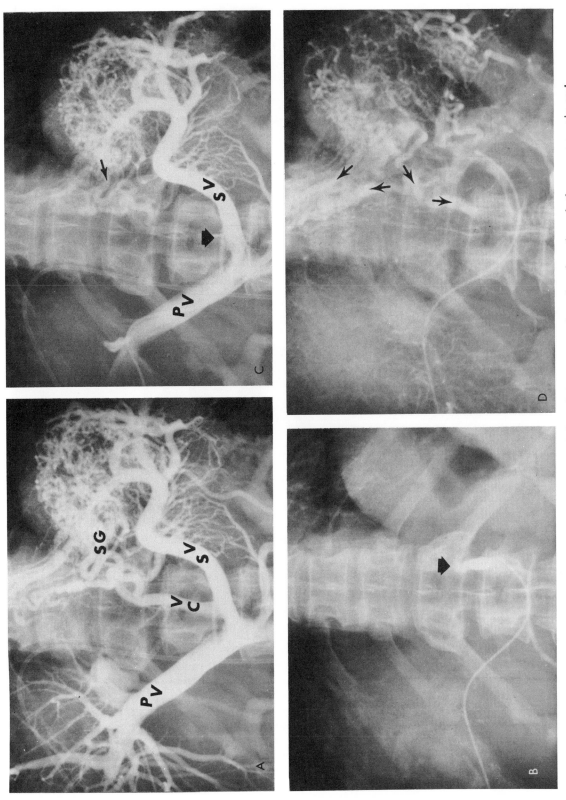

Fig. 12-48. **A.** Transhepatic splenoportogram shows filling of the gastroesophageal varices through the coronary vein and several short gastric veins. **B.** The proximal coronary vein is occluded (*arrow*). **C, D.** Postembolization splenoportogram shows occlusion of the coronary vein at its origin with peripheral filling of this vessel by the patent short gastric veins (*arrows*). PV, portal vein; CV, coronary vein; SV, splenic vein; SG, short gastric veins.

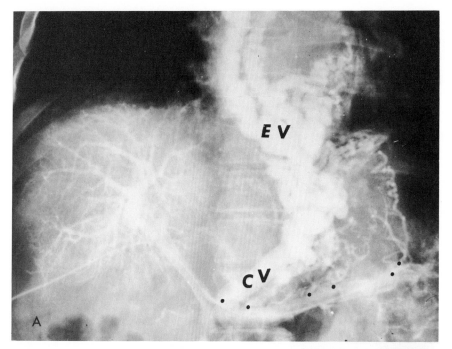

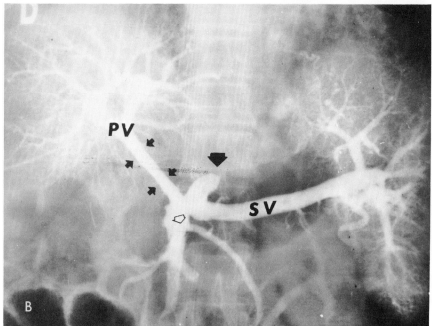

Fig. 12-49. A. Huge gastroesophageal varices (*EV*) are demonstrated on this transhepatic splenoportogram. Note the origin of the coronary vein (*CV*) and multiple short gastric veins (*multiple dots*). **B.** Total occlusion of the varices was attained by a single peripheral embolization of the coronary vein (*large arrow*). A mural thrombus (*small arrows*) involves the portal veins (*PV*). The flow of the mesenteric veins is reversed following embolization (*open arrow*). SV, splenic vein.

with multiple large side holes (Fig. 12-59*B*). A No. 8.3 and a No. 9.3 French polyethylene pig-tail catheter have also been used (Fig. 12-60).[108] Catheters as large as No. 12 French have been used to prevent dislocation from the liver and the abdominal wall (Fig. 12-61). They also allow the construction of large side holes, which delay occlusion with sludge substances.[29,68,92] Side holes are constructed in the catheter before its introduction so as to be located above and below the obstructive lesion (see Fig. 12-58). The most proximal side hole should be well within the biliary tree, because, if the side holes lie in the parenchyma of the liver, persistent bleeding through the catheter may

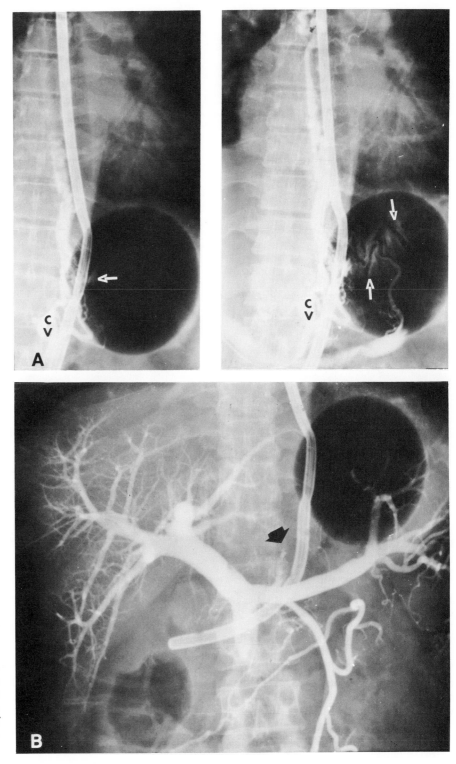

Fig. 12-50. A. Transhepatic injection into the coronary vein (*CV*) shows active bleeding into the gastric fundus (*arrows*) despite an SB tube. **B.** Control of bleeding after coronary vein occlusion (*arrow*).

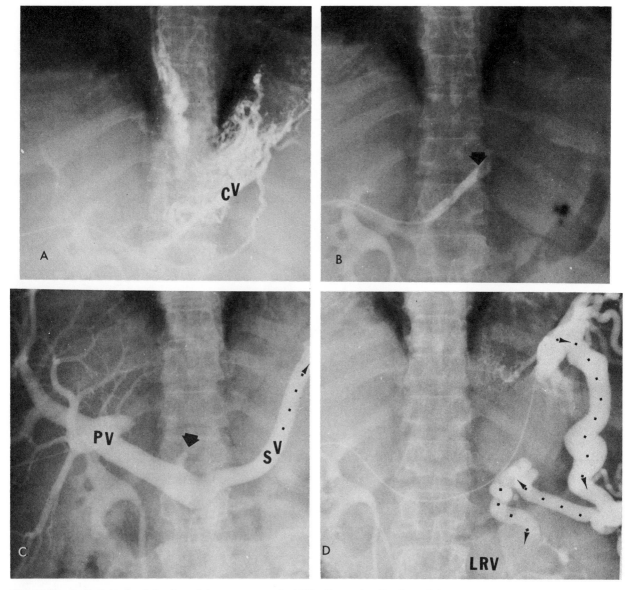

Fig. 12-51. A, B. Selective injection of the coronary vein (*CV*) allows visualization of the gastroesophageal varices before and after embolization (*arrow*). **C, D.** Postembolization study reveals the occluded coronary vein (*large arrow*) and a spontaneous splenorenal vein (*dotted arrowheads*). PV, portal vein; CV, coronary vein; SV, splenic vein; LRV, left renal vein.

occur from branches of the hepatic or portal veins that have been traversed by the track.[69,93,97] After catheterization, the catheter is fixed by gluing to a Molnar disk which is sutured to the skin. The catheter is connected to a bag and allowed to drain externally for a few days. Flushing of this catheter every 3 or 4 hours may be necessary for the first several days, especially if bleeding was a problem during the procedure. After this, internal drainage from the side holes is challenged by the clamping of the external tube. If the level of serum bilirubin does not rise or if it continues to fall, the catheter is left closed on the outside, thus producing internal drainage. Daily flushing with 20 ml of saline is recommended. It is also advised that the catheter be changed at 3-month intervals.

Internal Biliary Prosthesis

In percutaneous transhepatic biliary prosthesis, an internal (self-retained) prosthesis[95] or endoprosthesis[17,18] is placed

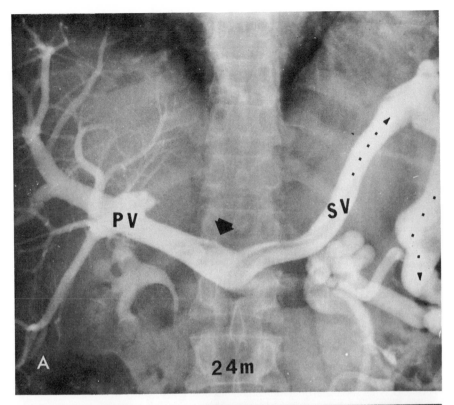

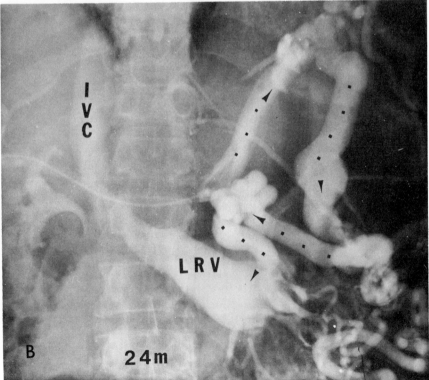

Fig. 12-52. An elective transhepatic splenoportogram was performed 24 months after the initial procedure. **A.** Obliteration of the coronary vein with Gelfoam and Sotradecol persists (*large arrow*). **B.** Note the huge spontaneous splenorenal shunt (*dotted arrowheads*), which is adequately decompressing the short gastric veins that were never embolized. PV, portal vein; SV, splenic vein, LRV, left renal vein; IVC, inferior vena cava.

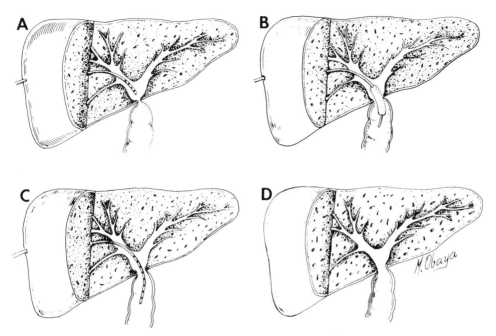

Fig. 12-53. A. The catheter is in position proximal to the strictured area for external drainage. **B.** The balloon catheter is introduced across the stricture, and dilatations are performed from 7 to 14 days later. **C.** After each dilatation session, an internal–external biliary drainage is left in place. **D.** After successful dilatation of a choledochoenterostomy stricture, the biliary drainage catheter is removed.

into the biliary tree, bridging an area of obstruction (Fig. 12-62). This has the great advantage over the previously described methods that no permanent external catheter is needed.

Technique

Percutaneous transhepatic cholangiography using the Chiba needle is first performed so that the exact site of obstruction can be determined and an estimate of the length of the prosthesis needed can be made.[17,18,95,97] A branch of the right hepatic duct is then entered with the standard sheathed trochar used for percutaneous transhepatic cholangiography. With the aid of a curved guidewire (0.025 in.), the Teflon sheath is passed through and beyond the stenotic segment (Fig. 12-62). The guidewire is then exchanged for a 0.038-in. wire, and the standard percutaneous transhepatic sheath is replaced by a No. 8 French catheter (outer diameter, 4 mm; inner diameter, 3 mm), which is advanced over the wire and the smaller catheter. The narrowed segment is next forcefully dilated to the desired diameter (Fig. 12-62), and the No. 12 French catheter is withdrawn.

A No. 12 French Teflon prosthesis (outer diameter, 4

mm; inner diameter, 3 mm) is constructed with a flared proximal end. The prosthesis measures 8 cm to 14 cm in length, depending upon the estimated length of the narrowed region. Using the No. 12 French catheter, the prosthesis is pushed over the No. 8 French catheter and guidewire until it bridges the site of narrowing (Fig. 12-62). The No. 12 French catheter and the guidewire are then withdrawn completely. Patency of the prosthesis is established by withdrawal of the No. 8 French catheter proximal to the prosthesis and injection of a small amount of contrast material. The No. 8 French catheter is then exchanged for a temporary drainage catheter (No. 7 French) with multiple side holes at the distal end. This catheter is left in place proximal to the prosthesis for 2 to 4 days. Care is taken to ensure that the side holes remain within the biliary system. The catheter is ordinarily removed at 2 days (Fig. 12-62) but is left in place for longer periods of time if cholangitis has complicated the situation. In patients with lesions involving the bifurcation area, several side holes are made in the proximal third of the prosthesis to help drainage from the left side and from branches of the right hepatic duct. For the last 3 years, all of our prostheses have been inserted with the tip within the duodenum to facilitate endoscopic exchange when plugging occurs. Also, two distal side holes and two barbs, such as

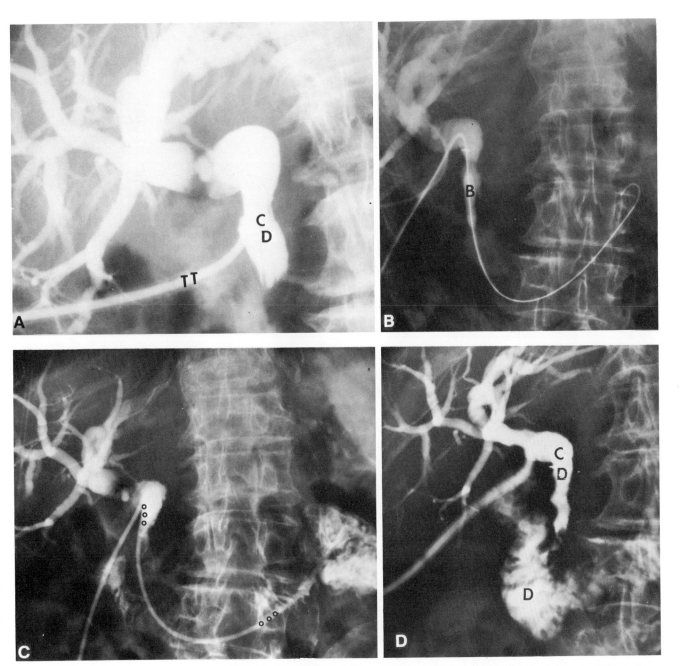

Fig. 12-54. Balloon dilatation of a benign distal common duct stricture. **A.** T-tube (*TT*) cholangiogram showing complete obstruction at the distal common bile duct (*CD*). **B.** Balloon (*B*) inflated at the site of stenosis. **C.** An internal–external biliary drainage catheter is left in place after each daily session of dilatation. **D.** T-tube cholangiogram 1 month postdilatation showing no recurrence of stenosis and a decompressed biliary tree. CD, common bile duct; D, duodenum.

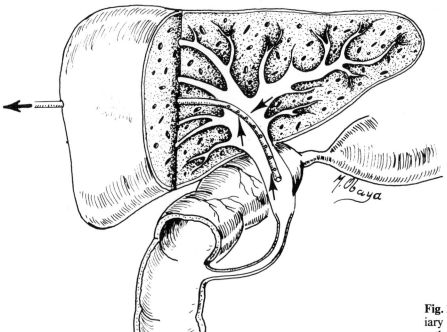

Fig. 12-55. Percutaneous external biliary drainage. Note position of the catheter with multiple side holes above stenosis within the biliary tree.

in a fish hook, are constructed in the duodenal segment of the prosthesis (Figs. 12-64, 12-65). The barbs will prevent proximal migration in distal lesions, and both the barbs and the side holes will facilitate endoscopic removal. All patients receive gross spectrum antibiotics I.V. for 24 hours before the procedure and for at least 72 hours thereafter, depending upon clinical condition. Sometimes it is difficult or impossible to introduce a No. 8 or No. 12 French dilating catheter over the 0.038-in. guidewire. In this situation, we recommend the use of a stiffening cannula.[93,97] The latter is introduced over the 0.038-in. wire to the point at which the guidewire angulates into the right branch of the hepatic duct. While the wire and the cannula are held with the right hand, the left can be used to advance the No. 8 French catheter through the stricture. Excellent results can also be obtained by use of a special hard guidewire with a 10-cm distal flexible tip.[57] Even with the aid of the stiffening cannula, it is not possible in some cases to perform the complete dilatation in a single day. If dilatation with a No. 12 French catheter is very difficult, it is advisable not to insert the prosthesis the first day. One should leave a No. 7 French internal–external catheter in place in the duodenum (see Fig. 12-59B). This facilitates insertion of the internal prosthesis in 2 to 3 days (see Fig. 12-59C). In patients with cholangitis, the insertion of the large prosthesis is not recommended in the first setting. We use a No. 7 French teflon catheter manufac-

tured by Cook for abdominal aortography as a temporary drainage until the cholangitis subsides. This catheter can be inserted with minimal trauma because of its construction and design. Although its tip is placed within the duodenum, it is only used as an external drainage, draining the bile into a bag to treat the infection. Additional side holes are constructed with a punch hole according to each patient's anatomy. If the wire cannot be manipulated because of stenosis, it is advised that an external catheter be left in place for several days. With the ducts decompressed, it is usually easier to cannulate the stenosis (see Fig. 12-59A).

Complications

The incidence of complications largely depends on the experience of the radiologist. Major acute complications such as intraperitoneal hemorrhage, septic shock, and bile peritonitis occur in 4% to 10% of cases.[10,29,68,78,98,100,138] The most frequent serious complication is sepsis.[30,68] A massive hemorrhage is rare, occurring in less than 2% of patients.[30] This can usually be prevented by correcting bleeding disorders, administering fresh frozen plasma, and platelets. If the bleeding source is from a hepatic artery pseudoaneurism, embolization is the treatment of choice. We have had 9 severe bleeding episodes in 450 biliary drainages. Two of these patients have died despite ag-

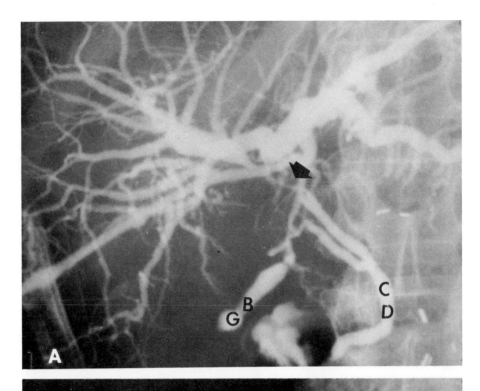

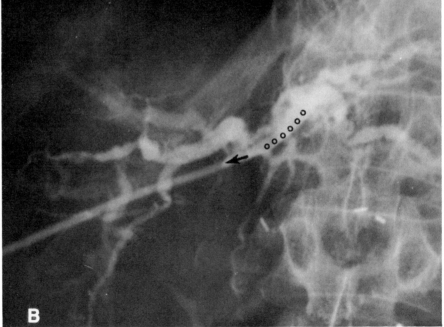

Fig. 12-56. Percutaneous transhepatic external biliary drainage. **A.** Skinny needle cholangiography showing short area of stricture at the common hepatic bifurcation (*arrow*) secondary to metastatic carcinoma. Note the small size of the gallbladder (*GB*). CD, common duct. **B.** Percutaneous external biliary drainage in place. The tip of the catheter was placed well into the left hepatic duct.

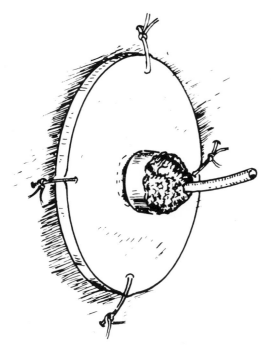

Fig. 12-57. A silicon disk is fixed to the drainage catheter. A permanent bond to the catheter is obtained with adhesive substances, and the disk is then sutured to the skin. After several weeks, the sutures are removed, and the skin–disk relationship is maintained with adhesives.

gressive surgical management. Severe bleeding into an external or internal–external biliary drainage catheter has occurred in two of our patients. In both cases, bleeding was controlled by external clamping of the catheter, which was eventually replaced by a new catheter. The catheter may pass through the lumen of a portal vein branch before it enters a major bile duct. If communication is established between these structures, bleeding may not be controlled without relocation of the course of the catheter. It is important that no side holes are in the vicinity of a hepatic blood vessel. This can be ascertained by injection of contrast material under fluoroscopic control. Minor acute complications such as pain, transient fever, or mild hematobilia have been reported in 20% to 50% of cases.[68,98,123] Mild abdominal pain was common during the first 24 hours and occurred in two thirds of our patients. Delayed in-hospital as well as long-term catheter-related problems are extremely common.[29,68,92,123] Meuller and associates[68] reported unsuccessful attempts at conversion to internal drainage by clamping a properly positioned catheter, the most common delay in-hospital complication. This was manifested by cholangitis (fever, chills) and occurred in 21 (63%) of their last 33 patients who underwent clamping of a properly positioned internal–external drainage tube. We have had the same experience as Ferrucci and Meuller and associates, who recommend replacing the initial 8.3 biliary catheter on the fifth or sixth day for a No. 12 French catheter.[29,68] We use a No. 7 French teflon aortography catheter made by Cook,

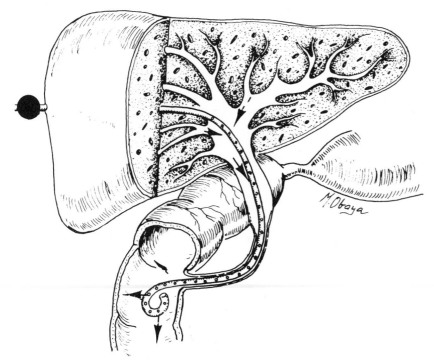

Fig. 12-58. Percutaneous internal–external biliary drainage. Note position of the catheter with multiple side holes and distal pigtail in the duodenum. Arrows show internal flow of bile when the tube is clamped.

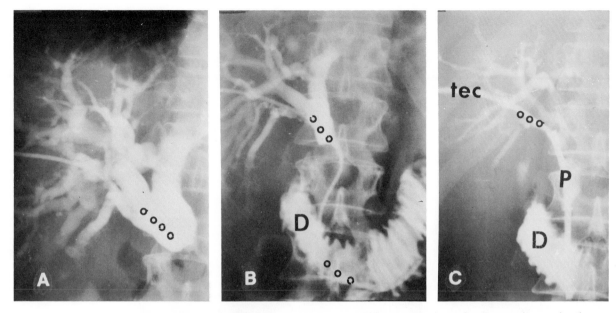

Fig. 12-59. Three-stage placement of internal biliary prosthesis. **A.** On day 1, an external catheter drainage was inserted; it was impossible to cannulate this stenosis. **B.** Internal–external catheter drainage with multiple side holes was successfully inserted on day 3. **C.** An internal prosthesis (*P*) with adequate emptying into the duodenum was introduced on day 6. TEC, temporary external catheter; D, duodenum.

Fig. 12-60. **A.** Carcinoma of the head of the pancreas causing complete obstruction of the distal common duct. **B.** Successful placement of internal–external biliary drainage with a distal pigtail configuration. D, duodenum.

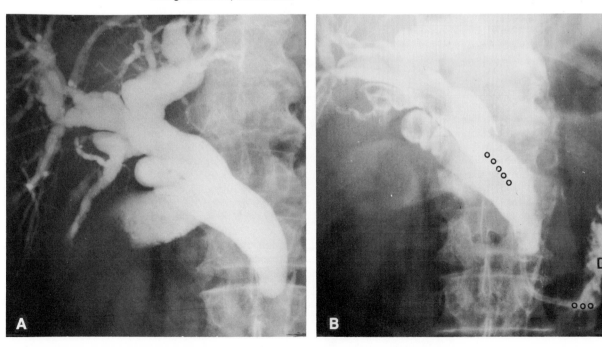

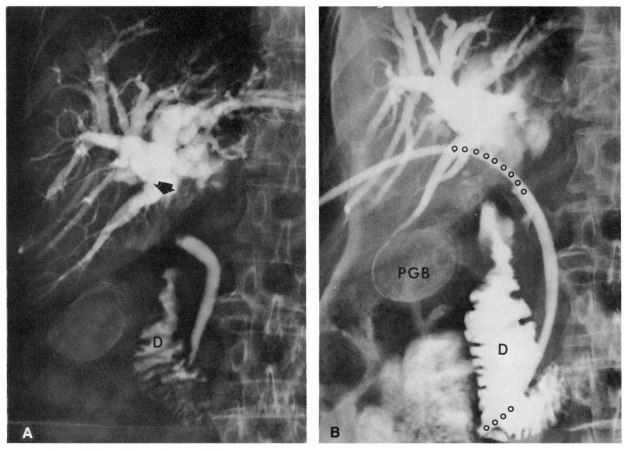

Fig. 12-61. Adenocarcinoma of the gallbladder causing almost complete obstruction of the common hepatic duct (*large arrows*). Note the porcelain gallbladder (*PGB*). A No. 12 French internal–external biliary drainage was successfully placed all the way into the duodenum (*D*).

which has a very long tapered tip to which we construct side holes according to the patient's anatomy. This catheter is extremely easy to insert and produces very minor trauma, reducing the complications of sepsis. We then exchange this catheter in 5 to 6 days for a No. 12 French catheter. In some cases, dilatation of the tract is needed.

We have had excellent results using the sump catheter designed by Eric van Sonnenberg for percutaneous abscess drainage. Additional large oval-shaped side holes are easily constructed using a sterile paper punch hole. The use of a large-bore internal–external catheter greatly reduces in-hospital postclamping complications.[35,68] In our experience, it has also greatly reduced outpatient chronic catheter care and complications, including obstruction and cholangitis. We, as Ferrucci, do not routinely perform quarterly catheter changes; we await indications of catheter occlusions or dysfunction. Most of our sump catheters

were never exchanged, because most of the patients died within 6 to 8 months. Several had lasted for more than a year without clogging, and one patient with metastatic disease of the colon that responded to chemotherapy is alive at 2 years with his original internal–external drainage.

Leakage of bile around the catheter occasionally occurs in external or internal–external drainage. Excessive bile drainage, although a rare complication, can be severe in external drainage. In one of our patients, it amounted to 5 liters or 6 liters of bile a day.

Complications unique to endoprosthesis are stent migration and occlusion. Cholangitis is much more common with external or internal–external drainage compared with endoprosthesis.[56,98,100] Burcharth reported only seven cases of cholangitis in 99 patients.[19] In a series of 71 stent placements, Coons reported only two instances of migration of the stent into the duodenum.[23] We have had only two

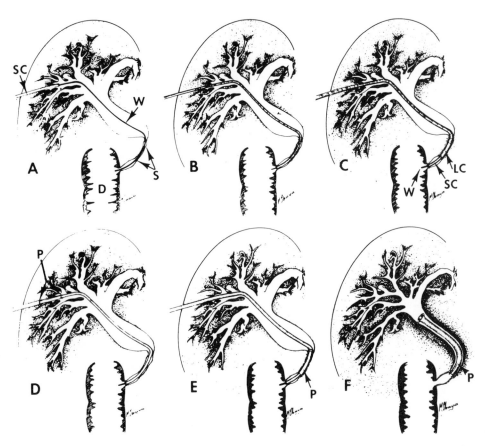

Fig. 12-62. Technique of insertion of an internal prosthesis. **A.** Wire (*W*) is placed through the right branch of the hepatic biliary tree and through the strictured segment (*S*) into the duodenum (*D*). SC, small catheter (No. 8 French) over wire. **B.** Wire and No. 8 French wire are now in place through the level of obstruction. **C.** Forceful dilatation of the strictured segment with a No. 12 French catheter inserted coaxially. LC, large catheter. **D.** Large catheter has been removed after dilatation and a Teflon prosthesis (*P*) pushed coaxially by the same large catheter. **E.** Prosthesis at the desired level with a small catheter distal to it. **F.** Prosthesis in place; the No. 8 French small catheter and wire have been removed.

instances in a total of 180 endoprostheses; in both instances, the stenosis was distal common duct and the migration was proximal, away from the duodenum. This should not occur with the type of prosthesis that we are now constructing, with distal barb-like fishhooks. We abandoned insertion of the prosthesis with multiple steps (Fig. 12-66) because its insertion was very difficult. In our experience, occlusion of a No. 12 French is unusual, because most patients die within 6 or 8 months. It is much more common in patients surviving for more than 1 year. We have had nine patients surviving longer than 12 months. Four of them had complete obstruction of their endoprosthesis between 12 and 14 months. Our longest survival with a patent endoprosthesis at the time of death was 17 months. With the new advancements in endoscopic

insertion of large-bore endoprostheses, we foresee that in a few years, occluded internal stents will be easily exchanged by the endoscopic route.

Discussion

Decompression of the biliary tree is often important as a palliative maneuver for treatment of malignant biliary tract obstruction. The initial symptoms and clinical problems encountered by these patients are usually directly related to the obstruction. The life span of these patients may be shortened by recurrent cholangitis, progressive hepatic decompensation aggravated by the obstruction, and nutritional deficiencies secondary to the interruption

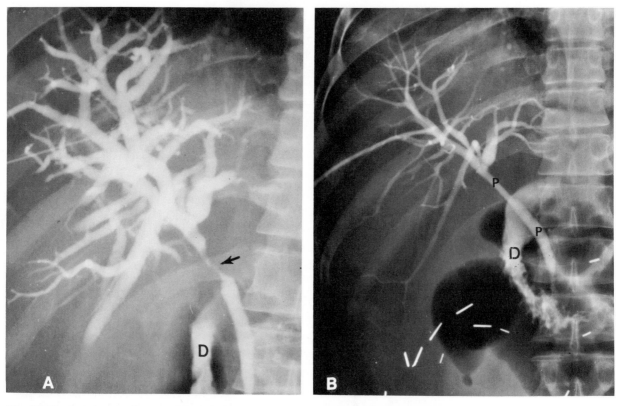

Fig. 12-63. A. Adenocarcinoma of the colon metastatic to liver hilum causing stricture of the common hepatic duct with marked dilatation of the biliary tree. **B.** Successful placement of a No. 12 French internal prosthesis (*P*) with its distal tip within the distal common bile duct. Adequate decompression of the biliary tree with good emptying into the duodenum (*D*).

of the flow of bile. Pruritus is frequently a devastating symptom unresponsive to usual medical therapy.

It has long been recognized that there is a high operative mortality in deeply jaundiced patients subjected to surgery of the biliary tree and pancreas. The operative mortality rate for pancreaticoduodenectomy has been reported to be from 20% to 50%.[13,17,23,33,79] Hepatic and renal failure and gastrointestinal hemorrhage are the most frequent causes of postoperative death in deeply jaundiced patients. A two-stage operation for extensively jaundiced patients has been recommended with satisfactory results.[21,42,61,103,112] Nakayama and associates[75] have demonstrated a reduction in operative mortality from 28% to 8% ($p = 0.05$) in patients with periampullary cancer with the use of temporary percutaneous biliary drainage to reduce the bilirubin level below 5 mg/dl.

Following Nakayama's work, there has been a controversy in temporary percutaneous transhepatic biliary drainage as a preoperative measure in jaundiced patients with malignant biliary obstruction. Hatfield and associates[40] and Norlander and co-workers[80] found no benefit in perioperative morbidity and mortality. Gunthrie and colleagues[35] reported on 50 patients and concluded that an operative mortality of 20% and a major morbidity of 52% was lowered to 4% and 8%, respectively, with preoperative temporary biliary drainage.

Dooley and co-workers[25] also found no statistical difference in mortality between groups drained and not drained preoperatively. We agree with Pogani and associates[100] in complication rates of the drainage procedures in the different institutions. Warechaw believes that preoperative decompression is unnecessary unless the bilirubin level is greater than 20 mg/dl.

Palliative surgical drainage procedures in jaundiced patients with malignant biliary obstruction carry an operative mortality rate that has been reported to be 23% to 33%,[27,74] rising to as high as 59% with extensive metastatic disease. In one study, half the patients with biliary cancer presented with jaundice.[27] In spite of numerous new diagnostic advances and the use of the potentially curative

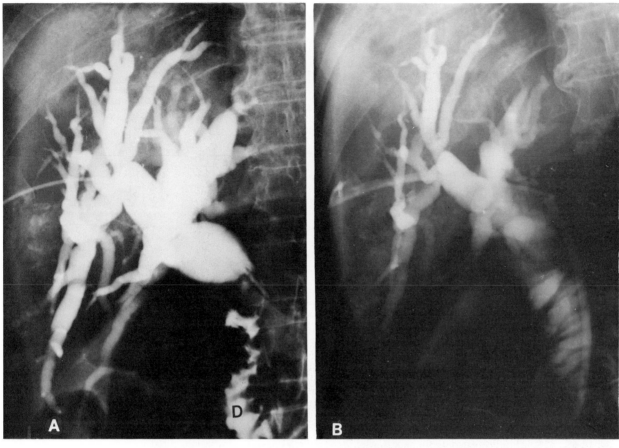

Fig. 12-64. A. Adenocarcinoma of the head of the pancreas causing almost complete obstruction of the distal common bile duct with marked dilatation of the biliary tree. **B.** A No. 12 French internal prosthesis was placed with its distal tip within the duodenum (*D*). Note large side holes in the duodenal segment of the internal prosthesis.

pancreaticoduodenectomy, the 5-year survival rate is still only 1%.[3] Most attempts at palliation consist of decompressive operations, but the benefit and justification of this kind of surgery are mitigated by the high surgical mortality rate and postoperative complications.

Permanent percutaneous external transhepatic biliary drainage techniques have been devised as an alternative to surgery.[72,75,124] These have proved to be successful with malignant and benign obstructions. The disadvantages of percutaneous external drainage include complicating cholangitis and sepsis,[38,56] persistent local pain at the entry point of the external catheter, accidental dislodgement of the tube, leaking of bile around the catheter, excessive external bile drainage, interruption of the enterohepatic circulation of bile with concomitant malabsorption, and the negative psychologic effects of an external catheter and a bag. Some of these problems should not occur with the internal–external drainage. If adequate, the internal drainage may prove successful,[7,44,69,107] but the side holes may become obstructed, decreasing the yield of the procedure. In that event, the patient is always left with an external catheter.

We recommend, when technically possible, the use of a permanent internal prosthesis for palliating malignant biliary obstructions, as the elimination of an external drainage tube dramatically improves the patient's quality of life.[17,23,95,98] In patients with very high lesions and especially those with involvement of multiple intrahepatic duct branches, an internal prosthesis is not recommended as the percutaneous drainage of choice. For this reason, we insert one internal prosthesis for every three to five internal–external biliary drains used. It may be a disadvantage that flushing of the internal prosthesis is impossible; however, clogging is a minor problem. Burcharth[18] used a small

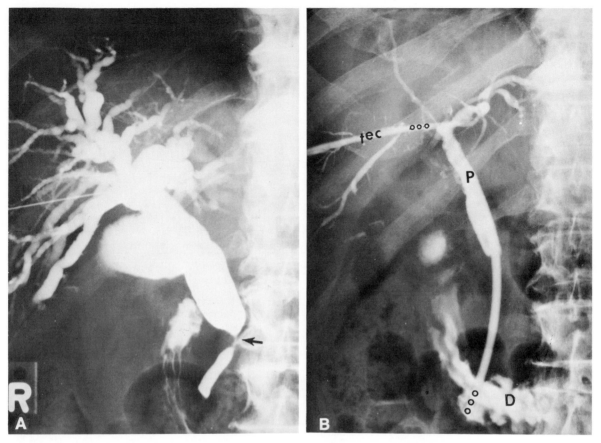

Fig. 12-65. A. Scirrhous cholangiocarcinoma causing short stricture of the common bile duct (*arrow*) with resultant dilatation of the biliary tree. This is the ideal case for an internal biliary prosthesis. **B.** Successful placement of a No. 12 French long internal biliary prosthesis (*P*) all the way into the duodenum. The length of this prosthesis is such that only very minimal dislodgement can occur; the prosthesis is anatomically anchored by the hepatic bifurcation and the duodenum. tec, temporary external catheter drainage.

No. 6 French polyethylene tube with multiple side holes and did not observe occlusion of the endoprosthesis. Coons had only one occluded endoprosthesis in his series of 71 stents.[23] In our experience, a No. 12 French or larger size endoprosthesis very rarely obstructs before 12 months. It is also recommended that the distal tip of the endoprosthesis be placed within the duodenum. This will also make possible endoscopic exchanges. If clogging occurs, it can be cleared by endoscopic flushing or by the use of a Fogarty balloon (Fig. 12-67).

The risk of cholangitis is less with an internal biliary prosthesis than with external or internal–external catheter drainage.[38,56,98] Burcharth[19] reported only two cases of cholangitis among 48 patients. Almost all patients with prolonged external or internal–external catheter drainage are noted to have at least one attack of cholangitis.[38] Dis-

lodgement of an internal prosthesis has been a minor problem.[17,18,93,95,97] In Coons' series of 71 stent placements, there were only two cases of migration into the duodenum.[23]

Percutaneous biliary drainage is a remarkable therapeutic advancement as an alternative to palliative surgical bypass for unresectable carcinoma of the pancreas, biliary tract, or metastatic disease. It is our opinion that a well-functioning endoprosthesis is preferable to bile drainage with an external or internal–external catheter. However, because patients with involvement of multiple intrahepatic branches are not usually treated by endoprostheses, the internal–external catheter drainage is the most commonly used. This technique should be the procedure of choice for patients who are poor surgical risks or who have lesions such as unresectable carcinoma of the pancreas. This

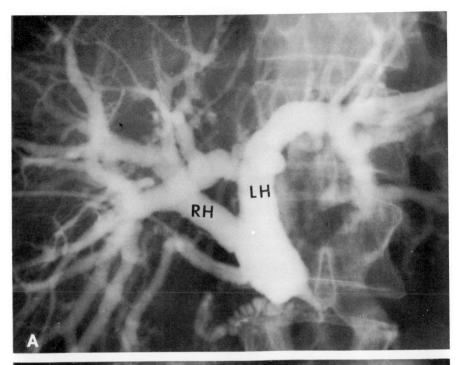

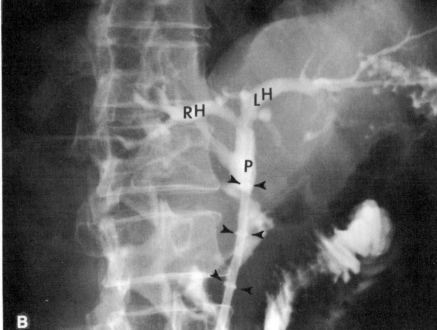

Fig. 12-66. A. Carcinoma of the head of the pancreas causing complete occlusion of the common bile duct with marked dilatation of the intrahepatic radicles. **B.** Successful placement of prosthesis (*P*) with multiple steps (*arrowheads*) to prevent dislocation. RH, right hepatic duct; LH, left hepatic duct.

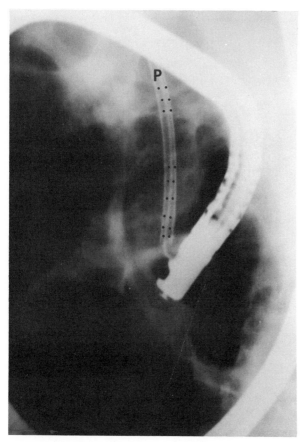

Fig. 12-67. Endoscopic cleaning of an obstructed internal biliary prosthesis (*P*). Note the small endoscopic catheter (*dots*) within the internal biliary prosthesis.

technique, in addition, avoids the pain, morbidity, and cost of a laparotomy for biliary tract bypass.

REFERENCES

1. Abrams RM et al: Angiographic features of cavernous hemangioma of the liver. Radiology 92:308–312, 1969
2. Adam YG et al: Malignant vascular tumors of the liver. Ann Surg 175:375, 1973
3. American Cancer Society: 1977 Cancer Facts and Figures, p. 7. New York, American Cancer Society, 1976
4. Andrew RC et al: The Hawkins needle system for percutaneous catheterization. AJR 142:1191–1195, 1984
5. Arner O et al: Percutaneous transhepatic cholangiography: Puncture of dilated and nondilated bile ducts under roentgen television control. Surgery 52:561–571, 1962
6. Ariyama J: Percutaneous transhepatic cholangiography. In Margulis AR: Alimentary Tract Radiology, pp 2229–2241. St Louis, CV Mosby, 1983
7. Baum S, Nusbaum M: The control of gastrointestinal hemorrhage by selective mesenteric arterial infusion of vasopresin. Radiology 98:497, 1971
8. Benner KG et al: Clinical outcome after percutaneous transhepatic obliteration of esophageal varices. Gastroenterology 85(1):146–153, 1983
9. Berk RN, Clemett AR: Radiology of the Gall Bladder and Bile Ducts. Philadelphis, WB Saunders, 1977
10. Berk RN et al: Radiography of the bile ducts. Radiology 145:1–9, 1982
11. Berman C: Primary Carcinoma of the Liver. A Study in Incidence, Clinical Manifestations, Pathology and Etiology. London, Lewis, 1951
12. Bonnel D et al: Surgical and radiological decompression in malignant biliary obstructions: A retrospective study using a multi-variate risk factor analysis. Radiology 152:347, 1984
13. Boysen E, Abrams HL: Roentgenologic diagnosis of primary carcinoma of the liver. Acta Radiol (Diagn) 3:52–77, 1965
14. Braasch JW et al: Progress in biliary stricture repair. Surgery 129:34,1975
15. Brown DB et al: Primary carcinoma of the extra hepatic bile ducts. Br J Surg 49:22, 1961
16. Burcharth F: Percutaneous transhepatic portography. 1. Technique and application. Am J Roentgenol 132:177–182, 1979
17. Burcharth F: A new endoprosthesis for nonoperative intubation of the biliary tract in malignant obstructive jaundice. Surg Gynecol Obstet 146:76, 1978
18. Burcharth F et al: Endoprosthesis for internal drainage of the biliary tract. Gastroenterology 77:133, 1979
19. Burcharth F et al: Nonsurgical internal biliary drainage by endoprosthesis. Surg Gynecol Obstet 153:857–860, 1981
20. Burhene MJ: Nonoperative roentgenologic instrumentation techniques of the postoperative biliary tract. Am J Surg 128:111, 1974
21. Cattell RB, Pyrtek LJ: An appraisal of pancreatoduodenal resection. Ann Surg 129:840, 1949
22. Clark RA: Percutaneous catheter biliary decompression. AJR 137, 1981
23. Coons HG, Cary BH: Large-bore biliary endoprosthesis for improved drainage. Radiology 148:89, 1983
24. Denning DA: Preoperative percutaneous transhepatic biliary decompression lowers operative morbidity in patients with obstructive jaundice. Am J Surg 141:61–65, 1981
25. Dooley JS, Dick N, Olney J, Sherlock S: Nonsurgical treatment of biliary obstructions. Lancet 2:1040–1044, 1979
26. Elias B Sc, et al: A randomized trial of P.T.C. with the Chiba needle versus E.R.C. for bile duct visualization in jaundice. Gastroenterology 71:439–443, 1976
27. Feduska NJ et al: Results of palliative operations for carcinoma of the pancreas. Arch Surg 102:330, 1971
28. Ferrucci JT, Wittenberg J: Refinements in Chiba needle transheptaic cholangiography. AJR 129:11–16, 1977
29. Ferrucci JT: Percutaneous transhepatic biliary drainage. Technique, results, and applications. Radiology 135:13, 1980
30. Ferrucci JT, Mueller PR: Interventional radiology of the biliary tract. Gastroenterology 82:974–985, 1982
31. Flemma RJ et al: Percutaneous transhepatic cholangiography in the differential diagnosis of jaundice. Surg Gynecol Obstet 116:559–568, 1963
32. Glenn F, Thorbjanarson B: Carcinoma of the pancreas. Ann Surg 159:954, 1964
33. Goldman ML et al: The transjugular technique of hepatic

venography and biopsy, cholangiography and obliteration of esophageal varices. Acta Radiol (Diagn) 128:325–331, 1978

34. Goldstein HM et al: Angiographic findings in benign liver cell tumors. Radiology 110:339–343, 1973

35. Gundry SR et al: Efficacy of preoperative biliary tract decompression in patients with obstructive jaundice. Arch Surg 119:703–709, 1984

36. Ham JM, Mackenzie DC: Primary carcinoma of the extrahepatic bile ducts. Surg Gynecol Obstet, 1964

37. Hanafee W, Weiner M: Transjugular percutaneous cholangiography. Radiology 88:35–39, 1967

38. Hansson JA: Clinical aspects of nonsurgical percutaneous transhepatic bile drainage in obstructive lesions of the extrahepatic bile ducts. Ann Surg, 1979

39. Harbin WP et al: Transhepatic cholangiography: Complications and use patterns of fine needle technique. Radiology 135:15–22, 1980

40. Hatfield ARW et al: Preoperative external biliary drainage in obstructive jaundice. Lancet 2:896–899, 1982

41. Herba MJ, Kiss J: Percutaneous transhepatic cholangiography—experience with 106 examinations. J Can Assoc Radiol 22:22–29, 1971

42. Hess W: Surgery of the Biliary Passages and the Pancreas, p. 474. Princeton, Van Nostrand, 1965

43. Hines C Jr et al: Percutaneous transhepatic cholangiography—experience with 102 procedures. Am J Dig Dis 17: 868–874, 1972

44. Hoevels J: Percutaneous transhepatic intubation of bile ducts for combined internal–external drainage in preoperative and palliative treatment of obstructive jaundice. Gastrointest Radiol 3:23, 1978

45. Hudson DG et al: Balloon dilatation of biliary strictures through a choledochojejuno cutaneous fistula. Ann Surg 199:637, 1984

46. Honjo J, Matsumurah: Vascular distribution of hepatic tumors, experimental study. Rev Int Hepat 15:681–690, 1965

47. Illescas FF et al: Ultrasound-guided transcholecystal cholangiography. Gastrointest Radiol 11:77–80, 1986

48. Ingis DA, Farmer RG: Adenocarcinoma of the bile ducts: Relationship of anatomic location to clinical features. Am J Dig Dis 20:253, 1975

49. Irish CR, Meaney TF: Percutaneous transhepatic cholangiography: Comparison of success and risk using 19 versus 22-gauge needles. AJR 134:137–140, 1980

50. Jaques TF et al: The failed transhepatic cholangiogram. Radiology 134:33–35, 1980

51. Kaude et al: Cholangiocarcinoma. Radiology 100:573, 1971

52. Keller FS: Transhepatic obliteration of gastroesophageal varices with absolute ethanol. Radiology 146:615–617, 1983

53. Kadir S et al: Percutaneous biliary drainage in the management of biliary sepsis. AJR 138:25–29, 1982

54. Krieger J et al: The roentgenologic appearance of sclerosing cholangitis. Radiology 95:369–375, 1960

55. La Russo et al: Primary sclerosing cholangitis. N Engl J Med 310:899, 1984

56. Lunderquist A: Unpublished data.

57. Lunderquist A: Guidewire for percutaneous transhepatic cholangiography. Radiology 132:228, 1979

58. Lunderquist A, Vang J: Transhepatic catheterization and obliteration of the coronary vein in patients with portal hypertension and esophageal varices. N Eng J Med 291: 646–649, 1974

59. Lunderquist A et al: Follow-up of patients with portal hypertension and esophageal varices treated with percutaneous obliteration of gastric coronary vein. Radiology 122:59–63, 1977

60. Lunderquist A et al: Isobutyl 2-cyanoacrylate (Bucrylate) in obliteration of gastric coronary vein and esophageal varices. Am J Roentgenol 130:1–6, 1978

61. Maki F et al: Pancreatoduodenectomy for periampullary carcinomas. Arch Surg 92:825, 1966

62. Marks WM et al: Hepatocellular carcinoma: Clinical and angiographic findings and predictability for surgical resection. AJR 132:7–11, 1979

63. Martin ED et al: Percutaneous dilatation in primary sclerosing cholangitis: two experiences. AJR 137:603–605, 1981

64. McLaughlin MJ et al: Focal nodular hyperplasia of the liver. Radiology 107:257–263, 1973

65. McLean, et al: Therapeutic alterations in the treatment of intrahepatic biliary obstruction. Radiology 145:289–295, 1982

66. Mendez G et al: Abandonment of endoprostatic drainage techniques in malignant biliary obstruction. AJR 143:617–622, 1984

67. Mendez G, et al: Gastrointestinal varices: percutaneous transhepatic therapeutic embolization in 54 patients. AJR 1935:1045–1050, 1980

68. Meuller DR et al: Percutaneous biliary drainage: Technique and catheter-related problems in 200 patients. AJR 138: 17, 1982

69. Molnar W, Stockum A: Relief of obstructive jaundice through percutaneous transhepatic catheter—a new therapeutic method. Am J Roentgenol 122:356, 1974

70. Molnar W, Stockum A: Transhepatic dilatation of choledochoenterostomy strictures. Radiology 129:59, 1978

71. Morettin LB, Dodd GD: Percutaneous transhepatic cholangiograph (methods and techniques). Am J Dig Dis 17: 831–845, 1972

72. Mori K et al: Percutaneous transhepatic bile drainage. Ann Surg 185:111, 1977

73. Muhletaler CA et al: The diagnosis of obstructive jaundice with non-dilated bile ducts. AJR 134:1149–1152, 1980

74. Nakase A et al: Surgical treatment of cancer of the pancreas and the periampullary region. Ann Surg 185:52, 1977

75. Nakayama T et al: Percutaneous transhepatic drainage of the biliary tract. Gastroenterology 74:554, 1978

76. Nebessar RA, et al: Celiac and Superior Mesenteric Arteries. A Correlation of Angiograms with Dissections. Boston, Little, Brown & Co., 1969

77. Nebessar RA et al: Angiographic diagnosis of malignant disease of the liver. Radiology 86:284, 1968

78. Nielssen U et al: Percutaneous transhepatic cholangiography and drainage. Risk and complications. Acta Radiologica 24:(6), 1983

79. Nilsson LA, Zettergren L: Blood supply and vascular pattern of diffuse hepatic carcinoma in rats. Acta Pathol Microbiol Scand 71:179–186, 1967

80. Norlander A et al: Effect of percutaneous transhepatic drainage upon liver function and postoperative mortality. Surg Gynecol Obstet 155:161–166, 1982

80a. Nunnerley HB: Diagnostic angiography of the liver. Clin Gastroenterol 14(2):331, 1985

81. Nunez, Diego et al: Portosystemic communications studied by transhepatic portography. Radiology 127:75–79, 1978

82. Ohnishi K et al: Transhepatic obliteration of esophageal

varices using stainless coils combined with hypertonic glucose and Gelfoam. J Clin Gastroenterol 7(3):200–207, 1985

83. Okuda K et al: Unpublished data presented at the American Association for the Study of Liver Diseases meeting, San Antonio, Texas, May 1975

84. Okuda K et al: Demonstration of hepatocellular carcinoma in the portal vein by celiac angiography: The thread and streaks sign. Radiology 117:303–309, 1975

85. Okuda K et al: Nonsurgical percutaneous transhepatic cholangiography: Diagnostic significance in medical problems of the liver. Am J Dig Dis 19:21–36, 1974

86. Oleaga JA et al: Selective hepatic arteriography in Herlingerh. Clinical Radiol of the Liver, pp 267–310. New York, Marcel Dekker, 1983

87. Pereiras R et al: Percutaneous transhepatic cholangiography utilizing the Chiba University needle. Radiology 121:219–221, 1976

88. Pereiras R et al: Percutaneous transhepatic cholangiography with the skinny needle. Ann Intern Med 86:562–568, 1977

89. Pereiras R et al. Percutaneous cholangiography with the Chiba University needle: A new safe and accurate method in the diagnosis of cholestatic syndromes. Rev Interam Radiol 1:17–19, 1976

90. Pereiras R et al: Transhepatic obliteration of gastroesophageal varices: Is it worth while? (In press)

91. Pereiras R et al: New technique for interruption of gastroesophageal venous blood flow. Radiology 124:313–323, 1977

92. Pereiras R: The practical management of obstructive jaundice. The transhepatic approach, diagnosis and therapy. British Society of Gastroenterology. Second International Teaching Day. Inst. of Education, April 1983

93. Pereiras R et al: Role of interventional radiology in diseases of the hepatobiliary system and the pancreas. Radiol Clin North Am 17:555, 1979

94. Pereiras R et al: Relief of obstructive jaundice by percutaneous transhepatic insertion of a permanent biliary prosthesis (in press).

95. Pereiras R et al: Relief of malignant obstructive jaundice by percutaneous insertion of a permanent prosthesis in the biliary tree. Ann Intern Med 89:589, 1978

96. Pereiras R et al: A new technique for transhepatic liver tract dilatation. Radiology 127:830–832, 1978

97. Pereiras R: Nonsurgical biliary decompression. In: Developments in Digestive Diseases, pp 243–258. Philadelphia, Lea & Febiger, 1980

98. Pereiras R: Percutaneous transhepatic decompression. In Wilkins RA (ed): Interventional Radiology, pp 309–326. Oxford, Blackwell Scientific Publications, 1982

99. Plecha FR et al: Percutaneous transhepatic cholangiography. Arch Surg 92:672–676, 1966

100. Pogani AC et al: Percutaneous biliary drainage. Clin Gastroenterol 14:87, 1985

101. Pollard JJ et al: Angiographic diagnosis of benign diseases of the liver. Radiology 86:276–283, 1966

102. Pollard JJ et al: Angiography of hepatic neoplasms. Radiol Clin North Am 8:31–41, 1970

103. Priestley JT, Wollaeger EE: Malignant lesions of the bile ducts and head of the pancreas—diagnosis and surgical treatment. Surg Clin North Am 41:963, 1961

104. Rabinowitz JG et al: Macroregenerating nodules of the cirrhotic liver. AJR 121:401–411, 1974

105. Redeker AC et al: Percutaneous transhepatic cholangiography. JAMA 231:386–387, 1975

106. Reuter SR et al: The spectrum of angiographic findings in hepatoma. Radiology 94:89–94, 1970

107. Ring E et al: Therapeutic application of catheter cholangiography. Radiology 128:333, 1978

108. Ring E et al: A multihole catheter for maintaining long-term percutaneous antegrade biliary drainage. Radiology 132:752, 1979

109. Roche A et al: Balloon catheter to central transhepatic obliteration of gastroesophageal varices. Am J Roentgenol 132:647–649, 1979

110. Rosch J et al: Experimental catheter obstruction of gastric coronary vein; possible technique for percutaneous intravascular tamponade of the gastroesophageal varices. Invest Radiol 10:206–211, 1975

111. Russell E et al: Dilatation of biliary strictures through a stomatized jejunal limb. Acta Radiol Diagnost 26:3, 1985

112. Ross DE: Cancer of the pancreas. Am J Gastroenterol 31:517, 1959

113. Salomowitz E et al: Biliary dilatation of benign biliary strictures. Radiology 151:613, 1984

114. Schiff ER: Diagnostic percutaneous transhepatic cholangiography. Semin Liver Dis 2(1): 1982

115. Scott J et al: Percutaneous transhepatic obliteration of gastro-oesophageal varices. Lancet 2:53–55, 1976

116. Seldinger SI: Catheter replacement of a needle in percutaneous angiography: A new technique. Acta Radiol 39:368–376, 1953

117. Shaldon S et al: Percutaneous transhepatic cholangiography (a modified technique). Gastroenterology 42:371–379, 1962

118. Shingleton WW, Bamburg D: Stenosis of the sphincter of Oddi. Am J Surg 119:35, 1970

119. Smith-Laing et al: Role of percutaneous transhepatic obliteration of varices in the management of hemorrhage from esophageal varices. Gastroenterology 80:1031–1036, 1981

120. Smith EC et al: Preoperative percutaneous transhepatic internal drainage in obstructive jaundice. A randomized controlled trial examining renal function. Surgery 97:641, 1985

121. Summerfield et al: The biliary system in primary biliary cirrhosis, a study by endoscopic retrograde cholangiopancreatography. Gastroenterology 70:240, 1976

122. Takada T et al: Percutaneous transhepatic cholangial drainage: direct approach under fluoroscopic control. J Surg Oncol 8:83, 1976

123. Teplick et al: Surg Clin North Am 64(1): 1984

124. Tylen U et al: Percutaneous transhepatic cholangiography with external drainage of obstructive biliary lesions. Surg Gynecol Obstet 144:13, 1977

125. Viamonte M Jr et al: Selective catheterization of the portal vein and its tributaries. Radiology 114:457–460, 1975

126. Viamonte M Jr et al: Pitfalls in transhepatic portography. Radiology 124:325–329, 1977

127. Viamonte M Jr et al: Transhepatic obliteration of gastroesophageal varices: Results in acute and non-acute bleeders. Am J Roentgenol 129:237–241, 1977

128. Voegeli DR et al: Percutaneous transhepatic cholangiography. Drainage and biopsy in patients with malignant biliary obstruction. An alternative to surgery. Am J Surg 150:243, 1985

129. Warren KW, McDonald WM: Facts and fiction regarding strictures of extrahepatic bile ducts. Ann Surg 159:966, 1964

130. Warren KW et al: A long-term appraisal of pancreatico-duodenal resection for periampullary carcinoma. Ann Surg 155:653, 1962

131. Weiner SN: Arterioportal fistula secondary to percutaneous transhepatic cholangiography. NY State J Med 86–87, 1984

132. Weichel KL: Percutaneous transhepatic cholangiography. Techniques and applications. Acta Quirurgica Scand (Suppl) 330:1–99, 1964

133. Whelan JG et al: Angiographic and radionuclear characteristics of hepatic angiosarcoma found in vinyl chloride workers. Radiology 118:549–557, 1976

134. Widrich WC et al: Pitfalls of transhepatic portal venography and therapeutic coronary vein occlusion. Am J Roentgenol 131:637–643, 1978

135. Widrich WC et al: Portal hypertension changes following selective splenorenal shunt surgery. Radiology 121:295–302, 1976

136. Widrich WC: Personal communication.

137. Williams RC, Wise RE: Infusion hepatic angiography. Asessment of hepatic malignancy via the infusion catheter. Radiol Clin North Am VIII, #1, April, 1979

138. Wong GH et al: Percutaneous transhepatic biliary decompression. Am J Surg 147:615, 1984

139. Yune HY et al: Absolute ethanol in thrombo therapy of bleeding esophageal varices. AJR 138:1137–1141, 1982

140. Zinberg SS et al: Percutaneous transhepatic cholangiography: Its use and limitations. Am J Dig Dis 10:154–169, 1965

chapter 13

Needle Biopsy of the Liver

KAMAL G. ISHAK, EUGENE R. SCHIFF, and LEON SCHIFF

"It is often only by the use of puncture biopsy of the liver that a precise diagnosis can be made, and when diagnosis is doubtful, treatment, advice and prognosis are apt to be hesitant, and perhaps in consequence, the handling of the patient ineffective."

(H. P. Himsworth)[123]

Needle biopsy of the liver remains an important diagnostic procedure in the management of hepatobiliary disorders. In recent years the trend has been away from blind percutaneous biopsies and more toward guided biopsies utilizing laparoscopy, ultrasound, and computed tomography (CT) for proper positioning of the needle. Regardless of how the specimen is obtained, tissue from the liver often provides the basis for a definitive diagnosis of hepatic and systemic disease processes. The establishment of an accurate diagnosis is dependent on sampling an adequate amount of tissue and, most importantly, on a histologic interpretation by someone well versed in liver histopathology.

HISTORICAL BACKGROUND

Although puncture of the liver has been practiced for many years in the diagnosis and the treatment of hepatic abscess, the first attempt at diagnostic aspiration of liver tissue by means of a syringe and a trocar is said to have been made by Lucatello in 1895.[196] Scattered reports on the aspiration of liver tissue fragments for diagnostic purposes between 1907 and 1928 are recorded by Roholm, Krarup, and Iversen.[264]

In 1939, Baron published his experience with 48 hepatic aspirations performed on 35 patients.[18] He used a 20-ml Luer-Lok or "Record" syringe and a 13-gauge needle about 9 cm long. The intercostal route was employed in several cases, but he preferred the subcostal approach, presuming this to offer less hazard of hemorrhage. He appended a note to his report indicating that he had one death from hemorrhage directly attributable to the procedure in a case of extensive metastatic carcinoma of the liver. He found the method of value in the recognition of metastatic carcinoma of the liver and in the differential diagnosis of jaundice. In the same year (1939), Iversen and Roholm[149] published their paper on aspiration biopsy of the liver and their studies on acute epidemic hepatitis.

These reports served as an important impetus to the use of the method. Needle biopsy is now employed throughout the world and has become an invaluable clinical tool for obtaining liver tissue both for histologic and biochemical analysis.[64,360]

PERFORMANCE OF LIVER BIOPSY

While various needles and procedural modifications have been proposed,[19,73,109,125,150,210–213,225,276,289,294,329,340,342,369] the transthoracic approach of Iversen and Roholm[149] remains the one of choice. The Vim-Silverman type of needle technique employs a cutting mechanism originally used by Tripoli and Fader[329] for hepatic biopsy by the subcostal route. Although still the needle of choice in some centers, it has largely been replaced by the Menghini type of needle, which is used with the aspiration or suction technique. There are now numerous disposable types of biopsy needles available, all of which have the advantage of always being sharp. The disposable feature prevents the unnecessary handling of contaminated needles by susceptible hospital-supply employees who may inadvertently stick themselves and in some cases develop viral hepatitis. Popular types of disposable needles include the Trucut, a variation of the Vim-Silverman needle. Fragmentation is more likely to occur with the Menghini technique, and some recommend using a Trucut needle if cirrhosis is suspected.[205,335]

Needle biopsy of the liver is usually carried out in the patient's room, and the intercostal approach is used almost exclusively. It provides the whole transverse depth of the right lobe for puncture, and intra-abdominal viscera are avoided. It does, however, involve puncture of the pleural cavity. The subcostal approach is applicable only if the liver is enlarged to at least 6 cm below the right costal margin or if there is a readily apparent mass on the anterior surface of the left lobe. It has the theoretic advantage of selecting for puncture a specific area on the surface of the liver. We infrequently use the subxiphoid approach.

It is not necessary to premedicate the patient before the biopsy. A light breakfast may be permitted to allow for gallbladder emptying, although many insist on an overnight fast to prevent aspiration if the patient vomits. Regardless of the needle technique used, the biopsy site is best selected by the placing of the patient in a supine position with the right hand under the head and the right side close to and parallel to the edge of the bed. The biopsy site is determined by percussing caudad over the right hemithorax between the anterior and the midaxillary lines until an intercostal space is reached where dullness is maximal at the end of expiration; the point of biopsy is selected one interspace below. If the liver is enlarged below the right costal margin, and particularly if there is evidence of a localized mass, a subcostal approach may be desirable. If there is uncertainty about the size of the liver and whether or not the biopsy site is accurately selected, ultrasound guidance should be employed. Some livers, often cirrhotic ones, are located posteriorly and superiorly and are more likely to be missed with a blind percutaneous approach to needle biopsy.[30] Prebiopsy screening with ultrasound will locate and allow one to avoid a gallbladder, which if lying laterally may be in the path of the originally planned biopsy tract. The detection of a previously unrecognized hemangioma will also alter the biopsy plans.

The skin is cleansed with an antiseptic agent such as povidone–iodine, and the biopsy site is draped with sterile towels. Approximately 5 ml of a local anesthetic agent, 1% lidocaine hydrochloride preferred, is infiltrated into the site of the biopsy, first subcutaneously, then into the intercostal area, and finally down to the peritoneum and liver capsule. Adequate local anesthesia is important in preventing severe reactions secondary to capsular pain. The skin is punctured with a stylet or nicked with the point of a No. 11 scalpel. The biopsy needle of choice is inserted through the skin incision.

SUCTION TECHNIQUE

Stressing the fact that the greatest risk of needle biopsy of the liver occurs while the needle is in the liver substance, Menghini[211–213] introduced a technique in which the needle remains in the liver only about one tenth of a second, instead of the usual 5 to 10 seconds with the original Vim–Silverman needle. He accomplishes this with the aid of suction and a specially designed needle that does not require rotation to cut loose the tissue specimen.

Since it is generally accepted that the risk of hemorrhage increases with increase in the diameter of the needle, the walls of the needle are ultrathin 90 μm to allow for a relatively wider specimen. The cannula is 6 cm long. The tip is oblique and slightly convex toward the outside. A needle with a penetration limiter is recommended for pediatric use.[213] Menghini has abandoned the wide (2-mm) gauge and employs 1.4-, 1.2-, and 1.0-mm needles only; he recommends the 1.2-mm needle for routine clinical practice and the 1-mm bore for beginners. The needle

without stylet is provided with a short stopping point in the shape of a nail with a blunted end 3 cm long. This prevents the tissue specimen from being sucked up into the syringe end and thus fragmented.

The Menghini technique as employed in the University of Miami Medical Center uses a disposable Jamshidi suction-type needle technique.[116] The biopsy needle is inserted about 4 mm into the intercostal muscle. When the internal fascia of the intercostal muscles has been perforated by the needle, a distinct popping sensation can be felt by the operator. Care should be taken at this point to avoid pushing the needle into the peritoneal cavity and causing a rent in the liver as the patient breathes. Saline (1 ml–2 ml) is infused to clear the needle of skin, subcutaneous tissue, and skeletal muscle. Steady suction is applied by pulling back the plunger of the syringe two to three notches and locking it into position. The patient is then asked to exhale and hold his breath in expiration. Then, with a quick to-and-fro movement, the needle is inserted into the liver and rapidly withdrawn. The biopsy specimen can be squirted out of the needle directly into the 10% formalin solution or into an appropriate receptacle. If a biopsy specimen is not obtained, one should check for leakage of air from the syringe during aspiration and make sure that the needle is tightly attached before repeating the biopsy. If it is apparent that the biopsy site is below the liver after confirming liver dullness with repeat percussion over the liver before and after inspiration, the biopsy can be repeated while the patient holds his breath in inspiration. This will displace the liver downward within the passage tract of the biopsy needle, but the biopsy tract must be below the lung.

Immediately following the biopsy, a bandage is placed over the puncture site, and the patient is placed in a right lateral decubitus posture, which is maintained for approximately 3 hours. The patient is monitored carefully for evidence of hemorrhage. This is particularly important during the first 12 hours. If vital signs are stable and the patient is experiencing no distress, the diet may be resumed within 2 hours of the biopsy. Bed rest should be maintained for 24 hours. The 1.9-mm needle is generally used, particularly if significant fibrosis of the liver is anticipated. In patients in whom there is a higher risk of bleeding, some prefer needles of a smaller diameter.

The Menghini technique has the virtue of simplicity, and because of the short interval during which the needle remains in the liver, this method allows for a great factor of safety. Furthermore, it lends itself to use in less cooperative patients, particularly children.

NONSUCTION TECHNIQUE

A commonly used disposable variation of the Vim–Silverman needle is a Trucut needle.[346] The biopsy needle is introduced into the skin incision with the outer sheath closed toward the tip and is advanced slowly through the intercostal muscle. After the patient has inhaled and exhaled deeply two or three times, he is instructed to hold his breath at the end of complete expiration. The needle assembly is inserted promptly a distance of approximately 2 cm to 3 cm within the substance of the liver in a slightly downward direction. Then the operator advances the inner trocar, holding the outer cutting sheath steady. Next, the outer cutting sheath is advanced to cut the liver in the biopsy notch, and the whole needle assembly is quickly withdrawn from the patient. The entire sequence should take 1 or 2 seconds within the liver substance. This bores a cylinder of hepatic tissue that is usually 1 mm in diameter and 1 cm to 2 cm in length.

OTHER TECHNIQUES

Laparoscopy is regaining popularity in some centers and is used more often at the University of Miami Medical Center. Although it is a more expensive technique than percutaneous liver biopsy and requires more time and manpower, it is clearly a more accurate means of detecting and diagnosing cirrhosis of the liver.[232,246] Sampling errors in patients with chronic hepatitis, left lobe enlargement, or focal anterior lesions of the liver will be avoided by employing laparoscopy with guided-needle biopsy.

The fine-needle biopsy has been used successfully for the diagnosis of neoplasms of the liver. The technique is enhanced by ultrasonic, angiographic, or CT localization of the biopsy target.[316,376] Few complications have been reported. CT provides the most precise localization of focal hepatic lesions and allows for verification of accurate placement of the biopsy needle within the lesion. Small-bore needles such as a 20-gauge modified Chiba needle either 10 cm or 15 cm long, depending on the depth of the lesion, is the preferred needle at Emory University Medical Center.[26] Once the needle tip is properly positioned in the target, the stylet is removed and constant suction applied with a 10-ml plastic syringe, while an "in and out" rotary excursion penetrating 1 cm to 2 cm into the lesions is performed to obtain a core of tissue. Adequate tissue specimens were obtained in 96% of 51 procedures performed on 50 patients. When tissue cores are not obtained, particularly with smaller gauge needles, smears for cytologic study will often be diagnostic depending on the skill of the histopathologists.

Rösch has described a transvenous method of liver biopsy that requires threading a needle through a catheter that is inserted into the right internal jugular vein and subsequently through the right atrium and into the hepatic vein.[110,269,270] The major drawback of this technique is the relatively small sample size obtained and the necessity for an operator with angiographic skills. This method is not commonly employed but can be used in the presence of ascites or impaired coagulation when percutaneous liver biopsy is contraindicated. Lebrec and co-workers report a large experience with transvenous liver biopsy. This procedure was attempted 1033 times in 932 patients. Tissue was obtained in 1000 of these attempts.[177] A fatal intraperitoneal bleed developed in one patient as a result of perforation of the liver capsule. Bull and associates obtained adequate specimens utilizing transjugular liver biopsy with a modified needle in 97% of 193 patients.[50] Bleeding occurred in two patients from puncture of the liver capsule. Supraventricular tachyarrhythmias developed in five patients, and the authors advise electrocardiographic monitoring when the transjugular technique is used.

A novel approach to liver biopsy reported by Andreoni and co-workers and recommended by these authors for obese patients or patients with coagulation defects is a technique of posterior percutaneous liver biopsy.[8] A Tru-cut needle is directed with the patient in the prone position. The biopsy site is generally over the upper edge of the 11th rib, about 8 cm to 9 cm from the spinous processes. In some cases the 12th rib is selected to avoid pneumothorax. A successful liver biopsy was performed in 98.6% of 500 patients, with a complication rate of less than 2%. One death resulted from a retroperitoneal hematoma.

Liver biopsy should not be attempted unless adequate facilities for blood transfusion are available. Some physicians type and crossmatch the blood of all patients before the biopsy, but this has not been our practice. Liver biopsy can be performed as an outpatient procedure if facilities are available for observation and hospital support.[170,238,352] Once discharged the patient must be accompanied home and should be within close proximity to the hospital. In one large series of patients who underwent liver biopsy, 18% of all complications and 26% of serious complications occurred more than 10 hours after the biopsy.[245] A recommendation from this study is not to perform liver biopsies on an outpatient basis in patients with cirrhosis or tumors, since these categories were the only ones associated with fatal complications, all of which were hemoperitoneum.

About one in ten patients requires medication for pain following the procedure, but it is most unusual for an analgesic to be required after 24 hours. The patient is permitted to leave the hospital after 24 to 48 hours.

Failure to obtain adequate tissue for proper interpretation may be a problem in unpracticed hands. However, with experience, failures of this type should be minimized. We do not hesitate in making an immediate second effort to procure a suitable specimen if the original yield appears to be grossly unsuitable. A biopsy core should be 2 cm in length and contain at least five portal areas; however, in practice, many specimens are smaller and yet still allow a diagnosis to be made. When searching for granuloma, as in cases of fever of unknown origin, redirection of the needle and obtainment of three consecutive specimens will increase the yield.[200]

Resistance to the biopsy needle is increased in any fibrotic process, especially cirrhosis, and in amyloidosis. The specimen in cirrhosis is more apt to crumble when the Menghini needle is used in place of the Vim–Silverman instrument.

The gross appearance of the liver specimen may prove of diagnostic value, as originally stressed by Terry.[320] The specimen must be examined without delay and before fixation in order for opacification to be avoided. The normal liver has a mild chocolate hue. The specimen is paler and uniformly icteric in viral and toxic hepatitis and when jaundice complicates cirrhosis. It is greenish and speckled in extrahepatic obstructive jaundice and may be so in cholestatic hepatitis. The gross speckling may sometimes be more striking than the microscopic confirmation of cholestasis, presumably because of some leaking of bile into the preserving fluid or variations in the quality of the hematoxylin and eosin (H & E) stain. A deep red color characterizes chronic passive congestion. In fatty liver, the whole core is pale and may float in the fixative; in metastatic carcinoma, the specimen appears white; in hemochromatosis, brown; and in the Dubin–Johnson syndrome, black. In Boeck's sarcoid and in miliary tuberculosis, the tubercles are not apparent on superficial examination, but if the specimen is transilluminated, the rounded granulomas usually are detected, for they are brightly translucent and contrast sharply with the opaque normal tissue.

CONTRAINDICATIONS

The following should be considered contraindications to needle biopsy of the liver.

The Uncooperative Patient was first emphasized by Sherlock. There must be a certain ability and willingness to follow instructions. This is particularly pertinent to the avoidance of breathing at the time the specimen is actually cut during transthoracic biopsy. Stuporous, delirious, psychotic, or comatose patients should be excluded.

Nevertheless, Foulk and associates[99] advocate the performance of transthoracic biopsy during a brief period of apnea (20–30 seconds) induced by the rapid intravenous administration of 4 ml to 6 ml of freshly prepared 2.5% solution of thiopental sodium (Pentothal sodium) in uncooperative psychotic patients. They procured specimens in this manner in 96 cases with only one minor complication—transient pleural pain. Equipment to provide the usual precautionary measures during anesthesia was immediately available, and the patient was observed carefully.

Impaired Coagulation. A blood prothrombin time of 4 seconds or more above the control time, a platelet count of less than 50,000/mm, or the presence of a blood dyscrasia with hemorrhagic tendency constitutes a serious hazard. Terry advised postponing the biopsy if cutaneous bleeding lasts more than 10 minutes.[319] Patients should be forewarned not to take any salicylates for at least one week before the biopsy, since salicylates can adversely affect the bleeding time. Zamcheck and Klausenstock abandoned the performance of biopsy when bleeding from

the preliminary nick of the skin was prolonged unduly.[369] We, too, have adopted this practice, although, on occasion, a second attempt on the following day may be unaccompanied by significant bleeding and thus permit completion of the procedure. If it is critical to obtain a liver biopsy in the presence of a prothrombin time greater than 4 seconds above the control time, fresh frozen plasma may be given to correct the impaired coagulation before and after the biopsy.[105]

Local Infection. Infectious organisms in the lower lobe of the right lung or the pleural cavity may be carried into the liver or the peritoneum. The presence of peritonitis is also a contraindication for similar reasons.

Ascites increases the difficulty of obtaining a satisfactory tissue specimen, particularly in cases of hepatic cirrhosis, and increases the chances of lacerating the surface of the liver. Paracentesis with reduction in the amount of abdominal fluid should be performed before the biopsy is attempted.

High-grade Extrahepatic Obstructive Jaundice is especially hazardous in elderly patients with enlarged palpable gallbladders. Intrahepatic biliary pressure is apt to be high under such circumstances. Nevertheless, with a modern approach to the differential diagnosis of jaundice, first using noninvasive screening methods such as ultrasonography and CT, then cholangiography, either percutaneously with a thin needle or endoscopically with retrograde cannulation of the ampulla, mechanical obstruction of the biliary tree should be readily recognized prior to consideration of liver biopsy. Bile leakage from the puncture wound in the liver or from a penetrated bile duct may result in bile peritonitis, but this is relatively uncommon, even in the presence of mechanical obstruction of the biliary tree.[164,217] Moreover, examination of the biopsy specimen, although establishing the presence of obstruction, rarely indicates its cause.

REACTIONS AND COMPLICATIONS

Pain at the Site of Entry may be referred to the right shoulder at the time of the biopsy procedure and persist thereafter. In our experience, this occurs in about one fourth of the patients and usually is mild and transient. Pain has been reported variously in 5% to 50% of patients.[80,125] The right shoulder pain probably is due to the presence of a small amount of blood on the undersurface of the diaphragm. Pain in the right hypochondrium may indicate a subcapsular accumulation of blood or bile.[150]

Epigastric Discomfort or Pain may be experienced during the time the needle is in the liver substance or for a period afterward and sometimes is described as a feeling of having one's "wind knocked out." A friction rub occasionally develops in the region of the biopsy site. While usually of short duration, the rub may last for several weeks.

Hemorrhage. Hemorrhage into the peritoneum, although uncommon, is a chief fatal complication of liver biopsy. Most cases of fatal hemorrhage have resulted from perforation of distended portal or hepatic veins or aberrant arteries.[370] In some cases, a tear in the liver occurs when the patient breathes deeply while the needles lies in the liver. Hemorrhage usually is manifest within 24 hours after performance of the biopsy. Fortunately, it ordinarily ceases spontaneously and should be controlled by blood transfusions.

Through the peritoneoscope, postbiopsy bleeding has been observed to consist of a thin trickle from the puncture wound in the liver. It lasts only 10 to 20 seconds and totals 5 ml to 10 ml. In two patients who died of unrelated causes 13 and 24 hours after biopsy, Roholm, Krarup, and Iversen[264] noted in each a small punctate wound in the liver and a tablespoonful of blood in the peritoneal cavity. After longer intervals in other cases, there was no stigma of the needle puncture, and no blood was visible in the abdominal cavity. In a patient with hepatic metastases from a carcinoma of the gallbladder, these observers found a "palm-sized" coagulum over the upper surface of the liver at necropsy performed 24 hours after the biopsy.

Terry[319] found serious significant hemorrhage recorded in 16 (0.2%) of 7532 reported biopsy cases that he reviewed. Laparotomy was required in four patients, transfusion alone in three, and expectant treatment sufficed in nine. Over a 4-year period at Rancho Los Amigos Hospital in Los Angeles, Redeker encountered significant postbiopsy bleeding in about 0.1% of patients. Lindner reported 67 instances of hemorrhage among 80,000 biopsies done with the Menghini technique (four requiring surgery), with 22 deaths.[190] Massive hemobilia has been reported within 1 to 10 days following percutaneous liver biopsy.[91,178,185,264,274] Characteristically, there is pain in the epigastrium or the right upper quadrant followed first by hematemesis, melena, or both, and later by jaundice. Endoscopic retrograde cholangiography and arteriography are most helpful in diagnosis. Selective angiography of the hepatic artery will help establish the diagnosis.[121] Embolism or balloon occlusion of the involved segmental artery at the time of catheterization may effectively stop the bleeding.[214,237] When the bleeding is severe, surgery may be necessary. Clinically apparent intrahepatic hematoma is a rare but serious complication of needle biopsy.[63] Fatal intrahepatic hemorrhage has occurred.[355] A liver scintiscan is helpful in the diagnosis of this complication.[155] Prospective screening with liver scans before and after the biopsy reveals otherwise unrecognized hematomas.[258] A rare manifestation of postbiopsy hematoma is the development of obstructive jaundice secondary to extrinsic mechanical blockage at the level of the bifurcation of the common hepatic duct.[57] Riley and co-workers have designed a method of plugging the needle tract with absorbable gelatin sponge to reduce the risk of bleeding from the biopsy site. Two methods are described, both of which are employed with the Trucut needle. The gelatin sponge material is injected into the biopsy tract after withdrawal of the needle.[262]

Bile Peritonitis is a complication most likely to occur in the presence of obstructive jaundice. It probably reflects the accompanying biliary tract infection. Lindner noted 12 fatalities from peritonitis among 80,000 biopsies performed with the Menghini technique.[190] Hoffbauer[126] stressed the importance of early recognition in order that prompt surgical decompression of the bile duct system may be initiated if necessary.[126] If peritonitis does occur following a liver biopsy, although bile leakage or a perforated viscus may be the cause, other unrelated processes should also be considered. A case of generalized peritonitis occurring 2 days after liver biopsy proved to be secondary to a perforated duodenal ulcer.[281] Asymptomatic bile leakage evolving into bilious ascites has been reported to develop following liver biopsy in a patient with mechanical obstruction of the biliary tree.[13] When the gallbladder is penetrated, bile quickly appears in the syringe if an aspiration technique is used. Within minutes, the patient develops abdominal pain and often hypotension. If underlying mechanical obstruction of the biliary tree is not present, the episode of pain and hypotension is usually self-limited and does not result in a bacterial peritonitis. Therefore, the initial approach should be a conservative one with supportive therapy and careful monitoring.

Hemorrhage into the Pleural Cavity or Pleural Effusion has been reported to result from injury to the pleura or penetration of an intercostal vessel. Arterial injury can be avoided by keeping the needle close to the lower border of the intercostal space. Passage of ascitic fluid into the thorax through a needle perforation of the right leaf of the diaphragm with mild respiratory embarrassment has been reported.[370] Bilious pleurisy has also been observed.[85,90]

Pneumothorax has occurred four times in our experience, and, in each instance the symptoms were mild and the pulmonary collapse did not exceed 10%. Pneumothorax occurred in 0.35% of one series of 68,276 liver biopsies.[245]

Severe Apprehension is associated with various nervous and hysterical manifestations and may be observed on rare occasions. When these become evident as the procedure is begun, biopsy should be postponed.

Shock occurs uncommonly after the procedure. Kleckner reported two cases of transient pleural shock lasting 1 to 2 hours after biopsy.[167] Fatal shock, not explainable on the basis of blood loss, has been described in two instances.[370] Roholm, Krarup, and Iversen encountered mild shocklike states three times in the performance of 297 biopsies.[264] These authors considered these to be similar to episodes exhibited by nervous and apprehensive patients following venipuncture. Kleckner[167] reported "pleural shock" in eight cases among a total of 145 consecutive liver biopsy procedures, some of which were carried out transabdominally. More recently, the term "neurogenic hepatic hypotension" has been coined for a form of acute transient hypotension, characterized by bradycardia that develops rapidly following biopsy and then disappears rapidly without residual complications.[310] The reaction is common in apprehensive patients. Atropine is usually not necessary because of the short duration of the episode. Anaphylactic shock occurred after a liver biopsy was performed in a patient with echinococcal disease.[318]

Bacteremia and Sepsis. Transient bacteremia has been noted in 6% to 13.5% of patients subjected to biopsy.[183,206] However, frank septic shock occurs infrequently, and, in such instances underlying cholangitis or malignancy should be suspected.[193] Liver abscess has been suspected as a late complication of liver biopsy in one case.[168]

Procaine Reactions have been reported by others[225] but have not been encountered in our own experience.

Fatal Pulmonary Bile Embolism has been reported following aspiration needle biopsy in a patient with carcinoma of the papilla of Vater.[47] This need not necessarily be considered a complication of needling, since we have observed two instances in which it occurred spontaneously in patients with high-grade biliary obstruction and infection.

Penetration of Abdominal Viscera. Theoretically, penetration of abdominal viscera is less likely to occur following transthoracic biopsy than with utilization of the anterior route. In Lindner's collected data, the kidney (77 cases) and gallbladder (27 cases) were the most often punctured; in addition, the biliary tract, colon, pancreas, adrenal, lung, and small bowel were occasionally penetrated.[190] Nephrectomy for renal hemorrhage has been reported by Blain.[31] On rare occasions, a neoplasm of the right kidney may push aside the right lobe of the liver, and the needle biopsy may be misinterpreted. Hoffbauer noted a case of perforation of the colon with fatal peritonitis following needling by the subcostal approach.[125]

Arteriovenous Fistula and Arterial Aneurysm have been reported and can be diagnosed by angiography.[231,275,345] These fistulas are primarily arterioportal and have been reported to occur in 5.4% of patients subjected to biopsy. Spontaneous disappearance of the fistula has been observed, and it is unusual for hemodynamically significant consequences to develop. Although portal hypertension may rarely develop, an unusual case of an iatrogenic omental arteriovenous fistula presented as rectal bleeding 3 years after the liver biopsy. Hemorrhagic complications are more likely to result from iatrogenic pseudoaneurysms

of the hepatic artery than from small arterioportal fistulas and may be controlled by selective arterial embolization.[283]

Fractured Needles. An unusual complication is that of a fractured Menghini needle resulting in the lodging of the distal fragment in the liver substance.[256]

Mortality. In a survey of the literature comprising over 10,000 needle biopsies, Terry listed a mortality rate of 0.12% and an incidence of major complications of 0.32%.[320] In a review of 20,016 needle biopsies of the liver, in which the large majority were carried out presumably with the Vim–Silverman needle, Zamcheck and Klausenstock reported a mortality rate of 0.17%.[369] Thaler reported a mortality rate of 0.017% among 20,382 percutaneous needle biopsies in which the Menghini needle was used.[323,324] Lindner reported a mortality rate of 0.015% among 123,000 percutaneous needle biopsies on the basis of a questionnaire to which 637 replies were obtained.[190] At the University of Cincinnati Medical Center, between 1944 and 1970, there was one death from bile peritonitis among 2500 biopsy procedures (0.04%), most of which were performed with the Vim–Silverman needle. Levy had no deaths in a total of 5066 biopsy specimens obtained with the Vim–Silverman needle from 1961 through 1971.[312] A multicenter retrospective study of 68,276 liver biopsies performed by Italian investigators yielded a mortality rate of .009% and an overall complication rate of 2.2%. Death, serious hemorrhagic complications, pneumothorax, and bile peritonitis were more frequent after biopsy with the Trucut needle than with the Menghini needle.[245] It appears likely that the true mortality rate following percutaneous needle biopsy of the liver is not known but is higher than the figures indicate. The evidence suggests that the risk is less with the use of the Menghini needle.

METHODOLOGY FOR PREPARATION OF SPECIMEN

Fixation and Sectioning

The ideal fixative for routine processing for light microscopy is 10% neutral formalin, whereas the best fixative for electron microscopy is glutaraldehyde. Special fixatives are needed in certain metabolic diseases in which the "stored" material is water soluble. Thus, hepatic material from patients with mucopolysaccharidoses should be fixed in Lindsay's dioxane picrate solution,[192] while material from patients with cystinosis is best fixed in alcohol. After routine processing several sections should be cut at 4 μm to 6 μm and stained with H & E. Serial sections are rarely necessary, but focal lesions such as granulomas can be searched for in such sections if the clinical findings strongly suggest their presence. Parasitic eggs or larvae may elude detection until multiple serial sections are studied.

While most pathologists continue to evaluate sections

of paraffin-embedded material, there has been increasing use of "thick" sections (actually thin sections 1 μm–2 μm in thickness) made from biopsy material embedded in water-soluble resins.[56,371] These provide excellent cytologic detail and can be used for special stains and for immunohistopathology.

Special Stains

Stains are very helpful in studying medical diseases of the liver. For the methodology of the majority of the stains cited, the reader is referred to *Manual of Histologic Staining Methods of the Armed Forces Institute of Pathology.*[197] A preparation stained for iron (*e.g.,* Mallory's stain for iron) is useful not only for demonstrating iron but also for bringing out the green color of bile and the golden brown color of lipofuscin, both of which can be masked by overstaining with either eosin or hematoxylin. A reticulin stain (*e.g.,* Wilder's or Manuel's stain) is useful for outlining areas of focal or zonal necrosis (Fig. 13-1), thick liver cell plates (Fig. 13-2), nodules of regeneration, septa linking portal areas to one another or to central veins, or septa partly or completely investing cirrhotic pseudolobules. The Masson trichrome is very useful for demonstrating the location and extent of fibrosis and in assessing changes involving veins or arteries, for example, the lesions of veno-occlusive disease and hepatic vein thrombosis. The Movat pentachrome stain is particularly useful for vascular lesions, since it stains elastica and acid mucopolysaccharide, in addition to collagen and smooth muscle. Elastic tissue can also be demonstrated clearly by orcein, Victoria blue, or aldehyde fuchsin, and these stains are essential for identification of the hepatitis B surface antigen (HBsAg) in liver cells.[290] These stains also identify

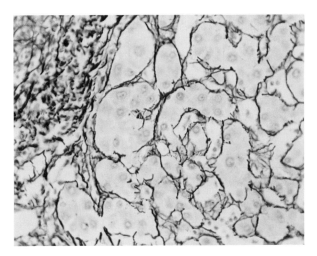

Fig. 13-2. Thick liver plates in a cirrhotic pseudolobule are outlined by reticulin fibers. (Manuel's reticulum stain; original magnification × 300)

so-called copper-binding protein,[151,297] but copper is best demonstrated specifically by the rubeanic or rhodanine stains.[132,191]

A periodic acid–Schiff (PAS) stain demonstrates glycogen; a much more useful stain that should be routinely employed is the PAS stain after pretreatment with diastase (DPAS). The DPAS stain strikingly demonstrates the presence of lipofuscin (and cell debris) and Kupffer cells and portal macrophages in acute hepatocellular injury. Dubin–Johnson pigment in liver cells stains variably with DPAS. In both type IV glycogenosis and Lafora's disease (myoclonus epilepsy), liver cells contain PAS-positive material that resists diastase digestion but can be digested by pectinase.[227] This appearance is also mimicked by cyanamide-induced hepatotoxicity. The globules of α_1-antitrypsin are strongly PAS positive and diastase resistant; they are of variable size (1 μm–40 μm) and, in the precirrhotic liver, are located largely in periportal hepatocytes (Fig. 13-3). The PAS stain is also useful for staining the basement membrane of interacinar bile ducts. Basement membrane changes include destruction in primary biliary cirrhosis (PBC) or thickening in primary sclerosing cholangitis (PSC). Other uses for the PAS stain include the demonstration of fibrin (*e.g.,* in eclamptic lesions in the liver or disseminated intravascular coagulopathy), amyloid, starch, amebae, and pathogenic fungi, although the latter are more readily identified by the Gomori methenamine silver stain.

Other stains that find occasional use in the study of hepatic biopsy material include the Rinehardt–Abulhaj colloidal iron stain, with and without pretreatment with hyaluronidase for acid mucopolysaccharide[192]; the Hall stain for bile; the Fontana stain for lipofuscin and the Dubin–Johnson pigment; the chromotrope aniline blue stain for Mallory bodies[268]; the phosphotungstic acid he-

Fig. 13-1. Collapse of reticulin fibers in acinar zone 3 helps to map the distribution and extent of antecedent ischemic necrosis. (Manuel's reticulum stain; original magnification × 60)

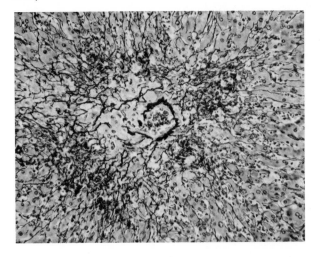

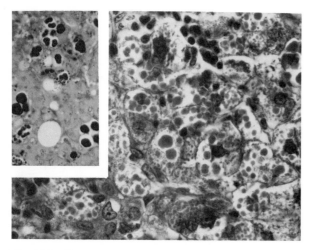

Fig. 13-3. Homozygous α_1-antitrypsin deficiency. Liver cells contain numerous eosinophilic globules of varied sizes. (H & E; original magnification × 630) Globules (*inset*) are intensely DPAS-positive. (Original magnification × 630)

matoxylin stain for fibrin or mitochondria; the Congo red, Sirius red, or crystal violet stains for amyloid; an acid-fast stain for tubercle bacilli, schistosome eggs, or the hooklets in the scoleces of echinococcal cysts; a Warthin–Starry or Levaditi stain for spirochetes or leptospira; a Giemsa stain for toxoplasma or leishmania; and a Brown–Hopps stain for bacteria. An acid-phosphatase stain is useful for Gaucher cells and cells of hairy cell leukemia.

Frozen sections are rarely used for rapid histologic diagnosis except when open-wedge biopsy specimens are available. Frozen sections of formalin-fixed biopsy material stained with oil red-O are useful for demonstration of neutral lipid in liver cells (*e.g.,* in Reye's syndrome) or cells of benign or malignant tumors, fat globules of perisinusoidal lipocytes (Ito cells), cholesterol crystals (which are also birefringent when examined under polarized light), and lipofuscin in liver or Kupffer cells. Lipid can be preserved in paraffin sections by postfixation in osmium tetroxide. Cholesterol can be specifically stained in frozen sections by the Schultz modification of the Liebermann–Burchardt reaction, a stain essential for the diagnosis of Wolman's disease or cholesterol ester storage disease. Baker's acid hematin with pyridine extraction is useful in identifying phospholipid in frozen sections, as in Niemann–Pick disease. Metachromatic granules in macrophage cells and bile duct epithelium (in metachromatic leukodystrophy) are best demonstrated in frozen sections with the use of such stains as toluidine blue or cresyl violet.

Immunohistopathology

Immunohistopathology has been used increasingly in the last few years in diagnostic and research pathology. It is of particular help in identifying tumor antigens (Table 13-1) but is also helpful in diagnosis of viral infections (*e.g.,* hepatitis B, delta agent, herpes simplex, cytomegalovirus) and at least one inherited metabolic disease, α_1-antitrypsin deficiency. The information on immunopathology in Table 13-1 is based on various sources.[46,95,102,114,145,160,161,171,209,234,250,317,327] Examples of diagnostic applications in the study of liver diseases are illustrated in Figures 13-4 to 13-8, as well as in several other sections.

Special Microscopy

Polarizing microscopy is useful in identifying talc in portal macrophages or Kupffer cells of abusers of intravenous drugs. It also identifies talc, starch, or suture material remaining on the surface of the liver from previous surgery. Silica particles in the liver are birefringent.[53,249] Both malarial and schistosomal pigments, which are brown to black, are birefringent under polarized light. Cholesterol crystals (*e.g.,* in the liver of patients with Wolman's disease and cholesterol ester storage disease) in frozen sections, whether stained or unstained, are birefringent, as are cystine crystals in cystinosis. Acicular uroporphyrin crystals in liver cells can be visualized by polarizing microscopy of unstained frozen or paraffin sections in porphyria cutanea tarda (PCT).[65] Red birefringent maltese crosses and amorphous material are characteristic of protoporphyrin accumulation in the liver in erythropoietic protoporphyria (EPP).[166] Collagen (type 1 collagen), as opposed to reticulin fibers (type III collagen), has a silvery birefringence under polarized light. A characteristic apple-green birefringence of amyloid is evident when sections stained with Congo red are examined by polarizing microscopy.

Ultraviolet (UV) microscopy is useful in studying the hepatic porphyrias. Unfixed air-dried frozen sections of the liver in PCT and EPP will reveal red autofluorescence when examined by UV microscopy.[65,166] Vitamin A that is stored in perisinusoidal lipocytes has a green autofluorescence in UV light.

A granular golden yellow autofluorescence is characteristic of lipofuscin examined by UV microscopy. UV microscopy has of course been used extensively in identifying various antigens in the liver (such as α_1-antitrypsin, hepatitis B surface and core antigens, [HBsAg and ABcAg] oncofetal proteins and other proteins synthesized by primary benign and malignant tumors), but the method has now been superceded by the immunoperoxidase or Avidin-biotin techniques.

Phase-contrast microscopy is of limited value in studying medical diseases of the liver but is useful in identifying Gaucher cells[42] and has been utilized in demonstrating Thorotrast in Kupffer cells[321] and silicone particles in portal macrophages of hemodialysis patients.[184]

Scanning Electron Microscopy

Scanning electron microscopy (SEM) has supplied considerable information regarding the microanatomy of the

TABLE 13-1. Immunohistochemistry: Hepatic Applications

TISSUE ANTIGEN	APPLICATION
Blood group antigens	Hemangioendothelioma; angiosarcoma
Factor VIII–related antigen	Hemangioma; hemangioendothelioma; angiosarcoma
Lectins	For potential applications see McMillan and co-workers[209]
Myoglobin	Embryonal rhabdomyosarcoma of bile ducts
Desmin	Tumors of muscle origin, *e.g.,* leiomyosarcoma
Vimentin	Tumors of mesenchymal origin, *e.g.,* fibrosarcoma
Actin	Identification of myofibroblasts
S-100	Malignant melanoma, metastatic; neurogenic tumors; granular cell tumors of extrahepatic bile ducts
Common leukocytic antigen	Lymphoma
Lysozyme	Kupffer cells; bile duct cells
Carcinoembryonic antigen	Cholangiocarcinoma; metastatic adenocarcinoma; hepatocellular carcinoma; normal and neoplastic bile canaliculi; bile ductules and ducts
α-fetoprotein	Hepatocellular carcinoma; hepatoblastoma
α_1-Antitrypsin	α_1-Antitrypsin deficiency; benign and malignant hepatocellular tumors; cholangiocarcinoma; tumors with histiocytic differentiation; bile ductules
Prekeratin	Cholangiocarcinoma; metastatic adenocarcinoma; lymphomas
Epithelial membrane antigen	Cholangiocarcinoma; metastatic adenocarcinoma; lymphomas
HBsAg	Hepatitis B carrier state
HBcAg	Hepatitis B carrier state
Delta agent	Delta agent co-infection or superinfection in acute or chronic infections with hepatitis B virus
Hepatitis A	Acute hepatitis A
Herpesvirus hominis	Identification of herpesvirus hominis types 1 and 2

liver,[218] but diagnostic applications have thus far been limited. On the other hand, the combination of SEM with energy-dispersive x-ray analysis has diagnostic applications in the localization and identification of a number of particulate substances,[133] such as Thorotrast,[41,133,321] silicone rubber,[35] and silica.[53,298] Deparaffinized (routinely processed) sections, usually coated with gold, can be used for SEM.[41]

Transmission Electron Microscopy

Ultrastructural studies have provided great insight into the normal structure of the liver and the pathology, pathogenesis, and etiology of many of its diseases. The chief application is in the diagnosis of the inborn errors of metabolism.[141,154,304,314] Use of transmission electron microscopy (TEM) in the diagnosis of neoplasms is likely to diminish in the future in view of the increasing utilization of immunohistochemistry. For further reading on applications of TEM to the study of the normal and diseased liver, several texts and papers are recommended,[141,154,304,314] in addition to Chapter 2.

Fig. 13-4. Same case as is shown in Figure 13-3. Globules are immunoreactive to α_1-antitrypsin antiserum. (Peroxidase-antiperoxidase technique; original magnification × 630)

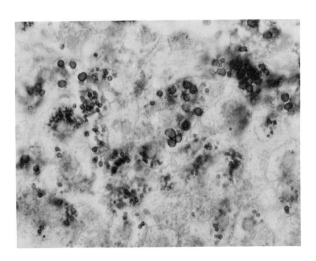

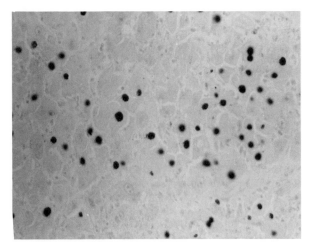

Fig. 13-5. HBcAg is demonstrated in nuclei of liver cells (*black*) by immunoperoxidase technique. (Original magnification × 250)

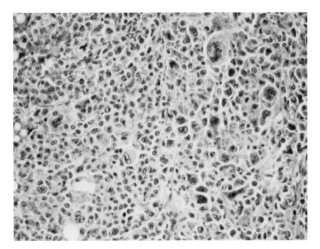

Fig. 13-7. Pleomorphic large cell lymphoma has infiltrated and destroyed hepatic parenchyma. (Original magnification × 250)

Morphometry

Although used in research and in the elucidation of baseline data (*e.g.,* normal and abnormal liver cell nuclei, quantitation of various organelles such as the nuclei, endoplasmic reticulum, glycogen, mitochondria, lysosomes), morphometry has few diagnostic applications, but they are likely to increase in the future.[14,15,62,122,156,259,265,266,338,348]

Aspiration Cytology

Aspiration cytology is especially useful in diagnosis of hepatocellular carcinoma.[44,315]

Flow Cytometry

Flow cytometry is a technique that already has diagnostic applications, particularly in hematopathology.[44,195] It has been applied to the study of experimental hepatocarcinogenesis[81] and recently to the study of mononuclear cells in the liver tissue and blood of patients with PSC.[354]

GENERAL APPROACH TO MORPHOLOGIC INTERPRETATION

Evaluation of diseases affecting the liver, whether intrinsic or secondary, requires a careful and methodical approach;

Fig. 13-8. Same case as is shown in Figure 13-7 reveals strong positive staining of lymphomatous infiltrates (darkly stained areas) for leukocyte common antigen. (Peroxidase-antiperoxidase technique; original magnification × 60)

Fig. 13-6. Factor-VIII-related antigen (darkly stained) in cells of epithelioid hemangioendothelioma. (Peroxidase-antiperoxidase technique; original magnification × 250)

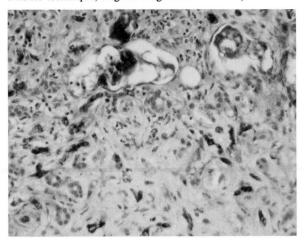

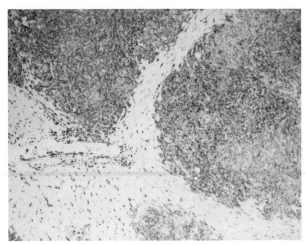

this applies in particular to medical diseases of the liver. At the light microscopic level, sections stained with H & E are evaluated first, followed by study of appropriate special stains. All fragments of a needle-biopsy specimen should be scanned at low-power magnification so that focal lesions, which may be present only in one fragment, are not missed. At low-power magnification, architectural distortion (*e.g.,* fibrosis, cirrhosis, nodular transformation) or various "space-occupying" lesions may be readily identified. If none are visualized, the medium- and high-power magnifications must be used. Inasmuch as many (particularly acute) lesions involve acinar zone 3, it is better to identify terminal hepatic venules (THVs) and then to proceed "centrifugally" to the portal areas. The THVs themselves should first be scrutinized for lesions (*e.g.,* phlebosclerosis, veno-occlusive changes, thrombi), after which the various "systems" should be carefully and methodically evaluated in zone 3, followed by zones 2 and 1. The evaluation should include hepatocytes (*e.g.,* ballooning ± necrosis with dropping-out of cells, acidophilic bodies, coagulative degeneration, Mallory body formation, fatty metamorphosis), bile canaliculi (*e.g.,* presence of deposits of protoporphyrin, bile plugs, dilatation with pseudogland formation), sinusoidal contents and lining cells, Kupffer cells, perisinusoidal lipocytes, and abnormalities in the spaces of Disse (*e.g.,* fibrosis, amyloid deposits).

After evaluation of the various systems within the acinus, the morphologist should turn his attention to the limiting plates and the portal areas. The periportal region should be carefully inspected for hemosiderin accumulation, glycogenated nuclei, storage material (*e.g.,* eosinophilic globules of α_1-antitrypsin, giant round or elongated mitochondria, Lafora bodies) and for evidence of acute necrosis (*e.g.,* hepatitis A, eclampsia, or toxic injury by phosphorous) or chronic "piecemeal" necrosis (*e.g.,* in chronic active hepatitis). Periportal fibrosis may accompany chronic necroinflammatory disease, chronic diseases of the biliary tract (whether extrahepatic or intrahepatic), and a variety of other conditions, and portal areas may be linked together or to THVs, depending on the etiology. Chronic cholestasis (*e.g.,* in PBC, PSC, prolonged extrahepatic biliary obstruction) leads to changes involving periportal liver cells; these include bile pigmentation, pseudoxanthomatous transformation, copper storage, and Mallory body formation. Regeneration is characterized by liver cells of two-cell thickness around portal areas. Cholangiolar proliferation (with or without neutrophilic infiltration and bile plugging) can occur in a variety of circumstances and must be assessed in light of all other changes affecting that particular liver.

Changes in the portal area connective tissue (*e.g.,* edema, focal scars) should be evaluated next, together with the types and distribution of inflammatory cells; the relative frequency of the various cell types should be noted. Lymphomas typically infiltrate portal areas and their contents (*e.g.,* vessels) but often extend beyond them to destroy adjacent parenchyma. Granulomas are frequently located in portal or periportal areas. Hypertrophied portal macrophages should be searched for and their contents identified; such cells may contain pigments (*e.g.,* hemosiderin, malarial or schistosomal pigment, lipofuscin), extraneous particulate matter (*e.g.,* talc, Thorotrast, silicone), mineral oil (with or without formation of lipogranulomas), and metabolites in several of the inherited metabolic diseases.

A variety of lesions may affect interacinar bile ducts; they may be acute (*e.g.,* suppurative cholangitis, dilatation, presence of bile plugs in the lumen) or chronic (*e.g.,* nonsuppurative destructive cholangitis or atrophy with periductal sclerosis). On the other hand, recognizing the *absence* of bile ducts in portal areas (*e.g.,* in arteriohepatic dysplasia in childhood or in PBC in adults) is just as important as evaluating changes in existing bile ducts (Fig. 13-9).

The vessels in portal areas always need careful assessment. Thus, portal vein branches may reveal phlebosclerosis, pylephlebitis, or pylethrombosis (recent or old) or may contain tumor emboli. Hepatic artery branches, on the other hand, may be involved by an arteritis (periarteritis, giant cell arteritis), endothelial hyperplasia (*e.g.,* in cystathioninuria or in women taking oral contraceptives), amyloidosis, or atherosclerotic changes.

After systematic appraisal of all the various systems in sections stained with H & E, the special stains should be evaluated. Minimally, these should include a connective tissue stain (*e.g.,* Masson trichrome), a stain for reticulin fibers, a PAS stain after diastase digestion, a stain for iron, and one of the "Shikata" stains (*e.g.,* orcein). Additional special stains and techniques, including immunohisto-

Fig. 13-9. Primary biliary cirrhosis. Expanded portal area is markedly inflamed and bereft of bile ducts. Junction of portal area with adjacent parenchyma is eroded. (H & E; original magnification × 250) Inset shows copper storage (*black granules*) in periportal liver cells. (Rhodanine; original magnification × 400)

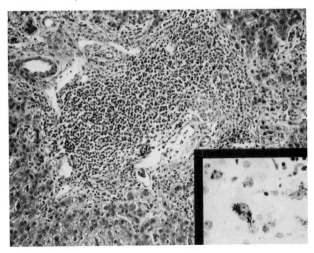

chemical stains and special microscopy, are discussed in the following paragraphs. Needless to say, after all the histopathologic changes are evaluated, the morphologist often must correlate them with the clinical, biochemical, and radiographic findings in order to arrive at the correct diagnosis.

MORPHOLOGIC PATTERNS OF INJURY

Morphologic patterns of injury are discussed under the following headings:

I. Cholestasis
II. Necroinflammatory diseases
III. Granulomatous diseases
IV. Storage diseases
V. Vascular diseases
VI. Fibrosis and cirrhosis

Infiltrative and space-occupying lesions, such as leukemias and lymphomas, primary benign and malignant tumors, metastatic tumors, cysts, and abscesses, are discussed elsewhere in this textbook.

Cholestasis

Bile initially accumulates in hepatocytes, canaliculi, and Kupffer cells in acinar zone 3 regardless of etiology or the site of obstruction. Today hepatic morphologists are rarely called upon to distinguish intrahepatic from extrahepatic obstruction, since radiographic studies (ultrasound, endoscopic retrograde cholangiography, CT, and nuclear magnetic resonance) have largely supplanted the liver biopsy in diagnosis. Matzen and co-workers[202] suggest that liver biopsy is still indicated in patients in whom ultrasonography fails to confirm the presence of large-duct obstruction when it is suspected clinically. Regardless of the indications for liver biopsy in the investigation of the jaundiced patient, the hepatic morphologist must be cognizant of the pathology of obstructive cholestasis, both intrahepatic and extrahepatic, and both acute or chronic. Careful assessment of the lesions accompanying the cholestasis is often crucial in morphologic differential diagnosis.

Acute Cholestasis

Cholestasis Unaccompanied by Other Significant Lesions ("bland cholestasis") is seen in benign recurrent cholestasis, intrahepatic cholestasis of pregnancy, intrahepatic cholestasis of Hodgkin's disease, drug-induced cholestasis (*e.g.*, during use of anabolic and contraceptive steroids) and cholestasis of sepsis, particularly *Escherichia coli* sepsis.[375]

Cholestasis Associated with Spotty Necroinflammatory Lesions, such as unicellular hepatocytic injury (acidophilic bodies, ballooning), focal necrosis, and variable

portal inflammation is typical of adverse reactions to several drugs, including the phenothiazines,[139] erythromycin derivatives,[365] and total parenteral nutrition.[353] The cholestatic form of acute viral hepatitis (usually attributable to epidemic non-A, non-B, [NANB] hepatitis) can incite similar changes. Other diseases include Kawasaki syndrome,[89] leptospirosis,[84] and the hemolytic uremic syndrome.[153]

Cholestasis with Pseudoglands and Marked Fatty Metamorphosis in newborns and young children occurs in galactosemia, tyrosinemia, and, to a lesser extent, in hereditary fructose intolerance.[141] These changes are followed by progressive fibrosis and cirrhosis in galactosemia (if untreated) and tyrosinemia. Typically, the latter disease is also associated with large adenoma-like regenerative nodules.

Cholestasis with Giant Cell Transformation is frequently observed in "neonatal hepatitis." Usually, this is also characterized by scattered acidophilic bodies, extramedullary hematopoiesis, and variable hemosiderosis. Neonatal hepatitis with giant cell transformation has many causes,[216] of which α_1-antitrypsin deficiency is one of the more important.[92,287] Giant cell transformation is also found in about one third of the cases of extrahepatic biliary atresia; cholangiolar proliferation and the presence of bile plugs in interacinar bile ducts help to distinguish these cases from neonatal hepatitis.

Giant cell transformation, usually without appreciable cholestasis, has been reported in children with hemolytic anemia[25] and in adults with chronic (and less often acute) NANB hepatitis[261,322] and autoimmune hepatitis.[325]

Cholestasis with Bile Plugs in Proliferating Cholangioles (ductular cholestasis) is characteristic of sepsis[17,179] (Fig. 13-10). In severe cases the portal areas are encircled by markedly dilated cholangioles, often containing inspissated bile. Neutrophils may surround and infiltrate the cholangioles. Interacinar ducts reveal no changes in this condition.

Cholestasis with Bile Plugs in Interacinar Bile Ducts is highly suggestive of extrahepatic obstruction. It may be accompanied by an acute cholangitis and sometimes by chronic lesions of the bile ducts (*e.g.*, periductal fibrosis) if the patient has had recurrent biliary tract obstruction. The bile plugs may be small and can be readily missed if not carefully sought. Additional findings seen in prolonged obstruction include marked dilatation of ducts with rupture and the formation of bile lakes, and variable periportal cholangiolar proliferation and fibrosis. Rupture of suppurating bile ducts can lead to cholangitic abscesses. Infection may spread to portal vein branches, thus inciting an acute portal pylephlebitis.

Cholestasis with an Acute Cholangitis is characteristic of ascending bacterial cholangitis and need not be accom-

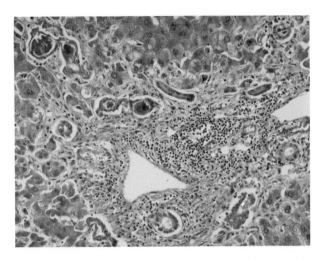

Fig. 13-10. Ductular cholestasis secondary to sepsis. Ductules in left upper corner are markedly dilated and filled with bile. Ductule in right upper corner is surrounded and infiltrated by neutrophils. (H & E; original magnification × 160)

panied by bile plugs in interacinar ducts. Unfortunately, acute cholangitis is not pathognomonic of ascending infection, since it has been observed in toxic shock syndrome[140] (Fig. 13-11), heat stroke[271] drug-induced injury (*e.g.,* chlorpromazine, chlorpropamide, allopurinol),[134] and toxic liver injury, such as that caused by 4,4-diaminophenylmethane, the cause of "Epping jaundice",[172] and Spanish toxic oil syndrome.[302]

Cholestasis with Bile Duct Degeneration and Necrosis, without significant inflammation, has been reported in acute paraquat toxicity[203,220] graft-versus-host disease,[24,292] and septicemia.[344]

Fig. 13-11. Acute cholangitis in toxic shock syndrome. (H & E; original magnification × 450)

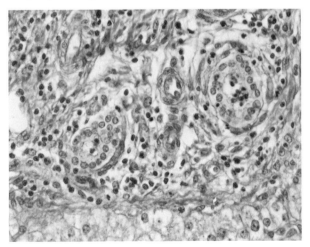

Chronic Cholestasis

Bile that is chronically retained in the lumen of canaliculi, cholangioles, and interacinar bile ducts undergoes inspissation and lamination, presumably as a result of absorption of water. In chronic cholestatic conditions, bile stasis tends to be mainly periportal. The lipid component of bile accumulates in the cytoplasm of liver cells (often around dilated canaliculi) and Kupffer cells, leading to pseudoxanthomatous and xanthomatous transformation, respectively. Affected cells display a foamy bile-tinged cytoplasm and pyknotic nuclei (Fig. 13-12). Accumulation of copper in periportal liver cells (see Fig. 13-9), as well as the formation of Mallory bodies, is characteristic of chronic cholestasis. Bile lakes are late manifestations of extrahepatic biliary obstruction. Other changes seen in chronic cholestasis include variable cholangiolar proliferation, periportal fibrosis with portal to portal linkage, and, eventually, a micronodular biliary cirrhosis.

Many of the diseases leading to chronic cholestasis are associated with loss of bile ducts. In extrahepatic biliary atresia, the destruction of bile ducts can continue despite satisfactory bile drainage following hepatoportoenterostomy.[4,103] Marked reduction of bile ducts is the hallmark of paucity of the intrahepatic bile ducts, which may be syndromatic (arteriohepatic dysplasia; Alagille's syndrome) or nonsyndromatic.[5] Cholangiodestructive lesions have been observed in early childhood in cases of arteriohepatic dysplasia, and the loss of bile ducts is progressive.[72,159] Distinctive ultrastructural changes involving the Golgi apparatus of liver cells have been reported recently.[332]

Reduction in the number of intrahepatic bile ducts has also been reported after intrauterine cytomegalovirus infection[98] and in α_1-antitrypsin deficiency,[117] coprostanic

Fig. 13-12. Cluster of pseudoxanthomatous cells (*center*) in liver biopsy from patient with primary biliary cirrhosis. (H & E; original magnification × 160)

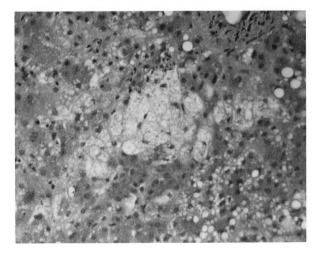

acidemia,[93,119] and several rare developmental syndromes.[142]

Progressive familial cholestatic disorders, not specifically associated with reduction of bile ducts, include some that are well characterized, such as Byler's disease[60,71,78] and the familial cholestasis of North American Indians[350,351] and others that are not.[157,163] These disorders usually culminate in cirrhosis; Byler's syndrome has also been complicated rarely by hepatocellular carcinoma.[71,331] Ultrastructural features of Byler's disease and the cholestasis of North American Indian children have been described by De Vos and co-workers[78] and Weber and co-workers,[350,351] respectively.

The two major chronic cholestatic disorders of adults are PBC and PSC. Both are associated with progressive loss of bile ducts, but the underlying lesions are fundamentally different. The nonsuppurative destructive cholangitis of PBC is characterized by necrosis of epithelial cells, destruction of the basement membrane, and lymphoplasmacytic infiltration of the epithelium of the affected ducts (Fig. 13-13). The distinctive lesion of PSC is progressive periductal fibrosis, with narrowing of the lumen and atrophy of the epithelium (Fig. 13-14). The basement membrane is not destroyed. Eventually, the ducts are transformed into solid fibrous cords (Fig. 13-15). Inflammation is generally more pronounced in the extrahepatic biliary ducts, including the gallbladder and cystic duct, and the pancreatic ducts. Granulomas, periductal and less often intra-acinar, are typical of PBC. The histopathologic markers of chronic cholestasis (see above) and its late sequelae (biliary fibrosis and cirrhosis) are identical in both diseases. Although the two diseases are chronic cholestatic syndromes, the main morphologic differential diagnosis of PBC is chronic active hepatitis, while that of PSC is extrahepatic (chronic and/or recurrent) biliary tract obstruction. Other diseases that, on occasion, require differentiation from PBC include sarcoidosis with protracted jaundice,[272] a syndrome with features overlapping those of PBC and sarcoidosis,[94] and chronic drug-induced or toxic cholestatic injury.[134,372] The most frequently reported association has been with the phenothiazines.[139] Recently reported drugs and toxins leading to chronic cholestasis include haloperidol,[82] oral contraceptives,[187] and Spanish toxic oil.[79] It is also important to emphasize that bile duct lesions resembling or indistin-

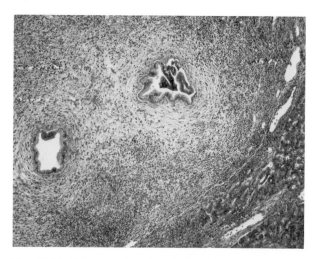

Fig. 13-14. Primary sclerosing cholangitis. Two bile ducts are surrounded by thick cuffs of collagen infiltrated by inflammatory cells. The surrounding portal connective tissue is heavily infiltrated with inflammatory cells. (H & E; original magnification × 60)

Fig. 13-13. Primary biliary cirrhosis. Interacinar bile duct shows extensive (nonsuppurative) necrosis. (H & E; original magnification × 400)

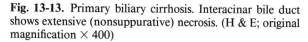

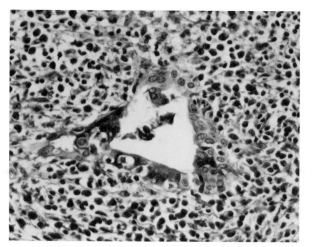

Fig. 13-15. Sclerosed bile duct has no lining epithelium. Instead the lumen is occupied by a tiny capillary. (H & E; original magnification × 160)

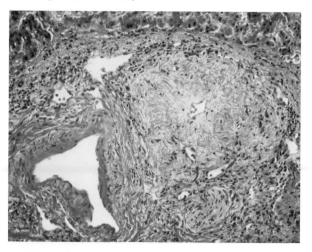

guishable from those of PBC, but not necessarily culminating in chronic cholestasis, have been identified in a number of diseases. They include sarcoidosis,[222] chronic (as well as acute) graft-versus-host disease,[23,97,300,339] acute and chronic rejection of human liver allografts,[97,301,339] Hodgkin's disease,[54] acute and chronic NANB, hepatitis,[130,174,175,282] and even autoimmune "lupoid" hepatitis.[180]

Necroinflammatory Diseases

Many diseases are characterized by degeneration and necrosis of liver cells, usually with an accompanying inflammatory response. Experience is needed in assessing these diseases, since different types of degeneration (*e.g.,* fat accumulation or ballooning, coagulative, acidophilic, or apoptotic degeneration) may have various patterns of distribution (*e.g.,* focal, zonal, panacinar, segmental, or lobar). The inflammatory response can also vary considerably and may be neutrophilic, lymphoplasmacytic, macrophagic, or granulomatous.

Acute Necroinflammatory Diseases

Acute Necroinflammatory Disease with Spotty Necrosis is the typical pattern of injury occurring in acute viral hepatitis B or NANB,[28,106,135,244] but it can also be seen in other viral infections (*e.g.,* rubella, rubeola). Many drug reactions, including those caused by rifampicin, isoniazid, methyldopa, papaverine, dantrolene sodium, disulfiram, and the sulfonamides, can induce a similar pattern of injury. Typically, there is haphazardly distributed degeneration and necrosis involving single or small groups of liver cells; affected cells may show ballooning (Fig. 13-16), acidophilic degeneration, or apoptosis (Figs. 13-17 and 13-18). Lysis of ballooned cells leads to focal necrosis,

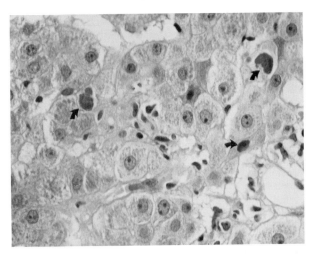

Fig. 13-17. Acute viral hepatitis A. There are several darkly stained acidophilic bodies (*arrow*). The remaining liver cells reveal mild ballooning. (H & E; original magnification × 630)

while the end-stages of acidophilic degeneration or apoptosis are acidophilic (hyaline) or apoptotic bodies located in sinusoids or, less often, in spaces of Disse. Kupffer cells and portal macrophages are usually hypertrophied and contain lipofuscin, hemosiderin, or both, as well as the cell fragments. Inflammatory cells in foci of necrosis and portal areas are usually lymphoplasmacytic, but hypersensitivity-related drug reactions may elicit an outpouring of eosinophils. Granulomas can be found in some acute necroinflammatory injuries with spotty necrosis; these injuries are caused by drugs such as phenylbutazone and, less often, diphenylhydantoin, hydralazine, methyldopa, or halothane.

Fig. 13-16. Acute viral hepatitis. Marked ballooning is associated with cytoplasmic rarefaction and lysis of nuclei and cell membranes. (H & E; original magnification × 630)

Fig. 13-18. Acute viral hepatitis. Globular sinusoidal acidophilic body is dark and has an eccentric nucleus. (H & E; original magnification × 1000)

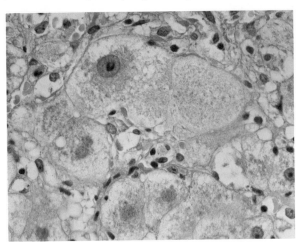

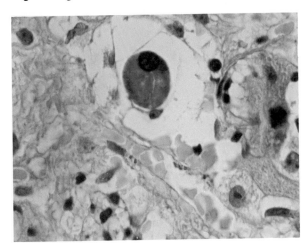

Acute Necroinflammatory Disease with Spotty Necrosis and Sinusoidal Lymphocytosis is characteristic of infectious mononucleosis hepatitis[143] but may also occur in NANB hepatitis,[16] cytomegalovirus mononucleosis[37,299] (Figs. 13-19 and 13-20), and toxoplasmic mononucleosis.[260] A similar response can be induced by several drugs, such as diphenylhydantoin,[219] para-aminosalicylic acid,[372] the sulfonamides,[372] and dapsone.[101] In addition to spotty necrosis (Fig. 19-20), the "mononucleosis hepatitides" are characterized by numerous mitotic figures, many lymphocytes in sinusoids (Fig. 13-19) (as well as in portal areas), and marked hypertrophy and hyperplasia of reticuloendothelial cells, with the formation of "retothelial nodules." True granulomas are rare in infectious mononucleosis but somewhat more frequent in cytomegalovirus mononucleosis.

Acute Necroinflammatory Disease with Focal Neutrophilic Necrosis and Macroabscesses occurs in some bacterial infections such as listeriosis[136] and melioidosis,[247] and in several disseminated mycotic diseases (*e.g.,* cryptococcosis and candidiasis). Focal neutrophilic infiltration is the typical response to ballooned liver cells harboring Mallory bodies when they undergo lysis. Focal necrosis, usually in the vicinity of THVs (Fig. 13-21), is a characteristic finding in surgical biopsy specimens and has been attributed to anoxia.[59]

Acute Necroinflammatory Disease with Focal Coagulative Necrosis is seen in some viral infections, such as coxsackievirus B4 and B9, and several of the hemorrhagic fevers.[144] The necrosis affects single or, more typically, groups of hepatocytes that are not enlarged and have a deeply eosinophilic and finely granular cytoplasm, as well

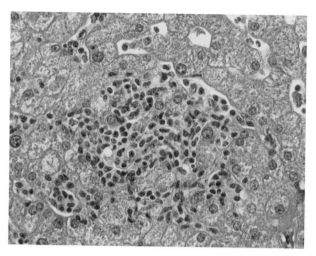

Fig. 13-20. Cytomegalovirus mononucleosis. Same case as is shown in Figure 13-19 reveals focal necrosis with mononuclear infiltration. (H & E; original magnification × 400)

as pyknotic or lysed nuclei. Viral inclusions are generally lacking, and the inflammatory reponse is often scanty.

Acute Necroinflammatory Disease with Large Areas of Patchy and Often Confluent Coagulative Necrosis is characteristic of disseminated herpes simplex hepatitis in neonates or adults.[115,257,296] Nuclear inclusions are usually readily identified and are of two types. In one type the

Fig. 13-21. Perivenular focal necrosis with neutrophilic infiltration is a characteristic finding in wedge biopsy specimens obtained at laparotomy. (H & E; original magnification × 350)

Fig. 13-19. Cytomegalovirus mononucleosis. Sinusoids contain numerous lymphocytes. (H & E; original magnification × 250)

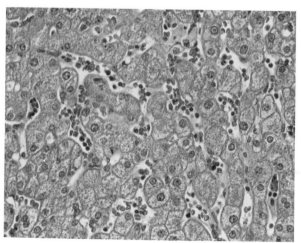

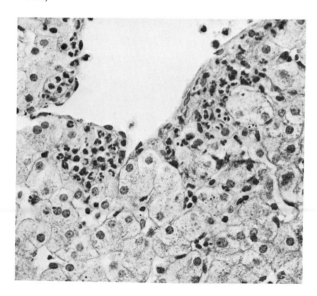

nuclear chromatin and nucleolus are replaced by a basophilic or amphophilic material, which gives the nucleus a "sanded" appearance. The other inclusion (Cowdry type A) is irregular and eosinophilic and is surrounded by a halo with margination of the chromatin (Fig. 13-22). Herpes-type viral particles can be identified in both types of inclusions by electron microscopic examination of biopsy (and even autopsy) material. Viral antigen is also readily demonstrable by immunohistochemical methods (Fig. 13-22).

Acute Necroinflammatory Disease with Submassive Necrosis can result from a number of insults. The necrosis can involve acinar zone 3 (central zone) (Fig. 13-23) with extension to zone 2 or zone 1 (peripheral zone). Linkage of the zones of necrosis is referred to as "bridging necrosis." Necrosis affecting acinar zones 3 and 2 can result from viral hepatitis (types B or NANB), idiosyncratic drug injury (*e.g.,* isoniazid, methyldopa, halothane [Fig. 13-23], penthrane, diphenylhydantoin, dihydralazine, ticrynafen, dantrolene, and many others), drug overdose or exposure to toxins (*e.g.,* acetaminophen, mushroom poisoning, and carbon tetrachloride or copper toxicity), and ischemia (*e.g.,* acute hepatic outflow tract obstruction, hypotensive shock, disseminated intravascular coagulopathy [DIC]). Necrosis of acinar zone 1 occurs in severe viral hepatitis A (Fig. 13-24), phosphorous poisoning, and, rarely, in Reye's syndrome.[48]

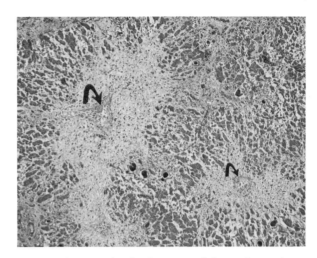

Fig. 13-23. Necrosis of acinar zone 3 (central zones) secondary to halothane injury. Terminal hepatic venules are indicated by arrows. (H & E; original magnification × 60)

It is important to emphasize that the type of degeneration that leads to the submassive necrosis can vary according to etiology. For example, the underlying injury in viral hepatitis and most idiosyncratic drug reactions is ballooning or acidophilic degeneration. Toxic liver injury (including acetaminophen overdose) and ischemic necrosis are characterized by coagulative degeneration. The inflammatory response also varies with the type of degeneration. Thus, the inflammatory cells in ballooning are predominantly mononuclear, while those in coagulative degeneration are neutrophilic. Clues to the etiology of ischemic necrosis in outflow tract obstruction include

Fig. 13-22. Nucleus of liver cell (*center*) contains Cowdry type A inclusion that is stained positively with antiserum to herpes simplex antigen. Other nuclei to the left are also positively stained but contain less viral antigen. (Peroxidase-antiperoxidase technique; original magnification × 630). Inset shows a liver cell with mirror image nuclei containing Cowdry type A inclusions. Note halos around inclusions and margination of the chromatin. (H & E; original magnification × 1000)

Fig. 13-24. Acute hepatitis A necrosis is periportal. Portal area is heavily infiltrated with inflammatory cells. (H & E; original magnification × 250)

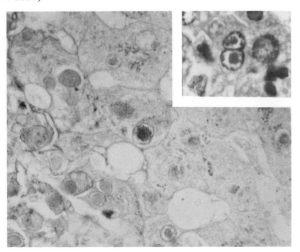

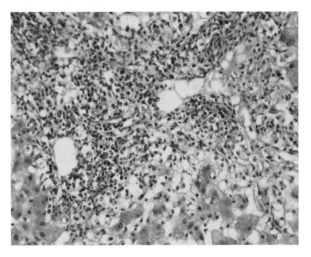

veno-occlusive lesions or thrombi of THVs and severe congestion.

Acute Necroinflammatory Disease with Massive Necrosis can be the result of severe viral hepatitis or toxic and drug-induced injury. Ischemic necrosis is usually submassive, with sparing of zone 1. When necrosis affects all acinar zones, morphologic study alone usually cannot elucidate an etiology except in instances of drug-induced injury based on a hypersensitivity-type mechanism, in which there may be an outpouring of many eosinophils.

A number of viral infections other than viral hepatitis B, NANB, or A can lead to massive necrosis. These include infectious mononucleosis, echovirus infections (type 7, 11, or 12), and adenovirus hepatitis. Only the latter disease has distinctive features, namely, large basophilic inclusions in nuclei of liver cells undergoing coagulative degeneration. It is worth noting at this juncture that yellow fever also leads to massive necrosis, although there is relative sparing of single or groups of liver cells throughout the acinus.[144] Affected cells also exhibit coagulative degeneration and microvesicular steatosis; sinusoidal Councilman bodies are also vacuolated. The inflammatory response is generally mild, and there is little or no cholestasis.

Chronic Necroinflammatory Disease

Traditionally, precirrhotic chronic necroinflammatory disease has been divided into chronic persistent and chronic active hepatitis. The term *chronic lobular hepatitis* has been used for acute viral hepatitis that has a protracted course lasting for months and sometimes years. The outcome is generally favorable, and progression to chronic active hepatitis has not been documented.[251,358]

Chronic Persistent Hepatitis is usually related to viral hepatitis, either type B or NANB. The former can be differentiated from the latter by the presence of ground-glass cells that can be specifically stained with orcein, aldehyde fuchsin, and Victoria blue. Portal areas show variable and often patchy inflammation, with predominance of mononuclear cells. There is little or no fibrous expansion of portal areas and no piecemeal necrosis. Intra-acinar changes include mild focal necrosis, scattered acidophilic or apoptotic bodies, and focal hypertrophy of Kupffer cells.

Chronic Active Hepatitis has a number of etiologies, the more frequent being hepatitis B and NANB. Other well-established causes include drugs such as oxyphenisatin, methyldopa, nitrofurantoin, and isoniazid[198,284,373]; autoimmunity (chronic active "lupoid" hepatitis); and some inherited metabolic diseases, such as α_1-antitrypsin deficiency[124] and Wilson's disease.[280] Cases with no obvious etiology are referred to as "cryptogenic."

The histopathologic hallmark of chronic active hepatitis is "piecemeal necrosis" (Fig. 13-25). It is a composite of several lesions that include apoptosis, ballooning with cytoplasmic dissociation, presence of lymphocytes and

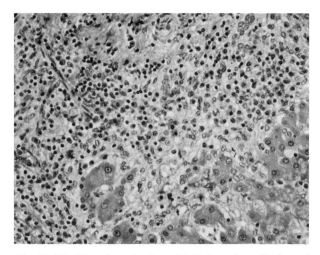

Fig. 13-25. Chronic active hepatitis B. Junction of inflamed portal area and the adjacent parenchyma is eroded and irregular. Detached liver cells are incorporated into the expanded portal area. (H & E; original magnification × 400)

plasma cells in spaces of Disse in close apposition to liver cells, separation of single or small islets of liver cells (that become incorporated into fibrotically expanded portal areas), increased fibrosis (often "stellate"), the deposition of basement membrane material in spaces of Disse, and the formation of "rosettes." Portal areas are moderately to markedly infiltrated with inflammatory cells, particularly plasma cells and lymphocytes (Figs. 13-25 and 13-26). Fibrosis is progressive, with portal-to-portal linkage (Fig. 13-26). Exacerbations in chronic active hepatitis are

Fig. 13-26. Chronic active hepatitis B. Two expanded portal areas, heavily infiltrated with inflammatory cells, are fused by fibrosis. (H & E; original magnification × 160)

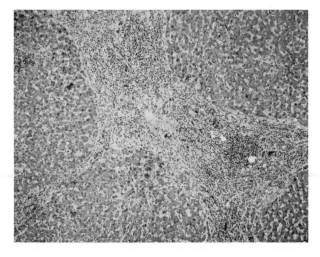

characterized by acute hepatitis-like necroinflammatory changes or by submassive or multiacinar necrosis. Healing leads to septa linking zone 3 with portal areas ("central-to-portal" bridging fibrosis) or to irregular multiacinar scars and, eventually, to the development of cirrhosis. Exacerbations in the chronic active hepatitis of hepatitis B may be spontaneous or secondary to rapid withdrawal of cytotoxic or steroid therapy[127] or to infection with delta agent.[75]

Etiologic clues not necessarily present in every case of a particular disease include the following: (1) The presence of ground-glass cells in chronic active hepatitis type B (Fig. 13-27). HBsAg can be identified in the cytoplasm by orcein, aldehyde fuchsin (Fig. 13-28), or Victoria blue stains, by immunohistopathologic techniques, or ultrastructurally. HBcAg can also be stained immunopathologically (see Fig. 13-5). In cases with delta agent superinfection, delta antigen can be immunostained in tissue sections, but the labeled antibody is not as yet available commercially. (2) Degenerative bile duct lesions, although not specific, are seen in chronic active hepatitis NANB. In some cases of chronic active hepatitis related to NANB, many multinucleated giant cells may be present.[322] (3) Variably sized eosinophilic globules are found in periportal hepatocytes in the chronic active hepatitis of α_1-antitrypsin deficiency, whether homozygous or heterozygous; they are strongly DPAS positive (see Fig. 13-3). The presence of α_1-antitrypsin in the globules should be confirmed by immunohistochemical methods (see Fig. 13-4). (4) Cytochemically demonstrable copper (rubeanic acid or rhodanine stains) is often present in periportal liver cells in the chronic active hepatitis of Wilson's disease. Other changes include variable fatty metamorphosis, glycogenated nuclei, and Mallory bodies in periportal hepatocytes.

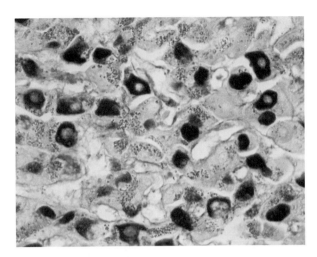

Fig. 13-28. HBsAg in liver cells is stained positively (black), but nuclei are unstained. Granular pigment is hemosiderin (Aldehyde fuschin; original magnification × 575)

Granulomatous Diseases

Granulomas of the liver have been the subject of several recent reviews.[22,137,152] Space does not permit a detailed discussion of this important response to liver injury. In the United States, the most frequent cause of hepatic granulomas is still sarcoidosis. Drug-induced liver injury is probably a more important cause than is generally realized; in a series of granulomas from one center, as many as one quarter of all cases were attributed to a drug etiology.[208] The more important drugs that can lead to hepatic granulomas include phenylbutazone (Fig. 13-29), di-

Fig. 13-27. Ground-glass cells of hepatitis B carrier. Ground-glass change involves varying portions of the cytoplasm of liver cells. Some nuclei are peripherally displaced. (H & E; original magnification × 575)

Fig. 13-29. Noncaseating granuloma in portal area in phenylbutazone-associated liver injury. (H & E; original magnification × 195)

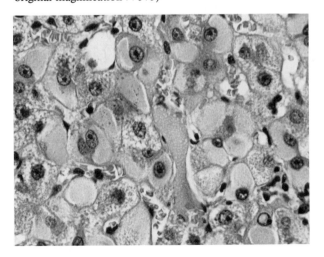

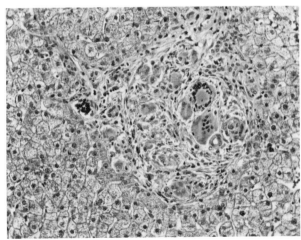

phenylhydantoin, quinidine, hydralazine, allopurinol, the sulfonamides, and the sulfonylurea compounds. Lipogranulomas are also frequently found incidentally in biopsy material; in two autopsy series they were identified in 45% and 48% of livers.[70,347] Infectious causes of granulomas include viral infections (such as infectious mononucleosis and cytomegalovirus hepatitis), rickettsial infections (boutonneuse fever, Q fever), bacterial infections (brucellosis, Whipple's disease), and mycobacterial infections, such as those caused by *Mycobacterium avium intracellulare* infections (particularly in patients with the acquired immune deficiency syndrome) and lepra bacilli. Granulomas occur in both secondary and tertiary syphilis. Systemic mycotic infections that can involve the liver with granulomas include histoplasmosis, blastomycosis, paracoccidioidomycosis, and coccidioidomycosis. Some systemic mycoses that not infrequently affect the liver, such as cryptococcosis, candidiasis, and aspergillosis, generally do not incite the formation of granulomas. Worldwide, parasitic diseases (particularly schistosomiasis) are the most important causes of hepatic granulomatosis. Other helminthic infections that are associated with granulomas include *Toxocara cati* or *canis* (the causes of most cases of visceral larva migrans), *Ascaris lumbricoides, Capillaria hepatica, Paragonimus westermani, Opisthorchis viverrini,* and *Clonorchis sinensis.* Several protozoal infections, including toxoplasmosis, visceral leishmaniasis, and giardiasis, also can lead to formation of granulomas in the liver.

Specific or diagnostic features of granulomas include the following: (1) The presence of gram-positive or gram-negative bacteria (*e.g.,* bacilli of Whipple's disease) or acid-fast bacilli in mycobacterial infections. Acid-fast bacilli are readily identified in untreated lepromatous leprosy and in *Mycobacterium avium intracellulare* infections (Fig. 13-30), rarely in miliary tuberculosis, and very infrequently in bacille Calmette-Guérin (BCG) infections or tuberculoid leprosy. The absence of caseation cannot be relied on for differentiation of hepatic tuberculosis from sarcoidosis or from other diseases with noncaseating granulomas; furthermore, caseation can occur in some systemic mycoses, including coccidioidomycosis (Fig. 13-31). (2) Fungal spores or hyphae in granulomas are best demonstrated by a Gomori methenamine silver stain (Fig. 13-31). (3) Protozoal organisms can be seen in reticuloendothelial cells of the liver in H & E sections, but special stains, such as a Giemsa or a reticulin stain, can be helpful in identification. Various parasitic eggs have characteristic morphologic features, but experience is required in their identification. Crumpled shells or fragments of schistosome eggs may be difficult to recognize in H & E sections but are readily identified in sections stained with an acid-fast stain (*e.g.,* Kinyoun's stain). (4) Rickettsial organisms are hardly ever present in Q fever granulomas, which, however, have a characteristic "doughnut" shape. The typical Q fever granuloma consists of a central vacuole (fat droplet) surrounded by a ring of fibrin and some macrophages and inflammatory cells.[305] The doughnut gran-

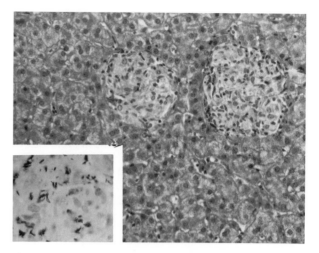

Fig. 13-30. Two noncaseating epithelioid granulomas caused by *Mycobacterium avium intracellulare* in liver of patient with AIDS. (Original magnification × 250) Numerous acid-fast bacilli (*inset*) were in the granulomas (Kinyoun's stain; original magnification × 630)

uloma is highly suggestive but not pathognomonic of Q fever; it has been described in Hodgkin's disease[341] and in allopurinol-related injury.[333] (5) Drug-induced granulomas have no specific features but may be associated with a combined hepatocellular-cholestatic or a pure hepatocellular injury and tissue eosinophilia. This combination of lesions is highly characteristic of hepatic injury related to phenylbutazone[146] but has also been reported with diphenylhydantoin.[225] (6) Lipogranulomas are easily recognized, since they generally consist of lipophages

Fig. 13-31. Coccidiomycosis. Large granuloma show caseation necrosis. (H & E; original magnification × 60) Fungal spores are readily identified by the Gomori methenamine silver stain. (Original magnification × 60)

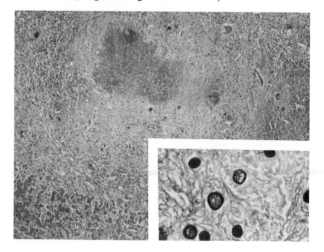

containing fat vacuoles, some inflammatory cells, and a variable quantity of fibrous tissue (Fig. 13-32). They may be located in portal areas or in the vicinity of THVs. (7) Granulomas associated with many eosinophils are typical of parasitic infections, particularly visceral larva migrans and schistosomiasis. As already noted, eggs or their chitinous remnants usually can be seen in schistosomal granulomas, but larvae are very rarely identified in the granulomas of visceral larva migrans. Additional features of hepatic schistosomiasis include the presence of a granular, brown, and birefringent pigment in reticuloendothelial cells, occlusive lesions of portal vein branches, and variable periportal fibrosis. The granulomas of visceral larva migrans are often confluent, have necrotic eosinophilic centers (composed of the granules of degenerated eosinophils), and frequently contain dipyramidal Charcot–Leyden crystals.

Ultimately, the diagnosis of a disease characterized wholly or in part by hepatic granulomas requires correlation of the pathologic features with all available clinical, laboratory, and radiographic findings. The hepatic morphologist must, however, use every available technique at his disposal (special stains, special microscopy, and so forth) to arrive at a morphologic diagnosis, whenever feasible.

Storage Diseases

The term *storage* is used broadly to include a variety of lesions and diseases characterized by the abnormal or excessive accumulation of a metabolite or substance in one of the "systems" of the liver, for example, liver cells, canaliculi, and reticuloendothelial cells.

Hepatocellular Storage

Pigment Accumulation occurs in many diseases and is best discussed on the basis of the type of pigment: (a) *Lipofuscin* pigment is increased in the liver of patients with Gilbert's disease and persons chronically using drugs such as chlorpromazine, phenacetin, and cascara sagrada[138]; (b) *Lipomelanin*, a term used to describe the pigment of the Dubin–Johnson syndrome, is coarsely granular and dark brown; it accumulates in all hepatocytes but tends to be more heavily concentrated in acinar zone 3 (Fig. 13-33). It shares some of the properties of lipofuscin and some of melanin. Thus it stains variably with PAS, is strongly argentaphilic, is sudanophilic in frozen sections, and exhibits yellow autofluorescence when excited by ultraviolet light. Ultrastructurally, the pigment is found in lysosomes; it is thought to have a more variegated appearance and less lipid than lipofuscin.[329]

Hemosiderin accumulates in liver cells in a large number of conditions that include primary hemochromatosis, neonatal hemochromatosis,[32,112] excessive dietary iron intake, and several of the hereditary anemias (*e.g.*, thalassemia major and minor). A slight to moderate quantity of iron storage is a frequent finding in alcoholic liver disease, but massive deposits of the metal are strongly suggestive of the hereditary form of hemochromatosis exacerbated by the consumption of alcohol.[255] Hepatic hemosiderosis has also been reported in patients on long-term hemodialysis who had received parenteral iron preparations.[173] Some pigment accumulates in liver cells in transfusional iron overload, in addition to its marked storage in reticuloendothelial cells.[277]

Hemosiderin is recognized by its coarse granularity and

Fig. 13-32. Three mineral oil granulomas are composed of clusters of lipid vacuoles and a few mononuclear cells. (H & E; original magnification × 250)

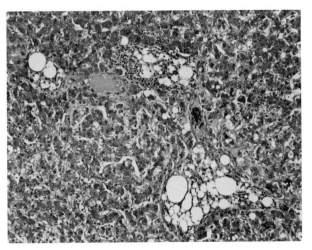

Fig. 13-33. Dubin-Johnson syndrome. Liver cells contain many pigment granules. Note THV in upper left corner. (H & E; original magnification × 300)

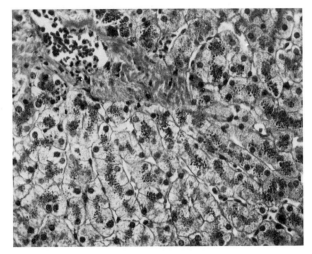

refractility, but special stains for iron should always be performed to confirm its identity. The pigment, regardless of causation, usually accumulates first in periportal hepatocytes and then progressively involves cells in acinar zones 2 and 3. There is usually good correlation between the histologic grading of stainable iron and quantitative determinations of the hepatic iron concentration.[45]

Copper storage occurs typically in Wilson's disease. In the precirrhotic stages the copper accumulates first in periportal liver cells. In the cirrhotic liver the copper is also concentrated in periportal and periseptal liver cells, but it may be stored in all liver cells in some, although not necessarily all, pseudolobules (Fig. 13-34).[309] Copper is not visible by light microscopy, but its presence can be suspected by the presence of "atypical" lipofuscin granules in periportal liver cells, a location where that pigment is ordinarily not present[309]; the copper is stored in the same lysosomes that contain the pigment.

Copper storage is a regular finding in all chronic cholestatic disorders. A cytochemical stain for copper should therefore be routinely performed in all cases of PBC, PSC, and other chronic cholestatic diseases. Copper also accumulates in many other conditions, among the most important of which is Indian childhood cirrhosis. The interested reader is referred to a recent review for further information.[311]

Carbohydrate Storage in liver cells occurs in the glycogenoses. Affected cells are swollen and have a rarefied cytoplasm due to the marked accumulation of glycogen. Subtle light microscopic differences between the various types have been described by McAdams and co-workers.[204] The glycogen is readily stained with the PAS reagent even in routinely processed material and is completely digest-

able by diastase. Type II glycogenosis is characterized ultrastructurally by storage of monoparticulate glycogen in lysosomes. Only type IV glycogenosis has distinctive light microscopic features, which will be described below. Fibrosis can be seen in types III, IV, and VI, and cirrhosis is a frequent complication of type IV.[141]

Protein Storage occurs in α_1-antitrypsin deficiency, fibrinogen storage disease, and within plasma inclusions. The accumulation of eosinophilic globules of variable size in the cytoplasm of liver cells is a well-recognized hallmark of homozygous and heterozygous (*e.g.,* MZ) α_1-*antitrypsin deficiency* (see Fig. 13-3). The globules are DPAS-positive and, in the precirrhotic liver, are periportal in location (see Fig. 13-3). Even in the cirrhotic liver they tend to be periportal and periseptal in distribution. The presence of α_1-antitrypsin in the globules should always be confirmed by immunohistochemical techniques (see Fig. 13-4). The globules may be present in the absence of overt clinical or pathologic evidence of liver disease. On the other hand, α_1-antitrypsin deficiency disease includes neonatal hepatitis, chronic active hepatitis, cirrhosis, and an increased incidence (in males) of hepatocellular carcinoma.[92,287] The main histopathologic differential diagnosis of α_1-antitrypsin globules is megamitochondria. Megamitochondria can be elongated or rounded; rounded ones, most frequently found in alcoholic liver disease, are usually present in acinar zone 3 (Figs. 13-35 and 13-36). All megamitochondria are readily distinguished from α_1-antitrypsin globules by their lack of staining with PAS.

In familial fibrinogen storage disease, liver cells contain polygonal eosinophilic structures that can be immunostained for fibrinogen and are weakly PAS positive.[243]

Plasma inclusions (intracisternal hyaline) impart a homogeneous ground-glass–like appearance to affected liver

Fig. 13-34. Wilson's disease. Marked copper accumulation (black granules) in cirrhotic liver. (Rhodanine; original magnification × 160)

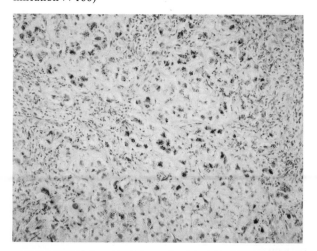

Fig. 13-35. Round megamitochondria are present in cytoplasm (*arrows*) of several liver cells. (H & E; original magnification × 400)

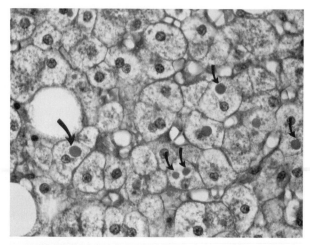

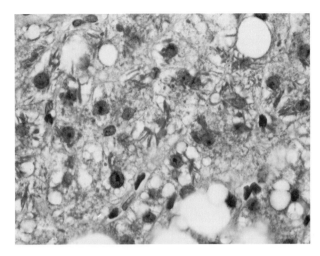

Fig. 13-36. Elongated megamitochondria are evident in the cytoplasm of periportal liver cells of an alcoholic. (H & E; original magnification × 630)

cells.[169] They may be small but can be large enough to occupy most of the cytoplasm and displace the nucleus to the periphery of the hepatocyte (Fig. 13-37). They are PAS negative or weakly PAS positive. A variety of plasma proteins have been identified in the inclusions by immunoperoxidase techniques.[223,307] The etiology and pathogenesis of plasma inclusions remain undetermined. Their chief significance is their possible confusion with the ground-glass cells of HBsAg carriers, from which they can be readily distinguished by their lack of staining with orcein, aldehyde fuchsin, or Victoria blue.

Other diseases and conditions that lead to ground-glass–like inclusions include hepatic injury induced by cyana-

mide (Fig. 13-38),[336] an alcohol-aversion drug (not used in the United States), and two inherited metabolic diseases, type IV glycogenosis and Lafora's disease.[141,227] In all three conditions the inclusions, which are lightly eosinophilic (but can be almost colorless in type IV glycogenosis), are more prominent in acinar zone 1 but can be found in other zones. They are intensely PAS positive, and some or all of the material in the inclusions resists diastase digestion.

There are two other lesions that can superficially resemble ground-glass inclusions. One is the appearance of liver cells in patients who are on long-term drugs (e.g., phenobarbital, phenytoin) or who are exposed to toxins that can lead to enzyme induction. The "induced" liver cells are seen mainly in acinar zone 3, but panacinar involvement also occurs. They are swollen from marked hypertrophy of the smooth endoplasmic reticulum and have a ground-glass or faintly vesiculated cytoplasm; nuclei of the liver cells remain in their central location. The other lesion that can affect liver cells in a variety of conditions is an "oxyphil" or "oncocytic" change that is the result of a marked increase of mitochondria in affected hepatocytes.[181] These cells resemble ground-glass cells only when the H & E sections are lightly stained with eosin. In a well-stained preparation the oncocytic liver cells have a more deeply eosinophilic and more coarsely granular cytoplasm than either ground-glass or normal hepatocytes. The pathogenesis and significance of the change remain to be elucidated.

Neutral Lipid Storage is one of the most common lesions seen in biopsy material. It may be the only change or it

Fig. 13-38. Ground-glass inclusions in liver cells in cyanamide-induced injury. Most are surrounded by empty (probably artifactual) spaces. (H & E; original magnification × 630) Inclusions in inset are strongly DPAS-positive. (Original magnification × 250)

Fig. 13-37. Numerous plasma inclusions in the cytoplasm of liver cells. (H & E; original magnification × 252)

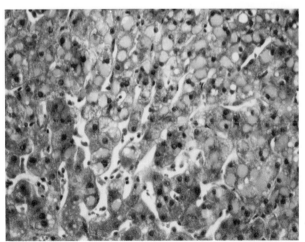

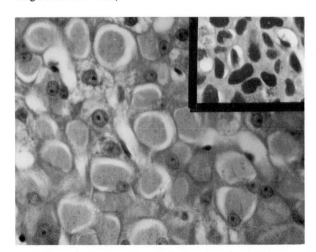

may be found in combination with a variety of other changes that merit separate consideration.

Fatty Metamorphosis as the Predominant Histopathologic Finding occurs in many diseases. Traditionally, two basic types of fat have been distinguished: macrovesicular and microvesicular. In the former the liver cell cytoplasm is replaced by one large or several medium-sized vacuoles, often with peripheral displacement of the nucleus (Fig. 13–40). The change varies in severity, and zonality is generally lacking except in some types of acute toxic injuries in which it can affect acinar zone 3 (carbon tetrachloride, tri-chlorethylene, and tetrachlorethylene) or zone 1 (yellow phosphorous toxicity) and is accompanied by necrosis. Examples of macrovesicular steatosis include alcoholic liver disease, obesity, diabetes mellitus, total lipodystrophy,[120] kwashiorkor, drugs (such as corticosteroids, asparaginase, minocycline),[51] chronic exposure to organic solvents,[86] and a number of inherited metabolic diseases,[141] such as hereditary fructose intolerance, urea-cycle disorders, homocystinuria, abetalipoproteinemia, primary carnitine deficiency (Fig. 13–40), Refsum's disease, and familial hepatosteatosis.

Microvesicular steatosis is characterized by small fat droplets that, in routinely processed material, give the cytoplasm a finely vacuolated appearance (see Fig. 13–39). However, fat globules may be so small that they cannot be resolved by light microscopy, as may occur in acute fatty metamorphosis of pregnancy[267] and Reye's syndrome[357]; in both these conditions it is essential that a piece of the biopsy specimen be saved for fat staining of frozen sections. Microvesicular steatosis is most often panacinar, but a periportal distribution has been reported in toxic shock syndrome.[140]

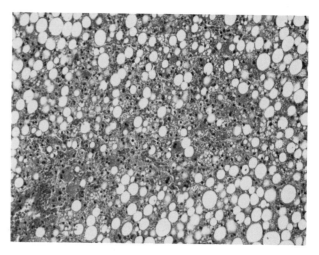

Fig. 13-40. Macrovesicular steatosis in child with primary carnitine deficiency. (H & E; original magnification × 160)

Among the more important causes of microvesicular steatosis are alcoholic foamy degeneration,[330] Reye's syndrome,[39,69] acute fatty metamorphosis of pregnancy[267] (see Fig. 13–39), salicylate toxicity,[39] and valproate-induced injury.[374] In both valporate toxicity[374] and acute fatty metamorphosis of pregnancy,[267] the microvesicular steatosis may be accompanied by necrosis of acinar zone 3. Conversely, in some cases of Reye's syndrome, the necrosis affects acinar zone 1.[20,48]

Fat and Cholesterol Storage is characteristic of Wolman's disease and cholesteroyl ester storage disease.[83,141,215] The fat vacuolization is small to medium sized and panacinar (Fig. 13-41). Cholesterol crystals are present both in liver and Kupffer cells but can be visualized only in frozen sections examined in polarized light, in which they appear as acicular birefringent crystals (Fig. 13-41). The cholesterol can also be specifically stained in frozen sections by the Schultz modification of the Lieberman–Burchardt reaction.

Fatty Metamorphosis with Mallory Bodies and Necroinflammatory Changes occurs most frequently in alcoholic liver disease, but the changes are not pathognomonic, since they can be found in a variety of other conditions. The most important of these conditions is nonalcoholic steatonecrosis (nonalcoholic steatohepatitis, fatty liver hepatitis) found in association with obesity or diabetes mellitus.[279] Others include Weber–Christman disease,[165] post–jejunoileal bypass,[118,201,241] and post–ileal resection.[68,242] Finally, several drugs can lead to a pattern of injury resembling alcoholic liver disease; they include synthetic estrogens[286]; glucocorticoids[147]; perhexilene maleate, a drug used in the treatment of angina (but not in the United States)[233,239,254]; and amiodarone, an antiarrhythmic drug.[253,295]

The pattern of injury in both alcoholic and nonalcoholic steatonecrosis is similar and affects predominantly acinar

Fig. 13-39. Microvesicular steatosis of acute fatty metamorphosis of pregnancy. (H & E; original magnification × 530) Frozen section stained with oil red-O (*inset*) from same liver confirms the marked small droplet (black) accumulation of triglyceride in hepatocytes. (Original magnification × 180)

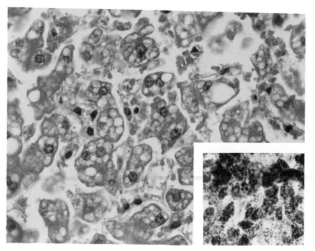

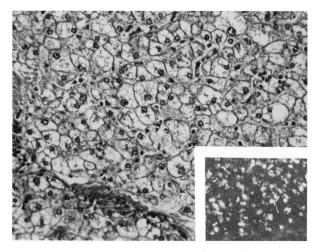

Fig. 13-41. Cholesterol ester storage disease. Liver cells are swollen and have a rarefied and faintly vacuolated cytoplasm. (H & E; original magnification × 250) Frozen section (*inset*) exhibits striking birefringence of cholesterol crystals. (Oil red-O; original magnification × 160)

zone 3. The skeinlike Mallory bodies are eosinophilic and are usually present in ballooned liver cells (Fig. 13-42). The inflammatory response to the degenerating cells harboring Mallory bodies is always neutrophilic (Fig. 13-42). Like alcoholic liver disease, many of the nonalcoholic entities mentioned above can be associated with severe fibrosis and can even progress to cirrhosis. At this juncture it is worth noting briefly some other conditions associated with Mallory body formation. Indian childhood cirrhosis

is one important cause of severe liver injury that is occasionally reported from the United States.[179] It is characterized by numerous Mallory bodies in liver cells of acinar zone 3, as well as other changes, but there is little or no associated fatty metamorphosis. As noted above, Mallory bodies in periportal liver cells are a frequent finding in chronic cholestatic diseases. In Wilson's disease, Mallory bodies are present in periportal–periseptal hepatocytes in the stages of chronic active hepatitis and cirrhosis.

Phospholipid Storage. In Niemann–Pick disease sphingomyelin is stored in both liver and Kupffer cells, giving the cells a foamy appearance. The drug-induced phospholipidoses resemble Niemann–Pick disease both histopathologically and ultrastructurally. Drugs implicated in phospholipidosis include 4,4′-diethylaminoethylhexestrol,[77,148,291] perhexilene maleate,[233,239] and amiodarone.[254,295]

Porphyrin Storage in liver cells occurs in PCT and EPP. In PCT needle-shaped uroporphyrin crystals can be identified by their silvery birefringence in unstained sections examined by polarized light.[65] Other changes in PCT include reticuloendothelial hemosiderosis, fatty metamorphosis, and variable periportal fibrosis. Cirrhosis can develop in one third of patients with PCT, and hepatocellular carcinoma is a recognized complication in elderly patients.[65]

In EPP, protoporphyrin is stored in canaliculi as rounded brown concretions, as a brown granular material in Kupffer cells, and to a lesser extent in liver cells (Fig. 13-43). Protoporphyrin is brilliantly birefringent in po-

Fig. 13-42. Mallory bodies (*arrows*) are present in ballooned hepatocytes. Degenerating liver cell containing a Mallory body (*inset*) is surrounded by neutrophils. (H & E; original magnification × 400)

Fig. 13-43. Erythropoietic protoporphyria. Dark protoporphyrin deposits are present in Kupffer cells and canaliculi. (H & E; original magnification × 250) Polarized section (*inset*) reveals Maltese-cross birefringence of protoporphyrin. (Original magnification × 250)

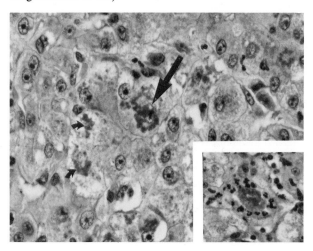

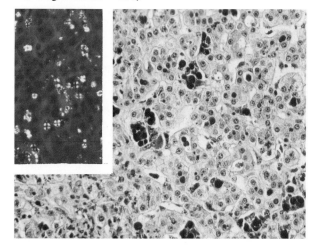

larized light; the canalicular concretions have a Maltese-cross shape and red birefringence, while the Kupffer cell aggregates have a silvery birefringence (Fig. 13-43).[33] Both protoporphyrin and uroporphyrin exhibit red autofluorescence by UV microscopy. Severe liver disease with cirrhosis, culminating in liver failure, has been reported in EPP.[36]

Ductular and Ductal Storage

Cystic fibrosis can be considered a ductular (cholangiolar) storage disease because of the abnormal accumulation of an inspissated secretion in the lumen of the ductules. The material is granular and pink and is PAS positive, but it is not carminophilic. Rupture of ducts containing the abnormal secretions, the nature of which remains to be elucidated, excites an inflammatory response and fibrosis and eventually leads to the characteristic "focal biliary fibrosis."[142]

Storage of iron in the epithelium of ductules and ducts is highly characteristic of primary hemochromatosis. Sulfatide typically accumulates in epithelial cells of intrahepatic and extrahepatic bile ducts and the gallbladder. Additionally, it is stored in hypertrophied macrophage cells in the tunica propria of the gallbladder, where it can lead to the formation of polyps and papillomas.[52,141]

Reticuloendothelial Storage

Pigment Storage. *Lipofuscin* accumulates in reticuloendothelial cells in acute necroinflammatory diseases of diverse etiology. It is released from lysed hepatocytes. After the wave of acute necrosis has subsided, the distribution of the hypertrophied Kupffer cells containing the pigment provides important clues to the pattern of the antecedent injury (*e.g.,* zonal, focal). The lipofuscin is light tan and finely granular and can be overlooked in an H & E section; a DPAS stain is very useful for better visualization and identification.

Lipofuscin pigment accumulation in reticuloendothelial cells is a highly characteristic finding of chronic granulomatous disease.[141] In addition to this feature, patients with the disease may also have hepatic granulomas and abscesses from the many infections that afflict them. Lipofuscin pigment is stored, along with sphingomyelin and ceramide trihexoside, in reticuloendothelial cells in Niemann–Pick disease and Fabry's disease, respectively.[141] A lipofuscin-like pigment accumulates in reticuloendothelial cells of patients given intravenous lipid emulsions[88,236] or infusions of parenteral nutrition not containing lipid.[21,61]

Hemosiderin is stored in reticuloendothelial cells in numerous conditions, particularly in hemolytic disorders such as hemolytic anemias and transfusion reactions.

Copper can accumulate in reticuloendothelial cells in Wilson's disease as a result of release from necrotic hepatocytes, as well as in acute copper toxicity. Histochemically identifiable copper is found in granulomas in the livers (and lungs) of vineyard sprayers occupationally exposed to copper sulfate.[249]

Bile pigment accumulates in reticuloendothelial cells in both acute and chronic cholestasis. In chronic cholestasis the storage of the lipid component of bile transforms the reticuloendothelial cells into xanthomatous and often bile-stained cells.

Other pigments stored in reticuloendothelial cells of the liver of which the hepatic morphologist should be aware include anthracotic pigment (black and not birefringent), schistosomal pigment (brownish black and birefringent), malarial pigment (black and birefringent), and melanin pigment (which can be positively stained with the Fontana stain and the Warthin–Starry stain at *p*H 3.8) in patients with metastatic malignant melanoma.

Crystal Storage occurs in several of the inherited metabolic diseases.[141] Cystine crystals typically accumulate in Kupffer cells (particularly in acinar zone 3) and portal macrophages. They are hexagonal or rectangular and brilliantly birefringent in polarized light. Protoporphyrin is stored in reticuloendothelial cells in EPP and has a reddish or silvery birefringence and red autofluorescence when examined by UV light microscopy. Cholesterol is stored in reticuloendothelial cells in Wolman's disease, cholesterol ester storage disease, and Tangier's disease. The crystals can be visualized in frozen sections because of their birefringence in polarized light and can be stained by the Schultz modification of the Liebermann–Burchardt reaction.

Numerous types of foreign crystals and materials can also accumulate in reticuloendothelial cells of the liver.[133,137] The most important of these is talc, which can be found (often in combination with starch) in adhesions on the surface of the liver from previous surgery, or in the reticuloendothelial cells of the liver of abusers of intravenous drugs. Talc is best visualized by its birefringence in polarized light. It can also be readily visualized by SEM and has a characteristic "flake-pastry" appearance (Fig. 13-44). The elements silica and magnesium in the crystals can be positively identified by energy-dispersive x-ray microanalysis. Other extraneous materials that can accumulate in reticuloendothelial cells of the liver include Thorotrast (Figs. 13-45 and 13-46), barium sulfate, silica (usually in association with anthracotic pigment), silicone, and polyvinyl pyrrolidone which are discussed in detail elsewhere.[133,137]

Storage of Metabolites other than crystals (such as cystine, protoporphyrin, and cholesterol) occurs in numerous inherited metabolic diseases. Examples include the storage of sphingomyelin in Niemann–Pick disease and glucocerebroside in Gaucher's disease, which impart a foamy or striated appearance to the cytoplasm of the affected reticuloendothelial cells, respectively. Other metabolites include glycosphingolipid (Fabry's disease), sulfatide (metachromatic leukodystrophy), and mucopolysaccharide (mucopolysaccharidoses and mucolipidoses).

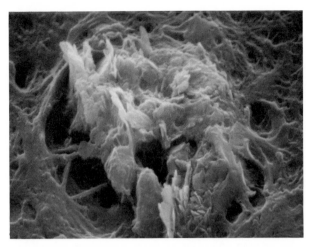

Fig. 13-44. Numerous talc crystals are present in a Kupffer cell. (Scanning electron micrograph; original magnification × 1250)

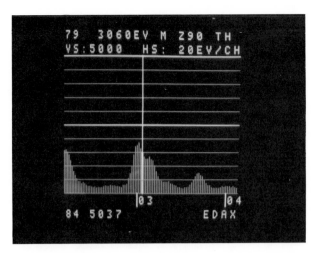

Fig. 13-46. Presence of element thorium in particles in Figure 13-45 is confirmed by energy dispensive x-ray microanalysis.

"Storage" of Infectious Agents in reticuloendothelial cells includes bacteria (*e.g.,* bacilli of Whipple's disease), mycobacteria (particularly in lepromatous leprosy and infections by *Mycobacterium avium intracellulare*), fungi (*e.g.,* in histoplasmosis and cryptococcosis), and protozoal organisms (*e.g.,* in toxoplasmosis or visceral leishmaniasis).[137]

Erythrophagocytosis (a form of "storage" of erythrocytes) occurs in leptospirosis,[84] Rocky mountain spotted fever,[2] extramedullary hematopoiesis, viral hemophagocytic syndrome, familial erythrophagocytic lymphohistiocyto-

sis,[356] and malignant histiocytosis.[87,158] Abnormally shaped erythrocytes (*e.g.,* sickle cells or acanthocytes) also are avidly phagocytosed by reticuloendothelial cells of the liver.

Perisinusoidal Storage

Storage in Spaces of Disse includes an increase in the amount of collagen in a variety of diseases. The collagen accumulation is often accompanied by the deposition of basement membrane material, a combination of lesions referred to as "capillarization'" by Schaffner and Popper.[278] The perisinusoidal fibrosis can affect acinar zone 3 (as occurs typically in alcoholic liver disease), acinar zone 1 (as is characteristic of chronic active hepatitis), or can be panacinar (as is typical of syphilis or type 1 insulin-dependent diabetes).[27]

Amyloid accumulates in spaces of Disse in a linear or "chicken-wire" pattern.[58] A rare type, globular amyloid, is also deposited in spaces of Disse but may be found in sinusoids (usually phagocytosed by Kupffer cells) and in portal connective tissue.[100,162] Both types of amyloid can be stained by Congo red and Sirius red and exhibit apple-green dichroism in polarized light. The fibrillar ultrastructure typical of amyloid is similar in both linear and globular types, but the three-dimensional appearance of globular amyloid on SEM is distinctive (Fig. 13-47).

Nonamyloid light-chain deposits have been identified in spaces of Disse.[189] Like amyloid deposits, these are DPAS positive but do not stain with amyloid stains. Furthermore, kappa light chain immunoglobulin has been identified in the deposits by immunohistochemical staining.[189]

Storage in Perisinusoidal Lipocytes (Ito cells) is characteristic of hypervitaminosis A. The excess vitamin A is

Fig. 13-45. Three-dimensional appearance of Thorotrast particles in a portal area. The particles are of varied size and opaque. (Scanning electron micrograph; original magnification × 5000)

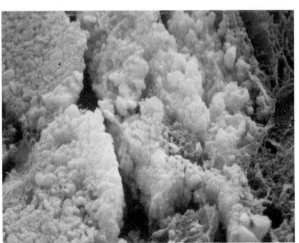

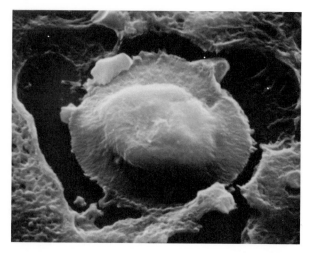

Fig. 13-47. Globular amyloid. "Globule" is not spherical but is hillock-shaped. (Scanning electron micrograph; original magnification × 2500)

stored in the fat globules of the lipocytes. During routine processing, the hypertrophied lipocytes are identified as a cluster of vacuoles jammed between the liver cell and the sinusoid. The lipid can be preserved by postfixation of formalin-fixed tissue by osmium tetroxide, and the lipid droplets in the cells can be stained in frozen sections by oil red-O or Sudan black B. The vitamin A in the fat globules is autofluorescent.

Vascular Diseases

Vessels of the liver may be involved by systemic diseases (*e.g.*, periarteritis nodosa, generalized amyloidosis) or primary diseases (*e.g.*, veno-occlusive disease or hepatic vein thrombosis). Additionally, many intrahepatic vessels may be secondarily involved in intrinsic liver diseases such as alcoholic liver disease, viral hepatitis, and graft-versus-host disease. The effects of vascular injury (particularly occlusion) depend on the site of occlusion, the type of vessel involved, and whether the injury is acute or chronic. In this section the vascular "diseases" encompass the contents of the vessels as well as the lesions actually involving their wall. Benign and malignant vascular tumors are not discussed.

Lesions of the Portal Vein and Branches

Sudden occlusion of the portal vein or its branches can cause true infarction[285] or the so-called infarct of Zahn (areas of sinusoidal dilatation and hepatocytic atrophy). Portal vein phlebitis may be complicated by "septic" infarcts or pylephlebitic abscesses. Cavernomatous transformation of the portal vein, an important cause of portal hypertension in children, is believed to result from thrombosis and recanalization. Subacute or chronic ob-

literative lesions of the intrahepatic portal vein branches can induce generalized atrophy of the liver, which may be followed by compensatory nodular transformation (nodular regenerative hyperplasia). Lobar (or segmental) atrophy is considered to be secondary to occlusion of the portal vein branch (usually the left) supplying the affected lobe.[104] The various diseases and lesions involving the portal vein and its branches are considered in the succeeding paragraphs.

Pylethrombosis can complicate a number of diseases, including myeloproliferative disorders, any type of cirrhosis, shunt surgery for relief of portal hypertension, trauma, or involvement by primary or metastatic neoplasms. According to Witte and co-workers,[363] the inciting factors include endothelial damage and blood hypercoagulability from trauma, infection, stagnant circulation, blood dyscrasia, and malignancy.

Pylephlebitis, with or without secondary thrombosis, is usually the result of intra-abdominal suppuration, such as colonic diverticulitis. In newborn infants it can complicate an acute omphalitis or umbilical vein catheterization. Other causes are discussed by Bolt.[34]

Hepatoportal Sclerosis is an important cause of noncirrhotic (idiopathic) portal hypertension, particularly in India and Japan.[229] Changes affecting the intrahepatic portal vein branches include phlebosclerosis (concentric or eccentric) and recent or old (and recanalized) thrombi (Fig. 13-48). Associated changes, which are variable, include periportal and intra-acinar fibrosis and acinar atrophy.

Fig. 13-48. Hepatoportal sclerosis. Lumen of half of vein in portal area is occluded by intimal fibrosis. Identification of the vessel is facilitated by an elastic stain demonstrating elastic fibers (*arrows*) in wall. (Movat pentachrome; original magnification × 160)

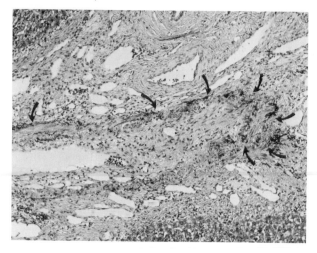

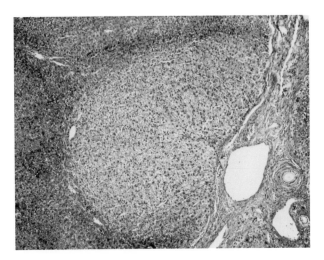

Fig. 13-49. Nodular regenerative hyperplasia. Periportal nodule is paler than the congested parenchyma surrounding it. (H & E; original magnification × 60)

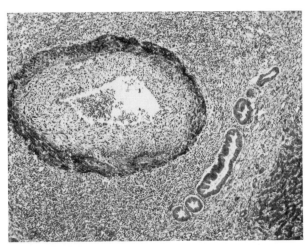

Fig. 13-50. Periarteritis nodosa involving artery (*left*) in portal area. (Masson, original magnification × 60)

The last change is recognized by approximation of portal areas to each other and to THVs. Nodular transformation (nodular regenerative hyperplasia) (Fig. 13-49) is considered to be secondary to atrophy, which in turn is caused by an obliterative venopathy of the intrahepatic portal venous system.[348] Recognition of the ill-defined regenerative nodules is facilitated by a reticulin stain; this demonstrates compression of the reticulin fibers around the periphery of the nodules and the two-cell-thick plates of cells that form the nodules.

Lesions of the Hepatic Artery and Branches

Occlusion of the hepatic artery and its branches may have either no adverse effect or may lead to ischemic necrosis and infarction. Ischemic necrosis affects predominantly acinar zone 3, often with confluence of adjacent zones. Infarcts can vary greatly in size; all affected acini are involved by ischemic necrosis and portal areas, and their contents are also infarcted and "ghostlike."

Thrombosis of the hepatic artery and its branches can complicate trauma, hepatic artery ligation, or perfusion by anticancer agents. Hyaline thrombi of intrahepatic arterioles are characteristic of thrombotic thrombocytopenic purpura.[67]

Arteritis of intrahepatic arteries can occur in polyarteritis nodosa (Fig. 13-50)[66] (which in turn can be related etiologically to hepatitis B infection[111]), the mucocutaneous or Kawasaki syndrome,[3] Rocky Mountain spotted fever,[2] and drug-induced hypersensitivity reactions (*e.g.,* those induced by phenytoin, allopurinol).[134] The liver can be involved by giant cell arteritis.[207]

Intimal Hyperplasia is a well-known complication of the long-term use of oral contraceptives.[131] In the liver the change is seen in portal areas adjacent to hepatocellular adenomas associated with oral contraceptives[138] but has also been observed in association with hemorrhagic necrosis in a woman taking a contraceptive steroid.[366] Intimal hyperplasia has been described in patients with cystathioninuria.[108]

Calcification of intrahepatic arterioles is rare but occurs in idiopathic arterial calcification of infancy and in hypercalcemia (*e.g.,* that secondary to parathyroid adenoma).

Arteriosclerosis is rarely seen in the liver, even when there is severe generalized disease.

Storage of amyloid, cholesterol (in Niemann–Pick disease), ceramide trihexoside (in Fabry's disease), and oxalate (in primary hyperoxaluria) has been noted above.

Lesions of Sinusoids

Sinusoidal Dilatation is typically seen in zone 3 (± extension to zone 2) in congestive heart failure and the Budd–Chiari syndrome. When chronic, it is accompanied by atrophy of liver cell plates and increased (pericellular) fibrosis in spaces of Disse. Severe fibrosis with fibrous linkage of acinar zone 3 leads to the so-called reversed lobulation of congestive cirrhosis.

Dilatation of sinusoids, with predominance in acinar zone 1, has been attributed to the long-term use of oral contraceptives.[303,361]

Patchy or panacinar sinusoidal dilatation has been observed in a number of conditions, including granulomatous diseases and various malignancies.[49]

Sinusoidal Dilatation with Abnormal Luminal Contents is observed in many conditions. Fibrin accumulation occurs in eclampsia and DIC. In the former it is periportal and is usually accompanied by hemorrhagic necrosis. In DIC the location of the fibrin accumulation may be similar to that of eclampsia but can also be haphazard (Fig. 13-51). The fibrin strands are lightly eosinophilic and can be readily overlooked, particularly when there is also severe congestion. They can be stained positively with DPAS and a phosphotungstic acid hematoxylin stain or by the immunoperoxidase technique.

Abnormally shaped erythrocytes can be identified in various diseases. Thus, sickled erythrocytes, often forming globi, can be seen in sinusoids throughout the acinus in sickle cell disease or trait. Acanthocytes and spherocytes can be identified in hepatic sinusoids.[12,133] SEM is useful for studying abnormally shaped erythrocytes (Figs. 13-52 and 13-53).

Sinusoidal neutrophilia and eosinophilia are frequent findings in patients with peripheral leukocytosis (with a shift to the left) and peripheral eosinophilia from multiple causes. The sinusoidal lymphocytosis that occurs in the mononucleosis hepatitides has been noted above. Sinusoidal lymphocytosis has also been reported in Felty's syndrome[326] and in the tropical splenomegaly syndrome.[129]

Other cells abnormally present in hepatic sinusoids can be recognized and identified by the experienced hepatic morphologist. They include hematopoietic cells, normal and abnormal plasma cells in multiple myeloma and Waldenström's macroglobulinemia, mast cells in systemic mastocytosis, and leukemic cells. Cells of hairy cell leukemia typically destroy sinusoidal lining cells and replace them.[224] Other cells include metastatic carcinoma (e.g.,

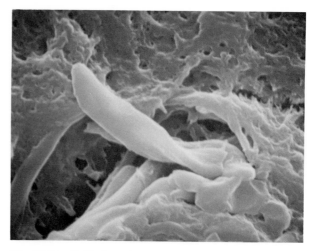

Fig. 13-52. Sickled erythrocytes in hepatic sinusoid are visualized by scanning electron microscopy. (Original magnification × 5000)

malignant melanoma and small cell carcinoma of the lung), and cells of primary malignant vascular tumors of the liver such as angiosarcoma and epithelioid hemangioendothelioma.

Parasites may inhabit or circulate in hepatic sinusoids. They include malarial parasites and babesia in parasitized red cells and parasitic larvae (e.g., Strongyloides stercoralis) in the lumen of sinusoids.

Sinusoidal Dilatation and Peliosis Hepatis. Peliosis hepatis is rarely diagnosed in hepatic biopsy material. It is generally manifested by cavities of varied size that have no endothelial lining (Fig. 13-54). Irregular and often

Fig. 13-51. Extensive deposition of fibrin (black) in sinusoids in periportal necrosis of disseminated intravascular coagulopathy. (Phosphotungstic acid hematoxylin stains; original magnification × 160)

Fig. 13-53. Acanthocytes in hepatic sinusoid. (Scanning electron micrograph; original magnification × 5000)

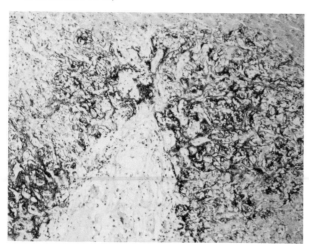

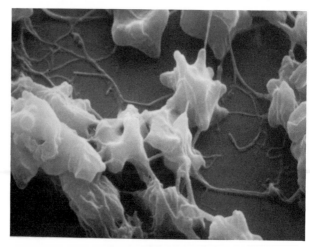

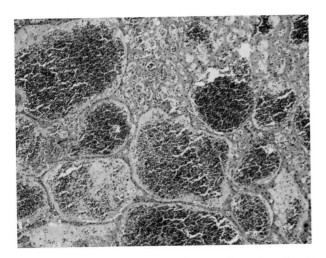

Fig. 13-54. Peliosis hepatis. Hepatic parenchyma is replaced by multiple cavities filled with blood. (H & E; original magnification × 60)

striking sinusoidal dilatation is a frequently associated finding. The majority of cases of peliosis hepatis are secondary to androgenic–anabolic steroid therapy.[221,367] Recently reported causes include tamoxifen,[194] danazol,[226] hypervitaminosis A,[368] and Thorotrast.[113,230]

Lesions of the Hepatic Outflow Tract

Phlebitis. An acute phlebitis ("endophlebitis") is a frequent finding in submassive or massive necrosis of diverse etiology. A "lymphocytic phlebitis" has been described in the precirrhotic and cirrhotic stages of alcoholic liver disease.[113] An "endothelialitis" is considered highly characteristic of graft-versus-host disease.[300] Recently, an endophlebitis of THV, associated with fibrous occlusion of sinusoids and cholestasis, has been attributed to the use of an intravenous vitamin E supplement (E-Ferol) in infants.[40]

Phlebosclerosis is a complication of congestive heart failure, alcoholic liver disease,[113] and graft-versus-host disease.[292,293] The lesion is thought to have prognostic significance in alcoholic liver disease.[364]

Hepatic Vein Thrombosis can induce acute as well as subacute and chronic changes. Often, lesions of various chronologic ages are seen in the same liver. Needle biopsy of the liver is an important adjunct in diagnosis. Acute thrombosis is associated with coagulative degeneration and marked sinusoidal congestion. Subacute and chronic thrombi, often with recanalization, are associated with atrophy of liver cell plates, in addition to the marked sinusoidal dilatation and the fibrosis in acinar zone 3. He-

patic vein thrombosis has many etiologies, which are reviewed by Maddrey.[199] Cases related to the use of oral contraceptives are discussed by Lewis and co-workers.[186]

Veno-occlusive Disease leads to partial or complete occlusion of THVs by intimal thickening (Fig. 13-55). Early lesions are associated with fluid accumulation in the intima and extravasation of erythrocytes. Older lesions are associated with collagenization of the intima. The acute and chronic parenchymal changes are similar to those of hepatic vein thrombosis.

Recognized etiologies are too numerous to mention in their entirety. Worldwide, the most important cause of veno-occlusive disease is ingestion of pyrrolizidine alkaloids, usually in the form of infusions ("bush teas") made from plants containing them.[38] Other well-recognized etiologies include radiation injury to the liver[96]; alcoholic liver injury (Fig. 13-55)[113]; cancer chemotherapy, particularly with dacarbazine[134,372]; hypervitaminosis A[273]; aflatoxin toxicity[313]; and prior administration of Thorotrast.[76]

Prolapse of Liver Cells into THVs is believed to result from hyperplasia and has been reported in patients on long-term anabolic–androgenic steroid therapy.[235] The prolapsed liver cells can be found dissecting the wall of THVs or in the lumen (Fig. 13-56).

Neoplastic Involvement of THVs, intercalated veins, and hepatic veins can be considered primary in malignant vascular tumors of the liver (*e.g.,* angiosarcoma and epithelioid hemangioendothelioma), or secondary in hepatocellular carcinoma or metastatic liver disease.

Fig. 13-55. Veno-occlusive lesion in patient with alcoholic liver disease. Terminal hepatic venule shows marked intimal thickening with narrowing of the lumen. (H & E; original magnification × 100)

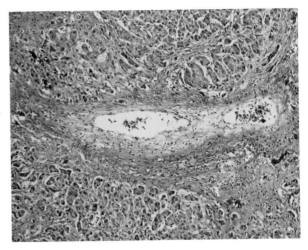

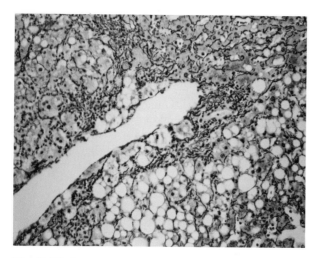

Fig. 13-56. Prolapse of liver cells into wall of THV. (Manuel's reticulum stain; original magnification × 160)

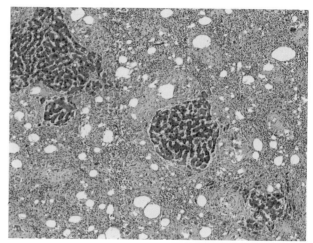

Fig. 13-57. Atrophy of left lobe of liver. Occasional small islets of surviving parenchyma appear to be floating in a sea of fibrosis. (H & E; original magnification × 75)

Fibrosis and Cirrhosis

Fibrosis

The presence or absence of fibrosis and its distribution are vital in histopathologic interpretation of hepatic biopsy material. The patterns of fibrosis are often highly characteristic of the ongoing or antecedent liver injury. Evaluation of hepatic fibrosis is facilitated by the use of connective tissue stains (*e.g.,* Masson trichrome, Van Geison, Movat pentachrome).

Capsular and Subcapsular Fibrosis may be seen in needle-biopsy specimens but is more likely to be observed in open "wedge" biopsy specimens. It may be diffuse (*e.g.,* from healed peritonitis), patchy (*e.g.,* exposure to vinyl chloride or Thorotrast), or localized (*e.g.,* healed traumatic injury, healed granulomas).

Focal Fibrosis within the liver may be very small (less than the size of a hepatic acinus) or multiacinar. Examples of the latter are healed granulomas. Multiacinar fibrosis can result from the healing of abscesses, syphilitic gummas, infarcts, tuberculomas, or conglomerate mycotic granulomas (*e.g.,* histoplasmosis). The healing of multiple gummas with extensive but irregular fibrosis and retraction of the scars can lead to a grossly distorted liver (hepar lobatum).

Segmented or Lobar Atrophy with Fibrosis (Fig. 13-57) may result from occlusion of a portal vein branch supplying that part of the liver.

Diffuse Intra-acinar Fibrosis can occur with or without associated nodule formation.

Diffuse Fibrosis Without Nodule Formation can develop in acinar zone 3 (*e.g.,* alcoholic liver disease, congestive heart failure, hypervitaminosis A) or acinar zone 1. Fibrosis of acinar zone 1 (periportal fibrosis) can be of developmental or metabolic origin, as is typical of congenital hepatic fibrosis (also characterized by proliferation of many small bile ducts) and the focal biliary fibrosis of cystic fibrosis. More frequently it is a complication of chronic necroinflammatory disease of diverse etiology and of chronic cholestatic diseases such as a primary biliary cirrhosis.

Diffuse panacinar fibrosis occurs in congenital syphilis, Zellweger syndrome, and Gaucher's disease.

Diffuse Fibrosis with Nodule Formation is by definition cirrhosis and is discussed in the next section.

It is worth noting at this juncture that fibrosis can involve various "systems" of the liver (*e.g.,* bile ducts, vessels) as discussed above and is an integral part of a number of primary benign (*e.g.,* focal nodular hyperplasia, bile duct adenoma, and sclerosed hemangioma) and malignant (*e.g.,* fibrolamellar carcinoma, cholangiocarcinoma, and epithelioid hemangioendothelioma) neoplasms of the liver.

Cirrhosis

Cirrhosis is diffuse hepatic fibrosis associated with nodule formation. It is classified histologically into micronodular, macronodular, and mixed types.[9] Establishing the diagnosis of cirrhosis in a needle-biopsy specimen may prove difficult. The following features are helpful in supporting a diagnosis of cirrhosis: (1) fragmentation of the biopsy specimen, (2) presence of fibrous septa partly surrounding some of the fragments (Fig. 13-58) or transecting them

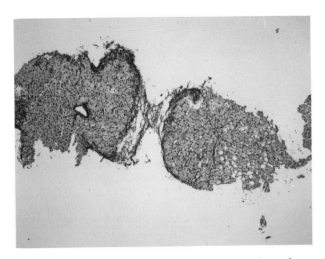

Fig. 13-58. Two fragments of needle biopsy specimen from cirrhotic liver are loosely held together by strands of fibrous tissue. Ends of fragments facing each other are invested by delicate septa. (Manuel's reticulum stain; original magnification × 30)

(Fig. 13-59), (3) absence of central veins or portal areas in some or all fragments, (4) liver cell plates that are two cells thick and (5) absence of lipofuscin pigment (which is present in normal liver cells but not in regenerating nodules).

In addition to classifying the cirrhosis, the hepatic morphologist should indicate the degree of "activity" (mild, moderate, marked) on the basis of the ongoing necroinflammatory changes and attempt to make an etiologic diagnosis. The etiologic diagnosis is based on the presence or absence of various changes in liver and bile duct cells.

A few examples will suffice. Thus, a micronodular cirrhosis associated with minimal activity and massive accumulation of iron in liver and bile duct epithelial cells is strongly suggestive of primary hemochromatosis. A macronodular cirrhosis with cytochemically demonstrable copper, glycogenated nuclei, Mallory bodies in periportal liver cells, and variable fatty metamorphosis should raise the possibility of Wilson's disease. A micronodular or mixed cirrhosis with features of chronic cholestasis as well as a marked reduction in the number of bile ducts should suggest PBC. A macronodular or mixed cirrhosis with numerous acidophilic globules (which are DPAS positive and immunoreactive for α_1-antitrypsin) in the cytoplasm of liver cells is consistent with homozygous or heterozygous α_1-antitrypsin deficiency. The presence of ground-glass cells staining positively for HBsAg (orcein, Victoria blue) in a cirrhosis that is macronodular or mixed supports a relationship of the cirrhosis to chronic hepatitis B infection. Cirrhosis complicating several of the inherited metabolic diseases (*e.g.,* type IV glycogenosis, EPP) may have distinguishing or pathognomonic features (see earlier sections) that are useful in establishing an etiologic diagnosis.

Finally, the hepatic morphologist should be cognizant of a number of conditions that can develop in a cirrhotic liver. These include ischemic necrosis (anoxic pseudolobular necrosis), superimposed acute viral hepatitis, drug-injury or extrahepatic biliary obstruction (in a cirrhosis that is not "biliary"), adenomatous regeneration,[240] and liver cell dysplasia. The last condition consists of a marked increase in the size of cells and nuclei in the cirrhotic pseudolobules (Fig. 13-60). Nuclei have prominent nucleoli and are hyperchromatic. The condition was originally described by Anthony and colleagues,[10] who noted

Fig. 13-59. Needle biopsy from cirrhotic liver is transected by two fibrous septa. (Masson; original magnification × 60)

Fig. 13-60. Liver cell dysplasia. Dysplastic cells (*right*) are larger and have very large and darkly stained nuclei in comparison to more normal liver cells to the left. (H & E; original magnification × 160)

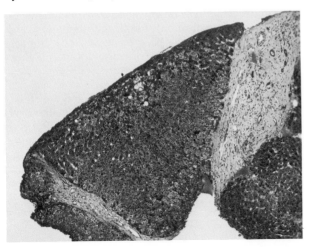

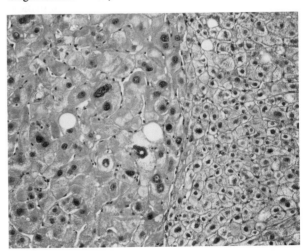

a frequent association with hepatitis B antigenemia and hepatocellular carcinoma; however, its precancerous nature remains a controversial issue.

CLINICAL APPLICATION

The development and refinement of many new techniques that aid in the diagnosis of liver disease, such as liver scans, ultrasound, CT, angiograms, percutaneous transhepatic cholangiography, and endoscopic retrograde cholangiopancreatography, have decreased the necessity for needle biopsies. However, this change has been offset to a degree by an increase in the frequency of some types of liver disease such as chronic viral hepatitis and neoplasms. In general, the knowledge gained from the study of a needle biopsy or repeated biopsies is the greatest value in diagnosis, following the course of chronic disease, and evaluating treatment.

Specifically, biopsies are particularly helpful in the following clinical problems.

Causes of Hepatomegaly. The liver may be enlarged as the result of many different lesions—a number of which may remain obscure without recourse to histologic study. Among these are amyloid disease, genetic metabolic disorders, alcoholic hepatitis, cirrhosis, and neoplasms. In addition, fatty liver, anicteric hepatitis, granulomatous disease, hemochromatosis, aleukemic leukemia, extramedullary hematopoiesis, fungus disease, parasitic disease, congenital hepatic fibrosis, and polycystic disease have been observed. In our experience, the needle-biopsy specimen has pinpointed repeatedly the nature of an ailment, or, equally important, has served to exclude one that was incorrectly believed to be present.

Distinction Between Medical and Surgical Jaundice. The diagnostic means now available, especially ultrasound, have made the performance of needle biopsy unnecessary in most cases of extrahepatic biliary obstruction. Occasionally, all diagnostic procedures are equivocal or negative, and a needle biopsy is done on a patient with incomplete or early extrahepatic biliary tract obstruction. However, there are many patients with medical jaundice who do have biopsies performed either for diagnostic purposes or in order that the course of their disease may be followed. Among the diseases in this category are drug-induced liver disease, neoplasms, PBC, benign recurrent cholestasis, postoperative jaundice, and pericholangitis accompanying inflammatory bowel disease. An ever-increasing number of pharmaceutical agents, including the phenothiazines, steroid compounds, nonsteroidal antiinflammatory products, newer antibiotics, and many other drugs, has led to the sporadic occurrence of jaundice with varying intensity. In spite of the fact that the changes seen on needle biopsy are often distinct from those in extrahepatic biliary tract obstruction, many patients with drug-induced cholestasis have undergone unnecessary surgery.

Patients with neoplasms of the liver, especially those with metastatic carcinoma, may be diagnostic problems when the first symptom is jaundice. The diagnosis of PBC in the early stage may be difficult because bile duct destruction may not be demonstrable. Microscopically, benign recurrent[128,359] and postoperative[308] jaundice differ sharply from obstructive jaundice.

Study of Familial Disease. The use of needle biopsy has given great impetus to the study of diseases of the liver that have a familial basis. These include hemochromatosis, Dubin–Johnson's disease, Gilbert's disease, glycogen storage disease, α_1-antitrypsin deficiency, tyrosinemia, sickle cell anemia, and Wilson's disease. Tissue may be taken not only for microscopic diagnosis but also for enzyme, biochemical, metal, and electron microscopic studies.

Value of Repeated Biopsies. The natural course of many liver diseases has been elucidated by repeated biopsies. These include the relationship of viral hepatitis to cirrhosis, and the courses of alcoholic liver disease and chronic active liver disease. Repeated biopsies are also used in the evaluation of the effectiveness of therapy. Notable among the conditions that may be investigated in this manner are fatty liver, hemochromatosis, tuberculosis, and Wilson's disease.

The Normal Biopsy. In the presence of a normal biopsy, the clinician may exclude hepatic disease in the patient who has apparent hepatomegaly. Normally the liver may extend 1 to 2 fingerbreadths below the costal margin and may be displaced downward in patients with pulmonary emphysema or right pleural effusion or may extend below this level in hyposthenic persons. The problem is even more urgent if the patient appears to have a history of alcoholism or is known to have had a malignant tumor. Furthermore, a patient may have abnormal liver function tests that are misleading, and a normal liver biopsy is clinically important.

Clinical Research. The potential value of transcutaneous biopsy in the investigation of both the normal and the disordered liver has long been recognized.[370] Although needle biopsies are performed primarily for morphologic diagnosis on patients with a wide variety of liver diseases, portions of the biopsy are also used for a wide range of studies related to biochemistry, enzymes, and the effects of therapeutic agents. Among these are biochemical investigations concerning lipids,[29,176] glycogen, and proteins, hepatic enzyme activity,[11,337,349] and the storage of copper and iron. The study of needle-biopsy material has contributed greatly to the rapid progress in the understanding of α_1-antitrypsin deficiency.[1,188,288] LIver biopsies have been used for direct immunofluorescence in the study of humoral immunity[74] and in the search for hepatitis B antigen.[55] A micromethod has been described that determines vitamin A content in the liver in human subjects.[362]

The effect of antibiotic therapy on active tuberculosis also has been evaluated.[263]

Although electron microscopy is widely used in the research laboratory, to date it has not found a place in the routine diagnosis of liver disease.[228] Tissue culture of the human liver has been undertaken and could prove to be an important research tool.[252]

Clinical Value. During a 14-year period (1944–1958) covering 1455 needle specimens obtained from 1324 patients, the biopsy specimens proved to be of significant aid in establishing a diagnosis in 72% to 85% of cases. The specimens confirmed the pre-biopsy clinical diagnosis in 49.8% to 55.7% and altered the clinical impression in 22% to 29.3% (Fig. 13-61).[281] The specimen proved to be noncontributory in 9.4% to 18.4%. In these instances, normal liver tissue or specimens with negligible alterations were obtained. In 3% to 4.4% of cases, the biopsy study failed to establish the correct diagnosis as shown at necropsy or surgical exploration or by subsequent clinical developments. The specimen obtained proved to be inadequate in 1.2% to 6.8% of cases. The needle specimens were particularly valuable in detecting unsuspected fatty degeneration and systemic granulomatous diseases and, in addition, often aided in establishing the presence or absence of cirrhosis and neoplasm of the liver, in distinguishing between hepatitis and obstructive jaundice, and in revealing hepatitis alone in alcoholics suspected of cirrhosis.

Fig. 13-61. Clinical evaluation of liver biopsy, showing analysis of positive aid in diagnosis. (Schiff L, Gall E, Oikawa Y: Proceedings of the World Congress of Gastroenterology. Baltimore, Williams & Wilkins, 1958)

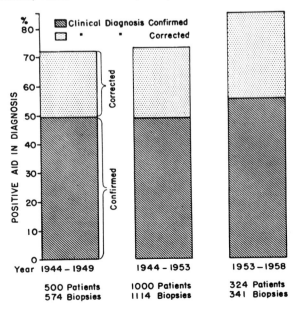

Obviously, the needle-biopsy method is not without limitations. The procedure is relatively safe, but deaths have followed its use.

With selective observance of the contraindications enumerated, serious complications should constitute a negligible risk. We have found that persons experienced in performing needle biopsy are much less prone to encounter difficulty or to provide unsuitable specimens. Therefore, in our own institution, only adequately trained and responsible persons carry out the needle biopsy.

The smallness of the specimen has been claimed by some to limit its value. Others[43] have found the narrow core of tissue to be representative in diffuse liver disorders. The Vim–Silverman type of instrument is preferable in procuring specimens during surgical exploration except in suspected cases of PBC, in which a wedge biopsy is preferred. The ordinary wedge section removed by the surgeon has the disadvantage of reflecting, on the one hand, the nonspecific distortions common to the subcapsular regions and, on the other, acute inflammatory reactions to the immediate surgical manipulations. A better appraisal of the status of the liver can be obtained from a specimen removed from its depths.

For a long time, disorders of the liver have been beclouded by inexact clinical pronouncements, by retrospective speculations derived from study of advanced lesions in a postmortem state, and by overly zealous faith in the results of so-called liver-function tests. The contribution that has been made to the modern dynamic concept of liver disease by the transcutaneous biopsy method is incalculable. One may not gainsay the value of intelligent clinical appraisal and the proper interpretation of accurately performed laboratory tests. Nonetheless, liver biopsy constitutes a keystone in the arch of the understanding of liver disease. Volwiler, Jones, and Mallory aptly remarked:

> The most careful clinical scrutiny of a patient with any chronic hepatitis may not permit one to predict with even moderate accuracy the histologic phase of the liver disease present. Neither do any laboratory tests, even when repeated serially, always correctly reflect the true histologic state of the liver at a given time, or the changes taking place during clinical observation; frequently the only means of determining this is microscopic examination of actual liver tissue.[343]

We are convinced that the procedure should be carried out only in institutions in which physicians are experienced with the technique, are aware of the risk entailed, and will follow the patients closely for at least twenty four[10] hours after the procedure is completed.

An adequate tissue yield and a minimum complication rate can be achieved only by experienced and properly trained physicians, with strict adherence to contraindications and careful observation of the patient after the biopsy is accomplished.

The clinician should always try to decide upon the type of liver disease present before being told of the pathologist's interpretation of the biopsy. The pathologist, in turn, will aid the clinician most by first interpreting the biopsy without any clinical data. By this practice, the diagnostic acumen of both will increase.

REFERENCES

1. Aagenaes O et al: Neonatal cholestasis in alpha-1-antitrypsin deficient children: Clinical, genetic, histological and immunohistochemical findings. Acta Paediatr Scand 61:632, 1972
2. Adams JS, Walker DH: The liver in fatal Rocky Mountain spotted fever. Am J Clin Pathol 75:156, 1981
3. Ahlstrom H et al: Infantile periarteritis nodosa or mucocutaneous lymph node syndrome. Acta Paediatr Scan 66:193, 1977
4. Alagille D: Extrahepatic biliary atresia. Hepatology, 4:75, 1984
5. Alagille D: Management of paucity of interlobular bile ducts. J Hepatol 1:561, 1985
6. Ali M et al: Hemosiderosis in hemodialysis patients: An autopsy study of 50 cases. JAMA 244:343, 1980
7. Alspaugh JP et al: CT directed hepatic biopsies: Increased diagnostic accuracy with low patient risk. J Comput Assist Tomog 7, No. 6:1012, 1983
8. Andreoni B et al: Liver biopsy and percutaneous cholangiography using a posterior approach. Am J Surg 143: No. 3:310, 1982
9. Anthony PP et al: The morphology of cirrhosis. J Clin Pathol 31:395, 1978
10. Anthony PP et al: Liver cell dysplasia: A pre-malignant condition. J Clin Pathol 26:217, 1973
11. Arias IM, London IM: Bilirubin glucuronide formation in vitro: Demonstration of a defect in Gilbert's disease. Science 126:563, 1957
12. Avigan MI et al: Morphologic features of the liver in abetalipoproteinemia. Hepatology 4:1223, 1984
13. Avner DL, Berenson MM: Asymptomatic bilious ascites following percutaneous liver biopsy. Arch Intern Med 139:245, 1979
14. Baak JPA: Basic points in and practical aspects of the application of diagnostic morphometry. Pathol Res Pract 179:193, 1984
15. Baak JPA, Ort J: A Manual of Morphometry in Diagnostic Pathology. Berlin, Springer–Verlag, 1983
16. Bamber M et al: Short incubation non-A, non-B hepatitis, transmitted by Factor VIII concentrates in patients with congenital coagulation disorder. Gut 22:854, 1981
17. Banks JO et al: Liver function in septic shock. J Clin Pathol 35:1249, 1982
18. Baron E: Aspiration for removal of biopsy material from the liver. Arch Intern Med 62:276, 1939
19. Beierwalter WH, Mallery OT Jr.: Liver biopsy: Clinical evaluation of a trephine needle. Univ Hosp Bull, Ann Arbor 12:13, 1946
20. Bentz MS, Cohen C: Periportal hepatic necrosis in Reye's syndrome. Am J Gastroenterol 73:49, 1980
21. Berger HM et al: Pathogenesis of liver damage during parenteral nutrition: Is lipofuscin a clue? Arch Dis Child 60:774, 1985
22. Berk JE, Cohen M: Hepatic granulomas. In Berk JE (ed): Bockus Gastroenterology, vol 5, pp 3189–3202. Philadelphia, WB Saunders, 1985
23. Berman D et al: Ultrastructural lesions of bile ducts in primary biliary cirrhosis: A comparison with the lesions observed in graft-versus-host disease. Hum Pathol 12:782, 1981
24. Berman MD et al: The liver in long-term survivors of marrow transplant-chronic graft-versus-host disease. J Clin Gastroenterol 2:53, 1980
25. Bernard O et al: Severe giant cell hepatitis with autoimmune hemolytic anemia in early childhood. J Pediatr 99:704, 1981
26. Bernardino ME. Percutaneous biopsy. AJR 142:41, 1984
27. Bernuau D et al: Ultrastructural aspects of the perisinusoidal space in diabetic patients with and without microangiopathy. Diabetes 31:1061, 1982
28. Bianchi L: Liver biopsy interpretation in hepatitis: Part II. Histopathology and classification of acute and chronic viral hepatitis/differential diagnosis. Pathol Res Pract 178:180, 1983
29. Billing BH et al: The value of needle biopsy in the chemical estimation of liver lipids in man. J Clin Invest 32:214, 1953
30. Bjork JT et al: Percutaneous liver biopsy in difficult cases simplified by CT or ultrasonic localization. Dig Dis Sci 26, No. 2:146, 1981
31. Blain C: Nephrectomy following liver biopsy. Am J Dig Dis 14:745, 1969
32. Blisard KS, Bartow SA: Neonatal hemochromatosis. Hum Pathol 17:376, 1986
33. Bloomer JR et al: Hepatic disease in erythropoietic protoporphyria. Am J Med 58:869, 1975
34. Bolt RJ: Diseases of the hepatic blood vessels. In Berk JE (ed): Bockus Gastroenterology, 4th ed, Vol. 5, LIver, pp 3259–3277. Philadelphia, WB Saunders, 1985
35. Bommer J et al: Silicone cell inclusions causing multiorgan foreign body reaction in dialyzed patients. Lancet 1:1314, 1981
36. Bonkowsky HL, Schned AR: Fatal liver disease in protoporphyria: Synergism between ethanol excess and the genetic defect. Gastroenterology 90:191, 1986
37. Bonkowsky HL et al: Acute granulomatous hepatitis: Occurence in cytomegalovirus mononucleosis. JAMA 233:1284, 1975
38. Bras G, Brandt KH: Vascular disorders. In MacSween RNM et al (eds): Pathology of the Liver, pp 315–334. Edinburgh, Churchill Livingstone, 1979
39. Bove KE et al: The hepatic lesion in Reye's syndrome. Gastroenterology 69:685, 1975
40. Bove KE et al: Vasculopathic hepatotoxicity associated with E-Ferol syndrome in low-birth-weight infants. JAMA 254:2422, 1985
41. Bowen JH et al: Energy dispersive X-ray detection of thorium dioxide. Arch Pathol Lab Med 104:459, 1980
42. Brady RO, King FM: Gaucher's disease. In Hers HG, Van Hoof F (eds): Lysosomes and storage Diseases, pp 381-393. New York, Academic Press, 1973
43. Braunstein H: Needle biopsy of the liver in cirrhosis: Diagnostic efficiency as determined by postmortem sampling. Arch Pathol 62:87, 1956
44. Braylan RC: Flow cytometry. Arch Pathol Lab Med 107:1, 1983
45. Brissot P et al: Assessment of liver iron content in 271 patients: A re-evaluation of direct and indirect methods. Gastroenterology 80:557, 1981
46. Brooks JJ: Immunohistochemistry of soft tissue tumors. Hum Pathol 13:969, 1982
47. Brown CY, Walsh GC: Fatal bile embolism following liver biopsy. Ann Intern Med 36:1529, 1952

48. Brown RE, Ishak KG: Hepatic zonal degeneration and necrosis in Reye syndrome. Arch Pathol Lab Med 100:123, 1976

49. Bruguera A et al: Incidence and clinical significance of sinusoidal dilatation in liver biopsy. Gastroenterology 75:474, 1978

50. Bull HJM et al: Experience with transjugular liver biopsy. Gut 24:1057, 1983

51. Burette A et al: Acute hepatic injury with minocycline. Arch Intern Med 144:1491, 1984

52. Burgess JH et al: Papillomatosis of the gallbladder associated with metachromatic leukodystrophy. Arch Pathol Lab Med 109:79, 1985

53. Carmichael GP et al: Hepatic silicosis. Am J Clin Pathol 73:720, 1980

54. Cavalli G et al: Changes in the small biliary passages in the hepatic localization of Hodgkin's disease. Virchows Arch Pathol Anat 384:295–306, 1979

55. Cerat G et al: Detection of Australia antigen in liver biopsies by immunofluorescence. Can Med Assoc J 108:981, 1973

56. Chi EY, Smuckler EA: A rapid method for processing liver biopsy specimens for 2 u sectioning. Arch Pathol Lab Med 100:457, 1976

57. Chiprut RO et al: Intrahepatic hematoma resulting in obstructive jaundice. Gastroenterology 74:124, 1978

58. Chopra S et al: Hepatic amyloidosis: A histopathologic analysis of primary (AL) and secondary (AA) forms. Am J Pathol 115:186, 1984

59. Christoffersen P et al: Focal liver cell necroses accompanied by infiltration of granulocytes arising during operation. Acta Hepato-Splenol 17:240, 1970

60. Clayton RJ et al: Byler disease. Am J Dis Child 117:112, 1969

61. Cohen C, Olsen MM: Pediatric total parenteral nutrition, liver histopathology. Arch Pathol Lab Med 105:152, 1981

62. Collan Y: Morphometry in pathology: Another look at diagnostic histopathology. Pathol Res Pract 170:189, 1984

63. Conn HO: Intrahepatic hematoma after liver biopsy. Gastroenterology 67:375, 1974

64. Conn HO: Liver biopsy in extrahepatic biliary obstruction and in other "contraindicated" disorders. Gastroenterology 68:817, 1975

65. Cortes JM et al: The pathology of the liver in porphyria cutanea tarda. Histopathology 4:471, 1980

66. Cowan RE et al: Polyarteritis nodosa of the liver: A report of two cases. Postgrad Med J 53:89, 1977

67. Craig JM, Gitlin D: The nature of the hyaline thrombi in thrombotic thrombocytopenic purpura. Am J Pathol 33:251, 1957

68. Craig RM et al: Severe hepatocellular reaction resembling alcoholic hepatitis after massive small bowel resection and prolonged total parenteral nutrition. Gastroenterology 79:131, 1980

69. Crocker JRS: Reye's syndrome. Sem Liv Dis 2:340, 1982

70. Cruickshank B, Thomas MJ: Mineral oil (follicular) lipidosis: II. Histologic studies of spleen, liver, lymph nodes, and bone marrow. Hum Pathol 15:731, 1984

71. Dahms BB: Hepatoma in familial cholestatic cirrhosis of childhood: Its occurrence in twin brothers. Arch Pathol Lab Med 103:30, 1979

72. Dahms BB et al: Arteriohepatic dysplasia in infancy and childhood: A longitudinal study of six patients. Hepatology 2:350, 1982

73. Davis WD et al: Needle biopsy of the liver. Am J Med Sci 212:449, 1946

74. Dawkins RL: Immunoglobulin deposition in liver of patients with active chronic hepatitis and in antibody against smooth muscle. Br Med J 2:643, 1973

75. De Cock KM et al: Fulminant delta hepatitis in chronic hepatitis B infection. JAMA 252:2746, 1984

76. Dejgaard A et al: Veno-occlusive disease and peliosis of the liver after Thorotrast administration. Virch Arch Pathol Anat 403:87, 1984

77. de la Inglesia FA et al: Morphologic studies of secondary phospholipidosis in human liver. Lab Invest 30:539, 1974

78. De Vos R et al: Progressive intrahepatic cholestasis (Byler's disease): Case report. Gut 16:943, 1975

79. Diaz de Rojas FD et al: Hepatic injury in the toxic oil syndrome. Hepatology 5:166, 1985

80. Dieulafoy G: Kystes hydatiques. Gaz D Hop 45:586, 1872 (quoted by Baron[18]).

81. Digernes V, Iversen OH: Flow cytometry of nuclear DNA content in liver cirrhosis and liver tumours in rats exposed to acetylaminofluorene. Virch Arch 47:139, 1984

82. Dincsoy HP, Saelinger DC: Haloperidol-induced chronic cholestatic liver disease. Gastroenterology 83:694, 1982

83. Dincsoy HP et al: Cholesterol ester storage disease and mesenteric lipodystrophy. Am J Clin Pathol 81:263, 1984

84. Dooley JR, Ishak KG: Leptospirosis. In Binford CH, Conner DH (eds): Pathology of Tropical and Extraordinary Diseases, vol 1, pp 101–106. Washington DC, Armed Forces Institute of Pathology, 1976

85. Dosik MH: Bile pleuritis: Another complication of percutaneous liver biopsy. Am J Dig Dis 20:91, 1975

86. Dossing M et al: Liver damage with occupational exposure to organic solvents in house painters. Eur J Clin Invest 13:151, 1983

87. Ducatman BS et al: Malignant histiocytosis: A clinical histologic and immunohistochemical study of 20 cases. Hum Pathol 15:368, 1984

88. DuToit DF et al: Fat emulsion deposition in mononuclear phagocyte system. Lancet 2:898, 1978

89. Edwards KM et al: Intrahepatic cholangitis associated with mucocutaneous lymph node syndrome. J Pediatr Gastroenterol Nutr 4:140, 1985

90. Ehrke D, Subert R: Gallige Pleuritis als Komplikation einer percutaner Leberbiopsie. Z Gesamte Inn Med 25:907, 1970

91. Elte PM et al: Hemobilia after liver biopsy. Arch Intern Med 140:839, 1980

92. Erikkson SG: Liver disease in alpha-1 antitrypsin deficiency: Aspects of incidence and prognosis. Scand J Gastroenterol 20:907, 1985

93. Eyssen H et al: Trihydroxycoprostanic acid in the duodenal fluid of two children with intrahepatic bile duct anomalies. Biochem Biophys Acta 273:212, 1972

94. Fagan EA et al: Multiorgan granulomas and mitochondrial antibodies. N Engl J Med 308:572, 1983

95. Falini B, Taylor CR: New developments in immunoperoxidase techniques and their application. Arch Pathol Lab Med 107:105, 1983

96. Fajardo LF, Colby TV: Pathogenesis of veno-occlusive liver disease after radiation. Arch Pathol Lab Med 104:584, 588, 1980

97. Fennell RH et al: Cellular damage in liver transplant rejection: Its similarity to that of primary biliary cirrhosis and graft-versus-host disease. Pathol Annu 16:289, 1981

98. Finegold MJ, Carpenter RJ: Obliterative cholangitis due to cytomegalovirus: A possible precursor of paucity of intrahepatic bile ducts. Hum Pathol 13:662, 1982

99. Foulk WT et al: A technic for liver biopsy applicable to

uncooperative psychotic patients. Proc Mayo Clin 34:8, 1959

100. French SW et al: Unusual amyloid bodies in human liver. Am J Clin Pathol 75:400, 1981

101. Gan TE, Van der Weyden MB: Dapsone-induced infectious mononucleosis-like syndrome. Med J Aust 1:350, 1982

102. Gatter KC et al: The differential diagnosis of routinely processed anaplastic tumors using monoclonal antibodies. Am J Clin Pathol 82:33, 1984

103. Gautier M et al: Histological liver evaluation 5 years after surgery for extrahepatic biliary atresia: A study of 20 cases. J Pediatr Surg 19:263, 1984

104. Gautier–Benoit C et al: Atrophie du lobe gauche du foie par thrombose de la branche gauche de la vein porte. Med Chir Dig 2:157, 1973

105. Gazzard BG et al: The use of fresh frozen plasma or a concentrate of Factor IX as replacement therapy before liver biopsy. Gut 16:621, 1975

106. Gerber MA, Thung SN: Viral hepatitis: Pathology. In Berk JE: (ed): Bockus Gastroenterology, 4th ed, Vol 5, The Liver, pp 2825–2855. Philadelphia, WB Saunders, 1985

107. Gerber MA, Thung SN: Hepatic oncocytes: Incidence, staining characteristics, and ultrastructural features. Am J Clin Pathol 75:498, 1981

108. Gibson JB et al: Pathological findings in homocystinuria. J Clin Pathol 17:427, 1964

109. Gillman T, Gillman J: A modified liver aspiration biopsy apparatus and technique, with special reference to its clinical application as assessed by 500 biopsies. S Afr J Med Sci 10:53, 1945

110. Gilmore IT et al: Transjugular liver biopsy. Br Med J 2: 100, 1977

111. Gocke DJ et al: Association between polyarteritis and Australia antigen. Lancet 2:1149, 1970

112. Goldfisher S et al: Idiopathic neonatal iron storage involving the liver, pancreas, heart, and endocrine and exocrine glands. Hepatology 1:58, 1981

113. Goodman ZD Ishak KG: Occlusive venous lesions in alcoholic liver disease: A study of 200 cases. Gastroenterology, 83:786, 1982

114. Goodman ZD et al: Combined hepatocellular cholangiocarcinoma: A histologic and immunohistochemical study. Cancer 55:124, 1985

115. Goodman ZD et al: Herpes simplex in apparently immunocompetent adults. Am J Clin Pathol (in press)

116. Greenwald R et al: Percutaneous aspiration liver biopsy using a large-caliber disposable needle. Dig Dis 22:1109, 1977

117. Hadchouel M, Gautier M: Histopathological study of the liver in the early cholestatic phase of alpha-1 antitrypsin deficiency. J Pediatr 89:211, 1976

118. Haines NW et al: Prognostic indicator of hepatic injury following jejunoileal bypass performed for refractory obesity: A prospective study. Hepatology 1:161, 1981

119. Hanson RF et al: The metabolism of 3X, 7X, 12X trihydroxy-5 cholestan-26-oic acid in two siblings with cholestasis due to intrahepatic bile duct anomalies: An apparent error of cholic acid synthesis. J Clin Invest 56:577, 1975

120. Harbour JR et al: Ultrastructural abnormalities of the liver in total lipodystrophy. Hum Pathol 12:856, 1981

121. Hellekant C: Vascular complications following needle puncture of the liver: Clinical angiography. Acta Radiol Diagn 17:209, 1976

122. Henmi A et al: Karyometric analysis of liver cell dysplasia and hepatocellular carcinoma. Cancer 55:2594, 1985

123. Himsworth HP: Lectures on the Liver and Its Diseases. Cambridge, Harvard University Press, 1950

124. Hodges TR et al: Heterozygous MZ alpha-1 antitrypsin deficiency in adults with chronic active hepatitis and cryptogenic cirrhosis. N Engl J Med 304:557, 1981

125. Hoffbauer FW: Needle biopsy of the liver. JAMA 134:666, 1947

126. Hoffbauer FW: Editorial: Needle biopsy of the liver. Surg Gynecol Obstet 92:113, 1951

127. Hoofnagle JH et al: Reactivation of chronic hepatitis B virus infection by cancer chemotherapy. Ann Intern Med 94:447, 1982

128. Hopwood D et al: Ultrastructural findings in idiopathic recurrent cholestasis. Gut 13:986, 1972

129. Hutt MSR: Idiopathic tropical splenomegaly in Uganda (big spleen disease). In Sommers SC (ed): Hematologic and Lymphoid Pathology Dicennial, 1966–1975, pp 31–44. New York, Appleton-Century-Crofts, 1975

130. Hyodo I et al: Clinical and histological features of sporadic non-A, non-B hepatitis. Acta Med Okayama 38:389, 1984

131. Irey NS, Norris HJ: Intimal vascular lesions associated with female reproductive steroids. Arch Pathol 96:227, 1973

132. Irons RD et al: Cytochemical methods for copper. Arch Pathol Lab Med 101:298, 1977

133. Ishak KG: Applications of scanning electron microscopy to the study of liver disease. In Poerr, H., Schaffner, F. (eds): Progressive Liver Diseases, Vol VIII, pp. 1–32. Orlando, Grune & Stratton, Inc. 1986.

134. Ishak KG: The liver. In Riddell RH (ed): Pathology of Drug-Induced and Toxic Diseases, pp. 457–513. New York, Churchill-Livingstone, 1982

135. Ishak KG: Light microscopic morphology of viral hepatitis. Am J Clin Pathol 65:787, 1976

136. Ishak KG: Listeriosis. In Binford CH, Connor DH (eds): Pathology of Tropical and Extraordinary Diseases, vol 1, pp 178–186. Washington DC, Armed Forces Institute of Pathology, 1976

137. Ishak KG: Liver granulomas. In Ioachim HL (ed): Pathology of Granulomas, pp 307–369. New York, Raven Press, 1983

138. Ishak KG: Hepatic neoplasms associated with contraceptive and anabolic steroids. In Lingeman CH (ed): Carcinogenic Hormones, pp 73–128. Berlin, Springer–Verlag, 1979

139. Ishak KG, Irey NS: Hepatic injury associated with the phenothiazines. A clinicopathologic and follow-up study of 36 cases. Arch Pathol 93:283, 1977

140. Ishak KG, Rogers WA: Cryptogenic acute cholangitis—Association with toxic shock syndrome. Am J Clin Pathol 76:619, 1981

141. Ishak KG, Sharp HL: Metabolic errors and liver disease. In MacSween RNM, Anthony PP, Scheuer PJ (eds): Pathology of the Liver, pp 88–147. Edinburgh, Churchill Livingstone, 1979

142. Ishak KG, Sharp HL: Developmental abnormalities and liver disease in childhood. In MacSween RNM, Anthony PP, Scheuer PJ (eds): Pathology of the Liver, pp 68–87. Edinburgh, Churchill-Livingstone, 1979

143. Ishak KG, Stromeyer FW: Medical diseases of the liver. In Silverberg SG (ed): Principles and Practice of Surgical Pathology, pp 937–994. New York, John Wiley & Sons, 1983

144. Ishak KG et al: Viral hemorrhagic fevers with hepatic involvement: Pathologic aspects with clinical correlations. In Popper H, Schaffner F (eds): Progress in Liver Diseases, vol 7, pp 495–515. New York, Grune & Stratton, 1982

145. Ishak KG et al: Epithelioid hemangioendothelioma of the

liver: A clinicopathologic and follow-up study of 32 cases. Hum Pathol 15:839, 1984.

146. Ishak KG et al: Granulomas and cholestatic hepatocellular injury associated with phenylbutazone: Report of two cases. Am J Dig Dis 22:611, 1977

147. Itoh S et al: Nonalcoholic fatty liver with alcoholic hyalin after long-term glucocorticoid therapy. Acto Hepato-Gastroenterol 24:415, 1977

148. Itoh S et al: Clinicopathological and electron microscopical studies on a coronary dilating agent, 4,4'-diethylaminoethoxyhexestrol-induced liver injuries. Acta Hepato-Gastroenterol 20:204, 1973

149. Iversen P, Roholm K: On aspiration biopsy of the liver with remarks on its diagnostic significance. Acta Med Scand 102:1, 1939

150. Iversen P et al: Biopsy studies of the liver and kidney. Adv Intern Med 6:161, 1954

151. Jain S et al: Histologic demonstration of copper and copper-associated protein in chronic liver disease. J Clin Pathol 31:784, 1978

152. James DG: Hepatic granulomas. In Brunner H, Thaler H (eds): Hepatology: A Festschrift for Hans Popper, pp 269–280. New York, Raven Press, 1985

153. Jeffrey G et al: Cholestatic jaundice in the haemolytic-uraemic syndrome: A case report. Gut 26:315, 1985

154. Johannessen JV (ed): Electron Microscopy in Human Medicine, Vol 8, The Liver. New York, McGraw Hill, 1979

155. Johnson RA et al: Intrahepatic hematoma following liver biopsy by the Menghini technic. Am J Gastroenterol 50:131, 1968

156. Jones AL, Schmuckler DL: Current concepts of liver structure as related to function. Gastroenterology, 73:833, 1977

157. Jones EA et al: Progressive intrahepatic cholestasis of infancy and childhood: A clinicopathological study of a patient surviving to the age of 18 years. Gastroenterology 71:675, 1976

158. Jurco S III et al: Malignant histiocytosis in childhood: Morphologic considerations. Hum Pathol 14:1059, 1983

159. Kahn EI et al: Arteriohepatic dysplasia: II. Hepatobiliary morphology. Hepatology 3:77, 1983

160. Kahn HJ et al: Categorization of pediatric neoplasms by immunostaining with antikeratin and antivimentin antisera. Cancer 51:645, 1983

161. Kahn HJ et al: Role of antibody to S-100 protein in diagnostic pathology. Am J Clin Pathol 79:341, 1983

162. Kanel GC et al: Globular hepatic amyloid: An unusual morphologic presentation. Hepatology 1:647, 1981

163. Kaplinsky C et al: Familial cholestatic cirrhosis associated with Kayser–Fleischer rings. Pediatrics 65:782, 1980

164. Kelley ML et al: Bile leakage following Menghini needle liver biopsy. JAMA 216:333, 1971

165. Kimura H et al: Alcoholic hyaline (Mallory bodies) in a case of Weber-Christian disease: Electron microscopic observations of liver involvement. Gastroenterology 78:807, 1980

166. Klatskin G, Bloomer JR: Birefringence of hepatic pigment deposits in erythropoietic protoporphyria. Gastroenterology 67:294, 1974

167. Kleckner MS Jr: Needle biopsy of the liver: An appraisal of its diagnostic indications and limitations. Ann Intern Med 40:1177, 1954

168. Klein B et al: Liver abscess as a late complication of percutaneous liver biopsy. Arch Surg 115:1233, 1980

169. Klinge O, Bannasch P: Zur Vermehrung des glatten endoplasmatischen Retikulum in hepatocytocyten menschlichter Leberpunktate. Verh Dtsch Ges Pathol 52:568, 1968

170. Knauer CM: Percutaneous biopsy of the liver as a procedure for outpatients. Gastroenterology 74:101, 1978

171. Kojiro M et al: Distribution of albumin and/or alpha-fetoprotein-positive cells in hepatocellular carcinoma. Lab Invest 44:221, 1981

172. Kopelman H et al: The liver lesion of the Epping jaundice. Q J Med 35:553, 1966

173. Kothari T et al: Hepatic hemosiderosis in maintenance hemodialysis (MHD) patients. Dig Dis Sci 25:363, 1980

174. Kryger P: Non-A, non-B hepatitis: Serological, clinical, morphological and prognostic aspects. Liver 3:176, 1983

175. Kryger P et al: Light microscopic morphology of acute hepatitis non-A, non-B: A comparison with hepatitis A and B. Liver 2:200, 1982

176. Laurell S, Lundquist A: Lipid composition of human liver biopsy specimens. Acta Med Scand 189:65, 1971

177. Lebrec D et al: Transvenous liver biopsy: An experience based on 1000 hepatic tissue samplings with this procedure. Gastroenterology 83, 1982

178. Lee SP et al: Traumatic hemobilia: A complication of percutaneous liver biopsy. Gastroenterology 72:941, 1977

179. Lefkowitch JH: Bile ductular cholestasis: An ominous histopathologic sign related to sepsis and "cholangitis lenta." Hum Pathol 13:19, 1982

180. Lefkowitch JH et al: Acute liver biopsy lesions in early autoimmune ("lupoid") chronic active hepatitis. Liver 4:379, 1984

181. Lefkowitch JH et al: Oxyphilic granular hepatocytes: Mitochondrion-rich liver cells in hepatic disease. Am J Clin Pathol 74:432, 1980

182. Lefkowitch JH et al: Hepatic copper overload and features of Indian childhood cirrhosis in an American sibship. N Engl J Med 307:271, 1982

183. LeFrock J et al: Transient bacteremia associated with percutaneous liver biopsy. J Infect Dis 131:S104, 1975

184. Leong ASY et al: Refractile particles in liver haemodialysis patients. Lancet 1:889, 1981

185. Levenson JD et al: Hemobilia secondary to percutaneous liver biopsy. Arch Intern Med 130:396, 1972

186. Lewis JH et al: Budd–Chiari syndrome associated with oral contraceptive steroids: Review of treatment of 47 cases. Dig Dis Sci 28:673, 1983

187. Lieberman DA et al: Severe and prolonged oral contraceptive jaundice. J Clin Gastroenterol 6:145, 1984

188. Lieberman J et al: Alpha-1-antitrypsin in livers of patients with emphysema. Science 175:63, 1972

189. Lindner J et al: Systemic kappa light-chain deposition: An ultrastructural and immunohistochemical study. Am J Surg Pathol 7:85, 1983

190. Lindner H: Das Risiko der perkutanen Leberbiopsie. Med Klin 66:924, 1971

191. Lindquist RR: Studies on the pathogenesis of hepatolenticular degeneration: II. Cytochemical methods for the localization of copper. Arch Pathol 87:370, 1969

192. Lindsay S et al: Gargoylism: Study of pathologic lesions and clinical review of twelve cases. Am J Dis Child 76:239, 1948

193. LoIudice T et al: Septicemia as a complication of percutaneous liver biopsy. Gastroenterology 72:949, 1977

194. Loomus GN et al: A case of peliosis hepatis in association with tamoxifen therapy. Am J Clin Pathol 80:881, 1983

195. Lovett EJ et al: Application of flow cytometry to diagnostic pathology. Lab Invest 50:115, 1984

196. Lucatello L: Sulla puncture del fegato a scopo diagnostico. In Lavori del congressi di medicina interna, p 327, Rome, 1895

197. Luna LG: Manual of Histologic Staining Methods of the Armed Forces Institute of Pathology, 3d ed. New York, McGraw-Hill, 1968

198. Maddrey WC, Boitnott JK: Drug-induced chronic liver disease. Gastroenterology 72:1348, 1977

199. Maddrey WC: Hepatic vein thrombosis (Budd–Chiari syndrome). Hepatology 4:445, 1984

200. Maharaj B et al: Sampling variability and its influence on the diagnostic yield of percutaneous needle biopsy of the liver. Lancet 1:523, 1986

201. Marubbio AT et al: Hepatic lesions of central pericellular fibrosis in morbid obesity, and after jejunoileal bypass. Am J Clin Pathol 66:684, 1976

202. Matsen P et al: Reproducibility and accuracy of liver biopsy findings suggestive of an obstructive cause of jaundice. In Brunner H, Thaler H (eds): Hepatology: A Festschrift for Hans Popper, pp 285–293. New York, Raven Press, 1985

203. Matsumoto T et al: A histopathological study of the liver in paraquat poisoning: An analysis of fourteen autopsy cases with emphasis on bile duct injury. Acta Pathol Jpn 30:859, 1980

204. McAdams AJ et al: Glycogen storage disease, types I to X: Criteria for morphologic diagnosis. Hum Pathol 5:464, 1974

205. McBateson et al: A comparative trial of liver biopsy needles. J Clin Pathol 80:131, 1979

206. McCloskey RV et al: Bacteremia after liver biopsy. Arch Intern Med 132:213, 1973

207. McCormack LR et al: Liver involvement in giant cell arteritis. Am J Dig Dis 23:725, 1978

208. McMaster KB, Hennigar GH: Drug-induced granulomatous hepatitis. Lab Invest 44:61, 1981

209. McMillan PN et al: Light and electron microscopic analysis of lectin binding in adult rat liver in situ. Lab Invest 50:408, 1984

210. Menghini G: Biopsia y microbiopsia del higado: Un effectivo progreso methodologico. Scientia Med Ital 6:212, 1957

211. Menghini G: One-second needle biopsy of the liver. Gastroenterology 35:190, 1958

212. Menghini G: Two-operator needle biopsy of the liver: A new, easier and safer version of the one-second technic. Am J Dig Dis 4:682, 1959

213. Menghini G et al: Some innovations in the technic of the one-second needle biopsy of the liver. Am J Gastroenterol 64:175, 1975

214. Merino-DeVillasante J et al: Management of post-biopsy hemobilia with selective arterial embolization. AJR 128:668, 1977

215. Miller R et al: Wolman's disease: Report of a case with multiple studies. Arch Pathol Lab Med 106:41, 1982

216. Montgomery CLK, Ruebner BH: Neonatal giant cell transformation: A review. Perspect Pediatr Pathol 3:85, 1976

217. Morris JS et al: Percutaneous liver biopsy in patients with large bile duct obstruction. Gastroenterology 68:750, 1975

218. Motta P et al: The Liver: An Atlas of Scanning Electron Microscopy. Tokyo, Igaku-Shoin, 1978

219. Mullick FG, Ishak KG: Hepatic injury associated with diphenyl-hydantoin therapy: A clinicopathologic study of 20 cases. Am J Clin Pathol 74:442, 1980

220. Mullick FG et al: Hepatic injury associated with paraquat toxicity in humans. Liver 1:209, 1981

221. Nadell J, Kosek J: Peliosis hepatis: Twelve cases associated with oral androgen therapy. Arch Pathol Lab Med 101:405, 1977

222. Nakanuma Y et al: Intrahepatic bile duct destruction in a patient with sarcoidosis and chronic intrahepatic cholestasis. Acta Pathol Jpn 29:211, 1979

223. Nakanuma Y et al: Cytoplasmic blood inclusions in human hepatocytes. Liver 2:212, 1982

224. Nanba K et al: Splenic pseudosinuses and hepatic angiomatous lesions: Distinctive features of hairy cell leukemia. Am J Pathol 64:417, 1977

225. Nelson RS: The development and function of a liver biopsy program: Training of personnel, description of a modified Vim-Silverman needle and clinical value of 500 biopsies. Am J Med Sci 227:152, 154

226. Nesher G et al: Hepatosplenic peliosis after danazol and glucocorticoids for ITP. Lancet 1:242, 1985

227. Nishimura R et al: Lafora's disease: Diagnosis by liver biopsy. Ann Neurol 8:409, 1980

228. Novikoff AB, Essner E: The liver cell: Some new approaches to its study. Am J Med 29:102, 1960

229. Okuda K, Omata M (eds): Idiopathic Portal Hypertension. Tokyo, University of Tokyo Press, 1983

230. Okuda K et al: Peliosis hepatis as a late and fatal complication of Thorotrast liver disease: Report of five cases. Liver 1:110, 1981

231. Okuda K et al: Frequency of intrahepatic arteriovenous fistula as a sequela to percutaneous needle puncture of the liver. Gastroenterology 74:1204, 1978

232. Pagliaro L et al: Percutaneous blind biopsy versus laparoscopy with guided biopsy in diagnosis of cirrhosis: A prospective, randomized trial. Dig Dis Sci 28, No. 1:39, 1983

233. Paliard P et al: Perhexilene maleate–induced hepatitis. Digestion 17:419, 1978

234. Palmer PE et al: Expression of protein markers in malignant hepatoma: Evidence for genetic and epigenetic mechanisms. Cancer 45:1474, 1980

235. Paradinas FJ et al: Hyperplasia and prolapse of hepatocytes into hepatic veins during long-term methyltestosterone therapy: Possible relationships of these changes to the development of peliosis hepatis and liver tumors. Histopathology 1:225, 1977

236. Passwell HH et al: Pigment deposition in the reticuloendothelial system after fat emulsion. Arch Dis Child 51:366, 1976

237. Pereiras R et al: The role of interventional radiology in disease of the hepatobiliary system and the pancreas. In Mackintosh PK, Thomson K (eds): Radiol Clin North Am 17, No. 3:555, 1979

238. Perrault J et al: Liver biopsy: Complications in 1000 inpatients and outpatients. Gastroenterology 74:103, 1978

239. Pessayre O et al: Perhexilene maleate induced cirrhosis. Gastroenterology 76:170, 1979

240. Peters RL: Pathology of hepatocellular carcinoma. In Okuda K, Peters RL (eds): Hepatocellular Carcinoma, pp 107–168. New York, John Wiley & Sons, 1976

241. Peters RL et al: Post-jejunoileal-bypass hepatic disease: Its similarity to alcoholic hepatic disease. Am J Clin Pathol 63:318, 1975

242. Peura DA et al: Liver injury with alcoholic hyaline after intestinal resection. Gastroenterology 79:128, 1980

243. Pfeifer U et al: Hepatocellular fibrinogen storage in familial hypofibrinogenemia. Virchows Arch Cell Pathol 36:247, 1981

244. Phillips MJ, Poucell S: Modern aspects of the morphology of viral hepatitis. Hum Pathol 12:1060, 1981

245. Piccinino F et al: Complications following percutaneous liver biopsy: A multicentre retrospective study on 68,276 biopsies. J Hepatol 2:165, 1986

246. Piciotto A et al: Percutaneous or laparoscopic needle biopsy in the evaluation of chronic liver disease? Am J Gastroenterol 79, No. 7:567, 1984

247. Piggott JA: Melioidosis. In Binford CH, Connor DH (eds): Pathology of Tropical and Extraordinary Diseases, vol 2, pp 169–174. Washington DC, Armed Forces Institute of Pathology, 1976

248. Pimentel JC, Menezes AP: Pulmonary and hepatic granulomatous disorders due to the inhalation of cement and mica dusts. Thorax 33:219, 1978

249. Pimentel JC, Menezes AP: Liver granulomas containing copper in vineyard sprayer's lung: A new etiology of hepatic granulomatosis. Am Rev Resp Dis 111:189, 1975

250. Pinkus GS: Diagnostic immunocytochemistry of paraffin-embedded tissues. Hum Pathol 13:411, 1982

251. Popper H, Schaffner F: Chronic hepatitis: Taxonomic, etiologic and therapeutic problems. Prog Liver Dis 5:531, 1976

252. Potter VR: Workshop in liver cell culture. Cancer Res 32:1998, 1972

253. Poucell S et al: Amiodarone-associated phospholipidosis and fibrosis of the liver: Light, immunohistochemical and electron microscopic studies. Gastroenterology 86:926, 1984

254. Poupon R et al: Perhexilene maleate–associated hepatic injury: Prevalence and characteristics. Digestion 20:145, 1980

255. Powell LW, Halliday JW: Hemochromatosis. In Berk JE (ed): Bockus Gastroenterology, Vol 5, Liver, pp 3203–3221. Philadelphia, WB Saunders, 1985

256. Purow E et al: Menghini needle fracture after attempted liver biopsy. Gastroenterology 73:1404, 1977

257. Raga J et al: Usefulness of clinical features and liver biopsy in diagnosis of disseminated herpes simplex infection. Arch Dis Child 59:820, 1984

258. Raines DR et al: Intrahepatic hematome: A complication of percutaneous liver biopsy. Gastroenterology 67:284, 1974

259. Ranek L et al: A morphometric study of normal human liver cell nuclei. Acta Pathol Microbiol Scand (Sect A) 83:467, 1975

260. Remington JS et al: Toxoplasmosis and infectious mononucleosis. Arch Intern Med 110:744, 1962

261. Richey J et al: Giant multinucleated hepatocytes in an adult with chronic active hepatitis. Gastroenterology 73:570, 1977

262. Riley SA et al: Percutaneous liver biopsy with plugging of needle track: A safe method for use in patients with impaired coagulation. Lancet 2:436, 1984

263. Ringleb O: Uber Retshelknotchen der Leber bei Tuberkulosen. Arch Pathol Anat 324:357, 1953

264. Roholm K et al: Aspirationsbiopsie der Leber. Mit einer ubersicht uber die Ergebnisse bei 297 Biopsien. Ergebn inn Med Kinderh 61:635, 1942

265. Rohr HP et al: Stereology of liver biopsies from healthy volunteers. Virchows Arch Pathol Anat 371:251, 1976

266. Rohr HP et al: Stereology: A new supplement to the study of human liver biopsy specimens. Prog Liver Dis 5:24, 1976

267. Rolfes DB, Ishak KG: Acute fatty liver in pregnancy: A clinicopathologic study of 35 cases. Hepatology, 5:1149, 1985

268. Roque AL: Chromotrope aniline blue method of staining Mallory bodies of Laennec's cirrhosis. Lab Invest 2:15, 1953

269. Rösch J et al: Transjugular approach to liver, biliary system and portal circulation. AJR Radium Ther Nucl Med 125:602, 1975

270. Rösch J et al: Transjugular approach to liver biopsy and transhepatic cholangiography. N Engl J Med 289:277, 1973

271. Rubel LR, Ishak KG: The liver in fatal exertional heatstroke. Liver 3:249, 1983

272. Rudzki C et al: Chronic intrahepatic cholestasis of sarcoidosis. Am J Med 59:373, 1975

273. Russell RM et al: Hepatic injury from chronic hypervitaminosis: A resulting in portal hypertension and ascites. N Engl J Med 291:435, 1974

274. Sandblom P: Hemobilia (Biliary Tract Hemorrhage): History, Pathology, Diagnosis, Treatment, p 80. Springfield, Charles C Thomas, 1972

275. Satava RM et al: Omental arteriovenous fistula following liver biopsy. Gastroenterology 69:492, 1975

276. Sborov VM: Simple guard for Vim-Silverman needle. J Lab Clin Med 36:773, 1950

277. Schafer AI et al: Clinical consequences of acquired transfusional iron overload in adults. N Engl J Med 304:319, 1981

278. Schaffner F, Popper H: Capillarization of hepatic sinusoids in man. Gastroenterology 44:239, 1963

279. Schaffner F, Thaler H: Nonalcoholic fatty liver disease. Prog Liver Dis 8:283, 1986

280. Scheinberg IH, Sternlieb I: Wilson's Disease. Philadelphia, WB Saunders, 1984

281. Schiff L et al: The clinical value of needle biopsy of the liver; selected case experiences: Proc World Congress. Gastroenterology 1958

282. Schmid M et al: Acute hepatitis non-A, non-B; Are there any specific light microscopic features? Liver 2:61, 1982

283. Schmidt B et al: Management of post-traumatic vascular malformations of the liver by catheter embolization. Am J Surg 140:332, 1980

284. Seeff LB: Drug-induced chronic liver disease, with emphasis on chronic active hepatitis. Sem Liver Dis 1:104, 1981

285. Seeley TT et al: Hepatic infarction. Hum Pathol 3:265, 1972

286. Seki K et al: "Nonalcoholic steatohepatitis" induced by massive doses of synthetic estrogen. Gastroenterol Jpn 18:197, 1983

287. Sharp HL: Inherited disorders with metabolic dysfunction. In Berk JE (ed): Bockus Gastroenterology, 4th ed, Vol 5, Liver, pp 3236–3258. Philadelphia, WB Saunders, 1985

288. Sharp HL: Alpha-1-antitrypsin deficiency. Hosp Pract 5:83, 1971

289. Sherlock S: Aspiration liver biopsy: Technique and diagnostic application. Lancet 2:397, 1945

290. Shikata T et al: Staining methods of Australia antigen in paraffin section: Detection of cytoplasmic inclusion bodies. Jpn J Exp Med 44:25, 1974

291. Shikata T et al: Phospholipid fatty liver: A proposal of a new concept and its electron microscopical study. Acta Pathol Jpn 20:457, 1970

292. Shulman HM et al: Chronic graft-versus-host syndrome in man: A long-term clinicopathologic study of 20 Seattle patients. Am J Med 69:204, 1980

293. Shulman HM et al: An analysis of hepatic veno-occlusive disease and centrilobular hepatic degeneration following

bone marrow transplantation. Gastroenterology 79:1178, 1980

294. Silverman I: Improved Vim-Silverman biopsy needle. JAMA 155:1060, 1954

295. Simon JB et al: Amiodarone hepatotoxicity simulating alcoholic liver disease. N Engl J Med 311:167, 1984

296. Singer DB: Pathology of neonatal herpes simplex viral infection. Perspect Pediatr Pathol 6:243, 1981

297. Sipponen P: Orcein positive hepatocellular material in longstanding biliary diseases: I. Histochemical characteristics. Scand J Gastroenterol 11:545, 1976

298. Slavin RE et al: Extrapulmonary silicosis: A clinical, morphologic and ultrastructural study. Hum Pathol 16:393, 1985

299. Snover DC, Horwitz CA: Liver disease in cytomegalovirus mononucleosis: A light microscopical and immunoperoxidase study of six cases. Hepatology 4:408, 1984

300. Snover DC et al: Hepatic graft-versus-host disease: A study of the predictive value of liver biopsy in diagnosis. Hepatology 4:123, 1984

301. Snover DC et al: Orthotopic liver transplantation: A pathological study of 63 serial liver biopsies from 17 patients with special reference to the diagnostic features and natural history of rejection. Hepatology 4:1212, 1984

302. Solis–Herruzo JA et al: Hepatic injury in the toxic epidemic syndrome caused by ingestion of adulterated cooking oil (Spain, 1981). Hepatology 4:131, 1984

303. Spellberg MA et al: Hepatic sinusoidal dilatation related to oral contraceptives: A study of two patients showing ultrastructural changes. Am J Gastroenterol 72:248, 1979

304. Spycher MA: Electron microscopy: A method for the diagnosis of inherited metabolic storage diseases. Pathol Res Pract 167:118, 1980

305. Srigley JR, et al: Q-fever: The liver and bone marrow pathology. Am J Surg Pathol 9:752, 1985

306. Starko KM, Mullick FG: Hepatic and cerebral pathology findings in children with fatal salicylate intoxication: Further evidence of a causal relationship between salicylate and Reye's syndrome. Lancet 1:326, 1983

307. Storch W: Immunohistological investigations of PAS-negative globular intracisternal hyalin in human liver biopsy specimens. Virchows Arch Cell Pathol 48:155, 1985

308. Strasberg SM, Silver MD: Postoperative hepatogenic jaundice. Surg Gynecol Obstet 132:81, 1971

309. Stromeyer FW, Ishak KG: Pathology of the liver in Wilson's disease: A study of 34 cases. Am J Clin Pathol 73:12, 1980

310. Sullivan S, Watson WC: Acute transient hypotension as complication of percutaneous liver biopsy. Lancet 1:389, 1974.

311. Sumithran E, Looi LM: Copper-binding protein in liver cells. Hum Pathol 16:677, 1985

312. Tamburro CH: Personal communication, 1974

313. Tandon HD et al: An epidemic of veno-occlusive disease of liver in Central India. Lancet 1:271, 1976

314. Tanikawa, K: Ultrastructural Aspects of the Liver and its Disorders. Tokyo, Igaku-Shoin, 1979

315. Tao LC et al: Cytologic diagnosis of hepatocellular carcinoma. Cancer 53:547, 1984

316. Tao LC et al: Percutaneous fine-needle aspiration biopsy of the liver. Acta Cytol 23:287, 1979

317. Taylor CR, Kledzik G: Immunohistologic techniques in surgical pathology: A spectrum of "new" special stains. Hum Pathol 12:590, 1981

318. Terpstra OT et al: An unexpected complication of a liver biopsy. Br J Surg 64:436, 1977

319. Terry R: Risks of needle biopsy of the liver. Br Med J 1: 1102, 1952

320. Terry R: Macroscopic diagnosis in liver biopsy. JAMA 154: 990, 1954

321. Terzakis JA et al: X-ray microanalysis of hepatic thorium deposits. Arch Pathol 98:241, 1974

322. Thaler H: Post-infantile giant cell hepatitis. Liver 2:393, 1982

323. Thaler H: Erfahrungen mit der Leberbiopsiemethode nach Menghini. Wien Klin Wschr 70:622, 1958

324. Thaler H: Ueber Vorteil und Risiko der Leberbiopsiemethode nach Menghini. Wien Klin Wschr 76:533, 1964

325. Thijs JC et al: Post-infantile giant cell hepatitis in a patient with multiple autoimmune features. Am J Gastroenterol 80:294, 1985

326. Thorne C et al: Liver disease in Felty's syndrome. Am J Med 73:35, 1982

327. Thung SN et al: Distribution of five antigens in hepatocellular carcinoma. Lab Invest 41:101, 1979

328. Toker C, Trevino N: Hepatic ultrastructure in chronic idiopathic jaundice. Arch Pathol 80:454, 1965

329. Tripoli CJ, Fader DE: The differential diagnosis of certain diseases of the liver by means of punch biopsy. Am J Clin Pathol 11:516, 1941

330. Uchida T et al: Alcoholic foamy degeneration: A pattern of acute alcoholic injury of the liver. Gastroenterology 86: 683, 1983

331. Ugarte N, Ganzalez–Crussi F: Hepatoma in siblings with progressive familial cirrhosis of childhood. Am J Clin Pathol 76:172, 1981

332. Valencia–Mayoral P et al: Possible defect in the bile secretory apparatus in arteriohepatic dysplasia (Alagille's syndrome): A review with observations on the ultrastructure of the liver. Hepatology 4:691, 1984

333. Vanderstigel M et al: Allopurinol hypersensitivity syndrome as a cause of hepatic fibrin-ring granulomas. Gastroenterology 90:188, 1986

334. VanSonnenberg E, Mueller PR: Ultrasound, CT, and fluoroscopic guidance for percutaneous abdominal biopsy. Applied Radiology, Nov/Dec 1981

335. Vargas-Tank L et al: Tru-cut and Menghini needles: Different yield in the histological diagnosis of liver disease. Liver 5:178, 1985

336. Vasquez JJ et al: Cyanamide-induced liver injury. Liver 3: 225, 1983

337. Verscheck J, Barbier F: Determination of copper in needle biopsies of the liver. Gastroenterology 69:279, 1975

338. Vidins EI et al: Sinusoidal caliber in alcoholic and nonalcoholic liver disease: Diagnostic and pathogenic implications. Hepatology 5:408, 1985

339. Vierling JM, Fennell RH: Histopathology of early and late human hepatic allograft rejection: Evidence of progressive destruction of interlobular bile ducts. Hepatology 5:1076, 1985

340. Voegtlin WL: An improved liver biopsy needle. Gastroenterology 11:56, 1948

341. Voigt JJ et al: Hepatite granulomateuse: A propos de 112 cas chez l'adults. Ann Pathol 4:78, 1984

342. Volwiler W, Jones CM: The diagnostic and therapeutic value of liver biopsies with particular reference to trocar biopsy. N Engl J Med 237:651, 1947

343. Volwiler W et al: Criteria for the measurement of results of treatment in fatty cirrhosis. Gastroenterology 11:164, 1948

344. Vyberg M, Poulsen H: Abnormal bile duct epithelium ac-

companying septicemia. Virchows Arch Pathol Anat 402: 451, 1984

345. Wallace S et al: Angiographic changes due to needle biopsy of the liver. Radiology 105:13, 1972

346. Walter JRF, Paton A: Liver biopsy. Br Med J 280:776, 1980

347. Wanless IR, Geddie IR: Mineral oil lipogranulomata in liver and spleen. Arch Pathol Lab Med 109:283, 1985

348. Wanless IR et al: Nodular regenerative hyperplasia of the liver in hematologic disorders: A possible response to obliterative portal venopathy. Medicine 59:367, 1980

349. Waterlow J: Enzyme activity in human liver, p 72, Tr. 11th Liver Injury Conference. New York, Macy, 1952

350. Weber AM et al: Severe familial cholestasis in North American Indian children: A clinical model of microfilament dysfunction. Gastroenterology 81:653, 1981

351. Weber AM et al: Cholestasis induced by microfilament dysfunction. In Daum F (ed): Extrahepatic Biliary Atresia, pp 203–213. New York, Marcel-Dekker, 1983

352. Westaby D et al: Liver biopsy as a day-case procedure: Selection and complications in 200 consecutive patients. Br Med J 281:1331, 1980

353. Whitington PF: Cholestasis associated with total parenteral nutrition in infants. Hepatology 5:683, 1985

354. Whitside TL et al: Immunologic analysis of mononuclear cells in liver tissue and blood of patients with primary sclerosing cholangitis. Hepatology 5:468, 1985

355. Whittle TS Jr: Fatal intrahepatic hemorrhage after percutaneous liver biopsy using a Menghini needle: A rare but real complication. South Med J 70:1355, 1977

356. Wieczorek R et al: Familial erythrophagocytic, lymphohistiocytosis: Immunophenotypic, immunohistochemical, and ultrastructural demonstration of the relation to sinus histiocytes. Hum Pathol 17:55, 1986.

357. Wigger HJ: Frozen section of liver in the diagnosis of Reye syndrome. Am J Surg Pathol 1:271, 1977

358. Wilkinson SP et al: Clinical course of chronic lobular hepatitis. Q J Med 71:421, 1978

359. Williams R et al: Idiopathic recurrent cholestasis: A study of functional and pathological lesions in four cases. Q J Med 33:387, 1964

360. Wilson JP et al: Percutaneous needle biopsies of the liver. Am Surg 37:155, 1971

361. Winkler K, Poulsen H: Liver disease with periportal sinusoidal dilatation: A possible complication to contraceptive steroids. Scand J Gastroenterol 10:699, 1975

362. With TK: Micromethod for the determination of vitamin A in liver biopsies in man and larger animals. Biochem J 40:249, 1946

363. Witte CL et al: Protean manifestations of pylethrombosis: A review of thirty-four patients. Ann Surg 202:191, 1985

364. Worner TM, Lieber CS: Perivenular fibrosis as precursor lesion of cirrhosis. JAMA 254:627, 1985

365. Zafrani ES et al: Cholestatic and hepatocellular injury associated with erythromycin derivatives: Report of nine cases. Am J Dig Dis 24:385, 1979

366. Zafrani ES et al: Focal hemorrhagic necrosis of the liver: A clinicopathologic entity possibly related to oral contraceptives. Gastroenterology 79:1295, 1980

367. Zafrani ES et al: Ultrastructural lesions of the liver in human peliosis: A report of 12 cases. Am J Clin Pathol 114:349, 1984

368. Zafrani ES et al: Peliosis-like ultrastructural changes of the hepatic sinusoids in human chronic hypervitaminosis A: Report of three cases. Hum Pathol 15:1166, 1984

369. Zamcheck N, Klausenstock O: Needle biopsy of the liver: II. The risk of needle biopsy. N Engl J Med 249:1062, 1953

370. Zamcheck N, Sidman RL: Needle biopsy of the liver: I. Its use in clinical and investigative medicine. N Engl J Med 249:1020, 1953

371. Zerpa H et al: Application of routine and immunohistochemical staining methods to liver tissue embedded in a water-soluble resin. Liver 1:62, 1981

372. Zimmerman HJ: Hepatotoxicity. New York, Appleton-Century-Crofts, 1978

373. Zimmerman HJ: Drug-induced chronic liver disease. In Farber E, Fisher MM (eds): Toxic Injury of the Liver, Part B, pp 687–737. New York, Marcel Dekker, 1980

374. Zimmerman HJ, Ishak KG: Valproate induced hepatic injury: Analyses of 23 fatal cases. Hepatology 2:591, 1982

375. Zimmerman HJ et al: Jaundice due to bacterial infection. Gastroenterology 77:362–365, 1979

376. Zornoza J et al: Fine-needle aspiration biopsy of the liver. AJR 134:331, 1980

chapter 14

Laparoscopy

H. WORTH BOYCE, JR.

Laparoscopy is the most reliable technique available for closing the diagnostic gap between clinical evaluation and surgical exploration. Anxiety over this method for intra-abdominal examination in the United States in past years apparently has resulted in its failure to be recognized as the valuable diagnostic procedure it is known to be in other countries of the world, particularly on the European continent and in Japan. Nevertheless, laparoscopy has become accepted as a simple and effective method for diagnosis of abdominal disorders.

HISTORY

Laparoscopy (originally called coelioscopy) was first performed by Kelling on a dog in 1901[42] and later on two humans.[43,59] In 1910, the procedure was named laparoscopy by Jacobaeus, who reported 45 examinations in his monograph.[33] The first report of transabdominal endoscopic diagnosis in the United States appeared in a 1911 report by Bernheim, an assistant in surgery at Johns Hopkins University.[6] He passed an ordinary proctoscope of one-half-inch bore through an epigastric incision, without the aid of pneumoperitoneum, and examined the surfaces of the upper abdominal viscera using illumination from an electric headlight. The patient was deeply jaundiced, and the examination revealed a distended gallbladder, later confirmed at laparotomy to have been caused by carcinoma of the pancreas obstructing the common bile duct.

Since 1913, many endoscopists have made significant contributions by devising new instruments and techniques for laparoscopy.[56] In 1920, Orndoff reported the first large series from the United States and named the procedure peritoneoscopy.[58] In Germany, Korbsch[44] and Kalk[38] published reports on the technique and clinical value of the procedure during the same decade.

In 1934, Ruddock presented the first of a series of papers that were to establish his position as the "father" of laparoscopy in the United States.[63] The instrument he described was the one most used in this country until the 1950s, when excellent instruments from Germany became available.

The diagnostic value of laparoscopy was greatly enhanced by the work of Kalk, who popularized the technique of guided liver biopsy.[39,40] During the past 25 years, others have made significant contributions that have re-sulted in a better understanding of the clinical value and improved technique for laparoscopy.[29,66,76,83,84] Steptoe has popularized both the diagnostic and therapeutic capabilities of laparoscopy in gynecology.[74]

INDICATIONS

Laparoscopy is a simple and safe procedure that has a diagnostic accuracy over 90% when performed for the proper indications.[45,66,70] General anesthesia is neither necessary nor desirable for medical laparoscopy.[8] The patient ordinarily is hospitalized no longer than 1 day following the procedure.

This technique should be considered an extension of physical diagnosis that has the added advantage of a direct-vision-guided biopsy of liver or peritoneum. Blind-needle liver biopsy has been shown to be inadequate for correct diagnosis in at least 40% of patients with carcinoma metastatic to the liver[16] and in 67% of patients with chronic active liver disease and known cirrhosis.[72]

The internist-gastroenterologist will find laparoscopy of most benefit in the evaluation of patients with liver disease.[30,35] In most instances, these patients have a history of alcoholism, suspected metastatic neoplasm,[22] jaundice,[17] hepatomegaly, abnormal liver function studies, or an abnormal radioisotope liver scan. Laparoscopy is helpful for a more complete evaluation of the liver before major surgery for malignant neoplasm.[27] It is of benefit in evaluation of ascites, obscure abdominal and pelvic pain, and certain abdominal masses.

A complete laparoscopy should include a thorough evaluation of pelvic structures. Consequently, the internist may use this technique for evaluation of pelvic pain, suspected endometriosis, salpingitis, and, in conjunction with the gynecologist, for the evaluation of amenorrhea, infertility, and other pelvic abnormalities.[24,65]

Ancillary diagnostic procedures that may easily be carried out by the internist in conjunction with laparoscopy include biopsy of the liver and parietal peritoneum, pneumoperitoneography, and collection of abdominal fluid for cytologic examination and culture.

The indications for diagnostic laparoscopy are as follows:

To examine the liver and perform guided biopsy for suspected focal or diffuse disease

To establish the etiology of ascites

To assess operability and staging of patients with malignant tumors (i.e., to determine the presence of abdominal metastasis)

To determine etiology of abdominal masses located in areas that can be visualized by this procedure

To examine pelvic organs for anomalies or disease

To evaluate chronic abdominal or acute and chronic pelvic pain suspected to originate from disease, infection, or adhesions of the parietal peritoneum or pelvic organs

To examine the gallbladder for disease or enlargement secondary to common bile duct obstruction

The contraindications for diagnostic laparoscopy are listed below:

Disorders of blood coagulation

Intestinal obstruction

Infection of the abdominal wall

History of generalized peritonitis

Uncooperative patient

Untrained, inexperienced operator

Severe cardiac or pulmonary disease (a relative contraindication)

Ascites, when severe and untreated in patients with portal hypertension (not when due to possible peritoneal carcinomatosis or tuberculosis)

Obesity of massive degree (a relative contraindication)

ANATOMIC LIMITATIONS

In the 1930s, when laparoscopy was first publicized widely in the United States, many instruments were purchased and many examinations were performed. It is apparent from talking to several clinicians in practice during those early days that laparoscopy was often performed on patients in whom it could not possibly achieve diagnostic success. This problem was the result of a failure of the laparoscopist to understand the anatomic limitations or the indications for the procedure.

Laparoscopy is a technique for the diagnosis of diseases that may be apparent by observation over the anterior and lateral aspects of the abdominal and pelvic viscera. Variations in the body position during examination and manipulation of structures by a transabdominal palpating wand will improve diagnostic accuracy. In most patients, the anterior and lateral parietal peritoneum, falciform ligament, anterior surface of the liver lobes, anterior greater curvature aspect of the stomach, greater omentum, variable portions of the large and small bowel, and pelvic organs may be examined. By the use of position changes, the spleen, appendix, and a larger area of the pelvis and lumbar peritoneal surfaces may also be examined. The use of a probe permits elevation of the liver for inspection of its anterior-inferior surface, palpation of the gallbladder

or other structures, and dislocation of the greater omentum to uncover small bowel, colon, or other organs. A properly applied cervical tenaculum and uterine sound enhance the diagnostic capability for pelvic disease.[54,74]

It is essential that the physician be aware of the usual causes of diagnostic failure (Table 14-1). Laparoscopy is of no value for the investigation of suspected disease on the posterior surfaces of the abdominal viscera or of the retroperitoneum or periaortic, renal, and adrenal areas. Until recently, the pancreas was considered inaccessible, but two reports indicate that accurate diagnosis of pancreatic disease is possible under certain conditions.[51,52] If there is a possibility that disease from the retroperitoneal area has extended directly or by metastasis to the anterior abdomen, laparoscopy may be helpful in establishing a diagnosis.

Laparoscopic success is also dependent on the degree of postinflammatory or postsurgical deformity of the abdominal structures. In individuals known to have had generalized peritonitis or multiple surgical procedures with known extensive peritoneal adhesions, it is obvious that chances for laparoscopic success are decreased, while the likelihood of complications is increased. On the other hand, patients who have had uncomplicated surgical procedures usually have adhesions localized to the region of the surgery. By selecting an insertion site away from abdominal incision scars, the endoscopist is able to avoid adhesions and successfully complete his examination. Thin, avascular, curtain-like adhesions are occasionally encountered and may be penetrated by the telescope to permit examination.[71]

Obesity of greater than moderate degree must be considered an anatomic limitation as well as a technical hindrance.[48] Massive obesity probably should be a contraindication for the procedure, since insertion of both pneumoperitoneum needle and trocar is difficult. After successful intraperitoneal placement of the telescope, the thick abdominal wall greatly restricts movement of the device in all directions except vertically in and out. Under these circumstances, the examination is limited to the region beneath the entry site and, in this area, the viscera are likely to be obscured by a sea of omental fat.

A special comment is needed for the patient who has had a cholecystectomy. In most instances, this operation is followed by a more dense adhesive peritonitis in the right upper quadrant than that associated with other uncomplicated surgical procedures. These extensive adhesions may prevent examination of the right hepatic lobe.

TABLE 14-1.   Reasons for Failure or Unsatisfactory Laparoscopy

Improper patient selection: failure to understand anatomic limitations of the procedure
Failure to biopsy
Inability to complete the examination
Incorrect interpretation of visual findings

Therefore, in the patient who is suspected of having a solitary right hepatic lobe lesion without apparent involvement of other areas of the abdomen, this possibility must be recognized and explained to the patient and referring physician before the procedure. If there is a chance that the disease process suspected in the right lobe also involves the left lobe, the laparoscopist may proceed with reasonable assurance of diagnostic success.

INSTRUMENTS

The laparoscope and its accessory instruments are basically very simple and sturdy. Excellent diagnostic instruments and accessories are available from American Cystoscope Makers Inc., Eder Instrument Company, Olympus Corporation, Karl Storz Endoscopy-America Inc., and Richard Wolf Medical Instrument Company. New powerful light sources provide excellent illumination through telescopes of large diameters (i.e., 7 mm to 10 mm). This "cold" light is sufficient in some systems to permit good laparoscopic photography, especially when ASA-400 color film is used. The Wolf photolaparoscope with distal flash, which provided optimum illumination for lower ASA film, color transparencies, and prints, as well as Polaroid prints, is no longer being produced. Instruments used for diagnostic and photolaparoscopy are shown in Figures 14-1 and 14-2.

A standard pack of surgical instruments and accessories should be available for each procedure. The set-up shown in Fig. 14-3 has proven satisfactory for diagnostic laparoscopy.

Sterilization of instruments and accessories is safely done by the ethylene oxide method available in most hospitals. Cold sterilization is also suitable with a solution such as 2% aqueous glutaraldehyde (Cidex) in an instrument tray or an acrylic, transparent sterilizing chamber (Eder Instrument Company). This chamber has a shelf that holds the instruments in a vertical position for easy retrieval from the solution after soaking for at least 20 minutes.

Camera equipment cannot be safely sterilized, so one must take suitable precautions to maintain sterility about the operative site during and after photography. This is easily done by clamping a sterile towel about the cannula before starting photography and by redraping and changing gloves before closing the skin incision.

TECHNIQUE

Preparation of the Patient

When the patient has an appropriate indication for laparoscopy, it is important that a standard group of laboratory tests be performed. These should include a white blood cell count, hematocrit, differential count, chest radiograph, and electrocardiogram. A platelet count, prothrombin

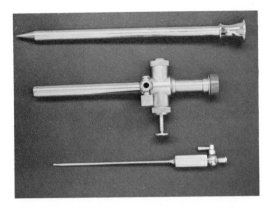

Fig. 14-1. Top to bottom: Conical trocar, cannula with trumpet valve, and Veres needle for pneumoperitoneum.

time, and partial thromboplastin time are sufficient for evaluation of coagulation. A negative bleeding history is most important in this regard. If the patient's coagulation status is marginal, or if he seems to have an increased risk of bleeding, it is wise to have a crossmatch completed for at least 1 unit of blood.

A thorough drug history should be obtained to determine medications presently being taken and any individual sensitivity or allergies to medications, as well as a history of tolerance for sedatives and narcotics.

If the patient has ascites due to cirrhosis, he should be managed by conservative medical means and laparoscopy delayed until optimum diuresis has been achieved. Rapid removal of a large volume of ascitic fluid is hazardous unless the patient's condition has been stabilized by a period of appropriate medical treatment. When laparoscopy is done in such patients, only enough fluid need be removed to permit examination of the anterior aspects of the viscera and peritoneal surfaces. The method for removing ascitic fluid is simple and is explained elsewhere.[8]

The physician should explain the indications for the procedure to the patient and briefly review the technique, the usual time required for complete examination, any

Fig. 14-2. Top to bottom: Wolf 180° forward-viewing telescope, 135° photolaparoscope with distal flash, and sheath containing fiberoptic light transmission system for use with photolaparoscope.

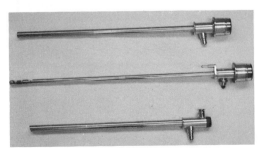

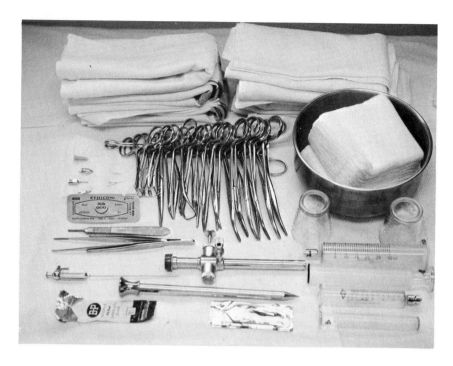

Fig. 14-3. Instrument pack containing accessories for laparoscopy.

special manipulations that are anticipated, the possible need for a biopsy, and what he should expect following the procedure, including mention of activity and diet. The patient must understand that he will have difficulty taking a normal deep breath during the time that the pneumoperitoneum is in place. He should be told that he should take shallow breaths and that this will allow him to accommodate comfortably to the elevated diaphragm.

The patient should be taught to elevate the anterior abdominal wall while keeping the lumbar spine flat on the examining table or bed. This maneuver is practiced before the procedure and is of considerable help during introduction of the pneumoperitoneum needle and the trocar by providing a tense abdomen for the operator to push against. Also, the anterior displacement of the abdominal wall away from the vertebrae, aorta, and vena cava is believed to add a measure of safety to insertion of the pneumoperitoneum needle and cannula trocar.

An operative permit should be signed after explanation of the procedure. The permit must include permission for both laparoscopy and liver or peritoneal biopsy. Patient cooperation is essential. There is no substitute for good rapport, verbal preparation, and compassion for the patient's expected anxiety.

Procedure

The incision site for laparoscopy is varied, depending on the purpose of the examination and the location and size of abdominal organs. Figure 14-4 illustrates the usual sites selected for examination of the right upper quadrant and liver, and the legend indicates the circumstances under which the various entry sites are selected. Site selection for pneumoperitoneum and trocar insertion perhaps is the most important part of the introduction procedure. Bad judgment at this stage can lead to major complications. The novice must remember that ptosis of the umbilicus is common in patients with alcoholic cirrhosis. This caudad displacement must be considered if the umbilicus is used as a guide for incision placement. An entry site for the laparoscope caudad to the ptotic umbilicus may position the telescope at too great a distance for complete liver examination.

Laparoscopy for medical diagnosis is best performed in the endoscopy room or any properly equipped similar area. There is no need for the internist to be competing for operating room space, since the procedure is done simply and safely in a nonsurgical environment. Good aseptic technique is far more important than location of the room used for laparoscopy.

Before premedication is given, the patient should be asked to void so that a distended urinary bladder will not interfere with the examination. If the patient is found by history or physical examination to be constipated, the administation of a mild laxative or enema the evening before laparoscopy will also be helpful.

Drug preparation ordinarily includes intramuscular meperidine hydrochloride (Demerol), 50 mg to 100 mg, and atropine sulfate, 0.6 mg, about 30 minutes before the procedure. Diazepam (Valium), 10 mg, may be given intramuscularly before laparoscopy or 3 mg to 10 mg slowly given intravenously as the pneumoperitoneum is instituted. In busy clinics, the meperidine and diazepam may be given intravenously by slow "clinical titration" based

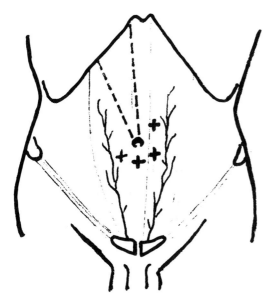

Fig. 14-4. Various sites for introduction of the laparoscope. Dark crosses indicate the most commonly used sites; location must be varied according to size of organs, operative scars, collateral vessels, and abdominal masses. The area between the broken lines indicates the region of the falciform and round ligaments, which must be avoided.

on the patient's response and tolerance. The onset of either hesitant or slurred speech or horizontal nystagmus are good indications of adequate diazepam dosage.

When enlarged organs, masses, or foci of chronic pain are present, the laparoscopist may desire to mark their precise location on the abdominal skin. A felt marking pen or gentian violet on a cotton applicator is used for this.

On the evening before laparoscopy, the chest from just below the breasts and the abdomen down to the pubic escutcheon may need to be shaved. Hospital personnel specifically should be told that there is no need to shave the pubic hair. The best way to ensure against such an unnecessary shave is simply to advise the patient that it is not to be done. The skin is cleansed by scrubbing with povidone-iodine surgical scrub (Betadine) and application of a prepping solution of the same material immediately before the patient is draped in a sterile fashion.

The major difference in medical-diagnostic and surgical-therapeutic laparoscopic technique is the type of anesthetic used. Manipulation and electrosurgical alteration of pelvic structures usually are painful and, for this reason, either general anesthesia or heavy sedative-analgesia preparation is required. Laparoscopy performed primarily for visual diagnosis and biopsy of liver or peritoneum is best done with the patient awake under mild sedative-analgesic drug preparation and local anesthesia. Thousands of laparoscopies have been performed under local anesthesia for over 50 years in many countries with a

superb record of patient tolerance, safety, and diagnostic accuracy.

Local 1% anesthetic solution without epinephrine is used (Figs. 14-5A and B). A volume of about 20 ml should provide adequate anesthesia along a path 3 cm to 5 cm in diameter from skin through parietal peritoneum. The most common mistake made by the operator during injection of the local anesthetic is the anesthetizing of too small an area of parietal peritoneum. The operator should ensure that the diameter of anesthetized tissue is the same at skin and peritoneal levels. If the patient complains of any discomfort about the cannula site as the examination progresses, additional anesthetic should be injected at peritoneal level about the cannula.

The Veres needle (Figs. 14-5E, F, G) is used for pneumoperitoneum. It has a blunt, spring-loaded tip that protrudes beyond the sharp bevel of the needle when the peritoneal space is entered. In past years, room air has been used for pneumoperitoneum. Air embolism is a threat, although it is rarely reported in the large series. Experience indicates that nitrous oxide is the gas of choice for diagnostic laparoscopy done under local anesthesia and that it is best administered by an insufflation unit (Fig. 14-5H). Carbon dioxide, a noncombustible gas, is used when electrosurgery is performed under general anesthesia by the gynecologist. This gas produces painful peritoneal irritation in the patient examined under local anesthesia.

A prospective controlled trial in 92 patients has shown that nitrous oxide is definitely less pain provoking than carbon dioxide. There is other evidence that nitrous oxide is absorbed faster, has an anesthetizing effect on the peritoneum, and is less often associated with cardiac arrhythmias than is carbon dioxide.[53] Although carbon dioxide has been reported least likely to support combustion, there is now substantial experience reported that electrosurgical procedures are safely done with nitrous oxide pneumoperitoneum in patients who have neither observed nor suspected lesions of the intestines.[23] This caveat is important since no study has yet been done in such cases to evaluate for possible hydrogen leakage through gut wall into the peritoneal cavity.

The photographs in Figure 14-5 illustrate the major steps in the procedure. Details of these techniques have been previously reported and will not be reviewed here.[8]

Any physician desiring to learn laparoscopic technique should review the literature, spend some time observing an experienced operator performing the procedure, and become an avid student of normal and pathologic anatomy. Training under direct supervision of an experienced laparoscopist is the ideal and proper way to learn this technique. It is to be hoped that more gastroenterology and hepatology training programs will be improved to offer such training in the future.

Atlases prepared by Wittman,[83,84] Beck and Schaefer,[5] Bruguera, Bordas, and Rodes,[10] and Dagnini,[18] and one be Henning soon to be published, are available to assist the laparoscopist in visual diagnosis. The excellent color

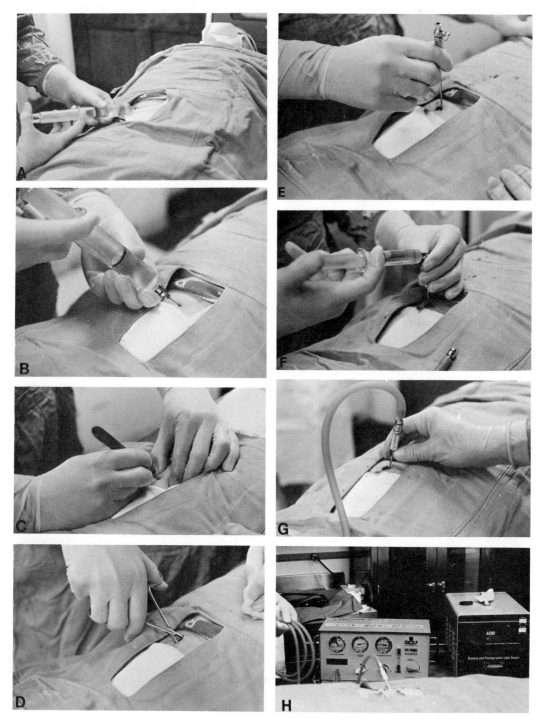

Fig. 14-5. A. Skin anesthesia using #25 gauge needle. **B.** Anesthesia of subcutaneous tissue down to and including peritoneum. **C.** Skin incision 11 mm in length using #15 surgical blade. **D.** Blunt dissection to separate subcutaneous fat. **E.** Passage of Veres needle with abdomen tense and elevated by the patient. **F.** After insertion of the pneumoperitoneum needle, gentle aspiration is attempted and followed by injection of sterile water or saline, the meniscus of which should promptly disappear down the needle by gravity if the tip is in free peritoneal space. **G.** Veres needle in position should be angled toward the horizontal to keep it out of omentum as air or nitrous oxide is injected. **H.** Insufflation unit for pneumoperitoneum is shown in background.

(Continued on facing page)

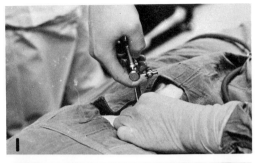

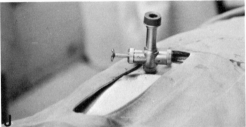

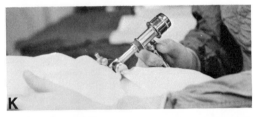

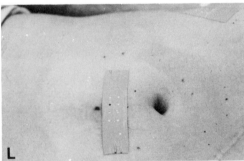

Fig. 14-5. *(Continued)* **I.** Trocar and cannula are introduced with the patient elevating and tightening the abdominal wall by Valsalva maneuver. **J.** Cannula in position with trocar removed; valve is closed to prevent loss of pneumoperitoneum. **K.** Telescope has been passed through cannula, and examination begins after fiberoptic light cable is attached. **L.** Adhesive strip covers introduction site after pneumoperitoneum is removed and skin incision closed.

photographs in these texts should be studied to learn the normal and gross pathologic anatomy that will be regularly encountered during laparoscopy. A return to anatomy and pathology texts, possibly not opened since medical school days, will reveal an amazing amount of useful information long since considered irrelevant and forgotten.

Most laparoscopists develop a routine sequence for examination. The falciform ligament is used as a starting or reference point because it is easy to locate. The examination should proceed in an orderly fashion through all quadrants, midabdomen, pelvis, and posterolateral lumbar areas, using position changes as needed. The head-up, head-down, and right and left decubitus positions are necessary for a complete examination.

A palpating-measuring probe may be passed through a second cannula to move the omentum about, to palpate the gallbladder and other organs, and to elevate the inferior liver margins for a good view. When hepatic metastases are suspected but not seen on the anterior aspect of the liver, it is imperative that a palpating probe be used to elevate the lobes and to examine their inferior surfaces. Failure to follow this procedure establishes the examination as incomplete.

On completion of the visceral examination, direct-vision liver biopsy may be done and photography used to document gross findings for correlation with histology and for teaching. A photolaparoscope (Figs. 14-2 and 14-6) is used for making superb 35-mm color transparencies, color Polaroid pictures (available in 1 minute for the clinical record), or black and white prints.

New photolaparoscopes with proximal flash from a powerful generator and ASA-400 film are proving a good combination for obtaining color transparencies of excellent quality.

The average duration of laparoscopy is 30 minutes or less for the experienced operator. Biopsy, photography, and teaching each requires an extra 10 minutes, so that, in most instances, 1 hour is sufficient time for a complete procedure.

The pneumoperitoneum is released and its expulsion aided by gentle kneading of the abdominal wall. The cannula is removed slowly to allow as much gas as possible to escape. The skin incision is closed with two 4-0 silk suture, clips, or adhesive strips.

If more than minimal ascites is present, it is best to avoid tight skin closure since the ascitic fluid may dissect through fascial planes into the abdominal wall, scrotum, or vulva when prevented from escaping through the skin incision. Usually it is difficult to suture the peritoneal opening, and generally it has proven best to cover the incision with sterile absorbent pads and allow the defect to heal secondarily. In most cases, the fluid drainage ceases in 3 to 5 days.

When no liver biopsy is done, the patient is allowed up as soon as he has recovered from premedication. Following liver biopsy, he is kept at bed rest, and vital signs are monitored for 24 hours, as is the standard procedure after blind liver biopsy.

In recent years both diagnostic and therapeutic laparoscopies are being performed as outpatient procedures, with the patient being allowed to return home the same day after an appropriate period of observation.

GUIDED LIVER BIOPSY

One of the distinct advantages of laparoscopy is its capability for biopsy of selected areas of the liver under direct

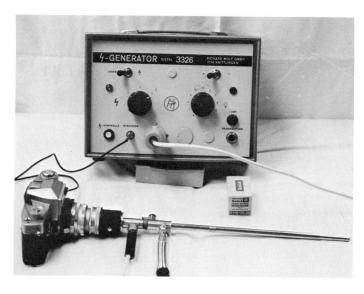

Fig. 14-6. Wolf flash generator with power cable and synchronization cable attached to the photolaparoscope and Leicaflex 35-mm camera, respectively.

visual control. Surface areas of increased vascularity, necrosis, and distended bile ducts may be avoided, and lesions far too small to be detected by physical examination, liver scan, sonography, computed tomography (CT), and arteriography may easily be biopsied. The work of Kalk and Wildhirt[40] and the reports of others[37,41,66,76–78] during the past 40 years have clearly established the simplicity, safety, and clinical value of this biopsy method.

Several types of needles may be used. The shaft of the needle must be sufficiently long to span the abdominal wall plus 6 cm to 10 cm of pneumoperitoneum. The Tru-Cut disposable biopsy needle (Travenol Laboratories) is ideal for this purpose (Fig. 14-7A). It has a 6-inch (15.2-cm) cannula and a 2-cm specimen notch in the trocar. A separate puncture site is selected subcostally as close as possible to the area to be biopsied (Fig. 14-7B). The subcostal approach is best, because passage through the pleural

space can lead to pneumothorax when pneumoperitoneum is present. In most cases, guided needle biopsy is done through the second puncture cannula, which has been used to pass the palpating wand.

After local anesthesia from skin to parietal peritoneum at the selected site, the biopsy needle is inserted through a 2-mm skin puncture, and its passage through the parietal peritoneum is observed through the laparoscope. When the needle tip is in proper position over the selected site, the patient is asked to hold his breath and the specimen is taken.

Bleeding ordinarily amounts to no more than 10 ml, and clotting can be detected at the site. If more than the expected bleeding should occur, the biopsy site may be occluded by tamponade with a blunt probe, or hemostatic agents such as topical thrombin or 1:1000 epinephrine may be injected into the site. Such artificial hemostasis

Fig. 14-7. A. Tru-Cut liver biopsy needle being passed through a second site under local anesthesia. **B.** Biopsy needle being guided by the laparoscopist under direct vision to a focal lesion in the liver.

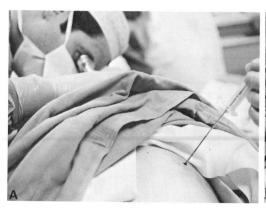
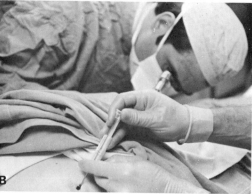

rarely has been needed in 22 years of personal experience with direct-vision biopsy.

Dagnini and co-workers have reported the routine use of a fibrin plug (Bioplug) to tamponade guided liver biopsies that are done under laparoscopic control.[19] A simple device, consisting of a cannula with a plunger, is used to discharge the cylindrical fibrin plug into the biopsy site under laparoscopic control.

We have been using a special cytology brush[47] and the Chiba needle to obtain tissue from hepatic metastases. These methods appear to have advantages in special situations, but either standard-needle or forceps biopsy remains the preferred method. Touch cytology specimens made from the liver biopsy can further improve diagnostic accuracy.[28]

GUIDED PERITONEAL BIOPSY

Direct-vision biopsy of lesions of the parietal peritoneum is performed in a fashion similar to liver biopsy by needle or, preferably, with a biopsy forceps passed through a second puncture. When lesions are large and protrude from the surface, the patient will not have pain with peritoneal biopsy. If small lesions on normal peritoneum are biopsied, the site must first be anesthetized.

OTHER ANCILLARY PROCEDURES

Other diagnostic procedures may be used in conjunction with laparoscopy, but some add additional hazards that probably outweigh their potential diagnostic benefit. These include endoscopic sonography, direct-vision cholecystocholangiography, transhepatic cholangiography, splenoportography, splenic biopsy, and portal manometry and venography of an omental vein.[85]

POSTMORTEM LAPAROSCOPY

The clinician should remember that laparoscopy may serve as a substitute when autopsy is refused by the patient's family. In this situation, laparoscopy may be acceptable, and much good information, especially about the liver, may be obtained by direct examination and biopsy. The instrument may also be used for postmortem thoracoscopy.

COMPLICATIONS

The complications one would expect from improper needle or trocar insertion into the abdomen are easy to predict and understand (Table 14-2).

The factors that most often affect the complication rates with this procedure deserve emphasis. Foremost among these is the experience of the operator. Inexperience with-

TABLE 14-2.   Complications of Laparoscopy

RELATED TO PNEUMOPERITONEUM
Subcutaneous emphysema
Mediastinal emphysema
Bleeding
Pneumothorax
Shock and/or cardiac arrest
Perforation of hollow viscus
Air embolism
Pain (abdominal and shoulder)

RELATED TO LAPAROSCOPY
Pain: usually transient and secondary to instrument
    pressure on parietal peritoneum
Bleeding
Perforation of hollow viscus
Puncture of solid organ or mass
Air embolism

RELATED TO LIVER BIOPSY
Bleeding
Bile peritonitis
Accidental puncture of abscess or hydatid cyst

out supervision in both technique and interpretation may be an awesome combination. Proper patient selection is essential for successful, uncomplicated laparoscopy. If the standard procedures recommended for patient selection, preparation, and technique are followed, the overall frequency of complications will lessen as the operator gains experience. The frequency of major complication should be quite low.

Overall complication rates reported in the literature vary between 1.2%[80] and 6%,[57] depending on whether or not an experienced operator or trainees are performing laparoscopy. Some authors, however, do not report minor complications, since they do not consider these of significance. The report by O'Kieffe and Boyce includes all complications regardless of degree (nearly all are minor) and probably reflects what one should expect in the way of complications in a training institution.[57] In their series, there were no deaths in 450 laparoscopies, and in only 1% of the procedures was the patient's hospital stay prolonged by complications.

Mortality rates for laparoscopy are low when compared with those for other major diagnostic procedures. Bruehl's review of 63,845 laparoscopies performed by 67 physicians revealed 1,594 complications (2.5%) and 19 deaths (0.029%),[9] certainly acceptable rates for a major diagnostic procedure. It is important to note, however, that this mortality rate is likely to be as much related to the 48,766 liver biopsies performed in these patients as to the laparoscopic procedures per se. Many of the reported instances of significant morbidity and mortality associated with laparoscopic technique are probably related to liver biopsy. It is to be hoped that future reports will provide an analysis indicating whether the complication was related to drug preparation, pneumoperitoneum, trocar insertion and laparoscopy, liver biopsy, or other associated procedures. Any physician who performs laparoscopy should have read all of the available reports concerning the complications of this procedure. Only selected references on complications can be included here.[9,50,57,60,62,63,65,66,80,83,87]

CLINICAL VALUE

Laparoscopy is an established method for abdominal examination, intermediate in complexity and safety between routine physical examination and exploratory surgical laparotomy. Modern techniques and instrumentation have progressively improved both its safety and its diagnostic capability. Although acceptance and application of laparoscopy in this country have lagged behind its extensive use in Europe and other areas of the world, it is now being introduced in many hospitals because its superb diagnostic and therapeutic advantages are finally being appreciated.

Laparoscopy was not available in many hospitals in the United States until the technique of laparoscopic tubal sterilization, popularized by Steptoe of England, was accepted as the simplest and safest method available.[74] The gynecologic literature on this subject has expanded rapidly and should be familiar to all who perform laparoscopy.

The indications for laparoscopy will expand as the physician using it gains experience and confidence. It seems wise for the internist to use laparoscopy in a medical setting in order for its diagnostic potential to be realized. The internist-gastroenterologist gains most for his patients by observation and direct-vision biopsy, while the gynecologist or surgeon is prepared by his training and experience to expand the indications to include therapeutic measures.

Examination of the liver and guided liver and peritoneal biopsy are the major advantages laparoscopy provides for the internist.[1,4] Hepatomegaly, jaundice, abnormal hepatic radioisotope scans, and abnormal liver tests appear in varied clinical situations and often require investigation beyond the usual blind liver biopsy for accurate evaluation. The fact that blind biopsy provides only a fraction of the hepatic mass for examination is well known, but the diagnostic deficiencies of blind liver biopsy have not yet been recognized by most physicians. About 10% of hepatic metastases are not in view of the laparoscope, while over 42% of metastases[15] and 67% of cases of macronodular cirrhosis[72] are not accurately diagnosed with blind liver biopsy alone.

One blind postmortem liver biopsy in patients who died of carcinoma revealed hepatic metastasis in less than 50% of those who were proven at autopsy to have metastases.[15] This report also revealed that a second blind liver biopsy increased the diagnostic yield to only 58%. Therefore, metastatic carcinoma in the liver likely will be missed by two blind biopsies in at least 40% of patients.

Jori and Peschle reported a 39.5% positive result for blind biopsy in patients suspected of having hepatic malignancy, whereas guided liver biopsy under laparoscopic control yielded a positive diagnosis in 69%.[37] When biopsy results by both methods were combined, the diagnosis of hepatic malignancy increased to 75%. The remaining 12 patients (25%) of the 48 studied were negative by both methods and presumed to have no hepatic metastases. This report indicates a much higher blind biopsy yield for primary hepatic carcinoma (70%) than for metastatic lesions (31%), a finding apparently not recognized in earlier investigations. Metastatic lesions are usually much smaller than clinically apparent hepatocellular carcinomas and therefore are less likely to be included in a blind biopsy specimen. Vilardell has reviewed the value of laparoscopy in the diagnosis of hepatocellular carcinoma.[81]

It has been estimated that about 10% of the livers proven later to contain metastases will have hidden metastases either deep within the liver substance or on the posterior surface with no chance of being detected by laparoscopy.[64] This 10% false-negative diagnosis rate for hepatic metastases is far superior to the 42% false-negative rate for metastatic carcinoma obtained when two blind liver biopsies are done.[15]

Most clinicians consider blind biopsy of the left liver lobe unsafe and, hence, lesions in this area may require a direct-vision or scan-directed biopsy approach. For this purpose, laparoscopy clearly is preferred over laparotomy. Whitcomb and co-workers have reported excellent results with laparoscopic-guided biopsy for diagnosis of left lobe lesions.[82]

Laparoscopy is of exceptional value to the patient with an extrahepatic malignancy who is scheduled for major surgery and particularly to the patient with no primary indication for laparotomy. Foremost among such patients are those with an intrathoracic or other malignant neoplasm who have an abnormality of the liver on physical examination, biochemical tests, radioisotope, sonographic, or CT scan. Appropriate therapy depends on whether hepatic metastases are present. If the patient with suspected liver metastases happens to be an alcoholic or has a past history of hepatic disease of a nonmalignant type, the problem is further compounded, but laparoscopy usually provides an accurate diagnosis. Laparoscopy can resolve this diagnostic dilemma in at least 90% of patients and thereby save them the discomfort and risks of a laparotomy.[64,68,76]

Another consideration is the frequency of hepatic metastases in patients who are known to have a malignancy but in whom there is no clinical evidence of liver involvement. Conn and Yesner found metastatic carcinoma in 20% of patients examined postmortem who had no antemortem clinical evidence of liver metastases.[16] Since their report, liver scans, and, more recently, sonography and CT scans have come into wide use and are helpful in diagnosis of metastases in such patients. These studies may also assist in the performance and accuracy of blind biopsy when metastases are of sufficiently large size to be detected and are within reach of the needle. However, these scans cannot be expected to detect lesions of less than 1 cm to 1.5 cm in diameter unless hepatic involvement is extensive. Metastatic lesions as small as 1 mm to 2 mm in diameter can be seen and biopsied under laparoscopic control.

Although the radioisotope liver scan has low specificity for metastatic neoplasms, it has been shown by Lightdale and associates to be a good screening study.[46] Radioisotope scans, sonography, and CT scans may provide information that is helpful by showing probable tumor location. This information may assist the laparoscopist in selecting the insertion site for the laparoscope and for biopsy of deep lesions when no surface metastases are present.

Currently the noninvasive scanning methods, sonography and CT, are used as the initial procedure(s) of choice to examine for focal hepatic lesions.[26,49] Improvements in equipment and guided biopsy methods have made ultrasound- and CT-directed biopsy the preferred approach for obvious hepatic metastases. They often are successful in revealing abnormalities suggestive of metastases but are diagnostic only when scan-guided needle biopsy provides a conclusive diagnosis. However, there are many patients with small, widely scattered metastases, fatty infiltration, cirrhosis, and benign hepatic tumors whose hepatic scans are equivocal or normal. These patients are best evaluated by laparoscopy with or without guided biopsy. Laparoscopy remains the most accurate method for diagnosis of small focal hepatic lesions, such as metastases and hemangiomas, cirrhosis, and peritoneal diseases. Studies using both CT scans and laparoscopy are in progress and should clarify the relative value of these methods for diagnosis of hepatic, peritoneal, and other abdominal disorders.

In 1983 Danielson and co-workers reported a retrospective record review comparison between CT and laparoscopy.[21] They reported sensitivity for detection of metastases to be 89% for CT and 62% for laparoscopy. This poor result for laparoscopy is lower than any reported in the literature and is more than worthy of challenge. The most bothersome aspect of this report is the likelihood of a nonstandardized and incomplete technique used for diagnostic laparoscopy. Any evaluation of laparoscopic accuracy for metastases to the liver must include use of a probe for moving the liver to examine the inferior surfaces. This report makes no mention of technique or use of such a palpating probe.

Ultrasonic laparoscopes are under investigation. The merit of the method is its ability to permit localization of lesions deep within the liver and serve as a guide for biopsy. High-resolution images are possible because the probe is applied directly to the liver surface. This technique also allows differentiation between hemangioma and hepatocellular carcinoma based on their sonographic features.[25]

Bleiberg and co-workers have reported on the use of laparoscopy to monitor the response of hepatic metastases to chemotherapy.[7] Direct observation with guided liver biopsy proved useful for documenting an objective response to treatment.

Laparoscopy has been shown of value in staging both Hodgkin's disease and non-Hodgkin's lymphoma.[2,14,73] For this purpose, laparoscopy again has proven more accurate than blind liver biopsy and safer than laparotomy.

Cirrhosis in patients with evidence of chronic active liver disease is often not detected by blind biopsy. Soloway and co-workers report a sampling error in their series in 67% of patients with previously proven macronodular cirrhosis. Confirmation of known cirrhosis by simultaneous or sequential blind biopsies was made in only 33% of their cases.[72] Vido and Wildhirt reported that blind liver biopsy failed to demonstrate cirrhosis in 51% of 254 patients in whom the diagnosis was made at laparoscopy.[79]

In 1982, Nord presented an excellent review of the literature comparing accuracy of blind versus laparoscopic-guided biopsy for diagnosis of cirrhosis.[55]

The sampling error in diagnosis of cirrhosis is significant, and only by observation of the liver surface and guided biopsy can this type of hepatic disease be accurately diagnosed. Ruddock reported 95.5% accuracy in the laparoscopic diagnosis of proven cases of cirrhosis, compared with 73.5% clinical accuracy in the same patients.[64] In addition, he found 84 clinical misdiagnoses of cirrhosis. Among these 84 patients were 50 with malignancy and 15 with normal livers confirmed by laparoscopy.

Kuster reported a high incidence of incorrect prelaparoscopic diagnoses (52.1%) in a series of 140 patients examined for obscure abdominal conditions not diagnosed by other examinations.[45] He also found 97.9% of the laparoscopic diagnoses correct when compared by biopsy, cholangiography, surgery, or autopsy.

The differential diagnosis between intrahepatic cholestasis and extrahepatic obstruction is crucial in the jaundiced patient. The newest and currently preferred initial procedures for diagnosis of extrahepatic jaundice are sonography and/or CT scan, percutaneous transhepatic cholangiography, or endoscopic retrograde cholangiography. Since these methods have proven safe and reliable, there is often no need for laparoscopy. However, if proof of abdominal metastases would influence decisions on further therapy, then laparoscopy may provide significant help.[17,76] Laparoscopic help for this problem will depend on the finding of an enlarged gallbladder or metastatic tumor. The appearance of the liver may be identical in both types of jaundice, unless an extrahepatic obstruction is of long standing, in which case dilated biliary ducts over the liver surface provide a diagnostic clue. When a collapsed, otherwise normal gallbladder is found, the laparoscopist can state that the cause of the jaundice is either intrahepatic or, less likely, extrahepatic due to obstruction of the common hepatic duct that prevents bile from reaching the gallbladder. Cholangiography by either the percutaneous transhepatic or endoscopic retrograde technique usually will resolve this problem efficiently.[62]

Hitanant and associates have reported 108 cases of liver abscess in a series of 4569 laparoscopies.[32] Eighty percent were in males, 73% were in the right lobe, 12% were in both lobes, 67% were amebic, 20% were pyogenic, and 12% were of unclassified etiology. Hepatic and perihepatic changes observed at laparoscopy were classified into six groups. These investigators claim that when needle aspiration is indicated the direct-vision laparoscopy-guided approach is the most safe and effective.

Laparoscopy should not be considered a substitute for laparotomy, since the purpose of these procedures should be different. When the limitations of laparoscopy are understood and the usual clinical evaluation suggests that a diagnosis is within the capability of laparoscopy, it should be considered the procedure of choice for reasons of comfort, safety, expense, and known diagnostic accuracy for the suspected condition.

There is considerable evidence in the literature to support the belief that, when properly applied, laparoscopy will permit exploratory laparotomy to be avoided in 43% to 70% of cases in which the two procedures have a common goal.[31,64,66] Trujillo emphasized the value of laparoscopy in 102 patients who had undergone all of the usual diagnostic studies for obscure abdominal diseases (including blind liver biopsy in nonjaundiced patients, if liver disease was suspected) and in whom exploratory laparotomy was considered the only other means of diagnosis.[76] Laparoscopy with guided liver biopsy obviated the need for surgical laparotomy in 92 of the 102 patients. In a series of 406 laparoscopies performed for gynecologic indications, Buckle and Grimewade reported that laparotomy was avoided in 120 patients.[11] On the other hand, diagnostic help from laparoscopy that confirms or changes a clinical diagnosis may be of value in preventing unnecessary delay when specific medical or surgical therapy is indicated.

In 1984, Dagnini and co-workers reported laparoscopic findings in 98 cases of primary carcinoma of the gallbladder.[20] Cano-Ruiz and colleagues described laparoscopic findings in seven patients with nodular regenerative hyperplasia of the liver in 1985.[12]

Other uses for diagnostic laparoscopy include the evaluation of ascites possibly due to peritoneal metastases or tuberculous peritonitis, splenomegaly, abdominal masses, congenital abnormalities of the female pelvic organs, ectopic pregnancies, infertility, chronic abdominal and pelvic pain, acute pelvic inflammatory disease, and various other gynecologic disorders.[3,13,34,36,61,66,67,69,74,75,77,86]

Meyer-Burg reported success with laparoscopy for the diagnosis of disease of the pancreas, an organ previously believed inaccessible to this procedure.[51,52] He visualized parts of the pancreas in 81 of 125 patients.[52] In order for this technique to be successful, the left lobe of the liver must be elevated by a probe and the gastrohepatic omentum must be tissue-paper thin to permit a view of portions of the pancreas.

Diagnostic success with laparoscopy depends primarily on proper clinical use of the procedure and the experience of the operator. It should follow in logical sequence after thorough clinical, laboratory, and radiographic studies, and perhaps blind liver biopsy, have failed to provide a satisfactory diagnosis. Anatomic limitations must be understood so that the procedure will not be expected to accomplish the impossible.

Laparoscopy is adaptable to either a medical or a surgical setting, but, in most situations, it is far more simply and inexpensively performed in the endoscopy room. Although it is in a sense diagnostically competitive with exploratory laparotomy, it is rare to find a well-informed internist or surgeon who does not welcome laparoscopy as the better first procedure to safely and promptly resolve diagnostic problems involving the peritoneum, liver, and other accessible abdominal organs.

REFERENCES

1. Anderson DA et al: Laparoscopy in hepatology. In Berci G (ed): Endoscopy, p 401. New York, Appleton-Century-Crofts, 1976
2. Anderson T et al: Peritoneoscopy: A technique to evaluate therapeutic efficacy in non-Hodgkin's lymphoma patients. Cancer Treat Rep 61:1017, 1977
3. Aronson AR, Parker GW: Peritoneoscopy: Its value as a diagnostic aid. Am J Dig Dis 5:931, 1960
4. Barry RE et al. Physicians use of laparoscopy. Br Med J 2:1276, 1977
5. Beck K, Schaefer HJ: Color atlas of laparoscopy. Stuttgart, FK Schattauer, 1970
6. Bernheim BM: Organoscopy: Cystoscopy of the abdominal cavity. Ann Surg 53:764, 1911
7. Bleiberg H et al: Peritoneoscopic evaluation of the effect of chemotherapeutic agents on liver metastases of breast cancer. Endoscopy 8:217, 1976
8. Boyce HW Jr, Palmer ED: Techniques of Clinical Gastroenterology. Springfield, IL, Charles C Thomas, 1975
9. Bruehl W: Incidence of complications during laparoscopy and liver puncture under direct vision: Results of a survey. Dtsch Med Wochenschr 91:2297, 1966
10. Bruguera M et al: Atlas of Laparoscopy and Biopsy of the Liver. Philadelphia, WB Saunders, 1979
11. Buckle AER, Grimwade JC: Clinical use of the laparoscope. Postgrad Med J 46:593, 1970
12. Cano-Ruiz A et al: Laparoscopic findings in seven patients with nodular regenerative hyperplasia of the liver. Am J Gastroenterol 80:796, 1985
13. Cohen MR: Culdoscopy versus peritoneoscopy. Obstet Gynecol 31:310, 1968
14. Coleman M et al: Peritoneoscopy in Hodgkin's disease. JAMA 236:2634, 1976
15. Conn HO: Editorial: Percutaneous versus peritoneoscopic liver biopsy. Gastroenterology 63:1074, 1972
16. Conn HO, Yesner R: A re-evaluation of needle biopsy in the diagnosis of metastatic cancer of the liver. Ann Intern Med 59:53, 1963
17. Cuschieri A: Value of laparoscopy in hepatobiliary disease. Ann R Coll Surg Engl, 57:33, 1975

18. Dagnini G: Clinical Laparoscopy. Padua, Picciu, 1980
19. Dagnini G et al: Tamponamento per via laparoscopica con spugna di fibrina negli incidenti da biopsia d'organo. Giorn Ital End Dig 4:339, 1981
20. Dagnini G et al: Laparoscopy in the diagnosis of primary carcinoma of the gallbladder: A study of 98 cases. Gastrointest Endosc 30:289, 1984
21. Danielson KS et al: Computed tomography and peritoneoscopy for detection of liver metastases: Review of Mayo Clinic experience. J Comput Assist Tomogr 7:230, 1983
22. Devita VT Jr et al: Peritoneoscopy in the staging of Hodgkin's disease. Cancer Res 31:1746, 1971
23. Drummond GB et al: Laparoscopy explosion hazards with nitrous oxide. Br Med J 1:586, 1976
24. Duignan NM et al: One thousand consecutive cases of diagnostic laparoscopy. J Obstet Gynaecol Br Commonw 79:1016, 1972
25. Fukuda M et al: Endoscopic sonography of the liver: Diagnostic application of the echolaparoscope to localize intrahepatic lesions. Scand J Gastroenterol 19(suppl 102):24, 1984
26. Gandolfi L et al: Indications for laparoscopy before and after the introduction of ultrasonography. Gastrointest Endosc 31:1, 1985
27. Gomel V: Laparoscopy in general surgery. Am J Surg 131:319, 1976
28. Grossman E et al: Cytological examination as an adjunct to liver biopsy in the diagnosis of hepatic metastases. Gastroenterology 62:56, 1972
29. Hegstrom GL et al: Peritoneoscopy. Gastroenterology 25:243, 1953
30. Henning N: Ein neues Lararoskop. Dtsch Z Verdau Stoffwechselkr 10:49, 1950
31. Herrera-Llerandi R: Peritoneoscopy: Endoscopic refinement par excellence. Br Med J 2:661, 1961
32. Hitanant S et al: Peritoneoscopy in the diagnosis of liver abscess. Gastrointest Endosc 30:235, 1984
33. Jacobaeus HC: Ueber Laparo- und Thorakoskopie. Beitr Klin Erforsch Tuberk 25:183, 1912
34. Jacobson L, Eström L: Objectivized diagnosis of acute pelvic inflammatory disease. Am J Obstet Gynecol 105:1088, 1969
35. Johnston IDA, Rodgers HW: Peritoneoscopy as an aid to diagnosis. Gut 5:485, 1964
36. Jori GP, Mazzacca G: Peritoneoscopic features of intra-abdominal vessels in cirrhosis of the liver. Gut 12:237, 1971
37. Jori GP, Peschle C: Combined peritoneoscopy and liver biopsy in diagnosis of hepatic neoplasm. Gastroenterology 63:1016, 1972
38. Kalk H: Erfahrungen mit der Laparoskopie (zugleich mit Beischreibung eines neuen Instrumentes). Z Klin Med 111:303, 1929
39. Kalk H, Bruhl W: Leitfaden der Laparoskopie und Gastroskopie, p 159. Stuttgart, Georg Thieme Verlag, 1951
40. Kalk H, Wildhirt E: Lehrbuch und Atlas der Laparoskopie und Leberpunktion, p 247. Stuttgart, Georg Thieme Verlag, 1961
41. Keil PG et al: Evaluation of the liver biopsy. Ann Intern Med 36:1278, 1952
42. Kelling G: Ueber Oesophagoscopie: Gastroskopie, und Koelioskopie. München Med Wochenschr 49:21, 1902
43. Kelling G: Ueber die Moeglichkeit, die Zystoskopie bei Undersuchungen seröser Hoehlungen anzuwenden. Munchen Med Wochenschr 57:2358, 1910
44. Korbsch R: Die Laparoskopie nach Jacobaeus. Berlin Klin Wochenschr 58:696, 1921
45. Kuster G, Biel F: Accuracy of laparoscopic diagnosis. Am J Med 42:388, 1966
46. Lightdale CJ et al: Laparoscopic diagnosis of suspected liver neoplasms. Dig Dis Sci 24:588, 1979
47. Lightdale CJ, Hajdu SI: Brush cytology of the liver and peritoneum at laparoscopy. Gastrointest Endosc 24:169, 1976
48. Loffer FD, Pent D: Laparoscopy in the obese patient. Am J Obstet Gynecol 125:104, 1976
49. Mansi C et al: Comparison between laparoscopy, ultrasonography, and computed tomography in widespread and localized liver diseases. Gastrointest Endosc 28:83, 1982
50. McQuaide JR: Air embolism during peritoneoscopy. S Afr Med J 46:422, 1972
51. Meyer-Burg J: The inspection, palpation and biopsy of the pancreas by peritoneoscopy. Endoscopy 4:99, 1972
52. Meyer-Burg J, Ziegler U: Supragastric pancreography. Dtsch Med Wochenschr 97:1969, 1972
53. Minoli G et al: The influence of carbon dioxide and nitrous oxide on pain during laparoscopy: A double-blind, controlled trial. Gastrointest Endosc 28:173, 1982
54. Neuwirth RS: Laparoscopy. Clin Obstet Gynecol 12:514, 1969
55. Nord HJ: Biopsy diagnosis of cirrhosis: Blind percutaneous versus guided direct vision techniques: A review. Gastrointest Endosc 28:102, 1982
56. Nordentoeft S: Ueber Endoscopie geschlossener Hohlem. Dtsch Med Wochenschr 39:1840, 1913
57. O'Kieffe DA, Boyce HW Jr: Peritoneoscopy: Has this procedure come of age? Med Ann DC 41:437, 1972
58. Orndoff BH: Peritoneoscope, pneumoperitoneum and x-rays in abdominal diagnosis. Ill Med J 39:61, 1921
59. Ott DO: Ventroscopic illumination of the abdominal cavity during pregnancy. Z Akus I Zhensk Bolezn, 1901
60. Palmer ED: Hemoperitoneum following peritoneoscopy without biopsy. Bull Gastrointest Endosc 10:7, 1963
61. Reichert JA, Valle RF: Fitz-Hugh-Curtis syndrome. JAMA 236:266, 1976
62. Royer M et al: Peritoneoscopic cholangiography with manometric control. Gastroenterology 26:626, 1954
63. Ruddock JC: Peritoneoscopy. West J Surg Obstet Gynecol 42:392, 1934
64. Ruddock JC: Peritoneoscopy. Southern Surgeon 8:113, 1939
65. Ruddock JC: The application and evaluation of peritoneoscopy: Review of 2,500 cases. Calif Med 71:110, 1949
66. Ruddock JC: Peritoneoscopy: A critical clinical review. Surg Clin North Am 37:1249, 1957
67. Ruddock JC, Hope RB: Coccidioidal peritonitis: Diagnosis by peritoneoscopy. JAMA 113:2054, 1939
68. Scott PJ et al: Benefits and hazards of laparotomy for medical patients. Lancet 2:941, 1970
69. Siegler AM: Trends in laparoscopy. Am J Obstet Gynecol 109:794, 1971
70. Smith VM: Clinical peritoneoscopy. Am J Gastroenterol 42:13, 1964
71. Smith VM, Cuevas AP: Peritoneoscopy and abdominal adhesions: Intentional perforation to improve visibility. Gastrointest Endosc 15:142, 1969
72. Soloway RD et al: Observer error and sampling variability tested in evaluation of hepatitis and cirrhosis by liver biopsy. Am J Dig Dis 16:1082, 1971

73. Spinelli P et al: Laparoscopy and laparotomy combined with bone marrow biopsy in staging Hodgkin's disease. Br Med J 4:554, 1975

74. Steptoe PC: Laparoscopy in Gynaecology, p 104. London, E & S Livingstone, 1967

75. Trujillo NP: Peritoneoscopy: A useful diagnostic technique. Med Ann DC 40:297, 1971

76. Trujillo NP: Peritoneoscopy and guided biopsy in the diagnosis of intra-abdominal disease. Gastroenterology 71:1083, 1976

77. Uhlich GA: Liver biopsy in the diagnosis of hepatic cancer. Gastroenterology 63:208, 1972

78. Uhlich GA, Haubrich WS: Laparoscopy (peritoneoscopy) and guided liver biopsy: II. Am J Gastroenterol 38:313, 1962

79. Vido I, Wildhirt E: Korrelation des laparoskopischen und histologischen Befundes bei chronischer Hepatitis und Leberzirrhose. Dtsch Med Wochenschr 94:1633, 1969

80. Vilardell F et al: Complications of peritoneoscopy: A survey of 1455 examinations. Gastrointest Endosc 14:178, 1968

81. Vilardell F: The value of laparoscopy in the diagnosis of primary cancer of the liver. Endoscopy 9:20, 1977

82. Whitcomb FF et al: Peritoneoscopy for the diagnosis of left lobe lesions of the liver. JAMA 138:126, 1978

83. Wittman I: Peritoneoscopy, vol I, p 171. Budapest, Akdemiai Kiado, 1966

84. Wittman I: Peritoneoscopy, vol II, p 187. Budapest, Akdemiai Kiado, 1966

85. Yamato S, Reynolds TB: Portal venography and pressure measurement at peritoneoscopy. Gastroenterology 64:602, 1964

86. Zoeckler SJ et al: Peritoneoscopy in malignant lesions of the abdomen. JAMA 152:1617, 1953

87. Zoeckler SJ: Peritoneoscopy: A reevaluation. Gastroenterology 34:969, 1958

chapter 15
Viral Hepatitis

RAYMOND S. KOFF and JOHN T. GALAMBOS

Viral hepatitis may be defined as a systemic viral infection in which hepatic cell necrosis and hepatic inflammation are responsible for a characteristic constellation of clinical, biochemical, immunoserologic, and morphologic features. It is caused by at least six viral agents with distinctive immunoserologic characteristics and specific epidemiologic attributes. The etiologically separate forms are called hepatitis A, hepatitis B, hepatitis D (delta hepatitis), and non-A, non-B viral hepatitis and indicate infection by hepatitis A virus (HAV), hepatitis B virus (HBV), hepatitis D virus (HDV), and the non-A, non-B hepatitis viruses (of which there appear to be three), respectively. Specific serologic identification of the two blood-borne forms of non-A, non-B hepatitis and the epidemic (fecal-oral) form of non-A, non-B hepatitis is not currently available.

Hepatic injury produced by other viruses is not described in this chapter; it differs from viral hepatitis in that, in general, clinical manifestations due to involvement of other organs are more prominent and more common than evidence of liver damage. In most instances the liver damage associated with these infections is trivial or entirely escapes clinical recognition, although occasionally it may be severe.

HISTORY

Hepatitis A

Outbreaks of jaundice were described as early as the fifth century BC in Babylonia, and the term *epidemic jaundice* appeared in the writings of Hippocrates in Greece.[166] Considerable circumstantial evidence supports the notion that hepatitis A has been a regular concomitant of warfare through recorded history.[190,381,931] The viral etiology of hepatitis was postulated by the first decade of the 20th century.[649,650] In 1912, acute yellow atrophy (now recognized as massive hepatic necrosis) was suggested to be a severe form of hepatitis (epidemic jaundice), which by then was distinguishable from Weil's disease.[166]

The development of percutaneous needle biopsy in the 1930s focused on the central role of hepatic parenchymal necrosis and inflammation in all forms of viral hepatitis. Early experiences with jaundice in clinical practice suggested that infectious jaundice was transmitted by person-to-person contact and that the incubation period was several weeks long.[767] During and after World War II human transmission experiments were undertaken. These indicated the existence of distinct agents with characteristic incubation periods, routes of transmission, and infectivity and provided a firm basis for understanding hepatitis A. In 1947, MacCallum suggested that the virus of infectious hepatitis should be called virus A.[605] The hepatitis A virus itself was discovered by immune electron microscopy in 1973.[275]

Hepatitis B and Non-A, Non-B Hepatitis

These two etiologic forms of viral hepatitis may be considered together because they share many historical, epidemiologic, and clinical characteristics. A form of viral hepatitis that was transmitted by direct inoculation of human blood or its derivatives cannot be identified before 1883.[481,603] Epidemiologic experience with postvaccinal jaundice culminated in 1941 when pooled human serum in vaccine produced by the United States Army caused at least 28,585 icteric cases.[480] The actual total was probably much larger.[752] Convalescent pooled serum for treatment or prevention of infectious diseases caused several epidemics.[73,616,787]

In 1947, MacCallum suggested that the virus that gives rise to serum hepatitis should be called virus B.[605] Throughout the 1950s and early 1960s the epidemiology of parenterally transmitted hepatitis was extensively studied, and a number of important human transmission studies were performed.

A new era in the history of viral hepatitis began with the discovery of Australia antigen by Blumberg and colleagues in 1963.[98] Confirmation of the existence of a third etiologic form of viral hepatitis required the development of specific methods to identify both hepatitis A and B. When this was achieved in the middle of the 1970s, non-A, non-B viral hepatitis was accepted as a third etiologic entity. Although there are probably at least three non-A, non-B hepatitis agents (two blood-borne and one epidemic form), the precise number remains controversial.[124]

Hepatitis D

Hepatitis D virus (HDV), or the delta virus, was first recognized in the mid-1970s in Turin, Italy. A nuclear antigen was detected in the livers of patients infected with HBV that clearly was not part of the antigenic component of HBV. Subsequently, evidence accumulated during the late 1970s that defined the delta agent as one distinct from HBV. This virus measured 35 nm to 37 nm and contained an inner core composed of delta antigen with an RNA genome and an outer cortex made up of hepatitis B surface antigen (HBsAg). The nucleotide sequence of HDV genome showed no similarity to any known RNA sequences. Furthermore, HDV was devoid of reverse transcriptase. This virus was infectious to experimental animals only if they carried HBsAg or, in the case of an eastern woodchuck, the woodchuck hepatitis virus, an agent that is analogous to human HBV. Whether there is an animal reservoir of HDV that can infect humans is theoretically possible but has not yet been documented. At first, delta hepatitis appeared to be confined to Italy, but subsequently, HDV infection was detected worldwide.[826,827]

ETIOLOGY

Identification and Transmissibility

McDonald had predicted a viral etiology for epidemic jaundice early in the 20th century.[649,650] Failure to identify a responsible bacterial agent led, in the 1920s and 1930s, to several attempts to transmit infection and isolate the etiologic agent by inoculating laboratory animals and embryonated hen's eggs with blood, nasopharyngeal washings, feces, and urine. These were uniformly unsuccessful.

Nevertheless an infectious etiology was strongly suggested by the fact that disease occurred in epidemic form. Transmission to a laboratory worker who worked with serum from a known case was reported in 1931.[289] Apparent transmission by a blood transfusion was observed by Yunet and Yunet in 1938.[1096]

The first experimental transmission may have been achieved by Japanese workers in 1940.[1091] Yoshibumi and Shigemoto administered filtered samples of blood, urine, and pharyngeal secretions to 20 children. Three of 10 subjects inoculated with blood developed jaundice 8, 11, and 23 days later. The unusually short incubation periods in two of the three cases, as well as mention of epidemic jaundice being prevalent in the area, create uncertainty about the validity of this work.

Comprehensive work to characterize adequately the etiology of epidemic and other forms of jaundice was carried out by British and American teams of investigators. Their work is the basis of present concepts, to which few significant additions were made until serologic tests were found in the late 1960s. MacCallum and co-workers in England, Havens and colleagues in New Haven, and Neefe and associates in Philadelphia identified two agents (HAV and HBV) having filterability characteristics as well as other properties consistent with those of viruses. The clinical illness and pathologic changes they produced were identical, but their epidemiologic behavior differed. Detailed immunoserologic characterization of hepatitis A and

B in the 1970s resulted in the recognition of other etiologic forms—non-A, non-B viral hepatitis and hepatitis D.

Terminology

Out of the etiologic clarification that emerged from the British and American experiments in World War II came the designations *infectious* and *serum* hepatitis. The term *infectious* hepatitis had been used for the etiologic form characterized by readily demonstrated fecal excretion, oral infectivity with the same incubation period observed after percutaneous administration, and community-wide epidemics due to person-to-person transmission. The term *serum* hepatitis had designated the etiologic form characterized by lack of fecal infectivity, negative evidence for transmission by the oral route, and the occurrence of epidemics only in instances of identifiable percutaneous exposure. The two types of infectious hepatitis described by Krugman and co-workers were actually the same as the classically delineated etiologic forms[545]; these investigators termed both *infectious* to emphasize their evidence for a low level of infectivity of *serum* hepatitis by mouth.

In proposing the names *infectious* and *serum* hepatitis, Neefe and co-workers in 1946 recognized the possibility that these etiologic terms would be confounded with epidemiologic background in instances in which both agents could be transmitted by a particular mechanism.[706] Their prediction was accurate. Review of cases reported in the 1960s as serum hepatitis revealed that most had a history of transfusion, not necessarily with an incubation period of 50 days or more, or a background of illicit self-injection.[671] Although infectious hepatitis was sometimes diagnosed on the basis of an appropriate setting, it was more often an assumption. For sporadic cases a specific diagnosis was seldom justified.

Experimental studies in World War II demonstrated that infectious hepatitis could be transmitted by injection of serum, as would be expected for any systemic viral infection. Serum hepatitis, therefore, could not be considered etiologically specific.

MacCallum's proposal that the terms *infectious hepatitis virus* and *serum hepatitis virus* be replaced by *hepatitis A* and *hepatitis B* was adopted in 1952 by the First Expert Committee on Hepatitis of the World Health Organization,[265] but there was limited acceptance of this nomenclature. When it was suggested that *Australia antigen* (now termed HBsAg) was actually specific for hepatitis B,[735,780] confusion resulted from the positive tests that occurred in cases diagnosed clinically as "infectious" hepatitis.[180,350,1085] It was for this reason that most investigators used the more noncommittal designation of *hepatitis-associated antigen* (HAA). The specificity of HBsAg for hepatitis B and consistent negativity in epidemiologically well-defined cases of hepatitis A have subsequently been amply demonstrated.[59,148,345,679] The presence of specific serologic markers of acute hepatitis A infection in epidemiologically bona fide cases of hepatitis A and their absence in serologically defined hepatitis B and epidemiologically defined non-A, non-B viral hepatitis cases, indicate that the term *HAA* is meaningless and should now be abandoned. There is no longer any rationale for the clinical diagnosis of infectious or serum hepatitis.

Other terms sometimes used as synonyms include *short incubation period* and *long incubation period* hepatitis, and *MS-1* and *MS-2* hepatitis. The distinction in incubation periods was based on the fact that there is relatively little overlap between the incubation periods of hepatitis A and B. However, the incubation period of non-A, non-B viral hepatitis encompasses that of both hepatitis A and B. Because incubation period does not therefore provide a consistent distinction, it is an unsuitable basis for nomenclature.

Etiologic Entities

Viral characteristics, serologic markers, patterns of immunity, susceptibility in nonhuman primates, and certain salient epidemiologic and clinical features, which are shown in Table 15-1, provide the current basis for distinction among the recognized etiologic entities of viral hepatitis.

Distinguishing viral characteristics include the size of the agents and their nucleic acid composition. HAV is smaller than HBV, and HAV is an RNA virus whereas HBV is a DNA virus. HDV, which is encapsulated by an outer coat of HBsAg, is a defective RNA virus that requires the helper function of HBV for its replication and expres-

TABLE 15-1.   Bases for the Differentiation of the Etiologic Forms of Viral Hepatitis

FEATURE	HEPATITIS A	HEPATITIS B	NON-A, NON-B VIRAL HEPATITIS	HEPATITIS D (DELTA HEPATITIS)
Viral characteristic				
Size of the virus	27 nm	42 nm	?20–37 nm	35–37 nm
Nucleic acid	RNA	DNA	Unknown	RNA
Serologic features				
Markers of hepatitis A	Yes	No	No	No
Markers of hepatitis B	No	Yes	No	Yes
Incubation period				
Range	15–49 days	28–160 days	15–160 days*	28–140 days
Mean	30 days	70–80 days	50 days†	?
Patterns of immunity				
Heterologous immunity	No	No	No	No
Homologous immunity	Yes	Yes	Second attacks may indicate two distinct agents	Unknown
Susceptible nonhuman primates				
Chimpanzees	Yes	Yes	Yes	HBsAg carriers
Marmosets	Yes	No	Yes	No
Epidemiologic features				
Infection by oral route	Yes	Experimentally demonstrated but low level	Epidemic form	Unknown
Viral excretion in feces	Yes	No	Epidemic form	Unknown
Fecal-oral transmission	Yes	No	Epidemic form	Unknown
Percutaneous transmission	Rare	Yes	Yes (bloodborne form)	Yes
Carrier state	No	Yes	Yes (bloodborne form)	Yes
Clinical features				
Risk of chronic hepatitis	No	Yes	Yes (bloodborne form)	Yes
Risk of primary hepatocellular carcinoma	No	Yes	Unknown	Unknown
Case-fatality rate	0.1–0.2%	Variable (0.3–37%) Mean 1%	Variable but lower than hepatitis B	Variable but higher than hepatitis B

* Incubation periods as short as 4 to 14 days are recorded.

† Shorter mean incubation periods (27 days) may reflect infection by one of the bloodborne non-A, non-B agents or by the epidemic form of non-A, non-B hepatitis.

sion. Its RNA is nonhomologous with the DNA of HBV. Preliminary studies of putative non-A, non-B agents suggest a size intermediate between that of HAV and HBV. The nucleic acid associated with the non-A, non-B viruses remains to be determined. Serologic markers of HAV infection are specific to hepatitis A whereas those of HBV infection are specific to hepatitis B. Since HDV can only infect HBV-infected persons, markers of HDV and HBV coexist in hepatitis D. Non-A, non-B viral hepatitis undoubtedly has its own specific set of serologic markers that are under study, but it is defined serologically, at present, by the absence of indicators of both hepatitis A and B. The various serologic measures are described in subsequent sections.

Historically, as previously indicated, the recognition of relatively little overlap in the incubation periods of hepatitis A and B provided a commonly used basis for distinction. In various experiments, orally and parenterally administered materials from hepatitis A patients resulted in symptoms from 15 to 49 days later in the recipients.[405,609] In contrast, injection of serum from individuals with hepatitis B resulted in onset of symptoms from 28 to 180 days later.[404,409,606,607,706,738] Route of inoculation could not explain this difference because serum from cases of hepatitis A resulted in disease 20 to 34 days later when given parenterally and 21 to 34 days when given by mouth.[398] The incubation period of non-A, non-B viral hepatitis following blood transfusion has a wide range, 15 to 160 days,[29,276] overlapping that of both hepatitis A and B. Hence, the distinction between the etiologic forms, based on incubation period, is now recognized to be imperfect.

The most fundamental immunologic basis for distinction among the etiologic forms is the lack of sufficient antigenic similarity to provide cross protection (heterologous immunity) on challenge. In two sets of experiments, volunteers rechallenged with HAV remained well.[400,706] In related studies, individuals who had recovered from hepatitis A developed disease when given the agent of hepatitis B.[607,706] Conversely, volunteers rechallenged with HBV were immune,[607,706,736] but when challenged with HAV became ill.[404,609,706] A number of studies have provided serologic evidence that past infection with HAV or HBV, or both, does not alter susceptibility to non-A, non-B viral hepatitis. The occurrence of two or rarely three episodes of non-A, non-B viral hepatitis[688,727] suggests either the existence of two or more antigenically dissimilar non-A, non-B agents or that homologous immunity is not a feature of infection by the non-A, non-B hepatitis virus(es). The latter seems unlikely because homologous immunity has been demonstrated in chimpanzees,[985] but this immunity may be overwhelmed by high dose inocula.[124]

Nonhuman primates are susceptible to human hepatitis virus infection; chimpanzees have been infected experimentally with each of the etiologic forms.[30,229,642,986] In contrast, marmosets (small South American monkeys) are susceptible to hepatitis A and non-A, non-B hepatitis agents[279,492] but resistant to hepatitis B and D.

Although a number of epidemiologic characteristics are common to the various etiologic forms of viral hepatitis (e.g., viremia), experiments performed in the 1940s clearly distinguished between hepatitis A and hepatitis B on the basis of fecal excretion and infectivity when ingested. Numerous volunteer studies demonstrated that administration of fecal suspensions by mouth readily transmitted hepatitis A. On the other hand, no illnesses occurred when feces from cases of hepatitis B were administered to volunteers by mouth in three separate sets of experiments.[404,606,711] Even *intramuscular* administration of a bacteria-free filtrate of pooled feces failed to induce definite disease; one of five volunteers did have slight abnormalities in some hepatic tests, but these were considered of questionable significance.[706] Further, serum of known infectivity (inducing hepatitis B in 60% of subjects when administered by injection) failed to provoke jaundice among adult volunteers in three sets of studies when given by mouth.[404,609,706] Subsequently Krugman and colleagues were able to show low levels of infectivity with a much longer incubation period when icterogenic hepatitis B serum was administered orally to children,[545] but they did not test feces. Thus, the distinction between hepatitis A and hepatitis B concerning oral infectivity is still relatively applicable and that based on fecal excretion has not been contravened. The epidemiologic behavior of non-A, non-B viral hepatitis appears to be dependent on the responsible agents. The blood-borne agents resemble hepatitis B in their behavior, while the epidemic and sporadic-endemic orally transmitted form of non-A, non-B hepatitis resembles hepatitis A.

A corollary of the preceding observations is the notion, supported by a large body of experimental studies and epidemiologic investigations, that fecal-oral transmission is the predominant mode of spread of hepatitis A. Furthermore, fecal-oral transmission of hepatitis B has never been documented and has not been accepted as an epidemiologic entity. Fecal-oral spread of the epidemic and sporadic-endemic form of non-A, non-B viral hepatitis appears likely, but the blood transfusion–and coagulation factor–associated forms do not appear to be enterically transmitted. In contrast, percutaneous transmission is characteristic of hepatitis B, hepatitis D, and non-A, non-B hepatitis but is rarely observed in the spread of hepatitis A.

Another major epidemiologic distinction between hepatitis A and the other etiologic forms concerns the existence of long-term carriers of the hepatitis viruses. Although two individuals with presumed chronic fecal excretion were described earlier,[961] more recent studies indicate that both had evidence of ongoing HBV infection.[441] The carrier state, which implies chronic infection and an epidemiologic reservoir of infection, has not been documented in hepatitis A since positive serologic identification became available in the 1970s.

In contrast, hepatitis B, hepatitis D, and non-A, non-

B hepatitis are associated with a viremic carrier state indicating chronic infection. The existence of infectious carriers serves to perpetuate the disease in any given population. The frequency of the carrier state in hepatitis B is variable. In the general population of the United States, perhaps 0.1% to 0.5% are carriers; a much higher frequency is seen in certain groups, for example, immigrants from Southeast Asia, parenteral drug abusers, promiscuous populations, and individuals with underlying immunologic disorders. HBV carrier rates as high as 20% have been described in some areas of the world. Chronic HDV infection, presumably with persistence of the infectious state, has been identified in some populations of hepatitis B carriers. The prevalence of chronic HDV infection appears to vary widely and remains poorly defined. The existence of carriers of non-A, non-B hepatitis has been documented by transmission studies, but the prevalence of the carrier state and its geographic distribution will not be established until specific serologic markers become available.

Clinical observations, including a number of follow-up studies, indicate that hepatitis A is not associated with the development of chronic hepatitis, whereas an appreciable number of patients with hepatitis B, with hepatitis D virus superinfection of hepatitis B carriers, and with non-A, non-B viral hepatitis are at risk. The association of hepatitis B with primary hepatocellular carcinoma provides another basis for distinction because there is no current evidence linking hepatitis A or hepatitis D with this hepatic malignancy. Whether non-A, non-B hepatitis is also implicated is unknown.

Mortality data provide another clinical distinction. The case-fatality rate in hepatitis A is very low, probably being no more than one or two deaths per 1000 icteric cases. Hepatitis B has a more variable[146] but usually higher case-fatality rate, probably averaging about 1%. The poorer prognosis of hepatitis B has been attributed in part to debility of the patient in the case of transfusion-associated disease.[78] Debility cannot, however, account for all instances in which mortality has been high. In one iatrogenic outbreak of hepatitis B among ambulatory psychiatric patients, 37% of those who became clinically ill died.[238] Children given icterogenic pooled serum had a case-fatality rate of 19% in one outbreak,[616] and in another, unrelated episode, soldiers had a rate of 17%.[146] On the other hand, among healthy soldiers given hepatitis B–contaminated yellow fever vaccine in World War II, the case fatality rate was 3 per 1000,[866] only slightly higher than that for hepatitis A. A similarly low rate was observed in Swedish track-finders who acquired hepatitis B through wound infections.[346] The case-fatality rate in non-A, non-B viral hepatitis also appears to be variable but is probably lower than that of hepatitis B. Fulminant hepatitis due to non-A, non-B agents, although less common than fulminant hepatitis B, had a more dismal prognosis in one study,[7] but not in another.[636] Coinfection of HDV infection with hepatitis B or HDV superinfection of HBV carriers may contribute importantly to the variable case-fatality rates attributed to hepatitis B in the past; fulminant co-primary HBV/HDV infection and fulminant HDV superinfection of hepatitis B carriers with case-fatality rates as high as 17% have been described.[384]

Hepatitis A Virus

The first successful experimental transmission of HAV to nonhuman primates was reported by Deinhardt and co-workers in 1967.[208] White-lipped marmosets inoculated intravenously with acute phase serum or plasma from patients with hepatitis A developed biochemical and hepatic morphologic alterations 3 to 5 weeks later. Clinical illness was not evident. Hepatitis could be transfered from marmoset to marmoset by inoculation of serum obtained during the acute phase of infection as reflected by elevation of serum enzymes. Parks and associates questioned the suitability of the marmoset as an experimental animal for the study of human hepatitis A because they had evidence that a latent marmoset hepatitis virus, unrelated to HAV, could affect these animals.[747,748] Part of this discrepancy was undoubtedly due to transmission of a virus, known as the GB agent, which is serologically distinct from HAV but can produce hepatitis in marmosets. Subsequently, Holmes and co-workers[442,443] and Provost and colleagues[791] described the reduction of both infectivity and pathogenicity of infective acute-phase marmoset serum following incubation with commercial immune serum globulin or convalescent phase serum. These and other studies using coded materials and serologic techniques for the identification of HAV and antibody to HAV (anti-HAV), have indicated that (1) marmosets are susceptible to hepatitis A; (2) they may be infected either by oral or parenteral inoculation of HAV; (3) HAV may be recovered from infected animals; and (4) HAV induces anti-HAV in infected animals. Unfortunately, marmosets are an endangered species, and importation restrictions have sharply curtailed the use of these animals.

Fortunately, chimpanzees are also susceptible to hepatitis A. Transmission of hepatitis A from newly imported chimpanzees to their human handlers was initially recognized in 1961 and suggested that this species could be infected.[422] Maynard and co-workers successfully transmitted HAV to chimpanzees that had been inoculated with a preparation of virus-like particles obtained from stool filtrates of patients with hepatitis A.[643] The chimpanzees developed a clinical illness with an incubation period of about 17 days. A virus-like particle morphologically identical to that in the inoculum was found in the stools of infected animals during the acute phase of the infection.[365] Subsequently, Dienstag and colleagues described successful transmission of hepatitis A to susceptible (anti-HAV negative) chimpanzees after oral or intravenous inoculation of acute-phase stool filtrates containing HAV particles.[229] After an incubation period of 3 to 4 weeks, biochemical, histologic, and clinical evidence of acute hepatitis was observed. Virus-like particles were seen in the stools of infected animals, and anti-HAV was identified in convalescent phase sera. Furthermore, HAV particles were identified in the liver and bile of infected chimpanzees.[879] Because the chimpanzee is also endangered and in short supply, alternative animal models have been sought. Both the owl monkey[570] and the stump-tailed macaque[624] are susceptible to hepatitis A and may be used in future studies.

In addition to ending the dependence upon human volunteers to demonstrate infectivity, the susceptibility of these nonhuman primates has permitted the development of a hepatitis A vaccine that can be tested extensively before human volunteers are studied.[789] Finally, tissues obtained from nonhuman primate sources have permitted the *in vitro* propagation of HAV. HAV has been propagated, without evidence of cytopathology, in marmoset liver explant cell cultures, in fetal rhesus monkey kidney cell lines, in African green monkey kidney cells, in human diploid lung and embryo fibroblasts, and in a variety of transformed cell lines.[192,304,325,790,795] HAV is thus unique among the viruses of hepatitis because it is the only agent that has been successfully grown *in vitro*.

In infected humans,[543] nonhuman primates,[229,365,879] explant cell cultures, and cell lines,[790] HAV has been identified as a spherical, nonenveloped particle 27 nm in diameter (Fig. 15-1) that demonstrates cubic symmetry and appears to be an icosahedron. The HAV capsid is probably composed of 32 capsomeres;[918] an internal core-like structure has been described but not yet confirmed. Staining of preparations of partially purified HAV particles with phosphotungstic acid reveals the particles to be either full (unpenetrated by the stain) or empty (penetrated by stain).[879] Full particles band at higher densities than empty particles in cesium chloride gradients.[113,115,919]

Although both high- and low-density particles appear

Fig. 15-1. Electron micrograph of antibody-coated aggregate of 27-nm HAV particles purified from the stool of a patient with acute hepatitis A. (Original magnification × 132,000; courtesy of Dr. Jules L. Dienstag)

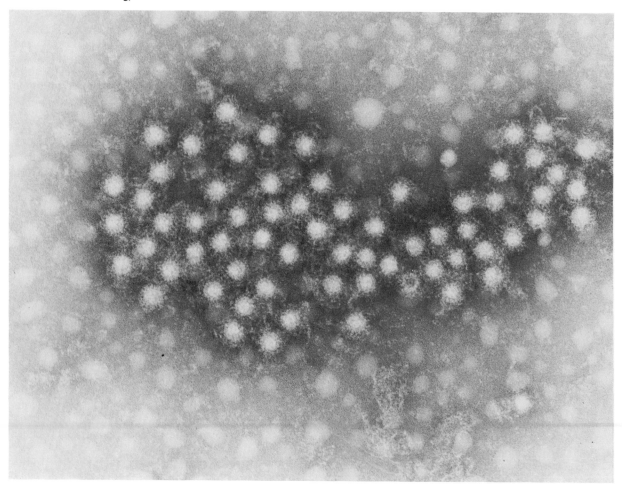

sensitive to RNAase treatment,[113] it seems likely that empty particles may be deficient in their nucleic acid content. As indicated previously, several populations of HAV particles, which band at densities between 1.28 g and 1.44 g/ml, have been described.[113,115,117,879,919] The major peak, banding at a density of 1.33 g to 1.34 g/ml,[794] appears to comprise full particles when examined by phosphotungstic acid staining and demonstrates maximal infectivity.[794]

The notion that HAV is a picornavirus with single-stranded RNA[113,794] was confirmed by a series of studies that indicated an intracytoplasmic localization of HAV particles in hepatocytes,[463,632,794] typical of the picornaviruses, partial inactivation of infectivity by treatment with pancreatic RNAase,[794] and finally, the isolation of RNA from HAV particles.[920] HAV-associated RNA appears to be linear, kinked, and single stranded with a molecular weight of 1.9 to 2.8 × 10^6 daltons.[920,921] The infectious RNA genome is 7,500 to 8,100 nucleotides long and contains a polyadenylic acid sequence at the 3′ terminus. Molecular cloning of RNA of HAV has been achieved and the nucleotide sequence partially characterized.[1002] Furthermore, the sequences that encode the structural polypeptides have been located.[591a]

HAV has therefore been categorized as enterovirus 72 in the picornavirus group.[655] Further support for this classification is provided by the observation that the polypeptides isolated from the intact HAV particle resemble those reported for enteroviruses.[113,181] Four major structural polypeptides with molecular weights between 10,000 and 32,000 daltons and a fifth minor "precursor" polypeptide with a molecular weight of 40,000 daltons have been characterized.[380] It should be emphasized that only one antigenic strain of HAV has been identified. Known characteristics of HAV are summarized in Table 15-2.

Serologic Tests for the Identification of HAV Infection. The routine use of nonhuman primates (marmosets or chimpanzees) for the identification of HAV is impractical because of limited availability, high costs, and the development of immunity after successful infection. Nonetheless, following experimental infection, these animals have served as sources of HAV used in the development of serologic methods for detection of HAV infection. The propagation of HAV and recovery of virus from explant and tissue culture systems should reduce dependence on intact animals and permit increased availability of HAV for further characterization of the virus and refinement of diagnostic laboratory procedures.

Identification of HAV. HAV particles in the feces of acutely infected patients with hepatitis A were visualized by immune electron microscopy as aggregates or single particles coated with antibody following incubation with either convalescent sera from other hepatitis A patients or immune serum globulin (immunoglobulin or γ-globulin) preparations.[275] HAV particles could not be detected in preinoculation or convalescent stool samples. Preino-

culation sera from patients with hepatitis A failed to aggregate HAV particles. Shortly after these observations were made, morphologically similar HAV particles were identified in the livers and sera of marmosets experimentally infected with the CR326 strain of HAV.[794]

To identify HAV in the liver of experimentally infected nonhuman primates, immunofluorescent, immunoperoxidase-staining and immune electron microscopic techniques have been used.[463,633,910] These studies have suggested that HAV is produced in the liver, which appears to be the sole site of HAV replication[633,635,693] despite the occasional detection of HAV in spleen, lymph nodes, and kidneys.[631] In infected chimpanzee hepatocytes, more than 90% of HAV antigenic activity (detected by solid-phase radioimmunoassay) was identified in cytosolic and microsomal fractions and less than 5% in the cell nucleus. In the microsomal fraction more than 75% of HAV was associated with smooth endoplasmic reticulum membranes.[507] In a patient with acute HAV infection, HAV was demonstrated in cytoplasmic vesicles of hepatocytes and Kupffer cells and the surrounding vesicle membranes demonstrated HAV activity.[911] These data suggest that HAV replication occurs predominantly within the cytoplasm of the hepatocyte, in close association with cellular membranes, a characteristic feature of enteroviruses.

Although far more sensitive than standard transmission electron microscopy for detecting HAV, immune electron microscopy is a cumbersome and time-consuming technique limited to research laboratories with experienced electron microscopists. Specific complement fixation (CF)[792] and immune adherence hemagglutination (IAH)[661] tests that could be employed for the detection of either HAV or its antibody (anti-HAV) were subsequently developed.

These techniques have been largely surpassed by the development of simple, widely available, radioimmunoassays (RIAs) and enzyme-linked immunosorbent assays (ELISAs) for the detection of HAV and anti-HAV. In the examination of fecal extracts for HAV, a microtiter solid-phase radioimmunoassay was shown to be highly sensitive and easy to perform. Liver, fecal, and serum specimens judged to be negative for HAV particles by immune electron microscopy were found to contain high levels of HAV when examined by radioimmunoassay.[434] Monoclonal antibodies specific for HAV have been produced and hold promise in the search for antigenic variants of HAV and further characterization of antigenic binding sites (epitopes) of the virus.[611] In fact, at least one neutralization epitope has been recognized on one of the major polypeptides.[464]

The major use of these techniques has been in the detection and quantification of HAV during purification procedures designed to provide reagents for serologic testing. Diagnosis of hepatitis A by detection of HAV in stool samples is impractical because viral shedding diminishes rapidly after the onset of jaundice. Only about half these patients have detectable shedding of HAV in the stool

TABLE 15-2.   Physicochemical Stability Characteristics of Hepatitis A Virus, Hepatitis B Virus, and the Non-A, Non-B Hepatitis Viruses

CHARACTERISTIC	HEPATITIS A VIRUS	HEPATITIS B VIRUS	NON-A, NON-B HEPATITIS VIRUSES
Ether stability	Survived 20% concentration at 4°C, for 18 hr	Survived triple extraction of serum [609]	Not done
Tween 80/ether (1%/20%, 4°C, 18 hr)	Not done	Inactivated [785]	Inactivated [785]
Acid stability	Survived *p*H 3.0 for 3 hr [791]	Not done	Not done
Heat stability			
Autoclaving, 15 psi, 30 min	Inactivated	Inactivated	Not done
Dry heat			
160°C, 60 min	Inactivated [856]	Inactivated [856]	Not done
100°C, 20 min	Inactivated [1065]	Inactivated [1065]	Not done
100°C, 5 min	Inactivated [794]	Not done	Inactivated [1093]
100°C, 1 min	Inactivated (98°C) [546]	Survived [543,549] Inactivated (98°C, 2 min) [524]	Not done
60°C, 10 hr	Survived (12 hr) [305]	Inactivated [328] Survived	Inactivated [440]
60°C, 4 hr	Survived [305]	Survived [696]	Not done
60°C, 1 hr	Survived [791]	Survived	Not done
Chlorination			
Water with high organic content			
Breakpoint chlorination	Inactivated [708]	Not done	Not done
1 ppm total residual, 30 min	Survived [708]	Not done	Not done
Water with low organic content			
1.1 ppm total residual, 30 min	Inactivated [708]	Not done	Not done
0.5–1.5 mg free residual chlorine/ liter/30 min	Partially inactivated [760]	Not done	Not done
2.0–2.5 mg free residual chlorine/ liter/30 min	Inactivated [760]	Not done	Not done
β-propiolactone	Not done	Inactivated [598]	Inactivated (0.05%, 4°C, 20 min) [1095]
Storage of plasma at 31.6°C, 6 mo	Not done	Survived [814]	Not done
Ultraviolet irradiation	Inactivated [794]	Survived irradiation of plasma [697]	Inactivated (with β-propiolactone and silicic acid adsorption) [786]
Tricresol 0.2%	Not done	Survived [287]	Not done
Thimerosal 1:2000	Not done	Survived [73]	Not done
Nitrogen mustard 500 mg/liter	Not done	Survived [240]	Not done

TABLE 15-2.—Continued

CHARACTERISTIC	HEPATITIS A VIRUS	HEPATITIS B VIRUS	NON-A, NON-B HEPATITIS VIRUSES
Formalin 1:4000 37°C, 72 hr	Inactivated[794]	Inactivated*[989]	Inactivated (1:1000, 37°C, 96 hr, or 1:2000, 37°C, 72 hr)[1093]
Glutaraldehyde 0.1 or 1%, 24°C, 5 min	Not done	Inactivated[524]	Not done
Chloroform extraction (10% vol/vol)	Survived[181]	Inactivated†[278]	Survived (one agent), Inactivated (one agent)[110,278]
Pepsin (1 mg/liter, pH 2.1, 37°C, 18 hr)	Not done	Inactivated[989]	Not done
Urea (8 M, 37°C, 4 hr)	Not done	Inactivated*[989]	Not done

* Inactivated 10^5 chimpanzee infectious doses of HBV per milliliter.
† Inactivated $10^{3.5}$ chimpanzee infectious doses of HBV per milliliter.

when studied within 1 week of the onset of dark urine.[182] Detection of HAV in sera[434] is also impractical because viral titers tend to be low and declining, or absent, when the diagnosis is likely to be considered.

Identification of Antibody to HAV. The serologic detection of fecal or circulating HAV is of limited value in the etiologic diagnosis of hepatitis A because samples are rarely available before the onset of illness and HAV may no longer be detectable in samples from jaundiced patients.[182,228,388,805] Anti-HAV can be detected early in the acute phase of illness and remains detectable for more than 10 years and probably indefinitely. The initial antibody response is composed of IgM anti-HAV, and the diagnosis of acute hepatitis A is established by the detection of anti-HAV of the IgM class in a single serum specimen obtained during the acute phase of illness. The IgM anti-HAV reaches peak levels within a few weeks of the onset of symptoms and declines progressively thereafter.[290] At 4 to 5 months after the onset of illness about 50% of patients no longer have detectable IgM anti-HAV.[397] Low levels of IgM anti-HAV reactivity have been found more than 200 days after the acute illness in about 13% of patients[493] and in a small proportion may persist for as long as 2 to 3 years.[129] The nature of this persistent reactivity is poorly defined and in some instances appears to represent false-positive reactions due to a rheumatoid factor–like substance unaffected by treatment with 2-mercaptoethanol.[129]

During the recovery phase, anti-HAV of the IgG class becomes the predominant antibody, reaching peak levels 3 to 12 months after the onset of illness. This IgG anti-HAV is not usually detected in acute-phase sera.[225,378] Relatively high levels of the IgG anti-HAV persist and are responsible for the prolonged presence of anti-HAV reac-

tivity. The presence of IgG anti-HAV indicates previous HAV infection and immunity to reinfection.

Radioimmunoassay and enzyme-linked immunosorbent assays for the detection of IgM and IgG anti-HAV have been developed.[200,247,597,634] Both employ sandwich techniques and have had widespread clinical application. The ELISAs are less expensive because they do not require radioactive materials and gamma counters and employ more stable reagents. Preliminary data suggest that they equal radioimmunoassays in sensitivity. The sequence of order of appearance of HAV, in liver, feces, and blood, and of anti-HAV in blood, is shown in Figure 15-2.

The detection of a fecal IgA-class anti-HAV has been described,[1092] but its use in diagnosis requires further study.

Fig. 15-2. Schema of the seroimmunologic events observed during the course of typical hepatitis A infection. In some patients, anti-HAV of the IgM class may persist longer and fecal shedding of HAV may be briefer than indicated below. (Koff RS: In Sanford JP [ed]: The Science and Clinical Practice of Medicine, vol 8. New York, Grune & Stratton, 1981)

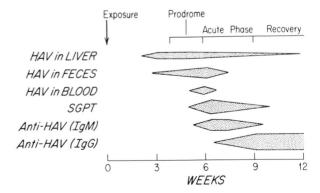

TABLE 15-3. Nomenclature in Hepatitis B

PREFERRED TERM	REPLACED TERM(S)	COMMENT
Hepatitis B	Serum hepatitis, homologous serum jaundice, inoculation hepatitis, long-incubation hepatitis, MS-2 hepatitis	Identifies a specific etiologic entity, defined serologically rather than epidemiologically; replaces epidemiologic terms
Hepatitis B virus (HBV)	Dane particle	The agent responsible for hepatitis B; a 42-nm spherical DNA virus, initially visualized by electron microscopy by Dane (hence Dane particle) in 1970
Hepatitis B surface antigen (HBsAg)	Australia antigen, SH antigen, hepatitis-associated antigen	The antigenic determinant on the surface of the HBV and also identified as smaller, 22-nm, spherical particles and tubular forms, representing excessively produced coat materials; replaces: Australia antigen, the designation coined by Blumberg following his discovery of the antigen in the serum of an Australian aborigine; SH antigen, the term used by Prince to indicate the association of the antigen with serum hepatitis when the latter was still used to describe hepatitis B; and hepatitis-associated antigen, a noncommittal term that failed to indicate a specific relationship to hepatitis B
HBsAg/adr or ayr or adwl-4, or aywl-4		Recognized subdeterminants of HBsAg include a group specificity labeled *a* and sets of subdeterminants designated *d*, *y*, *w1*, *w2*, *w3*, *w4,* and *r*. These and other less well-defined antigenic subdeterminants of HBsAg are found on HBV and the small spheres and tubular forms.

Hepatitis B Virus

A large number of terms have been used to describe hepatitis B, HBV, and HBV-associated antigenic components and their corresponding antibodies. The preferred terminology, indicated in Table 15-3, is employed throughout this chapter.

The host range of HBV appears to be limited to humans and chimpanzees.[56,57,627,1108] In the chimpanzee, experimental transmission results in a serologic pattern that appears similar to that of human HBV infection, and cloned HBV DNA has been shown to be infective.[1075] Extensive studies of seroimmunologic and immunopathologic responses to HBV infection have been undertaken in this species. Chimpanzees cannot be used in routine laboratory testing for detection of HBV infection in humans for the same reasons mentioned in the section on HAV infection in these primates. They have nonetheless played a critical

role in the efficacy and safety testing of HBV vaccines prior to studies in volunteers. This is described in a subsequent section.

HBV of humans and hepatitis B–like viruses found in woodchucks (*Marmota monax*), Beechey ground squirrels (*Spermophilus beecheyi*), and Pekin ducks (*Anas domesticus*) share many features and belong to a family of hepatotrophic DNA viruses called hepadnaviruses. Human HBV has been classified as hepadnavirus type 1.[655] Each of the hepadnaviruses has a double-shelled virion 42 nm to 47 nm in diameter, a 27-nm internal core, an excess of incomplete 22-nm spheres and, except for the duck hepatitis B virus, tubular forms, and circular partially double-stranded and partially single-stranded DNA, with a length varying between 3000 and 3300 base pairs. All four viruses contain endogenous DNA polymerase and protein kinase, share some DNA and virion polypeptide homology, replicate within the liver, and may be asso-

TABLE 15-3.—Continued

PREFERRED TERM	REPLACED TERM(S)	COMMENT
Antibody to HBsAg (anti-HBs)		Antibody to the surface determinants on HBV and the small spherical and tubular particles. Individual antibodies are designated anti-a, anti-d, anti-y, etc.
Hepatitis B core antigen (HBcAg)		The antigenic determinant associated with the core of HBV, detectable in the nucleus of the infected hepatocyte or following removal of the coat of HBV. HBcAg is not associated with the small HBsAg spheres or tubular forms.
Antibody to HBcAg (anti-HBc)		Antibody to the core antigen of HBV
Hepatitis B e antigen (HBeAg)		A soluble nonparticulate antigen immunologically distinct from HBcAg, HBsAg, and the latter's subdeterminants; associated with the core of HBV but not the small HBsAg particles. HBeAg appears to be a degradation product of HBcAg.
HBeAg/1, HBeAg/2, HBeAg/3		The three components of the HBeAg system that have been recognized
Antibody to HBeAg (anti-HBe)		Antibody to the hepatitis B e antigen. Individual antibodies to the three components are designated anti-HBe/1, anti-HBe/2, and anti-HBe/3.

ciated with acute or persistent infection, immune complex–mediated extrahepatic disease, and hepatocellular carcinoma.[838]

Multiple attempts to grow HBV in tissue or organ cultures have been reported, but *in vitro* cultivation has yet to be achieved. HBsAg was detected in cell extracts and supernatant fluid of a primary hepatocellular carcinoma cell line derived from an HBsAg-positive patient.[615] Subsequent studies of this cell line, termed PLC/PRF/5 have confirmed synthesis of HBsAg[10,433] and its polypeptides[626] and that HBV DNA is integrated into the host DNA of these cells.[210]

The major breakthrough in the study of HBV, which in fact immensely expanded knowledge of the various etiologic forms of viral hepatitis, resulted from unrelated work on genetically determined serum protein polymorphisms. In 1965, Blumberg and co-workers reported the identification of an antigen in the serum of an Australian aborigine that formed a precipitin line in an agar gel diffusion system with antibody in the serum of a multiply transfused patient with hemophilia.[98] The newly discovered antigen was called the Australia antigen and initially appeared to be linked with leukemia in the United States. The antigen subsequently was shown to be associated with several other disorders, including Down's syndrome and

viral hepatitis. A specific association with hepatitis B was independently postulated by Prince in the United States,[780] and the association was confirmed in Japan in 1968.[735] The relationship was obscured at first by the widespread practice of etiologically labeling cases on the basis of epidemiologic background. With the subsequent definitive association of the antigen with hepatitis B and its identification as the surface material of HBV, the term *hepatitis B surface antigen* (HBsAg) superseded the earlier nomenclature. For his discovery of HBsAg, Blumberg was awarded the Nobel Prize in Medicine in 1976.[97]

The presence of HBsAg in serum was found to be associated with three distinct circulating particles demonstrable by electron microscopy (Figs. 15-3 and 15-4). The first to be recognized and the most numerous (10^{13}/ml) are the small spherical particles with a diameter of about 22 nm (range 16 nm to 25 nm).[65] The second is a tubular, tadpole, or rodlike form with a diameter of 22 nm and a variable length ranging up to several hundred nanometers. The small 22-nm particles and the tubular forms are antigenically identical with the surface material of the HBV particle. The HBV particle, the third and last particle to be recognized, was initially described by Dane and co-workers in 1970 and became known as the Dane particle.[194] The Dane particle subsequently has been identified

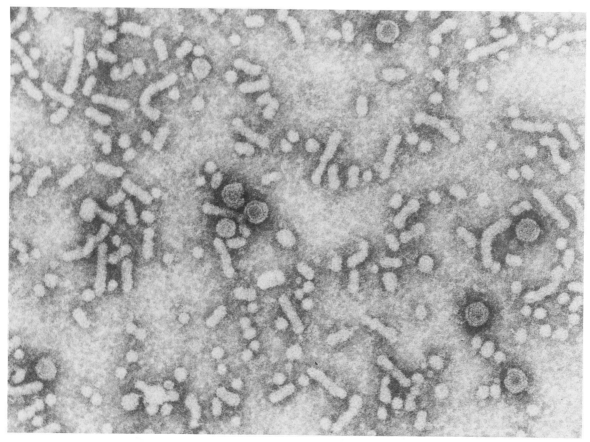

Fig. 15-3. Electron micrograph of the three morphologic forms of particles associated with HBV, purified from the serum of a carrier of HBsAg. (Original magnification × 132,000; courtesy of Dr. Jules L. Dienstag)

Fig. 15-4. Diagram of the three morphologic forms of the HBV-associated particles, the antigens of HBV, and their interrelationships. DNA and DNA polymerase in the core of the 42-nm HBV particle are shown. (Koff RS: In Sanford JP [ed]: The Science and Clinical Practice of Medicine, vol 8. New York, Grune & Stratton, 1981)

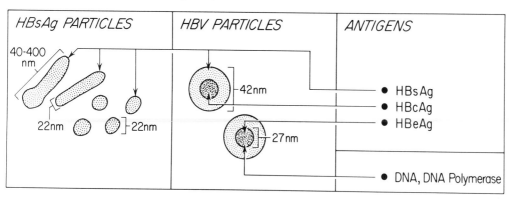

as the intact HBV particle, and the latter term has supplanted the eponymic designation. The HBV particle is spherical, 42 nm (range 40 nm to 45 nm) in diameter; it contains an inner core measuring 27 nm in diameter and an outer coat approximately 7 nm in thickness. The core differs antigenically and biochemically from the coat material.

Properties. HBV particles are found in the serum (10^{10}/ml)[194] and in hepatocytes[461] of humans and chimpanzees infected with HBV. The presence of HBV DNA in extrahepatic tissues, such as vascular endothelium, bile duct epithelium, bone marrow, and peripheral leukocytes, suggests but does not prove that HBV replication may occur in nonhepatocytes.[96] Within the hepatocyte the HBV DNA can be found in a freely replicating form or integrated into the host genome.[966] The physicochemical characteristics of this 42-nm, double-shelled virus are shown in Table 15-2. Identification of this particle as the intact HBV is based on a number of observations that include (1) the experimental transmission of serologically documented HBV infection to susceptible chimpanzees with an inoculum of purified particles[999]; (2) identification of the particle in serum shown to be infectious in human subjects[544]; (3) compatibility of the 42-nm particle with the estimated size of HBV based on human transmission studies[648]; (4) the presence of DNA[837] and DNA polymerase[496] in the 42-nm particle but not in the smaller 22-nm HBsAg particle; and (5) demonstration that inoculation of cloned HBV DNA induced hepatitis B in chimpanzees.[1075] The latter finding is consistent with the notion that the 42-nm particle is the intact DNA-containing HBV.

The structure and genetic organization of native HBV DNA extracted from the nucleocapsid core of the virus and HBV DNA cloned in bacterial, yeast, and mammalian cell vectors have been determined.[1004] HBV DNA is small, circular, and partly double stranded and partly single stranded, with a length of about 3200 nucleotides.[1005] A long, linear strand of complete genomic length nicked at a fixed position and a short strand of variable length ranging from 50% to 85% of the long strand comprise the complementary DNA strands.[211] A DNA polymerase, also localized to the nucleocapsid of HBV, appears to repair the gap in the short strand by filling in the missing nucleotides.[425] The two DNA strands are maintained in circular configuration by base-pairing of the 5′ ends of each strand that have a fixed position. The position of the 3′ end of the long strand is also fixed, but the position of the 3′ end of the short strand is variable.

Four regions (genes) of the HBV genome have been identified: the pre-S and S region, the C region, the P region, and the X region.[211] The pre-S and S gene encode for the major polypeptide of HBsAg and a polypeptide receptor for polymerized human serum albumin.[734] The latter may play a role in the attachment of HBV to hepatocytes. The C region encodes for the polypeptides of the nucleocapsid core, the HBcAg and the HBeAg. The P region encodes for the HBV DNA polymerase. The precise function and gene products of the X region remain poorly characterized. However a peptide encoded by the X region appears to be associated with HBV-induced hepatocellular carcinoma.[668]

The mechanisms of replication of HBV and the other members of the hepadnavirus family appear to be analogous to those of the RNA containing retroviruses in that a reverse transcriptase step is used.[967] Hybridization techniques have revealed that the replication of the DNA strands occurs asymmetrically in the hepatocyte cytoplasm[95] or nucleus,[296] with the formation of heterogenous DNA replicative intermediates,[889] possibly including a supercoiled form of DNA,[855] and a HBV RNA pregenome that is reverse transcribed to the long DNA strand.

HBV DNA also has been identified in the sera of HBV-infected individuals[81,122,1020]; its presence appears to be an index of ongoing viral replication. Examination of the molecular species of circulating HBV DNA shows considerable variation, suggesting that replicative intermediates may be released into serum.[295] Although it seems likely that measurements of specific molecular species of circulating HBV DNA will provide the most reliable test for infectivity, such testing is not currently available.

A population of HBV particles lacking DNA and DNA polymerase has been identified,[494] but the mechanism of production of these defective particles remains poorly understood. Defective HBV particles are likely to be noninfectious and may modify infection induced by intact HBV particles.

Core and Core-Associated Antigens. Treatment of HBV particles, obtained from serum or infected liver, with detergents[19] or subjecting the particles to shearing forces[428] disrupts or strips away the surface coat of HBsAg and exposes the inner core of HBV. The inner core is the nucleocapsid of HBV; DNA, DNA polymerase, and the DNA polymerase reaction product have been localized to the core. Exposed cores appear to be icosahedral particles with a diameter of approximately 27 nm.[55,131,461,594] Core particles are morphologically and antigenically similar whether derived from circulating HBV particles or isolated from liver tissue. Core particles have a buoyant density of 1.30 g to 1.40 g/ml in cesium chloride.[55,429,458,594]

In addition to the viral DNA found in the core, HBV-specific, DNA-dependent DNA polymerase activity[425] and protein kinase activity[15] have been identified in the core. HBV DNA polymerase activity is reduced by heat (60° C for 10 hr) and formalin (1:2000, at 37° C for 96 hr) treatment, and study of its biochemical characteristics suggests that it behaves like the β-DNA polymerase of eukaryotic organisms.[355] The HBV DNA polymerase appears to have unusual ionic requirements, and intact sulfhydryl groups are necessary for activity.[427] Variable activation patterns following exposure to different salt or nonionic detergent concentrations may be useful in identifying HBV specific enzyme.[428] HBV DNA polymerase activity is inhibited by intercalating agents such as ethidium bromide, chloroquine, quinacrine, and chlorpromazine.[426] HBV-specific DNA polymerase activity has been detected in the sera of patients[495] and chimpanzees[116] with hepatitis B and appears to be closely linked with the presence of intact HBV particles. Measurement of HBV-specific DNA polymerase activity has been used as a biochemical marker for HBV, identifies the period of HBV replication, and is correlated with the infectivity of sera[548] and patients.[755]

The protein kinase detected in HBV core particles appears to share many characteristics with protein kinase activity demonstrated in liver-derived core particles of the ground squirrel hepatitis virus.[15,280] It seems likely that these protein kinases are similar to those of other enveloped viruses. HBV-associated protein kinase has been shown to phosphorylate serine residues of the major core protein.[340a] Protein kinase activity appears to be associated with the presence of the HBeAg.[899]

The core contains specific immunologically reactive material termed the *HBcAg* and *HBeAg*. HBcAg reactivity and core particles do not circulate freely in infected patients or in nonhuman primates and are not detected in sera unless HBV particles are present in a nonintact, disrupted (chemically or physically) form. HBcAg and core particles have been found, using immunofluorescent techniques or electron and immunoelectron microscopy in the nucleus and in the cytoplasm of hepatocytes obtained from chronically infected subjects.[373,1087,1088] HBcAg has been detected in the liver during the late incubation period of hepatitis B in chimpanzees[450] and in the early acute phase of infection in chimpanzees and humans.[450,632]

HBeAg reactivity has been identified on a 22,000 molecular weight polypeptide isolated from the cytoplasm of infected human hepatocytes.[762] HBcAg determinants were present on the same protein. HBeAg determinants also have been found on a HBcAg polypeptide expressed in cloned *Escherichia coli*,[614] and monoclonal antibodies to HBeAg have been derived from denatured HBcAg.[284] These and other data indicate that HBcAg and HBeAg are intimately linked and that HBeAg may be a degradation product of HBcAg. HBeAg may occur in multimeric forms and may be a structural component of the HBV core.[899] HBeAg subtypes may reflect distinct polypeptides of similar molecular weights.[732]

Discovered in 1972 by Magnius and Espmark,[620] HBeAg is a soluble nonparticulate, thermolabile, lipid-free, carbohydrate-free material.[995] Three antigenic subtypes of HBeAg, labeled HBeAg/1-3, have been described.[692] HBeAg has been identified in the nucleus of the HBV-infected hepatocyte and infrequently in hepatocyte cytoplasm.[40] Intranuclear HBeAg may be identified in association with intranuclear HBcAg. HBeAg is found nearly exclusively in HBsAg-positive serum. The major exception to the co-occurrence of HBsAg and HBeAg is the identification of HBeAg without HBsAg in the venous blood of newborns of HBsAg- and HBeAg-positive mothers. In this instance HBeAg appears to cross the placenta without HBsAg.

HBeAg has been correlated with the presence of circulating intact HBV particles, HBV DNA, and HBV-specific DNA polymerase activity.[423,467,1010] It is an excellent but imperfect marker of infectivity.[31,257,755]

Initially, HBeAg appears in a free form in serum.[991] It subsequently is bound to an immunoglobulin to form immune complexes.[991,992]

HBV Surface Antigen. The coat or surface material of HBV is synthesized independently of the core of HBV, contains neither DNA nor DNA polymerase activity, and is immunogenic but noninfectious. Surface material exists in the serum of infected individuals in three antigenically identical forms that are recognized by electron microscopy (Fig. 15-4).[65,194] These include the outer coat of the intact HBV particle, the spherical 22-nm particles, and the tubular forms. The 22-nm spherical particle and rods represent the product of excessive synthesis of the coat material by infected hepatocytes. They are present in sera far in excess of intact HBV particles, reaching concentrations as high or higher than 20 mg/dl of HBsAg protein.[509] Immunoreactive HBsAg has been identified in infected hepatocytes in the cytoplasm,[252] endoplasmic reticulum[333] and adjacent to or on the cell membrane. Although HBsAg has been detected in extrahepatic sites in HBV-infected chimpanzees[694] and humans,[96,907] whether the accumulation of antigen in these tissues is a consequence of immune complex deposition or viral replication due to extrahepatic infection has yet to be determined. The identification of HBV DNA in some of these sites[96,841] supports but does not prove extrahepatic replication of HBV.

Purified preparations of the 22-nm spherical particle have a buoyant density of 1.20 g to 1.22 g/ml in cesium chloride.[338] The molecular weight of HBsAg has been estimated to be 2.4 to 4.6×10^6 daltons.[143] HBsAg has the chemical characteristics of a lipoprotein with carbohydrate components. Lipids comprise 20% to 30% of the surface material.[456] Major lipid components include cholesterol, phosphatidylcholine, sphingomyelin, and lysophosphatidylcholine.[953] Glycolipids have been described[953] but not confirmed.[912] Three percent to 8% of the surface material is carbohydrate[456] and is present in the form of glycoprotein. Galactose, mannose, fucose, glucosamine, and sialic acid have been demonstrated.[912] Removal of sialic acid residues does not reduce immunoreactivity.[716] The precise role of carbohydrate in the antigenic reactivity of HBsAg requires further definition.

Forty percent to 60% of HBsAg is protein[456] and 70% to 80% is in the form of an α helix.[965] Large amounts of tryptophan,[808] proline, leucine, cysteine, and phenylalanine have been recovered.[456] At least seven and possibly nine polypeptides with molecular weights varying from 10,000 to 120,000 daltons have been identified by several laboratories.[761,905,906] The two major polypeptides of HBsAg with molecular weights of 22,000 to 25,000 and

28,000 to 29,000 have been extensively studied. The heavier peptide is a glycosylated form of the smaller peptide. The complete sequence of the 226 amino acids that comprise the major HBsAg polypeptide has been deduced from both the nucleotide sequence of the S region of HBV DNA and amino acid sequencing data.[149,314,749,761,1025] The amino acids appear to be arranged in a series of alternating hydrophobic and hydrophilic areas. The antigenic domains that stimulate the neutralizing, protective antibody may be represented by amino acid sequences in the hydrophilic areas. Carbohydrate-binding sites are also linked to the hydrophilic regions. The hydrophobic regions may play a role in the positioning of the HBsAg polypeptide within the lipid component of the lipoprotein.[798]

Radiolabeling of the peptides indicates that they are neither exclusively internal nor external in position on the HBsAg particle.[905] Humoral and cell-mediated immunity to HBsAg have been elicited by inoculation of isolated HBsAg polypeptides. Among the higher molecular weight polypeptides that are minor components of HBsAg, a 33,000-dalton glycoprotein comprising the major polypeptide (25,000 daltons) and a 55 amino acid peptide encoded by the pre-S region,[612] has received considerable attention. This fusion protein appears to be preferentially expressed in viremic carriers,[415] suggesting a correlation with HBV replication, may be the site of the receptor for the binding of polymerized human albumin,[468,613] and may be more immunogenic than the S region encoded 25,000 dalton polypeptide.[658,717] Larger polypeptides have also been described, but their function is not known.[415]

HBsAg reactivity is stable after freezing for prolonged periods, exposure to 100° C for 1 minute, and after treatment with ether or acid. Treatment with periodate, butanol, or ethanol leads to losses of antigenicity.[466]

Subdeterminants of HBsAg. The basis for serologic recognition of HBsAg appears to be a group-specific antigenic determinant in the coat of HBV and in the small HBsAg particles to which the designation *a* has been given.[420,448,581] Additional specificities were suggested by Levene and Blumberg,[581] and subsequently defined by others.[49,343,566] Lines of partial identity could be demonstrated in agar gel diffusion when sera with different HBsAg specificities were compared using discriminating antisera. The antigenic subdeterminants, listed in Table 15-3, are present on individual particles, coded for by the genome of HBV, elicit specific antibodies, and do not change during the course of infection.[57] At least two subdeterminants from sets labeled *d* or *y* and *w* 1–4 or *r* have been extensively studied. Although these sets initially appeared to represent mutually exclusive subdeterminants, the existence of mixed subtypes in a few sera suggest mixed infection with two populations of HBV, virus recombination, or aggregation of mixed viral products into a single particle population.[343] Polypeptides isolated from HBsAg particles induce antibodies to both the *a* determinant and the specific subdeterminants.[761] The *a* determinant is specified by sequences within amino acid residues 110 to

137 and 139 to 147.[86] The *d/y* determinants, which differ by only one or two amino acid substitutions, are specified by amino acid residues 110 to 137.[340]

Infection with a specific subtype confers cross-protection.[684] Because the subdeterminants are virus determined they are useful as epidemiologic tools in tracing HBV infection.[682] Assessment of subdeterminants does not provide clinically useful information regarding either the severity of illness or the outcome of infection.[334] The various subtypes demonstrate definite differences in geographic distribution and may serve as markers of population migration patterns.[644,645,1089]

Other reactivities, designated g, n, q, x, t, and l, also have been described[62,567,913,946] but their importance remains to be established.

Serologic Tests for Identification of HBV Infection. Identification of serologic patterns of viral and host-induced immunologic markers has permitted the specific laboratory recognition of acute and persistent HBV infection as well as recovery following HBV infection. Although some variation in the time of appearance and duration of circulating serologic markers has been established in several studies both in humans and nonhuman primates, the patterns are nonetheless sufficiently consistent to be clinically useful in diagnosis. The sequential appearance and disappearance of the antigens and antibodies are illustrated schematically in Figure 15-5.

Identification of HBV Antigens. The first serologic marker to appear in the HBV-infected chimpanzee or human is HBsAg. HBsAg is present in the circulation 1 to 10 weeks after exposure to HBV and 2 to 8 weeks before the onset of symptoms or biochemical evidence of liver injury as reflected by a rise in serum aminotransferase levels.[543,548,549] HBsAg is detected by a widely available sensitive, polyvalent radioimmunoassay procedure.[592] An enzyme-linked immunosorbent assay may be equally sensitive.[387] Subtyping of HBsAg for epidemiologic purposes may be achieved by agar gel diffusion, counterimmunoelectrophoresis, or a highly sensitive radioimmunoassay.[448] HBsAg, measured by the polyvalent radioimmunoassay, persists for a variable period (several days to weeks) during the acute phase of the illness and is usually cleared during the convalescent phase following the formation of immune aggregates of HBsAg and its antibody, anti-HBs. Studies employing a monoclonal radioimmunoassay suggest that HBsAg may persist for several months before clearance.[1049] Failure to clear HBsAg may occur in about 5% of HBV infections in adults.[812] Individuals or chimpanzees with persistent circulating HBsAg for 6 or more months after acute infection are termed *HBsAg carriers.* Carriers invariably have high titers of anti-HBc,[251,446,447,548] and 10% to 40% may have anti-HBs. The anti-HBs detected is present in low titers and is directed at HBsAg subdeterminants other than those in the circulating HBsAg of the carrier.[293]

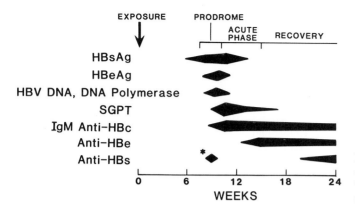

Fig. 15-5. Schema of the sequential seroimmunologic events observed during the course of typical hepatitis B. *Anti-HBs may be present early but cannot be detected as freely circulating antibody.

The second antigen of HBV that is regularly detected by a sensitive radioimmunoassay just after or within a week of the appearance of HBsAg is HBeAg.[549] HBeAg thus appears well before the onset of biochemical evidence of hepatic injury and usually disappears within 2 weeks, whereas HBsAg remains detectable.[549,699] In individuals who develop persistent HBV infection HBeAg may persist together with HBsAg. As previously indicated, HBeAg is rarely detected in sera in the absence of HBsAg. HBV-specific DNA-dependent DNA polymerase activity appears in serum at approximately the same time as HBeAg.[548,549] HBV-specific DNA polymerase activity is determined by measuring the incorporation of radiolabeled thymidine into DNA.[548] DNA polymerase activity is correlated with the presence of HBeAg and intact HBV particles[31,423,725] and is a measure of active HBV replication and infectivity. Activity persists in the sera of some individuals with chronic HBV infection.[548] The technique for detection of DNA polymerase activity is primarily a research tool and has not been adopted for routine clinical use.

HBV DNA has been detected by molecular hybridization techniques, in the serum of patients with persistent HBV infection.[81,590,890] As shown in Figure 15-5, serum HBV DNA also is present during the active phase of viral replication in typical acute hepatitis B and may persist throughout the period in which HBV DNA polymerase activity and HBeAg are present, and for some period thereafter.[1026] The precise duration of circulating HBV DNA in acute, self-limited HBV infection remains to be determined. Serum HBV DNA hybridization tests remain a research tool and are not widely available.

HBcAg is not regularly detected as a freely circulating antigen in HBV infection.

Identification of Antibodies to HBV. Anti-HBc develops regularly during acute HBV infection and usually is detected in serum just prior to or at the time that serum aminotransferase levels become elevated.[447] Although it has been suggested that anti-HBc may precede the appearance in sera of HBsAg in a few patients, this pattern has not been confirmed. Nonetheless, anti-HBc is the first

host-induced immunologic marker of HBV infection that can be measured. Anti-HBc persists throughout the acute phase of illness and for several years to decades (perhaps indefinitely) after recovery in most individuals.[549]

Anti-HBc belonging to both IgM and IgG classes has been described, and the IgM anti-HBc may be the sole detectable serologic marker of HBV infection during the interval between the disappearance of HBsAg and the appearance of detectable anti-HBs.[448,549,577] IgM anti-HBc appears before IgG anti-HBc, is present in high titer during the acute phase of infection, and persists at high titer for only a few months.[756] In patients with acute HBV infection a 19S IgM anti-HBc appears to be the predominant fraction while in patients with persistent HBV infection in whom IgM anti-HBc remains detectable, a 7S immunoglobulin is the major component.[925,1018] IgG anti-HBc develops during convalescence, replaces the IgM antibody, and is responsible for the persistence of anti-HBc long after acute HBV infection.[549] In most individuals who have recovered, radioimmunoassay or enzyme-linked immunosorbent assay reveals that anti-HBc is accompanied by anti-HBs. Over many years the titer of anti-HBc and anti-HBs may decline and in a small proportion of individuals one, or rarely both, of the antibodies may reach nondetectable levels.

In contrast to anti-HBs, anti-HBc is not a neutralizing antibody, and detection of anti-HBc does not necessarily signal recovery from HBV infection. In fact, individuals with persistent HBV infection who are identified as HBsAg carriers invariably have circulating anti-HBc. Immune complexes of anti-HBc with HBcAg[462,930] released from nonintact HBV particles may circulate in some HBsAg carriers. Persistent high titers of anti-HBc in the absence of HBsAg or anti-HBs may indicate the presence and continuing replication of HBV in the liver. Sera from such individuals may contain infectious amounts of intact HBV particles.[453,461]

Anti-HBe is the next antibody to appear after anti-HBc.[533] Anti-HBe does not react with intact HBV particles and plays no role in virus neutralization: HBV particles may be present in sera containing anti-HBe.[83,884,1062] Despite the latter observation, the presence of anti-HBe usually signifies reduced infectivity. Anti-HBe of the IgG immunoglobulin class is detected, by radioimmunoassay, as a freely circulating antibody during the acute phase of illness as early as the fourth week after the onset of symptoms.[549,991] Immune complexes of HBeAg-anti-HBe may precede the appearance of the free antibody.[991] These immune complexes appear to be short lived but may nonetheless result in the development of immune complex–mediated extrahepatic disease in some subjects.[932] Free anti-HBe may persist for several months after the clearance of HBeAg–anti-HBe complexes.[991]

Anti-HBs is the last antibody to appear during HBV infection and is usually detected during the late convalescent phase.[543] In typical patients anti-HBs may be detected by a simple, widely available and sensitive radioimmunoassay or enzyme immunoassay, 4 or more months after the onset of the acute illness, weeks to months after the disappearance of HBsAg.

There is considerable evidence that anti-HBs may be synthesized earlier in the course of acute HBV infection. In fact, circulating immune complexes of HBsAg and anti-HBs may be readily detected during the late incubation period and early acute phase of illness.[20,22,1045] During this period, anti-HBs is not detectable as freely circulating antibody because HBsAg is present in excess.

Anti-HBs is a neutralizing, protective antibody. It reacts with HBsAg on the surface of the intact HBV particle and HBsAg in the form of the small spherical or rodlike particle. A hepatitis B immune globulin containing high-titer, anti-HBs and a hepatitis B vaccine that stimulates production of anti-HBs are available for prophylaxis of hepatitis B.

Anti-HBs is found predominantly in IgM and IgG in sera[562] and as an IgA antibody in secretions.[730] IgM anti-

HBs is short lived, whereas the IgG anti-HBs persists for prolonged periods. The appearance of anti-HBs usually indicates recovery from infection and the development of immunity.[549] Individuals with preexisting anti-HBs are usually resistant to reinfection. When they are reexposed to HBV, such individuals develop an anamnestic response. This is signaled by a rise in the titer of anti-HBs without other serologic, biochemical, or clinical evidence of infection.[58,560] The appearance of anti-HBs without preceding HBsAg or anti-HBc is indicative of a primary immunization response following exposure to HBsAg.[452] This is the pattern that follows inoculation of HBsAg in the hepatitis B vaccines and occurs in the absence of viral replication.

Hepatitis D Virus

Identified in 1977 by immunofluorescent staining of liver tissue from Italian patients with chronic hepatitis due to persistent HBV infection,[832] HDV, also termed delta hepatitis virus (Table 15-4), is now recognized as a distinct hepatitis agent. Limited studies demonstrating antibody to hepatitis D antigen (anti-HD) in immune globulin prepared in the United States in 1944 indicate that HDV was introduced into human populations at least 4 decades ago.[772] In liver tissue HDV has been recognized as a 23-nm to 25-nm intranuclear or, occasionally, cytoplasmic particle with antigenic reactivity, hepatitis D antigen (HDAg), which can be detected by immunofluorescent or immunoperoxidase techniques. In serum, HDV exists as a 35-nm to 37-nm particle.[831] Disruption of the particle with detergent reveals the presence of internal components, including delta proteins (with HDAg reactivity) and a small, linear RNA molecule with 1750 nucleotides.[101]

TABLE 15-4.   Nomenclature of Hepatitis D

PREFERRED TERM	OTHER TERM(S)	COMMENTS
Hepatitis D	Delta hepatitis	Hepatitis due to infection by the hepatitis D virus; acute or chronic hepatitis is seen in patients with either acute or persistent HDV infection.
Hepatitis D virus (HDV)	Delta agent/virus	A defective RNA virus requiring the helper function of HBV for its expression and replication; HDV appears to be cytopathic.
Hepatitis D antigen (HDAg)	Delta antigen	The antigenic reactivity of the hepatitis D virus
Antibody to HDAg (Anti-HD)	Antibody to delta (anti-delta)	Antibody to the hepatitis D antigen; IgM and IgG antibodies have been described.

Purified HDV RNA has a molecular weight of 5.5×10^5, shows no homology with HBV DNA or host RNA, and has neither a poly A tail at its 3' end nor reverse transcriptase activity.[460] Complementary DNA prepared from HDV RNA has been used to determine nucleotide sequences of the genome.[214]

The external coat of HDV in serum is HBsAg. The complete HDV has a buoyant density of 1.25 g/cm^3 in cesium chloride and a sedimentation coefficient intermediate between those of the 22-nm particle and the intact HBV particle.[831]

HDV is believed to be a defective hepatotrophic pathogen that requires the helper functions of HBV for its expression, replication, and induction of hepatitis. Because HDV is dependent on the synthesis of HBsAg for its assembly, HDV infection is limited to HBsAg-positive humans or chimpanzees. Transmission experiments reveal that HDV is highly infectious: a 10^{-11} dilution of serum containing HDV induced infection in HBsAg carrier chimpanzees.[799] HDV also has been shown to be infectious on inoculation into woodchucks infected by the woodchuck hepatitis virus. The HDV particles identified in experimentally infected woodchucks are enveloped by the woodchuck hepatitis virus surface antigen.[771]

Although the mechanism of HDV replication is poorly understood, HDV appears to compete with HBV for its replication. As a result, HDV infection is accompanied by a reduction in both intrahepatic levels and serum titers of HBsAg, HBeAg, HBV DNA, and HBV DNA polymerase.[830] HDV and HBV may simultaneously infect a host (co-primary infection) or HDV may superinfect an existing HBsAg carrier. The duration of HDV infection appears to be dependent, in large part, on the duration of HBV infection. In co-primary infection, HDV replication is limited to the period in which HBsAg is produced. As a result, HDV infection is self-limited and in many instances resembles uncomplicated HBV infection.[932] In other cases, co-infection appears to induce severe, fulminant hepatitis.[357] In contrast, in patients with persistent HBV infection, HDV superinfection may result in an exacerbation of illness, suggesting superimposed acute hepatitis, which may be fulminant, or persistent HDV infection leading to severe chronic liver disease.[171,266,829]

Serologic Tests for Identification of HDV Infection. Initial studies of the hepatitis D antigen (HDAg) and antibody to HDAg (anti-HD) used indirect immunofluorescent techniques to identify the antigen and simple blocking assays for detection of antibody.[832] Subsequently, a sensitive, solid-phase radioimmunoassay for HDAg and anti-HD were developed by Rizzetto and colleagues,[828] using liver tissue obtained at autopsy as a source of HDAg. A simple, enzyme-linked immunosorbent assay, which also employed HDAg extracted from liver tissue, was reported to be less sensitive than radioimmunoassay for detection of anti-HD but more sensitive for the detection of HDAg.[188] More recently, sensitive and specific solid-phase radioimmunoassays and enzyme-linked immunosorbent

assays for HDAg and anti-HD that use serum as the source of HDAg have been developed.[235,901] Comparable sensitivity and specificity seem likely, but extensive evaluation is not yet available, and most tests for HDAg and anti-HD have been limited to research laboratories. The release of commercial assays should permit expansion of knowledge about HDV serology.

Identification of HDAg. The presence of HDV infection in HBsAg-positive patients can be identified by detection of HDAg in liver tissue or in serum or by demonstration of anti-HD seroconversion. Although HDAg may be present in hepatocyte nuclei in acute HDV infection before HDAg can be identified in sera, before the onset of liver injury, and before the development of anti-HD,[830] liver biopsy is an impractical means of establishing the diagnosis of HDV in patients with acute hepatitis. In early studies of HDV infection, HDAg was infrequently detected in the serum of patients with acute hepatitis and when present usually disappeared within a few days.[933] In subsequent studies, HDAg has been detected in as few as 2% and as many as 70% to 80% of patients with acute HDV infection.[459,476,901] This extraordinarily wide range may reflect differences in the sensitivity of assays or in the timing of specimen collections. The precise time of appearance and disappearance and changes in the serum titer of HDAg in acute HDV infection remains to be defined. Although the finding of HDAg in serum is consistent with active HDV infection, the absence of circulating HDAg does not exclude HDV infection, which may be recognized by the demonstration of anti-HD seroconversion. In patients with persistent HDV infection, circulating HDAg may be present but in many, if not most instances, it is below the detection limits of current assays. In contrast, demonstration of HDAg in the liver of patients with HBsAg-positive chronic hepatitis serves as a marker of HDV infection.

Identification of Antibody to Hepatitis D Antigen (Anti-HD). Acute HDV infection in either HBsAg-positive chimpanzees or humans elicits the production of an IgM anti-HD that is usually detectable in serum in low titer for a brief period.[934] In those instances in which HDV and HBV co-infection is self-limited, the IgM anti-HD rarely remains demonstrable after clearance of HBsAg and intrahepatic HDAg. In most patients with acute HDV infection IgG anti-HD, if present, is found in very low levels or cannot be detected.[846] However, in an unknown but presumably small number of patients low-level IgG anti-HD may remain detectable (without circulating HBsAg) long after HDV/HBV infection.[728] The mechanism leading to long-term persistence of anti-HD in HBsAg-negative patients is uncertain. Because circulating anti-HD has usually disappeared 3 or more months after acute infection in most patients, serodiagnosis of HDV infection in the past cannot be regularly detected with current assays. In contrast to acute HDV infection, persistent HDV infection of HBsAg carriers is characterized serologically by the presence of high titers of anti-HD. Both IgM and IgG anti-HD may be present, but anti-HD of the IgG class is the predominant immunoglobulin.[825]

Non-A, Non-B Hepatitis Virus(es)

Highly sensitive and specific techniques for the serologic identification of HAV and HBV infections made it clear that another set of agents, immunologically unrelated to either HAV, HDV, or HBV, also is responsible for viral hepatitis in humans. These agents, serologically distinct from HAV, HDV, HBV, and other viruses known to involve the liver (*e.g.,* cytomegalovirus, Epstein-Barr virus) have been termed the *non-A, non-B hepatitis viruses,* to indicate the absence of an etiologic relationship to either HAV or HBV. This nomenclature has been widely adopted. Two blood-borne and a third epidemic (and sporadic-endemic) non-A, non-B hepatitis agents have been postulated.[983]

The earliest evidence suggesting the existence of multiple non-A, non-B agents was the observation of sequential episodes of viral hepatitis that could not be attributed either to HAV, HBV, or to other recognized agents affecting the liver.[222,497,688] Although it was possible that second attacks of non-A, non-B viral hepatitis reflected failure of a single agent to induce homologous immunity, support for this concept is limited. In fact, most cross-challenge studies in susceptible chimpanzees indicated that recovery from infection provided protection against clinically apparent reinfection following inoculation with a presumably antigenically similar, if not identical, agent.[111,438,1094] In some studies reinfection has been described but may reflect the presence of more than one agent in the inoculum[132] or that immunity can be overwhelmed by the use of a very large inocula.[124] Human transmission studies are concordant with the chimpanzee studies showing homologous immunity.[449] Five recipients of plasma that had earlier been implicated in post-transfusion non-A, non-B viral hepatitis, developed non-A, non-B infection. After recovery, these individuals were reinoculated with the same plasma. None developed clinically apparent infection, suggesting that acquired immunity had developed.[449]

Another observation favoring the existence of more than one non-A, non-B hepatitis virus is the description of different incubation periods and different periods and patterns of serum aminotransferase elevations in groups of patients with non-A, non-B viral hepatitis.[449] Although biologic variability could be responsible, similar observations in experimentally infected chimpanzees suggest that the phenomenon reflects true differences among the etiologic agents.[30,986]

Further support for two distinct bloodborne non-A, non-B hepatitis viruses has been provided by limited studies of the physicochemical properties of agents isolated from inocula of known infectivity and by identification of ultrastructural alterations in the hepatocytes of infected chimpanzees. Both agents are inactivated by heating at 60° C for 10 hours and at least one and probably both are inactivated by exposure to formalin.[440,1093] Sensitivity to chloroform is a differential point: one agent is inactivated by exposure to chloroform, while the other is chloroform resistant.[110] The chloroform-sensitive virus passes through an 80-nm membrane filter[112] and is associated, in the infected chimpanzee, with the formation of cytoplasmic tubules in the hepatocyte. The chloroform-resistant agent does not induce cytoplasmic tubules. Although "strain-specific" nuclear alterations were postulated in early studies of chimpanzees infected with different inocula,[909] subsequent studies have failed to confirm a relationship of nuclear virus-like particles to non-A, non-B hepatitis, and even the specificity of nuclear particles to viral hepatitis seems unlikely.[219,366,948]

At least one of the non-A, non-B agents is resistant to inactivation by prolonged storage (for years) in lyophilized or frozen (−70° C) serum or plasma products.[986]

In contrast to the demonstrated susceptibility of chimpanzees to the blood-borne non-A, non-B hepatitis viruses, the epidemic form of non-A, non-B hepatitis has yet to be successfully transmitted to these animals.[492] The epidemic non-A, non-B agent as well as the blood-borne agents have been transmitted to marmosets[279,492] and the epidemic agent also has been transmitted to cynomolgus monkeys.[47] The epidemic non-A, non-B hepatitis virus has been transmitted to a single human volunteer by ingestion of a pooled stool extract prepared from patients during the acute phase of the illness.[47] Spherical particles 27 nm to 30 nm in diameter have been identified in stool samples from the volunteer, in patients with this disease,[492,950] and in experimentally infected marmosets.[492] In contrast to these data indicating fecal excretion of the epidemic non-A, non-B hepatitis virus, fecal excretion of at least one of the blood-borne agents has not been established in susceptible chimpanzees.[125]

Despite the repeated observation of 27- to 30-nm virus-like particles in the stools of patients with epidemic non-A, non-B hepatitis, the precise size and nucleic acid composition of the three postulated agents of non-A, non-B hepatitis remain uncertain. Virus-like particles ranging from 14 nm to 140 nm in diameter have been reported in serum and liver samples:[222] the specific relationship of any of these to the blood-borne agents of non-A, non-B hepatitis remains unsubstantiated. Putative 27-nm virus-like particles are shown in Figure 15-6. In one study a small fragment of DNA isolated from a human serum of known infectivity was cloned and used to detect the same DNA fragment in sera from chimpanzees experimentally infected by one of the blood-borne agents. These data suggest that one of the non-A, non-B agents is a DNA virus.[336] In contrast, particle-associated reverse transcriptase activity, characteristic of the RNA containing retroviruses, has been described in the sera of patients with blood-borne non-A, non-B hepatitis.[900] Each of these findings has yet to be corroborated by other investigators.

An additional and continuing controversy concerns the possible relationship of one or both of the non-A, non-B

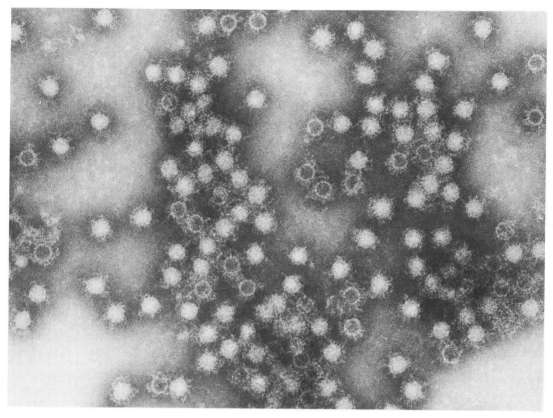

Fig. 15-6. Electron micrograph of 27-nm viruslike particles detected in liver homogenates of a chimpanzee experimentally infected with a putative non-A, non-B hepatitis virus. (Original magnification × 206,700; courtesy of Dr. Daniel W. Bradley)

blood-borne agents to HBV. It has been suggested that non-A, non-B hepatitis may be a unique form of HBV infection in which the typical serologic markers of HBV do not appear. Support for this concept includes descriptions of HBV-like particles in the plasma of affected patients,[394] reports of antigenic activity in non-A, non-B sera cross-reacting with HBV antigens,[1013,1034] the identification of HBV DNA in sera or liver samples of patients with chronic liver disease attributed to non-A, non-B hepatitis,[285] and the detection of HBV DNA in the serum of chimpanzees experimentally infected with non-A, non-B hepatitis.[1048] Other observations cast considerable doubt on the validity of this notion. These include epidemiologic considerations,[274] the lack of homologous immunity between HBV and non-A, non-B hepatitis,[976] evidence of viral interference (suppression of HBV DNA in HBsAg carrier chimpanzees superinfected with one of the blood-borne non-A, non-B viruses),[396] and the uncertain specificity of the laboratory techniques (monoclonal assays for HBsAg, molecular hybridization assays for detection of HBV DNA)[274] used in those studies suggesting a close relationship. The weight of currently available evidence fails to support the hypothesis that non-A, non-B hepatitis is a cryptic form of HBV infection.

A variety of conventional serologic techniques have been used by dozens of investigators in the search for non-A, non-B hepatitis antigens and antibodies. Among these are immunodiffusion, counterimmunoelectrophoresis, immunofluorescence and immune electron microscopy, radioimmunoassay, and enzyme-linked immunosorbent assay. Although several laboratories have described candidate antigen–antibody systems with each of these methodologies,[222,274,444] confirmation of their reproducibility, specificity, sensitivity, and diagnostic value has yet to be made. A number of assays appear to detect nonspecific rheumatoid factor–like materials or reactivity to host antigens present in the sera of patients with a spectrum of liver disorders unrelated to non-A, non-B viral hepatitis.[839] The difficulty in developing a specific and sensitive serologic test may be related, in large part, to the observation that the titer of circulating virus may be relatively low in non-A, non-B hepatitis. In a number of experimental transmission studies titers of less than 10^3 to 10^6 chimpanzee infectious doses per milliliter have been documented.[109] At such low levels, detection of particle-associated viral antigens may be impossible with conventional serologic techniques. It is also possible that specific antibody is produced in insufficient titers for optimal sensitivity in serologic testing. Confounding the issue, of course, is the existence of at least two blood-borne agents as well as the agent of epidemic non-A, non-B hepatitis. The multiplicity of agents suggests that multiple serologic tests will be required for specific identification of all non-A, non-B hepatitis virus infections.

Other approaches under current investigation for the identification of non-A, non-B agents have not yet been fruitful.[109] Propagation of virus in tissue culture systems yielding a cytopathic effect and detection of viral nucleic acids or viral-specific proteins in cell cultures or explants have not been achieved. Similarly, detection of non-A, non-B hepatitis virus nucleic acid sequences with specific molecular probes and detection of in vitro viral interference associated with non-A, non-B infections are under study, but definitive reports are not yet available.

Identification. The specific identification of non-A, non-B agents by serologic techniques is not yet available in the clinical laboratory. Identification of the disease remains dependent on serologic studies that exclude the presence of HAV and HBV infections. The absence of IgM anti-HAV, HBsAg, and IgM anti-HBc is the usual requirement before non-A, non-B hepatitis can be accepted. Confirmation of infection requires experimental infection of chimpanzees, an impractical procedure for the clinical laboratory. Diagnosis by exclusion will be superceded when candidate antigen-antibody systems are confirmed, sensitive techniques for their detection are developed, and the responsible agents are isolated and partially purified. Whether these can be propagated in tissue culture systems remains to be determined.

IMMUNOPATHOGENESIS OF VIRAL HEPATITIS

The mechanisms underlying the development of the necroinflammatory lesions characteristic of viral hepatitis remain incompletely defined. Host-mediated immunologic responses have received considerable attention because there is very little evidence that hepatitis viruses are directly cytotoxic to hepatocytes.

Hepatitis A

Classification of HAV as an enterovirus favors a cytopathic role because cytopathogenicity is characteristic of enteroviruses. The absence of an asymptomatic HAV viremic or fecal carrier state also supports, indirectly, the notion that HAV is cytopathic. Further indirect support for direct cytotoxicity is provided by the observation of a correlation between severity of the hepatitis and fecal shedding of HAV.[234,303] If fecal shedding is directly related to viral replication in the liver and viral replication is related to extent of hepatocyte necrosis, then hepatocyte necrosis

and severity of illness may be directly related to virus-induced cytotoxicity. Finally, in experimentally infected marmosets, it was observed that the incubation period of hepatitis A became progressively shorter on serial passage, reaching an interval as short as 7 days.[793] This brief incubation period is compatible with direct cytotoxicity induced by HAV but does not prove this mechanism.

In most primates, fecal shedding of virus occurs well before the clinical or histologic evidence of hepatitis. Both in the chimpanzee and in patients, fecal shedding rapidly drops and disappears at the peak of hepatitis. Indeed, HAV is usually not recoverable from stool after peak aminotransferase or bilirubin levels were reached. In vitro observation based on marmoset liver explant cultures and fetal rhesus monkey kidney cell lines in which HAV have been propagated have not shown that HAV is cytopathic.[90,192,304,790]

An immunologically mediated host contribution to the pathogenesis of hepatitis A is also supported by the detection of anti-HAV of the IgM class,[117] circulating immune complexes,[998] and depressed levels of serum complement during the early acute phase of the illness when hepatocyte injury is evident. It is not known whether this humoral response to HAV is related to cell necrosis or whether antibody-dependent lymphocyte cytotoxicity plays a role in the pathogenesis of liver injury in hepatitis A. Despite the detection of HAV in glomeruli of infected marmosets,[631] which suggests intrarenal deposition of immune complexes of HAV and anti-HAV, the contribution of immune complexes to the development of liver injury remains uncertain. Furthermore, evidence of extrahepatic immune complex disease in hepatitis A is scant. Current evidence indicates that the immunopathology of hepatitis A falls into two stages. The first one is viral replication in the liver with increasing viral shedding in the stool but without hepatocyte necrosis. In the second phase, hepatocyte necrosis appears, which is associated with the development of antibodies against HAV and a marked and progressive reduction and elimination of viral shedding at an equal rate with the development of immunity.

Cell-mediated immune mechanisms have been incompletely evaluated. A reduction of T lymphocytes has been noted in the peripheral blood of HAV-infected marmosets and humans,[206] but the specificity of this feature is doubtful because nonviral hepatic disorders may also be associated with peripheral T-lymphocytopenia. An inhibitor of T lymphocytes, the rosette-inhibitory factor (a serum lipoprotein) has been detected in some patients with delayed clinical resolution.[155] In other patients, an intrinsic defect in the ability of the T lymphocyte to form rosettes has been described.[155] The precise role of these lymphocyte alterations in the pathogenesis of hepatic injury in HAV infection remains uncertain. The suggestion that parenchymal necrosis in the liver in hepatitis A is mediated by an immunopathologic mechanism is strongly supported by the fact that NK lymphocytes preferentially kill monkey kidney cells that have been infected by the hepatitis A virus.[558]

Hepatitis B

HBV is not directly cytopathic either in infected humans or in experimentally infected chimpanzees. Failure of HBV to evoke cytopathic effects in tissue culture systems in which, nonetheless, HBsAg may be produced, suggests that intracellular production of HBsAg is not necessarily accompanied by cell injury. HBsAg containing hepatocytes in human liver biopsies often show no evidence of damage. The observation that persistent HBV infection in humans or chimpanzees, as ascertained by the identification of asymptomatic carriers of circulating HBsAg, is frequently unassociated with either biochemical or histopathologic evidence of liver injury lends further credence to the search for mechanisms of injury other than direct virus-induced cytotoxicity.

Therefore, immunologically mediated host responses have become the major focus of studies directed to elucidating the pathogenesis of liver injury in HBV infection. Humoral and cell-mediated immune mechanisms and their interaction have been considered to be critically important factors controlling hepatocyte injury directly or through modulation of HBV replication. Immune-mediated inhibition of virus synthesis or immune-mediated destruction of virus-infected hepatocytes is the likely mechanism. Immunologic responses appear to play key roles in the resolution or persistence of infection. It has been postulated that both acute hepatic injury and resolution of HBV infection are a reflection of an appropriate immune response. In contrast, infection without apparent cytotoxicity and persistent HBV replication appear to indicate failure of the host to mount an immune response capable of suppressing HBV replication or eradicating HBV-infected hepatocytes.

Immunologic responses directed to viral products of infection, for example, HBV antigens, appear to have a temporal but not necessarily a pathogenic relationship to hepatic injury. For example, anti-HBc, which is usually found in sera during the early acute phase of hepatitis B simultaneously with evidence of liver injury, is not readily implicated because it is almost always present, in high titers, in asymptomatic HBsAg carriers. Because carriers may be entirely free of hepatocyte injury, the role of anti-HBc *per se* in inducing hepatocyte damage must be minimal if any. It is also clear that the presence of HBsAg and HBcAg in hepatocytes does not necessarily provoke cell destruction. It is possible, however, that immunologic elimination of viral antigens is associated pathogenically with hepatocyte destruction. In experimental infection of chimpanzees with HBV, peak biochemical and morphologic alterations indicative of hepatocellular injury occurred at the time of disappearance or diminution of HBV antigens in the liver.[450]

It has been postulated that the pathogenic immunologic responses may be directed not merely to viral antigens but also to virus-induced or virus-modified membrane antigens or normal hepatocellular components. Viral antigen can be accessible when it is attached to or is incor-porated into the hepatocyte membrane. Immune response may be elicited to host antigen by the exposure or release of host hepatocyte antigens in a modified form. Both humoral and cell-mediated mechanisms have been implicated in the response to hepatocyte antigens. Antibodies to a liver-specific membrane lipoprotein (LSP) were found in most patients with HBV infection within 2 weeks of the onset of jaundice, and antibody titers decreased progressively during convalescence.[482] No correlation was found between titer and severity of illness. The antibody was also identified in cases of viral hepatitis due to agents other than HBV. The importance of this antibody in the pathogenesis of hepatitis remains uncertain.

Immunoglobulins with reactivity to HBV antigens, HBV antigens, and complement (immune complexes) have been identified in the livers of some patients with chronic liver disease associated with HBV but infrequently in individuals with acute HBV infection.[729] Immune complexes or cryoproteins containing anti-HBs and HBsAg immune complexes[652,914] or anti-HBe and HBeAg immune complexes[991] are often present in sera during the prodrome and early phase of hepatitis B. These are usually found in a state of antigen excess and disappear during the late stage or convalescent period coincident with the appearance of free anti-HBs in the circulation. The role of these immune complexes in the pathogenesis of hepatic injury is uncertain. Nevertheless it is possible that they contribute indirectly by altering humoral and cell-mediated responses. It has been unequivocally shown that immune complex–mediated responses to HBV infection play a pathogenic role in some of the extrahepatic manifestations of HBV infection. However, the presence of detectable immune complexes in HBV infection is not always accompanied by clinical manifestations of immune complex disease.[782,1045] In fact, only a small proportion of patients with acute hepatitis B develop clinically apparent manifestations of extrahepatic disease.

The usual clinical picture in affected patients is that of a syndrome resembling serum sickness and comprising urticaria,[233] angioneurotic edema,[22] other rashes,[1061] polyarthritis,[527] and rarely, glomerulonephritis,[173,743] or forme fruste of this syndrome with just one or two components. Deposition of immune complexes in skin,[233,1061] joints,[880] and glomeruli[173] appears to be responsible for the associated clinical manifestations. In contrast to the immune complexes seen in patients with hepatitis B who do not have extrahepatic manifestations, those isolated from sera of patients with the serum sickness–like syndrome appear to activate both the classic and alternate complement pathways.[1045] Complement components may be depressed in sera during the period in which immune complex disease is evident.[22] In summary, humoral immune reaction to HBsAg seems to be responsible for the extrahepatic manifestations of HBV infection but probably not for hepatitis.

Cell-mediated immune mechanisms in the induction of the hepatic injury of HBV infection have been studied in a number of laboratories.[246,572,718,1011,1046] The bulk of present evidence suggests that cell-mediated responses are more closely related to resolution of infection than to the development of hepatocyte injury. Depressed T-lymphocyte function, measured *in vitro* in the presence of HBV antigens,[246,572,1011] has been correlated with the development of persistent HBV infection. Absent or markedly reduced T-cell function may lead to the HBsAg carrier state, whereas a blunted response may result in chronic liver damage.[1011] It has been suggested that normal T-lymphocyte function is responsible for the self-limited course of most HBV infections. Despite these notions, there is considerable evidence that T-lymphocyte function is altered during HBV infection.

A transient decrease of T lymphocytes in peripheral blood has been observed during the acute phase of hepatitis B but is not invariably found.[250] Lymphocytotoxic IgG or IgM antibodies[205] and other factors (*e.g.*, rosette-inhibitory factor) that may depress T-lymphocyte function have been described.[155,1046] Rosette-inhibitory factor (RIF) can contribute to lack of production of anti-HBs during the acute phase of hepatitis B.[859] RIF, a low-density lipoprotein, suppresses immunoglobulin and anti-HBs synthesis by inhibiting specific helper T cell (OKT4) function but does not affect B cell function in response to soluble T helper factors.[860] A factor in sera of patients with acute hepatitis inhibited mitogen-induced transformation of normal lymphocytes. The serum inhibitory factor (SIF) titer decreased in those who recovered but tended to remain positive in those whose hepatitis remained active 1 year after its onset. In these patients, HBsAg remained positive and they failed to develop anti-HBs.[1069] SIF and RIF seem to be prognostic of outcome of acute viral hepatitis: SIF is related to the immune response and RIF is associated with hepatocellular injury.[364]

Circulating lymphocytes may directly damage HBV-infected hepatocytes. HBsAg or other HBV antigens on the hepatocyte membranes or induced alterations of the membrane may serve as a reactive site for HBsAg-binding lymphocytes that subsequently damage the membrane irreversibly, leading to hepatocyte death. K (killer) lymphocytes may also play a critical role. These cells, lacking surface immunoglobulin or receptors for sheep erythrocytes, are known to lyse IgG-coated target cells in the absence of complement. In acute hepatitis B, K-cell activity appears to be increased during the acute phase, falling to normal levels several weeks after the onset of illness.[250]

Hepatitis D

There are two clearly established characteristics of HDV infection: (1) it cannot cause disease by itself but causes infection only when HBV is present in the host and (2) any material that contains HDV will be infectious to susceptible individuals only if it also contains HBV. That means that anyone who is immune to HBV is automatically protected against HDV infection.

Serologic evidence of HDV infection was found commonly among Italians, whether they resided in Italy or elsewhere. However, outside of Italy, evidence of HDV infection in HBsAg carriers was found almost exclusively among drug addicts or polytransfused carriers. Although evidence of HDV infection can be found occasionally in HBsAg-negative individuals, it is found predominantly in those who are chronic carriers of HBsAg. The HBsAg-negative individuals, however, have either other serologic evidence of previous exposure to HBV or demonstrable sequential serologic changes indicating recovery from acute hepatitis B.[201,834,835]

When co-infection of HBV and HDV occurs, the usual sequence of events is a transient acute hepatitis. Under these circumstances, HDV replication is only transient and can be demonstrated by finding a transient increase of IgM anti-HD antibody. In this case, the transient HBV infection subsides and immunity develops following the seroconversion from HBsAg to anti-HBs. However, if hepatitis B viremia is not transient but is prolonged, then the co-infecting HDV is allowed to replicate. The consequences are either cumulative or sequential development of HDV hepatitis, co-occurring or following HBV hepatitis. In an area of Italy endemic for hepatitis D, the prevalence of anti-HD was low in patients with acute hepatitis (6.6%). In none of the 592 consecutive subjects was HD antigen (HDAg) detectable.[185]

In general, when HBV and HDV occur together, the disease is significantly more severe than when HBV is the sole infectious agent.[846,901] A co-infection of HBV and HDV can be the explanation for some of the fulminant hepatitis B cases.

Superinfection of HDV can occur in HBsAg carriers. Acute hepatitis B is more likely to become chronic with HDV superinfection than without it.[135] The presence of HBsAg amplifies the pathogenicity of HDV. Consequently, the most common clinical setting for HDV infection is in chronic carriers of HBsAg. This infection is characterized by a low titer HBsAg, the presence of anti-HBe, and a lack of IgM anti-HBc. HDV infection will cause an acute hepatitis in the "healthy" carrier or it can cause a deterioration and increased aggressiveness of chronic active hepatitis B.

Acute hepatitis B and acute hepatitis D co-infection are characterized by the following serologic markers: HBsAg, HBeAg, IgM anti-HBc, the absence of anti-HBe, positive IgM anti-HD and negative anti-HBs. On the other hand, the development of acute hepatitis D in a chronic HBsAg carrier is characterized by the following serologies: positive HBsAg, IgG anti-HBc, and negative anti-HBs, positive IgM anti-HD. The HBeAg may or may not be positive, and, conversely, the anti-HBe may or may not be positive.

When an HBsAg carrier becomes infected with HDV, an acute transient hepatitis is usually experienced. Occasionally, the surface antigenemia may be terminated by an acute HDV infection. HDV infection can also produce subclinical hepatitis. Such disease was identified in more than 30% of Italian blood donors positive for anti-HD. Greek workers found anti-HD in a high proportion of asymptomatic HBsAg carriers who had biopsy evidence of hepatitis. A person who had HBV infection but continues to have active hepatitis is much less susceptible to HDV infection. On the other hand, those whose HBV infection became inactive or dormant and developed anti-HBe are much more susceptible to HDV infection.[826]

HDAg is usually detectable prior to the clinical onset of hepatitis. HDAg rapidly clears during the course of acute hepatitis. It then rapidly converts to IgM anti-HD. The mechanism of clearance of HDV is not known. Protective antibody similar to anti-HBs in the case of HBV infection has not been identified for HDV.

If a person has an HBsAg-positive acute hepatitis, the diagnostic difference between acute hepatitis B and acute hepatitis D is the presence or absence of IgM anti-HBc: it is present in acute hepatitis B and is absent in hepatitis D.

Hepatitis D is due to a direct cytopathic mechanism, in contrast to an immunologic attack on the hepatocyte in the case of hepatitis B. Acute hepatitis produced by infection with HBsAg-associated HDV agent in experimental animals is associated with the development of intrahepatic deposits of immunoglobulins. The production of immune complexes that are detectable by *in vitro* complement fixation is of no pathogenetic significance in the production of acute hepatitis D but is an epiphenomenon.[833]

After recovery from acute hepatitis D, immunity can be overcome by a larger dose of the same plasma pool that caused the initial acute hepatitis in chimpanzees.*

Non-A, Non-B Hepatitis

The immunopathogenesis of non-A, non-B infections is poorly understood because available data are very limited. Because an asymptomatic non-A, non-B hepatitis virus carrier state has been recognized and because it has been demonstrated that acute infection may lead to chronic liver disease with persistence of the etiologic agent in peripheral blood and presumably in the hepatocyte, analogies to HBV infection have seemed reasonably well drawn. Whether persistent infection and prolonged viremia are reflections of properties inherent to these agents, or, as in the case of HBV infection, are indicative of an immune response that is not sufficient to terminate the infection, remains to be determined.

Anticomplementary activity has been detected in acute-phase sera of patients with non-A, non-B viral hepatitis following blood transfusion.[797] Subsequently, circulating immune complexes have been recognized in a majority of patients with non-A, non-B viral hepatitis studied prospectively after blood transfusion.[226] Immune complexes appeared just before, coincident with, or just after the development of increased serum aminotransferase levels. In a small number of patients who developed chronic liver disease following transfusion-associated non-A, non-B hepatitis, fluctuating levels of aminotransferases appeared

to parallel changes in levels of circulating immune complexes.[226] Because immune complexes were detected in a few individuals following transfusion without biochemical evidence of hepatitis, the specificity of the immune complexes requires further evaluation. Isolation and characterization of the antigenic components will be necessary in future studies.

EPIDEMIOLOGY

Despite the imprecision resulting from the lack of specific serologic markers of the hepatitis viruses, various factors provided an early foundation for the understanding of the epidemiology of the diseases. These factors included limited studies based on human transmission experiments, field investigations of hepatitis outbreaks, collections of hospitalized cases, and morbidity data obtained through the national viral hepatitis surveillance program. The development and widespread use of specific laboratory tests in the late 1960s and the 1970s resulted in increased epidemiologic sophistication and important revision of invalid concepts. Descriptions of the epidemiologic behavior of hepatitis A have changed but little, whereas those concerning hepatitis B have been altered extensively.

The epidemiologic features of hepatitis D are incompletely understood but appear to resemble those of hepatitis B. The epidemiologic attributes of blood-borne non-A, non-B hepatitis share many characteristics with hepatitis B, while the epidemic form of non-A, non-B hepatitis more closely resembles hepatitis A.

Hepatitis A, B, D, and non-A, non-B are worldwide in distribution. Geographic differences in the incidence of the acute disease, the prevalence of infection, the frequency of chronic infection (in the case of hepatitis B, D, and presumably non-A, non-B viral hepatitis), and in the distribution of the various etiologic forms have been described. Although biologic-ecologic factors may be largely responsible for variations in epidemiologic patterns, other factors appear to contribute to the lack of concordance reported from country to country. These include nonuniformity of reporting practices, of accessibility to medical care, and of thresholds for recognition of mild or asymptomatic infections. Serologic studies are not used universally, and relatively insensitive techniques may be employed in lieu of the expensive, highly sensitive procedures. Failure to distinguish the responsible agent by serologic testing and misdiagnosis also are responsible for part of the reported differences.

In the United States viral hepatitis has been a notifiable disease since 1952. Since 1974, notified cases have been classified by the reporting physician as hepatitis A, B, or unspecified, and since 1982, non-A, non-B hepatitis has been a separate category. However, even here use of serologic testing for diagnosis remains incomplete, and specific trends cannot be identified directly from categorization of physicians' diagnoses. Furthermore, reporting by physicians of viral hepatitis comprises less than 20%

---

* Purcell RH: Personal communication, 1985.

of all recognized cases.[531,625] In spite of these limitations, data obtained by the national hepatitis surveillance program appear to delineate adequately secular trends, age-specific attack rates, and alterations in patterns of infection that may be attributed circumstantially to specific etiologic agents.

Based on secular and seasonal patterns of reported cases between 1952 and 1965, hepatitis A was believed to be the predominant etiologic form of the disease. Between 1966 and 1970, highest age-specific attack rates shifted from children (aged 1 to 14) to young persons aged 15 to 29. This shift appeared to be associated with a dramatic increase in exposure to parenteral illicit drugs in this age-group,[127,236,320] presumably due to a true increase of hepatitis B and possibly non-A, non-B viral hepatitis, and a reduction in the frequency of hepatitis A in children. Seasonal variations have virtually disappeared since 1970. In the past decade, case rates have declined slightly to approximately 24 cases per 100,000, and an equal distribution between urban and rural areas has been recognized. Attack rates remained high in males 14 to 29 years of age.

The exact contribution of the four etiologic forms to hepatitis morbidity in the United States remains ill defined. In a series of hospitalized adults with viral hepatitis in Los Angeles, about 50% of patients had serologic evidence of hepatitis B.[223] The remainder were equally divided between hepatitis A and non-A, non-B hepatitis. Among veterans hospitalized in Boston in the mid 1970s, 65% had serologically documented hepatitis B and 35% were categorized as non-A, non-B viral hepatitis because serologic evidence of recent hepatitis A infection was absent.[528] In Baltimore, 48% of hospitalized hepatitis patients were confirmed hepatitis B, 10%, hepatitis A, and 42%, non-A, non-B hepatitis.[32] In Goteborg, Sweden, serologic studies revealed that 57% of acute cases were hepatitis B, 27%, hepatitis A, and the remainder, non-A, non-B.[726] In São Paulo, Brazil, 60% of hospitalized children and adults were serologically categorized as hepatitis A, 20% as hepatitis B, and 20% as non-A, non-B disease.[534] In Athens, 80% of sporadic hepatitis in adults was caused by hepatitis B, 11% by hepatitis A, and 9% by non-A, non-B agents.[744] Inapparent infections are common but have been less well categorized serologically. Less than 5% of individuals with serologic evidence of past HAV or HBV infection can recall an illness recognized to be hepatitis or jaundice. Seroepidemiologic studies in many, but not all, parts of the world indicate that HAV infections are more common than HBV infections.

Epidemiologic features generally attributed to hepatitis A[672] include highest age-specific attack rates in children aged 1 to 14; cyclic patterns reflecting in their nadirs the accumulation of a large number of susceptibles followed by wide-scale infections that at their peak result in a large immune population resulting in a subsequent decline in attack rates; seasonal peaks in late fall and winter; highest attack rates in rural regions; familial aggregation of cases; no recognized relationship to transfusion of blood or blood products; and low mortality rate.

In some but not all developing areas of the Third World, hepatitis A exhibits evidence of continuing hyperendemicity with extremely high inapparent infection rates in early childhood resulting in long-term immunity and very low attack rates in the adult population. Similar patterns have been recognized in closed institutions for the mentally retarded and in day-care centers in developed countries.

Because neither persistent viremia nor persistent fecal excretion of HAV has been established, it is believed that HAV is maintained in the population by serial transmission from acutely infected patients to susceptibles. No reservoir of infection has been documented in humans or nonhuman primates, although some species of the latter are susceptible to HAV infection and may transmit infection to humans. The predominant mode of HAV transmission is person-to-person contact involving fecal-oral spread. Hence, the intensity of fecal exposure as well as the number of susceptibles in a given population determine the attack rate of hepatitis A. Common-source transmission involving water or food vehicles, including mollusk-associated hepatitis A, is occasionally responsible for outbreaks but, with the possible exception of mollusk transmission, contributes minimally to the recognized morbidity of hepatitis A.

Transmission of hepatitis B was originally believed to require percutaneous exposure. Now it is also recognized in a variety of other settings as well. The existence of a variable but epidemiologically large reservoir of infected individuals and the documentation of person-to-person transmission by nonpercutaneous routes have been established unequivocally during the past decade. Because HBV produces both acute and chronic infections in humans and in some nonhuman primates, HBV is not dependent on transmission from acutely infected individuals to maintain itself in the population. Nonhuman primates are not believed to play a role in the perpetuation of HBV in humans; the reservoir of infection in humans is maintained by the existence of long-term carriers.

The prevalence of the HBsAg carrier state varies widely (see Table 15-5) from 0.3% to 1.0% in North America and western Europe, to 5% to 20% in some populations in sub-Saharan Africa, Asia, and the Mediterranean littoral.[723,1084] With some exceptions, carrier rates appear to be higher in the tropics or in urban areas, among children and males, and in low socioeconomic status groups. In a number of studies, males seemed to be more prone to develop either overt hepatitis B or the HBsAg carrier state. The latter reflects a genetic predisposition, which has also been postulated to account for the high infection rates found in some ethnic groups, although the primacy of genetic factors has not been definitively established. Other important determinants of HBsAg carrier rates include age at primary infection and the presence of immune deficiency states.

In general, carriers of HBV appear to have a milder disease than individuals with the acute disease. This is biologically advantageous because persistent infection appears to be an efficient means of perpetuating infection

TABLE 15-5.   Estimated World Prevalence of HBsAg Carrier State

REGION	ESTIMATED POPULATION (IN MILLIONS)	CARRIER PREVALENCE (%)	NUMBER OF CARRIERS (IN MILLIONS)
Asia	2,757	~4	110
Japan	118	~1.5	1.8
Europe	692	~1	7
USSR	269	~3	8.1
Africa	513	~6.6	33.9
North America	340	~0.5	1.7
South America	260	~2	5.2
World total	4,677	~3.5	165

in some populations because spread of infection is more likely from a chronically infected host. Persistent infection is not innocuous to the host however; chronic hepatitis and primary hepatocellular carcinoma appear to be sequelae of chronic HBV infection.

Nonpercutaneous "person-to-person" direct mucosal contact may result in transfer of HBV and is an important mode of transmission of HBV.

HDV infections, which occur only in individuals with HBV, appear to be spread by the same routes as HBV. Two major epidemiologic patterns are recognized. In countries in which HDV is endemic, such as those in southern Europe, north Africa, and the Middle East, infection is believed to be spread by intimate person-to-person contact. In nonendemic areas, such as the United States, HBV is transmitted by percutaneous routes and is most frequently detected in drug addicts and recipients of blood and blood products such as hemophiliacs.[846] From these populations, spread to intimate contacts has been described.[393] Explosive outbreaks of HDV may occur in endemic as well as nonendemic areas.[384,596,1022]

The epidemiology of non-A, non-B viral hepatitis remains incompletely defined in the absence of distinct serologic markers. Its existence has been recognized in virtually all parts of the world in which serologic testing for HAV and HBV can be achieved. The occurrence of multiple attacks of viral hepatitis in parenteral drug users that could not be attributed to HAV or HBV provided early evidence for the existence of the blood-borne non-A, non-B agents. These observations suggested that percutaneous transmission was the likely route of spread. Further support was derived from studies of post-transfusion viral hepatitis. The screening of blood donors for HBsAg almost eliminated transfusion-associated hepatitis B. However, this screening did not dramatically reduce the overall incidence of post-transfusion hepatitis. With rare exceptions, hepatitis A is not responsible for transfusion-associated hepatitis. Therefore, non-A, non-B viral agents were incriminated. At present, non-A, non-B infections appear to be responsible for more than 90% of transfusion-associated hepatitis.

These studies, as well as limited experimental transmission studies in humans and in nonhuman primates,

indicate that blood-borne non-A, non-B hepatitis strongly resembles hepatitis B in its epidemiologic characteristics. In addition to the identification of the percutaneous mode of transmission, they indicate the existence of a reservoir of chronically infected viremic individuals.[987] The carrier state in non-A, non-B infections appears to be more common in lower socioeconomic strata because transfusion of blood from paid donors, a low socioeconomic group, is more likely to produce non-A, non-B hepatitis in the recipient than is volunteer donated blood. Nonpercutaneous transmission from acutely infected individuals has been postulated, but the exact modes of nonpercutaneous spread remain to be determined.

Epidemic non-A, non-B hepatitis resembles HAV infections in its epidemiology. Fecal-oral transmission appears responsible for water-borne point-source outbreaks and person-to-person spread among household contacts. Persistent infection appears to be infrequent.

One further feature shared by blood-borne non-A, non-B viral hepatitis and hepatitis B is the risk of development of chronic liver disease associated with persistent infection.[806] Non-A, non-B viral hepatitis, however, has not been etiologically linked with primary hepatocellular carcinoma despite a few suggestive case reports.[45,820] This statement may require revision when serologic identification of the non-A, non-B agents is achieved and confirmed.

Incubation Period

Definition. The incubation period in viral hepatitis may be defined as the interval from exposure-infection to onset of symptoms. This definition conforms to that applied to other infectious disease, has been used in the literature with sufficient frequency to permit comparisons, and can be used in anicteric as well as icteric cases. In cases of inapparent infection, serum aminotransferase (transaminase) levels may be used to define the incubation period.

Hepatitis A. A large body of data accrued in naturally acquired outbreaks[300,591,767] and human transmission experiments[401,609] indicate that the mean incubation period of hepatitis A is approximately 30 days, with a range of 15 to 49 days. In most cases, the incubation period varies between 20 to 37 days. In clinical practice, the incubation period is most easily evaluated in common-source outbreaks in which exposure to a contaminated vehicle of infection is limited to a short period such as a day or two.[48,256,764,1019,1042]

The incubation period of hepatitis A is not influenced by the route of infection. In several transmission studies, materials containing HAV produced hepatitis with nearly identical incubation periods after percutaneous or peroral administration to volunteers.[399,706] No convincing evidence that size of the dose influences the incubation period is available.[400,1051]

Hepatitis B. The incubation period of hepatitis B, as determined in experimental transmission studies,[736–738] outbreaks of postvaccinal (smallpox,[481,603] yellow fever[866]) disease, and analysis of hepatitis B associated with transfusion of blood and blood derivatives,[17,360,675] is wide, ranging from 28 to 180 days. In most infections, the incubation period is 60 to 110 days with a mode of 70 to 80 days. However, in three series of post-transfusion hepatitis B, almost 20% of patients had an incubation period, from day of transfusion, of less than 45 days.[27,359,678] Viremia, however, may develop before HBsAg becomes detectable.[349]

Route of infection appears to affect the incubation period; in one study of experimental transmission, elevated levels of serum aminotransferase were observed 46 to 91 days after parenteral inoculation whereas peroral inoculation of a dose 50 times larger was associated with enzyme elevations at 88 to 108 days after ingestion.[545] Although early titration studies showed no effect of inoculum dilution on incubation period, it is likely that inoculum size

is inversely related to incubation period within the wide range described previously, that is, 28 to 180 days. In one study of HBV-contaminated plasma, the incubation period in recipients of undiluted plasma varied from 45 to 92 days with a mean of 77 days.[54] Two recipients of a 10^{-3} dilution of this plasma developed hepatitis 92 and 130 days later, and a third subject given a 10^{-4} dilution had the onset of clinical hepatitis 119 days later. HBsAg appeared in the sera of individuals receiving the diluted plasma significantly later than in those given undiluted plasma. This observation is in contrast to the observations made in 32 volunteers who were infected by blood obtained 30 days apart during the incubation period of hepatitis B. The incubation period of seroconversion in those who became infected was similar after the inoculation of these two batches. However, the incidence of infection (*i.e.*, seroconversion) was much lower after the inoculation of blood obtained earlier during the incubation period.

The modal incubation period of post-transfusion hepatitis in the era before HBsAg testing was 45 to 49 days (Fig. 15-7), shorter than that expected for hepatitis B (70 to 80 days). Although it had been postulated that variable inoculum size in the units transfused was responsible, it seems more likely that non-A, non-B viral hepatitis contributed importantly to the distribution of incubation periods found.

Ultraviolet irradiation of pooled plasma resulted in a lengthening of the modal incubation period from 70 to 79 days to 100 to 109 days presumably due to some reduction in titer of HBV.[697]

Hepatitis D. The incubation period of hepatitis D appears to overlap that of hepatitis B but has not been definitively established in humans. In chimpanzees, HBV/HDV coinfection appears to have an incubation period ranging

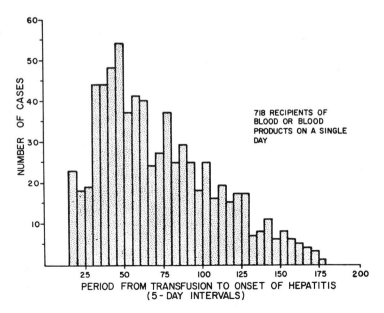

Fig. 15-7. Incubation periods of transfusion-associated viral hepatitis among 718 recipients of blood or blood products on a single day. (Mosley JW: Epatologia 12:527, 1966)

between 4 and 20 weeks. HDV superinfection of HBV carrier chimpanzees has an incubation period of 3 to 6 weeks.[830]

Non-A, Non-B Hepatitis. In studies conducted in the setting of transfusion-associated disease, non-A, non-B hepatitis has an incubation period that overlaps those of hepatitis A and B. A range of 15 to 160 days has been described with mean incubation periods of about 27 and 50 days. Although considerable variation may occur, the 50-day peak nearly coincides with the mode shown in Figure 15-7 for post-transfusion hepatitis before screening for HBsAg was available. In an outbreak of non-A, non-B hepatitis associated with blood platelet collection, the mean incubation period was shorter—27 days. It is not known whether route of infection or inoculum size influences the incubation period.

Epidemic non-A, non-B hepatitis appears to have a variable mean incubation period estimated to range between 15 and 40 days in water-borne outbreaks.[58,1079]

Period of Infectivity and Infective Materials in Hepatitis A

The presence of HAV has been demonstrated, by immunofluorescent techniques, in hepatocytes during the acute and early convalescent phase of hepatitis A in chimpanzees[693] and marmosets.[631] With a similar method, HAV has been detected in liver biopsies of about two thirds of patients with hepatitis A.[632] Positive immunofluorescent material was localized exclusively to the cytoplasm of hepatocytes and possibly in Kupffer cells. HAV was present as late as 3 to 4 weeks after the onset of symptoms. It is postulated that concomitantly with the presence of HAV in the liver, HAV may be shed in the feces of infected individuals for several weeks. It seems likely that the source of HAV in the intestine is hepatic bile, because HAV has been isolated from the bile of acutely infected chimpanzees,[879] and no evidence of intestinal or extrahepatic replication of HAV is available.[693] The precise mechanism by which HAV enters bile remains uncertain.

The presence of HAV in feces for a period of several weeks, which has been virologically documented,[182,388] might permit the assumption that patients are contagious throughout this period. Indeed, infectivity has been demonstrated with fecal filtrates obtained at various times from acutely infected individuals and administered to human volunteers under experimental conditions. Virologic and epidemiologic data indicate, however, that fecal shedding of HAV and communicability are not constant. In a number of studies maximal fecal excretion of HAV has been detected just before or at the onset of symptoms. Although an occasional outbreak of hepatitis A has been attributed to individuals incubating the disease, considerable data[805] support the notion that most infections are acquired at about the time of onset of symptoms, when fecal shedding approaches or reaches peak levels.

HAV in Feces. In human transmission studies undertaken before HAV had been isolated, the presence of infectious quantities of HAV in feces during the late incubation period and early acute phase of illness was established. In these experiments,[551] fecal suspensions collected 28 to 35 days before the onset of jaundice (about 21 to 28 days before the onset of symptoms) were noninfective, whereas stools collected 7 to 14 days before the onset of symptoms induced hepatitis A in other subjects. The presence of HAV during the acute phase of illness has been demonstrated in a number of transmission experiments. Stools collected on the first, third, and first through eighth day of jaundice were infectious,[409,551] but those obtained 19 to 43 days after onset of jaundice did not transmit hepatitis A.[403,550,711] These studies indicate that virus is present in feces as late as the onset of jaundice and for several days thereafter, but prolonged fecal excretion of HAV in infectious quantities is not a feature of this infection. Studies using immunoserologic techniques for the detection of HAV have failed to show chronic fecal excretion of HAV and have substantiated much of the information acquired in the transmission studies described previously and have permitted intensive study of nonhuman primates infected with HAV.

Experimental infection of marmosets by the parenteral route results in the appearance of HAV in feces simultaneously with serum aminotransferase elevations.[209] Peroral inoculation resulted in fecal excretion of HAV for several days, then a period in which HAV was absent, followed by its reappearance at the time that serum enzyme abnormalities were noted.[209] In chimpanzees, fecal HAV has been detected as early as 9 days after parenteral inoculation,[114] although virus recovery in other studies was limited to the period between onset of illness and peak serum aminotransferase levels.[229] Peak fecal HAV excretion concurrently with peak serum enzyme levels also has been described, and fecal HAV has been detected as long as 7 to 18 days after peak enzyme values.[434]

In experimentally infected human subjects, HAV was detected, by immune electron microscopy, 5 days before the initial serum aminotransferase abnormality but was no longer present after peak aminotransferase levels were reached.[228] In children with naturally acquired hepatitis A, fecal HAV was detected inconstantly a few days before or on the first day of abnormal aminotransferase levels, but peak excretion occurred early and HAV was no longer detectable when serum enzymes were at their maximum.[806] The presence of HAV in stool was described as early as 21 days before and as late as 14 days after peak enzyme values in another study in which maximal fecal excretion of HAV occurred 5 to 15 days before peak serum aminotransferase levels.[388] In a subsequent series of hospitalized patients with hepatitis A, 45% of fecal specimens obtained within the first week after onset of dark urine contained detectable HAV and 11% of those obtained in the second week were positive.[182] The number of particles of HAV in fecal specimens, measured by electron microscopy, diminished rapidly after the 5th day following the onset of dark urine. Because serum aminotransferase levels were falling in all patients, fecal shedding of HAV, in a substantial proportion of patients, continued for several days after peak enzyme values were attained.

HAV has been detected in the feces of anicteric patients,[388] but quantities of virus present and patterns of appearance and disappearance are incompletely understood.

HAV in Blood. Transmission studies with human volunteers and very rare instances of inadvertent transmission of hepatitis A by blood transfusion have provided incontrovertible evidence of viremia in HAV infections. The time course of viremia appears to be variable, but it presumably parallels the pattern described previously for fecal excretion of HAV. Viremia is present during the incubation period.[344] Specimens of blood, plasma, and pooled serum obtained from patients 1 to 3 weeks before the onset of symptoms (25 days,[344] 14 to 21 days,[550] and 3 to 7 days[550] before onset of jaundice) induced infection in inoculated volunteers. In other studies, viremia could not be demonstrated with specimens obtained 21 to 28 days before jaundice,[550] or 17 days prior to jaundice[403] (11 days prior to onset of symptoms). Blood transfusion–associated hepatitis A has resulted when blood was collected 3 and 11 days before the onset of symptoms in the donors.[299,395]

Viremia in the acute phase of illness was detected in transmission studies using pooled or single sample sera obtained either 1 to 8 days[403] after onset of symptoms or on the third day of jaundice.[551] Single specimens obtained during the first or second week of illness did not produce hepatitis.[707] Convalescent sera, taken 31 days[403] and 66 to 141 days[738] after the onset of hepatitis appeared to be noninfective. No experimental or epidemiologic evidence of chronic viremia is available. Furthermore, epidemiologic data suggest that HAV is rarely spread by parenteral routes.

Immunoserologic detection of HAV in the blood of infected chimpanzees has been correlated with peak serum aminotransferase activity.[434] The precise course of viremia in infected humans is probably similar, but few direct observations have been undertaken.

HAV in Urine. HAV is present in urine in low titers during the viremic phase of the illness. In early transmission studies, oral administration of large (30 ml to 50 ml) amounts of blood-contaminated urine induced hepatitis A in 5 of 17 volunteers.[286] In a later study, urine collected on the first day of jaundice produced evidence of hepatitis A in 1 of 12 subjects following oral inoculation.[344] Failure to transmit hepatitis with urine in three sets of experiments involving 29 volunteers suggests absence or low levels of HAV in urine.[403,608,707] HAV in urine is believed to be epidemiologically unimportant. Only in one outbreak,[489] in which an unstable mess hall worker with anicteric hepatitis appeared to have purposefully contaminated the mayonnaise used in a potato salad with his urine, has this unconventional route of infection been suspected. How-

ever, the more likely route of infection, namely, fecal contamination, could not be excluded.

HAV in Nasopharyngeal Secretions. Nasopharyngeal secretions from patients with presumed hepatitis A reportedly produced anicteric or inapparent infection in 2 of 7 volunteers.[608] However, in four other sets of experiments involving a total of 26 subjects, no evidence of transmission was found.[403,608,707] Although it is possible that HAV shedding into these secretions may occur in a few infected individuals and could be responsible for a few outbreaks in exceptional circumstances, for example, that in which a worker appeared to contaminate food items by wetting her hands with oropharyngeal secretions,[585] and suspected airborne transmission within a school bus,[2] transmission by this route appears to be epidemiologically inconsequential. HAV has not been demonstrated by immunoserologic techniques in nasopharyngeal secretions.

HAV in Intestinal Secretions. HAV is probably present within the intestinal lumen during the period in which HAV is excreted from the liver into bile. As previously indicated, HAV has been detected in the bile of chimpanzees infected with HAV.[879] The presence of HAV in gastric aspirates has not been studied.

HAV in Semen, Vaginal Secretions, and Menstrual Blood. The presence of HAV in these fluids during the viremic phase of illness seems a reasonable supposition. However, limited data suggest that venereal transmission is unlikely to be an important epidemiologic entity in the transmission of hepatitis A. Seroepidemiologic studies of HAV infection in New York City[972] and London[169] failed to demonstrate an increased prevalence of infection in male homosexuals. In contrast, in a study in Seattle,[176] the prevalence of anti-HAV was significantly higher in homosexual than in heterosexual humans. The acquisition of hepatitis A was closely correlated only with oral-anal sexual contact indicating a fecal-oral route of infection rather than semen-associated transmission.

Period of Infectivity and Infective Materials in Hepatitis B

In the era preceding the discovery of HBV's immunologic markers, limited numbers of human transmission experiments indicated that hepatitis B had a prolonged period of infectivity consistent with the prolonged incubation period recognized in this disease. Chronic viremia with an agent compatible with HBV was documented in the 1950s in studies with volunteers[710] and by observation of multiple cases of post-transfusion hepatitis caused by blood collected from certain donors over a period of years.[187,417,1107] With the development of serologic techniques for the identification of HBV infection, it was shown that the period of infectivity during the course of the illness varied widely from patient to patient. Furthermore, persistent HBV infection with prolonged viremia and infectivity could follow both subclinical and clinically apparent infection. Chronically infected individuals were recognized by the prolonged carriage of HBsAg. This population is critically important in the perpetuation of HBV infection.

Although prolonged infectivity may be an inherent feature of HBV infection, other contributory factors are incompletely understood. For example, host factors, such as age at the time of infection, may play an important role in the development of chronic infection. The immunobiology of HBV infection and recovery is complex. There are large gaps in knowledge of the control of hepatic HBV synthesis and release. Both HBsAg and HBcAg have been identified with immunofluorescent techniques in liver biopsies in about 30% of patients with acute HBV infection.[632] However, intact HBV particles are infrequently observed in the hepatocytes of acutely infected individuals. In chimpanzees infected with HBV, HBsAg and HBcAg are detected in hepatocytes before histologic or biochemical evidence of hepatitis is apparent.[450] Undoubtedly these antigens are present before as well as after HBsAg can be detected in serum, even by sensitive radioimmunoassay. Indeed, infectivity of HBsAg-negative blood was documented in volunteers during the incubation period of acute hepatitis. In self-limited HBV infection in the chimpanzee, HBsAg remains in hepatocytes until or shortly after HBcAg reactivity is lost. Serum aminotransferase levels diminish after the antigens are lost from hepatocytes.[450] The pattern of intrahepatic expression of antigens and its relationship to infectivity during the development of chronic infection has not been established. Two patterns of persistent HBV infection have been proposed. In some patients viral replication persists and is associated with continuing disease activity. In this case, HBV DNA is present in serum and in a nonintegrated, freely replicating form in the hepatocyte. In other patients viral replication does not occur, inflammatory disease activity is minimal or absent, and HBV DNA is integrated into the hepatocyte's DNA. HBV DNA is not present in the patient serum and infectivity is low level or absent.

A number of caveats are required in discussing infectivity of biologic materials. This is because the presence of HBsAg by itself has been used as a marker of infectivity, often without appropriate interpretation. It is now recognized that detection of HBsAg by itself is not synonymous with infectivity. The detection of HBsAg does not have the same meaning as that of detection of infectious HBV particles. Indeed, a study on the effectiveness of hyperimmune globulin to prevent needlestick-associated hepatitis had to be discontinued because not a single case of hepatitis developed in the control group of over 100 placebo recipients despite the fact that they had been inoculated percutaneously with HBsAg-positive material. Noninfectious HBsAg particles may be released from the liver into the circulation without HBV. Conversely, the lack of detectable HBsAg in blood or other materials does not necessarily indicate the absence of infectious HBV particles, which even in minute amounts are sufficient to induce infection. It has been recognized that in a small proportion of patients with acute HBV infection, the virus may remain in the serum despite the disappearance of HBsAg early in the acute phase of illness. HBV may also remain in the sera of chronically infected individuals in whom HBsAg cannot be identified, even by currently available highly sensitive techniques. Hence, HBsAg is an imperfect marker of infectivity. HBeAg and HBV DNA are more closely associated with the presence of intact HBV particles and are better correlates of infectivity.

Among all biologic material it is the liver and blood that contain the highest concentrations of HBV during the course of hepatitis B. HBsAg-positive semen and saliva may contain HBV particles and should be considered infectious. Other body fluids in which HBsAg has been identified may contain intact HBV and should be considered potentially infectious.

HBV in Feces and Intestinal Secretions. Fecal excretion of HBV could not be established in experimental studies of volunteers in the 1940s. These individuals received relatively large amounts of feces from other subjects with experimentally induced HBV infection. Both peroral and intramuscular administration of fecal filtrates failed to produce disease. After testing for HBsAg became available, conflicting data were reported concerning the presence of HBsAg in feces.[180,369,379,618,730,1017] In the majority of studies HBsAg could not be detected. Furthermore, HBsAg could not be detected in the feces of a carrier who had ingested 4 ml of his own serum.[273] It has been suggested that the immunoreactivity of HBsAg may be altered within the gastrointestinal tract because HBsAg becomes undetectable after admixture with homogenates of intestinal mucosa. Although early studies suggested that fecal suspensions also inhibited HBsAg reactivity,[766] confirmation was not obtained in a later investigation.[273] Although degradation of HBsAg is not synonymous with loss of infectivity, the evidence for loss of antigenicity is in accord with lack of fecal infectivity in studies in volunteers.

Gastric and duodenal aspirates free of gross blood have been consistently negative for HBsAg.[273] The reported detection of HBsAg in bile[13,21] has been confirmed,[432] and HBsAg has been found in pure pancreatic juice.[432] Incubation of HBsAg with bile acids and pronase was reported to change the appearance of HBsAg particles.[666] Incubation with bile alone or with pancreatic juice alone inhibited the detectability of HBsAg.[432]

HBV in Blood. Viremia occurs during the incubation period and acute phase of hepatitis B and may persist after convalescence in as many as 5% to 10% of adult patients. The latter are recognized indirectly by the persistence of HBsAg in their sera. In studies in volunteers, hepatitis B was transmitted with blood taken 87 days before onset of symptoms in one instance,[712] and with specimens collected 60 and 16 days before onset in two others.[404,753] HBsAg is usually detectable in serum 1 to 2 months prior to the onset of symptoms,[543] and may be found as early as 1 week after exposure.[549] It is usually still demonstrable in most patients at the onset of jaundice and persists in about 50% as late as 6 weeks following onset. A minor proportion of patients with hepatitis B may be HBsAg negative when first seen during the acute illness. Such patients can be identified by the presence of anti-HBc of the IgM type during the acute phase, in the absence of circulating anti-HBs. The appearance of anti-HBs in late convalescence also confirms the diagnosis of hepatitis B.

Retrospective studies of experimental subjects infected during the early 1950s revealed that 12 of 115 (10%) persistently had HBsAg positivity during the 6 to 34 months of observation.[53] Persistent infection and continued HBsAg positivity was documented in an experimentally infected child 45 months after exposure.[542] Retrospective analysis of sera from an individual implicated in multiple cases of transfusion-associated hepatitis B revealed the persistence of HBsAg for more than 20 years.[1108] It is estimated that there are 165 ± 30 million HBsAg carriers in the world. The prevalence of carriers varies widely, as shown in Table 15-5. Quantities of HBsAg and HBV in the sera of HBsAg carriers appear to be variable. It is likely that the individual with replicative infection and a high level of intact HBV particles is more likely to transmit infection than the person with nonreplicative infection and few particles. In the individual with low-grade viremia, large inocula may be necessary for contact transmission. However, the efficiency of parenteral transmission is such that the size of the inoculum is probably less critical.

HBV in Urine. HBsAg has been detected in the absence of recognized hematuria in concentrated urine specimens of a small number of patients with acute hepatitis B.[103,730,1017] Intact HBV was not seen. The presence of intact HBV particles in urine remains to be established. Although it has been postulated that urine may be a potential source of infection from diapered infants with HBV infection, firm epidemiologic support for this notion is not available, and the importance of infective urine in the spread of hepatitis B is unknown.

HBV in Nasopharyngeal Secretions and Saliva. Early human transmission studies failed to demonstrate infectivity of nasopharyngeal secretions or washings from patients with naturally acquired or experimentally induced hepatitis B when these were inoculated intranasally into volunteers. In two instances transmission appeared to have been achieved,[609] but salivary contamination of the materials may have occurred. Saliva, uncontaminated by detectable blood, has been shown to contain HBsAg.[123,513,1032,1050] Furthermore, HBV particles have been identified by electron microscopic examination of saliva from HBsAg carriers.[50,604] It has been suggested that HBsAg and HBV enter saliva from crevicular fluid.[759] In patients with hepatitis B, HBsAg was detected in saliva during the first 3 weeks after onset of symptoms[1032] and disappeared before serum became HBsAg negative.[1080] HBsAg may be intermittently present in the saliva and sneeze droplets of carriers.[1032] Percutaneous inoculation of saliva containing HBsAg and HBV in gibbons[50,888] and chimpanzees[28] induced infection but neither intranasal nor peroral inoculation was associated with infection. HBsAg-positive saliva from an HBsAg and HBeAg seropositive person did not produce infection in susceptible individuals by oral exposure.[1076] These data suggest that saliva may contain small numbers of intact HBV particles and that the magnitude of infectivity is low. Nonetheless, percutaneous introduction of HBsAg-positive saliva from the bite of a HBsAg-positive child resulted in HBV infection in the hapless victim—a teacher.[617]

HBV in Semen, Vaginal Secretions, and Menstrual Blood. HBsAg has been identified in semen,[28,414] vaginal secretions,[196] and menstrual blood.[470] The presence of infectious HBV in semen was demonstrated by the successful transmission of hepatitis B following intravenous inoculation of chimpanzees with semen obtained from human carriers of HBsAg[28] or intravaginal instillation of HBsAg-positive semen in gibbons.[888] The infectivity of HBsAg-positive semen by oral administration was not documented. A venereal route of infection appears to be an important mechanism of hepatitis B transmission in promiscuous heterosexual and homosexual populations. Serologic evidence of exposure to HBV is more common among sexual partners of HBsAg carriers than among their blood relatives.

HBV in Other Body Fluids. HBsAg has been detected with variable frequency and little consistency in body fluids in which occult blood may be absent. Positive reports have been described in tears, anterior chamber eye fluid, sweat, amniotic fluid, colostrum, cerebrospinal fluid, ascites, pleural effusions, and synovial fluid, to name but a few. Direct demonstration of HBV in these materials is limited, and transmission studies have not been undertaken. Although they are potentially infectious, their role in transmission of HBV appears unlikely to be important except in unusual circumstances.

Period of Infectivity and Infective Materials in Hepatitis D

Precise information on the period of infectivity and infective materials in HDV infection is not yet available. HDV particles have been identified in sera, in HBV/HDV co-infections, during the early acute phase of infection only after the appearance of HBsAg. In self-limited HBV/HDV co-infection the period of HDV viremia is likely to be very short and the titer of virus low; HDV disappears with clearance of HBsAg. In many cases, the viremic phase may be undetectable or missed. In contrast to this picture, in HDV superinfection of HBsAg carriers, HDV particles may be present in high titers for several weeks and in an uncertain but presumably large proportion may persist for months to years. Although the presence of HDV outside the liver or serum has yet to be unequivocally established, it is likely to be detected in those body fluids in which HBsAg has been identified.

Period of Infectivity and Infective Materials in Non-A, Non-B Hepatitis

Due to the limitations imposed by the absence of confirmed serologic markers, information about period of infectivity in non-A, non-B hepatitis and infective materials has been derived mainly by inference. The epidemiologic similarity of the blood-borne forms to hepatitis B suggests that patterns of the presence and duration of the agents in blood and other body fluids may resemble that found in HBV infection. Transmission studies using nonhuman primates have provided fragmentary data. Blood-borne non-A, non-B hepatitis virus is present in blood during the incubation period. Blood obtained 12 days before the onset of clinical disease transmitted infection to chimpanzees.[435] Serial transmission studies in chimpanzees established the presence of viremia near the time of onset of serum aminotransferase elevations and persistence of viremia until at least 1 week after peak enzyme levels were reached.[984] The persistence of viremia through the convalescent period and for a protracted period thereafter seems likely because carriers have been identified epidemiologically and by transmission studies. The frequency of chronic infection in humans or chimpanzees remains uncertain but appears to be high.

MODES OF TRANSMISSION

Contact

Hepatitis A. Contact transmission is the predominant mode of spread of hepatitis A. Fecal-oral transmission is

the major contact route. Person-to-person transmission of type A hepatitis is limited in most instances to close contacts. In community-wide outbreaks, the pattern of age-specific attack rates suggests that contact among children and within the household is usually the most important.

The time distribution of cases in households in relation to the index case is presented in Figure 15-8. The example is derived from a 1951 epidemic in Missouri,[519] but other investigations in the United States and abroad have demonstrated a similar pattern.[934,964] Other cases in the family occur as a large wave of secondary illnesses and a smaller group of tertiary infections. Household members in whom the onset is less than 15 days after that of the index case are usually regarded as having co-primary rather than secondary infections. Evidence for early fecal excretion is compatible with some such infections being secondary[551] and acquired 2 to 3 weeks before the first person in the family becomes ill. Most household cases, however, occur one incubation period or more after the index case.[805] This suggests that the patient is most infectious for close contacts about the time of onset of symptoms.

Spontaneous transmission 1 to 2 weeks prior to onset has been documented in instances in which exposure was to mentally retarded children.[63] The extent of fecal soiling of the environment by this group is a possible explanation of the ease with which they seem to transmit the disease relatively early and of the persistent hyperendemicity found in these institutions. Fecal contamination resulting from the presence of infants and non-toilet-trained toddlers also appears to be responsible for outbreaks of hepatitis A in day-care centers.[383a]

Sexual transmission of hepatitis A has been postulated,[175] but convincing evidence of venereal spread in the absence of a fecal-oral mechanism is not available. Oral-

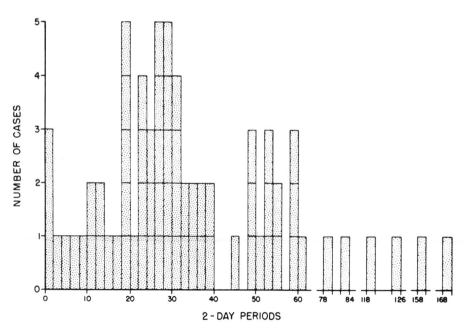

Fig. 15-8. Intervals between onset of symptoms in index and subsequent cases of hepatitis A in 37 families in Cooper County, Missouri, 1951. (Knight V et al: Am J Hyg 59:1, 1954)

anal contact, supporting a fecal-oral mechanism, was implicated in the spread of hepatitis A among male homosexuals studied in one clinic.[176]

It has been postulated from time to time that respiratory transmission may occur. This was the conclusion of Pickles, whose epidemiologic observations in rural England suggested that casual contact was sufficient.[767] Failure to demonstrate transmission by nasopharyngeal secretions administered to volunteers has led most observers to dismiss this possibility. Aach and co-workers observed an explosive epidemic in which airborne transmission seemed the only likely explanation.[2] Although there are occasional instances of transmission resulting from casual contact,[471] these seem to be the exception. In Figure 15-9 it is shown that there is no temporal relationship suggestive of intraschool or intraclass transmission. Residential distribution of childhood cases shows clusterings by neighborhood. Play contacts, therefore, are more likely to be important than cohabitation in classrooms.

Because transmission is limited to close contacts and the incubation period is relatively long, hepatitis A spreads leisurely through the community. Several months are usually required to reach the peak of the outbreak and a comparable period of time for the wave to recede.

Hepatitis B. Despite failure of early studies clearly to demonstrate contact spread of hepatitis B, a number of observations[119,301] supporting the concept of contact transmission were difficult to ignore in light of later experimental evidence that hepatitis B could be transmitted by peroral inoculation of large amounts of infectious serum.[454] With the development of serologic techniques for the identification of hepatitis B, HBV infections were identified in the absence of parenteral transmission. Contact transmission was recognized to be common and more important in the spread of hepatitis B than was previously believed. Contact-associated transmission of HBV is suggested by several sets of epidemiologic observations: (1) the very high proportion of persons in institutions for the retarded who become infected[436,971,975]; (2) a similarly high proportion of infection among persons living in the same households as an HBsAg carrier[755,924,978]; (3) episodes of transmission between sexual partners in which one is recognized as a carrier[1086] or to be acutely infected[414,419]; (4) a high prevalence of infection among sexually promiscuous individuals; (5) higher secondary attack rates in spouses of acutely or chronically infected persons than in other household contacts[533,672,755,815]; (6) the occurrence of outbreaks and an area-wide epidemic under circumstances in which a percutaneous mechanism could be excluded with reasonable certainty[321]; and (7) transmission among children in the absence of a percutaneous mechanism.[1030]

Contact transmission of hepatitis B occurs less readily than for hepatitis A. A direct comparison of an outbreak of contact-spread hepatitis B with an epidemic of contact-spread hepatitis A 3 years later revealed important differences.[1030] In the epidemic attributed to hepatitis B, all age-groups were affected, the disease appeared to spread very slowly, and the secondary attack rate was just 2.4%. In contrast, in the outbreak attributed to hepatitis A, children were affected predominantly, the disease appeared to disseminate at a more rapid rate within the affected communities, and the secondary attack rate was 7.3%.

Mechanisms of contact-associated HBV transmission are incompletely defined, and fecal-oral spread is unlikely to be important on epidemiologic grounds. Furthermore, no epidemic of hepatitis B attributable to fecal contami-

Fig. 15-9. Intervals between onset of symptoms in index and subsequent cases of hepatitis A in schools and classrooms having more than one case, Kenton County, Kentucky, 1956–1957.

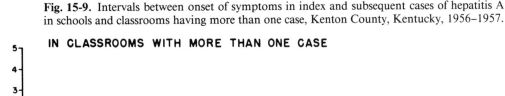

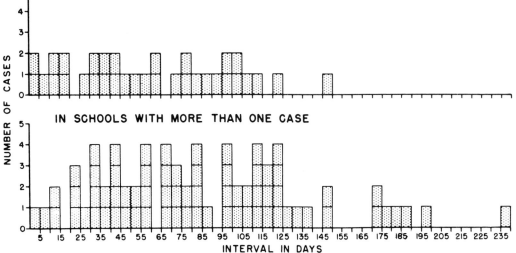

nation of food or water has been described. Contact spread is more likely to involve physical contact in which HBV is transferred to mucosal or cutaneous surfaces. Sexual and oral-oral contact appear to be the principal routes. Inapparent percutaneous transmission involving shared vehicles, such as razor blades, may play a role. Airborne transmission has also been suggested but appears to be limited to unique situations in which extremely heavy exposure occurs. The possibility of transfer of infection by passive vectors, such as tattoo needle or fluid, mosquitoes or bed bugs, must also be considered.

Hepatitis D. Contact spread has been postulated to be responsible for the spread of HDV from index cases to their sexual intimates.[393] Fecal-oral transmission appears to be unlikely.

Non-A, Non-B Hepatitis. Contact transmission of the blood-borne forms of non-A, non-B hepatitis has been postulated to be responsible for the spread of disease where parenteral exposure could not be demonstrated.[1031] Sporadic instances of non-A, non-B hepatitis have been attributed to close contact with individuals who either had acute hepatitis or those believed to be carriers of the non-A, non-B agents. Mechanisms of contact spread are presumed to be similar to those identified in the contact transmission of hepatitis B. The epidemic form of non-A, non-B hepatitis is believed to be transmitted by a fecal-oral route. The secondary attack rate in household contacts has yet to be definitively established.

Maternal-Neonatal

Maternal-neonatal transmission of viral hepatitis from mother to fetus or newborn may be considered a unique form of "contact" transmission occurring *in utero,* during birth, or in the early postpartum period. Perinatal transmission of hepatitis A has not been established as an epidemiologic entity, and serologic documentation of this route of hepatitis A spread is not available. Limited data suggest that the non-A, non-B hepatitis viruses can be transmitted perinatally,[1009] but the frequency and importance of this mode requires further study.

The notion of maternal-neonatal transmission of hepatitis B was suggested as early as 1951.[963] Serologic studies subsequently undertaken in many parts of the world have repeatedly documented perinatal transmission from acutely infected or HBsAg carrier women.[733,745,881,885,929,954] Transmission of HBV from a woman with acute infection appears to be dependent on the stage of pregnancy in which hepatitis B develops. When the acute infection occurs in the first two trimesters, neonatal infection rates are usually under 10%.[885,929] Infection during the third trimester or in the early postpartum period is associated with a higher neonatal infection rate that reaches 70% in some series.[571,881]

In the United States and other western societies, neonatal HBV infection rates are generally under 10% when the pregnant woman is an HBsAg carrier.[885,929] Higher infection rates approaching 90% have been documented in some Asian countries.[571,733,954] In these areas, it is believed that perinatal transmission resulting in infection early in life contributes importantly to the perpetuation of high HBV prevalence rates. The infected newborn may develop acute hepatitis B of variable severity or persistent HBV infection.[272,881] In some instances, chronic hepatitis develops during the first year of life.

A number of factors have been correlated with the risk of maternal-neonatal transmission. Positive predictors include the presence of HBeAg,[67,571,733] high titers of HBsAg in maternal sera,[571,954] and the race of the mother. In the United Kingdom the frequency with which infants born to HBsAg carrier mothers become carriers themselves was dependent on the race of the mother: 64% if the mother was Chinese, 31% if she was black but none if she was European.[217] Less powerful predictors are the presence of HBsAg in cord blood and the detection of HBsAg in siblings of the newborn.[954]

Transplacental infection *in utero,* maternal-fetal transfusion due to placental injury, and exposure during delivery have been postulated to play a role because amniotic fluid, cord blood, and gastric contents of the newborn may contain HBsAg.[571] The frequently delayed appearance of HBsAg in the newborn makes intrauterine infection less likely. Cesarean section does not prevent infection.[347] Instances of hepatitis B in the early postpartum period in the mother associated with subsequent HBV infection of the newborn[928] have suggested that mechanisms of contact transmission may be responsible. Breastfeeding has received considerable attention. Although breast milk may contain small quantities of HBsAg,[105,593] its infectivity has not been established. Indeed, breast feeding has been considered an unimportant mechanism for vertical transmission of HBV infection.[66]

Nonhuman Primates

Contact with nonhuman primates has been recognized as a mode of hepatitis A transmission since 1961,[422] and serologic evidence of recent HAV infection has been documented in human and nonhuman primate contacts of implicated animals.[227] Newly imported chimpanzees,[198,302,685,854] siamangs, woolly monkeys, gorillas, and Celebes apes have been incriminated in cases of hepatitis A developing in their human handlers. Veterinarians, zoo workers, research scientists, and other handlers exposed to these animals are at risk. Transmission of hepatitis A from human to primate and then back to human by a fecal-oral route seems likely. In most instances clinical illness is not recognized in the animal. Although hepatitis B has been implicated in an outbreak of infection in nonhuman primates in a London zoo,[1108] transmission to staff members could not be demonstrated. Whether nonhuman primates can transmit hepatitis B or non-A, non-B hepatitis to humans is not yet known.

Water

Water-borne hepatitis A was probably first recognized as an epidemiologic entity in England in 1895.[770] Other episodes have been reported repeatedly since that time,[35,677] and hepatitis A has been considered the predominant viral disease transmissable by the ingestion of contaminated water. This mode of transmission results from both contamination of the usual supplies of drinking water and ingestion of contaminated water not intended for consumption. Examples of the latter include inadvertent swallowing of water during swimming or accidental immersion in contaminated recreational water[128] and use of leaky plastic water-filled "freeze balls" to cool drinks in an instance in which the water within the balls was grossly contaminated with fecal organisms and HAV.[821] In the United States most cases of water-borne disease are produced by private supplies,[128,823,1019] but municipal systems have been involved in at least two instances.[687,777] In the instances in which a broad segment of the community is exposed, age-specific attack rates characteristically show a peak in young adults.[687] Whether this pattern will continue in light of the declining prevalence of HAV infection in this country remains to be determined.

It is surprising that water-borne hepatitis does not occur more frequently. Water-borne transmission is believed to play a minor role in the spread of hepatitis A in developed countries. Epidemic non-A, non-B hepatitis agents have been responsible for some outbreaks of water-borne hepatitis in India,[1079] North Africa,[74] the USSR,[47] and Asia[1090] but have yet to be described in the United States or western European countries. Water-borne hepatitis B is also theoretically possible but seems an unlikely probability except under extremely unusual circumstances.

Food

Epidemiologic and serologic data indicate that hepatitis A is the predominant agent of food-borne hepatitis.[165] Hepatitis B and non-A, non-B hepatitis transmission through contaminated food have not been established but are theoretically possible. Outbreaks of hepatitis A attributed to food-borne transmission have usually been explosive but short-lived, suggesting brief periods of contamination. Although a variety of food items have been implicated,[525] including alcohol-containing beverages,[764] the primary recognized source of contamination is the food handler responsible for the terminal preparation of food before serving.[525] Food-borne transmission requires that contamination be sufficient to provide infective doses of HAV to each susceptible individual who consumes that food and develops infection. Fecal contamination due to inadequate personal hygiene on the part of the food handler with HAV infection is generally assumed to be responsible. Milk-borne and mollusk-associated hepatitis represent different mechanisms.

Although food-borne transmission may fail to be recognized as such, in developed countries food-borne hepatitis appears to be a minor factor in the spread of hepatitis A.

Milk. Three cases of hepatitis were traced to ingestion of raw milk collected by a woman who developed hepatitis 30 days before the outbreak.[891] In two other episodes, contamination of water used to wash milk buckets[695] or in processing of milk for pasteurization[810] appeared responsible. The latter suggests that pasteurization may not inactivate HAV.

Mollusk. Mollusk-associated hepatitis was first recognized as a mode of hepatitis A transmission in Sweden in 1955 when raw oysters stored in sewage-contaminated waters were implicated in an outbreak that affected more than 600 persons.[316,842] Major outbreaks of oyster-or clam-associated hepatitis were recognized subsequently in the United States in 1961, 1964, and 1973, and minor episodes have been identified occasionally.[529] Although ingestion of raw mollusks has been responsible for most outbreaks,[249,529] inadequately cooked bivalves, steamed clams, and briefly boiled mussels[104,230] also have been implicated. In the far East ingestion of raw or partially cooked cockles has resulted in epidemics of hepatitis A.[351] In one study, the internal temperature of steamed clams, measured at the time of shell opening, was below that likely to inactivate HAV.[530]

Endemic mollusk-associated hepatitis has been documented and appears to result from low-level fecal contamination of coastal waters and the accumulation and concentration of HAV in bivalves.[532,959] Its epidemiologic importance is difficult to define because cases may be widely scattered in time and place of onset. Neither hepatitis B nor non-A, non-B viral hepatitis appears to be transmitted through ingestion of mollusks.

Insects

Mechanical transmission by externally contaminated insects has been suggested for HAV in some instances but firm evidence is lacking. Forty-seven cases of presumed hepatitis A in Port Sudan were seen in native men, but not in native women or Europeans who did not eat in the fly-infested market place.[1067] In the Sudan, outbreaks of hepatitis usually began when flies were most prevalent at the onset of the hot season. An epidemic of hepatitis was described in New Zealand troops at El Alamein in an area strewn with corpses and feces from the German troops previously encamped there.[511] The Germans had had a high incidence of hepatitis A, and flies were extremely prevalent. Hepatitis was not a problem in other sections of the line where flies were equally numerous but there were no human bodies or feces scattered over the ground. On the other hand, during a summer camp epidemic, infectivity could not be documented with flies collected from a trap adjacent to the camp kitchen.[707] The flies were homogenized and their filtrate administered orally to five volunteers. None of these developed clinical or laboratory evidence of hepatitis.

A role for cockroaches in transmitting hepatitis A in a Los Angeles housing project was postulated when the disease decreased following control measures directed against this insect.[994] Others, however, found no evidence for such association.[532] It has been suggested that HBV may multiply in cockroaches and that these insects may have a role in transmission.[1099] This work has not been confirmed.

Evidence that biting insects transmit hepatitis is also inconclusive. Blood-sucking sandflies, black flies, and tsetse flies did not contain detectable HBsAg,[126] but wild[783] and urban-caught mosquitoes[221] and engorged bed bugs[126] were found to be HBsAg positive in several studies. HBsAg positivity persists much longer in bed bugs[490,719,731] than in mosquitoes.[719] Even after consuming several HBsAg-negative blood meals, bed bugs remained HBsAg positive. Definitive evidence of HBV replication in these insects is not available, and attempts to transmit HBV by inoculating susceptible chimpanzees with mosquito tissues containing HBsAg or by allowing HBsAg-positive mosquitoes to feed on susceptible animals failed to transfer infection.[82] The role of biting insects in transmission of hepatitis A, hepatitis D, or non-A, non-B hepatitis also is uncertain.

Transfusions

In 1943, Beeson described the occurrence of hepatitis following transfusion of blood or plasma.[72] Since then, viral hepatitis has been recognized to be the major hazard of blood transfusion and administration of blood derivatives. In the era before serologic testing became available, hepatitis A and B were believed to be the principal etiologic agents of transfusion-associated hepatitis. Subsequently, it has been repeatedly shown that hepatitis A is rarely the cause. The wide application of sensitive tests for HBsAg in blood donors and the rejection of positive donors reduced the incidence of post-transfusion hepatitis B.[27,437,894] However, the anticipated dramatic decline of transfusion-associated hepatitis did not materialize. These observations provided circumstantial evidence for the existence and importance of the non-A, non-B hepatitis agents that appear to be responsible for over 90% of present cases of transfusion-associated hepatitis.[29,276,521] The persistence of transfusion-associated hepatitis B at a low rate undoubtedly reflects the imperfect sensitivity of current methods to detect infectious blood with low HBV content. Furthermore, blood and blood products that appear to lack HBsAg may transmit both HBV and HDV. Although the risk of HBV and HDV transmission to normal recipients has been shown to be very low, transfusion-associated HDV transmission to HBsAg carrier recipients is considerably more common.[846] Transfusion of coagulation factors produced from large pools of plasma carry the highest risk.[846]

The frequency of post-transfusion hepatitis is dependent on a number of factors. These have been elucidated, at least in part, by careful prospective studies of large numbers of transfused subjects. Characteristics of the donor population are major determinants of the hepatitis risk. It has been demonstrated that the commercial, paid blood donor presents a significantly greater hepatitis B and non-A, non-B hazard to the recipient than does the volunteer or family replacement donor.[29,894] Wide geographic variations in the United States in the rate of post-transfusion hepatitis have been attributed to differences in the utilization of commercial donors.[1] Attack rates of non-A, non-B, post-transfusion hepatitis in patients transfused exclusively with volunteer blood have varied between 5% and 10%, with a mean of about 7%.[1] In contrast, attack rates of 17% to 54% have been identified in recipients of commercial blood.[1] Variable methods used to define hepatitis probably play only a minor role in reported differences. Anicteric post-transfusion hepatitis is considerably more common than clinically apparent disease. In general, a ratio of 3 to 5 anicteric cases to each case with overt jaundice seems likely. Hence in those studies in which anicteric hepatitis is recognized by appropriate laboratory tests, the frequency of transfusion-association hepatitis is considerably higher than in studies in which jaundice is used to determine case rates.

Another factor influencing the risk of transfusion-associated hepatitis is the volume of blood transfused. The attack rate of hepatitis increases with the number of units of commercial blood transfused.[897] This relationship is not linear, however, and appears to be less prominent in recipients of volunteer blood.[894]

A high frequency of prior experience with viral hepatitis appears to account for the low frequency of transfusion-associated hepatitis reported from some areas.[150,152] Also, the development and clinical severity of post-transfusion hepatitis theoretically may be affected by the presence and titer of specific neutralizing antibodies in plasma infused in proximity with an infected unit of blood. The importance of this interaction remains to be established.

As indicated previously, hepatitis B, hepatitis D, and non-A, non-B hepatitis can be transmitted by blood derivatives as well as transfused blood. Human blood and blood derivatives in present use may be classified according to their risk of transmitting viral hepatitis (Table 15-6). Average-risk materials are whole blood itself and derivatives that are prepared without pooling of individual units. High-risk derivatives are produced when plasma or platelets from individual units are separated and pooled. Under these circumstances, a single unit containing the virus of human hepatitis could contaminate the entire batch. The frequency with which units from such pools are contaminated is much higher than that of an equivalent number of nonpooled units; and the frequency increases with the size of the pool. Fibrinogen and pooled plasma are no longer commercially available in the United States because of a very high hepatitis hazard. Safe materials are prepared by Cohn fractionation or are heat treated. Neither ultraviolet irradiation[697] nor storage at room temperature[814] is effective. As indicated in Table

TABLE 15-6. Classification of Human Blood and Blood Products According to Risk of Transmitting Viral Hepatitis

"AVERAGE-RISK" MATERIALS
Whole blood
Packed, washed, or frozen red blood cells
Fresh, frozen plasma
Single-donor platelet concentrates
Single-donor granulocyte concentrates
Single-unit cryoprecipitate

"HIGH-RISK" MATERIALS
Factor IX complex
Antihemophilic factor (factor VIII concentrates)
Multiple donor platelet concentrates

"SAFE" MATERIALS*
Albumin
Immune globulin†
Hyperimmune globulin (hepatitis B, Rh$_0$ (D))

---

* Heat-treated for 10 hours at 60°C or prepared by Cohn fractionation (cold ethanol).

† Preparations prepared by non-U.S. manufacturers are reported to transmit hepatitis.

15-6, immune globulin prepared by foreign manufacturers[485,763] has been reported to transmit hepatitis.

Transplantations

A case of hepatitis B in an untransfused patient receiving a bone graft has been reported.[915] Three of four susceptible recipients of transplanted kidneys from HBsAg-positive cadaver donors developed serologic evidence of HBV infection or an immune response to HBsAg in the absence of recent transfusion or other exposure to hepatitis.[1078] The increasing use of organ transplants suggests that transplantation-associated hepatitis should be sought in other instances, but it is difficult to document because of the frequency with which recipients are transfused with blood and icterogenic blood products.

Hemodialysis

High rates of acute and chronic HBV infection have been widely reported in patients with chronic kidney disease who undergo maintenance hemodialysis.[628,784,940,977] Non-A, non-B has been responsible for some outbreaks,[312,313] but hepatitis A has not been implicated.[973] In a few instances cytomegalovirus[704,1055] and Epstein-Barr virus[177] have been incriminated in hemodialysis-associated hepatitis.

Hepatitis B in hemodialysis patients is often subclinical but results in the carrier state and low-grade persistent hepatic injury more frequently than it does in the general population.[319,599] Non-A, non-B hepatitis may be responsible for a large proportion of instances of prolonged hepatic dysfunction seen in hemodialysis patients in the absence of serologic markers of HBV.[312,313] Dual infection with HBV and blood-borne non-A, non-B hepatitis viruses may be responsible for the extraordinary virulence noted in some hemodialysis-associated outbreaks.

It is likely that HBV and the non-A, non-B agents are introduced into hemodialysis units through blood transfusion or by the admission of infected new patients or staff.[319,628] However, evidence from subtyping of HBsAg indicates that intraunit transmission of HBV is more important than transfusion in the spread of infection.[568,942] A variety of mechanisms have been implicated in patient-to-patient and patient-to-staff transmission. These include dialysis machine malfunctions,[942] contamination of shared equipment,[177] exposure to patient's blood,[943] accidental tissue penetrations with contaminated needles,[943] and possibly air-borne spread[18] and environmental contamination.[195,271] Infected hemodialysis patients also may pose a hazard to their family members through contact transmission.[751] In addition, in one instance, close home contacts were readily infected by exposure to blood leaking from the site of a dialysis patient's shunt.[321]

Health Care Providers

Viral hepatitis is an occupational hazard for health care workers, and serologic evidence of HBV infection is found more commonly in these individuals than in the general population. Although an increased frequency of non-A, non-B hepatitis infections also seems likely, there is no evidence that hepatitis A is an occupational hazard except among personnel working in institutions for the mentally retarded and in day-care centers. Serologic evidence for past experience with HBV is significantly higher among health care workers in general and in physicians, in particular, than in blood donors. The prevalence of anti-HBs increases with years of practice among physicians.[213,588] The increased risk of hepatitis B for surgeons was exemplified by a description of a mini-epidemic among surgical house officers who operated on a HBsAg-positive patient.[844] Serologic evidence of HBV infection among health care workers was associated with their professional activity. It was more frequent among surgeons and pathologists and less common among those in family practice. The highest frequency is noted among those physicians who work on hemodialysis, renal transplant, or oncology services. In laboratory personnel, seropositivity was invariably associated with exposure to blood. It is highest among those who work in the blood bank, in the chemistry section, or among those doing blood gas determinations or working with multichannel analyzers and those on blood-drawing or intravenous teams.[586] A likely explanation for the high frequency of HBV infection among laboratory workers is derived from a survey of laboratories for HBV contamination.[565] HBsAg was detected in 34% of environmental surfaces and about half on the outside surfaces of blood or serum containers. There was splattering of minute amounts of blood around multichannel analyzers. These observations suggest that transmission of HBV in clinical laboratories is probably due to hand contact with contaminated surfaces that became polluted by inapparent spread of antigen-positive blood. The portal of entry of HBV is either through inapparent breaks in skin or by contact with mucous membranes.[565] Similar observations were made in Europe where a significantly higher proportion of health care workers were positive for both HBsAg and for anti-HBs than in the control group in the same city. On the average, 19% of 826 health care workers were positive for anti-HBs. In this group, serologic evidence of exposure to HBV was significantly higher in those who worked in operating rooms and laboratories and was significantly lower in those who worked in radiology and pediatric departments than among health care workers in general.[878]

The excess risk of hepatitis B for health care workers on hemodialysis units is now well established. Almost a third of the personnel in 15 hemodialysis centers in the United States had serologic evidence of current or past experience with HBV.[977] In a prospective investigation of 65 renal hemodialysis units, the incidence of hepatitis infection among staff was 3.4 per 100 persons at risk per year, only slightly lower than that observed among patients.[319] Infected dialysis patients expose health care workers to infection with HBV, and two thirds of their family contacts also had evidence of current or past experience with HBV.[977] HBV is transferred from patient to health care personnel most frequently by the percutaneous route. However, other nonpercutaneous transmission mechanisms must also occur.[319] Furthermore, in one instance a possible air-borne spread had been described in a hemodialysis unit.[18]

A high incidence of hepatitis among health care workers on an oncology unit was also described.[1047] The source of infection was believed, in one instance, to be a leukemic patient whose HBsAg titer increased during the period of exposure. The evaluation of 19 risk factors elicited only two significant variables among infected personnel: smoking and nail biting while on duty in the oncology unit.

Health care workers in institutions for the mentally handicapped are also at excess risk of developing HBV infection. This is particularly true for those workers who are exposed to children under 15 years of age.[1003]

Serologic evidence of past exposure to HBV among dentists is also significantly higher than that of the general population. The frequency of prior infection with HBV increases uniformly with years of practice of general dentistry in California.[680] In Florida, the frequency of serologic evidence of HBV infection also was significantly higher among dentists than in the control population.[281] The prevalence of HBsAg, however, is not increased among dentists when compared with blood donors. The increased risk of HBV infection among dentists was also demonstrated in the United Kingdom and New Zealand.[356,720]

These observations indicate that health care workers in general are infected by the patients they care for. There is one more group, probably as far removed from "health care" as any group possibly can be, but in whom exposure to an excess risk of HBV infection might be postulated. That group, undertakers, did not demonstrate an increased experience with HBV on serologic examination.[84]

Not only are health care workers at risk of being infected by HBsAg-positive patients, but these infected health care workers then in turn can infect their patients. This sequence is more likely if the subjects are also HBeAg positive.[944] The current evidence indicates that the risk to a patient of infection by an HBsAg-positive health care worker is small.[26,322] Although total safety from HBsAg-positive health care workers cannot be guaranteed, the risk is usually lower than that anticipated. The exception is the health care worker who can be implicated specifically in multiple cases of hepatitis. For example, several cases of hepatitis were traced to a resident in gynecologic surgery who had high titers of HBsAg and both HBeAg and intact HBV particles in his serum.[170] On the other hand, a "nonepidemic" was described when 49 patients, followed up after they were operated on by an orthopedic surgeon during the incubation period of his HBsAg-positive hepatitis, failed to develop disease.[656] Although in isolated instances general dentists or dental surgeons have been implicated as sources of hepatitis B infection, a broad indictment of HBsAg-positive dentists is not warranted. For example, apparently 12 patients were infected by two chronically HBsAg-positive dentists, one of whom had severe chronic active hepatitis B.[582] Fifty-five patients might have been infected during a 4-year period by another dental surgeon.[822] The mode of transmission of HBV in these cases was probably a hemo-oral route. On the other hand, the patient contacts of two dentists were followed prospectively for 6 months after exposure to the dentists during the incubation period of their acute HBsAg-positive hepatitis. There was no evidence of transmission of HBV to any of these patients by these dentists, despite the fact that the dentists undoubtedly had HBV in their blood during the incubation period.[811]

Syringes and Needles

It is clearly established that transmission from patient to patient may result from the common use of unsterilized instruments. Any instrument that breaks the skin of one person and then breaks the skin or mucosa of another without being sterilized has the potential for transmitting the hepatitis viruses. The variety of instruments implicated in transmission is wide and will undoubtedly be extended if epidemiologic alertness to the possibility is maintained. A number of outbreaks have been traced to improper technique, for example, the use of one syringe for multiple doses.[137,457,904]

The mechanism by which hepatitis is transmitted by syringe was demonstrated to be aspiration of needle contents into the syringe while the needle is being removed.[465]

Red cells were found in the syringe contents following 17 of 39 intramuscular injections, although no blood was grossly visible and aspiration was not attempted. Red cells migrated spontaneously from the tip of the needle into the syringe in as little as 45 seconds. In view of transmission of icteric hepatitis B to 5 of 10 volunteers by only 0.00004 ml of whole blood,[240] the frequency of syringe-associated hepatitis is not surprising.

With widespread adoption of adequate techniques for sterilization and use of disposable equipment for injections, syringe-associated hepatitis appears to be relatively infrequent in the United States.[532] Nevertheless, percutaneous transmission does occur whenever good technique is ignored. An outbreak in 1959 involved patients of a physician who had 41 cases among 329 patients in his practice, with 15 deaths.[238] Syringe-associated hepatitis is frequent in some areas outside the United States.

Acupuncture needles that can puncture small blood vessels and become contaminated have been implicated in the transmission of hepatitis when reused without sterilization.[106]

A history of an injection or dental procedure during the 6 months prior to onset is not of itself adequate to suggest that this was the source of infection. A frequency greater than that in a comparable population without hepatitis must be demonstrated also. Nevertheless, a detailed epidemiologic history is worth obtaining from each patient regarding visits to physicians, dentists, clinics, and hospitals. If several cases occur among patients of any given physician or facility, it is worthwhile to investigate.

Other Instruments

The frequency with which contaminated tattoo needles and vials of dye transmit hepatitis is probably greater than can be documented. In addition to cases related to professional parlors,[354,690,836,936] amateur efforts with improvised equipment may be responsible.[869]

A variety of other instruments used successively on members of open or closed populations may be responsible for transmission of viral hepatitis. Ear-piercing is one procedure for which this risk has been documented.[486] The barber's razor and the manicurist's nail file may also be suspected, although documentation will be difficult except under unusual circumstances.

A role for fiberoptic gastrointestinal endoscopy in the transmission of hepatitis is theoretically possible because standard sterilization procedures cannot be employed between uses. Available data do not support this mode of transmission.[44,647,669]

Illicit Self-Injection

Viral hepatitis may be acquired by one-time, casual, or repeated sharing of equipment for illicit self-injection of drugs. Although first described in Chicago,[952] this epidemiologic entity was most frequently recognized during the 1950s and early 1960s in New York City.[33,37,478,583]

Indeed, as early as 1954 the New York City Department of Health made addiction-associated hepatitis a separate category for its epidemiologic classification of notified cases. By the mid-1960s, however, an epidemiologic pattern similar to New York City's and also due to addiction-associated illnesses, was discerned for New Jersey as a whole.[236] Subsequently, groups of cases in drug users have been reported from most areas of the United States[199,487,651,845,1066] and abroad.[85,474]

Approximately half of cases in persons identified as self-injectors have been serologically documented as hepatitis B.[151,359,671] The majority of drug abusers studied have serologic evidence of HBV infection.[896] Hepatitis A and non-A, non-B hepatitis are also responsible for the acute hepatitis seen in this population.[474,688] The presence of chronic liver disease is common in the asymptomatic parenteral drug user and has been related to persistent HBV infection.[896] Non-A, non-B hepatitis has also been implicated.

Track-Finding

Since 1962, there have been several reports of an unusual frequency of viral hepatitis among participants in the Scandinavian sport of track-finding (orienteering).[308,824,1027] The competitors run a course of their own devising over rugged terrain, past a number of checkpoints located 1 to 2 kilometers apart. Clothing usually consists of short socks, shorts, and a short-sleeved shirt. Most meets are held in wooded areas; over 90% of the participants indicated frequent or occasional scratches and cuts. When facilities were limited, the track-finders washed in small pools of stagnant water, and used a small number of basins. An association began to be recognized late in 1957, and by 1963 an estimated 568 cases had occurred. The pattern of illnesses had the epidemiologic characteristics of hepatitis B rather than of hepatitis A. Hepatitis B subsequently was serologically confirmed when sera were tested, years later, for HBsAg.[77] By preventive measures, this epidemiologic entity was virtually abolished, although relaxation of these rules permitted a new epidemic of 41 cases in 1965–1966.[824]

PATHOLOGY

The role of histopathology in the diagnosis and management of viral hepatitis has evolved through several distinct phases during the past 40 years. Before World War II it was not generally recognized that injury to the hepatocyte itself was the cause of viral hepatitis. Various circumstances in World War II resulted in large numbers of cases of hepatitis, so that even low case-fatality rates resulted in accumulation of a considerable amount of necropsy material. Thus, Lucke based his 1944 study on specimens from 125 fatal cases in which the disease was acquired from hepatitis B virus-contaminated yellow fever vaccine.[601] Iversen and Roholm,[473] as well as Dible, McMichael, and Sherlock,[220] obtained large amounts of information on the histopathologic alterations during acute viral hepatitis by examining needle aspiration specimens from nonfatal cases. These autopsy and biopsy studies, comprising the first phase, permitted thorough delineation of the histopathologic features of viral hepatitis by the late 1940s. Relatively little has been added since that time to what can be learned by light microscopy.

Electron microscopy has not been clinically useful in the diagnosis of viral hepatitis. It does, however, identify the rough endoplasmic reticulum as one of the earliest sites of injury in the hepatocyte during viral hepatitis.[871]

The second phase was characterized by the central role that histologic examination of the liver played in the diagnosis of viral hepatitis. In contrast to other infectious diseases, biopsy of affected tissue held a far more important position in the diagnosis of viral hepatitis. This attitude reached its peak in the 1960s when liver biopsy was considered, by many, to be the *sine qua non* for the diagnosis of acute viral hepatitis. In the 1970s, this attitude was questioned. By the early 1970s, an informal survey among hepatologists resulted in a draw: Half of them considered liver biopsy essential for diagnosis in every patient with acute hepatitis in whom the procedure can be performed with minimum risk, whereas the other half even by then considered a routine liver biopsy unnecessary for the diagnosis and management of these patients. The two major arguments in favor of the biopsy diagnosis of viral hepatitis were that (1) the demonstration of confluent bridging necrosis identifies a more serious disease that requires a different mode of therapy and (2) the first clinical manifestations of a chronic active hepatitis can mimic acute viral hepatitis and the two could be readily separated by histologic examination.

The third phase was reached in the second half of the 1970s with the advent of serologic markers of both hepatitis A and hepatitis B. Serologic diagnosis of acute viral hepatitis made morphologic examination of the liver unnecessary for a firm diagnosis of these diseases. Furthermore, two additional developments made biopsy of the liver during the early stages of acute hepatitis less important. One of them was the recognition that in many instances histologic examination of liver biopsies could not differentiate with certainty an acute, self-limited hepatitis from that of chronic active hepatitis, and the second was the recognition that a similar clinical picture and histologic lesion complex can be produced by chemicals and drugs and, therefore, a liver biopsy could not separate, in most cases, drug hepatitis from viral hepatitis.

In recent years, the availability of serologic markers to HBV components opened a new field. Immunohistopathologic techniques, adopted to both light and electron microscopy provided valuable information in understanding various aspects of hepatitis B. In the future some of these techniques may even find a role in the diagnosis, classification, and clinical management of patients with HBV infection.

Although liver biopsy is resorted to for the diagnosis and management of acute viral hepatitis less frequently now, it nevertheless still plays a role in the care of patients suspected of having acute viral hepatitis. The histologic diagnosis of viral hepatitis depends on the coexistence of a group of morphologic abnormalities and on the distribution of these lesions within the hepatic lobules. No single histopathologic lesion is diagnostic of a viral hepatitis. To date there is no recognized histologic pattern that can differentiate hepatitis A from hepatitis B or from other non-A, non-B types of hepatitis.

The entire liver is involved in acute viral hepatitis. Despite the reasonably uniform distribution and uniform severity of the histopathologic lesions in some livers, in others the expressions of the acute hepatitis varies in different parts of the liver. This variation is manifested usually by minimal, but at times considerable, differences in the severity of hepatocellular destruction even in adjacent lobules.

Another problem with the histopathologic examination of biopsy specimens in acute viral hepatitis is that one cannot invariably predict the severity of the clinical illness on the basis of the severity of the histologic changes. Although in general, the more severe the histologic injury, the more likely that the clinical picture is correspondingly grave, this is by no means true in all cases. In a few patients, minimal histologic changes were associated with severe, indeed fulminant disease, and in others severe and extensive histologic changes were associated with a fairly mild clinical illness and good prognosis. It is not surprising therefore that the histologic manifestations of typical viral hepatitis are similar to those seen in anicteric or even subclinical viral hepatitis. Therefore, both of these are described together under typical viral hepatitis.

Typical Viral Hepatitis

The characteristic morphologic abnormality in "typical viral hepatitis" is a combination of portal, periportal, and lobular hepatitis. The classic and less common findings in the histologic diagnosis of viral hepatitis are shown in Table 15-7. The changes in inapparent and anicteric hepatitis are usually but not always less severe than those in icteric disease.

Portal Hepatitis. The portal tracts are enlarged by the accumulation of inflammatory cells and by edema. The severity of portal inflammation can vary from minimal to severe (Figs. 15-10 through 15-12). The portal inflammatory cells are predominantly lymphocytes and histiocytes with an admixture of various but usually small proportions of neutrophilic and eosinophilic leukocytes. Plasma cells are uncommon. In a few livers, however, polymorphonuclear leukocytes are the most numerous type of cell (Fig. 15-11). These leukocytes are more commonly seen in portal inflammation than in lobular hepatitis, and their dominance in portal triads is not as unusual as it is in the lobular parenchyma. Granulomas are rare; when they occur, they are usually associated with the intravenous use of illicit drugs. Occasionally, lym-

TABLE 15-7.   Histologic Diagnosis of Viral Hepatitis*

HISTOLOGIC FEATURE	HEPATITIS A	HEPATITIS B	NON-A, NON-B HEPATITIS
Portal (mononuclear) inflammation	Marked	Modest	Minimal
Limiting plate	Disrupted	Preserved	Preserved
Periportal inflammation	Simulate CAH†	Minimal	Minimal
Bile ductular lesions	Rare	Occasional	Common
Zone-3 cholestasis	Common	Occasional	Occasional
Parenchymal necrosis	Moderate	Marked	Mild
Pleocytosis	Moderate	Moderate	Mild
Sinusoidal lining cell activity	Minimal	Moderate	Marked
Sinusoidal inflammation	Mild	Mild	Marked
Fat	Rare	Rare	Common
Ground glass hepatocytes	Absent	Rare	Absent

* Data from references 4, 554, 765, and 996.
† CAH = chronic active hepatitis.

Fig. 15-10. Portal hepatitis—minimal. Portal tract contains three hepatic arterioles, two bile ducts, a large portal vein, and sparse portal connective tissue with a few mononuclear cells. The portal tract is not enlarged, and the intensity of inflammatory exudate is minimal. The limiting plate, that is, the demarcation between the portal tract and the parenchyma, is reasonably sharp. The periportal parenchyma shows lobular disarray with regenerative and degenerative activity, illustrated by liver cell fallout, spotty necrosis, and double-cell-thick liver cell plates. (H & E stained section; original magnification × 200)

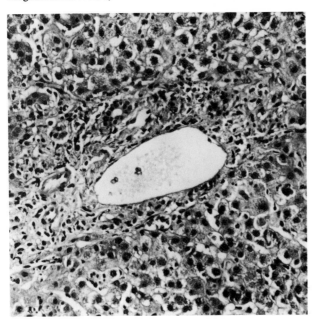

phocytes may aggregate in a follicle-like pattern (Fig. 15-13). The limiting plate, that is, the demarcation between portal tract and the surrounding hepatic parenchyma, is usually well preserved and may remain more or less sharp. The limiting plate becomes destroyed only when the inflammatory exudate spills out of the portal tracts into the periportal parenchyma. In the later stages of acute viral hepatitis, portal inflammation tends to persist, but the limiting plates are usually preserved and the portal tracts, therefore, are sharply delineated from the periportal parenchyma. Portal changes often persist for prolonged periods but, if so, they are very mild. In non-A, non-B hepatitis, portal inflammation is associated with mild and widely scattered lobular changes that may persist for months or years.

Bile ducts and ductules are usually unaffected. However, electron microscopy commonly detects lesions in the ductal epithelial cells in viral hepatitis.[138] In about 25% of livers, mild to severe changes are detectable by light microscopy (Figs. 15-13 and 15-14). Ductular proliferation may be seen in some portal tracts. An inflammatory exudate usually composed of lymphocytes and histiocytes may accumulate around the basement membrane of small bile ducts or ductules. The significance of this pericholangitis during the acute stage of illness is not clear; it may well be part of a generalized portal inflammation. In an occasional portal tract, ductular epithelial injury is prominent and is accompanied by infiltration of lymphocytes or histiocytes and even by polymorphonuclear leukocytes (see Fig. 15-14). The degenerative changes range from swelling, vacuolization, and irregularity of epithelial cells to necrosis of the epithelium. Although the ductular lesion in viral hepatitis is a type of nonsuppurative cholangitis

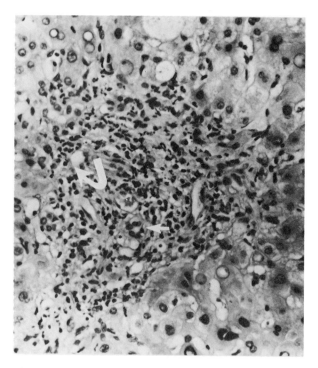

Fig. 15-11. Portal hepatitis and duct injury—moderate in severity. The terminal portal tract contains two bile ductules: One shows only mild epithelial swelling and vacuolization (*arrow*), whereas the other exhibits major changes, that is, part of its epithelium is destroyed and is invaded by predominantly PMN leukocytic inflammatory cells (*curved arrow*). This portal tract contains a predominantly PMN-leukocytic inflammatory exudate. The demarcation between portal tract and lobular parenchyma is fairly sharp. Many of the parenchymal cells contain vacuolated nuclei, and an occasional one has fatty vacuoles in the cytoplasm. This patient had diabetes and self-limited cholestatic hepatitis. (H & E stained section; original magnification × 240)

that resembles that of primary biliary cirrhosis (see Fig. 15-13), any relation of this lesion to primary biliary cirrhosis is obscure.[778] None of these ductular lesions, whether they are accompanied by periductular fibrosis or not, has a prognostic significance,[156] and progression to primary biliary cirrhosis has not been documented.

Periportal Hepatitis. Necrosis of periportal hepatocytes and the merger of portal and lobular inflammatory exudate may destroy the limiting plate (Figs. 15-15 and 15-16). The "piecemeal necrosis" in typical acute hepatitis may be indistinguishable from that of chronic active hepatitis (Figs. 15-17 and 15-18). Periportal necrosis of acute hepatitis has no prognostic significance. Piecemeal necrosis during acute hepatitis does not indicate an increased risk of chronic hepatitis. This lesion is a more reliable prognostic indicator if seen 3 to 6 months after the onset of

illness. The diagnosis of chronic active hepatitis, however, must not be made on the presence of piecemeal necrosis alone unless the duration of the hepatitis is known to have exceeded 6 months.

Lobular Hepatitis. The characteristic lesion of viral hepatitis is lobular disarray. This picture is produced by disruption of the liver cell plate by spotty necrosis and single-cell fallout, pleomorphism, and anisocytosis of hepatocytes due to concomitant degenerative and regenerative changes. There are accumulations of inflammatory cells in areas where groups of hepatocytes have vanished from the liver cell plates (Figs. 15-19 and 15-20). Although these spotty necroinflammatory changes are distributed randomly throughout the lobule, these are often more pronounced in the perivenular area that is the most distal portion of the hepatic microcirculation.[809] Phlebitis of the hepatic venule (central phlebitis) is the characteristic lesion of viral hepatitis. When seen, it is of help in arriving at the proper diagnosis. The endothelium of the efferent vein is unaffected, but the vessel wall becomes edematous because inflammatory exudate accumulates between the liver cell plate and the vein. Endophlebitis can develop with endothelial proliferation and accumulation of inflammatory cells in a proteinaceous meshwork. This reaction appears to be more severe when it coincides with necrosis of perivenular hepatocytes. Under these conditions, the inflammatory exudate evoked by parenchymal necrosis merges with the periphlebitis (Fig. 15-21).

The inflammatory exudate in the lobule is usually dominated by lymphocytes and histiocytes, but eosinophilic and neutrophilic leukocytes are also present and occasionally a few plasma cells may also be seen. Although eosinophils are commonly seen, their accumulation is not associated with eosinophilia in peripheral blood. In about 5% of biopsies, polymorphonuclear leukocytes are prominent in the inflammatory exudate. The mononuclear intralobular inflammatory exudate is not confined to the liver cell plates, but is also seen in the space of Disse and in the sinusoids where it is accompanied by hypertrophy of endothelial macrophages (see Fig. 15-20). In some biopsies, plasma cells are prominent in the inflammatory exudate without being associated with a chronic course of the hepatitis (see Fig. 15-34). Intrasinusoidal accumulation of mononuclear cells associated with some fatty vacuolization of hepatocytes and portal alterations may be characteristic of at least one of the non-A, non-B types of hepatitis.

The differences of staining qualities of adjacent liver cells may be marked. Some show mild degenerative changes, others undergo lytic necrosis and disappear. A variable proportion of cells shows regenerative activity characterized by more basophilic cytoplasm and by increased size, number, and staining intensity of nuclei and nucleoli. Some hepatocytes enlarge, others shrink. This varies in extent from cell to cell. When cellular enlargement is extreme, such cells contain only small fragments of thin strands of eosinophilic cytoplasm and are called

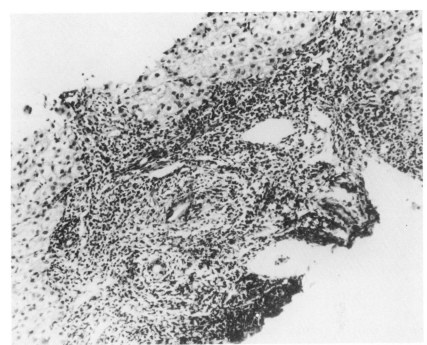

Fig. 15-12. Portal hepatitis—severe. The enlarged portal tract contains a dense inflammatory exudate that consists mostly of mononuclear cells. The limiting plate is intact because the demarcation between this portal tract and the parenchyma is reasonably well defined. (H & E stained section; original magnification × 90)

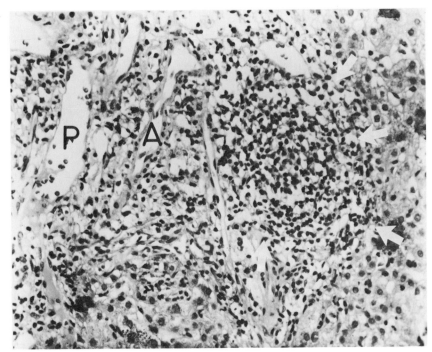

Fig. 15-13. Bile duct injury—severe. This interlobular portal tract has a portal vein (*P*) and a hepatic artery (*A*). A dense folliclelike aggregate of lymphocytes (*arrows*) replaced the bile duct. This picture is similar to that seen in primary biliary cirrhosis. (This patient had acute hepatitis and recovered completely. On followup, there was no evidence of biliary cirrhosis.) (H & E stain; original magnification × 200)

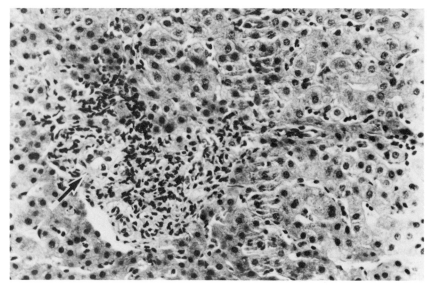

Fig. 15-14. Bile ductular injury—mild. The terminal portal tract shows a bile ductule and mild periportal hepatitis. The ductular epithelium shows swelling, vacuolization, and irregularity with pyknosis and cell dropout. The normally uniform pattern of epithelial nuclei is disrupted in this ductule (*arrow*). (H & E stain; original magnification × 200)

balloon cells. On electron microscopy, these ballooned cells show deglycogenation of the cytoplasm and degranulation, disruption, and dilatation of the cysternae of the endoplasmic reticulum with detachment of polysomes, a decrease in the number of ribosomes and wide separation of cytoplasmic organelles.[483,774,870,871] The disruption of the function of the endoplasmic reticulum in surviving cells suggests anatomic basis for impairment of several

functions such as protein and steroid synthesis, glucuronide conjugation, and detoxification.[870] Mitochondrial injury is usually a late occurrence.

When a single liver cell shrinks and its cytoplasmic basophilia disappears, the cytoplasm becomes "brick red" in hematoxylin-eosin stained sections. This acidophilic degeneration begins with shrinkage of the hepatocyte and the development of more intense cytoplasmic eosino-

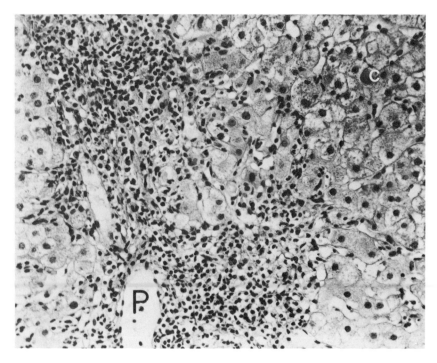

Fig. 15-15. Portal and periportal hepatitis—moderate in severity. The portal vein is cut tangentially (*P*), and a predominantly mononuclear inflammatory exudate extends into the periportal parenchyma and has destroyed the limiting plate. Some of the hepatocytes adjacent to the portal tract undergo ballooning. Acidophilic degenerative changes lead to the formation of a Councilman-like body (*C*). (H & E stained section; original magnification × 200)

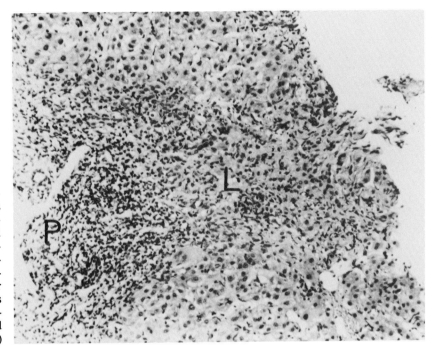

Fig. 15-16. Portal and periportal hepatitis—severe. The limiting plate is completely destroyed; thus the demarcation between the portal tract (*P*) and the parenchyma is no longer recognizable. The inflammatory exudate extends deep in the lobule (*L*) and consists of predominantly mononuclear cells, although many PMN leukocytes are seen in both the portal and periportal inflammation. (H & E stained section; original magnification × 160)

philia. The nucleus gradually becomes pyknotic, and nuclear vacuolization occasionally develops. These degenerating hepatocytes subsequently round off and are gradually extruded from the liver cell plates into the sinusoids. The typical eosinophilic (Councilman-like) body is found in the sinusoids (see Figs. 15-19 and 15-20). It

has sharply outlined margins and contains a pyknotic nucleus or nuclear fragments or no nuclear material at all. These bodies are eventually phagocytosed by sinusoidal macrophages. By electron microscopy, the eosinophilic hepatocytes appear as dark cells that have a dense hyaloplasm, although still recognizable but damaged organ-

Fig. 15-17. Portal hepatitis with periportal piecemeal necrosis—minimal. The margin of an enlarged portal tract with a number of entrapped hepatocytes is evident. The surrounding of single or small groups of periportal hepatocytes by inflammation is characteristic of piecemeal necrosis (*arrows*). The predominant inflammatory cells are lymphocytes. In addition to parenchymal hepatitis, bile plugs are seen (*curved arrows*) in the middle of pseudoductules. Acute hepatitis, piecemeal necrosis, and cholestasis are present. (H & E stain; original magnification × 200)

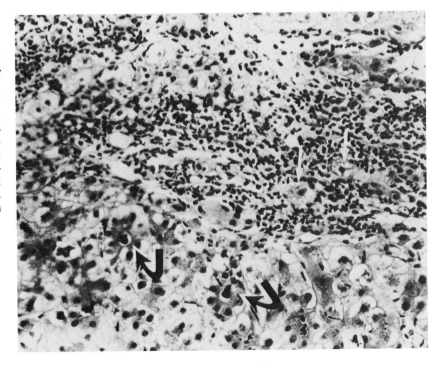

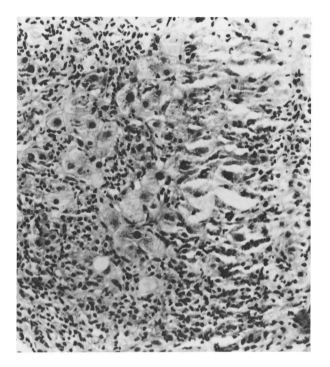

Fig. 15-18. Portal hepatitis with periportal piecemeal necrosis—severe. Single cells and small groups of hepatocytes are surrounded by predominantly mononuclear inflammatory exudate that contains numerous PMN leukocytes. Several of the lymphocytes are in contact with the membrane of entrapped hepatocytes. (H & E stained section; original magnification × 240)

elles.[516] These changes are due to cytoplasmic dehydration, to alteration of nuclear function leading to accelerated senescence, or to both.[472] These "acidophilic" bodies are called Councilman-like bodies because they resemble the acidophilic bodies found in zone 3 of the lobule in yellow fever. The acidophilic bodies are commonly seen in viral hepatitis but are not specific for it. They are also seen in other viral, bacterial, and parasitic infections[472] and in other disorders associated with hepatocyte necrosis. Electron microscopy suggests that the development of these acidophilic Councilman-like bodies is due to cytoplasmic dehydration.[154] In some patients with chronic hepatitis B but rarely in those with acute hepatitis B, the cytoplasm of parenchymal cells has a ground-glass appearance (Fig. 15-22).

Regeneration proceeds together with necrosis of the liver parenchyma. Groups of young or multinucleated hepatocytes are frequently seen adjacent to areas of necrosis and inflammation. Vigorous regenerative activity may be evidenced by the increased frequency of karyokinesis without cytokinesis and of hyperkaryokinesis. The former is manifested by increased numbers of multinucleated and even giant cells and the latter by more frequently occurring polyploid cells. Increased rate of mitosis is seen, and multipolar mitoses may be evident.[622]

The combination of degenerative enlargement and shrinkage and regeneration of more intensely staining hepatocytes potentiates the characteristic *pleocytosis* of viral hepatitis. Indeed, pleocytosis may be seen without disruption of the lobular architecture. Necrosis, degeneration, regeneration, and inflammation in proximity distort the normal architectural pattern and result in lobular disarray.

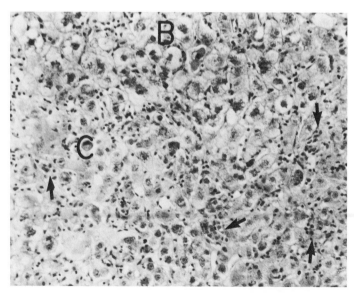

Fig. 15-19. Lobular hepatitis. The typical features of acute hepatitis are shown. Lobular disarray is caused by [1] pleocytosis, which is caused by marked variation of the size of the hepatocytes and their nuclei; and by [2] variation of both the thickness and arrangement of the liver cell plates, which is caused by single-cell fall-out, Councilman bodies (*C*), ballooning of hepatocytes (*B*), spotty necroinflammatory changes (*arrows*), pseudoductular changes, and regeneration of hepatocytes. (H & E stain; original magnification × 100)

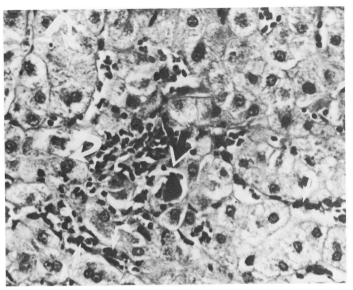

Fig. 15-20. Lobular hepatitis. The characteristic features of spotty necrosis are shown. A Councilman body (*large arrow*) is adjacent to a defect in the liver cell plate, from which a small group of hepatocytes is missing, and is replaced by a typical lymphocytic and histiocytic inflammatory exudate. In addition to the inflammatory cells in the liver cell plate, the same type of mononuclear cells also accumulates in the sinusoids along with hypertrophied endothelial macrophages (*small arrows*). Also shown are two-cell-thick liver cell plates that replaced the normal single-cell-thick ones (*curved arrow*) as a manifestation of regenerative activity in acute hepatitis. (H & E stain; original magnification × 240)

In some biopsies, scattered areas are seen where the liver cells arrange themselves in a ductlike pattern (see Figs. 15-19 and 15-22). Pseudoduct formation, also known as glandular transformation, is not limited to certain epidemics. This lesion is commonly seen with extensive parenchymal necrosis or with cholestasis, regardless of the specific etiologic agent.

Often, hepatocytes vanish from liver cell plates without a trace, and their absence is manifested by the collapse of the reticulum fibers with or without the accumulation of inflammatory cells (see Fig. 15-28).

Kupffer cells (endothelial macrophages) are increased in number and size (see Fig. 15-20). Many of these cells contain periodic acid–Schiff (PAS)–positive glycoproteins, such as γ-globulin. After several weeks of viral hepatitis, endothelial macrophages (Kupffer cells) show increased phagocytic activity. Consequently, these cells may contain dirty brown pigment and cell fragments. The pigment is

Fig. 15-21. Hepatic (central) phlebitis. Subendothelial inflammation is seen in a hepatic (central) venule that is surrounded by necroinflammatory changes and vacuolated hepatocytes in the adjacent parenchyma. The inflammatory exudate is a mixture of mononuclear and PMN leukocytic cells. (H & E stain; original magnification × 450)

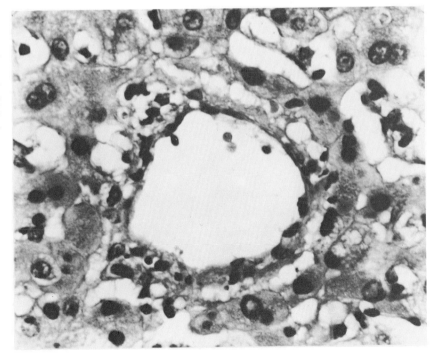

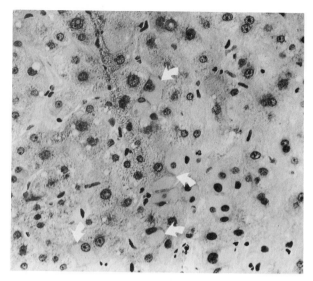

Fig. 15-22. Acute hepatitis B. The cytoplasm of the hepatocytes has a ground-glass appearance (*arrows*). This feature is rare in the acute disease. (H & E stained section; original magnification × 120)

called wear and tear pigment, is thought to be lipofuscin, and is acid fast.[601,935] It is suggested that this pigment is the result of digested organelles, such as mitochondria, in membrane-enclosed spaces (autophagosomes).[774] The lipofuscin pigment in the Kupffer cells is not characteristic of viral hepatitis. Its presence indicates previous paren-

chymal necrosis regardless of its causes. Nevertheless, its presence can be helpful in the differential diagnosis of jaundice during the subsiding stages of viral hepatitis, when only a few of the characteristic morphologic features remain.

Some patients with only minimal hepatocellular necrosis may be very ill (Fig. 15-23); others with extensive lobular alterations feel well and have good appetites. Symptoms and several abnormalities of liver tests (particularly aminotransferases) appear to be caused by injured rather than dead hepatocytes.

Immunohistopathology of Acute Hepatitis B. After HBV infection, the distribution of HBV antigens in the lobule can exhibit four distinct patterns.[89] In the well-developed stage of typical acute hepatitis B, which is characterized by spotty necrosis throughout the lobule, viral components are usually not detectable in most hepatocytes. Nevertheless, in widely scattered areas, occasional hepatocytes may have detectable amounts of intranuclear HBcAg. These findings are associated with a vigorous mononuclear inflammatory exudate both in scattered areas of spotty necrosis and in portal tracts. When the biopsy is obtained very early during the course of acute hepatitis B, occasional hepatocytes may show membrane-associated cytoplasmic HBsAg. This stage is associated with circulating HBV as well as HBsAg. During the incubation period of acute hepatitis B in the nonhuman primate, both HBcAg and HBsAg are demonstrable in the hepatocyte nuclei and cytoplasm, respectively.[232] Similar observations were made on liver biopsies obtained after HBV infection of patients.[251] The expression of both HBcAg and HBsAg in

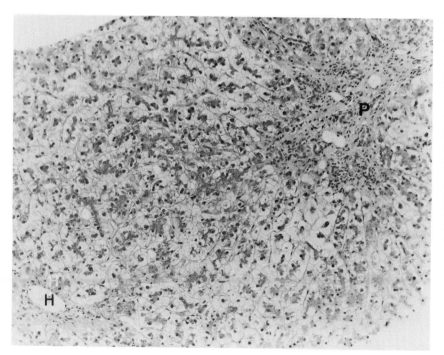

Fig. 15-23. Lobular hepatitis—atypical. This illustrates the wide discrepancy in the histologic clinical severity of hepatitis. The hepatic lobule is intact. There is widespread ballooning of hepatocytes, but little necroinflammatory activity is detectable. Many of the liver cell plates are thickened. The portal tract (*P*) shows little inflammatory reaction, and the limiting plate is mostly intact. The hepatic venule (*H*) is surrounded only by a few inflammatory cells. Despite the paucity of severe histologic lesions, this patient had fulminant hepatitis. (H & E stain; original magnification × 100)

hepatocytes represents the stage of viral replication that precedes the vigorous cell-mediated immunologic response to the infection in the normal host. This immunologic attack on infected hepatocytes leads to the spotty necrotic changes of typical acute viral hepatitis B. The likely explanation of the paucity of immunohistopathologic changes at the peak of typical acute hepatitis B is that the cell-mediated immunologic attack on the infected hepatocytes has successfully eradicated the infected hepatocytes. This immunologic attack clinically manifests itself with an acute illness, hepatomegaly, and high serum aminotransferase levels. It is followed by the decrease and disappearance of HBsAg from the serum and by the development of anti-HBc, in response to exposure of the core antigen from destroyed hepatocytes to immunocompetent cells. This process is believed to be responsible for the eradication of infection and the development of effective and permanent immunity manifested by the appearance of anti-HBs in the serum.

A second type of immunohistopathologic pattern emerges following HBV infection in immunologically suppressed patients. For example, patients receiving chemotherapy for malignant diseases or patients with chronic uremia undergoing hemodialysis or renal transplant recipients appear to be susceptible to this pattern.[375] A similar picture also develops in immunologically tolerant infants and children who acquire HBV infection from their mother at or near birth. This immunohistopathologic pattern is characterized by positive reaction for HBcAg of most hepatocyte nuclei. In only a few of these cells is HBsAg expressed on membranes. The specific immunofluorescence for anti-HBc gives the biopsy a honeycomb-like appearance. Clinically, this is often a mild disease and may be associated with only minimal to modest elevations of the serum aminotransferases. These patients are often contagious because HBV may be found in their circulation.[87]

A third type of immunohistopathologic pattern develops late in the course of HBV infection in patients who may have had no clinical evidence of an acute hepatitis. This is the typical picture seen in prolonged carriers of HBsAg who are either not contagious or have only very low grade infectivity. This pattern is manifested by the expression of HBsAg within numerous hepatocytes. This antigen is distributed uniformly throughout the cytoplasm. On the other hand, HBcAg-positive nuclei are absent or are uncommon and when seen usually are not associated with HBsAg-positive hepatocytes.[375]

Finally, the fourth type of immunohistopathologic pattern is characterized by the spotty distribution of both HBcAg and HBsAg in the liver. Up to 60% of the liver cell nuclei may contain HBcAg and up to 30% of the hepatocytes may be positive for HBsAg and, when so, HBsAg is usually associated with membranes.[374] The serum of these patients is often positive for HBV and for HBsAg-containing immune complexes. These patients may demonstrate confluent bridging necrosis in addition to spotty necrotic hepatitis on their biopsy.

Late Changes of Typical Viral Hepatitis. During the later stages of typical viral hepatitis, the same lesions are seen as during the acute phase. The extent and severity of the lesions, however, are usually milder. The characteristic findings are lipofuscin in the Kupffer cells; widely scattered areas of single cell or "spotty" necrotic lobular hepatitis associated with mononuclear inflammatory cells only; and irregularity of the liver cell plates. Hyperchromatic or multinucleated regenerating hepatocytes are also seen. Enlargement of portal tracts that contain increased numbers of lymphocytes, plasma cells, and histiocytes is characteristic of this stage, but periportal hepatitis is usually absent, the limiting plate is intact, and there is little or no fibrosis. These features are similar to that seen in chronic persistent and chronic portal hepatitis.[204,775] These types of histologic changes can be seen commonly up to 4 to 6 months and even years after recovery from the acute episode of viral hepatitis. Persistence of these mild histologic changes is particularly common after non-A, non-B hepatitis. The prognosis for this persistent or unresolved hepatitis is usually good, because chronic active hepatitis and cirrhosis are uncommon.[71] Nevertheless, follow-up biopsies are needed to detect either periportal extension of hepatitis or increased activity of the hepatic connective tissue, which would indicate the possibility of progression to a chronic active hepatitis.[88]

Cholestatic Hepatitis

Cholestasis is a term applied to the presence of bile plugs or microcalculi in canaliculi or in ductules. The same histologic picture may be produced by mechanical obstruction of a major bile duct (extrahepatic cholestasis) or in the absence of mechanical interference with bile flow (intrahepatic cholestasis). Therefore, this histologic finding, by itself, cannot differentiate extrahepatic obstruction (surgical jaundice) from intrahepatic cholestasis (medical jaundice).

A microcalculus or a bile plug is a bilirubin-containing coagulum that has precipitated in a dilated canaliculus. The canalicular microvilli are flattened or are absent. Microcalculi are seen most frequently in the perivenular region. Often several hepatocytes are arranged in a ductlike pattern surrounding a bile plug (see Fig. 15-17). Such a ductlike appearance of hepatocytes gave rise to the descriptive term *pseudoductule*. In addition to this intracanalicular bile stasis, golden yellow bilirubin-containing pigment also may be visible in hepatocytes and in Kupffer cells.

In severe forms of viral hepatitis, often in association with confluent necrosis, microcalculi may be seen in portal bile ductules. Rarely, such cholestasis may be associated with necrosis and inflammation (cholangitis) of the ductular epithelium (Fig. 15-24).

The distinct changes in the cholestatic type of viral hepatitis are canalicular and intracellular; there is formation of pseudoductules and prominence of polymorphonuclear leukocytes, both in the portal and periportal

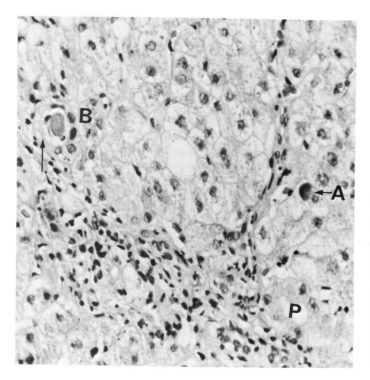

Fig. 15-24. Pseudoductule and cholangitis. The illness began 2 weeks after transfusions and had a severe course. Coma and ascites developed. Other areas of the specimen show submassive necrosis. Note an acidophilic body (*A*) and a pseudoduct (*P*). The portal tract contains a predominantly PMN leukocytic inflammatory exudate. A perilobular bile ductule (*B*) contains a large "microcalculus." A part of the ductular epithelium shows necrosis (*vertical arrow*) and is infiltrated with PMN leukocytes. This biopsy was obtained 7 weeks after the onset of transfusion-associated viral hepatitis in a 52-year-old man. (H & E stain; original magnification × 200)

inflammatory exudates. Ballooning degeneration of hepatocytes may be prominent. The degree of cholangiolar changes in the periportal region is variable. The dilated cholangioles may be infiltrated by polymorphonuclear leukocytes (see Fig. 15-22). Interlobular bile ducts are not affected by this process.[472] Cholestasis in viral hepatitis is commonly associated with the characteristic morphologic lesion complex described previously in the section on typical viral hepatitis. In a few cases, lesions other than cholestasis are difficult to find, although long and meticulous search may reveal an occasional focus of parenchymal cell necrosis. The portal areas contain many polymorphonuclear leukocytes that frequently aggregate around bile ducts. The differentiation of the cholestatic form of viral hepatitis from drug-induced cholestatic changes is difficult if not impossible.[851] If serologic documentation of viral hepatitis is absent, other etiologies should be considered.

The mechanism of intrahepatic cholestasis in viral hepatitis has not been defined. It may be related to primary damage of the microvilli of the bile canaliculi or secondary to abnormalities of the bile secretory apparatus of the hepatocyte itself. The latter would be manifested by a change of the physicochemical composition of freshly secreted bile that readily precipitates in the canaliculi.

In histologically confirmed cholestatic viral hepatitis, clinical features simulating extrahepatic bile duct obstruction may not be present. Liver biopsies obtained in two hepatitis epidemics disclosed that the histopathologic features of cholestasis were associated with clinically typical viral hepatitis rather than with the clinical picture of intrahepatic cholestasis.[243,244] Despite frequent mention of cholestatic viral hepatitis in the literature, clinical simulation of extrahepatic obstruction (surgical jaundice) appears to be rare.

Confluent Hepatic Necrosis

The term *confluent hepatic necrosis* was suggested by an international group of hepatopathologists[88] to designate parenchymal necrosis affecting substantial groups of adjacent hepatocytes. The lesion contrasts to the usual spotty distribution of necrosis in typical viral hepatitis. Confluent necrosis is zonal, that is, the affected hepatocytes are located in a microcirculatory zone of the simple or complex hepatic acinus. Spotty necrosis is focal, that is, the affected hepatocytes are randomly distributed in the lobules.

Confluent hepatic necrosis encompasses a spectrum of histologic changes. Depending on the severity and extent of necrosis, it is variably called bridging necrosis, subacute or submassive hepatic necrosis, and massive hepatic necrosis. These designations,[107,515,945,1006,1007] often used interchangeably, are also applied to changes seen in chronic active hepatitis[107,945] as well as to those found in the acute disease. The adjective "subacute," however, is confusing because it may be taken as having a temporal connotation that is inappropriate for describing a pattern of necrosis. Yet, "subacute" is still used by some to designate a certain type of hepatitis that usually is associated with confluent necrosis.[758] The various patterns of confluent (bridging)

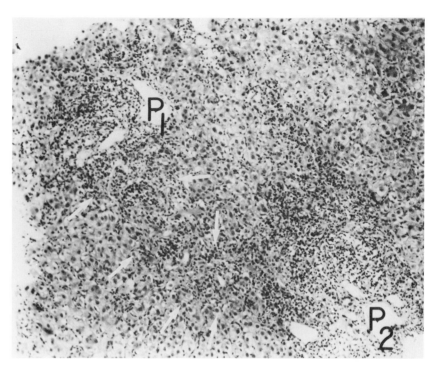

Fig. 15-25. Bridging between portal tracts (portal-to-portal bridging). Periportal necroinflammatory reaction (*arrows*) enlarged adjacent portal tracts (P_1, P_2) that fortuitously merged by a bridge of periportal hepatitis. This type of portal-to-portal bridging affects the most proximal portion of the terminal microcirculatory unit, the hepatic acinus (see Chap. 1). This type of bridging is not considered a histologic manifestation of severe hepatitis (beyond that implied by periportal hepatitis itself). (H & E stain; original magnification × 94)

necrosis in acute hepatitis are shown in Figures 15-25 through 15-29.

Confluent Necrosis: Bridging. When hepatocellular necrosis or a necroinflammatory process involves contiguous groups of hepatocytes that connect recognizable anatomic structures, then this confluent lesion appears to bridge these structures. The term *bridging* is a pictorial description of this type of confluent necrosis.[515] The importance of bridging necrosis depends on the location and extent of the injury and on the host's response to it (regeneration, fibrosis).

Fig. 15-26. Confluent necrosis between portal tract and hepatic venules (portal-to-venular [central] bridging). Confluent necrosis is seen in the most distal portion of the hepatic microcirculation, in zone 3 of the hepatic acinus. This biopsy was obtained 6 days after the onset and 2 days after recovery from deep coma due to fulminant acute hepatitis. The lytic necrosis is severe, but the inflammation is minimal around the hepatic venule (*H*). The portal tract (*P*) is enlarged, and the moderately severe periportal hepatitis abolished the limiting plate. In the inflammatory exudate, mononuclear cells predominate. (H & E stain; original magnification × 100)

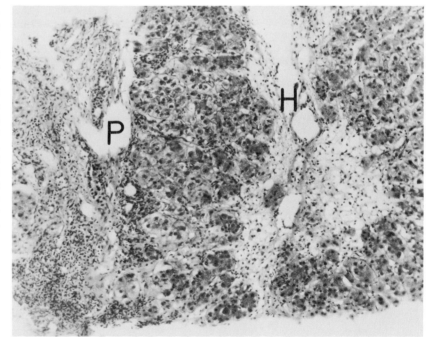

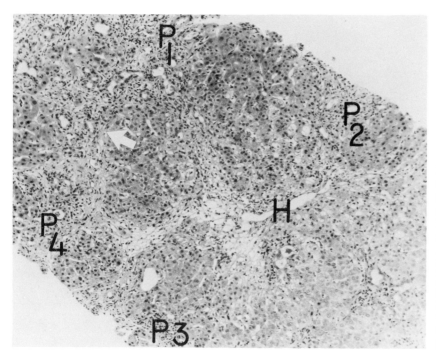

Fig. 15-27. Confluent bridging necrosis between multiple structures within adjacent lobules. There is a tangentially cut hepatic venule (*H*) from which bands of confluent necrosis extend to at least three portal tracts (P_1, P_2, P_3, P_4). This type of confluent (bridging) necrosis surrounds at least three adjacent hepatic lobules. In addition to portal-to-venular bridging, there is also portal (P_1)-to-portal (P_4) bridging (*arrow*), which gives the appearance of a nodule. (H & E stain; original magnification × 102)

Fig. 15-28. Reticulum collapse. The absence of hepatocytes from the liver cell plates is marked by the "collapse" of the reticulum fibers. These fibers normally lie between the liver cell plates and sinusoidal lining cells in close association with the latter; with light microscopy, they appear as single thin lines along both sides of the hepatocytes. When hepatocytes have disappeared, these reticulum fibers approach each other or "collapse." The biopsy was taken from a 26-year-old man during acute hepatitis. (Weigert's silver impregnation; original magnification × 200)

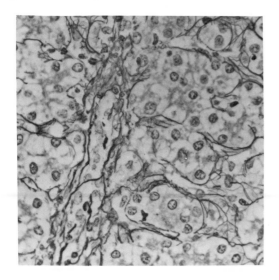

Portal-to-Portal Bridging. Periportal hepatitis increases the chances that random sections across the hepatic lobules produce apparent confluence of adjacent portal tracts. The meaning of this type of bridging necrosis may be the same as that of periportal hepatitis (see Fig. 15-25) except when linked to portal-to-venular bridging.

Portal-to-Venular (Central) Bridging (Confluent Necrosis Between Portal Tract and Hepatic Venule). In this type of lesion, the necroinflammatory process is in the periphery of the hepatic lobule; thus, it is in zone 3 of the hepatic acinus. This injury therefore involves the most distal portion of the hepatic microcirculation. This type of bridging necrosis may result in collapse and condensation of the remaining reticulum fibers and form a passive septum. Adjacent passive septa may give the appearance of a nodule. This is particularly likely when portal-to-portal bridging is associated with portal-to-hepatic venous bridging (see Figs. 15-26 and 15-27). The term *bridging* is excellent to describe this type of confluent necrosis.[515]

The most common type of bridging is the confluent necrosis between portal tract and hepatic venule. The cellular debris and necroinflammatory lesion may continue to separate reticulum fibers, and passive septum does not necessarily develop in these lesions (see Fig. 15-28). The necrosis usually is complete and eliminates all recognizable cellular structures in some livers (see Fig. 15-26). However, in other bridges of confluent necrosis, entrapped hepatocytes remain. This lesion may, in some respect, be similar to that of piecemeal necrosis in the periportal area.

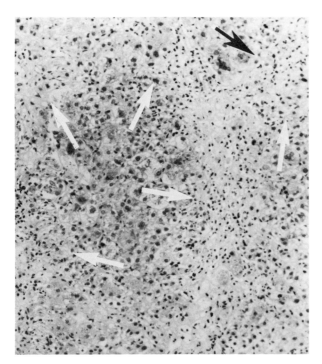

Fig. 15-29. Bridging adjacent to hepatic venules (central-to-central bridging). There is only sparse inflammatory exudate in confluent necrosis between neighboring hepatic venules (*arrows*). This type of confluent necrosis affects hepatocytes in a more proximal portion of the hepatic microcirculation than does portal-to-venular bridging. Here the lesion is in the periphery of the complex hepatic acinus of Rappaport. (H & E stain; original magnification × 160)

The extent and width of these bridging lesions vary. The remaining parenchyma in zone 1 of the affected lobule and the hepatocytes in adjacent lobules may show the spotty necrotic type of lesions described under lobular hepatitis. In some of these cases evidence of cholestasis may be prominent, and bile plugs may be seen both in the canaliculi and in portal bile ductules and ducts. These portal tracts commonly show edema, enlargement, and various degrees of ductular abnormalities. The inflammatory exudate in these portal tracts may contain a fair proportion of polymorphonuclear leukocytes. The diagnosis of confluent or bridging necrosis may be difficult because confluent lesions are usually widely separated from each other and the intervening lobules show no evidence of this type of extensive necroinflammatory process.

Bridging Adjacent Hepatic Venules (Central-to-Central Bridging).

When the injury affects a more proximal segment of the hepatic microcirculation, confluent necrosis can affect hepatocytes in the periphery of the complex hepatic acinus. This is manifested by confluent necrosis that bridges hepatic venules with each other (see Fig. 15-29).

In these livers both the areas of spotty and those with confluent necrosis contain numerous lymphocytes and variable numbers of plasma cells, histiocytes, and eosinophilic and polymorphonuclear leukocytes. A similar inflammatory exudate is seen in the enlarged and edematous portal areas. The prominent cellular exudate is not uniformly distributed in all areas of necrosis and collapse. In some areas the mononuclear cells tend to form follicle-like aggregates. They accumulate along blood vessels, bile ductules, or interlobular bile ducts.

Confluent necrosis during acute viral hepatitis in older patients indicates a more severe form of the disease. In a series of patients with confluent necrosis in which 63% were over 40 years of age, half died.[107] Confluent bridging necrosis is not associated with a more severe disease in patients under 30 years of age. Indeed, this lesion was seen in 34% of consecutive young soldiers with acute viral hepatitis, all of whom recovered.[1070] The mechanism of confluent bridging necrosis is not known. Ischemic and anoxic damage may contribute to the extent of lytic necrosis and can amplify the extent of parenchymal injury. The observations that confluent necrosis is localized to the microcirculatory periphery either of the simple hepatic lobule (portal-to-venular [central] bridging) or of the complex hepatic acinus (hepatic venule-to-venule bridging) support this suggestion. Furthermore, the appearance of the distal portion of confluent bridging necrosis is that of ischemic necrosis (see Fig. 15-26).

Confluent Necrosis: Submassive. A more severe injury leads not only to confluent necrosis of a portion of a lobule but also can result in the complete destruction of an entire lobule. If the necrosis affects the complex hepatic acinus, then a group of adjacent lobules is destroyed. The consequence of such severe injury is lobular or multilobular necrosis (Figs. 15-30 and 15-31).

This type of extensive confluent necrosis is referred to as submassive hepatic necrosis. The clinical counterpart of submassive necrosis is a severe hepatitis that may lead to fulminant hepatic failure and can be fatal. The fatal cases may run a fulminant or protracted course. The majority of fatal cases run a fulminant course, developing coma in a week or two of rapidly progressive illness. Submassive necrosis is the usual finding at autopsy of these patients who are over 40 years of age. However, about one in five of the fatal cases runs a protracted but progressively downhill course that terminates fatally after 2 to 5 months.

Confluent Necrosis: Massive. The most severe form of necrosis is the widespread and extensive destruction of the hepatic parenchyma, or massive hepatic necrosis. The clinical counterpart of massive necrosis is a rapidly progressive severe hepatitis that leads to a fulminant and fatal hepatic failure. Massive necrosis is the usual finding at autopsy of younger patients who die with fulminant hepatitis. Massive necrosis in acute viral hepatitis was first described by Rokitansky in 1842, who named it *acute*

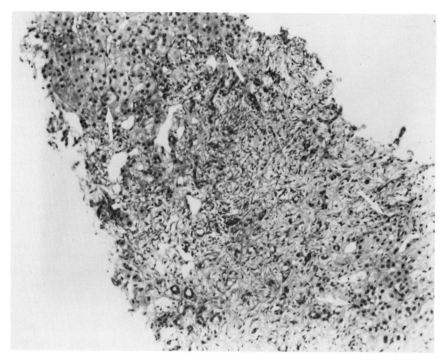

Fig. 15-30. Submassive necrosis—single lobule. In a more severe type of confluent necrosis, an entire lobule is destroyed. At the two margins of the illustration, the hepatic parenchyma of adjacent lobules is intact (*arrows*). Ductular proliferation and collapsed reticulum replaced the hepatocytes in the affected lobule. (H & E stain; original magnification × 94)

Fig. 15-31. Submassive necrosis—multiple lobules. Two enlarged portal tracts (*P*) and a hepatic venule (*H*) are shown. No recognizable hepatocytes remained in the affected lobules. In this case, the destruction involved a larger circulatory unit, which supplied a group of adjacent lobules, that is, a complete hepatic acinus. (H & E stain; original magnification × 90)

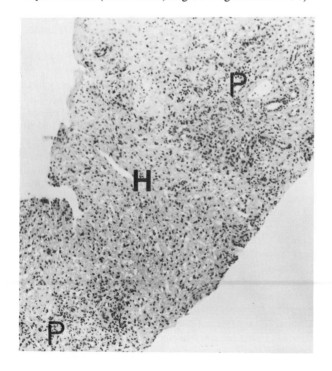

yellow atrophy.[840] The term is inaccurate because at autopsy these livers do not look yellow, but brownish, and are not atrophic, but necrotic. The most detailed morphologic study of the fatal form of viral hepatitis was reported by Lucké and Mallory.[602]

At autopsy, the liver capsule is usually finely wrinkled. As the liver is removed and placed on the table, it does not hold its shape because of its flabby consistency. Histologic examination shows that the lobular parenchyma is destroyed throughout the liver and that almost all the hepatocytes have disappeared. The reticulum framework is the only remnant of the hepatic lobule (Figs. 15-32 and 15-33). This reticulum framework is intact but in many areas it has collapsed because of the loss of supporting hepatocytes. The portal triads are preserved and the hepatic arteries, portal veins, and bile ducts in them show little change. The spaces between the sinusoids are filled with scavenger cells and necrotic debris. The sinusoids in some regions are congested with red and white blood cells. In widely scattered areas, single or small groups of lymphocytes may be seen (see Fig. 15-33). Here and there small groups of surviving hepatocytes can be found; these usually are close to portal tracts. The massive necrosis of the liver parenchyma is unexpectedly accompanied by little inflammatory reaction.

In the same portal tracts and periportal zones, moderate lymphocytic inflammatory exudate may accumulate, and this may be accompanied by ductular proliferation. Ductular structures may be seen scattered through the remnants of lobules, but these are not connected by portal bile ductules. These ductular structures are lined by he-

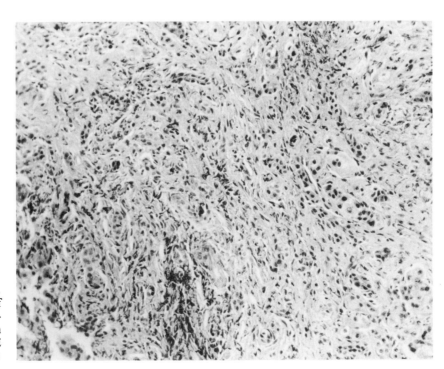

Fig. 15-32. Massive hepatic necrosis. A portion of widespread necrosis of hepatic parenchyma is shown. Inflammation is minimal or absent in areas of massive collapse. (H & E stain; original magnification × 200)

patocytes and not by ductular epithelium. Occasionally, hepatic endophlebitis may also be seen. When hypertrophy and hyperplasia of endothelial macrophages is marked, then these cells contain pigment having the characteristics of lipofuscin. On morphologic grounds, massive hepatic necrosis of viral hepatitis cannot be differentiated from that caused by drugs and anesthetic agents.

The absence of the usual mesenchymal changes that precede the development of fibrosis and cirrhosis argues in favor of restitutio integrum if complete recovery occurs. If death is delayed and a sufficient amount of parenchyma survives, then the liver cell plates can regenerate along preexisting reticulum fibers. Most young patients who survived submassive necrosis and did not use illicit drugs intravenously did not develop either chronic hepatitis or cirrhosis on follow-up liver biopsy. However, older patients who survived fulminant hepatitis and had confluent bridging necrosis did develop chronic active hepatitis and cirrhosis.[455]

PROGNOSIS

The prognosis of acute hepatitis can be based on features of the clinical illness, the serologic diagnosis, and the histopathology.

Fatal outcome is associated either with a fulminant hepatitis or hepatitis running a subacute course with progressive deterioration. Chronicity cannot be reliably predicted by the clinical features.

The *frequency* of a chronic course of typical viral hepatitis varies according to its serologic classification. Recovery is the rule after typical hepatitis A. Five percent to 10% of patients with acute hepatitis B develop chronic hepatitis. Only a minority of these patients have an aggressive lesion that leads to cirrhosis and disability. Up to 40% of patients developed chronic hepatitis after transfusion-associated non-A, non-B hepatitis. The vast majority of these patients have a mild disease.[80]

The *prognosis* based on histologic features is controversial. Bianchi[89] proposed the following five histologic observations in biopsies obtained during acute hepatitis that may indicate an increasing propensity for the development of chronic active hepatitis: (1) The demonstration of HBV antigenic components in liver tissue; (2) An unusually severe degree of predominantly lymphocytic portal and periportal inflammation, piecemeal necrosis, and formation of lymphoid follicles; (3) The predominance of plasma cells in the portal and lobular inflammation; (4) Confluent necrosis in zone 3 (portal-to-venular bridging necrosis) when associated with piecemeal necrosis; (5) Entrapped viable groups of hepatocytes within zones of confluent bridging necrosis. Peters, however, found that during typical acute viral hepatitis even a disproportionately severe degree of portal and periportal inflammation with piecemeal necrosis, enlargement of the portal tracts, follicular accumulation of lymphocytes, increased number of plasma cells, extension of collagen fibers from the portal tract into the periportal areas, and the development of portal-to-portal bridging are of no value in predicting the development of chronic active hepatitis.[758]

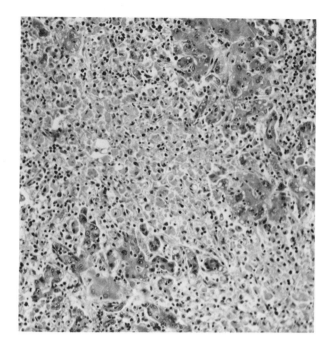

Fig. 15-33. Massive hepatic necrosis. One of the few small groups of surviving hepatocytes is shown. Some are vacuolated; others have two to four hyperchromatic nuclei, which suggests regenerative activity. This liver elsewhere contained only portal structures and necrotic parenchyma. Here, poorly stained cytoplasmic remnants, necrotic hepatocytes with pyknotic nuclei and proteinaceous coagulum, are filling the space between the surviving hepatocytes. "Scavenger" cells are seen in the necrotic debris where liver cell plates used to be. No significant inflammatory exudate can be seen, although, in widely scattered areas, small groups of lymphocytes accumulate. The morphologic picture is not characteristic of the etiology of massive hepatic necrosis. (H & E stain; original magnification × 100)

In general, one cannot predict with certainty the development of chronic active hepatitis following acute viral hepatitis on the basis of histologic examination of liver biopsy specimens obtained during the acute clinical illness. This is why one should not make a diagnosis of chronic active hepatitis from a liver biopsy obtained during the first 4 to 6 months of acute viral hepatitis. Nevertheless, there are certain histologic features of acute hepatitis that may increase the risk of chronic hepatitis. The combination of severe portal and periportal inflammation, piecemeal necrosis, enlargement of portal tracts, and portal-to-portal bridging are such features. Chronicity may be more likely in those cases of acute hepatitis in which the inflammatory exudate is predominantly lymphocytic and is associated with lymphoid follicle formation, particularly if a large number of plasma cells are also seen. However, patients who had follicle formation (see Fig. 15-13) or plasma cells (Fig. 15-34) during their acute hep-

atitis did not develop chronic active hepatitis. Such severe portal and periportal reaction has been seen in patients who abused illicit drugs intravenously. Birefringent foreign material was demonstrable in the portal tracts by polarized light in these patients.[758] This type of "hippy hepatitis" had been common in large American cities during the 1970s but is uncommon now. The extent to which chronicity in these patients is associated with morphologic damage and to repeated infections with other strains of hepatitis agents is not clear.

Another type of lesion that may increase the risk of chronic hepatitis is confluent bridging necrosis. The ominous prognosis of this lesion was first reported in 1970.[107] Nineteen percent of 51 patients with confluent bridging necrosis died, and 37% developed cirrhosis, in contrast to a group of 118 patients treated in the same institution for spotty necrotic viral hepatitis. None of the latter group died nor did they develop cirrhosis. The prior prognostic significance of the lesion was reemphasized by Ware and co-workers in 1975.[1054] However, these investigators changed their minds by 1978[1052] on the basis of their prospective studies of patients with severe hepatitis when compared with those without confluent bridging necrosis. The prognosis of this lesion may be related to the presence

Fig. 15-34. Mononuclear inflammatory exudate. At high magnification, many plasma cells can be seen among other mononuclear cells. The biopsy was taken from a 29-year-old man with self-limited acute hepatitis. (H & E stain; original magnification × 450)

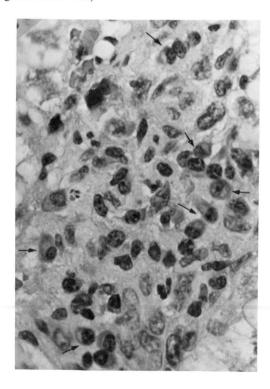

of certain specific features. When the etiology of confluent bridging necrosis is a drug, the outcome may be better than if the etiology is not known (*i.e.,* neither drug nor HBV).[659,949] Another feature may be the histologic characteristic of bridging necrosis. Bridging of adjacent portal tracts (portal-to-portal bridge) by itself appears to have little prognostic significance. Confluent hepatic necrosis that bridged portal tracts and hepatic venules or adjacent hepatic venules with each other, when associated with a considerable number of entrapped hepatocytes and piecemeal necrosis, may increase the risk of chronic active hepatitis. However, confluent necrosis in the absence of entrapped hepatocytes and piecemeal necrosis has no effect on the prognosis of the lesion. Furthermore, it was suggested that confluent necrosis at the periphery of the simple hepatic acinus (portal-to-venular bridging) is more likely to lead to chronicity than is confluent necrosis at the periphery of the complex hepatic acinus (hepatic venule-to-venule bridging).[89] In this respect, it is noteworthy that such confluent bridging necrosis had a different outcome depending on the severity of illness (fulminant hepatic failure) and age of patients.[455,498,758]

A problem in interpreting the development of chronic active hepatitis following an acute illness with biopsy evidence of piecemeal necrosis and confluent bridging necrosis is that it may be difficult to separate acute hepatitis from the initial acute exacerbation of chronic active hepatitis in the absence of clinical and laboratory evidence of preexisting liver disease.

Another problem is whether cirrhosis can develop as a result of acute hepatitis. It was claimed that submassive hepatic necrosis during acute hepatitis will lead to coarse nodular cirrhosis. It is likely that this lesion leads either to death or recovery or to chronic hepatitis but not to cirrhosis. Thus, cirrhosis develops not as a sequela of acute hepatitis and healing of submassive areas of collapse but through a stage of chronic active hepatitis. If acute hepatitis with confluent bridging necrosis progresses to cirrhosis directly, it is uncommon. Indeed, some suggest that it does not.[758] On the other hand, one of us observed a 16-year-old girl with severe acute hepatitis with submassive necrosis on biopsy who developed portal hypertension, bleeding duodenal varices, and cirrhosis in 8 months after the onset of illness. Others[1052] also described the development of severe hepatitis with bridging necrosis in 1 of 34 patients whose liver tests returned to normal. Hepatic architecture returns to normal after confluent bridging or submassive necrosis in young persons who survived fulminant hepatic failure.[498] However, both chronic hepatitis and cirrhosis developed following confluent bridging necrosis accompanying fulminant hepatic failure in older persons or in young patients who continue intravenous abuse of illicit drugs.[455]

One of the most important factors for survival in acute viral hepatitis is a prompt and appropriate regenerative response to hepatocellular necrosis. In fatal cases of submassive or massive necrosis, the most striking feature is the lack of appropriate hepatocellular regeneration. Lytic

necrosis is prominent but inflammatory response is poor (massive necrosis) or cellular inflammation is seen in and adjacent to portal tracts only. Peters pointed out that fatal outcome is probably due to inadequate hepatocellular regeneration in acute hepatitis.[758] The importance of hepatocellular regeneration was also emphasized by morphometric studies of liver biopsy specimens in patients with fulminant hepatic failure. Evidence of regeneration was associated with favorable prognosis whereas lack of regenerative activity was associated with mortality. However, evidence of impaired regeneration is not found invariably in fatal cases.[657]

CLINICAL FEATURES

Infection by the agents of viral hepatitis produces a spectrum of clinical features and laboratory manifestations. These range in severity from inapparent, asymptomatic infection to fulminant disease leading to death within a few days. The majority of patients with recognized viral hepatitis exhibit typical patterns of illness. Atypical patterns are seen in a small proportion. Although most patients with typical viral hepatitis recover completely, a small and variable number of patients with either typical or atypical clinical patterns develop self-limited or serious sequelae.

Typical Acute Viral Hepatitis

Typical viral hepatitis can be divided conveniently into inapparent, anicteric, and icteric hepatitis, headings that roughly correspond to the severity of infection. Such a classification should not be interpreted rigidly, because the category to which any patient may be assigned depends not only on the severity of the disease but also on the frequency of examination and astuteness of the examiner.

Inapparent Hepatitis

The term *inapparent hepatitis* refers to an infection that produces no symptoms. It can be recognized only by detecting one or more abnormalities in patients monitored because of exposure to the disease. The term *anicteric hepatitis* has often been used to describe inapparent hepatitis. It seems useful, however, to distinguish those persons with sufficient involvement to produce illness from those with no symptoms; in this discussion *anicteric hepatitis* is restricted to the former group.

Hepatitis, as a general rule, is milder in young than in older patients. Over 80% of very young children who transmitted hepatitis to family members remained asymptomatic.[75,382] In contrast, over three fourths of adult patients who acquired hepatitis A in epidemics were symptomatic.[75,569] As in hepatitis A, hepatitis B also tends to be more severe in older patients. This is well illustrated by the Yupik Eskimos in Alaska who have the highest prevalence of HBV infections in the United States. During a 5-year prospective study, the proportion of these Eskimos who developed symptomatic hepatitis B increased from 9.5% of infections in children under 4 years of age to one third of infected adults over 30 years of age.[654]

Inapparent infections were documented by abnormalities in liver chemistries and histopathologic examination during World War II. In addition, liver chemistries have been used to study institutional populations,[216,239,352,552,619] familial groups,[877] and recipients of blood and blood products.[186,391,908]

Such investigations have been considerably assisted by the availability since 1956 of a convenient assay for serum aminotransferase activity. Its superior sensitivity over serum bilirubin and flocculation procedures was demonstrated in an asymptomatic child with documented viremia.[551] It may be no more sensitive than measurement of sulfobromophthalein (BSP) retention, but the BSP test is inconvenient, sometimes dangerous, and affected by fever. The serum aminotransferase assay is readily available as an automated procedure and has displaced the flocculation and BSP tests. A fasting specimen is not needed.

Radioimmunoassay for detection of cholic acid conjugates in postprandial sera appears to be no more sensitive than aminotransferase determinations and is considerably more expensive.

The frequency of inapparent hepatitis detectable by aminotransferase abnormality in relation to symptomatic anicteric or icteric hepatitis has varied widely in published reports. Some investigators have found fewer than one inapparent infection for every clinically overt case.[877] Others have found 10 to 30 persons with aminotransferase elevation for every icteric patient.[216,391,908] The inapparent-to-overt case ratio seems to be high in transfusion-associated infections, in children, and also in groups or populations with a tendency to chronic infection with hepatitis B virus.

Aminotransferase elevations, particularly milder and transient elevations, do occur in a variety of infections. Aminotransferase abnormalities, therefore, must be interpreted with caution unless the observations are well controlled. This is particularly true when large numbers of "anicteric cases" are found in the presence of only a few icteric cases, especially among adults.

In some settings there is evidence that HAV infection is more likely to produce icteric disease than either HBV or non-A, non-B hepatitis virus infections.[807] However, anicteric infections are well known in hepatitis A and occasional infections without detectable hepatitis may be documented by serologic tests for hepatitis A markers. Hepatitis B often produces mild infections that are detected serologically in the absence of either clinical or laboratory features of hepatic dysfunction. It seems probable that non-A, non-B hepatitis viruses also produce at least occasional infections without detectable hepatitis. Serologic proof, however, is not yet available.

Symptomatic Acute Viral Hepatitis

When infection with the agents of hepatitis produces symptoms, the illness may be anicteric or icteric. The latter term does not imply hyperbilirubinemia alone; it should be restricted to patients with clinically detectable jaundice of the conjunctiva, mucous membranes, or skin.

The relative frequency of various symptoms in some 450 patients with icteric and anicteric illnesses in an epidemic setting was determined in the 1950s and 1960s by the Communicable Disease Center. The results are shown in Table 15-8.

Anicteric Viral Hepatitis. The symptoms of anicteric viral hepatitis are essentially the same as those of the icteric disease. The clinical course is qualitatively similar, but of lesser duration in most instances. The high percentage of bilirubinuria (see Table 15-8) in the patients recognized as having anicteric hepatitis during epidemic investigations is undoubtedly an exaggeration of its "true" frequency. In surveys in which this group of anicteric cases was identified, bilirubinuria itself was an important criterion leading to the diagnosis of what otherwise was an "undifferentiated" acute illness. In a study of hospitalized adults, a history of contact with a sick, nonjaundiced child was significantly more frequent among adults with icteric hepatitis than among controls.[532] This finding suggests that anicteric hepatitis in children is often not recognized as such. About one third of adult patients with symptomatic hepatitis A remain anicteric.[569]

Icteric Viral Hepatitis. Most persons with icteric viral hepatitis have symptoms, although jaundice is occasionally observed in an asymptomatic individual. The level of hyperbilirubinemia that produces clinically detectable jaundice varies with the alertness of the examiner, the conditions of the examination, and the natural pigmentation of the patient. In general, conjunctival jaundice becomes detectable at serum bilirubin concentrations of 2.0 mg to 4.0 mg/dl.[390]

Onset. The symptoms of HAV, HBV, HDV, and non-A, non-B infections are similar. One noteworthy exception may be in the mode of onset. When questioned, the patient with hepatitis A is sometimes able to recall having tired more easily during the several days prior to onset. It is uncommon, however, for this premonitory fatigability to have been sufficiently severe for him to have relinquished any of his usual activities. The transition from health to acute illness takes place within a period of 24 hours in about 60% of patients. It has been suggested that vigorous activity in the prodromal period may precipitate symptoms as well as worsen prognosis.[539] The onset of symptoms is usually more insidious in hepatitis B and non-A, non-B than in hepatitis A. The mode of onset, however, cannot be used to differentiate between the etiologic agents in the individual patient.

TABLE 15-8.   Symptoms Reported by 415 Icteric and 35 Anicteric Patients: Epidemics of Typical Hepatitis A: Hepatitis Unit, NCDC, 1955–1963

SYMPTOMS	ICTERIC PATIENTS			ANICTERIC PATIENTS		
	Number Questioned	Number Experiencing Symptom	% Experiencing Symptom	Number Questioned	Number Experiencing Symptom	% Experiencing Symptom
Brown urine	415	389	94	35	27	77
Lassitude	415	378	91	35	32	91
Loss of appetite	415	372	90	35	28	80
Nausea	415	360	87	35	21	60
Weakness	257	198	77			
Fever	415	316	76	35	21	60
Vomiting	415	295	71	35	19	54
Headache	415	294	70	35	19	54
Chilliness	381	250	66	31	10	32
Abdominal discomfort	415	271	65	35	29	83
Abdominal pain	257	168	65			
Whitish stools	415	217	52	31	8	26
Myalgia	158	82	52	35	13	37
Drowsiness	67	33	49	17	11	65
Irritability	92	40	43	22	9	41
Itching	395	164	42	31	8	26
Constipation	383	110	29			
Diarrhea	101	25	25			
Arthralgia	34	7	21			
Sore throat	138	27	20			
Nasal discharge	138	20	14	31	4	13
Cough	106	8	7			

In experimentally induced hepatitis B, a transient illness with mild symptoms was sometimes observed early in the incubation period. Headache, loss of appetite, nausea, and occasionally vomiting was found in eight of nine volunteers within 50 days after inoculation.[712] In seven of nine volunteers, the mild symptoms developed after 12 to 35 days. These complaints lasted one to several days and were accompanied by mild abnormalities of liver function tests. After the minor illness, the patient either was well or had one or more brief recurrences until the onset of the major phase of the illness 73 to 110 days after inoculation. The occurrence of minor illness is reminiscent of the premonitory symptoms and transient rash observed in measles, which is thought to be related to the initial viremia. The minor illness in hepatitis B is rarely observed clinically, presumably because patients are not under such careful scrutiny.

Acute Phase of Illness. Symptoms in hepatitis A usually last 2 to 7 days before the onset of jaundice. In one series in which children predominated, the median duration of the preicteric phase was 5 days.[665] However, the interval from first symptoms to jaundice exceeded 10 days in 14% of cases (Fig. 15-35). In a group of British servicemen, it exceeded 8 days in about 12% of patients.[1106]

The main features of the clinical disease are well known. The relative frequencies of complaints among icteric patients represented in Table 15-8 are similar to those reported by others.[589] Considering the varying circumstances under which such data have been collected, the uniformity is remarkable.

Flulike symptoms predominate in the early phase of the acute illness. Fever or feverishness occurs in two thirds to three fourths of patients with hepatitis A and is more prominent in the first few days of illness. The temperature is usually 37.5°C to 38.5°C (99.5°F to 101.3°F), but occasionally reaches 39°C to 40°C (102°F to 104°F). Chilliness accompanies the early phases in about half of those patients with fever, but shaking chills are rare. Headache is frequent but usually not severe.

Nasal discharge, sore throat, or cough is seen during the prodromata of 10% to 20% of patients and has been reported to occur more often among children.[406] These symptoms are mild and are not usually mentioned spontaneously by the patient. Bronchitis and pneumonitis attributable to the hepatitis agents have not been described.

Loss of appetite is one of the most frequent of all symptoms, as is true in other forms of parenchymal cell injury. Anorexia possibly is induced by a "toxin" produced by the impaired liver or by the failure of the hepatocyte to

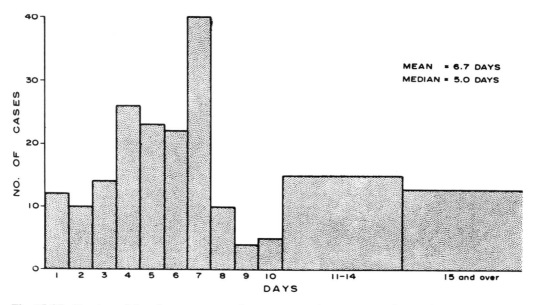

Fig. 15-35. Number of days between onset of symptoms and appearance of overt jaundice among 194 patients with hepatitis A, Detroit, 1937–1938. (Molner JG, Meyer KF: Am J Public Health 30:509, 1940)

"detoxify" an abnormal product. The patient not only lacks appetite but finds food repugnant when presented to him. Merely the smell of food often induces nausea. Greasy or "heavy" foods are tolerated poorly by most patients. Anorexia is usually more marked later in the day, so that it is common for a patient to eat well at breakfast but poorly at other meals. In addition to aversion to food, patients are also offended by cigarette smoke and other strong odors. Gustatory acuity, tested by measurements of detection and recognition thresholds, is impaired in early acute viral hepatitis and improves with clinical resolution.[418,938] A weight loss of 2 kg to 4 kg is typical.

Vomiting in typical viral hepatitis is neither severe nor protracted. Nausea, vomiting, and diarrhea are more common among children than among adults during acute hepatitis A.[575] When vomiting becomes progressively more severe for several days, it may indicate a more serious, atypical form. The mechanism of nausea and vomiting has not been defined. Acute superficial gastritis was found by gastroscopy during the preicteric and acute phases of the illness in seven of nine patients[520] and in three of six volunteers with experimentally induced hepatitis A.[410] The gastric mucosa was seen as normal in the latter group by gastroscopy before infection. Roentgenologic examination suggests antral gastritis and duodenitis.[410,776] Gastric acid secretory studies indicate that acid output is unaffected.[161]

Changes have been described in the intestinal mucosa,[42,175] but these are nonspecific, infrequent, and mild. A diffuse reduction in jejunal brush-border disaccharidase and alkaline phosphatase activities has been described in patients with acute viral hepatitis.[376] Disaccharide intol-

erance may contribute to the short-lived diarrhea seen in some patients. Steatorrhea is present in an occasional patient and is related to impaired bile flow leading to a reduction of bile salt concentrations within the intestinal lumen.[663] Constipation or diarrhea is seen in about one fourth of patients.

Abdominal discomfort or pain, particularly in the right upper quadrant, is common. Such discomfort may be increased by or noticed only on motions that produce jarring or "jogging" of the liver.

The urine becomes sufficiently brownish (dark) for the change in color to be noticed in 94% of patients with clinically detectable jaundice. This often occurs one to several days before jaundice of eyes or skin is noted. In 29 of 398 cases, bilirubinuria preceded jaundice by 7 to 14 days.[412] Similar observations were made in 1846 when Budd described the "colouring matter of bile" in the urine before "the skin becomes yellow."[130] Bilirubin concentration in the urine is initially too low to be detected by casual observation, but laboratory tests can correctly demonstrate its presence.

Patients are usually found to have become aware of their jaundice by having noticed that their "eyes turned yellow." This is due to icterus of their conjunctivae, and at onset it is not scleral. Jaundice can be detected in the mucous membrane before the skin becomes noticeably icteric. In some patients jaundice can be detected first by observing the tympanic membranes.

The onset of jaundice may be associated with progression, persistence, or rapid disappearance of all distressing symptoms. When symptoms persist or progress, malaise and gastrointestinal complaints are among those most likely to remain.

The duration of jaundice in hepatitis A in the majority of patients is exaggerated by reports in the literature. Most studies have been based largely on hospitalized cases, which ordinarily represent the more severe forms of the disease. In addition, in the past, concern with sequelae of hepatitis often prolonged hospitalization. Most children recover within 2 weeks and most adults within 4 to 6 weeks.[665] This is illustrated in Figure 15-36.

Gray or yellow stools are observed during the first week of jaundice by 20% to 40% of persons with clinical jaundice. The return of normal fecal color is one sign of recovery. In most patients this occurs during the second or third week of the illness.

Itching results in almost half of the patients;[589] it is usually transient and mild. A few patients, however, are severely distressed by pruritus and may have excoriations. Itching commonly occurs as jaundice begins to appear or as it begins to recede.

Transient rashes are noted by a small number of patients with acute viral hepatitis, regardless of the etiologic agent. The most common is a macular erythema; however, a papular rash is sometimes seen. Urticarial eruptions are uncommon;[292,412,1001] these usually develop during the preicteric phase of hepatitis B and may be associated with other extrahepatic manifestations, for example, arthritis. Deposition of immune complexes of HBsAg-anti-HBs in blood vessels of the skin appears to be responsible.[233] In some patients, cutaneous involvement may be the sole manifestation of circulating immune complexes in hepatitis B. Angioedema, Raynaud's phenomenon, digital vasospasm, and infarction of the fingertips are rare manifestations.[179]

An unusual skin lesion, termed *infantile papular acrodermatitis* or *Gianotti-Crosti syndrome,* has been described in infants and young children with hepatitis B. The disease, reported predominantly from Japan and Italy,[342,1008] is characterized by a nonpruritic papular erythematous eruption on the face and extremities that lasts for several weeks. Lymphadenopathy is common and the hepatitis is usually anicteric.

Rarely, erythema nodosum[412] and dermatomyositis[768] have been described in viral hepatitis.

Arthralgia, sometimes difficult to differentiate reliably from myalgia, occurs in 10% to 20% of cases of hepatitis A and B.[288,292] It probably occurs in a similar frequency in non-A, non-B hepatitis. Frank arthritis is observed in a small proportion (1% to 10%) of patients with hepatitis B[283,646,739] and rarely, if ever, in hepatitis A and non-A, non-B hepatitis. Arthritic manifestations usually precede the onset of systemic symptoms of hepatitis by many weeks to a few days and usually subside as jaundice develops.[14] Occasionally, the polyarthritis will not be accompanied or followed by jaundice; physicians should be aware of this possibility. The arthritis of hepatitis B resembles acute rheumatoid arthritis.[526] During the arthritic phase serum complement levels and complement com-

Fig. 15-36. Duration in days of overt jaundice among 194 patients with hepatitis A, Detroit, 1937–1938. Most of the patients (83.5%) were younger than 15 years of age. (Molner JG, Meyer KF: Am J Public Health 30:509, 1940)

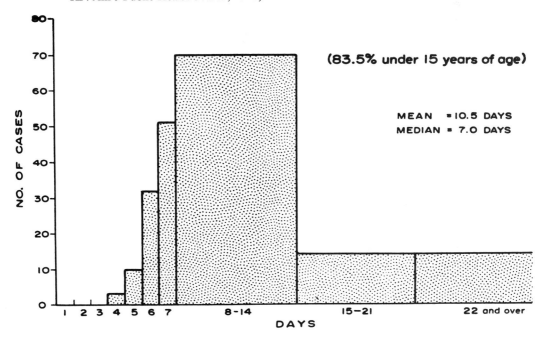

ponents are reduced,[22] synovial fluid complement levels are depressed,[739] and HBsAg and HBV-like particles may be seen in synovial tissue or fluid.[880] It is believed that the arthritis is related to the presence of circulating immune complexes of HBsAg and anti-HBs that fix complement and activate both the classic and alternate complement pathways.[1045]

An instance of severe myalgia associated with a lipid-storage myopathy has been described in hepatitis B.[750] The pathogenesis is unknown.

Irritability, querulousness, insomnia, and drowsiness may be early symptoms of impending hepatic coma; however, these symptoms may be seen early in about 10% of patients with typical viral hepatitis and do not necessarily denote the potentially serious form of the disease. Asterixis, however, is seen only in severe disease. Apathy may last into the icteric stage.

Depression is not uncommon. Any mature adult would be concerned if faced with the prospect of an illness lasting several weeks; in some patients, however, fear and depression are disproportionate to the situation. Such symptoms are self-limited and require no specific treatment, although depression may persist for weeks and extend into convalescence. Depression was profound in 2.8% of cases in one large series.[288] Frank delirium and psychosis are rare except as part of acute hepatic failure, but their occurrence has been described.[292,573] It is not clear whether or not these patients had psychologic disturbances prior to the onset of viral hepatitis.[38]

There are reported instances of meningitis,[292,876,1059] Guillain-Barré syndrome,[576,722,754,769,1102] myelitis,[133,1059] encephalitis,[120] cranial nerve involvement,[133,288,1024] and peripheral polyneuritis and very rarely mononeuritis.[580,623,960] The cerebrospinal fluid is usually normal but occasionally is icteric and contains lymphocytes.[843] The pathogenesis of these alterations is poorly understood. Although a role for immune complexes has been postulated, it is plausible that hepatitis viruses may occasionally be neurotropic, but other possible etiologies coincidentally present should be as carefully and thoroughly excluded as possible.[38]

Physical Examination. Almost all patients with acute viral hepatitis have tenderness over the liver. It may be elicited by palpation of the right upper quadrant of the abdomen or by fist percussion over the right hypochondrium. In most patients, only slight tenderness if found. Occasionally, however, tenderness is marked and may pose a problem in attempts to palpate the edge of the liver, for the patient is reluctant to breathe with his diaphragm. Even a cooperative patient will spontaneously use his thoracic muscles to "take a deep breath" if the physician's hand is pressing below his right rib cage. The greater the descent of the diaphragm, the more severe the discomfort. Unless the patient is explicitly shown how to breathe with his diaphragm and reassured about the discomfort that deep inspiration may cause, the examiner may not be able to palpate the enlarged liver.

In the average adult, the liver is commonly enlarged to 12 cm to 14 cm in the vertical axis. Its edge may be sharp or rounded but never irregular. Although the liver usually feels firmer than normal, it does not have the firm, rubbery consistency that it has in cirrhosis. Although hepatomegaly is common, it is rarely massive in viral hepatitis. Before the diagnosis of viral hepatitis is accepted in such cases, it should be confirmed by biopsy.

In some patients it is said that the liver is not palpable because it is "too soft." As a rule, inflammation and edema in the liver are sufficiently acute to make the capsule tense. These changes produce tenderness and an increase in firmness of the liver. Only massive necrosis leads to a small and soft liver.

The spleen is palpable in 5% to 15% of the patients, and the posterior cervical lymph nodes may be mildly enlarged. Generalized or marked lymphadenopathy is not a feature of viral hepatitis.

Spider angiomata may develop in patients during acute hepatitis; their frequency is generally underestimated because these lesions are not specifically sought. They disappear in convalescence[412] and do not indicate chronic liver disease. Palmar erythema also occurs without relation to severity. Transient gynecomastia has been described in convalescence.

A physical finding suggestive of the diagnosis of viral hepatitis in drug addicts is the occurrence of hematomas, ecchymoses, or scars along the course of veins. Most such lesions occur on the left forearm of a right-handed person. Occasional addicts, especially prisoners who would suffer punitive measures if their practice were discovered, use femoral or neck veins.

Abnormalities in Laboratory Tests. Despite shortened survival of erythrocytes labeled with chromium Cr 51 in a high percentage of patients with typical viral hepatitis,[139,175,258,500] the hematocrit and hemoglobin concentrations are usually within or close to normal limits.[398,431] A modest decline of 1.0 g to 2.0 g/dl, however, may be found on serial determinations and may be accompanied by reticulocytosis. In occasional cases, frank hemolytic anemia occurs.[392,514,801] Hemolysis is most frequently associated with glucose-6-phosphatase dehydrogenase (G-6-PD) deficiency,[147,157,162,857] which may not be detectable in the anemic patient due to destruction of most of the deficient red cells. Rapid hemolysis produces a sudden increase in jaundice, as does agglutination of erythrocytes in hepatic sinusoids among patients with SS or SC hemoglobin. Upper gastrointestinal tract bleeding is unusual in the absence of corticosteroid therapy. Occult gastrointestinal blood loss could not be detected by ^{51}Cr-labeled erythrocytes in five patients.[139]

Although a total white cell count within normal limits is usual in viral hepatitis, leukopenia was documented as early as 1923.[488] A decrease in leukocytes, although not necessarily to leukopenic levels, was found to develop with onset of fever in experimentally induced viral hepatitis.[407] The count returned to its usual level by the end of the first week of jaundice. The fall in white cell levels in the early stages of viral hepatitis is due to granulocytopenia, so that relative lymphocytosis results. Many of the lymphocytes appear large and atypical ("virucytes").[595] The relative lymphocytosis and atypical lymphocytes that are considered characteristic of infectious mononucleosis occur in viral hepatitis as well. The frequency of atypical lymphocytes, however, usually does not exceed 10%. T lymphocytes of peripheral blood may be reduced in number.[203,206,1068] Typical viral hepatitis should be diagnosed with caution when leukocytosis is present. The white cell count occasionally is slightly elevated in typical viral hepatitis, but levels over 12,000 are likely to denote a more severe, atypical form of hepatitis or an entirely different etiology of illness. Granulocyte function may be impaired.[865]

Rarely, agranulocytosis,[701] thrombocytopenia,[23] pancytopenia,[212,514] or aplastic anemia[574,587,937] develops during viral hepatitis. The latter is described under the heading Sequelae.

Examination of the urine occasionally shows a few red cells or mild proteinuria. The frequency of hematuria and proteinuria in the study of American soldiers in Korea is not typical of the usual urinary findings during viral hepatitis in this country.[175] The association of hepatitis B with membranous glomerulonephritis and the nephrotic syndrome is described under the heading Sequelae.

Bilirubinuria is often seen during the preicteric phase of viral hepatitis. Bilirubinuria during the early phase of hepatitis has been described at direct and total serum bilirubin concentrations much lower than those found later when bilirubin is no longer in the urine.[327] This disparity between serum and urine bilirubin levels is poorly understood. Percutaneous renal biopsy shows minor histopathologic changes in the kidney[175]; however, changes in renal histology have not been correlated with bilirubin excretion.

An alternative explanation for the disparate urine and serum bilirubin levels is based on a qualitative difference in the bilirubin metabolites presented to the kidneys during the early phase of viral hepatitis compared with those present later in the disease.[269] Bilirubin diglucuronide has a higher renal clearance than the monoglucuronide,[868] but serial determinations of these components have demonstrated no change in their relative proportions with convalescence.[91] The fraction of serum bilirubin represented by C-8 or C-12 monoconjugates, diconjugates, and total ester conjugates does not explain the disparity either.[872] On the other hand, in 15 patients with hepatitis, the urinary excretion of bilirubin was directly and linearly related to the estimated filtered load.[1041]

The mechanism of bilirubinuria during the early phase of hepatitis may be due to a rise of plasma concentration of bile salts, which increase the dialysability of direct bilirubin by reducing its binding to plasma proteins.[306] The dialysable serum bilirubin increased when its renal excretion was prevented by ureteral ligation.[307] An increase in the plasma bile salts during the early phase of hepatitis

but not during convalescence would explain bilirubinuria with low direct bilirubin plasma levels during the former and absence of bilirubinuria during the latter when plasma direct bilirubin levels are higher. The most likely explanation is that late in the course of acute hepatitis a large proportion of conjugated bilirubin is covalently bound to albumin and therefore cannot be excreted by the kidneys.[1060]

Renal failure is a rare complication of typical viral hepatitis.[1072] It is commonly seen in patients with severe disease, particularly fulminant hepatitis. The pathogenesis of renal failure in otherwise uncomplicated viral hepatitis is obscure.

The serum bilirubin determination is one of the most frequently used laboratory tests. It is also one of the most difficult to carry out reproducibly at levels within or near the normal range. In addition, the test should be carried out soon after venipuncture because bilirubin deteriorates quickly on storage. For both reasons, borderline or negative results may need to be interpreted with caution.

An increase is sometimes seen in the direct-reacting component of serum bilirubin when the total concentration is within normal limits. This abnormality may be found in some patients with anicteric hepatitis and in others during the preicteric phase of an icteric illness. With onset of the icteric phase, the serum concentration usually rises for 10 to 14 days in the average adult. The rate of decline from the peak level is more gradual and often requires 2 to 4 weeks during which the level decreases by slightly more than 50% per week.[850] In most patients the maximum concentration of bilirubin is less than 10 mg/dl,[970] although higher values up to 20 mg/dl may occasionally be observed in patients with typical viral hepatitis. It is unusual for the serum level to reach a high value or to remain constant for a prolonged period of time. If the serum bilirubin concentration reaches a plateau, the possibility of an atypical form of hepatitis should be considered. Particularly in older women, however, typical viral hepatitis may be associated with high levels of serum bilirubin that show little change for weeks. Liver biopsy reveals only the typical spotty necrosis of viral hepatitis, and liver function subsequently becomes normal.

Studies using prolonged infusions of BSP have been helpful in understanding the pathophysiology of viral hepatitis.[779] Hepatic storage (S) of the dye and the excretory function (Tm) are impaired early. Changes of both S and Tm correlated with the serum bilirubin concentration, but Tm alone correlated with alkaline phosphatase activity. During convalescence the storage function returned to normal before excretory function did. This could be interpreted as indicating a more rapid restoration of cellular function and vascular perfusion than biliary excretion.

The most popular laboratory test to detect parenchymal injury of the liver is assay of the serum aminotransferase activities.[163] This popularity is generally well founded on the experience accumulated thus far. The assays are sufficiently sensitive, are as specific an index as is generally needed, and are within the technical capability of every hospital laboratory.

Hyperaminotransferasemia may precede the onset of symptoms of hepatitis by 7 to 10 days,[352,619,877] but elevated levels may also coincide with symptoms.[99] The peak level is usually reached in the first week after symptoms begin. The height of the activity may have some statistical correlation with severity of the disease as judged by the presence or absence of clinical illness. There is, however, no necessary correlation, as is evident from finding levels as high as 2000 mU/ml in asymptomatic household contacts of patients with hepatitis A.[877] The height of aminotransferase activity should not, therefore, be regarded as prognostic. The peak aminotransferase level is highly variable but is usually in the range of 500 to 5000 mU/ml. The level of alanine aminotransferase is usually higher than that of aspartate aminotransferase throughout the illness.[850]

As the acute illness subsides, the serum aminotransferase activity usually returns to and remains within normal limits. The decrease in level may be more rapid than that of the serum bilirubin concentrations.[619] Aminotransferase levels decrease by about 75% per week.[850] This rate is not maintained and levels tend to plateau at slightly above normal limits in a small proportion of patients. However, in one fourth to one half of patients, after an initial fall, a secondary rise of the serum aminotransferase has been observed[621,681,818] and varies markedly in duration. The persistence of the serum aminotransferase elevation during the convalescent and postconvalescent phase is nevertheless compatible with complete clinical recovery.

Serum alkaline phosphatase activity may be normal in typical viral hepatitis patients, but in the majority of patients, it is slightly elevated.[318] Usually, it does not exceed twice the upper limit of normal for any of the usual assay procedures.[1106] Transient elevations are often seen concurrently with a transient decrease of the bile pigment content of the stool when sought during the early cholestatic phase of the typical disease. In association with intrahepatic cholestasis, marked elevations of serum alkaline phosphatase activities are observed. Elevated levels of the hepatic isoenzyme of alkaline phosphatase contribute to the increased serum levels. Although alkaline phosphatase elevations are the rule during the early acute phase of hepatitis, none of 625 soldiers studied had hypercholesterolemia.[318]

Nonetheless, elevated levels of serum cholesterol and serum triglycerides have been observed in some individuals with viral hepatitis.[667,997] In one patient studied sequentially before and during hepatitis B infection, the serum cholesterol level decreased in the preicteric period and then rose abruptly after the onset of jaundice.[864] Regardless of the level of serum cholesterol, the proportion of cholesterol esters is usually reduced presumably due to decreased levels of α-lipoproteins, impaired activation of lecithin-cholesterol-acyl-transferase, and lowered concentrations of this enzyme, which is produced in the liver.[923] The mechanisms leading to elevated serum triglyceride levels are poorly understood.

The electrophoretic separation of serum proteins shows no marked changes in most patients. In some cases of typical viral hepatitis and in prolonged or more severe hepatitis, decreased albumin and increased gamma globulin levels are seen. However, rates of albumin synthesis correlate poorly with serum albumin levels and with other liver chemistries.[638] The γ-globulin concentration may reach twice the normal limit without indicating a change to persistent or chronic disease. γ-Globulins over 3.5 g/dl, with albumin below 2.5 g/dl, however, indicate a disease other than typical viral hepatitis. The underlying disease should be confirmed by biopsy under such conditions.

The prothrombin time is usually within 5 seconds of the control value. Prolongation greater than 5 seconds may occasionally be seen in typical viral hepatitis but suggests the presence of a more severe variant.

Mild elevations of serum α-fetoprotein[506] and plasma carcinoembryonic antigen[664] levels are found in a variable proportion of patients with viral hepatitis. Interferon activity has not been detected in sera from hepatitis patients with any regularity.

Transient alterations in carbohydrate metabolism have been observed during viral hepatitis. During the postabsorptive state, hyperglycemia is more common than hypoglycemia.[1104] A "diabetic" glucose tolerance curve during viral hepatitis must be interpreted with caution. This abnormality is likely to be due to the poor carbohydrate intake rather than to diabetes mellitus. The insulin requirement may increase in a diabetic during acute hepatitis but returns to the previous level as the patient improves. Although it has been claimed that hepatitis runs a more stormy clinical course among diabetics, this finding may have been due to a greater frequency of hepatitis B among diabetics at the time of the study. The outcome of the disease in diabetics does not appear to be different from that in nondiabetic patients of similar age and state of general health.

Electrocardiographic changes during the acute phase of hepatitis include bradycardia, PR interval prolongation, and T-wave depression.[431,600] These changes returned to normal during convalescence.[862] One case of complete heart block has been reported.[535] Pericarditis and pericardial effusion have been described but rarely.[11] In typical hepatitis, however, important cardiac involvement is extremely unusual. An exudative pleural effusion with pleuritic chest pain may be a presenting feature of acute viral hepatitis in a few instances.[371,741] The effusion usually subsides with recovery from hepatitis.

In typical viral hepatitis, hepatic scintiscanning, performed with radiotracer colloids, for example, technetium-99m sulfur colloid, reveals a diffuse nonhomogeneous uptake pattern and mild hepatomegaly.[1040] The spleen appears to be enlarged in 20% to 30% of patients, and bone marrow uptake is increased in a similar proportion.[341] Infrequently, transient focal defects are noted within the liver.[1077] Their nature is poorly understood.

Elevated serum levels of iron,[1021] protein-bound iodide,[559] manganese,[1028] copper,[1028] and vitamin B_{12}[800] are commonly found in acute viral hepatitis. α_1-Antitrypsin and ceruloplasmin levels in serum are elevated during the acute phase, whereas haptoglobin, hemopexin, and prealbumin levels tend to be diminished.[510] Serum complement levels tend to be depressed during the acute phase of illness[537] owing to the presence of circulating complement-fixing immune complexes and decreased hepatic synthesis of complement components.

Diagnosis

The presence of typical viral hepatitis may be suspected on epidemiologic grounds if the patient's illness resembles and is temporally related to viral hepatitis in his associates. This association of the individual with others with recognized hepatitis also may permit identification of inapparent hepatitis that can be documented by laboratory and specific serologic tests. The search for a probable source of infection and time of exposure in groups of patients with hepatitis may help in the identification of the responsible etiologic agent. In the sporadic case of typical viral hepatitis, clinical and epidemiologic features are less helpful in etiologic differentiation; specific serologic tests are required. The diagnosis of typical viral hepatitis is usually established by recognition of the characteristic clinical features, laboratory tests, and course of the illness during a period of observation. No single clinical finding or test of hepatic function is absolutely diagnostic because they may be found in other disorders. The diagnosis is based on a constellation of clinical and laboratory features and a characteristic temporal pattern of disease evolution and subsidence.

In patients with atypical forms of viral hepatitis, diagnosis may be more difficult and may require, when possible, histologic examination of liver tissue. Diagnostic problems of atypical hepatitis are described below. In typical viral hepatitis, examination of liver tissue obtained by percutaneous needle biopsy is usually unnecessary. It is indicated only when the diagnosis remains uncertain or the presence of another liver disorder seems most likely. As described in the section on pathology of viral hepatitis, liver biopsy reveals a characteristic set of lesions that usually permits a definite diagnosis but may be indistinguishable from some forms of drug-induced hepatitis.

Serologic diagnosis of hepatitis A, B, D, and by exclusion, of non-A, non-B viral hepatitis is described in the section on Etiology. Other viral disorders affecting the liver are distinguished serologically in those few instances in which clinical differentiation is not possible. As mentioned previously, drug-induced hepatitis may closely resemble viral hepatitis. Hence a complete drug history is essential. Alcoholic liver disease, that is, alcoholic hepatitis, also may be considered in the differential diagnosis. The presence of signs of alcoholism, only moderate elevation of serum aminotransferases, particularly with aspartate aminotransferase higher than alanine aminotransferase, and of a distinctive lesion on liver biopsy, consisting of perivenular (zone 3) location of the lesion, polymorphonuclear leukocytic inflammation, megamitochondria, ballooning, "alcoholic hyaline," lack of regeneration of hepatocytes, and fatty infiltration, favors alcohol-induced disease. Rare patients with acute heart failure, prolonged hypotension, or shock may be misdiagnosed as having viral hepatitis. In most such patients, there are distinctive clinical features suggesting the presence of an underlying nonhepatic disorder, and the course of the "hepatitis" is abbreviated. The potential confusion of viral hepatitis with extrahepatic biliary tract obstruction is described below under the heading of Cholestatic Viral Hepatitis.

Atypical Viral Hepatitis

Atypical viral hepatitis can be divided into two major groups: (1) variants of a self-limited, benign disease and (2) the development of a serious, life-threatening, acute illness.

Benign Variants of Viral Hepatitis

The term *cholestatic viral hepatitis* is commonly used in two ways: (1) to refer to a clinical picture in which the course of the disease and the laboratory findings simulate those associated with mechanical obstruction of the bile ducts and (2) to describe a characteristic set of histopathologic findings in the liver. The latter findings are frequently but not necessarily associated with a clinical and laboratory picture suggestive of mechanical obstruction. It was initially assumed that the clinical picture and pathologic changes in the liver were *pari passu* because liver biopsy was carried out only in clinically atypical cases. Biopsy on a more routine basis in two epidemics, however, revealed that the histopathologic findings of cholestasis could be associated with clinically typical viral hepatitis.[243,244] The present discussion refers to the clinically atypical variant, which is exceedingly rare.

In cholestatic viral hepatitis, the clinical course is prolonged with more marked and persistent jaundice. Itching is often prominent and may be persistent. The serum bilirubin concentration is usually 10 mg to 20 mg/dl and may be higher; it rarely exceeds 30 mg/dl. The peak bilirubin level may be reached in the eighth week of illness or later. The serum aminotransferase levels are often in the same range as in typical viral hepatitis but decline despite the persistence of jaundice. The serum alkaline phosphatase level is almost invariably elevated, and at times the increase is marked. Serum cholesterol levels may be increased. Prolongation of the prothrombin time reflects impaired transport of bile salts and is responsive to administration of parenteral vitamin K.

In cholestatic viral hepatitis, jaundice may last from 2 to 8 months. During this period the patient usually feels well despite jaundice and pruritus and often regains the weight lost during the early phase of the illness.

Despite frequent reference to cholestatic viral hepatitis in the literature, the disorder is rare and infrequently simulates extrahepatic obstruction of the biliary tree. Furthermore ultrasonographic examination of the bile duct fails to reveal ductal dilatation in patients with cholestatic viral hepatitis. In those instances in which ultrasonographic studies are technically unsuccessful, radiologic visualization of the biliary tract by percutaneous transhepatic needle cholangiography or endoscopic retrograde cholangiography may exclude the presence of extrahepatic, mechanical obstruction.

The mechanism of transient intrahepatic cholestasis in typical viral hepatitis and prolonged cholestasis in cholestatic viral hepatitis is poorly defined. Specific serologic diagnosis of cholestatic viral hepatitis as hepatitis A has been reported,[353] but the roles of HBV, HDV, and the non-A, non-B agents remain to be established.

Life-Threatening Variants of Viral Hepatitis

Fulminant viral hepatitis is the term applied to the rare clinical picture in which acute viral hepatitis results in hepatic failure, manifested by encephalopathy and, often, death. Massive or submassive hepatic necrosis is the underlying lesion. The symptoms of fulminant hepatitis may be present from the beginning or may develop during the course of what appears to be typical viral hepatitis. Rarely, death occurs before jaundice becomes detectable. Among 196 cases collected during World War II, over half of the fatal cases terminated within 10 days of onset of symptoms, and three fourths of the patients died within 3 weeks.[602]

An altered state of consciousness within the first few days must be distinguished from the drowsiness and depression often seen in typical viral hepatitis. The danger signals that may indicate the development of fulminant hepatitis are hyperexcitability, irritability, insomnia, somnolence, impaired mentation, and severe vomiting. In fulminant hepatitis, these are followed by obtundation, asterixis, confusion, and coma. Convulsions (most often seen in children) may also occur. The most ominous signs heralding massive hepatic necrosis are the rapid decrease in size of a previously enlarged liver, the rapid shrinking of a normal-sized liver, and progressive prolongation of prothrombin time despite vitamin K administration. In rare instances, the one-stage prothrombin time remains within 5 seconds of control values until just before death. More commonly, the prothrombin time is prolonged because of the deficiency of clotting factors II, V, VII, and X.[315]

A shortened half-life of fibrinogen,[1029] increased serum fibrin degradation products,[421] and thrombocytopenia[802] suggest the presence of low-grade or moderately severe disseminated intravascular coagulation in many patients. Acquired dysfibrinogenemia due to defective fibrin polymerization[564] and an acquired abnormality of platelet function[853] have been described.

In view of these multiple hemostatic abnormalities it is not surprising that bleeding is a common complication. Gastrointestinal bleeding, usually from erosions in the esophagus, stomach, or duodenum, is noted in approximately 50% of patients.[610] Bleeding from the nasopharynx, respiratory tract, or into the retroperitoneal space is less common. Intracerebral hemorrhage is unusual.

Fever develops in most patients with fulminant viral hepatitis in the early phase of the illness. In late stages, hypothermia may be seen. Hypothermia may indicate the presence of hypoglycemia, the progression of neurologic involvement, or the imminence of death.

Cerebral edema is present in many cases although papilledema is infrequently detected.[326,1053] Tentorial herniation and brain stem compression may be evident. Central respiratory failure, cardiac arrest, hypothermia, and vasomotor depression, the latter leading to hypotension due to lowered peripheral resistance, appear to be closely associated with cerebral edema.[326] Hyperventilation leading to respiratory alkalosis is also believed to be mediated by involvement of the central nervous system. Terminal lactic acidosis may be responsible for the hyperventilation seen late in the course of fulminant hepatitis.

In addition to centrally mediated apnea and respiratory failure, hypoxemia is commonly observed regardless of ventilatory status and appears to reflect the development of intrapulmonary shunts.[1015] Bronchopneumonia, aspiration, fluid overload, and atelectasis also may contribute to hypoxemia. Clinical evidence of the adult respiratory distress syndrome is present in about a third of patients.[1014]

Hyponatremia, edema, and ascites reflect sodium and water overload. Oliguria and azotemia[1071] are common and may indicate the development of either the hepatorenal syndrome or acute tubular necrosis.

In 10% to 20% of patients with fulminant viral hepatitis, the course is further complicated by bacterial infection. Pneumonia, urinary tract infection, and septicemia related to intravenous lines and cutdown sites are characteristic.

Most patients with fulminant viral hepatitis are deeply jaundiced; serum bilirubin levels greater than 40 mg/dl may be seen. The serum aminotransferase levels may be indistinguishable from those observed in typical viral hepatitis. In many instances nearly normal levels may be found a few days before death. Leukocytosis with neutrophilia is a usual finding. This contrasts to the normal or low level of leukocytes, with relative lymphocytosis, in typical viral hepatitis. Hypoglycemia is present in about 5% of patients. Elevated serum levels of α-fetoprotein have been described in a large proportion of patients.[92]

Clinical staging of the encephalopathy in fulminant viral hepatitis indicates that the maximal degree of encephalopathy can be correlated with survival rate. Staging is not particularly useful in determining outcome prospectively because it is not possible to predict the maximal degree of encephalopathy from a single observation point.

The pathogenesis of fulminant viral hepatitis is poorly understood. Host factors appear to be potential determinants of the massive destruction of liver cells, but the precise mechanisms, which are presumed to be immunologically mediated, have not yet been elucidated. Both enhanced and impaired immune responses have been suggested. The mechanisms of encephalopathy and cerebral edema in fulminant viral hepatitis are ill defined. In a group of 32 fatal cases,[1053] 50% died with cerebral edema. Most of those who died with cerebral edema were under 30 years of age.

Although each of the etiologic agents of viral hepatitis has been associated with fulminant disease, hepatitis B and non-A, non-B are the predominant infections. Patients who were seen with fulminant hepatitis in Italy, France, and England had a significantly higher prevalence of serologic evidence of HDV infection than did those whose clinical course was benign. In about 40% of the patients who had markers for both HDV and HBV infections, fulminant hepatitis appeared to have been caused by HDV superinfection.[932] In the United States one third of 71 patients with fulminant hepatitis B also had evidence of HDV infection. Of these, 80% had evidence of simultaneous infection of HBV and HDV and 20% had evidence of HDV superimposed on chronic HBV infection.[357] On the other hand, in a population in which the HBsAg carrier rate is high, HDV superinfection was a much more common cause of fatal acute hepatitis.[384]

The diagnosis of fulminant viral hepatitis is established by recognition of severe alterations of central nervous system function in the patient with clinical and laboratory features of viral hepatitis. The differential diagnosis includes massive hepatic necrosis due to drugs, hepatotoxic chemicals, and mushrooms, extensive centrilobular hepatic necrosis due to hypoperfusion syndromes, and, less frequently, severe toxemia of pregnancy, Wilson's disease, and chronic active hepatitis in relapse. Acute hepatic failure due to Reye's syndrome, acute fatty liver of pregnancy, and fatty liver associated with intravenous tetracycline administration may be considered. In these three disorders, the major histologic alteration in the liver is fatty infiltration, although minor degrees of hepatocyte necrosis also may be present.

Prognostic factors influencing survival rates are only partially defined. Mortality is highly correlated with age, with survival occurring in an important number of young patients and being uncommon in individuals over age 45.[146] Survival rates are poorest in non-A, non-B fulminant hepatitis, intermediate in hepatitis B, and best in hepatitis A–associated disease.[7,636,804] The case-fatality rate of hepatitis A among patients hospitalized for this disease is about 0.14%.[377] Available data suggest that three other variables affect survival rate: (1) the extent of hepatic necrosis, (2) the development of complications that may be fatal, and (3) the induction and perpetuation of hepatic regeneration sufficient to restore hepatic function. In survivors, total hepatic architectural restitution and normal hepatic function are anticipated.[498]

Confluent (bridging) hepatic necrosis is the term used to designate an unusual variant of viral hepatitis in which specific histopathologic lesions may be found (see section on pathology). It is believed that confluent necrosis in viral hepatitis begins as such because transition from non-confluent necrosis in viral hepatitis to confluent necrosis has not been documented.[107] Confluent necrosis, on the other hand, can progress to fatal massive hepatic necrosis.[1056] Submassive hepatic necrosis is a synonymous histopathologic diagnosis, and although "subacute" hepatitis has been used in the past to describe the clinical disorder, it is no longer an acceptable term because it has chronologic and prognostic implications that do not necessarily apply to this condition. There are no clinical or epidemiologic features that predict the outcome of this form of hepatitis.[1056]

Confluent hepatic necrosis appears to be more common in hepatitis B[107] than in hepatitis A or non-A, non-B viral hepatitis. The frequency of this variant is poorly defined, but an incidence of 1% to 4% seems likely based on selected series in which liver biopsy was performed. Confluent hepatic necrosis developed more frequently in women than in men. Although women over 40 years of age were predominantly affected in one large study,[107] age was not a predictor of frequency or severity in another large series.[1054] In the former series,[107] complicating but unrelated disorders were present in about half of the affected patients.

The clinical course of confluent hepatic necrosis varies. Many patients subsequently found to have confluent hepatic necrosis begin their illness with symptoms and findings characteristic of typical viral hepatitis. The disease is often insidious in onset. In about 30% of cases, the prodrome is longer than expected, exceeding 2 weeks.[107] The frequency of anorexia, malaise, myalgia, arthralgia, pruritus, and fever is nearly identical to that found in typical hepatitis. In a small proportion of patients, the illness becomes progressively more debilitating during the preicteric phase. In these patients, in contrast to those with typical viral hepatitis, fever lasts longer than a few days, and anorexia, nausea, and vomiting are more persistent. Edema or ascites develops in 5% to 25% of patients,[107] and, occasionally, the first overt manifestation is unexplained ascites. Enlargement of the spleen is thought to be more frequent than in typical viral hepatitis.

Later phases of confluent hepatic necrosis may simulate typical viral hepatitis, but with a more protracted, stormy course. Hepatic encephalopathy may be observed in 15% to 20% of hospitalized patients. These clinical features, indicative of a more serious disease, may be the only diagnostic characteristics that are recognizable. In most patients, however, this variant is clinically indistinguishable from typical viral hepatitis.

No laboratory findings are diagnostic. Atypical patterns of laboratory abnormalities may raise the suspicion of the presence of confluent necrosis. The serum aminotransferase levels fluctuate during the disease and may persist at high levels rather than demonstrate a discrete peak. The alkaline phosphatase may be normal or markedly elevated. Prolongation of the prothrombin time may be seen, and the serum albumin concentration is usually lowered. In about 20% of patients leukocytosis is present. Conversely, leukocytosis during acute hepatitis, particularly when associated with a shift to the left, is almost always associated with confluent necrosis. Confluent hepatic necrosis has been recognized in anicteric patients although jaundice is a characteristic feature in most reported cases. Serum bilirubin levels are variably elevated with levels above 30 mg/dl in about 25% of cases.[107] In about 50% of patients, peak serum bilirubin elevations are reached more than 2 weeks after the initial elevation. In contrast to typical hepatitis, in which the serum bilirubin concentrations either rise or decline, in these cases, a prolonged plateau of serum bilirubin is common.[107]

As indicated previously, there is no unequivocal clinical or laboratory feature, nor is there a sufficiently typical combination of these abnormalities that would confirm the diagnosis of confluent hepatic necrosis. The only definitively diagnostic procedure is a liver biopsy.

Most patients with confluent hepatic necrosis, regardless of whether or not the variant is recognized, recover completely. Two percent to 20% may develop hepatic failure identical to that seen in fulminant viral hepatitis with poor survival rates.[107,455,1054] About 15% to 30% of patients develop clinical and biochemical features of chronic active hepatitis,[107,1054] which has the potential for progression to cirrhosis but does not invariably do so.

SEQUELAE

Each etiologic form of viral hepatitis is associated with sequelae; differences in their nature and incidence have been identified. Estimates of the frequency of the various sequelae have varied widely, depending on the responsible etiologic agent, the patient population studied, and diagnostic criteria used for classification. Extensive experience permits tabulation of the estimated frequencies of outcomes and sequelae shown in Table 15-9. Frequencies for outcomes and sequelae in hepatitis D and epidemic non-A, non-B viral hepatitis are less well defined.

In the patient with hepatitis B, hepatitis D, or blood-borne non-A, non-B viral hepatitis, prolonged or persistent infection appears to be intimately linked with the development of certain sequelae. In contrast, evidence of viral persistence is not available in the patient with sequelae following hepatitis A.

Benign Sequelae

Prolonged viral hepatitis (chronic lobular hepatitis) refers to rare cases of viral hepatitis that are atypically lengthy; laboratory abnormalities persist and symptoms and physical findings continue. The point in the clinical course at which "typical" becomes "prolonged" is entirely arbitrary, however. The duration of acute hepatitis is known to vary with age; the illness lasts longer in adults than in children. The duration of illness probably varies also with the strain of virus, although this opinion is difficult to document. Four months is the time limit beyond which adults would be considered to have a prolonged course.

In prolonged viral hepatitis, the initial symptoms and findings are identical with those of typical viral hepatitis but the disease may be evident for 12 months or longer. The symptoms are those seen in the latter part of typical viral hepatitis. Appetite is adequate; malaise is variable, but usually mild or absent. Lassitude and fatigability may be pronounced. Jaundice is usually not deep. The liver may remain palpable, but it usually returns to normal size after the first weeks of illness. The laboratory abnormalities may show some fluctuation, but the trend in general is toward slow improvement. Elevation of serum bilirubin and serum aminotransferase levels may punctuate the course. In some patients, antinuclear, antimitochondrial, or anti–smooth muscle antibodies are present in sera.[1073] Liver biopsy shows scattered areas of mononuclear cell infiltrate, spotty necrosis, and increased cellularity of portal areas, indistinguishable from the lesion of typical viral hepatitis.[1073] The difference lies in the fact that the lesion is "chronic" in patients with prolonged hepatitis.

Prolonged hepatitis appears to represent only a lengthening of the acute illness and does not constitute a separate entity. This attitude can be justified by available data. The length of illness in the large group of patients studied by Barker and associates conforms not to a bimodal curve but rather to a skewed unimodal distribution.[61] Mathematical analysis suggests that an illness lasting 4 months or longer would be expected in 3% to 5% of cases.[309] This self-limited variant of viral hepatitis must be differentiated from lengthier forms. Cirrhosis does not develop in affected patients.

TABLE 15-9. Estimated Frequency of Outcomes or Sequelae of Hepatitis A, Hepatitis B, and Blood-borne Non-A, Non-B Hepatitis in Adults

OUTCOMES OR SEQUELAE	ESTIMATED FREQUENCY (%)		
	Hepatitis A	Hepatitis B	Non-A, Non-B Hepatitis (Blood-borne)
Complete recovery	95–99	80–85	50–90
Fulminant hepatitis	<1	1	<1
Confluent hepatic necrosis	<1	1–4	? 1–5
Carrier state	0	5–10	? 10–20
Chronic hepatitis	0	5–10	10–50
Cirrhosis	0	<1	1–5
Primary hepatocellular carcinoma	0	<1	? <1
Aplastic anemia	<1	<1	<1
Glomerulonephritis	0	<1	?
Necrotizing vasculitis	0	<1	?

Relapsing hepatitis refers to an illness in which the patient who has apparently had complete recovery following an acute episode of viral hepatitis manifests a recurrence of the original symptoms and findings on one or more occasions, usually within 6 months of the original illness. Recurrences are, however, usually milder than the original attack. The rises of bilirubin and serum aminotransferase levels occasionally exceed the values found during the first episode. The relapse does not denote a different type of disease but probably means incomplete recovery from the original illness, despite an asymptomatic interval. In patients with suspected relapsing hepatitis A, sharp rises in aminotransferase levels have occurred 7 to 12 weeks after the onset of the original illness and persistently positive tests for IgM anti-HAV have been described.[178,372] In some patients a second and, rarely, a third relapse occurs in the succeeding weeks or months.

A small number of patients have been described in whom remissions lasting several months to as long as 5 years have been followed by severe clinical relapses.[1073] In these relapses, serum aminotransferase and bilirubin levels may exceed the values noted in the initial illness. Autoantibodies were present in sera, and serum globulin levels may be elevated. Liver biopsy in these rare patients reveals the lesion of chronic lobular hepatitis (see section on Prolonged Hepatitis). Complete serologic studies have not been undertaken in such individuals. Thus, the possibility that multiple separate infections are responsible for this unusual occurrence cannot be excluded.

Relapses sometimes are attributed to too early ambulation or excessive physical activity, but adequate documentation of a relationship is not available. At times they have been blamed on consumption of alcoholic beverages. An increased frequency of relapse has also been described in patients whose acute illness was treated with corticosteroids.[94,262,263]

The incidence of relapse has varied in different groups of patients. Depending on the frequency of observations, methods of examination, and criteria used to estimate the relapse, the incidence was 1.5% to 18%.[402,406,431] In general, clinical relapse occurs only in a small proportion of cases, but in some groups the relapse rate may be high. For example, in one group of 350 patients with a mean duration of illness of 56 days, the relapse rate was 13.4%.[557] These patients, like those with prolonged viral hepatitis, recover completely and cirrhosis is not seen.

In recent years, the frequency of relapsing hepatitis appears to be diminishing because serologic identification of the hepatitis viruses has become widely available.

Relapsing hepatitis must be differentiated from a second attack caused by a different agent. Infection by two agents may be acquired simultaneously, one with a shorter and the other with a longer incubation period, or a second infection can be acquired after the recovery from the first one.[1065] For example, a patient recovering from hepatitis B may have an "apparent relapse" due to HDV infection.[826] Such a patient will be positive for HBsAg and anti-HD, but the anti-HBc will be the IgG and not the IgM type, and the anti-HD will be the IgM type. The longer the interval between the two icteric illnesses, the more likely it is that the second illness is not a relapse but a separate infection.

Post-hepatitis unconjugated hyperbilirubinemia was found in a few patients who had apparently recovered from acute viral hepatitis and who had no symptoms or other biochemical abnormalities related to the disease.[1036] Most observations of this sequel of hepatitis were made in the era before measurement of serum aminotransferases was available. Unconjugated hyperbilirubinemia following viral hepatitis has been associated with the presence of chronic persistent hepatitis[282] (*see below*) that may be recognized principally by increased levels of serum aminotransferases. Whether or not unconjugated hyperbilirubinemia following viral hepatitis may be found in the absence of chronic persistent hepatitis remains uncertain. It seems probable that preexisting and coincidental Gilbert's syndrome, unrecognized prior to the episode of hepatitis, may be responsible for some instances of unconjugated hyperbilirubinemia identified after an attack of viral hepatitis.

Chronic persistent hepatitis is a term introduced by a group of pathologists organized in 1968 under auspices of the European Association for the Study of the Liver.[204] They offered criteria by which chronic hepatitis not actively progressing to serious disease could be differentiated from that showing "aggressive" features. Although *chronic* is redundant vis-a-vis *persistent,* their term has become the one most widely used for chronic infection having a benign course and good prognosis.

Chronic persistent hepatitis is believed to follow hepatitis B[721,812] and blood-borne non-A, non-B viral hepatitis[523,536] more frequently than hepatitis A or epidemic non-A, non-B hepatitis. It may also be a sequel of HDV superinfection of HBV carriers. In most affected patients an initial episode of typical viral hepatitis is recognized but does not resolve in the usual time frame. In some patients there is no history of a prior attack, and it is presumed that the initial episode was inapparent hepatitis. Serologic evidence of hepatitis B infection, HBsAg and anti-HBc, is present in many such patients and indicates a relationship to preceding inapparent hepatitis B and continuing viral infection. A similar sequence seems likely in blood-borne non-A, non-B viral hepatitis and hepatitis D, but documentation of chronic viral infection following hepatitis A is not available.

Most patients with chronic persistent hepatitis are asymptomatic[1064] and appear healthy. Mild fatigue and a sense of malaise are noted in a small number of individuals. Episodes of acute illness are infrequent, mild hepatomegaly may be the only physical finding, and the spleen is not usually enlarged. Ascites and edema are absent. Serum bilirubin levels are elevated in less than 10% of cases. Maximum bilirubin levels do not exceed 4 mg to 5 mg/dl, and unconjugated bilirubin comprises 70% or more of the total serum bilirubin.[282] Evidence of hemolysis is not present. Impaired bilirubin UDP-glucuronyl-transferase activity in liver biopsy specimens of affected patients has been described, but family studies do not support the notion that coexistence of Gilbert's syndrome is responsible.[282]

The most characteristic laboratory feature of chronic persistent hepatitis is fluctuating, low-level serum aminotransferase abnormalities. Peak levels infrequently exceed 400 mU/ml. Serum albumin levels, the prothrombin time, and serum alkaline phosphatase are typically within normal limits. Circulating immunoglobin levels are usually normal.

The persistence of laboratory abnormalities for long periods of time without progression to more severe hepatic dysfunction in an asymptomatic or only mildly symptomatic individual with or without serologic or historic evidence of a preceding bout of hepatitis should suggest the diagnosis. The patient suspected to have chronic persistent hepatitis may be recognized (1) as a result of routine follow-up after apparent clinical recovery from acute disease; (2) because of laboratory tests obtained for other reasons; (3) by referral as a result of blood bank screening of donors; or (4) through diagnostic evaluation of symptoms. The diagnosis is confirmed by follow-up examinations that show no evidence of disease progression and liver biopsy that reveals lymphocytic inflammatory infiltration of the portal tracts with little or no piecemeal necrosis, fibrosis, or architectural distortion. Diagnostic accuracy of liver biopsy increases with the length of follow-up and passage of time. Progression to chronic active hepatitis and the development of cirrhosis do not appear to be sequelae of bona fide chronic persistent hepatitis. Instances of progression suggest misdiagnosis of chronic active hepatitis in remission as chronic persistent hepatitis or superinfection by hepatitis D, converting HBsAg-positive chronic persistent hepatitis to more severe disease.

The abnormalities in chronic persistent hepatitis are often viewed with concern by the physician, who may restrict activity or even enforce bed rest for a person who feels well. The caution that has been exercised concerning serum aminotransferase abnormalities is understandable in view of emphasis on necrosis as the major or only mechanism for elevation of serum activity. Nonetheless, restriction of activity is not warranted because the course is benign. Although resolution may be delayed for many years, eventual recovery is likely without therapeutic intervention.

Carrier State Following Viral Hepatitis

There is no evidence that hepatitis A leads to persistent infection or to the development of a prolonged carrier state. Neither viremic nor fecal carriers of HAV have been identified.

A large body of information indicates that, in 5% to 10% of patients with hepatitis B, serum will remain HBsAg positive for a protracted period after acute infection. Although this criterion is arbitrary, persistence of HBsAg for more than six months after the acute illness is generally accepted as indicating the development of the HBsAg carrier state. However, in a number of individuals who are HBsAg positive at this time, HBsAg disappears after extended follow-up over a period of many months.[812] Because most HBsAg carriers are unable to recall an episode of acute hepatitis in the past, inapparent infections appear to be largely responsible for the initiating hepatitis B infections. In the asymptomatic individual identified as a probable HBsAg carrier, follow-up studies are necessary because a single positive test may indicate early infection that will be followed by typical viral hepatitis. Persistent HBsAg positivity for a period of six or more months in the absence of clinical or laboratory features of acute infection is characteristically found in the carrier state. Persistence of HBsAg may be detected for many years, and some carriers appear to be sources of infection for a prolonged period. The infectivity of the HBsAg carrier is correlated with the presence of circulating intact HBV particles and HBeAg.[641]

The frequency of life-long carriage of HBsAg is not known. In a number of studies, the prevalence of HBsAg appears to decline with increasing age.[974] These data suggest that the carrier state is not inevitably life-long but is often limited to a finite period of time.

HBsAg carriers almost always have detectable anti-HBc. IgG anti-HBc is the predominant immunoglobulin, but IgM anti-HBc may also persist, usually in low titer, in carriers with persistent viral replication.[926] Low titer anti-HBs is present in 10% to 40% of carriers, but subtyping indicates that the antibody is directed to subdeterminants not present on the HBsAg of the carrier.[293,863] In some instances the anti-HBs represents a false-positive test. HBeAg and anti-HBe are present in a variable proportion of HBsAg carriers.

The prevalence of the HBsAg carrier state varies widely. In the continental United States and most, but not all, western countries 0.1% to 0.5% of the general population are carriers. In southeast Asia, the South Pacific, sub-Saharan Africa, the Mediterranean littoral, and Eskimo villages of Alaska and Greenland prevalence rates greater than 5%, occasionally approaching 20%, have been described. The carrier state develops following acute hepatitis B more frequently in those who have a mild disease, and more often in younger people than in older patients. In the Yupik Eskimo study, carrier states developed in over 28% of infected children under 4 years of age in contrast to less than 8% of those who developed hepatitis B when they were 30 years old or older.[654] Cultural variations in exposure to HBV, age at infection, and ill-defined host factors that may be responsible for impaired clearance of HBsAg appear to be critical determinants of carrier rates.[974] In many areas higher carrier rates are observed in males than in females. In low-prevalence populations, peak carrier rates are found in individuals between 20 and 40 years of age, and in intermediate-prevalence areas peaks are seen in adolescence. In high-prevalence populations, peak carrier rates are found in childhood. Maternal-neonatal transmission of HBV, with infection in early life, appears to be an important factor in the perpetuation of the carrier state in high-prevalence areas whereas other mechanisms are operative in low- and intermediate-prevalence areas.

The HBsAg carrier state is usually readily differentiated from the clinical entities of chronic persistent and chronic active hepatitis because most carriers have neither symptoms nor signs of liver disease. When symptoms or signs are present, these disorders should be suspected before the patient is labeled a HBsAg carrier. In the asymptomatic HBsAg carrier in whom signs of liver disease are absent, serum aminotransferase levels may be mildly elevated or normal on sequential measurements. Other liver chemistries are usually within normal limits. As shown in Table 15-10, almost 40% of 682 HBsAg carriers, in whom clinical evidence of liver disease was absent, had elevated serum aminotransferase levels. Liver biopsy in asymptomatic HBsAg carriers reveals a spectrum of liver injury ranging from none to severe chronic active hepatitis with cirrhosis. The more serious lesions of chronic active hepatitis with or without cirrhosis were found in 22% of patients with abnormal aminotransferase levels (see Table 15-10), whereas only 1% of patients with normal enzyme levels had these lesions. The majority of carriers, regardless of aminotransferase level, had histologic evidence of chronic persistent hepatitis, minimal or nonspecific findings such as occasional foci of necrosis and inflammation, or presumably normal liver tissue. Ground-glass hepatocytes (see section on Pathology) may also be present in liver tissue of HBsAg carriers.

The long-term prognosis of most asymptomatic HBsAg carriers with or without liver biopsy evidence of hepatic injury is not defined. Limited follow-up studies indicate that the antigen may spontaneously disappear in 2% to 6% annually.[858] Short-term follow-up studies involving sequential liver biopsies suggest that progression of the hepatic process is unusual,[202,969] except in those individuals in whom HDV superinfection occurs. On the other hand there is considerable evidence relating the HBsAg carrier state and hepatic injury to the most serious potential sequel of HBV infection, namely, primary hepatocellular carcinoma. The latter is described subsequently.

Persistent HDV infection of HBsAg carriers has been associated with progressive liver disease but in an uncertain but presumably small proportion of patients, an asymptomatic dual (HBV/HDV) carrier state may exist.[846]

A viremic carrier state in non-A, non-B viral hepatitis has been established by transmission experiments in humans and in nonhuman primates.[1051] Although the precise prevalence is uncertain in the absence of a confirmed serologic marker, based on the frequency of post-transfusion non-A, non-B viral hepatitis, it is likely that carriers of non-A, non-B agents may be even more common than HBsAg carriers. The development of chronic hepatitis in as many as a third of individuals with tranfusion-associated non-A, non-B viral hepatitis[523,536] suggest that persistent infection may lead to chronic hepatic injury analogous to that seen in HBsAg carriers.

Serious Sequelae

Chronic active hepatitis refers to seriously destructive liver disease, which is due in some instances to chronic infection by HBV, HBV/HDV, or the blood-borne non-A, non-B hepatitis agents but not to HAV. It is an etiologically diverse clinical entity (nonviral forms are known) in which the underlying histopathologic changes are well defined.

The term *chronic aggressive hepatitis* was introduced by the European pathologists in 1968 to encompass histopathologic changes thought to indicate poor prognosis.[204] Apart from objection to the anthropomorphism of "aggressive," this designation has not been an accepted replacement for *chronic active hepatitis*. The defined changes are found in one or more biopsy specimens from many persons with no subsequent progression. It is also true that clinically overt chronic active hepatitis may revert to an inactive form in which the histopathologic changes are indistinguishable from those in chronic persistent hepatitis. Interpretation of liver biopsies obtained shortly after the onset of viral hepatitis may be difficult because in some instances features of chronic active hepatitis may be identified but have no prognostic importance.[270] Further clarification of nomenclature, of diagnostic criteria, and of prognostic features is clearly needed.

Evidence of HBV infection as an antecedent of chronic active hepatitis includes prospective studies in which acute hepatitis B evolved into chronic active hepatitis,[721,812] the finding that HBsAg occurs with a high frequency in many series of cases,[781] although not all, and the identification of HBV markers in liver biopsy specimens obtained from affected patients.[332] As previously indicated, HBV/HDV dual infections have also been associated with the development of chronic active hepatitis and cirrhosis. Prospective studies of patients with non-A, non-B viral

TABLE 15-10.   Hepatic Histologic Findings in HBsAg Carriers: Relationship to Serum Aminotransferase Elevations in 26 Studies of 682 Individuals

SERUM AMINOTRANSFERASE LEVELS	NORMAL, CHRONIC PERSISTENT, OR NONSPECIFIC HEPATITIS	CHRONIC ACTIVE HEPATITIS/ CIRRHOSIS	OTHER	TOTALS
Normal	401 (96%)	5 (1%)	12 (3%)	418 (61%)
Abnormal	197 (75%)	58 (22%)	9 (3%)	264 (39%)

hepatitis[523,536] indicate that chronic active hepatitis may be an important sequel of these infections.

Cirrhosis

Postnecrotic cirrhosis is a recognized sequel of acute viral hepatitis but appears to be a very infrequent outcome (see Pathology).[29,160,191,709,713,1101] Some studies of "cryptogenic" cirrhosis have demonstrated a moderate frequency of HBsAg positivity.[781] Whatever role HBV and HBV/HDV have in the etiology of chronic active hepatitis is presumably continued when that disease progresses to cirrhosis. Limited data suggest that cirrhosis is an uncommon denouement of chronic active hepatitis due to the non-A, non-B hepatitis viruses. Hepatitis A has not been linked with the development of cirrhosis.

Primary Hepatocellular Carcinoma

Neither HAV nor HDV have been implicated in the development of this malignancy. In contrast, an association of HBV infection with this carcinoma has been unequivocally established in seroepidemiologic studies. Furthermore, HBV antigens have been identified in the liver of affected patients, and HBV DNA appears to be integrated into the genome of the malignant hepatocyte. Whether HBV is oncogenic is no longer seriously questioned, but the identification of co-carcinogenic factors that may act together with HBV remains a goal. The role of the non-A, non-B agents requires further definition.

Aplastic Anemia Following Viral Hepatitis

The development of aplastic anemia has been described in over 200 patients with acute viral hepatitis.[386] Non-A, non-B hepatitis has been the presumptive disease in the majority of cases, but hepatitis A and B have been implicated in a few instances.[1100] Pancytopenia is noted, on the average, about 9 weeks after the onset of hepatitis during the recovery phase but may be seen within days of the onset of illness. All age-groups are susceptible, but more males than females are affected. The case-fatality rate is nonetheless higher in females, and about 85% of patients have succumbed. The cause of death is usually bleeding or infection and unrelated to the clinical course of the hepatitis, which is usually mild and uneventful until pancytopenia is recognized. No predictive clinical or laboratory features are known. Histologic examination reveals acute or resolving hepatitis and aplastic or hypoplastic bone marrow. Standard supportive therapy with blood and platelet transfusion, antibiotics, corticosteroids, anabolic androgens, immunosuppressive agents, and splenectomy have been employed in these patients. Bone marrow transplantation may be necessary if conventional measures fail.

Glomerulonephritis Following Viral Hepatitis

In patients with persistent HBV infection, membranoproliferative or membranous glomerulonephritis, often associated with the nephrotic syndrome, has been described. In Japan[993] and Europe[702] children with glomerulonephritis have been shown to have a considerably higher frequency of HBV infection, as measured by the prevalence of circulating HBsAg, than expected. The association of HBV infection with glomerulonephritis in adults also has been reported but is less prominent. Glomerulonephritis has been associated with the asymptomatic HBsAg carrier state and chronic persistent[173] and chronic active hepatitis[518] with circulating HBsAg. Examination of kidney biopsies from affected patients reveals the presence of immune complex deposits along the subepithelial surface of the glomerular basement membrane.[173,743] Immunofluorescent identification of HBsAg, anti-HBs, and complement in the nodular glomerular deposits suggests that the renal injury is related to deposition of immune complexes. In some patients with glomerulonephritis and positive tests for HBsAg and HBeAg in serum, HBeAg and immunoglobulin without HBsAg has been found in glomeruli.[992] Thus, in some circumstances, immune complexes of HBeAg and its antibody appear to be pathogenic.

The natural history of HBV-associated glomerulonephritis is incompletely understood. Renal involvement, as well as liver disease, may improve following clearance of HBsAg from blood,[518] but the frequency of spontaneous resolution is not known. No relationship of glomerulonephritis to preceding hepatitis A, hepatitis D, or non-A, non-B hepatitis has been recognized.

Necrotizing Vasculitis Following Viral Hepatitis

In a few patients, necrotizing vasculitis has developed either during or after typical hepatitis B.[242] Histopathologically, the vasculitis resembles that seen in polyarteritis nodosa or hypersensitivity angiitis. In other patients, manifestations of chronic liver disease associated with HBV infection have been recognized prior to the onset of symptoms and signs of vasculitis. Mild, subclinical, or no detectable liver disease may be noted in patients with necrotizing vasculitis associated with HBV infection.[248,898,1012] Twenty percent to 30% of patients with necrotizing vasculitis have circulating HBsAg. Immunofluorescent studies of affected blood vessels have indicated the presence of HBsAg, anti-HBs, and immune complexes in the arterial lesions. Necrotizing vasculitis associated with HBV infection appears to be a protracted disorder with a relatively high case-fatality rate. The response to treatment is unpredictable.

Mixed Cryoglobulinemia and Viral Hepatitis

HBsAg and anti-HBs have been identified in the sera and cryoprecipitates of some patients with mixed cryoglobulinemia,[584] a syndrome characterized by vasculitis, purpura, arthralgia, and progressive glomerulonephritis. The association of HBV infection with essential mixed cryoglobulinemia remains controversial.[773]

PREGNANCY AND VIRAL HEPATITIS

In developing countries in the Middle East,[102,331] Africa,[158] and Asia,[9] viral hepatitis may be disastrous for the pregnant woman and her fetus. The frequency of fulminant viral hepatitis is considerably more common in the pregnant than in the nonpregnant woman with viral hepatitis, and the occurrence of hepatitis in the third trimester of pregnancy increases the risk of development of this severe and often fatal variant. The frequency of fetal loss, including intrauterine and neonatal deaths, is strikingly increased in affected women. Premature spontaneous termination of pregnancy is a characteristic feature. The specific etiologic forms of viral hepatitis associated with the development of fulminant disease in the pregnant woman in these high-risk areas have not been serologically identified. In one study, hepatitis B could not be implicated in fatal cases of viral hepatitis in pregnancy,[158] suggesting that hepatitis A and/or non-A, non-B hepatitis were responsible. Although malnutrition has been postulated to play an important role in the development of severe hepatitis during pregnancy, the available evidence is entirely circumstantial and other factors, now poorly understood, may be critical.

In the United States and other developed nations, viral hepatitis during pregnancy is generally a mild disease without important effects on the course of the pregnancy or on the frequency of fetal wastage. Maternal viral hepatitis does not lead to increased rates of spontaneous abortion, stillbirth, or congenital malformation.[916,917] Fatal fulminant viral hepatitis is uncommon. Among 201 cases of viral hepatitis during pregnancy, reported from New York,[134] Dallas,[8] and Los Angeles,[882] only three fatalities, a case-fatality rate of 1.4%, were described. Severe hepatitis in the third trimester may influence the fetus. Low birth weights and early gestational age have been described,[883] but neither the frequency nor the clinical consequences of these observations are well defined.

The importance of maternal-neonatal transmission of viral hepatitis from the acutely infected or carrier mother to her fetus or newborn is described in the section on Epidemiology.

MANAGEMENT

None of the available therapeutic measures has a specific beneficial effect on hepatocellular necrosis or inflammation; what one can accomplish, therefore, is more accurately labeled "management" rather than "therapy" of hepatitis.

Management is based on (1) analogies with other forms of liver disease in humans or in the experimental animal, (2) clinical impressions gained during the management of individual patients with viral hepatitis, and (3) clinical studies of groups of patients. The most reliable data, of course, have been derived from adequately controlled clinical studies. However, one must use a degree of caution in applying conclusions, gained from studies that used as subjects otherwise healthy young men, to patients whose illness is caused by a different etiologic agent and whose age, sex, and general health vary from those of the study subjects. Nevertheless, the controlled clinical trials provide the firmest basis for principles of management.

In general, typical viral hepatitis is managed by rest, diet, and drugs. Various measures fall in these categories: (1) what the physician should do, (2) what the physician should not do, and (3) measures that probably make no difference.

Typical Viral Hepatitis

Restriction of Activity

It is usually not necessary to insist that a person severely ill with viral hepatitis remain in bed, for he feels too ill to stir about too much. Personal pressures due to business or family affairs, however, may cause the patient to be more active than he wishes at this stage of the illness. The patient should be in bed as long as he feels the need to rest. Physical separation from the household and office or factory is sometimes the only way to provide adequate rest.

Enforced rest until liver tests return to normal or stabilize at levels near normal was based on the experience in the Mediterranean Theater during World War II.[60,61,136,402] Hepatitis patients among troops who had been debilitated by the severe physical demands of war permitted early ambulation; this seemed, however, to increase the frequency of relapse and other serious sequelae. The concept that bed rest is necessary was reinforced by the theoretical consideration that the erect position itself decreases hepatic blood flow by 40%[118,189] and that exercise in the erect position decreases the flow by 80% to 85%.[849,1039] Strenuous physical activity in the early phase of the illness was incriminated for a fatal outcome in an occasional case.[539,540] Assuming that any decrease in hepatic blood flow lengthens the course of hepatitis, it follows that the upright position and physical exercise prolong hepatic debility.

The average duration of hospital bed rest for soldiers with viral hepatitis rose from 30 days in 1943–1944, to 50 days in the Mediterranean Theater in 1943–1945 to 60 days in Europe in 1947–1949, to 89 days in the Orient in 1949–1951.[401] Since the early 1950s, however, the emphasis on strict bed rest and prolonged confinement has been increasingly challenged. For patients who walked about the ward as they wished, regardless of the severity of jaundice, the course of the illness was not affected as long as they rested in bed after each meal.[144] Indeed, it has been claimed that even hard physical exercise during acute viral hepatitis had no deleterious effect.[714] Clinical deterioration followed exercise in patients with high serum bilirubin concentrations but not in those with serum bilirubin concentration less than 3 mg/dl in one study.[970] This deterioration was not confirmed, however, by others.[253,818] Post-hepatitis sequelae were attributed to lack of bed rest despite negative follow-up studies.[713,1098]

No evidence is available that recumbency-induced enhancement of hepatic blood flow accelerates the rate of recovery from viral hepatitis. Prolonged bed rest by itself results in physical debility, and in some patients it is emotionally disturbing and in others the long confinement may impose an unnecessary financial hardship. Prolonged bed rest, therefore, should be discouraged. Patients with good appetite and a sense of well-being, regardless of the depth of jaundice, may ambulate in and near their home within the limits of physical fatigue. Such limited activity has not been shown to be deleterious nor does an occasional visit to the physician's office impede recovery. During the acute illness, if the patient's physical strength permits, he may use the bathroom. When the patient's sense of well-being returns and laboratory abnormalities improve, one should determine whether increasing ambulation alters the rate of improvement. After performing an out-of-bed task, the patient should rest before proceeding to the next activity if fatigue is excessive. Gradual but progressive ambulation can hasten rather than slow recovery.

Generally, certain laboratory tests and physical findings are helpful indicators of disease activity. For the improving patient, the most useful tests are the serum aminotransferases and the serum bilirubin, and the most helpful physical finding is the decreased size and tenderness of the liver. In some patients, however, the serum aminotransferase levels show a secondary rise after 2 or 3 weeks of illness. Such later elevations do not *necessarily* indicate any deterioration of the clinical course and are entirely compatible with continued clinical improvement.

A diminution in symptoms together with results of physical examination of the liver and laboratory procedures permits progressive ambulation of the improving patient. When in doubt, one should reduce ambulation in an attempt to increase the rate of improvement. If increased rest does not prove superior to ambulation, then the patient may resume activities that will permit the rate of improvement obtainable with rest. These considerations are particularly important in prolonged hepatitis, which may last for months.

In the occasional patient who develops a relapse, a return to a program of rest with bathroom privileges is reasonable, but increasing ambulation is permitted again with clinical and laboratory improvement, provided that improvement continues during progressive ambulation.

Weakness and easy fatigability are not uncommon after viral hepatitis, particularly for patients who have been kept in bed for long periods of time. They result more often from prolonged bed rest than from the ravages of a self-limited disease. Nevertheless, in an occasional patient, post-hepatitis asthenia may persist for weeks to months. It may require a 30- to 60-minute rest period at lunch time. It invariably improves but usually subsides gradually.

Diet

Acutely ill patients with viral hepatitis should receive over 16 carbohydrate calories (4 g of glucose) per kilogram of ideal body weight. Early in the disease, anorexia, nausea, and vomiting may cause problems in achieving this goal. Although the patient is nauseated, he usually can take some food by mouth. Hard candy, carbonated drinks, and fruit juices are often retained when other foods are not. If oral intake is not retained, intravenous glucose is used to supplement the oral calories and also to provide hydration. Potassium and sodium chloride should be added to the glucose solution to correct losses induced by vomiting.

Because some patients with severe viral hepatitis cannot excrete a normal water load, the administration of large amounts of glucose in water may induce water intoxication. Excessive hydration is indicated by an unexplained rise in body weight and a decline of serum sodium concentration and hematocrit. Infusion of 25% glucose is needed only in submassive or massive hepatic necrosis for treatment of hypoglycemia. The value of intravenous amino acid therapy has not been evaluated in the nutritional management of acute hepatitis.

As vomiting subsides and appetite returns, the diet should equal or exceed 1 g of protein and 30 to 35 calories per kilogram of ideal body weight. This amount of food, divided into five or six small feedings rather than the usual three large meals, is more likely to be consumed by patients with such brittle appetites. Because nausea and vomiting may be progressive throughout the day and least troublesome in the morning, a hearty breakfast may be the most readily tolerated meal of the day. The physician, however, should not interfere with the patient's diet and should allow foods that the patient prefers.

In a well-nourished civilian population, a high-calorie, particularly of high protein, intake is of questionable value and should not be forced. A high-protein (150 g) and high-calorie (3,000) diet had a slight effect on the rate of convalescence of soldiers with non-B hepatitis. On the other hand, a similar diet did not compare favorably with an *ad libitum* diet in 67 volunteers with hepatitis B.[579] The duration of illness in the high-calorie diet group was either longer than or similar to that of controls in these experiments. The disadvantage of possible weight gain during inactivity outweighs by far the possible advantages of such culinary largesse.

The physician should not arbitrarily restrict fat in the diet. An ill patient with poor appetite may find "heavy" or "greasy" items unappealing. In such cases, eliminating fatty foods has its basis in common sense rather than in scientific observations. Furthermore, in a group of patients with viral hepatitis who consumed a high-fat diet, organic anion clearance by the liver did not improve any more slowly and probably did so more rapidly than that of controls.[430]

One of the traditionally important "do nots" in the dietary management of viral hepatitis is consumption of alcoholic beverages. However, this injunction against ethanol has also been without adequate evidence.[401] A single intravenous infusion of 80 mg of ethanol per kilogram of body weight (equivalent to two martinis for an average adult) during icteric acute hepatitis had no demonstrable effect on the activities of two serum aminotransferases or two dehydrogenases.[310] Administration of ethanol to chimpanzees during acute hepatitis B produced no changes in the course of the disease or in the titers of HBV markers.[988] A transient elevation of serum aminotransferases occurred but was similar to that seen in uninfected control chimpanzees. Nevertheless, larger amounts of ethanol are deleterious to hepatic metabolism and morphology in human subjects and should be avoided during hepatitis.[852]

After a patient recovers completely from viral hepatitis, alcohol ingestion has not been demonstrated to be more harmful than for the general population. The practice of forbidding alcoholic beverages for 1 year or more after full recovery from viral hepatitis is based more on the physician's likes and dislikes than on acceptable scientific observations. There was no relationship between the drinking habits of 114 soldiers and the appearance of residuals 6 to 12 months after recovery from viral hepatitis.[317] However, excessive intake of alcoholic beverages soon after jaundice subsided has been followed by apparent relapse of the hepatitis in a few cases.[193]

There is no evidence that vitamin supplements contribute to the therapy of viral hepatitis. The customary administration of water-soluble vitamins by mouth is useless in well-nourished individuals but may help patients with previously poor dietary habits. Although it has been argued that administration of some medication is psychologically comforting to both the patient and the physician, counseling, education, and reassurance are far more effective goals.

Vitamin K is usually administered in viral hepatitis whenever the prothrombin time is depressed. A single injection of 10 mg of menadione intramuscularly or the same amount of phytonadione (vitamin K_1) intramuscularly or 1 mg to 3 mg intravenously is justified because of the evidence for impaired absorption of fat during acute hepatitis.[172] If marked improvement in prothrombin time follows, the basis for the diagnosis should be reconsidered, because such a result is infrequently seen in patients with acute hepatocellular damage. Repeated injections in an attempt to force the prothrombin time to respond are not only useless but may be harmful. For some patients with hepatocellular disease the prothrombin time is further prolonged for 24 to 48 hours after large doses of vitamin K are administered.[1023]

Drugs

Corticosteroids. *Corticosteroid* administration in the typical form of viral hepatitis is likely to be harmful, despite occasional and transient acceleration of the decrease of the aminotransferase activity and bilirubin concentration in the serum. The first uncontrolled studies that attributed therapeutic benefits to ACTH and cortisone were published in the early 1950s.[168,867,1000] Following ACTH or corticosteroid therapy, serum bilirubin values strikingly decreased in one half to two thirds of patients with viral hepatitis ("whitewash" effect).[145,1074] When a rapid decrease was observed, it began within 1 to 2 days and lasted 1 to 3 days. The average decline was 32% per day, compared with 22% per day in the hyperbilirubinemia due to other causes. The initial, rapid decrease was followed by a second phase characterized by a much slower decline averaging 7.4% per day. Corticosteroids did not affect the slow phase of bilirubin decrease, the biliary or urinary excretion of bilirubin, or erythrocyte breakdown.[1074] A statistically significant difference in rate of overall decline of serum bilirubin, aminotransferase, and aldolase levels in prednisone-treated patients could not be demonstrated.[215]

There is no evidence that corticosteroids can either slow the rate of liver cell necrosis in typical viral hepatitis or can increase the rate of hepatocellular regeneration. It has been suggested that corticosteroids may convert a self-limited acute hepatitis B to chronic active hepatitis.[267] The incidence of relapse of viral hepatitis increased when the original illness was treated with corticosteroids.[94,262,263] Therefore, the physician should not give corticosteroid therapy in typical acute viral hepatitis.[875] Even until recently, the use of corticosteroids in atypical acute hepatitis was controversial. Recent evidence, however, failed to support earlier uncontrolled observations on the beneficial effect of corticosteroids on the course of even unusually severe viral hepatitis. It does not shorten the illness sufficiently to risk the complications of these agents.[94]

Estrogens. The severity of both hepatitis B and non-B acute hepatitis was similar in oral contraceptive users and nonusers hospitalized with the disease.[886] Furthermore, the nature and frequency of the sequelae of acute viral hepatitis were not influenced by oral contraceptive use before and during the course of the hepatitis.

On the basis of these data, it may be reasonable to continue administration of birth control pills during the acute phase of viral hepatitis unless this type of prophylaxis is no longer needed. After recovery from viral hepatitis, antiovulatory drugs may be instituted for the first time without undue concern.

Antiemetics. Nausea and vomiting in typical viral hepatitis usually subside within a few days. If medication is needed, metoclopramide appears to be the drug of choice. The major advantage of metoclopramide over phenothiazines is that the former can increase the rate of gastric emptying and has no deleterious effect on liver function whereas the latter group of drugs can impair hepatic excretory function and may produce cholestasis. Unfortunately, metoclopramide-associated side-effects, such as drowsiness and fatigue, may confuse the clinical picture and limit the drug's usefulness.

Immune Globulin in the Treatment of Active Acute Hepatitis. From experience with other viral diseases, it would be anticipated that immune globulin (IG) is not of value in the treatment of viral hepatitis. This was, in fact, the finding in the large-scale studies of both acute[330] and chronic hepatitis.[1035] As much as 45 ml of IG was of no demonstrable benefit. This experience was confirmed in a smaller series of patients also given corticosteroids at the United States Army Hepatitis Center in Germany.[261] Even hyperimmune serum globulin is ineffective in treatment. In a group of 148 patients, IG did not affect the course, the complication rate, or the development of chronic hepatitis in HBsAg-positive or HBsAg-negative patients who had follow-up liver biopsies.[255]

New Agents of Unproven Effectiveness. Because HBV infection becomes chronic more often in those patients who have been treated with immunosuppressive therapy or who have impaired immune responsiveness, the effectiveness of an immunostimulant was explored in the therapy of acute hepatitis B. Levamisole, a nonspecific immunostimulant, or a placebo was given to 24 patients with acute hepatitis B and 26 patients with non-B hepatitis.[746] Among patients with hepatitis B none of the 10 treated patients remained HBsAg-positive after 3 months, whereas 5 of the 14 placebo recipients were still HBsAg positive. Serum IgG and IgA levels showed significant increases in the levamisole-treated groups. Recovery from acute disease, as judged by normalization of serum aminotransferase levels, disappearance of HBsAg, and/or histologic appearances, was observed at the end of 3 months in 22 of 23 levamisole-treated and 19 of 27 placebo-treated patients. This difference was statistically significant. Further controlled studies are needed.

In a prospective, randomized, double-blind trial of transfer factor therapy versus placebo in 29 patients with hepatitis B, no significant differences in clinical or laboratory features of the illness were found.[257] It was concluded that the transfer factor employed in this study did not influence the course of the disease. Whether other preparations of transfer factor might have important effects in typical or severe hepatitis B cases remains uncertain.

A free radical acceptor, (+)-cyanidanol-3, an agent effective in the treatment of experimental liver disease, was also studied in a double-blind prospective clinical trial in 100 patients with acute hepatitis.[93] Seventy-five of these were HBsAg positive: 19 of the 42 were treated and 33 received placebo. Nineteen of the 42 treated patients became antigen negative in 1 month compared with only 7 of the 33 controls. Among the 100 patients, symptoms

persisted longer in the placebo group, and the serum bilirubin level declined faster in the treated group. However, the duration of hospitalization was not affected by drug therapy.

Reporting of Cases

Viral hepatitis is a notifiable disease in all states of the United States. The diagnosis of acute hepatitis A should be based on the presence of anti-HAV of the IgM class and of hepatitis B on serologic evidence rather than on epidemiologic background. Non-A, non-B hepatitis is strongly suggested by recent transfusions or by the absence of HBsAg, anti-HBc, and anti-HAV of IgM class. Each case should be reported to the local health authority on the postal card form used for acute communicable diseases. The physician in charge of care is responsible for making such reports. Control measures in the community are dependent on as complete a picture of hepatitis morbidity as can be obtained.

Relapsing or Prolonged Viral Hepatitis

The same measures used for acute hepatitis are applicable in relapsing or prolonged hepatitis. *Ad libidum* bed rest is intended to accelerate recovery. It is, however, debilitating of itself. If the clinical condition is not improved by rest, ambulation should be permitted. The extent of ambulation depends on the behavior of the clinical and laboratory manifestations of the disease. A liver biopsy may be necessary in these patients to help in the evaluation for the unlikely progression to chronic active hepatitis.

Cholestatic Viral Hepatitis

Cholestasis due to viral hepatitis is primarily a problem in differential diagnosis. The only therapeutic maneuver that is uniquely helpful in cholestatic hepatitis is the use of cholestyramine when pruritus becomes clinically significant. Patients with transient steatorrhea are helped by reducing intake of dietary fats. Steatorrhea is rarely severe enough to warrant supplementary administration of medium-chain fatty acids.

Corticosteroid therapy was associated with decrease of jaundice in some patients with this form of hepatitis,[740] but many others have not shown such gratifying responses. In a group of five patients with cholestatic hepatitis, only one failed to decrease the serum bilirubin concentration with either ACTH or corticosteroid treatment. In the remaining four, the initial rapid decrease of serum bilirubin averaged 10% per day and was followed by a slower rate of decrease. Neither corticosteroids nor ACTH had an apparent effect on the second, slow phase of bilirubin response in these patients.[968,1074] Corticosteroids should not be used in this form of hepatitis unless evidence of chronic active hepatitis with cholestasis can be documented.

Severe Hepatitis with Confluent (Bridging) Necrosis

A more severe form of acute viral hepatitis is characterized by confluent (bridging) necrosis and was called subacute hepatic necrosis.[107] In contrast to the acutely downhill course of fulminant hepatitis, these patients run a more prolonged, that is, subacute course that often terminates fatally or progresses to chronic hepatitis and cirrhosis. The term *subacute hepatitis* is an appropriate description of this illness. Peters[758] properly expressed his distress on finding the term *subacute hepatitis* omitted from the new nomenclature proposed by the Internation Association of the Study of Liver.[291] Confluent (bridging) hepatic necrosis is seen in approximately one third of patients who have undergone liver biopsy for acute viral hepatitis.[107,724,1054] It is likely that these patients were selected because of the unusually severe nature of the disease or because of some other complications. Subacute hepatitis is characterized clinically by severe clinical illness, by the development of complications, such as ascites, edema, or encephalopathy, by prolongation of the progressive rise of serum bilirubin concentrations beyond the usual 2 weeks and by the peaking of serum bilirubin at higher levels (over 15 mg/dl) than is seen in typical acute viral hepatitis, and by continued depression of the serum albumin concentrations, often below 3 g/dl. These features are particularly ominous when seen in patients over 40 years of age. In the initial report based on 52 patients, the mortality rate of subacute hepatitis was 19%. Chronic hepatitis and cirrhosis developed in 37% of these patients during a 4½-year follow-up period.[107] The course of subacute hepatitis lasts for several weeks to months and can end with recovery, development of chronic active hepatitis and cirrhosis, or death. It was thought that corticosteroid therapy in these patients would increase survival and the rate of recovery of patients with confluent (bridging) necrosis.[107] Although it is more likely for acute hepatitis to be clinically severe if it is associated with confluent bridging necrosis than with spotty necrosis, the converse is not necessarily true. That is, the clinical severity of hepatitis alone does not reliably identify patients with confluent (bridging) necrosis. For example, the severity of hepatitis was not significantly different in a group of patients who had confluent (bridging) necrosis as compared with those in whom the confluent necrosis was not demonstrable.[1052] Of course, sampling error could have accounted for missed bridging lesions because their patchy distribution is well recognized. Corticosteroid therapy had no beneficial effect in severe viral hepatitis whether or not this was associated with biopsy evidence of confluent necrosis.[367,1056] Indeed, when patients with severe hepatitis were separated according to HBsAg positivity and presence of confluent (bridging) necrosis, then the excess mortality in the steroid-treated patients with confluent (bridging) necrosis reached statistical significance ($p = .04$).[367] Although the data are not persuasive enough definitely to incriminate corticosteroids as harmful agents in the treatment of patients with sub-

acute hepatitis, randomized clinical trials in subacute hepatitis, as in fulminant hepatitis with confluent (bridging) necrosis, failed to show that this form of therapy can enhance survival.

Fulminant Hepatitis

Fulminant hepatitis is characterized by a 1- to 3-week course of hepatic failure, encephalopathy, and coma and terminates in death in 70% to 95% of patients.

There is no specific, effective therapy of this form of dramatic and overwhelming hepatic failure. Only general supportive measures are available for the care of the patient. Specific measures can be used only to treat specific complications of this illness.

There are effective measures for the expected complications that are of known or of likely benefit. It is probable that the apparent improvement from fewer than 10% survivors in the 1940s and 1950s[245,264] to 20% to 30% in the 1960s and 1970s[43,79,1016] is attributable to better supportive care, effective supportive measures, and specific measures for the management of complications.

In conformity with British, French, and American observations, the most serious of these complications and the most common cause of death is due to encephalopathy-associated neurologic complications. Approximately two thirds of the patients die because of coma, and half of these have cerebral edema at autopsy. Cerebral edema is more frequent among younger than older patients. Bacterial infection accounts for 10% to 20%, massive gastrointestinal hemorrhage for 5% to 12%, cardiac failure for about 5%, and vasomotor collapse for about 5% of deaths. Thrombocytopenia is common in those who experience hemorrhage, but there is no correlation between prolongation of prothrombin time and gastrointestinal hemorrhage.[79] Nonfatal life-threatening complications include cardiac arrhythmia or cardiac arrest, which developed in almost 40%, respiratory distress or arrest in a similar number, and gross gastrointestinal hemorrhage in about a third of such patients. Because of the high frequency of these life-threatening complications, patients with fulminant hepatic failure can be best treated in an intensive care unit.[79]

Nursing personnel should be in constant attendance so the patient can be closely supervised. The care team needs to anticipate and be prepared for emergency situations. There is no requirement for enteric isolation. Isolation requirements are confined to blood and saliva, which do not prevent handling in the usual intensive care unit.[674]

Blood pressure, cardiac rhythm, and respiratory rate should be monitored. If respiratory distress develops, arterial blood gases and *p*H should be monitored. Daily weights should be obtained, fluid intake and output recorded, and the serum BUN and creatinine values measured daily.

Electrolyte disturbances are common. Hypernatremia can develop as a result of impaired sodium excretion in patients receiving large amounts of fresh frozen plasma to correct coagulation defects or in those who receive osmotic diuretics in an attempt to correct cerebral edema.[1071] Hyponatremia can develop because of impaired free water clearance in these patients. Therefore, intravenous or enteral fluid and electolyte therapy has to be closely monitored to prevent excessive swings of serum osmolarity and electrolyte concentrations.

The hematocrit, BUN, and serum creatinine levels are measured daily. The level of blood glucose is measured every 12 to 24 hours because of the possibility that hypoglycemia will occur. Serum electrolytes should also be obtained daily or more frequently if problems develop. Lactic acidosis can progress rapidly unless treated with large amounts of bicarbonate, but the latter is contraindicated in patients with respiratory alkalosis.

Caloric balance can be maintained by giving 16 carbohydrate calories (4 g of glucose) per kilogram of ideal body weight per day. Twenty-five percent glucose may be given in a central vein or polycose by enteric alimentation through a small-bore feeding tube. Because of the possible deleterious effects of ammonia and related compounds produced by the intestinal flora, protein intake by mouth should be restricted to essential amino acids if enteric alimentation is used. Neomycin orally or by nasogastric tube in a dose of 4 g to 6 g per day is also used, although there is no definite evidence concerning its benefit in hepatic coma due to fulminant acute hepatitis. It should be discontinued, however, when oliguria or anuria develops. Cleansing enemas and rectal instillation of neomycin may be helpful. Lactulose also has no proven value in fulminant hepatic failure but may be used in lieu of neomycin. It can interfere with good nursing care if it produces diarrhea in a comatose patient.

The clotting factors produced by the liver are depressed, and thrombocytopenia is common in fulminant hepatitis, so gastrointestinal bleeding is a common danger in these patients. Blood replacement and the use of fresh frozen plasma may be required to maintain blood volume in bleeding patients. Clotting factor concentrates lack factor V and have been relatively ineffective in the treatment of these patients.[861] The incidence of upper gastrointestinal hemorrhage decreased significantly following cimetidine therapy of patients with fulminant hepatic failure caused by acetaminophen.[79,610] By analogy, cimetidine, 300 mg IV every 6 hours, is therefore recommended for patients with fulminant hepatitis. Limited personal experience suggests that it is less effective and does not influence survival of patients with fulminant viral hepatitis.

An uncertain and largely untested approach to therapy is predicated on the assumption that disseminated intravascular coagulation is responsible for or contributes importantly to bleeding in fulminant hepatitis. Heparin combined with fresh frozen plasma, therefore, has been used.[803] The hazards of this approach are obvious, and if tried at all, it should only be attempted by appropriately staffed major medical centers as part of a randomized clinical trial.

Vitamins are not needed in the management of ful-

minant hepatitis in otherwise well-nourished patients, although there may be defects in the metabolism of certain vitamins. For example, patients with fulminant hepatic failure have either impaired capacity to convert pyridoxine to pyridoxal-5′-phosphate (PLP) or there is an accelerated utilization of PLP in this condition.[847] Vitamin B complex and thiamine should be given during the period in which intravenous nutrition is required.

A patient with fulminant hepatic failure may require medication for control of seizures. Intravenous diazepam (Valium) seems to be suitable for this purpose.[698] Depressant drugs should not be used, however, for the treatment of delirium or maniacal behavior that is not associated with convulsions. Such behavior is usually of brief duration and wanes as the patient slips into increasingly advanced stages of encephalopathy. However, when the delirium is severe and prolonged, particularly when it is accompanied by convulsions, drug therapy becomes appropriate at that time. Schenker pointed out five of the requirements of an ideal drug for these patients[873]: (1) it should be possible to titrate the effect rapidly; (2) the duration of action should be very short; (3) it should have normal binding to plasma proteins; (4) it should not depress unduly cerebral receptors that are involved in the maintenance of consciousness; and (5) it should not interfere significantly with respiratory function or with the control of blood pressure. Unfortunately, there is no known drug that fulfills these requirements. Therefore, these patients should be given small and, if needed, repeated doses of sedation just to overcome the problem for which it is administered. If enteral alimentation is taking place with a tube or the patient can take drugs by mouth, then oxazepam (Serax) is the drug of choice. If intravenous therapy is required, then lorazepam (Ativan), if available, or diazepam (Valium) should be given slowly intravenously and the patient's response titrated. Both oxazepam and lorazepam are inactivated by glucuronidation, and therefore their half-life and clearance rates are not importantly affected by hepatocellular failure. On the other hand, diazepam requires hepatocellular metabolism before it is excreted, and therefore in acute hepatitis, let alone fulminant hepatic failure, its half-life and clearance rates are markedly prolonged. Furthermore, if serum protein concentrations are decreased, the proportion of unbound drug is increased and its effect is exaggerated. An additional consideration is that cerebral sensitivity to all these drugs increased in the presence of severe liver disease.[873]

Unproven (Experimental) Forms of Therapy

Some of these methods have been tried but were not proved effective to date; others are in various stages of their development.

Exchange Transfusions. Anecdotal reports claimed encouraging results because coma improved after exchange transfusions. Fulminant hepatic failure due to viral hepatitis has not been shown to be benefited by this method of therapy in a single controlled clinical trial.[813] The most extreme form of exchange transfusion is the "total body washout." This consists of total exsanguination of a comatose patient under hypothermia. The hematocrit is reduced to less than 1% by replacement of blood with physiologic salt solution, which then rapidly is replaced by fresh blood. Here again, the initial encouraging results were not supported by observations of others. In the experience of one of us (JTG), all 10 patients so treated died eventually. Where failure was not attributable to technical difficulties, the depth of coma invariably lightened, or the patient recovered consciousness. However, death ensued sooner or later because of hepatic failure or various complications, such as hemorrhage, sepsis, or, as in one patient who left the hospital alive but returned and died, aplastic anemia.

***Ex vivo* Liver Support Using Pig Liver or Baboon Liver.** *Ex vivo* liver support using pig liver or baboon liver did result in recoveries of a few patients in uncontrolled, anectodal studies. Here again, there is no convincing evidence that this mode of therapy has a beneficial effect on the rate of recovery of patients with fulminant viral hepatitis.

Cross Circulation of Patients. Cross circulation of patients in coma to a human volunteer with normal liver was thought to be effective on the basis of uncontrolled studies of 21 patients. However, a series of six consecutive cross circulations with a flow rate of 50 ml to 200 ml/min failed to elicit any benefit in a French study.[76] Failure of cross circulations may reflect the fact that under experimental conditions the systemic-to-portal exchange circuit at lower flow rates produced improved electroencephalographic findings whereas much higher flow rates induced by a systemic-to-systemic circuit failed to do so. Because the systemic-to-portal circuit is a clinically unsuitable mode of cross circulation, it is unlikely that this method will find clinical application even if one does not consider the potential major risks to the donor who is cross circulated with a fulminant hepatitis patient.

A number of therapeutic strategies were based on the premise that the removal of certain "toxins," which accumulate because of the destruction of functional hepatocytes, may permit survival long enough for hepatic regeneration to take place. These artificial hepatic support systems include the following:

1. Hemodialysis with the use of various membranes having particular permeability characteristics.
2. Various sorbants, which are supposed to serve as an artificial liver support system. These include charcoal hemoperfusion systems, resin hemoperfusion systems, albumin agarose gel, and an immunoabsorbant system for the removal of circulating immunoreactants.
3. Combination of hemoperfusion system with various absorbants.

4. Plasmapheresis, such as *ex vivo* blood separation with a flow-through centrifuge or on-line plasmapheresis.
5. The use of gel-entrapped microsomes. These include microsomes that are isolated by fractionation of liver cell homogenates.
6. Enzymes: the use of carrier-bound microsomal enzymes for extracorporeal hepatic support system or their use by microencapsulation of multienzyme systems with the recycling of cofactors. These are used in combination with microporous membranes and absorbants noted previously.
7. Liver cell cultures were used as artificial liver and were perfused through multiple parallel hollow fibers serving as artificial capillaries.

Because the specific neurotoxin or toxins have not been identified and because it is not clear whether fulminant hepatic failure induces coma and cerebral edema because of the presence of such a toxin rather than a lack of compounds that are not produced by the failing liver, these systems have not yet improved survival rates. These are experimental and are of great interest. They may become modified and become effective in the future. These have no immediate clinical applicability.[79]

In summary, heroic, complex, expensive measures, which are dangerous on their own account, have not proved to be of sufficient benefit to warrant their clinical use.

Forms of Therapy Found Useless

Two types of agents have undergone controlled clinical trials and were found useless in the therapy of fulminant hepatitis: hyperimmune globulin and corticosteroids.

Hyperimmune Globulin Therapy. With the ability to identify units of plasma rich in anti-HBs, it became feasible to treat patients with fulminant hepatitis B with this material or with hepatitis B immune globulin (HBIG) prepared from it. Encouraged by results with specific antibody in an animal model,[670] Gocke obtained an unexpectedly high survival rate with anti-HBs–rich plasma.[348] However, in a controlled study, large doses (1.32 g and 5.28 g) of HBIG were ineffective in the treatment of patients with fulminant hepatitis B.[6] There was no difference in the survival of 25 treated compared with 28 control patients. The mortality rate was related not to globulin therapy but to the stage of coma: it was lowest in those in stage II coma (7 of 13: 54%); it was higher in those in stage III (12 of 20: 60%), and highest in those in stage IV (16 of 20: 80%).

Corticosteroid Therapy. The use of corticosteroids (or ACTH) for the treatment of severe viral hepatitis was initially reported to be helpful by Thorn and co-workers in 1950[1000] and for fulminant hepatic failure by Ducci and Katz in 1952,[245] leading to their wide acceptance.[264,501,947] Indeed, since the 1960s, "massive" doses of corticosteroids have been customary. Hydrocortisone doses ranged from 200 mg to 1000 mg/day while patients were in coma. An occasional physician used as much as 1 g of prednisone per day. The two factors that recommended the use of corticosteroids in the treatment of fulminant hepatitis were the physician's deep-felt urge to do "something," and the enthusiasm based on uncontrolled observations.

In a prospective randomized clinical trial, the possible effectiveness of corticosteroid therapy in fulminant hepatic failure was first evaluated in a small group of patients in 1974.[1052] Two years later another small group of patients was evaluated in a similar manner.[816] The small number of subjects in these two clinical trials failed to show either benefit or definite harm attributable to corticosteroids in the treatment of fulminant hepatic failure. Another randomized clinical trial on the effectiveness of corticosteroid therapy on severe viral hepatitis was published in 1976 by Gregory and co-workers.[367] This study involved patients with severe hepatitis and confluent (bridging) necrosis and not with fulminant hepatic failure. A definitive answer on the effectiveness of corticosteroid therapy in the treatment of fulminant hepatitis can be based on two multicenter cooperative prospective randomized clinical trials. One was unblinded and was organized by the European Association for the Study of Liver Disease;[260] the other, a double-blind study, was directed by Mosley and conducted by the Acute Hepatic Failure Study Group (AHFSG).[7] These studies did not show any benefit attributable to corticosteroids in the treatment of fulminant hepatitis. The European study lasted for a 4-year period and was based on 40 patients of whom 33 had viral hepatitis: 26 were treated with corticosteroids and 14 with placebo. The groups were comparable and the survival of the two groups was 12% and 14%, respectively. Of the 33 patients with acute hepatitis, 18 had hepatitis B and these had a better survival regardless of therapy than the remainder. In the European study alone, the increased incidence of the steroid-induced harmful side-effects was not statistically significant. However, when the European data were pooled with those of comparable but not identical groups published elsewhere, the harmful effect of corticosteroids in the treatment of fulminant hepatic failure became significant at the 2% level of probability.[255] The AHFSG consortium consisted of 16 institutions from the United States and Canada. This group evaluated the effectiveness of high-dose (800 mg/day) and low-dose (400 mg/day) hydrocortisone therapy in a stratified randomized clinical trial. In 188 cases evaluated by the AHFSG, hepatitis A accounted for 2% of the patients, hepatitis B for 56%, and non-A, non-B hepatitis for 34%. A drug was incriminated as an etiologic agent in 6% of patients. The sex distribution of hepatitis B and non-A, non-B hepatitis patients was not significantly different ($p = .071$). There was a statistically significant difference in the age distribution of patients with fulminant hepatitis B: none was under 15 years of age, 84% of the patients were between the ages of 15 and 44 years, and 16% of the patients were over 45 years of age. In fulminant non-A, non-B hepatitis,

10% of the patients were under 15 years of age, 61% were between 15 and 44 years of age and 29% were over 45 years of age. The overall survival was 33% in fulminant hepatitis B, but only 13% in fulminant non-A, non-B hepatitis. The survival rates among men and women were comparable; however, age had an important effect on survival rates. The higher survival rate of patients with fulminant hepatitis B compared with that of those with non-A, non-B hepatitis was confined to the 15-year to 44-year age-groups, with a rate of $37 \pm 5\%$ vs. $13 \pm 5\%$ ($p = .06$). The survival rates in patients over age 45 were $12 \pm 6\%$ versus $16 \pm 9\%$ in the fulminant hepatitis B or non-A, non-B hepatitis group respectively, a difference that is not significant. Neither high-dose (800 mg/day) nor low-dose (400 mg/day) hydrocortisone therapy had any demonstrable beneficial effect either on fulminant hepatitis B or fulminant non-A, non-B hepatitis.

Glucagon-Insulin Therapy. In the same animal model in which, on at least two occasions, it was demonstrated that corticosteroids can be harmful in hepatitis, limited studies also indicated that glucagon in combination with insulin may be helpful.[268] These animals received 0.3 mg of glucagon and 20 units of insulin per kilogram per 24 hours. The infusion with glucagon significantly increased the rate of incorporation of tritiated thymidine into DNA of hepatocyte nuclei of virus-treated animals. Is the combination of these polypeptide hormones—insulin and glucagon—useful in the treatment of fulminant hepatitis in humans? To date, there is no evidence that these are helpful. Theoretically, there are several persuasive arguments in their favor. These hormones may be the portal venous "goodies" that were shown to promote hepatocellular regeneration under a variety of experimental conditions.[903] Both in fulminant hepatic failure and in subacute hepatitis with confluent (bridging) or submassive necrosis, it is the lack of hepatocellular regeneration that seems to be the key reason for fatal outcome rather than the pronounced inflammation associated with a vigorous immunologic mechanism that is responsible for the continued destruction of regenerating hepatocytes. Although these arguments are intellectually stimulating, they lack any documentation that it is indeed a hormone, let alone glucagon and insulin together, that is responsible for the benefits provided by portal venous perfusion of the liver.

A major issue is the desperation that clinicians manifested in selecting even dangerous therapeutic modalities in the treatment of this often fatal and dramatic clinical disaster. The use of corticosteroids now has been put to rest, along with exchange transfusions, but cross circulations with human or nonhuman primates or extracorporeal liver perfusion and various types of artificial livers masquerading as charcoal or resin-coated columns are lurking on the therapeutic horizon. The use of these treatments themselves carries risks of morbidity and mortality that are far more than negligible. Controlled clinical trials are required. Whether liver transplantation will become an accepted mode of therapy, in the absence of controlled trials demonstrating efficacy in fulminant hepatitis, remains uncertain at this time.

PREVENTION

General Preventive Measures

In an era of rapid advances in viral diseases, it is commonplace to think almost exclusively in terms of vaccination for prevention. Although active immunization against hepatitis B has been developed, for the immediate future no vaccine will be generally available against hepatitis A, hepatitis D, or non-A, non-B viral hepatitis. Nonetheless, there are many approaches to the prevention of viral infections other than active immunization. Instrument-associated hepatitis, for example, whether due to HBV, HBV/HDV, or one of the non-A, non-B viruses, is theoretically entirely preventable. Transfusion-associated hepatitis, at least in relation to whole blood and some blood products, cannot be eliminated until non-A, non-B agents can be identified. Nevertheless, there are ways to reduce its incidence greatly. Water- and food-borne hepatitis, although infrequent, represent epidemiologic forms of hepatitis A that can be controlled. Similarly, water-borne, epidemic non-A, non-B hepatitis may be controllable.

Each epidemiologic entity requires an approach suitable to the mode of transmission.[678] For example, measures that prevent instrument-associated hepatitis have no relevance to water-borne hepatitis. The way in which infection is acquired in each individual case, therefore, has implications for the prevention of other potential cases that may be derived from the same source. Preventive measures, if they are to be effective, must be based on a continuing search for those modes of transmission contributing to viral hepatitis in the particular community.

Table 15-11 indicates the preventive measures applicable to each epidemiologic form of hepatitis A, B, D, and non-A, non-B hepatitis. Certain aspects of these approaches deserve further comment.

Prevention of Contact Mode of Transmission (Personal and Environmental Hygiene)

Good personal hygiene should reduce the incidence of hepatitis as it does that of other diseases transmitted by the person-to-person route. With hepatitis A, fecal particles are presumably transferred to the mouth from hands contaminated by direct contact with the infected person or soiled indirectly through objects in the environment. Consistent with this concept are the high attack rates of hepatitis A often observed among young children, among groups in lower socioeconomic levels, and in institutions housing persons intellectually or emotionally incapable of practicing good hygiene, such as day-care centers for infants.

There seems no reason to doubt that poor hygienic habits on the part of either the infected person or his susceptible contacts contribute to an increased risk for the latter group. It is by no means clear, however, that compulsive cleanliness greatly reduces the likelihood of infection in a situation in which exposure is considered likely.

Most susceptible persons living in the same household as a patient with hepatitis A are infected by the time the diagnosis is made. They should receive immune globulin (IG) for prophylaxis. Rigid isolation, therefore, is not necessary. The patient's dishes and linens do not require separate handling, as long as soap and hot water are used routinely in the household. Separate toilet facilities are not needed.

Supervised hand washing at schools in the face of an epidemic may help reinforce a habit desirable from the standpoint of preventing all enteric infections; epidemiologic evidence suggests that the practice does little to alter the course or extent of an outbreak of hepatitis A. "Disinfection" of desks, door knobs, and other objects in the school room similarly contributes nothing.

In contrast, hand washing may be the most effective preventive measure for medical, nursing, and laboratory personnel, and the only one necessary to protect against transmission by direct contact. In laboratories where benches may become contaminated with feces, urine, serum, or other body fluids, regular washing with detergent is probably as effective as disinfection. No surface on which specimens are placed or work with contaminated materials carried out should be used as a table for eating.[271] Similarly, refrigerators used to store patient specimens should not be used by personnel to hold lunch bags or drinks. Smoking in patient care areas should be prohibited.

Because of good evidence for increased risk of transmission of hepatitis B infection from one sexual partner to the other, the prohibition of sexual activity among sexual partners will reduce the risk of infection of the susceptible partner (anti-HBs-negative). Either because infection might have taken place or sexual abstinence is unacceptable, immunization is necessary. Isolation precautions are not required. When non-A, non-B viral hepatitis is present in the family, the same types of precautions are advised as in the case of hepatitis B, but whether sexual contacts can be protected by IG remains uncertain.

Prevention of Primate-Associated Hepatitis

Recently imported nonhuman primates, particularly chimpanzees, are a potential source of hepatitis A (as well as other diseases). For at least 60 days after their entry into the United States contacts should be restricted to the minimum required for care. Several victims of chimpanzee-associated hepatitis acquired their infection during coffee breaks or lunch hours after unauthorized play with these animals.

If a person must handle a primate, he should wear protective clothing and wash his hands carefully after contact with the animal's paws, fur, or cage. In this situation good

TABLE 15-11. Approaches to Prevention of Viral Hepatitis Based on Mode of Transmission

EPIDEMIOLOGIC ENTITY (MODE OF TRANSMISSION)	ETIOLOGIC AGENT(S)	APPROACHES TO PREVENTION
Contact-associated hepatitis	HAV and HBV	Administer IG to household contacts of IgM anti-HAV positive cases. Administer HBIG to susceptible sexual contacts of HBsAg-positive cases.
Primate-associated hepatitis	HAV	Restrict contacts of nonhuman primates for 60 days after importation. House in animal quarters permitting good sanitation. Limit physical contact of handlers to minimum for care; wear protective devices to prevent fecal soiling of clothing; wash hands carefully after contact. Administer IG to persons having continued exposure to newly imported animals if above measures fail to achieve control.
Water-borne hepatitis	HAV and epidemic non-A, non-B	Monitor public and private water supplies for evidence of fecal pollution. Avoid uncertain or infrequently used supplies. Observe reported cases for unexpected clustering or shift in age distribution. Administer IG to persons exposed to supply when epidemic wave is recognized.
Mollusk-associated hepatitis	HAV	Vigorously police contaminated (closed) waters. Avoid raw or partially cooked mollusks, especially abroad. Question patients for history of ingestion of raw or steamed clams or oysters or mussels within 50 days of onset. Observe reported cases for clustering of cases with history of mollusk ingestion.
Food-borne hepatitis (other than mollusk-associated)	HAV	Enforce good food sanitation practices. Observe reported cases for unexpected clusterings or shift in age distribution. ? Administer IG to persons exposed to food when epidemic wave is recognized.
Blood-associated hepatitis	HBV, HDV, and non-A, non-B	Enforce high standards of donor quality. Test for HBsAg. ? Test for SGPT (ALT) and/or anti-HBc. Administer blood only when necessary. Administer no more blood than necessary. Report all cases of blood-associated hepatitis (10 to 180 days) to bank supplying blood and health department. Maintain donor registers with exclusion of recognized carriers (similar to typhoid carrier register in relation to food handling).
Clotting factor–associated hepatitis	HBV, HDV, and non-A, non-B	Administer only when deficiency is specific cause of bleeding. Substitute single-unit, fresh-frozen plasma if clinically appropriate. Administer all units from one lot. Record manufacturer and lot number for all recipients. Identify and withdraw contaminated (icterogenic) lots.
Syringe-associated hepatitis	HBV, HDV, and non-A, non-B	Sterilize any instrument that breaks the skin or mucous membranes or that is contaminated with blood or tissue fluids.

TABLE 15-11.—Continued

EPIDEMIOLOGIC ENTITY (MODE OF TRANSMISSION)	ETIOLOGIC AGENT(S)	APPROACHES TO PREVENTION
		a. Boil 30 minutes.
		b. Autoclave 15 psi for 30 minutes.
		c. Dry heat 160° C for 60 minutes.
		d. Ethylene oxide
		Use disposable equipment once only.
		Avoid multiple-dose-per-syringe technique.
Tattoo-associated hepatits	HBV, HDV, and non-A, non-B	Supervise sterilization practices of tattoo parlors. Educate to danger of sharing unsterilized equipment or dyes (often improvised).

personal hygiene and environmental sanitation do appear to be of value. Routine immune globulin (IG) is probably helpful[553] but should be administered to handlers only when the volume of newly imported animals is high and cleanliness fails.

Relatively few chimpanzees are carriers of HBsAg, and no cases of human infection are known to have occurred. No special precautions appear needed.

Prevention of Water- and Food-Borne Hepatitis (Water and Food Sanitation)

The same engineering practices that have contributed to safety of drinking water supplies from the standpoint of typhoid fever and gastroenteritis are applicable to prevention of hepatitis A and epidemic non-A, non-B hepatitis transmitted by drinking water. Early recognition of a water-borne epidemic is of importance from two standpoints: (1) Because the incubation period of hepatitis A and epidemic non-A, non-B hepatitis is at least 15 to 20 days, and often 30 to 40 days, in common-vehicle epidemics, contamination has often ended before cases begin to occur. In other instances, however, contamination is intermittent or persistent, so that detection of the fault can prevent further cases. (2) If an epidemic is recognized early, administration of IG may prevent disease in some persons exposed to HAV. The role of IG in the prevention or modification of epidemic non-A, non-B hepatitis remains uncertain at this time.

In some instances, water-borne epidemics of hepatitis A are preceded by "herald waves" of gastroenteritis. Water-borne epidemics of gastroenteritis occur far more frequently than those of hepatitis A and should not be considered in themselves an indication for IG administration.

Food-borne epidemics of hepatitis A have been recognized with increasing frequency in recent years; they are, nevertheless, uncommon. They undoubtedly are decreased in frequency by (1) good personal hygiene on the part of food handlers, (2) minimizing the extent that food is actually handled, and (3) preventing sewage contamination of foods in storage, especially those served without

cooking. In some food-borne epidemics, a food handler has been recognized to have had overt disease; in the remainder, no source of contamination could be identified.

No information is available concerning the frequency with which infection is transmitted by an overtly ill food handler, but it appears to be rare. It seems advisable, therefore, to withhold IG from persons eating food in the establishment unless it is clear that a person with poor hygienic habits has definitely handled food served without further cooking. A food handler who develops hepatitis A should be prohibited from handling food until fully recovered. There is no benefit, however, in exclusion beyond convalescence. To the extent that volunteer experiments are applicable, their results indicate that fecal excretion of virus peaks at the onset of illness and typically ends within a week after onset of jaundice. The food-handler who is acutely or chronically infected with hepatitis B virus is not known to pose a hazard. He should not work while acutely ill, but no other restrictions are justified by presently available information.

Mollusk-associated hepatitis is more difficult to prevent. Although shellfish sanitation practices undoubtedly have contributed to the decline of shellfish-borne typhoid fever, general sanitation improvements, with decrease in the frequency of the typhoid bacillus in sewage, must also have had a role. Application of quality standards to growing areas, patrol, and inspection, all contribute to shellfish safety. The problems of preventing illegal harvesting are so numerous, however, that other solutions must be found. Several hundred cases of mollusk-associated hepatitis occur each year in the United States; consumption of raw mollusks abroad may also result in an increased risk of disease. Purchase of mollusks to be eaten raw or with minimal heating from a supplier of known reputation is no guarantee.

Prevention of Transfusion-Associated Hepatitis

The anticipated decrease of post-transfusion hepatitis following elimination of HBsAg-positive blood did not materialize. It is now clear that the most common cause of post-transfusion hepatitis is that due to the non-A, non-B agents. Therefore, the same meticulous standards are required despite availability of serologic testing for HBV markers.

Enforcing Standards of Donor Quality

Physicians must generally rely on collection agencies rather than hospital blood banks to supply most of their patients' needs. The burden of endorsement of donor standards, therefore, falls primarily on regulatory agencies. The individual physician, however, has the responsibility of knowing the character of the blood used for his patients. It behooves him from the standpoint of his ethical and legal responsibility for his patients' welfare to be aware of the recruitment practices and quality of professional supervision at the agencies supplying his hospital.

Exclusion of Commercial Donors

In repeated studies, the use of blood supplied by commercial blood banks (those making cash payments for some or all of their donations) has carried an appreciably increased risk.[27,349,556,705,895] Indeed, it appears that the single most effective measure to prevent transfusion-associated hepatitis would be to eliminate paid donations, and a number of communities and states in the United States have initiated measures to accomplish this goal.

Blame for the higher rate of transfusion-associated hepatitis focused first on the "skid row" alcoholic and subsequently on the self-injecting drug abuser. Studies of patients with alcoholic cirrhosis have demonstrated a frequency of hepatitis B surface antigen positivity higher than that among volunteer blood donors, but not one that is extraordinarily high.[781] Persons practicing illicit self-injection have a higher incidence of HBsAg-positivity,[153] and in some circumstances their contributions to blood banks with poor enforcement policies have resulted in an appreciable amount of disease.[167] It is not entirely clear, however, that they are usually responsible for the higher risk that accompanies paid donations: (1) the small compensation is trivial in its support of his habit compared with that of the alcoholic; and (2) many if not most commercial banks, out of self interest, reject the user with obvious stigmata of his practice.[683]

The problem with donation at commercial blood banks may be related to the frequency of HBV and non-A, non-B virus infection in the population likely to donate at these establishments. Cherubin and co-workers in New York found an inverse relationship between socioeconomic level and the frequency of serologic evidence for HBV infection.[152] A similar trend among marriage-license applicants in Los Angeles County is known to exist. Thus, the impact of eliminating paid donations depends in part on the stratum of society from which the unpaid substitutes are derived.

Individuals who practice the parenteral administration of illicit drugs with associates and promiscuous homosex-uals should be considered in the same category as commercial donors. Indeed, these groups may be more likely to have experience with HBV or non-A, non-B agents.

Exclusion of Donors with History of Hepatitis

A history of hepatitis at any time in the past has been a basis for exclusion of donors in the United States for many years. The exclusion of subjects with known hepatitis A following recovery and development of immunity is hard to justify. Indeed, these individuals would contribute greatly to improving the anti-HAV titer of plasma pools. Furthermore, the evidence is good against HAV being present in the blood for prolonged periods of time in patients who have acute hepatitis A. There is no evidence for a carrier state of HAV in asymptomatic patients. With regard to hepatitis B virus infection, past history of an icteric episode of hepatitis has not seemed to be meaningful. Lewis and colleagues did not find HBsAg positivity significantly more frequent among health care or nonmedical personnel with a past history of hepatitis than among those without recollection of such a history.[588] Egoz and co-workers, however, did find a higher frequency of past hepatitis among implicated donors in Israel, where donation is allowed 5 years or more after the acute disease.[254] Individuals who had non-A, non-B hepatitis in the past should be excluded because they may be carriers of the non-A, non-B agents. Unfortunately, the history of icteric hepatitis is an inefficient way to exclude carriers of non-A, non-B agents.

Donors who have been transfused themselves are excluded only if they received blood within the previous 6 months. Egoz and associates, however, found a higher risk associated with blood from persons transfused at *any* time in their lives, compared with donors who had never been transfused.[254] Lewis and co-workers found a significantly higher incidence of HBsAg positivity in nonmedical workers at the National Institutes of Health who had received prior transfusions.[588] Reevaluation of risk, therefore, seems appropriate for this group.

Identification and Exclusion of Donors Who Are Carriers of Hepatitis

The HBsAg and non-A, non-B carrier state of viral hepatitis may persist over a prolonged period of time. It is extremely important, therefore, that carriers of hepatitis virus be identified and excluded from future donations.

It is impractical for most hospitals to conduct follow-up studies of all persons who receive blood from their banks. It is possible, however, for the physician to question all patients with viral hepatitis concerning prior transfusion of blood or blood products. Such cases should be reported specifically as transfusion-associated hepatitis to the local health department and to the blood bank that supplies the units administered.

Hospitals should notify the blood bank that supplies blood if the recipient develops transfusion-associated hepatitis. The blood bank should exclude such a person by a notation on its own records and inform the donor himself that his blood is potentially hazardous.

Carrier registries similar to those for food handlers who harbor the agent of typhoid fever have been advocated and a few exist on a citywide or statewide basis.

Nonspecific Laboratory Screening for the Exclusion of Carrier Donors

The intuitive supposition that the person with hepatitis viremia should have abnormal liver tests has led to a number of attempts to screen donors on this basis. Initial studies using the insensitive and nonspecific flocculation and turbidity tests were unsuccessful, and early studies of serum aminotransferase screening suggested limited, if any value.[51,121] Subsequent studies, undertaken after recognition of non-A, non-B hepatitis as the predominant form of transfusion-associated hepatitis, have focused on the measurement of serum alanine aminotransferase (ALT, SGPT) in screening blood donors. In these studies recipients of blood with elevated ALT levels appear to be at greater risk of non-A, non-B transfusion-associated hepatitis than are recipients of blood with normal ALT levels.[3,24] Estimates of the impact of ALT screening, using a variety of adjustments, have suggested that elimination of donor blood with elevated ALT levels might prevent one third to one half of non-A, non-B post-transfusion hepatitis.[956] Despite cost-effectiveness analysis suggesting that screening for ALT would be cost saving,[922] controlled clinical trials of the protective efficacy of ALT screening are not available, the nonspecificity of an elevated ALT level remains bothersome, and the major blood banking organizations have not supported routine ALT screening.

With regard to screening for serologic markers of hepatitis B virus carriers, the procedures thus far available have unquestionably contributed to the lowering of rates of transfusion-associated hepatitis B. It is obvious, however, that the presently used third-generation procedures miss some low-level infectious carriers of HBV. Screening for anti-HBc in HBsAg-negative blood may provide additional protection.[453] It is not clear whether such additional screening is cost effective in reducing the already low level of transfusion-associated hepatitis B. On the other hand, because HBV and blood-borne non-A, non-B hepatitis share many epidemiologic features, HBsAg-negative donors with markers of HBV infection appear to be exposed to non-A, non-B hepatitis viruses more often than donors without these markers. Retrospective studies have linked the presence of anti-HBc in HBsAg-negative donor blood with an increased risk of non-A, non-B hepatitis in recipients and suggest that screening for anti-HBc might prevent about one third of transfusion-associated non-A, non-B hepatitis.[956] Unfortunately, screening for anti-HBc might result in high discard rates, prospective, controlled clinical studies are not available, and anti-HBc is clearly not a specific marker of non-A, non-B hepatitis. Markers of non-A, non-B agents are needed, therefore,

before the problem can be reduced to an insignificant level or eliminated.

Use of Blood Only When Necessary

Potentially icterogenic materials should be used only if clearly necessary. If whole blood or other "average risk" materials must be used, the minimal amount that will accomplish the purpose should be given.

In general, it is agreed that initiation of transfusion *with the intention* of administering only a single unit within the patient's immediately forseeable course is a highly questionable practice. If, however, after tranfusion is begun it becomes apparent that only 1 unit is required, then 1 unit is all that should be given. Administering a second unit approximately doubles the patient's risk of developing hepatitis.

A high-risk blood derivative should not be used if a safer substitute (albumin or fresh frozen plasma) will accomplish the same purpose. If a high-risk derivative must be used, all unit numbers should be recorded in the event that transmission of hepatitis occurs.

Adequate Transfusion Records

The ability to identify the recipient of a given unit of blood, *and,* conversely, the identification numbers of units received by a given patient are both indispensable parts of defining the problem of transfusion-associated hepatitis. Non-A, non-B carriers and HBV carriers who are not detected by screening for HBsAg can be identified only if blood can be traced from donor to recipient and from recipient back to donor. The work of a hospital transfusion committee[1044] requires a list of recipients and the units of blood and blood derivatives administered to each. Although all hospitals keep some records concerning whole blood, such records are frequently unsatisfactory. The card or ledger entry usually indicates cross-matching of a unit for a given patient, but often does not state definitely whether blood was given to that patient. One may have to resort to the patient's chart to see whether the blood was administered. Even in the chart, the doctor's orders or the nurse's notes may have to be scrutinized. Occasionally, the only adequate indication that a transfusion was given will be found in the accounting office.

When clotting factor concentrates are used, the name of the manufacturer and the lot number should be recorded. The lot of these high-risk derivatives can then be identified if hepatitis develops subsequently. If the same lot is common to other cases, the unused units should be promptly withdrawn from the shelves. In many hospitals, however, these products are dispensed by the pharmacy instead of the blood bank, without adequate records being kept of recipients, the manufacturer, or the lot number. As a consequence, it is usually extremely difficult to establish attack rates due to these products or to incriminate specific lots so that the unused portion can be withdrawn. It is to be strongly urged, therefore, that clotting factor concentrates be dispensed only through hospital blood banks, with maintenance of similar records as for whole blood. It should be possible to identify recipients of a particular lot and to identify the lot and manufacturer for any given recipient.

It is advisable to dispense even "safe" blood derivatives through the blood bank rather than the pharmacy, keeping a record of the manufacturer and lot number. In the rare instances in which processing safeguards fail, it is then possible to identify the particular batches to be implicated.

Prevention of Instrument- and Equipment-Associated Hepatitis

Any instrument that breaks the skin or mucous membrane of one person or becomes contaminated with blood or any other body fluids, should be sterilized to eliminate the possibility that it can introduce a hepatitis virus into another person. This principle applies not only to syringes and needles, surgical instruments, and dental equipment, but also to a wide variety of other potential vehicles. As a result of recent medical developments, the surfaces over which the patient's blood moves in heart-lung and hemodialysis machines pose new difficulties. Also, everyday instruments, such as razors, clippers, ear-piercing equipment, and cuticle removers, should be considered, but only the tattoo artist's needle has received any attention. Many practical problems are involved in documentation of transmission of hepatitis by nonmedical instruments and in enforcement of their sterilization.

Many methods of sterilization have been and continue to be proposed. The methods dependent on heat are inconvenient because of the time required for their application, their destructive effect on some instruments and equipment, and their complete inapplicability in other instances (i.e., the sterilization of respirators). Furthermore, problems arise because of changed conditions or because of compromises made out of convenience or necessity. Some techniques appropriate for large institutions where their use can be monitored by microbiologists and engineers are completely inappropriate for the physician's or dentist's office.

Although the effect of various sterilization procedures on the hepatitis viruses could be tested in nonhuman primates, this is clearly not feasible because of the limited supply and high cost of the animals. It is practical to test for HBsAg, but the relationship of the denaturation of this protein to loss of infectivity of the virion is unknown. We are still dependent, therefore, on evidence derived from three major sources: (1) experimental studies in which viruses easily studied in the laboratory and bacterial spores are used as models, (2) epidemiologic observations of situations in which transmission of viral hepatitis is interrupted by changing some practice, and (3) practical experience in situations in which transmission of viral hepatitis would be expected if the sterilization procedure were not effective. As usual, the evidence is not as ample as one would like in order to make any of the decisions

necessary in everyday practice. The data are sufficient, however, to define acceptable standards in most instances.

Syringes, needles, and other equipment should be disassembled and cleaned of gross blood and other human proteins. This permits better heat penetration and removes protection to viruses by organic matter in the milieu. Such cleaning is potentially hazardous to persons carrying out the procedure,[424] and precautions should be taken. Rubber gloves, preferably of the heavy-duty type used for housecleaning, should be worn at all times in handling blood-contaminated equipment. In some hospitals instruments that can be autoclaved without damage are "presterilized" prior to cleaning; this heating, however, makes subsequent removal of coagulated protein extremely difficult.[197] Ultrasonication in the presence of a detergent is a more easily applicable and efficient process and safer than manual cleaning. Under no circumstances should the bare hands be placed in any solution containing contaminated instruments, even a liquid labeled as a "germicide." Even apparently unabraded fingers may have sufficient breaks in the skin, especially around the nails, to permit infection.

The use of conventional disinfectant solutions cannot be considered adequate under conditions of everyday practice even when combined with other measures such as ultrasound. Loss of virucidal potency occurs in the presence of any organic material[1043] or even from simple storage.[715] It is also probable that some virus particles are protected by sequestration in protein precipitates.

Boiling for 20 to 30 minutes appears to be effective in inactivating the hepatitis agents.[1065] On the other hand, allegedly boiling for 5 minutes was not adequate in at least one instance,[259] and the longer time should always be used. The effect of 98°C for 1 minute on infectivity of a dilute solution of serum[542] should not be misapplied to sterilization practices. Autoclaving at 15 psi for 30 minutes and dry heat at 160°C for 60 minutes were effective measures in venereal disease clinics in the 1940s. Any of the three methods of heat inactivation is acceptable. For metal cystoscopes and endoscopes, steam at subatmospheric pressure, especially when combined with formaldehyde, may be an appropriate procedure.

Fragile equipment that would be damaged by heating is now frequently sterilized by ethylene oxide, and it has been used under circumstances suggesting that it is effective against the hepatitis agents.[662] This sterilizing agent, however, must be used under carefully defined conditions (a concentration of 0.5 g to 1.0 g/dl for 6 to 10 hours at 60°C with humidity in the range 10% to 30%) to be effective. When mixed with air it is explosive, and materials must subsequently be exposed to air to permit absorbed gas to dissipate.[951]

Another approach of equal or perhaps greater efficacy is the disinfection of sensitive equipment (e.g., fiberoptic endoscopes) after thorough cleansing with glutaraldehyde-containing solutions.[100,524] These have been shown to inactivate HBV; their action on non-A, non-B agents has yet to be conclusively demonstrated.

Dialysis equipment presents special problems that are well discussed by Marmion and Tonkin.[628] HBsAg-positive patients should use separate dialysis equipment that is not shared with HBsAg-negative and anti-HBs-negative (and hence, susceptible) patients.

For the sterilization of biologic reagents that may contain the agent of hepatitis B, the use of β-propiolactone combined with ultraviolet radiation has been advocated.[598] The use of β-propiolactone alone for sterilization of arterial and bone grants was reported in the 1950s, but its effectiveness and safety have never been established.

Meticulous care should be exercised with instruments used in everyday life as well as with instruments used for the care of sick patients. Susceptible individuals should not use any razors, hair clippers, nail clippers, cuticle removers, or toothbrushes that are used by one who could be a carrier of HBV or of a non-A, non-B agent. It is strongly urged that one should avoid or use meticulous sterilization techniques before permitting the use of an ear-piercing instrument, tattoo artist's needle, or the needles of acupuncturists.

Prevention of Nosocomial Hepatitis

Under certain specific conditions, bidirectional transfer of HBV from patients to physicians, nurses, and other health care workers and vice versa can take place.[941] Effective measures to prevent all such transfer of hepatitis will have to await answers to several unsolved questions: What is the mechanism of spread of hepatitis B and non-A, non-B agents by routes other than percutaneous in this setting? What is the importance of low-level carriers in the spread of HBV? What serologic tests will accurately identify infectious carriers of the non-A, non-B agents? What is the effectiveness of cleansing procedures in inactivating the various hepatitis viruses?

Risk to the Patient

The HBsAg-positive physician, dentist, nurse, or health care worker is not a new kind of leper.[676] Although hepatitis B is communicable, even by nonpercutaneous routes, it is not readily transmitted. Considering the large number of health care workers who are HBsAg carriers and who are in contact with patients, there are extremely few reported cases of documented transmission of hepatitis from physician or nurse to patient. These reports include an acutely infected nurse who was thought to have infected 11 patients by giving them parenteral medications[322] and carrier dentists or oral surgeons who were incriminated in the transmission of infection to their patients.[383,582,817,822] Documented transmission of hepatitis B from an infected health care worker to patients, with some exceptions, involved individuals who did major dental-surgical procedures.[358,370] In order to transmit hepatitis B, reasonably intimate exposure is necessary. It seems evident that less overt contact rarely results in infection. It is probably the ungloved hand of the dentist that may be injured on the jagged edge of a dental prosthesis or tooth that could cause the seepage of serum into the patient's mouth, and when HBV reached the mucosal surface this could produce infection. This type of transmission can readily be prevented by the use of gloves. Gloves not only protect the patient from the dentist, but the dentist from the patient. Although puncture-proof gloves are not available, damage to the glove can readily be identified and cleansing can be instituted right away to prevent or at least reduce the risk of infection. Routine gloving by all dentists is suggested.

Currently, with a few exceptions, there is no evidence that would justify the removal of a persistently HBsAg-positive physician, nurse, or other health care worker from his current professional activity. Only those physicians, dentists, and nurses should be removed from direct patient care who have acute hepatitis or in whom transfer of hepatitis to their contacts was repeatedly documented. The recognition of acute hepatitis is simple enough and creates no difficulty either in its identification or in obtaining cooperation of the ill physician or nurse. Documented transmission of hepatitis by an asymptomatic physician or nurse is an entirely different problem. Physicians and nurses are working in an area in which the background frequency of hepatitis can fluctuate. The type of practice of different physicians and nurses varies; some are frequently exposed to patients who develop hepatitis, others very rarely. Therefore, a definition of "documented transmission" from physician or nurse to patient may be difficult. How many of the doctor's contacts must develop hepatitis to make it too many? Is one per year too few or too many? Is there a specific number of hepatitis cases among patient contacts per year that can be used as a criterion for removal of a physician or a nurse from professional activity. And what constitutes removal? Is avoiding surgical procedures, either oral surgery or general surgery, sufficient removal? Is the process of physical examination or oral interview sufficient exposure for contamination? An HBsAg-positive physician or nurse should avoid percutaneous procedures if another person is available to do that. A surgeon, however, may continue to work as long as no more of his patients develop hepatitis B than do those of his HBsAg-negative colleagues. Even when operations were performed during the incubation period of acute hepatitis B and even in the performance of difficult orthopedic surgical procedures, patients were not contaminated by their HBsAg-positive surgeon, who at the time was likely to have been HBeAg-positive as well.[656] On the other hand, an HBsAg- and HBeAg-positive resident in gynecology was responsible for infecting his patients during surgery because of a common technical flaw: punctures of glove and skin by sharp instruments during major surgical procedures. This puncture permits the transmission of HBV from surgeon to patient.[819] Double gloving or the instant removal of the hand with the punctured glove from the operating field and regloving may prevent or at least can reduce the risk of intraoperative infection.

Physicians and nurses who had acute hepatitis B and recovered from the acute infection but continue to remain HBsAg positive can resume their professional activities. The same precautions apply to them as to those who are incidently discovered to be carriers of HBsAg. Although there is an increased risk of being infectious if, in addition to HBsAg, the physician or nurse is also HBeAg positive, it must be remembered that all HBeAg-positive personnel do not transmit the disease, nor can it be assumed that HBeAg-negative persons will fail to do so.[361]

The routine screening of health care workers for HBsAg and anti-HBs is highly desirable. However, there are two major problems. One is that hospitals are resistant to routine screening of personnel because of its cost, and also personnel resist being identified as HBsAg carriers. Although desirable, routine screening is usually available only in high-risk areas: the dialysis and transplantation units and the cancer chemotherapy unit.

Although the management of the professional activity of the HBsAg-carrier health care worker who has been implicated in hepatitis B transmission to his patient contacts is exceedingly difficult, the following approach may be suggested but is subject to revision as new information becomes available. In the first place, other potential sources of infection, for example, blood transfusion, must be considered and excluded before attributing infection in the contact to transmission from the health care worker. Second, subtyping of the HBsAg of the carrier and the infected patient(s) should be performed. Although identical reactivity would be compatible with transmission between the affected individuals, disparate subtyping would exonerate the carrier and suggest other sources of infection. Third, an immediate review of the techniques of the health care worker must be undertaken to identify possible errors of omission or commission. Fourth, the roster of patient contacts must be assessed to determine whether or not other cases have been recognized. During this period of investigation, temporary suspension of patient-care activity may be necessary while appropriate procedures are relearned and injudicious habits are broken. The HBsAg-positive health care worker subsequently may return to his practice, provided that a formal surveillance program is undertaken and the techniques of patient care are monitored on a regular basis. If recurrent transmission is identified, restrictions on patient care activities must be reinstituted and the practice should be reviewed again. If the carrier continues to infect patient contacts and no technical errors are found on repeated observation, prohibition of practice may be necessary. The medicolegal, ethical, and financial problems associated with transmission of hepatitis from health care worker to patient and the prohibition of practice are enormous. The rights of patients to be free of disease and the civil rights of health professionals may be readily violated by arbitrary actions or lack of action unless extreme caution is exercised.

Risk to the Physician, Nurse, and Other Health Care Workers

Although soul searching among health care workers is important to find better means for reducing even the minimal risk of infecting a patient, the major and by far the most common problem of nosocomial hepatitis is the spread of infection in the other direction: from patients to physicians, nurses, or other health care workers. Therefore, the following recommendations can be made to prevent nosocomial viral hepatitis:

At all times, one must emphasize good personal hygiene when dealing with infected patients, particularly with their blood or blood products or secretions. The same hygienic measures must be enforced in the working environment. All surfaces and utensils potentially contaminated by patients' blood or body fluids must be kept meticulously clean.

In High-Risk Areas of the Hospital. In high-risk areas of the hospital, adequate washing facilities must be available to permit prompt cleansing of hands if contamination might have taken place. Abrasions or open lesions of the skin of health care workers must be reported at the beginning of the work period, not after questionable contamination "might have" occurred.

Food consumption or smoking should not be permitted in an area exposed to patients' secretions or blood or blood products. Foods and drinks must not be kept in refrigerators used for storage of blood or serum.

Gloves must be worn when there is potential exposure to blood (blood drawing) or to secretions of patients who have active hepatitis or who are HBsAg positive.

All needles used in patients with hepatitis or who are HBsAg positive must be discarded in specially labeled containers. Blood or material contaminated with blood must be handled specially and autoclaved before discarding.

In high-risk areas, such as dialysis, transplantation, or oncology-hematology units, surveillance of patients and personnel for HBsAg and anti-HBs should be done periodically; as often as once a month has been recommended.[941] Every patient new to the unit should be screened before assigning him to a health care worker. Where possible anti-HBs-positive health care workers should be assigned to the care of HBsAg-positive patients.

Dialysis equipment should be segregated according to the use of HBsAg-positive or HBsAg-negative patients, and they should not be crossed no matter how well they are cleaned and sterilized.

Patients with acute renal failure should be treated in an area separate from that where chronic renal failure patients receive care.

A record should be kept on all accidents or failures of machinery or equipment and the technicians and patient related to the malfunction. After each use, the nondisposable components of the dialysis machines should be thoroughly cleansed and treated chemically with disinfectants.

Patients with an arteriovenous fistula should be trained in aseptic technique for the care of their shunt and to cannulate their shunt to reduce the exposure of staff to patient's blood. Staff should be gloved whenever a procedure is performed on patients that might even remotely result in contamination with blood or with dialysis fluid or bloody secretions. The staff should wear a disposable uniform while working on the unit, and this should be covered by a clean outer garment whenever they leave the unit. Containers of blood from the dialysis or cancer chemotherapy unit should be so labeled.

The use of transfusions of blood, plasma, or blood products should be reduced to a minimum.

Sharing of food, cigarettes, or other items in the dialysis unit among patients or patients and staff should be avoided during the performance of dialysis.

Containers of blood from patients who have acute hepatitis or who are HBsAg-positive should have a bright, readily identifiable "hepatitis" caution label attached to the container.

In Low-Risk Areas of the Hospital. In low-risk areas of the hospital (general medical and surgical services) there is no need to segregate patients who have either acute hepatitis B or who are carriers of HBsAg. Indeed, as a practical matter, no effort is made to identify those HBsAg-positive patients not clinically suspected of having hepatitis. The anxiety level of administrators rises once the patient is identified as HBsAg positive. If these individuals should be segregated, then all patients and personnel should be routinely screened at frequent intervals. Because such segregation is not warranted, no effort is made to identify asymptomatic carriers. Those who come in contact with the secretions or blood of the HBsAg-positive carrier or patient with acute hepatitis should wear gloves (blood drawing should be done by gloved personnel). Mask and gown need not be worn unless a procedure is performed during which splattering of blood may take place. Food can be served on regular dishes and utensils. These can be handled in a routine manner. Commercial dishwashers are adequate to cleanse and decontaminate the dishes. The patient should be instructed not to share his razor or toothbrush with others.

In Clinical Laboratories. In clinical laboratories, containers that are smeared with blood should not be touched with ungloved hands, regardless of the presence or absence of the hepatitis precaution label on the container. "Hepatitis" label should be on all specimens from patients who are either acutely ill with hepatitis or are HBsAg-positive. This rule should be enforced throughout the hospital. The labeled container should be enclosed in a tough plastic bag.

Request forms soiled with blood should be considered contaminated.

All blood containers should be considered potentially contaminated. They must be opened carefully and handled in the manner to prevent splattering.

"Hepatitis," labeled specimens should be handled with special precautions, preferably by experienced personnel. These should be opened in a special area, preferably in a laminar flow hood. All equipment that comes in contact with blood should be considered contaminated. Gloves

and protective clothing must be used not only when handling patients' blood but also when cleaning or working on equipment, such as the autoanalyzer, in which sera or plasma have been analyzed.

Mouth pipetting of blood products must be avoided. Automatic pipetting devices should be used. Pooled sera should not be used as standards; commercial reference sera are available for this purpose. However, reference sera should be checked for HBsAg before use.

Finally, just as there is no such thing as an unloaded gun, there is no noninfectious blood or serum. There is no currently available technique to detect non-A, non-B agents. Therefore, all blood or sera should be handled as potentially contaminated.

The enforcement of such control measures was successful in reducing the attack rate of hepatitis to one fourth of that experienced in earlier years in British and Danish laboratories.[368,927]

IMMUNOPROPHYLAXIS OF HEPATITIS

Infection control strategies, while of considerable value, have been supplemented and to a large extent superseded by the development of effective and safe immunization techniques. Immunoprophylaxis may be passive, active, or passive-active. In passive immunization protective antibody is administered, in active immunization specific antigenic material (vaccine) is given to induce the formation of protective antibody, and in passive-active immunization both mechanisms are operative.

Principles of Passive Immunization

Serum immune globulins (IG), in the vernacular usually referred to as γ-globulins, were successfully used for the prevention of certain diseases but were much less effective in their therapy. In the case of tetanus, rabies, pertusis, and Rh incompatibilities, IG may be used both as treatment or as prevention. For the replacement of immune globulins in those who have either hypo- or agammaglobulinemia and in patients who are exposed to viral hepatitis, IG is used only as a prophylactic measure. Prophylaxis can be administered either before an anticipated exposure, in which case it is referred to as *preexposure prophylaxis*, or after an exposure has taken place, in which case it is referred to as *postexposure prophylaxis*. In the passive immunoprophylaxis of viral hepatitis, the most extensive experience is based on the prevention of hepatitis A. With the availability of markers for HBV infection and the manufacture of hyperimmune hepatitis B immunoglobulin, also termed hepatitis B immune globulin (HBIG), a great deal of new information became available on passive immunoprophylaxis for hepatitis B. In the absence of serologic markers for the non-A, non-B agents, some, though minimal, information is available concerning the immunoprophylaxis of non-A, non-B hepatitis with immune globulin. Immunoprophylaxis of hepatitis D is a long-term goal.

Immune globulin (IG) is produced in the United States from plasma obtained from outdated donor blood and from fresh plasma collected by plasmapheresis from commercial donors. Each production pool usually includes plasma from thousands of donors. All manufacturers of IG in the United States use modifications of the cold ethanol fractionation technique of Cohn for separation of plasma protein components. American preparations contain 10 g to 18 g of protein per deciliter of which at least 90% must have the electrophoretic characteristics of globulin. Plasma used for IG preparation must be HBsAg negative. Commercial IG consists mostly of immunoglobulins of the IgG class, but low levels of IgA and IgM are also found in most lots.[416] The immunoglobulin in the IG is stabilized with glycine, and thiomerosal (Merthiolate) is added as a preservative. Federal regulations require each lot to contain minimum titers of antibody against diphtheria toxin, measles, and polio type 1 viruses. There are no requirements for the antibody titer either against hepatitis A or hepatitis B virus markers (anti-HAV and anti-HBs). However, testing of IG manufactured in the United States indicates the presence of both antibodies in all lots prepared since 1977.

Satisfactory preparations of concentrated antibodies became available when techniques for large-scale separation of plasma protein components were developed in the early 1940s. The first trial of IG for prevention of hepatitis A was in 1944 during a common-vehicle epidemic at a summer camp in Pennsylvania.[707] Of 53 exposed persons who received the material, only 3, or 5.7%, subsequently experienced hepatitis with jaundice. In contrast, 45% of the other 278 persons had icteric disease. These results were quickly confirmed in two other studies.[329] Thus, the effectiveness of IG was established by field trials within a short time of becoming available. No serious question of its value for the prevention of hepatitis A has subsequently been raised.

The titer of anti-HAV in 62 lots of IG manufactured between 1962 and 1977 remained reasonably stable. The geometric mean titer was approximately 1:1000, with a range of 1:500 to 1:4000.[445]

IG was effective in protecting subjects against hepatitis A when passive immunization was provided by lots with anti-HAV titers ranging from 1:2000 to 1:3200 to 1:10,000, respectively.[389,541,807]

HBIG is manufactured from sera with high titers of anti-HBs. This is obtained from volunteers who acquired natural immunity or whose serum titer is boosted by HBsAg vaccine. While the anti-HBs titer in conventional IG, prepared since 1977 in the United States, is at least 1:100 by radioimmunoassay, in HBIG the titer is in excess of 1:100,000.

Mechanism of Protection

Hepatitis A. It is assumed that IG is protective because it contains type-specific neutralizing antibody to hepatitis A virus: IgG anti-HAV. Experience with hepatitis A indicates that immunity (as reflected by persistence of the protective antibody) in naturally infected populations is long lasting. It is of interest that IG from a population in one area of the world seems to protect adequately against hepatitis A that occurs in other, distant areas.[108,324,686,788]

Passive immunization can suppress either the infection itself or its clinical manifestations only. There is adequate evidence that in many cases, IG suppresses only the clinical illness caused by hepatitis A virus. This was first documented by Drake and Ming during an institutional outbreak.[239] Using conventional liver tests to detect inapparent hepatitis, they demonstrated that attack rates in immunized persons were similar to those in unimmunized persons. Inapparent infections occurred during the first 8 weeks after IG administration in persons who received a dose of 0.01 mg/kg, but continued for 13 weeks in the group that received 0.02 ml/kg. The incidence of anicteric hepatitis (illness without clinical jaundice) during the first 4 weeks after administration of IG was also lower in those who received the larger dose. These observations suggest that with a larger dose not only are the clinical manifestations suppressed, but the infection is prevented altogether.

By serum aminotransferase assay, inapparent infection in IG-protected persons has been extensively confirmed. Schneider and Mosley found that for household contacts who received IG in a community-wide epidemic, the incidence of serum aspartic aminotransferase abnormality was equivalent to that for those to whom protection had not been given.[877] Almost all such abnormalities were observed within 36 days after onset of the index case, which indicates that most of these persons were in the incubation phase at the time IG was given. Krugman and co-workers found, in an institutional study, that aminotransferase and other laboratory abnormalities occurred at the same rate among those who received IG on admission as residents who were not protected.[552] In this situation, infection followed passive immunization, which indicates that modification is also applicable to those not already effectively exposed to the agent.

The half-life of IG[411] is often used as a guide to the duration of protection and the time for administration of subsequent doses. The most frequently cited values are those obtained by Dixon and co-workers using ^{131}I: 20.3 days in children and 13.1 days in adults.[237] Results using ^{35}S labeling of autogenously synthesized γ-globulin indicate slower metabolism, a half-life of 33 to 37 days.[39,1037] Martin and co-workers, measuring antibody by biologic assay, found various rates of degradation for antibodies with different antigenic affinities.[630] The mean half-life of antibodies ranged from 21.7 days for coxsackie virus A 10 to 44.9 days for adenovirus type 2. The half-life of anti-HBs, after injection of HBIG was about 27 days,[362] in one study. In another study mean half-lives of anti-HBs varied between 17.5 and 25 days, with a range of 5.9 to 35 days.[874]

Inapparent infection was suspected by Stokes and associates on the basis of subsequent absence of icteric illness despite continued exposure. They suggested that partial passive immunity conferred by IG was supplanted by active immunity as a result of "low-grade" infection ("passive-active" immunization).[962] They challenged part of an institutional population protected by IG more than 1 year earlier and found a significantly lower rate of induced hepatitis A than in a control group. Such protection could be explained only on the basis of active immunity due to inapparent infection. The fact that IG permits asymptomatic infections does not exclude the possibility, however, that large doses administered before infection or early in the incubation period may suppress infection entirely.

Hepatitis B. Although there is general agreement that anti-HBs is the protective, neutralizing antibody against HBV and that an immune globulin containing high titers of anti-HBs is more effective for immunoprophylaxis than one that does not contain high titers of this antibody,[639] conflicting studies[475,757] indicate that our knowledge of this area is still fragmentary. Despite these caveats, most would agree that a prompt (within hours to a few days) injection of the immune globulin after exposure increases the likelihood of protection as compared with one given several days later.[673] One of the reasons why prompt immunoprophylaxis is necessary with a specific antibody-containing immune globulin is that the interval between exposure and antigenemia may be as short as 6 days,[549] and viremia can precede detectable HBs antigenemia. Absolute protection cannot be guaranteed even when immune globulin with large amounts of anti-HBs is administered. The incidence of typical hepatitis is 1.4% to 9.8% after HBIG therapy for incidental exposure to small-dose HBsAg-positive material.[174,362,892,1057] Following low-dose exposure (needlestick) to HBsAg-positive material, the risk of overt hepatitis is low, probably no more than 6% even in persons who do not receive anti-HBs containing globulin.[892]

The dose of anti-HBs required to provide an acceptable degree of protection remains controversial, at least in part because during the past 15 years, commercial IG lots have undergone major changes regarding their content of hepatitis B virus markers.[363,445] In one study, 62 lots of IG were tested that were manufactured between 1962 and 1977. The anti-HAV titers in these lots remained reasonably constant. However, striking changes took place in the anti-HBs content of IG lots that were manufactured after 1972. The percentage of lots that contained anti-HBs rose from 29% in the 1962 to 1972 decade to 100% in the 1972 to 1975 period. Furthermore, the mean anti-HBs titer ranged from less than 1:10 during the 1962 to 1972 decade but rose to an average of 1:500 in commercial IG lots manufactured after 1972.[445] The changing anti-HBs titer is only one of the variables that further complicates the interpretation of studies that compared commercial IG with HBIG. IG lots manufactured from sera collected before 1972 (when widespread screening for HBsAg began) not only contained no detectable or only low titers of anti-HBs, but also contained HBsAg in the form of immune complexes. Free HBsAg was rarely detectable in any of these IG lots. The HBsAg-containing immune complexes raise the possibility that the antigen could have been freed from the immune complex *in vivo* after injection of IG and could be responsible for the production of active immunity.[451] However, there is no experimental, clinical, or epidemiologic evidence to support this hypothesis by demonstrating the development of active immunity to HBsAg after IG injection in subjects not naturally exposed to HBsAg. Although it is clear that passive-active immunity developed after IG was given as immunoprophylaxis for HBV infection, it is not clear that it was due to the presence of small amounts of HBsAg in the IG, although this remains a distinct possibility.[25,445] However, this assumption fails to consider the presence of HBsAg inoculated by the initial exposure that led to the need for IG immunoprophylaxis. Furthermore, passive-active immunity developed also after immunoprophylaxis with HBIG, which did not contain any HBsAg.[549]

The selection of the immunoglobulin for postexposure prophylaxis is based on the interpretation of data collected by three prospective randomized clinical trials. The first was conducted in a small group of children and was published in 1973.[543] Here the infectious inoculum was high, HBIG was injected promptly (4 hours after infection), and four of the ten children developed hepatitis B. Importantly, there was clear-cut evidence for prolongation of the incubation period both for the clinical manifestations of hepatitis B and for the development of HBsAg in this optimally protected (HBIG) group compared with the IG-treated group, control, or untreated children. A similar prolongation of the incubation period of hepatitis B in HBIG-protected individuals was also noted in two other studies.[362] In the second study,[362] persons contaminated by needlestick were randomized into three categories and received (1) commercial IG with an anti-HBs titer of 1:50 (low) group, (2) HBIG with an anti-HBs titer of 1:500,000 (high), and (3) an intermediate titer group in which the immunoglobulin contained an anti-HBs titer of 1:5,000. Subjects received 3 ml of their respective globulins within 7 days of their needlestick and a second injection between 25 and 35 days. During the first 5 months there was significant protection in the group that received HBIG; however, by 9 months this difference disappeared. A third randomized clinical trial compared HBIG with commercial IG that had no detectable anti-HBs titer.[892] The HBIG had an anti-HBs titer of 1:100,000. Subjects received the respective globulins within 1 week of exposure and again 28 days later. There was a statistically significant reduction of clinically overt hepatitis B during the first 6 months of the follow-up period—in the HBIG-protected group 1.4% and in the commercial IG-treated group 5.9%—a significant difference. However, when seroconversion and clinical hepatitis cases were combined, there was no significant difference between the HBIG and IG-treated groups. In this study, therefore, HBIG modified but did not prevent HBV infection by needlestick in a higher proportion of patients than did IG that did not contain anti-HBs by radioimmunoassay.

A large body of data support the notion that HBIG is the globulin of choice for passive immunoprophylaxis of hepatitis B.[893] However, it is considerably more expensive, varying from $150 to $200 per injection, $300 to $400 for a course of two injections, as opposed to $10 to $25 for commercial IG, and the protective efficacy of HBIG has rarely exceeded 75% to 80%.

Hepatitis D. Passive immunization for the prevention of HDV infection is not available.

Non-A, Non-B Hepatitis. *Post-transfusion.* Table 15-12 lists three randomized double-blind studies on the efficacy of 10 ml IG versus albumin placebo injected within a week after the transfusions. One of the studies[555] failed to show any benefit attributable to IG. The other two studies[522,897] showed reduction of the incidence of icteric but not of nonicteric hepatitis. The three studies were of similar design. They included a total of 2678 transfused patients of whom 10.4% of placebo and 8.3% of IG treated recipients developed hepatitis. This difference is not significant.

The absence of clear evidence of benefit attributable to IG prophylaxis and the high cost of giving IG to each transfused patient[454,1058] are important arguments against the routine use of IG prophylaxis to prevent post-transfusion hepatitis. Furthermore, it is now well demonstrated that selection of blood donors has a profound effect on the incidence of post-transfusion hepatitis. Selection of volunteer donors, eliminating single unit transfusions (which are hardly if ever justifiable), rigorous restraint in the use of blood and blood products for transfusion when other forms of therapy would suffice, and, possibly, exclusion of donors with elevated serum alanine aminotransferase levels can more effectively reduce the frequency of post-transfusion hepatitis than IG immunoprophylaxis. Beyond these considerations there is the overriding consideration that to give 0.1 ml to 0.2 ml/kg of IG for each transfused patient would exhaust the immune globulin production potential of the world. In this setting, one must consider that the United States cannot import serum for IG production from other countries without providing those same countries with IG for their immunoprophylaxis programs.[477,499,1058]

Contact and Other Exposures. There is little information on the effect of IG or HBIG on post- or pre-exposure prophylaxis of blood-borne or the epidemic form of non-A, non-B hepatitis. It is possible that antibody titers to non-A, non-B agents are sufficient in IG to provide effective protection to exposed persons. Recommendations for immunoprophylaxis are presently arbitrary and will have to be evaluated when serologic markers for the non-A, non-B agents become available.[1033]

Side-Effects

Adverse reactions are generally limited to pain and tenderness at the injection site. Hematomas are seen occasionally, especially in patients who are receiving anticoagulants, especially if large amounts of globulin are given at a single site. The few reported cases of anaphylactic shock may have been due to inadvertent intravenous injection.

The frequency of adverse reactions is between 0.8% and 1.2% in recipients of intramuscular IG in three separate studies.[479,705,897] These side-effects to IG injections may not be unique for the immunoglobulin content of the injected material because 0.7% of 11,010 patients who received albumin placebo developed similar reactions. However, when IG injections are given repeatedly, such as in immunoglobulin-deficient children, then allergic reactions become increasingly more frequent.[1038] In contrast to the relative safety and freedom from toxic side-effects following intramuscular injection of IG, 3% of normals and 92% of immunodeficient individuals developed toxic reactions following the intravenous injection of IG.[52]

Despite the relative safety of intramuscular IG, anaphylactic shock or angioneurotic edema did develop in a few patients.[64,742]

The stimulation of antibodies to heterologous immunoglobulin types in the Gm system has been demonstrated.[16,958] On this basis, the question of later adverse reactions to IG administration has been raised, although no definitely documented case has been reported. An even more likely consequence would be the subsequent shortening of passive immunity, although this has not yet been demonstrated either.

TABLE 15-12. Effect of IG on the Incidence of Post-transfusion Non-A, Non-B Hepatitis

| NUMBER OF PATIENTS | PERCENT DEVELOPING NON-A, NON-B HEPATITIS | | | | REFERENCE |
| | Anicteric | | Icteric | | |
	IG	Placebo	IG	Placebo	
2204	6.9	7.7	0.8	1.8	897
279	4.9	5.3	1.1	7.4	522
195	11.8	8.8	6.4	7.8	555

Infectivity of Immune Globulin

Although immune globulins are used to prevent viral hepatitis, some contaminated lots can cause outbreaks of HBV or non-A, non-B hepatitis. HBV contamination may be due to the fact that the γ-globulin was isolated from massively infected lots of serum or that the production technique was improper. For example, free HBsAg has rarely been found in IG lots isolated by cold ethanol fractionation. γ-Globulin lots prepared by other techniques, such as zinc or ammonium sulfate precipitation, may not provide the safety against HBV contamination that the cold ethanol precipitation does. Outbreaks of hepatitis B infection have been reported after immunization with zinc- or ammonium sulfate–precipitated IG[485,763] produced by non-United States manufacturers. Furthermore, IG prepared by cold ethanol fractionation has twice the protection efficacy against hepatitis A of that prepared by ammonium sulfate precipitation.[686] Neither IG nor HBIG have been contaminated by the etiologic agent of the acquired immune deficiency syndrome (AIDS), the human T-lymphotropic virus type III/lymphadenopathy-associated virus (HTLV-III/LAV), and transmission of AIDS through IG or HBIG administration has not been reported.[140]

PRINCIPLES OF ACTIVE IMMUNIZATION

Hepatitis A Virus Vaccine

Inactivated HAV Vaccine. A formalin-inactivated HAV vaccine has been prepared from HAV-infected marmosets and tested in these animals.[789] The partially purified formalin-treated final vaccine preparation contained 1.4×10^{10} viral particles per milliliter and induced anti-HAV in all inoculated animals. Repeated subcutaneous administration of this inactivated vaccine provided complete protection against subsequent challenge with live HAV. Intravenous administration of this vaccine, given on a single occasion only, provided partial protection against HAV infection. Despite the success of these studies in demonstrating the feasibility of developing an inactivated HAV vaccine, the development of live, attenuated and genetic recombinant vaccines has become the major focus of research efforts.

Attenuated HAV Vaccine. Serial passage of HAV in fetal rhesus monkey kidney cells and human diploid embryonic lung fibroblasts resulted in attenuation of virulence for both marmosets[795] and chimpanzees.[277,796] Primates inoculated with appropriately attenuated HAV variants showed little or no alterations in serum enzymes or liver histopathology, indicating low degrees of viral replication. On subsequent challenge with live, virulent HAV, vaccinated animals were resistant to infection. Selected variants with suitable virulence/attenuation ratios will be studied in humans to determine the immunogenicity,

protective efficacy, and safety of these experimental vaccines. The ideal attenuated, live HAV vaccine should be cheap, induce high levels of protective antibody for prolonged periods, induce intestinal immunity on oral administration, remain stable on serial passage, and be easily distinguished serologically from wild HAV strains. Whether any of the present prototype vaccines will meet these criteria remains uncertain at this time.

Genetic Recombinant HAV Vaccines. The RNA genome of HAV has been molecularly cloned, and complementary DNA (cDNA) copies of the viral RNA have been used to determine the entire nucleotide sequence of the genome.[703] It should be possible to identify that segment responsible for the expression of immunogenic HAV antigens and introduce that segment into bacterial cells. The immunogenic peptides produced by the cloned DNA in the bacteria could be purified and used as vaccine. Another approach involves the splicing of antigenic HAV cDNA segments into the DNA genome of other, attenuated viruses used as vaccines, thereby forming chimeric, polyvalent vaccines. A third approach, also using recombinant techniques, would identify the amino acid sequences of the immunogenic peptides by analysis of the nucleotide sequences coding for these peptides. Chemical synthesis of immunogenic peptides could then be achieved and the synthetic peptides used as vaccine. Whether progress in the development of these molecular biology–derived vaccines will be sufficiently rapid to outpace the development of live, attenuated vaccines remains to be determined.

Impact of HAV Vaccines. Although HAV infection has no known link to chronic hepatitis, cirrhosis, or primary hepatocellular carcinoma, it is an important source of morbidity and economic losses. An effective, safe, and low cost vaccine would be highly beneficial. In the United States and other developed nations specific targeted populations would include health care workers caring for children, workers in institutions for the mentally retarded and in day-care centers, homosexual men, military and foreign service personnel stationed in endemic parts of the world, and missionaries and tourists visiting high-risk areas. Routine immunization of the general population may be considered if the cost–benefit ratio is highly beneficial.

Hepatitis B Virus Vaccine

Historical Background. The first attempts to develop a vaccine against hepatitis B were made in the early 1970s by Krugman and his associates. Heat-treated infective serum was used because it was known to contain HBV.[543,544,547] The tenfold diluted serum heated at 98° C for 1 minute was partially inactivated and produced sufficient immunity to prevent the development of hepatitis in 70% of susceptible children who were challenged with the original infectious serum 4 to 8 months after vaccination.

The immunizing antigen of this prototype vaccine appeared to be the 22-nm HBsAg particle. These studies indicated that the serum or plasma of HBV-infected individuals could serve as the source of HBsAg particles, which, after extraction, purification, and exposure to virus-inactivating agents, could serve as an immunogenic and protective HBV vaccine.

Production of Plasma-Derived Vaccine. The only HBV vaccine currently available in the United States (Heptavax B, Merck Sharp & Dohme, West Point, PA) is prepared from the pooled plasma of asymptomatic, healthy, high-titer HBsAg carriers. HBsAg particles in the plasma pool are concentrated, isolated, and partially purified by exposure to ammonium sulfate, isopycnic banding in sodium bromide, and rate-zonal sedimentation in a sucrose gradient. These biophysical separation procedures can remove 10^4 chimpanzee infectious doses per milliliter of HBV.[335] The partially purified HBsAg particles are treated with pepsin (1 mg/liter, pH 2.1, 37° C, 18 hr), which digests residual plasma proteins and inactivates rhabdoviruses, poxviruses, togaviruses, herpesviruses, coronaviruses, and reoviruses as well as 10^5 chimpanzee infectious doses per milliliter of HBV.[989] Treatment with 8 M urea for 4 hours, which inactivates myxoviruses, picornaviruses, and the slow viruses, follows, and after dialysis the HBsAg particles are further treated with a 1:4000 formaldehyde solution at 37° C for 72 hours. Formaldehyde inactivates parvoviruses, retroviruses, at least one (possibly both) of the blood-borne non-A, non-B hepatitis viruses, and the hepatitis D virus. Both the urea and formaldehyde treatment steps are capable of inactivating 10^5 chimpanzee infectious doses per milliliter of HBV.[989] All three treatment procedures (pepsin, urea, and formaldehyde) can inactivate all known classes of animal viruses.

The final product is adsorbed to an alum adjuvant, and thimerosol, 1:20,000, is added as a preservative. Prior to release each lot of vaccine is tested for sterility, pyrogenicity, and inactivation of adventitial infectious agents by inoculation into tissue culture systems, small animals, and chimpanzees. The final product contains 20 μg/ml of HBsAg protein.

Other plasma-derived HBV vaccines have been produced by foreign manufacturers.[184,637,990] The single or double inactivation procedures used in the preparation of these vaccines appears to increase their immunogenicity when compared with the triple inactivation used in the preparation of Heptavax B. Whether they are as safe as the triply inactivated vaccine remains to be determined. In any case, the bulk of clinical experience has been with the triple-inactivated plasma-derived vaccine.

Future HBV Vaccines. Alternative sources of HBsAg for vaccine production have received considerable attention in recent years.[798] These include the purification of HBsAg from genetically engineered eukaryotic and prokaryotic cells and the synthesis of immunogenic HBsAg polypeptides predicted from the nucleotide sequence of the HBV genome. Other approaches include the insertion of the HBsAg gene into live virus vectors (*e.g.,* vaccinia virus),[689] enhancement of immunogenicity by administration of specific anti-idiotype antibodies,[505] or the use of such antibodies as vaccines without HBsAg administration.[241] Considerable progress has been made in the development of a genetically engineered vaccine. Recombinant plasmids that induce yeast cells to produce HBsAg have been developed and the nonglycosylated HBsAg particles synthesized by the yeast have been formulated into a vaccine. Preliminary studies indicate that this recombinant-produced vaccine may be as immunogenic and safe as the plasma-derived vaccine.[484,887] Clinical availability will be dependent on efficacy trials that are currently underway.

Plasma-Derived Vaccine: Storage, Route of Administration, and Dose. The plasma-derived triple-inactivated vaccine must be stored at 2° C to 8° C (36° F–46° F). Freezing alters the consistency of the vaccine and reduces its immunogenicity.[653] Occasional instances of nonresponsiveness may be attributable to improper storage of vaccine vials. A variety of routes of administration have been studied: intramuscular, subcutaneous, and intradermal. Limited data suggest that all three routes elicit protective antibody, but intramuscular inoculation is the route of choice; subcutaneous and intradermal inoculation may lead to the formation of transient nodules or macules at the injection site, and the duration of protective antibody has not been established for either of these routes.[218,578,660,1105] However, because the reduced doses of vaccine used in these injections may lower the costs of vaccination, the intradermal and subcutaneous routes require further study. The recommended site for intramuscular injection is the deltoid in adults or the anterolateral thigh muscle in newborns and infants; injection in the buttock is associated with reduced immunogenicity.[142] In hemophiliacs, subcutaneous inoculation may be the preferred route in order to prevent muscle hemorrhage.

Intramuscular injections of vaccine preparations containing 5 μg to 40 μg HBsAg protein have elicited the development of anti-HBs in 90% to 100% of healthy, immune-competent recipients.[893] Although no important differences in seroconversion rates have been identified in these studies, in one study measurement of anti-HBs titer suggested a direct correlation between dose and titer of antibody elicited.[439] The recommended dose of the plasma-derived, triple-inactivated vaccine for adults and children over 10 years of age is currently 20 μg (1.0 ml).[141] Children under 10 years of age are vaccinated with 10 μg (0.5 ml) per dose. In patients on maintenance hemodialysis and in immunocompromised individuals, a 40-μg (2.0-ml) dose has been suggested despite seroconversion rates that are considerably lower (60% to 80%) than in healthy individuals.[893]

The currently recommended vaccination schedule is a three-dose regimen: the first dose is followed 1 month later by the second dose, and the third dose is given 6 months after the initial one.[141] The first two doses appear to act as "priming" doses that induce anti-HBs in 85% to 95% of healthy recipients. An additional 5% to 10% will seroconvert after the third (booster) dose. The third dose enhances the anti-HBs titer by 10-fold and appears to be critically important for the prolonged presence of circulating anti-HBs.[653] The third dose can be given at 9 or 12 months after the initial dose without impeding the enhancement of anti-HBs titers.

HBV vaccines containing one subtype of HBsAg (ad) protect against infection with HBV associated with another HBsAg subtype (ay).[981]

Immunogenicity and Protective Efficacy. Field trials of the triply-inactivated HBV vaccine have shown that among susceptible healthy individuals who develop anti-HBs after the full three-dose vaccine schedule, protective efficacy approaches 100%.[976,980] These data strongly support the notion that anti-HBs is the protective, neutralizing antibody and that vaccine-induced antibody confers protection against clinically apparent hepatitis B and the development of the HBsAg carrier state. In the best designed, executed, and analyzed trials, conducted by Szmuness and his colleagues,[976,980,981] protective efficacy could be correlated with the strength of the immune response to the vaccine. In a beautifully conceived and meticulously performed double-blind, randomized clinical trial, 1083 homosexual men known to be at high risk for HBV infection were studied.[976,980] Among the 549 HBV vaccine recipients, 95.4% developed measurable levels of anti-HBs. In 90.5% of vaccine recipients, anti-HBs levels were more than 20 sample ratio units (SRU) as measured by radioimmunoassay, 2.9% had levels between 10 and 20 SRU, and 2% had 2.2 to 9 SRU. A SRU of 2.1 is used to define a positive test result. Among the vaccinated men who developed HBV events after the third (booster) dose, 7 of 9 had failed to respond to the vaccine (<2.1 SRU), 1 had had a SRU less than 10, and only 1 had had a SRU greater than 10. These data suggest that vaccine-induced antibody levels greater than 10 SRU are generally associated with nearly complete protection. As a corollary, in prevaccination screening to identify immune individuals, anti-HBs levels of at least 10 SRU appear to serve as a practical, if imperfect, guide[1063]: individuals with levels below 10 SRU should be vaccinated, while withholding vaccine seems appropriate for those with higher levels.

In addition to demonstrating its protective efficacy when given prior to exposure, the landmark vaccine studies of Szmuness and his co-workers in homosexual men[976,980] also provided data supporting the concept that vaccination given after exposure may be partially effective. Although the frequency of HBV infection was nearly identical in vaccine and placebo recipients during the first 60 days of the study, the infection appeared to be modified to a milder form in vaccinated individuals. Thus vaccination given shortly after exposure may have some protective value.

Although a 40-μg HBsAg protein dose was employed in the initial studies, subsequent trials confirmed the immunogenicity and protective efficacy of a 20-μg, three-dose schedule.[298,981] In healthy individuals, the most important determinant of the immune response to vaccination appears to be the age of the recipient. In infants and children (aged 1 to 19 years) the seroconversion rate, measured 1 month after the third dose, was 100%. In those between 20 and 39 years of age the seroconversion rate was 98%. The rate fell to 91% in adults aged 40 to 59 years and to 85% in individuals aged 60 to 79 years. Although healthy women may have a better immune response to the vaccine than healthy men,[207] the differences appear to be slight and inconsequential. In fact, in some studies gender-related differences in immune responsiveness have not been detected among healthy subjects.[231] However, in immunocompromised individuals, such as hemodialysis patients, women have had a higher seroconversion rate and higher titers of vaccine-induced anti-HBs.[955]

Overall, the most important determinant of vaccine-induced immune responsiveness (and protective efficacy) is the immunologic status of the recipient. Immunocompromised individuals, such as patients undergoing maintenance hemodialysis, renal transplant recipients, developmentally disadvantaged persons, patients with malignant disease, and those receiving immunosuppressive chemotherapy have a reduced, delayed, or less persistent anti-HBs response, regardless of the dose employed.[893] Although failure to respond to the vaccine in otherwise healthy individuals might suggest the presence of an occult disorder of the immunologic system, there is no support for this notion. In fact, limited data suggest that 25% to 40% of nonresponders will produce adequate anti-HBs levels when revaccinated. Furthermore, nonresponders who subsequently become infected by HBV appear to have entirely typical responses to the acute infection and are not at increased risk of becoming HBsAg carriers.

Persistence of Protection. The duration of anti-HBs after vaccination has yet to be established. In limited studies of vaccinated children between 1 and 10 years of age, all had detectable anti-HBs, with a slight decline in titers, 3 years after the initial dose.[653] In adults, peak anti-HBs levels are reached 9 to 12 months after the initial dose. Subsequently, the titer of anti-HBs falls fairly briskly through the 18th month and then declines more gradually. At 3 to 4 years after vaccination 10% to 15% have lost detectable anti-HBs. Despite loss of anti-HBs, revaccination with a single booster dose results in a dramatic anamnestic response.[653] Furthermore, some individuals who have lost their vaccine-induced anti-HBs appear to be protected against clinical disease when exposed to HBV.[893] All in all, these data suggest that the majority of vaccinated individuals will retain anti-HBs and remain protected for at least 4 years. A single booster dose of 20 μg given in the fifth year may provide continuing protection for another 4 to 5 years.

Vaccination of HBsAg Carriers and Immune Individuals. Administration of the HBV vaccine to HBsAg carriers, with or without elevated serum aminotransferase levels, has failed to reduce the titer of circulating HBsAg or stimulate the development of anti-HBs.[224] No serious adverse reactions were recognized in vaccinated carriers. Vaccine administration in individuals with pre-existing anti-HBs may induce an anamnestic rise in titer but will not cause adverse reactions.[1063] The presence of passively acquired anti-HBs (*e.g., from* HBIG administration) will not interfere with the immune response to the vaccine.[979]

Adverse Reactions. The major immediate side-effect of vaccine administration has been transient pain or soreness at the injection site, which occurs in 10% to 15% of adult vaccines. Short-lived, low-grade fever is reported in less than 3%, and other minor side-effects such as headache, fatigue, malaise, nausea, rash, arthralgias, myalgias, and respiratory distress are seen in less than 1% of recipients. The Guillain-Barré syndrome and instances of aseptic meningitis, transverse myelitis, and grand-mal seizures have been reported in vaccine recipients but appear to represent background illness etiologically unrelated to the HBV vaccine.[893] Transmission of the acquired immune deficiency syndrome (AIDS) is not a consequence of vaccination.[5]

Although the safety of the vaccine in the pregnant woman has not been definitively established in field trials, there is no reason to believe that it has deleterious effects. Hence, pregnancy is not a contraindication to the use of the vaccine.

Hepatitis D Virus and Non-A, Non-B Hepatitis Vaccines

Vaccines for the immunoprophylaxis of HDV and non-A, non-B hepatitis virus infections are not available.

Principles of Passive-Active Immunization

Passive-active immunization refers to the production of immediate but short-term protection resulting from the administration of protective antibody usually in the form of immune globulin (IG) combined with the formation of long-lasting protective antibody resulting from either natural exposure to an infectious agent or vaccine-induced immunization.

Hepatitis A

In HAV infection passive-active immunization might develop if the passively administered anti-HAV in IG is capable of neutralizing the infecting dose of naturally acquired HAV just incompletely enough to prevent the clinical manifestations of hepatitis; yet HAV antigens are recognized sufficiently enough by immunocompetent cells to stimulate the production of active immunity. Although passive-active immunization occurs in HAV it appears to

be an infrequent event and the factors affecting its development, such as dose of antibody administered, timing, and virus inoculum size, remain poorly understood. For example, in one experimental study, only two of eight children who received the same mixture of HAV-containing serum and IG within the same time interval developed evidence of passive-active immunization, whereas the remaining six acquired only passive immunity.[541]

Hepatitis B

A number of studies of combined passive immunization with HBIG and active immunization with plasma-derived HBV vaccine have revealed that passively acquired anti-HBs does not interfere with the immune response to the vaccine and that the vaccine does not affect the level of circulating anti-HBs resulting from HBIG administration.[979,1097] Combined passive-active immunization appears to entail no additional risks, and no immune-complex mediated illness has been identified in individuals simultaneously inoculated with HBIG and vaccine.

The pioneering field trials of the combined regimen of HBIG and vaccine, undertaken in infants born to HBsAg- and HBeAg-positive mothers in Taiwan, have provided evidence that the protective efficacy of the combination (approaching 95%) is considerably greater than that of HBIG or vaccine alone (70% to 75%).[68-70] Subsequent trials of combined passive-active immunization of newborns at high risk for perinatal transmission of HBV in Hong Kong, Japan, Korea, and the United States (in Asian-American women) have confirmed these observations.[159,491,957,1081] The frequency of development of the carrier state was dramatically reduced by passive-active immunization of these infants and protective levels of anti-HBs appeared to persist for prolonged periods.[957] Prophylaxis failure has been attributed, at least in part, to infection *in utero*. Although differences in dose, dose schedule, and vaccine source may account for some of the variation in protective efficacy reported in these studies, and the ideal regimen has yet to be established, on theoretical grounds it seems reasonable to begin immunization as quickly as possible after birth.

Whether passive-active immunization is more effective than passive immunization alone in other settings in which postexposure prophylaxis is recommended has not yet been established.

Hepatitis D and Non-A, Non-B Hepatitis

Passive-active immunization is not available for the immunoprophylaxis of these infections.

Recommendations for Immunoprophylaxis of Hepatitis A

Pre-exposure Prophylaxis of Hepatitis A

Immune globulin prevents disease when administered prior to exposure. Its use for this purpose, particularly among Americans abroad, has increased greatly in recent years. In fact, international travel or residence abroad is the major indication for pre-exposure prophylaxis of hepatitis A.

The systematic use of IG to prevent hepatitis A among persons in high-risk areas was begun by the Swedish. As early as 1956, a contingent of Swedish troops serving under the auspices of the United Nations in the Gaza Strip received this material, and it was used regularly after 1957.[517] The incidence of viral hepatitis was reduced from 4.0% among unprotected Swedish soldiers to 0.1%. Marked reductions were achieved in other Scandinavian contingents for which the practice was adopted.

Through the late 1950s, the frequent occurrence of viral hepatitis among some Americans abroad was often mentioned, but no reports appeared in the medical literature. Some use of IG to protect individual travelers probably began during this time. By 1961, when the first groups of Peace Corps Volunteers went abroad, the possibility that hepatitis A could be a significant hazard was sufficiently well known that IG was made available for individual units on an optional basis. Some unprotected contingents remained free of the disease; two unprotected groups in South America, however, had rates of 14%. As a result, the measure became mandatory. Subsequent rates were

approximately one half of the previous rates and approximately one third of those in missionaries.[1083]

Data were collected on the incidence of viral hepatitis in American missionaries, who have generally served abroad without having IG prophylaxis. The overall risk for Protestant missionaries and their dependents was 1.6% per year in one study.[164] Rates were highest among younger adults and varied with the area of residence. The incidence per 100 adults per year ranged from 0.5 in Japan to 8.0 in North Africa and the Middle East. Other studies have shown similarly high rates.[297,1082] Geographic variations in incidence based on a survey of 8363 persons are shown in Figure 15-37.[504] All such studies have demonstrated that a high risk continues for 10 years or more.

On the other hand, short-term travelers have a relatively low risk. Two studies have demonstrated that the hazard of icteric disease is less than 1 per 1000 persons.[502,503] Travelers to highly developed countries in western Europe, to Japan, and to Australia appear to have no greater risk of hepatitis A than travelers visiting the United States.

From these data it is possible to state that Americans residing 4 months or more in countries in which the risk has been found to be high should receive 0.06 ml/kg of IG every 4 to 6 months; those remaining for 3 months or less need only 0.02 ml/kg on one occasion.[469,788] Although

Fig. 15-37. Case rates of icteric viral hepatitis per 100 person-years of experience abroad among American missionaries, 1950–1970. The highest incidence was in the Middle East, North Africa, and Latin America. (Kendrick MA: J Infect Dis 129:227, 1974)

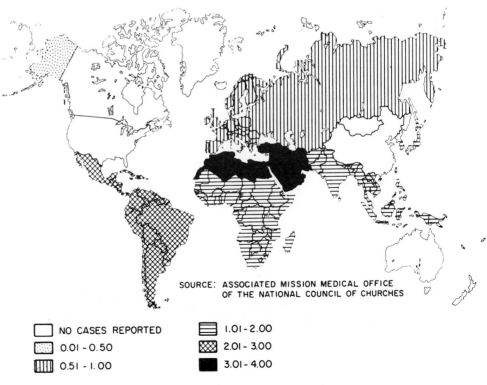

SOURCE: ASSOCIATED MISSION MEDICAL OFFICE OF THE NATIONAL COUNCIL OF CHURCHES

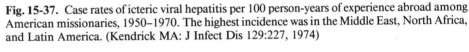

NO CASES REPORTED   1.01 - 2.00
0.01 - 0.50   2.01 - 3.00
0.51 - 1.00   3.01 - 4.00

susceptible travelers staying in the usual tourist accommodations may have a lower risk of infection than those who "go native," prophylaxis remains a reasonable measure for both groups.

Screening for IgG anti-HAV prior to travel to avoid the unnecessary administration of IG to immune individuals seems reasonable, particularly for frequent travelers to high-risk areas and those with a past history of "hepatitis."

Postexposure Prophylaxis of Hepatitis A

On the basis of controlled clinical trials, commercial IG reduced the attack rate of clinically recognizable hepatitis A by 80% to 90% in the United States,[563] by 80% in New Zealand,[36] and by 84% to 87% in the United Kingdom.[41] Experience indicates that 0.01 ml to 0.02 ml/kg protects as adequately as larger doses.[239,294] A single intramuscular dose of 0.02 ml/kg is recommended by the Immunization Practices Advisory Committee for postexposure prophylaxis of hepatitis A.[141]

Because the incubation period is relatively long, IG can be administered to many susceptibles before onset of symptoms. This is particularly true for household contacts. IG can be given to persons exposed to a common source if it is recognized sufficiently early. The course of several epidemics due to a common vehicle has been truncated by administration of IG to those known to have been exposed.[687,810] The earlier in the incubation period IG is given, the more likely it is to have a protective effect.[538] It is worthwhile, however, to administer IG up to 6 weeks after known exposure. The Immunization Practices Advisory Committee recommends that IG postexposure prophylaxis is not indicated if more than 2 weeks have elapsed after exposure to hepatitis A.[141]

Household Contacts. In the United States, the secondary attack rate among household contacts is frequently high. Rates of icteric disease have been as great as 45% among children. The incidence of secondary infections has been lower in adults but is nonetheless 5% to 20%. As a result, the usual practice in the United States is to administer IG to all household contacts as soon as the index case is diagnosed. Indeed, protection of susceptible household contacts is an integral part of the care of the patient. Determination of susceptible versus immune contacts by measurement of anti-HAV prior to IG injection is a valid notion but is not presently cost effective and would delay IG administration.

In some instances, it is considered unnecessary to administer IG to adults because of the low attack rate in this group. Although the incidence is lower in persons 20 years of age and over, it is sufficiently high after household exposure to warrant protection. The illness in adults is more serious and of greater economic consequences for the family. Even grandparents or other older adults living in the household should receive IG. Instances of severe or even fatal illnesses in older, unprotected persons have come to our attention.

School Contacts. Although school-centered epidemics occur in the United States, epidemiologic evidence suggests that neighborhood play contact among children of school age is of more importance than classroom contact. For this reason, it does not appear justified to administer IG on a school-wide or classroom-wide basis unless there is clear evidence that infections are being acquired at the school itself.

Day-Care Centers. IG has been shown to be effective in the control of hepatitis A in day-care centers.[385] Contact within the facility and the presence of diapered children appear to be responsible for the spread of HAV. IG should be given to all attending children and center employees if hepatitis A is recognized in either group or in the households of attending children. IG should also be considered for the household contacts of non-toilet-trained children attending a day-care center if hepatitis A is recognized in more than two or three households in which a child is attending the center.

Institutions. Institutions are comparable to households in the intimacy of contact, and high attack rates similar to secondary rates in households sometimes occur. Explosive epidemics are particularly likely when hygiene is poor, as among the mentally retarded or regressed psychiatric patients, or when sanitation is substandard, a common finding in some prisons. When hepatitis A threatens to become rampant, use of IG is justified.

In general, hepatitis A in institutions for custodial care shows three patterns: (1) freedom from disease for long periods, followed by explosive epidemics; (2) sporadic cases with occasional epidemics of limited extent; and (3) continuous endemic hepatitis. The third pattern is usually seen only in large institutions with high rates of admission and discharge.

In institutions largely or entirely free of the disease, IG is administered to cottage, dormitory, or ward mates having close contact with patients with hepatitis A in the hope of restricting the disease to one building. Such attempts, however, are often unsuccessful. Retarded patients appear to be the most likely persons to transmit the disease in the incubation period, and it is spread commonly by patients who work or visit in other parts of the institution before jaundice is recognized. Institution-wide administration whenever hepatitis A occurs in a resident, however, is expensive. Delay, therefore, is justified until the infection is clearly propagating itself, for cases sometimes remain isolated or are limited to small clusters. Whether institution-wide administration of IG in institutions with endemic infection can abolish the disease is unknown.

Hospitals and Medical and Paramedical Personnel. In general, in these situations one should rely on measures other than administration of IG for prevention of hepatitis A.

Chimpanzee Handlers. Routine administration of IG to personnel who care for recently imported chimpanzees has been advocated in the past. Good hygienic and sanitation practices in proper animal quarters probably provide adequate protection in most instances. When the disease cannot otherwise be controlled, 0.06 ml/kg of IG every 4 to 6 months should be used.

Work Contacts. Hepatitis A is infrequently transmitted by casual contact such as that which occurs in an office. Although use of common toilet facilities frequently causes concern to co-workers of the hepatitis patient, administration of IG is not justified by this circumstance.

Common-Vehicle Exposure. IG is indicated for persons exposed to a common vehicle such as water or food if it can be given early after exposure. Illnesses in such situations have undoubtedly been prevented by this measure. Prevention of cases is one of the major reasons for continual alertness to the possible occurrence of common-vehicle epidemics.

Water- and food-borne outbreaks of hepatitis A have been preceded by a "herald" wave of gastroenteritis. In contrast, however, water- and food-borne gastroenteritis is rarely followed by hepatitis A. Similarly, a few food-borne epidemics of hepatitis A have followed disease in a food handler; more commonly, no overt case was recognizable, or was recognized only in retrospect. In many instances a food handler has developed hepatitis without transmitting it. In some instances transmission to other food handlers results in prolonged or repeated contamination of food and relatively long-lasting outbreaks. The Immunization Practices Advisory Committee recommends IG administration to other food handlers when hepatitis A is recognized in an index food handler but does not recommend IG for patrons unless they can be identified and treated within 2 weeks of exposure.[141] The latter criterion may be too stringent since some cases can be prevented even if IG is given several weeks after exposure; furthermore, repeated exposures may have occurred, making the precise date of infection difficult to establish.

Recommendations for Immunoprophylaxis of Hepatitis B

Pre-exposure Prophylaxis of Hepatitis B

Active immunization with the HBV vaccine is the only recommended form of immunoprophylaxis for susceptible individuals who will be at risk of acquiring HBV. Pre-exposure prophylaxis with HBIG is not recommended because of its high cost and limited duration of protective efficacy.

Prevaccination screening to determine susceptibility is recommended, on the basis of estimates of cost-effectiveness, for those individuals in groups with the highest risk of HBV infection, such as homosexual men, parenteral drug abusers, Asian-Americans, health care workers who have had a high frequency of exposure to blood or blood products, and patients with hemostatic disorders who have received clotting factor concentrates in the past.[141,691,893] Serologic screening to identify susceptibles has marginal cost-effectiveness in intermediate risk groups and lacks cost-effectiveness in low-risk groups, such as first- and second-year medical students who have not yet been exposed to patient's blood.

The appropriate screening serologic test for determining susceptibility is controversial and dependent on the cost of testing and the population being screened. In groups with high HBV infection and high carrier rates, such as homosexual men and parenteral drug abusers, anti-HBc may be the preferred test. Anti-HBs is the preferred test in lower risk groups, but if used for this purpose, vaccine should be withheld only from those with high (in excess of 10 SRUs) levels of anti-HBs. Use of both tests would be in many circumstances, prohibitively expensive.

Although post-vaccination testing for immunity has not been recommended by the Immunization Practices Advisory Committee,[141] management of individuals in high-risk groups is dependent on knowledge of their immune status. Testing for anti-HBs at 7 to 9 months after the initial dose of vaccine would seem appropriate to identify nonresponders or low-level responders in whom re-vaccination should be attempted. Failure to test for post-vaccination immunity might have serious consequences for the individual who believed he was immune when, in fact, he remained susceptible.

Health Care Workers. There is considerable evidence that exposure to patient's blood is the major determinant of the HBV risk. Health care workers who have frequent contact with blood or blood products, such as surgeons, pathologists, blood bank technicians, operating room staff, clinical chemistry and hematology technicians, intensive care unit staff, intravenous infusion nurses, phlebotomists, emergency department staff, emergency medical personnel (including first-responders in the community), and cardiac catheterization teams, to name but a few, represent the highest risk groups. Exposure to oral secretions admixed with blood may be responsible for the spread of HBV from infected patients to dentists, dental hygienists, and dental assistants. Exposure to contaminated wire sutures appears to contribute to the high risk of HBV in oral surgeons. Health care workers not exposed to blood or blood products, such as administrators and food handlers, carry no increased risk of acquiring HBV. Ideally, HBV vaccination should be initiated early in the training of medical, dental, and nursing students, prior to exposure to patient blood.

Hemodialysis Staff and Patients. The risk of HBV transmission in hemodialysis units has been reduced by programs of routine serologic surveillance, control of environmental contamination, and segregation of HBsAg-positive patients. Vaccination of susceptible personnel and staff is recommended, nonetheless. As previously mentioned, dialysis patients are less likely to respond to the vaccine, even if the 40-μg triple-dose schedule is employed. Whether or not vaccination will be more effective for patients with chronic renal disease if initiated prior to the onset of hemodialysis remains to be determined. Susceptible household and sexual contacts of HBsAg-positive patients on hemodialysis or home dialysis treatment programs should be vaccinated.

Recipients of High-Risk Blood Products and Multiple Blood Transfusions. The risk of HBV in patients with clotting disorders, in whom high-risk blood products, such as factor VIII concentrates, are administered, is exceedingly high. Vaccination should be initiated as soon as the diagnosis of a clotting disorder likely to require high-risk replacement therapy has been established. Serologic screening to determine susceptibility prior to vaccination is reasonable for those patients who have received high-risk blood products in the past. Vaccination also seems appropriate for patients requiring repeated transfusion therapy, for example, those with refractory and aplastic anemias, hemoglobinopathies and the leukemias. The larger dose (40 μg) may be preferred in patients with the latter disorders.

Parenteral Drug Users. Screening is recommended for all users of illicit parenteral drugs because the HBV infection rate has been very high in this population. Vaccination of susceptibles is recommended and under ideal circumstances should be initiated immediately after parenteral drug abuse begins. In most instances this goal is impractical.

Homosexual Men and Promiscuous Populations. After screening to determine immune status, susceptible sexually active homosexual men should be vaccinated. Vaccination should be considered early after homosexual practices begin. Early immunization of prostitutes, both men and women, also is recommended but vaccination programs for lesbians are not indicated because such individuals do not have an increased risk of HBV. The Immunization Practices Advisory Committee[141] has suggested that vaccination be considered for individuals presenting with sexually transmitted diseases or who have histories of sexual activities with multiple partners.

Institutions for the Mentally Retarded. The increased risk of infection with HBV in these facilities is a consequence of exposure to blood, saliva, skin lesions, and other body fluids that may be infective. Susceptible residents and employees who are likely to be exposed to residents should be vaccinated. Vaccination should be considered for the classroom contacts (children, teachers, teachers' aides) of HBsAg-positive mentally retarded children attending schools, particularly if the child's classroom behavior might favor HBV transmission.

Prisoners. Homosexual activity and illicit parenteral drug use appear to be key factors facilitating the transmission of HBV in prisoners. Vaccination of susceptibles should be considered in those prisons in which HBV infection is recognized.

Sexual and Household Contacts of HBsAg Carriers. While all household contacts of individuals with persistent HBV infection are at risk of acquiring HBV infection, sexual contacts appear to have the highest risk. Nonetheless, vaccination is recommended for all household members, after screening for susceptibility, when a HBsAg carrier has been recognized in the family. In many instances the index HBsAg carrier has been identified incidentally and the existence of the carrier state was totally unanticipated. On the other hand, screening of high-risk populations, such as immigrants, refugees, and children adopted from areas with high HBV infection rates, seems to be an appropriate public health measure. If HBsAg carriers are identified, susceptible household members are candidates for vaccination. Casual contacts of HBsAg carriers in whom exposure occurs in the classroom, office, and factory do not appear to be at increased risk. For these individuals vaccination is not recommended.

Travelers to HBV Endemic Regions. Short-term travelers to regions in which HBV is endemic probably do not require vaccination for the usual casual contact such individuals are likely to have with the local populations. Individuals likely to have intimate contact with unrecognized HBsAg carriers in the local population (*e.g.,* military and foreign service personnel assigned to high risk areas and health care professionals directly exposed to the local population) are candidates for vaccination. Vaccination also should be considered for travelers who may require treatment (*e.g.,* venipuncture, injections, acupuncture, blood transfusion) in local medical facilities. In each of these instances vaccination should be initiated 6 months prior to departure for the high-risk area.

Postexposure Prophylaxis of Hepatitis B

Strategies for the immunoprophylaxis of hepatitis B after exposure to HBV are less well established and more controversial than those designed for pre-exposure prophylaxis. A number of controlled clinical studies have shown that passive immunization with HBIG given twice after accidental percutaneous (needlestick) exposure to HBsAg-positive blood or once after sexual exposure to an index case of acute hepatitis B may have a protective efficacy approaching 75%.[362,815,892] Conventional IG may also confer some protection for sexual contacts,[757] but confirmation of this important observation is not yet available.

The use of active immunization with the hepatitis B vaccine alone for postexposure prophylaxis of needlestick accidents has not been studied; the delay in the development of protective antibody resulting from active immunization is sufficiently long that little if any protective efficacy can be anticipated. Data on the efficacy of combined passive-active immunization (HBIG and HBV vaccine) for needlestick exposures are not yet available. The use of active immunization alone also has been studied in the sexual exposure setting. Postexposure vaccination of spouses of patients with acute hepatitis B failed to provide evidence of protection.[848] Whether HBIG and vaccine together are more efficacious than HBIG alone in the postexposure prophylaxis of sexual contacts remains to be determined. Trials of HBIG alone or vaccination alone given to newborns of HBsAg-positive mothers indicate a protective efficacy rate of 70% to 75%. In this setting a protective efficacy rate of 85% to 95% has been achieved with combined passive and active immunization.[68–70,159,491,957,1081]

The recommendations described below are largely adapted from those of the Immunization Practices Advisory Committee (ACIP).[141] Areas of disagreement are indicated.

Needlestick or Permucosal Exposure to Blood or High-Risk Body Fluids (Health Care Workers)

1. *Nonvaccinated exposed individual, immune status unknown.*
   A. *HBsAg-positive source.* Obtain serum sample from exposed person for anti-HBs testing and administer a single intramuscular dose of HBIG (0.06 ml/kg) as early as possible within 7 days of the exposure. The efficacy of later HBIG administration is uncertain. If the exposed individual has protective titers of anti-HBs in the tested sera, no further therapy is indicated. If anti-HBs testing confirms susceptibility, begin first dose of HBV vaccine (20 μg given intramuscularly at a different site) within 7 days of exposure and repeat at 1 and 6 months later. If vaccination is refused, a second dose of HBIG should be given 1 month after the first. If HBIG cannot be obtained, conventional IG given in a similar dose (0.06 ml/kg) may confer some protection. The degree of protection is controversial.
   B. *HBsAg-status of source unknown.*
      1) *Source available for testing.* The ACIP recommends that for high-risk sources, the exposed individual should receive the first dose of vaccine within 7 days. The source should be tested for HBsAg and if positive, the exposed person should be given HBIG (0.06 ml/kg) within 7 days of the exposure. For low-risk sources, the ACIP recommends vaccination only and suggests that testing of low-risk sources for HBsAg is unnecessary. We would suggest testing of the source for HBsAg in low as well as high-risk settings since a positive result would require early administration of HBIG.
      2) *Source unavailable for testing.* Vaccination is indicated for susceptibles based on the presumption that similar needlestick or permucosal exposures may occur in the future. Administration of HBIG is not suggested.
2. *Vaccinated exposed individual*
   A. *HBsAg-positive source*
      1) *Incomplete vaccination (<3 vaccine doses).* Test exposed individual for anti-HBs. If levels are adequate, complete vaccine series. If anti-HBs is not present or is present at low levels, give HBIG (0.06 ml/kg) as soon as possible, within 7 days of exposure and complete vaccine schedule.
      2) *Complete vaccination*
         a) If the exposed person has been shown to have protective levels of anti-HBs within 12 months prior to exposure, no treatment is indicated.
         b) If the exposed individual was not tested for anti-HBs post-vaccination, test now. If anti-HBs is adequate, no treatment is indicated. If anti-HBs is not present or is found in low titers, give HBIG (0.06 ml/kg) and a single dose of vaccine (20 μg) at separate sites. For the individual without detectable anti-HBs we would complete a second vaccine series.
         c) If the exposed person was vaccinated more than 1 year before exposure and had adequate anti-HBs levels post-vaccination, retest now. If levels are still high no treatment is required. If levels are low or absent give one dose of vaccine as soon as possible.
         d) If the exposed individual is a known nonresponder, the ACIP suggests one dose of HBIG and one dose of vaccine. We would complete the vaccine schedule in such individuals.
   B. *HBsAg-status of source unknown.* For high-risk sources, the ACIP suggests that additional immunoprophylaxis is only necessary if the exposed person is a known vaccine nonresponder, in which case the source is tested for HBsAg. If the source is HBsAg positive, HBIG and vaccine are given at separate sites. For low-risk sources, the ACIP recommends that neither the source nor the exposed individual should be tested and that no further treatment is indicated. The ACIP suggests that no treatment is needed when the source is unknown. We would suggest that the source and exposed individual be tested in high- and low-risk exposures since we would then follow the regimens outlined previously for HBsAg-positive sources in vaccinated individuals.

Newborns of HBsAg-Positive Mothers. The ACIP recommends that pregnant women belonging to groups known to be at high risk for HBV infection should be screened during prenatal visits. We would extend this recommendation to all pregnant women. The newborns of HBsAg-positive mothers should receive HBIG (0.5 ml) intramuscularly within 12 hours of birth, preferably within the first hour after birth. HBV vaccine, in a dose of 10 μg (0.5 ml), is given at the same time at a separate site, and is repeated at 1 and 6 months after the first dose. The child is tested for HBsAg and anti-HBs at 12 to 15 months of age to determine whether or not prophylaxis has been effective. Testing of the mother for HBeAg does not influence the decision to administer immunoprophylaxis to the newborn.

Household and Sexual Contacts. *Acute HBV Infection.* Sexual contacts of the acutely infected HBsAg-positive patient should be screened for susceptibility. A single dose of HBIG (0.06 ml/kg) should be given to susceptible sexual contacts if it can be given within 2 weeks of the last sexual exposure. Whether concurrent HBV vaccine administration increases postexposure prophylaxis efficacy in this setting is uncertain. The ACIP states that vaccination is optional in the initial treatment of heterosexual contacts of individuals with acute HBV infection. If vaccine is given and the index case remains HBsAg positive at 3 months, no further therapy is needed for the sexual contact. If vaccine is not given, a second dose of HBIG can be given to the regular sexual partner if the index case remains HBsAg-positive on follow-up. Nonsexual contacts in the household do not require immunoprophylaxis unless an identifiable blood exposure has occurred, in which case the regimen for sexual contacts may be used.

Persistent HBV Infection. If the index case is a HBsAg carrier, all susceptible sexual and household contacts should be protected by vaccination, using the three-dose schedule. The use of HBIG in this setting is not recommended.

Immunoprophylaxis of Hepatitis D

Neither pre-exposure nor postexposure immunoprophylaxis for hepatitis D virus infection is available.

Immunoprophylaxis of Non-A, Non-B Hepatitis

The value of IG in the prevention of the epidemic form of non-A, non-B viral hepatitis has not been demonstrated. Similarly, for blood-borne non-A, non-B hepatitis the efficacy of IG as pre-exposure prophylaxis remains ambiguous and recommendations for its use are arbitrary. In our view there is no evidence to justify this form of immunoprophylaxis for non-A, non-B hepatitis even in circumstances that are known to be associated with this illness, such as intravenous abusers of illicit drugs, renal dialysis and transplant patients, bone marrow transplant patients, repeatedly transfused subjects, and endemic disease in institutions. For postexposure prophylaxis of the blood-borne forms of non-A, non-B hepatitis, administration of IG in a dose of 0.06 ml/kg is an option of uncertain value. We would consider use of IG for the following exposures: (1) percutaneous (needlestick), if the donor has acute or chronic non-A, non-B hepatitis; (2) sexual, if the partner was in the incubation period of or has acute non-A, non-B hepatitis; (3) newborn of a mother with acute or chronic non-A, non-B hepatitis; and (4) institutional outbreaks of acute non-A, non-B hepatitis.

REFERENCES

1. Aach RD, Kahn RA: Post-transfusion hepatitis: Current perspectives. Ann Intern Med 92:539, 1980
2. Aach RD et al: An epidemic of infectious hepatitis possibly due to airborne transmission. Am J Epidemiol 87:99, 1968
3. Aach RD et al: Serum/alanine aminotransferase of donors in relation to the risk of non-A, non-B hepatitis in recipients: the Transfusion-Transmitted Viruses Study. N Engl J Med 304:989, 1981
4. Abe H et al: Light microscopic findings of liver biopsy specimens from patients with hepatitis type A and comparison with type B. Gastroenterology 82:938, 1982
5. ACIP: Hepatitis B vaccine: Evidence confirming lack of AIDS transmission. MMWR 33:685, 1984
6. Acute Hepatic Failure Study Group: Failure of specific immunotherapy in fulminant type B hepatitis. Ann Intern Med 86:272, 1977
7. Acute Hepatic Failure Study Group: Etiology and prognosis in fulminant hepatitis. Gastroenterology 77:A33, 1979
8. Adams RH, Combes B: Viral hepatitis during pregnancy. JAMA 192:195, 1965
9. Adams WH et al: Coagulation studies of viral hepatitis occurring during pregnancy. Am J Med Sci 272:139, 1976
10. Aden DP et al: Controlled synthesis of HBsAg in a differentiated human liver carcinoma-derived cell line. Nature 282:615, 1979
11. Adler R et al: Acute pericarditis associated with hepatitis B infection. Pediatrics 61:716, 1978
12. Adler VG et al: Disinfection of cystoscopes by subatmospheric steam and steam and formaldehyde at 80 degrees centigrade. Br Med J 3:677, 1971
13. Akdamar KA et al: SH antigen in bile. Lancet 1:909, 1971
14. Alarcon GS, Townes AS: Arthritis in viral hepatitis: Report of 2 cases and review of the literature. Johns Hopkins Med J 132:1, 1973
15. Albin C, Robinson W: Protein kinase activity in hepatitis B virus. J Virol 34:297, 1980
16. Allen JC, Kunkel HG: Antibodies to genetic types of gamma globulin after multiple transfusions. Science 139:418, 1963
17. Allen JG, Sayman WA: Serum hepatitis from transfusions of blood. JAMA 180:1079, 1962
18. Almeida JD et al: Possible airborne spread of serum hepatitis virus within a haemodialysis unit. Lancet 2:849, 1971
19. Almeida JD et al: New antigen-antibody system in Australia-antigen-positive hepatitis. Lancet 2:1225, 1971
20. Almeida JD, Waterson AP: Immune complexes in hepatitis. Lancet 2:983, 1969
21. Alp MH, Wright R: Immunoglobulins, virus-like particles and auto-antibodies in bile. Gut 12:859, 1971

22. Alpert E et al: The pathogenesis of arthritis associated with viral hepatitis: Complement-component studies. N Engl J Med 285:185, 1971

23. Alt HL, Swank RL: Thrombocytopenic purpura associated with catarrhal jaundice: Report of a case. Ann Intern Med 10:1049, 1937

24. Alter HJ et al: Donor transaminase and recipient hepatitis: Impact on blood transfusion services. JAMA 246:630, 1981

25. Alter HJ et al: Hepatitis B immune globulin: Evaluation of clinical trials and rationale for usage. N Engl J Med 293:1093, 1975

26. Alter HJ et al: Health-care workers positive for hepatitis B surface antigen: Are their contacts at risk? N Engl J Med 292:454, 1975

27. Alter HJ et al: Post-transfusion hepatitis after exclusion of commercial and hepatitis B antigen-positive donors. Ann Intern Med 77:691, 1972

28. Alter HJ et al: Transmission of hepatitis B to chimpanzees by hepatitis B surface antigen-positive saliva and semen. Infect Immun 16:928, 1977

29. Alter HJ et al: Clinical and serological analysis of transfusion-associated hepatitis. Lancet 2:838, 1975

30. Alter HJ et al: Evidence for a transmissable agent in non-A, non-B hepatitis. Lancet 1:459, 1978

31. Alter HJ et al: Type B hepatitis: The infectivity of blood positive for "e" antigen and DNA polymerase after accidental needle-stick exposure. N Engl J Med 295:909, 1976

32. Alter MJ et al: Sporadic non-A, non-B hepatitis: Frequency and epidemiology in an urban US population. J Infect Dis 145:886, 1982

33. Altschul A et al: Incidence of hepatitis among narcotic addicts in the Harlem Hospital, New York. Arch Intern Med 89:24, 1952

34. Andersen J, Vellar O: Viral hepatitis: A follow-up study of 373 notified cases in Oslo 1949–53. Acta Med Scand 182:691, 1967

35. Andersson O: Epidemic of jaundice. Nord Hyg T 2:252, 1921

36. Andrews DA: Immunoglobulin prophylaxis of infectious hepatitis. NZ Med J 73:199, 1971

37. Appelbaum E, Kalkstein M: Artificial transmission of viral hepatitis among intravenous diacetylmorphine addicts. JAMA 147:222, 1951

38. Apstein MD et al: Neuropsychological dysfunction in acute viral hepatitis. Digestion 19:349, 1979

39. Armstrong SH Jr et al: Comparison of the persistence in the blood of gamma globulin labeled with S^{35} and I^{131} in the same subjects. J Lab Clin Med 44:762, 1954

40. Arnold W: Localization of e antigen in nuclei of hepatocytes in HBsAg-positive liver diseases. Gut 18:994, 1977

41. Assessment of British gamma-globulin in preventing infectious hepatitis: A report to the Director of the Public Health Laboratory Service. Br Med J 3:451, 1968

42. Astaldi G et al: Intestinal biopsy in acute hepatitis. Am J Dig Dis 9:237, 1964

43. Auslander MO, Gitnick GL: Vigorous medical management of acute fulminant hepatitis. Arch Intern Med 137:599, 1977

44. Axon ATR et al: Disinfection of gastrointestinal fibre endoscopes. Lancet 1:656, 1974

45. Ayoola EA et al: Primary liver cancer (PLC) after non-A, non-B hepatitis (NANBH). Hepatology 2:154, 1982

46. Baer GM: Studies of acute hepatitis A: I. Complement level fluctuation. J Med Virol 1:1, 1977

47. Balayan MS et al: Evidence for a virus in non-A, non-B hepatitis transmitted via the fecal-oral route. Intervirology 20:23, 1983

48. Ballance GA: Epidemic of infective hepatitis in an Oxford college. Br Med J 1:1071, 1954

49. Bancroft WH et al: Detection of additional antigenic determinants of hepatitis B antigen. J Immunol 109:842, 1972

50. Bancroft WH et al: Transmission of hepatitis B virus to gibbons by exposure to human saliva containing hepatitis B surface antigen. J Infect Dis 135:79, 1977

51. Bang NU et al: Detection of hepatitis carriers by serum glutamic oxalacetic transaminase activity. JAMA 171:2303, 1955

52. Barandun S et al: Intravenous administration of human gamma globulin. Vox Sang 7:157, 1962

53. Barker LF, Murray R: Acquisition of hepatitis-associated antigen: Clinical features in young adults. JAMA 216:1970, 1971

54. Barker LF, Murray R: Relationship of virus dose to incubation time of clinical hepatitis and time of appearance of hepatitis associated antigen. Am J Med Sci 263:27, 1972

55. Barker LF et al: Hepatitis B core antigen: Immunology and electron microscopy. J Virol 14:1552, 1974

56. Barker LF et al: Transmission of type B viral hepatitis to chimpanzees. J Infect Dis 127:648, 1973

57. Barker LF et al: Hepatitis B virus infection in chimpanzees: Titration of subtypes. J Infect Dis 132:451, 1975

58. Barker LF et al: Antibody responses in viral hepatitis, type B. JAMA 223:1005, 1973

59. Barker LF et al: Transmission of serum hepatitis. JAMA 211:1509, 1970

60. Barker MH et al: Acute infectious hepatitis in the Mediterranean theater. JAMA 128:997, 1945

61. Barker MH et al: Chronic hepatitis in the Mediterranean theater: A new clinical syndrome. JAMA 129:653, 1945

62. Bastiaans MJS et al: A new antigenic determinant on HBsAg. Vox Sang 37:129, 1979

63. Batten PJ et al: Infectious hepatitis: Infectiousness during the presymptomatic phase of the disease. Am J Hyg 77:129, 1963

64. Baybutt JE: Hypersensitivity to immune serum globulin. JAMA 171:415, 1959

65. Bayer ME et al: Particles associated with Australia antigen in the sera of patients with leukemia, Down's syndrome and hepatitis. Nature 215:1057, 1968

66. Beasley RP et al: Evidence against breast feeding as a mechanism for vertical transmission of hepatitis B. Lancet 2:740, 1975

67. Beasley RP et al: The "e" antigen and vertical transmission of hepatitis B surface antigen. Am J Epidemiol 105:94, 1977

68. Beasley RP et al: Hepatitis B immune globulin (HBIG) efficacy in the interruption of perinatal transmission of hepatitis B virus carrier state: Initial report of a randomized double-blind placebo-controlled trial. Lancet 2:388, 1981

69. Beasley RP et al: Efficacy of hepatitis B immune globulin for prevention of perinatal transmission of the hepatitis B virus carrier state: Final report of a randomized double-blind, placebo-controlled trial. Hepatology 3:135, 1983

70. Beasley RP et al: Prevention of perinatally transmitted

hepatitis B virus infections with hepatitis B immune globulin and hepatitis B vaccine. Lancet 2:1099, 1983

71. Becker MD et al: Prognosis of chronic persistent hepatitis. Lancet 1:53, 1970

72. Beeson PB: Jaundice occurring one to four months after transfusion of blood or plasma. JAMA 121:1332, 1943

73. Beeson PB et al: Hepatitis following injection of mumps convalescent plasma. Lancet 1:814, 1944

74. Belabbes H et al: Non-A/non-B epidemic viral hepatitis in Algeria: Strong evidence for its water spread. In Vyas GN, Dienstag JL, Hoofnagle JH (eds): Viral Hepatitis and Liver Disease, p 637. Orlando, FL, Grune & Stratton, 1984

75. Benenson MW et al: A military community outbreak of hepatitis type A related to transmission in a child care facility. Am J Epidemiol 112:471, 1980

76. Benhamou J, cited by Berk PD, Popper H: Fulminant hepatic failure. Am J Gastroenterol 69:349, 1978

77. Berg R et al: Australia antigen in hepatitis among Swedish trackfinders. Acta Pathol Microbiol Scand 79:423, 1971

78. Berk JE: Hepatitis following transfusion. Gastroenterology 8:296, 1947

79. Berk PD, Popper H: Fulminant hepatic failure. Am J Gastroenterol 69:349, 1978

80. Berman M et al: The chronic sequelae of non-A, non-B hepatitis. Ann Intern Med 91:1, 1979

81. Berninger M et al: An assay for the detection of the DNA genome of hepatitis B virus in serum. J Med Virol 9:57, 1982

82. Berquist KR et al: Experimental studies on the transmission of hepatitis B by mosquitoes. Am J Trop Med Hyg 25:730, 1976

83. Berquist KR et al: Infectivity of serum containing HBsAg and antibody to e antigen. Lancet 1:1026, 1976

84. Berris B et al: Hepatitis in undertakers. JAMA 240:138, 1978

85. Bewley TH et al: Morbidity and mortality from heroin dependence: III. Relation of hepatitis to self-injection techniques. Br Med J 1:730, 1968

86. Bhatnagar PK et al: Immune response to synthetic peptide analogues of hepatitis B surface antigen specific for the common *a* determinant. Proc Natl Acad Sci USA 779: 4400, 1982

87. Bianchi L, Gudat F: Histologische Charakteristika und Nachweis von hepatitis-B-antigen-Komptonenten im Lebergewebe bei akuter und chronischer Virushepatitis. Immunitat Infektion 3:159, 1975

88. Bianchi L et al: Morphological criteria in viral hepatitis. Lancet 1:333, 1971

89. Bianchi L et al: Viral hepatitis. In MacSween NM et al (eds): Pathology of the Liver, p 164. Edinburgh, Churchill Livingstone, 1979

90. Binn LN et al: Primary isolation and serial passage of hepatitis A virus strains in primate cell cultures. J Clin Microbiol 20:28, 1984

91. Blacklidge VY: The clinical significance of Eberlein's method of determining the three main fractions of serum bilirubin. J Pediatr 62:666, 1963

92. Bloomer JR et al: Serum alpha-fetoprotein in patients with massive hepatic necrosis. Gastroenterology 72:479, 1977

93. Blum AL et al: Treatment of acute viral hepatitis with (+)-cyanidanol-3. Lancet 2:1153, 1977

94. Blum AL et al: A fortuitously controlled study of steroid therapy in acute viral hepatitis. Am J Med 47:82, 1969

95. Blum HE et al: Asymmetric replication of hepatitis B virus DNA in human liver: Demonstration of cytoplasmic minus-strand DNA by blot analyses and *in situ* hybridization. Virology 139:87, 1984

96. Blum HE et al: Detection of hepatitis B virus DNA in hepatocytes, bile duct epithelium, and vascular elements by *in situ* hybridization. Proc Natl Acad Sci USA 80:6685, 1983

97. Blumberg BS: Australia antigen and the biology of hepatitis B. Science 197:17, 1977

98. Blumberg BS et al: A "new" antigen in leukemia sera. JAMA 191:101, 1965

99. Boggs JD et al: Viral hepatitis: Clinical and tissue culture studies. JAMA 214:1041, 1970

100. Bond WS et al: Inactivation of hepatitis B virus by intermediate to high level disinfectant chemicals. J Clin Microbiol 18:535, 1983

101. Bonino F et al: Delta hepatitis agent: Structural and antigenic properties of the delta-associated particle. Infect Immun 43:1000, 1984

102. Borhanmesh F et al: Viral hepatitis during pregnancy: Severity and effect on gestation. Gastroenterology 64:304, 1973

103. Bose S et al: Australia antigen in body fluids other than serum. Gastroenterology 60:766, 1971

104. Bostock AD et al: Hepatitis A infection associated with the consumption of mussels. J Infect 1:171, 1979

105. Boxall EH: Breast feeding and hepatitis B. Lancet 2:979, 1975

106. Boxall EH: Acupuncture hepatitis in the West Midlands, 1977. J Med Virol 2:377, 1978

107. Boyer JL, Klatskin G: Pattern of necrosis in acute viral hepatitis: Prognostic value of bridging (subacute hepatic necrosis). N Engl J Med 283:1063, 1970

108. Brachott D et al: Fragmented IgG for post-exposure prophylaxis of type A hepatitis. Transfusion 12:389, 1972

109. Bradley DW, Maynard JE: Non-A, non-B hepatitis: Research progress and current perspectives. Dev Biol Stand 54:463, 1983

110. Bradley DW et al: Posttransfusion non-A, non-B hepatitis: Physicochemical properties of two distinct agents. J Infect Dis 148:254, 1983

111. Bradley DW et al: Non-A, non-B hepatitis in experimentally infected chimpanzees: Cross-challenge and electron microscopic studies. J Med Virol 6:185, 1980

112. Bradley DW et al: Posttransfusion non-A, non-B hepatitis in chimpanzees: Physicochemical evidence that the tubule-forming agent is a small, enveloped virus. Gastroenterology 88:773, 1985

113. Bradley DW et al: Biochemical and biophysical characterization of light and heavy density hepatitis A particles: Evidence HAV is an RNA virus. J Med Virol 2:175, 1978

114. Bradley DW et al: Cyclic excretion of hepatitis A virus in experimentally infected chimpanzees: Biophysical characterization of the associated HAV particle. J Med Virol 1:133, 1977

115. Bradley DW et al: CsCl banding of hepatitis A-associated virus-like particles. J Infect Dis 131:304, 1975

116. Bradley DW et al: Hepatitis B and serum DNA polymerase activities in chimpanzees. Nature 251:356, 1974

117. Bradley DW et al: Serodiagnosis of viral hepatitis A: Detection of acute-phase immunoglobulin M anti-hepatitis A virus by radioimmunoassay. J Clin Microbiol 5:521, 1977

118. Bradley SE: Effect of posture and exercise upon blood

flow through the liver. In Seventh Liver Injury Conference, p 53. New York, Macy, 1948

119. Bradley WH: Homologous serum jaundice. Proc R Soc Med 39:649, 1946

120. Brain R: Discussion on recent experiences of acute encephalomyelitis and allied conditions. Proc R Soc Med 36:319, 1943

121. Brandt KH et al: Data on the determination of SGOT and SGPT activity in donor blood for the possible prevention of post-transfusion hepatitis. Acta Med Scand 177:321, 1965

122. Brechot C et al: Detection of hepatitis B virus DNA in liver and serum: A direct appraisal of the chronic carrier state. Lancet 2:765, 1981

123. Brodersen M et al: Salivary HBsAg detected by radioimmunoassay. Lancet 1:675, 1974

124. Brotman B et al: Non-A, non-B hepatitis: Is there more than a single blood-borne strain. J Infect Dis 151:618, 1985

125. Brotman B et al: Blood-borne non-A, non-B hepatitis: Lack of infectivity of feces from chimpanzees infected with a strain producing cytoplasmic tubular alterations. J Infect Dis 147:535, 1983

126. Brotman B et al: Role of arthropods in transmission of hepatitis B virus in the tropics. Lancet 1:1305, 1973

127. Bryan JA, Gregg MB: Viral hepatitis in the United States, 1970–1973: An analysis of morbidity trends and the impact of HBsAg testing on surveillance and epidemiology. Am J Med Sci 270:271, 1975

128. Bryan JA et al: An outbreak of hepatitis-A associated with recreational lake water. Am J Epidemiol 99:145, 1974

129. Bucens ME et al: False-positive results occurring in a radioimmunoassay for hepatitis A antibody of the IgM class. J Virol Methods 7:287, 1983

130. Budd G: Diseases of the Liver, p 368. Philadelphia, Lea & Blanchard, 1846

131. Budkowska A: Immunochemical and morphological studies of hepatitis B core antigen isolated from the nuclei of hepatocytes. J Infect Dis 135:463, 1977

132. Burk KH et al: Long-term sequelae of non-A, non-B hepatitis in experimentally infected chimpanzees. Hepatology 4:808, 1984

133. Byrne EAJ, Taylor GF: An outbreak of jaundice with signs in the nervous system. Br Med J 1:477, 1945

134. Cahill KM: Hepatitis in pregnancy. Surg Gynecol Obstet 114:545, 1962

135. Caporaso N et al: Role of delta infection in the progression to chronicity of acute HBsAg positive hepatitis. Gastroenterol Clin Biol 8:646, 1984

136. Capps RB, Barker MH: The management of infectious hepatitis. Ann Intern Med 26:405, 1947

137. Capps RB et al: A syringe-transmitted epidemic of infectious hepatitis. JAMA 136:819, 1948

138. Cavalli G et al: Ultrastructural studies of bile ductules in the course of acute hepatitis. Acta Hepato-Spleno 18:355, 1971

139. Cawein MJ III et al: Anemia of hepatic disease studied with radiochromium. Gastroenterology 38:324, 1960

140. Centers for Disease Control: Provisional public health service inter-agency recommendations for screening donated blood and plasma for antibody to the virus causing acquired immunodeficiency syndrome. MMWR 34:1, 1985

141. Centers for Disease Control: Recommendation of the Immunization Practices Advisory Committee. Recommendations for protection against viral hepatitis. MMWR 34:313, 1985

142. Centers for Disease Control: Suboptimal response to hepatitis B vaccine given by injection into the buttock. MMWR 34:105, 1985

143. Chairez R et al: Comparative biophysical studies of hepatitis B antigen subtypes adw and ayw. J Virol 15:182, 1975

144. Chalmers TC et al: The treatment of acute infectious hepatitis: Controlled studies of the effects of diet, rest and physical reconditioning on the acute course of the disease and on the incidence of relapses and residual abnormalities. J Clin Invest 34:1163, 1955

145. Chalmers TC et al: Evaluation of a four day ACTH test in the differential diagnosis of jaundice. Gastroenterology 30:894, 1956

146. Chalmers TC et al: A note on fatality in serum hepatitis. Gastroenterology 49:22, 1965

147. Chan TK, Todd D: Haemolysis complicating viral hepatitis in patients with glucose-6-phosphate dehydrogenase deficiency. Br Med J 1:131, 1975

148. Chang LW, O'Brien TF: Australia antigen serology in the Holy Cross football team hepatitis outbreak. Lancet 2:59, 1970

149. Charnay P et al: Localization on the viral genome and nucleotide sequence of the gene coding for the two major polypeptides of the hepatitis B surface antigen (HBsAg). Nucleic Acids Res 7:335, 1979

150. Cherubin CE: Risk of post-transfusion hepatitis in recipients of blood containing S.H. antigen of Harlem Hospital. Lancet 1:627, 1971

151. Cherubin CE et al: The serum hepatitis related antigen (SH) in illicit drug users. Am J Epidemiol 91:510, 1970

152. Cherubin CE et al: Acquisition of antibody to hepatitis B antigen in three socioeconomically different medical populations. Lancet 2:149, 1972

153. Cherubin CE et al: Persistence of transaminase abnormalities in former drug addicts. Ann Intern Med 76:385, 1972

154. Child PL, Ruiz A: Acidophilic bodies. Arch Pathol 85:45, 1968

155. Chisari FV et al: Mechanisms responsible for defective human T-lymphocyte sheep erythrocyte rosette function associated with hepatitis B virus infection. J Clin Invest 57:1227, 1976

156. Christoffersen P et al: Clinical findings in patients with hepatitis and abnormal bile duct epithelium. Scand J Gastroenterol 5:117, 1970

157. Choremis C et al: Viral hepatitis in G-6-PD deficiency. Lancet 1:269, 1966

158. Christie AB et al: Pregnancy hepatitis in Libya. Lancet 2:827, 1976

159. Chung WK et al: Prevention of perinatal transmission of hepatitis B virus: A comparison between the efficacy of passive and passive-active immunization in Korea. J Infect Dis 151:280, 1985

160. Chuttani HK et al: Follow-up study of cases from the Delhi epidemic of infectious hepatitis of 1955–6. Br Med J 2:676, 1966

161. Cirillo NB et al: Gastric acid secretion in infectious hepatitis. Milit Med 137:64, 1972

162. Clearfield HR et al: Acute viral hepatitis, glucose-6-phos-

phate dehydrogenase deficiency, and hemolytic anemia. Arch Intern Med 123:689, 1969

163. Clermont RJ, Chalmers TC: The transaminase tests in liver disease. Medicine 46:197, 1967

164. Cline AL et al: Viral hepatitis among American missionaries abroad: A preliminary study. JAMA 199:551, 1967

165. Cliver DO: Implications of food-borne infectious hepatitis. Public Health Rep 81:159, 1966

166. Cockayne EA: Catarrhal jaundice, sporadic and epidemic and its relation to acute yellow atrophy of the liver. QJ Med 6:1, 1912

167. Cohen SN, Dougherty WJ: Transfusion hepatitis arising from addict blood donors. JAMA 203:427, 1968

168. Colbert JW et al: The use of ACTH in acute viral hepatitis. N Engl J Med 245:172, 1951

169. Coleman JC et al: Homosexual hepatitis. J Infect 1:61, 1979

170. Collaborative Study by the Communicable Disease Surveillance Centre and the Epidemiological Research Laboratory of the Public Health Laboratory Service Together With a District Control-of-Infection Service: Acute hepatitis B associated with gynaecological surgery. Lancet 1:1, 1980

171. Colombo M et al: Long-term delta superinfection in hepatitis B surface antigen carriers and its relationship to the course of chronic hepatitis. Gastroenterology 85:235, 1983

172. Colwell AR: Fecal fat excretion in patients with jaundice due to viral hepatitis. Gastroenterology 33:591, 1957

173. Combes B et al: Glomerulonephritis with deposition of Australia antigen–antibody complexes in glomerular basement membrane. Lancet 2:234, 1971

174. Combined Medical Research Council And Public Health Laboratory Service Report: The incidence of hepatitis B infection after accidental exposure and anti-HBs immunoglobulin prophylaxis. Lancet 1:6, 1980

175. Conrad ME et al: Infectious hepatitis: A generalized disease. Am J Med 37:789, 1964

176. Corey L, Holmes KK: Sexual transmission of hepatitis A in homosexual man. N Engl J Med 302:435, 1980

177. Corey L et al: HBsAg-negative hepatitis in a hemodialysis unit. N Engl J Med 293:1063, 1975

178. Cornu C et al: Persistence of immunoglobulin M antibody to hepatitis A virus and relapse of hepatitis A infection. Eur J Clin Microbiol 3:45, 1983

179. Cosgriff TM, Arnold WJ: Digital vasospasm and infarction associated with hepatitis B antigenemia. JAMA 235:1362, 1976

180. Cossart YE, Vahrman J: Studies of Australia-SH antigen in sporadic viral hepatitis in London. Br Med J 1:403, 1970

181. Coulepis AG et al: The polypeptides of hepatitis A virus. Intervirology 10:24, 1978

182. Coulepis AG et al: Detection of HAV in feces. J Infect Dis 141:151, 1980

183. Courouce-Pauty A-M et al: Simultaneous occurrence in the same serum of hepatitis B surface antigen and antibody to hepatitis B surface antigen of different subtypes. J Infect Dis 140:975, 1979

184. Coutinho RA et al: Efficacy of a heat-inactivated hepatitis B vaccine in male homosexuals: Outcome of a placebo-controlled double-blind trial. Br Med J 286:1305, 1983

185. Craxi A et al: Delta agent infection in acute hepatitis and chronic HBsAg carriers with and without liver disease. Gut 25:1288, 1984

186. Creutzfeldt W: Die Transfusions Hepatitis und ihre Vehrutung. Internist 7:1, 1966

187. Creutzfeldt W et al: Transmission of hepatitis over ten years by a blood donor with posthepatitis cirrhosis. German Med Monthly 8:30, 1963

188. Crivelli O et al: Enzyme-linked immunosorbent assay for detection of antibody to the hepatitis B surface antigen-associated delta antigen. J Clin Microbiol 14:173, 1981

189. Culbertson JW et al: The effect of the upright position upon the hepatic blood flow in normotensive and hypertensive subjects. J Clin Invest 30:305, 1951

190. Cullinan ER: In Cope VZ (ed): History of World War II, p 230. VK Medical Series, Medicine and Pathology. London, His Majesty's Stationery Office

191. Cullinan ER et al: The prognosis of infective hepatitis: Preliminary account of a long-term follow-up. Br Med J 1:1315, 1958

192. Daemer RJ et al: Propagation of human hepatitis A virus in African green monkey cell culture: Primary isolation and serial passage. Infect Immun 32:388, 1981

193. Damodaran K, Hartfall SJ: Infective hepatitis in garrison of Malta. Br Med J 2:587, 1944

194. Dane DS et al: Virus-like particles in serum of patients with Australia-antigen–associated hepatitis. Lancet 1:695, 1970

195. Dankert J et al: Hepatitis B surface antigen in environmental samples from hemodialysis units. J Infect Dis 134:123, 1976

196. Darani M, Gerber M: Hepatitis B antigen in vaginal secretions. Lancet 2:1008, 1974

197. Darmady EM et al: The cleaning of instruments and syringes. J Clin Pathol 18:6, 1965

198. Davenport FM et al: A common source multihousehold outbreak of chimpanzee-associated hepatitis in humans. Am J Epidemiol 83:146, 1966

199. Davis LE et al: Hepatitis associated with illicit use of intravenous methamphetamine. Public Health Rep 85:809, 1970

200. Decker RH et al: Serological studies of transmission of hepatitis A in humans. J Infect Dis 139:74, 1979

201. de Cock KM et al: Acute delta hepatitis without circulating HBsAg. Gut 26:212, 1985

202. DeFranchis R et al: Chronic asymptomatic HBsAg carriers: Histologic abnormalities and diagnostic and prognostic value of serologic markers of the HBV. Gastroenterology 79:521, 1980

203. DeGast GC et al: T-lymphocyte number and function and the course of hepatitis B in hemodialysis patients. Infect Immun 14:1138, 1976

204. Degroote J et al: A classification of chronic hepatitis. Lancet 2:626, 1968

205. DeHoratius RJ et al: Lymphocytotoxins in acute and chronic hepatitis: Characterization and relationship to changes in circulating T-lymphocytes. Clin Exp Immunol 26:21, 1976

206. DeHoratius RJ et al: T and B lymphocytes in acute and chronic hepatitis. Clin Immunol Immunopathol 2:353, 1974

207. Deinhardt F: Aspects of vaccination against hepatitis B, passive-active immunization schedules and vaccination responses in different ages groups. Scand J Infect Dis Suppl 38:17, 1983

208. Deinhardt F et al: Studies on the transmission of human viral hepatitis to marmoset monkeys: I. Transmission of

disease, serial passage, and description of liver lesions. J Exp Med 125:673, 1967

209. Deinhardt F et al: Hepatitis in marmosets. Am J Med Sci 270:73, 1975

210. Dejean A et al: Characterization of integrated hepatitis B viral DNA cloned from a human hepatoma and hepatoma-derived cell line PLC/PRF/5. Proc Natl Acad Sci USA 80:2505, 1983

211. Delius H et al: Structure of the hepatitis B virus genome. J Virol 47:337, 1983

212. Deller JJ Jr et al: Fatal pancytopenia associated with viral hepatitis. N Engl J Med 266:297, 1962

213. Denes AE et al: Hepatitis B infection in physicians: Results of a nationwide seroepidemiologic survey. JAMA 239: 210, 1978

214. Denniston KJ et al: cDNA cloning of delta agent–associated RNA and preliminary nucleotide sequence determination. In Vyas GN, Deinstag J, Hoofnagle J (eds): Disease, p 696. Orlando, FL, Grune & Stratton, 1984

215. DeRitis F et al: Negative results of prednisone therapy in viral hepatitis. Lancet 1:533, 1964

216. DeRitis F et al: Anicteric virus hepatitis in a closed environment as shown by serum transaminase activity. Bull WHO 20:589, 1959

217. Derso A et al: Transmission of HBsAg from mother to infant in four ethnic groups. Br Med J 1:949, 1978

218. Desmyter J et al: Hepatitis B vaccination of hemophiliacs. Scand J Infect Dis Suppl 38:42, 1983

219. DeVos R et al: Are nuclear particles specific for non-A, non-B hepatitis. Hepatology 3:532, 1983

220. Dible JH et al: Pathology of acute hepatitis: Aspiration biopsy studies of epidemic, arsenotherapy and serum jaundice. Lancet 2:402, 1943

221. Dick SJ et al: Hepatitis B antigen in urban-caught mosquitoes. JAMA 229:1627, 1974

222. Dienstag JL: Non-A, non-B hepatitis: I. Recognition, epidemiology, and clinical features: II. Experimental transmission, putative virus agents and markers, and prevention. Gastroenterology 85:439; 743, 1983

223. Dienstag JL et al: Etiology of sporadic hepatitis B surface antigen-negative hepatitis. Ann Intern Med 87:1, 1977

224. Dienstag JL et al: Hepatitis B vaccine administered to chronic carriers of hepatitis B surface antigen. Ann Intern Med 96:644, 1982

225. Dienstag JL et al: Quantitation of antibody to hepatitis A antigen by immune electron microscopy. Infect Immun 13:1209, 1976

226. Dienstag JL et al: Circulating immune complexes in non-A, non-B hepatitis. Lancet 1:1265, 1979

227. Dienstag JL et al: Nonhuman primate-associated viral hepatitis type A. JAMA 236:462, 1976

228. Dienstag JL et al: Fecal shedding of hepatitis A antigen. Lancet 1:765, 1975

229. Dienstag JL et al: Experimental infection of chimpanzees with hepatitis A virus. J Infect Dis 132:532, 1975

230. Dienstag JL et al: Mussel-associated viral hepatitis, type A: Serologic confirmation. Lancet 1:561, 1976

231. Dienstag JL et al: Hepatitis B vaccine in health care personnel: Safety, immunogenicity and indicators of efficacy. Ann Intern Med 101:34, 1984

232. Dienstag JL et al: The pathology of viral hepatitis types A and B in chimpanzees: A comparison. Am J Pathol 85: 131, 1976

233. Dienstag JL et al: Urticaria associated with acute viral hepatitis type B. Ann Intern Med 89:34, 1978

234. Dienstag JL et al: Foodhandler-associated outbreak of hepatitis type A. Ann Intern Med 83:647, 1975

235. Dimitrakakis M et al: Detection of delta infection using reagents obtained from the serum of patients infected with HBV. J Virol Meth 8:331, 1984

236. Dismukes WE et al: Viral hepatitis associated with illicit parenteral use of drugs. JAMA 206:1048, 1968

237. Dixon FJ et al: The half-life of homologous gamma globulin (antibody) in several species. J Exp Med 96:313, 1952

238. Dougherty WJ, Altman R: Viral hepatitis in New Jersey 1960–61. Am J Med 32:704, 1962

239. Drake ME, Ming C: Gamma globulin in epidemic hepatitis: Comparative value of two dosage levels apparently near the minimal effective level. JAMA 155:1302, 1954

240. Drake ME et al: Effect of nitrogen mustard on virus of serum hepatitis in whole blood. Proc Soc Exp Biol Med 80:310, 1952

241. Dreesman GR, Kennedy RC: Anti-idiotype antibodies: Implications of internal image-based vaccines for infectious diseases. J Infect Dis 151:761, 1985

242. Drueke T et al: Hepatitis B antigen-associated periarteritis nodosa in patients undergoing long-term hemodialysis. Am J Med 68:86, 1980

243. Dubin IN: Intrahepatic bile stasis in acute non-fatal virus hepatitis: Its incidence, pathogenesis and correlation with jaundice. Gastroenterology 36:645, 1959

244. Dubin IN et al: The cholestatic form of viral hepatitis: Experiences with viral hepatitis at Brooke Army Hospital during the years of 1951 to 1953. Am J Med 29:55, 1960

245. Ducci H, Katz R: Cortisone, ACTH and antibiotics in fulminant hepatitis. Gastroenterology 21:357, 1952

246. Dudley FJ et al: Cell-mediated immunity in patients positive for hepatitis-associated antigen. Br Med J 4:754, 1972

247. Duermeyer W, Van Der Veen J: Specific detection of IgM-antibodies by ELISA applied in hepatitis A. Lancet 2:684, 1978

248. Duffy J et al: Polyarthritis, polyarteritis and hepatitis B. Medicine 55:19, 1976

249. Earampamoorthy S, Koff RS: Health hazards of bivalve-mollusk ingestion. Ann Intern Med 83:107, 1975

250. Eckhardt R et al: K-lymphocytes (killer-cells) in Crohn's disease and acute virus B hepatitis. Gut 18:1010, 1977

251. Edgington TS, Chisari FV: Immunological aspects of hepatitis B virus infection. Am J Med Sci 270:213, 1975

252. Edgington TS, Ritt DJ: Intrahepatic expression of serum hepatitis virus-associated antigens. J Exp Med 134:871, 1971

253. Edlund A: The effect of defined physical exercise in the early convalescence of viral hepatitis. Scand J Infect Dis 3:189, 1973

254. Egoz N et al: Viral hepatitis in Israel: Transfusion-associated hepatitis. Transfusion 12:12, 1972

255. Eisenburg VJ et al: Gammaglobulin-therapie der akuten Virushepatitis. Fortschr Med 93:1085, 1975

256. Eisenstein AB et al: An epidemic of hepatitis in a general hospital. Probable transmission by contaminated orange juice. JAMA 185:171, 1963

257. Ellis-Pegler R et al: Transfer factor and hepatitis B: A double-blind study. Clin Exp Immunol 36:221, 1979

258. Enk B, Friss T: Red cell survival in acute hepatitis. Nord Med 86:1148, 1971

259. Epidemic of Homologous Serum Hepatitis: Foreign Letters. JAMA 137:209, 1948

260. European Association for the Study of the Liver: Randomized trial of steroid therapy in acute liver failure. Gut 20:620, 1979

261. Evans AS et al: Adrenal hormone therapy in viral hepatitis: IV. The effect of gamma globulin and oral cortisone in the acute disease. Am J Med 19:783, 1955

262. Evans AS et al: Adrenal hormone therapy in viral hepatitis: I. The effect of ACTH in the acute disease. Ann Intern Med 38:1115, 1953

263. Evans AS et al: Adrenal hormone therapy in viral hepatitis: II. The effect of cortisone in the acute disease. Ann Intern Med 38:1134, 1953

264. Evans AS et al: Adrenal hormone therapy in viral hepatitis: III. The effect of ACTH and cortisone in severe and fulminant cases. Ann Intern Med 38:1148, 1953

265. Expert Committee on Hepatitis: First report, Technical Report Series No. 62. Geneva, World Health Organization, 1953

266. Farci P et al: Delta hepatitis in inapparent carriers of hepatitis B surface antigen: A disease simulating acute hepatitis B progressive to chronicity. Gastroenterology 85:669, 1983

267. Farini R et al: La terapia corticosteoidea nell'epatite acute virale (E.V.A.). Rev Ospedali 4:103, 1972

268. Farivar M et al: Effect of insulin and glucagon on fulminant murine hepatitis. N Engl J Med 295:1517, 1976

269. Farquhar JD: Renal studies in acute infectious (epidemic) hepatitis. Am J Med Sci 218:291, 1949

270. Fauerholdt L et al: Significance of chronic aggressive hepatitis in acute hepatitis. Gastroenterology 73:543, 1977

271. Favero MS et al: Hepatitis-B antigen on environmental surfaces. Lancet 2:1455, 1973

272. Fawaz KA et al: Repetitive maternal-fetal transmission of fatal hepatitis B. N Engl J Med 293:1357, 1975

273. Feinman SV et al: Failure to detect hepatitis B surface antigen (HBsAg) in feces of HBsAg-positive persons. J Infect Dis 140:407, 1979

274. Feinstone SM, Hoofnagle JH: Non-A, may be -B hepatitis. N Engl J Med 311:185, 1984

275. Feinstone SM et al: Hepatitis A: Detection by immune electron microscopy of a virus-like antigen associated with acute illness. Science 182:1026, 1973

276. Feinstone SM et al: Transfusion-associated hepatitis not due to viral hepatitis type A or B. N Engl J Med 292:767, 1975

277. Feinstone SM et al: Live attenuated vaccine for hepatitis A. Dev Biol Standard 54:429, 1983

278. Feinstone SM et al: Inactivation of hepatitis B virus and non-A, non-B hepatitis by chloroform. Infect Immun 41:816, 1983

279. Feinstone SM et al: Non-A, non-B hepatitis in chimpanzees and marmosets. J Infect Dis 144:588, 1981

280. Feitelson MA et al: Core particles of hepatitis B virus and ground squirrel hepatitis virus: II. Characterization of the protein kinase reaction associated with ground squirrel hepatitis virus and hepatitis B virus. J Virol 43:741, 1982

281. Feldman RE, Schiff ER: Hepatitis in dental professionals. JAMA 232:1228, 1975

282. Felsher BF, Carpio NM: Chronic persistent hepatitis and unconjugated hyperbilirubinemia. Gastroenterology 76:248, 1979

283. Fernandez B, McCarty DJ: The arthritis of viral hepatitis. Ann Intern Med 74:207, 1971

284. Ferns RB et al: Monoclonal antibodies to hepatitis B e antigen (HBeAg) derived from hepatitis B core antigen (HBcAg). Their use in characterization and detection of HBeAg. J Gen Virol 65:899, 1984

285. Figus A et al: Hepatitis B viral nucleotide sequences in non-A, non-B or hepatitis B virus-related chronic liver disease. Hepatology 4:364, 1984

286. Findlay GM: Infective hepatitis in West Africa: I. Mon Bull Ministry Health 7:2, 1948

287. Findlay GM, MacCallum FO: Note on acute hepatitis and yellow fever immunization. Trans R Soc Trop Med Hyg 31:297, 1937

288. Findlay GM et al: Hepatitis after yellow fever inoculation: Relation to infective hepatitis. Lancet 2:301, 340, 365, 1944

289. Findlay GM et al: Observations on epidemic catarrhal jaundice. Trans R Soc Med Hyg 25:7, 1931

290. Flehmig B et al: A solid-phase radioimmunoassay for detection of IgM antibodies to hepatitis A virus. J Infect Dis 140:169, 1979

291. Fogarty International Center Proceedings No. 22: Diseases of the liver and biliary tract: Standardization of nomenclature, diagnostic criteria, and diagnostic methodology, DHEW publication No. (NIE) 76-725. Washington, DC

292. Ford JC: Infective hepatitis: 300 cases in an outer London borough. Lancet 1:675, 1943

293. Foutch PG et al: Concomitant hepatitis B surface antigen and antibody in thirteen patients. Ann Intern Med 99:460, 1983

294. Fowinkle EW, Guthrie N: Comparison of two doses of gamma globulin in prevention of infectious hepatitis. Public Health Rep 79:634, 1964

295. Fowler MJF et al: Analyses of the molecular state of HBV DNA in the liver and serum of patients with chronic hepatitis or primary liver cell carcinoma and the effect of therapy with adenine arabinoside. Gut 25:611, 1984

296. Fowler MJF et al: The mechanism of replication of hepatitis B virus: Evidence for asymmetric replication of the two DNA strands. J Med Virol 13:83, 1984

297. Frame JD: Hepatitis among missionaries in Ethiopia and Sudan. JAMA 203:819, 1968

298. Francis DP et al: The prevention of hepatitis B with vaccine: Report of the Center for Disease Control multi-center efficacy trial among homosexual men. Ann Intern Med 97:362, 1982

299. Francis T Jr et al: Demonstration of infectious hepatitis virus in presymptomatic period after transfer by transfusion. Proc Soc Exp Biol Med 61:276, 1946

300. Fraser R: A study of epidemic catarrhal jaundice. Can J Public Health 22:396, 1931

301. Freeman G: Epidemiology and incubation period of jaundice following yellow fever vaccination. Am J Trop Med 26:15, 1946

302. Friedmann CTH et al: Chimpanzee-associated hepatitis among personnel at an animal hospital. J Am Vet Med Assoc 159:541, 1971

303. Frosner GG et al: Seroepidemiologic investigations of patients and family contacts in an epidemic of hepatitis A. J Med Virol 1:163, 1977

304. Frosner GG et al: Propagation of human hepatitis A virus in a hepatoma cell line. Infection 7:303, 1979

305. Frosner GG: Zuchtung des Hepatitis A Virus in Gewebekultur: Moghckeit zur virus Produktion fur impfstpffe undtestzwercke, zur Untersuchung von Patienten auf In-

fektiositat und zur Prufung von Desinfektionsmitteln. Offentl Gesundh Wes 44:370, 1982

306. Fulop M, Sandson J: The effect of bile salts on the binding of bilirubin by plasma proteins. Clin Sci 33:459, 1967

307. Fulop M et al: Dialysability of conjugated bilirubin from plasma of jaundiced dogs and patients. Lancet 1:1017, 1964

308. Gabinus O, Jonsson T: Serum hepatitis through wound infection. Lancet 1:43, 1962

309. Galambos JT: Chronic persisting hepatitis. Am J Dig Dis 9:817, 1964

310. Galambos JT et al: The effect of intravenous ethanol on serum enzymes in patients with normal or diseased liver. Gastroenterology 44:267, 1963

311. Galambos JT et al: Unpublished observations, 1977

312. Galbraith RM et al: Non-A, non-B hepatitis associated with chronic liver disease in a haemodialysis unit. Lancet 1:951, 1979

313. Galbraith RM et al: Chronic liver disease developing after outbreak of HBsAg-negative hepatitis in haemodialysis unit. Lancet 2:886, 1975

314. Galibert F et al: Nucleotide sequence of the hepatitis B virus genome (subtype ayw) cloned in E. coli. Nature 281:646, 1979

315. Gallus AS et al: Coagulation studies in patients with acute infectious hepatitis. Br J Haematol 22:761, 1972

316. Gard S: Discussion. In Hartman FW et al (eds): Hepatitis Frontiers, Henry Ford Hospital International Symposium, p 241. Boston, Little, Brown, & Co, 1957

317. Gardner HT et al: Hepatitis among American occupation troops in Germany. Ann Intern Med 30:1009, 1949

318. Gardner HT et al: Serum cholesterol and cholesterol esters in viral hepatitis. Am J Med 8:584, 1950

319. Garibaldi RA et al: Hemodialysis-associated hepatitis. JAMA 225:384, 1973

320. Garibaldi RA et al: Impact of illicit drug-associated hepatitis on viral hepatitis morbidity reports in the United States. J Infect Dis 126:288, 1972

321. Garibaldi RA et al: Nonparenteral serum hepatitis: Report of an outbreak. JAMA 220:963, 1972

322. Garibaldi RA et al: Hospital-acquired serum hepatitis: Report of an outbreak. JAMA 219:1577, 1972

323. Garnier P, Harpey JP et al: Paralysie faciale au cours d'une hepatitie virale. Arch Fr Pediat 30:549, 1973

324. Gateau PH et al: Passive immunotherapy in HBsAg fulminant hepatitis: Results on antigenemia and survival. Digestion 14:304, 1976

325. Gauss-Muller V et al: Propagation of hepatitis A virus in human embryo fibroblasts. J Med Virol 7:233, 1981

326. Gazzard BG et al: Causes of death in fulminant hepatic failure and relationship to quantitative histological assessment of parenchymal damage. Q J Med 44:615, 1975

327. Gellis SS, Stokes J Jr: Methylene blue test in infectious (epidemic) hepatitis. JAMA 128:782, 1945

328. Gellis SS et al: Chemical, clinical, and immunological studies on the products of human plasma fractionation: XXXVI. Inactivation of the virus of homologous serum hepatitis in solutions of normal human serum albumin by means of heat. J Clin Invest 27:239, 1948

329. Gellis SS et al: The use of human immune serum globulin (gamma globulin) in infectious (epidemic) hepatitis in the Mediterranean theater of operations: I. Studies on prophylaxis in two epidemics of infectious hepatitis. JAMA 128:1062, 1945

330. Gellis SS et al: The use of human immune serum globulin (gamma globulin) in infectious (epidemic) hepatitis in the Mediterranean theater of operations: II. Studies on treatment in an epidemic of infectious hepatitis. JAMA 128:1158, 1945

331. Gelpi AP: Fatal hepatitis in Saudi Arabian women. Am J Gastroenterol 53:41, 1970

332. Gerber MA et al: Incidence and nature of cytoplasmic hepatitis B antigen in hepatocytes. Lab Invest 32:251, 1975

333. Gerber MA et al: Electron microscopy and immunoelectron microscopy of cytoplasmic hepatitis B antigen in hepatocytes. Am J Pathol 75:489, 1974

334. Gerety RJ et al: Hepatitis B surface antigen (HBsAg) subtypes and indices of clinical disease. Gastroenterology 68:1253, 1975

335. Gerety RJ et al: Summary of an international workshop on hepatitis B vaccines. J Infect Dis 140:642, 1979

336. Gerety RJ et al: Non-A, non-B hepatitis agents. In Vyas GN, Dienstag JL, Hoofnagle JH (eds): Viral Hepatitis and Liver Disease, p 23. Orlando, FL, Grune & Stratton, 1984

337. Gerin JL et al: Biochemical characterization of Australia antigen. Am J Pathol 81:651, 1975

338. Gerin JL et al: Biophysical properties of Australia antigen. J Virol 4:763, 1969

339. Gerin JL et al: Antigens of hepatitis B virus: Failure to detect HBeAg on the surfaces of HBsAg forms. J Gen Virol 38:561, 1978

340. Gerin JL et al: Chemically synthesized peptides of hepatitis B surface antigen duplicate the d/y specificities and induce subtype specific antibodies in chimpanzees. Proc Natl Acad Sci USA 80:2365, 1983

340a. Gerlich WH et al: Specificity and localization of the hepatitis B virus-associated protein kinase. J Virol 42:761, 1982

341. Geslien GE et al: The sensitivity and specificity of ^{99m}Tc-sulfur colloid liver imaging in diffuse hepatocellular disease. Radiology 118:115, 1976

342. Gianotti F: Papular acrodermatitis of childhood: An Australia antigen disease. Arch Dis Child 48:794, 1973

343. Gibson PE: Quantitiative analysis of the major sub-determinants of hepatitis B surface antigen. J Infect Dis 134:540, 1976

344. Giles JP et al: Early viremia and viruria in infectious hepatitis. Virology 24:107, 1964

345. Giles JP et al: Viral hepatitis: Relation of Australia/SH antigen to the Willowbrook MS-2 strain. N Engl J Med 281:119, 1969

346. Gille G et al: Serum hepatitis among Swedish track-finders: II. A clinical study. Acta Med Scand 82:129, 1967

347. Giraud P et al: Hepatitis B virus infection of children born to mothers with severe hepatitis. Lancet 2:1088, 1975

348. Gocke DJ: Fulminant hepatitis treated with serum containing antibody to Australia antigen. N Engl J Med 284:919, 1971

349. Gocke DJ: A prospective study of posttransfusion hepatitis: The role of Australia antigen. JAMA 219:1165, 1972

350. Gocke DJ, Kavey NB: Hepatitis antigen: Correlation with disease and infectivity of blood donors. Lancet 1:1055, 1969

351. Goh KT et al: An epidemic of cockles-associated hepatitis A in Singapore. Bull WHO 62:893, 1984

352. Goldberg DM, Campbell DR: Biochemical investigation of outbreak of infectious hepatitis in a closed community. Br Med J 2:1435, 1962

353. Gordon SC et al: Prolonged intrahepatic cholestasis secondary to acute hepatitis A. Ann Intern Med 101:635, 1984

354. Gostling JVT: Long-incubation hepatitis and tattooing. Lancet 2:1033, 1971

355. Goto Y et al: Characterization of hepatitis B virus DNA polymerase. Jpn J Med Sci Biol 37:9, 1984

356. Goubran GF et al: Hepatitis B virus infection in dental surgical practice. Br Med J 2:559, 1976

357. Govindarajan S et al: Fulminant B viral hepatitis: Role of delta agent. Gastroenterology 86:1417, 1984

358. Grady GF: Hepatitis B from medical professionals: How rare? How preventable? N Engl J Med 296:995, 1977

359. Grady GF et al: Eight years of surveillance of hospitalized hepatitis patients interpreted in light of epidemic parenteral drug abuse and availability of testing for hepatitis-associated antigen. J Infect Dis 126:87, 1972

360. Grady GF et al: Risk of post-transfusion viral hepatitis. N Engl J Med 271:337, 1964

361. Grady GF et al: Relation of "e" antigen to infectivity of HBsAg-positive inoculations among medical personnel. Lancet 2:492, 1976

362. Grady GF et al: Hepatitis B immune globulin for accidental exposure among medical personnel: Final report of a multicenter controlled trial. J Infect Dis 138:625, 1978

363. Grady GF et al: Hepatitis B antibody in conventional gamma-globulin. J Infect Dis 132:474, 1975

364. Grauer W et al: Immunosuppressive serum factors in viral hepatitis: III. Prognostic relevance of rosette inhibitory factor and serum inhibition factor in acute and chronic hepatitis. Hepatology 4:15, 1984

365. Gravelle CR et al: Hepatitis A: Report of a common-source outbreak with recovery of a possible etiologic agent: II. Laboratory studies. J Infect Dis 131:167, 1975

366. Gravelle CR et al: Temporal patterns of ultrastructural alterations in hepatocytes of chimpanzees with experimental non-A, non-B hepatitis. J Infect Dis 145:854, 1982

367. Gregory PB et al: Steroid therapy in severe viral hepatitis: A double-blind randomized trial of methylprednisolone versus placebo. N Engl J Med 294:681, 1976

368. Grist NR: Hepatitis in clinical laboratories 1975–6. J Clin Pathol 31:415, 1978

369. Grob PJ, Jemelka HI: Fecal SH-antigen in acute hepatitis. Am J Dis Child 123:400, 1972

370. Grob PJ, Moeschlin P: Risk to contacts of a medical practitioner carrying HBsAg. N Engl J Med 293:197, 1975

371. Gross PA, Gerding DN: Pleural effusion associated with viral hepatitis. Gastroenterology 60:898, 1971

372. Gruer LD et al: Relapsing hepatitis associated with hepatitis A virus. Lancet 2:163, 1982

373. Gudat F, Bianchi L: Evidence for phasic sequences in nuclear HBsAg formation and membrane-directed flow of core particles in chronic hepatitis. Gastroenterology 73:1194, 1977

374. Gudat F, Bianchi L: HBsAg: A target antigen on the liver cell? In Popper H et al (eds): Membrane Alterations as Basis of Liver Injury, p 171. Lancaster, MTP Press, 1977

375. Gudat F et al: Pattern of core and surface expression in liver tissue reflects state of specific immune response in hepatitis B. Lab Invest 32:1, 1975

376. Gudman-Hoyer E, Soeberg B: Jejunal brush-border disaccharidase and alkaline phosphatase activity in acute viral hepatitis. Scand J Gastroenterol 8:377, 1973

377. Gust ID: The epidemiology of viral hepatitis. In Vyas GN, Dienstag JL, Hoofnagle JH, (eds.): Viral Hepatitis and Liver Disease p 415. Orlando, FL, Grune & Stratton, 1984

378. Gust ID et al: Non-B hepatitis in Melbourne: A serological study of hepatitis A virus infection. Br Med J 1:193, 1977

379. Gust ID et al: Absence of Au antigen in faeces of patients with Au-positive sera. Lancet 1:797, 1971

380. Gust ID et al: Taxonomic classification of hepatitis A virus. Intervirology 20:1, 1983

381. Gutzeit K: Die Hepatitis epidemica. Munchen Med Wochenschr 92:1161, 1295, 1950

382. Hadler SC et al: Hepatitis A in day-care centers: A community-wide assessment. N Engl J Med 302:1222, 1980

383. Hadler SC et al: An outbreak of hepatitis B in a dental practice. Ann Intern Med 95:133, 1981

383a. Hadler SC et al: Risk factors for hepatitis A in day-care centers. J Infect Dis 145:255, 1982

384. Hadler SC et al: Delta virus infection and severe hepatitis: An epidemic in the Yucpa Indians of Venezuela. Ann Intern Med 100:339, 1984

385. Hadler SC et al: Effect of immunoglobulin on hepatitis A in day-care centers. JAMA 249:48, 1983

386. Hagler L et al: Aplastic anemia following viral hepatitis. Medicine 54:139, 1975

387. Halbert SP, Anken M: Detection of hepatitis B surface antigen (HBsAg) with use of alkaline phosphatase–labeled antibody to HBsAg. J Infect Dis 136:S318, 1977

388. Hall WT et al: Comparison of sensitivity of radioimmunoassay and immune electron microscopy for detecting hepatitis A antigen in fecal extracts. Proc Soc Exp Biol Med 155:193, 1977

389. Hall WT et al: Protective effect of immune serum globulin (ISG) against hepatitis A infection in a national epidemic. Am J Epidemiol 106:72, 1977

390. Hallgren R: Epidemic hepatitis in the country of Vasterbotten in Northern Sweden: II. Continued epidemiologial and clinical studies. Acta Med Scand 115:21, 1943

391. Hampers CL et al: Post transfusion anicteric hepatitis. N Engl J Med 271:747, 1964

392. Hansbarger EA, Hyun BH: Acute hemolytic anemia in viral hepatitis. Va Med Monthly 90:134, 1963

393. Hansson BG et al: Infection with delta agent in Sweden: Introduction of a new hepatitis agent. J Infect Dis 146:472, 1982

394. Hantz O et al: Non-A, non-B hepatitis: Identification of hepatitis-B-like virus particles in serum and liver. J Med Virol 5:73, 1980

395. Harden AG et al: Transmission of infectious hepatitis by transfusion of whole blood. N Engl J Med 253:923, 1955

396. Harrison TJ et al: Assay of HBV DNA in the plasma of HBV-carrier chimpanzees superinfected with non-A, non-B hepatitis. J Virol Methods 6:295, 1983

397. Hatzakis A et al: Sex-related differences in immunoglobulin and in total antibody response to hepatitis A virus observed in two epidemics of hepatitis A. Am J Epidemiol 120:936, 1984

398. Havens WP Jr: Elimination in human feces of infectious hepatitis virus parenterally introduced. Proc Soc Exp Biol Med 61:210, 1946

399. Havens WP Jr: Experiment in cross immunity between infectious hepatitis and homologous serum jaundice. Proc Soc Exp Biol Med 59:148, 1945

400. Havens WP Jr: Immunity in experimentally induced infectious hepatitis. J Exp Med 84:403, 1946

401. Havens WP Jr: Infectious hepatitis. Medicine 27:279, 1948

402. Havens WP Jr: Infectious hepatitis in the Middle East: A clinical review of 200 cases seen in a military hospital. JAMA 126:17, 1944

403. Havens WP Jr: Period of infectivity of patients with experimentally induced infectious hepatitis. J Exp Med 83:251, 1946

404. Havens WP Jr: Period of infectivity of patients with homologous serum jaundice and routes of infection in this disease. J Exp Med 83:441, 1946

405. Havens WP Jr: Properties of the etiologic agent of infectious hepatitis. Proc Soc Exp Biol Med 58:203, 1945

406. Havens WP Jr: Viral hepatitis: Clinical patterns and diagnosis. Am J Med 32:665, 1962

407. Havens WP Jr, Marck RE: The leukocytic response of patients with experimentally induced infectious hepatitis. Am J Med Sci 212:129, 1946

408. Havens WP Jr, Paul JR: Prevention of infectious hepatitis with gamma globulin. JAMA 129:270, 1945

409. Havens WP Jr et al: Experimental production of hepatitis by feeding icterogenic materials. Proc Soc Exp Biol Med 57:206, 1944

410. Havens WP Jr et al: Experimentally induced infectious hepatitis: Roentgenographic and gastroscopic observations. Arch Intern Med 79:457, 1947

411. Havens WP Jr et al: The half-life of ^{131}I labeled normal human gamma globulin in patients with hepatic cirrhosis. J Immunol 73:256, 1954

412. Hayman JM, Read WA: Some clinical observations on an outbreak of jaundice following yellow fever vaccination. Am J Med Sci 209:281, 1945

413. Heathcote J, Sherlock S: Spread of acute type B hepatitis in London. Lancet 1:1468, 1973

414. Heathcote J et al: Hepatitis B antigen in saliva and semen. Lancet 1:71, 1974

415. Heermann KH et al: Large surface proteins of hepatitis B virus containing the pre-S sequence. J Virol 52:396, 1984

416. Heiner DC, Evans L: Immunoglobulins and other proteins in commercial preparations of gamma globulin. J Pediatr 70:820, 1967

417. Heisto H, Julsrud AC: Silent carriers of hepatitis virus B. Acta Med Scand 164:349, 1959

418. Henkin RI, Smith FR: Hyposmia in acute viral hepatitis. Lancet 1:823, 1971

419. Hersh T et al: Nonparenteral transmission of viral hepatitis type B (Australia antigen-associated serum hepatitis). N Engl J Med 285:1363, 1971

420. Hess G et al: The demonstration of subtype (d or y)-specific determinants on the surface of the presumed hepatitis B virus. J Immunol 119:1542, 1977

421. Hillenbrand P et al: Significance of intravascular coagulation and fibrinolysis in acute hepatic failure. Gut 15:83, 1974

422. Hillis WD: An outbreak of infectious hepatitis among chimpanzee handlers at a United States Air Force base. Am J Hyg 73:316, 1961

423. Hindman SH et al: "e" antigen, Dane particles, and serum DNA polymerase activity in HBsAg carriers. Ann Intern Med 85:458, 1976

424. Hinton WA: Acute infectious hepatitis, a hazard for workers in blood testing laboratories. Public Health Lab 5:2, 1947

425. Hirschman SZ: The hepatitis B virus and its DNA polymerase: The prototype three-D virus. Mol Cell Biochem 26:47, 1979

426. Hirschman SZ, Garfinkel E: Inhibition of hepatitis B DNA polymerase by intercalating agents. Nature 271:681, 1978

427. Hirschman SZ, Garfinkel E: Ionic requirements of the DNA polymerase associated with serum hepatitis B antigen. J Infect Dis 135:897, 1977

428. Hirschman SZ et al: Differential activation of hepatitis B DNA polymerase by detergent and salt. J Med Virol 2:61, 1978

429. Hirschman SZ et al: Purification of naked intranuclear particles from human liver infected by hepatitis B virus. Proc Natl Acad Sci 71:3345, 1974

430. Hoagland CL et al: An analysis of the effect of fat in the diet on recovery in infectious hepatitis. Am J Public Health 36:1287, 1946

431. Hoagland CL, Shank RE: Infectious hepatitis: A review of 200 cases. JAMA 130:615, 1946

432. Hoefs JC et al: Hepatitis B surface antigen in pancreatic and biliary secretions. Gastroenterology 79:191, 1980

433. Hofschneider PH et al: Labeling of hepatitis B virus surface antigen (HBsAg) synthesized in a HBsAg producing hepatoma cell line. J Med Virol 4:171, 1979

434. Hollinger FB et al: Detection of hepatitis A viral antigen by radioimmunoassay. J Immunol 115:1464, 1975

435. Hollinger FB et al: Non-A, non-B hepatitis transmission in chimpanzees: A project of the Transfusion-Transmitted Viruses Study Group. Intervirology 10:60, 1978

436. Hollinger FB et al: Immune response to hepatitis virus type B in Down's syndrome and other mentally retarded patients. Am J Epidemiol 95:356, 1972

437. Hollinger FB et al: A prospective study indicating that double-antibody radioimmunoassay reduces the incidence of post-transfusion hepatitis B. N Engl J Med 290:1104, 1974

438. Hollinger FB et al: Transfusion-transmitted viruses study: Experimental evidence for two non-A, non-B hepatitis agents. J Infect Dis 142:400, 1980

439. Hollinger FB et al: Response to hepatitis B vaccine in a young adult population. In Szmuness W, Alter HJ, Maynard JE (eds): Viral Hepatitis, pp 451–466. Philadelphia, Franklin Institute Press, 1982

440. Hollinger FB et al: Reduction in risk of hepatitis transmission by heat treatment of a human factor VIII concentrate. J Infect Dis 150:250, 1984

441. Holmes AW: Chronic hepatitis A: An historical note. J Med Virol 15:101, 1985

442. Holmes AW et al: Transmission of human hepatitis to marmosets: Further coded studies. J Infect Dis 124:520, 1971

443. Holmes AW et al: Hepatitis in marmosets: Induction of disease with coded specimens from a human volunteer study. Science 165:816, 1969

444. Hoofnagle JH, Feinstone SM: Serological tests for non-A, non-B hepatitis: Controversy. Liver 1:177, 1981

445. Hoofnagle JH, Waggoner JG: Hepatitis A and B virus markers in immune serum globulin. Gastroenterology 78:259, 1980

446. Hoofnagle JH et al: Antibody to hepatitis B virus core in man. Lancet 2:869, 1973

447. Hoofnagle JH et al: Antibody to hepatitis B core antigen: A sensitive indicator of hepatitis B virus replication. N Engl J Med 290:1336, 1974

448. Hoofnagle JH et al: Subtyping of hepatitis B surface antigen

and antibody by radioimmunoassay. Gastroenterology 72: 290, 1977

449. Hoofnagle JH et al: Transmission of non-A, non-B hepatitis. Ann Intern Med 87:14, 1977

450. Hoofnagle JH et al: Immunofluorescence microscopy in experimentally induced, type B hepatitis in the chimpanzee. Gastroenterology 74:182, 1978

451. Hoofnagle JH et al: Passive-active immunity from hepatitis B immune globulin: A re-analysis of a Veterans Administration Cooperative Study of needlestick hepatitis. Ann Intern Med 91:813, 1979

452. Hoofnagle JH et al: Serologic responses in HB. In Vyas GN et al (eds): Viral Hepatitis, p 219. Philadelphia, Franklin Institute Press, 1978

453. Hoofnagle JH et al: Type B hepatitis after transfusion with blood containing antibody to hepatitis B core antigen. N Engl J Med 298:1379, 1978

454. Hoppe J, Schmidt K: Statische Analyse zur Wirkung der intravenosen Immunoglobulin-prophylaxe der Transfusionhepatitis. Dtsch Med Wochenschr 99:1092, 1974

455. Horney JT, Galambos JT: The liver during and after fulminant hepatitis. Gastroenterology 73:639, 1977

456. Howard CR, Burrell CJ: Structure and nature of hepatitis B antigen. Prog Virology 22:36, 1976

457. Howells L, Kerr JDO: Hepatitis after penicillin injections. Lancet 1:51, 1946

458. Hruska JF, Robinson WS: The proteins of hepatitis B Dane particle cores. J Med Virol 1:119, 1977

459. Hoy JF et al: Delta agent infection in Melbourne. J Med Virol 13:339, 1984

460. Hoyer B et al: Properties of delta-associated ribonucleic acid. In Verme G, Bonino F, Rizzetto M (eds): Viral Hepatitis and Delta Infection, p. 91. New York, Alan R. Liss, 1983

461. Huang SN: Structural and immunoreactive characteristics of hepatitis B core antigen. Am J Med Sci 270:131, 1975

462. Huang SN et al: A study of the relationship of virus-like particles and Australia antigen in liver. Hum Pathol 5: 209, 1974

463. Huang SN et al: Electron and immunoelectron microscopic study on liver tissues of marmosets infected with hepatitis A virus. Lab Invest 41:63, 1979

464. Hughes JV et al: Neutralizing monoclonal antibodies to hepatitis A virus: Partial localization of a neutralizing antigenic site. J Virol 52:465, 1984

465. Hughes RR: Postpenicillin jaundice. Br Med J 2:685, 1946

466. Imai M et al: Antigenicity of reduced and alkylated Australia antigen. J Immunol 112:416, 1974

467. Imai M et al: Hepatitis B antigen-associated deoxyribonucleic acid polymerase activity and e antigen/anti-e system. Infect Immun 14:631, 1976

468. Imai M et al: A receptor for polymerized human and chimpanzee albumins on hepatitis B virus particles co-occurring with HBeAg. Gastroenterology 76:242, 1979

469. Immune Globulins for Protection Against Viral Hepatitis: Recommendation of the Public Health Service Advisory Committee on Immunization Practices. Center for Disease Control. MMWR 26:52, 1977

470. Inaba N et al: Sexual transmission of hepatitis B surface antigen: Infection of husbands by HBsAg carrier-state wives. Br J Vener Dis 55:366, 1979

471. Ipsen J et al: Sociologic factors in the spread of epidemic hepatitis in a rural school district. J Hyg 50:457, 1952

472. Ishak KG: Viral hepatitis: The morphologic spectrum. In

Gall EA et al (eds): The Liver, p 218. Baltimore, Williams & Wilkins, 1973

473. Iversen P, Roholm K: On aspiration biopsy of the liver with remarks on its diagnostic significance. Acta Med Scand 102:1, 1939

474. Iwarson S et al: Multiple attacks of hepatitis in drug addicts: Immunochemical and histological characteristics. J Infect Dis 127:544, 1973

475. Iwarson S et al: Protection against hepatitis B virus infection by immunization with hepatitis B core antigen. Gastroenterology 88:763, 1985

476. Jacobson IM et al: Epidemiology and clinical impact of hepatitis D virus (delta) infection. Hepatology 5:188, 1985

477. Jakob G: Zur Prognose der Transfusionhepatis. Blut 26: 1, 1973

478. Jampol ML, Shahidi F: Prognosis in homologous serum hepatitis. NY State J Med 63:672, 1963

479. Janeway CA: Plasma fractionation. Adv Intern Med 3: 295, 1949

480. Jaundice following yellow fever vaccination. JAMA 119: 1110, 1942

481. Jehn: Icterusepidemie in wahrscheinlichem Zusammenhang mit vorausgegangener Revaccination. Dtsch Med Wochenschr 11:339, 354, 1885

482. Jensen DM et al: Detection of antibodies directed against a liver specific membrane lipoprotein in patients with acute and chronic active hepatitis. N Engl J Med 299:1, 1978

483. Jezequel AM et al: Les cellules clarifées dans l'hepatite parenchymateuse: Étude comparée en microscopie optique et electronique. Presse Med 68:567, 1960

484. Jilg W et al: Clinical evaluation of a recombinant hepatitis B vaccine. Lancet 2:1174, 1984

485. John TJ et al: Epidemic hepatitis B caused by commercial human immunoglobulin. Lancet 1:1074, 1979

486. Johnson CJ et al: Ear piercing and hepatitis: Nonsterile instruments for ear piercing and the subsequent onset of viral hepatitis. JAMA 227:1165, 1974

487. Johnson JS: Serum hepatitis and illicit drug use. Rocky Mt Med J 2:43, 1968

488. Jones CM, Minot GR: Infectious "catarrhal" jaundice: An attempt to establish a clinical entity. Boston Med Surg J 189:531, 1923

489. Joseph PR et al: An outbreak of hepatitis traced to food contamination. N Engl J Med 273:188, 1965

490. Jupp PG, McElligott SE: Transmission experiments with hepatitis B surface antigen and the common bedbug (Cimex lectularius L). S Afr Med J 56:54, 1979

491. Kanai K et al: Prevention of perinatal transmission of hepatitis B virus (HBV) to children of e antigen–positive HBV carrier mothers by hepatitis B immune globulin and HBV vaccine. J Infect Dis 151:287, 1985

492. Kane MA et al: Epidemic non-A, non-B hepatitis in Nepal: Recovery of a possible etiologic agent and transmission studies in marmosets. JAMA 252:3140, 1984

493. Kao HW et al: The persistence of hepatitis A IgM antibody after clinical hepatitis A. Hepatology 4:933, 1984

494. Kaplan PM et al: Demonstration of subpopulations of Dane particles. J Virol 17:885, 1976

495. Kaplan PM et al: Hepatitis B specific DNA polymerase activity during post-transfusion hepatitis. Nature 249:762, 1974

496. Kaplan PM et al: DNA polymerase associated with human hepatitis B antigen. J Virol 12:995, 1973

497. Karvountzis GG et al: Serologic characterization of pa-

tients with two episodes of acute viral hepatitis. Am J Med 58:815, 1975

498. Karvountzis GG et al: Long-term follow-up studies of patients surviving fulminant viral hepatitis. Gastroenterology 67:870, 1974

499. Katz R et al: Post-transfusion hepatitis-effect of modified gamma globulin added to blood in vitro. N Engl J Med 285:925, 1971

500. Katz R et al: Red cell survival estimated by radiochromium in hepatobiliary disease. Gastroenterology 46:399, 1964

501. Katz R et al: Corticosteroids in the treatment of acute hepatitis in coma. Gastroenterology 42:258, 1962

502. Kendrick MA: Study of illness among Americans returning from international travel, July 11–August 24, 1971 (preliminary data). J Infect Dis 126:684, 1972

503. Kendrick MA: Summary of study on illness among Americans visiting Europe, March 31, 1969–March 30, 1970. J Infect Dis 126:685, 1972

504. Kendrick MA: Viral hepatitis in American missionaries abroad. J Infect Dis 129:227, 1974

505. Kennedy RC et al: Immune response to hepatitis B surface antigen: Enhancement by prior injection of antibodies to the idiotype. Science 221:853, 1983

506. Kew MC et al: Serum alpha-fetoprotein levels in acute viral hepatitis. Gut 14:939, 1973

507. Khan NC et al: Localization of hepatitis A virus antigen to specific subcellular fractions of hepatitis-A–infected chimpanzee liver cells. Intervirology 21:187, 1984

508. Khuroo MS: Study of an epidemic of non-A, non-B hepatitis: Possibility of another human hepatitis virus distinct from post-transfusion non-A, non-B type. Am J Med 68:818, 1980

509. Kim CY, Tilles JG: Purification and biophysical characterization of hepatitis B antigen. J Clin Invest 52:1176, 1973

510. Kindmark CO, Laurell CB: Sequential changes of the plasma protein pattern in inoculation hepatitis. Scand J Clin Lab Invest 29(suppl 124):105, 1972

511. Kirk R: Spread of infective hepatitis. Lancet 1:80, 1945

512. Kissel P, Arnould G: Les Maladies á Virus Lymphotrope: Leurs Manifestations Nerveuses, p 160. Paris, Doin, 1952

513. Kistler GS et al: Hepatitis B antigen (HB-Ag, Australia antigen) in mixed saliva of patients with HB antigenemia. Pathol Microbiol 39:313, 1973

514. Kivel RM: Hematologic aspects of acute viral hepatitis. AM J Dig Dis 6:1017, 1961

515. Klatskin G: Subacute hepatic necrosis and post-necrotic cirrhosis due to anicteric infections with the hepatitis virus. Am J Med 25:333, 1958

516. Klion FM, Schaffner F: The ultrastructure of acidophilic "Councilman-like" bodies in the liver. Am J Pathol 48:755, 1966

517. Kluge T: Gamma-globulin in the prevention of viral hepatitis: A study on the effect of medium-size doses. Acta Med Scand 174:469, 1963

518. Knecht GL, Chisari FV: Reversibility of hepatitis B virus–induced glomerulonephritis and chronic active hepatitis after spontaneous clearance of serum hepatitis B surface antigen. Gastroenterology 75:1152, 1978

519. Knight V et al: Characteristics of spread of infectious hepatitis in schools and households in an epidemic in a rural area. Am J Hyg 59:1, 1954

520. Knight WA, Cogswell RC: Preliminary observations of the gastric mucosa in patients with infectious hepatitis. JAMA 128:803, 1945

521. Knodell RG et al: Etiological spectrum of post-transfusion hepatitis. Gastroenterology 69:1278, 1975

522. Knodell RG et al: Efficacy of prophylactic gamma globulin in preventing non-A, non-B post-transfusion hepatitis. Lancet 1:557, 1976

523. Knodell RG et al: Development of chronic liver disease after acute non-A, non-B post transfusion hepatitis: Role of gamma globulin prophylaxis in its prevention. Gastroenterology 72:902, 1977

524. Kobayashi H et al: Susceptibility of hepatitis B virus to disinfectants or heat. J Clin Microbiol 20:214, 1984

525. Koff RS: Epidemiology of viral hepatitis. Crit Rev Environmental Control 1:383, 1970

526. Koff RS: Immune-complex arthritis in viral hepatitis. N Engl J Med 285:229, 1971

527. Koff RS: Polyarthritis and viral hepatitis: A report of three cases with this relatively unusual association, and review of literature. Hepatitis Surveillance Report No. 28, p 20. Atlanta, National Communicable Disease Center, January 31, 1968

528. Koff RS: Unpublished observations, 1978

529. Koff RS: Viral Hepatitis, p 79. New York, John Wiley & Sons, 1978

530. Koff RS, Sears HS: Internal temperature of steamed clams. N Engl J Med 276:737, 1967

531. Koff RS et al: Under-reporting of viral hepatitis. Gastroenterology 64:194, 1973

532. Koff RS et al: Viral hepatitis in a group of Boston hospitals: III. Importance of exposure to shellfish in a non-epidemic period. N Engl J Med 276:703, 1967

533. Koff RS et al: Contagiousness of acute hepatitis B: Secondary attack rates in household contacts. Gastroenterology 72:297, 1977

534. Koff RS et al: Hepatitis A and non-A, non-B viral hepatitis in Sao Paulo, Brazil: Epidemiological, clinical, and laboratory comparisons in hospitalized patients. Hepatology 2:445, 1982

535. Kontaxis AN et al: Complete heart block in a child following infectious hepatitis: Treatment with permanent pacing: Case report. J Cardiovasc Surg 12:501, 1971

536. Koretz RL et al: Post-transfusion chronic liver disease. Gastroenterology 71:797, 1976

537. Kosmidis JC, Leader-Williams LK: Complement levels in acute infectious hepatitis and serum hepatitis. Clin Exp Immunol 11:31, 1972

538. Krasna V, Radkovsky J: Evaluation of the effectiveness of gamma globulin in the prevention of infectious hepatitis in Prague in 1953–1956. J Epidemiol Microbiol Immunol 6:295, 1957

539. Krikler DM: Hepatitis and activity. Postgrad Med J 47:490, 1971

540. Krikler DM, Zilberg B: Activity and hepatitis. Lancet 2:1046, 1966

541. Krugman S: Effect of human immune serum globulin on infectivity of hepatitis A virus. J Infect Dis 134:70, 1976

542. Krugman S, Giles JP: Viral hepatitis: New light on an old disease. JAMA 212:1019, 1970

543. Krugman S, Giles JP: Viral hepatitis, type B (MS-2 strain): Further observations on natural history and prevention. N Engl J Med 288:755, 1973

544. Krugman S et al: Characterization of MS-2 (hepatitis B) serum by electron microscopy. J Infect Dis 130:416, 1974

545. Krugman S et al: Infectious hepatitis: Evidence for two distinctive clinical, epidemiological and immunological types of infection. JAMA 200:365, 1967

546. Krugman S et al: Hepatitis virus: Effect of heat on the infectivity and antigenicity of the MS-1 and MS-2 strains. J Infect Dis 122:432, 1970

547. Krugman S et al: Viral hepatitis, type B (MS-2 strain): Studies on active immunization. JAMA 122:432, 1971

548. Krugman S et al: Viral hepatitis, type B: DNA polymerase activity and antibody to hepatitis B core antigen. N Engl J Med 290:1331, 1974

549. Krugman S et al: Viral hepatitis, type B: Studies on natural history and prevention re-examined. N Engl J Med 300:101, 1979

550. Krugman S et al: The natural history of infectious hepatitis. Am J Med 32:717, 1962

551. Krugman S et al: Infectious hepatitis: Detection of virus during incubation period and in clinically inapparent infection. N Engl J Med 261:729, 1959

552. Krugman S et al: Infectious hepatitis: Studies on the effect of gamma globulin and on the incidence of inapparent infection. JAMA 174:823, 1960

553. Krushak DH: Application of preventive health measures to curtail chimpanzee-associated infectious hepatitis in handlers. Lab Anim Care 20:52, 1970

554. Kryger P, Christoffersen P: Liver histopathology of the hepatitis A virus infection: A comparison with hepatitis type B and non-A, non-B. J Clin Pathol 36:650, 1983

555. Kuhns WJ et al: A clinical and laboratory evaluation of immune serum globulin from donors with a history of hepatitis: Attempted prevention of post-transfusion hepatitis. Am J Med Sci 272:255, 1976

556. Kunin CM: Serum hepatitis from whole blood: Incidence and relation to source of blood. Am J Med Sci 237:293, 1959

557. Kunkle HG et al: Chronic liver disease following infectious hepatitis: I. Abnormal convalescence from initial attack. Ann Intern Med 27:202, 1947

558. Kurane I et al: Human lymphocyte responses to hepatitis A virus-infected cells: Interferon production and lysis of infected cells. J Immunol 135:2140, 1985

559. Kydd DM, Man EB: Precipitable iodine of serum in disorders of the liver. J Clin Invest 30:874, 1951

560. Lander JJ et al: Viral hepatitis type B (MS-2 strain): Detection of antibody after primary infection. N Engl J Med 285:303, 1971

561. Lander JJ et al: Anticore antibody screening of transfused blood. Vox Sang 34:77, 1978

562. Lander JJ et al: Antibody to hepatitis-associated antigen: Frequency and pattern of response as detected by radioimmunoprecipitation. JAMA 220:1079, 1972

563. Landrigan PJ et al: The protective efficacy of immune serum globulin in hepatitis A: A statistical approach. JAMA 223:74, 1971

564. Lane DA et al: Acquired dysfibrinogenaemia in acute and chronic liver disease. Br J Haematol 35:301, 1977

565. Lauer JL et al: Transmission of hepatitis B virus in clinical laboratory areas. J Infect Dis 140:513, 1979

566. LeBouvier GL: The heterogeneity of Australia antigen. J Infect Dis 123:671, 1971

567. LeBouvier GL, Williams A: Serotypes of hepatitis B antigen (HBsAg): The problem of "new" determinants as exemplified by "t". Am J Med Sci 270:165, 1975

568. LeBouvier GL et al: Subtypes of Australia antigen and hepatitis B virus. JAMA 222:928, 1972

569. Lednar WM et al: Frequency of illness associated with hepatitis A virus infection in adults. Am J Epidemiol 122:226, 1985

570. LeDuc JW et al: Experimental infection of the new world owl monkey (Aotus trivingatus) with hepatitis A virus. Infect Immun 40:766, 1983

571. Lee AKY et al: Mechanisms of maternal-fetal transmission of hepatitis B virus. J Infect Dis 138:668, 1978

572. Lee WM et al: Immune responses to the hepatitis B surface antigen and liver-specific lipoprotein in acute type B hepatitis. Gut 18:250, 1977

573. Leibowitz S, Gorman WF: Neuropsychiatric complications of viral hepatitis. N Engl J Med 246:932, 1952

574. LeMoine Parker M: Aplastic anemia and infectious hepatitis. Lancet 2:261, 1971

575. Lemon SM: Type A viral hepatitis: New developments in an old disease. N Engl J Med 313:1059, 1985

576. Lemon SM, Binn LN: Serum neutralizing antibody response to hepatitis A virus. J Infect Dis 148:1033, 1983

577. Lemon SM et al: IgM antibody to hepatitis B core antigen as a diagnostic parameter of acute infection with hepatitis B virus. J Infect Dis 143:803, 1981

578. Lemon SM et al: Subcutaneous administration of inactivated hepatitis B vaccine by automatic jet injection. J Med Virol 12:129, 1983

579. Leone NC et al: Clinical evaluation of a high-protein, high-carbohydrate, restricted fat diet in the treatment of viral hepatitis. Ann NY Acad Sci 57:948, 1954

580. Lescher FG: The nervous complications of infective hepatitis. Br Med J 1:554, 1944

581. Levene C, Blumberg BS: Additional specificities of Australia antigen and the possible identification of hepatitis carriers. Nature 221:195, 1969

582. Levin ML et al: Hepatitis B transmission by dentists. JAMA 228:1139, 1974

583. Levine RA, Payne MA: Homologous serum hepatitis in youthful heroin users. Ann Intern Med 53:164, 1960

584. Levo Y et al: Association between hepatitis B virus and essential mixed cryoglobulinemia. N Engl J Med 296:1501, 1977

585. Levy BS et al: A large food-borne outbreak of hepatitis A: Possible transmission via oropharyngeal secretions. JAMA 234:289, 1975

586. Levy BS et al: Hepatitis B in ward and clinical laboratory employees of a general hospital. Am J Epidemiol 106:330, 1977

587. Levy RN et al: Fatal aplastic anemia after hepatitis. N Engl J Med 273:1118, 1965

588. Lewis TL et al: A comparison of the frequency of hepatitis B antigen and antibody in hospital and nonhospital personnel. N Engl J Med 289:647, 1973

589. Lichtman SS: Diseases of the Liver, Gall Bladder and Bile Ducts, vol. I, p 486. Philadelphia, Lea & Febiger, 1953

590. Lieberman HM et al: Detection of hepatitis B virus DNA directly in human serum by a simplified molecular hybridization test: Comparison to HBeAg/anti-HBe status in HBsAg carriers. Hepatology 3:285, 1983

591. Lindstedt F: Beitrag zur kenntnis des icterus catarrhalis mit besonderer rucksicht auf die incubationszeit dessen epidemischen formen. Nord. Med. 51:583, 1919

591a. Linemeyer, DL et al: Molecular cloning and partial sequencing of hepatitis A virus cDNA. J Virol 54:247, 1985

592. Ling CM, Overby LR: Prevalence of hepatitis B virus antigen as revealed by direct radioimmune assay with ^{125}I-antibody. J Immunol 109:834, 1972

593. Linnemann CC Jr, Goldberg S: HBAg in breast milk. Lancet 2:155, 1974

594. Lipman MB et al: Isolation of cores from hepatitis B Dane particles. J Infect Dis 128:664, 1973

595. Litwins J, Leibowitz S: Abnormal lymphocytes ("viruscytes") in virus diseases other than infectious mononucleosis. Acta Haematol 5:223, 1951

596. Ljunggren KE et al: Viral hepatitis in Colombia: A study of the "hepatitis of the Sierra Nevada de Santa Marta." Hepatology 5:299, 1985

597. Locarnini SA et al: Solid-phase enzyme-linked immunosorbent assay for detection of hepatitis A-specific immunoglobulin M. J Clin Microbiol 9:459, 1979

598. Logrippo GA: Human plasma treated with ultraviolet and propiolactone. JAMA 187:722, 1964

599. London WT et al: An epidemic of hepatitis in a chronic-hemodialysis unit: Australia antigen and differences in host response. N Engl J Med 281:571, 1969

600. Louis V: Elektrokardiographische befunde bei der Hepatitis epidemica. Schweiz Med Wochenschr 75:986, 1945

601. Lucke B: Pathology of fatal epidemic hepatitis. Am J Pathol 20:471, 1944

602. Lucke B, Mallory T: The fulminant form of epidemic hepatitis. Am J Pathol 22:867, 1946

603. Luerman: Eine Icterusepedemie. Berl Klin Wochenschr 22:20, 1885

604. Macaya G et al: Dane particles and associated DNA-polymerase activity in saliva of chronic hepatitis B carriers. J Med Virol 4:291, 1979

605. MacCallum FO: Early studies of viral hepatitis. Br Med Bull 28:105, 1972

606. MacCallum FO: Transmission of arsenotherapy jaundice by blood: Failure with faeces and nasopharyngeal washings. Lancet 1:342, 1945

607. MacCallum FO, Bauer DJ: Homologous serum jaundice: Transmission experiments with human volunteers. Lancet 1:622, 1944

608. MacCallum FO, Bradley WH: Transmission of infective hepatitis to human volunteers. Lancet 2:228, 1944

609. MacCallum FO et al: Infective hepatitis studies in East Anglia during the period 1943–47. Medical Research Council Special Rep. Series, No. 273. London, His Majesty's Stationery Office, 1951

610. MacDougall BRD et al: H^2-receptor antagonists and antacids in the prevention of acute gastrointestinal haemorrhage in fulminant hepatic failure: Two controlled trials. Lancet 1:617, 1977

611. MacGregor A et al: Monoclonal antibodies against hepatitis A virus. J Clin Microbiol 18:1237, 1983

612. Machida A et al: A polypeptide containing 55 amino acid residues coded by the pre-S region of hepatitis B virus deoxyribonucleic acid bears the receptor for polymerized human as well as chimpanzee albumins. Gastroenterology 86:910, 1984

613. Machida A et al: A hepatitis B surface antigen polypeptide (p31) with the receptor for polymerized human as well as chimpanzee albumins. Gastroenterology 85:268, 1983

614. Mackay P et al: The conversion of hepatitis B core antigen synthesized in E. coli in e antigen. J Med Virol 8:237, 1981

615. Macnab GM et al: Hepatitis B surface antigen produced by a human hepatoma cell line. Br J Cancer 34:509, 1976

616. MacNalty AS: Acute infective jaundice and administration of measles serum. Annual Report of the Chief Medical Officer, Ministry of Health, p 38. London, His Majesty's Stationery Office, 1938

617. MacQuarrie MB et al: Hepatitis B transmitted by a human bite. JAMA 230:723, 1974

618. Madden DL et al: Search for Ferris's fecal antigen and Australia antigen in stool samples obtained during a large outbreak of infectious hepatitis. Proc Soc Exp Biol Med 139:1028, 1972

619. Madsen S et al: Serum glutamic oxaloacetic transaminase in diseases of the liver and biliary tract. Br Med J 1:543, 1958

620. Magnius LO, Espmark JA: New specificities in Australia antigen positive sera distinct from the LeBouvier determinants. J Immunol 109:1017, 1972

621. Maitre P et al: Infectious hepatitis: I. Study of the variations of glutamic oxaloacetic transaminase (GPT):155 case studies. Sem Hop Paris 38:2790, 1962

622. Mallory TB: The pathology of epidemic hepatitis. JAMA 134:655, 1957

623. Mandal BK, Allbeson M: Trigeminal sensory neuropathy and virus hepatitis. Lancet 2:1322, 1972

624. Mao JS et al: Susceptibility of monkeys to human hepatitis A virus. J Infect Dis 144:55, 1981

625. Marier R: The reporting of communicable diseases. Am J Epidemiol 105:587, 1977

626. Marion PL et al: Polypeptides of hepatitis B virus surface antigen produced by a hepatoma cell line. J Virol 32:796, 1979

627. Markenson JA et al: Effects of cyclophosphamide on hepatitis B virus infection and challenge in chimpanzees. J Infect Dis 131:79, 1975

628. Marmion BP, Tonkin RW: Control of hepatitis in dialysis units. Br Med Bull 28:169, 1972

629. Marmion BP et al: Dialysis-associated hepatitis in Edinburgh, 1969–1978. Rev Infect Dis 4:619, 1982

630. Martin CM et al: Studies on gamma globulins: I. Distribution and metabolism of antibodies and gamma globulin in hypogammaglobulinemic patients. J Lab Clin Med 49:607, 1957

631. Mathiesen LR et al: Localization of hepatitis A antigen in marmoset organs during acute infection with hepatitis A virus. J Infect Dis 138:369, 1978

632. Mathiesen LR et al: Immunofluorescence studies for hepatitis A virus and hepatitis B surface and core antigen in liver biopsies from patients with acute viral hepatitis. Gastroenterology 77:623, 1979

633. Mathiesen LR et al: Detection of hepatitis A antigen by immunofluorescence. Infect Immun 18:524, 1977

634. Mathiesen LR et al: Enzyme-linked immunosorbent assay for detection of hepatitis A antigen in stool and antibody to hepatitis A antigen in sera: Comparison with solid-phase radioimmunoassay, immune electron microscopy, and immune adherence hemagglutination assay. J Clin Microbiol 7:184, 1978

635. Mathiesen LR et al: Hepatitis A virus in the liver and intestine of marmosets after oral inoculation. Infect Immun 28:45, 1980

636. Mathiesen LR et al: Hepatitis type A, B and non-A, non-B in fulminant hepatitis. Gut 21:72, 1980

637. Maupas P et al: Efficacy of hepatitis B vaccine in preven-

tion of early HBsAg carrier state in children: Controlled trial in an endemic area (Senegal). Lancet 2:289, 1981

638. Mayer G, Schomerus H: Synthesis rates of albumin and fibrinogen during and after acute hepatitis. Digestion 13: 261, 1975

639. Maynard JE: Passive immunization against hepatitis B: A review of recent studies and comment on current aspects of control. Am J Epidemiol 107:77, 1978

640. Maynard JE: Epidemic non-A, non-B hepatitis. Semin Liver Dis 4:336, 1984

641. Maynard JE et al: Relation of e antigen to hepatitis B virus infection in an area of hyperendemicity. J Infect Dis 133:339, 1976

642. Maynard JE et al: Experimental infection of chimpanzees with the virus of hepatitis B. Nature 237:514, 1972

643. Maynard JE et al: Preliminary studies of hepatitis A in chimpanzees. J Infect Dis 131:194, 1975

644. Mazzur S et al: Geographical distribution of Australia antigen determinants d, y, and w. Nature 247:38, 1974

645. Mazzur S et al: Geographical variation of the "w" subtype of Australia antigen. Nature 243:44, 1973

646. McCarty DJ, Ormiste V: Arthritis and HB Ag-positive hepatitis. Arch Intern Med 132:264, 1973

647. McClelland DBL et al: Hepatitis B: Absence of transmission by gastrointestinal endoscopy. Br Med J 1:23, 1978

648. McCollum RW: The size of hepatitis virus. Proc Soc Exp Biol Med 81:157, 1952

649. McDonald S: Acute yellow atrophy. Edinburgh Med J 15: 208, 1908

650. McDonald S: Acute yellow atrophy in syphilis. Br Med J 1:76, 1918

651. McGarry JD, Brumback CL: Hepatitis epidemic in the young drug-oriented society of Palm Beach County. J Fla Med Assoc 58:28, 1971

652. Mcintosh RM et al: The nature and incidence of cryoproteins in hepatitis B antigen (HBsAg) positive patients. Q J Med 45:23, 1976

653. McLean AA et al: Summary of world-wide experience with H-B-vax (B, MSD). J Infect 7:95, 1983

654. McMahon BJ et al: Acute hepatitis B virus infection: Relation of age to the clinical expression of disease and subsequent development of the carrier state. J Infect Dis 151: 599, 1985

655. Melnick JL: Classification of hepatitis A virus as enterovirus type 72 and of hepatitis B virus as hepadnavirus type 1. Intervirology 18:105, 1982

656. Meyers JD et al: Lack of transmission of hepatitis B after surgical exposure. JAMA 240:1725, 1978

657. Milandri M et al: Evidence for liver cell proliferation during fatal acute liver failure. Gut 21:423, 1980

658. Milich DR et al: Enhanced immunogenicity of the pre-S region of hepatitis B surface antigen. Science 228:1195, 1985

659. Miller DS, Klatskin G: Halothane hepatitis: Benign resolution of a severe lesion. Ann Intern Med 89:212, 1978

660. Miller KD et al: Intradermal hepatitis B virus vaccine: Immunogenicity and side-effects in adults. Lancet 2:1454, 1983

661. Miller WJ et al: Specific immune adherence assay for human hepatitis A antibody: Application to diagnostic and epidemiologic investigations. Proc Soc Exp Biol Med 149: 254, 1975

662. Miller WV et al: Ethylene oxide sterilization to prevent post-transfusion hepatitis. N Engl J Med 280:386, 1969

663. Modai M, Theodore E: Intestinal contents in patients with viral hepatitis after a lipid meal. Gastroenterology 58:379, 1970

664. Molnar IG, Gitnick GL: Hepatitis transmission by CEA positive blood. Gastroenterology 72:1103, 1977

665. Molner JG, Meyer KF: Jaundice in Detroit. Am J Public Health 30:509, 1940

666. Moodie JW et al: The problem of the demonstration of hepatitis B antigen in faeces and bile. J Clin Pathol 27: 693, 1974

667. Mordasini RC et al: Veranderungen der serumlipide und lipoproteine bei akuter hepatitis. Schweiz Med Wochenschr 106:1173, 1976

668. Moriarty AM et al: Antibodies to peptides detect new hepatitis B antigen: Serological correlation with hepatocellular carcinoma. Science 227:429, 1985

669. Morris IM et al: Endoscopy and transmission of hepatitis B. Lancet 2:1152, 1975

670. Morris TO et al: Exchange transfusion treatment of fulminating canine viral hepatitis: the role of specific antiviral antibody. Gastroenterology 61:885, 1971

671. Mosley JW: Epidemiologic implications of changing trends in type A and type B hepatitis. In Vyas GN et al (eds): Hepatitis and Blood Transfusion, p 23. New York, Grune & Stratton, 1972

672. Mosley JW: Epidemiology of viral hepatitis: An overview. Am J Med Sci 270:253, 1975

673. Mosley JW: Hepatitis B immune globulin: Some progress and some problems. Ann Intern Med 91:914, 1979

674. Mosley JW: Hepatitis B virus: The importance of "nonepidemics." Am J Dig Dis 23:289, 1978

675. Mosley JW: New patterns of transfusion-associated hepatitis. Epatologia 12:527, 1966

676. Mosley JW: The HBV carrier—A new kind of leper? N Engl J Med 292:477, 1975

677. Mosley JW: Transmission of viral diseases by drinking water. In Berg G (ed): Transmission of Viruses by the Water Route, p 5. New York, Interscience, 1967

678. Mosley JW: Viral hepatitis: A group of epidemiologic entities. Can Med Assoc J 106:427, 1972

679. Mosley JW et al: Failure to detect hepatitis-associated antigen in a community epidemic. Nature 225:953, 1970

680. Mosley JW et al: Hepatitis B virus infection in dentists. N Engl J Med 293:729, 1975

681. Mosley JW et al: Elevations of serum transaminase activities following infectious hepatitis. Gastroenterology 41: 9, 1961

682. Mosley JW et al: Subdeterminants d and y of hepatitis B antigen as epidemiologic markers. Am J Epidemiol 95: 529, 1972

683. Mosley JW et al: Subtypes ad and ay of hepatitis B virus among blood donors in the greater Los Angeles area. Transfusion 14:372, 1974

684. Mosley JW et al: Protection against d+ type B hepatitis from prior y+ infection. Gastroenterology 62:787, 1972

685. Mosley JW et al: Chimpanzee-associated hepatitis: An outbreak in Oklahoma. JAMA 199:695, 1967

686. Mosley JW et al: Comparison of two lots of immune serum globulin for prophylaxis of infectious hepatitis. Am J Epidemiol 87:539, 1968

687. Mosley JW et al: Infectious hepatitis in Clearfield County, Pennsylvania: I. A probable water-borne epidemic. Am J Med 26:555, 1959

688. Mosley JW et al: Multiple hepatitis viruses in multiple attacks of acute viral hepatitis. N Engl J Med 296:75, 1977

689. Moss B et al: Live recombinant vaccinia virus protects chimpanzees against hepatitis B. Nature 311:67, 1984

690. Mowat NAG et al: Outbreak of serum hepatitis associated with tattooing. Lancet 1:33, 1973

691. Mulley AG et al: Indications for use of hepatitis B vaccine, based on cost-effectiveness analysis. N Engl J Med 307:644, 1982

692. Murphy B et al: Third component, HBeAg/3, of hepatitis B e antigen system, identified by three different double-diffusion techniques. J Clin Microbiol 8:349, 1978

693. Murphy BL et al: Immunofluorescence of hepatitis A virus antigen in chimpanzees. Infect Immun 21:663, 1978

694. Murphy BL et al: Immunofluorescent localization of hepatitis B antigens in chimpanzee tissues. Intervirology 6:207, 1975/1976

695. Murphy WJ et al: Outbreak of infectious hepatitis apparently milk-borne. Am J Public Health 36:169, 1946

696. Murray R, Diefenbach WC: Effect of heat on the agent of homologous serum hepatitis. Proc Soc Exp Biol Med 84:230, 1953

697. Murray R et al: Effect of ultraviolet radiation on the infectivity of icterogenic plasma. JAMA 157:8, 1955

698. Murray-Lyon IM et al: Clinical and electroencephalographic assessment of diazepam in liver disease. Br Med J 4:265, 1971

699. Mushahwar IK et al: Radioimmunoassay for detection of hepatitis B e antigen and its antibody: Results of clinical evaluation. Am J Clin Pathol 76:692, 1981

700. Mushahwar IK et al: Interpretation of hepatitis B virus and hepatitis delta virus serologic profiles. Pathologist 38: October 1984

701. Nagaraju M et al: Viral hepatitis and agranulocytosis. Dig Dis 18:247, 1973

702. Nagy J et al: The role of hepatitis B surface antigen in the pathogenesis of glomerulopathies. Clin Nephrol 12:109, 1979

703. Najarian R et al: Primary structure and gene organization of human hepatitis A virus. Proc Natl Acad Sci USA 82:2627, 1985

704. Nakao T et al: Cytomegalovirus infection in patients receiving long-term hemodialysis. JAMA 217:697, 1971

705. National Transfusion Hepatitis Study: Risk of posttransfusion hepatitis in the United States: A prospective cooperative study. JAMA 220:692, 1972

706. Neefe JR: Homologous serum hepatitis and infectious (epidemic) hepatitis: Studies in volunteers bearing on immunological and other characteristics of the etiological agents. Am J Med 1:3, 1946

707. Neefe JR, Stokes J Jr: An epidemic of infectious hepatitis apparently due to a water-borne agent. JAMA 128:1063, 1945

708. Neefe JR et al: Inactivation of the virus of infectious hepatitis in drinking water. Am J Public Health 37:365, 1947

709. Neefe JR et al: Prevalence and nature of hepatic disturbance following acute viral hepatitis with jaundice. Ann Intern Med 43:1, 1955

710. Neefe JR et al: Carriers of hepatitis virus in blood and viral hepatitis in whole blood recipients: I. Studies on donors suspected as carriers of hepatitis virus and as sources of post-transfusion viral hepatitis. JAMA 154:1066, 1954

711. Neefe JR et al: Oral administration to volunteers of feces from patients with homologous serum hepatitis and infectious (epidemic) hepatitis. Am J Med Sci 210:29, 1945

712. Neefe JR et al: Hepatitis due to the injection of homologous blood products in human volunteers. J Clin Invest 23:836, 1944

713. Nefzger MD, Chalmers TC: The treatment of acute infectious hepatitis: Ten-year follow-up study of the effects of diet and rest. Am J Med 35:299, 1963

714. Nelson RS et al: Effect of physical activity on recovery from hepatitis. Am J Med 16:780, 1954

715. Neugeboren N et al: Control of cross-contamination. JAMA 85:123, 1972

716. Neurath AR et al: Sialyl residues in hepatitis B antigen: Their role in determining the life span of the antigen in serum and in eliciting an immunological response. J Gen Virol 27:81, 1975

717. Neurath AR et al: Hepatitis B virus contains pre-S gene-encoded domains. Nature 315:154, 1985

718. Newberry WM et al: Depression of lymphocyte reactivity to phytohemagglutinin by serum from patients with liver disease. Cell Immunol 6:87, 1973

719. Newkirk MM et al: Fate of ingested hepatitis B antigen in blood-sucking insects. Gastroenterology 69:982, 1975

720. Nicholas NK: Viral hepatitis among practicing dentists. N Z Med J 85:413, 1977

721. Nielsen JO et al: Incidence and meaning of persistence of Australia antigen in patients with acute viral hepatitis. N Engl J Med 285:1157, 1971

722. Niermeijer P, Gips HC: Guillain-Barré syndrome in acute HBsAg positive hepatitis. Br Med J 4:732, 1975

723. Nishioka K: Collaborating and cooperation crossing national boundaries in Asia, Africa and Oceania: An outline of WHO-assisted workshop on hepatitis B antigen 1973. Asian Cooperative Health 3:15, 1974

724. Nisman RM et al: Acute viral hepatitis with bridging hepatic necrosis: An overview. Arch Intern Med 139:1289, 1979

725. Nordenfelt E, Andrea-Sandberg M: Dane particle associated DNA polymerase and "e" antigen: Relation to chronic hepatitis among carriers of HBsAg. J Infect Dis 134:85, 1976

726. Norkrans G et al: The epidemiological pattern of hepatitis A, B. and non-A, non-B in Sweden. Scand J Gastroenterol 13:873, 1978

727. Norkrans G et al: Multiple hepatitis attacks in drug addicts. JAMA 243:1056, 1980

728. Novick DM et al: Hepatitis D virus antibody in HBsAg-positive and HBsAg-negative substance abusers with chronic liver disease. J Med Virol 15:351, 1985

729. Nowoslawski A et al: Immunopathological aspects of hepatitis type B. Am J Med Sci 270:229, 1975

730. Ogra PL: Immunologic aspects of hepatitis-associated antigen and antibody in human body fluids. J Immunol 110:1197, 1973

731. Ogston CW et al: Persistence of hepatitis B surface antigen in the bedbug. J Infect Dis 140:411, 1979

732. Ohori H et al: Immunological and morphological properties of HBeAg subtypes (HBeAg/1 and HBeAg/2) in hepatitis B virus core particles. J Gen Virol 65:405, 1984

733. Okada K et al: "e" antigen and anti "e" in the serum of asymptomatic carrier mothers as indicators of positive and negative transmission of hepatitis B virus to their infants. N Engl J Med 294:746, 1976

734. Okamoto H et al: Hemagglutination assay of polypeptide

coded by the pre-S region of hepatitis B virus with monoclonal antibody: Correlation of pre-S polypeptide with the receptor for polymerized human serum albumin in serums containing hepatitis B antigens. J Immunol 134:1212, 1985

735. Okochi J, Murakami S: Observations on Australia antigen in Japanese. Vox Sang 15:374, 1968

736. Oliphant JW: Infectious hepatitis: Experimental study of immunity. Public Health Rep 59:1614, 1944

737. Oliphant JW: Jaundice following administration of human serum. Bull NY Acad Med 20:429, 1944

738. Oliphant JW et al: Jaundice following administration of human serum. Public Health Rep 58:1233, 1943

739. Onion DK et al: Arthritis of hepatitis associated with Australia antigen. Ann Intern Med 75:29, 1971

740. Overhold EL, Hardin EB: Cholangiolitic hepatitis: Clinicopathologic studies and response to steroid therapy in four cases. Arch Intern Med 103:859, 1959

741. Owen RL, Shapiro H: Pleural effusion, rash, and anergy in icteric hepatitis. N Engl J Med 291:963, 1974

742. Owings WBJ: Hypersensitivity to gamma globulin. J Med Assoc State Ala 23:74, 1953

743. Ozawa T et al: Acute immune complex disease associated with hepatitis: Etiopathogenic and immunopathologic studies of the renal lesion. Arch Pathol Lab Med 100:484, 1976

744. Papaevangelou G et al: Differential serodiagnosis of sporadic acute viral hepatitis. Proc Soc Exp Biol Med 161:322, 1979

745. Papaevangelou G et al: Transplacental transmission of hepatitis B virus by symptom-free chronic carrier mothers. Lancet 2:746, 1974

746. Par A et al: Levamisole in viral hepatitis. Lancet 1:702, 1977

747. Parks WP, Melnick JL: Attempted isolation of hepatitis viruses in marmosets. J Infect Dis 120:539, 1969

748. Parks WP et al: Characterization of marmoset hepatitis virus. J Infect Dis 120:548, 1969

749. Pasek M et al: Hepatitis B virus genes and their expression in E. coli. Nature 282:575, 1979

750. Patten BM et al: Hepatitis-associated lipid storage myopathy. Ann Intern Med 87:417, 1977

751. Pattison CP et al: Serological and epidemiological studies of hepatitis B in haemodialysis units. Lancet 2:172, 1973

752. Paul JR, Gardner HT: Viral hepatitis. In Coates JB Jr (ed): Preventive Medicine in World War II, Vol V, Communicable Diseases Transmitted through Contact or by Unknown Means, p 411. Washington DC, Office of the Surgeon General, Department of the Army, 1960

753. Paul JR et al: Transmission experiments in serum jaundice and infectious hepatitis. JAMA 128:911, 1945

754. Penner E et al: Serum and cerebrospinal fluid immune complexes containing hepatitis B surface antigen in Guillain-Barré syndrome. Gastroenterology 82:576, 1982

755. Perrillo RP et al: Hepatitis B e antigen, DNA polymerase activity, and infection of household contacts with hepatitis B virus. Gastroenterology 76:1319, 1979

756. Perrillo RP et al: Anti-hepatitis B core immunoglobulin M in the serologic evaluation of hepatitis B virus infection and simultaneous infection with type B, delta agent, and non-A, non-B viruses. Gastroenterology 85:163, 1983

757. Perrillo R et al: Immune globulin and hepatitis B immune globulin: Prophylactic measures for intimate contacts exposed to acute type B hepatitis. Arch Intern Med 144:81, 1984

758. Peters RL: Viral hepatitis: A pathologic spectrum. Am J Med Sci 270:17, 1975

759. Petersen NJ et al: Hepatitis B surface antigen in saliva, impetiginous lesions, and the environment in two remote Alaskan villages. Appl Environ Microbiol 32:572, 1976

760. Peterson DA et al: Effect of chlorine treatment on infectivity of hepatitis A virus. Appl Environ Microbiol 45:223, 1983

761. Peterson DL et al: Partial amino acid sequence of two major component polypeptides of hepatitis B surface antigen. Proc Natl Acad Sci USA 74:1530, 1977

762. Petit MA, Pillot J: HBc and HBe antigenicity and DNA-binding activity of major core protein P22 in hepatitis B virus core particles related from the cytoplasm of human liver cells. J Virol 53:543, 1985

763. Petrelli FL et al: Hepatitis B in subjects treated with a drug containing immunoglobulins. J Infect Dis 135:252, 1977

764. Philip JR et al: Infectious hepatitis outbreak with mai tai as the vehicle of transmission. Am J Epidemiol 97:50, 1973

765. Phillips MJ, Powell S: Modern aspects of the morphology of viral hepatitis. Hum Pathol 12:1060, 1981

766. Piazza M et al: Hepatitis B antigen inhibitor in human feces and intestinal mucosa. Br Med J 2:334, 1973

767. Pickles WN: Epidemic catarrhal jaundice: An outbreak in Yorkshire. Br Med J 1:944, 1930

768. Pittsley RA et al: Acute hepatitis B simulating dermatomyositis. JAMA 239:959, 1978

769. Plough IC, Ayerle RS: The Guillain-Barré syndrome associated with acute hepatitis. N Engl J Med 249:61, 1953

770. Plowright CB: On an epidemic of jaundice in King's Lynn, 1895. Br Med J 1:1321, 1896

771. Ponzetto A et al: Transmission of the hepatitis B virus-associated delta agent to the eastern woodchuck. Proc Natl Acad Sci USA 81:2208, 1984

772. Ponzetto A et al: Antibody to the hepatitis B virus-associated delta-agent in immune serum globulin. Gastroenterology 87:1213, 1984

773. Popp JW Jr et al: Essential mixed cryoglobulinemia without evidence for hepatitis B virus infection. Ann Intern Med 92:379, 1980

774. Popper H: The pathology of viral hepatitis. Can Med Asoc J 106:447, 1972

775. Popper H, Schaffner F: The vocabulary of chronic hepatitis. N Engl J Med 284:1154, 1971

776. Poschl M: Roentgenuntersuchungen des magen-daruckanals bei icterus infectiosus. Rontgenpraxis 14:401, 1942

777. Poskanzer DC, Beadenkopf WG: Waterborne infectious hepatitis epidemic from a chlorinated municipal supply. Public Health Rep 76:745, 1961

778. Poulsen H, Christoffersen P: Abnormal bile duct epithelium in liver biopsies with histological signs of viral hepatitis. Acta Pathol Microbiol Scand 76:383, 1969

779. Preisig R et al: Changes in sulfobromophthalein transport and storage by the liver during viral hepatitis in man. Am J Med 40:170, 1966

780. Prince AM: An antigen detected in the blood during the incubation period of serum hepatitis. Proc Natl Acad Sci USA 60:814, 1968

781. Prince AM: Role of serum hepatitis virus in chronic liver disease. Gastroenterology 60:913, 1971

782. Prince AM, Trepo C: Role of immune complexes involving SH antigen in pathogenesis of chronic active hepatitis and polyarteritis nodosa. Lancet 1:1309, 1971

783. Prince AM et al: Hepatitis B antigen in wild-caught mosquitoes in Africa. Lancet 2:247, 1972

784. Prince AM et al: Hepatitis B immune globulin: Effectiveness in prevention of dialysis-associated hepatitis. N Engl J Med 293:1063, 1975

785. Prince AM et al: Inactivation of hepatitis B and Hutchinson strain non-A, non-B hepatitis viruses by exposure to tween 80 and ether. Vox Sang 46:36, 1984

786. Prince AM et al: Inactivation of a non-A, non-B virus infectivity by a beta-propiolactone/ultraviolet irradiation treatment and aerosol adsorption procedure used for preparation of a stabilized human serum. Vox Sang 46:80, 1984

787. Propert SA: Hepatitis after prophylactic serum. Br Med J 2:677, 1938

788. Prophylactic Gamma Globulin for Prevention of Endemic Hepatitis: Effects of US gamma globulin upon the incidence of viral hepatitis and other infectious diseases in US soldiers abroad. Arch Intern Med 128:723, 1971

789. Provost PJ, Hilleman MR: An inactivated hepatitis A virus vaccine prepared from infected marmoset liver. Proc Soc Exp Biol Med 159:201, 1978

790. Provost PJ, Hilleman MR: Propagation of human hepatitis A virus in cell culture in vitro. Proc Soc Exp Biol Med 160:213, 1979

791. Provost PJ et al: Etiologic relationship of marmoset-propagated CR.26 hepatitis A virus to hepatitis in man. Proc Soc Exp Biol Med 142:1257, 1973

792. Provost PJ et al: A specific complement-fixation test for human hepatitis A employing CR326 virus antigen. Proc Soc Exp Biol Med 148:962, 1975

793. Provost PJ et al: Suitability of the rufiventer marmoset as a host animal for human hepatitis A virus. Proc Soc Exp Biol Med 155:283, 1977

794. Provost PJ et al: Physical, chemical and morphologic dimensions of human hepatitis A virus strain CR326. Proc Soc Exp Biol Med 148:532, 1975

795. Provost PJ et al: Progress toward a live attenuated human hepatitis A vaccine. Proc Soc Exp Biol Med 170:8, 1982

796. Provost PJ et al: Studies in chimpanzees of live, attenuated hepatitis A vaccine candidates. Proc Soc Exp Biol Med 172:357, 1983

797. Purcell RH et al: Seroepidemiological studies of transfusion-associated hepatitis. J Infect Dis 123:406, 1971

798. Purcell RH, Gerin JL: Prospects for second and third generation hepatitis B vaccines. Hepatology 5:159, 1985

799. Purcell RH, Gerin JL: Experimental transmission of the delta agent to chimpanzees. In Verme G, Bonino F, Rizzetto M (eds): Viral Hepatitis and Delta Infection, p 79. New York, Alan R. Liss, 1983

800. Rachmilewitz M et al: Serum vitamin B_{12} binding proteins in viral hepatitis. Eur J Clin Invest 2:239, 1972

801. Raffensperger EC: Acute acquired hemolytic anemia in association with acute viral hepatitis. Ann Intern Med 48:1243, 1958

802. Rake MO et al: Intravascular coagulation in acute hepatic necrosis. Lancet 1:533, 1970

803. Rake MO et al: Early and intensive therapy of intravascular coagulation in acute liver failure. Lancet 2:1215, 1971

804. Rakela J et al: Hepatitis A infection in fulminant hepatitis and chronic active hepatitis. Gastroenterology 74:879, 1978

805. Rakela J, Mosley JW: Fecal excretion of hepatitis A virus in humans. J Infect Dis 135:933, 1977

806. Rakela J, Redeker AG: Chronic liver disease after acute non-A, non-B viral hepatitis. Gastroenterology 77:1200, 1979

807. Rakela J et al: Viral hepatitis: Enzyme assays and serologic procedures in the study of an epidemic. Am J Epidemiol 106:493, 1977

808. Rao KR, Vyas GN: Hepatitis B surface antigen (HBsAg): Tryptophan content and biological activity. J Gen Virol 24:571, 1974

809. Rappaport AM: Anatomic considerations. In Schiff L (ed): Diseases of the Liver, 4th ed, p 1. Philadelphia, JB Lippincott, 1975

810. Raska K et al: A milkborne infectious hepatitis epidemic. J Hyg Epidemiol Microbiol Immunol 10:413, 1966

811. Redeker AG: Hepatitis B: Risk of infection from antigen-positive medical personnel and patients. JAMA 233:1061, 1975

812. Redeker AG: Viral hepatitis: Clinical aspects. Am J Med Sci 270:9, 1975

813. Redeker AG, Yamahiro HS: Controlled trial of exchange-transfusion therapy in fulminant hepatitis. Lancet 1:3, 1973

814. Redeker AG et al: A controlled study of the safety of pooled plasma stored in the liquid state at 30°C–32°C for six months. Transfusion 8:60, 1968

815. Redeker AG et al: Hepatitis B immune globulin as a prophylactic measure for spouses exposed to acute type B hepatitis. N Engl J Med 293:1055, 1975

816. Redeker AG et al: Randomization of corticosteroid therapy in fulminant hepatitis. N Engl J Med 294:728, 1976

817. Reingold AL et al: Transmission of hepatitis B by an oral surgeon. J Infect Dis 145:262, 1982

818. Reisler DM et al: Transaminase levels in the post-convalescent phase of infectious hepatitis. JAMA 202:37, 1967

819. Report of a Collaborative Study by the Communicable Disease Surveillance Centre and the Epidemiological Research Laboratory Service Together with a District Control of Infection Service: Acute hepatitis B associated with gynaecological surgery. Lancet 1:1, 1980

820. Resnick RH et al: Primary hepatocellular carcinoma following non-A, non-B post-transfusion hepatitis. Dig Dis Sci 28:908, 1983

821. Reynolds RD et al: Freeze-ball hepatitis. Arch Intern Med 122:48, 1968

822. Rimland D et al: Hepatitis B outbreak traced to an oral surgeon. N Engl J Med 296:953, 1977

823. Rindge ME et al: Infectious hepatitis: Report of an outbreak in a small Connecticut school due to waterborne transmission. JAMA 180:33, 1962

824. Ringertz O, Zetterberg B: Serum-hepatitis among Swedish track-finders: I. An epidemiological study. N Engl J Med 276:540, 1967

825. Rizzetto M: The delta agent. Hepatology 3:729, 1983

826. Rizzetto M: Delta virus hepatitis. Fegato 30:73, 1984

827. Rizzetto M, Verme G: Delta hepatitis—present status. J Hepatol 1:187, 1985

828. Rizzetto M et al: The hepatitis B virus-associated delta antigen: Isolation from liver, development of solid-phase radioimmunoassays for delta antigen and anti-delta and partial characterization of delta antigen. J Immunol 125:318, 1980

829. Rizzetto M et al: Chronic hepatitis in carriers of hepatitis B surface antigen, with intrahepatic expression of the delta antigen: An active and progressive disease unresponsive

to immunosuppressive treatment. Ann Intern Med 98:437, 1983

830. Rizzetto M et al: Transmission of hepatitis B virus-associated delta antigen to chimpanzees. J Infect Dis 121:590, 1980

831. Rizzetto M et al: Delta antigen: The association of delta antigen with hepatitis B surface antigen and ribonucleic acid in the serum of delta infected chimpanzees. Proc Natl Acad Sci USA 77:6124, 1980

832. Rizzetto M et al: Immunofluorescence detection of a new antigen–antibody system (delta/anti-delta) associated with hepatitis B virus in liver and serum of HBsAg carriers. Gut 18:997, 1977

833. Rizzetto M: Experimental HBV and delta infections of chimpanzees: Occurrence and significance of intrahepatic immune complexes of HBcAg and delta antigen. Hepatology 1:567, 1981

834. Rizzetto M et al: Delta infection and liver disease in hemophilic carriers of hepatitis B surface antigen. J Infect Dis 145:18, 1982

835. Rizzetto M et al: Epidemiology of HBV-associated delta agent: Geographical distribution of anti-delta and prevalence in polytransfused HBsAg carriers. Lancet 1:1215, 1980

836. Roberts RH, Still H: Homologous serum jaundice transmitted by a tattooing needle. Can Med Assoc J 62:75, 1950

837. Robinson WS et al: DNA of a human hepatitis B virus candidate. J Virol 14:384, 1974

838. Robinson WS et al: The hepadna viruses of animals. Semin Liver Dis 4:347, 1984

839. Roggendorf M, Deinhardt F: Demonstration of a rheumatoid factor-like reaction in the acute phase of hepatitis non-A, non-B. In Viral Hepatitis: Second International Max von Pettenkofer Symposium, p 125. New York, Marcel Dekker, 1983

840. Rokitansky K: Handbuch der speciellen pathologischen Anatomie, vol 3, p 343. Vienna, Braumuller & Seidel, 1842

841. Romet-Lemonne JL et al: Hepatitis B virus infection in cultured human lymphoblastoid cells. Science 221:667, 1983

842. Roos B: Hepatitis epidemic conveyed by oysters. Sven Lak-Tidning 53:989, 1956

843. Rosenberg DG, Galambos JT: Yellow spinal fluid: Diagnostic significance of cerebrospinal fluid in jaundiced patients. Am J Dig Dis 5:32, 1960

844. Rosenberg JL et al: Viral hepatitis: An occupational hazard to surgeons. JAMA 223:395, 1973

845. Rosenstein BJ: Viral hepatitis in narcotics users: An outbreak in Rhode Island. JAMA 199:698, 1967

846. Rosina F et al: Risk of post-transfusion infection with the hepatitis delta virus: A multicenter study. N Engl J Med 312:1488, 1985

847. Rossouw JE et al: Plasma pyridoxal phosphate of parenteral supplementation. Scand J Gastroenterol 12:123, 1977

848. Roumeliotou-Karayannis A et al: Post-exposure active immunoprophylaxis of spouses of acute viral hepatitis B patients. Vaccine 3:31, 1985

849. Rowell LB et al: Indocyanine green clearance and estimated hepatic blood flow during mild to maximal exercise in upright man. J Clin Invest 43:1677, 1964

850. Rozen P et al: Computer analysis of liver function tests and their interrelationships in 347 cases of viral hepatitis. Isr J Med Sci 6:67, 1970

851. Rubin E: Interpretation of the liver biopsy: Diagnostic criteria. Gastroenterology 45:400, 1963

852. Rubin E, Lieber CS: Alcohol-induced hepatic injury in nonalcoholic volunteers. N Engl J Med 278:869, 1968

853. Rubin MM et al: Abnormal platelet function and ultrastructure in fulminant hepatic failure. Q J Med 46:339, 1977

854. Ruddy SJ et al: Chimpanzee-associated viral hepatitis in 1963. Am J Epidemiol 86:634, 1967

855. Ruiz-Opazo N et al: Evidence for super coiled hepatitis B virus DNA in chimpanzee liver and serum DNA particles: Possible implications in persistent HBV infection. Cell 29:129, 1982

856. Salaman MH et al: Prevention of jaundice resulting from antisyphilitic treatment. Lancet 2:7, 1944

857. Salen G et al: Acute hemolytic anemia complicating viral hepatitis in patients with glucose-6-phosphatase dehydrogenase deficiency. Ann Intern Med 65:1210, 1966

858. Sampliner RE: The duration of hepatitis B surface antigenemia. Arch Intern Med 139:145, 1979

859. Sanders GE, Perrillo RP: Rosette inhibitory factor: T-lymphocyte subpopulation specificity and potential immunoregulatory role in hepatitis B virus infection. Hepatology 2:547, 1982

860. Sanders GE, Perrillo RP: Suppression of T helper function: An immunoregulatory effect of rosette inhibitory factor in hepatitis B virus infection. Hepatology 5:392, 1985

861. Sandler SG et al: Prothrombin complex concentrates in acquired hypoprothrombinemia. Ann Intern Med 79:485, 1973

862. Saphir O et al: Myocarditis in viral (epidemic) hepatitis. Am J Med Sci 231:168, 1956

863. Sasaki T et al: Co-occurrence of hepatitis B surface antigen of a particular subtype and antibody to a heterologous specificity in the same serum. J Immunol 117:2258, 1976

864. Saudek CD: The effect of hepatitis B on plasma cholesterol and sterol balance. Am J Med 63:453, 1977

865. Saunders SJ et al: Serum factor affecting neutrophil function during acute viral hepatitis. Gut 19:930, 1978

866. Sawyer WA et al: Jaundice in the Army personnel in the western region of the United States and its relation to vaccination against yellow fever. Am J Hyg 39:337, 1944

867. Sborov VM et al: ACTH therapy in acute viral hepatitis. J Lab Clin Med 43:48, 1954

868. Schachter D: Estimation of bilirubin mono and diglucuronide in the plasma and urine of patients with nonhemolytic jaundice. J Lab Clin Med 53:557, 1959

869. Schafer IA, Mosley JW: A study of viral hepatitis in a penal institution. Ann Intern Med 49:1162, 1958

870. Schaffner F: Intralobular changes in hepatocytes and the electron microscopic mesenchymal response in acute viral hepatitis. Medicine 45:547, 1966

871. Schaffner F: The structural basis of altered hepatic function in viral hepatitis. Am J Med 49:658, 1970

872. Scharschmidt BF et al: Measurement of serum bilirubin and its mono- and diconjugates: Application to patients with hepatobiliary disease. Gut 23:643, 1982

873. Schenker S, cited by Berk PD, Popper H: Fulminant hepatic failure. Am J Gastroenterol 69:249, 1978

874. Scheiermann N, Kuwert EK: Uptake and elimination of hepatitis B immunoglobulins after intramuscular application in man. Dev Biol Standard 54:347, 1983

875. Schiff L: The use of steroids in liver disease. Medicine 45: 565, 1966

876. Schlenker H: Meningitis als auftakt zu Hepatitis epidemica und Poliomyelitis. Schweiz Med Wochenschr 74:47, 1944

877. Schneider AJ, Mosley JW: Studies of variations of glutamic-oxalacetic transaminase in serum in infectious hepatitis. Pediatrics 24:367, 1959

878. Schoppe WD et al: HBs-antigen und anti-HBs bei Krankenhauspersonal. Dtsch Med Wochenschr 102:1712, 1977

879. Schulman AN et al: Hepatitis A antigen particles in liver, bile, and stool of chimpanzees. J Infect Dis 134:80, 1976

880. Schumacher HR, Gall EP: Arthritis in acute hepatitis and chronic active hepatitis: Pathology of the synovial membrane with evidence for the presence of Australia antigen in synovial membranes. Am J Med 57:655, 1974

881. Schweitzer IL: Vertical transmission of the hepatitis B surface antigen. Am J Med Sci 270:287, 1975

882. Schweitzer IL, Peters RL: Pregnancy in hepatitis B antigen positive cirrhosis. Obstet Gynecol 48:535, 1976

883. Schweitzer IL et al: Viral hepatitis B in neonates and infants. Am J Med 55:762, 1973

884. Schweitzer IL et al: e antigen in HBsAg carrier mothers. N Engl J Med 293:940, 1975

885. Schweitzer IL et al: Factors influencing neonatal infection by hepatitis B virus. Gastroenterology 65:277, 1973

886. Schweitzer IL et al: Oral contraceptives in acute viral hepatitis. JAMA 233:979, 1975

887. Scolnick EM et al: Clinical evaluation in healthy adults of a hepatitis B vaccine made by recombinant DNA. JAMA 251:2812, 1984

888. Scott RM et al: Experimental transmission of hepatitis B virus by semen and saliva. J Infect Dis 142:67, 1980

889. Scotto J et al: Hepatitis B virus DNA in Dane particles: Evidence for the presence of replicative intermediates. J Infect Dis 151:610, 1985

890. Scotto J et al: Detection of hepatitis B virus DNA in serum by a single spot hybridization technique: Comparison with results for other viral markers. Hepatology 3:279, 1983

891. Seddon JH: An epidemiological survey of infectious hepatitis in a country town. NZ Med J 60:55, 1961

892. Seeff LB: Type B hepatitis after needle-stick exposure: Prevention with Hepatitis B immune globulin. Ann Intern Med 88:285, 1978

893. Seeff LB, Koff RS: Passive and active immunoprophylaxis of hepatitis B. Gastroenterology 86:958, 1984

894. Seeff LB et al: VA cooperative study of posttransfusion hepatitis, 1969–1974: Incidence and characteristics of hepatitis and responsible factors. Am J Med Sci 270:335, 1975

895. Seeff LB et al: VA cooperative study of gamma globulin prophylaxis of post-transfusion hepatitis. Gastroenterology 64:893, 1973

896. Seeff LB et al: Hepatic disease in asymptomatic parenteral narcotic drug abusers: A Veterans Administration collaborative study. Am J Med Sci 270:41, 1975

897. Seeff LB et al: A randomized double blind controlled trial of the efficacy of immune serum globulin for the prevention of post-transfusion hepatitis: A Veterans Administration Cooperative Study. Gastroenterology 72:111, 1977

898. Sergent JS et al: Vasculitis with hepatitis B antigenemia: Long-term observations in nine patients. Medicine 55:1, 1976

899. Serrano MA, Hirschman SZ: Properties of hepatitis B e antigen synthesized by rat cells transfected with circular viral DNA. J Gen Virol 65:1373, 1984

900. Seto B et al: Detection of reverse transcriptase activity in association with the non-A, non-B hepatitis agent(s). Lancet 2:941, 1984

901. Shattock AG et al: Increased severity and morbidity of acute hepatitis in drug abusers with simultaneously acquired hepatitis B and hepatitis D virus infections. Br Med J 290:1377, 1985

902. Shattock AG, Morgan BM: Sensitive enzyme immunoassay for the detection of delta antigen and anti-delta, using serum as the delta antigen source. J Med Virol 13: 73, 1984

903. Sherlock S: Portal venous "goodies" and fulminant viral hepatitis. N Engl J Med 295:1535, 1976

904. Sherwood PM: An outbreak of syringe-transmitted hepatitis with jaundice in hospitalized diabetic patients. Ann Intern Med 33:380, 1950

905. Shih JW-K, Gerin JL: Proteins of hepatitis B surface antigen. J Virol 21:347, 1977

906. Shih JW-K, Gerin JL: Proteins of hepatitis B surface antigen: Compositions of the major polypeptides. J Virol 21:1219, 1977

907. Shimada T et al: Light microscopic localization of hepatitis B virus antigens in the human pancreas. Gastroenterology 81:998, 1981

908. Shimizu Y, Kitamoto O: The incidence of viral hepatitis after blood transfusions. Gastroenterology 44:740, 1963

909. Shimizu YK et al: Non-A, non-B hepatitis: Ultrastructural evidence for two agents in experimentally infected chimpanzees. Science 205:197, 1979

910. Shimizu YK et al: Localization of hepatitis A antigen in liver tissue by peroxidase-conjugated antibody method: Light and electron microscope studies. J Immunol 121: 1671, 1978

911. Shimizu YK et al: Detection of hepatitis A antigen in human liver. Infect Immun 36:320, 1982

912. Shiraishi H et al: Carbohydrate composition of hepatitis B surface antigen. J Gen Virol 36:207, 1977

913. Shorey J: A new hepatitis B surface antigen. J Infect Dis 133:1, 1976

914. Shulman NR, Barker LF: Virus-like antigen, antibody, and antigen-antibody complexes in hepatitis measured by complement fixation. Science 165:304, 1969

915. Shutkin NM: Homologous-serum hepatitis following the use of refrigerated bonebank bone. J Bone Joint Surg [Am] 36:160, 1954

916. Siegel M: Congenital malformations following chickenpox, measles, mumps and hepatitis: Results of a cohort study. JAMA 226:1521, 1973

917. Siegel M et al: Comparative fetal mortality in maternal virus diseases: Prospective study on rubella, measles, chickenpox and hepatitis. N Engl J Med 274:768, 1966

918. Siegl G: Structure and biology of hepatitis A virus. In Szmuness W, Alter HJ, Maynard JE (eds): Viral Hepatitis, International Symposium, 1981, p 13. Philadelphia, Franklin Institute Press, 1982

919. Siegl G, Frosner GG: Characterization and classification of virus particles associated with hepatitis A: I. Size, density, and sedimentation. J Virol 26:40, 1978

920. Siegl G, Frosner GG: Characterization and classification of virus particles associated with hepatitis A: II. Type and configuration of nucleic acid. J Virol 26:48, 1978

921. Siegl G et al: The physiochemical properties of infectious hepatitis A virions. J Gen Virol 57:331, 1981

922. Silverstein MD et al: Should donor blood be screened for elevated alanine aminotransferase levels? A cost-effectiveness analysis. JAMA 252:2839, 1984

923. Simon JB, Scheig R: Serum cholesterol esterification in liver disease: The importance of lecithin-cholesterol acyltransferase. N Engl J Med 283:841, 1970

924. Singleton JW et al: Liver disease in Australia-antigen-positive blood donors. Lancet 2:785, 1971

925. Sjogren MH et al: Low molecular weight IgM antibody to hepatitis B core antigen in chronic infections with hepatitis B virus. J Infect Dis 148:445, 1983

926. Sjogren MH, Hoofnagle JH: Immunoglobulin M antibody to hepatitis B core antigen in patients with chronic type B hepatitis. Gastroenterology 89:252, 1985

927. Skinhoj P: Viral hepatitis in Danish clinical chemical laboratories 1968–1978: Incidence rates, aetiology and risk factors. Scand J Clin Lab Invest 40:23, 1980

928. Skinhoj P et al: Transmission of hepatitis type B from healthy HBsAg positive mothers. Br Med J 1:10, 1976

929. Skinhoj P et al: Hepatitis associated antigen (HAA) in pregnant women and their newborn infants. Am J Dis Child 123:380, 1972

930. Slusarczyk J et al: Membranous glomerulopathy associated with hepatitis B core antigen immune complexes in children. Am J Pathol 98:29, 1980

931. Smart C: The Medical and Surgical History of the War of the Rebellion, Part III, Vol I, p 874. Washington, DC, US Government Printing Office, 1888

932. Smedile A et al: Influence of delta infection on severity of hepatitis B. Lancet 2:945, 1982

933. Smedile A et al: Epidemiologic patterns of infection with the hepatitis B virus-associated delta agent in Italy. Am J Epidemiol 117:223, 1983

934. Smedile A et al: Radioimmunoassay detection of IgM antibodies to the HBV-associated delta antigen: Clinical significance in delta infection. J Med Virol 9:131, 1982

935. Smetana HF: The histopathology of acute nonfatal hepatitis. Bull NY Acad Med 28:482, 1952

936. Smith BF: Occurrence of hepatitis in recently tattooed service personnel. JAMA 144:1074, 1950

937. Smith D et al: Spontaneous resolution of severe aplastic anemia associated with viral hepatitis A in a 6-year-old child. Am J Hematol 5:247, 1978

938. Smith FR et al: Disordered gustatory acuity in liver disease. Gastroenterology 70:568, 1976

939. Snow DJR: Infective hepatitis: A discussion on its mode of spread in families. Med J Aust 2:139, 1953

940. Snydman DR et al: Hemodialysis-associated hepatitis in the United States, 1974. J Infect Dis 135:687, 1977

941. Snydman DR et al: Prevention of nosocomial viral hepatitis, type B (hepatitis B). Ann Intern Med 83:838, 1975

942. Snydman DR et al: Transmission of hepatitis B associated with hemodialysis: Role of malfunction (blood leaks) in dialysis machines. J Infect Dis 134:562, 1976

943. Snydman DR et al: Hemodialysis-associated hepatitis: Report of an epidemic with further evidence on mechanisms of transmission. Am J Epidemiol 104:563, 1976

944. Snydman DR et al: Nosocomial viral hepatitis B: A cluster among staff with subsequent transmission to patients. Ann Intern Med 85:573, 1976

945. Soloway RD et al: Clinical, biochemical, and histological remission of severe chronic active liver disease: A controlled study of treatments and early prognosis. Gastroenterology 63:820, 1972

946. Soulier JP, Courouce-Pauty AM: New determinants of hepatitis B antigen (Au or HB antigen). Vox Sang 25:212, 1973

947. Spellberg MA: Observations on the treatment of hepatic coma: The favorable effect of corticotropin and corticoids and the responsiveness of adrenal cortex to corticotropin during hepatic coma. Gastroenterology 32:600, 1957

948. Spichtin H et al: Nuclear particles of non-A, non-B type in healthy volunteers and patients with hepatitis B. Hepatology 4:510, 1984

949. Spitz RD et al: Bridging necrosis: Etiology and prognosis. Am J Dig Dis 23:1076, 1978

950. Sreenivasan MA et al: Non-A, non-B epidemic hepatitis: Visualization of virus-like particles in the stool by immune electron microscopy. J Gen Virol 65:1005, 1984

951. Stanley P et al: Toxicity of ethylene oxide sterilization of polyvinyl chloride in open-heart surgery. J Thorac Cardiovasc Surg 61:309, 1971

952. Steigmann F et al: Infectious hepatitis (homologous serum type) in drug addicts. Gastroenterology 15:642, 1950

953. Steiner S et al: Major polar lipids of hepatitis B antigen preparations: Evidence for the presence of a glycosphingolipid. J Virol 14:572, 1974

954. Stevens CE et al: Vertical transmission of hepatitis B antigen in Taiwan. N Engl J Med 292:771, 1975

955. Stevens CE et al: Hepatitis B vaccine: Immune responses in haemodialysis patients. Lancet 2:1211, 1980

956. Stevens CE et al: Hepatitis B virus antibody in blood donors and the occurrence of non-A, non-B hepatitis in transfusion recipients: An analysis of the Transfusion-Transmitted Viruses Study. Ann Intern Med 101:733, 1984

957. Stevens CE et al: Perinatal hepatitis B virus transmission in the United States: Prevention by passive-active immunization. JAMA 253:1740, 1985

958. Stiehm EF, Fudenberg HH: Antibodies to gamma-globulin in infants and children exposed to isologous gamma-globulin. Pediatrics 35:229, 1965

959. Stille W et al: Austern-hepatitis. Dtsch Med Wochenschr 97:145, 1972

960. Stokes J et al: Neurological complications of infective hepatitis. Br Med J 2:642, 1945

961. Stokes J Jr et al: The carrier state in viral hepatitis. JAMA 154:1059, 1954

962. Stokes J Jr et al: Infectious hepatitis: Length of protection by immune serum globulin (gamma globulin) during epidemics. JAMA 147:714, 1951

963. Stokes J Jr et al: Viral hepatitis in the newborn: Clinical features, epidemiology and pathology. Am J Dis Child 82:213, 1951

964. Strom J: A comparison between family infections during epidemics of poliomyelitis and hepatitis in Stockholm. Acta Med Scand. 165:49, 1959

965. Sukeno N et al: Conformational studies of Australia antigen by optical rotatory dispersion and circular dichroism. J Virol 10:157:1972

966. Summers J: Replication of hepatitis B viruses. In Vyas GN, Dienstag JL, Hoofnagle JH (eds): Viral Hepatitis and Liver Disease, p 87. Orlando, FL, Grune & Stratton, 1984

967. Summers J, Mason WS: Replication of the genome of a hepatitis B-like virus by reverse transcriptase of an RNA intermediate. Cell 29:403, 1982

968. Summerskill WHJ, Jones FA: Corticotrophin and steroids

in the diagnosis and management of "obstructive" jaundice. Br Med J 2:1499, 1958

969. Sun S-C et al: Serial liver biopsy observations in hepatitis B antigen carriers by light and electron microscopy. Am J Dig Dis 21:366, 1976

970. Swift WE Jr et al: Clinical course of viral hepatitis and the effect of exercise during convalescence. Am J Med 8:614, 1950

971. Szmuness W, Prince AM: The epidemiology of serum hepatitis (SH) infections: A controlled study in two closed institutions. Am J Epidemiol 94:585, 1971

972. Szmuness W et al: Distribution of antibody to hepatitis A antigen in urban adult populations. N Engl J Med 295:755, 1976

973. Szmuness W et al: Hepatitis Type A and hemodialysis: A seroepidemiologic study in 15 US centers. Ann Intern Med 87:8, 1977

974. Szmuness W et al: Sociodemographic aspects of the epidemiology of hepatitis B. In Vyas GN et al (eds): Viral Hepatitis, p 297. Philadelphia, Franklin Institute Press, 1978

975. Szmuness W et al: The serum hepatitis virus specific antigen (SH): A preliminary report of epidemiologic studies in an institution for the mentally retarded. Am J Epidemiol 92:51, 1970

976. Szmuness W et al: Hepatitis B vaccine: Demonstration of efficacy in a controlled clinical trial in a high-risk population in the United States. N Engl J Med 303:834, 1980

977. Szmuness W et al: Hepatitis B infection: A point-prevalence study in 15 US hemodialysis centers. JAMA 227:901, 1974

978. Szmuness W et al: Familial clustering of hepatitis B infection. N Engl J Med 289:1162, 1973

979. Szmuness W et al: Passive-active immunization against hepatitis B: Immunogenicity studies in adult Americans. Lancet 1:575, 1981

980. Szmuness W et al: A controlled clinical trial of the efficacy of the hepatitis B vaccine (Heptavax B): A final report. Hepatology 1:377, 1981

981. Szmuness W et al: Hepatitis B vaccine in medical staff of hemodialysis units: Efficacy and subtype cross-protection. N Engl J Med 307:1481, 1982

982. Szmuness W et al: Passive-active immunizations against hepatitis B: Immunogenicity studies in adult Americans. Lancet 2:675, 1981

983. Tabor E: The three viruses of non-A, non-B hepatitis. Lancet 1:743, 1985

984. Tabor E et al: Acute non-A, non-B hepatitis: Prolonged presence of the infectious agent in blood. Gastroenterology 76:680, 1978

985. Tabor E et al: Acquired immunity to human non-A, non-B hepatitis: Cross challenge of chimpanzees with three infectious human sera. J Infect Dis 140:789, 1979

986. Tabor E et al: Transmission of non-A, non-B hepatitis from man to chimpanzee. Lancet 1:463, 1978

987. Tabor E et al: Chronic non-A, non-B hepatitis carrier state. N Engl J Med 303:140, 1980

988. Tabor E et al: Effect of ethanol during hepatitis B virus infection in chimpanzees. J Med Virol 2:295, 1978

989. Tabor E et al: Inactivation of hepatitis B virus by three methods: Treatment with pepsin, urea, or formalin. J Med Virol 11:1, 1983

990. Tada H et al: Combined passive and active immunization for preventing perinatal transmission of hepatitis B virus carrier state. Pediatrics 70:613, 1982

991. Takahashi K et al: Shift from free "small" hepatitis B e antigen to IgG-bound "large" form in the circulation of human beings and a chimpanzee acutely infected with hepatitis B virus. Gastroenterology 77:1193, 1979

992. Takekoshi Y et al: Free "small" and IgG-associated "large" hepatitis B e antigen in the serum and glomerular capillary walls of two patients with membranous glomerulonephritis. N Engl J Med 300:814, 1979

993. Takekoshi Y et al: Strong association between membranous nephropathy and hepatitis B surface antigenaemia in Japanese children. Lancet 2:1065, 1978

994. Tarshis IB: The cockroach—a new suspect in the spread of infectious hepatitis. Am J Trop Med Hyg 11:705, 1962

995. Tedder RS, Bull FE: Characterization of 'e' antigen associated with hepatitis B. Clin Exp Immunol 35:380, 1979

996. Teixeira MR Jr et al: The pathology of hepatitis A in man. Liver 2:53, 1982

997. Thalassinos N et al: Plasma alpha-lipoprotein pattern in acute viral hepatitis. Dig Dis 20:148, 1975

998. Thomas HC et al: Immune complexes in acute and chronic liver disease. Clin Exp Immunol 31:150, 1978

999. Thomssen R et al: Aetiologie der hepatitis B-Borlaenfige Ergebnisse: einer kooperativen Studie. Zentralbl Bakteriol (I Orig. A), 235:242, 1976

1000. Thorn GW et al: The clinical usefulness of ACTH and cortisone. N Engl J Med 242:865, 1950

1001. Thorne EG et al: Urticaria with hepatitis associated antigen (HAA) positive hepatitis. Cutis 10:705, 1972

1002. Ticehurst JR et al: Molecular cloning and characterization of hepatitis A virus cDNA. Proc Natl Acad Sci USA 80:5885, 1983

1003. Tiku ML et al: Hepatitis B infection in health care personnel of an institution for mentally handicapped children and adults. J Clin Microbiol 3:469, 1976

1004. Tiollais P et al: Biology of hepatitis B virus. Science 213:406, 1981

1005. Tiollais P et al: Structure of hepatitis B virus DNA. In Vyas GN, Dienstag JL, Hoofnagle JH (eds): Viral Hepatitis and Liver Disease, p 49. Orlando, FL, Grune & Stratton, 1984

1006. Tisdale WA: Clinical and pathologic features of subacute hepatitis. Medicine 45:557, 1966

1007. Tisdale WA: Subacute hepatitis. N Engl J Med 268:85, 1963

1008. Toda G et al: Infantile papular acrodermatitis (Gianotti's disease) and intrafamilial occurrence of acute hepatitis B with jaundice: Age dependency of clinical manifestations of hepatitis B virus infection. J Infect Dis 138:211, 1978

1009. Tong MJ et al: Studies in infants born to mothers with type A hepatitis and acute non-A, non-B hepatitis during pregnancy. Gastroenterology 75:991, 1978

1010. Tong MJ et al: Correlation of e antigen, DNA polymerase activity, and Dane particles in chronic benign and chronic active type B hepatitis infections. J Infect Dis 135:980, 1977

1011. Tong MJ et al: Lymphocyte stimulation in hepatitis B infection. N Engl J Med 293:318, 1975

1012. Trepo CG et al: The role of circulating hepatitis B antigen/antibody immune complexes in the pathogenesis of vascular and hepatic manifestations in polyarteritis nodosa. J Clin Pathol 27:863, 1974

1013. Trepo CG et al: Non-A, non-B hepatitis virus: Identification of a core antigen–antibody system that cross reacts with hepatitis B core antigens and antibody. J Med Virol 8:31, 1981

1014. Trewby PN et al: Incidence and pathophysiology of pulmonary edema in fulminant hepatic failure. Gastroenterology 74:859, 1978

1015. Trewby PN et al: Intrapulmonary vascular shunts in fulminant hepatic failure. Digestion 14:466, 1976

1016. Trey C: The fulminant hepatic failure surveillance study: Brief review of the effects of presumed etiology and age of survival. Can Med Assoc J 106:525, 1972

1017. Tripatzis I: Australia antigen in urine and feces. Am J Dis Child 124:401, 1972

1018. Tsuda F et al: Low molecular weight (7S) immunoglobulin M antibody against hepatitis B core antigen in the serum for differentiating acute from persistent hepatitis B virus infection. Gastroenterology 87:159, 1984

1019. Tucker CB et al: Outbreak of infectious hepatitis apparently transmitted through water. South Med J 47:732, 1954

1020. Tur-Kaspa R et al: Detection and characterization of hepatitis B virus DNA in serum of HBe antigen-negative HBsAg carriers. J Med Virol 14:17, 1984

1021. Turnberg LA: Iron absorption in acute hepatitis. Am J Dig Dis 11:20, 1966

1022. Ukena T et al: Delta hepatitis—Massachusetts. MMWR 33:493, 1984

1023. Unger PN, Shapiro S: The prothrombin response to the parenteral administration of large doses of vitamin K in subjects with normal liver function and in cases of liver disease: A standardized test for the estimation of hepatic function. J Clin Invest 27:39, 1948

1024. Urban GE: Severe sensorineural hearing loss associated with viral hepatitis. South Med J 71:724, 1978

1025. Valenzuela P et al: Nucleotide sequence of the gene coding for the major protein of hepatitis B virus surface antigen. Nature 280:815, 1979

1026. van Ditzhuijsen TJM et al: Detection of hepatitis B virus DNA in serum and relation with the IgM class anti-HBc titers in hepatitis B virus infection. J Med Virol 15:49, 1985

1027. Vellar OD: Acute viral hepatitis in Norwegian track-finders: An epidemiological study in Norway 1962–63. Acta Med Scand 176:651, 1964

1028. Versieck J et al: Manganese, copper, and zinc concentrations in serum and packed blood cells during acute hepatitis, chronic hepatitis, and posthepatic cirrhosis. Clin Chem 20:1141, 1974

1029. Verstraete M et al: Excessive consumption of blood coagulation components as cause of hemorrhagic diathesis. Am J Med 38:899, 1965

1030. Villarejos VM et al: Identification of a type B hepatitis epidemic in Costa Rica: Comparative analysis of two outbreaks of viral hepatitis. Am J Epidemiol 96:372, 1972

1031. Villarejos VM et al: Evidence for viral hepatitis other than type A or type B among persons in Costa Rica. N Engl J Med 293:1350, 1975

1032. Villarejos VM et al: Role of saliva, urine and feces in the transmission of type B hepatitis. N Engl Med 291:1375, 1974

1033. Vitvitski L et al: Detection of virus-associated antigen in serum and liver of patients with non-A, non-B hepatitis. Lancet 2:1263, 1979

1034. Vitvitski L et al: Use of cross-reactivity between hepatitis B and non-A, non-B viruses for the identification and detection of non-A, non-B 'e' antigen. J Med Virol 1:149, 1980

1035. Volwiler W, Dealy JB Jr: Gamma globulin in treatment of chronic phase of epidemic infectious hepatitis. Gastroenterology 12:87, 1949

1036. Volwiler W, Elliott JA Jr: Late manifestations of epidemic infectious hepatitis. Gastroenterology 10:349, 1948

1037. Volwiler W et al: Biosynthetic determination with radioactive sulfur of turn-over rates of various plasma proteins in normal and cirrhotic man. J Clin Invest 34:1126, 1955

1038. Vyas GN et al: Anaphylactoid transfusion reactions associated with anti-IgA. Lancet 2:312, 1968

1039. Wade OL, Bishop JM: Cardiac Output and Regional Blood Flow, p 87. Oxford, Blackwell Scientific Publications, 1962

1040. Wagner H et al: Diagnosis of liver disease by radioisotope scanning. Arch Intern Med 107:324, 1961

1041. Wallace DK, Owen EE: An evaluation of the mechanism of bilirubin excretion by the human kidney. J Lab Clin Med 64:741, 1964

1042. Wallace EC: Infectious hepatitis: Report of an outbreak apparently water-borne. Med J Aust 1:101, 1958

1043. Wallis C et al: The ineffectiveness of organic iodine (Wescodyne) as a viral disinfectant. Am J Hyg 78:325, 1963

1044. Walz DV: An effective hospital transfusion committee. JAMA 189:660, 1964

1045. Wands JR et al: The pathogenesis of arthritis associated with acute hepatitis B surface antigen-positive hepatitis: Complement activation and characterization of circulating immune complexes. J Clin Invest 55:930, 1975

1046. Wands JR et al: Cell-mediated immunity in acute and chronic hepatitis. J Clin Invest 55:921, 1975

1047. Wands JR et al: Hepatitis B in an oncology unit. N Engl J Med 291:1371, 1974

1048. Wands JR et al: Detection and transmission in chimpanzees of hepatitis B virus–related agents formerly designated "non-A, non-B" hepatitis. Proc Natl Acad Sci USA 79:7552, 1982

1049. Wands JR et al: Monoclonal antibodies and hepatitis B: A new perspective using highly sensitive and specific radioimmunoassays. In Vyas GN, Dienstag JL, Hoofnagle JH (eds): Viral Hepatitis and Liver Disease, p 543. Orlando, FL, Grune & Stratton, 1984

1050. Ward R et al: Hepatitis B antigen in saliva and mouth washings. Lancet 2:726, 1972

1051. Ward R et al: Infective hepatitis: Studies of its natural history and prevention. N Engl J Med 258:407, 1959

1052. Ware AJ et al: Controlled trial of corticosteroid therapy in severe acute viral hepatitis. Gastroenterology 75:992, 1978

1053. Ware AJ et al: Cerebral edema: A major complication of massive hepatic necrosis. Gastroenterology 61:877, 1971

1054. Ware AJ et al: Prognostic significance of subacute hepatic necrosis in acute hepatitis. Gastroenterology 68:519, 1975

1055. Ware AJ et al: Etiology of liver disease in renal transplant patients. Ann Intern Med 91:364, 1979

1056. Ware AJ et al: A prospective trial of steroid therapy in severe viral hepatitis. Gastroenterology 80:219, 1981

1057. Wauters JP, Leski M: Delayed hepatitis after treatment with hepatitis B immune serum globulin. Br Med J 2:19, 1976

1058. Weidner J: Posttransfusions hepatitis und gamma-globulin-prophylaxe. Dtsch Med Wochenschr 101:755, 1976

1059. Weinstein L, Davison WT: Neurologic manifestations in the preicteric phase of infectious hepatitis. Am Pract 1:191, 1946

1060. Weiss JS et al: The clinical importance of a protein-bound fraction of serum bilirubin in patients with hyperbilirubinemia. N Engl J Med 309:147, 1983

1061. Weiss TD et al: Skin lesions in viral hepatitis: Histologic and immunofluorescent findings. Am J Med 64:269, 1978

1062. Werner BG et al: Association of e antigen with Dane particle DNA in sera from asymptomatic carriers of hepatitis B surface antigen. Proc Natl Acad Sci 74:2149, 1977

1063. Werner BG et al: Isolated antibody to hepatitis B surface antigen and response to hepatitis B vaccination. Am Intern Med 103:201, 1985

1064. Wewalka F: Protracted and recurrent forms of viral hepatitis. Am J Dis Child 123:283, 1972

1065. Wewalka F: Zur Epidemiologie des Ikterus bei der antisyphilitischen Behandlung. Schweiz Z Allg Pathol 16:307, 1953

1066. Whaley WH, Galambos JT: Race and risk of hepatitis in narcotic addicts. Am J Dig Dis 18:460, 1973

1067. Whitehead NT, Crouch HA: Infectious jaundice in the Sudan. J Trop Med 29:359, 1926

1068. Wicks RC et al: Thymus-derived lymphocytes in type B acute viral hepatitis and healthy carriers of hepatitis B surface antigen (HBsAg). Am J Dig Dis 20:518, 1975

1069. Wiedmann KH et al: Serum inhibitory factors (SIF) are of prognostic value in acute viral hepatitis. Lancet 1:309, 1985

1070. Wiener M et al: Bridging hepatic necrosis in acute viral hepatitis. Isr J Med Sci 20:33, 1984

1071. Wilkinson SP et al: Frequency and type of renal and electrolyte disorders in fulminant hepatic failure. Br Med J 1:186, 1974

1072. Wilkinson SP et al: Renal failure in otherwise uncomplicated viral hepatitis. Br Med J 2:338, 1978

1073. Wilkinson SP et al: Clinical course of chronic lobular hepatitis. QJ Med 47:421, 1978

1074. Williams R, Billing BH: Action of steroid therapy in jaundice. Lancet 2:392, 1961

1075. Will H et al: Cloned HBV DNA causes hepatitis in chimpanzees. Nature 299:740, 1982

1076. Wind, saliva and hepatitis B. Lancet 1:163, 1980

1077. Winston MA, Shapiro M: Pseudo-tumors in acute hepatitis. J Nucl Med 15:1039, 1974

1078. Wolf JL et al: The transplanted kidney as a source of hepatitis B infection. Ann Intern Med 91:412, 1979

1079. Wong DC et al: Epidemic and endemic hepatitis in India: Evidence for a non-A, non-B hepatitis virus aetiology. Lancet 2:876, 1980

1080. Wong ML et al: Detection of hepatitis B surface antigen in the saliva of patients with acute hepatitis B, and of chronic carriers. Med J Aust 2:52, 1976

1081. Wong VCW et al: Prevention of the HBsAg carrier state in newborn infants of mothers who are chronic carriers of HBsAg and HBeAg by administration of hepatitis B vaccine and hepatitis B in immunoglobulin. Lancet 1: 921, 1984

1082. Woodson RD, Cahill KM: Viral hepatitis abroad: Incidence in Catholic missionaries. JAMA 219:1191, 1972

1083. Woodson RS, Clinton JJ: Hepatitis prophylaxis abroad: Effectiveness of immune serum globulin in protecting Peace Corps volunteers. JAMA 209:1053, 1969

1084. World Health Organization Technical Report Series: Viral Hepatitis. Geneva, World Health Organization, 1975

1085. Wright R et al: Australia antigen in acute and chronic liver disease. Lancet 2:117, 1969

1086. Wright RA: Hepatitis B and the HBsAg carrier: An outbreak related to sexual contact. JAMA 232:717, 1975

1087. Yamada G et al: Electron and immunoelectron microscopic study of Dane particle formation in chronic hepatitis B virus infection. Gastroenterology 83:348, 1982

1088. Yamada G, Nakane PK: Hepatitis B core and surface antigens in liver tissue: Light and electron microscopic localization by the peroxidase-labeled antibody method. Lab Invest 36:649, 1977

1089. Yamashita Y et al: South-to-north gradient in distribution of the r determinant of hepatitis B surface antigen in Japan. J Infect Dis 131:567, 1975

1090. Yamauchi M et al: An epidemic of non-A/non-B hepatitis in Japan. Am J Gastroenterol 78:652, 1983

1091. Yoshibumi H, Shigemoto T: Human experiment with epidemic jaundice. Acta Paediatr Jpn 47:975, 1941

1092. Yoshizawa H et al: Diagnosis of type A hepatitis by fecal IgA antibody against hepatitis A antigen. Gastroenterology 78:114, 1980

1093. Yoshizawa H et al: Non-A, non-B (type 1) hepatitis agent capable of inducing tabular ultrastructures in the hepatocyte cytoplasm of chimpanzees: Inactivation by formalin and heat. Gastroenterology 82:502, 1982

1094. Yoshizawa H et al: Demonstration of two different types of non-A, non-B hepatitis by reinjection and cross-challenge studies in chimpanzees. Gastroenterology 81:107, 1981

1095. Yoshizawa H et al: Beta-propiolactone for the inactivation of non-A/non-B type 1 hepatitis virus capable of inducing cytoplasmic tubular ultrastructures in chimpanzees. Vox Sang 46:86, 1984

1096. Yunet R, Yunet W, cited by Corelli F: Beitrag zum Studium des alsuten Gelenkrheumatismus Bleituhentragung von akutem Gelenkrheumabsumsblut. Z Rheumatol 4: 544, 1941

1097. Zachoval R et al: Passive/active immunization against hepatitis B. J Infect Dis 150:112, 1984

1098. Zaversnik H, Petrovic S: Incidence of chronic hepatitis after epidemic of infectious hepatitis. Br Med J 3:220, 1970

1099. Zebe H et al: Insect vectors in serum hepatitis. Lancet 1: 1117, 1972

1100. Zeldis JB et al: Aplastic anemia and non-A, non-B hepatitis. Am J Med 74:64, 1983

1101. Zieve L et al: The incidence of residuals of viral hepatitis. Gastroenterology 25:495, 1953

1102. Zimmerman HJ, Lowry CF: Encephalomyeloradiculitis (Guillain-Barré syndrome) as a complication of infectious hepatitis. Ann Intern Med 26:934, 1947

1103. Zimmerman HJ et al: Infectious hepatitis: Clinical and laboratory features of 295 cases. Am J Med Sci 213:395, 1947

1104. Zimmerman HJ et al: Fasting blood sugar in hepatic disease with reference to infrequency of hypoglycemia. Arch Intern Med 91:577, 1953

1105. Zoulek G et al: Evaluation of a reduced dose of hepatitis B vaccine administered intradermally. J Med Virol 14: 27, 1984

1106. Zuckerman AJ: The clinical and laboratory features of acute hepatitis in the Royal Air Force. Monthly Bull Minist Hlth Lab Ser 24:340, 1965

1107. Zuckerman AJ, Taylor PE: Persistence of serum hepatitis (SH/Australia) antigen for many years. Nature 223:81, 1969

1108. Zuckerman AJ et al: Hepatitis B outbreak among chimpanzees at the London zoo. Lancet 2:652, 1978

chapter **16**

Hepatitis Caused by Viruses Other Than Hepatitis A, Hepatitis B, and Non-A, Non-B Hepatitis Viruses

GILBERT M. SCHIFF

In considering liver disease caused by viruses in humans, one naturally thinks of classic viral hepatitis caused by the infectious hepatitis or hepatitis A virus (HAV); the serum hepatitis or hepatitis B virus (HBV); or the recently recognized non-A, non-B hepatitis virus(es) (NANB). However, this is far from the complete story. Some viruses, such as the yellow fever virus, the etiologic agent of infectious mononucleosis, and a trio of newly described "exotic" viruses (Ebola, Marburg, and Lassa fever viruses), almost invariably produce liver disease. Some viruses, such as herpes hominis, cytomegalovirus, and rubella, frequently cause hepatitis when acquired transplacentally or neonatally, but do so less frequently or rarely when acquired later in life. Other common human viruses, such as adenoviruses and enteroviruses, have occasionally been associated with clinical liver disease, although their clinical presentations usually lack liver involvement. Indeed, such viruses are probably associated with human hepatitis more frequently than we realize. Rarely is there a laboratory search for viruses other than HAV or HBV in cases of hepatitis. Similarly, common clinical viral diseases, such as influenza, mumps, and measles, are not uncommonly associated with liver enzyme abnormalities. However, studies documenting the presence of liver disease are not pursued. The true etiologic role assumed by human viruses other than HAV, HBV, and NANB in causing hepatitis and other forms of liver disease has not yet been defined.

VIRUSES FREQUENTLY INVOLVED WITH LIVER DISEASE

Yellow Fever

Yellow fever virus is a known hepatotropic agent of humans. Two epidemiologic patterns of the disease occur in humans, the urban and sylvanic, or jungle type. The former is transmitted from human to human by certain domestic or semi-domestic species of Aedes mosquitoes; the latter involves a virus cycle of wild animals, particularly monkeys, and forest mosquitoes, with humans as incidental victims when intruding the jungle environment. History has recorded severe epidemics of the disease.[8] Today, yellow fever is enzootic in large areas of tropical Central America and South America and Africa.[29]

The yellow fever virus is a member of the group B arboviruses. It can be grown in several types of tissue culture cells and several laboratory animals including the rhesus monkey, white mouse, guinea pig, and chicken embryo.[8] The virus can be modified by tissue culture or intracerebral mouse passage, with the development of two effective vaccines.[69] Serologically, infection with the virus results in the development of neutralizing hemagglutination inhibition and complement fixation antibodies. The usual laboratory diagnosis consists of isolating the virus from an acute blood specimen by inoculation of mice or the detection of a significant neutralization or hemagglutination inhibition antibody rise in the serum.[41] Diagnosis can also be made by histologic examination of the liver.

The clinical features have been described in detail by Kerr.[34] The incubation period is 3 to 6 days. The disease spectrum ranges from inapparent infection to a fulminating disease with a fatal outcome after a few days. In the typical case, the onset is abrupt and followed by an initial phase of fever, severe headache, dizziness, muscular aches, nausea, and vomiting. A brief remission occurs followed by a second, toxic phase with high fever, bradycardia, jaundice, vomiting, hematemesis and other hemorrhagic manifestations, oliguria or anemia, and frequently hypotension and delirium or coma. The disease may appear as a uniphasic, influenza-like illness, or end in death. Mortality rates vary; in 1905, the southern United States experienced an outbreak with a 20% mortality rate.[8] Laboratory abnormalities include leukopenia, albuminuria, casts, elevated blood urea nitrogen, and altered liver function tests and prothrombin time. Terminal cases are associated with early, marked abnormalities in the serum bilirubin, urea, and prothrombin time.[12]

The pathologic findings have been described in detail by Bugher.[3] Icterus occurs and hemorrhagic manifestations involve various organs. Microscopically, the liver shows fatty degeneration and mid-zonal to complete lobular necrosis of hepatic cells with scattered Councilman bodies. Little inflammatory reaction is found. The virus has been found in both Kupffer and parenchymal cells.[41]

The treatment is nonspecific supportive care. Prophylactic and control measures have been highly effective. Urban yellow fever can be prevented by eradication of the Aedes species of mosquitoes. Jungle yellow fever can be prevented in humans by immunization. There are two strains of vaccines: the Dakar (French neurotropic), attenuated by mouse brain passage, and the 17D, grown in chick embryo tissue culture. The 17D strain is recommended over the Dakar strain because the latter has been associated with a relatively high incidence of meningoencephalitic reactions. Persons 6 months or older traveling or living in areas where yellow fever exists (currently Africa and parts of Central America and South America) and laboratory personnel who might be exposed to virulent yellow fever virus should receive a single subcutaneous injection of 0.5 ml of 17D vaccine.[47] Revaccination should be administered every 10 years.

Infectious Mononucleosis

Infectious mononucleosis is a disease of young adults that has a typical clinical syndrome consisting of severe, exudative pharyngitis, lymphadenopathy, a relative and absolute lymphocytosis, atypical peripheral mononuclear cells, and a positive heterophil antibody test. Liver involvement is frequent. There is a definite association between the disease and the Epstein–Barr virus (EBV).

The EBV has been classified in the herpes group of viruses. It was originally found in cell lines derived from Burkitt's lymphomas.[77] Circulating antibodies to EBV have been demonstrated in patients with Burkitt's lymphoma,[23] carcinoma of the posterior nasal space,[51] and infectious mononucleosis.[24] Several studies have confirmed the strong, positive serologic relationship in patients with infectious mononucleosis.[19,24,50] These patients lack EBV antibody in their sera prior to onset of the disease but rapidly develop EBV antibody during the acute stages of the disease. The EBV antibody persists indefinitely. In addition, it is possible to cultivate lymphoid cell lines that are chronically infected with EBV from infectious mononucleosis patients.[46]

Infectious mononucleosis is very common in childhood but seldom clinically apparent. Serologic surveys measuring EBV antibody have shown that in North America and western Europe, 50% to 60% of children have acquired antibodies by 5 years of age and by 20 years the incidence of antibodies is 80% to 90% or more.[19,27,54] In poorer populations, the incidence of antibodies is 80% to 90% in young children. In more privileged populations, the incidence in young adults may be as low as 25% to 50%. This lower incidence in the higher socioeconomic group

probably explains why the disease is frequently found in university students.

Clinical infectious mononucleosis occurs principally in adolescents and young adults between 15 and 25 years of age. It is especially prevalent in school and university, hospital, and military communities. Transmission of EBV infection is probably by close personal contact in young children and probably involves intimate oral contact in young adults.[15,27] Actual transfer of infected cells in saliva may be required.[5,55] Transmission by blood transfusion has also been documented.[53] The disease rarely, if ever, occurs in epidemics. The incubation period is generally between 4 and 7 weeks, although some have estimated a shorter period.[77]

The clinical course varies considerably in severity and length of time. The duration may be as short as a few days or protracted for weeks. The early symptoms include malaise, fatigue, and inability to concentrate followed by increasing fever with evening peaks of 103° to 105°F (39.4°–40.5°C), headache, sore throat, and cervical and axillary lymphadenopathy. Hoagland described the findings in more than 500 patients studied[19,26] which in general included lymphadenopathy, pharyngeal inflammation and exudation and, to a lesser extent, hepatosplenomegaly. Hepatosplenomegaly was found in 17%; jaundice occurred in 11%. Splenomegaly has been reported in up to 75% of patients. Palatal enanthem consisting of punctate and pinpoint petechiae occurred in 50%, periorbital edema in 33%, and a maculopapular rash in less than 5% of patients.

Complications are relatively rare and include spontaneous splenic rupture, central nervous system (CNS) involvement (aseptic meningitis, encephalitis, infectious polyneuritis), thrombocytopenic purpura, and pericarditis. Convalescence may be prolonged with frequent complaints of malaise and fatigue.

The laboratory findings in infectious mononucleosis consist of the following:

1. Absolute lymphocytosis 12 to 18 days after onset of illness
2. Relative lymphocytosis
3. Presence of atypical lymphocytes, usually more than 20%
4. A positive heterophil antibody test sometime during the illness

In addition, the development of specific EBV antibodies can now be added to the laboratory picture.

Although only 11% of patients with infectious mononucleosis develop jaundice, hepatitis occurs in close to 90%. There are abnormal flocculation and serum enzyme tests.[19] Peak abnormalities occur during the second to fourth week. Liver biopsies in patients with infectious mononucleosis have revealed portal exudates with mononuclear infiltration, sinusoidal invasion by monocytes, areas of scattered mononuclear necrosis, and proliferation of Kupffer cells.[77] There is an intense regeneration of hepatic cells. Rarely the hepatitis can be persistent for months. Cirrhosis is not a common sequela.

The laboratory diagnosis of the disease depends on the demonstration of the relative and absolute lymphocytosis, the atypical lymphocytes (Downey cells), and the development of a positive serum heterophil test (Paul–Bunnell–Davidsohn test). The last-named should include the differential absorption tests with guinea pig kidney and beef red blood cells.[9,19]

More recently, the demonstration of presence or change in antibody titers to various specific EBV antigens has been used for diagnostic purposes.[62] The test results must be interpreted with care and correlated to the time the patient presents himself to the physician.

The differential diagnosis of infectious mononucleosis can be difficult at times, particularly in differentiating it from infectious hepatitis. In infectious hepatitis, fever disappears when jaundice occurs (except in the fulminant forms), whereas fever often persists during jaundice in infectious mononucleosis. A widely-used and highly specific test is a slide test on which a drop of serum and formalin-treated horse red cells are mixed—the so-called monospot test. This test, however, can be positive in infectious hepatitis and serum sickness, but can be distinguished by the differential absorption tests alluded to above. The heterophil agglutination, unlike the falsely positive one that may occur in infectious hepatitis, persists after absorption by beef red cells. Other diseases that must be differentiated are adenovirus, rubella, toxoplasmosis, cytomegalovirus, streptococcal pharyngitis, and diphtheria. In all cases, reliance on laboratory tests is essential. Culturing the offending organisms and the use of specific serologic tests will permit a definitive diagnosis of the other diseases.

Treatment of infectious mononucleosis is generally supportive. Use of corticosteroids has been advocated in severe cases. More recently, routine use of short-term, low-dose corticosteriods has been associated with dramatic improvement in symptoms, especially pharyngitis.[39] Surgical intervention is required when splenic rupture occurs.

Currently, no vaccine exists. Not only has the virus been associated with oncogenic diseases, but inoculation with tissue culture affects the cells in a malignant fashion, and administration to animals results in tumor production.[19] Thus, only "subparticle" or "synthetic" vaccines produced by newer technologies (i.e., genetic engineering) are feasible.

"Exotic" Viruses

Since the late 1960s, explosive outbreaks of three "new" viruses have occurred in western and central Africa.[11,29] They have been labeled Lassa virus,[44,57] Marburg virus,[18,58] and Ebola virus.[25,59,72,73] The outbreaks have been characterized by fulminant illness and high mortality rates with the liver as a prime target. The multimammate rat (*Mastomys natalensis*) and the African green monkey (*Cercopithecus aethiopo*) trapped in Uganda have been identified as animal reservoirs for Lassa and Marburg viruses, respectively. However, person to person transmission occurs, primarily by exposure to body fluids, for all three viruses. Until these diseases are diagnosed and measures taken to effectively isolate the infected patients, a serious health hazard exists for persons exposed, especially in the hospital setting. Secondary cases in households have been documented, but the most cases have resulted from spread of the viruses within the hospital. The clinical illnesses include influenza-like signs and symptoms (headache, high fever, malaise, myalgia), rash and pharyngitis, gastrointestinal tract signs (vomiting or watery diarrhea), and usually bleeding manifestations. Jaundice has been reported in Ebola fever.

Because of the location of the outbreaks, there have been relatively few adequate histopathologic studies. All three viruses have a profound effect on the liver and appear to propagate in the hepatocytes.[74] Early comparisons of the liver pathology indicate that distinguishing patterns may be present.

Treatment is primarily supportive, although use of convalescent plasma has been promising if given early in the course of disease.[72,73] Ribavirin, a synthetic nucleoside resembling guanosine, has been reported to be effective in the treatment of Lassa fever when administered intravenously in relatively high doses.[42]

While these viruses appear to be restricted in their locale, the rapidly changing social and political status of these African countries and the availability of modern transportation systems make them a worldwide threat.

VIRUSES FREQUENTLY INVOLVED WITH LIVER DISEASE IN THE NEONATE

Rubella, herpes hominis, cytomegalovirus, and coxsackie type B virus frequently cause liver disease following intrauterine infection or acquisition of infection soon after birth. All except rubella have been associated with liver disease in later life.

Rubella

Rubella (German measles, 3-day measles) is a relatively mild exanthematous disease of childhood. It has serious implications during the first trimester of pregnancy with resultant fetal death or congenital anomalies. The rubella virus is an RNA virus that grows in several tissue culture lines and infects ferrets and monkeys.[60] The virus is easily recovered from the nasopharynx during active acquired infection and from the nasopharynx and various tissues of infants with congenital rubella. Both acquired and congenital infections stimulate active antibody development. Laboratory diagnosis is accomplished by isolation of the virus or demonstration of a significant rise in hemagglutination-inhibition, enzyme-linked immunosorbent assay (ELISA), or latex agglutination antibody levels between acute and convalescent serum specimens.

Acquired rubella is characterized by a three-day generalized maculopapular rash; cervical, occipital, and posterior auricular lymphadenopathy; and low-grade fever. Arthralgia or arthritis tends to occur in affected adults. Liver disease has been reported in acquired rubella.[76]

Congenital rubella is commonly manifested by one or more of the following: cataracts, deafness, anomalies of the heart, and mental retardation. Liver, blood, lung, and bone lesions occur less frequently. The congenital rubella infant may exhibit hepatosplenomegaly, but it is usually temporary.[38]

Jaundice and other manifestations of acute hepatitis may occur. The hepatic lesions vary from a mild hepatitis with minimal hepatocellular necrosis, periportal inflammation, and cholestasis to a severe, fatal neonatal giant cell hepatitis.[14] The virus has been recovered from the liver.

There is no specific treatment for rubella. Effective live, attenuated vaccines exist for control of the disease, but these should not be given to pregnant women.

Herpes Hominis

Herpes hominis (herpes simplex) virus infection of humans is very common. Serologic studies have shown that up to 80% of adults have detectable antibody to the virus, indicating previous infection sometime during their lifetime.[32] There are two strains of herpes hominis virus: type 1 and type 2 (genital). As a general rule, type 1 produces lesions above the waist and type 2 produces lesions below the waist and in the newborn. The viruses are relatively large DNA viruses, which can be grown in tissue culture cells, and are pathogenic for laboratory animals. Infection produces intranuclear inclusion bodies. Active infection is followed by an antibody response, which may be measured by neutralization and complement fixation tests. Laboratory diagnosis is accomplished by cultivation of the virus from lesions in tissue culture systems and demonstration of a rise in antibody titer.

Primary herpes infection usually occurs early in life and is subclinical 99% of the time. When clinical illness occurs, it usually is manifested by a vesicular, ulcerative, gingivostomatitis accompanied by regional lymphadenopathy, fever, and other constitutional symptoms. Less frequently, the primary infection is a keratoconjunctivitis, encephalitis, eczema herpeticum, or vesicles in a traumatized region. Very rarely will a generalized infection occur. Following primary infection, recurrent herpes infection may occur periodically, usually with vesicular lesions at mucocutaneous junctures, such as the lips, but may involve lesions of the genitalia or cornea. Recurrent herpes infections are usually not accompanied by systemic features. Various events may precipitate an active recurrent infection, such as sunburn, psychological stress, menstruation, fever, and so forth. In the premature infant and neonate, herpes infections tend to be generalized, causing multisystem involvement with a high fatality rate. Herpes virus type 2 is commonly responsible for neonatal herpes.

Liver involvement by the herpes virus is found in several situations. Generalized herpes infection of the neonate usually is associated with hepatic lesions. The liver shows extensive diffuse hepatocellular necrosis, sparse inflammatory cellular reaction, multinucleated hepatocytes, and intranuclear eosinophilic inclusion bodies. Becker and co-workers[2] described severe involvement of the liver in young children with kwashiorkor who had herpes infection. In addition, there have been a few reports of primary herpes infection of adults with hepatomegaly and elevated alkaline phosphatase and transaminase levels.[32] Flewett and colleagues[17] have described severe hepatitis in a 24-year-old pregnant woman with generalized herpes ir whom the virus was isolated from the liver. Acute hepatitis has been seen in an immunosuppressed renal transplant patient with recovery of the virus from a liver biopsy specimen.

Treatment usually has consisted of supportive measures. There is no vaccine. Recently, several drugs have been used to treat the more severe forms of herpes infections, such as encephalitis, eczema herpeticum, genital herpes and neonatal herpes. These drugs include 5-iodo-2-deoxyuridine, cytosine arabinoside, and adenine arabinoside, and acyclovir. The results have varied, but acyclovir appears most effective.[7]

Cytomegaloviruses

The cytomegaloviruses (CMV) are a group of species-specific agents infecting humans, monkeys, rodents, and other animals. Both in vivo and in vitro, they induce a cellular response characterized by cytomegaly and prominent intranuclear inclusion bodies. In humans, CMV infection produces a spectrum of disease but most frequently is subclinical. Liver involvement may be prominent.

The CMV resembles the herpes hominis virus and is classified as a member of the herpes group. The virus has an inner DNA core surrounded by a single lipoprotein-enveloping membrane. The virus is relatively labile and quickly loses infectivity on storage. The addition of sorbital will partially stabilize it.[71] CMV produces very large cells in the tissues. These so-called cytomegalic cells are up to 40 nm in diameter and contain a large nucleus with a large inclusion body. The inclusion body is separated from the nuclear membrane and gives an "owl's eye" appearance. The human CMV can be propagated only in human tissues and grows preferentially in cells of fibroblastic or myometrial origin.[70] The cells become swollen, rounded, and closely resemble cytomegalic cells observed in vivo, containing typical inclusion bodies. Because of the species-specificity of the viruses, human CMV has not been adapted to laboratory animals. This has resulted in failure to prepare reference antisera by the immunization of animals.

Infection with CMV results in a complement-fixation and neutralization antibody response in humans. This response seems to be somewhat specific, since frequently serum from infected infants will neutralize only the infecting virus, and complement fixation antibody to heterogenous human CMV cannot be detected until an older age. This has led to the establishment of several human types of CMV.

CMV is widely disseminated around the world. Serologic surveys have indicated that 5% to 10% of children acquire antibodies by 2 years, 20% by 15 years, and 50% to 80% by 30 to 35 years of age.[56,66] A higher incidence of antibodies was found in populations of lower socioeconomic status and in institutionalized persons. These findings suggest that CMV exposure is quite common. Indeed, cytomegalic cells have been found at autopsy in the salivary glands of 10% of children who died of unrelated causes.[71]

The viral excretion patterns of CMV-infected persons vary. Primary infection in healthy older children and adults is usually associated with transient viral excretion. However, prolonged viral excretion in the throat and urine occurs for months to years in congenital infection, in infection in pregnant women, and in active infection in immunosuppressed patients. The main sources of infection are probably the older children and adults with primary infection, and the most likely route of spread is by person-to-person contact. The virus has been recovered from the cervix; thus, sexual intercourse is a possible method of transmission.[45] Recently, blood transfusions have been demonstrated to spread infection,[33] since CMV has been isolated from the while cells of 5% of healthy blood donors. The risk of acquiring CMV infection by transfusion is greatest for those patients receiving massive transfusions from multiple donors. Studies have shown that up to 60% of patients lacking CMV antibody before surgical procedures requiring massive transfusion acquire antibody afterwards.[33]

Active CMV infection may result from primary inoculation with virus or reactivation of a latent viral infection similar to that occurring with herpes simplex infection. Reactivation of latent infection seems to be the most likely mechanism in patients who are immunosuppressed.

The pathology of CMV disease is highlighted by the presence of the cytomegalic cell with an intranuclear inclusion. The inclusions are located primarily in epithelial cells but may also involve endothelial and connective tissue cells.[78] In disseminated disease of infants, many organs are involved, including salivary glands, kidneys, liver, lungs, and brain. In adults, the lungs, adrenals, gastrointestinal tract, spleen, pancreas, and kidneys are likely to be affected.[16,75]

CMV causes a spectrum of disease. Infection of healthy children and adults is usually subclinical. Neonatal CMV infection can also vary in intensity from subclinical to fatal disease. The classic picture presents at or shortly after birth, with hepatomegaly, jaundice, thrombocytopenic purpura, hemolytic anemia, and brain damage with periventricular calcification and microcephaly.[20] The jaundice generally presents with cholestatic features and may persist for months. The hepatomegaly may persist for a year or more, long after liver function tests have become normal.

Liver biopsy findings may vary from fatty changes, through multifocal necrosis, to early interstitial and peripheral fibrosis.[65] There is an inflammatory response and marked bile stasis.[65] Cytomegalic cells can be found in parenchyma and bile duct epithelium.[65] Survivors may recover completely from the liver disease, but many have extensive brain damage.

CMV infection in early childhood may result in chronic infection with hepatomegaly and abnormal liver function. While liver dysfunction is usually asymptomatic, it may be associated with febrile disease, transient jaundice, and rising CMV antibody titer. In older children and adults, CMV infection is almost always subclinical. This is true of the pregnant woman who experiences primary infection and is at risk of producing a congenitally infected offspring. Diagnosis in the pregnant woman depends completely on the laboratory findings.

Cytomegalic mononucleosis occurs in adults and occasionally in older children. This is a febrile illness of 3 to 6 weeks duration, with malaise, anorexia, nausea, and vomiting. The blood picture exhibits a relative and absolute lymphocytosis and many abnormal or atypical mononuclear cells. The Paul–Bunnell test is negative, and exudative pharyngitis and lymphadenopathy are absent. There may be hepatosplenomegaly and abnormal liver function tests. Jaundice is unusual, but some patients have hepatitis and severe cholestatic jaundice.[65] Liver biopsy reveals a histologic picture compatible with viral hepatitis.[65] Cytomegalic cells are not found.

A similar disorder is the *postperfusion syndrome,* which is a common complication of open-heart surgery and other surgical or medical procedures that require massive transfusions of fresh blood from multiple donors. The disease occurs both in patients who lack or possess preexisting CMV antibody, the latter experiencing a rise in antibody titer.

Finally, active CMV disease can occur in patients with debilitating reticuloendothelial system illnesses or who are undergoing immunosuppression. The exact clinical significance of the CMV infection in these patients has not been determined, but some patients develop systemic disease with a fatal pneumonitis or liver dysfunction with jaundice.[65] Many of these patients have preexisting CMV antibody, and their active disease is felt to be reactivation of a latent infection. Frequently, these patients have mixed infections of which CMV is only one component.

Diagnosis of infection with CMV is best established by recovery of the virus from urine, saliva, or other body fluids, or from infected tissues by cultivation in human fibroblasts. Exfoliative cytology may also be used to demonstrate the typical cytomegalic cells. However, culture of the virus is more reliable.[71] Because of the ubiquitous distribution of CMV, virus recovery does not necessarily mean cause and effect of a disease. Care must be used in the interpretation of laboratory findings. Serologic procedures for diagnosis of active CMV have limited value because of the heterogeneity of the CMV group.

Currently, no specific treatment for CMV disease exists.

Certain antiviral agents have been used with rather poor results.[1] Management of patients is essentially symptomatic.

VIRUSES OCCASIONALLY ASSOCIATED WITH LIVER DISEASE

Adenoviruses

The adenoviruses, a group of DNA viruses, are common causes of upper and lower respiratory tract disease, lymphadenopathy, and conjunctivitis in humans and have been associated with gastroenteritis, intussusception, and hepatitis. Certain human adenoviral strains have been shown to induce tumors in newborn hamsters. There are 35 strains of human adenoviruses. The organisms grow well in tissue culture and elicit an antibody response in humans that can be measured by hemagglutination-inhibition, complement fixation, and neutralization tests. Zuckerman has grown several types of adenoviruses in tissue cultures of human embryo liver cells.[78] There are numerous animal adenoviruses, including the canine hepatitis virus of dogs.

Adenoviruses have been associated with hepatitis in humans. The most impressive incidence involves the San Carlos agents. These agents were isolated from fecal and plasma specimens from 14 of 22 Indian children during an epidemic in Eastern Arizona in 1959.[10] Acute blood specimens failed to neutralize the viruses while convalescent blood specimens did. Twelve of the fourteen strains were later identified as adenoviruses type 1, 2, or 3.[10]

Adenovirus type 5 was isolated from the liver of a young immunosuppressed adult who died of fulminant hepatitis.[4] Electronmicroscopy also revealed crystalline arrays of virions within hepatocytes. Adenovirus type 5 was also isolated from blood clots of 27 of 30 sporadic cases of infectious hepatitis.[21] This virus was recovered from all twelve family contacts of two of the patients, some of whom subsequently developed infectious hepatitis. Only one recovery of type 5 adenovirus was made from 70 control subjects. Adenovirus types 2, 11, and 16 have also been isolated from patients with infectious hepatitis.[67] A serologic survey among military personnel in Korea showed that adenovirus type 11 antibodies were significantly more common among soldiers with hepatitis than in healthy soldiers.[67]

The exact significance of proof of adenoviral infection in cases of infectious hepatitis must be considered with some reservation; the etiologic significance remains in doubt. Adenoviruses are known to be associated with latency, and their recovery from infectious hepatitis patients may be a result of reactivation of virus in the presence of a disease process. Whether or not adenoviruses can cause hepatitis or are reactivated in the presence of another virus or are merely common inhabitants of the gastrointestinal tract remains to be determined.

Treatment of adenoviral infections is symptomatic. No effective vaccines exist for the general population, although vaccines containing selected strains of adenoviruses are presently used in the military.

The Enteroviruses

The enteroviral group consists of poliomyelitis viruses, coxsackieviruses A and B, ECHO viruses, and the "higher enteroviruses" (types 68–72). Type 72 is HAV. Numerous reports have associated coxsackie viruses A and B and ECHO viruses with liver disease. The exact significance of these viruses as etiologic agents of liver disease remains in doubt, but their recovery or the subsequent antibody response to the viruses in patients with liver disease requires their consideration as etiologic agents. All three groups of viruses produce syndromes that usually are devoid of clinical liver involvement. However, in the occasional case or outbreak, hepatitis or hepatomegaly has been a prominent part of the illness.

There are 23 serotypes of group A coxsackieviruses. They are small, RNA viruses that produce distinctive lesions in suckling mice. Most strains require careful adaptation to grow in tissue culture. Although some strains of coxsackievirus A hemagglutinate, the most specific and most utilized method to demonstrate antibodies to the group requires neutralization of effects on suckling mice. Thus, routine diagnosis for most coxsackie A strains involves additional expense and is frequently not performed.

The group A coxsackieviruses produce several clinical features, which include herpangina, aseptic meningitis, rashes, respiratory infection, pericarditis, myocarditis, and, very rarely, paralytic disease.

Morris and associates[48] isolated a coxsackievirus A4 from the blood of a child with fever, rash, and a clinical picture of hepatitis. Neutralizing antibodies to the virus developed during convalescence. Embil and co-workers[13] isolated coxsackievirus A10 from the stools of 45 close contacts of patients involved in an outbreak of infectious hepatitis. The same virus was recovered from the blood of four contacts. Jezequel and Steiner[31] identified isolates from the stools of five patients with infectious hepatitis as reacting with coxsackieviruses A13 and A18 antisera.

There are six serotypes of coxsackievirus B. They are small RNA viruses that produce distinctive lesions in the brains of infant mice and in the pancreas and myocardium of older mice. They grow well in tissue culture cells and elicit antibody responses in humans that can be measured by neutralization, hemagglutination-inhibition, and complement fixation tests.

The coxsackieviruses B produce several clinical syndromes. These include myocarditis of the neonate, older children, and adults; pericarditis; pleurodynia; aseptic meningitis; acute febrile illnesses; vesicular and papular rashes; and respiratory illnesses.

Kibrick,[35] in his review, noted that the relationship between coxsackievirus B infection and hepatitis in the newborn was clear, and that suggestive evidence existed that both coxsackieviruses A and B may be related to hepatitis in patients beyond the newborn period. Kibrick and Benirschke[36] reported two fatal cases of generalized neonatal infection including hepatitis from which coxsackievirus B4 was isolated, including one isolation from the liver. Coxsackievirus B5 was isolated from a pregnant woman suffering from clinical hepatitis,[52] while the same virus strain was found in 19 young children with pleurodynia, pneumonia, and hepatomegaly.[64] Hosier and Newton[28] recovered various coxsackievirus B in patients with severe focal hepatic necrosis. Sun and Smith[68] described a case in which a 19-year-old woman developed pleurodynia, myocarditis, and hepatitis. A coxsackievirus B3 was isolated from the feces, and a specific antibody response developed. Liver biopsy on the 18th day of illness was interpreted as subacute portal triaditis with inflammation of the interlobar ducts and markedly cloudy swelling of central zone hepatocytes. Coxsackievirus B2 was isolated from an 8-year-old girl with anicteric hepatitis.[40] She developed a significant coxsackie B2 antibody titer. The child had previously had Reye's syndrome.

The ECHO viruses comprise 33 serotypes. They are small RNA viruses that are not pathogenic for laboratory animals. They grow well in tissue culture systems and elicit neutralization, hemagglutination-inhibition, and complement fixation antibody responses.

The ECHO viruses are frequently found in the feces of healthy children. However, they can cause a variety of clinical syndromes including aseptic meningitis, maculopapular rashes, respiratory disease, diarrhea, and acute febrile illnesses. Very rarely have they caused paralytic disease.

ECHO viruses have also been associated with liver disease. Kiseleva[37] reported that ECHO viruses types 1 and 8 were recovered from patients with infectious hepatitis in Turkmenia (USSR). Neutralizing antibody to these viruses developed in two thirds of the sera examined. ECHO virus type 6 was associated with two cases of severe infectious hepatitis in Finland. Virus particles were visualized and specific antibody developed. Sharlai and associates[63] isolated ECHO virus types 7 and 12 in children with nonactive forms of infectious hepatitis. Schleissner and Portnoy[61] described a woman with pneumonia and hepatitis from whom ECHO virus type 9 was recovered from pharyngeal swabs. This patient developed a significant rise in ECHO 9 antibody levels. Hughes and coworkers[30] reported on ECHO virus type 14 infection associated with hepatic necrosis in a neonate. At autopsy, 95% of the liver parenchyma was necrotic, although the reticulum network was largely intact. A few hepatocytes were present around the portal areas and contained numerous vacuoles in the cytoplasm and no inclusion bodies.

Enteroviruses types 68 to 71 have been associated with CNS disease, acute hemorrhagic conjunctivitis, and pneumonitis.[6] These viruses have caused explosive outbreaks in various parts of the world. In general, the US population lacks immunity to these viruses.

Treatment of enteroviral infections is symptomatic. No vaccines exist for coxsackieviruses A and B, ECHO viruses, and the higher enteroviruses. HAV (type 72) vaccines are being developed.

REFERENCES

1. Alford C: Personal communication
2. Becker W et al: Virus studies in disseminated herpes simplex infections: Association with malnutrition in children. S Afr Med J 37:74, 1963
3. Bugher JC: The pathology of yellow fever. In Stode GK (ed): Yellow Fever, pp 137–163. New York, McGraw Hill, 1951
4. Carmichael GP et al: Adenovirus hepatitis in an immunosuppressed adult patient. Am J Clin Pathol 71:352, 1979
5. Chang RS Golden HD: Transformation of human leukocytes by throat washings from infectious mononucleosis patients. Nature 234:359, 1971
6. Cherry J: Nonpolio enteroviruses: Coxsackieviruses, echoviruses, and enteroviruses. In Feigen R, Cherry J (eds): Textbook of Pediatric Infectious Diseases, pp 1316–1365. Philadelphia, WB Saunders, 1981
7. Chow S, Merigan TC: Antiviral chemotherapy. In Fields BN (ed): Virology, pp 323–348. New York, Raven Press, 1985
8. Clarke DH, Casals J: Arboviruses, group B. In Horsfall Tamm (eds): Viral and Rickettsial Infections of Man, 4th ed, pp 606–658. Philadelphia, JB Lippincott, 1965
9. Davidsohn J, Lee CL: Serologic tests for infectious mononucleosis. Med Clin North Am 46:234, 1962
10. Davis EV: Isolation of virus from children with infectious hepatitis. Science 133:2059, 1961
11. Dowdle WR: Exotic viral diseass. Yale J Biol Med 53:109, 1980
12. Elton NW et al: Clinical pathology of yellow fever. Am J Clin Pathol 25:135, 1955
13. Embil JA Jr et al: Coxsackie A 10 virus infection among infectious hepatitis contacts. Can Med Assoc J 93:740, 1965
14. Esterly JR et al: Hepatic lesions in the congenital rubella syndrome. J Pediatr 71:676, 1967
15. Evans AS: Infectious mononucleosis in University of Wisconsin students: Report of a five year investigation. Am J Hyg 71:676, 1967
16. Evans DJ, Williams ED: Cytomegalic inclusion disease in the adult. J Clin Pathol 21:311, 1968
17. Flewett RH et al: Acute hepatitis due to herpes simplex virus in an adult. J Clin Pathol 21:311, 1968
18. Gear JSS et al: Outbreak of Marburg virus disease in Johannesburg. Br Med J 4:489, 1975
19. Glade PR (ed): Infectious Mononucleosis. Philadelphia, JB Lippincott, 1973
20. Griffiths PD: Cytomegalovirus and the liver. Semin Liver Dis, 4:307, 1984
21. Hartwell WV et al: Adenovirus in blood clots from cases of infectious hepatitis. Science 152:1390, 1966
22. Hatch MH, Siem RA: Viruses isolated from children with infectious hepatitis. Am J Epidemiol 84:495, 1966
23. Henle G, Henle W: Immunofluorescence in cells derived from Burkitt's lymphoma. J Bacteriol 91:1248, 1966
24. Henle G et al: Relation of Burkitt's tumor-associated herpes-type virus to infectious mononucleosis. Proc Natl Acad Sci USA 59:94, 1968
25. Heymann DL et al: Ebola hemorrhagic fever, Zaire, 1977–1978. J Infect Dis 42:372, 1980
26. Hoagland RJ: Infectious Mononucleosis. New York, Grune & Stratton, 1967
27. Hoagland RJ: The transmission of infectious mononucleosis. Am J Med Sci 229:262, 1955
28. Hosier DM, Newton WA Jr: Serious Coxsackie infection in infants and children: Myocarditis, meningoencephalitis, and hepatitis. Am J Dis Child 96:251, 1968

29. Howard CR, Ellis DS, Simpson DIH: Exotic viruses and the liver. Semin Liver Dis 4:361, 1984

30. Hughes JR et al: Echovirus 14 infection associated with fatal neonatal hepatic necrosis. Am J Dis Child 123:61, 1972

31. Jezequel AM, Steiner JW: Some ultrastructural and histochemical aspects of Coxsackie virus-cell interactions. Lab Invest 18:1055, 1966

32. Juel-Jensen BE, MacCallum FO: Herpes Simplex, Varicella and Zoster. Philadelphia, JB Lippincott, 1972

33. Kaariainen L et al: Rise of cytomegalovirus antibodies in an infectious mononucleosis-like syndrome after transfusion. Br Med J 1:1270, 1966

34. Kerr JA: The clinical aspects and diagnosis of yellow fever. In Strode GK (ed): Yellow Fever, pp 385–425. New York, McGraw-Hill, 1951

35. Kibrick S: Current status of Coxsackie and ECHO viruses in human diseases. Prog Med Virol 6:27, 1964

36. Kibrick S, Benirschke K: Severe generalized disease (encephalohepatomyocarditis) occurring in the newborn period and due to infection with Coxsackie virus group B: Evidence of intrauterine infection with this agent. Pediatrics 22:857, 1958

37. Kiseleva NV: Contributions to the etiology of epidemic hepatitis in Turkmenia. In Stakhanova VM (ed): Abstracts of Papers, IX International Congress for Microbiology, p 393. Moscow, Organizing Committee of the Congress, 1966

38. Korones SB: Congenital rubella syndrome. Advances and new concepts. Gen Practitioner 35:78, 1967

39. Krugman S, Katz SL: Infectious mononucleosis. In Infectious Diseases of Children and Adults. St Louis, CV Mosby, 1981

40. Lansky LL et al: Anicteric Coxsackie B hepatitis. J Pediatr 94:64, 1979

41. Lennette EH, Schmidt NJ: Diagnostic Procedures for Viral and Rickettsial Infections. Washington, DC, American Public Health Association, 1979

42. McCormick JB, Webb PA, Johnson KM et al: Chemotherapy of acute Lassa fever with ribavirin. In Smith RA, Knight V, Smith JAD (eds): Clinical Applications of Ribavirin, pp 187–192. New York, Academic Press, 1984

43. McCracken GH Jr et al: Congenital cytomegalic inclusion disease. Am J Dis Child 117:522, 1969

44. Monath TP: Lassa fever: Review of epidemiology and epizootiology. Bull (WHO) 52:3386, 1975

45. Montgomery R et al: Recovery of cytomegalovirus from the cervix in pregnancy. Pediatrics 49:524, 1972

46. Moore GE et al: Culture of normal human leukocytes. JAMA 199:519, 1967

47. Morbidity and Mortality. ACIP Recommendation: Yellow Fever Vaccine, p 42. Washington, DC, DHEW Publication No. (HSM) 72-8154, 1972

48. Morris JA et al: Hepatitis associated with Coxsackie virus group A type 4. N Engl J Med 267:1230, 1962

49. Niederman JC et al: Prevalence, incidence, and persistence of EB virus in young adults. N Engl J Med 282:361, 1970

50. Niederman JC et al: Infectious mononucleosis: Clinical manifestations in relation to EB virus antibodies. JAMA, 203:205, 1968

51. Old LJ et al: Precipitating antibody in human serum to an antigen present in cultured Burkitt's lymphoma cells. Proc Natl Acad Sci USA, 56:1699, 1966

52. O'Shaughnessey WJ, Buechner HA: Hepatitis associated with a Coxsackie B5 virus infection during late pregnancy. JAMA 179:71, 1962

53. Paloheimo JA, Halonen PI: A case of mononucleosis-like syndrome after blood transfusion from a donor with asymptomatic mononucleosis. J Cardiovasc Surg 6:558, 1965

54. Pereira MS et al: EB virus antibody at different ages. Br Med J 4:526, 1969

55. Pereira MS et al: Evidence for oral excretion of EB virus in infectious mononucleosis. Lancet 1:710, 1972

56. Rowe WP et al: Cytopathogenic agent resembling human salivary gland virus recovered from tissue cultures of human adenoids. Proc Soc Exp Biol Med 92:418, 1956

57. Sanford J: Lassa fever. In Sanford J, Luby JP (eds): Infectious Diseases: The Science and Practice of Clinical Medicine, pp 152–154. New York, Grune & Stratton, 1981

58. Sanford J: Marburg virus disease. In Sanford J, Luby JP (eds): Infectious Diseases: The Science and Practice of Clinical Medicine, pp 154–156. New York, Grune & Stratton, 1981

59. Sanford J: Ebola virus hemorrhagic fever. In Sanford J, Luby JP (eds): Infectious Diseases: The Science and Practice of Clinical Medicine pp 156–157, New York, Grune & Stratton, 1981

60. Schiff GM, Sever JL: Rubella: Recent laboratory and clinical advances. Prog Med Virol 8:30, 1966

61. Schleissner LA, Portnoy B: Hepatitis and pneumonia associated with ECHO virus, type 9, infection in two adult siblings. Ann Intern Med 68:1315, 1968

62. Schooley RT, Dolin R: Epstein–Barr virus (infectious mononucleosis). In Mandell GL, Douglas RG, Bennett JE (eds): Principles and Practice of Infectious Diseases, pp 971–982. New York, John Wiley & Sons, 1985

63. Sharlai IV et al: The etiology of non-icteric forms of hepatitis in children. Sov Med 28:38, 1965

64. Siegel W et al: Two new variants of infection with Coxsackie virus group B type 5 in young children. N Engl J Med 268:1210, 1963

65. Stern H: Cytomegalovirus and EB virus infections of the liver. Br Med Bull 28:180, 1972

66. Stern H, Elek SD: The incidence of infection with cytomegalovirus in a normal population. J Hyg 63:79, 1965

67. Strong WB: Adenovirus isolations from patients with infectious hepatitis. CDC Hepatitis Surveillance Report, No. 22, p 17. Atlanta, 1965

68. Sun NC, Smith VM: Hepatitis associated with myocarditis: Unusual manifestation of infection with Coxsackie virus group B, type 3. N Engl J Med 274:190, 1966

69. Theiler M: The virus. In Strode GK (ed): Yellow Fever, pp 39–136. New York, McGraw-Hill, 1951

70. Weller TH: Cytomegaloviruses. In Horsfall, Tamm (eds): Viral and Rickettsial Infections of Man. Philadelphia, JB Lippincott, 1965

71. Weller TH, Hanshaw TB: Virologic and clinical observations on cytomegalic inclusion disease. N Engl J Med 266:1233, 1962

72. WHO International Study Team (1978): Ebola haemorrhagic fever in Sudan, 1976. Bull WHO 56:247, 1978

73. WHO International Commission (1978): Ebola haemorrhagic fever in Zaire, 1976. Bull WHO 56:271, 1978

74. Winn WC, Walker CJ: The pathology of human Lassa fever. Bull WHO 52:535, 1975

75. Wong T, Warner NE: Cytomegalic inclusion disease in adults. Arch Pathol 74:403, 1962

76. Zeldis JB, Miller JG, Dienstag JL: Hepatitis in an adult with rubella. Am J Med 79:S15, 1985

77. Zuckerman AJ: Virus Diseases of the Liver. London, Appleton-Century-Crofts, 1970

78. Zuckerman AJ, Fulton F: Adenovirus infection of human embryo liver cells. Nature 214:606, 1967

chapter 17
Toxic and Drug-Induced Hepatitis

HYMAN J. ZIMMERMAN AND WILLIS C. MADDREY

Many chemical agents produce hepatic injury. Some are intrinsic toxins; others are drugs that produce liver damage as an idiosyncratic reaction. Acute injury may consist of parenchymal damage (cytotoxic injury), mainly arrested bile flow and jaundice (cholestatic injury), or, most often, a mixture of the two. Chronic injury includes a number of lesions. The damage may be acquired as a toxicologic phenomenon or therapeutic misadventure or may be induced experimentally.

IMPORTANCE OF CHEMICAL HEPATIC INJURY

The relative importance of various toxins causing hepatic injury has changed considerably over the years. Acute toxic injury, at one time a predominantly occupational and domestic hazard, is now mainly a domestic one. Chlorinated hydrocarbons are an uncommon but still encountered cause of injury in the home.[20] Poisoning by yellow phosphorus has almost disappeared from the United States but remains a problem in parts of the world where suicidal or accidental ingestion of rodenticides or firecrackers containing it still occurs.[151,607,627] Mushroom poisoning accounts for several hundred cases of hepatic injury per year, most of them in Europe.[171] A recently emerged cause of hepatotoxicity, outstripping all others in England, and of increasing importance elsewhere, is the ingestion of large amounts of acetaminophen in suicide attempts.[108,124,264,567–573,623]

To most clinicians, hepatic injury caused by adverse reactions to medicinal agents is more important than that caused by other substances. Nevertheless, adverse reactions to drugs rank as a relatively minor cause of acute hepatic disease. Less than 5% of instances of jaundice in several series[54,368] have been attributable to drug reactions. As a cause of severe hepatic necrosis, however, drug-induced injury assumes a much more important role. In the United States, up to 25% of cases of fulminant hepatic failure may be the result of adverse reactions to medicinal agents.[740,741,806]

Drugs also are an important cause of chronic liver disease, including chronic active hepatitis, fatty liver, cirrhosis, and several vascular and neoplastic lesions of the liver.[438,641,663,807] Also of concern today is the possible risk of acquiring chronic hepatic disease, including hepatic neoplasm, as a result of prolonged occupational exposure to toxic chemicals[557,733] and of ingestion of mycotoxins and other natural hepatoxins.[388,440,790] Drugs are also an important cause of chronic hepatic disease, and therapeutic agents have been held responsible for instances of chronic active hepatitis, fatty liver, and cirrhosis as well as of several vascular and neoplastic lesions of the liver.[363,364,434,438,641,663,806,807]

SUSCEPTIBILITY OF LIVER TO CHEMICAL INJURY

The great susceptibility of the liver to damage by chemical agents is presumably a consequence of its primary role in the metabolism of foreign substances. The position of the liver as portal to the tissues for ingested agents and the concentration of xenobiotics in the liver may contribute to its special vulnerability. The role of the liver in metabolic conversions of foreign compounds is particularly important in its susceptibility to chemical injury.[18,811]

Biotransformation reactions have traditionally been considered protective as detoxifiers of potentially toxic foreign compounds. However, such reactions also can convert nontoxic agents to potentially toxic products. Indeed, it has become clear that the formation of reactive, and therefore toxic, metabolic intermediates within the hepatocyte accounts for the injury it sustains from many of the known toxic chemicals and drugs.[18,473–475]

Relevant to the effects of reactive intermediate molecules is the modification of the liver's ability to metabolize foreign chemicals. This results from exposure to a number of compounds. Administration of phenobarbital, insecticides, alcohol, and many other agents enhances the ability of the liver to metabolize a large number of compounds.[18,473–475,551] This induction of the drug-metabolizing enzyme system (mixed function oxidase [MFO]) enhances the hepatotoxicity of agents that are converted to toxic products by the MFO[18,473–475] It may, however, reduce the toxic effects of agents transformed along pathways that detoxify.[807]

The chief enzyme of the MFO, cytochrome P-450, consists of a number of isoenzymes.[18,486,487,627] These differ in their selective capacity to catalyze the metabolism of various compounds. Such differences may serve to explain selective modification of toxic effects by induction of the

591

MFO. For example, the cytochrome P-450 isoenzymes, which are most active in catalyzing conversion of acetaminophen to a toxic metabolite, are also the ones particularly induced by ethanol,[487] a phenomenon that may explain the enhancement of acetaminophen toxicity by ethanol.[810]

Host Factors

Individual susceptibility to chemical hepatic injury appears to be affected by genetic factors, age, sex, nutritional status, exposure to other drugs and chemicals, systemic disease, and other factors.[807] For the most part, the effect of these factors on vulnerability to hepatic injury appears to result from their effect on conversion of the respective agent to a toxic metabolite, or on detoxifying disposal of the metabolite.[18]

The importance of genetic factors is most clearly evident in the differences between various species in vulnerability to hepatotoxic effects of carbon tetrachloride (CCl_4), aflatoxin B_1, bromobenzene, acetaminophen, and other agents, differences that appear largely attributable to species differences in the metabolism of the toxic agents.[807] In humans, however, there are only hints of the importance of genetic factors. These include the reports that perhexiline maleate–induced hepatic injury appears to occur predominantly in patients who have a genetically diminished capacity to oxidize the drug[488] and that patients with a genetically limited capacity to convert an aryl epoxide to a nontoxic dihydriol seem predisposed to develop hepatic injury from phenytoin[696] and halothane.[198] HLA typing also has provided evidence of a genetic susceptibility to halothane injury.[519] Susceptibility to contraceptive steroid–associated cholestasis appears to have a strong genetic component.[433] Efforts to relate susceptibility to isoniazid-associated hepatic injury to genetic difference in metabolism of the drug have floundered on the conflicting attribution of increased susceptibility to "slow" and to "rapid" acetylator status.[18]

Sex appears to affect susceptibility to some agents. When differences have been noted, females have appeared to be more vulnerable than males to drug-induced disease. Methyldopa,[648] nitrofurantoin,[807] halothane,[807] benoxaprofen,[168,207,209,248,570,718] and, to a lesser extent, ticrynafen[816] have appeared to lead to hepatic injury more frequently in females than in males. Enhanced female susceptibility has been even more evident among patients with drug-induced chronic hepatitis.[438,650] For many of the instances of hepatic injury, however, the available data do not permit distinction between different degree of exposure to a drug and increased susceptibility to injury as the basis for the apparently differing incidences of liver damage.

Age can be seen to affect vulnerability. The incidence of isoniazid-induced hepatic injury increases with advancing age.[56] Halothane-induced injury[807] and ticrynafen-associated[816] liver disease are other examples of apparent age dependence of susceptibility to drug-induced

hepatic injury. A seemingly inverse relationship is also seen in some drugs. Aspirin-associated hepatic injury appears to involve children, especially those under the age of 10, more often than adults,[809] and valproate toxicity has appeared to involve patients under the age of 20, more than older ones.[812]

Nutritional status introduces several relevant factors. Foods (cabbage, brussel sprouts) and dietary regimens (high protein) can enhance activity of the cytochrome P-450 system and so increase the potential for converting a drug to its toxic metabolite, while the reverse is effected by a low protein intake.[9,18] Deficient intake of protein and of sulfur-containing animo acids can lead to depleted glutathione stores and so enhance toxicity.[18,608] It is also reasonable to infer that deficient intake of antioxidants such as vitamin E and selenium can lead to increased vulnerability to hepatotoxic agents that produce peroxidative injury.

Several systemic conditions affect vulnerability. Obesity appears to enhance susceptibility to halothane injury, perhaps because of storage of the agent in fat tissue or because obesity has other effects on vulnerability.[807] Experimental diabetes enhances vulnerability to some toxic agents (e.g., CCl_4) and decreases it to others (e.g., acetaminophen).[551] These dichotomous effects appear to be due to the enhancement of conversion of CCl_4 to a toxic metabolite by the inducing effects of ketosis on the MFO but to the inhibition of acetaminophen conversion to a toxic metabolite by enhancing the nontoxic pathway, glucuronidation.[571] Hyperthyroidism appears to enhance and hypothyroidism to inhibit the toxic effect of CCl_4.[807] Patients with active rheumatoid arthritis, systemic lupus erythematosus, and rheumatic fever seem distinctly more susceptible than those with inactive forms of the disease or normal individuals to aspirin-induced hepatic injury.[809]

Exposure to a variety of drugs, insecticides, and other chemicals that induce the MFO can enhance the hepatotoxic effects of drugs and other chemicals.[18,473,475] Particularly noteworthy is the enhancement by alcohol of the toxic effects of CCl_4[551,711,810] and other haloalkanes of acetaminophen and of a number of other agents.

CLASSIFICATION OF HEPATOTOXIC AGENTS

There are two main categories of agents that can produce hepatic injury. One consists of agents that are predictable (intrinsic) hepatotoxins; the other contains agents whose toxicity is nonpredictable, that is, they produce hepatic injury only in unusually susceptible persons (idiosyncratic "hepatotoxins") (Table 17-1).[363,556,641,663,807]

Intrinsic hepatotoxins are recognized by the high incidence of hepatic injury in persons exposed to them, the production of a similar lesion in experimental animals, and the dose dependence of the phenomena. Agents that produce hepatic damage in only a small proportion of exposed persons that is not dose related and not reproducible in experimental animals are recognized to depend in some way on host idiosyncrasy for their adverse effect. Each group is heterogeneous (see Table 17-1).

Intrinsic Hepatotoxins

The types of physiologic perturbation by which intrinsic toxins and their metabolic products produce hepatic injury appear to fall into two broad categories (Table 17-2, Fig. 17-1). One involves a direct, physicochemical destructive effect on hepatocyte membranes, exerted by peroxidation and associated changes. Peroxidation is produced by free radicals or by activated oxygen.[196] We have referred to this form of injury as direct hepatotoxicity. The other broad mechanism for intrinsic hepatotoxicity produces injury as an indirect consequence of distortion of cell molecules or membranes, depletion of essential molecules, or blockage of physiologic reactions or of biochemical pathways essential for cell integrity.[807] Distortion of cell molecules and membranes results from binding of the toxic agent or its products. The binding may be covalent, of an electrophilic metabolite of the toxic agent (e.g., acetaminophen, bromobenzene), or noncovalent of the unaltered toxin (e.g., phallodin) to hepatocyte membrane receptors (see Table 17-2).[390] Covalent binding has been the subject of considerable attention during the past decade and appears to be the most important form of indirect toxicity. It appears to be the mechanism by which acetaminophen[473-476,795] and bromobenzene[473-476] lead to necrosis and by which electrophilic metabolites of carcinogens distort molecules of DNA.[469,476]

Protection against the toxic effects of covalent binding is provided by glutathione, which itself binds covalently to the reactive electrophilic metabolites of toxic agents (e.g., acetaminophen), converting them to nontoxic products, which are then excreted.[18,473-476] In addition, glutathione serves to reduce peroxides and so provides protection against the peroxidation of activated oxygen.[18,196]

Direct toxicity, in which the effects of peroxidation are exerted first at the site of free radical (or activated oxygen) production, then apparently transmitted to other areas of the hepatocyte by secondarily activated molecules may be caricatured as analogous to shrapnel dispersion after explosion of an artillery shell (see Fig. 17-1). Indirect toxicity is a more selective, precisely targeted injury. In effect, direct hepatotoxicity may be characterized as, primarily, destruction of the structural bases of hepatocyte function, while indirect hepatotoxicity leads first to metabolic or other functional lesions that can result in cell injury.[807]

The direct and indirect categories are somewhat reminiscent of the "toxipathic" and "trophopathic" forms of toxicity proposed by Himsworth many years ago.[291] Most of the intrinsic hepatotoxins produce injury by indirect hepatotoxicity. Relatively few act mainly by direct toxicity; examples are CCl_4, several other halogenated hydrocarbons, and yellow phosphorus. It is not uncommon, however, for the injury to result from a mixture of both mechanisms. For example, the toxicity of CCl_4 that results mainly from peroxidation also includes some covalent binding of CCl_3.[196,580] Conversely, acetaminophen produces its characteristic injury mainly by covalent binding of its electrophilic metabolite.[18,473-475]; yet, peroxidative injury also has been implicated.[196] Nevertheless, it is possible to designate individual agents as mainly direct or indirect hepatotoxins.[807]

Direct Hepatotoxins

These agents, or their metabolic products, injure the hepatocyte and its organelles by a direct physicochemical effect, that is, peroxidation of the membrane lipids, and by other chemical changes that lead to distortion or destruction of the membranes. The membrane injury is the first stage in the injury that culminates in necrosis or steatosis.

Carbon tetrachloride is the prototype. This agent produces centrilobular (zone 3) necrosis and steatosis in humans and experimental animals. The mechanism for injury by CCl_4, involves damage to membranes of the hepatocyte and its intracellular organelles. The two chief histologic abnormalities, steatosis and necrosis, are dissociable and of individual pathogenesis.[581]

Steatosis develops because the pathway for movement of fat from the liver is blocked by disruption of the mechanism for coupling triglycerides to the appropriate apoprotein to form the lipoprotein "carrier" molecule (very low density lipoprotein [VLDL]) as well as by impaired synthesis of the apolipoprotein.[581] Contributing to the defect in the exit of fat from the liver may be the demonstrated inhibition of protein synthesis.[581] Although the main factor in the production of hepatic steatosis is this interference with movement of lipid from the liver, there is also evidence of increased arrival of lipid to the liver from peripheral depots during the acute phase of CCl_4 intoxication.[359,636]

The mechanism for hepatic necrosis remains uncertain.[193,195,581] Current views focus on alteration of cell membranes, particularly the plasma membrane, as the initiating, necrogenic event.[195,580] The membrane injury provokes release of calcium ion from mitochondria and smooth endoplasmic reticulum and entry from extracellular fluid. Furthermore, the injury appears to interfere with function of the "calcium ion pump," which normally serves to prevent cytosolic accumulation of calcium ion.[196] The deleterious effect on cell metabolism of accumulation of calcium ion in the cytosol, the additional metabolic chaos induced by loss of potassium ion, enzymes, and coenzymes from the cytoplasm, and loss of the essential energy source that results from mitochondrial injury may all contribute to the necrosis; some compounding of the effect may result from release of destructive hydrolytic enzymes from injured lysozomes.[807]

Most of the injurious effect results from the action of a metabolite of CCl_4.[580,581] Circumstances or manipulations that prevent metabolism of CCl_4 inhibit its hepatotoxicity while manipulations that enhance its metabo-

TABLE 17-1. Classification of Hepatotoxic Agents and Major Characteristics of Each Group

CATEGORY OF AGENT	INCIDENCE	EXPERIMENTAL REPRODUCIBILITY	DOSE-DEPENDENT	MECHANISM	HISTOLOGIC LESION	EXAMPLES
Intrinsic toxicity						
Direct	High	Yes	Yes	Direct physicochemical distortion and destruction of structural basis of cell metabolism	Necrosis (zonal) and/or steatosis	Carbon tetrachloride Chloroform Phosphorus
Indirect						
Cytotoxic	High	Yes	Yes	Interference with specific pathways leading to structural injury	Steatosis or necrosis	See Tables 17-2 and 17-3.
Cholestatic	High	Yes	Yes	Interference with hepatic excretory pathways leading to cholestasis	Bilirubin casts	
Host idiosyncrasy						
Hypersensitivity	Low	No	No	Drug allergy	Necrosis or cholestasis	Phenytoin, PAS, Sulfonamides, ? HALO,* CPZ, PBZ
Metabolic	Low	No	No	Production of hepatotoxic metabolites?	Necrosis or cholestasis	INH, VPA, HALO,* ? oral hypoglycemic agents

* Features suggestive of both hypersensitivity and metabolic idiosyncrasy.
(PAS, P-aminosalicylic acid; HALO, halothane; CPZ, chlorpromazine; PBZ, phenylbutazone; INH, isoniazid; VPA, valproic acid)

TABLE 17-2. Putative Biochemical Lesions Produced by Indirect Hepatotoxins

BIOCHEMICAL LESION	HISTOLOGIC LESION	AGENT
Attachment to membrane receptors	Necrosis	Phalloidin
Alkylation of molecules of nucleus and ? cytoplasm*†	Necrosis ± fat, Ca	DMN and other nitrosamines ? Thioacetamide
Arylation of cell proteins*†	Necrosis ± fat	Bromobenzene Acetaminophen
Binding or blockade of tRNA	Steatosis	Tetracycline Puromycin
ATP depletion	Steatosis	Ethionine‡ Orotic acid
UTP depletion	Necrosis Steatosis ± CA	GALN§
Thiol group binding†	Necrosis, Steatosis ± CA	As‖
Binding*† of active metabolites to molecules of nucleus and cytoplasm	Necrosis Steatosis Vascular injury Ca and Sarcoma	AFB, PAs‖ AFB₁ PAs, AFB₁‖ AFB₁, PAs,‖ vinyl chloride

* By active metabolite

† Covalent binding

‡ Ethionine also produces hepatic carcinoma perhaps as result of ethylation of nucleic acids.

§ El-Mofty and co-workers[187] have suggested that galactosemia also may lead to injury to plasma membrane by replacing the normal sugar component.

‖ Arsenic (As) not carcinogenic in animals.

(GALN, galactosamine; DMN, dimethylnitrosamine; PAs, tyrrolidizine alkaloids; AF, aflatoxin; Ca, carcinoma)

(Zimmerman HJ: Hepatotoxicity: Adverse Effects of Drugs and Other Chemicals on the Liver, p 98. New York, Appleton-Century-Crofts, 1978)

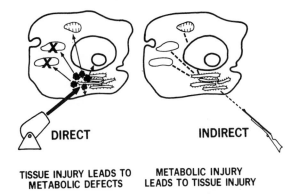

DIRECT   **INDIRECT**

TISSUE INJURY LEADS TO METABOLIC DEFECTS   METABOLIC INJURY LEADS TO TISSUE INJURY

Fig. 17-1. Sketch depicting difference between direct and indirect hepatotoxins. The direct type destroys the structural basis of metabolism; the indirect type produces a selective biochemical lesion that results in structural injury. (Zimmerman HJ: Hepatotoxicity. New York, Appleton-Century-Crofts, 1978)

There is reason to believe that native, nonmetabolized CCl_4 also may contribute to the injury,[159,804,810] particularly of the plasma membrane, and initiate the leakage of intracellular enzymes, coenzymes, and electrolytes from the hepatocyte and entry of calcium and other ions into the cytosol. The hypothetical scheme for the sequence of events after a toxic dose of CCl_4 is shown in Figure 17-2.

The yellow allomorph of phosphorus also appears to produce its hepatic damage by a direct attack on hepa-

Fig. 17-2. Hypothetical scheme for overall mechanism of CCl_4-induced hepatic necrosis. Increased cytosol levels of Ca^{2+} reflect leakage from organelles and entry from extracellular fluid secondary to early changes in membrane.

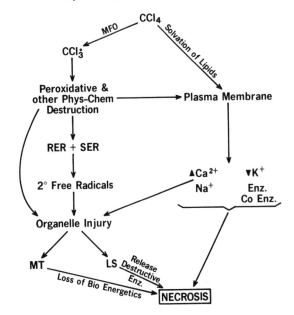

lism enhance its hepatotoxicity.[581] The centrilobular (zone 3) localization of CCl_4-induced hepatic necrosis can be attributed to the concentration in the central zone of the enzyme system responsible for its biotransformation.[679] There is evidence[581,679,680] that the responsible metabolite is a free radical (?CCl_3 that appears to produce peroxidation of the unsaturated lipids of cellular membranes and probably converts other cellular molecules to secondary free radicals that extend the injury.[581] There is also some covalent binding of CCl_3 to cell molecules, which presumably contributes to the injury.[580]

tocyte constituents. The injury consists of hepatic steatosis and necrosis, mainly in zone 1 of the lobule.[807] The membrane injury appears to involve direct physicochemical destruction, but the role of peroxidation is in dispute.[807]

Indirect Hepatotoxins

This category includes activated compounds, antimetabolites, and related compounds that produce hepatic injury by selective interference with a specific metabolic pathway or structural process (see Fig. 17-1, Table 17-2). The structural injury is secondary to a metabolic or other selective lesion (hence indirect), while that produced by direct hepatotoxins is primary and leads to metabolic derangement.[807] The hepatic damage produced by indirect hepatotoxins may mainly be cytotoxic (expressed as steatosis or necrosis) or cholestatic (expressed as arrested bile flow) (Table 17-3).

Cytotoxic Indirect Hepatotoxins. Cytotoxic indirect hepatotoxins cause hepatic injury by interfering with meta-

TABLE 17-3.   Types of Indirect Hepatotoxins

TYPE	MECHANISM	LESION	EXAMPLES OF AGENTS PRODUCING LESION
Cytotoxic	Selective interference with metabolic pathways by antimetabolites and related compounds or selective distortion of key molecules by covalent or other binding	Steatosis	MTX* a-Amanitin †‡§ Ethionine †‡ Ethanol*†‡ Tetracycline*† Puromycin*†‡ L-Asparaginase*† Azaserine*†‡ Azacytidine*† Azauridine*† AFB$_1$†‡§
		Necrosis	AFB$_1$†‡§ Acetaminophen*‡ α-Amanitin †‡§ Phalloidin †‡ Urethane* Thioacetamide‡ Bromobenzene*‡ PAs*†‡ 6-Mercaptopurine* Tannic acid*†‡§ DMN‡§ Mithramycin*†
		Carcinoma	Many agents
Cholestatic	Selective interference with bile excretory mechanisms	Bilirubin casts	Icterogenin †‡ C-17 alkylated and ethinylated steroids LCA †‡
	Selective interference with sinusoid-hepatocyte transport or with bilirubin conjugation	No lesion; only hyperbilirubinemia	Flavaspidic acid*†‡ Cholecystographic dyes* Rifamycin*†$^{||}$ Novobiocin*†$^{||}$

* Medicinal agent or other purposeful human exposure.
† "Natural" hepatotoxin.
‡ Experimental.
§ Relative prominence of fat and necrosis varies with agent, species, dose, and other circumstances.
$^{||}$ Cholestatic effect is dose related. In addition, drug can produce hepatocellular injury as rare, idiosyncratic reaction.
(DMN, dimethylnitrosamine; PAs, pyrrolizidine alkaloids; LCA, lithocholic acid; MTX, methotrexate; AF, aflatoxin)
(Zimmerman HJ: Hepatotoxicity: Adverse Effects of Drugs and Other Chemicals on the Liver, p 108. New York, Appleton-Century-Crofts, 1978)

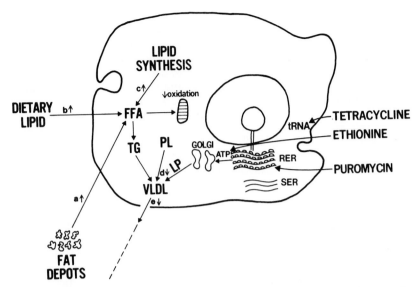

Fig. 17-3. Schema of lesions in lipid metabolism that can lead to hepatic steatosis. Fat in liver comes from peripheral depots (*a*), diet (*b*), and hepatic synthesis (*c*). Steatosis can result from increased mobilization of fatty acids from depots (*a*), decreased egress from liver (*e*) as a consequence of deficient or defective formation of the apoprotein of the very low density lipoprotein, or impaired union (*d*) of the apoprotein with phospholipid and triglyceride. Inhibition of synthesis of apoprotein results from selective lesions, for example, ethionine leading to ATP depletion, tetracycline binding to transfer RNA, and puromycin blocking access of activated amino acids to rough endoplasmic reticulum. FFA = free fatty acids; TG = triglyceride; PL = phospholipid; LP = apoprotein; VLDL = very low density lipoprotein; RER = rough endoplasmic reticulum; SER = smooth endoplasmic reticulum. (Zimmerman HJ: Hepatotoxicity. New York, Appleton-Century-Crofts, 1978)

bolic pathways essential for parenchymal cell integrity (Table 17-2, Fig. 17-3). They lead to diversion, competitive inhibition, or structural distortion of molecules essential for metabolism or to selective blockage of key metabolic pathways required to maintain the intact hepatocyte. The biochemical and physiologic lesions induced by these agents lead to steatosis, necrosis, or both (Table 17-3).[807]

The cytotoxic indirect hepatotoxins include compounds of experimental interest, drugs, and botanical hepatotoxins (see Table 17-3). Ethionine,[191] puromycin,[191] galactosamine,[138] and bromobenzene[475,593] are experimental tools, the study of which has thrown considerable light on the possible mechanisms for hepatotoxicity induced by specific metabolic lesions. Of greater clinical relevance are some antibiotics and antimetabolites employed as therapeutic agents, which are indirect hepatotoxins.[807] For example, tetracycline,[639] L-asparaginase,[103,254,276,564] methotrexate,[124,125,288] urethane,[83,775] 6-mercaptopurine,[177] and some of the other agents used in cancer chemotherapy can induce hepatic injury by mechanisms that presumably relate to their selective interference with cell metabolism.[807] Aflatoxin, ochratoxin, luteoskyrin, cycasin, pyr-

rolizidines, mushroom alkaloids, tannic acid, and other agents of plant origin produce hepatic injury by known or presumed mechanisms that warrant their categorization as indirect cytotoxic hepatotoxins (see Table 17-3).[807]

Many of these agents produce steatosis (ethionine, tetracycline, puromycin, asparaginase, methotrexate, aflatoxin*). Some produce necrosis (bromobenzene, thioacetamide, urethane, 6-mercaptopurine). Some produce both (toxins of *Amanita phalloides,* tannic acid, aflatoxin*).[807]

Necrosis produced by indirect hepatotoxins also is presumably initiated by membrane injury. The manner in which covalent binding of electrophilic metabolites of the toxic agents leads to necrosis is not clear,[196,473–476] however, nor is the manner in which distortion of the smooth endoplasmic reticulum membranes, the site of the biotransformation, leads to plasma membrane injury.[580] Nevertheless, distortion of intracellular environment, in-

---

* In some circumstances, aflatoxin produces steatosis; in others, necrosis or both steatosis and necrosis occur.[807]

cluding cytosol concentration of free calcium ion, presumably provokes necrosis.[196]

Hepatic steatosis caused by indirect hepatotoxins, like that of the direct hepatotoxins, may be of complex pathogenesis. It also is most often a consequence of defective egress of lipid from the liver.[150,191–193,639] The indirect cytotoxic hepatotoxins have the ability to interfere with protein synthesis by introducing selective biochemical lesions into the cell (see Table 17-2).

The consequent deficient[150,191–193] or defective[698] synthesis of the apoprotein moiety of VLDL or defective assembly of the triglyceride with apoprotein to form the VLDL by which lipid is transported from the liver to the depots can lead to steatosis (see Fig. 17-3). Increased mobilization of lipids from the depots and increased synthesis and decreased oxidation of fatty acids may contribute to the pathogenesis of steatosis.[150,191–193,413]

Ethionine is a good exemplary indirect hepatotoxin. It produces hepatic injury by competing with methionine for the available adenosine triphosphate (ATP), by interfering with the utilization of methionine, and by ethylating compounds that should be methylated.[191–193] In this example of "lethal synthesis" (as Peters[540] calls in vivo formation of toxic counterfeit compounds), S-adenosyl-ethionine is formed instead of S-adenosyl-methionine. The depletion of cellular ATP and the involvement of S-adenosyl-ethionine in the reactions that normally use S-adenosyl-methionine appear to be responsible for the deficient and defective synthesis of mRNA, and in turn for deficient synthesis of protein.[191–193] Impaired production of the apoprotein moiety of the VLDL needed to transport lipid from the liver results in steatosis.[191,192]

Puromycin, an antibiotic tested in cancer chemotherapy and of interest in experimental pathology, leads to a similar lesion. It also interferes with synthesis, by attachment to the ribosome at the "P" site, supplanting the activated tRNA that would normally be attached. The result is formation of incomplete proteins truncated by a terminal puromycin molecule.[192]

Tetracycline (and its derivatives) are antibiotics that in high doses lead to microvesicular steatosis (Fig. 17-4).[130,392,400,401,543,639] This lesion is dose related and reproducible in experimental animals.[401,639] It appears as an important lesion in humans, leading to clinical evidence of hepatic disease only when blood levels of the antibiotic are high.[130,535] Tetracycline-induced injury occurs when the agent is given intravenously in doses that exceed 1.0 g/day and seems particularly prone to occur if the recipient is in the last trimester of pregnancy or has renal disease.[130] Smaller intravenous doses or oral administration usually produce no clinical evidence of hepatic disease; although minor degrees of fat accumulation can be observed in biopsy sections of the liver even after oral doses.

The mechanism for steatosis involves inhibition by tetracycline of lipid movement from the liver.[639] Presumably this is related to its known ability to interfere with protein synthesis,[797] perhaps through binding of tRNA[713] or interference with some other element of the complex system

of apolipoprotein synthesis of VLDL. Other effects of tetracycline may contribute to its steatogenic effects.[639]

Parenteral administration of tetracycline is now rarely used. Derivatives of tetracycline, however, share its steatogenic properties. Furthermore, the hepatic lesion is a classic one that serves as a model of one form of toxic injury.

Ethanol also warrants classification as an indirect hepatotoxin. It leads to fatty metamorphosis by a number of adverse effects on hepatocyte metabolism.[413] It also can lead to necrosis, perhaps by the necrogenic effects of acetaldehyde[193] or by increasing oxygen requirements of hepatocytes.[758]

Ethanol also can potentiate the hepatotoxic effects of a number of known toxic agents, through induction of the MFO and consequent enhancement of biotransformation of the agents to toxic metabolites or by other mechanisms.[18,551,711,810] Of special clinical importance is the enhancement by ethanol of the hepatotoxic effects of chlorinated hydrocarbons[551,711] and of acetaminophen.[630,651,711]

A number of cytotoxic indirect hepatotoxins produce necrosis by selective biochemical lesions (see Table 17-3). Depletion of UTP, alkylation and arylation of macromolecules, or selective attachment (of the toxins or their metabolites) to membranes are among the reactions that appear to be responsible.[193,195,473,807]

Cholestatic Indirect Hepatotoxins. Cholestatic indirect hepatotoxins produce jaundice or impaired liver function by selective interference with hepatic mechanisms for excretion of substances into the bile canaliculus, by injury to bile ducts, or by inhibition of hepatocellular uptake from the blood of substances destined for biliary excretion (see Table 17-3).[807]

The prototypic cholestatic hepatotoxin interfering with excretion into the canaliculus is icterogenin, an alkaloid of the plant *Lippia rhemani*.[14,602] A clinical counterpart of icterogenin jaundice is the impairment of hepatic function and jaundice produced by methyltestosterone and a number of other C-17 alkylated anabolic steroids.[14,803] The effect of these agents is dose related but modified by the individual susceptibility of the recipient. Hepatic dysfunction is produced in most patients but jaundice in only a few.[803] Impairment of ability to excrete sulfobromophthalein (BSP) occurs promptly, often within a few days.[802] Continued administration of the agent usually leads to a plateau or even to some decrease in the degree of abnormality of hepatic function.[803] This would suggest that adjustment to the adverse effects of the agents occurs in most persons and that patients who develop jaundice after prolonged administration of one of these steroids are unable to make this adjustment, perhaps on a genetic basis.[803] Similar to this phenomenon is the high incidence of a relatively slight degree of hepatic dysfunction in women who take oral contraceptives, which contain C-17 ethinyl estrogen and progesterone derivatives.[1,179,226,363,462,518] Curiously, the oral contraceptive

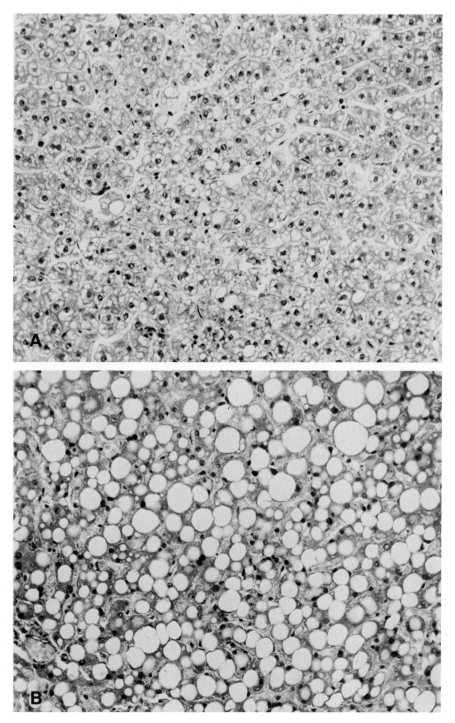

Fig. 17-4. A. Tetracycline-induced fatty liver with small droplet fat (microvesicular) that does not displace the hepatocyte nuclei. (H & E; original magnification × 215) **B.** Alcohol-induced fatty liver with large droplet fat displacing the hepatocyte nuclei. (H & E; original magnification × 215)

agents are particularly likely to produce jaundice in women who have had the benign cholestatic jaundice of pregnancy, a syndrome with a genetic basis.[297,462] Also probably related to this phenomenon is the impairment of liver function produced by estradiol and a number of other estrogenic agents.[226]

The mechanism for the impaired function induced by these anabolic, progestational, and estrogenic steroids is unknown. The available evidence indicates a precise structural requirement to induce injury, namely, an alkyl group at C-17. Testosterone, which lacks this type of substituent, does not lead to impaired function, while methyl testosterone, identical in structure save for the C-17 methyl substituent, does (Fig. 17-5).[807] A number of other agents with C-17 alkyl substituents also produce jaundice. The phenolic ring A of estrogenic steroids with[747] or without[226] an ethinyl group at C-17 also appears to enhance the ability of the steroid to interfere with biliary excretion of bile salts, bilirubin, and BSP.

Presumably the cholestatic effects result from alterations in the plasma membrane of the hepatocyte. Studies[592] suggest that the effect of ethinyl estradiol and presumably of other estrogenic steroids is mainly on the basolateral plasma membrane, leading to a decrease in fluidity and in the Na$^+$,K$^+$-ATPase activity. These changes lead to impaired hepatocyte uptake of bile acids and consequent decrease in bile flow. The anabolic steroid effect, however, may be on the canalicular plasma membrane. Curiously, the estrogenic injury appears to be reversed by administration of S-adenosyl-methionine,[592,632] acting to repair a steroid-induced defect in the lipids of the hepatocyte membrane or to methylate the abnormal phospholipid.[63]

A category of indirect hepatotoxins that might be considered a variant of the cholestatic type includes several agents that can produce unconjugated hyperbilirubinemia and interfere with uptake of BSP and other foreign dyes from sinusoidal blood.[807] It includes male fern extract (flavaspidic acid),[266] an antifungal agent (saramycetin),[12,789] novobiocin,[271] rifampicin,[99] and gallbladder dyes.[49,53]

There are several agents that produce cholestasis by selectively damaging the ductal system. α-Naphthyl-isothiocyanate has long served to provide an experimental model of cholestasis.[551] 4,4'-Diaminodiphenylmethane is a plastics hardener, employed in industry, which led to an epidemic of cholestatic jaundice in Epping, England, as a result of its presence as a contaminant of flour[385] and to similar hepatic injury in occupationally exposed individuals.[291] A similar lesion has been reported in Spain as the apparent result of ingestion of rapeseed oil contaminated with aniline.[690] Paraquat poisoning also can produce ductal destruction.[495] 5-Fluorouridine given by hepatic

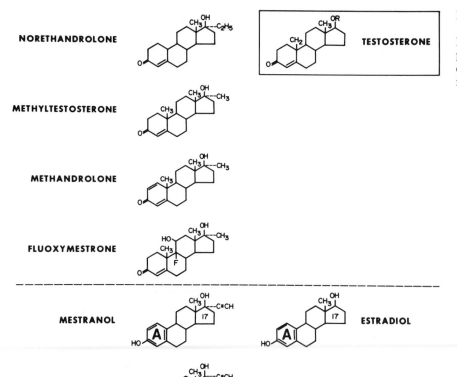

Fig. 17-5. Structures of several C-17 alkylated anabolic and ethinylated contraceptive steroids compared with those of testosterone and estradiol. Note unsaturated ring A in estrogenic steroids.

artery infusion in the treatment of metastatic carcinoma of the liver leads to injury of the biliary tree resembling sclerosing cholangitis.[294] Sporidesmin is a mycotoxin that also mainly causes ductal injury in some species.[681]

Carcinogenic Indirect Hepatotoxins. Many of the cytotoxic indirect hepatotoxins produce hepatic carcinoma as well as degeneration or necrosis of the liver. Indeed, hepatocarcinogens produce selective injury to the cell by exquisitely selective changes in the control macromolecules, usually alkylation or arylation of the DNA.[194,469] The selective and precise biochemical lesion produced by the hepatocarcinogens accordingly warrants designation of the compounds as indirect hepatotoxins.[807]

Idiosyncratic Hepatic Injury

Many drugs unpredictably produce hepatic injury in a small proportion of recipients. Some analyses have referred to the special, individual susceptibility of the injured patients as hypersensitivity, a designation that tacitly assumes or explicitly regards the mechanisms for hepatic injury to be that of drug allergy. Indeed, some instances of drug-induced injury probably are a manifestation of hypersensitivity. Others, however, appear to represent a different mechanism, presumably an aberrant metabolic pathway for the drug in the susceptible patient that permits the production or accumulation of hepatotoxic metabolites.[804] Accordingly, to avoid confusion, hepatic injury induced by a drug sporadically, unpredictably, and in low incidence should be designated as an idiosyncratic response to the drug. The term *hypersensitivity* should be reserved for hepatic injury for which there is at least clinical evidence of allergy to the drug. The clinical features distinguishing the two categories of idiosyncrasy are listed in Table 17-4.

Some drugs seem able to produce hepatic injury by either mechanism. For example, most cases of liver damage induced by isoniazid appear to result from toxic metabolites.[478] In a few cases, however, the liver damage is accompanied by fever and eosinophilia and may be presumed to result from hypersensitivity.[807]

Hypersensitivity Related

The inference that an idiosyncratic reaction is mediated by hypersensitivity has been based on clinical characteristics and response to readministration of the drug. Laboratory evidence of humoral or cell-mediated immune response to the drug has also been offered. Hypersensitivity is the presumptive mechanism for the hepatic injury that develops after a relatively fixed "sensitization" period of 1 to 5 weeks; recurs promptly on readministration of the agent; and tends to be accompanied by fever, rash, and eosinophilia, by lymphocytosis and circulating "atypical" lymphocytes, and by an eosinophil-rich or granulomatous inflammatory infiltrate in the liver. Support for this view is provided by a prompt recurrence of fever, rash, or hepatic abnormality on readministration of the drug. These features provide circumstantial evidence for hypersensitivity as the cause of hepatic disease. Efforts to demonstrate a role for humoral or cell-mediated immunity in clinical cases have yielded variable and inconclusive results for the most part. Antibodies to phenytoin have been found in patients with reactions to the drug. Lymphocytes from patients with reactions to some drugs have been reported to undergo lymphoblastic transformation[620] and to release macrophage migration inhibitory factor[620] or kinins that can inhibit bile flow,[483] but such reports have not been consistent or not studied in other laboratories. Furthermore, efforts to establish an immunologic basis for drug-induced hepatic disease are hampered by the probability that the putative antigen is an unknown metabolite of the suspected drug. Nevertheless, the circumstantial evidence seems sufficiently compelling to support the view that hypersensitivity plays an important role in the hepatic injury provoked by some drugs (*e.g.,* phenytoin, sulfonamides, halothane).[363,556,635,663,807] Indeed, some of these reactions resemble serum sickness and, by analogy, may be deduced also to be the result of circulatory antigen–antibody complexes. On the other hand, there are drugs that produce hepatic injury in an equally small proportion of cases without clinical features suggestive of drug hypersensitivity. Some of these respond promptly to a challenge dose, as illustrated by ticrynafen-associated hepatic injury.[813]

TABLE 17-4. Putative Types of Idiosyncratic Reactions to Drugs as Cause of Hepatic Injury

TYPE OF IDIOSYNCRASY	DURATION* OF EXPOSURE	CLINICAL FEATURES	RESPONSE TO CHALLENGE DOSE
Hypersensitivity	1–5 weeks	Hypersensitivity, (rash, fever, eosinophilia)	Prompt, after 1 or 2 doses
Metabolic aberration	Variable 1 week–12 months or more		Delayed, many days or weeks

* Prior to development of overt hepatic injury.

Others do not (*e.g.*, isoniazid-, valproic acid–, and perhexilene maleate–associated hepatic injury).

We suggest that those reactions that do not resemble serum sickness but are, nevertheless, reprovoked by a challenge dose are also the result of hypersensitivity but by a different immunologic mechanism. Those reactions that have neither clinical manifestations of hypersensitivity nor manifest prompt response on readministration of the drugs have been presumed to have resulted from metabolic idiosyncrasy, a view supported by recent studies.[807]

The concept that drug hypersensitivity per se can lead to hepatic injury warrants closer scrutiny (Fig. 17-6). Generalized hypersensitivity caused by some drugs (*e.g.*, penicillin) almost never includes liver injury,[130,807] while that caused by others (*e.g.*, phenytoin) includes liver disease with appreciable frequency.[91,149,272,367,397,443] Still other drugs (*e.g.*, chlorpromazine) may cause liver damage with or without associated features suggestive of drug allergy. Furthermore, while chlorpromazine causes overt liver disease in less than 1% of recipients, it can induce a much higher incidence (35%–50%) of hepatic dysfunction.[803] These figures are too high to permit the assumption that hypersensitivity alone is the mechanism for the hepatic abnormality. With other observations, they have led to the hypothesis that a mildly adverse effect of some agents on the liver, when accompanied by generalized hypersensitivity, may be expressed as overt hepatic injury.[804] The demonstrations that chlorpromazine can produce injury in *in vitro* models[166,167,804,813] and cholestatic injury in experimental animals[246,596,702] are consistent with this hypothesis.

Hypersensitivity Dependent on Metabolic Defect

That hypersensitivity-mediated reactions can result from a metabolic defect is also strongly suggested by the observations of Spielberg and co-workers.[696] They found that patients who had sustained hepatic injury in a hypersensitivity type reaction to phenytoin (and their relatives) had an apparent defect in converting the active metabolite

(arene oxide) to the inactive dihydriol. The active metabolite presumably could serve as a hapten or be cytotoxic.

Toxic Metabolite Dependent

Idiosyncratic hepatic injury that is not accompanied by clinical hallmarks of hypersensitivity and is not promptly reproduced by readministration of the drug and may appear after widely varying periods of exposure to the drug had long been assumed to result from metabolic rather than immunologic idiosyncrasy.[615] There is now convincing evidence that some of these do depend on metabolic idiosyncrasy. These include perhexilene maleate,[488] valproic acid,[360,409] isoniazid, and iproniazid.[474,475,478]

MORPHOLOGIC FORMS OF TOXIC HEPATIC INJURY

The main types of morphologic change in the liver produced by chemicals, drugs, and other agents are listed in Table 17-5. Definition of the forms of injury produced by the intrinsic hepatotoxins has been relatively simple since the hepatic damage can be reproduced in experimental animals.[621] Characterization of the forms of idiosyncratic injury, however, has been more difficult and depended on collation of material from reports of individual and groups of cases.[803]

Acute Injury

Toxic agents may lead to degeneration or necrosis of hepatocytes (cytotoxic injury) or to arrested bile flow (cholestatic injury). There is some relationship between the type of hepatotoxin and the form of injury. Most intrinsic toxins mainly produce cytotoxic injury.[363,557,807] Only a few lead to injury that is cholestatic.[807] Idiosyncratic injury caused by some drugs is cholestatic and by others is cytotoxic. Some drugs characteristically produce a mixed type of injury in which both cytotoxic and cholestatic injuries are prominent.[807]

ASSOCIATION BETWEEN HYPERSENSITIVITY TO DRUGS & HEPATIC INJURY INDUCED BY THEM

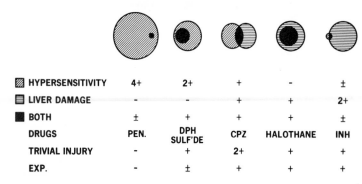

	PEN.	DPH SULF'DE	CPZ	HALOTHANE	INH
▨ HYPERSENSITIVITY	4+	2+	+	-	±
☰ LIVER DAMAGE	-	-	+	+	2+
■ BOTH	±	+	+	+	±
DRUGS	PEN.	DPH SULF'DE	CPZ	HALOTHANE	INH
TRIVIAL INJURY	-	+	2+	+	+
EXP.	-	±	+	+	+

Fig. 17-6. Penicillin (*PEN*) rarely produces hepatic injury and does so only in association with clinical evidence of hypersensitivity. Phenytoin (*DPH*) and sulfonamides (*Sulf'de*) produce hepatic injury more frequently but only in association with clinical features of hypersensitivity. Chlorpromazine (*CPZ*) may produce hepatic injury alone, hypersensitivity alone, or both. Halothane may produce hepatic injury alone or with hypersensitivity but rarely leads to hypersensitivity alone. Isoniazid (*INH*) usually leads to hepatic injury without hypersensitivity.

Cytotoxic Injury

Degeneration, necrosis, and steatosis of hepatocytes can occur in various combinations.[558,641] Indeed, toxic hepatic damage can cause virtually all of the morphologic lesions known in liver disease.

Necrosis. Necrosis may be zonal, massive, or diffuse. Massive hepatic necrosis, in which many entire lobules are destroyed, should be distinguished from the zonal type. The two appear to have a different pathogenesis, and agents are usually consistent in producing one or the other. Massive necrosis seems to be an extreme form of diffuse, but not of zonal, necrosis. Indeed, zonal necrosis, even when severe, usually leaves a rim of hepatocytes; even when the entire lobule is wiped out, lobular arrangement remains. In massive necrosis, however, lobules collapse and disappear (Fig. 17-7).

In general, the necrosis produced by *intrinsic* hepatotoxins is zonal while that produced by *idiosyncratic* injury is usually diffuse and, when extreme, massive. There are exceptions. The experimental necrosis produced by galactosamine, a hepatotoxin, is diffuse rather than zonal.[138] Also, the occupational hepatic injury induced by trinitrotoluene, chloronaphthalenes, and tetrachlorethane during World Wars I and II was, in many instances, apparently massive rather than zonal.[363] Conversely, the necrosis produced by halothane is often centrizonal (zone 3) despite its presumed idiosyncratic basis,[489,544] suggesting that it is produced by toxic metabolites of halothane formed in zone 3 by the cytochrome P-450 system.[807]

Zonal* necrosis may be in the central, (zone 3) peripheral, (zone 1) or midzone (zone 2) of the lobule, depending on the agent. Centrizonal (zone 3) necrosis (see Fig. 17-7) is the characteristic lesion produced by a number of intrinsic toxins. Some are mainly of experimental interest.[621,807] Those relevant to human disease include CCl_4, chloroform, copper salts, pyrrolizidine alkaloids, tannic acid, and the toxins of the mushroom *Amanita phalloides* and others.[363,621,641,807] In large overdoses, acetaminophen becomes an intrinsic hepatotoxin and causes centrizonal necrosis (see Fig. 17-7D). The central (zone 3) necrosis induced by some agents (*e.g.,* pyrrolizidine alkaloids and aflatoxin B_1 in some species) and by some agents used in cancer therapy is accompanied by injury to the hepatic veins or venules, which adds a hemorrhagic component to the necrosis.[456,621,807]

Some agents characteristically produce peripheral (zone 1) necrosis; in this category are known toxins such as allyl alcohol and its esters,[587] the endotoxin of *Proteus vulgaris,*[291] yellow phosphorus,[151] overdoses of ferrous sulfate,[363] as well as idiosyncratic injury due to some drugs. A few agents produce midzonal necrosis in experimental animals. These include beryllium, furosamide, and, in hyperthyroid animals, CCl_4 and chloroform.[475,621,807] Midzonal necrosis, however, is a rare lesion in humans.

* Zones 1, 2, and 3 designated by Rappaport.

The zonality of necrosis appears to be related to the mechanism of injury. The centrizonal location of the lesion induced by CCl_4,[679] by bromobenzene,[593] and by acetaminophen[473-476] appears to reflect the centrizonal concentration of the enzyme system responsible for the conversion of these agents to hepatotoxic metabolites.[473-476] The peripheral zone necrosis produced by allyl formate has been attributed to the location in that zone of the enzyme (alcohol dehydrogenase), which converts that compound to its toxic metabolite, acrolein.[587] This observation has been challenged recently.[41]

Diffuse necrosis, which is the usual form caused by idiosyncratic injury (see Fig. 17-7 *E* through *G*), resembles that produced by viral hepatitis although the injury may be more intense centrally.[641] The extreme form of diffuse injury is massive necrosis (see Fig. 17-7E). The idiosyncratic injury caused by halothane and other haloalkane anesthetics differs from that caused by other drugs in that the necrosis is often centrizonal and strikingly similar to that of CCl_4 or chloroform (see Fig. 17-7B).[419,489,544,598]

Degeneration of hepatocytes precedes actual necrosis and is seen in the nonnecrotic cells accompanying the necrosis. These prenecrotic degenerative changes may be the chief lesion. Throughout the zone destined to undergo necrosis or at its periphery, hepatocytes show "ballooning" and eosinophilic degeneration and "free" sinusoidal, acidophilic bodies. The free *acidophilic body,* a characteristic lesion of viral hepatitis, may also result from parenchymal injury induced by a number of drugs and chemicals (see Fig. 17-7F and G).

The Mallory body ("alcoholic hyaline") is a dramatic form of hyaline degeneration of hepatocytes (see Fig. 17-8A) seen in alcoholic liver disease and a number of other diseases, including Wilson's disease, primary biliary cirrhosis, liver damage after ileojejunal bypass for obesity, Indian childhood cirrhosis, and hepatocellular carcinoma.[219,542] In Western societies, alcoholic hepatitis remains the clinical setting in which the Mallory body is most regularly found. The relative importance of malnutrition and of the toxicity of ethanol in producing the hepatic disease of alcoholics remains uncertain. There is little doubt, however, that ethanol is an intrinsic hepatotoxin[413,758] and the liver disease is, at least in part, a form of hepatotoxicity and that the Mallory body is its characteristic, histologic marker. Furthermore, the recent report of the development of Mallory bodies in rats given toxic doses of griseofulvin confirms it as a histologic marker of toxicity.[143] Of additional interest is the recent report of "Mallory bodies" in patients with perhexiline-maleate–induced and amiodarone-induced[559] hepatic injury (see Fig. 17-8).[399,407,522,538]

Steatosis. Steatosis can be produced by a large number of agents. Although zonal steatosis has not commanded the attention of zonal necrosis, there are differences in the zonal distribution of fat of different toxic etiology. Some agents (*e.g.,* yellow phosphorus) mainly or initially lead to accumulation of fat in the peripheral zone. Others

TABLE 17-5. Morphologic Types of Toxic Hepatic Injury

TYPE OF INJURY	AGENT OR COMMENT
Acute	
Parenchymal	
Cytotoxic	
Necrosis*	
Zonal	
Central (zone 3)	CCl_4, acetaminophen, halothane
Mid (zone 2)	Ngaione, furosamide
Peripheral (zone 1)	Allyl formate, albitocin
Massive	TNT, Some drugs
Diffuse (panlobular)	Some drugs†
Focal	Some drugs†
Degeneration (ballooning, acidophilic)	
Acidophilic bodies	Large number of agents
Steatosis	
Microvesicular	Ethionine, tetracycline, phosphorus
Macrovesicular	Ethanol, MTX
Cholestatic	
Hepatocanalicular ("pericholangitic")	CPZ, Erythromycin estolate, organic arsenicals
Canalicular ("bland")	C-17 alkylated anabolic and contraceptive steroids
Vascular (hepatic veins and branches)	
Hepatic venule injury	PAs
Peliosis hepatis‡	Phalloidin; anabolic and contraceptive steroids
Hepatic vein thrombosis	Contraceptive steroids
Chronic	
Parenchymal	
Chronic necroinflammatory disease (chronic hepatitis)	Oxyphenisatin, α-methyldopa, nitrofurantoin, dantrolene, clometacine, papaverine, sulfonamides, PTU
Subacute necrosis	Same drugs listed under chronic necroinflammatory disease
Steatosis	Ethanol, MTX, glucocorticoids, antineoplastic agents, AF, CCl_4, PAs
Phospholipidosis	
Pseudoalcoholic liver disease (Mallory bodies)	Coralgil, perhexiline maleate, amiodarone, DES
Cirrhosis	Ethanol, MTX, and drugs listed in first five types of injuries in this section, except glucocorticoids
Cholestatic lesions	
Chronic intrahepatic cholestasis (primary biliary cirrhosis like)	CPZ, haloperidol, imipramine, organic As, thiobendazole, tolbutamide
Biliary sclerosis† (Resembles sclerosing cholangitis)	FuDR by hepatic artery perfusion
Vascular lesions	
Hepatic vein thrombosis	OCs, antineoplastic agents
Veno-occlusive disease	PAs, antineoplastic agents, OCs, x-ray, anabolic steroids
Peliosis hepatis	Medroxyprogesterone, vinyl cloride, As, Th-O, Aza-T

TABLE 17-5.—Continued

TYPE OF INJURY	AGENT OR COMMENT
Other sinusoidal lesions	
Sinusoidal dilatatic	OCs
Perisinusoidal fibrosis	As, vitamin A, CuSO$_4$, Th-O, antineoplastic agents, AZA-T
Hepatoportal sclerosis (portal vein and perisinusoidal)	
Granulomas	Many drugs
Neoplasms	
Adenoma	OCs, anabolic steroids
Carcinoma	Anabolic steroids, OCs, Th-O, vinyl cloride
Angiosarcoma	Th-O, vinyl cloride, As, CuSO$_4$ anabolic steroids, estrogen (?), OCs (?)

* Degenerative changes including acidophilic bodies, hyalinization, and ballooning precede necrosis.

† Small doses of toxic agents and drugs can lead to focal necrosis.

‡ Peliosis hepatis may be produced in experimental animals as acute lesion by phalloidin, or occurs in humans as chronic lesions induced by anabolic and contraceptive steroids.

(TNT, trinitrotoluene; CPZ, chlorpromazine; DMN, dimethylnitrosamine; PAs, pyrrolizidine alkaloids; MTX, methotrexate; AF, aflatoxin; INH, isoniazid; As, arsenic; PTU, propylthiouracil; Th-O, Thorotrast; AZA-T, azathioprine; OCs, oral contraceptives; DES, diethylstilbesterol)

(*e.g.,* tetracycline, ethanol) predominantly or initially lead to centrizonal steatosis.

Two main types of fatty change occur.[304,641] Some agents (*e.g.,* tetracycline) produce microvesicular steatosis. In this form of fatty liver the hepatocytes are filled with many tiny fat droplets that do not displace the nucleus (see Fig. 17-4). This is also the type of steatosis found in Reye's syndrome and in the fatty liver of pregnancy.[304] A similar lesion of Thai children has been ascribed to aflatoxins and has been produced in monkeys by aflatoxin.[66,67] Other agents (ethanol, methotrexate) lead to macrovesicular steatosis,[641] in which the hepatocyte contains a large fat droplet that displaces the nucleus to the periphery (see Fig. 17-4).

Some agents produce both necrosis and fatty metamorphosis.[621,807] For some (*e.g.,* CCl$_4$, chloroform, tannic acid), the necrosis is dominant and the steatosis is less prominent. For others (*e.g.,* α-amanitin, yellow phosphorus), the steatosis is more prominent than the necrosis.

Phospholipidosis is an additional form of lipid accumulation that may be drug induced.[430,514,666] It differs strikingly in pathogenesis and characteristics from the two classic forms of steatosis. Phospholipidosis was first recognized in Japan in 1969 to be the result of administration of the "coronary vasodilator" 4,4'-diethylaminoethoxyhexestrol (Coralgil),[514] and it has been recorded by Japanese authors in over 100 patients.[430] It is characterized by enlarged, foamy hepatocytes, as seen by light microscopy, and by lamellated or crystalloid inclusions, as seen by electron microscopy.[430] There are similar changes in Kupffer cells and in cells of extrahepatic sites.[514] The lesion, which resembles that of several inborn disorders of phospholipid metabolism,[430] is accompanied by a char-

acteristic clinical syndrome and has led to cirrhosis.[666] Perhexiline maleate[547] and amiodarone[559] have been reported to produce the lesion, and a number of amphiphilic compounds produce similar ultrastructural changes in experimental animals.[430] The full-blown lesion with the development of cirrhosis is a chronic change that requires several months to develop, but early changes occur after only several doses.

Cholestatic Injury

Some agents lead to injury that appears to spare the parenchyma and to cause only or mainly arrested bile flow.[363,556,641,663,807] The histologic manifestation of cholestatic injury consists mainly of bilirubin casts in the canaliculi (Fig. 17-9). Two main types of drug-induced cholestasis have long been recognized. One type is exemplified by chlorpromazine-induced jaundice and the other by steroid (anabolic and contraceptive)-induced jaundice (Table 17-6). Cholestatic injury induced by chlorpromazine is more likely to be accompanied by a minor degree of parenchymal injury and by portal inflammation than that induced by the anabolic and contraceptive steroids.[363,641,807] The chlorpromazine type has been referred to as hepatocanicular or hypersensitivity cholestasis and the steroid type as canalicular or bland cholestasis. A third type of cholestasis has recently been reported as a reaction to benoxaprofen. It is characterized by the presence in cholangioles of striking, inspissated casts apparently containing a bile-stained precipitate.[168,207,209,248] This form might be called cholangiolar cholestasis. A fourth type that could be designated ductal or cholangiodestructive is characterized by injury to interlobular or larger ducts. It

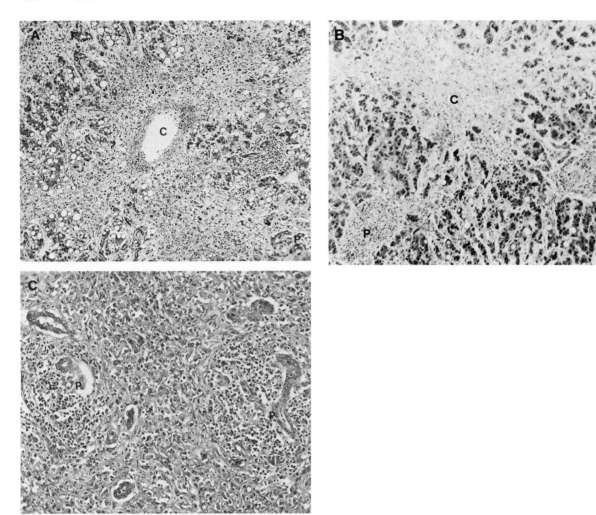

Fig. 17-7. A. Fatal centrizonal hepatic necrosis in carbon tetrachloride poisoning. Note islands of surviving, fatty cells at periphery of lobule. C = central vein; P = portal area. AFIP Neg. No. 72-8406. (H & E; original magnification × 90) **B.** Fatal, centrizonal, hepatic necrosis associated with halothane-induced anesthesia. C = central vein; P = portal area. (H & E; original magnification × 80) **C.** Massive hepatic necrosis due to phenytoin. Note loss of lobular structure. P = portal areas. AFIP Neg. No. 73-7313. (H & E; original magnification × 145) *(Continues on facing page)*

has been produced by rapeseed oil contaminated with aniline oil,[690] by poisonous doses of paraquat,[493] by phenylene diamine,[385] and, in animals, by α-naphthyl-isothiocyanate.[240]

Sequelae of cholestatic injury can occur. Just as acute cytotoxic injury can lead to chronic disease with distortion of hepatic parenchyma (cirrhosis), so can acute cholestatic disease, at times, eventuate in a chronic cholestatic lesion that mimics primary biliary cirrhosis.[323,363,405,556,641,663] A number of cases of acute cholestatic jaundice due to chlorpromazine, organic arsenicals, thiobendazole, ajmaline, and tolbutamide have failed to subside and have progressed to the chronic cholestatic syndrome.[807]

Patterns of Inflammatory Response

The hepatic injury induced by intrinsic hepatotoxins usually elicits little inflammation. When there is an inflammatory response, it usually includes neutrophils.[335,641] Necrosis induced by drugs is also accompanied by a slight or moderate degree of inflammatory infiltration consisting of lymphocytes and eosinophils. In general, it appears to be less prominent than the inflammatory response to necrosis of equal severity caused by viral hepatitis.[320,641] However, the cytotoxic injury induced by some drugs (*e.g.,* phenytoin, *p*-aminosalicylic acid) usually leads to a striking infiltration of mononuclear cells with or without eosin-

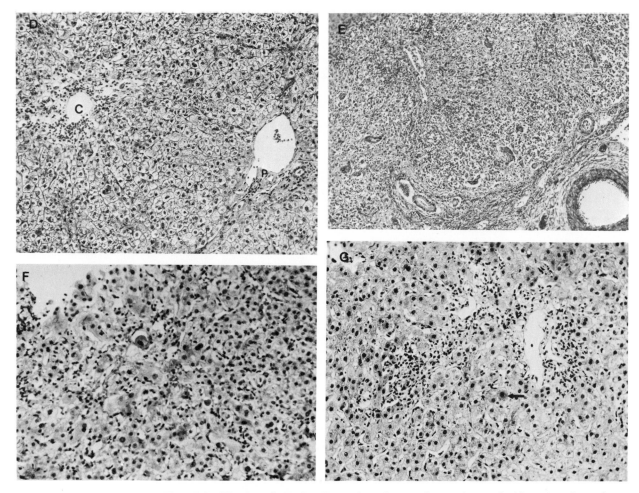

Fig. 17-7. *(Continued).* **D.** Small centrizonal area of necrosis seen in biopsy specimen from patient recovering from acetaminophen-induced necrosis. C = central vein; P = portal area. AFIP Neg. No. 73-5193. (H & E; original magnification × 130) **E.** Massive necrosis due to isoniazid. Note complete loss of lobular structure. AFIP Neg. No. 73-7310. (Masson; original magnification × 75) **F.** Hepatitislike injury in patient with α-methyldopa-jaundice showing diffuse degeneration, inflammation, and "free" sinusoidal, acidophilic body *(arrow).* (H & E; original magnification × 110) **G.** Hepatitislike injury in patient with isoniazid-jaundice. Note inflammatory infiltration, areas of necrosis, and developing acidophilic body *(arrow).* AFIP Neg. No. 70-5844 (H & E; original magnification × 110)

ophils (Fig. 17-10). These may be diffusely distributed throughout the parenchyma or aggregated around areas of necrosis. There are usually prominent aggregates in the portal area.[641] The inflammation accompanying phenytoin-induced hepatic injury may resemble that of infectious mononucleosis (see Fig. 17-10) and may include granulomas or granulomatoid lesions. Some drugs[325] may lead to granulomas with or without other manifestations of hepatic injury (Fig. 17-11, Table 17-6).[458] Sarcoid-like granulomas can also be found in the liver, lungs, and other organs as a result of chronic occupational exposure to heavy metals such as beryllium[707] and copper.[549] Indeed,

copper can be demonstrated histochemically in the hepatic and pulmonary granulomas of vineyard sprayers chronically exposed to a copper sulfate mixture.[549,550]

The character of the inflammatory response bears some relation to the apparent pathogenesis of the injury. Eosinophilic or granulomatous inflammation in a patient with drug-induced hepatic injury is generally taken as evidence that the mechanism for injury is hypersensitivity.[641] Prominence of eosinophils in the sinusoids is usually a reflection of peripheral eosinophilia.[323]

Inflammation mainly localized to the portal areas has a special relevance to cholestatic injury. In the intrahepatic

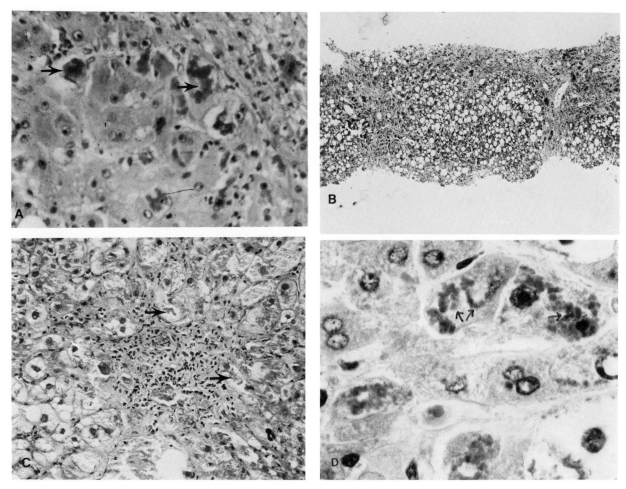

Fig. 17-8. A. Biopsy showing "alcoholic" hyaline (*arrows*) fat and necrosis in patient with alcoholic hepatitis. (H & E; original magnification × 300) **B,C.** Biopsy from patient with perhexiline-induced hepatic injury showing steatosis and fibrosis, (*B*) and elements in hepatocytes (*C*) resembling "alcoholic hyaline" (*arrows*). **B.** AFIP Neg. No. 79-12455. (H & E; original magnification × 60) **C.** AFIP Neg. No. 12450. (H & E; original magnification × 250) **D.** Biopsy from patient with amiodarone-associated hepatic injury showing Mallory bodies ("alcoholic" hyaline). AFIP Neg. No. 85-10212. (H & E; original magnification × 1000)

cholestasis caused by some drugs (*e.g.,* chlorpromazine or erythromycin estolate) there is a prominent portal infiltrate that may be rich in eosinophils. According to Scheuer,[641] the portal inflammatory lesion is only prominent early in the illness. Intrahepatic cholestasis accompanied by portal inflammation has been called the cholangiolitic or hypersensitivity type of cholestasis. In the intrahepatic cholestasis, which is induced by anabolic or contraceptive steroids, there is little or no portal inflammation. This has been called the bland or steroid type. It is more characteristic of the cholangiolitic than of the bland type of cholestatic injury to have some degree of overt hepatocyte injury. Accordingly, we have termed the

cholangiolitic type, *hepatocanalicular* and the bland type, *canalicular* injury (Table 17-7).[807]

SUBACUTE HEPATIC INJURY

There are two main forms of subacute toxic liver injury. One, subacute hepatic necrosis, lies midway between acute hepatic necrosis and chronic hepatic disease (cirrhosis), in clinical and histologic features. This term also has been applied to a form of viral hepatitis characterized by "bridging necrosis" and conveying the concept of severity

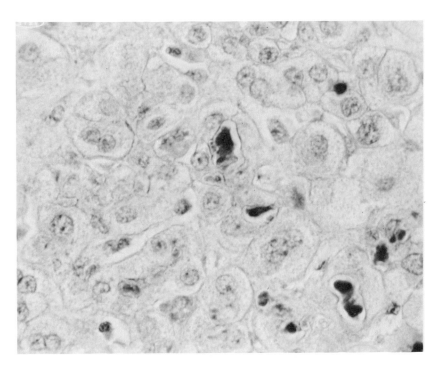

Fig. 17-9. Biopsy from patient with jaundice due to prochlorperazine (Compazine) showing bilirubin casts in distended canaliculi and mild hepatocyte abnormality. AFIP Neg. No. 65-3956. (H & E; original magnification × 70)

rather than duration. The other form, subacute veno-occlusive disease (VOD), is described in a later section.

Subacute hepatic necrosis was a dread occupational disease of the defense industries during World Wars I and II resulting from prolonged exposure to tetrachlorethane, trinitrotoluene, chlorinated biphenyl-chloronaphthalene mixtures, and dinitrobenzene.[79,291,363,470] Occupationally acquired subacute hepatic necrosis is now virtually obsolete. Subacute hepatic necrosis, however, can also result from long-term administration of isoniazid[56,436] or methyldopa[437,647] and has been described in recipients of cinchophen,[523,774] propylthiouracil,[465] and hydralazine.[31]

The histologic features of subacute hepatic necrosis have included varying degrees of necrosis, fibrosis, and regeneration (Fig. 17-12). In patients with a brief (2 to 3 weeks) clinical course of industrial subacute hepatic necrosis the changes have been largely those of extensive necrosis and collapse with relatively little cirrhosis.[79,470] The liver in these circumstances has been remarkably shrunken, weighing as little as 500 g. Patients with a prolonged course of several months or more usually develop a macronodular cirrhosis. Areas of extensive necrosis and parenchymal collapse, areas of surviving or regenerated parenchyma, and broad areas of fibrosis lead to architectural distortion and macronodular cirrhosis. Similar features can be seen in instances of subacute hepatic necrosis caused by drugs, although portal-portal, portal-central, and central-central bridging is more common with drug-induced disease (see Fig. 17-12).[315] In the subacute hepatic necrosis caused by occupational toxins, fat was prominent in surviving cells; its prominence seemed inversely proportional to the rate of necrosis. Fat has not been a part of the subacute hepatic necrosis caused by adverse reaction to drugs.[56,437,647,774]

CHRONIC HEPATIC INJURY

A number of chronic lesions can result from the subtle, continued, or repeated injury of prolonged exposure to hepatotoxic agents or drugs or can be a sequel to acute injury. These may be parenchymal, cholestatic, vascular,

TABLE 17-6.   Drugs That Can Lead to Hepatic Granulomas

Allopurinol	Nitrofurantoin[678]
Aspirin	Penicillin
Carbamazepine[404,406,479]	Phenylbutazone
Cephalexin	Phenytoin
Diazepam	Procainamide
Feprazone[782]	Procarbazine
Halothane	Oxyphenbutazone
Hydralazine	Quinidine
Isoniazid	Seatone*
Metahydrine	Sulfonamide
Methyldopa	Sulfonylurea derivatives
Metolazone	

* Proprietary drug derived from mussels and used to treat arthritis. See reference 6.

(Data from references 325, 429, and 458)

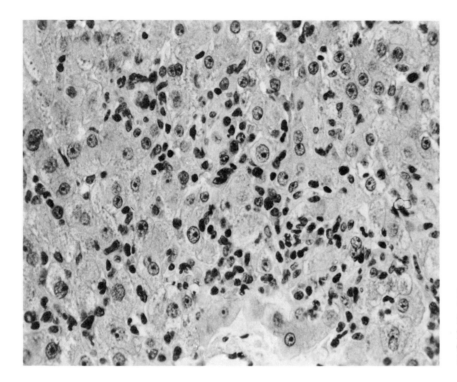

Fig. 17-10. Striking sinusoidal "beading" with mononuclear cells from patient with jaundice due to phenytoin. AFIP Neg. No. 73-11834. (H & E; original magnification × 395)

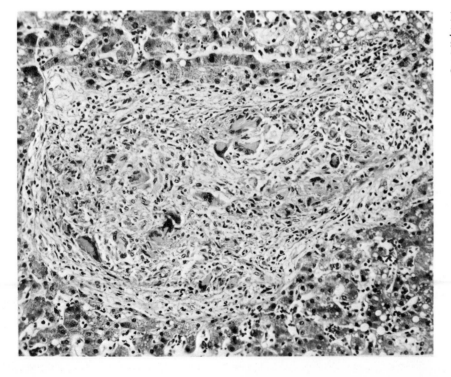

Fig. 17-11. Biopsy from patient with jaundice due to phenylbutazone showing granuloma. AFIP Neg. No. 79-15667. (H & E; original magnification × 160)

TABLE 17-7.   Types of Cholestatic Jaundice Caused by Drugs

FEATURES	CANALICULAR JAUNDICE	HEPATOCANALICULAR JAUNDICE
Etiology	C-17 alkylated steroids (anabolic, contraceptive)	Chlorpromazine Erythromycin estolate Some oral antidiabetic agents Some antithyroid drugs
Clinical evidence of hypersensitivity	0	Frequent
Biochemical features		
SGOT/SGPT	↑ (1–10×)	↑ (1–10×)
Alkaline phosphatase	↑ (1–2×)	↑ (3–10×)
Histology		
Bile casts	+	+
Portal inflammation	0	++ (esp. early)
Parenchymal injury	0–±	± – +
Other hepatic lesions*		
Adenoma	+	−
Carcinoma	+	−
Primary biliary cirrhosis–like syndrome	± or 0	+
Peliosis	+	−
Other terms	"Bland" cholestasis	"Cholangiolitic" cholestasis

* Produced by steroids but not by drugs that cause hepatocanalicular cholestasis.

neoplastic, or granulomatous (see Table 17-5). The parenchymal lesions include chronic active hepatitis, steatosis, phospholipidosis, pseudoalcoholic lesions, and cirrhosis.[241,291,363,435,589,599,621,641,663,807] The cholestatic lesions include prolonged intrahepatic cholestasis with a syndrome resembling primary biliary cirrhosis[807] and one resembling sclerosing cholangitis.[811]

Parenchymal Lesions

Chronic Active Hepatitis

A number of drugs have been incriminated in the production of chronic necroinflammatory disease that resembles chronic active hepatitis.[16,21,56,57,241,277,369,435,438,539,561,641,649,658,663] The lesion is characterized by dramatic portal and periportal inflammation composed of lymphocytes, plasma cells, and, often, eosinophils (Fig. 17-13). A cardinal histologic characteristic is the extension of the inflammation, often accompanied by fibrous strands into the periportal surrounding individual degenerating cells and groups of cells ("piecemeal necrosis").

The entity resembles "autoimmune" chronic active hepatitis ("lupoid hepatitis") histologically and clinically.

There is a striking female predominance among patients. A majority of patients have serologic features considered to be "autoimmune markers." Antinuclear antibodies, the "L.E. factor," smooth muscle antibodies, anti–single-strand DNA, and several other antibodies against cell organelles have been noted.[435,539,561,649,658] Frequently, there is also marked hyperglobulinemia. Drugs that have been incriminated in this lesion are listed in Table 17-8.

Several other drugs (propylthiouracil, sulfonamides) have been implicated less convincingly in the production of this entity, and several others can lead to a smouldering, subtle necrosis accompanied by little inflammation and no autoimmune serologic markers (isoniazid, acetaminophen). There is no evidence that any of these lesions have persisted after the drug had been withdrawn.

Steatosis

Chronic steatosis is mostly macrovesicular. It can be produced by several drugs including ethanol, glucocorticoids, and a number of antineoplastic agents, most notably, methotrexate and asparaginase.[807,811] Glucocorticoid-induced steatosis appears to have no sequelae, methotrexate steatosis can eventuate in cirrhosis, and asparaginase fatty liver may be accompanied by necrosis.

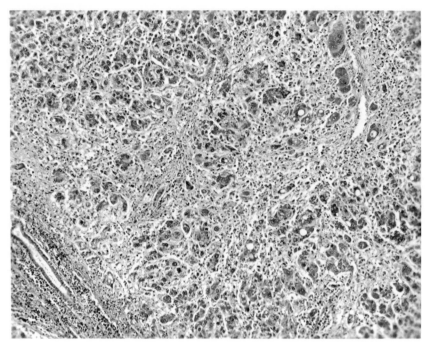

Fig. 17-12. Subacute hepatic necrosis induced by isoniazid. AFIP Neg. No. 4647. (H & E; original magnification × 75)

Phospholipidosis

Phospholipidosis was discussed in an earlier section. The lesion may be relatively acutely produced, but the syndrome is a chronic one. Often accompanied by Mallory body change, it may merge with and present with the syndrome of pseudoalcoholic liver disease (nonalcoholic steatonecrosis).[430,514,547,559]

Nonalcoholic Steatonecrosis

Nonalcoholic steatonecrosis (Fig. 17-8 *C* and *D*) is characterized by wasting, lassitude, hepatomegaly, ascites, and often peripheral neuropathy.[547,559] Biochemical changes consist of mildly elevated (twofold to fourfold) aminotransferase levels. Liver biopsy shows Mallory bodies, relatively slight steatosis, and portal mononuclear inflammation.[547,559] The foamy phospholipid-laden cells may not be appreciated on light microscopy and may require electron microscopy to identify the histologic marker.[559] In the Western World, the drugs chiefly responsible for the entity have been perhexiline (not used in the United States)[547] and amiodarone.[559]

Fibrosis

Changes ranging from portal and periportal fibrosis to frank cirrhosis occur in patients with chronic active hepatitis, with methotrexate injury, and with the phospholipidosis–nonalcoholic steatonecrosis lesion. Strategic deposition of collagen, in the periportal area and space of Disse, even without cirrhosis, can also lead to portal hypertension. This "noncirrhotic" portal hypertension has been termed *hepatoportal sclerosis*.[466] Reduction of the portal vein caliber also accompanies the hepatoportal sclerosis. Instances of noncirrhotic portal hypertension have been attributed to chronic exposure to inorganic arsenicals,[503,801] to vinyl chloride,[557] and to copper sulfate,[550] as well as to alcoholic liver disease.[466] A form of noncirrhotic portal hypertension can result from vitamin A intoxication.[626]

Periportal fibrosis occurs in drug-induced chronic active hepatitis and in the primary biliary cirrhosis–like syndrome that may follow chlorpromazine-induced jaundice. Methotrexate has led to periportal fibrosis when used in the treatment of leukemia[112,314] and to both periportal and intralobular fibrosis when used in the long-term therapy of psoriasis.[641] Alcoholic liver disease and hypervitaminosis A can lead to centrilobular fibrosis; in the latter condition, there is also marked hypertrophy of the perisinusoidal lipocytes (Ito cells) that store the vitamin A, atrophy of liver cells, and dilatation of sinusoids.[807]

Cirrhosis

Chemical hepatic injury can lead to all of the known morphologic types of cirrhosis. Macronodular and micronodular cirrhosis,[98,291,438] congestive hepatopathy,[83,86,252,456,484,706,712,719,775] resembling cardiac cirrhosis, and a biliary cirrhosis–like lesion[278,323,363,383,438,498,708,764,807] can all result from toxin- or drug-induced liver damage.

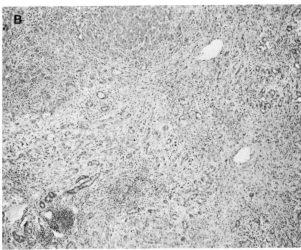

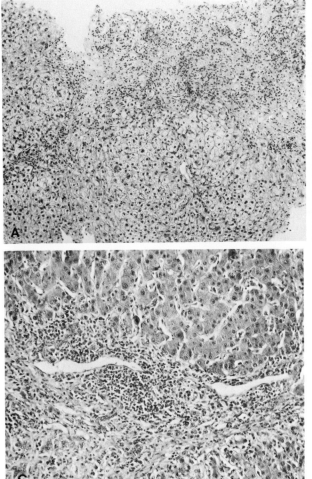

Fig. 17-13. **A.** Methyldopa-induced chronic active hepatitis showing marked anisocytosis, diffuse inflammation, and large areas of collapse. (H & E; original magnification × 100) **B.** Chronic active hepatitis due to nitrofurantoin. Note inflammatory aggregates in markedly expanded portal area and invading the parenchyma. AFIP Neg. No. 78-6715. (H & E; original magnification × 60) **C.** Area from biopsy shown in *B,* demonstrating portal inflammation, periportal expansion, and "piecemeal necrosis." AFIP Neg. No. 78-6735. (H & E; original magnification × 250)

Macronodular or Micronodular Cirrhosis

Either form of cirrhosis may be a sequel to continued or often-repeated subtle injury, the result of subacute necrosis, or of chronic necroinflammatory disease. Rarely, cirrhosis of the macronodular type may follow a single episode of necrosis.[363] In general, however, a single bout of zonal necrosis in experimental animals (*e.g.,* CCl₄ poisoning), even when extensive, is following by complete histologic restitution in surviving animals.[98,291] Given at intervals too short to permit recovery from each dose, CCl₄ can lead to cirrhosis.[98] Massive, but nonlethal, necrosis is more likely to leave architectural distortion and, perhaps, cirrhosis.[363] Many of the known hepatotoxins can lead to cirrhosis in experimental animals.[621] Presumably, they could also do so in humans, although epidemiologic evidence to support this possibility is limited to a few agents. Occupational exposure to CCl₄, tetrachlorethane, dimethylnitrosamine, and trinitrotoluene has been incriminated in instances of cirrhosis in humans.[363,621,805]

Inorganic arsenical compounds employed in the past for the treatment of leukemia and psoriasis, for example, have also been incriminated.[216,773] In a sense, history has repeated itself in the modern era as instances of cirrhosis have resulted from the use of methotrexate to treat these diseases.[807] The most important paths to cirrhosis as the

TABLE 17-8. **Drugs Incriminated as Possible Causes of Chronic Active Hepatitis**

MORE CONVINCING	QUESTIONABLE
Clometacine	Isoniazid
Dantrolene	Propylthiouracil
α-Methyldopa	Sulfonamides
Oxyphenisatin	
Papaverine	
Ticrynafen	

result of drug-induced injury are the lesions of chronic active hepatitis[435] and of phospholipidosis–nonalcoholic steatonecrosis.[430,514,547,559] The role of fungal and plant toxins in the production of cirrhosis in humans, remains inconclusive, although probable in some settings.[807]

Congestive cirrhosis may be a sequel to veno-occlusive disease or hepatic vein thrombosis.[807] Primary biliary cirrhosis may be mimicked by chronic intrahepatic cholestasis occurring as a sequel to acute intrahepatic cholestasis,[435,807] and an obstructive biliary cirrhosis type of injury might be a consequence of the biliary sclerosis produced by hepatic artery infusion of FuDR for treatment of metastatic carcinoma of the liver.[294]

Cholestatic Lesions

Chronic Intrahepatic Cholestasis

A syndrome that resembles primary biliary cirrhosis has followed acute cholestasis due to chlorpromazine and to several other phenothiazines, thiazides, imipramine, organic arsenicals, tolbutamide, ajmaline, and in one instance to methyltestosterone, alone, or with other drugs and to thiobendazole.[807] Table 17-9 contains a comparison of the features of the drug-induced primary biliary cirrhosis syndrome with those of "true" primary biliary cirrhosis.

TABLE 17-9. Comparison of Primary Biliary Cirrhosis (PBC) with Drug-Induced Chronic Cholestasis (DICC)

CHARACTERISTICS	PBC	DICC
Associated disease	Sicca syndrome other "collagen" disease	Irrelevant
Drug intake	Irrelevant	Phenothiazines Organic arsenicals Tolbutamide ? Other cholestasis-producing drugs
Symptoms		
Pruritus	+	+
Jaundice*	− or ±	+
Signs		
Melanoderma	+	±
Jaundice	− or ±	+
Xanthomas	+ or −	+ or −
Hepatomegaly	+ or −	+ or −
Splenomegaly	+ or −	+ or −
Laboratory		
Bilirubin	1-5 mg/dl	1-20 mg/dl
SGOT/SGPT	↑ (1-5)	↑ (1-5)
Alkaline phosphatase	↑ 3-10×	↑ 3-10×
Cholesterol	↑	↑
β-globulin	↑	↑
γ-M globulin	↑	?
Histology		
Nonsuppurative cholangitis†	+	−
Ductopenia	+	±
Hepatic granulomas	+	−
Copper in hepatocytes	+	+
Cirrhosis	±	±
Prognosis	Variable	Good

  * Jaundice is usually slight and tends to come relatively late in the course of PBC, while it is early in the course of DICC.

  † Refers to inflammatory response in portal area.

  (+, usually present; −, usually absent; ±, present but of slight degree)

  (Zimmerman HJ: Hepatotoxicity: Adverse Effects of Drugs and Other Chemicals on the Liver, p 356. New York, Appleton-Century-Crofts, 1978)

Duct destruction and portal inflammation are less prominent in the drug-induced syndrome than in "true" primary biliary cirrhosis but may be part of the lesion.[323]

Biliary Sclerosis

Biliary sclerosis has been applied to the biliary tree injury produced by therapy of hepatic metastatic carcinoma, with FuDR infused into the hepatic artery. The incidence appears to be high, and the lesion consists of blebs and edema in the duct epithelial surfaces and compression and distortion of the duct lumen. On cholangiography, the lesion resembles sclerosing cholangitis. Clinical features include upper abdominal aching, anorexia, weight loss, and jaundice.

Vascular Lesions

A number of important vascular lesions can be produced by drug injury (see Table 17-5). Two involve interference with efferent blood flow and lead to congestive hepatop-

athy (Fig. 17-14). They are thrombosis of the hepatic veins and occlusion of the hepatic venules. A third lesion is peliosis hepatis. Additional lesions include sinusoidal dilatation, perisinusoidal fibrosis, and hepatoportal sclerosis.[807]

Hepatic Vein Thrombotic Occlusion

Hepatic vein thrombotic occlusion leads to the Budd–Chiari syndrome. A number of instances of hepatic injury have been reported in patients taking oral contraceptives and have been attributed to the thrombogenic effects of contraceptive steroids.[410]

Veno-occlusive Disease

Injury and occlusion of the central hepatic venules has long been known to be produced by pyrrolizidine alkaloids.[86,456,712,719] The initial lesion is central necrosis accompanied and followed by progressive decrease in venule caliber.[712] It leads to hepatic congestion and can lead to

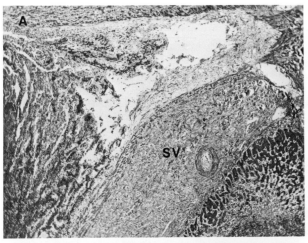

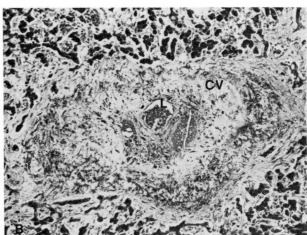

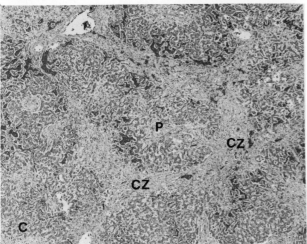

Fig. 17-14. Autopsy sections from patients with Budd–Chiari syndrome secondary to hepatic vein thrombosis. **A.** Thrombosis in sublobular vein (*SV*). AFIP Neg. No. 70-9626. (H & E; original magnification × 55) **B.** Thrombosis in central vein (*CV*) showing recanalized lumen (*L*) and central congestion and necrosis. AFIP Neg. No. 79-14020. (H & E; original magnification × 160) **C.** Section showing "reverse lobulation" with necrosis and fibrosis extending between centrizonal areas of original lobules. CZ = centrizonal areas; P = portal area. AFIP Neg. No. 79-13961. (H & E; original magnification × 40)

a fatal congestive cirrhosis, to an arrested lesion, or even to reversal.[86,456,712,807] The clinical features and hepatic congestion are similar to the Budd-Chiari syndrome produced by hepatic vein thrombosis. Causes, in addition to the alkaloids, include urethane, thioguanine, azathioprine, and a number of other oncotherapeutic agents, as well as x-irradiation.[811]

Peliosis Hepatis

Peliosis hepatis, which consists of large blood-filled cavities (Fig. 17-15), has long been of interest to pathologists but of recognized clinical significance only recently.[22,141,173,450,452,499,641,664,796] The lesion has also been produced in experimental animals by administration of lasiocarpine[8] and of phalloidin.[743] Since phalloidin has a special proclivity for injury to membranes,[743] its production of peliosis would be consistent with the theory that the lesion reflects "weakening" of sinusoidal supporting membranes. Necrosis also has been suggested as the initial injury.[796] Of practical import is the observation of marked sinusoidal dilatation in livers that show peliosis hepatis,[499,560] even in sites remote from the actual lesion. Furthermore, anabolic and contraceptive steroids can lead to sinusoidal dilatation even when no peliosis has developed[803] and a characteristic lesion of prominent dilatation of peripheral lobular sinusoids (Fig. 17-16) has been described.[560]

Neoplasms

Several types of benign and malignant hepatic neoplasm can result from administration of chemical agents. Ade-noma, a lesion almost restricted to females in the child-bearing years, was an extremely uncommon tumor until recently.[175] The observation during the past few years of many more cases than had formerly been encountered, almost all in recipients of contraceptive steroids, has led to the conclusion that the steroids can lead to the development of this benign tumor,[30,37,173,175,176,321,324,364] Perhaps the most convincing evidence for a relationship is the reported regression of this tumor following withdrawal of oral contraceptives.[176] Less convincing is the reported association between the development of focal nodular hyperplasia (hamartoma) and contraceptive steroids. There has been considerable confusion, however, regarding the terminology of benign hepatic tumors.[324]

Malignant neoplasms of the liver are discussed elsewhere in this volume. Nevertheless, both carcinomas and sarcomas warrant mention among the chronic hepatic lesions produced by toxic agents. The carcinoma with a generally accepted relation to chemical carcinogenesis is the hepatocellular type.[94] A large number of chemical and botanical toxins can produce hepatocellular carcinoma in experimental animals.[194,440,449,469] Most of the cholangio-carcinomas attributed to experimental hepatocarcinogens are probably variants of hepatocellular carcinoma,[94] although true cholangiocarcinomas have been induced in experimental animals.[583,621,705,730] In humans, Thorotrast has led to hepatocellular and cholangiocellular carcinoma as well as to angiosarcoma.[654] These effects may be due to the radioactivity rather than the chemical toxicity of the agent. The epidemiology of hepatocellular carcinoma in humans and the demonstrated experimental hepato-carcinogenicity of mycotoxins and other natural hepa-totoxins and of synthetic chemicals encountered occu-

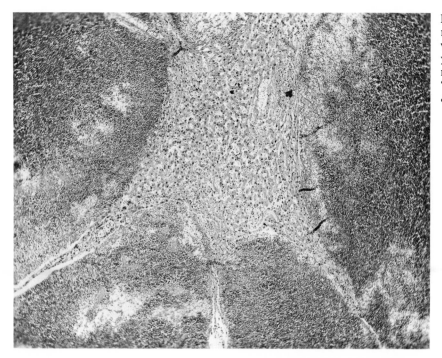

Fig. 17-15. Autopsy section showing marked peliosis hepatitis in patient with aplastic anemia treated with ox-ymethalone. Note compressed parenchyma surrounded by blood "lakes." AFIP Neg. No. 72-8401. (H & E; original magnification × 50)

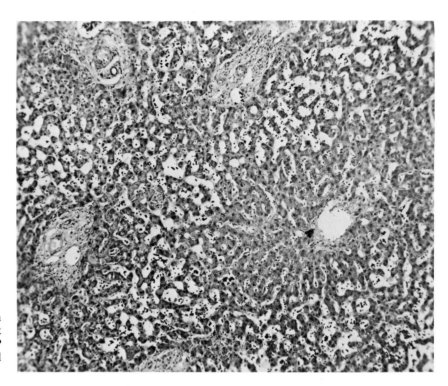

Fig. 17-16. Dilatation of sinusoids in peripheral zone of lobule in patient taking contraceptive steroids. AFIP Neg. No. 77-5119. (H & E; original magnification × 40)

pationally have raised the possibility that other xenobiotics may also be responsible for carcinoma of the liver in humans.[194,469]

Several medicinal agents have come under suspicion during the past few years as possible hepatocarcinogens. The development of hepatocellular carcinoma in a few long-term recipients of anabolic and of contraceptive steroids have made these agents suspect,[321] although the issue remains controversial.[13] Although griseofulvin[311] and isoniazid[616] are experimental hepatocarcinogens, there is no evidence of their carcinogenicity for humans.

Angiosarcoma (hemangioendothelial sarcoma) has recently come into sharp focus as a malignant tumor occurring in persons with occupational exposure to vinyl chloride.[281,557] Support for the etiologic role of vinyl chloride derives from the heretofore great rarity of the lesion,[557] the epidemiologic relationship to exposure to vinyl chloride,[281] and the ability to produce this vascular tumor in experimental animals by administration of vinyl chloride.[442] This rare tumor also has developed in vintners with long exposure to inorganic arsenic, in patients with psoriasis treated with Fowler's solution, and in patients who had been injected with Thorotrast.[319,654] A case of angiosarcoma in a 54-year-old man who had sprayed vineyards with copper sulfate for 35 years raises a possible etiologic relationship of this neoplasm to another heavy metal.[550] Anabolic steroids also have been incriminated in the etiology of this neoplasm.[322] Of interest in this context is the occurrence of several cases of angiosarcoma in patients with hemochromatosis.[319] Some chemical agents (*e.g.,* dialkylnitrosamines), which usually lead to hepa-

tocellular carcinoma in experimental animals, can also produce angiosarcoma in several species.[292,621]

Adaptive Morphologic Changes

Long-term drug therapy may cause the hepatocyte cytoplasm to develop a ground-glass appearance. This change has been observed in patients on long-term therapy with chlorpromazine and barbiturates,[371] azathioprine, steroids, phenytoin, resorcin, and some analgesics[787] and in some patients with chronic hepatitis, cirrhosis, or hepatocellular carcinoma. The ground-glass appearance reflects a marked, diffuse hypertrophy of the smooth endoplasmic reticulum.[371] It resembles that of hepatocytes containing the surface antigen of hepatitis B virus (HBsAg) carriers[261,372] or patients with chronic viral hepatitis;[642] but it differs in that the special reagents that stain the ground-glass hepatocyte containing HBsAg[667] do not stain the drug-induced ground-glass hepatocyte.[320,787]

The ground-glass appearance is apparently the light-microscopic equivalent of the smooth endoplasmic reticulum proliferation "induced" by the drugs and demonstrated by ultrastructural studies.[336] It is accompanied by elevated blood levels of γ-glutamyl transferase[524] and presumably accounts for the hepatomegaly seen in patients taking anticonvulsants and other drugs.[337] Presumably, the type and dosage of drug, the duration of therapy, age, sex, and other characteristics of the person affect the development of the ground-glass appearance.

The prognostic significance of the ground-glass transformation is not known. It is not associated with overt, acute, or chronic injury caused by the same drug. Nevertheless, the borderline between adaptation and toxicity remains uncharted.[203,336]

A striking form of ground-glass change has been described in patients undergoing aversion therapy.[754] Although it was originally attributed to disulfiram, it is now recognized to be caused by cyanamide. The ground-glass cells produced by cyanamide contain condensed "inclusion bodies" full of degenerated organelles and other cellular debris.

Pigment Deposits

Several types of pigmentary deposit may follow exposure to exogenous chemicals. Least significant is lipofuscin, the pigment of lysosomal origin seen in the normal liver. It becomes more prominent in elderly patients and in patients who had been taking phenacetin or chlorpromazine.[641] Although hepatocyte deposits have little clinical significance, Kupffer cells, seemingly engorged with lipofuscin, may be useful markers of recent necrosis nearby. Presumably they represent the engulfed debris of the necrotic cells. Pigment deposition also occurs in reticuloendothelial (RE) cells of the liver after intravenous infusion of fat emulsions,[381,529] conceivably leading to RE blockade and resultant depression of several immune functions.[529]

Hemosiderin deposits are seen in association with several forms of chemical hepatic injury, namely, alcoholic liver disease[432] and the porphyria cutanea tarda associated with alcoholism[432] or other chemical (e.g., hexachlorobenzene) injury.[644]

Copper overload is a regular concomitant of primary biliary cirrhosis. It is also seen in the secondary form induced by chlorpromazine.[323] It presumably will be found in all other forms of prolonged cholestasis. Copper has been histochemically demonstrated in Kupffer cells and within granulomas in patients occupationally exposed to copper salts.[549]

Thorotrast remains in the livers of patients many years after they received this radioactive material.[654] It appears as glistening, grayish-brown granules in engorged macrophages.

Bilirubin is, of course, the pigment most likely to be seen in patients with toxic hepatic injury. In intrahepatic cholestasis it is particularly prominent in centrolobular canaliculi. It may also be seen in Kupffer cells and in hepatocytes.

BIOCHEMICAL, FUNCTIONAL, AND CLINICAL MANIFESTATIONS OF INJURY

The clinical and biochemical manifestations of the hepatic injury caused by drugs and other chemicals reflect the histologic pattern of injury (Table 17-10). Necrosis leads to hepatocellular jaundice and a syndrome with clinical

TABLE 17-10.   Histologic Types of Acute Toxic Hepatic Injury and Associated Biochemical and Clinical Aspects

| HISTOLOGIC LESION | BIOCHEMICAL ABNORMALITIES IN SERUM* | | | CLINICAL ASPECTS | EXAMPLES |
	SGOT and SGPT	Alkaline Phosphatase	Cholesterol		
Cytotoxic					
Zonal necrosis	10–500×	1–2×	N or ↓	Hepatic and renal failure	Carbon tetrachloride, MSH, ACM, HALO
Diffuse necrosis	10–200×	1–2×	N or ↓	Severe hepatitis-like disease	INH, methyldopa, HALO
Steatosis	5–20×	1–2×	N or ↓	Resembles fatty liver of pregnancy and Reye's syndrome	Tetracycline
Cholestatic					
With pericholangitis (hepatocanalicular)	1–10×	1–10×	↑	Resembles obstructive jaundice	CPZ, EE
Without pericholangitis (canalicular)	1–5×	1–3×	N or ↑	Resembles obstructive jaundice	Anabolic and contraceptive steroids
Mixed (mixtures of cytotoxic and cholestatic	10–100×	1–10×	N or ↑	May resemble hepatitis or obstructive jaundice	PBZ, PAS, sulfonamides

* Degree of abnormality indicated as fold increases: N, normal; ↓ = reduced; ↑ = increased.
(PAS, *p*-aminosalicylic acid; MSH, poisonous mushrooms; ACM, acetaminophen; HALO, halothane; INH, isoniazid; CPZ, chlorpromazine; EE, erythromycin estolate; PBZ, phenylbutazone)

and biochemical features resembling viral hepatitis. Indeed, the pattern of injury is referred to as the hepatitic[663] or hepatocellular[806] type of drug-induced jaundice. Diffuse parenchymal degeneration with little necrosis, as in salicylate-induced hepatic injury, leads to a syndrome resembling anicteric hepatitis.[809] Toxic steatosis of the microvesicular type, as in tetracycline-induced hepatic injury, leads to a syndrome resembling in its clinical, histologic, and biochemical features, the fatty liver of pregnancy and Reye's syndrome.[304,807] Toxic, macrovesicular steatosis (e.g., methotrexate-or alcohol-induced steatosis) leads to a far smaller degree of biochemical abnormality. Drug-induced cholestasis leads to a syndrome resembling extrahepatic biliary tree obstruction.[807]

Necrosis leads to high levels in the blood of enzymes released from the damaged liver. Most extensively studied, in this regard, are the levels of the aminotransferases glutamic oxaloacetic transaminase (SGOT) and glutamic pyruvic transaminase (SGPT), which may be increased to values that are 10- to 500-fold the norm.[792,811] Values for serum alkaline phosphatase, 5' nucleotidase, and leucine aminopeptidase, all enzymes that reflect cholestasis, generally increase no more than 1- to 3-fold in response to necrosis.[803,807]

Depressed levels of plasma coagulation factors are characteristic of hepatic necrosis, and in the usual clinical setting, are reflected in the "one-stage" prothrombin time. Indeed, the most useful clinical clues to severity of necrosis are the prothrombin time and bilirubin level.[108,603,806]

Albumin levels do not change appreciably in the early phase of acute necrosis. Only late in the clinical course, or in subacute or chronic disease, does hypoalbuminemia ensue. Globulin levels also may stay unchanged in acute injury. In subacute and chronic drug-induced disease, the γ-globulin fraction may increase somewhat. Plasma cholesterol levels tend to be low or normal in acute hepatic necrosis.

The chief clinical manifestations of hepatocellular injury are fatigability, anorexia, and nausea, usually followed by jaundice, although jaundice may be the first manifestation of hepatic injury.[54] Severe cases may manifest all of the features of acute or subacute hepatic necrosis including deep jaundice, hemorrhagic phenomena, ascites, coma, and death.[603,741,807] Indeed, drug-induced hepatocellular jaundice is a serious entity with a case-fatality rate of 10% or more.

Toxic microvesicular steatosis leads to less dramatic biochemical evidence of hepatic injury than does acute necrosis. Values for the aminotransferases, in tetracycline toxicity, increase 5- to 20-fold the upper limit of normal. Bilirubin levels are only modestly increased. Values for alkaline phosphatase resemble those of hepatic necrosis in their slight degree of increase. Prolonged prothrombin times are characteristic. Hypoglycemia may be prominent.[807] The clinical features associated with the prototype, tetracycline toxicity, are discussed in a later section. Macrovesicular steatosis as in the usual methotrexate toxicity often leads to relatively slight elevation of aminotransferases,[124,552] although large, acute doses of methotrexate can lead to briskly elevated values.[288]

Cholestatic injury is clinically manifested by jaundice and itching. Biochemical features include relatively slight elevations of aminotransferases. The histologic differences between the two forms of cholestatic jaundice in humans described in an earlier section (hepatocanalicular and canalicular) have biochemical counterparts (see Table 17-7). While the aminotransferase levels of the two do not differ appreciably, alkaline phosphatase and cholesterol levels do. Levels for alkaline phosphatase are elevated more than threefold and cholesterol values are increased in hepatocanalicular (e.g., chlorpromazine-induced) but not in canalicular (e.g., methyltestosterone-induced) jaundice.[803,807] Almost all patients with drug-induced acute cholestasis recover. While death is rare, instances of acute cholestatic jaundice due to chlorpromazine, organic arsenicals, thiobendazole, ajmaline, and tolbutamide have progressed to a syndrome resembling primary biliary cirrhosis. The cholestatic jaundice that has occurred in patients taking benoxaprofen differs from other drug-induced cholestasis in that it was associated with renal failure and a high case-fatality rate (see section on antirheumatic drugs).

Some drugs produce a mixed form of hepatic injury with features of both hepatocellular and cholestatic jaundice. Predominantly hepatocellular injury, but with prominent cholestatic features, may be called mixed-hepatocellular; that which is predominantly cholestatic but includes parenchymal injury as well may be called mixed cholestatic.[803] A graphic formulation of the biochemical patterns of the several categories of drug-induced injury is shown in Figure 17-17.

Toxic porphyria may accompany several forms of hepatic injury.[463,644] The hepatic steatosis, necrosis, and cirrhosis produced in humans[644] and experimental animals[513] by hexachlorobenzene is accompanied by a form of porphyria resembling porphyria cutanea tarda. Griseofulvin-induced hepatic injury may also be accompanied by a similar defect in porphyrin metabolism.[311] Most cases of porphyria cutanea tarda are associated with alcoholism and alcoholic liver disease.[432]

Systemic and other extrahepatic clinical manifestations may be a prominent component of drug-induced hepatic injury. Fever, rash, and eosinophilia are hallmarks of the hypersensitivity type of drug-induced injury that may precede or accompany the hepatic injury.[363,803] Indeed, the "pseudomononucleosis" or serum sickness–like syndrome of fever, rash, lymphadenopathy, and lymphocytosis with "atypical" lymphocytes in the blood is the characteristic hypersensitivity reaction to a number of drugs (e.g., phenytoin, sulfonamides, aminosalicyclic acid).[803,807] Renal injury may occur as a result of nephrotoxic metabolites (methoxyflurane)[185] or as a manifestation of generalized hypersensitivity.[803]

Syndromes of injury produced by several well-known hepatotoxins tend to consist of three phases: (1) immediate, severe, neurologic, or gastrointestinal manifesta-

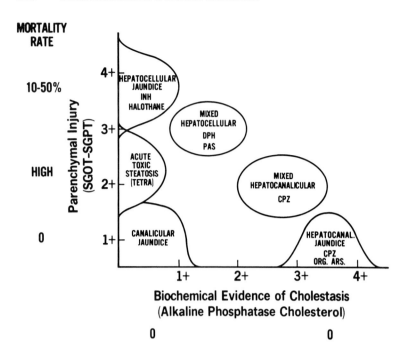

Fig. 17-17. Graph of types of drug-induced hepatic injuries. Note that the hepatocellular type is in the zone of high values of aminotransferase and of no or only modest elevation of alkaline phosphatase values. The hepatocanalicular type is in the zone of high alkaline phosphatase and cholesterol levels and modest levels of SGOT and SGPT. The canalicular type is also in the zone of low aminotransferase and alkaline phosphatase levels. See text for discussion of mixed categories and toxic steatosis. INH = isoniazid; PAS = para-aminosalicylic acid; DPH = phenytoin (diphenylhydantoin); CPZ = chlorpromazine; ORG, ARS = organic arsenicals; TETRA = tetracycline.

tions; (2) a period of relative well-being; and (3) the phase of overt hepatic injury that often includes renal failure.[806] This sequence is characteristic of poisoning due to CCl₄,[335] yellow phosphorus,[151] hepatotoxic mushrooms,[273] and, to some degree, of that due to acetaminophen (Table 17-11).[108]

ANALYSIS OF HEPATOTOXIC REACTIONS ACCORDING TO CIRCUMSTANCES OF EXPOSURE

Occupational and Domestic Hepatotoxins

Many agents with hepatotoxic potential have been employed in the munitions, rocketry, plastics, agricultural, paint, cosmetic, pharmaceutical, and other chemical industries.[807] Nevertheless, overt, acute hepatic injury is a rare consequence of occupational exposure to toxic chemicals today.

Hepatotoxins that may be encountered in the home include some of the industrial toxins (*e.g.,* CCl₄) and other toxic chemicals, such as yellow phosphorus, copper salts, mycotoxins and other botanical agents, and large overdoses of ordinarily safe drugs (*e.g.,* acetaminophen, ferrous salts). Ingestion of food accidentally or carelessly contaminated with toxic chemicals has led to dramatic epidemics of hepatic disease (see Table 17-11).

Poisonous mushrooms are still an important cause of acute hepatic injury in some parts of the world.[171,273,622] Food contaminated with aflatoxins has been implicated in the causation of acute hepatic disease[66,67,389] and, on epidemiologic grounds, in the etiology of hepatic carcinoma.[388,790] Consumption of plants containing pyrrolizidine alkaloids has long been known to cause acute and chronic hepatic disease[86,456,712] and continues to be responsible for epidemics of veno-occlusive disease.[484,719] Although long recognized to be a problem in other parts of the world, only recently has pyrrolizidine alkaloid toxicity been seen as a cause of hepatic disease in the United States. Some items obtained in "natural food" stores and some health remedies sold in pharmacies in southwestern states contain pyrrolizidine alkaloids.[601] Ingestion of the cycad nut can cause acute hepatic disease[223] and has the potential for causing chronic liver disease including carcinoma.[440] The possible consequences of the synthesis in the gastrointestinal tract of hepatotoxic (and hepatocarcinogenic) nitrosamines from ingested nitrites and secondary amines have been the subject of speculation.[416]

Widely employed insecticides include a number of chlorinated aromatic hydrocarbons, some of which are hepatotoxic in large doses. Exposure of humans to these agents may be widespread by way of foodstuffs, occupational exposure, and at times, accidental ingestion. Long-term storage in human tissues of DDT and other insecticides and their metabolites has been demonstrated.[51] Nevertheless, there is no significant evidence of hepatic injury from sustained occupational exposure to the chlorinated insecticides.[807] Accidental ingestion of large amounts of DDT (approximately 6 g),[687] and of paraquat (approximately 20 g),[90] however, has led to rare instances of centrizonal hepatic necrosis. Paraquat also has been reported to lead to destruction of intrahepatic bile ducts and cholestasis.[495] The clinical relevance of the known ability of DDT and related compounds to "induce" the

TABLE 17-11. Salient Features of Syndromes of Acute Toxic Hepatic Injury

	CCl$_4$	PHOSPHORUS	TOXIC MUSHROOMS	ACETAMINOPHEN
Phase I (1st 24 hr)				
Diarrhea	+	+*	−	−
Vomiting	±	+*	+	±
Pain	±	+	−	−
Hemorrhage	−	+	−	−
Shock	−	+	±	±
Phase II (24–72 hr)				
"Asymptomatic" period	−	+	+	+
Jaundice	+	−	−	−
Renal	±	±	+	−
CNS	−	−	+	−
Phase III (48–72 hr)				
Hepatic failure	+	+	+	+
Jaundice	4+	4+	4+	+
± Renal failure	+	+	+	±
± Hemorrhagic phenomena	+	+	+	+
Hepatic lesion	+	4+	4+	±
Necrosis	CZ (4+)‡	PZ (+)†‡	CZ (+)†	CZ (4+)
Death	10–20%	30–40%	50%	15%

* Phosphorescent appearance and garlic odor to vomitus and feces.
† Fat also prominent.
‡ CZ, centrizonal (zone 3); PZ, peripheral zone (zone 1).
(Zimmerman HJ: Hepatotoxicity: Adverse Effects of Drugs and Other Chemicals on the Liver. New York, Appleton-Century-Crofts, 1978)

drug-metabolizing enzyme system and thereby increase the rate of metabolism and conversion to toxic metabolites of many other compounds is open to speculation.[473]

The usual circumstances of exposure and the character of the injury produced by household hepatotoxins are summarized in Table 17-12. The toxicity of several of these agents, however, warrants description in more detail.

Carbon Tetrachloride Poisoning

Carbon tetrachloride was once widely used in many cleaning compounds, in fire extinguishers, and as a solvent. The agent was even used as an anthelmintic.[269] It has largely been replaced for these purposes because of the considerable number of toxic reactions following its use.

Instances of CCl$_4$ intoxication still occur but are now, fortunately, rare. Most victims are alcoholics; alcohol enhances susceptibility to this hepatotoxin and may lead to increased carelessness with its use.[269,485] Inhalation of the agent, usually during careless domestic use, or accidental ingestion of the toxin, during a state of alcoholic intoxication has been the usual mode of exposure.[269,335,485] There is little evidence to support an early view that poisoning by inhalation produces mainly renal injury and by ingestion leads mainly to hepatic injury.[363]

The amount of CCl$_4$ necessary to produce injury is quite small. Indeed, in experiments conducted many years ago on prisoners awaiting execution a dose as small as 5 ml was found to produce histologic evidence of damage.[155] The mechanism or mechanisms by which alcohol enhances the toxicity of CCl$_4$ is not known. Suggested explanations have included the possible additive effects of CCl$_4$-induced hepatic injury to that of alcohol, the enhancement of storage of CCl$_4$ by its solubility in the fat of the alcoholic fatty liver and the enhancement of absorption by the simultaneous presence of alcohol in the gastrointestinal tract.[807] All of these, however, fail to explain the enhancement of CCl$_4$ toxicity by a single dose of alcohol given hours before the CCl$_4$.[739] Even the attractive hypothesis[413,804] that ethanol, by inducing the microsomal metabolizing enzymes, potentiates CCl$_4$ toxicity by enhancing its conversion to a toxic metabolite seems somewhat belied by the demonstration that even a single dose of ethanol or a variety of other alcohols can also increase the toxicity.[739] At any rate there is no doubt that alcohol enhances the hepatotoxic effects of CCl$_4$. The nutritional status of the patient may also influence CCl$_4$ tox-

TABLE 17-12.   Hepatotoxic Agents to Which Household Exposure Is Known or Potential

AGENTS	EXPOSURE	LESION
Chlorinated hydrocarbons	Careless use, accidental "solvent sniffing"	Centrizonal necrosis, steatosis
Phosphorus (yellow)	Suicidal or accidental	Steatosis, periportal necrosis
Toxic chemicals as inadvertent contaminants of food:		
4 4'-Diaminodiphenylmethane	Contaminant of flour ("Epping jaundice")	Cholestatic jaundice
Hexachlorobenzene	Fungistatic added to wheat	Steatosis, necrosis, toxic porphyria
Chlorinated biphenyls	Contaminant of rice (Japan)	Steatosis, necrosis
Toxic foods of plant origin:		
Amanita phalloides and related species	Ingested as food in ignorance of toxicity	Centrizonal necrosis, steatosis
Cycad nut	Ingested as food in ignorance of toxicity	Necrosis, steatosis, cirrhosis, hepatocellular carcinoma
Senecio, heliotropium, crotolaria, and other plants that contain pyrrolidizine alkaloids	Ingested as additive to foods, as medicinal decoction, or as abortifacient	Centrizonal necrosis, veno-occlusive disease, congestive cirrhosis
Nutmeg	Ingested as abortifacient	Steatosis, midzonal necrosis
Mycotoxins Aflatoxins Ochratoxin Luteoskyrin	Present mainly in legumes and other foods of vegetable origin when climatic conditions permit	Steatosis, necrosis, cirrhosis, hepatocellular carcinoma

(Zimmerman HJ, Ishak KG: Hepatic injury due to drugs and other chemicals. In MacSween RNM, Anthony PP, Scheuer PJ [eds]: Pathology of the Liver, p 356. New York, Churchill Livingstone, 1979)

icity. In animals, starvation and high-fat diets increase the toxicity of CCl_4, whereas low-protein diets decrease it.[621]

The principal clinical manifestations of CCl_4 intoxication result from a combination of (1) general (including neurologic and gastrointestinal) toxic effects; (2) liver injury; and (3) renal injury.[269,335,803] The general toxic effect may be apparent within hours of exposure. Headache, dizziness, and confusion are usual, reflecting the anesthetic properties of CCl_4. Indeed a small proportion of deaths from CCl_4 poisoning are "anesthetic deaths."[335] Nausea, vomiting, diarrhea, and abdominal pain also occur during the first 24 hours. Severe abdominal pain and collapse occur in patients who have had large exposures.[269,335] The liver injury usually appears 2 to 4 days after intoxication (Fig. 17-18).[269,335,803] Jaundice and hepatic enlargement are usual. The histologic lesion in the liver is well developed when these signs appear. The renal injury is apparent at about the time the liver injury is detected but reaches its peak later and may dominate the clinical picture.[803] Azotemia, often accompanied by hypertension, is frequent.

Laboratory findings include neutrophilic leukocytosis, hemolytic anemia, and azotemia.[762] Urinary sediment abnormalities, which include hematuria and casts, reflect acute tubular necrosis.[762] Serum values of the aminotransferases can reach astronomical levels (>10,000 IU).[794]

Values for alkaline phosphatase are usually only slightly elevated. The prolonged prothrombin time reflects the usually depressed levels of plasma coagulation factors.

The chief histologic abnormalities are in the liver and kidney, but there are also changes in the lung, heart, pancreas, and brain.[269,335,485,762,807] The liver reveals centrolobular (zone 3) necrosis and some steatosis (see Fig. 17-7). The degree of steatosis is variable, presumably reflecting, at least in part, the effects of the often-associated alcoholism. Prominent ballooning of hepatocytes may precede the necrosis. Renal abnormalities include necrosis and fatty change of the tubules with heme and cellular casts.[762]

The lungs of patients with fatal cases show edema, an alveolar pseudomembrane, and thickened, fibrotic alveolar walls with epithelial proliferation. These changes may reflect renal failure rather than the pulmonary toxicity of CCl_4.[745] Myocardial degeneration also may be a complication of renal failure or of its treatment, or may reflect a toxic effect of CCl_4 on the myocardium. Focal pancreatitis is a frequent finding.[762]

The prognosis after CCl_4 intoxication is difficult to assess. Prior to the modern era of hemodialysis treatment for renal failure, the case-fatality rate appeared to be approximately 25%.[269,335] More recent figures appear to be lower.[167] Most patients who die of liver failure do so within

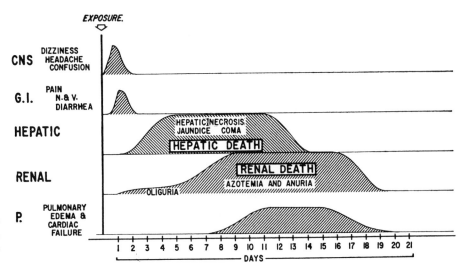

Fig. 17-18. Clinical sequence in CCl₄ poisoning. (Zimmerman HJ: Ann NY Acad Sci 104:954, 1963)

the first week.[335,803] Renal failure appears to be responsible for about 75% of the fatal cases,[335] but the renal deaths usually occur during the second week (see Fig. 17-18). Patients who survive acute injury generally recover completely with no residual liver damage, although instances of residual hepatic scarring have been described.[363] There is no specific treatment for CCl₄ intoxication other than dialysis for the renal failure. Corticosteroids are probably of no benefit.

Other chloroalkanes (*e.g.,* trichloroethylene)[20,762] may produce a similar syndrome and histologic changes. The relative toxicity of haloalkanes and the likelihood of their producing hepatic injury depends on the energy of the carbon–halogen bond of the respective compound and the relative ease of formation of the active metabolite.[581,680,807]

Mushroom and Phosphorus Poisoning

A somewhat similar clinical syndrome to that of CCl₄ poisoning occurs from ingestion of the hepatotoxic mushroom (*Amanita phalloides* and related species) or yellow phosphorus.[151,171,273,607,627] Mushroom poisoning leads to very prominent steatosis and some centrizonal necrosis. Yellow phosphorus poisoning may lead only or mainly to steatosis, at first in the periphery of the lobule and then throughout. Necrosis may, however, be present and is also predominantly in the peripheral zone.

Yellow phosphorus poisoning is characterized by more severe gastrointestinal symptoms and shock than is CCl₄ poisoning, and by phosphorescence and garlic-like odor of excreta and vomitus. The fully developed clinical picture is that of fulminant hepatic and renal failure.[151,607,627,807]

Mushroom poisoning presents as severe diarrhea, followed by amelioration and subsequently by severe hepatic and renal failure.[171,273,622] The mortality rates of yellow phosphorus[151,607,627] and mushroom[273,622] poisoning are higher (>50%) than that of CCl₄ intoxication (10%–25%).[806]

Acetaminophen Poisoning

Acetaminophen (Paracetamol) is a widely used analgesic-antipyretic that has few side-effects when taken in the usual therapeutic dose. When taken in large doses, it becomes a potent hepatotoxin, producing centrizonal (zone 3) necrosis.[55,809] Indeed, acetaminophen overdose has become one of the most popular means of attempting suicide and the most prominent cause of severe hepatic necrosis in the United Kingdom.[264,697] The incidence of suicidal overdose in the United States, fortunately, has lagged behind; but, by now, appreciable numbers of cases of acetaminophen-induced hepatic necrosis have been recorded in this country.[55] The phenomenon also has spread to other countries,[55,76,697] but the number of cases is small.[697]

The vast majority of instances of acetaminophen-related hepatic injury have resulted from large single overdoses, taken in an attempt at suicide.[55,108,133,264,567,568,569,573,623] A few cases have involved accidental rather than suicidal, single overdoses,[55,133] or apparently have resulted from large single or multiple doses taken with therapeutic intent.[28,651,766] The characteristic centrizonal (zone 3) necrosis of acetaminophen appears to be produced by an electrophilic metabolite of the drug (? quinoneimine) that binds covalently to tissue macromolecules.[473,474,476] The centrizonal location of the necrosis is a consequence of the location in that zone of the MFO, the enzyme system responsible for converting acetaminophen to its active metabolite.[474] Normally, the amount of metabolite formed is small, since the therapeutic dose of acetaminophen taken is not large and its metabolic fate is largely in the direction of conjugation with glucuronate and sulfate (Fig. 17-19). The small amounts of active metabolite formed

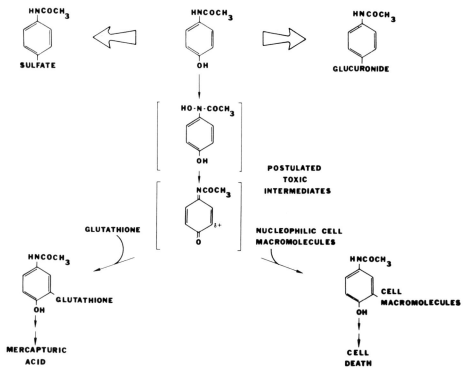

Fig. 17-19. Schema of acetaminophen metabolism. Increased dose and blood levels provide basis for increased amounts of active metabolite. Increased activity of mixed function oxidase leads to higher proportion of active metabolite. Depletion of glutathione stores leads to higher proportion of active metabolite that can bind to cytoplasmic proteins and produce necrosis. (Zimmerman HJ: Hepatotoxicity. New York, Appleton-Century-Crofts, 1978)

are readily detoxified by reacting with glutathione to form mercapturic acid.[476] Hepatic necrosis occurs only when the amount of active metabolite produced exceeds the binding capacity of the glutathione. This occurs when the dose of drug taken is large. Furthermore, the adverse effects of a large dose or even of smaller doses are enhanced by factors that increase the fraction of drug converted to an active metabolite or that decrease the availability of glutathione. The likelihood, accordingly, that a dose of acetaminophen will lead to hepatic injury depends on the quantity ingested, on the activity of the MFO, and on the adequacy of glutathione stores (see Fig. 17-19).

Doses have exceeded 15 g in about 80% of fatal cases and have ranged from 6 g to 15 g in the remaining instances of poisoning from a single overdose.[264] The reported relationship between dose and severity of injury, however, is far from exact. Quantities as small as 15 g have led to fatal hepatic disease, and those as large as 75 g have been followed by recovery.[807] Efforts to determine the dose, however, have been thwarted by inexact information from patients and the obscuring effects of early vomiting.

Blood levels of drug measured between 4 and 10 hours after ingestion are useful clues to the quantity of drug taken and helpful in predicting the probable severity of subsequent hepatic injury.[567-569] Patients with blood levels above 300 μg/ml at 4 hours are likely to develop overt, often severe injury, while those with values below 150 μg/ml are not.[567] Indeed, Prescott and co-workers[568] have developed a nomogram based on these observations (Fig. 17-20).

The activity of the MFO governs the rate of production of the active metabolite and affects the toxicity of the acetaminophen. Stimulation with phenobarbital enhances and inhibition with piperonyl butoxide decreases the hepatotoxicity of the drug for experimental animals.[474] The clinical parallel is seen in the greater toxicity of acetaminophen for patients who had been taking other drugs or alcohol, which presumably had, each, induced the MFO.[792] Although most workers accept the view that covalent binding leads to necrosis, peroxidative injury also has been proposed as the mechanism[196] generated by the biotransformation of the acetaminophen also. In either event, the rate and degree of metabolic conversion of

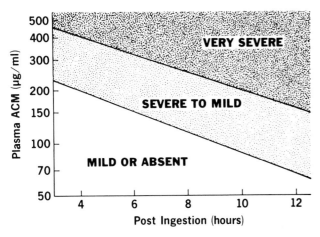

Fig. 17-20. Nomogram that can be used as a basis for treatment of acetaminophen (*ACM*) overdose. Levels of ACM in blood drawn between 4 and 10 hours after ingestion that fall in the lowest zone indicate that liver damage will be mild or will not eventuate, and that specific therapeutic measures are not needed. Blood levels in the uppermost zone are predictive of serious liver damage and mandate treatment with acetyl cysteine or related agents. Values in the intermediate zone offer less conclusive prediction but warrant similar treatment. (Zimmerman HJ: Hepatotoxicity. New York, Appleton-Century-Crofts, 1978)

acetaminophen to an active metabolite is a critical factor in the toxicity of acetaminophen.[18]

Tissue levels of glutathione are critical to the toxic effects of the drug. Acetaminophen leads to hepatic necrosis in experimental animals only when doses are large enough to lead to depletion of hepatic glutathione by more than 70% or when the glutathione levels have been depleted by diethyl maleate[476] or by fasting.[455] The parallel in humans is seen when doses smaller than the usual toxic ones are hepatotoxic in patients with alcoholism or another disease that may lead to depletion of glutathione.[809]

Clinical Features. The clinical course consists of the three phases seen with a number of other hepatotoxins (see Table 17-10). The first consists of acute gastrointestinal symptoms. Anorexia, nausea, and vomiting begin within several hours of ingestion and may be accompanied by vascular collapse. The second phase, characterized by abatement of the nausea and vomiting and by a relative well-being, continues for approximately 2 days. During this apparent subsidence of severity, biochemical evidences of hepatic injury appear, and there may be pain and tenderness in the right hypochondrium. Oliguria is usual. The third phase, that of overt hepatic damage, becomes clinically apparent by 3 to 5 days after ingestion, with the appearance of jaundice. Renal failure may occur.[108]

Severe hepatic failure, as evidenced by hemorrhagic phenomena and hepatic encephalopathy, has occured in up to one third of patients who develop jaundice in some series[108] and in a very small proportion of others. Early treatment with substitutes for, or that help replenish, glutathione has been effective in reducing the severity of hepatic injury from acetaminophen overdose.[565–569,623]

Biochemical Changes. Increased levels of serum enzymes, hyperbilirubinemia, and abnormal plasma levels of coagulation factors are evidence of hepatic necrosis.[108,264,565,569] Values for SGOT and SGPT are very high, reaching levels up to 20,000 IU. Despite the evident severity of injury in some patients, as reflected in the histology and the very high levels of serum aminotransferases, the bilirubin level is often only slightly elevated. Indeed, in one report,[108] serum levels needed only to exceed 4 mg/dl to indicate an adverse prognostic sign. Clotting abnormalities may be severe and the one-stage prothrombin time has appeared to be a useful prognostic indicator.[108]

Histologic Features. Histologic changes in the liver consist of zonal necrosis and sinusoidal congestion in zone 3. The kidney may show necrosis of proximal and distal tubules. There may be myocardial necrosis.[807]

Prognosis. The outlook for survival from the hepatic injury due to acetaminophen overdose is similar to that of acute hepatic necrosis induced by other drugs. Early reports described a case-fatality rate of 6% to 25% of patients with acetaminophen-induced hepatic disease. Today it is considerably lower, presumably in part because a greater range of severity has now been recorded.[623] Furthermore, the effective treatment that is now available for acetaminophen poisoning can prevent serious hepatic injury. When preventive treatment has not been given in time (first 16 hours) and hepatic necrosis has occurred, the prognosis depends on the severity of the liver failure. One report has noted that patients whose prothrombin time is more than twice the control value, whose bilirubin levels exceed 4 mg/dl, and who show any evidence of encephalopathy, appear to have a mortality rate above 30%.[108]

Treatment. Treatment with acetylcysteine during the first 16 hours after intake of the acetaminophen can minimize hepatic injury and can prevent fatal hepatic disease. While administration after that time seems innocuous, there is no evidence of benefit. The mechanisms of action of acetylcysteine appears to be enhancement of synthesis of glutathione.[566] Acetylcysteine is given orally in the United States and as an intravenous preparation in the United Kingdom. (The intravenous preparation is not approved for use in the United States and Canada.[623]

If possible, blood should be drawn for measure of the level of acetaminophen during the predictive period of 4 to 12 hours, before treatment has been started. If after the first dose or two the level is found to have been clearly predictive of no injury, the treatment can be stopped. If the level is borderline or predictive of toxicity, treatment should be completed.

The demonstration that cimetidine inhibits the MFO and, accordingly, the toxicity of acetaminophen in animals has led to the suggestion that it may be of use in the treatment of acetaminophen overdose in humans.[480] Cimetidine, however, would have to be given at least as early as acetylcysteine is now given, and the current results with acetylcysteine are excellent. Furthermore, cimetidine blocks the nontoxifying conjugation pathway as well as the toxifying cytochrome P-450 pathway, thus threatening to vitiate potential benefit[18]; nevertheless, the issue remains open.[482]

Supportive treatment and treatment of hepatic failure in patients who came to attention too late for acetylcysteine to be helpful are similar to that for other forms of fulminant hepatic failure.

Hepatotoxic Reaction as a Therapeutic Misadventure. There have also been reported instances of hepatic injury from therapeutic use of acetaminophen.[28,55,651,766,809] In some instances multiple doses taken with therapeutic intent in a sufficiently short period have reached a total dose of 10 g/day, one sufficiently large to produce hepatic injury.[55,651,809] Smaller total doses ranging from 2.6 g to 10 g/day also appear able to lead to hepatic injury in patients with enhanced susceptibility.[28,55,651,809] There have been a number of instances of alcoholic patients who have sustained hepatic necrosis after taking the drug in such daily doses for periods ranging from 1 day to several weeks.[55,453,651] Alcoholics seem to have enhanced susceptibility to large single and to multiple therapeutic doses[651] as a presumed[55,651,711] consequence of induction of the MFO by ethanol and, presumably, depletion of glutathione associated with their disease and life-style.[651]

Alcoholic patients have presented with hepatic injury after repetitive doses of acetaminophen in a short period for dental pain, the pain of pancreatitis, or headache, leading to daily doses ranging from 2.5 g to 10 g/day. The clinical picture in some of these patients has been consistent with characteristic alcoholic liver disease or pancreatitis, only to have the extraordinarily elevated aminotransferase levels serve as a clue to the complicating acetaminophen hepatotoxicity. Indeed, since alcoholic liver disease rarely leads to SGOT levels that are more than eightfold the upper limit of normal and to even lower SGPT levels, the appearance of very high levels of the aminotransferases is a clue to other etiology. Indeed, a syndrome of alcoholism-associated acetaminophen hepatic injury has emerged,[651] characterized by SGOT levels that are 40 to 500 times or more the normal. We are aware of at least 25 published examples of the acetaminophen hepatotoxicity[651] occurring as a therapeutic misadventure in the alcoholic.

Other authors, however, have not concurred with the impression that alcohol intake enhances the toxicity[47] of acetaminophen or have dismissed the relevance of alcoholic intake to the gravity or management of acetaminophen toxicity.[623] Experimental studies, however, have provided support for the clinical inference of enhancement of acetaminophen hepatotoxicity by alcohol. Chronic administration of ethanol to experimental animals enhances the toxicity of acetaminophen.[630] That this relates to the effect of alcohol on the biotransformation of acetaminophen is supported by the observation that administration of a dose of ethanol concurrently with the acetaminophen actually decreases the hepatotoxic effects of the drug.[631] The alcohol apparently protects by competing for metabolism of the acetaminophen. When given long enough before (over 18 hours), alcohol enhances acetaminophen toxicity.[631,711]

Instances of nonalcoholics who have developed acute hepatic injury from daily intake of 5 g to 8 g and even from daily doses as low as 3.9 g also have been reported.[28,809] The circumstances in patients in whom hepatic injury has developed as a result of therapeutic misadventure and, therefore, that may reflect factors able to enhance susceptibility to adverse effects of multiple therapeutic doses[28,766,809] include wasting disease and malnutrition that might lead to glutathione depletion. Underlying hepatic disease also has been invoked as the factor predisposing patients with infectious mononucleosis to hepatic injury from acetaminophen.[614] The view that underlying hepatic disease enhances the toxicity of acetaminophen has been challenged by Benson.[47]

Acetaminophen in usual therapeutic doses, over a prolonged interval, has been reported to produce chronic liver damage.[64,809] Bonkowsky and co-workers have described chronic hepatic necrosis with inflammation, collapse, and fibrosis in a man who had taken 4 g/day of acetaminophen for a year.[64] Following discontinuation of the drug, a fivefold elevation of aminotransferases returned to near normal. He subsequently resumed taking acetaminophen, and signs of liver damage reappeared. Later, when he had stopped the drug and had only minimal elevation of aminotransferases, a challenge dose (1325 mg) was given and there was a rise in aminotransferases within 12 to 18 hours. In another patient with underlying chronic active hepatitis, therapeutic doses of acetaminophen appeared to cause an exacerbation of the disease.[340]

HEPATIC INJURY CAUSED BY MEDICINAL AGENTS

There is an interesting and useful relationship between the pharmacologic category of a drug and the type of hepatic injury that it can produce. General anesthetics, most drugs used to treat rheumatic and musculoskeletal disease, antidepressants, and anticonvulsants, in general, produce cytotoxic injury. "Tranquilizing" drugs and some antithyroid and antidiabetic agents produce predominantly cholestatic injury. Other antithyroid and antidiabetic agents lead to cytotoxic injury. Anabolic and contraceptive steroids also produce cholestasis, albeit of a somewhat different category than do the "tranquilizers." The diversity of drugs employed in cardiovascular and microbial disease precludes such generalizations.[807]

Anesthetic Drugs

Volatile anesthetics that injure the liver produce the cytotoxic type of injury. None lead to cholestasis. Those that have seen clinical use fall into three groups (Table 17-13):

1. Known *intrinsic* hepatotoxins
2. Agents that produce *idiosyncratic* hepatic injury
3. Agents that do not injure the liver

Known hepatotoxins include chloroform, trichloroethylene, divinyl ether, and tribromomethanol. All can produce hepatic necrosis in experimental animals. None is used as an anesthetic today; and, accordingly, their toxicity is largely of historical and toxicologic interest. The toxicity of trichloroethylene, however, remains relevant, since it has caused hepatic injury as a drug of abuse[20] and as an occupational hazard.[421]

Multihalogenated Hydrocarbons

Idiosyncratic hepatic injury is produced by halothane, methoxyflurane, fluroxene, and enflurane. These multihalogenated hydrocarbons, introduced into clinical use about 3 decades ago, have experienced enormously wide use with a generally safe record. By now, however, these agents, especially halothane and methoxyflurane, have been incriminated in a large number of instances of hepatic injury.[65,316,317,343,366,419,420,489,492,541,544,736] Indeed, by

1976, at least 900 cases of "halothane jaundice" had been reported in the English literature.[807]

Halothane. Most observers today agree that halothane-induced hepatic injury is a real phenomenon, albeit of low incidence.[100,366,419,420,489,492] Dissenters remain,[676] and the issue (at least as it regards the incidence of adverse reactors) is still somewhat controversial.[634,676]

The incidence of hepatic injury is uncertain. Carney and Van Dyke[100] have estimated that halothane anesthesia probably causes fatal or non-fatal hepatitis in 1 of 9,000 recipients and fatal hepatitis alone in 1 of 40,000 recipients. Incidence is greater after multiple exposures than after a single one. Figures as high as 1 in 10,000 on first exposure and almost 1 in 1,000 on multiple exposure have been estimated.[807] Indeed, very high figures, in excess of 1% have been recorded among women treated for carcinoma of the cervix with repeated radium implantation under halothane anesthesia.[132,308,742,793] Despite the low incidence, the widespread use of halothane and the severity of halothane-induced injury has made it an important cause of acute hepatic failure during the past 2 decades.[740,741,806] Liver damage after occupational exposure to halothane[40,341,365] and in individuals who have "sniffed" halothane[347,366] has been reported. Halothane-induced liver injury also has been produced by halothane contamination of anesthesia machines in situations in which halothane had been purposely avoided.[755]

Susceptibility to hepatic injury from halothane appears to be somewhat greater in females, to be enhanced by advancing age and obesity, and to be low in children.[65,100,120,247,492,544,556] Many of the patients had had fever, with or without eosinophilia, after a previous exposure to halothane.[366,373,420,544,662]

TABLE 17-13.   Hepatotoxic Potential of General Anesthetics

HEPATOTOXICITY FOR HUMANS	AGENT*	LESION	
		Steatosis	**Necrosis**
Intrinsic hepatotoxins	Chloroform	+	CZ
	Trichlorethylene	+	CZ
	Vinyl ether	±	CZ
	Tribromoethyl alcohol	±	CZ
Agents hepatotoxic only as idiosyncratic reactions	Halothane	±	CZ, M, D
	Methoxyflurane	+	CZ, M, D
	Fluroxene	−	CZ
	Enflurane	−	CZ, M, D
	Isoflurane	?**	?**
Agents that seem virtually free of potential for significant hepatic injury in humans	Cyclopropane	−	−
	Ether	−	−
	Nitrous oxide	−	−

 * Distinction between weaker hepatotoxins in group I and agents in group II may be quite arbitrary.
 ** No injury reported in literature. Cases reported to FDA and AFIP remain to be fully established.
 (CZ, centrizonal; M, massive; D, diffuse and hepatitis-like; +, present; ±, variable and usually slight; −, absent.)
 (Data from references 411 and 807)

The syndrome of halothane-induced hepatic injury includes features that appear to reflect hypersensitivity in more than half of the reported cases, followed or accompanied by manifestations of severe hepatic disease.[247,366,373,420,492,807] Onset is usually abrupt with fever in approximately 90%, a diffuse rash in 10%, myalgia in 20%, and anorexia and nausea in about 50% of patients. The onset of symptoms may be as early as 3 days or as late as 15 days after initial exposure.[373] Chills may occur. Right upper quadrant abdominal discomfort is usual. Hepatomegaly is usually present. Jaundice appears within 3 to 4 days after onset of fever. The interval between anesthesia and onset of illness is shorter (average 3 days) in patients who have had prior exposure to halothane than in those who develop hepatic damage after the first exposure (average 6 days).[247,316,317,366,507,662,807] Fatal cases are characterized by progressively deepening jaundice, prolonged prothrombin times with hemorrhagic phenomena, ascites, and coma.[662] Serum bilirubin levels correlate somewhat with prognosis.[65,373,492] Marked prolongation of the prothrombin time is the most important adverse prognostic sign.

The hepatic injury is cytotoxic, consisting of necrosis and slight steatosis. There are some differences in the literature regarding the type of necrosis. A spectrum of histologic patterns of halothane-induced injury has been reported ranging from multifocal spotty necrosis resembling viral hepatitis to massive necrosis.[46] Massive necrosis, zonal necrosis, or diffuse hepatitis-like degeneration and necrosis have each been reported. Zone 3 (centrizonal) necrosis, resembling that of CCl_4 is the most characteristic lesion (see Fig. 17-7).[489,544] We have also seen instances of peripheral zone necrosis.[46] Progression of severity of injury from focal to massive necrosis appears to be related to multiple exposures to halothane and inversely to the duration of the intervals between exposures.[46] The type of surgical procedure does not appear to affect the type or severity of liver injury.[46,507]

Sections obtained by liver biopsy in mildly or moderately severe illness, however, may reveal diffuse acidophilic degenerations, sinusoidal ("free") acidophilic bodies, and mononuclear infiltration, changes that are said to be indistinguishable from those of viral hepatitis.[363] Even in moderately severe injury, however, liver biopsy sections may show zonal injury.[46,544] Furthermore, the sharp demarcation of the zones of necrosis that is often seen in halothane injury is a feature that is of infrequent occurrence in fatal cases of viral hepatitis. In general, inflammatory infiltration is much less prominent in halothane-induced injury than in viral hepatitis,[46,544,641] although the liver from some patients shows a prominent, eosinophilic inflammatory response. An instance of granulomatous inflammation in a patient with fatal halothane jaundice has been reported.[158] In view of its singularity, the granulomatous lesion was probably unrelated to the halothane injury.

Laboratory studies reflect the severe parenchymal injury. Values of aminotransferases are very high (elevated 10- to 200-fold). Alkaline phosphatase levels are normal or only moderately elevated (less than 3-fold) in most patients but may be higher in a few. Bilirubin levels may reach very high values, especially in patients with a fatal outcome. Hypoprothrombinemia is common and may be profound. Leukocytosis is usual, and eosinophilia occurs in over 50% of recognized cases.[247,366,373,419,420,492,586,736,807]

Prognosis of clinically recognized instances of patients with halothane-induced liver injury who become jaundiced has been grave, with estimates of 20% to 60% mortality.[100,120,316,317,419,420,492,586,807] Milder instances, however, probably go unrecognized. Cirrhosis has been reported to follow repeated occupational (anesthesiologist) exposures.[40,365] An instance of "chronic active hepatitis" has been attributed to halothane-induced injury.[725] It should be noted that follow-up of this patient was only for 3 months. Even extensive bridging hepatic necrosis found on liver biopsy in patients with halothane hepatitis usually completely subsides with no residual damage if the patient survives the acute illness.[468]

The mechanism of injury in halothane-induced injury, at least in part, appears to be the result of hypersensitivity to halothane or a metabolite[87,100,366,662,807] or to halothane-triggered released or altered hepatocyte membrane proteins.[507] The importance of multiple exposures, the prevalence of fever and eosinophilia, the demonstration of sensitivity to planned or inadvertent exposure, and reports of eosinophilic aggregates in the liver all support this view.[366,586,662] Some support also derives from experimental studies.[120,507,753] The zonal necrosis of halothane toxicity, however, resembles the lesion of known toxins, such as CCl_4,[544] but not that of apparent hypersensitivity-dependent hepatic injury. It supports the view that a toxic metabolite formed in zone 3 contributes to or is responsible for the hepatic injury.[120,804] Experimental studies support this possibility.[87,120,139,246,596,677,702] It has been proposed that free radicals are formed from halothane by cytochrome P-450 and that lipid peroxidation by these radicals or covalent binding of them to cell molecules, is at least one mechanism of injury.[120,139] Metabolism of halothane may occur by both oxidative (aerobic) and reductive (anaerobic) pathways.[87,139,736] It is the reductive pathway that appears to lead to hepatotoxic metabolites.

Vergani and colleagues reported circulating antibodies to a cell membrane antigen that was obtained from rabbits pretreated with halothane in 9 of 11 patients with severe halothane-induced liver injury.[756] Sera from these patients also demonstrated cytotoxicity mediated by normal lymphocytes toward hepatocytes from rabbits pretreated with halothane.

In summary, the available data suggest that the mechanism is idiosyncrasy. In some patients the idiosyncrasy is metabolic (i.e., due to a toxic metabolite). In others, it is immunologic.[120] In some patients, perhaps both are involved.

Farrell and colleagues have reported that patients with halothane-induced liver injury may have a genetic susceptibility to develop the injury.[198] Lymphocytes from 11 patients with halothane-induced liver injury showed an increase in cytotoxicity when incubated with metabolites of phenytoin, suggesting the lymphocytes were highly susceptible to damage from electrophilic drug intermediates. Healthy controls and patients with other types of liver disease did not differ in having a low percentage of the cell susceptibility factor. Family studies revealed an increased incidence of the cell susceptibility factor in family members. Further studies will be needed to confirm the observation and identify the exact nature of the presumed abnormality.

The management of halothane-induced liver injury is directed toward support of the patients and awareness and prevention of complications such as hepatic encephalopathy, bleeding, and bacterial infections. Corticosteroids have been often used as treatment, but a role for these agents is not established.

Methoxyflurane. Methoxyflurane is a halogenated ether closely resembling halothane in chemical structure and anesthetic properties. This agent also may produce hepatic necrosis resembling that following exposure to halothane.[78,120,343,351] The hepatic necrosis from methoxyflurane is also usually in zone 3 (centrizonal), although it may be massive. The syndrome also is similar to that observed in halothane-induced injury, differing only in the propensity for methoxyflurane to produce, in addition, renal injury, characterized by azotemia and a long-persisting defect in concentrating capacity. In addition, there is oxaluria and deposition of calcium oxalate crystals in the proximal tubules.[217] No apparent relation exists between the nephropathy and liver damage. The renal damage presumably results from the effects of fluride metabolites on the kidney. There are reports of cross-sensitivity between methoxyflurane and halothane.[344,363] Fluroxene also has been reported to cause zone 3 (centrizonal) necrosis.[598]

Enflurane. Enflurane is another halogenated anesthetic that occasionally is associated with clinical, biochemical, and histologic features similar to those found with halothane and methoxyflurane.[144,370,412] The incidence of enflurane-induced hepatic injury appears to be less than that from halothane, possibly because a smaller percentage of the drug undergoes transformation.[328] Prior exposure to another haloalkane anesthetic may increase the risk of enflurane administration.[412]

Isoflurane. A newer halogenated anesthetic, isoflurane, remains intact with only 0 to 1% metabolism, and instances of isoflurane hepatotoxicity have yet to be reported in the literature.

Cyclopropane, Divinyl Ether, and Diethyl Ether

These agents are essentially nonhepatotoxic anesthetics that have been extensively employed. In our opinion, there is no convincing evidence relating hepatic injury in humans to any of these anesthetics. Minor liver function abnormalities reported after the use of these agents is most likely secondary to circulatory changes or other intraoperative and postoperative problems.

Psychotropic Drugs and Anticonvulsants

There is a striking and useful correlation between the form of injury and the therapeutic category of the drugs in this group (Table 17-14). Chlorpromazine and other tranquilizers and antipsychotics including haloperidal[807] produce mainly a cholestatic lesion. Antidepressant hydrazines and the anticonvulsants cause cytotoxic injury. Hepatic injury caused by tricyclic antidepressants has been less consistent in their manifestations. A tetracyclic antidepressant has been reported to cause hepatotoxicity that appeared 3 weeks after a 63-year-old man began receiving the drug.[107] Liver biopsy showed portal inflammation and expansion, presumably cholestatic injury. All the biochemical abnormalities resolved when the drug was removed.

Despite its widespread use, diazepam has been remarkably free of hepatotoxicity. There is one report of a mild hepatitis that developed in a patient receiving diazepam and isoniazid and resolved when the drugs were withdrawn.[721] The hepatic abnormalities reappeared during a diazepam challenge. No evidence of hepatic injury was found during an isoniazid challenge. Haloperidol-associated cholestasis has been reported.[807]

Tranquilizers

Chlorpromazine. Jaundice occurs in 0.5% to 1% of all patients who receive chlorpromazine.[174,722,803,807] A period of 1 to 5 weeks of drug administration precedes the development of jaundice in 90% of cases.[803] Readministration of small doses leads to prompt recurrence of hepatic dysfunction or jaundice in approximately half of patients.[295,296,661]

Prodromal symptoms, which occur in 75% of patients, may include fever, chilliness, and abdominal distress. Eosinophilia occurs in about 60% of cases.[803]

The hepatic injury is primarily cholestatic (hepatocanalicular) in type. Severe itching is common. Serum alkaline phosphatase values are over threefold elevated and aminotransferase values are only slightly or moderately elevated (50 to 300 IU). Liver biopsy in most patients reveals prominent cholestasis in zone 3 with only mild hepatocyte degeneration and necrosis, and occasional sinusoidal acidophilic bodies (see Fig. 17-9).[323,363,558,803] The inflammatory response is mainly in the portal area, is usually rich in eosinophils,[641] and is prominent only early in the course of the illness. A small proportion of patients develop hepatic necrosis and high amino-transferase levels, as well as prominent cholestasis and high alkaline phosphatase levels (mixed hepatocanalicular jaundice).[802,803]

TABLE 17-14.   Hepatic Injury Produced by Various Psychotropic and Anticonvulsant Drugs

DRUG	TYPE OF INJURY	DRUG	TYPE OF INJURY
Tranquilizers		Isocarboxid (Marplan)	
Phenothiazines*		Nialamide (Niamid)	H-Cell
Chlorpromazine (Thorazine)†		Phenelzine (Nardil)	
Carphenazine (Proketazine)		Pheniprazine (Catron)	
Fluphenazine (Prolixin)		Phenoxypropazine	
Laevopromazine (Veratril)		(Drazine)	
Mepazine (Pacatal)		Pivaloylbenzylhydrazine	H-Cell
Perphenazine (Trilafon)		(Tersavid)	
Prochlorperazine (Compazine)	Ch or M	Mebanazine (Actomal)	
Promazine (Sparine)‡		Non-hydrazines	
Promethazine (Phenergan)§		Tranylcypromine	
Thiopropazate (Dartal)‡		(Parnate)‖	
Thioproperazine (Majepti)§		Tricyclic antidepressants*‖	
Thioridazine (Mellaril)		Amitryptiline (Elavil)	
Triflupromazine (Vesprin)		Desipramine (Pertofran)	
Thioxanthenes*‖		Doxepin (Sinequan)	Ch or M
Chlorprothixene (Taractan)		Imipramine (Tofranil)	
Chlorpenthixol (Sordinol)	Ch or M	Nortriptyline (Aventyl)	
Thiothixene (Navene)		Protriptyline (Vinactyl)	
Butyrophenones*‖		Iprindole (Prondol)	
Haloperidol (Haldol)	Ch or M		
Benzodiazepines*‖¶		Anticonvulsants	
Chloridiazepoxide		Phenacemide (Phenurone)	
(Librium)*‖¶	Ch or M	Trimethadione (Tridione)	
Diazepam (Valium)*‖		Mephenytoin (Mesantoin)	H-Cell-M#
Oxazepam (Serax)**		Paramethadione (Paradione)	
		Phenytoin (Dilantin)	
Antidepressants		Phenobarbital	H-Cell
Monoamine oxidase inhibitors		Valproate (Depekene)	
Hydrazines			
Iproniazid (Marsilid)			

* Hepatic injury produced by agents in this group is usually cholestatic.
† Rare instances of frank hepatic necrosis (Zelman[802]).
‡ 0 = No reports for injury according to review of Rees[588] and very few to our knowledge.
§ 0 = No cases of hepatic injury reported.
‖ Too few cases for clear picture.
¶ Rare instances of hepatocellular injury in recipients of chlordiazepoxide plus other drugs (Ebert and Shader[174]).
# Marked diffuse inflammation resembles lesion in viral hepatitis or infectious mononucleosis.
** Oxazepam has been reported to cause hepatic tumors and peliosis in rats.[807]
(Ch, cholestatic injury; consists mainly of bilirubin casts in canaliculi usually with portal inflammatory infiltrate and with or without mild parenchymal injury. H-Cell, hepatocellular lesion consists mainly of necrosis with or without inflammation. M, mixed)
(Data from references 1, 174, 363, 521, 562, 588, 635, 663, 722, 802, and 807)

The prognosis of chlorpromazine jaundice is generally good. Two thirds of the patients recover within 8 weeks. Most of the remainder require 2 to 12 months to return to normal.[803] There have been a number of reported instances of a prolonged cholestatic syndrome, with clinical and biochemical (marked hypercholesterolemia, xanthomatosis) and, in some patients, even histologic features that have resembled those of primary biliary cirrhosis (see Fig. 17-18).[310,323,363,383,405,498,579,764] Several of the patients have died.[498,764] Histologic changes interpreted as chronic active hepatitis were reported in a 59-year-old man 8 months after an overdose of chlorpromazine.[625] It is not clear that the histologic pattern in this case is different from those other reported cases of chronic or slowly resolving liver disease attributable to chlorpromazine. Furthermore the biochemical features resembled those of primary biliary cirrhosis rather than chronic active hepatitis.

Clinical features of chlorpromazine-induced jaundice and the prompt recurrence of hepatic abnormality in many of those given a "challenge" dose suggest that hypersensitivity is responsible for the hepatic injury.[804] There is considerable evidence, however, that the mechanism of injury also involves a toxic effect of the chlorpromazine on the liver.[69,184] It does produce a dose-related enzyme release from suspensions of Chang liver cells[163] and of rat hepatocytes[812] and from liver slices,[165] and inhibits bile salt independent bile flow in monkeys, and perfused rat livers.[69,184,612,807] The drug, and its derivatives, inhibits membrane Na^+,K^+-ATPase and alters membrane fluidity.[632] In addition, chlorpromazine forms free radicals on exposure to light, capable of binding to cellular components.[665] The manner in which intrinsic toxicity and hypersensitivity interact to produce the clinical cholestatic syndrome is not clear.

Other phenothiazines and related tranquilizers that produce hepatic injury are listed in Table 17-14. In general, the clinical and histologic features appear to resemble those of chlorpromazine.

Antidepressants

Iproniazid and Other Hydrazine Derivatives. Amine oxidase inhibitors that are hydrazine derivatives can produce hepatic injury in susceptible persons (see Table 17-14).[363,558,663,807] Their use was estimated by Rosenblum and co-workers[615] to produce jaundice in approximately 1% of recipients. Onset was insidious with anorexia, malaise, fatigability, and jaundice, the illness usually beginning 1 to 6 months after starting the drug. Biochemical, histologic, and clinical features indicated hepatocellular injury. The mortality rate was about 15%.[363,615,663]

The liver showed extensive, diffuse parenchymal degeneration and necrosis.[558,615,663,803] In some instances, there was centrilobular predominance. Cases of massive necrosis resembled the lesion of fatal viral hepatitis,[363] albeit the inflammatory response was usually sparse.

The suggestion of Rosenblum and co-workers[615] that the mechanism for the hepatic injury is the production of hepatotoxic metabolites of iproniazid has found support in the experimental studies of Mitchell and co-workers.[473–475] Presumably, the responsible metabolites are formed or accumulate in greater amounts in susceptible persons.

Other Antidepressants. Several antidepressants that are *not* hydrazine derivatives have been reported to produce jaundice. The jaundice produced by one of them (tranylcypromine) also is hepatocellular like that of the hydrazine derivatives.[25,807] That induced by the tricyclic antidepressants[670,807] may apparently be either cholestatic or cytotoxic and remains to be further evaluated. The number of cases available for analysis, however, has been small. A tetracyclic antidepressant, trazodone, has been incriminated in four instances of hepatic injury, apparently cholestatic or undefined.[107,423,660]

Anticonvulsants

Several anticonvulsant agents have led to "toxic hepatitis" (see Table 17-14).

Phenytoin. The incidence of jaundice in recipients of phenytoin (Dilantin) appears to be much lower.[807] The drug, however, is very widely used and by now, the number of reported cases of hepatic injury approaches 100. Most patients developing phenytoin hepatitis are adults. Despite widespread use of the drug in children, reports of adverse hepatic reactions are rare. In reviewing the reported cases there does appear to be an increased female susceptibility. The hepatic damage is mainly cytotoxic, as revealed by parenchymal necrosis, high aminotransferase values, and poor prognosis.[1,149,170,272,367,397,494,527] The characteristically high alkaline phosphatase values led one report[443] to describe the lesion as cholestatic. In another report, cholestatic jaundice was attributed to phenytoin in a 64-year-old woman who had used the drug for more than 40 years![720] The hepatic injury resolved when the drug was withdrawn and recurred on rechallenge. The usual hepatic injury is of the mixed hepatocellular type.

The liver shows diffuse degeneration, multifocal necrosis, and multiple acidophilic bodies accompanied by a rich inflammatory[272,397] response. The latter often includes clusters of eosinophils or lymphocytes and, at times, focal aggregates of hyperplastic Kupffer cells having a granulomatoid appearance. Frank granulomas have been described.[113,494] The hepatic lesion, with lymphocyte "beading" in sinusoids, granulomatoid changes, and frequent hepatocyte mitosis, may resemble that of infectious mononucleosis (see Fig. 17-10). In some instances, however, severe generalized hypersensitivity rather than hepatic failure *per se* appears responsible for the devastating clinical syndrome.[367] Almost all patients develop a generalized rash that often becomes exfoliative. Instances of periarteritis nodosa,[752] of curious lymph node changes,[227] and of bone marrow injury accompanying liver damage also have been described.[170]

The symptoms, signs, and laboratory features offer strong clinical support for the view that the hepatic injury is a manifestation of drug hypersensitivity.[272,367,443,695] Indeed, the "pseudomononucleosis" syndrome of lymphadenopathy, lymphocytosis, and circulating atypical lymphocytes, observed as a reaction to phenytoin resembles serum sickness,[807] a facet that suggests the presence of circulating immune complexes. There is some evidence that phenytoin may have mild intrinsic hepatotoxicity[90] and, in some patients, a combination of toxic and sensitization reactions may occur.[807]

The prognosis for reported cases of phenytoin hepatitis has been poor with a 40% to 50% mortality.[149,443,807] There are no documented instances of development of a chronic active hepatitis or cirrhosis in survivors.

Toxicity from phenytoin metabolic products may be the cause of the hepatic injury.[696] Phenytoin is metabolized by the cytochrome P-450 mixed function oxidase system, yielding highly reactive arene oxides. These arene oxides bond covalently to tissue macromolecules, unless further metabolized by a process involving the enzyme. The union with tissue proteins may provide antigens to provoke hypersensitivity or produce tissue injury. Spielberg and colleagues[696] have demonstrated a genetically determined deficiency in epoxide hydrolase activity in patients with phenytoin-induced hepatic injury and in their family members. These observations suggest that susceptibility to phenytoin-induced liver injury is metabolically dependent and genetically determined.

Sodium Valproate. Sodium valproate is particularly useful in the management of petit mal and other forms of intractable seizures. A number of instances of fatal liver disease in patients taking the drug, however, have been reported.[157,327,562,714,768,798,812] In contrast to the finding with most other drugs, children appear to be especially severely affected.[562,812] The reactions have been characterized by gradual onset of systems of disease, changes in mental status, increased seizures followed by profound jaundice, elevated aminotransferases, progressive encephalopathy, coagulopathy, and death. Histologic studies have revealed diffuse hepatocellular injury with submassive necrosis, microvesicular fat, and bile duct injury. Increases in aminotransferase levels are frequently found when large series of patients receiving sodium valproate are prospectively followed.[714] The mechanism of sodium valproate–induced liver injury is not known. It has been speculated that the 4-pentanoic derivative may be responsible.[117,360,409,812] Because serious liver damage may develop insidiously with few clinical or biochemical manifestations of hepatic injury, patients receiving sodium valproate should be monitored closely throughout the time the drug is being administered.

Carbamazepine. Carbamazepine is an iminostilbene derivative that is used to treat trigeminal neuralgia, refractory seizures, and paresthesias from peripheral neuropathies, as well as convulsive disorders. Aplastic anemia, agranulocytosis, and thrombocytopenia are established adverse effects. A number of instances of hepatitis from carbamazepine also have been reported.[298,406,479,555,575,689,819] The onset of liver injury is usually within a month of initiating therapy. The forms of injury reported include granulomatous hepatitis,[406,479,689] cholestatic jaundice,[575] and massive necrosis.[819] The mechanism for hepatic injury is unknown.

Anti-Inflammatory Agents and Other Drugs Used in Gout and Musculoskeletal Disease

A number of agents employed to treat arthritis, gout, and musculospastic disease have been reported to cause hepatic injury in low incidence (Table 17-15). Indeed, there has been a sharp increase in attention to the hepatic injury associated with use of nonsteroidal anti-inflammatory drugs (NSAIDs) generated by the instances of dramatic liver disease in patients taking benoxaprofen (Oroflex).[737,530] Focus on the instances of NSAID-associated hepatic injury has led the Arthritis Advisory Committee of the Food and Drug Administration (FDA) to conclude that liver injury should be considered a "class charac-

TABLE 17-15. Hepatic Injury Produced by Nonsteroidal Anti-inflammatory Drugs and Other Agents Used to Treat Rheumatic and Musculospastic Disease

AGENT	TYPE OF INJURY
Acetaminophen	H-Cell [565,566,809]
Allopurinal	H-Cell or Ch [7,71,93,190]
Benorilate	H-Cell [408,709]
Benoxaprofen ‡§	Ch [168,207,209,570,718]
Chlorzoxazone	H-Cell [563]
Cinchophen ‡	H-Cell [807]
Colchicine ‖	H-Cell [807]
Dantrolene ¶	H-Cell [748]
Diclofenac	H-Cell [169,215]
Diflunisal	Ch [769]
Fenbufen	LFT [122,408,709]
Fenclozic acid *	H-Cell [807]
Fenoprofen *	LFT [408]
Glafenine	H-Cell [709]
Ibufenac	H-Cell [807]
Ibuprofen	H-Cell [74,700,701]
Indomethacin	H-Cell [709,807]
Naproxen	Ch or H-Cell [394,709]
Penicillamine	Ch [408,709]
Phenylbutazone †	H-Cell or Ch [45]
Oxyphenbutazone †	H-Cell or Ch [123,709]
Piroxicam *	H-Cell or Ch [275,709]
Probenecid #	H-Cell [807]
Salicylates g	H-Cell [709,809]
Sulindac	Ch or H-Cell [5,709,781]
Tolmetin *	H-Cell [709]
Zoxazolamine (‡)	H-Cell [807]

* Too few cases reported for clear picture.
‡ Largely or completely withdrawn from clinical use.
‖ Hepatic injury observed mainly in experimental animals.
¶ Can also cause chronic active hepatitis.
† Can cause granulomas.
g) Usually anicteric.
So rare as to suggest that the reported cases may have been coincidental rather than caused by the drug.
(H-Cell, hepatocellular lesion; Ch, cholestatic lesion; LFTs, liver function test abnormality)

istic" of this group of drugs.[737] The hepatic injury induced by the NSAIDs, however, is not uniform with regard to character or mechanism of production (see Table 17-15). Some of the drugs produce cytotoxic injury; fewer lead to cholestatic injury. Some can produce either. Although the mechanism in all appears to be idiosyncrasy, for some of these drugs, it is immunologic (hypersensitivity) while for others it appears to be metabolic (see Table 17-15).

Antiarthritic Drugs

Cinchophen. Cinchophen, once used to treat rheumatic disease and gout, fell into disuse 3 decades ago.[307] Nevertheless, it remains of interest as the first agent reported to produce idiosyncratic hepatic injury and as the prototype of drug-induced hepatocellular jaundice.[807] The reported mortality for patients with clinically evident liver injury was high, approaching 50%.[523,807] Fatal cases showed acute or subacute hepatic necrosis.[523] In those with a prolonged course the liver was described as showing "toxic cirrhosis."[774]

Phenylbutazone. Phenylbutazone has been incriminated in instances of hepatic injury since shortly after its entry into clinical use 4 decades ago.[45,393,803] The mechanism of injury is clearly idiosyncrasy with an estimated incidence of 0.25[393] to 5%.[123] The idiosyncrasy appears to be immunologic hypersensitivity in most instances, as deduced from the frequency of rash or fever and onset of illness within 6 weeks of starting the drug.[45] The injury is cytotoxic in at least two thirds of patients.[45,803] In these patients, the liver shows parenchymal necrosis and the jaundice is hepatocellular.[45,803] However, instances of cholestatic jaundice due to phenylbutazone also occur.[45,641] These cases have shown high values of alkaline phosphatase and cholesterol, slightly elevated aminotransferase values, and an almost normal parenchyma. Some patients with phenylbutazone-induced injury have shown granulomas, especially in the portal areas.[45,325] Oxyphenbutazone apparently produces a similar injury.

Indomethacin. Indomethacin has been reported to produce several instances of jaundice, one of them associated with massive hepatic necrosis.[205,356] Hepatocellular and cholestatic type injuries have been reported. The incidence must be very low, however, since this agent has been widely used. Nevertheless, the report of Cuthbert,[123] suggests a higher incidence than can be inferred from the individually reported cases.

Sulindac. Sulindac is chemically related to indomethacin, but it has been incriminated in more cases of hepatic injury.[408] Approximately 15 cases of overt hepatic injury associated with use of this drug have been reported.[10,85,96,148,235,313,352,525,684,781,790] Both cholestatic and hepatocellular injury have been recorded, but cases of cholestatic injury outnumber those with the hepatocellular type. Death has been recorded in patients with hepatocellular injury. The mechanism in more than half of the published cases appears to have been hypersensitivity as judged from associated fever and rash and time of onset of injury.

Ibufenac. Ibufenac, which has been withdrawn from use, produced elevated aminotransferase levels in about 30% and jaundice in about 5% of recipients.[274,726] The injury was predominantly hepatocellular. There was liver biopsy evidence of necrosis. Several reports of fatal liver disease were recorded.

Ibuprofen. Ibuprofen, which is chemically closely related to ibufenac, appears to have a much lower incidence of hepatic injury, although a few cases have been reported.[408] The injury appears to be mild and hepatocellular. However, at least one fatal case attributed to ibuprofen has been reported,[74] a curious instance of massive hepatic steatosis and pleural effusion. The mechanism for hepatic injury is unknown. The association with Stevens-Johnson syndrome[700] and other hallmarks of hypersensitivity[691] suggests that it may reflect immunologic idiosyncrasy.

Naproxen. Naproxen has rarely been incriminated in the causation of hepatic injury. Only four cases of jaundice have been attributed to its use.[33,394,395,757] The jaundice in the three with sufficient description has appeared to be cholestatic[33,757] or mixed.[395] Hypersensitivity has been suggested as the mechanism,[395] but there is not enough information to define the type of idiosyncrasy responsible for the injury.

Piroxicam. Piroxicam has been incriminated in very few instances of hepatic injury.[408] Hepatic necrosis has been held accountable for four deaths.[709] Mild, transient elevation of SGOT and SGPT have been recorded.[408] It appears that the incidence of hepatic injury by this very widely used drug is low.[407,709]

Benoxaprofen. Benoxaprofen is a nonsteroidal anti-inflammatory drug that was briefly available in the US market but was withdrawn when a number of patients with evidence of hepatic and renal insufficiency died.[168,207,209,248,570,718] Most patients with benoxaprofen-induced injury were elderly females. The liver injury was predominantly cholestatic with little if any evidence of inflammation. The mechanism of injury and the exact cause of death remain unknown. It is clearly and probably metabolic rather than hypersensitivity mediated. The perplexing aspect of the reported cases was the high apparent case-fatality rate (11 fatal cases of 14 reported), a paradox in such overtly cholestatic injury. Prescott and co-workers have suggested that severe cholestasis and renal failure together blocked excretion of the drug so completely as to lead to fatal blood levels.[570] This interesting hypothesis is not subject to clinical proof in the absence of blood levels from the patients.

Clometacine. Clometacine is an analgesic agent used in France for rheumatic and other conditions that has led to both acute and chronic hepatic injury.[224,539] Acute injury is hepatocellular. Chronic injury resembles clinical, histologic, and serologic features, the "autoimmune" type of chronic active hepatitis. Discontinuation of the drug appears to be followed by rapid recovery, and readministration can lead to prompt and, in one instance, fatal recurrence.[539] Involvement has been virtually confined to elderly women.

Gold. Intrahepatic cholestasis is a rare complication of gold therapy for rheumatoid arthritis. The mechanism of the liver injury is apparently that of an idiosyncratic reaction.[105,172,199,267,640] Eosinophilia was present in two of the three middle-aged female patients reported by Favreau and associates.[199] Elevated IgE antibodies as well as eosinophilia were described in one patient.[136] In addition to cholestasis, there may be moderate hepatocellular injury. Evidence of liver toxicity has appeared after as little as 37.5 mg.[199,640] Fatal intrahepatic cholestasis and interstitial lung fibrosis following gold therapy was described in a 53-year-old female with rheumatoid arthritis. Jaundice has been reported in recipients of aurothioglucose as well as of sodium thiomalate. Auronofin, a new oral preparation, has not been reported to have produced any instances.[408]

The liver injury from gold generally resolves within 3 months of cessation of therapy. Older literature suggesting massive hepatic necrosis from gold therapy is difficult to interpret; in some instances[162] it may have represented needle-transmitted viral hepatitis.

Salicylates. Salicylates, long considered to be free of potential for producing hepatic injury, have been established to cause focal hepatic necrosis when blood levels are high.[346,516,600,624,648,649,744,809] Biochemical abnormalities have included high aminotransferase levels, ranging from slight elevation to values in the thousands, but little or no hyperbilirubinemia. Bilirubin levels have exceeded the normal in only 3% of reported cases.[809] Early reports suggested that hepatic injury was seen only with blood salicylate levels above 25 mg/dl. More recent analysis indicates that lower levels can lead to damage. Only 7% of reported instances of hepatic injury have involved blood levels below 15 mg/dl.[809] Hepatotoxic salicylate levels are achieved with the usual "full dosage" employed to treat rheumatic fever, acute rheumatoid arthritis, and systemic lupus erythematosus. The hepatic injury appears to depend on the salicylate moiety, since it has been observed with aspirin, choline salicylate, and sodium salicylate.[809] Histology has shown focal necrosis and inflammation.[809] Patients with juvenile rheumatoid arthritis and systemic lupus erythematosus seem particularly vulnerable to aspirin-induced injury, but normal subjects are also susceptible.[648] The hepatic damage induced by salicylates generally resolves rapidly on identification of the injury and withdrawal of the drug. We have not seen a chronic active hepatitis or other residual damage develop, although an instance of salicylate injury said to mimic chronic active hepatitis has been described.[649] Most likely the injury is the result of a toxic reaction.[732] Evidence has been presented suggesting that hepatic injury is more likely to occur in patients with decreased serum albumin levels because there is more free (unbound) salicylate in these patients.[236] It is not established as to whether patients with underlying liver disease are more susceptible to salicylate injury. Recent attention has focused on the evidence for a role of salicylates in enhancing the likelihood that Reye's syndrome will follow viral infections.[127]

Allopurinol. The xanthine oxidase inhibitor allopurinol has been incriminated in several types of hepatic injury. These include minor abnormalities of biochemical tests,[259] hepatic granulomas,[190,717] cholestasis,[673] and hepatocellular injury.[71,93] The liver injury generally rapidly disappears when the drug is withdrawn. Fulminant fatal hepatic failure associated with fever, eosinophilia, exfoliative dermatitis, and jaundice has been reported.[93,576] A clear view of the predominant form of injury has not yet emerged.

Probenecid. Probenecid is a widely used agent that has been incriminated in only one instance of jaundice to our knowledge, a case of fatal hepatic necrosis.[597] The rarity of the lesion, despite the extensive use of the drug, suggests that this case may have been a coincidence.

Muscle Relaxants

Zoxazolamine was briefly in use as a muscle relaxant several decades ago. Instances of severe hepatic necrosis in recipients led to its abandonment.[101,182,332,807] Chlorzoxazone, a derivative of zoxazolamine, also has led to instances of hepatic necrosis.[563]

Dantrolene, another drug in this group, also has led to instances of acute and subacute hepatic necrosis.[748] The subacute lesion may resemble chronic active hepatitis. Evidence of liver damage usually does not appear until at least 6 weeks after starting the drug.[748] Overt hepatic injury, which occurs in about 0.5% of recipients, tends to spare children under the age of 10 and adults taking daily doses below 200 mg/day.

Agents Used in the Treatment of Endocrine Disease

A number of hormones and their derivatives and other agents used in the treatment of endocrine disease produce hepatic dysfunction and jaundice (Table 17-16). These include the thiourea derivatives, some of the oral hypoglycemic agents, the C-17 alkylated anabolic steroids, and the oral contraceptive agents.

Thiourea Derivatives

Too few cases of hepatic damage attributable to these agents have been reported in sufficient detail to permit fully confident characterization of the type of injury. Nevertheless, there appear to be differences between the type of injury produced by the various derivatives of thiourea.[807] The instances of jaundice induced by thiourea, methimazole, and carbimazole and methylthiouracil appear to have been cholestatic (hepatocanalicular or mixed hepatocanalicular)[60,208,433,613,761] and those reported in recipients of propylthiouracil appear to have been hepatocellular.[202,208,465,613,668,807] Instances of fulminant hepatitis[202,208] and of chronic active hepatitis[202,465] have been attributed to propylthiouracil, and we have observed two instances of bridging necrosis on liver biopsy. Mech-

TABLE 17-16. Hepatic Injury Produced by Hormonal Derivatives and Other Agents Used in Endocrine Disease

AGENT	TYPE OF INJURY	OTHER LESIONS
Steroids		
Anabolic C-17	Ch-Can	Carcinoma
		Adenoma
		Peliosis hepatis
Oral contraceptives	Ch-Can	Adenoma
		? Carcinoma
		Hepatic vein thrombosis
		Peliosis hepatis
Tamoxifen	Ch	Peliosis hepatis[424]
Danazol	Ch[532]	
Glucocorticoids	Steatosis	
Oral hypoglycemics		
Acetohexamide	H-Cell-M	
Azepinamide	H-Cell-M	
Carbutamide	H-Cell-M	
Chlorpropamide	Ch-H-Can	
Glibenclamide	Ch-H-Can	
Metahexamide	H-Cell-M	
Tolazemide	Ch-H-Can	
Tolbutamide	Ch-H-Can	Can cause PBC-like disease
Antithyroid drugs		
Carbimazole	Ch-H-Can	
Methimazole	Ch-H-Can	
Methylthiouracil	Ch-H-Can	
Thiouracil	Ch-H-Can	
Propylthiouracil	H-Cell	Can cause CAH[465]

(H-Cell, hepatocellular lesion; CH, cholestatic lesion; M, mixed; Ch-Can, cholestasis without portal inflammation; CAH, chronic active hepatitis; PBC-like, chronic intrahepatic cholestasis with features resembling primary biliary cirrhosis)
(Data from references 709 and 807)

anism for hepatic injury can be deduced to be hypersensitivity as judged by the association of rash, fever, eosinophilia, and neutropenia, the response of patients to a challenge dose and of their lymphocytes to *in vitro* exposure to the drug.[60,465]

Oral Hypoglycemic Drugs

Hepatic injury has occurred in 0.5% to 1% of recipients of carbutamide, chlorpropamide, or metahexamide.[88,263,362,591,803,807] At least 20 instances of jaundice have been recorded among patients taking acetohexamide.[24,118,244] Tolbutamide, despite its extremely wide use, has been incriminated in only a few instances of jaundice.[23,251] There have been no reported instances of cross-reactions in diabetics who have had chlorpropamide-induced injury and are subsequently given tolbutamide.[263]

The jaundice of chlorpropamide has been cholestatic (hepatocanalicular); that of metahexamide, acetohexamide, and carbutamide appears to have been mixed he-

patocellular.[244,803,807] The few reported examples of tolbutamide jaundice have appeared to be cholestatic.[23,251] Gregory and associates[251] have described prolonged jaundice and features resembling those of primary biliary cirrhosis with a fatal outcome in a patient taking tolbutamide. We have seen two other unreported instances of chronic intrahepatic cholestasis in patients who had been taking tolbutamide. Sulfonylurea derivatives also can produce granulomas without other evidence of hepatic injury.[61]

Only scattered instances of hepatic injury have been ascribed to biguanides,[682] and those may have been coincidental. Phenformin, no longer available but formerly widely used, has not been reported to produce hepatic damage. This is somewhat surprising, since this compound is structurally related to the hepatotoxic agent synthalin.[121]

Anabolic and Contraceptive Steroids

The hepatic effects of the C-17 alkylated anabolic and of the oral contraceptive steroids have much in common (see Table 17-16). Both groups of drugs are intrinsic hepatotoxins capable of producing acute, cholestatic jaundice.[322,363,663,807] Both have led to instances of peliosis hepatis[22,450,452,499,560,645,763] and have been implicated in hepatic tumor production.[13,31,173,175,176,284,321,322,364,447,664,807] There are also differences. Anabolic steroids have been particularly incriminated in hepatocarcinogenesis, while contraceptive steroids have been far more clearly related to the development of benign hepatic tumors, especially adenomas.[13,173,321,322,447,664] Furthermore, hepatic vein occlusion and Budd-Chiari syndrome has been clearly related to the thrombogenic effect of the estrogenic component of the contraceptive preparations.[410,706]

The structure of these agents is important (see Fig. 17-5). The presence of an alkyl or ethinyl group on carbon-17 appears to be essential for the production of cholestatic jaundice. Testosterone does not lead to jaundice or impaired hepatic function[803,807] but can lead to peliosis hepatis. Unsaturation of ring A, a characteristic of native estrogens, appears to enhance the adverse effect of steroids on hepatic function in experimental animals,[226] as may also be deduced from the greater adverse potency in humans of the estrogenic than of the progestational component of contraceptive preparations.[747]

C-17 Alkylated Anabolic Steroids. The incidence of jaundice in patients who receive these agents appears to be very low, although some evidence of hepatic dysfunction occurs in almost all patients who take them in sufficiently large doses.

This may indicate that homeostatic adjustments to the adverse effect of the drug occurs and that jaundice may develop when these homeostatic adjustments fail. Most of the patients in whom jaundice has developed have been taking the respective agent for 1 to 6 months.[803]

Oral Contraceptives. The impression gained from the anabolic/androgenic steroid phenomenon that individual susceptibility permits a mildly adverse effect to be translated into jaundice development is even more apparent with respect to the contraceptive steroids. The latter are far more likely to lead to jaundice in women who have a personal or familial history of jaundice of pregnancy.[4,297,462,518] This and the clustering of cases of "pill jaundice" in Chile[518] and Scandinavia[35,664] suggest a genetic susceptibility to this type of hepatic injury.

The jaundice appears to result from the selective interference with excretion of bile[14] apparently secondary to impaired uptake of bile acids from sinusoidal blood and other effects on bile flow.[15] The impaired uptake may be attributed to the loss of fluidity and decrease in Na^+,K^+-ATPase of the plasma membrane produced by the estrogenic component of the contraceptive preparation.[592]

The jaundice has been characterized in an earlier section (see Table 17-7) as cholestatic, canalicular type.[803,807] There is no portal inflammation and little or no parenchymal injury. The prognosis is good. Contraceptive steroid jaundice usually has its onset within the first 1 to 6 months of treatment. Onset is insidious with pruritus and mild jaundice (serum bilirubin value less than 5 mg/dl). Occasionally, jaundice may be severe and persist months after the drugs are withdrawn.[415] Alkaline phosphatase levels remain normal or only slightly elevated. Aminotransferase levels are usually normal or only slightly increased, although it has been stated[462] that an occasional patient may have high levels mimicking viral hepatitis. The syndrome may recur in the third trimester of pregnancy. Death in canalicular jaundice has been reported only in patients who were debilitated or had other disease.[363,803]

Hepatocellular carcinoma has been reported in several recipients of the anabolic/androgenic steroids and in a few patients who had been taking contraceptive steroids.[225,284,321,322,447,778] Many of the patients with anabolic/androgenic steroid-related tumors have received the agents for various types of anemias, although tumors have been reported in athletes taking the drugs to increase strength.[322,520,778] In view of the large number of women who have taken contraceptives, and the relatively limited number of patients who have used anabolic/androgenic steroids, hepatocarcinogenesis would appear to be more readily attributable to anabolic than to contraceptive steroids. The atypical character of the carcinomas described in recipients of anabolic steroids, however, has led to a questioning of the true carcinomatous nature of the tumors.[13,447] In a review of 128 cases of hepatocellular carcinoma in women reported to the Armed Forces Institute of Pathology (AFIP), there was no evidence of an association between hepatocellular carcinoma and the oral contraceptive.[245]

Hepatic adenoma seems clearly related to the taking of contraceptive steroids. Over 500 cases have now been recorded.[30,321,364,377] Almost all have appeared since the introduction of oral contraceptives, and almost all patients with this tumor have been users of these steroids. Hepatic adenoma was first described as a complication of oral contraceptive therapy in 1973.[37] There is a direct relationship between the duration of oral contraceptive use and the incidence of adenoma.[611] The hepatic adenomas may present as a painless asymptomatic right upper abdominal mass, as a painful mass, or as hemoperitoneum secondary to rupture of the tumor.[447] Approximately 10% of the tumors are pedunculated. The tumor is usually solitary and on liver biopsy appears to be a collection of normal hepatocytes. No Kupffer cells are found in the adenoma; therefore, the lesion will not take up technetium on a liver scan. Characteristically, in symptomatic patients there is a hemorrhagic border around the adenoma, which explains the abdominal pain, and lesions on the surface of the liver may rupture, causing intra-abdominal hemorrhage.

Somewhat less convincingly related to the use of contraceptive steroids is the development of focal nodular hyperplasia.[322,377] The frequency of focal nodular hyperplasia has not apparently increased since the introduction of oral contraceptives. Focal nodular hyperplasia affects both sexes (85% women) and patients of all ages.

Antimicrobial Agents

Antibiotics

A number of agents in this category can produce hepatic dysfunction or jaundice. The form of injury and the presumed mechanism are listed in Table 17-17. A few of the agents warrant special comment.

Tetracyclines. The tetracyclines can lead to dose-related hepatic, renal, and pancreatic toxicity.[114] Tetracyclines produce a characteristic microvesicular form of hepatic steatosis (see Fig. 17-4), resembling the fatty liver of pregnancy or of Reye's syndrome.[130,304,392,807] Hepatocytes contain many small sudanophilic droplets. Rarely the steatosis may be macrovesicular.[92] There is little or no necrosis and little cholestasis. Initially described as an adverse reaction to chlortetracycline,[400,401] it also has followed administration of oxytetracycline and tetracycline[130] and presumably could result from any tetracycline derivative that shares the antimicrobial properties of the group and reaches the hepatocyte in sufficiently high concentration. The histologic pattern can be reproduced in experimental animals.[639]

The clinically significant syndrome of severe fatty liver with hepatic failure is dose-related and occurs in patients who have received the drug in a dose of 1.0 g/day or more, especially if the drug is administered intravenously, and, particularly, if the recipient is in the last trimester of pregnancy or has renal disease.[130] Although pregnancy appears to enhance susceptibility to tetracycline-induced hepatic injury,[130,304] non-pregnant females and male patients are also at risk.[400,543]

The clinical manifestations include nausea, vomiting, and abdominal pain, possibly related in part to the frequently associated pancreatitis and there is usually evidence of renal injury. Jaundice is rarely intense. Most of the recorded cases have died.[130,304] Less severe cases probably go unrecognized or unrecorded.

The biochemical features resemble those of fatty liver of pregnancy and of Reye's syndrome. Bilirubin levels are usually below 10 mg/dl. Levels of aminotransferases rarely exceed 500 IU and, in the majority of patients, are below 200 IU. Values for alkaline phosphatase are slightly elevated. Prothrombin time is usually strikingly prolonged.[304]

The mechanism for the hepatic injury is clearly that of indirect cytotoxic hepatotoxicity and appears to be mainly the result of inhibition of transport of lipid from the liver.[639]

Erythromycin Estolate. Until a recent[152,355,760,799] description of apparent erythromycin ethylsuccinate–associated liver damage, the only erythromycin derivative known to produce jaundice was the estolate.[152,382,604,807] Jaundice occurs in 1% to 2% of adult recipients but very rarely in children taking the drug.[73] The jaundice is usually hepatocanalicular with high values for alkaline phosphatase and modest aminotransferase values.[807] Liver biopsy

usually shows only bile casts and a prominent portal inflammatory infiltration, usually rich in eosinophils.[641,807] However, hepatic necrosis does occur in some patients.[279]

Typically jaundice, pruritus, abdominal pain, and elevated aminotransferase levels appear 2 to 21 days after initiation of the drugs.[363] The manifestations of hepatic injury may develop after a much shorter interval when susceptible individuals are reexposed to the drug.[73,152,799] The symptoms of liver disease usually subside promptly, when the drug is withdrawn, and chronic residual liver damage has not been reported.

The blood and tissue eosinophilia, fever, and rash that accompany the hepatic injury all suggest hypersensitivity. The high incidence of hepatic dysfunction in patients taking erythromycin estolate[780] and the demonstration that this compound is more damaging to isolated hepatocytes[165,166,812] and the ex vivo perfused liver[357] than are other erythromycin esters suggest that intrinsic hepatotoxicity of the agent may contribute to the hepatic injury.[804,807] In most instances, jaundice appears between the 2nd and 21st day of receiving the drug and there is usually associated abdominal discomfort.[73] The symptoms of liver disease rapidly subside when the drug is withdrawn, and chronic residual liver damage has not been reported.

Chloramphenicol. Jaundice has been reported in a number of recipients of chloramphenicol, but it is rare. The scanty data available suggest that both hepatic parenchymal necrosis and cholestasis can occur. The mechanism for the apparent hepatotoxicity is unclear.[807]

Triacetyloleandomycin. Triacetyloleandomycin produced jaundice in 4% and hepatic dysfunction in over 50% of one group of patients who had been taking 2 g/day for 2 or more weeks.[729] The histologic features and the pattern of hepatic dysfunction produced by this drug have been those of mixed hepatocellular jaundice. Mild parenchymal injury and bilirubin casts are seen. Triacetyloleandomycin or a metabolite appears to be a mild intrinsic hepatotoxin. Individual metabolic differences between different persons presumably determine the extent of hepatic injury.[729] An interesting report described 12 young females who were regularly taking oral contraceptives in whom intrahepatic cholestasis developed 2 to 20 days after beginning triacetyloleandomycin.[206] It was suggested the triacetyloleandomycin might interfere with the metabolism of the oral contraceptive, leading to the cholestasis.

Novobiocin. Novobiocin can produce unconjugated hyperbilirubinemia, apparently by blockage of conjugation of bilirubin.[271] Accordingly, it should be categorized as a mild indirect hepatotoxin. Rare instances of hepatic necrosis due to idiosyncrasy have been described.[81,537] This antibiotic, however, has fallen into disuse and its toxicity is of little importance.

Penicillin. Hypersensitivity reactions from penicillin, especially with fever and rashes, are common, but reports

TABLE 17-17.   Hepatic Injury Produced by Antimicrobial Agents

AGENT	TYPE OF INJURY	COMMENT
Antibiotics		
Amphotericin		See antifungal agents
Chloramphenicol †	H-Cell or M	
Cephalosporins †	Ch	
Clindamycin †	H-Cell	
Colimycin †	J	
Erythromycin estolate	Ch or M	
Erythromycin ethyl succinate	Ch	
5-Flurocytosine		See antifungal agents
Griseofulvin		See antifungal agents
Novobiocin †	H-Cell	Also ‡
Penicillins		
G †	H-Cell †	
Amoxicillin †	Anicteric †	
Ampicillin †	H-Cell †	
Carbenicillin	Anicteric	
Oxacillin †	Ch	
Cloxacillin	Ch	
Rifampicin	H-Cell	Also ‡
Spectinomycin †	Anicteric †	
Tetracyclines	Steatosis	Only with large intravenous doses
Triacetyloleandomycin	M	
Synthetic drugs		
Arsenicals, inorganic	Fat, necrosis §	
Arsenicals, organic	Ch	Can lead to PBC-like disease
Nitrofurans	Ch or mild H-Cell	Also can lead to CAH
Sulfonamides	H-Cell or M	Also can lead to CAH
Sulfones	H-Cell or M	
Sulfamethoxazole-trimethoprim	H-Cell, Ch or M	
Antifungal agents		
Amphotericin		Vague reference to hepatic injury but no cases reported
5-Fluorocytosine	Ch †	
Griseofulvin	Ch + H-Cell †	Causes necrosis, fat, Ca, and porphyria in experimental animals
Hydroxystilbamidine	H-Cell †	
Ketoconazole	H-Cell	
Saramycetin ‡	Hyperbilirubinemia	
Antimetazoal and antiprotozoal agents		
Antimonials	H-Cell	Fat, necrosis
Amodiaquine	H-Cell †	
Carbarsone		See organic arsenicals
Emetine		No apparent hepatotoxic effects in clinical use. Toxic for experimental animals ‖
8-Hydroxyquinolines		No apparent hepatotoxic effects in clinical use

TABLE 17-17.—Continued

AGENT	TYPE OF INJURY	COMMENT
Hycanthone	H-Cell	Can cause Ca in animals
Mepacrine †	H-Cell †	
Metronidazole		Mutagenic, and possibly carcinogenic
Niclofan	Ch	
Thiabendazole	Ch †	Can lead to PBC-like disease
Antituberculous agents		
Cycloserine †	Anicteric	
Ethionamide	H-Cell	
Isoniazid	H-Cell #	Also can lead to CAH
p-Aminosalicylic acid	H-Cell or M	
Pyrazinamide	H-Cell	
Rifampicin	H-Cell	Also ‡
Thiosemicarbazone	H-Cell	Fat and necrosis
Antiviral agents		
Cytarabine †	J	
Idoxuridine †	M	
Vidarabine	H-Cell	
Xenelamine †	Ch	

* Agents with general antimicrobial use shown alphabetically, others shown by category of use.
† Too few cases for clear picture. See text for references.
‡ Dose-related dysfunction leading to unconjugated hyperbilirubinemia.
§ Also can lead to cirrhosis, hepatoportal sclerosis, and angiosarcoma.
∥ Potent cause of fatty liver.
Overt injury approximately 1%; anicteric, 10–20%.
(Ch, cholestatic injury; bilirubin casts in canaliculi, with or without portal inflammation and with or without mild parenchymal injury. H Cell, hepatocellular injury, mainly degeneration and necrosis with or without inflammation. M, Mixed type. J, Jaundice, details not clear. Ca, carcinoma; PBC, primary biliary cirrhosis; CAH, chronic active hepatitis)
(Data from reference 807 and from Zimmerman HJ, Lewis JH: Hepatic toxicity of antimicrobial agents. *In* Antimicrobial Therapy, pp 153–202. New York, Churchill Livingstone, 1984)

of hepatic injury due to penicillin are rare.[130,807] Among the huge number of patients who have been given penicillin, very few instances of liver damage have been reported.[130,204,234,242,496,750,770,807]

Some have had reversible cholestatic hepatic injury.[242] Several semisynthetic penicillin derivatives (see Table 17-17), however, seem to produce jaundice or biochemical evidence of hepatic injury more commonly.[44,62,68,89,154,218,375,386,448,506,617,723,765,786] Carbenicillin caused eight episodes of a reversible anicteric hepatitis in 4 patients with a reappearance of the injury on rechallenge in all.[786] Liver biopsy showed focal hepatitis. Intravenous oxacillin has also been reported to cause a mild nonspecific hepatitis that returned on rechallenge.[89,154] Cloxacillin was associated with severe cholestasis in one patient.[189] Flucloxicillin has been implicated as the cause of reversible cholestatic liver damage occurring 4 and 7 weeks after treatment with the drug in two elderly (68- and 75-year-old) women.[44]

Synthetic Antimicrobials

Organic Arsenicals. "Intrahepatic obstructive" jaundice in patients given arsphenamine was first described by Hanger and Gutman.[268] Their careful description of the first clearly recognized cases of cholestatic jaundice, apparently resulting from drug allergy, is a milestone in the history of drug-induced hepatic disease. Based on the occurrence of fever and eosinophilia, they ascribed the syndrome to drug hypersensitivity and distinguished it from the hepatic parenchymal lesion (zonal or massive necrosis) produced by very large doses of arsenicals.

The pattern of biochemical abnormality in arsphenamine jaundice closely simulated that of obstructive jaundice. The alkaline phosphatase levels were more than fourfold increased. Hypercholesterolemia was common. The livers showed cholestasis and a variable prominent portal inflammatory infiltration.[268] A syndrome resembling that of primary biliary cirrhosis has also been reported to follow arsenical jaundice.[278,708]

Sulfonamides. Acute hepatitis has been most frequently reported in patients receiving sulfonamide therapy but definite instances of liver damage have been documented in patients on sulfathiazole, sulfadiazine, sulfamethoxypyridazine, sulfamethoxazole, and sulfadimethoxine.[164,221,363,439] Sulfonamides have also been implicated in the production of a chronic acute hepatitis.[734] Tonder and associates[734] have reported on a 54-year-old woman who developed symptoms of hepatitis while receiving sulfonamides on several occasions, including one deliberate rechallenge. A liver biopsy during her second bout of hepatitis showed changes compatible with chronic active hepatitis.

Over 100 instances of acute hepatic injury have appeared to be due to sulfonamides.[164] Most have shown hepatic necrosis and hepatocellular jaundice, although instances of cholestatic jaundice have been described.[164] Our analysis of the reported cases has led us to classify the hepatic damage caused by these agents as mixed-hepatocellular.[164,807] The rash, fever, eosinophilia, and tissue eosinophils and granulomas seen in many of the patients and the relatively fixed latent period of 5 to 14 days that has usually preceded the jaundice suggest that hypersensitivity is the mechanism for the hepatic damage.[164,807] One patient developed cholestatic jaundice from use of a sulfanilamide vaginal cream.[439]

Sulfonamide-Trimethoprim Combination. Jaundice caused by this preparation has been reported.[214,232,363] We have seen two instances of cholestatic jaundice and of mixed type with features of cholestasis and parenchymal injury. The clinical features were consistent with hypersensitivity as the mechanism.

Sulfasalazine (Azulfidine) is a sulfonamide widely used in the treatment of inflammatory bowel disease, but its use has been associated with only several instances of liver injury.[347,426,464,686,692] The syndrome resembles other instances of sulfonamide-induced injury in that fever, rash, arthralgias, and hepatitis develop within 1 to 4 weeks of starting the drug. Low serum complement and circulating immune complexes have been found, supporting the assumption of an allergic basis for the reaction.[464]

Sulfones. Sulfones, used in the treatment of leprosy, appear to produce hepatic injury more often than do the sulfonamides. The incidence has been reported to be about 5% in recipients of the prototypic compound, 4,4′-dapsone. Jaundice appears to be mixed hepatocellular, although the available data are scanty. The mechanism for the hepatic injury is not clear.

Nitrofurantoin. Most cases of hepatic injury from nitrofurantoin have been cholestatic, but hepatocellular damage has also been observed in recipients of this drug.[243] Clinical features suggest that the mechanism is that of hypersensitivity, although toxic metabolites may be responsible for some cases.[243] Perhaps even more important are the reports of approximately 25 instances of chronic active hepatitis that have been reported in recipients of the drug.[57,277,369,418,655,658,710] Females have been affected predominately and the syndrome has resembled the autoimmune type of chronic active hepatitis.[658] It has been reported in a male.[21]

Nitrofurantoin-induced chronic active hepatitis is most often found in women who have received the drug for months or years (up to 11 years).[658] The majority had taken the drug for longer than 6 months. Most patients have a slow resolution of the chronic active hepatitis–type lesion on drug withdrawal. Five patients had evidence of relapse when rechallenged.[658] The clinical illness in older females may closely resemble idiopathic chronic active hepatitis.[277,658] The mechanism for the liver injury is unknown. At least three patients have been reported to have HLA-B8 antigen,[277,330] and it is possible that patients with this particular HLA type are at increased risk of developing the syndrome.

Antituberculous Drugs

Clarification of the etiologic role of a particular agent in this group as the cause of hepatic injury has been complicated by the frequent use of several drugs in combination. Nevertheless, observations recorded from the period when p-aminosalicylic acid was employed alone or with streptomycin and the recent practice of treating "tuberculin-converters" with isoniazid alone have permitted some deductions regarding the ability of each of these agents to produce hepatic injury.[807] Streptomycin, dihydrostreptomycin, and ethambutal appear to be free of hepatotoxic potential, but p-aminosalicylic acid can cause liver damage. Rifampicin also has been implicated in cases of hepatic injury. According to some authors, rifampicin also appears to potentiate the ability of isoniazid to produce hepatic injury and *vice versa*. By far the most important member of the antituberculous drugs with regard to hepatotoxicity is isoniazid. Similar injury is caused by its congeners pyrazinamide and ethionamide.[807]

p-Aminosalicylic Acid. Hepatic injury in recipients of p-aminosalicylic acid occurs as part of a generalized hypersensitivity reaction that is found in 0.3 to 5% of patients taking the drug.[803] The reaction, which appears after 1 to 5 weeks of taking p-aminosalicylic acid, includes fever, rash, eosinophilia, lymphadenopathy, and often "atypical" circulating lymphocytes ("pseudomononucleosis"). Approximately 25% of patients with this generalized hypersensitivity develop jaundice and biochemical evidence of hepatic injury. High aminotransferase levels, high levels of alkaline phosphatase, as well as both parenchymal injury and prominent cholestasis seen in the liver warrant designation of the mixed hepatocellular injury.[285,803] The histologic changes include prominent inflammation accompanying the diffuse degeneration, necrosis, and cholestasis.[803] Necrosis may be massive in fatal cases. In some nonfatal cases, there may be striking periportal necrosis.[807] The drug, however, sees little use today.

Isoniazid. Isoniazid had appeared to show extraordinarily slight potential for producing hepatic injury during the initial 2 decades of its clinical use.[56,228,436] Despite the huge number of recipients of isoniazid, only a few instances of jaundice had been attributed to the drug prior to 1972, and these were usually in patients who also had been taking other drugs. In the late 1960s, isoniazid began to be used alone as a chemoprophylactic agent to prevent the later emergence of tuberculosis. The drug was used alone first in patients who were known "convertors" of their tuberculin skin tests and later in all patients who had a positive tuberculin skin test.[9] In 1972, Garibaldi and co-workers[228] reported 19 instances of hepatocellular injury, most of them accompanied by jaundice, out of 2321 patients taking isoniazid for "chemoprophylaxis." These authors also cited a number of other previously unreported instances of isoniazid hepatotoxicity described to them by other physicians. Many subsequent reports of isoniazid-induced liver injury have appeared, and isoniazid has been recognized as one of the most important causes of drug-induced liver injury.[56,434,436,807]

The incidence of jaundice among recipients of isoniazid approaches 1%. Manifest liver injury is very low under the age of 20 and rises to greater than 2% in patients above 50.[478,577] Females are apparently more susceptible. Alcoholics appear to be more susceptible to injury.

Minor elevations (less than threefold) of amino transferases may occur in 10% to 20% of patients during the first 2 months of isoniazid therapy.[434,637] In most of these the abnormality does not progress and may even subside despite continued administration of the drug.[478,637] Such patients do show minor histologic abnormalities on liver biopsy.[637]

Clinical features of isoniazid-induced liver injury resemble those of acute viral hepatitis. Anorexia, fatigue, nausea, and vomiting are important prodromal features. Jaundice and dark urine, however, may be the first evidence of injury. The hepatocellular injury may be severe with peak values for aminotransferases as high as 4000 IU. Continued administration of isoniazid after prodromal symptoms have appeared may enhance the severity of injury.[434,436] Biopsy of the liver has revealed diffuse degeneration, and necrosis and liver sections of fatal cases have shown massive necrosis.[56,436] In a few patients the liver biopsy has shown changes consistent with chronic active hepatitis and cirrhosis.[56,249] Ongoing chronic active hepatitis after the isoniazid is removed has not been reported. The fatality rate for jaundiced patients is in excess of 10%.[56,228,436]

The mechanism of isoniazid-induced hepatic necrosis is, at least in part, related to the production of toxic reactive intermediates, which are highly reactive compounds and bind covalently to cell macromolecules leading to cell necrosis.[478,505] Earlier studies[478] suggesting that rapid acetylators of isoniazid are at greater risk to develop hepatic injury have not been confirmed.[253,258] The production of toxic intermediates appears to explain the 10% to 20% incidence of elevated aminotransferases with minimal hepatic necrosis and may also well explain the 1% incidence of frank necrosis in patients receiving isoniazid. However, it is possible that a sensitization reaction to an isoniazid intermediate may contribute to the more serious injury. The rarity of clinical hallmarks of hypersensitivity, however, suggests that these are in the minority.[434,478]

Rifampicin. A number of patients have developed jaundice while taking rifampicin and isoniazid or rifampicin alone.[398] Hepatic injury due to rifampicin appears during the first month of therapy[643] in contrast to isoniazid injury in which most cases (85%) present 2 to 12 months after starting treatment.[56] Rifampicin-induced injury is mainly hepatocellular, although cholestasis may be present. Degeneration and necrosis are characteristic and tend to be most prominent in the centrizonal (zone 3) area.[643] The inflammatory response appears to be more intense than that of isoniazid injury.[643] The reports of Lesobre and associates[402] and of Pieron and associates[546] suggest that the prognosis is guarded in rifampicin-induced hepatitis, with a high case fatality. Scheuer and co-workers,[643] however, suggest that the disease is relatively mild.

Presumably unrelated to this hepatic injury is the ability of rifampicin to produce unconjugated hyperbilirubinemia and impaired BSP excretion in experimental animals and patients. Apparently the drug competes with other substances cleared by the liver for excretion into bile or uptake from sinusoidal blood by the hepatocyte.[99,110,358]

Several reports suggest that rifampicin and isoniazid together may be more hepatotoxic than either alone.[253,379,398,546] This view seems supported by the report of Hugues and associates,[309] who found that rats developed hepatic necrosis when given rifampicin and isoniazid together but not when given either drug alone. The potentiating effect on animal toxicity, however, is not supported by the studies of Newman and others.[509] Gronhagen-Riska and co-workers[253] reported some evidence of hepatic toxicity in 18% of patients receiving isoniazid-rifampicin. The majority (approximately 75%) of these patients had only a modest (fourfold) asymptomatic increase in aminotransferases, but 25% had larger increases. Females over the age of 50 appeared to have increased susceptibility to injury, as did alcoholics and patients with a history of previous liver disease. There seemed to be a greater prevalence of slow acetylators of isoniazid among more severely affected patients than would be expected by chance. These authors concluded that the toxicity of isoniazid plus rifampicin is greater than that of isoniazid alone.

The impression that there is a higher incidence of hepatic injury in recipients of the isoniazid-rifampicin regimen than in those who take isoniazid alone and the even stronger impression that isoniazid alone is much more likely to produce hepatic injury than when taken with p-aminosalicylic acid permits some intriguing speculation regarding possible mechanisms (Fig. 17–21). Taken alone, isoniazid presumably produces hepatotoxic metabolites, but in most patients the dominant pathway is to nontoxic metabolites, or detoxifying processes keep pace with pro-

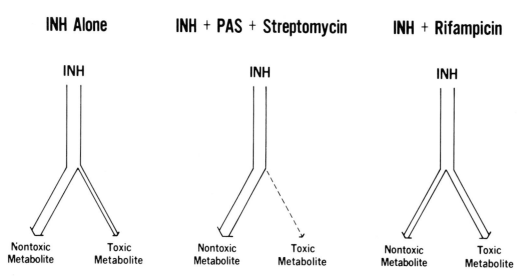

Fig. 17-21. Hypothetical explanation for greater incidence of hepatic injury induced by isoniazid (INH) alone or by INH with rifampicin than by INH with para-aminosalicylic acid (PAS) and streptomycin. (Zimmerman HJ: Hepatotoxicity. New York, Appleton-Century-Crofts, 1978)

duction of toxic metabolites. In the susceptible minority, the rate of production of toxic metabolites is greater or the detoxifying process is less effective. Presumably, when taken with *p*-aminosalicylic acid or streptomycin, production or accumulation of toxic metabolite is in some way inhibited, and conceivably when taken with rifampicin it is enhanced.

Antifungal Agents

Griseofulvin. Griseofulvin is an antifungal agent that is a known experimental hepatotoxin. It produces hepatic necrosis, hepatocellular carcinoma, and toxic porphyria in mice.[27,311,446] A report by Denk and others[143] has described lesions similar to alcoholic hyaline in mice given griseofulvin. Humans have developed porphyrinuria, and those with acute intermittent porphyria in remission may experience a relapse while taking the drug.[48,584,675] We are aware of only two reported cases of jaundice, both cholestatic.[77,104] Other vague references to liver damage in humans have appeared.[807]

Ketoconazole. Ketoconazole is used in the treatment of deep mycoses and candidiasis. Hepatocellular necrosis and frequent abnormalities in biochemical tests are found in patients receiving the drug.[283,333,411,716] Fatal instances have occurred. Symptomatic hepatic reactions occur mainly within the first few months of treatment.[333] Most reported instances of ketoconazole-induced liver injury have occurred in women over 40 years old.[411] There are no reports of rash or eosinophilia to suggest a hypersensitivity reaction, and the presumed mechanism of injury is toxicity via a metabolic product. The incidence of symptomatic hepatic injury appears to be very low. Nevertheless, it has

been recommended[411] that patients receiving ketoconazole be monitored regularly in order to detect evidence of liver injury at an early easily reversible stage.

Saramycetin. Saramycetin has a dose-related effect on bilirubin and BSP clearance. The effect appears to involve both uptake and excretions of anions by the hepatocytes.[12,789] It is of physiologic interest but of no clinical importance.

Flucytosine. Flucytosine is converted to 5-fluorouracil, a transformation on which its antifungal activity depends. Data on the hepatic effects of this drug are scanty; it appears to lead to transient elevations of aminotransferases in 10% of recipients and has been incriminated in the causation of hepatic necrosis.[35,211,582]

Antiviral Agents

Information on the hepatotoxicity of agents in this group is limited. Since these agents are antimetabolites, they may be expected to be indirect hepatotoxins. Idoxuridine has been reported to produce cholestatic jaundice,[137,671] as well as instances of aminotransferase levels elevated to a degree that suggests hepatocellular injury.[75] Xenelamine has led to instances of cholestatic jaundice[282,286] and cytarabine had led to jaundice of uncertain type.[306,738] Vidarabine also has resulted in elevated levels of bilirubin and aminotransferases.[510]

Antiprotozoal Agents

Most of the agents employed to treat malaria, amebiasis, and other protozoan disease have had little overt hepatotoxic effect.[807] A fatal case of multisystemic toxicity with evidence of hepatic necrosis as well as oliguric renal failure and bullous exfoliative dermatitis has been reported in a 60-year-old female taking pyrimethamine and sulfadoxine for prophylaxis against malaria.[652] Other instances of toxic reactions to pyrimethamine and sulfadoxine have been reported.[517,780]

Anthelmintics

Chlorinated hydrocarbons and organic antimonials, long used as anthelmintics are known to cause hepatic injury (see Table 17-17). Hycanthone, recently introduced for the treatment of schistosomiasis, has also been found to produce hepatocellular injury and, in some cases, fatal necrosis.[11,197] Thiobendazole has led to a few instances of intrahepatic cholestasis, one of which progressed to a syndrome resembling primary biliary cirrhosis.[331] A 55-year-old male was reported to develop intrahepatic cholestasis and a sicca complex after thiabendazole.[595] He recovered completely from the liver injury but the sicca complex persisted 1 year after the drug was withdrawn. One of the authors (WCM) has seen a patient with severe cholestasis after thiabendazole that has persisted for more than 2 years. Piperazine has recently been reported to cause acute hepatocellular injury.[265]

Drugs Used in Cardiovascular Disease

Among the drugs that are employed in treatment of cardiac disease, hypertension, and atherosclerosis are several that can produce hepatic injury (Table 17-18). A few warrant special comment.

Anticoagulants

Phenindione has led to well over 100 instances of generalized hypersensitivity. About 10% of these were accompanied by jaundice, which had both cholestatic and hepatocellular features.[257,270,533,534,803] The approximately 10% case-fatality rate, however, reflects generalized hypersensitivity rather than liver failure.[270,533,534] Other anticoagulants have rarely been incriminated in instances of hepatic disease in humans, although an instance of warfarin-induced cholestasis has been described.[590]

Antiarrhythmic Drugs

Quinidine. Despite 60 years of clinical use, quinidine had not been recognized to cause hepatic injury until 1969.[111] Since then, approximately 24 cases have been reported.[140,231,378,497] Presumably, previous instances had been overlooked. In the reported patients the syndrome has been ushered in with fever within 6 to 12 days of initiation of treatment. In most cases, readministration of a single dose of quinidine has led to prompt recurrence of fever and to elevated aminotransferase levels. Liver biopsy has shown granulomata in several patients.[102]

TABLE 17-18. Hepatic Injury Produced by Various Drugs Used to Treat Cardiovascular Disease

AGENT	TYPE OF INJURY
Ajmaline	Ch or M
Amiodarone	H-Cell*
Aprindine†	H-Cell-M
Benziodarone‡	H-Cell
Captopril	Ch
Chlorthalidone†	Ch
Clofibrate§	Minor§
Coralgil*	Phospholipidosis
Dihydralazine	H-Cell
Disopyramide	Ch
Furosemide**	H-Cell
Hydralazine†‖	H-Cell
Methyldopa¶	H-Cell
Nicotinic acid	H-Cell-M
Nifedipine	Ch
Papaverine¶	H-Cell
Perihexilene maleate	H-Cell
Phenindione	Ch-M
Procainamide‖	H-Cell-M
Pyridinol carbamate†	H-Cell
Quinethazone†	Ch
Quinidine‖	H-Cell-M
Thiazides†	Ch
Ticrynafen¶	H-Cell
Verapamil†	H-Cell, Ch

* Lesion may include "alcoholic hyaline" and phospholipidosis and may lead to cirrhosis.[559]
† Too few cases for clear picture.
‡ Largely or completely withdrawn from clinical use.
§ Hepatic injury trivial.
‖ Also leads to hepatic granulomas.
** Can cause midzonal necrosis in experimental animals.
(Ch, cholestatic injury; consists mainly of bilirubin casts in canaliculi, usually with portal inflammatory infiltrate and with or without mild parenchymal injury. H-Cell, hepatocellular lesion; consists mainly of necrosis with or without inflammation. M, mixed)
(Data from reference 807)

Blood eosinophilia has been specified as absent or has not been mentioned in the reports.[378] Injury is hepetocellular as manifested by degeneration and focal necrosis.[378]

Procainamide. Hepatic injury caused by this drug appears to be extremely rare. We are aware of only one case report[361] and of three unpublished instances. In these patients, the injury appeared to be mixed hepatocellular. The aminotransferase levels in one of them reached almost 500 IU and in the other two were above 200 IU. In all three patients, the alkaline phosphatase levels were in the cholestatic range. Granulomatous hepatitis has been attributed to procainamide.[458,618]

Aprindine. Aprindine has local anesthetic properties similar to those of procainamide. It has been reported to cause hepatic injury with both cytotoxic and cholestatic features.[72,183,287] Evidence of hepatic injury has appeared in most patients within 3 weeks of initiating therapy with the drug. Rechallenge with aprindine has led to a reappearance of the injury.[183,287]

Ajmaline. Ajmaline, which is derived from the root of *Rauwolfia serpentina,* is closely related to quinidine in structure and has similar clinical applications. It has been incriminated in at least 30 instances of jaundice.[54,156,329,501] In some of these patients, the jaundice has been cholestatic with high levels of alkaline phosphatase, modestly elevated aminotransferase values, and evidence of cholestasis on biopsy.[54,156] Other reports have described cholestatic injury in some patients and hepatocellular injury in others.[329,501] One report has described a syndrome resembling primary biliary cirrhosis as a sequel to cholestatic jaundice in a patient taking ajmaline, methyltestosterone, and ethinyl estradiol.[54]

Verapamil and Nifedepine. The calcium-channel blocking agents verapamil and nifedepine are used in the treatment of hypertension, angina pectoris, and supraventricular arrhythmias. Hepatocellular injury has been reported in a few patients receiving verapamil.[84,256,502,703] The onset of evidence of hepatotoxicity was 2 to 3 weeks after initiation of therapy. The relation of the drug to the production of the injury has been proven by rechallenge.[84] In one patient in whom a liver biopsy was available, there was cholestasis.[256]

Three instances of a predominantly cholestatic injury from nifedipine have been reported.[129,619,620] In one patient a rechallenge led to reappearance of the injury within 1 day.[620]

Antihypertensive Agents

α-Methyldopa. During almost 2 decades of widespread clinical use of this drug as an antihypertensive agent, there have been reports of hepatic injury in at least 80 patients.[95,605] Presumably, there are many additional unreported cases. The available data suggest that the incidence of overt hepatic disease is less than 1%, but that trivial injury reflected by biochemical abnormalities is more frequent.[807] Females, especially those who are postmenopausal, appear to have an increased incidence of injury.[438,807]

The hepatic disease has been acute in 85% of recorded cases and chronic in the remainder. The predominant acute injury has been hepatocellular and has resembled that of acute viral hepatitis.[95,303,437,605] There has usually been a prodromal period of anorexia, malaise, and fever, followed in a few days by frank jaundice. In about half

of the patients the hepatic injury has appeared within 2 to 4 weeks of beginning the agent. Values for aminotransferases in most patients have ranged up to 1500 IU. Levels of alkaline phosphatase have been elevated in almost all patients, but in 90% of them they have been less than threefold elevated over normal. The hepatic injury induced by methyldopa may result from a hypersensitivity reaction, although production of a toxic metabolite by microsomes has been demonstrated.[474]

The histologic changes also resemble those of acute viral hepatitis. Cell degeneration, "free" acidophilic bodies, and areas of necrosis are characteristic (see Fig. 17-7). The inflammatory response tends to be concentrated in the portal and periportal zones and consists mainly of lymphocytes and other mononuclear cells with some neutrophils. Tissue eosinophilia is uncommon.[807] Prominence of plasma cells is also not characteristic of the acute form of injury but, as described below, is seen in the patients with the chronic active hepatitis form of damage. "Bridging necrosis" extending between portal areas and from portal to central areas was prominent among the patients of Maddrey and Boitnott[437] and several reported patients have had severe subacute hepatic necrosis.[437,589,647]

Other laboratory data have revealed Coombs-positive hemolytic anemia in 3% of patients with hepatic injury, a figure similar to the incidence in all recipients of α-methyldopa, even those without hepatic injury.[605,807] The blood may contain the "L.E. factor" and antinuclear and anti–smooth muscle antibodies in a number of patients with acute hepatic injury, but these findings are also present in the absence of liver disease.[807] The majority of recipients of the drug who develop acute hepatocellular injury have not shown these serologic markers of "autoimmunity." Blood eosinophilia also has been rare.

The prognosis of the acute form of hepatocellular injury approximates that of other forms of drug-induced hepatocellular damage. Approximately 10% of the reported patients with acute hepatic injury have died.[605] In nonfatal cases, recovery is usually prompt after discontinuation of the drug, and jaundice is gone by 3 to 8 weeks.[437,605,807]

A chronic syndrome, which in all regards resembles that of the "autoimmune" type of chronic active hepatitis, has been attributed to α-methyldopa in a number of reports.[241,303,438,657,731,785,808] In one series, 2 of 20 patients with methyldopa-induced hepatitis had histologic evidence of chronic active hepatitis.[731] Biopsy has revealed confluent areas of lobular collapse, condensation of reticulum, an intense inflammatory response in the plasma cells, and varying numbers of eosinophils. Biopsy specimens from some patients have shown fibrous septa dissecting the lobule; several have had the pattern of frank macronodular cirrhosis in a setting of chronic necroflammatory disease.[438,659] Maddrey and Boitnott,[437] in their report of acute hepatocellular injury in recipients of α-methyldopa, have emphasized the prominence of bridging necrosis.

The clinical features, like those of other forms of chronic active hepatitis, have been a mixture of acute and chronic hepatic disease. Some patients had already developed clinical evidence of cirrhosis when first recognized to have hepatic disease. Others have presented with an apparent acute hepatocellular injury, only to have the biopsy reveal a histologic pattern of chronic active hepatitis.[785] There is little evidence that the hepatitis persists after the drug has been withdrawn, although patients may be left with some degree of scarring and even cirrhosis.[438]

Hydralazine. Hydralazine has been incriminated in very few instances of hepatic injury during the quarter century that it has been in clinical use. An early paper by Perry[535] referred to "hepatitis" in a patient taking hydralazine and reserpine but provided no details. In the next 1½ decades there was no further reference to the phenomena. During the past 3 years, however, there have been reports of hepatocellular injury with bridging necrosis and very high aminotransferase levels in two patients taking hyralazine[31,188] and in two others taking dihydralazine.[376,531] There has also been a report of hepatic granulomas accompanied by slight biochemical evidence of hepatic injury in a patient taking hydralazine.[342] In a patient who developed hepatitis after 3 years of therapy with phenobarbital, phenytoin, primidone, and hydralazine, the hydralazine was shown to be the inciting agent by a rechallenge study.[326]

Captopril. The antihypertensive angiotensin-converting enzyme inhibitor captopril has been reported to cause cholestatic hepatic injury.[526,574,753] The mechanism of injury is not established. Several of the affected patients had fever, rash, and eosinophilia, suggesting a hypersensitivity reaction. Usually jaundice, fever, pruritus, and evidence of liver injury disappeared rapidly on drug withdrawal.[574] No rechallenges with captopril in a patient with presumed drug-induced injury have been reported.

Diuretic Drugs

Rare instances of jaundice, apparently hepatocanalicular, have been observed in patients taking thiazide diuretics.[128,160] Quinethazine, ethacrynic acid, chlorthalidone, and furosamide have been reported to lead to instances of jaundice, perhaps as a result of hypersensitivity.[128,363] Mitchell and others,[473] however, have shown that large doses of furosamide lead to midzonal necrosis in rats. Their studies demonstrated clearly that the injury was caused by a metabolite of the drug. Nevertheless, we know of no instances of zonal necrosis that have been reported in humans.

Ticrynafyn (Selacryn), a diuretic agent with uricosuric properties was found to produce a number of instances of acute hepatic injury shortly after it entered clinical use in the United States and was promptly withdrawn from use in this country.[816] Analysis of 340 cases of ticrynafen-associated liver injury reported to the FDA by the manufacturer[816] revealed acute hepatocellular injury to be the characteristic lesion with a case-fatality rate of 10% (25 of 246 patients). The clinical and histologic pattern

in almost all was that of an acute hepatitis. A few showed histologic features of chronic hepatitis. The presumed mechanism of injury was metabolic idiosyncrasy as deduced from the absence of fever and eosinophilia and the variable duration of drug administration (usually greater than 30 days) before signs of hepatic injury appeared. However, the prompt response to challenge dose in 15 of 16 patients suggested that hypersensitivity may also have played a part.[816]

Antianginal Drugs

Perhexiline Maleate. Perhexiline is a lipophilic drug that has been reported to produce hepatic injury and death from cirrhosis.[212,280,399,407,522,538,547] Some patients have shown only mild to moderate fatty changes on liver biopsy. Others have shown a lesion closely resembling alcoholic hepatitis with intracellular inclusions similar to Mallory bodies (alcoholic hyaline). These patients also show, on electron microscopy, abnormal lysosomes reflecting phospholipid accumulation (phospholipidosis). It has been suggested that perhexiline forms drug–lipid complexes within lysosomes that may be important in promoting the deposition of the phospholipids.[430,431] Aminotransferase levels have been increased in 24% to 50% of patients taking the drug[229,300,302,490,508,538,548] with the incidence and degree of abnormality dependent on the dose.

The mechanism of injury remains to be defined, but it has been shown that perhexiline is metabolized by hepatic oxidation and that patients with peripheral neuropathy induced by the drug often have decreased clearance of perhexiline apparently due to impaired oxidative capacity; the defect is genetically determined.[488] Similarly, severely impaired oxidative capacity has been demonstrated in patients with perhexilene-induced liver injury by using debrisoquine as a test substance.[488] Accordingly, perhexiline-induced hepatic injury appears to be an example of metabolic idiosyncrasy-determined toxicity.

Amiodarone. Amiodarone is an iodine-containing benzofuran derivative that has been successfully used for the treatment of angina pectoris and for supraventricular and ventricular arrhythmias. Side-effects observed in patients from amiodarone include pulmonary infiltrates and interstitial fibrosis, hyperthyroidism and hypothyroidism, corneal deposits, peripheral neuropathy, cutaneous photosensitivity, and a bluish discoloration of the skin.[559,674] Pleomorphic lysosomal inclusions have been found in many tissues, including cornea, peripheral nerve, skeletal muscle, lung, heart, skin, lymphocytes, plasma cells, granulocytes, and tissue macrophages.[559,674] These inclusions reflect the phospholipidosis similar to that produced by perhexilene.

A variety of hepatic abnormalities have been associated with the use of amiodarone. Hepatomegaly is usual, and other signs or symptoms indicating chronic hepatic disease have been reported,[453,559,674] including moderate increases in serum aminotransferase levels (one- to fivefold) and alkaline phosphatase (onefold to twofold). Jaundice is unusual. The biochemical abnormalities generally resolve over several weeks to months after drug withdrawal. In some patients hepatic abnormalities remained present for up to a year after cessation of the drug, and the drug may be detected in the serum months after the drug is withdrawn as it is released from tissue stores.

Abnormalities found on the light microscopic examination of liver biopsy from a patient with amiodarone-induced hepatic injury often resemble changes found in patients with alcoholic hepatitis with enlarged hepatocytes, granular cytoplasm, and pericellular fibrosis. Particularly noteworthy are the Mallory bodies in hepatocytes (see Fig. 17-8D) and biliary epithelial cells, polymorphonuclear leukocytic infiltration, lipogranulomas, macrovesicular steatosis, proliferated bile ducts, and evidence of cholangitis. In some, a micronodular cirrhosis is found. Electron microscopic examination shows osmiophilic lysosomal inclusions, found most abundantly in the region of the bile canaliculi.[559] The inclusions have been found in hepatocytes, bile duct epithelial cells, Kupffer cells, and endothelial cells. Collagen fibers have been found in the space of Disse.

Similar light and electron microscopic changes to those found in amiodarone-induced liver injury have been observed in liver injury induced by other drugs, including perhexiline, chloroquine, and 4-4'-diethylaminoethoxyhexestrol.[407,431,538] These drugs are all amphiphilic and form drug–lipid complexes within lysosomes that may be important in promoting deposition of phospholipid.[559]

Benziodarone. This coronary vasodilator was introduced into clinical use in England approximately 20 years ago. A number of cases of hepatocellular jaundice, however, led to its early withdrawal.[807]

4,4'-Diethylaminoethoxyhexesterol (Coralgil). This "coronary dilator" was found to be one of the most frequent causes of drug-induced hepatic injury in Japan during the period of its active use. It was found to lead to a peculiar form of fatty metamorphosis in which there is an accumulation of phospholipids in the hepatic lysosomes, which gives the hepatocyte a foamy appearance.[430,666] Mallory bodies may be seen. This phospholipidosis leads to a syndrome characterized by a mild fever, malaise, anorexia, weight loss, and hepatomegaly. Values of SGOT are slightly elevated (one- to threefold); those for SGPT are even lower, and levels of alkaline phosphatase are negligibly increased.[514,666]

The pathogenesis of the lesion remains unclear. Lullman and co-workers[430] have attributed it to the binding of phospholipids by the reaction between their polar groups and the drug.

Antihyperlipidemia Agents

Clofibrate. Clofibrate, used to treat hypercholesterolemia, has appeared to have no important adverse effect on the liver.[646,777,807] Nevertheless, there is a reported low incidence of slight and transient elevations of aminotransferase (and creatine kinase) levels attributed to muscle injury[683] and there is evidence that clofibrate and its congeners can impair BSP excretion.[460] In experimental animals, large doses of this and several related compounds led to hepatomegaly, enlargement of individual hepatocytes,[38,289] a variable degree of fat accumulation, and increased number of lysozomes.[289,384] Individual instances of "granulomatous hepatitis"[545] and of intrahepatic cholestasis[749] have been attributed to this drug. An important adverse hepatobiliary effect of clofibrate is its alteration of composition of bile leading to greater lithogenicity and a higher incidence of gallstones.[36,115,353] When given to patients with primary biliary cirrhosis as treatment for the hypercholesterolemia, it leads to a further, paradoxical increase in cholesterol levels.[715]

Nicotinic Acid. Nicotinic acid and its derivatives, also employed to treat hypercholesterolemia, have caused hepatic dysfunction in about one third and jaundice in 3% to 5% of long-term recipients.[106,528] The demonstration of parenchymal degeneration and necrosis on biopsy, and the high serum levels of aminotransferases indicate the hepatocellular nature of the damage. Employment of huge doses of nicotinic acid to treat psychiatric disease has led to several instances of jaundice with features of hepatocellular injury and cholestasis.[178,788]

Pyridinol Carbamate. Pyridinol has been used in the treatment of atherosclerosis. Instances of hepatocellular injury have been reported.[363,501]

Papaverine. The convincing description by Ronnov-Jensen and Tjernbrund[610] of hepatotoxic effects of this drug in 4 of 15 recipients came as a surprise after 50 years of injury-free use of this smooth muscle relaxant in circulatory disease and other conditions. The hepatic injury appears to be hepatocellular with 10- or 20-fold elevation of the aminotransferase levels[610] and hepatocyte degeneration and necrosis seen on biopsy.[345] The clinical features suggest the mechanism to have been hypersensitivity, but the apparent high incidence suggests that intrinsic toxicity contributes to the pathogenesis.[805] Papaverine also has led to a syndrome of chronic active hepatitis.[561]

Antineoplastic Agents

The number of candidate oncotherapeutic agents studied in experimental animals and tested in patients is far too great and the data regarding the possible adverse effects of many of them on the liver far too scant to permit systematic analysis of the hepatotoxicity of cancer chemotherapeutic agents. Additional problems in assessing and ascribing an etiology to liver damage in patients receiving cancer chemotherapy are the frequent, multiple, possible etiologies including viral hepatitis (hepatitis B; non-A, non-B; herpes; cytomegalovirus), effects of the neoplasm

TABLE 17-19.   Some Hepatic Lesions Produced By Oncotherapeutic Agents

AGENT	STEATOSIS	NECROSIS	CHOLESTASIS	VASO-OCCLUSIVE DISEASE*	PELIOSIS HEPATIS
Amsacrine			+		
L-Asparaginase	+	(+)			
ARA-C		(+)		+	
Azathioprine†		(+)	+	+	+
Bleomycin	+				
Busulfan			+		
Chlorambucil		+			
Cisplatinum	+	+			
Cyclophosphamide		+			
Dactinomycin	+				
Daunorubicin				+	
Doxorubicin		+			
DTIC				+	
5-Fu		(+)†			
FuDR‡		(+)	+		
Hydrazines	+				
Hydroxyurea					+
Indicine-N-oxide		+		+	
Mercaptopurine		+	+		
Methotrexate	+	(+)			
Mithramycin		+			
Mitomycin	+			+	
Nitrosoureas		+			
Streptozocin		+			
Thioguanine		+		+	
Urethane		+		+	
Vinca alkaloids		(+)			

* Combination chemotherapy with or without irradiation or irradiation alone can lead to vaso-occlusive disease.
† Only when administered parenterally.
‡ Only when administered by infusion into hepatic artery.
(Data from references 195, 276, 445, 451, 459, 461, 472, 536, 638, and 811)

itself, and the multiple drugs the majority of these patients receive. Nevertheless, information on the effects of a number of agents on the liver is available (Table 17-19).[195,276,445,451,459,461,472,535,638,811] A number are hepatotoxic.[807] Others appear to spare the liver or to produce hepatic injury rarely as the result of host idiosyncrasy.[638,811]

For the most part, the forms of acute and chronic hepatic injury produced by oncotherapeutic agents are similar to those produced by other agents (see Table 17-5). There are, however, several forms of injury that are particularly prominent. Steatosis is much more frequently noted in the hepatic injury of anticancer agents than in that produced by other drugs. Cirrhosis attributable to intrinsic drug toxicity, seen with methotrexate therapy, is not seen with most other medicinal hepatic injury. Veno-occlusive disease, the dramatic lesion characteristically produced by pyrrolizidine alkaloids, (1) is produced by a number of cancer chemotherapy agents and protocols[811] (see Table 17-19) and not by other medicinals. Another unique drug-induced lesion is the ductal injury resembling

sclerosing cholangitis that is seen as a complication of "pump" infusion therapy of metastatic hepatic carcinoma.[294]

In general, antimetabolites and antibiotics are the oncotherapeutic agents most likely to cause hepatic injury, while the alkylating agents are least likely to do so.

Antimetabolites and Related Agents

Some antimetabolites, selective enzyme poisons, and antibiotics are intrinsic hepatotoxins with a dose-related ability to produce liver damage. In this category are methotrexate, some antipyrimidine and antipurine compounds, asparaginase, and a number of antineoplastic antibiotics (see Table 17-19).

Methotrexate. Shortly after the introduction of methotrexate for the treatment of leukemia 25 years ago, hints that it might be hepatotoxic appeared.[112,314] Subsequently even more convincing evidence of the hepatotoxicity of this agent came from its use for the treatment of psoriasis. By now more than 100 psoriatic patients treated with methotrexate have been reported to develop cirrhosis, fibrosis, or fatty liver.[124,125,471,512,552,609,772] The likelihood of liver damage seems directly related to duration of therapy and inversely related to the length of the interval between doses.[124,125] Daily small doses are more likely to lead to liver damage than are larger doses at weekly intervals.[125,471,512] The role of co-factors, such as age, obesity, and alcoholism has been especially emphasized in the studies of Nyfors and Poulsen.[512]

Histologic changes of methotrexate-induced liver damage include steatosis, ballooning degeneration, and necrosis of hepatocytes, fibrosis, and ultimately cirrhosis. An increase in the number of Ito cells (fat-laden lipocytes) has been reported in patients receiving methotrexate.[299] Portal inflammation is usually moderate and consists of lymphocytes, macrophages, and neutrophils. Nuclei of hepatocytes are usually hyperchromatic, pleomorphic, and vacuolated. The cirrhosis resembles somewhat that of the alcoholic.[641]

Biochemical changes provide insensitive reflections of the extent of hepatic injury. Mildly abnormal values for BSP excretion and slight elevations of aminotransferases are usually found for 1 or 2 days after a dose of methotrexate and may remain mildly abnormal. The values, however, may be so slightly abnormal as to be of little value in the recognition of hepatic injury.[363,512,552] Liver biopsy is essential for identification of damage and repeated biopsy necessary to follow a patient.[363,512]

Antipyrimidines. Azauridine and azacytidine are pyrimidine antagonists that have been shown to produce a fatty liver and some necrosis in experimental animals.[42,43,339] Cytarabine produces mild hepatocellular injury.[738]

Antipurines. Azaserine is a glutamine antagonist that inhibits purine synthesis. It produces steatosis, as well as some necrosis of the liver.[305,704]

6-Mercaptopurine, an agent employed for the treatment of leukemia and, to a small degree, for immunosuppression, has been reported to produce hepatic injury with jaundice in 6% to 40% of recipients.[177,186,669] While cholestasis is prominent in some patients, the predominant injury is hepatocellular, and even fatal hepatic necrosis has occurred. Possible potentiation of the hepatotoxicity of 6-mercaptopurine by doxorubicin (Adriamycin) has been suggested by Minow and co-workers[472] because of the frequency and severity of the hepatic injury when these two drugs are used in combination for the treatment of refractory leukemia.[472,606]

6-Chloropurine has led to similar hepatic injury.[186] Thioguanine has been reported to cause jaundice[119] and veno-occlusive disease.[252]

Azathioprine, a derivative of 6-mercaptopurine used mainly as an immunosuppressant, has led to a few reported instances of cholestatic injury.[146,161,250,694,735] It has also been incriminated in a number of instances of he-

patocellular injury among patients exposed to other causes of liver diseases.[82,318,441,467,767] The hepatotoxic role of azathioprine in these cases is not clear.

Fatal hepatic necrosis also has been attributed to aziothioprine.[800] An even more important observation is the recent attribution of the vascular lesions, veno-occlusive disease, and peliosis hepatis to this drug.[444,811] The mechanism of aziothioprine-related hepatic injury is unknown, but the parenchymal lesions may relate to the conversion of the drug to 6-mercaptopurine.

L-Asparaginase. This agent, although an enzyme, behaves like an antimetabolite. By catalyzing the deamination of asparagine it deprives the neoplastic cell of the amino acid and so blocks protein synthesis. Presumably, the steatosis, which asparaginase produces in 60% to 90% of recipients[254,255,276,564] depends on the same mechanism,[807] although some authors have attributed the hepatic injury to a contaminant of the enzyme.[103] Large doses lead to necrosis.

Antineoplastic Antibiotics

Some antineoplastic antibiotics produce necrosis. Others cause steatosis, presumably by mechanisms related to their antineoplastic effects.[807] Nevertheless, some potent cytostatic agents (dactinomycin d, cycloheximide, doxorubicin, daunorubicin) cause necrosis of bone marrow and intestinal mucosa but few hepatic lesions (see Table 17-19). The potentiation of hepatic injury of 6-mercaptopurine by doxorubicin has, however, been noted previously. Similarly, severe liver toxicity may follow the administration of dactinomycin after nephrectomy and irradiation for Wilms' tumor.[459]

Alkaloids

The Vinca alkaloids vincristine and vinblastine differ from each other somewhat in their toxic side-effects, but both lead to little instances of hepatic injury in humans, although rarely.[116,811] Coupled with x-irradiation these agents can lead to necrosis.[536]

Indocine-N-oxide can lead to vaso-occlusive disease and the associated zone 3 necrosis.[811] This is to be expected since the drug is in the family of pyrrolizidine alkaloids, classic causes of vaso-occlusive disease.[811]

Colchicine. There is no evidence that colchicine, in doses given humans, causes hepatic injury. Large doses, however, can lead to hepatic steatosis and necrosis in rats.[150] A derivative, demecolcine, has led to jaundice in humans.[807]

Emetine. Emetine, used mainly for the treatment of amebic abscess, has intermittently been tried as an anticancer agent but without success. It is an extremely powerful producer of hepatic steatosis in experimental animals.[150] Nevertheless, during its long years of use as an antiamebic drug, it has not been recognized to cause hepatic injury in humans.

Alkylating Agents

Four groups of alkylating agents have been used in the treatment of neoplastic diseases. As nearly as can be ascertained, from the available (and confusing) literature, the ethylenimine derivatives have not been incriminated in the production of liver damage. Among the nitrogen mustards, the prototypic mechlorethamine and melphalan also seem free of responsibility for hepatic injury, although several other members of the group have been incriminated in the production of liver damage. Chlorambucil and cyclophosphamide have been incriminated in several instances of hepatocellular jaundice with necrosis.[811] A case of cholestatic jaundice has been attributed[746] to an alkyl sulfonate (Busulfan). The most convincing evidence for some hepatotoxic potential applies to the nitrosoureas (see Table 17-19).

Nitrosoureas

Nitrosoureas have been found to have dose-related hepatotoxic effects in experimental animals. Of special note is the toxicity of dacarbazine (DTIC). This cytostatic drug used as adjuvant therapy in patients with malignant melanoma has been associated with frequent transient and important aminotransferase elevations. Reports of a number of instances of acute veno-occlusive disease,[811] however, are of greater importance.

Other Antitumor Agents

Urethane, formerly used to treat leukemia, and multiple myeloma, is a known hepatoxin and hepatocarcinogen.[621] It has produced centrizonal necrosis and fibrosis in association with injury to the efferent hepatic veins and venules. The histologic changes and syndrome resemble the veno-occlusive disease of pyrrolizidine toxicity.[83,775]

4'4-Diaminodiphenylamine (known as M&B 938) was tested for therapeutic value in multiple myeloma 2 decades ago and found to produce cholestatic jaundice.[145] Other agents incriminated in hepatic injury are listed in Table 17-19.

Miscellaneous Drugs

A large number of other agents are listed in Table 17-20. Some have been discarded because of known toxicity, after wide clinical use (*e.g.,* tannic acid)[807] or clinical trials (*e.g.,* lergotrile mesylate),[414] or are folk remedies that are hardly taken today. Nevertheless, a listing of several of these agents and the lesions they produce may be of some value. Several of these warrant additional comment.

Oxyphenisatin. Oxyphenisatin, which has been in use as a component of laxative preparations for many years has been recognized during the past decade to lead to hepatic disease.[17,599] By now more than 100 cases have been identified.[17,599,807] Of these about two thirds have presented with the syndrome of chronic hepatitis while the remainder had apparently acute disease.

The majority of patients have been women. Anorexia, fatigue, and jaundice, often accompanied by slight upper abdominal distress, have been presenting complaints in patients whose biochemical and histologic features had been those of acute disease. Some patients with these complaints, however, have shown histologic features of chronic disease. More often the syndrome of chronic active hepatitis in patients taking the drug presents insidiously. It is particularly likely to be found in patients who continue taking oxyphenisatin after jaundice has appeared and been ignored or the relationship to the drug overlooked.[599] Most patients with acute or chronic disease have shown rapid improvement when the drug has been withdrawn.

Values for aminotransferases in patients with acute injury are in the range typical for acute viral hepatitis, 750 to 1500 IU. Levels of alkaline phosphatase are only slightly or moderately elevated. Prothrombin levels are often depressed. Patients with the syndrome of chronic disease usually show biochemical values that are somewhat intermediate between those of acute and chronic liver disease. Hypoalbuminemia, hyperglobulinemia, hypoprothrombinemia, and variable degrees of hyperbilirubinemia are characteristic.[599]

Serologic features typical for "lupoid hepatitis" have been observed in a number of patients with the chronic syndrome.[599] They include the L.E. factor, antinuclear antibodies, and smooth muscle antibodies.

Histologic changes in oxyphenisatin-induced disease range from those typical for acute hepatitis, through changes classic for chronic active hepatitis, to frank cirrhosis. Patients with the acute syndrome show diffuse hepatocellular necrosis, acidophilic bodies, lobular disarray, Kupffer cell prominence, and inflammation, mainly portal.[363,599] The pattern resembles somewhat that of acute viral hepatitis, although cholestasis and steatosis appear to be more prominent in oxyphenisatin-induced jaundice. Ultrastructural differences have been cited.[363] Patients with the syndrome of chronic active hepatitis may show subacute hepatic necrosis.[241] More often the changes are those classic for chronic active hepatitis with "piecemeal necrosis," portal and periportal inflammation, which includes plasma cells and lymphocytes, "rosette" formation, and periportal architectural distortion.[599] A number of patients have had frank cirrhosis.[241,363]

The prognosis in most patients with acute injury is quite good. Withdrawal of the drug usually leads to prompt improvement, although instances of progression of disease even after stopping the drug have been described.[17] Even patients with chronic disease usually improve after the drug has been stopped, but they may continue to show active disease.[599] Cirrhosis once established, however presumably remains.

TABLE 17-20.   Hepatic Injury Produced by Miscellaneous Drugs

DRUGS	TYPE OF INJURY	REFERENCES
Analgesics		
Acetaminophen*	CZ-Necrosis	108, 565
Amidopyrine†	J	565
Propoxyphene	Ch	126, 368
Clometacine	Ch	239
Adrenergics		
Lergotrile mesylate	H-Cell	414
Levodopa*‡	H-Cell (?)	504
Carbamazepine‡	H-Can-M	807
Cimetidine	Ch	428, 761, 814
Disulfiram‡	H-Cell-M	180
Cholecystographic dyes		
Bunamiodyl	§	363
Iopanic acid	§	363
Iodipamid	§	363
Essential oils		
Apiol*‖	Steatosis	428
Myristicin*‖	Steatosis	262
Heavy metal antagonists		
BAL*‖	Steatosis	621
Penicillamine	Ch	32, 457, 578, 783
Iodide ion		
(Providone-iodine)	CZ-Necrosis	807
Oxyphenisatin¶	H-Cell	599, 807
Methyl methacrylate*‖	Steatosis	442
Phenazopyridine‡	H-Cell	807
Phenobarbital‡		521
Pyridine	H-Cell	554
Ranitidine	H-Cell-Ch	29, 58, 109, 290, 396, 572, 693
Salizopyridine‡	H-Cell-M	97, 464
Tannic acid*	H-Cell	807
Trimethobenzamide†‡	H-Cell-M	807
Tripellannamine†‡	Ch	807
Thorotrast		654
Vitamin A#	CZ degeneration, necrosis	626
X-Irradiation**	CZ necrosis, venous injury	472

  * Toxic only in overdose.

  † So rare as to suggest that the reported cases may have been coincidental rather than caused by the drug.

  ‡ Too few cases for clear picture.

  § Interferes with bilirubin clearance by competition for uptake.

  ‖ Hepatic injury observed mainly in experimental animals.

  ¶ Can also cause chronic-active hepatitis syndrome.

  # Can lead to angiosarcoma, hepatocellular carcinoma, and cholangiocarcinoma.

  ** Causes centrizonal fibrosis.

  (Ch, cholestatic injury; consists mainly of bilirubin casts in canaliculi, usually with portal inflammatory response, and with or without mild parenchymal injury. H-Cell, hepatocellular injury; consists mainly of degeneration and necrosis, with or without inflammation. M, mixed; CZ, Centrizonal)

Cimetidine. Cimetidine has been widely used for the reduction of gastric activity in several clinical settings with little evidence of overt hepatic injury.[220] Nevertheless, a number of cases of jaundice have been described.[142,334,417,649,759,761,814] Although the injury has been called cholestatic in several reports,[417,814] very high aminotransferase levels[417,761] and reference to centrizonal necrosis, albeit "mild," suggest that hepatocellular injury also occurs and the lesion appears to have both hepatocellular and cholestatic components. Ability of cimetidine to inhibit the mixed function oxidase has required attention to its effects on other drugs.[649]

Ranitidine. Instances of hepatotoxic effects of ranitidine, an H_2 antagonist, also have been reported.[29,58,109, 290,396,572,693] Both hepatocellular and cholestatic injury have been noted, and the frequency, character, and significances of the injury remain to be evaluated.

Streptokinase. One patient, a 27-year-old woman, developed evidence of hepatic injury 2 days after beginning streptokinase therapy for venous thrombosis.[628] After all biochemical abnormalities had resolved, streptokinase was again administered and evidence of hepatic injury returned within 24 hours.

D-Penicillamine. Occasionally instances of hepatic injury (predominantly cholestatic) have been reported from the use of D-penicillamine.[32,147,457,578]

Disulfiram. A few instances of hepatocellular injury have been reported in patients receiving disulfiram.[180,354,491,632] All but one, who died of fulminant hepatic failure,[632] recovered rapidly following withdrawal. Cyanamide, another drug used in aversion therapy, leads to striking degenerative changes with cytoplasmic inclusion bodies and can eventuate in cirrhosis.[754]

Quinine. One patient, a 65-year-old woman, developed granulomatous hepatitis with occasional eosinophils 5 months after beginning quinine therapy for leg cramps.[348] After the quinine was withdrawn, the biochemical abnormalities and clinical symptoms resolved and later reappeared within hours of a rechallenge.

CONCLUDING COMMENTS

Chemical hepatic injury can be acute and chronic. Acute injury may be mainly cytotoxic or cholestatic. Cytotoxic injury may be manifested by necrosis, steatosis, or both. Cholestatic injury may be associated with portal inflammation (hepatocanalicular jaundice) or may not be (canalicular jaundice). Chronic hepatic injury includes several forms of cirrhosis, chronic active hepatitis, steatosis, phospholipidosis, veno-occlusive disease, peliosis hepatitis, or hepatic neoplasms. The mechanism for injury may be intrinsic toxicity of the agent, an unusually susceptible host or mixtures of the two factors. Unusual susceptibility may be the result of hypersensitivity reaction to, or of toxic metabolite of, the drug.

REFERENCES

1. Aaron JS et al: Diphenylhydantoin-induced hepatotoxicity. Am J Gastroenterol 80:200, 1985
2. Acetaminophen hepatoxicity. Med Lett Drug Ther 20:61, 1978
3. Adler E et al: Cholestatic hepatic injury related to coumadin exposure. Arch Intern Med 146:1837, 1986
4. Adlercreutz H, Tenhunen R: Some aspects of the interaction between natural and synthetic female sex hormones and the liver. Am J Med 49:630, 1970
5. Ahern WJ et al: Granulomatous hepatitis and seatone. Med J Aust 2:151, 1980
6. Al-Kawas FH et al: Allopurinol hepatotoxicity: Report of two cases and review of the literature. Ann Intern Med 95:588, 1981
7. Allen JR, Carstens LA: Monocrotaline-induced Budd-Chiari syndrome in monkeys. Am J Dig Dis 16:111, 1971
8. American Thoracic Society: Chemoprophylaxis for the prevention of tuberculosis. Am Rev Respir Dis 96:558, 1967
9. Anderson KE et al: Nutritional influences on chemical biotransformation in humans. Nutr Rev 40:161, 1982
10. Anderson RJ: Letter: Severe reaction associated with sulindac administration. N Engl J Med 300:735, 1979
11. Andrade ZA et al: Letter: Lesoes hepaticas produzidas por hycanthone. Rev Inst Med Trop Sao Paulo 16:160, 1974
12. Andriole VT: Altered sulfobromophthalein metabolism in the dog induced by the antifungal agent X-5079C. J Lab Clin Med 61:730, 1963
13. Anthony PP: Hepatoma associated with androgenic steroids. Lancet 1:685, 1975
14. Arias IM: Effects of a plant acid (icterogenin) and certain anabolic steroids on the hepatic metabolism of bilirubin and sulfobromophthalein (BSP). Ann NY Acad Sci 104:1014, 1963
15. Arias IM: What is primary in cholestasis? In Brunner H, Thaler H (eds): Hepatology: A Festschrift for Hans Popper, pp 281–284. New York, Raven Press, 1985
16. Arranto AJ, Sotaniemi EA: Morphologic alterations in patients with alpha-methyldopa-induced liver damage after short- and long-term exposure. Scand J Gastroenterol 16:853, 1981
17. Australian Drug Evaluation Committee: Withdrawal of oxyphenisatin acetate diacetoxydiphenolisatin and triacetyldiphenolisatin from the Australian Market. Med J Aust 1:1051, 1972
18. Aw TY et al: Hepatic drug metabolism and drug induced liver injury. In Gitnick G (ed): Current Hepatology, vol 5, pp 113–196. New York, John Wiley, 1985
19. Bacon AM, Rosenberg SA: Cyclophosphamide hepatotoxicity in a patient with systemic lupus erythematosus. Ann Intern Med 97:62, 1982
20. Baerg RD, Kimberg DV: Centrilobular hepatic necrosis and acute renal failure in "solvent sniffers." Ann Intern Med 73:713, 1970
21. Baetens P, Ramboer C: Chronic active hepatitis due to hydroxymethyl-nitrofurantoin in a male patient. Acta Clin Belg 39:85, 1984
22. Bagheri SA, Boyer JL: Peliosis hepatis associated with androgenic-anabolic steroid therapy: A severe form of hepatic injury. Ann Intern Med 81:610, 1974
23. Baird RW, Hull JG: Cholestatic jaundice from tolbutamide. Ann Intern Med 53:194, 1960
24. Balodimos MC et al: Acetohexamide in the therapy of diabetes mellitus. Metabolism 17:669, 1968
25. Bandt C, Hoffbauer FW: Liver injury associated with tranylcypromine therapy. JAMA 188:752, 1964
26. Barcoff E et al: Ketoconazole-induced fulminant hepatitis. Gut 26:636, 1985
27. Barich LL et al: Toxic liver damage in mice after prolonged intake of elevated doses of griseofulvin. Antibiot Chemother 11:566, 1961
28. Barker JD Jr et al: Chronic excessive acetaminophen use and liver damage. Ann Intern Med 87:299, 1977

29. Barr GD, Piper DW: Possible ranitidine hepatitis. Med J Aust 2:421, 1981
30. Barrows GH, Christopherson WM: Human liver tumors in relation to steroidal usage. Env. Health Perspec 50:201, 1983
31. Bartoli E et al: Acute hepatitis with bridging necrosis due to hydralazine intake: Report of a case. Arch Intern Med 139:698, 1979
32. Barzilai D et al: Cholestatic jaundice caused by d-penicillamine. Ann Rheum Dis 37:98, 1978
33. Bass BH: Letter: Jaundice associated with naproxen. Lancet 1:998, 1974
34. Bastion PG: Occupational hepatitis caused by methylene diamine. Med J Aust 141:533, 1984
35. Bateman JR et al: 5-Fluorouracil given once weekly: Comparison of intravenous and oral administration. Cancer 28:907, 1971
36. Bateson MC et al: Clofibrate therapy and gallstone induction. Am J Dig Dis 23:623, 1978
37. Baum JK et al: Possible association between benign hepatomas and oral contraceptives. Lancet 2:926, 1973
38. Beckett RB et al: Studies on hepatomegaly caused by the hypolipidemic drugs nafenopin and clofibrate. Toxicol Appl Pharmacol 23:42, 1972
39. Beermann B et al: Transient cholestasis during treatment with ajmaline, and chronic xanthomatous cholestasis after administration of ajmaline, methyltestosterone and ethinylestradiol. Acta Med Scand 190:241, 1971
40. Belfrage S et al: Halothane hepatitis in an anesthetist. Lancet 2:1466, 1966
41. Belinsky SA et al: Rates of allyl alcohol metabolism in periportal and pericentral regions of the liver lobule. Mol Pharmacol 25:158, 1984
42. Bellet RE et al: Hepatotoxicity of 5-azacytidine: A clinical and pathologic study. Neoplasma 20:303, 1973
43. Bellet RE et al: Clinical trial with subcutaneously administered 5-azacytidine. Cancer Chemother Rep 58:217, 1974
44. Bengtsson F et al: Flucloxacillin-induced cholestatic liver damage. Scand J Infect Dis 17:125, 1985
45. Benjamin SB et al: Phenylbutazone liver injury: A clinicopathologic survey of 23 cases and review of the literature. Hepatology 1:255, 1981
46. Benjamin SB et al: The morphologic spectrum of halothane-induced hepatic injury: Analysis of 77 cases. Hepatology 5:1163, 1985
47. Benson GD: Hepatotoxicity following the therapeutic use of antipyretic analgesics. Am J Med 75 (suppl 5A):85, 1983
48. Berman A, Franklin RL: Precipitation of acute intermittent porphyria by griseofulvin therapy. JAMA 192:163, 1965
49. Berthelot P, Billing BH: Effect of bunamiodyl on hepatic uptake of sulfobromophthalein in the rat. Am J Physiol 211:395, 1966
50. Bezahler GH: Fatal methyldopa-associated granulomatous hepatitis and myocarditis. Am J Med Sci 283:41, 1982
51. Bick M: Chlorinated hydrocarbon residues in human body fat. Med J Aust 1:1127, 1969
52. Bickers JN et al: Hypersensitivity reaction to antituberculosis drugs with hepatitis, lupus phenomenon and myocardial infarction. N Engl J Med 265:131, 1961
53. Billing BH et al: Hepatic transport of bilirubin. Ann NY Acad Sci 111:319, 1963
54. Bjorneboe M et al: Infective hepatitis and toxic jaundice in a municipal hospital during a five-year period. Acta Med Scand 182:491, 1967
55. Black M: Acetaminophen hepatotoxicity. Ann Rev Med 35:577, 1984
56. Black M et al: Isoniazid-associated hepatitis in 114 patients. Gastroenterology 69:289, 1975
57. Black M et al: Nitrofurantoin-induced chronic active hepatitis. Ann Intern Med 92:62, 1980
58. Black M et al: Possible ranitidine hepatotoxicity. Ann Intern Med 101:208, 1984
59. Blackburn AM et al: Tamoxifen and liver damage. Br Med J 289:288, 1984
60. Blom H: A case of carbimazole-induced intrahepatic cholestasis. Arch Intern Med, 145:1513, 1985
61. Bloodworth JM Jr: Morphologic changes associated with sulfonylurea therapy. Metabolism 12:287, 1963
62. Bodey GP et al: Carbenicillin therapy for Pseudomonas infections. JAMA 218:62, 1971
63. Boelsterli UA et al: Modulation by S-adenosylmethionine of hepatic (Na+,K+)-ATPase membrane fluidity and bile flow in rats with ethinyl estradiol-induced cholestasis. Hepatology 3:12, 1983
64. Bonkowsky HL et al: Chronic hepatic inflammation and fibrosis due to low doses of paracetamol. Lancet 1:1016, 1978
65. Bottiger LE et al: Halothane-induced liver damage: An analysis of the material reported to the Swedish Adverse Drug Reaction Committee, 1966–1973. Acta Anaesth Scand 20:40, 1976
66. Bourgeois C et al: Acute aflatoxin B₁ toxicity in the macaque and its similarity to Reye's syndrome. Lab Invest 24:206, 1971
67. Bourgeois C et al: Encephalopathy and fatty degeneration of the viscera: A clinicopathologic analysis of 40 cases. Am J Clin Pathol 56:558, 1971
68. Boxerbaum B et al: Efficacy and tolerance of carbenicillin in patients with cystic fibrosis. In Hobby GL (ed): Antimicrobial Agents and Chemotherapy, pp 292–295. Baltimore, Williams & Wilkins, 1969
69. Boyer JL: Mechanisms of chlorpromazine cholestasis: Hypersensitivity or toxic metabolite? Gastroenterology 74:1331, 1978
70. Boyer JL, Klatskin G: Pattern of necrosis in acute viral hepatitis: Prognostic value of bridging (subacute hepatic necrosis). N Engl J Med 283:1063, 1970
71. Boyer TD et al: Allopurinol hypersensitivity and liver damage. West J Med 126:143, 1977
72. Brandes JW et al: Gelbsucht nach Aprindin: Eine hepatitsahnliche Arzneimittelschadigung. Dtsch Med Wochenschr 101:111, 1976
73. Braun P: Heptotoxicity of erythromycin. J Infect Dis 119:300, 1969
74. Bravo JF et al: Fatty liver and pleural effusion with ibuprofen therapy. Ann Intern Med 87:200, 1977
75. Breeden CJ et al: Herpes simplex encephalitis treated with systemic 5-iodo-2'(2') deoxuridine. Ann Intern Med 65:1050, 1966
76. Breen KJ et al: Paracetamol self-poisoning. Med J Aust 1:77, 1982
77. Breinstrup H, Sogaard-Andersen J: Cholestasis intrahepatica after griseofulvin-behandling. Ugeskr Laeger 128:145, 1966
78. Brenner A, Kaplan M: Recurrent hepatitis due to methoxyflurane anesthesia. N Engl J Med 284:961, 1971
79. Bridge JC et al: Discussion on trinitrotoluene poisoning. Proc R Soc Med 35:553, 1942

80. Bridges ME, Pittman FE: Tolazamide-induced cholestasis. South Med J 73:1072, 1980

81. Bridges RA et al: Serious reactions to novobiocin. J Pediatr 50:579, 1957

82. Briggs WA et al: Hepatitis affecting hemodialysis and transplant patients. Arch Intern Med 132:21, 1973

83. Brodsky I et al: Fibrosis of central and hepatic veins and perisinusoidal spaces of the liver following prolonged administration of urethane. Am J Med 30:976, 1961

84. Brodsky SJ et al: Hepatotoxicity due to treatment with verapamil. Ann Intern Med 94:490, 1981

85. Brogden RN et al: Sulindac: A review of its pharmacological properties and therapeutic efficacy in rheumatic disease. Drugs 16:97, 1978

86. Brooks SEH et al: Acute veno-occlusive disease of the liver. Arch Pathol 89:507, 1970

87. Brown BR, Sipes IG: Biotransformation and hepatotoxicity of halothane. Biochem Pharmacol 26:2091, 1977

88. Brown G et al: Hepatic damage during chlorpropamide therapy. JAMA 170:2085, 1959

89. Bruckstein AH, Attia AA: Oxacillin hepatitis. Am J Med 64:519, 1978

90. Buch-Andreassen P et al: Abnormalities in liver function tests during long-term diphenylhydantoin therapy in epileptic outpatients. Acta Med Scand 194:261, 1973

91. Bullivant CM: Accidental poisoning by paraquat: Report of two cases in man. Br Med J 1:1272, 1966

92. Burette A et al: Acute hepatic injury associated with minocycline. Arch Intern Med 144:1491, 1984

93. Butler RC et al: Massive hepatic necrosis in a patient receiving allopurinol. JAMA 237:473, 1977

94. Butler WH: Pathology of liver cancer in experimental animals. In Liver Cancer IARC. Scientific Publication 1, pp 30–41. Lyon, WHO International Agency for Research in Cancer, 1971

95. Cacace LG, Cohen M: Alpha-methyldopa (Aldomet) hepatitis: Report of a case and review of the literature. Drug Intell Clin Pharmacol 10:144, 1976

96. Calabro J et al: Sulindac in juvenile rheumatoid arthritis. Clin Pharmacol Ther 25:216, 1979

97. Callen JP, Soderstrom RM: Granulomatous hepatitis associated with salicylazosulfapyridine therapy. South Med J 71:1159, 1978

98. Cameron GR, Karunaratne WAE: Carbon tetrachloride cirrhosis in relation to liver regeneration. J Pathol Bacteriol 42:1, 1936

99. Capelle P et al: Effect of rifampicin on liver function in man. Gut 13:366, 1972

100. Carney FM, Van Dyke RA: Halothane hepatitis: A critical review. Anesth Analg 51:135, 1972

101. Carr HJ Jr, Knauer QF: Death due to hepatic necrosis in a patient receiving zoxazolamine: Report of a case and review of the literature. N Engl J Med 264:977, 1961

102. Chajek T: Quinidine and granulomatous hepatitis. Ann Intern Med 82:282, 1975

103. Chew BK et al: Fatty livers, adenosine triphosphate and asparagine. Biochem Pharmacol 17:2463, 1968

104. Chiprut RO et al: Intrahepatic cholestasis after griseofulvin administration. Gastroenterology 70:1141, 1976

105. Chishan FK et al: Intrahepatic cholestasis after gold therapy in juvenile rheumatoid arthritis. J Pediatr 93:1042, 1978

106. Christensen NA et al: Nicotinic acid treatment of hyper-cholesteremia. JAMA 177:546, 1961

107. Chu A et al: Trazodone and liver toxicity. Ann Intern Med 99:128, 1983

108. Clark R et al: Hepatic damage and death from overdose of paracetamol. Lancet 1:66, 1973

109. Cleator I: Adverse effects of ranitidine therapy. Can Med Assoc J 129:405, 1983

110. Cohn HD: Clinical studies with a new rifamycin derivative. J Clin Pharmacol 9:118, 1969

111. Colding H: Et tilfaelde af kinidinallergi med feber og leverpavirkning. Ugeskr Laeger 131:1657, 1969

112. Colsky J et al: Hepatic fibrosis in children with acute leukemia after therapy with folic acid antagonists. Arch Pathol 59:198, 1955

113. Combes B et al: Tetracycline and the liver: Clinical manifestations of tetracycline toxicity. Prog Liv Dis 4:589, 1972

114. Cook IF et al: Phenytoin induced granulomatous hepatitis. Aust NZ J Med 11:539, 1981

115. Cooper J et al: Clofibrate and gallstones. Lancet 1:1083, 1975

116. Costa G et al: Initial clinical studies with vincristine. Cancer Chemother Rep 24:39, 1962

117. Coulter DL et al: Valproic acid therapy in childhood epilepsy. JAMA 244:785, 1980

118. Council on Drugs: An oral hypoglycemic agent: Acetohexamide (Dymelor). JAMA 191:127, 1965

119. Council on Drugs: Evaluation of two antineoplastic agents. JAMA 200:619, 1967

120. Cousins MJ et al: Toxicity of volatile anesthetic agents. Clin Anesth 2:551, 1984

121. Creutzfeldt W, Soling HO: Oral Treatment of Diabetes (A Clinical and Experimental Review). Gless C (trans). Munich, Springer-Verlag, 1961

122. Crossley RJ: Side effects and safety data for fenbufen. Am J Med 75:84, 1983

123. Cuthbert MF: Adverse reactions to non-steroidal anti-inflammatory drugs. Curr Med Res Opin 2:600, 1974

124. Dahl MGC et al: Liver damage due to methotrexate in patients with psoriasis. Br Med J 1:625, 1971

125. Dahl MGC et al: Methotrexate hepatotoxicity in psoriasis: Comparison of different dose regimens. Br Med J 1:654, 1972

126. Daikos GK, Kosmidis JC: Propoxyphene jaundice. JAMA 232:835, 1975

127. Daniels SR et al: Scientific uncertainties in the studies of salicylates use and Reye's syndrome. JAMA 249:1311, 1983

128. Dargie HJ, Dollery CT: Adverse reactions to diuretic drugs. In Dukes MNG (ed): Meyler's Side Effects of Drugs, vol 8, pp 483–501. Amsterdam, Excerpta Medica, 1975

129. Davidson AR: Lymphocyte sensitization in nifedipine-induced hepatitis. Br Med J 281:1354, 1980

130. Davies GE, Holmes JE: Drug-induced immunological effects on the liver. Br J Anaesth 44:941, 1972

131. Davis J: Liver damage due to tetracycline and its relationship to pregnancy. In Meyler L, Peck HM (eds): Drug-Induced Diseases, pp 103–110. Amsterdam, Excerpta Medica, 1968

132. Davis M et al: Halothane hepatitis—toxicity and immunity. In Eddleston AL Weber JCP, Williams R (eds): Immune Reactions in Liver Disease, pp 235–246. Bath, England, Pittman Medical, 1979

133. Davis M et al: Metabolism of paracetamol after therapeutic and hepatotoxic doses in man. J Int Med Res 4(suppl 4): 40, 1976

134. Davis M et al: Drug Reactions and the Liver. London, Pitman Medical, 1981

135. Davis P, Holdsworth CD: Jaundice after multiple halothane anaesthetics administered during the treatment of carcinoma of the uterus. Gut 14:566, 1973

136. Davis P, Hughes GRV: A serial study of eosinophilia and raised IgE antibodies during gold therapy. Ann Rheum Dis 34:203, 1975

137. Dayan AD, Lewis PD: Idoxuridine and jaundice. Lancet 2:1073, 1969

138. Decker K, Keppler D: Galactosamine-induced liver injury. Prog Liver Dis 4:183, 1972

139. De Groot H, Noll T: Halothane hepatotoxicity: Relation between metabolic activation, hypoxia, covalent binding, lipid peroxidation and liver cell damage. Hepatology 3:601, 1983

140. Deissroth A et al: Quinidine-induced liver disease. Ann Intern Med 77:595, 1972

141. DeLage C, Lagace R: La peliose hepatique: Role etiologique possible des medicaments. Union Med Can 102:1888, 1973

142. Del Arbol LR et al: Bridging hepatic necrosis associated with cimetidine. Am J Gastroenterol 74:267, 1980

143. Denk H et al: Hepatocellular hyalin (Mallory bodies) in long term griseofulvin-treated mice: A new experimental model for the study of hyalin formation. Lab Invest 32:773, 1975

144. Denlinger J et al: Hepatocellular dysfunction without jaundice after enflurane anesthesia. Anesthesiology 41:86, 1974

145. Denman AM, Ward HWC: Jaundice during treatment of myelomatosis with M and B 938. Br Med J 1:482, 1960

146. DePinho RA et al: Azathioprine and the liver: Evidence favoring idiosyncratic, mixed cholestatic-hepatocellular injury in humans. Gastroenterology 86:162, 1984

147. Devogelaer JP et al: A case of cholestatic hepatitis associated with d-penicillamine therapy for rheumatoid arthritis. Int J Clin Pharmacol Res 5:35, 1985

148. Dhand AK et al: Sulindac (Clinoril) hepatitis. Gastroenterology 80:505, 1981

149. Dhar GJ et al: Diphenylhydantoin-induced hepatic necrosis. Postgrad Med 56:128, 1974

150. Dianzani MU: Toxic liver injury by protein synthesis inhibitors. Prog Liver Dis 5:232, 1976

151. Diaz-Riversa RS et al: Acute phosphorus poisoning in man: A study of 56 cases. Medicine 29:269, 1950

152. Diehl AM et al: Cholestatic hepatitis from erythromycin ethylsuccinate. Am J Med 76:931, 1984

153. Dincsoy HP, Saelinger DA: Haloperidol-induced chronic cholestatic liver disease. Gastroenterology 83:694, 1982

154. Dismukes WE: Oxacillin-induced hepatic dysfunction. JAMA 226:861, 1963

155. Dochert JF et al: Action of carbon tetrachloride on liver. Br Med J 2:907, 1922

156. Dolle W: Intrahepatische Cholestase durch Ajmalin. Med Klin Wochenschr 57:1648, 1962

157. Donat JF et al: Valproic acid and fatal hepatitis. Neurology 29:273, 1979

158. Dordal E et al: Fatal halothane hepatitis with transient granulomas. N Engl J Med 283:357, 1970

159. Dorling PR, LePage RN: Studies on in vitro treatment of rat liver plasma membranes with carbon tetrachloride. Biochem Pharmacol 21:2139, 1972

160. Drerup AL et al: Jaundice occurring in a patient treated with chlorothiazide. N Engl J Med 259:534, 1958

161. Drinkard JP et al: Azathioprine and prednisone in the treatment of adults with lupus, nephritis: Clinical, histological, and immunological changes with therapy. Medicine 49:411, 1970

162. Driver JR, Weller JN: Untoward results from use of gold compounds: Report of a fatal case. Arch Dermatol Syph 23:87, 1931

163. Dujovne CA, Zimmerman HJ: Cytotoxicity of phenothiazines on Chang liver cells as measured by enzyme leakage. Proc Soc Exp Biol Med 131:583, 1969

164. Dujovne CA et al: Sulfonamide hepatic injury: Review of the literature and report of a case due to sulfamethoxazole. N Engl J Med 277:785, 1967

165. Dujovne CA et al: Hepatotoxicity of phenothiazines in vitro as measured by loss of aminotransferases to surrounding media. Proc Soc Exp Biol Med 128:561, 1968

166. Dujovne CA et al: Experimental basis for the different hepatotoxicity of erythromycin preparations in man. J Lab Clin Med 79:832, 1972

167. Dume T et al: Klinik und Therapie der Tetrachlorkohlenstoff-vergiftung. Dtsch Med Wochenschr 94:1646, 1969

168. Duthie A et al: Fatal cholestatic jaundice in elderly patients taking benoxaprofen. Br Med J 285:62, 1982

169. Dux S et al: Anaphylactic shock induced by diclofenac. Br Med J 286:1861, 1983

170. Easton JD: Potential hazards of hydantoin use. Ann Intern Med 77:998, 1972

171. Ebert MH, Shader RI: Hepatic effects. In Shader RI, DiMascio A: Psychotropic Drug Side Effects: Clinical and Theoretical Considerations, pp 175–197. Baltimore, Williams & Wilkins, 1970

172. Edelman J et al: Liver dysfunction associated with gold therapy for rheumatoid arthritis. J Rheum 10:510, 1983

173. Editorial: Death-cap poisoning. Lancet 1:1320, 1972

174. Editorial: Liver tumours and steroid hormones. Lancet 2:1481, 1973

175. Edmondson HA et al: Liver-cell adenomas associated with use of oral contraceptives. N Engl J Med 294:470, 1976

176. Edmondson HA et al: Regression of liver cell adenomas associated with oral contraceptives. Ann Intern Med 86:180, 1977

177. Einhorn M, Davidsohn I: Hepatotoxicity of mercaptopurine. JAMA 188:802, 1964

178. Einstein N et al: Jaundice due to nicotinic acid therapy. Am J Dig Dis 20:282, 1975

179. Eisalo A et al: Hepatic impairment during the intake of contraceptive pills: Clinical trial with post-menopausal women. Br Med J 2:426, 1964

180. Eisen HJ, Ginsberg AL: Disulfiram hepatotoxicity. Ann Intern Med 83:673, 1975

181. Eisenhauer T et al: Favourable outcome of hepatic veno-occlusive disease in a renal transplant patient receiving azathioprine, treated by portacaval shunt. Digestion 30:185, 1984

182. Eisenstadt HB, Elster BB: Zoxazolamine hepatitis. JAMA 176:874, 1961

183. Elewaut A et al: Aprindine-induced liver injury. Acta Gastroenterol Belg 40:236, 1977

184. Elias E, Boyer JL: Chlorpromazine and its metabolites alter polymerization and gelation of actin. Science 206:1404, 1979

185. Elkington SG et al: Renal and hepatic injury associated with methoxyfluorane anesthesia. Ann Intern Med 69:1229, 1968

186. Ellison RR et al: Clinical evaluation of 6-chloropurine in leukemia of adults. Blood 13:705, 1958

187. El-Mofty SK et al: Early reversible plasma membrane injury in galactosamine-induced liver cell death. Am J Pathol 79:579, 1975

188. Enat K et al: Leberschaden durch Adelphan. Schweiz Med Wochenschr 107:657, 1977

189. Enat R et al: Cholestatic jaundice caused by cloxacillin: Macrophage inhibition factor test in preventing rechallenge with hepatotoxic drugs. Br Med J 2:982, 1980

190. Espiritu CR et al: Allopurinol-induced granulomatous hepatitis. Am J Dig Dis 21:804, 1976

191. Farber E: Biochemical Pathology. Annu Rev Pharmacol Toxicol 11:71, 1971

192. Farber E: In Farber E (ed): Biochemistry of Disease, Vol II, The Pathology of Transcription and Translation. New York, Marcel Dekker, 1972

193. Farber E: Some fundamental aspects of liver injury. In Khanna JM, Israel Y, Kalant H (eds): Alcoholic Liver Pathology, pp 289–303. Toronto, Addiction Research Foundation, 1975

194. Farber E: On the pathogenesis of experimental hepatocellular carcinoma. In Okuda K, Peters RL (eds): Hepatocellular Carcinoma, pp 3–24. New York, John Wiley & Sons, 1976

195. Farber JL, El-Mofty SK: The biochemical pathology of liver cell necrosis. Am J Pathol 81:237, 1975

196. Farber JL, Gerson RJ: Mechanisms of cell injury with hepatotoxic chemicals. Pharmacol Rev 36:71S, 1984

197. Farid Z et al: Hepatotoxicity after treatment of schistosomiasis with hycanthone. Br Med J 2:88, 1972

198. Farrell G et al: Halothane hepatitis: Detection of a constitutional susceptibility factor. N Eng J Med 313:1310, 1985

199. Favreau M et al: Hepatic toxicity associated with gold therapy. Ann Intern Med 87:717, 1977

200. FDA Drug Bulletin, vol. 12, no. 2

201. Feaux de Lacroix W et al: Acute liver dystrophy with thrombosis of hepatic veins: A fatal complication of dacarbazine treatment. Cancer Treat Rep 67:779, 1983

202. Fedotin MS, Lefer LG: Liver disease caused by propylthiouracil. Arch Intern Med 135:319, 1975

203. Feinman L et al: Adaptation of the liver to drugs. In Orlandi F, Jezequel AM (eds): Liver and Drugs, pp 41–83. London, Academic Press, 1972

204. Felder SL, Felder L: Unusual reaction to penicillin. JAMA 143:361, 1950

205. Fenech FF et al: Hepatitis with biliverdinaemia in association with indomethacin therapy. Br Med J 3:155, 1967

206. Fevery J et al: Severe intrahepatic cholestasis due to the combined intake of oral contraceptives and triacetyloleandomycin. Acta Clin Belg 38:242, 1983

207. Firth H et al: Side effects of benoxaprofen. Br Med J 284:1784, 1982

208. Fischer MG et al: Methimazole-induced jaundice. JAMA 233:1028, 1973

209. Fisher BM, McArthur JO: Side effects of benoxaprofen. Br Med J 284:1283, 1982

210. Fisher MM: Mechanisms of drug-induced cholestasis. Sem Liver Dis 1:151, 1981

211. Flucytosine (Ancobon): A new antifungal drug. Med Lett Drugs Ther 14:29, 1972

212. Forbes GB et al: Liver damage due to perhexiline maleate. J Clin Pathol 32:1282, 1979

213. Ford JM et al: Fatal graft-versus-host disease following transfusion of granulocytes from normal donors. Lancet 2:1167, 1976

214. Fowle ASE, Zorab PA: *Escherichia coli* endocarditis successfully treated with oral trimethoprim and sulfamethoxazole. Br Heart J 32:127, 1970

215. Fowler PD: A double-blind comparison of diclofenac sodium (Voltarol). Rehabilitation 2(suppl):75, 1979

216. Franklin M et al: Fowler's solution as an etiologic agent in cirrhosis. Am J Med Sci 219:589, 1950

217. Frascino JA et al: Renal oxalosis and azotemia after methoxyflurane anesthesia. N Engl J Med 283:676, 1970

218. Freedman MA: Oxacillin-apparent hematologic and hepatic toxicity. Rocky Mt Med J 62:34, 1965

219. French SW, Davies PL: The Mallory body in the pathogenesis of alcoholic liver disease. In Khanna JM, Israel Y, Kalant H (eds): Alcoholic Liver Pathology, pp 113–143. Toronto, Addiction Research Foundation, 1975

220. Freston JW: Cimetidine: II. Adverse reactions and patterns of use. Ann Intern Med 97:728, 1982

221. Fries J, Siraganian R: Sulfonamide hepatitis: Report of a case due to sulfamethoxazole and sulfisoxazole. N Engl J Med 274:95, 1966

222. Fuchs HA, Avant GR: Nitrofurantoin-induced liver disease. J Tenn Med Assoc 77:584, 1984

223. Fukunishi R: Acute hepatic lesions induced by cycasin. Acta Pathol Jpn 23:639, 1973

224. Furet Y, Bretaeau M: Accidents hépatique à la clométacine. Therapie 39:523, 1984

225. Gala KV, Griffin TW: Hepatomas in young women on oral contraceptives: Report of two cases and review of the literature. J Surg Oncol 22:11, 1983

226. Gallagher TF Jr et al: Estrogen pharmacology: Studies of the structural basis for estrogen-induced impairment of liver function. Medicine 45:471, 1966

227. Gams RA et al: Hydantoin-induced pseudolymphoma. Ann Intern Med 69:557, 1968

228. Garibaldi RA et al: Isoniazid-associated hepatitis: Report of an outbreak. Am Rev Respir Dis 106:357, 1972

229. Garson WP et al: Clinical experience with perhexiline maleate in forty-six patients with angina. Postgrad Med J 49(suppl 3):90, 1973

230. Gasparetto P: Un caso di ittero epatocellulare in corso di trattamento con ibuprofen. Minerva Pediatr 26:531, 1974

231. Geltner D et al: Quinidine hypersensitivity and liver involvement: A survey of 32 patients. Gastroenterology 70:650, 1976

232. Ghishan FK: Trimethoprim-sulfamethoxazole-induced intrahepatic cholestasis. Clin Ped 22:212, 1983

233. Gill RA et al: Hepatic veno-occlusive disease caused by 6-thioguanine. Ann Intern Med 96:58, 1982

234. Girard JP et al: Lupoid hepatitis following administration of penicillin. Case report and immunological studies. Helv Med Acta 34:23, 1967

235. Giroux Y et al: Cholestatic jaundice caused by sulindac. Can J Surg 25:334, 1982

236. Gitlin N: Salicylate hepatotoxicity: The potential role of hypoalbuminemia. J Clin Gastroenterol 2:381, 1980

237. Glober GA, Wilkerson JA: Biliary cirrhosis following the administration of methyltestosterone. JAMA 204:170, 1968

238. Goldberg JW, Lidsky MD: Cyclophosphamide-associated hepatotoxicity. South Med J 78:222, 1985

239. Goldfarb G et al: Clometacine hepatitis. Gastroenterol Clin Biol 3:537, 1979

240. Goldfarb S et al: Experimental cholangitis due to alpha-naphthyl-isothiocyanate (ANIT). Am J Pathol 40:685, 1962
241. Goldstein GB et al: Drug-induced active chronic hepatitis. Am J Dig Dis 18:177, 1973
242. Goldstein LI, Ishak KG: Hepatic injury associated with penicillin therapy. Arch Pathol 98:114, 1974
243. Goldstein LI et al: Hepatic injury associated with nitrofurantoin therapy. Am J Dig Dis 19:987, 1974
244. Goldstein MJ, Rothenberg AJ: Jaundice in a patient receiving acetohexamide. N Engl J Med 275:97, 1966
245. Goodman ZD, Ishak KG: Hepatocellular carcinoma in women: Probable lack of etiologic association with oral contraceptive steroids. Hepatology 2:440, 1982
246. Gopinath C et al: The effect of the repeated administration of halothane on the liver of the horse. J Pathol 102:107, 1970
247. Gottlieb LS, Trey C: The effects of fluorinated anesthetics on the liver and kidneys. Annu Rev Med 25:411, 1974
248. Goudie BM et al: Jaundice associated with the use of benoxaprofen. Lancet 1:1799, 1982
249. Graham WG, Dundas GR: Isoniazid-related liver disease: Occurrence with portal hypertension, hypoalbuminemia and hypersplenism. JAMA 242:353, 1979
250. Greaves MW, Dawber R: Azathioprine in psoriasis. Br Med J 2:237, 1970
251. Gregory DH et al: Chronic cholestasis following prolonged tolbutamide administration. Arch Pathol 84:194, 1967
252. Griner PF et al: Veno-occlusive disease of the liver after chemotherapy of acute leukemia: Report of two cases. Ann Intern Med 85:578, 1976
253. Gronhagen-Riska C et al: Predisposing factors in hepatitis induced by isoniazid-rifampin treatment of tuberculosis. Am Rev Respir Dis 118:461, 1978
254. Gross MA et al: Hepatic lipidosis associated with L-asparaginase treatment. Proc Soc Exp Biol Med 130:733, 1969
255. Grundmann E, Oettgen HF (eds): Experimental and Clinical Effects of L-Asparaginase. New York, Springer-Verlag, 1970
256. Guarascio P et al: Liver damage from verapamil. Br Med J 288:362, 1984
257. Gupta MC et al: Stomatitis, agranulocytosis and hepatitis due to phenindione sensitivity. J Indian Med Assoc 63:324, 1974
258. Gurumurthy P et al: Lack of relationship between hepatic toxicity and acetylator phenotype in three thousand South Indian patients during treatment with isoniazid for tuberculosis. Am Rev Respir Dis 129:58, 1984
259. Gutman AB: The past four decades of progress in the knowledge of gout, with an assessment of the present status. Arthritis Rheum 16:431, 1973
260. Haber E, Osborne RK: Icterus and febrile reaction to response to isonicotinic acid hydrazine. N Engl J Med 260:417, 1959
261. Hadziyannis S et al: Cytoplasmic hepatitis B antigen in "ground glass" hepatocytes of carriers. Arch Pathol 96:327, 1973
262. Hall RL: Toxicants occurring naturally in spices and flavours. In Toxicants Occurring Naturally in Foods, publication 1354, pp 164–173. Washington, DC, National Academy of Sciences, National Research Council, 1966
263. Hamff LH et al: The effects of tolbutamide and chlorpropamide on patients exhibiting jaundice as a result of previous chlorpropamide therapy. Ann NY Acad Sci 74:820, 1959
264. Hamlyn AN et al: The spectrum of paracetamol (acetaminophen) overdose: Clinical and epidemiological studies. Postgrad Med J 54:400, 1978
265. Hamlyn AN et al: Piperazine hepatitis. Gastroenterology 70:1144, 1976
266. Hammaker L, Schmid R: Interference with bile pigment uptake in the liver by flavaspidic acid. Gastroenterology 53:31, 1967
267. Hanissian AS et al: Gold: Hepatotoxic and cholestatic reactions. Clin Rheum 4:183, 1985
268. Hanger FM Jr, Gutman AB: Post-arsphenamine jaundice apparently due to obstruction of intrahepatic biliary tract. JAMA 115:263, 1940
269. Hardin BL Jr: Carbon tetrachloride poisoning—a review. Indust Med Surg 23:93, 1954
270. Hargreaves T, Howell M: Phenindione jaundice. Br Heart J 27:932, 1965
271. Hargreaves T, Lathe GH: Inhibitory aspects of bile secretion. Nature 200:1172, 1963
272. Harinasuta U, Zimmerman HJ: Diphenylhydantoin sodium hepatitis. JAMA 203:1015, 1968
273. Harrison DC et al: Mushroom poisoning in five patients. Am J Med 38:787, 1965
274. Hart FD, Boardman PL: Ibufenac (4-isobutylphenyl acetic acid). Ann Rheum Dis 24:61, 1965
275. Hartman H et al: Prolonged cholestatic jaundice and leukopenia associated with piroxicam. Z Gastroentererol 22:343, 1984
276. Haskell CM et al: L-Asparaginase: Therapeutic and toxic effects in patients with neoplastic disease. N Engl J Med 281:1028, 1969
277. Hatoff DE et al: Nitrofurantoin: Another cause of drug-induced chronic active hepatitis? Am J Med 67:117, 1979
278. Haubrich WS, Sancetta SM: Spontaneous recovery from hepatobiliary disease with xanthomatosis. Gastroenterology 26:658, 1954
279. Havens WP Jr: Cholestatic jaundice in patients treated with erythromycin estolate. JAMA 180:30, 1962
280. Hay DR, Gwynne JF: Cirrhosis of the liver following therapy with perhexiline maleate. NZ Med J 96:202, 1983
281. Heath CW et al: Characteristics of cases of angiosarcoma of the liver among vinyl chloride workers in the United States. Ann NY Acad Sci 246:231, 1975
282. Hecht Y et al: Hepatites cholostatiques dues à la Xénalamine. Arch Mal Appar Dig 54:615, 1965
283. Heiberg JK, Svejgaard E: Toxic hepatitis during ketoconazole treatment. Br Med J 283:825, 1981
284. Henderson BE et al: Hepatocellular carcinoma and oral contraceptives. Br J Cancer 48:437, 1983
285. Hensler NM et al: Hypersensitivity reactions due to para-aminosalicylic acid: Review of the literature and report of a case showing cholangiolitic hepatitis. Am Rev Tuberc 76:132, 1957
286. Herbeuval R et al: Hépatitis cholostatique à la xénelamine. Therapie 21:871, 1966
287. Herlong HF et al: Aprindine hepatitis. Ann Intern Med 89:359, 1978
288. Hersh EM et al: Hepatotoxic effects of methotrexate. Cancer 19:600, 1966
289. Hess R et al: Nature of the hepatomegalic effect produced by ethyl-chloro-phenoxy-isobutyrate in the rat. Nature 208:856, 1965
290. Hiesse C et al: Ranitidine hepatotoxicity in renal transplant patients. Lancet 1:1280, 1985

291. Himsworth HP: Lectures on the Liver and Its Disease. Cambridge, Harvard University Press, 1947

292. Hirao K et al: Primary neoplasms in dog liver induced by diethylnitrosamine: I. Cancer Res 34:1870, 1974

293. Hoft RH et al: Halothane hepatitis in three pairs of closely related women. N Engl J Med 304:1023, 1981

294. Hohn D et al: Biliary sclerosis in patients receiving hepatic arterial infusions of floxyuridine. J Clin Oncol 3:98, 1985

295. Hollister LE: Allergy to chlorpromazine manifested by jaundice. Am J Med 23:870, 1957

296. Hollister LE: Discussion. In Wolstenholme G, Porter R (eds): Drug Responses in Man, p 151. Boston, Little, Brown & Co, 1967

297. Holzbach RT, Sanders JH: Recurrent intrahepatic cholestasis of pregnancy: Observations on pathogenesis. JAMA 193:542, 1965

298. Hopen G et al: Fatal carbamazepine-associated hepatitis: Report of 2 cases. Acta Med Scand 210:333, 1981

299. Hopwood D, Nyfors H: Effect of methotrexate therapy in psoriatics on the Ito cells in liver biopsies, assessed by point-counting. J Clin Pathol 29:698, 1976

300. Horowitz JD et al: Perhexiline maleate in the treatment of severe angina pectoris. Med J Aust 1:485, 1979

301. Horst DA et al: Prolonged cholestasis and progressive hepatic fibrosis following imipramine therapy. Gastroenterology 79:550, 1980

302. Howard DJ, Rees RJ: Long-term perhexiline maleate and liver function. Br Med J 1:133, 1976

303. Hoyumpa AM Jr, Connell AM: Methyldopa hepatitis: Report of three cases. Am J Dig Dis 18:213, 1973

304. Hoyumpa AM Jr et al: Fatty liver: Biochemical and clinical considerations. Am J Dig Dis 20:1142, 1975

305. Hruban Z et al: Effect of azaserine on the fine structure of the liver and pancreatic acinar cells. Cancer Res 25:708, 1965

306. Hryniuk W et al: Cytarabine for herpesvirus infections. JAMA 219:715, 1972

307. Hueper WC: Cinchophen (Atophan): A critical review. Medicine 27:43, 1948

308. Hughes M, Powell LW: Recurrent hepatitis in patients receiving multiple halothane anesthetics for radium treatment of carcinoma of the cervix uteri. Gastroenterology 58:790, 1970

309. Hugues FC et al: Effets hépato-biliares de l'association rifampicine-isoniazide. Therapie 24:899, 1969

310. Hurst EW, Paget GE: Protoporphyrin, cirrhosis and hepatomata in the livers of mice given griseofulvin. Br J Dermatol 75, 1963

311. Hurt P, Wegmann T: Protracted Largactil jaundice developing into primary biliary cirrhosis. Acta Hepatosplen 8:87, 1961

312. Husebye KO: Jaundice with persisting pericholangiolitic inflammation in a patient treated with chlorothiazide. Dig Dis 9:439, 1964

313. Huskisson EC et al: Sulindac: Trials of a new anti-inflammatory drug. Ann Rheum Dis 7:89, 1978

314. Hutter RV et al: Hepatic fibrosis in children with acute leukemia: A complication of therapy. Cancer 13:288, 1960

315. Imoto S et al: Drug-related hepatitis. Ann Intern Med 91:129, 1979

316. Inman WHW, Mushin WW: Jaundice after repeated exposure to halothane: A further analysis of reports to the Committee on Safety of Medicines. Br Med J 1:5, 1974

317. Inman WHW, Mushin WW: Jaundice after repeated exposure to halothane: A further analysis of reports to the Committee on Safety of Medicines. Br Med J 2:1455, 1978

318. Ireland P et al: Liver disease in kidney transplant patients receiving azathioprine. Arch Intern Med 132:29, 1973

319. Ishak KG: Mesenchymal tumors of the liver. In Okuda K, Peters RL (eds): Hepatocellular Carcinoma, pp 247–307. New York, John Wiley & Sons, 1976

320. Ishak KG: Light microscopic morphology of viral hepatitis. Am J Clin Pathol 65:787, 1976

321. Ishak KG: Hepatic neoplasms associated with contraceptive and anabolic steroids. In Ligeman CH (ed): Recent results in Cancer Research, vol 66, pp 73–128. Berlin, Springer-Verlag, 1979

322. Ishak KG: Hepatic lesions caused by anabolic and contraceptive steroids. Semin Liver Dis 1:116, 1981

323. Ishak KG, Irey NS: Hepatic injury associated with phenothiazines: Clinicopathologic and follow-up study of 36 patients. Arch Pathol 93:283, 1972

324. Ishak KG, Rabin L: Benign tumors of the liver. Med Clin North Am 59:995, 1975

325. Ishak KG et al: Granulomas and cholestatic-hepatocellular injury associated with phenylbutazone: Report of two cases. Dig Dis 22:611, 1977

326. Itoh S et al: Hydralazine-induced liver injury. Dig Dis Sci 25:884, 1980

327. Itoh S et al: Sodium valproate-induced liver injury. Am J Gastroenterol 77:875, 1982

328. Ivanetich KM et al: Enflurane and methoxyflurane: Their interactions with hepatic cytochrome P450 in vitro. Biochem Pharmacol 28:785, 1979

329. Iwamura von K: Arzneimittelschadigung der Leber in Japan. Z Gastroenterol 11:365, 1973

330. Iwarson S et al: Nitrofurantoin-induced chronic liver disease: Clinical course and outcome of five cases. Scand J Gastroenterol 14:479, 1979

331. Jalota R, Freston JW: Severe intrahepatic cholestasis due to thiabendazole. Am J Trop Med Hyg 23:676, 1974

332. Jasper H: Jaundice in a patient receiving zoxazolamine (Flexin). Am J Gastroenterol 34:419, 1960

333. Janssen P, Symoens JE: Hepatic reactions during ketoconazole treatment. Am J Med 74:80, 1983

334. Jaundice with cimetidine. Med J Aust 1:394, 1980

335. Jennings RB: Fatal fulminant acute carbon tetrachloride poisoning. Arch Pathol 59:269, 1955

336. Jezequel AM, Orlandi F: Fine morphology of the human liver as a tool in clinical pharmacology. In Orlandi F, Jezequel AM (eds): Liver and Drugs, pp 145–192. London, Academic Press, 1972

337. Jezequel AM et al: Changes induced in human liver by long-term anticonvulsant therapy: Functional and ultrastructural data. Liver 4:307, 1984

338. Jick H, Walker AM, Porter J: Drug-induced liver disease. J Clin Pharmacol 21:359, 1981

339. Jiricka Z et al: Studies on 6-azauridine and 6-azacytidine: I. Toxicity studies of 6-azauridine and 6-azacytidine in mice. Biochem Pharmacol 14:1517, 1965

340. Johnson GK, Tolman KG: Chronic liver disease and acetaminophen. Ann Intern Med 87:302, 1977

341. Johnston G et al: Halothane hepatitis in a laboratory technician. Aust NZ J Med 2:171, 1971

342. Jori GP, Peschle C: Hydralazine disease associated with transient granulomas in the liver: A case report. Gastroenterology 64:1163, 1973

343. Joshi PH, Conn HO: The syndrome of methoxyflurane-associated hepatitis. Ann Intern Med 80:395, 1974

344. Judson JA et al: Possible cross-sensitivity between halothane and methoxyflurane: Report of a case. Anesthesiology 35:527, 1971

345. Kaier HW et al: Hepatotoxicity of papaverine. Arch Pathol 98:292, 1974

346. Kanada SA et al: Aspirin hepatotoxicity. Am J Hosp Pharm 35:330, 1978

347. Kanner RS et al: Azulfidine (sulfasalazine)-induced hepatic injury. Dig Dis 23:956, 1978

348. Kaplan HC et al: Hepatitis caused by halothane sniffing. Ann Intern Med 90:797, 1979

349. Kaplowitz N et al: Drug-induced hepatotoxicity. Ann Intern Med 104:826, 1986

350. Katz B et al: Quinine-induced granulomatous hepatitis. Br Med J 286:264, 1983

351. Katz S: Hepatic coma associated with methoxyflurane anesthesia. Dig Dis Sci 5:733, 1970

352. Kaul A et al: Hepatitis associated with use of sulindac in a child. J Pediatr 99:650, 1981

353. Kawamoto T et al: The influence of dietary cholesterol on the lithogenicity of bile in rats treated with clofibrate. Hiroshima J Med Sci 27:147, 1978

354. Keeffe EB, Smith FW: Disulfiram hypersensitivity hepatitis. JAMA 230:435, 1974

355. Keeffe EB et al: Hepatotoxicity to both erythromycin estolate and erythromycin ethylsuccinate. Dig Dis Sci 27:701, 1982

356. Kelsey WM, Scharyj M: Fatal hepatitis probably due to indomethacin. JAMA 199:586, 1967

357. Kendler J et al: Perfusion of the isolated rat liver with erythromycin estolate and other derivatives. Proc Soc Exp Biol Med 139:1272, 1972

358. Kenwright S, Levi A: Sites of competition in the selective hepatic uptake of rifamycin-SV, flavaspidic acid, bilirubin, and bromosulphthalein. Gut 15:220, 1974

359. Kessler JI: The role of adipose tissue fatty acids in the apthogenesis of acute fatty liver. In Paumgartner G, Preisig R (eds): The Liver, Quantitative Aspects of Structure and Function, pp 278–286. Basel, Karger, 1973

360. Kesterson JW et al: The hepatotoxicity of valproic acid and its metabolites in rats: I. Toxicologic, biochemical and histopathologic studies. Hepatology 4:1143, 1984

361. King JA, Blount RE Jr: An unexpected reaction to procainamide. JAMA 186:603, 1963

362. Kirtley WR: Occurrence of sensitivity and side reactions following carbutamide. Diabetes 6:72, 1957

363. Klatskin G: Toxic and drug-induced hepatitis. In Schiff L (ed): The Liver, 4th ed, pp 604–710. Philadelphia, JB Lippincott, 1975

364. Klatskin G: Hepatic tumors: Possible relationship to use of oral contraceptives. Gastroenterology 73:386, 1977

365. Klatskin G, Kimberg DV: Recurrent hepatitis attributable to halothane sensitization in an anesthetist. N Engl J Med 280:515, 1969

366. Klatskin G, Smith DP: Halothane-induced hepatitis. In Gerok W, Sickinger K (eds): Drugs and the Liver, pp 289–296. Stuttgart, FK Schattauer Verlag, 1975

367. Kleckner HB et al: Severe hypersensitivity to diphenylhydantoin with circulating antibodies to the drug. Ann Intern Med 83:522, 1975

368. Klein NC, Magida MG: Propoxyphene (Darvon) hepatotoxicity. Dig Dis 16:467, 1971

369. Klemola H et al: Anicteric liver damage during nitrofurantoin medication. Scand J Gastroenterol 10:501, 1975

370. Kline MM: Enflurane-associated hepatitis. Gastroenterology 79:126, 1980

371. Klinge O, Bannasch P: Zur Vermehrung des glatten endoplasmatischen Retikulum in Hepatocyten Menschlicher Leberpunktate. Verh Dtsch Ges Pathol 52:568, 1968

372. Klinge O et al: Feingewebliche Befunde an der Leber Klinisch gesunder Australia-Antigen-(HB Ag-) Trager. Virchows Arch 361:359, 1973

373. Klion FM et al: Hepatitis after exposure to halothane. Ann Intern Med 71:467, 1969

374. Kloss MW et al: Cocaine-mediated hepatotoxicity: A critical review. Biochem Pharmacol 33:169, 1984

375. Knirsch AK, Gralla EJ: Abnormal serum transaminase levels after parenteral ampicillin and carbenicillin administration. N Engl J Med 282:1081, 1970

376. Knoblauch M et al: Dihydralazin-induzierte akute Hepatitis bei IgM-Mangel. Schweiz Med Wochenschr 107:651, 1977

377. Knowles DM et al: The clinical, radiologic and pathologic characterization of benign hepatic neoplasms. Medicine 57:223, 1978

378. Koch MJ et al: Quinidine hepatotoxicity: A report of a case and review of the literature. Gastroenterology 70:1136, 1976

379. Kochman S et al: Apropos de 5 cas d'icteres a la rifampicine (I). Presse Med 79:524, 1971

380. Koff RS et al: Profile of hyperbilirubinemia in three hospital populations. Clin Res 18:680, 1970

381. Koga Y et al: Hepatic "intravenous fat pigment" in infants and children receiving lipid emulsion. J Pediatr Surg 10:641, 1975

382. Kohlstaedt KG: Propionyl erythromycin ester lauryl sulfate and jaundice. JAMA 178:89, 1961

383. Kohn NN, Myerson RM: Xanthomatous biliary cirrhosis following chlorpromazine. Am J Med 31:665, 1961

384. Kolde G et al: Effects of clofibrate (alpha-p-chlorophenoxyisobutyryl-ethyl-ester) on male rat liver. Virchows Arch 22:73, 1976

385. Kopelman H et al: The liver lesion of the Epping jaundice. Q J Med 35:553, 1966

386. Kosmidis J et al: Amoxycillin: Pharmacology, bacteriology and clinical studies. Br J Clin Pract 26:341, 1972

387. Krawitt EL et al: Mercaptopurine hepatotoxicity in a patient with chronic active hepatitis. Arch Intern Med 120:729, 1967

388. Kraybill HR: The toxicology and epidemiology of natural hepatotoxin exposure. Isr J Med Sci 10:416, 1974

389. Krishnamachari KAVR et al: Hepatitis due to aflatoxicosis: An outbreak in western India. Lancet 1:1061, 1975

390. Kroker R, Hegner D: Solubilization of phalloidin binding sites from rat liver hepatocytes and plasma membranes by trypsin. Naunyn Schmiedebergs Arch Pharmacol 279:339, 1973

391. Kumana CR et al: Herbal tea induced hepatic veno-occlusive disease: Quantitation of toxic alkaloid exposure in adults. Gut 26:101, 1985

392. Kunelis CT et al: Fatty liver of pregnancy and its relationship to tetracycline therapy. Am J Med 38:359, 1965

393. Kuzell WC et al: Phenylbutazone: Further clinical evaluation. Arch Intern Med 92:646, 1953

394. Larriga J: Naproxen icterica. Rev Sanid Mil Mexico 29:250, 1975

395. Lauritsen K et al: Ranitidine and hepatotoxicity. Lancet 2:1471, 1984

396. Law IP, Knight H: Letter: Jaundice associated with naproxen. N Engl J Med 295:1201, 1976

397. Lee TJ et al: Diphenylhydantoin-induced hepatic necrosis. Gastroenterology 70:422, 1976

398. Lees AW et al: Toxicity from rifampicin plus isoniazid and rifampicin plus ethambutol therapy. Tubercle 52:182, 1971

399. Lenoir C, Blanchon P: Hépatite due au maleate de perhixiline. Coeur Med Interne 17:69, 1978

400. Lepper MH et al: Effect of large doses of aureomycin on human liver. Arch Intern Med 88:271, 1951

401. Lepper MH et al: Effect of large doses of aureomycin, terramycin, and chloramphenicol on livers of mice and dogs. Arch Intern Med 88:284, 1951

402. Lesobre R et al: Les icteres au cours du traitement par la rifampicine. Rev Tuberc Pneumol 33:393, 1969

403. Levander DA: Selenium biochemical actions, interactions and some human health complications. *In* Prasad AS (ed): Clinical Biochemical and Nutritional Aspects of Trace Elements, pp 345–368. New York, Alan R Liss, 1982

404. Levander HG: Granulomatous hepatitis in a patient receiving carbamazepine. Acta Med Scand 208:333, 1980

405. Levine RA et al: Chronic chlorpromazine cholangiolitic hepatitis: Report of a case with immunofluorescent studies. Gastroenterology 50:665, 1966

406. Levy M et al: Granulomatous hepatitis secondary to carbamazepine. Ann Intern Med 95:64, 1981

407. Lewis D et al: Liver damage associated with perhexiline maleate. Gut 20:186, 1979

408. Lewis JH: Hepatic toxicity of nonsteroidal anti-inflammatory drugs. Clin Pharm 3:128, 1984

409. Lewis JH et al: Valproate-induced hepatic steatogenesis in rats. Hepatology 2:870, 1982

410. Lewis JH et al: Budd-Chiari syndrome associated with oral contraceptive steroids: Review of treatment of 47 cases. Dig Dis Sci 28:673, 1983

411. Lewis JH et al: Hepatic injury associated with ketoconazole therapy. Gastroenterology 86:503, 1984

412. Lewis JH et al: Enflurane hepatotoxicity: A clinicopathologic study of 24 cases. Ann Intern Med 98:984, 1983

413. Lieber CS: Alcohol and the liver. Transition from adaptation to tissue injury. In Khanna JM, Israel Y, Kalant H (eds): Alcoholic Liver Pathology, pp 171–189. Ontario, Addiction Research Foundation, 1975

414. Lieberman AN et al: Lergotrile in Parkinson disease: Further studies. Neurology 29:267, 1979

415. Lieberman DA et al: Severe and prolonged oral contraceptive jaundice. J Clin Gastroenterol 6:145, 1984

416. Lijinsky W, Greenblatt M: Carcinogen dimethylnitrosamine produced *in vivo* from nitrite and aminopyrine. Nature 236:177, 1972

417. Lilly JR et al: Cimetidine cholestatic jaundice in children. J Surg Res 24:384, 1978

418. Lindberg J et al: Trigger factors and HL-A antigens in chronic active hepatitis. Br Med J 4:77, 1975

419. Lindenbaum J, Leifer E: Hepatic necrosis associated with halothane anesthesia. N Engl J Med 368:525, 1963

420. Little DM: Effects of halothane on liver function. In Greene NM (ed): Clinical Anesthesia: Halothane, pp 85–137. Philadelphia, FA Davis, 1968

421. Little DM Jr, Wetstone HJ: Anesthesia and the liver. Anesthesiology 25:815, 1964

422. LoIndice TA, Lang JA: Tolazamide-induced hepatic dysfunction. Am J Gastroenterol 68:81, 1978

423. Longstreth GF, Hershman J: Trazodone-induced hepatotoxicity and leukonychia. J Am Acad Dermatol 13:149, 1985

424. Loomis JN et al: A case of peliosis hepatitis in association with tamoxifen. Am J Clin Pathol 80:881, 1983

425. Lorenzini I et al: Cimetidine-induced hepatitis: Electron microscopic observations and clinical pattern of liver injury. Dig Dis Sci 26:275, 1981

426. Losek JD, Werlin SL: Sulfasalazine hepatotoxicity. Am J Dis Child 135:1070, 1981

427. Lowdell CP, Murray-Lyon IM: Reversal of liver damage due to long-term methyltestosterone and safety of non-17 α-alkylated androgens. Br Med J 291:637, 1985

428. Lowenstein L, Ballew DH: Fatal acute hemolytic anemia, thrombocytopenic purpura, nephrosis and hepatitis resulting from ingestion of a compound containing apiol. Can Med Assoc J 78:195, 1958

429. Ludwig J, Axelsen R: Drug effects on the liver: An updated tabular compilation of drugs and drug-related hepatic diseases. Dig Dis Sci 28:651, 1983

430. Lüllmann H et al: Drug-induced phospholipidoses: II. Tissue distribution of the amphiphilic drug chlorphentermine. CRC Crit Rev Toxicol 4:185, 1975

431. Lüllmann H et al: Lipidosis induced by amphiphilic cationic drugs. Biochem Pharmacol 27:1103, 1978

432. Lundvall O: Alcohol and porphyria cutanea tarda. In Engel A, Larsson T (eds): Alcoholic Cirrhosis and Other Toxic Hepatopathies, pp 356–372. Stockholm, Nordiska Bokhandelns Forlag, 1970

433. Lunzer M et al: Jaundice due to carbimazole. Gut 16:913, 1975

434. Maddrey WC: Isoniazid-induced liver disease. Semin Liver Dis 1:129, 1981

435. Maddrey WC: Drug and chemical-induced hepatic injury. In Berk JE (ed): Bockus Gastroenterology, vol 5, pp 2922–2956. Philadelphia, WB Saunders, 1985

436. Maddrey WC, Boitnott JK: Isoniazid hepatitis. Ann Intern Med 79:1, 1973

437. Maddrey WC, Boitnott JK: Severe hepatitis from methyldopa. Gastroenterology 68:351, 1975

438. Maddrey WC, Boitnott JK: Drug-induced chronic liver disease. Gastroenterology 72:1348, 1977

439. Magee G et al: Cholestatic hepatitis from use of sulfanilamide vaginal cream. Dig Dis Sci 27:1044, 1982

440. Magee PN: Liver carcinogens in the human environment. In Liver Cancer, IARC Scientific Publication 1, pp 110–120. Lyon, International Agency for Research on Cancer, 1971

441. Malekzadeh MH et al: Hepatic dysfunction after renal transplantation in children. J Pediatr 81:279, 1972

442. Mallory TH et al: Potential hepatotoxic effects of methylmethacrylate monomer. Clin Orthop 93:366, 1973

443. Martin W, Rickers J: Cholestatische Hepatose nach Diphenylhydantoin. Wien Klin Wochenschr 84:41, 1972

444. Marubbio AT, Danielson B: Hepatic veno-occlusive disease in a renal transplant patient receiving azathioprine. Gastroenterology 69:739, 1975

445. Massey WH et al: Hepatic artery infusion for metastatic malignancy using percutaneously placed catheters. Am J Surg 121:160, 1971

446. Matilla A, Molland EA: A light and electron microscopic study of the liver in case of erythrohepatic protoporphyria and in griseofulvin-induced porphyria in mice. J Clin Pathol 27:698, 1974

447. Mays ET, Christopherson W: Hepatic tumors induced by sex steroids. Semin Liver Dis 4:147, 1984

448. McArthur JE, Dyment PG: Stevens-Johnson syndrome with hepatitis following therapy with ampicillin and cephalexin. NZ Med J 81:390, 1975

449. McCann J et al: Detection of carcinogens as mutagens in the Salmonella/microsome test: Assay of 300 chemicals. Proc Natl Acad Sci 72:5135, 1975

450. McDonald EC, Speicher CE: Peliosis hepatis associated with administration of oxymetholone. JAMA 240:243, 1978

451. McDonald GB et al: Intestinal and liver toxicity of neoplastic drugs. West J Med 140:250, 1984

452. McGiven AR: Peliosis hepatis: Case report and review of pathogenesis. J Pathol 101:283, 1970

453. McGovern B et al: Adverse reaction during treatment with amiodarone hydrochloride. Br Med J 287:175, 1983

454. McLain CJ et al: Potentiation of acetaminophen hepatotoxicity by alcohol. JAMA 244:251, 1980

455. McLean AE et al: Dietary factors in renal and hepatic toxicity of paracetamol. J Intern Med Res 4(suppl 4):79, 1976

456. McLean EK: The toxic actions of pyrrolizidine (Senecio) alkaloids. Pharmacol Rev 22:429, 1970

457. McLeond BD, Kinsella TD: Cholestasis associated with d-penicillamine therapy for rheumatoid arthritis. Can Med Assoc J 120:965, 1979

458. McMaster KR, Hennigar GR: Drug-induced granulomatous hepatitis. Lab Invest 44:61, 1981

459. McVeagh P, Ekert H: Hepatotoxicity of chemotherapy following nephrectomy and radiation therapy for right-sided Wilms' tumor. J Pediatr 87:627, 1975

460. Meijer DK et al: Effect on nafenopin (SU-13,437) on liver function: Influence on the hepatic transport of organic anions. Arch Pharmacol 290:235, 1975

461. Menard DB et al: Antineoplastic agents and the liver. Gastroenterology 78:143, 1979

462. Metreau JM et al: Oral contraceptives and the liver. Digestion 7:318, 1972

463. Meyer UA, Maxwell JD: Human and experimental porphyria: Relationship of defects in heme biosynthesis to drug idiosyncrasy. In Gerok W, Sickinger K (eds): Drugs and the Liver, pp 201–207. Stuttgart, FK Schattauer-Verlag, 1975

464. Mihas AA et al: Sulfasalazine toxic reactions: Hepatitis, fever and skin rash associated with hypocomplementemia and immune complexes. JAMA 239:2590, 1978

465. Mihas AA et al: Fulminant hepatitis and lymphocyte sensitization due to propylthiouracil. Gastroenterology 70:770, 1976

466. Mikkelsen WP et al: Extra- and intrahepatic portal hypertension without cirrhosis (hepatoportal sclerosis). Ann Surg 162:602, 1965

467. Millard PR et al: Azathioprine hepatotoxicity in renal transplantation. Transplantation 16:527, 1973

468. Miller DJ et al: Halothane hepatitis: Benign resolution of a severe lesion. Ann Intern Med 89:212, 1978

469. Miller EC, Miller JA: Hepatocarcinogenesis by chemicals. Prog Liver Dis 5:699, 1976

470. Miller J: Atrophy of the liver. Br Med J 2:581, 1920

471. Millward-Sadler GA et al: Methotrexate-induced liver disease in psoriasis. Br J Dermatol 90:661, 1974

472. Minow RA et al: Clinicopathologic correlation of liver damage in patients treated with 6-mercaptopurine and adriamycin. Cancer 38:1524, 1976

473. Mitchell JR, Jollow DJ: Metabolic activation of drugs to toxic substances. Gastroenterology 68:392, 1975

474. Mitchell JR et al: Metabolic activation: Biochemical basis for many drug-induced liver injuries. Prog Liver Dis 5:259, 1976

475. Mitchell JR et al: Toxic drug reactions. In Eichler O, Farah A, Herken H et al (eds): Handbook of Experimental Pharmacology, vol 283, pp 383–419. Berlin, Springer-Verlag, 1975

476. Mitchell JR et al: Acetaminophen-induced hepatic injury: Protective role of glutathione in man and rationale for therapy. Clin Pharmacol Ther 16:676, 1974

477. Mitchell JR et al: Increased incidence of isoniazid hepatitis in rapid acetylators: Possible reaction to hydrazine metabolites. Clin Pharmacol Ther 18:70, 1975

478. Mitchell JR et al: Isoniazid liver injury: Clinical spectrum, pathology and probable pathogenesis. Ann Intern Med 84:181, 1976

479. Mitchell MC et al: Granulomatous hepatitis associated with carbamazepine therapy. Am J Med 71:733, 1981

480. Mitchell MC et al: Cimetidine protects against acetaminophen hepatotoxicity in rats. Gastroenterology 81:1052, 1981

481. Mitchell MC et al: Budd-Chiari syndrome: Etiology, diagnosis and management. Medicine 61:199, 1982

482. Mitchell MC et al: Selective inhibition of acetaminophen oxidation and toxicity by cimetidine and other histamine H_2-receptor antagonists in vivo and in vitro in the rat and in man. J Clin Invest 73:389, 1984

483. Mizoguchi Y et al: Studies on intrahepatic cholestasis in drug-induced allergic hepatitis: Intrahepatic cholestasis induced in the rat by the culture supernatant of activated lymphocytes. Hepatogastroenterology 28:147, 1981

484. Mohabbat O et al: An outbreak of hepatic veno-occlusive disease in northwestern Afghanistan. Lancet 2:269, 1976

485. Moon HD: Pathology of fatal carbon tetrachloride poisoning with special reference to histogenesis of hepatic and renal lesions. Am J Pathol 26:1041, 1950

486. Morgan ET et al: Comparison of six rabbit liver cytochrome P-450 isoenzymes in formation of a reactive metabolite of acetaminophen. Biochem Biophys Res Commun 112:8, 1983

487. Morgan ET et al: Catalytic activity of cytochrome P-450 isozyme 3a, isolated from liver microsomes of ethanol-treated rabbits. J Biol Chem 257:13951, 1982

488. Morgan MY et al: Impaired oxidation of debrisoquine in patients with perhexiline liver injury. Gut 25:1057, 1984

489. Morgenstern L et al: Postoperative jaundice associated with halothane anesthesia. Surg Gynecol Obstet 121:728, 1965

490. Morledge J: Effects of perhexiline maleate in angina pectoris: A double-blind clinical evaluation with ECG-treadmill exercise testing. Postgrad Med J 49(suppl 3):64, 1973

491. Morris SJ et al: Disulfiram hepatitis. Gastroenterology 75:100, 1978

492. Moult PJ, Sherlock S: Halothane-related hepatitis: A clinical study of twenty-six cases. Q J Med 44:99, 1975

493. Muller SA et al: Cirrhosis caused by methotrexate in the treatment of psoriasis. Arch Dermatol 100:523, 1969

494. Mullick FG, Ishak KG: Hepatic injury associated with diphenylhydantoin therapy. Ann J Clin Pathol 74:442, 1980

495. Mullick FG et al: Hepatic injury associated with paraquat toxicity in humans. Liver 1:209, 1981

496. Murphy ES, Mireles M: Shock, liver necrosis and death after penicillin injection. Arch Pathol 73:355, 1962

497. Murphy PJ, Rymer W: Quinidine-induced liver disease? Ann Intern Med 76:785, 1973

498. Myers JD et al: Xanthomatous biliary cirrhosis following chlorpromazine, with observations indicating overproduction of cholesterol, hyperprothrombinemia and the development of portal hypertension. Trans Assoc Am Physicians 70:243, 1957

499. Nadell J, Kosek J: Peliosis hepatis: Twelve cases associated with oral androgen therapy. Arch Pathol Lab Med 101:405, 1977

500. Nakao NL et al: A case of chronic liver disease due to tolazamide. Gastroenterology 89:192, 1985

501. Namihisa T et al: Der Lymphozytentransformationstest bei allergischen Arzneimittelschaden der Leber. Leber Magen Darm 5:73, 1975

502. Nash DT, Feer TD: Hepatic injury possibly induced by verapamil. JAMA 249:395, 1983

503. Neale G, Azzopardi JG: Chronic arsenical poisoning and non-cirrhotic portal hypertension: A case for diagnosis. Br Med J 4:725, 1971

504. Nelemans FA: Drugs affecting adrenergic function. In Meyler L, Herxheimer A (eds): Side Effects of Drugs, vol VII, pp 224–238. Amsterdam, Excerpta Medica, 1972

505. Nelson SD et al: Isoniazid and iproniazid: Activation of metabolites to toxic intermediates in man and rats. Science 193:901, 1976

506. Neu HC, Swarz H: Carbenicillin: Clinical and laboratory experience with a parenterally administered penicillin for treatment of *Pseudomonas* infection. Ann Intern Med 71:903, 1969

507. Neuberger J, Williams R: Halothane anesthesia and liver damage. Br Med J 289:1135, 1984

508. Newberne JW: Assessment of safety data from patients on short- and long-term perhexiline therapy. Postgrad Med J 49(suppl 3):125, 1973

509. Newman R et al: Rifampin in initial treatment of pulmonary tuberculosis. Am Rev Respir Dis 109:216, 1974

510. Nicholson KG: Properties of antiviral agents. Lancet 2:503, 1984

511. Nuzzo JLJ et al: Peliosis hepatitis after long-term androgen therapy. Urology 15:518, 1985

512. Nyfors A, Poulsen H: Liver biopsies from psoriatics related to methotrexate therapy: I. Finding in 123 consecutive non-methotrexate treated patients. Acta Pathol Microbiol Scand 84:253, 1976

513. Ockner RK, Schmid R: Acquired porphyria in man and rat due to hexachlorobenzene intoxication. Nature 189:499, 1961

514. Oda T et al: Phospholipidosis der Leberzellen durch das Medikament "Coralgil." Acta Hepatol Jpn 10:530, 1969

515. Offit K, Sojka D: Letter: Ranitidine. N Engl J Med 310:1603, 1984

516. O'Gorman T, Koff RS: Salicylate hepatitis. Gastroenterology 72:726, 1977

517. Olsen VV et al: Serious reactions during malaria prophylaxis with pyrimethamine-sulfadoxine. Lancet 2:994, 1982

518. Orellana-Alcale JM, Dominguez JP: Jaundice and oral contraceptive drugs. Lancet 2:1278, 1966

519. Otsuka S et al: HLA antigens in patients with unexplained hepatitis following halothane anesthesia. Acta Anesthesiol 29:497, 1985

520. Overly WL et al: Androgens and hepatocellular carcinoma in an athlete. Ann Intern Med 100:158, 1984

521. Pagliaro L et al: Barbiturate jaundice: Report of a case due to barbital-containing drug, with positive rechallenge to phenobarbital. Gastroenterology 56:938, 1969

522. Paliard P: Perhexiline maleate-induced hepatitis. Digestion 17:419, 1978

523. Palmer WL et al: Cinchophen and toxic necrosis of liver: Survey of problem. Trans Assoc Am Physicians 51:381, 1936

524. Pamperl H et al: Influence of long-term anticonvulsant treatment in man. Liver 4:294, 1984

525. Park GD et al: Serious adverse reactions associated with sulindac. Arch Intern Med 142:1292, 1982

526. Parker WA: Captopril-induced cholestatic jaundice. Drug Intell Clin Pharm 18:234, 1984

527. Parker WA, Schearer CA: Phenytoin hepatotoxicity: A case report and review. Neurology 29:175, 1979

528. Parsons WB: Studies of nicotinic acid use in hypercholesteremia: Changes in hepatic function, carbohydrate tolerance and uric acid metabolism. Arch Intern Med 107:653, 1961

529. Passwell JH et al: Pigment deposition in the reticuloendothelial system after fat emulsion infusion. Arch Dis Child 51:366, 1976

530. Paulus HE: FDA arthritis advisory committee meeting. Arthritis Rheum 25:1124, 1982

531. Paumgartner G: Dihydralazine-induced hepatitis. Schweiz Med Wochenschr 107:649, 1977

532. Pearson K, Zimmerman HJ: Danazol and liver damage. Lancet 1:645, 1980

533. Perkins J: Phenindione jaundice. Lancet 1:125, 1962

534. Perkins J: Phenindione sensitivity. Lancet 1:127, 1962

535. Perry HM Jr: Multiple reactions to antihypertensive agents during treatment of malignant hypertension. Ann Intern Med 57:441, 1962

536. Perry MD: Hepatotoxicity of chemotherapeutic agents. Semin Oncol 9:65, 1982

537. Persico L: L'ittero da novobiocina. Policlinico 73:1607, 1966

538. Pessayre D et al: Perhexiline maleate-induced cirrhosis. Gastroenterology 76:170, 1979

539. Pessayre D et al: Chronic active hepatitis and multinucleated hepatocytes in adults treated with clometacin. Digestion 22:66, 1981

540. Peters R: Biochemical Lesions and Lethal Synthesis, p 88. New York, Macmillan, 1963

541. Peters RL: Halothane hepatitis. Lancet 2:790, 1978

542. Peters RL, Reynolds TB: Hepatic changes simulating alcoholic liver disease, post ileo-jejunal bypass. Gastroenterology 65:564, 1973

543. Peters RL et al: Tetracycline-induced fatty liver in non-pregnant patients. Am J Surg 113:622, 1967

544. Peters RL et al: Hepatic necrosis associated with halothane anesthesia. Am J Med 47:748, 1969

545. Pierce EH, Chesler DL: Possible association of granulomatous hepatitis with clofibrate therapy. N Engl J Med 299:314, 1978

546. Pieron R et al: Icteres et rifampicine, Sem Hop Paris 47:1286, 1971

547. Pieterse AS et al: Perhexiline maleate-induced cirrhosis. Pathology 15:201, 1983

548. Pilcher J et al: Long-term assessment of perhexiline maleate in angina pectoris. Postgrad Med J 49(suppl 3):115, 1973

549. Pimentel JC, Menezes AP: Liver granulomas containing copper in vineyard sprayer's lung: A new etiology of hepatic granulomatosis. Am Rev Respir Dis 111:189, 1975

550. Pimentel JC, Menezes AP: Liver disease in vineyard sprayers. Gastroenterology 72:275, 1977

551. Plaa GL: Toxic responses of the liver. In Doull J, Klaassen CD, Amdur MO (eds): Casarett and Doull's Toxicology: The Basic Science of Poisons, pp 206–231. New York, Macmillan, 1980

552. Podurgiel BJ et al: Liver injury associated with methotrexate therapy for psoriasis. Mayo Clin Proc 48:787, 1973

553. Pollock AA et al: Hepatitis associated with high-dose oxacillin therapy. Arch Intern Med 138:915, 1978

554. Pollock LJ et al: Toxicity of pyridine in man. Arch Intern Med 71:95, 1943

555. Ponte CD: Carbamazepine-induced thromboyctopenia, rash, and hepatic dysfunction. Drug Intell Clin Pharm 17:642, 1983

556. Popper H: Drug-induced hepatic injury. In Gall EA, Mostofi FK (eds): The Liver, pp 182–198. Baltimore, Williams & Wilkins, 1973

557. Popper H, Thomas L: Alterations of liver and spleen among workers exposed to vinyl chloride. Ann NY Acad Sci 246:172, 1975

558. Popper H et al: Drug-induced liver disease: A penalty for progress. Arch Intern Med 115:128, 1965

559. Poucell S et al: Amiodarone-associated phospholipidosis and fibrosis of the liver: Light, immunohistochemical and electron microscopic studies. Gastroenterology 86:926, 1984

560. Poulsen H, Winkler K: Liver disease with periportal sinusoidal dilatation. Digestion 8:441, 1973

561. Poupon R et al: Hépatite chronique associée à la prise prolongée de papavérine. Gastroenterol Clin Biol 2:305, 1978

562. Powell-Jackson PR et al: Hepatotoxicity to sodium valproate: A review. Gut 25:673, 1984

563. Powers BJ et al: Chlorzoxazone hepatotoxicity: An analysis of 21 identified or presumed cases. Arch Intern Med 146:1183, 1986

564. Pratt CB, Johnson WW: Duration and severity of fatty metamorphosis of the liver following L-asparaginase therapy. Cancer 28:361, 1971

565. Prescott LF: Paracetamol overdosage. Drugs 25:290, 1983

566. Prescott LF, Critchley AJH: The treatment of acetaminophen poisoning. Ann Rev Pharmacol Toxicol 23:87, 1983

567. Prescott LF et al: Plasma-paracetamol half-life and hepatic necrosis in patients with paracetamol overdosage. Lancet 1:519, 1971

568. Prescott LF et al: Successful treatment of severe paracetamol overdosage with cysteamine. Lancet 1:588, 1974

569. Prescott LF et al: Cysteamine, L-methionine and D-penicillamine in paracetamol poisoning. J Intern Med Res 4(suppl 4):112, 1976

570. Prescott LF et al: Side effects of benoxaprofen. Br Med J 284:1783, 1982

571. Price VF, Jollow DJ: Mechanism of ketone-induced protection from acetaminophen toxicity in the rat. Drug Metab Dispos 11:451, 1983

572. Proctor J: Hepatitis associated with ranitidine. JAMA 251:1554, 1984

573. Proudfoot AT, Wright N: Acute paracetamol poisoning. Br Med J 3:577, 1970

574. Rahmat J et al: Captopril-associated cholestatic jaundice. Ann Intern Med 102:56, 1985

575. Ramsay ID: Carbamezepine-induced jaundice. Br Med J 4:155, 1967

576. Raper R et al: Fulminant hepatic failure due to allopurinol. Aust NZ J Med 14:63, 1984

577. Rapp RS et al: Isoniazid hepatotoxicity in children. Am Rev Respir Dis 118:794, 1978

578. Rau R et al: Allergisch-toxische Leber-schadigung durch D-Penizillamin. Schweiz Med Wochenschr 102:1226, 1972

579. Read AE: Chronic chlorpromazine jaundice. Am J Med 31:249, 1961

580. Recknagel RO: A new direction in the study of carbon tetrachloride hepatotoxicity. Life Sci 33:401, 1983

581. Recknagel RO, Glende EA Jr: Carbon tetrachloride hepatotoxicity. An example of lethal cleavage. CRC Crit Rev Toxicol 2:263, 1973

582. Record CO et al: *Candida* endocarditis treated with 5-fluorocytosine. Br Med J 1:262, 1971

583. Reddy KP et al: Cholangiocarcinomas induced by feeding 3'-methyl-4-dimethyl-aminoazobenzene to rats: Histopathology and ultrastructure. Am J Pathol 87:189, 1977

584. Redeker AG et al: Effect of griseofulvin in acute intermittent porphyria. JAMA 188:466, 1964

585. Reed GR Jr, Cox AJ Jr: The human liver after radiation injury: A form of veno-occlusive disease. Am J Pathol 48:597, 1966

586. Reed WD, Williams R: Halothane hepatitis as seen by the physician. Br J Anaesth 44:935, 1972

587. Rees KR, Tarlow MJ: The hepatotoxic action of allyl formate. Biochem J 104:757, 1967

588. Rees L: Drugs used in treatment of psychiatric disease. Abstr World Med 39:129, 1966

589. Rehman OU et al: Methyldopa-induced submassive hepatic necrosis. JAMA 224:1390, 1973

590. Rehnqvist N: Intrahepatic jaundice due to warfarin therapy. Acta Med Scand 204:335, 1978

591. Reichel J et al: Intrahepatic cholestasis following administration of chlorpropamide. Am J Med 28:654, 1960

592. Reichen J, Simon F: Mechanisms of cholestasis. Int Rev Exp Pathol 26:232, 1984

593. Reid WD et al: Bromobenzene metabolism and hepatic necrosis. Pharmacology 6:41, 1971

594. Reshev R et al: Cholestatic jaundice in fascioliasis treated with niclofolan. Br Med J 285:1243, 1982

595. Rex D et al: Intrahepatic cholestasis and sicca complex after thiabendazole. Gastroenterology 85:718, 1983

596. Reynolds ES, Moslen MT: Liver injury following halothane anesthesia in phenobarbital-pretreated rats. Biochem Pharmacol 23:189, 1974

597. Reynolds ES et al: Fatal massive necrosis of the liver as a manifestation of hypersensitivity to probenecid. N Engl J Med 256:592, 1957

598. Reynolds ES et al: Massive hepatic necrosis after fluoroxene anesthesia: A case of drug interaction? N Engl J Med 286:530, 1972

599. Reynolds TB: Laxative liver disease. In Gerok W, Sickinger K (eds): Drugs and the Liver, pp 319–325. Stuttgart, FK Schattauer-Verlag, 1975

600. Rich RR, Johnson JS: Salicylate hepatotoxicity in patients with juvenile rheumatoid arthritis. Arthritis Rheum 16:1, 1973

601. Ridker PM et al: Hepatic veno-occlusive disease associated with the consumption of pyrrolizidine dietary supplements. Gastroenterology 88:1050, 1985

602. Rimington C et al: Studies on the photosensitization of animals in South Africa: The ictogeneric factor in gelldik-

kop: Isolation of the active principle from *Lippia rehmanni*. Onderstepoort J Vet Sci 9:225, 1937

603. Ritt DJ et al: Acute hepatic necrosis with stupor or coma: An analysis of thirty-one patients. Medicine 48:151, 1969

604. Robinson MM: Demonstration by "challenge" of hepatic dysfunction association with propionyl erythromycin ester lauryl sulfate. Antibiot Chemother 12:147, 1962

605. Rodman JS et al: Methyldopa hepatitis: A report of six cases and review of the literature. Am J Med 60:941, 1976

606. Rodriguez V et al: Combination 6-mercaptopurine-adriamycin in refractory adult acute leukemia. Clin Pharmacol Ther 18:462, 1975

607. Rodriguez-Iturbe B: Acute yellow-phosphorus poisoning. N Engl J Med 284:157, 1971

608. Roe D: Therapeutic significance of drug-nutrient interactions in the elderly. Pharmacol Rev 36(suppl):109S, 1984

609. Roenigk HH Jr et al: Hepatotoxicity of methotrexate in the treatment of psoriasis. Arch Dermatol 103:250, 1971

610. Ronnov-Jessen V, Tjernlund A: Hepatotoxicity due to treatment with papaverine. N Engl J Med 281:1333, 1969

611. Rooks JB et al: Epidemiology of hepatocellular adenoma. JAMA 242:644, 1979

612. Ros E et al: Effects of chlorpromazine hydrochloride on bile salt synthesis, bile formation and biliary lipid secretion in the Rhesus monkey: A model for chlorpromazine-induced cholestasis. Eur J Clin Invest 9:29, 1979

613. Rosenbaum H, Reveno WS: Agranulocytosis and toxic hepatitis from methimazole. JAMA 152:27, 1953

614. Rosenberg DM, Nealon FA: Acetaminophen and liver disease. Ann Intern Med 88:129, 1978

615. Rosenblum LE et al: Hepatocellular jaundice as a complication of iproniazid therapy. Arch Intern Med 105:583, 1960

616. Rosenkranz HS, Carr HS: Hydrazine antidepressants and isoniazid: Potential carcinogens. Lancet 1:1354, 1971

617. Ross S et al: Alpha-aminobenzylpenicillin: New broad-spectrum antibiotic: Preliminary clinical and laboratory observations. JAMA 182:238, 1962

618. Rotmensch HH et al: Granulomatous hepatitis: A hypersensitivity response to procainamide. Ann Intern Med 89:646, 1978

619. Rotmensch HH et al: Lymphocyte sensitization in nifedipine-induced hepatitis. Br Med J 281:977, 1980

620. Rotmensch HH et al: Experience with immunological tests in drug-induced hepatitis. Z Gastroenterol 19:691, 1981

621. Rouiller C: Experimental toxic injury of the liver. In Rouiller C (ed): The Liver, vol II, pp 335–476. New York, Academic Press, 1964

622. Rueff B, Benhamou JP: Acute hepatic necrosis and fulminant hepatic failure. Gut 14:805, 1973

623. Rumack BH: Acetaminophen overdose. Am J Med 75(5A):104, 1983

624. Russell AS et al: Serum transaminases during salicylate therapy. Br Med J 2:428, 1971

625. Russell RI et al: Active chronic hepatitis after chlorpromazine ingestion. Br Med J 1:655, 1973

626. Russell RM et al: Hepatic injury from chronic hypervitaminosis A resulting in portal hypertension and ascites. N Engl J Med 291:435, 1974

627. Ryan DE et al: Separation and characterization of highly purified forms of liver microsomal cytochrome P-450 from rats treated with polychlorinated biphenyls, phenobarbital and 3-methylcholanthrene. J Biol Chem 25:1365, 1979

628. Salfelder K et al: Fatal phosphorus poisoning: A study of forty-five autopsy cases. Beitr Pathol 147:321, 1972

629. Sallen MK et al: Streptokinase-induced hepatic dysfunction. Am J Gastroenterol 78:523, 1983

630. Sato C, Lieber CS: Increased hepatotoxicity of acetaminophen after chronic ethanol consumption in the rat. Gastroenterology 80:140, 1981

631. Sato C, Lieber CS: Mechanism of the preventive effect of ethanol on acetaminophen-induced hepatotoxicity. J Pharmacol Exp Therap 218:811, 1981

632. Schacter D: Fluidity and function of hepatocyte plasma membranes. Hepatology 4:190, 1984

633. Schade R et al: Fulminant hepatitis associated with disulfiram: Report of a case. Arch Intern Med 143:1271, 1983

634. Schaffner F: Halothane hepatitis. In Ingelfinger F, Ebert P, Finland M et al (eds): Controversy in Internal Medicine, 2nd ed, pp 465–584. Philadelphia, WB Saunders, 1974

635. Schaffner F, Raisfeld IH: Drugs and the liver. A review of metabolism and adverse reactions. Adv Intern Med 15:221, 1969

636. Schaffrir E, Khassis S: Role of enhanced fat mobilization in liver triglyceride accumulation in carbon tetrachloride-induced liver injury. Isr J Med Sci 5:975, 1969

637. Scharer L, Smith JP: Serum transaminase elevations and other hepatic abnormalities in patients receiving isoniazid. Ann Intern Med 71:1113, 1969

638. Schein PS, Winokur SH: Immunosuppressive and cytotoxic chemotherapy: Long-term complications. Ann Intern Med 82:84, 1975

639. Schenker S et al: Pathogenesis of tetracycline-induced fatty liver. In Gerok W, Sickinger K (eds): Drugs and the Liver, pp 269–289. Stuttgart, FK Schattauer-Verlag, 1975

640. Schenker S et al: Intrahepatic cholestasis due to therapy of rheumatoid arthritis. Gastroenterology 64:622, 1973

641. Scheuer PJ: Drugs and toxins. In Liver Biopsy Interpretation, 3rd ed, pp 88–101. Baltimore, Williams & Wilkins, 1980

642. Scheuer PJ: Chronic hepatitis: A problem for the pathologist. Histopathology 1:5, 1977

643. Scheuer PJ et al: Rifampicin hepatitis: A clinical and histological study. Lancet 1:421, 1974

644. Schmid R: Cutaneous porphyria in Turkey. N Engl J Med 263:397, 1960

645. Schonberg LA: Peliosis hepatitis and oral contraceptives. J Reprod Med 27:753, 1982

646. Schwandt P et al: Clofibrate and the liver. Lancet 2:325, 1978

647. Schweitzer IL, Peters RL: Acute submassive hepatic necrosis due to methyldopa: A case demonstrating possible initiation of chronic liver disease. Gastroenterology 66:1203, 1974

648. Seaman WE, Plotz PH: Effect of aspirin on liver tests in patients with rheumatoid arthritis or systemic lupus erythematosus and in normal volunteers. Arthritis Rheum 19:155, 1976

649. Sedman AJ: Cimetidine-drug interactions. Am J Med 76:109, 1984

650. Seeff LB: Drug-induced chronic liver disease with emphasis on chronic active hepatitis. Semin Liver Dis 1:104, 1981

651. Seeff LB et al: Acetaminophen hepatotoxicity as a therapeutic misadventure. Ann Intern Med 104:399, 1986

652. Seeverens H et al: Myocarditis and methyldopa. Acta Med Scand 211:233, 1982

653. Selby DC et al: Fatal multisystemic toxicity associated with

prophylaxis with pyrimethamine and sulfadoxine (Fansidar). Br Med J 290:113, 1985

654. Selinger M, Koff RS: Thorotrast and the liver: A reminder. Gastroenterology 68:799, 1975

655. Selroos O, Edgren J: Lupus-like syndrome associated with pulmonary reaction to nitrofurantoin: Report of three cases. Acta Med Scand 197:125, 1975

656. Shaban MR et al: Fatal intrahepatic cholestasis and interstitial lung fibrosis following gold therapy for rheumatoid arthritis. J R Soc Med 77:960, 1984

657. Shalev O et al: Methyldopa-induced immune hemolytic anemia and chronic active hepatitis. Arch Intern Med 143:592, 1983

658. Sharp JR et al: Chronic active hepatitis and severe hepatic necrosis associated with nitrofurantoin. Ann Intern Med 92:14, 1980

659. Shashaty GG: Cryptogenic cirrhosis associated with methyldopa. South Med J 72:364, 1979

660. Sheikh KH, Nies AS: Trazodone and intrahepatic cholestasis. Ann Intern Med 99:572, 1983

661. Sherlock S: In Wolstenholme G, Porter R (eds): Drug Response in Man, pp 151–153. Boston. Little, Brown & Co, 1967

662. Sherlock S: Progress report: Halothane hepatitis. Gut 12:324, 1971

663. Sherlock S: Drugs and the liver. In Diseases of the Liver and Biliary System, 5th ed, pp 295–322. Oxford, Blackwell Scientific Publications, 1981

664. Sherlock S: Progress Report. Hepatic adenomas and oral contraceptives. Gut 16:753, 1975

665. Sherlock S et al: Progress report: Hepatic reactions to drugs. Gut 20:634, 1979

666. Shikata T et al: Phospholipid fatty liver: A proposal of a new concept and its electron microscopical study. Acta Pathol Jpn 20:467, 1970

667. Shikata T et al: Staining methods of Australia antigen in paraffin section detection of cytoplasmic inclusion bodies. Jpn J Exp Med 44:25, 1974

668. Shipp JC: Jaundice during methimazole ("Tapazole") administration. Ann Intern Med 42:701, 1955

669. Shorey J et al: Hepatotoxicity of mercaptopurine. Arch Intern Med 122:54, 1968

670. Short MH et al: Cholestatic jaundice during imipramine therapy. JAMA 206:1791, 1968

671. Silk BR, Roome APCH: Herpes encephalitis treated with intravenous idoxuridine. Lancet 1:411, 1970

672. Silverblatt F, Turck M: Laboratory and clinical evaluation of carbenicillin (carboxybenzyl penicillin). In Hobby GL (ed): Anti-microbial Agents and Chemotherapy—1968, pp 279–285. Baltimore, Williams and Wilkins, 1969

673. Simmonds F et al: Granulomatous hepatitis in a patient receiving allopurinol. Gastroenterology 62:101, 1972

674. Simon JB et al: Amiodarone hepatotoxicity simulating alcoholic liver disease. N Engl J Med 311:167, 1984

675. Simon N et al: Der Einflus der Griseofulvin-Therapie auf die Leberfunktion und den Porphyrin-Stoffwechsel. Arch Dermatol Forsch 241:148, 1971

676. Simpson BR et al: Evidence for halothane hepatotoxicity is equivocal. In Ingelfinger FJ, Relman AS, Finland M (eds): Controversy in Internal Medicine II, p 580. Philadelphia, WB Saunders, 1974

677. Sipes JG et al: Halothane-associated hepatitis: Evidence for direct toxicity. In Davis M, Tredger JM, Williams R (eds): Drug Reactions and the Liver, pp 219–231. London, Pittman Press, 1981

678. Sippel PJ, Agger WA: Nitrofurantoin-induced granulomatous hepatitis. Urology 18:177, 1981

679. Slater TF: Necrogenic action of carbon tetrachloride in the rat: A speculative mechanism based on activation. Nature 209:36, 1966

680. Slater TF: In Free Radical Mechanisms in Tissue Injury, pp 118–163. Bristol, JW Arrowsmith, 1972

681. Slater TF et al: Sporidesmin poisoning in the rat. Res Vet Sci 5:450, 1964

682. Smetana HF: The histopathology of drug-induced liver disease. Ann NY Acad Sci 104:821, 1963

683. Smith AF et al: Clofibrate, serum enzymes, and muscle pain. Br Med J 2:86, 1970

684. Smith FE, Lindberg PJ: Life-threatening hypersensitivity to sulindac. JAMA 244:269, 1980

685. Smith JP et al: Hypogastric artery infusion and radiation therapy for advanced squamous cell carcinoma of the cervix. AJR 114:110, 1972

686. Smith MD et al: Combined hepatotoxicity and neurotoxicity following sulfasalazine administration. Aust NZ J Med 12:76, 1982

687. Smith NJ: Death following accidental ingestion of DDT; experimental studies. JAMA 136:469, 1948

688. Sodium valproate: A new anticonvulsant. Med Lett Drugs Ther 19:93, 1977

689. Soffer EE et al: Carbamazepine-induced liver injury. South Med J 76:681, 1983

690. Solis-Herruzo JA et al: Hepatic injury in the toxic epidemic syndrome caused by ingestion of adulterated cooking oil (Spain, 1980). Hepatology 4:131, 1984

691. Sonnenblick M, Abraham AH: Ibuprofen hypersensitivity in systemic lupus erythematosus. Br Med J 1:619, 1978

692. Sotolongo RP et al: Hypersensitivity reaction to sulfasalazine with severe hepatotoxicity. Gastroenterology 75:95, 1978

693. Souza-Lima MA: Hepatitis associated with ranitidine. Ann Intern Med 101:207, 1984

694. Sparberg M et al: Intrahepatic cholestasis due to azathioprine. Gastroenterology 57:439, 1969

695. Spechler SJ et al: Cholestasis and toxic epidermal necrolysis associated with phenytoin sodium ingestion: The role of bile duct injury. Ann Intern Med 95:455, 1981

696. Spielberg SP et al: Predisposition to phenytoin hepatotoxicity assessed *in vitro*. N Engl J Med 305:722, 1981

697. Spooner JB: Paracetamol-induced hepatic damage. Worldwide extent of the problem. In Davis M, Tredger JM, Williams R (eds) Drug Reactions and the Liver, pp 121–129. London, Pittman Medical, 1981

698. Stein O et al: Lipoproteins and the liver. Prog Liver Dis 4:45, 1972

699. Steinbrecher UP, Mishkin S: Sulfmethoxazole-induced hepatic injury. Dig Dis Sci 26:756, 1981

700. Steinlieb P, Robinson RM: Stevens-Johnson syndrome plus toxic hepatitis due to ibuprofen. NY State J Med 87:200, 1978

701. Stempel DA, Miller JJ: Lymphopenia and hepatic toxicity with ibuprofen. J Pediatr 90:657, 1977

702. Stenger RJ, Johnson EA: Effects of phenobarbital pretreatment on the response of rat liver to halothane administration. Proc Soc Exp Biol 140:1319, 1972

703. Stern EH et al: Possible hepatitis from verapamil. N Engl J Med 306:612, 1982

704. Sternberg SS, Phillips FS: Azaserine: Pathological and pharmacological studies. Cancer 10:889, 1957

705. Sternberg SS et al: Gallbladder and bile duct adenocarcinomas in dogs after long term feeding of aramite. Cancer 13:780, 1960

706. Sterup K, Mosbech J: Budd-Chiari syndrome after taking oral contraceptives. Br Med J 4:660, 1967

707. Stoeckle JD et al: Chronic beryllium disease: Long-term follow-up of sixty cases and selective review of the literature. Am J Med 46:545, 1969

708. Stolzer BL et al: Post arsenical obstructive jaundice complicated by xanthomatosis and diabetes mellitus. Am J Med 9:124, 1950

709. Stricker BH, Spoelstra P: Drug-Induced Hepatic Injury. Elsevier, Amsterdam, 1985

710. Stromberg A, Wengle B: Chronic active hepatitis induced by nitrofurantoin. Br Med J 2:174, 1976

711. Strubelt O: Alcohol potentiation of liver injury. Fundam Appl Toxicol 4:144, 1984

712. Stuart KL, Bras G: Veno-occlusive disease of the liver. Q J Med 28:291, 1957

713. Suarez G, Nathans D: Inhibition of aminoacyl-s RNA binding to ribosomes by tetracycline. Biochem Biophys Res Commun 18:743, 1965

714. Suchy FJ et al: Acute hepatic failure associated with the use of sodium valproate: Report of two fatal cases. N Engl J Med 300:962, 1979

715. Summerfield JA et al: Effects of clofibrate in primary biliary cirrhosis: Hypercholesterolemia and gallstones. Gastroenterology 69:998, 1975

716. Svjgaard E, Ranek L: Hepatic dysfunction and ketoconazole therapy. Ann Intern Med 96:788, 1982

717. Swank LA et al: Allopurinol-induced granulomatous hepatitis with cholangitis and a sarcoid-like reaction. Arch Intern Med 138:997, 1978

718. Taggart HM, Alderdice JM: Fatal cholestatic jaundice in elderly patients taking benoxaprofen. Br Med J 284:1372, 1982

719. Tandon BN et al: An epidemic of veno-occlusive disease of liver in central India. Lancet 2:271, 1976

720. Taylor JW et al: Cholestatic liver dysfunction after long-term phenytoin therapy. Arch Neurol 41:500, 1984

721. Tedesco FJ, Mills LR: Diazepam (Valium) hepatitis. Dig Dis Sci 27:470, 1982

722. Teller DN: Phenothiazines and butyrophenones in relation to neurochemistry and pharmacology. In Denber HCB (ed): Psychopharmacological Treatment: Theory and Practice, pp 28–42. New York, Marcel Dekker, 1975

723. Ten Pas A, Quinn EL: Cholestatic hepatitis following the administration of sodium oxacillin. JAMA 191:674, 1965

724. Thies PW, Dull WL: Trimethoprim-sulfamethoxazole-induced cholestatic hepatitis. Arch Intern Med 144:1691, 1984

725. Thomas FB: Chronic aggressive hepatitis induced by halothane. Ann Intern Med 81:487, 1974

726. Thompson M et al: Ibufenac in the treatment of arthritis. Ann Rheum Dis 23:397, 1964

727. Thor H et al: Potentiation of oxidative cell injury in hepatocytes which have accumulated Ca^{2+}. J Biol Chem 259:6612, 1984

728. Ticktin HE, Robinson MD: Effects of some antimicrobial agents on the liver. Ann NY Acad Sci 104:1080, 1963

729. Ticktin HE, Zimmerman HJ: Hepatic dysfunction and jaundice in patients receiving triacetyloleandomycin. N Engl J Med 267:964, 1962

730. Tilak TB: Induction of cholangiocarcinoma following treatment of a rhesus monkey with aflatoxin. Food Cosmet Toxicol 13:247, 1975

731. Toghill PJ et al: Methyldopa liver damage. Br Med J 3:545, 1974

732. Tolman KG et al: Hepatotoxicity of salicylates in monolayer cell cultures. Gastroenterology 74:205, 1978

733. Tomatis L: The IARC program on the evaluation of the carcinogenic risk of chemicals to man. Ann NY Acad Sci 271:396, 1976

734. Tonder M et al: Sulfonamide-induced chronic liver disease. Scand J Gastroenterol 9:93, 1974

735. Torisu M et al: Immunosuppression, liver injury, and hepatitis in renal, hepatic, and cardiac homograft recipients: With particular reference to the Australia antigen. Ann Surg 174:621, 1971

736. Touloukian J, Kaplowitz N: Halothane-induced hepatic disease. Semin Liver Dis 1:134, 1981

737. Toxicity of nonsteroidal anti-inflammatory drugs. Med Lett Drugs Ther 25:15, 1983

738. Traggis DG et al: Cytosine arabinoside in acute leukemia of childhood. Cancer 28:815, 1971

739. Traiger GJ, Plaa GL: Differences in the potentiation of carbon tetrachloride in rats by ethanol and isopropanol pretreatment. Toxicol Appl Pharmacol 20:105, 1971

740. Trey C et al: Fulminant hepatic failure: Presumable contribution of halothane. N Engl J Med 279:798, 1968

741. Trey C, Davidson CS: The management of fulminant hepatic failure. Prog Liver Dis 3:282, 1970

742. Trowell J et al: Controlled trial of repeated halothane anaesthetics in patients with carcinoma of the uterine cervix treated with radium. Lancet 1:821, 1975

743. Tuchweber B et al: Peliosis-like changes induced by phalloidin in the rat liver: A light and electron microscopic study. J Med 4:327, 1973

744. Ulshen MH et al: Hepatotoxicity with encephalopathy associated with aspirin therapy in rheumatoid arthritis. J Pediatr 93:1034, 1978

745. Umiker W, Pearce J: Nature and genesis of pulmonary alterations in carbon tetrachloride poisoning. Arch Pathol 55:203, 1953

746. Underwood JCE et al: Jaundice after treatment of lukaemia with busulfan. Br Med J 1:556, 1971

747. Urban E et al: Liver dysfunction with mestranol but not with norethynodrel in a patient with Enovid-induced jaundice. Ann Intern Med 68:598, 1968

748. Utili R et al: Dantrolene-associated hepatic injury: Incidence and character. Gastroenterology 72:610, 1977

749. Valdes M, Jacobs WH: Intrahepatic cholestasis following the use of atromid-s. Am J Gastroenterol 66:69, 1976

750. Valdivia-Barriga V et al: Generalized hypersensitivity with hepatitis and jaundice after the use of penicillin and streptomycin. Gastroenterology 45:114, 1963

751. Van Thiel OH et al: Tolazemide hepatotoxicity. Gastroenterology 67:506, 1974

752. Van Wyk JJ, Hoffmann CR: Periarteritis nodosa: A case of fatal exfoliative dermatitis resulting from "dilantin sodium" sensitization. Arch Intern Med 81:605, 1948

753. Vandenberg M et al: Hepatitis associated with captopril treatment. Br J Clin Pharmacol 11:105, 1981

754. Vaquez JJ et al: Cyanamide-induced liver injury: A predictable lesion. Liver 3:225, 1983

755. Varma RR et al: Halothane hepatitis without halothane: Role of inapparent circuit contamination and its prevention. Hepatology 5:1159, 1985

756. Vergani D et al: Antibodies to the surface of halothane-altered rabbit hepatocytes in patients with severe halothane-associated hepatitis. N Engl J Med 303:66, 1980

757. Victorino RMM et al: Jaundice associated with naproxen. Postgrad Med J 56:368, 1980

758. Videla L et al: Increased oxidative capacity in the liver following ethanol administration. In Khanna JM, Israel Y, Kalant H (eds): Alcoholic Liver Pathology, pp 331–340. Ontario, Addiction Research Foundation, 1975

759. Villeneuve JP, Warner HA: Cimetidine hepatitis. Gastroenterology 77:143, 1979

760. Viteri AL et al: Erythromycin ethylsuccinate-induced cholestasis. Gastroenterology 76:1007, 1979

761. Vitug AC, Goldman JM: Hepatotoxicity from antithyroid drugs. Horm Res 21:229, 1985

762. Von Oettingen WF: The Halogenated Hydrocarbons of Industrial and Toxicological Importance. Amsterdam, Elsevier, 1964

763. Wakabayashi T et al: High incidence of peliosis hepatis in autopsy cases of aplastic anemia with special reference to anabolic steroid therapy. Acta Pathol Jpn 34:1079, 1984

764. Walker CO, Combes B: Biliary cirrhosis induced by chlorpromazine. Gastroenterology 51:631, 1966

765. Walker SH, Standiford WE: The treatment of infants with oxacillin sodium. Am J Dis Child 114:64, 1967

766. Ware AJ et al: Acetaminophen and the liver. Ann Intern Med 88:267, 1978

767. Ware AJ et al: Spectrum of liver disease in renal transplant hepatitis. Gastroenterology 68:519, 1975

768. Ware S, Millward-Sadler GH: Acute liver disease associated with sodium valproate. Lancet 2:1110, 1980

769. Warren JS: Diflunisal-induced cholestatic jaundice. Br Med J 2:736, 1978

770. Waugh D: Myocarditis, arteritis, and focal hepatic splenic, and renal granulomas apparently due to penicillin sensitivity. Am J Pathol 28:437, 1952

771. Weinstein A et al: Low dose methotrexate treatment of rheumatoid arthritis. Am J Med 79:321, 1985

772. Weinstein G et al: Psoriasis-liver methotrexate interactions. Arch Dermatol 108:36, 1973

773. Weir JF: Cirrhosis associated with chronic inorganic arsenical poisoning. Proc Staff Meet Mayo Clin 5:173, 1930

774. Weir JF, Comfort MW: Toxic cirrhosis caused by cinchophen. Arch Intern Med 52:685, 1933

775. Weiss DL, De Los Santos R: Urethane-induced hepatic failure in man. Am J Med 28:476, 1960

776. Weiss M et al: Propylthiouracil-induced liver damage. Arch Intern Med 140:1184, 1980

777. Weiss P et al: Effects of SU-17437 on serum lipid in hyperlipoproteinemia patients. Clin Pharmacol Ther 11:90, 1970

778. Westably D et al: Androgen related primary hepatic tumors in non-Fanconi patients. Cancer 51:1947, 1983

779. White LB et al: Hepatotoxicity following enflurane anesthesia. Dig Dis Sci 26:466, 1981

780. Whitfield D: Presumptive fatality due to pyrimethamine-sulfadoxine. Lancet 2:1272, 1982

781. Whittaker SJ et al: Sulindac hepatotoxicity. Gut 23:875, 1982

782. Wiggins J, Scott DL: Hepatic injury following feprazone therapy. Rheum Rehab 20:44, 1981

783. Wildhirt E: Therapie chronischer Leberkrankheiten mit D-Penicillamin. Munch Med Wochenschr 116:217, 1974

784. Wilkinson SP et al: Hepatitis from dantrolene sodium. Gut 20:33, 1979

785. Williams ER, Khan MA: Liver damage in patients on methyldopa. J Ther Clin Res 1:5, 1967

786. Wilson FM et al: Anicteric carbenicillin hepatitis: Eight episodes in four patients. JAMA 232:818, 1975

787. Winckler K et al: Ground-glass hepatocytes in unselected liver biopsies: Ultrastructure and relationship to hepatitis B surface antigen. Scand J Gastroenterol 11:167, 1976

788. Winter SL, Boyer JL: Hepatic toxicity from large doses of vitamin B_3 (nicotinamide). N Engl J Med 289:1180, 1973

789. Witorsch P et al: The polypeptide antifungal agent (X-5079C): Further studies in 39 patients. Am Rev Respir Dis 93:876, 1966

790. Wogan GN: Aflatoxins and their relationship to hepatocellular carcinoma. In Okuda K, Peters RL (eds): Hepatocellular Carcinoma, pp 25–41. New York, John Wiley & Sons, 1976

791. Wolfe PB: Letter: Sulindac and jaundice. Ann Intern Med 91:656, 1979

792. Wright N, Prescott LF: Potentiation by previous drug therapy of hepatotoxicity following paracetamol overdose. Scott Med J 18:56, 1973

793. Wright R et al: Controlled prospective study of unexplained hepatitis following halothane anesthesia. Lancet 1:817, 1975

794. Wroblewski F: The clinical significance of alterations in transaminase activities of serum and other body fluids. Adv Clin Chem 1:313, 1958

795. Yamada T: Covalent binding theory for acetaminophen toxicity. Gastroenterology 85:202, 1983

796. Yanoff M, Rawson AJ: Peliosis hepatis. An anatomic study with demonstration of two varieties. Arch Pathol 77:1159, 1964

797. Yeh SDJ, Shils ME: Tetracycline and incorporation of amino acids into proteins of rat tissues. Proc Soc Exp Biol Med 121:729, 1966

798. Zafrani ES, Berthelot P: Sodium valproate in the induction of unusual hepatotoxicity. Hepatology 2:648, 1982

799. Zafrani ES et al: Cholestatic and hepatocellular injury associated with erythromycin esters. Dig Dis Sci 24:385, 1979

800. Zaraday Z et al: Irreversible liver damage after azathioprine. JAMA 222:690, 1972

801. Zeegan R et al: Prolonged survival after portal decompression of patients with non-cirrhotic intrahepatic portal hypertension. Gut 11:610, 1970

802. Zelman S: Liver cell necrosis in chlorpromazine jaundice (allergic cholangiolitis). Am J Med 27:708, 1959

803. Zimmerman HJ: Clinical and laboratory manifestations of hepatotoxicity. Ann NY Acad Sci 104:954, 1963

804. Zimmerman HJ: The spectrum of hepatotoxicity. Perspect Biol Med 12:135, 1968

805. Zimmerman HJ: Papaverine revisited as a hepatotoxin. N Engl J Med 281:1364, 1969

806. Zimmerman HJ: Hepatic failure. In Gall EA, Mostofi FK

(eds): The Liver, pp 384–405. Baltimore, Williams & Wilkins, 1973

807. Zimmerman HJ: Hepatotoxicity: The Adverse Effects of Drugs and Other Chemicals on the Liver. New York, Appleton-Century-Crofts, 1978

808. Zimmerman HJ: Drug-induced chronic hepatic disease. Med Clin North Am 63:567, 1979

809. Zimmerman HJ: Effects of aspirin and acetaminophen on the liver. Arch Intern Med 141:333, 1981

810. Zimmerman HJ: Effects of alcohol on other hepatotoxins. Alcoholism: Clin Exp Res 10:3, 1986

811. Zimmerman HJ: Hepatotoxic effects of oncotherapeutic agents. Prog Liver Dis 8:621, 1986

812. Zimmerman HJ, Ishak KG: Valproate-induced hepatic injury: Analyses of 23 fatal cases. Hepatology 2:591, 1982

813. Zimmerman HJ, Mao R: Cytotoxicity of carbon tetrachloride as measured by loss of cellular enzymes to surrounding media. Am J Med Sci 250:688, 1965

814. Zimmerman HJ, Seeff LB: Enzymes in hepatic disease. In Coodley, EL (ed): Diagnostic Enzymology, pp 1–38. Philadelphia, Lea & Febiger, 1970

815. Zimmerman HJ, et al: Hepatocyte suspensions as a model for demonstration of drug hepatotoxicity. Biochem Pharmacol 23:2187, 1974

816. Zimmerman HJ et al: Ticrynafen-associated hepatic injury: Analysis of 340 cases. Hepatology 4:315, 1984

817. Zimran A et al: Reversible cholestatic jaundice and hyperamylasaemia associated with captopril treatment. Br Med J 287:1676, 1983

818. Zuchner H: Cholestatische Hepatose unter Cimetidin. Dtsch Med Wochenschr 102:1788, 1977

819. Zucker P et al: Fatal carbamazepine hepatitis. J Pediatr 91:667, 1977

chapter 18
Alcoholic Hepatitis

CHARLES L. MENDENHALL

Simply stated, alcoholic hepatitis is a form of toxic liver injury associated with chronic excess ethanol consumption. Reports of clinical jaundice after excessive ethanol consumption were not unusual in the early literature. As far back as 1892,[135] Osler attributed "acute necrosis of the liver" to excessive alcohol consumption. These reports most likely represented instances of alcoholic hepatitis. "Progressive alcoholic cirrhosis," "subacute alcoholic cirrhosis,"[64,65] florid cirrhosis,[153] "sclerosing hyalin necrosis,"[37] fatty liver with hepatic failure,[152] acute hepatic insufficiency of the chronic alcoholic,[147] and steatonecrosis[67,68] were all terms used to describe the severe form of toxic alcoholic liver disease. Note that these early names all attempted to show the association of this form of alcoholic injury with various histologic and clinical manifestations of the disease, such as cirrhosis, necrosis, fatty liver (steatosis), and liver failure. The term "alcoholic hepatitis" was first used in 1961 by Beckett and co-workers,[7] who described the clinical features of the disease in seven jaundiced patients with moderate disease (mean bilirubin 10.5 mg/dl). The following year Beckett described an additional five cases.[8] This time the patients all had mild disease, were anicteric, and had the diagnosis made by liver biopsy. Thus the full clinical spectrum of alcoholic hepatitis was recognized, ranging from anicteric to deep jaundice and fulminant hepatic failure. In the anicteric cases, the authors point out that misdiagnosis was frequent in the absence of histology. This fact has not changed in the 20 or more years since then.

PATHOLOGY AND PATHOGENESIS

The amount of ethanol consumed necessary to produce clinically significant liver pathology varies markedly among individuals. For most patients this represents an excess of 80 g/day for 15 years or more.[96] When this quantity is converted to volumes of alcoholic beverages consumed, it represents more than eight 12-ounce 6% beers, a litre of 12% wine, or ½ pint of 80 proof whiskey per day. For some, the susceptibility to alcohol injury may be considerably less.[165] In the Veterans Administration Cooperative Study,[61,114] mean consumption even for clinically mild disease was 234 g/day for a mean duration of 22 years. However, pathology of a lesser nature may have been present for some time before the clinical diagnosis was made.

The spectrum of pathology associated with chronic alcoholism ranges from no abnormalities to far advanced cirrhosis. The four most important alcohol-induced liver lesions are fatty liver, alcoholic hepatitis, cirrhosis, and perhaps hepatocellular carcinoma.[74] By itself, alcoholic hepatitis represents a serious (frequently life-threatening) but often reversible stage in the disease process. However, association with some degree of fatty liver is almost universal, and cirrhosis is present in over half the cases.[110] Characterization of the pathologic changes of alcoholic hepatitis preceded the clinical definition of the disease by approximately 50 years. Mallory, in 1911,[103] first described in detail the changes in the liver that preceded the late end-stages of cirrhosis in the alcoholic.

Three obligatory features have been defined as essential for the histologic diagnosis of alcoholic hepatitis[74]:

Liver cell damage, typically as "ballooning degeneration" with areas of necrosis

Inflammatory cell infiltration, predominantly polymorphonuclear leukocytes

Fibrosis, both pericellular, producing a lattice-like or "chicken-wire" appearance, and perivenular (centrolobular)

"Ballooning degeneration" begins in the centrolobular area (zone three of Rappaport) and is characterized by large swollen hepatocytes with a pale granular-appearing cytoplasm. In some instances, finely dispersed particles are entrapped among "cobweb-like strands." Within such cells alcoholic hyalin or Mallory bodies can often be seen.[51,74] The incidence of Mallory body formation varies with the acumen of the pathologists and the severity of the disease. It is reported in up to 84% of the cases.[110] Histologically, Mallory bodies appear as irregular aggregates of purplish red material (as seen with hematoxylin and eosin stain), which are typically intracytoplasmic and perinuclear in location. In the centrolobular area, they are characteristic but not pathognomonic of alcoholic hepatitis.[58] When alcoholic cirrhosis has evolved with fibrotic distortion of the centrolobular areas, Mallory bodies are found at the periphery of the nodules. Although uncommon, Mallory bodies have been observed with Indian childhood cirrhosis,[127,164] Wilson's disease,[150,157,169] primary biliary cirrhosis,[57,123] chronic biliary obstruction,[57] diabetes mellitus,[48,91] after jejunoileal bypass surgery,[106,141] in morbid obesity,[1,126] with postnecrotic cirrhosis,[57] after certain drug-related injuries,[140] and in some hepatomas.[36,142]

The pathogenesis of the swollen balloon-like heptatocytes is believed to be related to an ethanol-induced impairment in the release into the serum of lipoproteins and serum proteins by the hepatocytes. Retention of these transport proteins and lipids results in cellular swelling.[6,47] The net result of these changes is the "hydropic" degenerative appearance of the cytoplasm,[6,37,38] which eventually progresses to the disintegration of the hepatocytes.

The antimicrotubular action of ethanol results in failure of the microtubular secretory apparatus of the cell. It appears likely that alcoholic hyalin or Mallory bodies are formed from intermediate filaments of this secretory apparatus.[45] The appearance of these Mallory bodies originally was classified as a form of hyalin degeneration occurring with hepatocyte damage[68,74]; associated with more severe clinical, biochemical, and histologic abnormalities[67]; and carrying a more serious prognosis[83,90,159]; however, survival does not appear to be adversely affected by their presence.[52,67,110,163] Furthermore, in tissue culture experiments[13] in which Mallory bodies were produced by hepatocytes, there was no association between Mallory bodies and degenerative changes in the hepatocyte. French[44] has suggested that the appearance of Mallory bodies in alcoholic hepatitis may result from the expression of a gene normally repressed in the adult that regulates the formation of intermediate filaments in the fetus (gene derepression phenomena). Activation of such a suppressed fetal gene would result in excessive intermediate filament formation and afford the appropriate conditions for Mallory body formation. This is not to say that Mallory bodies are without adverse biologic effects. Like intermediate filaments,[134] they bind nonspecifically to immunoglobulins.[143,173] Mallory bodies, extruded from dead or dying liver cells and complexed with serum and tissue carbohydrates and immunoglobulins, possess strong chemotactic properties,[95] which may account for part of the polymorphonuclear inflammatory response seen in alcoholic hepatitis. Indeed, inflammatory cells are frequently seen in close proximity to necrotic and Mallory body–containing liver cells.[74] Mallory body complexes have also been implicated in fibrogenesis by activating lymphocytes to secrete fibrogenic lymphokines.[188] Specific antibodies to Mallory bodies have been reported in the serum of patients with alcoholic hepatitis, and immune complexes have been found in their livers.[80] This raises the possibility that they may act as a neoantigen[175] for an autoimmune type liver injury.

The centrolobular location of the early injury may be related to hypoxia. This area of the liver lobule has the lowest oxygen content and hence is most susceptible to injury. Furthermore, animal studies[77,132] have shown that during the early phase of ethanol withdrawal a decrease in hepatic venous oxygen content is associated with a significant increase in oxygen consumption by the liver. Thus, the centrolobular area becomes more susceptible to hypoxic injury and necrosis.[77] The extensive loss of hepatocytes in this perivenular area is replaced by a relatively acellular confluent sclerotic area. This pathologic change has been termed "sclerosing hyalin necrosis"[37] and is believed by some to be an obligatory step in the natural evolution of alcoholic liver injury into cirrhosis.[81]

Although the sclerotic process may be sharply outlined in the pericentral area, necrosis and inflammation (active alcoholic hepatitis) frequently extend into the surrounding areas. In the more advanced cases, fibrosis and necrosis develop in the portal areas (perhaps by another mechanism to be discussed) so that they join to form central-central and central-portal bridging necrosis and fibrosis, which may rapidly lead to the development of cirrhosis.[74,151] The time required for the completion of the cirrhotic process is not well established and appears to be variable. In Galambos' series of 23 patients[50] in whom serial biopsies were performed at 3- to 4-month intervals, progression to cirrhosis was observed to have occurred prior to the initial follow-up biopsy in 61% (14/23).

Other mechanisms, in addition to anoxia and autoimmune injury, may also be operational in the alcoholic to explain the development of liver cell necrosis. Considerable indirect experimental evidence exists that suggests free radical formation is a contributing factor.[27,28,33,87,156] The theorized sequence of events leading to liver injury is graphically shown in Figure 18-1. Using in vitro microsomal preparations, reactive hydroxyl radicals can be generated from ethanol.[19,25] However, these radicals have not been detected in vivo.[35] Acetaldehyde, the first oxidation product of ethanol, may also result in the formation of destructive high-energy free radicals. In the presence of molecular oxygen, such radicals attack unsaturated fatty acids in membranes and organelles to produce lipid epoxides and peroxides. These unstable intermediates then undergo peroxidative degradation with loss of membrane permeability, changes in membrane fluidity, altered enzyme function, and, ultimately, cellular death and necrosis. Unfortunately, high-energy free radicals are very short lived and are present in low concentration so that evidence for their existence is mainly indirect. Studies from a number of different laboratories observed increases in peroxidative lipid degradation products, principally malonaldehyde, after ethanol consumption.[27,28,87] These products were markedly reduced when ethanol metabolism was blocked by pyrazole, which diminishes acetaldehyde formation, and were increased by disulfiram, an inhibitor that promotes acetaldehyde accumulation.[35] These studies suggest that acetaldehyde-generated free radicals are responsible for the injury. If lipid peroxidation is occurring after ethanol consumption, then a reduction in tissue antioxidants would be anticipated. When antioxidants were measured after ethanol treatment, mitochondrial concentrations were significantly reduced.[34] Furthermore, when a technique to quantify peroxidative degradation (diene conjugation absorption spectroscopy) was used,[12] ethanol treatment resulted in selective enhanced diene absorption in the mitochondria.[33] Such an organelle localization of injury might be anticipated, since acetaldehyde is metab-

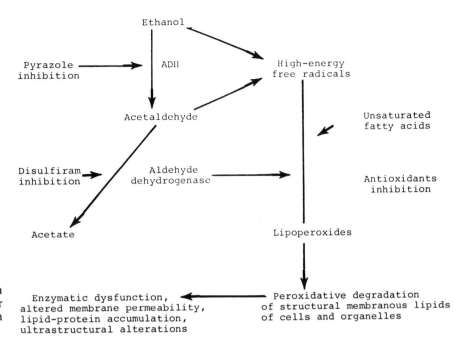

Fig. 18-1. Proposed sequence in the pathogenesis of alcoholic liver injury. (Mendenhall CL: Clin Gastroenterol 10:417, 1981)

olized primarily in the mitochondria.[63,104] Pathologically, mitochondrial abnormalities are known to occur frequently in alcoholic liver injury. In one large study,[21] 20% of 220 patients with alcoholic hepatitis had swollen deformed mitochondria (giant mitochondria). These are not unique to alcoholic hepatitis but have been reported in other forms of liver injury.[15,17,86,89,145] In the alcoholic, they appear to be more common in milder forms of liver disease.[21]

The inflammatory changes in alcoholic hepatitis are predominantly polymorphonuclear and may be focal or diffuse in distribution, depending on the severity of the disease and usually in relation to areas of necrosis and Mallory bodies, with their heaviest infiltration in the centrolobular areas. Other cell types (lymphocytes and plasma cells) also infiltrate and may have clinical importance. Although they too may be present in the centrolobular areas,[47] more often they are seen in the portal areas located at the limiting plate and in association with piecemeal necrosis. In the Veterans Administration Cooperative Study on alcoholic hepatitis,[110] piecemeal necrosis and limiting plate erosion were present in 89% of the biopsies. These findings suggest a cytotoxic role for lymphocytes, similar to that in chronic active hepatitis[82] or in orthotopic liver homograft rejection.[30] Phenotype identification of the lymphocytes has shown them to be T cells.[46,73,167] Since T lymphocytes tend to be decreased in the peripheral blood of alcoholic hepatitis patients,[9,73,167] sequestration into the liver has been postulated.[9,73,185] Lymphocytes with cytotoxic effects on hepatocytes have been found in the blood of baboons chronically fed ethanol,[136] as well as in patients with alcoholic hepatitis,[79] suggesting that chronic ethanol

ingestion leads to sensitization of lymphocytes to liver cell antigens.[80,95,167,187] Sensitized lymphocytes with cytotoxic potential adhere to target cells *in vitro*,[186] producing cell death. In the case of alcoholic hepatitis, such sensitized lymphocytes bind to hepatocytes and lead to hepatocellular destruction. Immunohistochemical analyses of liver in patients with alcoholic hepatitis have demonstrated such potentially cytotoxic T lymphocytes (T$_8$) in close proximity to portal areas of necrosis,[171] similar to that observed with chronic active hepatitis or rejection of liver allografts.[172] These observations may explain in part the chronicity associated with alcoholic hepatitis[50] and suggest the possibility of more than one mechanism operating concomitantly to produce injury.

Hepatic fibrosis associated with alcohol injury begins early and is an integral part of the pathology. Pericentral venous sclerosis has been observed to occur in the absence of the inflammatory changes of alcoholic injury. Such lesions were observed in the alcoholic fatty livers of both baboons and alcoholic patients.[180] This has suggested to some that cirrhosis may develop in the alcoholic without going through the "alcoholic hepatitis" phase.[172,180] This question is not yet resolved. In the Veterans Administration Cooperative Study on alcoholic hepatitis,[110] 100% of the 220 livers on which biopsy or autopsy had been performed had increased fibrosis, ranging from focal scarring (16%) to bridging fibrosis (28%) and established cirrhosis (56%). The overall incidence of established cirrhosis was most likely higher than the observed 56%, since histology was not available on 46% (200/435) of patients, predominantly in the group of severely ill patients in whom the prevalence of cirrhosis would be expected to be highest.

Mallory, in 1911, postulated that fibrosis in alcoholic liver disease resulted from the inflammatory exudate, which produced "mechanical injury" followed by proliferation of fibroblasts and the deposition of connective tissue.[103] The mechanism for increased collagen formation and deposition in the liver of the alcoholic appears to be much more complex than merely a response to inflammation. In part this may be related to Mallory body–activated secretion of lymphokines. However, ethanol does have a direct effect on the biochemistry of collagen-stimulating hepatocyte proline uptake[113] and collagen synthesis in the absence of inflammation and alcoholic hepatitis.[41,121,122,139] This may account for the early appearance of fibrosis in alcohol-induced liver injury.

Other pathologic changes common in alcoholic hepatitis, but not obligatory for its diagnosis include the following:

Fatty metamorphosis. This change is present, to some degree, in over 95% of the cases.[110] (The pathogenesis and clinical significance of fatty liver are discussed in detail Chapter 22).

Intrahepatic cholestasis. This may occur in a significant number of patients. Thirty-eight percent in the Veterans Administration series had histologic evidence of cholestasis. In some patients this may be attributed to large bile duct obstruction associated with sclerosing pancreatitis. In most, the cholestatic picture represents a part of the alcohol-induced injury and is associated with bile stasis, bile plugs, periportal necrosis, mixed inflammatory exudate, and destruction of intralobular bile ducts.[2]

Excessive iron deposits. These occur both in parenchymal cells and in Kupffer cells of livers of patients with alcoholic liver injury. In one series of 329 alcoholics studied histologically by liver biopsy, hemosiderosis was observed in 51% of patients.[24] It is said to be most commonly associated with cirrhosis[74]; however, in this series[24] no difference in prevalence was observed between cirrhotics and noncirrhotics. Iron overload may result through a variety of mechanisms, possibly due to increased iron absorption,[184] increased iron content in alcoholic beverages (especially wine), hemolytic episodes, or secondary to repeated episodes of liver cell necrosis.

INCIDENCE

The world incidence of alcohol-induced liver injury varies considerably among countries. In general, a significant correlation between alcohol consumption and deaths from cirrhosis has been reported within a given country,[96] but comparisons among countries show much more variation and suggest interactions with other local factors. For example, Austria ranks first on the list for reported deaths while ranking tenth for alcohol consumption. Similarly, Japan ranks 12th for deaths but only 24th for alcohol

consumption. Figure 18-2 shows the correlation between these two variables. These differences have been attributed to genetic predisposition,[4,107,170] malnutrition,[69,148] and concomitant viral hepatitis infections (especially hepatitis B).[56,144] Further studies are needed to confirm these interactions.

The true incidence of alcoholic hepatitis, especially of the milder forms, is unknown, since the persons may be asymptomatic and the diagnosis usually requires biopsy confirmation. Again the incidence appears to differ among countries.

In one European study on Danish alcoholics,[62] 329 consecutive patients admitted for alcoholism (>50 g/day) were studied by biopsy. The total incidence of changes consistent with alcoholic hepatitis was 19.8%, of which two thirds already had cirrhosis or biopsies suggestive of cirrhosis (see Fig. 18-3).

The spectrum of liver disease in the alcoholics of Japan is somewhat different.[129] In several large series of hepatitis B surface antigen (HBsAg)-negative alcoholics, the incidence of chronic inflammatory liver disease (chronic persistent and chronic active hepatitis) was much higher (10%–61%), as was the incidence of cirrhosis or hepatic fibrosis (16%–59%) and hepatocellular carcinoma in cirrhosis (16%). Fatty liver and alcoholic hepatitis were less frequent (1%–15% and 6%–11%, respectively). The incidence seemed to depend on the patient population (medical service vs. psychiatric service), with the higher incidence of inflammatory disease in the psychiatric patients. Although no evidence of hepatitis B viral infections could be detected, the possibility of hepatitis non-A, non-B infection could not be excluded. However, the high prevalence of these changes in alcoholics with liver disease in the absence of clinical or laboratory evidence of viral infection has suggested to some that this may be one of the pathologic changes induced by alcohol injury to the liver.[62]

In a recent epidemiologic study in the United States[53,55] based on discharge diagnoses (nongovernment hospitals), 136.5 hospitalizations for alcoholic hepatitis were observed per 100,000 population (0.14%). The ratio of alcoholic fatty liver to alcoholic hepatitis to alcoholic cirrhosis was 1.0:5.3:3.8. The high prevalence of alcoholic hepatitis and the low prevalence of fatty liver may reflect the more severe, sometimes life-threatening symptomatology of acute alcoholic hepatitis, which requires hospitalization more readily. It does not necessarily reflect the prevalence among all alcoholics.

These data suggest that the prevalence of acute alcoholic hepatitis in the United States is much higher than that reported in Denmark and Japan. In a prospective study of six Veterans Administration Medical Centers,[111] of the initial 995 alcoholics with liver disease who were screened, 33.8% of those studied by biopsy had alcoholic hepatitis. These observations reflect only the prevalence of alcoholic hepatitis among patients with existing liver disease severe enough to require hospitalization. The mild or asymptomatic disease would not be reflected in these studies; thus, the total prevalence is probably even higher. Of in-

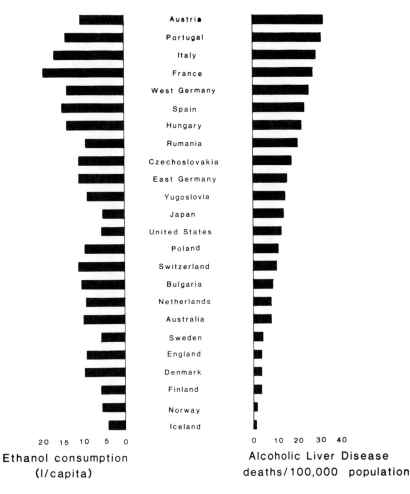

Fig. 18-2. Incidence of deaths from alcoholic liver disease in various countries with their corresponding consumption of ethanol. Countries are arranged in order of decreasing mortality. (Data are abstracted from Alcoholic Liver Disease: Pathology, Epidemiology, and Clinical Aspects).[54,96,129]

Ethanol consumption
(l/capita)

Alcoholic Liver Disease
deaths/100,000 population

terest was the observation that 55% of these patients already had established cirrhosis.

SYMPTOMATOLOGY

The spectrum of clinical signs and symptoms varies from very mild with minimal or no complaints to that of severe life-threatening liver failure. At the mild end of the spectrum, one of the earliest signs is the presence of some degree of liver enlargement. In the Veterans Administration Study,[110] a liver greater than 12 cm in the right midclavicular line was present in more than 85% of patients with even the mild cases. The presence of cirrhosis in combination with alcoholic hepatitis is a frequent occurrence seen in 55% (126/228) of all patients in whom histology was available.[110] Typically, patients with cirrhosis are said to have a small, shrunken liver. However, hepatomegaly was observed in nearly every patient regardless of clinical severity and was not helpful in differentiating the presence or absence of cirrhosis. In mild cases, only

the liver biopsy can establish the diagnosis and differentiate it from pure fatty liver, chronic persistent hepatitis, malignancy, or a variety of other liver pathologies. The presenting signs and symptoms depend to a great extent on the severity of injury. Shown graphically in Fig. 18-4 is the prevalence of observed findings in 16 reported studies on 1108 patients.[7,8,11,18,31,67,68,70,98,102,115,132,147,153,154,179] When certain of these symptoms occur in combination, pitfalls in the diagnosis may result and are worthy of comment. Alcoholic liver disease in general, and alcoholic hepatitis in particular, produce laboratory changes that are cholestatic in nature. (These will be discussed later under Laboratory Findings.) In a small but significant number of patients, symptoms of anorexia, nausea, vomiting, and right upper quandrant pain are associated with fever, jaundice, leukocytosis, and liver biochemistries consistent with cholestasis. In these instances, a false diagnosis of cholelithiasis and/or an acute abdomen may result. This may be disastrous for these patients, since surgery is very poorly tolerated and may be associated with a high morbidity and mortality.[8,70,111]

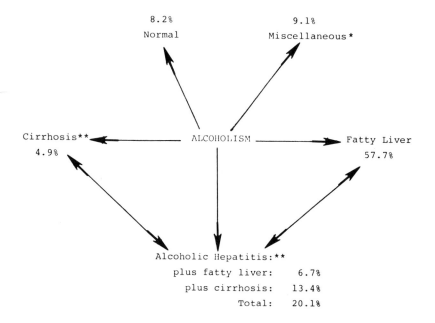

*   Miscellaneous changes include hemosiderosis (7%), "viral"
     hepatitis (0.9%), chronic active hepatitis (0.6%), and non-
     specific abnormalities (0.6%). (Christoffersen P. and Nielsen
     K.: <u>Acta Path Microbiol Scand</u>, (Section A), <u>80</u>:557, 1972.)

**   The 66 patients designated as "alcoholic hepatitis" frequently
      had fatty liver and/or Mallory bodies present (22 patients),
      and/or cirrhosis (44 patients). Although cirrhosis was present
      alone in 4.9% (13 patients), when patients with cirrhosis plus
      alcoholic hepatitis are combined the incidence of cirrhosis
      increased to 17.3% (57 patients).

Fig. 18-3. Prevalence of liver disease observed in 320 Danish alcoholics biopsied consecutively.

In some, signs and symptoms of liver failure predominate with ascites, portal hypertension, and hepatic encephalopathy. Symptomatology may not correlate well with histologic findings, so that an incorrect diagnosis of irreversible cirrhosis results, when in fact the condition is reversible. Portal hypertension with bleeding esophageal varices has been described with perivenular fibrosis, inflammation, and necrosis, but without cirrhosis.[37] Ascites and encephalopathy have been observed with minimal or no clinical jaundice and without cirrhosis. In the Veterans Administration Cooperative Study,[110] ascites was observed in 39% of cases in which, histologically, only alcoholic hepatitis was present and cirrhosis was absent. In these cases even tense ascites was observed in 5% of the cases. Changes consistent with portal systemic encephalopathy were reported in 33% of these cases. These changes were typically grade 1. However, 10% had clinical and physical findings of grades 2 to 4.

LABORATORY FINDINGS

The following laboratory changes shown in Table 18-1 are taken from the initial data on the 363 patients in the Veterans Administration Cooperative Study on alcoholic hepatitis.[110] The laboratory changes in these patients reflect the multisystem involvement by alcohol as well as the dysfunction present in the liver. Frequently several pathologic processes interact so that a variety of laboratory results may be seen, depending on which process predominates. Hematologic changes demonstrate this diversity of response. Leukocytosis was present in 41% of the patients, with the frequency increasing as the severity of the liver disease increased. Leukopenia, however, was observed in 8%, presumably as a result of direct bone marrow suppression by ethanol. A normal white cell count was observed in 51% of the cases. Chronic liver disease and malnutrition may result in anemia. Indeed, anemia was seen in over 90% of patients with severe alcoholic hepatitis. Typically this is a macrocytic type resulting from membrane alterations by ethanol. Folate deficiency may further complicate the picture and represents one of the most frequent vitamin deficiencies in the alcoholic. This has been reported to be present in 78% of alcoholics.[93] Less frequently, vitamin B_{12} deficiency may occur (25%) and contribute to the macrocytosis. More often, serum vitamin B_{12} levels are elevated in alcoholic hepatitis, reflecting

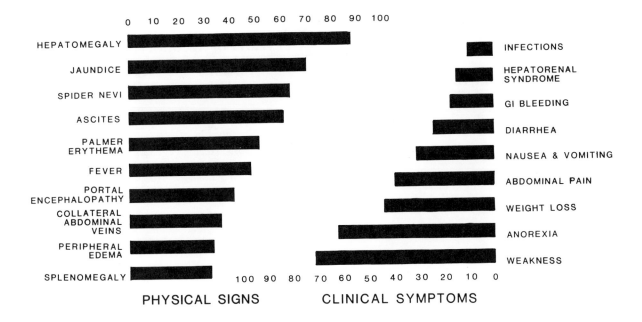

Fig. 18-4. Prevalence of physical signs and clinical symptoms is derived from 16 reported series containing 1108 patients with alcoholic hepatitis.[7,8,11,18,31,67,68,70,98,102,116,132,147,151,154,179]

acute liver cell injury and release from liver stores.[117] As a result of these two processes (direct toxicity of ethanol on red cells and vitamin deficiency), the mean corpuscular volume (MCV) is typically increased. Mean value in the Veterans Administration Cooperative study was 102.4 mm³. It should be noted that gastrointestinal tract blood loss is frequent in the alcoholic as a result of increased peptic ulcer disease, alcoholic gastritis, esophagitis, and esophageal varices. When this blood loss occurs with sufficient severity, iron deficiency anemia results, with a decrease in MCV. This phenomenon was seen in 2% of the Veterans Administration patients. Associated with severe liver disease, renal functional impairment was a frequent observation. Blood urea nitrogen (BUN) and serum creatinine levels both tended to be higher while urine volume tended to be lower. A low BUN (<5 mg/dl) is said to occur in severe liver disease because of decreased liver synthesis of urea by the failing liver. This was not observed in any of the 435 Veterans Administration patients. Although 6% (25/435) did have values below 5 mg/dl, these typically were patients with mild disease, good renal function, and reasonably good liver function (mean bilirubin 6.9 ± 1.7), rather than end-stage liver disease. None of those critically ill patients who died of their disease in the initial 30 days of hospitalization had a low BUN.

Abnormalities in the biochemical tests related to liver injury were usually diffusely abnormal. However, a pattern of change can be detected. Typically, the serum glutamic-oxaloacetic transaminase (SGOT) level is less than five times the upper limits of normal (depending on the laboratory, this is usually less than 200 µU/liter). Only 5% of the Veterans Administration patients had an SGOT level greater than 200 µU/liter, and most of these were terminal patients. Even in this seriously ill group, none of the levels were above 300 µU/liter. If one reviews other series of patients, scattered observations of high values have been observed, but they are infrequent,[68,166] so that in the presence of a high level of SGOT the diagnosis of alcoholic hepatitis should be suspect unless proven histologically. The serum glutamic-pyruvic transaminase (SGPT) reflects even less the degree of alcohol injury, and its serum levels are typically less than half those of the SGOT. Because of this relationship, a ratio (SGOT/SGPT) of greater than 2.0 has been suggested as a diagnostic test for this disease.[26] Results of the Veterans Administration Study suggest that although 93% of the patients had an SGOT level higher than that of the SGPT, the ratio exceeded 2.0 in only 58%. This was almost exclusively in the more severely ill patients, especially those with cirrhosis.[62] The explanation for the low levels of SGOT and SGPT in the face of cellular injury and necrosis is not proven. Certainly the magnitude of the changes does not parallel the degree of injury.[70] Vitamin deficiency, particularly pyridoxine, has been implicated,[128] but remains to be proven. Gamma glutamyltransferase (GGT) levels are almost invariably elevated in alcoholic hepatitis. However, increases may reflect microsomal enzyme induction rather than liver injury.[161,178] For that reason this enzyme is less

TABLE 18-1.   Laboratory Changes Associated with Alcoholic Hepatitis*

LABORATORY TESTS	SEVERITY OF ALCOHOLIC HEPATITIS†			
	Mild (113)	Moderate (124)	Severe (126)	Combined (363)
HEMATOLOGY				
Hemoglobin (14–18 g/dl)	12.7 ± 0.2	11.7 ± 0.2	11.2 ± 0.2	11.8 ± 0.1
% Abnormal	63%	90%	91%	80%
Hematocrit ($47 \pm 5\%$)	38.0 ± 0.5	35.1 ± 0.5	33.1 ± 0.5	35.3 ± 0.3
% Abnormal	65%	91%	94%	82%
MCV (80–94 mm³)	100.1 ± 0.7	103.4 ± 0.8	103.4 ± 0.8	102.4 ± 0.5
% Increased	64%	86%	85%	77%
% Decreased	2%	4%	1%	2%
WBC (5–10×10^9)	8.7 ± 0.3	11.2 ± 0.5	12.3 ± 0.6	10.8 ± 0.3
% Increased	23%	51%	53%	41%
% Decreased	8%	7%	9%	8%
GENERAL CHEMISTRY				
Blood glucose (75–120 mg/dl)	108 ± 3	108 ± 3	107 ± 3	107 ± 2
% Increased	22%	20%	27%	23%
% Decreased	0%	0%	1%	<1%
Amylase (60–160 Su/dl)	125 ± 8	157 ± 37	111 ± 9	131 ± 13
% Abnormal	19%	19%	21%	20%
BUN (4–20 mg/dl)	10 ± 1	16 ± 1	23 ± 2	16 ± 1
% Increased	6%	20%	37%	20%
% Decreased	4%	3%	0%	2%
Creatinine (0.6–1.7 mg/dl)	1.0 ± 0	1.5 ± 0.2	1.9 ± 0.2	1.5 ± 0.1
% Abnormal	3%	19%	31%	17%
IMMUNOGLOBULINS				
IgA (70–312 mg/dl)	556 ± 26	797 ± 33	1065 ± 44	802 ± 23
% Abnormal	89%	98%	97%	94%
IgG (639–1349 mg/dl)	1582 ± 65	1758 ± 67	2123 ± 73	1815 ± 41
% Abnormal	53%	71%	87%	70%
IgM (56–352 mg/dl)	229 ± 13	276 ± 15	312 ± 15	272 ± 9
% Abnormal	13%	25%	33%	23%
CHEMISTRIES RELATED TO LIVER INJURY				
SGOT (10–40 µU/ml)	82 ± 5	109 ± 5	115 ± 6	103 ± 3
% Abnormal	55%	97%	96%	80%
SGPT (10–30 µU/ml)	51 ± 5	45 ± 3	48 ± 5	48 ± 3
% Abnormal	45%	62%	64%	56%
SGOT/SGPT ratio	2.33 ± 0.15	3.27 ± 0.20	3.13 ± 0.16	2.93 ± 0.10
% > 2.0	35%	67%	74%	57%
% < 1.0	23%	2%	2%	10%
Total bilirubin (0.1–1.0 mg/dl)	1.5 ± 0.1	14.6 ± 0.8	17.1 ± 1.0	11.3 ± 0.6
% Abnormal	37%	100%	100%	76%
Prothrombin time (0 seconds above control)	1.0 ± 0.1	2.6 ± 0.2	5.8 ± 0.2	3.2 ± 0.1
% Abnormal	69%	95%	100%	87%
Albumin (3.5–5.0 g/dl)	3.7 ± 0.1	2.7 ± 0.1	2.4 ± 0.1	2.9 ± 0.0
% Abnormal	29%	93%	98%	70%
Cholyl glycine (0–60 µg/dl)	413 ± 48	1595 ± 86	1758 ± 97	1269 ± 58
% Abnormal	75%	100%	100%	91%

* Data derived from 363 patients in the Veterans Administration Cooperative Study.[110]

† The numbers in (   ) indicate the number of patients in each severity group.

MCV, mean corpuscular volume; WBC, white blood cell count; BUN, blood urea nitrogen; SGOT, serum glutamic-oxaloacetic transaminase; SGPT, serum glutamic-pyruvic transaminase.

Mendenhall CL, the VA Cooperative Study Group on Alcoholic Hepatitis: Unpublished observations.

useful for diagnosis and management of this disease. Typically, alcoholic hepatitis may be considered a cholestatic type of liver disease. The most commonly used laboratory tests for cholestasis are the serum alkaline phosphatase and bilirubin. Usually these tend to parallel each other and were observed to be abnormal in 82% (>120 IU/ml) and 78% (>1.1 mg/dl), respectively. Cholestatic laboratory changes in which SGOT and SGPT levels were normal or only minimally elevated relative to a disproportionately elevated alkaline phosphatase and/or bilirubin level were observed in 46% of the patients (mean bilirubin 18 mg/dl; mean alkaline phosphatase 253 IU/ml). The prognostic significance of these changes will be discussed below.

Prothrombin time and albumin concentration are both used as a measure of the liver's capacity to synthesize proteins. However, both may be altered during malnutrition. Abnormalities in these two parameters are frequently observed; thus they are of little use in the initial diagnosis. However, alterations in the liver function (protein synthesis) tend to develop more slowly, with normal or near normal values observed with clinically mild disease, while severe alterations are common with far advanced illness. Similar observations on the magnitude of the serum bilirubin have also been observed such that these parameters have been used to predict severity of disease.[22,102,115,133] Their accuracy in this regard will be discussed under Prognosis.

MALNUTRITION

Considerable data in the literature suggest a relationship between nutritional deficiency and alcoholic liver injury.[146] The mechanism for the deficiency state is multifaceted. In some instances chronic alcoholism may induce pancreatitis, cause malabsorption and diarrhea, and alter biochemical processes essential for nutrient utilization.[3,5,20,60,66,76,92,94,100,101,118–120] Of more importance is the very poor nutrient value of ethanol, providing mainly "empty calories" that are wasted as heat.[149] Thus, although total caloric intake may seem adequate or marginal, when ethanol constitutes 40% to 60% of these calories, a catabolic state can develop. When this is combined with a low dietary protein intake, inadequate cell repair after injury may occur. In addition, a vicious cycle may develop as the low intake of usable calories may be associated with an alcohol-induced hypermetabolic state.[18] Although additional calories are needed to meet metabolic needs, the alcoholic experiences anorexia, which results in decreased caloric intake.[116] It should not be surprising, then, that all of the initial 363 patients enrolled in the Veterans Administration Cooperative Study[114] had some evidence of protein-calorie malnutrition. Fat stores, creatinine height index, responsiveness to skin tests, and visceral protein depletions were the most commonly observed abnormalities in patients with severe disease (Fig. 18-5). Furthermore, if one considers the nutritional parameters collectively as a percent of normal, a highly significant

correlation ($P < 0.0001$) between the degree of nutritional deficiency and acute 30-day mortality was observed.[117] Although its frequent association is irrefutable, a cause and effect relationship is more difficult to establish. The mere presence of the malnutrition does not prove that it initiated or even potentiated the associated liver injury. This will be discussed more in association with therapy.

COURSE AND PROGNOSIS

It is not unusual for the illness to increase in severity during the initial 10 days to 2 weeks after hospitalization, at a time when alcohol consumption has been stopped and essential nutrients are restored to the diet.[105] This increased severity is manifest primarily by an 10% to 20% increase in serum bilirubin and SGOT levels. The apparent increasing severity may persist for as long as 3 weeks before improvement begins or the patient succumbs to his disease. Acute 30-day mortality varies considerably and depends upon the severity of the disease at the time of admission. In the Veterans Administration Study,[110] the overall acute 30-day mortality rate for all degrees of severity was 15% (55/358). This increased progressively to 39% (114/291) by one year.

Three major attempts have been made to assess disease severity on the basis of clinical and laboratory findings. To be useful, such an assessment must be simple to apply and give a reasonable estimate of prognosis. Child used five parameters (ascites, encephalopathy, nutritional state, albumin, and bilirubin) to evaluate the ability of alcoholic patients to tolerate shunt surgery.[22] This has subsequently been modified to assess survival in alcoholic cirrhosis[23] by assigning numerical values from 1 to 3 for each of the five parameters, with a maximum score of 15. Orrego has done more complex analyses consisting of 14 parameters, each weighted a variable amount from 1 to 3 so that the maximum score is 25.[133] Maddrey, using discriminant analysis, observed the bilirubin concentration and prothrombin time to be the two best indicators of survival,[102] where the discriminant function (DF) = 4.6 (prothrombin time) + bilirubin.

When these three estimates of disease severity were applied to the Veterans Administration Cooperative Study patients (using 30-day mortality as the "gold standard" for severity), all correlated significantly with survival. The Maddrey formula gave the best correlation. In addition, the Orrego and Child criteria suffered from their complexity, since they utilized 5 and 14 variables versus two for Maddrey. When one wishes to identify 90% of those who will die in 30 days with the fewest number of false positives (patients who by the various criteria are severely ill enough to die but who survive), then again Maddrey's DF is superior, with 32% false positives versus 34% and 41% for Orrego and Child, respectively.

Of interest is the observation that two individual parameters, bilirubin and creatinine alone, without applying any formula such as Maddrey's, gave a reasonable pre-

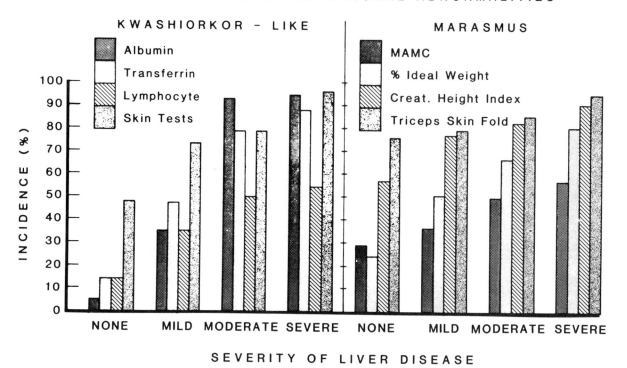

Fig. 18-5. Prevalence of abnormalities for each of the parameters used to diagnose protein-calorie malnutrition in 373 alcoholic patients with varying degrees of alcoholic hepatitis. MAMC = Midarm muscle circumference. (Mendenhall CL et al: Am J Med 76:211, 1984)

diction. For bilirubin and creatinine, a 90% accuracy for mortality was associated with a 39% and 37% incidence of false positives (superior to the Child criteria) and only slightly less precise than Orrego. Figure 18-6 *A, B,* and *C* shows the values for Maddrey's DF, bilirubin alone, and creatinine alone, and corresponding percent mortality. Other parameters that correlated with survival included encephalopathy, age, prothrombin time, and albumin. However, none were as accurate as the Maddrey DF, bilirubin, or creatinine. The enzymatic biochemical tests of liver injury, SGOT and SGPT, did not correlate significantly. Although typically bilirubin and alkaline phosphatase levels are elevated together, in those patients with a high acute mortality only the bilirubin level was markedly elevated. The alkaline phosphatase changes did not correlate significantly with survival.

Most of the early mortality from alcoholic hepatitis occurs in the initial 2 weeks after admission.[111] Clinical features of liver failure and portal hypertension (hepatic encephalopathy, ascites, and bleeding esophageal varices) were present in 91%, 63%, and 37% of the fatal cases, respectively. However, these features were not useful as prognostic indicators, since they were so frequently observed in surviving patients (false positives).

Beyond the initial acute mortality, few studies have been performed in which serial liver biopsies have established the natural course of the disease. In the Emory series,[49] complete recovery established by serial biopsy appeared to be unpredictable. If alcohol consumption continued, no patient recovered from his disease and a persistent alcoholic hepatitis resulted, with 38% progressing to cirrhosis within 18 months. Even abstinence from ethanol did not guarantee recovery. Only 27% of abstainers returned to normal by the seventh month, and 18% had progressed to cirrhosis. The remaining 55% still had active persistent alcoholic hepatitis that had neither returned to normal nor progressed to cirrhosis by 12 to 14 months. These observations suggest that alcoholic hepatitis, once initiated, is slow to resolve and that other factors capable of causing continuation and progression are present even after ethanol consumption has ceased.

TREATMENT

The essential role of ethanol in the initiation and potentiation of the morbidity, mortality, and progression of the

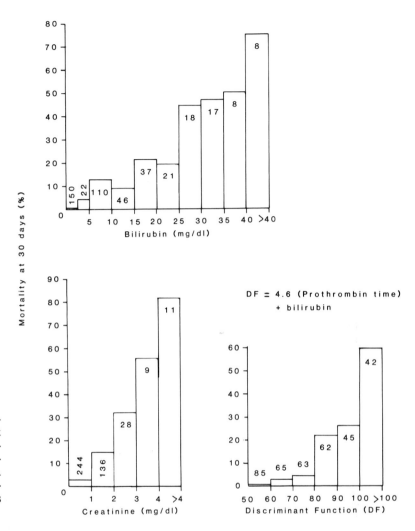

Fig. 18-6. Correlation between acute 30-day mortality and Maddrey's discriminant function (*DF*) (*A*),[102] admission serum bilirubin (*B*), and serum creatinine (*C*). Observations on mortality taken from the VA Cooperative Study.[111] The numbers in parentheses indicate the number of patients in each group.

alcoholic liver injury is undeniable.[16,99,111,168] Hence, abstinence should be the mainstay for any treatment program. Although there is no evidence that occasional drinking of small amounts is harmful, the psychodynamics of the chronic alcoholic makes complete abstinence the more desirable goal. Unfortunately, this is usually difficult to achieve.

Diet therapy represents the second most important mainstay for treatment. As indicated above, nutritional deficits are almost invariably present. Experimental evidence suggests that nutrition therapy results in improved nutritional status[116] and that repletion of the malnutrition is essential for improvement of the liver disease.[146–148] When alcohol consumption was stopped but malnutrition allowed to persist, only minimal improvement in the liver disease occurred. Conversely, alcohol administration did not prevent or delay improvement in the liver disease so long as nutritional support was adequate.[40,137,158,176,182]

In the Veterans Administration Study,[110–112,114–117] patients were hospitalized for 30 days of treatment, thus preventing (in most instances) ethanol consumption. Although multivitamins and minerals were provided along with a well-balanced 2500 kcal diet, the anorexia associated with the disease impaired adequate intake such that only 63% of the estimated energy requirements (EER) were consumed by the moderately ill patients and 53% of the EER by the severely ill patients. It is not surprising that after one month of hospitalization 19% showed some deterioration. This was not the case for those receiving active nutritional supplementation.[116] Older studies have reported on the therapeutic use of diets rich in protein and B-complex vitamins,[137,138] in which significant improvement in 5-year survival was observed. Unfortunately the comparison control group was obtained retrospectively from a different hospital. More recently several reports from Galambos and associates[54,125] have noted significant improvement in survival after more vigorous parenteral hyperalimentation with amino acid therapy. Although the number of patients evaluated under appropriate controlled conditions was small, these results strongly attest to the importance of nutritional therapy in this disease. It is suggested that when malnutrition is observed to be severe,[117] the prognosis is grave and vigorous replacement therapy should be provided. In the absence of hepatic encephalopathy, this therapy may consist of any high-calorie, high-protein nutrient. However, when encephalopathy is present, protein intake should be maintained using high branch-chain amino acid types of nutrients such as Hepatic-Aid, since these are well tolerated[116] and may be therapeutic for the encephalopathy.[72] Every effort should be made to meet the EER and produce a positive nitrogen balance.

Vitamin and mineral deficiencies in this population are frequent and typically multiple.[5,93,112] Since serum levels do not correlate well with the deficiency present in the tissues, replacement therapy is usually given empirically. A high-potency multivitamin preparation that includes B_{12}, folic acid, thiamin, pyridoxine, vitamin A, vitamin D, and such minerals as zinc, magnesium, calcium, and phosphorus should be provided. Unless iron loss is present, replacement of iron should be given with caution in view of the increased iron absorption seen in cirrhosis[184] and the high prevalence of hemosiderosis in alcoholic hepatitis.[24]

Assessment of the efficacy of specific therapy is considerably more controversial. Since alcoholic hepatitis is characterized by inflammation and necrosis, one theoretic approach to therapy is with glucocorticosteroids. Of the ten major studies[11,18,29,31,70,98,102,115,154,179] encompassing 449 patients, the acute 30-day mortality was uneffected by these corticosteroids (38% versus 33%, treated versus controls). Some have suggested a beneficial effect in a select population of severely ill patients with encephalopathy.[70,98] In the Veterans Administration Study, 70 patients met this criteria (severely ill with encephalopathy); unfortunately, no improvement in survival was effected by corticosteroid treatment. It appears that although corticosteroids did not increase the incidence of complications they did little to improve survival.

In an effort to stimulate protein synthesis and cell repair, androgenic anabolic corticosteroids have been used as therapy. With this form of treatment, liver fat is mobilized rapidly so that fatty liver rapidly undergoes restoration to a normal histology along with a return to normal of biochemical tests for liver injury.[108] In more severe disease, improvement in defective synthesis of coagulation factors has been reported after treatment with large doses.[177]

Of the ten published reports on the use of anabolic corticosteroids in alcoholic liver disease, nine reported clinical improvement.[42,43,59,71,75,85,109,124,162,183] Unfortunately, only the Veterans Administration Study was performed on sufficient numbers of patients with a randomized double-blind experimental design.[115] For reasons not well understood, perhaps related to differences in binding affinity at the target organ level,[14] a therapeutic effect after 80 mg of oxandrolone daily for 30 days was delayed so that no improvement in survival was observed in the initial 30 days during treatment. However, long-term effects on survival in the 6-month posttreatment period were observed. This was especially true for the moderately ill patients. In this group the 6-month conditional death rate for those patients treated with oxandrolone was 3.5% compared with a 19.7% mortality in the controls. By 12 months (11 months after treatment had been stopped), only 24% of the treated patients had died versus 55% of the controls ($P < 0.02$). Although impressive, additional studies are needed to confirm their efficacy and establish the optimum dose and duration of treatment. In addition, since anabolic corticosteroids increase protein utilization,[88,155] the combination of anabolic corticosteroids and vigorous nutrition therapy needs evaluation.

Several other forms of therapy have also been recommended for this condition. It is well known that chronic alcoholism can induce a hypermetabolic state in the liver.[10,181] In an effort to depress this hypermetabolic state, propylthiouracil has been suggested as therapy.[78,131,132] Using the Orrego "clinical severity index," a more rapid normalization was observed. However, the patients treated were only mildly ill, and no difference in mortality was observed. The efficacy of this form of therapy for alcoholic hepatitis remains to be established.

Since cirrhosis and hepatic fibrosis are frequent and early pathologic changes are associated with alcoholic hepatitis, agents that inhibit collagen synthesis have been used for therapy. D-Penicillamine, a drug that retards the cross linking of collagen, has been recommended.[157] Unfortunately, D-penicillamine has numerous undesirable side-effects, including nausea, vomiting, urticaria, skin eruptions, renal toxicity, and bone marrow suppression. Another less toxic agent is colchicine, which interferes with the transcellular movement and transport of collagen from the cytoplasm to the extracellular space.[32,39,130] In a preliminary 4-year study involving 43 cirrhotic patients,[84,160] mortality improved from 40% with placebo to 17% with colchicine (1 mg/day, 5 days/week). Clinical symptomatology (ascites, encephalopathy, splenomegaly) improved significantly ($P < 0.05$). Because of the small number of patients in each treatment group and the slow rate at which histologic improvement in fibrosis occurred (only 3/20 improved), statistical significance was not obtained histologically. More comprehensive studies are needed to confirm these encouraging preliminary observations. Perhaps even "irreversible" cirrhosis is reversible.

Alcoholic hepatitis is a common disease that is life threatening in nature, but one for which no universally accepted treatment exists. New approaches to therapy for long-term survival are encouraging. Additional well-controlled studies are needed to confirm their efficacy and optimize their application.

REFERENCES

1. Adler M, Schaffner F: Fatty liver and cirrhosis in obese patients. Am J Med 67:811, 1979
2. Afshani MD et al: Significance of microscopic cholangitis in alcoholic liver disease. Gastroenterology 75:1045, 1978
3. Arky RA: The effect of alcohol on carbohydrate metabolism: Carbohydrate metabolism in alcoholics. In Kissin B, Begleiter H (eds): The Biology of Alcoholism, vol 1, p 197. New York, Plenum Press, 1977
4. Bailey RJ et al: Histocompatibility antigens, autoantibodies, and immunoglobulins in alcoholic liver disease. Br Med J 2:727, 1976
5. Baker H et al: Effect of hepatic disease on liver B-complex vitamin titers. Am J Clin Nutr 14:1, 1964
6. Baraona E et al: Alcoholic hepatomegaly: Accummulation of protein in the liver. Science 190:794, 1975
7. Beckett AG et al: Acute alcoholic hepatitis. Br Med J 2:1113, 1961
8. Beckett AG et al: Acute alcoholic hepatitis without jaundice. Br Med J 2:580, 1962
9. Bernstein IM et al: Reduction in circulating T-lymphocytes in alcoholic liver disease. Lancet 2:488, 1974
10. Bernstein J et al: Metabolic alterations produced in the liver by chronic ethanol administration: Changes related to energetic parameters of the cell. Biochem J 134:515, 1973
11. Blitzer BL et al: Adrenocorticosteroid therapy in alcoholic hepatitis: A prospective double-blind randomized study. Dig Dis Sci 22:477, 1977
12. Bolland JL, Koch HP: The course of autoxidation reactions in polyisoprenes and allied compounds: IX. The primary thermal oxidation product of ethyl linoleate. J Chem Soc 19:445, 1945
13. Borenfreund E et al: In vivo initiated rat liver cell carcinogenesis studies in vitro: Formation of alcoholic hyalin-type bodies. Cancer Lett 3:145, 1977
14. Breuer CB, Florini JR: Amino acid incorporation into protein by cell-free systems from rat skeletal muscle: IV. Effects of animal age, androgens, and anabolic agents on activity of muscle ribosomes. Biochemistry 4:1544, 1965
15. Bruguera M et al: Giant mitochondria in hepatocytes: A diagnostic hint for alcoholic liver disease. Gastroenterology 73:1383, 1977
16. Brunt PW et al: Studies in alcoholic liver disease in Britain. Gut 15:52, 1974
17. Burns WA et al: Cytoplasmic crystalline regions in hepatocytes of liver biopsy specimens. Arch Pathol 97:43, 1974
18. Campra JL et al: Prednisone therapy of acute alcoholic hepatitis: Report of a controlled trial. Ann Intern Med 79:625, 1973
19. Cederbaum AI et al: The effect of dimethylsulfoxide and other hydroxyl radical scavengers on the oxidation of ethanol by rat liver microsomes. Biochem Biophys Res Commun 78:1254, 1977
20. Chang T et al: Effect of ethanol and other alcohols on the transport of amino acids and glucose by everted sacs of rat small intestine. Biochem Biophys Acta 135:1000, 1967
21. Chedid A et al: Megamitochondria: A parameter of reversible alcoholic liver injury. Hepatology 3:857, 1983
22. Child CG, Turcotte JG: Surgery and portal hypertension. In Child CG (ed): The Liver and Portal Hypertension, p 50. Philadelphia, WB Saunders, 1964
23. Christensen E et al: Prognostic value of Child–Turcotte criteria in medically treated cirrhosis. Hepatology 3:430, 1984
24. Christoffersen P, Nielsen K: Histologic changes in human liver biopsies from chronic alcoholics. Acta Pathol Microbiol Scand (Section A) 80:557, 1972
25. Cohen G, Cederbaum AI: Chemical evidence for production of hydroxyl radicals during microsomal electron transfer. Science 204:66, 1979
26. Cohen JA, Kaplan MM: The SGOT/SGPT ratio: An indicator of alcoholic liver disease. Dig Dis Sci 24:835, 1979
27. Comporti M et al: Effect of in vivo and in vitro ethanol administration on liver lipid peroxidation. Lab Invest 16:616, 1967
28. Comporti M et al: Studies on the in vitro peroxidation of liver lipids in ethanol-treated rats. Lipids 8:498, 1973
29. Copenhagen Study Group for Liver Diseases: Effect of prednisone on the survival of patients with cirrhosis of the liver. Lancet I:119, 1969
30. Cossel L et al: "Killer" lymphocytes in action: Light and electron microscopical findings in orthotopic liver homografts. Virchows Arch Pathol Anat 364:179, 1974
31. Depew W et al: Double-blind controlled trial of prednisolone therapy in patients with severe acute alcoholic hepatitis and spontaneous encephalopathy. Gastroenterology 78:524, 1980
32. Digelman RF, Peterkofsky B: Inhibition of collagen secretion from bone and cultured fibroblasts by microtubular disruptive drugs. Proc Natl Acad Sci USA 69:892, 1972
33. DiLuzio NR: Antioxidants, lipid peroxidation and chemical-induced liver injury. Fed Proc 32:1875, 1973
34. DiLuzio NR, Hartman AD: The effect of ethanol and carbon tetrachloride administration on hepatic lipid-soluble antioxidant activity. Exp Mol Pathol 11:38, 1969
35. DiLuzio NR, Stege NR: The role of ethanol metabolites in hepatic lipid peroxidation. In Fisher MM, Rankin JG (eds): Hepatology: Research and Clinical Issues, Vol 3, Alcohol and the Liver, p 45. New York, Plenum Press, 1977
36. Edmondson HA: Tumors of the liver and intrahepatic bile ducts. Armed Forces Institute of Pathology, Section 7, Part 25, p 49, 1958
37. Edmondson HA et al: Sclerosing hyalin necrosis of the liver in the chronic alcoholic. Ann Intern Med 59:646, 1963
38. Edmondson HA et al: The early stage of liver injury in the alcoholic. Medicine 46:119, 1967
39. Ehrlich HR, Bornstein P: Microtubules in transcellular movement of procollagen. Nature 238:257, 1972
40. Erenoglu E et al: Observations on patients with Laennec's cirrhosis receiving alcohol while on controlled diets. Ann Intern Med 60:814, 1964
41. Feinman L, Lieber CS: Hepatic collagen metabolism: Effect of alcohol consumption in rats and baboons. Science 176:795, 1972
42. Fenster LF: The nonefficacy of short-term anabolic steroid therapy in alcoholic liver disease. Ann Intern Med 65:738, 1966
43. Figueroa RB: Mesterolone in steatosis and cirrhosis of the liver. Acta Hepatogastroenterol 20:282, 1973
44. French SW, Burbige EJ: Alcoholic hepatitis: Clinical, morphologic, pathogenic, and therapeutic aspects. In Popper H, Schaffner F (eds): Progress in Liver Disease, vol 6, p 557. New York, Grune & Stratton, 1979

45. French SW, Davies PL: The Mallory body in the pathogenesis of alcoholic liver disease. In Khanna JM, Israel Y, Kalant H (eds): Alcoholic Liver Pathology, p 113. Toronto, Addiction Research Foundation of Ontario, 1975

46. French SW et al: Percent T and B cells in the liver in alcoholic hepatitis (abstr). Am J Pathol 86:20, 1977

47. French SW et al: Alcoholic hepatitis. In Fisher MM, Rankin JG (eds): Alcohol and the Liver, p 261. New York, Plenum Press, 1977

48. Fulchuk KR et al: Pericentral hepatic fibrosis in diabetes mellitus. Gastroenterology 78:535, 1980

49. Galambos JT: Natural history of alcoholic hepatitis: III. Histologic changes. Gastroenterology 63:1026, 1972

50. Galambos JT: Alcoholic hepatitis: Its therapy and prognosis. In Popper H, Schaffner F (eds): Progress in Liver Disease, vol 6, p 567. New York, Grune & Stratton, 1972

51. Galambos JT: Alcoholic hepatitis. In Schaffner F, Sherlock S, Leevy CM (eds): The Liver and Its Diseases, p 255. New York, Intercontinental Medical Book Corporation, 1974

52. Galambos JT: The course of alcoholic hepatitis. In Khanna JM, Israel Y (eds): Alcoholic Liver Pathology, p 97. Toronto, Addiction Research Foundation of Ontario, 1975

53. Galambos JT: Epidemiology of alcoholic liver disease: United States of America. In Hall P (ed): Alcoholic Liver Disease: Pathobiology, Epidemiology, and Clinical Aspects, p 230. New York, John Wiley & Sons, 1985

54. Galambos JT et al: Hyperalimentation in alcoholic hepatitis. Am J Gastroenterol 72:535, 1979

55. Garagliano CF et al: Incidence rates of liver cirrhosis and related diseases in Baltimore and selected areas of the United States. J Chronic Dis 32:543, 1979

56. Gerber MA et al: Hepatitis virus B and chronic alcoholic liver disease. Lancet 2:1034, 1972

57. Gerber MA et al: Hepatocellular hyalin in cholestasis and cirrhosis: Its diagnostic significance. Gastroenterology 64: 89, 1973

58. Gerber MA et al: Hepatocellular hyalin in cholestastis and cirrhosis: Its diagnostic significance. Gastroenterology 64: 89, 1973

59. Girolami M: Treatment of ascitic atrophic cirrhosis of the liver with high dosages of testosterone propionate. J Am Geriatr Soc 6:306, 1958

60. Goidsnohoven van EG et al: Pancreatic function in cirrhosis of the liver. Am J Dig Dis 8:160, 1963

61. Goldberg SJ et al: VA Cooperative Study on Alcoholic Hepatitis. IV: The significance of clinically mild alcoholic hepatitis—describing the population with minimal hyperbilirubinemia. Am J Gastroenterol (in press)

62. Goldberg SJ et al: "Non-Alcoholic" chronic hepatitis in the alcoholic. Gastroenterology, 72:598, 1977

63. Grunnet N: Oxidation of acetaldehyde by rat liver mitochondria in relation to ethanol oxidation and the transport of reducing equivalents across the mitochondrial membrane. Eur J Biochem 35:236, 1973

64. Hall EM, Morgan WA: Progressive alcoholic cirrhosis: A clinical and pathologic study of 68 cases. Arch Pathol 27: 672, 1930

65. Hall EM, Ophuls W: Progressive alcoholic cirrhosis: Report of 4 cases. Am J Pathol 1:477, 1925

66. Halsted CH et al: Intestinal malabsorption in folate-deficient alcoholics. Gastroenterology 64:526, 1973

67. Harinasuta U, Zimmerman HJ: Alcoholic steatonecrosis: Relationship between severity of hepatic disease and presence of Mallory bodies in the liver. Gastroenterology 60: 1036, 1971

68. Harinasuta U et al: Steatonecrosis: Mallory body type. Medicine 46:141, 1967

69. Hartroft WS: On the etiology of alcoholic liver cirrhosis. In Khanna JM, Israel Y, Kalant H (eds): Alcoholic Liver Pathology, p 189. Toronto, Addiction Research Foundation, 1975

70. Helman RA et al: Alcoholic hepatitis: Natural history and evaluation of prednisolone therapy. Ann Intern Med 74: 311, 1971

71. Hirayama C et al: Anabolic steroid effect on hepatic protein synthesis in patients with liver cirrhosis. Digestion 3:41, 1970

72. Horst D et al: Comparison of dietary protein with an oral, branched-chain enriched amino acid supplement in chronic portal-systemic encephalopathy: A randomized controlled trial. Hepatology 4:279, 1984

73. Husby G et al: Localization of T and B cells and alphafetoprotein in hepatic biopsies from patients with liver disease. J Clin Invest 56:1198, 1975

74. International Group: Review of alcoholic liver disease morphologic manifestations. Lancet I:707, 1981

75. Islam N, Islam A: Testosterone propionate in cirrhosis of the liver. Br J Clin Pract 27:125, 1973

76. Israel Y et al: Inhibitory effects of alcohol on intestinal acid transport in vivo and in vitro. J Nutr 96:499, 1968

77. Israel Y et al: Experimental alcohol-induced hepatic necrosis suppression by propylthiouracil. Proc Natl Acad Sci 72: 1137, 1975

78. Israel Y et al: Liver hypermetabolic state after chronic ethanol consumption: Hormonal interrelationships and pathogenic implications. Fed Proc 34:2052, 1975

79. Kakumu S, Leevy CM: Lymphocyte cytotoxicity in alcoholic hepatitis. Gastroenterology 72:594, 1977

80. Kanagasundaram N et al: Alcoholic hyalin antigen (AHAg) and antibody (AHAb) in alcoholic hepatitis. Gastroenterology 73:1368, 1977

81. Karasawa T, Chedid A: Sclerosis hyalin necrosis in noncirrhotic chronic alcoholic hepatitis. Am J Clin Pathol 66: 802, 1976

82. Kawanishi H: Morphologic association of lymphocytes with hepatocytes in chronic liver disease. Arch Pathol Lab Med 101:286, 1977

83. Kern WH et al: The significance of hyalin necrosis in liver biopsies. Surg Gynecol Obstet 128:749, 1969

84. Kershenobich D et al: Treatment of cirrhosis with colchicine: A double-blind randomized trial. Gastroenterology 77:532, 1979

85. Kinsell LW: Factors affecting protein balance in the presence of chronic viral liver damage. Gastroenterology 11: 672, 1948

86. Koch OR et al: Ultrastructural and biochemical aspects of liver mitochondria during recovery from ethanol-induced alterations. Am J Pathol 90:325, 1977

87. Koes M et al: Lipid peroxidation in chronic ethanol treated rats: In vitro uncoupling of peroxidation from reduced nicotine adenosine dinucleotide phosphate oxidation. Lipids 9:899, 1974

88. Kruskemper HL: Clinical application of anabolic steroids: Exogenous protein deficiency. In Kruskemper HL (ed): Anabolic Steroids, chap 6, p 126. New York, Academic Press, 1968

89. Lane BP, Lieber CS: Ultrastructural alterations in human hepatocytes following ingestion of ethanol with adequate diets. Am J Pathol 49:595, 1966

90. Lang AP et al: Preoperative liver biopsy and the prognosis of portosystemic shunt surgery (abstr). Lab Invest 38:353, 1978

91. Ledwig J et al: Nonalcoholic steato-hepatitis: Mayo Clinic experiences with a hitherto unnamed disease. Mayo Clin Proc 55:434, 1980

92. Leevy CM, Zetterman RK: Malnutrition and alcoholism: An overview. In Rothschild MA, Orztz M, Schreiber SS (eds): Alcohol and Abnormal Protein Biosynthesis, Biochemical, and Clinical, vol 1, p 3. New York, Pergamon Press, 1975

93. Leevy CM et al: Vitamins and liver injury. Am J Clin Nutr 23:493, 1970

94. Leevy CM et al: Alcoholism, drug addiction, and nutrition. Med Clin North Am 54:1567, 1970

95. Leevy CM et al: Liver disease of the alcoholic: Role of immunologic abnormalities in pathogenesis recognition and treatment. In Popper H, Schaffner F (eds): Progress in Liver Disease, vol 5, p 516. New York, Grune & Stratton, 1976

96. Lelbach WK: Epidemiology of alcoholic liver disease. In Popper H, Schaffner F (eds): Progress in Liver Disease. vol 5, p 494. New York, Grune and Stratton, 1976

97. Lelbach WK: Epidemiology of alcoholic liver disease: Continental Europe. In Hall P (ed): Alcoholic Liver Disease: Pathobiology, Epidemiology, and Clinical Aspects, p 130. New York, John Wiley & Son, 1985

98. Lesener HR et al: Treatment of alcoholic hepatitis with encephalopathy: Comparison of prednisolone with caloric supplements. Gastroenterology 74:169, 1978

99. Lieber CS et al: Fatty liver, hyperlipemia and hyperuricemia produced by prolonged alcohol consumption despite adequate dietary intake. Trans Assoc Am Physicians 76:289, 1963

100. Lindenbaum J, Leiber CS: Alcohol-induced malabsorption of vitamin B_{12} in man. Nature 224:806, 1969

101. Losowsky MS, Walter BE: Liver disease and malabsorption. Gastroenterology 56:598, 1969

102. Maddrey WC et al: Corticosteroid therapy of alcoholic hepatitis. Gastroenterology 75:193, 1978

103. Mallory FB: Cirrhosis of the liver: Five different types of lesions from which it may arise. Bull Johns Hopkins Hosp 22:69, 1911

104. Marjanen L: Intracellular localization of aldehyde dehydrogenase in rat liver. J Biochem 127:633, 1972

105. Marshall JB et al: Clinical and biochemical course of alcoholic liver disease following sudden discontinuation of alcoholic consumption. Alcoholism 7:312, 1983

106. Marubbio AT et al: Hepatic lesions of central pericelluar fibrosis in morbid obesity and after jejunoileal bypass. Am J Clin Pathol 66:684, 1976

107. Melendez M et al: Distribution of HLA histocompatibility antigens, ABO blood groups, and Rh antigens in alcoholic liver disease. Gut 20:288, 1979

108. Mendenhall CL: Anabolic steroid therapy as an adjunct to diet in alcoholic hepatic steatosis. Am J Dig Dis 13:738, 1968

109. Mendenhall C, Goldberg S: Risk factors and therapy in alcoholic hepatitis. Gastroenterology 72:1100, 1977

110. Mendenhall CL, The VA Cooperative Study Group on Alcoholic Hepatitis: Unpublished observations

111. Mendenhall CL, The Cooperative Study Group on Alcoholic Hepatitis: Alcoholic Hepatitis. Clin Gastroenterol 10:417, 1981

112. Mendenhall CL, The VA Cooperative Study on Alcoholic Hepatitis: Clinical and therapeutic aspects of alcoholic liver disease. In Seitz HK, Kommerell B (eds): Alcohol Related Diseases in Gastroenterology, p 304. Berlin, Springer–Verlag, 1985

113. Mendenhall CL et al: Altered proline uptake by mouse liver cells after chronic exposure to ethanol and its metabolites. Gut 25:138, 1984

114. Mendenhall CL et al: Protein-calorie malnutrition associated with alcoholic hepatitis: Veterans Administration Cooperative Study Group on Alcoholic Hepatitis. Am J Med 76:211, 1984

115. Mendenhall CL et al: Acute and long-term survival in patients treated with oxandrolone and prednisolone. N Engl J Med 311:1464, 1984

116. Mendenhall CL et al: VA Cooperative Study on Alcoholic Hepatitis III: Changes in protein-calorie malnutrition associated with 30 days of hospitalization with and without enteral nutritional therapy. JPEN 9:590, 1985

117. Mendenhall CL et al: VA Cooperative Study on Alcoholic Hepatitis II: Prognostic significance of protein-calorie malnutrition. Am J Clin Nutr (in press)

118. Mezey E: Intestinal function in chronic alcoholism. Ann NY Acad Sci 252:215, 1975

119. Mezey E, Potter JJ: Changes in exocrine pancreatic function produced by altered dietary protein intake in drinking alcoholics. Johns Hopkins Med J 318:7, 1976

120. Mezey E et al: Pancreatic function and intestinal absorption in chronic alcoholism. Gastroenterology 59:657, 1970

121. Mezey E et al: Hepatic fibrogenesis in alcoholism. In Khanna JM, Israel Y, Kalant H (eds): Alcoholic Liver Pathology, p 145. Toronto, Addiction Research Foundation of Ontario, 1975

122. Mezey E et al: Hepatic collagen proline hydroxylase activity in alcoholic liver disease. Clin Chim Acta 68:313, 1976

123. Monroe S et al: Mallory bodies in a case of primary biliary cirrhosis: An ultrastructural and morphological study. Am J Clin Pathol 59:254, 1973

124. Müting D: Die Wirkung einer Langzeitbehandlung mit einer anabolen Substanz (Nandrolondecanoat) auf Proteinsynthese und -abbau sowie Ausscheidungs- und Entgiftungsfunktion der Leber bei chronischen Leberkrankheiten und Diabetes mellitus. Klin Wochenschr 42:843, 1964

125. Nasrallah SM, Galambos JT: Aminoacid therapy of alcoholic hepatitis. Lancet 2:1276, 1980

126. Nasrallah SM et al: Hepatic morphology in obesity. Dig Dis Sci 26:325, 1981

127. Nayak NC et al: Indian childhood cirrhosis: The nature and significance of cytoplasmic hyalin of hepatocytes. Arch Pathol 88:631, 1969

128. Ning M et al: Reduction of glutamic pyruvic transaminase in pyridoxine deficiency in liver disease. Proc Soc Exp Biol Med 121:27, 1966

129. Ohnishi K, Okuda K: Epidemiology of alcoholic liver disease: Japan. In Hall P (ed): Alcoholic Liver Disease: Pathology, Epidemiology, and Clinical Aspects, p 167. New York, John Wiley & Son, 1985

130. Olmsted JB, Borisy GG: Microtubules. Annu Rev Biochem 42:507, 1973

131. Orrego H et al: Effect of propylthiouracil in treatment of alcoholic liver disease. Gastroenterology 73:A39, 1977

132. Orrego H et al: Effect of short term therapy with propylthiouracil in patients with alcoholic liver disease. Gastroenterology 76:105, 1979

133. Orrego H et al: Assessment of prognostic factors in alcoholic liver disease: Toward a global quantitative expression of severity. Hepatology 3:896, 1983

134. Osborn M et al: Visualization of a system of filaments 7–10 nm thick in cultured cells of an epithelioid line (PtK2) by immunofluorescence microscopy. Proc Natl Acad Sci USA 74:2490, 1977

135. Osler W: The Principles and Practice of Medicine, p 444. Edinburgh, Young J. Pentland, 1892

136. Paronetto F, Lieber CS: Cytotoxicity of lymphocytes in experimental alcoholic liver injury in the baboon. Proc Soc Exp Biol Med 153:495, 1976

137. Patek AJ, Post J: Treatment of cirrhosis of the liver by a nutritious diet and supplements rich in vitamin B complex. J Clin Invest 20:481, 1941

138. Patek AJ et al: Dietary treatment of cirrhosis of the liver: Results in 124 patients observed during a 10 year period. JAMA 138:543, 1948

139. Patrick RS: Alcoholism as a stimulus to hepatic fibrogenesis. J Alcoholism 8:13, 1973

140. Pessayre D et al: Perihexilen maleate-induced cirrhosis. Gastroenterology 76:170, 1979

141. Peters RL: Pathology of hepatocellular carcinoma. In Okuda K, Peters RL (eds): Hepatocellulary Carcinoma, p 107. New York, John Wiley & Son, 1976

142. Peters RL et al: Post-jejunoileal bypass hepatic disease. Am J Clin Pathol, 63:318, 1975

143. Petersen P: Alcoholic hyalin, microfilaments and microtubules in alcoholic hepatitis. Acta Pathol Microbiol Scand Section A, 85:384, 1977

144. Pettigrew NM et al: Evidence for a role of hepatitis B virus in chronic alcoholic liver disease. Lancet 2:724, 1972

145. Pfeifer U, Klinge O: Intracisternal hyalin in hepatocytes of human liver biopsies. Virchow Arch B Cell Pathol 16:141, 1974

146. Phillips GB: Acute hepatic insufficiency of the chronic alcoholic: Revisited. Am J Med 75:1, 1983

147. Phillips GB, Davidson CS: Acute hepatic insufficiency of the chronic alcoholic. Arch Int Med 94:585, 1954

148. Phillips GB et al: Comparative effects of a purified and an adequate diet on the course of fatty cirrhosis in the alcoholic. J Clin Invest 31:351, 1952

149. Pirola RC, Lieber CS: Hypothesis: Energy wasting in alcoholism and drug abuse: Possible role of hepatic microsomal enzymes. Am J Clin Nutr 29:90, 1976

150. Popper H: Comments: Wilson's disease. Birth Defects 4:103, 1968

151. Popper H: Pathogenesis of alcoholic cirrhosis. In Fisher MM, Rankin JG (eds): Alcohol and the Liver, p 289. New York, Plenum Press, 1976

152. Popper H, Szanto PB: Fatty liver with hepatic failure in alcoholics. J Mt Sinai Hosp 24:1121, 1957

153. Popper H et al: Florid cirrhosis: A review of 35 cases. Am J Clin Pathol 25:889, 1955

154. Porter HR et al: Corticosteroid therapy in severe alcoholic hepatitis: A double-blind drug trial. N Engl J Med 284:1350, 1971

155. Regoeczi E, Germer WD: Experimentelle Beobachtungen uber die Wirkung des Testosteron-Propionates bei diatetischer Lebernekrose. Dtsch Arch Klin Med 205:624, 1959

156. Reitz RC: A possible mechanism for the peroxidation of lipids due to chronic ethanol ingestion. Biochim Biophys Acta 380:145, 1975

157. Resnick RH et al: Preliminary observations of δ-penicillamine therapy in acute alcoholic liver disease. Digestion 11:257, 1974

158. Reynolds TB et al: Role of alcohol in pathogenesis of alcoholic cirrhosis. In McIntyre N, Sherlock S (eds): Therapeutic Agents and the Liver, p 131. Oxford, Blackwell Scientific Publications, 1965

159. Rice JD Jr, Yesner R: The prognostic significance of so-called Mallory bodies in portal cirrhosis. Arch Intern Med 105:99, 1960

160. Rojkind M et al: Colchicine and the treatment of liver cirrhosis (letter). Lancet 1:38, 1973

161. Rosalki SB et al: Plasma gamma-glutamyl transpeptidase elevation in patients receiving enzyme-inducing drugs. Lancet 2:376, 1971

162. Rosenak BD et al: Treatment of cirrhosis of the liver with testosterone propionate. Gastroenterology 9:695, 1947

163. Rouselot LM et al: Prognostic value of liver biopsy in the electively shunted patient (abstr). Gastroenterology 64:165, 1973

164. Roy S et al: An ultrastructural study of the liver in Indian childhood cirrhosis with particular reference to the structure of cytoplasmic hyalin. Gut 12:6931, 1971

165. Ryberg U, Skerfuing S: Toxicity of ethanol: A tentative risk evaluation. In Gross EM (ed): Alcohol Intoxication and Withdrawal, p 403. New York, Plenum Press, 1977

166. Sabesin SM et al: Alcoholic hepatitis. Gastroenterology 74:276, 1978

167. Sanchez-Tapias J et al: Lymphocyte populations in liver biopsy specimens from patients with chronic liver disease. Gut 18:472, 1977

168. Schaffner F, Popper H: Alcoholic hepatitis in the spectrum of ethanol-induced liver injury. Scand J Gastroenterol 5:69, 1970

169. Schaffner F et al: Hepatocellular changes in Wilson's disease. Am J Pathol 41:315, 1962

170. Shigeta Y et al: HLA antigens as immuno-genetic markers of alcoholism and alcoholic liver disease. Pharmacol Biochem Behav 13(Suppl 1):89, 1980

171. Si L et al: Lymphocyte subsets studied with monoclonal antibodies in liver tissues of patients with alcoholic liver disease. Alcoholism Clin Exp Res 1:431, 1983

172. Si L et al: Lymphocyte subpopulations at the site of "piecemeal" necrosis in end stage chronic liver diseases and rejecting liver allografts in cyclosporine treated patients. Lab Invest 50:341, 1984

173. Sims JS, French SW: Peroxidase-antiperoxidase complex: Binding by Mallory bodies by unfixed tissues. Arch Pathol Lab Med 100:550, 1976

174. Sorensen TIA et al: Prospective evaluation of alcohol abuse and alcoholic liver injury in men as predictors of development of cirrhosis. Lancet 2:242, 1984

175. Sorrell MF, Leevy CM: Lymphocyte transformation and alcoholic liver injury. Gastroenterology 63:1020, 1972

176. Summerskill WHJ et al: Response to alcohol in chronic alcoholics with liver disease: Clinical, pathological and metabolic changes. Lancet 1:335, 1957

177. Tamburro C, Leevy CM: Protein clotting factor synthesis in liver disease. Gastroenterology 52:325, 1967

178. Teschke R et al: Induction of hepatic microsomal gamma-glutamyltransferase activity following chronic alcohol consumption. Biochem Biophys Res Commun 75:718, 1977

179. Theodossi A et al: Controlled trial of methylprednisolone therapy in severe acute alcoholic hepatitis. Gut 23:75, 1982

180. Van Waes L, Lieber CS: Prognostic significance of pericentral venous sclerosis in alcoholic fatty liver (abstr). Fed Proc 36:332, 1977

181. Videla L et al: Metabolic alterations produced in the liver by chronic ethanol administration: Increased oxidative capacity. Biochem J 134:507, 1973

182. Volwiler W et al: Criteria for the measurement of results of treatment in fatty cirrhosis. Gastroenterology 11:164, 1948

183. Wells R: Prednisolone and testosterone propionate in cirrhosis of the liver: A controlled trial. Lancet 2:1416, 1960

184. Williams R et al: Iron absorption and siderosis in chronic liver disease. Q J Med 36:151, 1967

185. Wybran J et al: Alcoholic liver disease and the immune system. JAMA 232:57, 1975

186. Zagury D et al: Isolation and characterization of individual functionally reactive cytotoxic T-lymphocytes: Conjugation, killing and recycling at the single cell level. Eur J Immunol 5:818, 1975

187. Zetterman RK et al: Alcoholic hyalin and hepatic fibrosis. Clin Res 22:559A, 1974

188. Zetterman RK et al: Alcoholic hepatitis cell-mediated immunologic response to alcoholic hyalin. Gastroenterology 70:382, 1976

chapter 19
Chronic Hepatitis

JAMES L. BOYER and DENIS J. MILLER

The term "chronic hepatitis" encompasses a group of disorders that share a chronically active necroinflammatory process in the liver but differ with respect to etiology, natural history, and response to therapy. The diagnosis of chronic hepatitis is applicable when unresolved necrosis, inflammation, and fibrosis are present for at least six months. Both sexes and all age-groups are affected; clinical symptoms vary from the asymptomatic patient to those with advanced hepatic failure. Examination of hepatic histology is essential because other forms of chronic active liver disease must first be excluded and the morphologic stage of the disease process established. This chapter reviews the distinctive clinical, biochemical, and histologic features of the various subgroups of chronic hepatitis and the potential mechanisms and rationale for treatment.

Despite often conflicting literature and nomenclature, two major clinical forms of chronic hepatitis are generally recognized.

Chronic persistent hepatitis (CPH) is usually clinically mild and histologically nonprogressive and is therefore considered benign. The chronic carrier with hepatitis B infection who develops hepatoma many years later is an exception to this general rule.

Chronic active hepatitis (CAH) is characterized by the presence of symptoms and tests of liver function or histology that indicate a high expectation for the condition to progress to the stage of cirrhosis. Corticosteroid therapy may often prevent or retard this process in selected patients.

Each of these two major forms of hepatitis has several etiologic, histologic, and clinical presentations that are reflected in differences in the natural history of the disease process and that will either dictate or preclude therapeutic intervention. Therefore, it is crucial to distinguish CPH from CAH, since prognosis and therapy are very different.

The text describes the historical development, clinical features, and classification of chronic hepatitis in an attempt to aid the student and physician in perfecting clinical judgements. Etiologic factors, the immune response, differential diagnosis, and treatment are also discussed.

HISTORICAL DEVELOPMENT

Prior to World War II, physicians recognized that severe hepatic necrosis and cirrhosis could occur following endemic hepatitis.[26,67,174] However, the duration of hepatitis was relatively brief, apparently lasting no more than several months. Between 1944 and 1945, Scandinavian workers in Denmark focused attention on more chronic sequelae following epidemic hepatitis.[6,30,143,149] Characteristically, the illness was prolonged and was preceded by a 1- to 2-month preicteric phase. Over 99% of cases occurred in women, mostly postmenopausal, and mortality was extremely high (61%). Ascites and edema were observed after 5 to 6 months, and by 10 to 12 months, the disease usually terminated in hepatic coma. It seemed plausible that the disease was transmitted by contact, since in some instances these older women had nursed female relatives who had been suffering from chronic hepatitis.

Chronic sequelae of epidemic hepatitis lasting more than 4 months were also noted at that time (1945) in military servicemen.[16] However, Neefe and associates[224] (1955) noted that recovery often occurred within 1½ years following the initial illness. Debate then ensued as to whether "viral" forms of hepatitis could give rise to chronic progressive liver disease of more than a year's duration, particularly since long-term follow-up studies of patients with clinically symptomatic serum or epidemic hepatitis in World War II American and British veterans, and later Korean War veterans or civilians failed to document progression of hepatitis to cirrhosis.[39,51,224,225,373] In 1958 Klatskin described nine patients with histologic features of viral hepatitis who developed subacute hepatic necrosis (bridging and multilobular necrosis) and postnecrotic cirrhosis following prolonged anicteric infections presumably with the hepatitis virus.[162] Later, prospective studies of patients with severe viral hepatitis indicated that subacute hepatic necrosis was a necessary histologic prerequisite for the development of postnecrotic cirrhosis and CAH.[44]

A second form of chronic hepatitis, characterized by cirrhosis, plasma cell infiltration of the liver, and marked hypergammaglobulinemia (presumably unrelated to viral infection) was first described by Waldenstrom in 1950[343] in young women. Severe jaundice, acne, amenorrhea, and hepatosplenomegaly were also noted. In 1951 and 1956, Kunkel and associates emphasized the high frequency of amenorrhea–hirsutism, obesity, acne, arthritis, cushingoid facies, pigmented abdominal striae, as well as a postnecrotic form of cirrhosis and hypergammaglobulinemia.[20,176] In 1955 the finding of the lupus erythematosus (LE) cell phenomena in similar patients with CAH[152] led to the introduction of the term "lupoid hepatitis" by

MacKay and associates in 1956.[185] It is now clear that there is no relationship between systemic lupus erythematosus (SLE) and CAH with LE cells.

Although initially described in young women, this "autoimmune" form of hepatitis was subsequently described in males,[190,362] children,[236,237] and postmenopausal women.[265]* Thus, by the early 1960s, it was clear that chronic hepatitis could occur in all age-groups and present with a variety of clinical manifestations. Considerable confusion followed because of the focus by different authors on particular clinical, biochemical, or histologic features, and authors tended to accumulate series that reflected particular manifestations. For example, the term "lupoid hepatitis" referred to patients with positive LE cells,[4,9,17,18,27,128,175,185,190,265,334,360] "plasma cell hepatitis" was applied to patients in whom plasma cell infiltrates were a predominant histologic feature,[235–237] "autoimmune hepatitis" was used for cases in which serologic features (hypergammaglobulinemia and antinuclear antibodies [ANAs]) were particularly prominent.[151,189] "Active juvenile cirrhosis,"[259] "chronic liver disease" in young people,[362] "subacute hepatitis,"[329] and "subacute hepatic necrosis"[162] were additional terms that were promoted as clinical entities. Other clinical features such as thrombocytopenic purpura,[362] hemolytic anemia with positive Coomb's test,[189,239] eosinophilia,[360] hypersplenism, and portal hypertension were all noted.[190,214] Some authors emphasized extrahepatic manifestations such as the association of colitis, arthritis, thyroiditis, pulmonary fibrosis, and kidney and heart involvement,[190,191,214,259,333] emphasizing the multisystemic nature of the disease process.[116]

In 1960, Popper and co-workers demonstrated gamma globulin by immunocytochemical techniques within the parenchymal cells of the liver in patients with chronic hepatitis and cirrhosis.[240,247] The type of necrosis most often associated with these gamma globulin–containing cells was termed "piecemeal necrosis." This condition was characterized by the necrosis or disappearance of parenchymal cells found predominantly in the periphery of the lobule or along fibrous or inflammatory septae. The authors concluded that other types of hepatic necrosis were not associated with the local production of gamma globulin. Hence the term "piecemeal necrosis" was felt to reflect the development of chronic progressive liver disease. Subsequently, it became clear that this form of necrosis was also seen frequently in a variety of acute forms of liver disease, particularly in viral hepatitis and disorders of the biliary tract, including ascending cholangitis[2]; in these forms of liver disease, gamma globulin–containing cells were usually absent. Mistakenly, the term "piecemeal necrosis" came to be synonymous with progressive liver injury. In 1968, DeGroote and associates attempted to classify chronic forms of hepatitis by histologic features.[76] Since that time, the terms "chronic persistent hepatitis"

and "chronic aggressive hepatitis" (applied to patients with chronic hepatitis with piecemeal necrosis), appear in the literature. Others presented evidence that the histologic features of bridging hepatic necrosis (subacute hepatic necrosis) were essential for the progression of hepatitis to cirrhosis.[13,44] However, most studies lacked sufficient histologic material and careful characterization of the natural history of forms of hepatitis to provide definitive information. In 1972 the Mayo Clinic Group, in a prospective study, demonstrated that patients with symptomatic chronic hepatitis of more than 10 weeks' duration were at greatest risk to develop cirrhosis when bridging or mutilobular hepatic necrosis was present, whereas cirrhosis developed rarely in patients with "chronic aggressive hepatitis" (as defined by DeGroote and co-workers[13,311]).

It also became clear that various drugs, including laxatives containing oxyphenisatin;[266] methyldopa;[194] isoniazid;[193] aspirin;[289,365] and nitrofurantoin[32,91,125,163,296,317]* could also produce the clinical syndrome of CAH. Metabolic disorders such as Wilson's disease[315] and α_1-antitrypsin deficiency were also incriminated,[24] as well as some forms of alcoholic hepatitis,[114] where histologic features were reminiscent of viral or drug-initiated disease. Thus, in order to understand the natural history of chronic hepatitis, the etiology must be established—viral, drug, metabolic, or immunologic. With such information, the distinctive clinical and histologic features, prognoses, and response to treatment can usually be recognized.

ETIOLOGY

Viruses

Hepatitis B

A highly variable but nonetheless significant number of patients with chronic hepatitis have evidence of hepatitis B virus (HBV) infection. The frequency with which hepatitis B surface antigen (HBsAg) occurs in patients with CAH is low in Australia (3%),[62] approximately 15% in the United States[369] and United Kingdom,[263] and as high as 51% in the Mediterranean.[29,109] The incidental finding of HBsAg does not, however, imply serious liver disease, since the existence of a chronic carrier state is well known; in such cases it is more common to find minor histologic abnormalities[171,264,366] although virtually normal liver histology has been observed in some patients.[305,306] Only rarely does a "carrier" manifest potentially progressive chronic liver disease.

In contrast, chronic hepatitis follows documented acute viral hepatitis, type B, in approximately 10% of cases.[228,262] The proportion of patients who develop CAH and CPH when persistent HBs-antigenemia is present varies in these two studies.[228,262]

---

* Cattan R et al: Cirrhoses dysprotéinémiques d'origine inconnue chez la femme. Bull Soc Med Hop Paris 73:608, 1957.

* Tolman KG: Nitrofurantoin and chronic active hepatitis. Ann Intern Med 92:119, 1980.

Generally, chronic hepatitis is attributed to HBV infection if the serum consistently contains HBsAg. In a study of Redeker,[262] a group of more than 400 patients with acute hepatitis B showed absolute concordance between persistence of HBsAg and chronic hepatitis.[262] Loss of HBsAg was not associated with chronic hepatitis in any patient. The viral antigen may persist in the liver despite loss of serum HBsAg. In a study by Omata and associates,[232] the finding of anti-HBc in HBsAg-negative serum was associated with intrahepatic viral antigens in all cases. Kojima and co-workers[170] found the titer of anti-HBc to be important, since only levels greater than 2^{11} (by radioimmunoassay) were associated with intrahepatic HBcAg. Moreover, the presence of anti-HBs in conjunction with anti-HBc does not necessarily imply that viral antigens have been cleared, since both anti-HBs and anti-HBc were detected in the sera of some patients who had viral antigens in the liver.[232,314] Therefore, even in the presence of anti-HBs, the neutralizing antibody in the HBV system, high-titer anti-HBc appears to correlate with continued intrahepatic viral synthesis.

The neat and clinically convenient assumption, based in large part on Redeker's study,[262]—that HBsAg-negative chronic hepatitis is unlikely to be due to HBV—cannot be made in all cases, and persistence of HBsAg in the liver in the face of loss of serum HBsAg has been reported.[170] Therefore, in determining that HBV is not responsible for chronic hepatitis, absence of serum HBsAg is suggestive. However, because HBV nucleotide sequences have also been detected in DNA extracted from livers of a few patients with HBsAg-negative disease,[94] it remains to be determined how many RIA serum HBsAg-negative cases of chronic hepatitis might ultimately be related to HBV infection.

Non-A, Non-B Hepatitis

There is now compelling evidence that non-A, non-B hepatitis is an important cause of chronic hepatitis.[25,78,167,255,291] It is not clear whether one or more agents are responsible. Although various candidate antigen–antibody systems have been described, none of them has proven specific for the disease.[78]

The importance of non-A, non-B hepatitis agent(s) as a cause of chronic hepatitis has been emphasized by the rapidly growing evidence of its association with both parenteral and nonparenteral[158,338,339] forms of transmission. In addition to being responsible for up to 90% of posttransfusion hepatitis,[1,93,166] non-A, non-B hepatitis is also an important cause of sporadic hepatitis. In the Los Angeles area, for example, it accounts for approximately 20% of such hepatitis cases.[217]

The assessment of the overall contribution of non-A, non-B hepatitis to the spectrum of chronic hepatitis must await the widespread use of a reliable marker of infection. However, approximately 8%[7,115] of recipients of blood transfusions develop this condition; when commercial blood is used, this figure is fourfold to fivefold higher.[7,115,253,290] There is little doubt that the liver function abnormalities persist for a significantly longer period of time in this disease than in other forms of hepatitis. Whereas almost 90% of patients with hepatitis B lose their hepatitis surface antigen within 3 months of acquisition,[228] between 26% and 67% of patients with posttransfusion non-A, non-B hepatitis have transaminase abnormalities for 6 months and longer.[25,167,173,255,291]

Several histologic studies have been reported in patients with unresolved non-A, non-B hepatitis (see Table 19-3). Even when the histologic lesions have been diagnosed as CAH, the disease has resolved spontaneously in one third of the patients without therapy over a period of 1 to 3 years.[25] Chronic disease was more likely in anicteric patients with a peak serum glutamic-pyruvic transaminase (SGPT) level greater than 300 IU/ml.

The magnitude of the problem of the chronic carrier state of this virus (viruses) is unknown. Transmission studies from patients with chronic hepatitis to chimpanzees suggest that these patients are potentially infectious.[322] However, until the extent of the infection in the population and the number of viruses involved are known, the question remains open.

Several investigators have detected nucleotide sequences for HBV DNA in liver tissue from patients with non-A, non-B hepatitis,[94] and serum from such patients when transmitted to chimpanzees results in the development of HBV markers. Although these studies suggest that certain non-A, non-B hepatitis cases may be occult HBV diseases,[349] the weight of evidence indicates that they are unique agents.[79]

Other Viruses

Hepatitis A has not led to chronic hepatitis.[256] The Epstein–Barr virus, although a cause of acute hepatitis, has not been documented as an important factor in the development of chronic hepatitis.

Drugs

Hepatotoxic agents (*e.g.*, carbon tetrachloride and acetaminophen) produce acute hepatocellular injury and do not result in either acute or chronic hepatitis. (An isolated report of acetaminophen-associated CAH does exist.[38]) Although repetitive CCl_4 administration can cause cirrhosis in the experimental animal, this lesion is not consistent with that of chronic hepatitis.

Oxyphenisatin

Oxyphenisatin is used as a laxative and has been associated with the development of typical clinical, biochemical, and histologic features of CAH.[266] The drug has been removed from the US market but is still in widespread use in Europe and parts of North and South America. The relationship of drug consumption to the onset of liver damage is not clear-cut; many patients received the drug for years before clinical manifestations of liver disease appeared.[80,203] Typically, withdrawal of the drug is associated with subsidence of inflammation and improvement in clinical status.[117,266,364] The long duration of therapy in most of these patients suggests that a straightforward sensitization reaction is not operative and that a cumulative dose-related effect may play a role. Positive serologic abnormalities, including ANA, VDRL, and LE cell phenomena, have been described.[266]

Methyldopa

The importance of methyldopa in causing CAH has been emphasized,[194] predominantly because of the frequency with which the drug was used in treating hypertension. The disease is more common in older women. However, the incidence of hepatitis is very low. Because the features may be typical of CAH, and, moreover, because the lesion tends to regress with discontinuation of the drug, it should always be considered in taking a history in a patient with chronic hepatitis. In contrast to oxyphenisatin, hepatitis associated with methyldopa commonly occurs within weeks after starting therapy, suggesting a hypersensitivity reaction to the drug.

Isoniazid

The causal relationship of isoniazid to liver injury is a complex one. Isoniazid produces asymptomatic elevations of serum transaminase levels in up to 20% of patients[47] and severe hepatic injury, associated with a high mortality, in a considerably smaller number of persons (1%).[31,104,142,193,279] To compound the issue, some patients are simultaneously taking rifampin or para-aminosalicylic acid (PAS), agents which may also have an injurious effect, whether it be by inducing microsomal enzymes or liver injury. Severe CAH accompanied by cirrhosis has invariably been associated with persistent administration of isoniazid.[192] Discontinuation of the drug after the onset of hepatitis has not necessarily been associated with survival, since even the lesion of acute hepatitis associated with isoniazid has a high mortality,[193] but chronic hepatitis does not generally ensue if the drug is discontinued soon after the recognition of hepatitis.

Halothane

Halothane has been reported, in one instance, to cause CAH.[326] However, follow-up was only 3½ months, and therefore proof of chronicity was not established. In another study follow-up studies of three patients up to 14 months after acute hepatitis showed resolution of the disease without residual, chronic hepatitis.[211]

Nitrofurantoin

Nitrofurantoin, a commonly used antiseptic for the urinary tract, causes chronic hepatitis infrequently. The disorder ranges in expression from anicteric illness to severe hepatic necrosis and death,[32,91,163,296,317] and often mimics "lupoid" hepatitis. Nitrofurantoin-induced chronic hepatitis has been described in patients with HLA-B8 antigens,[125] supporting the hypothesis that drugs might be an initiator of "autoimmune" forms of chronic hepatitis.*

Putative Autoimmune-Mediated ("Lupoid") Chronic Active Hepatitis

CAH, unassociated with documented or recognizable viral infection, drugs, or any other known cause of liver disease, accounts for one of the two major groups of patients with chronic hepatitis. The hallmarks of this disease are as follows:[60,161,212,214,311]

Predominance in women, both young and menopausal.

Early evidence of hepatic decompensation with frequent peripheral stigmata of chronic liver disease.

Hyperglobulinemia.

High incidence of autoantibodies and associated autoimmune disease.[41,82,190]

A 10% to 15% incidence of LE cells.[214]

A higher than expected frequency of the histocompatibility antigen HLA-B8,[100,102,186,238] as well as HLA-A1.[186]

The finding of a genetic marker has led to the widespread support for a genetic contribution to the development and pathogenesis of this lesion. The very high female predominance suggests the effect of an immunoregulatory gene on the X chromosome. Although the number of multiple cases in families is rare,[188] family members have a higher incidence of immune-mediated disease,[102] as well as a higher prevalence of autoantibodies than the general population.[102,103]

HLA-B8 has been associated with other diseases—notably, juvenile-onset diabetes mellitus, myasthenia gravis, gluten-sensitive enteropathy, and Addison's disease; the association of this HL antigen thus seems clear, although the mechanism of its control of inappropriate antibody synthesis and the genesis of immune-mediated liver disease is not clear. An association with a B lymphocyte alloantigen, DRW$_3$, has also been demonstrated.[102] DRW$_3$ and B8 are in strong linkage disequilibrium, and, since the target antigens are extremely varied, the mechanism by which these genes operate is not restricted to a single antigen. It is thus possible that the genetic influence is on immunoregulation (i.e., T-B or T-T cell cooperation). For example, it has been suggested that an inadequate suppressor T cell response may be associated with this genetic influence.[88] Chronic hepatitis due to drugs has not usually been associated with an increased incidence of HLA antigens,[182] although studies have been few, and further analysis is necessary.

---

* Tolman KG: Nitrofurantoin and chronic active hepatitis. Ann Intern Med 92:119, 1980.

IMMUNOLOGIC RESPONSES

Hepatitis B

There is considerable evidence that the virus is not cytopathic and the resultant liver injury is caused by the host immune response to the virus antigens.[46,89,309,375] This evidence has been derived from clinical and histologic observations: The demonstration of cytoplasmic and nuclear involvement of cultures of primary human embryo liver cells after inoculation with serum containing HBV, in the absence of cytopathic changes[46,309] supports this contention. Patients may have HBV infection without any detectable liver injury,[366] and they may be entirely asymptomatic. In addition, different human volunteers given the same dose of HBV-containing serum may develop widely varying responses, which range from asymptomatic carriage of the HBsAg to fulminant hepatitis.[133]

Further evidence of a role for the immune response in the pathogenesis of liver injury derives from the observations that immunosuppressed patients (asymptomatic HBsAg carriers) receiving chemotherapy for malignancies may develop severe and fatal hepatitis when therapy is abruptly discontinued.[101,345] Thus, the host immune response may be a critical determinant in the pathogenesis of liver injury that develops with this infection, even though the mechanism of the immune reaction that causes liver injury is unknown. During the past decade numerous hypotheses have been put forward.

HBV-Related Hepatitis

Immune Complex Disease

Complexes of HBsAg, anti-HBs, and complement occur in hepatitis B infection. These complexes have been demonstrated in serum,[302] blood vessels,[112] and renal glomeruli.[59] The weight of evidence suggests that these complexes play a role in the pathogenesis of associated extrahepatic diseases such as arthritis and nephritis but not in liver injury.

T-Cell–Mediated Injury

Dudley and co-workers[84] proposed in 1972 that the adequacy of the cellular immune response determines the course of hepatitis B infection. It is now widely held that the T-cell response is crucial in the mediation of liver injury. However, since target cells analogous to infected human hepatocytes are not readily adaptable to *in vitro* testing against lymphocytes, the supportive evidence remains circumstantial; most studies have employed either tumor cells[56] or erythrocytes[5] or lymphocytes.[352] Furthermore, there has not been histocompatibility between effector and target cells, a requirement in terms of HLA restriction.[374] In a preliminary study, HBsAg was felt to be the principal target antigen for cytotoxic T cells in acute

hepatitis B[215] using peripheral blood lymphocytes and autologous hepatocytes isolated from the patients' own liver biopsies.

Studies with monoclonal antibodies directed toward peripheral blood lymphocytes in chronic hepatitis B disease have shown an increase in the "helper/suppressor" ratio correlated with active viral replication[326]; in a subsequent study, a low "helper/suppressor" ratio correlated with active viral replication and more severe histologic and biochemical activity. Peripheral blood studies are always subject to the criticism that they may not reflect mechanisms operative at the site of injury in the liver. Therefore studies showing the nature of T-cell subsets in the livers of patients with various forms of acute and chronic hepatitis B infection are of interest and may prove to be more informative in the evaluation of cytopathic mechanisms of cell death. In CAH T8[+] cells were found in areas of necrosis, whereas T8[+] and T4[+] cells were found in portal areas. In acute hepatitis B, cells of non–T-cell origin were found.[90] A third study in patients with chronic hepatitis found a subgroup of cytotoxic T cells or cells with natural killer (NK) properties (T5 positive, T1 negative), but there was no special relationship to the cellular expression of HBV antigens. These disparate results have not clarified the mechanisms of hepatitis injury but point the way for further study.[215]

Non–T-Cell Mechanisms

Antibody-Dependent Cellular Cytotoxicity (ADCC) Mediated by K Cells. This mechanism of tissue injury has been suggested to be important in the genesis of liver injury both in HBV-related and autoimmune CAH.[88] According to this theory, HBV or other initiating factors produce an abnormality in immune regulation, whereby B cells secrete antibody inappropriately against liver-specific protein (LSP). This IgG antibody, presumably anti-LSP, attaches to liver cells, and K cell–mediated killing of the antibody coated hepatocytes then occurs. Lymphocytes from patients with chronic hepatitis demonstrate cytotoxicity against rabbit hepatocytes[57,88,327] and against autologous liver cells[209,241] in support of this theory.

Natural Killer or Spontaneous Cell-Mediated Cytotoxicity. Cells with Leu 7[+] antigen markers, detectable with anti-Leu monoclonal antibody, characterized as NK cells,[328] predominate in the livers of patients with acute hepatitis B.[90] This suggests a role for NK cells in the genesis of liver injury in acute hepatitis B.

Hepatitis Unrelated to HBV ("Autoimmune" or Lupoid Hepatitis)

It has long been held that CAH (lupoid) is an autoimmune disease. Although it has been recognized for many years that nonspecific autoantibodies can be found in the serum of such patients,[84,332] there is no evidence that these antibodies play any pathogenetic role. However, with the isolation and purification of LSP,[207,208] against which autoantibodies may be directed, there have, at least on theoretic grounds, been putative antigens to invoke in the antibody-mediated destruction of hepatocytes. Antibody against LSP has been detected in the serum of patients with HBsAg-negative CAH;[139] in addition, linear deposition of IgG has been found on the surface of hepatocytes in these patients. It has thus been postulated[88] that in CAH a suppressor T-cell defect exists, allowing the production of autoantibody against normally occurring LSP. This defect, it is suggested, allows for antibody directed against the liver cell membrane to bind with the antigen and thus allow for ADCC mediation by K cells. T-cell subsets have been analyzed in liver tissue in patients with autoimmune CAH and "helper/suppressor" ratios are increased. This finding is consistent with a diminution of suppressor T cells in this disease.[90,215]

DIFFERENTIAL DIAGNOSIS

It is important that the diagnosis of chronic hepatitis be made only after the clinician has satisfactorily excluded other causes of chronic active liver disease. This distinction can usually be made after a careful history and physical examination or from specific chemical or radiologic tests; however, the liver biopsy is often the most helpful diagnostic discriminator. Other forms of chronic liver disease should be carefully excluded; at times this may be difficult if their clinical and biochemical features overlap with those of chronic hepatitis.

Alcoholic Liver Disease

More common in men, alcoholic liver injury is suspected in the patient who consumes more than 40 g to 80 g of alcohol daily.[178] However, if the serum aminotransferases are much greater than 300 and the SGPT/serum glutamic-oxaloacetic transaminase (SGOT) ratio is greater than 1, alcoholic liver injury is unlikely; a liver biopsy will resolve the issue.[180] Confusion may arise in the alcoholic when histologic evidence of chronic hepatitis is observed because the incidence of hepatitis B infection in the alcoholic patient is high[180,246] and alcohol may predispose the patient to chronic injury from hepatitis, perhaps by interfering with the normal cellular immune response.[114] Progression of the lesions seems to depend on the continued use of alcohol.[66] Alternatively, some authors believe that an immune response to alcoholic hyalin will result in "chronic hepatitis."[140,154,372] The issue has not been resolved, although the high incidence of exposure to hepatitis B favors the coincidental occurrence of chronic viral hepatitis in the alcoholic.[180]

Primary Biliary Cirrhosis

Primary biliary cirrhosis affects women nine times more frequently than men,[3,298] and classic cases are not easily confused with chronic hepatitis.[98,248] Typical cases begin with pruritus or isolated elevations in alkaline phosphatase levels and later progress to clinically overt cholestasis. Eighty-five percent have positive antimitochondrial antibodies,[155] and liver biopsies demonstrate degeneration of interlobular ducts, often in association with hepatic granulomata.[12,221,270,363] All of these typical features may not always be present in a given case, and the disorder may then be particularly difficult to distinguish from chronic hepatitis. Degenerative bile ducts typical of primary biliary cirrhosis may also be observed in chronic hepatitis,[250] most frequently non-A, non-B[15,283] and contribute to diagnostic confusion. Clinical responses to a challenge with corticosteroid therapy occasionally will resolve the issue, but in a small group of patients the clinical distinction remains unclear.[108,282] Since 12% of patients with chronic hepatitis may have antimitochondrial antibody in their sera,[155] the diagnosis of primary biliary cirrhosis must not be based on this serologic finding alone.

Metabolic Disorders

Wilson's Disease

The clinical, biochemical, and histologic features of chronic forms of hepatitis that result from Wilson's disease, an inherited disorder of hepatic copper metabolism, may be indistinguishable from CPH and CAH of other etiologies.[52,285,304,315] However, Wilson's disease is a potentially reversible disorder. It responds specifically to therapy with penicillamine, which chelates serum copper and excretes it in the urine. This therapy also prevents neurologic deterioration and may be lifesaving.[316] Therefore, the diagnosis must be excluded in every patient with chronic hepatitis who is under the age of 30. Most cases present during late childhood or adolescence and are recognized if the ceruloplasmin level is low, if Kayser–Fleischer rings are present on slit-lamp examination of the eye, or if copper determinations are performed on liver biopsy specimens. Each of these abnormalities has also been described in chronic liver disease unrelated to Wilson's disease, but such false-positive tests are distinctly unusual.[97,99,141,313,344] Hepatic copper levels may be elevated to Wilson's disease range (20 μg/g wet tissue) in chronic cholestatic disorders such as primary biliary cirrhosis because the bile is the primary route of copper excretion. Liver biopsy findings are never diagnostic of Wilson's disease, but the finding of glycogen nuclei in a patient without carbohydrate intolerance should raise this possibility.[281]

α_1-Antitrypsin Deficiency

α_1-Antitrypsin deficiency is associated with cirrhosis in childhood and is specifically diagnosed by abnormally low values of the α_1 globulin on protein electrophoresis and periodic acid-Schiff (PAS)-positive intracellular inclusions in the parenchymal cells of the hepatocytes. Protease inhibitor phenotyping defines the disorder more precisely (ZZ). The disorder is not usually confused with CAH of childhood but may manifest as cryptogenic cirrhosis unless recognized.[24,96] A heterozygote state has been found in chronic hepatitis (MZ).[96,130]

Hemochromatosis

Commonly presenting with minor abnormalities of liver function, hemochromatosis is more common in the adult male but is also seen in the postmenopausal female.[37,40] Cirrhosis is usually present, and the disorder is distinguished by the clinical constellation of bronzed skin, diabetes, and iron overload.[210,251] Hepatic parenchymal cells and portal triads are heavily infiltrated with iron, which also later deposits in the reticuloendothelial system, pancreas, cardiac tissue, joints, and pituitary glands, to mention a few. Saturation of the serum iron and elevations in serum ferritin levels suggest the diagnosis. Like certain patients with CAH, patients with hemochromatosis also develop arthritis and may initially seek medical help from rheumatologists.[120,210]

Biliary Tract Disease and Pancreatitis

Chronic cholelithiasis, choledocholithiasis, and pancreatitis may each result in minor abnormalities in liver function consisting of mild to moderate elevations in the aminotransferase levels and moderate and sometimes substantial increases in serum alkaline phosphatase. Jaundice may also occur but is usually transient unless common duct obstruction is present. These extrahepatic diseases result in an inflammatory reaction within and around the portal triad, characterized by an acute and chronic inflammatory cell infiltrate, varying degrees of bile duct proliferation and edema, and necrosis of hepatocytes adjacent to the triads. Occasionally, foci of inflammation and necrosis occur within hepatic lobules. Cholestasis may or may not be present. These histologic findings may be confused with an unresolved viral hepatitis or with CPH and, if the "pericholangitis" is severe, CAH may be mistakenly diagnosed.[2,42,76] If it is recognized that these conditions may occasionally lead to diagnostic error, tests such as ultrasonography and oral cholecystography will be performed and lead to the appropriate diagnosis. It must be remembered that patients with chronic hepatitis also develop both cholesterol and bilirubin gallstones; thus, the two disorders may occur simultaneously. In this instance it may be difficult to evaluate the cause of abnormalities in hepatic function, and surgical removal of the gallstones may be indicated. However, cholecystectomy in some cirrhotic patients with hypoprothrombinemia carries a mortality rate of up to 80%; therefore caution is warranted before undertaking surgery in this group of patients.[8]

Inflammatory Bowel Disease

CAH has been described in association with inflammatory bowel disease in up to 10% of cases,[212,214] but this coincidence is usually rare. It is likely that some of these cases represent "pericholangitis," which, like other biliary tract disorders, may at times be confused histologically with chronic hepatitis. Whereas nonspecific liver function abnormalities and histologic evidence of "triaditis" may occur in up to 25% of patients with inflammatory bowel disease (both ulcerative colitis and Crohn's disease),[213,243,244] a more severe disorder, sclerosing cholangitis, occurs less commonly.[53,353,354] Certain cases of sclerosing cholangitis may be distinguished clinically from chronic hepatitis by the history of recurrent episodes of right upper-quadrant pain, shaking chills, fever, and transient dark urine and clay-colored stools, which typically last for 24 to 72 hours. Jaundice and elevations in the aminotransferase and alkaline phosphatase levels may occur. Diagnosis is confirmed by radiographic demonstrations of focal strictures and dilatations of the extrahepatic and intrahepatic biliary tree. The condition may rarely lead to carcinoma of the bile ducts. Endoscopic retrograde cannulation procedures have also revealed cases in which sclerosing cholangitis is limited to the intrahepatic portion of the biliary tree.[28,33] Liver biopsy and cholangiography may be necessary to distinguish patients with these disorders from those with chronic hepatitis.

CLASSIFICATION

General Principles

The classification that we propose (Table 19-1) is based upon the premise that progressive forms of CAH can usually be distinguished from self-limited forms of the disease by combining clinical symptomatology and hepatic histology, together with knowledge of the etiologic agent. Transthoracic needle biopsies of the liver usually allow patients with chronic persistent or unresolved hepatitis to be distinguished from those with CAH.[2,42,76]

Liver biopsy material is also usually adequate to establish whether bridging necrosis, multilobular necrosis, or an established cirrhosis is present. However, the more advanced the fibrosis, the greater the potential for sampling error, so that it becomes increasingly difficult to judge the content of hepatic fibrosis accurately in a small 50-mg needle biopsy sample once the disease has progressed. If the specimen is fragmented or is less than 1.5 cm to 2 cm in length, the problem is compounded because of the inadequacy of the specimen.[284]

Several guidelines for biopsy preparation will increase the accuracy of histologic classification.

1. At least 2 cm of tissue must be obtained before attempting histologic classification.
2. A connective tissue stain, such as Mallory's trichrome, is required in addition to a silver reticulin stain to assess alterations in architecture and to distinguish between bridging necrosis and fibrosis, and the degree to which zones of parenchymal cell collapse have evolved toward the formation of fibrous septa.

TABLE 19-1.   Classification of Chronic Hepatitis

TYPE	ETIOLOGY	HISTOLOGIC SUBGROUPS	PROGNOSIS BASED ON HISTOLOGIC CRITERIA	TREATMENT
Chronic persistent hepatitis	Hepatitis B virus, non-A, non-B virus Drugs Unknown causes ("autoimmunity"? —"lupoid")	"Chronic persistent" or unresolved hepatitis	Nonaggressive	Reassurance Periodic follow-up
Chronic active hepatitis	Hepatitis B virus, non-A, non-B virus Drugs Unknown causes ("autoimmunity"? —"lupoid")	Chronic active hepatitis (without cirrhosis) A. Periportal piecemeal necrosis and inflammation only*	Probably nonaggressive	Periodic follow-up
		B. Bridging hepatic necrosis† and multilobular necrosis	Definitely precirrhotic	Corticosteroid therapy‡
		C. Periportal and piecemeal necrosis and bridging hepatic necrosis	Definitely precirrhotic	Corticosteroid therapy‡
		(With cirrhosis)	Cirrhosis established	Depends on activity

* Previously considered a major feature of the histologic spectrum of chronic aggressive hepatitis.
† Previously called "subacute hepatic necrosis."
‡ Usually restricted to "autoimmune" cases.

3. The more portal triads within a biopsy, the less the chances for sampling error.

Hepatic Morphology

Histologic classification of chronic hepatitis depends on morphologic criteria defining histologic patterns that predict a transition from acute to either self-limited or chronic disease. While knowledge of the pathogenesis of morphologic subtypes of hepatitis remains incomplete, a number of histologic features have now been defined that facilitate clinical diagnosis.

Chronic Persistent Hepatitis

CPH (Figs. 19-1 and 19-2) was initially defined by DeGroote and co-workers[76] as a "chronic inflammatory infiltration, mostly portal, with preserved lobular architecture and little or no fibrosis. Piecemeal necrosis is absent or slight. Features of acute hepatitis may be superimposed."

The lobular architecture in patients with CPH is always normal, and the limiting plate of hepatocytes surrounded by triads is usually intact; if necrosis is present, parenchymal cell injury is not extensive. There is universal agreement about these typical features of this histologic subtype, and when they are present, CPH can be readily distinguished from CAH. However, the degree of lobular

inflammation and necrosis may be variable, and there may be times when the histologic features may closely resemble an unresolved viral hepatitis. Some authors reserve the term "chronic persistent hepatitis" exclusively for patients in whom inflammation is limited to the portal triads and in whom the hepatic lobule is relatively normal, using terms such as "chronic lobular hepatitis" or "unresolved viral hepatitis" to describe more diffuse lobular necroinflammatory processes.[2,249]

The clinical significance of the varying degrees of lobular inflammation in patients with chronic persistent and chronic lobular hepatitis is probably not important, since this feature does not correlate with progression of the hepatic disease.[22,361] Occasionally, when the inflammatory process is limited to the portal triads, it may not always be possible to distinguish this form of chronic hepatitis from portal inflammation produced by extrahepatic biliary tract disorders such as gallstone disease, pancreatitis, and the triaditis associated with inflammatory bowel disease.

When CPH results from hepatitis B infection, little or no intranuclear core antigen may be present, whereas cytoplasmic surface antigen may be abundant.[122] However, occasionally nuclear core antigen is predominant. It is not clear whether or not these different expressions of nuclear antigen represent important differences in immune response to the infectious agent, which may subsequently alter the natural history of the chronic hepatitis. In chronic carriers of HBsAg, some of the hepatocytes

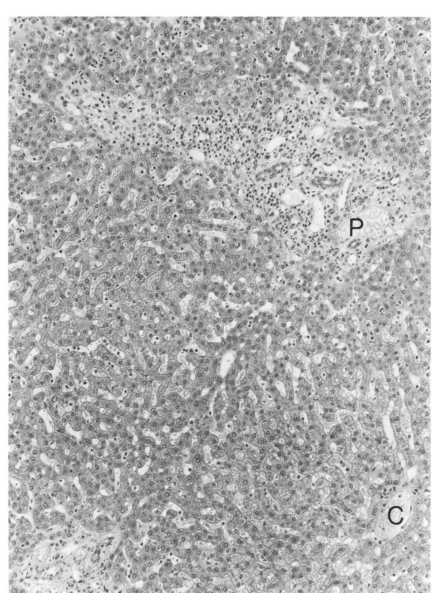

Fig. 19-1. Chronic persistent hepatitis. The lobular architecture is normal, and there is little cellular infiltrate or necrosis. An increase in inflammatory cells is seen within the portal triads (*P*). C = central vein. (H & E; original magnification × 100) (Boyer JL: Chronic hepatitis. A perspective on classification and determinants of prognosis. Gastroenterology 70:1161, 1976. © 1976, The Williams & Wilkins Co., Baltimore)

demonstrate a "ground-glass" appearance manifested by a granular homogeneous eosinophilia staining of the cytoplasm.[124] Ground-glass cells stain with orcein[301] and are more common in HBsAg-positive CPH but may also be seen in HBsAg-positive CAH and cirrhosis.

There are several pitfalls in diagnosing chronic hepatitis in patients in whom histologic evidence of CPH may be misleading.

1. Small fragmented specimens may not reveal a sufficient number of portal triads to differentiate CPH from CAH.
2. Anti-inflammatory treatment, particularly corticosteroids, may suppress histologic evidence of CAH, and hepatic histology may revert to the appearance of CPH during therapy.[71]
3. The lobular heterogeneity of fibrosis in a cirrhotic liver may result in a benign-appearing lesion if a nonrepresentative sample is obtained.
4. Finally, in some cases, it may be difficult to decide whether the periportal inflammation and necrosis or fibrosis is simply a more extensive version of CPH or whether CAH is present.[245] Because CPH has a benign prognosis, recognition of this type of hepatitis is clinically important, since these patients should not receive corticosteroids.

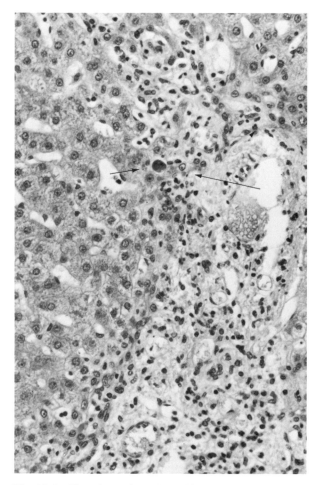

Fig. 19-2. Chronic persistent hepatitis. The limiting plate of hepatocytes surrounding a portal triad is interrupted only occasionally by extension of the portal infiltrate into the lobule or by acidophilic necrosis of bordering hepatocytes (*arrows*). (H & E; original magnification × 200) (Boyer JL: Gastroenterology 70:1161, 1976. © 1976, The Williams & Wilkins Co., Baltimore)

Chronic Active Hepatitis

Unlike CPH, there has been considerable debate over the histologic features of CAH and varying degrees of acceptance of definitions by international groups, including the International Association for the Study of the Liver.[2,42,76,282,336] Original emphasis was placed on the histologic features of "piecemeal necrosis," defined as "the destruction of liver cells at an interface between parenchyma and connective tissue, together with a predominantly lymphocytic or plasma cell infiltrate"[2] (Fig. 19-3). This process is often seen at the borders of portal triads or along the edges of either fibrous septa in cirrhotic livers or zones of necrosis. This form of cell necrosis (also known as "apoptosis"[157]) was initially observed in "autoimmune" forms of chronic hepatitis, particularly in association with

inflammatory infiltrates enriched in lymphocytes, macrophages, and plasma cells demonstrating immunoglobulins by immunocytochemical techniques.[240] Thus, the term "piecemeal necrosis" came to be synonymous with chronic progressive liver disease.

Although many believed that "piecemeal necrosis" was a pathognomonic sign for the development of CAH, it is now well recognized that reliance on this histologic feature alone often leads to diagnostic error. Such an error may have considerable adverse consequences for the patient, if it leads to unnecessary corticosteroid treatment and toxicity, when the diagnosis is based on this histologic feature alone.[2,42,282] The problem is significant, since the morphologic features of piecemeal necrosis are commonly present around the portal triad in patients with both acute and chronic forms of hepatitis; the extension of inflammatory and necrotic infiltrate into the lobule may easily be described as "piecemeal necrosis"[245] and overinterpreted. Second, a variety of biliary tract disorders may produce the same lesion, even though lymphocytic and plasma cell infiltrates may be relatively mild compared with those seen in most patients with CAH. Occasionally, other disorders such as primary biliary cirrhosis, Wilson's disease, inflammatory bowel disease, and sclerosing cholangitis may produce "piecemeal necrosis."

Others, including ourselves, believe that more reliable prognostic histologic features are confluent areas of necrosis that form zones of parenchymal collapse that bridge between portal triads and central veins or span lobules between portal triads.[42,44,162] This pattern of necrosis alters the underlying hepatic architecture; it was originally termed "subacute hepatic necrosis." However, because the word "subacute" has clinical rather than morphologic connotations, it has largely been replaced by the more descriptive term, "bridging hepatic necrosis" or "multilobular necrosis," where areas of confluent necrosis are more extensive such that complete lobular destruction is present (Figs. 19-4 to 19-6). Boyer and Klatskin emphasized the prognostic value of bridging hepatic necrosis in patients with viral hepatitis of less than 8 weeks' duration. In these cases, 13% developed CAH, requiring corticosteroids to suppress clinical symptoms and control liver function abnormalities; half of the remaining group developed a clinically inactive postnecrotic cirrhosis.[42] Others have also emphasized the prognostic importance of this histologic abnormality as a marker of potential chronicity[324,350] in the acute phases of hepatic injury, although some patients with bridging necrosis recover completely, including patients with acute massive hepatic necrosis.[156] Ware and colleagues[351] found that only 5 of 42 patients with bridging necrosis of less than one month's duration developed chronic liver disease. This lesion has greater prognostic significance when detected later in the course of viral hepatitis, since spontaneous recovery is much more frequent when the disease is less than 4 to 6 weeks in duration.

The most important evidence that bridging and multilobular necrosis are significant prognostic indicators for

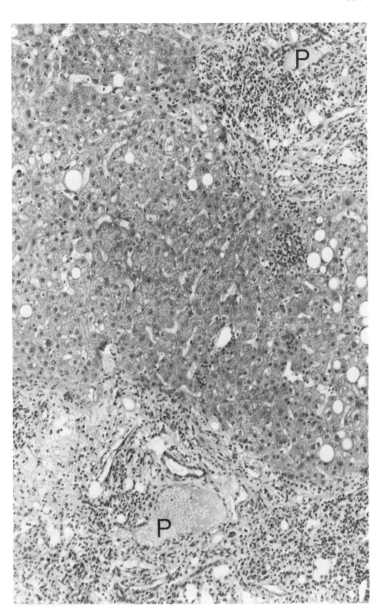

Fig. 19-3. Portal inflammation and piecemeal necrosis (apoptosis). In this field, two portal triads (*P*) are greatly expanded with chronic inflammatory cell infiltrates that erode the limiting plate. In the absence of bridging between portal triads or portal triads and central veins, it may be difficult at times to distinguish this lesion from chronic persistent hepatitis. (H & E; original magnification × 100) (Boyer JL: Gastroenterology 70:1161, 1976. © 1976, The Williams & Wilkins Co., Baltimore)

patients with CAH comes from a series of studies from the Mayo Clinic.[13,274,275,311] These studies clearly demonstrate that patients with liver biopsy evidence of bridging and multilobular necrosis are at high risk of progression to cirrhosis and death from hepatic failure. Others have subsequently confirmed these findings.[63,231]

An active postnecrotic cirrhosis may already be present when histologic material is first obtained in patients with chronic hepatitis and is distinguished by regenerating nodules, increases in hepatic fibrosis, and altered hepatic architecture (Figs. 19-6*A, B*). The activity of the cirrhosis is reflected by the degree of "piecemeal necrosis" and "bridging" or "multilobular hepatic necrosis." Bridging and multilobular necrosis are not always associated with

an ominous prognosis, and many patients with acute hepatitis, particularly when secondary to drug-induced liver injury, recover completely both clinically and histologically.[192,211]

The term "chronic aggressive hepatitis" was initially coined by the European Association for the Study of the Liver in 1968[76] and is often equated with the lesion of "piecemeal necrosis" (see Fig. 19-3). We do not like this term, however, since it implies progressive tissue damage and yet may be seen in a variety of self-limited forms of liver injury. Furthermore, subsequent studies also emphasize that piecemeal necrosis in the absence of bridging is a nonprogressive lesion in patients with chronic hepatitis.[63,231]

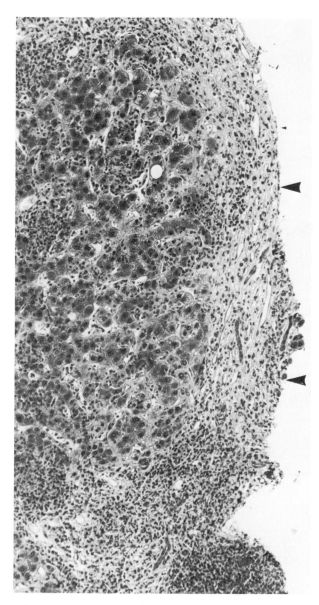

Fig. 19-4. Bridging necrosis (subacute hepatic necrosis). Two portal triads, which are expanded by inflammatory infiltrates and erosion of the limiting plate, are seen at either end of the field. A zone of parenchymal-cell collapse forms a bridge between the two triads at the edge of the biopsy (*arrowheads*). (Masson trichrome stain; original magnification × 100) (Boyer JL: Gastroenterology 70:1161, 1976. © 1976, The Williams & Wilkins Co., Baltimore)

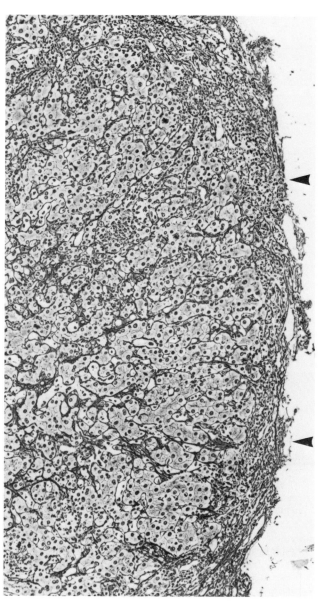

Fig. 19-5. Reticulum silver stain of the same area of bridging necrosis represented in Figure 19-4. Note the zone of cell collapse running along one edge of this biopsy specimen (*arrowheads*). (Original magnification × 100) (Boyer JL: Gastroenterology 70:1161, 1976. © 1976, The Williams & Wilkins Co., Baltimore)

CLINICAL FEATURES

Clinical features in patients with chronic hepatitis range from the asymptomatic patient with minor abnormalities of liver function who is healthy and has a normal physical examination to the patient who is bedridden with advanced hepatocellular failure. In the latter case, weakness, fatigue, weight loss, jaundice, ascites, and hepatic encephalopathy are prominent features.

In the first example, histologic examination usually reveals CPH, whereas an advanced cirrhosis or severe bridging necrosis and multilobular necrosis can almost always be predicted when clinical features of hepatocellular failure are obvious. Nevertheless, the degree of histologic im-

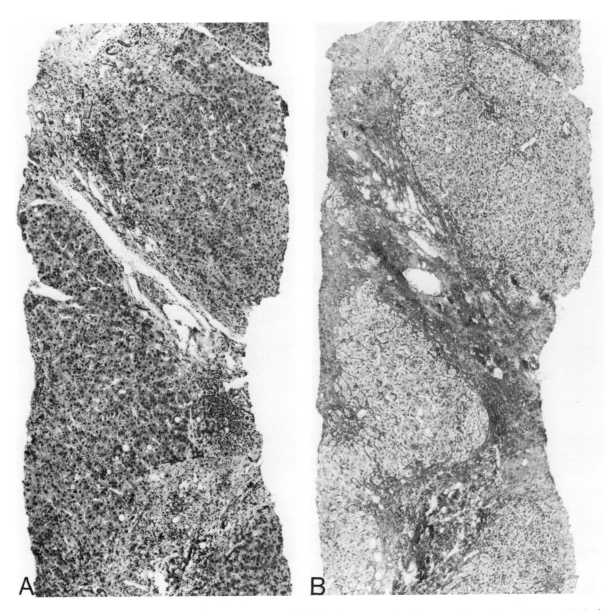

Fig. 19-6. A. Active postnecrotic cirrhosis, representing the most advanced stage in the pathologic spectrum of the clinical entity of chronic active hepatitis. (Masson trichrome stain; original magnification × 50) (Reproduced with permission of Gastroenterology[42]) **B.** Reticulin silver stain of the same area represented in Figure 19-6*A*, illustrating dense fibrous bridges that evolved from previous zones of parenchymal cell collapse such as those illustrated in Figures 19-4 and 19-5. (Original magnification × 50) (Boyer JL: Gastroenterology 70:1161, 1976. © 1976, The Williams & Wilkins Co., Baltimore)

pairment in chronic hepatitis does not always correlate with the clinical manifestation of hepatic derangement. More advanced disease, such as a minimally active postnecrotic cirrhosis, may be present in patients who are asymptomatic and who have few or no abnormalities on physical examination and only minor changes in tests of liver function. For this reason it is impossible to classify chronic hepatitis on the basis of clinical findings alone

and equally difficult to generalize about typical clinical features in the different subgroups.

Unresolved Viral Hepatitis

In 10% to 15% of patients with acute viral hepatitis (HBV and non-A, non-B), the disease fails to completely resolve within the first 2 to 3 months after the initial infection.[262]

Symptoms usually disappear but if not may consist of mild fatigue or malaise and occasional anorexia, but weight loss and other signs of hepatocellular failure are uncommon. If tests of liver function have returned to normal, the syndrome is known as "posthepatitis" syndrome[300] and is similar to other postviral asthenias. These patients may complain of right upper-quadrant pain, particularly if a biopsy has been performed, and symptoms are most common in patients who are hypochondriacal and who somatocize physical complaints. Reassurance often "cures" the disorder, which is not associated with any histologic abnormality.

More commonly, unresolved viral hepatitis is associated with fluctuations in serum aminotransferase activity twofold to 20-fold above the normal range. Physical examination may be normal, but tender hepatomegaly and a palpable spleen may be detectable. Liver biopsy demonstrates typical histologic features of CPH or lobular hepatitis. A clinical variant of chronic lobular hepatitis has been described that is characterized by a complete biochemical and clinical remission followed by a series of clinical relapses associated with elevations in aminotransferase levels ranging from 800 IU to nearly 3000 IU and recurrence of jaundice. Progression to chronic liver disease has not been observed. Although hepatitis B antigen is not detected, antinuclear antibodies and smooth muscle antibodies are present, suggesting that an altered immune response accounts for this uncommon clinical variant.[361]

Chronic Hepatitis B

Approximately 10% of patients with acute viral hepatitis B infection develop some form of chronic liver disease.[228,262] The majority take the form of an unresolved hepatitis or CPH, in which the major clinical manifestations are continued elevation in the serum aminotransferase levels and detection of HBsAg. Three percent to six percent develop chronic progressive disease that leads to cirrhosis.[262] Clinical features that characterized chronic hepatitis B in one large series are summarized in Table 19-2.[355] The reader is also referred to the work of Bradbear and co-workers[45] and Giusti and co-workers.[110]

Sex

The majority of patients with chronic hepatitis B are males; it is uncommon for women to present with this form of chronic hepatitis.[161,245,274,275] In the large referral population comprising the Mayo Clinic and Stanford[275,355] series, few of the chronic HBV patients were women. Women usually have less severe chronic disease. Rather, there is a predilection for the female to develop a progressive deterioration in hepatic function if she does not resolve the infection after a 4- to 6-week period. Peters describes this process as an "ineffective regenerative response," which leads to hepatic failure, coma, and death 4 to 6 months after the apparent onset of infection.[245]

TABLE 19-2. Clinical Features of Chronic Active Hepatitis B

	WITHOUT CIRRHOSIS	WITH CIRRHOSIS
Number	144	139
Male	87.5%	93%
Female	12.5%	7%
Age	39 ± 1*	43 ± 1
Acute onset	56%	51.5%
Duration of HB$_s$Ag positivity (months)	28 ± 2	31 ± 2
Homosexual	20%	18.5%
i.v. drug use	13%	9.2%
Alcoholic	2%	10%
Prior corticosteroid therapy	45%	54%
Symptoms	61%	73%
Liver ≥ 13 cm	16%	20%
Palpable spleen	14%	31.5%
Ascites	3%	21%
>2 Spider nevi	14%	38.5%
Total bilirubin (mg%)	0.99 ± 0.06	1.6 ± 0.14
Alkaline phosphatase	95 ± 5	127 ± 6
SGOT (IU)	109 ± 9	125 ± 13
Albumin (g%)	4.0 ± .05	3.5 ± .06
Hepatitis B DNA polymerase	60%	45%

* Mean ± SE.

(Weissburg JI et al: Survival in chronic hepatitis B: An analysis of 379 patients. Ann Intern Med 101: 613, 1984)

These women are usually in their sixth or seventh decade and appear to respond in much the same way as the elderly female patients described prior to the Second World War, when the clinical manifestations of hepatitis were often severe and rapidly progressive.[6,30,149,143]

Blumberg believes that genetic factors make the male more susceptible to continued viral infection with the HBV, possibly because of an immunoregulatory gene on the X-chromosome.[83] Males with chronic HBV infection are less likely to reject renal transplants than females, and chronic hepatitis has been described in male but not female members of families in which transmission is presumed to be from mother to son.[222]

Hepatitis B Carrier State

The incidence of the carrier state for HBV varies throughout the world and is also more common in males.[35,223] The incidence is as low as 0.1% in midwestern rural communities in the United States and some Eastern and Southern European countries, but rises to 4% to 5% in the ghettos of larger US urban areas, and to 10% to 20% in areas of Asia.[227,359] The frequency of hepatic abnormalities in carriers is variable; many have minor abnormalities of liver function. Findings from biopsy studies in such patients have ranged from nonspecific focal and reactive hepatitis to fully documented CAH or cirrhosis.[144,305,306,340] Considering that there are 150 to 200 million HBV carriers worldwide, a substantial reservoir of clinically undetected chronic liver disease exists that is related to chronic HBV infection. However, liver biopsies are not routinely recommended in carriers in whom tests of hepatic function are normal.[119,171] The risk of developing postnecrotic cirrhosis or primary liver cell carcinoma in the chronic HBsAg carrier is not known unless the infection is acquired at birth. Prospective studies from Taiwan estimate the risk of hepatocellular cancer to be 200 times greater than in persons who are not HBsAg carriers.[21]

Predisposing Factors

Chronic hepatitis B infection is particularly common in hemophiliacs because of multiple transfusions and the increasing use of Factor VIII concentrate.[179,197,252] The incidence of positive HBsAg or anti-HBsAb serology may be as high as 70%.[198] Chronic active liver disease is also frequent in these patients, but a liver biopsy is usually required to differentiate between CPH and CAH in patients who have liver function abnormalities. Chronic HBV infection is also prevalent in patients showing alterations in the cellular immune response, including those in hemodialysis units,[105,321] chronic drug users,[292] those with Down's syndrome, those with leukemia or lymphoma,[65] and those receiving chemotherapy on oncology units.[348] Clinical manifestations of the illness are minimal or absent, and histologic features usually demonstrate CPH or unresolved hepatitis rather than more serious forms of the disease. Male homosexuals are also prone to develop chronic hepatitis B infection as a result of the high prevalence of HBV in this population.[81,294] In contrast, chronic hepatitis B infection is rare in the female homosexual or prostitute.

Delta Infection

The discovery of the delta agent by Rizzutto has led to a reassessment of the role that this superinfection plays in the pathogenesis of hepatitis B disease.[267] The antigen can be detected by immunofluorescence studies in liver tissue, whereas antibody is detected in the serum. Serologic testing for antibody indicates a relatively high incidence of infection in patients with chronic HBV in Italy, Europe, and the United States. In contrast, the delta agent is rarely found in chronic liver disease in Taiwan or Japan, despite the high incidences of chronic HBV infection.[54]

The peak prevalence of the antigen is greatest in patients with active cirrhosis and is particularly common in patients with progressive disease.[58] However, there are conflicting reports about the prognostic significance of delta infection. Some studies find that rates of progression of disease are similar in patients with and without delta infection,[58,145,272] whereas others report that delta-infected patients with chronic active hepatitis without cirrhosis deteriorate and die more frequently than those uninfected by the agent.[272,*]

Presenting Features

Chronic hepatitis B infection begins with the typical clinical manifestations of acute viral hepatitis in one third of cases but may be clinically silent as in the chronic carrier, or present with only vague symptoms of fatigue and malaise, which may last for months before the patient seeks medical attention. Some patients present initially with biochemical and clinical evidence of cirrhosis without any antecedent history of hepatitis or clinical illness, and only the serologic markers of hepatitis B infection allow recognition of the cause of the cirrhosis.[43] Absence of HBsAg or HBsAb in the sera does not completely exclude the diagnosis since either anti-HB$_c$ or HBV DNA has been detected in a few cases that were otherwise serologically negative.[94]

Symptoms and Physical Findings

Anorexia, weakness, abdominal pain, arthralgia, amenorrhea, jaundice, hepatosplenomegaly, ascites, bleeding varices, and hepatic coma are the symptoms and physical findings recorded in most large series of patients with chronic hepatitis. However, only a minority of these cases are HBsAg-positive (4% of patients from King's College[219] and 14% from the Mayo Clinic series[311]). Experience from the Mayo Clinic indicates that patients with HBV and chronic hepatitis are older and more likely to have advanced stages of clinical disease and biopsy evidence of

---

* De Cock KM et al: Delta hepatitis in the Los Angeles Area: A report of 126 Cases. Ann Intern Med 105:108, 1986.

cirrhosis.[275] Yet, clinics drawing patients from large urban ghettos sample a different population with HBV-related chronic hepatitis. In these clinics the disease is found in younger patients who are often asymptomatic and whose physical findings are minimal or absent. HBsAg-positive chronic hepatitis is a more benign disease in this latter setting, and few patients appear to develop fatal or progressive disease.[131] A more representative series has been reported from Stanford. Symptoms and stigmata of chronic liver disease increased in frequency in patients with more advanced histologic disease.[355]

Laboratory Findings

Routine tests of liver function reflect the extent of parenchymal cell impairment but do not distinguish HBV-associated chronic hepatitis from other forms.[161,275] The persistence of HBsAg in serum over time suggests the diagnosis, although the antigen can eventually disappear even after many years.[320] Screening HBsAg and anti-HBs antibody-negative cases of chronic hepatitis for anti-HBc or HBV DNA yields only a few additional cases of HBV infection, indicating that serologic markers for HBV detect nearly all HBV related cases when the tests are performed by sensitive radioimmunoassay techniques.[170] HBV-associated chronic hepatitis varies in geographic distribution and accounts for as many as 60% of cases in countries such as Italy,[110] but is less prevalent in England and Australia.[29,45,62,109,263,369] In Western countries, Dane particles and HBeAg are observed more frequently in patients with chronic liver disease than in asymptomatic HBsAg carriers[195,229,310,331] and correlate with greater infectivity and derangement in hepatic function. However, the presence of HBeAg or Dane particles does not distinguish between CPH or CAH in an individual case; rather, their detection indicates only that there is viral replication and that the patient's serum is potentially infectious. However, in general, patients with HBV-associated chronic hepatitis do more poorly and are more refractory to therapy if e-antigen or high titers of Dane particles persist.[271,342]

Serologic markers of autoimmunity are found infrequently in chronic HBV infection[49,95,187,275,341,368] and high serum titers of antinuclear (ANA), anti–smooth muscle, or antimitochondrial antibodies should raise a question regarding etiology. However, low titers of smooth muscle antibody and ANA (<1 : 40) are not uncommon and occur in liver diseases of all types. Antiribosomal antibodies are also infrequent in HBsAg-positive chronic hepatitis and when reported are present in low titer.[106] The lupus erythematosus test (LE cell), once thought to be a specific marker of "lupoid hepatitis," has been reported, albeit infrequently, in HBsAg-positive chronic hepatitis.[201,312]* Gamma globulin levels are only mildly to moderately elevated in patients with HBsAg-positive hepatitis.[161,275]

* Kater L et al: HAA and ANA in chronic active hepatitis. Lancet 1:598, 1971.

Extrahepatic Involvement

A spectrum of extrahepatic manifestations occurs with both acute and chronic forms of HBV hepatitis,[116,212,214] including urticaria,[111,337] rash,[204] arthritis,[346,347] polyarteritis,[14,85,218,242,269,293] polyneuropathy,[92] glomerulonephritis,[48,164,165,168,220] cryoglobulinemia, pancreatitis, and pleural effusion.[181] Each has been attributed to HBsAg-antibody immune complex formation. Circulating immune complexes have been detected in cryoprecipitates from patients with HBsAg-positive CAH and both arthralgia and frank arthritis. Cryoprecipitates from patients with frank arthritis contain IgM, IgG, IgA, and complement components C_3, C_4, and C_5, as well as HBsAg. There is also evidence for activation of both classic and alternate complement pathways. The pathogenesis of the arthritis resembles a "serum-sickness–like" syndrome, since the presence of immune complexes correlates with the timing of the arthritis and disappears with resolution of the joint symptoms.[346,347]

A relationship between hepatitis and vasculitis has also been recognized since Paull described four cases of polyarteritis nodosa in Army officers following yellow fever vaccination in 1942.[242] Subsequently, it was recognized that some patients with polyarteritis nodosa have chronic hepatitis[218,269] and that chronic hepatitis B infection is a significant cause of necrotizing vasculitis in humans. The clinical manifestations of chronic hepatitis are usually mild; more than half the cases are anicteric, and CPH is detected histologically. CAH can also occur. There may be no consistent relationship between the onset of the liver disease and the manifestation of vasculitis. HBsAg has been detected in the synovial fluid and in immune complexes in the serum. In patients with multisystemic involvement, the progression of the vasculitis may be rapid, and death is the end result.[14,85,293]

Circulating immune complexes can also be detected in patients with chronic hepatitis and glomerulonephritis,[48,59,164,165,168,220] peripheral neuropathy,[92] or essential cryoglobulinemia.[181] Patients with cryoglobulinemia typically manifest purpura, arthralgias, or arthritis and weakness. Glomerulonephritis is frequently part of the multisystemic manifestations of immune complex formation, but renal involvement may be the primary clinical disorder. Both children and adults can present with the nephrotic syndrome, and the chronic hepatitis may not be clinically apparent. The disorder is manifested by glomerular deposits of IgG, Clq, and HBsAg. Spontaneous remission of glomerular disease has been reported in association with clearance of detectable HBsAg in the sera, suggesting that eradication of the HBV infection with antiviral agents might reverse the disease process.[164]

Clinical Sequelae

Postnecrotic cirrhosis is a known sequela of chronic hepatitis B infection and ultimately leads to the production of portal hypertension and esophageal varices.[43] Hepatocellular carcinoma is also a known sequela of HBV and occurs most frequently in countries in which the carrier state for chronic hepatitis B infection is high. Hepatoma is associated with serologic evidence of HBV infection in up to 75% of cases in nonalcoholics, and postnecrotic cirrhosis is often present.[233]

Spontaneous remission in the activity of chronic hepatitis B infection also occurs and has been estimated at rates of 10% to 30% per year.[138,260] Seroconversion from HBeAg to HBeAb is usually observed at this time and is often preceded by an abrupt increase in the aminotransferases. These episodes of biochemical relapse may be associated with an apparent acute episode of clinical hepatitis, possibly reflecting a spontaneous increase in the host immune response to the infection. Rarely (2%–3%) these spontaneous exacerbations may result in severe hepatic decompensation and death.[297] Some of these episodes may be initiated by intercurrent delta and possible non-A, non-B infections.

It is also clear that loss of hepatitis e-antigen and seroconversion to e-antibody do not necessarily connote permanent remission. In one study, 32% of patients with CAH who were converted spontaneously reactivated their disease within 1 year.[73] These patients were older and were more likely to have cirrhosis and disease of longer duration than the patients who did not relapse. CAH HBV disease can also be reactivated by chemotherapeutic[135] and immunosuppressive agents.[87]

Survival

Life expectancy for patients with chronic hepatitis B disease is dependent on the severity of the histologic lesion at the time of diagnosis. In a large follow-up study of 379 patients[355] (Fig. 19-7), 5-year survival rates were estimated at 97% for patients with histologic evidence of CPH and 86% for patients with CAH without bridging necrosis. In contrast, patients with CAH and cirrhosis had significantly lower 5-year survival rates of 55%, which were comparable to the 41% estimated rates for untreated "autoimmune" hepatitis in England.[60,160] Death usually was related to liver failure and its sequelae. A multivariate analysis determined that patients 40 years of age or older and those with bilirubin levels of 1.5 mg/dl or greater and ascites and spider nevi were at highest risk of death from chronic HBV disease.

Non-A,Non-B Chronic Hepatitis

Of posttransfusion hepatitis, 95% is now secondary to non-A,non-B hepatitis. Up to 46% of these patients develop chronic disease of more than a year's duration.[1,7,25,167,172,255] This form of hepatitis is also found in dialysis and oncology units[167] where exposure to blood products is common. The disease also occurs sporadically in the community, although the incidence of chronic infection appears to be less than following transfusion.[79] Unlike chronic hepatitis B, non-A,non-B chronic hepatitis is frequently anicteric, mildly symptomatic, and marked by periodic sharp rises in the serum aminotransferase activity followed by falls to normal.[78]

In one prospective follow-up study of 388 patients who underwent open-heart surgery, 7% developed non-A,non-B hepatitis that could not be attributed to drug toxicity

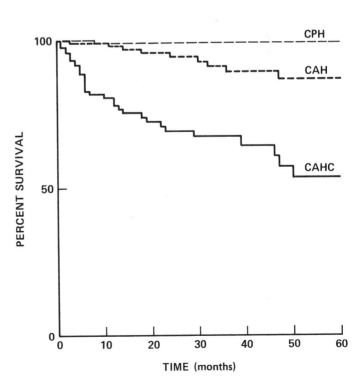

Fig. 19-7. Life-table survival curves for 379 patients with chronic hepatitis B. CAHC = chronic active hepatitis with cirrhosis (130 patients); CAH = chronic active hepatitis (128 patients); CPH = chronic persistent hepatitis (121 patients). Each survival curve is significantly different from the others (p < 0.001). (Weissberg JI et al: Ann Intern Med 101:613–616, 1984. Reproduced with permission of the authors and publisher)

or to other known viral infections.[25] Those who developed chronic hepatitis usually could not be distinguished clinically from those with only transient abnormalities in liver function, and they did not differ in terms of age (46 vs. 50 years), symptoms during the acute phase of hepatitis, or peak in aminotransferase levels (719 vs. 762). In one series, those who developed chronic hepatitis received more transfusions.[167] One third were transiently icteric in each group. Although acute hepatitis was seen equally in men and women, 75% of those who developed chronic disease were men. The mean incubation period was 8 weeks and ranged from 6 to 12 weeks. Most anicteric patients whose aminotransferase levels were higher than 300 IU/liter developed chronic hepatitis.[25] The most prominent symptoms are mild fatigue; but non-A,non-B hepatitis patients usually do not develop skin rash, arthritis, pruritus, or weight loss, and stigmata of chronic liver disease is rare. Results of other liver function tests are usually normal, and hypergammaglobulinemia, if present, is mild. Serum anti–smooth muscle and antinuclear antibodies, antimitochondrial antibodies, and other autoantibodies[196] are seldom detected.

Limited histologic data are available in this group of patients, but CAH is the most common lesion (usually without bridging necrosis or cirrhosis),[25,167,172,255] (Table 19-3).

There are also a limited number of long-term follow-up studies to determine the risk of developing progressive liver disease or liver failure.[126,173] However several studies suggest that progression to cirrhosis may be more common than initially believed. A 9-year study of 79 hemophiliacs with non-A,non-B hepatitis who received clotting factor concentrates revealed progressive liver disease in 21%, and 11% developed histologic evidence of cirrhosis.[126] Another 5- to 11-year follow-up study of 69 patients with post-transfusion non-A,non-B hepatitis revealed a minimal incidence of cirrhosis of 6%.[173] Despite these histologic studies, most patients with chronic non-A,non-B hepatitis remain asymptomatic, and symptoms of liver failure are extremely rare.

Despite the tendency to chronicity, some patients gradually resolve their biochemical abnormalities over time, falling to normal range within one to three years (4 of 12 patients in one series[25]). However, a chronic carrier state may remain, and the patient may still be potentially infectious.[322] There is no objective data regarding the efficacy of corticosteroids in non-A,non-B chronic hepatitis. However, in one study preoperative gamma globulin prophylaxis significantly reduced the incidence of transmission and progression to chronic liver disease.[167]

Chronic Active Hepatitis of Unknown Etiology ("Auto-immune" Chronic Hepatitis)

Chronic active hepatitis of unknown etiology represents the classic form of CAH in which the cause of the chronic liver disease cannot readily be attributed to sensitization from drug ingestion, infection with a virus, Wilson's disease, primary biliary cirrhosis, or a known metabolic defect. Initial reports by Waldenstrom in 1950[343] and Kunkel in 1951[176] emphasized the occurrence of this disease in young women with the clinical manifestations of amenorrhea, hepatosplenomegaly, hyperglobulinemia, cushingoid facies, pigmented abdominal striae, and arthritis, all in association with a postnecrotic form of cirrhosis. In 1955 Joske and King reported the LE cell phenomenon in patients with CAH,[152] and the term "lupoid hepatitis" became popular (see section on historical development). It is now known that this disease occurs in patients of all ages, and that the endocrine abnormalities and LE cells

TABLE 19-3.   Liver Biopsies in Non-A, Non-B Chronic Hepatitis

STUDY	NUMBER OF PATIENTS BIOPSIED	RESULTS
Koretz and co-workers[171]	15	9 CAH, without bridging necrosis 2 CPH 4 Unresolved hepatitis
Knodell and co-workers[166]	10	8 CAH 1 CPH 1 Cirrhosis
Berman and co-workers[25]	8	6 CAH (1 cirrhosis) 2 CPH
Rakela and co-workers[255]	14	4 CAH 10 CPH
Hay and co-workers[126]	34	21 CPH 9 CAH 4 Cirrhosis
Koretz and co-workers[173]	21	4 Cirrhosis

CAH, chronic active hepatitis; CPH, chronic persistent hepatitis.

occur in only a small minority of cases. Careful clinical studies in relatively large numbers of patients referred to centers for the study of liver disease (in Melbourne,[214] London,[60,219] Minnesota,[311] and New Haven[161]) demonstrate that this form of CAH is relatively similar throughout the world. These patients also share a number of common clinical characteristics and respond beneficially to corticosteroid therapy in a similar fashion.

Age, Sex, and Predisposing Factors

Characteristically, 70% to 80% of the patients are women.[60,161,214,259,299,311] The disease is usually detected in the third to fifth decade of life, but young children and adults in their 60s and 70s are also affected (see Table 19-4). No more than 15% of patients give a history of contact with jaundiced patients or are found to carry HBsAg in their sera, so that HBV does not appear responsible for this form of chronic hepatitis. Studies for HBsAg in liver tissue and sera and serum HBsAb have usually failed to detect a significant incidence of HBV infection, even though a few reports have detected hepatitis B core antibody in sera from as many as 40% and 38% of patients who are seronegative for HBsAg.[23,107,258] However, the more sensitive RIA was not always used for detection of HBsAg or HBsAb. In addition, evidence of sensitization to drugs has not been obtained, although a history of prior ingestion of drugs of hepatotoxic potential was reported in over 40% of patients in one large study.[311] It is still possible, therefore, that viral and drug exposure may account for a larger percentage of CAH than currently believed.[77]

As previously noted, genetically determined modifications in the host's immune response appear to influence both susceptibility to developing CAH and the manifestations of the clinical response and have led to the notion that this form of CAH is an "autoimmune" disease. However, no evidence for a primary immune disorder exists.

Presenting Features

In approximately one third of patients, the disease begins abruptly and is clinically indistinguishable from typical acute viral hepatitis. However, these patients fail to resolve the initial episode of hepatitis and after several months continue to manifest abnormalities in liver function and complain to a variable extent of fatigue and anorexia. The majority of patients develop the illness insidiously. In Mistilis' study,[214] clinical features at onset included progressive jaundice (61%), severe anorexia (46%), asymptomatic hepatomegaly (36%), abdominal pain (35%), epistaxis (21%), acne (19%), and persistent fever and arthralgia (11% each). Extrahepatic manifestations of the illness may predominate but do so less commonly (Table 19-5). Arthralgia and skin rashes are most common, occurring 20% to 25% of the time; ulcerative colitis, pleurisy-pericarditis, myocarditis, thyroiditis, leg ulcers, and pulmonary complications (including fibrosing alveolitis)

TABLE 19-4. Clinical Features of Chronic Active Hepatitis (Hepatitis B Surface Antigen-Negative)*

	ROYAL PRINCE ALFRED HOSPITAL[214] (SYDNEY, AUSTRALIA) 1968	ROYAL FREE HOSPITAL[60] (LONDON, ENGLAND) 1971	KINGS COLLEGE HOSPITAL[219] (LONDON, ENGLAND) 1973	MAYO CLINIC[311] (ROCHESTER, MN) 1972	YALE-NEW HAVEN HOSPITAL[161] (NEW HAVEN, CT) 1975
No. patients	82	49	47	63	67
Female	79%	76%		71%	69%
Age					
Range	8–72	3–61		12–75	
Mean	~30	39	46	41	>40
Duration of illness at time of diagnosis or treatment	>6 months	18 months	5 months	11 months	>5 months
Onset					
Insidious	68%	65%		44%	
Acute	32%	35%		56%	
Contact with jaundiced patients	7%	16%		<10%	1%
HBsAg		0/21	4%	14%	0
Cirrhosis on biopsy	35%	80%	68%	30–50%	73%

* A minority of patients (0–14%) have serologic evidence of HBsAg.

TABLE 19-5.   Systemic Manifestations of Chronic Active Hepatitis

	ROYAL PRINCE ALFRED HOSPITAL[214] (SYDNEY, AUSTRALIA) 1968	ROYAL FREE HOSPITAL[60] (LONDON, ENGLAND) 1971	KINGS COLLEGE HOSPITAL[219] (LONDON, ENGLAND) 1973	MAYO CLINIC[311] (ROCHESTER, MN) 1972	YALE-NEW HAVEN HOSPITAL[161] (NEW HAVEN, CT) 1975
Chronic diarrhea	28%				
Rash	20%				
Arthralgia-arthritis	18%	14%		25%	6%
Ulcerative colitis	11%	8%		8%	4%
Pleural-pericarditis	11%	6%			6%
Chronic glomerulo-nephritis	7%	2%			
Diabetes	6%	4%			
Myocarditis	4%				
Thyroiditis	4%	5%		3%	

occur less than 5% to 10% of the time.[116] Rare instances of uveitis, mixed connective tissue, disease, macroglobulinemia, and lichen planus have also been described.[34,148,261,268] This multisystemic involvement provides further clinical evidence for a generalized disorder of immune function in such patients. However, skin rashes, glomerulonephritis, neuropathy, and arthritis may also be secondary to HBV infection and immune complex formation (in some cases). In these early studies in the 1950s and 1960s, tests for HBsAg were not available.

Symptoms and Physical Findings

Despite the severity of hepatic damage in many patients, severe weight loss is not common and patients often look remarkably well. Jaundice is the most common physical finding (75%–85%), but is not severe, and serum bilirubin levels average around 5 mg/dl in most series.[60,161,214,219,311] (Table 19-6). Hepatomegaly is also common (70%–80%), and splenomegaly and palmar erythema can be detected 50% of the time. The liver may often be tender to palpation and can be a cause of abdominal pain. In premenopausal females, amenorrhea occurs in one third to one half of the patients, but other endocrine disturbances are much less frequent despite previous emphasis in the literature.[20,176] Cushingoid facies, hirsutism, pigmented striae, and gynecomastia in males occurs less than 10% of the time. Portal hypertension, as evidenced by esophageal varices, is detectable in 10% to 30% of patients at the time of initial diagnosis and increases in incidence slowly thereafter. Ascites is detectable with the same frequency, but portal systemic encephalopathy is present in less than 10% of cases at the time of initial diagnosis.[60,214,311]

Laboratory Findings

Hematology. Mild abnormalities in the blood count may be observed, although they are reported in the literature infrequently (Table 19-7). A normocytic normochromic anemia, mild leukopenia, and thrombocytopenia may be related to mild hypersplenism. Severe anemia, when present, is usually secondary to gastrointestinal tract bleeding or rarely from an autoimmune hemolytic anemia. Coombs'-positive hemolytic anemias have been reported infrequently, but Mackay noted this complication in 3 of 26 patients.[189] Leukocyte and platelet counts are usually either normal or in the low normal range, but an occasional patient may present with severe thrombocytopenia. Eosinophilia is uncommon, but patients with CAH and eosinophilia counts of 9% to 48% have been described.[189,239,362] The combination of Coombs'-positive hemolytic anemia and eosinophilia has also been noted.[239]

Liver Function Tests. Serum aminotransferase levels are elevated in 100% of patients, but the average values range between 200 IU and 300 IU liter.[60,161,214,219,311] Although correlating poorly with histologic evidence of cell necrosis, the aminotransferase is a relatively good reflector of disease activity during initial phases of the disease, but not so when advanced cirrhotic changes are present. Serum bilirubin levels and alkaline phosphatase values are increased in 80% to 90% of cases but are only mildly to moderately deranged. Increases in alkaline phosphatases during the course of the disease may reflect development of a hepatoma. Values of alkaline phosphatases may be increased disproportionately in the growing child. Cholestasis in CAH and postnecrotic cirrhosis has been described, but symptoms of pruritus are distinctly uncommon, and serum bile acid levels usually do not reach levels seen in cholestatic disorders.[61,72] When cholestasis occurs, the disorder may be difficult to distinguish from primary biliary cirrhosis. Hypoalbuminemia is frequently noted; in the Mayo Clinic series, it was less than 3.0 g/dl in 75% of the cases.[311] Hypergammaglobulinemia is also common and usually averages between 5 g and 6 g/dl. Prothrombin

TABLE 19-6. Clinical Features of Chronic Active Hepatitis

	ROYAL PRINCE ALFRED HOSPITAL[214] (SYDNEY, AUSTRALIA) 1968	ROYAL FREE HOSPITAL[60] (LONDON, ENGLAND) 1971	KINGS COLLEGE HOSPITAL[219] (LONDON, ENGLAND) 1973	MAYO CLINIC[311] (ROCHESTER, MN) 1972	YALE-NEW HAVEN HOSPITAL[161] (NEW HAVEN, CT) 1975
Anorexia	63%	Common		27%	
Weakness		Common		67%	
Jaundice	80%	84%		86%	48%
Hepatomegaly	75%	82%		70%	67%
Splenomegaly	49%	53%			54%
Spider nevi	45%	53%			22%
Palmar erythema	33%				
Hepatic tenderness or abdominal pain	30%	12%		40%	
Acne	21%				
Rash	9%				
Encephalopathy	9%	0		5%	
Ascites or edema	9%	27%		24%	24%
Esophageal varices	Infrequent	27%	28%	13%	
Hirsutism	8%				
Arthritis	8%	14%		25%	6%
Cushingoid features	5%				

time abnormalities are not as frequently reported but occur in 50% to 80% of cases and are not usually severe. In Mistilis' series only 10% were prolonged to values less than 50% of normal.[214]

Serologic Abnormalities. Hypergammaglobulinemia represents the most common immunologic abnormality in this form of chronic hepatitis. In the Mayo Clinic series (Table 19-8), 84% were associated with IgG, 57% with IgM, and 29% with IgA.[311] Antinuclear[41,82] and anti–smooth muscle,[150,190] and antiribosomal antibodies[106] are also frequently detected; these findings are helpful in distinguishing this form of hepatitis from HBsAg-positive disease, in which these antibodies are either absent or low in titer. Antithyroid antibodies have been described less frequently.[82] The LE cell phenomenon occurs in 12% to 32% of the larger reported series.[60,161,214,219,311] In one study,[312] LE-positive patients could be differentiated from LE-negative cases by a shorter anicteric period before onset of symptoms (more frequent hepatosplenomegaly; higher levels of bilirubin, gamma globulin and IgG; longer prothrombin time; lower levels of serum albumin). Histologic studies demonstrated a higher incidence of bridging but not multilobular necrosis or cirrhosis. Association of other serologic markers of immunity did not differ in the two groups and there was no difference in response to therapy with corticosteroids. Of patients who responded to corticosteroids, 92% converted to a negative test, whereas those who failed to enter a remission continued to manifest the LE cell phenomenon. Rather than identifying a unique subgroup of patients (formerly called "lupoid hepatitis"), the LE cell phenomenon indicated only that those patients with CAH were more likely to have a more active and severe disease than those in whom the test was negative.[312] In a subsequent study from the same institution, patients with classic autoimmune markers (LE cell or ANA) had responses to therapy similar to those of patients with chronic active hepatitis of uncertain etiology (remission, 77% vs. 69%; treatment failure, 16% vs. 14%). Furthermore, other associated autoimmune disease occurred with equal frequency in patients with or without LE cells or ANAs, and the serum levels of IgG were similar. Thus patients with these autoimmune markers do not seem to represent a clinical group distinct from CAH patients of less certain etiology.[68]

Unlike patients with lupus erythematosus, ANAs to double-stranded DNA have not been detected in patients with autoimmune "lupoid" hepatitis.[123]

Other serologic abnormalities have been described in patients with CAH of the autoimmune type but are of little clinical usefulness, including latex and sheep cell agglutinations,[11,113] biologically false-positive reactions for syphilis,[11,41] antibodies for gastric mucosa, and renal tubular epithelial cells.[82] Serum antibodies to liver-specific lipoproteins, a normal constituent of liver plasma membranes, may be found in up to 60% of patients with autoimmune CAH. Unfortunately, these antibodies are of little diagnostic use because they are found as frequently

TABLE 19-7. Biochemical and Hematologic Tests

	ROYAL PRINCE ALFRED HOSPITAL[214] (SYDNEY, AUSTRALIA) 1968	ROYAL FREE HOSPITAL[60] (LONDON, ENGLAND) 1971	KINGS COLLEGE HOSPITAL[219] (LONDON, ENGLAND) 1973	MAYO CLINIC[311] (ROCHESTER, MN) 1972	YALE-NEW HAVEN HOSPITAL[161] (NEW HAVEN, CT) 1975
BIOCHEMICAL					
Bilirubin (mean)	~80% † 5.1 mg/dl	82% 3.4 mg/dl	2.56 mg/dl	90%	57%
Alkaline phosphatase (mean)	80% 21 KA units	92% 31 KA units	168 IU/liter	89%	64%
Serum albumin (mean)	50% 3.4 g/dl	94% 2.9 g/dl	3.2 g/dl	75% (<3.0 g/dl)	34% (<3.0 g/dl)
Serum globulin* (mean)	~50% 5.5 g/dl	100% 5.1 g/dl	100% 5.1 g/dl	92%	76% (↑ IgG)
SGOT	200–300 IU	19–500 IU	X̄ 247	100%	96%
Prothrombin	10% (<50% of normal)	81% (abnormal)		50% (abnormal)	
HEMATOLOGY					
Hemoglobin		7.3–14.5 g/dl			
Leukocyte count		1,400–10,600			
Platelets		36,000–625,000			

*During course of disease.
† % = percent abnormal.

TABLE 19-8. Serologic Features

	ROYAL PRINCE ALFRED HOSPITAL[214] (SYDNEY, AUSTRALIA) 1968	ROYAL FREE HOSPITAL[60] (LONDON, ENGLAND) 1971	KINGS COLLEGE HOSPITAL[219] (LONDON, ENGLAND) 1973	MAYO CLINIC[311] (ROCHESTER, MN) 1972	YALE-NEW HAVEN HOSPITAL[161] (NEW HAVEN, CT) 1975
LE cells	15%	12%		32%	26%
ANA	83% (15 cases only)	57%	64%	23%	30%
SMA	66% (15 cases only)		43%	71%	46%
AMA			11%		11%
IMMUNOGLOBULIN ↑					
IgG				84%	
IgM				57%	
IgA				29%	

ANA, antinuclear antibody; SMA, smooth muscle antibody; AMA, antimitochondrial antibody.

in HBsAg-positive and HBsAg-negative disease. Titers of these antibodies are highest in CAH but may also be detected in acute viral hepatitis and CPH.[139,147,153,323]

Other Laboratory Tests. The Bromsulphalein (BSP) retention test is now performed infrequently. Retention of BSP in the sera 45 minutes after a 5 mg/kg dose has been used to follow the response of the disease to therapy once serum bilirubin levels have normalized. Studies have also demonstrated a markedly reduced transport maximum (Tm) and storage capacity with the single BSP infusion test in patients with CAH.[118] Although the Tm may return to normal, storage capacity reflects the functioning mass of remaining hepatic parenchyma and may remain reduced if the disease has progressed to the cirrhotic stage. The ^{14}C- or ^{13}C-aminopyrine breath test may be a more accurate assessment of functioning hepatic mass because the microsomal mass of the liver can be assessed.[129] Preliminary studies suggest that the test may be useful in judging response to corticosteroid therapy because values may continue to improve with further therapy after routine tests of liver function have normalized. As a noninvasive test that correlates well with the degree of morphologic impairment in chronic hepatitis (*e.g.,* CPH < CAH with piecemeal necrosis < CAH with bridging necrosis < cirrhosis), it deserves further critical evaluation in patients with chronic hepatitis.[50,216]

Clinical Course

The course of patients with autoimmune CAH is extraordinarily variable. It appears to be dependent on the severity of the underlying liver disease, as reflected by the histologic subtype, as well as therapy with corticosteroids (see Treatment).

In untreated patients, the course is unpredictable and may range from progressive deterioration in liver function over periods of weeks or months to spontaneous remissions and exacerbations. In one study, 20% of patients followed in a clinical trial on placebo sustained a spontaneous remission in clinical symptoms over a period of three years. Remission was accompanied by complete or partial resolution of biochemical abnormalities to normal or improvement of histologic abnormalities by reversion to nonspecific findings or to CPH.[311] However, the disease is usually progressive, and mortality rates are high in the untreated patient. Patients with bridging necrosis and multilobular necrosis are at high risk to develop cirrhosis (three of six, and four of four, respectively, in the Mayo Clinic placebo group[13,311]). Nearly one third of the patients died over a 3-year follow-up period (1 of 6 with bridging necrosis, 5 of 5 with multilobular necrosis, and 6 of 12 with cirrhosis on initial biopsy in the untreated patient). Patients with CAH and piecemeal necrosis without bridging or multilobular necrosis had a more benign prognosis in this study, with no deaths reported during the 3 years.[13] Hepatic encephalopathy and ascites developed in 12 of

19 untreated patients, and three had hemorrhages from esophageal varices.

Mortality rates have also been high in untreated patients or in those receiving only azathioprine in other studies. Fifty-six percent died over a 6-year period at London's Royal Free Hospital,[60] 28% over a 2-year period at King's College Hospital in London,[219] and 65% of untreated patients with CAH died over a 5-year period at Royal Prince Alfred Hospital in Sydney, Australia.[214] In this group of patients, the course was marked by recurrent episodes of disease ranging from malaise and moderate SGOT elevations to manifestations of severe hepatocellular failure. Symptoms usually developed insidiously over weeks and persisted for months in the absence of corticosteroid therapy. Jaundice was episodic, lasting from 2 weeks to 6 months. Ascites and encephalopathy were frequent, and reversible episodes of hepatic coma occurred in 31% of cases. Once cirrhosis was established, episodes of encephalopathy were precipitated by gastrointestinal tract hemorrhage, infection, or congestive heart failure. As signs of portal hypertension appear, the liver diminishes in size and the spleen enlarges. Esophageal varices and hypersplenism develop. Only 6 of 82 patients in this series survived for more than 10 years, with most untreated patients dying in the first 2 years of their illness.[214] Prognostic features that suggested a poor outcome included an abrupt hepatitis-like onset, persistent jaundice, associated colitis, ascites, and episodes of spontaneous or precipitated hepatic encephalopathy.

TREATMENT

Prior to the mid-1960s, the treatment for CAH was largely empirical and based on uncontrolled observations. Because of the uncertainty of the natural history and recognition of variable mortality and hepatic histology, several large randomized controlled trials were initiated. These therapeutic trials demonstrated that corticosteroid therapy has a significant beneficial effect on symptoms, hepatic histology, and survival. However, these conclusions can be applied only to a highly selected group of patients with chronic hepatitis, mainly those with symptomatic HBsAg-negative "autoimmune" type of chronic hepatitis in whom hepatic histology reveals bridging necrosis or multilobular necrosis and/or active postnecrotic cirrhosis. Other subgroups (those with viral- or drug-related chronic hepatitis) represented only a small percentage of the patients entered into these therapeutic trials. The efficacy of corticosteroid therapy in these patients thus remains untested.

Initial Response

Four controlled trials started between 1963 and 1968 were published in 1969, 1971, 1972, and 1973.[60,64,219,311] Three of these trials have been critically analyzed by Wright and co-workers.[367] In the largest of these studies (and the only one of the three in which detailed histologic features were correlated with outcome[13,311]), 63 patients were initially randomized to treatment regimes of prednisone, or prednisone and azathioprine or placebo. Prednisone alone or in combination was shown to be superior to azathioprine 100 mg alone and placebo. In this study, 20% of patients failed to respond to treatment with prednisone or combination; this group had longer duration of symptoms, longer prothrombin times, high SGPT levels, and histologic evidence of cirrhosis, indicating more advanced disease. A similar number, 20%, experienced remission without treatment. Most of the remaining 60% who responded to treatment had histologic evidence of bridging necrosis and multilobular necrosis.

Survival

All three therapeutic trials demonstrated that corticosteroid treatment significantly improved survival. In the initial 3½ year follow-up of the Mayo Clinic study, only 6% died in the treated group, compared with 30% in the azathioprine-alone or placebo group.[311] In a longer 10-year follow-up of the Royal Free group,[160] 63% of treated patients were alive at 10 years, compared with only 27% in the control group (Fig. 19-8). The median survival in this treatment group was 12.2 years, compared with 3.3 years in the control group. The effect of corticosteroids on mortality was most pronounced in the first 5 years of therapy, since most (87.5%) of the deaths in the placebo group occurred in this early period.

Histology

Many patients already had established postnecrotic cirrhosis at the time of entry into the therapeutic trials, but only the Mayo Clinic study[13,311] provides sufficient data to analyze the effect of corticosteroids on histologic subtypes in CAH. In these studies, corticosteroids were most effective in terms of improved survival or prevention of progression of liver injury in patients with bridging necrosis, multilobular necrosis, or active postnecrotic cirrhosis. Patients with advanced inactive postnecrotic cirrhosis were less responsive to therapy and demonstrated a high incidence of corticosteroid side-effects. The data do not permit a conclusion on the therapeutic effect of corticosteroids in patients with histologic evidence of CAH (piecemeal necrosis) in whom bridging necrosis or multilobular necrosis was absent because of the small number of patients in this subgroup in the original controlled trial.[13,311] However, several other studies indicate that this lesion does not result in progressive liver disease[63,231] so that it is unlikely that other therapeutic trials will ever be undertaken in this subgroup of patients.

The incidence of histologic cure in the initial Mayo Clinic trials was 12%, when defined as a lack of residual functional abnormality and of inflammatory changes on biopsy after long-term follow-up. Remission of disease occurred at a mean interval of 52 months of follow-up and 17 months after the last course of treatment. Several courses of treatment were generally required to reach this end-point.

Ten-year follow-up studies of patients without cirrhosis at the Mayo Clinic indicate that histologic evidence of cirrhosis will develop either during or after cessation of treatment in 37% of patients by 5 years and 47% within 10 years.[74] However, the development of cirrhosis did not appear to affect immediate morbidity, and subsequent 5-year survival estimates in these cirrhotic patients was 93%. Thus the prognosis of patients with CAH without cirrhosis who are treated with corticosteroids is extremely good, whether or not they subsequently develop histologic evidence of cirrhosis. The incidence of ascites, encephalopathy, and esophageal varices was less than 10% in either group.

Fig. 19-8. Life-table survival curves of control and prednisolone-treated patients. ⊙---⊙ controls; ×——× prednisolone. (Kirk AP et al: Gut 21:78, 1980)

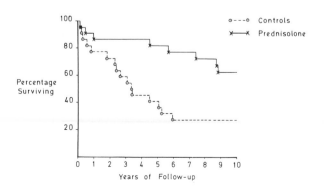

SURVIVAL BY TREATMENT GROUP

Therapeutic Regimen

From cumulative Mayo Clinic data,[273,275,311,318,319] a combination of 10 mg prednisone and 50 mg azathioprine (Imuran) appears to be the regimen that best minimizes side-effects and optimizes the clinical, biochemical, and histologic response and survival. Although the initial trial began with a dose of 100 mg Imuran, 50 mg in combination with prednisone was found to be optimal. This regimen gave a similarly high remission rate as prednisone in a dose of 20 mg per day. Even though the side-effects of the combination therapy were still appreciable, they were reduced in comparison with prednisone alone. Alternate day corticosteroids, equivalent to 10 mg of prednisone daily, were also used in the Mayo Clinic trials. Although clinical and biochemical remission occurred in nearly three quarters of the patients, only 19% had histologic evidence of remission. This is in contrast to the combined therapy group in which the histologic remission rate was 57%. Predictably, however, the incidence of side-effects was less than half that seen with prednisone 20 mg daily, and about two thirds of that observed when combination therapy was used. Alternate-day corticosteroids may have an advantage in children with chronic hepatitis, since linear growth may be stimulated.[55]

Penicillamine has been used successfully in a few patients when corticosteroids were unable to be administered.

Duration of Therapy

In the two largest studies, duration of treatment ranged from a mean of approximately 2 years at the Mayo Clinic,[70,311] to 4½ years in the London study.[60] In the Mayo Clinic study, 87% of those entering remission did so within 3 years. The risk of developing side-effects was 38% during the 3 years; this risk increased by only 4% during the next year. However, by continuing treatment beyond 4 years, the risk of side-effects was nearly twice the probability of remission (13% vs. 7%).[75]

In later reports from the Mayo Clinic, biochemical, histologic, and clinical remission was achieved in 60% of patients followed for 2.5 years and 83% followed for 4 years.[70]

Many patients with autoimmune CAH will relapse following withdrawal of immunosuppressive therapy.[69,128,202] In a Kings College study, 25 of 30 patients on long-term maintenance treatment developed reactivation of their disease with significant elevations in transaminase levels, severe symptoms, and histologic evidence of piecemeal necrosis and lobular hepatitis. These relapses occurred between 5 and 32 weeks after discontinuation of therapy and responded to reinstitution of treatment.[128]

In the Mayo Clinic series, only 3 of 32 patients in whom cirrhosis was present when treatment was initiated remained inactive after withdrawal of therapy 4 years later. Most of these patients respond to reinstitution of therapy. In patients who reverted to normal liver histology, 13 of 18 remained in remission after treatment withdrawal.[69] Cirrhosis is likely to develop in those that relapse off therapy.[70]

Relapse is also frequent in children with autoimmune CAH and cirrhosis, and treatment should be continued for several years before attempting withdrawal.[200] Therefore long-term immunosuppression at the lowest possible maintenance doses is usually necessary in patients with chronic active hepatitis of the autoimmune type or in whom etiology is uncertain.

Therapy of HBsAg-Positive CAH

The treatment of HBsAg-positive CAH has been frustrating to clinicians because of the lack of therapeutic agents with undisputed beneficial properties. Corticosteroid therapy is generally contraindicated in most patients with chronic hepatitis B disease because it is associated with serologic evidence of enhanced viral replication[257,286]

with an increase in complications and death rate.[177] In addition, corticosteroids do not improve suppressor cell activity in *in vitro* incubations of lymphocytes from HBsAg-positive patients in marked contrast to lymphocytes from patients with autoimmune hepatitis. Nevertheless, corticosteroids continue to be given as a therapeutic trial by some clinicians, and a favorable clinical response has been observed in highly selected cases with hyperimmune features and clinical deterioration.

Controversy over the use of corticosteroids in selected HBsAg-positive patients remains in part because the clinical and histologic features of this disease are much more heterogeneous than in the "autoimmune group," and careful distinctions have not always been made between patient subgroups when assessing therapeutic responses. For example, as clearly documented by the Stanford group,[355] the 5-year survival of patients with chronic hepatitis B disease and histologic evidence of CPH and CAH without cirrhosis is so good (97% and 86% respectively) that therapeutic intervention to alter the natural history of the disease would not be practical. In contrast, the prognosis for patients with chronic hepatitis B and active cirrhosis at presentation is as dire as that for untreated patients with autoimmune CAH (compare Figs. 19-7 and 19-8), and it is in this group that therapeutic intervention is most needed. Unfortunately, therapeutic trials of corticosteroids in chronic hepatitis B disease have usually not included clear-cut distinctions between the histologic subgroups seen in chronic active hepatitis B.

Initial corticosteroid trials contained only a few patients with chronic HBV disease. In the Mayo Clinic trial, 13 HBsAg-positive patients were treated, and higher treatment failure rates were observed than in HBsAg-negative patients. Clinical and biochemical improvement was observed intermittently when higher doses of prednisone were used. Nonetheless, complete remission did not result, and treatment failures were noted particularly when the HBeAg was also positive,[342] a finding also observed by others.[260] Meyer zum Buschenfelde[206] also reported a poorer response to corticosteroid treatment in HBsAg-positive patients with hypergammaglobulinemia. During a 2- to 5-year period, only 18% and 23% of these patients improved histologically and biochemically, respectively, in contrast to improvement in both these clinical features in 77% of HBsAg-negative patients.

In an often-quoted prospective randomized trial from Hong Kong, Lam and co-workers actually concluded that corticosteroids had an overall deleterious effect when administered to HBsAg-positive patients with CAH, resulting in an increased rate of complications and death.[177] In addition, progression to cirrhosis was not prevented by corticosteroids, and the treatment resulted in a significant increase in erosion of the limiting plate and a larger quantity of HBsAg and HBcAg in the liver biopsy specimens than in the control group.[370] Criticisms of this study include (1) a high carrier rate of HBV in their patient population, increasing the fortuitous association of HBsAg positively and chronic hepatitis; (2) a high incidence of cirrhosis (50%) upon entry into the trial, a patient group in which treatment failure is often observed; (3) a relatively low degree of activity of disease as assessed by the mean values of the SGPT levels; and (4) prior treatment of some of the study group with prednisone. Despite these concerns, we can conclude that corticosteroids are harmful in patients with advanced HBsAg-positive cirrhosis and relatively inactive disease and unnecessary in the larger number of patients with HBV who have mild disease in which CAH is observed without bridging necrosis or an active cirrhosis. It remains undetermined whether corticosteroids are beneficial in the selected subgroup of symptomatic patients with severe CAH secondary to HBV.

More favorable reports have been published from Italy. In one large uncontrolled multicenter retrospective study of 867 patients, the combination of prednisone and azathioprine resulted in more frequent improvement and less frequent deterioration than either treatment alone or placebo.[109] However, these studies were uncontrolled. A prospective randomized trial also reported clinical improvement and less frequent deterioration in patients treated with the combination of corticosteroids and imuran, but only in a subgroup of patients that had already developed antibody to e-antigen.[199]

Short-term high-dose corticosteroid therapy with abrupt withdrawal has been suggested in an effort to induce immune response to the replicating virus as the immune system rebounds from the corticosteroid suppression. Some exacerbation in disease activity has been observed after corticosteroid withdrawal, but remissions have been infrequent.[257] Recently corticosteroid withdrawal has been combined with antiviral therapy in a renewed effort to eliminate the ongoing viral infection[371] (see later section on antiviral therapy).

Corticosteroid therapy is also ineffective in altering the clinical deterioration of chronic hepatitis B disease with superimposed delta infection.[262,267]

Suggested Therapeutic Approach

HBsAg-Positive Chronic Active Hepatitis

In the absence of critical data, the rationale for therapy in HBsAg-positive patients is empiric. We believe that only symptomatic patients with life-threatening HBV e-antigen-negative-related disease and potentially progressive histologic lesions (bridging necrosis, multilobular necrosis, or active postnecrotic cirrhosis) should be treated with corticosteroids, recognizing that there is at present no evidence that this therapy either prevents progression of the lesion or alters survival. However, a few patients derive symptomatic relief and demonstrate biochemical improvement with a dosage schedule that minimizes corticosteroids' side-effects (see dosage schedules). Long-term therapy is not advocated if there is no improvement within 6 weeks, or if side-effects develop.

Because treatment is contingent on the subject's evaluation of symptoms, careful and meticulous assessment of these symptoms is imperative. Patients who are jaundiced and who have anorexia, nausea, or right upper-quadrant discomfort do not present problems in terms of evaluation; however, the more common complaints are lassitude, malaise, and easy fatigability. Patients should be questioned as to whether a full day's work can be completed; whether the symptoms have caused loss of job, change of job, or work-related problems; whether significantly more time is spent resting or sleeping; and whether effort tolerance is severely compromised. Patients often do not volunteer symptoms until directly questioned, and then only in retrospect realize that their entire lifestyle has changed because of lassitude, irritability, and easy fatigability. Because many of these symptoms are protean and may be caused by other disease processes, it is important to establish that the symptoms are secondary to liver disease before embarking on a therapeutic trial. Therefore, histologic evidence of chronic *active* disease is an essential prerequisite.

We recommend a therapeutic trial of corticosteroids only when symptoms and a progressive histologic lesion are present and the e-antigen is negative. The patient is reevaluated after 6 weeks and the therapeutic trial terminated if symptoms are not alleviated or if biochemical improvement does not occur (notably, a fall in bilirubin in the jaundiced patient), or corticosteroid side-effects develop. Otherwise, corticosteroid therapy should be continued in a dosage that does not cause significant side-effects. Serologic markers of viral replication increase with immunosuppressive therapy* so that increased infectivity is a side-effect of corticosteroids in patients who are e-antigen positive. Alternative therapeutic options (antiviral therapy) are reviewed in the final section.

HBsAg-Negative Autoimmune Chronic Active Hepatitis

In the presence of bridging necrosis or multilobular necrosis on biopsy, regardless of the existence of postnecrotic cirrhosis, treatment should be instituted. The vast majority of patients are jaundiced or otherwise symptomatic and have considerable elevations in transaminase levels, together with the other biochemical and serologic features described above. In the asymptomatic patient, liver function tests usually show minimal impairment, but if bridging necrosis or multilobular necrosis is present on biopsy, a therapeutic trial of corticosteroids appears to be indicated. Histologic reevaluation may be necessary 6 months after starting therapy to guide decisions about the duration of therapy.

---

* Scullard GH et al: The effect of immunosuppressive therapy on hepatitis B viral infection in patients with chronic hepatitis. Gastroenterology 77:40A, 1979.

Non-A, Non-B–Related Chronic Active Hepatitis

As pointed out above, chronic non-A, non-B hepatitis is often asymptomatic and a spontaneous biochemical and clinical resolution can occur.[25] It is therefore very difficult to evaluate the effect of corticosteroids, particularly since few patients have been treated, and there have been no controlled trials of corticosteroid therapy in this disease. We would, therefore, initiate a therapeutic trial only in symptomatic patients with severe histologic features (bridging or multilobular necrosis or active cirrhosis). More definitive recommendations must await more critical data.

Specifics of Therapy

Recognition of Side-Effects and of Absolute or Relative Contraindications

Before initiating therapy with corticosteroids (Table 19-9) (particularly since such therapy may well continue for a number of years), a review of potential contraindications to therapy should be followed. The presence of any single factor may not be an absolute contraindication to therapy, but the frequency of follow-up and attention to the relevant preexisting complications clearly permits more effective management of the patient. Major contraindications in which corticosteroids would not be given, or, if so, only with great care, are insulin-requiring diabetes and symptomatic osteoporosis. Leukocyte counts less than 2,500 or thrombocytopenia less than 50,000 are absolute contraindications to the use of azathioprine.

Initiation

Therapy is begun with prednisone or prednisolone (20–40 mg), with or without azathioprine (50 mg). Prednisone is metabolized to prednisolone in the liver and, for this

reason, prednisolone is the theoretically preferable drug. However, prednisolone is more expensive and is not uniformly available in all hospital formularies. Furthermore, adequate blood levels of prednisolone can be achieved with the less expensive prednisone even when administered to patients with severe hepatic insufficiency.[335] Also, it is important to administer the same preparation from the same manufacturer throughout the course of therapy, since the potency of the corticosteroid varies significantly from one manufacturer to another. Prednisone is therefore our choice of drug. Starting daily doses may vary from 15 mg to 60 mg, but it is our general practice to initiate therapy with 30 mg to 40 mg in the patient who is severely symptomatic and then reduce this dose over a 4- to 6-week period until a maintenance dose is found, usually less than 20 mg/day.

Maintenance

Most patients become asymptomatic and have a significant fall in transaminase and bilirubin levels within the first week or two of therapy. Later, serum globulin levels fall. It is ideal to obtain a state of remission in which biochemical normality is achieved. If this can be achieved at a daily dose of 10 mg, the side-effects of corticosteroids can be kept to a minimum. In some cases, enzyme and γ-globulin levels do not normalize, and the lowest possible dosage must be used which minimizes side-effects but keeps enzyme levels at a level preferably no greater than twice normal. Over the long term, this dose should be less than 15 mg/day to minimize side-effects, although susceptibilities of different patients can be quite variable. Once remission is achieved, the dosage can gradually be reduced, even to as low as 5 mg/day particularly if azathioprine is also used as maintenance therapy. Treatment should be continued for at least 6 months, even with earlier remission, since the rate of relapse is significantly higher if therapy is discontinued before this time.[318,319] Azathioprine is generally maintained at a dose of 50 mg per day. Hepatotoxic and bone marrow depression are uncommon at this dosage.

Liver Biopsy

Assessment of histologic response may be useful 6 to 12 months after initiation of therapy to monitor progress and help determine the need for further therapy. The need for follow-up liver biopsies is dependent on the patient's subsequent course and thus must be individualized. Once cirrhosis has been established histologically, there is less need to repeat the biopsy unless their is a major change in the patient's clinical course.

Exercise, Diet, Alcohol, Drugs

There have been no controlled trials addressing the questions of exercise, diet, alcohol, and drugs in patients with

TABLE 19-9.   Use of Corticosteroids

FACTORS FAVORING USE OF CORTICOSTEROIDS	INITIAL DOSE	MAINTENANCE DOSE
Symptoms		
HBsAg-Negative		
Autoantibodies	Azathioprine 50 mg	50 mg
↑ IgG		
Female sex	Prednisone 20–40 mg	10 mg
Histology:		
Multilobular		
necrosis		
Bridging necrosis		
Active postnecrotic		
cirrhosis		

CAH. The patient is encouraged to live as normal a life as possible; exercise and exertion are encouraged and limited by the point of fatigue, and the patient is otherwise not restricted from full activities. Alcohol is not forbidden, but we recommend that patients minimize alcohol intake to less than 2 ounces to 3 ounces per week, so that alcohol-induced fatty liver or abnormal liver tests will not obscure evaluation. There is no evidence that the liver is unable to metabolize these relatively small amounts of alcohol.

Aspirin is proscribed, both because of its erosive effect on the gastric mucosa and the abnormalities in platelet function that occur. Obviously, this recommendation is most important in patients who have esophageal varices. Acetaminophen may be administered up to a maximum dose of 1 g daily, since there are reports of therapeutic doses causing significant hepatotoxicity when taken chronically.[38] Drugs producing hypersensitivity reactions are not likely to cause liver injury in patients with preexisting liver disease more frequently, but if they do, the consequences may be considerably greater. The choice of common therapeutic agents such as Aldomet, Halothane, and Thorazine should be based on clinical judgment; we would use these agents when they are clearly the best drug and there is no suitable alternative. The one exception is isoniazid, since there is a 10% to 20% likelihood that it will produce elevations in transaminase levels, which could result in confusion in evaluating response to therapy.

Antiviral Agents and Other Alternative Forms of Treatment of HBsAg-Positive Chronic Active Hepatitis

Because of the detrimental effects of corticosteroid therapy in most patients with chronic hepatitis B infection, alternative forms of treatment have been sought, focusing particularly on the antiviral agents, interferon and adenine arabinoside (Table 19-10). Initial uncontrolled trials with human fibroblast, leukocyte, and lymphoblastoid interferons were associated with a suppression in serologic markers of active HBV replication, but the effect was usually transient and there was little or no improvement of disease activity.[121,159,183,205] Similar effects were observed in infected chimpanzees.[254] Controlled trials, necessitated

TABLE 19-10.   Antiviral Therapy and Other Alternative Therapies in Chronic Hepatitis B

Interferons
Adenine arabinoside
Acyclovir
Transfer factor
Levamizole
Quinicrine
Combination corticosteroid withdrawal and antiviral
    agents
Combination of two antiviral agents

by 10% to 30% annual spontaneous remission rates and loss of serologic markers of viral replication,[138,276,277] have been limited but show no alteration in the natural course of the disease.[276,277] Treatment with larger doses and for longer periods of time has recently been possible with the production of leukocyte interferon from *Escherichia coli* by recombinant DNA technology. This form of interferon also suppresses HBV replication,[86,121,234] but adequate controlled trials are not yet available. Side-effects include fever, chills, and flulike symptoms. Prednisone withdrawal combined with interferon therapy may prove to be more effective.[234]

More patients have been treated with adenine arabinoside, a purine nucleoside with antiviral activity against DNA-containing viruses.[295] Like the interferons, this antiviral agent also suppresses DNA polymerase.[19,137,287,288,356] However, even multiple courses do not induce significant remission.[234] Controlled trials have been limited, but treatment for up to 4 to 12 weeks has failed to induce long-term remission rates that exceed yearly spontaneous rates of HBeAg clearance of 10% to 30%.[136,138,184,276,288] Significant side-effects included malaise and a severe prolonged neuopathic pain syndrome.[136,184] Preliminary studies have also combined short-term corticosteroid withdrawal (which induces a decline in DNA polymerase activity)[257,286] with adenine arabinoside (ARA-A) therapy.[371] This combination appears to be more effective in stimulating seroconversion than ARA-A alone, but further analysis is necessary. The rationale is based on corticosteroid withdrawal lowering the virus load.[257,307]

Other therapeutic modalities have been tried with consistent lack of success. Transfer factor, an immunostimulant, has been administered to patients with chronic hepatitis B infection, but all results have been disappointing, since long-lasting therapeutic effects have not been observed.[146,169,303,330] Levamizole, an immunostimulant, has been administered to patients with chronic hepatitis of diverse etiologies in a multicenter double-blind trial that included patients with chronic hepatitis B disease. However no differences in therapeutic effects were obtained between controls and treatment groups. One case of agranulocytosis was observed.[230] Levamizole is also without effect in chronic delta hepatitis.[58] Quinicrine, a DNA intercalating agent that decreases DNA polymerase activity *in vitro,* was also found to be ineffective in a small randomized trial in chronic HBV infection.[36] Acyclovir, a virustatic agent that inhibits HBV-DNA polymerase, has received only limited trial in patients with chronic hepatitis B infection, but side-effects are significant and include renal impairment.[357,358] Preliminary uncontrolled studies indicate that the combination of interferon and acyclovir is more effective in reducing DNA polymerase and HBeAg levels than either therapy alone.[278]

Liver Transplantation

Patients with CAH have been candidates for liver transplantation when the disease process has progressed to cirrhosis and clinical signs of liver failure have developed that can no longer be reasonably managed by medical therapy. The optimum time for transplantation has not been established because of the relatively high mortality rates associated with this radical form of therapy. However most agree that an assessment of quality of life is helpful in making this decision. When patients no longer can work and are limited in their physical activity to the point that they are essentially housebound, transplantation is a viable option. Candidates include those with autoimmune chronic hepatitis and chronic non-A, non-B hepatitis. Most centers considered the presence of chronic hepatitis B infection a contraindication to autologous human liver transplants because the disease recurrence rates are high and may be facilitated by the immunosuppression[135] required to prevent organ rejection.

However, treatment with HBV hyperimmune globulin before, during, and immediately after transplantation has now been recommended by some to minimize recurrence of disease. Survival rates for patients receiving cyclosporin therapy following transplantation for CAH are estimated at 40% to 50% at 1 to 3 years after surgery.[280] Recurrence of disease in a transplanted patient with autoimmune hepatitis has been reported, emphasizing the role of the host immune response.[226]

REFERENCES

1. Aach RD et al: Transfusion-transmitted viruses: Interim analysis of hepatitis among transfused and non-transfused patients. In Vyas GN et al (eds): Viral Hepatitis, pp 383. Philadelphia, Franklin Institute Press, 1978
2. Acute and chronic hepatitis revisited—Review by an international group. Lancet 2:914, 1977
3. Ahrens EH Jr et al: Primary biliary cirrhosis. Medicine 29:299, 1950
4. Alarcon-Segovia D et al: Significance of the lupus erythematosus cell phenomenon in older women with chronic hepatic disease. Mayo Clin Proc 40:193, 1965
5. Alberti A et al: T-lymphocyte cytotoxicity to HBsAg-coated target cells in hepatitis B virus infection. Gut 18:1004, 1977
6. Alsted G: Studies on malignant hepatitis. Am J Med Sci 213:257, 1947
7. Alter HJ et al: Non-A, non-B hepatitis: A review and interim report of an ongoing prospective study. In Vyas GN et al (eds): Viral Hepatitis, p 359. Philadelphia, Franklin Institute Press, 1978
8. Aranha GV et al: Cholecystectomy in cirrhotic patients: A formidable operation. Am J Surg 143:55, 1982
9. Aronson AR, Montgomery MM: Chronic liver disease with a "lupus erythematosus-like syndrome." Arch Intern Med 104:544, 1959
10. Arrisoni A et al: Levamisole and chronic delta hepatitis. Ann Intern Med 98:1024, 1983
11. Atwater EC, Jacox RF: The latex-fixation test in patients with liver disease. Ann Intern Med 58:419, 1963
12. Baggenstoss AH et al: The pathology of primary biliary cirrhosis with emphasis on histogenesis, Am J Clin Pathol 42:259, 1964
13. Baggenstoss AH et al: Chronic active liver disease. The range of histologic lesions, their response to treatment, and evolution. Hum Pathol 3:183, 1972
14. Baker AL et al: Polyarteritis associated with Australia antigen positive hepatitis. Gastroenterology 62:105, 1972
15. Bamber M et al: Clinical, serological, and histological features of non-A, non-B (NANB) hepatitis. Gastroenterology 79:1098, 1980 (abstr)
16. Barker HM et al: Chronic hepatitis in the Mediterranean theater: A new clinical syndrome. JAMA 129:653, 1945
17. Bartholomew LG et al: Further observations on hepatitis and cirrhosis in young women with positive clot tests for lupus erythematosus. Gastroenterology 39:730, 1960
18. Bartholomew LG et al: Hepatitis and cirrhosis in women with positive clot tests for lupus erythematosus. N Engl J Med 259:947, 1958
19. Bassendine MF et al: Adenine arabinoside therapy in HBsAg-positive chronic liver disease: A controlled study. Gastroenterology 80:1014, 1981
20. Bearn AG et al: The problem of chronic liver disease in young women. Am J Med 21:3, 1956
21. Beasley RP et al: Hepatocellular carcinoma and HBV: A prospective study of 22,707 men in Taiwan. Lancet 2:1129, 1981
22. Becker MD et al: Prognosis of chronic persistent hepatitis. Lancet 1:53, 1970
23. Benhamou JP et al: Core antigen in chronic hepatitis. Lancet 1:817, 1976
24. Berg NO, Eriksson S: Liver disease in adults with alpha$_1$-antitrypsin deficiency. N Engl J Med 287:1264, 1972
25. Berman M et al: The chronic sequelae of non-A, non-B hepatitis. Ann Intern Med 91:1, 1979
26. Bergstrand H: Über die akute und chronische gelbe Leberatrophie mit besonderer Berucksichtigung ihres epidemischen Auftretens in Schweden im Jahre 1927, 114. Leipzig, Georg Thieme Verlag, 1930
27. Bettley FR: The "L.E. cell" phenomenon in active chronic viral hepatitis. Lancet 2:724, 1955
28. Bhathal PS, Powell LW: Primary intrahepatic obliterating cholangitis: A possible variant of sclerosing cholangitis, Gut 10:886, 1969
29. Bianchi P et al: Occurrence of Australia antigen in chronic hepatitis in Italy. Gastroenterology 63:482, 1972
30. Bjorneboe M, Brochner–Mortensen K: Om prognosen for hepatitis acuta. Ugeskr Laeger 107:715, 1945
31. Black M et al: Isoniazid-associated hepatitis in 114 patients. Gastroenterology 69:289, 1975
32. Black M et al: Nitrofurantoin-induced chronic active hepatitis. Ann Intern Med 92:62, 1980
33. Blackstone MD, Nemchausky BA: Cholangiographic abnormalities in ulcerative colitis—associated pericholangitis which resembles sclerosing cholangitis. Am J Dig Dis 23:579, 1978
34. Bloom JN, Rabinowicz IM, Shulman S: Uveitis complicating autoimmune chronic active hepatitis. Am J Dis Child 137:1175, 1983
35. Blumberg BS et al: Sex distribution of Australia antigen. Arch Intern Med 130:227, 1972
36. Bodenheimer HC Jr, Schaffner F, Vernace S et al: Randomized controlled trial of quinacrine for the treatment of HBsAg-positive chronic hepatitis. Hepatology 3:936, 1983
37. Bomford A, Williams R: Long-term results of venesection therapy in idiopathic haemochromatosis. Q J Med 45:611, 1976
38. Bonkowsky HL et al: Chronic hepatic inflammation and

fibrosis due to low doses of paracetamol. Lancet 1:1016, 1978

39. Bothwell PW, Martin D, Macara AW et al: Infectious hepatitis in Bristol 1959–1962. Br Med J 2:1613, 1963

40. Bothwell TH, Charlton RW: Hemochromatosis. In Schiff L (ed): Diseases of the Liver, 4th ed, p 971. Philadelphia, JB Lippincott, 1975

41. Bouchier IAD et al (eds): Serological abnormalities in patients with liver disease. Br Med J 1:592, 1964

42. Boyer JL: Chronic hepatitis: A perspective on classification and determinants of prognosis. Gastroenterology 70:1161, 1976

43. Boyer JL: The diagnosis and pathogenesis of clinical variants in viral hepatitis. Am J Clin Pathol 65:898, 1976

44. Boyer JL, Klatskin G: Pattern of necrosis in acute viral hepatitis. Prognostic value of bridging (subacute hepatic necrosis). N Engl J Med 283:1063, 1970

45. Bradbear RA, Robinson WN, Cooksley WG et al: Are the causes and presentation of chronic hepatitis changing? An analysis of 104 cases over 15 years. Q J Med 53:279, 1984

46. Brighton WD et al: Changes induced by hepatitis serum in cultured liver cells. Nature 232:57, 1971

47. Brummer DL: Isoniazid and liver disease. Ann Intern Med 75:643, 1971

48. Brzosko WJ et al: Glomerulonephritis associated with hepatitis B surface antigen immune complexes in children. Lancet 2:478, 1974

49. Buckley BH et al: Distinction in active chronic hepatitis based on circulating hepatitis-associated antigen. Lancet 2:1323, 1970

50. Carlisle R et al: The relationship between conventional liver tests, quantitative function tests, and histopathology in cirrhosis. Dig Dis 24:358, 1979

51. Chalmers TC et al: The treatment of acute infectious hepatitis: Controlled studies of the effects of diet, rest, and physical reconditioning on the acute course of the disease and on the incidence of relapses and residual abnormalities. J Clin Invest 34:1163, 1955

52. Chalmers TC et al: Hepatolenticular degeneration (Wilson's disease) as a form of idiopathic cirrhosis. N Engl J Med 256:235, 1957

53. Chapman RWG et al: Primary sclerosing cholangitis: Review of clinical, cholangiographic, and hepatic histological features. Gut 20(10):A954, 1979

54. Chen DS, Lai MY, Sung JL: Delta agent infection in patients with chronic liver diseases and hepatocellular carcinoma: An infrequent finding in Taiwan. Hepatology 4:502, 1984

55. Chisari FV, Bieber MS, Josepho CA et al: Functional properties of cytotoxic effector cell killing of targets that naturally express hepatitis B surface antigen and liver specific lipoprotein. J Immunol 126:45, 1981

56. Clark JH, Fitzgerald JF: Effect of exogenous corticosteroid therapy on growth in children with HBsAg-negative chronic aggressive hepatitis. J Pediatr Gastroenterol Nutr 3:72, 1984

57. Cochrane AMC et al: Antibody-dependent cell mediated (K cell) cytotoxicity against isolated hepatocytes in chronic active hepatitis. Lancet 1:441, 1976

58. Colombo M, Cambieri R, Rumi MG et al: Long-term delta superinfection in hepatitis B surface antigen carriers and its relationship to the course of chronic hepatitis. Gastroenterology 85:235, 1983

59. Combes B et al: Glomerulonephritis with deposition of Australia antigen-antibody complexes in glomerular basement membrane. Lancet 2:234, 1971

60. Cook GC et al: Controlled prospective trial of corticosteroid therapy in active chronic hepatitis. Q J Med 40:159, 1971

61. Cooksley WGE et al: Cholestasis in active chronic hepatitis. Dig Dis 17:495, 1972

62. Cooksley WGE et al: Australia antigen in acute chronic hepatitis in Australia: Results in 130 patients from three centers. Aust N Z J Med 2:261, 1972

63. Cooksley WGE et al: The prognosis of chronic active hepatitis without cirrhosis in relation to bridging necrosis. Hepatology 6:345–348, 1986

64. Copenhagen Study Group for Liver Diseases: Effect of prednisone on the survival of patients with cirrhosis of the liver. Lancet 1:119, 1969

65. Cowan DH et al: Occurrence of hepatitis and hepatitis B surface antigen in adult patients with acute leukemia. CMA Journal 112:693, 1975

66. Crapper RM, Bhathaland PS, Mackay IR: Chronic active hepatitis in alcoholic patients. Liver 3:327, 1983

67. Cullinan ER: Idiopathic jaundice (often recurrent) associated with subacute hepatic necrosis of the liver. St. Bartholomew's Hosp Rep 49:55, 1936

68. Czaja AJ et al: Autoimmune features as determinants of prognosis in steroid-treated chronic active hepatitis of uncertain etiology. Gastroenterology 85:713–717, 1983

69. Czaja AJ et al: Complete resolution of inflammatory activity following corticosteroid treatment of HBsAg-negative chronic active hepatitis. Hepatology 4:622, 1984

70. Czaja AJ et al: Clinical features and prognosis of severe chronic active liver disease (CALD) after corticosteroid-induced remission. Gastroenterology 78:518, 1980

71. Czaja AJ et al: Corticosteroid-treated chronic active hepatitis in remission: Uncertain prognosis of chronic persistent hepatitis. N Engl J Med 304:1, 1981

72. Datta DV et al: Postnecrotic cirrhosis with chronic cholestasis. Gut 4:223, 1963

73. Davis GL et al: Spontaneous reactivation of chronic hepatitis B virus infection. Gastroenterology 86:230, 1984

74. Davis GL et al: Development and prognosis of histologic cirrhosis in corticosteroid-treated hepatitis B surface antigen-negative chronic active hepatitis. Gastroenterology 87:1222, 1984

75. Davis GL, Czaja AJ: Prolonged steroid therapy for severe chronic active liver disease (CALD): A diminishing return (abstr)? Gastroenterology 78:1153, 1980

76. DeGroote J et al: A classification of chronic hepatitis. Lancet 2:626, 1968

77. Dienstag JL: Hepatitis B virus infection: More than meets the eye. Gastroenterology 75:1172, 1978

78. Dienstag JL: Non-A, non-B hepatitis: I. recognition, epidemiology and clinical features: II. Experimental transmission, putative virus agents and markers, and prevention. Gastroenterology 85:439, 743, 1983

79. Dienstag JL et al: Etiology of sporadic hepatitis B surface antigen-negative hepatitis. Ann Intern Med 87:1, 1977

80. Dietrichson O et al: The incidence of oxyphenisatin-induced liver damage in chronic non-alcoholic liver disease. A controlled investigation. Scand J Gastroenterol 9:473, 1974

81. Dietzman DE et al: Hepatitis B surface antigen (HBsAg) and antibody to HBsAg: Prevalence in homosexual men. JAMA 238:2625, 1977

82. Doniach D et al: Tissue antibodies in primary biliary cirrhosis, active chronic (lupoid) hepatitis, cryptogenic cirrhosis and other liver diseases and their clinical implications. Clin Exp Immunol 1:237, 1966

83. Drew JS et al: Cross-reactivity between hepatitis B surface antigen and a male-associated antigen. Birth Defects 14(6A): 91, 1978

84. Dudley FJ et al: Cellular immunity and hepatitis-associated Australia antigen liver disease. Lancet 1:723, 1972

85. Duffy J et al: Polyarthritis, polyarteritis, and hepatitis B. Medicine 55:19, 1976

86. Dusheiko G, Dibisceglie A, Bowyer S et al: Recombinant leukocyte interferon treatment of chronic hepatitis B. Hepatology 5:556, 1985

87. Dusheiko GM, Song E, Bowyer S et al: Natural history of hepatitis B virus infection in renal transplant recipients: A fifteen year follow-up. Hepatology 3:330, 1983

88. Eddleston ALWF, Williams R: Inadequate antibody response to HBAg or suppressor T cell defect in development of active chronic hepatitis, Lancet 2:543, 1974

89. Edgington TS, Chisari FV: Immunological aspects of hepatitis B virus infection. Am J Med Sci 270:213, 1975

90. Eggink HF, Houthoff HJ, Huitema S et al: Cellular and humoral immune reactions in chronic active liver disease: II. Lymphocyte subsets and viral antigens in liver biopsies of patients with acute and chronic hepatitis B. Clin Exp Immunol 56:121, 1984

91. Fagrell B et al: A nitrofurantoin-induced disorder simulating chronic active hepatitis. Acta Med Scand 199:237, 1976

92. Farivar M et al: Cryoprotein complexes and peripheral neuropathy in a patient with chronic active hepatitis. Gastroenterology 71:490, 1976

93. Feinstone SM et al: Transfusion-associated hepatitis not due to viral hepatitis type A or B. N Engl J Med 292:767, 1975

94. Figus A, Blum HE, Vyas GN et al: Hepatitis B viral nucleotide sequences in non-A, non-B or hepatitis B virus-related chronic liver disease. Hepatology 4:364, 1984

95. Finlayson NDC et al: Interrelations of hepatitis B antigen and autoantibodies in chronic idiopathic liver disease. Gastroenterology 63:646, 1972

96. Fisher RL et al: α_1-Antitrypsin deficiency in liver disease: The extent of the problem. Gastroenterology 71:646, 1976

97. Fleming CR et al: Pigmented corneal rings in non-Wilsonian liver disease. Ann Intern Med 86:285, 1977

98. Foulk WT et al: Primary biliary cirrhosis: Reevaluation by clinical and histological study of 49 cases. Gastroenterology 47:354, 1964

99. Frommer D et al: Kayser-Fleischer-like rings in patients without Wilson's disease. Gastroenterology 72:1331, 1977

100. Galbraith RM et al: Histocompatibility antigens in chronic hepatitis and primary biliary cirrhosis. Br Med J 3:604, 1974

101. Galbraith RM et al: Fulminant hepatic failure in leukemia and choriocarcinoma related to withdrawal of cytotoxic drug therapy. Lancet 2:528, 1975

102. Galbraith RM et al: Autoimmunity in chronic active hepatitis and diabetes mellitus. Clin Immunol Immunopathol 8:116, 1977

103. Galbraith RM et al: High prevalence of seroimmunologic abnormalities in relatives of patients with active chronic hepatitis or primary biliary cirrhosis. N Engl J Med 290: 63, 1974

104. Garibaldi RA et al: Isoniazid-associated hepatitis: Report of an outbreak. Ann Rev Respir Dis 106:357, 1972

105. Garibaldi RA et al: Hemodialysis-associated hepatitis. JAMA 225:384, 1973

106. Gerber MA et al: Antibodies to ribosomes in chronic active hepatitis. Gastroenterology 76:139, 1979

107. Gerber MA et al: Antibodies to hepatitis B core antigen in hepatitis B surface antigen -positive and -negative chronic hepatitis. J Infect Dis 135:1006, 1977

108. Geubel AP et al: Responses to treatment can differentiate chronic active liver disease with cholangitic features from the primary biliary cirrhosis syndrome. Gastroenterology 71:444, 1976

109. Giusti G, Piccinino F, Galanti B et al: Immunosuppressive therapy in chronic active hepatitis (CAH): A multicentric retrospective study on 867 patients. A report from a study group for CAH of the Italian Association for the Study of the Liver. Hepatogastroenterology 31:24, 1984

110. Giusti G, Ruggiero G, Galanti B et al: Chronic active hepatitis in Italy: A multicentric study on clinical and laboratory data of 1154 cases. A report from the study group for CAH of the Italian Association for the Study of the Liver. Hepatogastroenterology 30:126, 1983

111. Gocke DJ: Extrahepatic manifestations of viral hepatitis. Am J Med Sci 270:49, 1975

112. Gocke DJ et al: Vasculitis in association with Australia antigen. J Exp Med 134:330A, 1971

113. Göcken M: Autoimmunity in liver disease: Serologic investigations with clinical correlation. Lab Clin Med 59:533, 1962

114. Goldberg SJ et al: "Non-alcoholic" chronic hepatitis in the alcoholic. Gastroenterology 72:598, 1977

115. Goldfield M et al: The consequence of administering blood pretested for HBsAg by third generation techniques: A progress report. Am J Med Sci 270:335, 1975

116. Golding PL et al: Multisystem involvement in chronic liver disease: Studies on the incidence and pathogenesis. Am J Med 55:772, 1973

117. Goldstein G, Mistilis SP: Use of double infusion of BSP in estimating disease activity in active chronic hepatitis. Scand J Gastroenterol 7:737, 1972

118. Goldstein GB et al: Drug-induced active chronic hepatitis. Am J Dig Dis 18:177, 1973

119. Gonzales–Molina A et al: Liver biopsy in asymptomatic carriers of HBsAg. Gastroenterology 78:1652, 1980

120. Gordon DA, Little HA: The arthropathy of hemochromatosis. Arthritis Rheum 16:305, 1973

121. Greenberg HB et al: Effect of human leukocyte interferon on hepatitis B virus infection in patients with chronic active hepatitis. N Engl J Med 295:517, 1976

122. Gudat F et al: Pattern of core and surface expression in liver tissue reflects state of specific immune response in hepatitis B. Lab Invest 32:1, 1975

123. Gurwin LE, Rogoff TM, Ware AJ et al: Immunologic diagnosis of chronic active "autoimmune" hepatitis. Hepatology 5:397, 1985

124. Hadziyannis S et al: Cytoplasmic hepatitis B antigen in "ground glass" hepatocytes of carriers. Arch Pathol 96:327, 1973

125. Hatoff DE et al: Nitrofurantoin: Another cause of drug-induced chronic active hepatitis. Am J Med 87:117, 1979

126. Hay CRM, Triger DR, Preston FE et al: Progressive liver disease in haemophilia: An understated problem? Lancet 1:1495, 1985

127. Hegarty JE, Nouri-Aria KT, Portmann B et al: Relapse following treatment withdrawal in patients with autoimmune chronic active hepatitis. Hepatology 3:685, 1983

128. Heller P et al: The L.E. cell phenomenon in chronic hepatic disease. N Engl J Med 254:1160, 1956
129. Hepner GW, Vessell ES: Quantitative assessment of hepatic function by breath analysis after oral administration of (^{14}C) amino-pyrine. Ann Intern Med 83:632, 1975
130. Hodges JR et al: Heterozygous MZ alpha$_1$-antitrypsin deficiency in adults with chronic active hepatitis and cryptogenic cirrhosis. N Engl J Med 304:557, 1981
131. Hoefs JC et al: Chronic hepatitis B. Interdepartmental Conference, University of Southern California School of Medicine and the John Wesley County Hospital, Los Angeles. West J Med 128:305, 1978
132. Holborow EJ et al: Antinuclear factor and other antibodies in blood and liver diseases. Br Med J 1:656, 1963
133. Hoofnagle JH et al: Transmission of non-A, non-B hepatitis. Ann Intern Med 87:14, 1977
134. Hoofnagle JH et al: Treatment of chronic type B hepatitis with multiple ten-day courses of adenine arabinoside monophosphate. J Med Virol 15:121, 1985
135. Hoofnagle JH et al: Reactivation of chronic hepatitis B virus infection by cancer chemotherapy. Ann Intern Med 96:447, 1982
136. Hoofnagle JH et al: Randomized controlled trial of adenine arabinoside monophosphate for chronic type B hepatitis. Gastroenterology 86:150, 1984
137. Hoofnagle JA et al: Adenine arabinoside 5'-monophosphate treatment of chronic type B hepatitis. Hepatology 2:784, 1982
138. Hoofnagle JH et al: Seroconversion from hepatitis B e antigen to antibody in chronic type B hepatitis. Ann Intern Med 94:774, 1981
139. Hopf U et al: Detection of a liver-membrane autoantibody in HBsAg-negative chronic active hepatitis. N Engl J Med 294:578, 1976
140. Hsu CCS, Leevy CM: Inhibition of PHA-stimulated lymphocyte transformation by plasma from patients with advanced alcoholic cirrhosis. Clin Exp Immunol 8:747, 1971
141. Hunt AH et al: Relation between cirrhosis and trace metal content of liver with special reference to primary biliary cirrhosis. Br Med J 2:1498, 1963
142. Isoniazid-associated hepatitis: Summary of the report of the Tuberculosis Advisory Committee and Special Consultants to the Director, CDC MMWR, 23:97, 1974
143. Iversen P: Om hepatitis. Nord Med (Hospitalstid.) 30:733, 1946
144. Iwarson S et al: Hepatitis-associated antigen and antibody in Swedish blood donors. Vox Sang 22:501, 1972
145. Jacobson IM, Dienstag JL, Werner BG et al: Epidemiology and clinical impact of hepatitis D virus (delta) infection. Hepatology 5:188, 1985
146. Jain S et al: Transfer factor responses in the attempted treatment of patients with HBsAg-positive chronic liver disease. Clin Exp Immunol 30:10, 1977
147. Jensen DM et al: Detection of antibodies directed against a liver specific membrane lipoprotein in patients with acute and chronic active hepatitis. N Engl J Med 299:1, 1978
148. Jensen DM et al: Chronic liver disease manifesting as Waldenstrom's macroglobulinemia. Arch Intern Med 142:2318, 1982
149. Jersild M: Increasing frequency of chronic hepatitis. Ugeskf Laeger 107:819, 1945
150. Johnson GD et al: Antibody to smooth muscle in patients with liver disease. Lancet 2:878, 1965
151. Jones WA, Castlemen B: Liver diseases in young women with hyperglobulinemia. Am J Pathol 40:315, 1962
152. Joske RA, King WE: The L.E. cell phenomenon in active chronic viral hepatitis. Lancet 2:477, 1955
153. Kakumu S et al: Occurrence and significance of antibody to liver-specific membrane lipoprotein by double-antibody immunoprecipitation method in sera of patients with acute and chronic liver disease. Gastroenterology 76:665, 1979
154. Kakumu S, Leevy CM: Lymphocyte cytotoxicity in alcoholic hepatitis. Gastroenterology 72:594, 1977
155. Kantor FS, Klatskin G: Mitochondrial antibodies in primary biliary cirrhosis. Ann Intern Med 11:533, 1972
156. Karvountzis GG et al: Long-term follow-up of patient surviving fulminant viral hepatitis. Gastroenterology 67:870, 1974
157. Kerr JFR et al: Hypothesis—The nature of piecemeal necrosis in chronic active hepatitis. Lancet 2:827, 1979
158. Khuroo MS: Study of an epidemic of non-A, non-B hepatitis. Am J Med 68:818, 1980
159. Kingham JGC et al: Treatment of HBsAg-positive chronic active hepatitis with human fibroblast interferon. Gut 19:91, 1978
160. Kirk AP et al: Late results of the Royal Free Hospital prospective controlled trial of prednisolone therapy in hepatitis B surface antigen-negative chronic active hepatitis. Gut 21:78, 1980
161. Klatskin G: Persistent HB antigenemia: Associated clinical manifestations and clinical lesions. Am J Med Sci 270:33, 1975
162. Klatskin G: Subacute hepatic necrosis and postnecrotic cirrhosis due to anicteric infections with the hepatitis virus. Am J Med 25:333, 1958
163. Klemola H et al: Anicteric liver damage during nitrofurantoin medication. Scand J Gastroenterol 10:501, 1975
164. Knecht GL, Chisari FV: Reversibility of hepatitis B virus-induced glomerulonephritis and chronic active hepatitis after spontaneous clearance of serum hepatitis B surface antigen. Gastroenterology 5:1152, 1978
165. Knieser MR et al: Pathogenesis of renal disease associated with viral hepatitis. Arch Pathol 97:193, 1974
166. Knodell RG et al: Etiological spectrum of post-transfusion hepatitis. Gastroenterology 69:1278, 1975
167. Knodell RG et al: Development of chronic liver disease after acute non-A, non-B posttransfusion hepatitis: Role of γ-globulin prophylaxis in its prevention. Gastroenterology 72:902, 1977
168. Kohler PF et al: Chronic membranous glomerulonephritis caused by hepatitis B antigen-antibody immune complexes. Ann Intern Med 81:448, 1974
169. Kohler PF et al: Immunotherapy with antibody, lymphocytes, and transfer factor in chronic hepatitis B. Clin Immunol Immunopathol 2:465, 1974
170. Kojima M et al: Correlation between titer of antibody to hepatitis B core antigen and presence of viral antigen in the liver. Gastroenterology 73:664, 1977
171. Koretz RL et al: Hepatitis B surface antigen carriers: To biopsy or not to biopsy. Gastroenterology 75:860, 1978
172. Koretz RL et al: Post-transfusion chronic liver disease. Gastroenterology 71:797, 1976
173. Koretz RL et al: Non-A, and non-B posttransfusion hepatitis: A decade later. Gastroenterology 88:1251, 1985
174. Krarup NB, Roholm K: The development of cirrhosis of the liver after acute hepatitis elucidated by aspiration biopsy. Acta Med Scand 108:306, 1941

175. Krook H: Liver cirrhosis in patients with a lupus erythematosus-like syndrome. Acta Med Scand 169:713, 1961

176. Kunkel HG et al: Extreme hypergammaglobulinemia in young women with liver disease of unknown etiology (abstr). J Clin Invest 30:654, 1950

177. Lam KC et al: Deleterious effect of prednisolone in HBsAg-positive chronic active hepatitis. N Engl J Med 304:380, 1981

178. Lelbach WK: Epidemiology of alcoholic disease. In Popper H, Schaffner F (eds): Progress in Liver Diseases, Vol V, p 494. New York, Grune & Stratton, 1976

179. Lesesne HR et al: Liver biopsy in hemophilia. Ann Intern Med 86:703, 1977

180. Levin DM et al: Non-alcoholic liver disease: Overlooked causes of liver injury in patients with heavy alcohol consumption. Am J Med 66:429, 1979

181. Levo Y, Gorevic PD, Kassab HJ et al: Liver involvement in the syndrome of mixed cryoglobulinemia. Ann Intern Med 87:287, 1977

182. Lindberg J et al: Genetic factors in the development of chronic active hepatitis. Lancet 1:67, 1977

183. Lok ASF, Weller IVD, Karayiannis P et al: Thrice weekly lymphoblastoid interferon is effective in inhibiting hepatitis B viral replication. Liver 4:45, 1984

184. Lok AS, Wilson LA, Thomas HC: Neurotoxicity associated with adenine arabinoside monophosphate in the treatment of chronic hepatitis B virus infection. J Antimicrob Chemother 14:93, 1984

185. Mackay IR et al: Lupoid hepatitis. Lancet 2:1323, 1956

186. Mackay IR et al: Association of autoimmune active chronic hepatitis with HLA-A1, 8. Lancet 2:793, 1972

187. Mackay IR et al: Immunopathogenesis of chronic hepatitis: A review. Aust NZ J Med 1:79, 1973

188. Mackay IR et al: Associations with autoimmune-type chronic active hepatitis: Identification of B8-DRw3 haplotype by family studies. Gastroenterology 79:95, 1980

189. Mackay IR et al: Autoimmune hepatitis. Ann NY Acad Sci 124:767, 1965

190. Mackay IR et al: Lupoid hepatitis: A comparison of 22 cases with other types of chronic liver disease. Q J Med 31:485, 1962

191. MacLachlin MJ et al: Chronic active ("lupoid") hepatitis. A clinical, serological, and pathologic study of 20 patients. Ann Intern Med 62:425, 1965

192. Maddrey WC, Boitnott JK: Drug-induced chronic hepatitis and cirrhosis. In Popper H, Schaffner F (eds): Progress in Liver Diseases, Vol VI, pp 595. New York, Grune & Stratton, 1979

193. Maddrey WC, Boitnott JK: Isoniazid hepatitis. Ann Intern Med 79:1, 1973

194. Maddrey WC, Boitnott JK: Severe hepatitis from methyldopa. Gastroenterology 68:351, 1975

195. Magnius LO et al: A new antigen-antibody system: Clinical significance in long-term carriers of hepatitis B surface antigen. JAMA 231:356, 1975

196. Manns M, Arnold W, Meyer-zum-Buschenfelde KH: Significance of autoantibodies in the diagnosis of non-A, non-B hepatitis. Leber-Magen-Darm 14:211, 1984

197. Mannucci PM et al: Liver biopsy in hemophilia. Ann Intern Med 88:429, 1978

198. Mannucci PM et al: Asymptomatic liver disease in hemophiliacs. J Clin Pathol 28:620, 1975

199. Manzillo G, Piccinino F, Sagnelli E et al: Treatment of HB$_s$Ag-positive chronic active hepatitis with corticosteroids and/or azathioprine: A prospective study. Ric Clin Lab 13:261, 1983

200. Maggiore G, Bernard O, Hadchouel M et al: Treatment of autoimmune chronic active hepatitis in childhood. J Pediatr 104:839, 1984

201. Mathews JD, Mackay IR: Australia antigen in chronic hepatitis in Australia. Br Med J 1:259, 1970

202. McCullough AJ, Czaja AJ: Relapse following treatment withdrawal in autoimmune chronic active hepatitis. Hepatology 4:747, 1984

203. McHardy G, Balart LA: Jaundice and oxyphenisatin. JAMA 211:82, 1970

204. McIntosh RM et al: The nature and incidence of cryoproteins in hepatitis B antigen (HBsAg) positive patients. Q J Med 45:23, 1976

205. Merigan TC: Chemotherapy of hepatitis B virus infection. In Szmuness W, Alter HJ, Maynard JE (eds): Viral Hepatitis 1981. International Symposium, pp 537–541. Philadelphia, Franklin Institute Press, 1982

206. Meyer Zum Buschenfelde KH: Immunosuppressive therapy in HBsAg-positive and -negative chronic active hepatitis. In Eddleston ALWF et al (eds): Immune Reactions in Liver Disease, pp 305. London, Sir Isaac Pitman & Sons, 1979

207. Meyer Zum Buschenfelde KH: Untersuchungen zur immunologischen specifitat des leberparenchyms. Arch Klin Med 215:107, 1968

208. Meyer Zum Buschenfelde KH, Miescher PA: Liver-specific antigens: Purification and characterization. Clin Exp Immunol 10:89, 1972

209. Mieli–Vergani G, Vergani D, Jenkins PJ et al: Lymphocyte cytotoxicity to autologous hepatocytes in HBsAg-negative chronic active hepatitis. Clin Exp Immunol 38:16, 1979

210. Milder MS et al: Idiopathic hemochromatosis: An interim report. Medicine 59:34, 1980

211. Miller DJ et al: Halothane hepatitis: Benign resolution of a severe lesion. Ann Intern Med 89:212, 1978

212. Mistilis SP: Chronic active hepatitis. In Schiff L (ed): Diseases of the Liver, Vol 4, p 787. Philadelphia, JB Lippincott, 1975

213. Mistilis SP: Pericholangitis and ulcerative colitis. I. Pathology, etiology, and pathogenesis. Ann Intern Med 63:1, 1965

214. Mistilis SP et al: Natural history of active chronic hepatitis. I. Clinical features, course, diagnostic criteria, morbidity, mortality, and survival. Aust Ann Med 17:214, 1968

215. Mondelli M, Eddleston ALWF: Mechanisms of liver cell injury in acute and chronic hepatitis B. Sem Liver Dis 4:47, 1984

216. Monroe P et al: The aminopyrine breath test (ABT) predicts histology and correlates with course in patients with chronic hepatitis (CH) (abst). Gastroenterology 78:1314, 1980

217. Mosley JW et al: Multiple hepatitis viruses in multiple attacks of acute viral hepatitis. N Engl J Med 296:75, 1977

218. Mowrey FH, Lundberg EA: The clinical manifestations of essential polyangiitis (periarteritis nodosa) with emphasis on the hepatic manifestations. Ann Intern Med 40:1145, 1954

219. Murray–Lyon IM et al: Controlled trial of prednisone and azathioprine in active chronic hepatitis. Lancet 2:735, 1973

220. Myers BD et al: Membrano-proliferative glomerulonephritis associated with persistent viral hepatitis. Am J Clin Pathol 60:222, 1973

221. Nakanuma Y, Goroku O: Histometric and serial section

observations of the intrahepatic bile ducts in primary biliary cirrhosis. Gastroenterology 76:1326, 1979

222. Nasrallah SM et al: Genetic and immunological aspects of familial chronic active hepatitis (Type B). Gastroenterology 75:302, 1978

223. Nassar NT et al: The prevalence of hepatitis B surface antigen (HBsAg) among students and blood donors at the American University of Beirut (AUB). Johns Hopkins Med J 139:45, 1976

224. Neefe JR et al: Prevalence and nature of hepatic disturbance following acute viral hepatitis with jaundice. Ann Intern Med 43:1, 1955

225. Nefzger MD, Chalmers TC: The treatment of acute infectious hepatitis: Ten-year follow-up study of the effects of diet and rest. Am J Med 35:299, 1963

226. Neuberger J, Portmann B, Calne R et al: Recurrence of autoimmune chronic active hepatitis following orthotopic liver grafting. Transplantation 37:363, 1984

227. Nielsen JO: What shall we do with the HBsAg carrier? Scand J Gastroenterol 11:641, 1976

228. Nielsen JO et al: Incidence and meaning of persistence of Australia antigen in patients with acute viral hepatitis: Development of chronic hepatitis. N Engl J Med 285:1157, 1971

229. Nielsen JO et al: Incidence and meaning of the e determinant among hepatitis antigen-positive patients with acute and chronic liver diseases. Lancet 2:913, 1974

230. Nilius R, Schentke U, Otto L et al: Levamisole therapy in chronic hepatitis: Results of a multicentric double blind trial. Hepatogastroenterology 30:90, 1983

231. Okuno T, Okanoue T, Takino T et al: Prognostic significance of bridging necrosis in chronic active hepatitis. Gastroenterology 18:577, 1983

232. Omata M et al: Comparison of serum hepatitis B surface antigen (HBsAg) and serum anticore with tissue HBsAg and hepatitis B core antigen (HBcAg). Gastroenterology 75:1003, 1978

233. Omata M et al: Hepatocellular carcinoma in the USA: Etiologic considerations. Gastroenterology 6:279, 1979

234. Omata M et al: Recombinant leukocyte a interferon treatment in patients with chronic hepatitis B virus infection. Pharmacokinetics, tolerance, and biologic effects. Gastroenterology 88:870, 1985

235. Page AR et al: Suppression of plasma cell hepatitis with 6-mercaptopurine. Am J Med 36:200, 1964

236. Page AR, Good RA: Plasma-cell hepatitis. Lab Invest 11:351, 1962

237. Page AR, Good RA: Plasma-cell hepatitis, with special attention to steroid therapy. Am J Dis Child 99:288, 1960

238. Page AR et al: Genetic analysis of patients with chronic active hepatitis. J Clin Invest 56:530, 1975

239. Panush RS et al: Chronic active hepatitis associated with eosinophilia and Coomb's positive hemolytic anemia. Gastroenterology 64:1015, 1973

240. Paronetto F et al: Local formation of γ-globulin in diseased liver, and its relationship to hepatic necrosis. Lab Invest 11:150, 1962

241. Paronetto F, Vernace SJ: Immunological studies in patients with chronic active hepatitis. Cytotoxic activity of lymphocytes to autochthonous liver cells grown in tissue culture. Clin Exp Immunol 19:99, 1975

242. Paull R: Periarteritis nodosa (panarteritis nodosa) with report of four proven cases. Calif Med 67:309, 1947

243. Perrett AD et al: The liver in Crohn's disease. Q J Med 40:187, 1971

244. Perrett AD et al: The liver in ulcerative colitis. Q J Med 40:211, 1971

245. Peters RL: Viral hepatitis: A pathologic spectrum. Am J Med Sci 270:17, 1975

246. Pettigrew NM et al: Evidence for a role for hepatitis virus B in chronic alcoholic liver disease. Lancet 2:724, 1972

247. Popper H: Immunocytochemical study of gamma globulin in liver in hepatitis and postnecrotic cirrhosis, J Exp Med 111:285, 1960

248. Popper H et al: Editorial: The problem of primary biliary cirrhosis. Am J Med 33:807, 1962

249. Popper H, Schaffner F: The vocabulary of chronic hepatitis. N Engl J Med 284:1154, 1971

250. Poulsen H, Christoffersen P: Abnormal bile duct epithelium in chronic aggressive hepatitis and cirrhosis: A review of morphology and clinical, biochemical, and immunologic features. Hum Pathol 3:217, 1972

251. Powell L et al: Hemochromatosis: 1980 update. Gastroenterology 78:374, 1980

252. Preston FE et al: Percutaneous liver biopsy and chronic liver disease in hemophiliacs. Lancet 2:592, 1978

253. Prince AM et al: Post-transfusion viral hepatitis caused by an agent or agents other than hepatitis B virus or hepatitis A virus: Impact on efficiency of present screening methods. In Greenwalt TJ, Jamieson GA (eds): Transmissible Disease and Blood Transfusion, p 129. New York, Grune & Stratton, 1975

254. Purcell RH et al: Modification of chronic hepatitis B virus infection in chimpanzees by administration of an interferon inducer. Lancet 2:757, 1976

255. Rakela J, Redeker AG: Chronic liver disease after acute non-A, non-B viral hepatitis. Gastroenterology 77:1200, 1979

256. Rakela J et al: Hepatitis A virus infection in fulminant hepatitis and chronic active hepatitis. Gastroenterology 74:879, 1978

257. Rakela J et al: Effect of short-term prednisone therapy on aminotransferase levels and hepatitis B virus markers in chronic type B hepatitis. Gastroenterology 84:956, 1983

258. Ray MB et al: Hepatitis B surface antigen (HBsAg) in the liver of patients with hepatitis: A comparison with serological detection. J Clin Pathol 29:89, 1976

259. Read AE et al: Active "juvenile" cirrhosis considered as part of a systemic disease and the effect of corticosteroid therapy. Gut 4:378, 1963

260. Realdi G, Alberti A, Rugge M et al: Seroconversion from hepatitis B$_e$ antigen to anti-HB$_e$ in chronic hepatitis B virus infection. Gastroenterology 79:195, 1980

261. Rebora A, Rongioletti F: Lichen planus and chronic active hepatitis: A retrospective survey. Acta Derm Venereol 64:52, 1984

262. Redeker AG: Viral hepatitis: Clinical aspects. Am J Med Sci 270:9, 1975

263. Reed WD et al: Detection of hepatitis B antigen by radioimmunoassay in chronic liver disease and hepatocellular carcinoma in Great Britain. Lancet 2:690, 1973

264. Reinicke V et al: A study of Australia antigen-positive blood donors and their recipients, with special reference to liver histology. N Engl J Med 286:867, 1972

265. Reynolds TB et al: Lupoid hepatitis. Ann Intern Med 61:650, 1964

266. Reynolds TB et al: Chronic active and lupoid hepatitis caused by a laxative, oxyphenisatin. N Engl J Med 285:813, 1971

267. Rizzetto DM, Verme G, Recchia S et al: Chronic carriers of hepatitis B surface antigen, with intrahepatic expression of the delta antigen: An active and progressive disease unresponsive to immunosuppressive treatment. Ann Intern Med 98:437, 1983

268. Rolny P, Goobar J, Zettergren L: HB$_s$Ag-negative chronic active hepatitis and mixed connective tissue disease syndrome: An unusual association observed in two patients. Acta Med Scand 215:391, 1984

269. Rose GA: The natural history of polyarteritis. Br Med J 2:1148, 1957

270. Rubin E et al: Primary biliary cirrhosis. Am J Pathol 46:387, 1964

271. Sagnelli E et al: Dane particles—associated hepatitis B core antigen in patients with HBsAg-positive chronic hepatitis. Gastroenterology 75:864, 1978

272. Sagnelli E et al: Delta agent infection: An unfavourable event in HB$_s$Ag positive chronic hepatitis. Liver 4:170, 1984

273. Schalm SW et al: Failure of customary treatment in chronic active liver disease: Causes and management. Ann Clin Res 8:221, 1976

274. Schalm SW et al: Severe chronic active liver disease: Prognostic significance of initial morphologic patterns. Am J Dig Dis 22:973, 1977

275. Schalm SW et al: Contrasting features and responses to treatment of severe chronic active liver disease with and without hepatitis B$_s$ antigen. Gut 17:781, 1976

276. Schalm SW, Heijtink RA: Spontaneous disappearance of viral replication and liver cell inflammation in HBsAg-positive chronic active hepatitis: Results of a placebo vs. interferon trial. Hepatology 2:791, 1982

277. Schalm SW, Heijtink RA: Controlled observations on the long-term effect of leucocyte interferon therapy in HBsAg (+) chronic active hepatitis (abstr). Gastroenterology 80:1347, 1981

278. Schalm SW, Heijtink RA, van Buuren HR et al: Acyclovir enhances the antiviral effect of interferon in chronic hepatitis B. Lancet 2:358, 1985

279. Scharer I, Smith JP: Serum transaminase elevations and other hepatic abnormalities in patients receiving isoniazid. Ann Intern Med 71:1113, 1969

280. Scharschmidt BF: Human liver transplantation: Analysis of data on 540 patients from four centers. Hepatology 4:95S, 1984

281. Scheinberg IH, Sternlieb I: The liver in Wilson's disease. Gastroenterology 37:550, 1959

282. Scheuer PJ: Chronic hepatitis: A problem for the pathologist. Histopathology 1:5, 1977

283. Scheuer PJ et al: Pathology of acute hepatitis A, B, and non-A, non-B (abstr). Gastroenterology 79:1124, 1980

284. Schlichting P, Hlund B, Poulsen H: Liver biopsy in chronic aggressive hepatitis: Diagnostic reproducibility in relation to size of specimen. Scand J Gastroenterol 18:27, 1983

285. Scott J et al: Wilson's disease presenting as chronic active hepatitis. Gastroenterology 74:645, 1978

286. Scullard GH, Smith C, Merigan TC et al: Effects of immunosuppressive therapy on viral markers in chronic active hepatitis B. Gastroenterology 81:987, 1981

287. Scullard GH et al: Antiviral treatment of chronic hepatitis B virus infection: Improvement in liver disease with interferon and adenine arabinoside. Hepatology 1:228, 1981

288. Scullard GH et al: Antiviral treatment of chronic hepatitis B virus infection: Changes in viral markers with interferon combined with adenine arabinoside. J Infect Dis 143:772, 1981

289. Seaman WE et al: Aspirin-induced hepatotoxicity in patients with systemic lupus erythematosis. Ann Intern Med 80:1, 1974

290. Seeff LB et al: Post-transfusion hepatitis, 1973–1975: A V.A. cooperative study. In Vyas GN et al (eds): Viral Hepatitis, p 371. Philadelphia, Franklin Institute Press, 1978

291. Seeff LB et al: A randomized, double-blind controlled trial of the efficacy of immune serum globulin for the prevention of post-transfusion hepatitis: A Veterans Administration cooperative study. Gastroenterology 72:111, 1977

292. Seefe LB et al: Hepatic disease in asymptomatic parenteral narcotic drug abusers: A Veterans Administration collaborative study. Am J Med Sci 270:42, 1975

293. Sergent JS et al: Vasculitis with hepatitis B antigenemia: Long-term observations in nine patients. Medicine 55:1, 1976

294. Shah N, Ostrow D, Altman N et al: Evolution of acute hepatitis B in homosexual men to chronic hepatitis B: Prospective study of placebo recipients in a hepatitis B vaccine trial. Arch Intern Med 145:881, 1985

295. Shannon WM: Adenine arabinoside: Antiviral activity in vitro. In Pavan–Langston D, Buchanan RA, Alford CA (eds): Adenine Arabinoside: An Antiviral Agent, pp 1–43. New York, Raven Press, 1975

296. Sharp JR et al: Chronic active hepatitis and severe hepatic necrosis associated with nitrofurantoin. Ann Intern Med 92:14, 1980

297. Sheen I-S, Yun-fan L, Tai D-I et al: Hepatic decompensation associated with hepatitis B$_e$ antigen clearance in chronic type B hepatitis. Gastroenterology 89:732, 1985

298. Sherlock S: Primary biliary cirrhosis. In Popper H, Schaffner F (eds): Progress in Liver Diseases, Vol V, p 559. New York, Grune & Stratton, 1976

299. Sherlock S: Waldenstrom's chronic active hepatitis. Acta Med Scand (Suppl) 179:445, 1966

300. Sherlock S, Walshe VM: The post-hepatitis syndrome. Lancet 2:482, 1946

301. Shikata T et al: Staining methods of Australia antigen in paraffin section: Detection of cytoplasmic inclusion bodies. Jpn J Exp Med 44:25, 1974

302. Shulman NR, Barker LF: Virus-like antigen, antibody, and antigen-antibody complexes in hepatitis measured by complement fixation. Science 165:304, 1969

303. Shulman S et al: Transfer-factor therapy of chronic active hepatitis. Lancet 2:650, 1974

304. Silverberg M, Gellis SS: The liver in juvenile Wilson's disease. Pediatrics 30:402, 1962

305. Simon JB, Patel SK: Liver disease in asymptomatic carriers of hepatitis B antigen. Gastroenterology 66:1020, 1974

306. Singleton JW et al: Liver disease in Australia antigen-positive blood donors. Lancet 2:785, 1971

307. Smith CI, Merigan TC: Therapeutic approaches to chronic hepatitis B. In Popper H, Schaffner F (eds): Progress in Liver Disease, pp 481–494. New York, Grune & Stratton, 1982

308. Smith CI, Weissberg J, Bernhardt L et al: Acute Dane particle suppression with recombinant leukocyte A interferon

in chronic hepatitis B virus infection. J Infect Dis 148:907, 1983

309. Smith JA, Francis TI: Immunoepidemiological and in-vitro studies of possible relationships between Australia antigen and hepatocellular carcinoma. Cancer Res 32:1713, 1972

310. Smith JL et al: Studies of the "e" antigen in acute and chronic hepatitis. Gastroenterology 71:208, 1976

311. Soloway RD et al: Clinical, biochemical, and histological remission of severe chronic active liver disease: A controlled study of treatments and early prognosis. Gastroenterology 63:820, 1972

312. Soloway RD et al: "Lupoid" hepatitis, a nonentity in spectrum of chronic active liver disease. Gastroenterology 63:458, 1972

313. Spechler SJ, Koff RS: Wilson's disease: Diagnostic difficulties in the patient with chronic hepatitis and hypercer-uloplasminemia. Gastroenterology 78:803, 1980

314. Spero JA et al: Asymptomatic structural liver disease in hemophilia. N Engl J Med 298:1373, 1978

315. Sternlieb I, Scheinberg IH: Chronic hepatitis as a first manifestation of Wilson's disease. Ann Intern Med 76:59, 1972

316. Sternlieb I, Scheinberg IH: Penicillamine therapy for hepatolenticular degeneration. JAMA 189:748, 1964

317. Stromberg A, Wengle B: Chronic active hepatitis induced by nitrofurantoin. Br Med J 3:174, 1976

318. Summerskill WJH: Chronic active liver disease re-examined: Prognosis hopeful. Gastroenterology 66:450, 1974

319. Summerskill WJH et al: Prednisone for chronic active liver disease: Dose titration, standard dose, and combination with azathioprine compared. Gut 16:876, 1975

320. Szmuness WA: Recent advances in the study of the epidemiology of hepatitis B. Am J Pathol 81:629, 1975

321. Szmuness WA et al: Hepatitis B infection: A point prevalence study in 15 U.S. hemodialysis centers. JAMA 227:901, 1974

322. Tabor E et al: Chronic non-A, non-B hepatitis carrier state—transmissible agent documented in one patient over a six-year period. N Engl J Med 303:140, 1980

323. Tage–Jensen U et al: Liver-cell membrane autoantibody specific for inflammatory liver disease. Br Med J 1:206, 1977

324. Tandon BN, Nayak NC, Tandon HD et al: Acute viral hepatitis with bridging necrosis: Collaborative study on chronic hepatitis. Liver 3:140, 1983

325. Thomas FB: Chronic aggressive hepatitis induced by halothane. Ann Intern Med 81:487, 1974

326. Thomas HC et al: Inducer and suppressor T-cell in hepatitis B virus, induced liver disease. Hepatology 2:202, 1982

327. Thomson AD et al: Lymphocyte cytotoxicity to isolated hepatocytes in chronic active hepatitis. Nature 252:721, 1974

328. Timonen T et al: Characteristics of human B large granular lymphocytes and relationship to natural killer and K cells. J Exp Med 153:569, 1981

329. Tisdale WA: Subacute hepatitis. N Engl J Med 268:85 (part 1), 138 (part 2), 1963

330. Tong MJ et al: Failure of transfer factor therapy in chronic active type B hepatitis. N Engl J Med 295:209, 1976

331. Trepo CG et al: Detection of e-antigen and antibody: Correlations with hepatitis B surface and hepatitis B core antigens, liver disease, and outcome in hepatitis B infections. Gastroenterology 71:804, 1976

332. Triger DR et al: Viral antibodies and autoantibodies in chronic liver disease. Gut 15:94, 1974

333. Turner-Warwick M: Fibrosing alveolitis and chronic liver disease. Q J Med 37:133, 1968

334. Upjohn C: L.E. cell phenomenon associated with chronic hepatitis. Proc R Soc Med 51:742, 1958

335. Uribe M et al: Oral prednisone for chronic active liver disease: Dose responses and bioavailability studies. Gut 19:1131, 1978

336. U.S. Government Printing Office: Diseases of the Liver and Biliary Tract, Standardization of nomenclature, diagnostic criteria, and diagnostic methodology. Washington, DC, Fogarty International Center Proceedings No. 22, DHEW Publication No. (NIH) 76-725, 1976

337. Vaida GA, Goldman MA, Bloch KJ: Testing for hepatitis B virus in patients with chronic urticaria and angioedema. J Allergy Clin Immunol 72:193, 1983

338. Villarejos VM et al: Seroepidemiologic investigation of human hepatitis caused by A, B, and a possible third virus. Proc Soc Exp Biol Med 152:524, 1976

339. Villarejos VM et al: Evidence for viral hepatitis other than type A or B among persons in Costa Rica. N Engl J Med 293:1350, 1975

340. Villeneuve PJ et al: Chronic carriers of hepatitis B antigen (HBsAg). Histological, biochemical, and immunological findings in 31 voluntary blood donors. Am J Dig Dis 21:18, 1976

341. Vischer TL: Australia antigen and autoantibodies in chronic hepatitis. Br Med J 2:695, 1970

342. Vogten AJM et al: Behavior of e antigen and antibody during chronic active liver disease—relation to HB antigen-antibody system and prognosis. Lancet 2:126, 1976

343. Waldenstrom J: Leber, blutproteine and nahrungeweiss. Dtsch Z Verdau Stoffwechselkr 2:113, 1950

344. Walshe JM, Briggs J: Ceruloplasmin in liver disease. A diagnostic pitfall. Lancet 2:263, 1962

345. Wands JR: Subacute and chronic hepatitis after withdrawal of chemotherapy, Lancet 2:979, 1975

346. Wands JR et al: Arthritis associated with chronic active hepatitis: Complement activation and characterization of circulating immune complexes. Gastroenterology 69:1286, 1975

347. Wands JR et al: The pathogenesis of arthritis associated with acute HBsAg-positive hepatitis: Complement activation and characterization of circulating immune complexes. J Clin Invest 55:930, 1975

348. Wands JR et al: Hepatitis B in an oncology unit. N Engl J Med 291:1371, 1974

349. Wands JR et al: Detection and transmission in chimpanzees of hepatitis B virus-related agents formerly designed "non-A, non-B" hepatitis. Proc Natl Acad Sci 79:7552, 1982

350. Ware AJ et al: Prognostic significance of subacute hepatic necrosis in acute hepatitis. Gastroenterology 68:519, 1975

351. Ware AJ et al: A prospective trial of steroid therapy in severe viral hepatitis: The prognostic significance of bridging necrosis. Gastroenterology 80:219, 1981

352. Warnatz H et al: Antibody-dependent cell-mediated cytotoxicity (ADCC) and cell-mediated cytotoxicity (CMC) to HBsAg-coated target cells in patients with hepatitis B and chronic hepatitis (CAH). Clin Exp Immunol 35:133, 1979

353. Warren KW et al: Primary sclerosing cholangitis. Am J Surg 111:23, 1966

354. Weiser RH, LaRusso NH: Clinicopathologic features of the syndrome of primary sclerosing cholangitis. Gastroenterology 79:200, 1980

355. Weissberg JI, Andres LL, Smith CI et al: Survival in chronic

hepatitis B: An analysis of 379 patients. Ann Intern Med 101:613, 1984

356. Weller IVD et al: Successful treatment of HB$_s$ and HB$_e$Ag positive inhibition of viral replication by highly soluble adenine arabinoside 5'-monophosphate (ARA-AMP). Gut 23:717, 1982

357. Weller IV et al: Acyclovir in hepatitis B antigen-positive chronic liver disease: Inhibition of viral replication and transient renal impairment with IV bolus administration. J Antimicrob Chemother 11:223, 1983

358. Weller IVD et al: Acyclovir inhibits hepatitis B virus replication in man. Lancet 1:273, 1982

359. Wewalka F: Epidemiology of hepatitis B antigen. In Schaffner F et al (eds): The Liver and Its Diseases, pp 133. New York, Intercontinental Medical Book Corporation, 1974

360. Wilkinson M, Sacker LS: The lupus erythematosus cell and its significance. Br Med J 2:661, 1957

361. Wilkinson SP et al: Clinical course of chronic lobular hepatitis. Q J Med 47:421, 1978

362. Wilcox RG, Isselbacher KJ: Chronic liver disease in young people. Am J Med 30:185, 1961

363. Williams GEG: Pericholangitic biliary cirrhosis. J Pathol Bacteriol 89:23, 1965

364. Willing RL, Hecker R: Oxyphenisatin and liver damage. Med J Aust 1:1179, 1971

365. Wolfe JD et al: Aspirin hepatitis. Ann Intern Med 80:74, 1974

366. Woolf IL et al: Asymptomatic liver disease in hepatitis B antigen carriers. J Clin Pathol 27:348, 1974

367. Wright EC et al: Treatment of chronic active hepatitis: An analysis of three controlled trials. Gastroenterology 73:1422, 1977

368. Wright R: Australia antigen and smooth muscle antibody in acute and chronic hepatitis. Lancet 1:521, 1970

369. Wright R et al: Australia antigen in acute and chronic liver disease. Lancet 2:117, 1969

370. Wu PC, Lai CL, Lam KC et al: Prednisolone in HB$_s$Ag-positive chronic active hepatitis: Histologic evaluation in a controlled prospective study. Hepatology 2:777, 1982

371. Yokosuka O, Donata M, Imazeki F et al: Combination of short term prednisone and adenine arabinoside in the treatment of chronic hepatitis B: A controlled study. Gastroenterology 89:246, 1985

372. Zetterman RK et al: Alcoholic hepatitis: Cell mediated immunological response to alcoholic hyalin. Gastroenterology 70:382, 1976

373. Zieve L et al: The incidence of residuals of viral hepatitis. Gastroenterology 25:495, 1953

374. Zinkernagel RM et al: H-2 compatibility requirement for virus-specific T-cell mediated cytolysis: Evaluation of the role of H-2I region and onon-H-2 genes in regulating immune response. J Exp Med 144:519, 1976

375. Zuckerman AJ: The immunopathogenesis of liver damage in hepatitis B. In Zuckerman AJ: Human Viral Hepatitis, p 233. New York, Elsevier, 1975

chapter 20

Cirrhosis

HAROLD O. CONN and COLIN E. ATTERBURY

Dark monarch,
giver of syrups and of poisons,
regulator of salts,
from you I hope for justice:
I love life: Do not betray me! Work on!
Do not arrest my song.

Pablo Neruda
Ode to the Liver
Translation by Oriana J. Kalant

In his classic monograph, which has withstood the challenges of 1½ centuries, Laënnec described the pathologic picture of cirrhosis and some of its clinical features, and, in a footnote, proposed the name "cirrhosis" for the disorder.[486] *Cirrhosis* in Greek means orange or tawny. This first definitive description by Laënnec is a concise and lucid example of medical writing:

> The liver, reduced to a third of its ordinary size, was, so to say, hidden in the region it occupied; its external surface, lightly mamellated and wrinkled, showed a greyish yellow tint; indented, it seemed entirely composed of a multitude of small grains, round or ovoid in form, the size of which varied from that of a millet seed to that of a hemp seed. These grains, easy to separate one from the other, showed between them no place in which one could still distinguish any remnant of liver tissue itself: their color was fawn or a yellowish russet, bordering on greenish; their tissue, rather moist, opaque, was flabby to the touch rather than soft, and on pressing the grains between the fingers, one could not mash but a small portion: the rest gave to the touch the sensation of a piece of soft leather.*

This early description is an inspiring starting point from

---

* "This type of growth belongs to the group of those which are confused under the name of scirrhus. I believe we ought to des ignate it with the name of *cirrhosis,* because of its color. Its development in the liver is one of the most common causes of ascites, and has the peculiarity that as the cirrhosis develops, the tissue of the liver is absorbed, and it ends often, as in the subject, by disappearing entirely."

which to begin a discussion of cirrhosis. Laënnec's name has traditionally been an almost obligatory adjective for the most common type of cirrhosis, "Laënnec's alcoholic cirrhosis," but during the past decade it has fallen out of general use, and this type of cirrhosis is usually referred to simply as alcoholic cirrhosis.

DEFINITION AND HISTORY

Much more has been written about the definition of cirrhosis than is known. Much of the confusion and controversy about its definition is based upon the almost 734ontrollable compulsion of the definers of cirrhosis to include various aspects of pathogenesis, which is even less well understood than the definition.

Cirrhosis can best be defined in terms of what is pathoanatomically certain about the liver. *Cirrhosis is a chronic disease of the liver in which diffuse destruction and regeneration of hepatic parenchymal cells have occurred, and in which a diffuse increase in connective tissue has resulted in disorganization of the lobular and vascular architecture.* The altered vascular abnormalities of cirrhosis are at least as important as any of these other components. In fact, from the clinical point of view, the resultant portal hypertension causes the most serious and lethal complications. Although some observers have argued about whether the scar tissue represents *de novo* formation of connective tissue or whether collapse and condensation of preexisting structural tissue is responsible, all agree that the amount of connective tissue or scar is increased. Some authors feel that cirrhosis is a progressive disease and that cirrhosis should be defined as ". . . a chronic, *progressive* disease. . . ." Clearly, cirrhosis in its mature state must have progressed, but whether it has progressed or will progress continuously or continually in the absence of etiologic stimulation is not at all clear. In all cirrhotic patients, regardless of the presence, absence, or nature of individual clinical manifestations, the triad of parenchymal necrosis, regeneration, and scarring, which was first emphasized by Rössle,[793] is present. All other clinical, laboratory, or pathologic manifestations of cirrhosis are inconstant and represent either pathogenetic or consequential features that may be found at specific stages of the disease or in specific types of cirrhosis. Infiltration of the portal zones with leukocytes, mononuclear cells, or plasmacytes, for example, may represent inflammation associated with an initial injury, a response to continued necrosis, or part of the chronic reparative process. Similarly, hemosiderin deposition in patients with genetically determined hemochromatosis may represent an antecedent, pathogenetic feature of the development of the cirrhosis[728] but may also represent the subsequent deposition of iron in the cirrhotic liver, as is common in alcoholic cirrhosis.[1065] Certainly, no one clinical, laboratory, or pathological feature of cirrhosis need be seen in every patient with cirrhosis.

The classification of cirrhosis is slightly less obscure, although controversy exists about the overlapping of certain types. The major complication is the frequent lack of correlation between the etiologic and pathologic types of cirrhosis. Alcoholic cirrhosis, for example, is supposedly characterized by uniform, micronodular formation and fine, almost ubiquitous strands of connective tissue. Large, irregularly sized nodules and broad, dense bands of scar, characteristic of postnecrotic cirrhosis, especially in later stages, may appear. Both lesions often coexist in the same liver, the so-called mixed cirrhosis.[314,799] Conversely, micronodules may occur in posthepatitic cirrhosis. In fact, expert pathologists have frequently disagreed in differentiating alcoholic from postnecrotic and posthepatitic cirrhosis in the blind histologic classification of cirrhosis.[317,332] The observation that pathologists disagreed more frequently on surgical biopsies than on percutaneous needle samples[317] has led to the sarcastic suggestion that the more tissue available, the more the pathologists have to disagree about. This conclusion is unfair, since these studies demonstrate not that the pathologists are deficient, but rather that the histologic criteria are neither specific nor mutually exclusive. Histologically, the lesions, though usually characteristic of any one type of cirrhosis, are not specific for that type of cirrhosis. Typical lesions of each of the major types of cirrhosis may be seen to coexist in the same liver.[314,799] Furthermore, the gross appearance of the liver may often be more reliable than a small histologic sample. Postnecrotic cirrhosis, with its coarse nodules of variable size, is characteristic and quite different from alcoholic cirrhosis with its fine uniform nodularity and may be distinguished with the naked eye from the more intermediate posthepatitic type.[314,918]

The large number of classifications previously proposed testifies to the inadequacy of our knowledge of the basic aspects of cirrhosis. These numerous classifications represent a corollary of the facetious "first law of pharmacology," which states that the number of forms of therapy for a specific disease is inversely proportional to therapeutic efficacy. The profusion of classifications has led inevitably to the proposal that there is but a single type of cirrhosis that has many clinical and histologic variations. Neither this concept of "lumping" nor the opposite approach to classification of dividing and endlessly subdividing solves the problem.

The classification proposed here (Table 20-1) is based on the one recommended at the Fifth Pan-American Congress[761] and modified by the working group of the

TABLE 20-1. Classification of Cirrhosis

MORPHOLOGIC	Hemochromatosis
Micronodular	Hepatolenticular degeneration (Wilson's
Macronodular	disease)
Mixed	Autoimmune
	Syphilis
HISTOLOGIC	Drugs and toxins
Portal	Alpha$_1$-antitrypsin deficiency
Postnecrotic	Cystic fibrosis
Posthepatitic	Galactosemia
Biliary obstructive	Glycogen storage disease
Primary	Hereditary tyrosinemia
Secondary	Hereditary fructose intolerance
Venous-outflow obstructive	Other metabolic
	Hereditary hemorrhagic telangiectasia
ETIOLOGIC	Hypervitaminosis A
Alcohol	Sarcoidosis
Viral hepatitis	Copper
Biliary obstruction	Small-bowel bypass
Primary	Indian childhood cirrhosis
Secondary	Idiopathic
Venous-outflow obstruction	Unproved
	Malnutrition
	Mycotoxins
	Schistosomiasis

World Health Organization in 1978,[23] the International Association for the Study of the Liver,[505] and by the authors. This classification categorizes cirrhosis according to morphologic, histologic, and etiologic criteria. The arbitrary "functional" classification of the earlier system has been discarded.

The morphologic classification simply characterizes the gross appearance of the liver (Table 20-1). The morphologic diagnosis as made at surgery, laparoscopy, or autopsy is usually more reliable than the histologic diagnosis.[23]

The usefulness of the morphologic classification is that it allows patterns to be studied epidemiologically and to be correlated with etiologic agents.[23]

1. *Micronodular cirrhosis* is characterized by the uniformity of the size of the nodules, virtually all of which are less than 3 mm in diameter (Fig. 20-1). These micronodules, which are about one lobule in size, lack normal lobular organization and are surrounded by fibrous tissue (Fig. 20-2). These lobules rarely contain

Fig. 20-1. Micronodular cirrhosis. **A.** Grossly the liver is large, pale, and uniformly finely nodular. **B.** Sectioned surface of the cirrhotic liver shows the fine nodularity and regular disposition of the delicate fibrous tissue.

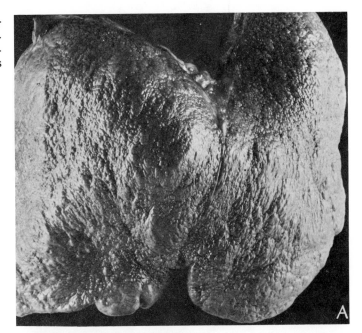

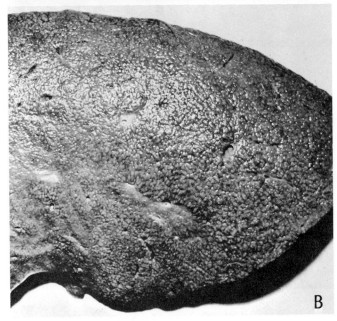

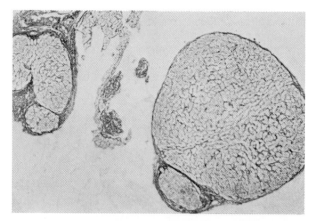

Fig. 20-2. Micronodular cirrhosis with characteristic fragmentation of a needle biopsy specimen. Micronodules are surrounded by fibrosis. (Reticulin stain; original magnification × 50) (Anthony PP et al: J Clin Pathol 31:395, 1978)

terminal hepatic (central) veins or portal tracts except in cardiac cirrhosis, in which they are characteristically present. Micronodular cirrhosis (Fig. 20-2) is seen in chronic alcoholism, biliary obstruction, hemochromatosis, venous outflow obstruction, small-bowel bypass, and Indian childhood cirrhosis.

2. *Macronodular cirrhosis* (Figs. 20-3 and 20-4) is characterized by variation in nodular size, but most nodules are greater than 3 mm in diamter and may measure several centimeters across. They contain both portal triads and efferent veins, but their orientation to each other varies. There are two subtypes of macronodular cirrhosis. In one, the liver is coarsely scarred and the large nodules are surrounded by broad fibrous septa (Fig. 20-4*B*). In this "postnecrotic" type of cirrhosis, numerous portal triads may be clumped together, presumably the consequence of the collapse of large areas of necrotic parenchyma. In the other, the so-called posthepatitic type, macronodules are separated by slender fibrous strands that connect individual portal areas to one another (Figure 20-5). This pattern has sometimes been called incomplete septal cirrhosis. Efferent veins are located eccentrically within these large lobules.

Macronodular cirrhosis may often be a later stage of micronodular cirrhosis. When serial biopsies were examined, up to 90% of the specimens that were originally classified as micronodular were found 10 years later to be macronodular. The mean time required for development of macronodular cirrhosis from micronodular cirrhosis was around 2 years.[266]

3. *Mixed cirrhosis* is a compromise term used when both macrolobules and microlobules are present with equal frequency.

The histologic classification of cirrhosis confirms the morphologic diagnosis and subdivides it into histologically discrete and sometimes etiologically precise categories. The postnecrotic and posthepatitic types are readily evident (Figs. 20-4 and 20-5). Characteristic histologic findings permit the differentiation of primary and secondary biliary cirrhosis, and establish the etiology of venous ob-

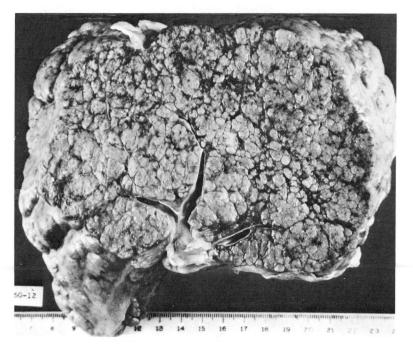

Fig. 20-3. Macronodular cirrhosis. Grossly the liver is coarsely nodular and shows marked variation in the pattern and character of nodulation. Broad bands of connective tissue distort the parenchyma into irregular nodules.

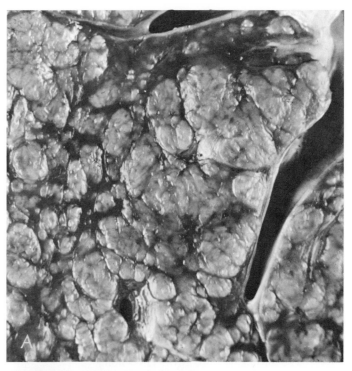

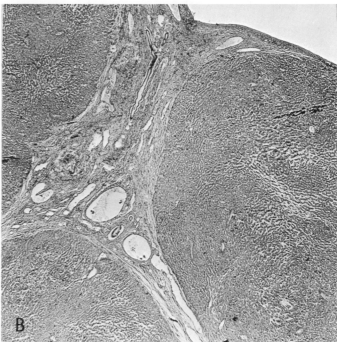

Fig. 20-4. Macronodular cirrhosis. **A.** Close-up of cross-section emphasizes the variable size of the large regenerative nodules and the irregular nature of the scarring. **B.** Photomicrograph shows characteristic broad septal scars. The large parenchymal nodules show no pseudolobulation but contain multiple distorted lobules, many portal areas, and asymmetrically located central veins.

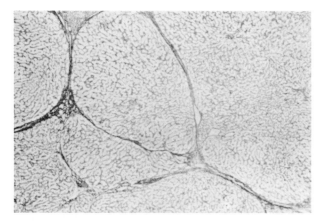

Fig. 20-5. Macronodular, posthepatitic cirrhosis. Slender, incomplete strands of fibrosis separate the macronodules. (Reticulin stain; original magnification × 24) (Anthony PP: J Clin Pathol 31:395, 1978)

struction, hemochromatosis and α_1-antitrypsin deficiency. Histologic findings may suggest other types of cirrhosis such as copper deposition in Wilson's disease or ground-glass cells in chronic hepatitis B virus infection.

The etiologic diagnosis includes established causative associations with cirrhosis; often, however, neither the precise nature of the association nor its pathogenetic mechanism is completely understood. Also included in this classification are several suspected but unproven types of cirrhosis and several cirrhoses of unknown origin. The etiologic category is designed to grow as new causes of cirrhosis are established.

PATHOLOGY

The pathologic classification of cirrhosis is in many ways the most satisfactory and definitive type of cataloguing. It represents a static, descriptive evaluation, often at the end stage of the disease. It permits gross and microscopic descriptions and categorization into several classic, obviously different, types of cirrhosis. It also provides an almost infinite variety of findings, which often encourage the subclassification of less clear-cut categories. In addition, it provides clues—sometimes misleading—about the pathogenesis.

The simplest, least controversial pathologic classification, as suggested in Table 20-1, is followed here.

Portal Cirrhosis

The liver in portal cirrhosis (also termed Laënnec's alcoholic, nutritional, and micronodular cirrhosis) is usually enlarged, ranging from less than 1000 g to 4000 g in weight. The small, shrunken, hard, nodular liver, so classically described in the earlier literature,[441,747] is seen much less

commonly now. In our experience, alcoholic cirrhotic livers at autopsy are usually moderately enlarged (1500–2000 g) and occasionally massive. Small livers are sometimes seen, most frequently in patients with advanced cirrhosis of long duration, often with severe degrees of portal hypertension. Large cirrhotic livers are most frequently found in patients with alcoholic cirrhosis with excessive fatty infiltration and active hepatic necrosis. These patients may die relatively early in the course of their cirrhosis of acute hepatic parenchymal failure or infection, rather than of the chronic consequences of progressive cirrhosis.

Grossly the liver is usually golden yellow, but the color varies greatly. Cirrhotic livers may be pale yellow when the liver is large and fat-filled. They may be tan, brown, or reddish depending on the degree of fatty infiltration, congestion, iron deposition, necrosis, and arterial oxygen saturation; and they may be gray or green, depending on the amount of scarring and the degree and duration of jaundice.

Usually the surface is pebbled by fine uniform nodulations that range from 1 mm to 5 mm in diameter separated by a delicate reticulum of scar tissue. Traditionally, this type of cirrhosis has been known as hobnail cirrhosis, but hobnails, defined as "short, large-headed nails for studding shoe soles," are not in style this century and are not known to present-day physicians. It is more appropriate nowadays to say that the liver surface resembles tanned pigskin in appearance (see Fig. 20-1). The cut surface also shows the uniform granular pattern. Sometimes in portal cirrhosis the liver shows both granularity and nodularity and, rarely, the liver is largely nodular. The nodules usually range from 5 mm to 12 mm in diameter, but nodules as large as 50 mm in diameter, separated by broad depressed scars, which resemble those of postnecrotic cirrhosis, may characterize all or part of the liver. In general, however, the nodules of alcoholic cirrhosis are small and uniform in size and are readily distinguishable from the large and variable nodularity of postnecrotic cirrhosis.

Microscopically, scar tissue distorts the normal architecture (Figs. 20-2 and 20-6). Portal zones are interconnected by bands of connective tissue that divide and subdivide the normal lobular structure into islands of parenchymal cells. In some areas stellate bands of connective tissue appear to isolate plates of cells and even individual cells. The typical nodules are generally less than one lobule in size, and many lobules are segmented into much smaller pseudolobules. Some nodules are larger and are formed by numbers of lobules. The strands of connective tissue are usually fine, 100 μm to 200 μm thick, and are rarely broader than 500 μm. Bands of connective tissue may connect portal areas to one another and often to central areas. The connective tissue appears to originate from the portal areas and to advance toward the center of the lobules from the peripheral areas. Often in early cases of alcoholic cirrhosis, the scar can be seen to be predominantly central and to involve the portal areas secondarily. In advanced cases, the scar appears predominantly portal, and

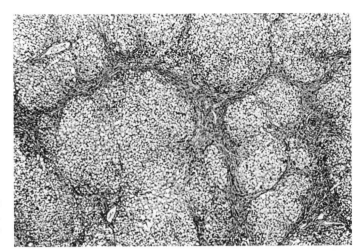

Fig. 20-6. Alcoholic cirrhosis. Microscopically the liver reveals fine fibrosis, micronodulation, and pseudolobule formation. Intracellular fat vacuolization is prominent.

it may be impossible to appreciate the morphogenetic development of the scar tissue. Sometimes scar may replace whole areas of parenchyma, as in postnecrotic cirrhosis, and may appear as broad areas of scar in which are enmeshed arteries, veins, bile ducts, proliferating ductules, occasional individual parenchymal cells or clumps of cells, macrophages, and inflammatory cells. At times it is a more delicate network of connective tissue that appears to be invading the lobules with fibrils of connective tissue that surround individual cells. Central veins may be centrally or eccentrically located or difficult to identify. Careful microscopic examination of many sites from the same liver will often show typical portal cirrhosis in some areas, and in other areas the characteristic postnecrotic pattern.[314,799] Interlobar bile ducts are unaffected, but proliferation of pseudoductules is typical.

Collagenization of the space of Disse has been shown to correlate closely with clinical decompensation and functional abnormalities.[658] This space is a lymphatic bed devoid of a basement membrane that permits maximal exposure of the hepatocytes to the circulation. The deposition of collagen in the space of Disse may be a critical pathologic lesion with functional and perhaps prognostic implications.

Hepatic parenchymal cells may appear normal, but often the cytoplasm shows altered tinctorial characteristics, sometimes staining more palely, and sometimes more densely, than normal cells. In alcoholic cirrhosis the cytoplasm may appear to be homogeneous or particulate, and sometimes hyaline clumping, which is usually eosinophilic but may occasionally be amphophilic or even basophilic, is prominent. Such alcohol hyalin, or "Mallory bodies,"[556] which are found in both the central portion of the lobule and in close proximity to the portal scars, are considered indices of alcoholic hepatitis, rather than of cirrhosis *per se*. They are so often present in active decompensated alcoholic cirrhosis as to represent a characteristic part of the histologic picture. Popper stresses the centrilobular localization of this hyaline material in alcoholic hepatitis[724] but in our experience alcoholic hyalin occurs at least as commonly in the peripheral portions of the lobule.

Mallory bodies have been seen in the absence of cirrhosis and, indeed, in the absence of alcoholic liver disease. They have been described in primary biliary cirrhosis, Wilson's disease and other diseases with prolonged cholestasis, in nonalcoholic nutritional liver disease, in hamartomas, in chronic drug therapy, and occasionally in a variety of other types of liver disease.[300,321,697]

Recent investigations have begun to clear up some of the mystery about alcohol hyalin, the homogeneous cytoplasmic bodies first described by Mallory in 1911[556] and known since as "Mallory bodies" (Fig. 20-7). Leevy and associates suggested that this hyaline material is immunologically important in the pathogenesis of alcoholic liver disease and that cell-mediated injury may contribute to the progression of alcoholic liver disease. It has been shown that alcohol, acetaldehyde, and alcohol hyalin all stimulate lymphocyte transformation and cell-mediated hyperreactivity and cytotoxicity to autologous liver tissue.[49,431,900,1056] Recently the presence of an alcoholic hyalin antigen and an antibody to it has been demonstrated in patients with alcoholic hepatitis.[435] Although this antibody is to Mallory bodies alone, it contains other types of antibody that bind to other structures as well.[299]

Denk and colleagues have produced Mallory bodies in mice by the chronic administration of griseofulvin,[220,221] an agent that has antimicrotubular and cell-activating properties and that can induce porphyria and cholestasis. Mallory bodies appear in all animals treated for 4 months with griseofulvin and disappear within a month after stopping griseofulvin. Mallory bodies do not appear if colchicine, another antimicrotubular agent, is administered. If griseofulvin or colchicine is given to a mouse in whom Mallory bodies have previously been induced by griseofulvin, Mallory bodies promptly reappear after 2 or

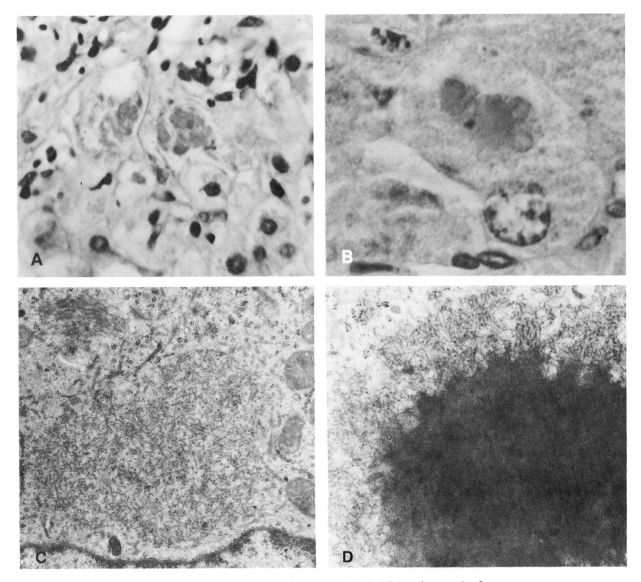

Fig. 20-7. Mallory bodies (MB). **A.** Light micrograph of a human MB. **B.** Light micrograph of a murine MB induced by griseofulvin. **C.** Electron micrograph of a portion of a hepatocyte showing in the upper left corner aggregates of filaments in parallel arrangements characteristic of type I MB and below it juxtanuclear clumps of moderately electron-dense intertwining filaments characteristic of type II MB **D.** Electron micrograph of an electron-dense, amorphous type III MB. Type II filaments surround and appear to merge with the clump. (Original magnification: A, $\times$ 440; B, $\times$ 980; C, $\times$ 23,700; D, $\times$ 36,400) These micrographs were made available by Dr. Z. Wessely. (Wessely Z: Ann Clin Lab Sci 9:24)

3 days.[219] These murine Mallory bodies, which appear to be identical to human Mallory bodies by ultrastructural, immunologic, and pharmacologic studies, seem to consist of intermediate size filaments (Fig. 20-7).

Mallory bodies have also been induced in hepatocytes after long-term feeding with dieldrin.[586] Both griseofulvin and dieldrin are carcinogens, and Mallory bodies are found in hepatomas induced by these agents.[300] The common denominator in Mallory body formation, whether it be induced by alcohol injury, the various liver disorders, drugs, or neoplasia, appears to be cellular injury followed by proliferation of hepatocytes.[300]

Franke and co-workers examined isolated purified Mallory bodies and identified them as containing prekeratin-like polypeptides assembled into unbranched, randomly oriented fimbriate rods 14 nm to 20 nm thick.[296]

These filaments differ from other intermediate filaments. On polyacrylamide gel electrophoresis they separate into six polypeptide bands, which appear to have molecular weights between 45,000 and 66,000. Antibody to prekeratin reacts immunofluorescently with Mallory bodies from griseofulvin-treated rats and from alcohol-abused human livers. Antibodies to actin or to tubulin do not react with Mallory bodies. Antisera against isolated human or murine Mallory bodies bind with the Mallory bodies in liver sections from either species.[301,872] Franke and co-workers concluded that Mallory bodies are composed of hollow, intermediate size tonofilaments that contain prekeratin.[296]

The source of the Mallory body appears to be the hepatocyte cytoskeleton, which has intermediate filaments located throughout the cytoplasm, especially at cell borders, attached to mitochondria, the nucleus, and other organelles, and connecting to centrioles.[299,300] It is known that keratin synthesis can be altered when the environment of the cell is changed, such as by drugs or carcinogens, and it is possible that Mallory body formation results from alterations in keratin polypeptide composition rather than from "toxic degeneration".[300,494] The result, whatever the mechanism, is the loss of the functions of the cytoskeleton. As shown in Figure 20-8, loss of intermediate filaments throughout the cytoplasm is accompanied by the massing of these filaments to form Mallory bodies.[299,300] Consequently, the cell becomes ballooned, it loses microvilli,

the nucleus is displaced, and organization of organelles is lost. Since cells containing Mallory bodies are prone to lysis owing to breaks in the plasma membranes, survival of the cell may be jeopardized.[299,699]

Another histologic trademark of alcoholic liver disease is the giant mitochondrion.[101] These spherical, hyaline, eosinophilic, cytoplasmic inclusions, which resemble erythrocytes in appearance, are clearly distinguishable from Mallory bodies. They vary in size from 2 μm to 10 μm and have been demonstrated on electron microscopy to be megamitochondria. They occur more frequently than alcohol hyalin but are not nearly so ominous.

Often there is variation in cellular and in nuclear size, altering dramatically the uniformity of the normal parenchymal structure. These regenerative changes are often accompanied by frequent binucleate cells and by increased mitotic activity. Regeneration appears to occur piecemeal in alcoholic cirrhosis compared with the large regenerating nodules characteristic of postnecrotic cirrhosis.

Necrosis is characteristically seen in the peripheral areas near the fibrous strands. When the lobular architecture is sufficiently preserved, necrosis may be prominent around the terminal hepatic (central) veins but may also be ubiquitous, although it may often be difficult to identify precisely normal landmarks in the distorted cirrhotic architecture. It is our impression that ballooning of hepatic parenchymal cells is more apt to occur near the central

Fig. 20-8. Artist's conception of the normal intermediate-filament cytoskeleton in a hepatocyte (*left*) compared to a hepatocyte that has undergone Mallory body transformation (*right*). The normal hepatocyte has microvilli, microfilaments in the ectoplasm, and intermediate filaments that form a guy wire-like framework holding organelles and the nucleus in place and maintaining the polygonal shape of the cell. In contrast, the Mallory-body-containing hepatocyte, attached at desmosomal connections, has lost both microfilaments and intermediate filaments, resulting in a change in shape of the hepatocyte to form a sphere (balloon degeneration). (Reproduced with permission of Dr. S. W. French; modified from figure presented previously in Reference 299)

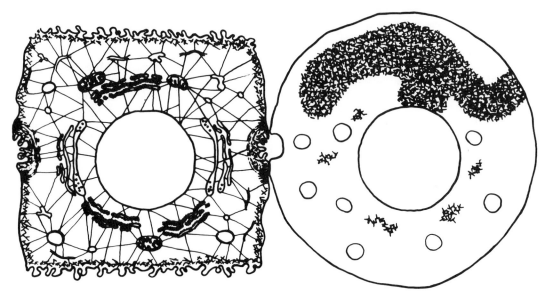

portion of lobules, while a more coagulative necrosis of cytoplasm, characterized by Mallory's alcohol hyalin, tends to be located along the peripheral fibrous strands; however, this pattern is very variable.

Areas of necrosis frequently contain polymorphonuclear leukocytes, which may surround or appear within necrotic or prenecrotic cells, and prominent Kupffer cells engorged with pigment. Portal areas may contain large numbers of inflammatory cells, which typically are predominantly lymphocytic and histiocytic but may sometimes contain large numbers of polymorphonuclear leukocytes, eosinophils, and sometimes plasma cells. The inflammatory reaction that accompanies alcoholic hepatic damage is unpredictable. There is little relationship between the type or extent of hepatocellular necrosis and the character, degree, or duration of inflammation.

Fatty infiltration, which is a common accompaniment of alcoholic cirrhosis, but not an obligatory part of the cirrhotic picture, tends to be centrally located. When intense, however, fatty infiltration may involve almost every cell. Hemosiderin, which is commonly deposited in the hepatic parenchymal cells of cirrhotic patients, is found earliest and most intensely in the periportal areas.

Postnecrotic Cirrhosis

The liver in postnecrotic cirrhosis (also termed posthepatitic cirrhosis, healed acute yellow atrophy, or coarsely nodular cirrhosis) is characterized grossly by a misshapen, often shrunken, liver (see Fig. 20-3). Broad bands of dense connective tissue divide the liver into nodules of varying size, which range from a few millimeters to 5 cm in diameter. Whole lobes may be replaced by dense, shrunken scar. The scar is grayish to greenish brown; the nodules may be tan, brown, or greenish-hued. The scarring is often eccentric and random (see Fig. 20-4).

Microscopically, the primary feature is scarring. Coarse, irregular scars are typical, but fine strands are also present. The overall architecture is distorted by displaced, but recognizable, portal areas and central veins. The areas of scar tissue contain abnormal collections of portal tracts that typify the lesion and that reflect the collapse and condensation of the hepatic stroma. It is widely felt that the juxtaposition of three or more portal triads abnormally placed within a single strand of scar is a hallmark of this lesion.[918] In long-standing postnecrotic cirrhosis, the cicatrized portal features may no longer be recognized.

Large regenerating nodules are the predominant parenchymal finding. Lymphocytic infiltration is typical, but plasma cells and polymorphonuclear leukocytes may be present, and often many eosinophils are seen. In the active phase, parenchymal necrosis—often piecemeal—may be present, but fatty infiltration is atypical and alcohol hyalin is rarely, if ever, present. Active necrosis reflects the changes associated with viral hepatitis, the most common cause of this type of cirrhosis. Eosinophilic Councilman-like bodies may accompany active necrosis.

Some authors consider posthepatitic cirrhosis (see Fig. 20-5) to be a discrete third type of cirrhosis. It appears to be intermediate between portal and postnecrotic cirrhosis in both gross and microscopic appearance, and its pathogenesis is similar to that seen in postnecrotic cirrhosis.

Biliary Cirrhosis

The liver in biliary cirrhosis is characteristically dark green, firm, and granular or nodular. The deep green color is more typical of secondary than of primary biliary cirrhosis.[227] Grossly it appears to be a green portal cirrhosis, but broad scars may predominate as in postnecrotic cirrhosis, with small or moderate-sized nodules, 1 mm to 10 mm in diameter. Microscopically, the cirrhosis shows broadened portal tracts that are linked with one another. In biliary cirrhosis secondary to prolonged obstructive jaundice, the major difference is the apparent *increase* in the number of interlobar bile ducts and the absence of ductular degeneration. The characteristic finding of primary biliary cirrhosis is *reduction* in the number of interlobular bile ducts and inflammation and degeneration of those that survive. The portal areas are heavily infiltrated with lymphocytes, plasma cells, and neutrophilic and eosinophilic leukocytes. Bile stasis is severe in both types, but bile lakes are typical of high-grade obstructive jaundice and are uncommon in primary biliary cirrhosis.

Cardiac Cirrhosis

Cardiac cirrhosis is a rare lesion that develops only after prolonged, severe, right-sided, congestive heart failure. For practical purposes, it develops only in patients with constrictive pericarditis or tricuspid insufficiency.[616] Unremittent, chronic congestion of the liver results in central cellular atrophy and necrosis. Congestion of sinusoids and dilatation of central veins are characteristic. Condensation of collapsed reticulum and new fiber formation combine to form fibrosis, which may connect the central areas of adjacent lobules. Sparing of the portal areas results in a reversal of the usual portal cirrhotic pattern (*i.e.,* central-to-central scarring, with virtual sparing of the portal triads, rather than portal-to-portal scarring, with relatively normal central areas). As the disease progresses, central-to-portal and even portal-to-portal scars develop and regenerative nodules form, which may obliterate the early, characteristic "central" cirrhotic pattern. The central predominance of the scar, however, usually permits recognition. Grossly, the liver shows a finely nodular appearance with some residual nutmeg pattern of chronic passive congestion, the underlying lesion.

Pathogenesis of the Pathologic Pattern

Morphogenetically, the development of the fibrosis is complex and not clearly understood. When large areas of parenchymal cells have undergone necrosis, as may occur in severe viral hepatitis, these "empty" necrotic areas collapse and undergo collagenization (Figs. 20-9 and 20-10).

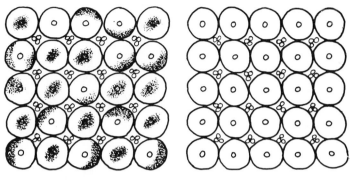

Viral hepatitis   Normal liver

Fig. 20-9. Diagrammatic relationship between focal necrosis and the absence of scarring in acute hepatitis. Necrosis in acute viral hepatitis of average severity involves individual cells diffusely throughout the lobule. It may be predominantly central or diffuse, but it is contained within individual lobules, as indicated by the stippling on the left. The basic lobular architecture of the liver is unimpaired, and healing takes place by regeneration. No scar tissue is formed. After recovery the liver is morphologically and histologically normal (*right*).

The *passive* septa thus formed represent merely the condensation of the collapsed reticular supporting framework of the hepatic parenchyma and its metamorphosis into scar tissue. This pattern is characteristic of bridging hepatic necrosis of viral hepatitis with the linkage of adjacent portal and/or central areas of collapsed, necrotic stromal elements, as described by Klatskin and Boyer.[87,464] A similar

pattern, occurring over a much longer period of time, develops in alcoholic liver injury (Fig. 20-11). Initially, this injury is centrilobular, but the process may extend in bridgelike fashion to the portal tracts. Massive necrosis of whole lobules, however, may also occur in alcoholic hepatitis and may thus cause broad areas of collapse that account for the postnecrotic pattern sometimes seen in

Fig. 20-10. Diagrammatic relationship between submassive (bridging) hepatic necrosis and subsequent scarring. In submassive hepatic necrosis, large areas of necrosis (indicated by *stippling*) involve whole lobules or groups of contiguous lobules or extend between the central areas of adjacent lobules or from central to portal areas. These "bridges" of necrosis disrupt the basic lobular structure of the liver. Wherever such large areas of necrosis develop, the empty stroma collapses and fibrous tissue formation is stimulated. As shown on the right, these areas of collapse may result in dense scar containing the condensed portal structures or in finer, more linear scars between adjacent lobules, giving rise to the patterns of postnecrotic and posthepatitic cirrhosis.

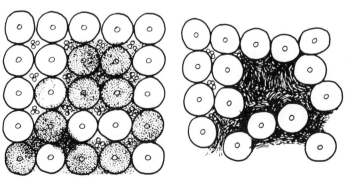

Submassive
hepatic necrosis   Postnecrotic cirrhosis

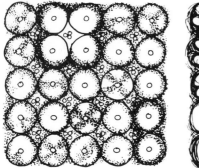 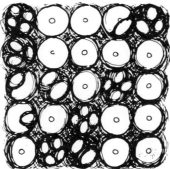

Alcoholic necrosis   Portal cirrhosis

Fig. 20-11. Diagrammatic relationship between alcoholic necrosis and portal cirrhosis. The distribution of necrosis in alcoholic hepatitis is predominantly central, but peripheral necrosis is common (indicated by *stippling* on left). The necrosis may be piecemeal, involving individual cells, or may bridge central-to-central zones or central-to-portal areas. The insidious development of scar tissue involves the centrilobular and portal areas and causes central sclerosis, portal cirrhosis, and, eventually, micronodular cirrhosis in which the lobules are subdivided into abnormal nodules and pseudolobules (*right*).

alcoholic cirrhosis.[799] In addition, active fibrogenesis is stimulated by alcoholic injury and inflammation of parenchymal, ductular, sinusoidal, and reticuloendothelial cells. This fibroplasia gives rise to *active* septa that radiate to the parenchyma primarily from the portal areas. These active septa, in contrast to passive septa, which give rise to static scar, represent a critical part of the process of the progression of cirrhosis.

Simultaneously, hepatic parenchymal necrosis stimulates regeneration. Potent stimuli for hepatic parenchymal hyperplasia, which occur at the same time, further distort the random, fibrous patterns. The complex interactions of the fibrogenic and regenerative stimuli, in relation to the altered vascular pattern, the inconstant and variable inflammatory response, and the impaired functional capacity of the liver, in the face of continued alcoholic injury result in the infinitely varied pathologic patterns seen in alcoholic cirrhosis.

ETIOLOGY AND PATHOGENESIS

The precise etiology of cirrhosis is not known. Although some of the settings in which cirrhosis develops are obvious, the mechanisms by which these situations or agents are translated to the clinicopathologic picture of cirrhosis are unclear. Circumstantially, it appears clear that cirrhosis is associated with excessive alcohol consumption, with viral hepatitis, with drug-induced hepatic injury, with prolonged extrahepatic biliary obstruction, with the late stages of certain parasitic diseases, and with some genetically transmitted metabolic disorders such as hemochro-

matosis and Wilson's disease (see Table 20-1). Despite the circumstantial indictment of malnutrition and the ritual use of the adjective "nutritional" to identify the most common type of cirrhosis, the development of cirrhosis as a consequence of pure dietary deficiency has never been established.

Studies in experimental animals, although productive of great volumes of data, have not provided until relatively recently a reliable animal model with which to study the problem. Investigations have suggested that cirrhosis may be induced in dogs[141] by the long-term administration of alcohol and intermittent feeding, conditions not unlike those associated with alcoholic cirrhosis in humans. Similar disorders have been produced by carbon tetrachloride in rats, by dimethylnitrosamine in rats and dogs,[521] by galactosamine or corticosteroids in rabbits,[549] and by bile duct ligation in dogs.[475]

The demonstration by Rubin and Lieber of the production of alcoholic cirrhosis in baboons is a landmark in liver disease.[798] These investigators showed for the first time that cirrhosis much like human alcoholic cirrhosis, can be reproducibly caused by the administration of alcohol in experimental animals. The authors solved the problem of the animals' natural dislike for excessive alcohol by offering them a liquid formula that provided normal amounts of high quality protein, carbohydrate, fat, vitamins, minerals, and water. It contained ethyl alcohol, which constituted 50% of the total calories. The baboons had no choice and took the diet in amounts that maintained normal body weight. They came to like the diet and averaged fropm 4.5 g to 8.3 g/kg of alcohol daily. This dose, which is approximately the equivalent of one to two quarts of whiskey per day for an average-sized man, caused intoxication and, perhaps, alcohol addiction. In several instances, withdrawal symptoms, much like delirium tremens, were observed when alcohol was discontinued.

This diet induced fatty infiltration, followed by hepatocellular necrosis, which was predominantly centrilobular in distribution, characteristic alcohol hyalin, the so-called Mallory bodies, fibrosis and, finally, cirrhosis. Histologically, the progression of hepatic pathology was similar to that of human alcoholic cirrhosis. The necrosis was predominantly central and the scarring was initially central and spread to involve the portal areas. Even the ultrastructural changes were similar to those seen in human alcoholic hepatitis. The most significant aspect of these studies is that the lesions that progressed to cirrhosis were induced *despite a normal* diet. Control animals who received a diet containing carbohydrate with the same number of calories as contained in the alcohol remained normal. Although a primary role for malnutrition now seems untenable, the importance of secondary malnutrition is being reaffirmed.[525] It is recognized that alcohol may impair nutrient digestion, absorption, or activation.[526] Selective nutrient depletion, such as vitamin A deficiency, which is associated with hepatic lysosomal lesions, may be produced by alcohol.[513]

There are several subtle differences between the cirrhosis produced in the baboons and that in humans. First, the disease developed in some after less than one year of alcohol administration, a much shorter time than in humans. Second, the disease developed in more than half of the experimental animals, compared with only a small percentage of human alcoholics. Both of these differences may be consequences of greater and more constant alcohol ingestion than the human condition permits in most instances. Finally, the early development of a centrilobular cirrhosis with fibrosis connecting the central portions of lobules and sparing the portal areas is characteristic of the reverse lobulation of cardiac cirrhosis. This pattern, in our experience, is unusual in alcoholic cirrhosis. It may occur early in the course of the disease, however, before the cirrhosis is evident clinically. These exciting findings, if confirmed, should help to answer many questions about the pathogenesis of alcoholic cirrhosis.

Differences among species and the inability to control an infinite number of variables, however, limit extrapolation of such preliminary animal data to humans. Until cirrhosis can be reproducibly induced by a single factor, presumably alcohol, in a number of species of experimental animals and can be unequivocally shown to be responsible for human cirrhosis, the etiology must remain unproved. Multiple factors, acting individually or in concert, may be responsible for cirrhosis, and multiple factors individually or collectively may satisfy such postulates. It is probable, in fact, that there are many causes of cirrhosis, each of which may act differently. In the hope of deriving some general mechanism, let us consider individually those factors that, like cigarette smoking in lung cancer, are guilty by association.

Alcohol

Alcoholism has been present throughout recorded history, but the relationship between excessive alcohol ingestion and cirrhosis was not recognized for several millennia. The association between alcohol and cirrhosis, which had apparently been recognized by Vesalius and was well known in the 17th century, is almost entirely circumstantial. It is based on the age-old observation that heavy drinkers frequently develop cirrhosis. This concept is supported primarily by repeated observations of a high prevalence of cirrhosis in alcoholic subjects, and by a low prevalence in moderate and nondrinkers. Jolliffe and Jellinek collected statistics from the literature that, although uncontrolled, appear to show that cirrhosis occurs seven times more frequently in alcoholics than in nondrinkers.[422] In addition, epidemiologic data show a close correlation between fatalities from cirrhosis and the per capita consumption of alcohol[422,465] (Fig. 20-12). Furthermore, unintentional social and political experiments, such as the institution and repeal of Prohibition in the United States (Fig. 20-13) and the abrupt, but transient decrease in wine consumption during the German occupation of France from 1940 to 1945,[502] provide epidemiologic evidence compatible with an etiologic association between alcohol consumption and cirrhosis. The Prohibition picture is particularly impressive, since the deprivation of alcohol was not accompanied by food deprivation, which occurred during the German occupation, and which usually coexists in patients who develop alcoholic cirrhosis. Such data, however, are national, not individual, and might well reflect agents other than alcohol.

Snapper, for example, rejected the alcohol hypothesis. He stated that in his opinion the national alcohol consumption levels do *not* correlate well with the incidence of cirrhosis and implied that nutritional and other toxic factors are responsible.[888] Furthermore, he argued persuasively that since cirrhosis takes 15 years or more to develop, the sharp changes in incidence observed during American Prohibition and the German occupation of France occurred too promptly to be related to alcohol consumption. His concept does not take into account, however, the effect of cumulative alcohol-induced damage (*i.e.*, the importance of the duration of excessive alcohol consumption in the development of cirrhosis). One might thus see less cirrhosis immediately after the long-term development of the lesion has been interrupted by the withdrawal of the offending agent, or a prompt rise in incidence after the resumption of alcohol in patients in whom the development of cirrhosis was transiently delayed during the obligatory abstinence.

Few present-day investigators go so far as to reject outright the relationship between excess alcohol ingestion and cirrhosis. There is, however, ongoing concern about accounting for why only some heavy drinkers seem predisposed to the development of cirrhosis. Explanations have arisen from two not necessarily mutually exclusive hypotheses. The first argues that the development of cirrhosis

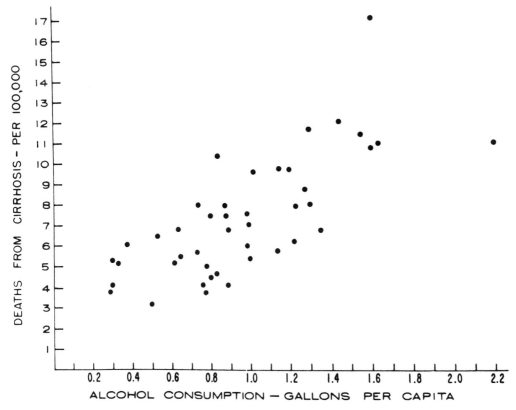

Fig. 20-12. Association between alcohol consumption and mortality rate from cirrhosis. These data show a close, positive correlation between national alcohol consumption and the incidence of death from cirrhosis. (Klatskin G: Gastroenterology 41:443, 1961. © 1961, American Gastroenterological Society)

is largely a function of alcohol consumed and the length of time over which it is ingested. The second hypothesis is that alcohol is only permissive and creates the setting for an additional factor to induce cirrhosis.[21]

The studies of Lelbach have most persuasively related the development of liver damage to the degree and duration of alcohol abuse in the individual patient. In studies of alcohol addicts of more than 15 years' duration, he found severe liver damage in 75% of those with a daily alcohol consumption in excess of 160 g (approximately 200 ml of ethanol or a pint of whiskey), compared with 17% of those who consumed less than this amount.[510] The time factor was equally important. The prevalence of severe liver damage after 15 years of excessive alcohol consumption was eight times greater than after only 5 years of heavy drinking. These data support our own clinical impression that a pint of whiskey per day for 15 years is the critical threshold. We refer to pint-years in a manner analogous to the pack-years of cigarette smoking associated with the development of lung cancer. Thus, 15 pint-years, which frequently culminate in alcoholic cirrhosis, may serve as a rough index to gauge the degree of alcohol-induced liver injury and to predict the possibility of de-

veloping cirrhosis. The prevalence of cirrhosis after 30 pint-years, accumulated at the rate of one pint per day for 30 years or a quart per day for 15 years, would probably be lower than in patients who consumed two quarts per day for 7½ years. It would be fascinating, but pure fantasy, to attempt to validate the linearity of this relationship prospectively in humans and to determine whether dose or duration predominates. There is evidence that women may be more susceptible than men. In women the threshold for increased likelihood to develop cirrhosis may be as low as 20 g/day.[827] Unfortunately, such data are retrospective and derived from patients who have already developed cirrhosis and consequently are not applicable to those actively engaged in accumulating pint-years. It is fascinating that only a small percentage of heavy drinkers actually develop cirrhosis. Is resistance to the ravages of alcohol absolute or relative? It is said that every man has his price. Does every liver have its critical pint-year requirement? It is probable that these questions can never be accurately answered.

On the other hand, no deleterious effects were observed when alcohol was administered in the hospital setting to patients recovering from alcoholic fatty liver.[929,986] In

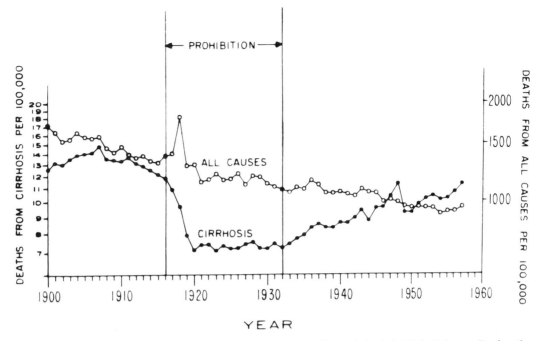

Fig. 20-13. Effect of Prohibition on mortality rate from cirrhosis in United States. During the period from 1900 to 1960 the overall mortality rate progressively decreased. The mortality rate from cirrhosis fell precipitously following enactment of the 18th Amendment to the Constitution in 1916. The decreased rate was sustained until 1932 when Prohibition was repealed, after which the mortality rate from cirrhosis progressively climbed. (Klatskin G: Gastroenterology 41:443, 1961. © 1961, American Gastroenterological Society)

larger amounts, however, it prevented the clearing of fat from the alcoholic fatty liver.[592] These findings again imply the existence of other cofactors that may act together with alcohol.

Orrego and colleagues have argued that consumption of alcohol above a threshold level is a necessary but not a sufficient condition for the development of cirrhosis.[659] They do not deny that in the setting of alcohol consumption the probability of developing cirrhosis increases linearly with time; they are impressed, however, that at whatever the dose or whatever the duration, many persons do *not* develop cirrhosis. They therefore wonder whether it is not possible that liver damage is produced by a simultaneous combination of a primary effect produced by alcohol and a precipitating factor, which occurs randomly, independent of alcohol consumption.[659]

Partial support for this view is to be found in a prospective study from Copenhagen.[898] These investigators found that neither the duration of alcohol abuse nor the average daily consumption was related to the subsequent incidence of cirrhosis. Noteworthy, however, is that their findings confirmed observations from Lelbach and others that above a 50 g/day threshold, the risk of developing alcoholic cirrhosis is about 15%.

The Copenhagen group does not identify factors that may be needed to induce cirrhosis. The hepatitis B virus

has been suggested from time to time as being such a factor. Several studies have found that in alcoholic cirrhosis there is either an increased prevalence of antibodies to hepatitis B surface antigen (HB_sAg),[387,601] evidence of cellular immunity to HB_sAg,[701] or an increased susceptibility of HB_sAg carriers to hepatic damage from alcohol.[981] These associations are intriguing but unproved.

A possible role for interactions with the histocompatibility antigens and other genetic factors is discussed in a later section of this chapter.

From time to time, the concept is raised that it is not alcohol *per se* but some other factor in the alcoholic beverage that is responsible for cirrhosis. It seems clear that alcohol-associated cirrhosis in the United States occurs predominantly in whiskey drinkers; in France, Italy, Chile, and in the German wine districts of Baden–Würtemberg and Rheinland–Pfalz in wine drinkers; and in Australia and in the vineyard-free parts of Germany, in beer drinkers. Alcohol is virtually the only factor common to these diverse beverages. This concept is supported by epidemiologic studies in Canada, where cirrhosis appears to be associated with the alcoholic beverage that provides alcohol at the lowest unit cost. Such observations have not altered the well-established convictions, unsubstantiated by hard data, that cirrhosis is associated with "rotgut" whiskey, not with "good stuff," that in northeastern France cirrhosis is associated with the consumption of red wine, but not with white, and that in Spain cirrhosis is associated with port wine, but not with sherry. It is fair to assume that Portuguese authorities have opposite opinions about the relative hepatotoxicity of sherry and port. Most data suggest it is the volume of alcohol consumed, rather than the type of beverage, that leads to cirrhosis. The ready availability of alcohol of all types in the American melting pot and the development of cirrhosis from the beverage of one's choice attests to one of the basic freedoms of American democracy.

Although it has been shown conclusively that alcohol, even in relatively small, socially acceptable, noninebriating quantities, induces fatty infiltration of the liver in humans,[527] there is no evidence that this lesion progresses to cirrhosis. In fact, fatty infiltration, which is almost invariably present after any alcohol ingestion, is rapidly reversible. Since only a small fraction—only 10% to 15%—of persons who drink alcohol to excess develop cirrhosis,[422,465,898] it seems clear that fatty infiltration *per se* is not an obligatory precirrhotic lesion. It certainly suggests that other factors, including genetic susceptibility, which is discussed subsequently, may act as a cofactor with alcohol.

Although fatty liver itself does not appear to be precirrhotic, there is evidence that there are lesions that can be present even at the fatty liver stage that may indeed presage the development of cirrhosis. The investigators from the Bronx Veterans Administration Hospital have offered evidence that perivenular fibrosis (thickening of the terminal hepatic vein) is a precursor lesion to cirrhosis.[631,973,1042] Other investigators have not been able to confirm the significance of thickening around the terminal hepatic vein.[81,636] One group of these investigators found instead that lobular fibrosis and sinusoidal fibrosis are markers for progressive fibrosis and development of cirrhosis.[636] Lieber has suggested that perivenular fibrosis and sinusoidal fibrosis may represent two aspects of a similar lesion surrounding vascular structures of different sizes, namely, venules and sinusoids.[525]

It is not yet certain whether alcoholic hepatitis, which is characterized histologically by active hepatic parenchymal necrosis, the presence of characteristic hyaline cytoplasmic inclusions, and inflammation,[312,365,365a] and which often is accompanied by fatty infiltration, can be induced in humans by alcohol *alone* or whether other cofactors are necessary. It seems clear, however, that alcoholic hepatitis is a precirrhotic lesion.[378] Galambos followed 61 such patients for a mean of 3 years and found that cirrhosis developed in 38%; even among the minority who stopped drinking, cirrhosis developed in 18%.[312] Sorensen and his group from Copenhagen found in their prospective study that the risk of subsequent development of cirrhosis was increased ninefold in patients with alcoholic hepatitis.[898] The critical difference between fatty liver and alcoholic hepatitis is that alcoholic hepatitis embodies hepatic necrosis, the *sine qua non* of the experimental production of cirrhosis by any agent, and alcoholic fat deposition does not. This concept was expressed by Moon in 1934,[607] and

50 additional years of research have not increased our understanding. He wrote,

> Alcohol, even in large amounts and long continued, had caused only parenchymatous degeneration and fatty changes. These have not resulted in necrosis nor in permanent hepatic changes. However, the probability that alcohol acts as a contributing or predisposing factor *has* received experimental support. Alcohol has been found to accentuate the injurious effects of bacteria, phosphorus, chloroform, and of carbon tetrachloride, upon the livers of animals. It is probable that alcohol may similarly accentuate the effects of injurious agents upon the human liver.

That is not to say that our knowledge has not advanced since Moon. Extensive studies have been carried out on the pathways of alcohol metabolism and on associated metabolic disturbances in an attempt to define the toxicity of ethanol. This research has identified toxic effects related to the generation of NADH by oxidation of ethanol via the alcohol dehydrogenase (ADH) pathway, the interaction of alcohol with liver microsomes, the generation of acetaldehyde in the metabolism of alcohol, the effects of ethanol on liver membranes, and the effects of an imbalance between oxygen delivery and the liver cells' requirements. These findings have been reviewed by Lieber,[524–526] and the role of each is discussed below.

Three pathways exist in the hepatocyte for ethanol metabolism: the ADH pathway of the cytosol, the microsomal ethanol oxidizing system (MEOS) in the endoplasmic reticulum, and the catalase pathway in peroxisomes. The major pathway is via ADH. In the process of oxidizing alcohol to acetaldehyde, the ADH pathway, which requires nicotinamide-adenine dinucleotide (NAD), generates an excess of reducing equivalents as free NADH.[525] The resulting altered redox state has multiple metabolic consequences, including hyperlipemia and changes in amino acid and protein metabolism. These changes may lead to cell injury and stimulation of collagen formation.

The interaction of ethanol with liver microsomes was first suggested by the morphologic observation that ethanol feeding resulted in proliferation of smooth endoplasmic reticulum (SER). Subsequently the SER was found to be the site of the MEOS. The activity of this system has been shown to be dependent on cytochrome P-450. The MEOS pathway of alcohol metabolism has particular importance in chronic ethanol ingestion and is a major mechanism for acceleration of ethanol metabolism at high ethanol concentrations. An ethanol-specific form of cytochrome P-450 has been postulated that is thought to increase in concentration with chronic alcohol ingestion. The interaction of drugs and environmental compounds with increased cytochrome P-450 content in hepatocytes may result in increased toxicity of these compounds to liver cells. Such increased susceptibility to their toxic effects has been demonstrated for acetaminophen and carbon tetrachloride.

The ADH and MEOS pathways, as well as the catalase pathway, generate acetaldehyde as a metabolic product.

Acetaldehyde has several toxic effects: it covalently binds to protein, it may impair protein secretion, and it also causes lipid peroxidation. Cell injury may result. For example, covalent binding to protein may directly injure hepatocytes or it may serve as an antigen that may initiate immunologic injury.

Alcohol's effect on cell membranes includes changes in their physical state and in their lipid composition. Membrane function and cell integrity may therefore be compromised.

Oxygen consumption after alcohol ingestion is known to show a greater increase in alcoholic patients than in nonalcoholic ones. This has been seen as "energy wastage." It is postulated that this increased oxygen demand, owing to either an enhanced role of the MEOS or to relative uncoupling of reoxidation of NADH, may aggravate alcohol hepatotoxicity.

Because biochemical evidence of hepatic injury often continues despite cessation of alcohol intake, a potential role for altered humoral and cellular immunity in the pathogenesis of alcoholic liver disease has been proposed.[548,681,900,1055,1056] Possible humoral mechanisms have included antibodies to Mallory bodies, antibodies to antigens on hepatocyte membranes that have been altered by alcohol or its metabolites, and the triggering of liver injury by immune complexes.[548] However, the pathogenetic role of these mechanisms remains unestablished.

The evidence for the role of altered cellular immunity in the pathogenesis of alcoholic liver disease is circumstantial. It includes changes in lymphocyte population and function, changes in the response of lymphocytes to mitogens, and occurrence of abnormal tests of delayed hypersensitivity. These changes are discussed below.

In alcoholic hepatitis and cirrhosis, there is a reduction in peripheral blood T lymphocytes coupled with an increased number of T lymphocytes in the liver. These changes are reversible when alcohol is withdrawn and the patient improves clinically. Cytotoxicity for liver cells by peripheral blood lymphocytes has been described in other studies.[151,431]

Sera from patients with alcoholic liver disease have been found to inhibit lymphocyte transformation *in vitro* when phytohemagglutinin, pokeweed mitogen, and concanavalin A were used.[548]

Suppression of delayed cutaneous hypersensitivity has been shown in acute alcoholic hepatitis.[891] *In vitro* studies using lymphocyte transformation studies and migration inhibition indices have found lymphocyte sensitization to alcohol and acetaldehyde in alcoholic hepatitis but not cirrhosis. Patients with alcoholic hepatitis as well as alcoholic cirrhosis have shown lymphocyte sensitization to Mallory bodies in some but not all studies.[548] Whether these immunologic alterations play a role in initiating alcoholic injury or are epiphenomena is yet to be elucidated.

Malnutrition

Malnutrition has long been claimed to be the cause of cirrhosis, or at least a major factor in its development.

The evidence to support this concept is of two types. First, the production of cirrhosis in experimental animals fed deficient diets, especially protein-, choline-, and vitamin-deficient diets, favors this concept. Hepatic lesions that resemble cirrhosis, both postnecrotic[384] and portal in type,[385] can be produced in rats and other experimental animals by protein- and vitamin-deficient diets.[367] It is not established, however, that these lesions represent true cirrhosis. Although histologically compatible, they are, unlike cirrhosis in humans, apparently reversible lesions and do not exhibit the vascular consequences commonly seen in human cirrhosis. It must always be kept in mind that data derived from animal experiments, although useful in suggesting and testing hypotheses and in indicating new directions for investigation, can only be extrapolated to humans at considerable risk.

Second, the beneficial response of malnutrition/alcohol-induced lesions to high-protein diets and diet supplements supports the nutritional pathogenesis.[684] In virtually all such instances, however, excessive alcohol ingestion had coexisted with malnutrition during the development of the lesion, and diet therapy in the hospital was almost invariably accompanied by abstinence from alcohol.

Until the present time, no one has been able to establish a causal relationship between malnutrition and human cirrhosis. The hepatic lesion closest to cirrhosis induced by protein malnutrition is kwashiorkor. This disease, which was first described by Williams in Africa,[1027] has also been reported, predominantly in infants and young children, in India, Indonesia, Central America, Jamaica, and many other impoverished areas. Although it is a generalized disease characterized by retarded physical and mental growth, edema, ascites and hypoalbuminemia, its hepatic characteristic is a large, fatty liver. There is no cirrhosis.[196,1000] Ramalingaswami reported that diffuse fibrosis, and perhaps cirrhosis, may occasionally be found in children suffering from prolonged kwashiorkor.[740] The disease is rapidly reversed by the administration of protein.[97] After recovery, the liver is normal, although in some cases a fine fibrosis may be found. This lesion appears to be similar to the lesions induced in experimental animals by dietary deficiencies. In adults, evidence for a malnutrition-induced lesion equivalent to kwashiorkor is scant.[862] The only indication of cirrhosis induced by malnutrition has been presented by Snapper, who observed epidemic cirrhosis associated with malnutrition in Peking during the Japanese occupation.[887] Other disorders may be responsible for, or predispose to, the development of cirrhosis. The prevalence of hepatitis is increased in many of the malnourished areas of the world, and underlying posthepatitic cirrhosis may account for some of the cirrhosis attributed to malnutrition. Aflatoxin, too, may play an unrecognized role in many of these areas.[755] A disorder indistinguishable from Indian childhood cirrhosis had been reported following chronic ingestion of food contaminated with aflatoxin B_1 derived from *Aspergillus flavus*.[18] Similarly, schistosomiasis and other parasitic infestations of the liver may be present in some of the tropical areas of malnutrition and may thus complicate the problem. Certainly, malnutrition could accelerate or exacerbate such underlying lesions.

The recognition that ileojejunal bypass operations for the treatment of obesity may induce progressive fatty infiltration of the liver and even cirrhosis[232] appears to challenge the concept that malnutrition does not cause cirrhosis in humans. Such small-bowel exclusion operations induce metabolically complex situations that alter absorption, enterohepatic circulation, and bile acid metabolism. Any of these abnormalities or other unrecognized consequences of these operations might conceivably induce liver damage and cirrhosis in a manner independent of malnutrition *per se*. Certainly total starvation, which is, in effect, an unbalanced and protein-deficient diet, causes no significant hepatic dysfunction and, in fact, is associated with the disappearance of the fatty infiltration of obesity.[232]

At the present time, the best conclusion is that malnutrition is undoubtedly associated with the pathogenesis of some types of cirrhosis and that famine, under certain complex, poorly studied, little understood situations, may cause cirrhosis in humans.

Viral Hepatitis

Hepatitis A has not been documented to result in either chronic liver disease or cirrhosis.[512] Perhaps this is because hepatitis A virus (HAV) infection is cytopathic, rather than immunogenic. There is less compelling evidence that HAV infection, in contrast to hepatitis B and non A, non B infection, requires a contribution from the host's immune system to cause hepatocellular injury.[325] Mediation of injury by an immunopathologic process, has been postulated, however.[512]

The progression of *hepatitis B* from acute to chronic occurs in about 10% of patients, but only about 3% develop potentially progressive disease.[156] Among patients with chronic active hepatitis, the progression to cirrhosis over 2 to 5 years may be as high as 70%.[217] This high frequency of development of cirrhosis is not necessarily limited to those with severe disease but may occur in patients who are not clinically ill, who have only piecemeal necrosis on biopsy, and who have only moderate biochemical abnormalities. There is no evidence that corticosteroid therapy alters the natural history of the histologic lesion. When chronic hepatitis B is histologically persistent (*i.e.*, limited to the portal tracts) rather than active hepatitis (*i.e.*, periportal hepatitis or confluent necrosis or both), cirrhosis is not a recognized consequence.[135] When hepatitis B progresses to cirrhosis, the 5-year survival is 55%, with liver failure or the complications of cirrhosis the most frequent cause of death.[1012]

Non A, non B hepatitis not only has a propensity to become chronic, but most reported series have documented the development of cirrhosis.[66,210,470,472,473,738,808] Cirrhosis has been reported as early as 4 months to 1 year after onset of non A, non B hepatitis,[226] but a larger number of cases appear to be found between the second and fourth years.[748] Cirrhosis has nonetheless been described as developing as late as 5 years after acute non A, non B hepatitis.[472] The prevalence of cirrhosis in most reported series has been between 5% and 10%,[470,472,473,484,738] but prevalences approaching 15% have also been reported.[748,808] The diagnosis of non A, non B hepatitis is one of exclusion and is nonspecific; estimates of its sequelae are therefore imprecise.

In some cases, the acute hepatitis has been symptomatic, cirrhosis has developed early, and death has occurred from liver failure,[226] but the more usual occurrence appears to be the slow development of cirrhosis in a clinically inapparent fashion.[210] Even when cirrhosis develops insidiously, some patients may subsequently develop encephalopathy, ascites, and variceal hemorrhage.[414] These latter patients have been predominantly elderly and have received large numbers of transfusions. Most patients progressing to cirrhosis have in fact acquired their preceding hepatitis by parenteral means (transfusions, parenteral drug use, or needle stick).

The number of patients who have been followed for long periods is not large, but available data suggest that when hepatitis B virus and hepatitis D virus (delta) infections are acquired simultaneously (*i.e.*, coinfection) the illness seldom progresses to chronicity.[753,878] This is not the case when patients chronically infected with hepatitis B virus develop delta superinfection. In such a setting, current knowledge suggests chronicity is likely to be the most frequent outcome. This is suggested by the observation that the prevalence of delta infection is three to five times higher in carriers with chronic hepatitis than in asymptomatic carriers.[780,781] It is further suggested by the finding that 90% of patients with delta infection in a Venezuelan epidemic among B virus carriers developed chronic hepatitis as opposed to only 10% of those with hepatitis B infection alone.[780] There is some evidence that chronicity is more likely in patients with inactive infections (presence of anti-HB_e in serum) than in patients who have active infection (characterized by HB_eAg in serum) who become superinfected.[780] In one large Italian series of patients who were chronic carriers of HB_sAg and had superimposed delta infection established by intrahepatic expression of delta antigen, cirrhosis was present at initial biopsy in 23% and developed in an additional 41% over a period of observation of 2 to 6 years.[781] One third of the patients who presented with cirrhosis and one fifth of those who developed cirrhosis died during the period of observation.[781] Nearly 60% of British HB_sAg carriers who were delta antibody–positive had cirrhosis as opposed to only 20% who had surface antigen alone.[1014] Even when carriers of HB_sAg with delta antibody are asymptomatic, 40% may have cirrhosis.[25]

The low prevalence of cirrhosis after hepatitis of all viral etiologies, relative to the large number of patients with presumed posthepatitic cirrhosis, poses a fascinating epidemiologic paradox. The demonstration that subacute hepatic necrosis and postnecrotic cirrhosis may follow anicteric hepatitis has raised the question of whether clinically mild, inapparent hepatitis may have a worse prognosis in terms of the development of cirrhosis[464] than overt hepatitis with jaundice. Complicating this whole problem is subjective, observer variability in the diagnosis of the presence[895] and type of cirrhosis[317,332] and evidence that the type of cirrhosis may differ in different portions of the liver.[314,799]

Obstruction of the Extrahepatic Biliary Tract

Any process that obstructs the biliary tree, including gallstones, neoplasms, benign strictures, extrinsic compression of any cause, or congenital or acquired atresia of the bile ducts, may in sufficient time result in secondary biliary cirrhosis. It is not, however, an invariable consequence of prolonged biliary obstruction. Fewer than 10% of patients with chronic biliary tract obstruction develop biliary cirrhosis.[329] Since the process takes from 3 months to more than a year to develop, it occurs more commonly with benign than with malignant causes of obstruction, since the latter may kill the patient before cirrhosis can develop. It is found more frequently with total than with partial obstruction, and this difference may explain the paradoxically less frequent occurrence of biliary cirrhosis in patients with ascending cholangitis, which is usually associated with incomplete obstruction.[227]

It is not clear exactly how biliary cirrhosis develops. Review of the consequences of obstruction of the extrahepatic biliary tree may shed some light on the problem. Acute biliary tract obstruction causes the prompt appearance of hepatomegaly and of dilated intrahepatic bile ducts. At first, the bile is dark but quickly becomes colorless, the so-called white bile, which results from the suppression of the secretion of bilirubin by increased intraductular pressure. Microscopically, bile duct regeneration occurs. The bile ductules, which are tortuous and distended, are lined by high cuboidal epithelium. Focal necrosis in the central areas occurs early in the process and is followed by peripheral necrosis. Periportal necrosis is more widespread and is characterized by bile lakes, which are bile-stained areas of parenchymal necrosis due, presumably, to the escape of bile from the interlobular bile ducts. Bile lakes are characteristic of high-grade mechanical obstruction of the biliary tree and are never seen in nonobstructive intrahepatic cholestasis. If infected, the bile may become purulent and the portal areas may show acute polymorphonuclear infiltration. If cholangitis or abscess formation develops, necrosis of the periportal areas may predominate.

Although the pathogenesis of secondary biliary cirrhosis is not fully understood, it is consistent with the pathogenetic patterns in other types of cirrhosis. The presence of periportal necrosis and inflammation may stimulate the development of portal scar. The concentric, onion-skin layering of scar tissue around the portal areas is compatible with this pathogenesis. It is not known whether infection is required to cause biliary cirrhosis. In humans,

infected biliary obstruction is less likely to be associated with biliary cirrhosis than is noninfected obstruction. Furthermore, experimental biliary cirrhosis can be produced in experimental animals with sterile biliary tract obstruction (i.e., in the absence of infection).

Histologically, it may be difficult to differentiate established secondary biliary cirrhosis from cirrhosis of other types, although the fibrous linkage from portal-to-portal areas tends to create a more regular pseudolobular pattern than the portal-to-central microlobularity of alcoholic cirrhosis or the macronodular appearance of postnecrotic cirrhosis. As the disease progresses, the pattern of necrosis-to-fibrosis proceeds and some portal-to-central scars develop. A dense cirrhosis may develop with unremittent biliary obstruction. Intense regenerative activity, which further distorts the pattern and makes it indistinguishable from other types of cirrhosis,[227] sometimes occurs. This type of cirrhosis is not functionally benign; approximately half the patients develop ascites, varices, and other evidence of portal hypertension,[848] although these complications occur only with longstanding obstructive disease in which much of the parenchymal tissue has been converted into regenerative nodules.[227]

In summary, the triad of necrosis, fibrosis, and regeneration in prolonged obstructive jaundice creates a pathologically characteristic form of portal cirrhosis, which in later stages may no longer be differentiable from advanced cirrhosis of other types.

Primary Biliary Cirrhosis

Primary biliary cirrhosis is discussed in Chapter 26.

Heart Failure and Outflow Obstruction

Cardiac cirrhosis is an uncommon consequence of chronic heart failure. It is most frequently seen in patients with longstanding cardiac decompensation, especially those with tricuspid insufficiency or with constrictive pericarditis. The disease is not overt clinically, and the diagnosis of cardiac cirrhosis may be difficult to make. It is rarely associated with deep jaundice or evidence of poor hepatic function, such as severe hypoalbuminemia or prolongation of prothrombin time, or manifestations of portal hypertension, such as bleeding esophageal varices or portal-systemic encephalopathy.

The liver in heart failure is enlarged, purplish, and rounded. It is rarely irregular or overtly nodular. On cut surface the veins are prominent and dilated. The characteristic "nutmeg" liver of alternating red and yellow areas represents the reddish centrilobular areas of congestion and the normal yellowish portions of the lobule.[991]

Microscopically, the liver shows distended central veins and engorgement of the sinusoids entering them. The radiating plates of liver cells are atrophic in the central areas. The rows of hepatocytes are smaller than in the periportal areas. When severe, there may be hemorrhage into the central areas, and centrilobular focal necrosis may be present. Lipofuscin pigment may be prominent in the central hepatocytes. The portal areas are relatively unaffected.

The pathogenesis of cardiac cirrhosis is compatible with the pathophysiology of heart failure and the histologic abnormalities noted above. In heart failure, reduction of cardiac output results in decreased perfusion pressure of the blood entering the liver. The oxygen content of blood is, of course, greatest in the periportal areas (area 1 of Rappaport) and falls progressively as it approaches the central portion of the lobules (Rappaport's area 3), which is metabolically the most susceptible portion of the lobule.[745] The metabolic susceptibility of the central portion of the lobule is shown by the peculiarly rapid postmortem autolysis of this area in patients with chronic congestive failure.[720] Similarly, the syndrome of massive elevations of serum transaminase levels in patients following a bout of hypotension is another clinical manifestation of this anatomically localized susceptibility.[461] Presumably, the hypoxic centrilobular hepatic cells become more so during a period of shock following myocardial infarction, pulmonary embolism, or transient arrhythmia. All of the injured cells simultaneously lose their enzymes into the serum, with a resultant sharp spike in transaminase activity that may reach levels of 5,000 units, 10,000 units, or even 20,000 units. Often this sequence of events is fatal, but if the hypotension is transient or promptly corrected, the enormous elevation in transaminase levels may be unaccompanied by other gross distortions of liver function and the patient may survive.

In addition, the increased central venous pressure of heart failure is transmitted backwards into the hepatic veins where congestion opposes the entry of portal and arterial blood to the central portion of the lobules. The localized centrilobular hypoxia results at first in congestion and atrophy of the hepatic cords with loss of cells and, later, in hemorrhage and necrosis. Loss of cells results in collapse and condensation of the reticulum. Active necrosis stimulates collagen production and collagenization of the collapsed reticulum and even of the central veins, giving rise to phlebosclerosis. It has been found in electron microscopic studies that initially atrophy of cells, rather than active necrosis, is the stimulus for fibrous tissue formation.[812] Finally, regenerative activity develops.

The pattern of cardiac cirrhosis fits this pathogenesis perfectly. The scar is initially centrilobular, and as it spreads into the lobule, the scars connect central areas to one another. In the presence of relatively unaffected portal areas, one sees the "reverse lobulation" of cardiac cirrhosis.[861] The portal areas appear to be "centrally" located and are surrounded by a ring of fibrous tissue bands that pass from central vein to central vein. The cirrhosis in this classic stage is characteristic and specific for cardiac cirrhosis, but later, as bile duct regeneration and portal fibrosis develop and as parenchymal regeneration takes place, the cirrhosis may lose its specific pattern.

Thus cardiac cirrhosis is a centrizonal cirrhosis that results in loss of cells from the central portion of the liver as a consequence of centrilobular hypoxia. Central deposition of scar produces a specific type of cirrhosis that reflects closely its pathogenesis.

A lesion indistinguishable from cardiac cirrhosis may occasionally be seen in patients with chronic hepatic venous obstruction (Budd–Chiari syndrome). The pathogenesis is similar to that seen in cardiac cirrhosis, except that the initial centrilobular congestion and hepatocellular atrophy are consequences of stasis *per se*. Since cardiac output in this situation is normal or elevated, the Budd–Chiari syndrome may give rise to *stasis* cirrhosis.

Similarly, in veno-occlusive disease, a type of the Budd–Chiari syndrome induced by ingesting *Senecio* or *Crotolaria* alkaloids, a centrilobular cirrhosis may develop.[91]

Hemochromatosis

The pathogenesis of the cirrhosis of hemochromatosis is discussed in the section devoted exclusively to this subject (see Chap. 27).

Hepatolenticular Degeneration

The pathogenesis of the cirrhosis of Wilson's disease is discussed in the section devoted exclusively to this subject (see Chap. 28).

Autoimmune Disorders

The pathogenesis of cirrhosis arising from altered immunity is discussed in Chapter 23.

Syphilis

Cirrhosis is a rare occurrence in syphilis and is seen only when syphilis is congenital. It is a fine intralobular cirrhosis with proliferation of connective tissue that surrounds small groups of cells or individual cells.[241,358,768]

In 10% of acquired secondary syphilis there is hepatitis, with or without granulomas.[267,504] Treatment resolves the hepatitis but may not prevent the accumulation of collagen in the walls of the sinusoids and in the spaces between the liver cells, but cirrhosis does not develop.[267,428]

Tertiary syphilis has erroneously been thought in the past to result in cirrhosis. Tertiary syphilis is characterized by widespread gummas that repair with fibrosis. As the fibrosis contracts, deep clefts may be produced in the liver that produce a pseudolobation of the liver, called *hepar lobatum*. These deep scars may divide the liver into masses of irregular size but do not produce true cirrhosis.[358,933] Previous reports of the occurrence of cirrhosis with syphilis often were based upon the finding of cirrhosis in syphilitic patients who had other epidemiologic associations or were based on series lacking appropriate control groups.[438,975]

Intrinsic Drug-Induced Hepatotoxicity

Carbon Tetrachloride

The solvent carbon tetrachloride represents the prototype of intrinsic hepatotoxicity. Intrinsic hepatotoxins are toxic to the livers of all species, following a short, predictable latent period. The minimal toxic dose is relatively reproducible, and the severity of hepatic injury, which is characteristic for the individual compound, is roughly proportional to dosage. No signs of hypersensitivity, such as fever, rash, or eosinophilia, accompany the liver injury. Carbon tetrachloride induces diffuse fatty degeneration and centrilobular necrosis. Although often fatal, the hepatic lesion is not often the cause of death. Usually, renal tubular injury is the lethal lesion, although the pancreatic and pulmonary lesions and other indirect consequences are sometimes fatal. Hepatic necrosis is usually not massive, and if the patient recovers, cirrhosis is rare.

The mechanism of action of carbon tetrachloride may explain this paradox. Carbon tetrachloride induces its hepatic lesion promptly, within a matter of hours after digestion. Carbon tetrachloride per se, however, is not the toxic material. Drug-metabolizing enzymes, presumably the P-450 microsomal enzyme system, remove one chlorine atom from the molecule, forming trichloromethane, which is extremely toxic to the hepatic endoplasmic reticulum and microsomal drug-metabolizing enzyme systems.[749,750] Lipoperoxidative destruction of these susceptible organelles prevents or diminishes further activation of carbon tetrachloride and, thus, further hepatic damage. Usually, patients who recover regain full hepatic function, and there are no pathologic sequelae. Occasionally, however, hepatic necrosis is massive. Several cases of subacute hepatic necrosis following carbon tetrachloride ingestion, which have gone on to develop postnecrotic cirrhosis, have been reported.[466] There are rare reports that recurrent or chronic exposure to carbon tetrachloride can cause cirrhosis.[717]

The terrible reputation of carbon tetrachloride, which is well deserved, has greatly restricted its commercial use. Consequently, this substance is not clinically important as a hepatotoxin or as a cause of cirrhosis but is of significance because of its well-studied mechanism of action.

Dimethylnitrosamine

Dimethylnitrosamine, an anticorrosive agent, like carbon tetrachloride can induce cirrhosis in experimental animals,[47,549] and, apparently, postnecrotic cirrhosis in humans.[302]

Methotrexate

Methotrexate is a widely used antimetabolite directed against folates, which are essential for DNA synthesis and cell division. It is used in combination chemotherapy in leukemia and diverse cancers as well as for suppression of graft-versus-host disease following bone marrow transplantation and finds an increasing role as a therapeutic agent for severe psoriasis that is not responsive to topical therapy.[421]

Its potential for hepatoxicity has been evident for nearly 30 years. Histologic changes attributed to methotrexate include steatosis, ballooning degeneration and necrosis of hepatocytes, fibrosis, and cirrhosis. The pathologic lesion is one of portal cirrhosis, which is in no way unique. Methotrexate is thought to be an intrinsic hepatotoxin; however, the inability to reproduce hepatic injury consistently in laboratory animals leaves this classification unestablished.[1063]

The extensive use of methotrexate in psoriatic patients has suggested that several factors tend to increase the propensity to liver damage. These include increased alcohol intake, obesity, diabetes mellitus, daily dosage schedules (as opposed to weekly), preexisting liver disease, treatment with arsenic, lowered renal function, and high cumulative dose, although agreement has not been uniform about the latter.[28,640,1010,1052]

Studies in patients with psoriasis treated with methotrexate for 2 or more years that have utilized pretreatment and post-treatment biopsies have suggested a prevalence of fibrosis and cirrhosis between 4% and 25%.[28]

A classification for liver biopsy findings in patients receiving methotrexate, which was developed for monitoring therapy in patients with psoriasis, is shown in Table 20-2.[785] The Psoriasis Task Force of the National Program of Dermatology recommends that liver biopsy be performed, when feasible, before starting methotrexate therapy and that patients be excluded from methotrexate therapy if there is significant preexisting liver disease. If methotrexate therapy is initiated, a repeat biopsy should

TABLE 20-2. Classification of Liver Biopsy Changes During Methotrexate Therapy

Grade I.	Normal; fatty infiltration, mild; nuclear variability, mild; portal inflammation, mild
Grade II.	Fatty infiltration, moderate-severe; nuclear variability, moderate-severe; portal tract expansion, portal tract inflammation, and lobular necrosis, moderate-severe
Grade III.	A. Fibrosis, mild; fibrotic septa extending into the lobules by connective tissue or reticulin stain
	B. Fibrosis, moderate to severe
Grade IV.	Cirrhosis

(Roenigk HH Jr: Methotrexate guidelines: Revised. J Am Acad Dermatol 6:145, 1982)

be considered after a total dose of 1 g. It is important to note that liver scans are of minimal value in identifying patients with methotrexate liver disease and that liver function tests will identify only a few cases of methotrexate toxicity.[785] The cirrhosis is often clinically silent, although portal hypertension may sometimes occur.[152]

Methotrexate can be continued if liver biopsy changes are no more severe than grade II, but repeat biopsies should be obtained after each additional 1.0 g to 1.5 g. Patients with grade IIIB or IV changes should not receive further methotrexate. Patients with grade IIIA changes may continue to receive methotrexate, but a repeat biopsy should be obtained after 6 months.[785]

The pathogenesis of methotrexate hepatotoxicity is unknown. It has been suggested that it may represent a toxic side-effect of its therapeutic mechanism of action. The major activity of methotrexate is its binding to dehydrofolic reductase, thus preventing the conversion of folic acid to its active form, folinic acid. This metabolic block may, in turn, slow the synthesis of nucleic acids, and some amino acids.

Drug-Induced Idiosyncratic Hepatotoxicity

Idiosyncratic hepatotoxicity, typified by α-methyldopa or halothane hepatitis, occurs rarely and after a variable, but prolonged, latent period. Its severity is not dosage-related. It occurs in only a single species—humans—and is associated with a variety of immunologic phenomena (*e.g.,* evidence of allergy, eosinophilia, and, often, abnormal immunologic reactions). Readministration of the offending drug is frequently followed by the prompt recurrence of hepatotoxicity.

It is striking that idiosyncratic hepatotoxins rarely cause cirrhosis, despite the fact that they often cause fatal hepatitis. Patients who survive massive or submassive hepatic necrosis, however, may conceivably develop postnecrotic cirrhosis, in a manner analogous to submassive necrosis in viral hepatitis. Several cases of α-methyldopa–associated cirrhosis have been reported.[856] It can be predicted with confidence that any of the drugs like α-methyldopa or oxyphenisatin that can cause chronic active hepatitis will occasionally cause cirrhosis.

Miscellaneous

Alpha-1-Antitrypsin Deficiency

Alpha$_1$-antitrypsin's (AAT) descriptive name identifies it with the α_1-globulins and correctly credits it with protection of cells against injury from trypsin and other proteases released from bacteria or dying cells. Its deficiency in serum was originally recognized as a cause of inherited liver disease in children and of an inherited predisposition to emphysema in adults.[316,855] Cirrhosis is now known also to occur in adults.

AAT deficiency results from amino acid substitution in the polypeptide core, which leads to secondary changes in the carbohydrate side-chains. These changes may impede release from the endoplasmic reticulum of the hepatocyte. There appear to be more than 30 different inherited alleles (see Chap. 38).

The pathogenesis of cirrhosis and liver injury is unknown, but it is hypothesized that the uninhibited action of proteases, perhaps from Kupffer cells, prevents control of liver damage once the process is initiated.[618]

Of children with homozygous AAT deficiency, 25% develop cirrhosis and portal hypertension and die of complications before age 10; another 25% die of the same process by the age of 20; and another 25% will have liver fibrosis and minimal liver dysfunction and live to adulthood, perhaps with later progression. The final 25% show no childhood evidence of progressive illness, but their fate in late adult life is uncertain.[618]

In a series of 246 adults with homozygous (ZZ in the proteinase inhibitor of Pi classification) AAT deficiency, 59% had chronic obstructive lung disease and 12% had cirrhosis of the liver. In homozygous AAT patients over the age of 50, the prevalence of cirrhosis was 19%.[493] An increased prevalence of steatosis and fibrosis was also reported but not quantified.[493] As many as two thirds of patients with liver disease are reported also to have lung disease.[619,954]

There has been interest in the possibility of increased prevalence of liver disease in adults with heterozygous AAT deficiency. A convincing study based on serum analysis and liver biopsy of 1055 adults, whose average age was 60, confirms an increased prevalence of at least the MZ phenotype in patients with non B chronic active hepatitis and in cryptogenic cirrhosis.[391]

In children liver disease related to AAT deficiency occurs only in Pi ZZ homozygous children.[8]

The presentation of adults with AAT-associated liver disease is usually that of hepatosplenomegaly or the overt manifestations of portal hypertension, such as variceal bleeding or ascites. An increased incidence of hepatocellular carcinoma is claimed by some to occur in AAT deficiency,[262,493] but the conclusion is not universally accepted at present.[346,854]

The diagnosis of AAT deficiency can be suggested by seeing eosinophilic globules on hematoxylin and eosin (H & E) stains in liver biopsy specimens. These lesions tend to be multiple, spheroidal, hyaline, acidophilic bodies of variable size in the cytoplasm of hepatocytes near the periphery of the lobule. The demonstration that these globules are positive with periodic acid-Schiff (PAS) stain and are diastase resistant increases the likelihood of AAT deficiency. These stains, however, are not pathognomonic.[737] For example, in alcoholic cirrhosis PAS-positive, diastase-resistant globules occurred in nearly one third of the patients in a series in which AAT deficiency had been excluded by phenotyping.[678]

The diagnosis of AAT deficiency is also suggested by the absence or diminution of the alpha$_1$-globulin band on the serum electrophoresis pattern. Serum electrophoresis will, however, detect only severely deficient patients.

When AAT deficiency is homozygous, its serum concentration is only 10% to 15% of normal. The association of increased hepatocellular deposition of the enzyme and its deficiency in the serum is analogous to that of copper in Wilson's disease. The association suggests that it may be a "storage" disease like familial hepatolenticular degeneration. Indeed, Ishak and colleagues have demonstrated increased copper pigment in the peripheral pseudolobular hepatocytes, the cells in which AAT bodies are most commonly found.[407] The significance of the copper accumulation is not known.

Functional assays of trypsin-inhibitory capacity or quantification of serum AAT concentration by immunologic techniques increase the precision of the diagnosis, but even these are not always adequate for diagnosing heterozygotes in periods of hormonal or medical stress.[854] Since AAT is an acute-phase reactant, concentrations obtained during these periods may be misleading. The gold standard for diagnosis is protease inhibitor phenotyping.

The only therapy for severe hepatic injury from AAT deficiency is liver transplantation.

Cystic Fibrosis of the Pancreas

Cystic fibrosis has long been known to the pediatrician but has had to be reckoned with only in recent years by physicians who treat adult patients. The increased longevity of cystic fibrosis patients into adulthood has resulted from improved nutritional management, improved use of pulmonary therapy, and the development of new antibiotics. The prevalence of hepatobiliary complications of cystic fibrosis has increased in parallel to survival.

Cystic fibrosis is the most common of the potentially lethal genetic disorders, occurring in 1 in 2000 white births. It affects the mucous secretory exocrine glands and electrolyte secretion in the eccrine sweat and parotid glands. Liver disease is thought to result from excessive intrahepatic bile duct secretion of mucus.

The pathognomonic lesion of cystic fibrosis, identifiable in 25% of patients living longer than a year, is characterized by bile duct proliferation, bile ducts containing eosinophilic plugs, an inflammatory infiltrate, and fibrosis. The lesion is present in some areas but absent in others. As patients live longer, the fibrosis extends to adjacent portal areas, and secondary biliary cirrhosis develops.[234]

The relationship between mucus plugging and the development of cirrhosis is not solid. In fact, with age, the prevalence of focal and diffuse cirrhosis increases while the presence of mucous plugging decreases.[797]

The prevalence of multilobular cirrhosis is about 10% in patients over the age of 25.[842] Conventional liver function tests are notoriously inadequate for the diagnosis of cirrhosis in cystic fibrosis. Portal hypertension frequently accompanies cirrhosis and may in some instances be the initial manifestation.[782,797]

The diagnosis of cystic fibrosis should be suspected in young adults with cirrhosis of inapparent etiology and can be confirmed by measuring elevated concentrations of sodium and chloride in sweat obtained by pilocarpine iontophoresis.

Galactosemia

The congenital absence of galactose-1-phosphate-uridyl transferase is a rare disorder responsible for galactosemia. It is transmitted as an autosomal recessive trait. Hepatomegaly and jaundice are usually seen in the first week of life. Progression of the disease may result in fibrosis or cirrhosis as early as 3 to 6 months of age, perhaps as a result of the accumulation of metabolites that are toxic to hepatocytes. The liver shows severe hepatic fatty infiltration. Although necrosis is not overt, regeneration is active, and a macronodular cirrhosis may develop. The presence of multinucleated syncytial cells and the development of ductular structures in the periportal areas probably represent nonspecific, infantile responses to liver injury, rather than specific responses or clues to the nature of the lesion. The cirrhosis may be associated with ascites and other evidence of portal hypertension.[879] Death may occur in the first year if galactose intake is not significantly curtailed.[406] Galactosemia may also result from deficiency of galactokinase, but this form does not lead to progressive liver disease.

Glycogen Storage Disease

Most enzymatic defects that cause hepatic glycogenesis are located in the sequence of enzymes that degrade glycogen to glucose-6-phosphate. As a result of these deficiencies, glycogen accumulates in varying tissues, including liver, kidney, intestine, heart, skeletal, and cardiac muscle. These enzymatic differences, however, result in similar clinical presentations, most of which include fasting-induced hypoglycemia.[351]

Liver failure and cirrhosis invariably develop only in patients with branching enzyme deficiency (Cori type IV), in which cirrhosis leads to death in early childhood. In debrancher enzyme deficiency (Cori type III), fibrosis may slowly progress to cirrhosis but is not inevitable. Other glycogenoses with predominant liver manifestations, but in which cirrhosis is not expected, are types I (von Gierke) and VI. Hepatic adenomas and hepatocellular carcinoma have complicated type I disease. Adenomas have also been reported with type III.[9]

Diagnosis of glycogen storage disease is confirmed by measuring enzyme activities in liver biopsy specimens. Therapy is usually dietary, but in several forms of glycogenoses types I, III, and VI, portacaval anastomosis has resulted in metabolic improvement. This may be on account of delivery of nutrients to peripheral tissues and correction of hypoinsulinism.[9,913]

Hereditary Tyrosinemia

Hereditary tyrosinemia (tyrosinemia I, tyrosinosis) is an autosomal recessive defect of fumaryl acetoacetate hydrolase and maleylacetoacetate hydrolase. Hereditary tyrosinemia occurs in acute and chronic forms. The acute form usually leads to death from liver failure by one year of age. The chronic form is associated with death in the first decade. Cirrhosis may be found in both forms but is more frequent in the chronic form.[335] The disorder is characterized by increased α-fetoprotein in serum and aminoaciduria. One third of patients with the chronic form have had associated hepatoma.[1008] Therapy has included diets low in tyrosine, phenylalanine, and methionine and liver transplantation.

Hereditary Fructose Intolerance

Hereditary fructose intolerance is an autosomal recessive, inherited deficiency of fructose-1-phosphate aldolase. The syndrome does not become manifest until breast or cow's milk is supplanted by fructose-containing foods. Death may occur in infancy, but some patients survive until childhood or early adulthood. In the more chronic form of the disease, cirrhosis may occur, but fibrosis is more common.[642]

Other Metabolic Cirrhoses of Infancy and Early Childhood

Cirrhosis has been reported in Niemann–Pick disease, Gaucher's disease, mucopolysaccharidosis, cystinosis, Wolman's disease, cerebrohepatorenal (Zellweger) syndrome, and neonatal adrenoleukodystrophy.[9,365]

Hereditary Hemorrhagic Telangiectasia

Cirrhosis, often of the coarse, nodular type, may be part of hereditary hemorrhagic telangiectasia.[565] The clue that suggests more than a fortuitous association is the observation that the scar tissue appears to contain large numbers of thin-walled telangiectases.[1054] The pathogenesis is obscure.

Hypervitaminosis A

Cirrhosis from hypervitaminosis A is usually the result of excessive ingestion of commercial vitamin A–containing preparations that are available without prescription in 25,000-unit and 50,000-unit doses. Vitamin A doses leading to hepatic toxicity range from 40,000 units to over 1 million units per day, which is far in excess of the recommended vitamin A intake of 5000 units.[339] Cirrhosis is usually preceded by clinical signs and symptoms of toxicity that include hepatomegaly, loss of hair, dermatologic changes, pruritus, and sometimes symptoms of increased intracranial pressure such as headache, nausea, and vomiting.[339,810a]

Vitamin A accumulates in Ito cells (lipocytes). Since perisinusoidal fibrosis is most evident near areas of increased Ito cell concentration, it has been suggested that such accumulation stimulates fibrogenesis. Ito cells may

be fibroblast precursors.[810a] Ultrastructural changes in the sinusoidal barrier, morphologically similar to peliosis hepatis, are also seen.[1053]

The diagnosis can be suggested by history and the finding of increased serum vitamin A levels; confirmation is by increased vitamin-A–like fluorescence on fluorescent microscopy or demonstration of increased vitamin A levels in liver tissue.

Sarcoidosis

Occasional cases of cirrhosis are confirmed in patients with chronic sarcoidosis and are often manifested by portal hypertension.[551] However, portal hypertension may occur in hepatic sarcoidosis without cirrhosis.[942] Other diseases may mimic sarcoidosis or may coexist with it.[264]

Copper

Copper-induced cirrhosis is an occasional occupational hazard of the wine industry.[708] Long-term inhalation of "Bordeaux mixture," a traditional fungicide spray made up of complex copper salts, may give rise to "vineyard workers' liver." This disease is characterized histologically by hyperplasia and hypertrophy of Kupffer cells, proliferation or sinusoidal lining cells, fibrosis, and occasionally micronodular cirrhosis and angiosarcoma. These lesions are similar to those attributed to arsenic, Thorotrast (colloidal thorium dioxide), and vinyl chloride. In Bordelaisian vineyard workers, it is safe to say that alcohol may be a potential cotoxin.

Small-Bowel Bypass

Primary jejunoileal and jejunocolic anastomoses have been introduced as therapy for massive intractable obesity. An unwelcome accompaniment to successful weight loss has been the recognition of liver disease that ranges from increased fatty infiltration, some of which is present before biopsy in the majority of patients, central sclerosis, hepatocellular disease resembling alcoholic hepatitis, and micronodular cirrhosis that sometimes results in death from hepatic failure.[232,609,697] Studies involving baseline biopsies and follow-up biopsies after 3 years or more suggest that as many as one-third of patients have new or progressive fibrosis, sclerosis or central inflammation on biopsy, including those with no symptomatic or biochemical evidence of liver dysfunction.[389] Ten percent of patients in this series developed cirrhosis, including one asymptomatic patient with normal liver function tests.[389] Similar prevalences of cirrhosis have been reported in other series for the initial years following bypass.[390,483,567] When cirrhosis develops, suggestive changes are usually seen in the first year after bypass but may not evolve until late in the postoperative period.[390] There is not uniform agreement on whether advancing age and degree of weight loss predispose to cirrhosis.[359,390,483] The only histologic marker before surgery that indicates a propensity to the development of cirrhosis is pericentral fibrosis.[359,568,637]

Although the pathogenesis of this problem remains a mystery, a number of imaginative hypotheses have been suggested. Among these are simple malnutrition, deficiency of essential amino acids[889] or of vitamin E,[723] a dietary imbalance in the ratio of carbohydrate to protein,[889] the absorbance of toxic peptides resulting from the maldigestion of enormous volumes of ingested food,[889] and the hepatotoxicity of lithocholic acid.[124] The last abnormality has been hypothesized to result from the impaired enterohepatic circulation of bile acids by virtue of which unabsorbed chenodeoxycholic acid is converted to lithocholic acid, a hepatotoxic substance.[722,889] A role in pathogenesis has been suggested for the excluded intestinal limb. Bacterial overgrowth may result in the release of endotoxin or endogenous ethanol or may result in changes in immune competence.[645] These intriguing explanations are at present completely hypothetical but may shed some light on the difficult question of the pathogenesis of cirrhosis.

Indian Childhood Cirrhosis

Indian childhood cirrhosis is a disorder occurring predominantly in India and Southeast Asia. However, similar cases have been reported from the western hemisphere, including the United States.[507] It occurs in children between 6 months and 4 years of age. It is characterized by severe hepatocellular degeneration with Mallory bodies. Deposits of copper may also be demonstrated. Liver cell damage is accompanied by a mixed inflammatory cell infiltrate and pronounced fibrosis, which isolates individual or small groups of hepatocytes. Micronodules may be seen, but regenerative nodules are not well developed. Clinically the disease may range from a continuing hepatitis to symptoms of decompensated cirrhosis. The etiology has not been established and may be multifactorial. The disease shows familial occurrence, but there is no clear evidence that it is inherited. The disease is generally fatal, and there is no known treatment.[768]

Idiopathic or Cryptogenic Cirrhosis

When morphologic cirrhosis is found and its etiology cannot be surmised from historical information, histologic findings, or laboratory data, either alone or in combination, the cirrhosis is said to be idiopathic or cryptogenic. Over the years the number of cases so labeled has tended to fall as markers have been found for viral hepatitis and immunologic disorders and as sophistication has increased in diagnosing metabolic disorders.

In urban North America, approximately 75% of cirrhotic patients are thought to have alcoholic cirrhosis. Cirrhosis follows viral hepatitis or other identifiable etiologies in another 15%, whereas 10% is cryptogenic or idiopathic. In Great Britain cryptogenic cirrhosis accounts for nearly one third of all cases.[931]

The natural tendency is for the physician to assume that the individual patient with cryptogenic cirrhosis has underestimated or remembered incorrectly alcohol intake. Although this may be true in some instances, occasionally the cirrhosis is macronodular and shows none of the histologic earmarks of alcoholic cirrhosis. Whether these patients represent posthepatitic cirrhosis after inapparent hepatitis, an environmental type of cirrhosis, a national constitutional susceptiblity to cirrhosis, some completely different cause, or erroneous diagnosis is not known.

In the final analysis, the pathogenesis of cirrhosis of any type is unknown. In some forms of cirrhosis, such as postnecrotic or cardiac cirrhosis, the precirrhotic hepatic lesion and the subsequent pathologic pattern suggest an apparent pathogenetic mechanism. Whether or not this is correct is another matter.

Genetic Predisposition to Cirrhosis

Although there is little proof of the presence of genetic susceptibility in the development of cirrhosis, a number of circumstantial factors repeatedly raise this question. The first is the well-established observation that not all abusers of alcohol develop cirrhosis. The great majority do not.[422] On the other hand, we have encountered alcoholic cirrhosis in eight pairs of brothers at our hospital. This prevalence seems higher than would be anticipated randomly. In addition, increased genetic susceptiblity appears to be a reasonable assumption in other situations. There are occasional families described in the literature in which several members have been found to have cirrhosis in the absence of viral infections, alcohol use, or metabolic defects. In another family several members were found to have the HLA haplotypes A24, B18, DRW 4X7.[14,550]

In addition to the possible association with HLA antigens in familial cirrhosis, there is a strong association between idiopathic hemochromatosis and A3, and a lesser association with B7 and B14.[52] Chronic active hepatitis has been associated with B8, CW3, or DR3. There are less well-established associations with geographical differences between alcoholic cirrhosis and the HLA antigens B8, B13, and B40.[547,548,828] An absence of A28 has been reported as well.[548] When Eddleston and Davis combined the results of seven published series, they found the frequencies of AW32, B8, B13, B27, and B37 to be higher in patients with alcoholic cirrhosis than in controls.[240] These data fail to give a cohesive account, at the present time, of the role of HLA antigens in cirrhosis.

Second, it is said that some ethnic, national, or racial groups are either predisposed to, or resistant to, the development of cirrhosis. The American Indian and the Irish are said to develop cirrhosis especially frequently, but blacks are thought to be relatively resistant, and alcoholic cirrhosis is said to occur only rarely in Jews. Again, good data are not available to support these statements. Even more bothersome is that such data may reflect alcohol consumption rather than predisposition to alcoholic cirrhosis.

Third, an association between alcoholic cirrhosis and color blindness has been suggested,[208] but some investigators have concluded that this association is an acquired, rather than a genetically determined defect.[275]

Fourth, there are several correlations of physical findings with cirrhosis that may suggest a genetic association. Loss of chest hair, for example, has long been considered an acquired sign in male cirrhotic patients. Some investigators have shown that chest hair is not lost, but rather that it has never been prominent in patients destined to develop cirrhosis.[935] Our own observations strongly support the latter concept, although others have reached opposite conclusions.[346a] This point needs controlled clarification in groups of patients with various types of cirrhosis.

The situation, then and now, was well summarized by Snapper:

When many decades ago we warned the 'diener' of the Department of Pathology in Vienna about the dangers of his alcoholic libations—after all, he even drank the alcohol in which the specimens had been fixed—he opened his shirt, beat his hairy chest and assured us in Viennese vernacular that hairy individuals never develop cirrhosis. Such an absolute pronouncement should probably be taken with a few grains of salt; nevertheless, it should not be disregarded completely.[886]

Fifth, Patek and colleagues have shown that not all rats of the same strain develop diet-induced cirrhosis and that resistance to this disease is genetically transmissible.[683,686] Finally, it has recently been observed that in alcoholic cirrhotic patients who have an increased incidence of diabetes,[206,627] the presence of a positive history of diabetes in the immediate family is far more frequent than expected.[191] This preliminary observation requires confirmation.

In summary, these diverse clues suggest that a number of genetically determined, pathogenic factors may be operative. Certainly, precedents for familial, ethnic, racial, and national susceptiblity to specific diseases are well es-

tablished. Assuming a genetic predisposition exists, it is not known whether genetically predisposed persons are destined to develop cirrhosis *de novo,* or whether they are merely more susceptible to any or all of the cirrhogenic stimuli discussed above. Even more to the point, it is not known whether any of these genetic factors is actually of clinical significance.

CLINICAL PRESENTATION

According to Feinstein's mathematical classification,[268] a disease can present in one of three ways. If one defines the universe of cirrhosis to include all patients with cirrhosis, the largest fraction or set, perhaps 60%, will consist of patients who seek treatment for symptoms or signs of cirrhosis (*i.e.,* complainant presentation) (Fig. 20-14). In a second set, which may account for 20%, the physician discovers cirrhosis coincidentally during evaluation of some other unrelated disease (*i.e.,* lanthanic or noncomplainant presentation. Lanthanic is derived from the Greek word meaning "to escape attention"). The patients in the third set are those in whom the diagnosis of cirrhosis is established at autopsy. These three sets are overlapping (*i.e.,* the three groups are not mutually exclusive). Some patients in whom cirrhosis is found at autopsy will have had the diagnosis of cirrhosis established clinically after a complainant presentation (*e.g.,* bleeding varices) or after a lanthanic presentation (*e.g.,* hepatomegaly noted during routine physical examination), but some will not have been recognized clinically. In our experience, clinically undetected cirrhosis is found at autopsy in approximately 30%. Others have found clinically unrecognized cirrhosis to occur in 40% of cirrhotic patients.[362] Finally, there is a fourth set, which does not overlap the other sets, in whom cirrhosis remains undiscovered (*i.e.,* cirrhosis is never recognized, neither during life nor after death).

The magnitude of the fourth group is by definition unknown, since the factors that determine its size are un-

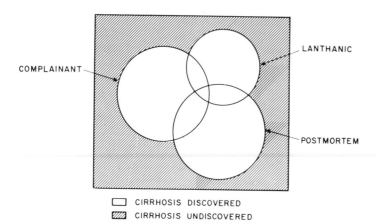

Fig. 20-14. Modes of clinical presentation of cirrhosis. The Venn diagram illustrates three intersecting modes of presentation. The *complainant* set comprises patients who see physicians because of symptoms of cirrhosis. The *lanthanic* or noncomplainant set contains patients in whom cirrhosis is discovered "accidentally" during investigation of other, noncirrhotic disease. The *postmortem* set comprises patients whose cirrhosis was unrecognized during life and is first discovered at autopsy. A fourth group, the *unrecognized* set, is composed of patients in whom cirrhosis is never discovered.

COMPLAINANT

LANTHANIC

POSTMORTEM

☐ CIRRHOSIS DISCOVERED
▨ CIRRHOSIS UNDISCOVERED

known and speculative. It is conceivable, for example, that medical care of the lowest socioeconomic class, which includes the indigent, alcoholic incumbents of skid row, is not so comprehensive as that of higher social classes and might thus permit a disproportionately large number of silent cirrhotic patients to escape detection. On the other hand, one of the paradoxes of American medicine is that the lowest socioeconomic group, which is often treated in large, urban, academic hospitals, may receive better medical care than some socioeconomically higher groups.

Clinically overt, decompensated cirrhosis in our experience presents in three general ways. In patients in the first group evidence of *hepatic parenchymal dysfunction* may predominate. This pattern is usually seen in relatively young patients—40 to 45 years of age—who drink excessive amounts of whiskey and, often, other alcoholic beverages as well. These patients enter the hospital acutely ill with the full syndrome of acute alcoholic hepatitis. They usually have deep jaundice, impaired coagulation, and hypoalbuminemia. If these patients survive they immediately resume heavy drinking and return to the hospital repeatedly until they die. They appear deliberately intent ondestroying themselves by their purposeful, unremitting drinking.

The second group presents with signs of *portal hypertension (i.e.,* vascular decompensation). In general, they are older patients, averaging about 55 to 60 years, who are more moderate drinkers. Often they have drunk large quantities of wine for many years, but are "ethnic alcoholics" rather than "abusive alcoholics" in the usual sense. They present often with ascites, esophageal varices, or portal-systemic encephalopathy and show little or no hepatic parenchymal damage.

The third group is admitted with both *parenchymal damage* and *portal hypertension* and has the worst prognosis. They are often patients from the first group who have survived long enough to develop the more slowly maturing vascular features of cirrhosis. At our institution patients with the vascular decompensation syndrome often were of Italian ancestry. They immigrated to the New Haven area early in the 20th century and made and consumed large quantities of red wine for many years. These patients are now seen very rarely. The patients with hepatic parenchymal decompensation tend to be of Middle European ancestry, come from the heavily industrial area around Bridgeport, and give a history of excessive consumption of whiskey, vodka, and beer.

Although these patterns are general and not mutually exclusive, they do have important therapeutic implications. The first group, if they survive the initial admission, might well benefit from intensive psychological care, since the progress of their liver disease may be reversible if the drinking can be controlled. The second group may benefit from some of the advances made in the treatment of complications of portal hypertension—they are often acceptable operative risks. The third group, of course, has the worst prognosis, and therapy must be directed toward immediate survival rather than more long-range goals.

CLINICAL FEATURES

Cirrhosis is characterized by a large number of specific findings. All may be present in some patients and any or all may be absent in others. Most of these signs can best be discussed in a review of systems, each of which exhibits abnormalities that are specific for cirrhosis or are involved in its differential diagnosis. Some, however, are constitutional factors and are considered next.

Constitutional

General Deterioration

The most common feature of cirrhosis is deterioration of health. This "failure to thrive" syndrome is typified by anorexia, weight loss, weakness, and ease of fatigability. The anorexia may be masked in alcoholic cirrhosis by heavy drinking, and indeed, so may the weight loss. The metabolism of alcohol, after all, supplies seven calories per gram, and a pint of whiskey per day therefore provides approximately 1500 calories. An equivalent amount of alcohol consumed as beer will furnish even more calories. With a small amount of food, an alcoholic patient may thus maintain his weight for a long period of time. Furthermore, the accumulation of edema or ascitic fluid may counterbalance the loss of tissue weight and may actually overcompensate, producing an absolute gain in weight. Muscle wasting may be evident peripherally despite the expansion in girth. When taking a nutritional history, it is essential for the physician to persevere and ask specifically about each meal of the past few days and the amount of each component of each meal. Similarly, one may not properly estimate the amount of alcohol consumed unless one establishes the patient's overall estimate by obtaining an hour-by-hour, glass-by-glass history, and confirming it by learning the frequency and volume of alcohol purchases, the amount of money spent on alcoholic beverages or, in the case of home winemakers, by the amount of grapes they purchase each fall. In obtaining either a dietary or a drinking history, it is wise to speak with members of the family, bartenders, or acquaintances. Friends, however, may compound the felony. The least reliable historical data in clinical medicine are obtained in trying to determine the type and volume of alcoholic beverage being consumed. Misdiagnoses of posthepatitic cirrhosis and metastatic cancer of the liver fill the records of physicians who take casual social histories. On the other hand, physicians tend to browbeat patients into exaggerating their alcohol intake and then apply a "correction" factor that raises the alcohol intake to the preconceived level. Nonalcoholic liver disease is not infrequently attributed to alcoholism on the basis of inaccurate histories.

Anorexia may be accompanied by abdominal unrest, nausea, or sometimes vomiting and diarrhea. Weakness and fatigue on mild exertion may be advanced despite the patient's failure to recognize them.

Jaundice

Jaundice is both a localized hepatic and a constitutional sign. It colors the skin and darkens the urine and is often the first evidence of ill health that the patient or the family recognizes. Jaundice results ultimately from the inability of the liver to metabolize bilirubin. Normally, the serum bilirubin is a reliable guide to the degree of hepatic damage. The liver's capacity to remove bilirubin may be overwhelmed by the increased bilirubin load of hemolysis. In both hepatitis and cirrhosis, hepatic parenchymal necrosis may occur in the absence of jaundice. The presence of jaundice does not necessarily correlate well with the histologic picture. In cirrhosis in which hepatic parenchymal damage is the most common cause of jaundice, in which hemolysis is common, in which biliary obstruction may develop in association with gallstones or pancreatitis, and in which any other cause of jaundice may also occur, the differential diagnosis is maximally challenging.

Fever

Fever is frequently present in decompensated cirrhosis.[741,951] Whenever it occurs, one is faced with another difficult differential diagnosis. Is the fever due to an unrecognized, self-limited disease, to an unrecognized bacterial infection that may be fatal if untreated, or is it a constitutional sign of decompensated cirrhosis? The fever of cirrhosis is usually low-grade and continuous, but it may sometimes reach levels of 102° to 103°F, often when alcoholic hepatitis is present. It may persist for weeks and thus qualify as a bona fide fever of unknown origin. Fever is common in alcoholic cirrhosis but is much less so in nonalcoholic forms of cirrhosis. Chills rarely accompany the fever. The syndrome of cirrhotic, necrotic fever is characterized by deep jaundice, elevated serum transaminase and alkaline phosphatase levels, and leukocytosis. The serum glutamic-oxaloacetic transaminase (SGOT) levels are almost invariably higher than serum glutamic-pyruvic transaminase (SGPT) activity in alcohol-induced liver disease, reflecting a higher concentration of SGOT in the hepatocytes.[154] Liver biopsy, which is an important procedure in the workup of fevers of unknown origin, shows alcoholic hepatitis with active necrosis. Unfortunately, the consequences of an erroneous diagnosis are too dire to risk, and an extensive search for an occult bacterial infection is mandatory. This requires examination and culture of all available body fluids, and if nothing is found, a diagnostic trial of broad-spectrum antibiotics may be indicated.

It has been postulated that the fever is due to products of hepatic necrosis, to the bypassing of the liver of enteric bacterial pyrogens, and to the failure of the liver to inactivate pyrogenic steroids such as etiocholanolone. It does not respond to antibiotic therapy and may disappear only when the liver disease begins to improve.

On the other side of the coin, cirrhotic patients may sometimes exhibit *hypothermia,* especially in the terminal stages, but not infrequently with bacterial peritonitis, with gram-negative bacteremia, with portal-systemic encephalopathy (PSE), or with the hepatorenal syndrome, all of which these patients are prone to develop.

Systemic

No system of the body is spared in the syndrome of cirrhosis.

Alimentary

Parotid Enlargement. Hypertrophy of the parotid gland is a frequent finding in cirrhosis,[82,905,1038] but is frequently overlooked. It may appear early, before any signs of cirrhosis *per se.* The parotidomegaly is painless and reversible and may decrease rapidly in size as hepatic decompensation wanes. The gland is soft, nontender, and not fixed to the skin. If often produces a trapezoid or lantern-jawed appearance to the face and causes distortion of the position of the ears in which the lobes tend to project at right angles to the face[94] (Fig. 20-15). Stenson's duct is patent. Sialographically, the duct system is normal or may show disappearance of the terminal branches, the so-called leafless tree appearance. Functionally, the parotids tend to be hypersecretory, and the amylase activity of the saliva is about twice normal. The hypersecretory state is supported by

Fig. 20-15. Parotid enlargement, bilateral. (Brick IB: Ann Intern Med 49:438, 1958)

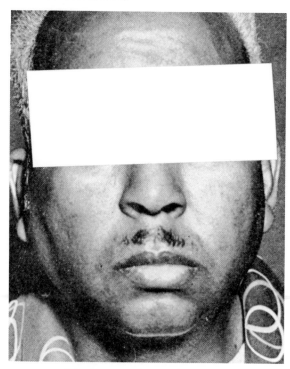

the histologic picture, which shows hyperplasia of the parotid parenchyma, hypertrophy of the individual cells and acini, and increased xymogen granulation of the parenchymal cells.[906] Fatty infiltration of the parenchymal cells and an increase in interlobar connective tissue may be seen in long-standing cases.

The cause of the parotid enlargement is not known. It occurs often with malnutrition of various types, but in careful studies in repatriated prisoners of war, parotid enlargement was found to appear not during starvation, but after refeeding. Some consider the parotid enlargement to be alcohol-induced; others believe that it is a natural consequence of increased salivary secretion, although the stimulus for the increased parotid activity is unknown. Malignant and other types of parotidomegaly should be excluded.

Varices. The gastrointestinal tract bears much of the brunt of cirrhosis, aside from abnormalities of the liver itself. Varices of the gastrointestinal tract develop as a consequence of the portal hypertension at the two ends of the intestinal tract—esophageal varices at the upper end and rectal varices at the nether end.

Esophageal varices are, in terms of hospitalization and ultimate mortality, the single most significant complication of cirrhosis. Admission for the management of hemorrhage from varices occupies an enormous amount of time and effort and complex techniques, as attested to by the massive bodies of literature that have accumulated regarding the diagnosis and treatment of variceal hemorrhage.[585] Despite the great amount of effort and research devoted to bleeding from varices, it continues to be the most lethal complication of cirrhosis.

Varices may be seen throughout the length of the esophagus and in the gastric fundus but tend to bleed predominantly from the distal esophagus. In this location they lie mainly in the lamina propria, whereas those of the stomach and the proximal esophagus lie predominantly in the submucosa. Their superficial location close to the lumen of the esophagus may therefore predispose them to rupture.[902]

Esophageal varices do not always imply cirrhosis. They may be seen in presinusoidal portal hypertension, such as schistosomiasis, splenic vein thrombosis, or portal arteriovenous fistulas.[216] Varices may also be seen in the absence of portal hypertension. "Downhill varices," which occur predominantly in the proximal esophagus, may result from obstruction of the superior vena cava, azygos vein, or inferior thyroid veins. Hemorrhage from these varices is rare, but it occurs.[287] Finally, there are rare reports of idiopathic varices in the absence of either portal hypertension or obstruction. Sometimes this finding may be a congenital anomaly.[216,953]

Rectal varices, which develop as part of the inferior mesenteric venous collateral system, may sometimes produce serious hemorrhage in cirrhotic patients. "Hemorrhoidal" hemorrhage, which is much less frequent and life-threatening than esophageal bleeding, may occasionally be extremely persistent and require the perverse use of rectal tamponade using a balloon tube analogous to the Sengstaken–Blakemore tube of esophageal fame.

Varices of more intermediate portions of the gastrointestinal tract are less well known. Duodenal varices, which have recently been found more frequently as a result of widespread use of duodenoscopy and arteriography, will probably be shown to cause bleeding more frequently than has been recognized previously. Other venous collateral vessels, including mesenteric and gallbladder varices, occasionally cause serious or even fatal bleeding in cirrhotic patients. Such lesions can be demonstrated *in vivo* by angiography, laparoscopy, surgery, or computed tomography (CT).

Gallstones. The prevalence of gallstones is increased in cirrhosis of both alcoholic and nonalcoholic origin.[86,638] Cholelithiasis is not, however, a direct complication of cirrhosis. Rather, it appears to be the complication of a complication; hypersplenism causes hemolysis. The resulting bilirubin probably exceeds its solubility in bile. There may also be a reduction in the solubilizing component, since bile acid concentrations have been found to be decreased in the bile of cirrhotic patients.[20,956] The resulting calcium bilirubinate stones are often amorphous and brittle.[956] This finding raises the possibility that they may cause obstruction less frequently than cholesterol stones.

Although recent investigations have suggested that cholesterol gallstones are actually the consequence of abnormal liver "function" (*i.e.,* the imbalance in bile of the normal components that maintain cholesterol in solution), cholesterol gallstones are not increased in cirrhosis. The relative absence of cholesterol gallstones in cirrhosis, despite decreased bile acid pool size,[985] presumably occurs because decreased cholesterol synthesis maintains the normal cholesterol/bile acid ratio. Conceivably, the normal solubility system of bilirubin in bile may be altered in cirrhotic patients, predisposing them to the development of gallstones, but it seems more likely that increased red cell turnover is the critical problem.

Peptic Ulcer. The prevalence of peptic ulcer is increased in cirrhotic patients.[462] Peptic ulcers occur in 4% to 7% of patients admitted to Veterans Administration hospitals, and in 10% to 15% of cirrhotic patients. Gastric acid secretion is not increased in cirrhotic patients.[544a] In experimental animals there is a sharp increase in gastric acid secretion after portacaval anastomosis.[374] In humans, however, a similar increment in gastric acid secretion has not been found.[1022] More recent prospective studies of the association of portacaval shunts with peptic ulcer employing appropriate control groups have shown that the prevalence of ulcers is no greater after shunt than in unshunted patients with equally advanced cirrhosis.[705] Although portal-systemic shunting, whether iatrogenic or spontaneous, appears important in the pathogenesis of peptic ulcer, the exact mechanism is not known.

Gastroesophageal Reflux is a controversial secondary manifestation in cirrhotic patients with ascites. Gastroesophageal reflux, like the heartburn of pregnancy, may result from increased abdominal pressure. In pregnancy the growing fetus is the problem; in cirrhosis it may be ascites. Regurgitation of gastric contents into the esophagus is rarely, if ever, seen in cirrhotic patients without hiatus hernia in the absence of ascites. In fact, gastroesophageal reflux, which may be present in cirrhotic patients with tense ascites has been reported to disappear after diuresis.[874] Manometric observations, show, however, that the lower esophageal sphincter is competent in cirrhosis, and that gastroesophageal reflux is uncommon.[239]

Gastritis is another common concomitant of alcoholic cirrhosis. It is most evident when it is the cause of upper gastrointestinal tract hemorrhage, but the diagnosis of gastritis is not usually made when the cirrhotic patient has only vague epigastric distress and/or vomiting. Gastritis results from the effects of both portal hypertension and alcohol ingestion. Clinical evidence of increased hemorrhage from gastritis in portal hypertension is suggestive but not definitive.[499] A review of the frequency of bleeding from gastritis in patients with and without portal hypertension who were endoscoped for upper gastrointestinal tract bleeding based on five published series, reveals that 38% of those with and without portal hypertension bleed from gastritis.[752] However, this comparison of percentages does not take into account the higher overall incidence of gastrointestinal tract bleeding in patients with portal hypertension.

The physiological basis for bleeding from gastritis in portal hypertension may be the high prevalence of morphologic alterations in the microcirculation of the stomach in cirrhotic patients, especially in those with esophageal varices. These alterations include arteriovenous anastomoses and dilatation of capillaries, precapillaries, and veins.[369a] These changes lead to low vascular resistance and high flow, which may play a permissive role in gastric bleeding.

Alcohol is an irritating, mildly corrosive substance. When taken with abandon as a concentrated solution, such as undiluted whiskey, and in the absence of protein or other adsorbent substances, it may at first induce self-protective emesis, later inflammation, and eventually, erosions that may bleed. A role for alcohol has been supported by studies in experimental animals that show alcohol potentiates mucosal abnormalities that occur in portal hypertension.[822]

Pitcher suggested that, in cirrhotic patients who bleed in the hospital, varices are the most likely site, while in those who are admitted bleeding, erosive gastritis is the best bet.[713]

Diarrhea. Along with vomiting, diarrhea is almost the *sine qua non* of the alcoholic cirrhotic syndrome. The cause is not known; a number of flimsy explanations have been offered. Pellagra, a niacin deficiency syndrome, has diarrhea as one of its prominent symptoms. It has been suggested that a *forme fruste* of pellagra, exhibiting only its intestinal component, may be responsible. It has also been suggested, rather glibly, that alcohol itself or other substances in alcoholic beverages can cause diarrhea. Actually alcohol infused chronically into the human jejunum and ileum in appropriate concentrations has been shown to diminish considerably the absorption of water and sodium by the small intestine.[587] The excess amount of saline solution in the intestinal lumen may induce a saline diuresis. Folate-deficient diets can also cause sodium and water malabsorption[363] and can exaggerate the defect induced by alcohol. Since both chronic alcohol ingestion and folate deficiency, which occur together clinically, cause malabsorption of glucose, amino acids, and other substances in addition to sodium and water, a severe, chronic, unresponsive, self-perpetuating diarrhea may result.

It has been shown that folate can be added to wine without affecting its taste noticeably in concentrations that can prevent the consequences of folate deficiency.[440] Beer is naturally rich in folic acid. Why, we wonder, do the authors discriminate against whiskey drinkers?

Hypomagnesemia, which is common in both chronic alcoholism and malnutrition, has been associated with diarrhea that may be eliminated by correction of the magnesium deficit.[1040] Whatever the explanation, these symptoms often complicate the management of cirrhosis.

Neurologic

Portal-Systemic Encephalopathy. PSE, the major neurologic manifestation of cirrhosis, is largely a consequence of portal-systemic shunting, and consequently, may be considered a secondary complication. In patients with portacaval anastomosis it represents a tertiary phenomenon. PSE, which is discussed in much greater detail elsewhere, is not considered further here.

Asterixis. The "flapping" tremor is the peripheral manifestation of a central nervous system metabolic abnormality. Although characteristic of PSE, it is not specific for PSE.[160] It is seen in the encephalopathy of a variety of other metabolic disorders including carbon dioxide narcosis, uremia, hypoglycemia, and barbiturate intoxication. The term "liver" flap is consequently a misnomer. "Lung" flap or "kidney" flap are equally inappropriate. Asterixis is usually accompanied by nonspecific slowing of the electroencephalogram, which also characterizes these other types of encephalopathy.

Asterixis, first described by Adams and Foley,[1] may be the consequence of metabolic suppression of the reticular activating system, which is extremely sensitive to a variety of metabolic depressants. Suppression of the ascending reticular system is associated with depression of consciousness and of arousal responses and is characterized by electroencephalographic slowing. Suppression of the descending reticular system, which is important in the maintenance of posture, muscle tone, and reflexes, may result in asterixis, rigidity, and abnormal pyramidal reflexes. Several observations provide insight into the nature of asterixis. Electromyographically, asterixis is associated with an electrical hiatus of both the active and opposing musculature.[2,495,957] It is bilaterally asynchronous and is not temporally associated with any specific electroencephalographic abnormality. We have observed unilateral asterixis in one patient as part of the prodrome of a contralateral cerebrovascular thrombosis and in another patient long after a stroke on the hemiparetic side. Such observations indicate that asterixis is centrally determined and involves the pyramidal tracts. Intermittent asterixis was observed in a patient with Cheyne–Stokes respiration. The asterixis was most marked during hyperventilation and least evident during apnea. Assuming a latent period for the delivery of neuronal hypoxia, asterixis appeared simultaneously with the nadir of intracellular oxygen content. Asterixis represents, therefore, a relatively acute and rapidly reversible phenomenon. Asterixis, which is often associated with hyperammonemia, can be elicited in cirrhotic patients by the administration of ammonium salts. An electromyographically similar lesion can also be produced in rabbits by the infusion of ammonium salts.

Long-Tract Neurologic Signs. These *exaggerated deep tendon reflexes,* the *Babinski sign,* and related eponymic signs occur unpredictably. Sometimes one may observe rigidity of the peripheral musculature and, rarely, the syndrome of hepatolenticular degeneration. In Wilson's disease, this neurologic syndrome is an inherited copper-associated metabolic defect, but a similar syndrome may be an acquired, noncuprogenic consequence of chronic PSE. *Portal-systemic myelopathy,* which in its most severe form presents as transverse myelitis, may occur in patients with severe recurrent PSE. This demyelinating lesion, first described by Zieve and colleagues,[1060] is depicted in Figure 20-16. It is most frequently seen in patients with portal-systemic anastomoses.[496]

Some neurologic findings that are often associated with alcoholic cirrhosis, such as *Wernicke's syndrome* or *peripheral neuritis,* are not consequences of cirrhosis at all, but merely other diseases associated with excessive alcohol consumption, dietary inadequacies, or both.

Hematologic

Impaired Coagulation is the major hematologic manifestation of cirrhosis. Most of the coagulation factors are synthesized in the liver. Decrease in the activity of any or all of these factors slows the coagulation process and, in conjunction with thrombocytopenia and a variety of potential bleeding sites, poses a lethal threat to decompensated cirrhotic patients. Plasma fibrinolysins, which are frequently increased in cirrhosis, may contribute to the bleeding tendency.

Impaired coagulation is more likely to occur when hepatic parenchymal dysfunction, as in acute alcoholic hep-

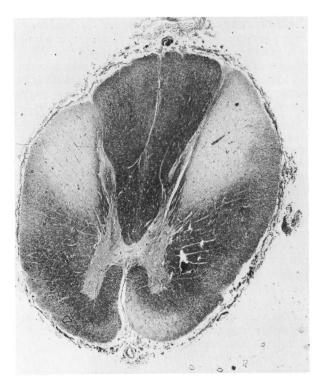

Fig. 20-16. Pyramidal tract demyelination. Cross-section of the dorsal region of the spinal cord of a cirrhotic patient with recurrent encephalopathy and spastic paraplegia. Demyelination of the pyramidal tracts is evident. (Luxol-fast H & E) (Provided by Dr. L. Zieve)

atitis, is coexistent with cirrhosis. Patients who have severe histologic cirrhosis and significant manifestations of portal hypertension, but who do not have parenchymal dysfunction, may have normal coagulation.

Disseminated Intravascular Coagulopathy (DIC) may occur in decompensated cirrhosis but is not frequently an overt manifestation. It is very common, however, in patients who have had peritoneovenous shunts. (See section on Ascites.)

Anemia is among the most frequent and important hematologic disorders of cirrhosis. *Microcytic hypochromic anemia* due to gastrointestinal blood loss is the most common type. *Macrocytic anemia* may be seen as a consequence of folic acid deficiency and may be associated with leukopenia or thrombocytopenia. *Hemolytic anemia* occurs more frequently than is generally recognized. Sometimes active splenic hemolysis can be demonstrated, but increased erythrocyte synthesis compensates and no anemia may be detectable. Other indices of hemolysis, such as reticulocytosis, hyperbilirubinemia, or increased serum levels of lactic dehydrogenase, may suggest, however, that active hemolysis is occurring. Often the anemia is minimal in degree, but rarely it may be severe enough to require blood transfusion. This form of anemia, which is almost always accompanied by splenomegaly, represents a form of hypersplenism. It is often associated with leukopenia or thrombocytopenia. Any of the formed elements may be suppressed individually or in any combination. Splenectomy may promptly correct these cytopenias. Severe hemolytic anemia may occasionally be precipitated by portacaval shunt, necessitating splenectomy in some instances. Low-grade hemolysis frequently follows portacaval shunts, but it is not clear in these instances whether the hemolysis is hypersplenic or whether it represents an intravascular consequence of portacaval vascular turbulence at the site of anastomosis, as may occur in patients with cardiac valvular prostheses or acquired valvular deformities, the so-called "Waring blender" syndrome. It has recently been reported in a controlled investigation of hypersplenism in association with portacaval anastomosis that preexistent anemia, leukopenia, thrombocytopenia, or any combination of these features of hypersplenism disappeared as frequently in shunted patients as they did in randomly selected, unshunted patients.[626] Furthermore, it was found that "new" hypersplenism developed as frequently in those unoperated, control patients as it did in those who had portacaval anastomosis.

The improvements in hypersplenism are often amazingly rapid and transient. Within minutes of constructing a shunt Schreiber reported increments in the formed elements that peaked within 2 days and that were usually gone after 1 month.[835]

Bone Marrow. In cirrhosis, bone marrow reflects hematologic disorders. Folic acid deficiency is associated with a megaloblastic marrow. In patients with blood-loss anemia, a hyperplastic, iron-depleted marrow is found. In chronic hepatocellular failure, a hyperplastic marrow is often found, reflecting anemia and the need for increased erythrogenesis. As might be expected in patients with hyperglobulinemia, bone marrow plasmacytosis is often present. Occasionally, it is so pronounced that myelomatosis is suspected. Rarely, multiple myeloma occurs in patients with underlying cirrhosis.[247] Whether this phenomenon represents coincidence or plasmacytotic stimulus gone awry is not known. In generalized iron-storage disease, excessive bone marrow hemosiderin usually accompanies the accumulation in the rest of the body.

Zieve's Syndrome is a complex disorder characterized by fatty infiltration of the liver, hyperlipemia, and hemolytic anemia.[1058] Although liver damage is implicit in this disorder, cirrhosis is not necessarily present. This syndrome is often difficult to differentiate from alcohol-induced pancreatitis.

Several rare cases of *spur cell anemia* have been reported in alcoholic cirrhosis.[869] In this serious disorder, which is associated with hemolytic anemia and hypercholesterolemia, the red cells have spurlike projections. This phenomenon may be a variant of Zieve's syndrome.

Hemosiderosis is another mysterious hematologic facet of cirrhosis. Modest deposition of hemosiderin occurs in the livers of 25% to 50% of patients with alcoholic cirrhosis.[167,1065] Occasionally however, massive amounts of iron distributed throughout the body may be associated with the classical clinical signs of hemochromatosis. Indeed, a background of excessive alcohol intake so often coexists in hemosiderotic patients as to question the hereditary concept of hemochromatosis. Accelerated hemosiderin deposition may occur following the construction of a portacaval shunt. More than 30 patients have been reported in whom disseminated iron deposition followed the construction of shunts. The full-blown syndrome of hemochromatosis has developed within 2 years after portacaval anastomosis in patients who were previously free of hepatic hemosiderin. This phenomenon has recently been shown to occur significantly more commonly in patients with portacaval anastomosis than in randomly selected, unshunted patients with cirrhosis of similar severity.[167] The pathogenesis of this association is unclear, although pancreatitis and hypersplenism, two causes of increased iron deposition, are frequently found in these hemosiderotic patients. Although portal-systemic shunting *per se* is related to the iron deposition, it cannot be the only factor.

Polycythemia is a paradoxical abnormality that is sometimes the clue to an occult hepatocellular carcinoma.[434]

Pulmonary

Pulmonary Oxygen Desaturation. The pulmonary manifestations of cirrhosis may include dyspnea on review of systems, cyanosis and clubbing on physical examination, and oxygen desaturation demonstrated in the laboratory.

Dyspnea is not a frequent complaint in cirrhotic patients except when severe ascites is present. Hyperventilation occurs, but the patient is seldom aware of it. Frank cyanosis is rare, but clubbing of the fingers can be found in many cirrhotic patients if carefully looked for. Cyanosis is always associated with clubbing, but the reverse is not necessarily the case[909]; even though oxygen desaturation always accompanies clubbing, there is no correlation with the degree of desaturation.

These findings of desaturation are generally attributed to reduced arterial oxygen concentration. Decreased arterial oxygen partial pressures have been observed in about half of decompensated cirrhotic patients, and PO_2 levels in the range of 60 to 70 mm Hg are not unusual.[588,784]

Multiple pathophysiological processes may contribute to decreased oxygen saturation. These factors are discussed below.

Right-to-Left Shunts. Arteriovenous anastomoses have been observed within the lung (usually in the lower lobes) and on the pleural surfaces at autopsy. They resemble the spider angiomata seen on the skin.[69,811] The existence of such shunts can sometimes be demonstrated antemortem when intravenous radio-labeled macroaggregated albumin, normally trapped in the capillary network, is seen by scan to pass quickly through the lungs and be taken up by organs with high blood flow, such as the brain, kidneys, and spleen.[41,450] In addition to these microcirculatory shunts, there is also evidence that some cirrhotic patients have right-to-left shunts involving larger vessels. Periesophageal veins in cirrhosis generally anastomose freely with mediastinal, pleuropericardial, and azygos veins. In some cirrhotic patients there is further anastomosis of the mediastinal venous plexus with bronchial veins and occasionally even pulmonary veins.[116,1028] In some instances, these portopulmonary anastomoses have been large enough to permit emboli to pass from a thrombosed portal vein with resulting pulmonary embolization.[560] For significant right to left shunting to occur, these anatomic anastomoses must be accompanied by a pressure elevation in the portal vein branches that exceeds pulmonary venous pressure. Significant oxygen desaturation almost always occurs in the setting of esophageal varices.

On conventional chest films intrapulmonary shunting may lead to the appearance of basilar infiltrates.[910]

In perhaps 5% of cirrhotic patients, intrapulmonary shunting is associated with debilitating *orthodeoxia,* that is, arterial deoxygenation accentuated in the upright position and reversed in recumbency, and *platypnea,* dyspnea induced in the upright position and relieved by recumbency.[449,482,783] It is presumed that increased hypoxia in the upright position is explained by the fact that vascular shunts occur predominantly at the lung bases. Their use increases when the upright position is assumed, leading to redistribution of blood to these areas.[482]

Altered Ventilation-Perfusion Relationships. In patients with cardiopulmonary disease, the most frequent cause of systemic arterial hypoxemia is uneven alveolar ventilation in relation to alveolar blood flow.[159] Such mismatches of gas and blood would therefore not be surprising as a contributory factor to cirrhotic hypoxemia. Nonuniform ventilation may result from elevated diaphragms in patients with ascites or from cirrhotic pleural effusions, which occur in 5% to 10% of patients with cirrhosis. These same processes may also impede flow in smaller pulmonary vessels. Because altered ventilation-perfusion relationships are also described in cirrhotic patients without ascites,[784] other factors must also participate in the imbalance. Premature airway closure has been described in cirrhosis with consequent gas trapping in lower lung zones and an associated low ventilation-perfusion ratio.[308,803] This may result from mechanical compression of small airways by bronchial blood vessels that have become engorged because of the azygos hypertension that accompanies portal hypertension.[803] An additional mechanism for gas and blood mismatching in cirrhosis is inappropriate pulmonary microvascular vasodilatation, which has been supported by anatomic studies from cirrhotic patients at autopsy.[213,629]

Alveolar Hypoventilation. General alveolar hypoventilation is a theoretic cause of arterial hypoxemia but is unlikely in most cases of cirrhosis because hyperventilation, accompanied by a mild respiratory alkalosis, is commonly seen.[375,376] It is postulated by some that hyperammonemia is the stimulus for hyperventilation, but there is a poor correlation between the ammonia content of arterial blood and the minute ventilation.[375,376]

Reduced Pulmonary Diffusing Capacity. Reduction in pulmonary diffusing capacity may play a role in the desaturation seen in some patients. Most patients in whom diffusing capacity has been measured have had normal values,[743] but appreciable abnormalities have been found in up to 20% of cirrhotic patients.[333,482] Diffusion defects should not be taken to imply interstitial disease. There may be instead an "alveolar–capillary oxygen disequilibrium," to use the term preferred by proponents. This is anatomically associated with tenfold increases in the diameter of thin-walled vessels in the lower lobes. It is postulated that layering of erythrocytes occurs so that only erythrocytes immediately adjacent to the capillary membrane equilibrate with alveolar gas. The problem is exacerbated when there is rapid transit as occurs in the high cardiac output state that accompanies some forms of cirrhosis.[215,1036]

Shifts in Oxyhemoglobin Dissociation Curve. Increased 2,3-diphosphoglycerate is reported in erythrocytes in cirrhotic patients.[29] These changes have been used to explain the decreased oxygen affinity of hemoglobin in cirrhotic patients. This decreased oxygen affinity results from a shift of the oxyhemoglobin dissociation curve to the right, which may contribute to the hypoxemia in cirrhosis.[117,460,1066]

Primary Pulmonary Hypertension. Pulmonary hypertension without demonstrable pulmonary or cardiac disease is not a common manifestation of cirrhosis. An unselected series of 17,901 autopsied patients revealed a prevalence of primary pulmonary hypertension of 0.13% and 0.73% ($p < 0.001$) in patients with cirrhosis.[581] These numbers suggest that, although infrequent, primary pulmonary hypertension occurs six to seven times more frequently in cirrhosis than in the general population.

In most cases in which primary portal hypertension is diagnosed clinically in cirrhotic patients, esophageal varices are present. Some reports emphasize the development of pulmonary hypertension after surgical portacaval shunts.[68,497,581]

Portal hypertension may be long standing before pulmonary hypertension develops, but it may also be diagnosed concurrently with cirrhosis. It is thought that subclinical portal hypertension precedes the onset of symptomatic pulmonary hypertension by months or years. Quantitative histologic studies suggest that severe hepatic injury is often associated with subclinical pulmonary hypertension that might become clinically manifest with long-term patient survival.[570]

The symptom most frequently associated with pulmonary hypertension is exertional dyspnea, but syncope, precordial pain, and hemoptysis have been reported.[497]

Accentuation of the pulmonic second sound, a murmur in the second or third intercostal space or along the left lower sternal border, cardiac enlargement, prominent main pulmonary arteries, and right ventricular hypertrophy occur frequently.[497]

The etiology of pulmonary hypertension accompanying cirrhosis is not yet established. Theories considered include the passing of emboli[853] or of humoral vasoconstrictors[497,570] from the portal to the pulmonary circulation, autoimmune mechanisms,[615] and effects of long-standing elevations in cardiac output and blood volume.[497]

Hypertrophic Pulmonary Osteoarthropathy. Periostitis, a common complication of bronchogenic carcinoma, is an occasional complication of cirrhosis. This bizarre finding, more common in biliary than alcoholic cirrhosis, is characterized by pain and tenderness along the distal long bones of the forearms and legs. Virtually all of these patients exhibit clubbing of the fingers, and some of them show gynecomastia. Radiographically, there is a thin opaque line of new bone, which is separated from the underlying denser cortex by a narrow radiolucent band along the distal end of the diaphysis of the long bones.[258] Serum calcium and phosphorus levels are normal. Alkaline phosphatase activity is almost invariably elevated, but it is not known whether the elevation is related to the underlying liver disease or the increased osteoblastic activity.

Relative bone and liver isoenzyme levels have not been reported. It has been suggested that stimuli to periosteal growth may escape pulmonary inactivation via right-to-left systemic shunts. Similarly, portal-systemic shunts have been proposed to explain the failure of the liver to inactivate such substances. No such substances have been identified, however. Pulmonary osteoarthropathy does not seem directly related to the presence or degree of hypoxemia, of right-to-left shunting, or of portal-systemic shunting, since only a rare patient with these disorders develops this syndrome. It is not associated with increased concentrations of growth hormone or of estrogen excretion. What causes it and why it is seen so much more commonly in primary biliary cirrhosis than in other types of cirrhosis are questions to be answered.

Cardiac

Between 30% and 60% of all cirrhotic patients develop a circulatory hyperdynamic state that is characterized by an increase in cardiac output and a reduction in peripheral resistance. These changes are present at rest and increase with exercise. The clinical correlates of this hyperkinetic state are bounding pulses, warm hands, and capillary pulsations.

Numerous factors contribute to these circulatory changes. The increase in cardiac output can be accentuated by concurrent anemia, expansion of blood volume, and an extensive collateral circulation. Increased blood flow to the extremities and to the splanchnic organs through low-resistance arterial beds also plays a role. On the other hand, ascites, which increases intra-abdominal pressure and decreases venous return, may decrease cardiac output as may diuretic therapy, recent hemorrhage, and underlying myocardial disease.[93]

The reasons for decreased peripheral resistance are not well explained. Both increased excretion and impaired hepatic inactivation of vasodilatory factors, such as glucagon or prostaglandins, have been suggested.[59,102] When arteriolar vasodilatation is present, aortic impedance is lessened and stroke output can increase without a change in myocardial contractility or in ventricular preload.[743]

In spite of increased cardiac output in many cirrhotic patients, systemic blood pressure is often slightly decreased because of the accompanying low systemic resistance.[93] Hypertension is not often seen in alcoholic cirrhotic patients, even though in noncirrhotic patients alcohol has a documented pressor effect[726] and the incidence of hypertension is increased in alcoholic patients.[467]

However, in alcoholic cirrhosis, alcohol may have hemodynamic consequences. Alcohol is known to be cardiotoxic. It might be expected that cirrhosis of alcohol-related etiology would be frequently accompanied by cardiomyopathy. It is usually claimed, however, that patients tend to develop either liver disease or cardiomyopathy, but not both.[756] One recent review found no evidence of either cirrhosis or alcoholic hepatitis in its series of patients with alcoholic cardiomyopathy.[506] Careful investigation, however, reveals that even though overt cardiomyopathy is infrequent in alcoholic cirrhosis, some patients have altered left ventricular function and are at risk of clinical decompensation in the presence of volume or pressure overload.[5]

Lymphatic

Dumont and the Wittes showed abnormalities of the lymphatic system in cirrhosis and suggested its importance.[235,1032] It has long been known that hepatic hilar lymphatics were distended in patients with portal hypertension and discharged large volumes of lymph when transected. These investigators have shown that in cirrhotic patients with portal hypertension, especially those with ascites, the thoracic duct is greatly enlarged and lymph flow through the thoracic duct is enormously increased, often 10 to 15 times greater than normal. They postulated that in portal hypertension, lymph flow may decompress the hepatic and/or splanchnic beds. When this lymphatic flow surpasses maximal capacity, ascites results, with elevated protein concentration in patients with hepatic venous outflow obstruction, low protein levels in extrahepatic portal venous obstruction, and intermediate levels when both types of venous hypertension coexist.[1031] They suggested that the size of the communication between the thoracic duct and the subclavian vein is critical in determining the occurrence and severity of ascites. Thoracic duct drainage either externally or by anastomosis into a systemic or pulmonary vein may promptly decrease ascitic volume and portal pressure.

Indeed, peritoneovenous shunts, which have proved effective in the management of intractable ascites, may be viewed as an accessory, man-made thoracic duct (see section on ascites).

Dermatologic

Jaundice. Many stigmata of cirrhosis are visible in the skin. Most obvious is the bilirubin staining of elastic tissue, which gives the skin its yellow color in jaundice. Depending on the type of pigment, the color may characteristically reflect the type of jaundice, as typified by the greenish biliverdin discoloration of long-standing obstructive jaundice. Since bilirubin pigments are transported bound to albumin, localized areas of edema may be differentially more jaundiced or less jaundiced than nonedematous areas. In patients with unilateral edema due to heart failure, which characteristically induces a low-protein edema fluid, contralateral jaundice may be observed.[664] When the edema fluid is relatively high in albumin, as in extravasated ascites, jaundice may be localized to the area of edema.[168] Similarly, hives, which are local inflammatory exudates high in protein concentration, often appear to be more jaundiced than the surrounding skin.

Spider Angiomata and Palmar Erythema probably represent cutaneous manifestations of endocrine imbalances in cirrhosis. Virtually all that is known about the arterial spiders (spider nevi), is discussed in Bean's classic monograph.[54] Histologically, spider angiomata resemble the short, corkscrew, endometrial arteries that develop and slough rapidly during the menstrual cycle. Similar spiders have been recognized on the pleural and pulmonary surfaces as well.[69] Other forms of telangiectasia, such as the "paper-money" facial skin have been described but are not specific for cirrhosis. Palmar erythema (liver palms), which characteristically involves the thenar and hypothenar eminences, the distal pads of the fingers, and often the circumungual areas on the dorsum of the fingers, usually sparing the central portion of the palm, represents an extensive collection of arteriovenous anastomoses.[871] These findings are not specific for cirrhosis, for they appear in rheumatoid arthritis (rheumatoid palms) and in pregnancy (palms of pregnancy). They occur with greater frequency in alcoholic cirrhosis than in cirrhosis of other etiologies.

Nail Changes. Nail changes of various sorts have been described in cirrhosis. Best known are Muehrcke's lines.[620] The transverse pale bands, also seen in the nephrotic syndrome, were initially said to be associated with hypoalbuminemia, but whether they represent a period of increased disease activity or other factors is open to speculation. Terry described white nails in cirrhosis.[946]

Dupuytren's Contracture. Contractions of palmar fascia occur more commonly in patients with alcoholic cirrhosis and with chronic alcoholism (Fig. 20-17) than in nonalcoholic persons. The cause of this contracture of the palmar fascia is not known.

Chest Hair is often absent or markedly decreased in cirrhosis. Its absence is not, as is so often stated, a loss of preexisting chest hair. When asked, "When did you lose the hair from your chest?" cirrhotic patients almost invariably answer, "I never had any!" We have been able to document this statement in many male cirrhotic patients by comparing photographs taken many years earlier,

Fig. 20-17. Dupuytren's contracture. Flexor tendons of third, fourth, and fifth digits are hypertrophied and incorporated into the thickened palmer fascia.

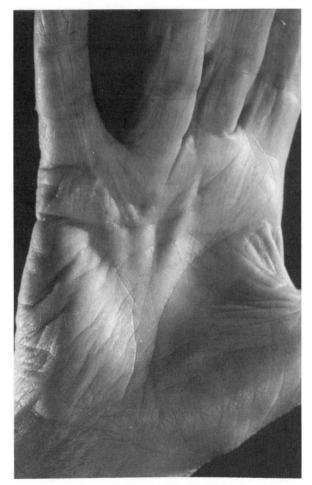

prior to development of the cirrhosis. Rarely have we encountered a patient who has lost his pectoral hair during or after the development of cirrhosis. The chest hair pattern, like gynecomastia, is of limited diagnostic value in women. Negroes, American Indians, and Orientals normally have scant chest hair, and its absence in cirrhosis is neither surprising nor meaningful. Other areas of hair distribution in the male do change, however. The pubic hair pattern frequently becomes inverted and resembles the feminine pattern, the so-called female escutcheon. Axillary hair may become quite scant both in men and women.

Vascular

Vascular phenomena cause many of the major consequences of cirrhosis. Esophageal varices are the most dangerous of the portal-systemic collaterals by virtue of their tendency to rupture, but this venous collateral system also gives rise to some of the major metabolic derangements of cirrhosis. The pathogenesis and treatment of these manifestations are discussed below.

Portal-Systemic Encephalopathy. PSE is largely a consequence of the passage of enteric, toxic substances from the gastrointestinal tract directly into the systemic circulation, instead of first passing through the liver where these substances are normally removed. Shunting of enteric bacteria through portal-systemic collaterals, instead of removal of the organisms by the hepatic reticuloendothelial system, results in bacteremia. Physiologic substances arising in the splanchnic bed, such as insulin or glucagon, may also bypass the liver with major metabolic consequences. It has been suggested that the post-portacaval shunt–hepatic failure syndrome is due to the shunting away from the liver of some hepatotrophic substances such as glucagon or insulin.[912]

Arteriovenous communications are known to be responsible for several abnormalities in cirrhosis. Palmar erythema, as described above,[871] represents a collection of local arteriovenous fistulas. Large numbers of such communications may exist in the lung and contribute to the severe right-to-left shunting so often seen in cirrhosis. The functional abnormalities seen in the renal lesion of cirrhosis, the so-called hepatorenal syndrome, appear to be related to shunting of arterial blood from the cortex of the kidney to the vessels of the medulla. Normally, arteriovenous fistulas occur with great profusion in the gastrointestinal tract. The purpose of these communications and the mechanism of their control are not clear, however.

Musculoskeletal

Even the motor system may be involved. *Alcoholic myositis,* a complication of excessive alcohol intake rather than cirrhosis *per se,* is characterized by pain and tenderness of the skeletal muscles accompanied by hyperkalemia, myoglobinuria, and elevated serum levels of glutamic ox-

aloacetic transaminase, creatine phosphokinase, and lactic dehydrogenase.[694] As cirrhosis advances, there is progressive reduction in lean body mass because of a high rate of muscle catabolism, which has been attributed to hyperglucagonemia.[563]

An interesting musculoskeletal manifestation of cirrhosis is seen secondary to massive ascites. In ascites, as in pregnancy, the accumulation of intra-abdominal weight must be counterbalanced by increased lordosis of the spine. This posture, which in pregnant women is called the pride of pregnancy, can be called, for poetic purposes, the lordosis of cirrhosis (Fig. 20-18).

Fig. 20-18. The lordosis of cirrhosis.

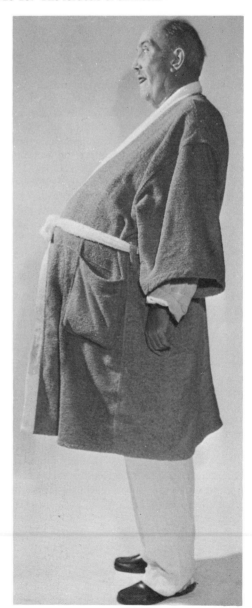

Another type of secondary musculoskeletal abnormality of ascites is the development of abdominal hernias. These include inguinal, ventral, umbilical, and hiatal, all of which are much more common in ascitic than in nonascitic patients. In addition, *diastasis recti* is virtually universal in ascitic patients.

The umbilical hernias are potentially the most dangerous. A knuckle of bowel can often become incarcerated and require surgical correction. In patients with ascites, surgical morbidity and mortality are increased, and there is a high incidence of hernia recurrence. Retrospective studies suggest that these risks may be significantly reduced when herniorrhaphy is preceded by placement of a peritoneovenous shunt.[514] In some series, repair of umbilical hernias in cirrhotic patients has been followed frequently by hemorrhage from esophageal varices due presumably to the elevation in variceal pressure resulting from the ligation of abdominal wall portal-systemic collateral vessels.[48] Not all studies have confirmed this claim.[695]

In patients with tense ascites, the umbilical hernias may sometimes rupture, giving rise to the so-called Flood syndrome, which is eponymic rather than descriptive.[291] In most cases the spontaneous perforation is heralded by ulceration of the skin overlying the hernia. Once perforation is established, operative management is usually indicated.[511] In addition to repair of the fascial defect, placement of a peritoneovenous shunt may be prudent to prevent reaccumulation of ascites during the immediate postoperative period.[641]

Hiatal hernias, which permit gastroesophageal reflux and may induce esophagitis, may, perhaps, predispose to and precipitate hemorrhage from esophageal varices.

Endocrine

Many endocrine abnormalities occur, most of them presumably as consequences of the failure of the liver to conjugate or otherwise metabolize hormones. These problems may arise from hepatic parenchymal cell injury, portal-systemic shunting, or both. Sometimes, in alcoholic cirrhosis, it is difficult to differentiate the changes induced by chronic alcoholism from those caused by the liver disease itself. Most of these abnormalities are subtle changes, such as secondary hypersomatotropism or hyperinsulinemia without overt physical signs. Others are evident functionally, for example, as hyponatremia in inappropriately increased antidiuretic hormone, or as hyperglycemia in diabetes. Some, such as gynecomastia, may be visible or palpable signs; others such as testicular or prostatic atrophy may be invisible, impalpable phenomena.

The sexual signs of cirrhosis in men are manifested by feminization and hypogonadism. The increase in femaleness and the decrease in maleness are separate syndromes.

Feminization. Feminization, which can occur in the absence of hypogonadism, is the acquisition of estrogen-induced characteristics. Feminization occurs in both alcoholic and nonalcoholic cirrhosis, but it is more common in the former. Feminization is manifested by gynecomastia, spider angiomata, palmar erythema, and changes in body hair patterns. Estradiol levels in cirrhotic men are either normal or only slightly increased. Plasma estrone levels are moderately increased.[971] Rather than resulting from significant increases in plasma estrogens, feminization is thought to result instead from the increased conversion of weakly androgenic steroids to estrogens in peripheral tissues (skin, adipose tissue, muscle, bone), where they have a local effect. Chronic alcoholism may result in adrenal overproduction of such androgens. In nonalcoholic cirrhosis, feminization occurs only when cirrhosis is sufficiently advanced to result in portal-systemic shunting.[971] Such shunting allows steroidal estrogen precursors to escape the enterohepatic circulation and undergo peripheral conversion. Thus peripheral estrogen effect is possible without altering systemic plasma estrogen levels.[967]

Gynecomastia in cirrhosis (Fig. 20-19) may sometimes have etiologies other than outlined above. It may, for instance, appear not during decompensation but as the patient improves, a phenomenon similar to "refeeding gynecomastia," which was observed in starved prisoners after liberation in World War II. Widespread clinical use of spironolactone, an aglycone, may, like digitalis, induce gynecomastia.

Hypogonadism. Hypogonadism in alcoholic cirrhosis is now generally thought to be a direct effect of alcohol and is not a manifestation of liver disease itself.[970] In nonalcoholic liver disease it is seen with increased frequency only in hemochromatosis. Since increased iron is sometimes seen in patients with hemochromatosis in the hy-

Fig. 20-19. Gynecomastia. The patient, who had alcoholic cirrhosis and persistent ascites, had required prolonged spironolactone therapy. Gynecomastia persisted for a year after the diuretic had been stopped.

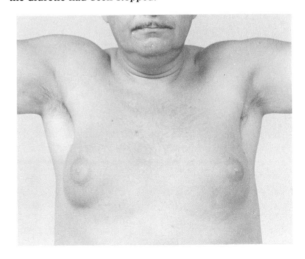

pothalamus, pituitary, and, rarely, the testes, in this disease, too, it is tissue injury rather than underlying liver disease that leads to hypogonadism. Hypogonadism is manifested by testicular atrophy (Fig. 20-20), high prevalence of infertility, changes in secondary sexual characteristics, loss of libido, and impotence. Even though testicular atrophy on physical examination occurs less frequently than textbooks imply, nonetheless the testes, even when not discernibly atrophic, may have a reduced number of germ cells, be oligospermic, or have many bizarre or inactive germ cells.[967] In 50% of alcoholic men there is a decrease in plasma testosterone levels.[968] Sex hormone–binding globulin is increased.[971] In addition to these indicators of gonadal failure, there is evidence of hypothalamic and pituitary dysfunction. Although plasma gonadotropins (follicle-stimulating hormone [FSH] and luteinizing hormone [LH]) are not actually decreased in concentration in alcoholic liver disease, they are inappropriately low for the degree of gonadal failure.[968] This indicates that there may be a hypothalamic defect, since in usual circumstances a reduction in a sex steroid level would leave hypothalamic sex steroid receptors unoccupied, and hypothalamic release of gonadotropin-releasing hormone (GnRH), which governs release of gonadotropin from the pituitary, would be enhanced.[967] Evidence for pituitary dysfunction also comes from diminished responses in most alcoholic men to a provocative stimulus with GnRH.[969] There are therefore defects in all components of the hypothalamic–pituitary–gonadal axis. In cirrhosis not of an alcoholic etiology, the few studies that have been done suggest that even when there is comparably severe liver disease, nonalcoholic cirrhosis, except hemochromatosis, is not characterized by reduced testosterone or by altered sperm concentration or volume.[967,970]

Fig. 20-20. Testicular atrophy. **A.** Testicular histologic specimen of normal adult man demonstrating active spermatogenesis in normal-sized seminiferous tubules with delicate basement membranes and minimal peritubular fibrosis. Leydig cells are scarce, being widely separated by seminiferous tubules. **B.** Testicular histologic specimen of a patient with alcoholic cirrhosis demonstrates germ cell aplasia, marked seminiferous tubular atrophy with prominent peritubular fibrosis, and condensation of Leydig cells around the seminiferous tubules. (Original magnification: *A, B* × 250) (Provided by Dr. D. H. Van Thiel)

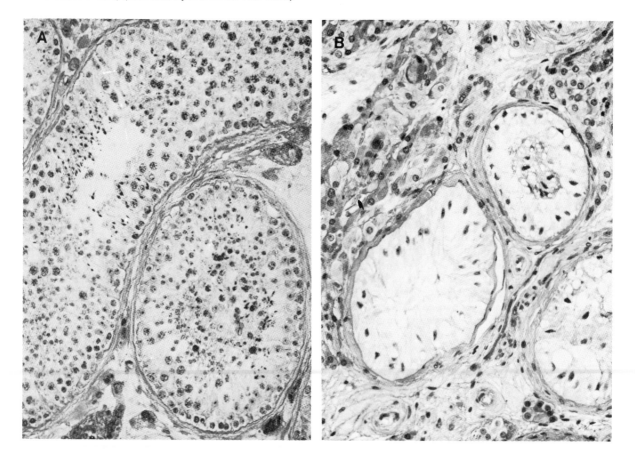

Impotence is a common complaint in cirrhosis. It is rarely, however, the initial complaint, since more pressing symptoms usually dominate the picture. Unless this information is specifically sought by the physician, it will not be commonly volunteered by the patient. Almost invariably, decreased sexual drive precedes the impotence, but poor performance is not appreciated due to the defect in desire. Often the symptom is recognized only in retrospect as sexual performance improves. Sexual capacity may return spontaneously after hepatic recompensation, and occasionally deficient activity becomes excessive. The pathogenesis of impotence is not well understood, and its therapy is unsatisfactory.

It has been demonstrated that the administration of testosterone enanthate to cirrhotic patients can increase plasma testosterone levels and normalize the male–female hormonal imbalance.[468] Unfortunately, the authors did not mention the clinical response in these patients. We and others have used injections of testosterone enanthate in sesame oil, usually with little improvement, but occasionally with resounding success.

Gonadal Failure in Women. Alcoholic cirrhotic women may show severe gonadal failure manifested by oligomenorrhea, loss of secondary sex characteristics, such as breast and pelvic fat accumulation, and infertility. Women still in the reproductive years have a marked decrease in developing follicles and few or no corpus lutea.[967] Plasma levels of estradiol and progesterone are reduced.[971] Amenorrhea may also occur in decompensated cirrhosis of other etiologies; normal menses may return with recovery. Pregnancies have been carried to successful conclusion in cirrhotic patients and even in those with portacaval anastomosis.[836]

Secondary Hyperaldosteronism. Increased secretion of aldosterone is the last in a series of steps initiated by increased intrahepatic sinusoidal pressure and is a key consequence of advanced cirrhosis. It is thought to be mediated by a decrease in effective plasma volume on the juxtaglomerular apparatus of the kidney, which stimulates the renin–angiotensin I–angiotensin II–aldosterone sequence. The factors that influence water balance, electrolyte concentration, and urine formation are discussed more fully in the sections on ascites and on the hepatorenal syndrome.

Diabetes. The prevalence of diabetes in patients with cirrhosis is increased.[206,627] Although "cirrhotic diabetes" is not a problem clinically, it is surprisingly common, occurring two to three times as frequently in patients with alcoholic cirrhosis as in noncirrhotic patients. Epidemiologically this type of diabetes is clearly secondary to the cirrhosis.[191] It usually occurs after the cirrhosis is well developed and is often found incidentally during evaluation of decompensated cirrhosis. It is usually manifested by hyperglycemia, mild glycosuria, glucose intolerance, hyperinsulinemia, and peripheral insulin resistance.[192,922]

There is rarely evidence of the vascular lesions of diabetes mellitus, and patients are resistant to diabetic ketoacidosis. Usually it can be treated with diet; occasionally it requires oral agents, but only rarely insulin. When a cirrhotic patient requires insulin the diabetes probably represents true diabetes mellitus of nonhepatogenous origin.

The pathogenesis of this metabolic disorder is not clear. It is characterized by insulin resistance, as in patients with obesity. It differs from the diabetes of obesity, which is characterized by hypoglucagonemia, by the presence of greatly increased plasma glucagon levels.[864] It does not appear to be related to pancreatitis, hemosiderosis, hypokalemia, or hyperadrenalcorticism.

The accompanying hyperinsulinemia is thought to result from decreased degradation of insulin by the liver, although increased secretion has also been demonstrated.[418] Current data suggest that the decreased degradation is primarily a result of a decrease in hepatic parenchymal function[922] rather than an effect of portal-systemic shunting, although the latter may contribute. Portal-systemic shunting appears to play a greater role in the hyperglucagonemia by means of pancreatic stimulation by some as yet unidentified factor.

Insulin resistance in cirrhotic patients may be contributed to by hormonal and nonhormonal antagonists, such as hypersomatotropism, hyperglucagonemia, and increased plasma levels of free fatty acids. Defects in target tissues for insulin action have been postulated.[646] Recent studies, for example, have suggested major roles for a decreased binding of insulin to adipocytes and for a post-receptor defect in the pathogenesis of insulin resistance in cirrhosis.[78,941]

The diabetes of cirrhosis occurs frequently in patients with inherited susceptibility to diabetes, and this suggests that these diabetogenic influences may precipitate diabetes in patients with a genetic predisposition.

Metabolic

Many of the metabolic derangements associated with cirrhosis are discussed elsewhere in this chapter but are mentioned here.

Potassium Deficiency. Hypokalemia is almost ubiquitous in alcoholic cirrhosis and quite common in nonalcoholic cirrhosis. Vomiting and diarrhea, which are frequently present in decompensated cirrhosis, may cause the loss of large amounts of potassium. In addition, secondary hyperaldosteronism favors the loss of potassium and interferes with the intrinsic and extrinsic attempts to correct the deficit. Finally, physicians may contribute a large iatrogenic component to the potassium deficit by the use of diuretic agents, the most potent of which are strongly kaliuretic substances. The inability of the renal tubules to conserve potassium as effectively as they do sodium contributes to this developing defect. Indeed, as metabolic alkalosis appears, the tubules may paradoxically and inappropriately secrete large amounts of potassium in the face of severe kaliopenia. The metabolic alkalosis and increased intracellular–extracellular pH gradient, which develops as intracellular potassium ions are exchanged for extracellular hydrogen ions (see section on hepatic coma), induces potentially comagenic shifts in ammonia and in amines.

Hyponatremia occurs as commonly as hypokalemia but is not so toxic. Both dilutional and natriopenic hyponatremia occur. Increased antidiuretic hormonal activity has long been recognized, although its source, nature, and pathogenesis have never been adequately elucidated.[739] This type of dilutional hyponatremia can be effectively treated by restricting water intake. The other type of hyponatremia, which is more complex and more disturbing, is rarely seen in untreated cirrhotic patients who have not been on salt-restricted diets or diuretic therapy. In this situation the hyponatremia results from sodium loss in excess of water and is often complicated by fluid retention. This combination creates the difficult dilemma of hyponatremia with edema and ascites. Water restriction in this situation often results in progressive azotemia, and the use of diuretic drugs may often exacerbate the hyponatremia. Sometimes it is difficult to tell whether fluid restriction, diuresis, or both are required. In most instances hyponatremia represents total body hypotonicity with expansion of the intracellular fluid volume and constriction of the extracellular volume with its attendant consequences—oliguria, azotemia, and hypotension. This syndrome may respond dramatically to the administration of hypertonic saline to correct the extracellular sodium concentration by shifting water into the extracellular fluid,[1015] which results in correction of the hyponatremia and, sometimes, in diuresis.

Hypoalbuminemia is an almost universal finding in cirrhosis, especially alcoholic cirrhosis. It is widely held that decreased hepatic synthetic capacity for albumin is responsible. Meticulous studies, however, have indicated that although albumin synthesis is sometimes decreased, it is often normal or even increased.[794] The albumin synthetic rate does not correlate well with the serum albumin concentration. Suppression of albumin production is closely correlated with elevated SGOT levels, decreased concentration of cholesterol esters, and prolonged prothrombin time, all indications of active hepatocellular dysfunction. Many other factors contribute to the decrease in albumin concentration.[795] Alcohol specifically inhibits albumin synthesis, and this inhibition can be reversed experimentally by tryptophan. Albumin synthesis may also be affected by the nutritional state, by changes in colloid osmotic pressure, by intrahepatic pressure relationships, and by altered metabolism of adrenal, genital, and thyroid hormones. The problem is extremely complex, since the albumin degradation rate is decreased in patients with hypoalbuminemia.[920]

Decreased serum albumin levels contribute greatly to the formation of edema and ascites and to the compensatory increase in serum globulins. In addition, decreased binding of the many substances that are bound to albumin, such as bilirubin, calcium, and many drugs, results in abnormal plasma/tissue ratios and a variety of metabolic derangements.

Oncologic

Oropharyngeal Cancer. Alcoholic cirrhosis is frequently complicated by the development of cancer of the mouth and pharynx.[444,446] Cancer of the floor of the mouth, uvula, and soft palate have also been associated independently with both alcohol consumption and smoking.[445] Since alcoholism is related to alcoholic cirrhosis by definition and to smoking by social mores, it is difficult to be certain whether oral cancer is associated with cirrhosis, alcoholism, smoking, or a combination of these factors. The association of oral cancer with alcoholism holds for the consumption of all types of alcoholic beverages—beer, wine, and whiskey—but for tobacco usage holds only for cigarette smoking, not for cigars or pipe.

Whenever such a positive association exists, one must wonder whether Berkson's bias may have been responsible for an artifactual relationship. Berkson's hypothesis suggests that any two diseases will occur more commonly together in hospitalized patients than their individual incidences would predict and that this comorbidity depends on the individual rates of admission to hospital for the two diseases.[65]

As Mainland has pointed out, any two lethal diseases will occur less commonly together than would be expected on the basis of their individual incidences.[554] The finding that oral cancer occurs *more* commonly in cirrhotic patients than in noncirrhotic patients at autopsy, despite the statistical expectation that it should occur less frequently in cirrhosis, supports the validity of the relationship.

Cancer Metastatic to the Liver. Several reports of a decreased incidence of hepatic metastases from nonhepatic cancers in cirrhotic patients[528,769] have been published. They may represent examples of the Berkson–Mainland postmortem principle.[554] On the other hand, one would expect that the portal-systemic venous collaterals of cirrhosis will decrease the frequency of hepatic metastases from cancers originating in the splanchnic organs that are disseminated by portal venous flow. Similarly, one might expect that intrahepatic arteriovenous anastomoses, which are common in cirrhosis, may reduce metastases that originate in other areas of the body and are spread by arterial dissemination. Carefully controlled investigations have failed to confirm the negative association between hepatic metastases and cirrhosis.[337] Indeed, one study suggests that hepatic metastases from gastrointestinal tumors occurred *more* often in cirrhotic than in noncirrhotic patients. On the other hand, nongastrointestinal tumors spread to the liver of cirrhotic patients less frequently than to those of noncirrhotic patients. It is worrisome, however, that in alcoholic cirrhosis the disproportionately frequent oropharyngeal cancers, which rarely metastasize to the liver, might falsely account for this negative relationship.

Hepatocellular Cancer. Hepatocellular carcinoma, which occurs with increased frequency in patients with most types of cirrhosis, is discussed in detail in Chapter 31. It is seen in ascending order of occurrence in alcoholic cirrhosis, posthepatitic cirrhosis, especially that associated with hepatitis B virus, and hemochromatosis. Although persistence of the virus intracellularly may allow abnormal oncogenic aberrations of the genetic code to develop, the increased incidence of hepatocellular carcinoma in cirrhosis appears teleologically to represent excessive regenerative activity gone awry.

DIAGNOSTIC PROCEDURES

A variety of diagnostic techniques are used in the diagnosis of cirrhosis and its complications. Some deal with the evaluation of the liver itself—its size, its shape and its composition. Some are biochemical "liver function tests," which are surprisingly useful in the differential diagnosis of liver disease,[193] and some are truly tests of liver function, which are valuable in assessing various hepatic functional capacities. Some deal with the diagnosis of the complications of cirrhosis, such as esophageal varices, portal hypertension, and ascites.

Liver Biopsy

Percutaneous liver biopsy is the procedure of choice for proving the diagnosis of liver disease. It is safe, simple, inexpensive, and readily acceptable to the patient. The Menghini needle,[591] which is the most widely used, has compiled an impressive safety record.[536] In generalized disease such as micronodular cirrhosis, it is a reliable, reproducible technique,[53] which provides adequate tissue for diagnostic studies. It may be somewhat less precise in patients with macronodular cirrhosis, in whom individual samples of tissue may not necessarily be representative. Like all other procedures that require subjective evaluation, it is subject to objective error.[317,332] It is useful in establishing the type and severity of cirrhosis and, within the limits of the clinical–histologic relationships, in estimating prognosis and response to therapy. It is effective in determining the cause of space-occupying lesions on liver scan, which are quite common in cirrhosis, by using scan-directed[169] or ultrasound-guided biopsies.[644]

Sometimes prolonged prothrombin time or thrombocytopenia increases the risk of percutaneous liver biopsy. One must here weigh the potential gains against the increased risks.[31,170] If the hazards seem disproportionately high, another option is to perform laparoscopy or a minilaparotomy under local anesthesia with surgical homeostasis. Laparoscopy has not, however, been shown to be

superior to percutaneous liver biopsy in the diagnosis of cirrhosis.[665]

Rösch and associates suggested transjugular liver biopsy (*i.e.,* through a catheter passing from the jugular vein into the hepatic vein through which the biopsy of the liver is performed).[788] Although this procedure is more difficult, it is reassuring to know that when postbiopsy hemorrhage occurs, the patient is bleeding into the bloodstream. A study based on 1000 tissue specimens found that enough tissue was available for evaluation of architecture in two thirds of cirrhotic livers and for almost all nonfibrotic or noncirrhotic livers.[500] Our more limited experience has been less consistent, with the tissue samples frequently too small for interpretation in suspected cirrhosis.

Ultrasonography

Ultrasound is one of the major technologic breakthroughs in the diagnosis of hepatobiliary disease. It is as noninvasive a technique as can be envisioned. At present its greatest value is in differentiating biliary obstruction from nonobstructive, parenchymal jaundice, a differential diagnosis that may involve cirrhosis and alcoholic hepatitis. In assessment of the cirrhotic liver *per se,* its value is limited. Textural differences and increased attenuation may provide diagnostic insight as shown in the gray-scale ultrasonograms from Taylor's fine atlas on the subject.[940] (Fig. 20-21). Liver volume can also be determined by ultrasonic scanning[746]

On occasion, an enlarged, tortuous portal vein can indicate the presence of portal hypertension (Fig. 20-21*C*). In addition, ultrasound has been used to determine the patency of portacaval anastomoses, to demonstrate postshunt dilatation of the inferior vena cava, and to demonstrate collateral pathways.[62,436]

Computed Tomography

Although computed tomographic (CT) evaluation of the liver can show liver size, shape, and density more precisely and in more familiar anatomic projections than ultrasound, its value in the diagnosis of cirrhosis is limited by its expense and relatively high radiation dosage.

The CT findings of cirrhosis are not diagnostic. Similar CT findings are observed in lymphomatous and granulomatous infiltrations as well as in alcoholic hepatitis.[702] It has been suggested that a ratio of the transverse widths of the caudate to right lobe greater than 0.65 on CT or ultrasound may be as accurate as the histologic diagnosis in cirrhosis. This phenomenon is based on shrinkage of the right lobe, which is postulated to be a consequence of more fibrous tissue in the right lobe than in the caudate lobe, and hypertrophy of the caudate lobe. Normal livers have a ratio less than 0.55.[364]

CT may be of use in confirming the etiology of cirrhosis when hemochromatosis is suspected. In the absence of contrast injection, increments in the average CT density

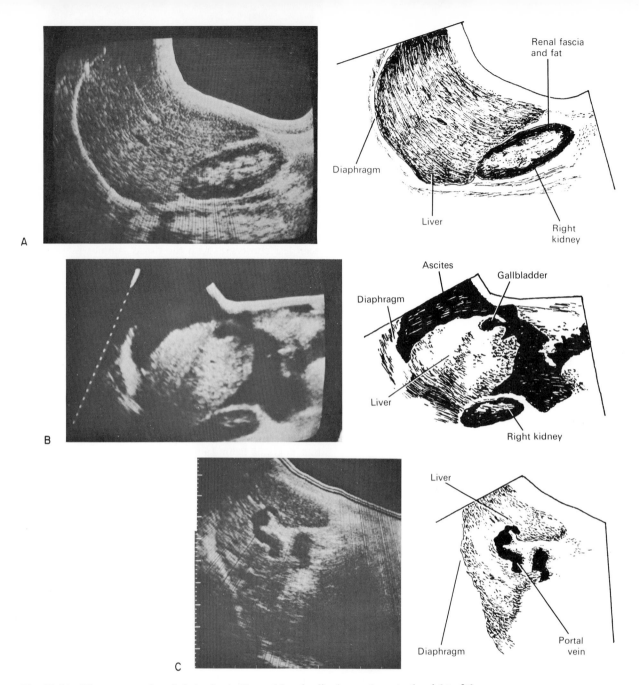

Fig. 20-21. Ultrasonography of cirrhosis. **A.** Normal longitudinal scan 4 cm to the right of the midline demonstrates the consistency of the liver. In this position, the liver is limited above by the right hemidiaphragm, anteriorly by the abdominal wall, and posteriorly by the right kidney, from which it is separated by the perirenal fat and fascia. These appear as a single, highly reflective interface. **B.** Parasagittal ultrasonogram through the right lobe of the liver and right kidney shows the liver to be surrounded by ascites both on its anterior aspect and between the visceral surface of the liver and right kidney (Morison's pouch). On the anterior surface of the liver, the lumen of the gallbladder is barely seen. The liver itself displays a highly abnormal consistency with dense white echoes and inadequate penetration to the deep surface, suggesting that there is both an increase in the echoes from the liver and increased attenuation within the liver. These findings are diagnostic of diffuse intrahepatic fibrosis and consistent with cirrhosis. **C.** A para-median scan through the liver substance 2 cm to the right of the midline shows a diffusely abnormal liver consistency with high-level echoes. Of note is a large, highly tortuous portal vein, which strongly suggests portal hypertension. (Taylor KJW: Atlas of Gray Scale Ultrasonography. New York, Churchill Livingstone, 1978)

to 75 Hounsfield units (H) to 132 H are seen in patients with hemochromatosis, whereas the normal CT density of the liver is 54H to 68H.[284]

Ultrasonography rather than CT is usually preferred when verification of the clinical impression of ascites is needed or when only small amounts are present. CT, however, has the additional capability of localizing the fluid collection to peritoneal, retroperitoneal, and extra-peritoneal compartments. Furthermore, it is claimed that benign transudative ascites has a CT density near that of urine or water, whereas malignant ascites has higher than normal CT density.[284]

In most clinical situations, the greater expense of CT probably does not justify its use in place of ultrasound.[1033]

Nuclear Magnetic Resonance Scans

Early claims for nuclear magnetic resonance (NMR) scans suggest that it is more sensitive than both ultrasound and radionuclide scans and comparable to CT scans in the diagnosis of cirrhosis.[230,881] NMR seems to be very effective in visualizing high flow vascular structures such as por-tacaval anastomoses. However, NMR technology has not yet been applied to large numbers of cirrhotic patients in a manner to determine its usefulness.

Radioisotopic Scans

Liver scans provide a simple and safe assessment of liver size, shape, and, to some degree, function. Technetium-99m-sulfur colloid, which is taken up by the reticuloen-dothelial tissue, shows liver size and homogeneity and spleen size and reticuloendothelial activity (Fig. 20-22). Typically the cirrhotic liver, by virtue of its irregular pa-renchymal pattern and uneven distribution of blood flow, shows a heterogeneous appearance. A significant corre-lation has been observed between the span of the liver determined by percussion–palpation and by radionuclide scan.[137] Since the liver is a three-dimensional organ that assumes an infinite variety of shapes,[617] it is often impos-sible to estimate liver size accurately. Liver volume and weight, the most valid indices, can be calculated easily and accurately from the anterior and right lateral scans.[786]

Some estimate of hepatic blood flow and of portal-sys-temic shunting can be made from the relative decrease in hepatic uptake and the increase in splenic and vertebral uptake.[130] Bircher and colleagues found that liver volume does not correlate well with functional capacity but does show a close correlation with hepatic blood flow and ox-ygen consumption.[75] It must be kept in mind, however, that liver volume in disease states may not be a reliable measure of hepatic parenchymal volume. The hepatic pa-renchymal tissue may represent a relatively small and widely variable fraction of the total liver weight.[540]

Endoscopy

The diagnosis of esophageal varices can best be made by endoscopy. However, endoscopic diagnosis of esophageal varices is not free of the uncertainties of observer vari-

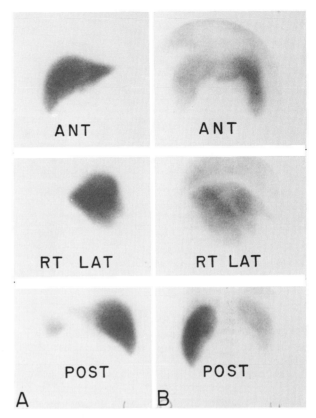

Fig. 20-22. Technetium-99m-sulfur colloid scans of the liver. **A.** A normal scan is shown on the left. Homogeneous uptake is shown on the anterior (*upper*), right lateral (*middle*), and posterior (*lower*) projections. The liver is of normal size and shape. A small spleen, which is not seen in the anterior view, is visible on the posterior scan. No uptake by the vertebrae is seen. **B.** An abnormal scan in a cirrhotic patient is shown on the right. Decreased and heterogeneous hepatic uptake is seen in the anterior and lateral projections. An enlarged spleen with greater uptake than the liver is seen. The clear area to the right and above the liver is caused by ascites. In the pos-terior scan increased vertebral uptake is visualized.

ability.[185] This technique has the advantage of visualizing the varices themselves, rather than their shadows, as is done radiologically. Certainly, when the patient is bleed-ing, endoscopic examination can establish unequivocally the site of hemorrhage.[667]

Barium-Contrast Esophagography

Barium-contrast esophagography is the time-honored method of demonstrating esophageal varices. It is safe, simple, and readily available. When the varices are large, the esophagogram shows the classic pattern (Fig. 20-23). Postprandial examination for esophageal varices appears to be more accurate than the traditional fasting study, since splanchnic blood flow is increased after meals, and varices are maximally distended at that time. Since ob-server variability can affect the diagnosis of varices ap-

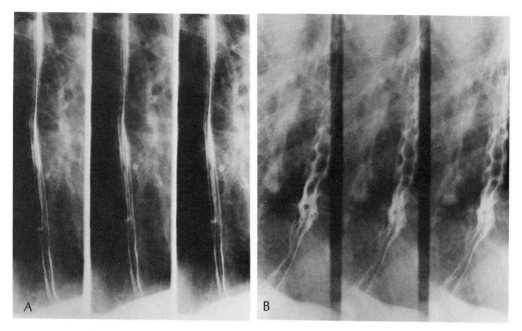

Fig. 20-23. Esophageal varices by barium swallow. **A.** A normal esophagogram shows delicate parallel mucosal folds. **B.** Large esophageal varices are seen in profile and *en face* on multiple films.

preciably,[186,189] several observers should interpret the films independently to establish a consensus diagnosis.

When the radiologic and endoscopic techniques for the diagnosis of esophageal varices were compared blindly, esophageal varices were found by each technique in approximately 50% of cirrhotic patients.[185,186,189] The two methods agreed with each other in 70% to 75% of patients.[185,189] The disagreements were evenly distributed, in a positive-negative sense, and appeared to be the consequence of observer error, rather than of intrinsic advantages of one method over the other.

Angiography

Visualization of the portal venous system, which had previously been done by splenoportography, is accomplished during the venous phase of arteriography. Arteriography may be helpful in determining the site of upper gastrointestinal tract hemorrhage. It can demonstrate leakage of contrast material from arterial or capillary lesions such as peptic ulcer or erosive gastritis. It rarely establishes bleeding from varices, however. Percutaneous transhepatic portography allows direct access to the portal venous system and definitive visualization of the portal vein and its collaterals.[1020] It is a more difficult and dangerous procedure than celiac or superior mesenteric arteriography. Umbilical vein catheterization has also been used to visualize the portal venous system,[977] but it requires surgical dissection of the umbilical vein, which is often unsuccessful.

The measurement of portal pressure can best be accomplished by hepatic vein catheterization. The correlation between the wedged hepatic venous pressure and the free portal venous pressure is almost perfect in alcoholic cirrhosis[89] (Fig. 20-24). This technique, which has been greatly simplified by the introduction of a balloon catheter, permits rapid serial measurements of wedged and free hepatic venous pressure[355] and calculation of the hepatic–portal venous pressure gradient, the most critical measurement in portal hypertension.

When hepatic arteries are visualized, cirrhosis can be suggested by the tortuous, corkscrew pattern formed by arterial branches. Arteriography can sometimes differentiate hepatomas, which occur with increased frequency in cirrhosis, from regenerating nodules.[965]

Splenoportography

For some years splenoportography had been the standard method of measuring portal (intrasplenic) pressure and of opacifying the portal venous system. It is used less frequently today because the technique does not allow for simultaneous determination of the ambient intra-abdominal venous presure (*i.e.,* a baseline level), and is associated with a small (around 1%) but definite risk of intrasplenic hemorrhage. When successful, the technique gives good visualization of the portal system. It is particularly useful for establishing the presence or absence of patency in the portal or splenic veins when thrombosis is suspected.[34] It is also useful in assessing the presinusoidal portal hyper-

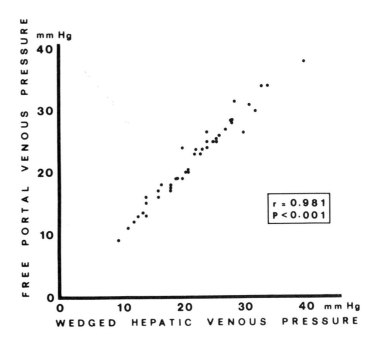

Fig. 20-24. Relationship between free portal venous pressure and wedged hepatic venous pressure. The correlation between these measurements in 43 patients with compensated alcoholic cirrhosis is almost perfect. (Viallet A et al: Gastroenterology 59:372, 1970)

tension of schistosomiasis and other disorders and the presinusoidal component of nonalcoholic cirrhosis.[718]

Transhepatic Portography

Because the wedged hepatic vein technique for measuring portal pressure is valid only in alcoholic cirrhosis, non-alcoholic cirrhosis, in which this technique underestimates portal pressure, necessitates a more direct measurement[89,718] (see Chap. 12). Visualization of the portal vein, its intrahepatic branches, the splenic vein, collateral vessels, and measurement of pressure within the portal venous system is possible by direct injection of contrast medium into the portal vein through a fine needle passed transhepatically. By redirecting the thin needle into a hepatic vein branch, a baseline pressure also can be measured for determining the portal–hepatic venous pressure gradient. Contrast injections into a hepatic vein branch can be useful in confirming Budd–Chiari syndrome, in which attempts at catheterization of hepatic veins are often unsuccessful.[751]

Paracentesis

Abdominal paracentesis is the standard procedure for examining ascitic fluid. It is simple when the volume of ascitic fluid is large. Fluid can be removed from the midline with the patient in the sitting position or from the flank with the patient supine or in the left lateral decubitus position. When the amount of ascitic fluid is small, paracentesis may be more difficult. In this situation, we prefer putting the patient on hands and knees and entering the abdomen from below. This abdomen-dependent position

has the advantage of puddling the fluid in the most dependent portion of the abdomen and floating loops of bowel away from the penetrating needle.

The usefulness of the differential analysis of ascitic fluid is suggested by Table 20-3.

MANAGEMENT OF MAJOR COMPLICATIONS

The course of cirrhosis is characterized by crisis, but the day-to-day management of cirrhosis is slow and tedious. The disease is gradually progressive and reaches clinical maturity slowly. There are no forms of therapy that rapidly reverse cirrhosis, although if the cause of continual injury, such as alcohol, is removed, self-reparative processes can ameliorate the lesion. There are, however, no documented cases of complete reversal of cirrhosis. Therapy consists of withdrawal of the toxic substance, (*e.g.,* alcohol in alcoholic cirrhosis or the offending drugs in drug-induced cirrhosis); the provision of a nutritious diet and vitamin supplements; the correction of anemia by the administration of iron, folic acid, or blood transfusions; the correction of fluid and electrolyte abnormalities; and the treatment of infections or other intercurrent problems. The treatment of cirrhosis for the most part is nondramatic, nonspecific, supportive therapy.

It has been reported that colchicine, which inhibits the deposition of collagen and stimulates its degradation, administered in small dosage (<0.6 mg/day) for long periods (>4 years) improves the clinical and histologic signs of cirrhosis.[454] In a recent, as yet unpublished report of a randomized clinical trial, these investigations have found

TABLE 20-3. Differential Analysis of Ascitic Fluid

TYPE OF ASCITES	APPEARANCE	PROTEIN (G/DL)		LEUKOCYTES*			CYTOLOGY	PERITONEAL BIOPSY	CULTURE	pH	AMYLASE	OTHER
		Mean	Range	PMN	MN	Total†						
Cirrhotic	Clear	1.8	0.6–6.0	75	225	300 ± 400	0	NS	0	7.45	Normal	Occasionally turbid; rarely bloody
Cardiac	Clear	2.2	1.5–5.5	50	200	250 ± 200	0	NS	0	7.40	Normal	Liver biopsy diagnostic
Neoplastic	Clear/bloody	2.2	0.6–6.0	340	360	700 ± 300	+ (30%)	+ (50%)	0	7.35	Normal	Occasionally chylous
Bacterial peritonitis	Cloudy	1.0	0.6–2.2	2200	300	2500 ± 2500	0	NS	+	7.25	Normal	Culture positive
Pancreatic	Clear/bloody	3.2	1.0–5.0	900	1000	1900 ± 800	0	NS	0	7.38	Elevated (80%)	Occasionally chylous
Tuberculous	Clear	3.4	1.5–7.0	125	875	1000 ± 600	0	+ (65%)	+ (65%)	7.30	Normal	Occasionally chylous
Nephrotic	Clear	0.9	0.3–1.8	45	175	220 ± 200	0	0	0	7.38	Normal	
Postdialysis	Clear	1.3	1.0–3.0	50	200	250 ± 200	0	0	0	7.40	Normal	

* Mean per mm³.
† Mean ± SD.
PMN, polymorphonuclear leukocytes; MN, mononuclear cells; NS, nonspecific; 0, negative; +, positive.

statistically significant improvement in survival after 10 years of colchicine therapy.[455]

Several reports have shown that transplantation of the liver for specific complications of cirrhosis, such as the hepatorenal syndrome[410] or hepatocellular carcinoma,[644a] not only replaces the cirrhotic liver with a noncirrhotic one, but eliminates the complication as well. Indeed, liver transplantation has been used in the treatment of end-stage primary biliary cirrhosis, posthepatitic cirrhosis, Wilson's disease, and other types of cirrhosis. Although available, transplantation is not yet standard therapy, but its use should be considered in specific situations while guidelines are being formulated.[33]

Much has been written about the mystique of the dietary treatment of cirrhosis. High-protein and low-fat diets supplemented by vitamins, choline, methionine, and other unproved dietary supplements have been authoritatively recommended. The high dietary protein is a double-edged sword that may well precipitate PSE in susceptible patients.[395,704] At the present time it seems reasonable to offer a normal, nutritious diet, supplemented with vitamins; if the patient exhibits anorexia, the diet can be adjusted to the patient's likes and dislikes to ensure adequate intake.

The dramatic aspects of the treament of cirrhosis take place in response to the development of major, life-threatening complications, such as bleeding esophageal varices, PSF, or the hepatorenal syndrome. The approach to these emergency situations should be based on the pathophysiology of the complication and tailored to the needs of the individual patient. In order to discuss rational management, it is necessary to consider each of these complications individually. Bleeding esophageal varices, hepatic encephalopathy, ascites, the hepatorenal syndrome, and spontaneous bacterial peritonitis are each considered separately in problem-oriented fashion.

Bleeding Esophageal Varices

Hemorrhage from esophageal varices is one of the most formidable emergencies in medicine. The mortality associated with variceal hemorrhage averages about 50% at the large medical centers in the United States.[882] There are many reasons for this awesome death rate.

1. Variceal bleeding usually occurs in decompensated cirrhotic patients who do not withstand well the consequences of massive hemorrhage. Cirrhotic patients often have abnormal coagulation, due either to impaired hepatic synthesis of clotting factors, to thrombocytopenia, or to circulating fibrinolysins or anticoagulants. Hemorrhage may be so massive that some patients exsanguinate even in the absence of clotting disorders. Some patients die in hepatic coma as a consequence of the bacterial breakdown of blood in the gastrointestinal tract, despite control of the hemorrhage. Others develop delirium tremens at a critical time. Electrolyte abnormalities are often present and include hyponatremia, hypokalemia, and hypomagnesemia, as well as respiratory and metabolic alkalosis. Hypotension may induce acute renal failure or acute hepatic necrosis.

2. The source of the hemorrhage is not readily evident. More than one third of cirrhotic patients with upper gastrointestinal tract hemorrhage bleed from sites other than varices.[95,713] This incidence is too high to permit the assumption that all cirrhotic patients are bleeding from varices, since the therapy of hemorrhage from varices is so different from that of nonvariceal hemorrhage.

3. Each of the methods of treating bleeding esophageal varices is itself dangerous. Each of the measures used in the management of variceal hemorrhage, such as balloon tamponade of the esophagus, vasopressin, endoscopic sclerosis, or percutaneous transhepatic obliteration of coronary veins is associated with significant hazards. More radical forms of therapy, which include transesophageal ligation of varices, gastroesophageal devascularization procedures, and emergency portacaval anastomosis, carry high operative mortality rates.

4. The standard form of definitive treatment, the creation of a portal-systemic anastomosis, has an elective operative mortality rate of 10% to 15%.[194] Portacaval anastomoses may be complicated by PSE, which may directly or indirectly cause or contribute to death.

This brief sketch paints a grim but realistic picture of the bleeding cirrhotic patient. When one considers the array of metabolic abnormalities and iatrogenic dangers that face the patient, it is surprising that even one-half survive. On the other hand, many of the defects outlined are correctable and most of the therapeutic hazards are avoidable. With prompt and precise diagnosis, rational therapy can be instituted.

Emergency Management

Emergency management is designed to correct as soon as possible those abnormalities that threaten the patient's life and to maintain the patient in optimal condition until more definitive therapy can be undertaken. It consists specifically of the administration of whole blood or other fluids to correct or prevent shock and to maintain the hematocrit at a reasonable level. An adequate airway is ensured. Finally, it is the phase in which nonspecific therapy is begun and in which preliminary diagnostic procedures may be initiated. During this phase, for example, one may confirm the presence of fresh blood in the stomach and remove this potentially toxic material by aspiration and catharsis.

Supportive Management

Wisely administered supportive therapy is probably the most important aspect of treatment. It may involve simply the administration of appropriate amounts of parenteral fluids, or it may require correction of specific electrolyte abnormalities. Routinely, vitamins, particularly B-complex, C, and K, are administered along with folic acid to correct deficiencies and to ensure availability of these substances. Sometimes paracentesis is required in patients with tense ascites to relieve pain or respiratory embarrassment and to decrease portal venous pressure. Antibiotics may be indicated to combat respiratory or other bacterial infection and to suppress the degradation of blood in the gastrointestinal tract and thereby to reduce the high incidence of bacterial infections that occur in cirrhotic patients after variceal hemorrhage.[269,778]

The most important factors in the supportive management of upper gastrointestinal tract hemorrhage are *blood transfusions,* and correction of the many abnormalities of coagulation that may exist in cirrhotic patients.

Another of the important aspects of the management of gastrointestinal tract hemorrhage in cirrhosis is the prevention of *ammonia intoxication.* Bacterial action on blood in the intestinal tract generates toxic amounts of ammonia and other nitrogenous substances that bypass the liver through portal-systemic collaterals and enter the systemic circulation. The increase in blood urea nitrogen, which frequently accompanies gastrointestinal tract bleeding, also provides substrate for bacterial ammonia production. Furthermore, the frequent occurrence in decompensated cirrhosis of respiratory and metabolic alkalosis, the latter associated with potassium depletion, potentiates ammonia toxicity.

This complication may be ameliorated or prevented by aspiration of blood from the stomach and by evacuation of the gastrointestinal tract. Vigorous catharsis should be carried out along with cleansing enemas. The mechanical removal of this potential source of ammonia, which is important in preventing encephalopathy, may be aided by the administration of neomycin or other antibiotics orally and enematically. As shown recently, oral antibiotics such as cefotaxime may also reduce the risk of bacterial infection after gastrointestinal tract hemorrhage.[269]

Lactulose is the ideal agent for preventing PSE, since it is a cathartic agent with potent antiammonia properties. It is given in frequent large doses (50 ml per 1 to 2 hours) until the patient has had two loose stools.[35] Intestinal cleansing procedures, however, tend to increase the potassium deficit and should be accompanied by the parenteral administration of potassium chloride. Soapsuds enemas or other alkaline enemas should be avoided, since they may adversely affect the *p*H gradient between the lumen of the bowel and the blood. Lactulose enemas may act favorably in this regard. Early attention to these details may avoid the difficulties and complications of treating a comatose patient.

Diagnosis

History and Physical Examination provide important information about the presence or absence of cirrhosis, presence and degree of portal hypertension, recency and magnitude of the hemorrhage, and potential sites of bleeding other than varices. This information may be complemented by aspiration of the gastric contents and examination of the stool. Although helpful, these leads are rarely definitive, however, and serve primarily as guides for determining the most rewarding order of diagnostic inquiry.

Emergency Endoscopy. Fiberoptic endoscopy performed during active bleeding can usually identify the bleeding site rapidly and accurately. Early establishment of the site of hemorrhage permits the immediate initiation of specific therapy and provides the basis for an orderly application of a therapeutic algorithm. Many alternative treatments are available for the control of active hemorrhage.

After hemorrhage has subsided, endoscopic examination can often identify the presumptive site of bleeding but can never prove unequivocally that any specific lesion was responsible. Thus, it is important to perform this examination while the patient is bleeding, although the presence of bleeding may make the procedure more difficult technically. Occasionally, massive hemorrhage will prevent demonstration of the lesion, although the approximate anatomic location of the bleeding can exclude certain possibilities and allow an educated guess.

Although fiberoptic endoscopy performed during active bleeding can identify the source of hemorrhage in over 90% of noncirrhotic patients, the percentage is much lower in cirrhotic patients. In the latter, in whom varices, ulcers, and mucosal erosive lesions are responsible for upper gastrointestinal tract bleeding with about equal frequency, more than one lesion may be present. Furthermore, bleeding from each of these sites may be intermittent, and in the absence of bleeding the responsible lesion may not be identifiable. Active bleeding from an esophageal varix can be seen in only 10% to 15% of the patients with such a source. Some (about 20%) are identified by the presence of an erosion or clot on a varix or of other putative markers of impending hemorrhage such as cherry red spots (Dagradi),[212] black points,[674] or red wales.[60] The remainder are inferential diagnoses in which nonbleeding esophageal varices are seen in the absence of any other potential site of hemorrhage.

Despite the logic of the early endoscopic diagnostic approach, its clinical value has never been established. In fact, investigations performed to establish the efficacy of emergency endoscopy have failed to confirm any clinical benefits for this rational type of diagnostic inquiry. These controlled investigations, which were undertaken to determine the efficacy of emergency endoscopy in patients with upper gastrointestinal tract hemorrhage (Table 20-4), showed no clinical benefits. None of eight studies, which include more than 1100 patients, has shown a reduction in the number of transfusions given, the need for surgery, the duration of hospitalization, or the mortality rate *despite prompt diagnosis of the bleeding site.* Unfortunately, these homogenous results apparently represent

TABLE 20-4. Controlled Investigations of Early Endoscopy in Upper Gastrointestinal Tract Hemorrhage That Failed to Show Benefits

FIRST AUTHOR	COMPARATIVE DIAGNOSTIC METHOD	NUMBER OF PATIENTS	MEAN AGE	SOURCE OF HEMORRHAGE		
				Peptic Ulcer*	Esophageal Varices*	Deaths*
Allan	Selective endoscopy (+UGI series)	100	54	19	1	8
Sandlow	Selective endoscopy at 1 week	150	49	46	5	8
Morris	UGI series	60	49	38	10	8
Keller	UGI series, then delayed endoscopy	76	54	26	16	—
Dronfield	UGI series	322	60	—	—	10
Graham	Early endoscopy (delayed diagnosis)	95	48	48	20	11
Peterson	Selective endoscopy	206	55	38	20	11
Giacosa	UGI series	104	53	21	12	17

* No. of patients.
UGI, upper gastrointestinal.

artefacts of patient selection and therapy. Over 90% of the patients included in these studies had bled from peptic ulcers or gastritis, sites from which the bleeding usually stops promptly with nonspecific, supportive therapy. Hemorrhages from such lesions are associated with a very low mortality. In patients bleeding from varices, the hemorrhage is unlikely to stop spontaneously, surgery is frequently required, and the mortality is high. The negative findings in these studies appear to represent a classic statistical paradox in which the positive findings in a small subgroup are obscured by the large number of negative observations in the remainder, that is, the silence drowns out the noise.[172] Furthermore, the treatment given did not differ in the variceal and nonvariceal subgroups; all received antacids only.[700] This results in another fallacious conclusion. Emergency endoscopy is found to be of no value *because* the endoscopic findings were not used to determine appropriate treatment. One should not fault a diagnostic technique for the faults of the therapy. It is our recommendation that in patients who have or may have cirrhosis or alcoholic liver disease or other types of portal hypertension, emergency endoscopy should be performed promptly and treatment administered in accord with the endoscopic findings. Although no controlled trial in such patients has established the therapeutic validity of this approach, it provides the opportunity for rational therapy. Almost certainly, this opened-eye attitude will give better results than the blind approach, which omits early endoscopy and which, in turn, requires treatment to be based on clinical guesses.

Selective Arteriography. When the site of hemorrhage cannot be established endoscopically, selective arteriography may be helpful. It can demonstrate leakage of radiopaque material only from lesions bleeding in excess of 0.5 ml per mIU, or one to two units per day, at the time of injection. Celiac arteriography is more effective in demonstrating bleeding from arterial or capillary lesions than from varices. Celiac arteriograms have been reported to show the bleeding site in 80% to 90% of bleeding gastric or duodenal lesions.[189a] However, fewer than 10% of bleeding esophageal varices can be so demonstrated because of the greater dilution and the long route for the injected contrast material to traverse the splanchnic organs and the sluggish flow through the tortuous portal-systemic collaterals. It is, therefore, not frequently used in the differential diagnosis.

Like emergency endoscopy, selective arteriography during active bleeding has therapeutic potential when combined with vasopressin infusions. Several investigations have shown that intra-arterial vasopressin infused into the mesenteric artery or a branch of the celiac artery can stop bleeding from varices and from nonvariceal sites.[52a,145,190,639a] There is no reason not to start an infusion of vasopressin after arteriography has shown the bleeding site.

Other Diagnostic Procedures. The age of the *barium contrast esophagogram* during active bleeding is past. It is a more difficult and less reliable procedure than fiberoptic endoscopy and provides, at best, an inferential diagnosis.

Treatment

The goal in the treatment of hemorrhage from esophageal varices is control of bleeding and preservation of life until definitive corrective therapy can be undertaken (Table 20-5). In addition to nonspecific measures, such as blood

TABLE 20-5.   Control of Hemorrhage

A. Endoscopic sclerotherapy*
B. Esophageal tamponade
C. Vasoconstrictive therapy
   1. Vasopressin
      a. Intravenous infusion*
      b. Intra-arterial infusion
   2. Vasopressin and nitroglycerin*
   3. Somatostatin
D. Angiographic transhepatic obliteration of coronary
   veins
   1. Sclerotherapy
   2. Embolization
E. Surgical
   1. Emergency portal decompression*
   2. Circular stapling transection of esophagus*
   3. Other

* Most important methods

transfusion, a number of specific methods are available to control hemorrhage, including pharmacologic, mechanical, angiographic, endoscopic and surgical techniques. Each is associated with hazards that can be justified by the excessive mortality of hemorrhage from varices. An overall scheme for the management of bleeding esophagogastric varices is shown in Figure 20-25. Our recommendations, which are based on our estimates of the benefits and risks of each of these types of treatment, start with the most benign and proceed in order to those of greater invasiveness. There are a number of therapeutic options for the control of active variceal bleeding (see Fig. 20-25). Each is discussed individually in terms of its rationale, efficacy, and complications. The interrelationships and sequencing of the therapies in the control of the bleeding are considered in algorithmic fashion. Finally, we attempt to integrate the application of those methods used to control bleeding with those definitive therapies designed to prevent the recurrence of variceal hemorrhage. In the absence of the proven superiority of any one of these techniques or any sequence of therapies over any other, our recommendations are based on the current state of our knowledge and experience. They are, thereby, subject to change as new information becomes available.

Acute endoscopic sclerotherapy represents the best therapeutic bargain. This statement is based on our commitment to the performance of emergency endoscopic examinations to establish the source of the bleeding[190] and the proved efficacy of emergency endoscopic sclerotherapy in promptly stopping the vast majority of variceal hemorrhages at least transiently.[133,199,288,420,943,1047] Indeed, it seems irrational not to try to stop the bleeding while the endoscope is in place and the precise site of bleeding has been identified. If the sclerotherapy is effective and the bleeding does not recur, definitive therapy can then be carried out (see below, Fig. 20-26).

Fig. 20-25. Management of acute hemorrhage from esophageal varices. If endoscopic sclerotherapy, the initial form of therapy, successfully stops bleeding, the patient is ready for definitive therapy (*long cross-hatched arrow*). If bleeding persists or recurs, any of the other therapies is available (indicated from left to right in order of increasing invasiveness). If these "secondary" forms of therapy are successful, the next step is definitive therapy (*short cross-hatched arrows*). If they are unsuccessful, other secondary forms of therapy are available (indicated by the *fine arrows*). The selection of these various forms of treatment should be tailored to the individual patient and to the skills and enthusiasm of the hospital and its staff.

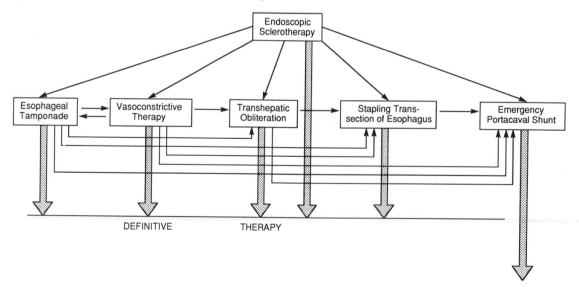

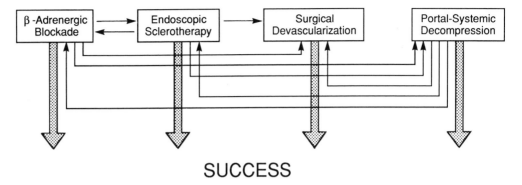

SUCCESS

Fig. 20-26. Definitive therapy of patients whose variceal hemorrhage has been controlled. Four forms of therapy are indicated from left to right roughly in order of ascending invasiveness. Successful prevention of recurrent hemorrhage is indicated (*cross-hatched arrows*). If any one form of therapy is unsuccessful, other therapeutic options are available (*fine arrows*).

If it does not stop the bleeding, little has been lost and one can try sclerotherapy again or any of the other options such as esophageal balloon tamponade, vasoconstrictive therapy, percutaneous obliteration of the coronary veins, esophageal transection, or emergency surgical portal decompression. We favor portacaval anastomosis by the process of exclusion. Both esophageal tamponade and vasoconstrictive therapy are complex, complicated, pragmatic forms of treatment that are only moderately effective in stopping bleeding. Furthermore, their effects are transient, bleeding usually recurs, and significant improvement in survival has not been established with either of these techniques. Thus, when used, one must expect that further therapy of acute bleeding will be required before definitive therapy can be instituted. Percutaneous transhepatic obliteration of coronary veins and the circular stapling transection of the esophagus are invasive techniques with a high morbidity that must be considered as only temporary therapy. They stop blood flow through varices by thrombosis, embolization, or ligation, but in each instance recanalization of the varices or the formation of new collaterals overcomes the obstruction and renews the risk of recurrent hemorrhage. The most rewarding form of therapy, therefore, appears to be emergency portacaval anastomosis. Although this procedure is associated with a very high operative mortality rate (about 50%), it effectively stops active bleeding and virtually eliminates the risk of recurrent bleeding.[57,656,657]

There are a number of therapeutic options for *definitive treatment after hemorrhage from varices has been controlled.* As emphasized in the presentation of the individual techniques, although each of these therapies has its proponents and has been shown to diminish the frequency and severity of recurrent hemorrhages, none has unequivocally been proven to prolong life. We favor the performance of surgical portal-systemic decompression using the end-to-side portacaval anastomosis in nonascitic patients and the side-to-side portacaval anastomosis in patients with long-standing ascites. We prefer portacaval

anastomosis to distal splenorenal shunt, since the former appears more effective than the latter in preventing recurrences of variceal hemorrhage; which is the *raison d'etre* of shunt operations. Furthermore, when compared in randomized trials, the complications of portal-systemic shunts—especially PSE—occur with about equal frequency with the two types of shunts. If the anatomy permits either type of shunt, we believe that the choice of the type of shunt should be the surgeon's, since it is always desirable to have surgeons enthusiastic about the operation they are performing. Mesocaval and mesorenal interposition grafts, which tend to undergo thrombosis and are associated with frequent rebleeding, should be avoided. We have no experience with the coronocaval shunt of Inokuchi, which allows portal blood flow to the liver to persist.[404] Despite the favorable Japanese experience with this operation, it is our opinion that this difficult surgical procedure, which requires the placement of a lengthy interposition graft, is not viable therapy in the West at the present time.

Beta-adrenergic blockade, which is by far the most acceptable form of therapy to patients, is as yet unproved. Lebrec and co-workers have reported it to be extremely effective in suppressing recurrent hemorrhage and in prolonging life,[501] but several other investigations have not confirmed these benefits.[111,982,982a] At the present time we believe that propranolol should be reserved for the performance of randomized clinical trials and for patients in whom the other procedures are contraindicated or not acceptable.

Endoscopic sclerotherapy is probably the most popular form of therapy at present. It is relatively simple to perform, and the equipment and the expertise to perform it are widely available. Although it has been shown repeatedly to reduce the frequency and severity of recurrent hemorrhages from varices, there is much controversy about whether it really reduces the mortality rate.[546,944] It should be kept in mind that endoscopic sclerotherapy is lifelong treatment that requires periodic endoscopic evaluations and the resumption of injections when varices recur.

Surgical devascularization procedures á la Sugiura have been restricted almost exclusively to Japan.[405] There is little experience and less enthusiasm for this procedure in the Western world.

Treatment of Active Bleeding from Varices

Endoscopic sclerotherapy which was introduced into medicine in 1939, became an effective method of treating actively bleeding varices during the 1960s and 1970s.[420,676] This technique, in which a sclerosing solution is injected into or around esophageal varices via a long, flexible needle that passes through an endoscope, is a difficult procedure for endoscopist and patient. It is not an easy task to identify a bleeding varix that waxes and wanes in size with respiration and that moves with peristalsis and with each beat of the adjacent heart. There is controversy about whether it is better to inject into the lumen of the varix or around the varix, but since many of the intravariceal injections are extravariceal and since both sites of injection appear to be effective in stopping bleeding, it is probably not an important issue. The procedures used also vary widely in the type of endoscopes, injectors, sclerosants, and adjuncts employed and in the site of injection, the amount of contrast, and the timing of the injections.[177]

In addition to many large consecutive series of patients,[51,288,420,676,944] several randomized, controlled trials have been reported.[50,133,199,398,675,892,1047] These studies indicate that this method can stop active bleeding in 72% to 93% of patients. It appears to be superior to balloon tamponade,[50,675] vasoconstrictive therapy with balloon tamponade,[892] and equal to emergency portacaval shunts[133] and to circular stapling transection[398] in the immediate cessation of bleeding. After bleeding has been controlled, the recurrence rate of hemorrhage was higher after sclerotherapy than after stapling transection ($P < 0.01$).[298] It therefore offers the opportunity to control the bleeding as soon as the site of bleeding is established and without undertaking any other procedure. Although effective, this procedure is not without hazards, which will be discussed below.

Esophageal Tamponade. During the past 37 years since Sengstaken and Blakemore described their ingenious tube (SBT) for the treatment of bleeding varices,[852] esophageal balloon tamponade has become a widely used form of therapy. Over the past 15 years, however, its popularity has decreased. Although the SBT controls bleeding in 50% to 90% of the patients in whom it is used, its effect is often transient, and recurrences of bleeding are common. Most disturbing is the high incidence of serious hazards attending its use. At our hospital, we observed fatal complications in about 20% of patients in whom it was used, despite awareness of the hazards and intensive attempts to avoid them.[164,184] The most common cause of death was vomiting with the inflated SBT in place, resulting in massive

pulmonary aspiration. This problem often occurred during the initial passage of the tube.[164]

In a more recent assessment we found a lower esophageal tamponade–associated mortality (8%) and a lower control of hemorrhage (40%), the latter probably reflecting patient selection.[146] Combining the results of all of the large reported series of esophageal tamponade in the past 15 years, one finds that among a total of 930 episodes of hemorrhage, bleeding was controlled in 78%.[146,164,184] Major complications occurred in 14%, and lethal complications in 3%. In the two randomized clinical trials in which balloon tamponade was compared with other forms of therapy, it was found to be less effective than endoscopic sclerotherapy[50,675] but as effective as intravenous vasopressin.[203] The hazards of balloon tamponade have been described in detail and are not discussed further here.

Pitcher has reported using a modified SBT with good therapeutic results and without serious complications.[712] Although he showed that this instrument can be safely employed with meticulous attention to detail, in our hands it remains a complex, complicated technique. More recently others have found SBT to be effective but associated with many serious complications despite meticulous care.[823]

Two groups have recently compared the SBT and the Linton–Nachlas balloon tube (LNT) in controlled clinical trials and found the SBT to be more effective and less hazardous (Fig. 20-27).[107,945] These investigators and others have found that the SBT is superior to the LNT for esophageal varices and imply the opposite for gastric varices.[108,945] Other modifications such as the Minnesota four-lumen tube,[604] the single esophagogastric balloon tube of Michel,[598] and the transparent tube of Idezuki[401] have been introduced. One large noncontemporaneous comparison of the LNT with the Michel tube showed the latter to be more effective and associated with fewer complications.[770] We still believe that this instrument is too dangerous for routine use in all patients with bleeding varices. It should be reserved for those patients proven unequivocally to be bleeding from esophageal varices, in whom bleeding continues despite active therapy including endoscopic sclerotherapy, and in whom surgical intervention is considered undesirable. It may also be used as a temporary measure during massive hemorrhage until definitive therapy can be undertaken. In such situations, one is justified in taking the high risks associated with its use. When the SBT is used, it should be placed and maintained in an intensive care unit by experienced personnel who are aware of its hazards and their prevention and treatment, ideally without traction, and it should be removed at the earliest time that definitive therapy can be undertaken. Detailed directions for its safe and sane use have been published and remain pertinent today.[164]

Vasoconstrictive Therapy. For the past 25 years vasopressin infusion, which is one of the most widely used and best studied forms of treatment, has been the first

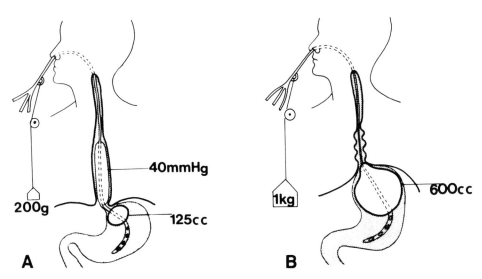

Fig. 20-27. Diagrams of (*A*) Sengstaken–Blakemore (SBT) and (*B*) Linton–Nachlas (LNT) balloon tubes. The SBT has an esophageal balloon; the LNT does not. The gastric balloon of the LNT is much larger and sturdier than that of the SBT. The traction weights depicted should not be used. (Burcharth F, Malmstrom J: Surg Gynecol Obstet 142:529, 1976)

line of therapy. Intravenous vasoconstrictor substances, which were introduced by Kehne and colleagues in 1956,[443] were thought to reduce portal pressure by constricting splanchnic arteries and thereby decreasing portal venous flow and pressure. This therapy was evaluated soon thereafter in a controlled trial in which single doses of posterior pituitary extract given intravenously were compared by Merigan and co-workers to a placebo injection.[593] They reported that although a single dose controlled hemorrhage transiently, it did not improve survival. Single bolus doses of posterior pituitary extract progressed to serial doses and were able to control bleeding in about 40% of cases.[180] Vasopressin replaced posterior pituitary extract and selective superior mesenteric arterial infusions replaced intravenous injections.[639a,787] This modified approach was effective in controlling bleeding[145,189a,190] but was not free of serious side-effects.[58,145,189a,190,566] In our own experience in 100 patients, in which we used infusions of 0.05 units to 0.5 units/min for periods up to 72 hours, control of hemorrhage, defined as no blood by gastric aspiration and stable vital signs and hematocrits for over 24 hours, was accomplished in 73% of patients, but survival was not significantly increased.[145,189a,190] Two small, controlled investigations have shown that intra-arterial and intravenous infusions of vasopressin are equally effective and induce complications with equal frequency[145,417] (Table 20-6).

Additional randomized controlled trials have now been published comparing vasopressin with placebo,[293] conventional therapy,[190,555] esophageal tamponade,[203] and triglycylvasopressin (tGVP)[297,415] (Table 20-6). In these studies control of bleeding varied from 10% to 90% with vasopressin and from 0 to 100% with the "other" treatment. In none of these studies did vasopressin reduce mortality significantly below that observed with the other form of therapy, whether it was placebo, somatostatin, or balloon tamponade. When reviewed objectively, vasopressin infusions appear to be able to control bleeding frequently, but only transiently, and not without the risk of serious complications. The serious systemic complications of vasopressin include cardiac arrest, heart failure, myocardial infarction, angina pectoris, arrhythmias, hypertension, and cerebrovascular accidents.[145,189a,190] Regional complications include necrosis of stomach or bowel, bacterial peritonitis, phlebitis, and peripheral necrosis.[19]

It seems clear that the role of vasopressin, if there is one, is as an early form of therapy in the hope of controlling hemorrhage in order to institute more definitive therapy. When used in this manner, it should be used in low dosage (0.2–0.6 units/min) for 2 to 6 hours to determine if it is effective. If not, it should be discontinued and other therapy instituted.

The failure of vasopressin to increase survival despite some success in stopping the bleeding has been attributed in part to the serious systemic side-effects of vasopressin. Several investigators have shown that isoproterenol,[875a] nitroprusside,[320a] and nitroglycerin[356] can reverse undesirable hemodynamic responses to vasopressin. Groszmann and co-workers recently showed that nitroglycerin can also potentiate the portal venous pressure–lowering effects of vasopressin and suggested that the simultaneous administration of vasopressin and nitroglycerin may en-

TABLE 20-6. Efficacy of Vasoconstrictor Substances in Hemorrhage from Esophageal Varices—Randomized Trials

FIRST AUTHOR	THERAPY		CONTROL OF HEMORRHAGE			SURVIVAL			COMPLICATIONS Vasopressin		
	Control	Vasoconstrictive	Control	Treatment	p	Control	Treatment	p	Mild	Severe	Fatal
Merigan	Placebo	IVVP	0/24 (0%)	16/29 (55%)	<0.01	3/15 (20%)	1/15 (7%)	NS	—	0	0
Johnson	IAVP	IVVP	7/14 (50%)	7/11 (64%)	NS	0/14 (71%)	6/11 (54%)	NS	2	0	0
Clanet	{ IAVP	IVVP	6/11 (55%)	14/15 (93%)	{ <0.05	2/11 (22%)	9/15 (60%)	{ NS	4	2	0
	LNT		14/18 (78%)		NS	6/18 (33%)		NS			
Chojkier	IAVP	IVVP	6/12 (50%)	5/10 (50%)	NS	3/12 (25%)	3/10 (30%)	NS	+	0	0
Fogel	Placebo	IVVP	7/19 (37%)	4/14 (29%)	NS	11/19 (58%)	7/14 (50%)	NS	7	1	1
Freeman	tGVP	IVVP	7/10 (70%)	1/11 (9%)	<0.02†	9/10 (90%)	7/11 (73%)	NS	0	0	0
Correia	SBT	IVVP	14/20 (70%)	11/16 (69%)	NS	13/17 (76%)	14/16 (88%)	NS	0	0	2
Kravetz	IVS	IVVP	16/30 (53%)	23/31 (74%)	NS	16/30 (53%)	17/31 (55%)	NS	14	8	0
Jenkins	IVS	IVVP	10/10 (100%)	4/12 (33%)	<0.01†	8/10 (80%)	8/12 (67%)	NS	0	2	0
Conn	Conventional	IAVP	4/16 (25%)	16/28 (60%)	<0.05	6/16 (38%)	8/17 (47%)	NS	7	0	2
Mallory	Conventional	IAVP	3/20 (15%)	8/18 (44%)	<0.05	11/20 (55%)	10/18 (56%)	NS	6	2	0

IVVP, intravenous vasopressin; IAVP, intra-arterial vasopressin; tGVP, triglycyl vasopressin; IVS, intravenous somatostatin; SBT, Sengstaken-Blakemore tamponade; LNT, Linton-Nachlas tamponade; NS, not statistically significant; , IVVP vs. LNT; +, present but not enumerated.
† Indicates that control therapy was significantly better than investigational therapy.

hance the efficacy and may decrease the toxicity of vasopressin.[356] Two randomized controlled trials have confirmed this hypothesis. Tsai and associates in Taiwan showed that sublingual nitroglycerin (0.6 mg every 30 min) plus intravenous vasopressin (0.7 units/min) was associated with more frequent control of bleeding (45% vs 21%) than vasopressin alone and decreased the frequency of both major and minor side-effects.[956a] Similarly, Gimson and co-workers in London showed that intravenous nitroglycerin (40–400 μg/min) plus vasopressin was more effective in stopping hemorrhage (68% vs 44%) than vasopressin alone (0.4 units/min) and virtually eliminated major complications.[329a] Unfortunately, the mortality was not reduced by nitroglycerin in either study. Our own investigation of nitroglycerin as an adjunct using transdermal disks was discontinued when we realized that the plasma levels of nitroglycerin achieved transdermally were below pharmacologic levels.

Two controlled trials have been performed with tGVP, a long-acting form of vasopressin.[297,415] This analogue of vasopressin has a triglycyl side-chain that reduces its vasoconstrictive activity and slows its degradation. As each glycyl residue is cleaved, the vasoconstrictive activity increases until the native vasopressin is released. In these studies tGVP appears to be equal or superior to vasopressin in controlling hemorrhage, but unfortunately, like vasopressin, it fails to enhance survival.

Somatostatin is a hormone that inhibits gastric and pancreatic secretions and reduces portal venous pressure,[85] although these effects are controversial.[897] On the basis of its pressure-reducing activity, somatostatin was tried as therapy in patients bleeding from varices. Two randomized clinical trials have compared vasopressin and somatostatin.[415,481] In both, somatostatin was more effective in stopping bleeding from varices than vasopressin, and in one of them this difference was statistically significant.[415] Furthermore, in both investigations, there were no complications in the patients treated with somatostatin, while the usual complications attributed to vasopressin were seen in those treated with vasopressin. Survival was slightly better in the somatostatin group. This agent is still not available commercially, but additional trials are in progress.

In our opinion, vasoconstrictive therapy with vasopressin has little to recommend it. It is only moderately effective in controlling hemorrhage, and this advantage is offset by the complications it causes. However, recent studies have shown that nitroglycerin appears to be a useful adjunct to vasopressin therapy that may enhance its therapeutic effects and diminish its side-effects. Similarly, intravenous infusions of somatostatin appear to be effective and safe in the treatment of bleeding varices. Both these treatments will require careful evaluation.

Percutaneous Transhepatic Obliteration of Coronary Veins. Percutaneous thrombosis of the coronary veins was introduced in 1974 by Lunderquist and Vang.[542] The procedure is performed by passing a fine, sheathed needle into a portal vein under fluoroscopy, replacing the needle with a guide wire, and advancing the catheter into the portal vein and then into the coronary collaterals. Ultrasonic guidance may be used to facilitate finding the porta hepatis.[108] In many ways this technique is the therapeutic equivalent of endoscopic sclerotherapy pathophysiologically: the goal of both methods is to occlude either the varices themselves or the coronary and/or short gastric veins, which bring blood to the varices (Fig. 20-28). Neither is definitive in that both are only transiently effective; when the coronary vein recanalizes, varices may recur and rebleed. Initially, thrombin was used to induce thrombosis until the introduction of isobutyl 2-cyanoacrylate, which is a synthetic liquid, plastic tissue adhesive that precipitates into a glasslike cast when it comes into contact with moisture.[542a] Gelfoam soaked in 3% sodium tetradecyl sulfate is used widely to embolize the varices,[978] as are autologous clots. Several investigators have used absolute alcohol as a more effective thrombotic–sclerosant but found that its lack of radiopacity allowed overinjection with regurgitation into and thrombosis of the portal vein.[959,1050] When the collaterals are very large, steel coils may be employed to obstruct the vessels and to prevent these coronary vein obliterants from becoming pulmonary emboli.[307] This procedure has also been attempted via the umbilical vein[938] and via the jugular vein, with the intrahepatic passage of the catheter from the hepatic to the portal vein,[334] a technique analogous to transjugular liver biopsy.[788]

Percutaneous obliteration of coronary veins has as many technical variations as endoscopic sclerotherapy,[177] but it is a more expensive, less available technique, and fewer investigators have been involved in introducing variations of this method.

Several large consecutive series of patients (>15 patients per series) with bleeding varices treated with transhepatic obliteration have been reported.[108,109,590,884,978,1051] In general, they show that in about 75% of the patients the hemorrhage can be controlled and that about 45% of the patients die. It has been found that bleeding could not be stopped in patients with retrograde portal venous flow.[590] In at least three fourths of the patients the coronary veins recanalize, and in about 25% of those whose bleeding had been stopped, bleeding recurs within 1 month. Recurrent hemorrhage develops in more than half within 12 months. Although the time of recurrence seems delayed by the procedure, the frequency of rebleeding does not.

Two randomized controlled trials that compared transhepatic obliteration with conventional therapy (esophageal tamponade and/or vasopressin[884] and with circular stapling transection of the esophagus[112] have been reported. In one it was found that conventional therapy was even more effective than the coronary vein obliteration in stopping bleeding; obliteration, however, delayed the time of recurrence, even though the frequency of bleeding was the same. In the other investigation transhepatic obliter-

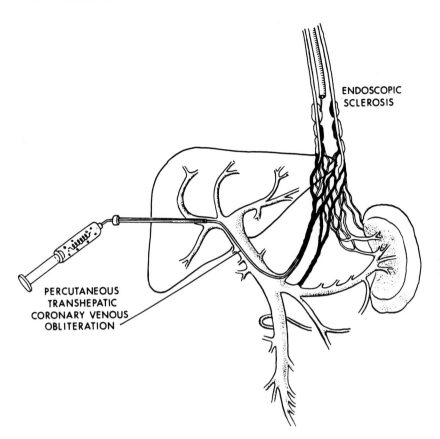

ENDOSCOPIC SCLEROSIS

PERCUTANEOUS TRANSHEPATIC CORONARY VENOUS OBLITERATION

Fig. 20-28. Diagram showing conceptual similarity of endoscopic sclerotherapy and percutaneous, transhepatic obliteration of varices. In sclerotherapy, varices are injected in the esophagus. With the portographic technique the coronary and short gastric veins are obliterated. Thrombosed vessels are shown in black. Theoretically gastric varices are not obliterated with the former technique, but with the latter technique blood flow to both gastric and esophageal varices is decreased.

ation and stapling transection of the esophagus were found to be about equally effective in controlling bleeding and in mortality.

Although transhepatic obliteration has the theoretic advantage over endoscopic sclerotherapy of blocking gastric as well as esophageal varices, it is less readily and less rapidly available and is more expensive and requires more sophisticated training and equipment. Complications are different in type, related primarily to the site of injection, but are no less frequent or severe than those seen with endoscopic sclerotherapy. With sclerotherapy the complications are mucosal erosions, esophageal perforations, and systemic effects of the sclerosant. With portographic obliteration, they are portal vein thrombosis or hepatic bleeding. Recanalization and rebleeding seem to occur earlier and more frequently with transhepatic obliteration than with sclerotherapy.

Circular Stapling Transection of the Esophagus. The introduction of the circular stapler gun converted surgical transection of the esophagus from a difficult, transthoracic procedure to a relatively simple laparotomy.[966] The circular stapler is a phallus-shaped cartridge that is invaginated into the esophagus from the stomach at laparotomy through an incision in the gastric wall. A circumesophageal ligature is tied firmly around the shaft of the stapler just below its corona, and the head of the stapler is retracted.

A circular blade transects the reduplicated esophageal wall, which is simultaneously reanastomosed by the ejaculation of a ring of staples (Fig. 20-29). A ring of esophageal wall about 0.5 cm in height is resected from just above the cardioesophageal junction.

The original instrument used for this purpose was a Russian stapler, but an American stapler that employs more than twice as many overlapping, automatically loaded staples is used much more widely now.[605] The procedure can be done as a basic, simple esophageal transection, which is performed several centimeters above the cardioesophageal junction and in which no attempt is made to preserve the vagus nerves, to devascularize the stomach, or to remove the spleen.[112] Transection can also be performed as a longer, more complex, procedure which is performed as close as possible to the cardioesophageal junction and in which preservation of the vagus nerves and devascularization of the lower esophagus and splenectomy are carried out.[419] Done in this manner the operation takes more than an hour longer and one transfusion more than the basic stapling transection does.

Several large consecutive series, each of which includes more than 15 patients, show that hemorrhage can be controlled in almost all patients, but that the operative mortality rate ranges from 33% to 73%.[419,903,995] The investigators who reported the higher mortality described many anastomotic leaks and resection of incomplete rings of

tensive operations. Although it is an effective procedure, it is not definitive therapy, since recanalization of the varices is common, and when recanalization occurs, recurrent hemorrhage cannot be far behind. Like many other "simple" procedures, this operation is most complex when performed on an occasional basis. Only a few hospitals have acquired much experience with it, and its use should be restricted to such institutions.

From the rings of the esophagus that have been examined histologically, it seems clear that esophagitis and esophageal reflux are rare precipitants of variceal hemorrhage.[719,904] These observations indicate that bleeding from varices is usually a consequence of portal hypertension rather than of mucosal erosion.

Emergency Portacaval Anastomosis. The concept of emergency portacaval anastomosis was developed in an attempt to salvage those patients who may have been reasonable operative risks shortly after hemorrhage had occurred, but who subsequently deteriorated as bleeding continued or recurred. The optimal time for performing portal decompression is 24 hours before the patient bleeds from varices. Such omniscient predictions are beyond the skills of present-day physicians. However, it is often true that during the first 24 hours after hemorrhage from esophageal varices has begun, cirrhotic patients are in the best physical condition they will ever again achieve. One may conclude that both temporally and functionally the ideal time for emergency shunts is as soon as the diagnosis of bleeding varices is established. Since 1967 Orloff and associates have proclaimed the efficacy of emergency portacaval anastomosis in a series of publications in which the number of patients has progressively increased.[57,649,650a,655,656] In this series of 180 patients, the operative mortality rate, which at the beginning was greater than 50%, has progressively decreased until the overall operative (30 days) mortality rate is 42% and the actuarial 12-year survival rate is 30%, a most impressive figure.[650a,656] For the past 5 years their operative mortality rate has been only 17%.[57] Obviously, these surgeons have either learned how to shunt better the patients they select or to select better the patients they shunt.[171] It should be emphasized that these 180 patients are "unselected" and include every patient admitted to their hospital who was proved to be bleeding from varices, "all comers" to use Orloff's phrase. Unfortunately, this procedure has never been reported in a randomized controlled trial, although these surgeons have stated that such a study was in progress. It is conceivable that such results reflect a referral bias.[175] A preliminary report of this randomized trial has recently been published and shows that emergency shunts prevent variceal hemorrhage and prolong survival.[657] Confirmation is needed.

Few other centers have performed emergency portacaval anastomosis, and no center has done so on all patients admitted with bleeding varices. Eleven reported series in which more than 25 patients had had emergency portacaval anastomosis[173,242,584a,599,656,1009] are shown in

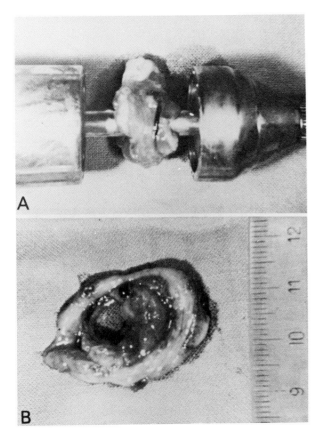

Fig. 20-29. Photographs of SPTU circular stapler gun. **A.** Just after stapling transection of the esophagus with the ring of transected esophagus within the apparatus. **B.** Transverse view of the ring of esophageal wall. (Vankemmel M: Nouv Pressé Med 5:1123, 1974).

esophageal wall that required repeated firing of the stapler gun. In general, stapling transection is equally effective as the other therapeutic techniques with which it was compared, but it is not superior to any of them. The mortality rates were very high because the patients studied were poor operative candidates, usually Child's class C.

Randomized clinical trials of stapling transection have compared it with percutaneous transhepatic obliteration of coronary veins,[112] emergency mesocaval anastomosis,[661] and endoscopic sclerotherapy.[132] Control of hemorrhage was achieved in virtually all patients with stapling transection, but bleeding recurred in one third of the patients, usually after a month or two. Although the mortality rates and cessation of bleeding rate were similar in stapling transection and sclerotherapy, the recurrence of bleeding was much lower after stapling (3%) than after sclerotherapy (49%).[398]

One may conclude that circular stapling transection is an effective procedure that should be reserved for actively bleeding patients who are poor candidates for more ex-

TABLE 20-7.   Emergency Portacaval Anastomosis: Results of Large Series

AUTHOR	NUMBER OF PATIENTS SHUNTED	NUMBER OF DEATHS (30 DAYS)	PERCENTAGE OF DEATHS
Mikkelsen	35	13	37
Preston	25	11	44
Weinberger	29	8	28
Adson	30	8	27
Conn	31	16	52
Megevand	30	9	30
Edmondson	50	24	48
Baird	31	9	29
Balasegaram	68	15	22
Langer	63	25	40
Orloff	180	76	42
Total	572	214	38%

Table 20-7. The operative mortality in this series of reports, all of which are uncontrolled, averages about the same as rates reported by Orloff and co-workers.

Two randomized controlled trials of emergency portacaval anastomosis have been performed. Malt and associates compared emergency portacaval anastomosis with emergency mesocaval anastomosis.[557] They found portacaval anastomosis to be superior in survival, prevention of recurrent hemorrhage, and postoperative patency of the shunts. Cello and his associates compared emergency portacaval anastomosis with emergency endoscopic sclerotherapy (plus chronic sclerotherapy).[133] Survival was similar in the two groups.

Others have recently reported that they were able to perform emergency DSRS, a much more difficult procedure than portacaval anastomosis, in 21 consecutive patients, with a respectable operative mortality rate of 29%.[727]

Emergency portacaval anastomosis remains an unproven form of therapy. Although it is a logical procedure in that it stops bleeding immediately in the overwhelming majority of patients with hemorrhage from varices (96%) and simultaneously reduces portal venous pressure, its efficacy has never been confirmed by controlled investigation. Despite an enormous operative mortality, the late mortality is surprisingly low, and long-term survival appears to be better than with other forms of therapy.[650a] The only controlled trial that compares emergency portacaval anastomosis with any other form of therapy, however, does not support the results of the uncontrolled reports.[133] *Caveat emptor.*

Definitive Therapy After Hemorrhage Has Been Controlled

The definitive forms of therapy available and their interrelationships are shown in Figure 20-26 and Table 20-8.

β-Adrenergic Blockade. The first investigation of β-adrenergic blockade in the treatment of portal hypertension by Lebrec and colleagues was a true breakthrough whether or not it ever becomes a major form of therapy.[499,501] These investigators administered propranolol because reduction in cardiac output should have reduced splanchnic arterial flow and, thereby, portal venous flow, and in cirrhotic patients, portal venous pressure. In their investigation they showed that propranolol significantly reduced the fre-

TABLE 20-8.   Definitive Therapy of Varices

A. Portal decompression
  1. Timing of surgery
    a. Therapeutic*
    b. Emergency*
  2. Type of surgery
    a. Portal venous–diverting
      (1) Portacaval anastomosis*
      (2) Mesocaval anastomosis
      (3) Other
    b. Portal venous–maintaining
      (1) Distal splenorenal anastomosis*
      (2) Coronocaval anastomosis
      (3) Other
B. Varices elimination
  1. Nonoperative
    a. Endoscopic sclerosis*
      (1) Intravariceal
      (2) Extravariceal
      (3) Intravariceal and extravariceal
    b. Percutaneous transhepatic obliteration
  2. Operative
    a. Transesophageal ligation
    b. Esophageal or gastric transection
    c. Esophageal and/or gastric resection
    d. Gastroesophageal devascularization
    e. Splenectomy-splenic devascularization
    f. Other

* Most important clinical procedures.

quency of hemorrhage compared with placebo-treated patients ($p < 0.0001$) as well as the mortality ($p < 0.02$), although the validity of the latter has been questioned.[178] In other studies they showed that virtually every cirrhotic patient studied showed a decrease in the hepatic venous pressure gradient after small doses of propranolol, a decrease that was sustained with prolonged therapy,[498] and that the reduction in the hepatic vein pressure gradient was proportionately greater than the reduction in cardiac output.[383] The clinical efficacy of propranolol has not been confirmed by two randomized trials,[111,982a] in which neither the frequency of variceal bleeding nor death was reduced. The explanation for these differences is not clear. The report of apparent confirmation of the Lebrec study reported in a letter to the editor was mysteriously withdrawn.[894]

It has been postulated that patients with mild alcoholic cirrhosis responded to β-blockade better than those with advanced or nonalcoholic cirrhosis. It has also been suggested that the tranquilizing effects of propranolol[90a] might be responsible,[178] but neither of these explanations seems likely in view of later observations.

One investigation compared propranolol therapy with sclerotherapy in a randomized trial.[228a] Prevention of recurrent hemorrhage and death were similar in the two groups.

The only other controlled trial of propranolol published thus far used propranolol as an adjunct to endoscopic sclerotherapy and showed no additional benefit.[1017a] In all likelihood the duration of therapy in that study was too short to be successful.

Propranolol is not completely benign. It sometimes reduces blood pressure to unacceptable levels. Since it blocks both β_1 and β_2 adrenergic receptors, it can prevent the adaptive response to stress.[111] Furthermore, its abrupt cessation can cause a rebound increase in portal venous pressure with the precipitation of variceal hemorrhage. It may precipitate asthmatic attacks by stimulating bronchial constriction. It can also cause hepatic encephalopathy.[937,1021]

Other β-blocking agents have been tried. Atenolol, a cardioselective agent, causes a smaller decrease in portal pressure than it does in cardiac output.[383] Metoprolol, another cardioselective β-blocker, does not appear to be effective in preventing rebleeding.[114,1017] Nadolol, a nonselective, nonlipophilic adrenergic blocker, which is less suppressive of the hepatic microsomal enzyme system than propranolol, may have theoretic advantages over propranolol.[679]

Although we are not convinced that propranolol is effective therapy, we accept that about one-third of patients with alcoholic cirrhosis who receive propranolol have a significant decrease in portal venous pressure[319] and believe that a sustained decrease in pressure should reduce the risks of recurrent hemorrhage. We do not, however, use it clinically, except in randomized investigations of its efficacy. We believe that in certain situations in which other accepted forms of therapy are contraindicated or

unavailable, propranolol may be tried as long as there are no contraindications to its use.

When propranolol is used, it should be administered in the smallest dosage that achieves the therapeutic goals. Ideally, the dosage should be determined by the degree of reduction of portal venous pressure induced by propranolol while the pressure is being measured.[319] We do so during hepatic vein catheterization and give 40 mg propranolol orally and measure the hepatic vein pressure gradient (HVPG) one hour later. If the HVPG has fallen to 12 mm Hg or below and the heart rate has not fallen below 55 per minute and the arterial blood pressure remains stable, we treat the patient with 40 mg propranolol twice per day. If not, we give a second 40-mg dose orally and remeasure the HVPG after one hour. If the HVPG is less than 12 mm Hg, 80 mg twice per day is prescribed. After removing the catheter, we maintain the patient on 80 mg twice daily for a few days, then reintroduce the catheter and complete the pressure titration using 40-mg increments of propranolol. We find, however, that patients who do not respond to the 80-mg dose of propranolol rarely exhibit a major decrease in HVPG with larger doses, although the heart rate is usually decreased by at least 25% of basal levels by 80 mg twice daily.[319] Most other investigators have used a 25% decrease in heart rate to determine propranolol dosage, although about half the patients who show such a drop in heart rate do not have a significant decrease in portal venous pressure. Patients should be warned of the dangers of sudden cessation of the drug and should be told to see their physicians promptly if they run out of the medication or cannot take it for any reason.

Chronic Endoscopic Sclerotherapy. Endoscopic sclerotherapy is a recently rediscovered technique for the eradication of esophageal varices. It was first introduced in 1939[205] but never achieved clinical importance until the development of fiberoptic endoscopes, which reopened the field. With this method a thrombosing–sclerosing solution is injected into or around esophageal varices in patients in whom active hemorrhage has been controlled. This procedure is repeated periodically at intervals of days or weeks until all the varices are eradicated. Once obliterated, the intervals between endoscopic examinations lengthen, but whenever new varices are detected they are injected. In this sense, chronic sclerotherapy is lifetime treatment.

Many techniques have been used. They vary in the type of endoscope used (flexible or rigid), which determines to some extent the type of anesthesia (topical or general), and the types of sclerosant (sodium morrhuate, tetradecyl sulfate, hypertonic glucose, ethanolamine, polydocanol, absolute alcohol, or isobutyl cyanoacrylate). The place and pattern of injection (lower 2–4 cm or lower half of esophagus, circular or spiral), the site of injection (intravariceal or paravariceal or both), the use of adjuncts to facilitate injection (balloons or sheaths) and the frequency of injection (every 3 or 4 days to every 2 weeks) vary from endoscopist to endoscopist.[177] The most important of these controversies deals with the intravariceal or extravariceal site of injection. Most endoscopists prefer the intravariceal approach, which blocks blood flow through the varices, and they go to great lengths to achieve it.[1017] Others believe that the extravariceal injections stimulate collagen deposition, which supports the varices without obstructing their pressure-lowering blood flow.[676,1035] Since many intravariceal injections are actually extravariceal[925] and intravariceal injections often leak into the paravariceal tissues, it is conceivable that extravariceal injections are responsible for the reduction in recurrent bleeding seen with both methods. In any event, either technique or purposeful combinations of the two are probably equally effective.[50,893]

Many endoscopists have reported large series of consecutive patients that provide documentation for the apparent efficacy of sclerotherapy.[420,523,674,876] These series indicate that chronic sclerotherapy reduces the frequency and severity of variceal hemorrhage and improves survival. They also identify a long list of complications, many of which are serious and some lethal.

The efficacy of endoscopic sclerotherapy can best be determined from randomized clinical trials, several of which have been published (Table 20-9). They tend to confirm the findings of the uncontrolled series in that the frequency of recurrent hemorrhage is reduced, but they do not provide confirmation for the enhancement of survival. The six controlled investigations published to date were performed in different ways. Most compared sclerotherapy with conventional therapy, but one compared it with emergency portacaval shunts.[133] Most include sclerotherapy of the initial bleeding episode as part of the course of therapy,[133,199,943,944,1047] but two do not.[474,1016] One study deals largely with patients with schistosomal liver disease,[1047] but most were performed in patients with alcoholic cirrhosis. Technical differences in endoscopes, sclerosants, and the type and timing of injections are typical. The critical factor of the time of initiating therapy varies from study to study.[882] The actual treatment schedules are probably not critical, as shown in one clinical trial.[1017] One study has attempted unsuccessfully to combine sclerotherapy with propranolol, to reduce portal pressure during the early stages before obliteration of the varices is accomplished.[1017a]

All show that variceal hemorrhage recurs less frequently after sclerotherapy than with conventional therapy except for the investigation that compares chronic sclerotherapy with emergency portacaval anastomosis.[133] It is well established that hemorrhage from varices is extremely uncommon after a successful portacaval anastomosis. It is interesting that in one of the other investigations in which survival was similar in the two groups, successful portacaval anastomosis appeared to be responsible for the relatively good survival rate in the conventional therapy group.[474] Exclusion from the calculations at the time of shunt surgery of those patients in the control group who bled from varices and had therapeutic portacaval anastomosis suggests that survival of the control group would have been worse if the shunts had not prevented recurrent bleeding.

In two studies cumulative survival was statistically improved by sclerotherapy.[1017a,1047] In two, cumulative survival was similar, although late survival (after 3 months) seemed better in the sclerotherapy-treated groups.[133,199] In the other four studies, survival was almost identical in the sclerotherapy and control groups (whether calculated by percentage of patients randomized or by cumulative survival.[331a,944] It seems clear that the trend is toward improved survival with sclerotherapy, but the efficacy of chronic sclerotherapy is still not established.

The complications, however, are common and diverse. An incomplete list of the complications reported to date is shown in Table 20-10. The most important ones are related to the endoscopic injections themselves. They include perforation of the esophagus with mediastinal infection or empyema.[814] Most common are the mucosal erosions and ulcerations, which are probably an inherent part of the procedure and, indeed, may be part of successful sclerotherapy.[99] They are often followed by esophageal strictures, which have occurred in more than half of some series.[899] Most worrisome are systemic complications, which include bacteremia[154a] and/or remote infection.[153] It has been suggested that the risk of bacteremia is related to the length of the injector needle.[885] Toxic effects of the sclerosants, which are complex substances, have affected the respiratory, cardiac, and central nervous system.[606] Finally when the esophageal varices are blocked, other varices may bleed; gastric, colonic, and rectal hemorrhages have been reported.[294]

Endoscopic sclerotherapy appears to be the treatment of choice for those patients whose variceal bleeding has been controlled and who are poor operative candidates. The decision as to sclerotherapy or other treatment should be made on an individual basis, taking into account the expertise of the physicians and the preferences of the patients.

Devascularization Procedures. A variety of nonshunting operations to prevent recurrent hemorrhage from varices have been devised. They include a number of procedures that involve esophageal or gastric transection, all of which share the disadvantage of being temporary procedures, since portal-systemic collaterals tend to reform after ligation. The combination of esophagogastric devascularization with splenectomy is a more rational procedure, since exclusion of splenic blood flow, which makes up one tenth to one third of portal venous blood flow, reduces the portal venous pressure and may thus play an important role in reducing the risk of recurrent hemorrhage. Hassab[370] and Sugiura[924] were the pioneers of this procedure. It has an operative mortality rate of 2% to 10%; it effectively reduces the prevalence of recurrent hemorrhage and has a 5-year survival rate of 93%.[218] One of its major advantages over shunt operations is that it is never followed by PSE.[1045]

TABLE 20-9. Controlled Clinical Trials of Chronic Endoscopic Sclerotherapy

AUTHOR	Control Therapy	CONTROL THERAPY				ENDOSCOPIC SCLEROTHERAPY				CUMULATIVE SURVIVAL
		Number of Patients	Number Who Died (%)	Number Who Re-bled (%)	Number with Complications	Number of Patients	Number Who Died (%)	Number Who Re-bled (%)	Number With Complications	
Terblanche	Conventional	38	24 (63%)	— (77%)*	9 (24%)	37	23 (62%)	— (58%)*	24 (65%)	NS
Yassin	Conventional	55	13 (42%)	16 (29%)	0 (0%)	53	5 (9%)	7 (13%)	4 (7%)	$p < 0.05$
Westaby	Conventional	60	32 (53%)	36 (60%)	—	56	18 (32%)	23 (41%)	24 (43%)	$p < 0.01$
Korula	Conventional	57	19 (33%)	14 (25%)†	—	63	21 (33%)	7 (11%)†	78‡ —	NS
Cello	Emergency PCA	24	20 (83%)§	5 (21%)	2 (8%)†‖	28	19 (68%)§	24 (86%)	0 (0%)†	NS
Copenhagen	Conventional	98	73 (75%)	51 (54%)	6 (6%)†	97	60 (65%)	45 (48%)	22 (23%)†	$p < 0.05$#

* Based on those who survived more than 1 month.
† Fatal complications.
‡ Total number of complications.
§ Includes deaths during acute bleeding.
‖ PCA failures.
Late survival only.
PCA, portacaval anastomosis; NS, not significant.

TABLE 20-10.   Complications of Endoscopic Sclerotherapy

I. Anesthetic
    A. Topical, hypnotic
        1. Allergy
        2. Encephalopathy
    B. General
        1. Allergy
        2. Hepatotoxicity
        3. Pulmonary
            a. Aspiration
            b. Pneumonia
        4. Miscellaneous
II. Endoscopic
    A. Rupture of esophagus
    B. Perforation of esophagus
        1. Mediastinitis
        2. Mediastinal granulomata
        3. Mediastinal abscess
        4. Empyema
        5. Bronchopleural fistula
        6. Esophagopleural fistula
        7. Esophagobronchial fistula*
        8. Pneumothorax
        9. Aortic rupture
      10. Chylothorax
      11. Pleural effusion
      12. Pseudodiverticulum
      13. Subcutaneous emphysema
    C. Laceration of esophageal mucosa
        1. Hemorrhage from varices
        2. Hemorrhage from esophageal wall
        3. Hemorrhage from other sites*
    D. Miscellaneous
III. Sclerosant
    A. Necrotic
        1. Erosion
            a. Hemorrhage
            b. Pain
            c. Dysphagia
        2. Ulceration
            a. Hemorrhage
            b. Hemorrhage from varix
            c. Hemorrhage from serosal vein
            d. Pain

III. Sclerosant (*continued*)
            e. Dysphagia
            f. Perforation of esophagus
        3. Gastric ulceration
        4. Pseudodiverticulum
    B. Thrombotic
        1. Periesophageal veins
        2. Portal vein
        3. Mesenteric veins
        4. Bowel infarction
    C. Pyelophlebitis
    D. Fibrotic stricture
    E. Functional dysphagia
    F. Systemic
        1. Allergy
        2. Fever
        3. Bacteremia
            a. Intrinsic
            b. Extrinsic
        4. Pulmonary edema
        5. Adult respiratory distress syndrome
        6. Cardiac-negative inotropism
        7. Disseminated intravascular coagulopathy
        8. Hemolysis
        9. Remote
            a. Brain abscess
            b. Hemiplegia, transient
            c. Paraplegia
            d. Spinal arterial thrombosis
      10. Redistribution of blood flow
            a. Hemorrhage from gastric varices
            b. Hemorrhage from colonic varices
            c. Hemorrhage from rectal varices
      11. Miscellaneous
IV. Endoscopist
    A. Allergy
    B. Infection
        1. Viral hepatitis
        2. Other
    C. Sclerosis
        1. Eye
        2. Other*

* Not yet reported

This operation is performed almost exclusively in Japan,[309,404,409,477,924,1045] although non-Japanese surgeons also perform it.[690] The recent investigation of *prophylactic* devascularization shows that it can be accomplished without operative mortality in good-risk patients and that it is extremely effective in preventing variceal hemorrhage.[405]

Portal Decompressive Surgery. Elective portal decompressive surgery is available to only a relatively small fraction of patients who have bled from esophagogastric varices. Approximately one fourth have such severe, un-

controlled hemorrhage that they either die quickly or require emergency operative therapy. Approximately one fourth are poor operative risks and are considered ineligible for elective shunt surgery. It is our recommendation that patients who have been shown to have bled from varices endoscopically, whose HVPG is greater than 12 mm Hg,[423] and who are relatively good candidates for major surgery have portal decompressive shunts.

Portacaval anastomosis, which was introduced in 1945, was the first definitive form of therapy used for the treatment of patients who had bled from varices (Fig. 20-30). It was quickly accepted and became the standard treat-

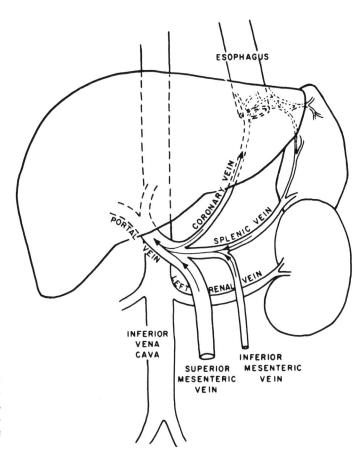

Fig. 20-30. Diagram of portal venous system and related vessels. The vascular pattern in cirrhotic patients with portal hypertension is depicted as a basis for diagrams of various types of splenorenal anastomoses shown in Figure 20-33. The arrows indicate the direction of blood flow.

ment by 1950. Its popularity began to wane in the 1970s, largely because of the frequency of PSE and the failure of randomized controlled trials to establish a statistically significant advantage in survival for shunted patients over those treated with conventional, supportive, nonoperative management. Each of the three American studies,[412,765,774] however, showed cumulative survival to be better for the shunted than for the nonshunted patients, and combination of the survival data from these studies shows a statistically significant advantage in survival for the shunted patients (Fig. 20-31).[171] The fourth study was different in design and execution. This French study,[802] which included patients who had bled from acute gastric erosions as well as those who had bled from varices, showed the opposite trend in survival and favored the unoperated control patients.

It is obvious, however, that the shunt operation in all studies virtually eliminated recurrent hemorrhage from varices. The failure of the shunt to enhance survival more impressively was attributed to complications of portacaval anastomosis—PSE and postshunt hepatic failure.[625]— plus, of course, the initial operative mortality in the shunted groups.

Mesocaval anastomoses are portal decompressive shunts in which an interposition graft is usually inserted

between the superior mesenteric vein and the inferior vena cava, creating in effect a side-to-side portacaval anastomosis (Fig. 20-32). This operation can be performed more easily and quickly than a portacaval anastomosis.[118,231] In this procedure, however, thrombosis of the graft and rebleeding occur commonly, and for this reason it is considered a less desirable procedure.[118,820] In one controlled clinical trial that compared DSRS with portal-systemic shunts, the DSRS appeared to be a better operation because the great majority of the portal-systemic shunts were mesocaval anastomoses or mesorenal shunts, many of which occluded and resulted in rebleeding from varices.[600] Other investigators, however, have objectively compared portacaval anastomosis with mesocaval anastomoses using an autologous jugular vein graft and found the two procedures to be equally effective.[921]

The DSRS was devised to preserve portal venous blood flow to the liver while decompressing esophagogastric varices via the spleen and splenic vein.[997] (Fig. 20-33) Six randomized clinical trials have been published in which conventional portal-systemic shunts were compared with DSRS in a total of 353 patients who had bled from varices.[194,277,366,489,600,758] The overall mortality and cumulative survival were similar in the six studies (Table 20-11). In five of the six, however, the operative mortality was higher

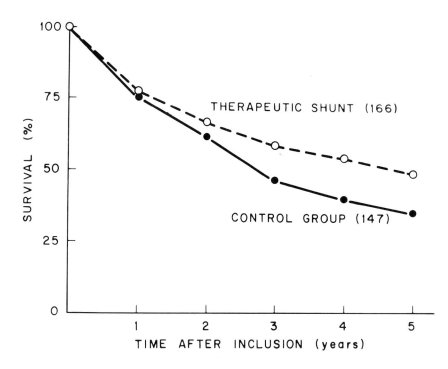

Fig. 20-31. Cumulative survival after therapeutic portacaval anastomosis. The data from the three American randomized controlled trials (Jackson,[412] Resnick,[765] Reynolds[774] and their co-workers) are consolidated. The difference in survival is statistically significant in favor of the shunted patients after four and five years of follow-up ($p < 0.05$). The numbers in parentheses indicate the combined totals of patients from the three trials.

Fig. 20-32. Diagram of mesocaval shunt with an interposition graft between the superior mesenteric vein and the inferior vena cava. The arrows indicate the direction of blood flow.

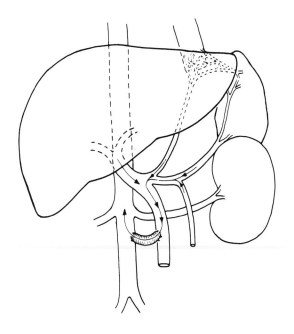

in the DSRS group than in the portal-systemic shunt group. The prevalence of postshunt PSE was appreciably lower in the DSRS group in three of the studies, and it was higher in the portal-systemic shunt group in two. Surprisingly, the frequency of recurrent hemorrhage from varices was higher in the DSRS group than in the portal-systemic shunt group in five of the six investigations. In the sixth, the controlled trial performed by the originators of the operation, rebleeding was more common in the portal-systemic shunt group because one third of the patients in that group developed thrombosis of the interposition grafts, and most of them bled from varices thereafter. It is surprising that these investigators selected the mesocaval shunt, which they had shown to be an inadequate operation[883] that is plagued by high incidence of shunt failure.[118,585]

We believe that the data from these six controlled studies indicate that the two operations are approximately equal in most ways. They both show similar mortality, which presumably is lower than in unshunted patients. Analysis of the three randomized trials in which the DSRS is compared with the predominantly end-to-side portacaval anastomosis in patients with alcoholic cirrhosis (Table 20-12) indicates that there is no real difference in mortality nor in the prevalence of PSE, but that the portacaval anastomosis is superior in the prevention of recurrent hemorrhage. It has been pointed out that alcoholic patients

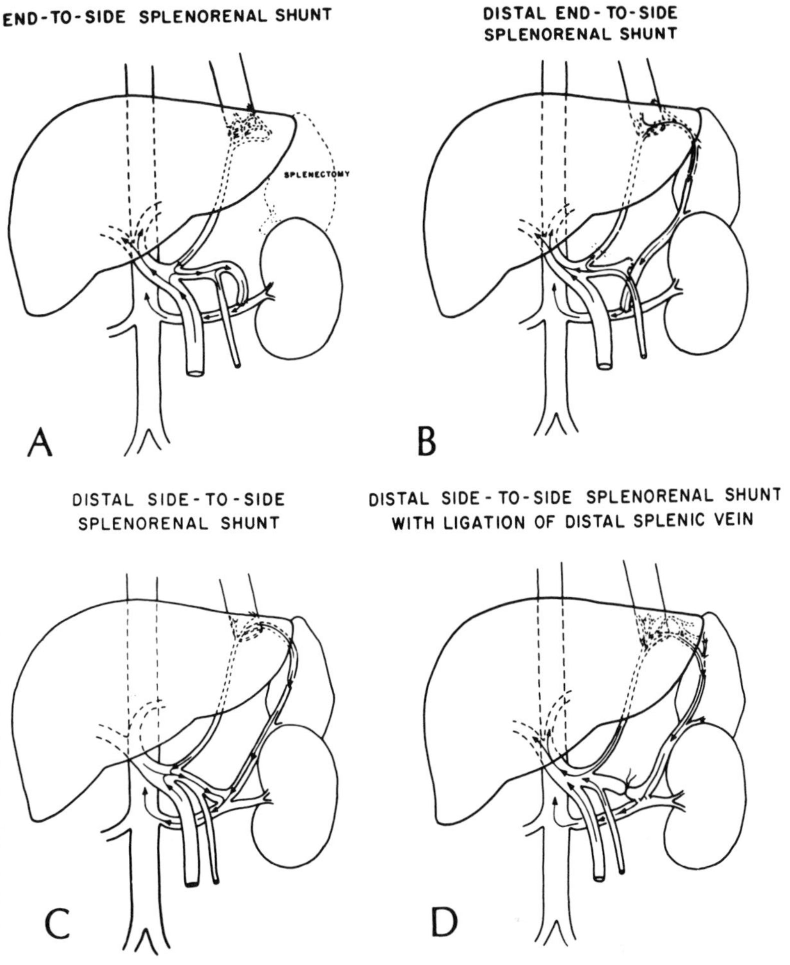

END-TO-SIDE SPLENORENAL SHUNT

DISTAL END-TO-SIDE
SPLENORENAL SHUNT

A

B

DISTAL SIDE-TO-SIDE
SPLENORENAL SHUNT

DISTAL SIDE-TO-SIDE SPLENORENAL SHUNT
WITH LIGATION OF DISTAL SPLENIC VEIN

C

D

Fig. 20-33. Diagrams of splenorenal anastomoses that preserve portal blood flow to the liver. **A.** Conventional splenorenal shunt involves splenectomy and an end-to-side anastomosis of the splenic vein with the renal vein. **B.** In the distal end-to-side splenorenal shunt (Warren–Zeppa) the spleen is preserved intact to serve as an outflow tract for blood from esophageal varices. The coronary vein is ligated to diminish blood flow to the varices. **C.** The central side-to-side splenorenal shunt (Britton) also uses the spleen to decompress esophageal varices, but this shunt also allows portal retrograde flow from the liver through the spleen. **D.** The central side-to-side splenorenal shunt with ligation of the splenic vein distal to the anastomosis (Britton, modified) functions the same as the distal end-to-side splenorenal shunt but may be technically simpler.

do poorly with the DSRS compared with nonalcoholic cirrhotic patients.[1054a] For this reason we believe that the portacaval anastomosis is the operation of choice in patients with alcoholic cirrhosis in whom the anatomy permits either procedure.

The coronocaval or left gastrocaval shunt is another shunt operation designed to maintain portal venous blood flow to the liver (Fig. 20-34).[404] In this operation an interposition graft connects the coronary vein with the inferior vena cava, thus reversing blood flow in the left gastric vein to its normal direction and decompressing the varices. Portal venous flow continues to perfuse the liver. This operation is very difficult technically and seems likely to have a high rate of graft thrombosis. Despite its theoretic value, this operation has not been widely accepted or used.

Prophylactic Therapy of Esophagogastric Varices

For many years physicians have treated varices only after they have ruptured. Many patients die during their first hemorrhages, and many others are poor candidates for the drastic forms of therapy then applied. It makes much more sense to treat patients prophylactically, that is, before they have the initial bleeding episode.

The time of starting therapy in relation to the onset of hemorrhage from varices has a great effect on the survival rate (Fig. 20-35). This concept was investigated almost 30 years ago using prophylactic portacaval anastomosis in stable cirrhotic patients with varices and portal hypertension. Unfortunately, three published randomized clinical trials showed that cumulative mortality was greater in the patients who received shunts than in unoperated control patients (Fig. 20-36).[188,411,763] When the data from these three studies are combined, the differences are statistically significant (Fig. 20-37). A fourth investigation, which was restricted to cirrhotic patients with portal hypertension, varices, and overt ascites, who have greater predilection to bleeding from varices, showed that survival in the shunted and control groups was similar.[183,188] Thus, the operative mortality and the late, lethal complications were too high compared with the relatively low risks of hem-

TABLE 20-11.   Comparison of Results of Six Randomized Studies of Distal Splenorenal Shunts

FIRST AUTHOR	% TOTAL MORTALITY		% VARICEAL HEMORRHAGE		% SHUNT OCCLUSION		% PSE	
	PSS	DSRS	PSS	DSRS	PSS	DSRS	PSS	DSRS
Millikan	72	58	31	22	29	14	76	26
Reichle	29	33	—	—	—	—	—	—
Langer	48	58	5	9	—	—	48	36
Conn	61	47	12	18	15	17	39	51
Harley	63	50	4	30	—	—	32	39
Fischer	19	24	7	11	12	23	16	8
Total	51	46	11	17	20	18	43	34

PSS, portal-systemic shunt; DSRS, distal splenorenal shunt; PSE, portal-systemic encephalopathy.

orrhage and death in unselected, cirrhotic patients, or even in ascitic, cirrhotic patients.

Other forms of prophylactic therapy have been reported and are in progress. In a randomized trial in patients with large varices and "black points," which are endoscopic markers of impending hemorrhage, prophylactic endoscopic sclerotherapy has been shown to reduce the risks of hemorrhage from varices and to improve survival.[674] Over a 3-year period almost 90% of the patients who satisfied the admission criteria bled from varices, indicating that these criteria correctly identified patients at increased risk of bleeding. It has also been shown that prophylactic endoscopic sclerotherapy prevented hemorrhage and improved survival in one investigation of *unselected* cirrhotic patients with varices.[1034] It is not clear why such a large percentage of these unselected patients, which included a sizable fraction of Child class A cirrhosis and patients with small varices, bled from varices. During the 2-year period of follow-up, 57% had bled, a percentage two to three times higher than that observed in the control groups of the four shunt studies (22% to 33%).[188,411,763] This unusually high rate of bleeding raises concern about their results. An additional half-dozen controlled studies are in progress, but the data are too few to comment further at this time.

Two controlled trials of beta blockade have been reported to date,[664a,682a] and several others are in progress. Both reported some reduction in the frequency of hemorrhage, and one found that propranolol improved survival.[117a]

Finally, a randomized, collaborative trial of prophylactic thoracicoabdominal devascularization has been reported by Inokuchi and colleagues in Japan.[405] One hundred twenty patients with varices and with endoscopic signs of imminent rupture, including the red wale sign,[60] were randomized. These complex operations, which include esophageal transection, gastric resection, and gastroesophageal resection with splenectomy, virtually eliminated hemorrhage from varices, while more than 35% of

TABLE 20-12.   Comparison of Results of Three Randomized Studies of Distal Splenorenal Shunt Versus Portacaval Anastomosis in Alcoholic Cirrhosis

FIRST AUTHOR	OPERATIVE MORTALITY		TOTAL MORTALITY		VARICEAL HEMORRHAGE		PSE*	
	PCA	DSRS	PCA	DSRS	PCA	DSRS	PCA	DSRS
Langer	0	5	19	17	2	3	19	12
Conn	5	4	18	16	4	7	13	20
Harley	2	3	15	10	1	7	8	9
Total	7	12	52	43	7	17	40	41
	7%	11%	49%	40%	7%	18%	41%	38%

* Percent of patients at risk, median follow-up 30–65 months.

PSE, portal-systemic encephalopathy; PCA, portacaval anastomosis; DSRS, distal splenorenal shunt.

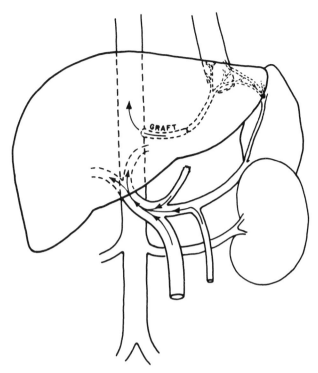

Fig. 20-34. Diagram of coronocaval (left gastrocaval) shunt. An interposition graft is placed between the divided coronary vein and the inferior vena cava. The varices are decompressed while antegrade portal venous flow to the liver persists.

the control group bled from varices during a 3-year period of follow-up. By this time 20% of the operated group had died compared with 45% of the control group, a statistically significant difference (Fig. 20-38).

Thoracicoabdominal devascularization, which is used almost exclusively in Japan, has not attracted serious attention elsewhere. We do not recommend its use at present outside of controlled clinical trials.

Prophylactic treatment of esophagogastric varices will certainly be the therapy of the future, but no specific type of treatment has yet been established.

Hepatic Coma

Difficulties in the management of hepatic coma reflect conceptual uncertainties about the pathogenesis of this syndrome. The literature abounds with discussion of whether or not ammonia is the cause of hepatic coma. The fallacy inherent in these controversies is the erroneous impression that hepatic coma is a discrete, etiologically homogeneous disease. Actually, hepatic coma is a readily recognized syndrome in patients with chronic liver disease, which consists of the concurrence of a number of individually nonspecific components, each of which may be induced by a variety of metabolic abnormalities.

When considered in this light one may rationally at-

tempt to determine which of these abnormalities is responsible for an individual episode of hepatic coma and to institute appropriate therapy. To treat rationally, however, requires a basic understanding of what is to be treated. Consequently, it is necessary to focus on the etiology and pathogenesis of these syndromes.

First, let us name and define this syndrome. The most widely used term is hepatic coma, although "coma" represents only one end of the spectrum. Some authors use "impending hepatic coma" or "precoma" to refer to the less advanced stages of this syndrome. "Hepatic encephalopathy" is a more formal version. Recently, as the pathogenesis has become better understood, the more meaningful, pathogenetically descriptive term portal-systemic encephalopathy has been employed. Sometimes the term ammonia intoxication is used. For those specific instances in which the disorder is caused by ammoniagenic substances, it is acceptable; when employed generically, it is presumptuous and often erroneous, since this syndrome may be mimicked by a variety of encephalopathic disorders of nonammoniacal origin. In dogs, the term "meat intoxication" is widely applied; it is not applicable to humans unless one is willing to give equal time to "cheese intoxication," "milk intoxication," or "fish intoxication."

Clinical Presentation

PSE is characterized by recurrent disturbances of consciousness, impaired intellectual function, neuromuscular abnormalities, metabolic slowing of the electroencephalogram (EEG), and elevated blood ammonia levels. The neuropsychiatric disturbances range from drowsiness to coma, from slowness of thinking to overt psychosis, and from asterixis to irreversible lesions of the central nervous system. The first clinical description of impending hepatic coma has been attributed to Hippocrates, who wrote: "Those who are mad on account of phlegm are quiet but those on account of bile are vociferous, vicious and do not keep quiet." That is a better description of the mental state of delirium tremens than of hepatic coma. Consequently, priority must be awarded to Shakespeare. In Twelfth Night, Sir Andrew Aguecheek, an alcoholic noble, says, "I'm a great eater of beef, but believe it does harm to my wit."[926] To our knowledge, this is the first clinical description of protein intoxication.

All the essential components of this characteristic syndrome are individually nonspecific. There is nothing specific about the delirium; it may occur in uremia, in carbon dioxide narcosis, or in barbiturate overdosage. One of the problems in managing patients with hepatic coma is the difficulty in quantitative assessment of the degree of encephalopathy. Assessment of mental state can be performed using simple, reproducible, semiquantitative grading systems.[187] Although coma and semicoma are easy to classify, subtle changes in mental state are more difficult to grade. A fast, simple, and reliable test, the Number Connection Test (NCT),[174] which permits serial, semi-

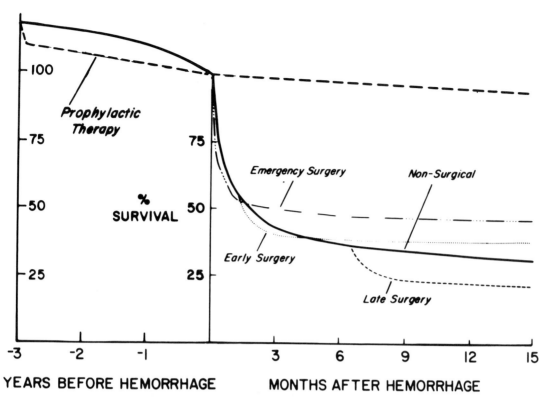

Fig. 20-35. Survival before and after hemorrhage from varices. On the right the heavy line shows cumulative survival with nonsurgical therapy starting at the time of hemorrhage (after Smith and Graham[882]). Note abscissa in months after hemorrhage. *Emergency surgery* performed during active bleeding has very high mortality but ultimately appears to improve long-term survival. *Early surgery* causes a small, transient decrease in survival and a small improvement in long-term survival. *Late surgery,* after the patient has reassumed a "normal" survival curve, induces an additional decrease in survival but no long-term survival benefits; it may induce a net decrease in cumulative survival. On the left the solid line shows the expected survival curve *before* variceal hemorrhage. Note abscissa in years before hemorrhage. *Prophylactic surgery* (*dashed line*) shows early operative mortality and a relatively large, long-term gain in survival.

quantitative assessment of minimal changes in intellectual capacity, has been described. The NCT, which is available to physicians from a pharmaceutical firm, has been objectively and successfully employed in a number of controlled clinical trials.[35,187,961] Several investigators using batteries of psychometric tests, including the NCT, have found that these tests detect significant intellectual impairment in cirrhotic patients, especially those with portacaval anastomosis, who appear normal to conventional evaluation and in whom EEGs are normal.[249,757,776,865] Asterixis represents a peripheral manifestation of impaired central nervous system metabolism, probably of the descending reticular system,[160] and is associated with a "coma" EEG abnormality.

Asterixis, the so-called flapping tremor or liver flap, is tested for by having the patient hold the hand in a dorsiflexed position (Fig. 20-39). When asterixis is present, the hand falls forward after a few seconds and then sharply resumes its dorsiflexed position. It can also be tested for by having the patient grip tightly two of the examiner's fingers and maintain the grip. Alternate relaxation and resumption of the clenched fist can be felt by the examiner. The intermittent interruptions of the sustained position correlate with brief lapses in electrical conductivity 75 msec to 200 msec in duration. Rarely the asterixis may be unilateral and may precede the signs of a contralateral cerebrovascular lesion.[259]

The EEG component of the PSE syndrome, the so-called metabolic EEG, is characterized by a progressive decrease in frequency and an increase in the amplitude of the brain waves as the encephalopathy develops and worsens. Some investigators believe that triphasic waves are specific for hepatic coma,[73] but it is clear that such complexes occur in a variety of situations including nonhepatic forms of encephalopathy.[182]

The temporal interrelationships of the state of con-

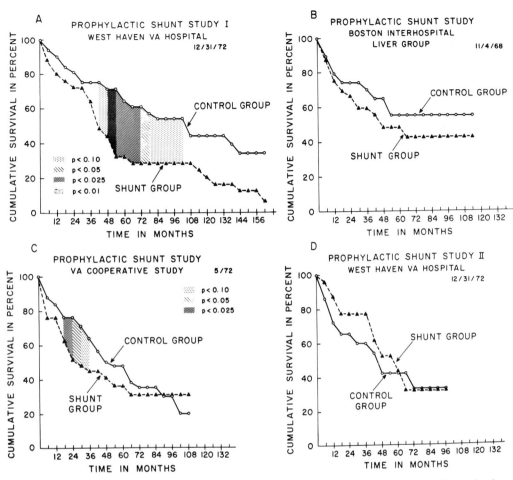

Fig. 20-36. Cumulative survival after prophylactic portacaval anastomosis—individual investigations. **A.** WHVAH Study I shows that survival was statistically worse in shunted patients than in the nonshunted control group from 48 to 78 months after inclusion. **B.** BILG Study found that survival tended to be better for the nonshunted group, although the differences were not significant statistically. **C.** VAC Study found survival to be significantly worse in the shunted group from 18 to 30 months after inclusion **D.** WHVAH Study II, which was performed in patients with overt ascites, showed a significant difference between the shunt and control groups, although the trend in survival favored the shunted patients. (Conn HO: In Schaffner F, Sherlock S, Leevy CM (eds): The Liver and Its Diseases. New York, Intercontinental Medical Book Corp, 1974)

sciousness, intellectual function, alterations in personality and behavior, and neuromuscular abnormalities in PSE are shown in Figure 20-40. The overlap in the time of appearance of the various components creates a broad spectrum of syndromettes.

Several indices have been devised to grade the PSE syndrome by semiquantitative assessment of its components, each weighted for its importance. These indices can be used to evaluate the effects of therapy or the severity of encephalopathy in the same patient at different times or to compare the severity of encephalopathy in different patients.[187] The *fetor hepaticus* is the only clinical sign specifically induced by a known precipitant of PSE, me-

thionine.[703] It is a common but inconstant component of the syndrome of hepatic coma. This sweetish odor, which has been described as fruity, fecal, or musty, can be detected on the breath and urine of many patients with PSE. It is not always present, however, and may be recognized in hepatic disorders unassociated with encephalopathy[113] and probably in nonhepatic disorders as well. Furthermore, all noses are not created equal, and the fetor hepaticus is not always differentiable from the odors of old wine, blood, acetone, uremia, or halitosis. For these reasons many physicians fail to find the fetor a useful physical sign. The biochemical basis of the fetor hepaticus has been attributed to mercaptans, primarily methanethiol (methyl

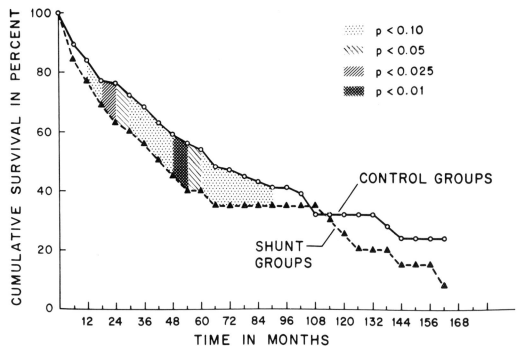

Fig. 20-37. Cumulative survival after prophylactic portacaval anastomosis—consolidated data. The survival data for the WHVAH-Study I, the BILG, and the VAC investigations were consolidated with permission of the investigators. Cumulative survival was statistically better, or nearly so, in the nonshunted control group than in the shunted group for the period from 1 to 7 years after inclusion. (Conn HO: In Schaffner F, Sherlock S, Leevy CM (eds): The Liver and Its Diseases, New York, Intercontinental Medical Book Corp, 1974)

mercaptan) and dimethyl sulfide.[136] It has long been known that orally administered methionine can induce encephalopathy[703] associated with an increase in blood ammonia levels, and that these changes can be prevented by the simultaneous administration of antibiotics.[1007] It has been shown that mercaptan derivatives are present in increased concentration on the breath of patients with decompensated cirrhosis and are further increased following gastrointestinal hemorrhage or the oral administration of methionine.[139] After methionine administration, the presence and intensity of the fetor hepaticus appears to correlate with the concentration of dimethylsulfide determined by gas chromatography.[228] The pathogenetic significance of these abnormalities of sulfur and nitrogen metabolism is not apparent and must await further developments. Zieve and his associates have reported that the individual toxic effects of methanethiol, short-chain fatty acids, and ammonia are synergistic and that individually subtoxic amounts of these agents in combination induce encephalopathy in experimental animals.[1061] These investigators have shown that these three substances vary in concentration from patient to patient with PSE, presumably reflecting a variety of precipitating substances.

PSE can present in ways other than the classic encephalopathic pattern. In its chronic form of *acquired hepatolenticular degeneration,* it may resemble the neurologic syndrome of Wilson's disease.[980] It sometimes presents with discrete neurologic abnormalities that may not suggest PSE, although they usually accompany the PSE syndrome. Among these lesions are cortical blindness, in which transient amblyopia appears in the presence of normal pupillary reflexes and in the absence of apparent ophthalmologic disease or opticokinetic nystagmus.[634] Conjugate deviation of gaze has also been reported as a clinical sign of PSE. Portal-systemic myelopathy may be seen occasionally as a late manifestation in patients with chronic recurrent PSE, most frequently in patients with portacaval anastomosis. It is characterized by spastic paraparesis with extensor plantar reflexes, hyperactive deep tendon reflexes, and demyelinization of the lateral corticospinal tracts.[204,496] Occasionally, it may present as peripheral neuritis, but usually this lesion is subclinical and requires specific testing to elicit.[610]

PSE may be precipitated by bacterial infections. It may occur in patients with urinary tract infections[817] in a manner analogous to that of ureterosigmoid implants, in which urea is degraded by urease-producing organisms. Although this syndrome is usually seen in cirrhotic patients,[870] it

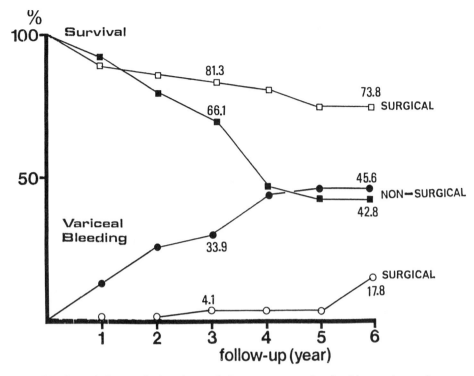

Fig. 20-38. Cumulative survival and cumulative percentage of variceal hemorrhage after prophylactic devascularization surgery (Japanese Society for Investigation of Portal Hypertension Collaborative Randomized Clinical Trial, June 1986). Survival is shown in the top two curves for the surgical and nonsurgical (control) groups. Survival is significantly better in the surgical group from 3 years onward ($p < 0.05$ to $p < 0.001$). Variceal hemorrhage is shown on the bottom two curves. The frequency of hemorrhage is significantly reduced in the surgical group from 2 years onward ($p < 0.01$ to $p < 0.001$). Actuarial percentages of cumulative survival and hemorrhage are shown after 6 years of follow-up. (Photograph provided by Professor K. Inokuchi)

may occur in the absence of liver disease.[439] The hyperammonemic encephalopathy that occurs so frequently in cirrhotic patients with spontaneous bacterial peritonitis may also reflect urea degradation in infected ascitic fluid, but the euammonemic encephalopathy in patients with spontaneous bacterial peritonitis probably represents a generalized catabolic reaction. It may also occur as a consequence of constipation.[515] PSE can also occur in the absence of cirrhosis in patients with large spontaneous portal-systemic shunts.[451]

PSE can be precipitated by some drugs, including *propranolol*[937,1021] and *valproate*.[1064] The mechanism is not known for either of these agents. Propranolol-induced PSE is thought to be related to the reduction in portal venous blood flow, while valproate is thought to represent a drug-induced type of Reye's hyperammonemic encephalopathy.

PSE is often latent and subclinical and in patients with normal mental state and EEGs may be detectable only by psychometric testing.[243,572,865] Indeed, employing a

battery of psychometric tests used to test the ability to drive cars, investigators found that most patients with portacaval shunts and many with cirrhosis were unfit to drive.[865]

Although it is extremely uncommon, PSE may occur in children, but it is usually seen in noncirrhotic children who have had portacaval anastomoses for portal vein thrombosis[988] or metabolic defects.[371] Presumably, young, noncirrhotic livers tolerate the consequences of portal-systemic shunting reasonably well.

The only biochemical test that is at all specific for PSE is an elevated blood ammonia concentration.[907a] This test, which is most accurately measured on arterial blood, is rarely elevated abnormally in the absence of PSE and is almost always increased in PSE. A normal arterial ammonia level requires that other, nonnitrogenous causes of encephalopathy, such as hypoglycemia or central nervous system depressants, be carefully excluded. Although the blood ammonia levels parallel the degree of encephalopathy, there is much overlap. Nevertheless, day-to-day

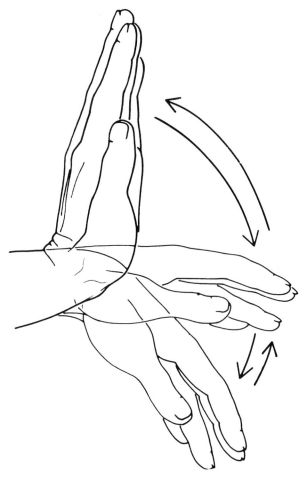

Fig. 20-39. Asterixis. The liver flap is demonstrated by having the patient hold the arm extended with the hand dorsiflexed. Within a few seconds the hand will involuntarily fall forward and then quickly resume the dorsiflexed posture. (Conn HO, Lieberthal MM: The Hepatic Coma Syndromes and Lactulose. Baltimore, Williams & Wilkins, 1979)

changes in arterial ammonia concentration in an individual patient permit assessment of the encephalopathy and its response to therapy.[187]

Elevations of cerebrospinal fluid glutamine concentration, which also reflect nitrogenous intoxication, are even more specific for PSE than hyperammonemia but are less readily available and impractical for serial measurements.[643,849]

Any disorder that interferes with metabolism of the brain—anoxia, hypoglycemia, or alkalosis—may induce encephalopathy. It is the very diversity of the causes of this syndrome that has created confusion about its pathogenesis. To start with a ridiculous example, assume a cirrhotic patient is brought into the emergency room in coma after trauma to the head, jaundiced but without any history; one must consider hepatic coma the prime diagnostic possibility. After subdural hematoma is discovered, hepatic coma is no longer a tenable diagnosis. Clinically, however, it may be difficult to differentiate such a traumatic encephalopathy from a metabolic disorder. Similarly, either hypoglycemia, which occurs occasionally in patients with liver disease, or a normal dose of meperidine hydrochloride (Demerol), which may produce delirium, asterixis, and a slow EEG in a cirrhotic patient, may induce a picture indistinguishable from classic, impending, hepatic coma. Failure to recognize the real cause of the encephalopathy in such cases may help to perpetuate the myth of the undiscovered, nonammoniacal cause of hepatic coma and to precipitate the death of the patient.

Epidemiology of PSE

The great majority of episodes of hepatic coma occur in cirrhotic patients, although other types of hepatic coma occur in noncirrhotic patients, including fulminant hepatic failure, deficiencies of urea cycle enzymes, and drug-induced hepatic injury. PSE occurs almost exclusively in the half of the cirrhotic population that has portal hypertension, and a disproportionately large percentage in patients with portal-systemic anastomoses. Approximately half of the cases of PSE occur in patients with surgical portal-systemic shunts, who comprise only about 5% of cirrhotic patients, and half in patients with spontaneous portal-systemic shunting.

The single most common cause of hepatic encephalopathy is azotemia, which accounts for about one third of cases (Fig. 20-41).[272] Brain-suppressing medications, such as tranquilizers, sedatives, and analgesics, cause one fourth. Gastrointestinal tract hemorrhage precipitates one fourth of the episodes of coma, and often the most severe ones by virtue of the large amount of toxic substrate in the intestinal tract. Smaller fractions are induced by dietary protein and hypokalemic alkalosis. Uncommon causes include constipation, infection, and severe hepatic parenchymal injury due to toxins, drugs, or viruses.

The fact that about half of all hepatic coma is iatrogenic has important implications for therapy.

Pathogenesis of PSE

The desire to find a single cause for all cases of hepatic coma has made PSE appear even more complex than it really is. In fact, ammonia intoxication, directly or indirectly, is responsible in part, at least, for a large majority of episodes of impending hepatic coma. The occurrence of PSE or its infantile equivalent in patients deficient in specific enzymes of urea synthesis[285,396,867] is strong evidence for the role of ammonia in PSE. Whether the encephalopathy is induced by ammonia per se, or its effects are mediated by other substances, is another question. Clearly, however, some episodes of "hepatic" coma are nonammoniacal in origin. A brief, oversimplified review of ammonia metabolism may help put some aspects of this syndrome in proper perspective.

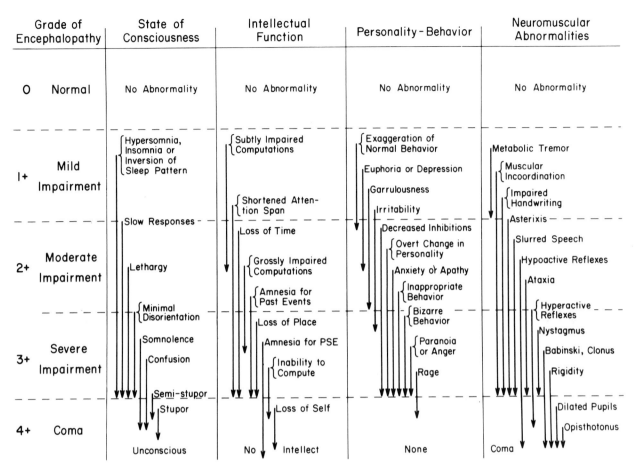

Grade of Encephalopathy	State of Consciousness	Intellectual Function	Personality-Behavior	Neuromuscular Abnormalities
0 Normal	No Abnormality	No Abnormality	No Abnormality	No Abnormality
1+ Mild Impairment	Hypersomnia, Insomnia or Inversion of Sleep Pattern / Slow Responses	Subtly Impaired Computations / Shortened Attention Span / Loss of Time	Exaggeration of Normal Behavior / Euphoria or Depression / Garrulousness / Irritability / Decreased Inhibitions	Metabolic Tremor / Muscular Incoordination / Impaired Handwriting / Asterixis
2+ Moderate Impairment	Lethargy / Minimal Disorientation	Grossly Impaired Computations / Amnesia for Past Events / Loss of Place	Overt Change in Personality / Anxiety or Apathy / Inappropriate Behavior / Bizarre Behavior	Slurred Speech / Hypoactive Reflexes / Ataxia / Hyperactive Reflexes
3+ Severe Impairment	Somnolence / Confusion / Semi-stupor	Amnesia for PSE / Inability to Compute	Paranoia or Anger / Rage	Nystagmus / Babinski, Clonus / Rigidity
4+ Coma	Stupor / Unconscious	Loss of Self / No Intellect	None	Dilated Pupils / Opisthotonus / Coma

Fig. 20-40. Temporal relationships of consciousness, intellectual function, personality-behavior, and neuromuscular disorders in PSE. As the degree of encephalopathy worsens, the manifestations of each component of mental state appear and become progressively more severe. The arrows indicate the stages of encephalopathy during which the individual abnormalities may occur. The interrelationships of these components vary widely in different individuals. (Conn HO, Lieberthal MM: The Hepatic Coma Syndromes and Lactulose. Baltimore, Williams & Wilkins, 1979)

Ammonia is the key intermediate in the metabolism of nitrogen. Nitrogen gains access to the body by the ingestion of protein or other nitrogenous substances and is excreted as urea, ammonium ion, and small amounts of other compounds in the urine and stool. Many organs participate in the maintenance of the ammonia concentration within relatively narrow limits[1004] (Fig. 20-42). The gastrointestinal tract is the major portal of entry of ammonia. The bowel, even in the fasting state, is a continuous source of ammonia, due primarily to bacterial enzymatic hydrolysis of urea and the deamidation of glutamine.[1004] Reports that nitrogenous substances induce hyperammonemia in germ-free animals, however, challenge traditional concepts.[632,633] Absorbed ammonia is carried by the tributaries of the portal vein to the liver, where ammonia, which is toxic in high concentrations, is converted

to glutamine, a nontoxic substance. At its leisure, the liver, which is the middleman in the removal of ammonia from the body, synthesizes urea for subsequent excretion. The ammonia concentration of the hepatic venous blood, which is slightly lower than that of peripheral blood, represents the sum of unextracted portal venous ammonia plus ammonia liberated by the liver in the degradation of nitrogenous substances. The liver, which has an enormous capacity for the extraction of ammonia, removes in a single passage about 80% of ammonia carried to it by the portal vein. The presence in cirrhosis of portal-systemic anastomoses permits large quantities of ammonia to bypass the liver and to elevate systemic blood ammonia concentration to toxic levels.

Studies using ^{13}N have demonstrated the regional distribution of ammonia in the body shortly after the intra-

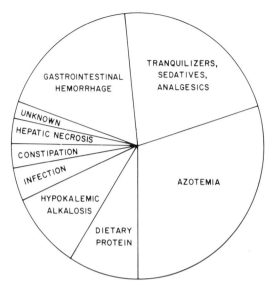

Fig. 20-41. The PSE pie. The distribution of the causes of 100 consecutive cases of PSE is shown.

Fig. 20-42. Diagram of blood ammonia concentration in various regions of the body in a normal subject. Arterial blood is shown in white; venous blood is stippled. The numbers represent ammonia concentration in μg per 100 ml by the Seligson–Hirahara method. Approximately 80% of the ammonia presented to the liver is removed in a single passage. The kidneys add ammonia to the blood. (Conn HO, Lieberthal MM: The Hepatic Coma Syndromes and Lactulose. Baltimore, Williams & Wilkins, 1979)

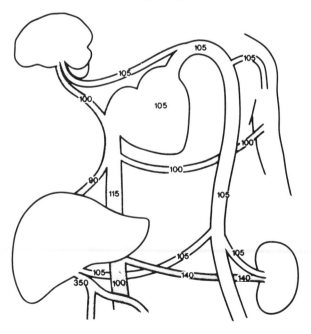

venous administration of ^{13}N-labeled ammonia.[538] Total body scans show that ammonia accumulates in the liver and brain and is rapidly concentrated in the urinary bladder (Fig. 20-43). These studies have also presented a dramatic scintigraphic visualization of hepatic encephalopathy. They show consistent abnormalities in the regional distribution of ^{13}NH$_3$ in the brains of patients developing PSE; the gray areas of the brain show little uptake (Fig. 20-44).

Although the kidney is the primary site of nitrogen excretion and the only organ that actually eliminates ammonium ion from the body, it is also an intrinsic source

Fig. 20-43. Distribution of ^{13}N-ammonia in a normal subject 20 minutes after intravenous injection of ^{13}NH$_3$. Body scan shows localization in liver, brain, and bladder. Cardiac and renal uptake are detectable. (Lockwood, AH et al: J Clin Invest 63:449, 1979)

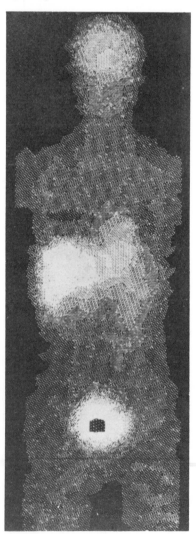

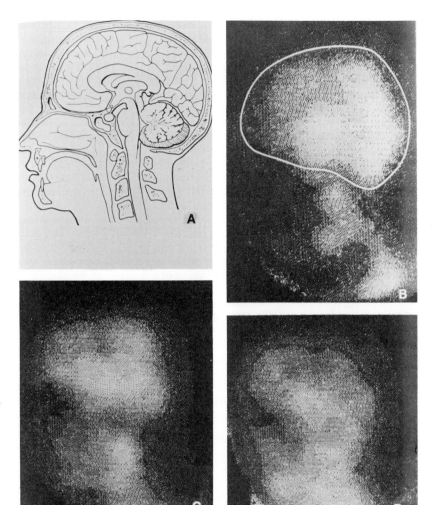

Fig. 20-44. ^{13}N-ammonia uptake by the head. A midsagittal drawing of the head is shown in (*A*) to facilitate comparisons with scintigraphs. Increasing dot densities indicate increasing levels of ^{13}N activity. A normal subject is shown in (*B*) with a line drawn to indicate the anatomic boundary of the brain. Salivary glands and muscle account for the increase in the activity near the angle of the jaw and shoulder, respectively. The effects of hepatic encephalopathy are seen in (*C*) and (*D*). In the time-interval between studies, encephalopathy progressed from grade 1 to 3. A decrease in the parietal ^{13}N-ammonia uptake is seen. (Lockwood AH et al: J Clin Invest 63: 449, 1979)

of ammonia. Renal venous ammonia concentrations are always higher than arterial levels and reach maximal levels in acidosis when increased NH_4^+ excretion takes place. Increased renal venous ammonia levels are associated with potassium depletion and with a variety of diuretic drugs.[311,402]

Under normal resting conditions there is a small uptake of ammonia by the peripheral tissues. During muscular activity, however, ammonia is liberated in large quantities.[12,539] In the face of rising blood ammonia levels, the extraction of ammonia by the muscles of the extremities may exceed 50% of the arterial level.[71]

Although the syndrome of hepatic coma can be induced by ammonium salts or ammoniagenic compounds such as ammonium-liberating cation-exchange resins, urea, or dietary protein, the failure of blood ammonia concentrations to correlate closely with the degree of coma has led many observers to conclude that ammonia is not responsible. There are, however, several reasons for the poor

correlation. First, most such observations have been based on venous ammonia levels, which do not reflect accurately the ammonia concentration of blood delivered to susceptible tissues, or to the intracellular ammonia concentration. *Arterial* ammonia levels correlate reasonably well with the severity of the encephalopathy despite overlap in groups of patients.[907a] Cerebrospinal fluid ammonia levels, which may reflect more accurately the intracellular ammonia concentration of the brain, correlate even more closely,[608] but are impractical for clinical use. Cerebrospinal fluid glutamine levels are elevated whenever blood ammonia levels are increased and show a more reliable correlation with the severity of encephalopathy.[643,849] Furthermore, ammonia levels increase in the veins draining exercising muscle. Even fist clenches used to distend antecubital veins may be enough to elevate appreciably the ammonia concentration in that arm.[12]

Second, since all patients do not respond with equal toxicity to the same blood ammonia concentration, serial measurements on the same patient are much more useful than absolute ammonia levels in different groups of patients.

Third, potassium depletion, which is extremely common in alcoholic cirrhosis as a consequence of vomiting, diarrhea, diuretics and the kaliuretic effects of secondary aldosteronism, causes major abnormalities in acid–base balance that alter the intracompartmental distribution of ammonia. Potassium lost from the extracellular fluid is replaced by potassium from the intracellular space in exchange for sodium and hydrogen. This phenomenon increases the pH of extracellular fluid and decreases the pH of intracellular fluid from the normal levels of about 7.4 and 7.0, respectively (Fig. 20-45).[907] The resultant increase in the pH gradient between the extracellular and intracellular compartments favors the volatilization of ammonia and its passage into the cells, where it exerts its toxic effects. Paradoxically, the shift of ammonia into the cells may decrease the ammonia concentration of blood, thus increasing the disparity between the degree of PSE and blood-ammonia levels. Simultaneous measurement of arterial ammonia and pH, or calculation of the partial pressure of NH_3 (pNH_3),[559] provides greater insight into this situation.

Fourth, the blood ammonia concentration, like blood glucose levels, rises after meals, the peak time and level depending on the type and amount of protein in the meal and the time of ingestion. Most reported blood ammonia levels have not been obtained from fasting patients, and correlation of clinical and laboratory findings is consequently impaired.

Finally, a temporal dissociation between blood ammonia levels and the symptomatology of ammonia intoxication may contribute to the clinical–laboratory disparity. Sustained changes in blood ammonia concentration sometimes precede appropriate clinical findings by 12 to 48 hours (Fig. 20-46).

When fasting arterial ammonia levels are used, the blood ammonia determination is an accurate, reproducible, useful test that correlates well with clinical signs of the presence or degree of PSE. Arterial ammonia levels are as useful in PSE as the blood urea nitrogen is in azotemia.

Although nonammoniacal substances such as short-chain fatty acids,[224,628,1061] amines,[278,279] phenols, as well as adenosine triphosphate (ATP) and nucleic acid deficiency have been implicated in hepatic coma, in the words of Walshe, "If the role of ammonia in the genesis of hepatic coma is not yet satisfactorily defined, there is no other theory that comes so near to conforming to the observed facts.[992]

One intriguing proposal for the pathogenesis of hepatic encephalopathy is the "multifactorial" hypothesis of Zieve and co-workers. They suggested that there is a round-robin synergism between ammonia, mercaptans, and short-chain fatty acids.[1061] They demonstrated in experimental animals that small amounts of any of these three substances greatly potentiated the coma-producing potential

Fig. 20-45. Effect of hypokalemia on the extracellular–intracellular pH gradient and ammonia equilibrium. Normally, the pH of extracellular fluid is 7.40 and of intracellular fluid, 7.00. The pH gradient is 0.4. The loss of K^+ from the extracellular fluid is replaced by the efflux of K^+ ions in exchange for Na^+ and H^+ ions. This exchange results in an increase in the pH of extracellular fluid and a decrease in the pH of intracellular fluid, thus increasing the pH gradient between extracellular and intracellular fluid to 0.65 and the ratio of NH_3/NH_4^+ in the extracellular fluid, which in turn favors the passage of NH_3 into the intracellular fluid. The predominant direction of flux is shown by the arrows.

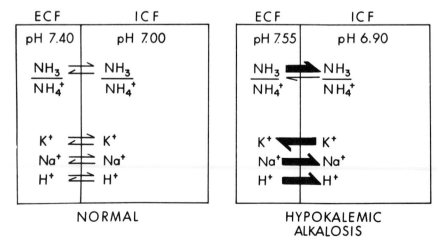

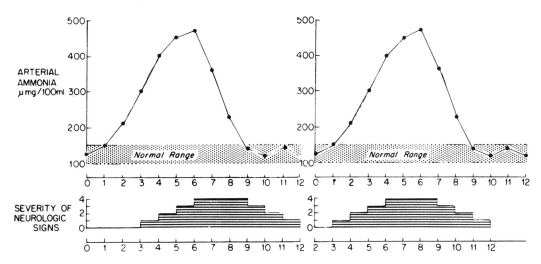

Fig. 20-46. Temporal dissociation between blood ammonia levels and clinical symptomatology of portal–systemic encephalopathy. In PSE, arterial ammonia levels may rise progressively. The clinical development of symptoms and signs of PSE may lag behind by 24 or more hours. Similarly, after therapy has been instituted, the blood ammonia level may reflect an effective antiammonia program, but clinical improvement may not appear for 24 or 48 hours, and occasionally even longer. If one compares the arterial ammonia concentration with the mental state on the same day, a poor correlation is noted (*left side*). If one takes this time-lag into account and corrects for this dissociation, a close correlation is achieved (*right side*).

of each of the others.[224,1057,1059,1061] Minute, subcomagenic doses of all these substances together can cause coma at subcoma plasma levels of each. Extrapolation to humans is, of course, hypothetic but suggests that in an individual patient any one of these three toxic substances may be the predominant toxin and that the pathogenetic pattern varies from patient to patient and from time to time in the same patient. In recent studies they indicated that these substances suppress hepatic regenerative activity as well as induce encephalopathy,[1062] and in fulminant hepatic failure they may both induce coma and interfere with regeneration, in effect interfering with recovery from coma.

Other explanations of the pathogenesis of PSE, which conform to the "observed facts," require serious consideration. Whether the induction of encephalopathy by methionine represents the consequences of ammonia liberation[1007] or abnormal mercaptan metabolism[139] or both[1061] is not clear.

The role of other amino acids such as tryptophan,[647] tyrosine[265] (perhaps by its extrahepatic conversion to octopamine and other toxic amines), or mixtures of amino acids by virtue of their contamination with[377] or generation of ammonia[357] must be considered.

Hyperaminoacidemia is thought to be the primary problem in the amino acid imbalance hypothesis of hepatic encephalopathy.[413] This theory is based on observations that plasma concentrations of aromatic amino acids (AAAs) such as phenylalanine, tyrosine and tryptophan are increased and those of branched-chain amino acids (BCAAs) such as leucine, isoleucine, and valine are decreased in PSE.[789] The hyperaromaticacidemia is thought to result from hyperglucagonemia-induced catabolism in the liver[621a] and the hypobranchedchainacidemia from insulin-induced metabolism in the periphery.[561] Infusion of somatostatin into cirrhotic patients reduces the plasma concentrations of both glucagon and insulin, thus reducing plasma levels of AAAs and increasing plasma concentrations of BCAAs.[535b] In the presence of excess ammonia the concentration of glutamine in the central nervous system increases. The AAAs and BCAAs share the same carrier system and therefore compete with each other for transport into the central nervous system in exchange for glutamine. The abundant AAAs, which are toxic, enter the brain in preference to the less available BCAAs, which are nontoxic, thus inducing encephalopathy. In experimental animals, the intracarotid infusion of phenylalanine and tryptophan precipitates hepatic encephalopathy, which can be prevented by the simultaneous administration of BCAAs. On this basis a number of investigations have administered BCAAs or BCAA-enriched, AAA-depleted amino acid mixtures to patients with hepatic encephalopathy.

Short-chain fatty acids, notably butyric, valeric, and octanoic acids, which may be produced by bacteria in the gut, have also been implicated.[628] Blood levels of these substances are increased in cirrhosis, achieve enormous levels in PSE, and return toward normal with therapy.[140,628] A similar syndrome can be induced in experimental animals by the administration of short-chain fatty acids.[1057,1061] These observations are compatible with the antibiotic-induced improvement in PSE. Similarly, Fischer and associates in their "false neurotransmitter hypothesis" have suggested that biogenic amines, either normal amines usually present in minute concentrations or abnormal amines, may induce PSE.[278] It is postulated that amines, such as octopamine, which are pharmacologically inert, may replace or dilute physiological, ert amines and thus suppress synaptic neurochemical transmission. Octopamine and β-phenylethanolamine have been found in increased concentration in the urine, serum and tissues of patients with PSE or in experimental animals.[122,487] Amines, which may arise from the bacterial degradation of protein in the intestinal tract and which therefore respond to antibiotic therapy, thus conform to the "observed facts" criterion. In addition, amines respond like ammonia to the increased extracellular–intracellular pH gradient.

γ-Aminobutyric acid (GABA), the principal inhibitory neurotransmitter of the mammalian brain, has been identified as a cause of hepatic encephalopathy. The cerebral concentration of GABA may be increased by the presence of excessive amounts of ammonia. When ammonia is abundant, it combines with α-ketoglutarate to form glutamate, which is then amidated to glutamine, an almost instantaneous reaction.[198] Some of the glutamate may be converted to GABA in the neuronal mitochondria, an irreversible reaction. GABA may reenter the tricarboxylic acid cycle through the GABA shunt, by mitochondrial metabolism.[182]

During the past 6 years Jones and associates have accumulated evidence to implicate GABA as a cause of the encephalopathy of galactosamine-induced hepatic injury in experimental animals.[424,830] They showed that GABA, which shares postsynaptic neuronal receptors with barbiturate and benzodiazepines, stimulates proliferation of receptor sites, accumulates on these receptors, and induces a specific visual-evoked potential pattern that is similar to that of barbituates and benzodiazepines but different from that induced by ammonia.[671,832] They have shown that GABA arises in the gut and can be produced by enteric bacteria.[831] In addition, they have demonstrated that serum GABA levels are increased in patients with hepatic encephalopathy, especially after gastrointestinal tract hemorrhage,[271] and in Reye's syndrome,[602] in which the mitochondrial injury may interfere with the degradation of GABA. Although the serum concentrations of GABA tend to parallel the degree of encephalopathy, the correlation is not close, but neither is it close for the blood ammonia concentration.* Finally, galactosamine-induced fulminant hepatic failure can be prevented by prior colectomy or the intravenous administration of large doses of lactulose[535] or galactose.[972]

Although these findings represent an impressive body of experimental evidence, they appear to reflect almost

exclusively an abnormality induced by a specific type of hepatic parenchymal injury, a syndrome that is much closer to viral or toxic fulminant hepatic failure than it is to the portal-systemic encephalopathy of cirrhosis, the prototype of hepatic encephalopathy. GABA has not yet been shown to play a role in human PSE. These experimental studies have shown that encephalopathy is ultimately caused by an increase in inhibitory neurotransmitter substances, a decrease in excitatory neurotransmitters, and/or alterations of the regulation of such substances.

A discussion of the therapy of hepatic coma can be simplified by classifying this disorder into two pathogenetic groups, those precipitated by nitrogenous substances and those unrelated to abnormalities of ammonia metabolism (Table 20-13). About two thirds of all instances of hepatic coma in cirrhotic patients are nitrogenous in origin, and these are almost always characterized by elevated arterial ammonia levels. Most are endogenous in origin; for example, bleeding into the gastrointestinal tract. Blood liberates much more ammonia and induces greater toxicity per gram of protein than does meat, milk,[70] or vegetable protein[350] in descending order of toxicity. Azotemia from any cause may give rise to the same syndrome as a consequence of the enterohepatic circulation of urea (i.e., degradation to NH_3 and CO_2 by bacterial ureases in the gut, synthesis of urea by the liver, diffusion of urea into the gut, ad infinitum). Bacterial infections caused by organisms that produce urease may break down urea in the urinary tract.[817] or in other infected fluid accumulations such as ascites in spontaneous bacterial peritonitis (SBP). "Prerenal hyperammonemia," which may occur as a consequence of prerenal azotemia in cirrhotic patients, may be effectively treated by the restoration of blood or plasma volume, the correction of profound hyponatremia, or by other appropriate measures.

---

* Recent observations have shown that the assay used in these measurements is nonspecific and that glutamine, which crossreacts in the GABA, was probably responsible for the elevated levels (Ferenci P: Personal communication).

TABLE 20-13.   Causes of Hepatic Coma Syndromes

NITROGENOUS	NON-NITROGENOUS
Endogenous	Pharmacologic agents
Blood in gastrointestinal	Sedatives
tract	Tranquilizers
Azotemia	Analgesics
Constipation	Metabolic
Exogenous	Hypoxemia
Dietary protein	Carbon dioxide
Ammonium salts	narcosis
Urea	Hypoglycemia
Cation-exchange resins	Myxedema
Amino acids	Anemia
Diuretic agents	Fulminant hepatic injury
Genetic (urea-cycle enzyme	Trauma
deficiency)	Potassium depletion
Bacterial infection	
Urease-producing bacteria	
Catabolic reaction	
Potassium depletion	
Reye's syndrome	

Exogenous sources of nitrogen, most commonly high-protein diets, may induce the same syndrome in cirrhotic patients. Ammonia intoxication associated with potassium depletion may, of course, be either endogenous, or exogenous, or may not require an increased nitrogen load. Diuretics such as hydrochlorothiazide, furosemide, and ethacrynic acid interfere with ammonia homeostasis by increasing the renal release of ammonia and/or by decreasing the arteriovenous uptake in muscle. In the clinical setting it is common for several of these factors to be operative simultaneously. Constipation may exaggerate these phenomena and in susceptible patients may itself induce PSE.[515]

Ammonia-induced hepatic coma is limited almost exclusively to patients with cirrhosis in whom extensive portal-to-systemic collateral communications exist. Portal-systemic shunting is more important in this disorder than hepatic parenchymal function *per se*. Patients with overt hepatitis rarely have elevated blood ammonia levels and usually metabolize added loads of ammonia normally. Patients with surgical portal-systemic anastomoses, on the other hand, usually exhibit susceptibility to ammonia intoxication despite good liver function. The role of hepatic function in ammonia intoxication, however, cannot be ignored. Patients with ureterosigmoid implants, who tolerate enormous endogenous loads of urea without difficulty, may develop profound ammonia intoxication when hepatic parenchymal injury occurs.[244,575]

Patients with schistosomiasis, who develop a presinusoidal type of portal hypertension without significant impairment of hepatic parenchymal function, may exhibit hyperammonemia and encephalopathy, but only after ingestion of large amounts of protein or after massive gastrointestinal tract hemorrhage. This situation suggests that good hepatic parenchymal function may compensate for portal-systemic shunting.

Among the few noncirrhotic situations in which nitrogenous encephalopathy occurs are the hereditary deficiencies of urea cycle enzymes, particularly ornithine transcarbamylase deficiency, which induce the equivalent hyperammonemic syndrome in homozygous infants or their heterozygous relatives.[182,285,396,867]

Another syndrome that may occur in noncirrhotic patients, hemodialysis encephalopathy, is seen when the ammonia liberated by urease degradation exceeds the capacity of the cation-exchange resin in the system to bind it.[121]

Treatment of Nitrogenous PSE

The principles involved in the treatment of acute ammonia-induced coma are rational, effective, and relatively simple (Table 20-13).[182] Most important is the prompt discontinuance of the offending substance. If, for example, the precipitant is dietary protein, the intake of protein should be sharply reduced. If blood in the intestinal tract is responsible, the bleeding must be controlled. If azotemia is the cause, vigorous treatment, particularly of prerenal

factors, is indicated. When appropriate, peritoneal or renal dialysis may be useful.

Second, the ammoniagenic material must be eliminated from the gastrointestinal tract. This may be accomplished by gastric emptying, by the administration of large doses of potent cathartics, and by the vigorous use of cleansing enemas. The physical removal of the contents of the colonic cesspool is by far the most important of these measures. Alkaline enemas, such as soapsuds enemas, create a *p*H gradient that favors the passage of ammonia or amines from the intestinal tract into the blood. Dilute acetic acid enemas, which introduce an acidified medium that traps ammonia and amines from the blood, are preferable. Lactulose enemas, which are acidic, trap ammonia and, after bacterial degradation, intensify the acidification, ammonia trapping, and catharsis.

Third, the activity of the bacterial flora of the intestinal tract may be suppressed by the oral administration of nonabsorbable antibiotic agents such as neomycin, paromomycin, sulfasuxidine, or sulfathalidine in doses cf 2 g to 6 g per day. Although it is traditional to use nonabsorbable antibiotic agents to treat PSE, any broad-spectrum antibiotic that is excreted in the bile in appreciable concentration, such as ampicillin, can be administered effectively by oral or parenteral routes.[595,930]

Fourth, general measures should not be overlooked. The intravenous administration of glucose around the clock minimizes protein breakdown. Vitamin B complexes may help to correct superimposed deficiencies. Correction of any abnormalities of electrolytes, particularly hypokalemia, may be essential to recovery. Oxygen should be administered in patients with arterial desaturation, a common finding in cirrhosis. When alkalosis is present—and respiratory or metabolic alkalosis or both are usually present in PSE—5% carbon dioxide and 95% oxygen (Carbogen) may be beneficial. All drugs that may directly or indirectly potentiate encephalopathy, particularly sedatives, tranquilizers, or analgesics, should be discontinued. Hepatic coma is often iatrogenic. We have found that 40% of the episodes of PSE at our hospital were associated with the administration of hypnotics, analgesics, or tranquilizers or with the use of diuretic drugs.

Finally, a number of specific measures have been used for the fixation of ammonia. Arginine has been used to prime the pump of urea synthesis.[771] Glutamic acid, which combines with ammonia to form glutamine, has also been employed.[578,992] Although theoretically effective, these applications of nature's own remedies add little to the measures outlined above. Recently introduced combinations of these and related substances such as arginine-glutamate[952] and ornithine-α-ketoglutarate[696] appear to be promising therapies that deserve objective evaluation. Cation-exchange resins have been used as oral medications and as extracorporeal columns, but the amounts of ammonia removable by such techniques are extremely small.

α-Keto analogues of amino acids, which are converted to amino acids by transamination reactions within the intestinal mucosa, incorporate ammonia. In urea-cycle enzyme deficiencies and in hyperammonemic encephalopathy, they may both reduce the ammonia content of the body and provide nutritional support.[382,990,990a]

In recurrent chronic PSE the same principles may be applied (Table 20-14). Long-term administration of neomycin, however, is undesirable. Neomycin may induce deafness,[63] intestinal malabsorption, predispose to staphylococcal enteritis, and result in neomycin blood levels high enough to cause renal tubular damage.[115] A number of imaginative alternative forms of therapy have been proposed. These include attempts to immunize patients against purified urease in order to decrease the ammonia derived from urea breakdown by intestinal bacteria. This technique has been reported to be successful in humans.[949] Other investigators have administered analogues of urea, which inhibit urease. Some of these analogues have been shown to be clinically effective.[386]

Some investigators have tried to replace putrefactive, ammoniagenic organisms with fermentative organisms by feeding *Lactobacillus acidophilus* milk, a technique that requires the prolonged administration of large quantities of the culture.[544]

The most dramatic development in the treatment of hepatic coma is lactulose.[74] This synthetic disaccharide, which is neither absorbed nor metabolized in the upper intestinal tract, is degraded by bacteria in the lower intestine, causing acidification of the lumen. The acid produced acts both as a stimulus to catharsis, as an inhibitor of coliform growth and ammonia production, and as a trap for ammonia. In fact, the acidified intestinal contents dialyze ammonia and other amphoteric, acidophilic substances from the blood into the bowel lumen (Fig. 20-47). It was originally thought that lactulose-induced acidification favored the replacement of urease-producing proteolytic bacteria with lactobacilli and other fermentative organisms, but quantitative stool cultures have failed to confirm this hypothesis. Actually, lactulose appears to stimulate the incorporation of ammonia into bacterial protein.[983,1002]

In double-blind, controlled clinical trials lactulose is as effective and as rapid in action as neomycin in the treatment of acute episodes of PSE.[35] It is effective in improving mental state, asterixis, and the EEG abnormality, in reducing the blood ammonia concentration, and in improving psychometric performance using tests such as the NCT.[174] As shown in Figure 20-48, lactulose improves the PSE Index, an integrated summation of the compo-

---

TABLE 20-14.   Treatment of Nitrogen-Induced Hepatic Coma

ACUTE NITROGENOUS ENCEPHALOPATHY	CHRONIC NITROGENOUS ENCEPHALOPATHY
Stop source of ammonia*	Decrease dietary protein intake
Remove substrate from gastrointestinal tract*	Substitute vegetable dietary protein
Catharsis	Suppress ammoniagenic intestinal flora*
Enemas	Neomycin or other antibiotics
Suppress intestinal bacterial flora*	*Lactobacillus acidophilus*
Replete potassium	Lactulose, oral*
Stimulate ammonia fixation	Inhibit bacterial urease
Glutamic acid	Immunization
Arginine	Urease inhibitors
Lactulose*	Lactulose (Lactitol, Lactose)
Oral	Lactulose plus antibiotics
Enematic	Exclude colon
Stimulate ammonia removal	Colectomy
Hemodialysis	Illeosigmoidostomy
Peritoneal dialysis	Ligate portacaval anastomosis
Extracorporeal perfusion	Stimulate ammonia fixation
Lactulose*	Hippuric acid synthesis (benzoic acid)
Oral	α-keto analogues of amino acids
Enematic	Bromocriptine (L-dopa)
Lactitol	Use of branched-chain amino acid mixtures
Lactose	General measures
Cation-exchange resins	Correct hypoxemia
Branched-chain amino acids	Correct anemia
α-keto analogues of amino acids	Correct electrolyte abnormalities
General measures	
Glucose	
Correct electrolyte abnormalities	
Oxygen	
Carbogen (95% O_2, 5% CO_2)	
Correct anemia	

* Most important measures.

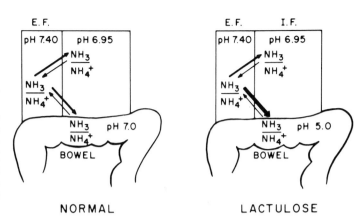

Fig. 20-47. Effect of lactulose in creating a pH gradient favoring the non-ionic diffusion of ammonia. Normally the pH of the intestinal contents is approximately 7.0, about the same as that of intracellular fluid. The pH gradient with the extracellular fluid is 0.4. When lactulose is administered, the pH of the intestinal contents drops to 5.0, which increases the pH gradient to 2.4. This massive increment in pH gradient favors the passage of ammonia into the acidified intestinal contents, which are excreted.

nents of the PSE syndrome.[187] In other clinical trials lactulose was shown to be at least as effective as neomycin in the management of chronic PSE.[187,648] Since lactulose induces few side-effects, it appears to be the treatment of choice for chronic PSE.

Lactulose has been used with impressive results as an enema in patients with acute PSE.[453,974] We, too, have found that lactulose enemas (500 ml plus 500 ml H_2O) are rapidly effective and especially useful as initial therapy of patients who are comatose and/or in whom oral administration is undesirable.[182]

Lactulose requires intestinal bacteria to be activated, but neomycin and other antibiotic agents inhibit bacterial growth. Despite this antagonism, the two agents have been used simultaneously with additive or synergistic effects.[403] Theoretically neomycin may prevent the degradation of

Fig. 20-48. Comparison of effect of lactulose and neomycin-sorbitol on PSE Index in acute PSE. The PSE Index is significantly and equally decreased by the two forms of therapy. The PSE Index, which is based on mental state, asterixis, EEG, NCT, and arterial ammonia concentration, indicates the degree of encephalopathic impairment.

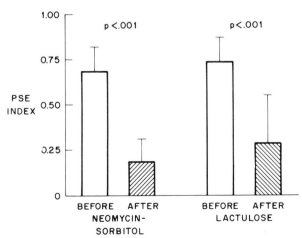

lactulose. Lactulose reduces urea synthesis and urea degradation, and the combination of lactulose and neomycin enhances this effect.[1002,1005] Lactulose can interfere with the effects of neomycin, since the antibiotic activity of aminoglycosides is progressively decreased as the pH falls.[1049] Both agents can be administered together without mutual inactivation, although the effects of each on the other may be diminished. Since the lack of a reduction of stool pH from its normal (pH 6-7) to that of lactulose-induced acidification (pH 5-6) shows that lactulose is not being degraded, one can determine functionally within 12 hours whether the two agents can be used together beneficially. We find that at least half of patients can degrade lactulose despite the simultaneous administration of neomycin.

The combination of lactulose and antibiotics should be used only when each of these agents alone has not given optimal results. The efficacy of the combination can be established only by comparing the therapeutic response in an impromptu crossover comparison of mental state, ammonia concentration, EEG, psychometric tests, and/or stool pH.

Uribe and his associates in a controlled clinical trial have shown that lactose is an effective therapeutic agent in lactase-deficient patients.[962] Although lactase deficiency is often asymptomatic or unrecognized in populations in which lactase deficiency is the rule rather than the exception (e.g., Mexico), a trial of lactose may be a reasonable approach to therapy.

Lactitol, β-galactosidosorbitol, is a disaccharide analogue of lactulose (β-galacosidofructose) that can be prepared in tablet form instead of syrup, like lactulose. It is metabolized in the same fashion as lactulose. In clinical use it is easier to store, less objectionable to the palate, and equally effective therapeutically.[76] It appears to be more consistent in its effect on bowel activity and to give more cathartic activity per gram than lactulose.[490]

Four randomized clinical trials of BCAA in the treatment of acute PSE have been published. One study by Rossi-Fanelli and co-workers compared BCAA (40 g–54 g/day) with *lactulose* (180 g–220 g) and found the BCAA to be superior.[792] In one third of the patients the PSE had been precipitated by hemorrhage and in one fourth by bacterial infections. Although the therapeutic response to BCAA was better than to lactulose, the treatment of the precipitating causes of the PSE was not presented. Unless gastrointestinal tract bleeding is controlled, no treatment can be successful, and no information is available about this aspect of the investigation. Similarly, antibiotic therapy of bacterial infections could inhibit the activation of lactulose, thus allowing BCAA therapy to appear superior.

A second study by Wahren and co-workers compared 40 g BCAA with placebo in acute PSE in patients with precipitating causes similar to those in the previous study.[989] In this investigation BCAA therapy had no beneficial effects, but the patients in the placebo group had received no nitrogen at all. The mortality rate was higher in the BCAA group than in the placebo group (40% vs 20%), and more died of PSE in the BCAA group. Exclusion of the patients who had received specific treatment for bleeding or hemorrhage did not change the results.

In a third investigation, Cerra and co-workers compared a BCAA-enriched mixture of amino acids (9 g–30 g/day) with neomycin plus glucose.[134] The precipitating causes of the PSE were not mentioned. Although both groups improved, more patients improved and improved more rapidly with BCAA than with neomycin; the latter group had received no protein. The mortality was significantly higher in the neomycin group than in the BCAA group (63% vs 35%; $P < 0.01$), but it is difficult to understand how BCAA therapy might have improved survival so promptly when the deaths were attributed to liver failure, sepsis, and hemorrhage.

In the fourth investigation Michel and co-workers compared a BCAA-enriched, AAA-depleted solution of amino acids with a conventional mixture of amino acids. Both groups received 36 g to 72 g of protein equivalent.[597] All patients received adequate carbohydrate and lipid. There was no difference in the two groups in the numbers of patients who improved, deteriorated, or died.

It is difficult to determine the efficacy of BCAA from these four investigations in which different amounts of BCAA were administered in different ways for different durations in comparison with four different forms of therapy. Two of the four studies showed BCAA to be beneficial, but two did not. In one additional investigation, BCAA plus lactulose was found to be better than BCAA or lactulose alone.[274]

BCAAs have also been used in the nutritional management of cirrhotic patients with chronic recurrent PSE. Several randomized trials have been reported.

One trial by Eriksson and co-workers studied a small number of patients in a randomized, double-blind crossover study.[261] The patients received either 30 g pure BCAA per day for 14 days orally or an equicaloric carbohydrate placebo. Similar percentages of patients improved, remained unchanged, or deteriorated under the two forms of therapy despite transient increments in plasma BCAA levels.

The second study, which was a double-blind trial by Horst and colleagues, compared progressive increments in dietary protein intake (up to 70 g per day) or a BCAA-enriched AAA-depleted mixture of essential amino acids (Hepatic Aid) in 37 stable cirrhotic patients who were prone to develop PSE.[395] In both groups nitrogen balance improved from negative to strongly positive. Dietary protein induced PSE in half the patients studied. The BCAA mixture caused PSE in only one patient ($p < 0.01$), but this patient died. It seems clear that the BCAA diet was less comagenic than conventional dietary protein.

In a similar study Christie and co-workers compared a different solution of BCAA-enriched amino acids (Travasorb-Hepatic), a casein diet.[148a] The BCAA content of the amino acid solution was 22 g/day compared with 9 g/day in the casein diet. In this double-blind trial no difference in the frequency of PSE was noted, although both groups that had been in negative nitrogen balance became strongly positive.

McGhee and co-workers studied the effects of 30 g casein per day or the nitrogenous equivalent of Hepatic Aid orally in a controlled, crossover study in four cirrhotic patients.[582] They found no difference between the two diets.

As in the studies of BCAA in acute PSE, there are no consistent benefits reported in the randomized clinical trials. The studies, however, use different amounts of BCAAs and compare them with different control diets. We believe that in patients who are intolerant to dietary protein, a trial on BCAA-enriched solutions of amino acids is indicated.

It has long been known that different sources of protein have different coma-producing potential. Meat protein is more comagenic than dairy protein, which is more so than vegetable protein. Vegetable protein, therefore, appears to be an ideal source of dietary nitrogen for cirrhotic patients who are frequently in negative nitrogen balance. There are several theories to explain why vegetable protein does not induce encephalopathy. The concentration of methionine, which can induce PSE and fetor hepaticus,[703] is low in vegetable protein. The content of AAAs is low in vegetable protein, and the content of BCAAs is high. Vegetable protein, therefore, is ideal food for the correction of the plasma amino acid patterns of PSE. Several crossover studies have been performed in cirrhotic patients with chronic PSE, and each has shown that vegetable protein diets induce less encephalopathy than equal amounts of meat protein.[350,963,964] Improvement was accompanied by reduction in asterixis and in blood ammonia concentration and improvement in EEG and psychometric tests. Doubling the amount of methionine by doubling the amount of vegetable protein did not make the diet more comagenic, nor did the addition of pure methionine to the vegetable protein diet. Furthermore, high-fiber vegetable diets reduced the glucose concentration and were especially useful in cirrhotic patients with diabetes,[964] a disorder that is unusually common in cirrhosis.[191] In one such study vegetable protein was better tolerated than meat protein, but there was no improvement in the BCAA/ AAA ratio.[456] Its mechanism of action remains a mystery. Vegetable protein has been shown to decrease the urea synthetic rate, urea excretion, and the blood urea nitrogen, and to increase fecal nitrogen excretion.[1006] Conceivably, vegetable fiber, which contains complex, unabsorbed, undigested carbohydrates, acts like lactulose, which is metabolized by bacteria in the lower bowel with the production of acid and catharsis.

Another therapeutic candidate is L-dopa. Fischer and Baldessarini have suggested that PSE may result from the accumulation in central nervous system neurons of abnormal, inert amines, instead of physiologic adrenergic amines, such as dopamine or norepinephrine.[278] Amines may, like ammonia, arise from the bacterial degradation of proteins in the gut, may, like ammonia, be adversely affected by an increased extra-intracellular *p*H gradient and may, like ammonia, be reduced by antibiotic or lactulose therapy or by the other "anti-ammonia" measures employed. L-Dopa has been used in hepatic coma with enthusiasm in uncontrolled series.[278,680] In controlled clinical trials of L-dopa in hepatic coma the results were unimpressive.[543,596] At present L-dopa is not considered viable therapy for PSE. Bromocriptine, a pharmacologic relative of L-dopa, may have met a similar fate. Although a preliminary anecdotal report of bromocriptine was enthusiastic,[611] the one clinical trial reported so far shows no beneficial results.[961]

Finally, surgical removal or short-circuiting of the colon (colectomy, ileosigmoidostomy) has been successfully employed. Unfortunately, the operative mortality is discouragingly high in patients with chronic recurrent PSE.[706,762] PSE in patients with surgical portal-systemic shunts may be improved by ligation of the anastomosis.[999]

Treatment of Non-Nitrogenous Encephalopathy

Hepatic coma induced by non-nitrogenous substances is characterized by essentially the same clinical picture as the nitrogenous type, except that blood ammonia levels are either normal or minimally elevated. Approximately one third of cases of hepatic encephalopathy are non-nitrogenous in origin. This syndrome may be induced by any substance or metabolic disorder that itself may depress consciousness. Among the most common substances are sedatives, depressants, and analgesics. Normal doses of barbiturates, for example, may produce overdose effects due to impaired drug catabolism by the liver. In one characteristic cirrhotic patient we found the explanation for episodic non-nitrogenous hepatic precoma in the nurses' notes. This patient was found on several consecutive mornings difficult to rouse, confused, and with asterixis. Review of the nurses' notes revealed that the "coma" was preceded each evening by conventional doses of medication for sleep. Discontinuation of these hypnotic drugs "cured" the hepatic coma.

Similarly, normal doses of preoperative medications

such as Demerol to cirrhotic patients before esophagoscopy or equivalent procedures will often induce surprisingly severe and prolonged hepatic encephalopathy with normal blood ammonia levels. We believe that patients with portacaval shunts are especially susceptible to such effects, and particularly to the postural abnormalities associated with phenothiazines and other tranquilizing drugs. These effects can be prevented by avoiding such drugs in patients with incipient hepatic coma or by administering one quarter or one half the usual dosage to cirrhotic patients who have previously experienced episodes of hepatic coma or who are suspected of being unduly sensitive. It is easier to add small doses than it is to remove overdoses. Similarly, small doses of analgesia after surgery in cirrhotic patients, especially after portacaval shunts, will avoid many episodes of postoperative "hepatic coma."

Primary treatment of such episodes consists of discontinuation of the offending drug. An antiammonia program may also be instituted, since the effects of ammonia intoxication and drug-induced coma appear to be additive or even synergistic in susceptible patients. Metabolic disorders such as hypoxemia, carbon dioxide narcosis, hypoglycemia, myxedema, or generalized infection seem to potentiate the toxic effects of ammonia or other precipitants of encephalopathy. Correction of the metabolic derangement in conjunction with the anti-ammonia program is usually effective.

In summary, the patient with hepatic coma should be carefully evaluated for the precipitating cause or causes. Eradication of the cause will usually reverse the encephalopathy. Therapy based on pathogenetic principles should be rationally designed for the individual patient. As our understanding of these disorders improves, so will our therapy.

Ascites

Ascites is the root of much hepatic evil. Hemorrhage from esophageal varices usually occurs in cirrhotic patients with ascites, and often when the abdomen is tightly distended. The classic hepatorenal syndrome, too, is a disorder that occurs almost exclusively in cirrhotic patients and rarely, if ever, in the absence of ascites.[927] Spontaneous bacterial peritonitis, for which ascites is the *sine qua non,* accounts for a small but appreciable fraction of mortality from cirrhosis.[181] In addition, ascites is indirectly responsible for much iatrogenic morbidity, such as azotemia, hypokalemia, and hepatic encephalopathy, precipitated by overzealous diuretic therapy. Ascites, however, is not invariably associated with dire consequences but may exist as a benign, concurrent, coincidental finding.

The mechanism by which ascites induces these problems is less clear. Ascites increases portal venous pressure as a simple function of increased intra-abdominal pressure.[120] Ascites may obstruct the inferior vena cava at the diaphragm[742,800] and may thus put additional burdens on the cardiac and renal circulatory systems. Ascites affects the lymphatic system, increasing manyfold the size of the thoracic duct[235] and the volume of lymph flow,[80] changes that are closely associated with ascites formation and that may compromise its bacteria-filtering function. In addition, ascites may cause anorexia by compressing the upper gastrointestinal tract, may predispose to atelectasis and pneumonia by elevation of the diaphragm and may produce hernias of all types—hiatal, umbilical, and inguinal—and sometimes incarceration of these hernias. Ascites may also, by virtue of its accompanying edema of the splanchnic tissues, alter the barrier against intestinal bacteria.[181]

Ascites influences physicians and their decisions in both direct and intangible ways. The diagnosis of the cause of ascites is often neither obvious nor simple. Ascites poses an almost irresistible challenge to the physician to deliver it. The methods for its delivery, however, are frequently antagonistic to other therapeutic aims. Furthermore, the presence of ascites may render more difficult the diagnosis of unrelated intra-abdominal disease and may contraindicate or complicate its surgical treatment. The attitude that if ascites is not bothering the patient, it should not be bothered, is a misleading concept and, sometimes, a dangerous one. The prognosis for cirrhotic patients with ascites is far worse than for those without.

Clinical Presentation

Although ascites seems to the patient to appear abruptly, usually as an increase in abdominal girth, it actually develops gradually and attracts attention only when it is voluminous. It is rarely painful unless the abdomen is tightly distended or unless bacterial peritonitis occurs. Indeed, the peritoneal surfaces often appear to be anesthetized after ascites has been present for some time.[105] Occasionally, bulging of inguinal or umbilical hernias is the first sign of ascites. Rupture of an umbilical hernia, the so-called Flood syndrome, is a late complication of ascites.[291] Sometimes ascites appears for the first time after abdominal surgery.[535a] Pleural effusions that are derived from the transdiaphragmatic transport of ascitic fluid appear early and sometimes are more apparent and symptomatic than the ascites itself.[801]

Diagnosis

For centuries the diagnosis of ascites has been based on physical examination. At present five signs are used: bulging flanks, flank dullness, shifting dullness, a fluid wave, and the puddle sign. Each of these signs is ideal when the ascites is obvious, but each leaves much to be desired when used to determine whether or not ascitic fluid is present.[131] At present ultrasonography is the simplest and most accurate way of establishing its absence or presence, although CT is also accurate but more expensive. Some-

times, the actual presence of ascitic fluid must be determined by paracentesis with the patient in an abdomen-dependent position.

Pathogenesis

Ascites represents the local consequence of an imbalance of those factors that favor the exudation of fluid from the vascular compartment over those that maintain vascular volume. Starling suggested that the transudation of fluid between capillaries and tissue spaces was determined by the equilibrium of hydrostatic and osmotic forces in the two compartments.[911] Normally, the higher hydrostatic pressure at the arterial end of a capillary favors the passage of protein-free fluid into the pericapillary space. At the venous end of the capillary, where the hydrostatic pressure is lower than the osmotic pressure and lower than the extravascular tissue pressure, reabsorption takes place. In the most simplistic sense, the advanced cirrhotic patient with portal hypertension has increased intravascular hydrostatic pressure (portal hypertension) and decreased vascular osmotic pressure (hypoalbuminemia) a combination of abnormalities that favors the loss of fluid into the extravascular space (the peritoneal cavity).

Others have expressed this relationship as the ratio of the colloidal osmotic pressure between plasma and ascitic fluid (π_A/π_P) and the transmural portal venous pressure, which is also known as the HVPG, and have shown that a mirror-image relationship exists between them (Fig. 20-49).[381a] Since albumin determines to a large extent the osmotic pressure of both plasma and ascitic fluid, as the HVPG increases the concentration of albumin in ascitic fluid decreases. This simplification of the osmotic–hydrostatic pressure relationship, however, is much less reliable than the osmotic–vascular pressure gradient. In addition, in cirrhosis the transcapillary escape rate of albumin from the splanchnic bed is increased.[381]

Practically, the problem is far more complex. Although the basic elements of Starling's equilibrium—portal hypertension and hypoalbuminemia—are valid, many additional factors participate. Many cirrhotic patients with portal hypertension do not have ascites. In fact, both clinically and experimentally portal vein thrombosis, which is associated with portal venous hypertension, does not usually cause ascites.[144] Many cirrhotic patients with hypoalbuminemia have no ascites. Peripheral edema is a far more common consequence of hypoalbuminemia than is ascites. Sometimes portal hypertension and hypoalbuminemia occur together without ascites.

Hepatic venous obstruction, however, is almost always associated with ascites. If the hepatic outflow obstruction is complete or nearly so, as occurs in advanced cirrhosis, hepatic vein thrombosis, or tumor compression (Budd–Chiari syndrome), the onset of ascites is swift and often intractable. Ascites, which may form rapidly before any changes in serum albumin concentration occur, does not develop, however, if the caval ligation is below the hepatic veins.[987] A similar syndrome, although less overt, may

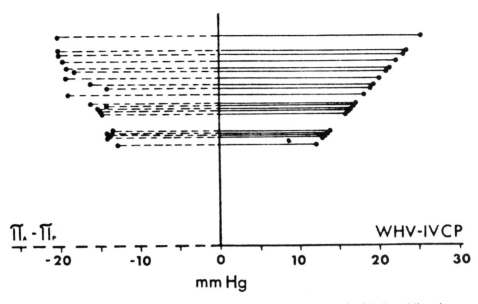

Fig. 20-49. The effective colloid osmotic pressure recorded on the left with dotted lines is seen to be a "mirror image" of the transmural portal pressure, that is, wedged hepatic venous pressure minus free hepatic venous pressure, the so-called hepatic venous pressure gradient. The effective colloid osmotic pressure is defined as the osmotic pressure in the ascitic fluid (π_A) minus the osmotic pressure in the plasma (π_P). (Reproduced from Hendrikson, JH: Scand J Gastroenterol 20:170, 1985)

occur in patients with severe cardiac disease such as constrictive pericarditis or advanced right-sided congestive heart failure.

The difference between "portal" and "hepatic" venous hypertension is critical to understanding the concepts that control ascites formation. When portal hypertension is caused, for example, by schistosomal ova that lodge in the small portal venules (presinusoidal obstruction or "inflow block"), the increase of pressure occurs upstream to the obstruction and is transmitted back to the splanchnic vessels and to the spleen. Although splanchnic venous hypertension may give rise to ascites,[1031] it does so only occasionally, as in end-stage schistosomiasis with "pipe stem" fibrosis, and the ascites, which tends to have a low albumin concentration, is rarely intractable.

On the other hand, if compressive obstruction of small hepatic venules is caused by regenerative nodular hypertrophy, the pressure elevation can be transmitted in retrograde fashion only to the intrahepatic sinusoidal bed (hepatic outflow obstruction or postsinusoidal obstruction). One of the major causes of increased pressure in alcoholic cirrhosis is obliteration of the intersinusoidal communications, which diminishes dissipation of pressure throughout the sinusoidal bed. The resultant increase in sinusoidal pressure is also aggravated by the hepatic arterial inflow, which flows directly into the obstructed hepatic sinusoidal bed (Fig. 20-50).

The increased sinusoidal pressure results in exudation of fluid from sinusoids into the perisinusoidal spaces. The hepatic lymph system carries as much of this excess fluid as possible, but the excessive exudation of fluid in complete hepatic venous occlusion results in extrusion of fluid from lymphatics on the surface of the liver into the peritoneal cavity.[399] The similarity of the fluid in appearance and composition to hepatic lymph[349] has led to the conclusion that the fluid exuded is largely hepatic lymph. Furthermore, transposition of the liver to the chest after inferior vena caval compression in experimental animals results in pleural effusions rather than in ascites,[6] thus establishing the liver itself as the source of the ascites.

The hepatic hilar lymphatics and lymph glands in patients with ascites are distended and edematous.[37] The thoracic duct is greatly distended and the lymph flow many times greater than normal.[80,235] It has been suggested that, in a sense, the inability of the lymphatic system to divert even more fluid from the liver may be "responsible" for the ascites, for when the thoracic duct is cannulated externally and large amounts of lymph drained, the portal hypertension and ascites are promptly ameliorated.[236] None of the forms of thoracic duct drainage, however, has provided a practical form of therapy. Paracentesis may actually accomplish the same thing.[673] Peritoneovenous shunts may be considered to be artificial thoracic ducts.

Although some of the primary concepts of ascites formation seem relatively clear-cut, there are other aspects that are much more complex and controversial. The most important of these is the role of the kidneys in ascites formation. In both ascitic patients and animals with ex-

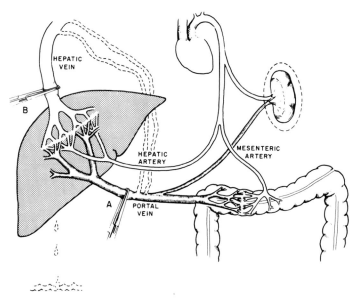

Fig. 20-50. Diagram of clinical consequences of presinusoidal and postsinusoidal obstruction. **A.** Presinusoidal block of the portal vein causes increased venous pressure in the portal vein and splanchnic venous beds. Inflow block results in the formation of portal–systemic collateral veins (*dotted varices*) and splenomegaly (*dotted spleen*). **B.** Postsinusoidal obstruction results in intrahepatic sinusoidal hypertension, which in effect causes inflow portal venous block as well. Outflow block causes ascites (*dotted drops*) plus the varices and splenomegaly of presinusoidal obstruction. (Conn HO: In Popper H, Schaffer F [eds]: Progress in Liver Diseases, 4th ed, pp 269–288. New York, Grune & Stratton, 1972)

perimental ascites, sodium excretion in the urine is virtually zero.

Aldosterone has been thought to be responsible for the intense sodium restriction. Indeed, increased aldosterone secretion, which is often greater in secondary aldosteronism than in primary, results in grossly elevated plasma aldosterone levels.[255,603,790] Studies showing dissociation between aldosterone levels and sodium retention have cast some doubt on the primacy of aldosterone in sodium retention. Some patients undergo diuresis while serum aldosterone levels remain high.[147,522,790] Reduction in serum aldosterone levels by inhibitors of aldosterone synthesis does not necessarily cause diuresis. In exciting studies Epstein showed that the effect of aldosterone was less potent than the effect of increasing the central blood volume induced by immersing the patient in water up to the neck.[255] When spironolactone alone is given to cirrhotic patients, there is minimal sodium excretion (Fig. 20-51). When patients on spironolactone are immersed, there is a prompt and impressive natriuresis. With immersion alone, despite a sharp decrease in aldosterone levels, some cirrhotic patients have a natriuretic response and some do not.[255,256] These observations suggest that aldosterone's role in sodium retention may be permissive rather than primary.

The traditional hypothesis supposes that as a consequence of a disruption of the Starling equilibrium, ascites forms and the resultant decrease in blood volume stimulates aldosterone secretion. Reexpansion of blood volume retriggers ascites formation, and reduced blood volume escalates aldosterone secretion, creating an endless cycle. Virtually all measurements, however, have shown the blood volume in ascitic cirrhotic patients to be increased,[531] leading to the hypothesis that the *effective* plasma volume is decreased. Effective plasma volume, which defies precise measurement, may be defined as that portion of the total plasma volume that effectively stimulates volume receptors. Lieberman and associates challenged the traditional view with provocative evidence that is inconsistent with the conventional concept.[533] They proposed, instead that sodium retention occurs first and that ascites forms as an overflow phenomenon after plasma volume has been increased.

Levy and colleagues have confirmed that fluid retention is, indeed, the original sin. In dimethylnitrosamine-induced cirrhosis in dogs they noted progressive sodium retention and increasing plasma volume for 7 to 10 days before ascites first appeared[521] (Fig. 20-52). This overload

Fig. 20-51. Effect of immersion and spironolactone on sodium excretion in a cirrhotic patient. The administration of spironolactone (400 mg/day for 5 days) was associated with a constant urinary sodium output. When the patient was immersed in water there was a prompt and profound increase in sodium excretion. (Epstein M: J Lab Clin Med 87:822, 1976)

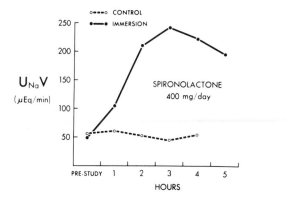

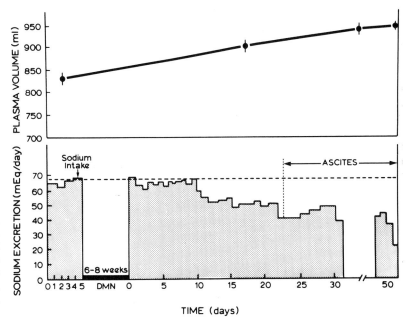

Fig. 20-52. Hypervolemia before ascites in experimental cirrhosis. Balance studies in five dogs given dimethylnitrosamine took from 6 to 8 weeks to induce cirrhosis. Sodium excretion decreased and plasma volume increased by 10% *before* ascites began to appear. (Levy M, Wexler MJ: J Lab Clin Med 91:520, 1978)

hypothesis is in keeping with the observation that posthemodialysis ascites is the consequence of chronic dialysis-induced overhydration.[345] More surprising was their demonstration that the same sequence occurs in dogs with end-to-side portacaval shunts, thus minimizing the role of portal hypertension in the pathogenesis of ascites.[522] When side-to-side portacaval anastomoses are constructed however, no ascites develops.[960] Furthermore, hypoalbuminemia, hyperaldosteronism, hepatic ischemia, and reduced renal perfusion did not appear important in initiating ascites in these experiments. These findings are at variance with those of Orloff and others, who showed that aldosterone secretion increases enormously in dogs within a few minutes after occlusion of the hepatic veins *before* appreciable ascites has formed and in the absence of any measurable decrease in plasma volume (Fig. 20-53).[653] This phenomenon, which does not occur in nephrectomized dogs, appears to be mediated by a humoral messenger triggered, presumably, by increased intrasinusoidal pressure.

Normal persons subjected to long-term administration of aldosterone escape fluid retention presumably by the elaboration of "third factor," which reduces sodium reabsorption in the proximal renal tubule in response to expansion of the effective extracellular fluid volume.[96] It is presumed that patients with primary aldosteronism do not develop edema for similar reasons. On the other hand, ascitic cirrhotic patients and experimental animals with inferior vena caval ligation given excess sodium usually retain it.[340] The explanation for the failure of this "escape" phenomenon is not known, but it is postulated that cirrhotic patients elaborate insufficient amounts of this substance. Several investigators have found that cirrhotic patients who had not developed ascites "escape" from

excessive mineralocorticoid administration, while those who had developed ascites do not.[1025] Furthermore, the urine and plasma of the group who escape contain natriuretic properties in various bioassay systems while the nonescapers do not.[479,1025]

Recent studies have shown that atrial natriuretic factor (ANF), which is a "third factor" that is important in volume homeostasis,[491] is greatly increased in patients with congestive heart failure and hypertension[253] but is not increased in cirrhotic patients with ascites.[24] However, plasma ANF levels are depressed by spironolactone therapy.[322] Furthermore, cirrhotic patients show only one half the normal increment in plasma ANF concentration when central venous volume and pressure are increased by head-out water immersion.[323] Cirrhotic patients with ascites show less than one fourth the normal increase in plasma ANF levels after immersion to the neck in water. These findings indicate that the ANF response to increasing the "effective plasma volume" is impaired in cirrhotic patients with ascites.

Plasma norepinephrine and epinephrine levels are increased in ascitic cirrhotic patients and are associated with increased plasma concentrations of aldosterone, renin, and vasopressin and a diminished diuretic response to an induced water load.[72,381] Since plasma norepinephrine secretion rates are increased and norepinephrine clearance rates are normal,[448,639] it appears that increased plasma catecholamine levels are the consequence of increased synthesis, which is stimulated by the decrease in effective plasma volume. Head-out water immersion, which increases central venous volume and, presumably, the effective arterial plasma volume and plasma ANF levels, reduces norepinephrine levels.[639] Conversely, assuming the standing position, which is the physiologic opposite of

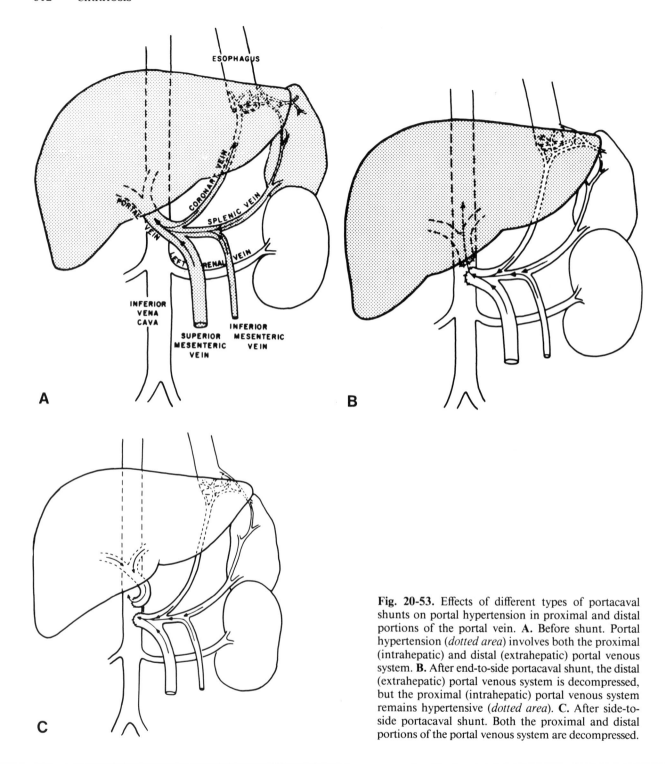

A

ESOPHAGUS

CORONARY VEIN

PORTAL VEIN

SPLENIC VEIN

LEFT RENAL VEIN

INFERIOR VENA CAVA

SUPERIOR MESENTERIC VEIN

INFERIOR MESENTERIC VEIN

B

C

Fig. 20-53. Effects of different types of portacaval shunts on portal hypertension in proximal and distal portions of the portal vein. **A.** Before shunt. Portal hypertension (*dotted area*) involves both the proximal (intrahepatic) and distal (extrahepatic) portal venous system. **B.** After end-to-side portacaval shunt, the distal (extrahepatic) portal venous system is decompressed, but the proximal (intrahepatic) portal venous system remains hypertensive (*dotted area*). **C.** After side-to-side portacaval shunt. Both the proximal and distal portions of the portal venous system are decompressed.

head-out water immersion, decreases central venous pressure and the effective plasma volume and increases plasma norepinephrine levels and presumably decreases plasma ANF concentrations.[67a]

Other factors also participate in the overall problem of ascites formation. Levels of antidiuretic hormone (ADH), which have been reported to be elevated in the serum and urine of cirrhotic patients with ascites by various bioassay methods, have been proved to be increased in plasma by highly sensitive radioimmunoassay.[663] It is postulated that increased release of ADH is a result of decreased "effective" plasma volume and a decrease in afferent parasympathetic activity.[837] Indeed, these patients have lower serum albumin and sodium concentrations, higher heart rates and plasma renin and aldosterone levels, and are less responsive to diuretic agents than patients without increased ADH activity.[72] Increased ADH activity may contribute to the retention of water in excess of sodium and the frequent occurrence of hyponatremia in ascitic cirrhotic patients.[373] Prostaglandins have been implicated in the problem of sodium retention and ascites formation. Indomethacin, a potent inhibitor of prostaglandin synthesis, decreases effective renal plasma flow and creatinine clearance in cirrhotic patients with sodium retention but not in those who are not retaining sodium.[88] Indomethacin also decreases plasma renin activity and aldosterone levels.[1070] These observations suggest that prostaglandins may be a determinant of renal plasma flow and sodium retention in decompensated cirrhosis, and may, in fact, be a beneficial compensatory mechanism. The *kallikrein-kinin system* may also be involved, since pre-kallikrein levels in the plasma of cirrhotic patients are decreased.[693] So might *vasoactive intestinal peptide* and increased *sympathetic nervous system* activity, but these are at the moment only dark horse candidates.

It has been shown that newly synthesized albumin appears directly in hepatic lymph and in ascites,[1069] evidence that abnormal mechanisms of albumin transport exist in ascitic cirrhotic patients. Similarly, it has been suggested that hepatic parenchymal metabolism of salt-retaining hormone may be impaired in patients with hepatic parenchymal damage,[138] but this mechanism can play only a minor role compared with the enormous aldosterone secretion rate.

Treatment

Paracentesis. Forty years ago large paracenteses were the accepted form of therapy for those patients in whom spontaneous diuresis did not occur after prolonged bed rest and sodium restriction. Large paracenteses were performed repeatedly, often on outpatients, the frequency depending on the rate of reaccumulation. Although the detrimental effects of repeated paracenteses have long been recognized, there were no reasonable alternatives. The major complications of paracentesis include perforation of abdominal viscera, hemorrhage due to penetration of abdominal wall vessels, introduction of infection, the induction of postparacentesis shock or hyponatremic syndromes, and the protein depletion caused by the loss of large amounts of proteins.

Recently, however, several groups have shown that large paracenteses (4–6 liters) can be employed without complication when performed slowly (over 30–90 min) and when serum albumin (40 g) is administered.[736] In fact, in a randomized clinical trial, large daily paracenteses were more effective, faster, cheaper, and as safe as conventional diuretic therapy. A second group reported that single, 5-liter paracenteses were free of complications in patients with peripheral edema, even without albumin administration.[437] These studies indicate that the deleterious consequences of large paracenteses may have been exaggerated that big taps are a viable, effective form of therapy. In the absence of peripheral edema large paracenteses without simultaneous albumin infusions have induced azotemia and are not recommended (Rodes J: Personal communication).

At present it is neither necessary nor desirable to perform paracenteses routinely in all cirrhotic patients. Indications for paracentesis include (1) diagnostic examination for unexplained fever, hypothermia, diarrhea, abdominal pain, or encephalopathy; (2) relief of abdominal pain; (3) relief of dyspnea or orthopnea; (4) reduction of intra-abdominal pressure in which a tense abdomen may be detrimental (*e.g.,* variceal hemorrhage, hepatorenal syndrome, incarceration of hernia); (5) facilitation of physical or radiologic examination or surgical procedures; (6) as a necessary part of peritoneal dialysis or ascites reinfusion. At the present time, paracentesis *per se* is not a standard method of treating ascites, but confirmation of the recent observations about large paracenteses may make big taps a treatment of choice in the future.

Medical Management. Before effective diuretic agents were available, conservative medical management consisted of bed rest and salt restriction. Although bed rest *per se* has never been proven effective, it has traditionally and unquestioningly been used. Bed rest in the hospital, however, may be assumed to be synonymous with abstinence from alcohol, a primary aspect of the therapy of alcoholic cirrhosis. Although dietary inadequacies have often been implicated in the pathogenesis of "nutritional" cirrhosis, their actual role in the development of or recovery from alcoholic cirrhosis has never been established.[465]

The keystone to the conservative treatment of ascites has long been salt restriction. The primacy of sodium in fluid retention is well established for all of the edematous diseases. Water will not be retained by the kidneys unless a sufficient quantity of salt is available to maintain an effective osmotic pressure in the extracellular fluid. The ingestion of a diet containing less salt than is excreted in the urine results in negative sodium balance. A negative balance of 140 mEq of sodium will be accompanied by a loss of approximately a liter of water, unless excessive ADH activity is present, in which case hyponatremia develops. A positive balance of 140 mEq of sodium can be predicted to cause retention of a liter of water and a 2-

pound weight gain. Often in cirrhotic patients with ascites, the urine is virtually free of sodium, and fluid retention gradually increases with even the most stringent sodium limitation. Strict sodium restriction will, however, retard the retention of the fluid.

It has been shown that with effective diuretic agents it is no longer necessary to restrict sodium.[225,773] In fact, less frequent and less severe hyponatremia and azotemia occur when excessive salt restriction is avoided. Using this philosophy, a patient with massive ascites may be given a palatable diet and thus provide the nutrition that strict salt restriction may prevent.

A small fraction of ascitic patients—perhaps 5%—promptly and spontaneously lose ascites after admission to hospital.[165,214,772] Another group—roughly 10%—quickly begin to mobilize ascites on salt restriction alone. As Patek, Davidson, and Reynolds have shown, prolonged salt restriction will result in the loss of the ascites in another 25% if it is continued for periods of 6 months or longer.[214,684,772] It is assumed that the delayed diuresis, which often starts suddenly, occurs when improvement in hepatic status takes place. This mysterious "turning the corner" may not correlate with apparent improvement of any clinical or laboratory manifestation of hepatic decompensation.

It is often recommended that fluid restriction be instituted along with sodium restriction in the management of massive ascites. In cirrhotic patients fluid restriction to levels less than output can guarantee progressively decreasing urine output, the "hepatorenal syndrome" and death. Lesser degrees of restriction tend to create lesser degrees of prerenal azotemia. Although such pseudohepatorenal syndromes can usually be reversed by volume repletion, the boundary between prerenal and renal azotemia is ill defined and not always recrossable. In the absence of hyponatremia caused by excessive water administration or inappropriate water retention, there is no place for water restriction. Fluid should be given *ad libitum* unless the patient exhibits excessive water retention.

Diuretics. The availability of potent diuretic drugs has obviated the need for prolonged hospitalization and has made the previously common problem of intractable ascites relatively rare. It should be kept in mind, however, that the use of diuretic therapy is directed not at the primary defect, but at a susceptible secondary site.

Since cirrhotic ascites is mediated largely by increased aldosterone secretion[17,201] inhibition of the renal effects by *spirolactones* is a rational, physiologic form of therapy. Actually spirolactones inhibit aldosterone synthesis, as well as its renal effects. This inhibition is histologically demonstrable by the presence of "watch spring" cytoplasmic inclusions in the cells of the zona glomerulosa of the adrenal gland (Fig. 20-54). These "spironolactone bodies" appear as plasma and urinary levels of aldosterone decrease and increase in number as the duration and dosage of spironolactone increase.[195] These bodies disappear gradually after spironolactone is stopped, and apparently have no untoward effects. Spironolactone (Aldactone), the

most effective of these synthetic corticosteroids, is remarkably free of side-effects. Although spironolactone alone is an effective diuretic, in practice it is usually used in conjunction with other diuretics, such as hydrochlorothiazide or furosemide, for several reasons.

1. There is a lag period of 3 or 4 days between the initiation of therapy and the onset of diuresis.
2. Spironolactone by itself may require large doses (>400 mg/day), which are relatively expensive.
3. Since spironolactone primarily decreases sodium reabsorption in the distal nephron, its combination with a diuretic, which decreases sodium absorption from the proximal tubule, enhances the effect.
4. The addition of a kaliuretic drug, such as furosemide or chlorothiazide, to antagonize the kalioretentive effect of spironolactone makes an attractive combination. Although theoretically ideal, in practice the combination of these drugs as initial therapy may be undesirable. The potassium deficit in patients with decompensated cirrhosis is as large as it is ubiquitous.[126,716] We have found a decrease of from 10% to 30% of the expected total body potassium in most patients with decompensated alcoholic cirrhosis. Furthermore, it is extremely difficult to replenish potassium despite administration of large supplements of potassium chloride plus spironolactone in these patients.[163,716]

Spironolactone can be employed more effectively and more rationally by adjusting the dose to the functional response. We recommend starting with 200 mg spironolactone per day, which may be given as a single daily dose or in divided doses. Urine electrolyte examinations performed before and daily during treatment are useful in assessing the response and in adjusting dosage. If by the fourth day there has been no weight loss and the urinary sodium concentration remains low (<10 mEq/liter), the dose of spironolactone should be doubled. If by the eighth day there is no diuretic response, one may either increase the dose of spironolactone still further or may add a small dose of one of the kaliuretic diuretic drugs. Spironolactone alone in response-determined dosage is an effective diuretic agent[245] and superior to furosemide or hydrochlorothiazide.[119] When used in the rational manner described, it is effective and safe even in patients with resistant ascites.[292,352]

There are advantages to this type of high spironolactone dosage as the primary form of therapy. First, at least 75% of our patients respond to the 400-mg dose of spironolactone in the absence of other diuretics. Only about one half of patients exhibit satisfactory diuresis with either furosemide or hydrochlorothiazide alone.[635,692,863] Second, this more physiologic approach avoids the frequent problem of over-diuresis by the more potent loop diuretic drugs, which often result in constricted plasma volume and prerenal azotemia. Third, it minimizes the complications associated with potassium depletion during a very susceptible period.

Hyperkalemia, however, is an occasional complication of spironolactone therapy. The patient may be taking large

Fig. 20-54. Spironolactone bodies. **A.** Histologic section of an aldosterone-producing adenoma. Pale, laminated, intracytoplasmic bodies are seen within a halo. (Original magnification × 750). **B.** Electron micrograph showing whorls of cytomembranes characteristic of a spironolactone body. (Original magnification × 23,000) (Conn JW, Hinerman DL: Metabolism 26:1293, 1977. Reproduced with permission)

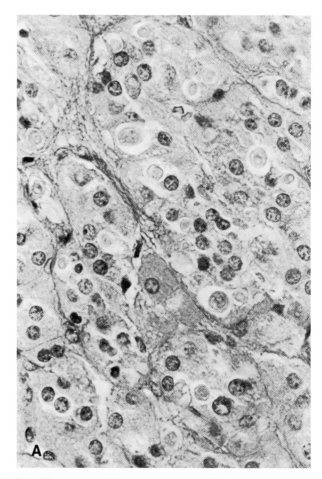

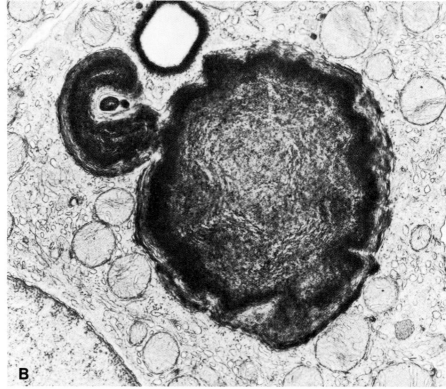

amounts of a salt substitute that contains mainly potassium chloride. Actually, in the absence of azotemia even the combination of potassium and spironolactone therapy rarely causes hyperkalemia. Another related complication of spironolactone therapy is hyperchloremic acidosis.[310] This uncommon but rarely fatal syndrome, which appears to be an acquired form of hypoaldosteronism, may be a consequence of the suppression of renal tubular ammonium excretion caused by hyperkalemia.

Symptomatic hyponatremia is a serious complication of spironolactone therapy that may occur as a consequence of overdiuresis. When large doses of spironolactone are inadvertently continued after the retained fluid has been lost, the patient may rapidly develop hyponatremia, decreased plasma volume, and azotemia, often with hepatic encephalopathy as the initial clinical manifestation. With any diuretic, one must carefully assess the situation as the patient approaches dry weight.

Non–Aldosterone-Inhibiting Diuretic Drugs. *Thiazide diuretic* agents, which interfere with sodium reabsorption at the distal loop of Henle and the distal tubule, cause chloriuresis and interfere with diluting capacity. They are potent diuretics that have the major advantage of oral administration and the major disadvantage of intense kaliuresis. Only one half of patients treated with hydrochlorothiazide alone exhibit satisfactory diuresis.[863]

Furosemide, piretanide, muzolimine[67a] *ibopamine and ethacrynic acid* are chemically dissimilar oral and parenteral agents, which act like powerful thiazides and interfere with sodium reabsorption proximal to the site of sodium–potassium exchange and, incidentally, with both the diluting and concentrating mechanisms. Their major disadvantage is their intense kalichloriuresis, which is roughly proportional to their diuretic activity. Since an effective diuresis is induced by furosemide and piretanide in only one half the patients,[27,635,691] loop diuretics should be used only in conjunction with spironolactone or when spironolactone alone is ineffective.

Ibopamine, a dopamine agonist, is as effective a diuretic agent as furosemide, but unlike furosemide, which tends to decrease creatinine clearance, it induces an increase in creatinine clearance.[589] The concept of inducing diuresis by improving renal function rather than by impairing it is a very attractive one. Ibopamine also reduces plasma vasopressin levels and thus may be especially effective in cirrhotic patients who are resistant to diuretic therapy and who often exhibit increased antidiuretic activity.[72]

Pteridine diuretics are nonsteroidal, potassium-retaining, natriuretic drugs, which act at the site of sodium–potassium and sodium–hydrogen ion exchange in the distal tubule. They do not inhibit aldosterone. The major advantage of these drugs (triamterene, amiloride) is their potassium-retaining properties, which, in combination with kaliuretic agents, make them desirable drugs for the diuresis of potassium-depleted patients.

These long-loop diuretic drugs are effective, and with

spironolactone, account for the decrease in the frequency of intractable ascites. They represent, however, a two-edged sword. In decompensated cirrhotic patients, these agents commonly precipitate or potentiate hypokalemia and azotemia.[530,635,863] The toxicity of these drugs is largely proportional to their efficacy as diuretics. The metabolic alkalosis and the increased pH gradient between the extracellular and intracellular fluids, which are part of the syndrome of potassium depletion, favor ammonia toxicity.[907] In the presence of azotemia, profound hepatic encephalopathy may develop. The frequency of this lesion may be in part explained by the increased renal release of ammonia caused by most of these agents.[402] It is no wonder that approximately 20% of cases of hepatic encephalopathy are diuretic-induced.[272]

Because of the frequency of these complications, we do not recommend the use of loop diuretic drugs alone or as primary therapeutic agents. We prefer to withhold their use until spironolactone has been tried. After the dangers of potassium depletion have been reduced, any of these diuretics in moderate dosage may be added. Although spironolactone may reduce the potassium loss of thiazide diuretics, it does not abolish it. If a good diuresis ensues with hydrodiuril, for example, excessive potassium loss may still occur despite the use of spironolactone.[791] In fact, diuresis induced by spironolactone alone may be associated with negative potassium balance.

Estimates of urinary potassium concentration provide insight into the situation and permit rational therapeutic adjuncts. It is sometimes necessary to give potassium chloride supplements as well as large doses of spironolactone. When renal function is impaired, however, kaliotherapy must be given only with great caution.

Whatever diuretic agents are used, a safe and sane rate of diuresis should be maintained. The maximal absorption rate of ascites from the peritoneum is approximately 900 ml/day—equivalent to a weight loss of just under 2 pounds daily.[860] A faster rate of diuresis can be achieved only by the loss of edema, which is much more easily mobilized than ascites, or by a reduction in plasma volume with impairment of renal function.[715] The dosage of diuretics should be adjusted to maintain the diuresis at less than 2 pounds per day. In the face of massive pools of ascites estimated to contain 20 to 40 liters, the prospect of a 4- or 6-week diuresis is not an appealing one. Impatience with such a deliberate program may paradoxically prolong the duration of the hospital stay or, even worse, end it abruptly.

Elevation of decreased serum albumin levels by *infusion of albumin* has been shown to promote diuresis in some cirrhotic patients with ascites and edema.[685,1024]

Ascites reinfusion has been used as an inexpensive, readily available albumin substitute for expanding plasma volume.[150,1044] The combination of plasma expansion plus paracentesis, which has the direct effect of reducing portal venous pressure,[469] may correct two of the derangements that favor ascites formation. A modification of this technique, which involves the reinfusion of a protein concentrate obtained by continuous ultrafiltration, has been reported to be effective.[677]

Intractable is defined as the inability to remove ascites by nonmechanical means without detrimentally distorting the internal milieu. We encounter only three or four such cases per year at our hospital.

A variety of surgical procedures including omentopexy, hepatopexy, ileoenterectomy, peritoneocalyceal anastomoses, and peritoneosubcutaneous fistulas have been tried and abandoned. The most rational form of surgery is decompression of the portal hypertension, the *sine qua non* of ascites. Portacaval anastomosis has been used for this purpose almost since its introduction in 1945. Both end-to-side and side-to-side shunts have been successfully employed, but the latter are physiologically more sound and therapeutically more effective.[650,960] End-to-side portacaval anastomoses relieve ascites when the portal venous inflow contributes to the intrahepatic sinusoidal hypertension. When high-grade sinusoidal or postsinusoidal hepatic venous obstruction is present, the flow in the portal vein may be retrograde.[998] The creation in such patients of end-to-side portacaval anastomosis which obliterates the escape valve, may result in the appearance of ascites in patients in whom it had not previously been present or its acceleration in those in whom it had. Side-to-side shunts in such patients do not interrupt such retrograde flow and thus decompress both the presinusoidal and postsinusoidal venous hypertension with the alleviation of ascites and the disappearance of varices[576,651] (see Fig. 20-53). The presence of retrograde flow and the necessity

for side-to-side anastomosis can be determined relatively simply during surgery. If the pressure in the portal vein is measured above and below occlusion of the portal vein, a decrease in pressure suggests that blood flow in the portal vein is antegrade, and that an end-to-side anastomosis will suffice (Fig. 20-55). A rise in portal venous pressure or its failure to fall after occlusion implies retrograde portal flow, and indicates the need for a side-to-side shunt (Fig. 20-55) if intractable ascites is to be avoided. The distal splenorenal shunt, which has some advantages over portacaval shunts, is not recommended for patients with severe ascites, in whom it may be considered a contraindication.[313]

Unfortunately, patients with intractable ascites are not ideal surgical candidates, and the operative mortality is often prohibitively high, although some investigators have accomplished side-to-side shunts with an acceptably low operative mortality rate.[650] It is recommended, therefore, that therapeutic side-to-side portacaval anastomosis be reserved for those patients with persistent, intractable massive ascites who cannot be effectively managed by more conservative forms of therapy.

Peritoneovenous Shunt. One surgical form of therapy that can be tolerated by decompensated cirrhotic patients is the placement of a *peritoneovenous shunt* although it is not free of hazard. A variety of tubes, buttons, and valves designed to return ascitic fluid to the systemic circulation have been tried and abandoned. The LeVeen valve has become the standard method of treatment of intractable ascites. This ascites drainage system consists of a Silastic

Fig. 20-55. Diagram showing pressure responses to portal venous compression useful in determining the optimal type of portacaval anastomosis. **A.** When occlusion of the portal vein results in a fall in portal pressure on the hepatic side of the clamp, antegrade portal venous flow is contributing to the portal hypertension, and an end-to-side anastomosis is indicated. **B.** With retrograde portal venous flow, partial pressure on the hepatic side of the occlusion rises, indicating a need for a side-to-side portacaval anastomosis that will allow systemic decompression of the increased intrahepatic portal pressure. (Conn HO: In Popper H, Schaffer F [eds]: Progress in Liver Diseases, 4th ed, pp 269–288. New York, Grune & Stratton, 1972)

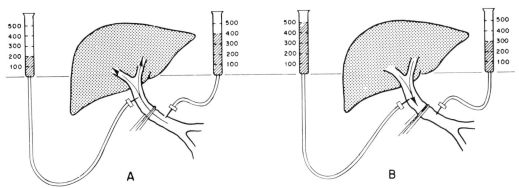

ANTEGRADE PORTAL VENOUS FLOW
END TO SIDE PORTACAVAL SHUNT

RETROGRADE PORTAL VENOUS FLOW
SIDE TO SIDE PORTACAVAL SHUNT

pressure-sensitive, one-way valve, which is implanted in the abdominal wall, and connected to the peritoneal cavity by a perforated, silicone rubber collecting tube (afferent limb) and to the venous system by a subcutaneous silicone rubber tube that enters the jugular vein (efferent limb) (Fig. 20-56). The valve is superior to previous valves in the lower pressure gradient required to permit the passage of fluid (3 cm H_2O) and its competency against backflow. Since 1974, when LeVeen and colleagues first described this apparatus, a series of reports by these investigators and by others have attested to the efficacy of this form of therapy in patients with resistant ascites.[518a,759,877]

Along with these enthusiastic reports of the alleviation of ascites and reversal of the hepatorenal syndrome by peritoneovenous shunts,[306,480,517,845] there are a number of reported diverse malfunctions and complications.[518a] Malfunction of the LeVeen shunt may be classified as follows.

1. Immediate failure to function usually represents malposition of the efferent limb, the distal end of which should be in the vena cava. If the tip of the tube is in the right ventricle or in the inferior vena cava, the higher pressure at these locations prevents the flow of ascites through the shunt. Similarly, kinking of the tube or bubbles introduced into the valve at the time of implantation may prevent the shunt from functioning properly.
2. Early failure of the shunt, which occurs from a few days to a few weeks after insertion, occurs abruptly

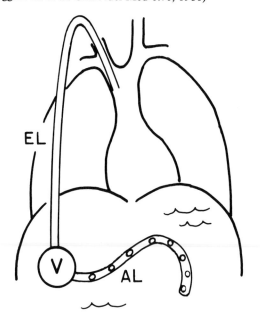

Fig. 20-56. Diagram of peritoneovenous shunt (LeVeen). The afferent limb (*AL*) carries ascitic fluid to the valve (*V*) and through the efferent limb (*EL*) to the superior vena cava (Taggart GJ et al: Clin Nucl Med 6:70, 1981)

after a period of normal function. In this situation the efferent limb is often found in the axillary or innominate vein encased in fibrin. Early malfunction may also occur when congestive heart failure develops after implantation and the pressure gradient across the valve is reduced to less than 3 cm H_2O.
3. Late malfunction occurs from several months to several years after surgery. This syndrome, which is characterized by the reaccumulation of ascites, may be called the "gummy valve syndrome," in which fibrin prevents the normal excursion of the Silastic diaphragm. Streptokinase has been used to dissolve fibrin in occluded shunts and to restore function.[857] Other apparent causes are obstruction of the collecting tube by the omentum or clots in the efferent tube. Occasionally, one or the other tube has become detached from the valve. Rarely, the malfunction cannot be explained.

A great variety of complications have been reported (Table 20-15). Several are consequences of greatly expanded plasma volume.

1. Congestive heart failure occurs in 2% to 4% of shunted patients, almost always in those who have shown evidence of previous cardiac decompensation or who are in borderline compensation at the time of implantation. Congestive heart failure may often be an overlooked contraindication rather than a true complication.
2. Bleeding from esophagogastric varices is another complication of expanded plasma volume. It is never clear in an individual patient whether the hemorrhage developed spontaneously or was caused by the shunt, since these patients are prone to bleed from varices anyway.
3. Disseminated intravascular coagulation (DIC) is a common and serious complication of peritoneovenous shunting. It probably occurs in the large majority of patients shortly after shunts and has been recorded in about two thirds of several prospective series.[480,516–518, 843,845,846] It is characterized in its minor form by a sharp reduction in plasma fibrinogen levels and platelet concentration and by prolongation of prothrombin, thrombin, and partial thromboplastin times. In about 25% of patients the DIC is symptomatic, and in about 5% it is lethal. The appearance of generalized bleeding is a true emergency that demands immediate occlusion of the shunt and replacement of depleted clotting factors and, perhaps, by anticoagulant therapy. Although the mechanism of postperitoneovenous shunt DIC is not clear, it is known that ascites often contains fibrin-split products, and that ascites reinfusions may induce DIC.[843,846] Determination of the incidence, pathogenesis, lethality, and therapy of this complication awaits prospective evaluation.

   The DIC associated with peritoneovenous shunts is their most common complication. Indeed, the absence of serologic evidence of DIC has been interpreted to mean that the shunt is not functioning.[328] Postshunt

TABLE 20-15. Complications of Peritoneovenous Shunt

I. Technical
   A. Obstruction of valve
   B. Obstruction of intra-abdominal tube
   C. Obstruction of subcutaneous tube
   D. Malposition of tube
      1. Malfunction
      2. Ventricular tachycardia
II. Operative
   A. Ascites leakage
   B. Bleeding
      1. Hemoperitoneum
      2. Hemothorax
      3. Incision sites
      4. Subcutaneous
   C. Pneumothorax
   D. Pleural effusion
   E. Subcutaneous emphysema
   F. Peritoneal
      1. Intestinal obstruction
      2. Fibroperitonitis
      3. Ileal cocoon
      4. Peritoneal pseudocyst
      5. Abdominal pain
   G. Miscellaneous: coronary sinus perforation
III. Systemic
   A. Cardiac
      1. Congestive heart failure
      2. Arrhythmia
      3. Right atrial thrombosis
   B. Vascular
      1. Hemorrhage from esophageal varices
      2. Thrombosis of superior vena cava
      3. Stenosis of superior vena cava
      4. Obstruction of superior vena cava
   C. Hematologic: disseminated intravascular coagulation

III. Systemic (*continued*)
   D. Infectious
      1. Bacterial peritonitis
      2. Bacterial endocarditis
      3. Septicemia
      4. Wound infection
      5. Intra-abdominal abscess
      6. Bacterial meningitis
      7. Bacterial nephritis (staphylococcal)
      8. Fever of unknown origin
   E. Pulmonary
      1. Pulmonary emboli
         a. Tumor
         b. Gas
         c. Air
         d. Cholesterol crystals
      2. Pulmonary metastases
      3. Pulmonary hypertension with pulmonary edema
   F. Gastrointestinal
      1. Intestinal obstruction
      2. Intestinal stenosis
   G. Metabolic
      1. Hypokalemia
      2. Hepatic encephalopathy
   H. Local metastatic cancer
      1. Pulmonary
      2. Subcutaneous tunnel
   I. Miscellaneous
      1. Pain
      2. Eventration of valve
      3. Erythema over tubing
      4. Erosion of tubing through skin
      5. Fibrous envelopes

DIC can be minimized or prevented by replacing the ascitic fluid with Ringer's solution before implanting the shunt, and DIC can be promptly improved by clamping the tubing of the peritoneovenous shunt. Recent studies have indicated that ascites contains a platelet-aggregating factor, which has been identified as collagen[815] and which activates both platelets and clotting factors. Collagen has been isolated from the ascitic fluid and shown to induce platelet aggregation in both rabbits and humans.[815] In rabbits the intravenous infusion of this material induces DIC, and the prior administration of aspirin or dipyridamole prevents these effects. Furthermore, the administration of aspirin (300 mg/day) and dipyridamole (400 mg/day) before implanting peritoneovenous shunts prevented DIC in six of eight patients so studied. Aspirin inhibits platelet cyclo-oxygenase, an essential enzyme in prostaglandin synthesis, and dipyridamole increases cyclic

adenosine monophosphate (cAMP) levels, thus interfering with platelet function. These fascinating observations indicate that DIC, the primary complication of peritoneovenous shunting, which also contributes to shunt occlusion and malfunction, may be a complication of the past.

4. Bacterial infection is another potentially lethal complication. It occurs in 4% to 8% of patients with peritoneovenous shunts and may be fatal in half of those who become infected.[843,846] If the ascitic fluid is infected at the time of implantation, peritonitis is almost unavoidable. Introduction of bacteria at surgery and postoperative wound infections are often fatal. The frequent occurrence of fever and abdominal tenderness after uncomplicated insertion may obscure the presence of peritonitis. The efficacy of prophylactic antibiosis awaits controlled investigation.

5. Another potentially lethal complication of peritoneo-

venous shunting is air embolism when patients require laparotomy. Clamping of the peritoneovenous shunt tubing before surgery can prevent this problem.[478]

Most reports of peritoneovenous shunting are concerned with the LeVeen valve, but two other shunts are commercially available. The Denver shunt, which employs a miter valve, appears to be more effective than the LeVeen shunt in patients with malignant ascites.[541] The Hakim shunt, which is implanted over the sternum, is accessible for determining where the shunt is obstructed when it malfunctions.[687] In a small randomized trial we found little difference between the LeVeen and Hakim instruments.

Shunt patency can be determined by the intraperitoneal injection of ^{99m}Tc-sulfur colloid. The injection of contrast material by inserting a fine needle into the subcutaneous tubing is often easier.[844] A noninvasive extracorporeal Doppler probe has been reported and appears to be ideal[594] but is probably too good to be true.

The precise place of peritoneovenous shunting in the treatment of ascites is not known. It is apparent that this relatively simple operation may make miracles; it is equally clear that it sometimes induces disaster. The failure rate is very high, and the complications are common, severe, and frequently lethal. It is difficult to be certain whether the gains outweigh the losses. Only time and clinical trials, which are in progress but as yet unreported, will tell.[908] When ascites is intractable, however, and further medical management offers little help, peritoneovenous shunting becomes the treatment of choice. It is also advocated in patients who have ruptured an umbilical hernia or are at risk of doing so[641] and those with persistent hepatic hydrothorax.[388] Criteria of operability are variable, but the bilirubin–creatinine guideline is useful.[331] It suggests that when the sum of the total serum bilirubin and the serum creatinine is less than 4 mg/dl, the chances of success are excellent. When the sum is greater than 4 mg/dl, the risks are greater and must be weighed against the possible gains.

In patients with the hepatorenal syndrome (see below), accumulating data indicate that the peritoneovenous shunting is frequently successful,[306,517,841,845,996] and when compared with the otherwise almost hopeless prognosis, it is a treatment to be tried. The serum bilirubin–creatinine guideline is of little value in the assessment for peritoneovenous shunt surgery in the hepatorenal syndrome, since the serum creatinine concentration alone may be 4 mg/dl. Indeed, it is to correct the gross elevation of the serum creatinine concentration that the surgery is being considered.

Hepatic Hydrothorax

Fluid that accumulates in the pleural cavity in cirrhotic patients is referred to as hepatic hydrothorax or cirrhotic pleural effusion. Although only 3% to 4% of all pleural effusions can be attributed to cirrhosis, the prevalence of hydrothorax in cirrhotic patients may approach 10% in patients with ascites.[416] Most are located on the right, but they frequently occur on both sides or, occasionally, only on the left. Transudation from increased thoracic duct lymphatic flow was once invoked as its cause. Present evidence suggests direct passage of ascitic fluid from the abdomen through defects in the diaphragm into the pleural space[519] (Fig. 20-57). Negative intrathoracic pressure also contributes to the peritoneal–pleural transfer of fluid. Ruptured blebs of pleuroperitoneum have been identified at autopsy.[529] These blebs may apparently also rupture from coughing or straining. Hepatic hydrothorax has been identified in patients without detectable ascites.[801,875] In such cases it is assumed that the negative intrathoracic pressure favors the transport of the ascitic fluid into the pleural space at a rate equivalent to its production in the abdomen.

Hepatic hydrothorax cannot always be distinguished from pleural effusions of other cause. It is not unusual for total protein, albumin, cholesterol, and total lipids to be higher in the pleural than in the peritoneal fluid, perhaps because water may be more rapidly absorbed from pleural vessels.[532] Since the dissimilarity of characteristics of ascitic and pleural fluids may raise questions about the etiology of the pleural effusion, the presence of a communication between the two cavities should be sought by the intraperitoneal injection of tracer amounts of ^{99m}Tc sulfur colloid.

Although hepatic hydrothorax is usually an incidental finding, on some occasions it may play a prominent role in causing respiratory embarrassment. The primary treatment of hepatic hydrothorax is the elimination of the ascites. If the pleural effusion causes respiratory embarrassment, thoracentesis may be necessary. An accompanying paracentesis to reduce intra-abdominal pressure may decrease the pressure differential on the two sides of the diaphragm that occurs when thoracentesis is performed alone. As the ascites is controlled, the diaphragmatic defect may heal. When repeated episodes of respiratory embarrassment occur as the result of recurrent pleural effusions, sclerosis of the diaphragmatic surface by instillation of nitrogen mustard or tetracycline into the chest cavity may be necessary. When hydrothorax persists, a peritoneovenous shunt may be required.[519]

The Hepatorenal Syndrome

The hepatorenal syndrome (HRS) is one of the primary causes of death from cirrhosis. In this syndrome patients with decompensated cirrhosis develop acquired, functional renal failure in which none of the usual causes of renal insufficiency are present and in which the kidneys themselves are normal. This disorder stubbornly resists attempts to improve renal function and usually ends in death. The single most frustrating aspect of this unique disorder is that the kidneys are anatomically and histologically normal and capable of normal function. The kidneys from patients who have died of the HRS can be transplanted into patients with chronic uremia, in whom

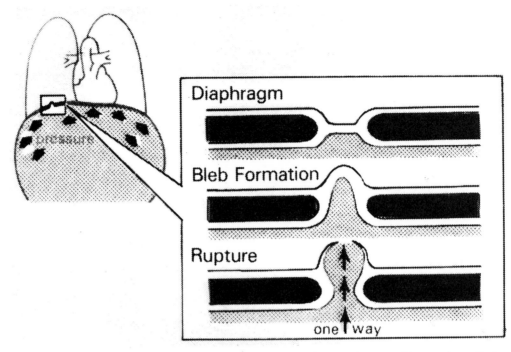

Fig. 20-57. A defect in the diaphragm is covered by pleuroperitoneum. Pressure beneath the diaphragm raises a bleb on its superior surface, and rupture of the bleb produces a one-way valve with fluid passing toward the pleural space. (Reproduced with permission from LeVeen HH et al: Am J Surg 148:210, 1984)

Fig. 20-58. Normal function of a kidney transplanted from a patient with the hepatorenal syndrome. The donor (*D-4*), who had the hepatorenal syndrome, died with rising BUN and serum creatinine levels and worsening oliguria. A cadaveric kidney was transplanted into the recipient (*R-4*) who had end-stage renal disease. After surgery, the patient underwent dialysis on five occasions, after which there was a progressive increase in urine volume and a decrease in BUN and serum creatinine concentrations. (Koppel MH et al: N Engl J Med 280:1367, 1969. Reproduced with permission)

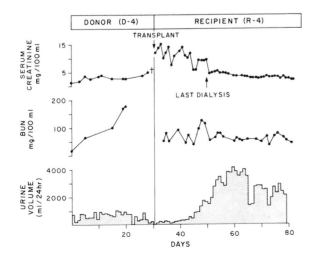

they function promptly and well[471] (Fig. 20-58). Conversely, transplantation of a liver into a patient with the HRS promptly restores renal function to normal (Fig. 20-59).

The term "hepatorenal syndrome" was first used in 1932 to describe postoperative renal failure in patients with biliary obstruction[379] and has since been used nonspecifically to describe any disorder with both hepatic and renal components. Despite opposition from the experts, however, this term has become established by common usage. A number of authors have used more precise, descriptive terms such as oliguric renal failure, functional renal failure, spontaneous impairment of renal function, and hemodynamic failure of the kidney, but none has caught on.

There are a number of diverse disorders that affect both the liver and kidney and, in effect, give rise to a variety of "hepatorenal" syndromes (Table 20-16). Clearly, however, these pseudohepatorenal disorders, which include leptospirosis, lupus erythematosus, carbon tetrachloride or toadstool poisoning, and disorders of many other etiologies, can be readily differentiated from the true HRS by recognition of the precipitating event or by characteristic clinical, laboratory, or functional features of the hepatic or renal lesions, or both.

The essential features of the HRS were first described by Austin Flint in a surprisingly up-to-date paper published over a century ago.[289] The HRS occurs almost in-

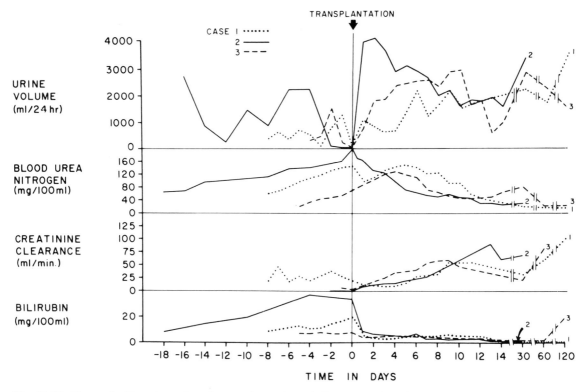

Fig. 20-59. Reversal of hepatorenal syndrome after orthotopic liver transplantation. All three patients had decreased urine volume and creatinine clearance and elevated BUN and serum bilirubin concentrations at the time of transplantation. Promptly after orthotopic transplantation, the four variables improved. (Iwatsuki S et al: N Engl J Med 289:1155, 1973)

variably in cirrhotic patients, usually alcoholic, the great majority of whom have decompensated liver disease characterized by jaundice, hepatosplenomegaly, hypoalbuminemia, and portal hypertension. Virtually all have ascites, which is often tense[40,531,673] and intense retention of sodium. Similar syndromes may be seen in metastatic liver disease[458] and in fulminant hepatitis in which ascites is prominent. Jaundice is usually marked, although neither jaundice nor ascites is always present. Although there is no evidence of preexisting renal disease and analysis of the urine is normal, a rather characteristic abnormal renal hemodynamic pattern is usually present. The onset of oliguria and azotemia usually occurs abruptly, often without evident precipitating factors, although oliguria is not invariably present. It frequently follows diuretic therapy, paracentesis, or gastrointestinal tract hemorrhage. Hyponatremia, hypokalemia, and hepatic coma frequently precede or accompany renal functional deterioration, but none of them is absolutely necessary. A modest decrease in systemic blood pressure is often present and is common terminally,[40,838] but profound hypotension is not part of the syndrome.

The prior presence of chronic renal disease, such as glomerulonephritis or pyelonephritis, should exclude this diagnosis. The HRS appears to be a disorder of reduced glomerular filtration rate and decreased renal blood flow, which probably precede by months the appearance of overt renal failure[40,838,858] and, perhaps, set the stage for its development. Paradoxically, this evidence of decreased renal blood flow usually exists in the presence of increased plasma volume and cardiac output.[531,955]

Renal tubular function is normal. These patients excrete urine that is practically sodium-free and retain the capacity to concentrate urine normally. They do have difficulty in excreting water loads,[488] but this feature may not be a result of renal tubular dysfunction *per se*. Although most patients with this constellation of findings die and recoveries are considered worthy of reporting in the literature, the mortality of this disease may be exaggerated by the paradoxical belief that patients who survive the HRS probably did not have it.

Physiological measures of *renal hemodynamics* in cirrhotic patients without ascites show normal glomerular filtration rates (GFR) and renal plasma flow (RPF), although in some patients with advanced cirrhosis without ascites they may be diminished.[40,673,955]

In ascitic cirrhotic patients without the HRS, the pattern is different. The GFR and RPF range from supernormal to moderately reduced, and in general parallel the severity of the cirrhosis and the amount of ascites.[40,252,340,672,858] In

TABLE 20-16.   Hepatorenal Syndromes

I. The hepatorenal syndrome
II. Pseudo-hepatorenal syndromes
  A. Generalized disorders
    1. Infectious
      a. Leptospirosis
      b. Yellow fever
      c. Reye's syndrome
      d. Viral hepatitis
      e. Sepsis
    2. Circulatory
      a. Shock
      b. Congestive heart failure
    3. Genetic
      a. Polycystic disease
      b. Sickle cell anemia
    4. Collagen vascular
      a. Disseminated lupus erythematosus
      b. Periarteritis nodosa
    5. Unknown etiology
      a. Toxemia of pregnancy
      b. Amyloidosis
      c. Sarcoidosis
      d. Waterhouse–Friderichsen syndrome
      e. Hyperthermia
  B. Toxins
    1. Direct
      a. Carbon tetrachloride
      b. Acetominophen
      c. Aspirin
      d. Copper sulfate
      e. Chromium
      f. Toadstool toxins
    2. Idiosyncratic or mixed
      a. Methoxyflurane
      b. Tetracycline
      c. Streptomycin
      d. Sulfonamides
      e. Iproniazid
  C. Neoplasms
    1. Metastatic
    2. Renal cell carcinoma

the presence of ascites tubular reabsorption is, of course, increased. The primacy of sodium retention in the formation of ascites is evident, especially in those ascitic patients who have maintained normal GFR. Impaired water excretion is sometimes found,[739] presumably associated with excessive antidiuretic activity, but many ascitic patients are able to excrete water loads promptly and to dilute urine normally.

A progressive correlation between the state of hepatic decompensation and the degree of renal functional impairment has been demonstrated.[40] Renal function is normal in compensated cirrhotic patients without ascites, mildly impaired in ascitic patients who are responsive to diuretic therapy, moderately abnormal in those with resistant ascites, and grossly deranged in patients with renal

insufficiency. The renal vascular resistance is increased and the renal fraction of the cardiac output is markedly reduced. This suggests that renal and systemic vasoconstriction results from diminished circulating volume.[955] This hypothesis has been confirmed in patients with reduced blood volume and cardiac output by expanding plasma volume, which causes decreased renal venous resistance, increased RPF, increased urine flow and sodium excretion. Urine flow rates are, of course, diminished in oliguric patients, as are sodium concentration in the urine and the response to water loads.[40,838,858] These parameters, too, become progressively more abnormal as the severity of the disease increases.

In patients with oliguria and azotemia (*i.e.,* the full-blown syndrome of functional renal failure), the pattern is relatively homogeneous. GFR and RPF are almost consistently and severely decreased. GFR may be in the range of 20 ml to 50 ml/min and RPF from 250 ml to 500 ml/min using a variety of techniques. Occasionally, however, patients who are markedly oliguric will have normal or even increased RPF.[955] Filtration fractions, although variable, tend to be decreased,[859] suggesting a relatively greater depression of cortical glomerular blood flow than of the total renal blood flow.[254,457] PAH extraction is reduced,[838,858] indicating that there is an internal redistribution of renal blood flow with a greater proportion of the blood flow perfusing the medulla, which extracts PAH poorly. The inability to concentrate urine maximally can be explained by increased medullary blood flow in the vasa recta, which leads to less efficient trapping of sodium, less hypertonicity of the medulla, and diminished ability to concentrate. The medullary shunting of blood was demonstrated directly using the ^{133}Xe wash-out technique; the rapid flow component (*i.e.,* perfusion of the outer renal cortex), is reduced[254,457] as graphically shown by gamma nephrograms and renal angiography.

Many pathogenic explanations of the HRS have been proposed but only a few deserve serious consideration. The traditional explanation for hemodynamic renal failure is based on the demonstration of diminished renal perfusion. It is tempting to conclude that in the presence of ascites, which is virtually the *sine qua non* of the HRS, *diminished plasma volume* is primarily responsible. Indeed, since ascitic fluid arises ultimately from plasma, it has been assumed that ascites formation, by definition, decreases plasma volume. This hypothesis is particularly attractive since the HRS often follows gastrointestinal tract hemorrhage, diuresis, or paracentesis, situations which have in common reduction of the circulating volume. In addition, a number of abnormalities that are commonly associated with the HRS, such as hypoalbuminemia, hyponatremia, and hypokalemia, can cause decreased extracellular volume.

Unfortunately for this lovely hypothesis, almost all studies have shown the plasma volume to be increased.[521,531,573] This awkward fact has led to a modified volume hypothesis that suggests that there is a "relative" decrease in plasma volume (*i.e.,* a diminution of *effective* plasma volume). Effective plasma volume is defined as that portion of the plasma volume that is involved in organ perfusion and that effectively stimulates volume receptors as opposed to the portion sequestered in the splanchnic bed. The most impressive evidence in favor of the plasma volume hypothesis is the observation that some patients with the HRS often have decreased plasma volume, which is associated with decreased cardiac output and increased renal vasoconstriction, as shown by increased renal vascular resistance and a reduced renal fraction of the cardiac output.[955] Expansion of the plasma volume with dextran or ascites reinfusions may increase cardiac output and improve the renal hemodynamics and urine flow. It has also been found that expansion of plasma volume will, at least transiently, improve the renal hemodynamics and urine output.[573,955,1044] Although long-term therapeutic implications of this technique are not known, it seems clear that this form of therapy requires objective evaluation.

A new hypothesis has been proposed about the pathogenesis of the HRS that appears to tie together a number of otherwise unexplained metabolic findings that are usually present.[16] It is known that the hepatic venous blood of various experimental animals contains a substance that stimulates the GFR and that is stimulated by dietary protein,[735] intravenous infusion of amino acids,[347] or glucagon.[689] Insulin suppresses the level of this substance. The GFR is increased in diabetes, which is also associated with hyperglucagonemia. Malnutrition, in which the hepatic uptake of amino acids is decreased, is characterized by decreased GFR,[463] which is increased by protein repletion.[13] It is proposed that normally the liver secretes a substance, *glomerulopressin*, which enhances the GFR and which is decreased in patients with advanced cirrhosis, who are characterized by negative nitrogen balance. Furthermore, it is suggested that glomerulopressin is required for the synthesis of prostaglandins, which also enhance GFR. The inhibition of prostaglandin synthesis by indomethacin or ibuprofen[88,1070] decreases GFR. Presumably, the postulated hypoglomerulopressinemia of cirrhosis also decreases GFR. One observation that does not fit this hypothesis is the hyperglucagonemia of patients with advanced cirrhosis, especially those with portal-systemic shunting.[561,864] The observation that glucagon administered intravenously induces little or no increase in GFR while intraportal infusions cause a potent stimulus to the GFR may help explain the role of portal-systemic shunting in the pathogenesis of the HRS. This hypothesis is under careful scrutiny.

Clearly, there are at least two types of hemodynamic patterns associated with oliguric hepatorenal failure—the uncommon, decreased plasma volume pattern, which may be reversed by expansion, and the typical high-output, increased plasma volume type. Unfortunately, it is not possible to differentiate on clinical or laboratory grounds those patients with the decreased plasma volume syndrome from those with increased plasma volume.[654]

The realization that functional renal failure that characterizes the HRS is reversible, as shown by normal function of "hepatorenal" kidneys after transplantation, is a landmark observation that is responsible for the resurgence of research in this area.[471] Epstein and co-workers demonstrated angiographic ". . . beading and tortuosity of the interlobar and proximal arcuate arteries . . . resembling, the aneurysmal dilatation of polyarteritis."[254] Postmortem angiograms in the same patients showed smooth, and regular interlobar and arcuate vessels (*i.e.,* the vasoconstrictive beading had disappeared) (Fig. 20-60). Investigators noted marked minute-to-minute variability and irregularity of the ^{133}Xe wash-out curves, which were often too unstable to allow interpretation, a pattern indicative of active vasoconstriction.[254,457] This *renal vasoconstriction* was confirmed directly by studies showing increased renal vascular resistance,[40,955] and frequent and extensive reflux into the aorta during renal angiography.

Although this vasoconstriction may be a sympathetic autonomic response to diminished effective plasma volume, increased renal sympathetic activity can be induced by other mechanisms. Attempts to induce β-adrenergic blockade, however, have given contradictory results. Some found no significant increase in RPF after phentolamine infusions in doses large enough to cause systemic hypotension.[254] Others reported significant increments in inulin and PAH clearance after intravenous phenoxybenzamine HCl (Dibenzyline) in doses that caused systemic hypotension.[39] The vasoconstriction may, of course, be humoral in origin, and serotonin, vasodepressor material (VDM), and angiotensin have been implicated.

Some workers who found hypotension, decreased peripheral resistance, diminished response to tyramine administration, and enhanced response to endogenous norepinephrine suggested that patients with the HRS behaved as if they were depleted of tissue norepinephrine.[569] This fascinating conjecture is compatible with the false neurotransmitter hypothesis that inert amines may replace active amines such as norepinephrine or dopamine in the HRS.[280] Some investigators reported that dopamine administered intravenously increased RPF, but not GFR or urine flow.[46] Others, at our institution, noted no significant changes in renal hemodynamics or function in cirrhotic patients with intractable ascites and azotemia after the prolonged administration of L-dopa at maximally tolerated oral doses.

The most attractive explanation for the renal hemodynamic alterations of the HRS is the *intrarenal shunting* of blood away from the cortex to the medulla. The kidneys act as if glomerular function were reduced and as if tubular function were maintained. Hemodynamic studies, which show proportionately greater reduction in GFR than in RPF, are compatible with this hypothesis. Studies with the ^{133}Xe wash-out technique for measuring renal blood flow and its intrarenal distribution have shown that the total renal blood flow is usually reduced, and the outer, cortical flow subnormal, while the juxtaglomerular and medullary flow is maintained.[254,457] Cortical perfusion is only occasionally and minimally reduced in patients with compensated cirrhosis, but in decompensated cirrhotic

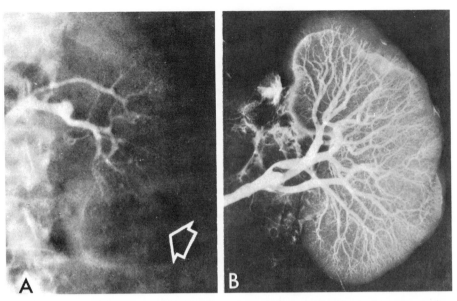

Fig. 20-60. Renal arteriograms in the hepatorenal syndrome. **A.** Renal arteriography during life shows decreased cortical perfusion and almost complete vasoconstriction of the interlobar and proximal arcuate arteries. **B.** Postmortem arteriogram shows a normal renal arterial system with uniform caliber of the arteries and normal cortical perfusion. (Epstein M et al: Am J Med 49:175, 1970)

patients with severe ascites and azotemia, it is al-most always severely reduced.[457] Plasma renin levels are elevated in cirrhotic patients with ascites, and the concentration of renin substrate (angiotensinogen), an α_2-globulin synthesized in the liver, is reduced, especially in patients with the HRS.[36,46] In renal perfusion experiments in dogs, reduced renin substrate was associated with decreased renal cortical blood flow, which can be reversed by repletion of this substance.[64] It has been suggested that failure of intrarenal angiotensin production may be responsible for the maldistribution of renal blood flow. This hypothesis requires critical investigation, since angiotensin II levels are increased in cirrhosis.

Based on the almost invariable association of ascites with the HRS, it has been proposed that the renal hemodynamic defect may be a consequence of increased abdominal and renal venous pressure.[707] It is well established that increased intra-abdominal pressure impairs renal function.[90] Increased intra-abdominal pressure in experimental animals and in humans causes decreased GFR and RPF, sodium conservation, and oliguria. Superficially, this pattern is not unlike the HRS, in which tense ascites is associated with similar hemodynamic and urinary changes.[621,707] However, the inferior vena caval pressure is increased in cirrhosis *with or without ascites,* although more commonly in the former, and is associated with impairment of renal function, which appears to be independent of the presence or absence of ascites. The increase in vena caval pressure has been attributed to in-

trahepatic compression of the inferior vena cava.[621] Others have shown that ascites *per se* can cause reversible compression of the inferior vena cava at the level of the diaphragm.[742,800]

This concept is supported by the observations that the renal hemodynamic alterations of cirrhosis were reversed by paracentesis.[344] Prompt and transient improvement in GFR and RPF and an increase in the filtration fraction, associated with decreased intra-abdominal and renal venous pressure and an increment in plasma volume and cardiac output, were noted. Other investigators reported a prompt increase in cardiac output after small paracenteses, but large paracenteses were associated with decreased cardiac output, presumably with reduction of plasma volume caused by the loss of plasma into the peritoneal cavity.[469]

The association of hepatic parenchymal failure and the HRS is almost entirely inferential. It is based largely on the observation that most patients with functional renal failure have jaundice and abnormal liver function indicative of hepatic parenchymal injury.[673,859] Furthermore, the occasional patient who recovers often shows simultaneous improvement in liver function.

A second reason for the association is the occurrence of "cholemic nephrosis" in patients who die of the HRS. At autopsy the typical renal lesion of bile nephrosis is characterized by intense staining of the epithelium of Bowman's capsule and of the proximal convoluted tubules and pigment casts in the tubular lumen of the lower nephron.[722] This histologic lesion, however, is seen in cholestasis of any type, appears to reflect the degree and duration of the jaundice, and is not normally associated with renal dysfunction.

It is almost an irresistible temptation to attribute the HRS to vasoactive substances that are either produced by the injured liver or not removed from the circulation by the liver. These substances include renin–angiotensin, prostaglandins, kinins, endotoxins, vasoactive intestinal peptide, and the vasoexcitor and vasodepressor substances postulated by Shorr.[866]

Renin-Angiotensin. This system is important in the control of blood pressure and in sodium homeostasis via aldosterone. Both aspects play roles in ascites formation and, by extrapolation, in the pathogenesis of the HRS. Renin is produced primarily in the renal cortex by specialized cells in the juxtaglomerular apparatus. It catalyzes the conversion of circulating renin substrate (angiotensinogen) to angiotensin I. Angiotensin I, in turn, is converted to angiotensin II, the most active endogenous vasoconstrictor substance known. It stimulates target organs in the lung (systemic effects) in the zona glomerulosa of the adrenal gland (aldosterone), and in the kidney (glomerular perfusion and volume of extracellular water). Both renin and aldosterone are degraded in the liver, the former to a much lesser degree than the latter. The renin–angiotensin–aldosterone axis is acutely activated by experimental obstruction of hepatic venous outflow,[653] and in cirrhotic patients plasma renin activity appears to be linearly related to the portal pressure.[84] Plasma renin activity, angiotensin II, and plasma aldosterone levels are all increased in cirrhotic patients with ascites.[824,851] There is an inverse relationship between elevated plasma renin activity (and concentration) and plasma renin substrate.[579] Renin substrate has been shown to be lower in renal venous blood than in arterial blood in the HRS, presumably because of its active conversion to angiotensin II.[1026]

The key to the HRS is the persistent hyperreninemia. Whether the persistence of high renin activity is a result of decreased effective plasma volume, increased portal pressure, or decreased feedback inhibition by angiotensin II is not clear. It is clear that spontaneous diuresis is usually accompanied by reduction in plasma renin and aldosterone levels.[790] Furthermore, plasma renin activity and aldosterone levels decrease after peritoneovenous shunts for ascites and for the HRS[64,79,841,996] and after side-to-side portacaval anastomoses,[840] both of which can mobilize ascites and reverse the HRS.

Prostaglandins. To elucidate the role of prostaglandins in the HRS would require a book—a book of speculation. Prostaglandins are into everything, and it is difficult to know whether prostaglandin-associated actions are primary prostaglandin effects, direct or indirect, or are secondary prostaglandin effects induced by other systems. Stimulation of the renin–angiotensin, kallikrein, and sympathetic nervous systems activates prostaglandins, which seem to serve as jack-of-all-trade, secondary messengers.

One study deals specifically with the role of prostaglandins in the HRS.[88] These investigators reasoned that since renal vasoconstriction is a primary aspect of the HRS and since prostaglandins E are potent intrarenal vasodilators, that increased prostaglandins might be a compensatory, beneficial response. Indeed, their studies, in which indomethacin (a potent inhibitor of prostaglandin synthetase) was given to cirrhotic patients, confirmed this hypothesis. Indomethacin appeared to induce a reasonable facsimile of the HRS. There was a decrease in effective renal plasma flow and creatinine clearance and an increase in serum creatinine levels. Surprisingly, plasma renin activity was decreased by indomethacin. All of these changes were reversed by infusions of prostaglandin A_1. These observations indicate that prostaglandins may play an impor-tant protective role in cirrhotic patients.[102] In a practical sense, they show that indomethacin and aspirin, another inhibitor of prostaglandin synthetase, are contraindicated in ascitic, cirrhotic patients.

Kallikrein–Kinin. Although bradykinin, the most potent endogenous vasodilator known, and related polypeptides are active in a variety of physiologic processes, their exact role in any system is not known. In normal subjects, plasma bradykinin levels respond in parallel with plasma renin and angiotensin II in response to sodium restriction or administration. In the HRS both plasma prekallikrein and bradykinin are greatly reduced.[693,1039] In addition, the kallikrein–kinin system may be modulated by prostaglandins. The normal interactions and interrelationships between these potent vasoactive systems are unknown, to say nothing of their possible perturbations in the HRS.

Endotoxins. These lipopolysaccharide components of the cell walls of gram-negative bacteria have been implicated in the HRS because of their potent renal vasoconstrictive properties. Absorbed into the portal venous blood, these substances are normally removed by the reticuloendothelial tissues of the liver but in cirrhosis may enter the systemic blood. About three fourths of patients with the HRS and 100% of those with acute tubular necrosis have endotoxins in the blood, compared with only 10% of cirrhotic patients without the HRS.[1026] The similarity of some aspects of the HRS with overwhelming sepsis gives seat-of-the-pants support for a relationship between endotoxins and the HRS, but inexplicable observations on regional vagaries of the presence or absence of endotoxins[936] leave the primary questions unanswered. Wilkinson and co-workers have suggested that the renal vasoconstriction of the HRS may be initiated by endotoxins and perpetuated by renin–angiotensin dysfunction.[1026]

Metabolic Abnormalities

Advanced cirrhosis is characterized by a number of metabolic abnormalities, which, when severe, may cause serious, even fatal, consequences and when mild, may predispose the patient to many other derangements including the HRS.

Hyponatremia. Reduced plasma concentrations of sodium, which are common in cirrhosis, may be dilutional, associated with increased antidiuretic activity, or may be due to sodium depletion caused by diuretics, diarrhea, or other abnormalities. The latter type is a profound disturbance of fluid balance, the major manifestation of which is decreased plasma volume, which results from a shift of water from the extracellular to the intracellular compartment to maintain isotonicity.[1015] It is characterized by azotemia, oliguria, decreased urinary sodium excretion, and may mimic completely the HRS. If not recognized as a reversible abnormality, it may remain uncorrected and end fatally.

Hypokalemia and Metabolic Alkalosis. Inseparably intertwined, hypokalemia and metabolic alkalosis are almost always present in cirrhosis, especially alcoholic cirrhosis.[127,630] The potassium deficit, which results from decreased dietary intake, vomiting, diarrhea, secondary aldosteronism, and diuretics, and which is aggravated by hypokalemia itself, may be enormous. When severe it may impair renal tubular concentrating ability and lead to dehydration, another syndrome that in the decompensated cirrhotic patient may be easily and erroneously mistaken for the HRS. The effect of increased arterial pH and of an increased pH gradient between the extracellular and intracellular fluids on ammonia, amines, or other substances that may affect renal hemodynamics is unknown.

Oxygen Desaturation. Almost always found in advanced cirrhosis,[784] oxygen desaturation has been attributed to right-to-left shunting of blood either through pulmonary arteriovenous anastomoses[142] or through portal-to-pulmonary venous shunts.[116] Although renal oxygen consumption was not significantly reduced in cirrhotic patients, there are suggestions that renal hypoxia may exist.

Portal-Systemic Shunting. Shunting may play a role in the pathogenesis of the HRS. In cirrhosis collateral veins carry portal blood around and through the liver and thus bypass hepatic extraction. Ammonia intolerance can be used as a rough index of the degree of such shunting.[162] This shunting mechanism is the basis for portal-systemic encephalopathy, which itself very commonly precedes or accompanies the development of the HRS. It is intriguing that the experimental infusion of ammonia into the renal artery causes prompt reduction in the GFR.[1019] Amines, which are also derived from bacterial action in the gut and which may also escape hepatic inactivation, have been implicated in the pathogenesis of both hepatic coma[278] and the HRS.[280] Vasoactive intestinal peptide, a polypeptide derived from the gut and, therefore, circumhepatically shuntable, has been shown to have potent properties and simulate some of the hemodynamic abnormalities of cirrhosis, including peripheral vasodilation, increased cardiac output, pulmonary right-to-left shunting, and hyperventilation.[813] Although portal-systemic shunting may play a

role in the pathogenesis of the HRS, it is obviously not the *sine qua non* of the syndrome, since portacaval anastomoses have reversed this disorder.[840]

Recovery from Advanced Hepatorenal Syndrome

It is generally agreed that very few patients with far-advanced HRS survive. Four patients were considered to have had spontaneous recoveries.[336] We have observed several recoveries, after cortisone administration, after portacaval shunt, after expansion of plasma volume, after implantation of peritoneovenous shunts, and spontaneously. Other spontaneous or "induced" recoveries have been reported occasionally. Some of the patients who recovered from "HRS" almost certainly represent cases of prerenal azotemia.

Treatment

Rational treatment of the HRS must be based on an understanding of the pathogenesis of the disease. Since our knowledge about the pathogenesis is anecdotal, inferential, and incomplete, we are forced to treat it in a pragmatic way. Thus, therapy may be considered to fall into four general categories.

1. Correction of those reversible uremic abnormalities that may be causing a pseudohepatorenal syndrome.
2. Provision of general supportive therapy.
3. Specific treatment of those features that may be pathogenetically related to the disorder.
4. When all else has failed, empiric measures, which have been sporadically employed successfully by others, may be tried.

Treatment of Reversible Uremic States. The practical principles of reversing reversible uremia have been beautifully outlined.[251] A number of reversible prerenal disorders such as urinary tract infection or obstruction, dehydration, hyponatremia, or hypokalemia may simulate or precipitate the HRS and should be corrected.

Supportive General Therapy includes the administration of appropriate amounts and types of fluids and electrolytes, low dietary protein and round-the-clock carbohydrate, the treatment or prevention of PSE, and cessation of any precipitating drug or disorder. Hypotension due to bleeding, dehydration, arrhythmia, or similar causes should be treated by eliminating the primary disorder. Anemia should be corrected. Any drugs that might adversely affect cardiac output or renal hemodynamics should be stopped, and no medication should be administered unless the indications are clear. Peritoneal or renal dialysis should be considered if a *reversible* precipitating cause of the HRS is known or suspected. These include correction of hyperkalemia, encephalopathy attributed to uremic toxins, acidosis, fluid overload, or elevated levels of dialyzable toxins.[682]

Specific Therapeutic Measures. Attempts to increase the effective plasma volume by *plasma volume expansion* have been made by a number of investigators. In more than one third of these patients the administration of dextran, albumin, or ascitic fluid has been associated with transient improvement in urine output and in some of the derangements of hemodynamic function. Volume-expansion therapy appears clearly beneficial in patients with plasma volume depletion. It would appear reasonable to try plasma expansion in all patients if measurements of plasma volume or cardiac output are not available and to continue it in those patients who respond.

Over a hundred years ago Flint noted increased urine output in some patients after *paracentesis.*[289] It seems clear that paracentesis may be associated transiently with an increase in cardiac output and plasma volume[344,469,476] in some patients. Whether paracentesis is beneficial by virtue of relieving compression of the inferior vena cava and thus increasing venous return, or by decreasing intra-abdominal and renal venous pressure or some other mechanism is not clear, but the potential benefits are apparent. Some observations suggest that small paracenteses of 500 ml provide optimal responses,[469] and daily paracenteses of this volume may be a rational basis of therapy.

Since both *paracentesis* and *plasma volume expansion* may work in the same or similar ways, combination of the two procedures is a logical step. Expansion of plasma volume guarantees prevention of volume constriction, which sometimes follows large paracenteses. Ascites reinfusion is probably the simplest and certainly the cheapest way of combining these therapies. Paracentesis combined with albumin infusions is an alternative way of accomplishing the same goals. Ascites reinfusion is a difficult procedure to maintain and can be used only for short periods. In those patients with the HRS in whom ascites reinfusion appears promising, placement of a peritoneovenous shunt seems justified. Reversal of the HRS has been reported in a small number of patients so treated[306,354,480,517,714,840] (Fig. 20-61), and this form of therapy deserves critical evaluation.

A number of *pharmacologic agents* have been used in attempts to correct or improve the altered renal hemodynamics. Octopressin appears to have the most promise. This synthetic phenylalanine lysine vasopressin (PLV-2) retains the pressor effects of vasopressin but has little or no antidiuretic activity. PLV-2 in small doses in humans causes a decrease in renal vascular resistance, an increase in RPF,[158] and dramatic transient improvement in patients with the HRS. In compensated cirrhosis, however, the changes induced by octopressin were not nearly so impressive.[459] This substance, which appears to correct specifically the renal hemodynamic disorder of cirrhosis, requires careful and critical clinical evaluation before its usefulness can be assessed.

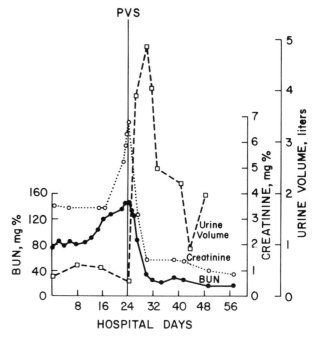

Fig. 20-61. Reversal of the hepatorenal syndrome after peritoneovenous shunt. On the 24th hospital day, when BUN and creatinine were increasing and urine output was decreasing, a LeVeen shunt was implanted. There was an enormous increase in urinary volume accompanied by a dramatic decrease in BUN, creatinine, and weight. (Pladson TR, Parrish RM: Arch Intern Med 137:1248, 1977. Copyright 1977, American Medical Association)

Several other drugs, including dibenzyline,[39] metaraminol,[46] dopamine,[46] and L-dopa, which may have some promise, have been used, but in each case the improvement was partial or transient.

The following agents have been reported to be of no value and of some potential harm; acetylcholine, phentolamine, papavarine, aminophylline, regitine, mannitol, angiotensin, and isoproteranol.

Portacaval anastomosis has resulted in dramatic recovery of patients with terminal HRS[840,841] (Fig. 20-62). Similar observations have been made after splenorenal shunt.[276] On the other hand, the HRS, or an indistinguishable syndrome, has been reported after end-to-side portacaval anastomosis, but only in the presence of ascites.[157] It should be kept in mind that these were end-to-side portacaval anastomoses, which decompress esophageal varices but do not necessarily reduce intrahepatic pressure or eliminate ascites (see Fig. 20-53). Clearly, if portal-systemic shunts are performed to relieve the HRS, they must be side-to-side in type. Portal decompressive therapy of the HRS deserves prospective, controlled investigative evaluation. Obviously, it can be considered

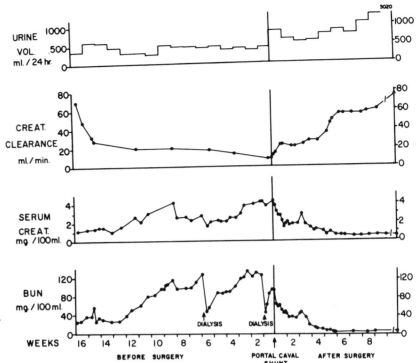

Fig. 20-62. Reversal of hepatorenal syndrome after portacaval anastomosis. Before PCA the patient had persistent oliguria, decreasing creatinine clearance, and increasing BUN and serum creatinine concentrations. All measures of renal function promptly improved after side-to-side PCA. (Schroeder et al: Ann Intern Med 72:923, 1970)

only in those patients in whom liver function is good enough to tolerate major surgery, and in whom less drastic forms of therapy have failed.

Adrenocortical steroids have been used empirically in the HRS, as in most other serious diseases, with retrospectively devised rationales and disappointing results.

Spontaneous Bacterial Peritonitis and Other Infections

Within the past 50 years, a hitherto rarely recognized complication of portal hypertension has appeared and taken a prominent place in our repertoire of complications of portal hypertension. Spontaneous bacterial peritonitis (SBP) is a syndrome that incorporates into its pathophysiology the basic hemodynamic abnormalities of portal hypertension. The first recorded victim of this disorder, diagnosed retrospectively, appears to have been Ludwig von Beethoven.[202] In the late 1950s Caroli and Platteborse found unexplained bacterial peritonitis in five patients with coliform septicemia.[125] In the mid-1960s Kerr and colleagues[452] and Conn[161] independently reported series of patients with this syndrome.

Clinical Presentation

Classic SBP is characterized by the abrupt onset of fever, chills, abdominal pain with rebound tenderness, absent bowel sounds, and leukocytosis. Paracentesis reveals cloudy ascitic fluid with many white blood cells, predominantly polymorphonuclear leukocytes, and acidified ascitic fluid. A single organism, usually enteric, is cultured from the ascitic fluid. The same organism is often recovered from the blood. Most of the patients die, many of the infection *per se*, others of its complications, and some from other hazards of cirrhosis such as bleeding varices or the HRS.

Although at first this syndrome was greeted with skepticism, sizable series of patients have been reported around the world.[181,202,209,709,818,1011] At the Veterans Administration Hospital in West Haven, Connecticut, alone, more than 140 bacteriologically proven cases have been seen (Fig. 20-63), involving approximately 10% of the cirrhotic patients with ascites. In other series the percentage of cirrhotic patients who develop SBP ranges from 3% to 30%.[273a,709,818]

This syndrome, which at first appeared to be a disorder of alcoholic cirrhosis, has been reported in posthepatitic cirrhosis[257] and in chronic active hepatitis.[1043] Individual cases have been reported in primary biliary cirrhosis,[202] hemochromatosis, cardiac cirrhosis,[805] viral hepatitis,[947] AAT deficiency,[492] pregnancy,[916] and in myeloid metaplasia[574] and myelofibrosis. Similar syndromes occur in patients with the nephrotic syndrome,[295,666] in cryptogenic cirrhosis, disseminated lupus erythematosus,[537] malignant ascites,[408] although very rarely,[485] and in patients with

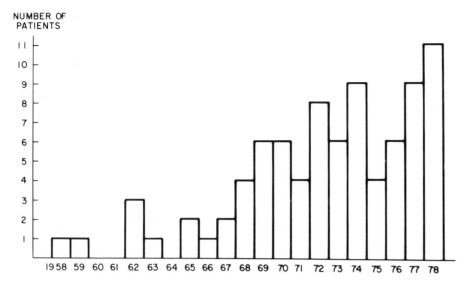

NUMBER OF
PATIENTS

Fig. 20-63. Increasing frequency of spontaneous bacterial peritonitis at a single hospital. During the period from 1958 to 1978, the number of patients with bacteriologically proven SBP has increased disproportionately to the number of patients admitted to the West Haven Veterans Administration Medical Center.

LeVeen shunts,[1041] ventriculoperitoneal shunts,[397] and chronic ambulatory peritoneal dialysis.[270]

The full-blown syndrome need not be present, and any one or all of its components may be missing (Fig. 20-64). The disease may be completely silent and discovered fortuitously. It may present as fever of unknown origin or as hypothermia with rectal temperatures below 96°F (35.5°C). Sometimes it emerges as encephalopathy of uncertain cause. Unexplained fever, hypothermia, hypotension, encephalopathy, or abdominal pain, or simply unexplained clinical deterioration should be considered indications for diagnostic paracentesis in ascitic cirrhotic patients.

Bacteria other than enteric types have been recovered from the ascitic fluid. Although approximately three fourths of the organisms isolated are enteric, the remainder are nonintestinal in origin (Fig. 20-65). A broad spectrum of organisms has been recovered and a flood of recent papers has described bacteria previously not incriminated in this syndrome, including meningococci, *Clostridia, Listeria, Pasteurella, Hemophilus, Pseudomonas, Arizonia, Campylobacter, Yersimia, Vibrio, Capnocytophaga* species and *Neisseria gonorrhoeae* (Table 20-17).[44,818,914,919] Although 90% of patients have single species isolated, multiple organisms have been recovered, especially in patients who are receiving vasopressin infusions that may compromise the intestinal barrier to bacteria and permit enteric species to escape.[43] In about 20% of cases of SBP the cultures are negative.[807]

Fig. 20-64. Frequency of signs and symptoms among 82 cirrhotic patients with SBP. (Vinel JP, Conn HO: Unpublished observations)

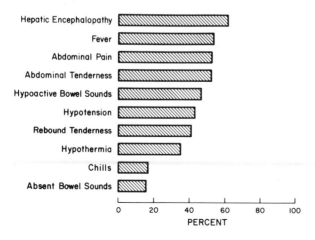

Fig. 20-65. Distribution of bacteria in *spontaneous bacterial peritonitis.* The major species of organisms isolated are shown, as is the breakdown of enteric and nonenteric organisms recovered.

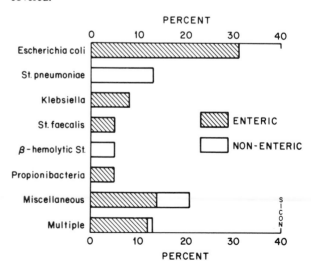

TABLE 20-17. Bacteria Isolated in Spontaneous Bacterial Peritonitis

Escherichia coli	*Streptococcus pneumoniae*
Klebsiella pneumoniae	*Streptococcus faecalis*
Proteus morgani	*Streptococcus viridans*
Proteus mirabilis	β-hemolytic streptococcus
Proteus freundii	γ-hemolytic streptococcus
Salmonella	Peptostreptococcus
Citrobacter species	*Streptococcus mitis*
Campylobacter jejuni	*Streptococcus sanguis*
Campylobacter fetus	*Streptococcus milleri*
Arizona hinshawii	*Staphylococcus aureus*
Yersinia enterocolitica	*Neisseria perflava*
Yersinia	*Neisseria meningitidis*
pseudotuberculosis	
Aeromonas liquefaciens	Propionibacteria
Clostridium perfringens	
Enterobacter cloaca	*Clostridium tertium*
	Bacteroides fragilis
Pseudomonas aeruginosa	Unidentified Group II-K$_2$
Pseudomonas	species
paucimobilis	
Hemophilus influenzae	*Candida albicans*
Listeria monocytogenes	*Chlamydia trachomatis*
Acinetobacter	
calcoaceticus	
Pasteurella multoceda	
Serratia marcescens	

Pathogenesis

The most important aspect of SBP is the insight it provides into the handling of bacterial infection by the liver, but it also furnishes clues about nonhepatic factors in the pathogenesis of bacteremia. Humoral antibody production in the cirrhotic patient is not impaired; it is at least normal and perhaps exuberant.[77] Although there is some evidence to indicate that the destruction of blood-borne bacteria by the reticuloendothelial system of the liver is deficient, the major defect in the handling of bacteria in cirrhotic patients is the presence of portal-systemic collateral vessels, which divert blood around and through the liver without passing through the hepatic reticuloendothelial filter. Other authors have demonstrated that intrahepatic anastomoses between hepatic arteries and portal veins and between portal and hepatic veins exist. Such portal-systemic shunts have been shown to diminish greatly the hepatic clearance of ammonia and other substances absorbed from the gastrointestinal tract.[303] These shunts are probably responsible for the decreased extraction of particulate matter by the liver of cirrhotic patients.[130] Presumably, these portal-systemic anastomoses permit circulating bacteria to bypass the hepatic reticuloendothelial filtering system, which has been shown to be a major site of removal of bacteria from the blood.[56] Decreased hepatic removal of circulating bacteria tends to perpetuate bac-

teremia and thus affords circulating organisms a greater opportunity to cause metastatic infections at susceptible sites such as ascitic collections. These speculations have been beautifully proved in patients with alcoholic cirrhosis.[777] It has been demonstrated that cirrhotic patients have an increased incidence of infections including SBP, bacteremia, and urinary tract infections. Furthermore, those patients who had decreased reticuloendothelial clearance of ^{99m}Tc sulfur colloid from the plasma suffered more bacterial infections than those who exhibited normal clearance. The size of the sulfur colloid particles is approximately the same as bacteria.

Ascites appears to be a critical part of this syndrome. The very abnormalities that cause portal hypertension and induce the development of portal collateral circulation are also important in formation of ascites. Spontaneous peritonitis in the absence of ascites probably does not occur. A few cases of "nonascitic" SBP have been reported but usually exhibit ascites later, suggesting that the ascitic fluid was inapparent rather than absent. The relative importance of ascites and of the circumhepatic shunting of blood may be estimated by considering patients with portacaval anastomosis. One might expect spontaneous peritonitis to be especially common in patients with portacaval anastomosis in whom portal-systemic shunting is total. On the other hand, patients with portacaval anastomosis are usually free of ascites because the shunt decreases the portal pressure. We have observed spontaneous peritonitis in several patients with portacaval anastomoses and ascites, but never in patients with patent portacaval anastomosis in the absence of ascites. Thus, ascites appears to be the *sine qua non* of this syndrome.

Ascitic fluid is a hospitable medium for bacteria. The peritoneal cavity is a moist, warm, dark environment, conditions that favor bacterial growth. Since phagocytes engulf bacteria in fluid accumulations by trapping them against a surface, the ratio of fluid to surface area is large and makes the ingestion of bacteria inefficient. Furthermore, several studies have shown the opsonification, the process of coating the surface of the organisms with IgG or the third component of complement, is essential to phagocytosis.[305,1048] The opsonic index of cirrhotic ascitic fluid has been shown to be decreased.[7,873] The concentrations of the third and fourth components of complement, which exist in normal peritoneal fluid at about half the concentration in serum, are found in cirrhotic ascites at half the level found in normal peritoneal fluid.[7,873] Thus decreased levels of complement appear to render cirrhotic patients especially susceptible to the development of SBP. It has also been shown that the protein concentration of ascitic fluid is lower in cirrhotic patients who develop SBP than in those who do not, and that there is a close correlation between opsonic activity and the protein and complement concentrations (Fig. 20-66).[806,809] Patients with ascitic fluid protein levels less than 1 g/dl are at increased risk of developing SBP. It has been noted that the protein concentration of ascitic fluid increases during diuresis.[393] If complement levels also increase with diuresis,

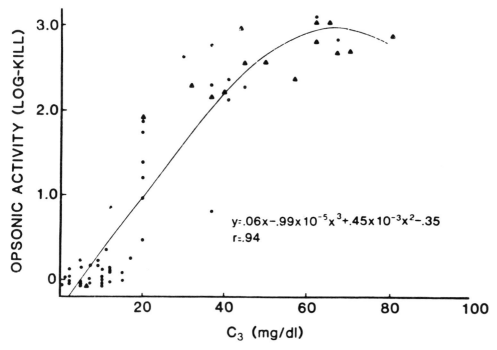

$$y = .06x - .99 \times 10^{-5} x^3 + .45 \times 10^{-3} x^2 - .35$$
$$r = .94$$

Fig. 20-66. Correlation between the opsonic activity of ascitic fluid and the concentration of complement (C3) in the ascitic fluid. Noncirrhotic patients are indicated by solid triangles and cirrhotic patients by solid dots. A close correlation is observed. (Reproduced with permission from Runyon BA et al: Hepatology 5:634, 1985)

as they appear to do, diuretic therapy may help prevent the development of SBP.[810]

One of the most surprising aspects of SBP is that a single species of bacteria causes the infection in virtually all instances. This indicates that the ascitic fluid is either infected by a single species or that a number of different bacteria invade the ascites but only one survives.

Another surprising aspect is that the number of bacteria in the ascitic fluid in SBP is extremely low,[432] ranging from 10 to 10,000 organisms/mm³. This is extremely low compared with urinary tract infections, in which less than 1,000,000 organisms/mm³ raises doubt about the diagnosis. Indeed, the small number of organisms may account for the frequent failure to obtain a positive culture in patients with clinically typical SBP. Larger volumes of ascitic fluid, about 30 ml, have been shown to increase the yield of positive cultures in SBP appreciably.[433]

For several reasons the hematogenous route appears to be the most reasonable mechanism to explain the spontaneous bacterial contamination of ascites. First, spontaneous bacteremia is a common event. Bacteremia occurs after the relatively mild trauma of teeth-brushing or food-chewing[624] or following massage of infected foci, such as furuncles,[775] or nonoperative instrumentation of the genitourinary tract.[731] Asymptomatic bacteremias have been found in association with menstrual periods and even in apparently healthy subjects, although enteric organisms were isolated only occasionally in these studies.

It is possible that portal bacteremias also occur spontaneously, but that the hepatic reticuloendothelial bacterial filter removes the organisms before they reach the systemic circulation. Normally the portal venous blood in humans is sterile,[833,939] but enteric bacteria can often be cultured from the portal blood and liver of dogs. In almost half the patients with ulcerative colitis, however, enteric bacteria can be recovered from the portal venous blood.[237] It may be assumed that portal bacteremia also occurs frequently with other disorders in which the intestinal mucosa is eroded. Manipulative examinations of the intestinal tract, either radiologic or endoscopic, or therapeutic enemas in PSE may precipitate the entry of bacteria into the bloodstream.

Bacteremia has been shown to occur after liver biopsy,[979] colonoscopy, sigmoidoscopy,[508] barium enema, rectal examination,[394] and endoscopic sclerotherapy.[154a] Indeed, in sclerotherapy it appears that the longer the injector needle the greater the risk of sclerotherapy-induced bacteremia.[885] Since many of these investigations were performed in noncirrhotic patients with normal hepatic bacterial clearance, the incidence and duration of bacteremia are minimal estimates. In cirrhotic patients with portal-systemic shunting, the incidence of bacteremia after any of these procedures must be higher. Conceivably, in cirrhotic patients, even defecation or the passage of flatus is a potentially catastrophic event.

Second, bacteremia provides a logical common pathway

for the great variety of bacteria and primary foci of infection encountered in patients with SBP. Other routes of infection, such as an unrecognized perforation of the intestinal or biliary tract, direct extension through the diaphragm or passage through the fallopian tubes,[100] however, must certainly occur. The majority of cases of SBP can be explained satisfactorily only by the common denominator of a bacteremia. For example, the occurrence of pneumococcal peritonitis in a patient with the same type of pneumococcal pneumonia, of β-streptococcal peritonitis in a patient with erysipelas, of meningococcal peritonitis in a patient with meningococcal meningitis[44] or of *Escherichia coli* peritonitis in a patient with a urinary tract infection caused by the same organism, all have in common a bacteremia. One might thus expect to see SBP caused by any organism that circulates in the blood of an ascitic patient. In principle, this concept is similar to the presumed pathogenesis of bacterial endocarditis. Indeed, it has been shown in a retrospective investigation that the prevalence of bacterial endocarditis is two to three times higher in cirrhotic than in noncirrhotic patients.[890] Furthermore, rheumatic and congenital valvular disease occurs in cirrhotic patients. Fewer γ-hemolytic streptococci and frequent enteric bacteria are characteristic of cirrhotic bacterial endocarditis. One group from an area where rheumatic heart disease is uncommon has failed to confirm the association between bacterial endocarditis and cirrhosis.[222]

Other susceptible sites apparently exist in cirrhotic patients. Spontaneous bacterial empyema,[286] spontaneous bacterial meningitis,[44] spontaneous bacterial arthritis[688] and spontaneous bacterial pericarditis[623] have all been reported in cirrhotic patients.

Organisms can come directly from the gastrointestinal tract, from the bloodstream, from the lymphatics or, in females, from the genital tract. The rarest route is through the fallopian tubes.[100] This route of entry has been implicated to explain the predominance of girls with primary peritonitis.[571] It is conceivable that this route may have been responsible in some of the cirrhotic women.

It is essential that *spontaneous* bacterial peritonitis be differentiated from *nonspontaneous* bacterial peritonitis (NSBP).[806] Although both are lethal infections in cirrhotic patients with ascites, nonoperative management of a perforated viscus or the surgical treatment of SBP carries a very high mortality rate. Surprisingly, SBP outnumbers NSBP 10 to 1. During a 21-year period in which more than 90 patients with SBP were observed at our hospital, only 9 patients with NSBP were encountered.

Successful differential diagnosis can be based on rational clinical principles (Table 20-18). A perforation of a peptic ulcer is often preceded by a history of worsening peptic ulcer symptoms. A perforated appendix may follow a history of acute and/or recurrent right lower quadrant pain. Perforation of a colonic diverticulum, however, is often silent. Perforation of the alimentary tract, especially the upper portion, is usually accompanied by gas in the peritoneal cavity. Gas is never present in SBP. Upright and lateral decubitus films may help detect gas. Similarly the use of a carbonated beverage orally or a diatrizoate meglumine (Hypaque) enema may document the nonspontaneous nature of the peritonitis. In NSBP multiple organisms are usually found in the ascitic fluid, and examination of a Gram stain of the sediment may indicate that the lesion is perforative. Anaerobic organisms from the intestine are characteristic of bowel perforation and rare in SBP, but this information is not available from culture for 24 to 48 hours. The odor of the ascitic fluid, which is putrid in mixed and anaerobic infections, may help in this differentiation. The ascitic fluid leukocytosis

TABLE 20-18. Differential Diagnosis of Spontaneous Bacterial Peritonitis (SBP) from Nonspontaneous Bacterial Peritonitis (NSBP)

FEATURE	SBP	NSBP
History of gastrointestinal tract disease	Usually negative	Often positive
Abdominal examination	Rebound tenderness	Pain, rigid abdomen
Free air	Absent	Usually present
Appearance of fluid	Frequently clear	Cloudy to purulent
Polymorphonuclear leukocytes (PMNs)	500–10,000/mm^3	1,000–100,000/mm^3
Ascitic fluid *p*H	7.0–7.4	6.5–7.3
Ascitic fluid glucose	Same as blood glucose	Much lower than blood glucose
Arterial-ascitic fluid *p*H gradient	0.02–0.30	0.10–1.00
Number of species of bacteria	Single	Multiple
Anaerobic organisms	Rare	Usual
Smear of ascitic fluid	PMNs, single type of bacteria	PMNs, multiple types of bacteria, vegetable fibers, feces
Blood in ascitic fluid	Rare	Common
Gastrointestinal tract enzymes in ascitic fluid	Absent	May be present

should be greater with perforations than with SBP. Leukocyte counts greater than 10,000/mm^3 should be viewed as NSBP until proven otherwise.[123,806]

Under certain conditions, bacteria may enter the peritoneal cavity by traversing the intact intestinal wall. Schweinburg and colleagues demonstrated that in dogs ^{14}C-labeled *E. coli* passed from the bowel into the peritoneal cavity after the introduction of hypertonic solutions into the peritoneum.[847] A similar mechanism may explain some of the enteric bacterial peritonitis that frequently complicates patients undergoing peritoneal dialysis. Clearly, this seems to be the mechanism of vasopressin-induced SBP.[43]

These hypotheses are based on the assumption that the intestinal mucosal barrier against the escape of bacteria in cirrhosis is normal. In fact, it may not be normal. Several abnormalities peculiar to decompensated cirrhosis may decrease local resistance of the intestinal mucosa to bacterial invasion. First, in patients with decompensated portal hypertension, the splanchnic veins and lymphatics are congested. Fluid retention associated with portal hypertension is not limited to the presence of ascites, but may cause edema of all splanchnic tissues, thus affecting adversely the mucosal barrier to bacterial invasion. Consequently, the bowel wall is edematous and often inflamed, and the intestinal mucosa is frequently severely degenerated.[26] Second, diarrhea is frequently present in cirrhosis.[747] Although there is no characteristic intestinal lesion associated with cirrhotic diarrhea, underlying mucosal inflammation or secondary irritation may alter the permeability of the mucosal barrier. Qualitative and quantitative abnormalities in the distribution of bacteria in the intestinal tract exist in cirrhosis.[290]

The lymphatic system may play an important role in the pathogenesis of SBP, and several areas of the lymphatic system may be involved. The engorged intestinal lymphatic system is the prime suspect.[37] Many more bacteria are carried from an infected site by lymphatics than by the bloodstream.[128] When bacteria penetrate the intestinal mucosa into the submucosal tissues, the intestinal lymphatics carry them to the major lymphatic channels and eventually into the the systemic circulation. In the ascitic cirrhotic patient both the hepatic and splanchnic lymphatics are distended and hypertrophied, and thoracic duct lymph flow, which is derived almost entirely from the hepatic and splanchnic beds, is greatly increased.[235]

It is possible that the hepatic lymphatics themselves may be involved in the pathogenesis of this syndrome. Hepatic lymph is the key to the formation of ascites. In cirrhotic patients with hepatic venous outflow obstruction[399] or in experimental animals with hepatic venous or superior vena caval obstruction, the production of hepatic lymph is increased, resulting in the formation of ascites, due largely to the exudation of hepatic lymph directly into the peritoneal cavity. In ascitic patients with bacteremia, organisms removed from the circulation by the liver may contaminate hepatic lymph and pass through the permeable lymphatic walls into the ascitic fluid. There

is, however, no experimental evidence to document the passage of bacteria from hepatic blood or reticuloendothelial cells to the lymphatics or into the ascitic fluid.

Whether other factors set the stage for this syndrome is not known. Diarrhea itself may in some way alter the host–bacterial relationship. Diarrhea of diverse etiologies may cause alteration in both the types of bacteria and in the physical distribution of flora in the intestinal tract.[155,342] Even in acute, experimentally induced diarrhea in normal subjects, coliform organisms may appear as high as the duodenum, where they are not usually present, and may be replaced by enterobacteria as the dominant organisms of the stools.[343] Such alterations alone or in combination with the abnormal distribution of intestinal bacteria in cirrhosis might result in replacement of nonvirulent bacteria by invasive organisms.

Neomycin, too, appears guilty by association. Neomycin, by altering the ecologic balance or by injuring the mucosal membrane, may change the microbial permeability of the intestinal wall. Other factors such as the almost invariable alkalosis, potassium depletion, or the arterial oxygen desaturation of decompensated cirrhosis may subtly alter the delicate balance between the host and its parasites. The instillation of alkaline solutions into the duodenum of dogs, for example, may cause the appearance of enteric organisms in the thoracic duct.[26]

The distribution of bacteria in SBP (Fig. 21-65) deserves comment. Virulence of intestinal bacteria has been defined as the ability to invade the epithelial cell. Whether or not virulence is inherent in the bacteria themselves or is affected by resistance of the epithelial cell or both is not clear. *E. coli* have been the organisms most commonly responsible, exhibiting normal cultural characteristics and the expected antibiotic sensitivity spectra. No typing or special studies were done to determine whether they were particularly pathogenic species.

A variety of other aerobic, enteric organisms have been found in other patients. It is remarkable that anaerobic organisms to not play a greater role in SBP. They are frequently found in secondary peritonitis due, for example, to a ruptured appendix or diverticulum. Obligative anaerobic bacteria, which make up the large bulk of the intestinal flora,[229,341] and particularly *Bacteroides,* which is the most common species in the feces of both normal and cirrhotic subjects, have been recovered in only a few patients with SBP in whom a special pathogenesis has been postulated.[43] Whether anaerobic organisms do not escape from the intact intestinal lumen, do not survive transit in the bloodstream, or do not grow well in large volumes of ascites is not known. It has been shown that normal peritoneal fluid has antimicrobial activity[61] and that cirrhotic ascitic fluid has potent antibacterial properties against gram-negative bacteria in general and *Bacteroides fragilis* in particular.[304] This inhibition may explain the infrequency of anaerobic infections in SBP.

The most common nonenteric organism recovered is the pneumococcus. The pneumococcus is, of course, a known pathogen that has, in addition to its pneumonia-genic properties, a special predilection for causing peritonitis in ascitic nephrotic[295] and cirrhotic patients[257] and also in nonascitic, noncirrhotic children.[571,666]

Epstein had observed pneumococcal SBP only in patients with posthepatitic cirrhosis.[257] An editorial that accompanied the report made a point of this association and the absence of reports of pneumococcal peritonitis in patients with alcoholic cirrhosis. Later observations indicate that the type of cirrhosis is not important in determining the species of the infecting organism.

Diagnosis

Since antibiotic therapy must be begun before the diagnosis of SBP can be established bacteriologically, it is necessary to use clinical and laboratory findings to make the diagnosis as early and accurately as possible.

Several groups of investigators have analyzed ascitic fluid to evaluate various conventional diagnostic determinants.[45,426,1029] It seems clear that gross appearance, specific gravity, and protein concentration of the fluid are not able to discriminate between infected and uninfected fluid although a low protein concentration is common in SBP. The number of leukocytes is the most reliable parameter. In the largest of these series—almost 400 patients—it was reported that the mean number of leukocytes in "normal," uninfected ascitic fluid was $281/mm^3$, but that in 5% it was above 1000. The leukocyte count was above $1000/mm^3$ in over 90% of patients with SBP. The granulocyte count was even more impressive; 97% of "normal" ascitic fluids had less than 500 PMN/mm^3 while 90% of patients with SBP had greater than 500. On the basis of these observations the following guidelines were devised.[45,426] Antibiotic therapy should be initiated whenever the clinical picture of SBP is present, regardless of the number of leukocytes in the ascitic fluid; whenever the number of polymorphonuclear leukocytes in the ascitic fluid is greater than $500/mm^3$ and the clinical picture is compatible with SBP (i.e., unexplained fever, encephalopathy, or abdominal pain); and whenever the number of granulocytes in the ascitic fluid is greater than $1000/mm^3$ even in the absence of any evidence of SBP. These recommendations are based on the premise that the ascitic fluid will be reexamined in 24 hours and that the antibiotic therapy will be discontinued or modified on the basis of the clinical, laboratory, and cultural findings.

Occasionally, periperitoneal inflammatory lesions such as cholecystitis or penetrating peptic ulcer may simulate SBP and may induce a sympathetic leukocytosis in the ascitic fluid.[368] Rarely, remote foci of infection may similarly give rise to a pseudo-SBP syndrome.[83]

Within the past 5 years it has been shown that metabolic changes induced by bacterial infections also provide diagnostic markers in the ascitic fluid. The metabolism of carbohydrate in the ascitic fluid by bacteria and/or by leukocytes increases the concentration of lactate[98] and other acids in the ascitic fluid and decreases the pH of the ascitic fluid.[330] Since the pH of arterial blood and that of ascitic fluid are identical or nearly so,[330] the arterial–ascitic fluid pH gradient (A–AFpHG) may be an important measurement. A number of investigators have undertaken studies to determine how accurate the ascitic fluid pH (AFpH) and A–AFpHG are in making the diagnosis of SBP, and to compare them with the ascitic fluid PMN (AFPMN) count.

Six trials have been published in which a total of 361 cirrhotic patients with sterile ascites were compared with 81 patients with bacteriologically proven SBP (Table 20-19).[30,320,710,829,915,1046]

In each of the six studies the AFPMN count was the most diagnostically accurate test. Ninety-eight percent of the patients with sterile ascites had less than 50 PMN/mm^3, whereas 86% of the patients with SBP had greater than 500 PMN/mm^3. In all six studies the A–AFpHG was slightly less accurate than the AFPMN and slightly more accurate than the AFpH. Ninety-nine percent of the uninfected patients had A–AFpHG less than 0.10, while 58% of those with SBP had gradients greater than 0.10. The A–AFpH was greater than 7.34 in 98% of the patients with sterile ascites and was less than 7.34 in 50% of those with SBP. These data indicate clearly that the PMN count in ascitic fluid is the most useful of the three laboratory tests. Its value is complemented by that of A–AFpHG and/or the AFpH. In patients in whom both the AFPMN and A–AFpHG are increased, the diagnosis is secure, and antibiotic treatment should be started promptly. If either is increased and the other normal, it is probable that the patient has SBP, but other disorders such as malignant or bloody ascites or tuberculous peritonitis should be excluded. Antibiotic therapy is advised during the period of diagnostic inquiry.

In addition, these studies demonstrated that malignant ascites with neoplastic cells in the ascitic fluid or bloody ascites or tuberculous peritonitis often exhibits decreased AFpH and increased A–AFpHG (and, often, increased ascitic fluid lactate and decreased ascitic fluid glucose levels), although the AFPMN is only occasionally increased in these disorders.[320,915,1046]

Treatment

Treatment of the full-blown syndrome must be prompt and vigorous. Antibiotics are, of course, the cornerstone of therapy. As in gram-negative sepsis, antibiotics must often be selected and administered on the basis of the clinical picture before the precise nature of the infecting organism and its antibiotic sensitivities are known. In half the cases, careful examination of the gram-stained ascitic fluid will provide morphologic information about the responsible organism that will be helpful in antibiotic selection. Similarly, smear of the buffy coat of the blood may provide a clue to the nature of the infectious agent. In the absence of any clinical or morphologic leads, the antibiotic program must be broad enough to cover the whole spectrum of possible bacteria. Conventional therapy is the combination of cephalothin or ampicillin and gen-

TABLE 20-19. Comparison of Studies of Ascitic Fluid Polymorphonuclear Leukocytes, *p*H, Arterial-Ascitic Fluid *p*H Gradient, and Lactate in Sterile, Ascitic Fluid and Spontaneous Bacterial Peritonitis

AUTHOR	NUMBER OF PATIENTS	AFPMN/mm^3		AFpH		A-AFpHG		AF LACTATE (mg%)	
		Mean	<500	Mean	<7.34	Mean	>0.10	Mean	<20
CONTROL SUBJECTS									
Attali	129	10	10/10	7.44	128/129*	0.02	128/129		
Garcia-Tsao	51	122	50/51	7.45	50/51†	0.02	50/51	15	50/51
Pinzello	54	102	52/54‡	7.41	52/54	0.02§	54/54	16	26/54‖
Scemama-Clergue	43	41	40/41	7.44	43/43	0.02	40/41		
Stassen	42	119	42/42	7.44	42/42	0.01	41/42	19	39/42#
Yang	42	41	39/42	7.50	40/42**	0.04	40/42	11	38/42††
Total	361	354/361 98%		355/361 98%		356/361 99%		153/189 81%	
SPONTANEOUS BACTERIAL PERITONITIS									
Attali	18	4,951	14/18	7.24	8/18*	0.21	12/18		
Garcia-Tsao	14	2,686	12/14	7.24	9/14†	0.22	9/14	45	9/14
Pinzello	18	7,247	18/18‡	7.30	8/18	0.12§	11/18	42	17/18‖
Scemama-Clergue	12	3,588	8/12	7.38	4/12	0.10	5/12		
Stassen	9	18,199	8/9	7.20	8/9	0.23	8/9	80	8/9#
Yang	10	9,522	10/10	7.34	3/10**	0.10	4/10	37	10/10††
Total	81	70/81 86%		42/81 52%		49/81 58%		44/51 86%	

* 7.32.
† 7.35.
‡ 450/mm^3.
§ 0.08.
‖ 15 mg/dl.
39 mg/dl.
** <7.31.
†† 25 mg/dl.
AFPMN, ascitic fluid polymorphonuclear leukocytes; AFpH, ascitic fluid *p*H; A-AFpHG, arterial-ascitic fluid *p*H gradient.

tamycin. The antibiotic program is made more specific as soon as the organism is identified and the antibiotic sensitivities are available. In addition, the treatment of shock and of PSE should be carried out promptly. Search for and treatment of any possible primary focus of infection demands immediate attention.

Because of the high prevalence of azotemia after the administration of aminoglycoside antibiotics,[115] to which cirrhotic patients are unusually susceptible, we prefer to use broad-spectrum cephalosporins such as cefotaxime sodium or mezlocillin sodium, which avoid the renal toxicity. A recent randomized trial has compared the effects of tobramycin plus ampicillin with cephotaxime in cirrhotic patients with serious infections.[269] Three-fourths of the patients had SBP, often with bacteremia. Although more than 90% of the bacteria isolated were sensitive to both antibiotic regimens, cefotaxime was more effective in curing those infections than tobramycin–ampicillin (85% vs 56%). Severe nephrotoxicity occurred in 8% of the patients treated with the aminoglycoside but was not seen in any of the patients treated with the cephalosporin.

This relatively low prevalence of aminoglycoside-induced nephrotoxicity may reflect the use of ampicillin rather than cephalothin, which is known to aggravate the renal toxicity of aminoglycoside antibiotics. Clearly, we have been shown the light and should take advantage of these results while awaiting confirmation.

When aminoglycosides are required, they should be used in smaller doses than are recommended, with careful monitoring of peak and trough plasma concentrations of the antibiotic and of the urinary excretion of β_2-microglobulin, which is an early laboratory sign of aminoglycoside toxicity.[115] Aminoglycosides should be stopped at the first sign of renal toxicity.

SBP, bacteremia, and other bacterial infections tend to occur in cirrhotic patients after gastrointestinal tract hemorrhage.[778] Oral aminoglycosides have been shown to be extremely effective in preventing these posthemorrhage infections.[778]

Several adjuncts to therapy may be considered. Although the antibiotic concentration of ascitic fluid, particularly in the presence of inflamed peritoneal surfaces, rapidly achieves bacteriocidal levels,[324] its equilibration is dependent on dosage, antibiotic binding, transport, and other factors. It is conceivable that there might be some advantage under special circumstances to administering a single initial dose of antibiotics directly into the ascitic fluid to achieve high antibiotic concentrations immediately. Bacitracin and other antibiotic agents are absorbed from the peritoneal cavity very rapidly and should be used with care, especially in patients with renal disease.

The concentration of antibiotics need not necessarily be the critical factor, however. We have observed patients in whom bacteria could still be recovered from the ascitic fluid after 2 or 3 days of appropriate dosage of antibiotics. In such a situation drainage of the infected ascitic fluid should be considered, just as one would drain a loculated abscess. Peritoneal lavage with an antibiotic solution, which has been recommended in the management of nonspontaneous peritonitis,[584] should also be considered.

In asymptomatic cases in which *bacterascites* is discovered, treatment may be postponed until the infecting organism is identified and its antibiotic sensitivities determined. Asymptomatic spontaneous bacterascites may represent an early stage in the development of SBP, or conceivably, a stalemate between the host and the parasite. Bacteria find ascitic fluid an optimal culture medium in

which the host defenses may have a handicap. The relatively low number of leukocytes found in the ascitic fluid of patients with SBP is surprising and may account, in part, for the difficulty in eradicating organisms from the ascitic fluid. The 500 PMNs to 10,000 PMNs/mm^3 seen in SBP are a small fraction of the number seen in the urinary tract infections or in abscesses. The bacteria may not be able to cause an acute peritonitis, but on the other hand, the host may not be able to eradicate them completely. Clinically silent bacterascites may persist until one or the other triumphs.

It is our experience, confirmed by others, that SBP is largely a nosocomial disease.[393] In the large majority of patients the syndrome develops at least one week after the patients are admitted to the hospital. The exact cause (or causes) is not known. Analysis of all of the procedures performed prior to the appearance of bacteriologically proven SBP in 82 cirrhotic patients and in 82 randomly selected cirrhotic patients with sterile ascites gave only a few clues (Fig. 20-67). The occurrence of recent bacterial infections was significantly more common in the SBP than in the uninfected group ($P < 0.02$). Similarly, diarrhea occurred much more frequently in those patients who had had sustained diarrhea ($P < 0.01$). Although many procedures other than those shown in Figure 20-68 had been

Fig. 20-67. Comparison of potential causes of bacteremia in 82 ascitic cirrhotic patients with SBP and in 82 ascitic cirrhotic patients with sterile ascites. Diarrhea had been present almost twice as frequently in those who developed SBP as in those who did not ($p < 0.01$). Recent bacterial infection had been more common among patients who developed SBP than among those who did not ($p < 0.02$). None of the other factors had occurred significantly more frequently among those who developed SBP, although the actual prevalence was usually higher among those who did when compared with those who did not. (Vinel JP, Conn HO: Unpublished observations)

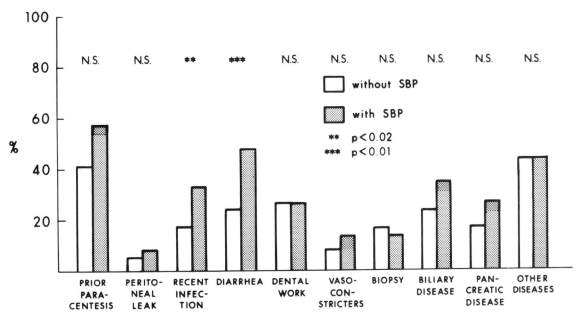

performed more frequently in the SBP group than in the non-SBP group, in none of them were the differences statistically significant.

Prophylactic therapy may prevent some instances of SBP. Certainly, patients with ascites should be considered relatively fragile and extremely susceptible to bacterial infections. Dental extractions should be postponed until the ascites is no longer present or, when this is impossible, should be performed after the institution of prophylactic antibiotics, just as one would do with a patient with rheumatic heart disease. Similarly, the drainage of abscesses, the placement of urinary or indwelling intravascular catheters, the performance of sigmoidoscopy, cystoscopy, and other potentially bacteremiagenic procedures should be avoided or performed after appropriate prophylactic antibiotic therapy has been begun.

The treatment of patients with cirrhosis and ascites can be devised to diminish the prevalence of SBP in several ways. First, SBP does not occur in the absence of ascites. Therefore, ascites should not be considered a cosmetic lesion, but rather a potential hazard that should be treated promptly and vigorously. Diuretic therapy may have the advantage over paracentesis or peritoneovenous shunts of concentrating the complement in the ascitic fluid, but these other therapies are often effective in their own right. Second, since 15% to 20% of SBP in cirrhotic patients is caused by the pneumococcus, it is logical that ascitic cir-

rhotic patients be vaccinated against pneumococci using polyvalent vaccine. Cirrhotic patients respond to pneumococcal vaccination with the development of high titers of effective antibody. Indeed, the prevalence of "primary" pneumococcal peritonitis in children with the nephrotic syndrome has been reduced by vaccination against pneumococci.[1023] Third, it may be possible to identify those patients who are most susceptible to the development of SBP by their failure to clear particulate material from their plasma normally[777] or perhaps by their low ascitic fluid protein concentration.[809] Such patients may well benefit from prophylactic antibiotics during their first 2 weeks in the hospital. Investigations of such prophylactic therapy are in progress.

Tuberculous peritonitis, which has a similar, but more indolent, clinical course, is not nearly so common as SBP. We observed only two instances of tuberculous peritonitis during the 25-year period during which we saw 140 cases of SBP. Almost half the cases of tuberculous peritonitis occur in patients with decompensated cirrhosis.[106] Although fever and abdominal pain are present, the course is usually less acute and dramatic. Most patients have evidence of active tuberculosis, primarily pulmonary. Peripheral blood leukocytosis is much less common than in SBP. The ascitic fluid leukocytes are predominantly lymphocytic rather than neutrophilic. The AFpH in tuberculous peritonitis is even lower than is seen in SBP, and

Fig. 20-68. Comparison of the frequency of common medical procedures in 82 ascitic cirrhotic patients with sterile ascites and 82 patients who developed SBP. Most of these varied procedures had been performed more frequently in the patients who subsequently developed SBP than in the control group, but none of the differences was statistically significant, except that SBP occurred less frequently in the group that had had intravenous infusions ($p < 0.01$). We believe this means that many procedures may contribute to bacteremia and to SBP but that no one procedure is primarily responsible. (Vinel JP, Conn HO: Unpublished observations)

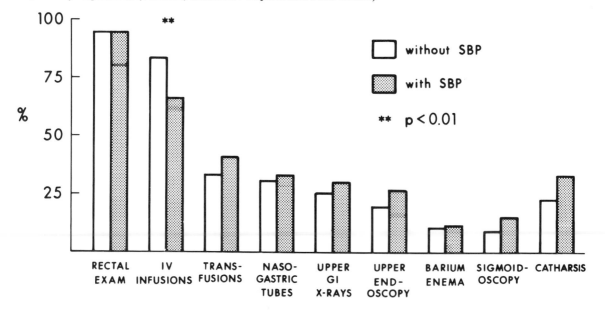

the ascitic fluid glucose concentration is frequently very low (<40 mg/dl). The pathogenesis of tuberculous peritonitis, however, may be similar to that of spontaneous, nontuberculous peritonitis. Although it may result from the direct entry into the peritoneal cavity of tubercle bacilli from lymph nodes, intestinal or genital tract in patients with active tuberculosis of these organs, it may also be disseminated hematogenously from remote foci of tuberculosis.

PROGNOSIS

It is difficult to make meaningful statements about the prognosis of cirrhosis unless its etiology, epidemiologic setting, clinical and laboratory manifestations, and histology are known, and unless the findings can be put into perspective by comparison with an appropriate control group.[32] Few studies provide all this information. Published series suggest that the 5-year survival may be as high as 90% in alcoholic cirrhosis in the absence of ascites, jaundice, hematemesis, or continued drinking,[730] and as low as 0% in patients with alcoholic cirrhosis who present with encephalopathy.[826] Intermediate 5-year survivals of 7%, 10%, and 19% are reported for patients with portal cirrhosis who present, respectively, with ascites, jaundice, and hematemesis.[747]

Surprisingly, the survival is reported to be higher for alcoholic cirrhosis than for nonalcoholic cirrhosis in some studies,[361,826,923] but others have found the opposite to be true.[318] On the other hand, abstinence appears to improve survival[683a,730,774,826] or has no apparent effect.[10,669,901] The effects of several factors such as alcohol consumption or abstinence and the presence or absence of esophageal varices are shown in Figure 20-69.

There is evidence from published papers that survival is also influenced by the patient's sex, although both males and females have had better survival in individual se-

Fig. 20-69. Effects of various factors on survival in alcoholic cirrhosis. **A.** Comparison of cumulative survival curves of two groups of cirrhotic patients 20 years apart showing poor survival[317,747] and three recent groups showing relative good prognosis.[730,901] The reasons for the differences are not known. **B.** Powell and Klatskin found continued alcoholic consumption associated with poor prognosis.[730] **C.** Soterakis and associates found no difference between those patients who abstained and those who continued to drink.[901] **D.** We found that the prognosis of cirrhotic patients without varices was better than those with varices. The slopes were parallel, however, and suggest that the two groups represented different degrees of advancement of the cirrhotic process.

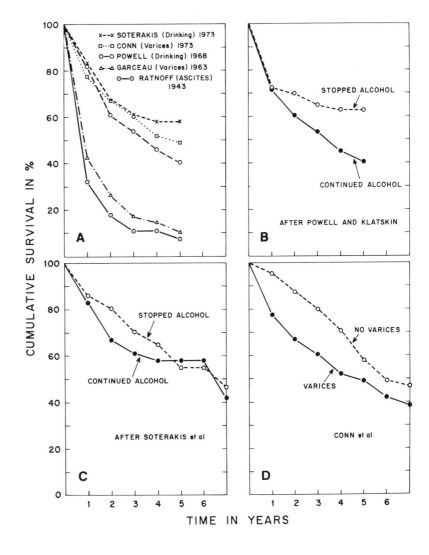

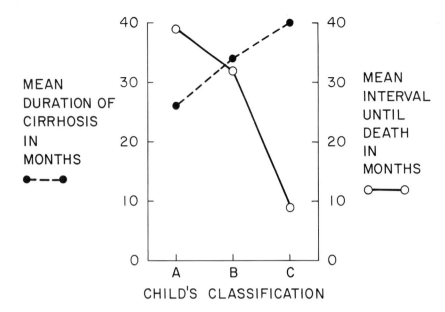

Fig. 20-70. The association of Child–Turcotte classification and survival. Child's classification is shown on the abscissa and time in months on the ordinates. On the left ordinate is plotted the mean interval between the clinical onset of cirrhosis and the time of classification (*open circles, dotted line*). The duration of cirrhosis increases as the severity of cirrhosis increases, that is, it takes longer to become Child's Class C than it does B. On the right ordinate is plotted the interval between classification and death (*open circles, solid line*). Survival is shortest for Class C patients (mean 8 months), longest for Class A patients (mean 39 months), and intermediate for Class B patients (32 months).

ries,[312a,318] race (higher mortality for blacks, especially women),[312a] social class (worse for "blue collar" workers),[312a] and therapy (adrenocortical steroids worsen prognosis in men without ascites, but improve it in women with ascites).[200] Clinical findings such as jaundice, ascites, varices, encephalopathy, or spider angiomata have been associated with worse prognosis.[10,200,312a,317,318,669,747,826,923] Laboratory findings such as serum bilirubin, hemoglobin, alkaline phosphatase, and albumin concentrations or serum prothrombin time show prognosis to be worse the more abnormal the value.[660,732,834] Histologic findings such as necrosis, inflammation, Mallory bodies, and eosinophilic parenchymal infiltrates are each associated with worse prognosis.[660,834] Provocatively, in one such study the presence of cirrhosis *per se* did not influence the mortality risk.[660]

Child and Turcotte devised a simple set of clinical and laboratory features to help select cirrhotic patients for portal-systemic shunt surgery.[143,148] These criteria graded patients on the basis of (1) serum bilirubin and (2) albumin concentration, and (3) severity of ascites and (4) encephalopathy and (5) the state of nutrition, each on a 3-point scale. Although the Child's classification appears to be a simple system, it is complex but surprisingly useful. We have found in systematic, prospective, unpublished studies that it is not only a useful predictor of survival in general (Fig. 20-70), it is also a reliable index of the occurrence of each of the complications of portal hypertension as well. Since several modifications of "Child's" criteria are in use[734] and each scheme can be calculated in a number of ways, one must use caution in interpreting and comparing results.[176]

Other studies have assessed prognosis by combining several features. A ratio of serum bilirubin to gamma-glutamyl transpeptidase was a better prognostic index than either value separately in alcoholic cirrhosis.[732] Some studies have presented complex computer-derived for-

mulas using multiple variables and variations of Cox model analysis.[660,834] Perhaps this approach holds promise for the future, but for the moment it is likely to remind clinicians of Aristotle's warning to bring no more science to a topic than the subject allows.

REFERENCES

1. Adams RD, Foley JM: The neurological changes in the more common types of severe liver disease. Trans Am Neurol Assoc 74:217,1949
2. Adams RD, Foley JM: The disorder of movement in the more common varieties of liver disease. Electroencephalogr Clin Neurophysiol 5 (Suppl 3):51, 1953
3. Adamsons RJ et al: Portacaval shunt with arterialization of the portal vein by means of a low flow arteriovenous fistula. Surg Gynecol Obstet 146:869, 1978
4. Admirand WH, Small DM: The physiochemical basis of cholesterol gallstone formation in man. J Clin Invest 47:1043, 1968
5. Ahmed SS et al: Cardiac function in alcoholics with cirrhosis: Absence of overt cardiomyopathy: Myth or Fact? J Am Coll Cardiol 3:696, 1984
6. Aiello RG et al: Experimental study of the role of hepatic lymph in the production of ascites. Surg Gynecol Obstet 111:79, 1960
7. Akalin G et al: Bactericidal and opsonic activity of ascitic fluid from cirrhotic and non-cirrhotic patients. J Infect Dis 147:1011, 1983
8. Alagille D: Alpha-1-anti-trypsin deficiency. Hepatology 4:11S, 1984
9. Alagille D, Odievre M: Liver and Biliary Tract Diseases in Children. New York, John Wiley & Sons, 1979
10. Alexander JF et al: Natural history of alcoholic hepatitis. Am J Gastroenterol 56:515, 1971
11. Allan R, Dykes P: A comparison of routine and selective endoscopy in the management of acute gastrointestinal hemorrhage. Gastrointest Endosc 20:154, 1974
12. Allen SI, Conn HO: Observations on the effect of exercise

on blood ammonia concentration in man. Yale J Biol Med 33:133, 1960

13. Alleyne GAO: The effect of severe protein calorie malnutrition on the renal function of Jamaican children. Pediatrics 39:400, 1967

14. Altman AR et al: Idiopathic familial cirrhosis and steatosis in adults. Gastroenterology 7:1211, 1979

15. Alves M et al: Gastric infarction: A complication of selective vasopressin infusion. Dig Dis Sci 24:409, 1979

16. Alvestrand A, Bergstom J: Glomerular hyperfiltration after protein ingestion, during glucagon infusion and in insulin-dependent diabetes is induced by a liver hormone. Lancet 1:195, 1984

17. Ames RP et al: Prolonged infusion of angiotensin II and norepinephrine and blood pressure, electroylte balance and aldosterone and cortisol secretion in normal man and in cirrhosis with ascites. J Clin Invest 44:1171, 1965

18. Amla I et al: Cirrhosis in children from peanut meal contaminated by aflatoxin. Am J Clin Nutr 24:609, 1971

19. Anderson JR, Johnston GW: Development of cutaneous gangrene during continuous peripheral infusion of vasopressin. Br Med J 287:1657, 1983

20. Angelin B et al: Biliary lipid composition in patients with portal cirrhosis of the liver. Scand J Gastroenterol 15:849, 1980

21. Anonymous: Who gets alcoholic cirrhosis? Lancet 2:263, 1984

22. Ansley DJ et al: Effect of peritoneo-venous shunting with the LeVeen valve on ascites, renal function, and coagulation in six patients with intractable ascites. Surgery 83:181, 1978

23. Anthony PP et al: The morphology of cirrhosis: Recommendations of definition nomenclature, and classification by a working group sponsored by the World Health Organization. J Clin Pathol 31:395, 1978

24. Arendt RM et al: Atrial natriuretic factor in plasma of patients with arterial hypertension, heart failure or cirrhosis of the liver. J Hypertension (Suppl) 4:5131, 1986

25. Arico S et al: Clinical significance of antibody to the hepatitis delta virus in symptomless HB$_s$Ag carriers. Lancet 2:356, 1985

26. Arnold L: Alterations in the endogenous enteric bacterial flora and microbic permeability of the intestinal wall in relation to the nutritional and meteorological changes. J Hyg 29:82, 1929

27. Arroyo V et al: Use of piretanide, a new loop diuretic, in cirrhosis with ascites: Relationship between the diuretic response and the plasma aldosterone level. Gut 21:855, 1980

28. Ashton RE et al: Complications in methotrexate treatment of psoriasis with particular reference to liver fibrosis. J Invest Dermatol 79:229, 1982

29. Astrup J, Rorth M: Oxygen affinity of hemoglobin and red cell 2,3-diphosphoglycerate in hepatic cirrhosis. Scand J Clin Lab Invest 31:311, 1973

30. Attali P et al: pH of ascitic fluid: Diagnostic and prognostic value in cirrhotic and noncirrhotic patients. Gastroenterology 90:1255, 1986

31. Atterbury CE: When not to do a liver biopsy. J Clin Gastroenterol 4:465, 1982

32. Atterbury CE: Prognosis in cirrhosis: Disbelieving Cassandra. J Clin Gastroenterol 5:359, 1983

33. Atterbury CE: The alcoholic in the lifeboat: Should drinkers be candidates for liver transplantation. J Clin Gastroenterol 8:1, 1986

34. Atterbury CE, Groszmann RJ: Portal venous pressure

measurement and its clinical significance. In Beker S (ed): Diagnostic Procedures in the Evaluation of Hepatic Disease, p 567. New York, Alan R Liss, 1983

35. Atterbury CE et al: Neomycin-sorbitol and lactulose in the treatment of acute portal-systemic encephalopathy. Am J Dig Dis 23:398, 1978

36. Ayers CR: Plasma renin activity and renin-substrate concentration in patients with liver disease. Circ Res 20:594, 1967

37. Baggenstoss AH, Cain JC: Further studies on the lymphatic vessels at the hilus of the liver of man: Their relation to ascites. Mayo Clin Proc 32:615, 1957

38. Baker HWG et al: A study of the endocrine manifestations of hepatic cirrhosis. Q J Med 45:145, 1976

39. Baldus WP: Etiology and management of renal failure in cirrhosis and portal hypertension. Ann NY Acad Sci 159:267, 1969

40. Baldus WP et al: The kidney in cirrhosis: II. Disorders of renal function. Ann Intern Med 60:366, 1964

41. Banks ER et al: Radionuclide demonstration of intrapulmonary shunting in cirrhosis. Am J Radiol 140:967, 1983

42. Bannayan GA, Hajdu SI: Gynecomastia: Clinicopathologic study of 351 cases. Am J Clin Pathol 57:431, 1972

43. Bar–Meir S, Conn HO: Spontaneous bacterial peritonitis induced by intraarterial vasopressin therapy. Gastroenterology 70:418, 1976

44. Bar–Meir S et al: Spontaneous meningococcal peritonitis: A report of two cases. Am J Dig Dis 23:119, 1978

45. Bar–Meir S et al: Analysis of ascitic fluid in cirrhosis. Am J Dig Dis 24:136, 1979

46. Barnardo DE et al: Renal function, renin activity and endogenous vasoactive substances in cirrhosis. Am J Dig Dis 15:419, 1970

47. Barnes JM, Magee PN: Some toxic properties of dimethylnitrosamine. Br J Ind Med 11:167, 1954

48. Baron HC: Umbilical hernia secondary to cirrhosis of the liver: Complications of surgical correction. N Engl J Med 263:824, 1960

49. Barry RE, McGivan JD: Acetaldehyde alone may initiate hepatocellular damage in acute alcoholic liver disease. Gut 26:1065, 1985

50. Barsoum MS et al: Tamponade and injection sclerotherapy in the management of bleeding esophageal varices. Br J Surg 69:76, 1982

51. Barsoum MS et al: The complications of injection sclerotherapy of bleeding oesophageal varices. Br J Surg 69:79, 1982

52. Bassett ML et al: Genetic hemochromatosis. Sem Liv Dis 4:217, 1984

52a.Baum S, Nusbaum M: The control of gastrointestinal hemorrhage by selective mesenteric arterial infusion of vasopressin. Diagn Radiol 98:497, 1971

53. Baunsgaard P et al: The variation of pathological changes in the liver evaluated by double biopsies. Acta Pathol Microbiol 87:51, 1979

54. Bean WB: The cutaneous arterial spider. Medicine 24:243, 1945

55. Beckman H: Treatment in General Practice, p 479. Philadelphia, WB Saunders, 1932

56. Beeson PB et al: Observations on the sites of removal of bacteria from the blood in patients with bacterial endocarditis. J Exp Med 81:9, 1945

57. Bell RH Jr et al: Outcome in cirrhotic patients with acute alcoholic hepatitis after emergency portacaval shunt for bleeding esophageal varices. Am J Surg 147:78, 1984

58. Beller BM et al: Pitressin-induced myocardial injury and depression in a young woman. Am J Med 51:675, 1971

59. Benoit JN et al: Role of humoral factors in the intestinal hyperemia associated with chronic portal hypertension. Am J Physiol 247:G486, 1984

60. Beppu K et al: Prediction of variceal hemorrhage by esophageal endoscopy. Gastrointest Endosc 27:213, 1981

61. Bercovici B et al: Antimicrobial activity of human peritoneal fluid. Surg Gynecol Obstet 141:885, 1975

62. Berger LA et al: The ultrasonic demonstration of portacaval shunts. Br J Surg 66:166, 1979

63. Berk DP, Chalmers T: Deafness complicating antibiotic therapy of hepatic encephalopathy. Ann Intern Med 73:393, 1970

64. Berkowitz HD et al: Improved renal function and inhibition of renin and aldosterone secretion following peritoneo-venous (LeVeen) shunt. Surgery 84:120, 1978

65. Berkson J: Limitations of the application of fourfold table analysis to hospital data. Biometric Bull 2:47, 1946

66. Berman M et al: The chronic sequelae of non A non B hepatitis. Ann Intern Med 91:1, 1979

67. Bernardi M et al: Renal function impairment induced by change in posture in patients with cirrhosis and ascites. Gut 26:629, 1985

67a. Bernardi M et al: Effects of a new loop diuretic (Muzolimine) in cirrhosis with ascites: Comparison with furosemide. Hepatology 6:400, 1986

68. Bernthal AC et al: Primary pulmonary hypertension after portocaval shunt. J Clin Gastroenterol 5:353, 1983

69. Berthelot P et al: Arterial changes in the lungs in cirrhosis of the liver-lung spider nevi. N Engl J Med 274:291, 1966

70. Bessman AN, Mirick GS: Blood ammonia levels following the ingestion of casein and whole blood. J Clin Invest 37:990, 1958

71. Bessman SP, Bradley JE: Uptake of ammonia by muscle: Its implications in ammoniagenic coma. N Engl J Med 253:1143, 1955

72. Bichet D et al: Role of vasopressin in abnormal water excretion in cirrhotic patients. Ann Intern Med 96:413, 1982

73. Bickford RG, Butt HR: Hepatic coma: The electroencephalographic pattern. J Clin Invest 34:790, 1955

74. Bircher J et al: Treatment of chronic portalsystemic encephalopathy with lactulose. Lancet 1:890, 1966

75. Bircher J et al: The significance of liver volume in patients with cirrhosis. In The Liver: Quantitative Aspects of Structure and Function, p 87. Basel, S Karger, 1973

76. Bircher J et al: Erstmalige von lactitol in der behandlung de porto-systemischen enzephalopathie. Schweiz Med Wochenschr 112:1306, 1982

77. Bjorneboe M et al: Tetanus antitoxin production and gamma globulin levels in patients with cirrhosis of the liver. Acta Med Scand 188:541, 1970

78. Blei AT et al: Insulin resistance and insulin receptors in hepatic cirrhosis. Gastroenterology 83:1191, 1982

79. Blendis LM et al: The renal and hemodynamic effects of the peritoneovenous shunt for intractable hepatic ascites. Gastroenterology 77:250, 1979

80. Blomstrand R et al: Observations on the thoracic duct lymph in patients with cirrhosis of the liver. Acta Hepatosplenol 7:1, 1960

81. Boitnott JK, Maddrey WC: Alcoholic liver disease: I. Interrelationships among histologic features and the histologic effects of prednisolone therapy. Hepatology 1:599, 1981

82. Bonnin H et al: Enlarged parotid glands in alcoholic cirrhosis. Pressé Med 62:1449, 1954

83. Borowsky SA et al: Dental infection in a cirrhotic patient: Source of recurrent sepsis. Gastroenterology 76:836, 1979

84. Bosch J et al: Hepatic hemodynamics and the renin-angiotensin-aldosterone system in cirrhosis. Gastroenterology 78:92, 1980

85. Bosch J et al: Effects of somatostatin on hepatic and systemic hemodynamics in patients with cirrhosis of the liver: Comparison with vasopressin. Gastroenterology 80:518, 1981

86. Bouchier IAD: Postmortem study of the frequency of gallstones in patients with cirrhosis of the liver. Gut 10:705, 1969

87. Boyer JL, Klatskin G: Pattern of necrosis in acute viral hepatitis: Prognostic value of bridging (subacute hepatic necrosis). N Engl J Med 283:1063, 1970

88. Boyer TD et al: Effect of indomethacin and prostaglandin A_1 on renal function and plasma renin activity in alcoholic liver disease. Gastroenterology 77:215, 1979

89. Boyer TD et al: Direct transhepatic measurement of portal vein presure using a thin needle: Comparison with wedged hepatic vein pressure. Gastroenterology 72:584, 1977

90. Bradley SE, Bradley GP: The effect of increased abdominal pressure on renal function in man. J Clin Invest 26:1010, 1947

90a. Brantigan CO et al: Effect of beta blockade and beta stimulation on stage fright. Am J Med 49:88, 1982

91. Bras G et al: Cirrhosis of the liver in Jamaica. J Pathol Bact 82:503, 1961

92. Brayton RG et al: The effect of alcohol and various diseases on leukocyte mobilization phagocytosis and intracellular bacterial killing. N Engl J Med 282:123, 1970

93. Bredfeldt JE, Groszmann RJ: Hemodynamic aspects of portal hypertension: The effect of increased intraabdominal pressure. In Epstein M (ed): The Kidney in Liver Disease, 2nd ed, p 281. New York, Elsevier, 1983

94. Brick IB: Parotid enlargement in cirrhosis of the liver. Ann Intern Med 49:438, 1958

95. Brick IB, Palmer ED: One thousand cases of portal cirrhosis of the liver: Implications of esophageal varices and their management. Arch Intern Med 113:501, 1964

96. Bricker NS: Extracellular fluid volume regulation: On the evidence for a biologic control system. In Epstein M (ed): The Kidney in Liver Disease, p 19. New York, Elsevier, 1978

97. Brock JF, Hansen JDL: The aetiology of kwashiorkor. Leech 37:35, 1958

98. Brook I et al: Measurement of lactate in ascitic fluid: An aid in the diagnosis of peritonitis with particular relevance to spontaneous bacterial peritonitis of the cirrhotic. Dig Dis Sci 26:1089, 1981

99. Brooks WS Jr: Variceal sclerosing agents. Am J Gastroenterol 79:424, 1984

100. Browne MK, Cassie R: Spontaneous bacterial peritonitis during pregnancy: Case report. Br J Obstet Gynecol 88:1158, 1981

101. Bruguera M et al: Giant mitochondria in hepatocytes: A diagnostic hint for alcoholic liver disease. Gastroenterology 73:1383, 1977

102. Bruix J et al: Effects of prostaglandin inhibition on systemic and hepatic hemodynamics in patients with cirrhosis of the liver. Gastroenterology 88:430, 1985

103. Brusilow S et al: Amino acid acylation: A mechanism of

nitrogen excretion in inborn errors of urea synthesis. Science 207:659, 1980

104. Bucher NLR, Swaffield MS: Regulation of hepatic regeneration in rats by synergistic action of insulin and glucagon. Proc Natl Acad Sci 72:1157, 1975

105. Buhac I, LoIudice TA: Verminderte peritoneale Schmerzempfindung bei patienten mit leberzirrhose und aszites. Schweiz Med Wochenschr 109:643, 1979

106. Burack WR, Hollister RM: Tuberculous peritonitis: A study of forty-seven proved cases encountered by a general medical unit in twenty-five years. Am J Med 28:510, 1960

107. Burcharth F et al: Experiences with the Linton-Nachlas and Sengstaken-Blakemore tubes for bleeding esophageal varices. Surg Gynecol Obstet 142:529, 1976

108. Burcharth F et al: Percutaneous transhepatic portography: I. Technique and application. AJR 132:177, 1979

109. Burcharth F et al: Percutaneous transhepatic portography: II. Comparison with splenoportography in portal hypertension. AJR 132:183, 1979

110. Burchell AR et al: A seven-year experience with side-to-side portacaval shunt in cirrhotic ascites. Ann Surg 168:655, 1968

111. Burroughs AK et al: Propranolol for the prevention of recurrent variceal hemorrhage in cirrhotic patients: Results of a controlled trial. N Engl J Med 309:1539, 1983

112. Burroughs AK et al: Randomised, controlled study of transhepatic obliteration of varices and oesophageal stapling transection in acute variceal haemorrhage. In Westaby D et al (eds): Variceal Bleeding, p 199. London, Pitman Press, 1982

113. Butt HR, Mason HL: Fetor hepaticus: Its clinical significance and attempts at clinical isolation. Gastroenterology 26:829, 1954

114. Bützow GH et al: Metoprolol in portal hypertension: A controlled study. Klin Wochenschr 20:1311, 1982

115. Cabrera J et al: Aminoglycoside nephrotoxicity in cirrhosis: Value of urinary β_2-microglobulin to discriminate functional renal failure from acute tubular damage. Gastroenterology 82:97, 1982

116. Calabresi P, Abelman WH: Portacaval and portopulmonary anastomosis in Laënnec's cirrhosis and heart failure. J Clin Invest 36:1257, 1957

117. Caldwell PRB et al: Oxyhemoglobin dissociation curve in liver disease. J Appl Physiol 20:316, 1965

117a. Cales P et al: Prophylaxis of first variceal bleeding in cirrhotic patients by propranolol: Final report of a multicenter randomized study (abstr). Gastroenterology 90:1717, 1986

118. Cameron JL et al: The mesocaval C shunt. Surg Gynecol Obstet 150:401, 1980

119. Campra JL, Reynolds TB: Effectiveness of high-dose spironolactone therapy in patients with chronic liver disease and relatively refractory ascites. Dig Dis 23:1025, 1978

120. Canter JW et al: The interrelationship of wedged hepatic vein pressure, intrasplenic pressure and intra-abdominal pressure. J Lab Clin Med 54:756, 1959

121. Canzanello VJ et al: Hyperammonemic encephalopathy during hemodialysis. Ann Intern Med 99:190, 1983

122. Capocaccia L et al: Influence of phenylethanolamine on octopamine plasma determination in hepatic encephalopathy. Clin Chim Acta 93:371, 1979

123. Caralis PV et al: Secondary bacterial peritonitis in cirrhotic patients with ascites. South Med J 77:579, 1984

124. Carey JB Jr et al: The metaboliasm of bile acids with special reference to liver injury. Medicine 45:461, 1966

125. Caroli J, Platteborse R: Septicemie portocave: Cirrhoses du foie et septicemie à colibacille. Sem Hôp Paris 34:472, 1958

126. Casey TH et al: Body and serum potassium in liver disease. II. Relationship to arterial ammonia, blood pH and hepatic coma. Gastroenterology 48:208, 1965

127. Casey TH et al: Body and serum potassium in liver disease: I. Relationship to hepatic function and associated factors. Gastroenterology 48:198, 1965

128. Casley–Smith JR: How the lymphatic system works. Lymphology 1:77, 1968

129. Castell DO, Conn HO: The determination of portacaval shunt patency: A critical review of methodology. Medicine 51:315, 1972

130. Castell DO, Johnson RB: ^{198}Au liver scan: An index of portalsystemic collateral circulation in chronic liver disease. N Engl J Med 275:188, 1966

131. Cattau EL et al: The accuracy of the physical examination in the diagnosis of suspected ascites. JAMA 247:1164, 1982

132. Cello JP et al: Endoscopic sclerotherapy versus esophageal transection in Child's class C patients with variceal hemorrhage: Comparison with results of portacaval shunt: Preliminary report. Surgery 91:333, 1982

133. Cello JP et al: Endoscopic sclerotherapy versus portacaval shunt in patients with severe cirrhosis and variceal hemorrhage. N Engl J Med 311:1589, 1984

134. Cerra FB et al: Disease-specific amino acid infusion (F080) in hepatic encephalopathy: A prospective, randomized, double-blind, controlled trial. JPEN 9:288, 1985

135. Chadwick RG et al: Chronic persistent hepatitis: Hepatitis B virus markers and histological follow-up. Gut 20:372, 1979

136. Challenger F, Walshe JM: Methyl mercaptan in relation to Foetor Hepaticus. Biochem J 59:372, 1955

137. Chalmers TC et al: Clinical estimation of liver and spleen size. In Preisis R, Paumgartner G (eds): The Liver: Quantitative Aspects of Structure and Function. p 76. Basel, S Karger, 1973

138. Chart JJ et al: Metabolism of salt-retaining hormone by surviving liver slices. J Clin Invest 35:254, 1956

139. Chen S et al: Mercaptans and dimethyl sulfide in the breath of patients with cirrhosis of the liver. J Lab Clin Med 75:628, 1970

140. Chen S et al: Volatile fatty acids in the breath of patients with cirrhosis of the liver. J Lab Clin Med 75:622, 1970

141. Chey WY et al: Effects of chronic administration of ethanol on the liver of dogs. Gastroenterology 65:533, 1973

142. Chiesa A et al: Role of various causes of arterial desaturation in liver cirrhosis. Clin Sci 37:803, 1969

143. Child CG (ed): The Liver and Portal Hypertension, p 50. Philadelphia, WB Saunders, 1964

144. Child CG et al: Pancreatico-duodenectomy with resection of the portal vein in the Macaca mulatta monkey and in man. Surg Gynecol Obstet 94:31, 1952

145. Chojkier M et al: A controlled comparison of continuous intraarterial and intravenous infusions of vasopressin in hemorrhage from esophageal varices. Gastroenterology 77:540, 1979

146. Chojkier M, Conn HL: Esophageal tamponade in the treatment of bleeding varices: A decadal progress report. Dig Dis Sci 25:267, 1980

147. Chomko AM et al: The role of renin and aldosterone in the salt retention of edema. Am J Med 63:881, 1977

148. Christensen E et al: Prognostic value of Child–Turcotte

criteria in medically treated cirrhosis. Hepatology 4:430, 1984

148a. Christie ML et al: Enriched branched-chain amino acid formula versus a casein-based supplement in the treatment of cirrhosis. JPEN 9:671, 1985

149. Clarke JS et al: Peptic ulcer following portacaval shunt. Ann Surg 148:551, 1958

150. Clermont RJ et al: Intravenous therapy of massive ascites in patients with cirrhosis: II. Long term effects on survival and frequency of renal failure. Gastroenterology 53:220, 1967

151. Cochrane AMG et al: Lymphocyte cytotoxicity for isolated hepatocytes in alcoholic liver disease. Gastroenterology 72:918, 1977

152. Coe RO, Bull FE: Cirrhosis and methotrexate treatment of psoriasis. JAMA 206:1515, 1968

153. Cohen FL et al: Solitary brain abscess following endoscopic injection sclerosis of esophageal varices. Gastrointest Endosc 31:331, 1985

154. Cohen JA, Kaplan MM: The SGOT–SGPT ratio: An indicator of alcoholic liver disease. Dig Dis Sci 24:835, 1979

154a. Cohen LB et al: Bacteremia after endoscopic injection sclerosis. Gastrointest Endosc 29:198, 1983

155. Cohen R et al: Microbial intestinal flora in acute diarrhea disease. JAMA 201:835, 1967

156. Cohen S, Soloway RD (eds): Chronic Active Liver Disease. New York, Churchill Livingstone, 1982

157. Cohn JN: Hepatorenal failure following portacaval shunt: Hemodynamic considerations and the application of ascitic fluid infusions. Med Ann DC 33:567, 1964

158. Cohn JN et al: Systemic vasoconstriction and renal vasodilator effects of PLV-2 (Octapressin) in man. Circulation 38:151, 1964

159. Comroe JH: Physiology of Respiration, 2nd ed. Chicago, Year Book Medical Publishers, 1974

160. Conn HO: Asterixis in nonhepatic disorders. Am J Med 29:647, 1960

161. Conn HO: Spontaneous peritonitis and bacteremia in Laënnec's cirrhosis caused by enteric organisms: A relatively common but rarely recognized syndrome. Ann Intern Med 60:568, 1964

162. Conn HO: Ammonia tolerance in the diagnosis of esophageal varices: Comparison of endoscopic, radiologic and biochemical techniques. J Lab Clin Med 70:442, 1967

163. Conn HO: Cirrhosis and diabetes: IV. Effect of potassium chloride administration on glucose and insulin metabolism. Am J Med Sci 259:394, 1970

164. Conn HO: Hazards attending the use of esophageal tamponade. N Engl J Med 259:701, 1958

165. Conn HO: The rational management of ascites. In Popper H, Schaffer R (eds): Progress in Liver Disease, 4th ed, pp 269–288. New York, Grune & Stratton, 1972

166. Conn HO: Lactulose: Comments on mechanism of action and current status. Conn Med 36:582, 1972

167. Conn HO: Portacaval anastomosis and hepatic hemosiderin deposition: A prospective, controlled investigation. Gastroenterology 62:61, 1972

168. Conn HO: Unilateral edema and jaundice following portacaval anastomosis. Ann Intern Med 76:459, 1972

169. Conn HO: Rational use of liver biopsy in diagnosis of hepatic cancer. Gastroenterology 62:142, 1972

170. Conn HO: Post liver biopsy hematoma and related phenomena. Gastroenterology 67:375, 1974

171. Conn HO: Therapeutic portacaval anastomosis: To shunt or not to shunt. Gastroenterology 67:1065, 1974

172. Conn HO: To scope or not to scope. N Engl J Med 304:967, 1981

173. Conn HO: The rational evaluation and management of portal hypertension. In Schaffner F et al (eds): The Liver and Its Diseases. New York, Intercontinental Medical Book Corp, 1974

174. Conn HO: The Trailmaking and Number Connection Tests in assessing mental state in portalsystemic encephalopathy. Am J Dig Dis 22:541, 1977

175. Conn HO: Emergency portacaval shunts in cirrhosis: A physician's perspective. In Hepatic, Biliary and Pancreatic Surgery, p 649–661. Miami, Symposia Specialists, 1980

176. Conn HO: A peek at the Child–Turcotte classification. Hepatology 6:673, 1981

177. Conn HO: Endoscopic sclerotherapy: An analysis of variants. Hepatology 3:769, 1983

178. Conn HO: Propranolol in portal hypertension: Problems in paradise? Hepatology 4:560, 1984

179. Conn HO, Brodoff M: Emergency esophagoscopy in the diagnosis of upper gastrointestinal hemorrhage. A critical evaluation of its diagnostic accuracy. Gastroenterology 47:505, 1964

180. Conn HO, Dalessio DJ: Multiple infusions of posterior pituitary extract in the treatment of bleeding esophageal varices. Ann Intern Med 57:804, 1962

181. Conn HO, Fessel JM: Spontaneous bacterial peritonitis in cirrhosis: Variations on a theme. Medicine 50:161, 1971

182. Conn HO, Lieberthal MM: The Hepatic Coma Syndromes and Lactulose. Baltimore, Williams & Wilkins, 1979

183. Conn HO, Lindenmuth WW: Prophylactic portacaval anastomosis in cirrhotic patients with esophageal varices and ascites. Am J Surg 117:656, 1969

184. Conn HO, Simpson JA: Excessive mortality with balloon tamponade. JAMA 202:587, 1967

185. Conn HO et al: Fiberoptic and conventional esophagoscopy in the diagnosis of esophageal varices: A comparison of techniques and observers. Gastroenterology 52:810, 1967

186. Conn HO et al: Balloon tamponade in the radiological diagnosis of esophageal varices. Gastroenterology 50:29, 1966

187. Conn HO et al: A comparison of lactulose and neomycin in the treatment of portal-systemic encephalopathy: A double-blind controlled trial. Gastroenterology 72:573, 1977

188. Conn HO et al: Prophylactic portacaval anastomosis: A tale of two studies. Medicine 51:27, 1972

189. Conn HO et al: A comparison of radiologic and esophagoscopic diagnosis of esophageal varices. N Engl J Med 265:160, 1961

189a. Conn HO et al: Selective intraarterial vasopressin in the treatment of upper gastrointestinal hemorrhage. Gastroenterology 63:634, 1972

190. Conn HO et al: Intraarterial vasopressin in the treatment of upper gastrointestinal hemorrhage: A prospective, controlled clinical trial. Gastroenterology 68:211, 1975

191. Conn HO et al: Cirrhosis and diabetes: I. Increased incidence of diabetes in patients with Laënnec's cirrhosis. Am J Dig Dis 14:837, 1969

192. Conn HO et al: Cirrhosis and diabetes: II. Association of impaired glucose tolerance with portal-systemic shunting in Laënnec's cirrhosis. Am J Dig Dis 16:227, 1971

193. Conn HO et al: The naked physician: The blind interpretation of liver function tests in the differential diagnosis of jaundice. In Preisig R, Bircher J (eds): The Liver:

Quantitative Aspects of Structure and Function, p 386. Aulendorf, Editio Cantor, 1979

194. Conn HO et al: Distal splenorenal shunt vs portal-systemic shunt: Current status of a controlled trial. Hepatology 1: 151, 1981

195. Conn JW, Hinerman DL: Spironolactone-induced inhibition of aldosterone biosynthesis in primary aldosteronism. Morphological and functional studies. Metabolism 26:1293, 1977

196. Cook GC, Hutt MS: The liver after kwashiorkor. Br Med J 3:454, 1967

197. Cooper AJ et al: A controlled trial of potensan forte ("Aphrodisiac") and testosterone combined in impotence. Ir J Med Sci 142:155, 1973

198. Cooper AJL et al: The metabolic fate of ^{13}N-labeled ammonia in rat brain. J Biol Chem 254:4982, 1979

199. Copenhagen Esophageal Varices Sclerotherapy Project: Sclerotherapy after first variceal hemorrhage in cirrhosis. N Engl J Med 311:1594, 1984

200. Copenhagen Study Group for Liver Diseases. Sex, ascites, and alcoholism in survival of patients with cirrhosis: Effect of prednisone. N Engl J Med 291:271, 1974

201. Coppage WS et al: The metabolism of aldosterone in normal subjects and in patients with hepatic cirrhosis. J Clin Invest 41:1672, 1962

202. Correia JP, Conn HO: Spontaneous bacterial peritonitis in cirrhosis: Endemic or epidemic? Med Clin North Am 59:963, 1975

203. Correia JP et al: Controlled trial of vasopressin and balloon tamponade in bleeding esophageal varices. Hepatology 4: 885, 1984

204. Cosnett JE et al: Shunt myelopathy: A report of 2 cases. S Afr Med J 62:215, 1982

205. Crafoord C, Frenckner P: New surgical treatment of varicose veins of the oesophagus. Acta Otolaryngol 27:422, 1939

206. Creutzfeldt W: Klinische beziehungen zwischen diabetes mellitus und leber. Acta Hepatosplenol 6:156, 1959

207. Crosby RC, Cooney EA: Surgical treatment of ascites. N Engl J Med 235:581, 1946

208. Cruz–Coke R: Colour-blindness and cirrhosis of the liver. Lancet 1:1131, 1965

209. Curry N et al: Spontaneous peritonitis in cirrhotic ascites. A decade of experience. Am J Dig Dis 19:685, 1974

210. Czaja AJ, Davis GL: Hepatitis non A non B. Mayo Clin Proc 57:639, 1982

211. Dagradi AE et al: The sources of upper gastrointestinal bleeding in liver cirrhosis. Ann Intern Med 42:852, 1955

212. Dagradi AE et al: Failure of endoscopy to establish a source for upper gastrointestinal bleeding. Am J Gastroenterol 72:395, 1979

213. Daoud FS et al: Failure of hypoxic vasoconstriction in patients with liver cirrhosis. JCI 51:1076, 1972

214. Davidson CS: Cirrhosis of the liver treated with prolonged sodium restrictions: Improvement in nutrition, hepatic function and portal hypertension. JAMA 159:1257, 1955

215. Davis HH et al: Alveolar-capillary oxygen disequilibrium in hepatic cirrhosis. Chest 73:507, 1978

216. Dawson JL. Oesophageal varices: Curiosities. Br Med J 286:826, 1983

217. Degroote J et al: Long-term follow-up of chronic active hepatitis of moderate severity. Gut: 19:510, 1978

218. Delaney JP, Quigley TM: Gastroesophageal devascularization for bleeding varices. In Najarian JS, Delaney JP

219. (eds): Advances in Hepatic Biliary and Pancreatic Surgery, pp 705–713. Chicago, Year Book Publishers, 1985

219. Denk H, Eckerstorfer R: Colchicine-induced Mallory body formation in the mouse. Lab Invest 36:563, 1977

220. Denk H et al: Experimental induction of hepatocellular hyalin (Mallory bodies) in mice by griseofulvin treatment: I. Light microscopic observations. Lab Invest 35:377, 1976

221. Denk H et al: Hepatocellular hyalin (Mallory bodies) in long term griseofulvin-treated mice: A new experimental model for the study of hyalin formation. Lab Invest 32: 773, 1975

222. Denton JH et al: Bacterial endocarditis in cirrhosis. Dig Dis Sci 26:935, 1981

223. Depew W et al: Double-blind controlled trial of prednisolone therapy in patients with severe acute alcoholic hepatitis and spontaneous encephalopathy. Gastroenterology 78:524, 1980

224. Derr RF, Zieve L: Effect of fatty acids on the disposition of ammonia. J Pharmacol Exp Ther 197:675, 1976

225. Descos L et al: Comparison of six treatments of ascites in patients with liver cirrhosis: A clinical trial. Hepatogastroenterology 30:15, 1983

226. Dienstag JL: Non A non B hepatitis: I. Recognition, Epidemiology, and Clinical Features. Gastroenterology 85: 439, 1983

227. Doehlert CA Jr et al: Obstructive biliary cirrhosis and alcoholic cirrhosis: Comparison of clinical and pathologic features. Am J Clin Pathol 25:902, 1955

228. Doizaki WM, Zieve L: An improved method for measuring blood mercaptans. J Lab Clin Med 90:849, 1977

228a. Dollet JM et al: Sclerotherapy versus propranolol after variceal hemorrhage in cirrhosis: A long-term controlled trial (abstr). Gastroenterology 90:1722, 1986

229. Donaldson RM Jr: Normal bacterial populations of the intestine and their relation to intestinal function. N Engl J Med 270:938, 1964

230. Doyle FH et al: Nuclear magnetic resonance imaging of the liver: Initial experience. AJR 138:193, 1982

231. Drapanas T: Interposition mesocaval shunt for treatment of portal hypertension. Ann Surg 176:435, 1972

232. Drenick EJ et al: Effect of hepatic morphology of treatment of obesity by fasting, reducing diets and small-bowel bypass. N Engl J Med 282:829, 1970

233. Dronfield MW et al: A prospective, randomized study of endoscopy and radiology in acute upper-gastrointestinal-tract bleeding. Lancet 1:1167, 1977

234. d'Sant'Agnese PA, Talamo C: Cystic fibrosis of the pancreas. N Engl J Med 277:1287, 1967

235. Dumont AE, Mulholland JH: Flow rate and composition of thoracic duct lymph in patients with cirrhosis. N Engl J Med 263:471, 1960

236. Dumont AE, Witte MH: Contrasting patterns of thoracic duct lymph foundation in hepatic cirrhosis. Surg Gynecol Obstet 122:524, 1966

237. Eade MN, Brocke BN: Portal bacteraemia in cases of ulcerative colitis submitted to colectomy. Lancet 1:1008, 1969

238. Eastwood GL: Does early endoscopy benefit the patient with active upper gastrointestinal bleeding? Gastroenterology 72:737, 1977

239. Eckardt VF, Grace ND: Gastroesophageal reflux and bleeding esophageal varices. Gastroenterology 76:39, 1978

240. Eddleston ALWF, Davis M: Histocompatibility antigens in alcoholic liver disease. Br Med Bull 38:13, 1982

241. Edington GM: Other viral and infectious diseases: In

Macsween RNM et al: Pathology of the Liver, p 202. Edinburgh, Churchill Livingstone, 1979

242. Edmondson HTR et al: Clinical investigation of the portacaval shunt: IV. A report of early survival from the emergency operation. Ann Surg 173:372, 1971

243. Egberts EH et al: Branched chain amino acids in the treatment of latent portosystemic encephalopathy: A double-blind placebo controlled crossover study. Gastroenterology 88:887, 1985

244. Egense J, Schwartz M: Recurrent hepatic coma following ureterosigmoidostomy. Scand J Gastroenterol (Suppl) 7: 149, 1970

245. Eggert RC: Spironolactone diuresis in patients with cirrhosis and ascites. Br Med J 4:401, 1970

246. Elashoff JD: Combining results of clinical trials. Gastroenterology 75:1170, 1978

247. Eliakim M et al: Gammopathy in liver disease. In Popper H, Schaffner F (eds): Progress in Liver Diseases, vol 4, p 403. New York, Grune & Stratton, 1972

248. Elkington SG et al: Lactulose in the control of portal-systemic encephalopathy. N Engl J Med 281:408, 1969

249. Elsass P et al: Encephalopathy in patients with cirrhosis of the liver: A neuropsychological study. Scand J Gastroenterol 13:241, 1978

250. Eppinger H: Die Leberkrankheiten. Wien, Springer, 1937

251. Epstein FH: Reversible uremic states. JAMA 161:494, 1956

252. Epstein FH et al: Renal function in decompensated cirrhosis of the liver. Proc Soc Exp Biol Med 75:822, 1950

253. Epstein M: Natriuretic hormone and the sodium retention of cirrhosis. Gastroenterology 81:395, 1981

254. Epstein M et al: Renal failure in the patient with cirrhosis. The role of active vasoconstriction. Am J Med 49:175, 1970

255. Epstein M et al: Characterization of the renin–aldosterone system in decompensated cirrhosis. Circ Res 41:818, 1977

256. Epstein M et al: Determinants of deranged sodium and water homeostasis in decompensated cirrhosis. J Lab Clin Med 87:822, 1976

257. Epstein M et al: Pneumococcal peritonitis in patients with postnecrotic cirrhosis. N Engl J Med 278:69, 1968

258. Epstein O et al: Hypertrophic hepatic osteoarthropathy. Am J Med 67:88, 1979

259. Ericson G et al: Unilateral asterixis in a dialysis patient. JAMA 240:671, 1978

260. Ericsson CD et al: Systemic absorption of bacitracin after peritoneal lavage. Am J Surg 137:65, 1979

261. Eriksson LS et al: Branched-chain amino acids in the treatment of chronic hepatic encephalopathy. Gut 23:801, 1982

262. Eriksson S, Hagerstrand I: Cirrhosis and malignant hepatoma in a alpha-l-anti-trypsin deficiency. Acta Med Scand 195:451,1974

263. Erlik D et al: Portorenal shunt: A new technique for portosystemic anastomosis in portal hypertension. Ann Surg 159:72, 164

264. Fagan EA et al: Multi-organ granulomas and mitochondrial antibodies. N Engl J Med 308:572, 1983

265. Faraj BA et al: Decarboxylation to tyramine: An important route of tyrosine metabolism in dogs with experimental hepatic encephalopathy. Gastroenterology 75:1041, 1978

266. Fauerholdt L et al: Conversion of micronodular cirrhosis into macronodular cirrhosis. Hepatology 3:928, 1983

267. Feher J et al: Early syphilitic hepatitis. Lancet 2:896, 1975

268. Feinstein AR: Clinical Judgment. Baltimore, Williams & Wilkins, 1967

269. Felisart J et al: Cefotaxime is more effective than is ampicillin–tobramycin in cirrhosis with severe infections. Hepatology 5:457, 1985

270. Fenton SS et al: Clinical aspects of peritonitis in patients on chronic ambulatory peritoneal dialysis. Peritoneal Dial Bull 1:S1, 1981

271. Ferenci P et al: Serum levels of gamma aminobutyric acid-like activity in patients with acute and chronic hepatocellular diseases. Lancet 1:811, 1983

272. Fessel JM, Conn HO: An analysis of the causes and prevention of hepatic coma. Gastroenterology 62:191, 1972

273. Fessel JM, Conn HO: Lactulose in the treatment of acute hepatic encephalopathy. Am J Med Sci 266:103, 1973

273a. Fiaccadori F: La peritonite bacterienne spontanee du cirrhotique. Med Chir Dig 12:167, 1983

274. Fiaccadori F et al: Selective amino acid solutions in hepatic encephalopathy treatment: A preliminary report. La Ricerca Clin Lab 10:411, 1980

275. Fialkow PJ et al: Cirrhosis and classical genetic color blindness. N Engl J Med 275:584, 1966

276. Fischer JE: Neurotransmitter and the hepatorenal syndrome. Conn Med 36:575, 1972

277. Fischer JE: Randomized comparison of proximal and distal splenorenal shunts. Unpublished observations

278. Fischer JE, Baldessarini RJ: False neurotransmitters and hepatic failure. Lancet 2:75, 1971

279. Fischer JE, Baldessarini RJ: Pathogenesis and therapy of hepatic coma. In Popper H, Schaffner F (eds): Progress in Liver Diseases, vol 5, p 363. New York, Grune & Stratton, 1976

280. Fischer JE, James JH: Treatment of hepatic coma and hepatorenal syndrome. Am J Surg 123:222, 1972

281. Fischer JE et al: Plasma amino acids in patients with hepatic encephalopathy. Am J Surg 127:40, 1974

282. Fischer JE et al: The effect of normalization of plasma amino acids on hepatic encephalopathy in man. Surgery 80:77, 1976

283. Fisher ER, et al: Rarity of hepatic metastases in cirrhosis: A misconception. JAMA 174:336, 1960

284. Fisher MR, Gore RM: Computed tomography in the evaluation of cirrhosis and portal hypertension. J Clin Radiol 7:173, 1985

285. Flannery DB et al: Current status of hyperammonemic syndromes. Hepatology 2:495, 1985

286. Flaum MA: Spontaneous colon bacillus bacterial empyema in cirrhosis. Gastroenterology 70:416, 1976

287. Fleig SW et al: Upper gastrointestinal hemorrhage from downhill esophageal varices. Dig Dis 27:23, 1982

288. Fleig WE et al: Emergency endoscopic sclerotherapy for bleeding esophageal varices: A prospective study in patients not responding to balloon tamponade. Gastrointest Endosc 29:8, 1983

289. Flint A: Clinical report of hydro-peritoneum, based on an analysis of forty-six cases. Am J Med Sci 45:306, 1863

290. Floch MH et al: Intestinal bacteriology: I. Qualitative and quantitative relationships of the fecal flora in normal subjects and cirrhotic patients. Gastroenterology 39:70, 1970

291. Flood FB: Spontaneous perforation of the umbilicus in Laënnec's cirrhosis with massive ascites. N Engl J Med 264:72, 1961

292. Fogel MR et al: Diuresis in the ascitic patient: A randomized controlled trial of three regimens. J Clin Gastroenterol 3:73, 1981

293. Fogel MR et al: Continuous intravenous vasopressin in active upper gastrointestinal bleeding. Ann Intern Med 96:565, 1982

294. Foutch PG, Sivak MV Jr: Colonic variceal hemorrhage after endoscopic sclerosis of esophageal varices: A report of three cases. Am J Gastroenterol 79:756, 1984

295. Fowler R Jr: Primary peritonitis. Aust NZ J Surg 26:204, 1957

296. Franke WW et al: Ultrastructural, biochemical, and immunologic characterization of Mallory bodies in livers of griseofulvin-treated mice. Lab Invest 40:207, 1979

297. Freeman JG et al: Controlled trial of terlipressin (glypressin) versus vasopressin in the early treatment of oesophageal varices. Lancet 2:66, 1982

298. Freeman S: Symposium on gastrointestinal diseases: Recent progress in physiology and biochemistry of liver. Med Clin North Am 37:109, 1953

299. French SW: Nature, pathogenesis, and significance of the Mallory body. Semin Liv Dis 1:217, 1981

300. French SW: Present understanding of the development of Mallory's body. Arch Pathol Lab Med 107:445, 1983

301. French SW et al: Thick microfilaments (intermediate filaments) and chronic alcohol ingestion. In Popper H et al (eds): Membrane Alterations as Basis of Liver Injury, p 311. Lancaster, England, St. Leonhard's House, MTP Press, 1977

302. Freund HA: Clinical manifestations and studies in parenchymatous hepatitis. Ann Intern Med 10:1144, 1937

303. Fritts HW Jr et al: Estimation of pulmonary arteriovenous shunt-flow using intravenous injections of T-1824 dye and Kr⁸⁵. J Clin Invest 39:1841, 1960

304. Fromkes JJ et al: Antimicrobial activity of human ascitic fluid. Gastroenterology 73:668, 1977

305. Fromkes JJ et al: Activation of the alternative complement pathway in ascitic fluid during spontaneous bacterial peritonitis. J Clin Gastroenterol 4:347, 1982

306. Fuller DW: Hepatorenal syndrome: Reversal by peritoneovenous shunt. Surgery 82:337, 1977

307. Funaro AH, et al: Transhepatic obliteration of esophageal varices using the stainless steel coil. AJR 133:1123, 1979

308. Furukawa T et al: Arterial hypoxemia in patients with hepatic cirrhosis. Am J Med Sci 287:10, 1984

309. Futagawa S et al: Emergency esophageal transection with paraesophagogastric devascularization for variceal bleeding. World J Surg 3:229, 1979

310. Gabow PA et al: Spironolactone-induced hyperchloremic acidosis in cirrhosis. Ann Intern Med 90:338, 1979

311. Gabuzda GJ, Hall PW III: Relation of potassium depletion to renal ammonium metabolism and hepatic coma. Medicine 45:481, 1966

312. Galambos JT: Natural history of alcoholic hepatitis: III. Histological changes. Gastroenterology 63:1026, 1972

312a.Galambos JT: Cirrhosis, p 357. Philadelphia, WB Saunders 1979

313. Galambos JT et al: Selective and total shunts in the treatment of bleeding varices: A randomized controlled trial. N Engl J Med 295:1089, 1976

314. Gall EA: Posthepatitic, postnecrotic and nutritional cirrhosis: A pathological analysis. Am J Pathol 36:241, 1960

315. Gall EA: Primary and metastatic carcinoma of the liver: Relationship to hepatic cirrhosis. Arch Pathol 70:226, 1960

316. Gans H et al: Antiprotease deficiency and familial infantile liver cirrhosis. Surg Gynecol Obstet 129:289, 1969

317. Garceau AJ et al: The natural history of cirrhosis: I. Survival with esophageal varices. N Engl J Med 268:469, 1963

318. Garceau AJ et al: The natural history of cirrhosis: II. The influence of alcohol and prior hepatitis on pathology and prognosis. N Engl J Med 271:1173, 1964

319. Garcia-Tsao G et al: Short term effects of propranolol on portal venous pressure. Hepatology 5:419, 1985

320. Garcia-Tsao G et al: The diagnosis of bacterial peritonitis: Comparison of pH, lactate concentration and leukocyte count. Hepatology 5:91, 1985

320a.Gelman S, Ernst S: Nitroprusside prevents adverse haemodynamic effects of vasopressen. Arch Surg 113:1465, 1978

321. Gerber MA et al: Hepatocellular hyaline in cholestasis and cirrhosis: Its diagnostic significance. Gastroenterology 64:89, 1973

322. Gerbes AL et al: Atrial natriuretic peptide, the sympathetic nervous system and decompensated cirrhosis. Lancet 1: 331, 1986

322a.Gerbes AL et al: Role of the atrial natriuretic factor (ANF) in volume regulation of healthy and cirrhotic subjects: Effects of water immersion (abstr). Gastroenterology 90: 1727, 1986

323 .Gerbes AL et al: Regulation of atrial natriuretic factor release in man: Effect of water immersion. Klin Wochenschr (in press)

324. Gerding DN et al: Antibiotic concentrations in ascitic fluid of patients with ascites and bacterial peritonitis. Ann Intern Med 86:708, 1977

325. Gerety RJ (ed): Hepatitis A. Orlando, Academic Press, 1984

326. Giascosa A et al: The emergency endoscopy in the haemorrhages of the oesophagus-stomach-duodenum. Acta Endoscopica 11:189, 1981

327. Gianturco C et al: Mechanical devices for arterial occlusion. AJR 124:428, 1975

328. Gibson PR et al: Disseminated intravascular coagulation following peritoneo-venous (LeVeen) shunt. Aust NZ J Med 11:8, 1981

329. Gibson WR, Robertson HE: So-called biliary cirrhosis. Arch Pathol 28:37, 1939

329a.Gimson AES et al: A randomized trial of vasopressin and vasopressin plus nitroglycerin in the control of acute variceal haemorrhage. Hepatology 6:410, 1986

330. Gitlin N et al: The pH of ascitic fluid in the diagnosis of spontaneous bacterial peritonitis in alcoholic cirrhosis. Hepatology 2:408, 1982

331. Gleysteen JJ, Klamer TW: Peritoneovenous shunts: Predictive factors of early treatment failure. Am J Gastroenterol 79:654, 1984

331a.Goff JS et al: A randomized trial of sclerotherapy vs standard therapy for bleeding esophageal varices. Long-term follow-up (abstr). Gastroenterology 90:1728, 1986

332. Goldblatt H: Report of pathologists on cirrhosis study. Transactions 6th Conference on Liver Injury, p 9. New York, Josiah Macy, Jr Foundation, 1947

333. Golding PL et al: Multisystem involvement in chronic liver disease: Studies on the incidence and pathogenesis. Am J Med 55:772, 1973

334. Goldman ML et al: The transjugular technique of hepatic venography and biopsy cholangiography and obliteration of esophageal varices. Radiology 128:325, 1978

335. Goldsmith LA: Tyrosinemia and related disorders. In Stanbury JB et al (eds): The Metabolic Basis of Inherited Disease, 5th ed, p 287. New York, McGraw Hill, 1983

336. Goldstein H, Boyle JD: Spontaneous recovery from the hepatorenal syndrome: Report of four cases. N Engl J Med 272:895, 1965

337. Goldstein MJ et al: Hepatic metastases and portal cirrhosis. Am J Med Sci 252:26, 1966

338. Gonzalez EM et al: Interposition left gastric-caval shunt

using internal jugular vein autograft in the treatment of portal hypertension. Br J Surg 65:115, 1978

339. Goodman DS: Vitamin A and retinoids in health and disease. N Engl J Med 310:1023, 1985

340. Goodyer, AVN et al: Salt retention in cirrhosis of the liver. J Clin Invest 29:973, 1950

341. Gorbach SL et al: Studies of intestinal microflora: I. Effects of diet, age and periodic sampling on numbers of fecal microorganisms in man. Gastroenterology 53:845, 1967

342. Gorbach SL et al: Studies of intestinal microflora: V. Fecal microbial ecology in ulcerative colitis and regional enteritis: Relationship to severity of disease and chemotherapy. Gastroenterology 54:575, 1968

343. Gorbach SL et al: Alterations in human intestinal microflora during experimental diarrhea. Gut 11:1, 1970

344. Gordon ME: The acute effects of abdominal paracentesis in Laënnec's cirrhosis upon exchanges of electrolytes and water renal function and hemodynamics. Am J Gastroenterol 33:15, 1960

345. Gotloib L, Servadio C: Ascites in patients undergoing maintenance hemodialysis: Report of six cases and physiopathologic approach. Am J Med 61:465, 1976

346. Govindarajans S et al: Alpha-1-antitrypsin phenotypes in hepatocellular carcinoma. Hepatology 1:628, 1981

346a.Grace WJ et al: Chest hair and cirrhosis of the liver. Am J Dig Dis 7:913, 1962

347. Graf H et al: Effect of amino acid infusion on glomerular filtration rate. N Eng J Med 308:159, 1983

348. Graham DY: Limited value of early endoscopy in the management of upper gastrointestinal bleeding: Prospective controlled trial. Am J Surg 140:284, 1980

349. Gray HK: Clinical and experimental investigation of circulation of liver: Moynihan lecture. Ann R Coll Surg Engl 8:354, 1951

350. Greenberger NJ et al: Effect of vegetable and animal protein diets in chronic hepatic encephalopathy. Am J Dig Dis 22:845, 1977

351. Greene HL: Glycogen storage disease. Sem Liv Dis 2:291, 1982

352. Gregory PB et al: Complications of diuresis in the alcoholic patient with ascites: A controlled trial. Gastroenterology 73:534, 1977

353. Grobe JL et al: Venography during endoscopic injection sclerotherapy of esophageal varices. Gastrointest Endosc 30:6, 1984

354. Grosberg SJ, Wapnick S: A retrospective comparison of functional renal failure in cirrhosis treated by conventional therapy or the peritoneovenous shunt (LeVeen). Am J Med Sci 276:287, 1978

355. Groszmann RJ et al: Wedged and free hepatic venous pressure measured with a balloon catheter. Gastroenterology 76:253, 1979

356. Groszmann RJ et al: Nitroglycerin improves the hemodynamic response to vasopressin in portal hypertension. Hepatology 2:757, 1982

357. Gullino P et al: Studies on the metabolism of amino acids and related compounds in vivo: I. Toxicity of essential amino acids, individually and in mixtures, and the protective effect of L-arginine. Arch Biochem Biophys 64:319, 1956

358. Hahn RD: Syphilis of the liver. Am J Syph 27:529, 1943

359. Haines NW et al: Prognostic indicators of hepatic injury following jejunoileal bypass for refractory obesity: A prospective study. Hepatology 1:161, 1981

360. Hales MR et al: Injection-corrosion studies of normal and cirrhotic livers. Am J Pathol 35:909, 1959

361. Hallén J, Kroak H: Follow-up studies on unselected ten year material of 360 patients with liver cirrhosis in one community. Acta Med Scand 173:479, 1963

362. Hällen J, Norđen J: Liver cirrhosis unsuspected during life: A series of 79 cases. J Chronic Dis 17:951, 1964

363. Halstead CH et al: Intestinal malabsorption in folate-deficient alcoholics. Gastroenterology 64:526, 1973

364. Harbin WP et al: Diagnosis of cirrhosis based on regional changes in hepatic morphology. Radiology 135:273, 1980

365. Hardwick DF, Dimmick JE: Metabolic cirrhoses of infancy and early childhood. In Rosenberg HS, Bolande RP (eds): Perspectives in Pediatric Pathology, vol 3, p 103. Chicago, Year Book Publications, 1976

365a.Harinasuta U, Zimmerman HJ. Alcoholic steatonecrosis: I. Relationship between severity of hepatic disease and presence of Mallory bodies in liver. Gastroenterology 60:1036, 1971

366. Harley H et al: A randomized trial of end-to-side portacaval shunt and distal splenorenal shunt in alcoholic liver disease with variceal bleeding. Gastroenterology 91:802, 1986

367. Hartroft WS: Experimental reproduction of human hepatic disease. In Popper H, Schaffner F (eds): Progress in Liver Disease, Vol 1, p 68. New York, Grune & Stratton, 1961

368. Harty RF, Steinberg WM: Noninfectious ascitic fluid leukocytosis associated with penetrating duodenal ulcer. Dig Dis 23:1132, 1978

369. Harvald B, Madsen S: Long-term treatment of cirrhosis of the liver with prednisone. Acta Med Scand 169:381, 1961

369a.Hashizume M et al: Morphology of gastric microcirculation in cirrhosis. Hepatology 3:1008, 1983

370. Hassab MA: Gastroesophageal decongestion and splenectomy in the treatment of esophageal varices in bilharzial cirrhosis: Further studies with a report on 355 operations. Surgery 61:169, 1967

371. Hassall E et al: Hepatic encephalopathy after portacaval shunt in a noncirrhotic child. J Pediatr 105:439, 1984

372. Havens WP Jr et al: The production of antibody by patients with chronic hepatic disease. J Immunol 67:347, 1951

373. Hecker R, Sherlock S: Electrolyte and circulatory changes in terminal liver failure. Lancet 2:1121, 1956

374. Hein MF et al: The effect of portacaval shunting on gastric secretion in cirrhotic dogs. Gastroenterology 44:637, 1963

375. Heinemann HO: Respiration and circulation in patients with portal cirrhosis of the liver. Circulation 22:154, 1960

376. Heinemann HO et al: Hyperventilation and arterial hypoxemia in cirrhosis of the liver. Am J Med 28:239, 1960

377. Heird WC et al: Hyperammonemia resulting from intravenous alimentation using a mixture of synthetic L-amino acids: A preliminary report. J Pediatr 81:162, 1972

378. Helman R et al: Alcoholic hepatitis: Natural history and evaluation of prednisolone therapy. Ann Intern Med 74:311, 1971

379. Helwig FC, Schutz CB: A liver kidney syndrome: Clinical, pathological and experimental studies. Surg Gynecol Obstet 55:570, 1932

380. Helzberg JH, Greenberger NJ: Peritoneovenous shunts in malignant ascites. Dig Dis Sci 30:1104, 1985

381. Henriksen JH et al: Noradrenaline and adrenaline concentrations in various vascular beds in patients with cirrhosis: Relation to hemodynamics. Clin Physiol 1:293, 1981

381a.Henriksen JH: Colloid osmotic pressure in decompensated cirrhosis: A "mirror image" of portal venous hypertension. Scand J Gastroenterol 20:170, 1985

382. Herlong HF et al: The use of ornithine salts of branched-

chain ketoacids in portal systemic encephalopathy. Ann Intern Med 93:545, 1980

383. Hillon P et al: Comparison of the effects of a cardioselective and a nonselective β-blocker on portal hypertension in patients with cirrhosis. Hepatology 2:528, 1982

384. Himsworth HP, Glynn LE: Massive hepatic necrosis and diffuse hepatic fibrosis (acute yellow atrophy and portal cirrhosis): Their production by means of diet. Clin Sci 5:93, 1944

385. Himsworth HP, Glynn LE: Toxipathic and trophopathic hepatitis. Lancet 1:457, 1944

386. Hirayama C, et al: A controlled clinical trial of nicotinohydroxamic acid and neomycin in advanced chronic liver disease. Digestion 25:115, 1982

387. Hislop WS et al: Serological markers of hepatitis B in patients with alcoholic liver disease: A multi-centre survey. J Clin Pathol 34:1017, 1981

388. Hobbs CL et al: Peritoneovenous shunt for hydrothorax associated with ascites. Arch Surg 117:1233, 1982

389. Hocking HP et al: Late hepatic histology after jejunoileal bypass for morbid obesity: Relation of abnormalities on biopsy and clinical course. Am J Surg 141:159, 1981

390. Hocking HP et al: Jejunoileal bypass for morbid obesity: Late follow-up in 100 cases. N Engl J Med 30:995, 1983

391. Hodges Jr et al: Heterozygous MZ alpha-1-antitrypsin deficiency in adults with chronic active hepatitis and cryptogenic cirrhosis. N Engl J Med 304:557, 1981

392. Hoefs JC: Increase in ascites white blood cell and protein concentrations during diuresis in patients with chronic liver disease. Hepatology 1:249, 1981

393. Hoefs JC et al: Spontaneous bacterial peritonitis. Hepatology 2:399, 1982

394. Hoffman BI et al: Bacteremia after rectal examination. Ann Intern Med 88:658, 1978

395. Horst D et al: Comparison of dietary protein with an oral, branched chain–enriched amino acid supplement in chronic portal-systemic encephalopathy: A randomized controlled trial. Hepatology 4:279, 1984

396. Hsia YE: Inherited hyperammonemic syndromes. Gastroenterology 67:347, 1974

397. Hubschmann OR, Countee RW: Gram-positive peritonitis in patients with infected ventriculoperitoneal shunts. Surg Gynecol Obstet 149:69, 1979

398. Huizinga WKJ et al: Esophageal transection versus injection sclerotherapy in the management of bleeding esophageal varices in patients at high risk. Surg Gynecol Obstet 160:539, 1985

399. Hyatt RE, Smith JR: The mechanism of ascites. A physiologic appraisal. Am J Med 16:434, 1954

400. Hyde GL, Moosnick FB: Treatment of intractable ascites by peritoneal-atrial shunt. JAMA 201:264, 1967.

401. Idezuki Y et al: Endoscopic balloon tamponade for emergency control of bleeding esophageal varices using a new transparent tamponade tube. Trans Am Soc Artif Intern Organs 23:646, 1977

402. Imler M et al: Importance de l'hyperammoniemie d'origine renale dans la pathogenie des comas hepatiques declenches chez les cirrhotiques par les diuretiques generateurs d'hypokaliemie. Pathol Biol 17:5, 1969

403. Imler M et al: Etude comparative du traitement de l'encephalopathie port-cave par le lactulose, les bacilles lactiques et les antibiotiques. Therapeutique 47:237, 1971

404. Inokuchi K: Selective decompression of esophageal varices by a left gastric venaocaval shunt. Surg Annu 10:215, 1978

405. Inokuchi K, Cooperative Study Group of Portal Hypertension of Japan: Prophylactic portal non-decompression

surgery in patients with esophageal varices: An interim report. Ann Surg 200:61, 1984

406. Ishak KG, Sharp HL: Metabolic errors and liver disease. In MacSween R et al (eds): Pathology of the Liver, p 28. Edinburgh, Churchill-Livingstone, 1979

407. Ishak KG et al: Cirrhosis of the liver associated with alpha-1-antitrypsin deficiency. Arch Pathol 94:445, 1972

408. Isner J et al: Spontaneous streptococcus pneumonia peritonitis in a patient with metastatic gastric cancer: A case report and etiologic consideration. Cancer 39:2306, 1977

409. Iwatsuki Y et al: Paradoxic elevation of serum growth hormone levels after splenectomy and/or paraesophagogastric devascularization in patients with portal hypertension. Metabolism 29:568, 1980

410. Iwatsuki S et al: Recovery from "hepatorenal syndrome" after orthotopic liver transplantation. N Engl J Med 289:1155, 1973

411. Jackson FC et al: A clinical investigation of the portacaval shunt: II. Survival analysis of the prophylactic operation. Am J Surg 115:22, 1968

412. Jackson FC et al: A clinical investigation of the portacaval shunt: V. Survival analysis of the therapeutic operation. Ann Surg 174:672, 1971

413. James JH et al: Hyperammonaemia, plasma aminoacid imbalance, and blood-brain aminoacid transport: A unified theory of portal-systemic encephalopathy. Lancet 2:772, 1979

414. Jeffers LJ et al: Post transfusion non B hepatitis resulting in cirrhosis of the liver. Hepatology 1:521, 1981

415. Jenkins SA et al: A prospective randomized controlled clinical trial comparing somatostatin and vasopressin in controlling acute variceal haemorrhage. Br Med J 290:275, 1985

416. Johnson RF, Loo RV: Hepatic hydrothorax: Studies to determine the source of the fluid and report of thirteen cases. Ann Intern Med 61:385, 1964

417. Johnson WC et al: Control of bleeding varices by vasopressin: A prospective randomized study. Ann Surg 186:369, 1977

418. Johnston DG et al: hyperinsulinism of hepatic cirrhosis: Diminished degradation or hypersecretion? Lancet 1:10, 1977

419. Johnston GW: Six years' experience of oesophageal transection for oesophageal varices using a circular stapling gun. Gut 23:770, 1982

420. Johnston GW, Rodgers HW: A review of 15 years experience in the use of sclerotherapy in the control of acute hemorrhage from oesophageal varices. Br J Surg 60:797, 1973

421. Jolivet J et al: The pharmacologic and clinical use of methotrexate. N Engl J Med 309:1094, 1983

422. Jolliffe N, Jellinek EM: Vitamin deficiencies and liver cirrhosis in alcoholism: VII. Cirrhosis of the liver. Q J Stud Alcohol 2:544, 1941

423. Joly JG et al: Bleeding from esophageal varices in cirrhosis of the liver: Hemodynamic and radiologic criteria for selection of potential bleeders through hepatic and umbilicoportal catheterization studies. Can Med Assoc J 104:576, 1971

424. Jones EA et al: The neurobiology of hepatic encephalopathy. Hepatology 4:1235, 1984

425. Jones SA et al: Arterialization of the human liver following portacaval anastomosis. West J Surg 63:574, 1955

426. Jones SR: The absolute granulocyte count in ascites fluid. West J Med 126:344, 1977

427. Joseph RR: A rational approach to the treatment of ascites in Laënnec's cirrhosis. Med Clin North Am 53:1359, 1963

428. Jozsa L et al: Hepatitis syphilitica: A clinico-pathological study of 25 cases. Acta Hepato-Gastroenterol 24:344, 1977

429. Juhl E et al: Liver morphology and biochemistry in eight obese subjects treated with jejunoilial anastomosis. N Engl J Med 285:543, 1971

430. Kakos GS et al: Subtotal portacaval shunt obliteration for chronic hepatic encephalopathy. Ann Surg 177:276, 1973

431. Kakumu S, Leevy CM: Lymphocyte cytotoxicity in alcoholic hepatitis. Gastroenterology 72:594, 1977

432. Kammerer J et al: Peritonites bacteriennes spontances du cirrhotique. Gastroenterol Clin Biol 3:709, 1979

433. Kammerer J et al: Apport des exams cytologiques et bacteriologiques du liquide d'ascite cirrhotique au diagnostic de peritonite bacterienne. Med Chir Dig 11:243, 1982

434. Kan YW et al: Further observations on polycythemia in hepatocellular carcinoma. Blood 18:592, 1961

435. Kanagasundaram N et al: Alcoholic hyalin antigen (AHAg) and antibody (AHAb) in alcoholic hepatitis. Gastroenterology 73:1368, 1977

436. Kane RA, Katz SG: The spectrum of sonographic findings in portal hypertension: A subject review and new observations. Radiology 142:453, 1982

437. Kao HW: Large volume paracentesis: A cause of hypovolemia? Hepatology 5:403, 1985

438. Karmi G et al: The association of syphilis with hepatic cirrhosis: A report of six cases and review of literature. Postgrad Med J 45:675, 1969

439. Kaufman JJ: Ammoniagenic coma following ureterosigmoidostomy. J Urol 131:743, 1984

440. Kaunitz JD, Lindenbaum J: The bioavailability of folic acid added to wine. Ann Intern Med 87:542, 1977

441. Karsner HT: Morphology and pathogenesis of hepatic cirrhosis. Am J Clin Pathol 13:569, 1943

442. Kearns PJ et al: Hepatorenal syndrome managed with hemodialysis, then reversed by peritoneovenous shunting. J Clin Gastroenterol 7:341, 1985

443. Kehne JH et al: The use of surgical pituitrin in the control of esophageal varix bleeding. Surgery 39:917, 1956

444. Keller AZ: The epidemiology of lip, oral and pharyngeal cancers and the association with selected systemic diseases. Am J Public Health 53:1214, 1963

445. Keller AZ: Cirrhosis of the liver, alcoholism and heavy smoking associated with cancer of the mouth and pharynx. Cancer 20:1015, 1967

446. Keller AZ, Terris M: The association of alcohol and tobacco with cancer of the mouth and pharynx. Am J Public Health 55:1578, 1965

447. Keller RT, Logan GM Jr: Comparison of emergent endoscopy and upper gastrointestinal series radiography in acute upper gastrointestinal haemorrhage. Gut 17:180, 1976

448. Keller U et al: Role of the splanchnic bed in extracting circulating adrenaline and noradrenaline in normal subjects and in patients with cirrhosis of the liver. Clin Sci 67:45, 1984

449. Kennedy TC, Knudson RJ: Exercise aggravated hypoxemia and orthodeoxia in cirrhosis. Chest 72:305, 1977

450. Keren G et al: Pulmonary arterio-venous fistula in hepatic cirrhosis. Arch Dis Child 58:302, 1983

451. Kerlan RK et al: Portal-systemic encephalopathy due to a congenital portocaval shunt. AJR 139:1013, 1982

452. Kerr DNS et al: Infection of ascitic fluid in patients with hepatic cirrhosis. Gut 4:394, 1963

453. Kersh ES, Rifkin H: Lactulose enemas. Ann Intern Med 78:81, 1973

454. Kershenobich D et al: Treatment of cirrhosis with colchicine: A double-blind randomized trial. Gastroenterology 77:532, 1979

455. Kershenobich D et al: Treatment of liver cirrhosis with colchicine: A double blind randomized trial from 1973 to 1983 (abstr). Hepatology 4:1061, 1984

456. Keshavarzian A et al: Dietary protein supplementation from vegetable sources in the management of chronic portal systemic encephalopathy. Am J Gastroenterol 79: 945, 1984

457. Kew MC et al: Renal and intrarenal blood-flow in cirrhosis of the liver. Lancet 2:504, 1971

458. Kew MC et al: Renal blood flow in malignant disease of the liver. Gut 13:421, 1972

459. Kew MC et al: The effect of octapressin on renal and intrarenal blood flow in cirrhosis of the liver. Gut 13:293, 1972

460. Keys A, Snell AM: Respiratory properties of the arterial blood in normal man and in patients with disease of the liver: Position of the oxygen dissociation curve. J Clin Invest 17:59, 1938

461. Killip T III, Payne MA: High serum transaminase activity in heart disease, circulatory failure and hepatic necrosis. Circulation 21:646, 1960

462. Kirk AP et al: Peptic ulceration in patients with chronic liver disease. Dig Dis 25:756, 1980

463. Klahr S, Tripathy K: Evaluation of renal function in malnutrition. Arch Intern Med 118:322, 1966

464. Klatskin G: Subacute hepatic necrosis and postnecrotic cirrhosis due to anicteric infections with the hepatitis virus. Am J Med 25:333, 1958

465. Klatskin G: Alcohol and its relation to liver damage. Gastroenterology 41:443, 1961

466. Klatskin G: Toxic and drug-induced hepatitis. In Schiff L (ed): Diseases of the Liver, p 517. Philadelphia, JB Lippincott, 1969

467. Klatsky AL et al: Alcohol consumption and blood pressure. N Engl J Med 296:1194, 1977

468. Kley HK et al: Effect of testosterone application on hormone concentrations of androgens and estrogens in male patients with cirrhosis of the liver. Gastroenterology 76: 235, 1979

469. Knauer CM, Lowe HM: Hemodynamics in the cirrhotic patient during paracentesis. N Engl J Med 276:491, 1967

470. Knodell RG et al: Development of chronic liver disease after acute non A non B post-transfusion hepatitis. Gastroenterology 72:902, 1977

471. Koppel MH et al: Transplantation of cadaveric kidneys from patients with hepatorenal syndrome: Evidence for the functional nature of renal failure in advanced liver disease. N Engl J Med 280:1367, 1969

472. Koretz RL: The long-term course of non A, non B post-transfusion hepatitis. Dig Dis Sci 79:893, 1980

473. Koretz RL et al: Non A non B post transfusion hepatitis: Disaster after decades? Hepatology 2:687, 1982

474. Korula J et al: A prospective, randomized controlled trial of chronic esophageal variceal sclerotherapy. Hepatology 5:584, 1985

475. Kountouras J et al: Prolonged bile duct obstruction: A

new experimental model for cirrhosis in the rat. Br J Exp Pathol 65:305, 1984

476. Kowalski HJ et al: The cardiac output in patients with cirrhosis of the liver and tense ascites with observations on the effect of paracentesis. J Clin Invest 33:768, 1954

477. Koyama K et al: Results of esophageal transection for esophageal varices: Experience in 100 cases. Am J Surg 139:204, 1980

478. Kozarek RA et al: Laparoscopy in a patient with LeVeen shunt: Prevention of air embolism. Gastrointest Endosc 30:193, 1984

479. Kramer HJ: Natriuretic activity in plasma following extracellular volume expansion. In Kaufmann W, Krause DK (eds): Central Nervous Control of Na$^+$ Balance-Relations to the Renin-Angiotensin System, p 126. Stuttgart, George Thieme Verlag, 1976

480. Kravetz D et al: Tratamiento de la ascitis refractaria mediante el shunt peritoneo-yugular: Eficacia, complicaciones y supervivencia. Gastroenterologia y Hepatolgia 5: 347, 1982

481. Kravetz D et al: Comparison of intravenous somatostatin and vasopressin infusions in treatment of acute variceal hemorrhage. Hepatology 4:442, 1984

482. Krowka MJ, Cortese DA: Pulmonary aspects of chronic liver disease and liver transplantation. Mayo Clin Proc 60:407, 1985

483. Kroyer JM, Talbert W: Morphologic liver changes in intestinal bypass patients. Am J Surg 139:855, 1980

484. Kryger P et al: The long-term prognosis of non-transfusion associated non A non B hepatitis. Scand J Gastroenterol 18:597, 1983

485. Kurtz RC, Bronzo RL: Does spontaneous bacterial peritonitis occur in malignant ascites? Am J Gastroenterol 77: 146, 1982

486. Laënnec RTH: Traité de l'auscultation mediate, p 196. Paris, Chaude, 1826

487. Lam KC et al: Role of a false neurotransmitter, octopamine in the pathogenesis of hepatic and renal encephalopathy. Scand J Gastroenterol 8:465, 1973

488. Lancestremere RG et al: Renal failure in Laënnec's cirrhosis: II. Simultaneous determination of cardiac output and renal hemodynamics. J Clin Invest 41:1922, 1962

489. Langer B et al: Further reports of a prospective randomized trial comparing distal splenorenal shunt to end-to-side portacaval shunt: An analysis of encephalopathy, survival, and quality of life. Gastroenterology 88:424, 1985

490. Lanthier PL, Morgan MY: Lactitol in the treatment of chronic hepatic encephalopathy: An open comparison with lactulose. Gut 26:415, 1985

491. Laragh JH: A trial natriuretic hormone, the renin-aldosterone axis, and blood pressure-electrolyte homeostasis. N Engl J Med 312:1130, 1985

492. Larcher VF et al: Spontaneous bacterial peritonitis in children with chronic liver disease: Clinical features and etiologic factors. J Pediatr 106:907, 1985

493. Larsson C: Natural history and life expectancy in severe alpha anti-trypsin, Pi Z. Acta Med Scand 204:345, 1978

494. Lazarides E: Intermediate filaments: A chemically heterogeneous, developmentally regulated class of proteins. Ann Rev Biochem 51:219, 1982

495. Leavitt S, Tyler HR: Studies in asterixis. Arch Neurol 10: 360, 1964

496. Lebovics E et al: Portal-systemic myelopathy after portacaval shunt surgery. Arch Intern Med 145:1921, 1985

497. Lebrec D et al: Pulmonary hypertension complicating portal hypertension. Am Rev Respir Dis 120:849, 1979

498. Lebrec D et al: The effect of propranolol on portal hypertension in patients with cirrhosis: A hemodynamic study. Hepatology 2:523, 1982

499. Lebrec D et al: Propranolol for prevention of recurrent gastrointestinal bleeding in patients with cirrhosis. N Engl J Med 305:1371, 1981

500. Lebrec D et al: Transvenous liver biopsy: An experience based on 1000 hepatic tissue samplings with this procedure. Gastroenterology 83: 330, 1982

501. Lebrec D et al: A randomized controlled study of propranolol for prevention of recurrent gastrointestinal bleeding in patients with cirrhosis: A final report. Hepatology 4:355, 1984

501a. Lebrec D et al: A randomized trial of nadolol for prevention of gastrointestinal bleeding in patients with cirrhosis: Results at one year (abstr). Gastroenterology 90:1740, 1986

502. Ledermann S: In Alcohol, Alcoholisme, Alcoholisation. Institut national d'etudes demographiques, Travaux et Documents, Cahier No. 14. Paris, Presses Universitaires de France, 1964

503. Lee FI: Cirrhosis and hepatoma in alcoholics. Gut 7:77, 1966

504. Lee RV et al: Liver disease associated with secondary syphilis. N Engl J Med 284:1423, 1971

505. Leevy CM et al: Disease of the Liver and Biliary Tract: Standardization of Nomenclature, Diagnostic Criteria, and Diagnostic Methodology. Fogarty International Center Proceedings, No. 22, DHEW Publication No. (NIH) 76-225. Washington DC, US Government Printing Office, 1976

506. Lefkowitch JH, Fenoglio JJ Jr: Liver disease in alcoholic cardiomyopathy: Evidence against cirrhosis. Hum Path 14:457, 1983

507. Lefkowitch JH et al: Hepatic copper overload and featuring Indian childhood cirrhosis in an American sibship. N Engl J Med 307:271, 1982

508. LeFrock JL et al: Transient bacteremia associated with sigmoidoscopy. N Engl J Med 289:467, 1973

509. Leger L et al: L'anastomose porto-renale: Justification et technique. Pressé Med 73:1587, 1965

510. Lelbach WK: Organic pathology related to volume and pattern of alcohol use. In Gibbons RJ et al (eds): Research Advances in Alcohol and Drug Problems, vol 1. New York, John Wiley & Sons, 1974

511. Lemmer JH et al: Management of spontaneous umbilical hernia disruption in the cirrhotic patient. Ann Surg 198: 30, 1983

512. Lemon SM: Type A viral hepatitis: New developments in an old disease. N Engl J Med 313:1059, 1985

513. Leo MA et al: Effect of hepatic vitamin A depletion on the liver in men and rats. Gastroenterology 84:562, 1983

514. Leonetti JP et al: Umbilical herniorraphy in cirrhotic patients. Arch Surg 119:442, 1984

515. Lerman BB et al: Hepatic encephalopathy precipitated by fecal impaction. Arch Intern Med 139:707, 1979

516. Lerner RG et al: Disseminated intravascular coagulation. JAMA 240:2064, 1978

517. Lerut JP et al: Peritoneo-venous drainage and hepatorenal syndrome. Acta Gastroenterol Belg 45:189, 1982

518. LeVeen HW, Wapnick S: Peritoneovenous shunt for ascites. Surg Annu 10:191, 1978

518a.LeVeen HH et al: Further experience with peritoneo-venous shunt for ascites. Ann Surg 184:574, 1976

519. LeVeen HH et al: Management of ascites with hydrothorax. Am J Surg 148:210, 1984

520. LeVeen HH et al: Peritoneovenous shunt occlusion: Etiology, diagnosis, therapy. Ann Surg 200:212, 1984

521. Levy M: Sodium retention and ascites formation in dogs with experimental portal cirrhosis. Am J Physiol 233:F572, 1977

522. Levy M, Wexler MJ: Renal sodium retention ascites formation in dogs with experimental cirrhosis but without portal hypertension or increased splanchnic vascular capacity. J Lab Clin Med 91:520, 1978

523. Lewis J et al: Sclerotherapy of esophageal varices. Arch Surg 115:476, 1980

524. Lieber CS: Medical Disorders of Alcoholism: Pathogenesis and Treatment. New York, WB Saunders, 1982

525. Lieber CS: Alcohol and the liver: 1984 update. Hepatology 4:1243, 1984

526. Lieber CS: Alcohol–nutrition interaction: 1984 update. Alcohol 1:151, 1984

527. Lieber CS, Rubin E: Alcoholic fatty liver. N Engl J Med 280:705, 1969

528. Lieber MM: The rare occurrence of metastatic carcinoma in the cirrhotic liver. Am J Med Sci 233:145, 1957

529. Lieberman FL, Peters RL: Cirrhotic hydrothorax: Further evidence that an acquired diaphragmatic defect is at fault. Arch Intern Med 125:14, 1970

530. Lieberman FL, Reynolds TB: The use of ethacrynic acid in patients with cirrhosis and ascites. Gastroenterology 49:531, 1965

531. Lieberman FL, Reynolds TB: Plasma volume in cirrhosis of the liver: Its relation to portal hypertension, ascites and renal failure. J Clin Invest 46:1297, 1967

532. Lieberman FL et al: Pathogenesis and treatment of hydrothorax complicating cirrhosis with ascites. Ann Intern Med 64:341, 1966

533. Lieberman FL et al: Effective plasma volume in cirrhosis with ascites: Evidence that a decreased value does not account for renal sodium retention, a spontaneous reduction in glomerular filtration rate (GFR), and a fall in GFR during drug-induced diuresis. J Clin Invest 48:975, 1969

534. Liebowitz HR: Hazards of abdominal paracentesis in the cirrhotic patient: Part III. NY State J Med 62:2223, 1962

535. Liehr H et al: Lactulose: A drug with antiendotoxin effect. Hepatogastroenterology 27:1, 1980

535a.Liel Y et al: Massive postoperative ascites: A presenting symptom of liver cirrhosis. Isr J Med Sci 21:634, 1985

535b.Limberg B et al: Correction of altered plasma amino acid pattern in cirrhosis of the liver by somatostatin. Gut 25:1291, 1984

536. Linder H: Grenzen und Gefahren der perkutanen leberbiopsie mit der Menghini-Nadel. Dtsch Med Wochenschr 92:1751, 1967

537. Lipsky PE et al: Spontaneous peritonitis and systemic lupus erythematosus: Importance of accurate diagnosis of gram-positive bacterial infections. JAMA 232:929, 1975

538. Lockwood AH et al: The dynamics of ammonia metabolism in man. Effects of liver disease and hyperammonemia. J Clin Invest 63:449, 1979

539. Lowenstein JM: Ammonia production in muscle and other tissues: The purine nucleotide cycle. Physiol Rev 52:382, 1972

540. Ludwig, Elveback LR: Parenchyma weight changes in hepatic cirrhosis: A morphometric study and discussion of the method. Lab Invest 26:338, 1972

541. Lund RH, Newkirk JB: Peritoneo-venous shunting system for surgical management of ascites. Comtemp Surg 14:31, 1979

542. Lunderquist A, Vang J: Transhepatic catheterization and obliteration of the coronary vein in patients with portal hypertension and esophageal varices. N Engl J Med 291:646, 1974

542a.Lunderquist A et al: Isobutyl 2-cyanoacrylate (bucrylate) in obliteration of gastric coronary vein and esophageal varices. AJR 130:1, 1978

543. Lunzer M: Treatment of chronic hepatic encephalopathy with levodopa. Gut 15:555, 1974

544. MacBeth WAAG et al: Treatment of hepatic encephalopathy by alteration of intestinal flora with Lactobacillus acidophilus. Lancet 1:399, 1965

544a.Macdougall BRD, Williams R: A controlled trial of cimetidine in the recurrence of variceal hemorrhage. Hepatology 3:69, 1983

545. Macdougall BRD et al: Increased long-term survival in variceal hemorrhage using injection sclerotherapy: Results of a controlled trial. Lancet 1:124, 1982

546. Macdougall BRD et al: A prospective randomized study of two sclerotherapy techniques for esophageal varices. Hepatology 3:681, 1983

547. Mackay IR: Genetic aspects of liver disease. Rec Adv Hepatol 1:11, 1983

548. MacSween RNM, Anthony RS: Immune mechanisms in alcoholic liver disease. In Hall P (ed): Alcoholic Liver Disease: Pathobiology, Epidemiology and Clinical Aspects, p 69. New York, John Wiley & Sons, 1985

549. Madden JW et al: Dimethylnitrosamine-induced hepatic cirrhosis: A new canine model of an ancient human disease. Surgery 68:260, 1967

550. Maddrey WC, Iber FL: Familial cirrhosis: A clinical and pathological study. Ann Intern Med 61:667, 1964

551. Maddrey WC et al: Sarcoidosis and chronic hepatic disease: A clinical and pathologic study of 20 patients. Medicine 49:375, 1970

552. Maddrey WC et al: Corticosteroid therapy of alcohol hepatitis. Gastroenterology 76:218, 1979

553. Maillard JN et al: Arterialization of the liver with portacaval shunt in the treatment of portal hypertension due to intrahepatic block. Surgery 67:883, 1970

554. Mainland D: The risk of fallacious conclusions from autopsy data on the incidence of diseases with applications to heart disease. Am Heart J 45:644, 1953

555. Mallory A, et al: Selective intraarterial vasopressin infusion for upper gastrointestinal tract hemorrhage: A controlled trial. Arch Surg 115:30, 1980

556. Mallory FB: Cirrhosis of the liver: Five different types of lesions from which it may arise. Johns Hopkins Med J 22:69, 1911

557. Malt RA et al: Randomized trial of emergency mesocaval and portacaval shunts for bleeding esophageal varices. Am J Surg 135:584, 1978

558. Mann JD et al: The vasculature of the human liver: A study by the injection cast method. Mayo Clin Proc 28:227, 1953

559. Manning RT: A nomogram for estimation of pNH$_3$. J Lab Clin Med 63:297, 1964

560. Mantz FA, Craige E: Portal axis thrombosis with spon-

taneous portacaval shunt and resultant cor pulmonale. Arch Pathol 52:91, 1951

561. Marchesini G et al: Insulin and glucagon levels in liver cirrhosis. Relationship with plasma amino acids imbalance of chronic hepatic encephalopathy. Dig Dis Sci 24:594, 1979

562. Marchesini G et al: Prevalence of subclinical hepatic encephalopathy in cirrhotics and relationship to plasma amino acid imbalance. Dig Dis Sci 25:763, 1980

563. Marchesini G et al: Muscle protein breakdown in liver cirrhosis and the role of altered carbohydrate metabolism. Hepatology 1:294, 1981

564. Martin WJ et al: Severe liver disease complicated by bacteremia due to gram-negative bacilli. Arch Intern Med 98: 8, 1956

565. Martini GA: Leber cirrhose bei Morbus Osler. Cirrhosis hepatic teleangiectatica. Gastroenterologia 83:157, 1955

566. Marubbio AT: Antidiuretic hormone effect of pitressin during continuous pitressin administration. Gastroenterology 62:1103, 1972

567. Marubbio AT: The liver in morbid obesity and following bypass surgery for obesity. Surg Clin North Am 59:1079, 1979

568. Marubbio AT et al: Hepatic lesion of central pericellular fibrosis in morbid obesity and after jejunoileal bypass. Am J Clin Pathol 66:684, 1976

569. Mashford ML et al: Studies of the cardiovascular system in the hypotension of liver failure. N Engl J Med 267: 1071, 1962

570. Matsubara O et al: Histometric investigation of the pulmonary artery in severe hepatic disease. J Pathol 143;31, 1984

571. McCartney JE, Fraser J. Pneumococcal peritonitis. Br J Surg 36:475, 1922

572. McClain CJ et al: The effect of lactulose on psychomotor performance tests in alcoholic cirrhotics without overt hepatic encephalopathy. J Clin Gastroenterol 6:325, 1984

573. McCloy RM et al: Effect of changing plasma volume, serum albumin concentration and plasma osmolality on renal function in cirrhosis. Gastroenterology 53:229, 1967

574. McCue JD: Spontaneous bacterial peritonitis caused by a viridans streptococcus or Neisseria perflava. JAMA 250: 3319, 1983

575. McDermott WV Jr: Diversion of urine to the intestines as a factor in ammoniagenic coma. N Engl J Med 256: 460, 1957

576. McDermott WV Jr: The treatment of cirrhotic ascites by combined hepatic and portal decompression. N Engl J Med 259:897, 1958

577. McDermott WV Jr: Evaluation of the hemodynamics of portal hypertension in the selection of patients for shunt surgery. Ann Surg 176:449, 1972

578. McDermott WV Jr et al: Treatment of "hepatic coma" with L-glutamic acid. N Engl J Med 253:1093, 1955

579. McDonald FD et al: Severe hypertension and elevated plasma renin activity following transplantation of "hepatorenal donor" kidneys into anephric recipients. Am J Med 54:39, 1973

580. McDonald RA, Mallory GK: Hemochromatosis and hemosiderosis. Arch Intern Med 105:686, 1960

581. McDonnell PJ et al: Pulmonary hypertension and cirrhosis: Are they related? Am Rev Respir Dis 127:437, 1983

582. McGhee A et al: Comparison of the effects of hepaticacid and a casein modular diet on encephalopathy, plasma

amino acids and nitrogen balance in cirrhotic patients. Ann Surg 197:288, 1983

583. McGiff JC et al: Modulation and mediation of the action of the renal kallikrein–kinin system by prostaglandins. Fed Proc 35:175, 1976

584. McKenna JP et al: The use of continuous postoperative peritoneal lavage in the management of diffuse peritonitis. Surg Gynecol Obstet 130:254, 1970

584a. Megavand R: Emergency treatment of bleeding esophageal varices. Digestion 3:372, 1970

585. Mehigan DG et al: The incidence of shunt occlusion following portal-systemic decompression. Surg Gynecol Obstet 150:661, 1980

586. Meirhenry EF et al: Mallory body formation in hepatic nodules of mice ingesting dieldrin. Lab Invest 44:392, 1981

587. Mekhjian HS, May ES: Acute and chronic effects of ethanol on fluid transport in the human small intestine. Gastroenterology 72:1280, 1977

588. Mellemgaard K et al: Sources of venoarterial admixture in portal hypertension. J Clin Invest 42:1399,1963

589. Melloni GF et al: Effectiveness of ibopamine in the management of ascitic liver cirrhosis: A controlled study of placebo and frusemide. Br J Clin Pharmacol 12:813, 1981

590. Mendez G Jr, Russell E: Gastrointestinal varices: Percutaneous transheptaic therapeutic embolization in 54 patients. AJR 135:1045, 1980

591. Menghini G: One second needle biopsy of the liver. Gastroenterology 35:190, 1958

592. Menghini G: L'aspect morpho-bioptique du foie de l'alcoolique (non-cirrhotique) et son evolution. Bull Schweiz Akad Med Wiss 16:36, 1960

593. Merigan TC Jr et al: Effect of intravenously administered posterior pituitary extract on hemorrhage from bleeding esophageal varices: A controlled evaluation. N Engl J Med 266:134, 1962

594. Metzler M et al: Noninvasive determination of LeVeen shunt patency. Surgery 87:106, 1980

595. Meyers S, Lieber CS: Reduction of gastric ammonia by ampicillin in normal and azotemic subjects. Gastroenterology 70:244, 1976

596. Michel H et al: Treatment of cirrhotic hepatic encephalopathy by L-dopa: A double-blind study of 58 patients. Digestion 15:232, 1977

597. Michel H et al: Treatment of acute hepatic encephalopathy in cirrhotics with a branched-chain amino acids enriched versus a conventional amino acids mixture: A controlled study of 70 patients. Liver 5:282, 1985

598. Michel J: Rupture de varices oesopgastriques: Traitement par une nouvelle sonde hemostatique. Nouv Presse Med 7:3245, 1978

599. Mikkelsen WP: Emergency portacaval shunt. Rev Surg 19:141, 1962

600. Millikan WJ Jr et al: The Emory prospective randomized trial: Selective versus nonselective shunt to control variceal bleeding: Ten year follow-up. Ann Surg 201:712, 1985

601. Mills PR et al: Evidence for previous hepatis B virus infection in alcoholic cirrhosis. Br Med J 282:437, 1981

602. Minuk GY et al: Elevated serum γ-aminobutyric acid levels in children with Reye's syndrome. J Pediatr Gastroenterol Nutr 4:528, 1985

603. Mitch WE et al: Plasma levels and hepatic extraction of renin and aldosterone in alcoholic liver disease. Am J Med 66:804, 1979

604. Mitchell K et al: Prospective comparison of two Sengstaken

tubes in the management of patients with variceal hemorrhage. Gut 21:570, 1980

605. Mittal VK et al: Esophageal transection for bleeding esophageal varices. Arch Surg 115:991, 1980

606. Monroe P et al: Acute respiratory failure after sodium morrhuate esophageal sclerotherapy. Gastroenterology 85:693, 1983

607. Moon VH: Experimental cirrhosis in relation to human cirrhosis. Arch Pathol 18:381, 1934

608. Moore EW et al: Distribution of ammonia across the blood-cerebrospinal fluid barrier in patients with hepatic failure. Am J Med 35:350, 1963

609. Morgan AP, Moore FD: Jejunoileostomy for extreme obesity: Rationale, metabolic observations, and results in a single case. Ann Surg 166:75, 1967

610. Morgan MH et al: Clinical and electrophysiological studies of peripheral nerve function in patients with chronic liver disease. Clin Sci 57:31, 1979

611. Morgan MY et al: Successful use of bromocriptine in the treatment of a patient with chronic portal-systemic encephalopathy. N Engl J Med 296:793, 1977

612. Morgan MY et al: Serum prolactin in liver disease and its relationship to gynaecomastia. Gut 19:170, 1978

613. Morgan MY et al: Plasma ratio of valine, leucine and isoleucine to phenylalanine and tyrosine in liver disease. Gut 19:1068, 1978

614. Morris DW et al: Prospective, randomized study of diagnosis and outcome in acute upper-gastrointestinal bleeding endoscopy versus conventional radiography. Am J Dig Dis 20:1103, 1975

615. Morrison EB et al: Severe pulmonary hypertension associated with macronodular (postnecrotic) cirrhosis and autoimmune phenomena. Am J Med 69:513, 1980

616. Moschcowitz E: The pathogenesis of splenomegaly in hypertension of the portal circulation: "Congestive splenomegaly." Medicine 27:187, 1948

617. Mould RF: An investigation of the variations in normal liver shape. Br J Radiol 45:586, 1972

618. Mowat AP: Hepatic disorders. Clin Gastroenterol 11:171, 1982

619. Mowat AP: Alpha-antitrypsin deficiency in liver disease. In Williams R, Maddrey W (eds): Liver, p 52. London, Butterworths, 1984

620. Muehrcke RC: The finger-nails in chronic hypoalbuminaemia: A new physical sign. Br Med J 1:1327, 1956

621. Mullane JR, Gliedman ML: Elevation of the pressure in the abdominal inferior vena cava as a course of a heptorenal syndrome in cirrhosis. Surgery 59:1135, 1966

621a. Munro HN: Insulin, plasma amino acid imbalance, and hepatic coma. Lancet 1:722, 1975

622. Murphy TL et al: Hepatic coma. Clinical and laboratory observations on 40 patients. N Engl J Med 239:605, 1948

623. Murray HW, Marks SJ: Spontaneous bacterial empyema, pericarditis, and peritonitis in cirrhosis. Gastroenterology 72:772, 1977

624. Murray M, Moosnick F: Incidence of bacteremia in patients with dental disease. J Lab Clin Med 26:801, 1941

625. Mutchnick MG et al: Portal-systemic encephalopathy and portal anastomosis: A prospective, controlled investigation. Gastroenterology 66:1005, 1974

626. Mutchnick MG et al: Effect of portacaval anastomosis on hypersplenism: A prospective controlled evaluation. Gastroenterology 68:1070, 1975

627. Muting D et al: Cirrhosis of the liver and diabetes mellitus. Ger Med Mon 11:385, 1966

628. Muto Y, Takahashi Y: Gas chromatographic determination of plasma short chain fatty acids in diseases of the liver. J Jpn Soc Int Med 53:828, 1964

629. Naeije R et al: Hypoxic pulmonary vasoconstriction in liver cirrhosis. Chest 80:570, 1981

630. Nagant de Deuxchaisnes C et al: Exchangeable potassium in wasting, amyotrophy, heart-disease and cirrhosis of the liver. Lancet 1:681, 1961

631. Nakano M et al: Perivenular fibrosis in alcoholic liver injury: Ultrastructure and histologic progression. Gastroenterology 83:777, 1982

632. Nance FC et al: Ammonia production in germ-free Eck fistula dogs. Surgery 70:169, 1971

633. Nance FC et al: Role of urea in the hyperammonemia of germ-free Eck fistula dogs. Gastroenterology 66:108, 1974

634. Naparstek Y et al: Transient cortical blindness in hepatic encephalopathy. Isr J Med Sci 15:854, 1979

635. Naranjo CA et al: Furosemide-induced adverse reactions in cirrhosis of the liver. Clin Pharmacol Ther 25:154, 1979

636. Nasrallah SM et al: Importance of terminal hepatic venule thickening. Arch Pathol Lab Med 104:84, 1980

637. Nasrallah SM et al: Liver injury following jejunoileal bypass. Ann Surg 192:726, 1980

638. Nicholas P et al: Increased incidence of cholelithiasis in Laënnec's cirrhosis: A postmortem evaluation of pathogenesis. Gastroenterology 63:112, 1972

639. Nicholls KM et al: Elevated plasma norepinephrine concentrations in decompensated cirrhosis: Association with increased secretion rates, normal clearance rates, and suppressibility by central blood volume expansion. Circ Res 56:457, 1985

639a. Nusbaum M et al: Clinical experience with the diagnosis and management of gastrointestinal hemorrhage by selective mesenteric catheterization. Ann Surg 170:506, 1969

640. Nyfors A: Liver biopsies from psoriatics related to methotrexate therapy. Acta Pathol Microbiol Scand 85:511, 1977

641. O'Connor M et al: Peritoneovenous shunt therapy for leaking ascites in the cirrhotic patient. Ann Surg 200:66, 1984

642. Odievre M et al: Hereditary fructose intolerance in childhood. Am J Dis Child 132:605, 1978

643. Oei LT et al: Cerebrospinal fluid glutamine levels and EEG findings in patients with hepatic encephalopathy. Clin Neurol Neurosurg 81:59, 1979

644. Okuda K et al: Frequency of intrahepatic arteriovenous fistula as a sequela to percutaneous needle puncture of the liver. Gastroenterology 74:1204, 1978

644a. Okuda K: Clinical aspects of hepatocellular carcinoma–analysis of 134 cases. In Okuda K, Peters RL: Hepatocellular Carcinoma, p 387. New York, John Wiley & Sons, 1976

645. O'Leary JP: Hepatic complications of jejunoileal bypass. Sem Liver Dis 3:203, 1983

646. Olefsky JM: Insulin resistance in humans. Gastroenterology 83:1313, 1982

647. Ono J et al: Tryptophan and hepatic coma. Gastroenterology 74:196, 1974

648. Orlandi F et al: Comparison between neomycin and lactulose in 173 patients with hepatic encephalopathy: A randomized clinical study. Dig Dis Sci 26:498, 1981

649. Orloff MJ: Emergency portacaval shunt: A comparative

study of shunt, varix ligation and nonsurgical treatment of bleeding esophageal varices in unselected patients with cirrhosis. Ann Surg 166:456, 1967

650. Orloff MJ: Pathogenesis and surgical treatment of intractable ascites associated with alcoholic cirrhosis. Ann NY Acad Sci 170:213, 1970

650a.Orloff MJ, Bell RH Jr: Long-term survival after emergency portacaval shunting for bleeding varices in patients with alcoholic cirrhosis. Am J Surg 151:176, 1986

651. Orloff MJ, Johansen KH: Treatment of Budd–Chiari syndrome by side-to-side portacaval shunt: Experimental and clinical results. Am Surg 188:494, 1978

652. Orloff MJ, Thomas HS: Pathogenesis of esophageal varix rupture. Arch Surg 87:301, 1963

653. Orloff MJ et al: Experimental ascites: VI. The effects of hepatic venous outflow obstruction and ascites on aldosterone secretion. Surgery 56:83, 1964

654. Orloff MJ et al: Experimental ascites: VII. The effects of external drainage of the thoracic duct on ascites and hepatic hemodynamics. Arch Surg 93:119, 1966

655. Orloff MJ et al: Emergency shunt for bleeding varices. Arch Surg 108:293, 1974

656. Orloff MJ et al: Long-term results of emergency portacaval shunt for bleeding esophageal varices in unselected patients with alcoholic cirrhosis. Ann Surg 192:325, 1980

657. Orloff MJ et al: Prospective randomized trial of emergency portacaval shunt and medical therapy in unselected cirrhotic patients with bleeding varices (abstr). Gastroenterology 90:1754, 1986

658. Orrego H et al: Collagenisation of the Disse space in alcoholic liver disease. Gut 20:673, 1979

659. Orrego H et al: Alcoholic liver disease: Information in search of knowledge? Hepatology 1:267, 1981

660. Orrego H et al: Assessment of prognostic factors in alcoholic liver disease. Hepatology 3:896, 1983

661. Osborne DR, Hobbs KEF: The acute treatment of haemorrhage from oesophageal varices: A comparison of oesophageal transection and staple gun anastomosis with mesocaval shunt. Br J Surg 68:734, 1981

662. Otte JB et al: Étude compareé de l'anastomose porto-cave avec et sans arterialisation de la veine porte. Acta Gastroenterol Belg 41:493, 1978

663. Padfield PL, Morton JJ: Application of a senstive radioimmunoassay for plasma arginine vasopressin to pathological conditions in man. Clin Sci Molec Med 47:16P, 1974

664. Page IH: Ipsilateral edema and contralateral jaundice associated with hemiplegia and cardiac decompensation. Am J Med Sci 177:273, 1929

664a.Pagliaro L et al: A randomized clinical trial of propranolol for the prevention of mitral bleeding in cirrhosis with portal hypertension. (correspondence) N Engl J Med 314:244, 1986

665. Pagliaro L et al: Percutaneous blind biopsy versus laparoscopy with guided biopsy in diagnosis of cirrhosis: A prospective, randomized trial. Dig Dis 28:39, 1983

666. Pahmer M: Pneumococcus peritonitis in nephrotic and non-nephrotic children: A comparative clinical and pathologic study with a brief review of the literature. J Pediatr 17:695, 1940

667. Palmer ED: Further experience with the vigorous diagnostic approach to upper gastrointestinal hemorrhage. Am J Med Sci 233:497, 1957

668. Palmer ED et al: Evaluation of clinical results of portal decompression in cirrhosis. JAMA 164:746, 1957

669. Pande NV et al: Cirrhotic portal hypertension: Morbidity of continued alcoholism Gastroenterology 74:64, 1978

670. Panes J et al: El taponamiento esofagico en el tratamiento de la hamorragia activa por varices esofagogastricas. Eficacia y complicaciones en una serie de 100 casos. Gastroenterologia y Hepatologia 8:13, 1985

671. Pappas SC et al: Visual potentials in a rabbit model of hepatic encephalopathy: Comparison of hyperammonemic encephalopathy, posital coma, and coma induced by syngeristic neurotoxins. Gastroenterology 86:546, 1984

672. Papper S: The role of the kidney in Laënnec's cirrhosis of the liver. Medicine 37:299, 1958

673. Papper S et al: Renal failure in Laennec's cirrhosis of the liver: I. Description of clinical and laboratory features. Ann Intern Med 51:759, 1959

674. Paquet KJ: Prophylactic endoscopic sclerosing treatment of the esophageal wall in varices: A prospective controlled randomized trial. Endoscopy 14:4, 1982

675. Paquet KJ, Feussner H: Endoscopic sclerosis and esophageal balloon tamponade in acute hemorrhage from esophagogastric varices: A prospective controlled randomized trial. Hepatology 5:580, 1985

676. Paquet, KJ, Oberhammer E: Sclerotherapy of bleeding oesophageal varices by means of endoscopy. Endoscopy 10:7, 1978

677. Parbhoo SP et al: Treatment of ascites by continuous ultrafiltration and reinfusion of protein concentrate. Gut 14:421, 1973

678. Pariente E-A et al: Hepatocytic PAS–positive diastase–resistant inclusion in the absence of alpha-1-antitrypsin deficiency: High prevalence in alcoholic cirrhosis. Am J Clin Pathol 76:299, 1981

679. Parker G et al: Do beta blockers differ in their effects on hepatic microsomal enzymes and liver blood flow? J Clin Pharmacol 24:493, 1984

680. Parkes JD et al: Levodopa in hepatic coma. Lancet 2:1341, 1970

681. Paronetto F: Immunologic factors in alcoholic liver disease. Semin Liver Dis 1:232, 1981

682. Parsons V et al: Use of dialysis in the treatment of renal failure in liver disease. Postgrad Med J 51:515, 1975

682a.Pascal JP et al: Prophylactic treatment of variceal bleeding in cirrhotic patients with propranolol: A multicentric randomized study (abstr). Hepatology 4:1092, 1984

683. Patek AJ Jr, de Fritsch NM: Evidence for genetic factors in the resistance of the rat to dietary cirrhosis. Proc Soc Exp Biol Med 113:820, 1963

683a.Patek AJ, Koff, RS: Predicting clinical recovery from alcoholic liver disease. J Clin Gastroenterol 5:303, 1983

684. Patek AJ Jr et al: The dietary treatment of cirrhosis of the liver: Results in 124 patients observed during a ten year period. JAMA 138:543, 1948

685. Patek AJ Jr et al: The effects of intravenous injection of concentrated human serum albumin upon blood plasma ascites and renal functions in three patients with cirrhosis of the liver. J Clin Invest 27:135, 1948

686. Patek AJ Jr et al: Strain differences in susceptibility of the rat to dietary cirrhosis. Proc Soc Exp Biol Med 121:569, 1966

687. Patino JF et al: El uso del "shunt" peritoneovenoso de Hakim en el tratamiento de la ascitis. Rev Argent Cirug 37:304, 1979

688. Pearson RD et al: Cirrhosis of liver with septic arthritis due to Escherichia coli: Unusual locus minoris resistenciae for bacteremic cirrhosis. NY State J Med 78:1762, 1978

689. Pek S et al: Effects upon plasma glucagon of infused and ingested amino acids and of protein meals in man. Diabetes 18:328, 1969

690. Peracchia A et al: A new technique for the treatment of esophageal bleeding in portal hypertension. Intern Surg 65:401, 1980

691. Perez-Ayuso RM et al: Eficacia de la furosemida en la cirrosis hepatica con ascitis: Relacion entre la respuesta diuretica y el grado de hiperaldosteronismo. Gastroenterologia y Hepatologia 4:402, 1981

692. Perez-Ayuso RM et al: Randomized comparative study of efficacy of furosemide versus spironolactone in non-azotemic cirrhosis with ascites. Gastroenterology 84:961, 1983

693. Perez-Ayuso RM et al: Renal kallikrein excretion in cirrhotics with ascites: Relationship to renal hemodynamics. Hepatology 4:247, 1984

694. Perkoff GT: Alcoholic myopathy. Annu Rev Med 22:125, 1971

695. Pescovitz MD: Umbilical hernia repair in patients with cirrhosis: No evidence for increased incidence of variceal bleeding. Ann Surg 199:325, 1984

696. Peter B et al: Influence de l'alpha-ceto-glutarate de L(+) ornithine sur l'hyperammoniémie provoquée des cirrhotiques. Ann Gastroenterol Hepatol 10:179, 1974

697. Peters RL, Reynolds TB: Hepatic changes simulating alcoholic liver disease postileojejunal bypass. Gastroenterology 65:564, 1973

698. Petersdorf RG, Beeson PB: Fever of unexplained origin: Report of 100 cases. Medicine 40:1, 1961

699. Petersen P. Alcoholic hyalin, microfilaments, and microtubules in alcoholic hepatitis. Acta Pathol Scand 85:384, 1977

700. Peterson WL et al: Routine early endoscopy in upper-gastrointestinal tract bleeding: A randomized, controlled trial. N Engl J Med 304:925, 1981

701. Pettigrew NM et al: Evidence for a role of hepatitis B virus in chronic alcoholic liver disease. Lancet 2:724, 1972

702. Phatak MC: Computed tomography of the liver. CT 8: 157, 1984

703. Phear et al: Methionine toxicity in liver disease and its prevention by chlortetracycline. Clin Sci 15:93, 1956

704. Phillips GB et al: The syndrome of impending hepatic coma in patients with cirrhosis of the liver given certain nitrogenous substances. N Engl J Med 247:239, 1952

705. Phillips MM et al: Portacaval anastomosis and peptic ulcer: A nonassociation. Gastroenterology 68:121, 1975

706. Picone SB Jr et al: Abdominal colectomy for chronic encephalopathy due to portal-systemic shunt. Arch Surg 118: 33, 1983

707. Pilkington LA et al: Intrarenal distribution of blood flow. Am J Physiol 208:1107, 1965

708. Pimentel JC, Menezes AP: Liver disease in vineyard sprayers. Gastroenterology 72:275, 1977

709. Pinzello G et al: Spontaneous bacterial peritonitis: A prospective investigation in predominantly nonalcoholic cirrhotic patients. Hepatology 3:545, 1983

710. Pinzello G et al: Is the acidity of ascitic fluid a reliable index in making the presumptive diagnosis of spontaneous bacterial peritonitis? Hepatology 6:244, 1986

711. Pirovino M et al: Pneumococcal vaccination: The response of patients with alcoholic liver cirrhosis. Hepatology 4: 946, 1984

712. Pitcher JL: Safety and effectiveness of the modified Sengstaken-Blakemore tube: A prospective study. Gastroenterology 61:291, 1971

713. Pitcher JL: Variceal hemorrhage among patients with varices and upper gastrointestinal hemorrhage. South Med J 70:1183, 1977

714. Pladson TR, Parrish RM: Hepatorenal syndrome: Recovery after peritoneovenous shunt. Arch Intern Med 137: 1248, 1977

715. Pockros PJ, Reynolds TB: Rapid diuresis in patients with ascites from chronic liver disease: The importance of peripheral edema. Gastroenterology 90:1827, 1986

716. Podolsky S et al: Potassium depletion in cirrhosis: Impaired growth-hormone and insulin response. N Engl J Med 288: 644, 1973

717. Poindexter CA, Greene CH: Toxic cirrhosis of the liver: Report of a case due to long continued exposure to carbon tetrachloride. JAMA 102:2015, 1934

718. Pomier-Layrargues G et al: Presinusoidal portal hypertension in non-alcoholic cirrhosis. Hepatology 5:415, 1985

719. Ponce J et al: Morphometric study of the oesophageal mucosa in cirrhotic patients with variceal bleeding. Hepatology 1:641, 1981

720. Popper H: Significance of agonal changes in the human liver. Arch Pathol 46:132, 1948

721. Popper H: Experimental ischemia of the liver and hepatic coma. Transactions 10th Conference on Liver Injury, p 171. New York, Josiah Macy Jr Foundation, 1951

722. Popper H, Schaffner F: Liver: Structure and Function, p 648. New York, McGraw-Hill, 1957

723. Popper H, Schaffner F: Nutritional cirrhosis in man. N Engl J Med 285:577, 1971

724. Popper H, Schaffner F: Alcoholic hepatitis: An experimental approach to a conceptual and clinical problem. N Engl J Med 290:159, 1974

725. Popper H et al: Florid cirrhosis: A review of 35 cases. Am J Clin Pathol 25:889, 1955

726. Potter JF, Beevers DG: Pressor effect of alcohol in hypertension. Lancet 1:119, 1984

727. Potts JR III et al: Emergency distal splenorenal shunts for variceal hemorrhage refractory to nonoperative control. Am J Surg 148:813, 1984

728. Powell LW: Iron storage in relatives of patients with hemochromatosis and in relatives of patients with alcoholic cirrhosis and haemosiderosis: A comparative study of 27 families. Q J Med 34:427, 1965

729. Powell LW, Axelsen E: Corticosteroids in liver disease: Studies on the biological conversion of prednisone to prednisolone and plasma protein binding. Gut 13:690, 1972

730. Powell WJ, Klatskin G: Duration of survival in patients with Laënnec's cirrhosis. Am J Med 44:406, 1968

731. Powers JH: Bacteremia following instrumentation of the infected urinary tract. NY J Med 36:323, 1936

732. Poynard T et al: Prognostic value of total serum bilirubin/gamma-glutanyl transpeptidase ratio in cirrhotic patients. Hepatology 4:324, 1984

733. Price JB Jr et al: Glucagon as the portal factor modifying hepatic regeneration. Surgery 72:74, 1972

734. Pugh RNH et al: Transection of the oesophagus for bleeding oesophageal varices. Br J Surg 60:646, 1973

735. Pullman TN et al: The influence of dietary protein intake

on specific renal functions in normal man. J Lab Clin Med 44:320, 1954

736. Quintero E et al: Paracentesis versus diuretics in the treatment of cirrhotics with tense ascites. Lancet 1:611, 1985

737. Quizilbash A, Young–Pong VA: Alpha-1-anti-trypsin liver disease differential diagnosis of PAS-positive diastase-resistant globules in liver cells. Am J Clin Pathol 79:697, 1983

738. Rakela J: Chronic liver disease after acute non A non B viral hepatitis. Gastroenterology 79:1200, 1979

739. Ralli EP et al: Studies of the serum and urine constituents in patients with cirrhosis of the liver during water tolerance tests. Am J Med 11:157, 1951

740. Ramalingaswami V: Perspectives in protein malnutrition. Nature 201:546, 1964

741. Rankin JGD et al: Alcoholic liver disease: The problem of diagnosis. Alcohol Clin Exp Res 2:327, 1978

742. Ranniger K, Switz D: Local obstruction of inferior vena cava by massive ascites. AJR 93:935, 1965

743. Rapaport E: Cardiopulmonary complications of liver disease. In Zakim D, Boyer TD (eds): Hepatology: A Textbook of Liver Disease, p 531. Philadelphia, WB Saunders, 1982

744. Rapaport SI et al: Plasma clotting factors in chronic hepatocellular disease. N Engl J Med 263:278, 1960

745. Rappaport AM: Acinar units and the pathophysiology of the liver. In Rouiller C (ed): The Liver: Morphology, Biochemistry, Physiology, vol 1, p 266. New York, Academic Press, 1963

746. Rasmussen SN: Liver volume by ultrasonic scanning. Br J Radiol 45:579, 1972

747. Ratnoff OD, Patek AJ Jr: The natural history of Laënnec's cirrhosis of the liver: An analysis of 286 cases. Medicine 21:207, 1942

748. Realdi G: Long term follow-up of acute and chronic non A non B post-transfusion hepatitis: Evidence of progression to liver cirrhosis. Gut 23:270, 1982

749. Recknagel RO, Ghoshal AK: Lipoperoxidation as a vector in carbon tetrachloride hepatotoxicity. Lab Invest 15:132, 1966

750. Recknagel RO et al: A new insight into pathogenesis of carbon tetrachloride fat infiltration. Proc Soc Exp Biol Med 104:608, 1960

751. Rector WG, Redeker AG: Direct transhepatic assessment of hepatic vein pressure and direction of flow using a thin needle in patients with cirrhosis and Budd-Chiari syndrome. Gastroenterology 86:1395, 1984

752. Rector WG, Reynolds TB: Risk for haemorrhage from oesophagel varices and acute gastric erosions. Clin Gastroenterol 14:139, 1985

753. Redeker A: Delta agent and hepatitis B. Ann Intern Med 98:542, 1983

754. Redeker AG et al: Randomization of corticosteroid therapy in fulminant hepatitis. N Engl J Med 294:728, 1976

755. Rees KR: Aflatoxin. Gut 7:205, 1966

756. Regan TJ, Haider B. Ethanol abuse and heart disease. Circulation 64 (suppl 3):14, 1981

757. Rehnstrom SH et al: Chronic hepatic encephalopathy: A psychometrical study. Scand J Gastroenterol 121:305, 1977

758. Reichle FA et al: Prospective comparative clinical trial with distal splenorenal and mesocaval shunts. Am J Surg 137:13, 1979

759. Reinhardt GF, Stanley MM: Peritoneo-venous shunting for ascites. Surg Gynecol Obstet 145:419, 1977

760. Reith AF, Squire TL: Blood cultures of apparently healthy persons. J Infect Dis 51:336, 1932

761. Report of the Board for Classification and Nomenclature of Cirrhosis of the Liver. Fifth Pan-American Congress of Gastroenterology, La Habana, Cuba. Gastroenterology 31: 213, 1956

762. Resnick RH et al: A controlled trial of colon bypass in chronic hepatic encephalopathy. Gastroenterology 54: 1057, 1968

763. Resnick RH et al: A controlled study of the prophylactic portacaval shunt: A final report. Ann Intern Med 70:675, 1969

764. Resnick RH et al: Renal function and fecal flora after colon bypass. Arch Surg 101:353, 1970

765. Resnick RH et al: A controlled study of the therapeutic portacaval shunt. Gastroenterology 67:843, 1974

766. Resnick RH et al: Distal splenorenal shunt (DSRS) vs. portalsystemic shunt (PSS): Current status of a controlled trial. Gastroenterology 77:A 33, 1979

767. Reubner BH, Miyai K: The low incidence of myocardial infarction in hepatic cirrhosis. Lancet 2:1435, 1961

768. Reubner BH, Montgomery CK: Pathology of the Liver and Biliary Tract. New York, John Wiley & Sons, 1982

769. Reubner BH et al: The rarity of intrahepatic metastasis in cirrhosis of the liver: A statistical explanation with some comments on the interpretation of necropsy data. Am J Pathol 39:739, 1961

770. Reynaert M et al: Traitement de l'hemorragie par rupture de varices oesophagiennes au moyen de la sonde de Michel. Acta Gastroenterol Belg 46:142, 1983

771. Reynolds TB et al: A controlled study of the effects of L-arginine on hepatic encephalopathy. Am J Med 25:359, 1958

772. Reynolds TB et al: Spontaneous decrease in portal pressure with clinical improvement in cirrhosis. N Engl J Med 263: 734, 1960

773. Reynolds TB et al: Advantages of treatment of ascites without sodium restriction and without complete removal of excess fluid. Gut 19:549, 1978

774. Reynolds TB et al: Results of a 12-year randomized trial of porta-caval shunts in patients with alcoholic liver disease and bleeding varices. Gastroenterology 80:1005, 1981

775. Richard JH: Bacteremia following irritation of foci of infection. JAMA 99:1496, 1932

776. Rikkers L et al: Subclinical hepatic encephalopathy: Detection, prevalence, and relationship to nitrogen metabolism. Gastroenterology 75:462, 1978

777. Rimola A et al: Reticuloendothelial system phagocytic activity in cirrhosis and its relation to bacterial infections and prognosis. Hepatology 4:53, 1984

778. Rimola A et al: Oral, nonabsorbable antibiotics prevent infection in cirrhotics with gastrointestinal hemorrhage. Hepatology 5:463, 1985

779. Rinzler DM et al: Diabetes and portacaval anastomosis: A prospective controlled investigation. Gastroenterology 75:956, 1978

780. Rizzetto M: The Delta agent. Hepatology 3:729, 1983

781. Rizzetto M et al: Chronic hepatitis in carriers of hepatitis B surface antigen, with intrahepatic expression of the delta antigen. Ann Intern Med 98:437, 1983

782. Roberts WC: The hepatic cirrhosis of cystic fibrosis of the pancreas. Am J Med 32:324, 1962

783. Robin ED et al: Platypnea related to orthodeoxia caused by true vascular lung shunts. N Engl J Med 294:941, 1976

784. Rodman T et al: Arterial oxygen unsaturation and the ventilation-perfusion defect of Laënnec's cirrhosis. N Engl J Med 263:73, 1960

785. Roenigk HH Jr: Methotrexate guidelines: Revised. J Am Acad Dermatol 6:145, 1982

786. Rollo FD, Deland FH: The determination of liver mass from radionuclide images. Radiology 91:1191, 1968

787. Rösch J et al: Selective arterial infusions of vasoconstrictors in acute gastrointestinal bleeding. Radiology 99:27, 1971

788. Rösch J et al: Transjugular approach to liver biopsy and transhepatic cholangiography. N Engl J Med 289:227, 1973

789. Rosen HM et al: Plasma amino acid patterns in hepatic encephalopathy of differing etiology. Gastroenterology 72:483, 1977

790. Rosoff L Jr et al: Studies of renin and aldosterone in cirrhotic patients with ascites. Gastroenterology 69:698, 1975

791. Ross EJ: Importance of potassium supplements during the use of spironolactone and thiazide diuretics. Br Med J 1:1508, 1961

792. Rossi–Fanelli F et al: Branched-chain amino acids vs. lactulose in the treatment of hepatic coma: A controlled study. Dig Dis Sci 27:929, 1982

793. Rössle R: In Henke F, Lubarsch O (eds): Handbuch der Spezillen Pathologischen Anatomie und Histologie, vol 5, part 1. Berlin, Julius Springer, 1930

794. Rothschild MA et al: Albumin synthesis in cirrhotic subjects with ascites studied with carbonate-^{14}C. J Clin Invest 48:344, 1969

795. Rothschild MA et al: Albumin synthesis. N Engl J Med 286:748, 816, 1972

796. Rowland M: Eosinophilic peritonitis: An unusual manifestation of spontaneous bacterial peritonitis. J Clin Gastroenterol 7:369, 1985

797. Roy CC et al: Hepatologic disease in cystic fibrosis: A survey of current issues and concepts. J Pediatr Gastroenterol Nutr 1:469, 1982

798. Rubin E, Lieber CS: Fatty liver, alcoholic hepatitis and cirrhosis produced by alcohol in primates. N Engl J Med 290:128, 1974

799. Rubin E et al: Pathogenesis of postnecrotic cirrhosis in alcoholics. Arch Pathol 73:288, 1962

800. Rubinson RM et al: Intra-abdominal pressure and vena caval obstruction. Arch Surg 94:766, 1967

801. Rubinstein D et al: Hepatic hydrothorax in the absence of clinical ascites: Diagnosis and management. Gastroenterology 88:188, 1985

802. Rueff B et al: A controlled study of therapeutic portacaval shunt in alcoholic cirrhosis. Lancet 2:655, 1976

803. Ruff F et al: Regional lung function in patients with hepatic cirrhosis. J Clin Invest 50:2403, 1971

804. Rumpelt HJ: Ultrastructure of alcoholic hyalin and fate of the affected hepatocytes. Virchows Arch 23:339, 1977

805. Runyon BA: Spontaneous bacterial peritonitis associated with cardiac ascites. Am J Gastroenterol 79:796, 1984

806. Runyon BA, Hoefs JC: Ascitic fluid analysis in the differentiation of spontaneous bacterial peritonitis from gastrointestinal tract perforation into ascitic fluid. Hepatology 4:447, 1984

807. Runyon BA, Hoefs JC: Culture-negative neurocytic ascites: A variant of spontaneous bacterial peritonitis. Hepatology 4:1209, 1984

808. Runyon BA, Peters RL: Non A non B post transfusion hepatitis: Natural history and response to corticosteroids. Gastroenterology 88:1690, 1985

809. Runyon BA et al: Opsonic activity of human ascitic fluid: A potentially important protective mechanism against spontaneous bacterial peritonitis. Hepatology 5:634, 1985

810. Runyon BA et al: Diuresis of cirrhotic ascites increases its opsonic activity and may help prevent spontaneous bacterial peritonitis. Hepatology 6:396, 1986

810a. Russell RM et al: Hepatic injury from chronic hypervitaminosis A resulting in portal hypertension and ascites. N Engl J Med 291:435, 1974

811. Rydell R, Hoffbauer FW: Multiple pulmonary arteriovenous fistulas in juvenile cirrhosis. Am J Med 21:450, 1956

812. Safran AP, Schaffner F: Chronic passive congestion of the liver in man: Electron microscopic study of cell atrophy and intralobular fibrosis. Am J Pathol 50:447, 1967

813. Said SI, Mutt V: Polypeptide with broad biological activity: Isolation from small intestine. Science 169:1217, 1970

814. Saks BJ et al: Pleural and mediastinal changes following endoscopic injection sclerotherapy of esophageal varices. Radiology 149:639, 1983

815. Salem HH, et al: Coagulopathy of peritoneovenous shunts: Studies on the pathogenic role of ascitic fluid collagen and value of antiplatelet therapy. Gut 24:412, 1983

816. Samson FE Jr et al: A study on the narcotic action of the short chain fatty acids. J Clin Invest 35:1291, 1956

817. Samtoy B, DeBeukelaer MM: Ammonia encephalopathy secondary to urinary tract infection with *Proteus mirabilis*. Pediatrics 65:294, 1980

818. Sanchez–Tapias JM et al: Spontaneous peritoneal infection in cirrhosis with ascites: Five years of experience. Gastroenterologia y Hepatologia 1:15, 1978

819. Sandlow LJ et al: A prospective randomized study of the management of upper gastrointestinal hemorrhage. Am J Gastroenterol 61:282, 1974

820. Sarfeh IJ: Comparative study of portacaval and mesocaval interposition shunts. Am J Surg 142:511, 1981

821. Sarfeh IJ et al: Clinical significance of erosive gastritis in patients with alcoholic liver disease and upper gastrointestinal hemorrhage. Ann Surg 194:149, 1981

822. Sarfeh IJ et al: Portal hypertension and gastric mucosal injury in rats. Gastroenterology 84:987, 1983

823. Sarin SK, Mundy S: Balloon tamponade in the management of bleeding oesophageal varices. Ann R Coll Surg Engl 66:30, 1984

824. Saruta T et al: Regulation of aldosterone in cirrhosis of the liver. In Epstein M (ed): The Kidney in Liver Disease, p 271. New York, Elsevier North-Holland, 1978

825. Sauerbruch T et al: Bacteriaemia associated with endoscopic sclerotherapy of oesophageal varices. Endoscopy 17:170, 1985

825a. Sauerbruch T et al: Endoscopic sclerotherapy (ST) for prophylaxis of first variceal bleeding in liver cirrhosis: Early results of a prospective randomized trial (abstr). Gastroenterology 90:1765, 1986

826. Saunders JB et al: A 20 year prospective study of cirrhosis. Br Med J 282:263, 1981

827. Saunders JB et al: Do women develop alcoholic liver disease more readily than men? Br Med J 282:1140, 1981

828. Saunders JB et al: Accelerated development of alcoholic cirrhosis in patients with HLA B-8. Lancet 1:1381, 1982

829. Scemama–Clergue J et al: Ascitic fluid pH in alcoholic

cirrhosis: A re-evaluation of its utility in the diagnosis of spontaneous bacterial peritonitis. Gut 26:332, 1985

830. Schafer DF, Jones EA: Hepatic encephalopathy and the γ-aminobutyric acid neurotransmitter system. Lancet 1:18, 1982

831. Schafer DF et al: Colonic bacteria: A source of γ-aminobutyric acid in blood. Proc Soc Exp Biol Med 167:301, 1981

832. Schafer DF, et al: Visual evoked potentials in a rabbit model of hepatic encephalopathy: I. Sequential changes and comparisons with drug-induced comas. Gastroenterology 86:540, 1984

833. Schatten EW et al: A bacteriologic study of portal vein blood in man. Arch Surg 71:404, 1955

834. Schlichting P et al: Prognostic factors in cirrhosis identified by Cox's regression model. Hepatology 3:889, 1983

835. Schreiber HW: Klinische und tierexperimentelle untersuchungen zum verhalten der splenpathischen blutzell-depression (hypersplenismus) nach Durchfuhrung einer porto-cavalen anastomose. Langenbecks Arch Chir 300:669, 1962

836. Schreyer P et al: Cirrhosis: Pregnancy and delivery: A Review. Obstet Gynecol Surv 37:304, 1982

837. Schrier RW, Bert T: Mechanism of the antidiuretic effect associated with interruption of parasympathetic pathways. J Clin Invest 51:2613, 1972

838. Schroeder ET et al: Renal failure in patients with cirrhosis of the liver: III. Evaluation of intrarenal blood flow by para-aminohippurate extraction and response to angiotensin. Am J Med 43:887, 1967

839. Schroeder ET et al: Plasma renin level in hepatic cirrhosis: Relation to functional renal failure. Am J Med 49:186, 1970

840. Schroeder ET et al: Functional renal failure in cirrhosis: Recovery after portacaval shunt. Ann Intern Med 72:923, 1970

841. Schroeder ET et al: Effects of a portacaval or peritoneovenous shunt on renin in the hepatorenal syndrome. Kidney Int 15:54, 1979

842. Schwachman H: Cystic fibrosis: A new outlook: 70 patients over 25 years of age. Medicine 56:129, 1977

843. Schwartz ML: Complications of the LeVeen shunt. In Najarian S, Delaney JP (eds): Hepatic, Biliary, and Pancreatic Surgery, p 493. Miami, Symposia Specialists, 1980

844. Schwartz ML, Miller RP: Angiographic assessment of peritoneovenous shunt malfunction. Arch Surg 116:435, 1981

845. Schwartz ML, Vogel SB: Treatment of hepatorenal syndrome. Am J Surg 139:370, 1980

846. Schwartz ML et al: Consumptive coagulopathy following peritoneovenous shunting. Surgery 85:671, 1979

847. Schweinburg FB, et al: Transmural migration of intestinal bacteria: A study based on the use of radioactive *Escherischia coli*. N Engl J Med 242:747, 1950

848. Scobie BA, Summerskill WHJ: Hepatic cirrhosis secondary to obstruction of the biliary system. Am J Dig Dis 10:135, 1965

849. Seegmiller JE et al: The plasma ammonia and glutamine content in patients with hepatic coma. J Clin Invest 33:984, 1954

850. Seeley JR: Death by liver cirrhosis and the price of beverage alcohol. Can Med Assoc J 83:1361, 1960

851. Sellars L et al: The renin-angiotensin-aldosterone system in decompensated cirrhosis: Its activity in relation to sodium balance. Q J Med 56:485, 1985

852. Sengstaken RW, Blakemore AH: Balloon tamponade for the control of hemorrhage from esophageal varices. Ann Surg 131:781, 1950

853. Senior RM et al: Pulmonary hypertension associated with cirrhosis of the liver and with portacaval shunts. Circulation 37:88, 1966

854. Sharp HL: Alpha-1-antitrypsin: An ignored protein in understanding liver disease. Sem Liver Dis 2:314, 1982

855. Sharp HL et al: Cirrhosis associated with alpha-1-antitrypsin deficiency: A previously unrecognized inherited disorder. J Lab Clin Med 73:934, 1969

856. Shashaty GG: Cryptogenic cirrhosis associated with methyldopa. South Med J 72:364, 1979

857. Shaw RB: Use of a fibrinolytic agent to restore function in a clotted LeVeen shunt. South Med J 75:1285, 1982

858. Shear L et al: Renal failure in patients with cirrhosis of the liver: II. Factors influencing maximal urinary flow rate. Am J Med 39:199, 1965

859. Shear L et al: Renal failure in patients with cirrhosis of the liver: I. Clinical and pathological characteristics. Am J Med 39:184, 1965

860. Shear L et al: Compartmentalization of ascites and edema in patients with hepatic cirrhosis. N Engl J Med 282:1391, 1970

861. Sherlock S: The liver in heart failure: Relation of anatomical, functional and circulatory changes. Br Heart J 13:273, 1951

862. Sherlock S, Walshe V: Effect of under-nutrition in man on hepatic structure and function. Nature 161:604, 1948

863. Sherlock S et al: Complications of diuretic therapy in hepatic cirrhosis. Lancet 1:1049, 1966

864. Sherwin R et al: Hyperglucagonemia in Laënnec's cirrhosis: Role of portal systemic shunting. N Engl J Med 290:239, 1974

865. Schomerus H et al: Latent portasystemic encephalopathy: I. Nature of cerebral functional defects and their effect on fitness to drive. Dig Dis Sci 26:622, 1981

866. Shorr E: Hepatorenal vasotropic factors in experimental cirrhosis. In Liver Injury. Transactions of the 6th Conference, p 33. New York, Josiah Macy Jr Foundation, 1947

867. Short EM et al: Evidence for x-linked dominant inheritance of ornithine transcarbamylase deficiency. N Engl J Med 288:7, 1973

868. Shumaker JB et al: A controlled trial of 6-methylprednisolone in acute alcoholic hepatitis. Am J Gastroenterol 69:443, 1978

869. Silber R et al: Spur-shaped erythrocytes in Laënnec's cirrhosis. N Engl J Med 275:639, 1966

870. Silberman R: Ammonia intoxication following ureterosigmoidostomy in a patient with liver disease. Lancet 2:937, 1958

871. Silverstein E: Peripheral venous O_2 saturation in patients with and without liver disease. J Lab Clin Med 47:513, 1956

872. Sim JS et al: Mallory bodies compared with microfilament hyperplasia. Arch Pathol Lab Med 101:401, 1977

873. Simberkoff MS et al: Bactericidal and opsonic activity of cirrhotic ascites and non-ascitic peritoneal fluid. J Lab Clin Med 91:831, 1978

874. Simpson JA, Conn HO: The role of ascites in gastro-

esophageal reflux. With comments on the pathogenesis of bleeding esophageal varices. Gastroenterology 55:17, 1968

875. Singer JA et al: Cirrhotic pleural effusion in the absence of ascites. Gastroenterology 73:575, 1977

875a.Sirinek K, Thomford N: Isoproterenol in offsetting adverse effects of vasopressin in cirrhotic patients. Am J Surg 129: 130, 1975

876. Sivak MV Jr et al: Endoscopic injection sclerosis of esophageal varices. Gastrointest Endosc 27:52, 1981

877. Smadja C, Franco D: The LeVeen shunt in the elective treatment of intractable ascites in cirrhosis: A prospective study on 140 patients. Ann Surg 201:488, 1985

878. Smedile A et al: Infection with the HBV associated delta agent in HBsAg carriers. Gastroenterology 81:992, 1981

879. Smetana H, Olen H: Hereditary galactose disease. Am J Clin Pathol 38:3, 1962

880. Smith AN: Peritoneocaval shunt with a Holter valve in the treatment of ascites. Lancet 1:671, 1962

881. Smith, FW et al: Nuclear magnetic resonance tomographic imaging in liver disease. Lancet 1:963, 1984

882. Smith JL, Graham DY: Variceal hemorrhage: A critical evaluation of survival analysis. Gastroenterology 82:968, 1982

883. Smith RB et al: Dacron interposition shunts for portal hypertension: An analysis of morbidity correlates. Ann Surg 192:9, 1980

884. Smith–Laing G et al: role of percutaneous transhepatic obliteration of varices in the management of hemorrhage from gastroesophageal varices. Gastroenterology 80:1031, 1981

885. Snady H et al: The relationship of bacteremia to the length of injection needle in endoscopic variceal sclerotherapy. Gastrointest Endosc 31:243, 1985

886. Snapper I: Bedside Medicine, New York, Grune & Stratton, 1960

887. Snapper I: Chinese Lessons to Western Medicine, 2nd ed, p 9. New York, Grune & Stratton, 1965

888. Snapper I: Geographical aspects of alcohol induced liver injury: In Alcohol and the Liver, p 449. New York, Grune & Stratton, 1971

889. Snodgrass PJ: Obesity, small bowel bypass and liver disease. N Engl J Med 282:870, 1970

890. Snyder N et al: Increased concurrence of cirrhosis and bacterial endocarditis: A clinical and postmortem study. Gastroenterology 73:1107, 1977

891. Snyder N et al: Depressed delayed cutaneous hypersensitivity in alcoholic hepatitis. Am J Dig Dis 23:353, 1978

892. Söderlund C, Ihre T: Endoscopic sclerotherapy vs conservative management of bleeding oesophageal varices: A 5-year prospective controlled trial of emergency and long-term treatment. Acta Chir Scand 151:449, 1985

893. Soehendra N et al: Morphological alterations of the esophagus after endoscopic sclerotherapy of varices. Endoscopy 15:291, 1983

894. Søgaard PE: Letter: Propranolol in portal hypertension. Lancet 1:1204, 1981

895. Soloway RD et al: Observer error and sampling variability tested in evaluation of hepatitis and cirrhosis by liver biopsy. Am J Dig Dis 16:1082, 1971

896. Soloway RD et al: "Lupoid" hepatitis, a nonentity in the spectrum of chronic active liver disease. Gastroenterology 63:458, 1972

897. Sonnenberg GE et al: Effect of somatostatin on splanchnic

hemodynamics in patients with cirrhosis of the liver and in normal subjects. Gastroenterology 80:526, 1981

898. Sorensen TIA et al: Prospective evaluation of alcohol abuse and alcoholic liver injury in men as predictors of development of cirrhosis. Lancet 2:241, 1984

899. Sorensen TIA et al: Oesophageal stricture and dysphagia after endoscopic sclerotherapy for bleeding varices. Gut 25:473, 1984

900. Sorrell MF, Leevy CM: Lymphocyte transformation and alcoholic liver injury. Gastroenterology 63:1020, 1972

901. Soterakis J et al: Effect of alcohol abstinence on survival in cirrhotic portal hypertension. Lancet 2:65, 1973

902. Spence RAJ: The venous anatomy of the lower esophagus in normal subjects and in patients with varices: An image analysis study. Br J Surg 71:739, 1984

903. Spence RAJ, Johnston GW: Results in 100 consecutive patients with stapled esophageal transection for varices. Surg Gynecol Obstet 160:323, 1985

904. Spence RAJ et al: Oesophagitis in patients undergoing oesophageal transection for varices: A histological study. Br J Surg 70:332, 1983

905. Sposito M: The enlargement of the parotid glands in liver cirrhosis. Riforma Med 58:1311, 1942

906. Sposito M, Cheli R: Significance of the enlargement of the parotid gland in liver cirrhosis. Riforma Med 65:1250, 1951

907. Stabenau JR et al: The role of pH gradient in the distribution of ammonia between blood and cerebrospinal fluid, brain and muscle. J Clin Invest 38:373, 1959

907a.Stahl J: Studies of the blood ammonia in liver disease: Its diagnostic, prognostic, and therapeutic significance. Ann Intern Med 58:1, 1963

908. Stanley MM, Members of VA Cooperative Study #142: Peritoneovenous shunting vs medical treatment of alcoholic cirrhotic ascites (abstr). Hepatology 5:980, 1985

909. Stanley NM, Woodgate DJ: The circulation, the lung, and finger clubbing in hepatic cirrhosis. Br Heart J 33:469, 1971

910. Stanley NM, Woodgate DJ: Mottled chest radiograph and gas transfer defect in chronic liver disease. Thorax 27:315, 1972

911. Starling EH: On the absorption of fluids from the connective tissue spaces. J Physiol 19:312, 1896

912. Starzl TE et al: The origin, hormonal nature, and action of hepatotrophic substances in portal venous blood. Surg Gynecol Obstet 137:179, 1973

913. Starzl TE et al: Portal diversion for the treatment of glycogen storage disease in humans. Ann Surg 178:525, 1973

914. Stassen WN et al: Spontaneous bacterial peritonitis caused by Neisseria gonorrhoeae: Evidence for a transfallopian route of infection. Gastroenterology 88:804, 1985

915. Stassen WN et al: Immediate diagnostic criteria for bacterial infection of ascitic fluid: Evaluation of ascitic fluid polymorphonuclear leukocyte count, pH, and lactate concentration, alone and in combination. Gastroenterology 90:1247, 1986

916. Stauffer RA et al: Spontaneous bacterial peritonitis in pregnancy. Am J Obstet Gynecol 144:104, 1982

917. Stearns EL et al: Effects of coitus on gonadotropin, prolactin and six steroid levels in man. J Clin Endocrinol Metab 37:687, 1973

918. Steiner PE: Precision in the classification of cirrhosis of the liver. Am J Pathol 37:21, 1960

919. Stephens CG et al: Spontaneous peritonitis due to *Hemophilus influenzae* in an adult. Gastroenterology 77: 1088, 1979

920. Sterling K: Serum albumin turnover in Laënnec's cirrhosis as measured by I^{131}-tagged albumin. J Clin Invest 30:1238, 1951

921. Stipa S et al: A randomized controlled trial of mesentericocaval shunt with autologous jugular vein. Surg Gynecol Obstet 153:353, 1981

922. Stone BG, Van Thiel DH: Diabetes mellitus and the liver. Semin Liver Dis 5:8, 1985

923. Stone WD et al: The natural history of cirrhosis. Q J Med 37:119, 1968

924. Sugiura M, Futagawa S: Further evaluation of the Sugiura procedure in the treatment of esophageal varices. Arch Surg 112:1317, 1977

925. Sukigara M et al: Systemic dissemination of ethanolamine oleate after injection sclerotherapy for esophageal varices. Arch Surg 120:833, 1985

926. Summerskill WHJ: Aguecheek's disease. Lancet 2:288, 1955

927. Summerskill WHJ: Hepatic failure and the kidney. Gastroenterology 51:94, 1966

928. Summerskill WH, Shorter RG: Progressive hepatic failure: Its association with undifferentiated renal tumor. Arch Intern Med 120:81, 1967

929. Summerskill WHJ et al: Response to alcohol in chronic alcoholics with liver disease: Clinical, pathological and metabolic changes. Lancet 1:335, 1957

930. Summerskill WHJ et al: The management of hepatic coma in relation to protein withdrawal and certain specific measures. Am J Med 23:59, 1957

931. Summerskill WHJ et al: Cirrhosis of the liver: A study of alcoholic and nonalcoholic patients in Boston and London. N Engl J Med 262:1, 1960

932. Swisher WP et al: Peptic ulcer in Laënnec's cirrhosis. Am J Dig Dis 1:291, 1955

933. Symmers D: Hepar lobatum. Arch Pathol 42:64, 1946

934. Taggart GJ et al: Percutaneous transtubal scintigraphic assessment of patency of peritoneovenous shunts. Clin Nuc Med 6:70, 1981

935. Tanyol H: A hitherto undescribed finding in patients with primary varicose veins: Generalized scantiness of body hair. Implications of this observation for possible vascular origin of hypotrichosis in patients with portal cirrhosis. Angiology 15:539, 1964

936. Tarao K et al: Detection of endotoxin in plasma and ascitic fluid of patients with cirrhosis: Its clinical significance. Gastroenterology 73:539, 1977

937. Tarver D et al: Precipitation of hepatic encephalopathy by propranolol in cirrhosis. Br Med J 287:585, 1983

938. Tauber JW et al: Emergency transumbilical embolization of bleeding esophageal varices. Arch Surg 117:624, 1982

939. Taylor FW: Blood-culture studies of the portal vein. Arch Surg 72:889, 1956

940. Taylor KJW: Atlas of Gray Scale Ultrasonography. New York, Churchill Livingstone, 1978

941. Taylor R et al: Insulin action in cirrhosis. Hepatology 5: 64, 1985

942. Tekeste H et al: Portal hypertension complicating sarcoid liver disease: Case report and review of the literature. Am J Gastroenterol 79:389, 1984

943. Terblanche J et al: Acute bleeding varices: A five year prospective evaluation of tamponade and sclerotherapy. Ann Surg 194:521, 1981

944. Terblanche J et al: Failure of repeated injection sclerotherapy to improve long-term survival after esophageal variceal bleeding. Lancet 2:1328, 1983

945. Teres J et al: Esophageal tamponade for bleeding varices. Controlled trial between the Sengstaken–Blakemore tube and the Linton-Nachlas tube. Gastroenterology 75:566, 1978

946. Terry R: White nails in hepatic cirrhosis. Lancet 1:757, 1954

947. Thomas FB, Fromkes JJ: Spontaneous bacterial peritonitis associated with acute viral hepatitis. J Clin Gastroenterol 4:259, 1982

948. Thomford NR, Sirinek KR: Intravenous vasopressin in patients with portal hypertension: Advantages of continuous infusion. J Surg Res 18:113, 1975

949. Thomson A, Visek WJ: Some effects of induction of urease immunity in patients with hepatic insufficiency. Am J Med 35:804, 1963

950. Tisdale WA: Spontaneous colon bacillus bacteremia in Laënnec's cirrhosis. Gastroenterology 40:141, 1961

951. Tisdale WA, Klatskin G: The fever of Laënnec's cirrhosis. Yale J Biol Med 33:94, 1960

952. Tobe BA: The metabolism of the volatile amines: II. Observations on the use of L-arginine L-gluamate in the therapy of acute hepatic encephalopathy. Can Med Assoc J 85:591, 1961

953. Trenker SW et al: Idiopathic esophageal varix. AJR 141: 43, 1983

954. Triger DR, Millward–Sadler GH: α_1-Antitrypsin deficiency and liver disease. In Wright R et al (eds): Liver and Biliary Disease, p 805. London, WB Saunders, 1979

955. Tristani FE, Cohn JN: Systemic and renal hemodynamics in oliguric hepatic failure: Effect of volume expansion. J Clin Invest 46:1894, 1967

956. Trotman BW: Pigment gallstone disease. Semin Liver Dis 3:112, 1983

956a. Tsai YT et al: Controlled trial of vasopressin plus nitroglycerin versus vasopressin alone in the treatment of bleeding esophageal varices. Hepatology 6:406, 1986

957. Tsukiyama K et al: Electromyographic studies on the flapping tremor, especially its relationship to hyperammonemia. Folia Psychiatr Neurol Jpn 15:21, 1961

958. Turcotte JG, Lambert MJ III: Variceal hemorrhage, hepatic cirrhosis and portacaval shunts. Surgery 73:810, 1973

959. Uflacker R: Percutaneous transhepatic obliteration of gastroesophageal varices with absolute ethanol. Radiology 146:621, 1983

960. Unikowsky B et al: Dogs with experimental cirrhosis of the liver but without intrahepatic hypertension do not retain sodium or form ascites. J Clin Invest 72:1594, 1983

961. Uribe M et al: Treatment of chronic portal systemic encephalopathy with bromocriptine. Gastroenterology 76: 1347, 1979

962. Uribe M et al: Controlled study of lactose versus neomycin plus cathartics in the management of chronic portal-systemic encephalopathy. Gastroenterology 76:1300, 1979

963. Uribe M et al: Treatment of chronic portal systemic encephalopathy with vegetable and animal protein diets: A controlled cross-over study. Dig Dis Sci 27:119, 1982

964. Uribe M et al: Beneficial effect of vegetable protein diet supplemented with *Psyllium plantago* in patients with he-

patic encephalopathy and diabetes mellitus. Gastroenterology 88:901, 1985

965. Van Breda A, Waltman A: Diagnostic hepatic angiography: Mass and diffuse disease. In Bernardino ME, Sones PJ (eds): Hepatic Radiography, p 214. New York, MacMillan, 1984

966. Vankemmel M: Resection-anastomose de l'oesophage suscardiol rupture de varices oesophagiennes: Bilan d'une technique nouvelle. Nouv Presse Med 5:1123, 1974

967. Van Thiel DH: Endocrine function. In Arias I et al (eds): The Liver: Biology and Pathbiology, p 717. New York, Raven Press, 1982

968. Van Thiel DH et al: Hypogonadism in alcoholic liver disease: Evidence for a double defect. Gastroenterology 67: 1188, 1974

969. Van Thiel DH ete al: Evidence for a defect in pituitary secretion of luteinizing hormone in chronic alcoholic men. J Clin Endocrinol Metab 47:499, 1978

970. Van Thiel DH et al: Pattern of hypothalamic–pituitary–gonadal dysfunction in men with liver disease due to differing etiologies. Hepatology 39:1, 1981

971. Van Thiel DH et al: Liver disease and the hypothalamic pituitary gonadal axis. Semin Liver Dis 5:35, 1985

972. VanVugt H et al: Galactosamine hepatitis, endotoxemia, and lactulose. Hepatology 3:236, 1983

973. Van Waes L, Lieber CS: Early perivenular sclerosis in alcoholic fatty liver: An index of progressive liver injury. Gastroenterology 73:646, 1977

974. Van Waes L et al: Emergency treatment of portal-systemic encephalopathy with lactulose enemas, a controlled study. Acta Clin Belg 34:122, 1979

975. Veeravahu M: Diagnosis of liver involvement in early syphilis: A critical review. Arch Intern Med 145:132, 1985

976. Viallet A et al: Comparison of free portal venous pressure and wedged hepatic venous pressure in patients with cirrhosis of the liver. Gastroenterology 59:372, 1970

977. Viallet A et al: Hepatic and umbilicoportal catheterization in portal hypertension. Ann NY Acad Sci 170:177, 1970

978. Viamonte M Jr et al: Transhepatic obliteration of gastroesophageal varices: Results in acute and nonacute bleeders. AJR 129:237, 1977

979. Vicente VF et al: Septicemia as a complication of liver biopsy. Am J Gastroenterol 76:145, 1981

980. Victor M et al: The acquired (non-Wilsonian) type of chronic hepatocerebral degeneration. Medicine 44:345, 1965

981. Villa E: Susceptibility of chronic symptomless HB$_s$Ag carriers to ethanol-induced hepatic damage. Lancet 2:1243, 1982

982. Villa E et al: Propranolol for the prevention of recurrent variceal hemorrhage: A controlled trial (abstr). Dig Dis Sci 28:381, 1983

982a. Villeneuve JP et al: The aminopyrine breath test in cirrhosis: Sophisticated but useless. Hepatology 5:1053,1985

983. Vince A et al: Effect of lactulose on ammonia production in a fecal incubation system. Gastroenterology 74:544, 1978

984. Vincent RG et al: Incidence of cirrhosis in oral cancer. NY State J Med 64:2174, 1964

985. Vlahcevic ZR et al: Bile acid metabolism in patients with cirrhosis: II. Cholic and chenodeoxycholic acid metabolism. Gastroenterology 62:1174, 1972

986. Volwiler W et al: Criteria for the measurement of treatment in fatty cirrhosis. Gastroenterology 11:164, 1948

987. Volwiler W et al: The relation of portal vein pressure to the formation of ascites: An experimental study. Gastroenterology 14:40, 1950

988. Voorhees AB et al: Portal-system encephalopathy in the non-cirrhotic patient. Arch Surg 107:659, 1973

989. Wahren J et al: Is intravenous administration of branched chain amino acids effective in the treatment of hepatic encephalopathy? A multicenter study. Hepatology 3:475, 1983

990. Walker S et al: The use of ornithine salts of branched-chain acids in hyperammonemia in patients with cirrhosis of the liver. A double-blind crossover study. Digestion 24: 105, 1982

990a. Walker S et al: Oral keto analogs of branched-chain amino acids in hyperammonemia in patients with cirrhosis of the liver: A double-blind crossover study. Digestion 24: 105, 1982

991. Wallach HF, Popper H. Central necrosis of the liver. Arch Pathol 49:33, 1950

992. Walshe JM: The effect of glutamic acid on the coma of hepatic failure. Lancet 1:1075, 1953

993. Walshe JM: Hepatic coma. Postgrad Med J 32:467, 1956

994. Walshe JM et al: Some factors influencing cerebral oxidation in relation to hepatic coma. Clin Sci 17:11, 1958

995. Wanamaker et al: Use of the EEA stapling instrument for control of bleeding esophageal varices. Surgery 94:620, 1983

996. Wapnick S et al: Randomized prospective matched pair study comparing peritoneovenous shunt and conventional therapy in massive ascites. Br J Surg 66:667, 1979

997. Warren WD et al: Selective trans-splenic decompression of gastroesophageal varices by distal splenorenal shunt. Arch Surg 166:437, 1967

998. Warren WD et al: Spontaneous reversal of portal venous blood flow in cirrhosis. Surg Gynecol Obstet 126:315, 1968

999. Warren WD et al: Ten years of portal hypertension surgery at Emory: Results and new perspectives. Ann Surg 195: 530, 1982

1000. Waterlow JC, Weisz T: The fat, protein and nucleic acid content of the liver in malnourished human infants. J Clin Invest 36:346, 1956

1001. Webb LJ, Sherlock S: The aetiology, presentation and natural history of extra-hepatic portal venous obstruction. Q J Med 192:627, 1979

1002. Weber FL Jr: The effect of lactulose on urea metabolism and nitrogen excretion in cirrhotic patients. Gastroenterology 77:518, 1979

1003. Weber FL, Reiser BJ: Relationship of plasma amino acids to nitrogen balance and portal-systemic encephalopathy in alcoholic liver disease. Dig Dis Sci 27:103, 1982

1004. Weber, FL Jr, Veach GI: The importance of the small intestine in gut ammonium production in the fasting dog. Gastroenterology 77:235, 1979

1005. Weber FL Jr et al: Effects of lactulose and neomycin on urea metabolism in cirrhotic subjects. Gastroenterology 82:213, 1982

1006. Weber FL Jr et al: Effects of vegetable diets on nitrogen metabolism in cirrhotic subjects. Gastroenterology 89:538, 1985

1007. Webster LT Jr, Gabuzda GJ: Effect of portal blood ammonium concentration and of administering methionine to patients with hepatic cirrhosis. J Lab Clin Med 50:426, 1957

1008. Weinberg AG et al: The occurrence of hepatoma in the

chronic form of hereditary tyrosinemia. J Pediatr 88:454, 1976

1009. Weinberger HA: Emergency portacaval shunt for esophagogastric hemorrhage. Arch Surg 91:333, 1965

1010. Weinstein G et al: Psoriasis-liver-methotrexate interactions. Arch Dermatol 108:36, 1973

1011. Weinstein MP et al: Spontaneous bacterial peritonitis: A review of 28 cases with emphasis on improved survival and factors influencing prognosis. Am J Med 64:592, 1978

1012. Weissberg JI et al: Survival in chronic hepatitis B: An analysis of 379 patients. Ann Intern Med 101:613, 1984

1013. Welch HF et al: Prognosis after surgical treatment of ascites: Results of side-to-side shunt in 40 patients. Surgery 56:75, 1964

1014. Weller IVD et al: Significance of delta agent infection in chronic hepatitis B virus infection: A study in British carriers. Gut 24:1061, 1983

1015. Welt LG: Edema and hyponatremia. Arch Intern Med 89:931, 1952

1016. Westaby D, Williams R: Follow-up study after sclerotherapy. Scand J Gastroenterol 19 (suppl 102):71, 1984

1017. Westaby D et al: A prospective randomized study of two sclerotherapy techniques for esophageal varices. Hepatology 3:681, 1983

1017a.Westaby D et al: Selective and non-selective beta receptor blockade in the reduction of portal pressure in patients with cirrhosis and portal hypertension. Gut 25:121, 1984

1018. Whipple RL Jr, Harris JF: E coli septicemia in Laënnec's cirrhosis of the liver. Ann Intern Med 33:462, 1950

1019. Wickham JEA, Sharma GP: Endogenous ammonia formation in experimental renal ischaemia. Lancet 1:195, 1965

1020. Widrich WC et al: Esophagogastric variceal hemorrhage. Arch Surg 113:1331, 1978

1021. Wiesner RH: Does propranolol precipitate hepatic encephalopathy? J Clin Gastroenterol 8:74, 1986

1022. Wilkenson FOW, Riddell AG: Studies on gastric secretion before and after portacaval anastomosis. Br J Surg 52:530, 1965

1023. Wilkes JC et al: Response to pneumococcal vaccination in children with nephrotic syndrome. Am J Kid Dis 2:43, 1982

1024. Wilkinson P, Sherlock S: The effect of repeated albumin infusions in patients with cirrhosis. Lancet 2:1125, 1962

1025. Wilkinson SP et al: Renal retention of sodium in cirrhosis and fulminant hepatic failure. Postgrad Med J 51:527, 1975

1026. Wilkinson SP et al: Renal failure in liver disease: Role of endotoxins and renin-angiotensin system. In Epstein M (ed): The Kidney in Liver Disease, p 113. New York, Elsevier-North Holland, 1978

1027. Williams CD: Nutritional disease of childhood associated with maize diet. Arch Dis Child 8:423, 1933

1028. Williams JH, Abelmann WH: Portopulmonary shunts in patients with portal hypertension. J Lab Clin Med 62:715, 1963

1029. Wilson JAP et al: Characteristics of ascitic fluid in the alcoholic cirrhotic. Dig Dis Sci 24:645, 1979

1030. Wise JK et al: Evaluation of alpha-cell function by infusion of alanine in normal, diabetic and obese subjects. N Engl J Med 288:484, 1973

1031. Witte CL et al: Dual origin of ascites in hepatic cirrhosis. Surg Gynecol Obstet 129:1027, 1969

1032. Witte MH et al: Lymph circulation in hepatic cirrhosis: Effect of portacaval shunt. Ann Intern Med 70:303, 1969

1033. Wittenberg J: Computed tomography of the body. N Engl J Med 309:1160, 1983

1034. Witzel L et al: Prophylactic endoscopic sclerotherapy of esophageal varices. Lancet 1:773, 1985

1035. Wodak E: Die konservative Behandlung von Oesophagusvarizen. HNO; Beihefte fur Zeitschrift fur hals-, nasen-, und ohrenheilfunfe 13:131, 1958

1036. Wolfe JD et al: Hypoxemia of cirrhosis. Detection of abnormal small pulmonary vascular channels by a quantitative radionuclide method. Am J Med 63:746, 1977

1037. Wolfe SJ et al: Thickening and contraction of the palmar fascia (Dupuytren's contracture) associated with alcoholism and hepatic cirrhosis. N Engl J Med 255:559, 1956

1038. Wolfe SJ et al: Parotid swelling, alcoholism and cirrhosis. N Engl J Med 256:491, 1957

1039. Wong PY et al: Kallikrein-kinin and renin-angiotensin systems in functional renal failure of cirrhosis of the liver. Gastroenterology 73:114, 1977

1040. Woodard JC et al: Primary hypomagnesemia with secondary hypocalcemia, diarrhea and insensitivity to parathyroid hormone. Dig Dis 17:612, 1972

1041. Wormser P, Hubbard RC: Peritonitis in cirrhotic patients with LeVeen shunts. Am J Med 71:358, 1981

1042. Worner TM, Lieber CS: Perivenular fibrosis as precursor lesion of cirrhosis. J Am Med Assoc 254:627, 1985

1043. Wyke RJ et al: Spontaneous bacterial peritonitis: A common complication of chronic active hepatitis. Abstract of European Assoc Study Liver, Dusseldorf, Sept 13, 1979

1044. Yamahiro HS, Reynolds TB: Effects of ascitic fluid infusion on sodium excretion, blood volume and creatinine clearance in cirrhosis. Gastroenterology 40:497, 1961

1045. Yamamoto S et al: The late results of terminal esophagoproximal gastrectomy (TEPG) with extensive devascularization and splenectomy for bleeding esophageal varices in cirrhosis. Surgery 80:106,

1046. Yang CY et al: White count, pH and lactate in ascites in the diagnosis of spontaneous bacterial peritonitis. Hepatology 5:85, 1985

1047. Yassin YM, Sherif SM: Randomized controlled trial of injection sclerotherapy for bleeding oesophageal varices: An interim report. Br J Surg 70:20, 1983

1048. Young L, et al: Gram-negative rod bacteremia: Microbiologic, immunologic and therapeutic considerations. Ann Intern Med 86:456, 1977

1049. Young LS, Hewitt WL: Activity of five aminoglycoside antibiotics in vitro against gram-negative bacilli and Staphylococcus aureus. Antimicrob Agents Chemother 4:617, 1973

1050. Yune HY et al: Absolute ethanol in thrombotherapy of bleeding esophageal varices. AJR 138:1137, 1982

1051. Yune HY et al: Ethanol thrombotherapy of esophageal varices: Further experience. AJR 144:1049, 1985

1052. Zachariae H et al: Methotrexate induced liver cirrhosis. Br J Drm 102:407, 1980

1053. Zafrani ES et al: Peliosis-like ultrastructural changes of the hepatic sinusoids in human chronic hypervitaminosis A: Report of three cases. Human Pathology 15:1166, 1984

1054. Zelman S: Liver fibrosis in hereditary hemorrhagic telangiectasia. Arch Pathol 74:66, 1962

1054a.Zeppa R et al: Survival after distal splenorenal shunt. Surg Gynecol Obstet 145:12, 1977

1055. Zetterman RK, Sorrell MF: Immunologic aspects of alcoholic liver disease. Gastroenterology 81:616, 1981

1056. Zetterman RK et al: Alcoholic hepatitis: Cell-mediated immunological response to alcoholic hyalin. Gastroenterology 70:382, 1976

1057. Zieve FJ et al: Synergism between ammonia and fatty acids in the production of coma: Implications for hepatic coma. J Pharmacol Exp Ther 191:10, 1974

1058. Zieve L: Jaundice, hyperlipemia and hemolytic anemia heretofore unrecognized syndrome associated with alcoholic fatty liver and cirrhosis. Ann Intern Med 48:471, 1958

1059. Zieve L: Hepatic encephalopathy: Summary of present knowledge with an elaboration on recent developments. In Popper H, Schaffner F (eds): Progress in Liver Diseases. vol 6, pp 327–341. New York, Grune & Stratton, 1981

1060. Zieve L et al: Shunt encephalomyelopathy: II. Occurrence of permanent myelopathy. Ann Intern Med 53:53, 1960

1061. Zieve L et al: Synergism between mercaptans and ammonia or fatty acids in the production of coma: A possible role for mercaptans in the pathogenesis of hepatic coma. J Lab Clin Med 83:16, 1974

1062. Zieve L et al: Ammonia, octanoate and mercaptan depress regeneration of normal rat liver after partial hepatectomy. Hepatology 5:28, 1985

1063. Zimmerman HJ: Hepatotoxicity, pp 525–527. New York, Appleton-Century-Crafts, 1978

1064. Zimmerman HJ, Ishak KG: Valproate-induced hepatic injury: Analyses of 23 fatal cases. Hepatology 2:591, 1982

1065. Zimmerman HJ et al: Hepatic hemosiderin deposits: Incidence in 558 biopsies from patients with and without intrinsic hepatic disease. Arch Intern Med 107:494, 1961

1066. Zimmon DS: Oxyhemoglobin dissociation in patients with hepatic encephalopathy. Gastroenterology 52:647, 1967

1067. Zimmon DS, Kessler RE: Regulation of portal pressure in man. Gastroenterology 60:169, 1971

1068. Zimmon DS, Kessler RE: Hepatic hemodynamic factors reflect prognosis after portacaval shunt. Gastroenterology 64:166, 1973

1069. Zimmon DS et al: Albumin to ascites: Demonstration of a direct pathway bypassing the systemic circulation. J Clin Invest 48:2074, 1969

1070. Zipser RD et al: Prostaglandins: Modulators of renal function and pressor resistance in chronic liver disease. J Clin Endocrinol Metab 48:895, 1979

chapter 21

Peritoneojugular Shunt for Treatment of Ascites

HARRY H. LeVEEN, P. R. RAJAGOPALAN, and ERIC G. LeVEEN

PROGNOSIS

The development of ascites marks a serious turning point in the course of cirrhosis. Life expectancy is considerably reduced. Patek's experience in 1942 revealed that only 32% of the patients surveyed with ascites survived more than one year.[37] Advancement in medical therapy has not substantially improved these statistics; Sherlock found 25 years later that 24 of 80 patients died in one year.[45] If patients are refractory to diuretic therapy, they succumb within a year. To place therapy in perspective, it is necessary to briefly review available therapy prior to the introduction of the peritoneojugular shunt. This should shed light on the extent of expectations from medical or alternative surgical therapy.

Influencing Risk Factors

As ascites progresses, nutritional depletion becomes more marked. As the intraperitoneal pressure increases, there is little room for food, which would raise the pressure even further. This leads to semistarvation. The experiments of Keyes and others have shown that during starvation there is a basal urinary loss of nitrogen in the form of urea. The urinary output of nitrogen often rises just before death. The increased nitrogen loss is due to the depletion of body fat, which has been totally consumed for energy needs. Protein then becomes the sole source of energy. Many patients with ascites, like persons suffering from starvation, have exhausted their supply of subcutaneous fat. Yet the significance of the subcutaneous fat loss is rarely appreciated. Many cirrhotic patients have a terminal episode of liver failure with jaundice or die in semicoma. Renal shutdown is not uncommon. Serious nutritional impairment heralds imminent death in cirrhosis.

Most patients with ascites die with an episode of renal failure, the primary or secondary cause of death.[6,44] This has not been averted by repeated infusions of plasma, ascitic fluid, or both during the course of their illness.[6] The renal failure is often hastened by diuretics. At this stage in the disease, there is often a decrease in the circulating blood volume and intense renal arterial vasoconstriction, which leads to a diminution in the glomerular filtration rate.[3,43] As renal perfusion decreases and glomerular filtration drops, the proximal tubule necessarily absorbs from the glomerular filtrate a proportion of salt and water larger than 80%, thereby leaving little tubular urine available for facultative reabsorption by the distal tubules. Given that most usable diuretics exert their action on the distal tubule or at the loop of Henley, diuretics become ineffective. In addition, sodium retention late in the course of ascites is influenced by an overactive renin–angiotensin system.[7,39] There is also hypersecretion of antidiuretic hormone (vasopressin), which leads to water retention. Occasional patients survive the hepatorenal syndrome,[17] but the condition is usually fatal. Reynolds reports that only 8 of 54 patients survived their hospital stay.[38]

Death can be linked to acute hepatic failure often provoked by acute alcoholic hepatitis, which can be precipitated by mental depression secondary to the failure of therapy to relieve the ascites. This phenomenon has been observed in a number of patients who make a conscious effort to "drink themselves to death."

The number of patients who die of perforated hernia is never included in mortality statistics, largely because an umbilical hernia is usually the only clinically recognized hernia that ruptures (with subsequent peritonitis). Yet 5% of patients develop hydrothorax from perforation of a minute hernial sac on the superior surface of the diaphragm. Tension hydrothorax is due to the development of this small leak through the diaphragm. As is described below, this condition is an urgent indication for an emergency peritoneojugular shunt.

Nutritional depletion predisposes to infection. Occult primary peritonitis is an infrequent but not rare complication of ascites.

Therapy Other Than Peritoneojugular Shunt

Treatment for ascites has been centered around mobilizing the ascitic fluid to reduce girth, increasing urine output and salt excretion, improving the nutrition of the patient, permitting freer breathing and mobility, and avoiding renal failure. Various treatment methods proposed over the years to accomplish these aims have achieved a modicum of success for conscientious physicians and tractable patients.

Diuretics and salt restriction are useful for patients who are not overly dehydrated. However, in more refractory patients, hospital stays are prolonged and success less predictable. Diuretics may not be totally effective in correcting excessive sodium retention if the sodium is primarily held in an inaccessible third space. Ascites recurs more and more frequently with increasing resistance to treatment. Azotemia by itself causes encephalopathy and coma. Hepatorenal syndrome may develop as the terminal event. Paracentesis is occasionally helpful to temporarily relieve respiratory distress, but it depletes the body of protein, may precipitate a further decline in effective peripheral perfusion, and is frequently associated with infection. Therefore, paracentesis with reinfusion of ascitic fluid has been given consideration.[11,18]

Reinfusion of unmodified autogenous ascitic fluid replaces depleted proteins and provides better kidney perfusion, but its effects are still not permanent. Ascites recurs in more than 70% of patients within 2 months.[20] Repeated reinfusions may have decreased benefits and increase the risk of infection.

Albumin has been used with mixed success to replenish the intravascular fluid volume after paracentesis, but the therapy is costly and the effects temporary.[10,52]

Reinfusion of protein concentrate from autogenous ascitic fluid replaces depleted protein but does not provide a permanent increase in kidney perfusion. Given that the results are evanescent, this treatment has not solved the problem of progressive renal failure, although it has been reported to be of value in shortening the hospital stay, especially for patients resistant to diuretic therapy.[52] To be of real benefit, the reinfusion must be continuous.

Side-to-side portacaval shunt carries a 12% mortality rate, and one third of the survivors have encephalopathy. Portacaval shunts adversely affect liver function.[5] Surgeons have strived to create shunts such as the distal splenorenal shunt to keep the portal pressure high so that the liver will be perfused with portal vein blood. Encephalopathy and death from liver failure doom procedures that shunt the major portion of portal vein blood into the systemic circulation. A portacaval shunt is not suitable therapy for ascites regardless of etiology, since it creates a portoprival syndrome.

PERITONEOJUGULAR SHUNT

The concept of continuous reinfusion of ascitic fluid into the venous system has attracted the attention of many surgeons.[7,34,36,46] However, the valves that were first employed were not designed for this purpose, and the operations came to early failure after initial success. The

ascites valve was developed in 1972 after a careful study of the hydrodynamic requirements. The system consists of an intraperitoneal collecting tube attached to a specially constructed one-way, pressure-sensitive valve. The valve is attached to a tube leading to the superior vena cava through an access vein, such as the jugular, axillary, or femoral.

The rigid valve casing is constructed of polypropylene and contains a silicone rubber, funnel-shaped valve seat (Fig. 21-1). Respiration supplies the driving force that moves the fluid and opens the valve. The valve normally remains closed but opens when the differential pressure between the peritoneum and the intrathoracic vena cava rises above 3 cm H_2O.

Types of Ascites Treated by Peritoneojugular Shunt

The shunt has now been inserted in more than 40,000 patients throughout the United States and Europe. Most of these patients have had ascites secondary to cirrhosis caused by alcoholism (85%), but in a number of patients cirrhosis was secondary to schistosomiasis depending on the region of the world.

The second largest group of shunt recipients has been patients with malignant ascites who die of cachexia and nutritional depletion rather than from an excessive tumor burden. The shunt improves nutrition and comfort and apparently extends life. Definitive studies on the extent of prolongation of life are scanty. Nonetheless, patients with malignant ascites have actually gained weight and returned to work after shunt implantation. Moribund patients with ovarian carcinoma and ascites have temporarily recovered and lived for as long as 2 or more years after shunt insertion.

In a small number of patients, the ascites is noncirrhotic and has diverse causes. All patients with ascites have been responsive to peritoneojugular shunt surgery regardless of the cause of the ascites. A number of cases of Budd–Chiari syndrome have been treated by such surgery, which may be the only form of therapy applicable to the problem, given that the vena cava is often occluded at or above the liver, making any form of portacaval shunt impractical.

Patients with chylous ascites of various causes have also been successfully treated. The largest number of such cases has been treated without incidence by Kinmounth.[21]

Nephrogenic ascites is unassociated with liver disease, and liver biopsies have proved to be normal. The peritoneum is also uninvolved. The etiology of the ascites is cryptogenic. Patients with nephrogenic ascites include anephric patients and persons with impaired renal function who are being treated by hemodialysis.[9] Cases of nephrogenic ascites have been successfully treated by peritoneojugular shunt by us and others.[53]

Although cardiac disease was first thought to contraindicate shunt surgery, a number of cardiac patients have been shunted for cardiac ascites with remarkable success. These patients require intensive medical care, including

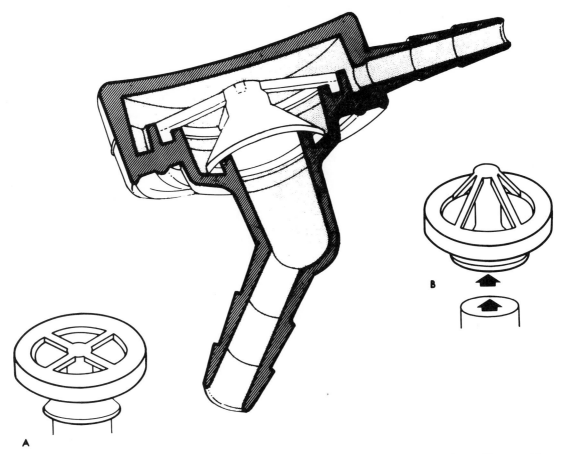

Fig. 21-1. Rigid valve casing is constructed of polypropylene and contains a silicone rubber, funnel-shaped valve seat.

digitalis, bed rest, diuretics, a salt-restricted diet, and consistent performance of breathing exercises against inspiratory resistance. In cardiac patients, the ascitic fluid is removed from the abdomen and discarded at the time of surgery. These patients are unable to excrete a salt and water load.

Finally, a number of cirrhotic patients develop ascites following some form of portacaval shunting. Many of these patients develop rapid, unrelenting ascites after vascular decompression for esophageal varices. The protein and fat content of their ascitic fluid is usually high, indicating that the ascites is due to continuous leakage of lymph from a transected lymph vessel into the peritoneal cavity. The leakage may be life-threatening and may require the insertion of a peritoneojugular shunt.[50]

Contraindications

Liver decompensation induced by jaundice with a serum bilirubin value greater than 5 mg/dl is best treated conservatively until the jaundice subsides. Patients with oliguria, an elevated blood urea nitrogen (BUN) level, and low urinary sodium concentration are exceptions and urgently require surgery; they will die in acute renal failure if a peritoneojugular shunt is delayed. Of 14 patients with jaundice and hepatorenal syndrome, 2 have survived for longer than 2 years and have made a complete recovery.[48] Patients with encephalopathy without azotemia are poor candidates for a shunt, given that this condition is an indication of advanced liver failure. Each day, 20% of all the urea in the body diffuses into the colon, where it is converted to ammonia.[47] Azotemia increases the amount of ammonia formed in this manner and may precipitate hepatic coma. A peritoneojugular shunt brings patients with azotemia, in contrast to those without, out of coma and ammonia intoxication; the BUN falls after the shunt and reduces endogenous ammonia formation in the colon.

Patients with ascites who have had bleeding varices bleed again from their varices postoperatively. At the conclusion of surgery, such patients require treatment for the varices and the insertion of an ascites valve. It is necessary that the abdomen be refilled with saline to avoid the occurrence of air embolism. Several patients have been successfully treated with combined surgery in this manner, but the number is too small to form a basis for firm conclusions. In one patient with hepatorenal syndrome, turbid fluid with a high white cell count was encountered at surgery and emptied from the peritoneal cavity, which was then irrigated with 10,000 ml of saline. More saline was instilled in the peritoneum to expel air at the conclusion of the washing. This patient made a good recovery.

Indications

The exact indications for a peritoneojugular shunt in cirrhotic ascites are undetermined. If the patient is refractory to medical therapy, it is too late, and fatal hepatorenal syndrome can intervene before the decision has been made that the patient is truly refractory. Also, many patients who require a protracted period of hospitalization to render them ascites-free should be treated by a shunt, since experience shows that these patients return with recurrences soon after discharge. The best indication for peritoneojugular shunt in cirrhotic ascites is the failure of a low-salt diet to bring about relief.

This belief is consonant with the work of Arroyo and Rodes,[2] who performed careful renal studies on 55 patients with ascites. Twenty-one of these patients had good renal function and responded with natriuresis. All of the patients in this group left the hospital alive. The patients who did not respond to salt restrictions were divided into two groups according to their free water clearance; of these, 17 had a free water clearance greater than 1 ml/minute, but although they responded to diuretics, 4 of the 17 died in the hospital. The 17 remaining patients with free water clearance below 1 ml/minute did not respond to diuretics, and 11 of them died in the hospital. The in-hospital mortality rate was 44% for patients who did not respond to salt restriction, and the ultimate mortality must have been considerably higher. Similarly, patients with resistant ascites but normal concentrations of blood chemical constituents demonstrated impairment of renal hemodynamics before the onset of azotemia.[4] A rising BUN in ascites is a poor prognostic sign that may therefore be a late indication of a fatal outcome.

Given that there is such a strong relationship between renal function and ascites, and given that the kidney plays such a vital role in survival, logic tells us that a good indication for surgery might have a renal basis. For this reason, failure to respond to a sodium-restricted diet may be the best indicator that exists. The abnormal parameters of renal function return to normal and remain normal immediately after a peritoneojugular shunt.[22]

Salt retention in cirrhotics with ascites has been proven to be a circulating volume deficit.[13] Yet, because disseminated intravascular coagulation (DIC) was a serious problem in the past, it was advised to consider the peritoneojugular shunt only as a last resort. This precaution is no longer necessary. Peritoneojugular shunt permanently expands the plasma volume to normal, rendering it the most physiologic therapy that can be offered.

Shunt implantation should be considered before a diuretic regimen in patients who do not respond to a salt-restricted diet.[30] This conclusion has been supported by a randomized study in which medical therapy (diet restriction and diuretics) was compared with surgical therapy (shunt implantation) in patients unresponsive to salt-restricted diets. The shunted patients survived longer than the medically treated patients; the usual cause of death was the advent of hepatorenal syndrome during the course of medical therapy.[49]

Emergency Indications

Hepatorenal Syndrome

Patients with hepatorenal syndrome require an immediate shunt because death usually ensues within weeks. This indication takes precedence over any contraindication to the shunt. Patients with hepatorenal syndrome may be clinically distinguished from those with acute tubular necrosis (ATN) by measurement of urinary sodium concentration or salt clearance. In hepatorenal syndrome, urinary sodium concentration is low, typically less than 10 mEq/liter, despite azotemia, confirming the presence of functioning renal tissue. Urinary sodium clearance is less than 0.2 ml/minute and is uninfluenced by diuretics. In ATN, urinary sodium concentration is high (above 40 mEq/liter) because the injured tubules are unable to resorb sodium. The kidneys of patients with hepatorenal syndrome are transplantable and function well in recipients.[23] Spontaneous recovery in jaundiced patients after pharmacologic manipulation of renal blood flow or after portacaval shunting is extremely rare unless associated with recovery from the underlying liver disease. Hepatorenal syndrome untreated by peritoneojugular shunting may progress to ATN. An elevated urea nitrogen level is an urgent indication for surgery even in jaundiced patients. Of 14 jaundiced patients with hepatorenal syndrome, 2 survived more than 2 years and are now relatively well. *Although the rate of survival with surgery is low, any survival in this situation is a dramatic salvage.*

There is extensive evidence that a peritoneojugular shunt reverses the hepatorenal syndrome and that patients who receive such a shunt survive. This has occurred so consistently that there is no reason to delay surgery.[15,28,29,35] Patients with ATN may not respond to peritoneojugular shunt in spite of volume expansion. Volume expansion is a necessary part of therapy for hepatorenal syndrome but should be done with albumin or plasma, since excessive expansion with ascitic fluid predisposes to DIC.

Tension Hydrothorax

Patients with hydrothorax associated with ascites should be suspected of having tension hydrothorax. The intrapleural pressure should be measured at the time the chest is tapped. The cause of the hydrothorax is usually a congenital defect on the right side of the diaphragm. It appears on the left side in only about 1 of 12 patients. Hydrothorax was present in 5.4% of 330 cases; this complication carries a high mortality and few patients leave the hospital alive. The defect consists of tiny holes in the diaphragm with a membranous pleuroperitoneal covering.[12,40] In ascites, this membrane is stretched and a bleb forms on the upper surface of the diaphragm. With increasing ascitic fluid pressure, the bleb finally ruptures, forming a one-way valve into the chest. Thus, if serum albumin labeled with radioactive iodine is injected into the pleural cavity, it does not appear in the peritoneal cavity. But if the tracer is injected into the peritoneal cavity, it appears in the pleural fluid. One way to confirm the communication is to inject air into the peritoneal cavity. The appearance of pneumohydrothorax is almost immediate.[32] The recommended way to prove that there is a communication between the thorax and the peritoneal cavity is the intraperitoneal injection of albumin particles containing technetium 99. The same material used for lung scans is preferable. The rate at which the isotope enters the pleural cavity gives an estimate of the size of the defect. Patients requiring 4 to 6 hours or more to transfer a diagnosable quantity of the isotope have small defects, which often cannot be detected unless an antecedent thoracocentesis is done. Small defects can be sclerosed by intrapleural tetracyline administration after a thoracocentesis. The management of patients with hydrothorax requires special knowledge, and one should consult the literature.[25] The defect in the diaphragm is small and often overlooked at autopsy unless the abdomen is distended under pressure with water.[31]

Tension hydrothorax can start with mild ascites. Once the diaphragm bleb ruptures, fluid drains into the chest and is absorbed by lung surfaces. The patient may complain of respiratory distress, and fluid in the pleural cavity may be evident radiographically, even though the ascites is not severe.

Excess fluid eventually crowds the heart and great vessels, and increasing positive pressure ultimately results in lung collapse. To prevent this, patients should be shunted immediately. It is tempting to place a drainage tube in the pleural cavity, but as long as ascitic fluid builds up in the peritoneum, this will simply result in ascitic fluid being pushed into and continually drained out of the chest. The chest should be tapped to remove existing ascitic fluid and a shunt implanted to keep ascitic fluid levels and pressure low enough to prevent leakage into the chest.

Acute Ascites After Surgery

A major lymphatic vessel may be opened at the time of abdominal surgery. In a normal person, this would not result in ascites, but in patients with portal hypertension, the lymph vessels are distended with fluid under high pressure, and the leakage is so great and so rapid that closure does not occur spontaneously.

Perforation of an Umbilical Hernia

Perforation of an umbilical hernia in patients with ascites often results in peritonitis or sepsis, leading to death. In such patients, the hole in the umbilical hernia should be clamped and a shunt inserted to decompress the peritoneal cavity.

PREOPERATIVE CARE

Hematocrit levels should be restored in patients with severe anemia. The severity of the anemia may not be apparent until the plasma volume is restored to normal in the postoperative period. Patients should be transfused with packed cells, if indicated, and given prophylactic antibiotics (*i.e.,* the same type of prophylactic antibiotic treatment administered in heart valve surgery). In addition, those patients with elevated central venous pressure or cardiac disease should be digitalized.

SURGERY

Shunt insertion takes place under local anesthesia.[26] The peritoneum is exposed through a right transverse incision just medial to the anterior axillary line. A purse-string suture is placed in the peritoneum, and an incision is made in its center. The perforated collecting tube is inserted into the peritoneal cavity and the purse-string is tied around the valve stem. The venous tube is brought through a small incision in the abdominal musculature, and the abdominal muscles are closed over the valve.

A watertight and airtight closure is important to prevent leakage, which might lead to infection. The venous tube is tunneled subcutaneously to the neck, where it is placed into the access vein (Fig. 21-2). Leakage from the incision into the tunnel area may cause a hernia-like sac lined with peritoneal membrane. The inner diameter of the tunnel must be close to the tubing outer diameter, and careful attention must be paid to the incision closure. There must be no leakage from the skin. If peritoneal infection or sepsis occurs, the valve system should be removed.

POSTOPERATIVE MANAGEMENT

Postoperatively, a binder and inspiratory effort against resistance are essential to accentuate the pressure differential between intraperitoneal and intrathoracic pressure. It is mandatory that the patient perform these exercises from a recumbent position. The exercises must be done several times a day for 10 to 15 minutes, as necessary.

Once the ascites has been eliminated, the patient may not require continued diuretic therapy. Diuretics should be reserved for patients with peripheral edema. Wexler, in a study of ascitic dogs with cirrhosis, noted that ascites did not recur after valve placement even when the dogs were salt loaded. Instead, peripheral edema resulted from salt loading.[51] Patients who are concealed cardiacs may require continued cardiac therapy.

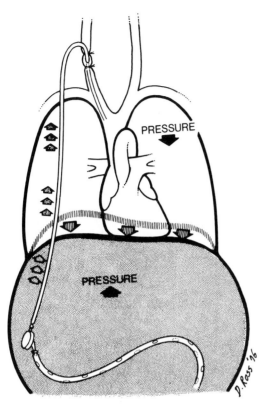

Fig. 21-2. Venous tube is tunneled subcutaneously to the neck, where it is placed into the access vein.

REVERSAL OF PATHOLOGIC PHYSIOLOGY BY SHUNT

Shunt insertion generally results in dramatic diuresis with fluid mobilization and loss of ascites. There is increased mean sodium clearance, reduced girth, improved venous return, increased cardiac output, reduction of respiratory effort, gain in appetite, and positive nitrogen balance with reformation of muscles mass, resulting in a dramatic improvement in physical appearance.[15,28] This is especially significant because some ascitic patients are in the terminal phases of starvation (Fig. 21-3). Renal function, as measured by renal perfusion and excretion of salt and water, remains normal for prolonged periods after shunt placement.

Hyperaldosteronism disappears with a return to normal plasma renin and aldosterone levels within 4 days.[42] In patients with hepatorenal syndrome, elevated creatinine and blood urea concentrations return to normal.[19] Hospitalization is reduced, and the risks associated with long-term diuretic and diet therapy are avoided. Mean sodium clearance in patients with truly refractory ascites and preoperative oliguria improves when furosemide is administered postoperatively, even though avid sodium retention is not usually overcome before shunt insertion. In one study, shunt placement alone resulted in an increase in mean sodium clearance from 0.16 ml/minute to 0.35 ml/minute (p = 0.025). The administration of furosemide resulted in even greater clearance in shunted patients (0.64 ml/minute, p = 0.001).[22] Because of severe hyperaldosteronism, patients must be given a maximum of diuretics immediately after surgery until the ascites disappears. This also tends to preserve the serum potassium levels.

The shunt appears to improve renal perfusion and decrease renal tubular reabsorption of salt. Withdrawal of ascitic fluid with infusion of albumin or saline produces only a water diuresis without an increase in salt excretion. Moreover, the hemodynamic effects of these treatments may not persist with repeated infusions.[22] It seems unlikely that reinfusion in itself can overcome the potent renal reabsorption of salt and water that occurs in refractory ascites. In fact, reinfusion of ascitic fluid may not be a reliable preoperative test of renal function, given that infusion of 1500 ml of ascitic fluid in a nonshunted patient may not be adequate to change the renal plasma flow (RPF) and the glomerular filtration rate and may produce no effect on salt excretion. More favorable responses occur when larger amounts of fluid are continually shunted. A test infusion should not be used as an indicator of which patients are likely to be responsive to shunt insertion.

HEMODYNAMIC CHANGES AFTER SHUNT INSERTION

The consequences of the volume expansion and hemodilution produced by the inflow of ascitic fluid contribute to the improvement that occurs in renal hemodynamics. Blood volume expansion with ascitic fluid increases cardiac output; this contributes to an increase in RPF and glomerular filtration rate, reestablishing normal sodium absorption in the proximal renal tubules.

However, these changes may not explain why renal perfusion increases so dramatically. Therefore, the role of blood viscosity, especially in states of low renal perfusion, has been investigated. Blood viscosity is directly related to the blood hematocrit level. A drop in hematocrit resulting from reinfused ascitic fluid causes a reduction in blood viscosity. This partially accounts for the measured increase in renal blood flow in spite of a vasospastic renal bed being part of the hepatorenal syndrome. Renal blood flow levels as low as 90 ml/minute have increased to 2000 ml/minute after shunt implantation. Renal perfusion levels have approached normal for as long as 20 days postoperatively.

Contrary to expectations, hemodilution and subsequent increased cardiac output do not necessarily result in a rise in portal vein pressure as measured by hepatic wedge pressure. In a study of nine patients, hepatic wedge pressure fell after shunt insertion, even though cardiac output increased by an average of about 50%. The drop in portal vein pressure was approximately 1 cm H_2O for each drop of a point in hematocrit (Fig. 21-4).[51]

The reduction in blood viscosity decreases the resistance

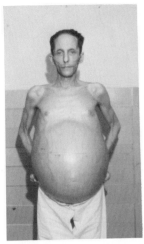
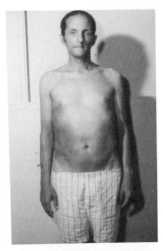
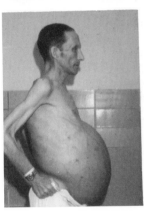
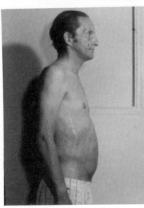

Fig. 21-3. Ascitic patients in the terminal phases of starvation.

to venous flow. Blood viscosity is greatest where the shear rates are low, such as in venous blood. The resistance to venous outflow is, therefore, greatly reduced by hemodilution. Blood inflow increases less, since the blood is less viscid in the arterial tree where shear rates are higher. Even though cardiac output increases, portal vein pressure falls. This conclusion is supported by experiments in which portal hypertension was produced in dogs by embolization of the portal system with silicone oil. Isovolumic hemodilution consistently lowered portal vein pressure in direct proportion to the lowering of the hematocrit. This hemodilution effect may significantly reduce the danger of rupturing esophageal varices in the immediate postoperative period.

COMPLICATIONS

Fluid Leakage

Fluid leakage may occur as the result of improper closure of the peritoneal cavity or fascia or from a large tunnel around the venous tube. Leakage may form a self-contained hydrocele, or it may form a hernial sac that empties into the peritoneum when the patient is lying down. Such leakage can be avoided with good surgical technique. Leakage through the skin requires immediate attention to prevent infection.

Fever

Fever is a common complication occurring in about half of all shunted patients. It is easily controlled by aspirin or cortisone and is usually not associated with positive bacterial cultures or other evidence of sepsis such as elevated white blood cell count. Fever usually abates as the shunt drains the ascitic fluid. Fever may possibly be related to the presence of endotoxins in the peritoneal fluid. Fever rarely lasts more than one week and is responsive to small doses of corticosteroids.

Postshunt Coagulopathy

Ascitic fluid always contains fibrin split products that have anticoagulant effects. The addition of ascitic fluid to a thromboelastogram causes prolongation of the reaction time and often clot lysis. Clot lysis is the primary problem after a peritoneojugular shunt, but severe postshunt coagulopathy (PSC) is a relatively rare complication. Although the mechanism of this coagulopathy is not clearly understood, it has received great attention in the literature, which tends to exaggerate its significance.[1,24]

Although 17% of our early patients developed ecchymoses, serious bleeding episodes were infrequent. Only 3

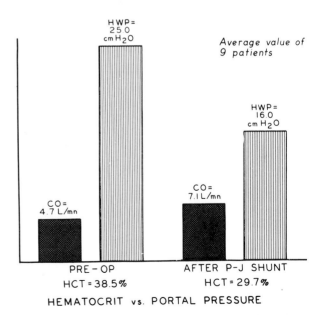

Fig. 21-4. The drop in portal vein pressure was about 1 cm H_2O for each drop of a point in hematocrit.

of 160 earlier patients died of PSC. The probability that there was some substance in the peritoneal fluid that caused the coagulopathy stimulated us to empty and discard all of the ascitic fluid. This procedure has been followed for the past 8 years in more than 230 cases. Only two mild cases of PSC have occurred in this interval. Both were manageable without interruption of the shunt, and only one patient required blood. This experience and our laboratory experiments confirm that PSC is a preventable syndrome different from DIC, which it does not resemble. Our first belief was that PSC might be caused by intraperitoneal endotoxin. However, many cirrhotics who have intraperitoneal endotoxin also have circulating endotoxin but do not exhibit any coagulopathy. Also, patients with PSC may not have circulating endotoxin. Logic told us that the fate of blood injected into the peritoneal cavity should be identical to the fate of the circulating blood exposed to large amounts of ascitic fluid. Blood placed into the peritoneal cavity immediately clots, with utilization of the platelets and clotting factors in the injected blood.[33] The protocoagulant in the ascitic fluid may be soluble collagen.[41] Fibrin in the clotted blood undergoes immediate lysis, with the formation of fibrin split products. Thus, blood entering into the peritoneal cavity becomes immediately incoagulable. The lysis is caused by a high concentration of plasminogen activator secreted by the endothelial cells of the peritoneum. Inactivation of the tissue plasminogen activator by epsilon amino caproic acid (EACA) prevents the lysis, and clot will form. PSC has been completely controlled by emptying of the peritoneal cavity and irrigation with saline. If PSC has occurred, bleeding should be controlled by administration of platelets, fibrinogen, and EACA. Heparin is not necessary but may be added in small amounts without danger. Since DIC has been said to be the main deterrent to a peritoneojugular shunt,[14] it now appears that peritoneojugular shunt should be given early consideration for ascitics rather than being considered as a last resort. DIC is a misnomer; the condition should be called PSC.

Pulmonary Edema

Pulmonary edema is a relatively rare complication, although it has occurred twice in our experience. In both cases, maximum diuresis with furosemide was not initiated; although the drug was ordered, it was never administered. Usually, increased venous pressure is sufficient to close the valve and prevent pulmonary edema, but if the ascites is tense, this protective mechanism may not be evoked. If the hematocrit count falls below 30, the patient should be put in an erect position until the excretion of urine is allowed to catch up to the level of fluid introduced through the shunt. Positive-pressure breathing may be necessary. It must be remembered that patients with ascites have severe hyperaldosteronism and therefore require diuretics postoperatively. Most do not require them thereafter.

Sepsis

Prophylactic antibiotic coverage preoperatively and postoperatively and irrigation of the wound with an aminoglycoside have eliminated operative wound infection, providing the skin closure does not leak ascitic fluid. Skin closure must be meticulous.

Infection may occur long after surgery during an intercurrent infection. Conn has shown that spontaneous occult peritonitis occurs in 9% of cirrhotics with ascites.[8] Conn describes the pathogenesis as being caused primarily by the failure of the liver to remove bacteria from portal vein blood, allowing access of enteric bacteria into the systemic circulation. The portal bacteremia usually follows a nonspecific episode of enterocolitis. Venous bypasses around the liver are also contributory. The bacteria, which have entered the systemic circulation, then enter the peritoneal cavity through the liver. Peritoneojugular shunt does not prevent this type of peritonitis and would actually spread the sepsis. Fortunately, the valve occludes in these cases as a result of necrotic debris, usually described by surgeons as "fibrin flecks in the valve." Although the infection is usually enteric, it can also follow tooth extraction.[16] All intercurrent infections must be treated with prophylactic antibiotics just as patients with an artificial heart valve should be protected by antibiotics. Later infection may result in late valve failure and can also progress to cause a fibroplastic peritoneal obliteration with the intestines wrapped in a cocoon-like fibrous bundle. These complications must be anticipated and prevented with prophylactic antibiotics.

Bleeding Varices

Patients with a preoperative history of bleeding varices bleed postoperatively unless surgical therapy is directed at the varices. Rupture of esophageal varices is infrequent immediately after a peritoneojugular shunt without a previous history of bleeding, but late bleeding is a not infrequent cause of death.

Superior Vena Cava Thrombosis

Clotting in the vena cava may be a cause of shunt failure. Nevertheless, a superior vena caval syndrome has occurred in only one of our patients 1½ years after shunt insertion. Superior vena caval syndrome cannot be relied on as an indication of superior caval thrombosis. The patient with caval syndrome responded well to removal of the shunt and the insertion of a shunt through the femoral vein up through the vena cava to the superior vena cava. In six patients with access problems, it was necessary to enter the femoral vein and extend the tubing up to the superior vena cava. If the venous tubing is disconnected from the valve and attached to a manometer, the pressure in the inferior vena cava will always be found to be positive and to rise further with respiration. As soon as the intrathoracic vena cava is reached, there is a prompt fall in venous pressure, which becomes negative on inspiration. Once thrombosis or shunt failure has occurred, patients must all be heparinized after reinsertion of another shunt. Heparinization is continued for 2 weeks with low-dose heparin therapy. Once thrombosis has occurred, it must be presumed that it will happen again unless the patient is heparinized.

In one patient with the Budd–Chiari syndrome, both the superior and the inferior venae cavae were obliterated. The venous tubing was placed directly into the right atrium.

Shunt Failure

Shunt failure occurs in about 10% of patients. It is heralded by the return of ascites, particularly in patients who have been ascites free.[27]

Patency of the shunt system can be tested by injection of colloidal radioactive material into the peritoneal cavity. This should be followed by a scan for appearance of the material in the tubing or its collection in the liver and spleen. However, radioactive scanning is not of great value, since the information it provides is rarely greater than that of the clinical history and is of no value in borderline cases in which the failure may be due to occult heart disease. Its use is almost always limited to the immediate postoperative period. Many shunt malfunctions are due to failure of the patient to wear an elastic binder and perform respiratory exercises in a recumbent position.

Shunt failure may also be due to a concealed cardiac failure with elevated central venous pressure. Such cardiac patients require frequent respiratory exercise, bedrest, digitalis, and diuretics.

If after a clinical trial of the recommended postoperative regimen, a patient does not respond adequately, venography is performed. The patency of the superior vena cava is checked by simultaneous injection of contrast agent into both arm veins. If there is no blockage of the superior vena cava, a contrast agent is injected into the venous tube by transcutaneous puncture with a 25-gauge needle. A small needle is required to prevent leakage. After 5 ml to 10 ml of contrast material has been injected into the tube, the patient should perform a Valsalva maneuver (inspire against resistance). If the shunt is patent, the dye will leave the tubing immediately. The pressure in the shunt should be measured with a spinal manometer.

If the dye is not removed by this forced breathing, blockage has occurred in the peritoneum or at the valve. Although fibrin clots, emboli, and fat globules sometimes clog the peritoneal tubing or the valve, blockage by the omentum has not been a significant problem.

A portion of early shunt failures are due to malplacement of the tubing. Most commonly, the venous tubing is placed into the subclavian vein. This can happen if the patient's head is bent too far to the left and the chin is flexed, bringing the internal jugular into a direct line with the subclavian. Failure to insert the proper length of tubing may cause failure. Excess tubing can reach the inferior vena cava or extend into the heart, whereas inadequate insertion fails to reach the superior vena cava. Shunt failure has also occurred because the tubing was punctured at the time of surgery.

Ninety-eight percent of all shunt failures are correctable if the cause is determined. Some patients may benefit from a new shunt placed on the opposite side or reintroduced into another vessel. For instance, the axillary vein may be used for access and tied off for shunt insertion; edema is rare because collateral vessels are sufficient, especially if the cephalic vein is not disturbed during surgery.

LATE RESULTS

The longest patient survival after shunt implantation has been 12 years. Expectancy of survival after shunt insertion depends on the status of the liver disease. In patients with alcoholic cirrhosis, prognosis is excellent if alcohol ingestion is terminated. Most deaths are due to esophageal bleeding or hepatic failure. Operative mortality has been 3%, but many of these deaths were early cases, and we expect this rate to fall. In the last 150 procedures we have performed, there was only one death, and this was in a complicated case that involved a bilateral hydrothorax.

REFERENCES

1. Ansley JD et al: Effect of reinfusion of ascitic fluid with LeVeen shunt on fibrinogen and platelet survival. Surg Forum 29:483, 1978
2. Arroyo V, Rodes J: A rational approach to the treatment of ascites. Postgrad Med J 51:558, 1975
3. Baldus WP et al: Renal circulation in cirrhosis: Observations based on catheterization of renal vein. J Clin Invest 43:1090, 1964
4. Baldus WP et al: The kidney in cirrhosis: I. Disorders of renal function. Ann Clin Med 60:366, 1964
5. Burchell AR et al: A seven year experience with side-to-side portocaval shunt for cirrhotic ascites. Ann Surg 168:655, 1968
6. Clermont RJ et al: Intravenous therapy of massive ascites in patients with cirrhosis: II. Long term effects on survival and frequency of renal failure. Gastroenterology 53:220, 1967
7. Clowdus BF et al: Treatment of refractory ascites with a new aldosterone antagonist in patients with cirrhosis. Proc Staff Meet Mayo Clin 35:97, 1960
8. Correia JP, Conn HO: Spontaneous bacterial peritonitis in cirrhosis: Endemic or epidemic. Med Clin North Am 59:979, 1975
9. Craig R et al: Nephrogenic ascites. Arch Intern Med 134:276, 1974
10. Dykes PA: A study of the effects of albumin infusions in patients with cirrhosis of the liver. Q J Med 30:297, 1961
11. Eknoyan G et al: Combined ascitic fluid and furosemide infusion in the management of ascites. N Engl J Med 282:713, 1970

12. Emerson PA, Davies JH: Hydrothorax complicating ascites. Lancet 1:487, 1955
13. Epstein M: Renal sodium handling in cirrhosis: A reappraisal. Nephron 23:215, 1979
14. Epstein M: The LeVeen shunt for ascites and hepatorenal syndrome. N Engl J Med 302:629, 1980
15. Fullen WD: Hepatorenal syndrome: Reversal by peritoneovenous shunt. Surgery 82:337, 1977
16. Gilas T, Langer B, Taylor BR et al: Hematogenous infection of peritoneovenous shunts after dental procedures. Can J Surg 25:215, 1982
17. Goldstein H, Boyle JD: Spontaneous recovery from the hepatorenal syndrome: Report of four cases. N Engl J Med 272:895, 1965
18. Graziano JL et al: Clinical experience with autogenous ascitic fluid infusion for chronic ascites. Am Surg 43:520, 1977
19. Grosberg S et al: Hepatorenal syndrome-reversal with LeVeen shunt. NY State J Med 78:637, 1978
20. Hacker LC et al: Intractable ascites treatment for continuous autogenous ascitic infusion. Rev Surg 31:449, 1974
21. Kinmounth J: Personal communication, 1978
22. Kinney MJ et al: Cirrhosis, ascites and impaired renal function: Treatment with the LeVeen-type chronic peritoneal-venous shunt. In Epstein M (ed): The Kidney in Liver Disease, p 349. New York, Elsevier, 1978
23. Koppel MH et al: Transplantation of cadaveric kidneys from patients with hepatorenal syndrome: Evidence for the functional nature of renal failure in advanced liver disease. N Engl J Med 280:1367, 1969
24. Lerner RG et al: Disseminated intravascular coagulation complication of LeVeen peritoneovenous shunt. JAMA 240:2064, 1978
25. LeVeen HH, Piccone VA, Hutto RB: Management of ascites with hydrothorax. Am J Surg 148:210, 1984
26. LeVeen HH, Wapnick S: Operative details of continuous peritoneovenous shunt for ascites. Bull Soc Int Chirurg 6:579, 1975
27. LeVeen HH, Vujic I et al: Peritoneovenous shunt occlusion: Etiology, diagnosis, therapy. Ann Surg 200 No. 2:212, 1984
28. LeVeen HH et al: Peritoneovenous shunting for ascites. Ann Surg 180:580, 1974
29. LeVeen HH et al: Further experience with peritoneovenous shunt for ascites. Ann Surg 184:574, 1976
30. LeVeen HH et al: Indications for peritoneojugular shunt for ascites. World J Surg 2:367, 1978
31. Lieberman FL, Peters RL: Cirrhotic hydrothorax: Further evidence that an acquired diaphragmatic defect is at fault. Arch Intern Med 125:114, 1970
32. Lieberman FL et al: Pathogenesis and treatment by hydrothorax complicating cirrhosis with ascites. Ann Intern Med 64:341, 1966
33. Moore KL, Bang NU, Broadie TA et al: Peritoneal fibrinolysis: Evidence for the efficiency of the tissue type plasminogen activator. J Lab Clin Med 101:927, 1983
34. Mortenson RA, Lawton RL: Surgical treatment for intractable ascites. Am J Surg 116:929, 1968
35. Pladson T, Parrish RM: Hepatorenal syndrome, recovery after a peritoneovenous shunt. Arch Intern Med 137:1248, 1977
36. Pollock AV: The treatment of resistant malignant ascites by the insertion of a peritoneo-atrial Holter valve. Br J Surg 62:104, 1975
37. Ratnoff OD, Patek AJ Jr: The natural history of Laennec's cirrhosis of the liver: Analysis of 386 cases. Medicine 21:207, 1942
38. Reynolds TB et al: The hepatorenal syndrome. In the Liver and Its Diseases, p 307. New York, Intercontinental Medical Book Corp, 1973
39. Rosoff L Jr et al: Studies of renin and aldosterone in cirrhotic patients with ascites. Gastroenterology 69:698, 1976
40. Rubin EH: Diseases of the Chest, p 532. Philadelphia, WB Saunders, 1947
41. Salem HH, Koutts J, Handley C et al: The aggregation of human platelets by ascitic fluid: A possible mechanism for disseminated intravascular coagulation complicating LeVeen shunts. Am J Hematology 2:156, 1981
42. Sampliner JE et al: Intractable ascites: Surgical management with reduction in secondary hyperaldosteronism. JAMA 236:483, 1976
43. Schroeder ET et al: Renal failure in patients with cirrhosis of the liver: III. Evaluation of intrarenal blood flow by para-aminohippurate extraction and response to angiotensin. Am J Med 43:887, 1967
44. Shear L et al: Renal failure in patients with cirrhosis of liver: I. Clinical and pathologic characteristics. Am J Med 39:184, 1965
45. Sherlock S et al: Complications of diuretic therapy in hepatic cirrhosis. Lancet 1:1049, 1966
46. Smith AN et al: The drainage of resistant ascites by a modification of the Spitz–Holter valve technique. J R Coll Surg 7:289, 1962
47. Walser M, Bodenlos LJ: Urea metabolism in man. J Clin Invest 38:1617, 1959
48. Wapnick S et al: LeVeen continuous peritoneojugular shunt: Improvement of renal function in ascitic patients. JAMA 237:131, 1977
49. Wapnick S et al: Prospective matched pair study comparing peritoneovenous shunt (LeVeen) and conventional therapy for massive ascites.
50. Warren D: Ascites and portosystemic shunts. Am J Surg 135:607, 1978
51. Wexler MJ, Levy M: Sodium retention in cirrhosis and ascites: Effects of continuous peritoneovenous shunting. Surg Forum 29:473, 1978
52. Wilkenson P, Sherlock S: The effects of repeated albumin infusions in patients with cirrhosis. Lancet 2:1125, 1962
53. Wooldridge TD et al: LeVeen shunt long-term therapy for idiopathic ascites of chronic renal failure. Rev Interam Radiol 6:36, 1976

chapter 22
Portal Hypertension

TELFER B. REYNOLDS

ANATOMY OF THE PORTAL VENOUS SYSTEM

The portal vein collects blood from the splanchnic area, which includes the abdominal portion of the digestive tube, the pancreas and the spleen, and transports it to the liver. The arteries supplying this blood are the nonhepatic branches of the celiac axis and the superior and inferior mesenteric arteries. There are frequent variations in the anatomy of the branches of the portal venous system, but the portal vein itself begins rather constantly at the level of the second lumbar vertebra, posterior to the head of the pancreas, at the junction of the splenic and superior mesenteric veins (Fig. 22-1). It is approximately 6 cm to 8 cm long and 1.2 cm in diameter and contains no valves. At the liver hilum, it separates into a right branch that supplies the right lobe and a left branch that supplies the left, caudate, and quadrate lobes. The ligamentum teres joins the left branch of the portal vein and contains within it one or more potential lumina (umbilical or paraumbilical veins) that are remnants of the fetal circulation running from the umbilicus to the left portal vein. The most frequent variations in portal system anatomy are in the inferior mesenteric vein, which may join the superior mesenteric instead of the splenic, and in the left gastric (coronary) vein, which may join the splenic instead of the portal.

Portal venous blood passes through one capillary system in the splanchnic viscera and leads to another capillary system, the hepatic sinusoids. Portal venous blood differs from most other venous blood in being under slightly higher pressure in order to overcome the resistance of the hepatic sinusoids, in being less depleted in oxygen because of the relatively high blood flow through the splanchnic area, and in containing many nutrients and bacterial waste products that are enroute to the liver from the digestive tube.

Normal fasting hepatic blood flow approximates 1500 ml/minute. The high-pressure hepatic arterial and low-pressure portal venous streams unite at the level of the hepatic sinusoid. The best estimates available indicate that about two thirds of the hepatic blood flow and about half of the total oxygen consumption is supplied by the portal vein, while the hepatic artery contributes the remainder.[178,211,213]

DEFINITION

Normal portal vein pressure is said to be 5 mm to 10 mm Hg. It is difficult to be certain of this value, however, since indirect pressure measurements are only approximate, and for direct measurements the subject must be anesthetized. Although the resistance to the flow of portal blood through the hepatic sinusoids is low, some pressure head in the portal vein is required to overcome it. By definition, portal hypertension implies a persistent increase above normal in portal vein pressure. Barring technical errors in measurement, direct portal system pressures at surgery over 30 cm of saline, intrasplenic pressures over 17 mm Hg, and wedged hepatic vein pressures in excess of 4 mm Hg above inferior vena caval pressure are reliable indications of portal hypertension. In most instances, this condition appears to be due to a primary increase in vascular resistance somewhere in the portal circuit and is accompanied by dilatation of the venous bed behind the obstruction, with stasis and a decrease in rate of blood flow. There is a decrease in the amount of blood flowing through the normal vascular channels with a reciprocal increase in collateral blood flow around the liver. The final level of pressure in the portal bed depends on the degree of vascular obstruction, the resistance in the collateral vessels, and the rate of inflow of blood into the splanchnic bed. Since the stimulus for collateral blood flow is the increase in portal tension, the latter can never be entirely relieved by the collateral flow.

HISTORY

Portal hypertension was probably recognized in the early decades of the 20th century. Investigators such as McIndoe[111] and McMichael[113] used the term portal hypertension in their publications. The first manometric measurements in the portal circulation were reported by Thompson and co-workers from the Presbyterian Hospital in New York in 1937.[207] In America, surgical therapy for portal hypertension was initiated in 1945 by Blakemore and Whipple working with this same group.[21] Whipple divided portal hypertension into intrahepatic and extrahepatic types.[235] Hemodynamic studies of the portal circulation followed the introduction of hepatic vein

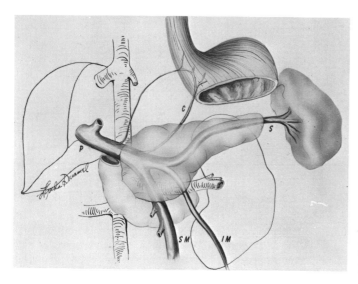

Fig. 22-1. Portal vein and its major tributaries. *C*, coronary (left gastric); *IM*, inferior mesenteric; *P*, portal; *S*, splenic; *SM*, superior mesenteric.

catheterization by Warren and Brannon in 1944,[229] the development of a method for measuring hepatic blood flow by Bradley and co-workers in 1945,[29] and the method for measuring hepatic wedge pressure by Friedman and Weiner,[64] Myers and Taylor,[123] Krook,[96] and Sherlock and co-workers[143] in the early 1950s.

ETIOLOGY

In all varieties of portal hypertension, there is a measurable increase in portal vascular resistance. In at least three conditions associated with portal hypertension, it is possible that the increased resistance to portal flow is a secondary response to increased portal flow and not a primary event. When portal hypertension accompanies splanchnic arteriovenous fistula, an increased portal flow is probably the primary abnormality followed by the development of increased intrahepatic portal vascular resistance and subsequent rise in portal vein pressure. The same sequence of events may occur in "hematologic" portal hypertension, since patients with this condition invariably have large spleens and rarely have any obvious abnormality on liver biopsy. In idiopathic portal hypertension, it is possible that increased splanchnic inflow is the primary event. However, recent studies of hepatic vascular casts and portograms suggest that the cause of the portal hypertension is more likely diffuse clotting of blood in the smaller radicles of the portal vein. Studies of splanchnic hemodynamics using radioactive microspheres in animal models of portal hypertension strongly suggest that increased splanchnic arterial inflow is an important factor in the maintenance of all portal vein hypertension, after the appearance of portal-systemic collaterals.[225,226] This could be regarded as a normal compensatory response to try to maintain portal blood flow to the liver.

METHODS FOR INVESTIGATION OF THE PORTAL SYSTEM

Portal Venography and Manometry

Because it is separated from both the arterial and systemic venous trees by capillary beds, the portal vein is not easily catheterized for angiography and pressure measurement. It can be opacified for radiologic examination indirectly, however, by celiac and superior mesenteric arteriography.[23] The arterial tree is entered with a catheter using the technique of Seldinger.[181] With a preformed curve on the tip, the catheter can be inserted into the celiac axis and later into the orifice of the superior mesenteric artery. Serial films taken after rapid injection of 80 ml to 100 ml of 76% contrast medium into the celiac axis show opacification of the hepatic, left gastric, and splenic arteries and, several seconds later, the splenic vein and portal vein (Fig. 22-2). Similarly, after injection of contrast into the superior mesenteric artery, late films show opacification of the superior mesenteric and portal veins (Fig. 22-3). With gradual improvement in radiologic equipment and increasing use of subtraction films and, now, computerized digital subtraction, the larger veins of the portal system can usually be clearly outlined and the major collateral vessels in portal hypertension can be identified. This is the method used today in most centers for radiographic investigation of portal hypertension. The risk of arteriography is small except in older persons, in whom atherosclerotic disease of the aorta may result in the dissection of intimal plaques by the catheter tip.

In splenic venography, the spleen is needled percutaneously and contrast medium is injected rapidly into the splenic substance.[2,138] Serial films show progressive opacification of the splenic and portal veins and the liver. Images of the veins ordinarily are sharper than with arterial

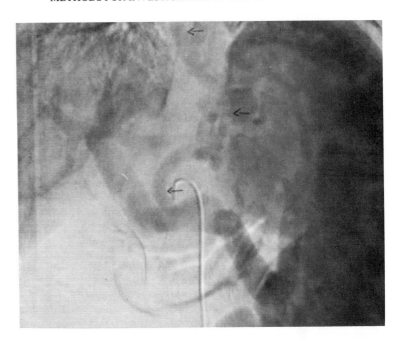

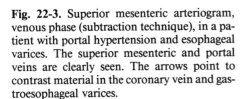

Fig. 22-2. Splenic arteriogram, venous phase (subtraction technique), in a patient with portal hypertension, splenomegaly, and esophageal varices. The splenic and portal veins are clearly outlined. The arrows point to contrast material in the coronary vein and gastric and esophageal varices.

portography because of the greater density of contrast medium. Intrasplenic pressure can be measured before contrast injection, and this pressure relates well to portal pressure. There is a risk of splenic hematoma and bleeding of approximately 5% after splenic venography; thus this technique is rarely used today unless high-quality radiographs of the portal vein are required for therapeutic decisions.

Fig. 22-3. Superior mesenteric arteriogram, venous phase (subtraction technique), in a patient with portal hypertension and esophageal varices. The superior mesenteric and portal veins are clearly seen. The arrows point to contrast material in the coronary vein and gastroesophageal varices.

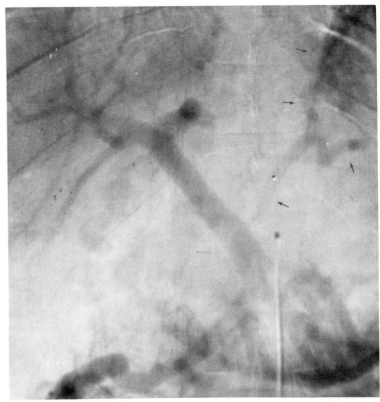

The portal vein can be catheterized transhepatically and, depending on the catheter position when contrast medium is injected, this allows high-quality images of the superior mesenteric, splenic, and portal veins.[107,130,190] Initial entry into the portal vein is with a thin needle, as in transhepatic cholangiography, with location in a portal vein branch ascertained by injection of a small amount of contrast medium that shows a flow pattern consistent with a portal vein branch. A guide wire with a flexible tip is then inserted through the needle and the needle is removed and replaced with a catheter. This method requires technical skill, and there is a small risk of bleeding from the puncture site on the liver surface. The procedure provides excellent radiographs and allows measurement of portal vein pressure and sampling of portal blood, and the catheter can be left in place for a few hours for serial studies, if needed.

The portal vein can also be catheterized by means of the umbilical vein remnant.[11,89,220] This is a surgical procedure in which the umbilical vein is identified in the preperitoneal fat cephalad of the umbilicus. In portal hypertension, the vein is occasionally patent and dilated and serves as a collateral vessel from the portal system. If not dilated, a potential lumen can be identified and enlarged with dilators to the point at which a catheter can be inserted along the vein into the left intrahepatic portal vein. Usually the catheter can then be manipulated back into the main portal trunk for injection of contrast medium, pressure recording, and blood sampling, as desired. The procedure has proven to be surprisingly free of major complications, but because it requires considerable technical skill, it is rarely used today.

Demonstration of Esophageal Varices

Radiographically, varices may appear as nodular filling defects in the partially barium-filled lower esophageal lumen. Multiple films are important because varices may be evident in one but not in several other exposures. Endoscopy is a more reliable technique for demonstrating varices, which appear as tortuous linear channels under the mucosa. If large, they bulge into the esophageal lumen. Experience is required to differentiate varices from esophageal folds; observer error and variation must be recognized,[47,49] especially when there is blood in the lumen of the esophagus.

Hepatic Vein Catheterization and Hepatic Blood Flow Measurement

The venous system can be catheterized by exposure of an arm or neck vein or by the Seldinger approach to a femoral vein. Hepatic vein catheterization may be difficult in the patient with advanced liver disease and ascites, possibly because of a change in the normal angle that the hepatic vein makes with the vena cava. However, failure to enter a hepatic vein is rare. There is virtually no morbidity from the procedure.

Wedged hepatic vein pressure (WHVP) is obtained by wedging the catheter into a peripheral hepatic venule. The catheter tip is in effect extended into the hepatic parenchyma by this maneuver insofar as an area of vascular stasis is achieved. For a zero reference point for WHVP, one can use the externally estimated right atrial position (5 cm below the sternal angle with the patient supine), or one can use the pressure measurement in the inferior vena cava or in the free hepatic vein. We prefer an internal zero reference point because we often find small pressure gradients between the vena cava and the right atrium that we feel have no relationship to portal hypertension and therefore should be included in the WHVP measurement. If the right atrial zero reference point is used, pressures up to 10 mm Hg are considered normal for WHVP, whereas with vena caval pressure as a baseline, we consider anything over 4 mm Hg to be abnormal.[35]

Regardless of which zero point is used, the pressure must be recorded during withdrawal of the catheter from the wedged position. Any abrupt fall in pressure under these circumstances is abnormal. Because the catheter fails to advance on occasion when it is not wedged, it is a useful precaution to confirm wedging by injection of a small amount of contrast medium. Wedged pressures in different areas of the liver, including the left lobe, often vary a few millimeters of mercury but are seldom widely divergent.

An alternative method of recording WHVP introduced by Groszmann and co-workers is a balloon catheter passed into a major hepatic vein after entrance into the femoral vein by the Seldinger approach.[70] WHVP is obtained by inflation of the catheter balloon until flow in the hepatic vein is completely obstructed. This method has the advantage of allowing repeated measurements of WHVP and free hepatic vein pressure without the need for moving the catheter in and out of the wedged position.

It has been assumed that a catheter wedged in a hepatic venule produces stasis in the vasculature only as far into the liver as the hepatic sinusoid, where multiple intersinusoidal anastomoses are present. Any elevation of WHVP has been ascribed to increased resistance in this area of vascular stasis, which has been assumed to be "postsinusoidal." It seems evident, however, that wedging of a catheter into a hepatic venule obstructs blood flow in a relatively large segment of the hepatic vasculature. In Figure 22-4, contrast medium has been allowed to flow into a wedged catheter, by gravity, at a pressure that is just sufficient to allow for slow flow. It is clear that stasis extends well back into the sinusoidal bed of the segment drained by the blocked hepatic vein. Anastomoses with unblocked hepatic sinusoids are around the periphery of the stagnant area, tending to decompress it, but it seems likely that the catheter will record a pressure close to that of the portal blood entering the sinusoidal bed. Increased sinusoidal as well as postsinusoidal resistance will then be

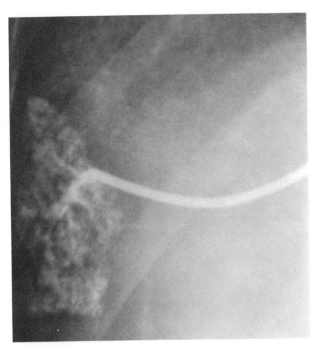

Fig. 22-4. Large area of vascular stasis resulting from the wedging of a catheter into a small hepatic vein; 8 ml of 50% Hypaque was administered over a 2-minute period by gravity drip at a pressure just sufficient to allow flow into the liver. (Popper H, Schaffner F [eds]: Progress in Liver Disease. New York, Grune & Stratton, 1965)

reflected by WHVP increase. It is correct to speak of portal hypertension accompanied by normal wedge pressure as "presinusoidal." We think it is incorrect, however, to assume that elevation of wedged pressure indicates only "postsinusoidal" resistance increase. Increased resistance in either the sinusoids or the postsinusoidal area causes elevation of WHVP.

Hepatic blood flow can be measured by the Fick principle after the catheter has been withdrawn to one of the larger hepatic veins. Hepatic extraction of the test substance, usually sodium sulfobromophthalein (Bromsulphalein [BSP]) or indocyanine green, is measured during a continuous infusion or after a single injection. Calculations of hepatic blood flow from arterial levels of test substances assuming a constant hepatic extraction are not reliable because hepatic extraction decreases considerably with liver disease. The potential error of calculation of hepatic blood flow becomes proportionally much larger when hepatic extraction of the test substance is reduced as it is in states of poor hepatic function. Measurement of hepatic blood flow then becomes progressively less reliable as liver disease increases. Cohn and colleagues have measured hepatic blood flow by the indicator dilution principle, injecting ^{131}I albumin into the hepatic artery beyond the origin of the gastroduodenal artery and sampling in the hepatic vein.[40] This method can be utilized in patients with impaired liver function in whom dye extraction is inadequate for application of the Fick principle.

Splanchnic oxygen consumption can be calculated as the product of hepatic blood flow and the arterial–hepatic venous oxygen difference. Hepatic oxygen consumption cannot be calculated unless portal blood is sampled by the umbilical approach in order to differentiate between intestinal and hepatic oxygen uptake.

Direct Transhepatic Measurement of Portal Pressure

Using a thin Chiba needle, it is relatively easy and safe to enter intrahepatic branches of the portal vein for pressure measurement (Fig. 22-5).[28] The approach is similar to that used for transhepatic cholangiography.[131] The only drawback to this otherwise ideal method for portal pressure measurement is lack of an internal zero reference point. This can be overcome by simultaneous catheterization of the inferior vena cava by the Seldinger approach to the femoral vein or by transhepatic needling of the hepatic vein.[158]

The same method of entry to the portal vein can be used to insert a guide wire, after which a larger catheter is passed percutaneously and transhepatically over the guide wire into the main portal vein. Portal venograms of high quality can be obtained by this approach, and sclerosis of venous collaterals can be performed.[107,132,180,221,237]

Direct Measurement of Intrahepatic Pressure

A large-bore needle, such as a Silverman liver biopsy needle, is inserted into the liver substance and filled with saline. "Tissue pressure" is then recorded with a strain gauge. Two groups have found good correlation between tissue pressure and portal pressure in relatively small numbers of patients.[217,222]

Ultrasound and Computed Tomography

High-resolution real-time ultrasound is a useful noninvasive modality for evaluation of the major vessels of the portal system and for assessment of portal hypertension.[76] In normal subjects, the entire length of the main portal vein can be identified by scanning obliquely. The normal diameter is 9 mm to 13 mm.[24] The proximal portion of the superior mesenteric vein and the entire length of the splenic vein are normally visible. The coronary vein, 2 mm to 3 mm in diameter, can be identified in 50% to 60% of normal subjects, and the remnant of the umbilical vein in the falciform ligament is usually identifiable as an echogenic, round structure 0.5 cm to 1.0 cm in diameter. In normal subjects, the portal vein and its major branches

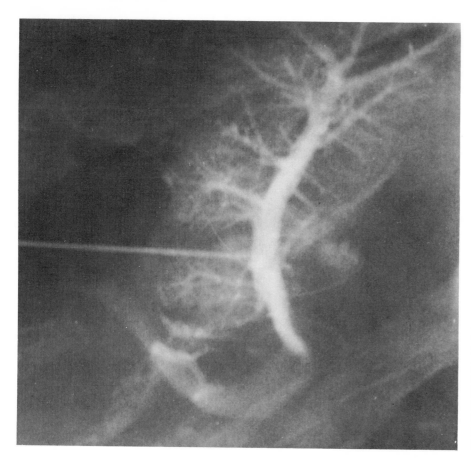

Fig. 22-5. Transhepatic puncture of a small portal vein branch with a thin needle for pressure measurement. Peripheral flow of contrast medium indicates that the vessel is a portal branch. (Boyer TD et al: Gastroenterology 72:584, 1977. © 1977, The Williams & Wilkins Co., Baltimore)

increase in size during inspiration as the diaphragm descends and flow in the hepatic vein is damped. In portal hypertension the most consistent sonographic finding is failure of the normal dilatation of the portal system to occur on inspiration.[24] A less consistent finding is an increased diameter of the portal vein.[24,98] Portal-systemic collaterals are often discernible on careful search and are a reliable indication of portal hypertension. The coronary vein and esophageal varices are frequently visible as hypoechoic channels with a coronary vein diameter greater than 5 mm. Splenorenal collaterals may be visible as irregular sonolucent channels between the splenic hilum and the left renal vein.[199] A dilated umbilical vein in the falciform ligament may give a "bull's eye" appearance[176]; the patent vessel often can be traced to the abdominal wall and thence subcutaneously to the area of the umbilicus.[85]

In extrahepatic portal vein occlusion, the main portal vein is usually invisible or consists of a group of small collateral channels.[86,232] In patients with surgical portal-systemic shunts, ultrasound can be used with considerable success to document patency of the anastomosis.[98]

Computed tomography (CT) with contrast enhancement is useful for demonstration of portal collateral flow. Large tortuous low-density tubular structures that enhance with contrast administration are often visible in the area near the splenic hilum, higher in the abdomen near the base of the esophagus, and on the anterior wall of the abdomen.[39] There may be well-defined round or tubular densities along the posteromedial wall of the gastric fundus. Their visualization can be facilitated by filling the stomach with water.[8]

Measurement of Portal Collateral Flow

Measurement of portal collateral flow has potential importance in understanding the metabolism of drugs, given that bioavailability is increased when hepatic "first-pass" removal is reduced by shunting. Quantitation of portal collateral flow may aid in evaluating patients for surgical portal-systemic shunt. All methods thus far devised have some drawbacks. By comparing count rates over liver and lung or heart after isotope injection into the spleen, it is possible to estimate the amount of collateral flow from the splenic vein that bypasses the liver.[198,233] If the isotope is attached to particles of an appropriate size (i.e., 20-μm albumin microspheres or small albumin macroaggregates), an estimate of intrahepatic shunt flow can be obtained in addition, given that isotope counts over the liver will decrease after an initial peak because some of the particles are able to bypass sinusoids.[193,212] Injection of isotope-labeled macroaggregated albumin or microspheres in the portal vein at the liver hilum allows calculation of intra-hepatic shunt by external counting over the lung.[132] Hoefs and associates have injected ^{99m}Tc-coated microspheres of a diameter of 20 μm into intrahepatic portal vein branches while sampling blood by catheter from a hepatic vein draining the region of injection. The microspheres are too large to pass through normal sinusoids; their appearance in the hepatic vein indicates intrahepatic shunting of blood, which can be quantitated if a nonextracted reference material such as ^{125}I-labeled albumin is included in the injection.[77] Porchet and Bircher have quantitated portal-systemic shunting by using digital plethysmography to measure the systemic effect of oral glyceryl trinitrate.[151] Systemic availability of oral glyceryl trinitrate is only 2 $\pm$ 4.0% in normal subjects because of virtually complete metabolism of the drug during its "first pass" through the liver after absorption into the portal system.

Ammonium Tolerance

Many investigators have demonstrated an abnormal rise in blood ammonium after patients with chronic liver disease ingest an ammonium salt. As shown by hepatic vein catheterization, the rise may be due either to poor hepatic function and failure to metabolize portal blood ammonium or to portal hypertension with portal-systemic collateral flow.[236] There is general agreement that the latter mechanism is the most common reason for a marked blood ammonium rise. One test for portal hypertension is to give 3 g of ammonium chloride orally and to consider a rise of arterial ammonium above 150 μg/dl at 45 minutes to be an abnormal result.[43]

Portal Vein and Hepatic Artery Flow

The square-wave electromagnetic flowmeter can be used at laparotomy to measure blood flow in the portal vein or hepatic artery. Considerable data have been accumulated on anesthetized patients with portal hypertension who are undergoing portacaval shunt. Values for hepatic artery flow have been variable (91–1100 ml/min) in 54 reported cases, with a mean value of 414 ml/min.[33,58,139,153] This is probably within the normal range, although few measurements have been made at surgery in subjects without liver disease.

Portal vein flow tends to be moderately reduced in portal hypertension.[58,119,153,163,178] Although pressure changes on both sides of a clamp placed across the portal vein suggest that blood flow occasionally is reversed,[116,153,230] flowmeter studies indicate that this is a rare event, despite the fact that, in about 10% of cases, there is portal stasis with little or no hepatic inflow.[119]

A number of techniques have been developed for portal blood flow measurement in the nonanesthetized patient. They are relatively complex and are invasive in that they depend upon portal blood sampling by the umbilical vein approach.[78,161,194,196]

Radionuclide angiography is a technique that attempts to quantitate hepatic arterial and portal venous flow non-invasively. After intravenous injection of a bolus of ^{99m}Tc-pertechnetate and sequential recording by a gamma camera, a computer generates time-activity curves over regions of interest that include liver, heart, and kidney. The liver activity curve usually can be separated into an early hepatic–arterial component followed by a portal–venous component. Either the total radioactivity under each segment of the curve or the slope of the accumulation curve can be used to calculate relative hepatic artery and portal venous flow, although neither can be quantitated absolutely.[19,175] The method may prove useful for selection of patients for portal-systemic shunt surgery and for following portal perfusion after distal splenorenal shunt.

A promising new noninvasive method for measuring portal blood flow employs the pulsed Doppler flowmeter. The cross-sectional area of the portal vein is measured by imaging the vein with an ultrasonic real-time sector scan. Portal flow velocity is calculated with a Doppler probe. A correction factor is used to estimate average flow velocity, since the Doppler probe measures the maximum velocity in the center of the vein. Portal vein flow is then calculated from the mean velocity and the cross-sectional area.[32,68,120,128,173] Mean velocity of flow correlated well with that of Lipiodol droplets observed cineangiographically.[128] This technique has great potential for enhancing our knowledge of portal hypertension and the effect of various treatments.

Small Doppler ultrasound probes can now be inserted through endoscopes to evaluate velocity and direction of flow in esophageal varices.[97,110] Cephalad flow is the rule, increasing during inspiration, but sometimes there is caudal flow in different locations in the same varix, suggesting the presence of valveless perforating veins connecting with periesophageal veins.

Azygos Vein Blood Flow

Bosch and Groszmann have used a double thermistor catheter (Webster Laboratories, Altadena, California) to catheterize the azygos vein from a femoral vein approach.[25] The catheter has a thermally insulated lumen containing an internal thermistor close to the distal end. Five percent glucose solution at room temperature is infused via the distal lumen at 30 ml to 60 ml/min, and a second thermistor located 2 cm proximally on the external surface of the catheter records the temperature change of the blood, which allows calculation of blood flow in the vein by the principle of thermal dilution. Ideally there should be greater distance between the thermistors to ensure adequate mixing of the indicator with the blood, but the length of the catheterizable portion of the azygos vein does not permit this. Reproducible data were obtained showing twice as much azygos blood flow in patients with varices (596 $\pm$ 78 ml/min) as in patients who had had portacaval shunt, and over four times as much as in a small group of six patients without portal hypertension (131 ± 17 ml/min). Others have confirmed a high value for this measurement in patients with cirrhosis, with a fall after administration of propranolol.[36]

DISEASES ASSOCIATED WITH PORTAL HYPERTENSION

Traditionally, portal hypertension is divided into three major types—suprahepatic, intrahepatic, and extrahepatic—based on the location of the presumed increase in vascular resistance. Imanaga and co-workers[80] and Sherlock[184] proposed classifications that incorporate both the site of the vascular block and the findings at hepatic vein catheterization. Intrahepatic portal hypertension is divided into types with normal WHVP (presinusoidal, portal vein obstruction) and with raised WHVP (postsinusoidal, hepatic vein obstruction). As mentioned, we object to the use of the word "postsinusoidal" (see Hepatic Vein Catheterization and Hepatic Blood Flow Measurement). Because in many of the syndromes accompanied by portal hypertension there are insufficient hemodynamic data available to be certain of the precise location of the increased vascular resistance, we have not attempted a classification in this chapter.

Block of the Hepatic Veins or Inferior Vena Cava (Budd–Chiari Syndrome)

When the major hepatic veins or the vena cava above the orifice of the hepatic vein is occluded, the liver becomes swollen and congested and develops sinusoidal hypertension and often hemorrhagic infarction of the areas around the central veins. Arterial blood must leave the liver by way of the portal vein and collateral veins, and pressure in the portal vein rises.

Known causes of hepatic vein obstruction include venous thrombosis, tumors, and hepatic abscess or cyst. More often, there is an unexplained fibrous obliteration of main hepatic veins. Membranous obstruction of the vena cava above the hepatic vein orifices is another frequent cause of the Budd–Chiari syndrome, particularly in the Orient and South Africa.

The clinical consequences of obstruction of the vena cava or major hepatic veins include hepatomegaly (sometimes painful, if the occlusion is acute), ascites, esophageal varices with hematemesis, and, if the vena cava is occluded, the appearance of vena cava collateral vessels on the abdominal wall. Unless the vena cava is closed, diagnosis is difficult and is usually achieved only by recognition of the characteristic histologic changes on liver biopsy. If a patient survives the acute phase, the liver may show only diffuse scarring that is misinterpreted as cirrhosis. Splenoportography usually fails to opacify the portal vein because of reverse blood flow. Failure to enter the hepatic veins with the catheter is not diagnostic, given

that it is sometimes impossible to do this in a patient with cirrhosis and an open hepatic vein.

If the vena cava is occluded, as it is in the majority of cases in Japan and about in one third of the cases in the United States, the diagnosis is much easier. Femoral vein pressure is above normal. Vena caval catheterization from below should demonstrate both the site of occlusion and marked collateral flow on venography. If vena caval occlusion is long-standing as with the web lesion, there will usually be characteristic vena caval collaterals on the trunk that can be differentiated from portal collaterals by their presence on the back and by the sugar test (see section on clinical assessment of portal hypertension). It is important to diagnose this treatable cause of portal hypertension.

Veno-occlusive Disease

Bras and colleagues have pointed out that approximately one third of the "cirrhosis" seen at autopsy in their department in Jamaica is a nonportal type of fibrosis with occlusion of centrolobular hepatic veins and subsequent centrolobular fibrosis.[30] Most patients with this lesion are under 20 years of age. Ascites and severe portal hypertension with bleeding from esophageal varices are prominent clinical manifestations. These investigators believe that the acute form of the disease is due to occlusion of small branches of the hepatic veins, with resulting severe centrolobular congestion and loss of hepatocytes in the center of the lobule. Various pyrrolizidine alkaloids from *Crotalaria* and *Senecio* plants are suspected as etiologic agents because they are used in native "bush-tea" and produce somewhat similar lesions in experimental animals.[31,112]

Similar lesions are seen after bone marrow transplant in patients with leukemia. It is uncertain whether they are due to intensive chemoradiotherapy[187] or are manifestations of graft-versus-host disease.[17]

Parenchymal Liver Disease

Cirrhosis

Distortion of the intrahepatic vasculature is a constant accompaniment of cirrhosis. Corrosion casts of the liver show a decrease in volume of both the portal venous and hepatic venous trees.[72] Portography usually shows a "winter-tree" appearance of the portal vessels. Serial sections demonstrate that the regenerative nodule compresses and distorts the hepatic veins.[87] Portal fibrosis and scarring may cause narrowing of the peripheral portal venules. Although these features seem to provide an adequate anatomic basis for increased vascular resistance in the cirrhotic liver, some investigators argue that increased flow from the hepatic artery into the portal vein may be the primary cause of portal hypertension. Postmortem perfusions and corrosion casts show a relative increase in hepatic artery mass in cirrhosis,[72,74] and abnormal communications can be seen between the smaller ramifications of the hepatic artery and the portal vein.[150] It would seem more logical to regard these as compensatory phenomena for reduced portal-vein flow rather than a primary cause of portal hypertension. However, any increase in hepatic arterial inflow is bound to contribute to portal hypertension if the principal resistance to blood flow is in the hepatic sinusoids or hepatic venules.

Many investigators have studied hepatic hemodynamics in cirrhosis by hepatic vein catheterization. Results from many publications were summarized in a review by La-Croix and Leusen in 1965.[99] Most values for hepatic blood flow have been normal or decreased. The inherent errors in the standard BSP method for measuring liver blood flow tend to give an artifactually high result when hepatic extraction of BSP is poor, as it often is in liver disease. This probably explains the relatively few high values reported for hepatic blood flow. If portal hypertension were due primarily to increased splanchnic inflow, hepatic blood flow measurements should tend to be high in cirrhosis, whereas if vascular obstruction is the major problem, they should tend to be low, as they appear to be.

WHVP is elevated in cirrhosis, roughly proportional to the stage of the disease. In alcoholic cirrhosis, WHVP is approximately equal to simultaneously measured portal vein pressure.[28,168,218] This suggests that most of the increased vascular resistance in alcoholic cirrhosis is sinusoidal or postsinusoidal, rather than presinusoidal. In nonalcoholic liver diseases with portal hypertension, WHVP tends to be variably lower than portal vein pressure.[28] There have not been enough comparisons made and published to tell us whether there are different patterns for different diseases. Of four patients with Wilson's disease studied by Taylor and co-workers,[201] three had only minor elevations of wedge pressure in spite of severe portal hypertension, implying a marked increase in presinusoidal resistance. This is not a consistent finding in Wilson's disease, as indicated by one of their patients and two patients of our own with considerable WHVP elevation. More comparisons between WHVP and portal pressure are needed in the various types of nonalcoholic cirrhosis to determine the frequency of increase in predominantly presinusoidal vascular resistance.

Alcoholic Liver Disease Without Cirrhosis

Severe acute liver damage may develop in the alcoholic without cirrhosis. Histologically, there is usually fatty infiltration, liver cell injury with "ballooning," necrosis, alcoholic hyaline and polymorphonuclear infiltration. This lesion has been variously called "alcoholic hepatitis,"[12] "florid cirrhosis,"[149] and "sclerosing hyaline necrosis."[55] Our pathologists have drawn our attention to the predominantly centrilobular location of the cellular injury and the collagen formation that accompanies it. Extensive centrilobular collagen deposition may greatly distort the hepatic architecture without the development of any regenerative nodules (Fig. 22-6).

We have found, by WHVP measurements, that portal hypertension develops early in this lesion. Ascites often accompanies the acute stage. In the subacute and chronic stages of the lesion, collagen formation in the liver is diffuse, predominantly in the central areas, somewhat reminiscent of the "centrilobular cirrhosis" described by Bras and colleagues in veno-occlusive disease.[30] Many of our alcoholic patients in Los Angeles die in the subacute stages of this lesion with a smooth liver surface, with all of the clinical features of portal hypertension including esophageal varices, and without regenerative nodules microscopically. If not too severe, acute sclerosing hyaline necrosis may resolve, leaving minimal hepatic scarring, or it may progress to cirrhosis with regenerative nodules.

Fig. 22-6. Predominantly centrilobular fibrosis without regenerative nodules as seen in chronic sclerosing hyaline disease caused by alcoholism. This patient had a smooth liver surface and elevated wedged hepatic vein pressure. (Sommers SC [ed]: Pathology Annual: 1967. New York, Appleton-Century-Crofts, 1967)

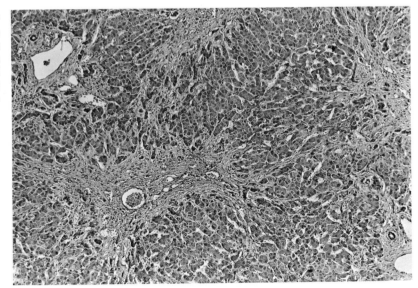

Sarcoidosis

Scattered in the literature are reports of hepatic sarcoidosis with manifest ascites and esophageal varices. The cause of the portal hypertension has not been determined. Hunt considered it to be a manifestation of increased inflow through the large spleen.[79] It has been postulated that the granulomas obstruct the portal venules, hepatic venules, or sinusoids.[118] Alternatively, periportal fibrosis and disruption of lobular architecture caused by the healing phase of the granulomatous lesions could cause portal hypertension. Our own catheterization experience includes only three patients with ascites, all of whom had moderate elevation of wedge pressure. From histologic examination in two of them, we were unable to decide the cause of portal hypertension.

Cystic Disease of the Liver

The liver lesion commonly called "congenital hepatic fibrosis"[88] is a form of cystic disease involving the small bile ducts. The liver surface does not have a cystic appearance; microscopic sections show marked bile duct hyperplasia in broad fibrous bands in the portal areas. Liver function is good, and portal hypertension is prominent, often causing variceal bleeding in childhood. The disorder is hereditary, with a pattern resembling that of an autosomal recessive trait. There is frequent association with some form of renal cystic disease. Kerr and colleagues found a considerable gradient (11 mm Hg) between portal vein pressure and WHVP in one patient and postulated that portal hypertension is due to compression or reduction of the portal venous radicles in the fibrous portal bands.[88] However, data on hepatic vein catheterization from six additional patients, summarized by Fauvert and co-workers, do not favor a predominantly presinusoidal vascular obstruction.[57]

The usual type of polycystic disease of the liver is probably rarely, if ever, associated with portal hypertension.

Partial Nodular Transformation of the Liver

Sherlock and associates have described four patients with portal hypertension apparently due to an unexplained nodular transformation of the perihilar portion of the liver, without appreciable fibrosis.[186] Hemodynamic studies in one patient demonstrated a high wedge pressure. Whether the portal hypertension is due to compression of the hepatic outflow by the nodules or to disease of the hepatic veins is unknown.

Nodular Regenerative Hyperplasia

Nodular regenerative hyperplasia is an uncommon, poorly understood disorder characterized by diffuse 1-mm to 2-mm nodules of regenerative-appearing hepatocytes that compress the intervening hepatic parenchyma. Unlike cirrhosis, there is no excess collagen surrounding the nodules. These nodules are often visible on the external liver surface and on the cut surface. They are most easily discerned on reticulin stain, which shows condensed reticulin fibers at the periphery of the nodules and widely separated strands in their centers. The regenerative character of the nodules is suggested by irregular cell plates, often more than one cell thick, prominent nucleoli, and occasional double nuclei and mitotic figures. There is an association with a wide variety of conditions including Felty's syndrome, macroglobulinemia, tuberculosis, myeloproliferative syndrome, and collagen vascular diseases.[22,191,197,228] The cause of the portal hypertension that frequently accompanies nodular regenerative hyperplasia is unknown. WHVP was reported to be substantially elevated in two patients and mildly increased in a third.[22,171]

Hematologic Disorders

Portal hypertension with ascites, esophageal varices, and an open portal vein has been reported in occasional patients with the myeloproliferative syndrome, Hodgkin's disease, leukemia, Gaucher's disease, and osteopetrosis. Some authorities have held that increased splenic arterial inflow is the cause of portal hypertension in these situations.[113,142,144] Considerably increased values for hepatic blood flow have been recorded by Benhamou and colleagues in one patient with Gaucher's disease[13] and by Rosenbaum and co-workers in five patients with the myeloproliferative syndrome.[170]

An alternate view is that portal hypertension is caused by vascular obstruction from the portal or intrasinusoidal infiltrate of the hematologic disease. In support of this, a normal hepatic blood flow with portal hypertension was found by Shaldon and Sherlock in two patients, one with Hodgkin's disease and one with myelosclerosis,[182] and by Dal Palu in one patient with leukemia.[52] The increased vascular resistance seemed to be presinusoidal in Shaldon and Sherlock's patients and in one we reported[53] and intrahepatic in Dal Palu's patient.

The mechanism for portal hypertension in hematologic disorders is unknown. It is uncertain whether removal of the spleen is beneficial.

Metastatic or Primary Carcinoma of the Liver

Ascites not due to peritoneal implants, together with splenomegaly and esophageal varices, may complicate metastatic carcinoma in the liver[172] or primary hepatocellular carcinoma.[124] Portal hypertension in this situation seems to be due to tumor emboli in the portal or hepatic venules or both. Hepatic vein catheterization measurements have been performed on a number of patients with metastatic liver carcinoma, but none had evidence of portal hypertension. Presumably, WHVP is high if the predominant obstruction is in the hepatic venules and low if it is in the portal venules.

Intrahepatic Portal Vein Obstruction Caused by Schistosomiasis

The ova of *Schistosoma mansoni* and *Schistosoma japonicum* are laid in the submucosa of the colon and rectum. Some pass into the portal bloodstream and lodge as emboli in the intrahepatic portal venules. A foreign body "pseudotubercle" tissue reaction with granulomatous change and eosinophilic infiltrate develops in the portal area with eventual healing and scarring. Portal hypertension follows, with splenomegaly and esophageal varices and relatively good preservation of liver function. The site of obstruction to blood flow appears to be the portal venules. On hepatic vein catheterization, one would predict a relatively normal wedge pressure level with this type of presinusoidal obstruction; several studies have recorded such findings.[3,121,154] When wedge pressure is moderately elevated, it usually accompanies greater distortion of hepatic architecture as a result either of a more advanced stage of the disease or of complicating liver cirrhosis of another cause.

Arteriovenous Fistulas in the Splanchnic Bed

The published experience with splanchnic arteriovenous fistulas has been reviewed by Stone and colleagues[195] and Van Way and co-workers.[216] Many patients demonstrated ascites, esophageal varices, and gastrointestinal tract bleeding. Portal hypertension was often documented by operative manometry.

The usual causes of acquired splanchnic arteriovenous fistulas are trauma or rupture of aneurysms of the splenic or hepatic artery. Congenital arteriovenous fistulas occur in hereditary hemorrhagic telangiectasia. It seems logical to ascribe the portal hypertension to increased flow of blood into the portal system. The hepatic vasculature must resist the increased flow sufficiently for portal hypertension to develop and thus prevent the onset of high-output heart failure, which seems to be a rare finding in this disorder. One would expect a moderate or marked increase in hepatic blood flow, depending upon how much compensatory increase in hepatic vascular resistance developed. Unfortunately, hepatic hemodynamic data in this important prototype of portal hypertension are sparse.

A patient of ours with clinical portal hypertension, esophageal varices, and a right hepatic artery–portal vein fistula due to an old gunshot wound had a portal vein pressure of 57 cm of saline at laparotomy. At hepatic vein catheterization, hepatic blood flow was within normal limits (1650 ml/min by the indocyanine green technique), and WHVP was only mildly elevated (9 mm Hg above inferior vena caval pressure).[54] Liver biopsy showed definite changes in the portal areas similar to what we have called "hepatoportal sclerosis,"[115] with sclerosis of the portal radicles and increased portal collagen. If these hemodynamic findings are typical for this type of portal hypertension, we can no longer exclude increased portal inflow as a cause of portal hypertension simply because of a failure to find increased hepatic blood flow. Perhaps our patient did have increased hepatic blood flow before the development of portal venous thickening and sclerosis. It is also possible that a functional increase in portal venous resistance could keep hepatic blood flow within the broad range of normal before the development of organic vascular pathology.

In dogs, portal vein arterialization can cause anatomic changes in portal venules, including thickening of the wall, hypertrophy of the muscularis, and fibrinoid necrosis.[59,155] Hemodynamic data in this type of animal preparation are limited. Siderys and co-workers found a marked increase in hepatic blood flow and moderate portal hypertension in six dogs 6 weeks after constructing a fistula between the aorta and splenic vein.[188] These findings are different than those in our patient referred to above. Further hemodynamic studies in this type of portal hypertension should be of great interest.

Idiopathic Portal Hypertension

Portal hypertension without any apparent cause is a relatively uncommon but vexing problem. Patients with this disorder have normal or nearly normal hepatic function, a smooth liver surface, minor histologic abnormality, and an open portal vein. Recognizable pathologic changes are limited to varying degrees of portal fibrosis, usually slight, and intimal thickening and eccentric sclerosis of the portal vein walls. Often there are large, thin-walled vascular or lymphatic channels in the portal areas. This type of portal hypertension is found occasionally in the United States,[73,147,208] and more frequently in India,[27,126,174] England,[240] and Japan.[80] In the latter two countries, it has been reported to be the pathologic process that accounts for portal hypertension in from 17%[240] to 33%[80] of patients undergoing portal decompression surgery. Its relationship to tropical splenomegaly in Africa is uncertain. Probably it is a universal disorder and has been lumped in with cirrhosis in some countries.

Terminology is varied, consistent with our lack of understanding of its pathogenesis. Various labels include hepatoportal sclerosis,[115] intrahepatic presinusoidal (portal vein) obstruction,[80] noncirrhotic portal fibrosis,[174] obliterative portal venopathy,[126] Banti's syndrome, and idiopathic portal hypertension.[27] Until the pathogenesis is better understood, the last term is probably the best.

Hemodynamic studies in Japanese patients consistently show normal or nearly normal WHVP and hepatic blood flow.[80] In Indian patients, WHVP was usually elevated, though to a lesser extent than in cirrhotic patients studied by the same investigators.[27] Hepatic blood flow varied from slightly below to slightly above normal. One patient investigated by Benhamou and colleagues had normal hepatic blood flow and slight elevation of wedge pressure.[14]

We could obtain only limited hemodynamic data in our own patients. WHVP was normal in three, and hepatic blood flow was moderately decreased in two.[115] This hemodynamic pattern is similar to that found in schistosomiasis with portal hypertension, suggesting that the intrahepatic radicles of the portal vein are the site of increased vascular resistance. It seemed that the subtle changes in the portal venules of our patients might indicate a primary lesion at this site. Nayak and Ramalingaswami[126] favor an obliterative portal venopathy, and Boyer and co-workers suggest the role of previously unrecognized pyelophlebitis.[27] Extensive studies from Japan support intrahepatic portal venous occlusion as the basis for the pathology.[65,129]

The prognosis in idiopathic portal hypertension is much better than in patients with cirrhosis. A Japanese series estimated survival at 77% 10 years after diagnosis,[129] and a British group projected 30-year survival to be 55%.[90] In spite of relative good liver function, there is an appreciable incidence of recurring encephalopathy after surgical portal-systemic shunt.[90]

Extrahepatic Portal Hypertension

In extrahepatic portal hypertension, the portal or splenic vein or both are occluded and are replaced by a fibrous cord or a collection of collateral channels called "cavernous transformation." The spleen is enlarged, and there are esophageal or gastric varices or both. Liver biopsy looks normal or nearly normal, and hepatic function tests are usually normal, with the exception of prothrombin time, which is sometimes inexplicably decreased. WHVP is normal, hepatic blood flow is mildly or moderately reduced, and intrasplenic pressure is raised. Portography fails to opacify the obstructed segments of the portal circulation and shows numerous collateral channels. Sometimes there is a short segment of normal portal vein on the hepatic side of the occluded area that opacifies via bridging collaterals. Portal vein occlusion can be diagnosed by ultrasound with reasonable confidence.[232]

The clinical manifestations of extrahepatic portal hypertension consist of episodes of hematemesis, often appearing early in childhood or young adulthood, and recurring irregularly, sometimes at widely spaced intervals. In childhood, bleeding episodes often seem related to respiratory infections. Whether this is due to coughing or to aspirin ingestion is unknown. Ascites appears temporarily after bleeding episodes in one third to one half of the patients.[114,231] Some patients have occasional episodes of hepatic encephalopathy,[114] presumably as a consequence of extensive collateral circulation. The hematologic manifestations of hypersplenism are often present to a moderate degree but seldom cause symptoms.

The cause of extrahepatic portal block is usually unknown.[61,114,206] A few patients give a history compatible with neonatal omphalitis. Localized splenic vein thrombosis produces a syndrome called "sinistral" portal hypertension and can be related to an episode of acute pancreatitis.[106,210] In this situation the varices may be entirely in the stomach and are easily missed at endoscopy. In an occasional patient, the portal clot can be blamed on an associated Budd–Chiari syndrome, polycythemia vera, or paroxysmal nocturnal hemoglobinuria. Portal vein thrombosis also may be a complication of cirrhosis of the liver, presumably as a consequence of stasis in the portal bed, or it may develop from invasion by hepatocellular carcinoma.

The cause of portal hypertension with portal block may seem obvious. Nevertheless, some facts are disconcerting. It is difficult to produce anything that resembles hypersplenism or permanent portal hypertension by ligating any branch of the portal system in animals.[37] Ravenna has pointed out that many examples of portal or splenic vein thrombosis in humans are not accompanied by splenomegaly or esophageal varices.[156] For these reasons, we should not be too confident of our understanding of extrahepatic portal hypertension.

CONSEQUENCES

Collateral Circulation

A natural consequence of stasis and increased pressure in any venous bed is the development of connections to neighboring low-pressure veins. The collateral circulation in long-standing portal hypertension is well developed, although the size and location of the major collaterals vary considerably from patient to patient. It has been proposed that a well-developed collateral flow can relieve portal hypertension, and patients have been described with large collaterals and relatively normal intrasplenic pressures.[209] However, since the stimulus for the development of collateral vessels is portal hypertension, it seems unlikely that the latter can ever be completely relieved by the collateral flow.

Portal collateral blood flow alters the pharmacokinetics of drugs that are metabolized by the liver. When drugs with high "first-pass" removal are taken orally, their systemic availability is increased in proportion to the amount of collateral flow. Another potential consequence of portal collateral flow is hepatic encephalopathy, which results when intestinally derived toxic substances bypass the liver.

The natural sites for the development of portal collateral vessels are areas in which veins draining into the portal system are in juxtaposition to veins draining into the caval system. The major locations for this are described below.

Submucosa of the Esophagus. Anastomoses form between the tributaries of the coronary vein (portal drainage) and azygos vein (superior vena cava drainage). This results in submucosal varices of the lower esophagus and upper stomach (Fig. 22-7). Collaterals from the spleen to the stomach contribute to this anastomotic plexus.

Submucosa of the Rectum. The lower portion of the rectum normally drains into the inferior vena cava through the inferior hemorrhoidal veins, whereas the upper portion of the rectum drains into the portal system through the

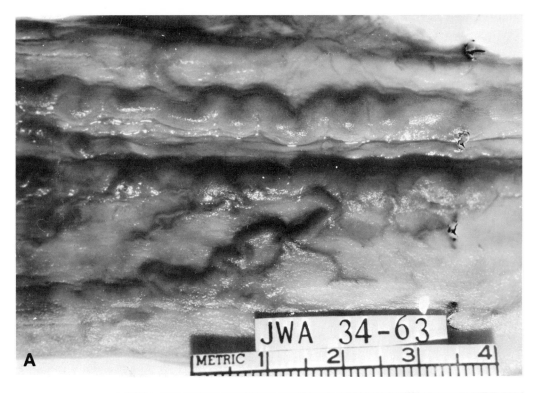

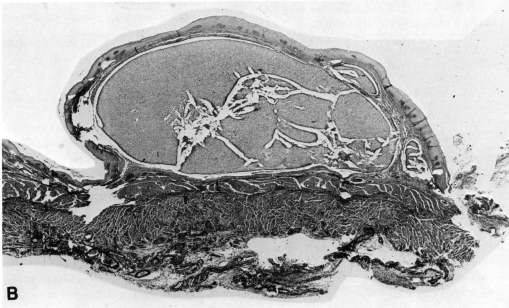

Fig. 22-7. A. Varices in the lower esophagus at autopsy in a patient with alcoholic liver disease. The veins have been injected with a blood–agar mixture. **B.** Cross-section through an injected varix.

middle and superior hemorrhoidal veins. Anastomoses between these venous systems result in hemorrhoids.

Anterior Abdominal Wall. The umbilical vein remnant of the fetal circulation in the falciform ligament normally carries little or no blood but remains probe-patent. In portal hypertension, it can serve as an anastomosis between the main left portal vein and the normotensive epigastric veins of the anterior abdominal wall that drain ultimately into the superior and inferior cavae.

Parietal Peritoneum. Connections between the portal and caval systems form in the posterior abdominal wall (veins of Retzius) and between the capsule of the liver and diaphragm (veins of Sappey).

Left Renal Vein. Large connections sometimes form between the splenic vein or other neighboring portal tributaries and the left renal vein. On rare occasions, these are nearly as large as a surgical splenorenal shunt.[100]

Increased Lymphatic Flow

The normal flow of hepatic lymph is toward the hilum; from there, lymphatics traverse the hepatoduodenal and hepatogastric ligaments to join the cisterna chyli and thoracic duct. In portal hypertension of intrahepatic cause, the flow of hepatic lymph is greatly increased. On postmortem studies, hilar lymphatics can be shown to be enlarged.[6] In life, the thoracic duct is dilated, lymph flow is markedly increased, and lymphatic pressure is raised. We have seen thoracic duct lymph flow as great as 15 ml/minute and pressures that rise as high as 30 mm Hg after 30 to 40 seconds of duct occlusion. Presumably, most of this lymph flow is from the liver, although, in ascites, some of the increase may come from the peritoneum or omentum. The thoracic duct lymph is often blood-tinged in portal hypertension; the highest hematocrit we have observed is 19 mm. There is no good explanation for the sanguineous lymph, although it has been suggested that it results from peripheral venolymphatic connections rather than from leakage at the hepatic sinusoid.[56]

Given that a natural response to the obstruction of venous return from any area of the body is an increase in lymph flow, the increased thoracic duct lymph flow in portal hypertension could be regarded as a manifestation of congestion of the liver. Because the major vascular obstruction in intrahepatic portal hypertension seems to be in the sinusoids or hepatic venules, the sinusoidal area can be considered congested and capable of forming more than the usual amount of hepatic lymph.

It would be interesting to know the thoracic duct pressure and lymph flow in extrahepatic portal hypertension; to my knowledge, this has not been measured.

Ascites

Portal hypertension is a major factor in ascites formation. The leading current theory, which has much experimental backing, is that ascites forms as a consequence of sinusoidal hypertension and hepatic lymph formation in excess of what can be carried away by the hepatic lymphatics. Witte and co-workers have pointed out the probable additional role of mesenteric and intestinal capillary stasis in ascites formation.[238] Portacaval shunting usually relieves ascites and, in our experience, when it does not do so, the residual hepatic sinusoidal pressure remains relatively high as assessed by WHVP.[75] Nevertheless, another factor is operative in the production of ascites, since at no fixed level of portal hypertension does ascites regularly appear. Whether this factor is the serum albumin level or something much more complex is unknown.

Increased Plasma Volume

A regular finding in chronic liver disease with portal hypertension, increased plasma volume has been documented by many investigators.[56,105,122,145] This is not a measurement artifact; we found the same degree of plasma volume increase in patients with and without ascites and no evidence of any significant loss of iodinated albumin into either the ascitic fluid or the thoracic duct lymph space during the 20 minutes required for equilibration.[105] Portal hypertension seems to provide a logical explanation for hypervolemia, since it is invariably accompanied by dilatation of the entire portal venous bed and adjacent collateral veins.

We found the greatest increases in plasma volume in patients with esophageal varices and previous hemorrhage. We also found a reasonably good correlation between plasma volume and level of portal hypertension as assessed by WHVP. However, portal hypertension may not be the only reason for increased plasma volume in chronic liver disease. In our experience, some degree of hypervolemia persists after portacaval shunting, even after the side-to-side variety.[105] Also, the degree of hypervolemia is apparently less in extrahepatic than in intrahepatic portal hypertension. Murray and associates found normal values for plasma volume in extrahepatic block,[122] whereas we found moderate increases. Unfortunately, Bradley's method for measuring splanchnic blood volume is not readily applicable to patients with extensive portal collateral circulation, and it has proved technically difficult to measure the volume of the splanchnic venous bed at autopsy. If the volume of the dilated portal venous bed were great enough to account for the observed increase in plasma volume in portal hypertension, it would be unnecessary to seek another explanation of hypervolemia.

CLINICAL ASSESSMENT

Physical Findings

Most of the physical findings of chronic liver disease have some bearing on the presence of portal hypertension. Those with specific importance include those described below.

Splenomegaly. Portal hypertension is not the only reason for splenic enlargement in chronic liver disease, since the size of the spleen does not correlate well with the level of portal pressure. However, palpable enlargement of the spleen is noted in a majority of patients with significant portal hypertension. Palpability of the spleen is enhanced for most examiners by use of light pressure in the left upper quadrant while the patient lies on his right side and inhales deeply.

Ascites. Ascites is suggestive of portal hypertension unless explained by carcinoma, heart failure, or inflammatory disease of the peritoneum. Shifting dullness is the best indicator of a moderate amount of ascites. Ultrasound is highly reliable in deciding about the presence of ascites.

Dilated Abdominal Veins. Many patients with portal hypertension have dilated veins in the flanks as a result of portal venous–parietal peritoneum connections, or on the anterior abdominal wall as a result of umbilical vein–epigastric vein connections. Minor degrees of increased abdominal wall collateral circulation may be indistinguishable from circulation in normal veins made more prominent by stretching and thinning of the overlying skin in the patient without portal hypertension whose abdomen is distended. Abdominal collaterals are often seen more easily in infrared photographs (Fig. 22-8) or through the red goggles used by radiologists. Occasionally, an extremely dilated and tortuous vein creates a lump on the abdominal wall that is best seen in lateral profile (Fig. 22-9). On one of our patients, such a vein was mistaken for an umbilical hernia. Rarely, the collateral veins take the shape of a "caput medusae" around the umbilicus.

When the veins are large, one can often hear the characteristic Cruveilhier–Baumgarten murmur. This is a continuous bruit varying from low to high pitch and most often heard somewhere between the umbilicus and the lower portion of the sternum. It is pathognomonic of intrahepatic portal hypertension with a large collateral vein in the falciform ligament. In some patients, the bruit comes and goes, resulting in disputes between examiners as to its presence. It is often enhanced by raising intraabdominal pressure, and it usually disappears completely when pressure is applied immediately above the umbilicus. There is often a palpable thrill over the area where the murmur is loudest.

Portal collateral veins must be differentiated from collateral vessels that form after obstruction of the inferior vena cava. Vena cava collaterals tend to be more prominent in the flanks and less so in the central areas of the abdomen (Fig. 22-10). There are often dilated vessels over the back that are never seen with portal obstruction. In vessels below the umbilicus, the direction of flow is upward in vena caval collaterals and downward in portal collaterals. However, the valves in dilated veins may become ineffective, and one cannot always ascertain the direction of the blood flow in a vessel by the usual technique of stripping it between two fingers. In vena caval obstruction,

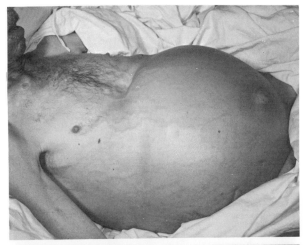

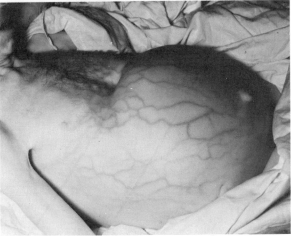

Fig. 22-8. Collateral abdominal veins on the anterior abdominal wall in a patient with alcoholic liver disease as recorded by black and white photography (*top*) and infrared photography (*bottom*).

bruits are not heard over the dilated vessels, and the femoral vein pressure should be elevated.

The sugar test has been reliable in our experience. During absorption of glucose from the gastrointestinal tract, sugar concentration should be higher in the portal vein and any of its collaterals than in the remainder of the circulatory system. Peripheral vein and abdominal vein glucose concentrations are compared 30 minutes after ingestion of 50 g of glucose by a fasting patient. If the abdominal vessels are portal collaterals, the sugar concentration should be substantially higher (usually 20 mg–50 mg/dl). Both values should be above normal to indicate that glucose is actually being absorbed.

Demonstration of Esophageal Varices

Demonstration of esophageal varices is almost but not quite pathognomonic of portal hypertension. "Downhill

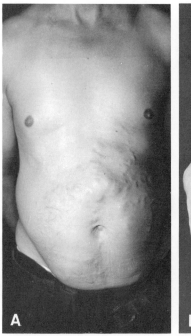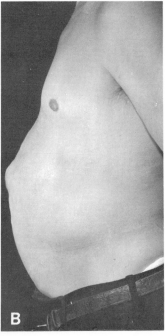

Fig. 22-9. Large abdominal collateral veins as seen anteriorly (*A*) and in profile (*B*). Cruveilhier–Baumgarten murmur was heard over this vein.

varices" can occur when the superior vena cava is obstructed below the azygos vein. Palmer has pointed out that dilated veins are sometimes seen in the lower esophagus in patients with hiatus hernia without portal hyper-

Fig. 22-10. Abdominal collateral veins resulting from long-standing inferior vena caval obstruction.

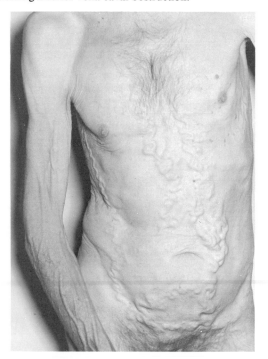

tension.[136] A few patients have been reported with esophageal varices that are unexplained.[137,177]

In looking for varices, endoscopy by an experienced endoscopist is preferable to barium swallow because false-negative reports are less frequent.

Supplementary Techniques

In many patients, if definite esophageal varices are demonstrated by barium swallow or esophagoscopy, and if the clinical picture is not complicated, further evaluation of the portal system is unnecessary. When more information is desired, the clinician has a wide choice of additional techniques as described in the first portion of this chapter. The most useful of these is celiac and superior mesenteric angiography. Morbidity with this technique is low, except in elderly patients with sclerotic arteries. The splenic, superior mesenteric, and portal veins usually are visualized clearly enough for determination of their size and patency, and collateral circulation, if present, usually is demonstrated. Splenoportography ordinarily provides sharper images of the splenic and portal veins and the esophageal and gastric collateral vessels, but there is small risk (about 5% in some series) of splenic bleeding that will require transfusion or splenectomy.

Transhepatic portography and umbilical portography are more invasive procedures than either angiography or splenoportography. They are most useful when portal blood sampling for physiological studies is needed in addition to anatomic information.

Hepatic vein catheterization is of limited usefulness. One of its major advantages, however, is the lack of any morbidity or significant discomfort to the patient. A definite elevation of WHVP is proof of portal hypertension, although a normal wedge pressure does not eliminate the possibility of presinusoidal or extrahepatic portal hypertension. The finding of portal hypertension, however, does not necessarily imply the presence of esophageal varices. Furthermore, the level of wedge pressure does not correlate directly with the likelihood of bleeding from varices, although data collected by Viallet and colleagues indicate that variceal hemorrhage rarely occurs if the gradient of pressure between wedged and free hepatic vein is less than 12 mm Hg.[219] For us, the major clinical application of hepatic vein catheterization has been to determine the presence of portal hypertension and to follow its level over a period of time. The procedure also has research applications.

HEMORRHAGE FROM ESOPHAGEAL VARICES

Risk Factors

If the factors that predispose to variceal bleeding were known, prophylactic treatment in highly susceptible patients could be considered. Unfortunately, the pathogenesis of variceal hemorrhage is uncertain. The bulk of the evidence does not support an erosive mechanism from acid reflux. Postmortem esophageal mucosal changes are frequently observed in patients who die of variceal hemorrhage, but these changes may be iatrogenic or agonal. Study of esophageal rings removed during stapling operations for variceal bleeding does not suggest esophagitis as the mechanism precipitating hemorrhage.[148,192] There is general agreement that large varices are more likely to bleed than small varices.[7,51,102] Debate exists concerning the relationship of portal vein pressure to variceal bleeding.[42,164] Clearly, portal hypertension is required in order for esophageal varices to develop. However, in patients who already have demonstrable varices, the data relating portal pressure and bleeding propensity are equivocal, although, in my opinion they favor the lack of a close relationship.[66,95,102,159,165,189,224] Intravariceal pressure, which should be lower than portal pressure due to interposed vascular resistance, has been little studied. Palmer found no relationship between directly measured intravariceal pressure and bleeding.[134] A more recent study showed a higher pressure in varices of grade 3 size (22.7 mm Hg) than grade 2 size (15.7 mm Hg).[193]

Several endoscopists have described localized abnormalities on the walls of varices that may predispose to hemorrhage. These include "cherry-red spots," "red wale markings," "hemocystic spots," and "varices upon varices."[15,51] Histologic study of esophageal rings removed at stapling operations suggests that these are angiomatous changes.[192] The fact that needle puncture of a varix for pressure measurement or sclerotherapy rarely causes sig-

nificant bleeding suggests that either structural defects of the vessel wall or local problems with hemostasis are required to allow bleeding to continue once rupture has occurred.

Diagnosis

Bleeding esophageal varices have to be suspected in all patients with upper gastrointestinal tract hemorrhage. If alcoholic liver disease is confirmed, the differential diagnosis is narrowed to four major considerations: esophageal varices, alcoholic gastritis, peptic ulcer, or the Mallory–Weiss syndrome. The first two occur with about equal frequency in most series; peptic ulcer is somewhat less frequent, and the Mallory–Weiss syndrome accounts for only 2% to 5% of cases. In a patient with known chronic nonalcoholic liver disease, varices are about four times as likely a source of bleeding as peptic ulcer.

The type of bleeding is not very helpful in differential diagnosis, except in the Mallory–Weiss syndrome, in which it sometimes follows repeated vomiting. Although there is usually hematemesis with varix bleeding, some patients have only melena. Bleeding from varices is not always voluminous and may be protracted, being evident only through strongly positive occult blood reactions in the feces.

The usual historic and physical evidences of chronic liver disease are sought. Most important are jaundice, firmness of the liver edge, palpability of the spleen, ascites, auscultation of a Cruveilhier–Baumgarten murmur, spider angiomata, hepatic fetor, and asterixis. In the alcoholic, epigastric tenderness is more often due to hepatic inflammation than to peptic ulcer. Rarely in chronic liver disease, none of these findings is present, although more often than not, this absence of findings results from hurried or inadequate examination. In extrahepatic portal hypertension, enlargement of the spleen is usually the only abnormal physical finding, and this can be missed as a consequence of splenic contraction from the hemorrhage.

In the laboratory, liver disease is detected and its severity assessed by hepatic tests. The most useful tests are serum proteins, bilirubin, and prothrombin. It is important to draw blood for these before multiple transfusions are given. Values may be normal in extrahepatic portal hypertension and in occasional patients with well-compensated cirrhosis.

Emergency endoscopy is extremely useful in experienced hands[45,51,135] and has been simplified by constant improvement in fiberoptic instrumentation. However, observer error remains a problem, and interpretation of the findings during active bleeding is somewhat more difficult than when endoscopy is done electively. Gastric varices can be hard to detect.

When there is failure to demonstrate a site of bleeding or when multiple potential sites are found, selective angiography is useful.[127] For success, the patient must be actively bleeding, and the patient's condition must permit transport to the radiology department.

Prognosis

In alcoholic liver disease, mortality following upper gastrointestinal tract hemorrhage is high. An average mortality rate of 73% was calculated by Orloff and colleagues from a total of eight reports in the literature, which included slightly more than 100 patients.[133] The mortality rate was 46% at our hospital (Los Angeles County-USC Medical Center) in a group of 59 patients. It should be remembered that published reports undoubtedly include patients bleeding from alcoholic gastritis as well as patients bleeding from varices, since it is often difficult to decide which of these two lesions is responsible for upper gastrointestinal tract hemorrhage. It is interesting that the mortality rate from episodes of bleeding was only 12% in a group of our patients with alcoholic liver disease who were treated medically in a controlled trial of portacaval shunt.[163] This marked difference in mortality clearly indicates that it is the deteriorated state of hepatic function that determines the very high mortality in alcoholic patients.

Much less documented information is available in the literature concerning nonalcoholic cirrhosis. Sherlock reports a 33% mortality rate within one year of hemorrhage from varices in 120 patients, 75% of whom were nonalcoholic.[185] In extrahepatic portal block, mortality from variceal hemorrhage is low.

Death following variceal hemorrhage is often not due directly to exsanguination or shock. Hepatic failure is the more common cause of death and is frequently complicated by aspiration pneumonia, sepsis, or renal failure. Many patients bleed terminally as a manifestation of hepatic failure, whereas in others, bleeding seems to precipitate lethal hepatic coma even when it has been controlled successfully.

For many years, we lacked information on the natural history of patients with esophageal varices after recovery from an episode of bleeding because such patients usually underwent portacaval shunt surgery. Recent reports of controlled trials of portacaval shunting provide some data. Five-year survival of patients randomized to medical therapy has ranged from 30% (Veterans Administration Study)[81] to 38% (Boston Interhospital Liver Group Study).[162] However, from 30% to 33% of these medically treated patients had surgical shunt performed when bleeding occurred during follow-up. In a similar trial that we conducted at Los Angeles County-USC Medical Center, only 16% of our "medical" patients received portacaval shunt, and 5-year survival was 25%.[163] A few patients have done well with infrequent episodes of bleeding; however, most have shown a pattern of recurring variceal hemorrhage with eventual death from bleeding or from hepatic failure precipitated by bleeding. The median survival time was 32 months. Spontaneous reduction in portal hypertension and improvement in esophageal varices may occur in acute alcoholic liver disease,[104,166] but this seems unlikely in any significant number of patients who have hemorrhaged from esophageal varices.

Medical Management of Acute Variceal Bleeding

Patients with liver disease and upper gastrointestinal tract bleeding are best managed in an intensive care unit. The general measures that we use in the USC liver unit are as follows: Blood is drawn for serum electrolytes, creatinine, and evaluation of liver function before blood transfusion is started. Since patients with decompensated liver disease sometimes have sepsis accompanying bleeding, cultures of blood and ascitic fluid are done if the clinical circumstances are appropriate. A central venous line is placed via a peripheral vein or the internal jugular vein for pressure monitoring and blood replacement. Blood is administered to replace the estimated loss, attempting to keep the hematocrit at 30% to 35%. Overtransfusion is to be avoided because hypervolemia raises portal pressure, which might encourage rebleeding. Fresh frozen plasma is given intermittently to support clotting factors. A rubber or plastic tube is placed in the stomach via the nares to facilitate gastric lavage and removal of as much of the shed blood as possible. The gastric tube is left in place to monitor bleeding and to allow administration of medications to patients who are unable to swallow. Magnesium sulfate or lactulose is given after gastric lavage to speed the elimination of intestinal blood and thus reduce the likelihood of hepatic encephalopathy. Lactulose administration is continued during the next 48 to 72 hours with the dosage adjusted to maintain mild diarrhea. Neomycin is given in addition, since its action is often synergistic.

General supportive care includes parenteral glucose, potassium, and magnesium; avoidance of a positive water balance; and supplemental vitamins, including at least one dose of vitamin K and folic acid. The use of sedatives poses a problem because of the frequent development of hepatic coma in bleeding patients. Discomfort from the tamponade tube, irritable and irrational behavior at the onset of encephalopathy, and incipient delirium tremens are all frequent events that require consideration of sedation in patients with bleeding varices. We know of no drugs that are entirely safe in this setting; if drug therapy is necessary, it is best to use small doses at short intervals to avoid cumulative effect.

Bleeding often ceases spontaneously within a few hours. If not, vasopressin therapy should be considered. Vasopressin causes a decrease in splanchnic blood flow and a reduction in portal pressure that has been documented by hepatic vein catheterization and by umbilical cannulation of the portal vein.[117,167,179,183] Hepatic arterial flow is little affected.[48] Bolus dosage of vasopressin has been largely abandoned in favor of continuous administration in a peripheral vein at 0.1 units to 0.6 units/minute, depending on effect. It has been difficult to show greater benefit from selective administration into the superior mesenteric artery,[9,38,62,83,117] and complications are more frequent. Side-effects of vasopressin include blanching, intestinal cramps, bradycardia, hypertension, and decreased cardiac output. Vasospasm can result in angina, myocardial infarction, and skin or bowel necrosis. Attempts to overcome the disagreeable cardiovascular effects of vasopressin include use of the triglycyl hormonogen of vasopressin-glypressin,[63,227] and the combined administration of vasopressin and nitroprusside[67] or vasopressin and nitroglycerin.[69] Nitroglycerin actually increases the drop in portal pressure. Although many consider vasopressin treatment to be moderately effective, it has been difficult to prove this in controlled trials.[60]

Somatostatin given intravenously also decreases portal pressure and has no obvious unfavorable cardiovascular side-effects. While some reports show less lowering of portal pressure than with vasopressin,[191] one controlled trial has shown it to be as effective as vasopressin in arresting variceal bleeding when given at 250 μg to 500 μg/hour after an initial bolus dose of 50 μg.[94] Bosch and colleagues have shown substantial falls in azygos vein blood flow after somatostatin administration as well as after administration of vasopressin.[26]

Balloon tamponade is used in many centers after vasopressin has failed or in place of vasopressin or in conjunction with it. Two standard tubes available are the Sengstaken–Blakemore and the Linton–Nachlas tubes. We prefer the latter, because it is somewhat simpler to handle and there is no danger of tracheal occlusion from the esophageal balloon should the tube slip partially out of the esophagus. Both seem to stop variceal bleeding effectively. The gastric balloon of the Linton–Nachlas tube directly compresses varices in the lower esophagus, and blood flow into the upper vessels is probably markedly reduced by the pressure on the cardiac end of the stomach. When we use tamponade, we remove the monitoring tube and pass the deflated ballon tube through the lubricated nostril into the stomach. Some physicians prefer to pass it through the mouth after applying topical anesthesia to lessen the gag reflex. The gastric balloon is inflated before passage to test for leaks. It is inflated again after the tube is well into the stomach, following which the tube is withdrawn until the balloon presses tightly against the cardia. If possible, the position of the tube should be checked radiographically after placement.

Pressure is maintained by attachment of the tube to a face mask of some sort (Fig. 22-11) or to a 1- to 2-pound weight by means of a pulley system slung from the top of the bed. If traction on the tube causes great distress in the patient, it is best to start with a 1-pound weight and add more later. If bleeding is controlled, we maintain pressure for 8 to 16 hours and then discontinue traction and remove the air from the gastric balloon, leaving the tube in place. If bleeding recurs, the balloon is reinflated and tension is again applied. If tamponade fails to stop the bleeding, it may be helpful to add 100 ml of air to the gastric balloon and increase the tension on the tube. If bleeding continues after this, we consider the possibility that it is from gastric varices outside the area covered by the balloon or from some other lesion, such as peptic ulcer, gastritis, or the Mallory–Weiss syndrome. We have seen instances, however, in which balloon tamponade was ineffective and yet

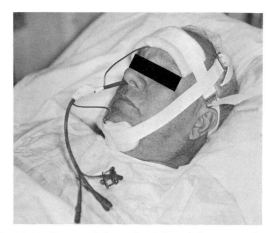

Fig. 22-11. Face mask for maintaining tension on esophageal tamponade tube. The tube is taped to the mask after it has been withdrawn far enough to achieve the desired tension on the gastric cardia.

no lesion other than esophageal varices was found at autopsy.

Both types of tamponade tubes can cause a wide range of complications, including pneumonitis, aspiration, esophageal ulceration, or rupture and asphyxia.[42] Complications are more frequent with inexperience, inadequate nursing care, and prolonged use of the tube. While Conn and Simpson maintain that balloon tamponade is too hazardous for routine use,[46] Pitcher reported only a moderate and acceptable number of complications in a prospective trial in 50 patients.[146] In summarizing the results reported in the literature in the use of balloon tamponade in 311 patients, Orloff and colleagues point out that, although bleeding was controlled in a high percentage of patients, the overall mortality rate was 74%.[133] It seems clear that hemorrhage from varices often sets in motion a chain of events that culminates in fatal hepatic failure whether or not the bleeding is controlled.

If the above measures fail to arrest the bleeding, one can resort to endoscopic sclerotherapy (see Chap. 11). Some centers use this for initial management of variceal bleeding. Other alternatives include a variety of surgical procedures (see Chap. 13). Still another approach is embolization of esophageal varices through a catheter inserted into the portal vein transhepatically. Introduced by Lunderquist and Vang in 1974,[107] this procedure has been employed by several groups with varying success.[130,180,190,221] Needle entry into the portal vein at an angle that permits guide wire and catheter introduction often is difficult and requires repeated punctures with the potential of bleeding from the liver surface. There may also be a large number of collaterals from the spleen and splenic vein leading toward gastric and esophageal varices, and, if these are not all found and injected, the treatment may be unsuccessful. Late follow-up suggests a high incidence of recanalization and recurrent bleeding.[108]

Long-term Medical Management

Pharmacologic Treatment

Vasopressin and the combination of vasopressin and nitroglycerin cause a modest reduction in portal pressure and have been used for short-term treatment of patients with variceal bleeding. Obviously, they are not suitable for long-term prophylaxis of bleeding. In 1967, Price and co-workers showed that propranolol, a β-adrenergic blocker, caused an increase in splanchnic vascular resistance.[152] This finding was not applied to patients with esophageal varices until 1980, when Lebrec and co-workers in Paris showed that WHVP was lowered an average of 25% in patients with alcoholic cirrhosis by doses of propranolol sufficient to lower the resting pulse rate 25%.[103] When continuous propranolol treatment was applied to patients who had been admitted to hospital for an upper gastrointestinal tract bleeding episode ascribed to either varices or gastritis, there was a remarkable reduction in rebleeding frequency over a 2-year follow-up in comparison with control patients treated with placebo.[101] During the trial, 21% of propranolol-treated patients had a rebleeding episode, compared with 68% of the control patients. Lebrec and colleagues noted no deleterious effects from long-term propranolol treatment. In a series of related studies they showed that the fall in WHVP averaged about 30%, probably due to a fall in portal outflow resulting from blockade of β-adrenergic vasodilator tone in the splanchnic bed and not directly correlated to fall in cardiac output. Although there was a tendency for hepatic blood flow to fall, this tendency was not statistically significant. Several studies by the French workers and others have shown that selective beta$_1$ blockers (atenolol, metoprolol) are less effective than propranolol in lowering WHVP. New beta blockers that depend more on renal excretion than hepatic metabolism for detoxification may prove to be better than propranolol.[20] Dosage selection determined by blood level or by response to isoproterenol infusion may prove to be more precise than by lowering of resting pulse rate.[16]

Enthusiasm for propranolol treatment as a means of preventing variceal bleeding has been tempered by recent findings. For unexplained reasons,[214] the fall in portal pressure is only about 50% of the fall in WHVP and is not seen in all patients.[41,125,157] Some deleterious effects of propranolol in patients with liver disease have been reported, including hepatic encephalopathy, increase in blood ammonium level, and reduced effect of diuretics.[160,200,215] Most importantly, second and third controlled trials with propranolol conducted in London[34] and in Montreal[223] have shown no reduction in bleeding frequency from treatment. There are no obvious explanations for the diametrically opposite results of the controlled trials. Additional trials are needed before a decision can be made about the value of propranolol treatment.

Endoscopic Sclerotherapy

Injection of sclerosing agents into esophageal varices through an endoscope was first carried out by Crafoord and Freckner in 1939.[50] Although a few surgeons continued to use this technique,[84,109] its popularity waned during the 1940s and 1950s, when portacaval shunting became the treatment of choice. There has been a recent resurgence of interest in variceal sclerosis due to failure of controlled trials of portacaval shunting to show significant prolongation of life. Terblanche and colleagues described injection of sclerosant directly into varices through a rigid esophagoscope with the patient under general anesthesia.[202] The barrel of the endoscope was used to compress the injection site to prevent postinjection bleeding. They used this as emergency treatment for bleeding varices and advocated repeated injections as long-term therapy to prevent recurrent variceal bleeding.[202] Paquet and Oberhammer recommended repeated injection of the sclerosing agent into the submucosa of the esophagus adjacent to the varices in order to thicken and strengthen the esophageal mucosa covering the veins.[141] Others began to use the fiberoptic endoscope for injection sclerotherapy, at first with a semirigid plastic sheath over the endoscope and with general anesthesia, and later without the sheath and without general anesthesia. This is still an evolving technique with no unanimity of opinion as to the relative value of intravariceal versus paravariceal injection, the best sclerosant (ethanolamine, polidocanol, morrhuate, or tetradecyl) or the frequency of injections. Injection sclerotherapy is technically difficult during active variceal bleeding because of poor visualization, but a number of studies have indicated a high degree of effectiveness in arresting hemorrhage.[1,10,18,82,202] After recovery from a bleeding episode, repeated sclerotherapy treatments at 1- to 3- week intervals can be undertaken with the objective of variceal clotting and eventual obliteration (Fig. 22-12). All studies to date indicate that varices will reform with the passage of time[203,234] so that follow-up endoscopy and variceal injection may have to be continued indefinitely.

Potential complications of endoscopic sclerotherapy include esophageal perforation, bleeding from the needle puncture site, esophageal ulceration, esophageal stenosis, mediastinitis, pleural effusion, and pulmonary abnormalities from embolization. Retrosternal pain immediately after sclerotherapy is a frequent complaint, and some patients have fever for 24 to 48 hours. Perforation is very rare unless a rigid endoscope or a plastic sheath is used. Important variceal bleeding after withdrawal of the injection needle is very unusual, and in patients whose general condition permits, treatments are done in an outpatient setting.[93] Esophageal ulceration is common after sclerotherapy, presumably as a consequence of the irritant properties of the sclerosant. The ulcers usually heal within 2 to 3 weeks; it is uncertain as yet which of the various sclerosants are most likely to cause ulceration. Rebleeding has been blamed by some on ulceration into still patent

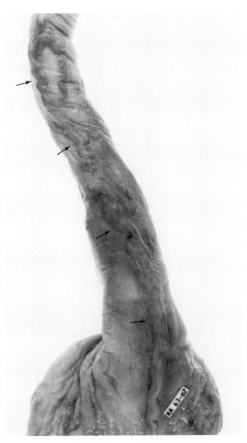

Fig. 22-12. Esophagus turned inside out at autopsy showing extensively clotted esophageal varices (*arrows*), the result of endoscopic sclerotherapy performed 4 days earlier for variceal hemorrhage. The patient died of hepatic failure.

varices.[4] We have shown pulmonary embolization of sclerosant by lung scanning after including ^{99m}Tc-labeled macroaggregated albumin with the sclerosant. Nevertheless, we have been unable to demonstrate significant changes in pulmonary function tests after sclerotherapy.[92] Pleural effusion has been reported by some groups,[5] most likely as a result of irritation and inflammation of the parietal pleura.

Several controlled trials have shown that repeated sclerotherapy treatments, attempting to eradicate varices, reduce bleeding frequency and blood transfusion requirement.[10,91,140,205,234,239] In a controlled study in the USC liver unit, the bleeding risk factor (episodes of upper gastrointestinal tract bleeding/patient/month) was reduced from 0.8 to 0.2, and the average number of blood transfusions required during follow-up was lowered from 13.2 to 3.5 pints by repeated sclerotherapy treatments.[91] It has been difficult, however, to show that repeated sclerotherapy significantly prolongs life. Our 38-month study at USC

did not show increased survival for patients randomized to receive sclerotherapy (Fig. 22-13). However, 28% of the control group eventually had surgical portal-systemic shunt performed because of recurrent bleeding, compared with only 6% of the sclerotherapy group, so the overall survival figures are difficult to interpret. When patients receiving surgical shunt were considered as withdrawn alive at the time of this event, there was a significant survival advantage for sclerotherapy. Similarly, Terblanche and colleagues were unable to show survival prolongation by repeated sclerotherapy, but the control subjects in their study were treated with sclerotherapy each time they had a bleeding episode.[203]

In an investigation of chronic sclerotherapy at Kings College Hospital in London, 116 patients were followed for a median of 37 months; 17% were removed for other treatments. There was a statistically significant prolongation of life in the sclerotherapy group as well as a marked reduction in bleeding frequency.[234] Two trials of prophylactic sclerotherapy from Germany[140,239] show significant life prolongation in the treated group. Controlled trials of sclerotherapy versus surgical shunt are now in progress at several centers, as well as additional trials of sclerotherapy begun prophylactically, before the first variceal bleeding episode.

FUTURE RESEARCH

Prevention of portal hypertension by control of chronic liver disease has become more feasible with the development of the hepatitis B vaccine and the discovery of an

Fig. 22-13. Cumulative survival curves from a controlled trial of chronic variceal sclerotherapy. Curves A and B depict survival in sclerotherapy and control groups, respectively, and are not significantly different. Curves C and D show survival of sclerotherapy and control groups when patients receiving portal–systemic shunt surgery were removed (defining surgery as the end point in the survival analysis). A significant difference, $p < 0.05$ (F ratios), between curves C and D is noted (Korula J et al: Hepatology 5:584, 1985)

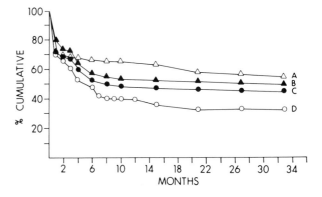

effective new drug for schistosomiasis, Praziquantel. However, in the western world, the problem of alcohol abuse is likely to remain indefinitely. Probably there are other toxic or immunologic causes for chronic liver disease that remain to be identified and that may be preventable.

Although increased vascular resistance is clearly the major direct cause of portal hypertension, increased splanchnic inflow may be an important factor in some diseases, and methods for evaluating this possibility should be devised.

From the standpoint of treatment of portal hypertension, no miracles are likely. Variceal hemorrhage is only one facet of the problem posed by advanced chronic liver disease, and there is little prospect of a really effective treatment for the underlying liver disease. Liver transplantation will undoubtedly be performed with increased frequency. For the immediate future, controlled trials to determine whether endoscopic sclerotherapy is preferable to surgical shunt are urgently needed.

The opinions expressed in this chapter inevitably reflect those of a group of the author's associates at the University of Southern California with long-standing interest in portal hypertension. This group includes internists Alan Redeker and Oliver Kuzma; pathologists Hugh Edmondson and Robert Peters; and surgeons William Mikkelsen, Fred Turrill, Arthur Donovan, and Albert Yellin.

REFERENCES

1. Alwmark A et al: Emergency and long-term transesophageal sclerotherapy of bleeding esophagel varices: A prospective study of 50 consecutive cases. Scand J Gastroenterol 17:409, 1982
2. Atkinson M et al: The clinical investigation of the portal circulation, with special reference to portal venography. Q J Med 24:77, 1955
3. Aufses AH Jr et al: Portal venous pressure in "pipestem fibrosis" of the liver due to schistosomiasis. Am J Med 17:807, 1959
4. Ayres SJ et al: Esophageal ulceration and bleeding after flexible fiberoptic esophageal vein sclerosis. Gastroenterology 83:131, 1982
5. Bacon BR et al: Pleural effusion following endoscopic variceal sclerotherapy. Gastroenterology 88:1910, 1985
6. Baggenstoss AH, Cain JC: The hepatic hilar lymphatics of man: Their relation to ascites. N Engl J Med 256:531, 1957
7. Baker LA et al: The natural history of esophageal varices. Am J Med 26:228, 1959
8. Balthazar EJ et al: Computed tomographic recognition of gastric varices. Am J Radiol 142:1121, 1984
9. Barr JW et al: Similarity of arterial and intravenous vasopressin on portal and systemic hemodynamics. Gastroenterology 69:13, 1975
10. Barsoum MS et al: Tamponade and injection sclerotherapy in the managment of bleeding oesophageal varices. Br J Surg 69:76, 1982
11. Bayly JH, Carbalhaes OG: The umbilical vein in the adult: Diagnosis, treatment and research. Am Surg 30:56, 1964
12. Beckett AG et al: Acute alcoholic hepatitis. Br Med J 2:1113, 1961
13. Benhamou JP et al: Etudes sur l'hemodynamique porto-hepatique. Rev Frac Etud Clin Biol 7:524, 1962
14. Benhamou JP et al: Hypertension portale essentielle. Presse Med 70:2397, 1962
15. Beppu K et al: Prediction of variceal hemorrhage by esophageal endoscopy. Gastrointest Endosc 27:213, 1981
16. Bercoff E et al: Assessment of B-adrenergic blockade with propranolol in patients with cirrhosis. Hepatology 4:451, 1984
17. Berk PD et al: Veno-occlusive disease of the liver after allogeneic bone marrow transplantation. Ann Intern Med 90:158, 1979
18. Bernau J, Rueff B: Treatment of acute variceal bleeding. Clin Gastroenterol 14:185, 1985
19. Biersack HJ et al: Determination of liver and spleen perfusion by quantitative sequential scintigraphy: Results in normal subjects and in patients with hypertension. Clin Nucl Med 6:218, 1981
20. Bihari D et al: Reductions in portal pressure by selective B2-adrenoceptor blockade in patients with cirrhosis and portal hypertension. Br J Clin Pharmacol 17:753, 1984
21. Blakemore AH: Portacaval shunt in surgical treatment of portal hypertension. Ann Surg 128:825, 1948
22. Blendis LM et al: Nodular regenerative hyperplasia of the liver in Felty's syndrome. Q J Med 43,169:25, 1974
23. Boijsen E et al: Coeliac and superior mesenteric angiography in portal hypertension. Acta Chir Scand 125:315, 1963
24. Bolondi L et al: Ultrasonography in the diagnosis of portal hypertension: Diminished response of portal vessels to respiration. Radiology 142:167, 1982
25. Bosch J, Groszmann RJ: Measurement of azygous venous blood flow by a continuous thermal dilution technique: An index of blood flow through gastroesophageal collaterals in cirrhosis. Hepatology 4:424, 1984
26. Bosch J et al: Azygous vein blood flow in cirrhosis: Effects of balloon tamponade, vasopressin, somatostatin and propranolol. Hepatology 3:855, 1983
27. Boyer JL et al: Idiopathic portal hypertension. Ann Intern Med 66:41, 1967
28. Boyer TD et al: Direct transhepatic measurement of portal vein pressure using a thin needle: Comparison with wedged hepatic vein pressure. Gastroenterology 72:584, 1977
29. Bradley SE et al: The estimation of hepatic blood flow in man. J Clin Invest 24:890, 1945
30. Bras G et al: Cirrhosis of the liver in Jamaica. J Pathol Bact 82:503, 1961
31. Bras G et al: Plants as aetiological factor in veno-occlusive disease of the liver. Lancet 1:960, 1957
32. Bru C et al: Noninvasive measurement of portal venous blood flow in man by combined doppler-real time ultrasonography: Effects of propranolol. Hepatology 3:855, 1983
33. Burchell AR et al: A seven-year experience with side-to-side portacaval shunt for cirrhotic ascites. Ann Surg 168:655, 1968
34. Burroughs AK et al: Propranolol for the prevention of recurrent variceal hemorrhage in cirrhotic patients: Results of a controlled trial. N Engl J Med 309:1539, 1983
35. Bynum TE et al: Wedged hepatic vein pressure (WHVP) in normal human subjects. Gastroenterology 64:177, 1973
36. Cales P et al: Superior porto-systemic collateral circulation estimated by azygous blood flow in patients with cirrhosis. J Hepatology 1:37, 1984
37. Child CG: The Hepatic Circulation and Portal Hypertension. Philadelphia, WB Saunders, 1954

38. Chojkier M et al: A controlled comparison of continuous intra-arterial and intravenous infusions of vasopressin in hemorrhage from esophageal varices. Gastroenterology 77: 540, 1979

39. Clark KE et al: CT evaluation of oesophageal and upper abdominal varices. J Comput Assist Tomogr 4:510, 1980

40. Cohn JN et al: Hepatic blood flow in alcoholic liver disease measured by an indicator dilution technique. Am J Med 53:704, 1972

41. Colman JC et al: Propranolol in decompensated alcoholic cirrhosis. Lancet 2:1040, 1982

42. Conn HO: Hazards attending the use of esophageal tamponade. N Engl J Med 259:701, 1958

43. Conn HO: Ammonia tolerance as an index of portal-systemic collateral circulation in cirrhosis. Gastroenterology 41:97, 1961

44. Conn HO: The varix volcano connection. Gastroenterology 79:1333, 1980

45. Conn HO, Brodoff M: Emergency esophagoscopy in the diagnosis of upper gastrointestinal hemorrhage. Gastroenterology 47:505, 1964

46. Conn HO, Simpson JA: Excessive mortality with balloon tamponade. JAMA 202:587, 1967

47. Conn HO et al: Fiberoptic and conventional esophagoscopy in the diagnosis of esophageal varices. Gastroenterology 52: 810, 1967

48. Conn HO et al: Hepatic arterial escape from vasopressin induced vasoconstriction: An angiographic investigation. AJR 119:102, 1973

49. Conn HO et al: Observer variation in the endoscopic diagnosis of esophageal varices. N Engl J Med 272:830, 1965

50. Crafoord C, Freckner P: New surgical treatment of varicose veins of the oesophagus. Acta Otolaryngol 27:422, 1939

51. Dagradi AE et al: Bleeding esophago-gastric varices. Arch Surg 92:944, 1966

52. Dal Palu C et al: Postsinusoidal portal hypertension in a patient with chronic lymphatic leukemia. Am J Dig Dis 8: 845, 1963

53. Denison EK et al: Portal hypertension in a patient with osteopetrosis: A case report with discussion of the mechanism of portal hypertension. Arch Intern Med 128:279, 1971

54. Donovan AJ et al: Systemic-portal arteriovenous fistulas: Pathological and hemodynamic observations in two patients. Surgery 66:474, 1969

55. Edmondson HA et al: Sclerosing hyaline necrosis of the liver in the chronic alcoholic. Ann Intern Med 59:646, 1963

56. Eisenberg S: Blood volume in patients with Laennec's cirrhosis of the liver as determined by radioactive chromium-tagged red cells. Am J Med 20:189, 1956

57. Fauvert R et al: Fibrose hepatique congenitale. Rev Int Hepat 14:395, 1964

58. Ferguson DJ: Hemodynamics in surgery for portal hypertension. Ann Surg 158:383, 1963

59. Fisher B et al: Further experimental observations on animals with arterialized livers. Surgery 38:181, 1955

60. Fogel MR et al: Continuous intravenous vasopressin in active upper gastrointestinal bleeding: A placebo-controlled trial. Ann Intern Med 96:565, 1982

61. Fonkalsrud EW: Surgical management of portal hypertension in childhood. Arch Surg 115:1042, 1980

62. Freedman AR et al: Primate mesenteric blood flow: Effects of vasopressin and its route of delivery. Gastroenterology 74:875, 1978

63. Freeman JG et al: Controlled trial of terlipressin (Glypressin) versus vasopressin in the early treatment of oesophageal varices. Lancet 2:66, 1982

64. Friedman EW, Weiner RS: Estimation of hepatic sinusoidal pressure by means of venous catheters and estimation of portal pressure by hepatic vein catheterization. Am J Physiol 165:527, 1951

65. Futagawa S et al: Hepatic venography in non-cirrhotic idiopathic portal hypertension: Comparison with cirrhosis of the liver. Diagn Radiol 141:303, 1981

66. Garcia-Tsao G et al: Portal pressure, presence of gastroesophageal varices and variceal bleeding. Hepatology 5:419, 1985

67. Gelman S, Ernst EA: Nitroprusside prevents adverse hemodynamic effects of vasopressin. Arch Surg 113:1465, 1979

68. Gill RW et al: Portal and splenic circulation studied by Doppler ultrasound. J Ultrasound Med 2, No. 10 (suppl): 56, 1983

69. Groszmann RJ et al: Nitroglycerin improves the hemodynamic response to vasopressin in portal hypertension. Hepatology 2:757, 1982

70. Groszmann RJ et al: Wedged and free hepatic venous pressure measured with a balloon catheter. Gastroenterology 76:253, 1979

71. Groszmann RJ et al: Hemodynamic effect of combined infusion of vasopressin and nitroglycerine in normal and cirrhotic dogs. Gastroenterology 77:A15, 1979

72. Hales MR et al: Injection-corrosion studies of normal and cirrhotic livers. Am J Pathol 35:909, 1959

73. Hallenbeck GA, Adson MA: Esophagogastric varices without hepatic cirrhosis. Arch Surg 83:370, 1961

74. Herrick FC: Experimental study into cause of increased portal pressure in portal cirrhosis. J Exp Med 9:93, 1907

75. Hidemura R, Reynolds TB: Ascites following portacaval shunting: Relationship between wedged hepatic venous pressure and ascites. Nagoya J Med Sci 35:133, 1973

76. Hill MC et al: Ultrasonography in portal hypertension. Clin Gastroenterol 14:83, 1985

77. Hoefs JC et al: A new method for the measurement of intrahepatic shunts. J Lab Clin Med 103:446, 1984

78. Huet PM et al: Simultaneous estimation of hepatic and portal blood flows using Cr-51 labelled red cells indicator dilution curves in dogs (abstr). Gastroenterology 64:183, 1973

79. Hunt AH: A Contribution to the Study of Portal Hypertension. Edinburgh, Livingstone, 1958

80. Imanaga H et al: Surgical treatment of portal hypertension according to state of intrahepatic circulation. Ann Surg 155:42, 1962

81. Jackson FC et al: A clinical investigation of the portacaval shunt: V. Survival analysis of the therapeutic operation. Ann Surg 175:672, 1971

82. Johnson AG: Injection sclerotherapy in the emergency and elective treatment of oesophageal varices. Ann R Coll Surg 59:497, 1977

83. Johnson WC et al: Control of bleeding varices by vasopressin: A prospective randomized study. Ann Surg 186: 369, 1977

84. Johnston GW, Rodger HW: A review of 15 years experience in the use of sclerotherapy in the control of acute hemorrhage from oesophageal varices. Br J Surg 60:797, 1973

85. Juttner HU et al: Ultrasound demonstration of portosys-

temic collaterals in cirrhosis and portal hypertension. Radiology 142:459, 1982

86. Kane RA, Katz SG: The spectrum of sonographic findings in portal hypertension: A subject review and new observations. Radiology 142:453, 1982

87. Kelty RH et al: The relation of the regenerated hepatic nodule to the vascular bed in cirrhosis. Proc Mayo Clin 25: 17, 1950

88. Kerr DNS et al: Congenital hepatic fibrosis. Q J Med 30: 91, 1961

89. Kessler RE, Zimmon DS: Umbilical vein catheterization in man. Surg Gynecol Obstet 124:594, 1967

90. Kingham JGC et al: Non-cirrhotic intrahepatic portal hypertension: A long term follow-up study. Q J Med 199: 259, 1981

91. Korula J et al: A prospective, randomized controlled trial of chronic esophageal variceal sclerotherapy. Hepatology 5:584, 1985

92. Korula J et al: Lung function in patients undergoing esophageal variceal sclerotherapy (abstr). Hepatology 3:825, 1983

93. Korula J et al: Outpatient esophageal variceal sclerotherapy: Safe and cost effective: A prospective study. Gastrointest Endosc (in press)

94. Kravetz D et al: Comparison of intravenous somatostatin and vasopressin infusions in treatment of acute variceal hemorrhage. Hepatology 4:442, 1984

95. Krook H: Circulatory studies in liver cirrhosis. Acta Med Scand (Suppl 318) 156:55, 1957

96. Krook H: Estimation of portal venous pressure by occlusive hepatic vein catheterization. Scand J Clin Lab Invest 5: 285, 1953

97. Kurtz W, Classen M: Messung des blutflussess in Osophagusvarizen mit einem endoskopischen ultraschall-Doppler (Assessment of blood flow in oesophageal varices with an endoscopic Doppler ultrasound probe). Dtsch Med Wochenschr 109:824, 1984

98. LaBella A: Evaluation of the portal system, porta-caval anastomosis and spleen size in liver cirrhosis: An ultrasonographic study with clinical correlations. Ital J Gastroenterol 13:179, 1981

99. LaCroix E, Leusen I: La circulation hepatique et splanchnique. J Physiol 57:115, 1965

100. Lam KC et al: Spontaneous portosystemic shunt: Relationship to spontaneous encephalopathy and gastrointestinal hemorrhage. Dig Dis Sci 26:346, 1981

101. Lebrec D et al: A randomized controlled study of propranolol for prevention of recurrent gastrointestinal bleeding in patients with cirrhosis: A final report. Hepatology 4:355, 1984

102. Lebrec D et al: Portal hypertension, size of esophageal varices and risk of gastrointestinal bleeding in cirrhosis. Gastroenterology 79:1139, 1980

103. Lebrec D et al: Propranolol: Medical treatment for portal hypertension? Lancet 2:1280, 1980

104. Leevy CM et al: Observations on influence of medical therapy on portal hypertension in hepatic cirrhosis. Ann Intern Med 49:837, 1958

105. Lieberman FL, Reynolds TB: Plasma volume in cirrhosis of the liver: Its relation to portalhypertension, ascites and renal failure. J Clin Invest 46:1297, 1967

106. Longstreth GE et al: Extrahepatic portal hypertension caused by chronic pancreatitis. Ann Intern Med 75:903, 1971

107. Lunderquist A, Vang J: Transhepatic catheterization and obliteration of the coronary vein in patients with portal hypertension and esophageal varices. N Engl J Med 291: 646, 1974

108. Lunderquist A et al: Isobutyl-2-cyano-acrylate (Bucrylate) in obliteration of gastric coronary vein and esophageal varices. AJR 130:1, 1978

109. Macbeth R: Treatment of oesophageal varices in portal hypertension by means of sclerosing injections. Br Med J 2: 877, 1955

110. McCormack TT et al: Perforating veins and blood flow in oesophageal varices. Lancet 2:1442, 1983

111. McIndoe AH: Vascular lesions of portal cirrhosis. Arch Pathol 5:23, 1928

112. McLean E et al: Veno-occlusive lesions in livers of rats fed *Crotalaria fulva.* Br J Exp Pathol 40:242, 1964

113. McMichael J: The portal circulation. J Physiol 75:241, 1932

114. Mikkelsen WP: Extrahepatic portal hypertension in children. Am J Surg 111:333, 1966

115. Mikkelsen WP et al: Extra- and intrahepatic portal hypertension without cirrhosis (hepatoportal sclerosis). Ann Surg 162:602, 1965

116. Mikkelsen WP et al: Portacaval shunt in cirrhosis of the liver: Clinical and hemodynamic aspects. Am J Surg 104: 204, 1962

117. Millette B et al: Portal and systemic effects of selective infusion of vasopressin into the superior mesenteric artery in cirrhotic patients. Gastroenterology 69:6, 1975

118. Mino RA et al: Sarcoidosis producing portal hypertension: Treatment by splenectomy and splenorenal shunt. Ann Surg 130:951, 1949

119. Moreno AH et al: Portal blood flow in cirrhosis of the liver. J Clin Invest 46:436, 1967

120. Moriyasu F et al: Quantitative measurement of portal blood flow in patients with chronic liver disease using an ultrasonic duplex system consisting of a pulsed Doppler flowmeter and B-mode electroscanner. Gasteroenterol Jpn 19:529, 1984

121. Mousa AH, El-Garen A: The haemodynamic study of Egyptian hepatosplenic bilharziasis. J Egypt Med Assoc 42: 444, 1959

122. Murray JF et al: Circulatory changes in chronic liver disease. Am J Med 24:358, 1958

123. Myers JD, Taylor WJ: An estimation of portal venous pressure by occlusive catheterization of an hepatic venule. J Clin Invest 30:662, 1951

124. Nakashima T: Vascular changes and hemodynamics in hepatocellular carcinoma. In Okuda, Peters (eds): Hepatocellular Carcinoma, pp 169–203. New York, John Wiley & Sons, 1976

125. Nakayama T et al: Effects of propranolol on portal vein pressure, portal blood flow and cardiac output in patients with chronic liver disease. Hepatology 3:812, 1983

126. Nayak NC, Ramalingaswami V: Obliterative portal venopathy of the liver. Arch Pathol 87:359, 1969

127. Nusbaum M et al: Clinical experience with the diagnosis and management of gastrointestinal hemorrhage by selective mesenteric catheterization. Ann Surg 170:506, 1969

128. Ohnishi K et al: Pulsed Doppler flow as a criterion of portal venous velocity: Comparison with cineangiographic measurements. Radiology 154:495, 1985

129. Okuda K et al: Clinical study of eighty-six cases of idiopathic portal hypertension and comparison with cirrhosis and splenomegaly. Gastroenterology 86:600, 1984

130. Okuda K et al: Percutaneous transhepatic portography and sclerotherapy. Semin Liver Dis 2:57, 1982

131. Okuda K et al: Nonsurgical, percutaneous transhepatic cholangiography: Diagnostic significance in medical problems of the liver. Am J Dig Dis 19:21, 1974

132. Okuda K et al: Percutaneous transhepatic catheterization of the portal vein for the study of portal hemodynamics and shunts. Gastroenterology 73:279, 1977

133. Orloff MJ et al: The complications of cirrhosis of the liver. Ann Intern Med 66:165, 1967

134. Palmer ED: On correlations between portal venous pressure and the size and extent of esophageal varices in portal cirrhosis. Arch Surg 138:741, 1953

135. Palmer ED: Diagnosis of Upper Gastrointestinal Hemorrhage. Springfield, IL, Charles C. Thomas, 1961

136. Palmer ED: Esophageal varices associated with hiatus hernia in the absence of portal hypertension. Am J Med Sci 235:677, 1958

137. Palmer ED, Brick IB: Varices of the distal esophagus in the apparent absence of portal and of superior caval hypertension. Am J Med Sci 230:515, 1955

138. Panke WF et al: Technique, hazards and usefulness of percutaneous splenic portography. JAMA 169:1032, 1979

139. Panke WR et al: A sixteen-year experience with end-to-side portacaval shunt for variceal hemorrhage. Ann Surg 168:957, 1968

140. Paquet KJ: Prophylactic endoscopic sclerosing treatment of the esophageal wall in varices: A prospective controlled randomized trial. Endoscopy 14:4, 1982

141. Paquet KJ, Oberhammer E: Sclerotherapy of bleeding oesophageal varices by means of endoscopy. Endoscopy 10:7, 1978

142. Parof A et al: Manometric splenique et splenoportographique dans les affections du systeme hemopoietique, les pyelophlebites, les cirrhoses du foie. Rev Int Hepat 5:617, 1955

143. Paton A et al: Assessment of portal venous hypertension by catheterization of hepatic vein. Lancet 1:918, 1953

144. Patrassi G et al: Pletora portale. Policlinico Sez 68:1920, 1961

145. Perera GA: The plasma volume in Laennec's cirrhosis of the liver. Ann Intern Med 24:643, 1946

146. Pitcher JL: Safety and effectiveness of the modified Sengstaken–Blakemore tube: A prospective study. Gastroenterology 61:291, 1971

147. Polish E et al: Idiopathic presinusoidal portal hypertension (Banti's syndrome). Ann Intern Med 56:624, 1962

148. Ponce J et al: Morphometric study of the esophageal mucosa in cirrhotic patients with variceal bleeding. Hepatology 1:641, 1981

149. Popper H et al: Florid cirrhosis, a review of 35 cases. Am J Clin Pathol 25:889, 1955

150. Popper H et al: Vascular pattern of cirrhotic liver. Am J Clin Pathol 22:717, 1952

151. Porchet H, Bircher J: Noninvasive assessment of portal-systemic shunting: Evaluation of a method to investigate systemic availability of oral glyceryl trinitrate by digital plethysmography. Gastroenterology 82:629, 1982

152. Price HL et al: Control of the splanchnic circulation in man: Role of beta-adrenergic receptors. Circ Res 21:333, 1967

153. Price JB et al: Operative hemodynamic studies in portal hypertension. Arch Surg 95:843, 1967

154. Ramos OL et al: Portal hemodynamics and liver cell function in hepatic schistosomiasis. Gastroenterology 47:241, 1964

155. Rather LJ, Cohn R: Some effects on the liver of the complete arterialization of its blood supply: III. Acute vascular necrosis. Surgery 34:207, 1953

156. Ravenna P: Splenoportal venous obstruction without splenomegaly. Arch Intern Med 72:786, 1943

157. Rector WG Jr: Propranolol for portal hypertension: Evaluation of therapeutic response by direct measurement of portal pressure. Arch Intern Med 145:648, 1985

158. Rector WG Jr, Redeker AG: Direct transhepatic assessment of hepatic vein pressure and direction of flow using a thin needle in patients with cirrhosis and Budd–Chiari syndrome: An effective alternative to hepatic vein catheterization. Gastroenterology 86:1395, 1984

159. Rector WG Jr, Reynolds TB: Risk factors for haemorrhage from oesophageal varices and acute gastric erosions. Clin Gastroenterol 14:139, 1985

160. Rector WG Jr, Reynolds TB: Propranolol in the treatment of cirrhotic ascites. Arch Intern Med 144:1761, 1984

161. Reichle FA et al: A method of portal vein flow determination in the unanesthetized patient (abstr). Gastroenterology 62:185, 1972

162. Resnick RH et al: A controlled study of the therapeutic portacaval shunt. Gastroenterology 67:843, 1974

163. Reynolds TB: Hepatic circulatory changes after shunt surgery. Ann NY Acad Sci 170:379, 1970

164. Reynolds TB: Interrelationships of portal pressure, variceal size and upper gastrointestinal bleeding. Gastroenterology 79:1333, 1980

165. Reynolds TB et al: Wedged hepatic venous pressure: A clinical evaluation. Am J Med 22:341, 1957

166. Reynolds TB et al: Spontaneous decrease in portal pressure with clinical improvement in cirrhosis. N Engl J Med 263:734, 1960

167. Reynolds TB et al: The effect of vasopressin on hepatic hemodynamics in patients with portal hypertension. J Clin Invest 39:1021, 1960

168. Reynolds TB et al: Measurement of portal pressure and its clinical application. Am J Med 19:649, 1970

169. Reynolds TB et al: Results of a 12-year randomized trial of portocaval shunt in patients with alcoholic liver disease and bleeding varices. Gastroenterology 80:1005, 1981

170. Rosenbaum DL et al: Hemodynamic studies of the portal circulation in myeloid metaplasia. Am J Med 41:360, 1966

171. Rougier P et al: Nodular regenerative hyperplasia of the liver. Report of six cases and review of the literature. Gastroenterology 75:169, 1978

172. Ruprecht AL, Kinney TD: Esophageal varices caused by metastasis of carcinoma to the liver. Am J Dig Dis 1:145, 1956

173. Saito M et al: Ultrasonic measurements of portal and splenic vein blood flows and their velocities in normal subjects and patients with chronic liver disease. Hepatology 3:812, 1983

174. Sama SK et al: Non-cirrhotic portal fibrosis. Am J Med 51:160, 1971

175. Sarper R et al: A noninvasive method for measuring portal venous/total hepatic blood flow by hepatosplenic radionuclide angiography. Nucl Med 141:179, 1981

176. Schabel SI et al: The "bull's-eye" falciform ligament: A sonographic finding of portal hypertension. Radiology 136:157, 1980

177. Schaefer JW et al: Gastroesophageal variceal bleeding in

the absence of hepatic cirrhosis or portal hypertension. Gastroenterology 46:583, 1965

178. Schenk WG Jr et al: Direct measurement of hepatic blood flow in surgical patients. Ann Surg 156:463, 1962

179. Schwartz SI et al: The use of intravenous Pituitrin in treatment of bleeding esophageal varices. Surgery 45:72, 1959

180. Scott J et al: Percutaneous transhepatic obliteration of gastro-oesophageal varices. Lancet 2:53, 1976

181. Seldinger SI: Catheter replacement of the needle in percutaneous arteriography: A new technique. Acta Radiol 39:368, 1953

182. Shaldon S, Sherlock S: Portal hypertension in the myeloproliferative syndrome and the reticuloses. Am J Med 32:758, 1962

183. Shaldon S et al: Effect of pitressin on the splanchnic circulation in man. Circulation 24:797, 1961

184. Sherlock S: Diseases of the Liver and Biliary System, 3rd ed. Oxford, Blackwell Scientific Publications, 1963

185. Sherlock S: Hematemesis in portal hypertension. Br J Surg 51:746, 1964

186. Sherlock S et al: Partial nodular transformation of the liver with portal hypertension. Am J Med 40:195, 1966

187. Shulman HM et al: An analysis of hepatic venocclusive disease and centrilobular hepatic degeneration following bone marrow transplantation. Gastroenterology 79:1178, 1980

188. Siderys H et al: The experimental production of elevated portal pressure by increasing portal flow. Surg Gynecol Obstet 120:514, 1965

189. Simert G et al: Correlation between percutaneous transhepatic portography and clinical findings in 56 patients with portal hypertension. Acta Chir Scand 144:27, 1978

190. Smith-Laing G et al: Percutaneous transhepatic portography in the assessment of portal hypertension: Clinical correlations and comparison of radiographic techniques. Gastroenterology 78:197, 1980

191. Sonnenberg GE et al: Effect of somatostatin on splanchnic hemodynamics in patients with cirrhosis of the liver and in normal subjects. Gastroenterology 80:526, 1981

192. Spence RAJ et al: Oesophagitis in patients undergoing oesophageal transection for varices: A histological study. Br J Surg 70:332, 1983

193. Staritz M et al: Intravascular oesophageal variceal pressure (IOPV) assessed by endoscopic fine needle puncture under basal conditions, Valsalva's maneuver and after glyceryltrinitrate application. Gut 26:525, 1985

194. Stone EM et al: Portal venous blood flow: Its estimation and significance (abstr). Gastroenterology 62:186, 1972

195. Stone HH et al: Portal arteriovenous fistulas: Review and case report. Am J Surg 109:191, 1965

196. Strandell T et al: Simultaneous determinations of portal vein and hepatic artery blood flow by indicator dilution technique in awake man. Acta Med Scand 191:139, 1972

197. Stromeyer FW, Ishak KG: Nodular transformation (nodular "regenerative" hyperplasia) of the liver: A clinico-pathologic study of 30 cases. Hum Pathol 12:60, 1981

198. Syrota A et al: Scintillation splenoportography: Hemodynamic and morphological study of the portal circulation. Gastroenterology 71:652, 1976

199. Takayasu K et al: Sonographic detection of large spontaneous spleno-renal shunts and its clinical significance. Br J Radiol 57:565, 1984

200. Tarver D et al: Precipitation of hepatic encephalopathy by propranolol in cirrhosis. Br Med J 287:585, 1983

201. Taylor WJ et al: Wilson's disease, portal hypertension and intrahepatic vascular obstruction. N Engl J Med 260:1160, 1959

202. Terblanche J et al: A prospective evaluation of injection sclerotherapy in the treatment of acute bleeding from esophageal varices. Surgery 85:239, 1979

203. Terblanche J et al: Failure of repeated injection sclerotherapy to improve longterm survival after oesophageal variceal bleeding. Lancet 2:1328, 1983

204. Terblanche J et al: A prospective controlled trial of sclerotherapy in the long term management of patients after esophageal variceal bleeding. Surg Gynecol Obstet 148:323, 1979

205. The Copenhagen Esophageal Varices Sclerotherapy Project: Sclerotherapy after first variceal hemorrhage in cirrhosis: A randomized multicenter trial. N Engl J Med 311:1594, 1984

206. Thompson EN, Sherlock S: The aetiology of portal vein thrombosis, with particular reference to role of infection in exchange transfusion. Q J Med 33:465, 1964

207. Thompson WP et al: Splenic vein pressures in congestive splenomegaly (Banti's syndrome). J Clin Invest 16:571, 1937

208. Tisdale WA et al: Portal hypertension and bleeding esophageal varices: Their occurrence in the absence of both intrahepatic and extrahepatic obstruction of the portal vein. N Engl J Med 261:209, 1959

209. Turner MD et al: Splenic venography and intrasplenic pressure measurement in the clinical investigation of the portal venous system. Am J Med 23:846, 1957

210. Turrill FL, Mikkelsen WP: "Sinistral" (left sided) extrahepatic portal hypertension. Arch Surg 99:365, 1969

211. Tygstrup N et al: Determination of the hepatic arterial blood flow and oxygen supply in man by clamping the hepatic artery during surgery. J Clin Invest 41:447, 1962

212. Ueda H et al: Detection of hepatic shunts by the use of 131I-macroaggregated albumin. Gastroenterology 52:480, 1967

213. Ueda H et al: Measurement of hepatic arterial and portal blood flow and circulation time via hepatic artery and portal vein with radioisotope. Jpn Heart J 3:154, 1962

214. Valla D et al: Discrepancy between wedged hepatic venous pressure and portal venous pressure after acute propranolol administration in patients with alcoholic cirrhosis. Gastroenterology 86:1400, 1984

215. Van Buuren HR et al: Propranolol increases arterial ammonia in liver cirrhosis. Lancet 2:951, 1982

216. Van Way CW et al: Arteriovenous fistula in the portal circulation. Surgery 70:876, 1971

217. Vennes JA: Intrahepatic pressure: An accurate reflection of portal pressure. Medicine 45:445, 1966

218. Viallet A et al: Comparison of free portal venous pressure and wedged hepatic venous pressure in patients with cirrhosis of the liver. Gastroenterology 59:372, 1970

219. Viallet A et al: Hemodynamic evaluation of patients with intrahepatic portal hypertension: Relationship between bleeding varices and the portohepatic gradient. Gastroenterology 69:1297, 1975

220. Viallet A et al: Hepatic and umbilicoportal catheterization in portal hypertension. Ann NY Acad Sci 170:177, 1970

221. Viamonte M et al: Transhepatic obliteration of gastroesophageal varices: Results in acute and nonacute bleeders. AJR 129:237, 1977

222. Vidins EI et al: Sinusoidal caliber in alcoholic and non-

alcoholic liver disease: Diagnostic and pathogenic implications. Hepatology 5:408, 1985

223. Villenueve JP et al: Propranolol for the prevention of recurrent variceal hemorrhage: A controlled trial (abstr). Hepatology 5:1053, 1985

224. Vinel JP et al: Clinical and prognostic significance of portohepatic gradients in patients with cirrhosis. Surg Gynecol Obstet 155:347, 1982

225. Vorobioff J et al: Hyperdynamic circulation in portal hypertensive rat model: A primary factor for maintenance of chronic portal hypertension. Am J Physiol 224, G52, 1983

226. Vorobioff J et al: Increased blood flow through the portal system in cirrhotic rats. Gastroenterology 87:1120, 1984

227. Vosmik J et al: Action of the triglycyl hormonogen of vasopressin (glypressin) in patients with liver cirrhosis and bleeding esophageal varices. Gastroenterology 72:605, 1977

228. Wanless IR et al: Nodular regenerative hyperplasia of the liver in hematologic disorders: A possible response to obliterative portal venopathy. A morphometric study of nine cases with an hypothesis on the pathogenesis. Medicine 59: 367, 1980

229. Warren JV, Brannon ES: A method of obtaining blood samples directly from the hepatic vein in man. Proc Soc Exp Biol Med 55:144, 1944

230. Warren WD, Muller WH Jr: A clarification of some hemodynamic changes in cirrhosis and their surgical significance. Ann Surg 150:413, 1959

231. Webb LJ, Sherlock S: The aetiology, presentation and natural history of extra-hepatic portal venous obstruction. Q J Med 48:627, 1979

232. Webb LJ et al: Grey-scale ultrasonography. Lancet 2:675, 1977

233. Weits J et al: Percutaneous HAM-splenoportoscintography, porta-systemic shunting and hepatic sinusoidal pressure in cirrhosis of the liver. Neth J Med 18:176, 1975

234. Westaby D et al: Improved survival following injection sclerotherapy for esophageal varices: Final analysis of a controlled trial. Hepatology 5:827, 1985

235. Whipple AO: The problem of portal hypertension in relation to the hepatosplenopathies. Ann Surg 122:449, 1945

236. White LP et al: Ammonium tolerance in liver disease: Observations based on catheterization of the hepatic vein. J Clin Invest 34:158, 1955

237. Widrich WC et al: Long-term follow-up of distal splenorenal shunts. Radiology 134:341, 1980

238. Witte MH et al: Progress in liver disease: Physiological factors involved in the causation of cirrhotic ascites. Gastroenterology 61:742, 1971

239. Witzel L et al: Prophylactic endoscopic sclerotherapy of oesophageal varices: A prospective controlled study. Lancet 1:773, 1985

240. Zeegen R et al: Prolonged survival after portal decompression of patients with non-cirrhotic intrahepatic portal hypertension. Gut 11:610, 1970

chapter 23

Renal Complications in Liver Disease

MURRAY EPSTEIN

Liver disease is frequently accompanied by a variety of alterations in renal function and electrolyte metabolism (Table 23-1).[40] These complications of liver disease are diverse and vary from those that have little clinical significance to others that constitute serious complications that require therapeutic intervention.

Providing an overview of such a large and complex subject has made it necessary to select the information presented and to establish rather arbitrary priorities concerning which areas receive more detailed discussion. In this review, emphasis is placed on abnormalities of renal sodium and water handling and on the syndromes of acute intrinsic renal failure (acute tubular necrosis [ATN]) and the hepatorenal syndrome (HRS), which often supervene in patients with severe liver disease.

RENAL SODIUM HANDLING

Clinical Features

Patients with Laennec's cirrhosis manifest a remarkable capacity for sodium chloride retention; indeed, such patients frequently excrete urine that is virtually free of sodium.[30,55,58,62,69] As a result, there is excessive accumulation of extracellular fluid that eventually becomes evident as clinically detectable ascites and edema. It should be emphasized that cirrhotic patients who are unable to excrete sodium will continue to gain weight and accumulate ascites and edema as long as the dietary sodium content exceeds the maximal urinary sodium excretion. If access to sodium is not curtailed, the relentless retention of sodium may lead to the accumulation of vast amounts of ascites (on occasion up to 30 liters). By contrast, weight gain and ascites formation promptly cease when sodium intake is restricted to a level below that of the maximal renal sodium excretion.

The abnormality of renal sodium handling in cirrhosis should not be regarded as a static and unalterable condition. Rather, cirrhotic patients in whom salt retention has occurred may undergo a spontaneous diuresis, followed by a return to avid salt retention.[58,69] While a significant number of patients who are maintained on a so-dium-restricted dietary program may demonstrate a spontaneous diuresis,[10] there is inadequate information about the incidence with which this occurs. Sometimes spontaneous diuresis occurs within a few days but more often within a few weeks after hospital admission. There is no reliable way of predicting which patients will demonstrate it and which will not.

Although ascites is often considered to be an indicator of decompensated hepatic disease, such is not always the case. The onset of ascites often can be related directly to an increased dietary sodium intake and is more a reflection of salt loading than of progressive alterations in hepatic function. Occasionally, a history of increased intake of salted foods in the period prior to the development of ascites can be elicited. The use of sodium-containing remedies such as antacids must be considered in these persons.

Even when such precipitating events are ruled out, it is evident that there is a poor relationship between abnormalities in renal sodium handling and the presence or absence of "compensation." While it is frequently stated that the abnormalities in renal sodium handling are restricted to the patient with frankly "decompensated" cirrhosis (*i.e.*, presence of clinically demonstrable ascites or edema), a review of the available data attempting to correlate renal sodium handling with a degree of "compen-

TABLE 23-1. Renal Abnormalities in Liver Disease

Parenchymal liver disease with secondary impairment
    of renal function
    Deranged renal sodium handling
    Impaired renal water excretion
    Impaired renal concentrating ability
    Hepatorenal syndrome (HRS)
    Acute renal failure (ATN)
    Glomerulopathies, associated with
        Cirrhosis
        Acute viral hepatitis
        Chronic viral hepatitis
    Impaired renal acidification
Extrahepatic biliary obstruction with secondary
        impairment of renal function: acute renal
        failure (ATN)

sation" lends little support to this concept. It is not possible to predict the presence or magnitude of the impairment of renal sodium handling in the cirrhotic patient merely on the basis of the absence of ascites and/or edema.

Finally, it should be emphasized that the primary renal excretory abnormality causing fluid retention is a disturbance of sodium, rather than of water excretion. Many sodium-retaining patients with ascites and edema are still capable of excreting large volumes of dilute urine when given excessive amounts of water without sodium. When the water is ingested with sodium, however, it is not excreted.[86,113]

In contrast to the wealth of available data on renal sodium handling in cirrhosis, there is a paucity of information in *humans* on this subject in hepatic conditions other than cirrhosis.[32,37] In contradistinction to patients with Laennec's cirrhosis, in whom renal sodium retention is common, patients with primary biliary cirrhosis (PBC) do not appear to manifest this abnormality. Chaimovitz and co-workers[15] have assessed the natriuretic and diuretic response to extracellular fluid volume expansion (ECVE) in patients with PBC and demonstrated that the natriuretic and diuretic response exceeded that observed in both healthy normal volunteers and in edema-free patients with Laennec's cirrhosis. The authors suggested that a common mechanism may underlie both the augmented natriuretic response to volume expansion in their PBC patients and the rarity of fluid retention observed in this type of cirrhosis.

Pathogenesis

The pathogenetic events leading to the deranged sodium homeostasis of cirrhosis are exceedingly complex and remain the subject of continuing controversy. Rather than an exhaustive review of the diverse alterations in liver structure and function and the perturbations in circulatory homeostasis that may contribute to the renal sodium retention of liver disease, this discussion considers two major concepts that have received much recent attention.

An examination of the pathogenetic events leading to the deranged sodium homeostasis of cirrhosis is simplified by a consideration of "afferent" events and "efferent" events. A discussion of "afferent" events usually includes consideration of the detector element responsible for the recognition of the degree of volume alterations as well as a consideration of the extracellular fluid translocations or sequestration into serous spaces or interstitial fluid compartments that characterizes advanced liver disease. Since the afferent derangements that supervene in advanced liver disease have recently been reviewed in depth,[32,38] I will review the concepts of a diminished effective volume and the "overflow" theory of ascites formation only briefly. The major emphasis is placed on the efferent events mediating sodium retention.

In considering the "afferent" events, it is worthwhile to consider two concepts that have been frequently cited in the pathogenesis of the abnormal sodium retention of liver disease: the role of a diminished "effective" volume and the "overflow" theory of ascites formation.

Afferent Events

Role of Diminished "Effective" Volume ("Underfill" Theory). Traditionally, it has been proposed that ascites formation in cirrhotic patients begins when a critical imbalance of Starling forces develops in the hepatic sinusoids and splanchnic capillaries. This causes the formation of an excessive amount of lymph, exceeding the capacity of the thoracic duct to return lymph to the circulation.[5,21,116] Consequently, excess lymph accumulates in the peritoneal space as ascites, with a resultant contraction of circulating plasma volume. Thus, as ascites develops, there is a progressive redistribution of plasma volume. While *total* plasma volume may be increased in this setting, the physiologic circumstance may mimic a reduction in plasma volume (a reduced "effective" plasma volume). The diminished "effective" volume is thought to constitute an afferent signal to the renal tubule to augment salt and water reabsorption. The traditional formulations thus suggest that the renal retention of sodium is a *secondary* rather than a primary event.

In this context, it is important to underscore that the term "effective" plasma volume refers to that part of the total circulating volume that is effective in stimulating volume receptors. The concept is somewhat elusive, since the actual volume receptors remain incompletely defined. A diminished "effective" volume may reflect subtle alterations in systemic hemodynamic factors such as decreased filling of the arterial tree, a diminished central blood volume, or both. Since the stimulus is unknown and the afferent receptors are incompletely elucidated, alterations in "effective" volume must be defined in a functional manner, such as the kinetic response to volume manipulation.

"Overflow" Theory of Ascites Formation. Over the past decade, an alternative hypothesis has been proposed. Lieberman and Reynolds and their associates[73,74] proposed the "overflow" theory of ascites formation. In contrast to the traditional formulation, the "overflow" theory suggests that the initiating or primary event is the inappropriate retention of excessive amounts of sodium by the kidneys, with a resultant expansion of plasma volume. In the setting of abnormal Starling forces (both portal venous hypertension and a reduction in plasma colloid osmotic pressure) in the portal venous bed and hepatic sinusoids, the expanded plasma volume is sequestered preferentially in the peritoneal space as ascites. Thus, according to this formulation, renal sodium retention and plasma volume expansion *precede* rather than follow the formation of ascites.

Since the promulgation of the "overflow" theory of ascites formation, controversy has centered on which of the

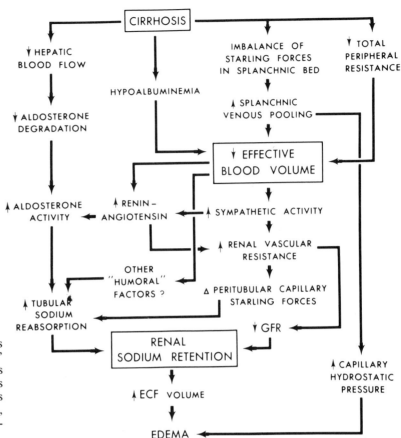

Fig. 23-1. Schematic drawing of the factors operative in the traditional or "underfill" theory of sodium retention in cirrhosis. As can be seen, an imbalance of Starling forces in the hepatosplanchnic microcirculation is not the sole mechanism. Acting in concert, these factors promote a reduction in effective plasma volume.

two hypotheses is correct. Evidence cited in support of the overflow theory includes the demonstration that plasma volume is increased in cirrhosis with ascites, and the finding that increases in measured plasma volume have not been observed in cirrhotic patients with ascites undergoing a spontaneous diuresis has been cited as evidence in support of the overflow hypothesis. Additional support derives from a series of elegant investigations carried out during the past decade by Levy[71,72] on dogs with experimental portal cirrhosis, investigations that demonstrate that renal sodium retention is the initial event and precedes the formation of ascites.

Although these observations collectively support the overflow theory of ascites formation, a number of clinical observations in *humans* are inconsistent with such a formulation. Thus, rapid volume expansion with exogenous solutions including saline, mannitol, and albumin frequently results in a transient improvement in renal sodium and water handling.[98,111,115] The results of many earlier studies must be considered inconclusive because of the confounding effects of the experimental designs. Studies from our laboratory over the past 16 years have circumvented many of the experimental problems of earlier studies by applying a unique investigative tool, the water

immersion model, to the assessment of renal function and volume–hormonal relationships.[36,50,53] Specifically, in contrast to saline administration, (1) water immersion is associated with a decrease in body weight, rather than the increase that attends saline infusion; (2) the "volume stimulus" of immersion is promptly reversible after cessation of immersion, in contrast to the relatively sustained hypervolemia that follows saline administration, and thus constitutes an important attribute in minimizing any risk to the patient; and (3) the "volume stimulus" of immersion occurs in the absence of changes in plasma composition.[36,50,53]

Studies in 32 patients with decompensated cirrhosis demonstrated a striking "normalization" of renal sodium handling following water immersion. As shown in Figure 23-2, immersion resulted in marked natriuresis and kaliuresis in the majority of these patients. During the final hour of immersion, $U_{Na}V$ was 20-fold greater than it was during the pre-study hour. Thus, the marked antinatriuresis of cirrhosis was promptly reversed by a manipulation that merely altered the distribution of plasma volume without increasing (and often decreasing) total plasma volume. Indeed, in many instances the natriuresis of such patients exceeded markedly the response mani-

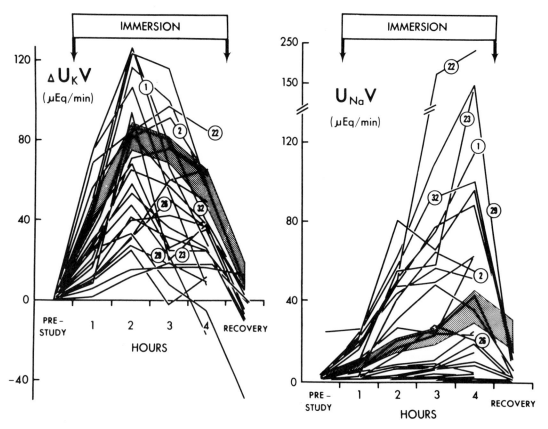

Fig. 23-2. Effects of water immersion after 1 hour of quiet sitting (prestudy) on rate of sodium excretion ($U_{Na}V$) and potassium excretion (U_KV) in a large group of patients with alcoholic liver disease. The circled numbers represent individual patients. Data for U_KV are expressed in terms of absolute changes from prestudy hour (ΔU_KV). The shaded area represents the SEM for 14 normal control subjects undergoing an identical immersion study while ingesting an identical diet of 10 mEq sodium/100 mEq potassium/day. More than half of the cirrhotic patients manifested an appropriate or "exaggerated" natriuretic response. In general, the increase in $U_{Na}V$ was associated with a concomitant increase in ΔU_KV.

fested by normal subjects to the identical procedure. Taken together, these studies lend strong support to the concept that a diminished *effective* intravascular volume is a major determinant of the enhanced tubular reabsorption of sodium in patients with established cirrhosis.

Although I believe that the currently available evidence favors a prominent role for a diminished effective volume in mediating the avid sodium retention of many cirrhotic patients, it is important to underscore that these two formulations (*i.e.,* diminished effective volume and "overflow" theory) may not be mutually exclusive. It is worth remembering that virtually all the available clinical studies of deranged sodium homeostasis were carried out at a time when decompensation was well *established,* with little information available during the incipient stage of sodium retention. The two ostensibly differing formulations may be reconciled by viewing the pathogenesis of abnormal sodium retention in cirrhosis as a complex clinical con-

stellation in which differing forces participate in varying degrees as the derangement in sodium homeostasis evolves. Thus, it is quite conceivable that a primary defect in renal sodium handling may assume a more prominent role in the early stages of cirrhosis and a diminished effective volume may constitute the major determinant of sodium retention in many patients once the derangement is established.

Effectors of Renal Sodium Retention

The initial attempts to explain the abnormalities of renal sodium handling focused on the decrement in glomerular filtration rate (GFR), which occurs frequently in patients with advanced liver disease. A number of observations indicate, however, that a decrease in GFR cannot constitute the major determinant of the abnormalities in renal sodium handling. Many observers have reported derangements in renal sodium handling despite preserved GFR. In fact, avid sodium reabsorption has been observed even in the face of supranormal GFR.[16,69]

Although the weight of evidence demonstrates that the renal sodium retention accompanying cirrhosis is attributable primarily to enhanced tubular reabsorption rather than to alterations in the filtered load of sodium, the precise nephron sites that are operative remain the subject of continuing controversy.[16,18,52,69]

The mediators of the enhanced tubular reabsorption of sodium in cirrhosis and their relative participation in the avid sodium retention have not been elucidated completely. Several mechanisms have been implicated or suggested, including hyperaldosteronism, alterations in intrarenal blood flow distribution, an increase in sympathetic nervous system activity, alterations in the endogenous release of renal prostaglandins, the possible role of a humoral natriuretic factor, and, more recently, atrial natriuretic factor. These mechanisms and their interrelationships are summarized schematically in Figure 23-2.

Role of Hyperaldosteronism. Cirrhosis is frequently associated with increased levels of aldosterone in the urine and in peripheral plasma as well. The elevation of plasma aldosterone levels is attributable to both an increased adrenal secretion and decreased metabolic degradation of the hormone.[23,31,45,97] The rate of hepatic degradation is related directly to hepatic blood flow, which is markedly decreased in patients with decompensated cirrhosis.

Nevertheless, the etiologic relationship between the hyperaldosteronism and the encountered sodium retention is uncertain. The traditional viewpoint held that aldosterone is a *major* determinant of the sodium retention.[31] In contrast to this long-held traditional view, many lines of evidence have challenged the etiologic role of elevated plasma aldosterone levels in mediating the sodium retention of cirrhosis: First, it should be noted that the widely held view that plasma aldosterone levels are usually elevated in advanced liver disease is probably an oversimplification.[31] Furthermore, increasing evidence demonstrates a dissociation between sodium excretion and plasma aldosterone in diverse clinical and experimental conditions,[31,97] thereby challenging the predominance of elevated plasma aldosterone levels in mediating the sodium retention of cirrhosis. Unfortunately, none of these studies attempted to assess in a kinetic manner the responses of plasma aldosterone and renal sodium excretion to acute volume manipulation. Recently, my co-workers and I investigated the role of aldosterone in mediating the abnormal renal sodium handling in cirrhosis by carrying out studies utilizing a newly developed investigative tool, the model of head-out water immersion. Immersion studies during chronic spironolactone administration permitted a further elucidation of the relative contribution of aldosterone to the sodium retention.[51] Spironolactone administration without immersion resulted in only a modest increase in sodium excretion. In contrast, there was a marked increase in sodium excretion when immersion was carried out during chronic spironolactone administration, thereby indicating that the major contribution to the natriuresis was an enhanced distal delivery of filtrate.[51]

More compelling evidence mitigating against a predominant role for aldosterone in prompting the antinatriuresis of cirrhosis is derived from recent immersion studies kinetically assessing the relationship of plasma aldosterone responsiveness to renal sodium handling.[45] Despite profound suppression of plasma aldosterone to comparable nadir levels in 16 cirrhotic patients, half of the patients manifested an absent or markedly blunted natriuretic response during immersion.[45] This demonstration of a dissociation between the suppression of circulating aldosterone and the absence of the natriuresis in these subjects lends strong support to the interpretation that aldosterone is not the primary determinant of the impaired sodium excretion of cirrhosis.

Role of Renal Prostaglandins and Renal Sodium Handling. The possibility that prostaglandins participate in mediating the sodium retention of cirrhosis should be considered. Since several studies indicate that alterations in prostaglandin release constitute a determinant of the natriuretic response to extracellular fluid volume expansion,[46] it is probable that alterations in renal prostaglandin synthesis may contribute to the derangements in renal sodium handling. Several studies have demonstrated that the administration of nonsteroidal anti-inflammatory drugs (which act as inhibitors of prostaglandin synthetase) to patients with decompensated cirrhosis results in profound decrements of renal hemodynamics, GFR, and sodium excretion.[11,118] These provocative observations suggest a role for renal prostaglandins as determinants of the abnormal sodium retention of cirrhosis.

Since the above-cited studies have examined the effect of inhibiting endogenous production of renal prostaglandins, it was of great interest to assess an opposite experimental manipulation, namely, augmentation of endogenous prostaglandins.[46] We utilized water immersion to the neck, which redistributes blood volume with concomitant central hypervolemia and enhances prostaglandin E (PGE) excretion in normal persons.[47] It was demonstrated that decompensated cirrhotic patients manifested an increase in mean PGE excretion that was threefold greater than that observed in normal subjects studied under identical conditions.[46] This is attended by a marked natriuresis and an increase in creatinine clearance. Collectively, these observations suggest that derangements in renal PGE production appear to contribute to the renal dysfunction of cirrhosis, including sodium retention. It is tempting to postulate that in the setting of cirrhosis of the liver, enhancement of prostaglandin synthesis is a compensatory or adaptive response to incipient renal ischemia.

Recently, it has been suggested that sulindac differs from

other nonsteroidal anti-inflammatory drugs (NSAIDs) by sparing *renal* but inhibiting *systemic* prostaglandins.[14,19] This is reflected by the lack of an effect on urinary PGE_2 excretion and on other putative endpoints of renal prostaglandin synthesis such as renin release and response to furosemide, whereas inhibition of systemic prostaglandins is reflected by the decreased production of thromboxane by platelets.[12] If such findings are extrapolated to cirrhotic patients, one might anticipate that sulindac would be associated with the lowest incidence of sodium retention. Despite these impressive preliminary results, it is unsettled whether sulindac is indeed renal-sparing in cirrhotic patients. Indeed, Brater and associates[12] have recently reported that sulindac did not differ from ibuprofen in its ability to decrease urinary PGE_2 and that both decreased the pharmacodynamics of response to furosemide. Daskalopoulos and co-workers[24] compared the effects of sulindac and indomethacin on furosemide-induced augmentation of PGE_2 and on renal sodium and water handling. Although only indomethacin reduced creatinine clearance, urinary volume, sodium, and PGE_2 *before* furosemide administration, these differences were virtually abolished after furosemide administration. That is, indomethacin appeared only slightly more potent in reducing the diuresis (55% vs. 38%), natriuresis (67% vs. 52%), and PGE_2 release (81% vs. 74%). Thus, under conditions of furosemide-enhanced prostaglandin activity, sulindac does affect renal function. To the extent that the ability to augment renal prostaglandin synthesis constitutes an important adaptive response in disorders characterized by decreased renal perfusion, the observations of Daskalopoulos and associates[24] merit attention. Additional studies are necessary to define the differences between sulindac and indomethacin in patients with cirrhosis, both under basal conditions and during maneuvers that alter (*i.e.,* augment) renal prostaglandin production.

Role of Sympathetic Nervous System Activity. An increase in sympathetic nervous system activity may also contribute to the sodium retention in cirrhosis.[29] Thus, the decrease in central blood volume could increase renal sympathetic activity.[29,110] Furthermore, recent studies have demonstrated that an increase in sympathetic tone promotes an antinatriuresis by altering intrarenal hemodynamics and by a direct tubular effect.[29]

Although these theoretic considerations suggest a role for the sympathetic nervous system in the sodium retention of cirrhosis, relatively little data are available that bear directly on this possibility. Bichet and co-workers[8] have reported that patients with advanced cirrhosis manifest elevated concentrations of plasma catecholamines. These investigators proposed that the encountered catecholamine changes accounted for the impaired sodium and water handling in their patients.

Although most observers agree that mean peripheral norepinephrine levels are elevated in cirrhotic patients,[45-47] it is an oversimplification to suggest that such alterations in catecholamine metabolism affect all cirrhotic patients with deranged sodium and water homeostasis. Recently we examined the relationship between plasma norepinephrine levels and renal sodium and water handling during immersion-induced central blood volume expansion.[43] Although mean norepinephrine levels were elevated for the group as a whole, more than half of the patients with decompensated cirrhosis manifested appropriate (nonelevated) norepinephrine levels. Furthermore, norepinephrine levels did not correlate with alterations in renal sodium or water excretion[43] (Figs. 23-3 and 23-4).

The available data regarding the role of the sympathetic nervous system may be summarized as fragmentary and inconclusive. More direct indices of autonomic activity (such as renal venous norepinephrine levels rather than

Fig. 23-3. Relationship between renal sodium excretion (*upper panel*) and alterations in plasma norepinephrine (NE) (*lower panel*) during immersion in 16 cirrhotic patients. The numbers along the horizontal axis designate individual patients. As can be seen, the magnitude of the natriuresis, as assessed by peak $U_{Na}V$, varied independently of ΔNE ("nadir" minus prestudy NE) during immersion (r = 0.256; NS). (Reproduced with permission from Epstein M et al: Mineral Electrolyte Metab 11:25–34, 1985)

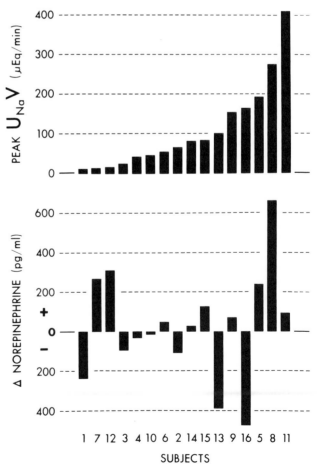

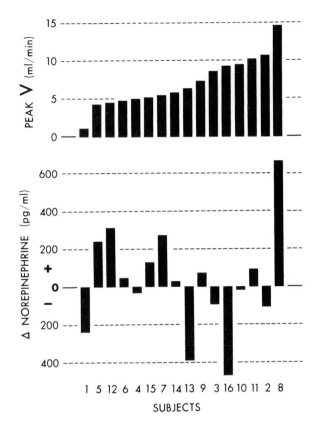

Fig. 23-4. Relationship between renal water handling (*upper panel*) and alterations in plasma norepinephrine (NE) (*lower panel*) during immersion in 16 cirrhotic patients. The numbers along the horizontal axis designate individual patients. As can be seen, the magnitude of the diuresis, as assessed by peak V, varied independently of ΔNE ("nadir" minus prestudy NE) during immersion (r = 0.239; NS). (Reproduced with permission from Epstein M et al: Mineral Electrolyte Metab 11:25–34, 1985)

peripheral plasma levels) are required to determine whether diminished effective volume with a concomitant increase in sympathetic activity, both in the kidney and in other regional vascular beds, contributes to the sodium retention of cirrhosis.[57]

Role of Humoral Natriuretic Factor. Several lines of evidence have suggested the possibility that a circulating natriuretic factor constitutes a component part of the biologic control system regulating sodium excretion in humans.[13] Recently the presence of this natriuretic factor has also been demonstrated in *normal* subjects during immersion-induced volume expansion[42] and during mineralocorticoid escape. Since this natriuretic factor is operative in uremia and since it has also been proposed to play a role in the regulation of sodium excretion in *normal* physiologic states, it is conceivable that deficiencies of this hormone could mediate at least in part the sodium retention of cirrhosis (see Fig. 23-2). Implicit in this concept is the

hypothesis that sodium retention results from a failure to elaborate natriuretic hormone when extracellular fluid volume increases in response to renal sodium retention.

Several preliminary observations utilizing bioassay systems are consistent with such a formulation.[56,80] Additional studies are needed to assess the precise role of a natriuretic factor in the pathogenesis of sodium retention in cirrhosis.

Role of Atrial Natriuretic Factor (Auriculin). It has been recently shown that mammalian atria contain potent natriuretic and vasoactive peptides, which have been referred to as atrial natriuretic factor (ANF) and auriculin.[27,76] Several laboratories have purified, sequenced, and synthesized atrial peptides that have the natriuretic and vasoactive properties of crude atrial extract. Studies in intact animals have demonstrated that ANF decreases blood pressure and increases GFR and sodium excretion without a sustained increase in renal plasma flow. In addition, synthetic auriculin decreased renin secretory rate, plasma renin levels, and plasma aldosterone levels. Taken together, these observations suggest an important potential role for auriculin in the regulation of blood pressure, renal function, and sodium-volume homeostasis.

In light of several lines of evidence suggesting that stretch receptors residing in the atria may participate in regulating volume homeostasis,[59] it is tempting to attribute a cardinal role to this peptide in modulating renal sodium handling in both normal persons and in patients with edematous disorders including chronic liver disease. Specifically, the sodium retention and activation of the renin–angiotensin–aldosterone system in patients with cirrhosis may result from a failure to elaborate auriculin when ECF volume increases in response to renal sodium retention. In light of active investigations in many laboratories with these peptides,[48] it is hoped that the role of this putative effector in mediating sodium retention in cirrhotic patients will be delineated.

It is apparent that the renal sodium retention of advanced liver disease is a complex pathophysiological constellation with numerous and diverse causes, each one of which may be operative to a varying degree during the course of the disease. Figure 23-5 represents an attempt to integrate these diverse findings and to summarize some of the mechanisms whereby these diverse hormonal mediators may act in concert to induce sodium retention.

Management of Ascites and Edema

It is well established that ascites is associated with many unwanted side-effects in the patient with liver disease.[20] Clearly the marked accumulation of ascites is associated with significant discomfort. Ascites enhances the two prime precipitants of variceal bleeding: high portal pressure, which favors rupture of the varices; and gastroesophageal reflux, which may lead to erosion of the varices. Furthermore, it has been suggested that ascites is the *sine qua non* of spontaneous bacterial peritonitis.[22] Finally,

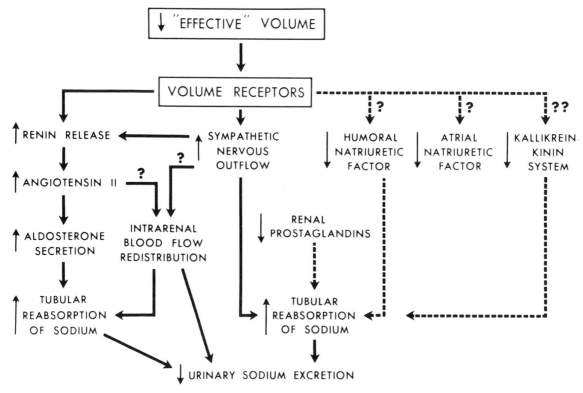

Fig. 23-5. Schematic drawing of possible mechanisms whereby a diminished *effective* volume results in sodium retention. The solid arrows indicate pathways for which evidence is available. The dashed lines represent proposed pathways, the existence of which remains to be established. (Reproduced with permission of the American Gastroenterological Association, Inc., from Epstein M et al: Gastroenterology 76:622–635, 1979)

the frequent association of ascites with the development of HRS raises the possibility that ascites may play an essential role in its pathogenesis.

While ascites is indeed the ". . . root of much evil," the decision to relieve ascites with diuretic agents should not be automatic. On the one hand, several studies have suggested that diuretic therapy in the cirrhotic patient may be associated with a substantial risk of adverse effects. Sherlock[105] surveyed diuretic-related complications occurring in a group of cirrhotic patients treated from 1962 to 1965 and reported an incidence of encephalopathy varying from 22% to 26% (depending on the diuretic used), hyponatremia varying from 40% to 49%, and azotemia (blood urea nitrogen [BUN] > 40 mg/dl) ranging from 20% to 40%. The incidence of hypokalemia was marked (as high as 64%), and this complication persisted, albeit at a much lessened frequency, even when potassium-sparing diuretics such as spironolactone and amiloride were added. While it may be argued that this 14-year old survey may be unrepresentative and that this study was uncontrolled in nature, a more recent report by Naranjo and coworkers[81] utilizing a prospective drug surveillance program suggests that diuretic-induced complications in the

cirrhotic patient continue to constitute formidable problems even today.

A Rational Approach

The approach to the cirrhotic patient with ascites should be grounded on the realization that ascites, unless massive, may not require treatment *per se*. While ascites has been implicated in the pathogenesis of a number of complications of liver disease, its removal has not been demonstrated to increase life expectancy. The initial goal of any treatment program should be an attempt to induce weight loss resulting from a spontaneous diuresis by consistent and scrupulous adherence to a well-balanced diet with rigid dietary sodium restriction (250 mg/day). It should be emphasized that the sodium intake prescribed for cardiac patients (1200–1500 mg daily) is not sufficiently restrictive for the cirrhotic patient, who continues to gain weight on such a regimen. While the frequency with which such dietary management successfully relieves ascites is unsettled, a sodium restricted diet still should be prescribed to all patients, since it is impossible to predict which patients will respond.

In some symptomatic patients, however, less rigid sodium restriction may be advisable for several reasons. First, as a consequence of the anorexia, the patient will eat only part of the meals offered and thus only a fraction of the daily sodium allowance. Second, in malnourished patients, nutrition must have a priority over rigid sodium restriction.

When the response to dietary management is inadequate or when the imposition of rigid dietary sodium restriction is not feasible owing to cost or unpalatability of the diet, the use of diuretic agents may be considered.

The rational basis of diuretic therapy lies in an understanding of the mechanisms and sites of action of the diuretic agent, coupled with an understanding of the pathophysiology of sodium retention in cirrhosis. Since the attributes and efficacy of the varying diuretic agents are reviewed in detail elsewhere,[34] I will focus solely on therapeutic considerations that are unique to the cirrhotic patient. When diuretics are used, the therapeutic aim is a slow and gradual diuresis not exceeding the capacity for mobilization of ascitic fluid. Shear and associates,[101] have demonstrated that ascites absorption averages about 300 ml to 500 ml/day during spontaneous diuresis and has as its upper limits 700 ml to 900 ml/day. Thus, any diuresis that exceeds 900 ml/day (in the ascitic patient without edema) must perforce be mobilized at the expense of the plasma compartment, with resultant volume contraction.

Finally, the dangers of diuretic-associated hypokalemia should be emphasized.[89] Since total body potassium depletion is frequently associated with cirrhosis, the use of any diuretic that acts proximal to the distal potassium-secretory site may result in profound hypokalemia. Because of the frequently observed temporal relationship between diuretic therapy and the development of hepatic encephalopathy and the probability that the enhanced renal ammonia production of hypokalemia may be related to the encephalopathy,[89] great care should be exercised in monitoring and correcting potassium derangements in the cirrhotic patient receiving diuretics. The overriding consideration in diuretic therapy, however, is that its use as the sole indication of cosmetic improvement be clearly contraindicated.

Choice of a Diuretic Agent

As discussed above, there is considerable sodium retention at both proximal and distal tubular sites in patients with liver disease. Although at first glance one may consider the therapeutic use of agents that act primarily by inhibiting proximal tubular reabsorption, such as carbonic anhydrase inhibitors or osmotic diuretics, their use is not advocated. In general, despite their ability to promote proximal tubular rejection of filtrate, these agents, when administered *alone,* are only weakly natriuretic. This is attributable primarily to an enhancement of sodium reabsorption at distal tubular sites, which tends to counteract the proximal tubular effect of the drug.

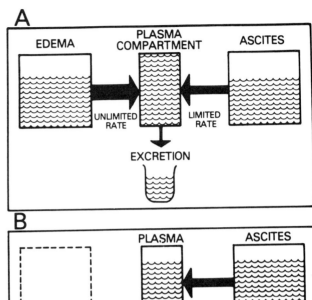
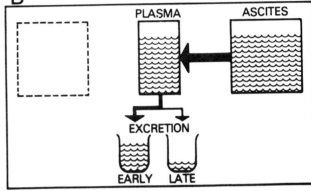

Fig. 23-6. Schematic depiction of the mobilization and formation of fluid in ECF compartments in patients with fluid retention. The key to understanding this diagram is the realization that the rate of ascites mobilization is limited, whereas that of edema is relatively unlimited. In the presence of ascites *and edema* (A), edema is recruited in an unlimited manner to equal the rate of diuresis. In the ascitic patient *without edema* (B), the rate of mobilization of ascitic fluid is limited (700–900 ml/day). Thus any diuresis that exceeds 900 ml/day must be mobilized at the expense of the plasma compartment. (Adapted with permission from a drawing by A. Miller, in Gabuzda GJ: Cirrhotic ascites: An etiologic approach to management. Hosp Pract 8[8]:67–74, 1973)

If there is no compelling reason for rapidly mobilizing excessive fluid, I favor *initiating* therapy with one of the distal potassium-sparing diuretics. Although such diuretics induce merely a modest natriuresis, this feature in a sense commends their use. With such drugs the physician is less likely to exceed the guidelines suggested by Shear and co-workers.[101]

One can start with spironolactone, 100 mg/day twice daily. If this dosage of spironolactone does not induce a natriuresis, the dosage may be increased in stepwise fashion every 3 to 5 days to a maximum of 400 mg/day. It should be remembered that spironolactone's onset of action is slow, requiring 3 to 5 days for the peak effect to become manifest, and thus a natriuresis will not occur during the initial 2 to 3 days of therapy. Such a regimen will result in a natriuresis in approximately 50% of the patients.*

Unfortunately, spironolactone is not free of side-effects. It causes gynecomastia in a large fraction of cirrhotic patients who receive large doses. To circumvent this problem, it has been suggested that the other potassium-sparing diuretics, triamterene or amiloride, may constitute alternative medications for such patients. Both are nonsteroidal, natriuretic, potassium-sparing agents that both promote sodium excretion and limit potassium excretion even in the absence of mineralocorticoids. All three potassium-sparing diuretics have the potential to induce hyperkalemia (and hyperchloremic acidosis), which sometimes is of serious proportions.

If no natriuresis occurs with the maximal dosage of spironolactone, furosemide (Lasix), 40 mg to 80 mg/day, should be added. If no natriuresis is observed on this regimen, the physician should reassess dietary intake to ensure that the patient is not "cheating." If dietary sodium intake is being restricted and if hepatic and renal function show no deterioration, one should consider increasing furosemide dosage in a stepwise fashion to a maximum of 240 mg/day.

Finally, in an attempt to minimize the complications of diuretic therapy, it has been proposed that intermittent administration, is safer than continuous treatment. From the limited data available, such "rest" periods appear advisable. At the very least, they provide adequate time to observe and detect any adverse effects and discontinue the therapy if so indicated.

Drug–Diuretic Interactions

For patients receiving spironolactone therapy, it would be wise to avoid the use of aspirin as an analgesic.[112] Although the interfering effect of aspirin on spironolactone-induced diuresis in cirrhotic ascitic patients has not been evaluated, observations made in normal subjects are sufficiently striking to advise that no aspirin-containing analgesics be used in patients who are undergoing spironolactone therapy. In normal subjects who were receiving exogenous mineralocorticoids, 600 mg of aspirin markedly blunted the effect of spironolactone.[112]

The detrimental effects of NSAIDs merit emphasis. NSAIDs are potent inhibitors of prostaglandin synthesis. In light of suggestions that the renal effects of loop diuretics may be attributable, at least in part, to an increased renal production of PGE_2,[17,25,106] it might be anticipated that the administration of NSAIDs may affect the natriuretic effect of loop diuretics. Recent studies have confirmed such suggestions.[4]

* It should be emphasized that the choice of spironolactone does not imply a predominant role for aldosterone in mediating the sodium retention of cirrhosis. As noted earlier in this chapter, I believe that the hyperaldosteronism of cirrhosis plays a permissive role in promoting sodium retention.

Studies in edematous patients with cirrhosis and cardiac failure have demonstrated that NSAID agents decreased the natriuretic response to furosemide.[79,117] Although NSAID agents cause a concomitant reduction of creatinine clearance, the available evidence suggests that these agents exert their effect primarily by an inhibition of the tubular action of furosemide rather than by an impairment of renal hemodynamics.[91] Regardless, the clinical importance is founded in a realization that NSAIDs often impair the natriuretic effects of *all* diuretics.

Combined Therapy with Thiazide-Type and Loop Diuretic Agents for Resistant Sodium Retention

True resistance to conventional diuretic regimens is unusual.[44] When true resistance is encountered, one proposed approach to management is the combined use of a thiazide-type diuretic with a loop diuretic. The addition of a relatively small dose of a diuretic agent that acts mainly in the cortical diluting segment of the distal nephron (*e.g.*, metolazone or thiazides) to a very large but apparently ineffective dose of a potent loop diuretic agent (*i.e.*, furosemide, bumetanide, or ethacrynic acid) might not be expected to produce a massive natriuretic response. Nevertheless, a synergistic effect of such a combination has been documented in several reports, and successful fluid removal has occurred in patients with previously resistant severe sodium retention associated with diverse disorders, including hepatic cirrhosis.[44]

There is no question that diuretic combinations can constitute a highly efficacious means to relieve refractory edema. Nevertheless, despite the positive aspects of these regimens, increasing experience has resulted in disturbing observations regarding morbidity. Specifically there is a growing awareness that the use of such combinations may be attended by a wide array of complications, including massive fluid and electrolyte losses and circulatory collapse.[83] Of particular concern in the cirrhotic patient is a major risk of profound hypokalemia that may occur with an alarming rapidity. Furthermore, such patients with a diminished effective volume are at risk of developing the HRS, ATN, and hepatic encephalopathy if an overly rapid diuresis occurs. As we explained in a recent editorial,[83] the potential risk may be only rarely justifiable in patients with liver disease. Rather, if there are compelling reasons for mobilizing excessive fluid (as discussed above), one should resort to the use of the peritoneojugular shunt.

RENAL WATER HANDLING IN CIRRHOSIS

Clinical Features

The serum sodium level is determined by the balance of water in relation to that of sodium: too much water causes hyponatremia; too little causes hypernatremia. Hyponatremia connotes a serum sodium concentration (S_{Na}) below the lower limit of normal, that is, less than 135 mEq/liter. In the cirrhotic patient, exchangeable sodium is increased. Therefore, if the patient is hyponatremic, the amount of water retained must be disproportionally greater than that of sodium. That is, there must be a specific defect in renal water excretion (*i.e.,* diluting capacity).

Impairment of renal diluting capacity occurs frequently in cirrhosis.[33,113] Hyponatremia, the expression of this impaired capacity to excrete water, is a commonly encountered clinical problem in cirrhotic patients. Indeed, hyponatremia probably represents the single most common electrolyte abnormality that confronts the physician treating patients with cirrhosis of the liver. For example, 20 of 50 (40%) patients with cirrhosis admitted to a liver unit in one year by Arroyo and associates[2] were found to have a serum sodium concentration below 130 mEq/liter.

Although it has been suggested that this abnormality correlates with the severity of the hepatic disease, a critical review of the available data suggests that it is difficult to relate the capacity of water diuresis with specific clinical features.[102,113] Whereas the majority of compensated patients (*i.e.,* those without clinical evidence of ascites or edema, or both) excrete water normally, decompensated patients (those with ascites or edema, or both) manifest widely varying responses to oral water loading. Furthermore, prospective studies have indicated that the transition from compensation to decompensation, or vice versa, is not necessarily accompanied by concomitant changes in renal water handling.[113]

Aside from the increased frequency of spontaneous hyponatremia, it should be noted that there is an increased propensity for patients with decompensated cirrhosis to develop hyponatremia in association with diuretic administration. Indeed, in an earlier survey of diuretic-related complications, Sherlock and co-workers[104] observed that hyponatremia occurred in over 40% of cirrhotic patients treated with chlorothiazide, furosemide, or chlorothiazide plus spironolactone. Subsequent studies have confirmed the heightened susceptibility of cirrhotic patients to develop this complication.

The symptoms of hyponatremia associated with severe liver disease do not differ from those found in dilutional hyponatremia of other etiologies. Therein lies a diagnostic dilemma. These symptoms (difficulty in mental concentration, anorexia, headache, apathy, nausea, vomiting, and, occasionally, seizures) can also be observed in patients with hepatic coma or precoma, but with normal serum sodium concentration. Thus, not infrequently, it is difficult to ascertain if symptoms relate to the hyponatremia itself or to severe liver disease. In addition, one may observe an increase in serum sodium levels without significant changes in symptoms.

Pathogenesis

The mechanisms responsible for the impairment in renal water excretion in cirrhosis have not been elucidated completely, but several possibilities have been proposed.

The two principal mechanisms are a decreased delivery of filtrate to the diluting segments of the nephron and enhanced antidiuretic hormone (ADH) activity. Additional mechanisms include a decrease in the release of endogenous renal prostaglandins and an increase in sympathetic nervous system activity.

Decreased Delivery of Filtrate to Diluting Segments of the Nephron

Theoretic considerations suggest that a decreased delivery of filtrate to the diluting segments of the nephron contribute to the impaired water excretion of cirrhotic patients. Many decompensated cirrhotic patients manifest a decrease in GFR.[32,38] Furthermore, much evidence suggests avid reabsorption of filtrate along the proximal tubule.[18,38,98] The demonstration that free-water generation is improved in some cirrhotic patients following expansion with infusions of hypotonic saline or isotonic mannitol or saline and albumin[38,98,115] supports a role for increasing distal delivery of filtrate in the enhancement of water excretion.

Elevated Levels of Antidiuretic Hormone

Several lines of evidence suggest that the impairment in water excretion is attributable to increased levels of ADH, with a resultant increased back-diffusion of free water in the collecting tubule. Most of the experimental evidence supporting a role for vasopressin has been indirect, involving an assessment of the responses to the administration of agents that either alter ADH release or interfere with its peripheral actions. Thus, the ingestion of alcohol increased urine flow and decreased urine osmolality in severely decompensated cirrhotic patients with normal GFR.[109] Subsequently, the administration of demeclocycline, a tetracycline derivative that appears to antagonize the peripheral action of ADH, has been shown to enhance free water generation in patients with cirrhosis and ascites.[28]

The development of sensitive and specific radioimmunoassays for ADH has provided a more precise delineation of the frequency with which ADH levels are elevated. The available reports suggest that decompensated cirrhosis is associated with a wide spectrum of ADH levels varying from normal to elevated values.[6,54,93] The possible mechanisms for increased vasopressin levels in cirrhosis are multiple. It has been proposed that enhanced vasopressin activity may be mediated by known nonosmotic stimuli, including a decrease in peripheral resistance and arterial pressure.[7] Alternatively, abnormalities in the metabolic clearance of vasopressin may contribute to the increase in the vasopressin activity.

Alterations in Renal Prostaglandin Metabolism

Alterations in renal prostaglandins may contribute to the antidiuresis of cirrhosis by several mechanisms.[87,92] Prostaglandins have been shown to exert a number of functional effects on urinary concentrating and diluting mechanisms, and these have been reviewed in depth by Stokes[108] and by Raymond and Lifschitz.[92] The overall action of prostaglandins appears to be that of promoting free water excretion, and several mechanisms have been proposed to account for this effect. Although the role of renal prostaglandins is not yet fully established, the majority of studies suggest that a "relative" diminution of renal prostaglandins may contribute to the antidiuresis of cirrhosis.[33,87,92] It should be underscored that such a formulation does not necessarily imply an absolute decrease in renal prostaglandins. Rather, a relative deficiency characterized by levels that may be appropriate in absolute terms but insufficient in light of the marked elevation of vasoconstrictor hormones may contribute to the pathogenesis of renal water retention.

Increase in Sympathetic Nervous System Activity

It is possible that an increase in efferent renal sympathetic nerve activity (ERSNA) may also contribute to the water retention of cirrhosis. Alterations in adrenergic nervous activity can modify renal water handling by several mechanisms.[29,110] Several studies have attempted to demonstrate a correlation between peripheral plasma norepinephrine levels and the impairment in renal water excretion[8] and demonstrated negative correlations between plasma norepinephrine and renal water excretion. Conversely, we have assessed kinetically the relationship of plasma catecholamines to changes in renal water handling during a well-defined volume expansive maneuver, namely, head-out water immersion, and have failed to demonstrate a relationship between suppression of norepinephrine and renal water excretion.[43]

In summary, it is apparent that the available data regarding the role of the sympathetic nervous system are fragmentary and inconclusive. Although most observers agree that mean peripheral norepinephrine levels are elevated in many cirrhotic patients, it would appear to be an oversimplification to suggest that such alterations in catecholamine metabolism affect all cirrhotic patients with deranged sodium and water homeostasis. Clearly, more direct indices of autonomic activity are required to determine whether a diminished effective volume with concomitant increase in sympathetic activity, both in the kidney and in other areas, contributes to the water retention of cirrhosis.

Treatment

The impaired diluting ability afflicting many patients with advanced liver disease may have important implications for management. As has been emphasized, hyponatremia connotes a dilutional state secondary to an impaired capacity to excrete water. A *sine qua non* of this observation is that the rational basis for treating hyponatremia is fluid restriction. Regardless of the degree of dilutional impair-

ment, appropriate fluid restriction will eventually repair this abnormality.

As a caveat, it must be emphasized that in many hospitals it is difficult to adhere to the physician's orders for fluid restriction. As examples, paramedical and nursing personnel may not consider the fluids administered with medication as part of the fluid restriction. We are often dismayed to observe pitchers of water and several containers of juice inadvertently placed at the bedside of patients thought to be severely fluid restricted. Thus, patients who ostensibly are on rigid fluid restriction may indeed be receiving 1500 ml or even 2000 ml of fluid per day. It is not surprising that the serum sodium level of such patients does not increase or may even decrease. Because of this problem, it is not infrequently necessary to resort to absolute fluid restriction with levels approaching 0 ml to 200 ml/day for the first few days in order to initiate the return of the serum sodium level toward normal.

Even though hyponatremia is frequently attributed to diuretic therapy, it should be noted that such an inference is somewhat simplistic. Although diuretics impair renal diluting ability, the diuresis that follows diuretic administration is characterized by a urine that is hypotonic relative to plasma. Therefore, hyponatremia will not ensue if concomitant water restriction is sufficient. Nevertheless, if the patient becomes severely hyponatremic while receiving diuretics, diuretic administration may have to be discontinued. This is particularly true in an outpatient setting because fluid restriction cannot be rigidly controlled.

Since many patients with advanced liver disease manifest an impairment of renal diluting ability, one may inquire when therapy should be instituted to normalize this disturbance. In light of experimental evidence suggesting that hyponatremia of even moderate degree (125 mEq/liter or less) may result in irreversible neurologic deficits if allowed to persist, it seems reasonable to treat hyponatremia in all liver disease patients in whom the serum sodium level is less than 130 mEq/liter.

Another major consideration sometimes not given sufficient attention is the inappropriate use of drugs that may adversely affect renal diluting capacity. Specifically, there may be numerous drugs administered to the cirrhotic patient that could impair renal diluting capacity. Examples include NSAIDs and chlorpropamide. For a more complete listing, the reader is referred to another source.[33]

The use of agents that block the hydrosmotic effect of ADH, such as demeclocycline, for the correction of hyponatremia in cirrhosis has been suggested by various investigators.[28,78] In view of the numerous recent reports of the appearance of renal failure in such patients treated with demeclocycline,[28,78] this drug should not be administered to cirrhotic patients.

Finally, in rare circumstances, one may be forced to consider the use of dialysis for the correction of severe hyponatremia in cirrhosis.[94] Such heroic measures, however, rarely are necessary, even in the most severely decompensated cirrhotic patient.

Another development that holds promise is the imminent availability of vasopressin antagonists. The discovery of diuretic vasopressin analogs by Manning and Sawyer has spurred interest in designing vasopressin receptor antagonists as potential specific water diuretic (aquaretic) agents.[68,107] The mechanism of action is most probably antagonism of vasopressin at the renal epithelial receptor. The future availability of such vasopressin antagonists heralds a new class of potent aquaretic agents that may be potentially useful for the treatment of dilutional hyponatremia in patients with liver disease.

SYNDROMES OF ACUTE AZOTEMIA

ATN occurs with increased frequency in patients with hepatic and biliary disease. While acute azotemia may often represent classic ATN, cirrhotic patients may also develop a unique form of renal failure for which a specific cause cannot be elucidated—the hepatorenal syndrome (HRS). The following section reviews the spectrum of acute azotemic syndromes, including HRS and ATN in the setting of hepatic and biliary disease.

Hepatorenal Syndrome

Progressive oliguric renal failure commonly complicates the course of patients with advanced hepatic disease.[35,85] While this condition has been designated by many names, including "functional renal failure" and "the renal failure of cirrhosis," the more appealing albeit less specific term hepatorenal syndrome has been commonly used to describe this syndrome. For the purposes of this discussion, the HRS may be defined as unexplained progressive renal failure occurring in patients with liver disease in the absence of clinical, laboratory, or anatomic evidence of other known causes of renal failure.

Clinical Features

A review of the clinical features of HRS reveals marked variability regarding both the clinical presentation and clinical course.[35,85] In the United States, HRS occurs usually in cirrhotic patients who are alcoholic, although cirrhosis is not a *sine qua non* for the development of HRS. HRS may complicate other liver diseases, including acute hepatitis and hepatic malignancy.[49,96,114] Renal failure may develop with great rapidity, often occurring in patients in whom normal serum creatinine levels have been previously documented within a few days of onset of HRS. Recently, Papadakis and Arieff[84] have suggested that the serum creatinine level may be a poor index of renal function in patients with chronic liver disease, often masking markedly reduced GFRs. Implicit in such a formulation is the concept that HRS represents a progression in patients who already have markedly impaired renal function.

Numerous reports have emphasized the development of renal failure following events that reduce effective blood volume, including abdominal paracentesis, vigorous diuretic therapy, and gastrointestinal tract bleeding, although it can occur in the absence of an apparent precipitating event. In this context, several careful observers have recently noted that HRS patients seldom arrive in the hospital with preexisting renal failure. Rather, HRS seems to develop in the hospital, raising questions as to whether events in the hospital might precipitate this syndrome.[85] Virtually all HRS patients have ascites, which is often tense, and clinical stigmata of portal hypertension are usually present. The degree of jaundice is extremely variable. Although the majority of reports suggest that HRS occurs in patients who manifest evidence of severe hepatocellular disease, it is quite apparent that HRS can occur with minimal jaundice and with little evidence of severe hepatic dysfunction.

The majority of patients have a modest decrease in systemic blood pressure, but significant hypotension occurs usually as a terminal event. Most patients die within 3 weeks of onset of azotemia, although occasional recoveries occur.[60] Rare patients have survived for several months with mild azotemia.

HRS patients manifest a rather characteristic urine excretory pattern, voiding urine that is practically sodium free and retaining the capacity to concentrate urine to a modest degree.

Pathogenesis

Several lines of evidence have lent strong support to the concept that the renal failure in HRS is functional in nature. Despite the severe derangement of renal function, pathologic abnormalities are minimal and inconsistent.[35,85,103] Furthermore, tubular functional integrity is maintained during the renal failure as manifested by an unimpaired sodium reabsorptive capacity and concentrating ability. Finally, more direct evidence is derived from the demonstration that kidneys transplanted from patients with HRS are capable of resuming normal function in the recipient.[70]

Despite extensive study, the precise pathogenesis of HRS remains obscure. Many studies utilizing diverse hemodynamic techniques have all documented a significant reduction in renal perfusion.[41,66,100] Since a similar reduction of renal perfusion is compatible with urine volumes exceeding 1 liter in many patients with chronic renal failure,[64] it is unlikely that a reduction in mean blood flow *per se* is responsible for the encountered oliguria.

Our laboratory has applied the ^{133}Xe washout technique and selective renal arteriography to the study of HRS and has demonstrated a significant reduction in both mean renal blood flow and preferential reduction in cortical perfusion.[41] In addition, we carried out simultaneous renal arteriography to delineate further the nature of the hemodynamic abnormalities.[41] Selective renal arteriograms disclosed marked beading and tortuosity of the interlobar and proximal arcuate arteries and an absence of both distinct cortical nephrograms and vascular filling of the cortical vessels (Fig. 23-7, *A*). Postmortem angiography carried out on the kidneys of five patients studied previously during life disclosed a striking normalization of the vascular abnormalities, with reversal of all the vascular abnormalities in the kidneys (Fig. 23-7, *B*). The peripheral vasculature filled completely, and the previously irregular vessels became smooth and regular. These findings provide additional strong evidence for the functional basis of the renal failure, operating through active renal vasoconstriction.

Although renal hypoperfusion with preferential renal cortical ischemia has been shown to underly the renal failure of HRS, the factors responsible for sustaining the reductions in cortical perfusion and the suppression of filtration in HRS have not been elucidated. Several major

hypotheses have been implicated or suggested, including the renin–angiotensin system, alterations in the endogenous release of renal prostaglandins, an increase in sympathetic nervous system activity, changes in the kallikrein–kinin system, and endotoxemia. These proposed mechanisms and their interrelationships are summarized schematically in Figure 23-8.

Renin–Angiotensin System. Several lines of evidence have suggested a role for the renin–angiotensin axis in sustaining the vasoconstriction in HRS.[63] Patients with decompensated cirrhosis with or without HRS frequently manifest marked elevations of plasma renin–angiotensin levels attributable to both decreased hepatic inactivation of renin and increased renin secretion by the kidney[63,99] (Fig. 23-

Fig. 23-7. Left. Selective renal arteriogram performed in a patient with oliguric renal failure and cirrhosis. Note the extreme abnormality of the intrarenal vessels, including the primary branches off the main renal artery and the interlobar arteries. The arcuate and cortical arterial system is not recognizable, nor is a distinct cortical nephrogram present. The arrow indicates the edge of the kidney. (Reproduced with permission from Epstein M, Berk DP, Hollenberg NK et al: Renal failure in the patient with cirrhosis. The role of active vasoconstriction. Am J Med 49:175–185, 1970) **Right.** Angiogram performed postmortem on the same kidney with the intra-arterial injection of micropaque in gelatin as the contrast agent. Note filling of the renal arterial system throughout the vascular bed to the periphery of the cortex. The peripheral arterial tree that did not opacify *in vivo* now fills completely. The vascular attenuation and tortuosity are no longer present. The vessels were also histologically normal. (Reproduced with permission from Epstein M, Berk DP, Hollenberg NK et al: Renal failure in the patient with cirrhosis. The role of active vasoconstriction. Am J Med 49:175–185, 1970)

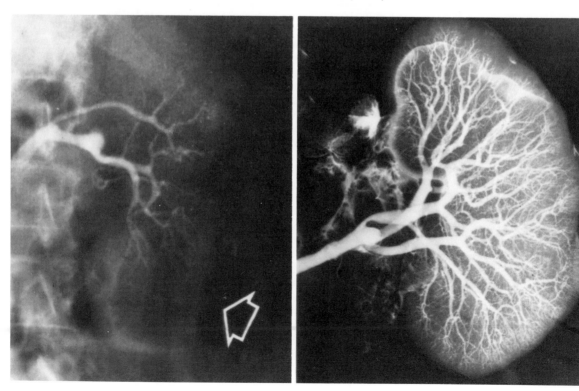

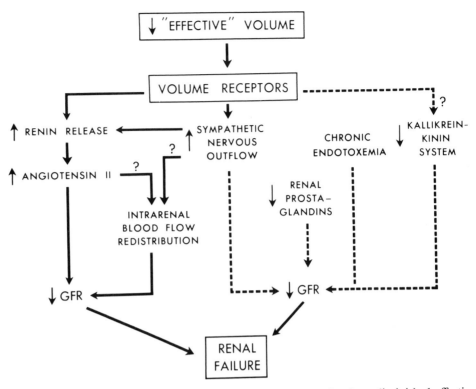

Fig. 23-8. Schematic representation of possible mechanisms whereby a diminished effective volume might modulate a number of hormonal effectors, eventuating in renal failure. Solid arrows indicate pathways for which evidence is available; dashed arrows represent proposed pathways, the existence of which remains to be established.

9). Often, the elevation of plasma renin–angiotensin occurs despite the presumed failure of hepatic synthesis of the α_2-globulin, renin substrate. There are at least two alternative explanations for the persistence of high renin levels in cirrhosis. First, it is possible that the renal hypoperfusion is the primary event, with a resultant activation of the renin–angiotensin system. Alternatively, the activation of the renin–angiotensin system (perhaps in response to a diminished effective blood volume) may constitute the primary event. In light of compelling experimental evidence that angiotensin plays an important role in the control of the renal circulation,[64] it is tempting to speculate that enhanced angiotensin levels contribute to the renal vasoconstriction and reduction in filtration rate of renal failure in cirrhosis (Fig. 23-9).

Renal Prostaglandins. It is probable that renal prostaglandins participate in mediating the renal failure of cirrhosis. Initially, this possibility was assessed by examining the renal hemodynamic response to the administration of exogenous prostaglandins.[1] Unfortunately, the relevance of such studies in cirrhotic persons is tenuous, since recent studies suggest that any action of prostaglandins on the kidney must be as a local tissue hormone.[77] Thus,

any evaluation of the physiologic role of prostaglandins on renal function necessitates an experimental design in which the endogenous production of the lipids is altered. Indeed, subsequent investigations of the role of prostaglandins on renal function have focused on comparisons before and after the administration of inhibitors of prostaglandin synthetase. Such studies have demonstrated that the administration of inhibitors of prostaglandin synthetase (both indomethacin and ibuprofen) resulted in a lowering of plasma renin–angiotensin and plasma aldosterone levels and marked decrements in GFR.[11,118]

Thromboxanes and Renal Function in Cirrhosis. Studies conducted by Zipser and co-workers[120] suggest that the ratio of the vasodilator PGE_2 to the vasoconstrictor prostaglandin thromboxane A_2 (TxA_2) (*i.e.,* E_2/TxA_2) rather than the absolute levels of PGE_2 may modulate the renal vasoconstriction of HRS. Urinary excretion of PGE_2 and thromboxane B_2 (TxB_2) (the nonenzymatic metabolite of Tx_2) was measured in 14 patients with HRS. It was observed that whereas PGE_2 levels were decreased in comparison with those of healthy controls and patients with ATN, TxB_2 levels were markedly elevated. The authors interpreted their data to suggest that an imbalance of va-

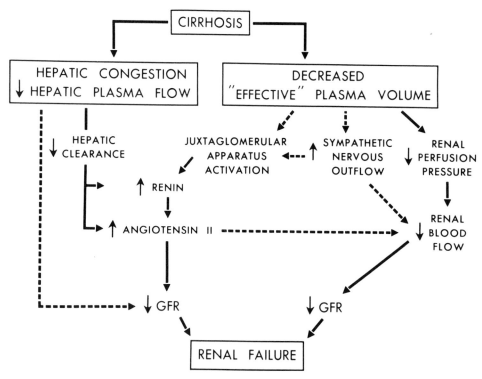

Fig. 23-9. Schematic drawing of probable mechanisms whereby the renin–angiotensin system and the sympathetic nervous system interact to produce renal failure. Both a diminished effective volume and impaired hepatic clearance of renin–angiotensin result in a marked enhancement of circulating PRA with a resultant decrease in GFR. An increase in sympathetic nervous system activity (possibly attributable to decreased effective volume) decreases GFR both by diminishing renal perfusion and by activating the renin–angiotensin system.

sodilator and vasoconstrictor metabolites of arachidonic acid contributes to the pathogenesis of HRS. Additional studies are needed to confirm such alterations.

Of interest, there has been a recent attempt to modify the course of HRS by administration of selective inhibitors of thromboxane synthesis.[119] Whereas *nonspecific* cyclooxygenase inhibitors, such as indomethacin and aspirin, reduce both thromboxane and prostaglandin synthesis to varying degrees in different biologic systems, *selective* inhibitors of thromboxane synthesis preserve or possibly increase the production of other metabolites of arachidonic acid, such as the potent vasodilator prostacyclin. Zipser and associates[119] administered the thromboxane synthetase inhibitor, dazoxiben, to patients with alcoholic hepatitis and progressive azotemia. Although administration of dazoxiben reduces the urinary excretion of the thromboxane metabolite, TxB_2 by approximately 50%, PGE_2 and 6-keto PGF_{1a} were essentially unaltered. Despite reduction in thromboxane excretion, there was no consistent reversal of the progressive renal deterioration.[119] Unfortunately, most of the patients had far advanced disease and may not have been capable of responding to therapeutic interventions. Additional studies with selective

thromboxane inhibitors in patients with widely varying degrees of acute renal insufficiency will be required to establish definitively the role of TxA_2 as a major determinant of the renal vasoconstriction in HRS.

Kallikrein–Kinin System. The available evidence suggests that bradykinin and other kinins synthesized in the kidney may participate in the modulation of intrarenal blood flow and renal function. Measurements of plasma prekallikrein levels in patients with HRS disclosed undetectable levels in many such patients,[82] raising the possibility that the decrease in prekallikrein levels results in diminished kinin formation. Since bradykinin has been suggested to be a physiologic renal vasodilator, it is possible that failure of bradykinin formation may contribute to the renal cortical vasoconstriction encountered in HRS.

Endotoxins. It has been proposed that systemic endotoxemia may participate in the pathogenesis of the renal failure of cirrhosis.[75] The increased endotoxin levels might result from incomplete hepatic inactivation and portal-systemic shunts of material of gastrointestinal origin in cirrhotic patients. Since several investigators have indeed demonstrated a high frequency of positive Limulus assays in cirrhotic patients with renal failure, but not in the absence of renal failure, it is conceivable that endotoxins might contribute to the pathogenesis of the renal failure. This interesting hypothesis awaits additional study and confirmation.

Acute Vasomotor Nephropathy

Although much attention has been directed to HRS, it must be emphasized that cirrhotic patients are no less vulnerable than noncirrhotic patients to the development of ATN. Indeed, a review of several published series discloses that among liver disease patients who developed renal failure, the etiology of the renal failure was more commonly ATN than HRS.[35] The increased frequency of ATN relates to the hypotension, bleeding dyscrasias, infection, and multiple metabolic disorders that often complicate the course of the patients.

Finally, the association between obstructive jaundice and ATN merits comment. Dawson noted that of patients undergoing operation for the relief of obstructive jaundice, the incidence of ATN was many times greater than that encountered in a comparable group of nonjaundiced patients.[26] It was further noted that the greater the degree of jaundice, the greater the risk of ATN. The demonstration that the risk of ATN is higher in the most deeply jaundiced patients prompted an investigation of the mechanisms in the Gunn rat (a species unable to conjugate bilirubin).[3] These studies suggest that circulating *conjugated* bilirubin was responsible for the increased proclivity of jaundiced animals to develop renal failure. It should be noted, however, that there is a lack of unanimity of opinion regarding the uniqueness of the association of biliary tract disease and ATN.[9]

Diuretic-Induced Azotemia

As noted earlier, cirrhotic patients who are being treated with diuretics frequently develop azotemia. While there is every reason to believe that this complication develops as a consequence of overly vigorous therapy in which negative fluid balances are attained, exceeding the maximal rate at which ascites can be mobilized, it has been proposed that mechanisms other than volume depletion *per se* may be causative.

Differential Diagnosis

The abrupt onset of oliguria in a cirrhotic patient does not necessarily imply the presence of HRS. Pre-renal causes are important to differentiate, particularly since they constitute reversible conditions if recognized and treated in the incipient phase. Volume contraction or cardiac pump failure may present as a "pseudohepatorenal" syndrome. Furthermore, as already mentioned, it is common for patients with alcoholic cirrhosis to develop classic ATN. In many instances the differentiation from HRS can be made readily by recognition of the precipitating event and by characteristic laboratory findings. Table 23-2 lists laboratory features helpful in differentiating the three principal causes of acute azotemia in the patient with liver disease. The most uniform finding in the urine of HRS patients is a strikingly low sodium concentration, usually less than 10 mEq/liter, and occasionally as low as 2 mEq to 5 mEq/liter. Similarly, pre-renal azotemia is associated with low urinary sodium concentrations. In contrast, patients with oliguric ATN frequently have urinary sodium concentrations exceeding 30 mEq/liter and usually even higher. Both HRS and pre-renal azotemia manifest well-maintained urinary concentrating ability characterized by a urine to plasma osmolality ratio (U/Posm) greater than 1.0, whereas ATN patients excrete an isosmotic urine. Urine to plasma creatinine ratio (U/P creatinine) is greater than 30 in both pre-renal failure and HRS, whereas U/P creatinine is less than 20:1 in ATN. Proteinuria is absent or minimal in HRS.

In summary, the finding of a low urinary sodium concentration in the presence of oliguric ATN precludes the diagnosis of ATN. Only when pre-renal failure and ATN are excluded can one establish the diagnosis of HRS.

Treatment

The management of the HRS is discouraging in view of the absence of any effective treatment modality. Since

---

TABLE 23-2.   Differential Diagnosis of Acute Azotemia in the Patient with Liver Disease: Important Differential Urinary Findings

	PRERENAL AZOTEMIA	HEPATORENAL SYNDROME (HRS)	ACUTE RENAL FAILURE (ATN)
Urine sodium concentration (mEq/liter)	<10	<10	>30
Urine to plasma creatinine ratio	>30:1	>30:1	<20:1
Urine osmolality	At least 100 mosm > plasma osmolality	At least 100 mosm > plasma osmolality	Equal to plasma osmolality
Urine sediment	Normal	Unremarkable	Casts, cellular debris

knowledge about the pathogenesis of HRS is inferential and incomplete, therapy must be primarily supportive. The initial step in management is not to equate decreased renal function with HRS, but rather to search diligently for and treat correctable causes of azotemia such as volume contraction, cardiac decompensation, and urinary tract obstruction. The diagnosis of ATN should be considered, since cirrhotic patients with ATN may recover if supported with dialytic therapy.

Once the correctable causes of renal functional impairment are excluded, the mainstay of therapy is careful restriction of sodium and fluid intake. While a number of specific therapeutic measures have been attempted, none has proved to be of practical value. Attempts at volume expansion with different exogenous expanders and exchange transfusion have resulted in only transient improvement in renal hemodynamics and function without significant improvement in the outcome.[35,65,111] Similarly, attempts at reinfusion of ascites utilizing peritoneal fluid that has been concentrated have not provided any lasting improvement.

Dialysis has been reported to be ineffective in the management of HRS. My own experience, however, suggests that such a sweeping condemnation should be qualified. Although most of the published literature indeed suggests a dismal prognosis for patients who are dialyzed, such reports have dealt with patients with chronic end-stage liver disease.[88] Our experience suggests that in selected patients, that is, patients with *acute* hepatic dysfunction in whom there is reason to believe that the renal failure may reverse coincident with resolution of the acute hepatic insult, dialytic therapy is indicated.

The most recent development in the management of HRS is the introduction of the peritoneojugular shunt.[39,67,90] The past several years have witnessed a flurry of enthusiasm for the use of the peritoneojugular shunt (LeVeen shunt) in the management of HRS. Unfortunately, many reports have been anecdotal with insufficient details to allow critical assessment. Even where sufficient data were available, we must conclude that the majority of putative "successes" occurred in patients who were not clearly documented to have HRS; rather, many patients probably had reversible azotemia secondary to a diminished effective blood volume. Furthermore, there is increasing awareness that the widespread utilization of the peritoneojugular shunt has been attended by a wide array of complications.[39,61]

In my opinion, a few well-documented cases in which the peritoneojugular shunt was successful in reversing HRS does not justify the growing and uncritical trend to resort to this modality in the treatment of virtually any cirrhotic patient with azotemia. The peritoneojugular shunt cannot yet be viewed as established therapy until its value is determined by appropriate peer-reviewed clinical trials. At present, I would consider its use in hemodynamically stable HRS patients in whom hypovolemia has been clearly excluded. It is hoped that in the next few years several ongoing clinical trials will assist us in selecting those HRS candidates who stand to benefit most from such a procedure.

CONCLUSION

In summary, it is apparent that the renal functional abnormalities in patients with advanced liver disease constitute complex pathophysiologic constellations with numerous and diverse causes. Although our understanding of the many ways by which the liver affects renal processes is inevitably incomplete, it is apparent that the past several years have witnessed much progress in the delineation of the abnormalities of renal sodium and water handling that characterize advanced liver disease. Advances in the measurement of renal vasoactive hormones (including renal licosanoids), which have recently been demonstrated to affect renal hemodynamics and renal sodium handling, are providing a basis for a more complete understanding of the mechanisms that promote sodium retention in cirrhosis. These insights provide a more rational basis for the management of the patient with liver disease who has impairment of renal sodium and water excretion.

Although there has been some progress in characterizing the pathogenesis of HRS, therapy of this disorder is largely empirical. It is apparent that any future breakthroughs in the definitive treatment of HRS will be predicated on greater clarification of mechanisms and delineation of mediators. The role of hemodialysis has recently undergone reappraisal, and it is apparent that dialysis may be warranted as a supportive measure in some patients with reversible hepatic dysfunction. Preliminary studies suggest that the peritoneojugular shunt may have a role in the management of selected patients with HRS.

Portions of this chapter have been modified and adapted from an earlier review by the author: Epstein ME: Renal sodium handling in liver disease. In The Kidney in Liver Disease, 2nd ed, pp 25–53. New York, Elsevier, 1982.

REFERENCES

1. Arieff AI, Chidsey CA: Renal function in cirrhosis and the effects of prostaglandin A_1. Am J Med 56:695, 1974
2. Arroyo V, Rodes J, Gutierrez–Lizarraga MA et al: Prognostic value of spontaneous hyponatremia in cirrhosis with ascites. Digest Dis 21:249, 1976
3. Baum M, Stirling GA, Dawson JL: Further study into obstructive jaundice and ischaemic renal damage. Br Med J 2:229, 1969
4. Benet LZ: Pharmacokinetics/pharmacodynamics of furosemide in man: A review. J Pharmacokinet Biopharm 7:1, 1979
5. Better OS, Schrier RW: Disturbed volume homeostasis in patients with cirrhosis of the liver. Kidney Int 23:303, 1983
6. Bichet D, Szatalowicz V, Chaimovitz C et al: Role of vasopressin in abnormal water excretion in cirrhotic patients. Ann Intern Med 96:413, 1982
7. Bichet DG, Groves BM, Schrier RW: Mechanisms of improvement of water and sodium excretion by immersion

in decompensated cirrhotic patients. Kidney Int 24:788, 1983

8. Bichet DG, VanPutten VJ, Schrier RW: Potential role of increased sympathetic activity in impaired sodium and water excretion in cirrhosis. N Engl J Med 307:1552, 1982

9. Bismuth H, Kuntziger H, Corlette MB: Cholangitis with acute renal failure. Ann Surg 181:881, 1975

10. Bosch J, Arroyo V, Rodes J et al: Compensacion espontanea de la ascites en la cirrosis hepatica. Rev Clin Esp 133:441, 1974

11. Boyer TD, Zia P, Reynolds TB: Effect of indomethacin and prostaglandin A_1 on renal function and plasma renin activity in alcoholic liver disease. Gastroenterology 77:215, 1979

12. Brater DC, Anderson S, Baird B et al: Effects of ibuprofen, naproxen, and sulindac on prostaglandins in men. Kidney Int 27:66, 1985

13. Buckalew VM Jr, Gruber KA: Natriuretic hormone. In Epstein M (ed): The Kidney in Liver Disease, 2nd ed, pp 479–499. New York, Elsevier, 1983

14. Bunning RD, Barth WF: Sulindac: A potentially renal-sparing nonsteroidal antiinflammatory drug. JAMA 248:1864, 1982

15. Chaimovitz C, Rochman J, Eidelman S et al: Exaggerated natriuretic response to volume expansion in patients with primary biliary cirrhosis. Am J Med Sci 274:173, 1977

16. Chaimovitz C, Szylman P, Alroy G et al: Mechanism of increased renal tubular sodium reabsorption in cirrhosis. Am J Med 52:198, 1972

17. Chennavasin P, Sciwell R, Brater DC: Pharmacokinetic-dynamic analysis of the indomethacin-furosemide interaction in man. J Pharmacol Exp Ther 215:77, 1980

18. Chiandusi L, Bartoli E, Arras S: Reabsorption of sodium in the proximal renal tubule in cirrhosis of the liver. Gut 19:497, 1978

19. Ciabottoni G, Cinotti GA, Pierucci A et al: Effects of sulindac and ibuprofen in patients with chronic glomerular disease: Evidence for the dependence of renal function on prostacyclin. N Engl J Med 310:279, 1984

20. Conn HO: Diuresis of ascites: Fraught with or free from hazard. Gastroenterology 73:619, 1977

21. Conn HO: The rational management of ascites. In Popper H, Schaffner F (eds): Progress in Liver Disease, vol 4, pp 269–288. New York, Grune & Stratton, 1972

22. Conn HO, Fessell JM: Spontaneous bacterial peritonitis in cirrhosis: Variations on a theme. Medicine 50:161, 1971

23. Coppage WS Jr, Island DP, Cooner AE et al: The metabolism of aldosterone in normal subjects and in patients with hepatic cirrhosis. J Clin Invest 41:1672, 1962

24. Daskalopoulos G, Kronborg I, Katkov et al: Sulindac and indomethacin suppress the diuretic action of furosemide in patients with cirrhosis and ascites: Evidence that sulindac affects renal prostaglandins. Am J Kidney Dis (in press)

25. Data JL, Rane A, Gerkens J et al: The influence of indomethacin on the pharmacokinetics, diuretic response and hemodynamics of furosemide in the dog. J Pharmacol Exp Ther 207:431. 1978

26. Dawson JL: The incidence of postoperative renal failure in obstructive jaundice. Br J Surg 52:663, 1965

27. De Bold AJ, Borenstein HR, Veress AT et al: A rapid and potent natriuretic response to intravenous injection of atrial myocardial extracts in rats. Life Sci 28:89, 1981

28. DeTroyer A, Pilloy W, Broeckaert I et al: Demeclocycline

treatment of water retention in cirrhosis. Ann Intern Med 85:336, 1976

29. DiBona GF: Renal neural activity in hepatorenal syndrome. Kidney Int 25:841, 1984

30. Eisenmenger WJ, Blondheim SH, Bongiovanni AM et al: Electrolyte studies on patients with cirrhosis of the liver. J Clin Invest 29:1491, 1950

31. Epstein M: Aldosterone in liver disease. In Epstein M (ed): The Kidney in Liver Disease, 2nd ed, pp 377–394. New York, Elsevier, 1983

32. Epstein M: Deranged sodium homeostasis in cirrhosis. Gastroenterology 76:622, 1979

33. Epstein M: Derangements of renal water handling in liver disease. Gastroenterology (in press)

34. Epstein M: Diuretic therapy in liver disease. In Eknoyan G, Martinez–Maldonado M (eds): The Physiological Basis of Diuretic Therapy in Clinical Medicine. Orlando, Grune & Stratton, 1986

35. Epstein M: Hepatorenal syndrome, In Berk JE (ed): Bockus Gastroenterology, 4th ed, pp 3138–3149. Philadelphia, WB Saunders, 1985

36. Epstein M: Renal effects of head-out water immersion in man: Implications for an understanding of volume homeostasis. Physiol Rev 58:529, 1978

37. Epstein M: Renal sodium handling in cirrhosis: A reappraisal. Nephron 23:211, 1979

38. Epstein M: Renal sodium handling in cirrhosis. In Epstein M (ed): The Kidney in Liver Disease, 2nd ed, pp 35–53. New York, Elsevier, 1983

39. Epstein M: The LeVeen shunt for ascites and hepatorenal syndrome. N Engl J Med 302:628, 1980

40. Epstein M (ed): The Kidney in Liver Disease, 2nd ed. New York, Elsevier, 1983

41. Epstein M, Berk DP, Hollenberg NK et al: Renal failure in the patient with cirrhosis: The role of active vasoconstriction. Am J Med 49:175, 1970

42. Epstein M, Bricker NS, Bourgoignie JJ: The presence of a natriuretic factor in urine of normal men undergoing water immersion. Kidney Int 13:152, 1978

43. Epstein M, Larios O, Johnson G: Effects of water immersion on plasma catecholamines in decompensated cirrhosis: Implications for deranged sodium and water homeostasis. Mineral Electrolyte Metab 11:25, 1985

44. Epstein M, Lepp BA, Hoffman DS et al: Potentiation of furosemide by metolazone in refractory edema. Curr Ther Res 21:656, 1977

45. Epstein M, Levinson R, Sancho J et al: Characterization of the renin-aldosterone system in decompensated cirrhosis. Circ Res 41:818, 1977

46. Epstein M, Lifschitz M, Hoffman DS et al: Relationship between renal prostaglandin E and renal sodium handling during water immersion in normal man. Circ Res 45:71, 1979

47. Epstein M, Lifschitz M, Ramachandran M et al: Characterization of renal PGE responsiveness in decompensated cirrhosis: Implications for renal sodium handling. Clin Sci 63:555, 1982

48. Epstein M, Loutzenhiser R, Friedland E et al: Stimulation of plasma ANF in normal humans by immersion-induced central hypervolemia. Kidney Int 1985 (abstr)

49. Epstein M, Oster JR, DeVelasco RE: Hepatorenal syndrome following hemihepatectomy. Clin Nephrol 5:128, 1976

50. Epstein M, Pins DS, Arrington R et al: Comparison of water

immersion and saline infusion as a means of inducing volume expansion in man. J Appl Physiol 39:66, 1975

51. Epstein M, Pins DS, Schneider N et al: Determinants of deranged sodium and water homeostasis in decompensated cirrhosis. J Lab Clin Med 87:822, 1976

52. Epstein M, Ramachandran M, DeNunzio AG: Interrelationship of renal sodium and phosphate handling in cirrhosis. Mineral Electrolyte Metab 7:305, 1982

53. Epstein M, Re R, Preston S et al: Comparison of the suppressive effects of water immersion and saline administration on renin-aldosterone in normal man. J Clin Endocrinol Metab 49:358, 1979

54. Epstein M, Weitzman RE, Preston S et al: Relationship between plasma arginine vasopressin and renal water handling in decompensated cirrhosis. Mineral Electrolyte Metab 10:155, 1984

55. Faloon WW, Eckhardt RD, Cooper AM et al: The effect of human serum albumin, mercurial diuretics, and a low sodium diet on sodium excretion in patients with cirrhosis of the liver. J Clin Invest 28:595, 1949

56. Favre H: Role of the natriuretic factor in the disorders of sodium balance. Adv Nephrol 11:3, 1981

57. Folkow B, DiBona G, Hjemdahl P et al: Measurements of plasma norepinephrine concentrations in human primary hypertension: A word of caution concerning their applicability for assessing neurogenic contribution. Hypertension 5:399, 1983

58. Gabuzda GJ: Cirrhosis, ascites, and edema: Clinical course related to management. Gastroenterology 58:546, 1970

59. Gauer OH: Mechanoreceptors in the intrathoracic circulation and plasma volume control. In Epstein M (ed): The Kidney in Liver Disease, 1st ed, pp 3–17. New York, Elsevier, 1978

60. Goldstein H, Boyle JD: Spontaneous recovery from the hepatorenal syndrome: Report of four cases. N Engl J Med 272:895, 1965

61. Greig PD, Langer B, Blendis LM et al: Complications after peritoneovenous shunting for ascites. Am J Surg 139:125, 1980

62. Hippocrates. Cited in Atkinson M: Ascites in liver disease. Postgrad Med J 32:482, 1956

63. Hollenberg NK: Renin, angiotensin and the kidney: Assessment by pharmacological interruption of the renin-angiotensin system. In Epstein M (ed): The Kidney in Liver Disease, 2nd ed, pp 395–411. New York, Elsevier, 1983

64. Hollenberg NK, Epstein M, Basch RI et al: Acute oliguric renal failure in man: Evidence for preferential renal cortical ischemia. Medicine 47:455, 1968

65. Horisawa M, Reynolds TB: Exchange transfusion in hepatorenal syndrome with liver disease. Arch Intern Med 136:1135, 1976

66. Kew MC, Varma RR, Williams HS et al: Renal and intrarenal blood flow in cirrhosis of the liver. Lancet 2:504, 1971

67. Kinney MJ, Wapnick S, Ahmed N et al: Cirrhosis, ascites, and impaired renal function: Treatment with the LeVeen-type chronic peritoneal-venous shunt. In Epstein M (ed): The Kidney in Liver Disease, 1st ed, pp 349–364. New York, Elsevier, 1978

68. Kinter LB, Huffman WF, Wiebelhaus VD et al: Renal effects of aquaretic vasopressin analogs in vivo. In Puschett JB (ed): Diuretics, pp 75–81. New York, Elsevier, 1984

69. Klingler EL Jr, Vaamonde CA, Vaamonde LS et al: Renal function changes in cirrhosis of the liver. Arch Intern Med 125:1010, 1970

70. Koppel MH, Coburn JW, Mims MM et al: Transplantation of cadaveric kidneys from patients with hepatorenal syndrome: Evidence for the functional nature of renal failure in advanced liver disease. N Engl J Med 280:1367, 1969

71. Levy M: Observations on renal function and ascites formation in dogs with experimental portal cirrhosis. In Epstein M (ed): The Kidney in Liver Disease, 1st ed, pp 131–142. New York, Elsevier, 1978

72. Levy M, Wexler MJ, McCaffrey C: Sodium retention in dogs with experimental cirrhosis following removal of ascites by continuous peritoneovenous shunting. J Lab Clin Med 94:933, 1979

73. Lieberman FL, Denison EK, Reynolds TB: The relationship of plasma volume, portal hypertension, ascites and renal sodium retention in cirrhosis: The overflow theory of ascites formation. Ann NY Acad Sci 170:202, 1970

74. Lieberman FL, Ito S, Reynolds TB: Effective plasma volume in cirrhosis with ascites: Evidence that a decreased value does not account for renal sodium retention, a spontaneous reduction in glomerular filtration rate (GFR) and a fall in GFR during drug-induced diuresis. J Clin Invest 48:975, 1969

75. Liehr H, Jacob AI: Endotoxin and renal failure in liver disease. In Epstein M (ed): The Kidney in Liver Disease, 2nd ed, pp 535–547. New York, Elsevier, 1983

76. Maack T, Marion DN, Camargo MJF et al: Effects of auriculin (atrial natriuretic factor) on blood pressure, renal function, and the renin-aldosterone system in dogs. Am J Med 77:1069, 1984

77. McGiff JC, Itskovitz HD: Prostaglandins and the kidney. Circ Res 33:479, 1973

78. Miller PD, Linas SL, Schrier RW: Plasma demeclocycline levels and nephrotoxicity: Correlation in hyponatremic cirrhotic patients. JAMA 243:2513, 1980

79. Mirouze D, Zipser RD, Reynolds TB: Effect of inhibitors of prostaglandin synthesis on induced diuresis in cirrhosis. Hepatology 3:50, 1983

80. Naccarato R, Messa P, D'Angelo A et al: Renal handling of sodium and water in early chronic liver disease. Gastroenterology 81:205, 1981

81. Naranjo CA, Pontigo E, Valdenegro C et al: Furosemide-induced adverse reactions in cirrhosis of the liver. Clin Pharmacol Ther 25:154, 1979

82. O'Connor DT, Stone RA: The renal kallikrein-kinin system: Description and relationship to liver disease. In Epstein M (ed): The Kidney in Liver Disease, 2nd ed, pp 469–475. New York, Elsevier, 1983

83. Oster JR, Epstein M, Smoller S: Combined therapy with thiazide-type and loop diuretic agents for resistant sodium retention. Ann Intern Med 99:405, 1983

84. Papadakis MA, Arieff AI: Progressive deterioration of renal function in non-azotemic cirrhotic patients with ascites: A prospective study. Kidney Int 27:149, 1985 (abstr)

85. Papper S: Hepatorenal syndrome. In Epstein M (ed): The Kidney in Liver Disease, 2nd ed, pp 87–106. New York, Elsevier, 1983

86. Papper S, Saxon L: The diuretic response to administered water in patients with liver disease: II. Laennec's cirrhosis of the liver. Arch Intern Med 103:750, 1959

87. Perez-Ayuso RM, Arroyo V, Camps J et al: Evidence that renal prostaglandins are involved in renal water metabolism in cirrhosis. Kidney Int 26:72, 1984

88. Perez GO, Oster JR: A critical review of the role of dialysis in the treatment of liver disease. In Epstein M (ed): The Kidney in Liver Disease, 1st ed, pp 325–336. New York, Elsevier, 1978

89. Perez GO, Oster JR: Altered potassium metabolism in liver disease. In Epstein M (ed): The Kidney in Liver Disease, 2nd ed, pp 147–182. New York, Elsevier, 1983

90. Pladson TR, Parrish RM: Hepatorenal syndrome: Recovery after peritoneovenous shunt. Arch Intern Med 137:1248, 1977

91. Planas R, Arroyo B, Rimola A et al: Acetylsalicyclic acid suppresses the renal hemodynamic effect and reduces the diuretic action of furosemide in cirrhosis with ascites. Gastroenterology 84:247, 1983

92. Raymond KH, Lifschitz MD: Effects of prostaglandins on renal salt and water excretion. Am J Med (in press)

93. Reznick RK, Langer B, Taylor BR et al: Hyponatremia and arginine vasopressin secretion in patients with refractory hepatic ascites undergoing peritoneovenous shunting. Gastroenterology 84:713, 1983

94. Ring–Larsen H, Clausen E, Ranck L: Peritoneal dialysis in hyponatremia due to liver failure. Scand J Gastroenterol 8:33, 1973

95. Ring–Larsen H, Hesse B, Henriksen JH et al: Sympathetic nervous activity and renal and systemic hemodynamics in cirrhosis: Plasma norepinephrine concentration, hepatic extraction and renal release. Hepatology 2:304, 1982

96. Ritt DJ, Whelan G, Werner DJ et al: Acute hepatic necrosis with stupor or coma. Medicine 48:151, 1969

97. Rosoff L Jr, Zia P, Reynolds T et al: Studies of renin and aldosterone in cirrhotic patients with ascites. Gastroenterology 69:698, 1975

98. Schedl HP, Bartter FC: An explanation for and experimental correction of the abnormal water diuresis in cirrhosis. J Clin Invest 39:248, 1960

99. Schroeder ET, Eich RH, Smulyan H et al: Plasma renin level in hepatic cirrhosis. Am J Med 49:186, 1970

100. Schroeder ET, Shear L, Sancetta SM et al: Renal failure in patients with cirrhosis of the liver: III. Evaluation of intrarenal blood flow by para-amino-hippurate extraction and response to angiotensin. Am J Med 43:887, 1967

101. Shear L, Ching S, Gabuzda GJ: Compartmentalization of ascites and edema in patients with hepatic cirrhosis. N Engl J Med 282:1391, 1970

102. Shear L, Hall PW, Gabuzda GJ: Renal failure in patients with cirrhosis of the liver: II. Factors influencing maximal urinary flow rate. Am J Med 39:199, 1965

103. Shear L, Kleinerman J, Gabuzda GJ: Renal failure in patients with cirrhosis of the liver: I. Clinical and pathologic characteristics. Am J Med 39:184, 1965

104. Sherlock S: Ascites formation and its management. Scand J Gastroenterol 7(suppl):9, 1970

105. Sherlock S: Ascites formation in cirrhosis and its management. Scand J Gastroenterol 7(suppl):9, 1970

106. Smith DE, Brater DC, Lin ET et al: Attenuation of furosemide's diuretic effect of indomethacin: Pharmacokinetic evaluation. J Pharmacokinet Biopharm 7:265, 1979

107. Stassen FL, Heckman GD, Schmidt DB et al: Actions of vasopressin antagonists: Molecular mechanisms. In Schrier RW (ed): Vasopressin. New York, Raven Press

108. Stokes JB: Integrated actions of renal medullary prostaglandins in the control of water excretion. Am J Physiol 9: F471, 1981

109. Strauss MB, Birchard WH, Saxon L: Correction of impaired water excretion in cirrhosis of the liver by alcohol ingestion or expansion of extracellular fluid volume: The role of the antidiuretic hormone. Trans Assoc Am Physicians 69:222, 1956

110. Thames MD: Neural control of renal function: Contribution of cardiopulmonary baroreceptors to the control of the kidney. Fed Proc 37:1209, 1977

111. Tristani FE, Cohn JN: Systemic and renal hemodynamics in oliguric hepatic failure: Effect of volume expansion. J Clin Invest 46:1894, 1967

112. Tweeddale MG, Ogilvie RI: Antagonism of spironolactone-induced natriuresis by aspirin in man. N Engl J Med 289: 198, 1973

113. Vaamonde CA: Renal water handling in liver disease. In Epstein M (ed): The Kidney in Liver Disease, 2nd ed, pp 55–86. New York: Elsevier, 1983

114. Vesin P, Roberti A, Viguie RR: Defaillance renale fonctionnelle terminale chez des malades atteints de cancer du foie, primitif ou secondaire. Sem Hop Paris 26:1216, 1965

115. Vlahcevic ZR, Adam NF, Jick H et al: Renal effects of acute expansion of plasma volume in cirrhosis. N Engl J Med 272:387, 1965

116. Witte MH, Witte CL, Dumont AE: Progress in liver disease: Physiological factors involved in the causation of cirrhotic ascites. Gastroenterology 61:742, 1971

117. Yeung Laiwah AC, Mactier RA: Antagonists effect of nonsteroidal anti-inflammatory drugs on furosemide-induced diuresis in cardiac failure. Br Med J 283:714, 1981

118. Zipser RD, Hoefs JC, Speckart PF et al: Prostaglandins: Modulators of renal function and pressor resistance in chronic liver disease. J Clin Endocrinol Metab 48:895, 1979

119. Zipser RD, Kronborg I, Rector W et al: Therapeutic trial of thromboxane synthesis inhibition in the hepatorenal syndrome. Gastroenterology 87:1228, 1984

120. Zipser RD, Radvan GH, Kronborg KJ et al: Urinary thromboxane B2 and prostaglandin E2 in the hepatorenal syndrome: Evidence for increased vasoconstrictor and decreased vasodilator factors. Gastroenterology 84:697, 1983

chapter 24

Hepatic Encephalopathy

LESLIE ZIEVE

This chapter is designed to give a comprehensive overview of hepatic encephalopathy and coma but will not attempt to provide a similar comprehensive citation of the primary literature that has made this synthesis possible. During the past 2 decades, several extensive reviews of hepatic coma appeared that cited the primary literature in detail and presented different perspectives on the subject.[31,57,62,86,122,136,170,175] Anyone seeking specific details on any facet of hepatic encephalopathy or coma mentioned in the following synthesis will benefit from these reviews, which provide additional information and the references desired.

DEFINITION

Hepatic encephalopathy leading to coma is a disorder of mentation, neuromuscular function, and consciousness occurring in patients with liver disease. It is a neuropsychiatric disturbance resulting primarily from metabolic abnormalities, the anatomic changes being insufficient to account for the manifestations, which are potentially entirely reversible. Episodes of hepatic encephalopathy may occur spontaneously or be induced by some precipitating factor. They may be endogenous or exogenous. Whatever the basis, the clinical manifestations are similar, allowing for variations due to the acuteness or intensity of the process. The spontaneous cases have no apparent precipitating factor, being the final consequence of extensive liver cell destruction. The induced cases are precipitated by known agents or abnormalities. The distinction has been losing its significance as our knowledge of the interplay among abnormal processes associated with hepatic failure has increased. As liver destruction proceeds, circulatory and metabolic alterations are produced that enhance the susceptibility of the individual to inducing agents. Therefore, the patient who is most likely to lapse into spontaneous hepatic coma is also most likely to have his coma induced by an extrahepatic abnormality or an exogenous agent. However, encephalopathy and coma may be induced in patients with fairly good hepatic function.

The predisposition to encephalopathy from exogenous agents is a result of the development of portal-systemic collaterals (shunts), electrolyte and acid–base imbalances, and hypoxemia and hypoxia, in addition to hepatic insufficiency. Aside from the liver damage, the portal-sys-temic shunts, which develop naturally in the course of cirrhosis or are produced surgically in an attempt to decompress the portal venous system, are of greatest importance. In fact, hepatic encephalopathy may be looked on as a portal-systemic encephalopathy resulting from the shunting of blood from the intestine around the liver as a whole or around viable hepatic cells during passage through the damaged liver. The liver is unable to metabolize normally such cerebrotoxic substances as ammonia and mercaptans originating in the intestine. The effects of shunting of blood around the liver and of hepatic cell dysfunction cannot be differentiated completely even in patients with a portacaval bypass and an apparently normal liver by histologic examination. Following an Eck fistula in normal animals, the liver urea cycle enzyme activities are reduced by 40% to 50%,[29] and liver cell function as reflected sensitively in the biliary transport maximum for sulfobromophthalein (BSP) is reduced by two thirds.[92]

VARIANTS

Hepatic or portal-systemic encephalopathy has various guises, depending on (1) the abruptness of onset and the severity and extent of the liver damage; (2) the extent of the portal-systemic collaterals or diversion; (3) the quantity and frequency of generation of noxious agents such as ammonia; (4) the degree of abnormality of predisposing factors; and (5) the severity (or excess) of some precipitating factor. A spectrum of presentations is seen, varying in the extremes from a brief hyperacute course to a chronic permanent state. Despite the wide variation in patterns that is seen, there is probably a common underlying pathogenetic mechanism that is multifactorial. The variant patterns of hepatic encephalopathy may be conveniently classified into four types:

1. Acute or subacute encephalopathy
2. Acute or subacute recurrent encephalopathy
3. Chronic recurrent encephalopathy
4. Chronic permanent encephalopathy or myelopathy

The distinction between the acute and subacute states is an arbitrary one, the acute cases being those with a rapid onset and short and intense course generally lasting only a few days. Patients with acute fulminant viral or toxic hepatitis and patients with Reye's syndrome have the most acute courses. However, patients with chronic liver diseases such as cirrhosis may follow an acute course once encephalopathy supervenes. The subacute cases have a more insidious onset with slower appearance of the fully manifested encephalopathy or coma and a less intense and more prolonged course often lasting more than a week. This is the typical pattern observed in the cirrhotic patient with terminal liver failure.

The acute or subacute recurrent type includes patients having more than one but not more than a few distinct episodes of hepatic encephalopathy of variable length and severity, with intervening periods when they have no overt manifestations of encephalopathy. Specific precipitating factors can usually be identified in association with the recurrent episodes.

Patients with the third type, chronic recurrent encephalopathy, are cirrhotics with an extensive portal collateral circulation who have many recurrences or, if untreated, prolonged persistence of mental, emotional, or neurologic abnormalities over a period of months or years but whose findings are reversible and controllable with suitable therapy.[143]

The fourth type is demonstrated by patients with chronic permanent encephalopathy or myelopathy; most but not all are cirrhotics with an extensive portal collateral circulation or a surgically created portal-systemic shunt. Most of the patients in this group develop a permanent neurologic abnormality resembling that seen in Wilson's disease but without the abnormality in copper metabolism. This syndrome, which has been called acquired chronic hepatocerebral degeneration, usually follows chronic recurrent episodes of hepatic encephalopathy associated with chronic hyperammonemia.[150] However, sometimes the neurologic syndrome precedes the first occurrence of a recognizable episode of overt encephalopathy. Thus, an abnormality other than that ordinarily associated with hepatic encephalopathy may be involved in the development of this neurologic syndrome, which follows a progressive course. A few of the patients of the fourth type develop a myelopathy in association with chronic recurrent episodes of hepatic encephalopathy. The spinal cord involvement is progressive and affects the lateral pyramidal tracts primarily.[63,150,176]

NEUROPATHOLOGY

Any disease of the liver that becomes destructive of liver parenchyma or results in abnormal shunting of blood around functioning liver tissue may predispose to hepatic encephalopathy. An occasional disease such as Reye's syndrome, with its selective mitochondrial injury, has biochemical effects leading to encephalopathy out of proportion to the apparent anatomic alterations in the liver. Other syndromes resulting in the accumulation of ammonia or fatty acids as a result of congenital hepatic enzyme deficiencies belong to this category. The pattern of cerebral dysfunction varies depending on the selective factors or on the acuteness or chronicity of the liver process and its associated complications. Thus, the liver pathology predisposing to hepatic encephalopathy varies widely.

In all of the variants of hepatic encephalopathy except the uncommon type with chronic permanent encephalopathy, the neuropathologic alterations are insufficient to account for the clinical manifestations. Thus, metabolic rather than anatomic abnormalities are the likely bases of this syndrome. In acute fulminant hepatic failure and in Reye's syndrome the only life-threatening abnormality in the brain at autopsy is cerebral edema, which is present in a high proportion of patients and may be the cause of death, especially in Reye's syndrome.[44,64,154] Although an important focus of therapy in these diseases, cerebral edema is in itself a nonspecific abnormality found in patients dying of various fulminant diseases affecting the brain.

In chronic liver diseases terminating with hepatic coma, changes in the glial cells are distinctive.[1] The protoplasmic astrocytes increase in number and size, taking on a characteristic appearance identified as the Alzheimer type II astrocyte. These cells frequently occur in pairs or clusters. Their nuclei are enlarged and have a watery or bubble-like appearance because they seem devoid of chromatin. A thin rim of cytoplasm surrounds the nucleus, so only the nuclei of these cells may be clearly visible in the sections. Mitoses are not seen, but the nuclei often contain periodic acid–Schiff (PAS)-positive inclusion bodies and may be deformed or lobulated. These distinctive cells are more numerous in all parts of the cerebral cortex, the basal ganglia, cerebellum, and brain stem, approaching twice the number seen in patients with chronic liver disease without overt encephalopathy or in normal controls. Similar increases in Alzheimer type II astrocytes have been observed in chronic hyperammonemia associated with congenital urea cycle enzyme deficiencies[17] or produced in animals experimentally by portacaval shunts, repeated infusions of an ammonium salt, or injections of urease.[31]

In cases of acquired hepatocerebral degeneration, one finds a diffuse increase in number and size of the protoplasmic astrocytes (Alzheimer type II cells), many of which have intranuclear PAS-positive inclusion bodies. In addition, in the deep layers of the cerebral cortex and subcortical white matter, the basal ganglia, and the cerebellum, there is diffuse but patchy laminar or pseudolaminar necrosis with degeneration of nerve cells and medullated fibers and zones of microcavitation giving a spongy appearance.[1,150] These abnormalities are similar to those seen in Wilson's disease, in which the changes in the basal ganglia are generally more marked and the degree of cerebral atrophy more noticeable. However, these two forms of hepatocerebral degeneration cannot be distinguished on the basis of neuropathology alone.

A rare patient with evidence of acquired hepatocerebral degeneration may have an associated myelopathy. Pyramidal tract demyelination resulting in spastic paraplegia is the usual finding, although, in some instances, demyelination of both the lateral and posterior columns is observed. Pyramidal tract demyelination has been observed in patients with chronic recurrent encephalopathy who showed no evidence of brain lesions other than proliferation of Alzheimer type II astrocytes.

Brain proteins measured in a few patients with cirrhosis within 24 hours of death following hepatic coma were found reduced by approximately one third, particularly in the gray matter.[15] In rats with portacaval shunts of 8 weeks' duration brain protein synthesis was reduced by 50%.[157]

The blood–brain barrier may be altered in hepatic encephalopathy. No data from patients are available. In totally hepatectomized rats, the blood–brain barrier remained intact for at least 18 hours.[72] As the encephalopathy progressed to its terminal phase the barrier became permeable to substances such as inulin, D-sucrose and trypan blue, which do not ordinarily cross into the brain.[66] Capillary endothelial vesicle formation and cerebral edema were associated with the increase in permeability.[124] Similar permeability results were observed after fulminant ischemic hepatic necrosis and severe galactosamine hepatitis.[163] Toxins that accumulate during hepatic failure (NH_4^+, mercaptan, octanoate, phenol) also increased blood–brain barrier permeability to inulin in rats.[162] In the foregoing studies, changes in cerebral blood volume, which might account for the results observed, were not measured or controlled. The brain uptake of neutral amino acids, especially tryptophan, was increased in conventional and germ-free rats after a portacaval shunt.[58,85] Studies using quantitative autoradiography indicated that the changes were most marked in several limbic structures and the reticular formation and least evident in the hypothalamus.[98] The observed amino acid uptakes and apparent permeability may possibly be artifactual results of the techniques used.[82] Thus the implications of the foregoing permeability studies are at present uncertain.

METABOLIC ABNORMALITIES

A host of abnormalities, which may be seen in the following list, occur in patients with liver failure progressing to hepatic encephalopathy and coma:

1. Respiratory or metabolic alkalosis or both (infrequently metabolic acidosis)
2. Electrolyte deficits
3. Decreased affinity of hemoglobin for oxygen
4. Hypoxemia and hypoxia
5. Hyperglycemia or hypoglycemia
6. Increased blood and cerebrospinal fluid (CSF) pyruvate, lactate, citrate, and α-ketoglutarate
7. Cerebral blood flow increased early, decreased late
8. Cerebral oxygen and glucose utilization normal early, decreased late
9. Reduced brain α-ketoglutarate, fumarate, malate, and oxaloacetate

10. Maintenance of balance between energy production and utilization by brain
11. Increased ammonia in blood, and increased ammonia, glutamine, and α-ketoglutaramate in brain and CSF
12. Increased brain and muscle ammonia utilization rates
13. Ammonia utilized and glutamine formed in small active brain compartments
14. Poor correlation between blood ammonia and severity of encephalopathy
15. Good correlation between CSF glutamine or α-ketoglutaramate and severity of encephalopathy
16. Increased short- and medium-chain fatty acids in plasma; decreased ketones
17. Mercaptans increased in blood, breath, brain and urine—probable cause of fetor hepaticus
18. Amino acids generally increased in blood, brain, CSF, and urine:
    a. Highest plasma levels: Met, Phe, Tyr, free Tyr, Asp, Glu
    b. Increased tyrosine derivatives (tyramine, phenols)
    c. Decreased branched-chain AA (Leu, Isoleu, Val)
19. Neurotransmitters generally decreased in brain and muscle, their metabolites increased in CSF, and false neurotransmitters increased in brain, muscle, blood, and urine:
    a. Increased CSF glutamine, asparagine, homovanillic acid, normetanephrine, indoleacetic acid (IAA), and 5-hydroxyindoleacetic acid (5-HIAA)
    b. Increased octopamine and phenylethanolamine in tissues and urine.
20. Through synergism, coma-producing potentials in animals of the toxins (ammonia, mercaptans, fatty acids, and phenols) and of the endogenous abnormalities (hypoxia, hypovolemia, and hypoglycemia) are increased. In combination, smaller doses and lower blood levels (or less abnormality) of each is required to produce coma.

None of the above abnormalities is pathognomonic. Some become most distinctive when encephalopathy supervenes. Others develop simultaneously with encephalopathy but are clearly unrelated to the presence of encephalopathy. This is particularly apparent in acute fulminant hepatic failure, a rapidly progressive illness in which many organ systems develop abnormalities in parallel with but independent of the occurrence of hepatic encephalopathy.[9,86] These complications include pulmonary edema, cardiac arrhythmias and other abnormalities, hypotension, functional renal failure or acute tubular necrosis, gastric erosions, hemorrhage, disorders of coagulation, intravascular coagulation and fibrinolysis, sepsis, endotoxemia, and acute pancreatitis. Some of these abnormalities, for example, sepsis and endotoxemia, may be causes as well as consequences of fulminant hepatic failure. The discussion that follows focuses on the abnormalities that become most distinctive with the development of encephalopathy.

Acid–Base and Electrolyte Balance

Acid–base imbalance probably plays an auxiliary role in the progression and outcome of hepatic encephalopathy. The abnormalities observed during encephalopathy are usually present before the development of encephalopathy. Depending on the extent and duration of respiratory or electrolyte abnormalities, the patient may have respiratory alkalosis, metabolic alkalosis, mixed respiratory and metabolic alkalosis, or metabolic acidosis.[167] The respiratory center is stimulated in the presence of hepatic failure, and hyperventilation leading to hypocapnia is present before it becomes clinically evident. This in itself significantly reduces cerebral blood flow. If hypokalemia is absent, the patient will generally have a compensated or uncompensated respiratory alkalosis. If hypokalemia is present, he will have a mixed respiratory and metabolic alkalosis. This is the usual variant seen. The hypocapnia is associated with a progressive accumulation of pyruvate, lactate, and other organic acids. If the process is severe enough, a metabolic acidosis will supervene. Cases with acidosis are usually complicated by circulatory and renal failure.

Theoretically, anything that increases the pH gradient between the extracellular and intracellular fluids favors the movement of ammonia into cells, because the partial pressure of ammonia, which is a function of pH, is lower at the lower pH of intracellular fluid. Thus, the usual alkalotic state observed in patients with hepatic encephalopathy would supposedly enhance the toxicity of ammonia that accumulates in the extracellular fluid.[31] Direct measurements do not support this hypothesis. Studies of hyperventilated and ammonia-infused rats showed a good correlation between cerebral intracellular ammonia and arterial blood ammonia concentrations. However, the intracerebral ammonia concentration was well above what would be predicted from the CSF ammonia concentration and the pH gradient between the two compartments.[74]

Several additional observations cast further doubt on the practical significance of the pH effect. First, dogs have had both acid and alkaline ammonium salts infused into the carotid artery over a period of several hours, producing a phase of excitement, then depression to the point of coma, with no detectable differences in the rapidity or severity of nervous system effects.[49] Second, infusions of sodium bicarbonate intravenously in patients with acute hepatic coma and patients with chronic recurrent encephalopathy resulted in significant improvement in cerebral blood flow, cerebral oxygen consumption, and the oxygen/glucose utilization index.[83] Third, hydrochloric acid was infused intravenously into patients in hepatic precoma or coma without beneficial effect.[156]

No pattern of electrolyte abnormality is characteristic of hepatic encephalopathy. The course of the underlying disease before the onset of encephalopathy largely determines the abnormalities found during encephalopathy. In the typical patient with chronic liver disease (usually cirrhosis) and encephalopathy as a precipitated or a terminal event, hyponatremia and hypochloremia are frequent. Cellular potassium, magnesium, and zinc depletion are also frequent, and hypokalemia resulting in metabolic alkalosis is common. Correction of body potassium and magnesium deficits in these patients requires care and persistence. During an early phase of hepatic encephalopathy, patients will often perk up considerably simply on improvement of their electrolyte deficiencies. Occasionally, the deficit in sodium, potassium, or magnesium is so severe that a state of lethargy, apathy, stupor, or even coma results at least in part from the deficit. It can be corrected by replacement therapy. Patients with chronic liver failure are more predisposed to this complication than those without liver disease but with equivalent cation depletion.

Some patients with severe cirrhosis have renal tubular acidosis with impaired renal potassium conservation. They are more predisposed to the development of encephalopathy than patients without renal tubular acidosis.[139] Cirrhotics with advanced disease commonly develop encephalopathy associated with functional renal failure, the so-called hepatorenal syndrome, which is characterized by renal vasoconstriction, low glomerular filtration and reduced renal plasma flow, oliguria, azotemia, and hypotonicity of body fluids. The hyponatremia is intractable, ascites is usually present, and the effective extracellular fluid volume is reduced. Although renal failure in cirrhosis is usually associated with intact tubular function, some patients may develop acute tubular necrosis.

Hypocalcemia and hypophosphatemia are also frequent complications of chronic decompensated liver disease and are therefore also found in association with hepatic encephalopathy.

Blood Oxygen

Hypoxemia is commonly seen in cirrhosis and has been related to right-to-left shunting of blood. Patients have a low pulmonary vascular resistance and seem to have defective hypoxic pulmonary vasoconstriction.[39] They also have a slight shift to the right in the oxyhemoglobin dissociation curve, a decreased affinity of hemoglobin for oxygen that contributes somewhat to the oxygen unsaturation.[89] This is due to an increase in red cell 2,3-diphosphoglycerate (2,3-DPG).[54] When hepatic encephalopathy develops, the red cell 2,3-DPG increases further and the oxygen affinity of hemoglobin decreases a little more, unless other complicating factors are present.[54,119] These abnormalities are rapidly reversible if the encephalopathy improves. Presumably, the presence of hypoxemia and hypoxia augments the effects of abnormalities causing the encephalopathy. In mice, hypoxia has been shown to increase the acute toxicity of ammonia.[155]

Blood Glucose and Metabolites

Hypoglycemia often occurs with extensive destruction of the liver, as in acute fulminant hepatic failure, or with specific cellular (mitochondrial) injuries interfering with gluconeogenesis, as in Reye's syndrome. However, in the most frequently seen cases of hepatic encephalopathy, that is, cirrhotics with advanced liver failure, hyperglycemia is more likely to be present, since glucose tolerance is impaired. The decrease in glucose tolerance is probably related to a disproportionate increase in serum glucagon over insulin. In dogs becoming encephalopathic after portacaval shunts, the molar ratio of glucagon to insulin in serum increased approximately threefold, probably reflecting the catabolic state present.[142]

Products of glucose metabolism, that is, pyruvic acid, lactic acid, citric acid, and α-ketoglutaric acid, accumulate in the blood and CSF.[167] The blood levels reflect the muscle, not the brain, content of these metabolites. The rise in blood pyruvate and lactate particularly is closely correlated with and at least partially due to a reduction in carbon dioxide tension resulting from hyperventilation. The elevated blood levels are usually a consequence of severe liver dysfunction, not the occurrence of encephalopathy. In the totally hepatectomized dog, increases in blood pyruvate and lactate are shown to reach maximal levels within 1 hour (α-ketoglutarate within 6 hours) of removal of the liver, before encephalopathy developed.[46] Thus, the increased blood levels reflected the absence of the liver rather than the presence of encephalopathy. Other derivatives of pyruvate such as acetoin and butylene glycol are also increased in the blood.

Brain

Blood flow to the brain is closely correlated with arterial PCO_2 and pH.[167] Normally, it is approximately 55 ml/100 g/min, with an oxygen uptake of 3.5 ml/100 g/min. The arteriovenous oxygen difference is 6 vol%, and the respiratory quotient is 0.99, indicating that the brain is metabolizing carbohydrate exclusively. Glucose utilization is 7 mg or 8 mg/100 g/min. In cirrhotics with a portacaval shunt and no evidence of encephalopathy, the cerebral blood flow is increased by about 75%, oxygen utilization by about 10%, and glucose utilization by about 25%,[123] A similar increase in cerebral blood flow (about 70%) is seen in unselected cirrhotics with acute hepatic coma of less than 24 hours' duration. These patients have normal cerebral oxygen and glucose utilization,[96] This is the best evidence that hepatic coma cannot be due to depression of brain energy metabolism. Experimental studies in rats of the brain adenylate energy charge after total hepatectomy or massive ischemic hepatic necrosis and of brain adenine nucleotides after portacaval shunt and ammonium ion infusions support this conclusion.[170]

Beyond 24 hours of hepatic encephalopathy or coma, cerebral blood flow, oxygen consumption, and glucose utilization decrease.[96] The average reduction of cerebral blood flow in the presence of encephalopathy with or without coma is approximately 25%. The average reductions in oxygen and glucose utilization are 40% to 50% in encephalopathy without coma and slightly more than 50% when coma ensues. In these patients, the correlation

between cerebral blood flow and oxygen utilization (0.66) is significant but not close. Because of extensive variability among individuals, there is no apparent correlation between cerebral oxygen utilization and severity of the encephalopathy.

Decreased utilization of oxygen characterizes all nonconvulsive or preconvulsive coma states. This is not due to lack of oxygen but to a reduced demand for oxygen. The balance between energy production and utilization by the brain is maintained. Oxidation is coupled normally to phosphorylation in acute experimental hepatic coma and, presumably, in human hepatic encephalopathy. Therefore, the reduced demand for oxygen must reflect decreased utilization of adenosine triphosphate (ATP).[175]

The decrease in cerebral glucose utilization in human hepatic encephalopathy is associated with a nonspecific abnormality in glucose metabolism, as judged from animal experiments. Brain analyses in totally hepatectomized dogs in hepatic coma revealed normal concentrations of glycolytic substrates and ATP but reduced concentrations of the citric acid cycle substrates, α-ketoglutarate, fumarate, malate, and oxaloacetate. These reductions were no different from those observed in normal dogs or mice receiving sedatives or anesthetics. Thus, there is nothing unique about cerebral glucose metabolism in experimental hepatic coma.[178]

Ammonia and Glutamine

Ammonia is increased in blood, and ammonia and glutamine are increased in muscle, brain, and CSF. Glutamine is derived from ammonia and glutamate in the tissues. Most of the ammonia in blood and tissues is of dietary origin. The major sources of blood ammonia are ammonia in the food eaten, small intestinal digestion of dietary protein and metabolic utilization of the absorbed glutamine, metabolic utilization of endogenous glutamine by the small intestine, and colonic bacterial metabolism of dietary protein or its products and of urea secreted into the intestine (25% to 30% of all the urea formed). It appears from studies of germ-free animals and studies with isolated bowel segments that about one half (or less) of the ammonia coming from the gut is a result of bacterial action, with the remainder coming from the small intestine. This applies to both fasting and nonfasting conditions.[118] In the presence of azotemia, increased amounts of ammonia are generated from the breakdown of increased urea in the intestine.

Nitrogenous food substances have varying effects on blood ammonia or encephalopathy, depending on the protein source and amino acid content.[31,175] Milk and cheese protein is better tolerated than meat protein by patients susceptible to encephalopathy. Dogs with portacaval shunts also tolerate milk protein better than meat protein. In cirrhotics, blood in the gut causes a greater rise in blood ammonia than equivalent amounts of casein and milk. Amino acids have varying ammoniagenic potency in cirrhotics susceptible to hepatic encephalopathy.

Those that raise the blood ammonia most are threonine, serine, glycine, glutamine, histidine, lysine, and asparagine. Alanine, phenylalanine, tyrosine, proline, leucine, isoleucine, and valine have about one eighth the effect of the highest group. Arginine, aspartic acid, glutamic acid, tryptophan, and urea have only a comparatively slight effect.

Under fasting conditions, ammonia coming from kidney, muscle, and brain, which are ordinarily relatively minor sources, has more significance. Ammonia release from kidney is greater than normal in patients with encephalopathy and is further increased in the presence of hypokalemia. Ammonia is released from muscle with exercise. The amount released for a given amount of exertion is greater than normal in encephalopathic patients.[40,118]

When blood ammonia levels are increased, brain and muscle uptake of ammonia is increased. The amount taken up is proportional to the arterial blood level. The brain ammonia utilization rate is also closely correlated ($r = 0.93$) with the arterial blood level.[95] The ammonia utilization reactions apparently take place in a compartment that includes less than one fifth of all brain ammonia. In encephalopathic patients, the brain ammonia utilization rate is increased by two thirds. The primary disposition of ammonia is by the formation of glutamine. Studies in normal cats receiving labeled ammonia by carotid artery infusion indicate that the newly formed glutamine is derived from a small but metabolically active compartment of glutamic acid.[10] The observation of a small active compartment of ammonia utilization in humans and of glutamine formation from a small active compartment of glutamic acid in cats is probably more than coincidence. In rats with portacaval shunts, there is a close correlation ($r = 0.90$) between blood ammonia and brain glutamine.[159]

In patients with liver disease, there is a fairly good correlation between blood (arterial or venous) and CSF ammonia, but those with hepatic coma cannot be differentiated from those not in coma. In general, the correlation between blood ammonia and degree of hepatic encephalopathy is poor, and a single blood ammonia determination is of little clinical value. This poor correlation probably stems from the fact that skeletal muscle is a much larger metabolic site than brain for circulating ammonia.[95] Thus, under constant conditions of formation of ammonia, muscle removal largely determines blood levels. This is particularly true in the presence of portal-systemic shunts. However, in an individual patient, fluctuations in blood ammonia often correlate fairly well with changing neuropsychiatric status, so serial blood ammonia determinations may be of value.

Acute ammonia intoxication in animals stimulates oxidative metabolism of the brain, but brain energy balance is maintained.[175] Studies of isolated cerebral or spinal cord neurons in the cat indicate that ammonium ions abolish the hyperpolarizing action of postsynaptic inhibition by blocking the active outward extrusion of chloride ions.

The effect is a loss of postsynaptic inhibition, depending to some extent on previous depolarization of the neuron.[125]

Chronic hyperammonemia associated with prolonged infusion of ammonium salts or with a portacaval shunt results in Alzheimer type II astrocytosis in the brain and diffuse slowing on the electroencephalogram (EEG) similar to those seen in hepatic coma.[31] Brain α-ketoglutarate levels are reduced.[28] Animals that are chronically hyperammonemic following a portacaval shunt are more susceptible than nonshunted animals to the toxic effects of an additional acute ammonia load. A smaller dose of ammonia causes coma, and cerebral depression lasts longer. Cerebral dysfunction occurs before any evidence of primary energy failure as reflected by changes in the brain adenine nucleotides.[75] Cerebral blood flow and oxygen consumption are reduced, and the concentrations of glutamate and aspartate in the brain are decreased.[67] The EEG develops high-voltage slow waves.

Experimental evidence relating increased blood ammonia to cerebral dysfunction dates back to 1877, when Eck first created a portacaval shunt. In the 1930s, van Caulert and Kirk described mental disturbances in cirrhotics receiving ammonium salts.[62] However, it was not until 1952 that Gabuzda, Phillips, Schwartz, and Davidson[61,121] recognized that symptoms and EEG changes indistinguishable from hepatic encephalopathy could be produced in cirrhotics orally given ammonium-containing cation-exchange resins, ammonium salts, urea, or protein. Two years later, a patient with a normal liver who had a portacaval shunt following a Whipple procedure for carcinoma of the pancreas was reported by McDermott and Adams to have recurrent episodes of irrationality, confusion, disorientation, incontinence, drowsiness, apathy, stupor, and sometimes coma.[104] Blood ammonia and EEG abnormalities were correlated with the manifestations, which were reproducible by feeding the patient meat, urea, ammonium-containing cation-exchange resin, or ammonium chloride. Such observations in cirrhotics and in patients with portacaval shunts have been confirmed many times since these early reports, so a relationship between ammonia and the clinical syndrome of hepatic coma is well established.

The formation of glutamine and of urea are the two ways of disposing of ammonia. The capacities of the urea and glutamine-synthesizing systems for ammonia removal are approximately equivalent in the presence of a large excess of ammonia. When there is excess ammonia, ornithine becomes rate limiting for the urea cycle with diversion of carbamyl phosphate into the pyrimidine pathway. Orotic aciduria reflects this diversion. Supplemental ornithine (or arginine) enhances the conversion of ammonia to citrulline and urea by increasing carbamyl transferase activity.[68] Dynamic studies in humans using isotopically labeled ammonia indicate the importance of the glutamine pathway, because about 50% of the arterial ammonia was metabolized by muscle, and the fraction going to the brain was approximately equivalent to that going to the liver.[95] If the urea pathway is lost, as in the totally hepatectomized dog, glutamine synthesis expands to largely, but not entirely, handle the increased ammonia load.[106] In patients with moderate or severe liver disease, in whom the maximum rate of urea synthesis is depressed,[4] glutamine synthesis presumably expands similarly.

In patients with hepatic encephalopathy, the correlation between CSF glutamine and the clinical severity of the encephalopathy or the degree of EEG abnormality is good, although not perfect.[81,113] CSF glutamine is presumably the spillover from brain glutamine, which accumulates as brain ammonia increases, α-Ketoglutaramate is derived from glutamine by removal of an amino group from the α-carbon. Like glutamine, it is increased in the CSF in hepatic encephalopathy and has at least as good a correlation as glutamine with severity.[47,122] The CSF concentration of glutamine in patients with hepatic encephalopathy is 30 to 50 times that of α-ketoglutaramate, which has the same significance as glutamine. There is no good evidence that either has a role in pathogenesis. However, no parameter has correlated better with severity of encephalopathy than these two substances, and any hypothesis of pathogenesis must account for this correlation.

Fatty Acids and Ketones

The significance of fatty acids in hepatic encephalopathy is presently an enigma. Plasma concentrations of short-, medium-, and long-chain free fatty acids are increased in chronic liver disease with or without encephalopathy.[175] There are difficulties in interpreting the long-chain fatty acid values because of extraneous factors that affect the measurements. Short-chain fatty acid values may run higher in patients with encephalopathy; however, this observation requires further verification.[170] Incomplete β-oxidation of long-chain fatty acids is probably the predominant source of the short-chain fatty acids.[170] In a small sample of patients with acute fulminant hepatic failure, no relationship could be demonstrated between the clinical course and the plasma level of the short-chain fatty acids.[170] In Reye's syndrome, plasma short- and medium-chain fatty acids may be markedly elevated, at times to levels that would be lethal if maintained.[97,145] In this disease, fatty acidemia is of major significance.

Experimentally, short- and medium-chain fatty acids cause coma that is reversible.[172] The longer the fatty acid chain, the more potent is the effect. Slow, high-amplitude waves are evoked on the EEG, with the changes correlating with the concentration of fatty acid in the CSF perfusing the brain.[170] Central hyperventilation is prominent, and the blood ammonia level increases threefold within a few hours.[145] In pathologic concentrations, fatty acids depress enzymes involved in the formation of urea and of glutamine, thus interfering with the disposition of ammonia.[43] At very low concentrations *in vitro,* fatty acids also depress a variety of other enzymes, including several glycolytic

enzymes and Na^+,K^+-ATPase of brain microsomal membranes.[2,158] *In vivo,* fatty acids augment the coma potential of ammonia and mercaptans.[170] They also augment the brain uptake of tryptophan by displacing free tryptophan from its binding sites on albumin. Free fatty acids enhance the release of insulin and depress glucagon, predisposing the animal to hypoglycemia.[138,180] Cumulatively, these experimental data suggest that fatty acids are important in hepatic encephalopathy despite the lack of clear-cut evidence from blood measurements. The role of fatty acids in usual cases of hepatic encephalopathy is perhaps secondary and indirect.

Ketone production is decreased. This reflects the presence of liver damage rather than encephalopathy per se.[167]

Mercaptans

Mercaptans are thioalcohols.[174] Like ammonia, they are toxic products largely generated in the gastrointestinal tract and normally efficiently removed by the liver. The association of mercaptans and hepatic coma was established in 1955 by the isolation of methyl mercaptan (methanethiol, CH_3SH) and dimethyl disulfide (CH_3S-SCH_3) from the urine of a patient in coma with massive hepatic necrosis and a prominent fetor hepaticus.[25] Mercaptans are increased in blood, breath, urine, and brain in hepatic encephalopathy.[170] Fetor hepaticus is probably due to a mixture of the three related volatile compounds methanethiol, dimethyl sulfide (CH_3SCH_3), and dimethyl disulfide. This presumption has never been verified by direct measurements of breath. However, direct measurements have established that mercaptans are normally present in breath and that in hepatic failure they increase about fourfold.[175] Cirrhotics fed methionine have a distinctive breath odor due to dimethyl sulfide, which is similar to but not identical with fetor hepaticus. Dimethyl sulfide is the primary metabolic derivative of methanethiol.

Blood methanethiol in moderate or severe liver disease without overt encephalopathy is approximately one and one-half times normal. In the presence of encephalopathy, it is approximately two and one-half times normal.[102] The average value observed in patients in hepatic coma and in animals with experimentally induced hepatic coma are similar, approximately 1000 pmol/ml.[45] The concentration of methanethiol in the brain of such animals is increased about fivefold.[181] As with blood ammonia, serial determinations of blood methanethiol are more valuable than a single measurement. The changing stages of encephalopathy in a given patient are reflected fairly well by the changing concentrations of blood methanethiol.[102]

Mercaptans cause reversible coma in animals. They also enhance the coma-producing potential of ammonia and fatty acids.[177] Like fatty acids, they depress enzymes involved in urea synthesis, interfering with the disposition of ammonia.[43] Methanethiol in low concentrations has been found to inhibit mitochondrial respiration in liver, carbonic anhydrase activity in red blood cells, and

Na^+,K^+-ATPase activity in the brain of experimental preparations.[174] Like anesthetics, they protect erythrocytes against hypotonic hemolysis, supporting the idea of a direct membrane effect.[3] All of these experimental effects are reversible.

Amino Acids

Amino acid levels are increased in blood, brain, CSF, and urine.[23,169,175] In *chronic liver failure* without encephalopathy, many of the straight chain amino acids are increased in the plasma, and, with the occurrence of encephalopathy, they increase further.[4] The highest concentrations are observed with methionine, phenylalanine, tyrosine, free tryptophan, aspartate, and glutamate; the increases are twofold to fourfold.[175] The levels of the branched-chain amino acids leucine, isoleucine, and valine are significantly decreased, as are those of threonine and arginine. In contrast to that of arginine, the citrulline concentration is increased.[167] This and the increase in aspartate can be related to disproportionate depression of liver argininosuccinate synthetase activity, one of the rate-limiting enzymes in the urea cycle.[90] The increments in plasma amino acids are associated with reductions in the ratio of acetoacetate to β-hydroxybutyrate in blood, which reflects the cellular mitochondrial redox potential.[119]

The plasma-free, but not the total, tryptophan is increased in association with increased free fatty acids and depressed albumin.[117] The concentration of free tryptophan and the ratio of free tryptophan to branched-chain amino acids have been correlated with the grade and evolution of the encephalopathy.[22] However, tryptophan has been found elevated in the plasma and brain in many circumstances other than hepatic failure.[38] An example is food deprivation. Tyramine, a derivative of tyrosine, is increased in the plasma, correlating closely with tyrosine.[52] Phenols derived from both tyrosine and tyramine are also increased in plasma and CSF, with the increase correlating with severity of encephalopathy.[111] This old observation takes on added significance as a result of recent studies of coma induction with phenol in rats, and its synergistic interaction with ammonia, octanoate, and mercaptans in the process of coma induction.[160,174] Also, phenols extracted from plasma of patients with acute fulminant hepatic failure depressed various brain and liver enzymes.[174] The elevated plasma tyrosine levels are associated with an increased plasma tyrosine flux and a reduced capacity for hepatic amino acid oxidation.[116] Tyrosine tolerance is abnormal. Deficiencies in the enzymes tyrosine transaminase, *p*-hydroxyphenylpyruvic acid oxidase, and homogentisic acid oxidase have been demonstrated.

Glutamine is the predominant amino acid in the CSF and, as already noted, is the most specific biochemical indicator of hepatic encephalopathy presently available. Asparagine[175] and tryptophan[117] also increase in the CSF and correlate fairly well with glutamine levels. There is a good correlation in the CSF between the concentration

of the end products of tryptophan metabolism 5-HIAA and IAA and the severity of hepatic encephalopathy.[111,161]

In *acute fulminant hepatic failure,* the plasma concentration of all except the branched-chain amino acids increases.[170] Methionine increases more than tenfold; phenylalanine, tyrosine, and tryptophan threefold to fivefold; and the others generally increase less than threefold. The branched-chain amino acids are normal or decreased. Correlations have been observed between the rise and fall of plasma amino acids and the progression or improvement of the encephalopathy.[27] A close correlation has been demonstrated between the plasma tyrosine concentration and the transaminase activity in patients with acute necrosis of the liver, suggesting that the damaged liver may be a source of the greatly increased circulating amino acids.

In the brain and CSF, glutamine is by far the predominant amino acid, its absolute concentration being at least 15 to 20 times that of any other amino acid. However, the relative increases in methionine, phenylalanine, tyrosine, and histidine particularly are greater.[170] Most of the others, including the branched-chain amino acids, are increased to a lesser extent. The concentration of taurine is not increased. The branched-chain amino acids have an increased brain-to-plasma ratio. However, the plasma concentration appears to be the main factor controlling brain concentrations of the straight-chain amino acids.

In both acute and chronic liver disease with or without encephalopathy, the molar ratio of plasma branched chain to aromatic amino acids is reduced and it cannot be used as an indicator of encephalopathy.[109]

Most of our insight into the abnormalities in amino acids stems from *experimental studies in animals,* particularly the rat and dog. In the totally hepatectomized dog, the plasma straight-chain amino acid levels increase threefold within 24 hours, whereas the branched-chain amino acid levels decrease slightly.[106] Plasma glutamine increases ninefold; tyrosine, sixfold to ninefold; and tryptophan, twofold.[106,147] Similar results are seen in the totally hepatectomized rat. The changes are less marked when the animal is also eviscerated.[60] Brain and muscle glutamine, tyrosine, and tryptophan increase about fourfold or more, whereas aspartate and glutamate decrease. Their concentrations do not vary greatly among the major subdivisions of the brain. Unlike tryptophan, from which they are derived, brain serotonin levels remain normal and those of 5-HIAA increase only twofold.[147]

In coma following massive ischemic hepatic necrosis, brain levels of glutamine, phenylalanine, tyrosine, tryptophan, threonine, and histidine increase greatly while aspartate and glutamate levels decrease.[101] These results are associated with a decrease in the ratio of insulin to glucagon. In pigs and rats, coma produced this way has been associated with increases in tryptophan in all parts of the brain studied.[35,38] The correlation between brain tryptophan and plasma-free tryptophan has been high (0.84–0.96), and the correlation between plasma-free tryptophan and free fatty acids has been high (0.90).[37]

The tryptophan derivatives serotonin and 5-HIAA have also been increased in various parts of the brain, especially the midbrain, pons, and medulla.[35] Their elevations have been less consistent and less prominent than those of tryptophan. Medium-sized molecules that have tyrosine-like fluorescence and pass through a polyacrylonitrile dialysis membrane have also been associated with ischemia-induced hepatic coma in pigs.[42]

In portacaval-shunted rats, the uptake of phenylalanine, tyrosine, tryptophan, and leucine by the brain is increased, whereas the uptake of arginine is decreased.[84] The total brain tryptophan value cannot be accounted for by the plasma concentration of free tryptophan and amino acids known to compete with tryptophan for brain uptake or by the ratio of insulin to glucagon. Thus, some additional factor, probably ammonia, must influence the brain concentration of tryptophan.[12] The rate of formation and release of glutamic acid by the brain is increased.[110] With the shunt alone the content of glutamate and glutamine in the striatum and cerebellum increase, but during severe encephalopathy induced with additional ammonium acetate they decrease selectively.[65] With time, portacaval-shunted dogs deteriorate and develop manifestations of encephalopathy. Such animals have an increase in plasma and CSF aromatic and sulfur-containing amino acids and a decrease in branched-chain amino acids.[140] Their plasma and CSF tyramine levels increase about 5- to 6-fold. The midbrain tyramine also increases 5-fold while its dopamine and norepinephrine content fall by one half.[53] After a loading dose of tyrosine, their peak ratio of tyramine to tyrosine concentration in plasma increases 50-fold. In the brain as well as the CSF of shunted dogs, glutamine accounts for about 80% of the total free amino acids.[13]

The toxicity of amino acids has been studied in some detail in rats. Lethal doses injected intraperitoneally are in the order of 2 g to 10 g/kg.[168] Tryptophan is the most toxic, and branched-chain amino acids are the least toxic. Mixtures of amino acids are less toxic because of the presence of arginine. About one half of the amino acid nitrogen appears in the blood as ammonia. Lethargy and coma occur with mixtures of amino acids if arginine is absent. The house cat is particularly susceptible. The rise in blood ammonia after injection of amino acids and the toxicity are prevented by the addition of enough arginine to process the excess ammonia. This effect of arginine has been demonstrated in humans.[51] Other amino acids, such as ornithine, which aid in the disposition of ammonia, have similar effects.

Ingestion of large amounts of tryptophan by patients may result in headache, dizziness, nystagmus, drowsiness alternating with euphoria, disturbances in gait, and abnormal reflexes.[141] Cirrhotics are more predisposed to this effect of tryptophan.[76] An exaggeration of the gait and visual disturbances have been observed in a dog with a portacaval shunt who was given a huge dose of tryptophan orally.[114] Monkeys given 800 mg/kg/day have shown no abnormalities.[36]

Intracarotid infusion in dogs of tryptophan plus phenylalanine has been reported to cause coma, which could be prevented with branched-chain amino acids.[132] The average plasma and CSF levels of tryptophan were, respectively, 28 and 5 times those observed in dogs in coma following portacaval shunts. Average plasma and CSF levels of phenylalanine were 2 and 3 times greater, respectively. Coma did not occur at the concentrations observed in shunted dogs with encephalopathy. Furthermore, dogs that received branched-chain amino acids along with tryptophan and phenylalanine remained normal clinically and by EEG when their average CSF phenylalanine and tryptophan concentrations were greater than those observed in the shunted dogs with encephalopathy. These data do not support a direct pathogenetic role for tryptophan or phenylalanine in hepatic encephalopathy.

Neurotransmitters and False Neurotransmitters

Information is available on aspartate, glutamate, dopamine, norepinephrine, serotonin, and γ-aminobutyric acid (GABA).[175] Only a small proportion of central nervous system synapses have transmission mediated by biogenic amines. In patients with encephalopathy resulting from fulminant hepatic failure or chronic liver disease, the neurotransmitters (dopamine, norepinephrine, serotonin, and GABA) and the neurotransmitter metabolites (asparagine, glutamine, homovanillic acid, normetanephrine, 5-HIAA, and IAA) are increased in CSF.[14] There was no decline in brain dopamine or norepinephrine in a sample of cirrhotics who died in hepatic coma.[34] Plasma concentrations of norepinephrine, and to a lesser extent epinephrine, are increased.[79] The false neurotransmitters, octopamine (norepinephrine minus a hydroxyl group) and, to a lesser extent, phenylethanolamine (octopamine minus a hydroxyl group), are increased in brain, muscle, blood, and urine.[18,56] There is no consistent net flux of these false neurotransmitters into and out of the brain.[19] The correlation of severity of encephalopathy with serum octopamine is fair. The arterial concentrations of octopamine and ammonia are apparently unrelated.[20] The extent to which platelets fail to take up octopamine is also significantly related to severity of encephalopathy.[170] By direct infusion of octopamine into a lateral cerebral ventricle of rats, brain octopamine has been raised artificially to fantastic heights and brain dopamine and norepinephrine depressed to less than 10% of controls without causing coma.[170] This experiment reminds us that correlations that have been observed between brain or tissue fluid concentrations of various substances and the presence of hepatic coma do not necessarily reflect cause and effect.

A possible role for the inhibitory neurotransmitter GABA has been postulated.[133] Several interesting observations have been made. The density of receptors for GABA are increased in neural synaptic membranes isolated from rabbits and rats with galactosamine-induced hepatic failure.[5,134] Such animals have increased serum levels of GABA-like activity and their serum inhibits the binding of ^{3}H-GABA to neural membranes obtained from normal animals. The GABA-like activity of portal vein blood in normal rabbits is about twice that of arterial blood. Finally, certain human colonic bacteria make GABA. Thus, GABA from the intestine that bypasses the liver is presumed to pass through a damaged blood–brain barrier and to bind to synaptic membranes. In portacaval-shunted rats and in rabbits infused with ammonium chloride receptors for GABA do not change.[55,164] However in the portacaval-shunted dog whose liver was first damaged with dimethylnitrosamine, an increase in GABA receptors was seen in the cortex and cerebellum.[6] The same workers found a similar increase in GABA receptors in brain of rats made comatose with a mixture of ammonium chloride, octanoic acid, and dimethyl disulfide acting synergistically.[7]

In the galactosamine-injured rabbit the number of receptors for excitatory amino acids decreases, that for inhibitory amino acids increases, and that for other neurotransmitters is unchanged. The mechanisms responsible for these changes and their exact significance is unknown. Although these recent observations are of great interest, "it is necessary to be cautious in extrapolating from data obtained using ligand-receptor binding assays in vitro to neurological events and behavioral changes in vivo."[87] In vivo studies of the effects of specific GABA agonists and antagonists on experimental hepatic encephalopathy may clarify the relevance of the foregoing observations to human or experimental hepatic coma.[130]

Another ubiquitous compound, cholecystokinin, which has excitatory effects in the brain and may function as a neuromodulator, was decreased significantly in the cerebral cortex and hypothalamus in acute fulminant failure of rats due to hepatic ischemia* and of rabbits due to galactosamine hepatitis.†

Other Measurements

Plasma bile acid concentrations have been similar in patients with or without encephalopathy. However, in fulminant hepatic failure, the rate of disappearance of free cholic acid after a bolus intravenous injection was slower in comatose patients who did not recover than in those who recovered.[77] Endotoxemia has been observed in fulminant hepatic failure, usually in the presence of renal failure, but its association with encephalopathy is not clear and there is only indirect evidence that it may have a role in producing some forms of fulminant hepatic failure.[93]

---

* Salerno F et al: Brain cholecystokinin and beta-endorphin immunoreactivity in rats with different experimental models of liver failure. In Kleinberger G et al (eds): Advances in Hepatic Encephalopathy and Urea Cycle Diseases, pp 402–410. Basel, Karger, 1984.
† Meryn S et al: Big and small immunoreactive brain cholecystokinin in experimental hepatic encephalopathy in the rabbit. In Kleinberger G et al (eds): Advances in Hepatic Encephalopathy and Urea Cycle Diseases, pp 411–416. Basel, Karger, 1984.

The serum prolactin level was three times normal in a sample of cirrhotics with hepatic encephalopathy and twice that of cirrhotics without encephalopathy.[103] Substance P, a potent vasodilating compound, was found elevated about fivefold in plasma of patients in hepatic coma over that seen in critically ill patients without liver disease.[80] It correlated significantly (0.66) with plasma norepinephrine concentrations.

Synergism

The coma-producing potential of toxic substances or abnormal metabolic states may be increased severalfold when they are present together as a result of their interdependent metabolisms or interrelated effects. Such synergism has been demonstrated experimentally for ammonia, mercaptans, fatty acids, hypoglycemia, and phenols.[171,175] Much smaller doses and lower blood levels of ammonia, mercaptans, fatty acids, and phenols are required in combination than singly to produce coma. The incidence of coma in normal rats can be raised from 0 to 100% by injection of subcoma doses of any two of these substances. Even less of each is required if the animals have liver damage. In the presence of hypoglycemia and hypoxia, two metabolic abnormalities that predispose the animal to encephalopathy, the doses of the toxins required to cause coma are reduced.[155,180]

Mercaptans, phenols, and fatty acids, as well as hypoglycemia, increase the blood level of ammonia resulting from the injection of a subcoma dose of NH_4^+. This effect on blood ammonia has been demonstrated with dimethyl sulfide as well as methanethiol and with long-chain as well as short-chain fatty acids.[168] An exogenous coma-producing substance such as pentobarbital, not primarily related to liver failure, does not have this synergistic effect on blood ammonia, although it does have an additive effect on production of coma. The effects of fatty acids and methanethiol on blood ammonia can be related to their inhibitory effects on urea synthesis or glutamate dehydrogenase activity.[170] A similar converse effect of ammonium salts and fatty acids on the blood methanethiol has also been demonstrated.[175]

The average blood levels of ammonia, free fatty acids, and methanethiol in rats with hepatic coma following massive ischemic hepatic necrosis are much lower than blood levels required to produce coma in normal rats with each of these substances individually. Normal rats become comatose when they are given a combination of doses of ammonium salt, fatty acid, and methanethiol, which give blood and brain levels of ammonia and methanethiol in the range of those observed in rats with ischemia-produced hepatic coma.[181] Thus, the encephalopathy that occurs following experimental ischemic fulminant hepatic failure in rats can be explained by the synergistic interaction of these toxic substances without invoking other factors. This evidence of synergism in animals suggests that similar interrelationships should be sought among variables reflecting the effects of suspected toxins in patients with hepatic encephalopathy. The multifactorial nature of hepatic encephalopathy has been accepted conceptually. It follows that a multifactorial approach to pathogenesis is required.

Most of the biochemical abnormalities that have been reported in blood and CSF of patients with hepatic encephalopathy are indicated in the metabolic map of Figure 24-1.

PATHOGENESIS

It is apparent from the previous section that many abnormalities are associated with the occurrence of hepatic encephalopathy. The problem is to distinguish which among these correlations reflect causation. To be considered pathogenetic, an abnormality must be present consistently when encephalopathy is present. The abnormality should correlate with the severity of encephalopathy in patients and should cause coma in animals. An abnor-

mality may be so intimately a part of the encephalopathy that an etiologic role is presumed. This was the case with brain oxidative metabolism until it was shown that coma occurred before brain oxygen and glucose utilization decreased.

Four candidate toxins seem likely pathogenetic factors because they are present in excess in patients with liver failure and they cause coma experimentally in animals. These are ammonia, mercaptans, phenols, and fatty acids. Of these, ammonia is probably most important and has the most cumulative evidence supporting its role as an etiologic factor. In patients with cirrhosis, ammonium salts and substances that generate or release ammonia cause encephalopathy or coma. Removal of the ammonia producers or releasers results in improvement in the encephalopathy. Patients without liver disease who have portacaval shunts have been observed to develop encephalopathy that worsened or improved in relation to the rise or fall in blood ammonia. A good correlation is observed

Fig. 24-1. Blood or cerebrospinal fluid abnormalities that have been observed in patients with hepatic encephalopathy. The heavy arrows show the direction of change. Double-headed arrows indicate that values have been found to be increased as well as decreased in different circumstances. (Zieve L, Nicoloff D: Ann Rev Med 26:143–157, 1975. © 1975, Annual Reviews Inc. Reproduced with permission.)

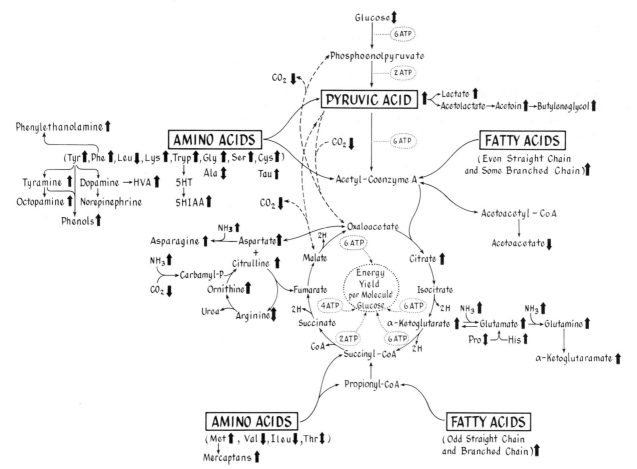

in unselected patients between severity of encephalopathy and the CSF concentration of glutamine or α-ketoglutaramate, substances that reflect brain ammonia levels. In diseases characterized by urea cycle abnormalities, that is, Reye's syndrome and congenital hyperammonemic states, encephalopathy occurs in association with high blood ammonia levels. The conclusion that disturbed ammonia metabolism is a basic causal factor in hepatic encephalopathy is unavoidable. However, from observed clinical inconsistencies and from experimental observations, it is clear that ammonia excess alone cannot entirely account for the encephalopathy in the typical case.

Like ammonia, mercaptans that accumulate during hepatic encephalopathy come largely from the gut. The most suggestive evidence that mercaptans actually have an etiologic role stems from observations in cirrhotics fed methionine; these patients become encephalopathic and develop a breath odor reminiscent of but not identical to fetor hepaticus. The encephalopathy disappears when the methionine is discontinued and can be prevented if a broad-spectrum antibiotic is given before the methionine feeding. An intense fetor hepaticus may be seen in patients with acute liver failure and encephalopathy. Although never proved by direct breath measurements, it is highly likely that methanethiol and its derivatives, dimethyl sulfide and dimethyl disulfide, cause the odor. Methanethiol was isolated from the urine of a woman in acute hepatic failure with coma and an intense fetor hepaticus.[25] Animals from whom the odor of methanethiol or its derivatives emanates following injections of methanethiol or dimethyl disulfide are encephalopathic. It is therefore likely that these substances are contributing to the encephalopathy of patients with fetor hepaticus.

As with mercaptans, phenol and its derivatives are products of metabolism normally largely removed by the liver or excreted in the urine. In human hepatic and renal failure they accumulate in blood and tissues. A significant correlation has been found between the serum or CSF content of phenols and the severity of hepatic encephalopathy.[111] In animals, pharmacologic doses of phenol cause a reversible encephalopathy including deep coma.[160] Phenols extracted from serums of patients with acute fulminant hepatic failure inhibit a variety of enzymes when added to rat liver or brain homogenates.[174] Phenols may thus have a pathogenic role in hepatic encephalopathy while interacting with the abnormal accumulations of ammonia and mercaptans.

The evidence for a pathogenetic role of fatty acids is less direct. An association has been observed between short- or medium-chain fatty acids and encephalopathy in chronic liver disease but not in fulminant hepatic failure. In Reye's syndrome, the abnormalities in short- and medium-chain fatty acids appear to be critical. Values of medium-chain fatty acids in plasma have been as much as 500 times normal.[97] Such a high concentration is enough to cause coma in animals with the fatty acids alone. While increments in the fatty acids are usually much less than this extreme, they occur in the presence of sub-

stantial hyperammonemia and significant hypoglycemia, with which they interact to produce encephalopathy. In the usual case of liver disease with encephalopathy, the role of fatty acids may be primarily as an augmenter or modulator of the encephalopathic effects of ammonia and mercaptans.

The synergistic interaction among these toxins and endogenous metabolic abnormalities such as hypoxia, hypoglycemia, electrolyte depletion (sodium and potassium particularly), and acid–base disturbances is probably of prime importance. The presence of several such abnormalities, which is the rule in liver failure, is more than additive. Thus, encephalopathy often occurs without evidence of extreme abnormality of any single variable. The apparent increased susceptibility of the cirrhotic patient to encephalopathy can be explained by the presence of a state of chronic low-grade ammonia or mercaptan intoxication onto which other precipitating factors are superimposed. Thus, given such a state of chronic intoxication, a comparatively small increase in one or the other of these toxins or an intensification of hypoxia, hypoglycemia, or electrolyte and acid–base disturbances may be enough to precipitate overt encephalopathy. The variable interplay among these factors as well as the rates of their accumulation probably account for the apparent differences between the encephalopathy of chronic liver disease and that of fulminant hepatic failure or Reye's syndrome. The same basic pathogenetic factors are probably involved in each of these three states; however, the relative importance and intensity of specific factors vary. The intensity of the effect of ammonia and mercaptans is probably greater in fulminant hepatic failure than in chronic liver disease. The fatty acids are of lesser significance, and hypoglycemia may play but a small role. In Reye's syndrome, unlike fulminant hepatic failure, fatty acids and ammonia have a prominent role. Hypoglycemia is also important, while mercaptans are probably unimportant.

The etiologic role of amino acids is uncertain at present. Amino acid abnormalities are associated with the development of encephalopathy in patients, and recession of the encephalopathy is associated with reduction in the amino acid abnormalities. Phenylalanine, tyrosine, and tryptophan are the amino acids of primary interest. What has not been clearly established is whether one or a combination of these amino acids causes coma in animals unrelated to the accumulation of ammonia. Tryptophan in excess reduces sleep latency and may cause drowsiness and gait disturbances in otherwise normal patients; however, it has not caused coma in psychiatric patients receiving doses large enough to raise blood levels 100-fold.[36] The highest increment seen in hepatic coma has been 10-fold. The ultimate consequence of the buildup of brain phenylalanine and tyrosine is the accumulation of false neurotransmitters and reduction of brain dopamine and norepinephrine. Dopamine and norepinephrine have been artificially reduced by about 90% in brains of rats without causing encephalopathy or coma. The maximum reduction in experimental hepatic coma has been 50%. Another consequence of excess tyrosine is the accumulation of phenols, which cause coma in animals.

The development and severity of encephalopathy in a patient with liver disease thus appear to depend on a balance between toxic and protective substances, coma producers and coma preventers. Toxic substances such as ammonia, mercaptans, fatty acids, and possibly certain amino acids accumulate with liver failure and act in a milieu that is less resistant to their toxic effects because of the depletion of various protective substances. Among the protective substances are oxygen, glucose, albumin, sodium, potassium, and arginine or ornithine, the depletion of which intensifies or augments the encephalopathy-generating effects of the toxins when they are present in small amounts. The relative significance of any single substance varies from case to case, but the net result depends on a variable quantitative balance between the combined effects of the coma producers and the coma preventers. The precise locus and mechanism of action of the toxins in the brain is unknown; however, damage by the toxins may alter the balance between inhibitory and excitatory amino acid neurotransmitters; may increase neuronal susceptibility to the inhibitory effects of GABA; may depress microsomal Na^+,K^+-ATPase activity; or may inhibit mitochondrial electron transfer. These fundamental effects have been demonstrated *in vitro*. Each might be variably altered *in vivo*.

PRECIPITATING FACTORS

The distinction between spontaneously occurring hepatic encephalopathy and that precipitated by some recognizable extrahepatic abnormality has been losing its significance as our knowledge of abnormal processes associated with hepatic failure has increased. Only infrequently are we unable to point to some specific abnormality as a precipitating event. The patient with liver disease is predisposed to the effects of extrahepatic abnormalities because of the presence of portal-systemic shunts, chronic hypoxia, varying degrees of electrolyte depletion, and acid–base imbalances, in addition to hepatic insufficiency. Most episodes of hepatic encephalopathy occur in patients with cirrhosis because of the frequency of this disease, its chronicity, and the common development of the predisposing abnormalities.

Most important among the precipitating factors is nitrogenous overload. This may be endogenous or exogenous in origin. Among the endogenous precipitants, azotemia is common. An increased quantity of urea passes into the bowel, where it is broken down to form ammonia, which is absorbed. Constipation is another precipitant that results in increased absorption of both ammonia and mercaptans. The kidney is also an endogenous source of ammonia. Potassium deficiency increases the renal vein ammonia output, which may become substantial. One of the causes of encephalopathy by this route is renal tubular acidosis occurring in cirrhosis.

Among the exogenous nitrogenous precipitants, gastrointestinal hemorrhage is most important. Bleeding, which may be from varices, gastritis, or peptic ulcer, not only results in excess ammonia and mercaptan formation from protein breakdown but also commonly is associated with hypovolemia, shock, and hypoxia, all of which augment the predisposition to encephalopathy. In addition, ammonia in transfused blood raises the recipient's blood ammonia by about 30 μg/dl for every bottle received. Blood proteins are more ammoniagenic than milk protein or its products. Azotemia due to blood in the gut results in turn in more intestinal urea with further increase in ammonia production. Dietary protein precipitates encephalopathy about one half as often as gastrointestinal hemorrhage. Patients with portacaval shunts or marked development of portal-systemic collaterals are most susceptible to the toxic effects of protein in the gut.

Next in frequency to nitrogenous overload as precipitating factors are sedatives, tranquilizers, and narcotic analgesics. These have an additive depressant effect on the brain to that produced by toxins such as ammonia and mercaptans. Those drugs that are metabolized or excreted by the liver accumulate in the blood and are retained longer in patients with liver dysfunction. The patient who does not have acutely decompensated liver disease tolerates these drugs surprisingly well. However, the patient who is acutely decompensated has little tolerance. Excitement is frequent in the precomatose state of hepatic failure, and one must resist the temptation to quiet the patient with sedatives.

Fluid and electrolyte abnormalities have been both predisposing and precipitating factors. Dehydration and hypovolemia are poorly tolerated by the patient predisposed to encephalopathy. Paracentesis was at one time a common precipitant of hepatic coma. However, it is now generally realized that little is gained by massive paracenteses, while needed protein and electrolytes are lost. Hyponatremia and hypokalemia were common consequences. Excessive diuresis may have a similar effect with electrolyte depletion, hypovolemia, prerenal azotemia, and increased ammonia generation by the gut and kidney. In the patient with hepatic failure, hyponatremia or hypokalemia is often associated with encephalopathy or coma, which is reversed simply by correction of the electrolyte abnormality. Equivalent abnormalities of these electrolytes in patients without liver disease are generally not associated with encephalopathy.

Encephalopathy may occur with the development of a severe infection. This is usually bacterial pneumonia, pyelonephritis, spontaneous bacterial peritonitis, or septicemia. The infections result in tissue breakdown, increasing the nitrogenous load. They also have other systemic effects, such as fever, dehydration, hypoxia, compromised renal function, and so on, all of which may potentiate the toxic effects of ammonia and mercaptans. Shock or hypovolemia unrelated to gastrointestinal hemorrhage may precipitate encephalopathy by compromising cerebral blood flow and other organ functions as well as intensifying the already existent hypoxia. Surgery, whether for a complication of the liver disease or not, commonly precipitates encephalopathy by a compounding of factors already mentioned, that is, hypnotics, anesthesia, hypoxia, hypovolemia, shock, and water and electrolyte imbalance. Superimposition of another disease such as acute pancreatitis may also precipitate encephalopathy by a combination of factors already mentioned.

CLINICAL MANIFESTATIONS

The appearance of hepatic encephalopathy is highly variable, depending on the rate and extent of occurrence of hepatic damage, the extent and duration of portal-systemic shunts, and the degree of abnormality of predisposing and precipitating events. The onset may be insidious, as in the cirrhotic who has gradually progressive hepatic de-

compensation, or abrupt, as in the patient with fulminant hepatic failure. The development or progression of the encephalopathy may also be slow or rapid. Fluctuations in severity of manifestations are to be expected. The subdivision of cases of encephalopathy into four types in the introduction to this chapter was based on the different patterns manifested. Even within each type, however, many variations in symptoms and signs are found. Despite differences that are readily recognizable, there is an underlying common aspect to all cases of all four types that justifies a general discussion of clinical manifestations; this will be the reference point from which deviations can be described.

A comprehensive list of symptoms and signs that occur in hepatic encephalopathy is given in Table 24-1. The abnormalities that reflect mental and personality changes are distinguished from those reflecting neuromuscular

TABLE 24-1.   Symptoms and Signs of Hepatic Encephalopathy

STAGE	MENTAL STATE-PERSONALITY	NEUROMUSCULAR
I	Exaggerated normal behavior patterns (moods, attitudes) Inverted sleep patterns Lowered perception Short attention span Subtle confusion Impaired calculations Euphoria, garrulousness Restlessness Aimless wandering Anxiety Agitation Irritability Apathy	Incoordination Tremor Impaired handwriting
II	Obvious personality change Decreased inhibitions Inappropriate behavior Picking and rearranging of bedclothes Disobedience, sullenness Slow responses Disorientation for time Poor memory Lethargy	Asterixis Ataxia Deliberate movements Expressionless facies Dysarthria Yawning, sucking, grasping Blinking, grimacing Abnormal muscle tonus Resistance to passive movement Feeble voluntary movement Flexion of legs
III	Bizarre behavior Obvious confusion Disorientation for place Delirium Paranoia, anger Somnolence, stupor	Hyperactive reflexes Muscle rigidity Seizures—focal and general Multifocal random muscle twitching Abnormal Babinski's sign Hyperpnea Hypothermia Incontinence
IV	Coma—responsiveness Coma—unresponsiveness	Oculocephalic and oculovestibular responses Decerebrate postures

changes. The manifestations of both types are listed in the order, more or less, in which they are apt to occur. Those near the top of each list occur early and those near the bottom occur late in the development of encephalopathy. Thus, as one goes down the list of manifestations, the encephalopathy is progressively more severe. The sequence can only be considered approximate, since from case to case the order of development of manifestations will vary. Not every patient has all these manifestations no matter how slowly the encephalopathy develops. Patients with a fulminant course may go quickly from the earliest manifestations to stupor and coma without displaying most of the behavioral and many of the neuromuscular findings listed. The sequences listed are not invariably progressive, there being fluctuations up and down the scale of manifestations. Speed of progression is highly variable.

For convenience of discussion of the encephalopathy, the manifestations are grouped into four stages of severity. These stages are somewhat arbitrary, but they conform more or less to criteria that have been used widely in the literature concerned with hepatic encephalopathy. Stage I includes patients who are restless, irritable, agitated, or apathetic and have muscular incoordination, tremor, and a short attention span. Stage II includes patients with inappropriate behavior, slow responses, disorientation for time, lethargy, asterixis, dysarthria, abnormal facial movements, and resistance to passive movement. Stage III includes patients with confusion, general disorientation, somnolence or stupor, hyperpnea, muscle rigidity, or a positive Babinski sign. Stage IV includes patients that are semiconscious or unconscious.

In Table 24-1 overt manifestations of encephalopathy are listed. Although many of these are overlooked in individual patients, if one is familiar enough with a patient's background and personality and assiduous enough to see the patient frequently and examine him carefully, these manifestations can be recognized at the bedside. Before any of these manifestations becomes apparent, however, patients predisposed to development of encephalopathy have abnormalities in psychometric tests.[31] If tests of psychomotor function were routinely given to patients with chronic liver disease, particularly cirrhotics, one could add a stage of incipient encephalopathy, stage O-I, falling between a true absence of encephalopathy and stage I. Any of a variety of tests may be used, as long as they are appropriately standardized. Of particular importance are age standards, because psychomotor function deteriorates progressively with age alone. Some of the tests that have been found of value are block designs,[66,127] digit symbol,[66,129] speed of writing words or numbers,[66] reaction time to light or sound,[66,127] Reitan trail-making,[66,129] color-word,[127] visual retention,[127] and canceling letters.[129] Based on such psychomotor tests, approximately 85% of cirrhotics were found unfit to drive an automobile or had questionable driving capacity.[137] At least two of these tests and the Reitan trail-making test should be included in any test battery designed to detect stage O-I or covert encephalopathy.

The most frequently seen cases of overt encephalopathy are those of *cirrhotics with acute or subacute encephalopathy.* The onset is insidious. Immediate relatives recall distortions of the patient's usual behavior. He may stay up at night and sleep during the day. His level of awareness seems stunted, and he may appear garrulous and euphoric. He becomes restless and has difficulty focusing on anything very long. He is more than usually irritable and may be anxious and agitated. He may be found wandering around the hospital or ward aimlessly. On examination, a tremor and muscular incoordination are usually detected. His handwriting is more jerky and less precise than usual, his signature recognizable but clearly abnormal. He may seem apathetic, and one suspects an element of confusion. His ability to make calculations has deteriorated.

After a few days, a change in his personality becomes more evident. He is less inhibited and often displays inappropriate behavior. He is less obedient and may become sullen. He responds slowly to requests, and his movements are deliberate. On testing, asterixis is evident. His muscle tone is not normal. He resists passive movement and will grab and hold onto the bed rails or examiner's arm. His voluntary movement seems weaker than expected, and he may be ataxic. As one observes him, he may yawn or blink and grimace repeatedly and may make sucking movements of his mouth. Occasionally one sees him picking at or rearranging the bed covers. If he is checked at this point, he appears lethargic, has lost his sense of time, and cannot remember even recent events very well.

Unless there is reversal of the manifestations in response to therapy or removal of some precipitating event, the encephalopathy progresses more rapidly into the next phase. Behavior may be bizarre, and confusion is obvious. The patient has no sense of time and does not know where he is or has been. He becomes angry easily, and he becomes inappropriately suspicious. He sleeps much of the time. Hyperventilation can be readily recognized. His body temperature is below normal unless he has a superimposed infection. He may be incontinent. His reflexes are generally hyperactive, and the Babinski sign or other tests of plantar response are positive. He shows muscle rigidity on passive or active movement. On rare occasions, a seizure may occur. However, more typically, he becomes somnolent and then stuporous. This progresses to a semiconscious state from which he can be aroused. Unconsciousness follows, at first with and then without response to painful stimuli. During this phase, the patient's breathing is usually stertorous, rapid, and deep.

In the patient with *acute encephalopathy due to fulminant hepatic failure,* the developmental process of the encephalopathy is condensed and most of the early and subtle behavioral aberrations are not manifest or cannot be recognized. However, a gross personality change may be seen. An excitement phase is evident and intense, and delirium and even mania are likely to occur. Violent behavior may be noted. Seizures, which may be focal or general, may also occur. Multifocal random twitching of muscles is often seen before the patient becomes comatose.

Asterixis is uncommon. Deep coma develops rapidly, while abnormalities of other organ systems than the brain or liver complicate the picture. Preterminally, dysconjugate eye movements as well as decerebrate rigidity may be seen. A prominent fetor hepaticus is most likely to be seen in these patients.

Children with *Reye's syndrome* present a distinctive clinical picture that differs from that of adult fulminant hepatic failure while having elements in common. The course is usually hyperacute. After an upper respiratory tract infection with fever and malaise, there may be an abrupt onset of profuse vomiting followed quickly by restlessness, irritability, dullness, and lethargy interspersed with wild delirium, slurred speech, and inappropriate language. Focal muscle twitching and tetanic spasms occur, and multifocal or general seizures may be seen. Sympathetic overactivity is prominent. Respirations are rapid, deep, and irregular. Reflexes are variable. The excitement is followed by stupor and light coma, during which decorticate posturing is seen. Then follows deep coma with decerebrate posturing, opisthotonus, and ocular palsies. Finally, flaccidity occurs with loss of pupillary reflexes and circulatory collapse. Fortunately, this frightening sequence is becoming less frequent with early and vigorous therapy.

In the various *hyperammonemic syndromes of childhood,* which will not be included in the review, the manifestations are more selectively those of ammonia toxicity.[8,59]

The episodes seen in *acute or subacute recurrent encephalopathy* are similar to those described above for cirrhosis with a single acute episode; however, the encephalopathy is not so fully developed and is more readily reversed with treatment.

Patients with *chronic recurrent encephalopathy* have many episodes more or less like that described for the cirrhotic with a single acute episode. Their episodes, which tend to appear, develop, and remit quickly, are exacerbations superimposed on a chronic abnormal state in which the motor disorder is prominent. Variability of the manifestations is a typical feature, and wide fluctuations are seen. Psychotic or psychoneurotic reactions occur commonly. Varying degrees of personality change, some extreme, are seen. Mood may fluctuate widely and abruptly. During intervals of improvement, the patients are at ease, pleasant, cooperative, and generally cheerful. They have little drive or initiative. In essence, these patients have a chronic organic reaction characterized by a motor disturbance, personality change, mood disorder, and intellectual defect that fluctuate in severity and are largely reversible. During exacerbations, they may resemble patients with chronic toxic psychoses or organic dementias. They are differentiated from these by the fluctuations in episodes, encephalographic changes typical of hepatic encephalopathy, and the presence of liver disease.

Patients with *chronic permanent encephalopathy* or hepatocerebral degeneration have a chronic unremitting motor disorder superimposed on a baseline of chronic recurrent encephalopathy in which the motor disturbance predominates.[150] The liability to the permanent neurologic

syndrome increases with repeated and prolonged episodes of recurrent hepatic encephalopathy. All of these patients have prominent portal-systemic collaterals, and about one half have had surgical portal-systemic shunts. Their neurologic manifestations are long lasting and fluctuate somewhat. The patients are generally mildly demented and careless in dress and appearance. They have changing moods, intermittent confusion and episodes of agitation and bizarre and boisterous behavior. They are generally mentally slow and apathetic, with little interest in their surroundings. Their memory and perception are defective. Some may have transient abnormalities of somatic cerebral functions, such as visual defects or hemiplegias. The motor abnormalities may vary from a combination of tremor, extrapyramidal rigidity, and reflex changes to advanced cerebellar, extrapyramidal, and pyramidal dysfunction. While a fine tremor is typical, asterixis is not prominent. An irregular, coarse parkinsonian-like postural tremor that disappears at rest may be present. There is resistance to passive stretch of muscles that becomes frank muscle rigidity with episodes of encephalopathy. Oral-facial dyskinesia may be prominent, and dysarthria is often present. Most patients have ataxia on walking, and some have choreoathetosis. Brisk reflexes and a positive Babinski sign are common.

Patients with myelopathy, who are rare, have episodes of chronic recurrent encephalopathy before and after the development of a spastic paraplegia. Some also have hepatocerebral degeneration. All but a few have previously had a surgical portal-systemic shunt, and in addition, some have previously had gastrectomies for bleeding peptic ulcers.

DIAGNOSIS

The diagnosis of hepatic encephalopathy is made primarily by recognition of the pattern of clinical neuropsychiatric changes occurring in a patient with known liver disease. In the classic and most frequently observed case, a cirrhotic whose liver disease has been followed for some time, the diagnosis becomes readily apparent with development of several of the features listed in Table 24-1. Similarly, the patient with acute fulminant hepatic failure and jaundice who quickly develops somnolence, stupor, and coma after a brief phase of restlessness and agitation offers no problem in diagnosis. However, when liver disease is not recognized or suspected, the nonspecific nature of the neuropsychiatric manifestations listed in Table 24-1 becomes more apparent. Although encephalopathy may be recognized, the differential diagnosis broadens to include space-occupying intracranial lesions, toxic or other metabolic encephalopathies, and various psychiatric disorders. In some patients whose liver disease is recognized, the usual pattern of development of encephalopathy does not occur. One or two behavioral or neurologic manifestations may be so dominant that the association with the liver disease is not even considered. Examples are patients with an apparent dementia, an apparent psychosis, or an apparent seizure disorder. Patients with chronic recurrent encephalopathy are particularly likely to be misdiagnosed, because their neurologic and behavioral abnormalities appear to be their primary ailments. Such patients may become residents on chronic neurologic wards or in mental institutions.

Laboratory Findings

Several laboratory procedures may be helpful in supporting a diagnosis of hepatic encephalopathy or, if encephalopathy is unsuspected, in alerting the physician to the possibility of this diagnosis. The *electroencephalogram* (EEG) develops abnormalities that, while not pathognomonic of hepatic encephalopathy, are fairly characteristic (Fig. 24-2). The changes usually precede the clinical deterioration. At first, the normal alpha rhythm is disturbed by random waves occurring at a frequency of 5 to 7/sec (theta waves). The slowing is symmetrical, appearing in the frontal areas and then spreading laterally and posteriorly as the encephalopathy progresses. These are followed by the appearance of larger triphasic waves with a frequency of 4 to 5/sec, which displace some of the theta waves. The alpha waves are usually gone at this time. The triphasic waves predominate in the frontal and central areas. As coma deepens, large random and arrhythmic waves with a frequency of 2 to 3/sec (delta waves) appear and dominate the EEG. These large waves begin over the frontal lobes and spread backward over the hemispheres. As the encephalopathy improves, the sequence of slowing is reversed.

The correlation between the staging of encephalopathy by clinical criteria and the severity of changes in the EEG is only fair, although significant.[120] No correlation has been observed between EEG changes and the blood or CSF ammonia levels. Attempts to develop EEG-provocative tests for the assessment of predispostion to encephalopathy using protein loading, ammonium salts, or morphine have been unrewarding.[70,88] The EEG has often been looked on as a reference yardstick for the presence of hepatic encephalopathy; however, it is no substitute for careful clinical assessment and staging of the encephalopathy and probably not as valid. An attempt has been made to objectify the EEG using an automated analysis based on the mean dominant frequency and the relative powers of the delta and theta bands.[149]

Distinctive visually evoked potentials have been found in small animals with hepatic encephalopathy.[135,165] Evoked potentials, visual or auditory, may prove to be useful when applied in patients.[100,166]

Many *blood measurements* have been made and correlations with encephalopathy described as indicated in the section on metabolic abnormalities. However, little of practical diagnostic value has resulted. Results of the usual liver function tests are no different in the patient with encephalopathy than in the same patient without encephalopathy. It is important to assess the patient's acid–base and electrolyte status, although not for purposes of diagnosis. Two measurements with potential diagnostic value are those of blood ammonia and methanethiol. The measurement of methanethiol is not practical for routine

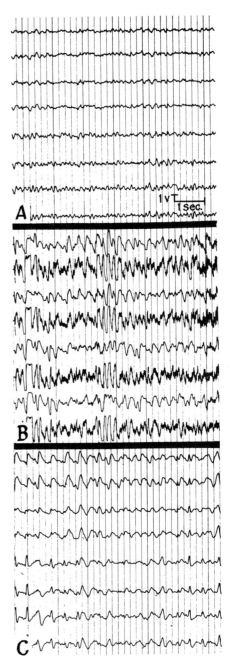

Fig. 24-2. Three EEG tracings from a patient with chronic recurrent encephalopathy. Tracing *A* was taken during stage I clinical encephalopathy and shows 5- to 7-per-second theta waves and some alpha rhythm. Tracing *B,* made a few days later, was taken during stage III clinical encephalopathy and shows 4- to 5-per-second triphasic waves. Tracing *C,* taken a day later during stage II clinical encephalopathy, shows a mixture of triphasic and theta waves. (Zieve L, Mendelson DF, Goepfert M: Ann Intern Med 53:33–52, 1960)

use. In contrast, the blood ammonia value is easily determined, especially with the use of an ammonia electrode. However, an isolated blood ammonia (or methanethiol) determination is of little diagnostic value in a patient with known liver disease, because of the great variability observed from patient to patient. It is of more value in the exceptional case without previously known liver disease. Serial measurements in a given patient with liver disease are a little more useful in following the course of an episode of encephalopathy.

The *CSF glutamine* determination, also easily determined with an ammonia electrode, is of much greater value than the blood ammonia level in assessing a suspected episode of encephalopathy. The correlation between the severity of the clinical or EEG indicators of encephalopathy and the CSF glutamine is good.[81,113] This measurement has been underused, probably because of previous complexities in the determination and the necessity of a spinal tap. In institutions regularly using the procedure, a small percentage of patients with hepatic encephalopathy are diagnosed for the first time after a CSF glutamine determination. The concentration of CSF α-ketoglutaramate (glutamine minus an amino group) also correlates well with the presence of encephalopathy.

Differential Diagnosis

The mental, personality, and neuromuscular manifestations of hepatic encephalopathy are nonspecific. Therefore, if, in a given patient, liver disease is unsuspected, the diagnostic possibilities are greatly enlarged. *Intracranial lesions* of various kinds may be considered, including brain tumor or abscess, cerebrovascular accident, or meningeal infection or irritation. A history of headache and signs of lateralizing or focal neurologic abnormalities that persist usually differentiate these lesions from hepatic encephalopathy. If the patient shows stupor or coma, *other metabolic encephalopathies* due to hypoxia, hypoglycemia, diabetic acidosis, or uremia must be considered. These can be excluded by the obviously indicated laboratory determinations.

In the presence of liver disease, *cerebral depression from drugs* such as sedatives, tranquilizers, or narcotics is likely to occur. The stuporous or comatose state is often confused with hepatic encephalopathy. However, it is usually a quiet flaccid coma without hyperpnea, in contrast to hepatic coma. Since alcoholism is so commonly associated with liver disease, *alcohol withdrawal syndromes* such as delirium tremens or Wernicke's syndrome may be confused with hepatic encephalopathy, especially since acute hepatic decompensation with jaundice may be present simultaneously. The alcohol withdrawal syndromes show a more constant relationship to the discontinuation of drinking. A fully conscious patient with total insomnia, sympathetic overactivity, greatly increased psychomotor activity, prominent fear and anxiety, aggressive and destructive behavior, great muscular strength, rapid elided speech, and hallucinations is more likely to have delirium tremens. Similarly, a confused alcoholic with ophthalmoplegia, nystagmus, and ataxia that respond to thiamine is more likely to have Wernicke's syndrome.

Because alcoholics are susceptible to trauma, *cerebral trauma* leading to encephalopathy may be confused with hepatic encephalopathy. The most important diagnosis to consider is *subdural hematoma.* The presence of headache, lateralizing neurologic abnormalities, radiographic findings, and CSF alterations of pressure and protein favor the diagnosis of trauma.

Sodium or potassium depletion of rather severe degree is commonly seen in cirrhotics with acute decompensation. These patients may be somnolent, stuporous, or comatose when hospitalized but often promptly improve when the electrolyte deficiencies are corrected.

Patients with chronic recurrent encephalopathy may masquerade as cases of *psychosis,* particularly manic depression or paranoia, or as cases of *psychoneurosis.* Their neurologic manifestations have been confused with diseases such as multiple sclerosis, Parkinson's disease, and Wilson's disease. *Wilson's disease* is more likely to be confused with hepatocerebral degeneration, which is essentially identical in its manifestations except for the absence of the abnormality in copper metabolism.

TREATMENT

Preventive Measures

Most episodes of hepatic encephalopathy occur in cirrhotics and have specific precipitating factors or events. Therefore, preventive measures are important. Stools should be kept soft with lactulose or sorbitol. Constipation is thereby avoided, and an acidic stool *p*H reduces the generation of ammonia and mercaptans. One should be aware of the patient's tolerance for protein and set a limit as a guide for him to follow. If, concurrent with stool softening as above, there is protein intolerance to a level of 60 g/day, the patient should avoid meat proteins. If he becomes symptomatic on more than 40 g of protein, eliminate animal protein entirely and use vegetable proteins such as soybean.[69]

One should anticipate the possibility of gastrointestinal hemorrhage by regular checking of stools for blood with one of the simple procedures that involves mailing a stool sample to the physician. These tests should be performed as often as one's index of suspicion or apprehension in the individual case warrants. However, a regular and systematic approach is desirable. Major gastrointestinal hemorrhage may often be avoided by early therapy. If hemorrhage occurs, it should be treated vigorously with avoidance of hypovolemia and hypoxia and with gentle catharsis to clear the bowel of blood as quickly as possible.

Sedatives, tranquilizers, and narcotic analgesics should be avoided, especially in the acutely decompensated patient. If unavoidable, they should be used with circumspection. Potassium, magnesium, and zinc deficits should be corrected by persistent replacement, because cellular loss is common and often marked. Zinc supplementation has been shown to improve psychomotor test performance of a sample of cirrhotics with covert encephalopathy.[126] Hyponatremia must also be anticipated and prevented.

Diuresis should not be vigorous, and paracenteses, except for diagnostic purposes, should be shunned. Alertness to potential infections in lungs, genitourinary tract, and ascitic fluid may reduce the likelihood of infection or at least encourage early treatment. If surgery is contemplated, every attempt should be made to minimize operating time, anesthesia, trauma, hypoxia, hypnotics, narcotics, blood loss, hypovolemia, and electrolyte imbalance.

Removal or correction of precipitating factors is a necessary first step if encephalopathy is already present when the patient is first seen.

Acute or Subacute Hepatic Encephalopathy

The patient with acute or subacute hepatic encephalopathy requires meticulous nursing care, good respiratory toilet, and attention to details of intake and output. A sequential tabulation of clinical, laboratory, and therapeutic data is valuable. This should include staging of the severity of the encephalopathy (at least daily) and a record of the patient's handwriting, at least his signature, at the time of each staging. Dietary protein should be stopped and calories provided as glucose, 300 g to 500 g/day orally or parenterally as appropriate. Thorough retention enemas with 20% lactose or with 1% neomycin solution adjusted to a pH of 4 should be given promptly until one can be confident that the entire colon has been cleansed of fecal matter. At the same time, catharsis with magnesium sulfate or citrate may be started. If the patient has not been taking lactulose, it should be given in sufficient dosage to keep the stools soft and continued after the episode is reversed. While the encephalopathy is present, 1 g to 2 g of neomycin is given orally every 6 hours. An alternative to neomycin is absorbable antibiotics such as ampicillin or tetracycline, which effectively destroy colonic bacteria and have a systemic action. These are preferable to neomycin in the presence of renal insufficiency. If definite improvement of the encephalopathy occurs, the antibiotics are discontinued, lactulose maintained and proteins reintroduced at a low level (20 g/day) and gradually increased.

Treatment so far has attempted to reduce the formation of ammonia and mercaptans or their absorption from the gut. Efforts have also been made to increase the removal of ammonia by providing an excess of glutamate to combine with ammonia to form glutamine or an excess of arginine or ornithine to enhance the conversion of ammonia to urea. Uncontrolled observations in selected patients in hepatic coma suggested that the coma could often be reversed with intravenous arginine (or arginine glutamate), although the ultimate outcome of the encephalopathy was determined by other factors.[112] Doses of arginine or ornithine in the range of 5 g to 10 g/hr infused intravenously in 10% dextrose for a maximum of 12 hours are recommended. The treatment is only appropriate for patients with a functional urea cycle; therefore, those with severe liver dysfunction are not likely to respond.[128] The rationale for this therapy and some supportive experimental data have been presented elsewhere.[173,182]

In uncontrolled therapeutic trials, L-dopa has appeared to have an arousal effect in almost two thirds of patients with hepatic coma.[58] L-Dopa was given as a water suspension of 0.5 g through a nasogastric tube every 4 hours or rectally every 6 hours. The favorable effect was related to early use of this therapy after onset of coma and to renal responsiveness. In those patients who responded to L-dopa, urinary volume and sodium increased twofold and threefold, respectively. In those who did not respond to L-dopa, they were unchanged. In normal rats, L-dopa prevents ammonia coma in association with increased renal excretion of ammonia and urea and reduction of brain ammonia.[179] After nephrectomy, this effect of L-dopa on ammonia coma is lost and the brain ammonia level is unchanged. It thus seems likely that the beneficial effect of L-dopa in patients is related to enhanced renal function. A controlled trial, which did not find any benefit from L-dopa, did not pair treatment and control groups with respect to renal function. The argument also applies to bromocriptine, a dopamine agonist that has had arousal effects in selected patients.

Branched-chain amino acids have been actively studied for their therapeutic value in patients with acute or subacute encephalopathy, and much has been written during the past few years.[21,91,152] The subject is confusing and controversial, even if one only considers controlled studies that have been reported. The difficulties arise from the highly variable nature of the underlying hepatic abnormality that is being treated, and the forces of selection that determine the structure of the sample of patients being treated. It appears that improvement in encephalopathy has been seen generally when the branched-chain amino acid mixture contained increased amounts of arginine (ammonia processor) and reduced amounts of glycine (ammonia generator), in addition to the increased amounts of branched-chain amino acids. A controlled multi-institution study that used branched-chain amino acids alone found no improvement in hepatic encephalopathy.[151] However, another controlled multi-hospital study found branched-chain amino acids alone as effective as lactulose in reversing hepatic encephalopathy.[131] The issue of effectiveness of branched-chain amino acids in treatment of acute hepatic encephalopathy is thus unsettled at this time. However the tolerance of patients with liver failure for branched-chain amino acids, and the nutritional benefits of such an amino acid mixture given in a glucose solution to such patients is unequivocal. Nitrogen balance is improved and protein breakdown is reduced while synthesis is enhanced.[21,24,91,115]*

Acute or Subacute Recurrent Encephalopathy

Each of the episodes in patients with acute or subacute recurrent encephalopathy is treated as outlined previously for the nonrecurrent cases. The reversible episodes do not

---

* Cerra F et al: Disease specific amino acid infusions (F080) and hepatic encephalopathy: A prospective randomized double blind control trial. J Parenteral Enteral Nutr 9:288, 1985.

generally require vigorous therapy to correct the process. Attention to the preventive measures will reduce the number of recurrences.

Chronic Recurrent Encephalopathy

Patients with chronic recurrent encephalopathy are particularly sensitive to protein and other nitrogenous products.[33] If an acute exacerbation of the encephalopathy occurs, they are treated like the patients with acute or subacute encephalopathy described previously. On a permanent basis, they need continuous attention to prevention of toxicity from dietary proteins yet provision of the minimum requirements of nitrogen for sustenance of body proteins. They should be seen at regular intervals by the physician, at which time their treatment should be reviewed and their mental and neuromuscular state assessed using some systematic scheme of rating, including psychomotor tests. The patient should be maintained on lactulose or sorbitol in a dosage sufficient to keep the stools soft. Constipation is to be avoided. If he still requires protein restriction to avoid symptoms of encephalopathy, several additional forms of treatment that have additive effects should be tried. One is placement on a vegetable protein diet.[41,148] A second is administration of intermittent 14-day courses of neomycin, 1 g every 6 hours for a total of 3 g each day. A third is administration of intermittent 14-day courses of metronidazole, 0.5 g every 6 hours for a total of 1.5 g each day.[108] A fourth is supplementation with oral ornithine or arginine, 10 g/day.[173]

A careful study of 13 patients of this type who were symptomatic despite animal protein restriction and lactulose showed that ornithine branched-chain keto analogues of the branched-chain amino acids were effective in improving the encephalopathy, whereas an equivalent dose of the branched-chain keto analogues alone or twice as much branched-chain amino acids alone were not.[73] If the ornithine alone proves ineffective, a trial with the ornithine branched-chain keto analogue should be undertaken.

Oral supplementation with branched-chain amino acids has been reported to be beneficial in such patients.[48,78] Again controlled studies with contradictory results have been published.[50,105] The branched-chain amino acids were well tolerated, and positive nitrogen balance was maintained. Such supplementation at least provides a way of increasing nitrogen intake without worsening the encephalopathy.

Acute Fulminant Hepatic Failure

By vigorous general medical management in an intensive care unit, the recovery rate from acute fulminant hepatic failure has reached 30% to 40%.[86] Special procedures such as charcoal hemoperfusion, polyacrylonitrile membrane hemodialysis, exchange transfusion, and extracorporeal hepatic perfusion have intrinsic problems and have not yielded higher recovery rates, although they can clearly reverse the comatose state.[9,16,26,170] The so-called conser-

vative medical management must be aggressive with respect to fluid, electrolyte, and acid–base status, blood volume and oxygenation, coagulation defects, pulmonary, cardiac, renal, and gastrointestinal status, and infections.[153] Monitoring various vital functions is crucial. A central venous catheter or pulmonary artery (Swan-Ganz) catheter and arterial line are inserted to measure corresponding pressures. The electrocardiogram and pulse are also monitored continuously. A nasogastric tube is inserted. Acid–base, oxygen, electrolyte, and osmolality status, blood glucose values, prothrombin time, and a chest roentgenogram are obtained daily. As a first step in therapy, the gastrointestinal tract is cleared of protein and bacteria with an osmotic cathartic such as magnesium sulfate or citrate and retention enemas with 20% lactose or 1% neomycin solution adjusted to a pH of 4. Lactulose or sorbitol is started by nasogastric tube. All sedatives and tranquilizers are prohibited.

General intensive care nursing procedures are employed with regular turning of the patient, oral and bronchial toilet, oxygen therapy, humidification, and physiotherapy. Fluids, electrolytes, and plasma or blood are given to maintain balance. Arginine hydrochloride is given intravenously along with potassium to correct alkalosis. Overloading is carefully avoided, but hypovolemia and hypotension must be prevented. Calories are given as glucose. Fresh frozen plasma and platelet packs are given to correct coagulation defects. Cimetidine is given prophylactically to prevent gastrointestinal bleeding. If bleeding occurs, vigorous replacement with fresh blood should be immediate and catharsis with magnesium salts prompt. Early endotracheal intubation is often required. Assistance from a mechanical respirator may be needed. Cardiac abnormalities are treated as they occur. Early peritoneal dialysis is used for renal failure and, if necessary, replaced with hemodialysis. Infections are looked for and treated promptly with antibiotics as appropriate. If there is no infection, hypothermia is usually present. This is not corrected, because the lowered temperature slows metabolic processes, a desirable consequence in these patients. If cerebral edema is suspected, hyperosmolar solutions of mannitol are given intermittently as long as urine flow is maintained. If renal function is compromised, fluid may be removed by artificial ultrafiltration.[30,71] This may be life saving. An intracranial device to monitor intracranial pressure has revolutionized therapy for cerebral edema in Reye's syndrome and, it is hoped, may have a similar beneficial effect in cases of fulminant hepatic failure when bleeding can be controlled.

Reye's Syndrome

Aggressive therapy has had a remarkable effect on the mortality from Reye's syndrome. The general intensive care approach to therapy outlined for fulminant hepatic failure applies as well to these patients. Monitoring the intracranial pressure with an intracranial device has resulted in more vigorous hyperosmolar therapy and improved survival in the severe cases. Death has usually been from cerebral edema. Mortality rates, which were as high as 70%, have been markedly reduced as a result of earlier diagnosis and more vigorous treatment.[32,44,99]

REFERENCES

1. Adams RD, Foley JM, Merritt HH, Hare CC (eds): The neurological disorder associated with liver disease. In Metabolic and Toxic Diseases of the Nervous System, vol 32, pp 198–237. Baltimore, Williams & Wilkins, 1953

2. Ahmed K, Thomas BS: The effects of long-chain fatty acids on sodium plus potassium ion–stimulated adenosine triphosphatase of rat brain. J Biol Chem 246:103, 1971

3. Ahmed K et al: Effects of methanethiol on erythrocyte membrane stabilization and on Na^+, K^+-adenosine triphosphatase: Relevance to hepatic coma. J Pharmacol Exp Ther 228:103, 1984

4. Ansley JD et al: Quantitative tests of nitrogen metabolism in cirrhosis: Relation to other manifestations of liver disease. Gastroenterology 75:570, 1978

5. Baraldi M, Zeneroli ML: Experimental hepatic encephalopathy: Changes in the binding of γ-aminobutyric acid. Science 216:427, 1982

6. Baraldi M et al: Portal-systemic encephalopathy in dogs: Changes in brain GABA receptors and neurochemical correlates. In Kleinberger G et al: (eds): Advances in Hepatic Encephalopathy and Urea Cycle Diseases, pp 353–359. Basel, Karger, 1984

7. Baraldi M et al: Toxins in hepatic encephalopathy: The role of the synergistic effect of ammonia, mercaptans and short chain fatty acids. Arch Toxicol Suppl 7:103, 1984

8. Batshaw ML et al: Treatment of inborn errors of urea synthesis: Activation of alternative pathways of waste nitrogen synthesis and excretion. N Engl J Med 306:1387, 1982

9. Berk PD, Popper H: Fulminant hepatic failure. Am J Gastroenterol 69:349, 1978

10. Berl S et al: Metabolic compartments *in vivo:* Ammonia and glutamic acid metabolism in brain and liver. J Biol Chem 237:2562, 1962

11. Bernardini P, Fischer JE: Amino acid imbalance and hepatic encephalopathy. Ann Rev Nutr 2:419, 1982

12. Bloxam DL, Curzon G: A study of proposed determinants of brain tryptophan concentration in rats after portacaval anastomosis or sham operation. J Neurochem 31:1255, 1978

13. Bollman JL et al: Coma with increased amino acids of brain and cerebrospinal fluid in dogs with Eck's fistula. Arch Surg 75:405, 1957

14. Borg J et al: Neurotransmitter modifications in human cerebrospinal fluid and serum during hepatic encephalopathy. J Neurol Sci 57:343, 1982

15. Brun A et al: Brain proteins in hepatic encephalopathy. Acta Neurol Scand 55:213, 1977

16. Brunner G, Schmidt FW: Artificial Liver Support. New York, Springer-Verlag, 1981

17. Bruton CJ et al: Hereditary hyperammonemia. Brain 93:423, 1970

18. Cangiano C et al: Plasma phenylethanolamine in hepatic encephalopathy. Eur J Clin Invest 8:183, 1978

19. Cangiano C et al: Plasma levels of false neurotransmitters across the brain in portal-systemic encephalopathy. Eur J Clin Invest 12:51, 1982

20. Capocaccia L et al: Octopamine and ammonia plasma levels in hepatic encephalopathy. Clin Chim Acta 75:99, 1977

21. Capocaccia L, Fischer JE, Rossi-Fanelli F: Hepatic Encephalopathy in Chronic Liver Failure. London, Plenum Press, 1984

22. Cascino A et al: Plasma amino acid imbalance in patients with liver disease. Dig Dis Sci 23:591, 1978

23. Cascino A et al: Plasma and cerebrospinal fluid amino acid patterns in hepatic encephalopathy. Dig Dis Sci 27:828, 1982

24. Cerra FB et al: Cirrhosis, encephalopathy, and improved results with metabolic support. Surgery 94:612, 1983

25. Challenger F, Walshe JM: Methyl mercaptan in relation to foetor hepaticus. Biochem J 59:372, 1955

26. Chamuleau RAFM et al: Problems in treating experimentally induced acute hepatic failure by hemoperfusion or cross circulation. Hepatology 3:596, 1983

27. Chase RA et al: Plasma amino acid profiles in patients with fulminant hepatic failure treated by repeated polyacrylonitrile membrane hemodialysis. Gastroenterology 75:1033, 1978

28. Clark GM, Eiseman B: Studies in ammonia metabolism: IV. Biochemical changes in brain tissue of dogs during ammonia-induced coma. N Engl J Med 259:178, 1958

29. Colombo JP et al: Liver enzymes in the Eck fistula rat: I. Urea cycle enzymes and transaminases. Enzyme 14:353, 1973

30. Colton CK et al: Kinetics of hemofiltration: I. *In vitro* transport characteristics of a hollow-fiber blood ultrafilter. J Lab Clin Med 85:351, 1975

31. Conn HO, Lieberthal MM: The Hepatic Coma Syndromes and Lactulose. Baltimore, William & Wilkins, 1979

32. Crocker JFS: Reye's syndrome. Semin Liver Dis 2:340, 1982

33. Crossley IR, Williams R: Progress in the treatment of chronic portasystemic encephalopathy. Gut 25:85, 1984

34. Cuilleret C et al: Changes in brain catecholamine levels in human cirrhotic hepatic encephalopathy. Gut 21:565, 1980

35. Cummings MG et al: Regional brain study of indoleamine metabolism in the rat in acute hepatic failure. J Neurochem 27:741, 1976

36. Curzon G, Knott PJ: Environmental, toxicological, and related aspects of tryptophan metabolism with particular reference to the central nervous system. CRC Crit Rev Toxicol 5:145, 1977

37. Curzon G et al: The biochemical, behavioral and neurologic effects of high L-tryptophan intake in the Rhesus monkey. Neurology 13:431, 1963

38. Curzon G et al: Plasma and brain tryptophan changes in experimental acute hepatic failure. J Neurochem 21:137, 1973

39. Daoud FS et al: Failure of hypoxic pulmonary vasoconstriction in patients with liver cirrhosis. J Clin Invest 51:1076, 1972

40. Dawson AM: Regulation of blood ammonia. Gut 19:504, 1978

41. DeBruijn KM et al: Effect of dietary protein manipulations in subclinical portal-systemic encephalopathy. Gut 24:53, 1983

42. Denis J et al: Respective roles of ammonia, amino acids, and medium-sized molecules in the pathogenesis of experimentally induced acute hepatic encephalopathy. J Neurochem 40:10, 1983

43. Derr RF, Zieve L: Methanethiol and fatty acids depress urea synthesis by the isolated perfused rat liver. J Lab Clin Med 100:585, 1982

44. Devivo DC, Keating JP: Reye's syndrome. Adv Pediatr 22:175, 1976

45. Doizaki WM, Zieve L: An improved method for measuring blood mercaptans. J Lab Clin Med 90:849, 1977

46. Drapanas T et al: Intermediary metabolism following hepatectomy in dogs. Ann Surg 162:621, 1965

47. Duffy TE et al: α-Ketoglutaramate in hepatic encephalopathy. Res Publ Assoc Nerv Ment Dis 53:39, 1974

48. Egberts E-H et al: Branched chain amino acids in the treatment of latent portosystemic encephalopathy: A double-blind placebo-controlled crossover study. Gastroenterology 88:887, 1985

49. Eiseman B, Clark GM: Studies of ammonia metabolism: III. The experimental production of coma by carotid arterial infusion of ammonium salts. Surgery 43:476, 1958

50. Eriksson LS et al: Branched-chain amino acids in the treatment of chronic hepatic encephalopathy. Gut 23:801, 1982

51. Fahey JL: Toxicity and blood ammonia rise resulting from intravenous amino acid administration in man: The protective effect of L-arginine. J Clin Invest 36:1647, 1957

52. Faraj BA et al: Hypertyraminemia in cirrhotic patients. N Engl J Med 294:1360, 1976

53. Faraj BA et al: Evidence for central hypertyraminemia in hepatic encephalopathy. J Clin Invest 67:395, 1981

54. Farber MO et al: The oxygen affinity of hemoglobin in hepatic encephalopathy. J Lab Clin Med 98:135, 1981

55. Ferenci P et al: Neurotransmitter receptor changes in experimental hyperammonemia in the rabbit. In Kleinberger G et al (eds): Advances in Hepatic Encephalopathy and Urea Cycle Diseases, pp 368–372. Basel, Karger, 1984

56. Fischer JE: False neurotransmitters and hepatic coma. Res Publ Assoc Nerv Ment Dis 53:53, 1974

57. Fischer JE, Baldessarini RJ: Pathogenesis and therapy of hepatic coma. In Popper H, Schaffner R (eds): Progress in Liver Diseases, vol 5, pp 363–397. New York, Grune & Stratton, 1975

58. Fischer JE et al: L-Dopa in hepatic coma. Ann Surg 183:386, 1976

59. Flannery DB et al: Current status of hyperammonemic syndromes. Hepatology 2:495, 1982

60. Flock EV et al: Utilization of U-^{14}C glucose in brain after total hepatectomy in the rat. J Neurochem 13:1389, 1966

61. Gabuzda GJ et al: Reversible toxic manifestations in patients with cirrhosis of the liver given cation-exchange resins. N Engl J Med 246:124, 1952

62. Gabuzda GJ: Hepatic coma: Clinical consideration, pathogenesis, and management. In Dock W, Snapper I (eds): Advances in Internal Medicine, vol 11, pp 11–73. Chicago, Year Book, Medical Publishers, 1962

63. Gauthier G, Wildi E: L'Encephalomyelopathic porto-systemique. Rev Neurol 131:319, 1975

64. Gazzard BG et al: Causes of death in fulminant hepatic failure and relationship to quantitative histological assessment of parenchymal damage. Q J Med 44:615, 1975

65. Giguere JF, Butterworth RF: Amino acid changes in regions of the CNS in relation to function in experimental portal-systemic encephalopathy. Neurochem Res 9:1309, 1984

66. Gilberstadt S et al: Psychomotor performance defects in cirrhotics without overt encephalopathy. Arch Intern Med 140:519, 1980

67. Gjedde A et al: Cerebral blood flow and metabolism in chronically hyperammonemic rats: Effect of an acute ammonia challenge. Ann Neurol 3:325, 1978

68. Goodman MW et al: Mechanism of arginine protection against ammonia intoxication in the rat. Am J Physiol 247:G290, 1984

69. Greenberger NJ et al: Effect of vegetable and animal protein diets in chronic hepatic encephalopathy. Dig Dis Sci 22:845, 1977

70. Hawkes CH et al: EEG-provocative tests in the diagnosis of hepatic encephalopathy. Electroenceph Clin Neurophysiol 34:163, 1973

71. Henderson LW et al: Kinetics of ultrafiltration: II. Clinical characterization of a new blood cleansing modality. J Lab Clin Med 85:372, 1975

72. Herlin PM et al: The blood–brain barrier is intact eighteen hours after total hepatectomy. Hepatology 1:515, 1981

73. Herlong HF et al: The use of ornithine salts of branched-chain ketoacids in portal-systemic encephalopathy. Ann Intern Med 93:545, 1980

74. Hindfelt B: The distribution of ammonia between extracellular and intracellular compartments of the rat brain. Clin Sci Mol Med 48:33, 1975

75. Hindfelt B et al: Effect of acute ammonia intoxication on cerebral metabolism in rats with portacaval shunts. J Clin Invest 59:386, 1977

76. Hirayama C: Tryptophan metabolism in liver disease. Clin Chim Acta 32:191, 1971

77. Horak W et al: Kinetics of ^{14}C-cholic acid in fulminant hepatic failure: A prognostic test. Gastroenterology 71:809, 1976

78. Horst D et al: Comparison of dietary protein with an oral branched chain–enriched amino acid supplement in chronic portal-systemic encephalopathy: A randomized controlled trial. Hepatology 4:279, 1984

79. Hortnagl H et al: Plasma catecholamines in hepatic coma and liver cirrhosis: Role of octopamine. Klin Wochenschr 59:1159, 1981

80. Hortnagl H et al: Substance P is markedly increased in plasma of patients with hepatic coma. Lancet 1:480, 1984

81. Hourani BT et al: Cerebrospinal fluid glutamine as a measure of hepatic encephalopathy. Arch Intern Med 127:1033, 1971

82. Huet PM et al: Blood–brain transport of tryptophan and phenylalanine: Effect of portacaval shunt in dogs. Am J Physiol 241:G163, 1981

83. James IM et al: Effect of induced metabolic alkalosis in hepatic encephalopathy. Lancet 1:1106, 1969

84. James JH et al: Blood–brain neutral amino acid transport activity is increased after portacaval anastomosis. Science 200:1395, 1978

85. Jeppsson B et al: Increased blood–brain transport of tryptophan after portacaval anastomosis in germ-free rats. Metabolism 32:4, 1983

86. Jones EA, Schafer DF: Fulminant hepatic failure. In Zakim D, Boyer TD (eds): Hepatology: A Textbook of Liver Disease, pp 415–445. Philadelphia, WB Saunders, 1982

87. Jones EA et al: The neurobiology of hepatic encephalopathy. Hepatology 4:1235, 1984

88. Jones DP et al: The contingent negative variation and psychological findings in chronic hepatic encephalopathy. Electroenceph Clin Neurophysiol 40:661, 1976

89. Keys A, Snell AM: Respiratory properties of the arterial blood in normal man and in patients with disease of the liver: Position of the oxygen dissociation curve. J Clin Invest 17:59, 1938

90. Khatra BS et al: Activities of Krebs-Henseleit enzymes in normal and cirrhotic human liver. J Lab Clin Med 84:708, 1974

91. Kleinberger G, Ferenci P, Riederer P et al: Advances in Hepatic Encephalopathy and Urea Cycle Diseases. Basel, S Karger, 1984

92. Lauterburg BH et al: Hepatic functional deterioration after

portacaval shunt in the rat: Effects on sulfobromophthalein transport maximum, indocyanine green clearance, and galactose elimination capacity. Gastroenterology 71:221, 1976

93. Liehr H et al: Endotoxemia in acute hepatic failure. Acta Hepatogastroenterol 23:235, 1976

94. Livingstone AS et al: Changes in the blood–brain barrier in hepatic coma after hepatectomy in the rat. Gastroenterology 73:697, 1977

95. Lockwood AH et al: The dynamics of ammonia metabolism in man: Effects of liver disease and hyperammonemia. J Clin Invest 63:449, 1979

96. Maiolo AT et al: Brain energy metabolism in hepatic coma. Exp Biol Med 4:52, 1971

97. Mamunes P et al: Fatty acid quantitation in Reye's syndrome. In Pollack JD (ed): Reye's Syndrome, pp 245–253. New York, Grune & Stratton, 1975

98. Mans AM et al: Regional blood–brain barrier permeability to amino acids after portacaval anastomosis. J Neurochem 38:705, 1982

99. Marshall LF et al: Pentobarbital therapy for intracranial hypertension in metabolic coma: Reye's syndrome. Crit Care Med 6:1, 1978

100. Martines D et al: Brain stem auditory-evoked responses (baers) in the clinical evaluation of hepatic encephalopathy. In Kleinberger G et al (eds): Advances in Hepatic Encephalopathy and Urea Cycle Disease, pp 430–435. Basel, Karger, 1984

101. Mattison WJ Jr et al: Brain amino acid in acute hepatic coma. Surg Forum 19:331, 1968

102. McClain CJ et al: Blood methanethiol in alcoholic liver disease with and without hepatic encephalopathy. Gut 21:318, 1980

103. McLain CJ et al: Hyperprolactinemia in portal-system encephalopathy. Dig Dis Sci 26:353, 1981

104. McDermott WV, Adams RD: Episodic stupor associated with an Eck fistula in the human with particular reference to the metabolism of ammonia. J Clin Invest 33:1, 1954

105. McGhee A et al: Comparison of the effects of Hepatic-Aid and a casein modular diet on encephalopathy, plasma amino acids, and nitrogen balance in cirrhotic patients. Ann Surg 197:288, 1983

106. McMenamy RH et al: Amino acid and α-keto acid concentrations in plasma and blood of the liverless dog. Am J Physiol 209:1046, 1965

107. Michel H et al: Treatment of cirrhotic hepatic encephalopathy with L-dopa: A controlled trial. Gastroenterology 70:207, 1980

108. Morgan MH et al: Treatment of hepatic encephalopathy with metronidazole. Gut 23:1, 1982

109. Morgan MY et al: Plasma ratio of valine, leucine and isoleucine to phenylalanine and tyrosine in liver disease. Gut 19:1068, 1978

110. Moroni F et al: The release and neosynthesis of glutamic acid are increased in experimental models of hepatic encephalopathy. J Neurochem 40:850, 1983

111. Muting D, Reikowski H: Protein metabolism in liver disease. In Popper H, Schaffner F (eds): Progress in Liver Disease, vol 2, pp 84–94. New York, Grune & Stratton, 1965

112. Najarian JS, Harper HA: Clinical study of the effect of arginine on blood ammonia. Am J Med 21:832, 1956

113. Oei LT et al: Cerebrospinal fluid glutamine levels and EEG findings in patients with hepatic encephalopathy. Clin Neurol Neurosurg 81:59, 1979

114. Ogihara K et al: Tryptophan as a cause of hepatic coma. N Engl J Med 275:1255, 1966

115. O'Keefe SJD et al: Protein turnover in acute and chronic liver disease. Acta Chir Scand Suppl 507:91, 1981

116. O'Keefe SJD et al: Increased plasma tyrosine concentrations in patients with cirrhosis and fulminant hepatic failure associated with increased plasma tyrosine flux and reduced hepatic oxidation capacity. Gastroenterology 81:1017, 1981

117. Ono J et al: Tryptophan and hepatic coma. Gastroenterology 74:196, 1978

118. Onstad GR, Zieve L: What determines blood ammonia? Gastroenterology 77:803, 1979

119. Ozawa K et al: Contribution of the arterial blood ketone body ratio to elevated plasma amino acids in hepatic encephalopathy of surgical patients. Am J Surg 146:299, 1983

120. Parsons-Smith BG et al: The electroencephalograph in liver disease. Lancet 1:867, 1957

121. Phillips GB et al: The syndrome of impending hepatic coma in patients with cirrhosis of the liver given certain nitrogenous substances N Engl J Med 247:239, 1952

122. Plum F, Hindfelt B: The neurological complications of liver disease. In Vinken PH, Bruyn GW (eds): Handbook of Clinical Neurology, Vol 27, Metabolic and Deficiency Diseases of the Nervous System, Part I, pp 349–377. New York, American Elsevier, 1976

123. Polli E et al: Cerebral metabolism after portacaval shunt. Lancet 1:153, 1969

124. Potvin M et al: Cerebral abnormalities in hepatectomized rats with acute hepatic coma. Lab Invest 50:560, 1984

125. Raabe W, Gumnit RJ: Disinhibition in cat motor cortex by ammonia. J Neurophysiol 38:347, 1975

126. Reding P et al: Oral zinc supplementation improves hepatic encephalopathy: Results of a randomized controlled trial. Lancet 2:493, 1984

127. Rehnstrom S et al: Chronic hepatic encephalopathy: A psychometrical study. Scand J Gastroenterol 12:305, 1977

128. Reynolds TB et al: A controlled study of the effects of L-arginine on hepatic encephalopathy. Am J Med 25:359, 1958

129. Rikkers L et al: Subclinical hepatic encephalopathy: Detection, prevalence, and relationship to nitrogen metabolism. Gastroenterology 75:462, 1978

130. Roberts E: The γ-aminobutyric acid (GABA) system and hepatic encephalopathy. Hepatology 4:342, 1984

131. Rossi-Fanelli F et al: Branched-chain amino acids vs lactulose in the treatment of hepatic coma: A controlled study. Dig Dis Sci 27:929, 1982

132. Rossi-Fanelli F et al: Induction of coma in normal dogs by the infusion of aromatic amino acids and its prevention by the addition of branched-chain amino acids. Gastroenterology 83:664, 1982

133. Schafer DF, Jones EA: Hepatic encephalopathy and the γ-aminobutyric acid neurotransmitter system. Lancet 1:18, 1982

134. Schafer DF et al: Gamma-aminobutyric acid and benzodiazepine receptors in an animal model of fulminant hepatic failure. J Lab Clin Med 102:870, 1983

135. Schafer DF et al: Visual evoked potentials in a rabbit model of hepatic encephalopathy: I and II. Gastroenterology 86:540, 1984

136. Schenker S et al: Hepatic encephalopathy: Current status. Gastroenterology 66:121, 1974

137. Schomerus H et al: Latent portasystemic encephalopathy: I. Nature of cerebral functional defects and their effect on fitness to drive. Dig Dis Sci 26:622, 1981

138. Seyffert WA, Madison LL: Physiologic effects of metabolic fuels on carbohydrate metabolism: I. Acute effect of ele-

vation of plasma free fatty acids on hepatic glucose output, peripheral glucose utilization, serum insulin, and plasma glucagon levels. Diabetes 16:765, 1967

139. Shear L et al: Renal tubular acidosis in cirrhosis: A determinant of susceptibility to recurrent hepatic precoma. N Engl J Med 280:1, 1969

140. Smith AR et al: Alterations in plasma and CSF amino acids, amines and metabolites in hepatic coma. Ann Surg 187:343, 1978

141. Smith B, Prockop DJ: Central nervous system effects of ingestion of L-tryptophan by normal subjects. N Engl J Med 267:1338, 1962

142. Soeters PB et al: Insulin, glucagon, portal-systemic shunting and hepatic failure in the dog. J Surg Res 23:183, 1977

143. Summerskill WHJ et al: The neuropsychiatric syndrome associated with hepatic cirrhosis and an extensive portal collateral circulation. Q J Med 25:245, 1956

144. Trauner DA: Treatment of Reye syndrome. Ann Neurol 7:2, 1980

145. Trauner DA, Huttenlocher PR: Short-chain fatty acid–induced central hyperventilation in rabbits. Neurology 28:940, 1978

146. Trauner DA et al: Short-chain organic acidemia and Reye's syndrome. Neurology 25:296, 1975

147. Tyce GM et al: 5-Hydroxyindole metabolism in the brain after hepatectomy. Biochem Pharmacol 16:979, 1967

148. Uribe M et al: Treatment of chronic portal-systemic encephalopathy with vegetable and animal protein diets: A controlled crossover study. Dig Dis Sci 27:1109, 1982

149. VanDerRijt CCD et al: Objective measurement of hepatic encephalopathy by means of automated EEG analysis. Electroenceph Clin Neurophysiol 57:423, 1984

150. Victor M et al: The acquired (non-Wilsonian) type of chronic hepatocerebral degeneration. Medicine 44:345, 1965

151. Wahren J et al: Is intravenous administration of branched-chain amino acids effective in the treatment of hepatic encephalopathy? A multicenter study. Hepatology 3:475, 1983

152. Walser M, Williamson JR (eds): Metabolism and Clinical Implications of Branched-Chain Amino Acids and Ketoacids. New York, Elsevier-North Holland, 1981

153. Ward ME et al: Acute liver failure: Experience in a special unit. Anaesthesia 32:228, 1977

154. Ware AJ et al: Cerebral edema: A major complication of massive hepatic necrosis. Gastroenterology 61:877, 1971

155. Warren KS, Schenker S: Hypoxia and ammonia toxicity. Am J Physiol 199:1105, 1960

156. Warren KS et al: Effect of alterations in blood pH on distribution of ammonia from blood to cerebrospinal fluid in patients in hepatic coma. J Lab Clin Med 56:687, 1960

157. Wasterlain CG et al: Chronic inhibition of brain protein synthesis after portacaval shunting. Neurology 28:233, 1978

158. Weber G et al: Feedback inhibition of key glycolytic enzymes in liver: Action of free fatty acids. Science 154:1357, 1966

159. Williams AH et al: The glutamate and glutamine content of rat brain after portacaval anastomosis. J Neurochem 19:1703, 1972

160. Windus-Podehl G et al: Encephalopathic effect of phenol in rats. J Lab Clin Med 101:586, 1983

161. Young SN, Lal S: CNS tryptamine metabolism in hepatic coma. J Neural Transmission 47:153, 1980

162. Zaki AEO et al: Potential toxins of acute liver failure and their effects on blood–brain barrier permeability. Experientia 39:988, 1983

163. Zaki AEO et al: Experimental studies of blood–brain barrier permeability in acute hepatic failure. Hepatology 4:359, 1984

164. Zanchin G et al: GABA and dopamine receptors after chronic portacaval shunt in the rat. In Kleinberger G et al (eds): Advances in Hepatic Encephalopathy and Urea Cycle Diseases, pp 360–367. Basel, Karger, 1984

165. Zeneroli ML et al: Comparative evaluation of visual evoked potentials in experimental hepatic encephalopathy and in pharmacologically induced coma-like states in rat. Life Sci 28:1507, 1981

166. Zeneroli ML et al: Visual evoked potential: A diagnostic tool for the assessment of hepatic encephalopathy. Gut 25:291, 1984

167. Zieve L: Pathogenesis of hepatic coma. Arch Intern Med 118:211, 1966

168. Zieve L: Metabolic abnormalities in hepatic coma and potential toxins to be removed. In Williams R, Murray-Lyon IM (eds): Artificial Liver Support, pp 11–25. Tunbridge Wells, Pitman Medical Publishing, 1975

169. Zieve L: Amino acids in liver failure. Gastroenterology 76:219, 1979

170. Zieve L: Hepatic encephalopathy: Summary of present knowledge with an elaboration on recent developments. In Popper H, Schaffner F (eds): Progress in Liver Diseases, vol 6, pp 327–341. New York, Grune & Stratton, 1979

171. Zieve L: Synergism among toxic factors and other endogenous abnormalities in hepatic encephalopathy. In Brunner G (ed): Artificial Liver Support, pp 18–24. Berlin, Springer-Verlag, 1981

172. Zieve L: Encephalopathy due to short- and medium-chain fatty acids. In McCandless DW (ed): Cerebral Energy Metabolism and Metabolic Encephalopathy, pp 163–177. New York, Plenum Press, 1985

173. Zieve L: Conditional deficiencies of ornithine or arginine. J Am College Nutr 5:167, 1986

174. Zieve L, Brunner G: Encephalopathy due to mercaptans and phenols. In McCandless DW (ed): Cerebral Energy Metabolism and Metabolic Encephalopathy, pp 179–201. New York, Plenum Press, 1985

175. Zieve L, Nicoloff DM: Pathogenesis of hepatic coma. Ann Rev Med 26:143, 1975

176. Zieve L et al: Shunt encephalomyelopathy: II. Occurrence of permanent myelopathy. Ann Intern Med 53:53, 1960

177. Zieve L et al: Synergism between mercaptans and ammonia or fatty acids in the production of coma: A possible role for mercaptans in the pathogenesis of hepatic coma. J Lab Clin Med 83:16, 1974

178. Zieve L et al: Effect of total hepatectomy on selected cerebral substrates and enzymes of the glycolytic pathway and Krebs cycle. Surgery 78:414, 1975

179. Zieve L et al: Reversal of ammonia coma in rats by L-dopa: A peripheral effect. Gut 20:28, 1979

180. Zieve L et al: Toxicity of a fatty acid and ammonia: Interactions with hypoglycemia and Krebs cycle inhibition. J Lab Clin Med 101:930, 1983

181. Zieve L et al: Brain methanethiol and ammonia concentrations in experimental hepatic coma and coma induced by injections of various combinations of these substances. J Lab Clin Med 104:655, 1984

182. Zieve L et al: Ammonia toxicity: Comparative protective effect of various arginine and ornithine derivatives, aspartate, benzoate and carbamyl glutamate. Brain Metabolic Disease 1:25, 1986

183. Zimmon DS: Oxyhemoglobin dissociation in patients with hepatic encephalopathy. Gastroenterology 52:647, 1967

chapter 25

Fatty Liver: Biochemical and Clinical Aspects

DAVID H. ALPERS and SEYMOUR M. SABESIN

The liver subserves many important functions in plasma lipoprotein metabolism, including the biosynthesis of very low density lipoprotein (VLDL).[82] VLDL formation is related directly to the availability of free fatty acids. Free fatty acids are transported to the liver bound to albumin and then quantitatively taken up by hepatocytes, where they are used for triglyceride synthesis. Next the triglycerides are combined with specific proteins (apoproteins), forming lipoprotein particles that are secreted into the circulation. There they undergo extensive alterations in composition during their metabolism.

The availability of free fatty acids for hepatic triglyceride synthesis is dependent on many factors, which include nutritional status (*i.e.,* type and quantity of diet), hormonal influences (*i.e.,* insulin availability and pituitary and adrenocortical hormones), and exogenous factors such as alcohol. Within the hepatocyte the availability of free fatty acids for triglyceride synthesis is also dependent on the status of complex regulatory mechanisms such as mitochondrial fatty acid oxidation, ketone body formation, endogenous fatty acid synthesis, and availability of precursors for glycerol synthesis. VLDL synthesis and secretion are also regulated precisely by the availability of apoprotein B (apo B); the assembly of apo B with triglyceride, phospholipid, and cholesterol; the glycosylation of the apoproteins; and the transport of the nascent (newly formed) VLDL particles sequentially through several subcellular compartments culminating in secretory vesicle formation and exocytosis of nascent VLDL into the perisinusoidal space of Disse.[154]

It is apparent that derangements in one or more of the metabolic regulatory steps leading to hepatic triglyceride synthesis, alterations in nutritional or hormonal status, as well as toxic influences on hepatocyte function could lead to imbalances in the biosynthesis, assembly, intracellular transport, or secretion of VLDL. Put another way, the constant cycling of fatty acids between liver and adipose tissue is easily distorted, and in the direction of hepatic deposition. There are limits to the rate of oxidation, but not esterification, and there is relatively limited triglyceride secretion as VLDL. The net result of such derangements leads to an excessive accumulation of triglyceride within hepatocytes. This is reflected clinically by hepatomegaly and abnormalities of hepatic function, termed variously *fatty liver, fatty degeneration,* or *fatty metamorphosis.*

The normal liver contains approximately 5% of its weight as fat, including triglycerides, fatty acids, phospholipids, cholesterol, and cholesteryl esters; however, when fat accumulates, it is almost all triglyceride and then 40% to 50% of the weight may be due to lipid. At the microscopic level, excessive triglyceride can be visualized as small droplets. These droplets are observed easily when special lipid stains are used. The lipid droplets result from the gradual coalescence of retained triglyceride, within the confines of the endoplasmic reticulum. Thus in early stages of fatty liver, electron microscopy reveals individual lipid droplets surrounded by membranes of the endoplasmic reticulum; however, with progressive triglyceride accumulation, the droplets coalesce into large masses that breach the membrane barrier of the endoplasmic reticulum.[155]

Although many chemicals, pharmacologic agents, and hormonal imbalances may cause fatty liver, most times the accumulation of fat is only one facet of a broader metabolic derangement, which often includes significant hepatocellular necrosis. In fact, the severity of the clinical manifestations resulting from deranged hepatic function is dependent more on the extent of hepatocellular injury than on the presence of fat. Even if quite excessive, necrosis and fatty infiltration are separate processes with differing pathogenesis and can develop and resolve independently. Thus, fatty liver can occur before necrosis and then resolve while hepatocellular necrosis persists.

In this chapter the pathogenesis of fatty liver is described based on current knowledge of peripheral and hepatic fatty acid metabolism and hepatic lipoprotein synthesis, secretion, and metabolism. Also, the clinical and laboratory manifestations of several human diseases characterized by fatty liver are explained. Since hepatic lipoprotein formation is so important for triglyceride secretion (and animal studies indicate a critical role for deranged lipoprotein metabolism in many types of drug- or toxin-induced fatty liver), composition and metabolism of plasma lipoproteins and subcellular aspects of lipoprotein synthesis and secretion will be emphasized.

PLASMA LIPOPROTEINS

The lipoproteins isolated from fasting plasma are the end-products of the metabolism of lipoproteins secreted by the liver and intestine.[13,31,57,82,105,156] The most commonly used separation procedure involves the sequential ultracentrifugation of plasma at increasing solution densities and isolation of each fraction within a predetermined density range (Table 25-1).

Composition

The main function of lipoproteins is the transport of lipids in the plasma. Except for the intestinal synthesis of chylomicrons after a fatty meal, the liver is the major source of plasma lipoproteins. Electrophoresis has been used for the separation and identification of lipoproteins in whole plasma, leading to a nomenclature used widely in clinical applications. Chylomicrons do not move electrophoretically, whereas low density lipoprotein (LDL) migrates with β-, VLDL migrates with pre-β-, and high density lipoprotein (HDL) migrates with α_1-globulins. Each of these lipoprotein classes has a characteristic lipid and apoprotein composition (see Table 25-1).

The apoproteins subserve several critical functions in lipoprotein metabolism.[162] Structurally they comprise the surface layer of the spherical lipoprotein particles, allowing the hydrophobic lipids (triglycerides, cholesteryl esters) to occupy the core. This spatial arrangement permits the transport of lipids in the aqueous environment of the blood. Specific apoproteins are also critical for various aspects of lipoprotein metabolism, functioning as cofactors for enzymes involved in triglyceride hydrolysis (apo C-II), and in cholesterol esterification (apo A-I) and as ligands for receptor-mediated uptake of lipoproteins by various tissues (apo B, apo E).

The isolated lipoproteins have a characteristic particle diameter. However, a rather broad range exists within each density class, reflecting, in part, different stages of catabolism at the time of their isolation (see Table 25-1). The particles can be visualized directly by so-called negative staining techniques applied to electron microscopic preparations. By electron microscopy the lipoproteins in each density class appear as dense spherical particles without any obvious substructure (Fig. 25-1). Although lipoprotein classes can be segregated because of their average composition or physical properties, the particles within a class are somewhat heterogeneous, reflecting the state of metabolic transformations occurring in the circulation.

In addition to classification based on criteria of density or electrophoretic mobility, it is useful to classify lipoproteins on the basis of their probable function. Currently, three major functions are believed to be provided by plasma lipoproteins:

1. Transport of a prime energy source, triglyceride, from biosynthetic sites in the intestine and liver to peripheral cells (chylomicrons and VLDL).
2. Transport of cholesterol required for cell membrane and steroid hormone synthesis from the liver to peripheral cells (LDL).
3. Transport of excess tissue cholesterol from peripheral cells to the liver for disposition into the bile or reutilization (HDL).

Sources

Chylomicrons synthesized by the small intestinal absorptive cells, in response to the absorption of dietary lipid,

TABLE 25-1.   Properties of Plasma Lipoproteins

	CHYLOMICRONS	VLDL	LDL	HDL
Source	Intestine	Liver	Plasma	Intestine, liver
Diameter (Å)	800–5000	280–800	200–250	50–150
Density (g/ml)	<0.95	<1.006	<1.063	<1.21
Electrophoretic mobility	Origin	Pre-β	β	α
Lipid content	≃98%	≃90%	≃75%	≃50%
Lipid classes (% of total lipid)	≃90 TG ≃8 PL ≃5 CH	≃60 TG ≃20 PL ≃17 CH	≃60 CH ≃30 PL ≃10 TG	≃50 PL ≃32 CH ≃10 TG
Protein content	0.5–2.5%	10–13%	20–25%	45–55%
Major apoproteins	B, C-I, C-II, C-III	B, C-III, E	B	A-I, A-II
Function	Exogenous TG transport	Exogenous TG transport	CH transport to peripheral cells	LCAT substrate, CH transport from peripheral cells to liver

(TG, triglycerides; PL, phospholipids; CH, cholesterol)

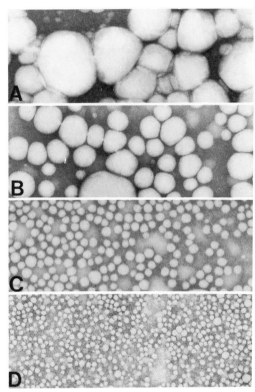

Fig. 25-1. Electron microscopic appearance of human plasma lipoproteins isolated by ultracentrifugation. **A.** Chylomicrons; **B.** VLDL; **C.** LDL; **D.** HDL. (Original magnification: *A,* × 72,000; *B–D,* × 95,000)

are large triglyceride-rich particles that are secreted directly into the lymph.[13,157] The newly secreted (nascent) chylomicrons undergo rapid metabolic transformations and are cleared from the circulation within a few minutes. Thus chylomicrons are not detected normally in fasting plasma. When secreted into lymph, the chylomicrons contain a low molecular weight form of apoprotein B, apo A-I, other A peptides, apo E, and some low molecular weight apoproteins of the C group (Fig. 25-2). As will become evident later, the A, C, and E apoproteins subserve important functions in lipoprotein metabolism, but the availability of apo B is essential for the secretion of chylomicrons from the intestinal absorptive cells and of VLDL from hepatocytes. Apo B deficiency due either to hereditary absence (abetalipoproteinemia) or to decreased synthesis because of drug or toxic inhibition (tetracycline, carbon tetrachloride) is associated with severe impairment of chylomicron and VLDL secretion and thus intracellular triglyceride accumulation. There is now evidence that the liver and intestine synthesize separate apo B's, which differ in molecular weight; however, their physiologic functions appear to be similar.

In the absence of dietary lipid, the intestinal absorptive cells also synthesize some VLDL-size particles. Studies in the rat indicate the intestinal production of lipoprotein particles with the characteristics of newly formed (nascent) HDL.[13,64] In support of the production of nascent HDL by the intestine is the observation that most of the intestinal apo A_1 is not associated with the HDL particle until it reaches the lamina propria, after the secretion from the enterocyte.[5] Most of the endogenously formed triglycerides in plasma are present in the VLDL, synthesized primarily in the liver. Studies using liver perfusion indicate that nascent VLDL is different in composition from circulating plasma VLDL (see Fig. 25-2). The apoprotein content of circulating VLDL includes apo C, apo B, and apo E, whereas nascent VLDL consists almost entirely of apo B.[162] Thus it appears that most of the apo C and most of the apo E acquired after the nascent VLDL is secreted from the hepatocyte (see Fig. 25-2).

The major lipoprotein of human plasma, LDL, is not synthesized by the liver but is formed in plasma as a product of VLDL catabolism.[31] The principal lipid component of LDL is esterified cholesterol, and it contains only apo B (see Fig. 25-2). The other lipoprotein synthesized and secreted by the liver is nascent HDL, which is strikingly different in structure and composition from the HDL found in fasting plasma (see Fig. 25-2). Evidence for the synthesis of nascent HDL is the isolation, from rat liver perfusates,[69] of a discoidal particle enriched in apo E, phospholipid, and unesterified cholesterol. Further evidence for the hepatic formation of nascent HDL is the accumulation of a similar discoidal particle in patients with severe alcoholic hepatitis[138,152,185] in whom cholesteryl esters are greatly decreased in plasma because of deficiency of the cholesterol esterifying enzyme lecithin:cholesterol acyltransferase (LCAT).[139] In these patients the HDL fractions contain considerable apo E and relatively little apo A-I, which is normally the major apoprotein (85%) of circulating HDL.

Enzymatic Modification

Lecithin: Cholesterol Acyltransferase

Since LCAT is responsible for the formation of all of the cholesteryl esters found in plasma, the hepatic synthesis and secretion of LCAT are very important in lipoprotein metabolism. LCAT transfers a fatty acyl group from lecithin to cholesterol to form cholesteryl esters. Nascent HDL is the principal substrate for LCAT and, as a result of its enzymatic activity, discoidal nascent HDL is converted to spherical particles, which are rich in cholesteryl esters. The cholesteryl esters formed by the LCAT reaction are then transferred to the metabolic pathway in which VLDL is converted to LDL (see Fig. 25-2). Apo A-I required for LCAT activation is the major apoprotein of plasma HDL. Although some apo A-I is synthesized by

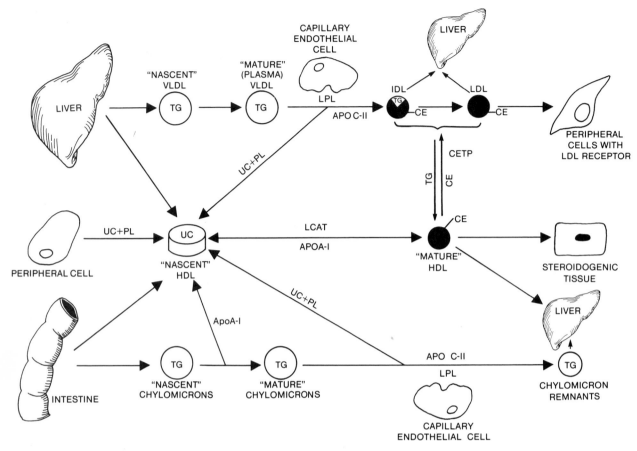

Fig. 25-2. Sources and metabolism of plasma lipoproteins. TG, triglycerides; CE, cholesteryl esters; UC, unesterified cholesterol; PL, phospholipids; LPL, lipoprotein lipase; LCAT, lecithin: cholesterol acyltransferase; CEP, cholesterol ester transfer protein. Details of the metabolic pathways and the transfer of lipids and apoproteins between the various lipoproteins are described in the text.

the liver, it is not a principal secretory product. Studies using immunofluorescent techniques have shown that apo A-I is synthesized by the small intestinal epithelial cells during lipid absorption and that it is the major apoprotein of mesenteric lymph chylomicrons.[58]

Lipoprotein Lipase

Lipoprotein lipase is also a key enzyme involved in plasma lipoprotein metabolism since it hydrolyzes chylomicron and VLDL triglycerides (see Fig. 25-2).[48] Apo C-II, required for lipoprotein lipase activation, is secreted by the liver in association with nascent HDL. After hydrolysis of VLDL and chylomicron triglycerides by lipoprotein lipase, and their acquisition of cholesteryl esters by transfer from HDL, remnant lipoproteins are formed. VLDL remnants are metabolized to intermediate density lipoprotein (IDL) and then to LDL through further hydrolysis of triglycerides by lipoprotein lipase. As this is accom-

plished, most of the apoproteins, other than apo B, are removed. The loss of apo C-II from the VLDL and chylomicron particles leads to a cessation of triglyceride hydrolysis by lipoprotein lipase. In humans the remnants of chylomicron metabolism are cleared by the liver by a receptor-mediated process that recognizes apo B and E on the remnant surface. The residual triglycerides in the chylomicron remnants are used by the liver in various metabolic pathways, and the chylomicron remnant cholesterol helps to regulate hepatic cholesterol synthesis. Evidence indicates that the intestinal epithelial cells also synthesize some C apoproteins, thereby providing a convenient source of lipoprotein lipase activators for chylomicron triglyceride hydrolysis.[14]

Metabolism

Lipoproteins should be thought of as dynamic particles that are constantly in a state of synthesis, degradation, and removal from the plasma compartment, rather than as static transport vehicles whose lipid and apoprotein composition is uniform and unvarying.[17,31,57,59,82,105] Figure 25-2 depicts a somewhat simplified version of the major pathways involved in lipoprotein catabolism, emphasizing the role of lipoprotein lipase and LCAT and the transfer of lipids and apoproteins between density classes. Figure 25-3 emphasizes the flux of fatty acids between plasma and tissues. During the process of lipoprotein catabolism the nascent (secretory) particles of intestinal or hepatic origin undergo triglyceride hydrolysis, acquire new apoproteins (which subserve physiologic functions), lose apoproteins of endogenous origin, and thus become altered drastically in size and composition. The end-products of these complex transformations also perform important functions. For example, LDL is a major source of cholesterol for peripheral cells and transports cholesterol to the liver, and other tissues, for excretion (in bile), degradation, and reutilization.

The first step in the catabolism of triglyceride-rich lipoproteins (chylomicrons and VLDL) is the hydrolysis of triglyceride by lipoprotein lipase located in vascular endothelial cells (see Figs. 25-2 and 25-3).[48] After VLDL and chylomicrons are secreted they become enriched in apo C peptides by transfer from HDL. This is important since apo C-II is required for lipoprotein lipase activation. As seen in Figures 25-2 and 25-3 the gradual lipolysis of chylomicron triglyceride results in formation of a progressively smaller particle, the chylomicron remnant.

The chylomicron remnants, depleted of triglycerides and enriched in cholesteryl esters, are removed by the liver as intact particles by a receptor-mediated process.[31,32] The cholesteryl ester contained in chylomicron remnants regulates (decreases) the activity of β-hydroxy-β-methylglutaryl-CoA (HMG-CoA) reductase, the rate-limiting enzyme of cholesterol synthesis.[105] Only a small amount

of chylomicron–apo B appears to become LDL–apo B[45]; therefore, it appears that most of chylomicron remnants are removed by the liver, whereas the end products of VLDL metabolism circulate longer as LDL.

The mechanism by which chylomicron remnants are removed by the liver and their remaining triglyceride hydrolyzed is unclear. A lipolytic enzyme, hepatic triglyceride lipase (H-TGL), that has activity against monoglycerides, diglycerides, and triglycerides has been postulated to have a role in both processes.[31] It has been suggested that H-TGL resides on hepatocytes near a lipoprotein remnant receptor and that it is interiorized during remnant endocytosis, where it can function in lysosomal triglyceride hydrolysis.[23]

A study of chylomicron cholesteryl ester hydrolysis comparing the activities of different cholesteryl ester hydrolases in liver cells led to the conclusion that hydrolysis of chylomicron cholesteryl esters was not required before their uptake by hepatocytes.[52] Furthermore, it appears that cholesteryl esters could be hydrolyzed without prior triglyceride hydrolysis and that lysosomal enzymes could degrade both cholesteryl esters and triglycerides of chylomicron remnants taken up by endocytosis.

During chylomicron catabolism in plasma, the surface lipids, phospholipids, and unesterified cholesterol are removed and replenish nascent HDL while the apo A-I of the "fresh" chylomicrons in lymph are also removed and transferred to HDL. Apo C peptides are probably exchanged back and forth between HDL and chylomicrons.

The replenishment of nascent HDL during chylomicron (and VLDL) catabolism is extremely important for other aspects of lipoprotein metabolism.[43] Since nascent HDL is the substrate for LCAT, the replenishment of HDL provides a means by which additional cholesterol can be esterified and then shunted into the pathway leading to LDL formation. Alternatively, cholesteryl esters in HDL can

Fig. 25-3. Sources and metabolism of plasma fatty acids (*FA*) emphasizing the role of the liver in fatty acid uptake and triglyceride synthesis and secretion.

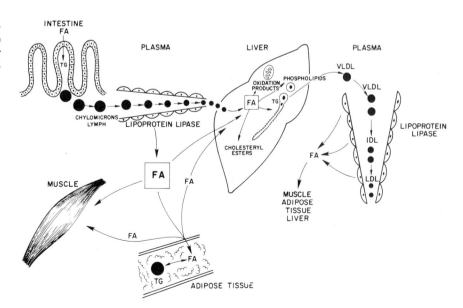

be removed from the plasma as HDL is taken up by the liver, or other tissues, and catabolized. At the same time, the transfer of apo A-I from chylomicrons to nascent HDL provides the cofactor for LCAT activity while transfer of apo C-II between HDL and the triglyceride-rich lipoproteins ensures lipoprotein lipase activation.

The triglycerides in VLDL are also hydrolyzed by lipoprotein lipase, and nascent VLDL likely receives almost all of its complement of C apoproteins from HDL. As in chylomicron catabolism, concurrent with depletion of the triglyceride core is loss of VLDL surface constituents that replenish HDL. The VLDL is degraded to a smaller particle—intermediate density lipoprotein—which is also subjected to triglyceride hydrolysis but is gradually enriched in cholesteryl esters. It seems most likely that cholesteryl esters are acquired by VLDL and IDL by transfer from HDL, perhaps in conjunction with apo E. Apo E, a major constituent of VLDL, is not present in plasma HDL; however, nascent HDL is enriched in apo E whereas nascent VLDL does not contain apo E.[139]

As the triglyceride of IDL is hydrolyzed, the C-apoproteins and apo E are removed. This results in the formation of a small particle composed almost entirely of cholesteryl esters and apo B. This lipoprotein is LDL. LDL is removed from plasma by peripheral tissues, a process that depends on the binding of apo B to high-affinity receptors. The binding and subsequent internalization of LDL are crucial for the intracellular regulation of cholesterol synthesis and for the control of plasma cholesterol concentration.[17,105] It is noteworthy that the liver is of major importance in the receptor-mediated uptake of LDL and that the liver can also directly remove IDL from the plasma by a similar process.

As indicated earlier when HDL is secreted by the liver, or intestine, it contains mostly unesterified cholesterol and phospholipid and appears by electron microscopy as a bilamellar disk. The LCAT reaction, using nascent HDL as substrate, converts the discoidal HDL to a spherical particle as the apolar cholesteryl esters form the hydrophobic core covered on the surface by apoproteins, unesterified cholesterol, and phospholipids. HDL may transport unesterified cholesterol from peripheral cells, thus preventing excessive accumulation of cellular cholesterol and providing a source of cholesterol for subsequent esterification. Kupffer cells possess a high capacity to degrade HDL, which accounts for more than 50% of the liver's capacity for HDL protein breakdown and cholesteryl ester hydrolysis. Hepatic HDL catabolism probably involves a sequence of binding, uptake, and proteolytic degradation, perhaps occurring in liver lysosomes, as is the case with chylomicron remnants.

It is important to emphasize that many diseases characterized by fatty liver are associated with derangements in plasma lipoprotein metabolism and concomitant alterations in the concentration of plasma lipids and composition of lipoprotein classes. Particularly noteworthy in this regard is alcoholic fatty liver, which is frequently associated with hyperlipidemia and abnormal plasma lipoproteins.

LIPID METABOLISM

Fatty Acid Metabolism

In fatty liver, the major lipid fractions that increase in amount are the fatty acids and triglycerides. Phospholipids, cholesterol, and cholesteryl esters usually increase to a limited extent. It is important to consider the physiology of fatty acid and triglyceride metabolism within the hepatocyte, since the pathogenesis of fatty liver is related intimately to derangements in the regulation of these metabolic processes. Figure 25-3 is a scheme of hepatic fatty acid and triglyceride metabolism emphasizing the sources of hepatic fatty acids and their fate in the liver.

As discussed, the triglyceride-rich lipoproteins of exogenous (dietary) origin, chylomicrons, are metabolized in the capillary bed of tissues throughout the body where lipoprotein lipase is located on vascular endothelial surfaces. The fatty acids formed during chylomicron triglyceride lipolysis can be used directly as a source of energy (i.e., muscle); taken up by adipocytes where they are esterified again to triglycerides and stored; or transported to the liver where they enter various biochemical pathways. The stored triglyceride in adipose tissue is an important potential source of energy that can be mobilized at time of need by once again undergoing hydrolysis, releasing fatty acids into the blood. The control of triglyceride lipolysis in adipose tissue is under exquisite hormonal regulation and provides a prime source of fatty acid influx into the liver under various changes in nutritional and hormonal status.[145] Thus, fatty acids entering the liver, in the fasting state, are derived from the hydrolysis of adipose tissue triglyceride. In the postprandial state, the fatty acids are derived mostly from the hydrolysis of dietary triglycerides, either from peripheral degradation of chylomicron triglyceride by lipoprotein lipase or by the direct uptake of chylomicron remnants with subsequent hydrolysis by hepatic triglyceride lipase. Within the hepatocyte the fatty acids may then be oxidized and used for energy, converted to phospholipids, used for the formation of cholesteryl esters, or used for triglyceride synthesis (see Fig. 25-3). The release of triglyceride as newly synthesized VLDL provides another source of fatty acids that can be oxidized in muscle, stored as triglyceride in adipose tissue, or returned once again to the liver (see Fig. 25-3).

Biosynthesis and Secretion of Lipoproteins by the Liver

Studies using *in vitro* techniques, or isolated hepatic perfusion, have shown that the liver is the major site of VLDL synthesis.[31,57] The sequential steps involved in hepatic

VLDL formation and intracellular transport and secretion, emphasizing the translocation of nascent particles through subcellular compartments, is shown schematically in Figure 25-4, whereas actual electron micrographs are illustrated in Figure 25-5. After uptake by the hepatocyte, fatty acids are reesterified to triglycerides, used for cholesterol or phospholipid synthesis, or oxidized. Acetate may also serve as a fatty acid precursor. The initial step involved in apoprotein synthesis involves the genetic transcription of the messenger RNA involved in apoprotein synthesis. Specific genes code for each individual apoprotein, but it is only within the past few years that the molecular biology of apoprotein formation has been extensively investigated.[24,61,162,189] After formation on the polyribosomes of the rough endoplasmic reticulum, the nascent apoproteins are translocated into the cisternae of the rough endoplasmic reticulum where they commence a vectorial transport through the endoplasmic reticulum channels toward their assembly with the lipid moieties.[26]

The enzymes involved in triglyceride, cholesterol, and phospholipid synthesis are located in the smooth endoplasmic reticulum, and presumably the newly formed lipids are then directed into the cisternae of the smooth endoplasmic reticulum. Assembly of the lipid and the apoprotein moieties probably occurs at the junction of the smooth and rough endoplasmic reticula (Fig. 25-5A), with the final assembly, concentration, and glycosylation of lipoproteins occurring within the Golgi apparatus.

The exact structural relationship between the transport of nascent proteins from the endoplasmic reticulum and the Golgi apparatus components is not known. One concept suggests continuous connections between endoplasmic reticulum and the Golgi components with passage of nascent particles directly into the Golgi cisternae. Alternatively, it has been suggested that nascent proteins may be transported in so-called shuttling vesicles derived from transitional elements of the smooth-surfaced extensions of the endoplasmic reticulum (Fig. 25-5B).[158] After final assembly of nascent VLDL in the Golgi (Fig. 25-5C), smooth-surfaced secretory vesicles derived from the Golgi (Fig. 25-5C) and containing nascent VLDL migrate through the cytoplasm where they merge with the lateral plasmalemma of the hepatocyte (Fig. 25-5D) and secrete the VLDL into the space of Disse by exocytosis (Fig. 25-5E). Biochemical evidence for this sequence of assembly and transport to the Golgi complex resides in subcellular fractionation studies in which Golgi vesicles have been isolated and their contents purified, demonstrating lipoprotein particles strikingly similar to VLDL in size and composition.[79]

Evidence suggests that transport of nascent lipoproteins into the Golgi apparatus is obligatory for their final assembly and secretion; however, the exact function of the Golgi apparatus, in this regard, has not been established. The Golgi apparatus may serve to complete the assembly of nascent proteins, perhaps by the addition of sugar moieties catalyzed by glycosyl transferases located in Golgi membranes. The final result of this process is the formation of secretory vesicles that bud off from the Golgi apparatus and transport the secretory product to the plasmalemma where secretion into the perisinusoidal space occurs by exocytosis (see Fig. 25-5C through E).

There is still relatively little information available concerning the mechanism by which nascent lipoproteins, in secretory vesicles, are directed toward the space of Disse for secretion. Colchicine and some other related alkaloids can inhibit hepatic VLDL secretion.[174] The inhibitory effects of colchicine on secretion may be due to its interference with the formation of another class of subcellular organelles, the microtubules.[153] Although microtubules

Fig. 25-4. Steps in the hepatic synthesis, intracellular transport, and secretion of VLDL. *SER,* smooth endoplasmic reticulum; *RER,* rough endoplasmic reticulum; *SV,* secretory vesicle; *MT,* microtubule. See text for description.

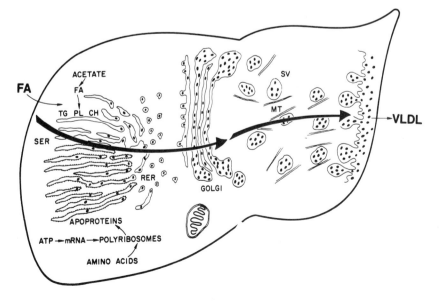

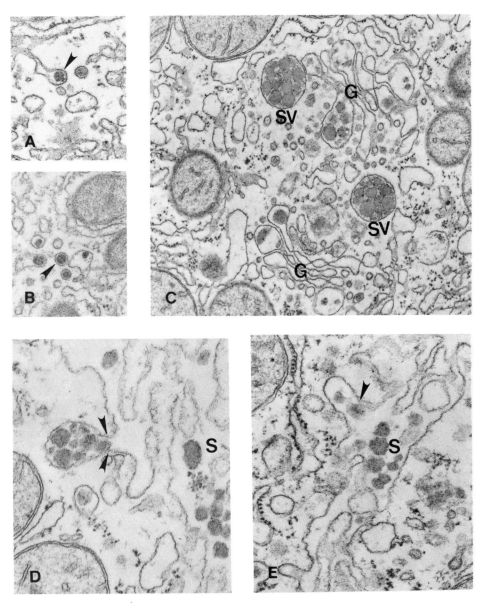

Fig. 25-5. Electron micrographs illustrating various aspects of the assembly, intracellular transport, and secretion of VLDL by rat liver. **A.** Formation of nascent VLDL in the endoplasmic reticulum (*arrow*). **B.** Vesicular transport of nascent VLDL (*arrow*) from the endoplasmic reticulum to the Golgi complex. **C.** VLDL in Golgi cisternae (*G*) and in secretory vesicles (*SV*). **D.** Exocytosis of VLDL. The arrows point to areas of fusion of a secretory vesicle, containing VLDL, with the hepatocyte sinusoidal membrane. Note the presence of VLDL in the perisinusoidal space of Disse (*S*). **E.** Secretion of VLDL (*arrow*) into the space of Disse (*S*). (Original magnification: *A,* × 44,000; *B,* × 40,800; *C,* × 30,000; *D,* × 50,490; *E,* × 50,400)

probably subserve several functions, they may direct the vectorial movement of secretory vesicles toward the cell membrane, thereby controlling the secretory process (see Fig. 25-4).

A specialized subcellular component has been described that, although located in proximity to the Golgi apparatus, can be distinguished from it by the specificity of its histochemical staining for acid phosphatase.[123] The acronym GERL has been applied to this region (*G*olgi, *e*ndoplasmic *r*eticulum, *l*ysosomes) although the organelle is probably the same as that referred to as endosomes or receptosomes. GERL can be distinguished cytochemically from the endoplasmic reticulum and the innermost elements of the Golgi apparatus by the specificity of its staining for acid phosphatase.[123] VLDL-size particles have been demonstrated in the smooth-surfaced cisternae and tubules of GERL. This suggests direct entry of VLDL from the endoplasmic reticulum into GERL, thereby "bypassing" the Golgi apparatus. Transformation of the VLDL within GERL has been suggested, since the VLDL, which always appear spherical within the Golgi, assume other configurations in GERL, appearing irregular in size and shape. Furthermore, so-called residual bodies containing homogeneous electron-dense material imply catabolism of the VLDL, perhaps related to apoprotein degradation or partial triglyceride lipolysis. These ultrastructural differences between VLDL morphology in GERL and the Golgi apparatus suggest a degradative function for GERL, perhaps related to lipoprotein catabolism. There appears to be good evidence for such a function, since GERL contains lysosomal enzyme activity and experimental studies have shown a marked distention of GERL with VLDL during the reversal of fatty liver.[122]

ADIPOSE TISSUE METABOLISM

Triglyceride Synthesis

Both exogenous and endogenous sources contribute free fatty acids for triglyceride synthesis by the liver; however, the relative contribution from each source varies under different physiologic and hormonal conditions. In the fasting state, the majority of free fatty acids used in hepatic triglyceride production are derived from peripheral adipose tissue.[57] These free fatty acids are the products of triglyceride hydrolysis within adipose tissue cells. This reaction, under the influence of a hormone-sensitive lipase, results in the liberation of free fatty acids and glycerol in the adipose cells.

The amount of free fatty acids released from adipose tissue may be measured by several techniques. These include direct measurement of free fatty acid concentration in plasma, determination of venous-arterial differences in free fatty acid concentration across adipose tissue, or changes in triglyceride content of the liver. The amount of glycerol released by the tissues can also be used as a measure of the rate of triglyceride hydrolysis. This is because partial hydrolysis is uncommon and glycerol cannot be used by adipose tissue for new triglyceride synthesis since adipose tissues lack glycerol kinase required for α-glycerol phosphate synthesis. The uptake or release of free fatty acids by adipose tissue is regulated by neural and hormonal stimuli. This process is enhanced by the rich vascular supply of adipose tissue and its direct contiguity with autonomic nerve endings.

In the fed state, when caloric intake exceeds the immediate metabolic needs of the animal, chylomicrons supply free fatty acids to the liver. The amount of free fatty acids extracted by the liver is proportional to the free fatty acid concentration in portal venous blood. Obviously an increase in exogenous triglyceride intake increases the quantity of fatty acids available for immediate energy needs and also provides a potential excess that is taken up by the liver or adipocytes.

Free fatty acids entering the adipose tissue cells can be used directly for triglyceride synthesis provided glucose is available for glycerol formation. Glucose is essential in many respects for fat formation in adipose tissue. As indicated previously, glucose forms α-glycerol phosphate and thus regulates the use of free fatty acids for triglyceride synthesis. Free fatty acids may also be synthesized directly from glucose using acetyl CoA as an intermediate. Via the pentose phosphate shunt, glucose generates NADPH, which enhances fatty acid synthesis. Thus, despite an adequate supply of free fatty acids, fat synthesis in adipose tissue does not occur unless glucose is available. This has implications both for the disposition of free fatty acids arriving from peripheral triglyceride lipolysis as well as of those resulting from adipocyte lipolysis by hormone-sensitive lipase.

Insulin is crucial in the regulation of adipose tissue triglyceride synthesis by promoting glucose entry into adipocytes and by inhibiting cyclic adenosine monophosphate (AMP) formation, the so-called second messenger, which regulates the activity of the hormone-sensitive lipase. Thus, the insulin response to alterations in blood glucose concentration determines whether fat synthesis and storage occur or whether triglyceride lipolysis is dominant in adipose tissue. Insulin deficiency, by promoting lipolysis, is an important cause of fatty liver in patients with poorly controlled diabetes mellitus. In that situation, massive lipolysis results in an enormous mobilization of free fatty acids, which are taken up by the liver and used, in part, for triglyceride synthesis. It is possible, although not yet proven, that excessive adipose tissue lipolysis also occurs in acute fatty liver of pregnancy and Reye's syndrome, thereby providing a massive supply of free fatty acids to the liver.

Fatty Acid Mobilization

Mobilization of fatty acids from adipose tissue is subject to numerous regulatory mechanisms that determine the rate at which free fatty acids enter the blood.[145] The hormone-sensitive lipase is responsive to hormonal, nutritional, chemical, or nervous factors, thereby providing a means of increasing the plasma free fatty acid concentration to satisfy energy requirements in various tissues (Table 25-2). Epinephrine, norepinephrine, adrenocorticotropic hormone, thyroid stimulating hormone, adrenocortical steroids, thyroxine, and glucagon all stimulate activation of cyclic AMP. Since cyclic AMP activates hormone-sensitive lipase, the hormonal activation of cyclic AMP provides a mechanism promoting triglyceride lipolysis.

Hormonal factors that increase lipid mobilization may act on adipose tissue by stimulation of the lipolytic process (catecholamines and glucagon). Thyroid hormones appear

TABLE 25-2. Factors Affecting Mobilization of Fatty Acids from Adipose Tissue

FACTORS	INCREASED MOBILIZATION	DECREASED MOBILIZATION
Nutritional	Low glucose availability	High glucose availability
Hormonal	ACTH TSH Growth hormone Corticosteroids Thyroid hormone Glucagon	Insulin
Nervous	Sympathetic stimulation	Cordotomy Sympathetic blocking agents Hypophysectomy Adrenalectomy
Chemical	Epinephrine Norepinephrine	Prostaglandins Nucleotides Nicotinic acid Salicylates Tranquilizers Adenosine triphosphate Chlorphenoxyisobutyrate (Atromid)

to sensitize adipose tissue to the stimulatory action of catecholamines on lipolysis. Adrenocortical hormones potentiate the lipolytic action of catecholamines by inhibiting carbohydrate metabolism in adipose tissue.

Low glucose availability is thought to increase lipid mobilization indirectly as the body seeks alternative means of energy. Additionally, fasting hypoglycemia is characterized by low insulin levels. Thus, the inhibition of adipose tissue lipolysis exerted by insulin is removed and an increase in free fatty acid mobilization occurs. Conversely, in states of high glucose availability and increased insulin levels, inhibition of adipose tissue lipolysis occurs and free fatty acid mobilization is decreased. It should be noted that experimentally, at least, glucose loading may stimulate free fatty acid production by the liver and may lead to an increase in hepatic triglyceride content.

The mode of action of the sympathetic nervous system in lipid mobilization relates to release of catecholamines (epinephrine), which stimulate adipose tissue lipolysis, regulate hepatic glycolysis, impair peripheral glucose uptake, and suppress insulin release. Histochemical studies have failed to show sympathetic nerve endings in direct contact with adipocytes; thus the locally released catecholamines may exert their effects via the rich blood supply surrounding the fat cells. Cordotomy or administration of sympathetic or adrenergic blocking agents would, by direct interference with catecholamines, be expected to reduce peripheral fat mobilization. Of recent interest is the fact that prostaglandins have an inhibitory effect on catecholamine-stimulated lipid mobilization in animals.

Certain nucleotides also exert a similar inhibitory effect. Whether these effects are important in basal or physiologic situations is unknown.

Obviously, fat feeding with an increase in portal venous chylomicrons results in a tremendous increase in fatty acid influx into the liver. If indeed the rate of hepatic triglyceride synthesis is proportional to the concentration of free fatty acid delivered in the portal venous blood, then an increase in lipid accumulation within the liver would be expected. This could lead to fatty liver if an imbalance between triglyceride availability and lipoprotein assembly and/or secretion occurred.

Other chemicals, notably adenosine triphosphate, appear to decrease the fat accumulation produced by agents such as ethionine, carbon tetrachloride, and ethanol (see Table 25-2).[81] Administration of adenosine triphosphate (ATP) leads to a decrease in circulating free fatty acids, which appears to be secondary to the relative hypothermia following ATP injections. Numerous other chemicals, including salicylates, propranolol,[53] and tranquilizers, decrease fatty acid mobilization.[22] Whether these drugs can improve liver histology in many by reducing fatty infiltration is not known. Chlorphenoxyisobutyrate (Atromid) has been used to induce hypolipidemia. In animals, this drug causes a decrease in plasma triglycerides and inhibits the release of newly formed triglycerides from the liver. This decreased rate of secretion of hepatic triglyceride has been confirmed in isolated perfused livers. However, in the intact animal the liver does not become fatty, presumably because plasma free fatty acid levels decrease also.

FATTY ACID UPTAKE AND USE

Fatty acids liberated from adipose tissue are carried in the bloodstream bound to albumin (see Fig. 25-3). Approximately one third of the circulating fatty acids is removed by the liver, a third by skeletal muscle, and the rest by other tissues, especially myocardium.[137,166] Hepatic triglyceride formation or accumulation is greatly affected by the rate at which fatty acids are presented to the liver. Fatty acids released from adipose tissue have a short half-life in the plasma, about 2 minutes. Normal levels of plasma free fatty acids are less than 500 mEq/liter, and the liver can extract 30% of circulating free fatty acids in a single cycle. In considering the transport, synthesis, and metabolism of fatty acids, it must be kept in mind that these include the essential fatty acids, such as linoleic acid, which cannot be synthesized by mammalian organisms. When tissues such as liver are called on to synthesize fatty acids from two carbon precursors, the main products are saturated long-chain fatty acids, such as palmitic acid.

The mechanism of fatty acid uptake by the liver is not well understood. Agents such as norepinephrine, however, tend to diminish fatty acid uptake by the isolated liver. Following hepatic uptake, fatty acids may be metabolized (*i.e.*, oxidized) or reesterified to triglycerides, phospholipids, and cholesteryl esters. Quantitatively most of the fatty acids reaching the liver are resecreted into the blood as triglycerides in the form of VLDL.

After uptake of exogenously or endogenously derived fatty acids, hepatic triglyceride esterification occurs rapidly. The rate of esterification may be measured by the administration of radiolabeled fatty acids into the blood and measurement of labeled fatty acids in hepatic tissue. Within 2 minutes after the injection of radiolabeled fatty acids, most fatty acids recovered from the liver are in esterified form. Electron microscopy reveals lipid droplets within rough and smooth endoplasmic reticulum soon after injection of fatty acids, and radiolabeled fatty acids may be found in the endoplasmic reticulum.

The rate of hepatic triglyceride synthesis from fatty acids can be estimated by two techniques. In the first, an intravenous injection of Triton is used to block peripheral lipolysis of VLDL, the main excretory vehicle for triglycerides leaving the liver. Thus, by measuring the increase in VLDL after infusion of a known amount of fatty acid, the rate of hepatic triglyceride and VLDL synthesis can be calculated. This process presumes that no other mechanisms are available for VLDL catabolism and that all fatty acids infused are incorporated into triglyceride and VLDL. A second technique, radiolabeled fatty acid infusion, allows determination of radioactivity in plasma triglycerides and may give a more accurate estimate of hepatic VLDL and triglyceride synthesis. These two techniques show that hepatic triglyceride synthesis is roughly proportional to the concentration of fatty acids entering the liver.

The esterification process is closely linked to hepatic oxidative phosphorylation and is dependent on a ready supply of α-glycerophosphate, the precursor of glycerol, supplied almost exclusively from glucose, and the availability of fatty acyl CoA. As with adipose tissue, glucose and insulin are extremely important in the regulation of hepatic fat formation. It is noteworthy in this regard that the liver is considerably more active than adipose tissue in triglyceride synthesis. The liver is the major site of glucose removal. This is controlled in part by insulin; but, in addition, a major effect of insulin is the inhibition of hepatic glucose release. Insulin also determines the fate of glucose in the hepatocyte, by regulating the activity of glucokinase essential for glucose phosphorylation, by increasing fatty acid synthesis from glucose, and by promoting hepatic triglyceride secretion.[119]

In addition to triglyceride synthesis, other fates exist for fatty acids in the hepatocyte.[10] In the fasting state, or when metabolic demands are great, fatty acids are oxidized to acetoacetate and other ketone bodies, which then may be used for energy. Fatty acid oxidation is important in removing excess lipid from the liver so that accumulation within the organ does not occur ordinarily. Finally, fatty acids may be incorporated into phospholipids and other lipids within the hepatocyte. They are thus stored in the formed membrane lipids or in the exchangeable phospholipid pools.

The synthetic rate of hepatic triglyceride synthesis is usually regulated by approximately equal hepatic secretion of triglyceride, but acute stresses of the system, such as mobilization of fatty acid from adipose tissue or a rapid and prolonged increase in dietary chylomicron triglyceride, can result in increased hepatic triglyceride synthesis. Hepatic triglyceride formation or accumulation is greatly affected by the rate at which fatty acids are presented to the liver,[172] but undoubtedly, other factors affect this also.[175]

Minor contributions of fatty acids for hepatic triglyceride synthesis also stem from *de novo* fatty acid production by the liver and from triglyceride and phospholipid "pools" in the liver. The relative contribution from these sources is minor in the basal state, but in certain clinical and experimental conditions, they may assume more importance. Thus, experimental animals fed diets high in carbohydrates but poor in fat convert a portion of the carbohydrate to fatty acids. Fatty acids may also be synthesized in the liver from amino acid precursors.

The liver may respond to an increased fatty acid influx by increasing the rate of lipoprotein and ketone body synthesis, but there is a limit to the extent to which the activity of these pathways may increase. If the rate at which fatty acids are brought to the liver exceeds the ability of the liver to metabolize and/or resecrete the fatty acids into the circulation, as lipoproteins, storage of fat within the hepatocyte will ensue. Although fatty acids are incorporated into phospholipids and cholesteryl esters, when a fatty liver is produced, the predominant lipid that accumulates is triglyceride.

Thus, the liver can be thought of as a tissue that can respond to multiple stimuli with a common pathway, the accumulation of triglycerides in hepatic parenchymal cells. Increased delivery of fatty acids to the liver related to intestinal triglyceride absorption, increased peripheral triglyceride lipolysis, or decreased hepatic VLDL secretion can result in the clinical syndrome of fatty liver. In all likelihood, a combination of factors may be necessary. Therefore, the discussion of experimental and clinical entities will try to suggest a reasonable mechanism in each case.

MECHANISMS OF THE PRODUCTION OF FATTY LIVER

The numerous theories proposed for the pathogenesis of fatty liver are based on derangements of the normal physiology of hepatic triglyceride synthesis and secretion.[57,158] These theories include not only abnormalities of physiologic and biochemical regulation but also derangements in the series of steps by which the VLDL lipid and apoproteins are synthesized, assembled into nascent particles, transported sequentially through subcellular compartments, and finally secreted. Singly or in combination, derangements of these events can be involved in the pathogenesis of fatty liver, as illustrated in the representation of VLDL synthesis and secretion in Figure 25-6. Thus an increased supply of fatty acids leading to an imbalance between triglyceride synthesis and secretion could result (see Fig. 25-6) from enhanced fatty acid mobilization from adipose tissue or diet, increased fatty acid synthesis, or decreased mitochondrial fatty acid oxidation. The secretion of triglycerides might be impaired secondary to inhibition of apoprotein synthesis or to inadequate apoprotein synthesis when a large triglyceride load is available for lipoprotein formation.

Defects in one or more of the steps involved in the assembly, intracellular transport, or secretion of nascent VLDL can also lead to fatty liver. These include inhibition of nascent VLDL transport from the endoplasmic reticulum to the Golgi complex, impaired Golgi function preventing the final glycosylation of nascent VLDL apoproteins or decreased secretory vesicle formation, interference with the migration of secretory vesicles to the plasmalemma membrane, possibly secondary to microtubule dysfunction, and impaired exocytosis of nascent VLDL.

Although there are no definitive data concerning the relative importance of these mechanisms, some are undoubtedly more important than others, depending on the agent directly responsible for the production of a fatty liver. Some of the pharmacologic or toxic agents for which a mechanism has been produced in animals are discussed next. These mechanisms form a framework into which the limited knowledge concerning human fatty liver may be placed.

Ultrastructural Aspects of Fatty Liver

Electron microscopic studies of human, or experimental, fatty liver reveal a monotonous engorgement of the cytoplasm with triglyceride droplets that are intensely stained with the osmium tetroxide used for fixation (Fig. 25-7). Since the triglycerides and apoproteins are synthesized in relationship to the membranes of smooth and rough endoplasmic reticula, and since the secretory particle is transported within the channels formed by these tubular organelles, an accumulation of triglyceride, either due to an imbalance between synthesis and secretion or inhibition of secretion, results in vesiculation of the endoplasmic reticulum (see Fig. 25-7). The vesiculation is caused by the gradual coalescence of triglyceride molecules into larger and larger lipid droplets. At higher magnification with the electron microscope, it is obvious that the retained

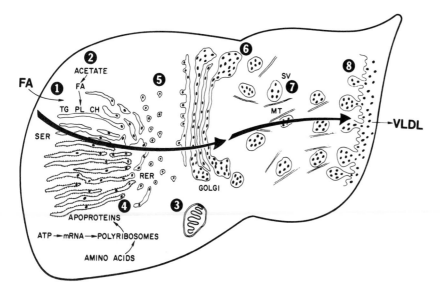

Fig. 25-6. Postulated mechanisms by which alterations in triglyceride synthesis and derangements in VLDL assembly, intracellular transport, and secretion can lead to fatty liver. The numbers refer to possible sites of such abnormalities. See text for details.

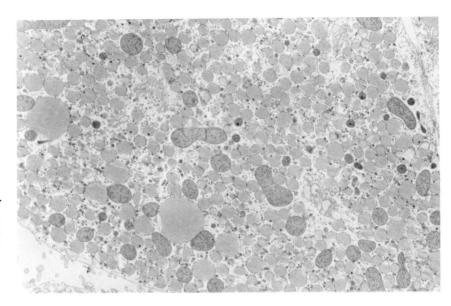

Fig. 25-7. Electron micrograph of rat liver obtained 10 days after having been fed a semisynthetic diet containing 1% orotic acid. The hepatocyte contains a massive accumulation of triglyceride droplets. (Original magnification × 5865)

triglyceride is surrounded by membranes of the smooth (Fig. 25-8A) or the rough (Fig. 25-8B) endoplasmic reticulum.[155]

In certain clinical conditions, fat accumulation appears, by light microscopy, as small discrete microvesicular fat droplets (*e.g., tetracycline fatty liver, Reye's syndrome, acute fatty liver of pregnancy*) whereas other disorders (*e.g., alcoholic fatty liver*) may be characterized by massive cytoplasmic fat droplets (macrovesicular fat droplets). This distinction implies a different pathogenesis for the two conditions, but in reality it is an expression of the severity and duration of the fat accumulation. With prolonged steatosis there is progressive aggregation of triglyceride into very large droplets. These droplets eventually assume enormous proportions and impinge on the barriers imposed by the endoplasmic reticulum membranes, resulting in the formation of massive lipid aggregates. Ultrastructural studies of several experimental models of fatty liver have provided some insight into the mechanism by which certain toxins or drugs may interfere with lipoprotein

Fig. 25-8. Higher magnification electron micrographs of orotic acid-induced fatty liver illustrating the vesiculation of the smooth endoplasmic reticulum (*A*) and the rough endoplasmic reticulum (*B*). In *B*, arrows point to ribosomes with retained triglyceride. (Original magnification: *A*, × 10,780; *B*, × 16,800)

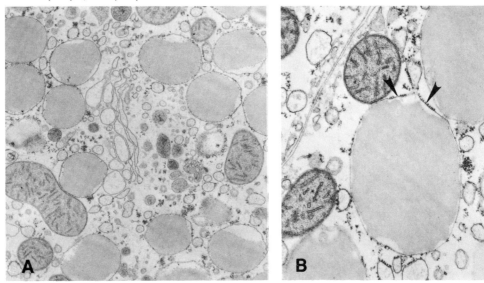

synthesis, intracellular transport, or secretion and thus produce fatty liver.[57] Thus, experimental alcoholic fatty liver is characterized initially by excessive triglyceride synthesis, engorgement of the Golgi complexes with VLDL, and active secretion. In this instance the accumulation of fat appears to represent an imbalance between triglyceride synthesis and the ability of the hepatocyte to package and rapidly secrete VLDL. In toxic states associated with inhibition of protein and presumably apoprotein synthesis (e.g., tetracycline), there is extreme accumulation of triglyceride droplets in the vesiculated endoplasmic reticulum but no evidence of VLDL secretion.

Abnormalities in other steps in the pathway leading to VLDL secretion have also been described for other experimental models of fatty liver. Feeding 1% orotic acid, incorporated into a semisynthetic diet, produces a profound accumulation of triglycerides in rat liver, associated with a specific defect in VLDL secretion.[148,188] Since orotic acid does not interfere specifically with protein or lipoprotein synthesis, it has been suggested that it may prevent the assembly and/or secretion of lipoproteins by the liver.[188] Apparently, the hepatic synthesis of the apoproteins involved in VLDL formation is not prevented following orotic acid feeding; however, there is a marked decrease in plasma triglyceride, cholesterol, and LDL concentration. The isolated, perfused rat liver, obtained from animals treated with orotic acid, cannot release lipoproteins containing apo B (VLDL, LDL) but can secrete HDL, albumin, and other plasma proteins.[148]

Ultrastructural analysis of the alterations in rat hepatic subcellular organelles following orotic acid feeding strongly suggests that orotic acid induces a VLDL secretory block within the Golgi apparatus.[155] This interpretation is based on the distention of Golgi cisternae and vesicles with lipid droplets at various phases during the development of fatty liver. The presence of VLDL-size droplets within elements of the Golgi apparatus is accompanied by a progressive distention of the endoplasmic reticulum owing to the presence of triglyceride droplets that presumably cannot be transported into the already lipid-filled Golgi stacks. The retention of triglycerides within endoplasmic reticulum cisternae causes vesiculation of the cisternae as the small droplets aggregate into increasingly large triglyceride-rich droplets.

These ultrastructural observations of the orotic acid–induced fatty liver suggest that the primary defect in lipoprotein transport may be related to interference with normal Golgi function. In the early phases of orotic acid–induced fatty liver, the Golgi cisternae are distended with lipid, secretory vesicles do not form, and there is no evidence of VLDL exocytosis.[155] After 10 or more days of orotic acid feeding, the Golgi complexes appear flattened and somewhat devoid of lipoprotein particles, suggesting secondary effects that prevent entrance of nascent VLDL into the Golgi apparatus.[122]

Ultrastructural studies of the effects of colchicine and other microtubular inhibitory agents on VLDL secretion indicate a role for microtubules in the secretory process.[174] The administration of colchicine is associated with a marked defect in VLDL secretion, disappearance of hepatocyte microtubules, diminished secretory vesicle formation, and vesiculation of the endoplasmic reticulum owing to triglyceride retention. Although colchicine has many effects on the cell, its inhibition of microtubule formation may be of major importance in the pathogenesis of fatty liver caused by this drug. In this regard microtubules may subserve an essential function in guiding the movement of secretory vesicles, containing nascent VLDL, to the plasma membrane for exocytosis (see Step 8, Fig. 25-6).

Studies with other agents have also provided some insight into possible subcellular sites of synthetic and/or secretory VLDL inhibition. The administration of 4-aminopyrazolopyrimidine (4-APP) causes fatty liver in the rat secondary to a VLDL secretory defect. Electron microscopic studies of the 4-APP–induced fatty liver show movement of the nascent VLDL particles from the endoplasmic reticulum to the Golgi apparatus; however, there is an impairment of Golgi function since secretory vesicles are decreased in number and evidence of exocytosis is rare.

Increased Fatty Acid Supply and Enhanced Triglyceride Synthesis

The data on fatty livers produced acutely by a number of agents suggest that much of the lipid that accumulates in the liver is derived from adipose tissue.[10] This is not surprising since most acute studies have been performed on fasting animals and under these conditions the plasma free fatty acids are predominantly those released from peripheral lipid depots. Many of the hormonal and experimental manipulations that interfere with the mobilization of fatty acids from adipose tissue are also effective in blocking development of fatty liver. By varying the supply of fatty acids to the liver, one can influence directly the amount of fat that accumulates in the liver. Thus, if the rate of fatty acid influx in the liver is reduced, less fat will accumulate.

It is likely that the hepatic steatosis that develops under conditions of enhanced supply of free fatty acids reflects an imbalance between triglyceride synthesis and the assembly and secretion of VLDL. This imbalance may be due to an inability of the hepatocyte to synthesize apoprotein B rapidly enough to accommodate the increase in triglyceride awaiting assembly into lipoproteins or to a relative deficiency in the secretory process. The latter could involve the final formation of nascent VLDL in the Golgi, inadequate secretory vesicle formation or movement, or the exocytotic process itself. In many conditions characterized by fatty liver, secondary to increased supply of free fatty acids, there is concomitant hypertriglyceridemia indicating active VLDL secretion even while fat accumulates in the liver. The secreted VLDL is larger and enriched in triglyceride compared with VLDL isolated from plasma under basal conditions.[159,160] The secretion of large triglyceride-rich particles implies an adaptive response by the hepatocyte, enabling the secretion of more triglyceride with less apoprotein.

Decreased Synthesis or Release of Lipoproteins

In earlier studies the inhibitory effect of certain drugs and hepatotoxins on hepatic VLDL secretion provided reasonable support for the hypothesis that hepatic triglycerides accumulate secondary to a lipoprotein secretory defect.[47,147] This concept was supported by many studies of hepatic lipoprotein synthesis that showed that the apoprotein moiety of VLDL is actually synthesized within the hepatocytes and that the final secretory product is assembled within the liver.[57]

The demonstration that inhibitors of protein synthesis can interfere with VLDL biosynthesis led to the conclusion that a lipoprotein secretory defect is the main cause of fatty liver. Despite the fact that some protein synthesis inhibitors produce fatty liver, it is evident that many of these agents cause only a moderate increase in hepatic triglyceride content. Thus, the hepatic triglyceride concentration following ethionine[47] or puromycin[147] administration is slight when compared with the massive fatty liver induced by orotic acid.[155,188] The discrepancy between protein synthesis inhibition and extent of fat accumulation in the liver is even more striking in the case of cycloheximide[83,181] or acetoxycycloheximide,[151] which produce only a twofold increase in hepatic triglyceride content despite their ability to inhibit protein synthesis almost completely. It is of interest that ethionine and D-galactosamine both also induce hypoglycemia and a secondary elevation of plasma free fatty acids.[152] Many of the hepatotoxic effects of ethionine can be prevented by glucose infusions or by feeding the animals throughout the experiment.[21,115] Thus, despite the inhibition of secretion produced by ethionine, or D-galactosamine,[159] fatty liver does not occur unless there is a stimulus for fatty acid influx into the liver.

The plasma lipoproteins are actually glycolipoproteins; however, the role of glycosyl moieties in determining the structure, secretion, and metabolism of lipoproteins is not known. Since there is evidence that the final assembly of lipoproteins occurs within the Golgi apparatus, and since this subcellular organelle is thought to be the site of important terminal glycosylations in glycoprotein synthesis, it is possible that the secretion of lipoproteins by hepatic Golgi complexes depends on the addition of the carbohydrate moiety.

It is tempting to speculate that the orotic acid–induced secretory block may be related to a defect in the glycosylation of certain VLDL apoproteins within the Golgi apparatus. Since it has been shown that the B- and C-apoproteins of VLDL are present within hepatic triglyceride droplets after orotic acid feeding, it is conceivable that certain sugar moieties cannot be added to these apo-

proteins after the nascent VLDL enter the Golgi apparatus.[133] Orotic acid is known to produce an imbalance in hepatic nucleotide levels, causing an increase in uridine and a decrease in adenine and cytidine nucleotides.[108] The decreased availability of specific sugars for transfer to incompletely glycosylated apoproteins within the Golgi apparatus might conceivably cause the secretory block. In this regard there is some evidence that a defect in glycoprotein formation may be important in the pathogenesis of the orotic acid–induced effect in VLDL secretion. Thus, liposomes isolated from the orotic acid fatty liver contain three of the four VLDL apoproteins normally found in plasma VLDL and the missing VLDL band is defective in its carbohydrate moiety but not in its peptide content.[135] Orotic acid might regulate synthesis of the enzyme required to glycosylate this apoprotein, or the enzyme may be inhibited by UDP-N-acetylglucosamine, which accumulates in the liver of the orotic acid–fed rats. It has also been shown that the VLDL apoproteins, derived from the orotic acid liver liposomes, are deficient in N-acetylglycosamines, galactose, and N-acetylneuraminic acid, perhaps due to a lack of exposure of the apoproteins to glycosylating enzymes in the Golgi.

In considering the mechanisms by which orotic acid might alter normal glycosylation reactions, it is noteworthy that orotic acid produces a decrease in hepatic levels of adenine and cytidine nucleotides.[108] The decrease in cytidine nucleotides may have very important implications for the pathogenesis of fatty liver since the hepatic Golgi complexes contain a sialyltransferase that catalyzes the incorporation of sialic acid from CMP-N-acetylneuraminic acid into a sialidase-treated apo C peptide isolated from VLDL.[187] A decrease in the availability of this sugar nucleotide might prevent adequate sialylation of C peptides in the Golgi apparatus and could explain the observations discussed previously. If one assumes that VLDL secretion is dependent on the presence of the sugar moieties of the VLDL apoproteins, then defective sialylation of the C peptides could cause the secretory block. It is of interest in this regard that the addition of adenine to the orotic acid diet not only reverses the hepatic triglyceride accumulation but also specifically restores to normal the balance of uridine and adenine nucleotides in the liver.

Fatty liver has been produced by a variety of agents that bring about decreased hepatic ATP concentration, inhibition of protein synthesis, and impaired lipoprotein formation. Ethionine is a prototypic agent in this respect.[47] The administration of ATP or an ATP precursor such as adenine completely protects against ethionine-induced fatty liver in rats, and reverses the ethionine-induced inhibition of protein synthesis. In other models (e.g., azaserine and carbon tetrachloride), administration of ATP also reverses the hepatic triglyceride accumulation. However, fatty liver production by these two models is not specifically dependent on inhibition of protein synthesis since ATP repletion does not alter the inhibition of protein synthesis evoked by these agents. The effects may be due to inhibition of fatty acid mobilization.

In the case of carbon tetrachloride, one of the earliest lesions noted microscopically is at the level of the endoplasmic reticulum, and biochemically protein synthesis is dramatically decreased.[142] This is associated with a breakdown of polyribosomes (needed for protein synthesis) to single ribosomes. The exact mechanisms whereby this occurs is unknown. Recknagel has suggested that in some way carbon tetrachloride forms peroxides of lipids, which then damage cellular membranes. Peroxidation of lipids, including microsomal lipids, is increased following ingestion of carbon tetrachloride, and it is possible that microsomal membrane function is affected by this process.[143] Peroxidation is the oxidative degradation of unsaturated fatty acids in the presence of oxygen. None of the many agents used to prevent carbon tetrachloride–induced fatty liver or necrosis in animals (adrenergic blocking agents, antihistamines, antioxidants) has proved useful clinically since they must all be given before the toxin is administered. Increased lipid peroxidation has been found in human liver at autopsy after carbon tetrachloride ingestion, but its pathogenetic significance is still unclear.

Nutritional deficiencies or imbalances of various types have led to fatty liver in animals, presumably related to a decrease in packaging or secretion of lipoproteins. The best studied of the deficiencies is that of choline.[103] Choline deficiency is characterized by growth failure, weakness, hemorrhagic lesions, myocardial and renal lesions, as well as fatty liver and cirrhosis. Choline is a precursor of phosphoryl choline and is therefore important in lipoprotein production. However, its effect is nonspecific; methionine and cysteine can replace choline. Moreover, choline is metabolized very poorly in humans owing to the almost total absence of choline oxidase.

FATTY LIVER OF THE ALCOHOLIC

Biochemical Mechanisms

Fatty liver can follow either acute or chronic administration of alcohol in laboratory animals and in humans. Many of the mechanisms postulated in Figure 25-6 have at some time been proposed for the alcoholic fatty liver by various investigators since it is clear that alcohol alters a number of processes that affect triglyceride accumulation in the liver. Alcohol apparently does not affect intestinal absorption of lipids, hepatic chylomicron uptake, hepatic protein synthesis, or lipoprotein formation. It does, however, increase lipolysis and thus influx of fatty acids to the liver (step 1), increase synthesis (step 2) and decrease oxidation of fatty acids (step 3), and increase triglyceride formation and decrease release of lipoproteins from the liver (steps 5–8).[95] Ethanol decreases the intracellular NAD/NADH ratio.[120] However, the change in this ratio is unlikely to be the only factor in the production of fatty liver. First, the ratio decreases early after ingestion of ethanol and returns to normal when fat is accumulating. Second, sorbitol changes the ratio but does not cause fatty liver.[141] Finally, antioxidant treatment reduces the fatty liver but does not alter the NAD/NADH ratio.[149] Moreover, the metabolism of ethanol itself produces metabolites (e.g., acetate) that can be used for fatty acid synthesis.

In reviewing the many studies on the effect of alcohol on lipid metabolism, numerous reports on first inspection appear to give conflicting results and to be contradictory. Many of the discrepancies, however, are perhaps explained by the fact that the effects of alcohol vary within a variety of experimental or clinical conditions. Different *in vitro* preparations, perfused livers, intact animals, and normal alcoholic human subjects have all been used for study. Different sampling times have been used. Since a high-fat diet suppresses fatty acid synthesis, the nutritional state of the subjects is another important variable. The dose of ethanol is significant, since at high doses nonspecific neural or endocrine responses may be evoked. Most authors now favor a direct toxic effect of ethanol on hepatic triglyceride metabolism.[95]

Results of acute experiments performed with large doses of alcohol differ from those of chronic experiments when alcohol is given in smaller amounts and other dietary nutrients are provided. Gender is also important, since the female animal is much more susceptible to hepatic fat accumulation than the male. It is clear that fatty liver can develop at blood alcohol levels in humans considered to be legal intoxication. Dietary deficiencies are not required for the production of such an acute fatty liver but clearly seem to play a modifying role in the more chronic syndromes associated with ethanol ingestion.[96,130] In humans the degree of fatty liver seems to correlate with the severity of dietary deficiency.[94] Patients with the lowest protein intake have the most hepatic steatosis. On the other hand, prospective studies in volunteers with initially normal livers showed that ingestion of 150 g to 200 g of ethanol per day for 10 to 12 days produced fatty livers, regardless of the content of the rest of the diet.[99] In addition to the variations in dose and time of ingestion and nutritional status, other factors such as genetic and metabolic differences may account for the presence or absence of hepatic fat.[133]

Fatty Acid Mobilization

The fatty acids present in hepatic triglycerides after acute alcohol administration are derived from the blood and hence are of extrahepatic origin. Under fasting conditions, during acute alcohol intoxication, most of the plasma fatty acids that reach the liver are derived from adipose tissue. Mobilization of fatty acids occurs only in the presence of adrenocortical and pituitary hormones. Thus, with acute intoxication, the fatty acid mobilization may be a nonspecific result of a stress reaction. On the other hand, when alcohol and food are administered chronically, the fatty acids in the plasma reflect the fatty acids present in the triglycerides absorbed from the intestinal tract.[98]

In acute experiments with single large doses of alcohol, the fatty acid composition of the liver suggests that much of the lipid is derived from extrahepatic sources.[99,164] The fatty acid derives from increased lipolysis, probably related to activation of adenyl cyclase. Epinephrine, norepinephrine, cortisol, adrenocorticotropic hormone, and prostaglandins among other hormones, can mediate this enhanced enzyme activity and lead to increased cyclic AMP concentrations in adipocytes. When mobilization of fatty acids from adipose tissues is interfered with as by adrenalectomy, cordotomy, hypophysectomy, and adrenergic blocking agents, the amount of fat that accumulates in the liver after alcohol is markedly reduced.[141]

In chronic experiments in rats and humans, in which alcohol plus food is administered, the fatty acids in the liver tend to reflect the lipids in the diet.[98,99] These acute and chronic experiments are not contradictory but simply reflect the importance of hepatic influx of fatty acids and the relationship of lipid that accumulates to the plasma composition. The latter is in turn influenced by whether the animal or subject is fasting or is ingesting fat. Therefore, while mobilization of free fatty acids may *increase* only with very high blood alcohol levels, influx of fatty acids to the liver must be at least *normal* for significant hepatic fat accumulation to occur.

When alcohol is highly concentrated in the blood (*i.e.,* greater than 250 mg/dl), the free fatty acids in the serum increase markedly.[163] However, at lower blood levels (*i.e.,* 80 mg to 100 mg/dl) no significant changes in serum free fatty acids are detected.[100] Hepatic uptake is proportional to the plasma free fatty acid concentration. Since a fatty liver may develop with prolonged alcohol administration and normal serum fatty acid concentrations, hepatic steatosis may result from an increased plasma flux of fatty acids or from intracellular events.

Increased Hepatic Fatty Acid Synthesis

Ethanol inhibits the tricarboxylic acid (TCA) cycle in hepatocytes, in part by damaging mitochondria, by increasing the NADH/NAD ratio, and by shuttling NADH into mitochondria for oxidation. By decreasing the condensation of maleate to oxaloacetate, the production of pyruvate (and acetate) is increased and the acetate is available for fatty acid synthesis. High levels of acetate also inhibit fatty acid oxidation.

The hydrogen ion used to reduce NAD comes from ethanol rather than from fatty acids via the citric acid cyle. Thus, fatty acids that normally serve as an energy source are replaced. In fasted animals ethanol does not increase fatty acid synthesis,[125] whereas in the fed state lipogenesis increases.[62] The changes in hepatic redox become attenuated with time, and fat does not continue to accumulate.[40]

Ethanol stimulates hepatic fatty acid synthesis *in vivo* and *in vitro*.[97] Ethanol is largely metabolized in the liver (90% to 98%) and hepatic alcohol dehydrogenase converts NAD to NADH as ethanol is metabolized to acetaldehyde. However, in the *de novo* synthesis of fatty acids from acetate, NADPH rather than NADH is required. Some fatty acids are produced by elongation, and the NADH as well as NADPH may serve as hydrogen donors in the elongation of fatty acid chain lengths and in the conversion of saturated to unsaturated fatty acids.[78] Thus, the effect of altered NADH/NAD ratios on fatty acid synthesis may be nonspecific.[141]

Glucose and sorbitol increase fatty acid synthesis without the concomitant formation of a fatty liver. In cordotomized rats ethanol increases hepatic fatty acid synthesis but does not produce a fatty liver. Thus, while the acute administration of ethanol may, under certain conditions, increase hepatic fatty acid synthesis, it is unclear whether this is a major factor in the production of the alcohol-induced fatty liver. Few data are available on the effect of chronic ethanol administration on hepatic fatty acid synthesis

Decreased Fatty Acid Oxidation

In humans, ingestion of alcohol decreases oxidation of lipids under conditions that do not affect carbohydrate or protein metabolism. Oxidation of long-chain fatty acids after ethanol ingestion is impaired to a greater extent than that of medium-chain fatty acids, perhaps accounting for the greater accumulation of long-chain fatty acids after ethanol ingestion.[101]

Acetaldehyde, the major metabolic product of ethanol, increases in concentration after ethanol ingestion in humans.[114] In rats, acetaldehyde metabolism is decreased in the presence of acetaldehyde administration. Acetaldehyde raises serum free fatty acids and triglyceride levels. Thus, the production of acetaldehyde may provide a vicious cycle in which damage to mitochondria further increases acetaldehyde and free fatty acid levels. Other hepatotoxins (carbon tetrachloride, phosphorus, ethionine, and choline) cause mitochondrial damage, which contributes to maintenance of high triglyceride levels in the liver but probably does not alone explain the onset of fat accumulation.[38]

The evidence that decreased oxidation is the major factor in the alcoholic fatty liver must be examined further. *In vitro*, ethanol can decrease oxidation of lipids, but so can other substances that do not lead to the development of a fatty liver (glucose, sorbitol, xylitol, and nicotinamide).[141] In fact, ethanol has been reported to increase the oxidation of lipids by the mechanism of peroxidation.[30]

Increased Esterification of Fatty Acids to Triglycerides

When fatty acids are presented to the liver they are esterified to triglycerides, phospholipids, and cholesterol esters. Alcohol could lead to increased conversion of fatty acids to triglycerides either directly or indirectly by inhibiting their incorporation into phospholipids and cholesterol esters. Acute alcohol administration to rats alters the esterifying system in liver microsomes. Microsomes isolated from rats 16 hours after an acute alcohol load show a fourfold increase in the conversion of ^{14}C-palmitate to triglyceride.[164] Enhanced esterification of fatty acids has been associated with an increased hepatic level of α-glycerophosphate, a substrate for triglyceride formation.[186] α-Glycerophosphate production is increased by NADH and the ethanol induced activity of the microsomal enzyme α-L-glycerophosphate transferase, which catalyzes the first step of triglyceride formation.[114] Few studies have been performed with chronic alcohol administration.

Decreased Hepatic Release or Secretion of Triglycerides

There has been no demonstrated effect of alcohol on protein synthesis, or on the interaction of lipid and apoprotein to form lipoprotein, as has been demonstrated in orotic acid fatty liver. Many other toxic agents leading to a fatty liver cause a decreased synthesis of protein and lipoprotein, and as a consequence decreased release of lipid into the blood. When alcohol is administered to humans, plasma triglycerides initially increase.[163] However, this increased release of lipoproteins from the liver is not sufficient to compensate for increased triglyceride production, so that fatty liver develops. When blood alcohol reaches high levels (i.e., greater than 250 mg/dl), plasma triglycerides decrease, accompanied by an increase in plasma free fatty acids. Since hepatic lipid first accumulates at lower levels of blood alcohol, and since at these levels decreased hepatic lipid release has not been demonstrated, one must assume that this mechanism is not a primary one but possibly a contributory factor.

In summary, alcohol administration both acutely and chronically affects many aspects of lipid metabolism. Some of these actions may be primary or major in regard to production of a fatty liver. Others may be minor or serve only to contribute to or affect the extent of the fatty liver.

CLINICAL ASPECTS

Diagnosis

Fatty liver can occur when fatty acid mobilization increases and either hepatic oxidation or triglyceride synthesis is decreased. As discussed previously, these tend to be the rate-limiting steps in hepatic triglyceride accumulation. With this pathophysiologic framework in mind, the diagnosis of fatty liver is often suspected clinically when a history of toxin exposure is elicited; obesity or diabetes, prolonged fasting, or steroid usage is present; and hepatomegaly is observed. The definitive diagnosis has required liver biopsy until recently. A number of additional techniques now offer noninvasive methods for assessing total hepatic lipid content and thus providing an explanation for the hepatomegaly. Because of its lower density, intrahepatic lipid alters the density of the hepatic parenchyma analyzed by computed tomography. The portal venous system then appears as higher density linear structures within a background of lower density parenchyma.[173] Hepatic steatosis can also be detected by the degree of hepatic ^{133}Xe retention as measured during pulmonary ventilation studies.[3] Furthermore, the degree of hepatic xenon retention correlates with the degree of steatosis found histologically.

Magnetic resonance imaging has been performed using a modified spin echo technique (simple proton spectroscopic imaging) that is designed to exploit the difference in the rate of procession between the protons in water and fatty acid molecules.[92] In the conventional spin echo technique, the image intensity is the sum of the signal produced by water and fat protons. With proton spectroscopic imaging, the opposed image intensity is the difference between the water and fat signals. It seems likely that this method will be quantitatively useful in the near future. In addition, the technique can distinguish hepatic metastases from focal fatty infiltration.[91]

The standard liver function tests (transaminase, alkaline phosphatase, and bilirubin) are helpful as screening parameters in identifying the presence of some liver disease but do not identify fatty liver as the cause, nor do they usually assess the severity of the process.[2,55] Increased sulfobromophthalein (BSP) retention is the most frequent abnormal test reported in fatty liver. However, this test is not performed now except for research purposes.

Steatosis, when discovered by any of the methods discussed, is often not the only pathologic lesion present. Inflammation, fibrosis, and even cirrhosis may be present, depending on the offending agent and the duration of the injury.

Fat accumulation in the liver is associated initially with normal hepatic function. This is the result of the fact that the liver is merely involved as an innocent bystander. More triglyceride precursors arrive than the liver can metabolize. However, with time and increased triglyceride accumulation, secondary changes can occur. Theories for these changes include decreased secretory ability secondary to pressure or contact inhibition or to enhanced peroxidation from an increase in lipid substrates.[38] The relationship of these secondary changes in hepatic function to inflammation, necrosis, and fibrosis is unknown. It is possible that the accumulation of fat in the liver is the appropriate response to increased peripheral mobilization of fatty acids. Since no lipotropes are known to be effective in humans, it is uncertain if hepatic triglyceride itself is pathogenetically important. Treatment of fatty liver depends on correction of the primary problem. The important clinical assessment is whether the fatty liver is appropriate under the circumstances.

Pathology

The liver is usually large, and the bulk of the fat is triglyceride, comprising up to 25% of the liver wet weight. The cut surface is yellow, due to the accumulation of carotenes and other lipochromes. Hepatic lipid is usually present as large or small droplets. Initially the droplets are small and are surrounded by membranes of the endoplasmic reticulum. As the droplets enlarge and merge, the membranes become difficult to see. When large globules are present, the hepatocytes look like adipocytes with flattened peripheral nuclei. This pattern can be seen in metabolic disorders or following administration of ethanol or steroids. Although alcoholic steatosis is characteristically centrilobular (zone 3 of Rappaport's acinus), the distribution of fat as pericentral or diffuse is not usually helpful in assigning an etiology. Small droplets with centrally placed nuclei are seen in some drug reactions (*e.g.*, tetracycline, valproic acid) or in acute fatty liver of pregnancy. Reye's syndrome and Jamaican vomiting sickness demonstrate small droplet fat in hepatocytes as well.

Microscopically, in addition to fatty hepatocytes, there is the accumulation of lipid- and lipofuscin-containing macrophages. These may be included in lipogranulomas along with lymphocytes and eosinophils.[25] When the severe fatty accumulation subsides, the lipid droplets in the macrophages diminish and the lipogranulomas may be difficult to distinguish from other granulomas. Usually, however, the fat in these periportal granulomas persists long after the hepatocellular steatosis and may raise the suspicion of preceding steatosis.

Focal fatty change has been reported at postmortem examination in a variety of disorders.[15] These lesions can measure up to 4 cm in diameter and might be mistaken for space-occupying lesions. Diffuse steatosis is not always present in the rest of the liver but may be present and not appreciated by standard radiologic techniques. Thus, focal change sometimes may be an artificially apparent variant of diffuse steatosis.

Many of the characteristics of alcoholic steatosis are the same as for any cause of fatty liver. Grossly the liver is extremely enlarged, often weighing up to 6000 g. The external and cut surfaces are smooth and pale yellow. Microscopically the liver cells are filled with fat vacuoles. Within days after alcohol ingestion, vacuolization of the endoplasmic reticulum occurs along with distorted mitochondrial cristae and an increase in free polyribosomes and autophagic vacuoles.[150] The exact significance of these changes is not clear.

Alcoholic hyalin is often seen. This lesion is nearly specific for alcoholic liver disease, with or without fat, but has been seen in the livers of malnourished children in India[170] and in some other nonalcoholic-induced liver disorders including jejunoileal bypass,[127] prolonged cholestatic jaundice, cirrhosis, hepatoma,[121] and Wilson's disease. When lobular architecture is intact, centrilobular hyalin is still specific to ethanol.[56] By light microscopy these bodies are eosinophilic, coarsely granular, usually perinuclear in distribution, and always intracellular. On electron microscopy they seem to be composed of intermediate filaments[169] of the prekeratin type.[37]

In alcohol-damaged livers pathologic findings range from only fat in the liver to marked necrosis with polymorphonuclear infiltration and bile stasis with only moderate fat in hepatocytes. Both extremes may be seen in the same patient at various stages of his illness. In addition, many patients who present with acute alcoholism have not eaten for days, and some of the hepatic fat may be related to starvation.

CLINICAL AND LABORATORY FEATURES FOLLOWING ALCOHOL INGESTION

Alcoholic Fatty Liver

The diagnosis is often suspected by a recent or excessive exposure to alcohol, absence of signs or symptoms of acute liver disease, and the presence of a big, smooth, normally shaped liver (in 73%). One third of asymptomatic alcoholics will have fatty liver.[19] A small percentage of patients have jaundice, ascites, peripheral edema, or signs of vitamin deficiency. The more severe the hepatic fat accumulation, the more likely is vitamin deficiency. Splenomegaly is uncommon unless hepatic fibrosis or frank cirrhosis is present.[94] If alcohol is withheld, splenomegaly and early fibrotic changes may be reversible. When the patient presents with hepatic decompensation, the prevalence of fatty liver is much lower.[12] Thus, the two clinical syndromes associated with the ethanol-induced fatty liver are the asymptomatic enlarged liver and alcoholic hepatitis and/or cirrhosis. This second group more often presents with pain and tenderness in the right upper quadrant, but pain and tenderness are present in some patients with fatty liver alone.[94]

Fatty liver has become a major pathologic condition reported by medical examiners.[36,90] Most of the fatal cases of fatty liver have no cirrhosis or other obvious cause of death. In a study of 268 autopsies of chronic alcoholics, 78% of these patients with fatty liver had fat embolism, especially in the lungs.[104] Thus, fat embolism may be a more important complication that was previously recognized. Sudden death in alcoholics with fatty liver may also occur due to hypoglycemia, adrenergic hypersensitivity, or alcohol withdrawal.[140] A different cause of death is found in patients with huge livers (up to 4 kg in weight) who die after an acute illness with jaundice, usually in association with nutritional deficiency. Centrilobular necrosis and alcoholic hyalin with only scattered focal leukocyte infiltration and intact lobular architecture is seen.[132] Obese females, aged 30 to 40, are most often affected.

The serum albumin level is often normal, and the globulin value is elevated. Hyperbilirubinemia up to 8 mg/dl is seen in about 25% of cases. The serum aspartate transaminase (AST) is usually less than 300 U/liter. Prothrombin time is prolonged by 2 seconds in about half the patients. The alkaline phosphatase level is elevated in only about 15% and usually only modestly (up to 200 IU/dl). The leukocyte count is usually normal, but rarely a leukemoid reaction may be seen.[28] However, the laboratory findings and clinical features depend very much on whether fatty liver alone is present or whether there is also some degree of necrosis or intrahepatic cholestasis. Moreover, the amounts of fat and necrosis in the liver usually vary independently. Therefore, the amount of fat in the liver may not correlate well with the degree of abnormality in liver function tests.[72] A better correlation is found with imaging techniques. Fatty liver alone usually resolves without important sequelae. No long-term studies regarding the prognosis of alcoholic fatty liver are available. It is unlikely, however, that the lesion is precirrhotic.

Alcoholic Hepatitis

Alcoholic hepatitis is not a syndrome separate from alcoholic fatty liver. Necrosis is merely another manifestation of hepatic injury related to alcohol. On liver biopsy one usually sees much fat, but fat may also be almost totally absent. In addition, the "unit lesion" is present (*i.e.,* necrosis of cells often containing alcoholic hyalin, rimmed with polymorphonuclear leukocytes). Sharply focal involvement of cells in centrilobular regions, with or without sclerosis of terminal hepatic veins, is common.[42] This perivenular sclerosis may precede cirrhosis.[180] The lesion is usually diffuse. In rare cases of alcoholic hepatitis, periportal hepatocytes are affected primarily.

When this pathologic picture is seen, patients present with hepatomegaly and abdominal pain just as they do with a fatty liver alone.[54,83] However, anorexia, nausea, vomiting, fever, and jaundice tend to be more frequent. Anemia and leukocytosis are usually present, and the alkaline phosphatase level is more frequently elevated, but in most cases only up to 200 IU/liter. Usually this syndrome is found after a prolonged bout of drinking.

Most of the reported patients have had a history or past evidence of chronic liver disease. Hepatomegaly is found in about 80% of patients, with splenomegaly, jaundice, abdominal pain, and fever in one third to one half.[54] AST levels are elevated in most but not all patients. Despite the necrosis seen on liver biopsy, the transaminase level is usually not above 500 U/liter. Alkaline phosphatase is elevated in 60% to 80% of patients but need not correlate with the degree of cholestasis on biopsy.[63] This condition is a frequent cause of undiagnosed fever in alcoholic liver disease. Although the fatty liver of the alcoholic may be associated with a variable degree of necrosis, necrosis is sometimes seen in the absence of fat. Although the degree of necrosis does not correlate well with the amount of fat or with liver function tests, the more severe the necrosis, the more serious is the clinical course.

Acute Fatty Liver with Cholestasis

Rarely, alcoholic fatty liver presents as obstructive jaundice.[9,116] Typically, these patients have a history of marked alcohol ingestion for years, with an increase in intake before hospitalization. The presenting symptoms are frequently identical to those seen in alcoholic hepatitis—in fact, acute inflammatory changes in the liver can complicate this form of fatty liver. However, acute right upper quadrant pain can be seen with a rigid epigastrium. Over half the patients are febrile (>38.3° C [101° F]) and one

third have leukocytosis. About 10% have splenomegaly and ascites. The liver is very large and tender, and liver function tests indicate the presence of cholestasis. Alkaline phosphatase is two to eight times normal. Serum cholesterol may be above 400 mg/dl and about half the patients have jaundice. AST is more than 100 U/liter in most cases. Grossly the liver is large and yellow, and microscopically practically every liver cell is filled with microvesicular fat. Cholestasis may be difficult to detect because of the severe fatty changes. Central zones often show necrosis. The syndrome of increased alkaline phosphatase (greater than four times normal) and a clinical picture of extrahepatic biliary obstruction may also occur without a fatty liver or even hepatomegaly.[126]

These patients are often thought to have biliary tract disease because of fever, right upper quadrant pain, and obstructive liver chemistries. A large tender liver and radiologic confirmation of a normal biliary tract (ultrasound or computed tomography) may be clues to the correct diagnosis. Other causes of cholestasis in alcoholic patients include severe alcoholic hepatitis and superimposed drug-induced or viral hepatitis, in none of which will hepatic fat or ductal dilatation occur. Of course, gallstones and pancreatitis or pancreatic tumors may produce ductal dilatation. When surgical intervention is contemplated, the possibility of alcoholic liver disease, with or without fat, must be considered beforehand.

Treatment

All of the acute changes induced by ethanol (fatty liver, alcoholic hepatitis, and acute fatty liver with cholestasis) are potentially reversible. The diagnosis can be suspected clinically or by imaging techniques but is best made by needle biopsy of the liver. However, when the cause of presumed steatosis is obvious, a biopsy is not always needed.

Although the lesions are reversible, the change may occur very slowly. It is not unusual for recovery to begin after only 2 to 3 weeks of hospitalization and for total recovery to require months. Treatment is supportive. The mainstay of therapy is abstinence from ethanol.

OTHER CLINICAL DISORDERS OR TREATMENTS CHARACTERIZED BY FATTY LIVER

Starvation

During starvation, serum free fatty acids increase and the plasma flux of these fatty acids is enhanced.[22] This can be associated with a moderate increase in liver fat. The mechanism seems to be related to the lack of availability of glucose, increase in growth hormone, and heightened sympathetic nervous activity, all of which mobilize free fatty acids from adipose tissue. Liver function tests are usually normal, except for BSP retention, which has been reported to be as high as 44% during starvation. However, prolonged fasting can also reduce fat within the liver.[34] This apparent paradox can be explained by the following mechanism[20]: During prolonged fasting, the brain, which usually requires glucose, uses ketone bodies resulting from fatty acid oxidation. Other tissues adapt likewise, so that fat supplies 95% of body energy needs. Hepatic gluconeogenesis is markedly decreased, essential amino acids are conserved, and fat does not accumulate in the liver. If small amounts of carbohydrate are ingested, this adaptation does not occur, lipids are mobilized but not oxidized, and fatty liver results. Thus, the development of hepatic steatosis depends on the completeness of starvation.

Protein-Calorie Malnutrition

Most workers recognize two distinct syndromes, kwashiorkor and marasmus, and believe that the former is related to a relative deficiency of protein, the latter to deficiency of both protein and calories. However, dietary history is of little help in distinguishing these two syndromes. If one defines kwashiorkor by gross edema, hepatomegaly, and depigmentation of skin, 11% of cases of malnutrition can be so classified.[183] When marasmus is defined as body weight less than half expected, with no edema or skin changes, 21% of the cases fall into this category. Lipid changes in marasmatic children are much less striking, and fatty liver does not occur in this syndrome. The remainder are mixed cases clinically. For this reason, many workers prefer the comprehensive term of *protein-calorie malnutrition.* This group of disorders is worldwide in distribution but occurs uncommonly in the United States in its overt clinical form. Liver function is only mildly impaired; AST values are usually less than 100 U/liter, but may be over 500, possibly related to secondary changes from marked steatosis.[184]

Fatty liver is only one aspect of the syndrome. The liver is enlarged and yellow, and there is a striking degree of fatty infiltration. The earliest deposition of fat is in the cells at the periphery of the lobules, but as the condition progresses, the cells of the middle and central areas of the lobules become involved.[112] When a high-protein diet is administered, fat disappears first from the center of the liver lobule and last from the peripheral cells.[113] The condition does not progress to cirrhosis, which suggests that fat alone is an insufficient stimulus for the formation of fibrosis.

The hepatic concentration of palmitic acid is increased, and that of linoleic acid is decreased.[111] Because these findings resembled those in animals fed a high-carbohydrate diet, it seemed that the fat was originally synthesized from carbohydrate, since the fat intake of these children is low.[112] In rodents it is clear that glucose administration triggers hepatic lipid synthesis, but the sugar acts indirectly via lactate or glycogen as the precursor.[89] When fatty liver is severe, the serum triglyceride and VLDL levels are very low. The serum free fatty acids are increased, which suggests that increased mobilization of fat is also important.

The rate of albumin synthesis is diminished, and it has been suggested that lipoprotein synthesis is also affected, impairing the release of triglyceride from the liver. No evidence for lipotrope deficiency exists. With ingestion of dietary protein there is a marked rise in VLDL, accompanied by a rise in triglyceride, phospholipid, and cholesterol in that fraction.[52]

Obesity

The frequency of fatty liver in obese patients is well recognized and ranges from 66% to 99%.[33,80] Enhanced fatty acid synthesis and altered partition of fatty acids between oxidation and esterification are the major causes of hypersecretion of triglyceride-rich lipoprotein in genetically obese rats.[7] Presumably hepatic accumulation of triglyceride exceeds secretion rate. Fatty liver may also be related to an increase in free fatty acid supply from the peripheral fat depots. As the mass of adipose tissue increases, free fatty acid release increases. These substrates diminish glucose utilization and increase serum glucose concentrations. Insulin secretion is stimulated and thus tends to lower free fatty acid levels. Although insulin decreases the rate of release of free fatty acids per kilogram of adipose tissue, the increased mass of adipose tissue overcomes this regulatory effect. Thus, insulin resistance and increased supply of free fatty acids may be secondary to the increased adipose tissue mass.[49]

The majority of obese patients with fatty liver have abnormal glucose tolerance tests but are not severely diabetic (see Diabetes Mellitus). Mildly elevated AST and alkaline phosphatase levels are the most frequent abnormal result of liver function tests.[107] Liver biopsy has revealed, in addition to fat, periportal inflammation and fibrosis and occasional areas of necrosis (Fig. 25-9).[2] In most cases the fat is diffusely distributed, but in milder cases it is centrilobular.[177] There seems to be no clear correlation between the degree of obesity and the amount of hepatic fat,[177] although the fatty infiltration can be reversed by weight reduction. Long-term follow-up of nonalcoholic, nondiabetic patients reveals no progression from fatty liver to cirrhosis.[74]

Bypass Surgery for Obesity

Jejunoileal bypass for obesity leads to a variety of pathologic changes in the liver, including increased steatosis and fibrosis, inflammation, granulomas, and cirrhosis.[67] No relationship has been detected between the amount of pre-bypass hepatic lipid or fibrosis and the subsequent development of cirrhosis or hepatic failure.[129] Perivenular sclerosis has been suggested as a prognostic indicator of cirrhosis,[109] but this correlation has not been confirmed.[177] The most consistent change after bypass is increasing steatosis.

The clinical features may range from only abnormal liver test results to frank hepatic failure in 2% to 5%.[67] If results of hepatic tests fail to return to preoperative levels (see obesity above) one should look for serious hepatic disease. Elevated AST and alkaline phosphatase levels are most commonly present.

Nearly all patients demonstrate increasing hepatic fat for the first 6 months after bypass.[131] After that the degree of steatosis diminishes until it reaches pre-bypass amounts of 2 or 3 years postoperatively.[161] These changes in hepatic fat are not associated with predictable changes in liver function test results. In fact, the only certain means of following the hepatic disease is by repeated liver biopsies.[55] Increased mobilization of adipose tissue fat is partially responsible for the increased steatosis after bypass. More than this explanation is involved, since morbidly obese patients who lose weight by dieting or by gastric bypass operations do not deposit increased fat in the liver. While fat is accumulating in the liver, serum essential amino acid levels fall.[118] This is similar to the situation seen in protein-calorie malnutrition. However, the distribution of fat in kwashiorkor is periportal, a pattern seen rarely after bypass surgery. Bacterial toxins or toxic bile acids (lithocholic acid) may also play a role in the production of post-bypass liver disease.[46,124] Tetracycline prevents steatosis in dogs,[124] and removal of the excluded loop in rats decreases liver toxicity.[179] Bacterial overgrowth in the bypass segment could help to explain the hepatic necrosis and fibrosis that sometimes develop.

Patients with progressive liver disease after bypass surgery have morphologic changes beyond fatty liver. The most consistent other feature is increased fibrosis with foamy degeneration of hepatocytes (Fig. 25-10). This change appears to varying degrees (27%–49%),[69,127] but becomes almost universal when frank cirrhosis occurs.[128] Alcoholic hyalin has been found with severe progressive hepatic disease[128] along with neutrophil infiltration. When progressive hepatic disease develops, reversal of the bypass is necessary.[68] Criteria for reversal include the onset of icterus and prolongation of prothrombin time. Oral amino acid supplementation[102] or parenteral alimentation[6,8] is probably advisable before reanastomosis is performed, especially if the patient is severely ill. Although most hepatic failure develops in the first 24 months after bypass, occasionally patients present at a later time with a change in hepatic function. The finding of steatosis at that time, by itself, does not imply progressive fibrosis or impending hepatic failure. If the patient is otherwise doing well, continued surveillance with periodic biopsy is indicated.

Diabetes Mellitus

Fatty liver occurs in diabetics, but the etiology and the importance attached to the observation remain unclear. Hepatomegaly occurs frequently in untreated diabetics but does not always mean fatty infiltration. Diabetes mellitus occurs in 4% to 46% of patients with fatty liver, with an average of 25%.[33] It does not matter whether the diabetes is chemical or overt. On the other hand, about 50% of patients with diabetes have fatty liver.[33,88,93] In addition, 50% to 80% of adult-onset diabetics are obese, and fatty

Fig. 25-9. Fatty liver with chronic inflammatory changes in obese patient before jejunoileal bypass. Note the few areas of focal cellular infiltrate and cell dropout. (Original magnification × 390)

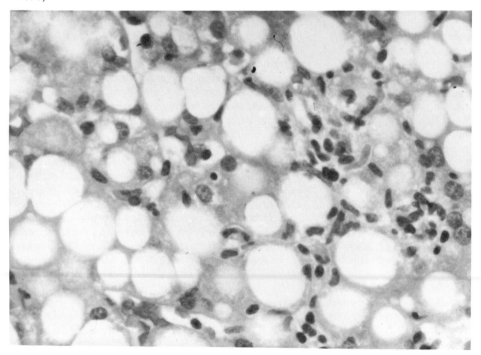

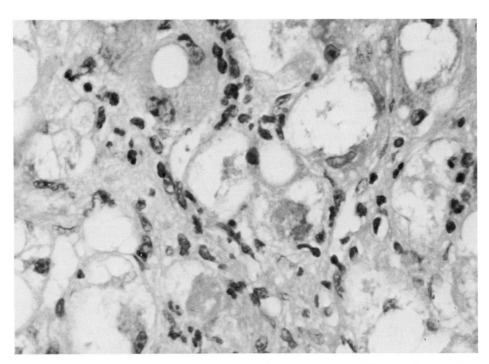

Fig. 25-10. Fatty liver with severe degeneration of hepatocytes and Mallory hyaline in obese patient after jejunoileal bypass. (Original magnification × 390)

liver was found at autopsy in 51% of patients with diabetic ketoacidosis. It seems that obesity is the major factor in the fatty infiltration seen in adult-onset diabetics and not the diabetes mellitus itself. Fatty liver is uncommon (4.5%) in insulin-deficient juvenile diabetics.[178] The incidence of fatty liver in diabetics over age 60 is about 45%.[178] No correlation exists between the degree of control or duration of the diabetes and the fatty infiltration. In about 75% of the cases the fat is either centrilobular or diffuse in distribution.[71]

It is possible that decreased glucose tolerance in some patients with fatty liver is a consequence of the hepatic involvement. After alcohol withdrawal, abnormal glucose tolerance and fatty liver have both been seen to disappear. Other primary liver diseases can also be associated with abnormal glucose tolerance. Certainly, if fat in the liver is significant in a stable, adult diabetic, causes other than the diabetes should be sought.

The presence of hepatic steatosis has little effect on the prognosis of the diabetes mellitus. Treatment should include weight reduction with a low-carbohydrate, high-protein diet. Insulin therapy alone is of little value in the steatosis of the adult onset diabetic.

Fatty Liver of Pregnancy

Fatty liver of pregnancy often cannot be easily differentiated clinically from fulminant viral hepatitis. However, the laboratory features and pathology are clearly not the same as those in hepatitis. Fifty cases have been collected and reviewed.[34] In this series the age at onset was 16 to 42 years. Almost all reported cases involve patients during their first pregnancy. The syndrome begins with the sudden onset of vomiting and abdominal pain, usually during the 36th to 40th week of pregnancy. There is a rapid progression to jaundice, hematemesis, tachycardia, premature labor, oliguria, coma, convulsions, and death. Occasionally jaundice is absent. Hematemesis results from mucosal ulcerations of the esophagus or stomach and is aggravated by coagulation defects. The liver is not palpable. The total illness usually lasts 1 to 2 weeks. Only six of the reported cases survived. Although the child usually is stillborn, some children survive with spontaneous delivery.[87] In some of these surviving cases cesarean section was performed early. Therefore, it has been suggested that the syndrome might be reversible if recognized early enough.[65] Of the more than 25 cases reported since 1980, maternal mortality was only 22%.[146] Greater awareness and prompt delivery seem to be responsible for improved survival.

Laboratory results show a bilirubin value that is usually about 10 mg/dl, alkaline phosphatase increased two to four times, and an AST modestly elevated (<300 U/liter) and greater than the alanine transaminase (ALT). Leukocytosis is marked and usually greater than 20,000/mm³. Azotemia is a frequent finding. In fulminant hepatitis the AST is usually greater than 1000 U/liter. Thrombocytopenia (<100,000/mm³) occurs in 80% of patients with acute fatty liver of pregnancy[1] but is uncommon in hepatitis. Severe bleeding is often due to disseminated intravascular coagulopathy, and fibrinogen levels (as well as platelet counts) are low. Grossly the liver is yellow and soft. Microscopically the fat is deposited first centrally, then spreads to involve the entire lobule. The cells often show fine fat vacuoles. It is usually stated that there is no necrosis or inflammation, although at least one case of hepatic necrosis has been reported.[34] In the presence of coagulopathy, the diagnosis should be made from typical symptoms, signs, and laboratory tests, so that delivery can proceed. If biopsy is performed, a frozen section stained with Oil Red O can identify the fine lipid droplets. Acute pancreatitis is sometimes present, and fat can be found in the pancreas, brain, and kidneys. Multiple systems may be involved (pancreas, kidney, intestine), and the cause of death may be unrelated to hepatic failure.[73] Moreover, profound hypoglycemia may be a complicating factor. When recovery has occurred, it is noted first at the periphery of the lobule. The mechanism of fatty infiltration during pregnancy is unknown.

Drugs and Toxins

Tetracycline

The administration of large intravenous doses (>2 g/day) of tetracycline and its derivatives is associated with a fine, fatty vacuolization of the liver. This injury has also been seen with oral administration and in any setting in which the blood levels of tetracycline are unusually high.[128] A few cases have been reported using parenteral doses of only 1 g/day, so that during pregnancy an upper limit of 1 g/day should be used. Many early cases occurred when tetracycline, which is excreted primarily in the urine, was given to patients with renal dysfunction. This condition has been seen usually in pregnant females but has been reported in nonpregnant females and males. In either case, the pathology is similar to that seen in fatty metamorphosis of pregnancy. A number of cases of fatty liver have been reported in association with tetracycline administration during pregnancy.[41] The fatty liver was reversible when tetracycline was discontinued.

Pathologically the fatty accumulation is localized to the central and midzonal areas, with fine foamy infiltration of the cell, and the nucleus of the hepatocyte in the center,[29] not pushed to the edge as is seen with alcoholic fatty liver. Necrosis is uncommon.

Approximately 75% of the reported patients have died. In a typical case, 3 to 12 days after tetracycline has been given, there is an abrupt onset of jaundice, nausea, and vomiting, spontaneous delivery, renal failure, gastrointestinal bleeding, coma, and finally death 1 to 2 weeks after the first dose of tetracycline. The laboratory findings and pathology in tetracycline-induced fatty liver are similar to those in fatty metamorphosis of pregnancy, except that jaundice is not so common. Leukocytosis, lactic aci-

dosis, and rising blood urea nitrogen, bilirubin, and AST usually occur. Fewer than half the patients develop a high AST of more than 400 U/liter.[29] Some patients have recovered, but only when the tetracycline administration was stopped. Tetracycline inhibits protein synthesis when used in large doses, but mechanisms other than impaired hepatic VLDL output probably are also responsible for tetracycline-induced fatty liver.[16]

Valproic Acid

Valproic acid is a branched medium-chain fatty acid that is used in the treatment of petit mal epilepsy. Overt liver damage is uncommon, but a variable increase in serum bilirubin, alkaline phosphatase, or SGOT activity is common, occurring 2 to 3 months after onset of therapy.[18] Fever, nausea, anorexia, and jaundice are the usual symptoms when they occur. The liver histologically shows centrilobular necrosis with small fat droplets in hepatocytes. Bile duct injury and submassive necrosis have been seen.[165] Recovery is usually spontaneous when the drug is withdrawn.

The etiology of the liver damage is unknown. The drug might be converted into an analog of 4-pentenoic acid, an agent that causes derangements similar to hypoglycin (*i.e.,* impaired fatty acid oxidation and decreased available coenzyme A and carnitine, along with fine droplets of fat in hepatocytes). A hypoglycin metabolite is the cause of Jamaican vomiting sickness, another disorder associated with small droplets of hepatocyte lipid.

Methotrexate

Methotrexate is used as long-term treatment for psoriasis. Appreciation of its toxicity was complicated by the high incidence of pretreatment liver lesions, especially among those consuming excess alcohol. The drug causes a wide variety of hepatic changes, including fatty deposition, ballooning degeneration, fibrosis, and cirrhosis.[44] The effects are dose related and can be minimized if the drug dose is adjusted to the lowest effective level.[35] Liver function tests are not sensitive enough to detect this damage, and liver biopsy at periodic intervals (6 to 12 months) is often carried out during treatment. Development of significant liver disease, more than fatty infiltration alone, would constitute a relative contraindication to the further use of the drug.

Perhexilene Maleate

Perhexilene maleate is an antianginal drug not presently available in the United States that has been reported to produce elevated transaminase levels, jaundice, encephalopathy, and ascites. Liver biopsy shows lesions such as in alcoholic hepatitis, including fat, necrosis, and alcoholic hyalin.[136] Since the drug causes change in total liver gangliosides, its effects may be related to a drug-induced defect in glycolipid metabolism.[77]

Corticosteroids

In Cushing's syndrome moderate to severe fatty infiltration of the liver is reported not uncommonly.[171] Fatty liver has been reported in patients receiving high doses of exogenous steroids over a period of weeks. In animals, plasma free fatty acids increase when high doses of cortisol are given,[76] suggesting that increased mobilization of fatty acid is involved. However, with low doses of steroids, all the increase in fatty acids can be accounted for by a decreased esterification of fatty acids in the liver.[84] Clinically, fatty liver occurs only with higher doses of steroids. Steroids given during viral hepatitis in the dose of 30 to 40 mg prednisone per day can result in a moderate fatty infiltration that is rarely seen in hepatitis in the absence of steroids. Systemic fat embolism has been reported after abrupt cessation of steroid therapy,[75,86] and fatty liver has been implicated as a possible source.

Chlorinated Hydrocarbons

Carbon tetrachloride has attracted more attention in recent years as an experimental hepatotoxin than as a cause of fatty liver in humans. Its former presence in fire extinguishers and cleaning fluids made it available for toxicity in humans. In recent years most commercial preparations that had contained carbon tetrachloride now contain another chlorinated hydrocarbon, trichloroethylene, which also has excellent solvent properties. Hepatotoxicity due to this solvent is much rarer than with carbon tetrachloride.[27,182] Chronic use has been reported to result in hepatitis, renal failure, myocarditis, or cranial nerve palsies. Ethanol potentiates the hepatic effects. However, chronic liver disease due to these compounds has never been reported in the absence of ethanol use.

Trichloroethylene is usually inhaled but may be ingested accidentally. Clinically, trichloroethylene often produces dizziness, nausea, vomiting, and headache as early symptoms. The time of onset depends on the dose. A burning sensation in the mouth, esophagus, and stomach is often present very early after ingestion. Subsequently, abdominal cramps, confusion, decreased consciousness, delirium, restlessness, choreiform movements, muscle pain, diarrhea, vasomotor collapse, and even coma may ensue. Neither jaundice or hepatomegaly need occur, even after ingestion, and deaths have been reported without much evidence of liver failure. When death occurs, it is usually the result of respiratory muscle paralysis, pulmonary edema, or cardiac involvement.

Laboratory data usually reveal elevated transaminases, prolongation of the prothrombin time, and normal or slightly elevated alkaline phosphatase levels. Hepatic pathology shows mild fatty change, often midzonal, with centrilobular necrosis. Many acute inflammatory cells are present, especially in the centrilobular areas. The fat may be present in cells as fine vacuoles or large cysts. Treatment is only supportive.

Phosphorus

Of the three forms of elemental phosphorus, only yellow phosphorus is toxic appreciably to the liver. It is a common component of many roach and rat poisons. After ingestion, frequently a burning sensation is felt in the mouth and throat. Abdominal pain and vomiting of violent nature follow. Within 1 or 2 days jaundice appears, and death can occur fairly rapidly. A fatal dose for humans is about 60 mg. The majority of patients recover in 1 to 3 days or progress to a syndrome of generalized toxicity involving liver, kidney, heart, and central nervous system.[51]

The mechanism of action of phosphorus and halogenated hydrocarbons is similar.[38] Hepatic protein (and apolipoprotein) synthesis is impaired, leading to decreased protein secretion. This can lead to a bleeding tendency and may account for the only moderate serum transaminase levels in some cases. In addition, these substances are potent toxins and produce cellular damage and inflammatory lesions. If recovery occurs, liver histology and function return to normal.

Pathologically the liver shows periportal necrosis and fat at early times, with the center of the lobule relatively spared. With severe poisoning the entire liver is rapidly involved. Gastric lavage is the treatment of choice.

Hepatic Resection

After a two-thirds hepatic resection in animals, steatosis develops almost immediately.[11] Hepatic lipid increases twofold within 10 hours, the majority being triglyceride. In humans the serum triglyceride, phospholipid, and cholesterol all fall acutely after resection and recover within 2 to 3 weeks.[4] The marked decrease is presumably due to impaired synthesis and release of lipoproteins by the liver. Although jaundice often occurs postoperatively, there is no indication of any functional impairment due to steatosis. Moreover, the steatosis has been more apparent in experimental animals than in humans, in whom its demonstration has been limited by the availability of biopsy material within the immediate postoperative period.

Systemic Disorders

As stated previously, fatty liver is commonly found on liver biopsy in patients with and without intrinsic liver disease. This results from the fact that fatty acid flux from adipose tissue to liver is constantly changing and the hepatic uptake depends on their rate of delivery. Since the capacity of the liver to oxidize, esterify, and secrete fatty acid in the form of VLDL is limited, accumulation often occurs. The presence of conditions such as diabetes mellitus or corticosteroid or alcohol ingestion may be superimposed on systemic illnesses that produce hepatic fat accumulation. By itself, fatty liver tells nothing of the other functional capacities of the liver.

Inflammatory Bowel Disease

Fat accumulation has been found in livers from patients with both ulcerative colitis and Crohn's disease, with a range from 0 to 80%. The fat is in large droplets and is usually diffusely distributed. The cause of the fatty liver is multifactorial. Many patients are malnourished and chronically ill. The incidence in autopsied livers is higher than at biopsy but is also higher than in patients dying with other diseases.[117] Thus, malnutrition is not the sole cause. Many patients are taking corticosteroids. However, many patients have had fatty liver while not receiving corticosteroids. Alcohol ingestion remains a possible factor, and no study has adequately addressed this issue. The possibility of some bacterial toxin has been suggested. However, the frequency of fatty liver was the same after colectomy for ulcerative colitis as before resection. Generally patients are asymptomatic from fatty liver itself, but fatty liver may occur with other hepatic lesions. Thus, abnormal laboratory tests and symptoms cannot be attributed usually to fatty liver alone. (See Chapter 44, part 5 for further discussion and references.) Total parenteral nutrition, if used, can also lead to fatty liver. (See Parenteral Alimentation below).

Primary Liver Disease

In distinction from other forms of viral hepatitis, non A, non B hepatitis can produce microvesicular steatosis.[39] Moderate microvesicular fat can also be seen in Wilson's disease, especially in the early stages of the hepatic dysfunction.[176] In this stage the cells can appear pleomorphic, but no other distinctive biopsy changes may be seen, so that the suspicion of Wilson's disease must be raised.

Diseases in Infancy and Childhood

The conditions that may demonstrate fatty liver on histology include Reye's syndrome, Wolman's disease, cholesterol storage disease, galactosemia, hereditary fructose intolerance, familial hepatosteatosis, and abetalipoproteinemia. These disorders are discussed in Chapter 43.

Parenteral Alimentation

Elevated serum AST, alkaline phosphatase, and bilirubin levels have been observed along with occasional pathologic evidence of fatty liver during intravenous alimentation.[85] Cholestasis and periportal inflammation have been found along with fatty changes.[167] In children, cholestasis with mild fibrosis has also been seen. In adult patients, fatty metamorphosis is associated most commonly with excessive caloric infusion (4000 to 6000 kcal) for over 6 weeks.[106] In this case the calorie-to-nitrogen ratio may be excessive and hepatic fatty acid synthesis may outstrip the ability of the liver to secrete lipids (see Protein-Calorie Malnutrition). In animals, parenteral feeding causes steatosis by enhanced hepatic synthesis of fatty acid and reduced triglyceride secretion.[66] Rarely, essential fatty acid deficiency secondary to prolonged intravenous feeding may cause fatty metamorphosis. In children, steatosis is found commonly with premature infants or in the presence of infection or intrinsic liver disease. When protein malnutrition is the cause of steatosis, as in obese patients after bypass surgery, treatment with parenteral nutrition actually causes a decrease in hepatic fat.

FATTY LIVER AND CIRRHOSIS

The role of fat per se in the production of cirrhosis has been discussed extensively in the literature. Most of the evidence in favor of this stems from experiments using the choline-deficient rat as a model.[135] Choline deficiency in animals with a low-protein diet leads to cirrhosis. That the two conditions might be related was further supported by the fact that both fatty change and fibrosis began centrilobularly. Choline deficiency produces fatty liver in animals that could be maintained for months without the production of cirrhosis.[70] On the other hand, severe choline deficiency leads to necrosis. Thus, the more severe amounts of fat would be associated with the most necrosis and this lesion could progress to cirrhosis. When another animal model is examined that produces fatty liver without necrosis (orotic acid feeding), no cirrhosis is seen, even after prolonged feeding.[168]

The closest counterpart in humans to choline deficiency in animals is kwashiorkor, and cirrhosis is rare in kwashiorkor.[183] Long-term follow-up studies of patients with kwashiorkor, including liver histology, demonstrate no cirrhosis,[183] although the cases investigated had been treated. Many of the other clinical conditions associated with fatty liver are so regularly accompanied by necrosis that the relation of fatty liver alone to cirrhosis cannot be demonstrated. Conditions that are most often seen with necrosis (alcohol, carbon tetrachloride) most often lead to cirrhosis. Tetracycline-induced fatty liver and fatty liver of pregnancy, although sometimes fatal, rarely lead to hepatic necrosis, and when there is recovery do not appear to have resulted in cirrhosis. Long-term follow-up of lesser degrees of fatty infiltration in obesity also has demonstrated no cirrhosis.[36,110] Thus, there is no evidence that hepatic fat accumulation by itself leads to cirrhosis. It seems more likely that the accumulation of fat is merely the most obvious manifestation of the pathologic process that eventually proceeds to cirrhosis.

REFERENCES

1. Adams WH, Shrestha M, Adams DA: Coagulation studies of viral hepatitis occurring during pregnancy. Am J Med Sci 272:129, 1976
2. Adler M, Schaffner F: Fatty liver hepatitis and cirrhosis in obese patients. Am J Med 67:811, 1979
3. Ahmad M et al: Xenon-133 retention in hepatic steatosis: Correlation with liver biopsy in 45 patients. J Nucl Med 20:397, 1979

4. Almersjo O et al: Serum lipids after extensive liver resection in man. Acta Hepatosplen 15:1, 1968

5. Alpers DH et al: Distribution of apolipoproteins A-I and B among intestinal lipoproteins. J Lipid Res 26:1, 1985

6. Ames FC, Copeland E, Leib D et al: Liver dysfunction following small bowel bypass for obesity. JAMA 235:1249, 1976

7. Azain MJ, Fukuda N, Chai FF et al: Contributions of fatty acid and sterol synthesis to triglyceride and cholesterol secretion by the perfused rat liver in genetic hyperlipidemia and obesity. J Biol Chem 260:174, 1985

8. Baker AL, Elson CO, Gaspan J et al: Liver failure with steatonecrosis after jejunoileal bypass. Arch Intern Med 239:239, 1979

9. Ballard H et al: Fatty liver presenting as obstructive jaundice. Am J Med 30:196, 1961

10. Baraona E et al: Effects of ethanol on lipid metabolism. J Lipid Res 20:289, 1979

11. Bengmark S: Liver steatosis and liver resection. Digestion 2:304, 1969

12. Bhathal PS et al: The spectrum of liver disease in an Australian teaching hospital: A prospective study of 205 patients. Med J Aust 2:1085, 1973

13. Bisgaier CL, Glickman RM: Intestinal secretion and transport of lipoproteins. Ann Rev Physiol 45:625, 1983

14. Blaufuss MC, Gordon JI, Schonfeld G et al: Biosynthesis of apolipoprotein C-III in rat liver and small intestinal mucosa. J Biol Chem 259:2452, 1984

15. Brawer MK, Austin GE, Lauren KJ: Focal fatty change of the liver, a hitherto poorly recognized entity. Gastroenterology 78:247, 1980

16. Brean KJ et al: Fatty liver induced by tetracycline in the rat. Gastroenterology 69:714, 1975

17. Brown MS, Goldstein JL: Lipoprotein receptors in the liver: Control signals for plasma cholesterol traffic. J Clin Invest 72:743, 1983

18. Browne TR: Valproic acid. N Engl J Med 302:661, 1980

19. Brugerera M, Borda JM, Rodes J: Asymptomatic liver disease in alcoholics. Arch Pathol Lab Med 101:644, 1977

20. Cahill GF Jr: Starvation in man. N Engl J Med 282:668, 1970

21. Campagnari-Visconti L et al: Inhibition by glucose of the ethionine-induced fatty liver. Proc Soc Exp Biol Med 111:479, 1962

22. Carlson LA et al: Some physiological and clinical implications of lipid mobilization from adipose tissue. In Renold AE, Cahill GR Jr (eds): American Physiology Society: Adipose Tissue, Handbook of Physiology, section 5, p 625. Baltimore, Williams & Wilkins, 1965

23. Chajek R et al: Effect of colchicine, cycloheximide and chloroquine on the hepatic triacylglycerol hydrolase in the intact rat and perfused liver. Biochim Biophys Acta 488:270, 1977

24. Chan L: Hormonal control of gene expression. In Arias IM, Schacter D, Shafritz DA (eds): The Liver: Biology and Pathobiology, pp 143–167. New York, Raven Press, 1982

25. Christofferson P, Braerstrup O, Juhl E et al: Lipogranulomas in human liver biopsies with fatty change: A morphological, biochemical and clinical investigation. Acta Pathol Microbiol Scand 79:150, 1971

26. Claude A: Growth and differentiation of cytoplasmic membranes in the course of lipoprotein granule synthesis in the hepatic cell: I. Elaboration of elements of the Golgi complex. J Cell Biol 47:745, 1970

27. Clearfield HR: Hepatorenal toxicity from sniffing spot remover (trichloroethylene). Am J Dig Dis 15:851, 1970

28. Coleman RW, Shein HM: Leukemoid reaction, hyperuricemia, and severe hyperpyrexia complicating a fatal case of acute fatty liver of the alcoholic. Ann Intern Med 57:110, 1962

29. Combes B et al: Tetracycline and the liver. Prog Liver Dis 4:589, 1972

30. Composti M et al: Studies on in vitro peroxidation of liver lipids in ethanol-treated rats. Lipids 8:498, 1973

31. Cooper A: Role of the liver in the degradation of lipoproteins. Gastroenterology 88:192, 1985

32. Cooper AD: The metabolism of chylomicron remnants by isolated perfused rat liver. Biochim Biophys Acta 488:464, 1977

33. Creutzfeldt W et al: Liver diseases and diabetes mellitus. Prog Liver Dis 3:371, 1970

34. Czernobilsky B, Bergnes MA: Acute fatty metamorphosis of the liver in pregnancy with associated liver cell necrosis. Obstet Gynecol 26:792, 1965

35. Dahl MGC, Gregory MM, Scheuer PJ: Methotrexate hepatotoxicity in psoriasis: Comparison of different dosage regimens. Br Med J 1:654, 1972

36. DeLint J, Schmidt W: Mortality from liver cirrhosis and other causes in alcoholics: A follow-up study of patients with and without a history of enlarged fatty liver. Q J Stud Alcohol 31:705, 1970

37. Denk H, Franke WW, Cherstorfer R et al: Formation and involution of Mallory bodies in murine and human liver revealed by immunofluorescence microscopy with antibodies to prekeratin. Proc Natl Acad Sci USA 76:4112, 1979

38. Dianzani MU: Biochemical aspects of fatty liver. In Slater TF (ed): Biochemical Mechanisms of Liver Injury, pp 45–96. New York, Academic Press, 1978

39. Dienes HP, Popper H, Arnold W et al: Histologic observations in human hepatitis non A-non B. Hepatology 2:562, 1982

40. Domschke S, Domschke W, Lieber CS: Hepatic redox state: Attenuation of the acute effects of ethanol induced by chronic ethanol consumption. Life Sci 15:1327, 1974

41. Dowling HF, Lepper MH: Hepatic reactions to tetracycline. JAMA 188:307, 1970

42. Edmondson HA et al: Sclerosing hyaline necrosis of the liver in the chronic alcoholic: A recognizable clinical syndrome. Ann Intern Med 59:646, 1963

43. Eisenberg S: High density lipoprotein metabolism. J Lipid Res 25:1017, 1984

44. Epstein EH, Croft JD Jr: Cirrhosis following methotrexate administration for psoriasis. Arch Dermatol 100:531, 1969

45. Faergeman O et al: Metabolism of apoprotein B of plasma very low density lipoproteins in the rat. J Clin Invest 56:1396, 1975

46. Faloon WW et al: Lithogenic and hepatotoxic potential in intestinal bypass. Gastroenterology 68:1073, 1975

47. Farber E et al: Biochemical pathology of acute hepatic adenosine triphosphate deficit. Nature 203:34, 1964

48. Fielding PE et al: Lipoprotein lipase: Properties of the enzyme isolated from post-heparin plasma. Biochemistry 13:4318, 1977

49. Flatt JP: Role of the increased adipose tissue mass in the apparent insulin insensitivity of obesity. Am J Clin Nutr 25:1189, 1972

50. Fletcher FG, Galambos JT: Phosphorus poisoning in humans. Arch Intern Med 112:846, 1963
51. Floren CH et al: Binding, interiorization and degradation of cholesteryl ester-labelled chylomicron-remnant particles by rat hepatocyte monolayers. Biochem J 168:483, 1977
52. Flores H et al: Lipid transport in kwashiorkor. Br J Nutr 24:1005, 1970
53. Fredholm B, Russell S: Effect of adrenergic blocking agents on lipid mobilization from canine subcutaneous adipose tissue after sympathetic nerve stimulation. J Pharmacol Exp Ther 159:1, 1968
54. Galambos J: Alcoholic hepatitis: Its therapy and prognoses. Prog Liver Dis 4:567, 1972
55. Galambos JT, Wills CE: Relationship between 505 paired liver tests and biopsies in 242 obese patients. Gastroenterology 74:1191, 1978
56. Gerber MA, Orr W, Denle H et al: Hepatocellular hyaline in cholestasis and cirrhosis: The diagnostic significance. Gastroenterology 64:89, 1973
57. Glickman RM, Sabesin SM: Lipoprotein metabolism. In Arias IM, Popper H, Schacter D et al (eds): The Liver: Biology and Pathology, pp 123–142. New York, Raven Press, 1982
58. Glickman RM et al: The intestine as a source of apolipoprotein Al. Proc Natl Acad Sci USA 74:1569, 1977
59. Goldstein JL, Kita T, Brown MS: Defective lipoprotein receptors and atherosclerosis. N Engl J Med 309:288, 1983
60. Goldstein JL et al: The low density lipoprotein pathway and its relation to atherosclerosis. Ann Rev Biochem 46:897, 1977
61. Gordon JI, Smith DP, Alpers DH et al: Proteolytic processing of the primary translation product of rat intestinal apolipoprotein A-IV mRNA. J Biol Chem 257:8418, 1982
62. Graham M, Taketomi S, Fumno K et al: Metabolic studies on the development of ethanol induced fatty liver in KK-A4 mice. J Nutr 105:1500, 1975
63. Green J et al: Acute alcoholic hepatitis: A clinical study of 50 cases. Arch Intern Med 11:67, 1963
64. Green PHR et al: Rat intestine secretes discoid high density lipoproteins. J Clin Invest 61:528, 1978
65. Haemmerli UP: Jaundice during pregnancy. Acta Med Scand Suppl 179:1, 1966
66. Hall RI, Grant JP, Ross LH et al: Pathogenesis of hepatic steatosis in the parenterally fed rat. J Clin Invest 74:1658, 1984
67. Halverson JD et al: Jejunoileal bypass for morbid obesity: A critical appraisal. Am J Med 64:461, 1978
68. Halverson JD et al: Reanastomosis after jejunoileal bypass. Surgery 84:241, 1976
69. Hamilton RL et al: Discoidal bilayer structure of nascent high density lipoproteins from perfused rat liver. J Clin Invest 58:667, 1976
70. Handler P, Dubin IN: The significance of fatty infiltration in development of hepatic cirrhosis due to choline deficiency. J Nutr 31:141, 1946
71. Hano T: Pathohistological study on the liver cirrhosis in diabetes mellitus. Kobe J Med Sci 14:87, 1968
72. Harinasuta U et al: Steatonecrosis–Mallory body type. Medicine 46:161, 1967
73. Hatfield AK et al: Idiopathic acute fatty liver in pregnancy: Death from extrahepatic manifestations. Am J Dig Dis 17:167, 1972
74. Hilden M et al: Fatty liver persisting for up to 33 years: A

follow-up of the Iverson-Roholm liver biopsy material. Acta Med Scand 194:485, 1973
75. Hill RB Jr: Fatal fat embolism from steroid-induced fatty liver. N Engl J Med 265:318, 1961
76. Hill RB Jr et al: Hepatic lipid metabolism in the cortisone treated rat. Exp Mol Pathol 4:320, 1965
77. Hoenig N, Warner F: Effect of perhexilene maleate on lipid metabolism in the rat. Pharmacol Res Commun 12:29, 1980
78. Holloway PW et al: On the biosynthesis of dienoic fatty acids by animal tissues. Biochem Biophys Res Commun 12:300, 1963
79. Howell KE, Palade GE: Heterogeneity of lipoprotein particles in hepatic Golgi fractions. J Cell Biol 92:833, 1982
80. Hoyumpa AM et al: Fatty liver: Biochemical and clinical considerations. Am J Dig Dis 20:1142, 1975
81. Hyams DE et al: The prevention of fatty liver by administration of adenosine triphosphate. Lab Invest 16:604, 1967
82. Jackson RL et al: Lipoprotein structure and metabolism. Physiol Rev 56:259, 1976
83. Jazcilevich S et al: Induction of fatty liver in the rat after cycloheximide administration. Lab Invest 23:590, 1970
84. Jeanrenaud B: Effect of glucocorticoid hormones on fatty acid mobilization and reesterification in rat adipose tissue. Biochem J 103:627, 1967
85. Jeejeebhoy KN et al: Total parenteral nutrition at home: Studies in patients surviving four months in five years. Gastroenterology 71:943, 1976
86. Jones JP Jr et al: Systemic fat embolism after renal homotransplantation and treatment with corticosteroids. N Engl J Med 273:1453, 1965
87. Joske RA et al: Acute fatty liver of pregnancy. Gut 9:489, 1968
88. Kalk H: The relationship between fatty liver and diabetes mellitus. Germ Med Monthly 5:81, 1960
89. Katz J, McGarry JD: The glucose paradox: Is glucose a substrate for liver metabolism? J Clin Invest 74:1901, 1984
90. Kramer K et al: The increasing mortality attributed to cirrhosis and fatty liver in Baltimore (1957–1966). Ann Intern Med 69:273, 1968
91. Lee JKT, Heiken SP, Dixon WT: Detection of hepatic metastases by proton spectroscopic imaging: Work in progress. Radiology 156:428, 1985
92. Lee JKT et al: Fatty infiltration of the liver: Demonstration by proton spectroscopic imaging. Radiology 153:195, 1984
93. Leevy CM: Diabetes mellitus and liver dysfunction. Am J Med 8:290, 1950
94. Leevy CM: Fatty liver: A study of 270 patients with biopsy proven fatty liver and the pathogenesis of fatty liver. Am J Clin Nutr 15:161, 1964
95. Lieber CS: Metabolism and metabolic effects of ethanol. Semin Liver Dis 1:189, 1981
96. Lieber CS: Alcohol-nutrition interaction—1984 update. Alcoholism 1:151, 1984
97. Lieber CS, Schmid R: The effect of ethanol on fatty acid metabolism; stimulation of hepatic fatty acid synthesis in vitro. J Clin Invest 40:394, 1961
98. Lieber CS, Spritz N: Effects of prolonged ethanol intake in man: Role of dietary, adipose, and endogenously synthesized fatty acids in the pathogenesis of the alcoholic fatty liver. J Clin Invest 45:1400, 1966
99. Lieber CS et al: Effects of prolonged ethanol intake: Production of fatty liver despite adequate diets. J Clin Invest 44:1009, 1965

100. Lieber CS et al: Effect of ethanol on plasma free fatty acids in man. J Lab Clin Med 59:826, 1962

101. Lieber CS et al: Difference in hepatic metabolism of long and medium chain fatty acids. J Clin Invest 146:1451, 1967

102. Lockwood DH et al: Effect of oral amino acid supplementation on liver disease after jejunoileal bypass for morbid obesity. Am J Clin Nutr 30:58, 1977

103. Lucas CL, Ridout JH: Fatty liver and lipotropic phenomena. Prog Chem Fats Other Lipids 10:1, 1967

104. Lynch MJC et al: Fat embolism in chronic alcoholism. Arch Pathol 67:68, 1959

105. Mahley RW, Innerarity TL: Lipoprotein receptors and cholesterol homeostasis. Biochim Biophys Acta 737:197, 1983

106. Maini P et al: Cyclic hyperalimentation: An optimal technique for preservation of visceral protein. J Surg Res 20:515, 1976

107. Manes JL et al: Relationship between hepatic morphology and clinical and biochemical findings in morbidly obese patients. J Clin Pathol 26:776, 1973

108. Marchetti M et al: Metabolic aspects of orotic acid fatty liver: Nucleotide control mechanisms of lipid metabolism. Biochem J 92:46, 1964

109. Marubio A, Buchwald H, Schwartz MZ et al: Hepatic lesions of central protocellular fibrosis in morbid obesity and after jejunoileal bypass. Am J Clin Pathol 66:684, 1976

110. Massarat S et al: Five-year follow up study of patients with non-alcoholic and non-diabetic fatty liver. Acta Hepatogastroenterol 21:176, 1976

111. McDonald I et al: Liver depot and serum lipids during early recovery from kwashiorkor. Clin Sci 24:55, 1963

112. McLaren DS et al: Protein calorie malnutrition and the liver. Prog Liver Dis 4:527, 1972

113. McLaren DS et al: The liver during recovery from protein calorie malnutrition. J Trop Med Hyg 71:271, 1978

114. Mezey E: Metabolic effects of ethanol. Fed Proc 44:134, 1985

115. Miyai K et al: Effects of glucose on the subcellular structure of the rat liver cells in acute ethionine intoxication. Lab Invest 23:268, 1970

116. Morgan NY, Sherlock S, Scheuer PJ: Acute cholestasis, hepatic failure, and fatty liver in the alcoholic. Scand J Gastroenterol 313:299, 1978

117. Mouto AS: The liver in ulcerative colitis of the intestinal tract: Functional and anatomic changes. Ann Intern Med 50:1385, 1959

118. Moxley RT et al: Protein nutrition and liver disease after jejunoileal bypass for morbid obesity. N Engl J Med 290:921, 1974

119. Newsholme EA: Role of the liver in integration of fat and carbohydrate metabolism and clinical implications in patients with liver disease. In Popper H, Schaffner F (eds): Progress in Liver Disease, vol V, pp 125–135. New York, Grune & Stratton, 1976

120. Nikkila EA, Ojala K: Role of hepatic L-α glycerophosphate and triglyceride synthesis in production of fatty liver by ethanol. Proc Soc Exp Biol Med 113:814, 1963

121. Norkin SA, Compagna-Pinto D: Cytoplasmic hyaline inclusions in hepatoma. Arch Pathol 86:25, 1968

122. Novikoff PM et al: Production and prevention of fatty liver in rats fed clofibrate and orotic acid diets containing sucrose. Lab Invest 30:732, 1974

123. Novikoff PM: Intracellular organelles and lipoprotein metabolism in normal and fatty livers. In Arias IM, Popper H, Schacter D et al (eds): The Liver: Biology and Pathobiology, pp 143–167. New York, Raven Press,1982

124. O'Leary JP et al: Pathogenesis of hepatic failure following jejunoileal bypass. Gastroenterology 66:859, 1974

125. Olivecrona T, Hernall O, Johnson O et al: Effect of ethanol on some enzymes inducible by free refeeding. J Stud Alcohol 33:1, 1972

126. Perrillo RP et al: Alcoholic liver disease presenting with marked elevation of serum alkaline phosphatase. Am J Dig Dis 23:1061, 1978

127. Peters RL: Hepatic morphologic changes after jejunoileal bypass. Prog Liver Dis 6:581, 1979

128. Peters RL, Edmondson HA, Mikkelsen WP et al: Tetracycline-induced fatty liver in nonpregnant patients: A report of six cases. Am J Surg 113:622, 1967

129. Peters RL et al: Postjejunal bypass hepatic disease: Its similarity to alcoholic hepatic disease. Am J Clin Pathol 63:318, 1975

130. Phillips GB: Acute hepatic insufficiency of the chronic alcoholic—revisited. Am J Med 75:1, 1983

131. Pie P et al: Fatty metamorphosis of the liver following small intestinal bypass for obesity. Arch Pathol Lab Med 101:411, 1977

132. Popper H, Thung SN, Gerber MA: Pathology of alcoholic liver disease. Semin Liver Dis 1:203, 1981

133. Porta EA: Nutrition and diseases of the liver and gallbladder. Prog Food Nutr Sci 1:289, 1975

134. Pottenger LA et al: Serum lipoprotein accumulation in the livers of orotic acid-fed rats. J Lipid Res 12:450, 1971

135. Pottenger LA et al: Carbohydrate composition of lipoprotein apoproteins isolated from rat plasma and from livers of rats fed orotic acid. Biochem Biophys Res Commun 54:770, 1973

136. Poupon R, Rosensztajn C, de Saint-Maur RD et al: Perhexilene maleate–associated hepatic injury: prevalence and characteristics. Digestion 20:145, 1980

137. Quarfordt SH, Goodman DeWS: Metabolism of doubly-labelled chylomicron cholesteryl esters in rat. J Lipid Res 8:264, 1967

138. Ragland JB et al: The role of LCAT defiency in the apoprotein metabolism of alcoholic hepatitis. Scand J Clin Lab Invest 38:208, 1978

139. Ragland JB et al: Identification of nascent high density lipoprotein containing arginine-rich protein in human plasma. Biochem Biophys Res Commun 80:81, 1978

140. Randall B: Sudden death and hepatic fatty metamorphosis. JAMA 293:1723, 1980

141. Reboucas G, Isselbacher JJ: Studies on pathogenesis of ethanol-induced fatty liver: I. Synthesis and oxidation of fatty acids by liver. J Clin Invest 40:1355, 1961

142. Recknagel RO: Carbon tetrachloride hepatotoxicity. Pharm Rev 19:145, 1967

143. Recknagel RO et al: Lipoperoxidation as a vector in carbon tetrachloride hepatotoxicity. Lab Invest 15:132, 1966

144. Reinberg MH, Lipson M: The association of Laennec's cirrhosis with diabetes mellitus. Ann Intern Med 33:1195, 1950

145. Renold AR et al: Metabolism of isolated adipose tissue, a summary. In Renold AE, Cahill GR Jr (eds): Adipose Tissue, Handbook of Physiology, section 5, p 483. Baltimore, Williams & Wilkins, 1965

146. Riely CA: Acute fatty liver of pregnancy–1984. Dig Dis Sci 29:456, 1984

147. Robinson DS et al: The development in the rat of fatty

livers associated with reduced plasma-lipoprotein synthesis. Biochim Biophys Acta 62:163, 1962

148. Roheim PS et al: Alterations of lipoprotein metabolism in orotic acid-induced fatty liver. Lab Invest 15:21, 1966

149. Rossiter P, Slater TF: The effects of antioxidants on the concentrations of reduced and oxidized nicotinamide-adenine dinucleotide and of triglyceride in rat liver after the administration of ethanol. Biochem Soc Trans 1:933, 1973

150. Rubin E, Lieber CS: Early fine structural changes in the human liver induced by alcohol. Gastroenterology 52:1, 1967

151. Sabesin SM: Effects of acetoxycycloheximide on the metabolism of hepatic triglycerides in the rat. Exp Mol Pathol 25:227, 1976

152. Sabesin SM: Lipid and lipoprotein abnormalities in alcoholic liver disease. Circulation 64:(III):72, 1981

153. Sabesin SM: Editorial: Microtubules: Biological machines at the molecular level. Gastroenterology 81:810, 1981

154. Sabesin SM et al: Lipoprotein metabolism in liver disease. In Stollerman C (ed): Advances in Internal Medicine, vol 25, pp 117–146. Chicago, Year Book Medical Publishers, 1980

155. Sabesin SM et al: Accumulation of nascent lipoproteins in rat hepatic Golgi during induction of fatty liver by orotic acid. Lab Invest 37:127, 1977

156. Sabesin SM et al: Lipoprotein disturbances in liver disease. In Popper H, Schaffner F (eds): Progress in Liver Diseases, vol VI, pp 243–262. New York, Grune & Stratton, 1979

157. Sabesin SM et al: Electron microscopic studies of the assembly, intracellular transport and secretion of chylomicrons by rat intestine. J Lipid Res 18:496, 1977

158. Sabesin SM et al: Biogenesis of rat hepatocyte Golgi during the induction of lipoprotein secretion by sucrose feeding. Gastroenterology 75:985, 1978

159. Sabesin SM et al: D-Galactosamine hepatotoxicity: IV. Further studies of the pathogenesis of fatty liver. Exp Mol Pathol 24:424, 1976

160. Sabesin SM et al: D-Galactosamine hepatotoxicity: V. Role of free fatty acids in the pathogenesis of fatty liver. Exp Mol Pathol 29:82, 1978

161. Salmon PA, Reedy KL: Fatty metamorphosis in patients with jejunoileal bypass. Surg Gynecol Obstet 141:75, 1975

162. Scanu AM, Edelstein C, Gordon JI: Apolipoproteins of human plasma high density lipoproteins: Biology, biochemistry and clinical significance. Clin Physiol Biochem 2:111, 1984

163. Schapiro RH et al: Effect of prolonged ethanol ingestion on the transport and metabolism of lipids in man. N Engl J Med 272:610, 1965

164. Scheig R, Isselbacher KHJ: Pathogenesis of ethanol-induced fatty liver: III. In vivo and in vitro effects of ethanol on hepatic fatty acid metabolism in rat. J Lipid Res 6:269, 1965

165. Seichy FJ, Balistreri WF, Buchino JJ et al: Acute hepatic failure associated with the use of sodium valproate. N Engl J Med 300:962, 1979

166. Shapiro B: Lipid metabolism. Ann Rev Biochem 36:247, 1967

167. Sheldon GF, Peterson SR, Sanders R: Hepatic dysfunction during hyperalimentation. Arch Surg 113:504, 1978

168. Sidransky H, Verney E: Chronic fatty liver without cirrhosis induced in the rat by dietary orotic acid. Am J Pathol 46:1007, 1965

169. Sim JS, Franks KE, French SW: Comparative electrophoretic study of Mallory body and intermediate filament protein. J Med 9:211, 1978

170. Smetana HG et al: Infantile cirrhosis: An analytical review of the literature and a report of 50 cases. Pediatrics 28:107, 1961

171. Soffer LJ et al: Cushing's syndrome, a study of 50 patients. Am J Med 30:129, 1961

172. Spitzer JJ, McElroy WT Jr: Some hormonal effects on uptake of free fatty acids by the liver. Am J Physiol 199:876, 1960

173. Stanley RJ et al: Computer tomography of the liver. Radiol Clin North Am 5:331, 1978

174. Stein O et al: Colchicine-induced inhibition of lipoprotein and protein secretion into the serum and lack of interference with secretion of biliary phospholipids and cholesterol by rat liver in vivo. J Cell Biol 62:90, 1974

175. Steinberg D, Vaughan M: Release of free fatty acids from adipose tissue in vitro in relation to rates of triglyceride synthesis and degration. In American Physiologic Society: Adipose Tissue, Handbook of Physiology, vol 5, p 335. Baltimore, Williams & Wilkins, 1965.

176. Sternlieb I: Mitochondrial and fatty change in hepatocytes of patients with Wilson's disease. Gastroenterology 55:354, 1980

177. Szilagyi A, Le Compte P, Goosens J et al: Comparison of liver injury and alcoholism and post jejunoileal bypass surgery. In Bank PD, Chalmers TC (eds): Frontiers in Liver Disease, pp 156–166. New York, Thieme-Stratton, 1981

178. Takac A et al: Leberverfettung bei diabetes mellitus. Michen Med Wochenschr 107:1148, 1965

179. Vander Hoof JA, Tuma DJ, Sorrell MF: Role of defunctionalized bowel in jejunoileal bypass–induced liver disease in rats. Dig Dis Sci 24:916, 1979

180. Van Waes L, Lieber C: Early perivenular sclerosis in alcoholic fatty liver: An index of progressive liver injury. Gastroenterology 73:646, 1977

181. Verbin RS et al: The biochemical pathology of inhibition of protein synthesis in vivo. Lab Invest 20:529, 1969

182. Von Oettingen WF: The Halogenated Hydrocarbons of Industrial and Toxicological Importance, p 107. Amsterdam, Elsevier, 1964

183. Waterlow JC, Alleyne GAD: Protein malnutrition in children: Advances in knowledge in the last 10 years. Adv Protein Chem 25:117, 1971

184. Webber BL, Freiman L: The liver in kwashiorkor. Arch Pathol 98:400, 1974

185. Weidman SW, Ragland JB, Sabesin SM: Plasma lipoprotein composition in alcoholic hepatitis: Accumulation of apolipoprotein E–rich high density lipoprotein and preferential reappearance of HDL$_2$ during recovery. J Lipid Res 23:556, 1982

186. Wene JD et al: The development of essential fatty acid deficiency in healthy man fed fat-free diets intravenously and orally. J Clin Invest 56:127, 1975

187. Wetmore S et al: Incorporation of sialic acid into sialidase-treated apolipoprotein of human very low density lipoprotein by pork liver sialytransferase. Can J Biochem 52:655, 1974

188. Windmueller HG, Levy RI: Total inhibition of hepatic β-lipoprotein production in the rat by orotic acid. J Biol Chem 242:2246, 1967

189. Zannis VI, Kurmit DM, Breslow JL: Hepatic apo A-I and apo E and intestinal apo A-I are synthesized in precursor isoprotein forms by organ cultures of human fetal tissues. J Biol Chem 257:536, 1982

chapter 26
Primary Biliary Cirrhosis

SHEILA SHERLOCK

Primary biliary cirrhosis was first described in 1851 by Addison and Gull and later by Hanot.[1,52] The association with high serum cholesterol levels and skin xanthomas led to the term *xanthomatous biliary cirrhosis.* Ahrens and colleagues[2] termed the condition *primary biliary cirrhosis.* However, in the early stages, nodular regeneration in the liver is inconspicuous and the anatomic criteria needed for the diagnosis of cirrhosis are not fulfilled.[109] Recent pathologic studies make the term *chronic nonsuppurative destructive cholangitis*[101] a better one, although it is unlikely that it will replace the shorter, more popular one in use.

In this disease, the small intrahepatic bile ducts are involved in a granulomatous reaction so that they are progressively damaged and ultimately disappear. The etiology is unknown. Any answer must take into account the predilection of the disease for women, usually between 40 and 60 years of age.[106] Earlier diagnosis at an asymptomatic stage lowers the age at presentation. Any answer must also explain the association of the disease with other conditions with disturbed immunity. The regular, consistent demonstration, in high titer, of serum mitochondrial antibodies is virtually confined to three liver diseases: primary biliary cirrhosis, chronic active hepatitis, and cryptogenic cirrhosis—particularly in women.

PATHOLOGY

The liver is large and green (Fig. 26-1). At operation or laparoscopy the surface appears smooth, but, as time passes, it becomes nodular. The gallbladder and bile ducts are normal. Enlarged fleshy lymph glands in the porta hepatis and along the common bile duct often lead to a mistaken diagnosis of reticulosis. Such lymph nodes show only a reticulum cell hyperplasia with phagocytes loaded with bile pigment. The spleen shows pulp hyperplasia and the changes associated with portal hypertension.

Hepatic Histology

The disease begins with damage to the epithelium of small bile ducts and a cellular reaction, which includes lymphocytes, plasma cells, eosinophils, and histiocytes.[48,101,109] Granulomas commonly form.

As the bile ducts become destroyed, their sites are marked by aggregates of lymphoid cells and bile ductules

begin to proliferate. Fibrosis extends from the portal tracts, and there is a variable degree of piecemeal necrosis. At this stage it may be difficult to distinguish primary biliary cirrhosis from chronic active hepatitis. Helpful features suggesting the correct diagnosis include loss of bile ducts, lymphoid aggregates, ductular proliferation, granulomas, and the appearance of substantial amounts of copper and copper-associated protein.

Biliary piecemeal necrosis, characterized by vacuolated periportal hepatocytes invaded by foamy macrophages, is frequent in the later stages when large hypocellular scars are also a characteristic feature.[91]

It is useful to recognize four stages,[74,104] although the interpretation and differentiation may be difficult. The changes in the liver are focal and evolve at different speeds in different parts of the liver. The stages also overlap, and in over one half of patients more than one stage may be present at one time. It is particularly difficult to separate stages 2 and 3.[104] Stages also show a poor correlation with the clinical state. Moreover, serial liver biopsies have shown that the same stage may persist for many years.

The fibrous septa gradually come to distort the normal architecture of the liver, and regeneration nodules form. These are often irregular in distribution, and there may be an appearance of cirrhosis in one part of the biopsy and not in another. This is also diagnostically useful. In some places lobular architecture may be preserved for some periods.

Histometric and serial sections show that bile ducts with lumens below 70 μm to 80 μm mm are destroyed.[85] The smaller the ducts, the more they are destroyed.

Copper may be shown histochemically in the liver by Shikata's orcein or, preferably, by the Rhodanine method.[57] Scanning proton microprobe analysis confirms its periportal location.[124]

Stage 1: Florid Duct Lesion (Portal Hepatitis)

This is pathognomonic. Septal and larger interlobular bile ducts are damaged and surrounded by a dense infiltrate of lymphocytes, large histiocytes or epithelioid cells, plasma cells, and a few eosinophils (Fig. 26-2). Lymphoid aggregates may be found. Granulomas are usually near a damaged duct in the portal tract. They decrease as bile ducts are lost.[86] This damage is seen as swelling, proliferation and crowding of epithelial cells, and rupture.

979

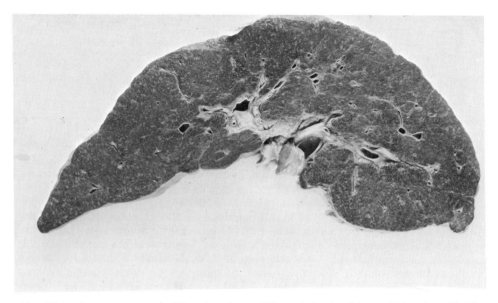

Fig. 26-1. Gross appearance of liver in primary biliary cirrhosis of 3 years' duration. Weight at autopsy is 1855 g.

Fig. 26-2. Stage 1. Primary biliary cirrhosis. The portal zone shows a damaged bile duct with a surrounding lymphocytic granulomatous reaction. This appearance is diagnostic. (H & E; original magnification × 120)

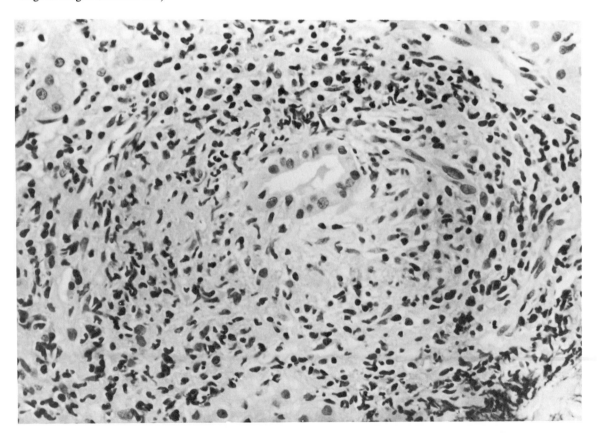

The portal tract is otherwise normal, and the limiting liver cell plates are intact. Within the lobules, there may be slight mononuclear cell infiltration and regenerative hyperplasia seen as double liver cell plates. Centrizonal cholestasis may be seen but is often absent and is rarely severe.

Stage 2: Ductular Proliferation (Periportal Hepatitis)

The lesions are now more widespread throughout the expanded portal tracts but are less specific. There is fibrosis, acute and chronic inflammatory infiltration, and ductular proliferation. Ducts are reduced and their place is taken by ill-defined lymphoid aggregates (Fig. 26-3). The appearances are often compatible with or suggestive of primary biliary cirrhosis rather than being diagnostic. Granulomas are less common.

Stage 3: Scarring (Septal Fibrosis)

Inflammation subsides and relatively acellular septa extend from the portal tracts into and around the lobules. Lymphoid aggregates are still seen and periportal cholestasis may be severe (Fig. 26-4). The appearances are not pathognomonic but can be interpreted as highly suggestive and compatible.

Stage 4: Cirrhosis

Regeneration nodules are seen, and the picture is of end-stage liver disease. The diagnosis may still be suggested by paucity of bile ducts or by accumulations of lymphocytes.

Hyaline Deposits

Hyaline inclusions, similar to those found in alcoholic disease, occur in the hepatocytes in about 25% of cases.[75] They are usually adjacent to portal tracts and connective tissue septa.

Ultrastructural Changes

Some of the changes observed in the bile ducts are also seen to a mild degree in other pathologic entities, but their prominence and progression are distinctive. They are particularly noted in the bile duct epithelium, which shows coagulative and lytic necrosis. A more specific change is the detachment of several adjoining biliary cells from the

Fig. 26-3. Stage 2. Fibrosis, ductular proliferation, and lymphoid aggregates are seen. These appearances are compatible rather than diagnostic. (H & E; original magnification × 48) (Sherlock S, Scheuer PJ: N Engl J Med 289:674, 1973)

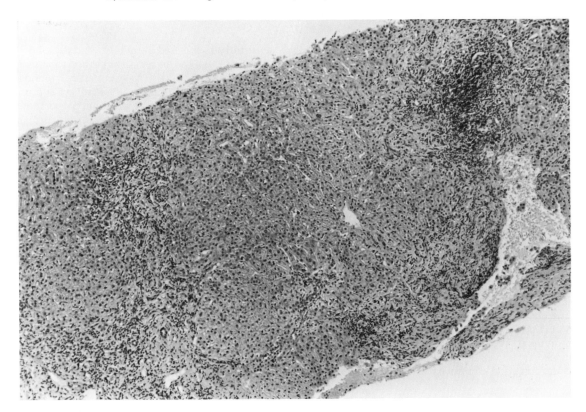

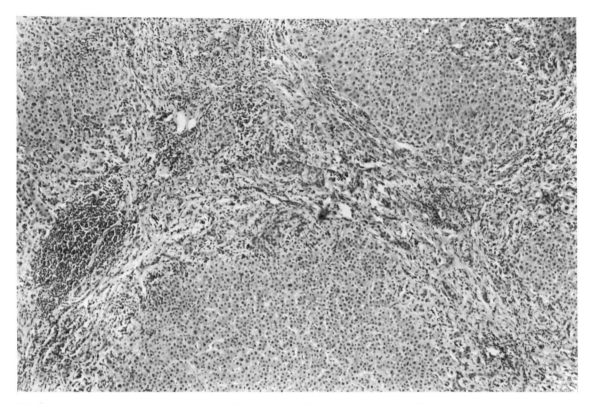

Fig. 26-4. Stage 3. Scarring and septa containing lymphoid aggregates are seen. Hyperplastic "regeneration" nodules are beginning to develop. (H & E; original magnification × 48) (Sherlock S, Scheuer PJ: N Engl J Med 289:674, 1973)

basement membrane and from neighboring biliary cells.[87] Focal cytoplasmic necrosis and apoptosis, a special form of cell death in which condensation and fragmentation of the cytoplasm and nucleus are followed by degradation of these fragments by other cells, are also found.[12] This is also a feature of graft-versus-host disease.

IMMUNOLOGIC CHANGES

The patient with primary biliary cirrhosis presents with many immunologic abnormalities—for example, depressed skin energy, granuloma formation, circulating immune complexes, complement activation, and reduction of regulator suppressor cells—so much so that it is difficult to distinguish the primary causative events from the epiphenomena. Cell-based immunity is considerably disturbed in primary biliary cirrhosis. This suggests that sensitized T cells might be the basis of the bile duct injury. The histologic reaction around injured bile ducts is predominantly monocytic with lymphocytic accumulations prominent. Well-formed granulomas are included, and, indeed, extrahepatic granulomas are found in lymph nodes, lung, and even bone marrow.[41] Granulomas suggest

disturbed cell-based immunity. Skin tests show that many patients with primary biliary cirrhosis are anergic.[41] Phytohemagglutinin (PHA)-stimulated lymphocytes show impaired transformation in patients with primary biliary cirrhosis.[41] There is no correlation between the histologic stage of the disease and degree of impairment. Indeed, two presymptomatic patients had normal mechanisms of delayed hypersensitivity.[40] This raises the possibility that the anergy was the result rather than the cause of the disease. Similarly, abnormal cell-mediated responses in the leukocyte migration test have been found.

In a further study, the humoral and cellular immune response to hemocyanin was measured in normal subjects and in patients with primary biliary cirrhosis.[39] Positive skin tests were reduced, and a poor antibody response was also noted. Both impaired T-cell function and a poor humoral response were therefore found, and lack of T- and B-cell cooperation was postulated.

The final event seems to be an attack by cytotoxic lymphocytes on biliary epithelium. The antigen might be the individual's own human leukocyte antigens (HLA-ABC glycoproteins), which are present in high concentration on biliary epithelium. It is unclear why the reaction should be to normal rather than to foreign proteins. Perhaps the patient's own lymphoid system is at fault so that "self" and "self-antigens" are not recognized. This could be due to failure of schooling by cytotoxic T cells in the thymus. These cells are regulated by suppressor cells, which have been shown to be diminished both in number and function in primary biliary cirrhosis (Fig. 26-5).[115] Alternatively, and perhaps more likely, the HLA proteins may have become foreign due to an extrinsic environmental factor. The identification of such a factor is an ongoing challenge to all those investigating primary biliary cirrhosis. Finally, patients with primary biliary cirrhosis have diminished natural killer activity due to a functional defect of cytolytic effector cells.[60]

Class 2 antigens of the major histocompatibility complex (HLA-DR) are glycoproteins that play an important role in presenting antigens and regulating the immune response. Aberrant expression of HLA-DR antigens on bile duct epithelium in primary biliary cirrhosis may enable these cells to present self-antigen to sensitized T cells and to promote autorecognition, possibly in response to environmental triggers.[5]

There is no relationship between the various serologic autoantibody markers, and particularly between the positive mitochondrial antibody test, and the etiology of the disease. Similarly, disturbances in cell-based immunity seem to bear little relationship to severity. Studies of a daughter who was symptomatic and a mother with primary biliary cirrhosis who was not showed strikingly similar immunologic changes.[120]

Immune Complexes

The bile duct destruction may be mediated via immune complex formation. The sera of most patients with primary biliary cirrhosis show immune complexes.[128] The large complexes may fix complement and be responsible for tissue damage. Large complexes of this type, when injected into animals, result in granuloma formation. It has been more difficult to demonstrate immune complexes in the liver parenchyma.

In primary biliary cirrhosis, C3 is probably activated by the classic pathway, since the catabolism of C1q (a component exclusive to the classic pathway) is five times greater than normal, but neither normal or slightly increased in other forms of chronic liver disease.[63,69,92] The immune complexes are probably produced in the walls of bile ductules or surrounding tissue—a reaction in many ways analogous to an Arthus reaction. An antigen absorbed through the bile may combine with antibody derived from the portal circulation and result in formation of complexes in the bile ductule wall and interstitial space of the portal tracts.[116] A spillover of complexes into the systemic circulation is incidental to the primary pathogenetic process but may explain the association of primary biliary cirrhosis with extrahepatic conditions such as arthritis, vasculitis, and glomerulonephritis. Such immune complexes might also contribute to the state of anergy.

Although this hypothesis describes a possible mechanism of bile duct damage and granuloma formation in primary biliary cirrhosis, the antigen involved and the way in which it enters the tissues of the portal zones of the liver are unknown.

Fig. 26-5. Evidence for defective immunoregulation in primary biliary cirrhosis. T suppressor (*Ts*) cells are reduced, allowing cytotoxic T cells (*Tc*) and B cells (*B*) to effect immunologic bile duct damage. TH, T-helper cells.

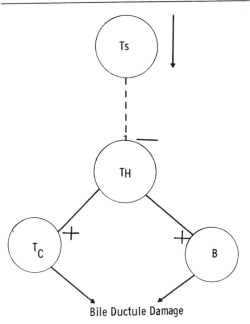

PBC - EVIDENCE FOR DEFECTIVE IMMUNOREGULATION

Primary Biliary Cirrhosis as Chronic Graft-Versus-Host Disease

Primary biliary cirrhosis is part of a disease complex characterized by dry eyes, dry mouth,[45] and both biliary and pancreatic hyposecretion.[29] It is a "dry gland syndrome," resulting from damage to ductular epithelium.[29] Identical ductular and extraductular features, including abnormalities of the immune system, are seen in chronic graft-versus-host disease after bone marrow transplantation. In primary biliary cirrhosis, ductular lesions and severe disturbance of the immune system, including macroglobulinemia and immune complex formation, might result from an immune response to the histocompatibility (HC) complex antigens present in high density on ductular epithelial cells of the biliary tree.[29] This response could be caused by altered antigenicity of epithelial cell HC antigen or by failure of the HLA-dependent T cell.[60]

The decrease in the ratio of inducer (helper) to suppressor T cells in the peripheral blood[99] is similar to that described in chronic-graft-versus host disease.

ROLE OF COPPER

Approximately 80% of absorbed copper is normally excreted in the bile. It is not surprising, therefore, that hepatic copper concentrations increase in cholestasis. In primary biliary cirrhosis, hepatic copper levels can reach those found in Wilson's disease. However, it is doubtful whether the copper retention is injurious to the liver cell.[33] Copper concentration does not correlate with the hepatocyte damage. Electron microscopy shows the copper to be contained in lysosomes, and the characteristic organelle changes associated with copper toxicity in Wilson's disease are not observed. In primary biliary cirrhosis the copper is probably retained within the hepatocyte in a nontoxic form.

GENETIC AND EPIDEMIOLOGIC ASPECTS

Familial instances of primary biliary cirrhosis are recorded. Two sisters have been reported, one of whom had fairly typical disease and the other a picture very suggestive of primary biliary cirrhosis.[126] Both had high titers of serologic mitochondrial antibodies. Other instances, in brothers and in twin sisters are noted.[19] In one family, four sisters of six suffered from primary biliary cirrhosis.[61] Their father may also have suffered. The sisters' children showed raised immunoglobulin levels without signs of any disease.

The possible familial nature is emphasized by surveys of serum autoimmune tests in family members of sufferers. Feizi and co-workers noted a significant increase in mitochondrial antibodies among the relatives of 26 patients with primary biliary cirrhosis.[37] In a larger study, 260 family members of sufferers from chronic active hepatitis or primary biliary cirrhosis were studied. Mitochondrial and smooth muscle antibodies were much more frequent than in controls matched for age and sex.[43] Surprisingly, the prevalence of positive mitochondrial antibody tests was not greater in the primary biliary cirrhosis relatives than in those with chronic active hepatitis. Seven to 8% of symptomless relatives of patients with primary biliary cirrhosis showed a positive mitochondrial antibody test, which is 10% more than that found in the general population. The reason for this familial incidence is uncertain. Equally unsure is the trigger that leads to clinically overt primary biliary cirrhosis in some but not all of these susceptible family members. Some factor or factors presumably sensitize the biliary epithelium to injury.

There is no excess of any particular ABO blood group, or HLA-ABC antigen.[7,51]

The disease has been reported from all parts of the world. Chinese, Europeans, Indians, Jews, and blacks are among those affected. The death rates from primary biliary cirrhosis in various countries are difficult to assess but are probably of the order of 0.6% to 2% of those dying with cirrhosis.[50] In an epidemiologic study conducted in England, it was concluded that primary biliary cirrhosis predominantly affects middle-aged women of social classes 1 and 2, living in an urban situation.[50] There is an undoubted sampling error in such studies. Further detailed epidemiologic surveys are essential in different parts of the world.

Environmental factors are suggested by a report of the disease in a daughter, her mother, and a related close friend who nursed the daughter in her terminal illness.[28] In a 3-year study (1977–1979) of primary biliary cirrhosis in Sheffield, England, 90% of patients came from an area that had only 4% of the population and one particular reservoir.[120] No one has so far matched this experience, and an environmental factor in the water supply could not be identified.

CLINICAL FEATURES

Criteria for Diagnosis

Clinically, primary biliary cirrhosis is a disease of middle-aged women who present with a slow onset of cholestasis.[107] The serum mitochondrial antibody test is positive. Needle liver biopsy histology shows small bile duct destruction, which is diagnostic, or features that are compatible with the diagnosis. The main bile ducts have to be shown to be patent by some form of cholangiography. Additional presence of diseases known to be associated with primary biliary cirrhosis may add diagnostic weight. This description is of the "ideal" case. In practice, of course, all these criteria may not be met.

Presentation

In the past, the patient presented at a late, icteric stage. One or more laparotomies had usually been performed to exclude surgical jaundice. Now, the disease can usually be recognized earlier and without surgery. In a series published in 1959,[106] 20% of the patients diagnosed were anicteric. This proportion had risen to 41% by 1973. By 1985, 36 patients could be diagnosed at a stage when they were asymptomatic.[13] Clinical features, histology, and biochemistry are in general similar in males and females.[100]

About 90% of the patients are female,[109] but male sex should not exclude the diagnosis. Nevertheless, more detailed investigations are necessary. The main bile ducts, in particular, must be shown to be patent before a diagnosis of primary biliary cirrhosis in males, compared with females, is made. The reason for the sex preference is unknown. The disease usually presents between the ages of 40 and 60 but has been diagnosed at the age of 23 in an asymptomatic patient,[71] and even up to the age of 72.[109]

The usual onset is as insidious, diffuse pruritus. It is enhanced by warm weather, or at night, or by wearing coarse, woolen underwear. This symptom usually brings the patient to her physician and often to the dermatologist. Unless the medical attendant is alert to the possibility of primary biliary cirrhosis, many months of local skin treatment can ensue before the underlying cholestasis is recognized.

The pruritus may appear during pregnancy, especially during the last trimester. Primary biliary cirrhosis may be confused with cholestatic jaundice of the last trimester. In contrast to that condition, however, the pruritus usually persists after the patient gives birth. Occasionally, the itching of primary biliary cirrhosis disappears after delivery only to return months or years later. Similarly, the pruritus of primary biliary cirrhosis may become manifest when the asymptomatic patient is given birth control pills containing cholestatic hormones.

Jaundice may appear at the same time as the pruritus but very rarely antedates it. The jaundice usually appears 6 months to 2 years after the itching, but delays of 10 to 20 years can occur. The jaundice is rarely deep at presentation. It is cholestatic in type with darkening of the urine and pallor of the stools. Jaundice without itching is very rare.

Although bleeding from esophageal varices has been reported as an initial complaint,[130] it is rare.[66] Portal hypertension develops as the disease advances.

Primary biliary cirrhosis may be diagnosed when the patient is under investigation for another condition known to be associated with it, such as rheumatoid arthritis, sclerodactyly, dermatomyositis, keratoconjunctivitis sicca, familial hyperparathyroidism, pernicious anemia, or telangiectasia.[71] Such patients tend to be younger than those diagnosed when symptomatic. The increasing use of biochemical screening procedures that include serum alkaline phosphatase values allows more patients to be diagnosed at an early stage. Any elevation of such values in a middle-aged woman should always raise the suspicion of primary biliary cirrhosis. Confirmation that the raised alkaline phosphatase is of hepatic origin is done either by isoenzyme techniques or by showing a raised serum γ-glutamyl transpeptidase value. Routine screening for serum autoantibodies and the finding of a positive mitochondrial antibody may be another mode of presentation.

The patient is usually pigmented (Fig. 26-6). The liver is variably enlarged and nontender, and the edge has a firm consistency. The spleen is usually enlarged. Xanthomas are never marked at presentation and, if present, are usually seen only as xanthelasma (Fig. 26-7).

Associated Diseases

In one series, 69% of 47 patients had a nonhepatic association.[44] The most common was with the collagen diseases. Articular symptoms were found in 4% of one series[44] and rheumatoid arthritis in 5% of 100 patients in another.[109] In general, the severity of the arthritic symptoms is the inverse of that of the primary biliary cirrhosis.[18] Serologic tests for rheumatoid factor are positive. Circulating immune complexes may be involved in the development of the arthritis.[24]

Primary biliary cirrhosis may be found described with scleroderma.[102] Later, the association of the whole CRST

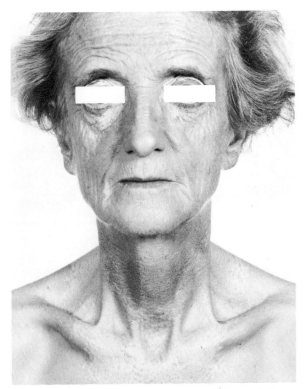

Fig. 26-6. Elderly pigmented woman with xanthelasma around eyes and xanthomas in necklace area.

syndrome (calcinosis cutis, Raynaud's phenomenon, sclerodactyly, and telangiectasia) was noted.[96] The telangiectasia is on finger pads and lips, and occasionally on the mucosa of the upper gastrointestinal tract. Concomitant polymyositis has also been noted.[122] The association of CRST syndrome with primary biliary cirrhosis was noted in 3 of 100 patients[109]; conversely, primary biliary cirrhosis was found in 11 of 29 patients with CRST.[67] The underlying hepatic disease is more likely to determine the prognosis than is the scleroderma. Such patients usually have a nuclear centromere antibody.[76]

Associated skin lesions include immune complex capillaritis and lichen planus, which is also a feature of graft-versus-host disease.[47]

The sicca complex of dry eyes and mouth, with or without the arthritis completing the Sjögren syndrome, is found in about 75% of patients with primary biliary cirrhosis.[45] Specimens of salivary gland may show appearances similar to those seen in hepatic ducts.[82] Investigations of this sicca component of the Sjögren syndrome show abnormalities that do not correlate with the duration or degree of liver disease, presence of autoantibodies, or serum immunoglobulin levels.

Steatorrhea may be related to pancreatic hyposecretion and to lack of bile or bile salts in the intestine.[30,98]

Autoimmune thyroiditis also correlates significantly

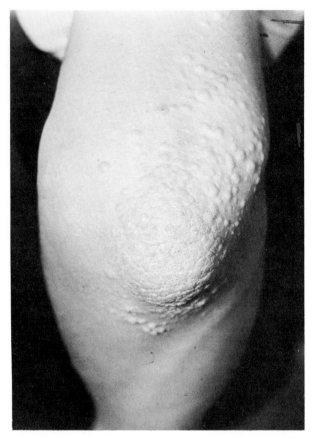

Fig. 26-7. Elbows showing tuberous xanthomas.

with lacrimal gland dysfunction.[23] Systemic lupus erythematosus may be associated.[49]

Renal tubular acidosis is attributed to copper deposits in the distal renal tubule.[90] Hypouricemia and hyperuricosuria are further expressions of renal tubular damage.[56] Bacteriuria develops in 35% of patients and may be asymptomatic.[17] It is unexplained, but it has been postulated that urinary organisms might be invoked in the pathogenesis of the primary biliary cirrhosis. Circulating antibodies to the loop of Henle have been seen in one patient. IgM-associated membranous glomerulonephritis has been reported.[93] Finger clubbing is common, and occasionally there is hypertrophic osteoarthropathy.[31]

Primary biliary cirrhosis and jejunal villous atrophy resembling celiac disease have been reported in five cases.[55,70]

There may be an increased incidence of breast cancer.[46,129]

Biochemical Changes

Serum bilirubin values are rarely very high at the outset; in about one half of patients, they are less than 2 mg/dl. The serum alkaline phosphatase value is always markedly raised. The serum bilirubin levels may fluctuate and may be within normal limits for many months. The serum alkaline phosphatase level, however, continues elevated. Asymptomatic patients may have normal or only minimally raised alkaline phosphatase, cholesterol, and aspartate transaminase levels, while the serum bilirubin level may be normal.[71]

Serum bile acid levels may be a more sensitive index of cholestasis than the serum alkaline phosphatases.[96]

The total serum cholesterol concentration increases, but not constantly, and is an unreliable diagnostic test. The total serum lipids are greatly increased, and this particularly involves the phospholipid and total cholesterol fractions. Neutral fat is very slightly increased. The serum is characteristically clear and not milky.

The serum albumin level is usually normal at presentation, and the total serum globulin may be moderately increased. Serum lipoproteins are increased owing to a rise in the low-density (α_2,β) fraction. The high-density lipoproteins are decreased. The increase consists largely of an abnormal lipoprotein containing a high proportion of unesterified cholesterol and phospholipid called lipoprotein X.

Serum lipoprotein X is usually found in patients with primary biliary cirrhosis in the icteric stage.

Serum IgM is usually raised, often to very high values.[36] The estimation has even been suggested for diagnosis.[14] However, in about 25% of patients, values do not exceed the upper limit of 1.95 g/liter (195 mg/dl).[109] Serum IgM levels can in no sense be regarded as reliable for diagnosis of primary biliary cirrhosis. However, increased values are found in 84% of asymptomatic cases so that high values in the presence of slightly raised serum bilirubin levels are supporting evidence for the diagnosis.

Hematologic Changes

In general hematologic changes are noncontributory. The erythrocyte sedimentation rate is usually markedly increased. The erythrocytes show reduced osmotic fragility. Target cells have been related to an accumulation of cholesterol in the erythrocyte membrane. Macrocytosis and folate deficiency may suggest associated jejunal villous atrophy. Thrombocytopenia is related to hypersplenism and occasionally to immunologic injury by platelet-associated immunoglobulins.[6]

MITOCHONDRIAL ANTIBODIES

In 1965, it was recognized that patients with primary biliary cirrhosis had in their serum an antibody against mitochondria.[125] This was shown by granular fluorescence in an immunofluorescent technique on tissue sections. The staining reactions were neither organ nor species specific.

The antigen is a component of the mitochondrial inner membrane.[10] It is a lipoprotein and has been purified.[9] This has led to a radioimmunoassay for diagnosis, although it is not generally available.[77] An enzyme-linked immunosorbent assay has also been developed.[65] Mitochondrial antibodies are not confined to primary biliary cirrhosis, being detected in 30% of patients with chronic active hepatitis (HbsAg negative) and 3% of those with connective tissue disease. They are absent in patients with mechanical obstruction to the bile ducts and in primary sclerosing cholangitis.

The mitochondrial antigens are heterogeneous.[8] The ATPase-associated antigen in the inner mitochondrial membrane is termed M2, and a positive immunoassay for this may be specific for primary biliary cirrhosis.[11] A further antigen found on the outer mitochondrial membrane and termed M4 is associated with chronic active hepatitis, granulomas, and bile duct proliferation and must be distinguished from that found with classic primary biliary cirrhosis. Yet another antigen also found on the outer mitochondrial membrane is termed M9 and has been found in increased numbers over controls, not only in sufferers from primary biliary cirrhosis but also in their spouses and in technicians handling blood from patients with primary biliary cirrhosis. M9 may be found in presymptomatic patients and is a good prognostic index.

The etiologic importance of the antibody is unknown but is probably slight, for it is not related either to the stage of the disease or to other immunologic phenomena.[41] It is possibly related to a cross-reaction with an unknown microorganism whose primitive enzyme systems resemble those of mitochondria. The test is positive in over 96% of patients with primary biliary cirrhosis.[27,67,83] It is negative in mechanical obstruction to bile ducts, however prolonged (Fig. 26-8).

The practical diagnostic importance of the mitochondrial antibody test is twofold. In a patient with cholestasis, a negative result always arouses suspicion that primary biliary cirrhosis is not the correct diagnosis. Second, a positive result in an icteric patient throws considerable doubt that the jaundice is due to a mechanical block to main bile passages.

Fig. 26-8. Percentage of positive serum mitochondrial antibodies in primary biliary cirrhosis and other diseases.

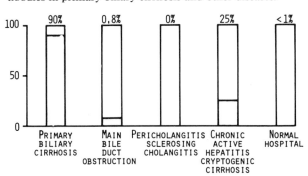

CHOLANGIOGRAPHY

If the diagnosis is in doubt, particularly in a male with a negative serum mitochondrial antibody, the main bile ducts should be demonstrated to be patent. In the anicteric or mildly jaundiced, the intravenous cholangiographic perfusion technique is often successful. In the more deeply jaundiced, endoscopic retrograde cholangiography or percutaneous cholangiography is required.

Endoscopic Retrograde Cholangiography

If the endoscope head is used as a standard of reference, the approximate maximum and minimum size of the main bile ducts can be assessed. The calibers of the common bile duct, right hepatic duct, and left hepatic duct do not differ from those observed in control subjects.[114] However, differences from control subjects may be seen in the main intrahepatic bile ducts that are irregular in caliber and run a tortuous course. These duct irregularities correlate well with histologically proven biliary cirrhosis.[114] Narrowing and tortuosity indicate that cirrhosis has developed. A filling defect in the common bile duct at the hilum indicates enlarged lymph glands.

Endoscopic retrograde cholangiography is also useful in diagnosing gallstones and in defining their location, whether in gallbladder or common bile duct. The high incidence of gallstones in patients with primary biliary cirrhosis is discussed later.

Percutaneous Cholangiography

This technique frequently succeeds in the patient with primary biliary cirrhosis who has nondilated ducts in the liver. It is less costly and technically easier than endoscopic retrograde cholangiography. It is playing an increasing role in establishing patent bile ducts in patients with primary biliary cirrhosis.

Scanning Procedures

Ultrasound or computed tomography may be used. Such techniques can demonstrate dilated intrahepatic ducts and thus diagnose obstruction to main bile ducts and exclude the diagnosis of primary biliary cirrhosis.

The Place of Laparotomy

With the advent of endoscopic and percutaneous cholangiography and more widespread availability of the mitochondrial antibody test, laparotomy with biopsy and cholangiography is rarely needed for the diagnosis of primary biliary cirrhosis. Indications include early deep jaundice and persistent pain and fever. Primary biliary cirrhosis in the presence of a negative mitochondrial antibody test always demands visualization of the bile ducts, and if this is impossible by endoscopic or percutaneous cholangiography, laparotomy may be needed.

GALLSTONES

In one series of 23 patients with primary biliary cirrhosis studied by endoscopic cholangiography, 39% had gallstones in the gallbladder but not in the common bile duct.[114] Cirrhotic patients are known to have an increased frequency of gallstone formation. In one autopsy study, 29.4% of all cirrhotics and 30.8% (4 of 13) of patients with primary biliary cirrhosis had gallstones, compared with 12.8% of the noncirrhotic population.[15] In contrast to the findings in noncirrhotic patients, most of the gallstones were of pigment type. Analysis of the last 21 autopsies on patients with primary biliary cirrhosis at the Royal Free Hospital showed that eight of 21 (38%) had gallstones.[114]

The decision whether to recommend surgical exploration in patients with primary biliary cirrhosis who also have gallstones is extremely difficult. If the gallstones are asymptomatic, and in the gallbladder, they are best left alone. If they are in the common bile duct, surgical intervention or endoscopic papillotomy is probably indicated. If the gallstones in the gallbladder are producing symptoms, the decision is particularly difficult. Patients with underlying chronic liver disease, even if it is only primary biliary cirrhosis, tolerate surgery poorly. In the presence of primary biliary cirrhosis, liver histology obtained by needle biopsy is not particularly helpful in making the distinction between gallstone obstruction and primary biliary cirrhosis. Indeed, liver biopsy may confuse the decision as to whether gallstones are, or are not, causing biliary obstruction. Each case has to be decided on its merits, and great clinical experience is needed for the decision making.

NEEDLE LIVER BIOPSY

The only hepatic lesion pathognomonic of primary biliary cirrhosis is the injured septal or interlobular bile duct. Such ducts are not often seen in sections of liver obtained by needle biopsy. Histopathologic diagnosis of primary biliary cirrhosis is more confident with operative biopsies than with needle ones. Yet the number of such specimens is decreasing, with the use of cholangiography for demonstration of main bile ducts and hence fewer laparotomies. Great importance is being placed in the reading of the needle biopsy section and the experience of the histopathologist.[104] Local, portal zone lymphocyte accumulations with a "biliary-type" of fibrosis and peripheral cholestasis are very suggestive of primary biliary cirrhosis. The distinction between diagnostic changes (*i.e.,* destructive lesions of larger bile ducts) and compatible ones is very helpful. The report of a compatible histology can be slotted into place with the clinical, biochemical, and immunologic findings to provide a diagnostic whole.

The florid lesion of stage 1 must be distinguished from the peribiliary infiltration of longstanding large duct obstruction in which duct damage is generally absent and granulomas are rare. In the pericholangitis associated with ulcerative colitis, the ducts are not destroyed, granulomas are absent, and the infiltrate is predominantly lymphocytic with few or no plasma cells. Piecemeal necrosis in the later stages may make it difficult to distinguish between primary biliary cirrhosis and chronic active hepatitis, and there are mixed forms. Features favoring primary biliary cirrhosis include intact lobules, slight piecemeal necrosis, periseptal cholestasis, lymphoid aggregates, and irregular fibrosis. Bile ducts are absent, and arteries exceed bile ducts. When cirrhosis has developed and clinical features are atypical, cryptogenic cirrhosis may be wrongly diagnosed.

PORTAL HYPERTENSION

Bleeding from esophageal varices is generally believed to be a late feature of primary biliary cirrhosis. This is not always so, and presentation as bleeding varices was noted in 15 of 23 patients in one series.[130] These patients, however, were highly selected, being referred to a surgeon for possible relief of portal hypertension. Nevertheless, if portal hypertension is sought, it is frequently demonstrated even quite early in the course. In one series of 109 patients, 50 showed esophageal varices radiologically.[66]

In only 4 patients of 50 with varices was bleeding the initial manifestation of disease. In another 17, however, it was recognized within 2 years of the first symptom. The presence of bleeding varices considerably worsens the prognosis, particularly when ascites is an associated factor.

In general, portal hypertension is related to nodular regeneration in the liver and to cirrhosis. Nodules are late features of primary biliary cirrhosis and, in fact, the portal hypertension frequently antedates nodule formation.[66,130] The mechanism of the early portal hypertension in these patients is therefore difficult to understand. It could be related to obstruction to portal venous flow by portal tract lesions and hence be at a presinusoidal level.[130] However, marked or moderate portal fibrosis is not more common in patients with varices; there is no difference in other factors, such as cellular infiltration or lymphoid aggregates in portal tracts or septa, which might cause obstruction at a presinusoidal level.[66] Nor is there a difference in the number of thin-walled vessels or arterioles in the portal tracts of patients with and without varices. Obstruction to efferent veins or at a sinusoidal level by mononuclear cell infiltration, hypertrophy of Kupffer cells, or narrowing of sinusoids by twin hepatocyte plates cannot be demonstrated. The mechanism of the portal hypertension therefore remains obscure.

BONE CHANGES AND CALCIUM METABOLISM

Bone changes may be seen in longstanding primary biliary cirrhosis.[4] In the early stages, these present simply as pain, particularly backache. Later, the vertebral bodies become crushed and wedge shaped and kyphosis is gross. The thoracic cage is decalcified, and pseudofractures are frequent. Ribbon-like areas of decalcification (Looser's zones), often symmetrical, are found, particularly in the axillary border of the scapula, in the pelvis (Fig. 26-9), femoral neck and ribs. Pain over the ribs may indicate a pathologic fracture. The hands also show rarefaction. The lamina dura around the teeth disappears, and the teeth loosen and fall out. Proximal myopathy may be associated and can be related to vitamin E deficiency.

The bony lesion is usually osteomalacia but can be osteoporosis. Osteomalacia is characterized by reduced mineralization and excessive production of osteoid. Osteoporosis is characterized by diminished bone volume. Using a computerized technique, 18 of 25 patients with chronic cholestatic disease had osteomalacia, and 10 of 25 had osteoporosis.[73]

The diagnosis of the type of bone change is very difficult without bone biopsy. There is no correlation of biopsy findings with clinical data, plasma calcium, phosphorus, magnesium, or bone alkaline phosphatase isoenzyme.[73] Clinical evidence of bone disease is slow to develop and unlikely unless the cholestasis is deep and has lasted longer than 2 years. Ill-advised prednisolone therapy may hasten the progress of bone changes.

Painful osteoarthropathy may develop in wrist and ankles usually in association with finger clubbing.[34] The cause is unknown.

When the serum cholesterol levels are very high for a long time, erosions are seen in the heads of the digits on the roentgenogram. These represent bone xanthomas.

Mechanisms of the Bone Changes

Where intestinal fat is excessive, dietary calcium forms insoluble soaps and is not absorbed. Bile acids are essential for the absorption of vitamin D in humans; hence this vitamin will not be absorbed properly in cholestasis. A poor diet and lack of sunshine adds to the vitamin D deficiency. Osteomalacia in primary biliary cirrhosis is usually reported from Europe and the Northern United States but not from sunnier areas.

After synthesis in the skin or absorption from the gut, ergocalciferol (vitamin D_2) and cholecalciferol (vitamin D_3) are transported to the liver. Hydroxylation in the C25 position takes place predominantly in the liver by a 25-hydroxylase enzyme with the formation of 25-hydroxy derivatives. With chronic hepatocellular disease, this metabolism could be disturbed and might account for the osteomalacia seen in some patients. Low levels of 25-hydroxy vitamin D (including both 25-hydroxy D_2 and 25-hydroxy D_3) are found in cholestatic liver disease (Fig. 26-10).[72] These low levels are returned to normal by regular monthly (high-dose) injections of vitamin D, indicating that the liver in primary biliary cirrhosis is usually able to hydroxylate vitamin D adequately if sufficient

Fig. 26-9. Radiogram of pelvis shows bilateral Looser's zones in inferior rami of pubis caused by osteomalacia.

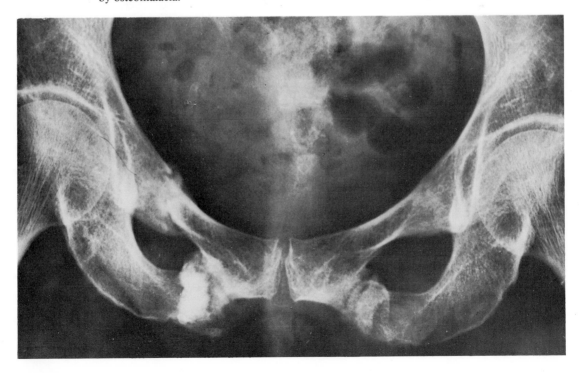

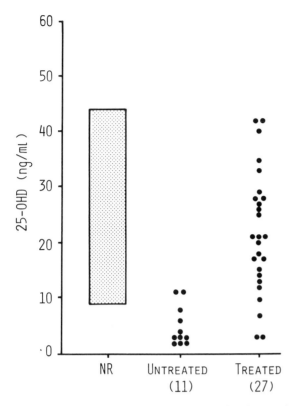

Fig. 26-10. Serum 25-(OH) vitamin D values in primary biliary cirrhosis. Values from 27 treated patients are contrasted with values from 11 patients untreated with parenteral vitamin D_2. NR, normal range. (Skinner RK et al: Lancet 1: 720, 1977)

amounts of substrate are provided.[110] In the later stages of liver failure, this hydroxylation may become inadequate. The 25-hydroxy vitamin D undergoes enterohepatic circulation, and deficiency of this metabolite may be increased by failure of intestinal reabsorption. This could be further interrupted by the administration of cholestyramine.

Increased bone resorption and turnover can be present without histomorphometric evidence of osteoporosis or osteomalacia; this is corrected by parenteral vitamin D_2.[25]

Parathyroid hormone, measured by radioimmunoassay, is normal in cholestatic patients with liver disease.

The osteoporosis is not adequately explained. It is presumably related to the general failure of protein synthesis as the liver cell fails. The osteoporosis may progress despite 25-hydroxy vitamin D_3 in doses sufficient to increase serum levels to normal.[54,80] The proximal myopathy is due to vitamin D and E deficiency.

Kayser-Fleischer Rings

The Kayser-Fleischer ring is a light brown ring at the periphery of the cornea. During the early stages it may be seen only by slit lamp examination. The granules contain copper and may consist of copper chelates. In view of the increased copper concentration in the liver in chronic cholestasis generally, it is perhaps not surprising that Kayser-Fleischer rings have been reported in primary biliary cirrhosis[38] and in a patient whose disease resembled primary biliary cirrhosis in some respects but in others was nearer to chronic active hepatitis.[42]

Other Vitamin Deficiencies

Vitamin A deficiency, with appreciable night blindness and low serum vitamin A concentrations, can develop in deeply jaundiced patients.[127] Vitamin E deficiency with neuromuscular weakness in the lower limbs is rare in the adult.

COURSE

The course of the disease is marked by all the complications of cholestasis. These include pruritus, xanthomas, and various other skin lesions. The effects of diminished bile salt concentration in the intestinal lumen include diarrhea, steatorrhea, and fat-soluble vitamin and calcium deficiency. Ultimately, hepatocellular failure becomes overt. The course is afebrile, and abdominal pain is, in general, unusual, although occasionally pain over the liver, in the absence of gallstones may be a problem. In spite of the jaundice, patients feel surprisingly well and have a good appetite. Weight loss is slow.

Jaundice is variable. It tends to fluctuate for the first 5 years or so and then deepens progressively during the last year of illness (Fig. 26-11). Skin pigmentation is progressive. It is particularly marked in those with a racial or other predisposition to pigmentation. The increase in pigment is particularly obvious in the face, in flexures, and in the scars of trauma or previous surgery.

Pruritus results in scratch marks on the skin, and these may become secondarily infected. A butterfly area over the back may be devoid of scratch marks as it is usually inaccessible to the fingers.[95] The skin becomes thickened over fingers, ankles, and legs.

Xanthomas develop frequently and sometimes acutely, but many patients remain in the prexanthomatous state throughout their illness. The planous variety occurs characteristically as xanthelasma around the eyes and on the upper lip (see Fig. 26-6). They may also be seen in the palmar creases, below the breasts, and on the neck, chest, or back. The tuberous lesions appear later and are characteristically found on extensor surfaces, especially the wrists, elbows, knees, ankles, and buttocks, on pressure points, and in scars (see Fig. 26-7). The xanthomas associated with cholestatic jaundice rarely affect tendon sheaths. The development of skin xanthomas is in proportion to the level of the total serum lipids. If the level is greater than 18 g/liter (1800 mg/dl) for longer than 3 months then skin xanthomas become generalized. Local

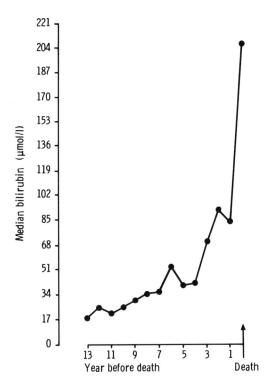

CONCLUSION

EXPECTED survival for any given bilirubin can be extrapolated from this nomogram

ie	Bilirubin (µmol/l)	Expected survival (years)
	< 34	8-13
	35-100	2-7
	> 100	< 2

Fig. 26-11. The evolution of liver failure in primary biliary cirrhosis. This nomogram is derived from the medians of pooled serum bilirubin results in patients followed serially from diagnosis to death. (Serum bilirubin 17 µmol/liter equals 1 mg/dl.)

xanthelasma may develop at levels of 13 g to 18 g/liter (1300 mg to 1800 mg/dl). Lowering of the serum lipid and cholesterol values results in disappearance of the xanthomas. In the later stages, hepatocellular failure results in a fall of serum lipid and cholesterol levels and the xanthomas disappear.

Pain in the fingers, especially on opening doors, and in the toes may be due to xanthomatous involvement of peripheral nerves causing a xanthomatous neuropathy.[118]

Easy bruising with minimal trauma is related to hypoprothombinemia following vitamin K deficiency.

Diarrhea is related to steatorrhea. The fingers show clubbing in the later stages.

Duodenal ulcer is frequent in patients with primary biliary cirrhosis. The defect in blood coagulation adds to the severity of bleeding.

Hepatocellular carcinoma is a very rare complication. This may be because of the female preponderance and the fact that cirrhosis is a late development. However, serial serum α-fetoprotein levels may predict the development of hepatocellular carcinoma, which has been reported in five patients.[81] It is probably of similar frequency to that found in other forms of cirrhosis.

DIAGNOSIS

Diagnosis is usually easy if all ancillary diagnostic tests are available. These must include the serum mitochondrial antibody test, needle liver biopsy, cholangiography (whether endoscopic or percutaneous), and hepatic scanning.

In the presymptomatic stage, the diagnosis must be made from other causes of a raised serum alkaline phosphatase, such as Paget's disease. The raised serum 5'-nucleotidase value in primary biliary cirrhosis usually makes the distinction. Before jaundice appears, distinction from other causes of chronic pruritus must be made.

In the later stages, the diagnosis from chronic active hepatitis and cryptogenic cirrhosis may be difficult. The pattern of biochemical tests of liver function and the liver biopsy appearances are usually diagnostic.

Ulcerative colitis with pericholangitis and/or sclerosing cholangitis may cause diagnostic difficulty. In sclerosing cholangitis, the mitochondrial antibody test is always negative or in low titer and cholangiography demonstrates the typical bile duct irregularities. Investigation of the large bowel by sigmoidoscopy, biopsy, and radiology establishes the presence of chronic inflammatory bowel disease.

Chronic drug jaundice, particularly that related to chlorpromazine, may simulate primary biliary cirrhosis. The onset, however, is much more acute, with rapidly deepening jaundice occurring 4 to 6 weeks after the drug is first used.

Widespread tissue granulomas may suggest sarcoidosis.[112] Chronic intrahepatic cholestasis has been described in sarcoidosis.[102] In sarcoidosis, however, the Kveim skin test is positive (75%) and the mitochondrial antibody test is negative.

PROGNOSIS

Prognosis is extremely variable. The outlook when the patient is first seen may be unpredictable, except that the disease is not curable at present. There seems to be no correlation between extent and severity of the histologic liver lesions and duration of symptoms. In 1959, the mean duration of 35 fatal cases was 5½ years (range 3 to 11 years) from diagnosis.[106] This applied to patients symptomatic at presentation and jaundiced before diagnosis was made. They were already far along the course of the disease. Over the years, diagnosis has become possible at an asymptomatic stage, and it has become apparent that

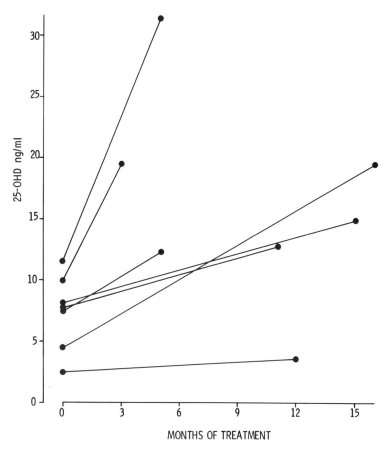

Fig. 26-12. Serum 25-OHD values in primary biliary cirrhosis before and after treatment of varying duration with monthly intramuscular califerol. (Long RG et al: Gastroenterology 72: 1204, 1977)

primary biliary cirrhosis runs a much longer course (see Figs. 26-13, 26-14).

The course of asymptomatic patients is variable and unpredictable, and counseling the patient and the family is very difficult. The life expectancy of some asymptomatic patients may not differ from that of the general population.[97,107] In general, therefore, the asymptomatic patient can be reassured. The time from diagnosis to development of symptoms differs widely. In one series 10 asymptomatic patients survived 1 to 10 years without developing symptoms referable to primary biliary cirrhosis.[71] In another series of 93 patients, diagnosed in the northeast of England, almost half were symptom free.[59] Sex, duration of symptoms, and the character of the first symptom or sign have no independent prognostic influence.[20] The serum bilirubin level is the most important prognostic factor.[32,105] When the serum bilirubin value rises rapidly, prognosis is poor (Table 26-1). Hepatomegaly and cirrhosis on liver biopsy are also bad signs.[97] The appearance of hepatic granulomas suggests a good prognosis.[68] Patients with primary biliary cirrhosis seem to be living considerably longer, perhaps related to earlier diagnosis. The mean survival of asymptomatic patients is 11.9 years. Many patients never enter a symptomatic stage and die of an unrelated

TABLE 26-1. Prognostic Profiles in PBC

CLINICAL FEATURES	EXCELLENT	INTERMEDIATE	POOR
Symptoms	Absent	Present	Present
Signs	Normal liver span	Hepatosplenomegaly	Hepatosplenomegaly ± ascites and encephalopathy
Liver histology	Stage 1 or 2 granulomas	Stage 3 or 4 ± granulomas	Stage 4 No granulomas
Serum bilirubin (μmol/liter)	<34	34–100	100
Expected survival (yr)	8–13	2–7	<2

cause. The rapid development of cholestasis, independent of the histologic stage, is a most important indication of a seriously progressing disease.

The final year or so of the disease is marked by progressive liver failure. Jaundice deepens rapidly. Total serum cholesterol levels fall, and xanthomas disappear. Pruritus is no longer experienced. Serum albumin values decrease, and edema and ascites appear. Fluid retention becomes less and less responsive to diuretic therapy and dietary sodium restriction. The hepatorenal syndrome may ensue. The intellect deteriorates and episodes of frank encephalopathy are seen. Death results from liver failure marked by the ominous triad of bleeding, ascites, and coma, usually with renal failure. Septicemias, particularly gram-negative, may be terminal.

TREATMENT

General Measures and Nutrition

In the jaundiced patient the problem is essentially of intestinal bile salt deficiency. Calorie intake should be maintained, and protein must be adequate. Neutral fat is poorly tolerated and badly absorbed, and steatorrhea reduces calcium absorption. Dietary fat should be restricted to 40 g/day. Additional fat is supplied by medium-chain triglycerides (MCT), which are digested and absorbed quite well, in the absence of bile salts, presumably into the portal vein as free fatty acids. They can be given as Portagen (Mead Johnson) or as MCT (coconut oil).

If there is evidence of bruising or hemorrhage associated with a prolonged prothrombin time, vitamin K, 10 mg, may be administered intramuscularly daily until the deficiency is corrected. It is then given in a dose of 10 mg intramuscularly every 4 weeks. Vitamin A, 100,000 units, should be given every 4 weeks intramuscularly. The problem of bone thinning is discussed later. Vitamin E, 20 mg/day is given orally.

Patients must be encouraged to lead as normal a life as possible, since the disease is compatible with a full domestic and professional life, often for many years. Skillful makeup may be necessary to conceal facial icterus. Plasmapheresis has been used to relieve xanthomatosis with intractable neuropathy.[121] It is given every 1 to 2 weeks and also improves the sense of well-being.[22]

Control of Pruritus

Cholestyramine is used to control pruritus. This drug will have its maximum benefit when bile salt concentrations in the small bowel are greatest. This is at breakfast time, when the gallbladder discharges its overnight reservoir of bile into the duodenum.[62] Cholestyramine should therefore be given as one sachet immediately before and another after the first meal of the day and one sachet before the midday and one before the evening meal. Cholestyramine may also be beneficial as a choleretic in increasing bile salt flow and perhaps in reducing the injurious effects of

retained (toxic) bile salts on the liver cell. Phenobarbital also increases bile flow but is not as effective as cholestyramine.

Other drugs that may be tried may be antihistaminics, terfenadine (an H_1 blocker), paroven (hydroxyethylutruside), and naloxone. Phototherapy has not proved effective. Plasmapheresis may be temporarily effective in controlling intractable pruritus.

On no account must clofibrate be given as a cholesterol-reducing agent. In primary biliary cirrhosis, there is a paradoxic increase in serum cholesterol, the mechanism being uncertain.[103] Xanthomas become more severe. Gallstones may form in the bile ducts.[113]

Treatment of Bone Changes

Patients should be encouraged to be in sunlight as much as possible. An ultraviolent lamp may be helpful. Immobilization must be avoided. The diet should be generally nutritious. The patient should take extra calcium (preferably low-fat or skimmed milk, at least 500 ml/day).

In most patients, osteomalacia will be prevented by 100,000 IU of vitamin D_2 intramuscularly every 4 weeks. This is adequate to maintain normal serum 25-hydroxycholecalciferol levels (see Fig. 26-12).[94,110] It will restore intestinal absorption to normal. Alternatively, 25-hydroxycholecalciferol, which is more potent and the naturally occurring form in humans, may be given in a daily dose of 50 μg to 100 μg orally. In the rarer patient, who still suffers bone pain and myopathy and whose bone biopsy gives evidence of osteomalacia, 1,25-dihydroxycholecalciferol may be given. This is formed in the kidney from the hepatic metabolite 25-hydroxy vitamin D. A dosage of 15 μg to 30 μg is given intramuscularly every 4 weeks.[73] In some patients this may relieve bone pain and resolve myopathy while the bone biopsy shows healing of osteomalacia.

Osteoporosis is more difficult to prevent and treat. Calcium supplements provide the best help. Jaundiced patients should take at least 1.5 g of elemental calcium daily in the form of calcium gluconate, effervescent calcium, ossopan, or Os-Cal.

A course of intravenous calcium injections may afford relief for 2 to 3 months from intractable pain.[3] Fifteen milligrams of calcium per kilogram of body weight is given as calcium gluconate in 500 ml 5% dextrose over 4 hours. The infusion is given daily for about 7 days and repeated as necessary.

Specific Measures

Primary biliary cirrhosis is marked by a profound immunologic disturbance, by increasing hepatic fibrosis, and by copper retention in the liver. Measures have been tried to treat all these developments. In every instance good results have been reported but, unfortunately, they are short term and limited. Serum biochemistry and liver histology may improve, but beneficial effects on symptoms and survival have been difficult to establish. Two problems exist in analyzing the results of any trial of therapy in primary biliary cirrhosis. First, in the presymptomatic patient, the life of the patient may exceed that of the investigator and benefit for any therapy is difficult to establish. In the symptomatic patient, marginal benefit means that very large numbers of patients are required to establish statistical significance. Multicenter trials are necessary. Nevertheless the symptomatic patient must be offered some therapy, and this should be one with minimal side-effects.

Asymptomatic

At the present time it is difficult to justify any treatment in which the prognosis is so long and unpredictable, and no particular therapy has been established of definite benefit. The patient should be reassured and examined and have serum biochemical tests performed every year.

Symptomatic

A choice has to be made between the various drugs that alter the immunologic responses and/or are antifibrotic.

Corticosteroids. Corticosteroids may reduce inflammation and the activity of cytotoxic K lymphocytes and may also relieve pruritus. Unfortunately corticosteroids can accentuate the bone thinning, and indeed some of the most disastrous examples of skeletal crumbling that I have seen have been in patients with late-stage primary biliary cirrhosis who had been treated with prednisolone for many years. Corticosteroids might be useful in the anicteric patient in whom the problem of bone thinning would never arise, but this has never been subjected to controlled clinical trials.

Azathioprine. In a controlled, prospective clinical trial performed at the Royal Free Hospital in London of 45 patients with primary biliary cirrhosis, azathioprine did not improve the results of liver function tests. Serial hepatic biopsies showed the development of cirrhosis equally in treated and untreated groups and survival was similar.[53] A larger multinational double-blind randomized trial of 248 patients showed reduction in the risk of dying and azathioprine also reduced the rate at which patients became incapacitated by the disease.[21] The dose was 80 mg/day for a 70-kg man. Disadvantages are the side-effects and cost. Certainly the disease is not cured, neither is its course substantially altered.

D-Penicillamine. D-Penicillamine would be expected to reduce hepatic copper levels, act immunologically by depressing the inflammatory response, and conceivably might reduce hepatic fibrosis.[58] A randomized controlled trial at the Royal Free Hospital showed that D-penicillamine therapy increased survival in primary biliary cirrhosis.[34] Improvement in survival only became apparent after 18 months of treatment. Those dying early probably

had irreversible liver disease. In surviving patients, D-penicillamine treatment was associated with improved biochemical tests and a fall in liver copper levels (Fig 26-14).[35] D-Penicillamine often reduces hepatic inflammation and piecemeal necrosis, but hepatic fibrosis progresses.

Side-effects unfortunately lead to noncompliance and to withdrawal of therapy. The most frequent is dyspepsia with nausea and vomiting. Taste may be lost, but this returns whether or not the drug is discontinued. Serious reactions include rashes, proteinuria, and blood dyscrasias such as thrombocytopenia and neutropenia. These usually lead to permanent withdrawal of therapy. Various autoimmune syndromes include myasthenia, polymyositis, systemic lupus erythematosus, and a Goodpasture syndrome–like picture.[78]

D-Penicillamine is begun in a daily dose of 125 mg, which is increased by 125 mg every 2 weeks until a maintenance dose of 500 mg/day is reached. Hemoglobin and white blood cell counts are measured and proteinuria sought every week for the first 4 weeks and then every

Fig. 26-13. The course of 20 patients presenting with asymptomatic primary biliary cirrhosis. The duration of follow-up and asymptomatic and symptomatic disease is indicated. (Long RG et al: Gastroenterology 72:1204, 1977)

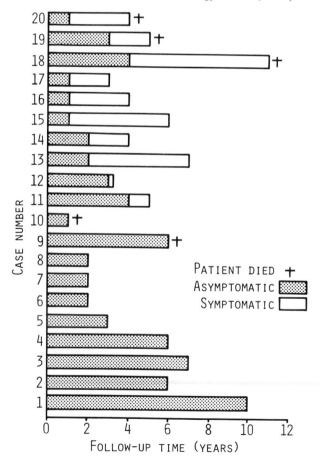

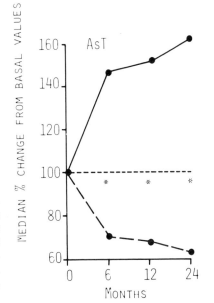

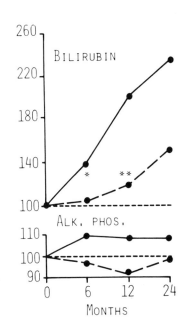

Fig. 26-14. Bilirubin, alkaline phosphatase, and aspartate transaminase concentrations in control (● —— ●) and penicillamine-treated (● - - - ●) patients. The median increase (+) or decrease (−) from basal values is shown. (Epstein O et al: N Engl J Med 300:274, 1979)

month. The drug should be continued unless there is a serious complication or a manifestation of late primary biliary cirrhosis, such as hematemesis, ascites, or precoma.

Researchers from Boston have concluded that D-penicillamine in a dose of 1000 mg/day is not effective in the treatment of primary biliary cirrhosis and is associated with a high incidence of serious side-effects.[79] The dose, however, was larger than that given in the Royal Free Hospital trial and was given for only 28 months.

In a further prospective, controlled trial from the Mayo Clinic, D-penicillamine, given for histologically advanced primary biliary cirrhosis, did not result in an overall improvement in survival compared with placebo.[26] Clinical symptoms and results of serial laboratory tests and liver

biopsies did not differ between treated and controlled patients. Those with earlier histologic disease were not included. Results in a further trial were not dramatically beneficial for the drug.[88] Nevertheless, D-penicillamine is worth a trial in those who are symptomatic with a rising serum bilirubin level and who are unsuitable or have not reached the stage of consideration for liver transplantation. There is little else to offer. D-Penicillamine should not be given to the asymptomatic patient.

Cyclosporin A. Cyclosporin A has a marked effect on the suppressor-inducer T cells and primary biliary cirrhosis.[99] However, the drug is nephrotoxic and difficult to justify for long-term use. Less toxic derivatives are awaited.

Fig. 26-15. Survival probability in early and late histologic stage primary biliary cirrhosis. Early primary biliary cirrhosis—stages 1 and 2, late PBC stages 3 and 4. (Epstein ME et al: Lancet 1: 1275, 1981)

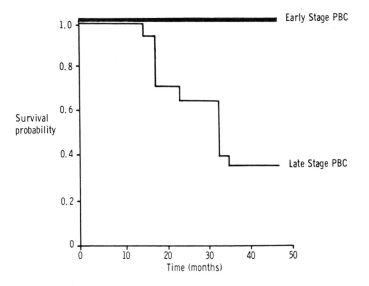

Chlorambucil. Chlorambucil is being studied in a controlled trial from the National Institutes of Health. Bone marrow suppression is a serious side-effect.

Colchicine. Preliminary results of two controlled trials have shown that colchicine, 500 μg, given twice daily results in improved biochemical tests, particularly γ-globulin, bilirubin, and albumin.[15,64] Effects on survival are uncertain. Liver histology and copper content together with serum immune complexes do not change.

Conclusions

Beneficial results for all the above drugs remain inconclusive. In the symptomatic patient with rising serum bilirubin levels, penicillamine, azathioprine, or colchicine is worth trying. This therapy must also be considered for those who are unsuitable for or who have not reached the stage for liver transplantation. There is little else to offer. The asymptomatic patient should not be treated.

Bleeding Esophageal Varices

Bleeding is usually easily controlled by standard measures. The varices may need to be obliterated by esophageal sclerotherapy. Portal-systemic shunts should be considered for recurrent severe bleeding in those without hepatocellular failure.[111] Such operations are tolerated well, and the incidence of encephalopathy is low, perhaps due to the preservation of hepatocellular function until late in the course of the disease.

Liver Transplantation

When the patient with primary biliary cirrhosis has developed hepatocellular failure, particularly ascites and rapidly deepening jaundice, the outlook is extremely grave and survival is unlikely to exceed 1 year. Survival can also be predicted on the serum bilirubin level (see Fig. 26-11). Persistent values above 100 IU/ml (6 mg/dl) are usually associated with death within 2 years. In such patients the question of hepatic transplantation must be considered.[108] This should be sooner rather than later, since malnutrition, coma, and ascites considerably worsen the chances of post-transplant survival. Age should preferably be under 50 years. In well-chosen patients the 1-year survival is about 75%.[123] In one series three patients were alive more than 3 years later and developed a syndrome resembling a recurrence of primary biliary cirrhosis.[89] Serum mitochondrial antibodies do in fact persist. It remains uncertain whether this was indeed primary biliary cirrhosis or a variant of the graft-versus-host disease of chronic liver rejection. If primary biliary cirrhosis does recur, it is likely to be in a mild form and controlled by the immunosuppressants needed to control rejection.

REFERENCES

1. Addison T, Gull W: On a certain affection of the skin—vitilogoidea α plana β tuberosa. Guys Hospital Rep 7:265, 1851
2. Ahrens EH Jr et al: Primary biliary cirrhosis. Medicine 29:299, 1950
3. Ajdukiewicz AB et al: The relief of bone pain in primary biliary cirrhosis with calcium infusions. Gut 15:788, 1974
4. Atkinson M et al: Malabsorption and bone disease in prolonged obstructive jaundice. Q J Med 25:299, 1956
5. Ballardini G, Mirakian R, Bianchi FB et al: Aberrant expression of HLA-DR antigens on bile duct epithelium in primary biliary cirrhosis: Relevance to pathogenesis. Lancet 2:1009, 1984
6. Bassendine MF, Collins JD, Stephenson J et al: Platelet associated immunoglobulins in primary biliary cirrhosis: A cause of thrombocytopenia? Gut 26:1074, 1985
7. Bassendine MF, Dewar PJ, James OFW: HLA-DR antigens in primary biliary cirrhosis: Lack of association. Gut 26:625, 1985
8. Baum H, Berg PA: The complex nature of mitochondrial antibodies and their relation to primary biliary cirrhosis. Semin Liver Dis 4:309, 1984
9. Ben-Joseph Y et al: Further purification of the mitochondrial inner membrane autoantigen reacting with primary biliary cirrhosis sera. Immunology 26:311, 1974
10. Berg PA et al: Mitochondrial antibodies in primary biliary cirrhosis. III. Characterization of the inner membrane complement fixing antigen. Clin Exp Immunol 4:511, 1969
11. Berg PA et al: ATPase-associated antigen (M2): Marker antigen for serological diagnosis of primary biliary cirrhosis. Lancet 2:1423, 1982
12. Bernuau D, Feldman G, Degott C et al: Ultrastructural lesions of bile ducts in primary biliary cirrhosis: A comparison with the lesions observed in graft-versus-host disease. Hum Pathol 12:782, 1981
13. Beswick DR, Klatskin G, Boyer JL: Asymptomatic primary biliary cirrhosis: Long-term follow-up and natural history. Gastroenterology 89:267, 1985
14. Bevan G et al: Serum immunoglobulin levels in cholestasis. Gastroenterology 56:1040, 1969
15. Bodenheimer H, Schaffner F, Pezzulo J: A randomized double-blind controlled trial of colchicine in primary biliary cirrhosis. Hepatology (in press)
16. Bouchier IAD: Postmortem study of the frequency of gallstones in patients with cirrhosis of the liver. Gut 10:705, 1969
17. Burroughs AK, Rosenstein IJ, Epstein O et al: Bacteriuria and primary biliary cirrhosis. Gut 25:133, 1984
18. Child DL et al: Arthritis and primary biliary cirrhosis. Br Med J 2:557, 1977
19. Chohan MR: Primary biliary cirrhosis in twin sisters. Gut 14:213, 1973
20. Christensen E et al: Clinical pattern and course of disease in primary biliary cirrhosis based on an analysis of 236 patients. Gastroenterology 78:236, 1980
21. Christensen E, Neuberger J, Crowe J et al: Beneficial effect of azathioprine and prediction of prognosis in primary biliary cirrhosis: Final results on an International Trial. Gastroenterology 89:1084, 1985
22. Cohen LB, Ambinder EP, Wolke AM et al: Role of plasmapheresis in primary biliary cirrhosis. Gut 26:291, 1985

23. Crowe JP et al: Primary biliary cirrhosis: The prevalence of hypothyroidism and its relationship to thyroid autoantibodies and sicca syndrome. Gastroenterology 78:1437, 1980

24. Crowe JP et al: Increased C1q binding and arthritis in primary biliary cirrhosis. Gut 21:418, 1980

25. Cuthbert JA, Pak CYC, Zerwerh JE et al: Bone disease in primary biliary cirrhosis: Increased bone resorption and turnover in the absence of osteoporosis or osteomalacia. Hepatology 4:1, 1984

26. Dickson ER, Fleming TR, Wiesner RH et al: Trial of penicillamine in advanced primary biliary cirrhosis. New Engl J Med 312:1011, 1985

27. Doniach D et al: Tissue antibodies in primary biliary cirrhosis, active chronic (lupoid) hepatitis, cryptogenic cirrhosis and other liver diseases and their clinical implications. Clin Exp Immunol 1:237, 1966

28. Douglas JC, Finlayson NDC: Are increased individual susceptibility and environmental factors both necessary for the development of primary biliary cirrhosis? Br Med J 2: 419, 1979

29. Epstein O, Arborgh B, Sagiv M et al: Is copper hepatotoxic in primary biliary cirrhosis? J Clin Pathol 34:1071, 1981

30. Epstein O, Chapman RWG, Lake-Bakaar G et al: The pancreas in primary biliary cirrhosis and primary sclerosing cholangitis. Gastroenterology 83:1177, 1982

31. Epstein O, Dick R, Sherlock S: Prospective study of periostitis and finger clubbing in primary biliary cirrhosis and other forms of chronic liver disease. Gut 22:203, 1981

32. Epstein O, Fraga E, Sherlock S: The value of staging for prognosis in primary biliary cirrhosis. In preparation 1986.

33. Epstein O et al: Primary biliary cirrhosis is a dry gland syndrome with features of chronic graft-versus-host disease. Lancet 1:1166, 1980

34. Epstein O et al: Reduction of immune complexes and immunoglobulins induced by D-penicillamine in primary biliary cirrhosis. N Engl J Med 300:274, 1979

35. Epstein O et al: D-Penicillamine treatment improves survival in primary biliary cirrhosis. Lancet 1:1275, 1981

36. Feizi T: Immunoglobulins in chronic liver disease. Gut 9: 193, 1968

37. Feizi T et al: Mitochondrial and other tissue antibodies in relatives of patients with primary biliary cirrhosis. Clin Exp Immunol 10:609, 1972

38. Fleming CR et al: Pigmented corneal rings in a patient with primary biliary cirrhosis. Gastroenterology 69:220, 1975

39. Fox RA et al: The primary immune response to haemocyanin in patients with primary biliary cirrhosis. Clin Exp Immunol 14:437, 1973

40. Fox RA et al: Asymptomatic primary biliary cirrhosis. Gut 14:444, 1973

41. Fox RA et al: Impaired delayed hypersensitivity in primary biliary cirrhosis. Lancet 1:959, 1969

42. Frommer D et al: Kayser-Fleischer-like rings in patients without Wilson's disease. Gastroenterology 73:1331, 1977

43. Galbraith RM et al: High prevalence of seroimmunologic abnormalities in relatives of patients with active chronic hepatitis or primary biliary cirrhosis. N Engl J Med 290: 63, 1974

44. Golding PL et al: Multisystem involvement in chronic liver disease. Am J Med 55:772, 1973

45. Golding PL et al: 'Sicca complex' in liver disease. Br Med J 2:340, 1970

46. Goudie BM, Burt AD, Boyle P et al: Breast cancer in women with primary biliary cirrhosis. Br Med J 291:1597, 1985

47. Graham-Brown RAC, Sarkany I, Sherlock S: Lichen planus and primary biliary cirrhosis. Br J Dermatol 106:699, 1982

48. Hadziyannis S et al: Immunological and histological studies in primary biliary cirrhosis. J Clin Pathol 23:95, 1970

49. Hall S, Axelsen PH, Larsen DE et al: Systemic lupus erythematosus developing in patients with primary biliary cirrhosis. Ann Intern Med 100:388, 1984

50. Hamlyn AN, Sherlock S: The epidemiology of primary biliary cirrhosis: A survey of mortality in England and Wales. Gut 15:473, 1974

51. Hamlyn AN et al: ABO blood groups: Rhesus negativity and primary biliary cirrhosis. Gut 15:480, 1974

52. Hanot V: Etude sur une Forme de Cirrhose Hypertrophique du Foie (Cirrhose Hypertrophique avec Ictere Chronique). Paris, JB Ballière, 1876

53. Heathcote J et al: A prospective controlled trial of azathioprine in primary biliary cirrhosis. Gastroenterology 70:656, 1976

54. Herlong HF, Recker RR, Maddrey WC: Bone disease in primary biliary cirrhosis: Histologic features and response to 25-hydroxy vitamin D. Gastroenterology 83:103, 1982

55. Iliffe GD et al: An association between primary biliary cirrhosis and jejunal villous atrophy resembling celiac disease. Dig Dis Sci 24:802, 1979

56. Izumi N, Hasumur Y, Takeuch IJ: Hypouricemia and hyperuricosuria as expressions of renal tubular damage in primary biliary cirrhosis. Hepatology 3:719, 1983

57. Jain S et al: Histological demonstration of copper and copper-binding protein in chronic liver diseases. J Clin Pathol 31:784, 1978

58. James OFW: D-Penicillamine for primary biliary cirrhosis. Gut 26:109, 1985

59. James O, Macklon AF, Watson AJ: Primary biliary cirrhosis: A revised clinical spectrum. Lancet 1:1278, 1981

60. James SP, Jones EA: Abnormal natural killer cytotoxicity in primary biliary cirrhosis: Evidence for a functional deficiency of cytolytic effector cells. Gastroenterology 89:165, 1985

61. Jaup BH, Zettergren LSW: Familial occurrence of primary biliary cirrhosis associated with hypergammaglobulinaemia in descendants: A family study. Gastroenterology 78:549, 1980

62. Javitt NB: Timing of cholestyramine doses in cholestatic liver disease. N Engl J Med 23:1328, 1974

63. Jones EA et al: Primary biliary cirrhosis and the complement systems. Ann Intern Med 90:72, 1979

64. Kaplan MM, Alling DW, Wolfe HJ et al: Colchicine is effective in the treatment of primary biliary cirrhosis. Hepatology (in press)

65. Kaplan MM, Gandolfo JV, Quaroni EQ: An enzyme-linked immunosorbent assay (ELISA) for detecting antimitochondrial antibody. Hepatology 4:727, 1984

66. Kew MC et al: Portal hypertension in primary biliary cirrhosis. Gut 22:830, 1971

67. Klatskin G, Kantor FS: Mitochondrial antibodies in primary biliary cirrhosis and other diseases. Ann Intern Med 11:533, 1972

68. Lee RG, Epstein O, Jauregui H et al: Granulomas in primary biliary cirrhosis: A prognostic feature. Gastroenterology 81:983, 1981

69. Lindgren S, Laurell AB, Eriksson S: Complement com-

ponents and activation in primary biliary cirrhosis. Hepatology 4:9, 1984

70. Logan RFA et al: Primary biliary cirrhosis and coeliac disease. Lancet 1:230, 1978
71. Long RG et al: Presentation and course of asymptomatic primary biliary cirrhosis. Gastroenterology 72:1204, 1977
72. Long RG et al: Serum 1-25-hydroxy-vitamin-D in untreated parenchymal and cholestatic liver disease. Lancet 2:650, 1976
73. Long RG et al: Parenteral 1-25-dihydroxy cholecalciferol in hepatic osteomalacia. Br Med J 1:75, 1978
74. Ludwig J, Dickson ER, McDonald GSA: Staging of chronic nonsuppurative destructive cholangitis (syndrome of primary biliary cirrhosis). Virchow's Arch 379:103 1978
75. MacSween RNM: Mallory's ('alcoholic') hyaline in primary biliary cirrhosis. J Clin Pathol 23:95, 1973
76. Makinen D, Fritzer M, Davis P et al: Anticentromere antibody in primary biliary cirrhosis. Arthritis Rheum 26:1914, 1983
77. Manns M, Meyer zum Buschenfelde R-H: A mitochondrial antigen–antibody system in cholestatic liver disease detected by radioimmunoassay. Hepatology 2:1, 1982
78. Matloff DS, Kaplan MM: D-Penicillamine-induced Goodpasture-like syndrome in primary biliary cirrhosis: Successful treatment with plasmapheresis and immunosuppressives. Gastroenterology 78:1046, 1980
79. Matloff DS, Alpert E, Resnick RH et al: A prospective trial of D-penicillamine in primary biliary cirrhosis. N Engl J Med 306:319, 1982
80. Matloff DS, Kaplan MN, Neer RM et al: Osteoporosis in primary biliary cirrhosis: Effects of 25-hydroxy vitamin D$_3$ treatments. Gastroenterology 83:97, 1982
81. Melia WM, Johnson PJ, Neuberger J et al: Hepatocellular carcinoma in primary biliary cirrhosis: Detection by alphafetoprotein estimation. Gastroenterology 87:660, 1984
82. Miller F et al: Primary biliary cirrhosis and scleroderma: The possibility of a common pathogenetic mechanism. Arch Lab Med 103:505, 1979
83. Munoz L et al: Is mitochondrial antibody diagnostic of primary biliary cirrhosis? Gut 22:136, 1980
84. Murray-Lyon IM et al: Scleroderma and primary biliary cirrhosis. Br Med J 3:258, 1970
85. Nakanuma Y, Ohta G: Histometric and serial section observations of the intrahepatic bile ducts in primary biliary cirrhosis. Gastroenterology 76:1326, 1979
86. Nakanuma Y, Ohta G: Quantitation of hepatic granulomas and epithelioid cells in primary biliary cirrhosis. Hepatology 3:423, 1983
87. Nakanuma Y, Ohta G, Kono N et al: Electron microscopic observation of destruction of biliary epithelium in primary biliary cirrhosis. Liver 3:238, 1983
88. Neuberger J, Christensen E, Portmann B et al: Double blind controlled trial of D-penicillamine in patients with primary biliary cirrhosis. Gut 26:114, 1985
89. Neuberger J, Portmann B, MacDougall BRD et al: Recurrence of primary biliary cirrhosis after liver transplantation. N Engl J Med 306:1, 1982
90. Pares A, Rimola A, Bruguera M et al: Renal tubular acidosis in primary biliary cirrhosis. Gastroenterology 80:681, 1981
91. Portmann B, Popper H, Neuberger J et al: Sequential and diagnostic features in primary biliary cirrhosis based on histologic study in 209 patients. Gastroenterology 88:1777, 1985
92. Potter BJ et al: Hypercatabolism of the third component

of complement in patients with primary biliary cirrhosis. J Lab Clin Med 88:427, 1976
93. Rai GS et al: Primary biliary cirrhosis, cutaneous capillaritis and IgM-associated membranous glomerulonephritis. Br Med J 1:817, 1977
94. Reed JS et al: Bone disease in primary biliary cirrhosis: Reversal of osteomalacia with oral 25-hydroxy-vitamin D. Gastroenterology 78:512, 1980
95. Reynolds TB: The 'butterfly' sign in patients with chronic jaundice and pruritus. Ann Intern Med 78:545, 1973
96. Reynolds TB et al: Primary biliary cirrhosis with scleroderma, Raynaud's phenomenon and telangiectasia. Am J Med 50:302, 1971
97. Rolls J, Boyer JL, Barry D et al: The prognostic importance of clinical and histological asymptomatic and symptomatic primary biliary cirrhosis. N Engl J Med 308:1, 1983
98. Ros E, Garcia-Puges A, Rexiach M et al: Fat digestion and exocrine pancreatic function in primary biliary cirrhosis. Gastroenterology 87:180, 1984
99. Routhier G et al: Suppressor and inducer T-lymphocytes in primary biliary cirrhosis: The effects of cyclosporin A. Lancet 2:1223, 1980
100. Rubel LR, Rabin L, Seeff LB et al: Does primary biliary cirrhosis in men differ from primary biliary cirrhosis in women? Hepatology 4:671, 1984
101. Rubin E et al: Primary biliary cirrhosis: Chronic nonsuppurative destructive cholangitis. Am J Pathol 46:387, 1965
102. Rudzki C et al: Chronic intrahepatic cholestasis of sarcoidosis. Am J Med 59:373, 1975
103. Schaffner F: Paradoxical elevation of serum cholesterol by clofibrate in patients with primary biliary cirrhosis. Gastroenterology 57:253, 1969
104. Scheuer PJ: Primary biliary cirrhosis. In Liver Biopsy Interpretation, 4th ed, p 47. Baltimore, Williams & Wilkins, 1986
105. Shapiro JM et al: Serum bilirubin: A prognostic factor in primary biliary cirrhosis. Gut 20:137, 1979
106. Sherlock S: Primary biliary cirrhosis (chronic intrahepatic obstructive jaundice). Gastroenterology 31:574, 1959
107. Sherlock S: Primary biliary cirrhosis: Critical evaluation and treatment policies. Scand J Gastroenterol [Suppl] 77:63, 1982
108. Sherlock S: Hepatic transplantation: The state of play. Lancet 2:778, 1983
109. Sherlock S, Scheuer PJ: The presentation and diagnosis of 100 patients with primary biliary cirrhosis. N Engl J Med 289:674, 1973
110. Skinner RK et al: 25-Hydroxylation of vitamin D in primary biliary cirrhosis. Lancet 1:720, 1977
111. Spisni R, Smith-Laing G, Epstein O et al: Results of portal decompression in patients with primary biliary cirrhosis. Gut 22:345, 1981
112. Stanley NN et al: Primary biliary cirrhosis or sarcoidosis or both. N Engl J Med 287:1282, 1972
113. Summerfield JA et al: Effects of clofibrate in primary biliary cirrhosis, hypercholesterolemia and gallstones. Gastroenterology 69:998, 1975
114. Summerfield JA et al: The biliary system in primary biliary cirrhosis. Gastroenterology 70:240, 1976
115. Thomas HC: Potential pathogenic mechanisms in primary biliary cirrhosis. Semin Liver Dis 1:338, 1981
116. Thomas HC et al: Is primary biliary cirrhosis an immune complex disease? Lancet 2:1261, 1977

117. Thomas HC et al: Immune complexes in acute and chronic liver disease. Clin Exp Immunol 31:150, 1978

118. Thomas PK, Walker JG: Xanthomatous neuropathy in primary biliary cirrhosis. Brain 88:1079, 1965

119. Tong MJ et al: Immunological studies in familial primary biliary cirrhosis. Gastroenterology 71:305, 1976

120. Triger DR: Primary biliary cirrhosis: An epidemiological study. Br Med J 281:772, 1980

121. Turnberg LA et al: Plasmapheresis and plasma exchange in the treatment of hyperlipaemia and xanthomatous neuropathy in patients with primary biliary cirrhosis. Gut 13:976, 1972

122. Uhl GS et al: Primary biliary cirrhosis in systemic sclerosis (scleroderma) and polymyositis. Johns Hopkins Med J 135:191, 1974

123. Van Thiel DH et al: Liver transplantation in adults. Gastroenterology 90:211, 1986

124. Vaux DJT, Watt F, Grime GW et al: Hepatic copper distribution of primary biliary cirrhosis shown by scanning protein microprobe. J Clin Pathol 38:653, 1985

125. Walker JG et al: Serological tests in the diagnosis of primary biliary cirrhosis. Lancet 1:827, 1965

126. Walker JG et al: Chronic liver disease and mitochondrial antibodies: A family study. Br Med J 1:146, 1972

127. Walt RP, Kemp CM, Lyness L et al: Vitamin A for night blindness in primary biliary cirrhosis. Br Med J 288:1030, 1984

128. Wands JR et al: Circulating immune complexes and complement activation in primary biliary cirrhosis. N Engl J Med 289:233, 1978

129. Wolke AM, Schaffner F, Kapelman B et al: Malignancy in primary biliary cirrhosis: High incidence of breast cancer in affected women. Am J Med 76:1075, 1984

130. Zeegan R et al: Bleeding oesophageal varices as the presenting feature in primary biliary cirrhosis. Lancet 2:9, 1969

chapter 27

Hemochromatosis

THOMAS H. BOTHWELL and ROBERT W. CHARLTON

The association between diabetes mellitus and pigmentation of the liver and pancreas was recognized by Troisier in 1871. It was Von Recklinghausen, however, who first noted, in 1889, that some patients with cirrhosis exhibited marked accumulations of hemosiderin and who coined the term *hemochromatosis*.[149]

Since that time there have been many descriptions of the clinical and pathologic features associated with the presence of excessive iron in the body. The literature was reviewed in 1935 by Sheldon,[377] and his observations have been updated on several subsequent occasions.[28,51,61,149,157,224,283,292,333,334,386,412] As years passed, Sheldon's concept—that hemochromatosis is the result of a specific metabolic abnormality—has been expanded to include a number of other forms of iron overload. In particular, it has become apparent that massive iron overload can develop in association with certain refractory anemias and can result from the ingestion of excessive quantities of absorbable iron in the diet. In addition, iron overload of varying degrees has been reported with porphyria cutanea tarda and following portacaval shunts. To understand the significance of these various conditions it is first necessary to have some idea of the normal content and distribution of iron in the body, and of iron balance regulation. When iron overload occurs, no matter what its cause, this regulatory mechanism has become disturbed in some way or has been bypassed.

FUNCTIONAL AND STORAGE IRON

The body of a healthy adult male normally contains between 3 g and 4 g of iron.[61] Two thirds of the iron is present in compounds such as hemoglobin, myoglobin, and tissue enzymes that are actively participating in metabolic functions. The remainder represents a surplus that is stored in various sites.

Storage iron exists in two forms: (1) as a diffuse soluble fraction called ferritin, in which the molecules are dispersed, and (2) as insoluble aggregates of hemosiderin. Ferritin, the primary iron storage protein, is found in all cells, being present in the cytoplasm and within lysozomes. The apoprotein has a molecular weight of 473,000 daltons and is made up of an approximately spherical protein shell, which contains 24 subunits.[106,165,197,198] The central cavity can accommodate as many as 4500 atoms of iron as an inorganic "hydrous ferric oxide-phosphate." When

laden with iron the protein has a half time of only a few days. Its continuous turnover thus provides an available iron pool. The observation that tissues contain a number of ferritins with different isoelectric points[130,131,282] excited considerable interest, since it raised the possibility that their biologic behavior might differ. There is, however, as yet no evidence that isoferritins have physiologic significance. Although more basic ferritins are synthesized in states of iron overload and more acidic ones by tumors, this pattern is by no means uniform. The most likely reason for the variations in isoelectric mobility is one propounded by Drysdale and co-workers. They have produced evidence that there are two subunits, one (H) with a molecular weight of 21,000 daltons and another (L) with a molecular weight of 19,000 daltons and that these are present in differing proportions in the variants. The H subunit predominates in the more acidic ferritins present in the heart and the L subunit in the more basic ferritins of liver and spleen.

Hemosiderin is a degraded form of ferritin in which the iron cores are no longer associated with an intact protein shell.[435] The ratio of ferritin to hemosiderin in storage organs varies according to the amount of iron present. At lower concentrations ferritin predominates, but at higher concentrations most iron is found as hemosiderin.[299] The iron cores of ferritin molecules are visible on electron microscopy but not normally on light microscopy. In contrast, the insoluble golden-yellow hemosiderin is readily seen. Hemosiderin stains intensely blue with potassium ferrocyanide, and the quantity seen has traditionally been used as a means of gauging the size of the body iron stores.[61] Although the liver is regarded as the most important storage organ for iron, it normally contains only about a fourth to a third of the total body iron content.[61] Most of the visible iron in the liver is within reticuloendothelial cells, but small amounts can also be seen in parenchymal cells. The quantitative importance of these two storage sites is difficult to estimate, since the number of parenchymal cells is very high in relation to the reticuloendothelial cells. Deposits in the reticuloendothelial system are largely derived from the breakdown of red blood cells; hepatocyte stores originate from the iron bound to transferrin,[160] and to a lesser extent from hemoglobin–haptoglobin[208,408] and heme–hemopexin complexes.[208] Although the plasma ferritin is selectively taken up by hepatocytes, it normally contains very little iron.[438]

The quantities of storage iron present in other organs

are less well documented. Studies in dogs and in humans suggest that as much as one third of the body stores may be present in skeletal muscles.[399] In addition, it has been clear for a number of years that the reticulum cells of the bone marrow contain a further iron store that closely mirrors the iron status of the individual.[61] The quantitative importance of the bone marrow as a storage organ has been confirmed by *in vitro* and *in vivo* studies indicating that about 300 mg of iron is stored in this site in normal males and approximately half this figure in normal females.[170] These quantities are similar to the amounts stored in the liver.[332]

Plasma Ferritin as a Measure of Body Iron Stores

The discovery of minute amounts of ferritin circulating in the plasma has provided a noninvasive and moderately accurate way of assessing the total amount of the iron stored in the body.[437] Although all body cells probably secrete ferritin, its main source appears to be the reticuloendothelial system. Plasma ferritin differs from tissue ferritin in that it is virtually iron free and partly glycosylated. Despite this, its concentration reflects the size of body iron stores, with 1 μg of ferritin per liter of plasma being roughly equivalent to about 140 μg of storage iron per kilogram of body weight.[158] The plasma ferritin concentration thus follows the physiologic changes in iron nutrition. Immediately after birth it rises while superfluous red cells are being destroyed and their iron stored. It then falls as the iron stores are mobilized to supply an expanding red cell mass during infancy and childhood. In young adult life menstruation and childbearing are responsible for lower plasma ferritin concentrations in females than in males, but after the menopause the levels in women rise and eventually the sex difference virtually disappears.

The chief restriction to the clinical use of the plasma ferritin concentration for assessing iron nutrition is the fact that it is influenced by other factors. Concentrations higher than justified by the amount of stored iron are found in inflammatory states, in neoplastic disorders, and in liver disease.[437] A raised ferritin concentration is therefore a relatively nonspecific finding in clinical situations. On the other hand, a low plasma ferritin concentration of less than 12 μg/liter can only be due to iron deficiency.

QUANTITATIVE ASPECTS OF IRON BALANCE

From a functional standpoint, the iron stores represent a buffer that can be drawn on when the need arises, and there is some evidence to show that gastrointestinal iron absorption is regulated to maintain these stores at an optimal level. The rate of absorption is greater than normal when the stores are depleted and is diminished when the stores are increased.[61,90] During childhood and adolescence there is a positive iron balance, with more iron being ab-

sorbed than is excreted. In this way the demands of the growing body for functional iron are met and the storage depots gradually build up. In the adult, however, the amounts of iron in stores remain relatively constant.[93] In the average male the accumulation of storage iron slows appreciably after adulthood is reached until it becomes barely perceptible; in the female there is a spurt after the menopause until equilibrium is approached.[102] In view of this, the considerable variation in the percentage of iron absorbed by apparently healthy subjects almost certainly represents individual adjustments to preserve the equilibrium. The homeostasis is, however, at best incomplete, and this is largely attributable to the fact that the bioavailability of the iron in food is so limited. Iron stores therefore tend to be less than normal when there are added losses from the body or when dietary deficiency is present. Factors such as this account not only for the smaller stores present in females but also for the differences in iron stores that have been noted in various population groups.[61,93]

The quantity of iron that must be absorbed from the diet clearly depends on the amounts that are lost from the body. Data obtained from chemical and isotopic studies indicate that the obligatory daily iron losses are of the order of 1.0 mg in adult males.[182] Approximately two thirds of this is via the gut, with most of the remainder being lost in the urine and desquamated skin cells. These obligatory losses are reduced by about half in iron deficiency[133] and may rise to figures of two to three times normal in states of iron overload.[182]

In the female there are, in addition, the extra losses incurred through menstruation and pregnancy. The mean normal menstrual losses when expressed in terms of daily iron balance are approximately 0.5 mg, but there is a considerable variation. In 5% of normal women the figure is greater than 1.4 mg.[189] During pregnancy the requirement is even greater, since an expanding maternal red blood cell mass, a growing fetus, and a placenta must be supplied. When these various requirements are added to the normal obligatory losses that continue throughout the gestation period, it has been calculated that about 1 g of iron is needed for each pregnancy.[61,96] To meet this requirement an average of between 5 mg and 6 mg must be absorbed each day throughout the last two trimesters.

Iron lost from the body must be replaced from food, and absorption by the intestine is under delicate control so that balance is maintained. However, both the quantity of iron in the diet and its availability for absorption vary. Of the two, the variation in the bioavailability of dietary iron is more significant for iron nutrition. Heme iron in food is easily absorbed regardless of the other components present in the diet, and the virtual disappearance of meat from the diet of the majority of the world's population is largely responsible for the high prevalence of iron deficiency in many countries.[50,61] In contrast, non-heme food iron absorption is seldom as efficient, since it is profoundly influenced by the nature of the various dietary ingredients. This can be ascribed to the fact that non-heme iron present in food enters a common pool in the lumen of the gastrointestinal tract where it is susceptible to numerous competing ligands. Some of these, such as tannins and phytates, form unabsorbable complexes, while ascorbic acid and factors in meat and fish are among those that facilitate absorption.[173] The amount of ascorbic acid in the diet of populations consuming little meat or fish becomes the limiting factor: if no ascorbic acid is present, not more than 1% to 7% of the iron in staples such as rice, maize, beans, and wheat can be absorbed. Four times as much iron can be absorbed from a meal containing reasonable quantities of heme and ascorbic acid as from one containing little of each but with an identical protein, calorie, and total iron content.[298] About 20% of the iron in the average American diet can be absorbed by the iron-deficient individual. With the diet containing about 6 mg of iron per 1000 calories, the maximum absorption from the 2500 calories per day ingested by most adult males is only 3 mg to 4 mg.[298] In the female the figure is even lower, since calorie intake, and hence iron intake, is usually smaller. It is therefore, apparent that the possible range of absorption from a normal diet is not wide, extending from less than 0.5 mg daily in the iron-replete individual to 3 mg to 4 mg in iron deficiency.

DEFINITIONS

As mentioned, when iron stores are increased, most of the additional iron is in the form of hemosiderin. The term *hemosiderosis* thus implies an increase in the amount of storage iron. *Siderosis* is used in exactly the same sense. It is important to realize that this does not necessarily mean that the total iron content of the body is increased. In any anemia not due to blood loss or dietary iron deficiency, there is a redistribution of body iron, with less in hemoglobin and more in the stores. In other words, there is a *relative hemosiderosis*. Under such circumstances, iron stores may increase to as much as two or three times normal. Hemosiderosis may also be localized to specific organs, for example, the lungs in idiopathic pulmonary siderosis and the kidneys in paroxysmal nocturnal hemoglobinuria. The hemosiderin deposited in these organs is not reutilized for blood formation, and the anomalous situation may arise that the body as a whole is iron deficient while the affected organs are loaded with iron.[61]

The term *absolute hemosiderosis* indicates that there is a true increase in total body iron. This is also often referred to as *iron overload*. Absolute hemosiderosis is uncommon; its presence implies that the regulatory mechanisms for controlling the iron content of the body are deranged or have been bypassed.

Before discussing the ways in which this can occur, it is important to define a second term, *hemochromatosis*. This term is essentially one based on pathologic criteria and has been applied in the past when the organs contain grossly excessive amounts of storage iron in parenchymal

cells and show evidence of damage, usually in the form of diffuse fibrotic change. Unfortunately much confusion has resulted from the designation of cirrhosis of the liver with slight to moderate amounts of hemosiderin as "hemochromatosis." This problem is considered elsewhere in the chapter, but at this stage it should be made clear that the pathologic term *hemochromatosis* should only be applied to the condition in which there are very large amounts of iron in the cirrhotic liver, usually more than 0.5 g/100 g wet weight.

Hemochromatosis may arise in a number of ways. The idiopathic or primary form that was initially recognized in the last century and that was so admirably described in 1935 by Sheldon[377] is now known to result from an inherited error of metabolism that is associated with excessive absorption of iron from the diet. Absorption inappropriate to body needs is also feature of a number of inherited and acquired refractory anemias, and in such circumstances the degree of loading with iron may be compounded by transfusion therapy. Finally, excessive absorption of iron may occur in normal subjects exposed to large amounts of absorbable iron in the diet. Because of its varied etiology it is therefore helpful to prefix the term *hemochromatosis* with an adjective describing its origin (*e.g.,* idiopathic, transfusional).

A further semantic problem has arisen in the recent past. The availability of techniques for detecting individuals homozygous for the idiopathic hemochromatosis gene has widened considerably the spectrum of presentation. Many individuals are now diagnosed at a time prior to the development of appreciable iron overload and thus have no organ damage. Currently they are designated as examples of *preclinical idiopathic hemochromatosis,* but this is a clumsy and unsatisfactory term. Although no general agreement has been reached on alternative ways of describing such individuals, certain suggestions in this regard are included later in the section concerned with the genetic transmission of the disorder.

CLASSIFICATION OF IRON OVERLOAD

Oral iron overload is due to a failure of the normal homeostatic mechanisms. This may occur with the consumption of a normal diet, as in idiopathic hemochromatosis, in certain anemias characterized by increased but largely ineffective erythropoiesis, and perhaps also after portacaval anastomosis. On the other hand, exposure for long periods of time to a diet containing excessive quantities of bioavailable iron may result in a positive balance in otherwise normal subjects. This condition has been most extensively studied in black South Africans, in whom the iron overload is frequently as severe as in fully developed idiopathic hemochromatosis. In other parts of the world excessive dietary iron is very rarely, if ever, the sole cause of severe iron overload, but it may play a part in the pathogenesis of other varieties of hemosiderosis (*e.g.,* the inappropriate administration of medicinal iron preparations in refractory anemias).

Parenteral iron overload results from multiple blood transfusions for nonhemorrhagic anemias but could theoretically also be due to repeated courses of treatment with injectable iron preparations.

More than one mechanism may be responsible for the iron overload in individual patients. A subject with thalassemia major, for example, may have absorbed inappropriately large amounts of iron from a normal diet and may have also been treated with oral iron preparations and multiple blood transfusions.

IDIOPATHIC HEMOCHROMATOSIS

In this form of iron overload the accumulation of the 20 g to 40 g of iron that is present in the body at the time of clinical diagnosis usually takes many years. Cirrhosis is often present, classically together with diabetes mellitus, skin pigmentation, and cardiac failure. The early stages are characterized by a high plasma iron concentration, a high percentage saturation of the plasma transferrin, and, with the passage of time, increasing concentrations of ferritin in the plasma and deposits of hemosiderin in the liver and other organs. Only after the concentration of storage iron has risen markedly does pathologic, biochemical, and clinical evidence of organ damage appear.

Prevalence

Fully developed idiopathic hemochromatosis is an uncommon but not excessively rare disease. By 1935, 350 well-documented cases had been reported,[377] and during the next 20 years there were another 800.[157] Since 1955 there have been many additional reports.[61,149] Phenotypic expression of the disease obviously depends not only on the frequency with which the gene occurs in a given population but also on the general standard of iron nutrition. Hemochromatosis is likely to be encountered much more commonly in patients in diabetic, endocrine, cardiac, arthritis, or liver clinics than in the general population, since it is the clinical manifestations that bring the hemochromatotic patient to the physician. The infrequent occurrence of any variety of iron overload in most communities was underlined by a study in which hepatic storage iron concentrations were estimated in almost 4000 specimens from 18 different countries: only 3 were found to be more than five times normal,[93] and none of these was anywhere near the hemochromatotic range of 20 to 50 times normal. In addition, none of more than 3000 apparently normal individuals in the Seattle, Washington, area had a plasma ferritin concentration approaching that found in idiopathic hemochromatosis.[102,161]

Early estimates of the prevalence of idiopathic hemochromatosis were 1/20,000 hospital admissions and 1/7,000 hospital deaths,[157] 2.5/10,000 necropsies per-

formed in Johannesburg,[33] and 4/100,000 necropsies performed in Olmstead County, Minnesota.[149] However, more recent studies indicate that iron metabolism is abnormal in a considerable proportion of the relatives of patients with the fully developed disease. The evidence is reviewed in the following text, but it is clear that for every individual with the full clinical and pathologic expression of idiopathic hemochromatosis, there are a number of subjects with latent or subclinical disease. The prevalence of the inborn error of metabolism that sometimes leads to the development of massive iron overload is thus much higher than the prevalence of the classic syndrome of bronzed diabetes.

The clinical manifestations of idiopathic hemochromatosis occur most commonly between the ages of 40 and 60 years,[157] but a number of cases have been reported in younger patients. Males develop clinical manifestations of the disease approximately ten times as frequently as females. This can be explained, at least in part, by the quantities of iron the female loses through menstruation, pregnancy, and lactation. It has been calculated that this amounts to a lifetime total of between 5 g and 15 g.[61] Although the absorptive mechanism is geared to make good such losses, the quantities of iron in the diet are rarely sufficient to allow for complete compensation. On this basis it would be expected that affected females would develop clinical manifestations of idiopathic hemochromatosis later than males. Data collected by Finch and Finch[157] suggest that this is so. Of all the male patients, 35% to 40% developed symptoms before the age of 46, compared with only 20% to 25% of the females. However, a complicating feature is that many females who do develop the disease give a history of scanty menstruation for several years preceding the onset of symptoms.

Pathogenesis

By the time clinical manifestations appear, the total body iron content is between 5 and 10 times normal. All the extra iron is contained within storage compounds, so that the iron stores of the body are increased between 20 and 50 times normal. The presence of this quantity of iron implies that iron balance must have been disturbed for many years, since the amount that can be absorbed from a normal diet is not more than 3 mg to 5 mg/day.[37,40,48] If the diet contains extraneous iron, it is obvious that greater rates of absorption may occur, and the amounts present in the fully developed condition accumulate sooner. Conversely, increased losses of iron from the body, whether physiologic or pathologic, delay or even prevent the buildup of sufficient quantities of storage iron.

Figures for radiolabeled iron absorption at the time of diagnosis have varied widely. In a number of early studies increased iron absorption was noted,[88] but since such results were obtained using the radioisotopic balance method, they should be treated with some reserve. On reviewing the evidence at the present time, it would appear that although iron absorption may be raised,[267] it is usually within the normal range by the time clinical manifestations appear.[59,149] Since the body's requirement for iron normally determines the absorption rate, it is apparent that a normal absorption rate is inappropriately high in the presence of grossly enlarged iron stores. During venesection therapy, absorption rises to high levels and may remain above the normal range for years after phlebotomies are discontinued.[37,293] This suggests that iron absorption in these subjects is influenced by the usual controlling factors, but that the whole mechanism is geared at a higher level than normal.

Etiologic Factors

In light of his extensive analysis of the literature, Sheldon[377] concluded that idiopathic hemochromatosis was the result of a specific inborn metabolic error. This conclusion was based on the characteristic nature of the clinical and pathologic findings, the lack of any obvious environmental factors, and the several reports of involvement of more than one member of a family. Twenty years later the understanding of the quantitative aspects of iron metabolism had become much clearer, and Finch and Finch[157] deduced that the subjects with clinically manifest disease represented only a proportion of affected individuals. They argued that the degree of overload in a particular individual must be influenced by several factors such as age, the amount of iron in the diet, and the rate of iron loss. They also concluded that the massive iron deposits were noxious to the tissues but that the presence of other hepatotoxins in the diet, particularly alcohol, would aggravate the condition and lead to the clinical presentation of the disease at an earlier age.

Although the need to postulate a genetic abnormality was seriously challenged during the 1960s,[276] the evidence that Sheldon[377] was correct is now irrefutable. Nevertheless, the environmental factors identified by Finch and Finch[157] play important roles in the phenotypic expression of the inherited abnormality.

Genetic Factors

The early evidence for a genetic etiology was the occurrence of the clinical disease in more than one member of a family.[61] Although it could have been argued that the condition was familial rather than genetic, and that the occurrence of the disease in siblings represented familial exposure to excessive dietary iron, other members of the household were frequently unaffected.[124,152,167,196,235,264,318] In addition, in some individuals at least there was no question of the consumption of excessive iron or alcohol.

It should be stressed that families in which more than one member is affected with the full-blown disease form only a small minority of the total number of cases reported.[276] When evidence of less extreme degrees of iron overload is sought among the relatives of patients, however, it is found much more frequently.[16,54,118,327,366,367,429]

The frequency of the HLA antigen A3 is increased in subjects with the disease.[45,381] Other associations include an excess of subjects with the HLA-B7 antigen and a higher prevalence of HLA-B14. In one study, the frequency of HLA-A3 and HLA-B14 was increased and the haplotype A3B14 carried a relative risk of 23.4[354] Simon and coworkers[380] believe it unlikely that the alleles themselves are directly concerned in the transmission of idiopathic hemochromatosis. It is more probable that the gene for hemochromatosis is located on the short arm of chromosome 6 tightly linked to the HLA-A locus.[141] In a study in which iron loading and HLA types were assessed in 24 siblings of patients with idiopathic hemochromatosis, a highly significant association ($p < .0001$) was noted between the presence of hemochromatosis in affected siblings and possession of the same two HLA haplotypes (Fig. 27-1).[379] These results support an autosomal recessive mode of transmission of the overt disease in these families. Similar findings have been supported in several extensive studies.[24,25,31,80,140,143,244,257,263,314,315,404]

The results of these studies indicate that the gene frequency is high. Current data based on HLA studies in affected families suggest that 8.4% of subjects in Utah and

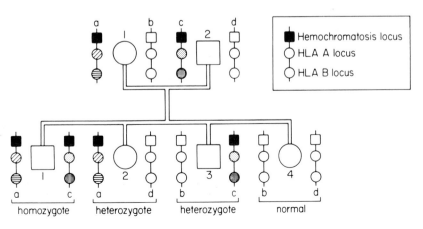

Fig. 27-1. Hypothetical distribution of iron-loading alleles, each designated by an HLA haplotype, among family members of a patient (*1*) with fully developed idiopathic hemochromatosis. The topographic relationships between the gene (■) and the HLA loci (○) are diagrammatic approximations. The two number 6 chromosomes of the mother of the patient are designated "a" and "b," of which "a" carries the mutant iron-loading allele. In the father the mutant allele occurs on the sixth chromosome, designated "c." The patient has inherited both mutant genes and is a homozygote.[51]

10.5% of those in Brittany are heterozygous carriers, yielding calculated homozygous frequencies of 1 in 319 and 1 in 400, respectively.[31,80] A similar frequency was found in Scotland on the basis of necropsy findings.[286] It might be argued that such estimates may have been inflated by biased ascertainment, but the results of two epidemiologic studies in central Sweden suggest that this is not so. In one, the transferrin saturation and the plasma ferritin concentration were screened in 718 male government employees and those with abnormal findings were investigated further.[314] The heterozygous frequency was calculated to be 13.8%, with one in 200 being homozygous. A second investigation was carried out on 8750 patients and blood donors in a country hospital, and one in 417 was found to be homozygous.[315] When these results are taken together, they suggest that the HLA-linked iron-loading gene is extremely common in several white populations. This explains a number of reports in which an apparently dominant inheritance has been noted,[54,118,138,177] since the mating of a homozygote with a heterozygote would not be an excessively rare occurrence.[26,143,382]

Another important point has emerged from these various studies. It is clear that homozygosity for the HLA-linked iron-loading gene is only associated with tissue damage and severe iron overload in a proportion of patients. Indeed, Finch and Huebers[158] have estimated that only one in five homozygotes progresses to overt tissue damage and symptomatic disease. Whether variation in phenotypic expression results from different genetic defects is not known, but some evidence that this may be so has been reported.[303]

It is of interest to speculate why the HLA-linked iron loading gene occurs so frequently in white populations. It is possible that in the past heterozygotes had a selective advantage if they were protected against the deleterious effects of iron deficiency by absorbing more dietary iron.[51] Better iron nutrition in times of deprivation may have been associated with improved survival during infancy, childhood, and pregnancy. Alternatively, it is possible that the gene reached a high frequency because of "hitchhiking" with the closely linked HLA complex, with the relative advantage not being related to the iron-loading gene but to some other gene or genes in the HLA cluster.

The nature of the metabolic disorder (or disorders) responsible for idiopathic hemochromatosis remains to be defined, although many hypotheses have been proposed.

Luke and co-workers[268] described a glycoprotein in gastric secretions that normally inhibits iron absorption and that is absent in subjects with idiopathic hemochromatosis, but this has not been confirmed by other workers.[300,439] In addition, no other abnormalities in gastric secretions have been found.[37]

Cox and Peters[104] have reported an increased uptake of iron by duodenal mucosa from patients with idiopathic hemochromatosis, but the reason for this has not been elucidated. Crosby[108] reported the finding of less mucosal ferritin in affected subjects: while this has not been confirmed by other workers[192] it has been shown that a larger proportion than normal of the iron taken up by mucosal cells is transferred into the body.[43,337]

The possibility that the liver might have an abnormal affinity for iron has been considered. A suggestion that xanthine oxidase deficiency might be the fundamental lesion[289] is no longer tenable, since the enzyme seems not to be involved in the physiologic release of iron from ferritin,[105] and inhibiting it with allopurinol has no measurable effect on iron metabolism.[13,62,117,183] Indeed, iron stored in the hemochromatotic liver is very readily mobilized in response to venesection, which does not support the suggestion that this organ has any increased tendency to sequestrate iron.[329]

Transferrin has also been studied; it was reported as being abnormal,[355] but this has not been confirmed.[55,428] Compelling evidence against a primary etiologic role for transferrin is the demonstration that the transferrin type does not segregate with the HLA type in families with variation at the transferrin locus.[232] These latter observations have been confirmed by the recent finding that the transferrin gene is on chromosome 3[443] and not on chromosome 6, which is the one associated with iron loading.

The demonstration of an abnormal hepatic isoferritin pattern in idiopathic hemochromatosis[338] aroused initial interest, but similar changes were later found in other varieties of iron overload,[9,339] with the pattern reverting to normal after removal of the excess iron.[190] Current evidence indicates that ferritin is biochemically normal in the disease[410] and ferritin synthesis appears to be normal in a variety of tissues.[27,32,192,229] Finally, there is recent evidence that one of the subunits of ferritin (H) is encoded on chromosome 19[83] and the other (L) on the short arm of chromosome 1.[281]

Both histologic and chemical studies indicate that the storage iron content of reticuloendothelial cells is inappropriately low in idiopathic hemochromatosis.[57,66,402] These findings have led to the suggestion that the reticuloendothelial and intestinal mucosal cells do not store iron normally, and there is evidence from kinetic studies that this may be so.[156] As a result, increased amounts of iron are delivered to hepatocytes and other parenchymal cells. The attraction of this as yet unproven hypothesis lies in its compatibility with a number of observed features of the condition, namely the lack of increased iron in mucosal and reticuloendothelial cells, the increased iron absorption, and the saturation of circulating transferrin with iron. According to this hypothesis deposition of iron in hepatocytes and parenchymal cells occurs only as a passive consequence of the saturated transferrin.[101]

Extrinsic Factors

Two extrinsic factors have received much attention: the amount of iron in the diet and alcohol. It is obvious that the amount of absorbable iron in the diet determines the rate at which iron can be accumulated in the body. The larger per capita consumption of meat seems likely to account for the apparently higher prevalence and earlier age at onset in Australia,[333,335,360] while the scanty bioavailable iron in the average diets of countries such as India makes the accumulation of excess iron stores difficult even for hemochromatotic homozygotes. In any population the absorbable iron intake may vary from person to person; factors other than those influencing bioavailability include the use of iron cooking utensils, which may add significant amounts, and the consumption of iron-containing tonics and medications.

The most severe test of the ability of the intestinal mucosa to protect the body against iron overload would be the consumption of medicinal iron for long periods. Unfortunately the information on this is quite inadequate at the present time and comprises only a few case reports. A number of anemic individuals have developed hemochromatosis after long-continued iron ingestion,[82,233,326, 401,413,414] but since the rate of absorption of iron may be enhanced by anemia, such reports are not relevant to the assessment of the risk to nonanemic subjects. Wheby[426] documented the presence of fully developed hemochromatosis with more than 20 g of storage iron in a non-anemic woman who had been taking iron therapy for a long time, while Hennigar and co-workers[204] reported the development of severe iron overload in a health faddist who had ingested large amounts of iron and vitamins over many years. In contrast, in a 55-year-old woman who had consumed 4644 g of iron in a tonic over a number of years the transferrin saturation was normal and there was no evidence of any of the tissue manifestations of hemochromatosis, although a liver biopsy was not performed.[304] A similar case has been described in which only mild hepatic siderosis was present after years of oral iron treatment.[154] The evidence is therefore confusing, and questions concerning the capability of the normal intestinal mucosa to withstand large amounts of oral iron will probably only be answered by serial measurements of plasma ferritin concentrations carried out over a period of years. Idiopathic hemochromatosis genes may play a part in those who do develop iron overload.

Other sources of excessive dietary iron include wines, which may contain large amounts. Concentrations as high as 90 mg/liter have been reported,[319] but it would appear that the usual figure is in the region of 5 mg/liter.[8,20,319] The iron is exogenous, and the variation can be ascribed to different methods of preparation. The bioavailability of such iron is probably low, since red wines contain polyphenolic compounds that inhibit iron absorption.[39]

It is well recognized that a significant proportion of subjects with hemochromatosis give a history of excessive alcohol consumption. The figure can be expected to vary according to social customs in the community and has ranged from 10% to 40%.[157,180,292,377] It appears that the alcohol may accelerate both the accumulation of iron and the damage to the tissues. In one study the average store of iron in alcoholic hemochromatotic patients was 24 g, compared with 16 g in nonalcoholic patients.[292] The sig-

nificant iron content of many wines has already been mentioned, but most alcoholic drinks have little or none; this is underscored by the finding of normal or even diminished iron stores in several studies of alcohol abusers.[269,270,277] Only 7% of 157 British alcoholics had significant hepatic siderosis as assessed histologically.[230] Other possible reasons for the association therefore deserve consideration.

It has been shown in acute experiments that alcohol enhances the absorption of ferric iron.[91] The importance of this is doubtful, however, since it appears to do so by stimulating acid secretion in the stomach, and many alcoholic subjects have hypochlorhydria from chronic gastritis.

There is evidence that iron absorption is increased in some patients with cirrhosis.[77,94,169,184,431] In the study described by Williams and co-workers,[431] one third of 47 cirrhotic patients absorbed increased amounts of iron, although they were not iron deficient. Some hemosiderosis was present in half of them, but it was generally slight and bore no relation to the absorption rate.

The possibility that alcohol might lead to increased iron absorption through pancreatic damage has also been considered. Davis and Badenoch[115] reported an increase in iron absorption in subjects with chronic pancreatic disease, but later studies have not substantiated this finding.[17,239,305]

A more likely reason for the strong association between symptomatic hemochromatosis and alcohol is that organ damage is accelerated. Alcohol is an accepted hepatotoxin, and it seems reasonable to conclude that individuals who do not drink may tolerate more iron than those who do. The descriptions of asymptomatic relatives with body iron burdens greater than 10 g[80,177,191,292] support this view. At the same time, there is no doubt that full-blown hemochromatosis can develop in individuals who have never drunk alcohol; this is most clearly demonstrated in very young patients.[92]

Although it is therefore clear that the presence of extraneous iron in the diet and the drinking of excessive alcohol may be expected to accelerate the accumulation of iron in susceptible individuals, it seems equally clear that hemochromatosis can develop in individuals who have never been exposed to anything but a normal diet containing a normal amount of iron.

Pathologic Findings

In established hemochromatosis the total iron content of the body is usually between 15 g and 40 g.[61,157,180,305,377] Storage iron concentrations are highest in the liver and pancreas, where they are between 50 and 100 times normal. In the thyroid the concentration is usually about 25 times normal, and in the heart and adrenals between 10 and 15 times normal. Lower concentrations of about 5 times normal are found in organs such as the skin, spleen, kidney, and stomach. Most of the iron present in these organs is visible histologically in the form of hemosiderin. In addition to hemosiderin, another pigment, "hemofuscin," has been observed. It is probably one of the lipo-fuscins and is not specific to hemochromatosis since it is found in old age and in cachectic states.[134] There is also an increase in the concentrations of other trace metals in hemochromatosis.[76] Of some interest is the observation that there is a relationship between the concentrations of manganese and iron in the livers of subjects with the disease,[4] since there is experimental evidence suggesting that the two metals are absorbed by similar mechanisms.[123]

Skin

It is often assumed that the pigmentation of the skin (a characteristic feature of patients with idiopathic hemochromatosis) is due to iron; however, it is present in increased amounts in only approximately half of the cases. When present, the hemosiderin is most obvious in the sweat glands, but deposits can also be seen in vascular endothelium and in the connective tissue of the corium. The majority of patients, including those with no excessive hemosiderin, show increased amounts of melanin in the deeper layers of the epidermis. Other features are atrophy of the epidermis, hair, and sebaceous glands.

Liver

The liver is usually considerably enlarged (average weight 2,400 g) and appears rusty red. A fine monolobular cirrhosis is almost invariably present, except in young subjects with the disease where lesser degrees of fibrous reaction have been found.[92] Rarely hepatic fibrosis may be absent despite massive iron overload and damage to other tissues.[292] In the typical advanced case the lobules are separated by wide bands of fibrous tissue, and sometimes a multinodular cirrhosis of the postnecrotic type is seen.[241] A characteristic pattern of fibrosis and lobular disruption of the liver has been recognized in nonalcoholic subjects.[335] Areas of partial preservation of the lobular structure may be found, with the central veins still identifiable in a fairly normal position. Bile duct proliferation is prominent and contrasts to the paucity of inflammatory cells. The bile duct epithelium invariably contains heavy deposits of hemosiderin, and although deposits are also present in Kupffer cells and in the fibrous connective tissue, there is far less than in some other forms of iron overload. The striking feature is the heavy deposition of hemosiderin granules in hepatocytes. These deposits are scattered throughout the lobules but tend to be heaviest in the periphery. The degree of hemosiderosis may vary from zone to zone and from lobule to lobule, tending to be less in areas of regeneration.[134] The hepatocytes are mostly normal in size and staining quality, but at the edge of the lobules they may be larger, with more prominent nucleoli and chromatin.[42] This is especially so in subjects with a history of excessive alcohol intake, in whom fatty change may also be present. As the cells degenerate, their nuclei become pyknotic and the iron released by them is taken up by the fibroblasts at the lobular periphery and in the portal spaces.

Carcinoma occurs as a complication in a proportion of cases,[157] usually in the form of hepatoma, but cholangiomas have also been reported.[134]

Information about the pathologic findings during the long asymptomatic period has been obtained from relatives of subjects with the disease on whom liver biopsies have been performed.[54,65,140,191,366] The histology has varied from total normality to the fully developed disease. In the early stages the iron is found as discrete granules of hemosiderin in the hepatocytes, either finely dispersed throughout the liver lobules or in focal scattered areas. Deposits tend to be greater at the periphery of the lobules. With larger quantities of iron it is aggregated into coarser masses and is more uniformly distributed. When hemosiderosis is marked, there is a slight to moderate increase in portal tract fibrosis, whereas true monolobular cirrhosis is seen only in association with the fully developed clinical disease.

Information about findings in other organs during the early stages of the disease is lacking, but it seems probable that most of the extra storage iron is initially located in the liver. This is certainly the pattern that has been found in experimental studies.[159,172,202] In animal experiments the iron delivered from the portal circulation appears to be incorporated first into cytoplasmic ferritin in the cells at the periphery of the hepatic lobules. As the concentration of ferritin increases it is converted into hemosiderin, which becomes the major compound in the cell.

Pancreas

The pancreas appears rust colored and is very firm. Fibrosis is almost invariably present with resulting disorganization of the gland. There is degeneration of acinar epithelium, and the islets of Langerhans are usually decreased in number.[377] Hemosiderin deposits are present in both the exocrine and endocrine cells but are more marked in the former.

Spleen

The spleen is usually somewhat enlarged, with an average weight of about 400 g, and it often shows congestive changes secondary to portal hypertension.[377] Although hemosiderin deposits may be seen, they are not prominent and are usually confined to the capsule, blood vessel walls, and trabeculae. Chemical analyses have confirmed that the iron concentrations in the spleen are relatively low.[92]

Bone Marrow

Chemical analysis of bone marrow trephine samples from subjects with idiopathic hemochromatosis has established that the concentrations are not significantly raised.[66] This emphasizes once again how minimal is the reticuloendothelial involvement in the disease.

Endocrine System

In addition to the islets of Langerhans, hemosiderin deposits are prominent in several endocrine glands, especially the epithelial cells of the thyroid, parathyroid, and anterior pituitary. In the adrenal they are usually confined to the zona glomerulosa. Testicular atrophy, particularly of the germinal epithelium, is present in about a fourth of patients, but hemosiderin deposits are usually scanty. Fibrosis is not a feature in any of these organs.

Gastrointestinal Tract

Hemosiderin is usually found in the mucosal cells of the stomach, and gastric biopsy has been suggested as a diagnostic procedure.[5] Deposits in the upper small bowel are, however, minimal or absent. This is another striking point of difference from dietary iron overload.

Joints

Synovial lining cells have been shown to be heavily laden with hemosiderin, and some fibrous thickening of the synovium has been described in certain cases.[11,129,193,243,369] The synovial fluid is normal.[243] Associated degenerative changes include separation of the superficial cartilage and clumping of the chondrocytes, as well as calcification of the fibrocartilage and hyaline cartilage.[11]

Heart

The pathology of the heart in hemochromatosis has been well described.[75] The weight of the heart is often two or three times normal. The ventricular walls are thickened, and iron pigment is visible in the myocardial fibers, espe-cially in the perinuclear region. Deposits tend to be more extensive in the ventricular than in the atrial myocardium, and also in contracting rather than in conducting tissue. In addition, degeneration, fragmentation, and necrosis of myocardial cells with myocardial fibrosis and interstitial edema have been described.[61,75,421]

Other Organs

Only small amounts of iron are present in the kidneys, in the convoluted tubules.[377] Small amounts of hemosiderin have also been described in striated muscle and in the choroid plexus. On the other hand, the deposits in the salivary and lacrimal glands, and in the submucous glands of the respiratory tract, are usually heavy. Iron may also be found in lymph nodes, especially those draining organs containing large quantities of iron.

Clinical Features

The clinical features associated with fully developed idiopathic hemochromatosis are shown in Figure 27-2.

Diabetes

Symptoms related to the onset of diabetes, including weight loss, lassitude, and weakness, are frequently present at the time of diagnosis. If diabetes is not overt, some degree of glucose intolerance can usually be demonstrated.[292] Although impaired exocrine pancreatic function may be demonstrable on special investigation, clinical evidence of exocrine pancreatic insufficiency is rare.[61] Insulin was formerly required by most patients with overt diabetes, but the proportion may be declining, perhaps as a result of earlier diagnosis.[292]

Fig. 27-2. The frequency with which various symptoms and signs occur in idiopathic hemochromatosis. (Bothwell TH et al: Iron Metabolism in Man. Oxford, Blackwell Scientific Publications, 1979)

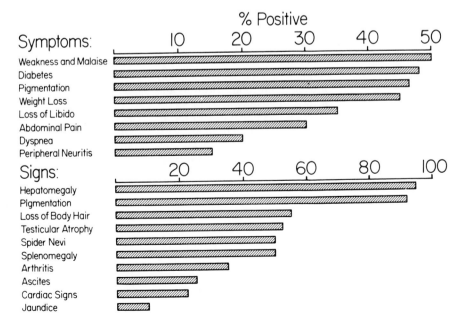

It was formerly assumed that the diabetes of hemochromatosis is the result of pancreatic islet failure, and low levels of circulating insulin have indeed been demonstrated in some patients.[136] The situation is more complicated, however, and at least two other factors may be implicated. Dymock and co-workers[136] found overt diabetes in 63% of 115 hemochromatotic patients; 25% of those with diabetes had a diabetic first-degree relative compared with only 4% of the nondiabetic group. An abnormal oral glucose tolerance test was found in one third of the remaining patients, and in some of these elevated serum insulin levels were demonstrated. Similar results were reported by Pozza and Ghidoni.[341] Balcerzak and colleagues[18] also showed that the incidence of diabetes in the relatives of subjects with hemochromatosis was high. It occurred in the absence of iron overload and was associated with high levels of circulating insulin. Another factor leading to the development of diabetes may be liver disease, since both insulin resistance[291] and hyperglucagonemia[378] are associated with cirrhosis. However, the iron overload may possibly exert a direct influence, since insulin resistance has been demonstrated in eight noncirrhotic individuals with idiopathic hemochromatosis whose glucose tolerance and glucagon concentrations were normal.[308] Stocks and Powell[393] found that the features of the disordered carbohydrate metabolism in idiopathic hemochromatosis and in other varieties of cirrhosis were similar, except for evidence of insulin deficiency in a proportion of the former.

On the basis of all of this evidence, it appears that at least three factors may play a part: (1) familial predisposition to develop diabetes; (2) diminished insulin sensitivity, due to cirrhosis and perhaps to iron overload as such; and (3) pancreatic insufficiency.

It has been stated that the vascular complications of diabetes are not common in idiopathic hemochromatosis,[377] although early vascular lesions of diabetic retinitis and intercapillary glomerulosclerosis have been described.[61] However, nephropathy, neuropathy, and peripheral vascular disease, either singly or together, were found in 22% of the patients studied by Dymock and co-workers,[136] and a similar number showed mild retinopathy with microaneurysms or exudates or both. Griffiths and co-workers[185] found diabetic retinopathy in 11 of 49 hemochromatotic patients, and it was noted in 6 of the 10 individuals who have been diabetic for 10 or more years, an incidence comparable to that found in diabetes mellitus. There is, however, evidence that the retinopathy may be milder than in idiopathic diabetes.[317]

Liver Involvement

The symptoms associated with involvement of the liver are nonspecific and include cachexia, weight loss, and weakness. Palmar erythema and spider angiomas are frequently present. Gynecomastia is unusual, but impotence, loss of libido, loss of body hair, and testicular atrophy are common; they are probably more often a manifestation of the endocrinopathy of hemochromatosis than of hepatic insufficiency. Splenomegaly is found in about 50% of subjects, but severe portal hypertension is much less common than with Laennec's cirrhosis, and esophageal varices are seen less frequently. Clinical evidence of ascites is also unusual.

The liver is almost always enlarged and firm, but hepatic function is often surprisingly good, provided the individual does not drink alcohol excessively.[157] Sulfobromophthalein excretion is normal in more than half of the patients, and abnormalities of turbidity tests are usually mild. The prothrombin time is abnormal in only one fourth of the cases, and the alkaline phosphatase is raised in about 20%. The serum albumin level is often normal; in one study the mean concentration was 3.3 g/dl[352] and in another, 3.7 g/dl.[292] The plasma glutamic oxalacetic transaminase concentration was raised in 15 of 28 patients, but in only 6 was it more than double the normal value, and the plasma bilirubin concentration was less than 1.3 mg/dl in all but 2. Minor changes in protein patterns have been recorded but are usually nonspecific and merely reflect impaired liver function or diabetes.

Liver disease in idiopathic hemochromatosis usually runs a prolonged and benign course, presumably because the majority of subjects do not consume alcohol excessively and do eat well. However, episodes of acute hepatic failure may occur, often provoked by blood loss or surgical procedures, and 25% of subjects eventually die of complications such as coma or gastrointestinal hemorrhage. In those patients whose liver function is more than mildly deranged when the diagnosis of hemochromatosis is made, the prognosis is poor. The median survival of four of seven patients whose serum albumin concentrations were less than 3.0 g/dl seen by Milder and co-workers[292] was 1.3 years; the other three were lost to follow-up. Ten of their patients had sulfobromophthalein retentions of more than 15%, and eight of these had encephalopathy, hepatoma, or congestive cardiac failure. The median survival of the seven who were followed was 2.1 years. It is noteworthy that six of the ten with marked sulfobromophthalein retention and five of the seven with hypoalbuminemia were alcoholics.

Hepatoma is an important late complication, and cholangiomas have also been reported.[61,348] The average incidence in a number of series is about 14%, but the risk appears not to be diminished by removal of the iron.[432] With the reduction in deaths due to cardiac and hepatic failure, the figure may be expected to rise. Six of 34 patients in one study[292] and no fewer than 29% of treated patients in another died of hepatoma.[44] The development of a hepatoma is suggested by the onset of unexplained weight loss, fever, nodular enlargement of the liver, ascites, jaundice, abdominal pain, anemia, or insulin insensitivity in a subject with previously well-controlled hemochromatosis.[157] There is suggestive evidence that nonhepatic carcinomas also occur more frequently than would be expected.[7]

Abdominal Pain

Abdominal pain occurs quite frequently and is sometimes the presenting symptom. Several types of pain have been described.[61] The most common is an aching sensation in the epigastrium or right hypochondrium, which may persist for long periods. The cause has been the subject of speculation, but one study[292] revealed a variety: in three patients it was ascribed to peptic ulceration; in four, to hepatoma; in three, to variceal bleeding; in three, to ascites; in three, to cholecystitis; and in one, to nephrolithiasis. More puzzling are the descriptions of the acute onset of excruciating pain in the disease, often associated with shock so that an abdominal emergency is simulated. The condition has been extensively reviewed by MacSween.[285] Later studies[12,349] have not supported the suggestion[290] that the release of ferritin into the circulation could be responsible through a vasodepressor action. It seems more likely that such episodes are due to gram-negative septicemia,[236] and *Escherichia coli* or *Pasteurella pseudotuberculosis* has been cultured from the blood or the peritoneum of several patients.[285,442] The possibly increased susceptibility of subjects with idiopathic hemochromatosis to such episodes has been attributed to the saturation of transferrin, since unsaturated transferrin has a bacteristatic effect that has been ascribed to its sequestration of iron required for the multiplication of iron-dependent microorganisms.[424] In experimental infections the injection of iron enhances bacterial virulence[61]; there is little clinical evidence, however, that individuals with saturated transferrin are more susceptible to infection. Furthermore, once an infection is present, the transferrin saturation falls.

Hypogonadism

Hypogonadism is a frequent finding in idiopathic hemochromatosis. Loss of libido, impotence, amenorrhea, sparse body hair, and testicular atrophy are common and almost invariable in young subjects. These are typical features of cirrhosis, but in hemochromatosis they may be present before liver function is significantly impaired. The body hair may be sparse for many years before other manifestations of the disease appear. Moreover, the gynecomastia that is characteristic of other varieties of cirrhosis is extremely uncommon in idiopathic hemochromatosis. Although cirrhosis may obviously play a part, it has now become clear that pituitary insufficiency is responsible for the hypogonadism in many subjects with idiopathic hemochromatosis. In a number of studies low circulating gonadotropin levels have been demonstrated and inadequate responses to gonadotrophin releasing hormone have also been noted.[6,38,87,292,392,393] In addition, a decrease in prolactin reserve has been described in some patients.[256,416] In contrast, the secretion of other trophic hormones is not impaired. Although mild hypothyroidism or hypoadrenalism has occasionally been demonstrated,[61] no functional abnormalities were found in three recent studies.[86,292,413] The nature of the lesion affecting gonadotrophic function, and whether it is at the pituitary or hypothalamic level, has not been elucidated.

Heart Complications

Cardiac complications in the form of right- and left-sided decompensation or arrhythmias are common. Twelve of 34 patients in one series developed congestive cardiac failure, and nine of these had significant arrhythmias; the average age at onset of cardiac symptoms was 56 years.[292] In young subjects cardiac complications are more frequently the presenting feature and almost always the cause of death, which follows within a year unless specific venesection therapy is instituted.[46,84] However, the cardiac symptoms and signs may initially be aggravated by venesection, and caution should be exercised.[231] In the older age-group it may be difficult to separate the contributions of hemochromatosis and ischemic heart disease to the pathogenesis of cardiac failure.

The onset may be acute, with the development of cardiac failure within a few days. Extreme degrees of pulmonary congestion and peripheral edema may be observed. Clinically, the picture is usually that of a congestive cardiomyopathy,[61] but restrictive features have also been described.[111,423] Both ventricles are usually dilated, and on radiographic investigation the cardiac profile has a globular appearance with decrease in the amplitude of the cardiac pulsations.

The presence of arrhythmias is a poor prognostic sign. The most common are ventricular extrasystoles, but supraventricular and ventricular tachycardias, ventricular fibrillation, and varying degrees of heart block may occur.[61] Other rather nonspecific electrocardiographic changes such as low voltage, left axis deviation, and flattening or inversion of T waves may be noted.

Skin Findings

Skin pigmentation is present in almost all subjects with the disease, especially in exposed areas and old scars, although it may not be so marked as to attract attention. When it is due to increased quantities of melanin, the skin has a bronze color, but in those individuals in whom iron deposits are also present, the color is slate-gray. Pigmentation of the conjunctiva and lid margin is found in about one third of patients; and of the oral mucosa in 10% to 15%.[113] The skin is typically fine and soft, and facial, pubic, and axillary hair are usually scanty, often for many years before the other features of the disease appear.[5]

Joint Involvement

Although arthropathy was recognized relatively recently to be a complication of idiopathic hemochromatosis,[369] it is frequently present. The reported prevalence has ranged from 25% to 75%,[121,129,149,166,193,365,422] and it rises the longer patients are kept under observation in spite of venesection therapy.[194] Arthritis may be the presenting feature.[10,178,213,302,365] Arthropathy has also been reported in other varieties of iron overload, including hereditary spherocytosis,[35,135] sideroblastic anemia,[163] and transfusional siderosis.[1,374]

Although virtually any joint may be affected, the most common symptoms are stiffness and pain in the hands, typically the second and third metacarpophalangeal joints and the proximal interphalangeal joints. The knees are also often affected. Involvement of other large joints may occasionally be disabling.

Superimposed on this chronic arthropathy may be acute attacks of inflammatory synovitis, which have been ascribed to the liberation of calcium pyrophosphate crystals into the synovial fluid.[3,193] Although the pathogenesis has not been firmly established, it has been suggested that the iron in the joint tissues may inhibit pyrophosphatase. Since this enzyme normally hydrolyzes pyrophosphate to soluble orthophosphate, deposition of pyrophosphate may result. Chondrocalcinosis and arthritis may progress or appear in spite of venesection treatment.[193,194] In some cases deposits of hemosiderin persist in the synovium and articular cartilage after venesection therapy.[243] Perhaps damage to the articular cartilage, once induced, is irreversible. However, the mechanism by which the cartilage is damaged has not been established, and indeed iron is not always visible in chondrocyte lacunae or in the synovium.[370]

Blood Findings

Changes in the blood are not remarkable in subjects with idiopathic hemochromatosis. The rates of red blood cell production and destruction are normal, and erythropoiesis is effective.[160] There may be mild macrocytosis consistent with the liver disease.[157] Iron-containing macrophages have been demonstrated in buffy-coat preparations of venous blood in approximately 50% of cases.[440] Occasional mild leukopenia and thrombocytopenia may be present, presumably as a result of hypersplenism. A rise in the leukocyte count, if unrelated to infection, uncontrolled diabetes, or cardiac failure, should raise suspicion of a developing hepatoma.[61] Blood coagulation studies are usually normal except for the hypoprothrombinemia that may accompany the liver disease. The relative normality of the blood findings in idiopathic hemochromatosis serves to distinguish it from a number of secondary forms of iron overload in which anemia is a constant and prominent feature.[61]

Diagnosis

The diagnosis of idiopathic hemochromatosis is usually suspected on the basis of the clinical history and the characteristic physical findings and may be missed unless it is considered "in every patient with cirrhosis of the liver, strange pigmentation of the skin, intractable heart disease, whether failure or arrhythmia or both, impotence or sterility, and, of course, diabetes mellitus."[109] To this list ar-

thritis must be added. Once suspected, the presence of grossly increased iron stores and any associated organ damage is confirmed by laboratory investigations. However, a detailed discussion of the special tests used for the assessment of hepatic, cardiac, endocrine, and pancreatic function is beyond the scope of this chapter.

In establishing the presence of iron overload it is useful to carry out the investigations in a certain order. The plasma iron concentration, the percentage saturation of the transferrin, and the plasma ferritin concentration should first be estimated. In normal subjects the plasma iron concentration is usually between 80 μg and 120 μg/dl and the unsaturated iron-binding capacity approximately 200 μg/dl. In untreated idiopathic hemochromatosis the total amount of circulating transferrin is usually less than normal because of the associated liver disease, but it is almost completely saturated with iron.[61] As a result, the plasma iron concentration is typically over 200 μg/dl, and the unsaturated iron-binding capacity appears to be up to 30 μg to 40 μg/dl; however, this is due to methodologic deficiencies since the transferrin is actually fully saturated.[99] The only exceptions are due to the presence of intercurrent infection or a hepatoma. In very rare instances a very high plasma iron concentration has been reported, and under such circumstances the iron is not bound to transferrin.[217] It is usually a terminal event, associated almost certainly with the release of ferritin from an anoxic liver, but it has also been observed in one subject during a phlebotomy program; at the time he appeared to be well.[61]

Although the finding of a high plasma iron concentration with saturation or near-saturation of the transferrin is thus almost invariable in subjects with idiopathic hemochromatosis, it is not diagnostic. It is also a feature of any anemia associated with ineffective erythropoiesis, and, in addition, occurs in affected relatives of patients with idiopathic hemochromatosis at a time when the stores are normal or only moderately increased. Further tests are therefore necessary in order to establish the quantities of storage iron present in the tissues.

The plasma ferritin concentration reflects the quantity of iron stored in the body in subjects with idiopathic hemochromatosis[30,261,340] and other forms of iron overload,[221,255,344] as well as in normal and iron-deficient subjects.[61] In untreated idiopathic hemochromatosis the values are typically several thousand micrograms per deciliter and there is a reasonably good correlation with the hepatic iron concentration.[342] As the iron is removed by venesection therapy, the plasma ferritin concentration decreases in parallel.[292] However, several families have been described in which the asymptomatic relatives of patients with idiopathic hemochromatosis had normal plasma ferritin concentrations in spite of considerably increased iron stores.[357,417] Halliday and co-workers[191] have observed this phenomenon in about 5% of relatives, although we have yet to encounter it. Whether these inconsistencies represent a different variety of hemochromatosis, an impairment in the production of plasma ferritin, or an antigenic variation resulting in a falsely low estimate, is not yet clear.

A noninvasive means of distinguishing between high plasma ferritin concentrations due to increased body iron stores and due to acute liver injury, inflammation, or neoplasia is the measurement of the chelator-induced urinary iron excretion. The two agents that have been used most extensively are the iron-specific desferrioxamine[19,21,110,153,201,222,266,328,388,389] and less often the nonspecific chelator diethylenetriamine penta-acetic acid (DTPA).[336,415] The chelating agent is injected intramuscularly, all urine passed over the following 6 to 24 hours is collected, and its iron content measured. A good correlation between the quantity of iron excreted and the amount of mobilizable storage iron in the body has been established.[389,413] Several variations of the basic procedure have been described, such as the concurrent administration of ^{59}Fe-ferrioxamine, which allows for calculation of the total amount of iron mobilized as the chelate.[153,155] However, these elaborations do not seem to have altered the general conclusions that have been reached.[61,195]

Although there is evidence from animal experiments that iron in both reticuloendothelial cells and hepatic parenchymal cells is chelated,[260] it has been suggested that the amount of iron mobilized by desferrioxamine correlates best with the quantity of storage iron in parenchymal tissue rather than in reticuloendothelial cells. Harker and co-workers[195] were able to show a moderately clear-cut separation between subjects with idiopathic hemochromatosis and those with other forms of iron overload. The average urinary iron excretion was 11 mg in idiopathic hemochromatosis, 6.0 mg in cirrhosis with parenchymal overload, 2.6 mg in cirrhosis with reticuloendothelial overload, and 1.2 mg without iron overload. Milder and co-workers[292] found a 24-hour urinary iron excretion of more than 8 mg of iron in 18 of 20 untreated patients with idiopathic hemochromatosis. One of the patients with a lower excretion had terminal hepatoma and the other had renal disease.

The total amount of storage iron in the body can also be estimated by performing weekly phlebotomies. The iron in the blood removed by venesection is replaced from the stores until these are exhausted, when the rate of red blood cell production falls and anemia develops. In normal subjects this occurs between the third and fourth weeks, after the removal of about 1 g of iron as hemoglobin. By the seventh week the anemia is severe. When iron overload is present, on the other hand, the hemoglobin concentration may remain near normal for many months. The quantity of iron removed, and hence the amount of storage iron originally present, may be estimated from the volume of blood removed and its hemoglobin concentration.[157]

Most of the superfluous iron is in the liver, and several new ways of assessing how much is present there have been described. The hepatic density quantitated by computed tomography correlates with the iron content.[85,176,216,265] An automated image analysis technique,[122] the nuclear resonance scattering of gamma rays,[407] and the measurement of magnetic susceptibility[69] have also been shown to provide a good indication of the amount present. Wherever the necessary equipment and expertise is available these techniques may prove useful.

In addition to establishing that iron overload is present, it is important to determine whether the parenchymal cells contain excessive amounts or whether it is predominantly the reticuloendothelial cells that are involved, since iron in the latter site is relatively innocuous. Parenchymal cell loading is found in idiopathic hemochromatosis, and the reticuloendothelial cells contain much less iron.[58] Needle biopsy of the liver provides this information, and in addition allows the extent of hepatic fibrosis to be assessed. However, as has been pointed out previously, iron deposits become visible histologically in suitably stained sections of liver at relatively low concentrations. Although it is therefore possible to suspect that a patient has idiopathic hemochromatosis from the degree of siderosis visible on the liver biopsy section, one of the methods described above must be employed to verify that the quantities of storage iron present in the body are indeed grossly increased. It has been shown that this can also be achieved by estimating the iron concentrations in the liver biopsy specimen, either by simple chemical methods[21,168] or by atomic absorption spectrophotometry.[36,398]

The measurement of the ferritin content of the red blood cells has been claimed to provide an estimate of iron overload[406] and deserves further study.

Other methods of diagnosis have been used in the past. These include the demonstration of hemosiderin in the urine, in the skin, in the stomach mucosa, and in the reticuloendothelial cells of the bone marrow.[157] However, none of these methods is even semiquantitative and they may give misleading results. For this reason they are not recommended at the present time.

A number of ferrokinetic studies have also been done in idiopathic hemochromatosis. It has been suggested that ferrokinetic measurements allow the differentiation of cirrhosis with hyperferremia from idiopathic hemochromatosis, there being a greater nonerythroid iron turnover in the latter condition. However, kinetic studies in which the early hepatic uptake of iron was measured have not shown any significant differences. It has been suggested that the reported lower red blood cell utilization was due to incomplete transferrin binding of the injected radiolabeled iron.[160]

Before leaving the question of diagnosis, the place of radiolabeled iron absorption studies should be considered. The disease is due to the inappropriate absorption of increased amounts of iron from a normal diet, and this increase in iron absorption presumably occurs over extended periods. Although results obtained in subjects during the clinical phase of the condition have been variable, the majority have been within the normal range.[149] Radiolabeled iron absorption is therefore not a useful method of diagnosing established hemochromatosis, but it may be helpful in uncovering affected relatives. However, iron absorption is so profoundly affected by the body storage iron content of the individual that the results should be considered in conjunction with information on the size of the stores.[59,403] Milder and co-workers[293] have described a test that distinguishes affected individuals from normal subjects by relating the plasma ferritin concentration to the plasma iron concentration after the ingestion of a meal.

The responsibility of the physician does not end with the diagnosis of hemochromatosis in his patient; it is mandatory to track down every blood relative and to identify those who are also affected before they have accumulated enough iron to cause organ damage. The combination of plasma ferritin and transferrin saturation measurements provides the best screen for this purpose. The amount of superfluous iron present can then be estimated in those with high values by the techniques described previously. Since the whole question of preclinical iron overload has become such an important one in the recent past, it is discussed more fully in a later section.

Differential Diagnosis

Although it is customary to mention Addison's disease, argyria, and various other conditions in the differential diagnosis of fully developed idiopathic hemochromatosis, there are only two real problems.

The first lies in its separation from alcoholic cirrhosis with some degree of iron overload. Many individuals with idiopathic hemochromatosis are also alcoholic, and reasons for the association have been considered previously. Many of the features of alcoholic liver disease are similar to those of hemochromatosis, namely the hepatomegaly, the carbohydrate intolerance, the hypogonadism, and the pigmentation. The plasma ferritin concentration and the transferrin saturation are elevated, although out of proportion to the body iron content. Subjects with alcoholic cirrhosis normally have greater impairment of hepatic function and may have other stigmata such as peripheral neuropathy, while cardiac manifestations are much less common. On histologic examination of the liver the hemosiderin loading is less and it is predominantly the Kupffer cells rather than the parenchymal cells that are affected. Features of alcoholic liver disease such as fatty degeneration of the hepatocytes and partial inflammatory infiltrates are unusual in idiopathic hemochromatosis. On the basis of an extensive study, Powell and Kerr[335] concluded that the findings in idiopathic hemochromatosis were distinctive. Areas could be found where the lobular architecture was partially preserved with central veins identifiable in fairly normal position. Other useful diagnostic features included the relatively smooth contours of the nodules and lobules, the absence of piecemeal necrosis, and the structural normality of the hepatocytes. In the majority of those patients with idiopathic hemochromatosis who drank excessively a similar pattern was noted. It cannot be overemphasized, however, that the major differentiating point relates to the degree of iron overload. As mentioned previously, it is extremely uncommon for subjects with other forms of cirrhosis to accumulate very large quantities of iron. It is of course possible for the two conditions to co-exist; this can be elucidated by HLA typing and by investigation of the family members.

The second problem arises if the quantity of iron is indeed in the hemochromatotic range, when the idiopathic disease must be distinguished from the other varieties of iron overload. It is usually simple enough to detect the presence of thalassemia or one of the other chronic anemias that may lead to iron loading, and the only real difficulty arises in the rare patient (outside southern Africa) in whom the combination of alcohol or liver disease and the prolonged consumption of large amounts of absorbable iron have resulted in a picture that can be very similar to that of idiopathic hemochromatosis. The possibility exists that those alcoholic subjects who develop iron overload are heterozygous for the mutant gene for idiopathic hemochromatosis, although determination of HLA-A and HLA-B antigens in such individuals and their families does not support this hypothesis.[384] On the basis of the findings in black South Africans (discussed in a subsequent section of this chapter), it would be reasonable to expect a much greater involvement of the reticuloendothelial system, and histologic examination of the liver may enable them to be distinguished from idiopathic hemochromatosis.

Whether subjects who have had portacaval shunts represent a special group is still a matter of debate. The presence of portacaval anastomosis has been reported to lead rapidly to the development of iron overload.[70,126,138,179,311,358,401] The exact significance of so-called hemochromatosis after shunt operations is, however, still very unclear. Although the development of such features as pigmentation and diabetes mellitus within relatively short periods after the operation has been reported, there is virtually no information on how much iron was present in the bodies of such individuals. In the four patients in whom the hepatic iron content has been recorded, it was less than 4 g, a figure lower than would be expected in the idiopathic disease. Furthermore, the degree of siderosis found in the careful study by Williams and co-workers[431] was slight and the iron absorption was not different from that of unoperated patients. It therefore seems that judgment should be suspended until more quantitative data have been collected.

Treatment

The treatment of idiopathic hemochromatosis can be considered under two major headings: supportive and definitive. Supportive therapy consists of the control of diabetes and hepatic and cardiac failure along conventional lines, although the value of β-adrenergic blocking agents for the control of supraventricular arrhythmias should be mentioned. In addition, loss of libido and secondary sexual characteristics is often benefited by an androgen.[61]

The definitive therapy of idiopathic hemochromatosis is to remove the excess iron. The most effective method is by repeated venesection.[157] Each pint of blood contains approximately 200 mg of iron, and a similar quantity must then be mobilized from the tissues to replace it. Many studies have confirmed that most patients can tolerate the removal of a pint of blood per week for prolonged periods. In fact, there are those who advocate even more frequent venesections. Crosby[107] was able to demonstrate a maximum hemopoietic response of three to six times normal in a subject from whom over 50 liters were removed in 1 year. However, patients with hemochromatosis usually maintain a hemopoietic rate of only two to three times normal during venesection therapy.[160] Before initiating the venesection program it is important to assess the degree of cardiac involvement, using radiography, electrocardiography, and echocardiography.[206] If there is evidence of cardiac irritability, it is advisable to give continuous infusions of desferrioxamine while the initial venesections are cautiously performed in order to protect the myocardium from free iron that may be mobilized.

During a course of weekly phlebotomies the hemoglobin concentration initially falls somewhat, but once the erythrocyte production rate has increased the hematocrit returns to within 10% of its initial level (Fig. 27-3). It is customary to estimate the hematocrit before each phlebotomy and the plasma iron concentration and the plasma ferritin concentration once a month. The depletion of the superfluous tissue iron stores can be effectively monitored via the serial plasma ferritin estimations. Weekly venesections must usually be continued for 2 to 3 years in order to remove 20 g to 40 g of iron, but in some patients the quantity present is not as great as this.[431] In most subjects the plasma iron concentration remains high dur-

Fig. 27-3. Serial changes in the hematocrit, plasma iron concentration, total iron-binding capacity, and plasma ferritin concentration in a subject with idiopathic hemochromatosis on repeated venesection therapy. (Bothwell TH et al: Iron Metabolism in Man. Oxford, Blackwell Scientific Publications, 1979)

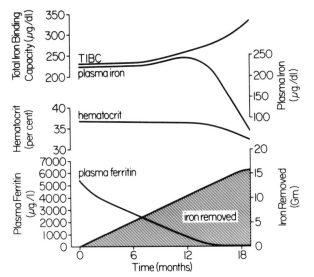

ing the course of venesection therapy, and only begins to fall when tissue iron stores are reaching exhaustion. However, occasionally an apparent iron-deficient state may occur early, presumably because the release of iron from stores is somewhat defective. Ascorbic acid deficiency, which inhibits the mobilization of hemosiderin iron,[258] may be responsible and the effect of ascorbic acid supplements can be assessed. Caution should, however, be exercised, since there is some evidence that the too-rapid mobilization of free iron in response to the repair of ascorbic acid deficiency may result in parenchymal cell damage; the myocardium is particularly vulnerable,[205] and it is possible that the ascorbic acid deficiency, which is a consequence of iron overload,[67,418] is actually protective. Instead of administering ascorbic acid, the rate of venesection may be slowed for a period, when a satisfactory response usually returns.[107] Another possible reason for the development of anemia early in the course of venesections is the presence of a hepatoma, and this should always be considered.

Subjects with idiopathic hemochromatosis withstand repeated venesections surprisingly well. A moderately high-protein diet is recommended, but usually the plasma albumin concentration remains within the normal range. In alcoholic subjects, however, this program may have to be modified and plasma may have to be replaced if hypoproteinemia is to be avoided. We have treated a patient with the restrictive form of cardiomyopathy who developed hypovolemic shock each time he underwent venesection. This was prevented by administering plasma at the same time as the venesection was carried out, and eventually a very satisfactory result was obtained. In passing, it should be mentioned that an iron-free diet is unnecessary. Such diets are unpalatable, and the amount absorbed from a normal diet is small in relation to the quantities removed by a vigorous venesection program. Once all mobilizable stores have been removed, the patient can be kept in iron balance by phlebotomies at intervals of 2 to 3 months.

The alternative to venesection therapy is the use of a chelating agent, but the rate of removal of iron from the body is much slower than with venesection.[203] In addition, the chelator has to be administered by daily injection. The average daily urinary iron excretion when DTPA is used would appear to be about 10 mg, a figure severalfold less than would be achieved by removing 500 ml blood weekly. In addition, severe toxic reactions, including renal damage, have been reported. Desferrioxamine has the advantage of being virtually nontoxic, but again the daily urinary iron excretion is only between 10 mg and 20 mg. Although there is evidence that some iron is also lost in the feces,[195] chelating agents should currently only be used in the cardiac patient who cannot tolerate phlebotomies, or as an adjunct to phlebotomy therapy in such patients. Under these circumstances, continuous or subcutaneous infusion is more effective than repeated injections. The technique is discussed in the section on the iron-loading anemias.

There is no longer room for serious doubt that the removal of excessive iron stores improves the symptoms, signs, and long-term prognosis. Bomford and Williams[44] compared the clinical effects in 85 treated and 26 untreated patients. Hepatic function improved in 28% of them. Other workers have noted impressive improvements in hepatic histology, with apparent regression of hepatic fibrosis,[71,180,240,242,426] and objective evidence of regression of the cardiopathy has been reported on a number of occasions.[2,44,78,137,148,186,226,250,275,386,432] All in all, the most impressive evidence for the beneficial effects of venesection therapy in idiopathic hemochromatosis is the survival figures reported by Bomford and Williams.[44] Life table data showed that the percentage survival 5 and 10 years after diagnosis was 66% and 32%, respectively, for the treated patients, and 18% and 6%, respectively, for the untreated patients (Fig. 27-4). After correcting for differences between the two groups by the use of covariant analysis, log survival values of 4.15 and 2.88, respectively, for the treated and untreated patients were obtained, equivalent to 63.4 months and 17.8 months. However, portal hypertension, testicular atrophy, and arthropathy are not improved, and despite the longer survival with venesection therapy, the incidence of hepatoma and of other malignant neoplasms remains high. Bomford and Williams[44] reported that hepatoma was the cause of death in 29% of subjects and other tumors in 22%, in spite of the fact that the excess iron had in many cases been removed a number of years before the neoplasms became manifest. The necessity of identifying affected relatives of probands, and instituting venesection treatment during the asymptomatic phase of the disease, is underlined by these findings.

The Widening Clinical Spectrum of Idiopathic Hemochromatosis

A number of workers have used the HLA system as a linked marker to detect homozygous and heterozygous relatives of subjects with fully developed hemochromatosis.[24,25,31,80,98,112,128,140,141,142,143,244,314,316,382,383,386,404] Information has been gathered on the degree of iron overload present, usually by means of the transferrin saturation and the plasma ferritin concentration. The transferrin saturation was found to be above 62% in 92% of adult homozygous subjects,[112] and it has also been shown to be increased in a proportion of heterozygotes.[25,80] However, the specificity of this test is reduced by the relatively high proportion of both false positives and false negatives.[191] In an unselected population a transferrin saturation greater than 70% was found in 1.7% of samples[315]; it was caused by physiologic fluctuations in 44%, liver disease in 22%, blood disorder in 10%, iron therapy in 10.5%, and parenchymal iron overload in only 11.5%. For this reason it is customary to combine the measurement of the transferrin saturation with that of the plasma ferritin concentration, since the latter is usually above the normal age adjusted range before there is any evidence of morphologic liver damage.[25]

Homozygotes

Family studies have revealed that the majority of homozygous individuals are asymptomatic[80] and that the classic hemochromatosis syndrome of hepatomegaly, skin pigmentation, and diabetes is uncommon.[301] Adult male siblings with the same two HLA haplotypes as a patient suffering from the clinical disease can be expected to have a transferrin saturation greater than 70% and a raised ferritin concentration. Ferritin concentrations are usually lower in females and may be within the normal range.[25,142] In one study of 35 homozygotes, half the subjects had hepatomegaly, cirrhosis, and skin pigmentation, while diabetes was present in less than 10% and cardiac failure in none.[142] Moreover, the prevalence of pathology in this study was considerably inflated by the fact that 14 of the subjects were probands. In another investigation only affected individuals who were younger than 35 years were studied; 29 of 34 of them were relatives diagnosed in family studies. Sixty-five percent of the males and 82% of the females were asymptomatic, while 26% of the males and 55% of the females showed no abnormal signs at all.[23] The most prevalent abnormalities were hepatomegaly (70% of males and 27% of females) and skin pigmentation (61% of males and 36% of females). Of interest was the fact that neither diabetes nor arthropathy was present in any subject. It was noted that the plasma ferritin concentration correlated well with the size of the initial iron stores, as judged by the amount of iron subsequently removed by venesection. Furthermore, all subjects with significant hepatic fibrosis or cirrhosis had plasma ferritin concentrations greater than 700 μg/dl. Another analysis was carried out on 60 subjects, the majority of whom had been identified in screening surveys. The hepatic architecture was found to be normal in 19, while slight to moderate fibrosis was present in 22 and cirrhosis in 4. A striking correlation was found between the degree of iron overload and the serum SGOT.[316] On the basis of their findings

Fig. 27-4. Life-table survival curves after diagnosis in treated and untreated groups of patients with idiopathic hemochromatosis. The vertical lines at each time interval represent ± 1 SE. (Bomford A, Williams R: Q J Med (New Series) 45:611, 1976)

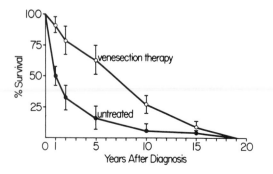

these workers suggested that any patient, and especially a male, with unexplained "transaminitis" should be investigated for iron overload.

Heterozygotes

Phenotypic expression in heterozygotes has been characterized in family studies in which affected individuals have been identified by HLA typing. Mean values for plasma iron concentration, transferrin saturation, and plasma ferritin concentration tend to be somewhat higher than in normal subjects, but there is a good deal of overlap.[25,31,80] In one study there was a tendency for hepatic iron concentrations to rise slightly with age so that a minor iron load had accumulated by middle age,[31,80] but in another investigation in which affected individuals were followed over a number of years, no such tendency was noted.[25] No clinical manifestations of hemochromatosis have been noted in heterozygotes.

The possibility exists that such extraneous factors as alcoholism, porphyria cutanea tarda, and accelerated erythropoiesis might lead to the clinical expression of iron overload in individuals heterozygous for the HLA-linked iron-loading gene. However, the HLA antigens that are associated with the disorder have been reported not to occur with increased frequency in subjects with the combination of iron overload and alcoholic liver disease.[385] The subject is nevertheless one that merits more study, since there is some suggestion that iron loading may tend to occur in those subjects with refractory sideroblastic anemia who also carry a single iron-loading gene.[81] Similar observations have been made in hereditary spherocytosis.[41,444] Finally, a significant correlation has been noted between the presence of HLA antigens A3, B7, and B14 and a raised plasma ferritin concentration in patients with chronic renal failure on maintenance hemodialysis.[64]

IRON OVERLOAD IN SOUTH AFRICAN BLACKS

Marked siderosis resulting from the presence of excessive absorbable iron in the diet is certainly rare in all populations that have been studied, with the single exception of the blacks of southern Africa. Strachan[394] first drew attention to the high incidence of iron overload in black South Africans. Subsequently it has become apparent that it also occurs in blacks in other parts of Africa south of the Sahara, including Zimbabwe, Malawi, Zambia, Botswana, Ghana, and Tanzania.[57,73,74,171] These people have been referred to as "Bantu" in most publications, but this is not linguistically correct. Dietary iron overload in people of East Indian or European descent in these countries is as rare as it is elsewhere in the world.

The prevalence of hepatic siderosis in black South Africans dying in Johannesburg hospitals was reported in 1962 to be as high as 70% of adult males and 25% of adult females.[53] In 20% of the males the hepatic iron concen-

trations were above 0.5 g/100 g wet weight, a figure comparable with that found in idiopathic hemochromatosis. The prevalence and the severity increased with age. A similar study carried out in 1979 revealed that both the prevalence and the severity had decreased by as much as 50%.[284] This has been ascribed to a decline in the consumption of the home-brewed alcoholic drinks that are the major source of the iron. They have largely been replaced by conventional beers, spirits, and wines and by commercial sorghum beers of low iron content.

Etiology

The iron content of the diet is very high.[56,411] Although some of the exogenous dietary iron may be derived from iron cooking pots, the major source is the iron drums used for the preparation of fermented sorghum and maize alcoholic beverages. The low pH of these brews leads to the ready solution of the iron, and the average concentration in a number of different samples was found to be 4 mg/dl; many contained a good deal more than this.[56] The alcohol content is low, and large volumes are consumed. Calculations based on these data and on the analysis of feces indicate that many males ingest in beer alone between 50 mg and 100 mg of iron daily. This is severalfold greater than the total of 10 mg to 30 mg of poorly bioavailable iron consumed by most people living in Western countries.

Iron is poorly absorbed from porridge made from maize or sorghum, presumably because of the formation of nonabsorbable complexes,[287] but absorption from beers made from these cereals is significantly better, and equivalent to that from a solution of ferric chloride.[56] The bioavailability of the iron improves at each stage of the brewing process, and it appears that the formation of lactic acid and alcohol and the removal of grits all play some part.[120]

Distribution of Iron

In the earliest stages there is an increase in the number of hemosiderin granules in the parenchymal and Kupffer cells of the liver.[47] When the hepatic iron concentrations are 5 to 10 times normal the deposits in these cells become denser, and at this stage the portal tract macrophages are also involved. When the concentrations reach 20 times normal, heavy deposits are seen in all three sites. Hemosiderin is visible in the spleen from an early stage, and with more severe degrees of iron overload the concentration in this organ may even exceed those in the liver. Reticuloendothelial involvement is also apparent in the bone marrow, which may contain as much as 10 g of storage iron.[170] There is a moderately close correlation between the amounts of storage iron in the marrow and in the liver over a wide range. The amount of iron located in the skeletal muscle also increases, about 6-fold in subjects with a 30-fold increase in liver iron.[399] Some of this iron is present within the muscle fibers, but the remainder is in tissue histiocytes lying between them.[405] In the duodenum and upper jejunum there are dense deposits in the lamina propria near the tips of the villi.[396] It is not clear whether this iron is in transit into or out of the body, but if it is the former, the turnover is slow, since no change could be detected after several weeks on a low-iron diet.[60]

Iron deposits elsewhere in the body are relatively scanty in the majority of subjects, so that the hepatocyte and the reticuloendothelial cell are principally involved. This distribution is notably different from that in idiopathic hemochromatosis, in which reticuloendothelial deposits are not prominent. In addition, the involvement of parenchymal cells in such structures as the pancreas, endocrine glands, and heart—a characteristic feature of idiopathic hemochromatosis—is rare in siderotic South African blacks and is found only under very special circumstances.

The difference between the localization of the iron in the two conditions is well illustrated by findings in the liver itself. In idiopathic hemochromatosis the major deposits are in parenchymal cells, and there is little iron present in portal tract phagocytes, whereas the Kupffer cells and portal tract phagocytes are heavily involved in siderotic South African blacks.[57] The contrasting patterns of iron distribution in the liver are apparent under both light microscopy (Fig. 27-5) and electron microscopy (Fig. 27-6). The difference is also striking in the spleen, in which the amount of iron is severalfold greater than in the idiopathic disease.

The reason for these differences has excited much interest, and while there are several clues, it must be accepted that there is as yet no certainty. Which distribution can,

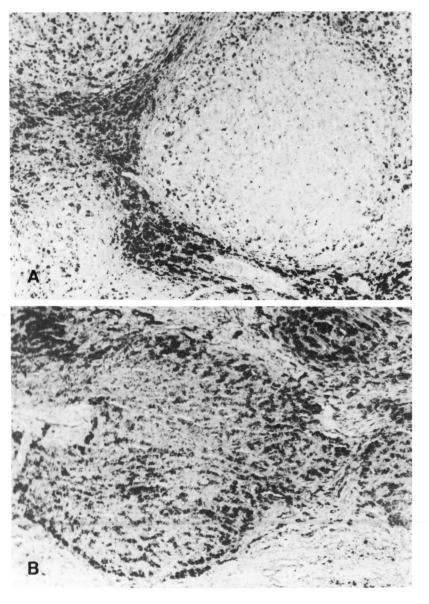

Fig. 27-5. Comparison between the distributions of hepatic hemosiderin in a black South African with iron overload (*A*) and in a patient with idiopathic hemochromatosis (*B*). In the black subject, the major deposits are in Kupffer cells and in the portal tracts, whereas in the patient with idiopathic hemochromatosis they are in hepatocytes. (Original magnifications × 30)

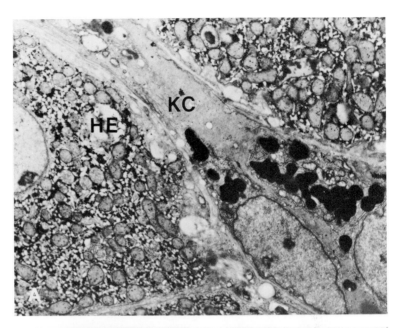

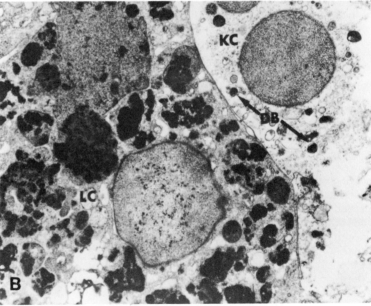

Fig. 27-6. Electron microscopic findings in a black South African with iron overload (*A*) and in a patient with idiopathic hemochromatosis (*B*). In *A,* it can be seen that the Kupffer cell (*KC*) contains an abundance of iron in the form of complex hemosiderin bodies. Some iron is present also in hepatocytes (*HE*), although there is much less than in the Kupffer cell. *B* shows the iron distribution in idiopathic hemochromatosis. An abundance of iron is seen in the liver cell (*LC*). The Kupffer cell contains dense bodies (*DB*); however, these do not contain iron. (Original magnification: *A,* × 9000; *B,* × 14,000) (Photographs courtesy of Dr. Geoffrey Kent)

in fact, be regarded as "normal?" A pointer to the answer may be that the distribution found in Africans resembles that described in many animal experiments in which iron overload has been created by feeding excess iron.[159,172,202] It has therefore been suggested that the marked involvement of parenchymal cells in idiopathic hemochromatosis is due to the release by the reticuloendothelial cells of excessive quantities of iron into the plasma. In favor of this concept is the experimental evidence indicating that the uptake of iron by parenchymal cells is facilitated by a high percentage saturation of circulating transferrin. This has been observed in some relatives of subjects with id-

iopathic hemochromatosis long before significant iron accumulation has occurred,[54] suggesting that defective reticuloendothelial function is one manifestation of the fundamental biochemical defect. If this supposition is right, then the massive reticuloendothelial iron deposits in dietary iron overload might result from the utilization for erythropoiesis of more newly absorbed iron than is normal. Less iron from catabolized red blood cells would be returned to the plasma, and the balance would be retained as hemosiderin within the reticuloendothelial cells.

A second possible explanation is that the excessive accumulation of reticuloendothelial iron in the dietary form of iron overload is due to a defect in iron release. Evidence has been obtained that ascorbic acid is necessary for the release of iron by reticuloendothelial cells[258] and ascorbic acid deficiency is widespread among severely siderotic blacks.[372] Furthermore, it has been shown that the administration of ascorbic acid to such subjects produces an immediate rise in the plasma iron concentration.[420] The further implications of these findings are discussed in a later section.

The hepatic parenchymal iron deposits found with all degrees of overload in the dietary condition can be explained if due attention is paid to the fact that the superfluous iron has been absorbed from the gut. The percentage saturation of the transferrin in portal venous blood may well be high in conditions where increased quantities of iron are being absorbed, and this would be expected to lead to deposition of iron in the hepatocytes during the first passage of the blood through the liver.

Direct Sequelae of Iron Overload

Most siderotic blacks do not have very large concentrations of iron in the body, and there is no evidence that any harm results. In fact, just the opposite occurs since the prevalence of iron deficiency anemia is low compared with similar population groups elsewhere. Iron deficiency is relatively uncommon even in pregnant women. It is only in the infants and children that iron deficiency is a problem and that iron overload is unknown.

Pathologic features ascribable to iron overload are, however, encountered in many of those individuals in whom the siderosis is severe. Since a large proportion of the superfluous iron is present in the liver, most attention has been paid to this organ. Several studies have shown a correlation between the degree of siderosis and the presence of portal fibrosis or cirrhosis.[53,63,210,225] Portal fibrosis is the usual finding, but in a small proportion of severely siderotic subjects frank micronodular cirrhosis develops. When this type of cirrhosis is present at necropsy there is almost invariably also severe siderosis, as judged by both histologic and chemical criteria. In contrast, no correlation has been found between the presence of macronodular cirrhosis and the quantity of iron.[225] It should be emphasized, however, that portal fibrosis or micronodular cirrhosis is by no means invariably present in individuals with severe siderosis. In one study as many as one third of subjects over the age of 50 with iron concentrations above 0.5 g/100 g wet weight did not even have significant portal fibrosis.[53] It is also noteworthy that the decline in the prevalence of severe siderosis in Johannesburg blacks has been accompanied by an increase in the prevalence of cirrhosis.[284] It seems probable that both phenomena can be ascribed to the switch from the traditional brews to Western-type liquor containing no iron but more alcohol.

One other point of interest relates to the association between portal cirrhosis in siderotic South African blacks

and the presence of significant hemosiderin deposits in the parenchymal cells of a number of other organs. As mentioned previously, this is not normally a feature of the condition, but when micronodular cirrhosis is present, iron may be seen in the pancreas (where both acinar and islet cells are involved), thyroid, adrenals, pituitary, and myocardium.[63,225] The findings are therefore very similar to those described in idiopathic hemochromatosis, the only difference being the large quantities of hemosiderin in the reticuloendothelial cells of the liver and spleen. The incidence of this dietary form of hemochromatosis is difficult to gauge. However, necropsy data suggest that in 1961 the figure was about 3% of adult blacks dying in hospitals in the Johannesburg area.[225] The different distribution of the hemosiderin deposits in the presence of cirrhosis is not merely a function of the degree of overload, which is often no greater than in noncirrhotic individuals. It is associated with a change in the percentage saturation of circulating transferrin. In subjects with siderosis but no cirrhosis, plasma iron levels are often not raised[420] and the percentage saturation is usually normal. With the development of cirrhosis, however, less transferrin is produced, and the percentage saturation is often considerably above normal; why it should rise is not clear. In any event, parenchymal cell uptake of iron has been shown to increase in parallel with the transferrin saturation.[100]

The resemblance to idiopathic hemochromatosis extends also to an association with diabetes. In one necropsy study, more than 20% of subjects with these pathologic features had been diabetic[225] while in a survey of living diabetics about 7% were found to have dietary hemochromatosis.[371] These individuals were mainly underweight middle-aged males. A firm hepatomegaly was always present, and features of portal hypertension and liver failure were often obvious. Tuberculosis and porphyria cutanea tarda with increased urinary excretion of uroporphyrin were common complications. The diabetes was typically severe and labile, and hypoglycemic episodes were common. Prognosis was found to be poor, mainly because of the severity and progression of the cirrhosis. Data concerning growth hormone and insulin levels are not yet available. This clinical picture is quite different from the more common form of diabetes encountered in South African blacks. As in whites, most of these individuals are middle-aged obese females, and the condition responds well to weight reduction alone or to oral hypoglycemic agents.

Siderosis, Scurvy, and Osteoporosis

Two other conditions have been noted in association with severe siderosis in South African blacks, namely, ascorbic acid deficiency and osteoporosis. The results of a number of studies suggest that these three conditions are causally related.[372] This evidence warrants brief consideration, since the association may be found in other forms of iron overload.

Siderosis and Scurvy

Ascorbic acid deficiency is extremely rare in black infants in spite of the fact that other nutritional disorders occur commonly, and siderosis also does not occur in this age-group. In contrast, biochemical evidence of ascorbic acid deficiency is present in virtually all black adults with iron overload, and frank scurvy is not uncommon.[372] Although it might be argued that each is merely the consequence of alcoholism and malnutrition, there are reasons for believing that this is not so. First, it has been possible to show that ascorbic acid metabolism is abnormal in blacks with severe iron overload. Repeated administration of large doses of ascorbic acid to normal subjects results after 1 or 2 days in most of the administered vitamin being excreted unchanged in the urine. In severely siderotic individuals, on the other hand, only a small fraction is recoverable in the urine, but the excretion of its irreversible oxidation product, oxalic acid, increases markedly.[273,368] The oxidation of the ascorbic acid has been ascribed to the large ferric iron deposits in the tissues, since there is in vitro evidence that ferric iron catalyzes the first step in the oxidative sequence. Another pointer to a direct relationship is the fact that low leukocyte ascorbic acid values have also been noted in well-nourished white subjects with other forms of iron overload, including idiopathic hemochromatosis and transfusional siderosis.[67,296,312,418] In addition, guinea pigs made siderotic by injecting iron dextran become scorbutic even though their diet contains adequate ascorbic acid.[421]

Siderosis and Osteoporosis

Spinal osteoporosis is common in middle-aged black males.[372] For example, in one survey of 110 asymptomatic manual laborers, 17 were found to have radiologic evidence of the condition.[272] In a small proportion of subjects, the osteoporosis is severe enough to produce vertebral collapse with resultant clinical symptoms. Although the usual presentation is low back pain, there is also an unduly high frequency of femoral head collapse.[390] The frequency of osteoporosis in this age- and sex-group is of considerable interest, since it is extremely rare in other populations. Furthermore, the common variety of osteoporosis seen in elderly women is rare in South African blacks.

An association between this form of bone disease and the presence of severe iron overload has been demonstrated.[372] In addition, the chemical analysis of necropsy specimens indicates that there is an inverse correlation between the hepatic iron concentration and the mineral density of iliac crest bone.[272]

The frequency of osteoporosis in other forms of iron overload has not been well documented, although there are descriptions in both the American and French literature[119] of its occurrence in patients with idiopathic hemochromatosis. There is also one report from New Zealand of beef cattle exposed to water with a high iron content (up to 20 mg/ml); they developed not only a form of siderosis very similar to that seen in South African blacks, but also osteoporosis of the vertebrae, sternum, and ribs.[200]

Osteoporosis and Scurvy

There is a significant association between osteoporosis and scurvy in South African blacks.[188,372] It has also been shown that leukocyte ascorbic acid concentrations are extremely low in osteoporotic blacks even in the absence of frank scurvy.[272]

Pathogenetic Relationships Among Iron Overload, Ascorbic Acid Deficiency, and Osteoporosis

The findings suggest that severe iron overload in South African blacks leads to a state of chronic ascorbic acid deficiency, and that this in turn is one of the factors involved in the production of osteoporosis.[372] The evidence that iron overload interferes with the metabolism of ascorbic acid seems strong. The dietary ascorbic acid content is also usually low in such individuals.[273] There is some evidence, although not completely conclusive, that the ascorbic acid deficiency in its turn may be responsible for the osteoporosis. Scurvy has been shown to cause osteoporosis in children and in experimental animals.[372] This has been ascribed to the fact that ascorbic acid is necessary for osteogenesis, including the synthesis of bone collagen, osteoblast maturation, and osteoid formation. Semiquantitative microradiography of the osteoporotic bone of scorbutic guinea pigs revealed the expected decrease in bone formation surface, but also an increase in bone resorption surface.[421] An increase in bone resorption surface was observed in osteoporotic blacks with severe iron overload. Experiments using radioactive calcium suggest both decreased bone formation and increased bone resorption.[274] In addition, it has been possible to show that repletion with ascorbic acid diminishes the urinary excretion of calcium.[274]

Although the fact that South African blacks with severe iron overload usually drink alcohol excessively and eat little animal protein obviously cannot be disregarded, ascorbic acid deficiency may play a central role, leading to both reduced osteogenesis and the formation of bone that is resorbed at a greater rate than normal. Support for this concept has been obtained by experiments with guinea pigs.[421] Iron overload was produced by injections of iron dextran, and the animals were kept on a balanced diet, including the normal daily requirements of ascorbic acid. The control animals remained healthy, but those with iron overload developed ascorbic acid deficiency; when killed several months later, they were found to have diminished bone mineral density. Both the ascorbic acid deficiency and the osteoporosis were prevented by large parenteral supplements of ascorbic acid.

Diagnosis and Management

A background history of an appreciable intake of home-brewed beer is most helpful. Subjects with this type of iron overload of mild or moderate severity do not usually complain of any symptoms and usually no signs are present, although modest hepatomegaly may sometimes be found. The clinical features in those with severe overload but no cirrhosis are usually related to secondary ascorbic acid deficiency. A small proportion develop classic scurvy, especially in late winter and early spring.[372] Some present with backache and spinal collapse due to osteoporosis. The patient is usually a middle-aged male working as a manual laborer, who on examination may exhibit evidence of shortening of the vertebral column; a lumbar or lower dorsal gibbus is sometimes present, and tenderness over the lower spine with spasm of paravertebral muscles is invariably found. Most patients exhibit firm hepatomegaly, and one third have splenomegaly.[372] In patients with fully developed dietary hemochromatosis other features may be present, including diabetes and the various complications of cirrhosis.

The diagnosis of iron overload rests on the same tests as are used in idiopathic hemochromatosis. There are, however, certain qualifications. Although the plasma iron concentration is raised and the transferrin is close to saturation in subjects with the acquired hemochromatosis syndrome,[371] this is not so in noncirrhotic subjects,[199,211,420] since the associated ascorbic acid deficiency blocks the release of iron from reticuloendothelial cells.[258] A more accurate reflection of the iron status can, however, be obtained if ascorbic acid is given. Under such circumstances there is a prompt rise in the plasma iron concentration.[420] Similarly, the urinary excretion of iron after giving desferrioxamine is misleadingly low, unless ascorbic acid stores have been repleted.[419] These reservations fortunately do not apply to the plasma ferritin concentration, which appears to bear a close relationship to iron stores, as in other varieties of iron overload.[59] In addition, since reticuloendothelial stores of iron are markedly increased, histologic examination of a bone marrow smear or the chemical estimation of the non-heme iron content of a specimen obtained by trephine biopsy is useful.[66]

The primary aim is to prevent the condition by reducing the iron content of the traditional beers. This has largely been achieved by substituting aluminum containers for iron ones. In addition, drinking habits are changing, with conventional liquors being increasingly consumed. Specific therapy in the form of repeated venesections has been carried out,[391] although not yet in many individuals because the more severely affected are the heaviest drinkers, and as such are both unreliable and unwilling to submit to the discipline of such treatment. Supportive treatment includes insulin for diabetes and conventional measures for liver failure. Ascorbic acid has also been given for both clinical and subclinical osteoporosis, but there is no objective evidence of its value.

IRON OVERLOAD IN REFRACTORY ANEMIAS

Clinical and pathologic features similar to those found in idiopathic hemochromatosis have been reported in a number of patients suffering from a variety of chronic anemias.[61] Analysis of the reported literature indicates that they fall into two distinct groups on the basis of the degree of erythropoietic activity in the bone marrow.

First, patients with hypoplastic anemia may accumulate enormous quantities of iron if they are given many transfusions, since there is 25 g of iron in 100 pints of blood. Tissue concentrations in the range found in idiopathic hemochromatosis are often reached and may even be exceeded. When reports of 20 such individuals were analyzed, one had developed cirrhosis of the liver, four had impaired glucose tolerance, and five had overt diabetes.[52] The findings were therefore similar to those in idiopathic hemochromatosis, except for the relative infrequency of cirrhosis. Two reasons for this seem plausible. First, the time of follow-up in such individuals has almost invariably been relatively short compared with the oral forms of iron overload. Second, the primary localization of the iron is reticuloendothelial, and although redistribution does occur with time, the major impact is still on the reticuloendothelial system rather than on the hepatic parenchymal cells.

The second group of chronic anemias in which large amounts of iron may accumulate in the body are those associated with a hyperplastic bone marrow. Iron overload is particularly liable to occur in anemias in which erythropoiesis is very active but largely ineffective in terms of the delivery of viable red blood cells into the circulation.[61,218] It is thus most often seen in thalassemia major but may also occur in refractory sideroblastic anemias (even when not severe),[322] pyridoxine-responsive anemias, refractory normoblastic anemias and a variety of anemias associated with blocks in the inclusion of iron into hemoglobin, and erythemic myelosis.

The pathogenesis of the iron overload in these subjects is more complex than in the hypoplastic anemias. Although transfusion therapy is also often an important source of iron in these conditions, especially in Western countries, it is not the only one. Markedly increased but ineffective erythropoiesis is accompanied by a considerable rise in the absorption rate, so that significant amounts of iron may be accumulated from the diet. Why iron overload should occur so predictably in conditions like thalassemia major and so rarely in the classic hemolytic syndromes is not known, although the erythropoietic rate does tend to be higher in thalassemia.[218] The relative contribution of donated blood and of dietary iron to the overload varies in different parts of the world. Donated blood is the important source of Western countries where transfusion therapy is freely available, while dietary iron is often the only source in countries such as Thailand.[90]

There are a number of factors that affect the distribution

and hence the toxic effects of the iron deposits in thalassemia major and related conditions. First, the iron is present over long periods, since the diseases are mainly inherited ones. Second, a variable proportion of the surplus iron enters via the oral route. Iron is absorbed from the gut despite the fact that the transferrin is saturated. The free iron present in the portal blood is then deposited in hepatocytes.[427] Third, internal iron kinetics are significantly different from what occurs in hypoplastic anemias; the plasma iron turnover is greatly increased and this may well facilitate hepatocyte loading.[208] Fourth, the significant degree of intravascular hemolysis that is frequently associated with ineffective erythropoiesis results in the uptake of increased amounts of hemoglobin iron by the hepatocytes.[218] The complexity of the problem is underlined by the observation that parenchymal overload has been reported to be particularly striking in subjects with thalassemia major who have been splenectomized.

From the previous discussion it is apparent that subjects with major thalassemic syndromes tend to accumulate massive amounts of iron whether they have received blood transfusions or not.[51,61,412] As a consequence, they develop many of the clinical and pathologic features of hemochromatosis, including cirrhosis, diabetes, and cardiac failure. The pathologic findings are striking. In one study of five transfused patients with thalassemia major aged 8 to 16 years the iron concentrations in the organs were found to be in the range described in idiopathic hemochromatosis.[434] Cirrhosis was present in all of them, and in three there was significant pancreatic fibrosis. Cardiac hypertrophy and hyaline degeneration of myocardial fibers were noted, although there was very little fibrosis. In a second study of 41 patients, 26 had developed congestive cardiac failure and 19 had pericarditis.[146] Eleven had widespread iron deposition and fibrosis in the tissues at necropsy, especially the liver, pancreas, gonads, thyroid, pituitary, and adrenal glands. The heart was dilated and hypertrophied and on microscopy large amounts of iron were present in muscle cells and histocytes, with extensive fibrosis and focal degeneration. In a third study, 32 liver biopsies were performed on children with thalassemia major. There was a good correlation between the severity of the fibrosis and both the age and the liver iron concentration.[353] At iron concentrations of less than 0.6 g/100 g progression was relatively slow, but thereafter it accelerated. Somewhat surprisingly, the severity of the fibrosis correlated more closely with the degree of reticuloendothelial siderosis than with the degree of parenchymal involvement. In an analysis of a further 207 patients, the majority of the 37 deaths that had occurred at an early age could be ascribed to inadequate transfusion therapy and/or hypersplenism.[295] The eight older subjects who had received an average of 277 pints of blood (range 145 to 402) all died of cardiac failure. In spite of this there was no fibrosis in the heart, although it was present in the liver and pancreas. Ultrastructural studies have revealed mitochondrial damage in the heart[361] and loading of the liver

lysosomes with iron.[227] Deposition of iron in the cytoplasm and in lysosomes is found in heavily transfused subjects even in infancy and is followed by pericellular collagen deposition and later by fibrosis.[224]

Clinical manifestations due to iron overload in thalassemia major resemble those in young and very severely affected patients with idiopathic hemochromatosis. Cardiac manifestations are the most serious for survival; they become particularly prominent in the second decade of life, and are essentially those of a cardiomyopathy.[295] The clinical course may be punctuated by attacks of pericarditis, while death usually occurs in the late teens or early 20s as a result of intractable arrhythmias with or without cardiac failure.[144,310] If the teens are reached, endocrine failure becomes prominent.[22,280] Failure or severe retardation of puberty is the most common manifestation of iron toxicity and is associated with absence or retardation of the adolescent growth spurt. Severe growth retardation becomes obvious between 9 and 11 years of age.[234,295,297] While maintaining the hemoglobin concentration at higher levels may improve the growth rate somewhat, stunting is not prevented.[238,307,436] It is not due to growth hormone deficiency,[253,297] and there is some evidence of somatomedin deficiency.[207,359] On this basis it has been suggested that the hepatic response to growth hormone is impaired.[207] Overt diabetes mellitus occurs in about a fifth of older transfused patients[445] and even when it is not present, abnormal glucose tolerance tests, insulin responses to glucose infusions, and glucagon responses to alanine infusions[252,253] can be demonstrated in the majority of patients.

Liver disease is a constant feature. In one study, hepatomegaly was prominent in the first decade and cirrhosis was uniformly found in heavily transfused patients.[434] Serum hepatitis is common and may aggravate the liver damage.[313] However, synthetic function is usually well maintained and the hepatic disease is rarely the cause of death.[294]

The management of thalassemia major altered following the demonstration in 1964 that children transfused frequently in order to maintain a higher hemoglobin concentration were a good deal healthier and lived just as long.[436] Although more iron is administered in the additional units of blood, absorption of dietary iron is diminished at higher hemoglobin concentrations, with the result that the net effect may not be much different.[295] In patients on such therapy growth is normal until about 9 years of age, but then the complications resulting from the iron overload appear. It is obviously desirable to remove as much of this iron as possible, and chelating agents, especially desferrioxamine, have been increasingly used for this purpose in recent years. There is evidence that worthwhile results have been achieved.[97,375] Although it does not appear to be possible with daily intramuscular injections of 0.5 g to 1 g of desferrioxamine to prevent the accumulation of iron during the first few years of life, an equilibrium can be reached at tissue iron concentrations significantly lower than in patients not given desferriox-amine.[22,296] Hepatic fibrosis may be arrested, and prelim-inary results suggest that cardiotoxicity may be diminished and survival prolonged. In this context, it is perhaps note-worthy that desferrioxamine may have effects other than those relating to the removal of iron from the body, since it has been shown that it inhibits collagen synthesis in fibroblast culture.[219] Whatever the reason for its effects, desferrioxamine holds some promise in the treatment of thalassemia major. Because of this, a number of workers have tried to develop more effective ways of delivering the drug to the patient. It has been known for a long time that continuous intravenous infusion mobilizes more iron than intramuscular injections, but this route of admin-istration is obviously not feasible for long-term daily treatment. An important observation has been that the subcutaneous route gives results very similar to those ob-tained with intravenous infusions.[323,344] The availability of small infusion pumps has made the method a partic-ularly attractive one, especially since almost as good results can be obtained when the desferrioxamine is given for only 12 of the 24 hours.[103,220,323,343,344,425] On such therapy it has been possible for the first time to induce a negative iron balance in the condition.[215] This occurs even in young children.[344]

Subcutaneous infusions of desferrioxamine have been given in doses ranging between 15 mg and 70 mg/kg/day,[344] usually about 25 mg/kg/day. It is worthwhile to establish the patient's dose response curve, since there is considerable individual variation. The sites of loss are in-fluenced by the rate of erythropoiesis. When erythropoiesis is suppressed by raising the hemoglobin level, fecal losses rise, while urinary losses rise as the rate of erythropoiesis increases.[324] At higher desferrioxamine doses urinary losses eventually reach a peak, but stool losses continue to rise and at doses of 150 mg/kg account for up to 40% of total losses.[324] However, such large doses are only indicated when life-threatening cardiac complications are present, since they can lead to severe (although reversible) retini-tis.[114] Since there is evidence that other iron chelators may have different sites of action, the use of combinations ap-pears logical, and diethylene-triamine penta-acetic acid (DTPA) in a dose of 1 g to 3 g may be added to the transfused blood, although it is too toxic for continuous administration.

There is some controversy concerning the place of ascorbic acid in therapy. It has been shown that the sub-clinical ascorbic acid deficiency that is commonly asso-ciated with iron overload reduces the response to desfer-rioxamine.[419] The correction of this deficiency leads on average to a twofold increase in iron excretion, and be-cause of this, ascorbic acid is now widely used as an adjunct to chelator therapy.[49,61,95,205,214] However, misgivings have been voiced concerning the wisdom of such an ap-proach.[89,205] The ascorbic acid deficiency causes a partial block in the release of iron from reticuloendothelial cells.[259] It is therefore theoretically possible that its ad-ministration in a disease such as thalassemia major may promote the relocation of iron from the reticuloendothelial system, where it is relatively innocuous, to parenchymal tissues, where it is toxic. Some evidence in support of this hypothesis has been provided by Henry and Nienhuis, who demonstrated objective deterioration in cardiac function in 8 of 11 thalassemic subjects treated with ascorbic acid.[205,309,310] Function improved in 5 of them when the ascorbic acid was stopped. Although other workers have not found evidence that ascorbic acid has deleterious effects,[215,220] it should only be administered under controlled conditions with careful cardiac moni-toring, preferably by echocardiography.[206] This is espe-cially so in subjects with massive iron overload.

A significant source of iron in thalassemia is the diet, since absorption is enhanced. It can be effectively coun-tered by the simple means of taking tea with meals,[117] because the tannins in tea are potent inhibitors of iron absorption.[125]

In an attempt to increase the interval between trans-fusions patients have been transfused with young red cells,[345] but the approach has not proved a useful one.[95] A more effective way of reducing blood requirements is to remove the spleen in subjects in whom splenomegaly is associated with significant red cell trapping.[95]

Preliminary results of modern treatment are promising, and reductions in serum ferritin, liver iron, and trans-aminase concentrations have been noted.[215] In a longer follow-up study, liver iron concentrations dropped to normal even in children who had received chelation ther-apy for 7 to 10 years.[95] In addition, transaminase levels fell and hepatic fibrosis was arrested. There is also evidence that cardiac function can improve on desferrioxamine therapy, although relatively large doses may be needed.[139]

Although current therapeutic approaches using iron chelators are promising, it must be pointed out that they are expensive and complicated. It is hoped that in the future there will be combinations of chelators with dif-fering and complementary modes of action, which can be given in depot form, or preferably orally.[181,228,325]

RELATIONSHIP BETWEEN IRON OVERLOAD AND TISSUE DAMAGE

It has proved difficult to investigate experimentally the relationship between high tissue concentrations of storage iron and the associated organ damage.[61] Various ap-proaches have been tried and several species used. A major problem until recently has been that simple dietary sup-plementation with iron produces only trivial hemosidero-sis. Methods to increase absorption have included reducing the phosphate content of the diet, ligating the pancreatic duct, and administering such substances as dl-ethionine, Tween 20, and d-sorbitol. Even then the con-centrations of iron have usually been much lower than those found in idiopathic hemochromatosis, but they have occasionally been comparable.[61] Bacon and co-workers have succeeded in producing hepatic iron concentrations in the hemochromatotic range within 44 days by feeding rats a diet containing 2.5% carbonyl iron, a highly purified form of elemental iron.[15] The iron was located in the hepatocytes as well as in Kupffer cells. In most animal experiments the iron has been confined to the liver and reticuloendothelial system, but slight deposits in other organs have been noted. Cirrhosis of the liver and pancreatic fibrosis have not been produced, however.

High concentrations of tissue iron have been achieved by administering large doses of parenteral iron in various forms and by various routes.[68,72,79,127,330,331,356] In most studies the iron has initially been located in the reticuloendothelial system, but with time a minor degree of redistribution has occurred. Certain pathologic changes have been produced in this way. When massive doses of parenteral iron (approximately 3 g/kg) were given to dogs, they died after some months, although no evidence of hepatic or pancreatic fibrosis was noted.[72] In one investigation a number of dogs were given large doses of iron dextran intravenously, and after 3 to 4 years the majority of the survivors had developed hepatic cirrhosis with massive siderosis.[262] On the other hand, Domellof[127] found that rats subjected to very large doses of parenteral iron remained in good health. The only morphologic changes noted were proliferation and hypertrophy of the hepatocytes, and it was concluded that excess iron stimulates the synthesis of protein. Parenchymal iron loading can be achieved by injecting the small-molecular iron chelate iron-nitriloacetate, and diabetes has been produced in rats in this way.[14,288]

In other experiments cellular injury has been produced in some way in addition to siderosis. For instance, Kent and co-workers[241] showed that massive doses of iron dextran promote hepatic fibrosis in rats exposed to carbon tetrachloride. Rats fed a choline-deficient diet with iron developed a fatty liver, with progressively increasing cirrhosis.[278] These changes could be prevented by the administration of folic acid.[279] However, the concentrations of iron in the liver were relatively modest (only six times normal), and the relationship of these findings to what occurs in idiopathic hemochromatosis is thus questionable. They do, however, support the concept that iron overload makes hepatocytes more susceptible to other insults.[174] Unfortunately, contradictory findings continue to be reported.[306] For example, after 110 weeks no hepatic fibrosis had been produced in rhesus monkeys given iron dextran (0.5 g/kg) intravenously and then exposed to alcohol, alcohol plus a low-protein diet, or carbon tetrachloride.

No final verdict can, therefore, be given concerning the relevance of these various studies. First of all, it has not been possible in any animal experiment to duplicate the long latent period, which in humans extends over half a lifetime. In addition, until the recent advent of iron-nitriloacetate and carbonyl iron, respectively, the impact with parenteral loading has been primarily on the reticuloendothelial cells, while in those studies in which the siderosis has been produced orally, the concentrations reached have been relatively low. It is also entirely possible that there is species variation in susceptibility to any noxious effects of iron overload. Certainly, many animal species are able to excrete iron much more rapidly than can humans,[162] and this may help to prevent parenchymal tissue loading with iron. A notable exception seems to be birds, several species of which have developed hepatic hemosiderosis in captivity. This has on occasion been associated with primary liver neoplasms or hepatic decompensation.[347,409] Finally, the fact that deficiencies in the diet, or the consumption of other toxic agents, sometimes potentiate the noxious effects of iron in animal experiments is perfectly compatible with clinical observations that symptomatic hemochromatosis occurs relatively commonly in subjects who consume large amounts of alcohol.

In contrast to the equivocal results in animals, in humans there is a good correlation between heavy parenchymal iron deposits and secondary pathologic changes. This is true irrespective of the cause of the iron overload. However, the relationship is by no means a simple one since other factors are often involved. For example, all forms of iron overload are characterized by liver damage, but in subjects with idiopathic hemochromatosis and in the blacks of South Africa, alcohol is often a complicating factor, while chronic anemia and serum hepatitis may potentiate the effect of iron in subjects with thalassemia major. In spite of these complicating factors, there is no doubt that excessive parenchymal iron deposits are toxic. The relationship between the iron and the disordered function is particularly striking in the heart, since a number of reports have confirmed the reversal of intractable heart failure after the removal of the iron deposits by repeated venesections.[88]

The mechanism by which iron damages tissues remains the subject of speculation. When excess iron is present within cells, it accumulates in the lysosomes. This has been shown in the livers of iron-loaded rats.[351,400] Studies on liver biopsies from subjects with hemochromatosis have also revealed dense deposits of ferritin and hemosiderin in structures tentatively characterized as lysosomes. Increased total, but decreased latent, activities of high-density hepatic lysosomal enzymes have been shown in subjects with various types of iron overload,[376] and the lysosomes were more fragile than normal.[320] On the basis of this latter finding, it has been suggested that iron accumulation damages the lysosomal membrane, releasing large amounts of acid hydrolases into the cytoplasm, thus initiating cell damage. The fact that these abnormalities return to normal after removal of the excessive iron from the liver suggests that it is iron that causes them.[321] However, the mechanism by which it does so is not known. It has been suggested that the iron promotes the formation of free radicals. Ferrous iron ligated with either adenosine diphosphate or triphosphate has been shown to catalyse hydrogen peroxide to yield hydroxyl free radicals.[164] Free radicals may promote lipid peroxidation and thereby damage the membrane of lysosomes and other subcellular organelles.[320] In addition, ferrous iron itself has a potent lipid-oxidizing potential and may cause membrane damage.[433] *In vivo* evidence of liver mitochondrial and microsomal lipid peroxidation has been obtained in iron-loaded rats.[15] In this context, the demonstration[29,209] that appreciable quantities of nontransferrin-bound iron are present in the plasma of hemochromatotic and of thalassemic patients whose transferrin is saturated with iron raises questions concerning its toxicity relative to that of the bound iron. At present it is not known whether the presence of this fraction in plasma correlates with the development of tissue damage. In rats a single injection of iron-nitrilotriacetate sufficient to produce circulating non-transferrin iron produces lipid peroxidation in the liver and release of hepatic enzymes into the circulation.[441] Such observations are clearly relevant to acute iron poisoning, if not also to chronic iron overload. Of some interest in this connection is the observation that the concentrations of the naturally occurring antioxidant vitamin E seem to be reduced in experimental iron overload[175] and in thalassemia major.[223] As mentioned, ascorbic acid deficiency is another common sequela of iron overload, and here, too, it has been suggested that lack of its nonspecific antioxidant action may lead to damage of susceptible tissues. However, no abnormalities in the subcellular distribution or the activity of glutathione reductase, superoxide dismutase, catalase, or glutathione peroxidase, enzymes implicated in the protection of cells from free-radical mediated damage, could be found in liver obtained by biopsy from individuals with iron overload,[373] although increased activity of selenium-independent glutathione peroxidase activity has been noted in the livers of rats in a high iron diet.[254]

PORPHYRIA CUTANEA TARDA

Porphyria cutanea tarda is the most common form of porphyria. It is manifested clinically by blistering and mechanical fragility of the sun-exposed skin; these lesions result from a combination of the deposition of porphyrins in the skin and chronic exposure to ultraviolet light. The condition appears to be due to a deficiency of the enzyme uroporphyrinogen decarboxylase in the liver,[151,247,248] with levels of the enzyme in erythrocytes being normal[145] or decreased.[248] Biochemically, porphyria cutanea tarda is characterized by the increased urinary excretion of uroporphyrin 1,7-carboxyl-porphyrin and coproporphyrin.[150,187] Coproporphyrin and sometimes protoporphyrin excretion in the feces may also be increased.[271,346]

Although the basic defect in porphyria cutanea tarda is the deficiency of uroporphyrinogen decarboxylase, there is evidence suggesting that both alcohol and iron overload play important parts in causing phenotypic expression of the disease.[212,249] The majority of patients give a history of prolonged consumption of excessive quantities of alcohol, and many affected individuals have varying degrees of hepatic siderosis.[150,212] In addition, the condition is common in South African blacks suffering from iron overload.[251] Support for the suggestion that siderosis plays a part is provided by reports that a marked decrease in porphyrin excretion has followed the treatment of the iron overload by repeated venesections.[147,237,363] The administration of desferrioxamine has also been beneficial in some hands,[397] but not in others.[364]

The etiology of the iron overload in porphyria cutanea tarda has not been completely elucidated and may vary in different settings. Increased iron absorption and an increased plasma iron turnover were reported in one study.[350] These findings may have relevance to the observation that there is an association between porphyria cutanea tarda and certain HLA haplotypes,[245] since they raise the possibility that patients with porphyria cutanea tarda who develop clinical manifestations may be heterozygous for the HLA-linked iron-loading gene.

There are several possible mechanisms by which iron can affect porphyrin metabolism. Taljaard and co-workers[395] found that rats fed hexachlorobenzene became porphyric much more readily if they had been given large doses of iron dextran intraperitoneally. It has been reported that the rate of uroporphyrin synthesis *in vitro* is significantly increased by the addition of ferritin and cysteine.[246] Ferrous iron stimulates porphyrin synthesis and inhibits the deficient enzyme uroporphyrinogen decarboxylase.[247,248] At the same time, it must be emphasized that iron overload is not invariably present, and that starting a program of phlebotomies may be followed by clinical and biochemical improvement before significant amounts of iron have been removed.[237]

The association with alcoholism may be a direct one or may merely reflect the association between iron overload and the consumption of alcohol, which is discussed in an earlier section of the chapter. It nevertheless seems clear that both the enzyme deficiency and an acquired factor must be present and that the latter is frequently iron overload, with or without alcohol. In this context, it is of interest that the relative importance of different exogenous factors may be changing and that estrogen-containing oral contraceptives now represent a significant etiologic factor.[187]

Although there is still controversy concerning the exact mode of inheritance, there is now good evidence that porphyria cutanea tarda is usually an inherited disease, and pedigrees have been collected in which abnormal porphyrin excretion has been found in individual members of several generations.[34,248] It seems that the enzyme defect is restricted to the hepatocyte in some pedigrees, while it is expressed in several tissues in others.[249] At the same time it remains possible that the enzyme defect may also be acquired as a result of exposure to unidentified toxins.[249]

REFERENCES

1. Abbott DF, Gresham GA: Arthropathy in transfusional siderosis. Br Med J 1:418, 1972

2. Acar J et al: Coeur et hemochromatose: Aspects particuliers. Coeur Med Intern 6:17, 1967

3. Adamson TC et al: Hand and wrist arthropathies of hemochromatosis and calcium pyrophosphate deposition disease: Distinct radiographic features. Radiology 147:377, 1983

4. Alstatt LB et al: Liver manganese in hemochromatosis. Proc Soc Exp Biol Med 124:353, 1967

5. Althausen TL et al: Hemochromatosis: An investigation of twenty-three cases with special reference to nutrition, to iron metabolism, and to studies of hepatic and pancreatic function. Arch Intern Med 88:553, 1951

6. Altman JJ et al: The GnRH test in idiopathic hemochromatosis. J Endocrinol Invest 3:223, 1980

7. Ammann RW et al: High incidence of extrahepatic carcinomas in idiopathic hemochromatosis. Scand J Gastroenterol 15:733, 1980

8. Anguissola AB: The nutritional value of wine as regards its iron content. In Harwerth H-G, Vannotti A (eds): Iron Deficiency, Pathogenesis, Clinical Aspects, Therapy, p 71. New York, Academic Press, 1970

9. Arosio P et al: Characterization of serum ferritin in iron overload: Possible identity to natural apoferritin. Br J Haematol 36:199, 1977

10. Askari AD et al: Arthritis of hemochromatosis: Clinical spectrum, relation to histocompatibility antigens, and effectiveness of early phlebotomy. Am J Med 75:957, 1983

11. Atkins CJ et al: Chondrocalcinosis and arthropathy: Studies in haemochromatosis and in idiopathic chondrocalcinosis. Q J Med 39:71, 1970

12. Aungst CW: Ferritin in body fluids. J Lab Clin Med 71:517, 1968

13. Awai M, Brown EB: Examination of the role of xanthine oxidase in iron absorption by the rat. J Lab Clin Med 73:366, 1969

14. Awai M et al: Induction of diabetes in animals by parenteral administration of ferric nitrilotriacetate. Am J Pathol 95:663, 1979

15. Bacon B et al: Hepatic lipid peroxidation *in vivo* in rats with chronic iron overload. J Clin Invest 71:429, 1983

16. Balcerzak SP et al: Idiopathic haemochromatosis: A study of three families. Am J Med 40:857, 1966

17. Balcerzak SP et al: Iron absorption in chronic pancreatitis. Gastroenterology 53:257, 1967

18. Balcerzak SP et al: Diabetes mellitus and idiopathic hemochromatosis. Am J Med Sci 255:53, 1968

19. Balcerzak SP et al: Measurement of iron stores using deferoxamine. Ann Intern Med 68:518, 1968

20. Barry M: Iron overload: Clinical aspects, evaluation and treatment. In Callender S (ed): Clinics in Haematology, vol 2, No. 2, p 405. Philadelphia, WB Saunders, 1973

21. Barry M, Sherlock S: Measurement of liver-iron concentration in needle biopsy specimens. Lancet 1:100, 1971

22. Barry M et al: Long-term chelation therapy in thalassaemia major: Effect on liver iron concentration, liver histology and clinical progress. Br Med J 2:16, 1974

23. Bassett ML: Haemochromatosis: Diagnostic and Metabolic Studies, thesis. University of Queensland, Australia, 1983

24. Bassett ML et al: Early detection of idiopathic hemochromatosis: Relative value of serum ferritin and HLA typing. Lancet 2:4, 1979

25. Bassett ML et al: HLA typing in idiopathic hemochromatosis: Distinction between homozygotes and heterozygotes with biochemical expression. Hepatology 1:120, 1981

26. Bassett ML et al: Idiopathic hemochromatosis: Evidence of homozygous-heterozygous mating by HLA typing of families. Hum Genet 60:352, 1982

27. Bassett ML et al: Ferritin synthesis in peripheral blood monocytes in idiopathic hemochromatosis. J Lab Clin Med 100:137, 1982

28. Bassett ML et al: Genetic hemochromatosis. Semin Liver Dis 4:217, 1984

29. Batey RG et al: A non-transferrin-bound serum iron in idiopathic hemochromatosis. Dig Dis Sci 25:340, 1980

30. Beamish MR et al: Transferrin iron, chelatable iron and ferritin in idiopathic haemochromatosis. Br J Haematol 27:219, 1974

31. Beaumont C et al: Serum ferritin as a possible marker of the hemochromatosis allele. N Engl J Med 301:169, 1979

32. Beaumont C et al: Hepatic and serum ferritin concentrations in patients with idiopathic haemochromatosis. Gastroenterology 79:877, 1980

33. Becker BJ, Chatgidakis CB: Cirrhosis of the liver in Johannesburg. Acta Int Cancer 17:639, 1961

34. Benedetto AV et al: Porphyria cutanea tarda in three generations of a single family. N Engl J Med 298:358, 1978

35. Berry EM, Miller JP: Hereditary spherocytosis, haemochromatosis, diabetes mellitus and chondrocalcinosis. Proc R Soc Med 66:9, 1973

36. Bezkorovainy A, Zschocke RH: Structure and function of transferrins I. Physical, chemical and iron-binding properties. Arzneim Forsch (Drug Res) 24:476, 1974

37. Bezwoda WR et al: Patterns of food iron absorption in iron-deficient white and Indian subjects and in venesected haemochromatotic patients. Br J Haematol 33:265, 1976

38. Bezwoda WR et al: An investigation into gonadal dysfunction in patients with idiopathic hemochromatosis. Clin Endocrinol 6:377, 1977

39. Bezwoda WR et al: Iron absorption from red and white wines. Scand J Hematol 34:121, 1985

40. Bjorn-Rasmussen E et al: Food iron absorption in man: Applications of the two-pool extrinsic tag method to measure haem and non-haem iron absorption from the whole diet. J Clin Invest 53:247, 1974

41. Blacklock HA, Meerkin M: Serum ferritin in patients with hereditary spherocytosis. Br J Haematol 49:117, 1981

42. Block M et al: Histogenesis of the hepatic lesion in primary hemochromatosis: With consideration of the pseudo-iron deficient state produced by phlebotomies. Am J Pathol 47:89, 1965

43. Boender CA, Verloop MC: Iron absorption, iron loss and iron retention in man: Studies after oral administration of a tracer dose of $^{59}FeSO_4$ and $^{131}BaSO_4$. Br J Haematol 17:45, 1969

44. Bomford A, Williams R: Long term results of venesection therapy in idiopathic haemochromatosis. Q J Med 45:611, 1976

45. Bomford A et al: Histocompatibility antigens as markers of abnormal iron metabolism in patients with idiopathic haemochromatosis and their relatives. Lancet 1:327, 1977

46. Bothwell TH, Alper T: The cardiac complications of haemochromatosis. S Afr J Clin Sci 2:226, 1951

47. Bothwell TH, Bradlow BA: Siderosis in the Bantu: A combined histopathological and chemical study. Arch Pathol 70:279, 1960

48. Bothwell TH, Charlton RW: Absorption of iron. In DeGraff AC (ed): Annual Review of Medicine, vol 21, p 145. Palo Alto, CA, Annual Reviews, 1970

49. Bothwell TH, Charlton RW: Current problems and iron overload. In Gross R, Hellriegel K-P (eds): Strategies in Clinical Hematology, p 87. Berlin, Springer-Verlag, 1979

50. Bothwell TH, Charlton RW: A general approach to the problems of iron deficiency and iron overload in the population at large. Semin Hematol 19:54, 1982

51. Bothwell TH, Charlton RW, Motulsky AG: Idiopathic hemochromatosis. In Stanbury JB et al (eds): The Metabolic Basis of Inherited Disorders, 5th ed, p 1269. New York, McGraw-Hill, 1983

52. Bothwell TH, Finch CA: Iron Metabolism. Boston, Little, Brown & Co, 1962

53. Bothwell TH, Isaacson C: Siderosis in the Bantu: A comparison of the incidence in males and females. Br Med J 1:522, 1962

54. Bothwell TH et al: A familial study in idiopathic hemochromatosis. Am J Med 27:730, 1959

55. Bothwell TH et al: Studies on the behaviour of transferrin in idiopathic haemochromatosis. S Afr Med Sci 27:35, 1962

56. Bothwell TH et al: Iron overload in Bantu subjects: Studies on the availability of iron in Bantu beer. Am J Clin Nutr 14:47, 1964

57. Bothwell TH et al: Idiopathic and Bantu hemochromatosis: Comparative histological study. Arch Pathol 79:163, 1965

58. Bothwell TH et al: Oral iron overload. S Afr Med J 39:892, 1965

59. Bothwell TH et al: Can iron fortification of flour cause damage to genetic susceptibles (idiopathic haemochromatosis and β-thalassaemia major)? Hum Genet (Suppl) 1:131, 1978

60. Bothwell TH et al: Unpublished data, 1978

61. Bothwell TH et al: Iron Metabolism in Man. Oxford, Blackwell Scientific Publications, 1979

62. Boyett JD et al: Allopurinol and iron metabolism in man. Blood 32:460, 1968

63. Bradlow B et al: The effect of cirrhosis on iron storage. Am J Pathol 39:221, 1961

64. Bregman H et al: HLA-linked iron overload and myopathy in maintenance hemodialysis patients. Trans Am Soc Artif Intern Organs 26:366, 1980

65. Brick IB: Liver histology in six asymptomatic siblings in a family with hemochromatosis: Genetic implications. Gastroenterology 40:210, 1961

66. Brink B et al: Patterns of iron storage in dietary iron overload and idiopathic hemochromatosis. J Lab Clin Med 88:725, 1976

67. Brissot P et al: Ascorbic acid status in idiopathic hemochromatosis. Digestion 17:479, 1978

68. Brissot P et al: Experimental hepatic iron overload in the baboon: Results of a two-year study. Dig Dis Sci 28:616, 1983

69. Brittenham GM et al: Magnetic-susceptibility measurement of human iron stores. N Engl J Med 307:1671, 1982

70. Brodanova M, Hoenig V: Iron metabolism in patients with porta-caval shunts. Scand J Gastroenterol 1:167, 1966

71. Brody JI et al: Therapeutic phlebotomies in idiopathic hemochromatosis. Am J Med Sci 244:575, 1962

72. Brown EB Jr et al: Studies in iron transportation and metabolism: X. Long-term iron overload in dogs. J Lab Clin Med 50:862, 1957

73. Buchanan WM: Bantu siderosis: A review. Central Afr J Med 15:105, 1969

74. Buchanan WM: The importance of protein malnutrition in the genesis of Bantu siderosis. S Afr J Med Sci 36:99, 1971

75. Buja LM, Roberts WC: Iron in the heart: Etiology and clinical significance. Am J Med 51:209, 1971

76. Butt EM et al: Trace metal patterns in disease states: I. Hemochromatosis and refractory anemia. Am J Clin Pathol 26:225, 1956

77. Callender ST, Malpas JS: Absorption of iron in cirrhosis of liver. Br Med J 2:1516, 1963

78. Candell-Riera J et al: Cardiac hemochromatosis: Beneficial effects of iron removal therapy: An echocardiographic study. Am J Cardiol 52:824, 1983

79. Cappell DF: The late results of intravenous injection of colloidal iron. J Pathol 33:175, 1930

80. Cartwright GE et al: Hereditary hemochromatosis. N Engl J Med 301:175, 1979

81. Cartwright GE et al: Association of HLA-linked hemochromatosis with idiopathic refractory sideroblastic anemia. J Clin Invest 65:989, 1980

82. Case Records of the Massachusetts General Hospital: Case 38512. N Engl J Med 247:992, 1952

83. Caskey J et al: Human ferritin gene is assigned to chromosome 19. Proc Natl Acad Sci 80:482, 1983

84. Cazzola M et al: Juvenile idiopathic haemochromatosis: A life threatening disorder presenting as hypogonadotrophic hypogonadism. Hum Genet 65:149, 1983

85. Chapman RWG et al: Computed tomography for determining liver iron content in primary haemochromatosis. Br Med J 280:440, 1980

86. Charbonnel B et al: Adrenocortical function in idiopathic haemochromatosis. Acta Endocrinol 95:67, 1980

87. Charbonnel B et al: Pituitary function in idiopathic haemochromatosis: Hormonal study in 36 male patients. Acta Endocrinol 98:178, 1981

88. Charlton RW, Bothwell TH: Hemochromatosis: Dietary and genetic aspects. In Brown EB, Moore CV (eds): Progress in Hematology, vol 5, p 298. New York, Grune & Stratton, 1966

89. Charlton RW, Bothwell TH: Iron ascorbic acid and thalassemia. In Bergsma D et al (eds): Iron Metabolism in Thalassemia, p 63. New York, Alan R Liss, 1976

90. Charlton RW, Bothwell TH: Iron absorption. In Creger WP et al (eds): Annual Review of Medicine, p 55. Palo Alto, CA, Annual Reviews, 1983

91. Charlton RW et al: Effect of alcohol on iron absorption. Br Med J 2:1427, 1964

92. Charlton RW et al: Idiopathic hemochromatosis in young subjects: Clinical, pathological and chemical findings in four patients. Arch Pathol 83:132, 1967

93. Charlton RW et al: Hepatic storage iron concentrations in different population groups. Am J Clin Nutr 23:358, 1970

94. Charlton RW et al: Liver iron stores in different population groups in South Africa. S Afr Med J 45:524, 1971

95. Cohen A et al: Treatment of iron overload. Semin Liver Dis 4:228, 1984

96. Committee on Iron Deficiency of the AMA Council on Foods and Nutrition: Iron deficiency in the United States. JAMA 203:407, 1968

97. Constantoulakis M et al: Combined long-term treatment of hemosiderosis with desferrioxamine and DTPA in homozygous β-thalassemia. Ann NY Acad Sci 232:193, 1974

98. Conte WJ, Ritter JI: The use of association data to identify family members at high risk for marker-linked diseases. Am J Hum Genet 36:152, 1984

99. Cook JD: Methods to determine plasma iron and total iron-binding capacity. In Hallberg L et al (eds): Iron Deficiency: Pathogenesis, Clinical Aspects, Therapy, p 397. New York, Academic Press, 1969

100. Cook JD, Finch CA: Iron nutrition. West J Med 122:474, 1975

101. Cook JD et al: Iron kinetics with emphasis on iron overload. Am J Pathol 72:337, 1973

102. Cook JD et al: Evaluation of the iron status of a population. Blood 48:449, 1976

103. Cooper B et al: Treatment of iron overload in adults with continuous parenteral deferrioxamine. Am J Med 63:958, 1977

104. Cox TM, Peters TJ: *In vitro* studies of duodenal iron uptake in patients with primary and secondary iron storage disease. Q J Med 195:249, 1980

105. Crichton RR: The biochemistry of ferritin. Br J Haematol 24:677, 1973

106. Crichton RR et al: Ferritin comparative structural studies, iron deposition and mobilization. In Brown E et al (eds): Proteins of Iron Metabolism, p 13. New York, Grune & Stratton, 1977

107. Crosby WH: Treatment of haemochromatosis by energetic phlebotomy: One patient's response to the letting of 55 litres of blood in 11 months. Br J Haematol 4:82, 1958

108. Crosby WH: Editorial review: The control of iron balance by the intestinal mucosa. Blood 22:441, 1963

109. Crosby WH et al: Hemochromatosis (iron-storage disease). JAMA 228:743, 1974

110. Cumming RLC et al: Clinical and laboratory studies on the action of desferrioxamine. Br J Haematol 17:257, 1969

111. Cutler DJ et al: Hemochromatosis heart disease: An unemphasized cause of potentially reversible restrictive cardiomyopathy. Am J Med 69:923, 1980

112. Dadone MM et al: Hereditary hemochromatosis: Analysis of laboratory expression of the disease by genotype in 18 pedigrees. Am J Clin Pathol 78:196, 1982

113. Davies G et al: Deposition of melanin and iron in ocular structures in hemochromatosis. Br J Ophthalmol 56:338, 1972

114. Davies SC et al: Ocular toxicity of high-dose intravenous desferrioxamine. Lancet 2:181, 1983

115. Davis AE, Badenoch J: Iron absorption in pancreatic disease. Lancet 2:6, 1962

116. Davis PS, Deller DJ: Effect of a xanthine-oxidase inhibitor (allopurinol) on radio-iron absorption in man. Lancet 2:470, 1966

117. De Alarcon PA et al: Iron absorption in the thalassemia syndromes and its inhibition by tea. N Engl J Med 300:5, 1979

118. Debre R et al: Genetics of haemochromatosis. Ann Hum Genet 23:16, 1958

119. Delbarre F: L'ostéoporose des hémochromatoses. Sem Hop Paris 36:3279, 1960

120. Derman DP et al: Iron absorption from maize (*Zea mays*) and sorghum (*Sorghum vulgare*) beer. Br J Nutr 43:271, 1980

121. De Seze S et al: Joint and bone disorders and hypoparathyroidism in hemochromatosis. Semin Arthritis Rheum 2:71, 1972

122. Deugnier Y et al: Comparative study between biochemical and histological methods and image analysis in liver iron overload. J Clin Pathol 35:45, 1982

123. Diez-Ewald M et al: Interrelationship of iron and manganese metabolism. Proc Soc Exp Biol Med 129:448, 1968

124. Dillingham CH: Familial occurrence of hemochromatosis: Report of four cases in siblings. N Engl J Med 262:1128, 1960

125. Disler PB et al: The effect of tea on iron absorption. Gut 16:193, 1975

126. Doberneck RC et al: Hepatic iron storage and erythrokinetics after portacaval shunt. Surgery 57:800, 1965

127. Domellof L: Effects of Parenteral Iron Overload on the Rat Liver. Gotebörg, Elanders, Boktryckeri Aktiebolag, 1972

128. Doran TJ et al: Idiopathic hemochromatosis in the Australian population: HLA linkage and recessivity. Hum Immunol 2:191, 1981

129. Dorfmann H et al: Les arthropathies des hémochromatoses. Sem Hop Paris 45:516, 1969

130. Drysdale JW: Microheterogeneity in ferritin molecules. Biochem Biophys Acta 207:256, 1970

131. Drysdale JW: Heterogeneity in tissue ferritins displayed by gel electrofocussing. Biochem J 141:627, 1974

132. Drysdale JW et al: Human isoferritins in normal and diseased states. Semin Haematol 14:71, 1977

133. Dubach R et al: Studies in iron transportation and metabolism: IX. The excretion of iron as measured by the isotope technique. J Lab Clin Med 45:599, 1955

134. Dubin IN: Idiopathic hemochromatosis and transfusion siderosis: Review. Am J Clin Pathol 25:514, 1955

135. Dymock IW et al: Arthropathy of haemochromatosis: Clinical and radiological analysis of 63 patients with iron overload. Ann Rheum Dis 29:469, 1970

136. Dymock IW et al: Observations on the pathogenesis, complications and treatment of diabetes in 115 cases of haemochromatosis. Am J Med 52:203, 1972

137. Easley RM Jr et al: Reversible cardiomyopathy associated with hemochromatosis. N Engl J Med 287:866, 1972

138. Ecker JA et al: The development of post-shunt hemochromatosis: Parenchymal siderosis in patients with cirrhosis occurring after portasystemic shunt surgery: A review of the literature and report of two additional cases. Am J Gastroenterol 50:13, 1968

139. Editorial: High-dose chelation therapy in thalassaemia. Lancet 1:373, 1984

140. Edwards CQ et al: Hereditary hemochromatosis: Diagnosis in siblings and children. N Engl J Med 297:7, 1977

141. Edwards CQ et al: Genetic mapping of the hemochromatosis locus on chromosome 6. Hum Immunol 1:19, 1980

142. Edwards CQ et al: Homozygosity for hemochromatosis: Clinical manifestations. Ann Intern Med 93:519, 1980

143. Edwards CQ et al: Hereditary hemochromatosis: Contributions of genetic analysis. Prog Hematol 12:43, 1981

144. Ehlers KH et al: Longitudinal study of cardiac function in thalassemia major. Ann NY Acad Sci 344:397, 1980

145. Elder KH et al: Decreased activity of hepatic uroporphyrinogen decarboxylase in sporadic porphyria cutanea tarda. N Engl J Med 299:274, 1978

146. Engle ME et al: Late cardiac complications of chronic, severe, refractory anemia with hemochromatosis. Circulation 30:698, 1964

147. Epstein JH, Redeker AG: Porphyria cutanea tarda: A study of the effect of phlebotomy. N Engl J Med 279:1301, 1968

148. Evans J: Treatment of heart failure in haemochromatosis. Br Med J 1:1075, 1959

149. Fairbanks VF et al: Clinical Disorders of Iron Metabolism. New York, Grune & Stratton, 1971

150. Felsher BF, Kushner JP: Hepatic siderosis and porphyria cutanea tarda: Relation of iron excess to the metabolic defect. Semin Hematol 14:242, 1977

151. Felsher BF et al: Decreased hepatic uroporphyrinogen decarboxylase activity in prophyria cutanea tarda. N Engl J Med 306:766, 1982

152. Felts JH et al: Hemochromatosis in two young sisters: Case studies and a family survey. Ann Intern Med 67:117, 1967

153. Fielding J: Desferrioxamine chelatable body iron. J Clin Pathol 20:668, 1967

154. Fielding J: Personal communication, 1978

155. Fielding J et al: Differential ferrioxamine test in idiopathic haemochromatosis and transfusional haemosiderosis. J Clin Pathol 19:159, 1966

156. Fillet G, Marsaglia G: Idiopathic hemochromatosis (IH): Abnormality in RBC transport of iron by the reticuloendothelial system (RES). Proceedings of the XVIIIth Meeting of the American Society of Hematology, p 53, 1975

157. Finch SC, Finch CA: Idiopathic hemochromatosis, an iron storage disease: I. Iron metabolism in hemochromatosis. Medicine 34:381, 1955

158. Finch CA, Huebers H: Perspectives in iron metabolism. N Engl J Med 306:1520, 1982

159. Finch CA et al: Iron metabolism: The pathophysiology of iron storage. Blood 5:983, 1950

160. Finch CA et al: Ferrokinetics in man. Medicine 49:17, 1970

161. Finch CA et al: Effect of blood donation on iron stores as evaluated by serum ferritin. Blood 50:441, 1977

162. Finch CA et al: Body iron loss in animals. Proc Soc Exp Biol Med 159:335, 1978

163. Fitzcharles MA et al: Sideroblastic anaemia with iron overload presenting as an arthropathy. Ann Rheum Dis 41:97, 1982

164. Floyd RA, Lewis CA: Hydroxyl free radical formation from hydrogen peroxide by ferrous iron-nucleotide complexes. Biochemistry 22:1645, 1983

165. Ford GC et al: Ferritin design and formation of an iron storage molecule. Phil Trans R Soc Lond 304:551, 1984

166. Francon F et al: Contribution a l'étude des arthropathies de l'hémochromatose. Presse Med 76:1809, 1968

167. Frey WG et al: Management of familial hemochromatosis. N Engl J Med 265:7, 1961

168. Frey WG et al: Quantitative measurement of liver iron by needle biopsy. J Lab Clin Med 72:52, 1968

169. Friedman BI et al: Increased iron-59 absorption in patients with hepatic cirrhosis. J Nucl Med 7:594, 1966

170. Gale E et al: The quantitative estimation of total iron stores in human bone marrow. J Clin Invest 42:1076, 1963

171. Gillman J, Gillman T: Perspectives in Human Malnutrition. New York, Grune & Stratton, 1951

172. Gillman T et al: Experimental dietary siderosis. Am J Pathol 35:349, 1959

173. Gillooly M et al: The effects of organic acids, phytates and polyphenols on the absorption of iron from vegetables. Br J Nutr 49:331, 1983

174. Golberg L, Smith JP: Iron overloading and hepatic vulnerability. Am J Pathol 36:125, 1960

175. Golberg L et al: The effects of intensive and prolonged administration of iron parenterally in animals. Br J Exp Pathol 38:297, 1957

176. Goldberg HI et al: Non-invasive quantitation of liver iron in dogs with hemochromatosis using dual-energy CT scanning. Invest Radiol 17:375, 1982

177. Goossens JP et al: Iron stores in familial haemochromatosis. Neth J Med 19:279, 1976

178. Gordon DA et al: The chondiocalcific arthropathy of iron overload. Arch Intern Med 134:21, 1974

179. Grace ND, Balint JA: Hemochromatosis associated with end-to-side portacaval anastomosis. Am J Dig 11:351, 1966

180. Grace ND, Powell LW: Iron storage disorders of the liver. Gastroenterology 64:1257, 1974

181. Grady RW: The development of new drugs for use in iron chelation therapy. In Bergsma D et al (eds): Iron Metabolism in Thalassemia, p 161. New York, Alan R Liss, 1976

182. Green R et al: Body iron excretion in man: A collaborative study. Am J Med 45:336, 1968

183. Green R et al: The effect of allopurinol on iron metabolism. S Afr Med J 42:776, 1968

184. Greenberg MS et al: Studies in iron absorption: III. Body radioactivity measurements of patients with liver disease. Gastroenterology 46:651, 1964

185. Griffiths JD et al: Occurrence and prevalence of diabetic retinopathy in hemochromatosis. Diabetes 20:766, 1971

186. Grosberg SJ: Hemochromatosis and heart failure: Presentation of a case with survival after three years treatment by repeated venesection. Ann Intern Med 54:550, 1961

187. Grossman MF et al: Porphyria cutanea tarda: Clinical features and laboratory findings in 40 patients. Am J Med 67:277, 1979

188. Grusin H, Samuel E: A syndrome of osteoporosis in Africans and its relationship to scurvy. Am J Clin Nutr 5:644, 1957

189. Hallberg L et al: Menstrual blood loss: A population study: Variation at different ages and attempts to define normality. Acta Obstet Gynecol Scand 45:320, 1966

190. Halliday JW et al: Serum ferritin in haemochromatosis: Changes in the isoferritin composition during venesection therapy. Br J Haematol 36:395, 1977

191. Halliday JW et al: Serum ferritin in diagnosis of haemochromatosis. Lancet 2:621, 1977

192. Halliday JW, Mack U, Powell L: Duodenal ferritin content and structure: Relationship with body iron stores in man. Arch Intern Med 138:1109, 1978

193. Hamilton E et al: The arthropathy of idiopathic haemochromatosis. Q J Med 37:171, 1968

194. Hamilton EBD: The natural history of arthritis in idiopathic haemochromatosis: Progression of the clinical and radiological features over ten years. Q J Med 199:321, 1981

195. Harker L et al: Evaluation of storage iron by chelates. Am J Med 45:105, 1968

196. Harris OD: Haemochromatosis: A family study. Med J Aust 49:755, 1962

197. Harrison PM: Ferritin: An iron-storage molecule. Semin Hematol 14:55, 1977

198. Harrison PM et al: Ferritin structure and function. In Jacobs A, Worwood M (eds): Iron in Biochemistry and Medicine, vol II, p 131. London, Academic Press, 1980

199. Hathorn M et al: Plasma iron and iron-binding capacity in African males with siderosis. Clin Sci 19:35, 1960

200. Hartley WJ et al: Nutritional siderosis in the bovine. NZ Vet J 7:99, 1959

201. Hedenberg L: Studies on iron metabolism with desferrioxamine in man: Experimental and clinical studies. Scand J Haematol (Suppl) 6:5, 1969

202. Hegsted DM et al: The influence of diet on iron absorption: II. The interrelation of iron and phosphorus. J Exp Med 90:147, 1949

203. Heilmeyer L, Wohler F: The treatment of haemochromatosis with desferrioxamine. German Med Monthly 8:133, 1963

204. Hennigar GR et al: Hemochromatosis caused by excessive vitamin iron intake. Am J Pathol 96:611, 1979

205. Henry WL, Nienhuis AW: Possible adverse effects of ascorbic acid on cardiac function in patients with myocardial iron overload. Blood 5:993, 1977

206. Henry WL et al: Echocardiographic abnormalities in patients with transfusion-dependent anaemia and secondary myocardial iron deposition. Am J Med 64:547, 1978

207. Herington AC et al: Studies on the possible mechanism for deficiency of non-suppressible insulin-like activity in thalassemia major. J Clin Endocrinol Metab 52:393, 1981

208. Hershko C et al: Storage iron kinetics: II. The uptake of hemoglobin iron by hepatic parenchymal cells. J Lab Clin Med 80:624, 1972

209. Hershko C et al: Non-specific serum iron in thalassemia: Abnormal serum iron fraction of potential toxicity. Br J Haematol 40:255, 1978

210. Higginson J et al: Hepatic fibrosis and cirrhosis in man in relation to malnutrition. Am J Pathol 33:29, 1957

211. Higginson J et al: Serum iron levels in siderosis due to habitually excessive iron intake. J Clin Invest 36:1723, 1957

212. Hines JD: Effects of alcohol on inborn errors of metabolism: Porphyria cutanea tarda and hemochromatosis. Semin Hematol 17:113, 1980

213. Hirsch JH et al: The arthropathy of hemochromatosis. Radiology 118:591, 1976

214. Hoffbrand AV: Transfusional siderosis and chelation therapy. In Jacobs A, Worwood M (eds): Iron in Biochemistry and Medicine, vol II, p 499. London, Academic Press, 1980

215. Hoffbrand AV et al: Improvement in iron status and liver function in patients with transfusional iron overload with long-term subcutaneous desferrioxamine. Lancet 1:947, 1979

216. Houang MTW et al: Correlation between computed tomographic values and liver iron content in thalassaemia major with iron overload. Lancet 1:1322, 1979

217. Howard RB et al: Extreme hyperferremia in two instances of hemochromatosis with notes on treatment of one patient by means of repeated venesection. J Lab Clin Med 43:848, 1954

218. Huebers HA, Finch CA: Transferrin: Physiologic behaviour and clinical implications. Blood 64:763, 1984

219. Hunt J et al: The effect of desferrioxamine on fibroblasts and collagen formation in cell cultures. Br J Haematol 41:69, 1979

220. Hussain MAM et al: Effect of dose, time and ascorbate on iron excretion after subcutaneous desferrioxamine. Lancet 1:977, 1977

221. Hussain MA et al: Value of serum ferritin estimation in sickle cell anaemia. Arch Dis Child 53:319, 1978

222. Hwang Y-F, Brown EB: Evaluation of deferoxamine in iron overload. Arch Intern Med 114:741, 1964

223. Hyman CB et al: dl-Alpha-Tocopherol, iron and lipofuscin in thalassemia. Ann NY Acad Sci 232:211, 1974

224. Iancu TC: Iron overload. Mol Aspect Med 6:1, 1982

225. Isaacson C et al: Siderosis in the Bantu: The relationship between iron overload and cirrhosis. J Lab Clin Med 58:845, 1961

226. Jachuck SJ et al: Cardiac involvement in idiopathic haemochromatosis and the effect of venesection. Postgrad Med J 50:276, 1974

227. Jacobs A: Iron overload: Clinical and pathologic aspects. Semin Hematol 14:89, 1977

228. Jacobs A: Iron chelation therapy in iron loaded patients. Br J Haematol 43:1, 1979

229. Jacobs A, Summers MR: Iron uptake and ferritin synthesis by peripheral blood leucocytes in patients with primary idiopathic haemochromatosis. Br J Haematol 49:649, 1981

230. Jakobovits AW et al: Hepatic siderosis in alcoholics. Am J Dig Dis 24:305, 1979

231. Jaquet P et al: Accident mortel après deux saignées au cours du traitment d'une hemachromatose. Diabete 15:70, 1967

232. Jenkins T et al: Is transferrin normal in idiopathic haemochromatosis? Br J Haematol 52:493, 1982

233. Johnson BF: Hemochromatosis resulting from prolonged oral iron therapy. N Engl J Med 278:110, 1968

234. Johnson FE, Krogman WM: Patterns of growth in children with thalassemia major. Ann NY Acad Sci 232:667, 1974

235. Johnson GB, Frey WG: Familial aspects of idiopathic hemochromatosis. JAMA 179:747, 1962

236. Jones NL: Irreversible shock in haemochromatosis. Lancet 1:569, 1962

237. Kalivas JT et al: Phlebotomy and iron overload in porphyria cutanea tarda. Lancet 1:1184, 1969

238. Kattamis C et al: Growth of children with thalassemia: Effects of different transfusion regimes. Arch Dis Child 45:502, 1970

239. Kavin H et al: Effect of the exocrine pancreatic secretions on iron absorption. Gut 8:556, 1967

240. Kent G, Popper H: Liver biopsy in diagnosis of hemochromatosis. Am J Med 44:837, 1968

241. Kent G et al: Effect of iron loading upon the formation of collagen in the hepatic injury induced by carbon tetrachloride. Am J Pathol 45:129, 1964

242. Knauer CM et al: The reversal of hemochromatotic cirrhosis by multiple phlebotomies: Report of a case. Gastroenterology 49:667, 1965

243. Kra SJ et al: Arthritis with synovial iron deposition in a patient with hemochromatosis. N Engl J Med 272:1268, 1965

244. Kravitz K et al: Genetic linkage between hereditary hemochromatosis and HLA. Am J Hum Genet 31:601, 1979

245. Kuntz BME et al: HLA-types in porphyria cutanea tarda. Lancet 1:155, 1981

246. Kushner JP et al: The role of iron in the pathogenesis of porphyria cutanea tarda. J Clin Invest 51:3044, 1972

247. Kushner JP et al: The role of iron in the pathogenesis of prophyria cutanea tarda: II. Inhibition of uroporphyrinogen decarboxylase. J Clin Invest 56:661, 1975

248. Kushner JP et al: An enzymatic defect in porphyria cutanea tarda: Decreased uroporphyrinogen decarboxylase activity. J Clin Invest 58:1089, 1976

249. Kushner JP et al: The enzymatic defect in prophyria cutanea tarda. N Engl J Med 306:799, 1982

250. Lamon JM et al: Idiopathic hemochromatosis in a young female. Gastroenterology 76:179, 1979

251. Lamont NM, Hathorn M: Increased plasma iron and liver pathology in Africans with porphyria. S Afr Med J 34:279, 1960

252. Lassman MN et al: Carbohydrate homeostasis and pancreatic islet cell function in thalassaemia. Ann Intern Med 80:65, 1974

253. Lassman MN et al: Endocrine evaluation in thalassemia major. Ann NY Acad Sci 232:226, 1974

254. Lee YH et al: Response of glutathione peroxidase and catalase to excess dietary iron in rats. J Nutr 111:2195, 1981

255. Letsky EA: A controlled trial of long-term chelation therapy in homozygous β-thalassaemia. In Bergsma D et al (eds): Iron Metabolism and Thalassemia, p 31. New York, Alan R Liss, 1976

256. Levy CL, Carlson HE: Decreased prolactin reserve in he-mochromatosis. J Clin Endocrinol Metab 47:444, 1978

257. Lipinski M et al: Hemochromatose idiopathique liaison avec le système HLA. Diabete Metab 4:109, 1978

258. Lipschitz DA et al: The role of ascorbic acid in the metab-olism of storage iron. Br J Haematol 20:155, 1971

259. Lipschitz DA et al: Some factors affecting the release of iron from reticuloendothelial cells. Br J Haematol 21:289, 1971

260. Lipschitz DA et al: The site of action of desferrioxamine. Br J Haematol 20:395, 1971

261. Lipschitz DA et al: A clinical evaluation of serum ferritin. N Engl J Med 290:1213, 1974

262. Lisboa PE: Experimental hepatic cirrhosis in dogs caused by chronic massive iron overload. Gut 12:363, 1971

263. Lloyd DA et al: Histocompatibility antigens as markers of abnormal iron metabolism in idiopathic hemochromatosis. Can Med Assoc J 119:1051, 1978

264. Lloyd HM et al: Idiopathic haemochromatosis in men-struating women: A family study, including the use of di-ethylene triamine penta-acetic acid. Lancet 2:555, 1964

265. Long JA Jr et al: Computed tomographic analysis of beta-thalassemic syndromes with hemochromatosis: Pathologic findings with clinical and laboratory correlations. J Comput Assist Tomogr 4:159, 1980

266. Losowsky MS: Effects of desferrioxamine in patients with iron-loading with a simple method for estimating urinary iron. J Clin Pathol 19:165, 1966

267. Losowsky MS, Wilson AR: Whole-body counting of the absorption and distribution of iron in haemochromatosis. Clin Sci 32:151, 1967

268. Luke CG et al: Gastric iron binding in haemochromatosis, secondary iron overload, cirrhosis and diabetes. Lancet 2:844, 1968

269. Lundvall O, Weinfeld A: Iron stores in alcohol abusers: II. As measured with the desferrioxamine test. Acta Med Scand 18:271, 1969

270. Lundvall O et al: Iron stores in alcohol abusers: I. Liver iron. Acta Med Scand 185:259, 1969

271. Lundvall O et al: Iron storage in porphyria cutanea tarda. Acta Med Scand 188:37, 1970

272. Lynch SR et al: Osteoporosis in Johannesburg Bantu males: Its relationship to siderosis and ascorbic acid deficiency. Am J Clin Nutr 20:799, 1967

273. Lynch SR et al: Accelerated oxidative catabolism of ascorbic acid in siderotic Bantu. Am J Clin Nutr 20:641, 1967

274. Lynch SR et al: Some aspects of calcium metabolism in normal and osteoporotic Bantu subjects with special ref-erence to the effects of iron overload and ascorbic acid de-pletion. S Afr J Med Sci 35:45, 1970

275. McAllen PM et al: The treatment of haemochromatosis with particular reference to the removal of iron from the body by repeated venesection. Q J Med 26:251, 1957

276. MacDonald RA: Hemochromatosis and Hemosiderosis. Springfield, IL, Charles C Thomas, 1964

277. MacDonald RA, Pechet GS: Tissue iron and hemochro-matosis: Comparative geographic studies in Ireland, Israel, Japan, South Africa and the United States. Arch Intern Med 116:381, 1965

278. MacDonald RA, Pechet GS: Experimental haemochro-matosis in rats. Am J Pathol 46:85, 1965

279. MacDonald RA et al: Folic acid deficiency and hemochro-matosis. Arch Pathol 80:153, 1965

280. McIntosh N: Endocrinopathy in thalassemia major. Arch Dis Child 51:195, 1976

281. McGill JR et al: Localization of human ferritin H (heavy) and L (light) subunits by in situ hybridization. Am J Hum Genet 36(suppl):1465, 1984

282. McKeering LV et al: Immunological detection of isoferritins in normal human serum and tissue. Clin Chim Acta 67:189, 1976

283. McLaren GD et al: Iron overload disorders: Natural history, pathogenesis, diagnosis and therapy. CRC Rev Clin Lab Sci 19:205, 1984

284. MacPhail AP et al: Changing patterns of dietary iron over-load in black South Africans. Am J Clin Nutr 32:1272, 1979

285. MacSween RNM: Acute abdominal crises, circulatory col-lapse and sudden death in haemochromatosis. Q J Med 35:589, 1966

286. MacSween RNM, Scott AR: Hepatic cirrhosis: A clinico-pathological review of 520 cases. J Clin Pathol 26:936, 1973

287. Martinez-Torres C, Layrisse M: Interest for study of dietary absorption and iron fortification. World Rev Nutr Diet 19:51, 1974

288. May ME et al: Iron nitrilotriacetate-induced experimental diabetes in rats. J Lab Clin Med 95:525, 1980

289. Mazur A, Sackler M: Haemochromatosis and hepatic xan-thine oxidase. Lancet 1:254, 1967

290. Mazur A, Shorr E: Hepatorenal factors in circulatory ho-meostasis: IX. The identification of the hepatic vasode-pressor substance, VDM, with ferritin. J Biol Chem 176:771, 1948

291. Megyesi C et al: Glucose tolerance and diabetes in chronic liver disease. Lancet 2:1051, 1967

292. Milder MS et al: Idiopathic hemochromatosis, an interim report. Medicine 59:34, 1980

293. Milder MS et al: The influence of food iron absorption on the plasma iron level in idiopathic hemochromatosis. Acta Haematol 60:65, 1978

294. Modell B: Total management of thalassemia major. Arch Dis Child 52:489, 1977

295. Modell CB: Transfusional haemochromatosis. In Kief H (ed): Iron Metabolism and its Disorders, p 230. Amsterdam, Excerpta Medica, 1975

296. Modell CB, Beck J: Long-term desferrioxamine therapy in thalassemia. Ann NY Acad Sci 232:201, 1974

297. Modell CB, Matthews R: Thalassemia in Britain and Aus-tralia. In Bergsma D et al (eds): Iron Metabolism and Thal-assemia, p 13. New York, Alan R Liss, 1976

298. Monsen ER et al: Estimation of available dietary iron. Am J Clin Nutr 31:134, 1978

299. Morgan EH, Walters MNI: Iron storage in human disease: Fractionation of hepatic and splenic iron into ferritin and haemosiderin with histochemical correlations. J Clin Pathol 16:101, 1963

300. Morgan OS et al: Studies on iron-binding component in human gastric juice. Lancet 1:861, 1969

301. Motulsky AG: Biased ascertainment and the natural history of disease. N Engl J Med 298:1197, 1978

302. M'Seffar A et al: Arthropathy as the major clinical indicator of occult iron storage disease. JAMA 238:1825, 1977

303. Muir WA et al: Evidence for heterogeneity in hereditary hemochromatosis: Evaluation of 174 persons in nine fam-ilies. Am J Med 76:806, 1984

304. Murphy KJ: 4,644 grammes of oral ferrous sulphate (over 19 years) without apparent damage. Med J Aust 1:1051, 1968

305. Murray MJ, Stein N: Does the pancreas influence iron ab-

sorption? A critical review of information to date. Gastro-enterology 51:694, 1966

306. Nath I et al: Experimental siderosis and liver injury in the rhesus monkey. J Pathol 106:103, 1972

307. Necheles TF et al: Intensive transfusion therapy in thalassemia major: An eight year follow-up. Ann NY Acad Sci 232:179, 1974

308. Niederau C, Berger M, Stremmel W, Strohmeyer G: Insulin resistance in hemochromatosis patients without liver cirrhosis. Gastroenterology 84:1387, 1983

309. Nienhuis AW et al: Thalassemia: Molecular and clinical aspects. Ann Intern Med 91:883, 1979

310. Nienhuis AW et al: Evaluation of cardiac function in patients with thalassemia major. Ann NY Acad Sci 344:384, 1980

311. Nixon DD: Spontaneous shunt siderosis. Am J Dig Dis 11:359, 1966

312. O'Brien RT: Ascorbic acid enhancement of desferrioxamine-induced urinary iron excretion in thalassemia major. Ann NY Acad Sci 232:221, 1974

313. O'Brien RT: Iron overload: Clinical and pathologic aspects in pediatrics. Semin Hematol 14:115, 1977

314. Olsson KS et al: Prevalence of iron overload in central Sweden. Acta Med Scand 213:145, 1983

315. Olsson KS et al: Screening for iron overload using transferrin saturation. Acta Med Scand 215:105, 1984

316. Olsson KS et al: Liver affection in iron overload studied with serum ferritin and serum aminotransferases. Acta Med Scand 8:58, 1984

317. Passa P et al: Retinopathy and plasma growth hormone levels in idiopathic hemochromatosis with diabetes. Diabetes 26:113, 1977

318. Perkins KW et al: Idiopathic haemochromatosis in children: Report of a family. Am J Med 39:118, 1965

319. Perman G: Hemochromatosis and red wine. Acta Med Scand 182:281, 1967

320. Peters TJ, Seymour CA: Acid hydrolase activities and lysosomal integrity in liver biopsies from patients with iron overload. Clin Sci Mol Med 50:75, 1976

321. Peters TJ, Seymour CA: Analytical subcellular fractionation of needle biopsy specimens from human liver. Biochem J 174:435, 1978

322. Peto TEA et al: Iron overload in mild sideroblastic anaemias. Lancet 2:375, 1983

323. Pippard MJ et al: Intensive iron-chelation therapy with desferrioxamine in iron-loading anaemias. Clin Sci Mol Med 54:99, 1978

324. Pippard MJ et al: Ferrioxamine excretion in iron-loaded man. Blood 60:288, 1982

325. Pitt CG et al: The selection and evaluation of new chelating agents for the treatment of iron overload. J Pharmacol Exp Ther 208:12, 1979

326. Pletcher WD et al: Hemochromatosis following prolonged iron therapy in a patient with hereditary nonspherocytic hemolytic anaemia. Am J Med Sci 246:27, 1963

327. Ploem JE et al: Idiopathic haemosiderosis. Scand J Haematol 2:3, 1965

328. Ploem JE et al: Sideruria following a single dose of desferrioxamine-B as a diagnostic test in iron overload. Br J Haematol 12:396, 1966

329. Pollycove M et al: Transient hepatic deposition of iron in primary hemochromatosis with iron deficiency following venesection. J Nucl Med 12:28, 1971

330. Polson CJ: The storage of iron following its oral and subcutaneous administration. Q J Med 23:77, 1929

331. Polson CJ: The fate of colloidal iron administered intravenously: II. Long experiments. J Pathol Bacteriol 32:247, 1929

332. Powell LW: Normal human iron storage and its relation to ethanol consumption. Aust Ann Med 15:110, 1966

333. Powell LW: Changing concepts in haemochromatosis. Postgrad Med J 46:200, 1970

334. Powell LW, Halliday JW: Idiopathic haemochromatosis. In Jacobs A, Worwood M (eds): Iron in Biochemistry and Medicine, vol II, p 461. New York, Academic Press, 1980

335. Powell LW, Kerr JFR: The pathology of the liver in hemochromatosis. In Loachim HL (ed): Pathobiology Annual, p 317. New York, Appleton-Century-Crofts, 1975

336. Powell LW, Thomas MJ: Use of diethylenetriamine pentaacetic acid (DTPA) in the clinical assessment of total body iron stores. J Clin Pathol 20:896, 1967

337. Powell LW et al: Intestinal mucosal uptake of iron and iron retention in idiopathic haemochromatosis as evidence for a mucosal abnormality. Gut 11:727, 1970

338. Powell LW et al: Abnormality in tissue isoferritin distribution in idiopathic haemochromatosis. Nature 250:333, 1974

339. Powell LW et al: Alterations in serum and tissue isoferritins in disease states: II. Hemochromatosis and malignant disease. In Brown EB et al (eds): Proteins of Iron Metabolism, p 61. New York, Grune & Stratton, 1977

340. Powell LW et al: Relationship between serum ferritin and total body iron stores in idiopathic haemochromatosis. Gut 19:538, 1978

341. Pozza G, Ghidoni A: Studies on the diabetic syndrome of idiopathic haemochromatosis. Diabetologia 4:83, 1968

342. Prieto J et al: Serum ferritin in patients with iron overload and with acute and chronic liver disease. Gastroenterology 68:525, 1975

343. Propper R, Nathan D: Clinical removal of iron. In Gregie WP et al (eds): Annual Review of Medicine, vol 33, p 509. Palo Alto, CA, Annual Reviews, 1982

344. Propper RD et al: Continuous subcutaneous administration of deferoxamine in patients with iron overload. N Engl J Med 297:418, 1977

345. Propper RD et al: New approaches to the transfusion management of thalassemia. Blood 55:55, 1980

346. Ramsay CA et al: The treatment of porphyria cutanea tarda by venesection. Q J Med 43:1, 1974

347. Randell MG et al: Hepatopathy associated with excessive iron storage in mynah birds. J Am Veterinary Assoc 179:1214, 1981

348. Raphael B et al: The trial of hemochromatosis, hepatoma and erythrocytosis. Cancer 43:690, 1979

349. Reissmann KR, Dietrich MR: On the presence of ferritin in the peripheral blood of patients with hepatocellular disease. J Clin Invest 35:588, 1956

350. Reizenstein P et al: Iron metabolism in porphyria cutanea tarda. Acta Med Scand 198:95, 1975

351. Richter GW: Studies of iron overload: Rat siderosome ferritin. Lab Invest 50:26, 1984

352. Rigas DA, Finch SC: Electrophoretic studies of serum proteins in hemochromatosis. Am J Med Sci 237:566, 1959

353. Risdon RA et al: Transfusional iron overload: The relationship between tissue iron concentration and hepatic fibrosis in thalassaemia. J Pathol 116:83, 1975

354. Ritter B et al: HLA as a marker of the hemochromatosis gene in Sweden. Hum Genet 886:1, 1984

355. Ross J et al: Kinetics of iron transferrin complex formation. Blood 24:850, 1964

356. Rous P, Oliver J: Experimental hemochromatosis. J Exp Med 28:629, 1918

357. Rowe JW et al: Familial hemochromatosis: Characteristics of the precirrhotic stage in a large kindred. Medicine 56:197, 1977

358. Sabesin SM, Thomas LB: Parenchymal siderosis in patients with pre-existing portal cirrhosis: A pathologic entity simulating idiopathic and transfusional hemochromatosis. Gastroenterology 46:477, 1964

359. Saenger P et al: Depressed serum somatomedin activity in beta-thalassemia. J Pediatr 2:214, 1980

360. Saint EG: Haemochromatosis. Med J Aust 50:137, 1963

361. Sanyal SK et al: Fatal "iron-heart" in an adolescent. Pediatrics 55:336, 1975

362. Sargent T et al: Iron absorption in hemochromatosis before and after phlebotomy therapy. J Nucl Med 12:660, 1971

363. Sauer GF, Funk DD: Iron overload in cutaneous porphyria. Arch Intern Med 124:190, 1969

364. Saunders SJ: Iron metabolism in symptomatic porphyria. S Afr J Lab Clin Med 9:277, 1963

365. Schattenkirchner M et al: Arthropathie bei der idiopathischen Hämochromatose. Klin Wochenschr 61:1199, 1983

366. Scheuer PJ et al: Hepatic pathology in relatives of patients with haemochromatosis. J Pathol 84:53, 1962

367. Scheuer PJ et al: The inheritance of idiopathic haemochromatosis: A clinical and liver biopsy study of 16 families. Q J Med 31:249, 1962

368. Schulz EJ, Swanepoel H: Scorbutic pseudoscleroderma: An aspect of Bantu siderosis. S Afr Med J 36:367, 1962

369. Schumacher HR Jr: Hemochromatosis and arthritis. Arthritis Rheum 7:41, 1964

370. Schumacher HR: Articular cartilage in the degenerative arthropathy of hemochromatosis. Arthritis Rheum 25:1460, 1982

371. Seftel H et al: Siderosis in the Bantu: The clinical incidence of hemochromatosis in diabetic subjects. J Lab Clin Med 58:837, 1961

372. Seftel HC et al: Osteoporosis, scurvy and siderosis in Johannesburg Bantu. Br Med J 1:642, 1966

373. Selden C et al: Activities of some free-radical scavenging enzymes and glutathione concentrations in human and rat liver and their relationship to the pathogenesis of tissue damage in iron overload. Clin Sci 58:211, 1980

374. Sella EJ, Goodman AG: Arthropathy secondary to transfusion haemochromatosis. J Bone Joint Surg [Am] 55:1077, 1973

375. Seshadri R et al: Long-term administration of desferrioxamine in thalassaemia major. Arch Dis Child 49:621, 1974

376. Seymour CA, Peters TJ: Organelle pathology in primary and secondary haemochromatosis with special reference to lysosomal changes. Br J Haematol 40:239, 1978

377. Sheldon JH: Haemochromatosis. London, Oxford University Press, 1935

378. Sherwin R et al: Hyperglucagonemia in Laennec's cirrhosis. N Engl J Med 290:239, 1974

379. Simon M, Bourel M: Heredite de l'hemochromatose: Idiopathique demonstration de la transmission recessive et mise en evidence du gene responsable porte par le chromosome 6. Gastroenterol Clin Biol 2:573, 1978

380. Simon M et al: The genetics of hemochromatosis. Prog Med Genet 4:135, 1980

381. Simon M et al: Association of HLA-A3 and HLA-B14 antigens with idiopathic haemochromatosis. Gut 17:332, 1976

382. Simon M et al: Hereditary idiopathic haemochromatosis: A study of 106 families. Clin Genet 11:327, 1977

383. Simon M et al: Idiopathic hemochromatosis: Demonstration of recessive transmission and early detection by family HLA typing. N Engl J Med 297:1017, 1977

384. Simon M et al: Idiopathic hemochromatosis and iron overload in alcoholic liver disease: Differentiation by HLA phenotype. Gastroenterology 73:655, 1977

385. Simon M et al: Heredite recessive de l'hemochromatose idiopathique: Deux observations de transmission pseudo-dominate reconnue comme recessive par l'étude de la surcharge en fer et des genotypes HLA dans les familles. Nouv Presse Med 8:421, 1979

386. Simon M et al: Les hemochromatoses. Ann Med Interne 132:413, 1981

387. Skinner C, Kenmore ACF: Haemochromatosis presenting as congestive cardiomyopathy and responding to venesection. Br Heart J 35:466, 1973

388. Smith PM et al: Assessment of body-iron stores in cirrhosis and haemochromatosis with the differential ferrioxamine test. Lancet 1:133, 1967

389. Smith PM et al: The differential ferrioxamine test in the management of idiopathic haemochromatosis. Lancet 2:402, 1969

390. Solomon L: Personal communication, 1974

391. Speight ANP, Cliff J: Iron storage disease of the liver in Dar-es-Salaam: A preliminary report on venesection therapy. East Afr Med J 51:895, 1974

392. Stocks AE, Martin FIR: Pituitary function in haemochromatosis. Am J Med 45:839, 1968

393. Stocks AE, Powell LW: Pituitary function in idiopathic haemochromatosis and cirrhosis of the liver. Lancet 2:298, 1972

394. Strachan AS: Haemosiderosis and haemochromatosis in South African natives, with a comment on the aetiology of haemochromatosis, thesis. University of Glasgow, 1929

395. Taljaard JJF et al: Porphyrin metabolism in experimental hepatic siderosis in the rat: II. Combined effect of iron overload and hexachlorobenzene. Br J Haematol 23:513, 1972

396. Theron JJ, Mekel RCPM: Ultrastructural localization of iron in the human jejunum in iron overload (Bantu siderosis). Br J Haematol 21:165, 1971

397. Thivolet J et al: Traitement des porthyries cutanés tardives par les chelateurs du fer (E.D.T.A., Desferal). Lyon Med 218:225, 1967

398. Torrance JD, Bothwell TH: Tissue iron stores. In Cook JD (ed): Methods in Hematology, vol 1, p 9. New York, Churchill Livingstone, 1980

399. Torrance JD et al: Storage iron in "muscle." J Clin Pathol 21:495, 1968

400. Trump BF et al: The relationship of intracellular pathways of iron metabolism to cellular iron overload and the iron storage diseases. Am J Pathol 72:295, 1973

401. Tuttle SG et al: Development of hemochromatosis in a patient with Laennec's cirrhosis. Am J Med 26:655, 1959

402. Valberg LS et al: Distribution of storage iron as body iron stores expand in patients with hemochromatosis. J Lab Clin Med 86:479, 1975

403. Valberg LS et al: Iron absorption in idiopathic hemochromatosis: Relationship to serum ferritin concentration in asymptomatic relatives. Clin Invest Med 2:1, 1979

404. Valberg LS et al: Clinical and biochemical expression of the genetic abnormality in idiopathic hemochromatosis. Gastroenterology 79:884, 1980

405. Vallat JM et al: Hemosiderin deposition in muscle: Report of three cases. Acta Neuropathol 42:153, 1978

406. Van der Weyden MB et al: Erythrocyte ferritin content in idiopathic haemochromatosis and alcoholic liver disease with iron overload. Br Med J 286:752, 1983

407. Vartsky D et al: Nuclear resonant scattering of gamma rays: a new technique for *in vivo* measurement of body iron stores. Phys Med Biol 24:689, 1979

408. Wada T et al: Autoradiographic study on the site of uptake of the haptoglobin-hemoglobin complex. J Reticuloendothel Soc 8:185, 1970

409. Wadsworth PF et al: Hepatic haemosiderosis in birds at the Zoological Society of London. Avian Pathol 12:321, 1983

410. Wagstaff M et al: Iron and isoferritins in iron overload. Clin Sci 62:529, 1982

411. Walker ARP, Arvidsson UB: Iron "overload" in the South African Bantu. Trans R Soc Trop Med Hyg 47:536, 1953

412. Walker RJ, Williams R: Haemochromatosis and iron overload. In Jacobs A, Worwood M (eds): Iron in Biochemistry and Medicine, p 589. London, Academic Press, 1974

413. Walker RJ et al: Relationship of hepatic iron concentration to histochemical grading and to total chelatable body iron in conditions associated with iron overload. Gut 12:1011, 1971

414. Wallerstein RO, Robbins SL: Hemochromatosis after prolonged oral iron therapy in a patient with chronic hemolytic anaemia. Am J Med 14:256, 1953

415. Walsh RJ et al: The use of DTPA in the diagnosis and management of idiopathic haemochromatosis. Aust Ann Med 12:192, 1963

416. Walton C et al: Endocrine abnormalities in idiopathic haemochromatosis. Q J Med 205:99, 1983

417. Wands JR et al: Normal serum ferritin concentrations in precirrhotic hemochromatosis. N Engl J Med 294:302, 1976

418. Wapnick AA et al: Effects of iron overload on ascorbic acid metabolism. Br Med J 3:704, 1968

419. Wapnick AA et al: The effect of ascorbic acid deficiency on desferrioxamine-induced urinary iron excretion. Br J Haematol 17:563, 1969

420. Wapnick AA et al: The relationship between serum iron levels and ascorbic acid stores in siderotic Bantu. Br J Haematol 19:271, 1970

421. Wapnick AA et al: The effect of siderosis and ascorbic acid depletion on bone metabolism with special reference to osteoporosis in the Bantu. Br J Nutr 25:367, 1971

422. Wardle EN, Patton JT: Bone and joint changes in haemochromatosis. Ann Rheum Dis 28:15, 1969

423. Wasserman AJ et al: Cardiac hemochromatosis simulating constrictive pericarditis. Am J Med 32:316, 1962

424. Weinberg ED: Iron withholding: A defence against infection and neoplasia. Physiol Rev 64:65, 1984

425. Weiner M et al: Cooley anaemia: High transfusion regimen

426. Weintraub LR et al: The treatment of hemochromatosis by phlebotomy. Med Clin North Am 50:1579, 1966

427. Wheby MS, Umpierre G: Effect of transferrin saturation on iron absorption in man. N Engl J Med 271:1391, 1964

428. Wheby MS et al: Brief report: Clearance of iron from hemochromatotic and normal transferrin *in vivo*. Blood 24:765, 1964

429. Williams R et al: Iron absorption in the relatives of patients with idiopathic haemochromatosis. Lancet 1:1243, 1965

430. Williams R et al: Iron absorption in idiopathic haemochromatosis before, during and after venesection therapy. Br Med J 2:78, 1966

431. Williams R et al: Iron absorption and siderosis in chronic liver disease. Q J Med 36:151, 1967

432. Williams R et al: Venesection therapy in idiopathic haemochromatosis: An analysis of 40 treated and 18 untreated patients. Q J Med 38:1, 1969

433. Wills ED: Lipid peroxide formation in microsomes: The role of non-heme iron. Biochem J 113:325, 1969

434. Witzleben CL, Wyatt JP: The effect of long survival on the pathology of thalassaemia major. J Pathol Bacteriol 82:1, 1961

435. Wixom RL et al: Hemosiderin: Nature, formation and significance. Int Rev Exp Pathol 22:193, 1979

436. Wolman IJ: Transfusion therapy in Cooley's anemia: Growth and health as related to long range hemoglobin levels, a progress report. Ann NY Acad Sci 119:736, 1964

437. Worwood M: Serum ferritin. In Jacobs A, Worwood M (eds): Iron in Biochemistry and Medicine, vol II, p 203. London, Academic Press, 1980

438. Worwood M et al: The characteristics of ferritin from human tissues, serum and blood cells. Clin Sci Mol Med 48:441, 1975

439. Wynter CVA, Williams R: Iron-binding properties of gastric juice in idiopathic haemochromatosis. Lancet 2:534, 1968

440. Yam LT et al: Circulating iron-containing macrophages in hemochromatosis. N Engl J Med 279:512, 1968

441. Yamanoi Y et al: Mechanism of iron toxicity in the liver and pancreas after a single injection of ferric nitrilotriacetate. Acta Haematol Jpn 45:47, 1982

442. Yamashiro KM: *Pasteurella pseudotuberculosis:* Acute sepsis with survival. Arch Intern Med 128:605, 1971

443. Yang F et al: Human transferrin: cDNA characterisation and chromosomal localization. Proc Nat Acad Sci 81:2752, 1983

444. Zimelman AP, Miller A: Primary hemochromatosis with hereditary spherocytosis. Arch Intern Med 140:983, 1980

445. Zuppinger K et al: Increased risk of diabetes mellitus in beta-thalassemia major due to iron overload. Helvet Paed Acta 34:197, 1979

and chelation therapy, results and perspective. J Pediatr 92:653, 1978

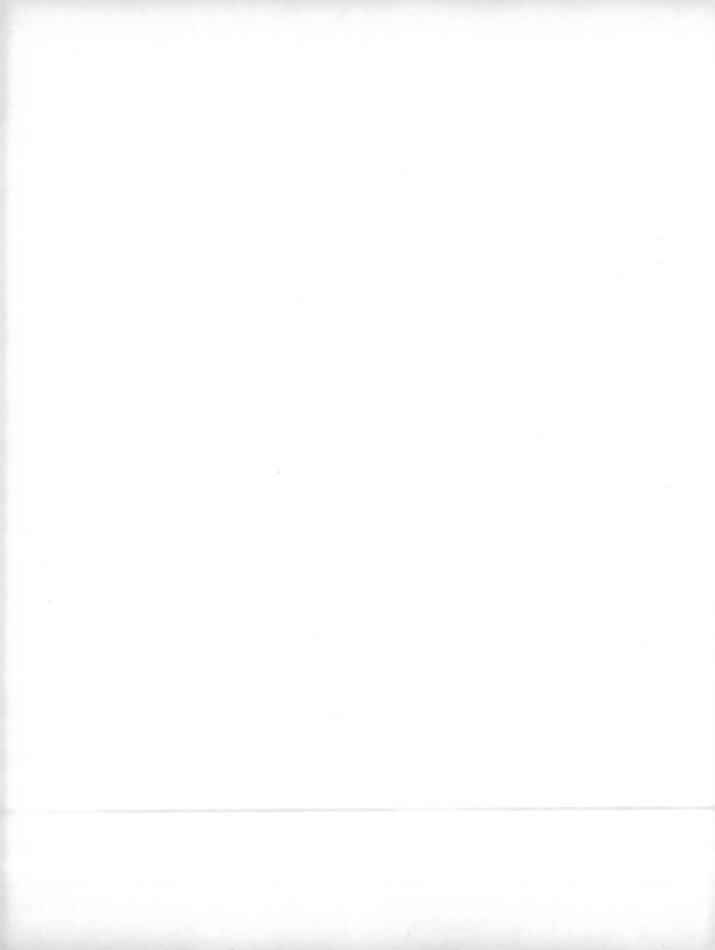

chapter 28

The Liver in Wilson's Disease (Hepatolenticular Degeneration)

J. M. WALSHE

There are few diseases of the liver for which there are specific and effective forms of treatment. One is Wilson's disease (hepatolenticular degeneration), which is an inherited metabolic disease, with the abnormal gene probably being carried on chromosome 13.[10] Although nothing is known about the abnormal gene or about the presumed enzyme or protein defect,[18] it is now established that this leads to an accumulation of copper in the tissues, principally the liver and the brain, and that the clinical picture of the disease is secondary to the toxic effects of the metal on these organs. The present available evidence supports the hypothesis that the biochemical defect is a failure of copper excretion via the bile[9,13] rather than excess absorption from the gut.

INCIDENCE

Once believed to be one of the rarest of the inherited metabolic diseases, Wilson's disease is now known to be relatively common, with an incidence of approximately 30 per million of the population[2,34] and a carrier rate approaching 1 in 100. In the relevant population subgroups it is, of course, found much more often, that is, in children and adolescents with liver disease and in adolescents and young adults with neurologic or psychiatric symptoms. In such patients the possibility that Wilson's disease may indeed be the correct diagnosis must always be borne in mind, especially since this is an eminently treatable illness provided the diagnosis is made before irrevocable damage has been inflicted on the target organs.

CLINICAL PICTURE

The clinical picture is based on an analysis of some 220 cases, 119 in males and 101 in females. This shows the slight male-to-female preponderance found in most large series, but the male-to-female preponderance is not as high as in the unaffected siblings. In 23 of the families studied the patient was an only child; in the remaining 129 families in which there were multiple births more than one child was affected in 48, and in two families there were no less than four affected siblings. On subtracting the propositi from the total number of children, we are left with 62 patients and 243 unaffected individuals, giving an incidence of 20.3%, which is close to the theoretical figure of 25% for recessive inheritance.

Generalizations about Wilson's disease are always dangerous because the next patient presenting at the clinic will not conform to previous findings; however, it is fair to say that the great majority will fall into one of two broad categories: those with a predominantly hepatic symptomatology and those presenting with a neurologic picture. There is no doubt, however, that a certain number of patients will give a history of an earlier episode of ill health for which no satisfactory diagnosis was made but that was, in all probability, related to their Wilson's disease: for instance the girl who at 13 years of age was found to be quite severely anemic (hemoglobin. 9 g/dl) and who 3 years later developed extensive bruising, leg vein thromboses, and gangrene of the toes of both feet. This episode resolved spontaneously, and she remained well until the age of 21 when she became dysarthric, and this was soon followed by tremor. Other patients have complained of bone and joint symptoms and attended rheumatologic clinics for some time before more characteristic signs of Wilson's disease drew attention to the correct diagnosis. Another problem in trying to categorize patients is that many who present with a typical neurologic picture give a history of an earlier, relatively brief, episode of jaundice, which, at the time, was called "hepatitis." Others who give no such history are found, on examination, to have severe and advanced hepatic disease of which they are largely unaware. However, in an attempt to separate patients into these two main groupings for diagnostic purposes the initial symptom of which they complained, relating either to the liver or the brain, has been selected and not the clinical picture at the time diagnosis was made. The result of this classification is shown in Figure 28-1. It will be seen that of the 217 patients included in this histogram, 101 presented with hepatic symptoms and 90 with neurologic symptoms and 28 were presymptomatic, having been found on screening the affected families. It must be mentioned that in considering these so-called presymptomatic patients a certain number had abnormal

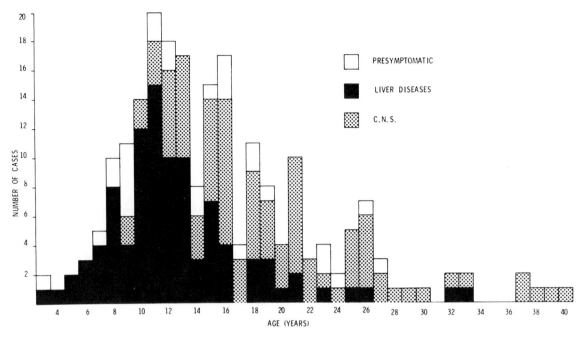

Fig. 28-1. Histogram showing distribution by age and first symptoms of 217 patients with Wilson's disease; 101 patients were hepatic in onset, 90 were neurologic, and 28 were presymptomatic.

physical signs that left no doubt as to the diagnosis while in others this depended on a detailed biochemical study, often requiring chemical analysis of liver biopsy tissue. Two such patients had dense complete Kayser-Fleischer rings, one with associated sunflower cataracts; six other patients had lightly pigmented rings; and ten patients had raised serum aminotransferases with or without hepatosplenomegaly. Only eight could be called truly free of abnormal signs or laboratory tests, other than those specifically aimed to determine disturbances of copper metabolism.

The age at which hepatic symptoms first appeared in this series varied from 3 to 33 years, although one such case has been reported in which the patient presented with cirrhosis in the sixth decade.[7] There is nothing in any way peculiar to the hepatic form of Wilson's disease; the picture can be acute, subacute, or chronic, and the occasional patient is found to have a symptomless splenomegaly on routine examination, the significance of this finding only becoming apparent later. Acute hepatic Wilson's disease has a very high mortality, and the diagnosis is usually only made at postmortem examination or even later when a second sibling falls ill with a similar, although usually less acute illness. Acute hepatic Wilson's disease is almost invariably associated with severe hemolysis, and the mode of death may be secondary renal failure. Apart from these acute cases hemolysis is a well-documented feature of Wilson's disease. In the present series, 25 patients gave a clear-cut history of one or more previous episodes of hemolysis, although only 2 were actually seen at the time of a hemolytic crisis. Of these 25 patients, 10 had a predominantly hepatic disease but no less than 15 recovered from the hemolysis only for the diagnosis of Wilson's disease to be made months or years later when the typical neurologic picture developed. The age range for this particular syndrome was from 7 to 21 years; thus, whenever hemolysis is seen in this particular age-group Wilson's disease must be placed high on the list of differential diagnoses. Coombs' test is always negative, and the disease is not associated with increased osmotic fragility of the red cells. Hemolysis may occur as a single acute episode, it may be recurrent at approximately monthly intervals, or it may be low grade and chronic.

Another feature of Wilson's disease associated with liver dysfunction is the presence of calcified pigment gallstones, which are occasionally large and single but usually multiple and faceted (Fig. 28-2). These were seen in 11 patients, 4 with a predominantly hepatic and 7 with a neurologic illness, but of the latter, 4 gave a clear-cut history of an earlier episode of hemolysis. In 4 patients the gallstones eventually caused symptoms requiring surgery. It is of interest that the copper content of the gallstones found in patients with Wilson's disease is lower by an order of magnitude than that in pigment gallstones found in patients without Wilson's disease.* The mean for 5 patients with Wilson's disease was 52.1 μg/g (range 5.2 μg to 85.4 μg) compared with a mean of 1072.5 μg/g in the control series (range 571.7 μg to 1951.8 μg).

* The copper content of cholesterol stones is very low.

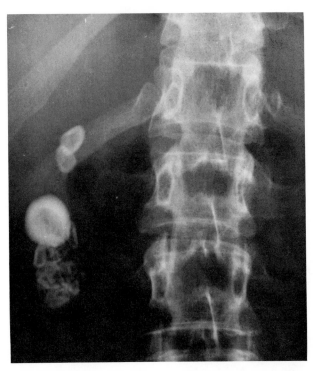

Fig. 28-2. Multiple-faceted gallstones from a woman with Wilson's disease. Between the ages of 7 and 10 years she had had repeated episodes of hemolysis. Symptomless calcified gallstones were found on radiologic survey at the age of 20 years. When she was 34 years of age, biliary colic and infection necessitated their removal.

It has been noted that primary carcinoma develops only very rarely in the cirrhotic liver of Wilson's disease,[23,34] in comparison with other forms of cirrhosis, possibly only five cases having been reported. The hypothesis has therefore been put forward that copper actually protects the liver against malignant change.[21] However a more likely explanation is that in the pretreatment era for Wilson's disease the patients died before this could occur while in well-treated patients the liver lesion becomes so quiescent that the stimulus to carcinoma formation is removed. The patient described by Madden and his associates[23] would seem to support this hypothesis; he had a prolonged history of a neurologic deficit beginning at the age of 35 but only required hospital admission at the age of 61 when he presented with hepatic failure "undoubtedly caused by the development of hepatocellular carcinoma," which presumably had time to develop during the long period of untreated copper overload.

If it is true that there is nothing characteristic in the evolution of hepatic Wilson's disease, the same can also be said for the findings on physical examination, that is, with the exception of the Kayser-Fleischer pigment ring. Any or all of the signs of acute, subacute, or, more commonly, chronic liver disease may be found. However, so important is the Kayser-Fleischer ring as a diagnostic sign

that it merits a more detailed description. In Wilson's disease it is always copper (probably copper proteinate), it is always deposited in Descemet's membrane of the cornea, it always appears first as a top crescent then as a lower crescent, and these grow laterally and spread medially until they join to form complete rings. As they reabsorb with treatment they leave behind a characteristic beaten silver appearance.[3] It is part of their natural history also that the rings spread centrally, becoming broader and more densely pigmented as the disease progresses. Dense, broad, complete rings are always evidence of heavy copper overload but not necessarily of advanced clinical signs or symptoms. On slit lamp examination the rings can also be seen to be granular; the color is usually brown, but when very dense they may appear gray, and it is reported that they are occasionally green.[46] The rings are always present in the neurologic stages of the disease, almost invariably in the hepatic stage (if sought by an experienced ophthalmologist using a gonioscope), and, as has been mentioned earlier, quite commonly in the presymptomatic stages of the illness. It can no longer be claimed that this particular physical sign is 100% diagnostic of Wilson's disease. However, a broad, complete granular ring probably is, but small brown pigmented crescents have been seen in other forms of liver disease associated with longstanding retention of biliary components as in primary biliary cirrhosis and severe, familial intrahepatic cholestasis.[8] Unfortunately in none of the patients was it possible to make histologic or chemical studies of the pigmented zones.

Another physical sign peculiar to Wilson's disease (in the absence of penetrating injury to the globe with a copper-containing foreign body) is the so-called sunflower cataract. This is not a true cataract since the changes are confined to the lens capsule and not to the body of the lens. Originally this was believed to be a rare and late manifestation of the disease, but in the present series 15 examples have been observed and 11 were found early in the course of the illness. The changes consist, typically, of a disk of chalcosis in the anterior lens capsule and petal-like fronds on the posterior capsule. Sometimes the disk of chalcosis is readily visible to naked eye inspection, but more often it requires slit lamp examination to demonstrate its presence. It may well be that a routine search for this would reveal that it is more common than is presently believed (Fig. 28-3).

As has already been stated, the clinical course of hepatic Wilson's disease may be an acute illness leading rapidly to death in liver failure[33] but more commonly the picture is of chronic active hepatitis or cirrhosis of the liver. Sometimes the picture is typical of acute hepatitis that resolves clinically, although careful follow-up will show that the results of the liver function tests do not return to normal. If no action is taken at this stage it is probable that neurologic signs and symptoms will appear in the course of the next few years. The most common of these are dysarthria, drooling, and tremor of one or more limbs, but the picture can be quite pleomorphic and involve al-

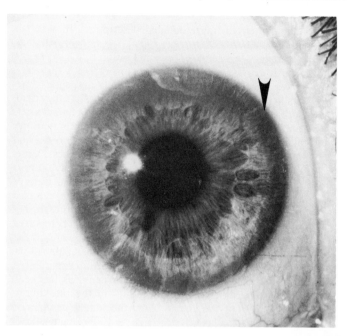

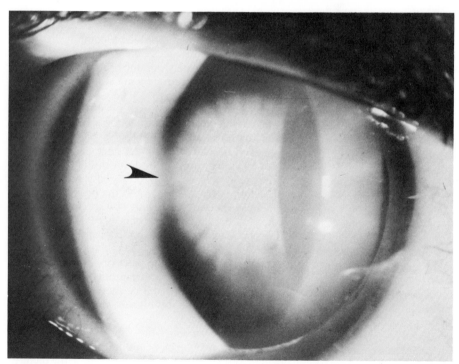

Fig. 28-3. The eye in Wilson's disease. **Top.** Dense, complete Kayser–Fleischer ring (arrow). The pigment can be seen in the photograph as a dark homogeneous ring encircling the periphery of the iris and obscuring the muscular pattern. **Bottom.** Sunflower cataract, as viewed under the slit lamp, showing the disk of chalcosis (arrow) on the anterior lens capsule; the fronds on the posterior capsule are visible on the right of the picture.

most any motor function so that patients may show chorea, parkinsonism, dystonia, and a wide variety of spontaneous movements, and these, too, may fluctuate in severity. Personality changes are also very common; there may be antisocial or inappropriate behavior, childishness, diminished attention span, and a general falling off in performance at school. The sensory nervous system is never involved, but occasionally hyperhidrosis, exophthalmos, and vasomotor instability suggest that the autonomic nervous system has suffered damage. In patients with severe chronic liver disease and portal hypertension and an early parkinsonism the picture may mimic portal-systemic encephalopathy, and this differential diagnosis must always be borne in mind, particularly in the younger age-groups.

In addition to the classic lesions of the brain and liver the abnormal copper deposits also involve the skeleton and the kidneys. The skeletal lesions are now well documented[6,16] and occasionally it is these that first take the patient to the clinic. One patient in the present series attended a rheumatologic clinic for several years with severe painful condylar erosions of his knees (Fig. 28-4A) while another was treated for low back pain (Fig. 28-4B) and yet a third for osteomalacia and pseudofractures. Radiologic skeletal surveys have shown that many changes can be found, of which perhaps the most common is a poorly calcified skeleton (and indeed fractures from inadequate trauma are rather common in patients with Wilson's disease) and a wide variety of degenerative joint changes.

Renal disease as a presenting symptom is almost unknown,[34] but proteinuria, mellituria (not necessarily glucose, since many sugars have been identified), phosphaturia, aminoaciduria, and peptiduria are not uncommon,

Fig. 28-4. A. Roentgenogram of the knee joint showing condylar erosions and fragmentation of the patella (*arrows*). A 22-year-old man with a short history of tremor and a speech defect. For 5 years he had had pain in his knees. **B.** Roentgenogram of the lumbar spine showing "squared" vertebral bodies, loss of the lumbar lordosis, and Schmorl's nodes (*arrows*) in a 13-year-old boy. At the age of 10 and again at 12 years, he had had hemolytic crises, neurologic signs, drooling, a speech defect, and a falling off in his school work were first noted at the age of 11 years.

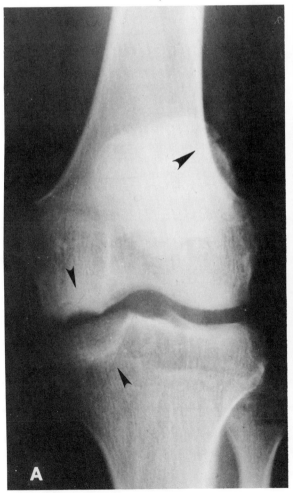
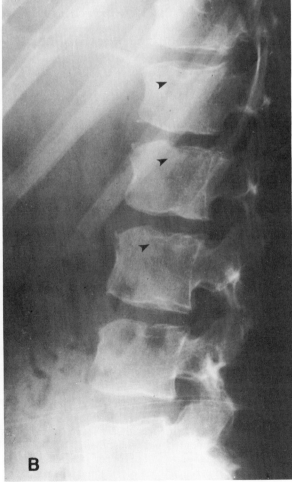

as are also microscopic hematuria and failure to acidify the urine. Hypercalciuria can lead to renal stone formation, and the renal leakage of calcium and phosphorus may lead to renal osteodystrophy, as mentioned previously.[25]

DIAGNOSIS

Correct diagnosis inevitably rests on the ability of the clinician to suspect Wilson's disease on a basis of clinical skills. Thereafter, it must be confirmed by laboratory means. The parameters on which a biochemical confirmation of the diagnosis must be based are the finding of an increased urinary excretion of copper and a reduced concentration of ceruloplasmin and copper in the blood. In a significant number of patients, one or more of these parameters may not be abnormal.

There are a number of different methods of estimating copper in blood, urine, and tissues. It is unlikely that any one of these is significantly superior to any other; what really matters is the experience and expertise of the laboratory undertaking the estimation. The simpler the method, the more likely it is to give highly reproducible results that, in the long run, is more important than striving for absolute truth. It cannot be stressed too strongly that results must be interpreted in light of information of the clinical stage of the illness. The more saturated the tissues are with copper, the more abnormal the results will be. In the very early presymptomatic stage, there may be little or no excess copper in the urine; but at this stage, the serum copper and ceruloplasmin are probably also very low unless the patient happens to have come from one of those rare kinships in which the ceruloplasmin approaches the normal range. In practice, there is always a wide range of overlap between patients and carriers and between carriers and normals for serum copper and ceruloplasmin values; the problems of interpreting these have been discussed in some detail elsewhere (Fig. 28-5).[11]

Another difficult differential diagnosis is between patients with severe liver disease and a secondary fall in the ceruloplasmin concentration[56] and patients with Wilson's disease whose liver damage has resulted in raised endogenous steroid levels and a secondary rise in the serum ceruloplasmin value. In such cases it is helpful to screen the parents and siblings (this should be done in all families of patients suspected of having Wilson's disease). The finding of a relatively low ceruloplasmin concentration in one or more close relatives strongly points to a diagnosis of Wilson's disease.

If these three simple tests fail to clinch the diagnosis, a liver biopsy should be performed. Not less than 10 mg of tissue should be sent for copper determination by an experienced laboratory that has already been consulted as to how the specimen should be handled. The finding of more than 60 μg/g wet weight of copper, unless the patient has biliary cirrhosis or cholestasis of some other etiology,

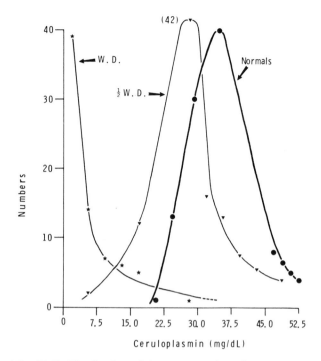

Fig. 28-5. Distribution of the concentration of serum ceruloplasm (mg/dl) in patients with Wilson's disease (*W.D.*), obligate heterozygotes (½ *W.D.*), and normal controls. Note the considerable degree of overlap between the three groups (see also Reference 12).

is almost diagnostic of Wilson's disease. Staining the histologic preparation for copper can be very misleading, and false-negative results are not uncommon. Again, the value of this procedure depends on the experience of the laboratory. The demonstration of copper-associated protein in the hepatocytes by the orcein stain is a further pointer to an excess load of copper in the liver.[20,36] The first histologic change to be found in the liver is glycogen nucleation of the hepatocytes and fatty droplets widely scattered in the lobules. This is followed by the appearance of inflammatory cells in the periportal tracts and may progress either to postnecrotic cirrhosis or chronic aggressive hepatitis. Preferably, the diagnosis will be made before this stage of the illness is reached (Fig. 28-6).

As a last resort, radiolabeled copper may be used. This is an expensive and time-consuming method of making the diagnosis but one that can, again with experience, give a great deal of information of diagnostic value. When ^{64}Cu is used, it is possible to define the pattern of uptake by the liver both by profile scanning[57] and by scintiscanning[26,27] and to estimate the incorporation of copper into ceruloplasmin.[42] Much valuable information can also be obtained from determination of the rate of excretion of the radiolabeled copper in the urine; this is particularly high in the first 8-hour period after injection of the isotope.[14]

Again, it must be remembered that the results obtained will depend on the stage of the disease the patient has reached.[26] It is always preferable that these tests be carried out in a laboratory familiar with the use of radiolabeled copper.

Additional studies of renal function, a blood cell count, and skeletal roentgenograms are essential in the long-term management of the disease and must always precede treatment. Knowledge of these factors is unlikely to be of great diagnostic value in a difficult case, but the finding of abnormal results of liver function tests, particularly the aminotransferases, is certainly of value in screening a sibship of presymptomatic cases.

PATHOGENESIS

The nature of the primary abnormal gene product in Wilson's disease remains unknown.[18] Yet it is established that copper accumulates in certain tissues in great excess, principally the liver, brain, kidney, cornea, and occasionally the lens; its presence in these organs is associated with pathologic changes that are reversible when the copper is removed. It seems reasonable, therefore, to assume that copper is the pathogenic agent in this disease. For copper to exert its toxic action, however, it appears that some normal protective mechanism must be deficient. It is the nature of this missing metabolic step that remains so enigmatic. The evidence for this protective mechanism is indirect. In humans, copper is found in great excess in the liver only in Wilson's disease, primary biliary cirrhosis, severe familial intrahepatic cholestasis,[11,53] and Indian childhood cirrhosis.[4,44] It is by no means clear in the latter two conditions whether the copper is related to the liver damage as cause or effect. Equally, there is no convincing evidence that, in these latter diseases, removal of the copper results in a significant clinical improvement. Although the biologic turnover time for copper in the liver is greatly prolonged in primary biliary cirrhosis it is less so than in Wilson's disease. Moreover, the mechanism for incorporation of copper into ceruloplasmin in primary biliary cirrhosis (unlike that involved in Wilson's disease) remains intact.[11] This may relate to the reduced vulnerability of the hepatocytes to copper compared with the situation in Wilson's disease. In certain animal species, the mechanism for storing copper in the liver is so well developed that concentrations, very high by human standards, can be reached with no apparent ill effects. Copper concentrations are ten times higher in dogs than in humans,[39] while in the Dominican toad (*Bufo marinus*) and the mute swan (*Cygnus orlo*) the concentration may be more than 100-fold higher. Other animals are very vulnerable to the metal, particularly oysters, goldfish, chickens, and sheep; in the latter two, hemolysis and liver damage dominate the clinical picture, while the central nervous system seems to remain uninvolved.

The exact site of the biochemical lesion induced by copper in humans has not been defined. Many isolated enzyme systems, particularly those with an —SH group at the catalytic center, are inhibited by copper, but in the intact cell, they seem to be at least in part protected. Indeed, Peters and Walshe,[31,32] working on the pigeon brain, were able to demonstrate only inhibition of the membrane ATPase by copper in the intact cell, although isolated mitochondria mediating the tricarboxylic acid cycle were easily inhibited by the metal *in vitro*. Similarly, Seymour, working on liver biopsy material from my patients with Wilson's disease, has found that the mitochondria are the first organelles to show damage following copper overload. Other possible sites of copper toxicity are the sulfhydryl proteins present in the cytosol where copper is diffusely present in high concentration in the early stages when hepatic damage is most prominent.[15] One such protein that may be involved is tubulin. Damage to this protein in turn may result in degradation of the microtubules and deposition of Mallory's hyalin in the cells. This aspect of copper toxicity has been reviewed in detail by Sternlieb.[39] Excess copper might also deplete the stores of reduced glutathione by oxidation of the —SH to S—S linkages and also by damage to the lysosomal membrane. However, the latter hypothesis appears unlikely, since this organelle is the main site of copper deposition in those animals with the highest liver copper levels and also has been found by Seymour to remain intact in patients with Wilson's disease.

The excess copper that accumulates in the liver may be due to increased absorption from the gut; the presence of an abnormal binding protein in the liver, with an increased affinity for the metal; or a defective excretory mechanism for copper into the bile.

The first mechanism has never seriously been entertained, and there is no evidence to support it. The second hypothesis has been a source of much controversy since first propounded by Uzman and associates in 1956[45,47] and again more recently by Evans.[5] It is difficult to follow the logic of this theory, for if the liver metallothionein has an increased affinity for copper, it should render the metal nontoxic even in greatly increased amounts. The third hypothesis of a defective excretory mechanism has the best experimental basis to support it,[9,13] and the evidence has been reviewed in some detail.[50] Moreover, there is no evidence for an abnormal enterohepatic circulation of the metal; there appears to be no reabsorption of copper from the gut once it has been excreted in the bile both in normal subjects and in patients with Wilson's disease.

Whatever the mechanisms of copper deposition in the liver and its hepatotoxic action, the unique state of affairs in Wilson's disease is, in fact, the overflow of the metal into the brain, occurring, presumably, when the liver binding sites for the metal have become saturated. Why this should occur in only about 50% of patients before disastrous liver damage occurs is yet another unsolved mystery. Once deposition commences in the brain, the copper continues to accumulate until it reaches toxic concentrations. This appears to be somewhere in excess of 40 μg/g wet weight, compared with a normal concentra-

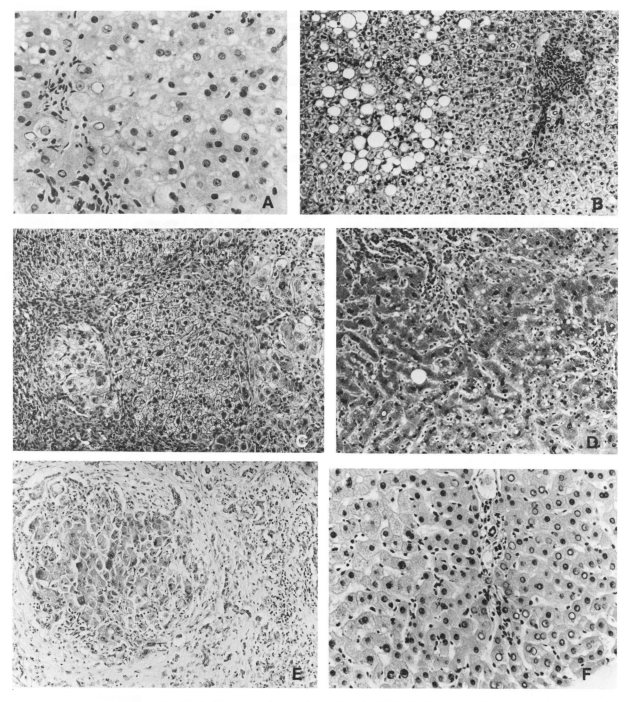

Fig. 28-6. Histologic changes in the liver in Wilson's disease. **A.** Eleven-year-old patient with marked elevation of the serum aminotransferases. This figure shows the earliest lesion, fatty droplets in the hepatocytes, early infiltration with inflammatory cells, and glycogen nuclei. **B.** Nineteen-year-old patient. No incorporation of radiocopper into ceruloplasmin; liver copper 63.5 µg/g wet weight. This patient had more advanced lesion than that of the patient in *A* but with similar features. **C.** Eight-year-old girl with anemia and jaundice. She recovered from this spontaneously, but at age 12 she developed a choreic syndrome. Wilson's disease was diagnosed, and treatment was started with penicillamine. She is now well controlled at the age of 34. Photograph shows an advanced hepatic lesion with pleomorphic hepatocytes, piecemeal necrosis,

(*continued*)

tion for cerebral gray matter of 5 μg to 10 μg/g wet weight. It is interesting that in patients dying of hepatic Wilson's disease, without clinical cerebral damage, the copper concentration is usually raised but is below 40 μg/g; this is in keeping with the findings of minor abnormalities in computed tomographic brain scans in patients with purely hepatic Wilson's disease (Fig. 28-7).[58] Although the cerebral symptoms of Wilson's disease are almost invariably motor or psychiatric, all areas of the brain appear to be equally involved in the accumulation of the copper. Although the sensory nervous system always appears to escape injury, it carries as high an abnormal load of the metal as do the motor centers; this presents yet another unsolved problem.

In many patients, the kidneys are also involved with increased copper loads. Abnormalities of glomerular and tubular function are common, including proteinuria, reduced glomerular filtration rate, failure of renal acidification, and a low threshold aminoaciduria and phosphaturia.[38] In the past there has been controversy about the nature of the aminoaciduria and peptiduria and its relationship to the pathogenesis of the disease. Uzman and Hood[45] believed that this was very closely linked to the primary gene defect and was an expression of the abnormal protein metabolism that resulted in a consecutive deposition of copper in the tissues. The most recent evidence, however, has shown that, using modern chromatographic techniques, the increased loss of free amino acids and peptides in the urine of patients with Wilson's disease is purely quantitative; qualitatively the pattern was similar to normal and it was not possible to show any relationship between aminoaciduria and peptiduria and copper excretion in the urine and the abnormalities returned to normal with treatment.[1] It would appear, therefore, that the renal damage observed is secondary to deposition of copper in the renal tubules; this is supported by the observation that renal function, particularly acidification, improves with treatment. This further supports the theory that excess copper is the cause of tissue damage in Wilson's disease.

GENETICS

Wilson's disease is transmitted via a recessive gene now believed to be located on chromosome 13.[10] Both parents

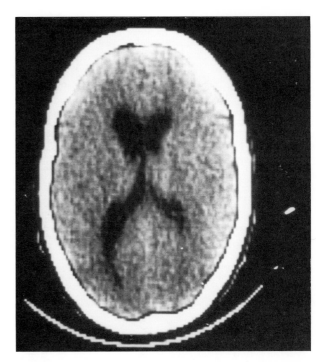

Fig. 28-7. CT brain scan of a 14-year-old girl who presented with chronic active hepatitis and was being treated for this at the time her sister was diagnosed as having Wilson's disease but was being treated in another hospital for "chorea." Both girls had dense, complete Kayser–Fleischer rings and the typical biochemistry of Wilson's disease. The scan shows asymmetrical dilatation of the lateral ventricles.

must carry one abnormal gene for the control of copper metabolism; hence parental consanguinity in affected families is more common than in the general population. In any such Wilson's disease family, the statistical risk is that one child in four will be affected with the disease, two will be carriers, and one will be normal. Strictly speaking, statistics are of little value to any given individual who suffers the same one-in-four risk of receiving the two abnormal genes irrespective of the status of his siblings. Every child, therefore, in a known Wilson's disease family must be screened for the disease; it is highly desirable that all close relatives should also be so studied, particularly if there is any history of consanguinity in the family tree.

and a severe inflammatory reaction. **D.** Twenty-five-year-old man, elder brother of the patient in *B,* had fatal neurologic Wilson's disease but no hepatic symptoms. A rather active-looking liver lesion with fatty hepatocytes, occasional glycogen nuclei, separation of the liver cell plates, and extensive infiltration with inflammatory cells but no fibrosis. **E.** Eight-year-old patient with fatal hepatic Wilson's disease. Figure shows the terminal stages of the liver lesion with a small necrotic nodule of liver cells surrounded by collapsed reticulin containing scattered necrotic hepatocytes and inflammatory cells. **F.** Fifteen-year-old girl with no hepatic signs or symptoms. She had a 3-year history of a rapidly progressive neurologic lesion that had left her bedridden and totally helpless. The histologic preparation shows the very earliest liver lesion like that seen in *A.* The patient made an excellent recovery on penicillamine therapy.

TABLE 28-1.   Comparative Copper Status for Patients with Wilson's Disease and Various Control Groups

GROUP	SERUM CERULOPLASMIN (mg/dl ± SE)	SERUM CU (μg/dl)	URINE CU (μg/24 hr)	LIVER CU (μg/g wet weight)	PLASMA ^{64}CU (24 hr/2 hr ratio)	RADIOACTIVE COPPER (^{64}Cu) ^{64}Cu—% intravenous dose excreted in urine per period		
						0–8 hours (mean ± SE)	8–24 hours (mean ± SE)	24–30 hr after penicillamine (mean ± SE)
Wilson's disease								
Presymptomatic	6.3 ± 1.0	<60	>50	>50	<0.4	0.92 ± 0.17	0.17 ± 0.04	0.84 ± 0.11
Symptomatic						1.22 ± 0.21	0.70 ± 0.16	3.45 ± 0.45
Heterozygote	25.4 ± 1.1	>60	<50	<50	>0.4	0.10 ± 0.01	0.05 ± 0.01	1.20 ± 0.17
Hepatic disease*	38.0 ± 2.9	>100	<50	<50	>0.6	0.20	0.17	1.94
Controls, male	33.3 ± 0.7	>80	<30	<10	>0.8	0.14 ± 0.02	0.07 ± 0.01	2.36 ± 0.33
Controls, female	36.6 ± 1.0							

* Excluding patients with primary biliary cirrhosis in whom figures for liver and urine copper may be found in the Wilson's disease range.
(Data from Gibbs K et al: The urinary excretion of radiocopper in presymptomatic and symptomatic Wilson's disease, heterozygotes and controls: Its significance in diagnosis and management. QJ Med 47:349, 1978, and Gibbs K, Walshe JM: A study of ceruloplasmin concentration found in 75 patients with Wilson's disease, their kinships and various control groups. QJ Med 48: 447, 1979)

As a first test, an estimation of the serum ceruloplasmin is the most useful, although it can by no means be considered infallible. Occasionally patients are seen with normal or near normal concentrations of the protein, and heterozygotes are seen with ceruloplasmin concentrations well down in the Wilson's disease range (see Fig. 28-5). This can result in one of the most difficult differential diagnoses in clinical medicine, because it is just as wrong to treat for life, with a potentially toxic drug, a heterozygote when no therapy is needed as it is to withhold treatment from a presymptomatic patient who may later develop rapidly progressive liver failure complicated by massive hemolysis. In such a situation, it is helpful to know the ceruloplasmin concentration of the propositus before any treatment has been given and the concentration of this protein in the parents (obligatory heterozygotes). The concentration of ceruloplasmin usually runs true to type in any one family. If the propositus has a low or very low concentration, it is highly probable that any affected sibling will have a similar concentration; the same applies if the propositus has a relatively high concentration of the protein. In some families the gene can be traced through the kinship with some success; in others it may be very difficult to identify. When doubt arises, as it often does, other tests that may help are estimation of the urine copper excretion and a search for evidence of hepatic or renal damage. A slit lamp examination of the eyes for Kayser-Fleischer rings is also useful. Normal findings, unfortunately, do not definitely rule out the possibility of Wilson's disease. When in doubt, it is necessary to resort either to radiolabeled copper studies, which are time consuming and expensive and require familiarity with the methods, or to a liver biopsy, making sure that enough tissue is available for biochemical and histologic examination (histology alone is not enough). Again, much experience is necessary for making accurate copper determinations on a few milligrams of liver. It is most desirable that such tests should be done in a specialist center familiar with the performance and interpretation of results. Figures for liver copper concentration are given in Table 28-1.

While on the subject of genetics, it is necessary to mention genetic counseling. The patient with Wilson's disease who has responded to treatment and contemplates marriage or who, if already married, considers the prospects of raising children may well seek advice as to the risks for the child. The parent, by definition, carries two abnormal genes for copper metabolism, one of which will, of necessity, be transmitted to the child whether from father or mother. The child will, therefore, be a carrier for Wilson's disease, but this, of itself, is no hazard. Where the risk really becomes significant is if a patient or known carrier marries a first cousin who will have a 1 in 4 chance of carrying the affected gene; as the relationship becomes more distant, the risk becomes smaller. It is for each individual to decide what degree of risk is acceptable. The risk at random mating, is low, probably of the order of 1 in 100.[2] Should the patient have the misfortune to mate with a carrier, the risk to each child is 1 in 2 for developing Wilson's disease. The first screening test should be carried out on cord blood. Ceruloplasmin is low in the newborn because this synthetic function is immature in the neonatal liver. Interpretation of results thus presents difficulties; the normal range at birth is from 10 mg to 20 mg/dl so that the reading would need to be zero or a little above it to cause real concern. A further test must therefore be carried out after 4 months of age when ceruloplasmin and liver copper levels will have reached the adult range. If doubt remains, it may be necessary to carry out liver biopsy and estimate the copper concentration in the liver. In children between 2 and 5 or 6 years of age, the normal ceruloplasmin concentration may be twice the upper limits of the adult normal, and this again may cause problems in interpretation. There is no information available as to what happens to the serum ceruloplasmin level in Wilson's disease children at this period in their development.

It is always my policy, when asked for genetic advice, to inform the prospective parents of the risks and the statistical chances, as to what steps I propose to take to screen children, and to what action I should advise if I considered the child was a probable or even possible case for Wilson's disease. The number of pregnancies that I have seen successfully completed in such families now approaches 50; one of these children appears to be homozygous for the Wilson's disease gene.

MANAGEMENT

The immediate objective of treatment in patients with Wilson's disease is to establish and maintain a negative copper balance, for only in this way can the disease process be arrested and reversed. In view of the occasionally fulminant nature of hepatic Wilson's disease, every effort should be made in suspected cases to establish the diagnosis as quickly as possible and start treatment before the disease has reached an irreversible stage. It must be remembered, however, that Wilson's disease demands lifelong treatment. It is important, therefore, not only that the diagnosis be established per adventure beyond all possibility of error but also that certain basic facts about the patient's biochemical status be established before any treatment is given. There is no place for the philosophy of giving some penicillamine to a patient with obscure symptoms in the hope that he will get better. This is inexcusable, for not only does it hazard the patient to the wrong diagnosis but it will also alter his biochemical status to such an extent that it might, at a later date, be very difficult to establish the correct diagnosis.

Once this is established, however, the following must be documented: serum copper and ceruloplasmin levels, basal urine copper excretion, and urine copper excretion in response to a single test dose of penicillamine. (It is my custom to give 500 mg of penicillamine and collect urine for 6 hours.) It is desirable, although not essential, to know the liver copper concentration. The blood cell count, differential leukocyte count, and platelet count must be known, since penicillamine can affect these; but so can hypersplenism, which is common in Wilson's disease. It is a common mistake to do the first blood cell count after penicillamine has been started and then blame the drug for an abnormal count that may have preceded therapy.

Renal function should be recorded, particularly the presence or absence of sugar and protein in the urine and the creatinine clearance or some similar measurement. A suitable battery of liver function tests should also be performed. A radiologic skeletal survey is of value since bone disease is not uncommon in these patients, particularly at the hands, wrists, elbows, knees, hips, and lumbar spine, where osteochondritis is perhaps the most common osteoarticular abnormality to be found (see Fig. 28-4). Demineralization of the skeleton is also common, with many patients giving a history of fractures from apparently minor trauma.

Finally, it is my policy to arrange for computed tomography of the brain; changes are occasionally found even when there is no obvious clinical evidence of central nervous system involvement (see Fig. 28-7). These changes, in such cases, consist of cortical atrophy and ventricular dilatation: low density areas in the regions of the basal ganglia and thalamus are found only in the neurologic stage of the illness.[58] Once this information has been gathered, treatment may be started.

The drug of choice is penicillamine,[48] and 30 years after its introduction its continued use proves its efficacy.[51] For an adolescent or adult, an initial dose of 500 mg three times a day before meals is usually sufficient. A very large man or a very sick patient might need more, and occasionally as much as 3 g/day might be given, although never for more than 3 months. Similarly, 2 g/day should never be given for more than 1 year because there is a real risk of inducing a typical hemorrhagic penicillamine dermatopathy from failure to form cross-linkages in collagen, which is normally mediated through the copper-dependent enzyme lysyl oxidase.

About 20% of patients with neurologic symptoms may undergo deterioration of their disease for several months before improvement sets in. Patients should always be warned of this possibility to avoid grave distress and loss of confidence in the physician, something to be avoided at all costs in a disease that requires lifelong management. Sometimes, indeed, the progression of symptoms is rapid and alarming at this stage so that the situation may appear to be hopeless. This, however, is seldom the case. In the great majority, improvement eventually occurs. Sometimes development of a feeling of well-being and a change in the general appearance is so striking that the start of recovery can be dated accurately even though a measurable improvement in neurologic performance may be more difficult to document. A very small number of patients fail to respond to treatment and suffer a steady progressive deterioration with a complete breakdown of physical and intellectual function until they die of infection, inanition, or wasting; such a sequence of events is infinitely distressing to both relatives and staff.

Once a useful improvement in neurologic performance or hepatic function has been established, it may be possible to reduce the penicillamine dose to a maintenance level of 500 mg or 750 mg/day. This should not be done until there has been a significant fall in the serum copper and ceruloplasmin levels and the urine copper excretion has returned to the normal range. If the dose is then reduced, it is important to monitor these parameters regularly; if the dose is inadequate or the patient stops or becomes irregular with his treatment, one or all will start rising back to the pretreatment level. This is a clear warning to increase the dose. It must be noted, however, that in a small number of patients, the serum copper and ceruloplasmin levels may rise after treatment has been started, even when all other markers, both clinical and biochemical, point to adequate and effective treatment.[12] The significance and mechanisms involved are far from obvious. The truth is that no single measurement in Wilson's disease can be considered in isolation; all have to be weighed in the balance in arriving at a final decision.

It is advisable to monitor the red blood cell count, sedimentation rate, and leukocyte and platelet counts and to test the urine for protein and erythrocytes for evidence of penicillamine toxicity. If there is a change in these values, if the sedimentation rate rises, or if there are unexplained musculoskeletal pains, fever, or weight loss, then it is not unlikely that an immune complex or collagen disease has been initiated.[17] The following should therefore be measured: the antinuclear antibody factor, DNA binding, and immune complexes. A search should be made for lupus erythematosus cells. These tests should reveal the most important and most dangerous manifestations of penicillamine toxicity, although not perhaps the most common, which is an acute allergy at or about 10 days after starting treatment. Penicillamine toxicity has been discussed in some detail, at no less than three specialist conferences.[28–30] Allergy at 10 days is most commonly manifest as a morbilliform rash starting on the face and chest, and, if the drug is not stopped, it can spread widely. The rash is itchy and may be associated with fever and sometimes even hematuria.[43] It is usually well controlled by stopping or greatly reducing the dose and giving an antihistamine cover; corticosteroids are seldom needed.

Occasionally penicillamine intolerance is so severe that the drug has to be withdrawn and cannot be restarted without return of the toxic manifestations. In a disease that is 100% fatal when left untreated, alternative therapy is needed. This is now available in triethylene tetramine dihydrochloride. There is no doubt that this is a highly effective therapy resulting in a full restoration of the neurologic deficit, even in severely disabled patients.[52] This is associated with disappearance of the Kayser-Fleischer corneal rings and biochemical evidence of depletion of the body stores of copper[49] and a return of liver function to normal. Unfortunately, patients who have shown a severe lupus reaction to penicillamine may have this reactivated by trientine.* Triethylene tetramine dihydrochloride can be given in a dose of up to 800 mg three times a day, apparently indefinitely, although once there has been a good clinical response a smaller maintenance dose will usually suffice.[52] This drug has now been granted a license in both the United Kingdom and the United States.

Recently the use of zinc sulfate as an anticopper agent has been much advocated.[19,35] The theoretical basis for this is that zinc completely blocks the absorption of copper from the gut and this establishes a negative copper balance with consequent depletion of the abnormal stores of the metal; improvement was reported to be apparent within a week of starting this treatment. Moreover zinc is claimed to be completely nontoxic and is said not to lead to the temporary clinical deterioration of neurologic signs, which may be seen after the administration of chelating agents. The reason for this difference is difficult to understand if the method of benefit resulting from either form of therapy depends on the removal of copper from the affected organs. The dose of zinc sulfate advocated is 200 mg three times a day, but the relationship of the timing to meals is debated.[19] My own experience with zinc sulfate therapy is that the majority of patients complain of severe epigastric burning pain whether the dose is taken before, during, or after food. Most have refused this treatment after only a few weeks, and this may explain why benefit has not been observed. A new alternative anticopper agent, possibly the most powerful available, is ammonium tetrathiomolybdate, although much work needs to be done before this treatment can be said to have passed the investigative stage.[53,55]

Dimercaprol (BAL) has not proved to be a practical long-term therapy since it must be given by painful intramuscular injection and because of frequent toxic reactions. However, its water-soluble analogue 2,3-dimercaptopropane-1-sulfonate (Rx Dimaval) looks promising.[54]

Those patients in whom liver function is irreparably destroyed before the diagnosis has been made may be considered as candidates for liver transplantation; if this is successful the patient gains the extra benefit that the metabolic lesion is cured at the same time and no further chelation therapy will be necessary.[34]

Once the diagnosis has been established, presymptomatic patients should be treated in exactly the same way as symptomatic patients.[40]

Any well-treated female patient with Wilson's disease is equally at risk to pregnancy as are her normal sisters. There is no medical contraindication to pregnancy, provided the patient has been adequately "decoppered" before conception. It has been my custom to advise such patients to stop penicillamine therapy until the pregnancy has reached 12 weeks; but a number have not been seen until

after this date. Of 45 pregnancies seen so far, there have been no mishaps attributable to the disease or to therapy. In my experience, neither penicillamine nor triethylene tetramine has proved to be teratogenic. There are two case reports in the literature, however, that have caused some concern. One was of a patient with cystinuria treated with penicillamine who was delivered of a fetus with connective tissue defect.[24] A similar mishap has been reported for a patient with rheumatoid arthritis,[37] but a survey of 27 pregnancies in other rheumatoid and cystinuric patients revealed no similar abnormality.[22] It seems, therefore, that pregnant patients with Wilson's disease should be managed as normal unless their neurologic deficit or liver damage necessitates more specific care. The child, once born, should be screened for the Wilson's disease gene on cord blood and again after 3 months of age.

CONCLUSION

Wilson's disease is an inborn error of metabolism and is one of the causes of juvenile or adolescent hepatic disease. It may be acute, subacute, or chronic and may present with or as an hemolytic crisis. The diagnosis must always be considered in patients presenting with liver damage in this age-group. The finding of Kayser-Fleischer rings is not a sine qua non of diagnosis before neurologic signs develop.

The diagnosis must be confirmed by demonstrating the classic biochemical disturbances of copper transport and storage. Once the diagnosis has been made, all siblings should be screened and appropriate treatment started with penicillamine or triethylene tetramine dihydrochloride. With either of these two drugs the great majority of patients will make a good recovery. Treatment must be continued for life.

REFERENCES

1. Asatoor AM et al: Urinary excretion of peptides and hydroxyproline in Wilson's disease. Clin Sci Mol Med 51:369, 1976
2. Bachmann H et al: Die Epidemiologie der Wilsonschen Erkrankung in der DDR und die derzeitige Problematik einer populationgenetischen Bearbeitung. Psychiat Neurol Med Psychol 31:393, 1979
3. Cairns JE, Walshe JM: The Kayser-Fleischer ring. Trans Ophthalmol Soc UK 90:187, 1970
4. Dang HS, Somasundaram S: Copper levels in Indian childhood cirrhosis. Lancet 2:246, 1976
5. Evans GW: Copper homeostasis in mammalian system. Physiol Rev 53:535, 1973
6. Finby N, Bearn AG: Roentgenographic abnormalities of the skeletal system in Wilson's disease (Hepatolenticular degeneration). AJR 79:603, 1958
7. Fitzgerald MA et al: Wilson's disease (hepatolenticular degeneration) of late adult onset. Mayo Clin Proc 50:438, 1975
8. Fleming CR et al: Pigmented corneal rings in a patient with primary biliary cirrhosis. Gastroenterology 69:220, 1975
9. Frommer D: Defective biliary excretion of copper in Wilson's disease. Gut 15:125, 1974

---

* Triethylene tetramine is the full chemical name of the compound. It is usually referred to by chemists by the shortened name "trien." It is registered as a pharmaceutical in the United Kingdom as "trientine" and in the United States as "cuprid."

10. Frydman M et al: Assignment of the gene for Wilson's disease to chromosome 13: Linkage to the esterase D locus. Proc Natl Acad Sci USA 82:1819, 1985
11. Gibbs K, Walshe JM: Studies with radioactive copper (^{64}Cu and ^{67}Cu): The incorporation of radioactive copper into caeruloplasmin in Wilson's disease and in primary biliary cirrhosis. Clin Sci 41:189, 1971
12. Gibbs K, Walshe JM: A study of the caeruloplasmin concentration found in 75 patients with Wilson's disease, their kinships and various control groups. Q J Med 48:447, 1979
13. Gibbs K, Walshe JM: Biliary excretion of copper in Wilson's disease. Lancet 2:538, 1980
14. Gibbs K et al: The urinary excretion of radiocopper in presymptomatic and symptomatic Wilson's disease, heterozygotes and controls: Its significance in diagnosis and management. Q J Med 47:349, 1978
15. Goldfischer S, Sternlieb I: Changes in the distribution of hepatic copper in relation to the progression of Wilson's disease (hepatolenticular degeneration). Am J Pathol 53:883, 1968
16. Golding D, Walshe JM: Arthropathy of Wilson's disease. Ann Rheum Dis 36:99, 1977
17. Golding D, Walshe JM: Penicillamine-induced arthropathy in Wilson's disease. Proc R Soc Med 70(suppl):4, 1977
18. Harris H: Genetics and orphan diseases. In Scheinberg IH, Walshe JM (eds): Orphan Diseases/Orphan Drugs, Manchester University Press (in press)
19. Hoogenraad TU et al: Effective treatment of Wilson's disease with oral zinc sulphate: Two case reports. Br Med J 289:273, 1984
20. Jones EA et al: Progressive intrahepatic cholestasis of infancy and childhood: A clinicopathological study of a patient surviving to the age of 18 years. Gastroenterology 71:675, 1976
21. Kamamoto Y et al: The inhibitory effect of copper on dl-ethionine carcinogenesis in rats. Cancer Res 33:1129, 1973
22. Lyle WH: Penicillamine in pregnancy. Lancet 1:606, 1978
23. Madden JW et al: An unusual case of Wilson's disease. Q J Med 55:63, 1985
24. Mjølnerød OK et al: Congenital connective tissue defect probably due to penicillamine in pregnancy. Lancet 1:673, 1971
25. Morgan HG et al: Wilson's disease and the Fanconi syndrome. Q J Med 31:361, 1962
26. Osborn SB, Walshe JM: Studies with radioactive copper (^{64}Cu and ^{67}Cu) in relation to the natural history of Wilson's disease. Lancet 1:346, 1967
27. Osborn SB et al: Studies with radioactive copper (^{64}Cu and ^{67}Cu): Abdominal scintiscans in patients with Wilson's disease. Q J Med 38:467, 1969
28. Penicillamine. Postgrad Med J 44(suppl):1968
29. Penicillamine: Recent work. Postgrad Med J 50(suppl 2):1974
30. Penicillamine at 21: Its place in therapeutics now. Proc R Soc Med 70(suppl):1977
31. Peters RA et al: Studies on the toxicity of copper: II. The behaviour of microsomal membrane ATPase of the pigeon's brain tissue to copper and some other metallic substances. Proc R Soc London 166:285, 1966
32. Peters RA, Walshe JM: Studies on the toxicity of copper: I. The toxic action of copper in vivo and in vitro. Proc R Soc Lond 166:273, 1966
33. Roche-Sicot J, Benhamou J-P: Acute intravascular haemolysis and acute liver failure as a first manifestation of Wilson's disease. Ann Intern Med 86:301, 1977
34. Scheinberg IH, Sternlieb I: Wilson's disease. In Smith LH (ed): Major Problems in Internal Medicine, vol 23. Philadelphia, WB Saunders, 1984
35. Schouwink G: De hepato-cerebrale degeneratie, thesis, University of Amsterdam. G. W. Van Der Wiel, Arnhem 1961
36. Sipponen P: Orcein positive hepatocellular material in long standing biliary disease: I. Histochemical characteristics. Scand J Gastroenterol 11:545, 1970
37. Solomon L et al: Neonatal abnormalities associated with D-penicillamine treatment during pregnancy. N Engl J Med 296:54, 1977
38. Stein WH et al: The amino acid content of the blood and urine in Wilson's disease. J Clin Invest 33:410, 1954
39. Sternlieb I: Copper and the liver. Gastroenterology 78:1615, 1980
40. Sternlieb I, Scheinberg IH: Prevention of Wilson's disease in asymptomatic patients. N Engl J Med 278:352, 1968
41. Sternlieb I et al: Bleeding oesophageal varices in patients with Wilson's disease. Lancet 1:638, 1970
42. Sternlieb I et al: Detection of the heterozygous carrier of the Wilson's disease gene. J Clin Invest 40:707, 1961
43. Strickland GT: Febrile penicillamine eruption. Arch Neurol 26:474, 1972
44. Tanner MS et al: Increased hepatic concentration in Indian childhood cirrhosis. Lancet 1:1203, 1979
45. Uzman LL, Hood B: The familial nature of the amino-aciduria of Wilson's disease (hepatolenticular degeneration). Am J Med Sci 223:932, 1952
46. Uzman LL, Jakus MA: The Kayser-Fleischer ring: A histochemical and electron microscope study. Neurology 7:341, 1957
47. Uzman LL et al: The mechanism of copper deposition in the liver in hepatolenticular degeneration (Wilson's disease). Am J Med Sci 231:511, 1956
48. Walshe JM: Penicillamine, a new oral therapy for Wilson's disease. Am J Med 21:487, 1956
49. Walshe JM: Copper chelation in patients with Wilson's disease: A comparison of penicillamine and triethylene tetramine dihydrochloride. Q J Med 42:441, 1973
50. Walshe JM: Wilson's disease (hepatolenticular degeneration). In Klawans HL (ed): Handbook of Clinical Neurology, Vol 27, Metabolic and Deficiency Diseases of the Nervous System. Amsterdam, North Holland, 1976
51. Walshe JM: Brief observations on the management of Wilson's disease. Proc R Soc Med 70(suppl 3):1, 1977
52. Walshe JM: Treatment of Wilson's disease with trientine (triethylene tetramine) dihydrochloride. Lancet 1:643, 1982
53. Walshe JM: Copper: Its role in the pathogenesis of liver disease. Semin Liver Dis 4:252, 1984
54. Walshe JM: Unithiol in Wilson's disease. Br Med J 290:673, 1985
55. Walshe JM: Tetrathiomolybdate (MoS$_4$) as an "anticopper" agent in man. In Scheinberg IH, Walshe JM (eds): Orphan Diseases/Orphan Drugs. Manchester University Press (in press).
56. Walshe JM, Briggs J: Caeruloplasmin in liver disease: A diagnostic pitfall. Lancet 2:263, 1962
57. Walshe JM, Potter G: The pattern of whole body distribution of radioactive copper (^{67}Cu and ^{64}Cu) in Wilson's disease and various control groups. Q J Med 46:445, 1977
58. Williams FJB, Walshe JM: Wilson's disease: An analysis of the cranial computerized tomographic appearances found in 60 patients and the changes in response to treatment with chelating agents. Brain 104:735, 1981

chapter 29

The Liver in Circulatory Failure

SHEILA SHERLOCK

A rise in pressure in the right atrium is readily transmitted to the hepatic veins. Liver cells are particularly vulnerable to diminished oxygen supply so a failing heart, lowered blood pressure, or reduced hepatic blood flow are reflected in impaired hepatic function. The left lobe of liver may suffer more than the right.

HEPATIC CHANGES IN ACUTE HEART FAILURE AND SHOCK

Hepatic changes are particularly common in acute heart failure and in shock due to trauma, burns, hemorrhage, sepsis, peritonitis, or black water fever.[3] Light microscopy shows congested central areas with local hemorrhage (Fig. 29-1). Focal necrosis with eosinophilic hepatocytes, hydropic change, and polymorphonuclear infiltration is usually centrizonal. Midzonal necrosis may be due to tangential section cutting, but in some instances is unexplained.[7] The reticulin framework is preserved within the necrotic zone. With recovery, particularly after trauma, mitoses may be prominent.

Hepatic calcification can develop in zone 3 areas following shock.[26] This might be related to the disturbance of intracellular calcium homeostasis as a result of ischemic liver injury.

Changes can be related to the duration of the shock: if longer than 24 hours hepatic necrosis is almost constant; if less than 10 hours it is unusual.

The fall in systemic blood pressure leads to a reduction in hepatic blood flow, and the oxygen content of the blood is reduced. Hepatic arterial vasoconstriction follows the fall in systemic blood pressure. The centrizonal (zone 3) cells receive blood at a lower oxygen tension than the peripheral (zone 1) cells[12] and therefore more readily become anoxic and necrotic (Fig. 29-2).

Some patients show mild icterus. Jaundice has been recorded in severely traumatized patients. Serum transaminase levels increase markedly, and the prothrombin time rises.[3]

ISCHEMIC HEPATITIS

Ischemic hepatitis refers to acute circulatory failure of the liver[10,13]; *acute hepatic infarction* might be a preferable term.[10] The picture simulates acute viral hepatitis.

The patient usually suffers from cardiac disease, which is often ischemic. He has an acute fall in cardiac output, often due to an arrhythmia or myocardial infarction. Zone 3 necrosis without inflammation results. Clinical evidence of hepatic failure is absent. Congestive cardiac failure is inconspicuous.

Serum bilirubin and alkaline phosphatase values increase slightly, but serum transaminase levels rise rapidly and strikingly to levels eight to ten times normal. These return speedily toward recovery in less than 1 week. Tests for hepatitis A and B are negative, and hepatotoxic drugs cannot be incriminated.

The outcome depends entirely on the cardiovascular status of the patient. The hepatic course is usually benign. However, if the liver has been previously damaged by chronic congestive heart failure, acute circulatory failure may lead to the picture of fulminant hepatic failure.[21]

POSTOPERATIVE JAUNDICE

Jaundice developing soon after surgery may have multiple causes.[14,15] Increased serum bilirubin follows blood transfusion, particularly of stored blood. The hemoglobin in 500 ml of blood contains about 250 mg of bilirubin, the normal daily production. Extravasated blood in the tissues gives an additional bilirubin load.

Impaired hepatocellular function follows operation, anesthetics, and shock. Severe jaundice develops in approximately 2% of patients, with shock resulting from major trauma.[22] Hepatic perfusion is reduced. This will be particularly evident if the patient is in incipient circulatory failure and the cardiac output is already reduced. Renal blood flow also falls.

Halothane anesthetics, especially if multiple, may be followed by a hepatitis-like picture. This is rare less than 7 days after a first operation. Other drugs used in the operative period, such as the promazines, must also be considered. Sepsis, per se, can produce deep jaundice, which may be cholestatic.[16]

In the United States glucose-6-phosphatase dehydrogenase deficiency affects approximately 10% of blacks. In such patients the administration of the many drugs at the time of surgery may precipitate hemolysis and jaundice.

Rarely a cholestatic jaundice may be noted on the first or second postoperative day. It reaches its height between 4 and 10 days and disappears by 14 to 18 days. Serum

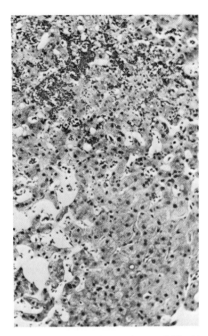

Fig. 29-1. Ischemic heart failure. Serum bilirubin 2.1 mg/100 ml. Liver cells have disappeared from the center of the lobule and are replaced by frank hemorrhage. (H & E; original magnification × 120). (Sherlock S: The liver in heart failure; relation of anatomical, functional and circulatory changes. Br Heart J 13:273, 1951)

biochemical changes are variable. Sometimes, but not always, the alkaline phosphatase and transaminase levels are increased.[24] The serum bilirubin value can rise to levels of 23 mg to 39 mg/dl. The picture simulates extrahepatic biliary obstruction.[11] Patients have all had an episode of shock, been transfused, and suffered heart failure of recent onset. Centrizonal hepatic necrosis, however, is not con-

spicuous and hepatic histology shows only minor abnormalities. The mechanism of the cholestasis is uncertain. This picture must be recognized[12] and if necessary needle biopsy of the liver performed. Surgical intervention to relieve a nonexistent biliary obstruction would be disastrous. The prognosis is good.

JAUNDICE AFTER CARDIAC SURGERY

Jaundice is frequent and develops in 20% of patients having cardiopulmonary by-pass surgery.[5,6] It carries a poor prognosis. The jaundice is detected by the second postoperative day. Serum bilirubin is conjugated, suggesting failure of canalicular biliary excretion. The serum alkaline phosphatase value may be normal or only slightly increased, and transaminase levels are raised, often becoming very high.[17] Patients over age 50 are particularly at risk. Jaundice is significantly associated with multiple valve replacement, high blood transfusion requirements, and a longer by-pass time.

Many factors contribute. The patient may have a liver that has already suffered from prolonged heart failure. Operative hypotension, shock, and hypothermia may have occurred. Infections, drugs (including anticoagulants), and anesthetics must be considered. The serum bilirubin load is increased by blood transfusion[2] and hemolysis due to mechanical prostheses. The pump may contribute by decreasing erythrocyte survival and by adding gaseous microemboli and platelet aggregates and debris to the circulation.

Non-A, non-B hepatitis is now the most common cause of post-transfusion hepatitis. The acute attack may be virtually asymptomatic, and the patient may present months or years later with a chronic hepatitis or cirrhosis. Hepatitis B is rare since blood has been screened routinely. Cytomegalohepatitis may develop after cardiac surgery.

THE LIVER IN CONGESTIVE HEART FAILURE

Pathology

Hepatic autolysis is particularly rapid in the patient dying of heart failure.[25] Autopsy material is therefore unreliable for the assessment of the effects of cardiac failure on the liver in life.

The liver is usually enlarged and purplish with rounded edges. As cardiac cirrhosis develops, the liver shrinks. Nodularity is never as great as with other types of cirrhosis. The cut surface shows prominent hepatic veins, which may be thickened. The liver drips blood. Central zones are prominent with alteration of yellow (fatty change) and red areas (centrizonal hemorrhage) giving a nutmeg-like appearance (Fig. 29-3).

The central vein is always dilated, and the sinusoids entering it are engorged for a variable distance toward the

Fig. 29-2. Factors leading to cardiac cirrhosis and zone 3 hemorrhage in patients with cardiac failure.

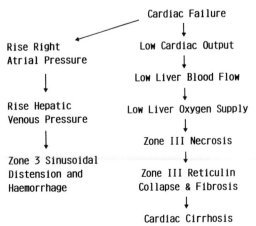

Cardiac Failure

Cardiac Failure → Rise Right Atrial Pressure

Cardiac Failure → Low Cardiac Output → Low Liver Blood Flow → Low Liver Oxygen Supply → Zone III Necrosis → Zone III Reticulin Collapse & Fibrosis → Cardiac Cirrhosis

Rise Right Atrial Pressure → Rise Hepatic Venous Pressure → Zone 3 Sinusoidal Distension and Haemorrhage

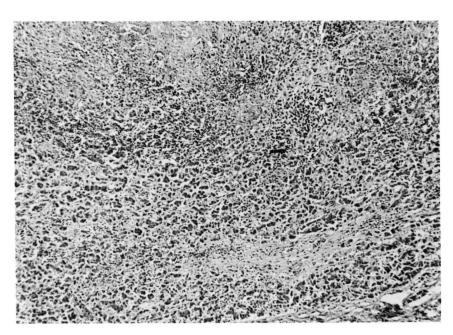

Fig. 29-3. Cut surface of liver from patient dying of congestive heart failure. Note dilated hepatic veins. Light areas corresponding to peripheral fatty zones alternate with dark areas corresponding to central zonal congestion and hemorrhage.

periphery (Fig. 29-4). In severe cases, there is frank hemorrhage with focal necrosis of liver cells. The liver cells show a variety of degenerative (zone 1) changes, but each portal tract (zone 3) is surrounded by relatively normal cells to a depth that varies inversely with the extent of the atrophy. Surviving cells usually retain their glycogen. Biopsy sections show significant fatty change in about one third. The absence of fat in biopsy material contrasts with the usual postmortem material. Cellular infiltration is inconspicuous.

The zone 3 degenerating cells are often packed with brown lipochrome pigment. As they disintegrate, pigment lies free amid cellular debris. Bile thrombi, particularly periportally, may be seen in deeply jaundiced patients.

Zone 3 reticulin condensation follows loss of liver cells (Fig. 29-5). Then reticulin and collagen increase and the

central vein shows phlebosclerosis. If the heart failure continues or relapses, bridges develop between central veins so that the unaffected portal zone is surrounded by a ring of fibrous tissue (reversed lobulation) (Fig. 29-6). Later the portal zones are involved and a complex cirrhosis results. A true cardiac cirrhosis is rare.

Electron microscopy shows atrophy of zone 3 cells,

Fig. 29-5. Same section as in Figure 29-4. Reticulin stains show condensation at the lobular center. (H & E; original magnification × 120) (Sherlock S: The liver in heart failure; relation of anatomical, functional and circulatory changes. Br Heart J 13:273, 1951)

Fig. 29-4. Factors leading to jaundice in patients with cardiac failure.

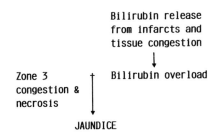

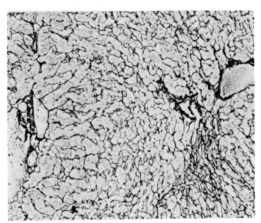

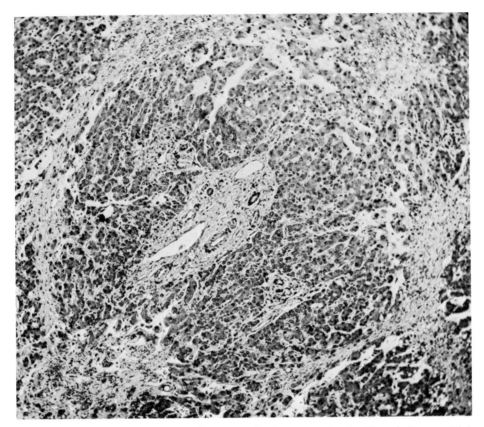

Fig. 29-6. Fibrous tissue bands pass from central vein to central vein. There is "reversed lobulation" and a fully developed cardiac cirrhosis. Portal tracts show only slight fibrosis. (H & E; original magnification × 90)

probably related to new fibers in the space of Dissë, which interfere with blood–hepatocyte transfer.[23] Canaliculi may dilate and rupture.

Mechanism

Zone 3 hepatocytes receive blood at a lower oxygen tension than those in zone 1. Hypoxia causes degeneration of zone 3 liver cells, dilatation of sinusoids, and slowing of bile secretion. The liver attempts to compensate by increasing the oxygen extracted as the blood flows across the sinusoidal bed. Collagenosis of the space of Dissë may play a minor role in impairing oxygen diffusion.

Necrosis correlates with a reduced systemic blood pressure and hence with a low cardiac output. The hepatic venous pressure increases in proportion to the rise in central venous pressure, and this correlates with zone 3 congestion.[1]

Clinical Features

Mild jaundice is common, but deeper icterus is particularly associated with chronic congestive failure, due, for example, to coronary artery disease or mitral stenosis.[20] In hospitalized patients, cardiorespiratory disease is the most common cause of a raised serum bilirubin level. Jaundice increases with prolonged and repeated bouts of congestive heart failure. Edematous areas escape, since bilirubin is protein bound and does not enter edema fluid with a low protein content.

Jaundice is partly hepatic because the greater extent of zone 3 necrosis, the deeper is the icterus (Fig. 29-7).[25]

Cholestasis due to bile thrombi or to pressure on bile ducts by distended veins is unlikely.

Bilirubin released from infarcts, whether pulmonary, splenic, or renal, or simply from pulmonary congestion, provides an overload on the anoxic liver. Patients in cardiac failure who become jaundiced with minimal hepatocellular damage usually have clear evidence of pulmonary infarction.[25] In keeping with bilirubin overload, the serum shows unconjugated bilirubinemia and the urine and the feces show excess of urobilinogen.

The patient may complain of right abdominal pain probably due to stretching of the nerve endings in the capsule of the enlarged liver. The firm, smooth, and tender lower edge may reach the umbilicus.

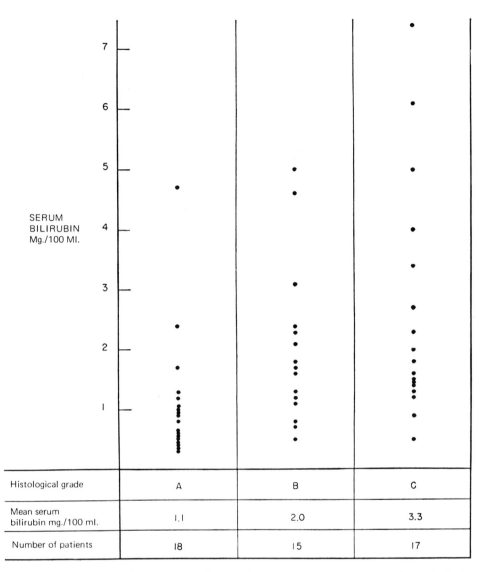

Histological grade	A	B	C
Mean serum bilirubin mg./100 ml.	I.I	2.0	3.3
Number of patients	18	15	17

Fig. 29-7. Relationship of extent of hepatic necrosis to serum bilirubin concentration. (Sherlock S: The liver in heart failure; relation of anatomical, functional and circulatory changes. Br Heart J 13:273, 1951)

A rise in right atrial pressure is readily transmitted to the hepatic veins. This is particularly so in tricuspid incompetence when the hepatic vein pressure tracing resembles that obtained from the right atrium. Palpable systolic pulsation of the liver can be related to this transmission of pressure. Presystolic hepatic pulsation occurs in tricuspid stenosis. The expansion may be felt bimanually with one hand over the liver anteriorly and the other over the right lower ribs posteriorly. This expansibility distinguishes it from the palpable epigastric pulsation due to the aorta or a hypertrophied right ventricle. Correct timing of the pulsation is important.

In heart failure, pressure applied over the liver increases the venous return and the jugular venous pressure rises due to the inability of the failing right heart to handle the increased blood flow.

The reflux is of value for the better identification of the jugular venous pulse and to establish that venous channels between the hepatic and jugular veins are patent.

The reflux is absent if the hepatic veins are occluded or if the main mediastinal or jugular veins are blocked. It is useful in diagnosing tricuspid regurgitation.[19]

Ascites is associated with a particularly high venous pressure, a low cardiac output, and severe, zone 3 necrosis. This description applies to patients with mitral stenosis and tricuspid incompetence or constrictive pericarditis. In such patients the ascites may be out of proportion to the edema and to the symptoms of congestive heart failure.

The ascitic fluid may have a high protein content similar to that observed in the Budd-Chiari syndrome.

Confusion, lethargy, and coma are occasional accompaniments of heart failure and are related to cerebral anoxia. Occasionally the whole picture of impending hepatic coma may be seen.[20]

Splenomegaly is frequent. Other features of portal hypertension are usually absent except in very severe cardiac cirrhosis associated with constrictive pericarditis. However, at autopsy, 6.7% of 74 patients with congestive heart failure showed esophageal varices, although in only 1 was there evidence of bleeding.

Cardiac cirrhosis should be suspected in patients with prolonged, decompensated mitral valve disease with tricuspid incompetence or in patients with constrictive pericarditis. The prevalence has fallen since both the conditions are now relieved surgically.

In congestive heart failure the serum bilirubin level usually exceeds 1 mg/dl, and in about one third it is more than 2 mg/dl.[25] The jaundice may be deep, exceeding 5 mg/dl and even up to 26.9 mg.[9,25] The serum bilirubin level corresponds to the degree of heart failure.

The serum alkaline phosphatase value is usually normal or slightly increased. Serum albumin values may be mildly reduced and globulin raised.[25] Protein loss from the intestine may contribute.

Serum transaminases are higher in acute than chronic failure and are proportional to the degree of shock and to the extent of zone 3 necrosis. The association of very high values with jaundice may simulate acute viral hepatitis.[4]

The urine shows excess urobilinogen, and fecal stercobilinogen is increased. Rarely, gray stools accompany deep icterus.

Prognosis

The prognosis of the liver changes is that of the underlying heart disease causing them. Cardiac jaundice, particularly if deep, is always a bad omen.

Cardiac cirrhosis per se does not carry a bad prognosis, and if the heart failure responds to treatment, the cirrhosis can be expected to become compensated.

HEPATIC DYSFUNCTION AND CARDIOVASCULAR ABNORMALITIES IN PEDIATRIC PATIENTS

Infants and children with heart failure and cyanotic heart disease show liver dysfunction.[18] Hypoxemia, systemic venous congestion, and a low cardiac output are associated with increased prothrombin time, serum bilirubin, and transaminase values. The most severe changes are found with a low cardiac output. Liver function correlates with cardiac status.

THE LIVER IN CONSTRICTIVE PERICARDITIS

The clinical picture and hepatic changes in constrictive pericarditis are those of the Budd-Chiari syndrome. Cardiac cirrhosis is frequent and marked thickening of the liver capsule simulates sugar icing (*Zuckergussleber*). Microscopically the picture is of cardiac cirrhosis. Jaundice is absent. The liver is enlarged and hard. Ascites is gross.

Diagnosis must be made from ascites due to cirrhosis or to hepatic venous obstruction. This is done by determination of the paradoxic pulse and the venous pulse, radiology showing the calcified pericardium, echocardiography, electrocardiography, and cardiac catheterization.

Treatment is that of the cardiac condition. If pericardectomy is possible, prognosis as regards the liver is good, although recovery may be slow. Within 6 months of a successful operation, results of liver function tests improve and the liver shrinks. The cardiac cirrhosis cannot be expected to resolve completely, but fibrous bands become narrower and avascular.

THORACOABDOMINAL ANEURYSM

A large thoracoabdominal aneurysm can cause congestive hepatomegaly by compressing the confluence of hepatic veins and the inferior vena cava.

REFERENCES

1. Anderson MD, Gabrieli E, Zizzi JA: Chronic hemolysis in patients with ball valve prosthesis. J Thorac Cardiovasc Surg 50:510, 1981
2. Arcidi JM Jr, Moore GW, Hutchins P: Hepatic morphology in cardiac dysfunction: A clinicopathologic study of 1000 subjects at autopsy. Am J Pathol 104:159, 1965
3. Birgens HS, Henriksen J, Matzen P et al: The shock liver. Acta Med Scand 204:417, 1978
4. Bloth B, De Faire U, Edhag O: Extreme elevation of transaminase levels in acute heart disease: A problem in differential diagnosis: Acta Med Scand 200:281, 1976
5. Chu CM, Chang CH, Liaw YF et al: Jaundice after open heart surgery: A prospective study. Thorax 39:52, 1984
6. Collins JD, Bassendine MR, Ferner R et al: Incidence and prognostic importance of jaundice after cardiopulmonary bypass surgery. Lancet 1:1119, 1983
7. De La Monte SM, Arcidi JM, Moore GW et al: Midzonal necrosis as a pattern of hepatocellular injury after shock. Gastroenterology 86:627, 1984
8. Dunn GD, Hayes P, Breen KJ et al: The liver in congestive heart failure: A review. Am J Med Sci 265:174, 1973
9. Gadeholt H, Haugen J: Centrilobular hepatic necrosis in cardiac failure: One case with severe acute jaundice. Acta Med Scand 176:525, 1964
10. Gibson PR, Dudley FJ: Ischemic hepatitis: Clinical features, diagnosis and prognosis. Aust NZ J Med 14:822, 1984
11. Gourley GR, Chesney PJ, Davis JP et al: Acute cholestasis

in patients with toxic-shock syndrome. Gastroenterology 81:928, 1981

12. Gumucio JJ, Miller DL: Functional implications of liver cell heterogeneity. Gastroenterology 80:393, 1981

13. Ischaemic hepatitis. Lancet 1:1019, 1985

14. Kantrowitz PA, Jones WA, Greenberger NJ et al: Postoperative hyperbilirubinemia simulating obstructive jaundice. N Engl J Med 276:591, 1967

15. Lamont JT, Isselbacher KJ: Current concepts: Postoperative jaundice. N Engl J Med 288:305, 1973

16. Lefkowitch JH: Bile ductular cholestasis an ominous histopathologic sign related to sepsis and "cholangitis lenta." Hum Pathol 13:19, 1982

17. Lockey E, McIntyre N, Ross DN et al: Early jaundice after open heart surgery. Thorax 22:165, 1967

18. Mace S, Borkat G, Liebman J: Hepatic dysfunction and cardiovascular abnormalities: Occurrence in infants, children, and young adults. Am J Dis Child 139:60, 1985

19. Maisel AS, Atwood JE, Goldberger AL: Hepatojugular reflux: Useful in the bedside diagnosis of tricuspid regurgitation. Ann Intern Med 101:78, 1984

20. Moussavian SN, Dincsoy HP, Goodman S et al: Severe hyperbilirubinemia and coma in chronic congestive heart failure. Dig Dis Sci 27:175, 1982

21. Novel O, Henrion J, Bernuau J et al: Fulminant hepatic failure due to transient circulatory failure in patients with chronic heart disease. Dig Dis Sci 25:49, 1980

22. Nunes G, Blaisdell FW, Margaretten W: Mechanism of hepatic dysfunction following shock and trauma. Arch Surg 100:646, 1970

23. Safran AP, Schaffner F: Chronic passive congestion of the liver in man: Electron microscopic study of cell atrophy and introlobular fibrosis. Am J Pathol 50:447, 1967

24. Schmid M, Hefti ML, Gattiker R et al: Benign post-operative intrahepatic cholestasis. N Engl J Med 272:545, 1965

25. Sherlock S: The liver in heart failure; relation of anatomical, functional and circulatory changes. Br Heart J 13:273, 1951

26. Shibuya A, Unuma T, Sugimoto M et al: Diffuse hepatic calcification as a sequela to shock liver. Gastroenterology 89:196, 1985

27. Sigal E, Pogany A, Goldman IS: Marked hepatic congestion caused by a thoracoabdominal aneurysm. Gastroenterology 87:1367, 1984

chapter 30

The Liver in Pregnancy

CAROLINE A. RIELY

For a variety of reasons, liver disease in pregnancy is poorly understood by many practitioners of internal medicine. First, medical problems arising during the course of gestation are usually cared for by the obstetrician. Many of the reports of liver diseases in pregnancy have appeared in the obstetric literature. As a consequence, most medical specialists have little familiarity with medicine in pregnancy. In addition, the pregnant state is accompanied by striking alterations in physiology, most of which are unfamiliar to the specialist in internal medicine. Finally, there are medical diseases that are unique to pregnancy (most notably the toxemias, preeclampsia and eclampsia) and that are often overlooked or misunderstood by the medical specialist.

Similarly, pregnancy is not commonplace in clinics specializing in liver disease. It does occur, however, and is not rare among women who are reformed alcoholics or who have adequately treated "autoimmune" chronic active hepatitis. Good, prospectively collected data on the incidence of pregnancy in patients with liver disease are not available. The incidence of liver disease occurring in pregnancy has been estimated, usually from collation of reported cases, but the figures are only rough estimates, at best. The reported incidence of jaundice (implying fairly severe liver disease) in pregnancy ranges from 1/1500 or 1/1600[56,100] to 1/2500.[72] The incidence of subicteric hepatic dysfunction must be higher.

Nevertheless, the study of liver diseases in pregnancy is a rewarding one, as is reflected by the many excellent reviews available on this topic.[43,50,56,67,74,94,127,142,145,154] Of particular interest to the hepatologist are the diseases that are unique to pregnancy (*e.g.,* cholestasis of pregnancy or acute fatty liver of pregnancy) that have interesting parallels or contrasts to liver disorders occurring in the nonpregnant population. Complete elucidation of the pathogenesis of these diseases is as of yet unavailable but will be based in a thorough understanding of the normal physiologic changes in pregnancy.

ALTERATIONS ASSOCIATED WITH THE PREGNANT STATE

Physiologic Changes

Normal pregnancy is associated with a series of dramatic hemodynamic changes (Table 30-1). The blood volume increases by an average of 48%, with a wide range but with an increase that is consistent over consecutive gestations for each individual.[121] This change, consisting ultimately of an average increase of 1.5 liters of plasma and 0.5 liter of red blood cells, begins in the first trimester, is more marked in the second trimester, and increases only slightly more in the third trimester. There is an associated increase in cardiac output and in heart rate.[162] The stroke volume increases gradually to reach a peak at 32 weeks of gestation, then decreases back to the prepregnancy norm. There is an attendant decrease in mean peripheral vascular resistance.[133] Renal blood flow increases, particularly in the second trimester. Hepatic blood flow does not change when compared with prepregnancy levels, but the fractional blood flow to the liver drops from 35% in the nonpregnant state to 29% during pregnancy.[111] The gravid uterus presents an increasing obstruction to blood return via the inferior vena cava as term approaches.[88] There is increased return to the heart via the azygous system, and esophageal varices may occur in as many as 66% of normal pregnant women near term. Also as term approaches, there is an increasingly hypercoagulable state.[73] The hemodynamic changes are magnified by Valsalva maneuvers during labor, and a peak in cardiac output is reached during the second stage.[169] In the days to weeks following delivery, these hemodynamic alterations revert to normal, aided by the blood loss at delivery.

Normal pregnancy is also associated with changes in gastrointestinal physiology. There is a decrease in lower esophageal sphincter tone, which may be the cause of the heartburn that so frequently affects pregnant women.[30] There is an increase in fasting gallbladder volume and an increase in residual volume after contraction, the so-called sluggish gallbladder of pregnancy.[18,42] These changes in smooth muscle motility correlate with increases in serum progesterone values and may be related etiologically to this putative smooth muscle relaxant. Studies of biliary lipids and bile acid kinetics during pregnancy have shown an increase in the lithogenic index of bile, associated with an increase in biliary cholesterol secretion and a decrease in both the synthesis of chenodeoxycholic acid relative to cholic acid and the rate of enterohepatic cycling of the bile acid pool.[87,171] These changes may reflect sequestration of the bile acid pool in the distended gallbladder as well as changes in bile acid synthesis modulated by gestational hormones.

TABLE 30-1. Changes Associated with Normal Pregnancy

PHYSIOLOGY
↑blood volume, cardiac output
↓mean peripheral vascular resistance
↑renal blood flow
↑azygous vein flow
Hypercoagulable state
↓lower esophageal sphincter tone
↑gallbladder volume
↓cheno/cholate synthesis
↑cholesterol secretion in bile
↑lithogenicity of bile
↓rate of enterohepatic cycling of bile acid pool

PHYSICAL EXAMINATION
Blood pressure: ↓ in second trimester, returns to
   prepregnancy norm at term
↑pulse
Spider angiomas
Palmar erythema
Impalpable liver

Physical Findings

During pregnancy, the findings on physical examination change (see Table 30-1). Serial measurements of blood pressure show a decrease in the second trimester, which is followed by an increase back toward the values of early pregnancy as term approaches. The pulse rate increases. Pregnant women often develop typical spider angiomas, which fade after delivery. Palmar erythema is also commonly found. The expanding uterus makes physical examination of the liver difficult, and hepatomegaly can rarely be detected.

Laboratory Values

The normal range for many laboratory values changes during pregnancy (Table 30-2).[40] The increase in blood volume and resulting hemodilution are reflected in a decrease in hemoglobin concentration and serum albumin. This hemodilution, together with an increase in fractional renal blood flow, results in a decrease in blood urea ni-

trogen and in uric acid levels, which normalize as term approaches. During normal pregnancy there is a decrease in serum levels of carnitine, perhaps implying relative carnitine deficiency.[9] Increases are found in the normal levels of white blood cells and of various proteins such as fibrinogen, ceruloplasmin, and α_2-globulins. Serum lipids change strikingly, with a 50% increase in serum cholesterol and a threefold increase in serum triglycerides.[119] Urinary excretion of the porphyrin precursors δ-aminolevulinic acid and porphobilinogen increase slightly during pregnancy.[22,36] Urinary orotic acid excretion appears to be unchanged.[52]

The question of the existence of a physiologic cholestasis of pregnancy has long been debated. Studies of serum bile acid levels during gestation show either normal values[136] or small but significant increases, usually within the range of normal.[47,59] The metabolism of another organic anion, sulfobromophthalein (BSP) has been investigated extensively. Estrogenic steroids are known to increase the retention of BSP after a simple bolus intravenous injection.[93,126] More sophisticated studies using infusion techniques have shown a decrease in the transport maximum for BSP and an increase in hepatic storage capacity as gestation advances.[31] Other studies, however, have shown unexpected changes in the albumin binding of BSP during pregnancy.[32] This compound is no longer available commercially in this country, although the agent is still useful for research purposes.[126]

Standard "liver function tests" are normal during the entire course of pregnancy with a single exception: the alkaline phosphatase level rises as term approaches. This is due to the presence of a heat-stable fraction of placental origin. Tests of "hepatic" alkaline phosphatase, such as 5′nucleotidase or γ-glutamyl transpeptidase (GGTP), remain normal throughout pregnancy or rise only minimally toward term.[40,160] Any consistent elevation in transaminase or bilirubin should warn the clinician of possible liver disease in the pregnant female.

Hepatic Histology

Hepatic histology is not altered by pregnancy.[10,76] Ultrastructure of the liver reveals no significant abnormalities,

TABLE 30-2. Changes in Laboratory Values During Normal Pregnancy

DECREASED	INCREASED	UNCHANGED
Hemoglobin	White blood cell count	Transaminases
Albumin	Fibrinogen	Serum bile acids
Blood urea nitrogen	Ceruloplasmin	5′Nucleotidase, GGTP
Uric acid	α_2-Globulins	
	Cholesterol	
	Triglycerides	
	BSP retention	
	Alkaline phosphatase	
	Urinary porphyrins	

with proliferation of the smooth endoplasmic reticulum and other nonspecific and nonpathologic changes.[117]

The Syndrome of Preeclampsia/Eclampsia

Any clinician who cares for pregnant women should be conversant with the syndrome of toxemia of pregnancy, now designated preeclampsia/eclampsia.[26,129,170] This syndrome is usually quite foreign to internists and gastroenterologists since it is unique to the pregnant state in humans or, rarely, concurrent with hydatidiform mole. It occurs in the third trimester of pregnancy and is more common in, although not limited to, the primiparous female. It is more common in multiple gestations. It is not rare, occurring in approximately 7% of all pregnancies. Once it has occurred, it is not more likely to complicate subsequent pregnancies. It is a multisystemic disease, most typically characterized by edema, proteinuria, and hypertension. There may be involvement of the central nervous system with hyperreflexia and, defining eclampsia, seizures. There is no direct correlation between the severity of the various manifestations: for example, seizures are not limited to cases with severe hypertension. Hypertension should be judged relative to the individual patient's previous blood pressure determinations. An elevation of 30 mm Hg systolic or 15 mm Hg diastolic over midtrimester levels should be considered pathologic. Any blood pressure of greater than 140/90 mm Hg in a pregnant female is pathologic. The serum uric acid level is often elevated relative to pregnancy norms, and any value over 6 mg/dl should be considered to be suggestive of this syndrome.[139] Treatment is delivery, after which the process abates. The infants of affected pregnancies have an increased incidence of being small for gestational age or stillborn. The pathogenesis of this disorder is unknown, although it is known to be associated with failure of the normal expansion of intravascular volume[121] and with an exaggeration of the activated state of coagulation and fibrinolysis normally seen in pregnancy.[73] The prevalence of this condition among family members has suggested genetic factors, possibly with inheritance as an autosomal recessive. Many possible etiologies have been proposed,[6] but none proven. Most obstetricians favor the postulate of vasospasm with enhanced vasoconstrictor tone, associated with vascular injury and microangiopathy, possibly due to alterations in eicosanoid (prostaglandin, prostacyclin, thromboxane) homeostasis.

PREGNANCY OCCURRING IN WOMEN WITH PREEXISTING LIVER DISEASE

In the usual practice of hepatology, pregnancy is rarely encountered. Most patients with liver disease are not women of childbearing age. In addition, most women with serious liver disease are infertile because of the associated anovulatory state. Nevertheless, pregnancy can occur in women with preexisting liver disease and, when it does, it presents some special problems.

Cirrhosis and Portal Hypertension

Worsening jaundice with progressive liver failure, ascites, and hepatic coma have been reported during the course of pregnancy in cirrhotic women.[16,140] Whether this exacerbation of hepatic dysfunction is caused by the gestation or merely coincident with it is unclear. It is clear, however, that cirrhotic women can sustain pregnancy without any worsening of hepatic function.[16,167] Published reports document an increase in the incidence of stillbirths and premature delivery in cirrhotic women.[16,25,138]

Worsening of preexisting portal hypertension might be anticipated in the setting of the marked increase in blood volume and in azygous flow seen in normal pregnancy. Prospective surveys of the course of pregnancy in patients with portal hypertension, either cirrhotic or noncirrhotic in origin, are not available. Published reports probably are biased toward complications occurring in this setting. Variceal hemorrhage during pregnancy or labor has been reported with some frequency.[25,138,151] Spontaneous rupture of a splenic artery aneurysm has been reported as a complication of pregnancy in women with portal hypertension,[12] but it is also a known complication of pregnancy in normals. Patients with a past history of variceal hemorrhage who have been shunted before the beginning of pregnancy have a lower incidence of hemorrhage during the pregnancy than do comparable women who have not had surgery. It is not clear, however, that the incidence of variceal hemorrhage is increased during pregnancy when compared with the incidence in nonpregnant patients with known varices, nor does the history of hemorrhage in one gestation predict the outcome of subsequent pregnancies.[21] There are many reports of successful shunt surgery without fetal wastage during gestation in women who have bled from varices. Elective ablation of varices by sclerotherapy in the pregnant woman has been proposed, but, given the uncertainty about its effectiveness and about the significance of the problem during pregnancy, such a suggestion seems premature.

Specific Liver Diseases

Hepatitis B. The major problem for women with hepatitis B is the risk of maternal-infant transmission of the infection at delivery. If the infection has been identified in the mother by a previous history and by appropriate prenatal screening, this transmission can be interrupted and the newborn protected by use of hepatitis B immune globulin and hepatitis B vaccine.[27] Although exacerbation of the disease during pregnancy has been reported, such worsening must be unusual.[140]

Chronic Persistent Non-A, Non-B Hepatitis. Uneventful pregnancy without worsening disease or fetal complications has been reported in patients with chronic persistent non-A, non-B hepatitis.[75]

Chronic Active Hepatitis ("Immunopathic"). Women appropriately treated for chronic active hepatitis with corticosteroids and azathioprine have been reported to have successful pregnancies, without any increase in fatality.[155] Flare-up of the underlying disease has been reported during pregnancy, but it is unclear that this is related to the pregnant state.[167] Cessation of therapy during pregnancy in such patients has been associated with relapse of the disease. Azathioprine has not been reported to be teratogenic in this setting of low-dose therapy. Such women are at increased risk, however, for obstetric complications such as preeclampsia and stillbirth or prematurity.[155]

Primary Biliary Cirrhosis. Pregnancy in women affected with primary biliary cirrhosis has been reported and may be associated with an increase in cholestasis, which resolves after delivery.[167]

Wilson's Disease. Women under treatment with penicillamine for Wilson's disease should continue therapy with this agent at a dosage of 0.75 g to 1 g/day during gestation. In this setting, this drug has not been associated with problems in the newborn.[161] Discontinuation of therapy has clearly been associated with hemolysis or worsening hepatic function.[137]

Hepatic Adenoma or Focal Nodular Hyperplasia. Hepatic adenomas or tumors of focal nodular hyperplasia associated with previous therapy with oral contraceptive agents have been reported to enlarge or to rupture during subsequent pregnancy.[86,141] Surgical removal prior to conception or during pregnancy has been successful.

Familial Hyperbilirubinemia. The unconjugated hyperbilirubinemia of Gilbert's syndrome is not exacerbated by the pregnant state.[46] In Dubin-Johnson syndrome, however, the conjugated hyperbilirubinemia worsens during gestation but returns to prepregnancy levels after delivery.[29]

Familial Intrahepatic Cholestatic Syndromes. Reported experience with pregnancy in these rare syndromes is meager. In arteriohepatic dysplasia (Alagille's syndrome)[131] and in Byler's syndrome, the underlying cholestasis is said to worsen during pregnancy.

Porphyria Cutanea Tarda. A genetic disorder, which may be exacerbated by estrogenic hormones, porphyria cutanea tarda has been rarely reported to have its initial presentation during pregnancy.[122]

After Liver Transplantation. Two successful, uncomplicated pregnancies have been reported in a liver transplant recipient who was on maintenance immunosuppression with azathioprine and prednisone.[110]

Given this rather incomplete picture of the outcome of pregnancy in women with liver disease, what advice should the clinician give to the patient who is, or desires to be, pregnant? First, such women should expect to have dif-ficulty conceiving. They should be informed that if they have cirrhosis they may be at increased risk for variceal hemorrhage, which could be life threatening during gestation, particularly if they are known to have esophageal varices or have had a past history of variceal bleeding. There is no increased incidence of congenital malformations in the offspring of cirrhotic women, but there is a greater likelihood of stillbirth or prematurity. There is little evidence that pregnancy worsens the underlying liver disease. Should such women desire to have children despite these risks and succeed in getting pregnant, they should be referred to obstetricians specializing in high-risk pregnancy who are well versed in the complications to be anticipated.

USUAL LIVER DISEASES COMPLICATING PREGNANCY

Common liver diseases, unrelated pathophysiologically to the pregnant state, may occur concurrently with it. Since pregnancy itself is common, one might anticipate that the most common diseases of the liver seen in pregnancy are in this group.

Viral Hepatitis

In general, viral diseases are neither more common nor more severe in pregnancy.[70] The few exceptions to this rule include infection with herpes simplex, which has been associated with fulminant hepatic failure in pregnant women.[54,166] Alterations in T-cell function have been reported in pregnancy and may relate to this enhanced susceptibility.[152] Infection with the hepatotrophic viruses is also reported to be more frequent in pregnant women. Hepatitis is reported to occur more frequently in pregnant females than in nonpregnant females or in males.[51,91] Within the course of gestation, hepatitis occurs most commonly in the third trimester as contrasted to the first two trimesters.[1,13,17,63,84,100,106] In the Third World, hepatitis is more likely to follow a fulminant, fatal course in pregnant women than in nonpregnant women or in men, particularly during the third trimester.[17,28,51,84,91,106] This predisposition to increased fatality has not been reported from the United States or France.[63,100,149] Most of these studies were done without serologic testing for hepatitis A or B. Where testing for hepatitis B was available, pregnant women with "hepatitis" had a lower than expected incidence of hepatitis B virus positivity.[28,84,100] This finding, in conjunction with the finding that the hepatic dysfunction resolved after delivery, raises the possibility that some of the patients diagnosed as having "viral hepatitis" could perhaps have had an illness associated etiologically with pregnancy instead. Indeed, autopsy demonstrated that one patient diagnosed as having hepatitis A during an epidemic actually had acute fatty liver of pregnancy.[3] An interesting study from an infectious disease hospital in Australia confirms this premise by demonstrating that among pregnant women thought to have viral hepatitis, positive serologies for either hepatitis A or B were much less commonly found in the second half of pregnancy when compared with the first.[13] The authors of this study concluded that their series of pregnant women with hepatitis had probably been expanded by inclusion of some women with cholestasis of pregnancy. The question of the true incidence and severity of viral hepatitis in pregnant women will have to await the development of testing for non-A, non-B hepatitis as well as further prospective studies done using modern serologic testing.

In patients with documented infection with hepatitis B virus, pregnancy was not associated with an increased mortality.[28,63,84,100] During epidemics of presumed hepatitis A[3] or non-A, non-B hepatitis[90,91] pregnancy, particularly during the third trimester, was associated with increased morbidity and mortality in comparison with nonpregnant patients. Again, these studies suffer from the lack of firm serologic proof of viral infection.

Drug Hepatitis

Because of concern about teratogenicity in the fetus, pregnant women in general take fewer medications than the nonpregnant population. When they do take medications, however, they run the same risk for adverse drug reactions as others. Typical hepatitic reactions have been reported to anesthetic agents (halothane[66] and methoxyflurane[134]). Adverse reactions to erythromycin estolate have been documented in pregnancy.[108] On the other hand, there is no documented increased incidence of such adverse reactions during pregnancy. For example, 1300 pregnant women took isoniazid for tuberculosis without ill effect.[148]

Biliary Tract Disease and Pancreatitis

As mentioned previously, pregnancy decreases gallbladder motility and increases the lithogenicity of bile. Acute cholecystitis may occur in pregnancy, and cholecystectomy may be accomplished during gestation without an increase in either maternal or fetal morbidity. In large studies of cholecystectomy in women, this procedure was only rarely performed during pregnancy,[64,120] suggesting that acute cholecystitis unresponsive to conservative medical management is not a common occurrence in pregnancy.

Acute pancreatitis may complicate pregnancy. Usually this occurs in the setting of cholelithiasis.[82,109] Alternatively, it may be associated etiologically with acute fatty liver of pregnancy or with preeclampsia.[168]

As in the nonpregnant state, cholecystitis due to *salmonella* infection may occur during pregnancy.[146]

Choledochal cyst may present during pregnancy with abdominal pain, a mass, and jaundice.[156] Such patients may represent cases of congenital choledochal cyst that was exacerbated by the effects of pregnancy on biliary motility.

Other Complicating Illnesses

Severe systemic infections with sepsis, particularly urinary tract infections, may be associated with jaundice in the pregnant female[100] as also occurs in the nonpregnant state. Amebic abscess of the liver has also been reported to occur in pregnancy.[159]

LIVER DISEASES ASSOCIATED ETIOLOGICALLY WITH PREGNANCY

Within this category are diseases that are unique to the pregnant state or conditions that are similar to diseases encountered in nonpregnant patients but are clearly related pathophysiologically to the pregnancy.

Hyperemesis Gravidarum

Nausea and vomiting are common in pregnancy, particularly in the first trimester. When this condition becomes protracted and severe, requiring hospitalization, abnormalities in liver function may occur.[2,98] These abnormalities include a mild elevation in bilirubin in one third of such patients, a mild increase in transaminase values in one fourth, and a prolongation of BSP clearance in over one half. The hepatic histology is normal or shows modest cholestasis with hepatocyte necrosis. There are no hepatic sequelae.

Cholestasis of Pregnancy

The diagnosis of cholestasis of pregnancy includes the conditions previously known as pruritus gravidarum, recurrent intrahepatic jaundice of pregnancy, and obstetric hepatosis. It is a syndrome of intrahepatic cholestasis, similar to other cholestatic syndromes more familiar to the clinician (primary biliary cirrhosis, drug-induced cholestasis, familial intrahepatic cholestasis) but atypical in that it occurs in otherwise healthy women only during pregnancy, or during oral contraceptive therapy and then resolves, leaving no sequelae.[56,68,157]

Clinical Hallmarks

This disease is a variable one in all aspects.[124] The classic symptom is pruritus, which typically begins in the third trimester but may start at any time after the second or third month of gestation. In severe cases there is progression to frank jaundice. The gallbladder becomes even more distended than it is normally in pregnancy.[171] The total serum bile acids rise,[59,147] although there may be wide fluctuation in the values. Even in the absence of jaundice or elevations in the serum bilirubin value, the urine specimen may be positive for bilirubin. Liver biopsy (Fig. 30-1) shows pure cholestasis with minimal nonspecific abnormalities.[4] The pruritus may fluctuate and occasionally becomes intolerable. Treatment is similar to that em-

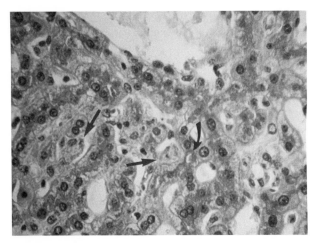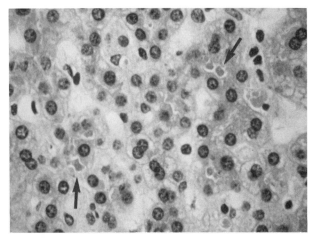

Fig. 30-1. Cholestasis associated with oral contraceptive therapy in a 33-year-old woman with a history of pruritus beginning in the 5th month of each of her six gestations. She was well between pregnancies. This biopsy was performed 2 weeks after she started therapy with oral contraceptives, and 1 week after the onset of pruritus and dark urine. **Left.** Centrolobular vein with adjacent parenchyma demonstrating swollen, bile stained Kupffer cells (*straight arrows*) and canalicular bile plugs (*curved arrow*). (Masson's trichrome; original magnification × 25) **Right.** Centrizonal parenchyma demonstrating numerous bile and protein plugs (*arrows*) without inflammation or hepatocellular necrosis. (H & E; original magnification × 40)

ployed in any other cholestatic syndrome, including cholestyramine and/or phenobarbital.[41,96] Both are safe to use during gestation, although cholestyramine may aggravate the fat malabsorption seen in affected patients. Some patients have responded favorably to ultraviolet light therapy. The cholestasis subsides promptly after delivery. In general, this is a benign condition for the mother. Because of the attendant fat malabsorption, affected patients should receive parenteral vitamin K before delivery. The condition may recur with subsequent pregnancies, although it is not possible to predict from one gestation to the next the clinical behavior of the syndrome. Follow-up studies of the originally described patients have shown a slight increase in the incidence of biliary tract disease.[48,135] One patient with cholestasis of pregnancy was later found to have primary biliary cirrhosis.[7] For the fetus, however, this may not be a benign condition, and some[123,124] but not all[58] authors report an increase in stillbirths and in the rate of prematurity. Therefore, any pregnancy complicated by cholestasis should be treated as high risk, with careful monitoring of both mother and child.

Pathophysiologic Considerations

The close association in affected patients between the cholestasis and pregnancy has led to the supposition that it is caused by the hormonal changes associated with gestation. Affected women may give a history of pruritus or jaundice while taking oral contraceptives and have been shown to respond to challenge with ethinyl estradiol by developing cholestasis.[93] This estrogen is known to cause cholestasis in experimental animals. The experimental agent *S*-adenosyl-L-methionine reverses this cholestasis in

rats and was effective in affected women in preliminary trials.[45] Epidemiologic studies have shown that this syndrome is most common in certain ethnic groups, including Scandinavians and the Araucanian Indians of Chile, who have a prevalence of 27% for this syndrome.[125] Family studies have shown an enhanced susceptibility to the cholestatic effect of ethinyl estradiol as measured by BSP clearance not only in patients known to have cholestasis of pregnancy but also in their female and male family members when compared with nonaffected families.[126] Studies in another large kinship have suggested that this disorder is inherited as an autosomal dominant trait, which may be transmitted by phenotypically normal males who never experience the cholestatic challange of pregnancy.[69] Autosomal dominant inheritance is suspected for some of the other familial intrahepatic cholestatic syndromes, most notably arteriohepatic dysplasia (Alagille's syndrome)[97] and benign recurrent intrahepatic cholestasis (BRIC). Studies in a large kindred affected with BRIC have shown a high incidence of cholestasis of pregnancy, suggesting that perhaps these two syndromes may be interrelated.[37]

In summary, the exact pathogenic mechanisms underlying cholestasis of pregnancy are not fully understood. One may postulate that it is an inherited disease that renders the individual particularly susceptible to cholestatic stress, such as that of pregnancy.

Liver Disease Associated with the Syndrome of Preeclampsia/Eclampsia

This group of disorders is particularly foreign to most gastroenterologists because it is made up of conditions unique to the pregnant state that have no counterparts in the wider patient population. In addition, there is a good deal of unresolved confusion in the literature about these conditions. This stems, in part, from the fact that preeclampsia is a multisystemic disease that may have a broad clinical spectrum.[53] The confusion is compounded by widely held tenets, for example, that necrosis is not seen in acute fatty liver of pregnancy, or that viral hepatitis is more common in pregnancy, which may not be true.[128] As a result, the reported cases are difficult to interpret and to categorize.[92] These conditions probably exist as part of a wide clinical spectrum of disease or diseases. For simplicity's sake, however, they will be discussed here as if they were distinct entities. For all of these entities, therapy is guided by good obstetric practice with the understanding that the disease is related etiologically to the pregnancy. In mild forms, when the life of the mother is not immediately at risk, timing of delivery is dependent on maturity and intrauterine well-being of the fetus. In women with severe hepatic dysfunction, delivery is accomplished with all due speed, since recovery will not begin until the pregnancy is interrupted. As is true for preeclampsia in general, there is no reason to anticipate recurrence of the condition with subsequent pregnancies.

Fibrinogen Deposition in Asymptomatic Preeclampsia

Studies using immunofluorescence to fibrinogen have shown its presence lining the hepatic sinusoids in women with uncomplicated preeclampsia, even in the absence of any abnormality of hepatic histology on routine light microscopy.[11] This finding has also been reported in patients with acute fatty liver of pregnancy.[128] Similar fibrinogen deposits are typical of the renal lesion of preeclampsia.

The Syndrome of Hemolysis, Hepatic Dysfunction, and Thrombocytopenia

The triad of microangiopathic *h*emolytic anemia, *e*levated *l*iver enzymes, and *l*ow *p*latelets, which has been called the HELLP syndrome, is seen in patients with epigastric pain who often lack the more conventional signs of severe preeclampsia.[164] Although it has been called a distinct syndrome, it is more probably a part of the spectrum of hepatic involvement in preeclampsia[53] and may be found in as many as 12% of patients with preeclampsia[104] and in patients with typical acute fatty liver of pregnancy.[128] The attendant thrombocytopenia may present some difficulties in differentiating this disorder from idiopathic thrombocytopenic purpura.[85]

Periportal Hemorrhage

Periportal hemorrhage is the lesion classically associated with preeclampsia/eclampsia. It is characterized histologically by periportal fibrin deposition and hemorrhage (Fig. 30-2).[77] It is rarely encountered today, perhaps because of improvement in the therapy of the underlying toxemia. Often this lesion was discovered at autopsy in women dying of eclampsia who were not recognized to have severe hepatic involvement. It may be present in patients presenting with jaundice,[101] and, like other preeclampsia-associated syndromes, may be complicated by disseminated intravascular coagulation. A similar lesion has been reported in an experimental model of preeclampsia.[6]

Fig. 30-2. Periportal hemorrhage and fibrinoid necrosis in fatal eclampsia in a 42-year-old woman who presented at term after no prenatal care with seizures and hypertension. Shortly thereafter she developed jaundice and died. At autopsy, a subcapsular hematoma of the liver was found. Histologic findings showed (*left*) portal triad with adjacent areas of necrosis and fibrin deposition (Masson's trichrome; original magnification × 4) and (*right*) a smaller triad demonstrating no inflammatory infiltrate but a contiguous area of hepatocyte dropout and fibrin deposition (Masson's trichrome; original magnification × 16).

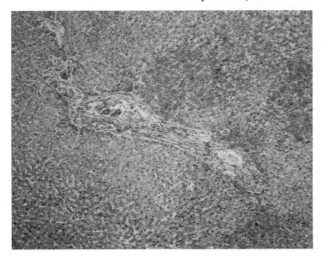
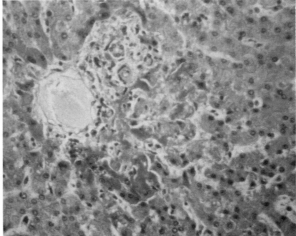

Spontaneous Rupture of the Liver

This catastrophic complication of pregnancy occurs in women who have no predisposing lesion (*e.g.,* hepatic adenoma) except preeclampsia, and it is thought to be consequent to the periportal hemorrhages discussed previously. This condition is more common in older women and in women who are multiparous.[15,62,79,113] It presents with right upper quadrant pain in a patient with preeclampsia. Hemorrhage under the capsule of the liver without frank rupture into the peritoneum may be detected by CT scanning and treated with close observation without surgery (Fig. 30-3).[107] When the capsule ruptures, the patient goes into shock, usually with the death of the fetus, and requires vigorous resuscitative efforts. The diagnosis may be confirmed by angiography[150] and, in some cases, the problem can be successfully treated with hepatic arterial embolization.[61] Most patients will require surgery, with packing with Gelfoam or with an omental pedicle, hepatic artery ligation, or lobectomy. In frank rupture, patients treated surgically fared better than those treated conservatively.[60] This syndrome should be distinguished from rupture of a splenic artery aneurysm, which is another catastrophe associated with pregnancy at term.[116]

Acute Fatty Liver of Pregnancy

Many aspects of this pregnancy-associated condition remain controversial. It has been accepted as a distinct pathologic entity characterized by microvesicular fatty infiltration (Fig. 30-4)[38,115,143] associated with severe, often fatal, hepatic failure.[83] It may occur in association with other complications typical of any form of fulminant hepatic failure, such as disseminated intravascular coagu-

Fig. 30-3. Subcapsular hematoma of the liver without rupture in a 25-year-old woman who presented at 30 weeks' gestation with preeclampsia and abdominal pain. Abdominal CT scan shows a hematoma contained between hepatic capsule and the surface of the right lobe (*arrow*). (Reproduced with permission from Manas KJ et al: N Engl J Med 312:426, 1985)

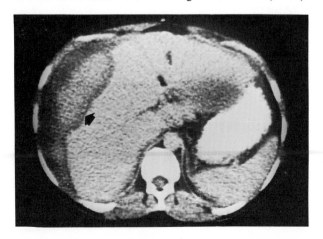

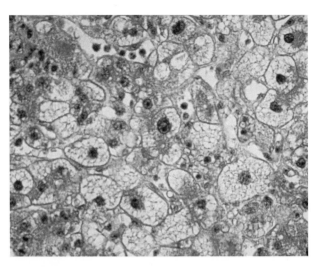

Fig. 30-4. Typical acute fatty liver of pregnancy in a 37-year-old primipara who delivered after the spontaneous onset of labor at 33 weeks of gestation. One week before delivery she had experienced the onset of abdominal pain, nausea and vomiting, and a feeling of restlessness and distress. After delivery she developed renal failure and jaundice. Needle biopsy was done 9 days postdelivery. Photomicrograph shows typical microvesicular fatty infiltration in centrizonal hepatocytes that were positive for fat on oil red O stain. (Masson's trichrome; original magnification × 40)

lation,[24] acute pancreatitis,[57] or hypoglycemia.[19] Although not originally thought to be associated with preeclampsia/eclampsia, review of the literature demonstrates a high incidence of signs of preeclampsia in affected patients, including hypertension,[23,34,57,81,114,118,128,153] hyperuricemia,[103] and thrombocytopenia.[23,34,57,128] Reports indicate that the very high maternal mortality initially reported may have been exaggerated[5,14,19,23,34,39,71,103,111,118,128,130] and that it is more common than previously thought, with a clinical spectrum that is broad, including asymptomatic patients.[128] The histologic appearance in affected patients also covers a broad spectrum and may include material originally interpreted as compatible with viral hepatitis or obstructive cholangitis, with ballooned vacuolated cells that are not obviously fat filled (Fig. 30-5).[128,130] In biopsies from affected patients, one may also demonstrate fibrinogen deposits along the sinusoids as seen in asymptomatic preeclampsia.[128]

The clinical presentation of acute fatty liver of pregnancy may be quite varied but typically includes signs of preeclampsia and features such as epigastric pain, headache, malaise, nausea and vomiting, and restlessness. The patient may become jaundiced and encephalopathic. Fetal wastage is high. After delivery, the liver function improves (normalization of prothrombin time, transaminases) but the patient may go on to experience any of the complications of acute hepatic failure. With early recognition of this condition and prompt delivery, the mother should be

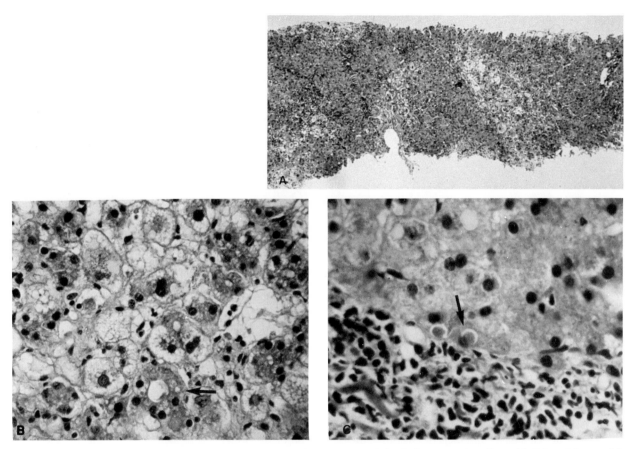

Fig. 30-5. Acute fatty liver of pregnancy, originally interpreted as "hepatitis," in a 25-year-old primipara. The patient was noted to be jaundiced and hypertensive when she went into labor at 37 weeks' gestation. After delivery, she developed ascites, coagulopathy, and renal failure. Needle biopsy was done 9 days after delivery, as she was recovering. **A.** Intact lobular architecture with scattered pale areas, predominately in the central regions. (Masson's trichrome; original magnification × 4) **B.** Central area showing lobular disarray with rosette formation (*arrow*) and pale, ballooned, vacuolated hepatocytes but without typical microvesicular fat. (Masson's trichrome; original magnification × 40) **C.** Portal region demonstrating portal infiltrate and periportal acidophilic bodies (*arrow*). (Masson's trichrome; original magnification × 40)

expected to return to full health with no hepatic sequelae. CT scanning of the liver without contrast media may be helpful when the condition has to be differentiated from fulminant hepatitis, particularly when needle biopsy of the liver is contraindicated.* Affected patients have been reported to complete subsequent pregnancies with no recurrence of liver disease,[20,128] although such patients should be followed as high-risk pregnancies.

The pathogenic mechanisms underlying this condition have long been debated. An early association with intravenous tetracycline therapy for urinary tract infections was made,[8,35,95] but the association was inconstant, and the disorder continues to occur after the discontinuation

of this form of antibiotic therapy. The possibility that low-dose, oral tetracycline used for acne may be contributing to present-day cases has been raised[165] but seems unlikely. The possibility of an interaction between the antibiotic and pregnancy-induced choline deficiency has also been raised.[55] The histologic similarity between this condition and other microvesicular fatty infiltration syndromes, such as Reye's syndrome, has given rise to speculation that these conditions may be interrelated.[144] Electron microscopic evidence would suggest, however, that these processes are not identical.[105,163] Systemic carnitine deficiency may have some similarities to acute fatty liver of pregnancy, and a relationship has been suggested.[44] The exact pathogenic mechanism remains unknown, although it is becoming increasingly clear that this disorder is among the hepatic abnormalities associated with preeclampsia.

* Bova JG et al: Acute fatty liver of pregnancy. N Engl J Med 313:1608, 1985.

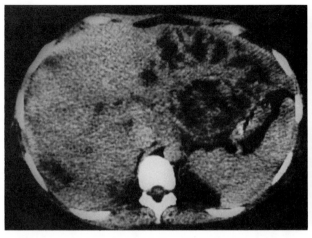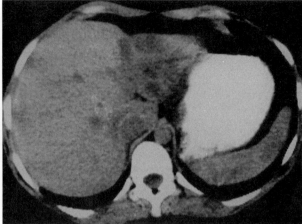

Fig. 30-6. Hepatic arterial thrombosis associated with pregnancy in a 22-year-old woman who presented in the 29th week of gestation in premature labor. After delivery she developed fever, abdominal pain, and renal failure. Needle aspiration of the lesion in the left lobe yielded only necrotic debris, negative on culture. Her recovery was uneventful. **Left.** Abdominal CT scan done 2 weeks after delivery, showing lesions in the right and left lobe. **Right.** Follow-up scan done 5 months later showing persistent defects in the left lobe.

Vascular Thrombosis

Both pregnancy and therapy with oral contraceptive agents are associated with a hypercoagulable state.[73,102] The Budd-Chiari syndrome (veno-occlusive disease of the major hepatic veins or the smaller intrahepatic venous radicles) occurs with increased frequency in women taking oral contraceptives.[99,158] Reports from India suggest that it is also more common in pregnant women, occurring usually immediately after delivery.[90] Similar cases have been reported from Spain[49] and Israel.[132] The prognosis for this syndrome when it occurs in the setting of pregnancy is ominous, as it is for idiopathic veno-occlusive disease. Nevertheless, successful uncomplicated pregnancy has been reported in a patient who had had Budd-Chiari syndrome associated with oral contraceptives.[158]

Thrombosis of the hepatic artery or its radicles has also been reported at the end of gestation, resulting in massive hepatic infarction.[33] A similar process has been reported in women taking oral contraceptives.[78] This complication can best be visualized by CT scanning, which produces dramatic images (Fig. 30-6). Presumed small arteriole thrombosis with resulting localized infarction has also been reported in pregnancy in a woman who subsequently was found to have ulcerative colitis.[65]

Primary Hepatic Pregnancy: On exceedingly rare occasions, the inferior surface of the right lobe of the liver is the site for implantation of an ectopic pregnancy. Such patients may present early in gestation with hemoperitoneum from hepatic hemorrhage.[92a] If the gestation progresses toward term, the patient presents with a mass in the liver[102a] as seen in Figure 30-7.

TABLE 30-3.   Usual Clinical Hallmarks of the Most Frequently Encountered Liver Diseases in Pregnancy

HALLMARK	VIRAL HEPATITIS	LIVER DISEASE WITH PREECLAMPSIA	CHOLESTASIS OF PREGNANCY
Positive family history	None	Often	Often
Trimester of onset	1, 2, or 3	3	2 or 3
Nausea and vomiting	Often	Often	None
Abdominal pain	Rare	Often	None
Pruritus	Rare	None	Always
Increased blood pressure	No	Usually	No
Thrombocytopenia	None	Often	None
Transaminase level	>1000 units	>100 units	<300 units
Cholestatic tests	Rare	No	Always
Positive hepatitis serologies	Often	No	No

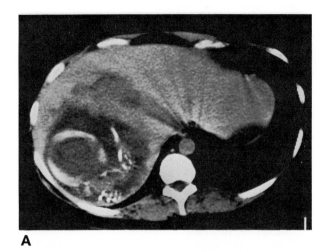

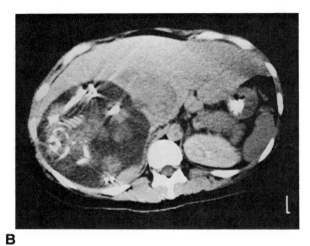

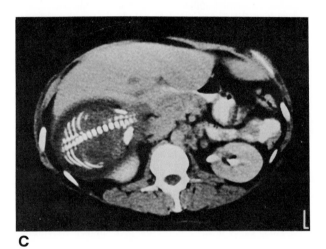

Fig. 30-7. Intrahepatic pregnancy demonstrated by CT scan. **A.** A cut from below the dome of the liver showing skull bones of the fetus and the placenta invading the hepatic substance. **B, C.** Lower cuts, demonstrating that the fetus was positioned with the spine protruding from the inferior surface of the liver.

A DIAGNOSTIC APPROACH TO THE PREGNANT WOMAN WITH LIVER DISEASE

The pregnant woman with liver disease presents a challenge to the consulting clinician. The three most important diagnoses to consider are characterized in Table 30-3, but many other conditions, indeed any liver disease, must be considered in the differential diagnosis. A careful history will provide many diagnostic clues. A history of previous liver disease would be expected in a patient bleeding from esophageal varices, although hemorrhage due to portal hypertension may initially present during gestation. A good family history is important, and patients with cholestasis of pregnancy or with preeclampsia may have similarly affected female family members. A medication history may reveal ingestion of a possibly toxic or sensitizing drug. A history of possible exposure to hepatitis, such as illicit drug use, an at-risk sexual partner, or blood transfusions, would suggest epidemiology compatible with viral hepatitis. The history of the pregnancy is very important. When is the due date? Cholestasis of pregnancy occurs in

either the second or third trimester, preeclampsia and its associated disorders in the third trimester, and viral hepatitis in any trimester. In order to evaluate the possibility of preeclampsia, the clinician should know the blood pressure, not only at the time of presentation but also at the beginning of pregnancy and in mid term. The history of the present illness should elicit symptoms such as nausea and vomiting, present in both acute fatty liver of pregnancy and viral hepatitis, and abdominal pain, which is more prominent in the liver diseases associated with preeclampsia. Severe generalized pruritus is the classic symptom of cholestasis of pregnancy, but is not a complaint in other conditions.

The physical examination is also important. An elevated blood pressure relative to mid trimester, but often within the range commonly accepted as normal in the practice of internal medicine, is very suggestive of preeclampsia and its associated liver disorders. A falling blood pressure or cardiovascular instability is suggestive of intraperitoneal hemorrhage, such as that seen in rupture of the liver or of a splenic artery aneurysm. Other physical signs of preeclampsia include edema and hyperreflexia. The presence of jaundice, ascites, or encephalopathy confirms that the liver dysfunction is severe and suggests the possibility of either hepatitis or preeclampsia/eclampsia-associated conditions.

Because liver disease in the pregnant woman implies risk not only to the patient but also to her fetus, the evaluation should be rapid, with the intent to establish quickly whether the disease is associated etiologically with pregnancy, in which case termination of the pregnancy should be considered. The usual indices of hepatic function, including prothrombin time and ammonia and bilirubin levels are useful to establish the presence or absence of acute hepatic failure, as seen in either hepatitis or preeclampsia-associated conditions. Thrombocytopenia, particularly in the absence of hypoprothrombinemia and in combination with microangiopathic changes on peripheral smear strongly suggests preeclampsia and its associated conditions. The level of the transaminases are helpful: very high levels (over 1000 units) are suggestive of hepatitis or arterial infarction. More moderate, but significant elevations are seen in the preeclampsia-associated disorders, including acute fatty liver of pregnancy. The transaminases are normal or only modestly increased in cholestasis of pregnancy. In that syndrome, indicators of cholestasis, including 5'nucleotidase, GGTP, and serum bile acids, are useful. Serologies for hepatitis A and B are important in excluding these two forms of viral hepatitis.

More extensive testing may be done if time and the patient's condition allow it. An abdominal ultrasound is useful in the evaluation of possible biliary tract disease. The CT scan is the most reliable way to detect both subcapsular hemorrhage and hepatic infarction. Liver biopsy remains the "gold standard" in the assessment of these as well as other forms of liver disease. However, interpretation of the specimen may be difficult, particularly in patients with acute fatty liver of pregnancy.[130] In the pregnant woman near term, the most important consideration is not the specificity of diagnosis but rather time, since the life of both mother and child may depend on rapid recognition that the liver disease is secondary to the pregnant state.

Once a diagnosis has been chosen, appropriate therapy must be considered. In pregnant patients with viral hepatitis there is no evidence that early delivery affects the course of the disease. However, the clinician should be very wary of accepting this diagnosis, especially in the third trimester, since preeclampsia and its associated liver diseases are common and require delivery as therapy. Therapy for cholestasis of pregnancy is similar to that for any cholestatic syndrome but must include careful obstetric monitoring, given the reported increased fetal risk, and parenteral vitamin K at or before delivery. The pruritus resolves with delivery. Mild transaminase elevations associated with preeclampsia should be taken as an indication of a potentially serious situation and treated conservatively with bed rest in the hospital and close monitoring of both mother and fetus. Severe disease, either acute fatty liver of pregnancy or subcapsular hemorrhage or rupture, should be recognized as caused by the pregnancy, and it should be interrupted with all due haste by whatever route is chosen by the obstetricians as most expeditious. A contained subcapsular hemorrhage may be treated with observation or angiographic embolization, but rupture requires emergency surgery. Patients affected with any of these conditions may experience a series of serious complications and will require prolonged multi-specialty care in an intensive care unit setting. With improved recognition and understanding of these conditions, both maternal and fetal mortality will decrease.

REFERENCES

1. Adams RH, Combes B: Viral hepatitis during pregnancy. JAMA 192:195, 1965
2. Adams RH et al: Hyperemesis gravidarum: I. Evidence of hepatic dysfunction. Obstet Gynecol 31:659, 1968
3. Adams WH et al: Coagulation studies of viral hepatitis occurring during pregnancy. Am J Med Sci 272:139, 1976
4. Adlercreutz H et al: Recurrent jaundice in pregnancy: I. A clinical and ultrastructural study. Am J Med 42:335, 1967
5. Ahola SJ et al: Acute fatty liver of pregnancy: Increased survival by early recognition and aggressive therapy. Diag Gynecol Obstet 4:69, 1982
6. Aladjem S et al: Experimental induction of a toxemia-like syndrome in the pregnant beagle. Am J Obstet Gynecol 195:27, 1983
7. Albot G et al: Ictère récidivant de la grossesse et cholangiolite chronique isolée ou maladie de Hanot et MacMahon. Sem Hop Paris 48:3425, 1972
8. Allen ES, Brown WE: Hepatic toxicity of tetracycline in pregnancy. Am J Obstet Gynecol 95:12, 1966
9. Angelini C et al: Carnitine deficiency: Acute postpartum crisis. Ann Neurol 4:558, 1978
10. Antia FP et al: Liver in normal pregnancy, preeclampsia, and eclampsia. Lancet 2:776, 1958
11. Arias F, Mancilla-Jimenez R: Hepatic fibrinogen deposits in pre-eclampsia: Immunofluorescent evidence. N Engl J Med 295:578, 1976
12. Barrett JM, Caldwell BH: Association of portal hypertension and ruptured splenic artery aneurysm in pregnancy. Obstet Gynecol 57:255, 1981
13. Bennett NMcK et al: Viral hepatitis and intrahepatic cholestasis of pregnancy. Aust NZ J Med 9:54, 1979
14. Bernuau J et al: Acute fatty liver of pregnancy: An often non-fatal disease. Hepatology 2:158, 1982
15. Bis KA, Waxman B: Rupture of the liver associated with pregnancy: A review of the literature and report of 2 cases. Obstet Gynecol Surv 31:763, 1976
16. Borhanmanesh F, Haghighi P: Pregnancy in patients with cirrhosis of the liver. Obstet Gynecol 36:315, 1970
17. Borhanmanesh F et al: Viral hepatitis during pregnancy: Severity and effect on gestation. Gastroenterology 64:304, 1973
18. Borman DZ et al: Effects of pregnancy and oral contraceptive steroids on gallbladder function. N Engl J Med 302:362, 1980
19. Breen KJ et al: Idiopathic acute fatty liver of pregnancy. Gut 11:822, 1970
20. Breen KJ et al: Uncomplicated subsequent pregnancy after idiopathic fatty liver of pregnancy. Obstet Gynecol 40:813, 1972

21. Britton RC: Pregnancy and esophageal varices. Am J Surg 143:421, 1982

22. Brodie MJ et al: Pregnancy and the acute porphyrias. Br J Obstet Gynecol 84:726, 1977

23. Burroughs AK et al: Idiopathic acute fatty liver of pregnancy in 12 patients. Q J Med 204:481, 1982

24. Cano RI et al: Acute fatty liver of pregnancy: Complication by disseminated intravascular coagulation. JAMA 231:159, 1975

25. Cheng Y-S: Pregnancy in liver cirrhosis and/or portal hypertension. Am J Obstet Gynecol 128:812, 1977

26. Chesley LC: History and epidemiology of preeclampsia-eclampsia. Clin Obstet Gynecol 27:801, 1984

27. Chin J: Prevention of chronic hepatitis B virus infection from mothers to infants in the United States. Pediatrics 71:289, 1983

28. Christie AB et al: Pregnancy hepatitis in Libya. Lancet 2:827, 1976

29. Cohen L et al: Pregnancy, oral contraceptives, and chronic familial jaundice with predominantly conjugated hyperbilirubinemia. Gastroenterology 62:1182, 1972

30. Cohen S: The sluggish gallbladder of pregnancy. N Engl J Med 302:397, 1980

31. Combes B et al: Alterations in sulfobromophthalein sodium removal mechanisms from blood during normal pregnancy. J Clin Invest 42:1431, 1963

32. Crawford JS, Hooi HWY: Binding of bromsulphthalein by serum albumin from pregnant women, neonates and subjects on oral contraceptives. Br J Anaesth 40:723, 1968

33. Dammann HG et al: *In vivo* diagnosis of massive hepatic infarction by computed tomography. Dig Dis Sci 27:73, 1982

34. Davies MH et al: Acute liver disease with encephalopathy and renal failure in late pregnancy and the early puerperium: A study of fourteen patients. Br J Obstet Gynecol 87:1005, 1980

35. Davis JS, Kaufman RH: Tetracycline toxicity: A clinicopathologic study with special reference to liver damage and its relationship to pregnancy. Am J Obstet Gynecol 95:523, 1966

36. De Klerk M et al: Urinary porphyrins and porphyrin precursors in normal pregnancy. S Afr Med J 49:581, 1975

37. de Pagter AGF et al: Familial benign recurrent intrahepatic cholestasis: Interrelation with intrahepatic cholestasis of pregnancy and from oral contraceptives? Gastroenterology 71:202, 1976

38. Duma RJ et al: Acute fatty liver of pregnancy. Ann Intern Med 63:851, 1965

39. Ebert EC et al: Does early diagnosis and delivery in acute fatty liver of pregnancy lead to improvement in maternal and infant survival? Dig Dis Sci 29:453, 1984

40. Elliott JR, O'Kell RT: Normal clinical chemical values for pregnant women at term. Clin Chem 17:156, 1971

41. Espinosa J et al: The effect of phenobarbital on intrahepatic cholestasis of pregnancy. Am J Obstet Gynecol 119:234, 1974

42. Everson GT et al: Gallbladder function in the human female: Effect of the ovulatory cycle, pregnancy, and contraceptive steroids. Gastroenterology 82:711, 1982

43. Fallon HJ: Liver diseases. In Burrow GN, Ferris TF (eds): Medical Complications during Pregnancy, 2nd ed, p 278. Philadelphia, WB Saunders, 1982

44. Feller A et al: Acute fatty liver of pregnancy: A possible disorder of carnitine metabolism. Gastroenterology 84:1150A, 1983

45. Frezza M et al: Reversal of intrahepatic cholestasis of pregnancy in women after high dose S-adenosyl-L-methionine administration. Hepatology 4:274, 1984

46. Friedlaender P, Osler M: Icterus and pregnancy. Am J Obstet Gynecol 97:894, 1967

47. Fulton IC et al: Is normal pregnancy cholestatic? Clin Chem Acta 130:171, 1983

48. Furhoff AK, Hellstrom K: Jaundice in pregnancy: A follow-up study of women originally reported by L. Thorling: Present health of the women. Acta Med Scand 196:181, 1974

49. Gatell Artigas JM et al: Letter: Pregnancy and the Budd-Chiari syndrome. Dig Dis Sci 27:89, 1982

50. Geall MG, Webb MJ: Liver disease in pregnancy. Med Clin North Am 58:817, 1974

51. Gelpi AP: Viral hepatitis complicating pregnancy: Mortality trends in Saudi Arabia. Int J Gynaecol Obstet 17:73, 1979

52. Glasgow AM, Larsen JW: Urinary orotic acid in pregnancy. Am J Obstet Gynecol 149:464, 1984

53. Goodlin RC: Severe pre-eclampsia: Another great imitator. Am J Obstet Gynecol 125:747, 1976

54. Goyert GL et al: Anicteric presentation of fatal herpetic hepatitis in pregnancy. Obstet Gynecol 65:585, 1985

55. Gwee MCT: Can tetracycline-induced fatty liver in pregnancy be attributed to choline deficiency? Med Hypothesis 9:157, 1982

56. Haemmerli UP: Jaundice during pregnancy. Acta Med Scand Suppl 444:1, 1966

57. Hatfield AK et al: Idiopathic acute fatty liver of pregnancy: Death from extrahepatic manifestations. Dig Dis 17:167, 1977

58. Heikkinen J: Serum bile acids in the early diagnosis of intrahepatic cholestasis of pregnancy. Obstet Gynecol 61:581, 1983

59. Heikkinen J et al: Changes in serum bile acid concentrations during normal pregnancy, in patients with intrahepatic cholestasis of pregnancy and in pregnant women with itching. Br J Obstet Gynaecol 88:240, 1981

60. Henny CP et al: Review of the importance of acute multidisciplinary treatment following spontaneous rupture of the liver capsule during pregnancy. Surg Gynecol Obstet 156:593, 1983

61. Herbert WNP, Brenner WE: Improving survival with liver rupture complicating pregnancy. Am J Obstet Gynecol 142:530, 1982

62. Hibbard LT: Spontaneous rupture of the liver in pregnancy: A report of eight cases. Am J Obstet Gynecol 126:334, 1976

63. Hieber JP et al: Hepatitis and pregnancy. J Pediatr 91:545, 1977

64. Hill LM et al: Cholecystectomy in pregnancy. Obstet Gynecol 46:291, 1975

65. Hirsh EH et al: Hepatic infarction in ulcerative colitis during pregnancy. Gastroenterology 78:571, 1980

66. Holden TE, Sherline DM: Hepatitis and hepatic failure in pregnancy. Obstet Gynecol 40:586, 1972

67. Holzbach RT: Jaundice in pregnancy—1976. Am J Med 61:367, 1976

68. Holzbach RT, Sanders JH: Recurrent intrahepatic cholestasis of pregnancy. JAMA 193:542, 1965

69. Holzbach RT et al: Familial recurrent intrahepatic cholestasis of pregnancy: A genetic study providing evidence for transmission of a sex-limited, dominant trait. Gastroenterology 85:175, 1983

70. Horstmann DM: Viral infections. In Burrow GN, Ferris

TF (eds): Medical Complications during Pregnancy, 2nd ed, p 333. Philadelphia, WB Saunders, 1982

71. Hou SH et al: Acute fatty liver of pregnancy: Survival with early cesarean section. Dig Dis Sci 29:449, 1984

72. Hurwitz MB: Jaundice in pregnancy: A 10-year study and review. S Afr Med J 44:219, 1970

73. Hyde E et al: Intravascular coagulation during pregnancy and the puerperium. J Obstet Gynaecol Br Common 80:1059, 1973

74. Iber FL: Jaundice in pregnancy—a review. Am J Obstet Gynecol 91:721, 1965

75. Infeld DS et al: Chronic persistent hepatitis and pregnancy. Gastroenterology 77:524, 1979

76. Ingerslev M, Teilum G: Biopsy studies on the liver in pregnancy: I. Normal histological features of the liver as seen on aspiration biopsy. Acta Obstet Gynecol Scand 25:352, 1945

77. Ingerslev M, Teilum G: Biopsy studies on the liver in pregnancy: III. Liver biopsy in albuminuria of pregnancy, eclampsism, and eclampsia. Acta Obstet Gynecol Scand 25:361, 1945

78. Jacobs MB: Hepatic infarction related to oral contraceptive use. Arch Intern Med 144:642, 1984

79. Jewett JF: Eclampsia and rupture of the liver. N Engl J Med 297:1009, 1977

80. Johnson P et al: Studies in cholestasis of pregnancy: I. Clinical aspects and liver function tests. Acta Obstet Gynecol Scand 54:77, 1975

81. Joske RA et al: Acute fatty liver of pregnancy. Gut 9:489, 1968

82. Jouppila P et al: Acute pancreatitis in pregnancy. Surg Gynecol Obstet 139:879, 1974

83. Kaplan MM: Current concepts: Acute fatty liver of pregnancy. N Engl J Med 313:367, 1985

84. Karouf M et al: Hépatite et grossesse à Tunis: A propos de 103 cas comparés à 100 cas en dehors de la grossesse. J Gynaecol Obstet Biol Repr 9:887, 1980

85. Kelton JG: Management of the pregnant patient with idiopathic thrombocytopenic purpura. Ann Intern Med 99:796, 1983

86. Kent DR et al: Effect of pregnancy on liver tumor associated with oral contraceptives. Obstet Gynecol 51:148, 1978

87. Kern FJ et al: Biliary lipids, bile acids, and gallbladder function in the human female. J Clin Invest 68:1229, 1981

88. Kerr MG et al: Studies of the inferior vena cava in late pregnancy. Br Med J 1:532, 1964

89. Khuroo MS: Study of an epidemic of non-A, non-B hepatitis: Possibility of another human hepatitis virus distinct from post-transfusion non-A, non-B type. Am J Med 68:818, 1980

90. Khuroo MS, Datta DV: Budd-Chiari syndrome following pregnancy. Report of 16 cases, with roentgenologic, hemodynamic and histologic studies of the hepatic outflow tract. Am J Med 68:113, 1980

91. Khurro MS et al: Incidence and severity of viral hepatitis in pregnancy. Am J Med 70:252, 1981

92. Killam AP et al: Pregnancy-induced hypertension complicated by acute liver disease and disseminated intravascular coagulation: Five case reports. Am J Obstet Gynecol 123:823, 1975

92a. Kirby NG: Primary hepatic pregnancy. Br Med J 1:296, 1969

93. Kreek MJ et al: Idiopathic cholestasis of pregnancy: The response to challenge with the synthetic estrogen, ethinyl estradiol. N Engl J Med 277:1391, 1967

94. Krejs GJ: Jaundice during pregnancy. Semin Liver Dis 3:73, 1983

95. Kunelis CT et al: Fatty liver of pregnancy and its relationship to tetracycline therapy. Am J Med 38:359, 1965

96. Laatikainen K: The effect of cholestyramine and phenobarbital on pruritus and serum bile acid levels in cholestasis of pregnancy. Am J Obstet Gynecol 132:501, 1978

97. LaBrecque DR et al: Four generations of arteriohepatic dysplasia. Hepatology 2:467, 1982

98. Larrey D et al: Recurrent jaundice caused by recurrent hyperemesis gravidarum. Gut 25:1414, 1984

99. Lewis JH et al: Budd-Chiari syndrome associated with oral contraceptive steroids: Review of treatment of 47 cases. Dig Dis Sci 28:673, 1983

100. Levy VG et al: Les ictères au cours de la grossesse: A propos de 95 cas. Med Chir Dig 6:111, 1977

101. Long RG et al: Pre-eclampsia presenting with deep jaundice. J Clin Pathol 30:212, 1977

102. Lowe GDO et al: Increased blood viscosity in young women using oral contraceptives. Am J Obstet Gynecol 137:840, 1980

102a. Luwuliza–Kirunda JMM: Primary hepatic pregnancy. Case report. Br J Obstet Gynaecol 85:311–313, 1978

103. MacKenna J et al: Acute fatty metamorphosis of the liver: A report of two patients who survived. Am J Obstet Gynecol 127:400, 1977

104. MacKenna J et al: Preeclampsia associated with hemolysis, elevated liver enzymes, and low platelets: An obstetric emergency? Obstet Gynecol 62:751, 1983

105. Malatjalian DA, Badley BWD: Acute fatty liver of pregnancy: Light and electron microscopic studies. Gastroenterology 84:1384, 1983

106. Mallia CP, Narncekivell AF: Fulminant virus hepatitis in late pregnancy. Ann Trop Med Parasitol 76:143, 1982

107. Manas KJ et al: Hepatic hemorrhage without rupture in preeclampsia. N Engl J Med 312:424, 1985

108. McCormack WM et al: Hepatotoxicity of erythromycin estolate during pregnancy. Antimicrob Agents Chemother 12:630, 1977

109. McKay AJ et al: Pancreatitis, pregnancy, and gallstones. Br J Obstet Gynecol 87:47, 1980

110. Meyers RL, Schmid R: Letter: Childbirth after liver transplantation. Transplantation 29:432, 1980

111. Moldin P, Johansson O: Acute fatty liver of pregnancy with disseminated intravascular coagulation. Acta Obstet Gynecol Scand 57:179, 1978

112. Munnell EW, Taylor HC: Liver blood flow in pregnancy: Hepatic vein catheterization. J Clin Invest 26:952, 1947

113. Nelson EW et al: Spontaneous hepatic rupture in pregnancy. Am J Surg 134:817, 1977

114. Nixon WCW et al: Icterus in pregnancy: A clinico-pathological study including liver-biopsy. J Obstet Gynaecol Br Emp 54:642, 1947

115. Ober WB, LeCompte PM: Acute fatty metamorphosis of the liver associated with pregnancy. Am J Med 19:743, 1955

116. O'Grady JP et al: Splenic artery aneurysm rupture in pregnancy: A review and case report. Obstet Gynecol 50:627, 1977

117. Perez VS et al: Ultrastructure of human liver at the end of normal pregnancy. Am J Obstet Gynecol 110:428, 1971

118. Pockros PJ et al: Idiopathic fatty liver of pregnancy: Findings in ten cases. Medicine 68:1, 1984

119. Potter JM, Nestle PJ: The hyperlipidemia of pregnancy in

normal and complicated pregnancies. Am J Obstet Gynecol 153:165, 1979

120. Printen KJ, Ott RA: Cholecystectomy during pregnancy. Am Surg 44:432, 1978

121. Pritchard JA: Changes in blood volume during pregnancy and delivery. Anesthesiology 26:393, 1965

122. Rajka G: Pregnancy and porphyria cutanea tarda. Acta Derm Venereol 64:444, 1984

123. Reid R, Ivey KJ: Fetal complications of obstetric cholestasis. Br Med J 1:870, 1976

124. Reyes H: The enigma of intrahepatic cholestasis of pregnancy: Lessons from Chile. Hepatology 2:86, 1982

125. Reyes H et al: Prevalence of intrahepatic cholestasis of pregnancy in Chile. Ann Intern Med 88:487, 1978

126. Reyes H et al: Sulfobromophthalein clearance tests before and after ethinyl estradiol administration, in women and men with familial history of intrahepatic cholestasis of pregnancy. Gastroenterology 81:226, 1981

127. Riely CA: Pregnancy and the liver. In Creasy RK, Resnik R (eds): Maternal-Fetal Medicine: Principles and Practice, p 992. Philadelphia, WB Saunders, 1984

128. Riely CA et al: Acute fatty liver, toxemia and viral hepatitis: A proposed reassessment based on observations in 9 pregnant patients (submitted for publication)

129. Roberts JM: Pregnancy-related hypertension. In Creasy RK, Resnik R (eds): Maternal-fetal Medicine, pp 703–752. Philadelphia, WB Saunders, 1984

130. Rolfes DB, Ishak KG: Acute fatty liver of pregnancy: A clinicopathologic study of 35 cases. Hepatology 5:1149, 1985

131. Romero R et al: Arteriohepatic dysplasia in pregnancy. Am J Obstet Gynecol 147:108, 1983

132. Rosenthal T et al: The Budd-Chiari syndrome after pregnancy: Report of two cases and a review of the literature. Am J Obstet Gynecol 113:789, 1972

133. Rovinsky JJ, Jaffin H: Cardiovascular hemodynamics in pregnancy: III. Cardiac rate, stroke volume total peripheral resistance, and central blood volume in multiple pregnancy: Synthesis of results. Am J Obstet Gynecol 95:787, 1966

134. Rubinger D et al: Hepatitis following the use of methoxyflurane in obstetric analgesia. Anesthesiology 43:593, 1975

135. Samsioe G et al: Studies in cholestasis of pregnancy: V. Gallbladder disease, liver function tests, serum lipids and fatty acid composition of serum lecithin in the non-pregnant state. Acta Obstet Gynecol Scand 54:417, 1975

136. Samuelson K, Thomassen PA: Radioimmunoassay of serum bile acids in normal pregnancy and in recurrent cholestasis of pregnancy. Acta Obstet Gynecol Scand 59:417, 1980

137. Scheinberg IH, Sternlieb I: Wilson's Disease. Philadelphia, WB Saunders, 1984

138. Schreyer P et al: Cirrhosis—pregnancy and delivery: A review. Obstet Gynecol Surv 37:304, 1982

139. Schuster E, Weppelmann B: Plasma urate measurements and fetal outcome in preeclampsia. Gynecol Obstet Invest 12:162, 1981

140. Schweitzer IL, Peters RL: Pregnancy in hepatitis B antigen positive cirrhosis. Obstet Gynecol 48:535, 1976

141. Scott LD et al: Oral contraceptives, pregnancy, and focal nodular hyperplasia of the liver. JAMA 251:1461, 1984

142. Seymour CA, Chadwick VS: Liver and gastrointestinal function in pregnancy. Postgrad Med J 55:343, 1979

143. Sheehan HL: The pathology of acute yellow atrophy and delayed chloroform poisoning. J Obstet Gynaecol Br Emp 47:49, 1940

144. Sherlock S: Acute fatty liver of pregnancy and the microvesicular fat diseases. Gut 24:265, 1983

145. Simon JA: Biliary tract disease and related surgical disorders during pregnancy. Clin Obstet Gynecol 26:810, 1983

146. Sinapolice RX et al: Hemoglobin SD disease associated with cholecystitis and cholelithiasis in pregnancy. Obstet Gynecol 60:388, 1982

147. Sjovall K, Sjovall J: Serum bile acid levels in pregnancy with pruritus. Clin Chim Acta 13:207, 1966

148. Snider DE et al: Treatment of tuberculosis during pregnancy. Am Rev Respir Dis 122:65, 1980

149. Snydman DR: Current concepts: Hepatitis in pregnancy. N Engl J Med 313:1398, 1985

150. Somner DG et al: Hepatic rupture with toxemia of pregnancy: Angiographic diagnosis. AJR 132:455, 1979

151. Soto-Albors CE et al: Portal hypertension and hypersplenism in pregnancy secondary to chronic schistosomiasis: A case report. J Reprod Med 29:345, 1984

152. Sridama V et al: Decreased levels of helper T cells: A possible cause of immunodeficiency in pregnancy. N Engl J Med 307:352, 1982

153. Stander HJ, Cadden JF: Acute yellow atrophy of the liver in pregnancy. Am J Obstet Gynecol 28:61, 1934

154. Steven MM: Pregnancy and liver disease. Gut 22:592, 1981

155. Steven MM et al: Pregnancy in chronic active hepatitis. Q J Med 48:519, 1979

156. Taylor TV et al: Choledochal cyst of pregnancy. J Coll Surg 22:424, 1977

157. Thorling L: Jaundice in pregnancy: A clinical study. Acta Med Scand [Suppl] 302:1, 1955

158. Tsung SH et al: Budd-Chiari syndrome in women taking oral contraceptives. Ann Clin Lab Sci 10:518, 1980

159. Wagner VP et al: Amebic abscess of the liver and spleen in pregnancy and the puerperium. Obstet Gynecol 45:562, 1975

160. Walker FB et al: Gamma glutamyl transpeptidase in normal pregnancy. Obstet Gynecol 43:745, 1974

161. Walshe JM: Pregnancy in Wilson's disease. Q J Med 46:73, 1977

162. Walters WAW, Lim YL: Changes in the maternal cardiovascular system during human pregnancy. Surg Gynecol Obstet 131:765, 1970

163. Weber FL et al: Abnormalities of hepatic mitochondrial urea-cycle enzyme activities and hepatic ultrastructure in acute fatty liver of pregnancy. J Lab Clin Med 94:27, 1979

164. Weinstein L: Syndrome of hemolysis, elevated liver enzymes, and low platelet count: A severe consequence of hypertension in pregnancy. Am J Obstet Gynecol 142:159, 1982

165. Wenk RE et al: Tetracycline-associated fatty liver of pregnancy, including possible pregnancy risk after chronic dermatologic use of tetracycline. J Reprod Med 26:135, 1981

166. Wertheim RA et al: Fatal herpetic hepatitis in pregnancy. Obstet Gynecol 62:38s, 1983

167. Whelton MJ, Sherlock S: Pregnancy in patients with hepatic cirrhosis: Management and outcome. Lancet 2:995, 1968

168. Wilkinson EJ: Acute pancreatitis in pregnancy: A review of 98 cases and a report of 8 new cases. Obstet Gynecol Surv 28:281, 1973

169. Willson JR, Carrington ER: Obstetrics and Gynecology, 6th ed. St. Louis, CV Mosby, 1979

170. Worley RJ: Pathophysiology of pregnancy-induced hypertension. Clin Obstet Gynecol 27:821, 1984

171. Ylostalo P et al: Gallbladder volume and serum bile acids in cholestasis of pregnancy. Br J Obstet Gynaecol 89:59, 1982

chapter **31**
Hepatic Porphyrias

D. MONTGOMERY BISSELL and RUDI SCHMID

The porphyrias are unusual diseases. Although encountered relatively rarely in clinical practice, they are objects of enduring fascination to physicians and basic scientists alike. The term "porphyrin" was coined to describe the purple color ("hematoporphyrin") that developed when a solution of hemoglobin was treated with concentrated sulfuric acid.[125] In a patient with red-purple urine and severe cutaneous photosensitivity, extraction and purification of the colored substances led to chemical characterization of the first naturally occurring porphyrin, called uroporphyrin.[64] Subsequent work, which showed that heme is a metalloporphyrin (iron-protoporphyrin IX), established a relationship of porphyrin to heme but left undecided whether porphyrins are precursors or catabolites of heme. This question eventually was resolved by a series of elegant radioisotopic experiments that led to the almost complete elucidation of the biochemical pathway of heme synthesis.[153] It was established that porphyrins (or their reduced forms, porphyrinogens) are *precursors* of heme (Fig. 31-1), which is the prosthetic moiety of hemoproteins functioning at the center of oxidative respiration; porphyrins also serve as precursors of chlorophyll and vitamin B$_{12}$.[112] It further was shown that physiologic catabolism of heme involves irreversible cleavage of the protoporphyrin ring, resulting in formation of biliverdin and bilirubin.[127]

CLASSIFICATION OF PORPHYRIAS

The term "porphyria" was first applied to patients with cutaneous manifestations who excreted large amounts of porphyrins and were believed to suffer from a hereditary disease.[79] However, porphyria was noted also in persons taking ethylsulfone hypnotics (Sulfonal) marketed in Europe at the end of the 19th century; this appeared to be an acquired disorder.[126] To these types of porphyria was added in the 1920s a disease characterized by excessive urinary excretion of a porphyrin precursor (porphobilinogen) rather than porphyrins. In contrast to porphyria with predominantly cutaneous manifestations, the latter disease involved solely acute neuropsychiatric attacks.[168] Subsequent reports concerned types in which the clinical features of the purely cutaneous form and those with acute attacks were combined. "Latent" porphyria was described in persons with biochemical markers of porphyria but without clinical manifestations.[168] Several systems of nomenclature emerged, and the total number of discrete types of porphyria remained unclear.

Developments over the past 25 years have made it possible to bring order to this proliferation of clinical and chemical types of porphyria. Hereditary deficiencies of individual enzymes in the pathway have been identified and firmly associated with specific types of clinical porphyria. Cases of acquired porphyria have been traced to a direct inhibitory effect of environmental factors (drugs, toxins) on the heme synthetic pathway. In both instances, the appearance of excessive amounts of porphyrins or porphyrin precursors in excreta appears to be a byproduct of metabolic efforts to overcome the enzymatic blocks and provide heme required by the organism. With the development of sensitive techniques for the measurement of these compounds, it has been recognized also that asymptomatic *porphyrinuria* is common, particularly in patients with liver disease or with intoxication by heavy metals. This presumably reflects either minimal impairment of heme synthesis or failure of the liver to normally excrete porphyrins, leading to their diversion from bile to urine.

Current classification of the porphyrias takes into account the existence of genetic and acquired forms, as well as clinical manifestations and chemical characteristics. An additional consideration is the principal tissue site of porphyrin overproduction. Experimental work in the 1950s demonstrated that chemically induced porphyria involves bone marrow or liver as the major sites of porphyrin overproduction.[149] Both tissues have relatively high rates of heme production—the bone marrow for synthesis of hemoglobin, and the liver for microsomal cytochromes (cytochromes b$_5$ and P-450); the latter uses at least 50% of hepatic heme synthesis.[115] In the hereditary porphyrias, the specific genetic defect presumably is present in all cells of the body. However, for reasons that are not clear, abnormal porphyrinogenesis is confined largely to either bone marrow or liver. The classification presented in Table 31-1 accordingly separates the porphyrias into erythropoietic or hepatic types. Other organs also may elaborate excess porphyrin, but their contribution to the total appears to be small.

Of the erythropoietic group (Table 31-1), only protoporphyria (PP) is relatively common; at times it also gives rise to hepatic manifestations. An asymptomatic increase in red blood cell porphyrins is observed in iron defi-

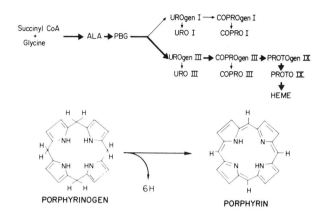

Fig. 31-1. Pathway of hepatic heme synthesis. (Modified from Bissell DM: Heme metabolism and the porphyrias. In Wright R et al [eds]: Liver and Biliary Disease. London, WB Saunders, 1979)

ciency,[133] lead intoxication,[93] and certain refractory anemias.[88] The hepatic group (Table 31-1) includes both hereditary and acquired types. Three of the hereditary conditions have major clinical and biochemical features in common, which justifies their treatment as a group; these are acute intermittent porphyria (AIP), hereditary coproporphyria (HCP), and variegate porphyria (VP). Porphyria cutanea tarda (PCT) clearly is separable, in terms of both pathogenesis and clinical manifestations. Each of these is a discrete genetic entity with a characteristic excretory pattern of heme precursors reflecting the position of the enzymatic defect in the pathway of heme synthesis.

METABOLIC PATHWAYS

Hepatic Heme Synthesis

In the biosynthesis of heme (ferriprotoporphyrin IX), all of the carbons for the porphyrin macrocycle are supplied by glycine and succinic acid. Condensation of these two compounds (succinic acid as the CoA derivative) results in formation of δ-aminolevulinic acid (ALA), the first committed intermediate in heme synthesis (step 1, Fig. 31-2). An alternative precursor of ALA is 4,5-dioxovaleric acid, a 5-carbon compound that is converted to ALA by transamination. Liver extract contains an enzyme mediating this conversion, with alanine as the amino donor, and intact cells *in vitro* utilize 4,5-dioxovalerate for heme and porphyrin synthesis.[118] However, the intracellular concentration of this ALA precursor is unknown, and it is unlikely that this pathway of ALA formation is of metabolic importance in intact mammals. On the other hand, it may represent the sole route of ALA formation in plants.[74]

The condensation of glycine and succinyl CoA, to form ALA, is catalyzed by a mitochondrial enzyme, ALA synthetase, and requires pyridoxal phosphate. In the liver, ALA synthetase is inducible, increasing rapidly when new heme synthesis is required and decaying with a half-life of approximately 70 minutes, which is very brief for a mammalian protein.[109] This finding suggests that formation of ALA is the rate-controlling step in hepatic heme synthesis.[66] This concept is supported by *in vitro* exami-

TABLE 31-1.   Classification of Human Porphyrias

	MODE OF INHERITANCE	DEMONSTRATED OR SUSPECTED ENZYME DEFECT*
Erythropoietic		
Congenital erythropoietic porphyria	Autosomal recessive	UROgen-I synthetase and/or UROgen-III cosynthetase
Protoporphyria	Autosomal dominant	Ferrochelatase
Hepatic		
Acute intermittent porphyria	Autosomal dominant	UROgen-I synthetase
Hereditary coproporphyria	Autosomal dominant	COPROgen oxidase
Variegate porphyria	Autosomal dominant	PROTOgen oxidase
Porphyria cutanea tarda	Autosomal dominant	UROgen decarboxylase
δ-Aminolevulinic aciduria	Autosomal recessive	PBG synthetase
Toxic porphyria	(Acquired)	(Variable)

* Abbreviations as in Figure 31-1.

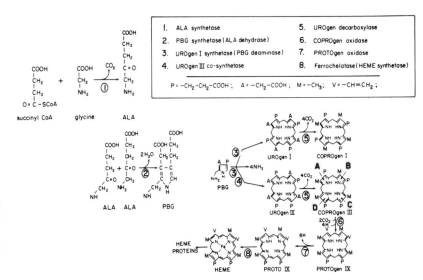

Fig. 31-2. Chemical intermediates and enzymes of heme synthesis. (Modified from Bissell DM: Heme metabolism and the porphyries. In Wright R et al [eds]: Liver and Biliary Disease. London, WB Saunders, 1979)

nation of the reaction kinetics of the individual enzymes in the pathway.[115]

Subsequent steps occur extramitochondrially, up to the formation of COPROgen. Two molecules of ALA condense (with elimination of H_2O) to form one molecule of porphobilinogen (PBG) in a reaction that is catalyzed by PBG synthetase (step 2, Fig. 31-2). The enzyme requires zinc for full activity and is particularly sensitive to inactivation by lead and other heavy metals.

The first porphyrin-like structure in the pathway, UROgen, is a macrocycle comprising four molecules of PBG, joined by meso-bridge carbons that represent the δ-carbon of ALA. A two-enzyme reaction occurs, in which four molecules of ammonia are released (steps 3 and 4, Fig. 31-2). Because PBG is asymmetric, having both acetic and propionic substituents, four isomeric forms of UROgen are possible. Of these, only type III serves as an intermediate in heme synthesis. Small amounts of type I are formed (step 3, Fig. 31-2) and are present in urine or bile; the other isomers do not occur in nature.

A mechanism for the formation of the physiologically "correct" UROgen-III isomer appears to have arisen early in evolution, in that the III isomer is a precursor of plant pigments (chlorophyll) as well as protoheme and vitamin B_{12}.[112] The principal enzyme, UROgen-I synthetase (also known as PBG deaminase or, more accurately, hydroxymethylbilane synthase, E.C. 4.3.1.8), catalyzes a regular head-to-tail condensation of four PBG, yielding a linear tetrapyrrole, hydroxymethyl-bilane, which forms UROgen I upon ring closure. In the presence of UROgen-III cosynthetase (UROgen-III synthase, E.C. 4.2.1.75), ring closure is preceded by reversal of the final pyrrole (ring D), which thus condenses with the first pyrrole (ring A) in a head-to-head relationship.[5] The cosynthetase normally is present in excess, relative to UROgen-I synthetase, which ensures almost quantitative conversion of PBG to the III isomer of UROgen.

The conversion of UROgen III to subsequent intermediates and finally to PROTO IX involves sequential decarboxylation and oxidation of the side chains of the porphyrin nucleus, leading to compounds of increasing hydrophobicity.* The octacarboxylic UROgen is converted enzymatically through heptacarboxylic, hexacarboxylic, and pentacarboxylic intermediates to the tetracarboxylic COPROgen; these reactions are mediated by the cytosolic enzyme UROgen decarboxylase (step 5, Fig. 31-2). Present evidence indicates that all four decarboxylations of the I and III isomers are catalyzed by a single enzyme. Purified UROgen decarboxylase consists of two subunits, each with a molecular weight of approximately 46,000 daltons.[40,59,84] The active center of the enzyme has at least one thiol group, which may render it susceptible to inhibition by iron (see discussion of PCT, below). Attempts to document an effect of iron on the enzyme *in vitro,* however, have led to divergent results.[40,120]

Formation of PROTOgen (by decarboxylation and oxidation of the propionic substituents on the A and B pyrrole units of COPROgen) requires a mitochondrial enzyme, COPROgen oxidase (step 6, Fig. 31-2). Also occurring within the mitochondrion is the oxidation of PROTOgen to PROTO (step 7) and insertion of iron to form ferriprotoporphyrin-IX, or heme (step 8).

Regulation of the heme synthetic pathway, while only partially understood at present, clearly is central to the pathogenesis of porphyria. As mentioned above, formation of ALA is the rate-limiting reaction in the pathway, a step controlled by ALA synthetase. The regulation of ALA synthetase has been subjected to scrutiny in a variety of experimental systems.[115] The findings provide com-

---

* Of the possible structural isomers of protoporphyrin, those with asymmetric pyrrole substituents were designated I-XV by Fischer: isomer IX belongs to the III series of uroporphyrin and is the physiologic intermediate in heme synthesis (Figs. 31-1 and 31-2).

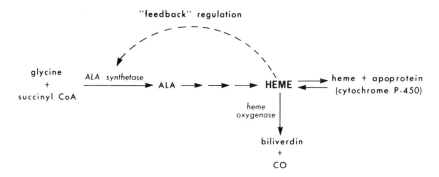

Fig. 31-3. Regulation of hepatic heme synthesis by heme. (Bissell DM, Hammaker LE: Cytochrome P-450 heme and the regulation of δ-aminolevulinic acid synthetase in the liver. Arch Biochem Biophys 176:103, 1976)

pelling albeit indirect evidence for the existence of a small labile heme pool in the liver, which regulates the amount (or activity) of ALA synthetase.[115] This pool may represent newly formed heme as well as that exchanging with specific cellular heme-proteins.[11] Because it is relatively insoluble in aqueous media at neutral pH, heme is believed to exist in a protein-bound state in cells[121]; its transfer among various postulated carriers and acceptor apoproteins may involve points at which heme utilization is regulated. In the liver, the pool of "free" or unassigned heme appears to flow principally to apocytochrome, notably for the synthesis of cytochrome P-450. A demand for heme, as during induction of cytochrome P-450, is met promptly by an increase in ALA synthetase and accelerated heme synthesis.[108] Thus, a "feedback" loop is established (Fig. 31-3), which adjusts the rate of heme synthesis to the prevailing needs of the cell.[10] Although usually reflecting the flux of endogenous heme, it also may be activated by exogenous heme.[110] Exogenously administered heme in experimental animals suppresses hepatic ALA synthetase activity,[110] suggesting that it enters in part the regulatory pool and is therefore available for cytochrome formation. This inference has been confirmed by studies in intact rats.[31]

Excretion and Pharmacologic Properties of Heme Precursors

The route of excretion of heme precursors reflects largely the water solubility of the individual compounds. ALA and PBG are highly water soluble at neutral pH, are filtered by the kidney, and excreted in the urine. URO likewise appears very largely in urine, whereas COPRO is excreted to a greater extent in bile than in urine and PROTO exits solely by the fecal route.

Characteristic of the porphyrins (but not of ALA, PBG, or porphyrinogens) is their excitation by near-ultraviolet light. Excited-state porphyrins *in vitro* yield their energy as fluorescence; *in vivo,* they effect a variety of alterations in accessible membranous structures. Various mechanisms of porphyrin-induced cutaneous pathology have been proposed, including the generation by light-activated porphyrin of singlet oxygen[154] and complement-derived peptides.[98] The light-mediated effects of uroporphyrin (as

in PCT) differ from those of protoporphyrin (in PP). Whether this reflects a property of the individual porphyrins or their distribution within the dermis is unclear. The extent of light-induced damage is proportional to the porphyrin content in skin[27] and also to its level in plasma, urine, or feces.

HEPATIC PORPHYRIA WITH NEUROLOGIC MANIFESTATIONS

The diseases in this group—AIP, HCP, and VP—are clinically the most important of the hereditary hepatic porphyrias. In all three, acute attacks occur consisting of abdominal pain and neuropsychiatric manifestations; ALA and PBG are excreted in abnormally large amounts; and intravenous administration of hematin provides effective therapy. The specific genetic defect in each type is expressed as an autosomal dominant trait, which is much more widespread than the apparent incidence of acute attacks, implying a large popualtion of "latent" carriers. Many carriers are completely asymptomatic while others complain of intermittent or chronic low-grade symptoms without acute exacerbations. The ethnic and geographic distribution of these genetic traits varies. In Europe and the United States, AIP is believed to be present in about 0.01% of the population but is much less common in blacks and Orientals than in whites. HCP reportedly is more often latent than is AIP, and the number of reported cases is few. Prevalence figures are not available, but the trait may be at least as common as AIP. The distribution of VP is worldwide; the type is notably prevalent in persons of Dutch ancestry dwelling in the Cape province of South Africa, affecting about one of 300 persons in this group.[37]

The difference among AIP, HCP, and VP, apart from genetic distinctions *per se,* consists largely of the characteristic excretion pattern of heme precursors associated with each type. This in turn is responsible for secondary clinical manifestations—in particular, photosensitivity—that distinguish HCP and VP from AIP. In HCP and VP, porphyrins (as well as ALA and PBG) are present in excess and cutaneous manifestations occur, whereas these are absent in AIP.

Clinical Presentation

Acute Intermittent Porphyria

Acute attacks of AIP consist of abdominal pain, initially subacute but usually progressing over a period of 24 to 48 hours until it may suggest acute cholecystitis, appendicitis, or other surgically remediable processes. While typically in the abdomen, the site of pain in some patients may be the back or extremities. Anorexia, nausea, and vomiting are frequent. Constipation often is a long-standing problem, worsening at the onset of an attack. Accompanying minor symptoms range from headache to paresthesias and are present to a variable extent (Table 31-2).

The physical findings associated with acute attacks are nonspecific (Table 31-2). In evaluating pain, the examiner may be impressed that the severity of symptoms is out of proportion to the abdominal findings. Unlike acute inflammatory processes of the abdomen, rebound tenderness is seldom, if ever, present. A moderate degree of fever may be noted. Tachycardia is a frequent finding and is useful in monitoring the course of an acute attack. Presenting neuropsychiatric symptoms include seizures, usually generalized, and mental abnormalities that range from confusion to frank psychosis. Motor and sensory deficits appear with prolonged attacks; these may be distal or proximal and may be asymmetric,[140] progressing in severe cases to quadriplegia, respiratory paralysis, and death. Pathologic examination reveals patchy demyelination or axonal degeneration of peripheral nerves as well as degenerative changes in elements of the autonomic nervous system.[160]

Routine laboratory findings in AIP generally are unremarkable, and this is useful for differentiating the disease from other abdominal processes. A moderate leukocytosis may be present, but the differential count usually is normal in the absence of a coexisting infectious process. Anemia is not associated with the hepatic porphyrias, and apart from a slight elevation of serum transaminase activity, liver function tests commonly are normal; hepatic histology shows minor, nonspecific changes.[8] In a series of 46 patients, 30% exhibited a significant elevation of blood urea nitrogen on admission.[155] Hyponatremia occurs in a minority of patients and occasionally may be striking: in some instances it appears to be due to inappropriate secretion of antidiuretic hormone.[166] Serum thyroxine levels may be elevated, but this appears to reflect largely an increase in thyroid-binding globulin.[81]

In a florid acute attack, the diagnosis often suggests itself. More troublesome is the evaluation of chronic or intermittent subacute symptoms in relatives of known cases of AIP or in persons in whom the diagnosis is suspected because of obscure abdominal or neurologic symptoms. These complaints typically are nonspecific and often appear neurotic. Indeed, in known carriers, it may be difficult to establish whether minor symptoms are due to AIP or to an unrelated problem. In all instances, how-

TABLE 31-2. Presentation of AIP, HCP, and VP

PATIENTS PRESENTING WITH SYMPTOM OR SIGN			
Symptom	%	Sign	%
Abdominal pain	90	Tachycardia	83
Vomiting	80	Hypertension	55
Constipation	80	Motor neuropathy	53
Pain in limbs	51	Pyrexia	38
Pain in back	50	Leukocytosis (>12,000)	20
Confused state	32	Bulbar involvement	18
Seizures	12	Sensory loss	15
Diarrhea	8	Cranial nerve involvement	9

Data are from a study of VP[50]; the findings in AIP[155] and HCP[70] are similar.

ever, it is important to document the presence of the carrier state, so that appropriate preventive measures can be taken to avoid precipitation of acute attacks (see following text).

The biochemical hallmark of AIP, whether acute or latent, is increased urinary excretion of PBG, consistent with the demonstrated enzymatic defect in the conversion of PBG to UROgen (Fig. 31-4). ALA, which is one step removed from the block, also is excreted in increased amounts. Excess urine URO would not be expected on theoretical grounds but does occur, presumably as a result of extrahepatic conversion of PBG to URO. In addition, in standing urine (in the urinary bladder or collection vessel) colorless PBG slowly polymerizes to a dark porphyrin-like compound ("porphobilin") that appears in the URO fraction after solvent extraction of urine.[169] This process is accelerated by sunlight, providing the basis for the observation that urine from persons with AIP acquires a dark color when illuminated in air. When the diagnosis of AIP is suspected, determination of urinary PBG should be carried out, preferably with a 24-hour collection. PBG and ALA are measured by ion-exchange chromatography.[35] The Watson–Schwartz test[170] is a rapid qualitative test for urinary PBG: urine mixed with Ehrlich's reagent (dimethylaminobenzaldehyde in HCl) forms an immediate red complex. While lack of color formation constitutes a negative test, it should be emphasized that a red color reaction is nonspecific. Endogenous urinary substances (notably, urobilinogen) as well as drugs or drug metabolites give a red color reaction.[170] However, after addition of sodium acetate (to $pH = 4$) and extraction with n-butanol, the pink PBG complex remains in the aqueous phase, while colored complexes due to the presence of urobilinogen or other substances are extractable. When performed in this manner, a positive Watson–Schwartz test is diagnostic. This requires that urinary PBG be at least 5 mg to 10 mg/liter, and in acute attacks of AIP, PBG excretion invariably exceeds this level. On the other hand, this qualitative test is unsuitable for screening

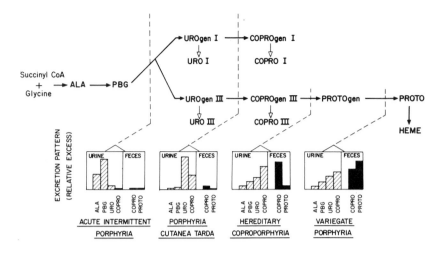

Fig. 31-4. Excretion pattern of porphyrins and other heme precursors in AIP, HCP, VP, and PCT. The vertical dashed lines indicate the known or suspected site of the genetically determined enzymatic defect for each type of porphyria. (Modified from Bissell DM: Heme metabolism and the porphyrias. In Wright R et al [eds]: Liver and Biliary Disease. London, WB Saunders, 1979)

possible carriers, who may exhibit only marginally elevated urinary PBG (Table 31-3). Thus, its usefulness is limited largely to the evaluation of patients with acute abdominal pain in whom AIP is one of the diagnostic possibilities and rapid information is required. In less urgent circumstances and for evaluation of the carrier state, the quantitative column assay should be performed. It may be noted that the "urinary porphyrin screen" commonly available in clinical laboratories does not measure PBG but only porphyrins and therefore has no place in the evaluation of patients with acute abdominal pain.

While an acute neuropsychiatric attack of porphyria is readily confirmed by measurement of PBG, identification of carriers on occasion proves difficult. When urinary PBG is quantitated by ion-exchange column chromatography, it is found to be elevated in the majority of adult carriers but will be normal in some, variously estimated as 10% to 40% of the total[4,114,168,175] and is normal in virtually all juvenile carriers. Because of the sizable number of false-negative results by this test, assay of UROgen-I synthetase ("urosynthetase") activity is a useful adjunct in screening for carriers. This enzyme is detectable in circulating erythrocytes and is decreased in the red blood cells of persons with AIP.[116] As noted (see Table 31-1, Fig. 31-4), decreased activity of this enzyme is characteristic of AIP and is apparent regardless of the age of the patient or the presence or absence of symptoms.

Several methods of measurement have been published and are suitable for routine clinical use.[106,131] Although assay of this activity would appear to be an ideal screening test for AIP, false-negative tests do occur.[123] The cellular content of enzyme varies with the age of circulating erythrocytes, young cells having the highest and senescent cells the lowest activity,[147] so that reticulocytosis in a carrier of AIP may raise blood urosynthetase activity into the normal range. An additional albeit small number of carriers exhibit enzyme activity that is considered in the normal range but still is significantly lower than that in unaffected family members.[4,146,166] Because of this difficulty, screening of relatives in parallel with the index case is a useful approach. In a recent study, the combined use of quantitative urinary PBG determinations, erythrocyte urosynthetase activity, and pedigree analysis permitted unequivocal classification of 90% of a group of known porphyrics and family members.[94]

Hereditary Coproporphyria

The spectrum of acute manifestations in HCP is indistinguishable from that of AIP or VP[25,70]; this is the reason for grouping these three genetic entities together. Since HCP involves overproduction of porphyrins as well as porphyrin precursors (Fig. 31-4), 20% to 30% of the patients with this disease exhibit photocutaneous manifes-

TABLE 31-3.   Normal Laboratory Values for Heme Precursors

URINE	(24 HOURS)	FECES (DRY WEIGHT)	ERYTHROCYTES
ALA	0–7.5 mg		
PBG	0–2.0 mg		
URO	10–50 μg	0–0.5 μg/g	
COPRO	50–250 μg	0–50 μg/g	0.5–1.5 μg/100 ml
PROTO		0–120 μg/g	25–75 μg/100 ml

Data are from the authors' laboratories. ALA and PBG[35] and porphyrins[152] are determined by the methods referenced.

tations.[25] The diagnosis of HCP requires quantitative measurement of both urinary and fecal porphyrins as well as urinary ALA and PBG. During acute attacks, the entire array of heme precursors is present in excess in urine, the increase in COPRO being most pronounced. While this pattern clearly excludes AIP, the differential diagnosis between HCP and VP requires measurement of fecal porphyrins. In contrast to the latter disease, the former exhibits excess fecal COPRO with normal or only slightly increased PROTO (Fig. 31-4).

As in AIP, elevation of urinary levels of PBG during acute neurologic attacks is sufficient to yield a positive Watson–Schwartz test, useful in the evaluation of acute abdominal pain. Although a urinary porphyrin "screen" also is positive (Fig. 31-4), it fails to distinguish between hereditary porphyria and nonspecific porphyrinuria associated with hepatic disease or other acquired intra-abdominal processes. The appropriate screening test is quantitative measurement of fecal COPRO, which is the most consistently positive finding in asymptomatic carriers.[25,70] The enzymatic defect in this disease is decreased COPROgen oxidase activity (see Table 31-1), which is a mitochondrial enzyme not present in mature erythrocytes. Enzyme assay therefore requires leukocytes or cultures of skin fibroblasts, and at present this is a research procedure.[25,55]

Variegate Porphyria

Acute attacks in VP are clinically similar to those of the other two types of hereditary hepatic porphyria.[37,50,122] Porphyrin overproduction generally is more marked than in HCP; the characteristic biochemical abnormality is excessive excretion of both COPRO and PROTO in feces (Fig. 31-4). Also increased is an ether-insoluble porphyrin fraction ("porphyrin X"), which may represent porphyrin–peptide complexes.[54,142] Cutaneous photosensitivity or unusual mechanical fragility of light-exposed skin is present in at least 80% of patients with symptomatic VP and commonly is a chronic process occurring in the absence of acute manifestations.[122] The approach to the diagnosis of acute attacks is the same as that for AIP or HCP (see preceding discussion). Carriers may be identified by quantitative assay of fecal PROTO. The enzymatic defect in this type of porphyria appears to be a partial deficiency of PROTOgen oxidase.[22] Although reduced activity of ferrochelatase also has been reported, its significance is uncertain. A marked reduction is present also in patients with PP,[17,22] a disease with clinical and biochemical characteristics quite different from those of VP (Table 31-4).

Pathogenesis

The patterns of heme precursor excretion that characterize AIP, HCP, and VP can be rationalized as reflecting the hereditary defect of heme synthesis for each of these types. Theoretically, a 50% decrease in enzyme activity at any one step results in a partial block of the flow of heme precursors, and heme synthesis is potentially—or actually—compromised. Indeed, from studies of the catalytic capacity in vitro of the various component enzymes of the pathway, it appears that a 50% reduction in UROgen-I synthetase activity significantly restricts the flow of ALA and PBG in AIP.[116] On the other hand, the biochemical consequences of deficient COPRO oxidase activity in HCP are less clear. The enzyme exhibits a catalytic activity in vitro far in excess of that required for normal heme synthesis; moreover, a patient homozygous for HCP and exhibiting only 2% of normal COPRO oxidase activity has been reported,[72] indicating that profound deficiency of this enzyme is compatible with life. It is possible that expression of the characteristic precursor pattern in HCP involves a secondary effect of the hereditary deficiency on UROgen-I synthetase.

Evidence for genetic heterogeneity of these clinically defined porphyrias is emerging. In studies of UROgen-I synthetase from persons with AIP, two distinct types of catalytic defect have been identified, suggesting failure of expression of one allele in one case and a structural mutation, leading to production of altered enzyme, in the other.[2] With cloning of a cDNA sequence for the UROgen-I synthetase gene,[73] molecular analysis of this apparent heterogeneity should proceed rapidly.

Regardless of the mechanisms by which the heme pathway is affected in these different conditions, cellular deficiency of heme ensues when requirements for hepatic heme production exceed the capacity of the restricted

---

TABLE 31-4.   Manifestations in the Hereditary Porphyrias

TYPE OF PORPHYRIA	NEUROLOGIC	CUTANEOUS	HEPATIC
AIP	++	0	0
HCP	+	+	0
VP	++	++	0
PCT	0	++	+
PP	0	+	(+)*

* Clinically apparent liver disease is a rare occurrence in PP associated with high levels of plasma PROTO (see text).

pathway. This leads to release of ALA synthetase from end-product regulation (see Fig. 31-3) and results in overproduction of ALA and PBG.

Although these deductions account satisfactorily for the chemical abnormalities present in these types of porphyrias, they fail to explain the variability in clinical expression. Even among siblings, manifestations vary from minimal to life-threatening acute attacks, which indicates that precipitating factors play an important role. These include certain types of drugs, fasting, infection, and gonadal hormones. While all may act similarly in precipitating acute attacks, induction of attacks by drugs—exemplified by barbiturates—is the most clearly delineated. Barbiturates induce hepatic cytochrome P-450, thereby increasing the requirement for hepatic heme synthesis. If the genetically compromised pathway is unable to meet the requirement, a porphyric attack ensues.

Inducers of hepatic heme synthesis, as a group, may be dangerous in these types of porphyria. This raises the issue of whether the potential of a given drug for precipitating an acute attack can be assessed prior to its clinical use. For this purpose, the intact rat[163,165] and chick embryo liver culture[135] have been used, and lists of potentially hazardous compounds have been compiled.[49,166,173] In general, the substances listed in Table 31-5 should be avoided in AIP, HCP, and VP, unless the clinical indications are compelling and adequate substitutes are unavailable. It should be noted, however, that direct extrapolation of experimental findings to humans may not be appropriate because of species differences; also, the response of patients with porphyria to drugs is highly variable.[49]

In addition to drug administration, decreased caloric intake—either deliberate or as a result of infection or anorexia—may precede acute attacks. The metabolic milieu of the liver during fasting apparently is conducive to the precipitation of attacks; specific factors are as yet undefined.[16] Other putative endogenous precipitants of acute attacks include 5-β-steroids and ovarian hormones. It has been reported that patients in acute attacks excrete increased amounts of 5-β-steroids and exhibit a deficiency of 5-α-steroid reductase.[1,83] However, this abnormality appears to be acquired rather than hereditary[1]; its relationship to the pathogenesis of acute porphyria is uncertain. Circumstantial evidence implicates ovarian steroids in the genesis of acute attacks: attacks are virtually unknown prior to puberty and, in adults, are much more common in women than in men. Women with AIP may experience cyclical exacerbations occurring premenstrually.[177] These observations notwithstanding, it has been difficult to assign a definite porphyrogenic role to any single gonadal steroid or to a specific hormonal milieu, in part because of the variable response among individual patients. In some women oral contraceptives clearly aggravate porphyria but in others provide relief from premenstrual symptoms.[130,174,177] Similarly, the effect of pregnancy is unpredictable; although porphyric exacerbations occur, a benign course or even decreased manifestations during pregnancy are not unusual.[24,155]

The pathogenesis of the neurologic manifestations in AIP, HCP, and VP remains a major unresolved problem. Three hypotheses have been advanced, none necessarily the sole explanation for the neurologic manifestations. Excess production of ALA (+PBG) is common to all acute

TABLE 31-5. Hazardous and Safe Drugs for Patients with AIP, HCP, or VP*

MAY PRECIPITATE ACUTE ATTACKS	BELIEVED TO BE SAFE
Apronalide	Aspirin
Barbiturates	Bromides
Chlordiazepoxide	Chlorpromazine
Chloroquine	Chloral hydrate
Chlorpropamide	Corticosteroids
Dichloralphenazone	Diazepam
Ergot preparations	Dicoumarol
Estrogens	Digoxin
Ethanol	Diphenhydramine
Glutethimide	Ether
Griseofulvin	Guanethidine
Hydantoins	Meperidine
Imipramine	Morphine
Meprobamate	Neostigmine
Methprylon	Nitrous oxide
Methsuximide	Penicillins
Methyldopa	Propranolol
Novonal	Tetracyclines
Sulphonamides	

* Data are taken from the authors' experience and other sources.[49,125,166,173]

hepatic porphyrias and may cause neurotoxicity or false neurotransmission. Support for this concept is the fact that in two unrelated conditions—lead poisoning and hereditary tyrosinemia—abdominal colic and/or encephalopathy are prominent, together with elevation of serum and urinary ALA levels.[61,99] ALA is similar structurally to the inhibitory neurotransmitter, gamma-aminobutyric acid (GABA), and has been reported to act as a partial GABA agonist.[21] GABA may function as a neurotransmitter in the peripheral nervous system,[82] in which case high circulating levels of ALA might explain the intestinal hypomotility and colic commonly associated with acute porphyric attacks. This hypothesis has been explored with studies of synaptic transmission *in vitro* in the presence of ALA. The results are difficult to interpret. On the whole, detectable effects are observed only with unphysiologically high concentrations of ALA.[19] Relatively unexplored is the possibility that ALA may affect neuronal function at sites other than the synapse. In a study of glucose transport in avian-cultured cerebral neurons, relatively low concentrations of ALA (0.01 mM) significantly inhibited transport of 2-deoxyglucose.[144] This result notwithstanding, the clinical data argue against any direct role of ALA in the neurologic syndrome of acute porphyria, in that serum levels of ALA or PBG correlate poorly with symptoms. Although excretion of these porphyrin precursors generally rises during acute attacks in individual patients, the range within a group of patients is broad and unrelated to the presence or absence of symptoms. Moreover, in a single study, removal of ALA and PBG from the circulation of a patient (by charcoal hemoperfusion and hemodialysis) had no observable effect on symptoms.[92]

According to a second hypothesis, neurologic symptoms may be due to neuronal heme deficiency. The inherited defect in heme synthesis in these porphyrias presumably is present in all tissues. If expressed in brain, the result might be a deficiency of heme essential for cellular heme proteins such as cytochromes. However, present evidence suggests that the regulation of heme formation in brain differs from that in liver: in the rat, porphyria-inducing compounds have no effect on the activity of ALA synthetase in brain.[128,129] Also, while hematin administration reverses acute neurologic symptoms in porphyria, evidence that circulating hematin is taken up by neural tissues is lacking.

Finally, recent studies have linked hepatic deficiency of tryptophan pyrrolase to neurologic dysfunction in porphyria. Tryptophan pyrrolase is a heme enzyme with a relatively low affinity for its prosthetic group, heme, and it exists in liver normally as both holoenzyme and (inactive) apoenzyme. Its activity in liver fluctuates with the level of available heme, and in acute porphyria, heme deficiency presumably causes a reduced level of the holoenzyme. The result is decreased conversion of tryptophan to kynurenine, increased plasma tryptophan, and conversion of the amino acid by an alternate pathway to the neurotransmitter serotonin. In rats with experimentally induced porphyria and hepatic heme deficiency, turnover of brain tryptophan and serotonin is increased, and the animals demonstrate an altered response to morphine analgesia, consistent with increased serotonergic tone.[100,101] The clinical relevance of these findings remains to be determined. A report of increased urinary excretion of 5-hydroxyindoleacetic acid in acute porphyria[102] provides indirect support for the hypothesis.

The remarkable efficacy of administered hematin (see text following) is consistent with any of these proposed mechanisms for the neuropsychiatric manifestations of porphyria. Exogenously administered hematin has been shown to enter hepatocytes,[31] where it suppresses the production of ALA and PBG and increases the activity of tryptophan pyrrolase.

Management

For all three porphyrias in this group, prevention of acute attacks is the cornerstone of management. In families with a known case of porphyria, identification of asymptomatic carriers is mandatory, using the screening procedures outlined in the preceding sections. Prenatal diagnosis of AIP also is feasible.[147] However, identification of a carrier *in utero* under normal circumstances is not an indication for termination of the pregnancy, since clinical disease occurs in only a minority of carriers and can largely be prevented. Prophylactic measures for carriers include avoidance of drugs implicated in acute attacks (Table 31-5) and of fasting or fad diets. With respect to the role of diet, caloric intake sufficient to maintain a normal body weight appears to be optimal. There is no evidence that a diet high in carbohydrate prevents attacks.

In acute attacks, administration of carbohydrate and/or hematin is combined with supportive care to bring about a remission. Carbohydrate is given to reverse the fasting state and, by itself, has been associated with remission of attacks.[62,155,172] The dose of dextrose should approach 500 g/day and usually is given intravenously because of nausea or vomiting in ill patients. This entails administration of relatively large volumes of water, which may cause dilutional hyponatremia. Use of hypertonic solutions of dextrose, given through a central catheter, circumvents this problem.

If an acute attack does not respond in 48 hours to carbohydrate administration or if neurologic manifestations develop or progress, treatment with hematin is indicated. Infusion of hematin (hydroxy-heme) presumably compensates for the genetically determined impairment in heme synthesis in AIP, HCP, and VP, suppressing ALA synthetase and, hence, overproduction of ALA and PBG. Although a controlled study is not available, there is little doubt regarding its efficacy in unequivocal acute attacks.[15,44,95,171] In the reported failures,[113] decayed hematin may have been used (this problem is discussed below); in some of these patients, also, the excretion of porphyrin precursors was only marginally abnormal, suggesting that the acute manifestations may have been due to problems other than porphyria. Hematin is prepared by dissolving crystalline ferriprotoporphyrin-IX chloride (hemin) in sodium carbonate solution (10 g/liter), which then is adjusted to pH 8.0 with HCl and sterilized by membrane filtration.[44] It should be infused promptly. Hematin in solution decays in a time- and temperature-dependent fashion to products that fail to suppress experimental porphyria[69] and therefore are probably ineffective in humans. At 4° C (39.2° F), the solution has an apparent half-life of about 30 hours (prepared solutions are stored at 4° C and discarded after 12 hours). Hematin solution that has been lyophilized is stable,[95] providing a preparation that may be stored and reconstituted as needed, and is now available commercially as Panhematin. A heme-arginate preparation (Normosang), which appears equal to hematin in efficacy and is more stable in solution, is being marketed in Europe.

An effective dose of hematin is 1.5 mg/kg given once daily; this is less than was previously recommended.[44] It must be given intravenously; it is ineffective after oral administration probably because of its degradation by heme oxygenase in the intestinal mucosa.[136] Similarly, intramuscularly or subcutaneously administered hematin probably is degraded largely *in situ.* After an intravenous dose, the decrease in serum hematin is biphasic ($t\frac{1}{2}$ is approximately 7 and 40 hours for the early and late phases, respectively).[95] Although prolonged administration of hematin might be expected to induce hepatic heme oxygenase,[161] this apparently is not associated with accelerated elimination of hematin from the circulation or with diminished clinical efficacy.[95]

The adequacy of treatment with hematin is assessed by the patient's clinical response and by decreased excretion of ALA and PBG; improvement generally is apparent within 72 hours after initiation of hematin therapy. The biochemical response to hematin persists only as long as hematin is present in the circulation, and excretion of heme precursors generally rises shortly after cessation of treatment. By contrast, the clinical response to hematin tends to be longer lasting.

Side-effects of hematin consist of a chemical phlebitis at the site of infusion and a transient anticoagulant effect. At very high doses, renal toxicity may occur.[29] In the single reported case of acute renal failure, the condition was reversible.[45] Phlebitis is due to the alkalinity of the infusate and occurs in approximately 4% of cases.[95] It is minimized by use of a large peripheral vein and a slow infusion rate (1–2 ml/min). The anticoagulant effect of hematin, which may be due to a decay product rather than to hematin itself,[69] is manifest as thrombocytopenia and reduced activity of several clotting factors.[75,124] These effects parallel the plasma hematin concentration: they are maximal 10 minutes after hematin administration, declining rapidly thereafter and disappearing after 48 hours.[68] Although plasma fibrinogen (as well as the platelet count) is reduced, disseminated intravascular coagulation is excluded by the absence of fragmented red cells and by normal plasminogen and antithrombin III.[68] Clinically significant bleeding after hematin administration appears to be uncommon[132]

but may have occurred in three patients,[68,78,117] one of whom was also receiving heparin. On the basis of the limited data available, hematin should be used cautiously, if at all, in patients with a known bleeding tendency and in those receiving anticoagulants or undergoing surgery.

As part of the initial evaluation of an acute attack, precipitating conditions—ingestion of an "inducing" drug, intercurrent infection, or fasting—need to be identified and treated. Supportive measures include correction of electrolyte abnormalities, control of seizures, and administration of analgesics. Seizures generally occur early in the course of an attack, are transient, and may be treated with parenteral diazepam, or magnesium.[159] Virtually all patients in acute attacks require symptomatic relief of pain while carbohydrate or hematin is introduced. Although the specificity of its effects is uncertain, chlorpromazine has been given for this purpose[166]; excessive sedation and other side-effects limit its usefulness. Propranolol counters the tachycardia accompanying acute attacks and, in occasional patients, appears to relieve pain.[6] It should be introduced conservatively, since hypotensive reactions occur.[14] In many patients, narcotic analgesics (*e.g.,* meperidine) are required despite the danger of addiction in patients with chronic disease.

The management of recurrent seizures and of surgical anesthesia poses special problems in AIP, HCP, or VP. The commonly used anticonvulsants (barbiturates or structurally related compounds) are contraindicated.[97,107] Nonbarbiturates useful in seizure disorders include clonazepam, carbamazepine, valproic acid, and bromides. Clonazepam has been administered without adverse effects in AIP[97] but failed to control seizures in one reported case.[18] The available data suggest that carbamazepine[97,107] and valproic acid[18] are inducers of hepatic heme synthesis and should be used cautiously, if at all. Bromides have been effective in controlling seizure activity, do not induce heme synthesis, and toxicity has not been a problem.[18,107]

Surgical anesthesia represents a dual hazard to persons with porphyria. Induction of anesthesia commonly involves intravenous administration of a barbiturate (*e.g.,* thiopental), and the routinely imposed preoperative fast increases the porphyrogenic potential of those anesthetics. Porphyria patients requiring surgery should receive intravenous carbohydrate to counter the lack of oral intake, and for induction of anesthesia, agents other than barbiturates should be used. Diazepam and ketamine have been given for this purpose.[143] Propanidid has been used with impunity in patients with VP in South Africa,[36] but at present this drug is not available in the United States.[36]

Prognosis

In older series, acute porphyric attacks resulted in a substantial mortality: among patients with advanced neurologic (paralytic) manifestations, approximately 50% died.[164] With the advent of hematin therapy and of modern intensive care for complications such as respiratory failure, mortality has been sharply reduced. The peak incidence of acute attacks is during the third and fourth decades of life,[168] which suggests that the frequency of recurring attacks may diminish with advancing age. In patients in whom exposure to barbiturates or other drugs has been a precipitating factor and this has been eliminated, subsequent attacks are unusual. Neurologic deficits may require months or several years to clear, but complete recovery is observed in a substantial proportion of cases.[140] Although mental abnormalities are a component of acute attacks, these are neither persistent nor progressive. Studies of VP have suggested that longevity and reproduction are unaffected by the carrier state.[37]

δ-AMINOLEVULINIC ACIDURIA

On theoretic grounds, a deficiency of PBG synthase, the second enzyme of the heme pathway, would be expected to lead to heme deficiency, overproduction of ALA, and a clinical syndrome similar to that of a heme-deficient porphyria, as described above. However, the fact that this enzyme is present normally in large excess, relative to ALA synthetase or UROgen-I synthase, suggests that only a profound deficiency would be associated with porphyria. In line with this reasoning, partial deficiencies of PBG synthase have been documented and appear not to produce symptoms.[9] Two patients with severe deficiency (<3% of normal activity) and porphyric symptoms have been reported.[42] They appear to produce immunologically reactive but enzymatically inactive protein and probably represent rare homozygous cases of a defect that is clinically silent in the heterozygous state. The urine contains increased amounts of ALA and coproporphyrin. The basis for the latter finding is unclear, unless it represents low-level exposure to lead. It has been suggested that partial deficiencies of this enzyme may confer an unusual sensitivity to lead intoxication.[48]

PORPHYRIA CUTANEA TARDA

Clinical Presentation

PCT probably is the porphyria most commonly encountered in clinical practice. It is characterized by mechanical fragility and blistering of light-exposed skin, is not associated with acute, drug-related attacks and, as such, is readily distinguishable from the group with neurologic manifestations (see Table 31-4). The onset of manifestations is almost always insidious, and only a minority of patients associate cutaneous problems with exposure to sunlight. Over a period of months or years, patients note that the skin on the arms, backs of hands, face or feet is unusually susceptible to injury. Seemingly trivial physical trauma at these sites leads to vesicles of varying size and then to an open sore that heals poorly with eventual scar

formation. Sclerodermoid changes may be present, and some of these patients have coexisting lupus erythematosus.[32] Without treatment, the problem often is progressive, becoming mutilating and disabling for manual workers. Infectious complications including septic arthritis have been reported.[148] Biopsy of the skin reveals an accumulation of periodic acid-Schiff (PAS)–positive material (IgG) at the dermal–epidermal junction.[30] About 15% of patients have diabetes mellitus.[77]

A history of chronic liver disease and/or substantial intake of ethanol is obtained frequently, and liver disease is clinically or biochemically evident in 70% to 90% of patients.[77] The pathologic changes seen in liver biopsies from patients with PCT are nonspecific, but almost all biopsy specimens exhibit an increase in stainable iron.[8,80,167] Freshly obtained tissue is fluorescent under ultraviolet light because of its high URO content.[149]

Porphyrin studies of urine from patients with PCT reveal a pathognomonic pattern of heme precursors. URO levels are strikingly elevated (greater than tenfold increased), whereas ALA excretion and PBG excretion are within the normal range unless there is massive overproduction of URO. Urinary COPRO levels also are increased but to a much lesser extent than URO; fecal COPRO excretion and PROTO excretion are normal (see Fig. 31-4). The urinary URO is largely type I isomer, rather than type III, the physiologic heme precursor (see Fig. 31-2). The COPRO fraction from urine contains both type III and type I isomers as well as isocoproporphyrins.[53] Serum iron is increased but usually without complete saturation of the iron-binding capacity.[103]

Pathogenesis

In PCT, hepatic iron virtually always is increased, and the disease responds uniformly to phlebotomy, which presumably brings about mobilization of the excess iron in the liver. Also, many cases are associated with ingestion of alcohol or estrogens, and discontinuation of this exposure may result in a remission of the disease. On this basis—and because familial occurrence is rare—it formerly was believed that PCT was an acquired type of porphyria, in which iron, alcohol, certain drugs, or other environmental factors exerted a direct inhibitory effect on heme synthesis. In humans[12,104,148] and in experimental animals, specific chemicals induce a porphyria that closely mimics PCT. However, there is strong evidence to implicate genetic factors in the pathogenesis of PCT. Among patient populations with hepatic iron overload (e.g., hemochromatosis) or with alcohol-related liver disease, PCT is unusual. Also, there is no direct correlation between the severity of hepatic siderosis or the extent of chronic liver disease and manifestations of PCT. Finally, studies of the heme synthetic pathway in PCT have revealed an apparently fixed deficiency of URO decarboxylase, the enzyme catalyzing the conversion of UROgen to COPROgen (see Figs 31-2 and 31-4). This deficiency has been noted in both hepatic tissue and erythrocytes of some patients with PCT, the latter providing a convenient approach to family studies, which have demonstrated that PCT is an inherited (probably autosomal dominant) disorder.[63,90] In other patients, enzyme deficiency has been detected in liver but not in erythrocytes.[39,55] It is unclear at present whether the latter cases (termed "sporadic" PCT) represent variable tissue expression of a single genetic defect, a different genetic disease, or an acquired deficiency.

On the basis of the available data, it may be inferred that decreased hepatic UROgen decarboxylase activity is present in all patients with PCT. A partial block in the conversion of UROgen to COPROgen accounts for the characteristic preponderance of URO in the urine of these patients. However, it fails to explain the overproduction of isomer type I porphyrins (Fig. 31-5) and the clinical response to phlebotomy and/or withdrawal of precipitating environmental factors. Overproduction of type I isomers points to a possible defect at the level of UROgen-III cosynthetase (see Fig. 31-2), and studies of this enzyme *in vitro* have suggested that it is sensitive to iron[89] and possibly to URO itself[52]; this may explain the apparently additive effect of the genetic lesion and hepatic iron in the clinical expression of PCT (Fig. 31-5).

New insight into the possible pathogenesis of this type of porphyria has emerged from studies linking it to hemochromatosis. For several parameters of iron metabolism, values in persons with symptomatic PCT fall in the same range as those in persons heterozygous for hemochromatosis.[103] Transferrin saturation is elevated, with a mean value of 60%, and body iron stores are 2 g to 4 g, which are moderately increased but well below the levels associated with clinically significant (homozygous) hemochromatosis.[51] In PCT, serum ferritin, in the absence of significant hepatocellular disease, is at the upper limits of normal or moderately elevated and declines progressively with iron-depletion therapy, as in hemochromatosis.[87,157] Finally, recent HLA typing of patients with PCT is consistent with their being heterozygous for hemochromatosis.[86,87] The latter analysis has been conducted with few persons and only one family,[87] and a chance codistribution of PCT and the hemochromatosis allele (which is common in the general population) cannot be excluded.[56] Nonetheless, the hypothesis that clinical expression of PCT requires a defect both in URO decarboxylase and in iron metabolism provides an attractive explanation for the hepatocellular siderosis commonly associated with symptomatic PCT and for the finding that carriers of the URO decarboxylase defect frequently show no overt signs of PCT.

In contrast to AIP, HCP, and VP, drug sensitivity in PCT is limited to a chronic effect of those compounds mentioned above. Acute reactions to inducers of hepatic heme synthesis—notably to barbiturates—do not occur. This suggests that in PCT significant impairment of heme synthesis does not exist, which may account for the lack of neurologic manifestations in this disease.

Differential Diagnosis

In VP, the cutaneous findings are indistinguishable from those of PCT and may occur as a chronic syndrome in the absence of acute neurologic attacks.[119] The two diseases are differentiated on the basis of fecal porphyrin analysis (see Fig. 31-4).

A mild form of congenital erythropoietic porphyria, in which symptoms resembling severe PCT occur in adulthood, has been reported.[43] In contrast to PCT, erythrocyte uroporphyrin levels are markedly elevated.

A rare cutaneous porphyria, with increased erythrocyte protoporphyrin and PCT-like skin lesions, was described in 1975 and termed "hepatoerythropoietic porphyria." Patients exhibit a profound deficiency of URO decarboxylase, consistent with homozygous PCT.[41,58]

Hepatic tumors may develop in the setting of alcoholic liver disease, and rarely these contain high concentrations of porphyrin. Porphyrins released by the tumor appear to be responsible for cutaneous manifestations.[77,162] PCT has been reported also in association with lymphoma.[91] Patients with porphyrin-producing hepatic tumors are generally over 60 years of age, and the pattern of urinary porphyrins is atypical for PCT.[76] The question of whether patients with PCT should be screened for hepatic tumors has been raised. In the case of relatively young patients with typical urinary porphyrin findings, such screening would appear to be unnecessary.

Patients with chronic renal failure who are on dialysis may develop a cutaneous syndrome identical to PCT,[67]

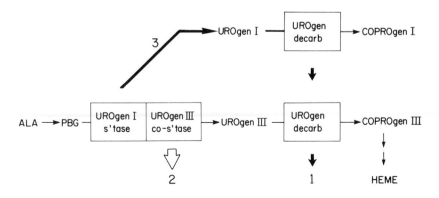

Fig. 31-5. Enzymatic alterations in PCT. The black arrow (*1*) indicates the site of the primary enzyme defect and the open arrow (*2*), the apparent secondary decrease in URO-III cosynthetase, which gives rise to increased formation of isomer type I uroporphyrin (*3*).

the basis for which is obscure. Only a minority exhibit increased plasma porphyrins[134] despite the fact that porphyrins are not readily dialyzed. Plasmapheresis may be helpful as therapy.[46] Phlebotomy usually is contraindicated because of anemia.

Management

Alcohol, estrogen, administered iron and, on occasion, occupational exposure underlie manifestations of PCT in many patients, and these should be eliminated. Phlebotomy is carried out at the rate of 500 ml to 1000 ml once or twice monthly, with monitoring of the patient's hemoglobin level. Chloroquine causes depletion of hepatic URO, apparently by forming a water-soluble complex with the porphyrin that is excreted in urine,[151] but serious hepatotoxic reactions are associated with its use in the commonly employed therapeutic dosage. While these appear to be mitigated with lower doses of chloroquine[3,158] or with concomitant phlebotomy,[156] the drug should be reserved for patients suffering disabling manifestations and unable to tolerate phlebotomy. Plasmapheresis may be an alternative in such patients.[77] In patients with both PCT and lupus erythematosus, withdrawal of aggravating exogenous factors is the only indicated therapy.[32] Topical sunscreens and β-carotene are of no proven value for symptomatic relief of cutaneous manifestations.[111]

Urinary excretion of URO is useful for following the disease. As a rule, cutaneous manifestations are present when excretion exceeds 800 μg/24 hours. The response to therapy is variable, sometimes requiring a year or more of serial phlebotomy.[60,77] When URO excretion has significantly decreased from pretreatment levels, the course of phlebotomies may be interrupted with the expectation of continued improvement, although hypertrichosis and hyperpigmentation may respond much more slowly than cutaneous fragility.[80] Complete remissions with normal URO excretion are achieved in some patients and may be long-lasting in the absence of the original aggravating factors.[60,77,80,137]

Screening of families with PCT requires assay of UROgen decarboxylase, since urine URO levels are elevated in only a minority of family members with decreased erythrocyte UROgen decarboxylase activity.[90] The assay is a research procedure at present.[39,56,90] Familial occurrence of sporadic PCT (with normal levels of erythrocyte URO decarboxylase) has been reported.[57] but may be uncommon and probably does not justify screening of family members for the disease. If the postulated association of clinical PCT and the hemochromatosis gene is confirmed, iron studies and HLA typing of family members may be warranted for the early detection of homozygous hemochromatosis[51] and for genetic counseling.

PROTOPORPHYRIA

PP is a cutaneous condition that is relatively common, although prevalence figures for the carrier state are not available. It appears to be inherited in autosomal dominant fashion; many carriers are asymptomatic.[141] Synonyms for the disease are *erythropoietic* or *erythrohepatic* protoporphyria.

Clinical Presentation

Although both PCT and PP are characterized largely (or solely) by cutaneous manifestations (see Table 31-4), the two diseases are readily separable on clinical grounds. Whereas in PCT manifestations are insidious in onset, in PP the cutaneous reaction to light is immediate, occurring during or just following exposure. It consists of a burning or tingling sensation that is followed shortly by edematous swelling (solar urticaria).[105] Repeated reactions may be well tolerated or may lead to cutaneous thickening and fibrosis (solar eczema).[138] The fragility, blistering, and hirsutism typical of PCT are rare in PP, and acute neurologic manifestations, as in AIP, HCP, and VP, are absent. In patients with marked elevation of erythrocyte or plasma PROTO levels, hepatic disease may appear.[47] Although unusual, this complication is serious, involving early hepatic decompensation and death. PROTO-containing gallstones occur in approximately 10% of patients with PP.

The laboratory diagnosis of PP depends on demonstration of elevated PROTO in erythrocytes, plasma, and feces.[141] Erythrocyte and fecal COPRO levels may be moderately elevated also, but those of other heme precursors are not. Microscopically, erythrocytes under blue light exhibit red fluorescence (this is fleeting, owing to degradation of the light-exposed porphyrin). Biopsy of involved skin reveals deposition of PAS-positive material in and around dermal capillaries.[145] In patients with liver disease, hepatic biopsy yields tissue that is grossly dark or black and exhibits intense red fluorescence.[13] PROTO is found in sinusoidal cells, in bile canaliculi, and occasionally in parenchymal cells and may be present as crystalline inclusions that are birefringent under polarized light.[13,26] Inflammatory exudate, cell necrosis, and findings characteristic of cholestasis, including periportal fibrosis and bile ductular proliferation, may be present. Abnormalities of liver function often do not appear until the hepatic disease is far advanced, suggesting that unsuspected histologic alterations may be present in many patients with PP.[33]

Pathogenesis

The characteristic overproduction of PROTO in this disease suggests a defect at the level of conversion of PROTOgen to heme, and ferrochelatase activity has been found to be deficient both in marrow cells[20] and in cultured skin fibroblasts[17] from patients with PP. While this genetic defect explains satisfactorily the laboratory features, controversy exists as to the tissue sites of PROTO overproduction in individual patients. In some carefully studied cases, the plasma concentration and fecal output of PROTO were matched by the rate of porphyrin loss from erythrocytes, suggesting that erythroid cells are the sole source of PROTO overproduction.[133] In other cases, fecal PROTO clearly was in excess of that derived from circulating erythrocytes, and tracer studies suggested a hepatic origin of at least part of the excess PROTO.[150] The current view is that these differences in the site of protoporphyrin production define two distinct groups of patients: those in whom protoporphyrin is derived from the erythron (with a negligible hepatic component) and those with significant hepatic production.[96] It remains to be determined whether the risk of cholestatic liver disease differs for the two groups. Interestingly, patients with PP either are not anemic or exhibit only a slight hypochromic anemia,[38] suggesting that PROTO in this disease is produced in excess of that required for hemoglobin formation.

The pathogenesis of liver disease associated with PP is uncertain; the early clinical abnormalities are cholestatic in type. While substantial deposition of PROTO in the liver may be common in PP,[33] progressive or fatal hepatic decompensation is rare. It would be of interest to determine whether, in those patients with liver disease, a large component of PROTO overproduction is hepatic in origin. Factors other than PROTO deposition in the liver also may play a role.

Cutaneous manifestations are proportional to the concentration of PROTO in plasma and, therefore, in skin. The sensitivity to light appears to be mediated by the porphyrin, since the peak wavelength for light-induced injury corresponds to the absorption maximum of PROTO (about 400 nm).[105] In PP, PROTO undergoes diffusion out of erythrocytes, and this appears to account in large part for the high concentration of PROTO in plasma.[133] By contrast, in disorders such as lead intoxication or iron deficiency in which excess erythrocyte PROTO occurs, the porphyrin is bound within the red blood cell as a zinc complex; consequently, plasma PROTO concentrations are normal and photosensitivity is absent.[93]

Management

Assay of ferrochelatase activity provides a means of screening for potential carriers, although this requires nucleated cells (*e.g.,* skin fibroblast cultures). Erythrocyte and fecal PROTO levels are inconstantly elevated, although increased numbers of fluorescent red blood cells may be present in most carriers.[139,176] Cutaneous manifestations are prevented or minimized with oral β-carotene,[111] presumably because this compound quenches singlet oxygen, which may be the mediator of skin damage[154] induced by light and porphyrin. The only side-effect of this therapy is a dose-related yellow discoloration of the skin (carotenodermia). Because hepatic complications of PP can develop insidiously, all patients should undergo tests of liver function, and sulfobromophthalein retention may be the most sensitive for this purpose.[13] In those with abnormal test results, liver biopsy may be required to evaluate the nature and extent of hepatic damage.

Therapy for the liver disease of PP is based on anecdotal information. Oral administration of cholestyramine[34,85] or activated charcoal[65] may be helpful in binding PROTO in the intestinal lumen and preventing its enterohepatic recirculation. Hematin caused a reduction in plasma and/or fecal PROTO in three reported cases[96]; however, its overall efficacy in the treatment of PP is uncertain, and chronic administration is impractical because of the need for an intravenous route of administration. Red cell transfusion, by reducing erythropoiesis, theoretically should suppress production of PROTO by the bone marrow; it appeared to be useful in one reported case.[28] Successful treatment with carbonyl iron also has been reported.[71]

TOXIC PORPHYRIA

Toxic porphyria occurred on a large scale in Turkey in 1959, when several thousand persons ingested seed grain that had been treated with the fungicide hexachlorobenzene.[148] It has resulted also from accidental or industrial exposure to hepatotoxins.[12,104] The manifestations are clinically and biochemically indistinguishable from those of PCT, suggesting that the toxic chemical directly attacks UROgen decarboxylase and/or UROgen-III cosynthetase. Management involves elimination of the toxic insult and attention to possible associated hepatic injury.

SUMMARY

The hepatic porphyrias comprise a group of five genetically determined diseases, together with acquired ("toxic") porphyria. These must be distinguished from asymptomatic, or incidental *porphyrinuria,* which accompanies a variety of disturbances of liver function.

AIP, HCP, and VP, while caused by discrete genetic defects in specific enzymes of the heme synthetic pathway, have in common acute attacks. In such attacks, neurologic manifestations are prominent and often are related to the ingestion of barbiturates or other drugs that induce hepatic heme synthesis. During attacks, excretion of ALA and PBG is elevated, and acute manifestations respond to intravenously administered hematin.

PCT is a cutaneous disease in which urinary URO— and, to a lesser extent, COPRO—are elevated. Many patients exhibit biochemical or clinical signs of chronic liver disease. A deficiency of UROgen decarboxylase probably is present in all cases, and environmental factors (iron, ethanol, estrogen) appear to be required for clinical expression of the disease. Manifestations respond to serial phlebotomy, which presumably acts by mobilizing excess hepatic iron.

PP is a cutaneous disorder characterized biochemically by excess PROTO in erythrocytes, plasma, and feces. PROTO deposition in the liver occurs and, rarely, leads to fatal liver disease; PROTO-containing gallstones are relatively frequent. Cutaneous manifestations are prevented by administration of β-carotene.

Toxic porphyria results from exposure to chemicals that appear to directly inhibit enzymes of heme synthesis. The clinical manifestations are indistinguishable from those of PCT.

REFERENCES

1. Anderson KE et al: Studies in porphyria: VIII. Relationship of the steroid hormones to clinical expression of the genetic defect in acute intermittent porphyria. Am J Med 66:644, 1979
2. Anderson PM, Reddy RM, Anderson KE et al: Characterization of the porphobilinogen deaminase deficiency in acute intermittent porphyria: Immunologic evidence for heterogeneity of the genetic defect. J Clin Invest 68:1, 1981
3. Ashton RE, Hawk JLM, Magnus IA: Low-dose oral chloroquine in the treatment of porphyria cutanea tarda. Br J Dermatol 3:609, 1984
4. Astrup EG: Family studies on the activity of uroporphyrinogen I synthase in diagnosis of acute intermittent porphyria. Clin Sci Mol Med 54:251, 1978
5. Battersby AR, Fookes CJR, Matcham GWJ et al: Biosynthesis of the pigments of life: Formation of the macrocycle. Nature 285:17, 1980
6. Beattie AD et al: Acute intermittent porphyria: Response of tachycardia and hypertension to propranolol. Br Med J 3:257, 1973
7. Becker DM et al: Reduced ferrochelatase activity: A defect common to porphyria variegata and protoporphyria. Br J Haematol 36:171, 1977
8. Biempica L et al: Hepatic porphyrias: Cytochemical and ultrastructural studies of liver in acute intermittent porphyria and porphyria cutanea tarda. Arch Pathol 98:336, 1974
9. Bird TD, Hamernyik P, Nutter JY et al: Inherited deficiency of delta-aminolevulinic acid dehydratase. Am J Hum Genet 31:662, 1979
10. Bissell DM: Heme metabolism and the porphyrias. In Wright R et al (eds): Liver and Biliary Disease, p 387. Philadelphia, WB Saunders, 1985
11. Bissell DM, Hammaker LE: Cytochrome P-450 heme and the regulation of δ-aminolevulinic acid synthetase in the liver. Arch Biochem Biophys 176:103, 1976
12. Bleiberg J et al: Industrially acquired porphyria. Arch Dermatol 89:793, 1974
13. Bloomer JR et al: Hepatic disease in erythropoietic protoporphyria. Am J Med 58:869, 1975
14. Bonkowsky HL, Tschudy P: Hazard of propranolol in treatment of acute porphyria. Br Med J 4:47, 1974
15. Bonkowsky HL et al: Repression of the overproduction of porphyrin precursors in acute intermittent porphyria by intravenous infusions of hematin. Proc Natl Acad Sci USA 68:2725, 1971
16. Bonkowsky HL et al: The glucose effect in rat liver: Studies of δ-aminolevulinate synthase and tyrosine amino-transferase. Biochim Biophys Acta 320:561, 1973
17. Bonkowsky HL et al: Heme synthetase deficiency in human protoporphyria: Demonstration of the defect in liver and cultured skin fibroblasts. J Clin Invest 56:1139, 1975
18. Bonkowsky HL et al: Seizure management in acute hepatic porphyria: Risks of valproate and clonazepam. Neurology 30:588, 1980
19. Bornstein JC, Pickett JB, Diamond I: Inhibition of the evoked release of acetylcholine by the porphyrin precursor δ-aminolevulinic acid. Neurology 5:94, 1979
20. Bottomley S et al: Diminished erythroid ferrochelatase activity in protoporphyria. J Lab Clin Med 86:126, 1975
21. Brennan MJW, Cantwill RC: δ-Aminolevulinic acid is a potent agonist for GABA autoreceptors. Nature 280:514, 1979
22. Brenner DA, Bloomer JR: The enzymatic defect in variegate porphyria: Studies with human cultured skin fibroblasts. N Engl J Med 302:765, 1980
23. Brivet F et al: Porphyria cutanea tarda-like syndrome in hemodialyzed patients. Nephron 20:258, 1978
24. Brodie MJ et al: Pregnancy and the acute porphyrias. Br J Obstet Gynaecol 84:726, 1977
25. Brodie MJ et al: Hereditary coproporphyria. Q J Med 46:229, 1977
26. Bruguera M et al: Erythropoietic protoporphyria: A light, electron, and polarization microscopical study of the liver in three patients. Arch Pathol Lab Med 100:587, 1976
27. Burnett JW, Pathak MA: Pathogenesis of cutaneous photosensitivity in porphyria. N Engl J Med 268:1203, 1963
28. Conley CL, Chisolm JJ: Recovery from hepatic decompensation in protoporphyria. Johns Hopkins Med J 145:237, 1979
29. Corcoran AC, Page IH: Renal damage from ferroheme pigments myoglobin, hemoglobin, hematin. Tex Rep Biol Med 3:528, 1945
30. Cormane RH et al: Histopathology of the skin in acquired and hereditary porphyria cutanea tarda. Br J Dermatol 85:531, 1971
31. Correia MA et al: Incorporation of exogenous heme into hepatic cytochrome P-450 in vivo. J Biol Chem 254:15, 1979
32. Cram D et al: Lupus erythematosus and porphyria: Coexistence in seven patients. Arch Dermatol 108:779, 1973
33. Cripps DJ, Goldfarb SS: Erythropoietic protoporphyria: Hepatic cirrhosis. Br J Dermatol 98:349, 1978
34. Davidson DL et al: Therapy of hepatic disease in erythropoietic protoporphyria. Gastroenterology 65:535, 1973
35. Davis R, Andelman L: Urinary delta-aminolevulinic (ALA) levels in lead poisoning: I. A modified method for the rapid determination of urinary delta-aminolevulinic acid using disposable ion-exchange chromatography columns. Arch Environ Health 15:53, 1967
36. Dean G: A report on propanidid, an intravenous anaesthetic in porphyria variegata. S Afr Med J 43:227, 1969
37. Dean G: The Porphyrias: A Story of Heredity and Environment, 2nd ed. London, Sir Isaac Pitman & Sons, 1971
38. de Leo VA et al: Erythropoietic protoporphyria: Ten years experience. Am J Med 60:8, 1976
39. de Verneuil H et al: Familial and sporadic porphyria cutanea: Two different diseases. Hum Genet 44:145, 1978
40. de Verneuil H et al: Purification and properties of uroporphyrinogen decarboxylase from human erythrocytes. J Biol Chem 258:2454, 1983
41. de Verneuil H et al: Enzymatic and immunological studies of uroporphyrinogen decarboxylase in familial porphyria cutanea tarda and hepatoerythropoietic porphyria. Am J Hum Genet 36:613, 1984
42. de Verneuil H et al: Hereditary hepatic porphyria with delta aminolevulinate dehydrase deficiency: Immunologic characterization of the non-catalytic enzyme. Hum Genet 69:174, 1985
43. Deybach JC, de Verneuil H, Phung N et al: Congenital erythropoietic porphyria (Gunther's disease): Enzymatic

studies on two cases of late onset. J Lab Clin Med 97:551, 1981

44. Dhar GJ et al: Effects of hematin in hepatic porphyria. Ann Intern Med 83:20, 1975

45. Dhar GJ et al: Transitory renal failure following rapid administration of a relatively large amount of hematin in a patient with acute intermittent porphyria in clinical remission. Acta Med Scand 203:437, 1978

46. Disler P, Day R, Burman N et al: Treatment of hemodialysis-related porphyria cutanea tarda with plasma exchange. Am J Med 72:989, 1982

47. Donaldson EM et al: Erythropoietic protoporphyria: Two deaths from hepatic cirrhosis. Br J Dermatol 84:14, 1971

48. Doss M, Becker U, Sixel F et al: Persistent portoporphyrinemia in hereditary porphobilinogen synthase (δ-aminolevulinic acid dehydrase) deficiency under low lead exposure. Klin Wochenschr 60:599, 1982

49. Eales L: Acute porphyria: The precipitating and aggravating factors. S Afr J Lab Clin Med 17:120, 1971

50. Eales M: Porphyria as seen in Cape Town: A survey of 250 patients and some recent studies. S Afr J Lab Clin Med 9: 151, 1963

51. Edwards CQ, Skolnick MH, Kushner JP: Hereditary hemochromatosis: Contributions of genetic analyses. Prog Hematol 14:227, 1981

52. Elder GH: Porphyria cutanea tarda and HLA-linked hemochromatosis. Gastroenterology 88:1276, 1985

53. Elder GH: Porphyrin metabolism in porphyria cutanea tarda. Semin Hematol 14:227, 1977

54. Elder GH et al: Faecal "X porphyrin" in the hepatic porphyrias. Enzyme 17:29, 1974

55. Elder GH et al: The primary enzyme defect in hereditary coproporphyria. Lancet 2:1217, 1976

56. Elder GH et al: Decreased activity of hepatic uroporphyrinogen decarboxylase in sporadic porphyria cutanea tarda. N Engl J Med 299:274, 1978

57. Elder GH et al: Identification of two types of porphyria cutanea tarda by measurement of erythrocyte uroporphyrinogen decarboxylase. Clin Sci 58:477, 1980

58. Elder GH et al: Hepatoerythropoietic porphyria: A new uroporphyrinogen decarboxylase defect of homozygous porphyria cutanea tarda? Lancet 2:916, 1981

59. Elder GH et al: Purification of uroporphyrinogen decarboxylase from human erythrocytes. Biochem J 215:45, 1983

60. Epstein JH, Redeker AG: Porphyria cutanea tarda: A study of the effect of phlebotomy. N Engl J Med 279:1301, 1968

61. Feldman RG et al: Lead neuropathy in adults and in children. Arch Neurol 34:481, 1977

62. Felsher BF, Redeker AG: Acute intermittent porphyria: Effect of diet and griseofulvin. Medicine 46:217, 1967

63. Felsher BF et al: Red-cell uroporphyrinogen decarboxylase activity in porphyria cutanea tarda and in other forms of porphyria. N Engl J Med 299:1095, 1978

64. Fischer H et al: Zur Kenntnis der natuerlichen Porphyrine: Chemische Befunde bei einem Fall von Porphyrinurie (Petry). Z Physiol Chem 150:44, 1925

65. Ghandi SN, Pimstone NR: Charcoal is superior to cholestyramine in blocking enterohepatic circulation of porphyrins: A major therapeutic tool in porphyria. Gastroenterology 84:1372, 1983

66. Gidari AS, Levere RD: Enzymatic formation and cellular regulation of heme synthesis. Semin Hematol 14:145, 1977

67. Gilchrest B et al: Bullous dermatosis of hemodialysis. Ann Intern Med 83:480, 1975

68. Glueck R, Green D, Cohen I et al: Hematin: Unique effects on hemostasis. Blood 61:243, 1983

69. Goetsch CA, Bissell DM: Instability of hematin used in the treatment of acute hepatic porphyria. N Engl J Med 315: 235, 1986

70. Goldberg A et al: Hereditary coproporphyria. Lancet 1: 632, 1967

71. Gordenk VR et al: Iron therapy for hepatic dysfunction in erythropoietic protoporphyria. Ann Intern Med 105:27, 1986

72. Grandchamp B et al: Homozygous case of hereditary coproporphyria. Lancet 2:1348, 1977

73. Grandchamp B et al: Molecular cloning of a cDNA sequence complementary to porphobilinogen deaminase mRNA from rat. Proc Natl Acad Sci USA 81:5036, 1984

74. Granick S, Beale SI: Hemes, chlorophylls, and related compounds: Biosynthesis and metabolic regulation. Adv Enzymol 46:33, 1978

75. Green D, Reynolds N, Klein J et al: The inactivation of hemostatic factors by hematin. J Lab Clin Med 102:361, 1983

76. Grossman ME, Bickers DR: Porphyria cutanea tarda: A rare cutaneous manifestation of hepatic tumours. Cutis 21: 782, 1978

77. Grossman ME et al: Porphyria cutanea tarda: Clinical features and laboratory findings in 40 patients. Am J Med 67: 277, 1979

78. Guidotti TL, Charness ME, Lamon JM: Acute intermittent porphyria and the Kluver-Bucy syndrome. Johns Hopkins Med J 145:233, 1979

79. Günther H: Die Haematoporphyrie. Dtsch Arch Klin Med 105:89, 1911

80. Haberman HF et al: Porphyria cutanea tarda: Comparison of cases precipitated by alcohol and estrogens. Can Med Assoc J 113:653, 1975

81. Hollander CS et al: Increased protein-bound iodine and thyroxine-binding globulin in acute intermittent porphyria. N Engl J Med 277:995, 1967

82. Jessen KR, Mirsky R, Dennison ME et al: GABA may be a neurotransmitter in the vertebrate peripheral nervous system. Nature 281:71, 1979

83. Kappas A et al: Abnormal steroid hormone metabolism in the genetic liver disease acute intermittent porphyria. Ann NY Acad Sci 179:611, 1971

84. Kawanishi S, Seki Y, Sano S: Uroporphyrinogen decarboxylase. J Biol Chem 258:4285, 1983

85. Kniffen JC: Porphyrin removal in intrahepatic porphyrastasis. Gastroenterology 58:1027, 1970

86. Kuntz BME, Goerz G, Merk H et al: HLA-A3 and -B7 in porphyria cutanea tarda. Tissue Antigens 24:67, 1984

87. Kushner JP, Edwards CQ, Dadone MM et al: Heterozygosity for HLA-linked hemochromatosis as a likely cause of the hepatic siderosis associated with sporadic porphyria cutanea tarda. Gastroenterology 88:1232, 1985

88. Kushner JP et al: Idiopathic refractory sideroblastic anemia: Clinical and laboratory investigation of 17 patients and review of the literature. Medicine 50:139, 1971

89. Kushner JP et al: The role of iron in the pathogenesis of porphyria cutanea tarda, an in vitro model. J Clin Invest 51:3044, 1972

90. Kushner JP et al: An inherited enzymatic defect in porphyria cutanea tarda: Decreased uroporphyrinogen decarboxylase activity. J Clin Invest 58:1089, 1976

91. Lai CL, Wu PC, Lin HJ et al: Case report of symptomatic

porphyria cutanea tarda associated with histocytic lymphoma. Cancer 53:573, 1984

92. Laiwah ACY, Junor B, Macphee GJA et al: Charcoal haemoperfusion and haemodialysis in acute intermittent porphyria. Br Med 287:1746, 1983

93. Lamola AA et al: Erythropoietic protoporphyria and lead intoxication: The molecular basis for difference in cutaneous photosensitivity: II. Different binding of erythrocyte protoporphyrin to hemoglobin. J Clin Invest 56:1528, 1975

94. Lamon JM et al: Family evaluations in acute intermittent porphyria using red cell uroporphyrinogen I synthetase. J Med Genet 16:134, 1979

95. Lamon JM et al: Hematin therapy for acute porphyria. Medicine 58:252, 1979

96. Lamon JM et al: Hepatic protoporphyrin production in human protoporphyria. Gastroenterology 79:115, 1980

97. Larson AW et al: Posttraumatic epilepsy and acute intermittent porphyria: Effects of phenytoin, carbamazepine, and clonazepam. Neurology 28:824, 1978

98. Lim HW, Perez HD, Poh-Fitzpatrick M et al: Generation of chemotactic activity in serum from patients with erythropoietic protoporphyria and porphyria cutanea tarda. N Engl J Med 304:212, 1981

99. Lindblad B et al: On the enzymic defects in hereditary tyrosinemia. Proc Natl Acad Sci USA 74:4641, 1977

100. Litman DA, Correia MA: Tryptophan: A common denominator of biochemical and neurological events of acute porphyria? Science 22:1031, 1983

101. Litman DA, Correia MA: Elevated brain tryptophan and enhanced 5-hydroxytryptamine turnover in acute hepatic heme deficiency: Clinical implications. J Pharmacol Exp Ther 232:337, 1984

102. Ludwig GD, Epstein IS: A genetic study of two families having the acute intermittent type of porphyria. Ann Intern Med 55:81, 1961

103. Lundvall O et al: Iron storage in porphyria cutanea tarda. Acta Med Scand 188:37, 1970

104. Lynch RE et al: Porphyria cutanea tarda associated with disinfectant misuse. Arch Intern Med 135:549, 1975

105. Magnus IA et al: Erythropoietic protoporphyria: A new porphyrin syndrome with solar urticaria due to protoporphyrinaemia. Lancet 2:448, 1961

106. Magnussen C et al: A red cell enzyme method for the diagnosis of acute intermittent porphyria. Blood 44:857, 1974

107. Magnussen C et al: Grand mal seizures and acute intermittent porphyria: The problem of differential diagnosis and treatment. Neurology 25:1121, 1975

108. Marver HS: The role of heme in the synthesis and repression of microsomal protein. In Gillette JR et al (eds): Microsomes and Drug Oxidations, p 495. New York, Academic Press, 1969

109. Marver HS et al: δ-Aminolevulinic acid synthetase: II. Induction in rat liver. J Biol Chem 241:4323, 1966

110. Marver HS et al: Heme and methemoglobin: Naturally occurring repressors of microsomal protein. Biochem Biophys Res Commun 33:969, 1968

111. Mathews–Roth MM et al: Beta carotene therapy for erythropoietic protoporphyria and other photosensitivity diseases. Arch Dermatol 113:1229, 1977

112. Mauzerall D: Chlorophyll and photosynthesis. Philos Trans R Soc Lond (Biol) 273:287, 1976

113. McColl KEL, Moore MR, Thompson GG et al: Treatment with haematin in acute hepatic porphyria. Q J Med 198:161, 1981

114. Meyer UA: Intermittent acute porphyria: Clinical and biochemical studies of disordered heme biosynthesis. Enzyme 16:334, 1973

115. Meyer UA, Schmid R: The Porphyrias. In Stanbury JB et al (eds): The Metabolic Basis of Inherited Disease, 4th ed, pp 1166–1220. New York, McGraw-Hill, 1978

116. Meyer UA et al: Intermittent acute porphyria: Demonstration of a genetic defect in porphobilinogen metabolism. N Engl J Med 286:1277, 1972

117. Morris DL, Dudley MD, Pearson RD: Coagulopathy associated with hematin treatment for acute intermittent porphyria. Ann Intern Med 95:700, 1981

118. Morton KA, Kushner JP, Burnham BF et al: Biosynthesis of porphyrins and heme from γ,δ-dioxovalerate by intact hepatocytes. Proc Natl Acad Sci USA 78:5325, 1981

119. Muhlbauer JE, Pathak MA, Tishler PV et al: Variegate porphyria in New England. JAMA 247:3095, 1982

120. Mukerji SK, Pimstone NR, Burns M: Dual mechanism of inhibition of rat liver uroporphyrinogen decarboxylase activity by ferrous iron: Its potential role in the genesis of porphyria cutanea tarda. Gastroenterology 87:1248, 1984

121. Muller–Eberhard U, Vincent SH: Concepts of heme distribution within hepatocytes. Biochem Pharmacol 34:719, 1985

122. Mustajoki P: Variegate porphyria. Ann Intern Med 89:238, 1978

123. Mustajoki P: Normal erythrocyte uroporphyrinogen: I. Synthetase in a kindred with acute intermittent porphyria. Ann Intern Med 95:162, 1981

124. Neely SM, Gardner DV, Reynolds N et al: Mechanism and characteristics of platelet activation by haematin. Br J Haematol 58:305, 1984

125. Nencki M, Sieber N: Ueber das Haematoporphyrin. Arch Exp Pathol Pharmakol 24:430, 1888

126. Neubauer O: Haematoporphyrin und Sulfonalvergiftung. Arch Exp Pathol Pharmakol 43:456, 1900

127. Ostrow JD et al: The formation of bilirubin from hemoglobin in vivo. J Clin Invest 41:1628, 1962

128. Paterniti JR, Simone JJ, Beattie DS: Detection and Regulation of δ-aminolevulinic acid synthetase activity in the rat brain. Arch Biochem Biophys 189:86, 1978

129. Percy VA, Shanley BC: Studies on heme biosynthesis in rat brain. J Neurochem 33:1267, 1979

130. Perlroth MG et al: Oral contraceptive agents and the management of acute intermittent porphyria. JAMA 194:1037, 1965

131. Peterson LR et al: Erythrocyte uroporphyrinogen I synthetase activity in diagnosis of acute intermittent porphyria. Clin Chem 22:1835, 1976

132. Pierach CA, Bossenmaier I, Cardinal R et al: Hematin, an anticoagulant. Hepatology 1:536, 1981

133. Piomelli S et al: Erythropoietic protoporphyria and lead intoxication: The molecular basis for difference in cutaneous photosensitivity: I. Different rates of disappearance of protoporphyrin from the erythrocytes, both in vivo and in vitro. J Clin Invest 56:1519, 1975

134. Poh–Fitzpatrick MB, Masullo AS, Grossman ME: Porphyria cutanea tarda associated with chronic renal disease and hemodialysis. Arch Dermatol 116:191, 1980

135. Racz WJ, Marks GS: Drug-induced porphyrin biosynthesis: IV. Investigation of the differences in response of isolated liver cells and the liver of the intact chick embryo to porphyria-inducing drugs. Biochem Pharmacol 21:143, 1972

136. Raffin B et al: Intestinal absorption of hemoglobin iron-

heme cleavage by mucosal heme oxygenase. J Clin Invest 54:1344, 1974

137. Ramsey CA et al: The treatment of porphyria cutanea tarda by venesection. Q J Med 43:1, 1974

138. Redeker AG, Berke M: Erythropoietic protoporphyria with eczema solare: Report of a case. Arch Dermatol 86:569, 1962

139. Reed WB et al: Erythropoietic protoporphyria: A clinical and genetic study. JAMA 214:1060, 1970

140. Ridley A: The neuropathy of acute intermittent porphyria. QJ Med 38:307, 1969

141. Rimington C et al: Porphyria and photosensitivity. Q J Med 36:29, 1967

142. Rimington C et al: The excretion of porphyrin–peptide conjugates in porphyria variegata. Clin Sci 35:211, 1968

143. Rizk SF et al: Ketamine as an induction agent for acute intermittent porphyria. Anesthesiology 46:305, 1977

144. Russell VA, Lamm MCL, Taljaard, JJF: Effects of δ-aminolaevulinic acid, porphobilinogen and structurally related amino acids on 2-deoxyglucose uptake in cultured neurons. Neurochem Res 7:1009, 1982

145. Ryan EA: Histochemistry of the skin in erythropoietic protoporphyria. Br J Dermatol 78:501, 1966

146. Sassa S et al: A microassay for uroporphyrinogen I synthase, one of three abnormal enzyme activities in acute intermittent porphyria, and its application to the study of the genetics of this disease. Proc Natl Acad Sci USA 71:732, 1974

147. Sassa S et al: Studies in porphyria: IV. Expression of the gene defect of acute intermittent porphyria in cultured human skin fibroblasts and amniotic cells: Prenatal diagnosis of the porphyria trait. J Exp Med 142:722, 1975

148. Schmid R: Cutaneous porphyria in Turkey. N Engl J Med 263:397, 1960

149. Schmid R et al: Porphyrin content of bone marrow and liver in the various forms of porphyria. Arch Intern Med 93:167, 1954

150. Scholnick P et al: Erythropoietic protoporphyria: Evidence for multiple sites of excess protoporphyrin formation. J Clin Invest 50:203, 1971

151. Scholnick P et al: The molecular basis of the action of chloroquine in porphyria cutanea tarda. Invest Dermatol 61:226, 1973

152. Schwartz S et al: Determination of porphyrins in biological materials. Methods Biochem Anal 8:221, 1960

153. Shemin D, Rittenberg D: The biological utilization of glycine for the synthesis of the protoporphyrin of hemoglobin. J Biol Chem 166:621, 1946

154. Spikes JD: Porphyrins and related compounds as photodynamic sensitizers. Ann NY Acad Sci 244:496, 1975

155. Stein JA, Tschudy DP: Acute intermittent porphyria: A clinical and biochemical study of 46 patients. Medicine 49:1, 1970

156. Swanbeck G, Wennersten G: Treatment of porphyria cutanea tarda with chloroquine and phlebotomy. Br J Dermatol 97:77, 1977

157. Sweeney GD, Jones KG: Porphyria cutanea tarda: Clinical and laboratory features. Can Med Assoc J 120:803, 1979

158. Taljaard JJF et al: Studies on low dose chloroquine therapy and the action of chloroquine in symptomatic porphyria. Br J Dermatol 87:261, 1972

159. Taylor RL: Magnesium sulfate for AIP seizures. Neurology 31:1371, 1981

160. Ten Eyck FW et al: Acute porphyria: Necropsy studies in nine cases. Proc Mayo Clin 36:409, 1961

161. Tenhunen R et al: The enzymatic catabolism of hemoglobin: Stimulation of microsomal heme oxygenase by hemin. J Lab Clin Med 75:410, 1970

162. Thompson RPH et al: Cutaneous porphyria due to a malignant primary hepatoma. Gastroenterology 59:779, 1970

163. Treece G et al: Exacerbation of porphyria during treatment of pulmonary tuberculosis. Am Rev Respir Dis 113:233, 1976

164. Tschudy DP: Porphyrin metabolism and the porphyrias. In Bondy P, Rosenberg L (eds): Duncan's Diseases of Metabolism, 7th ed, p 775. Philadelphia, WB Saunders, 1974

165. Tschudy DP, Bonkowsky L: Experimental porphyria. Fed Proc 31:147, 1972

166. Tschudy DP et al: Acute intermittent porphyria: Clinical and selected research aspects. Ann Intern Med 83:851, 1975

167. Turnbull A et al: Iron metabolism in porphyria cutanea tarda and in erythropoietic protoporphyria. Q J Med 42:341, 1973

168. Waldenström J: The porphyrias as inborn errors of metabolism. Am J Med 22:758, 1957

169. Waldenström J, Vahlquist B: Studien ueber die Entstehung der roten Harnpigmente (Uroporphyrin and Porphobilin) bei der akuten Porphyrie aus ihrer farblosen Vorstufe (Porphobilinogen). Z Physiol Chem 260:189, 1939

170. Watson CJ et al: Urinary porphobilinogen and other Ehrlich reactors in diagnosis. JAMA 175:1087, 1961

171. Watson CJ et al: Postulated deficiency of hepatic heme and repair by hematin infusions in the "inducible" hepatic porphyrias. Proc Natl Acad Sci USA 74:2118, 1977

172. Welland FH et al: Factors affecting the excretion of porphyrin precursors by patients with acute intermittent porphyria: I. The effect of diet. Metabolism 13:232, 1964

173. Wettenberg L: Report on an international survey of safe and unsafe drugs in acute intermittent porphyria. Supplement to the Proc. of the First International Porphyrin Meeting, "Porphyrias in Human Disease," Freiburg, p 191. Freiburg, Falk, 1975

174. Wettenberg L: Oral contraceptives and acute intermittent porphyria. Lancet 2:1178, 1964

175. With TK: Acute intermittent porphyria: Family studies on the excretion of porphobilinogen and δ-aminolevulinic acid with ion-exchange chromatography. Z Klin Chem Klin Biochem 1:134, 1963

176. Wuepper KD, Epstein JH: Erythrocyte fluorescence in relatives of patients with erythropoietic protoporphyria. JAMA 200:70, 1967

177. Zimmerman TS et al: Onset of manifestations of hepatic porphyria in relation to the influence of female sex hormones. Arch Intern Med 118:229, 1966

chapter 32

Amyloidosis of the Liver

ALAN S. COHEN and MARTHA SKINNER

BACKGROUND

In the early 19th century, Rokitansky and others observed a unique disorder causing a waxy, enlarged liver and, occasionally, similar changes in the spleen.[95] Virchow subsequently observed that the "lardaceous" liver and spleen stained with iodine and sulfuric acid and, because of his belief that it had a certain similarity to cellulose, named it amyloid.[25,27] This substance was studied for about 60 years at the autopsy table and in experimental animals until direct biopsy procedures (1928) and the Congo red test and stain were introduced in the 1920s.[10–12,135] In the subsequent 30 years, a wide variety of studies, both clinical and experimental, were carried out on what was then considered an extremely rare "degenerative" condition. It has become apparent, however, that amyloidosis is far more common than had been thought, that it very often is of great clinical significance, that it is associated with an extraordinarily wide variety of diseases, and, in the past several decades, that a number of genetically determined amyloidoses exist.[29]

Amyloidosis may be defined as the extracellular deposition of the fibrous protein amyloid in one or more sites of the body. A more modern definition would include the fact that this protein shows green birefringence on polarization microscopy after Congo red staining, 70-nm to 100-nm fibrils on electron microscopy, and a cross-beta pattern on x-ray diffraction analysis. The substance may be local and isolated with no clinical consequences, may grossly involve virtually any organ system of the body, leading to severe pathophysiologic changes, or may fall between these two extremes. The natural history is poorly understood, and the clinical diagnosis is often not made until the disease is far advanced.

Although early studies showed that amyloid was often an accompaniment of chronic suppuration, it became apparent over 100 years ago that amyloidosis could also occur without predisposing disease. This led to a variety of classifications of amyloidosis, starting with that of Lubarsch (typical, common, or secondary variety vs atypical, uncommon, or primary variety)[78] and leading to the popular classification proposed by Reimann and co-workers of primary amyloidosis (no antecedent or coexisting dis-

ease; mesodermal tissue involvement; variability of staining; tendency to nodular deposits), secondary amyloidosis (chronic disease associated; liver, spleen, kidney, adrenal involvement; constant staining properties), tumor-forming amyloidosis (single or multiple masses of amyloid in eye, genitourinary or respiratory tract), and amyloidosis associated with multiple myeloma.[94] King subsequently commented on the overlap in organ involvement and staining properties and proposed that amyloid be called typical (one or many focal deposits) with or without associated disease.[67] Dahlin returned to the use of primary (systemic or focal), secondary (systemic or focal), and myeloma-related disease.[43] Symmers emphasized the overlap in the many parameters and suggested division into generalized amyloidosis associated with a recognizable predisposing disease (generalized secondary amyloidosis), generalized amyloidosis without a recognized predisposing disease (generalized primary amyloidosis), and localized amyloidosis.[124]

In recent years, it has become apparent that the heredofamilial amyloidoses, with their varying clinical manifestations, are not accommodated in the above schemes. A new system of classification has therefore been devised based on the polarization optical properties of amyloid as defined by Missmahl and Hartwig.[84] These investigators, who reaffirmed the green birefringence of amyloid after Congo red staining, believed that amyloid is laid down along either reticulin fibers or collagen fibers and classified it accordingly.[59,60]

As information has accrued regarding the basic chemical and immunologic properties of amyloid, it has seemed reasonable and clinically useful to classify the various types according to these new data. Thus, a nomenclature has been established that uses the letter A to designate amyloid fibril proteins.[37] This is modified by a second letter indicating the nature of the protein and the tissue, organ system, or disorder with which it is associated (Table 32-1). Primary and multiple myeloma-associated amyloid, which has an N-terminal sequence homologous with a portion of the variable part of immunoglobulin light chains, is designated AL. Secondary amyloidosis has a unique N-terminal sequence termed A-protein and is called AA. Heredofamilial types of amyloid with polyneuropathy are

TABLE 32-1. Chemical and Clinical Classification of Amyloid

NOMENCLATURE	CLINICAL ASSOCIATION
AL	Primary amyloid—multiple myeloma
AA	Chronic infectious or inflammatory disease
	Familial Mediterranean fever
AF	Familial or hereditary amyloid
AS	Senile amyloidosis
AE	Endocrine organ-related amyloid

classified AF and formed from the protein prealbumin. Senile types of amyloid are AS, and endocrine organ–related are AE, although, as yet, precise biochemical data are lacking for these types. Another component in amyloid known as the plasma or pentagonal component (see below) has been termed AP. The serum counterpart of each of these tissue proteins is identified by addition of the letter S as a prefix, for example, SAA for the serum component related to AA.

The incidence of amyloidosis in the population at large is not known. The only data available are those based on postmortem studies, which, for the most part, give a falsely low indication of the autopsy incidence (because special stains without which many cases of amyloid would be missed are not routinely carried out). There are a few studies on selected populations (patients with known leprosy, chronic tuberculosis, and so on) in which an exceedingly high incidence (up to 50%) of amyloid disease has been observed at postmortem examination. In the heredofamilial form of amyloid associated with familial Mediterranean fever, for which clinical and postmortem data have been carefully assessed, evidence of amyloidosis has been obtained in 26.5% of 470 patients.[118]

Amyloid of the Liver

Since the liver was possibly the first organ in which amyloid was described, the association has been well known to pathologists and clinicians alike. It has, however, attracted remarkably little detailed attention because (1) many reports were isolated case histories, (2) many cases undoubtedly went undetected, and (3) even when involved, hepatic amyloid was believed to be rarely of great clinical consequence. Until the 1920s, the diagnosis of hepatic amyloid disease was rarely, if ever, made while the patient was alive.

In 1928, Waldenstrom demonstrated the value of biopsy when he performed the procedure on a patient with hepatomegaly and demonstrated the presence of amyloid.[135] The role of the liver in the general pathophysiology of amyloid disease remained minor, and in one review in 1936, it was stated that jaundice never occurred in amyloidosis.[85] Despite the fact that amyloid was usually secondary in origin when classified as parenchymal (kidney, spleen, liver, lymph node distribution) and was usually regarded as primary when classified as mesenchymal (heart, blood vessels, gastrointestinal tract), the literature suggested that there was little diffuse parenchymal liver involvement in secondary amyloid. Indeed, one group in 1941 studied 30 cases of secondary amyloid and found the liver function tests to be virtually normal in all.[130] Before that, Rosenblatt had reviewed 100 cases of amyloidosis without finding a single case of jaundice.[96]

In 1933, one of the earliest cases of amyloidosis associated with hepatomegaly and severe ascites was reported by Bannick and co-workers.[3] Although jaundice was not initially present, it developed one week after the patient's hospitalization, the bilirubin rose to 9.4 mg/dl, and the patient died in hepatic coma. At autopsy, the liver weight was 3187 g. Subsequently, Tiber and associates in 1941 noted that, although the 30 patients they studied had no jaundice, a review of 100 records of patients with amyloid who came to autopsy indicated one instance of clinical jaundice.[130] In 1944, Spain and Riley reported a case of jaundice in a patient with amyloidosis secondary to tuberculosis.[121] They found that of the previous 12,000 autopsies at Bellevue Hospital, there were 78 recorded cases of amyloidosis, 50 with liver disease and none with jaundice. Orloff and Felder in 1946 described a patient with primary amyloidosis with jaundice who at autopsy was found to have a liver weighing 5900 g.[87] Their review of 2260 autopsy cases at Montefiore Hospital recorded 102 cases of amyloid disease, none with jaundice.

Over the next few years, it became clear that, although severe liver dysfunction leading to jaundice was an unusual accompaniment of amyloidosis, it was not as rare as had been previously thought. Jaundice with evidence of portal hypertension (ascites and esophageal varices) was found in a patient with massive amyloid hepatomegaly (liver weight 5540 g)[2]; a similar case (liver weight 3200 g) was reported in 1947,[140] and severe jaundice and hemorrhage were found in another patient in 1949 (liver weight 3250 g).[14]

In some cases in which hepatomegaly was associated with evidence of portal hypertension, classic cirrhosis was mimicked, and only when tissue was obtained was the issue clarified.[57] Hepatomegaly and evidence of portal hypertension were reported in a number of other series.[19,40,58,66,90,137] In more recent studies, jaundice has not been as rare. For example, Levine reported it in 3 of 13 patients (23%) with primary hepatic amyloid and in 1 of 34 patients (3%) with secondary amyloid.[72] In our reported series of 42 patients, ascites was found in 4 and portal hypertension in 1.[17] Recently, Levy and co-workers reported clinical ascites in 14% of 21 patients with amyloidosis but in 47% of these patients at autopsy.[74] Recently, we reviewed our experience and found that of 78 patients with primary amyloidosis, 4 (5.3%) developed severe intrahepatic cholestasis (see below for further details).[98] More recent analysis of the histopathology has led to a clearer understanding of the distribution and overlap of the various types of systemic amyloidosis.[24]

PATHOLOGY

General Characteristics

Gross Appearance

Amyloid is an amorphous, eosinophilic, glassy, hyaline, extracellular substance that is ubiquitous in its distribution. Grossly, it may be identified by the classic iodine and diluted sulfuric acid stain first used by Virchow. When successful, this stain imparts a blue–purple color to the amyloid. It is, however, inconstant and currently only of historical interest. When small amounts of amyloid are present, no gross organ abnormalities are demonstrable. With larger amounts, the involved organs take on a rubbery, firm consistency. They may have a waxy pink or gray appearance. Organ enlargement (especially liver, kidney, spleen, and heart) may be prominent when the deposits are large. In patients with long-standing renal involvement, however, the kidneys may become small and pale. Gastrointestinal ulcerations are not uncommon. The heart, in addition to being enlarged because of interstitial myocardial involvement, may have nodular elevations on its pericardial and endocardial surfaces as well as lesions on the valves. Nerves are often normal, even when involved, but at times are described as thickened and nodular. Other gross findings are variable and depend upon the presence of local nodular deposits of amyloid.

Tinctorial Properties

Microscopically, amyloid is pink with the hematoxylin and eosin stain and shows crystal-violet or methyl-violet "metachromasia," although it is orthochromatic when stained with toluidine blue. The van Gieson stain for collagen stains the latter red and most of the background yellow but imparts a khaki color to amyloid. The periodic acid-Schiff (PAS) stain gives amyloid a violaceous hue.

Congo red remains one of the most widely used stains. It is not completely specific because it stains elastic tissue and, unless carefully decolorized, stains dense bundles of collagen. However, when formalin-fixed Congo red–stained sections are viewed in the polarizing microscope, a unique green birefringence is present. This is the single most useful procedure for establishing the presence of amyloid. Amyloid has also been stained with fluorochromes to produce a secondary fluorescence, and thioflavine dyes in particular have been found to be very sensitive indicators of amyloid. The lack of specificity of these dyes, however, makes it mandatory for them to be employed primarily for screening and to be followed by more specific stains. Cotton dyes, especially Sirius red, have also been found to be useful and specific. A comparative evaluation of these stains has borne out the high degree of sensitivity and specificity of the green birefringence after Congo red or Sirius red staining.[39]

Light and Electron Microscopic Appearance

In the light microscope, amyloid is almost invariably extracellular in the connective tissue. The deposits may be focal in almost any area of the body, but most often perivascular amyloid is present. The amyloid may involve bone marrow, spleen, capillaries, venules, veins, arterioles, or arteries. The heart may have focal or diffuse interstitial deposits in the myocardium, endocardium, or pericardium. In the kidney, the glomerulus is primarily affected, although interstitial, peritubular, and vascular amyloid may be prominent. In early lesions, small nodular or diffuse deposits near the basement membrane appear, and as the disease progresses, the glomerulus may be massively laden with apparent occlusion of the capillary bed. Atrophic glomeruli laden with amyloid may show marked thickening in the area of Bowman's capsule, and rarely the glomerulus may be almost replaced by connective tissue. Tubular dilatation, casts, and interstitial amyloid deposits may be found in the medulla.

In the gastrointestinal tract, there may be perivascular deposits only, or irregular or diffuse deposits may be found in the submucosa, muscularis mucosa, or subserosa. The amyloid may appear at any level or portion of the gastrointestinal tract, including gallbladder and pancreas. Hepatic deposits may be perivascular only; more commonly, diffuse amyloid is found between the Kupffer and parenchymal cells (see Liver Pathology). In the nervous system, amyloid has been described along peripheral nerves and in autonomic ganglia, senile plaques, and vessels of the central nervous system. It may be found in any portion of the orbit, including the vitreous humor and cornea.

The bronchopulmonary tract may be involved focally or extensively. The unique aspect of pulmonary or pleural involvement is that, whereas amyloid in virtually all areas of the body remains without any evidence of resorption or foreign-body reaction, pulmonary amyloid deposits may be accompanied by large numbers of macrophages about and within the lesions. These deposits may also contain islets of cartilage and ossification. Thus, there is virtually no area of the body that is spared. This ubiquitous distribution elicits a wide variety of clinical symptoms and signs.

In 1959, Cohen and Calkins found upon direct examination of amyloid tissues in the electron microscope that the amyloid itself consists of fine fibrils.[30] This has been amply confirmed, and it is now known that all types of human amyloid—primary, secondary, heredofamilial—[27,34] no matter how classified consist of these fine, nonbranching rigid fibrils measuring in tissue sections approximately 100 nm in diameter. They are usually arranged randomly when distal to the cell, but proximally they may be parallel or perpendicular to the plasmalemma, with which they occasionally appear to merge. Intracellular fibrils with dimensions comparable to those outside the cell are also occasionally observed. Their precise nature has not yet been established.

In the kidney, amyloid fibrils are usually first seen closest to mesangial cells[103]; as deposits enlarge, they appear closer to endothelial and, finally, epithelial cells. In the liver, they first border the Kupffer cells but finally fill the space of Disse and abut the hepatic cells as well. In many other locations, they have been found close to blood vessels, pericytes, and endothelial cells. Thus, although the cells that form amyloid fibrils appear in many instances to be in the reticuloendothelial or macrophage family, it is possible that, under some circumstances or in advanced disease, the ability to produce these fibrils may be a more ubiquitous phenomenon. The probable production of amyloid fibrils by reticuloendothelial cells in isolated spleen explants[35] and cultures[4] has been suggested by autoradiographic techniques at the light and electron microscopic levels. It is now clear that secondary amyloid (AA) has as its precursor SAA, which is produced in the liver as an acute-phase reactant in response to the monokine interleukin 1.[11,126]

The amyloid fibrils thus visualized can be extracted from amyloid-laden tissues in a variety of ways for more definitive ultrastructural, chemical, and immunologic study. When isolated, they can be specially stained (positively or negatively with phosphotungstic acid) and their delicate, thin, nonbranching fibrous character illustrated. The individual fibril has a diameter of about 70 nm, and the fibrils tend to aggregate laterally. Each fibril is made up of filaments, and subunit protofibrils (about 30 nm–35 nm in diameter) have been defined. The protofibril is beaded, may consist of two subunits, and exists in spirals of five protofibrils or multiples of two such subunits.[102]

A second protein, P-component (AP), which has a pentagonal ultrastructure and unique chemical characteristics, has been isolated from amyloid and shown to be identical to a circulating alpha globulin present at a level of 5 mg to 7 mg/dl in all sera.[109,113] Protein AP is bound to all forms of amyloid thus far investigated by a calcium-dependent ligand.[88] It was originally thought to be present in only minute amounts but recently has been measured and found in varying amounts averaging 5% of fibril weight; however, it is not responsible for the characteristic tinctorial properties or ultrastructure of amyloid.[114] It has been shown to have many similarities to C-reactive protein (CRP) in that both are pentagonal in appearance and have some sequence homology. However, AP is antigenically distinct from CRP and is of unknown significance in the pathogenesis of amyloid. Its molecular weight is twice that of CRP, and it appears as doublets in the electron microscope.

Liver Pathology

The incidence of amyloid of the liver in association with generalized primary and secondary amyloidosis has undergone reassessment in recent years as better staining techniques have become available. In our opinion, the most sensitive and specific method is the properly used Congo red stain on formalin-fixed tissues (with appropriate controls) and the assessment of such tissues by means of polarization microscopy. The green birefringence observed under such conditions is characteristic of amyloid.[33]

In 1949, Dahlin found parenchymal amyloid infiltration in two of six cases of primary disease leading to severe atrophy of the hepatic cords.[42] The amyloid was laid down between the sinusoids and cords of liver cells. Two additional patients had lesser amounts, and two showed no parenchymal amyloid. All six, however, had small-vessel infiltration of amyloid, especially in the arteries of the portal triads. The livers with moderate or severe amyloid were firm and rubbery and had an average weight of 2880 g. In his study of 30 cases of secondary amyloid, the same author found that 26 demonstrated liver involvement, one with massive amyloid (liver weight 2900 g).[41] As with primary amyloid, the substance was deposited between the hepatic cords and sinusoids and was present in artery and vein wells.

Eisen collected 48 cases of primary amyloid from the literature up to 1945 and found 8 with hepatic involvement.[46] Subsequently, Mathews updated his review to 1954 and found hepatic amyloid in 27 of 50 cases.[80] In 1957, Bero stated that liver involvement was almost universal in secondary amyloidosis and that it occurred in 30% to 40% of cases of primary disease.[13] In his series, eight of nine livers (in 12 cases) whose weights were recorded were enlarged, many massively so; one weight was recorded as 5900 g. Symmers found amyloid in all five cases of primary amyloid studied, although, in most, the deposits were small and solely vascular.[123] Briggs noted that the liver was most commonly involved in secondary amyloidosis (52 of 53 cases positive), although hepatic involvement in primary amyloid was also common (17 of 20 cases).[18] In three of his cases, liver weights of over 4000 g were recorded. Six previous cases of amyloid liver weights from 5000 g to 9000 g have been reported.[99] Levine found the liver to be the third most commonly involved organ in 84 patients affected (i.e., 47 of 84, 56% had hepatic amyloid).[72] Kuhlback and Wegelius found amyloid in 17 of 20 patients with the secondary type,[69] while Hallen and Rudin found it in all but 3 of 15 cases of primary amyloidosis.[59]

In our earlier study of 42 patients with biopsy-proved amyloid disease,[17] tissue was available from 17 patients with hepatomegaly and from 6 with no liver enlargement. All specimens had amyloid present in either parenchyma or blood vessels or both. In our more recent analysis of liver tissue from 54 amyloidotic patients,[32] amyloid deposits were again found to be a universal phenomenon, although the distribution and magnitude varied. Two of our hepatic amyloid specimens were massive and weighed 7200 g and 8200 g, respectively. Both were from patients with primary amyloidosis. Other isolated instances of massive hepatomegaly have been reported with liver weights of 3050 g, 6125 g, and 8500 g.[64,82,91]

In a more recent study, we analyzed the histopathology of the liver to evaluate the spectrum of morphologic changes in primary (AL) and secondary (AA) amyloidosis and to determine whether these two forms are distinguishable based on such analysis.[24] Thirty-eight patients with systemic amyloid (25 primary or myeloma [AL] and 13 secondary, reactive [AA]) were evaluated. Overall architectural distortion, alterations of portal triads, as well as predilection for topographic deposition in the parenchyma and/or blood vessel walls were noted. Significant histopathologic differences in AL or AA amyloid liver involvement included (1) portal fibrosis, seen in 7 of 25 (28%) AL patients and 8 of 13 (62%) AA patients; (2) parenchymal amyloid deposition, seen in 25 of 25 (100%) AL amyloid and 10 of 13 (77%) AA amyloid patients; and (3) vascular amyloid deposition, found in 17 of 25 (68%) with AL amyloid and 13 of 13 (100%) patients with AA amyloid. These data varied from the widely held concept that deposition of amyloid is predominantly vascular

in the AL form and parenchymal in amyloid AA. Clearly, however, in individual cases significant overlap occurred, and characterization of amyloid types based on morphologic distribution of amyloid deposits, may be possible in only a minority of cases. In most cases, differentiation of amyloid AL and amyloid AA forms will require clinical, histochemical, immunochemical, and sometimes more elaborate laboratory amino acid sequence studies for accurate identification.

Thus, amyloid of the liver is extremely common whether the patient has primary or secondary disease. Postmortem, the involved organ will be found enlarged, smooth, and of a waxy, rubber consistency. It may be massive. Microscopic study of the amyloid shows that it is close to the Kupffer cells and that it lies between the sinusoids and the parenchymal cells (Fig. 32-1 and 32-2). Vascular deposits about arteries and veins, especially in the portal area, are common (Figs. 32-3 and 32-4). Periportal and pericentral area distribution has been described. The progress of the hepatic amyloid is unpredictable and has on serial biopsy appeared to be stable in some cases and rapidly progressive in others.[72]

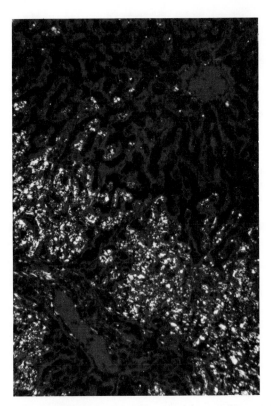

Fig. 32-1. Amyloidosis of the liver secondary to rheumatoid arthritis. Although the amyloid is diffusely present, its concentration is more marked in the periportal area. Deposits are localized between the Kupffer cells and parenchymal cells when the lesions are small, whereas diffuse distortion of the architecture occurs when the lesions are more massive. (Original magnification × 120; Congo-red stain)

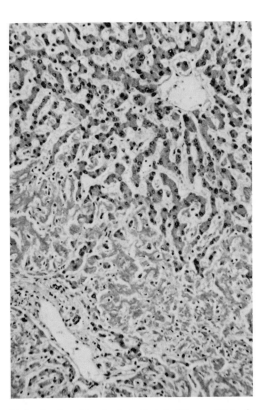

Fig. 32-2. Section identical to that in Figure 32-1 viewed through the polarizing microscope, demonstrating the birefringence of the amyloid deposits. In color, the birefringence has a clear-cut green appearance. (Original magnification × 120)

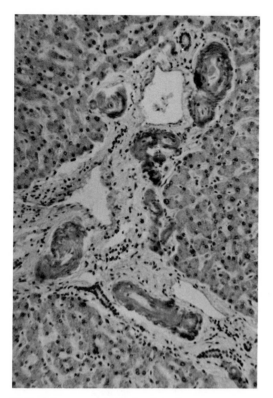

Fig. 32-3. Primary amyloidosis of the liver. Pattern of massive amounts of amyloid in the blood vessel walls and virtually none in the hepatic parenchyma. (Original magnification × 120; Congo-red stain)

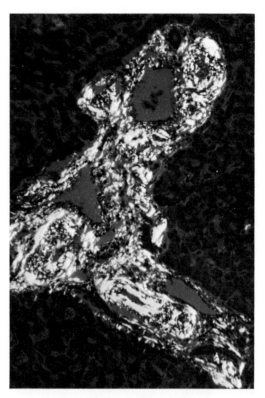

Fig. 32-4. Section identical to that in Figure 32-3 but viewed in the polarizing microscope. Again, the striking birefringence of the amyloid is noted. (Original magnification × 120)

Hepatic amyloid has also been studied by electron microscopy. Thiery and Caroli reported on the fibrous ultrastructure of human hepatic amyloid in 1961.[129] Manitz and Themann in 1962 analyzed the ultrastructure of several amyloid liver biopsy specimens.[79] The fine fibrils were found within but not completely confined to the space of Disse. Amyloid extended between seemingly normal parenchymal cells. Skinner and co-workers reported on the fine structure of hepatic amyloid associated with multiple myeloma.[117] They found fine fibrils filling and distending the spaces of Disse. The fibrils frequently were oriented at right angles to the plasma membrane of the hepatic parenchymal cells and the adjacent sinusoidal lining cells. These findings are comparable to those seen in experimental animals, in which the ultrastructure of hepatic amyloidosis has been extensively studied.[5,20,31,51,119,120,123] Representative electron microscopy of hepatic amyloid demonstrates the fine rigid fibrils and close relationship to Kupffer cells as well as to parenchymal cells (Figs. 32-5 and 32-5). In one study, a liver biopsy from a patient with primary amyloidosis was found to show degenerative changes in the cytoplasmic periphery of hepatocytes. These were interpreted as indicating shedding of peripheral parts

of the cytoplasm (1) with protrusion and sequestration of hernia-like blebs of cytoplasm and (2) with shedding of vesicles derived from degenerated endoplasmic reticulum. This resulted in an increased fractional volume of mito chondria (which were retained in the cell) and was felt to represent the mechanism by which the cell adapts to the unfavorable environment created by the amyloid.[89]

Deposits in the form of round amyloid bodies between or within hepatocytes have been reported and are felt to be of benign nature.[50,77] A more extensive study of 14 cases with globular hepatic amyloid suggested that it is not clinically distinguishable from other forms of classic hepatic amyloid and in 7 patients on whom autopsy was performed, extensive systemic (nonglobular) amyloid was found.[65]

A freeze-etched liver specimen of mice with casein-induced amyloid showed the feltlike structure of the amyloid fibrils, amyloid bundles, and globular profiles among amyloid fibrils. Amyloid bundles enveloped by the cytoplasmic membrane of Kupffer cells projected from the concave surface of the cytoplasmic membrane into Disse's space and had a stone column-like appearance. The amyloid bundles projecting from the invaginated cytoplasmic membrane were in close contact with it and deeply rooted in the Kupffer cell cytoplasm.[63] Scanning electron microscopy (SEM) of the mouse amyloid liver showed amyloid bundles in close contact to the Kupffer cell cytoplasm and projecting from the cell into the space of Disse on three-dimensional figures.[125]

PATHOGENESIS

The etiology of amyloidosis is not known. Throughout the years, however, amyloid has been regarded as (1) a disorder of serum proteins with associated hyperglobulinemia; (2) a disorder of protein metabolism; (3) a disorder related to an abnormality of the reticuloendothelial system; (4) the result of chronic immunologic stimulation leading to excessive antibody production and the deposition of antibody or antibody–antigen complexes as amyloid; (5) a disorder of delayed hypersensitivity; or (6) a combination of the above mentioned. These hypotheses are not mutually exclusive, and because the etiology is unknown, it is difficult to be certain as to when a specific abnormality is present and whether it is of primary significance or represents a secondary phenomenon.

Early observations suggested to many that amyloid might be related to a specific serum protein because of its association with multiple myeloma and its known plasma protein aberrations and because of the potential for intense antigenic stimulation in the many inflammatory disorders complicated by amyloid. The pendulum of scientific opinion swung away from this hypothesis when several studies showed the lack of identity of serum proteins with whole amyloid fibrils and when increasing numbers of patients with primary amyloid and no form of other disease and no M-components were apparent.

Extracts of amyloid that were prepared in a number of laboratories demonstrated the absence of gamma globulin and other serum constituents even in very purified preparations. Thus, until several years ago, amyloid was regarded as a unique fibrous protein immunologically distinct from gamma globulin. Chemical studies showed it to have a high nitrogen content and no unique amino acids and to lack the components of both collagen and elastin (hydroxyproline, hydroxylysine, desmosine, isodesmosine, lysinonorleucine).[26,28]

Neutral sugars are present in small amounts; whether glycosaminoglycans are present as part of the molecule or in the milieu in which the fibril is embedded is not known. X-ray diffraction studies have demonstrated that the amyloid fibril has a cross-beta pattern, suggesting the pleated sheet morphology of Corey and Pauling.[16,45]

The interesting observation that primary amyloid fibrils are predominantly immunoglobulin light chains or the variable segments thereof is consistent with the clinical observation of an abnormal serum protein or M-component in these patients.[54,106,107] In addition, patients may have Bence–Jones proteinuria and increased bone-marrow mature plasma cells (15%–20%) but no overt myeloma. Extensive deposits of amyloid are frequently present in the spleen, liver, heart, intestines, tongue, blood vessels, and other organs.

Also, a proportion of patients with clear-cut multiple myeloma manifested by sheets of immature plasma cells in the bone marrow and lytic lesions in bones develop amyloidosis. For reasons yet unknown, only a limited number of such patients do so. Although this type of amyloid is biochemically indistinguishable from primary amyloid, the mean survival is much shorter and clinically separates these forms of disease from each other.

Biochemically, various sizes of light-chain fragments make up the major portion of the amyloid fibril; N-terminal sequence studies suggest that it is always the variable portion of the light chain with or without part or all of the constant segment. Various types of light chains have been identified thus far, including kappa I, kappa II, and lambda chains with blocked amino terminals. One unique type of light chain, a lambda VI with an aspartic amino terminus, has been found only in association with amyloid and may be implicated etiologically (Table 32-2).[111] In some instances, the Bence–Jones protein and the amyloid protein from the same patient have been found to be identical.

However, not all amyloid is related to immunoglobulin. Protein AA and its serum counterpart SAA have been associated with the type of amyloidosis known to be secondary to chronic inflammatory or infectious disease. Protein AA is the main constituent of the amyloid fibrils in secondary amyloidosis in humans, as well as in animals, and has been identified in tissue extracts from the amyloid of patients with rheumatoid arthritis, bronchiectasis, and tuberculosis, as well as the amyloid associated with familial Mediterranean fever. It is approximately 8000 daltons in size with a unique 76 residue sequence.[7,71]

SAA is an acute-phase reactant induced by interleukin 1 that is the putative precursor of protein AA and is found in the blood plasma as a polypeptide of about 12,500 daltons. It has been found to be one of the apoproteins of the high-density lipoproteins.[89] Studies have shown a marked increase in the liver content of SAA after stimulation with casein or lipopolysaccharide (LPS) in the mouse model. It is speculated that the liver may be one site of synthesis of this apoprotein.[11,126] Isoelectric focusing has identified several SAA bands, some of which may be partially degraded forms of others.[6] In the murine model, molecular biological studies have shown two major gene products (SAA_1 and SAA_2), one of which (SAA_2) has sequence identity with amyloid protein AA, suggesting a selective deposition of only one gene product.*

The comparative N-terminal sequence data of AA and SAA in various species are summarized in Table 32-3. An N-terminal heterogeneity can be noted in spite of the obvious sequence homology.

---

* Hoffman JS et al: Only one apo SAA isotype is the precursor to murine amyloid fibril protein A. Fed Proc 43:468, 1984.

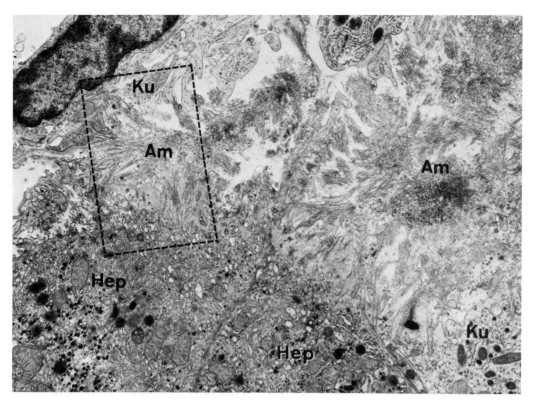

Fig. 32-5. Low-power electron micrograph of mouse liver with amyloidosis induced by repeated casein injections. Amyloid (*Am*) deposits in two areas surrounded by Kupffer cells (*Ku*) and hepatocytes (*Hep*). Amyloid fibrils deposit densely and in random array in the central portion of the amyloid mass, whereas in the peripheral portion they form bundles of amyloid fibrils well oriented perpendicularly to the cell border. This area appears stellar under the light microscope, the so-called amyloid star. The area surrounded by dotted lines is seen at higher magnification in Figure 32-6. (Original magnification × 7000)

The AP of amyloid, as mentioned above, is completely distinctive from the amyloid fibril components (both the AL and the AA proteins) and has distinctive morphologic, tinctorial, immunologic, and biochemical properties.[109] It is made up of a parallel pair of pentagonal units with a subunit size of approximately 23,000 daltons. It shares several characteristics with CRP, including its ultrastructure, calcium-dependent binding properties, and a 60% sequence homology.[86,114] AP is synthesized by the liver, has a relatively short half-life of 7 to 8 hours, and is maintained at a stable serum concentration of approximately 5 mg/dl.[116,126] The hamster female protein (FP) has structural similarities to AP and CRP, giving the name pentraxins to the three proteins.

The amyloid fibrils in the dominantly inherited familial amyloid polyneuropathies (FAP) have been found to be composed of the protein prealbumin with variant molecular structures. In the FAP type I kinships of Swedish, Portuguese, and Japanese origins, a methionine is substituted for valine at position 30.[44,101,108,127] In a Jewish patient, glycine for threonine was found at position 49, and in two patients with FAP type II a substitution of serine for isoleucine has been identified at position 84.[12,92] Senile and endocrine types of amyloidosis await more precise biochemical definition.

The actual pathogenesis of the various types of amyloidosis is probably very complex. Recent studies have shown variations in the ability of monocytes and polymorphonuclear leukocytes to degrade the SAA protein, suggesting genetic differences.[70,105] Such differences in degrading ability may be an important factor in understanding why the development of amyloid occurs in some but not all persons with elevated SAA levels. It is also possible that differences in degrading M-components may account for some but not all persons with multiple myeloma developing amyloidosis.

CLINICAL ASPECTS

General Considerations

Whether a patient has primary, secondary, or heredofamilial amyloidosis, the clinical manifestations depend

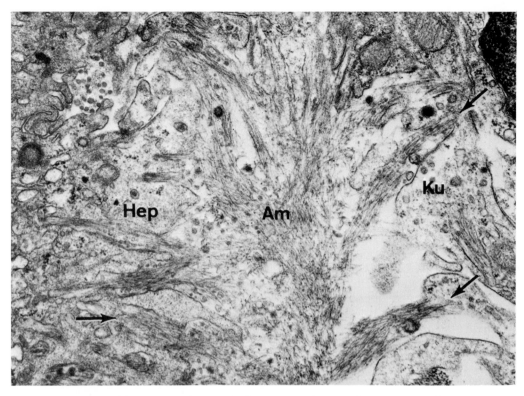

Fig. 32-6. Higher-power micrograph of the area outlined in Figure 32-5. Kupffer cell (*Ku*) and the hepatocyte (*Hep*) form many deep invaginations that contain bundles of well-oriented amyloid fibrils (*Am*). At the amyloid–cell border, especially at the bottom of the invagination containing the bundle of amyloid fibrils, the plasmalemma appears indistinct (*arrows*). (Original magnification × 24,000)

upon the anatomic site of the deposit and the degree of interference with normal organ function.[27] The genetically determined forms, in which clinical patterns are usually recognizable, are the subject of another report.[29] Renal involvement is potentially the most serious manifestation of the disease and the major cause of death in most series. Despite this, renal amyloid may be present and asymptomatic for many years, and the disorder does not inevitably progress rapidly. Most patients, however, exhibit proteinuria, possibly massive, and a classic nephrotic syndrome may be the presenting manifestation or may develop. Patients with renal amyloid may also have hematuria. Radiologically, the kidneys may be large, but with increased duration of disease, small, shrunken kidneys develop. Hypertension is rare early in the course, but as patients with renal amyloid survive longer, the incidence of hypertension increases.

When present, cardiac amyloid also may be asymptomatic but on occasion may be severe enough to cause congestive heart failure. Electrocardiographic abnormalities include a wide variety of conduction abnormalities, especially heart block but including flutter and fibrillation.

TABLE 32-2.   Examples of N-Terminal Sequence of AL Amyloid Fibril Proteins

AMYLOID	TYPE	1	2	3	4	5	6	7	8	9	10
Lep	AL Kappa I	Asp-	Ile-	Gln-	Met-	Thr-	Gln-	Ser-	Pro-	Ser-	Ser[75]
	BJP Kappa I	Asp-	Ile-	Gln-	Met-	Thr-	Gln-	Ser-	Pro-	Ser-	Ser[15]
Tew	AL Kappa II	Asp-	Ile-	Val-	Met-	Thr-	Glu-	Ser-	Pro-	Leu-	Ser[128]
	BJP Kappa II	Asp-	Ile-	Val-	Met-	Thr-	Gln-	Ser-	Pro-	Leu-	Ser[93]
Mcg	BJP Lambda	PCA-	Ser-	Ala-	Leu-	Thr-	Gln-	Pro-	Pro-	( )-	Ser[48]
Jam	AL Lambda VI	Asp-	Phe-	Met-	Leu-	Thr-	Glu-	Pro-	His-	Ser-	Val[111]

( ), not identified.

TABLE 32-3.   N-Terminal Sequence of AA and SAA Proteins

PROTEIN							1	2	3	4	5	6	7	8	9	10
Human	AA						Arg	Ser	Phe	Phe	Ser	Phe	Leu	Gly	Glu	Ala[71]
	SAA						Arg	Ser	Phe	Phe	Ser	Phe	Leu	Gly	( )	Ala[97]
Mouse	AA						Arg	Ser Gly	Phe	Phe	Ser	Phe	Ile	Gly	Glu	Ala[47,112]
	SAA							Gly	Phe	Phe	Ser	Phe	Val Ile	Gly	Glu	Ala[1]
Monkey	AA						Arg	Ser	Trp	Phe	Ser	Phe	Leu	Gly	Glu	Ala[61]
Guinea pig	AA	His	Ala	Lys	Gly	Gly	Arg	Ser	Ile	Phe	Ser	Phe	Leu	Lys	Glu	Ser Ala[110]
Duck	AA	Asp	Asn	Pro	Phe	Thr	Arg	Gly	Gly	Arg	Phe	Val	Leu	Asp	Ala	Ala[56]

( ), not identified.

Patients with cardiac amyloid may have arrhythmias precipitated by digitalis, and this drug should be used with caution. The electrocardiogram in cardiac amyloid may indicate coronary artery disease without clinical symptoms. The reading is usually that of anterior or anteroseptal infarction and often shows decreased voltage. The recent use of M-mode and two-dimensional echocardiography has led to a more precise definition of the extent of amyloid cardiomyopathy.

Gastrointestinal symptoms in amyloidosis are very common. They may result from direct involvement of the gastrointestinal tract at any level or from infiltration of the autonomic nervous system with amyloid. The symptoms include those of obstruction, ulceration, malabsorption, hemorrhage, protein loss, and diarrhea. Whereas hepatic involvement is common, liver function abnormalities are unusual and occur late in the disease. The two tests most useful in indicating hepatic amyloid are sodium sulfobromophthalein (Bromsulphalein [BSP]) extraction and the level of serum alkaline phosphatase activity. Signs of portal hypertension occur but are uncommon. Because amyloidosis can involve any level of the respiratory tract, symptoms vary widely and include hoarseness, hemoptysis, epistaxis, and dysphagia. Neurologic symptoms are especially prominent in several of the heredofamilial amyloidoses, and a patient may show an asymmetric or symmetric sensory or motor neuropathy, severe autonomic nervous dysfunction, or even isolated cranial nerve lesions. Amyloid of the eye or orbit may cause proptosis, decreased visual acuity, muscle weakness, or ptosis. Thus, virtually any organ of the body may be involved, and the symptoms depend upon the site of the deposit and its size.

There are no laboratory abnormalities specific to or unique for amyloid. Routine blood studies (hematocrit, white cell count, and differential) are within normal limits unless there is blood loss or complicating disease. The erythrocyte sedimentation rate (ESR) and other nonspecific indices of inflammation may or may not be elevated. The ESR may be markedly elevated in primary amyloidosis with the nephrotic syndrome. Occasionally, the fi-brinogen level is nonspecifically elevated (especially in familial Mediterranean fever). No uniform changes in serum complement have been found. There are no specific changes in serum proteins. Urinary abnormalities include mild or severe proteinuria, hematuria, and the occasional presence of granular casts. Levels of cerebrospinal fluid proteins may be elevated in certain heredofamilial forms. Serum prealbumin levels appear to be decreased in FAP.[38]

The occasional bleeding reported is usually due to injury to amyloid-infiltrated blood vessels, although disseminated intravascular coagulation has been observed. In severe hepatic amyloid, however, the prothrombin time may be slightly elevated, and the literature has documented an acquired selective factor-X (Stuart factor) deficiency.[52] Although selective factor-X deficiency is most common, multiple clotting-factor deficiencies may exist in patients with a rapidly progressing form of primary amyloidosis. Our *in vitro* experimentation has shown that when clotting factors are incubated with amyloid fibrils and calcium, a clotting-factor activity can subsequently be eluted from the fibrils with citrate.[115] It is presumed that such calcium-dependent binding can occur *in vivo* and that clinical deficiencies of clotting factors in amyloidosis are not due to decreased hepatic synthesis of clotting factors but rather to their calcium-dependent adsorption to the amyloid fibrils.

Diagnosis

The diagnosis of amyloidosis rests first on one's clinical acumen, that is, the recognition of a patient with a predisposing disorder such as rheumatoid arthritis in whom proteinuria and hepatomegaly develop, or the recognition of a typical pattern of symptoms and signs attributed to a heredofamilial amyloid syndrome. Inevitably, however, the diagnosis depends largely upon biopsy, use of the appropriate stain (Congo red), and observation of such stained tissue in the polarizing microscope for the characteristic green birefringence.[33]

Biopsy has been shown to be safe if an accessible site (gingiva, rectum, abdominal fat) is used and simple precautions taken.[53,132] In general, to cope with the potential problem of bleeding, it is preferable to perform biopsy on sites that can be visualized directly. The abdominal fat aspiration technique is currently the method of choice because of its sensitivity (80% of patients known to have amyloid are positive) and because it is a procedure easily performed at the bedside.[76,136] Amyloid deposits lend a tissue a certain amount of rubbery rigidity, which makes it prone to hemorrhage. This is seen with the ecchymoses associated with amyloid of the skin, the hematuria seen in renal amyloid, and the startling gastrointestinal bleeding that may occur when amyloid is present in the intestinal tract. With appropriate precautions, however, and with knowledge of the platelet count, prothrombin time, and bleeding and clotting times, closed biopsies can be undertaken with relative impunity. Renal biopsy has been successfully performed in many cases of suspected or known amyloid of the kidney. Hepatic biopsy is usually safe, although the procedure should be approached with caution in patients with massive hepatomegaly (see below). Peroral small intestinal biopsy has been performed as well as splenic biopsy. In patients with respiratory tract masses, direct biopsy of laryngeal or bronchial lesions may determine the diagnosis. Nerve biopsy is indicated whenever amyloid neuropathy is suspected.

Treatment and Prognosis

There is no specific treatment for any variety of amyloidosis. Eradication of the predisposing disease apparently slows the progress of secondary amyloidosis, and, in rare cases, serial biopsy in some organs suggests that reabsorption takes place. The cure of the underlying disease does not guarantee freedom from amyloid, however; there are a number of recorded cases of its appearance many years after activity of the primary disorder has ceased. In most of the reported cures of amyloid, direct biopsy proof is lacking, and judgment is made on the basis of a clinical diagnosis (i.e., hepatomegaly). In some of these cases, however, the circumstantial evidence for amyloid and its regression is quite strong. It is of interest that in one series of four cases of massive hepatic amyloid (liver weights 4200 g, 3600 g, 2300 g, and 2000 g), two showed clinical hepatomegaly without cholestasis and the other two less pronounced hepatomegaly but severe and progressive intrahepatic cholestasis.[81]

Various agents that have been used or recommended include whole liver extract, adrenal-cortical steroids, ascorbic acid, and immunosuppressive agents. None has caused clear-cut improvement. However, it is important to emphasize that, with conservative supportive measures (i.e., treatment of complicating infections), the prognosis is far better than was once thought.[17] We have followed patients with renal amyloid for over 12 years. In selected instances, renal transplantation has been performed with surprisingly good results.[31,36] Ten-year survival has been reported after such transplantation. Colchicine has been shown to be effective in preventing acute febrile attacks in familial Mediterranean fever and possibly the amyloid associated with it. In the casein-induced amyloid model in the mouse, inhibition of amyloid development has been reported,[104] and it is possible that colchicine may be effective in preventing new amyloid deposits. Clinical studies are in progress, but no definitive results are available. Dimethyl sulfoxide (DMSO) is under study both experimentally and in patients with amyloid and thus far has produced varied results.

Hepatic Amyloid

Amyloidosis of the liver is one of the most common manifestations of the disease. It can occur at any age and has been reported in children as a complication of juvenile rheumatoid arthritis and de novo in a child of 9 years.[55] In most modern series, as already noted, amyloid is present at least in the blood vessels in the great majority of cases, whether primary, secondary, or myeloma-related. In all 54 cases of our series from which tissue was available, amyloid was present, occasionally in massive amounts, occasionally as a minor finding near blood vessel walls. Liver weights of up to 9000 g have been reported.

The clinical presentation of amyloid liver disease may be nonspecific, and often the patient appears with vague abdominal complaints. In many of these patients, hepatomegaly is the only positive physical finding. Clinical signs such as spider angiomas, clubbing, gynecomastia, and alopecia are rare. Several series recorded no such findings.[68,74] Levine found that although 29 of 47 patients (62%) had symptoms or physical findings suggesting hepatic involvement, none showed peripheral stigmata of cirrhosis (i.e., spider angiomas, abdominal collaterals, palmar erythema, or testicular atrophy).[72] Presenting complaints were referable to the liver in only three patients, one with ascites and two with an abdominal mass. One of Levine's patients developed signs of hepatic coma (with stupor and flapping). Death was attributed to hepatic amyloid in that case and in two others, both with intractable ascites unassociated with renal failure.

In our previous report of 42 patients, spider angiomas were found in only 1 patient, Dupuytren's contractures (long-standing) were found in 1, and clubbing was present in 2 (1 with associated bronchiectasis and 1 with granulomatous ileitis). Unilateral gynecomastia developed in one patient. Palmar erythema, asterixis, and alopecia were not observed. Jaundice was present in one, ascites in four (two of whom also had congestive heart failure), and portal hypertension in one.[17] The multiple case reports of patients with jaundice (see section on amyloid of the liver) and the increasing longevity of patients with amyloid suggest that jaundice, while not a common presenting sign, may be observed more frequently in the future.

One reviewer noted an incidence of jaundice of 4.7% in 490 patients with hepatic amyloid, although serum bilirubin rarely exceeded 5 mg/dl.[73] Severe obstructive jaundice is rarer; a limited number of patients with such cholestatic jaundice has been reported.[83,98] All of these persons had a very poor prognosis and died within months of the diagnosis. The more serious complications secondary to portal hypertension, fortunately, are late manifestations, but they do occur and, in our experience, are seen progressively more frequently. An unusual association, congenital dilatation of the intrahepatic bile ducts and amyloidosis, has recently been reported in two cases.[49] Focal intrahepatic mass lesions, comprising extensive amyloid infiltration of the liver, and spontaneous rupture of the liver are the most rarely reported manifestations.[62,131]

Laboratory abnormalities in amyloidosis of the liver are surprisingly sparse. Levine assessed the value of ten liver function tests in 47 cases and found the most common abnormalities to be hypoalbuminemia, elevated BSP retention, alkaline phosphatase, cholesterol, and thymol turbidity.[72] However, these tests were felt to be of little value because they did not clearly distinguish those patients with and those without hepatic amyloid or differentiate one type of amyloid from another. Furthermore, no correlation was found between the degree of functional abnormality and the extent of hepatic amyloid infiltration. Some patients with massive amounts of amyloid had normal liver function tests, whereas others with minimal vascular deposits had abnormal tests.

Our previous study[17] and those of others[74] are in general agreement with the detailed analyses of Levine.[72] We noted occasional mild hypoprothrombinemia, rare elevations in serum lactic acid dehydrogenase and glutamic-oxaloacetic transaminase levels, and rare mild elevations in bilirubin. Abnormal BSP excretion and elevated serum alkaline phosphatase levels proved to be very useful, but even these did not correlate well with the true extent of the disease.

Although liver biopsy in the diagnosis of amyloid liver disease was introduced in 1928,[135] it did not receive extensive use until the 1950s.[137] In a detailed review, Volwiler and Jones reported one death from hemorrhage after amyloid liver biopsy.[134] This tended to temper the use of liver biopsy as a diagnostic procedure; however, although this precaution is reasonable, it is our experience that the procedure is more than routinely dangerous only in patients with massive hepatomegaly, who often are in the terminal stages of their illness. A second death after liver biopsy in a patient with extensive hepatic amyloid was also reported.[22] At about the same time, another patient with jaundice and liver disease of unknown etiology was reported to have been subjected to an open liver biopsy. The patient died 48 hours postoperatively, and although there was widespread amyloid and diffuse focal hemorrhage throughout the body, there also occurred extensive retroperitoneal hemorrhage, with 450 ml of free blood in the peritoneal cavity.[100]

In 1961, however, Stauffer and co-workers reported a series of 18 needle biopsies of the liver in patients with amyloid liver disease.[122] No difficulties were encountered in 17, but, in one, intraperitoneal bleeding probably occurred, requiring one transfusion. They concluded that the procedure was important in reaching the conclusive diagnosis of amyloidosis. Certainly, if the diagnosis has already been established in other organs (e.g., by rectal biopsy), one would have to have a special indication for doing a liver biopsy in addition. In a patient with hepatomegaly of unknown etiology, liver biopsy is a reasonable procedure to consider for the diagnosis of amyloidosis in conjunction with measures noted above. Liver scans have been performed on a number of patients with amyloid and produced variable results. No diagnostic pattern is demonstrated, and the appearance varies from normal scan with patchy cold spots to cirrhotic liver with decreased liver and increased splenic and bone-marrow uptake. Peritoneoscopy is said to be of help when it reveals a light-colored liver with a rosy-violet appearance.[21]

We evaluated the bone-scanning radionuclides technetium 99m pyrophosphate and methylene diphosphonate to delineate soft tissue amyloidosis. Of 23 patients, 6 had abnormal soft tissue uptake of radionuclide. The most common soft tissue abnormality observed was diffuse hepatic uptake, which occurred in three of eight patients with biopsy-proved hepatic amyloidosis (Fig. 32-7). It was concluded that this procedure is not sensitive enough for definitive diagnosis but that amyloidosis should be considered in patients with diffuse hepatic or other soft tissue uptake of bone-seeking radionuclides.[139] Angiographic findings in one case of hepatic amyloid included narrowing of the intrahepatic vessels, mimicking an intrahepatic mass.[138]

Personal Observations

Between 1965 and 1975, 80 patients with biopsy-proven systemic amyloidosis have been studied by the members of the Boston University Arthritis and Connective Tissue Section at the University Hospital and in the Thorndike Memorial Laboratory of the Boston City Hospital. Data on some of these patients have already been reported, with emphasis on clinical presentation and prognosis in 42 cases[17] and immunoglobulin abnormalities in 62 cases.[23]

Data on some patients were reported to us by other institutions, and because liver disease was occasionally not suspected, liver function studies are not available in these cases. A number of patients are alive and have not had liver biopsies. Several patients were brought to our attention only on the basis of an autopsy diagnosis, so that, again, clinical information is lacking. However, in 73 patients with biopsy-proved amyloidosis (any site), some data concerning the liver were available. This information included (1) histologic material from a biopsy or postmortem examination, (2) adequate clinical evaluation of liver size or postmortem liver weight, or (3) two or more laboratory studies of liver functions (from alkaline phosphatase, BSP extraction, serum glutamic-oxaloacetic acid level, lactic acid dehydrogenase level, bilirubin, prothrombin time, and serum albumin).

Several preliminary conclusions can be drawn from these data. In 54 patients, tissue was available for exam-

jaundice in four, and spider angiomata in six. Ascites was present in eight patients but was associated with generalized anasarca and renal failure. Two patients with primary amyloid who had markedly infiltrated livers histologically developed esophageal varices with bleeding. In one of these, the condition was terminal. Hepatic coma occurred and was the cause of death in only one patient.

As has been noted in other series, elevated alkaline phosphatase levels and increased BSP extraction seem to be among the earliest and most useful chemical determinations. The remarkable degree to which the liver parenchyma can be replaced by amyloid is indicated by one patient who had a liver that was palpable below the iliac crest and that weighed 7200 g at postmortem examination; his liver function tests showed a BSP of 17% with only moderately elevated alkaline phosphatase level. Others with significant liver involvement had normal liver function tests in all respects.

One patient with amyloid (small amounts) proved by biopsy had a normal liver scan, whereas six others were abnormal. The scans generally showed a diffuse decrease in uptake, but there was some variation.

Despite the above comments, detailed liver function tests showed mild abnormalities in 75% of cases. Most frequent were elevation of alkaline phosphatase level, BSP retention, and prolongation of the prothrombin time. Occasionally, there was minor elevation in the levels of serum glutamic-oxaloacetic transaminase, lactic dehydrogenase and bilirubin. Serum albumin was often low (in 75% of the patients tested); however, this was nearly always associated with elevated levels of serum cholesterol and renal failure. We found in a more recent analysis that 4 of 78 patients (5.3%) had severe intrahepatic cholestasis.[98] Data were reviewed on an additional eight patients recorded in the literature. Criteria for inclusion were a tissue diagnosis of amyloidosis, a serum bilirubin level greater than 5 mg/dl, histopathologic evidence of cholestasis, and no extrahepatic biliary obstruction. Hepatomegaly was present in 12 patients (100%), ascites in 9 (75%), and pruritus in 8 (67%). Serum bilirubin ranged from 9 mg to 44 mg/dl, serum alkaline phosphatase was markedly increased in 10 patients (83%), and hypercholesterolemia occurred in 7 (58%). Microscopic examination of the liver revealed diffuse amyloid deposition and compression atrophy in 12 patients (100%). The amyloid was prominent in the periportal regions, and some sparing of the centrilobular areas was observed. Bile thrombi and bilirubin staining of hepatocytes were predominantly in the centrilobular zones. Liver cell necrosis, fibrosis, and nodularity were uncommon.

The pathogenesis of intrahepatic cholestasis is these patients was probably related to the deposition of amyloid in a manner that interferes with the passage of bile from the canaliculi or the small intrahepatic bile ducts to the septal bile ducts. Obstructive jaundice carried a poor prognosis. Of 12 patients, 9 (75%) died of renal failure 3 weeks to 2 months after the onset of jaundice. Amyloidosis should be considered in the patient with unexplained in-

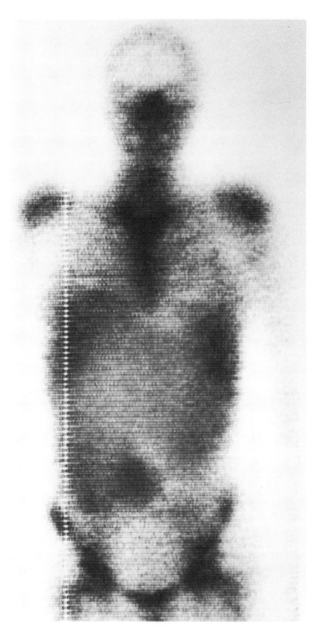

Fig. 32-7. Technetium-99m-pyrophosphate bone scan (anterior view) of a 47-year-old woman with primary amyloidosis. Note the intense diffuse hepatic uptake of radionuclide.

ination. All 54 had some amyloid present either in the parenchyma or about blood vessels. Information on clinical estimation of liver size was available in 42 patients, and in 39 hepatomegaly was believed to be present. Among the remaining 19 patients in whom no tissue was available, hepatomegaly was present in only 12.

Clinical stigmata of liver disease were unusual in this series of patients. Palmar erythema occurred in two cases,

trahepatic cholestasis, and liver tissue should be stained with Congo red and viewed under polarized microscopy.

In the group of patients in whom tissue histology was available, only a rough correlation could be made between the degree of liver involvement with amyloid and the liver function test abnormalities. Elevated BSP and alkaline phosphatase levels and slightly prolonged prothrombin time occurred in 50% of the patients in whom only blood vessels were involved with amyloid. More of the patients with marked parenchymal infiltration had the same abnormalities (80%–90% of those tested). Patients with either primary or secondary disease had patterns of parenchymal or blood vessel involvement that were indistinguishable from each other except for the above-noted rare intrahepatic cholestasis.

REFERENCES

1. Anders R et al: Amyloid-related serum protein SAA from three animal species: Comparison with human SAA. J Immunol 118:229, 1977
2. Atkinson AJ: Clinical pathological conference. Gastroenterology 7:477, 1946
3. Bannick EG et al: Diffuse amyloidosis. Three unusual cases: A clinical and pathologic study. Arch Intern Med 51:978, 1933
4. Bari WA et al: Electron microscopy and electron microscopic autoradiography of splenic cell cultures from mice with amyloidosis. Lab Invest 20:234, 1969
5. Battaglia S: Elektronenoptische Untersuchungen am Leberamyloid in der Maus. Beitr Pathol Anat 126:300, 1962
6. Bausserman LL et al: Heterogeneity of human serum amyloid A proteins. J Exp Med 152:641, 1980
7. Benditt EP et al: The major proteins of human and monkey amyloid substance: Common properties including unusual N-terminal amino acid sequences. FEBS Lett 19:169, 1971
8. Benditt EP et al: Amyloid protein SAA is associated with high density lipoprotein from human serum. Proc Natl Acad Sci USA 74:4025, 1977
9. Benditt EP et al: Amyloid protein SAA is an apoprotein of mouse plasma high density lipoprotein. Proc Natl Acad Sci USA 76:4092, 1979
10. Bennhold H: Eine spezifische Amyloidfarbung mit Kongorot. Munchen Med Wochenschr 69:1537, 1922
11. Benson MD et al: Synthesis and secretion of serum amyloid protein A (SAA) by hepatocytes in mice treated with casein. J Immunol 124:495, 1980
12. Benson MD et al: Identification of a new amino acid substitution in plasma prealbumin associated with hereditary amyloidosis. Clin Res 33:590A, 1985
13. Bero GL: Amyloidosis: Its clinical and pathologic manifestations, with a report of 12 cases. Ann Intern Med 46:931, 1957
14. Berris B, Wolff HJ: Primary systemic amyloidosis with jaundice and hemorrhage. Gastroenterology 13:67, 1949
15. Block PJ et al: The identity of a peritoneal fluid immunoglobulin light chain and the amyloid fibril in primary amyloidosis. Arthritis Rheum 19:755, 1976
16. Bonar L et al: Characterization of the amyloid fibril as a cross-β protein. Proc Soc Exp Biol Med 131:1373, 1969
17. Brandt K et al: A clinical analysis of the course and prognosis of 42 patients with amyloidosis. Am J Med 44:955, 1968
18. Briggs GW: Amyloidosis. Ann Intern Med 55:943, 1961
19. Bürgi W: Primäre und sekundäre Leberamyloidose. Dtsch Arch F Klin Med 207:585, 1962
20. Caesar R: Die Feinstruktor von Milz und leber bei experimentellen Amyloid Z. Zellforsch. Mikroskop. Anat Abt Histochem 52:653, 1960
21. Carroll J et al: Les formes hepatique de l'amylose. Rev Med Chir Mal Foie 31:1, 1956
22. Castleman B: Case records of the Massachusetts General Hospital. Case 44461. N Engl J Med 259:979, 1958
23. Cathcart ES et al: Immunoglobulins and amyloidosis. Am J Med 52:93, 1972
24. Chopra S et al: Hepatic amyloidosis: A histopathologic analysis of primary (AL) and secondary (AA) forms. Am J Pathol 115:186, 1984
25. Cohen AS: The constitution and genesis of amyloid. In Ritcher GW, Epstein MA (eds): International Review of Experimental Pathology, vol 4, pp 159–243. New York, Academic Press, 1965
26. Cohen AS: Preliminary chemical analysis of partially purified amyloid fibrils. Lab Invest 15:66, 1966
27. Cohen AS: Amyloidosis. N Engl J Med 277:522, 574, 628, 1967
28. Cohen AS: Chemical and immunological characterization of 2 components of amyloid. In Balacz EA (ed): Chemistry and Molecular Biology of the Intercellular Matrix, vol 3, pp 1517–1536. New York, Academic Press, 1970
29. Cohen AS: Inherited systemic amyloidosis. In Stanbury JB et al (eds): Metabolic Basis of Inherited Disease, 3rd ed. New York, McGraw-Hill, 1972
30. Cohen AS, Calkins E: Electron microscopic observations on a fibrous component in amyloid of diverse origins. Nature 183:1202, 1959
31. Cohen AS, Cathcart ES: Casein-induced experimental amyloidosis: I. Review of cellular and immunologic aspects. In Bajusz E, Jasmin G (eds): Methods and Achievements in Experimental Pathology. Montreal, Karger, 1972
32. Cohen AS, Skinner M: Amyloidosis of the liver. In Schiff LB (ed): Diseases of the Liver, p 1003. Philadelphia, JB Lippincott, 1976
33. Cohen AS, Skinner M: Diagnosis of amyloidosis. In Cohen AS (ed): Laboratory Diagnostic Methods in the Rheumatic Disease, 3rd ed, pp 377–399. New York, Grune and Stratton, 1985
34. Cohen AS et al: A study of the fine structure of the amyloid associated with familial Mediterranean fever. Am J Pathol 41:567, 1962
35. Cohen AS et al: The light and electron microscopic autoradiographic demonstration of local amyloid formation in spleen explants. Am J Pathol 47:1079, 1965
36. Cohen AS et al: Renal transplantation in 2 cases of amyloidosis. Lancet 2:513, 1971
37. Cohen AS et al: Nomenclature. In Wegelius O, Pasternack A (eds): Amyloidosis, p IX. New York, Academic Press, 1976
38. Connors LH et al: Nephelometric measurement of human serum prealbumin and correlation with acute phase proteins, CRP and SAA: Results in familial amyloid polyneuropathy. J Lab Clin Med 104:538, 1984
39. Cooper JH: An evaluation of current methods for the diagnostic histochemistry of amyloid. J Clin Pathol 22:410, 1969
40. Czyzyk A, Caroli J: Primary hepatic amyloidosis: I. Clinical

study with presentation of 6 cases. Rev Intern Hepat 11: 589, 1961

41. Dahlin DC: Secondary amyloidosis. Ann Intern Med 31: 105, 1949

42. Dahlin DC: Primary amyloidosis, with report of 6 cases. Am J Pathol 25:105, 1949

43. Dahlin DC: Classification and general aspects of amyloidosis. Med Clin North Am 34:1107, 1950

44. Dwulet FE, Benson MD: Primary structure of an amyloid prealbumin and its plasma precursor in a heredofamilial polyneuropathy of Swedish origin. Proc Natl Acad Sci USA 81:694, 1984

45. Eanes ED, Glenner GG: X-ray diffraction studies on amyloid filaments. J Histochem Cytochem 16:673, 1968

46. Eisen HN: Primary systemic amyloidosis. Am J Med 1: 144, 1946

47. Eriksen N et al: Mouse amyloid protein AA: Homology with nonimmunoglobulin protein of human and monkey amyloid substance. Proc Natl Acad Sci USA 73:964, 1976

48. Fett JW et al: Primary structure of the Mcg λ chain. Biochemistry 13:4102, 1974

49. Fevery J et al: Congenital dilation of the intrahepatic bile ducts associated with the development of amyloidosis. Gut 13:604, 1972

50. French SW et al: Unusual amyloid bodies in human liver. Am J Clin Pathol 75:400, 1981

51. Fruhling L et al: Sur les modifications histologiques liees a la formation des depots de substance amyloide. Etude au microscope electronique. Compt Rend Soc Biol 155:1563, 1961

52. Furie B et al: Syndrome of acquired factor X deficiency and systemic amyloidosis. N Engl J Med 297:81, 1977

53. Gafni J, Sohar E: Rectal biopsy for diagnosis of amyloidosis. Am J Med Sci 240:332, 1960

54. Glenner GG et al: Amyloid fibril proteins: Proof of homology with immunoglobulin light chains by sequence analyses. Science 172:1150, 1971

55. Goldberg S: Primary amyloidosis: Report of a case and review of the literature. S Afr Med J 24:801, 1950

56. Gorevic PO et al: The amino acid sequence of duck amyloid A (AA) protein. J Immunol 118:1113, 1977

57. Graham W: Primary amyloidosis simulating cirrhosis of the liver. Can Med Assoc J 66:58, 1952

58. Gregg JA et al: Ascites in systemic amyloidosis. Arch Intern Med 116:605, 1965

59. Hallen J, Rudin R: Peri-collagenous amyloidosis: A study of 51 cases. Acta Med Scand 179:483, 1966

60. Heller H et al: Amyloidosis: Its differentiation into peri-reticulin and pericollagen types. J Pathol Bacteriol 88:15, 1964

61. Hermodson MA et al: Amino acid sequence of monkey amyloid protein A. Biochemistry 11:2934, 1972

62. Hurd WW, Katholi RE: Acquired functional asplenia. Arch Intern Med 140:844, 1980

63. Ishihara T et al: Pathological study on amyloidosis—the fine structure of amyloid-laden liver as revealed by freeze-etching. Acta Pathol Jpn 26:357, 1976

64. Itescu S: Hepatic amyloidosis. Arch Intern Med 144:2257, 1984

65. Kanel GC et al: Globular hepatic amyloid: An unusual morphologic presentation. Hepatology 1:647, 1981

66. Kapp JP: Hepatic amyloidosis with portal hypertension. JAMA 191:497, 1965

67. King LS: Atypical amyloid disease; with observations on a new silver stain for amyloid. Am J Pathol 24:1095, 1948

68. Kleckner MS Jr, Magidson J: Amyloidosis of the liver: Correlation of clinical and pathologic features. Gastroenterology 29:56, 1955

69. Kuhlback B, Wegelius O: Secondary amyloidosis: A study of clinical and pathological findings. Acta Med Scand 180: 737, 1966

70. Lavie G et al: The degradation of serum amyloid A protein by peripheral blood monocytes. J Exp Med 148:1020, 1978

71. Levin M et al: The amino acid sequence of a major nonimmunoglobulin component of some amyloid fibrils. J Clin Invest 51:2773, 1972

72. Levine RA: Amyloid disease of liver: Correlation of clinical, functional and amorphologic features in 47 patients. Am J Med 33:349, 1962

73. Levy M et al: Intrahepatic obstructive jaundice due to amyloidosis of the liver. Gastroenterology 61:234, 1971

74. Levy M et al: The liver in amyloidosis. Isr J Med Sci 8: 1848, 1972

75. Lian JB et al: Fractionation of primary amyloid fibrils: Characterization and chemical interaction of the subunits. Biochem Biophys Acta 491:167, 1977

76. Libbey CA et al: Familial amyloid polyneuropathy: Demonstration of prealbumin in a kinship of German/English ancestry with onset in the seventh decade. Am J Med 76: 18, 1984

77. Livni N et al: Unusual amyloid bodies in human liver. Isr J Med Sci 13:1163, 1977

78. Lubarsch O: Zur Kenntnis Ungewoehnlicher Amyloid Ablagerungen. Virchows Arch Pathol Anat 271:867, 1929

79. Manitz G, Themann H: Elektronenmikroskopischer Beitrag zur Feinstruktur menschlichen leberamyloids. Beitr Pathol Anat UZ Allg Pathol 128:103, 1962

80. Mathews WH: Primary systemic amyloidosis. Am J Med Sci 228:317, 1954

81. Melato M et al: Different morphologic aspects and clinical features in massive hepatic amyloidosis. Digestion 29:138, 1984

82. Melkebeke P et al: Huge hepatomegaly, jaundice and portal hypertension due to amyloidosis of the liver. Digestion 20: 351, 1980

83. Mir-Madjlessi SH et al: Cholestatic jaundice associated with primary amyloidosis. Clev Clinic Q 39:167, 1972

84. Missmahl HP, Hartwig M: Polarisationsoptische untersuchungen an der amyloid-substanz. Virchows Arch Pathol Anat 324:489, 1953

85. Moschcowitz E: The clinical aspects of amyloidosis. Ann Intern Med 10:73, 1936

86. Oliveira EB et al: Primary structure of C-reactive protein. J Biol Chem 254:489, 1979

87. Orloff J, Felder L: Primary systemic amyloidosis: Jaundice as a rare accompaniment. Am J Med Sci 212:275, 1946

88. Pepys MB et al: Bind of serum amyloid P. component (SAP) by amyloid fibrils. Clin Exp Immunol 37:284, 1979

89. Pfeifer U et al: Shedding of peripheral cytoplasm: A mechanism of liver cell atrophy in human amyloidosis. Virchows Arch Cell Pathol 29:229, 1979

90. Pocock DS, Dickens J: Paramyloidosis with diabetes mellitus and gastrointestinal hemorrhage. N Engl J Med 248: 359, 1953

91. Pras M et al: Idiopathic AL-(Kappa iv) amyloidosis presenting as giant hepatomegaly. Isr J Med Sci 18:866, 1982

92. Pras M et al: A variant of prealbumin from amyloid fibrils in familial polyneuropathy of Jewish origin. J Exp Med 154:989, 1981

93. Putnam FW et al: Amino acid sequence of a Bence Jones

protein from a case of primary amyloidosis. Biochemistry 12:3763, 1973

94. Reimann HA et al: Primary amyloidosis limited to tissue of mesenchymal origin. Am J Pathol 11:977, 1935

95. Rokitansky C: Handbuch der Pathologischen Anatomie, vol 3, p 311. Vienna, Braumuller & Seidel, 1842

96. Rosenblatt MB: The clinical manifestations of amyloidosis. Ann Intern Med 8:678, 1934

97. Rosenthal CJ et al: Isolation and partial characterization of SAA—and amyloid-related protein from human serum. J Immunol 116:1415, 1976

98. Rubinow A et al: Severe intrahepatic cholestasis in primary amyloidosis. Am J Med 64:937, 1978

99. Rukavina JG et al: Primary systemic amyloidosis: A review and experimental, genetic and clinical study of 29 cases with particular emphasis on the familial form. Medicine 35:239, 1956

100. Sanders R, Child CG III: Primary amyloidosis with jaundice. JAMA 174:1202, 1960

101. Saraiva MJM et al: Amyloid fibril protein in familial amyloidotic polyneuropathy, Portuguese type: Definition of molecular abnormality in transthyretin (prealbumin). J Clin Invest 74:104, 1984

102. Shirahama T, Cohen AS: High resolution electron microscopic analysis of the amyloid fibril. J Cell Biol 33:679, 1967

103. Shirahama T, Cohen AS: The fine structure of the glomerulus in human and experimental renal amyloidosis. Am J Pathol 51:869, 1967

104. Shirahama T, Cohen AS: Blockage of amyloid induction by colchicine in an animal model. J Exp Med 140:1102, 1974

105. Silverman SL et al: A pathogenetic role for polymorphonuclear leukocytes in the synthesis and degradation of SAA protein. In Glenner GG et al (eds): Amyloid and Amyloidosis, pp 420–425. Amsterdam, Excerpta Medica 1980

106. Skinner M, Cohen AS: N-terminal amino acid analysis of the amyloid fibril protein. Fed Proc 27:476, 1968

107. Skinner M, Cohen AS: N-terminal amino acid analysis of the amyloid fibril protein. Biochem Acta 236:183, 1971

108. Skinner M, Cohen AS: The prealbumin nature of the amyloid protein in familial amyloid polyneuropathy (FAP): Swedish variety. Biochem Biophys Res Commun 99:1326, 1981

109. Skinner M et al: P. component (pentagonal unit) of amyloid: Isolation, characterization and sequence analysis. J Lab Clin Med 84:604, 1974

110. Skinner M et al: Isolation and identification by sequence analysis of experimentally induced guinea pig amyloid fibrils. J Exp Med 140:871, 1974

111. Skinner M et al: Amyloid fibril protein related to immunoglobulin lambda chains. J Immunol 114:1433, 1975

112. Skinner M et al: Murine amyloid protein AA in casein-induced experimental amyloidosis. Lab Invest 36:420, 1977

113. Skinner M et al: Serum amyloid P-component levels in amyloidosis, connective tissue diseases, infection and malignancy as compared to normal serum. J Lab Clin Med 94:633, 1979

114. Skinner M et al: Studies of amyloid protein AP. In Glenner GG et al (eds): Amyloid and Amyloidosis. Amsterdam, Excerpta Medica, 1980

115. Skinner M et al: The calcium dependent interaction of blood clotting factors with primary amyloid fibrils. In Glenner GG et al (eds): Amyloid and Amyloidosis, pp 361–365. Amsterdam, Excerpta Medica, 1980

116. Skinner M et al: Characterization of P-component (AP) isolated from amyloidotic tissue: Half-life studies of human and murine AP. Ann NY Acad Sci 389:190, 1982

117. Skinner MS et al: Electron microscopic observations of early amyloidosis in human liver. Gastroenterology 50:243, 1966

118. Sohr E et al: Familial Mediterranean fever: A survey of 470 cases and review of the literature. Am J Med 43:227, 1967

119. Sorenson GD et al: Experimental amyloidosis: II. Light and electron microscopic observations of liver. Am J Pathol 44:629, 1964

120. Sorenson GD et al: Experimental amyloidosis. In Bajusz E, Jasmin G (eds): Methods and Achievements in Experimental Pathology, vol I, pp 514–543. New York, S Karger, 1966

121. Spain D, Riley R: Jaundice in amyloidosis of the liver. Am J Clin Pathol 14:284, 1944

122. Stauffer MH et al: Amyloidosis: Diagnosis with needle biopsy of the liver in 18 patients. Gastroenterology 41:92, 1961

123. Symmers W St C: Amyloidosis: Five cases of primary generalized amyloidosis and some other unusual cases. J Clin Pathol 9:212, 1956

124. Symmers W St C: Primary amyloidosis: A review. J Clin Pathol 9:187, 1956

125. Takahashi M et al: Ultrastructural evidence for the synthesis of serum amyloid A protein by murine hepatocytes. Lab Invest 52:220, 1985

126. Tatsuta E et al: Different regulatory mechanisms for serum amyloid A and serum amyloid P synthesis by cultured mouse hepatocytes. J Biol Chem 258:5414, 1983

127. Tawara S et al: Amyloid fibril protein in type 1 familial amyloidotic polyneuropathy in Japanese. J Lab Clin Med 98:811, 1981

128. Terry WD et al: Structural identity of Bence Jones and amyloid fibril proteins in a patient with plasma cell dyscrasia and amyloidosis. J Clin Invest 52:1276, 1973

129. Thiery JP, Caroli J: Etude au microscope electronique de l'amylose hepatique primaire de l'homme. Sem Hop Paris 37:29, 1961

130. Tiber AM et al: Hepatic function in patients with amyloidosis. Arch Intern Med 68:309, 1941

131. Totterman KJ, Manninen V: Tumefactive liver infiltration in amyloidosis. Ann Clin Res 14:11, 1982

132. Trieger N et al: Gingival biopsy as a diagnostic aid in amyloid disease. Arch Oral Biol 1:187, 1959

133. Uchino F: Pathological study on amyloidosis: Role of reticuloendothelial cells in inducing amyloidosis. Acta Pathol Jpn 17:49, 1967

134. Volwiler W, Jones CM: The diagnostic and therapeutic value of liver biopsies: With special reference to trocar biopsy. N Engl J Med 237:651, 1947

135. Waldenstrom H: On the formation and disappearance of amyloid in man. Acta Chir Scand 63:479, 1928

136. Westermark P et al: Demonstration of protein AA in subcutaneous fat tissue obtained by fine needle biopsy. Ann Rheum Dis 38:68, 1979

137. Wollaeger EE: Primary systemic amyloidosis with symptoms and signs of liver disease: Diagnosis by liver biopsy. Med Clin North Am 34:1113, 1950

138. Yaghoobian J et al: Angiographic findings in liver amyloidosis. Radiology 136:332, 1980

139. Yood RA et al: Soft tissue uptake of bone seeking radionuclide in amyloidosis. J Rheumatology 8:760, 1981

140. Zetzel L: Hepatomegaly with jaundice due to primary amyloidosis. Gastroenterology 8:783, 1947

chapter 33
Neoplasms of the Liver

HUGH A. EDMONDSON† and JOHN R. CRAIG

Over the past 20 years, interest in liver tumors has increased because of identification of new etiologic factors and an apparent increase in the frequency of hepatocellular carcinoma (HCC) in many parts of the world. The occurrence of neoplasms related to hepatitis B virus (HBV) after exposure to vinyl chloride, the use of oral contraceptives, and the injection of thorotrast many years ago have all contributed to the increased interest in the subject. New diagnostic methods and more radical approaches to treatment have led to considerable progress.

It is important for all physicians interested in liver disease to have some understanding of the gross features of hepatic neoplasms and of lesions that simulate tumors. Angiograms, scans, echograms, and computerized tomography (CT) are all helpful in determining the number, size, and location of tumors of the liver, but gross and microscopic pathology are necessary for final diagnosis. Upon inspection, the following features should be considered: How many distinct lesions are there? Is umbilication present? Is the tumor hard, soft, or cystic? What is its color? Are there tumors in other organs?

Each of the above features is important. Adenomas are usually solitary but may be multiple; HCC is usually a single mass when it develops in the noncirrhotic liver but multinodular in cirrhosis. Metastatic carcinoma and sarcoma usually consist of multiple nodules, but either may be large and solitary. Focal nodular hyperplasia (FNH) is ordinarily a single mass.

Metastatic carcinoma is often umbilicated, whereas adenoma, HCC, and sarcoma are not. Cholangiocarcinoma may form a large single mass but is never smooth. Sclerosing carcinomas, sarcomas, and FNH range between firm and hard; HCC, most metastatic carcinomas, and adenomas are palpably softer. Cyst formation occurs in the solitary nonparasitic cyst, polycystic disease, and multilocular cystadenoma. The color is helpful in diagnosing melanomas, choriocarcinomas, hemangiomas, and bile-forming HCC. A clinicopathologic classification including both tumors and tumor-like conditions is used in this chapter to bring together lesions with a similar gross appearance at surgery or autopsy and those that may yield similar results on ultrasound and liver scan. Some tumors can be distinguished from one another by angiographic or other *in vivo* studies. This chapter is concerned primarily with the frequency of neoplasms of the liver and

† Deceased.

the clinical problems related to them. Our classification of liver tumors will be published elsewhere.[72] The natural history of liver tumors has been reviewed.[40]

METASTATIC TUMORS OF THE LIVER

Among all malignant tumors of the liver, metastatic neoplasms constitute by far the largest number. The reasons for this are rather complex and have been the subject of numerous articles and reviews.[251] There is evidence that metastases result from the growth of subpopulations of specialized cells that are shed into the circulation by primary tumors. There are probably many factors concerned with the trapping followed by growth of malignant cells within the environment of the human liver.

During the 62-year period from 1918 to 1980, 94,556 autopsies were performed at the Los Angeles County-University of Southern California Medical Center (LAC-USCMC) and the John Wesley County Hospital (JWCH). In 19,208, 20.4% of the cases, there was an extrahepatic primary malignant tumor. In 7299, 38% of those with tumors, hepatic metastases were present. Table 33-1 shows the frequency of metastases in 17 of the more common tumors. Metastatic carcinoma is frequently diagnosed on liver biopsy. Of the total liver biopsies submitted to us from 1960 to 1980, 1025, or 3.8%, included metastatic carcinoma.

Clinical Features

In our series, some 52% of the patients dying with metastatic carcinoma to liver had some hepatic signs or symptoms; in 31% of those with hepatic metastases at autopsy, the only physical sign was hepatomegaly. Although 14.5% of the patients were icteric at death, 90% of the icteric patients had one of the 11 tumors listed in Table 33-2. The cause of jaundice differed; duct obstruction was the most important in patients with carcinoma of the pancreas, gallbladder, or bile ducts (Table 33-2).

Among all patients with hepatic metastases who were jaundiced during their final hospitalization, 21% had pancreatic carcinoma as the primary tumor. This equals the percentage with jaundice from colon carcinoma, even though liver involvement by metastatic colon carcinoma is more common than metastatic pancreatic carcinoma (see Table 33-1). Of those with pancreatic carcinoma

TABLE 33-1.   Seventeen Most Common Nonlymphoma Metastatic Malignant Tumors in Liver and Development of Jaundice

TUMOR	NUMBER OF PRIMARY TUMORS	NUMBER WITH HEPATIC METASTASES	PERCENTAGE WITH HEPATIC METASTASES	PERCENTAGE OF PATIENTS WITH HEPATIC METASTASES WHO WERE ICTERIC
Bronchogenic	682	285	41.8	9
Colon	323	181	56.0	34
Pancreas	179	126	70.4	51
Breast	218	116	53.2	30
Stomach	159	70	44.0	60
Unknown primary	102	59	57.0	35
Ovary	97	47	48.0	0
Prostate	333	42	12.6	0
Gallbladder	49	38	77.6	60
Cervix	107	34	31.7	10
Kidney	142	34	23.9	15
Melanoma	50	25	50.0	13
Urinary bladder and ureter	66	25	37.9	11
Esophagus	66	20	30.3	29
Testis	45	20	44.4	14
Endometrial	54	17	31.5	<20
Thyroid	70	12	17.1	14

(Data obtained at Los Angeles County University of Southern California Medical Center [1970–1979] and John Wesley County Hospital [1960–1976].)

metastatic to liver, 34% were icteric at the time of final hospital admission. In contrast, bronchogenic carcinoma, four times more common than pancreatic carcinoma and one and one-half times as common a cause of hepatic metastasis, was the cause of jaundice much less than half as often as pancreatic carcinoma.

Of the total number of patients with a malignant tumor, including all primary sites, 18% had ascites, whether or not there were hepatic metastases. Of patients with hepatic metastases from stomach, ovary, and gallbladder, 60% had ascites. When liver metastases were present, 45% of all tumors were associated with ascites. Varices were recog-

TABLE 33-2.   Metastatic Carcinoma to Liver: Relative Frequency and Cause of Icterus

PRIMARY TUMOR PER 100 ICTERIC TUMOR PATIENTS		CAUSES OF ICTERUS		
		>75% Hepatic Replacement	Duct Involvement by Tumor	<60% Hepatic Replacement, Unknown
Colon	21	86%	6%	9%
Pancreas	21	11%	45%	43%
Stomach	14	33%	11%	56%
Breast	12	72%	17%	11%
Unknown primary	9	83%	<1%	17%
Bronchogenic	8	30%	20%	50%
Gallbladder	3	21%	43%	36%
Hodgkin's	3	0	3%	97%
Bile duct	3	<1%	100%	<1%
Melanoma	1	67%	33%	<1

nized in only 1% of those with liver involvement, most frequently with the pancreas as the primary site.

Occasionally, carcinoma is first recognized by its hepatic metastases without determination of the primary site until later, possibly not until autopsy. The most common "occult" primary site is the pancreas; occasionally, asymptomatic stomach or lung carcinoma may prove to be the origin of hepatic metastases. It is very uncommon for either colon or breast to serve as occult primary sites, but liver involvement may be the first sign of recurrence in either after resection of the primary tumor. The liver is the classic recurrence site of melanoma, particularly that of ocular origin—even as late as 20 years after removal of the primary tumor.

Metastatic tumors to liver originating in some organs never give rise to hepatic symptoms, whereas others produce hepatic symptoms or jaundice with less than 60% replacement of the liver (stomach, lung). Certain tumors (colon, breast, melanoma) typically replace 90% of the liver before jaundice develops. Melanomas are associated with such minimal tissue reaction that almost complete hepatic replacement is required before hepatic symptoms develop. The liver of one patient in our series involved by melanoma weighed 9.1 kg.

The auscultation of arterial bruits over the liver that do not change character with shift of position may be helpful in identifying patients with hepatic tumor. A coexisting hepatic rub due to fibrin deposited over a subcapsular tumor focus is considered strong evidence of hepatic neoplastic involvement.[291]

Gross Appearance

Depending upon the primary source, metastases do vary with respect to size, uniformity of growth pattern, consistency, vascularity, and stromal response. They may be expansive or infiltrative. The major gross morphologic patterns are described in Table 33-3 and shown in Figure 33-1.

About one half of the patients with hepatic metastases die without hepatic signs or symptoms. Although the involvement is usually similar though less extensive than in

TABLE 33-3. Morphologic Patterns of Metastatic Tumors to Liver

	CHARACTERISTIC OF PRIMARY IN	HEPATIC SIGNS OR SYMPTOMS
1. Expanding		
a. Massive (solitary, with satellites or multiple foci)	colon gallbladder testis	+ or −
b. Uniform nodular	lung melanoma pancreas	−
2. Infiltrative		
a. Massive	lung breast pancreas urinary bladder melanoma	+ or −
b. Uniform multifocal	breast pancreas lung melanoma	−
c. Diffuse	breast pancreas lymphomas	+ or −
3. Surface spreading	colon ovary occasionally, stomach	−
4. Incidental	any	−
5. Miliary	prostate occasionally, any	−
6. Mixed or indeterminate	any	+ or −

The patterns of 1a, 1b, 2b, and 2c are shown in Figure 33-1 *A–E*.

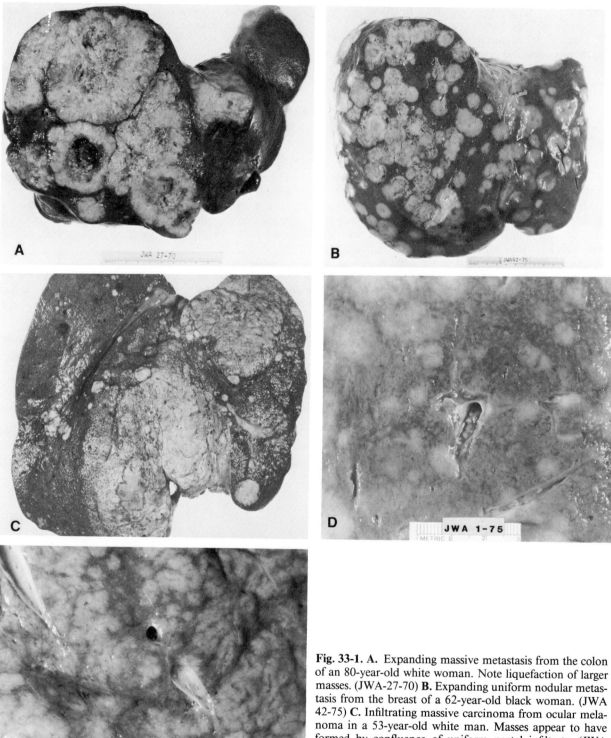

Fig. 33-1. A. Expanding massive metastasis from the colon of an 80-year-old white woman. Note liquefaction of larger masses. (JWA-27-70) **B.** Expanding uniform nodular metastasis from the breast of a 62-year-old black woman. (JWA 42-75) **C.** Infiltrating massive carcinoma from ocular melanoma in a 53-year-old white man. Masses appear to have formed by confluence of uniform portal infiltrate. (JWA 93-71) **D.** Infiltrative uniform multifocal metastases from carcinoma of pancreas in a 78-year-old black woman. (JWA 1-75) **E.** Infiltrative diffuse metastases from the breast of a 54-year-old white woman. Note that the lobular pattern of the liver is preserved. (JWA 220-65)

symptomatic patients, there may be only one or more incidental foci, too small to characterize further, or there may be a miliary pattern of 1- to 2-cm foci heavily seeding the entire liver (Fig. 33-2) or 1- to 3-cm nodules throughout. Metastases from some tumors almost never result in sufficient replacement to cause symptoms, possibly because some neoplasms may release a shower of metastases only in the preterminal state or because they do not grow well in the liver. Prostatic carcinoma is an example of a tumor that metastasizes to the liver in relatively few cases (12.6%); but even when it does, it almost never results in hepatic signs or symptoms, in spite of the long survival of prostatic carcinoma patients.

Metastatic adenocarcinomas, particularly from gallbladder and colon, are often recognizable by mucin production, which results in a glistening, often slimy, cut surface. Metastases from colon carcinoma are usually the expanding, massive type and frequently have central liquefactive necrosis (see Fig. 33-1A). Because of necrosis and fibrosis, many subcapsular tumors retract, producing an umbilicated pattern on the liver capsular surface (Fig. 33-3). The umbilication is a helpful diagnostic feature because hepatocellular carcinomas rarely, if ever, umbilicate, although umbilication is sometimes found on the surface of cholangiocarcinoma and primary carcinomas with mixed hepatocellular–cholangiolar components.

Squamous cell carcinomas often have a granular, central portion with a cheesy appearance, lacking the shiny character of most adenocarcinomas. Poorly differentiated tumors (in contrast to pleomorphic tumors) tend to be uniformly soft and like "fish flesh" (see Fig. 33-1C). Ex-

amples of the latter characteristic are seen particularly in oat cell carcinomas, non-Hodgkin's lymphomas, undifferentiated sarcomas, and seminomas.

The cut surface of hepatic metastases in liver may vary greatly in the same liver, depending upon the differences in blood supply as well as hemorrhage, necrosis, fibrosis, and cellular differentiation from one focus to another (Fig. 33-4). Choriocarcinoma, carcinoid tumors, bronchogenic carcinoma, and renal carcinomas may all have such a variable pattern.

A peculiar zone of venous stasis surrounds tumor metastases in about 25% of livers so involved. At times, the zone may be striking and up to about 1 cm wide. The congested zone is not a reflection of pressure occlusion of hepatic venous outflow, because the zones are uniformly circumferential, and either all or none of the metastatic foci in a particular liver are involved. Among the common neoplasms, this hyperemia is seen most frequently in metastatic bronchogenic carcinoma (Fig. 33-5) and least frequently in livers involved by carcinoma of the colon.

Microscopically, most metastatic tumors retain the features of the primary site, including the degree of stromal growth. For example, bronchogenic carcinoma usually excites a minimal stromal response (Fig. 33-6). Tumor cells from undifferentiated primary tumors, particularly bronchogenic oat cell carcinoma, often intermingle with the liver plates and give the appearance of blending with hepatocytes (Fig. 33-7). It has been demonstrated that it is possible for a metastatic bronchogenic cancer cell to form a desmosome at the intercellular boundary formed with an hepatocyte.[135] More commonly, however, tumor

Fig. 33-2. Miliary spread of bronchogenic carcinoma in a 52-year-old white woman. (JWA 121-76)

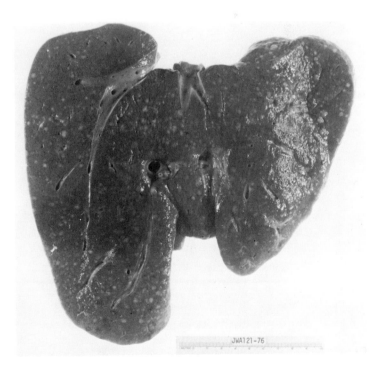

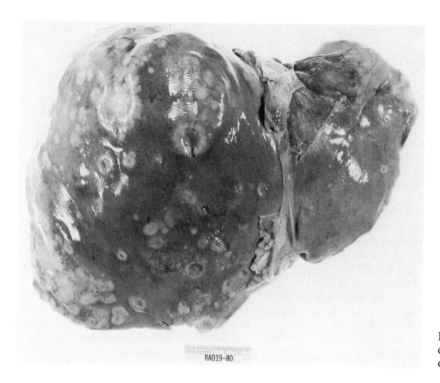

Fig. 33-3. Umbilication of metastatic carcinoma from pancreas in a 41-year-old black man. (RA 19-80).

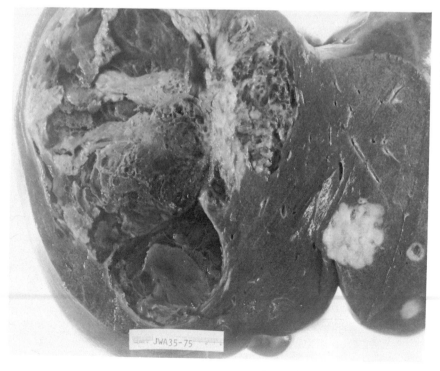

Fig. 33-4. Differences in growth pattern produce multicoloration and variation in the multiple tumor foci. From carcinoma of uncertain primary in a 37-year-old black woman. (JWA 35-75)

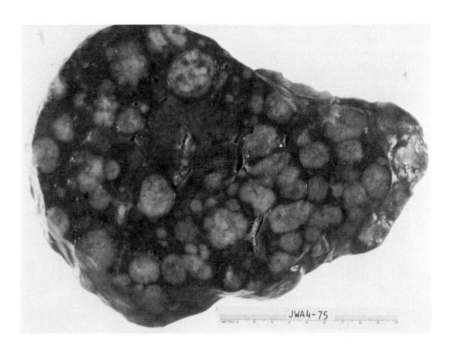

Fig. 33-5. Ring of congestion around metastatic pancreatic carcinoma in a 74-year-old white woman. (JWA 4-75)

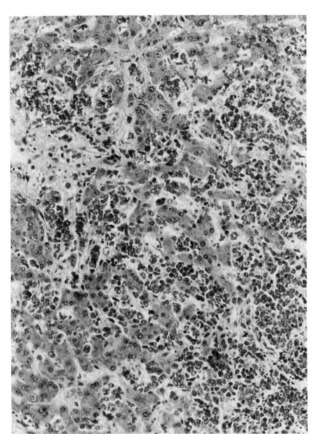

Fig. 33-6. Oat-cell carcinoma infiltrating among hepatocytes with little reaction to tumor. (JWA 111-76) (Original magnification × 216; H&E)

cells that excite little or no stromal response grow within the sinusoidal spaces while the adjacent hepatic plates atrophy and ultimately disappear. Intrasinusoidal growth may result in the tumor retaining the pattern of the sinusoidal bed, thus imparting a false appearance of a ductal carcinoma to a metastatic bronchogenic carcinoma, bladder carcinoma, or other tumor that has no organoid pattern in the primary site. Occasionally, such intrasinusoidal growth pattern of a metastatic tumor that excites little or no stromal response may result in a resemblance to hepatocellular carcinoma. Malignant melanoma on occasion produces such a pattern (Fig. 33-8).

In an opposite type of stromal response that usually develops with metastatic carcinoma of the pancreas or breast ductal origin, an intense fibrous or sclerosing reaction occurs around all of the tumor acini. This reaction often results in wide separation of the ductal elements by collagen, leading to dense scarification.

Microscopically, metastatic foci are usually poorly delineated because there is no barrier between tumor and liver. In most metastatic colon carcinomas, a thin collagenous pseudocapsule is often situated between the tumor margin and compressed liver but does not surround individual tumor glands or ducts.

Hepatic metastases occasionally lead to tumor thrombi that occlude the portal or hepatic veins. Nontumor thrombi of the small intrahepatic portal vein radicals may also occur. When the hepatic veins are involved, there is usually abdominal pain, ascites, and massive hepatomegaly. Successful surgery has been performed on some of these patients.[91]

According to Willis, metastases that penetrate the large portal veins provide a mechanism for dissemination throughout peripheral portal branches. Similar growth

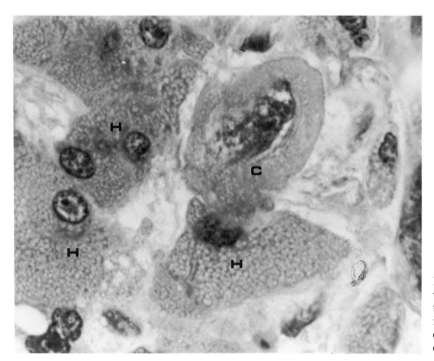

Fig. 33-7. Blending of the tumor cells with the hepatocytes may occur, particularly with bronchogenic carcinoma. H, hepatocyte; C, carcinoma cell. (JWA 111-76) (Original magnification × 2160; H&E)

within the hepatic veins is a source of extensive pulmonary metastases.[355]

Calcification occurs in a small percentage of the tumors of patients with metastatic liver disease. Usually, such calcification is radiologically detectable.[143] Some metastatic tumors, particularly mucinous adenocarcinoma of the colon, have a tendency to undergo calcification. Microscopically, the calcification is in the mucinous or necrotic centers of the deposits. The presence of necrosis, mucin, and phosphatase activity has been considered in the etiology of calcification.[110]

In recent years there has been a more aggressive approach to the surgical treatment of secondary tumors of the liver.[199] Wedge resection, segmentectomy, lobectomy, and even hepatectomy have been performed for both solitary and multiple tumors. The long-term survival of over 10 years is not unusual. The survival ratio of patients with multiple hepatic metastases is similar to that of those with isolated metastases.

Vascular Supply

The blood supply to metastatic tumors in the liver is arterial, forming the basis for certain modes of therapy of metastatic carcinoma, including arterial ligation, arterial embolization, arterial chemotherapeutic perfusion, and arterial ligation followed by portal vein chemotherapeutic infusion.[166] Apparently, hepatic metastases from cancer originating in the splanchnic bed initially derive their blood supply from the portal vein. As the metastatic nodule grows, the blood supply becomes progressively arterial.

After arterial ligation has been performed as a therapeutic measure, the blood supply reverts to portal origin.[323]

Duct Involvement by Tumor

Although tumor metastases to periportal lymph nodes is often suggested as a cause of jaundice in the 14.5% of terminal cancer patients who become icteric, in only rare instances can the cause be attributed to node involvement, despite the fact that node metastases are common. The causes of jaundice in 191 icteric patients with metastatic carcinoma to the liver are listed in Table 33-2. The majority of patients with carcinoma of breast or colon were jaundiced when over 75% of the liver was replaced. Patients with carcinoma of the lung or stomach often had jaundice when 50% or less of the liver was involved. Gallbladder and pancreatic carcinoma involve the biliary tract by direct invasion, but metastasis to the extrahepatic duct wall with duct obstruction occurs most often with bronchogenic carcinoma and melanomas.

Metastatic carcinoma of the breast may involve the wall of the common duct at any point from the hilum of the liver to the head of the pancreas, often producing jaundice.[78,248,258] The point of obstruction is often obvious by the use of percutaneous cholangiography. The liver is usually involved either by small deposits or extensive metastatic disease. Prognosis is poor in these patients.

Lymphoma, Leukemia

The liver is frequently involved by lymphomatous disorders, but only rarely is the initial diagnosis made on

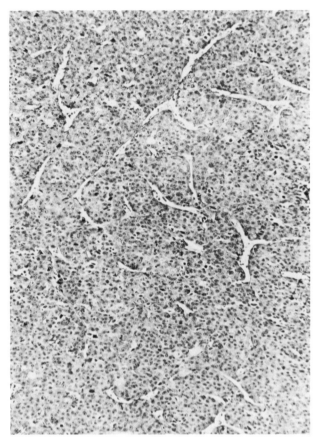

Fig. 33-8. Metastatic melanoma from a 65-year-old woman simulating the trabecular growth of hepatocellular carcinoma. (LUS 3148-78) (Original manuscript × 130; H&E)

liver biopsy. In liver biopsies of patients with untreated lymphoma, about 15% to 25% of those with histiocytic lymphoma and a similar percentage of those with lymphocytic lymphoma have hepatic infiltration, in contrast to only 7.8% of those with Hodgkin's disease.[88,276,327] In our material, 50% of patients with lymphomas had hepatic involvement at autopsy; 28% had nodular or mass lesions and 72% infiltrative lesions.

Lymphoma and lymphocytic leukemia first involve the lymphoid tissue in the portal areas, which becomes tightly packed with monotonously similar cells; the portal collagenous component becomes effaced, leaving the arteriole, portal vein, and bile duct afloat in a crowded sea of lymphocytes or histiocytes. The portal area expands, but the limiting plate remains intact until late in the course of the untreated disease, when a flow of lymphocytes into the parenchyma sometimes occurs. Nodules apparently develop from confluence of portal areas. Chemotherapy often causes resolution of lymphomatous infiltrate. Liver biopsies in partially treated patients or patients going into relapse are particularly difficult to evaluate because the portal infiltrate includes several cell types and no longer has the uniformity characteristic of that seen in the untreated disease. The hepatic sinusoids may be packed with abnormal cells during a leukemic phase or, in other cases, contain only sparse lymphosarcoma cells.

In hairy cell leukemia, the circulating histiocytes have tiny cytoplasmic projections that first adhere to the sinusoidal lining cells, then insinuate their cytoplasmic processes through the network of endothelial pores (Fig. 33-9) and ultimately displace and replace the lining cells. The replacement phenomena may produce pseudosinusoids in liver and spleen.[206]

Patients with mycosis fungoides or the Sézary syndrome (shown to be T-cell lymphomas[37,173] and appropriately renamed *cutaneous T-cell lymphomas* [CTCL],[173]) have been shown to have hepatic involvement in 45% at autopsy[79,168,170,261] and in 14% to 16% by liver biopsy.[111,125,233] Hepatic involvement consists of irregular involvement of some of the portal areas by loosely arranged convoluted lymphocytes mixed with other lymphoid elements rather than by tightly packed monotonously similar cells. Other portal areas or parts of the portal area are free of involvement. In addition to portal changes, focal punched-out lesions within the lobules contain an aggregated mixture of convoluted lymphocytes, histiocytes, normal-appearing lymphocytes, and even plasma cells. In one study, 64% of liver biopsies of patients with CTCL, although considered nondiagnostic, nonetheless included scattered foci of convoluted cell aggregates in either sinusoids or portal areas. Epithelioid granulomas were found in 20%.[219]

Patients with lymphomatous liver disease have an increased incidence of chronic B viral disease and chronic non-A, non-B disease. Persistent hepatitis is reported in 19% and chronic active hepatitis in 4.2% of lymphoma patients.[276] Most of the hepatitis infection is now of the non-A, non-B type. Chronic forms of hepatitis type B have been decreased with appropriate screening of blood-donor source. Siderosis is common in hepatocytes of lymphoma patients, particularly in those with marrow involvement and chronic anemia. Patients with non–iron deficient chronic anemia absorb increased amounts of iron, which become deposited in hepatocytes. Transfusions, hemolysis, and hepatocyte necrosis, also common in the lymphoma patient, result in Kupffer cell iron deposition.

It has been suggested that patients with chronic liver disease have an increased tendency to develop lymphoma.[207] The reverse, chronic liver disease developing in patients with lymphomas, has long been recognized as a potential sequela of posttransfusion hepatitis.

Hepatic involvement has been observed in 7.8% of initial liver biopsies of patients with Hodgkin's disease,[276] but, in our material, 72% had liver involvement at autopsy. Liver and spleen involvement occurs together, with rare exceptions.[89]

Although nonspecific microscopic changes such as Kupffer cell hyperplasia, scattered focal necrosis, and even

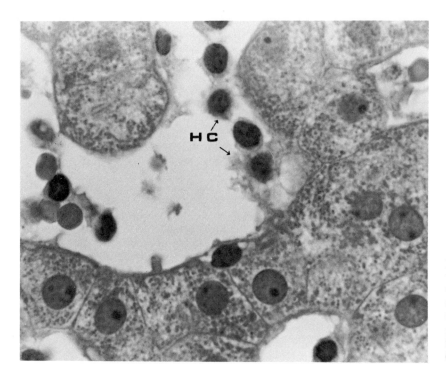

Fig. 33-9. Hairy-cell leukemia lining the sinusoids in liver of a 66-year-old white man. The processes of the circulating cells insinuate themselves through the endothelial lining and replace the lining cells. HC and arrows indicate two hairy cells. (RS 1039-79) (Original magnification × 1080; H&E)

epithelioid granulomas may be seen in Hodgkin's disease, specific hepatic involvement by Hodgkin's disease consists of a destructive lesion of the portal areas in which lymphocytes, collagen, and a background of young mesenchymal cells are present. The limiting plate is usually destroyed, and interlobular bile ducts are often effaced. The portal cellular infiltrate usually produces ductal distortion but not proliferation in anicteric patients, whereas in those with icterus, there is collagenous deposition and ductal proliferation.[42] Reed–Sternberg (R–S) cells are sparse in liver biopsies, but primitive reticulum cells, some with prominent nucleoli, and eosinophils may be numerous. In advanced disease, the portal structures may be destroyed as the widened portal infiltrate becomes confluent. At autopsy, R–S cells are often abundant.

Icterus is reported in 13% to 14% of patients with Hodgkin's disease.[240] It was present in 32% of our patients by time of death. The most common cause of jaundice is the widespread portal destruction at the lobular level as described above. A second cause is Hodgkin's involvement around and in the wall of the major duct structures. Such involvement produces a radiologic pattern resembling that of hilar cholangiocarcinoma. The involvement usually extends intrahepatically about major ducts. We have found this in only 3% of our patients. A third, the most puzzling type of icterus, occurs in a small number of patients with episodes of unexplained jaundice on more than one occasion, even before recognition of Hodgkin's disease. On liver biopsies, only cholestasis is found, without portal reaction or Kupffer cell hyperplasia. The jaundice usually subsides, and the recognition of Hodgkin's disease generally is delayed until months or years after the initial episode of jaundice, in spite of vigorous diagnostic efforts to explain the cause of the jaundice.[239,245]

PRIMARY MALIGNANT TUMORS

Hepatocellular Carcinoma

Not only is HCC the most common primary malignancy in liver on a worldwide basis, but HCC has been and continues to be one of the most common malignant tumors in internal organs. This is particularly true in Africa, the Orient, and the South Pacific Islands.[7,13,22,61,96,119,254,302,304,313,337,342] The pathology and clinical aspects were well known by 1902, and as knowledge about the disease increased, it became evident that HCC arises often in a cirrhotic liver.[275] Over the last decade, there has been increased interest in HCC because of its relationship to HBV, possibly to mycotoxins, and to certain industrial agents.[43,53,65,113,126,138,149,162,172,176,210–213,241,243,255,264,297,316,318,319,325,332,342,343,359] It has long been recognized that there is a tendency for HCC to develop predominantly in male cirrhotic patients, whereas there is equal sex incidence when HCC arises in a normal liver.

Distribution and Incidence

Geographic differences in the incidence of HCC are well known, but because of problems in reporting from different countries, the statistics collected by the World

TABLE 33-4.   Incidence per 100,000 of Liver Tumor* and Cirrhosis

COUNTRY	LIVER TUMORS	CIRRHOSIS	TUMORS/ CIRRHOSIS
USA	1.4	22.5	6%
UK	1.2	3.05	39%
Australia	1.4	8.82	16%
France	7.1	48.04	14%
Italy	11.3	44.73	25%
Japan	12.2	22.36	54%

* Incidences include all primary liver tumors and liver tumors not specified.
(Aoki K: Cancer of the liver: International mortality trends. World Health Stat Rep 31:28, 1978)

Health Organization (WHO) have certain recognized deficiencies due to information available from various sources. Thus, WHO must tabulate hepatic tumors for each country into two categories: those reported as "liver cancer" and those representing "primary liver cancer plus unspecified." With the data available, WHO cannot separate HCC from peripheral cholangiocarcinoma (PCC), the latter tumor constituting an inconsequential fraction of liver cancer in countries with a high rate of HCC. However, cholangiocarcinoma may represent 25% of cases of liver cancer in patients from countries with a low rate of HCC. A few countries with a high rate of HCC also have a significant portion of PCC. WHO statistics accumulated from 1963 to 1972 show no significant change in incidence of liver cancer during that period in any of the countries studied. However, the occurrence of HCC at autopsy has been increasing at several institutions.[174,179,257] It is not settled, therefore, whether the risk of acquiring HCC has changed because incidence figures and autopsy occurrence rates are both subject to variation based on other factors. The incidence per 100,000 population from WHO data is listed in Table 33-4.

Our data in this section were derived from a study of the 339 patients with HCC that were encountered in the 94,556 autopsies performed at LAC-USCMC (1918–1980) and the JWCH (1960–1979) (Table 33-5). HCC occurred five times as frequently in men, but HCC in normal liver occurred equally in men and women. Ninety percent of the men with HCC had preexisting chronic liver disease,

TABLE 33-5.   Incidence of Malignant Tumors Primary in Liver

	NUMBER	PERCENT	COMPARISON AS A PERCENTAGE OF
Autopsies	94,556	30.0*	total deaths
Cirrhosis	5,368*	5.7	total autopsies
No. with HCC	284	5.2	cirrhotics
Malignant tumors, primary in liver	405	.4	total autopsies
Hepatocellular	339	.35	total autopsies
Cirrhotic and precirrhotic	284	84.0	total HCC
Alcoholic	176*	52.0*	total HCC
B viral	71*	21.9*	total HCC
Hemochromatotic	6	1.8	total HCC
Other	31	9.0	total HCC
Normal liver	55	16.0	total HCC
Cholangiolocellular	4	1.0	total primary malignant hepatic tumors
Peripheral cholangiocarcinoma	45	11.0	total primary malignant hepatic tumors
Hilar cholangiocarcinoma	11	2.7	total primary malignant hepatic tumors
Angiosarcoma	1	.2	total primary malignant hepatic tumors
Sarcoma	4	1.0	total primary malignant hepatic tumors
Carcinosarcoma	1	.2	total primary malignant hepatic tumors

* Extrapolated from less than total material.
(Data obtained at Los Angeles County University of Southern California Medical Center [1918–1979] and John Wesley County Hospital [1960–1976]. Other source materials for study not included in Table 33-5 obtained from the California Tumor Tissue Registry and through a survey of private hospitals in Los Angeles County (1971–1974), the Surgical Pathology Services of LAC-USCMC and the USC Liver Unit, referral material to the authors from the United States, Japan, Taiwan, and Gambia, Africa.)

whereas only 50% of the women did. The average age of cirrhotic patients with HCC was 63 years in both men and women, whereas the average age with HCC arising in normal livers was 59 years in men and 57 years in women.

In the United States, the percentage of autopsies in which HCC is found varies considerably, not only from city to city, but also within each city from one hospital to another. Fig. 33-10 charts the changing pattern of HCC occurrence at LAC-USCMC in the autopsy series with relative distribution of the tumor among the four major racial-ethnic groups.

The racial distribution of patients studied at autopsy at LAC-USCMC changed between 1950 to 1954, when it was 72% white, 13% black, 14% Mexican, and 0.8% Oriental, and 1975 to 1979, when it was 41% white, 22% black, 33% Mexican, and 2% Oriental. By 1965 to 1969, Orientals, only 1% of the autopsy total, contributed over 11% of the HCC. By 1975 to 1979, when Orientals were 2% of the population, 16% of the cases of HCC were in Oriental patients.

Reports from autopsy series throughout the United States suggest an increase in HCC that may have started in the 1930s. Although local differences are great, at least two series other than those at LAC-USCMC showed increased numbers of HCC per 100 autopsies at the same institution at two different periods.[174,179,257]

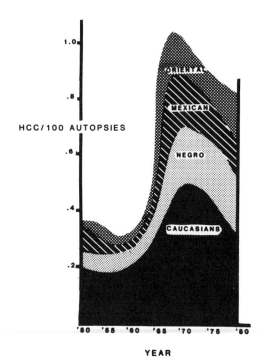

Fig. 33-10. Pattern of HCC occurrence over a 30-year period in the autopsy series at LAC-USCMC. Distribution of HCC among the four major racial–ethnic groups is shown.

Etiology

Multiple etiologies of HCC are currently proposed.[115] Because of remarkable variation in prevalence of these etiologic factors within high and low HCC prevalence areas, a multifactorial etiology is likely. Important etiologic factors include HBV, alcoholic cirrhosis, aflatoxin, and hemochromatosis.

Viral Hepatitis. *Hepatitis A.* A relationship between HCC and viral hepatitis was suggested by early investigators.[302] Before the 1970s, hepatitis A ("infectious" hepatitis) was suspected as a precursor of cirrhosis and HCC, but current data indicate that hepatitis A virus (HAV) is associated with no chronic disease and bears no relationship to cirrhosis.[67] Although there is no way to disprove the carcinogenic potential of a virus that produces only acute infection and that is acquired by 60% to 100% of the population sometime during their lives, there is nothing to favor the relationship.[317]

Hepatitis B. Studies have shown that, in some regions of Asia and Africa, chronic infection with HBV is present in at least as many as 91% of patients with HCC.[148] An additional 10% of patients with HCC may be infected with HBV in a fashion such that the hepatocyte nuclei contain hepatitis B core (HBc), but the hepatitis B surface antigen (HBsAg) in blood is present in quantities too small to detect.[154,225,316] In 97 consecutive autopsy cases of HCC, 21% were based on B viral disease at our institution. The incidence of HCC has a direct relationship to the incidence of chronic HBV infection in most ethnic groups and geographic locations. Exceptions include Greenland, where it has been reported that, in spite of a HBsAg carrier rate of 7% to 25% of the population, the incidence of HCC is about the same as in Denmark, where the HBsAg carrier rate is less than one tenth that found in Greenland.[297] The possibility of cocarcinogenic effects between hepatitis B and certain hepatotoxins has been raised in an effort to explain the varied incidence of HCC in different geographic and socioeconomic settings. A large multisite case-control study in Los Angeles County of 78 patients with HCC indicated that risk factors are cigarette smoking, alcohol consumption, and history of hepatitis and blood transfusion.[362] Increasing alcohol consumption in Japan also appears to promote liver cirrhosis and HCC even in HBsAg carriers.[215] However, in our material from the indigent population of Los Angeles County, 40% of 55 patients dying with B viral cirrhosis had HCC at autopsy. HCC is found in 40% of patients dying of B viral cirrhosis in Japan.* Steiner indicated that HCC was found in 44% of cirrhotic livers in native Africans,[302] and in Hong Kong, 52% of 353 B viral cirrhotics had HCC at autopsy.† Thus, the major factor determining the number of cases of HCC in a population appears to be incidence of B viral cirrhosis

---

* Okuda K: Personal communication, 1983.
† Lam KC: Personal communication, 1982.

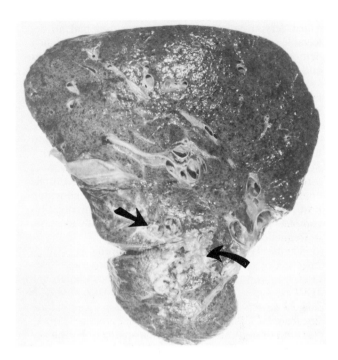

Fig. 33-11. Precirrhotic chronic active hepatitis B with HCC in a 45-year-old white man. Symptoms developed as a result of intraductal growth. Top arrow indicates tumor; lower arrow indicates intraductal foci radiating from the primary site. (JWA 31-70)

in that population, although other factors including exposure to toxins such as aflatoxin may promote HCC development in the HBV-infected patient.[115]

In our material, only 14% of the patients with HCC arising in B viral cirrhosis could recall having had an illness that, in retrospect, might have been viral hepatitis or chronic active hepatitis.[242] Most patients have had chronic hepatitis B infection for many years before HCC becomes evident. Redeker studied five Chinese-born patients with HCC arising in B viral cirrhosis. The patients had left China as small children and never returned. At ages ranging between 32 and 57 years, when HCC became evident, all five had HBsAg subtype "r," a subtype not found in hepatitis acquired in the United States. Thus, it appears that their infection occurred in the Orient up to 50 years earlier.* Similar results have been obtained in Chinese Americans in New York. It is believed that many patients born in areas of high incidence of chronic hepatitis B acquire the infection perinatally from infected mothers. Such early infection may partially explain the appearance of HCC at an earlier age in patients from both the Orient and Africa than in patients from the United States and Western Europe, where perinatal infection by HBV is less common. If the major mode of infection is perinatal, and if the maternal infection rate is the same, it remains unclear why first-generation American-born Chinese have a lower incidence of chronic hepatitis B and HCC than those born in the Orient.

Usually, HCC becomes clinically manifest after cirrhosis is well formed, but there is some evidence that the carcinoma may arise even before cirrhosis is completely developed, much earlier in the course of B viral chronic liver disease than previously believed. This is supported by the finding that the mean age of patients dying from HCC in B viral cirrhosis is 52; the mean age of patients dying of B viral cirrhosis alone is 50, nearly the same. In Africa, patients with only cirrhosis had an average age at death of 38.2 years. Those with cirrhosis and HCC had an average age of 37 at death.[242,302] Occasionally, a complication of HCC results in the early discovery of the disease when the liver is only finely granular, before nodules have developed (Fig. 33-11). Many patients ultimately proved to have HCC have increased α_1-fetoprotein (AFP) levels for years before symptoms become manifest.[220]

It is equivocal whether HCC develops with increased frequency in livers of patients who have persistent hepatitis type B any more than it does in patients with normal livers that are HBsAg-negative. Unfortunately, most investigators have separated the underlying hepatic condition in their series into cirrhosis and noncirrhosis, whereas the separation should be between chronic liver disease (cirrhotic or precirrhotic) and essentially normal liver. Of 15 patients with HBsAg-positive HCC in our material in Los Angeles, only 1 (6.7%) was interpreted as having persistent hepatitis type B, 3 (20%) were classified as precirrhotic, and 11 had frank cirrhosis.[242]

HBsAg becomes undetectable in sera of some patients with B viral cirrhosis, but most patients retain the B viral core antigen (HBcAg) in liver cell nuclei. We found that nearly one third of the autopsy patients we had previously

---

* Redeker AG: Personal communication, 1983.

called "cryptogenic" cirrhotic because they had no detectable serum levels of HBsAg by the time of death had demonstrable HBcAg in their liver and anti-HBc without anti-HBs in their serum.[235] We have called the disease of such patients *latent B viral cirrhosis*. Of six patients with latent B viral cirrhosis, three had HCC, essentially in the same frequency of HCC as in patients who have overt B viral cirrhosis.[226,227]

The HBV genome has been identified within the host hepatic DNA (*integration*) of tumor and nontumor liver.[30] Such detection has occurred in patients with and *without* serum HBsAg and even in those with anti-HBs. Multiple copies of HBV-DNA have been proven integrated within host hepatic DNA. This integration process involves incomplete portions of HBV-DNA and apparently increases in frequency with time of carrier state.

Whether HCC is related directly to chronic hepatitis B infection or instead nonspecifically develops as a consequence of chronic liver disease is unsettled. Usually the HBV cannot be demonstrated within the HCC, but with diligent search, it can be found,[149] and a tissue culture line from HCC has been established that produces HBsAg but not HBcAg.[176] If the carcinoma arising in B viral cirrhosis is the simple sequela of cirrhosis, the occurrence of HCC in the livers of 40% to 44% of patients with B viral cirrhosis is much higher than the association of HCC with other types of cirrhosis.

Naturally occurring hepatitis virus–HCC association is now recognized in woodchucks, California ground squirrels, and Chinese ducks.[314] These models will aid investigation of maternal–fetal transmission of hepatotropic virus.

Delta Hepatitis Virus. A common chronic infection with HBV, delta hepatitis virus (HDV) appears unrelated to HCC. In our material in Los Angeles, 39 patients with HCC associated with HBV were tested for anti-HDV and only 1 patient was positive, whereas 31.5% (18 of 57) of chronic HBV patients with HCC had antibody to HDV.[107] However, exposure to HDV varies widely throughout the world, with low incidence in the Far East despite a very high incidence of HBV. Because of the perinatal transmission of HBV from mother to infant, the familial incidence of HCC is high in patients with B viral cirrhosis.[65,214,226]

Hepatitis Non-A, Non-B. There is increasing evidence of the cirrhotogenic potential of hepatitis non-A, non-B, particularly in relation to posttransfusion acquisition of the infection.[260] There is no concrete evidence that hepatitis non-A, non-B is related to carcinoma; however, the possibility cannot be excluded. Substantial numbers of HCC in cryptogenic cirrhotic livers in countries such as Japan mean that some other etiology of HCC exists. In Taiwan, however, HCC in cryptogenic cirrhosis is uncommon; HBV accounts for nearly all of the HCC. In the United States, alcohol, HBV, and a few other recognized entities form the basis of the majority of HCC in cirrhosis.

Alcoholic Cirrhosis. Alcoholic cirrhosis is a major predisposing lesion for HCC in the United States and in some European countries where alcoholic liver disease is prevalent. The percentage of patients with alcoholic cirrhosis who develop HCC is much lower than of those with B viral cirrhosis who acquire HCC. However, alcoholic cirrhosis is so common in some countries that it forms an important underlying disease. Of our HCC patients, 52% had alcoholic cirrhosis. Most of the societies in which B viral cirrhosis is common have a low incidence of alcoholic cirrhosis, although there are exceptions.

Development of HCC in alcoholic cirrhosis, unlike that in B viral cirrhosis, is restricted to advanced cirrhosis and is rarely found in the finely granular alcoholic cirrhotic liver and almost never in the fatty cirrhotic liver. Thus, the stated percentage of autopsies of patients with alcoholic cirrhosis in which HCC may be encountered varies among reports and depends upon which of the following is used as the denominator: (1) all stages of alcoholic liver disease, resulting in 3% to 4% occurrence; (2) alcoholic cirrhosis only, resulting in 4% to 6% occurrence; or (3) advanced alcoholic cirrhosis only, resulting in 8% to 10% occurrence. A tendency in the past to classify cirrhotic livers with discrete nodules and dense fibrous scars as postnecrotic (*i.e.*, nonalcoholic by inference) has resulted in reports that incorrectly reflect a diminutive HCC frequency in patients with alcoholic cirrhosis. The cirrhotic nodules of the alcoholic patient who has stopped drinking may become larger as the dense, restricting collagen characteristic of alcoholic cirrhosis undergoes vascularization and softening. One study indicated that 55% of alcoholic cirrhotic patients who had discontinued the use of alcohol had HCC at autopsy.[165] The cessation of alcoholism allows the alcoholic patient to live long enough to develop HCC. In some countries such as the United States, alcoholism is often characterized by nearly continual inebriation, bringing about the demise of many patients either by hepatic failure in early stages of alcoholic liver disease or by one of the many other consequences of alcoholism. In other countries such as France and Italy, where alcohol is consumed in large, regular amounts, often without significant outward evidence of intoxication, cirrhosis is acquired more insidiously, and a greater degree of advancement may be attained. The alcoholic cirrhotic liver in which HCC is more likely to develop is the insidiously acquired variety. France and Italy, with twice the incidence of cirrhosis found in Japan or the United State, have HCC in cirrhotic livers intermediate in number between the United States, where most cirrhosis is alcoholic, and Japan, where carcinoma arises predominantly in B viral cirrhosis (see Table 33-4).

Among the alcoholic cirrhotic patients with HCC at our unit on whom such data were available, 85% had never been in the hospital for liver disease, although they may have had hospital admissions related to other aspects of alcoholism. Twenty-one percent had discontinued alcoholism for varied periods of time before development of HCC.[242]

HCC develops in the alcoholic cirrhotic at an average age of 60, later in life than B viral cirrhosis. Patients dying of HCC in alcoholic cirrhosis are on an average 10 years older than those dying of alcoholic cirrhosis without tumor.[242]

Hemochromatosis. A high percentage of patients with hemochromatosis develop either HCC or cholangiocarcinoma (Table 33-6). Variability in frequency, at least in the United States, may relate to differences in definition between alcoholic cirrhosis with increased iron stores and idiopathic hemochromatosis. Many of the HCC in hemochromatotic livers have ductal features. One third of the HCC in hemochromatosis in our material had such ductal changes. Cholangiocarcinoma also arises in hemochromatosis: 9% of our hemochromatosis patients had cholangiocarcinoma. The rare occurrence of separate HCC and PCC in the same liver is encountered more often in hemochromatosis than in other conditions antedating liver tumors.

The risk of developing HCC is higher in patients with B viral cirrhosis than in those with hemochromatosis. Hemochromatosis is reported to underlie between 0.8% and 15% of cases of HCC (Table 33-6.).

The removal of hemosiderin stores by venesection has reduced much of the hepatic, cardiac, and pancreatic dysfunction in hemochromatosis. Reports differ regarding the effect of hemosiderin removal on the risk of development of HCC. In one series, 13 of 45 treated hemochromatosis patients died of HCC[31]; in another, only 4 of 44 had HCC.[263]

Aflatoxins. Aflatoxins, products of *Aspergillus flavus*, have been implicated as a cause of HCC in those parts of the world in which there is heavy aflatoxin contamination of foodstuff. Aflatoxins are very potent carcinogens in experimental animals. The *Aspergillus flavus* mold has been recognized on peanuts, wheat, rice, soybean, corn, bread, milk, and cheese as well as in tropical soils. Although aflatoxin is not produced in similar amounts on all media or under all conditions, it is present in substantial amounts on ground nuts (peanuts), a major food staple in parts of Africa. Although there are several aflatoxins, the most potent is aflatoxin B_1, which is invariably present when any other of the aflatoxins are found.[358] The aflatoxins are highly substituted coumarins, having an effect almost exclusively on liver. In the hepatocyte, the initial effect is a profound inhibition of DNA and RNA polymerases, resulting perhaps from aflatoxin effect on the chromatin template, but aflatoxins also apparently act upon endoplasmic reticular basement membrane. Suitable levels of aflatoxins produce HCC in 100% of some animal species. In contrast, some inbred mouse strains are completely resistant to aflatoxin induction of HCC, even when substantial quantities of aflatoxin are administered. Differences in the carcinogenic effect of aflatoxins on subhuman primates are considerable, not allowing an accurate extrapolation to the carcinogenic effect on humans. Experiments designed to study the effect of a high- or low-protein diet on the carcinogenic potential of aflatoxins have produced disparate results.[103,178,210–213,263,271,273,358,359]

The amount of aflatoxins consumed in a population is roughly correlated with HCC incidence.[4,144,237,286–288] An exception is Thailand, where, in spite of a huge dietary intake of aflatoxins, the incidence of HCC is lower than that reported in African studies (Fig. 33-12). One puzzling feature is the young age at which the tumors occur in geographic areas where HCC is common. The average age of 222 Africans with HCC was 37.2 years,[302] compared with an average age of 52 for patients in the United States with B viral cirrhosis. It may be that a major cocarcinogenic effect of aflatoxins on chronic hepatitis B is to bring about tumor induction at a younger age or to affect the immune system adversely to the extent that chronic infection with HBV is allowed or encouraged.[172]

Other Mycotoxins and Plant Alkaloids. Food contaminants by other mycotoxins and plant toxins have not received the study given to aflatoxins alone. Lasiocarpine, a pyrrolizidine alkaloid given with aflatoxins to rats, produces HCC in cirrhotic liver, whereas aflatoxin alone induces formation of HCC without cirrhosis.[263] Outbreaks of veno-occlusive disease in Afghanistan and India, induced by plant alkaloids, indicate that the alkaloids are present in the environment, often in substantial amounts,[193,321] but their impact upon the development of HCC is unknown.

Hormones. *Oral Contraceptives.* Many hepatocellular adenomas and a few HCCs have been reported in young women taking oral contraceptives for several years.[34,49,114,]

TABLE 33-6.   Importance of Hemochromatosis in Genesis of HCC

LOCALE	HEMOCHROMATOSIS		TOTAL HCC IN HEMOCHROMATOSIS AND NONHEMOCHROMATOSIS
	Total	Number with HCC	
Australia[188]	15	4 (27%)	26
Boston[174]	204	16 (8%)	108
Los Angeles[242]	14	3 (21%)	225
Los Angeles[71]	28	3 (17%)	81
Africa[304]	47	7 (15%)	863
Cincinnati[93]	27	1 (3%)	76
Total	335	34 (10%)	1379

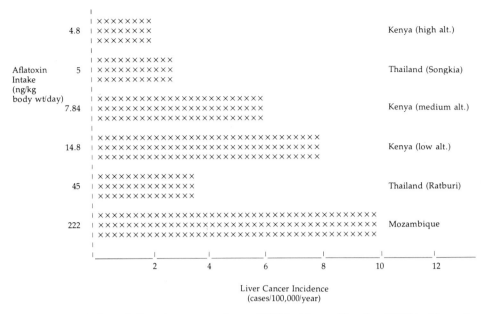

Fig. 33-12. Relation of aflatoxin consumption to HCC incidence. Note low HCC incidence in Thailand, whereas aflatoxin intake is high.

[185,209,244] From a review of the reports and tissue of several cases, some of the tumors appear to be adenomas that were overdiagnosed, a few resemble metastatic carcinomas, and others are HCCs. Some of the carcinomas are a variety of carcinoma that we have called *fibrolamellar carcinoma*. Fibrolamellar carcinomas characteristically develop in adolescents or adults under 35 years of age (average age, 26.4) and occur with equal sex incidence.[57] It is possible that isolated examples of fibrolamellar carcinoma are reported as being etiologically related to oral contraceptives simply because the latter are used by such a sizable number of women in the under 35 age-group. It is difficult to accept that such a tumor is a consequence of only a few months of contraceptive use, as has been reported.[185] The most acceptable cases of HCC being related to oral contraceptives are those that arise within adenomas, particularly in patients who have been taking oral contraceptives for several years.[209] Although it seems that some HCC has occurred relative to contraceptives, the exact risk is unclear. Considering the tendency of pharmaceutical companies toward reduction of the amount of hormonal contents of oral contraceptives, adenomas may again become curiosities, and the few HCCs that may be related to estrogen therapy may also disappear.

Androgens. In 1971, Bernstein and co-workers reported the first case of a 21-year-old man with Fanconi's anemia who developed a hepatic tumor after prolonged treatment with an anabolic steroid.[25] Several additional cases of hepatic tumor in androgen-treated boys or men were reported in the next few years.[25,118,137,191,280,289,363] Most were a result of steroids given as part of therapy for aplastic anemia, usually Fanconi's anemia. In contrast to the case of HCC and birth control pills, in which exposure of a huge population has resulted in a small incidence of adenoma and a miniscule occurrence of HCC, only a very small porportion of the adolescent and young adult male population is taking androgens for chronic anemia. The use of androgenic steroids by moderate numbers of athletes has resulted in only a few reported cases of liver tumors, but cases have been reported in which anabolic steroids were given for non-Fanconi aplastic anemias[84,167,191,363]; thus, some factor other than either androgenic steroids or the genetic aberration of Fanconi's anemia alone must be implicated. Atlhough chronic anemia patients receive multiple transfusions, patients with hemophilia, thalassemia, and hemoglobinopathies, who are at the same risk of posttransfusion hepatitis as are aplastic anemic patients, do not have a comparable incidence of hepatic tumor, and a transfusion factor therefore cannot be implicated.

An unusual feature of the androgen-related HCC-like tumors is their high degree of hormone dependence. Most of the tumors have been incidental autopsy findings. Others, found at surgery, regressed with cessation of androgenic steroids. Two were reported to have ruptured into the abdominal cavity.[26,38,136] There is no evidence that biologically malignant liver tumors have yet resulted from androgen use in spite of the malignant histologic appearance.

Alpha₁-Antitrypsin (AAT). Since the first reports of HCC occurring in adult patients with protease inhibitor type

Z-,[21] many single case reports have appeared in which histochemical demonstration of AAT in the liver, of HCC, or of both has been described, implying a relationship between AAT abnormality and HCC.[48,145,231,232,265,266,326] Lack of AAT association with HCC has been reported in numerous reviews including those from South Africa, Dakar, and Greece.[54] Furthermore, tissues and serum phenotypes of 127 patients were studied at our unit, and the incidence of protease inhibitor type MZ was found to be equal in the normal population, the cirrhotic population, and in patients with HCC. Patients with fibrolamellar HCC were a possible exception; three of five were type MZ. No ZZ patients were found among the 127 patients with HCC, and only one of over 1000 adult cirrhotic patients autopsied at the USC Liver Unit was found to be type ZZ. Thus, if middle-aged patients with ZZ cirrhosis have an increased incidence of HCC, at least in the United States, such patients are too rare to identify and were not included in our series of more than 127 patients with HCC.[106,145,242] If MZ is related to HCC, it is related to a variety of HCC that constitutes only about 2% of total HCC cases.

Other Etiologic Considerations

Several case reports deal with diseases, usually rare, in which HCC occurs more often than expected by chance alone (Table 33-7).

Chronic Cirrhotic Conditions. Certain types of cirrhosis are rarely complicated by HCC. *Wilson's disease,* in which long survival is attained even after development of a coarsely nodular liver, has no documented relationship to HCC. Shikata mentions having seen a case but does not describe it.[292]

Chronic Active Autoimmune (Lupoid) Hepatitis and Cirrhosis. HCC is rare in chronic active autoimmune cirrhosis. Lupoid hepatitis, which appears to be diminishing in incidence, results in coarsely nodular cirrhosis. We have encountered one example of HCC in 16 autopsies of patients with lupoid cirrhosis in the 25 years since the condition was first recognized and have seen no reports in the literature.

Primary Biliary Cirrhosis. Primary biliary cirrhosis (PBC) is not associated with HCC.

Clinical Features

The most common symptoms of HCC are an enlarging right upper quadrant mass, often accompanied by pain and epigastric fullness and discomfort. Less often, acute abdominal symptoms or esophageal hemorrhage occurs. Clinical symptoms differ in various parts of the world. In South Africa, weight loss was the most prominent initial feature.[23] In African patients, HCC formed a much larger mass, replacing a greater amount of the liver than in American or Asiatic patients. Most of the latter two groups

TABLE 33-7. Conditions Associated with HCC

PREDISPOSING CONDITION	CIRRHOSIS +/-
Alcoholic cirrhosis[73,138,165,242]	+
B viral cirrhosis[3,138,216,292]	+
Hemochromatosis[347]	+
Cryptogenic cirrhosis (adults)	+
Aflatoxins[4,144,237,286,288]	?
Oral contraceptives[34,49,114,185,209,256,324]	−
Androgens and aplastic anemia[25,118,191,280-289,313]	−
Thorotrast[136]	−
Inflammatory bowel disease[299]	?
Radiation[50]	−
Immunodeficiency[10,295]	+
Prolonged Phenobarbitone[282]	−
Cystothiouria[97]	−
Hemihypertrophy[97]	−
Budd–Chiari disease[296]	−
Familial cholestasis[59]	+
Congenital biliary atresia[66,156]	+
Alpha antitrypsin[95,106,307]	+
Plant alkaloids[99]	−
Congenital[217]	−
Porphyria cutanea tarda[330]	−,+
Fanconi's anemia without androgens[41]	+
Transfusional hemochromatosis, HBsAg-negative	−
Methotrexate[279]	−
Idiopathic portal hypertension—late	−
Parasitic infestation[205]	−
Congenital hepatic fibrosis[180]	−
Water-borne carcinogens	−
Immunosuppressants[10]	−
No known predisposing lesion	+,−
Arsenic, chronic[56]	−

had cirrhosis, many with small atrophic livers. Okuda has separated the clinical patterns into nine types listed in Table 33-8.[222]

The cirrhotic type of HCC seems to be the most common in the United States. HCC should be considered high on the list of diagnostic probabilities in patients who have alcoholic cirrhosis but who have stopped drinking for a long period and, without starting to drink again, have rapidly developed signs of hepatic failure and jaundice. Since the arterial blood that enters HCC egresses into portal vein branches, a frequent initial symptom is bleeding from esophageal varices due to an abrupt increase in portal pressure.

Paraneoplastic. Many functional alterations associated with HCC have been reported since the first description of hypoglycemia and HCC in 1929 (Table 33-9).[201]

α_1 **Fetoprotein.** One paraneoplastic product, AFP, an oncofetoprotein, deserves special mention because of its di-

TABLE 33-8. Classification of Clinical Presentation of HCC

CLASSIFICATION	DESCRIPTION	OCCURRENCE (%)[219b]
Frank	Epigastric discomfort, fullness, mass	61.6
Cirrhotic	Ascites, hepatic failure, variceal bleed	21.1
Occult	Incidental autopsy or surgical findings	3.0
Febrile	High fever, abdominal pain, rapid worsening	3.0
Metastatic	Metastases produce first symptoms	3.0
Hepatic	Rapid onset of jaundice, high SGOT, SGPT	3.0
Acute abdominal	Sudden pain, peritoneal reaction	2.2
Cholestatic	Severe jaundice (Ca obstruction of duct)	0.7
Other (unclass)		3.0

SGOT, serum glutamic-oxaloacetic transaminase; SGPT, serum glutamic-pyruvic transaminase.

agnostic value.[1,17] It has a molecular weight between 64,000 daltons and 74,000 daltons, is present during fetal development, and, for a short time, is the major serum protein. After reaching peak serum levels in the first fetal trimester, it drops to levels of about 10 μg to 14 μg/ml at time of birth, 1000 times the adult level. It normally decreases rapidly after birth and, in a child one year of age,

TABLE 33-9. Paraneoplastic Manifestations of HCC*

Serum protein abnormalities
  Fetoprotein
  Abnormal globulin
  Increased hepatoglobin
  Increased ceruloplasmin
  Increased alpha$_1$-antitrypsin
  Aberrant alkaline phosphatase
  Abnormal isoferratins
  Increased levels of chorionic gonodotrophins
  Increased levels of chorionic somatotrophins
Hematologic abnormalities
  Dysfibrinogenemias, cryofibrinogenemia
  Antifibrinolysis
  Plasmacytosis
  Hemolytic processes
  Erythrocytosis
Lipid abnormalities
  Hypercholesterolemia
  Hypertriglyceridemia
Other abnormal serum factors
  Porphyria
  Cystathioninuria
  Ethanolaminuria
Functional and hormone-like abnormalities
  Hypoglycemia
  Pseudohyperparathyroidism
  Precocious puberty
  Gynecomastia
  Hypertrophic pulmonary osteoarthropathy

* See references[9,12,18,24,51,108,151,163,186,189,196,202,218,224,242,250, 253,290,329,341,349,351]

is at the normal adult level of 10 ng/ml or less. A few *in utero* conditions such as fetal distress or neural tube defects produce elevated levels of AFP both in the amniotic fluid and in the maternal blood.[35,36,263,308,344]

Any one of many medical or surgical diseases of the liver may be associated with elevated levels of AFP during infancy. Infants or children with ataxia telangiectasia,[294,345] hereditary tyrosinosis,[17] Indian childhood cirrhosis,[208] and hepatoblastomas have elevated levels of AFP.

In the adult, AFP detection is a helpful screening test for HCC. In a few other conditions, AFP is found in levels of over 400 ng/ml. Lesser levels in the range of 25 ng to 100 ng/ml may be found in acute viral hepatitis, particularly hepatitis B, in chronic liver disease, and in some cases of metastatic carcinoma.[277] Young adult patients with fulminant hepatitis type B may occasionally have levels of 1000 ng to 4000 ng/ml.[142] Higher levels in the range of 1,000 ng to 1,000,000 ng/ml are encountered in patients with teratocarcinomas with embryonal elements and yolk-sac tumors[161,194,238,320] and, very rarely, in patients with hepatic metastatic carcinomas from stomach or pancreas.[278,331,335] We have found no patients with cholangiocarcinoma to have increased AFP. However, a report from Japan indicates that 20% of 268 patients with cholangiocarcinoma had AFP elevation.[219]

In Japan, among 177 cases of HCC, AFP was above 400 ng/ml in 71.7%.[221] In a larger multicenter report of 2411 cases of HCC, AFP levels were found to be higher than 200 ng/ml in 70%.[219] In our material in Los Angeles, 75% of the patients with HCC arising in B viral cirrhosis have AFP levels over 400 ng/ml, but 65% of those whose carcinomas arise in alcoholic cirrhosis and only 33% with carcinoma arising in noncirrhotic liver have AFP levels above 400 ng/ml.

Pathology

Gross Pathology. The gross appearance of HCC depends upon the presence or absence of cirrhosis, encapsulation, fibrosis (including pattern), and growth pattern. These features differ in HCC arising in Japan, the United States,

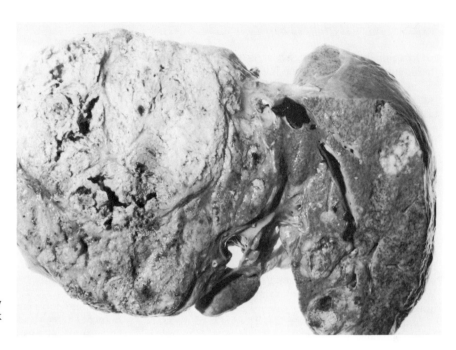

Fig. 33-13. HCC in previously normal liver of a 47-year-old black woman. (JWA 221-65)

and South Africa.[222] For example, only 17% of 90 cases of HCC were of the expanding type in our series, yet 36% to 38% were of that type in the Japanese and South African series.[222]

Carcinoma arising in a normal liver grows as a fairly homogeneous mass, compressing the surrounding parenchyma and later developing satellite nodules that may blend with the primary (Fig. 33-13). In contrast, carcinoma arising in cirrhotic or precirrhotic liver tends to mimic cirrhosis and is referred to as *cirrhotomimetic* (Fig. 33-14A). Some carcinomas arising in cirrhotic liver, however, form a pseudoencapsulated, sharply defined mass of nodular tissue. Others arising in cirrhotic liver gradually blend into the parenchyma with a transition between the hyperplastic nodules of the nontumor liver and the neoplastic nodules (Fig. 33-14B). In the center of the tumor, the

Fig. 33-14. A. External surface of cirrhotic liver showing tumor nodules and replacing the cirrhotic right lobe with scattered small tumor foci in the left. The tumor grows as in an exaggerated cirrhotic process. (JWA 22-73) **B.** Cirrhotomimetic HCC arising in cirrhotic liver of a 58-year-old alcoholic cirrhotic man. The pale nodules are carcinoma.

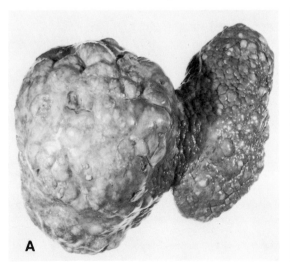

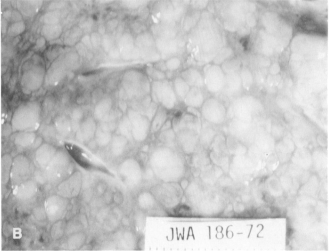

nodular or pseudolobular pattern is often effaced by necrosis.

Occasionally, HCC is invasive at its margins, destroying the nodular pattern. This type is called *invasive.*

The question remains unsettled as to whether the intrahepatic spread of HCC is entirely by intrahepatic metastases or partly by the concurrent development of neoplastic change of tissue under the same etiologic stimulus that produced the original lesion.

In support of multiple origins is a gross type of HCC characterized by scattered nodules of similar size, each resembling an adenomatous hyperplastic focus, and called *multifocal* HCC. It has not been established whether this represents multiple foci of neoplastic development or spread from a single focus. The ultimate example of multifocal carcinoma is *diffuse* HCC, in which the entire liver is composed of relatively uniform nodules of carcinoma resembling and often grossly mistaken for cirrhosis. In such livers, a larger single primary focus is not identified. We have identified only one example of diffuse HCC in noncirrhotic liver.[242]

Improved detection methods, especially ultrasound, have stimulated identification of "minute" HCC (maximum size varies from less than 4.5 cm diameter to 2.0 cm).[293] Because serum AFP and HBsAg are less often abnormal in this group and most patients are asymptomatic,

identification may allow surgical treatment and longer survival. Intra–bile duct growth by HCC occasionally produces prominent presenting symptoms and occurred in approximately 10% of one Japanese autopsy series yet in only 2% of our HCC series.[154]

Pedunculated HCC, possibly arising in an accessory lobe or ectopic liver, is a recently described variant reported from Japan but rare in the United States.[121]

Gross examination of an HCC in a mass reveals variegated patterns of bright yellow, gray, and white with hemorrhage. The parenchyma of HCC is soft in most cases unless there is fibrosis. Rarely HCC is fibrous and may resemble metastatic carcinoma (sclerosing hepatic carcinoma), and the fibrolamellar carcinoma often has a prominent fibrous scar and thus resembles FNH.

Vascular Changes. All HCCs receive their blood supply from the hepatic arterial branches. The arterioles that supply the capillary plexus in the portal tract and around the bile ducts are shunted into the developing tumor nodule,[204] and the egress of blood is into the portal vein branches rather than into the hepatic vein structures. In large tumors, this constitutes an arterioportal shunt. However, since most of the portal blood flow is centripetal, angiograms in the portal venous phase do not show portal vein filling, since the contrast material is flushed into the

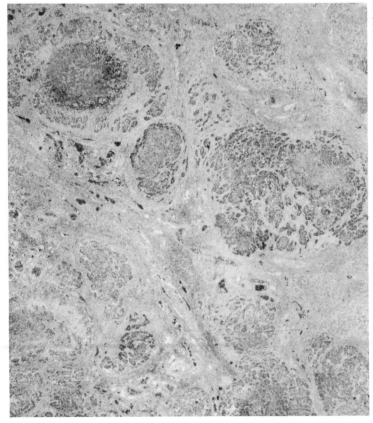

Fig. 33-15. Photomicrograph of cirrhotomimetic pattern of HCC in a 62-year-old black woman with nonalcoholic cirrhosis. (LUA 42-77) (Original magnification × 22; H&E)

nontumor liver. When the major branch of the portal vein becomes occluded by the tumor, blocking centripetal flow, hepatic arteriograms show the shunting into the portal vein. Often the initial complaint of a patient with HCC is sudden esophageal hemorrhage.

The egress of blood from HCC arising in normal livers has not been studied. Portal vein thromboses and varices have not been encountered in our patients with HCC arising in normal liver.

Rarely, an HCC has a highly vascular pattern that results in a gross similarity to angiosarcoma. This has been called *atypical hemorrhagic malignant hepatoma.*[158] We have seen only one such example in 339 adult patients with HCC studied from 1918 to 1980.

Histopathology. HCC arising in cirrhotic or precirrhotic liver usually mimics cirrhosis in growth pattern, hence the term *cirrhotomimetic.* By low-power microscopy, multiple variably sized nodules of HCC are defined by fibrous septa (Fig. 33-15). HCC arising in normal liver, however, grows as an expanding mass, usually without a capsule.

The characteristic trabecular pattern, which is most frequently observed in the cirrhotomimetic form, may appear as an exaggeration of hepatic cord growth (Fig. 33-16*A*). The finger-like trabeculae have no stroma but are covered with a thin, widely spaced layer of endothelial lining cells (Fig. 33-16*B*). Although the spaces around the trabeculae are vascular and apparently communicate freely with the arterial vessels,[204] there is little blood microscopically. Most commonly, trabeculae are arranged in solid cores three to four cells thick. Occasionally, a *macrotrabecular* pattern will develop in which there is multiple cell thickness, widening each trabecula to a plump peninsular structure (Fig. 33-17).

The trabeculae often have a central canalicular-like space that becomes dilated by secretory material with or without bile pigment, giving an acinar configuration. As the acinar or glandlike areas develop, a fibrous stroma occasionally becomes associated with the trabeculae, resulting in a loss of the characteristic trabecular appearance and making identification of HCC more difficult (Fig. 33-18*A*, *B*). Sometimes a follicle-like transformation develops that we call *adenoid* (Fig. 33-18*C*).

At higher magnification, the neoplastic cells may closely resemble normal hepatocytes. They generally have an eosinophilic granular cytoplasm and nuclei that are more primitive than in the nonneoplastic hepatocytes; the

Fig. 33-16. A. Photomicrograph of microtrabecular HCC showing separate fingers of tumor that resemble an exaggeration of cord pattern. (RS 1667-80) (Original magnification × 1080; H&E) **B.** The tumor cords are lined by a thin layer of endothelial cells (*arrow*). (RS 1667-80) (Original magnification × 2160; H&E)

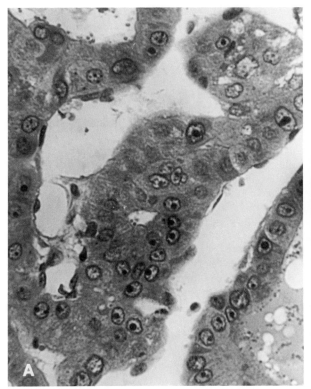

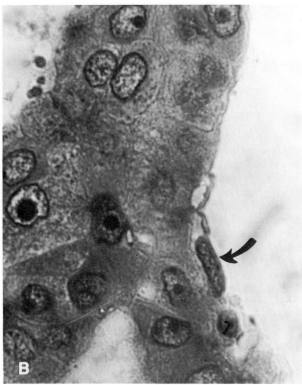

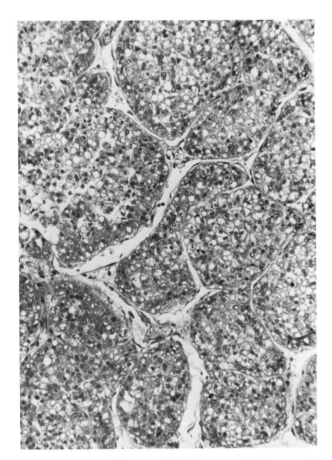

Fig. 33-17. The trabeculae of HCC are occasionally several tumor cells thick; the tumor pattern is then called macrotrabecular. (RS 2180-80) (Original magnification × 216; H&E)

chromatin is more clumped than normal, and the chromatin–parachromatin demarcation is distinct. The nucleoli are usually prominent, and their absence should cause hesitation in making the diagnosis of HCC. The tumor cells lose the ability to incorporate hemosiderin into their cytoplasm early in neoplastic transformation, but other functional activities may persist. Bile secretion often occurs, fat and glycogen may accumulate, and alcoholic hyaline is occasionally found. HCC frequently has hyaline bodies. Some of these bodies give a staining reaction that suggests AAT accumulation,[266] but they frequently do not contain glycoprotein. Structures that resemble megamitochondria are often found, and pale bodies that superficially resemble ground-glass cells of Hadziyannis but are HBsAg-negative are infrequently found. The pale bodies have a granular pattern on electron microscopy, and some contain fibrinogen.[312] Staining for AFP by immunofluorescent or immunoperoxidase techniques demonstrates the proteins in those tumors that are actively producing the material.[112,155,230,242]

HCC often varies widely in degree of differentiation from one area to another. A large series of HCC and bile duct carcinoma has been studied by electron microscopy.[229] Occasionally, the tumors are undifferentiated, often quite pleomorphic. Clear-cell areas may be found in many HCCs, and occasionally the entire tumor will be made up of clear cells (Fig. 33-19A, B). In such instances, it may be difficult to differentiate the tumor from a clear-cell carcinoma of the kidney (Fig. 33-19B). There have been suggestions of a relationship of the clear-cell type of HCC to improved prognosis, but there are conflicting reports in this regard.[39,71,75,159]

Large bizarre pleomorphic cells may constitute a part or most of an HCC. This is the giant cell type. A pure giant cell HCC is rare, accounting for 1.8% of our series. Up to 15% of HCCs have some areas of giant cell change. A few reported cases of osteoclast-like giant cell HCC also have osseous metaplasia.[157,201] We have one example of osteoclastoma-like HCC. Such a tumor has abundant spindling "stromal" cells.

HCC commonly invades portal vein branches and, less frequently, the hepatic veins. When the portal vein is involved, the carcinoma may spread throughout the liver, growing in a treelike fashion. Occasionally, the main growth is into the extrahepatic portal vein.

Trabecular HCC is typically characterized by lack of stroma, but HCC in which the pattern is acinar, pseudoglandular, or adenoid often has variable amounts of stroma. Occasionally, the stromal response may be dense enough to be called *sclerosing hepatic carcinoma.* The cords, because of the surrounding collagen, resemble duct structures. In patients with sclerosing hepatic carcinoma, we found that 69% had serum calcium levels that were elevated without bone metastases. Although some sclerosing hepatic cancers are truly ductal, others appear predominantly hepatocellular.[228]

Fibrolamellar HCC. Young adults with HCC commonly have a characteristic histologic variant we have called *fibrolamellar carcinoma.*[57] Lamellar strands and bundles of collagen separate thin cords of pink hepatocytes. Pale bodies and periodic acid-schiff (PAS)–positive diastase-resistant globules are noted in one half. A pelioid pattern is also present in one third. The clinical behavior is also distinctive because of origin in young adults (15–30 years, mean 26 years), origin in normal liver, equal sex origin, prolonged survival, and frequent surgical resection. AAT phenotype MZ occurred in three of five patients tested. Extraordinarily high serum vitamin B_{12} binding capacity has been reported in this variant.[339]

This tumor is only 2% of our autopsy series but often accounts for 25% to 50% of HCC in young adults. Geographic distribution of this variant indicates cases in the United States, western Europe (England, France, Spain), Taiwan, and Australia, but it has not been reported in South Africa or Japan (Fig. 33-20).

Metastatic Pattern. The metastatic patterns of HCC arising in normal livers and in cirrhotic livers, of PCC, of

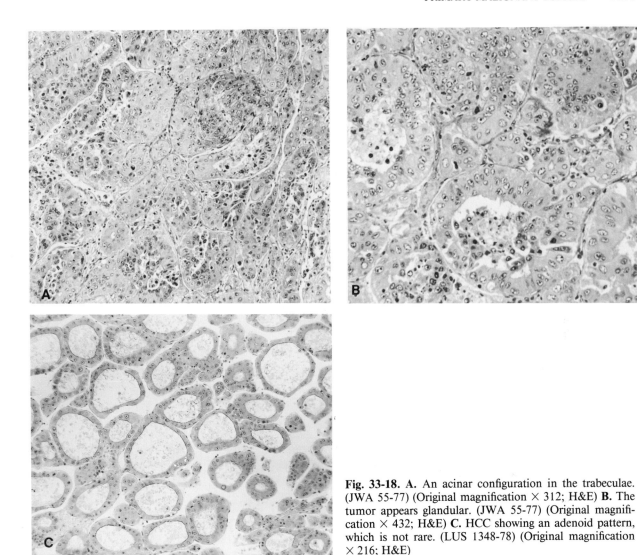

Fig. 33-18. A. An acinar configuration in the trabeculae. (JWA 55-77) (Original magnification × 312; H&E) **B.** The tumor appears glandular. (JWA 55-77) (Original magnification × 432; H&E) **C.** HCC showing an adenoid pattern, which is not rare. (LUS 1348-78) (Original magnification × 216; H&E)

hilar cholangiocarcinoma, and of mixed cholangiohepatocellular carcinoma are all somewhat different, as shown in Table 33-10. Rarely, the metastases may produce the precipitating, initial symptoms of disease.[242]

Metastases are absent at autopsy in a higher percentage of patients with HCC arising in cirrhotic liver than in those with HCC in normal liver. However, the latter patients probably live longer after HCC develops. Carcinoma arising in previously normal or precirrhotic liver usually becomes quite large and may even replace most of the liver before symptoms develop. Patients with carcinoma arising in cirrhotic liver have little hepatic reserve, and the replacement by carcinoma of a small portion of the liver brings about hepatic failure or features of portal hypertension because of the increased flow of arterial blood into the portal vein by way of HCC.

Preneoplastic Change. In the cirrhotic liver with HCC, there are areas that apparently correspond to the "initiated cell" described in experimental induction of HCC by chemical carcinogens.[82,83] These are called "paraplastic changes."[242] The paraplastic changes that occur in the nonalcoholic cirrhotic liver differ from those in alcoholic cirrhosis. Patients with HCC in B viral cirrhosis have large numbers of dysplastic cells but also subtle areas of accentuated cell growth that are recognized by larger, more hydropic cells compressing the surrounding hepatocytes. Much of the liver appears to have varying degrees of regenerative stimulus (Fig. 33-21). In alcoholic cirrhotic livers with carcinoma, the nontumor hepatocytes have a uniform, shrunken cord arrangement within the nodules. Within such quiescent nodules, an abrupt change to an accelerated growth pattern is often recognizable (Fig. 33-

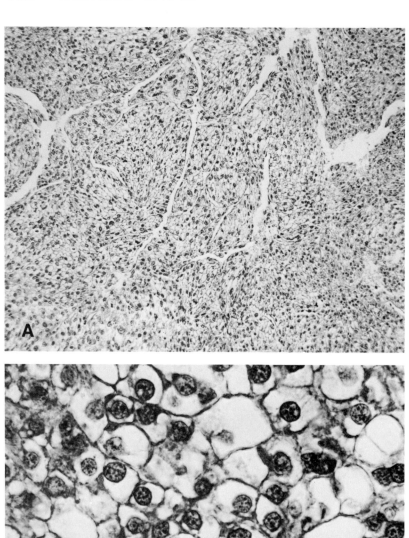

Fig. 33-19. A. HCC is occasionally made up of clear cells, as shown here. (LUS 1345-78) (Original magnification × 216; H&E) **B.** Higher-power magnification shows resemblance to carcinoma of the kidney. (LUS 1345-78) (Original magnification × 1018; H&E)

22). Occasionally, some of the accelerated growth structures are neoplastic.

Cholangiohepatocellular Carcinoma

Of 405 primary cancers of the liver diagnosed in our material from 1918 to 1979, 19, or 4.7%, were combined, or "cholangiohepatocellular," carcinomas. However, more than 20% of HCC had glandular or ductal transformation of neoplastic hepatocytes that, nonetheless, still retained the cytologic features of hepatocytes with granular, pink cytoplasms and prominent nucleoli. The term cholangiohepatocellular carcinoma is readily exemplified by the few cases that harbor ductal carcinoma in one area of liver

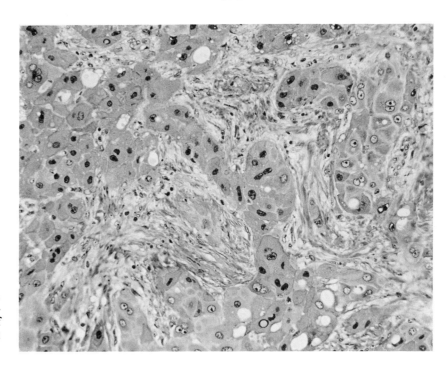

Fig. 33-20. Fibrolamellar HCC. Note the clusters of acidophilic hepatocytes separated by bundles of collagen. (Original magnification × 432; H&E)

remote from a separate HCC. We have always considered most tumors with ductal and hepatocellular components in the same mass to be variants of HCC because of behavioral similarities to HCC and because glandular transformation of neoplastic hepatocytes is so common (see Fig. 33-18*B*). The sex ratio of cholangiohepatocellular carcinoma patients has been 3:1, with male predominance; 73.7% have arisen in cirrhotic livers. The metastatic pattern has been intermediate between ductal and HCC (see Table 33-10).

Goodman and co-workers[105] reported 24 cases of combined cholangiohepatocellular carcinoma and distinguished three major groups: collision tumors (*i.e.,* two separate carcinomas); transitional tumors with transition of the two tumor types; and fibrolamellar tumors, which had mucin-producing pseudoglands. Immunohistochemical staining revealed keratin reaction in 90% of cholangiocarcinomas and 52% of combined cholangiohepatocellular carcinomas. On the other hand, AFP was noted in 50% of HCC and 29% of combined tumors but was absent in cholangiocarcinoma.

Carcinoma of the Intrahepatic Bile Ducts

In our series of 405 primary liver tumors, 56 originated in the intrahepatic bile-duct system. Such tumors are called *intrahepatic cholangiocarcinoma.* The true occurrence of cholangiocarcinoma on a national basis is frequently buried under the designation of primary hepatic cancer. Even in autopsy series, many carcinomas that are classified as cholangiocarcinomas at one institution may

be called "mixed cholangiohepatocellular carcinoma," "adenocarcinoma," or "hepatocellular carcinoma with ductal transformation" at others.

Intrahepatic cholangiocarcinomas may arise at any point from the hilum of the liver to Glisson's capsule. They may be separated into PCCs, the major duct cholangiocarcinomas, and hilar cholangiocarcinoma (HCLC). PCC arises from small bile ducts within the liver, whereas HCLC arises from the major hepatic ducts near or at the juncture of the right and left hepatic ducts. The two principal types, PCC and HCLC, differ both in symptomatology and in progressive neoplastic growth. Two rare tumors that do not fit into the categories of PCC or HCLC but are of ductal origin are biliary papillomatosis and cholangiolocellular carcinoma.

Peripheral Cholangiocarcinoma

PCC, which was found in only 0.05% of our 96,625 autopsies, represents 9% of primary malignant hepatic tumors. In our material, 62% of the patients were men. The mean age of the patients is 61 years. Compared with the racial distribution of the autopsy population from which these patients were drawn, there is a slight preponderance of whites, as seen in Table 33-11.

Twenty-four percent of the patients with PCC had cirrhosis, in contrast to 5.7% of the entire autopsy population and 84% of the patients with HCC.

Etiology. PCC has been reported to occur coincidentally with certain other conditions. The coincident disorders

TABLE 33-10.   Metastatic Patterns of HCC, Cholangiocarcinoma, and Cholangiohepatocellular Carcinoma

	HCC, NON-CIRRHOTIC (39 CASES) (%)	HCC, CIRRHOTIC (188 CASES) (%)	PERIPHERAL CHOLANGIO-CARCINOMA (18 CASES) (%)	HILAR CHOLANGIO-CARCINOMA (6 CASES) (%)	CHOLANGIO-HEPATO-CELLULAR CARCINOMA (14 CASES) (%)
No metastases	33	54.8	25.0	66	21.4
Single metastases	25.0	19.1	18.8	0	21.4
Lung	41.0	38.8	25.0	33	21.4
Lymph node (portal)	43.6	16.5	68.8	17	42.0
Portal vein	23.0	37.2	12.5	0	35.7
Hepatic vein	18.0	22.9	18.8	0	21.4
Skin	0	2.7	0	0	0
Serosa	23.1	7.4	25.0	17	35.7
Adrenal gland	3.0	6.9	18.0	0	21.5
Bone marrow	7.7	8.0	25.0	17	14.3
Heart	2.6	1.6	0	0	0
Spleen	7.7	2.1	6.3	0	7.1
Pancreas	0	1.1	0	0	0
Central nervous system	0	0	0	0	0
Kidney	2.6	3.7	0	0	0
Diaphragm	2.6	3.7	6.3	0	21.4
Gallbladder	10.3	5.3	0	0	14.3
Other	5.1	3.2	6.3		

are principally those that involve chronic cholestasis; however, 90% of patients with PCC have no recognized antecedent disorder or etiology other than cirrhosis. Cirrhosis was present in 24% of our cases, but, of those, 28% had hemochromatosis.

Duct Anomalies. Cystic disease of the liver in one of its many varieties, including Meyenburg complexes and Caroli's disease, has been reported in association with cholangiocarcinoma in 47 cases (Fig. 33-23).[58,120,140,267,354] However, Meyenburg complexes are such common anomalies that their occurrence in livers involved or not involved by cholangiocarcinoma is undoubtedly often overlooked. Some patients with congenital cystic diseases of the liver have HCC rather than PCC. Cholangiocarcinomas do not seem to arise from the cystic structures, however. Carcinoma actually arising within the simple cyst walls has been squamous cell carcinoma.[27,28] Investigators have hypothesized that, because of the liver's usual function of excretion of toxins, including carcinogens, conditions resulting in slowly flowing bile cause prolonged exposure of the duct system to hypothetical biliary carcinogens.[94,160,171,348] Carcinoma arising in congenital hepatic fibrosis is less common than carcinoma arising in a liver involved by simple cysts or by congenital dilatation of the intrahepatic ducts. The reported instances of PCC in association with congenital hepatic fibrosis have been identified in patients who were asymptomatic with respect

to portal hypertension or hepatic disease and developed the carcinoma late in life.[60,86,187,234]

Biliary Atresia. There are a few reports linking PCC with congenital biliary atresia.[156] However, HCC is a more common complication. The cases identified as cholangiocarcinoma were actually described as mixed cholangiocarcinoma and HCC, a group we usually consider a variant of HCC. Carcinoma arising in biliary atresia has been described in patients from 5 months to 12 years of age. The incidence of this complication may increase in patients who have undergone the Kasai operation and have increased life spans.

Chronic Cholangitis. Cholangitis and hepatolithiasis have been reported to lead to PCC.[153] As might be anticipated, the largest series is from the Orient, where cholangiohepatitis and hepatolithiasis are relatively common. The etiology of cholangiohepatitis is still a mystery.[81,281,360]

Clonorchis sinensis. *Clonorchis sinensis* infestation of the hepatic duct has been related to cholangiocarcinoma, particularly in Hong Kong, where both *Clonorchis* infestation and PCC are more common than in the west.[101,123,124] More than 90% of cholangiocarcinomas in Hong Kong are associated with *Clonorchis* infestation, whereas one third of the control patients without bile-duct carcinoma also have *Clonorchis* infection. The flukes are associated with a generalized duct inflammatory reaction with epithelial hyperplasia and *in situ* atypia of the

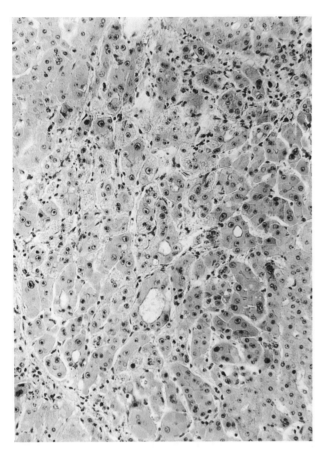

Fig. 33-21. Paraplastic change in nonalcoholic cirrhotic liver with HCC elsewhere. Note variation in cellular pattern with the acidophilic cells compressing the adjacent parenchyma. (Original magnification × 312; H&E)

ductal epithelium. Apparently, a majority of cholangiocarcinomas that arise in association with clonorchiasis are hilar in position, but in others the parasite may be associated with PCC.

Chronic Ulcerative Colitis. The incidence of cholangiocarcinoma has been reported to be tenfold higher in patients with chronic ulcerative colitis than in the general population. The tumor may be peripheral or hilar.[198,235,262,338,346] Only one of 45 patients with cholangiocarcinoma of the peripheral type in our series had ulcerative colitis; that patient was only 25 years old. Carcinoma of the biliary tree, when it arises in a patient with chronic ulcerative colitis, develops 20 years earlier than the average age for PCC.

Cirrhosis. PCC is usually stated to be unrelated to cirrhosis, yet, in nearly all reports, patients with PCC are more frequently cirrhotic than the rest of the autopsy population. In our material, 24% of the patients had cirrhosis; most was of the advanced alcoholic type, but 28% of the cirrhotics had hemochromatosis. In a large series

from Japan, 25% of the patients with cholangiocarcinoma had chronic liver disease of the nonalcoholic type. No increased coincidence of hepatitis B has been associated with cholangiocarcinoma in our material, but one study reports that 14.5% of 268 patients with PCC were HBsAg-positive.[219]

Thorotrast. One third of all cases of malignant tumors associated with thorotrast are angiosarcomas, and the remainder are divided between tumors of the bile-duct system and HCC.[15,102] There is one case report of combined cholangiocarcinoma and angiosarcoma in a patient who received thorotrast.[356]

Hemochromatosis. Hemochromatosis has been associated with both cholangiocarcinoma and HCC. The tumor arising in hemochromatosis frequently has features of both metaplasia and HCC and is referred to as "mixed." In our experience, the predominant tumor type has been hepatocellular with ductal transformation but 9% of our hemochromatosis patients had PCC, compared with 18% who had HCC. Hemochromatosis was the underlying disease of 6.7% of the PCC cases.

Gross Pathology. Cholangiocarcinomas are sclerosing gray tumors with infiltrative margins. The borders are irregular, and the tumor does not produce the compression of adjacent liver tissue that is often seen in metastatic lesions. Usually, there are satellite tumor nodules. There is rarely extensive necrosis or liquefaction of the carcinoma (see Fig. 33-23).

Histopathology. Cholangiocarcinomas are made up of ductal structures with variable degrees of differentiation. Most are well differentiated, forming ducts and fairly dense fibrous stroma (Fig. 33-24). Occasionally, they have larger glandlike structures and well developed columnar epithelial cells. It is possible that such carcinomas may have arisen from major intrahepatic ducts. The demarcation between the carcinoma and the surrounding liver is usually distinct microscopically. Often, there is a border of inflammatory cells that forms an interface between the liver parenchyma and the proliferating ductal structures (Fig. 33-25). Some carcinomas that had predominantly ductal features in some areas may have HCC in others. These have often been called mixed hepatocellular cholangiocarcinomas and have been thought to arise from cells that have the potential to form either hepatocytes or duct cells. Alternatively, these tumors may represent metaplastic change from HCC. Because of a presumed association with cholangioles, some of these tumors have been referred to as cholangiolocellular carcinomas.[5] However, cholangiocellular carcinoma is originally a designation that Steiner assigned to carcinoma in which the entire tumor resembles cholangioles throughout (see section on cholangiocellular carcinoma).

Metastatic Pattern. Of the patients with PCC in our series, 25% had no metastases. Sometimes, because of involvement of the right lobe of the liver and the bed of the

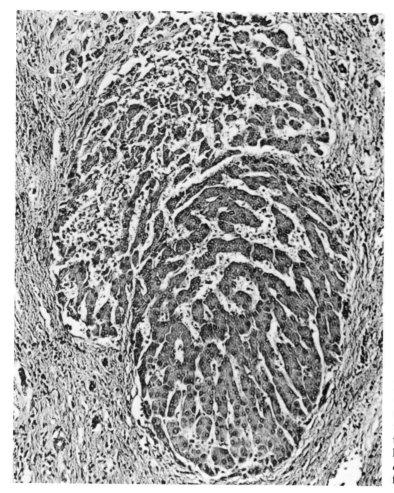

Fig. 33-22. Paraplastic change in alcoholic cirrhotic liver with a spurt of growth from a small inactive nodule. Note the trabecular development in the new nodule. (Courtesy of Peters RL: In Okuda K, Peters RL: Hepatocellular Carcinoma, p 120. New York, John Wiley & Sons, 1976) (JWA 77-66) (Original magnification × 160; H&E)

gallbladder, it may be impossible to distinguish PCC from carcinoma of the gallbladder invading the liver. Metastases in the portal lymph nodes occurred in 69% of the cases. Although cholangiocarcinoma does not invade the extrahepatic portal vein as readily as HCC, about 8% of patients with PCC have portal vein thrombosis, and, occasionally, the carcinoma may invade or occlude the hepatic vein radicles or even the inferior vena cava.

Major duct hepatic cholangiocarcinomas arise from a grossly discernible major duct tributary. These are extraordinarily rare. Their pathology differs little from that of PCC.

TABLE 33-11.   Racial Distribution of Peripheral Cholangiocarcinoma

	AUTOPSY POPULATION (%)	CHOLANGIO-CARCINOMA POPULATION (%)	HEPATOCELLULAR CARCINOMA POPULATION (%)
White	64.5	76	52
Black	20.5	4	24
Mexican	13.8	10	15
Oriental	0.9	4	9
Other	0.3		

(Data obtained at Los Angeles County University of Southern California Medical Center and John Wesley County Hospital [1918–1979].)

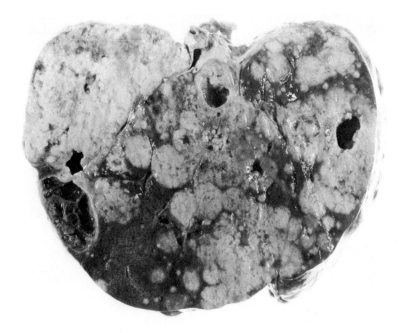

Fig. 33-23. Gross photograph of PCC in liver with multiple simple cysts. (RA 37-80)

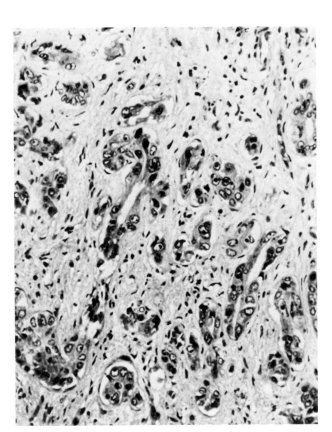

Fig. 33-24. PCC with fibrosis. (RA 22-79) (Original magnification × 432; H&E)

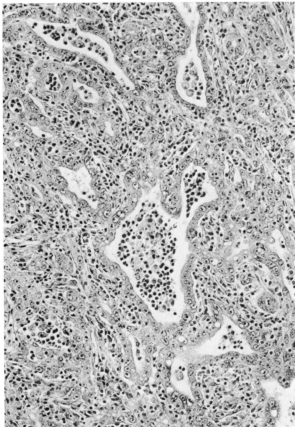

Fig. 33-25. PCC with acute inflammatory infiltrate. (LUS 1347-78) (Original magnification × 312; H&E)

Hilar Cholangiocarcinoma

HCLC arises from the hepatic duct or near its bifurcation (Fig. 33-26). The location of the lesion produces a unique set of symptoms separating it from other carcinomas of the biliary tree. The tumor represented 25% of intrahepatic cholangiocarcinomas in our series, but in a Japanese study in which HCLC was found in 0.4% of autopsies and in 10% of primary hepatic malignancies, 29 of 57 intrahepatic cholangiocarcinomas were hilar. In our material, the tumor was found in 0.01% of autopsies, 0.06% of all malignant tumors encountered at autopsy, and 2.7% of all primary liver tumors. The average age of the patients was 62.8 years, with 2:1 predominance of women over men. There is no explanation for the difference between the two population groups.

HCLC has an insidious onset and progresses slowly. In about one half of the patients, jaundice is not an initial symptom, but abdominal pain, malaise, fever, abdominal distention, and pruritus are usually part of the initial manifestations. Patients develop signs of bile-duct obstruction, which, before the ready availability of percu-

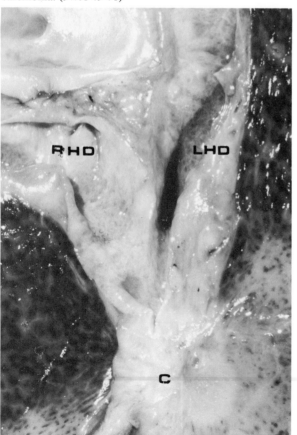

Fig. 33-26. Sclerotic tumor arising at bifurcation of hepatic duct. RHD, right hepatic duct; LHD, left hepatic duct; C, carcinoma. (JWA 49-71)

taneous cholangiograms, presented difficult diagnostic problems. The carcinoma is often too well hidden between the recesses of the right and left lobes and the quadrate and caudate lobes for adequate biopsy or even duct curettement. Since the tumors classically remain small, extension into the liver parenchyma is usually insufficient to allow diagnosis by means of a liver biopsy, scan, or angiogram. The alert surgeon, however, should note the shrunken gallbladder and common duct as well as the pale duct mucosa. Given these and the biopsy findings of mechanical obstruction, one could surmise a diagnosis of either sclerosing cholangitis or HCLC. As rare as is HCLC, extrahepatic sclerosing cholangitis is even less common. In one 10-year study of surgical investigation of 13 patients with sclerosing lesions of the hepatic duct thought to be sclerosing cholangitis clinically, 8 patients were found at surgery to have carcinoma of the hepatic duct. Five could not be diagnosed at surgery, but four of those five were ultimately found at autopsy to have HCLC.[236]

Many patients with HCLC may have a protracted clinical course and often are considered to have PBC. A clinical survival of 3 years is not rare.

Etiology. The coincidental relationships of other conditions to HCLC are similar to those in patients with PCC; however, there is no relationship of HCLC to cirrhosis, hemochromatosis, or thorotrast. Many cases of HCLC have been associated with chronic ulcerative colitis. In one report of 15 patients who had carcinoma of the biliary tract associated with ulcerative colitis, 4 patients had HCLC.[272] Patients with ulcerative colitis who develop HCLC, like patients who develop PCC, tend to be much younger than those who do not have inflammatory bowel disease.

Cystic diseases of liver and biliary tree may be associated with HCLC as well as with PCC.

Carcinoma may arise from the hilum in patients with *Clonorchis sinenesis* infestation.

Pathology. HCLC is most frequently a sclerosing lesion that involves the duct wall and occludes the lumen, extending only 1 cm or so into the surrounding tissue (see Fig. 33-25). Occasional tumors apparently start as superficial adenocarcinomas and proliferate as solid tumors arising from the duct mucosa to occlude the lumen. Such tumors tend to be associated with atypical epithelial changes in other parts of the duct. Sometimes HCLC infiltrates more extensively into the surrounding parenchyma. In such instances, it is usually difficult or impossible to ascertain whether the carcinoma actually originated in the main hepatic duct juncture or whether it represents a PCC that secondarily obliterates the hilar area.

Biliary Papillomatosis

Papillary growth in the biliary tract is rare, but several individual cases have been reported. The pathology consists of papillary proliferation of the epithelial lining filling the biliary passages, sometimes involving most of the entire bile-duct system. Although the tumor rarely infiltrates outside of the duct or even into the duct wall, it has a malignant course.[76,117,134,177,223,274]

Cholangiolocellular Carcinoma

In 1957, Steiner introduced the concept of cholangiolocellular carcinoma, a tumor with a growth pattern that resembles cholangioles, although there is no definite evidence that the tumor actually arises from those structures (see Fig. 33-26).[303] Approximately 1% of primary malignant tumors of the liver in our series have had the morphology that Steiner described. It is not uncommon to encounter areas of either HCC or cholangiocarcinoma that have the appearance of cholangioles, but a tumor in which the entire differentiated portion resembles cholangioles is rare. The neoplastic cells retain the configuration usually associated with cholangioles in that they form double-layered cuboidal epithelial cell cords that have a tiny lumen and a basement membrane (Fig. 33-

Fig. 33-27. Cholangiolocellular carcinoma. Note resemblance of tumor ductules to cholangioles. (JWA 123-74) (Original magnification × 216; H&E)

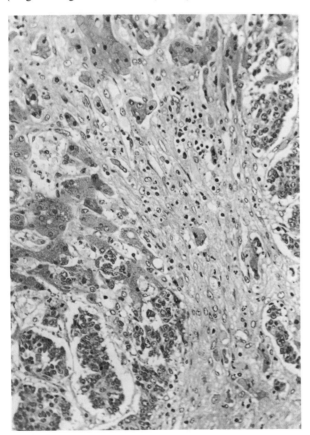

27). The cytoplasm is scanty, forming a narrow clear zone around the dark oval nuclei. The nuclei lack the prominent nucleoli usually found in HCC.[242,305]

Sarcoma of the Liver

Sarcomas of the liver may be easily divided into two groups, the soft blood-filled vascular tumors and the solid tumors. Angiosarcoma has received much publicity because of its relationship to known etiologic factors such as vinyl chloride and thorotrast.[169,249] No specific etiologic agents have been identified in the reported cases of solid sarcomas, although a few have arisen within cirrhotic livers. The solid sarcomas have certain features more or less in common. Most are large, some of massive size before they are clinically recognized. They are usually gray–white and fairly firm. Occasionally, more undifferentiated forms occur that are softer and may contain areas of hemorrhage and necrosis. Both sarcoma and HCC produce large nonumbilicated tumors. However, HCC is much softer and more likely to be discolored. In our collection, there are 57 sarcomas of the liver principally submitted in consultation. A definite microscopic diagnosis may be very difficult. The recognition of angiosarcoma, leiomyosarcoma, fibrosarcoma, and rhabdomyosarcoma is possible. In addition, there are many undifferentiated tumors that, for want of a better term, we choose to call mesenchymal sarcomas. Several types of sarcomas are represented by a single case. These include malignant schwannoma, hemangiopericytoma, and a liposarcoma. The use of immunohistochemistry is becoming more important in the microscopic diagnosis of sarcomas.[14] The possibility of metastatic sarcoma must be considered whenever sarcoma is present in liver.

Angiosarcoma

Angiosarcomas are vasoformative tumors in which the vascular spaces are lined with malignant endothelial cells and carry blood. We believe in strict adherence to this definition because other highly vascular tumors of the liver, both primary and metastatic, enter into the differential diagnosis. Many cases of angiosarcoma have been reported in vinyl chloride workers and in patients who have had injections of thorotrast.[122,249,283] The average latent period in vinyl chloride workers who developed angiosarcoma was 19 years, with a range of 11 to 37 years[164,169]; after injection of thorotrast, the average was 24 years, with a range of 12 to 35 years. Both long-term and short-term use of arsenic has resulted in hepatic angiosarcoma.[169,269] It is of further interest that patients with idiopathic hemochromatosis may develop angiosarcoma.[315] One patient developed angiosarcoma after exposure to a radium needle.[169] In our material, there are 18 examples of angiosarcoma, one of which was associated with thorotrast injection, one of which followed long continued use of Fowler's solution, and one of which was

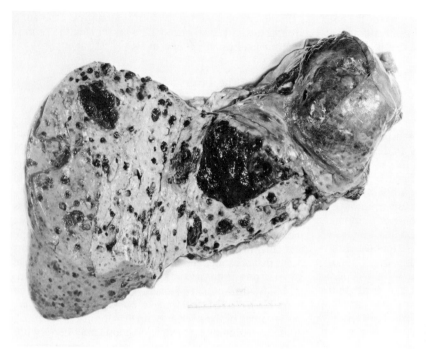

Fig. 33-28. Hepatic angiosarcoma with sharply circumscribed hemorrhagic nodules. Cavernous spaces are present in the larger nodules. The patient was a 57-year-old white woman who died of hemorrhage from one of the larger nodules. (ASC 120)

present in a patient with apparent idiopathic hemochromatosis. The group consisted of 14 men and 4 women. In the literature, the ratio of men to women is 4:1.

The most common complaint in patients with angiosarcoma is abdominal pain. Weakness, weight loss, anorexia, and abdominal swelling are also symptoms. A large liver, ascites, and jaundice are the most prominent findings.

The laboratory abnormalities include elevated levels of serum alkaline phosphatase, serum glutamic-pyruvic transaminase (SGPT), serum bilirubin, and serum globulin; anemia; a prolonged prothrombin time; and thrombocytopenia. Arteriography is the most valuable diagnostic procedure. The course of the disease is usually short, averaging less than 6 months. Hepatic failure, gastrointestinal bleeding, and renal failure are the most common complications.

A majority of angiosarcomas present as multiple nodules of variable size. A few are solitary. As a rule, the liver is greatly enlarged (Fig. 33-28). The nodules have a hemorrhagic appearance, sometimes cavernous, particularly in their central portions, whereas the margin tends to be more cellular and not so congested. Microscopically, angiosarcomas are composed of newly formed vascular channels that are lined with malignant cells. At least three types of lining cells occur, each tumor having a fairly uniform population. In most cases, the cells are rather plump and have a large hyperchromatic nucleus and a moderate amount of cytoplasm, and mitoses are observed (Fig. 33-29). In a few cases, the lining cells are rather large, and even giant cell forms are seen. In another variant, the cells

are spindle-shaped. Usually, in these cases the spindle cells form septa composed of thick bundles. At the margin of the lesion, the malignant endothelial cells invade adjacent liver, replacing normal sinusoidal cells (Fig. 33-30). Near the growing margin, there is often a highly cellular angiosarcoma. In the older, central portions of the nodules, large cavernous spaces may form with rather thin septa, but the spaces are always lined with malignant cells. Thrombosis of the central areas may occur. The metastatic deposits are similar in appearance to the primary liver tumor. Delorme has described a solid sarcomatous type of angiosarcoma.[64]

We have also included among the angiosarcomas another solid tumor that has a prolonged clinical course and is known by a multitude of names. Among these are epithelioid hemangioendothelioma, pseudocartilaginous sarcomas, mixed tumor, sclerosing endothelioid angiosarcoma, and sclerosing interstitial vascular sarcoma.[72] However, we have chosen to call this tumor *vasoablative endotheliosarcoma (VABES)* with pseudocartilaginous change. It grows slowly but aggressively and gradually forms a fibrous hyalinized replacement of much of the liver tissue. The stroma of the tumor strongly resembles cartilage. The duration of survival after diagnosis is usually 5 to 10 years. Microscopically, there is great variation in appearance depending upon the age of the tumor. At the margin of the growth, rather large, plump tumor cells may fill the sinusoids while the center of the growth has a fibrous stroma. Factor VIII is often demonstrable within the tumor cells. Metastases most often occur in bone, lymph nodes, and pleura.

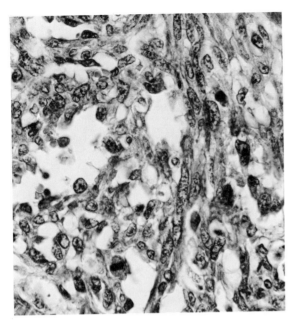

Fig. 33-29. Highly cellular angiosarcoma with capillary-sized lumens. Note mitoses near the bottom. (ASC 3329) (Original magnification × 420)

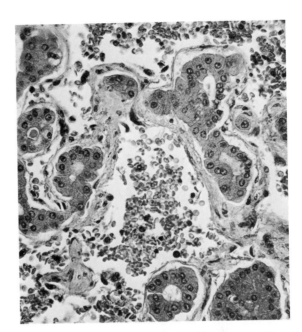

Fig. 33-30. Dilated sinusoids lined with plump malignant endothelial cells. Cord pattern is still present. (ASC 3329) (Original magnification × 260)

Solid Sarcoma

Solid sarcomas that can be identified on microscopic examination include leiomyosarcoma, rhabdomyosarcoma, fibrosarcoma, and rare examples of other sarcomas. However, in our collection, the undifferentiated mesenchymal sarcomas accounted for the largest group.

Leiomyosarcoma. Fifteen cases of leiomyosarcoma have been reported in the literature.[46] In our material there are five cases that we consider to be leiomyosarcoma, all in white men 24 to 64 years of age, with an average age of 50 years. Leiomyosarcomas of the liver are massive, slow-growing tumors that arise in adults.[183] The chief complaints are abdominal swelling and pain. On physical examination there is hepatomegaly, sometimes extreme. Ascites may also be present. Liver scans performed in three reported cases disclosed one or more cold areas. Surgery has been recommended even if metastases are present.[183] The prognosis is better than that observed in HCC. A patient with leiomyosarcoma may live for more than a year, occasionally for several years.[69]

Grossly, the liver may weigh as much as 11,200 g.[90] Leiomyosarcomas are most often solitary, rarely multiple. Microscopically, they consist of interlacing bundles of spindle cells with a variable amount of cytoplasm (Fig. 33-31). Elongated cigar-shaped nuclei are characteristic, as is mitotic activity. Leiomyosarcomas arising within the hepatic veins and producing the Budd–Chiari syndrome have been reported.[175]

Electron microscopy has proven to be helpful in the diagnosis of smooth-muscle tumors.[28,195] Morales lists ultrastructural criteria of leiomyosarcoma as follows: the presence of intracytoplasmic myofilaments; dense bodies, both in cytoplasm and in association with the plasma membrane; pinocytic vesicles and invaginations of the plasma membranes; and remnants of basal lamina or an extensive cell coat. Bloustein noted that ten cases of leiomyosarcoma have been reported in the literature.

Fibrosarcoma. Fibrosarcoma is a rare entity. Only 21 cases have been reported,[247] mostly in men. We have three in our collection, making a total of 24. Fibrosarcomas form large firm tumors, some undergo central necrosis with hemorrhage, and, in one case, there was rupture and hemoperitoneum. Cirrhosis was present in three cases. One of our patients, a 59-year-old man, continues to survive after 10 years; moreover, he has had repeated episodes of severe hypoglycemia. A similar case has recently been published.[98] The microscopic criteria for the diagnosis included a herringbone pattern, close association of long spindle-shaped cells with collagen fibrils, and envelopment of the cells by reticulin. The nuclei in fibrosarcoma tend to have rather angulated ends (Fig. 33-32). Metastases occur most often in the abdominal lymph nodes.

Rhabdomyosarcoma. Rhabdomyosarcoma in the adult has recently been reported in a 76-year-old man with cirrhosis who had a positive AFP test.[197] A massive tumor

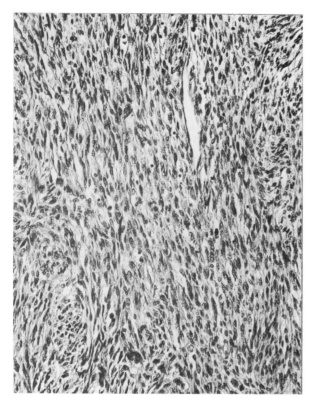

Fig. 33-31. Densely cellular sarcoma in the left lobe of the liver of a 64-year-old man. Patient died of recurrence 6 months after resection. (ASC 2457) (Original magnification × 220)

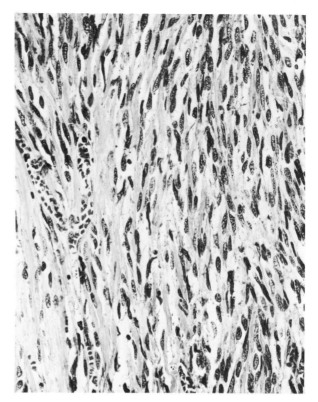

Fig. 33-32. Tumor removed from the left lobe of the liver of a 58-year-old man. Patient is alive 10 years later with a mass in the right lobe. Note that the nuclei have angulated ends and are closely apposed to heavy bands of collagen. (ASC 1759) (Original magnification × 250)

of the left lobe was noted at autopsy. In infants and children, rhabdomyosarcomas are most often of the embryonal type.[62] These have a characteristic microscopic appearance. The nuclei have an eccentric location within the cell, and cross-striations are often present in the cytoplasm.

Mesenchymal Sarcoma. Mesenchymal sarcomas are undifferentiated tumors that grow rapidly and have a poor prognosis.[45,68,310] They usually occur in children and only occasionally in adults. These sarcomas often reach huge proportions. Among the 57 sarcomas of the liver in our collection, 14 were termed mesenchymal sarcoma. Grossly, they are gray–white to yellow, and nearly all have one or more degenerative areas such as a cystic change, necrosis, and hemorrhage.

Microscopically, although there is considerable variation in cell type, most of the tumors have rather short, plump nuclei and a paucity of intercellular fibers. Many have a myxoid stroma (Fig. 33-33). This is especially true of mesenchymal sarcomas in young girls. Some mesenchymal sarcomas contain giant cells. Necrosis and hemorrhage are common. PAS-positive diastase-resistant bodies have been described in the tumor cells,[77] as have

remnants of bile ducts. Hepatic artery ligation and systemic therapy have been used in treatment of nonresectable tumors.[322]

The use of immunohistochemistry stains has made the diagnosis of solid sarcomas somewhat easier inasmuch as Desmin will stain tumors of muscle origin and Vimentin will stain the mesenchymal tumors.[15]

Although extremely rare, HCC and sarcoma may arise together, forming a single tumor.[336] In the case reported by Tsujimoto and co-workers, only the sarcoma metastasized.

Sarcoma in Cirrhosis

Sarcoma in cirrhosis is another rare entity. In HCC complicating cirrhosis, there may be areas that have the gross and microscopic features of sarcoma. Microscopically, the sarcomatous portion is composed of undifferentiated spindle cells. Some of these tumors are separate and distinct from one another, whereas, in other cases, bridging forms are evident between the carcinoma and sarcoma. The first may be called carcinoma and sarcoma while the

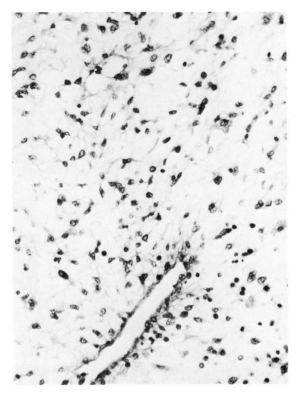

Fig. 33-33. Myxoid appearance of mesenchymal sarcoma. This tumor occurred in a 7-year-old girl who had the right lobe of the liver resected. (ASC 1327) (Original magnification × 225)

latter is HCC, spindle-cell variant. Only ten cases of carcinoma and sarcoma occurring together in the cirrhotic liver have been reported.[300] In nine of these, HCC was present, and, in one case, cholangiocarcinoma was diagnosed. In addition, some cirrhotics developed only a spindle-cell sarcoma[6] that differs little from those associated with HCC. The true nature of these sarcomas may well be elucidated more clearly by electron microscopy and immunohistochemistry in the future.

BENIGN EPITHELIAL TUMORS AND TUMOR-LIKE LESIONS

Benign epithelial tumors and tumor-like lesions most commonly arise from hepatocytes. The majority of these are composed of adenomas and FNH, although the bile duct epithelium does rarely give rise to a benign tumor. A general review of benign tumors has been published by Ishak and Rabin.[129] The epithelial lesions are conveniently divided into adenomas and the hyperplasias. The latter consist of focal nodular, adenomatous, and nodular regenerative types.

Hepatocellular Adenoma

In the era before the use of oral contraceptives, that is, before 1960, liver cell adenomas were among the rarest of tumors. For example, there were only two recognized at the LAC-USMC among the first 50,000 autopsies. Some 13 years after the advent of oral contraceptives, examples of liver cell adenomas began to be published.[16] After reviewing all of our material on adenomas of the liver, we propose the clinicopathologic classification presented in Table 33-12. Many of the tumors included in this classification are extremely rare, but all possible etiologic factors should be considered by the pathologist when studying an adenoma of the liver. In our files there are 52 cases of adenoma that followed the use of oral contraceptives; 39 of these were solitary and 13 were multiple. The largest tumor in our series was 38 cm in diameter and weighed 2700 g. Usually the multiple tumors are small to moderate in size, but occasionally they are rather large (Fig. 33-34). The typical adenoma is encapsulated, somewhat lighter in color than the surrounding liver (perhaps yellow as a result of bile formation), and has a homogeneous appearance. Adenomas are prone to hemorrhage and necrosis, especially in their central portions, which lead to pain and discomfort in the right upper quadrant in about one third of all patients. In less than one third, rupture and intraperitoneal bleeding that require emergency surgery occur. The remaining one third of patients have only a palpable mass. Patients who have an unresected adenoma that follows the use of oral contraceptives are at considerable risk if they become pregnant because hemorrhage and rupture may follow.[146] Excellent reviews of the clinical, radiologic, and pathologic aspects of liver cell adenoma and FNH have been published by Knowles and co-workers and Kerlin and co-workers.[147,152]

Microscopically, adenomas are composed of neo-hepatocytes that are usually arranged in closely approxi-

TABLE 33-12.   A Useful Clinicopathologic Classification of Hepatocellular Adenoma

I. Women
   A. Associated with the use of oral contraceptives and other corticosteroids
   B. Spontaneous
II. Pediatric age-group
   A. Spontaneous
   B. In glycogen-storage disease, tyrosinemia, galactosemia
III. Men
   A. Spontaneous
   B. Estrogen
IV. Adenomas associated with
   A. Diabetes mellitus
   B. Cirrhosis
   C. Siderosis
   D. Miscellaneous
V. Androgen-induced adenomas

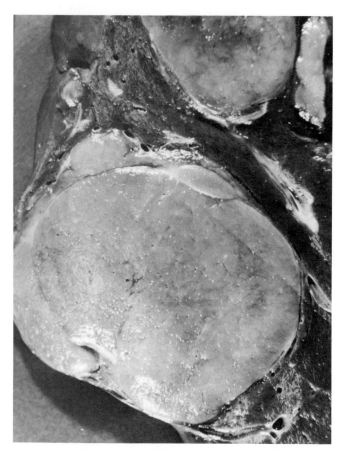

Fig. 33-34. Large encapsulated gray-white tumors surgically removed from a 30-year-old woman who had been taking oral contraceptives for more than four years. Numerous blood vessels are noted on the cut surface. Two closely adjacent adenomas are included in the specimen. (ASC 2141)

mated cords. Several types of hepatocytes may be distinguished. Among these are acidophilic cells, hydropic-type cells, extraordinarily large cells, and clear cells that are apparently filled with glycogen. The most common type is the hydropic cell that has a somewhat vacuolated base that borders on the sinusoid (Fig. 33-35). The cytoplasmic granules are present in opposite poles of the cells and surround the small canaliculi that may contain variable amounts of bile pigment. The canaliculi are not always visible. An occasional adenoma is composed chiefly of cells filled with fat vacuoles. In others, an excess of lipochrome is present. At the margin of some adenomas in adjacent liver, small areas of hepatocytes occur that are similar to the adenoma cells. These appear to arise by transformation of existing hepatocytes, but new formation of cells may also be taking place. The centers of adenomas may undergo various degenerative changes including vascular dilatation (peliosis), necrosis, fibrosis, and hemorrhage. A variable degree of hemosiderin deposit may occur. Adenomas have an abundant blood supply; often the arteries and veins accompany one another throughout the tumor. Large, thick-walled arteries may be noted in the capsular area. Ultrastructure studies have shown adenoma cells to be similar to normal hepatocytes but oversimplified,[240] whereas in FNH, the hepatocytes are like those of hyperplastic but otherwise normal liver. In our collection, there was one tumor that contained large areas of adenoma and also a component of fibrolamellar carcinoma. A similar case, in which there appeared to be both adenoma and carcinoma, has been reported by Neuberger and associates.[209]

Large liver cell adenomas have been known to disappear when oral contraceptives are discontinued.[74] On rare occasions, liver cell adenomas occur in women and children not receiving estrogen compounds. Microscopically, these do not differ significantly from those adenomas that arise in pill users. Adenomas in infant girls may grow to great size and, as in one of our cases, may regress spontaneously.[353]

In men, liver cell adenoma is one of the rarest of tumors. It consists of an encapsulated tumor that has rather uniform hepatocytes. Some of these adenomas are associated with androgen therapy and typically form acinar structures that are different from other adenomas in men or in women.[52] Hemorrhage and rupture do not appear to be a complication of adenomas in men. However, in a large adenoma that arose in a transsexual taking methyltestosterone, rupture did occur and required a right lobectomy.[55] For reasons unknown, adenomas may arise in men who are diabetics.[92]

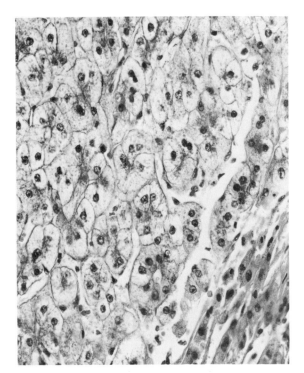

Fig. 33-35. Liver cell adenoma, the hepatocytes of which have a trabecular arrangement and form canaliculi. The bases of the cells are vacuolated. Normal hepatocytes at lower right. (ASC 2141) (Original magnification × 250)

Adenomas apparently grow by amitotic cell division. Many of the cells are binucleated and mitoses are rarely seen. Adenomas have a scanty connective tissue framework, the only tissue being that which accompanies the blood vessels. Degenerative changes, including hemorrhage and necrosis, were present in 36 of our 52 cases. Old central necrotic lesions may become fibrotic and contain hemosiderin. A few of the adenomas contained central blood-filled lakes consistent with the diagnosis of peliosis hepatis.

In our material there were only four cases of liver cell adenoma in men. All the tumors were solitary and encapsulated and varied from 2½ cm to 12 cm in diameter. Septa were present and gave them a nodular appearance, thus differing from adenomas in women. Microscopically, the tumors were composed of acidophilic hepatocytes. Although many of the androgen-associated tumors have been considered malignant, we have seen proven metastases in only one case, and it is not recognizable as hepatocellular origin.

Focal Nodular Hyperplasia

FNH is a tumor-like lesion that has been given various names and has been confused with liver cell adenoma. FNH occurs most often in women and may also be associated with the use of oral contraceptives.[147,150] Usually, these tumor-like lesions do not produce symptoms, and complications are almost unknown. A few reach a large size and become palpable, and surgery is performed. Most are found incidentally at surgery or autopsy. In our surgical material, there were 35 cases, 34 in women and one in a man, age 51. The age range of the 34 women was 20 to 74, with the average age of 38. In only 11 of the 34 women was surgery performed for symptoms for physical findings related to FNH. FNH may also occur in the pediatric age-group.[309]

Grossly, FNH has a characteristic appearance because of its central stellate-like scar with small linear projections to the periphery of the lesion (Fig. 33-36). There is no true encapsulation, and the line of demarcation between FNH and the liver is due mostly to a difference in color. The nodules are often present beneath Glisson's capsule, where they form a gray–brown bosselated mass. Rarely, the nodule is pedunculated and easily removed surgically. Hemorrhage is rarely a complication of FNH. Malignant change has not been reported. Both with the light microscope and electron microscope, the hepatocytes in FNH appear similar to normal hepatocytes. The characteristic microscopic feature is the small anatomic unit that is seen best at the periphery of the lesion. This comprises a central connective tissue core that contains blood vessels and bile duct radicles wih surrounding hepatocytes, usually about the size of a normal liver lobule (Fig. 33-37A). Another feature of FNH is the abundance of thick-walled blood vessels in the central area. These often have a myxomatous appearance. Angiograms have shown that the blood supply to FNH comes from central arteries, and the flow is centrifugal, whereas in liver cell adenomas, the flow is centripetal.[85] The predominant arterial supply has been emphasized by Whelan and co-workers.[328]

Other Benign Tumors

Other types of hyperplasia may be recognized, one of which is adenomatous hyperplasia, which may occur in livers that have undergone submassive necrosis or in which cirrhosis has developed. An area of adenomatous hyperplasia may have the gross appearance of an adenoma, but it is subdivided by septa that contain small bile ducts and blood vessels, thus distinguishing it from adenomas. It may be diagnosed by arteriograms and liver scans.[259] Although unusual, similar but smaller nodules arise in cirrhotic livers.

Another rare disorder is *nodular regenerative hyperplasia (NRH),*[311] which is characterized by hyperplastic foci of hepatocytes that form throughout the liver. When small, these are easily missed on microscopic examination but are easily demonstrated with the reticulum stain. A thin rim of reticulum fibers surrounds each of the tiny nodules in a characteristic fashion (Fig. 33-37B). NRH may occur as a complication of any one of several diseases, including Felty's syndrome, heart disease, drug therapy, and other disorders. NRH is sometimes associated with a noncirrhotic portal hypertension, varices, and hemorrhage.

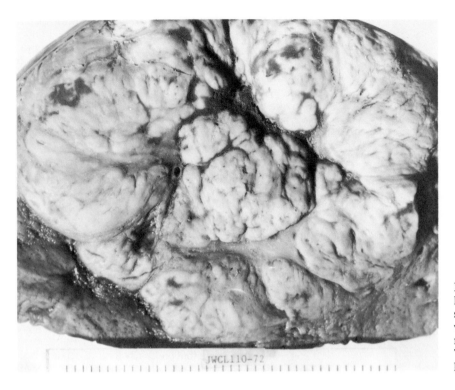

Fig. 33-36. Typical focal nodular hyperplasia with central stellate scar. Patient was a 21-year-old woman who was operated on for a mass in the middle upper abdomen. Tumor was removed from the left lobe of the liver. (ASC 1427A)

Fig. 33-37. Left. Anatomic subunit of focal nodular hyperplasia with central vessels and bile ducts. Adjacent liver at upper right. The nodule was an incidental finding in the left lobe, removed during cholestectomy. Patient was a 20-year-old woman. (ASC 1708) (Original magnification × 50) **Right.** Small nodules of hyperplasia with thickening of reticulum around the margins. (ASC 3900) (Original magnification × 104; Gridley reticulum)

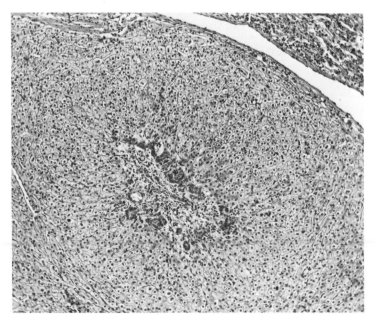

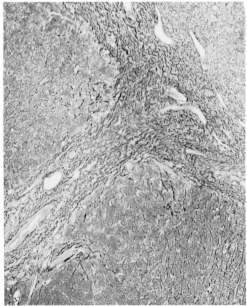

Bile ducts may rarely give rise to a benign tumor. Usually these are fairly small, white nodules less than 1 cm in diameter just beneath Glisson's capsule. They are composed of fairly abundant stroma and a bile ductular component that shows no evidence of malignancy. Most often bile duct adenomas are noted incidentally during upper abdominal surgery. They may be diagnosed by arteriograms and liver scans.[259] Although unusual, similar but smaller nodules arise in cirrhotic livers.

BENIGN MESENCHYMAL TUMORS

Vascular Tumors

Hemangiomas are, by far, the most common benign tumor of mesenchymal origin. They are circumscribed tumors comprising closely adjacent vascular channels, capillary to cavernous in size, that are lined with a single layer of endothelium. Solitary capillary angiomas are extremely rare and do not have clinical significance. In hereditary telangiectasia (Rendu–Osler–Weber disease), vascular spaces of capillary size are often widespread throughout the liver, notable especially along the portal tracts. Hepatic cavernous hemangiomas do occur in an occasional patient with hereditary telangiectasia.

Cavernous Hemangiomas

Cavernous hemangiomas occur in all age-groups but are most frequent in the elderly. Among 91,000 autopsies at the LAC-USCMC, cavernous hemangiomas were noted in 904: 575 men and 329 women. However, of those under 40, 37 were men and 53 were women. Cavernous hemangiomas often grow during pregnancy. Ultrasonography[32,181] and CT, are now being used successfully in the diagnosis of hemangiomas.[233]

A useful clinicopathologic classification of cavernous hemangiomas is given in Table 33-13.

Cavernous hemangiomas are most often solitary but may be multiple, and occasionally similar lesions occur in other organs. Most hemangiomas are small and symptomless, but others grow to a large size and become manifest both to the patient and to the clinician. Cavernous hemangiomas may be present beneath Glisson's capsule

TABLE 33-13. Cavernous Hemangiomas

CLASSIFICATION	DESCRIPTION
Solitary or multiple	Usually symptomless when under 4 cm in diameter
Solitary or multiple	With symptoms
Giant hemangiomas	Small percentage of all hemangiomas of liver
Hemangiomatosis	Diffuse of liver only, or with extrahepatic sites

or deep within the liver. They have a characteristic red–purple or blue–purple appearance, and their cavernous nature is easily seen on gross examination (Fig. 33-38). They may or may not be sharply delineated by connective tissue. With aging, they often undergo fibrosis, beginning in their central portion, that may completely replace the angioma. More rarely, there are multiple small angiomas throughout the liver known as hemangiomatosis, or the liver may be greatly enlarged by a giant hemangioma. These have been defined as 4 cm or more in greatest dimension.[2] We believe that 10 cm or 12 cm might be a more appropriate criterion. Hemangiomas may reach enormous size, the liver edge intruding into the pelvis (Fig. 33-39). In diffuse hemangiomatosis, the normal liver tissue may be almost completely replaced. Lastly, there is a type of hemangiomatosis that involves multiple organs.[141] In this disorder, destructive tumors occur in the lungs, bone, liver, and other structures. Although the hemangiomas have a benign microscopic structure, the patient's course may be like that of a patient with a malignancy.

Microscopically, the loculi of hemangiomas are lined by large, rather flat endothelial cells. The septa are composed of poorly cellular fibrous tissue that often has a myxomatous appearance. Many septa are incomplete and project into the vascular spaces like fingers (Fig. 33-40). Blood vessels and small bile ducts may be present in the larger septa. Some of the thick-walled blood vessels with small lumina are probably hepatic vein branches and likely contribute to the fibrosis that often occurs in hemangiomas. Large dilated portal vein radicles seen in cavernous hemangiomas and diffuse hemangiomatosis are probably the result of arterial–portal venous shunting.[132,357] Calcification occurs rarely in the septa or within the vascular lumina. This may be seen on radiographs.[246]

Among the complications are spontaneous rupture, which has been reported in 11 cases[182,285] and thrombosis of the cavities, which, when severe, may cause thrombocytopenia.

In diffuse hemangiomatosis, the angiomatous clusters may lie in close proximity to the blood vessels in the portal tracts, but they also appear adjacent to the outflow veins, where severe phlebosclerosis and thrombosis may follow. Small foci of capillary angiomatous change are frequent in diffuse hemangiomatosis.

Several instances of cavernous hemangioma and of infantile hemangioendothelioma have been reported in the newborn.[298] Most often, a palpable tumor is noted in the right upper quadrant the first day of life. The use of intravenous urograms and of arteriograms has led to prompt diagnosis and successful surgery in several instances. When an early diagnosis is not made, rupture of the hemangioma, congestive failure due to arteriovenous shunts, or consumptive coagulopathy may be fatal.

A biopsy of a cavernous hemangioma should never be attempted because it may lead to uncontrollable hemorrhage. The treatment of hemangiomas depends upon the size, location, and the risk of surgical removal. Trastek

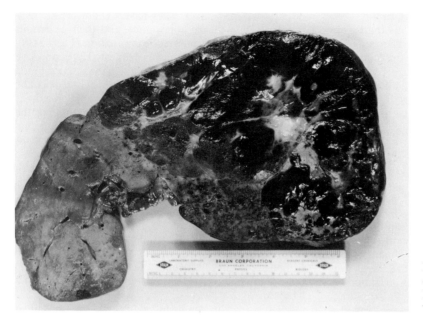

Fig. 33-38. Giant cavernous hemangioma of the liver. Weight was 13,000 g. Patient was a 57-year-old white woman who had borne many children. (ASC 684)

and co-workers have studied the successful removal in 49 patients.[334]

Infantile Hemangioendothelioma

Infantile hemangioendothelioma is a rare vasoformative cellular tumor that appears during the first 2 years of life.[63,70,87,133] The tumor is usually multiple and is often accompanied by similar tumors in the skin and other parts of the body. Grossly, the vascular reddish white lesions are usually present throughout the liver. A few of them are solitary and have been successfully resected. The presence of arteriovenous shunts within the tumors often causes congestive failure and death. Microscopically, there are many newly formed blood vessels lined by one or more layers of endothelial cells (Fig. 33-41). The growing nodule has in its center larger vessels and more cavernous change, whereas at the periphery, the lumina of the newly formed vessels are small and the proportion of cells to the vascular lumina is greater than at the center. With growth, the vasoformative component tends to infiltrate along the sinusoids, sometimes forming long columns of hepatocytes that have been converted to a bile duct–type of epithelium. In a few cases, malignant change has occurred, leading to angiosarcomas that metastasize to other organs. It is of interest that malignant change has been observed only in the liver and not in the extrahepatic sites. Successful treatment with prednisone has been reported.[333]

Others

The other benign mesenchymal tumors are most infrequent and usually not recognized during life. These include lipomas, fibromas, leiomyomas, and myxomas. Li-

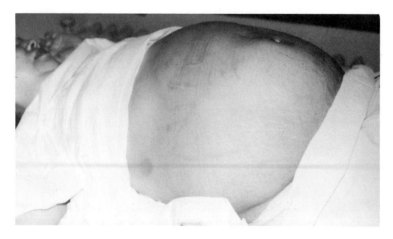

Fig. 33-39. Abdominal distension owing to giant hemangioma of the liver. Patient survived for 17 years. (ASC 3557)

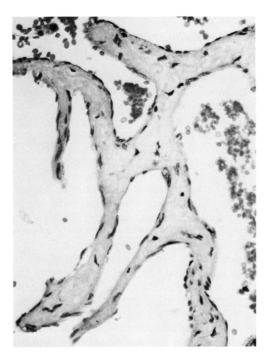

Fig. 33-40. Cavernous spaces of hemangioma with fingerlike projections. (ASC 3557) (Original magnification × 250)

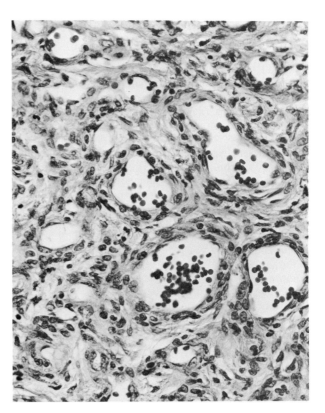

Fig. 33-41. Infantile hemangioendothelioma with congeries of newly formed vessels with a multilayered endothelial lining. The patient was a girl 6 months of age in whom a laparotomy revealed multiple nodules of the liver. She was treated with steroids, and 3 years later the left lobe of the liver was resected for a hemangioendothelial sarcoma. (ASC 3181) (Original magnification × 320)

pomas are sharply circumscribed and are composed of rather large fat-filled cells. Angiomyolipomas have been reported.[104] These tumors are usually small but may grow to 18 cm to 20 cm in diameter and produce right upper quadrant pain. As the name implies, they are composed of thick-walled blood vessels, lipocytes, and smooth-muscle cells. Ishak also has reviewed the subject of lipomatous tumors of the liver[127] for a small group that includes not only lipoma but myelolipoma, angiomyolipoma, and angiolipoma.[127] Ishak noted that two patients in this group had clinical manifestations and had their tumors removed surgically. One patient had a myelolipoma 12 cm to 13 cm in diameter. In another patient, there were two tumors, each 8 cm in diameter, one an angiolipoma and the other a lipoma. Areas of focal fatty change must be considered in differential diagnosis of lipomatous tumors.[33] Rare examples of other benign mesodermal tumors have been reported. These include fibromas of the liver,[127] solitary leiomyomas,[116] a massive myxoma of the liver,[80] and a lymphangioma.[11] In our files there is one fibroma that occurred in a 21-year-old man. The tumor weighed 4500 g.

Cystic Tumors and Tumor-like Lesions

Cystic masses constitute another recognizable group because of their gross appearance and because of characteristic findings with the use of ultrasound. They are, of course, avascular on angiograms. The entities under consideration are cystadenoma with mesenchymal stroma (CMS), polycystic disease, Caroli's disease, mesenchymal hamartoma, and, for purposes of differential diagnosis, echinococcus cysts.

CMS[130,352] are mucin-filled cystic lesions that usually grow to a large size before detection and excision. The tumors occur exclusively in women. In our material there were 17 cases. The mean age of 13 patients with benign cystadenoma was 41.7 years, whereas the 4 patients with cystadenocarcinoma were older, with a mean age of 51.5 years. Abdominal discomfort of some variety was noted in 13 patients, and pain had occurred in 8. The sole physical finding is an upper abdominal mass. Nearly all of the cystadenomas were present in the left lobe. They may reach a diameter of 20 cm or more and weigh up to 4000 g. The size of the cysts varies considerably. Sometimes there is one large one and only a few smaller cysts. More frequently, they are of variable size and are separated by dense stroma. The cysts are most often filled with clear mucinous fluid but may contain a cloudy or brownish liquid. Evidence of old hemorrhage is often seen in the submucosal tissue.

Microscopically, the cysts are lined with tall columnar cells that have an undulating pattern (Fig. 33-42) and sometimes show papillary formations. The lining cells have centrally placed, rather clear cytoplasm that stains positive for mucin. Macrophages laden with hemosiderin or lipofuscin are often present in the submucosal tissue. The stroma is characteristically composed of closely packed mesenchymal cells that form few fibrils. In some respects, the stroma of cystadenomas is similar to that of the ovary. Only one of the cystadenomas is a true tumor, namely, CMS, yet all of the pseudotumors enter into the differential diagnosis of masses within the liver; thus, their diagnostic features must be kept in mind. The four tumors in our series that were malignant were papillary adenocarcinomas.

Surgical removal of cystadenomas can usually be accomplished but was impossible in one of our patients. The prognosis is good in the benign tumors.

A number of *developmental cysts* and tumor-like anomalies are worthy of discussion. Some of these may be seen not only in the liver but are accompanied by similar cysts in other organs or in the extrahepatic ducts. These various entities have been considered as ductal plate malformations and have been reviewed by Jorgensen and others.[139]

Anomalous ductal microcystic changes known as Meyenburg complexes are usually noted in the lobules, often in close proximity to the smallest portal radicles.[200] These tiny lesions vary from a fraction of a millimeter to 5 mm in diameter. They are usually imbedded in rather dense adult-type connective tissue with sharply defined borders.

They are thought to represent developmental failure between the interlobular ducts and the cholangioles. The tiny gray granules or nodules may be seen beneath Glisson's capsule.

Microscopically the portal tracts are widened by a combination of adult connective tissue and bile duct structures. Many of the latter may form tiny cysts, and it is not unusual for some of these cysts to contain bile. Usually there is a fairly sharp line of demarcation between the complexes and the periphery of the lobules.

About one half of the large simple cysts are not solitary but are associated with polycystic disease. Solitary simple cysts may also be associated with multiple Meyenburg complexes and infrequently with congenital hepatic fibrosis. The simple or nonparasitic cysts of the liver may rarely give rise to a neoplasm.[27] These may be either squamous cell carcinomas or adenocarcinomas.[350]

Caroli's disease entails a variable degree of cystic dilation of the intrahepatic bile ducts.[192] The disease may involve all or a portion of the duct system and may be accompanied by a choledochal cyst. Hepatic resection is now being performed for Caroli's disease.[203]

Mesenchymal hamartomas[131,301] are cystlike congenital abnormalities in which a portion of liver is extremely edematous, often increases in size, and may produce death by respiratory embarrassment. Although these hamartomas usually occur in children younger than 2 years of age, one case has been reported in an adult.[109] Grossly, a mesenchymal hamartoma has a lobulated appearance with large bleblike areas separated by thin connective tissue septa. Upon sectioning, the entire mass tends to collapse because of loss of its light yellow fluid content. Microscopically, most of the tumor consists of interstitial edema

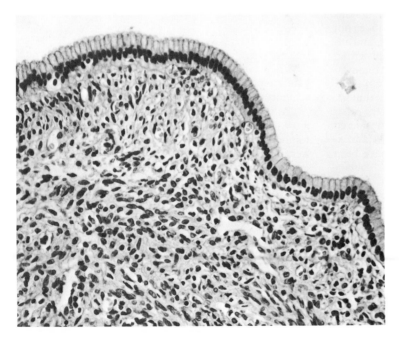

Fig. 33-42. Cystadenoma lined with tall columnar epithelium. The underlying mesenchyme is densely cellular. The cyst was successfully removed from a 46-year-old woman. Before excision, the surgeon removed 4200 ml of mucinous dark brown fluid. The tumor occupied all of the left lobe and extended into the right lobe. (ASC 2156) (Original magnification × 312)

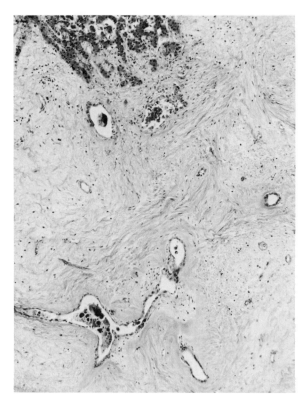

Fig. 33-43. Portal tract with intense fibrosis, distorted bile ducts, and island of hepatocytes. (ASC 3677) (Original magnification × 150)

and connective tissue septa in which there are a few bile ducts, blood vessels, and often a small remnant of hepatocytes (Fig. 33-43). A mature form of dense connective tissue is noted along these triadal remnants, usually with a semiwhorled arrangement.

Echinococcus cysts are usually diagnosed without difficulty before surgery. Their pathology, particularly their chitinous wall, differs sharply from that of any neoplasms of the liver.

Another rare noncystic entity is inflammatory pseudotumor of the liver,[47] which must be carefully studied to distinguish it from VABES.

REFERENCES

1. Abelev GI: Alpha-fetoprotein in ontogenesis and its association with malignant tumors. Adv Cancer Res 14:295, 1971
2. Adam YG et al: Giant hemangiomas of the liver. Ann Surg 172(2):239, 1970
3. Almersjo O et al: Liver metastases found by follow-up of patients operated on for colorectal cancer. Cancer 37:1454, 1976
4. Alper ME et al: Association between aflatoxin content of food and hepatoma frequency in Uganda. Cancer 28:253, 1971
5. Alpert L et al: Cholangiocarcinoma: A clinicopathologic study of 5 cases with ultrastructural observation. Hum Pathol 5:709, 1974
6. Alrenga DP: Primary fibrosarcoma of the liver: Case report and review of the literature. Cancer 36:446, 1974
7. Anthony PP: Primary carcinoma of the liver: A study of 282 cases in Ugandan Africans. J Pathol 110:37, 1973
8. Aoki K: Cancer of the liver: International mortality trends. World Health Stat Rep 31:28, 1978
9. Araki E, Okazaki N: Lipid metabolism in patients with hepatocellular carcinoma. In Okuda K, Peters RL (eds): Hepatocellular Carcinoma, New York, John Wiley & Sons, 1976
10. Arbus GC, Hung RH: Hepatocarcinoma and myocardial fibrosis in 8¾ year old renal transplant recipient. Can Med Assoc J 107:431, 1972
11. Asch MJ et al: Hepatic and splenic lymphangiomatosis with skeletal involvement: Report of a case and review of the literature. Surgery 76(2):334, 1974
12. Barr RD et al: Dysfibrinogenaemia and liver cell growth. J Clin Pathol 31:889, 1978
13. Barrera B et al: An analysis of malignant tumors among Filipinos seen in the UP-PGH Medical Center during 10 years (1947–1956). Phil J Cancer 2:189, 1958
14. Battifora H: Recent progress in the immunohistochemistry of solid tumors. Semin Diagn Pathol 1(4):11, 1984
15. Battifora HA: Thorotrast in tumors of the liver. In Okuda K, Peters RL (eds): Hepatocellular Carcinoma. New York, John Wiley & Sons, 1976
16. Baum JK et al: Possible association between benign hepatomas and oral contraceptives. Lancet 2:926, 1973
17. Beilby JOW et al: Alpha-fetoprotein, alpha-1-antitrypsin, and transferrin in gonadal yolk-sac tumours. J Clin Pathol 32:455, 1979
18. Bell W et al: Cryofibrinogenemia, multiple dysproteinemias and hypervolemia in patient with primary hepatoma. Ann Intern Med 64:658, 1966
19. Belmaric J: Intrahepatic bile ducts carcinoma and *C. sinensis* infection in Hong Kong. Cancer 31(2):468, 1973
20. Belmaric J: Malignant tumors in Chinese. Int J Cancer 4:560, 1979
21. Berg NO, Eriksson S: Liver disease in adults with alpha-1-antitrypsin deficiency. N Engl J Med 287:1264, 1972
22. Berman C: Primary carcinoma of the liver in the Bantu races of South Africa. S Afr J Med Sci 5:54, 1940
23. Berman C: Primary carcinoma of the liver: A study in incidence, clinical manifestations, pathology, and etiology. London, HK Lewis, 1951
24. Berman J, Braun A: Incidence of hepatoma in porphyria cutania tarda. Rev Czech Med 8:290, 1962
25. Bernstein MS et al: Hepatoma and peliosis hepatis developing in a patient with Fanconi's anemia. N Engl J Med 284:1135, 1971
26. Blattner WA et al: Malignant mesenchymoma and birth defects: Prenatal exposure to phenytoin. JAMA 238:334, 1977
27. Bloustein PA: Association of carcinoma with congenital cystic conditions of the liver and bile ducts. Am J Gastroenterol 67(1):40, 1977
28. Bloustein PA: Hepatic leiomyosarcoma: Ultrastructural study and review of the differential diagnosis. Hum Pathol 9(6):713, 1978

29. Bloustein PA, Silverberg SG: Squamous cell carcinoma originating in an hepatic cyst: Case report with a review of the hepatic cyst—Carcinoma Association. Cancer 38:2002, 1976

30. Blumberg DS, London WT: Hepatitis B virus: Pathogenesis and prevention of primary cancer of the liver. Cancer 50:2657, 1982

31. Bomford A et al: Treatment of iron overload including results in a personal series of 85 patients with idiopathic haemochromatosis. In Kief H (ed): Iron Metabolism and Its Disorders, pp 324–331. New York, Elsevier, 1975

32. Bondestam S et al: Sonography and computed tomography in hepatic haemangioma. Acta Med Scand (suppl) 668:68, 1982

33. Brawer MK et al: Focal fatty change of the liver, a hitherto poorly recognized entity. Gastroenterology 78:247, 1980

34. Britton WJ et al: Liver tumours associated with oral contraceptives. Med J Aust 2:223, 1978

35. Brock DJ: Review: Prenatal diagnosis of neural tube defects. Eur J Clin Invest 7:465, 1977

36. Brock DJH: Mechanisms by which amniotic-fluid alpha-fetoprotein may be increased in fetal abnormalities. Lancet 2:345, 1976

37. Brouet SC et al: Indication of thymus-derived nature of the proliferating cells in six patients with Sezary's syndrome. N Engl J Med 289:341, 1973

38. Bruguera M: Hepatoma associated with androgenic steriods. Lancet 1:1294, 1975

39. Buchanan TF, Huvos AG: Clear cell carcinoma of the liver. Am J Clin Pathol 61:529, 1974

40. Cady B: Natural history of primary and secondary tumors of the liver. Sem Oncol 10(2):127, 1983

41. Cattan D et al: Liver tumors and steroid hormones. Lancet 1:878, 1974

42. Cavalli G et al: Changes in the small biliary passages in the hepatic localization of Hodgkin's disease. Virchows Arch Pathol Anat 384:295, 1979

43. Chainuvati T et al: Relationship of hepatitis B antigen in cirrhosis and hepatoma in Thailand. Gastroenterology 68(5):1261, 1975

44. Chang HP, Hou PC: Pathological changes in the intrahepatic bile ducts of cats (Felis catus) infested with *Clonorchis sinesis.* J Pathol Bacteriol 89:357, 1965

45. Chang WWL: Primary sarcoma of the liver in the adult. Cancer 51:1510, 1983

46. Chen KTK: Hepatic leiomyosarcoma. J Surg Oncol 24:325, 1983

47. Chen KTK: Inflammatory pseudotumor of the liver. Hum Pathol 15(7):694, 1984

48. Chio L-F, Oon C-J: Changes in serum alpha-1-antitrypsin, alpha-1-acid glucoprotein and beta-2-glycoprotein 1 in patients with malignant hepatocellular carcinoma. Cancer 43:596, 1979

49. Christopherson WM et al: Hepatocellular carcinoma in young women on oral contraceptives. Lancet 2:38, 1978

50. Chudeckj B: Primary cancer of the liver following treatment of polycythemia vera with radioactive phosphorus. Br J Radiol 45:770, 1972

51. Cochrane M, Williams R: Humoral effects of hepatocellular carcinoma. In Okuda K, Peters RL (eds): Hepatocellular Carcinoma. New York, John Wiley & Sons, 1976

52. Cocks JR: Methyltestosterone-induced liver cell tumours. Med J Aust 2:617, 1981

53. Cohen C et al: Hepatitis B antigen in black patients with hepatocellular carcinoma. Cancer 41:245, 1978

54. Cohen C et al: Alpha-1-antitrypsin deficiency in Southern African hepatocellular carcinoma patients: An immunoperoxidase and histochemical study. Cancer 49:2537, 1982

55. Coombes GB et al: An androgen-associated hepatic adenoma in a transsexual. Br J Surg 65:869, 1978

56. Cowlishaw J et al: Liver disease associated with chronic arsenic ingestion. Aust NZ J Med 9(3):301, 1978

57. Craig JR et al: Fibrolamellar carcinoma of the liver: (A tumor of adolescents and young adults with distinctive clinico-pathologic features). Cancer 46:372, 1980

58. Cruickshank AH: The pathology of 111 cases of primary hepatic malignancy collected in the Liverpool region. J Clin Pathol 14:120, 1961

59. Dahms BB: Hepatoma in familial cholestatic cirrhosis of childhood: Its occurrence in twin brothers. Arch Pathol Lab Med 103:30, 1979

60. Darioca PJ et al: Cholangiocarcinoma arising in congenital hepatic fibrosis. Arch Pathol 99:592, 1975

61. Davies JNP: Incidence of primary liver carcinoma in Kampala. Acta Unio Internat Contra Cancerum 13:606, 1957

62. Dehner LP: Hepatic tumors in the pediatric age group: A distinctive clinicopathologic spectrum. In Rosenberg HS, Boland RP (eds): Perspectives in Pediatric Pathology, vol 4. Chicago, Year Book Medical Publishers, 1978

63. Dehner LP, Ishak KG: Vascular tumors of the liver in infants and children. Arch Pathol 92:101, 1971

64. Delorme F: Dix ces Canadiens d' angiosarcomes du foie chez des ouvriers du chlorure de vinyle. Annal Anat Pathol 23(2):98, 1978

65. Denison EK et al: Familial hepatoma with hepatitis associated antigen. Ann Intern Med 74:391, 1971

66. Deoras MP, Dicus W: Hepatocarcinoma associated with biliary cirrhosis. Arch Pathol 86:338, 1968

67. Dienstag J et al: Hepatitis A virus infections: New insights from seroepidemiology. J Infect Dis 137:328, 1978

68. Donnelly WH et al: Malignant undifferentiated stromal tumor of liver (mesenchymoma): An ultrastructural study. Lab Invest 38:385, 1978

69. Echeverria RA et al: Hepatic tumors of long duration with metastases. Am J Clin Pathol 69(6):624, 1978

70. Edmondson HA: Differential diagnosis of tumors and tumor-like lesions of the liver in infancy and childhood. Am J Dis Child 91:168, 1956

71. Edmondson HA: Tumors of the liver and intrahepatic bile ducts. Atlas of Tumor Pathology, Sect 7, Fasc 25. Washington, DC, Armed Forces Institute of Pathology, 1958

72. Edmondson HA, Peters RL: Armed Forces Institute of Pathology (in press)

73. Edmondson HA, Steiner PE: Primary carcinoma of the liver: A study of 100 cases among 48,900 necropsies. Cancer 7:462, 1954

74. Edmondson HA et al: Regression of liver cell adenomas associated with oral contraceptives. Ann Intern Med 86:180, 1977

75. El-Domeiri AA, Huvos AG: Clear cell carcinoma of the liver. Am J Clin Pathol 61:529, 1974

76. Eliss S et al: Multiple papillomas of the entire biliary tract. Ann Surg 152:320, 1960

77. Ellis IO, Cotton RE: Primary malignant mesenchymal tumour of the liver in an elderly female. Histopathology 7:113, 1983

78. Engel JJ et al: Metastatic carcinoma of the breast: A cause of obstructive jaundice. Gastroenterology 78:132, 1980

79. Epstein EH et al: *Myuycosis fungoides:* Survival prognostic features, response to therapy, and autopsy findings. Medicine 51:61, 1972

80. Evans N, Hoxie HJ: Primary myxosarcoma of liver. Am J Cancer 31:290, 1973

81. Falchuk KR et al: Cholangiocarcinoma as related to chronic intrahepatic cholangitis as in hepatolithiasis. Am J Gastroenterol 66:57, 1976

82. Farber E: Pathogenesis of experimental hepatocellular carcinoma. In Okuda E, Peters RL (eds): Hepatocellular Carcinoma. New York, John Wiley & Sons, 1976

83. Farber E et al: Newer insights into the pathogenesis of liver cancer. Am J Pathol 89:477, 1977

84. Farrell HC et al: Androgen-induced hepatoma. Lancet 1:430, 1975

85. Fechner RE, Roehm JOF Jr: Angiographic and pathologic correlations of hepatic focal nodular hyperplasia. Am J Surg Pathol 1(3):217, 1977

86. Fee JP et al: Halothane and anicteric hepatitis. Lancet 1:361, 1980

87. Feldman PS et al: Ultrastructure of infantile hemagioendothelioma of the liver. Cancer 42:521, 1978

88. Ferguson DJ et al: Surgical experience with staging laparotomy in 125 patients with lymphoma. Arch Intern Med 131:356, 1973

89. Fialk MA et al: Hepatic Hodgkin's disease without involvement of the spleen. Cancer 43:1146, 1979

90. Fong JA, Ruebner BH: Primary leiomyosarcoma of the liver. Hum Pathol 5:115, 1974

91. Fortner JG et al: Surgical management of hepatic vein occlusion by tumor. Arch Surg 112:727, 1977

92. Foster JH et al: Familial liver cell adenomas and diabetes mellitus. N Engl J Med 299(5):239, 1970

93. Gall EA: Primary and metastatic carcinoma of the liver. Arch Pathol 70:226, 1960

94. Gallagher PJ et al: Congenital dilation of the intrahepatic bile ducts with cholangiocarcinoma. J Clin Pathol 25:804, 1972

95. Ganrot PO et al: Obstructive lung disease and trypsin inhibition in alpha-1-antitrypsin deficiency. Scand J Clin Lab Invest 19:205, 1967

96. Geddes EW, Falkson G: Malignant hepatoma in the Bantu. Cancer 25:1271, 1970

97. Geiser CH et al: Epithelial hepatoblastoma associated with congenital hemihypertrophy and cystathioninuria: Presentation of a case. Pediatrics 46:66, 1970

98. Gen E et al: Primary fibrosarcoma of the liver with hypoglycemia. Acta Pathol Jpn 33(1):177, 1983

99. Gibson JB: Parasites, liver disease, and liver cancer. In Publication No. 1: Liver Cancer, pp 42–50, Lyon, International Agency for Research on Cancer, 1971

100. Gibson JB, Chan WC: Primary carcinoma of the liver in Hong Kong: Some possible etiological factors. Cancer Res 39:107, 1972

101. Gibson JB, Sun T: Clonorchiasis. In Marcial–Rojas RA (ed): Pathology of Protozoal and Helminthic Disease, pp 564–566. Baltimore, Williams & Wilkins, 1971

102. Gokel JM et al: Hemangiosarcoma and hepatocellular carcinoma of the liver following vinyl chloride exposure: A report of two cases. Virchows Arch Pathol Anat 372:195, 1976

103. Goodall CM, Butler WH: Aflatoxin carcinogenesis: Inhibition of liver cancer induction in hypophysectomized rats. Int J Cancer 4:422, 1969

104. Goodman ZD, Ishak MG: Angiomyolipomas of the liver. Am J Surg Pathol 8:745, 1984

105. Goodman ZD et al: Combined hepatocellular-cholangiocarcinoma: A histologic and immunohistochemical study. Cancer 55:124, 1985

106. Govindarajan S et al: Alpha-1-antitrypsin phenotypes in hepatocellular carcinoma (abstr). Gastroenterology 79:1022A, 1980

107. Govindarajan S et al: Prevalence of delta antigen/antibody in B-viral associated hepatocellular carcinoma. Cancer 53:1692, 1984

108. Gralnick HR et al: Dysfibrinogenemia associated with hepatoma: Increased carbohydrate content of fibrinogen molecule. N Engl J Med 291:226, 1978

109. Grases PJ et al: Mesenchymal hamartomas of the liver. Gastroenterology 76:1466, 1979

110. Green PA, Stephens DH: Hepatic calcification in cancer of the large bowel. Am J Gastroenterol 55:466, 1971

111. Griem ML et al: Staging procedures in mycosis in fungoides. Br J Cancer (suppl) 37:1454, 1976

112. Guillouzo A et al: Cellular and subcellular immunolocalization of alpha-fetoprotein and albumin in rat liver: Reevaluation of various experimental conditions. J Histochem Cytochem 26(11):948, 1978

113. Hadziyannis S, Merikas G: Australia antigen in primary liver cell carcinoma and cirrhosis (abstr). Digestion 8:72, 1973

114. Ham JM et al: Hepatocellular carcinoma possibly induced by oral contraceptives. Am J Dig Dis (suppl) 23(5):383, 1978

115. Harris CC, Sun T: Multifactorial etiology of human liver cancer. Carcinogenesis 6(5):697, 1984

116. Hawkins EP et al: Primary leiomyoma of the liver: Successful treatment by lobectomy and presentation of criteria for diagnosis. Am J Surg Pathol 4:301, 1980

117. Helpap B: Malignant papillomatosis of the intrahepatic bile ducts. Acta Hepatogastroenterol 24:419, 1977

118. Henderson JT et al: Letter: Androgenic-anabolic steroid therapy and hepatocellular carcinoma. Lancet 1:934, 1972

119. Higginson J: Pathogenesis of liver cancer in Johannesburg area (S. Africa). Acta Unio Internat Contra Cancerum 13:590, 1957

120. Homer LW et al: Neoplastic transformation of Von Meyenburg complexes of the liver. J Pathol Bacteriol 96:499, 1968

121. Horie Y et al: Pedunculated hepatocellular carcinoma: Report of three cases and review of literature. Cancer 51:746, 1983

122. Horta J: Late effects of thorotrast on the liver and spleen, and their efferent lymph nodes. Ann NY Acad Sci 145:676, 1967

123. Hou PC: Relationship between primary carcinoma of the liver and infestation with *Clonorchis sinesis.* J Pathol Bacteriol 72:239, 1956

124. Hou PC, Pang LSC: *Clonorchis sinensis* infestation in man in Hong Kong. J Pathol Bacteriol 87:254, 1964

125. Huberman MS et al: Hepatic involvement in the cutaneous T-cell lymphomas: Results of percutaneous biopsy and peritoneoscopy. Cancer 45:1683, 1980

126. Ichida F et al: Fetoprotein and hepatitis B antigen in hepatoma and hepatitis. Ann NY Acad Sci 259:259, 1975

127. Ishak KG et al: Mesenchymal tumors of the liver. In Okuda K, Peters RL (eds): Hepatocellular Carcinoma. New York, John Wiley & Sons, 1976

128. Ishak KG, Glunz PR: Hepatoblastoma and hepatocarcinoma in infancy and childhood. Cancer 20(3):396, 1967

129. Ishak KG, Rabin L: Benign tumors of the liver. Med Clin North Am 59(4):995, 1975

130. Ishak KG et al: Biliary cystadenoma and cystadenocarcinoma. Cancer 39:322, 1977

131. Ito H et al: Hepatic mesenchymal hamartoma of an infant. J Pediatr Surg 59(4):995, 1975

132. Itzchak Y et al: Intrahepatic arterial portal communications: Angiographic study. AJR 121:384, 1974

133. Jackson C et al: Hepatic hemangioendothelioma. Am J Dis Child 131:74, 1977

134. Jakimowicz JJ, Stockmann CHJ: Diffuse papillomatosis of the biliary tract. Arch Chir Neerl 29:255, 1977

135. Jesudason ML, Iseri OA: Host-tumor cellular junctions: An ultrastructural study of hepatic metastases of bronchogenic oat cell carcinoma. Hum Pathol 11:67, 1980

136. Johnson FL: Androgenis-anabolic steroids and hepatocellular carcinoma. In Okuda K, Peters RL (eds): Hepatocellular Carcinoma. New York, John Wiley & Sons, 1976

137. Johnson FL et al: Association of androgenic-anabolic steroid therapy with development of hepatocellular carcinoma. Lancet 2:1273, 1972

138. Johnson PJ et al: Hepatocellular carcinoma in Great Britain: Influence of age, sex, HBsAG status and aetiology of underlying cirrhosis. Gut 19:1022, 1978

139. Jorgensen MJ: The ductal plate malformation. Acta Pathol Microbiol Scand (A) (Suppl) 257:1, 1977

140. Kagawa Y et al: Carcinoma arising in a congenitally dilated biliary tract: Report of a case and review of the literature. Gastroenterology 74:1286, 1978

141. Kane RC, Newman AB: Diffuse skeletal hepatic hemangiomatosis. Calif Med 118(3):41, 1973

142. Karvountzis G, Redeker AG: Relations of alpha-fetoprotein in acute hepatitis to severity and prognosis. Ann Intern Med 80:156, 1974

143. Katragadda CS et al: Gray scale ultrasonography of calcified liver metastases. AJR 129:591, 1977

144. Keen P, Martin P: Is aflatoxin carcinogenic in man? The evidence in Swaziland. Trop Geogr Med 23:44, 1971

145. Kelly JK et al: Alpha-1 antitrypsin deficiency and hepatocellular carcinoma. J Clin Pathol 32:373, 1979

146. Kent DR et al: Effects of pregnancy on liver tumor associated with oral contraceptives. Obstet Gynecol 51(2):148, 1978

147. Kerlin R et al: Hepatic adenoma and focal nodular hyperplasia: Clinical, pathologic, and radiologic features. Gastroenterology 84:994, 1983

148. Kew MC: Clinical, pathologic, and etiologic heterogeneity in hepatocellular carcinoma: Evidence from South Africa. Hepatology 1(4):366, 1981

149. Kew MC et al: Hepatitis B surface antigen in tumour tissue and nontumorous liver in black patients with hepatocellular carcinoma. Br J Cancer 41:399, 1980

150. Kinch R, Lough J: Focal nodular hyperplasia of the liver and oral contraceptives. Am J Obstet Gynecol 132:717, 1978

151. Knill–Jones RP et al: Hypercalcemia and increased para-thyroid hormone activity in a primary hepatoma. N Engl J Med 282:704, 1970

152. Knowles DM II et al: The clinical, radiologic, and pathologic characterization of benign hepatic neoplasms: Alleged association with oral contraceptives. Medicine 57:223, 1978

153. Koga A et al: Hepatolithiasis associated with cholangiocarcinoma: Possible etiologic significance. Cancer 55:2826, 1985

154. Kojiro M et al: Hepatocellular carcinoma presenting as intrabile bile duct tumor growth: A clinicopathologic study of 24 cases. Cancer 49:2144, 1982

155. Kukman RJ et al: Cellular localization of alpha-fetoprotein and human chorionic gonadotropin in germ cell tumors of the testis using an indirect immunoperoxidase technique. Cancer 40:2136, 1977

156. Kulkarni PB, Beatty EC: Cholangiocarcinoma associated with biliary cirrhosis due to congenital biliary atresia. Am J Dis Child 131:442, 1977

157. Kuwano H et al: Hepatocellular carcinoma with osteoclast-like giant cells. Cancer 54:837, 1984

158. L'Esperance ES: Atypical hemorrhagic malignant hepatoma. J Med Res 32:225, 1915

159. Lai CL et al: Histologic prognostic indicators in hepatocellular carcinoma. Cancer 44(5):1676, 1979

160. Landais P et al: Cholangiocellular carcinoma in polycystic kidney and liver disease. Arch Intern Med 144:2274, 1985

161. Lange PH et al: Serum alpha-fetoprotein and human chorionic gonadotropin in the diagnosis and management of non-seminomatous germ-cell testicular cancer. N Engl J Med 295:1237, 1976

162. Larouze B et al: Host responses to hepatitis B infection in patients with primary hepatic carcinoma and their families. Lancet 2:534, 1976

163. Laurell CB et al: Glycoproteins in serum from patients with myeloma, macroglobulinemia and related conditions. Am J Med 22:24, 1957

164. Lazlo M et al: Clinical and morphologic features of hepatic angiosarcoma in vinyl chloride workers. Cancer 37(1):149, 1976

165. Lee FL: Cirrhosis and hepatoma in alcoholics. Gut 7:77, 1966

166. Lee Y-TN: Non-systemic treatment of metastatic tumors of the liver: A review. Med Pediatr Oncol 4:185, 1978

167. Lesna M et al: Liver nodules and androgens. Lancet 1:1124, 1976

168. Levi JA, Wiernick PH: Management of mycosis fungoides: Current status and future prospects. Medicine 54:73, 1975

169. Locker GY et al: The clinical features of hepatic angiosarcoma: A report of four cases and a review of the English literature. Medicine 58(1):48, 1979

170. Long JC, Mihm M: Mycosis fungoides with extra cutaneous dissemination: A distinct clinicopathologic entity. Cancer 34:1745, 1974

171. Ludwig J et al: Focal dilatation of intrahepatic bile ducts (Caroli's disease), cholangiocarcinoma, and sclerosis of extrahepatic bile ducts: A case report. J Clin Gastroenterol 4:53, 1982

172. Lutwick LI: Relations between aflatoxin, hepatitis-B virus, and hepatocellular carcinoma. Lancet 1:755, 1979

173. Lutzner M et al: Cutaneous T-cell lymphomas: The sezary syndrome, mycosis fungoides, and related disorders. Ann Intern Med 83:534, 1975

174. MacDonald RA: Cirrhosis and primary carcinoma of the

liver: Changes in their occurrence at the Boston City Hospital 1897–1954. N Engl J Med 255:1179, 1956

175. MacMahon HE, Ball HG: Leiomyosarcoma of hepatic vein and the Budd–Chiari syndrome. Gastroenterology 61:239, 1971

176. MacNab GM et al: Hepatitis B surface antigen produced by a human hepatoma cell line. Br J Cancer 34:509, 1976

177. Madden JJ, Smith GW: Multiple biliary papillomatosis. Cancer 34:1316, 1974

178. Madhavan TV, Gopalan C: The effect of dietary protein on carcinogenesis of aflatoxin. Arch Pathol 85:133, 1968

179. Mallory FB: Cirrhosis of liver. N Engl J Med 205:1231, 1932

180. Manes JL et al: Congenital hepatic fibrosis, liver cell carcinoma and adult polycystic kidneys. Cancer 39:2619, 1977

181. Marchal G et al: Ultrasonography of liver haemangioma: A report of 35 patients totalizing 53 lesions. ROFO 138(2):201, 1983

182. Massaki K et al: Hemangioma of the liver: Diagnosis of combined use of laparoscopy and hepatic arteriography. Am J Surg 129:698, 1975

183. Masur H et al: Primary hepatic leiomyosarcoma. Gastroenterology 69:994, 1975

184. Matilla S et al: Primary non-differentiated sarcoma of the liver. Acta Chir Scand 140:303, 1974

185. Mays ET et al: Hepatic changes in a young woman ingesting contraceptive steroids. JAMA 235:730, 1976

186. McArthur JW et al: Sexual precocity attributable to ectopic gonadotrophin secretion by hepatoblastoma. Am J Med 54:390, 1973

187. McCarthy LJ et al: Congenital hepatic fibrosis. Gastroenterology 49:27, 1965

188. McCaughan G et al: Primary hepatocellular carcinoma in Australia. Med J Aust 1:304, 1979

189. McKee PA et al: Incidence and significance of cryofibrin. Lab Clin Med 61:203, 1963

190. McLean AEM, Marshall A: Reduced carcinogenic effects of aflatoxin in rats given phenobarbitone. Br J Exp Pathol 52:322, 1971

191. Meadows AT et al: Hepatoma associated with androgen therapy for aplastic anemia. J Pediatr 84:109, 1974

192. Mercadier M et al: Caroli's disease. World J Surg 8:22, 1984

193. Mohabbat O et al: An outbreak of hepatic venoocclusive disease in North Western Afghanistan. Lancet 2:269, 1976

194. Moore MR et al: The use of human chorionic gonadotropin (HCG) and alpha-fetoprotein (AFP) in evaluation of testicular tumors. Proc Am Soc Clin Oncol 17:239, 1976

195. Morales AR et al: The ultrastructure of smooth muscle tumors with a consideration of the possible relationship of glomangiomas, hemangiopericytomas and cardiac myxomas. Pathol Annu 10:65, 1975

196. Morgan AG et al: A new syndrome associated with hepatocellular carcinoma. Gastroenterology 63:340, 1972

197. Mori H et al: Alpha-fetoprotein producing rhabdomyosarcoma of the adult liver. Acta Pathol Jpn 29(3):485, 1979

198. Morowitz DA et al: Carcinoma of the biliary tract complicating chronic ulcerative colitis. Cancer 27(2):356, 1971

199. Morrow CE et al: Hepatic resection for secondary neoplasm. Surgery 92(4):610, 1982

200. Moschowitz E: Non-parasitic cysts (congenital) of the liver, with a study of aberrant bile ducts. Am J Med Sci 131:674, 1985

201. Munoz PA et al: Osteoclastoma-like giant cell tumor of the liver. Cancer 1(48):771, 1980

202. Nadler WH, Wolfer JA: Hepatogenic hypoglycemia associated with primary liver cell carcinoma. Arch Intern Med 44:700, 1929

203. Nagasue N: Successful treatment of Caroli's disease by hepatic resection: Report of six patients. Ann Surg 300:718, 1984

204. Nakashima T: Vascular changes and hemodynamics in hepatocellular carcinoma. In Okuda K, Peters RL (eds): Hepatocellular Carcinoma. New York, John Wiley & Sons, 1976

205. Nakashima T et al: A minute hepatocellular carcinoma found in a liver with clonorchis sinensis infection: Report of two cases. Cancer 39:1306, 1977

206. Namba K et al: Splenic pseudosinuses and hepatic angiomatous lesions. Am J Clin Pathol 67:415, 1977

207. Naparstek J, Eliakim M: Malignant lymphoproliferative disorders in chronic liver disease. Dig Dis 23:887, 1978

208. Nayak NC et al: Alpha fetoprotein in Indian childhood cirrhosis. Lancet 1:68, 1972

209. Neuberger J et al: Oral-contraceptive associated liver tumors: Occurrence of malignancy and difficulties in diagnosis. Lancet 1:273, 1980

210. Newberne PM, Williams G: Inhibition of aflatoxin and carcinogenesis of diethylstilbestrol in male rats. Arch Environ Health 19:489, 1969

211. Newberne PM, Wogan GN: Potentiating effects of low-protein diets on effect of aflatoxin in rats. Toxicol Appl Pharmacol 11:51A, 1969

212. Newberne PM et al: Effects of cirrhosis and other liver insults on induction of liver tumors by aflatoxin in rats. Lab Invest 15:962, 1966

213. Newberne PM et al: Neoplasms in the rat associated with administration of urethane and aflatoxin. Exp Mol Pathol 6:285, 1967

214. Ohbayoshi A et al: Familial clustering of asymptomatic carriers of Australia antigen and patients with chronic liver disease or primary liver cancer. Gastroenterology 42(4):618, 1972

215. Ohnishi K: The effect of chronic habitual alcohol intake on the development of liver cirrhosis and hepatocellular carcinoma: Relation to hepatitis B surface antigen carriage. Cancer 49(4):672, 1982

216. Ohta Y: Viral hepatitis and hepatocellular carcinoma. In Okuda K, Peters RL (eds): Hepatocellular Carcinoma. New York, John Wiley & Sons, 1976

217. Okayasu I et al: An autopsy case of congenital hepatic cell tumor. Acta Pathol Jpn 24:387, 1974

218. Okazaki N et al: Hepatocellular carcinoma associated with erythrocytosis: A nine year survival after successful chemotherapy and left lateral hepatectomy. Acta Hepatogastroenterol 26:238, 1979

219. Okuda K: The Liver Cancer Study Group of Japan: Primary liver cancers in Japan. Cancer 45:2663, 1980

219b.Okuda K: Clinical aspects of hepatocellular carcinoma—analysis of 134 cases. In Okuda K, Peters RL (eds): Hepatocellular Carcinoma. New York, John Wiley & Sons, 1976

220. Okuda K et al: Serum alpha-fetoprotein in the relatively early stage of hepatocellular carcinoma and its relationship to gross anatomic type. Ann NY Acad Sci 259:248, 1975

221. Okuda K et al: Clinical aspects of intrahepatic bile duct carcinoma including hilar carcinoma. Cancer 39:232, 1977

222. Okuda K et al: Gross anatomic features of hepatocellular carcinoma from three disparate geographic areas: Proposal of new classification. Cancer 54:2165, 1984

223. Okulski EG et al: Intrahepatic biliary papillomatosis. Arch Pathol Lab Med 103:647, 1979

224. Olmer J et al: Le retentissement hepatique de la macroglobulinemie de Waldenstrom. Presse Med 65:524, 1957

225. Omata M et al: Comparisons of serum hepatitis B surface antigen (HBsAg) and serum anti-core with tissue HBsAg and hepatitis B core antigen (HBcAg). Gastroenterology 75:1003, 1978

226. Omata M et al: Letter: Hepatocellular carcinoma and hepatitis B virus markers in Europe and U.S.A. Lancet 1:433, 1979

227. Omata M et al: Hepatocellular carcinoma in the USA: Etiology considerations. Gastroenterology 76:279, 1979

228. Omata M et al: Sclerosing hepatic carcinoma, a relationship to hypercalcemia. Liver 1:33, 1981

229. Ordonze NG, Mackay B: Ultrastructure of liver cell and bile duct carcinomas. Ultrastr Pathol 5:201, 1983

230. Palmer PE, Wolfe HJ: Immunocytochemical localization of oncodevelopmental proteins in human germ cell and hepatic tumors. J Histochem Cytochem 26(7):523, 1978

231. Palmer PE, Wolfe HJ: Alpha-1-antitrypsin deposition in primary hepatic carcinomas. Arch Pathol Lab Med 100, 1976

232. Palmer PE et al: Alpha-1-antitrypsin, protein marker in oral contraceptive-associated hepatic tumors. Am J Clin Pathol 68(6):736, 1977

233. Parienty R, Freeny PC: Computer tomography in the diagnostic approach to cavernous hemangioma of the liver. Radiology 134(2):553, 1980

234. Parker RGF: Fibrosis of the liver as a congenital anomaly. J Pathol 71:359, 1956

235. Parker RGS, Kendall EJC: The liver in ulcerative colitis. Br Med J 2:1031, 1954

236. Peck JJ et al: Sclerosis of the extrahepatic bile duct. Arch Surg 108:798, 1974

237. Peers FG, Linsell CA: Dietary aflatoxin and liver cancer: A population-based study in Kenya. Br J Cancer 27:473, 1973

238. Perlin E et al: The value of serial measurements of both human chorionic gonadotropin and alpha-fetoprotein for monitoring germinal cell tumors. Cancer 37:215, 1976

239. Perra DR et al: Cholestasis associated with extrabiliary Hodgkin's disease: Report of three cases and review of four others. Gastroenterology 67:680, 1974

240. Perrin D: Foie et Maladie de Hodgkin. Sem Hop (Paris) 46:1732, 1970

241. Peters RL: Hepatitis B antigen and chronic hepatic conditions. In Blumberg BS (ed): Australia Antigen. Baltimore, University Park Press, 1972

242. Peters RL: Pathology of hepatocellular carcinoma. In Okuda K, Peters RL (eds): Hepatocellular Carcinoma. New York, John Wiley & Sons, 1976

243. Peters RL et al: The changing incidence of association of hepatitis B with hepatocellular carcinoma in California. Am J Clin Pathol 68(1):1, 1977

244. Phillips MJ et al: Benign liver cell tumors: Classification and ultrastructural pathology. Cancer 32:463, 1973

245. Piken EP et al: Investigation of a patient with Hodgkin's disease and cholestasis. Gastroenterology 77:145, 1979

246. Plachta A: Calcified cavernous hemangioma of the liver: Review of the literature and report of 13 cases. Radiology 79:783, 1962

247. Pollak ER et al: Fibrous mesenchymal tumor liver associated with hypoglycemia (in press)

248. Popp JW et al: Extrahepatic biliary obstruction caused by metastatic breast carcinoma. Ann Intern Med 91:568, 1979

249. Popper H et al: Development of hepatic angiosarcoma in man induced by vinyl chloride, thorotrast and arsenic. Am J Pathol 92:349, 1978

250. Portugal ML et al: Serum alpha feto-protein and variant alkaline phosphatase in human hepatocellular cancers. Int J Cancer 6:383, 1970

251. Poste G, Fidler IJ: The pathogenesis of cancer metastases. Nature 283:139, 1980

252. Powell LW: Tissue damage in haemachromatosis: An analysis of the roles of iron and alcoholism. Gut 11:980, 1970

253. Prat JR et al: Anaemia hemolytica asociada a hepatocarcinoma. Revista Espanola de las Enfermedades del Aparato Digestivo 39:577, 1973

254. Prates MD: On etiology of primary cancer of liver in natives of Mozambique. Acta Unio Internat Contra Cancerum 13: 662, 1957

255. Prince AM et al: A case control study of the association between primary liver cancer and hepatitis B infection in Senegal. Int J Cancer 16:376, 1975

256. Pryor AC et al: Hepatocellular carcinoma in a woman on long term oral contraceptives. Cancer 40:884, 1977

257. Purtilo DR, Gottlieb LS: Cirrhosis and hepatoma occurring at Boston City Hospital (1917–1968). Cancer 32:458, 1973

258. Rabin MS, Richter IA: Metastatic breast carcinoma presenting as obstructive jaundice: A report of 3 cases. S Afr Med J 388, 1979

259. Rabinowitz JF et al: Macroregenerating nodules in the cirrhotic liver. Radiologic features and differential diagnosis. AJR Radiat Ther Nucl Med 121:401, 1974

260. Rakela J, Redeker AG: Chronic liver disease after acute non-A non-B viral hepatitis. Gastroenterology 77:1200, 1979

261. Rallaport H, Thomas LB: Mycosis fungoides: The pathology of extracutaneous involvement. Cancer 34:1198, 1974

262. Rankin JG et al: Liver in ulcerative colitis: Obstructive jaundice due to bile duct carcinoma. Gut 7:433, 1966

263. Reddy JK, Svoboda D: Effect of lasiocarpine on aflatoxin B-1 carcinogenicity in rat liver. Arch Pathol 93:55, 1972

264. Reed WD et al: Detection of hepatitis B antigen by radioimmunoassay in chronic liver disease and hepatocellular carcinoma in Great Britain. Lancet 2:690, 1973

265. Reintoft I, Hagerstrand IE: Does the gene variant of alpha-1-antitrypsin predispose to hepatic carcinoma? Hum Pathol 10(4):419, 1979

266. Reintoft I et al: Demonstration of antitrypsin in hepatomas. Arch Pathol Lab Med 103:495, 1979

267. Richmond HG: Carcinoma arising in congenital cysts of the liver. J Pathol 72:681, 1956

268. Rios–Dalenz JL: Leiomyoma of the liver. Arch Pathol 79: 54, 1956

269. Roat JW et al: Hepatic angiosarcoma associated with short-term arsenic ingestion. Am J Med 73:933, 1982

270. Rogers AE, Newberne PM: Aflatoxin B-1 carcinogenesis in lipo trope-deficient rats. Cancer Res 29:1965, 1969

271. Rogers AE, Newberne PM: Nutrition and aflatoxin carcinogenesis. Nature (Lond) 229:62, 1971

272. Rogers AE et al: Absence of an effect of partial hepatectomy on aflatoxin B-1 carcinogenesis. Cancer Res 31:491, 1971

273. Rogers AE et al: Absence of an effect of partial hepatectomy on aflatoxin B-1 carcinogenesis. Cancer Res 31:491, 1971

274. Rogers KE: A papillary cystadenoma of the common hepatic duct. Can Med Assoc J 55:597, 1946

275. Rolleston HD: Diseases of the Liver, Gallbladder and Bile Ducts, 2nd ed. New York, McMillan, 1912

276. Roth A et al: Histologic and cytologic liver changes in 120 patients with malignant lymphomas. Tumori 64:45, 1978

277. Ruoslahti E et al: Serum alpha-fetoprotein: Diagnosis significance in liver disease. Br Med J 2:527, 1974

278. Ruoslahti E et al: Radioimmunoassay of alphafetoprotein in primary and secondary cancer of the liver. J Natl Cancer Inst 49:623, 1972

279. Ruymann FB et al: Hepatoma in a child with methotrexate-induced hepatic fibrosis. JAMA 238:2632, 1977

280. Sale GE, Lerner KG: Multiple tumors after androgen therapy. Arch Pathol Lab Med 101:600, 1977

281. Sanes S, MacCallum JD: Primary carcinoma of the liver: Cholangioma in hepatolithiasis. Am J Pathol 18:675, 1942

282. Schneiderman MA: Phenobarbitone and liver tumors. Lancet 2:1085, 1974

283. Selinger M, Koff RS: Thorotrast and the liver: A reminder. Gastroenterology 68:799, 1975

284. Seppala M: Immunologic detection of alphafetoprotein as a marker of fetal pathology. Clin Obstet Gynecol 20:737, 1977

285. Sewell JH, Weiss K: Spontaneous rupture of hemangioma of the liver. Arch Surg 83:105, 1961

286. Shank RC et al: Dietary aflatoxins and human liver cancer: IV. Incidence of primary liver cancer in two municipal populations of Thailand. Food Cosmet Toxicol 10:171, 1972

287. Shank RC et al: Dietary aflatoxins and human liver cancer: III. Field survey of rural Thai families for ingested aflatoxins. Food Cosmet Toxicol 10:71, 1972

288. Shank RC et al: Dietary aflatoxins and human liver cancer: II. Aflatoxins in market foods and foodstuff of Thailand and Hong Kong. Food Cosmet Toxicol 10:61, 1972

289. Shapiro P et al: Multiple hepatic tumors and peliosis hepatis in Fanconi's anemia treated with androgens. Am J Dis Child 131:1104, 1977

290. Shaw JW et al: Urinary cyclic AMP analyzed as a function of the serum calcium and parathyroid hormone in the differential diagnosis of hypercalcemia. J Clin Invest 59:14, 1977

291. Sherman HI, Hardison JE: The importance of co-existent hepatic rub and bruit: A clue to the diagnosis of cancer of the liver. JAMA 241:1495, 1979

292. Shikata T: Primary liver carcinoma and liver cirrhosis. In Okuda K, Peters RL (eds): Hepatocellular Carcinoma. New York, John Wiley & Sons, 1976

293. Shinagawa T et al: Diagnosis and clinical features of small hepatocellular carcinoma with emphasis on the utility of real-time ultrasonography: A study in 51 patients. Gastroenterology 86:495, 1978

294. Simons MJ, Hosking CS: AFP and ataxia-telangiectasia. Lancet 1:1234, 1974

295. Simons MJ et al: Immunodeficiency to hepatitis B virus infection and genetic susceptibility to development of hepatocellular carcinoma. Ann NY Acad Sci 259:2181, 1975

296. Simson IW, Middlecote BD: The Budd–Chiari syndrome in the Bantu. In Saunders SJ, Terblanche J (eds): Liver. London, Isaac Pitman & Sons, 1973

297. Skinhoj P et al: Occurrence of cirrhosis and primary liver cancer in an Eskimo population hyperendemically infected with hepatitis B virus. Am J Epidemiol 108:121, 1978

298. Slovis TL et al: Hemangiomas of the liver in infants: Review of diagnosis, treatment and course. AJR Rad Ther Nucl Med 123:791, 1975

299. Smith PM: Hepatoma associated with ulcerative colitis: Report of a case. Dis Colon Rectum 17:554, 1975

300. Sonoda T et al: Simultaneous occurrence of primary carcinoma and chondrosarcoma in the liver: A case report and a review of the literature. Acta Pathol Jpn 34(4):919, 1984

301. Srouje MN et al: Mesenchymal hamartomas of liver in infants. Cancer 42:2483, 1978

302. Steiner PE: Cancer of the liver and cirrhosis in Trans-Saharan Africa and the United States of America. Cancer 13(6):1085, 1960

303. Steiner PE: Carcinoma of liver in the United States. Acta Unio Int Contra Cancerum 13:628, 1957

304. Steiner PE, Davies JNP: Cirrhosis and primary liver carcinoma in Uganda Africans. Br J Cancer 11:523, 1957

305. Steiner PE, Higginson J: Cholangiocellular carcinoma of the liver. Cancer 12(2):753, 1959

306. Steinherz PG et al: Hepatocellular carcinoma, transfusion-induced hemochromatosis and congenital hypoplastic anemia (Blackfan–Diamond syndrome). Am J Med 60:1032, 1976

307. Sternlieb L: Evolution of the hepatic lesion in Wilson's disease (hepatolenticular degeneration). Prog Liver Dis 4:511, 1972

308. Stewart CR et al: Amniotic fluid alpha-l-fetoprotein in the diagnosis of neural tract malformations. Br J Obstet Gynaecol 82:257, 1975

309. Stocker JT, Ishak KG: Focal nodular hyperplasia of the liver: Study of 21 pediatric cases. Cancer 48:336, 1981

310. Stocker JT, Ishak KG: Undifferentiated (embryonal) sarcoma of the liver: Report of 31 cases. Cancer 42:336, 1978

311. Strohmeyer FM, Ishak KG: Nodular transformation (nodular "regenerative" hyperplasia) of the liver: A clinicopathologic study of 30 cases. Hum Pathol 12(1):60, 1981

312. Strohmeyer FW et al: Ground glass cells in hepato-cellular carcinoma may contain fibrinogen (abstr). Gastroenterology 77(5):A42, 1979

313. Strong GF, Pitts HH: Primary carcinoma of the liver. Arch Intern Med 46:105, 1930

314. Summers J: Three recently described animal virus models for human hepatitis B virus. Hepatology 1(2):179, 1981

315. Sussman EB et al: Hemangioendothelial sarcoma of the liver and hemochromatosis. Arch Pathol 97:39, 1974

316. Szmuness W: Hepatocellular carcinoma and the hepatitis B virus: Evidence for a causal association. Prog Med Virol 24:40, 1978

317. Szmuness W et al: The prevalence of antibody of hepatitis A antigen in various parts of the world: a pilot study. Am J Epidemiol 106:392, 1977

318. Szmuness W et al: Prevalence of hepatitis B virus infection and hepatocellular carcinoma in Chinese-Americans. J Infect Dis 1376:822, 1978

319. Tabor E et al: Hepatitis B virus infection and primary hepatocellular carcinoma. J Natl Cancer Inst 58:1197, 1977

320. Talerman A et al: Alpha-l-antitrypsin (AAT) and alpha-

foetoprotein (AFP) in sera of patients with germ-cell neoplasms. Int J Cancer 19:741, 1977

321. Tandon BN et al: An epidemic of venoocclusive disease of liver in Central India. Lancet 2:271, 1976

322. Tanner AR et al: Primary sarcoma of the liver. Gastroenterology 74(1):121, 1978

323. Taylor I et al: The blood supply of colorectal liver metastases. Br J Cancer 39:749, 1979

324. Thalassinos NC, Lyberatos C: Liver cell carcinoma after long-term estrogen-like drug. Lancet 1:270, 1974

325. Theodoropolulos G et al: Australia antigen and malignant hepatoma. Ann Inter Med 82(6)809, 1975

326. Theodoropolulos G et al: Serum trypsin inhibitory capacity and alpha-l-antitrypsin levels in liver cirrhosis and hepatoma. Acta Hepatogastroenterol 26:195, 1979

327. Thomas FB: Chronic aggressive hepatitis induced by halothane. Ann Intern Med 81:487, 1974

328. Thomas J et al: Focal nodular hyperplasia of the liver. Ann Surg 177(2):150, 1973

329. Thompson RPH et al: Cutaneous porphyria due to a malignant primary hepatoma. Gastroenterology 59:797, 1970

330. Tio TH et al: Acquired porphyria from a liver tumor. Clin Sci 16:517, 1957

331. Todorov V et al: Alpha-fetoprotein in the serum of patients with neoplasms of the gastrointestinal tract. Neoplasma 23:179, 1976

332. Tong MJ et al: Evidence for clustering of hepatitis B virus infection in families of patients with primary hepatocellular carcinoma. Cancer 44:2338, 1979

333. Touloukian RJ: Hepatic hemangioendothelioma during infancy: Pathology, diagnosis and treatment with prednisone. Pediatrics 45(1):71, 1970

334. Trastek VF et al: Cavernous hemangioma of the liver: Resect or observe? Am J Surg 145:49, 1983

335. Trichopoulos D et al: Alphafetoprotein levels of liver cancer patients and control in an European population. Cancer 46:736, 1980

336. Tsujimoto K et al: Hepatocellular carcinoma with sarcomatous proliferation showing an unusual and wide-spread metastasis. Acta Pathol Jpn 34(4):839, 1984

337. Tull DC: Primary carcinoma of the liver: A study of one hundred and thirty-four cases. J Pathol 35:557, 1932

338. Van Herden JA et al: Carcinoma of the extrahepatic bile ducts. Am J Surg 113:49, 1967

339. van Tonder S et al: Serum vitamin B-12 binders in South African blacks with hepatocellular carcinoma. Cancer 56:789, 1985

340. Variakojis D et al: *Mycosis fungoides:* Pathologic findings in staging laparotomies. Cancer 33:1589, 1974

341. Viallet A et al: Les manifestations paraneoplasiques des cancers primitifs du foie. Rev Fr Etud Clin Biol 6:1087, 1961

342. Vogel CL et al: Hepatitis-associated antigen in Ugandan patients with hepatocellular carcinoma. Lancet 2:621, 1970

343. Vogel CL et al: Hepatitis associated antigen and antibody in hepatocellular carcinoma. J Natl Cancer Inst 46:1583, 1972

344. Wald NJ et al: Amniotic fluid alphaprotein measurement in antenatal diagnosis of anencephaly and open spina bifida in early pregnancy. Lancet 1:651, 1979

345. Waldman TA, McIntire KR: Serum alpha-fetoprotein levels in patients with ataxiatelangiectasis. Lancet 2:1112, 1972

346. Warren KW et al: Primary sclerosing cholangitis: A study of forty-two cases. Am J Surg 111:23, 1966

347. Warren S, Drake EL: Primary carcinoma of the liver in hemochromatosis. Am J Pathol 27:573, 1951

348. Weber BB et al: Carcinoma arising in a choledochal cyst. Dig Dis 16:1019, 1971

349. Weintraub BD, Rosen SW: Ectopic production of chorionic somatomammatropin by non-trophoblastic cancers. J Clin Endocrinol Metab 32:94, 1971

350. Wellwood JM et al: Large intrahepatic cysts and pseudocysts (pitfalls in diagnosis and treatment). Am J Surg 135:57, 1978

351. Wepsic HT, Kirkpatrick A: Alpha-fetoprotein and its relevance to human disease. Gastroenterology 77:767, 1979

352. Wheeler DA, Edmondson HA: Cystadenoma with mesenchymal stroma (CMS) in the liver and bile ducts: A clinicopathologic study of 17 cases, 4 with malignant change. Cancer 56:1434, 1985

353. Wheeler DA et al: Spontaneous liver cell adenoma in children Am J Clin Pathol 85:6, 1986

354. Willis RA: Carcinoma arising in congenital cysts of the liver. J Pathol Bacteriol 55:492, 1943

355. Willis RA: Pathology of Tumours, 45th ed, pp 181–182. New York, Appleton-Century-Crofts, 1967

356. Winberg CD, Ranchod M: Thorotrast induced hepatic cholangiocarcinoma and angiosarcoma. Hum Pathol 10(1):108, 1979

357. Winograd J, Pallubinskas AJ: Arterial-portal venous shunting in cavernous hemangioma of the liver. Diagn Radiol 122:331, 1977

358. Wogan GN: Aflatoxins and their relationship to hepatocellular carcinoma. In Okuda K, Peters RL (eds): Hepatocellular Carcinoma. New York, John Wiley & Sons, 1976

359. Wogan GN et al: Structure activity relationships in toxicity and carcinogenicity of aflatoxins and analogs. Cancer Res 31:1936, 1971

360. Yamigawa K: Zurkeentins des primaren parenchymatosen leberkarazinoms ("Hepatoma"). Virchows Arch Pathol Anat 206:436, 1911

361. Yoshiaki N et al: Hepatic sarcoma associated with hepatoma. Acta Pathol Jpn 28(4):645, 1978

362. Yu MC et al: Hepatitis, alcohol consumption, cigarette smoking, and hepatocellular carcinoma in Los Angeles. Cancer Res 49:6077, 1983

363. Ziegenfuss J, Carabasi R: Letter: Androgens and hepatocellular carcinoma. Lancet 1:262, 1973

chapter 34

Management of Primary and Metastatic Cancer of the Liver

CHARLES J. LIGHTDALE and JOHN DALY

Cancer of the liver, primary and metastatic, is usually incurable and rapidly lethal. New surgical techniques, however, make resection of malignant liver disease a possibility for more patients. Medical treatments can provide palliation, and supportive care is of major importance in patient management.

EVALUATION FOR TREATMENT

Since malignant liver disease has such serious implications for survival, the first consideration in management is to be certain of the diagnosis. All imaging methods and blood tests have limited specificity in diagnosing malignant liver disease.[30,85] False-positive results may be related to such benign entities as hemangioma, fatty liver, and cirrhosis. A cytologic or histologic tissue diagnosis is usually needed to guide therapy and establish prognosis.[84]

Optimal management includes an assessment of resectability along with confirmation of malignant disease. This is usually accomplished by liver imaging. The radionuclide scan is now being replaced by ultrasound and computed tomography (CT) (Figs. 34-1 and 34-2). If multiple focal defects are evident in both liver lobes, disease is considered unresectable and biopsy is the next logical step. Biopsy directed by ultrasound, CT, or laparoscopy will be of higher yield than standard percutaneous biopsy.[15,91,136]

In some cases, the pathologist can ascertain that a biopsy shows malignant disease but cannot differentiate primary hepatocellular carcinoma (PHC) from metastatic disease. Serum α_1-fetoprotein (AFP) immunoassay may be helpful in this setting. In PHC, AFP is usually greater than 1000 ng/ml. Germ cell tumors and pregnancy must be ruled out. An AFP level of less than 10 ng/ml excludes PHC with an accuracy of 90% to 95%. In patients with metastatic liver cancer, AFP may be increased, but elevations are usually less than 100 ng/ml. If biopsy material is adequate, it may be stained for AFP by immunohistologic technique; a positive result indicates a very high likelihood of PHC.[69,101]

In patients with liver cancer of unknown origin, some workup for a possible source of metastatic disease is worthwhile. Clinical clues may direct the search. In female patients, breast and ovarian primary cancers have a better prognosis than other adenocarcinomas, and these areas should be carefully evaluated.

If there is a solitary liver defect on scan, or if the disease appears to be confined to one lobe, the patient is potentially resectable. Malignant disease must be differentiated from benign disease, and primary from metastatic cancer. If a resection for cure is to be done, it is preferable not to perform a biopsy preoperatively. Although it is a rare complication, a percutaneous biopsy carries the risk of spreading cancer cells in the needle tract or peritoneum.[45] However, performance of a preoperative biopsy need not preclude an attempt at curative resection.

Determination of resectability involves a search for disease within and outside the liver. As a single test, CT usually provides the most information.[30] However, ultrasound and selective arteriography are often needed as well. CT with contrast is often effective in determining tumor vascularity. PHC tends to be a particularly hypervascular neoplasm; this helps differentiate it from most metastatic adenocarcinomas, which tend to be hypovascular. Hemangiomas may resemble PHC. Arteriography or special CT scans (timed, dynamic) and magnetic resonance imaging facilitate this distinction.[52] The most common sites of metastases from PHC, the lungs, bones, and central nervous system, should be evaluated, particularly if there are localizing symptoms.[25]

Malignant foci on the liver of less than 1 cm are usually not seen on CT scans. However, lesions as small as 1 mm to 2 mm may be visualized and a biopsy performed using the laparoscope. Small peritoneal and diaphragmatic metastases are common in PHC; these can also be accurately assessed by biopsy at laparoscopy. Under direct vision, biopsy of hemangiomas or apparently resectable lesions can be avoided. If a biopsy is performed, vascular tumors such as PHC are likely to bleed, and at laparoscopy that bleeding can be directly controlled with pressure, hemostatic agents, or electrocautery. Laparoscopy can also establish the presence of cirrhosis and portal hypertension, and these findings may weigh significantly in the decision to proceed with a major hepatic resection.[86,116]

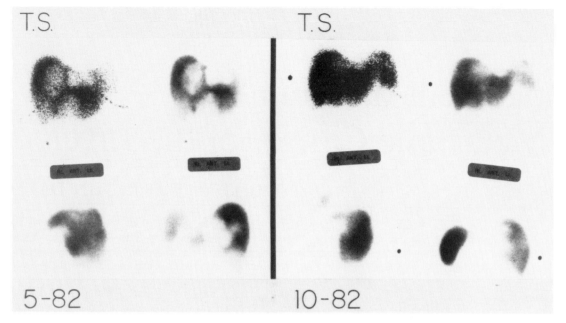

Fig. 34-1. Malignant liver disease can sometimes be well defined on radionuclide scan of the liver, illustrated by the abnormalities caused by metastatic colon cancer in the [99mTc] study dated 5/82. An excellent partial response to chemotherapy is documented by a subsequent examination dated 10/82. (Courtesy of Dr. N. Kemeny, Memorial Sloan–Kettering Cancer Center)

MEASURING RESPONSE

At first glance, objectively measuring the response of malignant liver disease to therapy would seem relatively easy. However, aside from the crucial parameter of survival, the response of hepatic lesions is difficult to quantify.[89]

Survival can be accurately measured from the time of diagnosis, surgery, or onset of therapy. Disease-free interval, while often inexact, is another important criterion of response, particularly following surgery or surgical adjuvant therapy. Palliation of symptoms and quality of life in advanced disease are much more difficult to assess, although the quantification of performance status, as developed by Karnofsky, has been useful.[73]

When malignant tissue is not surgically resected, objective measurement of tumor size is the key in assessing the effectiveness of therapy. Particularly in chemotherapy, response has been classified as complete, partial, or minor depending on the degree of tumor reduction. Complete response (the disappearance of all measurable disease) and partial response are emphasized in evaluating treatment, since these categories often correlate with improved survival. Minor response and stabilization of tumor growth have considerably lower clinical significance, representing an antitumor effect of far less magnitude. High-quality reports do not lump minor responses into a general response category. Reports from different investigators must be carefully compared in terms of how responses are measured and categorized.[75]

The response of malignant liver disease to therapy has been measured by physical examination, radionuclide scan, ultrasound, and CT (see Figs. 34-1 and 34-2). Blood tests of liver enzymes and specific tumor markers have also been used. On physical examination, a partial response is often taken to be a greater than 30% decrease in the sum of measurements of the liver edge to the costal margin. Measurements are made at the xiphoid and at the midclavicular line bilaterally.[108] At Memorial Sloan-Kettering Cancer Center, the measurements are made at the xiphoid and at 5 cm, 10 cm, and 15 cm to its left and right. A partial response is defined as a greater than 50% reduction in the sum of these measurements.[75]

The use of imaging techniques to assess response has proven much more difficult than expected. To be classified as a partial response, a greater than 50% reduction in the greatest diameter of a scan defect is widely used. While reduction in size may be clear in some cases, a statement of a greater than 50% reduction cannot always be achieved. When evaluating change in the size of lesions, CT tends to be more reliable than ultrasound (see Fig. 34-2). Even with CT, however, slight variations in technique may cause the tumor diameter to be incorrectly measured.[30,75]

Standard blood tests of liver function, such as serum bilirubin, alkaline phosphatase, and aminotransferase, are notably nonspecific and are usually not very helpful in judging the response of malignant liver disease to therapy. Activities of liver-specific enzymes may be relevant in some patients, for example, in the presence of coexistent

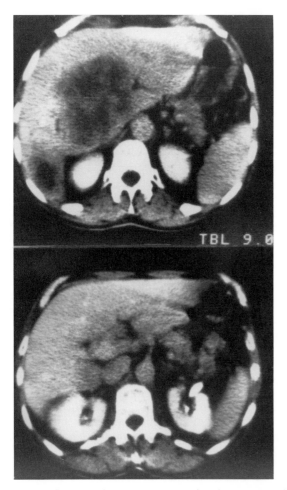

Fig. 34-2. CT scan above shows a massive liver metastasis in a patient with colorectal cancer. The scan below, performed 6 months later after chemotherapy, illustrates a nearly complete response. (Courtesy of Dr. N. Kemeny, Memorial Sloan–Kettering Cancer Center)

bone metastases. Tumor-specific secretory products in the blood seem to be better parameters of response. Carcinoembryonic antigen (CEA) has been most often used for this purpose, particularly for evaluating the response of colon cancer metastases in the liver. The use of CEA as a major determinant of response remains controversial, and instances of disagreement between CEA and other clinical parameters have been reported. A widely accepted definition of an objective partial response is a reduction in CEA by at least 25% from a baseline level of 50 ng/ml or greater.[96,97,130]

In patients being treated for PHC, serial measurements of AFP have been used as a guide to response. After successful surgical resection of PHC, AFP levels fall to normal. Persistent elevations of AFP indicate residual tumor.[69,104] The same is true with less specificity for CEA elevations after resection of PHC or liver metastases. CEA

has been most thoroughly studied in relation to liver metastases from colorectal cancer. Certainly, rising tumor secretory antigens in the blood indicate that the curative hepatic surgery has not been successful.[9]

In unresectable PHC, there have been conflicting data on the prognostic significance of AFP levels. A recent study has shown median survival of 12.8 months in patients with normal levels of AFP, 8.9 months in patients with AFP levels of less than 10,000 ng/ml, and 4.0 months in patients whose AFP levels exceed 10,000 ng/ml.[29] Other tumor markers evaluated in PHC include alpha-antitrypsin, alpha acid glycoprotein, ferritin, vitamin B_{12}–binding protein, and an abnormal prothrombin, (des)-carboxyprothrombin, but so far these have not proven specific enough to be clinically useful.[25,83] AFP and human chorionic gonadotropin are used in following the response to treatment of liver metastases from germ cell tumors that secrete these products.[69] Other hepatic metastases and PHC may secrete endocrine or exocrine hormones such as serotonin, gastrin, adrenocorticotropin, and erythropoietin. These can be measured with precision but do not always correlate with tumor mass and can only be considered a rough guide to response.[75]

In the evaluation of any group of patients with specific liver malignancies, it is often useful to stratify into subgroups.[73,75,89] One of the most important criteria is the amount of normal liver replaced at the time of treatment.[67,153,157] This is usually assessed by imaging techniques or at the time of surgery. Patients are often divided into three groups: those with less than 20% of liver replaced, those with 20% to 70% replaced, and those with massive disease or greater than 70% replacement.[6] Liver function tests may also be used for stratification.[78] In PHC, bilirubin elevation before treatment is a poor prognostic sign. In a recent series, the median survival of patients with a slightly elevated bilirubin level (less than 2.0 mg/dl) was only 1.1 months.[25] Positive hepatitis B surface antigen also tends to make the prognosis worse. Pathological classification of tumor subgroups is of great importance in PHC.[25] Age, sex, nutrition, and performance status may also need to be considered in evaluating overall response rates of hepatic tumors to therapy.

SYSTEMIC CHEMOTHERAPY

Metastatic liver disease is most often treated with systemic chemotherapy. Drugs are administered by mouth or intravenously and carried to the liver by the hepatic arterial and portal venous routes. Other metastatic sites are simultaneously treated. The drugs selected are those that have been shown to be of value in treating the primary cancer. Combinations of chemotherapeutic agents are often used.[39] Complete response to systemic chemotherapy and apparent cures have been reported in patients with disease metastases from such responsive primary tumors as testicular cancer, Hodgkin's disease, and non-Hodgkin's lymphoma. Partial responses and prolongation of survival are also commonly achieved in many soft tissue sarcomas, in cancers of the breast and ovary, and in small cell carcinoma of the lung. Unfortunately, the most common metastases to the liver in western societies are from primary cancers that are poorly responsive to chemotherapy, including the gastrointestinal adenocarcinomas, lung cancer (other than small cell), and melanoma. These are tumors with slow growth rates, low rates of cell division and DNA synthesis, and a high degree of cell heterogeneity. Chemotherapeutic drugs are most effective against homogenous cell populations undergoing rapid division and actively making DNA.[24,51,87,88,137]

PHC falls squarely into the class of tumor that is inherently resistant to chemotherapeutic attack. At the present time, there is no satisfactory or standard effective chemotherapy for PHC.[28,43]

The agents most often used in the past 2 decades for systemic chemotherapy of PHC have been 5-fluorouracil (5-FU) and its analog, 5-fluoro-2-deoxyuridine (FUDR). Benefit has been reported in the range of 0% to 30%.[107] Doxorubicin (Adriamycin) activity against PHC was described in 1973, and a great deal of interest in this drug as single-agent therapy followed a report from Uganda in 1975 of improvement in all of 11 patients treated.[119] Subsequent results with Adriamycin, however, have been disappointing. A follow-up study from Uganda reported 44% of 50 patients responding,[118] but other investigators found responses in only 0% to 24%.[27,28] Response tended to last only a few weeks or months, and survival time has not been significantly prolonged. Adriamycin analogs have shown similar low-level activity against PHC in initial trials.[25,44] Another of the newer agents, cisplatinum, has shown some activity in PHC, but initial results do not indicate it to be more effective than Adriamycin.[105] Various combinations of agents have not yet been shown to be more beneficial than Adriamycin alone.[28,118] Combination of agents that show only little activity individually against PHC is unlikely to provide major synergism. It is of note that the level of hepatitis B surface antigen may rise dramatically after chemotherapy in antigen-positive patients.[93]

The idea of bonding drugs to other agents designed to localize in malignant areas in the liver has not yet shown impressive utility.[36,70,115] The search for an *in vitro* system to predict reliably which tumors will respond to which drugs is another area of experimentation not currently applicable clinically.[68,134,152] Finally, the identification of more effective drugs is a continuing area of active research.

SURGICAL APPROACHES

Resection

Surgery offers the only chance for cure of primary and metastatic liver cancer. There has been enormous progress in liver resection for cancer as a result of better anesthesia,

new methods in vascular surgery, improved drainage techniques, and experience derived from liver transplantation.[16,48,113]

The extent of liver resection is tailored to the size and nature of the cancer. The minimum procedure that removes all tumor is sufficient, with no additional benefit evident for more extended resections. The simplest procedures, wedge and segmental resections, are associated with a mortality rate of less than 5%. Hemihepatectomy and trisegmentectomy have a mortality rate of less than 10% in recent series.[4,16,48,49,66,113,134,150] In the United States about 10% of primary malignancies of the liver are resectable.[2,16,94] In children, 5-year survival after resection of hepatoblastoma is in the range of 50%.[100,128] Survival rates after 5 years average about 40% in PHC. The natural history of PHC is usually measured in months.[4,13,26,48,66,150]

Cirrhosis is a common accompaniment of PHC and limits the prognosis. Operative risks are increased, liver regeneration is less than normal, and the cancer tends to be multicentric.[84,94,100,101] In a report from Hong Kong, where 85% of patients resected for PHC had cirrhosis, the operative mortality rate was 20% and the 5-year survival 20%.[79]

In metastatic liver cancer, the main surgical experience has been with metastases from colorectal cancer. The liver becomes the sole initial site of colorectal metastases in about 2000 patients annually in the United States.[16] The lack of successful medical treatment for colorectal cancer has spurred an increasingly aggressive surgical approach to metastases in the liver. Many large series are now available documenting 5-year survival of 20% to 40% after hepatic resection for colorectal metastases.[1,3,5,47–49,66,150,158] Without resection there are no reports that document 5-year survival in patients with biopsy-proven colon cancer metastatic to the liver.

Patient selection undoubtedly has a major effect on benefit from hepatic resection. The best results seem to be achieved if there is a solitary metastasis or single lobe involvement, although multiple and bilobar metastases have been successfully resected with apparent long-term benefit.[5,21] Initially it was hypothesized that liver metastases appearing after a long interval from resection of primary colon cancer had a better prognosis. More recent experience has demonstrated no clear-cut difference in survival between patients with liver metastases resected at the time of primary colon resection (synchronous) and those resected later (metachronous).[16,49,155] The natural history of the disease must be considered in analyzing surgical palliation. With or without resection, patients with small solitary liver metastases will survive longer on the average than those with extensive bilobar disease.[13,14,67,153,157] Randomized prospective studies have not been done, but only resection offers the potential for 5-year survival equated with cure.[16,49,113]

The improved safety of liver resection is evident from the experience of the Colorectal Surgery Service at Memorial Sloan-Kettering Cancer Center, where from 1950 to 1967 the operative mortality rate was 24%; from 1968 to 1981 it was only 2%.[20] It has been estimated that about 10% of patients with liver metastases from colorectal cancer can expect surgery to prolong their lives.[1,3,47]

Metastases to sites in addition to the liver are a major limitation to the benefit of hepatic resection. Experience in resection of liver metastases other than colorectal has been small and discouraging. There have been good results in children with Wilms' tumor who have received effective systemic therapy.[16,49,128] Some success has been achieved in partially resecting liver metastases from carcinoid, adrenocortical, and pancreatic islet cell cancers for palliation of otherwise uncontrollable endocrine or metabolic syndromes.[38,102,144]

The ultimate liver resection for malignant disease is total hepatectomy with liver transplantation. The expense, morbidity, and mortality of transplantation remain high, and with chronic immunosuppression, malignancy recurs in the majority.[23,65] In patients with PHC, Starzl in the United States and Calne in Great Britain will selectively consider transplantation if resection is not possible and intensive evaluation reveals no extrahepatic metastases.[23,65] In Starzl's experience, the longest survivors have been children undergoing transplantation for other incurable liver conditions who have incidental foci of PHC.[141] Transplantation is generally not indicated for metastatic disease because cancer nearly always recurs after immunosuppression.[16]

Hepatic Arterial Occlusion

Most liver cancers probably receive the bulk of their blood supply and oxygen from the hepatic arteries.[17,147] Normal hepatocytes derive 75% of their blood supply and 50% of their oxygen from the portal vein. This has led to the idea of deliberate ligation of the main hepatic arterial system at surgery or occlusion by selective angiographic embolization. Specific necrosis of liver tumors after hepatic artery occlusion has been achieved in a majority of patients.[59,99,110,122,140] However, the morbidity of the procedure is high, with mortality rates averaging 10% to 15%. Patients with poor hepatic function are at high risk, and in patients with portal vein compromise there is an increased risk of major liver infarction. As a result of the rapid development of collateral arterial circulation, survival is not significantly prolonged.[126] More aggressive attempts at nearly complete hepatic dearterialization at surgery are associated with an even higher operative mortality, and this procedure has been generally abandoned.[11]

REGIONAL CHEMOTHERAPY

Disappointment with systemic chemotherapy for liver cancer has prompted investigators to evaluate the effects of direct infusion of antineoplastic agents into the hepatic circulation. The basis for this method of treatment lies in the dose-response relation of drug to tumor, which can be demonstrated in the laboratory.[50] The greater the concentration of drug, the greater the antitumor effect. Clinically, however, there is a fine line between beneficial effect and toxicity, which limits drug dosage. By injecting drugs directly into the hepatic circulation, higher concentrations are achieved in the liver, with lower levels systemically.[156] The liver metabolizes some agents, (including the fluorinated pyrimidines) into less active compounds, in theory further decreasing systemic toxicity.[41]

The hepatic artery has been principally used for regional infusion of chemotherapy, but the best route has not been established.[156] Portal vein infusion may also be effective.[48] Primary and metastatic liver cancers seem to draw the bulk of their blood supply from the hepatic artery, but their vascularity can be complex.[17,147]

There have been numerous reports of small series of patients with PHC treated with regional chemotherapy, but the benefits over systemic therapies have not been clearly demonstrated. The greatest experience with regional chemotherapy has been in metastatic colorectal cancer. Beneficial response has been reported in almost all series, ranging from 29% to 83% objective tumor regression with median patient survivals of 9 to 12 months.[7,18,22,31,32,54,57,106,113,131,145,146] These reports, however, are all retrospective in type, lack controls against systemic therapy, or use historical controls, leaving their findings in doubt. One prospective study carried out by the Central Oncology Group in 1979 compared results with 5-FU infused into the hepatic artery with the same drug administered intravenously in 74 patients with liver metastases from colorectal cancer. No significant difference in objective response rate or survival was found between the two groups.[53]

The potential benefits of hepatic artery infusion must be balanced against significant morbidity. Much of this morbidity has been associated with external arterial catheters. Most of the initial studies involved surgical placement of indwelling catheters that emerged from the abdomen to be connected to portable external pumps. Another method involved percutaneous placement of temporary catheters using angiographic techniques via the axillary or femoral arteries. Thrombosis of hepatic and other intra-abdominal arteries, catheter displacement, sepsis, and hemorrhage were common complications.[53,54] A representative series had an operative mortality rate of 12% and a catheter-related morbidity rate of 24%.[131]

An important advance in regional chemotherapy has been the development of an implantable pump (Infusaid).[18,32,40] The drug used most often in the pump has been FUDR (Fig. 34-3). The implantable pump offers several advantages over external catheter methods. There is a major reduction in catheter-related complications and greater patient acceptance with the elimination of bulky external pumps (Fig. 34-4). The pump is placed subcutaneously, and drug injections are administered easily through a resealable diaphragm into the pump reservoir.

Anomalies in hepatic circulation must be analyzed preoperatively with angiography for optimal catheter placement (Fig. 34-5). Postimplantation studies using contrast

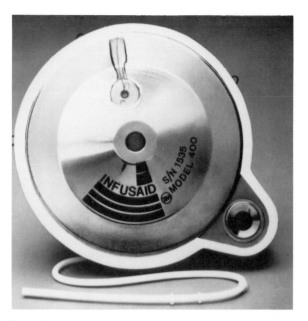

Fig. 34-3. Use of an implantable Infusaid pump has increased patient comfort and minimized septic and technical complications of regional infusion chemotherapy for malignant liver disease.

and radionuclide materials are useful to confirm perfusion and study response.[113] In a pilot study of Infusaid pump therapy at Memorial Sloan-Kettering Cancer Center, a partial response was achieved in 41% of patients.[37] There was a partial response of 31% in patients who failed prior systemic chemotherapy, which is encouraging considering the very dismal prognosis after initial treatment failure.[74]

The median response duration was only 4 months in the previously treated group versus 8 months in the responding patients in whom hepatic artery infusion was the initial treatment. Previous reports with external catheters have suggested that hepatic artery infusion might achieve responses in patients failing systemic therapy.[7,19] Similar results have been reported in other series using the Infusaid pump, with increased response and survival compared with historical controls of systemic treatment.[18,32,113] Degree of liver involvement and patient performance status are important variables in all such studies. Several randomized, prospective trials of implantable pump intra-arterial chemotherapy versus systemic treatments are in progress, with initial results showing no advantage for pump therapy.[76,82]

Operative morbidity associated with pump implantation has been less than 2%. The surgery also provides an opportunity for optimal staging, since progression of non-hepatic intra-abdominal disease is a major limitation of hepatic artery infusion therapy. Pump- or catheter-related complications have been in the range of 0% to 10%, and complications requiring reoperation have been less than 5%.[12,18,32,37,113]

The major toxicity from hepatic artery infusion has been related to chemotherapy, but complications have been very different from those associated with systemic treatment, in which the most serious problems have been marrow suppression and diarrhea.[74] The most common side-effects of implantable pump hepatic artery infusion have been gastroduodenal ulceration and inflammation, which develop in 48% to 68% of patients.[37,113] Serious ulcer complications such as perforation and hemorrhage have not been unusual.[35,112] Prophylactic treatment with cimetidine or sucralfate has been of no apparent benefit. Healing has occurred with decrease or cessation of che-

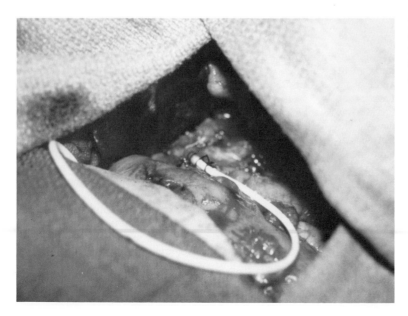

Fig. 34-4. After cannulation of the gastroduodenal artery for regional infusion chemotherapy to the liver, the catheter can be seen to lie freely within the abdomen with a gentle curve.

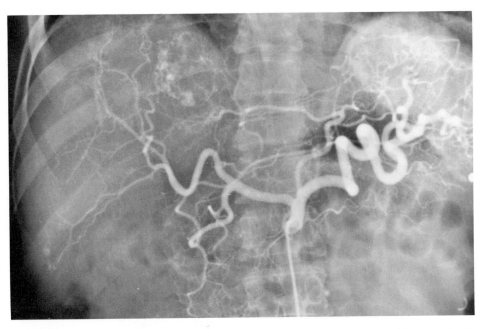

Fig. 34-5. A hepatic arteriogram is necessary to outline the arterial supply to the liver in all patients in whom regional infusion therapy is anticipated. In this study, the blood supply to the right liver lobe arises from the common hepatic artery, whereas the blood supply to the left lobe arises from the left gastric artery. Access to the entire hepatic arterial system could be obtained by proximal cannulation of the splenic artery. (Courtesy of Dr. J. Botet, Memorial Sloan–Kettering Cancer Center)

motherapy treatment. Toxicity appears to be related to the drug reaching the gastroduodenal mucosa via arterial collaterals.

Liver toxicity (which rarely occurs with systemic therapy) has been another common side-effect of hepatic artery infusion with FUDR.[37,76,113] There have been two major types of toxic reactions. The most common has been hepatocellular inflammation, with tripling of baseline aminotransferase levels occurring in 45% to 65% of those treated. Bilirubin has increased to greater than 3 mg/dl in 20% to 25%. Decrease or cessation of FUDR has resulted in return to baseline serum levels in most patients. A second type of liver toxicity resembles sclerosing cholangitis. This complication, affecting primarily extrahepatic bile ducts, has occurred in 1% to 2% of patients.

SURGICAL ADJUVANT CHEMOTHERAPY

Following hepatic resection of primary and metastatic liver cancer, chemotherapy is usually recommended. This can be given systemically or via the hepatic artery. The rationale is to attack microscopic disease at a time when the relatively small number of cancer cells may be more vulnerable to drug therapy.[39,87,137] Cell cycle–specific chemotherapy agents may be more effective against prolif-

erating cells, and as tumors become larger their growth fraction becomes lower. In addition, chemotherapeutic agents act according to first-order kinetics: a fixed proportion of sensitive cells is killed with each dose of drug. Thus, the smaller the number of cells, the greater the possibility of eradicating the disease. While these theoretic advantages make surgical adjuvant chemotherapy seem like good sense, the limitation for PHC and most metastatic liver disease is again the lack of highly active drugs. There are no good data establishing benefit from the use of currently available agents following surgery in terms of increased cure rates or delay in clinical recurrence.[107,114,142] An exception in children is Wilms' tumor, against which chemotherapy is effective.[49,128]

Since metastases to the liver from colorectal cancer are common, there have been various adjuvant treatments used following resection of the primary cancer to prevent spread to the liver. Most often 5-FU has been given systemically to those patients with pathologic stage Dukes C (lymph node metastases), but numerous studies have found minimal or no benefit.[74] Peritoneal lavage or "belly bath" with 5-FU has also been performed at the time of surgery without clear-cut advantage.[10] Another adjuvant approach has been 5-FU infusion into the portal vein via a temporary catheter. Cancer cells most commonly reach the liver from the colon through the portal circulation and might be best treated at an early stage using the portal vein. Initial results using this method were encouraging but need confirmation.[148]

RADIATION THERAPY

Radiation has played a relatively minor role in the treatment of malignant liver disease. The problem has been that the most common cancers that affect the liver are relatively radioresistant, and the normal liver is susceptible to radiation damage.[125] Patients receiving over 3500 rad to the whole liver are at risk for hepatic damage, and in some instances much lower doses have caused severe toxicity.[63] The risk of hepatic damage is greater in younger patients who have received chemotherapy.[149]

PHC has been among the cancers most resistant to radiation therapy. Cholangiocarcinoma may be more responsive, and radiation has been used in selected cases for relief of obstructive jaundice.[124] Few studies have specifically evaluated radiation treatment for metastatic liver disease. Most of the cancers that are radiosensitive also respond to systemic chemotherapy, and since metastases are often widespread, chemotherapy is used preferentially.

While objective response and prolongation of survival are infrequently achieved with hepatic radiation, some patients may experience palliation of symptoms.[127] Even patients with relatively radioresistant liver metastases may receive symptomatic benefit. Upper abdominal pain due to advanced liver metastases has been relieved in a majority of those completing a course of more than 2000 rad to the liver.[151] Toxicity, usually low at these doses, includes mild and transient anorexia and nausea. Higher doses may cause a type of veno-occlusive disease, producing a Budd–Chiari–like syndrome of varying severity.[81,92]

There have been a variety of experimental approaches to the delivery of radiation therapy to hepatic metastases. Radioactive agents have been injected into the hepatic artery,[55,149] and radioactive wires have been placed into the bile ducts percutaneously and via endoscopy.[123] A combination of radiation and chemotherapy has been used with slightly increased toxicity to treat malignant liver disease, but it has as yet shown no major clinical advance.[8,80,98,139] Hyperthermia has also been used experimentally in combination with chemotherapy and radiation therapy with no important benefit evident.[56,109]

IMMUNOTHERAPY

There have been many attempts to harness immune functions for antitumor effects. Patients with primary or metastatic liver cancer, like most patients with advanced malignancies, are generally immunosuppressed.[60,154] However, nonspecific immunostimulants, such as bacille Calmette Guérin (BCG), C parvum, and Levamisole, have shown little or no activity against primary or metastatic liver disease.[64,77,133]

The administration of circulatory factors such as interferon, transfer factor, complement components, lymphokines, and tumor necrosis factor is in an active phase of laboratory and human experimentation, with potential for treatment in malignant liver disease.[58]

A promising area of research is the use of specifically developed monoclonal antibodies. Order and colleagues have developed an antiferritin immunoglobulin that localizes to the ferritin often present in PHC and some other cancers.[120] Using a combination of immunotherapy and radiation therapy, they have radiolabeled the antiferritin with ^{131}I, safely delivering enough radiation to produce major objective tumor regression in some patients with PHC.[42] Anti-AFP antibodies have been produced, labeled with ^{131}I, and tested for activity in advanced PHC.[95] Isotopes other than ^{131}I are being tested. These early studies may be accelerated by the recent improvement in hybridoma methods for producing large amounts of monoclonal antibodies.[62,117]

GENERAL SUPPORT

Malignant liver disease, unresectable or recurrent, is likely to be incurable and the limiting factor in patient survival. While treatment aimed directly at the responsible cancer may be helpful, there is a great deal that can be done in terms of supportive measures to relieve symptoms and provide good quality prolongation of survival.

The physician managing a patient with incurable liver cancer must attempt to communicate sensitively and accurately the nature of the disease, while at the same time affirming a program of continuing treatment. The patient's fear of being abandoned should be overcome by frequent physician reassurance.

A firm commitment to maintain comfort should be stressed. There has been some tendency in past years to underdose patients with malignant liver disease. Even in jaundiced patients, analgesics, antiemetics, sedatives, tranquilizers, and antidepressants can be used if carefully titrated. Recent work has shown that pain control is better if patients have access to oral analgesics. This may provide better pain control with the use of less medication than fixed time and dosage schedules. The avoidance of anxiety and frequent reassessment of the quality and effectiveness of pain control are important. When narcotic analgesics are needed, clinicians and patients should not confuse drug tolerance and physical dependence with addiction or psychological dependence, the latter being infrequent in patients with cancer pain. Inappropriate fear of addiction may lead to inadequate pain control.[46] The cause of pain should be specifically treated whenever possible.

Anemia is common in malignant disease of the liver. Correction of severe anemia will add considerably to patient comfort. Anemia is usually due to bone marrow suppression from the tumor and from chemotherapy. However, specific causes of anemia should be considered, especially occult gastrointestinal tract bleeding.[90] Portal hypertension can occur in both primary and metastatic disease of the liver, and bleeding may occur from esophageal varices. A large hepatic cancer may sometimes directly invade the distal stomach or proximal duodenum, presenting as a malignant ulcer. More commonly, gastrointestinal tract bleeding is from benign sources, many specifically treatable, such as peptic ulcer, gastritis, monilial esophagitis, or pseudomembranous colitis. If possible, the hematocrit should be kept greater than 30% for patient comfort. Replacement of iron, folic acid, or vitamin B_{12} is sometimes indicated, but most often periodic blood transfusions will be needed.

Anorexia is present to some degree in almost all patients with malignant liver disease. Strict diets are of dubious benefit; to maximize caloric intake, patients should be urged to eat what they like when they feel most like it. Therapeutic doses of vitamins have not proven to be of value. High-calorie supplements may be useful between meals. Weight loss, particularly of muscle mass, contributes to a feeling of weakness and illness.

The benefit of nutritional support in patients with advanced cancer receiving chemotherapy remains controversial. It does seem that a good response to chemotherapy is less common in malnourished patients. Supplementation by nasogastric tube or the intravenous route can be employed. Certainly patients feel better when serious malnutrition is corrected and seem better able to tolerate the side-effects of chemotherapy.[33,138]

Ascites may develop in patients with malignant liver disease secondary to portal hypertension, Budd–Chiari syndrome, malnutrition, hypoalbuminemia, or peritoneal implants. Transudates can be controlled with diuretic therapy and spironolactone. High-protein exudates can often be managed by periodic paracentesis. A surgically placed peritoneovenous shunt can provide symptomatic relief in patients with chronic ascites associated with advanced liver cancer. However, shunts tend to be less successful than in patients with ascites due to cirrhosis.[129,143]

Jaundice is a grave prognostic sign in malignant liver disease and usually signifies extensive progression of the tumor in the liver. However, other causes of jaundice must also be considered. Hepatitis due to blood transfusion is a common occurrence. A reaction to any of multiple medications being received should be a primary concern, since this cause of jaundice is often reversible if the causative agent is stopped. In some cases, jaundice is due to a relatively small malignant lesion that invades or metastasizes to the porta hepatis, compromising the major bile ducts. Ultrasound or CT examinations of the liver may suggest this diagnosis, which can be confirmed by retrograde endoscopic or percutaneous cholangiography.[103] Drains or internal stents may be placed with about 80% success at the time of cholangiography to mechanically relieve the jaundice and attendant pruritus. Complications from these procedures, primarily hemorrhage and sepsis, are in the range of 5%, which is acceptable considering the severity of the problem and absence of good alternative treatment. Internal drainage avoids bile acid deficiency, cutaneous fistula, and collection devices and is clearly preferable but not always possible in patients with obstruction at the porta hepatis.[121,132]

CONCLUSION

One of the most feared diagnoses in medicine, primary or metastatic liver cancer usually presages an early death. Until recently, surgical resection of primary liver cancer was considered highly risky and resection of metastatic disease almost unthinkable. Technical improvements have markedly increased the safety of hepatic resection, and there is mounting evidence that selected patients may benefit considerably from surgery. For the majority of patients with unresectable liver cancer, effective therapy does not exist. Methods are not yet available to identify the occasional patient with a generally resistant cancer who will have a major response to medical therapy. Thus, an attempt at treatment is usually indicated, preferably in the setting of a controlled trial. With alertness for complications and attention to detail, supportive treatment can do a great deal to alleviate symptoms and improve the quality of survival.

REFERENCES

1. Adson MA: Hepatic metastases in perspective. AJR 140: 695, 1983
2. Adson MA, Farnell MB: Hepatobiliary cancer: Surgical considerations. Mayo Clin Proc 56:686, 1981
3. Adson MA, Van Heerden JA: Major hepatic resections for metastatic colorectal cancer. Ann Surg 191:576, 1980
4. Adson MA, Weiland LH: Resection of primary solid hepatic tumors. Am J Surg 141:18, 1981
5. Adson MA et al: Resection of hepatic metastases from colorectal cancer. Arch Surg 119:647, 1984
6. Almersjo et al: Evaluation of hepatic dearterialization in primary and secondary cancer of the liver. Am J Surg 124: 5, 1972
7. Ansfield FJ et al: Further clinical studies with intrahepatic arterial infusion with 5-fluorouracil. Cancer 36:2413, 1975
8. Ariel IM, Padula G: Treatment of symptomatic metastatic cancer to the liver from primary colon and rectal cancer by the intraarterial administration of chemotherapy and radioactive isotopes. J Surg Oncol 10:327, 1978
9. Attiyeh RR, Stearns MW Jr: Second-look laparotomy based on CEA elevations in colorectal cancer. Cancer 47:2119, 1981
10. August DA et al: Hepatic resection of colorectal metastases: Influence of clinical factors and adjuvant intraperitoneal 5-fluorouracil via Tenckhoff catheter on survival. Ann Surg 201:210, 1985
11. Balasegaram M, Lumpur K: Complete hepatic dearterialization for primary carcinoma of the liver. Am J Surg 124: 340, 1972
12. Balch CM et al: A prospective phase II clinical trial of continuous FUDR regional chemotherapy for colorectal metastases to the liver using a totally implantable drug infusion pump. Ann Surg 198:567, 1983
13. Bengmark S, Hafstran L: The natural history of primary and secondary malignant tumors of the liver. Cancer 23: 198, 1969
14. Bengstsson G et al: Natural history of patients with treated liver metastases from colorectal cancer. Am J Surg 14:586, 1981
15. Bernadino M: Percutaneous biopsies. AJR 142:41, 1984

16. Bouwman DL, Walt AJ: Current status of resection for hepatic neoplasms. Sem Liver Dis 3:193, 1983

17. Breedis C et al: The blood supply of neoplasms in the liver. J Pathol 30:969, 1954

18. Buchwald H et al: Intraarterial infusion chemotherapy for hepatic carcinoma using a totally implantable infusion pump. Cancer 45:866, 1980

19. Buroker T et al: Hepatic artery infusion of 5-FUDR after prior systemic 5-fluorouracil. Cancer Treat Rep 60:1277, 1976

20. Butler J et al: Hepatic resection for colorectal metastases. Surg Gynecol Obstet 162:109, 1986

21. Cady B, McDermott WV: Major hepatic resection for metachronous metastases from colon cancer. Ann Surg 201:204, 1985

22. Cady B et al: Regional infusion chemotherapy of hepatic metastases from carcinoma of the colon. Am J Surg 127:220, 1974

23. Calne RY: Liver transplantation for liver cancer. World J Surg 6:76, 1982

24. Chabner BA et al: The clinical pharmacology of antineoplastic agents. N Engl J Med 292:1107, 1159, 1975

25. Cheng EW, Lightdale CJ: Primary liver cancer: Diagnosis and laboratory findings in hepatic and biliary cancer. In Wanebo H (ed): Surgical and Clinical Management. New York, Marcel Dekker, 1985

26. Cheng E et al: Phase II trial of (m-AMSA) 4'-9 (Acridinylamino) methanesulfon-m-amiside in primary liver cancer. A J Clin Oncol 6:211, 1983

27. Chiebowski RT et al: Doxorubicin (75 mg/m^2) for hepatocellular carcinoma: Clinical and pharmacokinetic results. Cancer Treat Rep 68:487, 1984

28. Choi T et al: Chemotherapy for advanced hepatocellular carcinoma: Adriamycin vs. quadruple chemotherapy. Cancer 53:401, 1984

29. Chun H et al: Hepatocellular carcinoma (HC): Statistical analysis of 78 consecutive patients (PTS). Proc ASCO, C23, 1984

30. Clark RA, Matsui O: CT of liver tumors. Semin Roentgenol 18:149, 1983

31. Clarkson B et al: Effects of continuous hepatic artery infusion of antimetabolites on primary and metastatic cancer of the liver. Cancer 15:472, 1962

32. Cohen AM et al: Regional hepatic chemotherapy using an implantable drug infusion pump. Am J Surg 145:529, 1983

33. Copeland EM III et al: Nutrition and cancer. Int Adv Surg Oncol 4:1, 1981

34. Cotton PB: Duodenoscopic placement of biliary prostheses to relieve malignant obstructive jaundice. Br J Surg 69:501, 1982

35. Crowley ML: Penetrating duodenal ulcer associated with an operatively implanted arterial chemotherapy infusion catheter. Gastroenterology 83:118, 1982

36. Dakhil S et al: Improved regional selectivity of hepatic arterial BCNU with degradable microspheres. Cancer 50:631, 1982

37. Daly JM et al: Long-term hepatic arterial infusion chemotherapy. Arch Surg 119:936, 1984

38. Danforth DN Jr et al: Metastatic insulin-secreting carcinoma of the pancreas: Clinical course and the role of surgery. Surgery 96:1027, 1984

39. DeVita VT, Schein PS: The use of drugs in combination for the treatment of cancer: Rationale and results. N Engl J Med 288:998, 1973

40. Ensminger W et al: Totally implanted drug delivery system for hepatic arterial chemotherapy. Cancer Treat Rep 5:393, 1981

41. Ensminger WD et al: A clinical-pharmacological evaluation of hepatic arterial infusions of 5-fluoro-2-deoxyuridine and 5-fluorouracil. Cancer Res 38:3784, 1978

42. Ettinger DS et al: Phase I-II study of isotopic immunoglobulin therapy for primary liver cancer. Cancer Treat Rep 66:289, 1982

43. Falkson G et al: Primary liver cancer: An Eastern Cooperative Oncology Group Trial. Cancer 54:970, 1984

44. Falkson G et al: A phase II study of m-AMSA in patients with primary liver cancer. Cancer Chemother Pharmacol 6:127, 1981

45. Ferrucci JT Jr et al: Malignant seeding of needle tract after thin needle aspiration biopsy: A previously unrecorded complication. Radiology 130:345, 1979

46. Foley KM: The treatment of cancer pain. N Engl J Med 313:84, 1985

47. Fortner JG et al: Multivariate analysis of a personal series of 247 consecutive patients with liver metastases from colorectal cancer. Ann Surg 199:306, 1984

48. Fortner JG et al: The seventies evolution in liver surgery for cancer. Cancer 47:2162, 1981

49. Foster JH, Lundy J: Liver metastases. Curr Probl Surg 18:157, 1981

50. Frei E III, Canellos G: Dose: A critical factor in cancer chemotherapy. Am J Med 69:585, 1980

51. Frei E III: Modification of host defense. In Holland JF, Frei E III (eds): Cancer Medicine, pp 720–730, Philadelphia, Lea & Febiger, 1982

52. Glazer G et al: Hepatic cavernous hemangioma: Magnetic resonance imaging. Radiology 155:417, 1985

53. Glouse ME et al: Complications of long-term transbrachial hepatic arterial infusion chemotherapy. AJR 129:799, 1977

54. Goldman ML et al: Complications of indwelling chemotherapy catheters. Cancer 36:1983, 1975

55. Grady ED: Internal radiation therapy of hepatic cancer. Dis Colon Rectum 22:371, 1979

56. Grady ED et al: Combination of internal radiation therapy and hyperthermia to treat liver cancer. South Med J 76:1101, 1983

57. Grage TB et al: Results of a prospective randomized study of hepatic artery infusion with 5-fluorouracil versus intravenous 5-fluorouracil in patients with hepatic metastases from colorectal cancer: A Central Oncology Group study. Surgery 86:550, 1979

58. Gutterman JL, Hersh E: Immunotherapy. In Holland JF, Frei E III (eds): Cancer Medicine, pp 1100–1133. Philadelphia, Lea & Febiger, 1982

59. Hafstrom L et al: Hepatic artery occlusion for liver cancer. Ann Chir Gynaecol 72:239, 1983

60. Hersh EM et al: Immunocompetence, immunodeficiency and prognosis in cancer. Ann NY Acad Sci 276:386, 1976

61. Hubregtse K, Tytgat GN: Palliative treatment of obstructive jaundice by trans-papillary introduction of large-bore bile duct endoprosthesis. Gut 23:371, 1982

62. Hwang KM et al: Selective antitumor effect on L10 hepatocarcinoma cells of a potent immunoconjugate composed of the A chain of abrin and a monoclonal antibody to a hepatoma-associated antigen. Cancer Res 44:4578, 1984

63. Ingold JA et al: Radiation hepatitis. AJR 93:200, 1965

64. Israel L et al: Brief communication: Daily intravenous infusions of *Corynebacterium parvum* in twenty patients with

disseminated cancer: A preliminary report of clinical and biologic findings. J Natl Cancer Inst 55:29, 1975

65. Iwatsuki S et al: Total hepatectomy and liver replacement (orthoptic liver transplantation) for primary hepatic malignancy. World J Surg 6:81, 1982

66. Iwatsuki S et al: Experience with 150 liver resections. Ann Surg 197:247, 1983

67. Jaffe BM et al: Factors influencing survival in patients with untreated hepatic metastases. Surg Gynecol Obstet 127:1, 1968

68. Johnson PA, Rossof AH: The role of the human tumor stem cell assay in medical oncology. Arch Intern Med 143:111, 1983

69. Johnson PJ et al: Alpha-fetoprotein concentrations measured by radioimmunoassay in diagnosing and excluding hepatocellular carcinoma. Br Med J 2:661, 1978

70. Kanematsu T et al: Selective effects of lipodolized antitumor agents. J Surg Oncol 25(3):218, 1984

71. Kanematsu T et al: Limited hepatic resection effective for selected cirrhotic patients with primary liver cancer. Ann Surg 199:51, 1984

72. Kaplan HS, Bagshaw MA: Radiation hepatitis: Possible prevention by combined isotopic and external radiation therapy. Radiology 91:1214, 1968

73. Karnofsky DA et al: Selection of patients for evaluation of chemotherapeutic procedures in advanced cancer. Cancer Chemother Rep 16:73, 1962

74. Kemeny N: Systemic chemotherapy of hepatic metastases. Sem Oncol 10:148, 1983

75. Kemeny N, Yagoda A: Chemotherapy of colorectal cancer: A critical analysis of response criteria and therapeutic efficacy. In Lipkin M, Good R (eds): Gastrointestinal Tract Cancer, pp 551–572. New York, Plenum Press, 1978

76. Kemeny N et al: Randomized study of intrahepatic vs systemic infusion of fluorodeoxyuridine in patients with liver metastases from colorectal carcinoma (preliminary results). Dev Oncol 26:85, 1984

77. Kreider JW et al: Immunotherapeutic effectiveness of BCG inactivated by various modalities. Cancer 46:480, 1980

78. Lahr CJ et al: A multifactorial analysis of prognostic factors in patients with liver metastases from colorectal carcinoma. J Clin Oncol 1:720, 1977

79. Lee NW et al: The surgical management of primary carcinoma of the liver. World J Surg 6:66, 1982

80. Leibel SA et al: Palliation of liver metastases with combined hepatic irradiation and misonidazole: Results of a radiation therapy oncology group phase I-II study. Cancer Clin Trials 4:285, 1981

81. Lewin K, Millis RR: Human radiation hepatitis. Arch Pathol 96:21, 1973

82. Lewis BJ et al: Intra-arterial vs intravenous FUDR for colorectal cancer metastatic to the liver: A Northern California oncology group study. Dev Oncol 26:77, 1984

83. Liebman HH et al: Des-v-carboxy (abnormal) prothrombin as a serum marker of primary hepatocellular carcinoma. N Engl J Med 310:1427, 1984

84. Lightdale CJ: Laparoscopy and biopsy in malignant liver disease. Cancer 50:2672, 1982

85. Lightdale CJ: Screening for diffuse and focal liver disease: A gastroenterologist's viewpoint. J Clin Ultrasound 12:85, 1984

86. Lightdale CJ: Laparoscopy in the age of imaging. Gastrointest Endosc 31:47, 1985

87. Lightdale CJ, Lipkin M: Cell division and tumor growth. In Becker FF (ed): Cancer: A Comprehensive Treatise, vol 3, pp 201–215. New York, Plenum Press, 1975

88. Lightdale CJ, Sherlock P: Chemotherapy of gastrointestinal cancer. Drug Ther 9:105, 1979

89. Lightdale CJ, Sherlock P: Management of Metastatic Liver Disease. In Popper H, Schaffner F (eds): Progress in Liver Diseases, pp 649–662. New York, Grune & Stratton, 1982

90. Lightdale CJ et al: Cancer and upper gastrointestinal tract hemorrhage: Benign causes of bleeding demonstrated by endoscopy. JAMA 226:139, 1973

91. Lightdale CJ et al: Laparoscopic diagnosis of suspected liver neoplasms: Value of prior liver scans. Dig Dis Sci 24:588, 1979

92. Lightdale CJ et al: Anticoagulation and high dose liver radiation. Cancer 43:174, 1979

93. Lightdale CJ et al: Primary hepatocellular carcinoma with hepatitis B antigenemia: Effects of chemotherapy. Cancer 46:1117, 1980

94. Lim RC Jr, Bongard FS: Hepatocellular carcinoma: Changing concepts in diagnosis and management. Arch Surg 119:637, 1984

95. Liu YK et al: Letter: Treatment of advanced primary hepatocellular carcinoma by 131-I-anti-AFP. Lancet 1:531, 1983

96. Lokich J: Determination of response in treatment of hepatic neoplasia. Semin Oncol 10:228, 1983

97. Lokich J et al: Lack of effectiveness of combined 5-fluorouracil and methyl-CCNU therapy in advanced colorectal cancer. Cancer 40:2792, 1977

98. Lokich J et al: Concomitant hepatic radiation and intraarterial fluorinated pyrimidine therapy: Correlation of liver scan, liver function tests, and plasma CEA with tumor response. Cancer 48:2569, 1981

99. Madding GF, Kennedy PA: Hepatic artery ligation. Surg Clin North Am 52:719, 1972

100. Mahour GH et al: Improved survival in infants and children with primary malignant liver tumors. Am J Surg 145:236, 1943

101. Maltz C et al: Hepatocellular carcinoma. Am J Gastroenterol 74:361, 1980

102. Martin JK Jr et al: Surgical treatment of functioning metastatic carcinoid tumors. Arch Surg 118:537, 1983

103. Matzen P et al: Accuracy of direct cholangiography by endoscopic or transhepatic route in jaundice: A prospective study. Gastroenterology 81:237, 1981

104. McIntire KR et al: Effect of surgical and chemotherapeutic treatment on alpha-fetoprotein levels in patients with hepatocellular carcinoma. Cancer 37:677, 1976

105. Melia WM et al: Diamminodichloride platinum (cis-platinum) in the treatment of hepatocellular carcinoma. Clin Oncol 7:275, 1981

106. Misra NC et al: Intrahepatic arterial infusion of combination of mitomycin-C and 5-fluorouracil in treatment of primary and metastatic liver carcinoma. Cancer 39: 1425, 1977

107. Moertel CG: The liver. In Holland JF, Frei E III (eds): Cancer Medicine, pp 1774–1781. Philadelphia, Lea & Febiger, 1982

108. Moertel CG, Reitmeier RJ: Advanced Gastrointestinal Cancer: Clinical Management and Chemotherapy. New York, Harper & Row, 1969

109. Moffat FL et al: Effect of radiofrequency hyperthermia and chemotherapy on primary and secondary hepatic malignancies when used with metronidazole. Surgery 94:536, 1983

110. Mori W et al: Hepatic artery ligation and tumor necrosis in the liver. Surgery 59:359, 1966

111. Nagasue N et al: Hepatic resection in the treatment of he-

patocellular carcinoma: Report of 60 cases. Br J Surg 72: 292, 1985

112. Narset T et al: Gastric ulceration in patients receiving intrahepatic infusion of 5-fluorouracil. Ann Surg 186:734, 1977

113. Niederhuber JE, Ensminger WD: Surgical considerations in the management of hepatic neoplasia. Semin Oncol 10: 135, 1983

114. O'Connell MJ et al: Clinical trial of adjuvant chemotherapy after surgical resection of colorectal cancer metastatic to the liver. Mayo Clin Proc 60:517, 1985

115. Ohnishi K et al: Arterial chemoembolization of hepatocellular carcinoma with mitomycin C microcapsules. Radiology 152:51, 1984

116. Okamoto E et al: Prediction of the safe limits of hepatectomy by combined volumetric and functional measurements in patients with impaired hepatic function. Surgery 95:586, 1984

117. Oladapo JM et al: In vitro and in vivo cytotoxic activity of native and ricin conjugated monoclonal antibodies to HBs antigen for Alexander primary liver cell carcinoma cells and tumors. Gut 25:619, 1984

118. Olweny CLM et al: Further experience in treating patients with hepatocellular carcinoma in Uganda. Cancer 46:2717, 1980

119. Olweny CLM et al: Treatment of hepatocellular carcinoma with adriamycin. Cancer 36:1250, 1975

120. Order S et al: Antiferritin IgG antibody for isotopic cancer therapy. Oncology 38:154, 1981

121. Pereiras RV et al: Relief of malignant obstructive jaundice by percutaneous insertion of a permanent prosthesis in the biliary tree. Ann Intern Med 89:589, 1978

122. Petrelli NJ et al: Hepatic artery ligation for liver metastasis in colorectal carcinoma. Cancer 53:1347, 1984

123. Phillip J et al: Endoscopic intraductal radiation therapy of proximal carcinomas of the common bile duct. Dtsch Med Wochenschr 109:422, 1984

124. Phillips R, Murikami K: Primary neoplasms of the liver. Cancer 13:714, 1960

125. Phillips R et al: Roentgen therapy of hepatic metastases. AJR 71:826, 1954

126. Plengvanit V et al: Colateral arterial blood supply of the liver after hepatic ligation: Arteriographic study of 20 patients. Ann Surg 180:305, 1974

127. Prasad B et al: Irradiation of hepatic metastases. Int J Radiat Oncol Biol Phys 2:129, 1977

128. Price JB Jr et al: Major hepatic resections for neoplasia in children. Arch Surg 117:1139, 1982

129. Raaf JH, Stroehlein JR: Palliation of malignant ascites by the LeVeen peritoneo-venous shunt. Cancer 45:1019, 1980

130. Ravry M et al: Usefulness of serial serum carcinoembryonic antigen (CEA) determinations during anti-cancer therapy or long term follow-up of gastrointestinal cancer. Cancer 34:1230, 1974

131. Reed MAL et al: The practicality of chronic hepatic artery infusion therapy of primary and metastatic hepatic malignancies: Ten-year results of 124 patients in a prospective protocol. Cancer 47:402, 1981

132. Ring EJ et al: Therapeutic applications of catheter cholangiography. Radiology 128:333, 1978

133. Rojas AF et al: Levamisole in advanced human breast cancer. Lancet 1:211, 1976

134. Ryan WH et al: Reduction in the morbidity and mortality of major hepatic resection: Experience with 52 patients. Am J Surg 144:740, 1982

135. Salmon SE et al: Quantitation of differential sensitivity of human tumor stem cells to anticancer drugs. N Engl J Med 296:1321, 1978

136. Schwerk WB, Schmitz-Moorman P: Ultrasonically guided fine-needle biopsies in neoplastic liver disease: Cytohistologic diagnoses and echo pattern of lesions. Cancer 48:1469, 1981

137. Shackney SE et al: Growth rate patterns of solid tumors and their relation to responsiveness to therapy. Ann Intern Med 89:107, 1978

138. Shils ME: Principles of nutritional therapy. Cancer 43:2093, 1979

139. Smith BJ et al: Inefficacy of dacarbazine, mitomycin C, and hepatic irradiation in patients with metastatic adenocarcinoma of the gastrointestinal tract. J Clin Oncol 2:578, 1984

140. Sparks FC et al: Hepatic artery ligation and postoperative chemotherapy for hepatic metastases: Clinical and pathophysiological results. Cancer 35:1074, 1975

141. Starzl TE et al: Changing concepts: Liver replacement for hereditary tyrosinemia and hepatoma. J Pediatr 106:604, 1985

142. Steele G Jr et al: Patterns of failure after surgical cure of large liver tumors: A change in the proximate cause of death and a need for effective systemic adjuvant therapy. Am J Surg 147:554, 1984

143. Straus AK et al: Peritoneo-venous shunting in the management of malignant ascites. Arch Surg 114:489, 1978

144. Strodel WE et al: Surgical therapy for small-bowel carcinoid tumors. So Arch Surg 118:391, 1983

145. Sudqvist K et al: Treatment of liver cancer with regional intraarterial 5-FU infusion. Am J Surg 136:328, 1978

146. Sullivan R et al: Chemotherapy of metastatic liver cancer by prolonged hepatic-artery infusion. N Engl J Med 270: 3211, 1964

147. Suzuki T et al: Study of vascularity of tumors of the liver. Surg Gynecol Obstet 134:27, 1972

148. Taylor I et al: A randomized controlled trial of adjuvant portal vein cytotoxic perfusion in colorectal cancer. Br J Surg 72:359, 1985

149. Tefft M et al: Irradiation of the liver in children: Acute effects enhanced by concomitant chemotherapeutic administration? AJR 111:165, 1971

150. Thompson HH et al: Major hepatic resection: A 25-year experience. Ann Surg 197:375, 1983

151. Turek–Maischeider M, Kazem I: Palliative irradiation for liver metastases. JAMA 232:625, 1975

152. Von Hoff DD: "Send this patient's tumor for culture and sensitivity." N Engl J Med 308:154, 1983

153. Wagner JS et al: The natural history of hepatic metastases from colorectal cancer. Ann Surg 199:502, 1984

154. Wanebo H et al: Immune reactivity in patients with colorectal cancer: Assessment of biologic risk by immunoparameters. Cancer 45:1254, 1980

155. Wanebo HJ et al: Surgical management of patients with primary operable cancer and synchronous liver metastases. Ann J Surg 135:81, 1978

156. Watkins E Jr et al: Surgical basis for arterial infusion chemotherapy of disseminated carcinoma of the liver. Surg Gynecol Obstet 130:581, 1970

157. Wood CB et al: A retrospective study of the natural history of patients with liver metastases from colorectal cancer. Clin Oncol 2:285, 1976

158. Woodington GF, Waugh JM: Results of resection of metastatic tumors of the liver. Am J Surg 105:24, 1963

chapter **35**

Parasitic Diseases of the Liver

MANUEL A. MARCIAL and RAÚL A. MARCIAL–ROJAS

Our aim in this chapter is to mention briefly the most important highlights in the parasitology and epidemiology of parasitic diseases that involve the liver and to concentrate on the clinical and pathological changes resulting from their hepatic involvement. Several reference textbooks are available for greater in-depth information.[8,100,177] In order to correlate histopathological changes with clinical manifestations, the various parasitic entities are grouped into categories based upon the type and extension of the pathologic process.[101]

PROTOZOAL DISEASES

Parenchymal Involvement (Localized)

Amebiasis

Amebiasis is caused by *Entamoeba histolytica,* a protozoan whose life cycle involves several consecutive morphological changes occurring within the host's intestinal lumen. Of these, the cyst and the trophozoite stage are the most important clinically. Transmission to humans is by way of the cyst, which may remain viable in water up to 4 weeks. The more frequent mode of spread is through vegetables and fruits handled by carrier persons (cyst passers) with poor hygienic habits or through washing of these foodstuffs with water containing the cysts. When the ingested cyst reaches the small intestine, the multinucleated ameba emerges from its cyst wall and its cytoplasm divides as many times as the number of nuclei present in the cell. Each one of these small amebae, known as metacystic trophozoites, will grow and mature to become a trophozoite. The adult trophozoite or motile form moves downstream and colonizes the large intestine, particularly the cecal region. Once in the colon, *E. histolytica* can behave either as a commensal or as a highly invasive pathogen. Although the determinants of which host–parasite interaction will be established have not been completely elucidated, the specific protozoal strain and its virulence seem to be the major factors. The pathogenicity and the spectrum of virulence of amebic strains have been determined *in vivo* using experimental animals such as the hamster.[105,111] In addition, by studying the electrophoretic patterns of four enzymes isolated from amebic trophozoites, characteristic isoenzyme patterns have been identified as markers of pathogenicity.[149] The degree of virulence, as determined by bioassays, has been correlated with both cytotoxic and proteinase activity present in the amebic trophozoite of that particular strain.[90,95,111,149] Furthermore, a positive correlation between the degree of virulence and the rate of erythrophagocytosis has been observed.[121] Host defense mechanisms against protozoal invasion include both humoral and cellular immune responses. The induced circulating antibodies, mostly of the IgG class, have protective effects, since they have *in vitro* amebicidal properties, and passive immunity in animal models partially protects the host against invasion.[155]

The pathogenic effect of *E. histolytica* is thought to be the result of a lectin-mediated, cytoskeleton-dependent adhesion of trophozoites to epithelial cells followed by the release of cytotoxins and the eventual phagocytosis of lysed cells by the ameba.[77,141,155] However, no specialized attachment organelle has been unequivocally identified by ultrastructural methods.[54] Cytotoxic–enterotoxic substances isolated from lysates of axenic cultures of *E. histolytica* have included proteolytic enzymes such as cathepsin and collagenase and neurohumoral substances such as serotonin.[47,88,89,96,111] Their cytopathic effects have been determined in monolayer cultures of mammalian cells, and their enterotoxic properties have been assayed in ligated intestinal loops and in Ussing chambers by demonstrating toxin-induced fluid secretion.

Incidence and prevalence rates of amebiasis are difficult to estimate, since the majority of infected persons are asymptomatic. Furthermore, false-positive and false-negative results are not uncommon when unskilled laboratory technologists perform stool examination for intestinal protozoa.[78] In the United States, although the prevalence in the general population is probably less than 5%, prevalence rates in populations of homosexual men have ranged from 21% to 36%.[102,122,131,137] *E. histolytica* is usually found in association with other intestinal pathogens, and its presence as part of the gay bowel syndrome correlates with oral–anal sexual practices.[102,131] Fortunately for these persons, it seems that the strains of amebae colonizing their large intestines are of low virulence. A large number of these patients are asymptomatic, and the presence of symptoms does not correlate with amebic infection.[102,122,131,137] The isoenzyme patterns of the amebae isolated from homosexual men have been of the zymodeme type regarded as non-pathogenic.[97] Moreover, erythrophagocytosis is seldom detected in the trophozoite-containing stools of these patients.[102] Thus, although amebiasis is an endemic infection among homosexual men, these persons are not at a high risk of developing invasive complications such as amebic liver abscess. Whether asymptomatic patients (cyst passers) should be treated, especially if they belong to an endemic population, is controversial, and some physicians limit treatment to food handlers and to those in contact with immunodeficient persons.[116]

In invasive intestinal amebiasis the most frequently mentioned lesion is the typical flask-shaped ulcer. Several such ulcers may coalesce and produce extensive areas of ulceration and hemorrhage. Patients present with the clinical manifestations of a dysentery with bloody, mucous stools. It is important to keep amebiasis in the differential diagnosis of inflammatory bowel disease since immunosuppression in these patients can lead to great morbidity and mortality.

Amebic liver abscess represents the most frequent form of extraintestinal dissemination. Its incidence in fatal cases of invasive amebiasis is extremely high. Hepatic amebiasis is more frequent in males, and liver abscesses, although found in all age groups, are more common in young and middle age adults. Intestinal involvement can be documented only in a few of the patients with amebic liver abscess.[26]

Amebae gain access to the liver via the portal venous system. Hepatic amebiasis can be produced experimentally in hamsters by injecting pathogenic amebae intraportally.[27] Animal models of amebic liver abscess have permitted the elucidation of the sequence of morphologic changes taking place during abscess formation.[27,28] The initial host response to the invasive trophozoite consists of a polymorphonuclear reaction surrounding the sinusoidal localized amebae. Many of these polymorphonuclear leukocytes undergo lysis with release of lysosomal enzymes, a process that apparently results in the necrosis of adjacent hepatocytes. Subsequently there is a decrease in neutrophils and an increase in mononuclear cells, lymphocytes, and macrophages, with the formation of a rim of granulomatous inflammation around these necrotic foci. The trophozoites are always located at the edge of this necrotic zone. The coalescence of multiple foci results in extensive areas of necrosis circumscribed by a layer of atrophied compressed hepatocytes and a zone of fibrosis.

In humans, the pathologic changes of amebic liver abscess are characteristic and only rarely are confused with such other lesions as pyogenic abscesses or liquefied metastatic tumors. The right lobe is involved in 50% to 70% of the cases, and the abscesses are multiple in 40% of the cases. They are usually between 8 cm and 12 cm in diameter and are frequently located close to the dome of the right lobe of the liver. The abscess is usually well delimited grossly, although not so clearly microscopically (Figs. 35-1 and 35-2).

In uncomplicated liver abscess, the content simulates anchovy paste or, when the exudate is admixed with blood, is chocolate colored. Amebae are practically never seen in the necrotic debris but are usually evident near its periphery. Nearby liver plates are attenuated and disorganized, frequently disclosing intervening fibrosis.

Clinically, amebic liver abscess usually exhibits a gradual onset. Fever is usually not a prominent feature unless the abscess becomes secondarily infected. Jaundice is very unusual. The initial localizing symptom is usually pain in the right upper quadrant, which starts as a dull ache but later becomes sharp and stabbing. When the abscess is near the diaphragm, referral of pain to the shoulder and accentuation of the pain by deep breathing may be present. Liver function tests are usually normal, with the exception of an occasional elevation of the alkaline phosphatase level. Leukocyte count values range between 13,000 and 16,000, with 70% to 80% neutrophils. The abscess is frequently located in the anterior–superior portion of the liver, thus producing a bulge in the anteromedial part of the right diaphragm. This also produces obliteration of the cardiophrenic angle anteriorly and of the anterior costophrenic angle laterally, a useful radiologic feature. With subphrenic abscess, the cardiophrenic angle is usually obliterated in its posterior lateral region.

Hepatic abscesses can be diagnosed and localized by nuclear scans using ^{67}Ga-citrate or radioactive colloids. The most commonly used is the ^{99m}Tc-sulfur colloid. Multiple scans should be made looking for filling defects or cold areas. The combination of posterior, anterior, and right lateral scans allowed a 98.6% diagnostic efficiency in an analysis of 4286 amebic abscesses.[27] Ultrasonography has also been used for the diagnosis of amebic liver abscesses. They appear usually as peripherally located homogeneous lesions that are hypoechogenic and show slight distal sonic enhancement.[139] Since ultrasound has an accuracy very similar to that of nuclear scanning and is fairly cheap and free of ionizing radiation, it is becoming the preferred method for diagnosis of amebic liver abscesses.[72] Computed tomography (CT) can also be used to accurately diagnose hepatic amebiasis.

The serologic diagnosis of amebiasis depends on the detection of the IgG antibodies that arise as the result of invasive amebiasis. Since these antibodies remain in circulation for a long period, their detection does not always mean infection. Available methods for serodiagnosis include complement fixation (CF), indirect hemagglutination (IHA), indirect immunofluorescence, latex agglutination, counterimmunoelectrophoresis, the enzyme-linked immunosorbent assay (ELISA), and a gel-diffusion precipitin test.[4,104,126,168] The IHA is the test most widely used, and it is the standard method performed at the Centers for Disease Control. The IHA test is considered positive if circulating antibodies are present in a dilution titer of 1:128 or greater. Once positive, the IHA test results remain so for a long period of time. This property, although of value for epidemiologic studies, sometimes makes interpretation of seropositivity difficult. Thus, al-

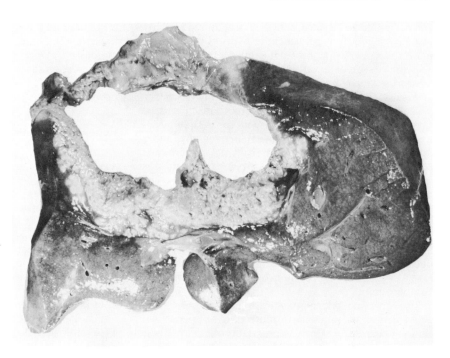

Fig. 35-1. A large amebic abscess of the liver. More than one half of the organ has been destroyed. (Pérez–Tamayo R, Brandt H: In Marcial–Rojas RA [ed]: Pathology of Protozoal and Helminthic Disease, p 166. Baltimore, Williams & Wilkins, 1971)

though very sensitive and specific, this test has a lower positive predictive value than other tests, such as the gel-diffusion precipitin test.[126] This test, like the latex agglutination test, is a sensitive, inexpensive, and a very simple test to perform. The remaining methodologies have comparable sensitivities, ranging from 95% to 99% for amebic liver abscess diagnosis.[125] Thus the methodology to be used is dependent largely on the laboratory director's personal preference. Recently a radioimmunoassay for the detection of circulating amebic antigens was reported.[132] It is very sensitive and specific for ongoing hepatic and/or intestinal amebiasis. Although the methodology is complex, the test could be of great diagnostic help in endemic populations.

Amebic abscess may follow three different courses: healing, rupture, or dissemination. If the abscess is prop-

Fig. 35-2. Multiple amebic abscesses of the liver. (Pérez–Tamayo R, Brandt H: In Marcial–Rojas RA [ed]: Pathology of Protozoal and Helminthic Diseases, p 166. Baltimore, Williams & Wilkins, 1971)

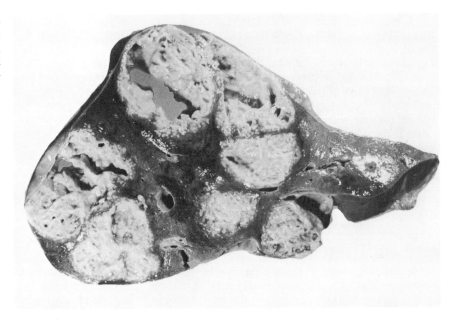

erly diagnosed and treated, cure may be achieved in many instances. Clinical improvement is evident by a decrease in liver size and by disappearance of many of the radiologic and clinical signs of hepatic involvement. Only a residuum of scar tissue may remain; this is usually of stellate shape and is associated with sub-capsular retraction. Occasionally, a residual cavity surrounded by fibroconnective tissue may persist. In a follow-up study with sonographic evaluation, 23 of 32 abscesses resolved after therapy, and a normal sonographic hepatic parenchymal pattern was achieved.[140] In six other abscesses a cystic residuum was seen with the sonographic appearance of simple cysts. The natural tendency for amebic abscess is to continue growing until it ruptures. Rupture into the peritoneal cavity may produce acute peritonitis. Rupture into other abdominal viscera, such as the stomach, duodenum, and colon, is also possible, as is rupture into the thoracic cavity, producing pleuropulmonary amebiasis. Rupture into the right lower or middle lobes is the most common of thoracic complications.[68]

The most frequent cause of death in amebic abscess is acute peritonitis following rupture into the peritoneal cavity. On a recent report, the mortality rate in patients with this complication was 42%.[40] Rarely, attachment to the abdominal wall may permit perforation through the skin, producing extensive ulceration and fistula formation. Hematogenous dissemination of amebae is practically never seen without involvement of the liver. Distribution of this type accounts for the production of pulmonary parenchymal and cerebral abscesses.

Secondary infection with pyogenic organisms is an important complication of amebic liver abscess. Aspiration reveals changes in appearance and color of the abscess content, and causative organisms may be recovered. Specific antibiotic treatment for the secondary organism should be instituted.

Treatment for amebic liver abscess consists of the administration of one or more of the following tissue amebicides; metronidazole, emetine hydrochloride, or its synthetic derivative dehydroemetine and chloroquine.[76] The drug of choice is metronidazole (750 mg tid p.o. for 5–10 days).[38] Although metronidazole has both tissue and luminal amebicidal properties, cure rates in intestinal disease have been as low as 80%.[133] Thus, to prevent relapse in those patients with both intestinal and hepatic amebiasis, iodoquinol (diiodohydroxyquin) 650 mg three times per day for 20 days is added to the metronidazole regimen.[38] Although emetine is cardiotoxic, it is sometimes used because it is the most potent amebicide and is active in all tissues.[76] It is of particular use whenever there is amebic peritonitis, which as stated above has a very high mortality. Dehydroemetine is probably as effective as emetine and is less cardiotoxic.[38] Either one may be administered intramuscularly for 5 days to be followed by a course of chloroquine.

The role of therapeutic needle aspiration in the treatment of amebic liver abscess is controversial. Although some experts recommend drainage whenever the abscess is painful and a point of maximal tenderness can be defined, it seems that most abscesses will resolve with chemotherapy alone.[2] Furthermore, therapeutic aspiration does not seem to improve resolution time.[156] Thus, most physicians would reserve aspiration for very large abscesses in which rupture is imminent.

Reticuloendothelial Involvement (Diffuse)

Malaria

Malaria is caused by protozoa of the genus *Plasmodium*. There are four species that commonly affect humans: *P. malariae, P. vivax, P. ovale,* and *P. falciparum.* In spite of the large sums of money that have been spent on insecticides and other public health control measures, malaria remains the most widespread of all infectious diseases. The immigration of refugees from Southeast Asia, where the disease is endemic, is bringing this disease to the forefront in our environment.

The life cycle of the malaria parasite consists of two phases: the asexual cycle, or schizogony, which takes place in humans, and the sexual cycle, or sporogony, which occurs in the female anopheline mosquito. The end result of the sexual reproductive cycle in the mosquito is the formation of sporozoites, which migrate through the body cavity of the mosquito to the salivary glands. These are then injected with the salivary secretion when the mosquito bites a human. Sporozoites in the human bloodstream circulate for approximately 30 minutes and then invade liver cells, beginning the preerythrocytic cycle. How the sporozoites gain access to the hepatocyte is presently unknown. A recent study has raised the possibility that sporozoites reach the hepatocytes not by diapedesis or sinusoidal fenestrae, but by Kupffer cell passage.[106] Whatever the mechanism of entry, once inside the hepatocyte the process of shizogony ensues. At the end of approximately one week for *P. falciparum,* the schizonts rupture the liver cells and free merozoites into the bloodstream. This damage to the liver parenchyma does not give rise to any significant functional alteration.

The erythrocytic cycle, the most important pathogenetically, begins with the merozoite invasion of red blood cells. The merozoites attach to the red blood cell membrane by specific receptors, such as the Duffy blood group determinant for *P. vivax* and glycophorin A and B for *P. falciparum.*[41,108,109] Subsequently, a "junction" is formed between the cell membranes of the host and parasite, and the protozoan enters the cell via a cytoskeleton-mediated process.[3] The merozoites become trophozoites, which in turn undergo either shizogony or gametogony within the erythrocyte. During its development the sporozoan digests hemoglobin, which becomes the malarial pigment hemozoin, an iron porphyrin proteinoid complex. When the erythrocyte ruptures, the merozoites liberated will parasitize other red blood cells and the hemozoin pigment will be phagocytized by reticuloendothelial cells. In addition to hemolysis of parasitized erythrocytes, by rupture of schizonts, other mechanisms are thought to contribute to the anemia in malaria, mainly, diminished erythrocyte production due to depression of erythropoiesis, increased phagocytosis of erythrocytes due to an altered sodium pump, and hemolysis of both normal and parasitized erythrocytes by immunologically mediated mechanisms.[130] The debris of the ruptured cells, together with the merozoites and their metabolic by-products, acts as a pyrogen, producing the characteristic high fever and chills. The interval between mosquito bite and fever ranges from 1 to 4 weeks, with an average of 2 weeks for *P. falciparum*. In addition to anemia, thrombocytopenia is the other frequent hematologic finding in patients with malaria. This results from a combination of platelet sequestration in the spleen, consumption coagulopathy, and immune-mediated destruction, not by immune complexes but by IgG specific against platelet-bound malarial antigens.[74,159]

The most serious complications of malaria include acute renal failure (blackwater fever) and cerebral dysfunction. These usually occur in *P. falciparum* infections when the parasitemia reaches very high levels. Alterations in host cell-mediated responses have been documented in patients with cerebral malaria and high parasitemia.[15] Mechanisms proposed for the induction of the immunosuppression in malaria have included clonal deletion of antigen-specific cells, responses to polyclonal activation, antigenic competition, and nonspecific activation of suppressor cells.[188] *P. falciparum* is capable of evading the host's immune system by a combination of mechanisms to include antigenic variation, antigenic complexity, and intracellular development.[94]

Malaria stimulates the reticuloendothelial system with ensuing phagocytosis and development of hepatosplenomegaly. The hepatic sinusoids are congested by parasitized erythrocytes, and there is diffuse Kupffer cell hyperplasia. These phagocytic cells are prominent and contain dark brown hemozoin granules, phagocytosed erythrocytes, and small amounts of hemosiderin (Fig. 35-3). There is focal ischemic degeneration of the centrilobular or acinar zone III hepatocytes. A lymphoplasmacytic infiltrate is prominent in the portal areas, and occasionally sinusoidal lymphocytosis may occur. Hepatic fibrosis is not a feature of malaria.

The diagnosis of malaria depends on the demonstration of malarial parasites on a Giemsa-stained thick or thin blood smear. Erythrocytes containing multiple ring forms and the presence of banana-shaped gametocytes are diagnostic of *P. falciparum*. Because of fluctuations in the degree of parasitemia, multiple periodic blood-smear examinations should be performed. Furthermore, followup of parasitemia is very important in the rapid recognition of a drug-resistant organism. When the parasites are not detected in several carefully examined smears but the diagnosis of malaria is strongly suspected, a therapeutic trial should be started and the diagnosis corroborated by serologic tests. The methods currently available include the IHA, the ELISA, the indirect fluorescent antibody test

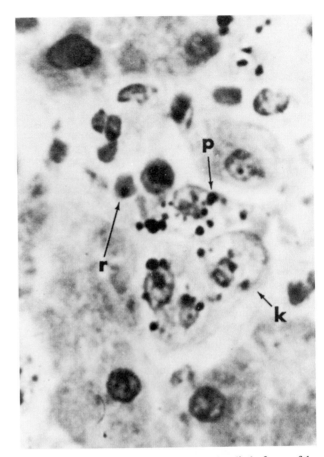

Fig. 35-3. Liver of a 21-year-old man who died of acute falciparum malaria. Several enlarged Kupffer cells appear in the center of the photograph (*arrow at k*); these contain many fine globules of malaria pigment. One globule is shown at p. A parasitized red cell is evident within the sinusoid at r. (AFIP Neg. 66-6167-2) (Original magnification × 900; H&E)

IFA, and the CF test.[161,162,187] The IFA test, because of its specificity and sensitivity, is the preferred method for serodiagnosis and the one presently used by the Centers for Disease Control.[184] A titer of 1:64 is considered indicative of past or present malaria. Serodiagnosis is also very useful for epidemiologic studies and for the investigation and identification of donors responsible for transfusion-related malaria cases. Even with the strict criteria for donor selection, there were 26 cases of transfusion-related malaria reported in the United States from 1972 through 1982.[58] In other countries, where posttransfusion malaria is a bigger problem, methods are being developed to screen serologically for the presence of malaria in potentially dangerous donors.[36,160]

The choice of antimalarial agents for the prevention and therapy of infection depends upon the specific parasite involved. Chemoprophylaxis for travelers should be tailored to the geographic region to be visited. The Centers for Disease Control publish guidelines that take into account risk of infection and presence of drug-resistant strains. Failure to adhere to these guidelines has been responsible for more than 90% of the cases of malaria among US travelers in the past decade.[20] These 2575 cases represented only 33% of the total imported cases of malaria in the United States, most of whom were foreign nationals.[20] Overwhelmed by the high incidence of malaria in the incoming Southeast Asian refugees, some countries have established prophylactic-therapeutic regimens for these immigrants.[56]

The drug of choice for the treatment of all uncomplicated cases of malaria, except for chloroquine-resistant *P. falciparum,* is chloroquine phosphate p.o., 1 g initially, then 500 mg in 6 hours, followed by 500 mg/day for 2 days.[38] Quinine sulfate (650 mg tid for 10 days) plus pyrimethamine (25 mg bid for 3 days) plus sulfadiazine (500 mg qid for 5 days) are used for uncomplicated cases involving chloroquine-resistant strains.[38,177] The latter two drugs are available in a fixed-dose combination under the trade name Fansidar (Roche). Since resistance and severe adverse reactions to Fansidar have recently been reported,[21,61] alternative drug therapies are already being evaluated.[142,152]

Treatment of severe complicated malaria requires slow intravenous infusion of 600 mg quinine dihydrochloride in 300-ml normal saline.[38] This dose is repeated every 8 hours until oral therapy can be instituted. Although quinine is potentially toxic, its use in complicated cases should not be delayed for this reason.[181,182] In cases in which renal and cerebral involvement accompany high parasitemia, some investigators have advocated the use of exchange blood transfusions.[42] Finally, to prevent relapses in *P. vivax* and *P. ovale,* primaquine phosphate is used after screening the patient for glucose 6-phosphate dehydrogenase (G6PD) deficiency. This drug is necessary to eliminate the low-level extra-erythrocytic infection common in these two strains. The hope for the future is that molecular biology will allow the development of a vaccine that will provide immunity against malarial infection.

Babesiosis

Babesiosis is a zoonosis caused by tick-transmitted parasites of the genus *Babesia.* The most common species to infect humans are *B. bovis* in Europe and *B. microti* in North America. Within the vertebrate host, *Babesia* merozoites invade erythrocytes with an entry process that requires the presence of complement factors[69,174] in a manner similar to the blood group determinant requirements of some plasmodia.[41,108,109] The protozoan multiplies inside the red blood cell by budding rather than by schizogony. The absence of schizonts and gametocytes and the lack of hemozoin pigment in *Babesia*-parasitized erythrocytes are the fundamental points in its differential diagnosis with malarial infections.[60] No exoerythrocytic cycle has been documented in babesiosis. A handful

of transfusion-mediated infections have been documented.[55,186] The incubation period ranges from 1 to 5 weeks.

The initial cases reported occurred in splenectomized patients. Their clinical course was one of hemoglobinuria, jaundice, anemia, and renal failure. Both serum glutamic-oxaloacetic transaminase (SGOT) and serum glutamic-pyruvic transaminase (SGPT) levels are usually elevated, and histopathological examination of the liver reveals fatty infiltration and Kupffer cell hyperplasia. Parasitized erythrocytes are usually seen distending the sinusoids. Other postmortem findings may include pulmonary edema and acute tubular necrosis.[30]

Recent cases in nonsplenectomized patients have presented a spectrum in symptomatology ranging from asymptomatic to severe illness.[144] That the absence of the spleen leads to a more severe illness has been confirmed in experimental animals.[145] In addition, the competence of the host's cell-mediated immune system is thought to play a major role in the control of parasitemia and the development of immunity.[11,143]

The diagnosis of babesiosis is confirmed by identifying the ring and tetrad forms in Giemsa-stained thick or thin blood smears. As in malaria, multiple examinations increase the yield of diagnosis. Smears are also helpful in quantitation of parasitemia to follow response to drug therapy. In cases of high suspicion in which parasites are not seen in smears, the patient's blood can be injected into a hamster for confirmation. This bioassay has also been used in the evaluation of drug therapy to distinguish complete eradication from lowering of parasitemia to undetectable levels by blood-smear examination.[46] Serodiagnosis for babesiosis, based on an IFA, is now available.[24]

The drug regimen of choice for the treatment of babesiosis is clindamycin (1.2 g bid parenterally or 600 mg tid orally for 7 days) plus quinine (650 mg tid orally for 7 days).[38] With therapy, parasitemia disappears, there is a decline in the antibody titers by the IFA test, and the patient's blood becomes uninfective as tested in hamsters.[186] Exchange transfusion has been useful in patients with very high parasitemia.[24]

Kala-azar (Visceral Leishmaniasis)

Visceral leishmaniasis or kala-azar (Hindi for black fever) is caused by parasites of the genus *Leishmania.* It is essentially a disease of the reticuloendothelial system, endemic in parts of Asia, the Middle East, the Mediterranean basin, Africa, and South America. The various species of *Leishmania* are virtually indistinguishable morphologically and have very similar life cycles. *L. donovani, L. infantum,* and *L. chagasi* are regarded as the causative agents of Old World, Mediterranean, and New World kala-azar, respectively.[180] However, some authors regard the latter two as subspecies of *L. donovani* and refer to them as *L. d. infantum* and *L. d. chagasi.*[81] It is hoped that the use of newly developed biochemical and immunologic methods will clarify the taxonomic classification in the very near future. The parasite is transmitted to humans by the bite of a sandfly of the genus *Phlebotomus* in the Old World and *Lutzomya* in the New World. The disease can rarely be transmitted by blood transfusion. *Leishmania* are dimorphic organisms, existing as flagellated extracellular promastigotes in the sandfly and as aflagellar obligate intracellular amastigotes in humans. The promastigotes, injected by the sandfly during its blood meal, rapidly change to the oval-shaped amastigote. After colonizing the dermis of humans, the amastigotes gain access to the bloodstream or lymphatics and are transported to the viscera, where they parasitize macrophages of the reticulo-endothelial system.

The process of entry of the amastigote into a host macrophage begins with attachment of the parasite to the host cell membrane, an interaction that is thought to depend on surface protein determinants.[189] The protozoan then enters the macrophages by phagocytosis and multiplies in them by binary fission. The amastigote has developed mechanisms for survival within the phagolysosome. These include inactivation of the microbicidal lysosomal enzymes and the capacity for parasite-specified phagocytosis. Through the latter mechanism these organisms are able to parasitize nonactivated macrophages without triggering a respiratory burst, and thus no leishmanicidal oxygen metabolites are produced.[71,112] The host's immune system reacts with both humoral and cellular responses.[129]

The disease is heralded by loss of weight, weakness, enlargement of the abdomen due to prominent splenomegaly and hepatomegaly, fever, cough, and pain over the spleen. The onset is insidious, and the course is chronic. The incubation period varies from 2 weeks to 18 months.

The main morphologic manifestations of kala-azar are those secondary to the dissemination and multiplication of the leishmania within phagocytic cells of the reticulo-endothelial system. This leads to splenomegaly (Fig. 35-4), hepatomegaly, and enlargement of lymph nodes, especially those in the mesentery. The bone marrow is replaced by parasitized macrophages. In the liver there is hyperplasia of Kupffer cells, the cytoplasm of which contains numerous Leishman–Donovan bodies. Phagocytic mononuclear cells, many of them with intracytoplasmic protozoa, are also seen in the portal areas. Inflammatory cells, including eosinophils, are also usually numerous here, especially adjacent to degenerating liver cells.

The definite diagnosis of kala-azar is made by identifying the parasite in tissue sections or smears. *Leishmania* is distinguished from other intracellular organisms, like *Histoplasma,* by its two basophilic dots, its nucleus and its kinetoplast (Fig. 35-5). Bone marrow aspiration yields a diagnosis in 90% of the cases, while liver biopsy is positive in 70% of them. Splenic puncture is a very high yield procedure with positive results in 95% of the cases. Although most physicians would prefer the bone marrow aspirate, for safety reasons, in expert hands splenic aspiration is a low-risk procedure that allows quantitation of

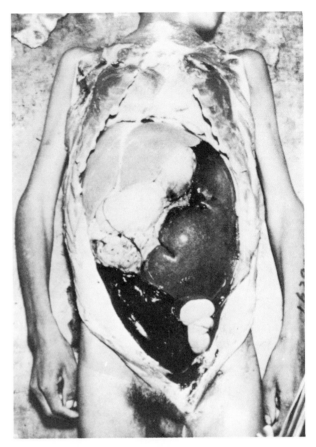

Fig. 35-4. Patient with kala-azar who died as a result of intraperitoneal hemorrhage following diagnostic puncture of the spleen. Note massive hepatosplenomegaly. Postmortem photograph. (AFIP Neg. A-45364)

parasite load.[25] Culture of aspirated samples increases the yield of diagnosis.[84]

Serodiagnosis of kala-azar is possible by several methods, including the IHA test, the IFA test, ELISA, CF, and direct agglutination (DA) test.[6,91] Both IFA and DA are available in the United States through the Centers for Disease Control. The DA test is the most sensitive of all. A dilution titer of 1:64 or more is considered positive.

The drug of choice for the treatment of kala-azar is sodium stibogluconate, a pentavalent organic antimonial. The usual dosage is 10 mg/kg/day IM or IV for 6 to 10 days.[38] For the African form of kala-azar, therapy may be extended to 30 days[38] or the dose may be given every 8 hours for 10 days.[157] This regimen resulted in good response as measured by reduction of spleen size and decrease in splenic aspirate parasite count with no increase in toxicity.[26] An alternative is pentamidine isethionate (2–4 mg/kg/day IM for up to 15 doses).[38] This drug has been useful in the treatment of antimonial-resistant kala-azar.[70]

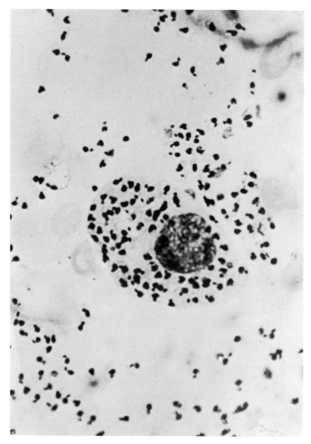

Fig. 35-5. Diagnostic smear for kala-azar showing many intracellular and extracellular leishmania. Note the two basophilic dots, the nucleus, and the kinetoplast. (AFIP Neg. 55-17580) (Original magnification × 1000; Giemsa stain)

HELMINTHIC DISEASES

Obstructive Biliary Lesions

Ascariasis

Ascariasis is a helminthic infection caused by the nematode *Ascaris lumbricoides.* It is a cosmopolitan parasite and the most prevalent and largest of human helminths. The infection is acquired by the ingestion of fertilized ova and is more frequent and severe in children, especially in areas with poor sanitary facilities. When the ingested embryonated egg reaches the small intestine, the larva hatches and penetrates into the intestinal mucosa, thereafter invading either lymphatics or portal venules. In experimental animals no inflammatory reaction is usually elicited in the liver sinusoids by the migrating larvae. However, in animals previously exposed to infection, larvae may be seen surrounded by an acute inflammatory infiltrate composed of eosinophils and neutrophils. This can lead to the death of the larvae and subsequent granuloma formation around the degenerated parasite. The final destination of the *Ascaris* larvae, whether by way of lymphatics or veins, is the pulmonary alveoli. Larvae pierce the alveolar lining, thus gaining access to the alveolar sacs. During pulmonary larva migration, cough, pneumonitis, and symptomatology suggestive of asthmatic bronchitis may become evident. Two weeks after arriving in the lung, the larvae ascend through the respiratory bronchioles, trachea, and pharynx, are swallowed, and finally reach the small intestine. Two or three months after the egg is ingested, the larva becomes an adult localized in the small intestine.

In addition to *A. lumbricoides,* the closely related pig roundworm, *Ascaris suis,* can sometimes infect humans. In humans, *A. suis* develops to the larval tissue-migratory stages and rarely reaches the adult intestinal stage.[127] The true incidence of *A. suis* infection in humans is unknown. In a recent report from a nonendemic rural area, four of five children with ascariasis were infected with *A. suis.*[86] Thus, in such communities the *A. suis* may be of epidemiologic importance.

Severe complications, such as intestinal obstruction, result from large numbers of adult parasites in the intestinal lumen and their tendency to wrap themselves around one another in tight bundles. Localization in the appendix may give rise to acute appendicitis and even to perforation with extrusion of the parasite into the peritoneal cavity.

The tendency of adult ascarids to enter small openings is also responsible for the invasion of the biliary or pancreatic duct system (Fig. 35-6). Most cases of biliary ascariasis have been reported from areas in which the prevalence of infection is high.[75] Clinical manifestations vary in severity, depending upon the number of parasites migrating into the biliary tree. Patients may be seized suddenly by acute agonizing epigastric or right upper quadrant pain that radiates to the shoulder, back, or hypogastrium. This is accompanied by nausea and vomiting. Vomiting of roundworms occurs in a large number of cases. Fever develops after several days and may be associated with chills and enlargement of the liver, the latter becoming tender to palpation. However, jaundice is rarely observed. This might be due to the intermittent nature of the obstruction, since the parasite is able to migrate in and out of the common bile duct. Leukocytosis ranging from 12,000 to 20,000, with eosinophils comprising 5% or less, is frequent. Symptoms subside in the great majority of patients when the worms migrate out of the biliary tract or are removed from the bile ducts by endoscopy. Eggs deposited in the intrahepatic biliary radicles induce a granulomatous response. Moderate destruction of surrounding parenchyma with repair by collagen deposition delimits these foci. Ultimately, the granulomas are transformed into hyalinized scars occasionally containing multinucleated giant cells. At this stage the ova are no longer identifiable.

However, when the adult parasite is trapped in the intrahepatic bile ducts, thousands of eggs are released upon

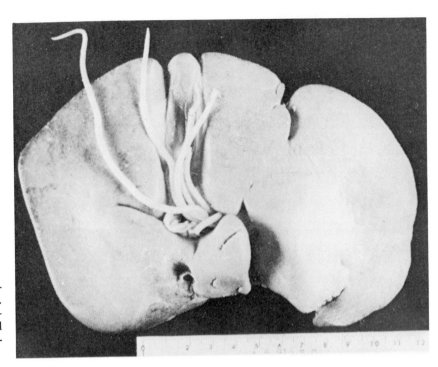

Fig. 35-6. Several *Ascaris* worms protruding from the common bile duct. (Areán VM, Crandall CA: In Marcial–Rojas RA [ed]: Pathology of Protozoal and Helminthic Diseases, p 788. Baltimore, Williams & Wilkins, 1971)

disintegration of the worm, giving rise to an acute suppurative cholangitis. If several adult worms are trapped within the liver, numerous abscesses may be formed and the organ becomes markedly enlarged, nodular, and tender. Occasionally, the abscesses may rupture into the peritoneal cavity or into the subdiaphragmatic space. The worms may then reach the pleural space and cause an empyema. Patients suffering from extensive ascaridic cholangitis have a very ominous prognosis.

At laparotomy or necropsy, the liver is markedly enlarged. Its surface is nodular and exhibits areas of grayish discoloration, some of which are covered by fibrinous or fibrous adhesions. Adult parasites may be noted under the capsule in these areas or in sections (Fig. 35-7); the parasites may be markedly degenerated or intact. When the infection is severe, many irregular cavities are found to contain an abundance of foul-smelling pultaceous material within which portions of adult parasites are identified. The lining of the abscesses is irregular and friable, and in the periphery a granulomatous response composed of epithelioid cells, multinucleated giant cells, eosinophils, plasma cells, and lymphocytes is identified.

There are reported instances of adult ascaris worms perforating the gallbladder or the common bile duct, giving rise to bile peritonitis. The worm can also migrate into the pancreatic duct, leading to acute pancreatitis.

One of the most dreaded complications of ascaridic cholangitis is extension of the inflammatory process to the hepatic or portal veins, leading to inflammation and thrombosis (pylephlebitis).

The diagnosis of ascaris is difficult to make during the phase of larval migration. Occasionally, the larvae may be found in the sputum or gastric contents. Once the parasite has reached the intestinal lumen and attained maturity, the diagnosis is easily established by the finding of the characteristic eggs when worms of both sexes are present. In biliary and pancreatic ascariasis, ova may not appear in the stool, but diagnosis can be made by identifying adult worms by endoscopy or eggs in duodenal aspirates. An accurate diagnosis of biliary ascariasis requires either direct visualization of the worm migrating through the ampulla of Vater or radiologic identification of ascaris inside the biliary tree in cholangiograms. Endoscopic retrograde cholangiopancreatography (ERCP) has been the method of choice.[75,185] Ultrasonography has also been helpful in the diagnosis and follow-up evaluation of biliary ascariasis.[150] Blood eosinophilia in ascariasis after the development of the mature worms is relatively insignificant; the highest eosinophil reaction occurs during the period of larval migration. The clinical pattern during larval migration may simulate that of the visceral larva migrans of toxocariasis. The most effective coprologic techniques available are the Kato and Muira thick smear and simple sedimentation. Immunodiagnostic tests available are of little help, since cross reactivity with other helminths makes them not specific for the diagnosis of ascariasis.

The drugs of choice for the treatment of intestinal ascariasis are mebendazole (100 mg bid p.o. for 3 days) or pyrantel pamoate (11 mg/kg once).[38] Since pyrantel pamoate costs less and only one dose is needed, it should

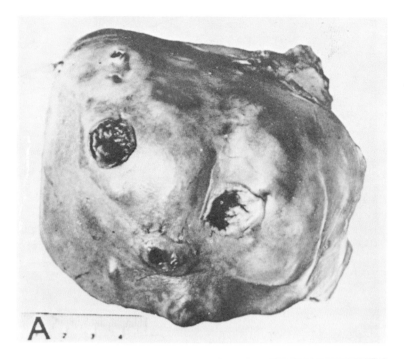

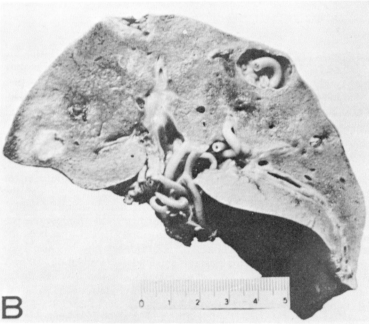

Fig. 35-7. A. Upper surface of the liver exhibiting multiple subcapsular liver abscesses. **B.** Cut surface of the liver. *Ascaris* worms may be noted in the abscess cavities and in bile ducts at hilum. (Areán VM, Crandall CA: In Marcial–Rojas RA [ed]: Pathology of Protozoal and Helminthic Diseases, p 790. Baltimore, Williams & Wilkins, 1971)

be the drug recommended for wide use in endemic areas. However, these populations usually have mixed nematode infections for which treatment with mebendazole is especially useful and effective.[158]

Liver Fluke Disease (Distomiasis)

Humans are subject to infection with several species of liver flukes. *Fasciola hepatica, Clonorchis sinensis, Op-* *isthorchis felineus, Opisthorchis viverrini,* and *Dicrocoelium dendriticum* have many features in common in respect to the structure of the parasite, the life cycle, accidental infection in humans, and pathologic alterations in the liver and biliary tree. The flukes are digenetic trematodes, since they undergo both sexual (in the definitive host) and asexual (in the intermediate host) reproduction. In all, when the helminth gains access to the human liver, either via the peritoneal lining or by ascent through the biliary tree, there is fever, right upper quadrant tenderness, and marked eosinophilia during the migratory phase. When the worms reach the biliary passages, they may cause obstruction, hyperplasia of bile duct epithelium, and suppurative cholangitis.

Fascioliasis. *F. hepatica* is most commonly found in middle and western Europe, in South America, and in the Caribbean area. Sheep and cattle are the usual definitive host; humans are accidental hosts. The nonembryonated eggs of *F. hepatica* are passed in the feces of the definitive or other host and hatch a miracidium, which escapes from the egg in fresh water and penetrates the first intermediary host, a lymnaead snail. Within the snail it goes through a further developmental cycle, becoming a cercaria. Cercariae leave the snail, swim about, attach themselves to the leaves of freshwater plants, such as watercress, and encyst as metacercariae. The encysted forms are ingested by definitive hosts and on occasion by humans.

In humans, excystment occurs in the duodenum. The metacercaria migrates through the wall of the gut, penetrates the liver capsule, and traverses the parenchyma, producing numerous tracts. In the course of this migration, hemorrhage, inflammation, and subsequent fibrosis occur.[1] During this period of migration eosinophilia is extremely high and is accompanied by fever, right upper quadrant pain, and hepatomegaly. The diagnosis of acute fascioliasis is difficult, since eggs of *F. hepatica* are not present in coprologic specimens at this stage of infection.[153] The metacercariae finally gain access to the intrahepatic bile ducts, where they mature as adult fasciolae. There, *F. hepatica* produces biliary epithelial hyperplasia supposedly by both mechanical irritation and by the release of chemical mediators.[45] However, the degree of proliferation is less than that seen with other flukes. Aberrant migration of Fasciola larvae can occasionally lead to ectopic fascioliasis, with abscess formation involving almost any organ. These complications are not seen in other liver fluke diseases because their excysted larvae reach the biliary tree via the ampulla of Vater.

In chronic phases of the disease, there may be biliary duct obstruction leading to a cholangitis. As a result, there is fibrous thickening of periductal tissues, occasionally accompanied by calcification. Peribiliary fibrosis is not as marked in humans as in the usual definitive hosts, probably the result of a lower parasitic burden. In cattle and sheep infected with *F. hepatica,* severe hepatic fibrosis with alterations in the intrahepatic vasculature can lead to chronic liver failure and portal hypertension.[113]

Diagnosis of biliary fascioliasis can be made by identifying eggs in duodenal aspirates or in stool specimens. Immunodiagnostic tests are not specific.[62] They can be useful as supportive evidence when a radiologic diagnosis of *F. hepatica* is suggested either by nuclear scans, by CT, or by ERCP.[19,35]

The drug of choice for fascioliasis is praziquantel, which has recently been approved for use in the United States.[38,128] The adult dose is 25 mg/kg p.o. three times per day for one day.

Clonorchiasis. In contrast to other flukes that affect the biliary tree, clonorchiasis has humans as its most suitable definitive hosts. The disease affects millions of persons over a wide area from Indochina to Japan. The disease is being recognized among immigrants to the United States. The eggs of *C. sinensis* are passed in human feces in an embryonated state. They can only hatch, however, when they are ingested along with food and dirt by a hydrobiid snail. In the snail, the initial intermediate host, a hatched miracidium emerges, and numerous cercarial forms are eventually produced. The latter are freed in fresh water and attach to a cyprinoid fish, usually a grass or black carp. Encysted metacercariae develop in the muscles of this secondary intermediate host. When the fish, containing the live encysted metacercariae, is eaten by a person or another definitive host, the metacercarie excyst in the duodenum and gain access to the biliary passages by way of the ampulla of Vater. The disorder is thus usually acquired by the ingestion of raw fish.

The lesions in the liver vary with the severity of parasitism. In some areas of Japan most infections observed at necropsy are mild or moderate, whereas in the Hong Kong area they are severe. The liver is usually slightly enlarged, and its surface exhibits minor irregularities. However, in the case of heavy infection, grayish white foci are noted through the capsule; these correspond to dilated cystic bile ducts, the seat of marked periductal fibrosis (Fig. 35-8). The bile duct epithelium undergoes hyperplasia and goblet cell metaplasia (Fig. 35-9). These changes are thought to be the result of both mechanical injury, caused by the suckers of the parasite, and chemical stimulation by parasitic metabolic products.[164] Most patients, especially those with low parasite burdens, are asymptomatic. Jaundice and alterations in liver function tests appear only in severe or complicated cases. The combination of parasite fragments or eggs and the highly mucous bile due to goblet cell secretion can lead to cholestasis and intrahepatic pigment gallstone formation. The development of biliary calculi is usually accompanied by some degree of cholangitis and cholangitic abscess formation. The bile can become infected by coliforms, especially *Escherichia coli,* resulting in repeated episodes of cholangitis. This entity, referred to as recurrent pyogenic cholangitis or Oriental cholangiohepatitis, is the most common complication in clonorchiasis and one of the most common causes of surgical emergency in many Oriental nations.[164,167] Although strongly associated with clonorchiasis and ascariasis, some investigators believe that the etiology of recurrent pyogenic cholangitis is unclear and that parasitic infestation can be excluded as a cause except in a few isolated cases.[167] There also appears to be no etiologic connection between primary liver carcinoma and clonorchiasis.[115,136] Their association is a result of the high incidence of both parasitism and hepatitis B infection in the same communities. The postnecrotic type of cirrhosis

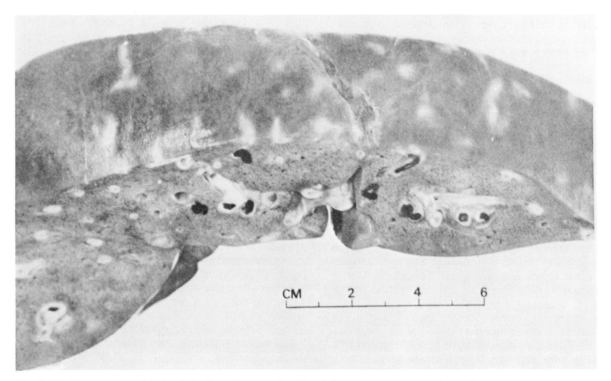

Fig. 35-8. Severe clonorchiasis of the liver. Many pale dilated ducts appear as cysts beneath the capsule. The cut surface exhibits several dilated thick-walled bile ducts filled with flukes. (Gibson JB, Sun T: In Marcial–Rojas RA [ed]: Pathology of Protozoal and Helminthic Diseases, p 557. Baltimore, Williams & Wilkins, 1971)

commonly seen in the cases of hepatoma is the result of viral or toxic injury and not of clonorchiasis. In contrast, the etiologic role of *C. sinensis* in the development of cholangiocarcinoma is supported by both epidemiologic and experimental data.[43] Pancreatitis may also develop as a result of worm migration into the pancreatic duct.

The diagnosis of clonorchiasis depends on the identification of eggs in stool or duodenal aspirate specimens.[153] Radiologic examination of the biliary tree is sometimes helpful in the diagnosis of clonorchiasis.[170] The drug of choice is praziquantel (25 mg/kg p.o. tid for 1 day).[38] The drug is highly effective, as determined by follow-up coprologic examination. Egg counts have been reported to be reduced by approximately 90% after the treatment.[66,87]

Opisthorchiasis. In humans, opisthorchiasis is caused by two important species of *Opisthorchis, O. felineus* and *O. viverrini. O. felineous* infection is found mainly in India, Vietnam, Korea, Japan, and the Philippines; *O. viverrini,* in Thailand and Laos. When the egg of *Opisthorchis* is deposited by its natural host, usually the cat, dog, or pig, it contains a fully developed miracidium. Hatching, however, does not occur in water; the egg is first ingested by a snail, the initial intermediate host. Within the snail, the miracidium proceeds to the cercarial stage, after which

access to fresh water is attained. The cercaria attaches itself to the scales of cyprinoid fish and penetrates the tissue. Encystment as metacercariae occurs within this secondary intermediate host. When the fish is ingested by the natural host or by humans, excystment occurs in the duodenum and metacercariae migrate through the ampulla of Vater to the smaller bile ducts. Here, after attachment to the biliary epithelium, they mature into adult flukes.

In most cases of opisthorchiasis, especially in cases with massive infestation, the liver is enlarged. The bile ducts are usually dilated with diameters up to 6 mm. The epithelium reveals hyperplastic changes similar to those seen in clonorchiasis. Experimental data have suggested that in addition to the mechanical and chemical effects from the fluke, the host's immunologic response may be important in the pathogenesis of the disease.[13] The symptomatology is similar to that of clonorchiasis, and the severity of right upper quadrant pain correlates with the intensity of the infection.[171] The degree of cholangitis and cholangiohepatitis is intimately related to the severity of the parasitic infection. Suppurative cholangitis is a frequent end result, and there are numerous pyogenic cholangitic abscesses. Cholangiocarcinoma is a frequent concomitant, as is the case in clonorchiasis.[43,80] The parasite

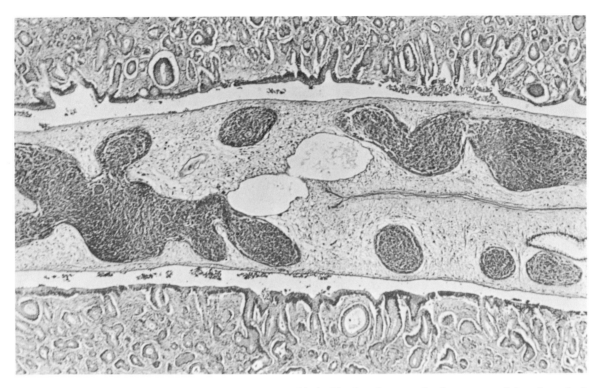

Fig. 35-9. Bile duct, human clonorchiasis. The ductal mucosa is edematous, and there is marked epithelial hyperplasia. Glandular overgrowth and goblet cell metaplasia are evident. (Original magnification × 54; H&E) (Gibson JB, Sun T: In Marcial–Rojas RA [ed]: Pathology of Protozoal and Helminthic Diseases, p 558. Baltimore, Williams & Wilkins, 1971)

supposedly renders the biliary epithelium more susceptible to chemical carcinogens.[44] The diagnosis of opisthorchiasis is made by finding the ova in the feces or duodenal contents. Stool quantitative methods allow estimates of the degree of infection.[171] Typical cholangiographic findings have been described. The drug of choice is praziquantel, in the same dosage as in clonorchiasis.[38,66,87]

Dicroceliasis. The fluke in dicroceliasis is *D. dendriticum,* primarily a parasite of cattle and sheep. Only a few cases of dicroceliasis have been reported in humans, and there have been no reports of pathologic findings.

Obstructive Vascular Lesions: Schistosomiasis (Bilharziasis)

Schistosomiasis in humans is due mainly to three species of digenetic trematodes: *Schistosoma haematobium, Schistosoma japonicum,* and *Schistosoma mansoni.* Occasionally, infection may be caused by *Schistosoma intercalatum* and *Schistosoma mekongi.*[17]

Schistosomes are the only trematodes affecting humans that dwell in the human vascular system and whose adult worms are of two sexes. They are frequently referred to as blood flukes, and the importance of the vascular local-

ization cannot be overemphasized. The lesions reflect the habitat of the parasites, and the dissemination of eggs is determined by the location.

Human infections occur in the course of bathing in or wading through contaminated streams, ponds, or irrigation canals. The schistosomal cercaria penetrates the skin or mucous membranes after leaving the intermediate molluscal host. While entering the skin, the cercariae undergo morphologic, antigenic, and biochemical changes in order to become schistosomulae.[175] The latter remain in the skin for a few days and then migrate via the lymphatics and venules to reach the right side of the heart. They then pass through the pulmonary circuit and finally enter the systemic circulation. Those entering arterial channels other than the mesenteric arteries do not survive. Those entering mesenteric vessels pass through capillaries into the portal venous system and mature within intrahepatic portal radicles.

The major component of the host immune response against the schistosomula is the eosinophil. Prominent eosinophilia characterizes the stages of larvae migration, especially in a previously sensitized host. Eosinophils have been shown to adhere to the surface of the schistosomula in the presence of antibody and/or complement. This is followed by degranulation with the release of lysosomal hydrolytic enzymes, peroxidase and major basic protein, the main effector of schistosomal damage.[18] The schistosomula attempts to evade the host's immune system by several mechanisms. It loses some of its surface antigens and masks others with a coat of host molecules that include blood group and major histocompatibility antigens.[157] Furthermore, the outer tegument of the schistosomula is resistant to immune damage.[157]

After a period of maturation in the intrahepatic portal radicles, the young adult migrates, against the inflow of incoming portal blood, into mesenteric venules adjacent to the intestine. For the most part, the adult forms of *S. japonicum* live in the small venules of the superior mesenteric vein; in the case of *S. mansoni*, it is the inferior mesenteric venules; and in *S. haematobium*, the vesical plexus of veins. There the adult female worms begin oviposition, which occurs intravascularly. The female worm produces an average of 239 eggs per day in *S. haematobium*, 300 in *S. mansoni*, and 3000 in *S. japonicum*.[98] The eggs can either work their way into the lumen of the bowel or bladder, be retained in the tissues of these organs, or be swept by the venous circulation to be deposited in the liver. It is during this period of oviposition that the clinical syndrome of acute schistosomiasis or Katayama fever is seen in patients with heavy infections with *S. mansoni* and *S. japonicum*. This syndrome is characterized by fever, chills, sweating, lymphadenopathy, eosinophilia, and hepatomegaly and is usually self-limited. In the liver, the classic bilharzial pseudotubercles with centrally located ova and pronounced portal eosinophilic infiltrates are noted. Although the etiology of Katayama fever remains unknown, the syndrome is thought to be a form of serum sickness, the result of immune complex formation that follows soluble antigen release by the egg.[98]

Hepatosplenic schistosomiasis is seen in a small subset of patients chronically infected with *S. mansoni* and *S. japonicum*. The ova lodged in the small intrahepatic portal radicles contain a living embryo that can survive for a period of 2 to 3 weeks.[176] During this period it continues to secrete soluble antigens that induce a granulomatous type of reaction. The granulomatous response in *S. mansoni* is an immunologic reaction of the cell-mediated type with delayed sensitivity.[176] The host's response interferes with the egg metabolic and immunologic activities.[32] The most frequently encountered vascular lesion is that in which the intrahepatic portal radicle is totally replaced by a granuloma that occludes the lumen. An acute endophlebitis of the intrahepatic radicles with subsequent thrombosis may be encountered. This is the principal cause of the intrahepatic vascular block. Lesions in which the hepatic artery and bile duct are preserved in the enlarged and fibrosed portal space but in which the portal vein has been destroyed are pathognomonic of schistosomiasis, even in the absence of the ova (Fig. 35-10).

The increased portal hypertension, as assessed by the comparison of wedged hepatic vein pressures with those of the portal vein or splenic pulp, has been shown to be of a presinusoidal nature. The hepatic artery manages to

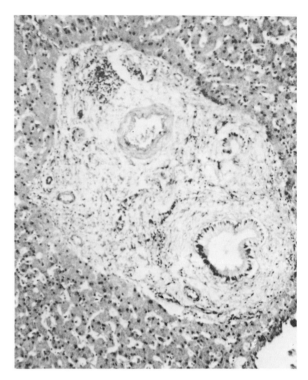

Fig. 35-10. Bile duct and hepatic artery preserved in an enlarged and fibrosed portal space; the portal vein has undergone total destruction. (Original magnification × 150; H&E) (Andrade ZA, Cheever AW: In Mostofi FK [ed]: Bilharziasis, p 162. New York, Springer-Verlag, 1967)

maintain almost a normal blood flow throughout the liver. Because of the vascular and fibrotic changes in the portal area, the latter are moderately broadened and lengthened and stand out in cross section, justifying the gross descriptive term of "pipestem" fibrosis (Fig. 35-11).

It is apparent that the reparative fibrosis that follows the destruction caused by the intravascular and perivascular portal granulomas is not sufficient to explain the extensive fibrosis seen in the classic pipestem pattern. However, a positive correlation between worm burden, fecal egg counts, and hepatic fibrosis has been documented.[23] Thus, it seems that the egg granulomas can induce collagen formation through a mechanism other than necrosis followed by reparative fibrosis. *In vitro* studies have shown that egg granulomas can secrete soluble products that alter collagen metabolism.[39,166,190]

Persons in the hepatosplenic phase of the disease come to attention after an episode of gastrointestinal tract bleeding or by the existence of hepatosplenomegaly on physical examination. Other findings usually attributed to liver disease, such as spider angiomas, gynecomastia, ascites, edema of the legs, testicular atrophy, and loss of body hair, are not prominent. Jaundice is characteristically absent except in terminal stages. Laboratory evaluation of liver function is often a helpful adjuvant to diagnosis.

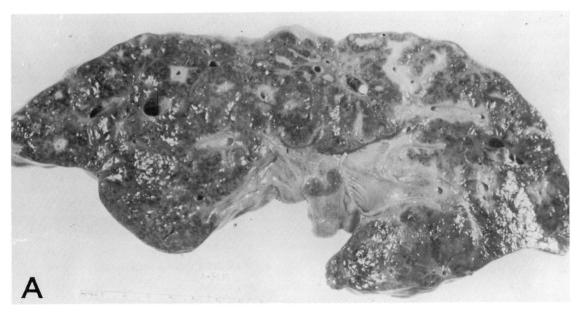

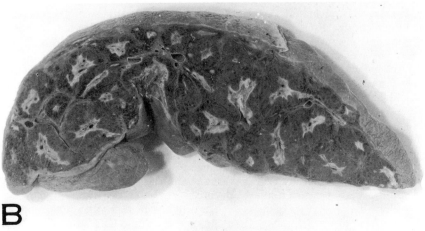

Fig. 35-11. A, B. The usual appearance of "pipe-stem" fibrosis. The surface of the liver is slightly bosselated. Note the enlargement of the portal spaces by the increase in fibrous connective tissue. (Marcial–Rojas RA [ed]: Pathology of Protozoal and Helminthic Diseases, p 396. Baltimore, Williams & Wilkins, 1971)

Hypoalbuminemia is encountered in one fourth of cases, and hyperglobulinemia is present in most instances. The prothrombin time may occasionally be prolonged but usually returns to normal following the administration of vitamin K. The serum alkaline phosphatase level is frequently elevated, but serum bilirubin, SGPT, and SGOT levels are usually within normal limits.

The most striking symptoms are hematemesis or melena secondary to variceal bleeding.[134] Medical management of these patients includes iced water lavage and esophageal tamponade with a Sengstaken–Blakemore tube. Sclerotherapy has been used with good results in controlling the initial bleed and reducing the incidence of

rebleeding.[12] The existence of esophageal varices is easily corroborated by esophagogram, esophagoscopy, and occasionally by splenoportography. The latter is particularly useful in evaluating patients being considered for shunt surgery and is especially valuable in the detection of portal and splenic vein thrombosis. Since a portacaval shunt may lead to the development of encephalopathy, the use of selective portal decompression procedures is recommended as the best alternative for the surgical treatment of bilharzial portal hypertension.[118,120,138] Unlike patients with intrahepatic portal hypertension from other causes, patients with the schistosomal variety may tolerate multiple episodes of upper gastrointestinal tract hemorrhage without developing hepatic encephalopathy and coma. The resistance to the development of hepatic encephalopathy in uncomplicated cases of hepatosplenic schistosomiasis with gastrointestinal tract bleeding is due to the presence of normal hepatic parenchyma. Ammonia levels in these patients remain within normal limits even during episodes of repeated hematemesis.[178] However, any patient can develop concomitant parenchymal disease either as the result of viral or toxin exposure or as result of ischemic damage during the episodes of gastrointestinal tract bleeding. In such a patient the liver would reveal postnecrotic fibrosis and nodular regeneration and the hepatic vein wedge pressure would be elevated consistent with sinusoidal portal hypertension. In these patients with complicated or decompensated hepatosplenic schistosomiasis, signs and symptoms of chronic liver disease are not uncommon. The presence of chronic active hepatitis or chronic hepatitis B carrier state has been documented in many of these patients.[14,93] Therefore, although schistosomal granulomas may be found in a cirrhotic liver, their presence is not related etiologically to the cirrhosis.[23] Also, no etiologic relationship has been documented between schistosomiasis and hepatocellular carcinoma.[103,114]

Splenomegaly is manifest in practically all cases of hepatosplenic schistosomiasis; in some instances the lower border reaches the iliac crest. The average weight of the spleen is 1000 g. The changes are those of congestive splenomegaly, with moderate degrees of pulp fibrosis. Foci of infarction, perisplenitis, and Gamna Gandy body formation are common. Neither parasites nor ova are seen. Hypersplenism is evident in most patients who have bled from varices as a result of portal hypertension. Although thrombocytopenia may become very severe, spontaneous bleeding is practically never seen. Anemia is frequent and may be attributable to hypersplenism and blood loss.

The portal systemic anastomoses that open as a result of portal hypertension allow direct passage of eggs to the right side of the heart and from there to the pulmonary arterial tree. The intravascular granulomatous reaction leads to pulmonary endarteritis, pulmonary hypertension, and finally cor pulmonale.[146] Cardiopulmonary schistosomiasis is seen almost exclusively in patients with hepatosplenic schistosomiasis.

The definitive diagnosis of schistosomiasis can be made only by finding schistosome eggs in feces or urine or in a biopsy specimen, usually from the rectum. Quantitative stool examination techniques are strongly recommended in order to assess the intensity of the infection.[179] The quick Kato smear technique is very suitable for this type of examination.

Immunodiagnostic methods are available for the diagnosis of schistosomiasis and include indirect immunofluorescence, the circumoval precipitin test, radioimmunoassays, and ELISA.[63,64,85] However, because of cross reactivity with other helminthic antigens, the tests are not specific enough for individual patient management. Furthermore, in endemic areas they cannot distinguish past from present infection. Radioimmunoassays and ELISA

are considered the most sensitive techniques. Currently the main use of these methods is for epidemiologic studies. In one such recent study, 97% of the patients tested had circulating antibodies against schistosomula antigens, and the antibody levels matched known age prevalence data.[37]

The drug of choice for the treatment of schistosomiasis caused by any of the three major species of schistosomes is praziquantel p.o.[33,38] The dosage for *S. haematobium* and *S. mansoni* is 40 mg/kg once, while that for *S. japonicum* is 20 mg/kg three times in one day.[38] The drug is very effective and has very low toxicity.[128] Oxamniquine is an alternative drug for infections with *S. mansoni* and was the best drug available until the advent of praziquantel.[33] The dosage varies for the different geographic regions, and the most frequently reported side-effects have been drowsiness, vomiting, and dizziness.[33,163]

Parenchymal Lesions

Cystic Lesions

Echinococcosis (Hydatidosis). Echinococcosis or hydatidosis is one of the most important zoonoses. The disease is caused by cestodes (tapeworms) of the genus *Echinococcus*. The species *E. granulosus* is the cause of cystic hydatid disease, the hydatid disease most commonly seen throughout the world. Areas of high incidence include North Africa, Spain, Greece, the Middle East, Iran, western Australia, Chile, Argentina, and Uruguay. *E. multilocularis* causes alveolar hydatid disease that is seen mostly in Alaska, Canada, the Soviet Union, and central Europe. A third species, *E. vogeli,* has recently been identified as the cause of polycystic hydatid disease in Colombia, a disease with features similar to those of alveolar hydatid disease.[28]

The definitive hosts for the adult cestode are carnivores, commonly the domestic dog for *E. granulosus* and the fox for *E. multilocularis.* The adult tapeworms, which may number several thousands in the heavily infected dog intestine, shed both eggs and gravid proglottids, which can be found in the host's stool. Human and the natural intermediate hosts become infected when they swallow these immediately infective eggs. In the duodenum the larvae or oncospheres are freed and, using their hooklets, find their way through the intestinal mucosa into the lumen of blood vessels. They are then carried by the blood until they lodge in capillaries at almost any site. In 60% of cases, the larvae are retained in the sinusoids of the liver. The remainder pass through the hepatic circulation, and 20% are retained in the lung; the others gain access to the systemic circulation.

The oncospheres of *E. granulosus* that survive can become encysted and develop a germinal membrane within a few days. From this inner germinal layer, which is supported by a semipermeable laminated cuticle, many brood capsules develop containing numerous scolices. These scolices represent the future head of the adult tapeworm.

The growing hydatid isolates itself from adjacent tissues by inciting a connective tissue wall, the adventitial membrane. The thickness and cellular composition of this membrane, which forms a true sac for the cyst, depend upon the consistency of the affected organ, the immunologic response of the host, and the duration of the cyst. Calcification of the adventitial wall of old cysts is an occasional occurrence.

In *E. multilocularis,* the daughter cysts, which arise from the germinal membrane by budding, develop on the outside of the original (mother) cyst. This results in invasion of surrounding parenchyma by the new scolices, which are not contained by the laminated cuticular membrane. The pattern of growth resembles that of malignant neoplastic lesions. The disease is fatal in the vast majority of untreated patients and in a significant percentage of those treated with surgery.[65,183]

The hydatid cyst caused by *E. granulosus* grows at a rate of approximately 1 cm per year. Clinical symptoms do not usually develop until the cyst has attained a diameter of at least 10 cm, and a mass is rarely palpated until the diameter reaches 20 cm.

The symptoms of hydatidosis are attributable to two factors: mechanical effects brought about by the space-occupying cyst, and the generalized toxic or allergic reactions secondary to absorption of the parasitic products. Over one half of the cases reported affect the liver, and hepatic manifestations are thus quite common (Fig. 35-12). Approximately 80% of the hydatid cysts of the liver are localized in the right lobe. The cyst may be located deep in liver substance or superficially beneath the capsule. Deep-seated lesions exhibit the well-ordered zonal arrangement of the adventitial layer described above (Fig. 35-13). The surrounding liver tissue undergoes compression atrophy. Compression of blood vessels and biliary canaliculi adjacent to the cyst causes mechanical disturbance of blood and biliary flow with congestion and cholestasis. Superimposed secondary infection may lead to cholangitis. Cyst rupture into the biliary system is a common complication seen in patients with hydatid cysts of the liver.[7] In patients suffering from this complication, jaundice and pain are the most common symptoms.[92]

Cysts located beneath Glisson's capsule are dome-shaped and grow away from the liver, even to the point

Fig. 35-12. Solitary hydatid cyst of the liver. Daughter cysts are shown on section. (Poole JB, Marcial–Rojas RA: In Marcial–Rojas RA [ed]: Pathology of Protozoal and Helminthic Diseases, p 646. Baltimore, Williams & Wilkins, 1971)

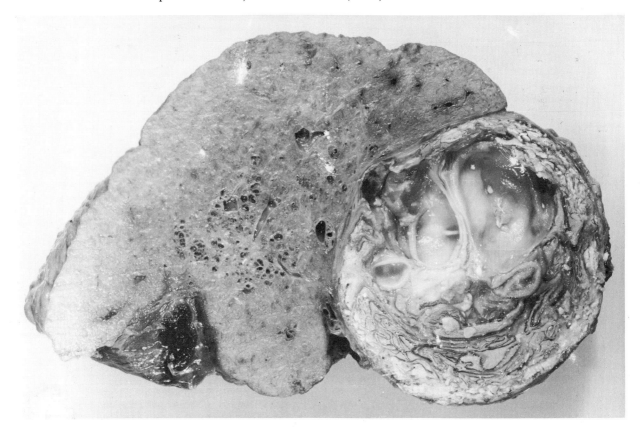

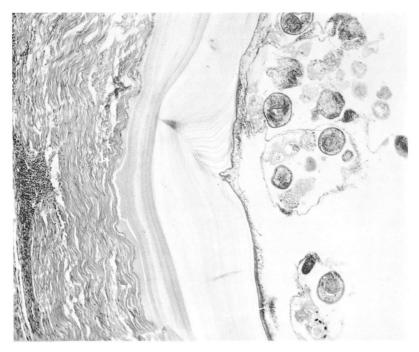

Fig. 35-13. Hydatid cyst of liver. The adventitial and germinal layers and brood capsules with scolices are evident. (AFIP Neg. 65-6462) (Original magnification × 90; H&E)

of becoming pedunculated. Those cysts beneath the diaphragm may erode and perforate into the pleural or pericardial cavities, the pulmonary parenchyma, or bronchi. Those projecting into the peritoneal cavity may perforate into the duodenum, colon, right renal pelvis, or the free peritoneum. Cysts located near the porta hepatis may lead to obstructive jaundice.

The diagnosis of cystic hydatid disease of the liver is suggested by the presence of an abdominal mass detected by palpation and confirmed by radiographic studies. A plain film of the abdomen will be helpful in those cases in which the cyst has undergone calcification. Ultrasound is very useful, not only for diagnosis, but also for the follow-up of medically treated cases.[59] CT is becoming a widely used technique for the diagnosis of hepatic hydatid cysts.[34,99,124] The sensitivity of CT has been reported to be as high as 98%.[34] The diagnosis of echinococcal cyst can be made by finding one or more spherical or oval, sharply delineated lesions of water density in which cyst wall calcification or daughter cysts are identifiable.[124]

Serodiagnosis can be helpful in confirming the clinicoradiologic impression. However, a negative test result does not rule out the diagnosis of echinococcosis. Of the several immunoserologic products available, immunoelectrophoresis, latex agglutination, and indirect hemagglutination are considered the best choices for the diagnosis of hydatid cyst.[79,173]

The treatment of hydatid disease is surgical, preferably the complete removal of the intact cyst. Marsupialization should be performed only when complete resection is impossible.[10] The use of a special suction cone has decreased spillage of the highly infectious hydatid cyst contents.

Sterilization of these contents is also routinely done using a 0.5% silver nitrate solution or 1% cetrimide solution.[79] Formalin is no longer used because it can lead to sclerosis of the biliary ducts that usually communicate with the hydatid cyst.

Medical treatment of hydatid disease with mebendazole and related benzi-imidazole compounds has been advocated as safe and effective therapy.[9] However, results of recent trials have raised doubts about the validity of these initial impressions. Not only has toxicity been documented with the dosages of mebendazole used, but the therapy has failed in the vast majority of cases.[50,83] Most recent reviews on the management of hepatic hydatid disease recommend medical management only for those patients in whom surgical resection is impossible or in whom surgical risk is too high.[31,147] This is usually the case with hepatic alveolar hydatid disease. The use of a new benzi-imidazole compound, albendazole, may be helpful in this subset of patients.[148] In addition, percutaneous biliary drainage to relieve intrahepatic bile duct obstruction has been proposed as a useful procedure in the management of patients with hepatic alveolar echinococcosis.[16]

Cysticercosis. Cysticercosis is acquired through ingestion of food or water containing the ova of the cestode *Taenia solium.* It is an important zoonosis in Mexico, Central America, and many countries of Europe, Asia, and Africa. The larva or oncosphere, after leaving the egg, pierces the intestinal mucosa and gains access to the bloodstream. The cysticerci are then disseminated to various tissues of the body, where they grow and form characteristic cystic structures, giving rise to symptomatology related to their location. Most localize in muscle, subcutaneous tissues, meninges, and brain.[117] Only rarely is the liver affected, and hepatic manifestations are most uncommon.

Granulomatous Lesions

Systemic Toxocariasis (Visceral Larva Migrans). Toxocariasis is a zoonotic disorder caused by the second larval stage of dog and cat ascarids, *Toxocara canis* and *Toxocara catis*. However, only *T. canis* represents a significant cause of visceral larva migrans.[51] The larvae are not habitual parasites of humans but under certain circumstances may invade the human organism, giving rise to disease with varying degrees of severity.

Toxocara infections are ubiquitous in the canine and feline world, the highest rates occurring in puppies and kittens during the first trimester of life. Infection is more frequent in rural areas. The eggs are deposited by the female worm in the small intestine of the habitual host and are passed with the stools in unsegmented forms. Embryonation takes place in the soil under appropriate environmental conditions of moisture and temperature. Transmission to the human subject is acquired by the ingestion of the infective eggs. The disorder is prevalent under substandard sanitary conditions in children between the ages of 1 and 4 years who have dirt-eating habits (pica). When the eggs hatch in the small intestine, the larvae migrate throughout the body. However, since they are not habitual parasites of man, they do not mature but die after migration into the tissues. Clinically, most infections are unassociated with systemic manifestations and are discovered accidentally in the course of medical investigation for other reasons.

The most severe forms of the disease are encountered among small children. Their symptoms may include high fever, anorexia, weight loss, urticarial rashes, asthma, irritability, and even convulsions. Hepatosplenomegaly and generalized lymphadenopathy may also be observed, and there may be vomiting and abdominal pain. Pulmonary symptoms may be very severe and derive from larvae migrating through the lungs, where they produce miliary granulomas. A leukocytosis, which may attain levels as high as 80,000, is accompanied by eosinophilia ranging from 20% to 90%. There is usually evidence of a hypergammaglobulinemia, including anti-A and anti-B isohemagglutinins stimulated by *T. canis* surface antigens that mimic human ABO blood groups.[51] The process lasts for several months and eventually regresses in the absence of reinfection. Larvae entering the eye may lead to blindness due to a posterior endophthalmitis.

The clinical syndrome of visceral larva migrans may also be produced by migrating larva of other helminths and by *Capillaria hepatica*.

Macroscopically, grayish white miliary granulomas are noted in the liver, some coalescent and forming lesions averaging 2 cm to 3 cm in diameter (Fig. 35-14). This gross appearance of the liver is not unlike that encountered in *C. hepatica* infestation. Histologically, the granulomas exhibit extensive eosinophilic necrosis surrounded by macrophages, round cells, and eosinophils. The kinetics of granuloma formation has been studied in experimental animal models and is consistent with a T lymphocyte–dependent cell-mediated process of the delayed hypersen-

Fig. 35-14. Visceral larva migrans. Multiple, confluent gray-white granulomas appear in the liver. (Marcial–Rojas RA: In Schiff L [ed]: Diseases of the Liver, 1st ed, p 800. Philadelphia, JB Lippincott, 1963)

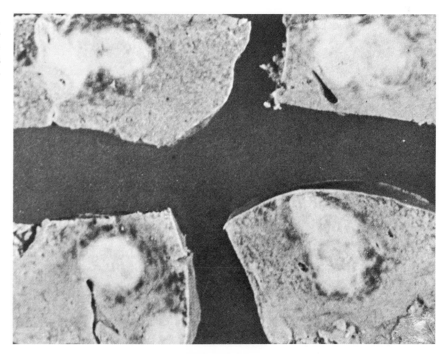

sitivity type.[73] Identification of the larvae may be difficult and usually requires multiple serial sections.

The diagnosis may be suspected in patients with the clinical syndrome, especially if they are children who have a history of geophagia and close contact with puppies. Definitive diagnosis can be made only by identifying the toxocara larvae in a biopsy. Liver biopsy, although a very specific method for diagnosis, has a very low sensitivity. Immunodiagnostic tests have been developed to improve the diagnostic yield.[52] An ELISA, which uses larval rather than adult antigens, has been proposed as a highly specific and fairly sensitive diagnostic method.[53,172]

Treatment for toxocariasis is indicated whenever the infection compromises organ function or whenever the larvae migrate to a critical site and thus interrupt normal physiologic function. The best drugs available are thiabendazole (25 mg/kg p.o. bid for 5 days) and diethylcarbamazine (2 mg/kg tid for 7 to 10 days). These drugs are not fully effective and are considered investigational drugs for this condition by the US Food and Drug Administration.[38]

Hepatic Capillariasis. Hepatic capillariasis is caused by the nematode *C. hepatica* or *Hepaticola hepatica*. This helminth is common in the liver of rats and, less frequently, of mice, hares, dogs, muskrats, beavers, and some species of monkey. The nonembryonated eggs of *C. hepatica* are released from the decaying carcasses of affected animals or are discharged in the feces of animals that prey upon or scavenge infected animals. The ova develop and become infective in damp soil. Humans acquire the disease by ingesting food or dirt contaminated with embry-

onated ova. Human infections are rare; fewer than 30 authenticated cases are reported in the world's literature.[5] The infective ova hatch in the cecum and the free larvae migrate to the liver by way of the portal system. Maturation to the adult stage occurs in the hepatic parenchyma. After a few weeks the female worm dies, liberating eggs into the surrounding liver tissue. The eggs induce a granulomatous response in the hepatic parenchyma.

The majority of cases of human infection have occurred in patients who live in substandard sanitary conditions, especially children or institutionalized mental patients, both of whom are prone to geophagia. The clinical features are those of an acute illness continuing for several days, weeks, or months. Patients are undernourished and dehydrated and usually exhibit nocturnal fever and diaphoresis. Anorexia, nausea, and vomiting are frequent. The abdomen is distended, and hepatomegaly is evident. There is a leukocytosis ranging between 30,000 and 80,000, with an eosinophil content ranging from 18% to 85%. Hyperglobulinemia is the rule, and the hepatic biochemical profile usually shows elevated levels of alkaline phosphatase, SGOT, and SGPT. The young age of the patient, the enlarged liver, and a high grade of eosinophilia constitute a clinical picture that must be differentiated from that of systemic toxocariasis or visceral larva migrans.[48]

Macroscopically the liver is enlarged, its surface is smooth, and beneath the capsule one notes many grayish or yellowish white nodules measuring 0.1 cm to 0.2 cm. Many of these coalesce and form lesions 2 cm to 3 cm in diameter. These granulomas are composed of epithelioid cells and multinucleated giant cells surrounding parasites or ova. The ova of *C. hepatica* are barrel-shaped, as are those of *Trichuris trichiura*, but possess a double shell

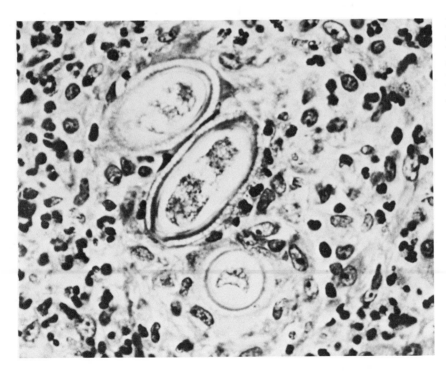

Fig. 35-15. Well-preserved *Capillaria hepatica* eggs appear in a portion of the liver infiltrated by eosinophils and macrophages. (Original magnification × 550; H&E) (Areán VM: In Marcial–Rojas RA [ed]: Pathology of Protozoal and Helminthic Diseases, p 670. Baltimore, Williams & Wilkins, 1971)

containing visible radiations between the two layers (Fig. 35-15).

The diagnosis of this disease can be established only by liver biopsy, since ova are present only in the liver substance and are not detectable in intestinal content. The severity of symptoms may be improved temporarily with supportive therapy, but there is no specific treatment for the disease. Although most of the cases reported have been fatal, there are probably unreported infections with mild and nonspecific manifestations.

Strongyloidiasis. Strongyloidiasis, caused by the nematode *Strongyloides stercoralis,* is an intestinal parasitic infection of very high prevalence in the tropics and subtropics. In immunosuppressed patients, large numbers of noninfective rhabditiform larvae, which develop in the upper small intestine, metamorphose into infective filariform larvae within the intestinal lumen and penetrate through the mucosa of the colon. This process, known as endogenous autoinfection, leads to disseminated, overwhelming strongyloidiasis, also known as hyperinfection.[151,187] In these patients the nematode larva migrates to the liver, where it may elicit a granulomatous response (Fig. 35-16). Clinical evidence of liver involvement with jaundice and elevated levels of alkaline phosphatase and bilirubin occurs in some of these patients.[151]

The diagnosis of strongyloidiasis rests on the identification of the rhabditiform or the infective filariform larvae in the stools, duodenal aspirates, or small-bowel biopsies. Serologic methods of diagnosis include IHA, CF, ELISA, and immunofluorescence. The latter two methods appear to be the most sensitive and specific.[49,57,119] The drug of choice for strongyloidiasis is thiobendazole (25 mg/kg p.o. bid for 2 days).[38] In overwhelming infection, therapy should be continued for 5 to 7 days.[107]

Enterobiasis. Enterobiasis, caused by the nematode *Enterobius vermicularis,* is a disease of worldwide distribution. Rarely this intestinal parasite can migrate to produce ectopic lesions; the most commonly reported occur along the female genital tract. Three cases of pinworm granulomas in the liver have been reported.[29] Hematogenous spread, facilitated by intestinal mucosal neoplasms, has been suggested as the probable access route to the liver.

Fig. 35-16. Filariform larva of *Strongyloides stercoralis* coiled in a portal space next to a granuloma. (Original magnification × 365; H&E) (Marcial–Rojas RA [ed]: Pathology of Protozoal and Helminthic Diseases, p 730. Baltimore, Williams & Wilkins, 1971)

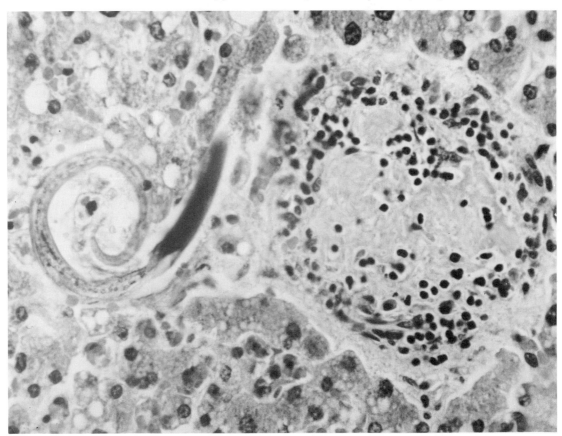

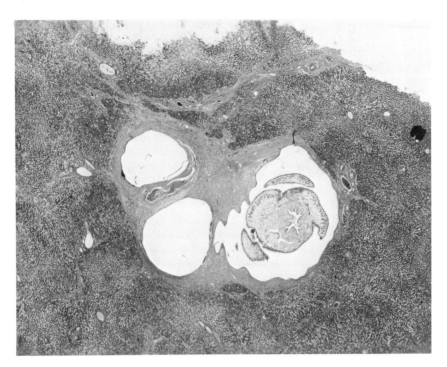

Fig. 35-17. Encysted third-stage larva of a pentastomiasis parasite in the liver. Portions of the coiled larva drop out of conventionally prepared paraffin sections, leaving empty cavities as shown here. (AFIP Neg. 69-2543) (Original magnification × 10; H&E)

Combined Cystic and Granulomatous Lesions

Paragonimiasis. Paragonimiasis affects primarily the lungs but may occasionally involve the liver. The usual method of human infection with *Paragonimus westermani* is undoubtedly the ingestion of raw or improperly cooked freshwater crabs or crayfish, the intermediate hosts of this parasite. Ingested metacercariae excyst in the small intestine and thereafter penetrate its wall. Young larvae may float in the peritoneal cavity and enter abdominal wall muscles. After maturing here for approximately 7 days, they reenter the peritoneal cavity, penetrate the diaphragm and pleura, and finally appear in the pulmonary parenchyma. Deviation from this usual path of migration may result in extrapulmonary lesions.

The liver, when affected, exhibits peanut-sized, soft, yellowish brown cystic structures scattered over its surface. These contain purulent exudate in which occasional parasites may be found. Microscopically, these abscesses are characterized by central necrosis with neutrophils, eosinophils, and Charcot–Leyden crystals. The zone of necrosis is surrounded by a zone of mononuclear cell infiltrate that extends into the adjacent compressed hepatic parenchyma. *Paragonimus* eggs are identifiable in the interphase between the two zones. The patients usually have biochemical evidence of hepatic necrosis, with SGOT and SGPT elevations.

The diagnosis is established by examination of the feces or sputum, looking for the characteristic operculated egg. Immunodiagnostic tests available include the CF test, countercurrent electrophoresis, and ELISA, all of which are sensitive and specific enough to be used for diagnositic purposes. The drug of choice for the treatment of paragonimiasis is praziquantel (25 mg/kg p.o. tid for 1–2 days).[38,110,123] An alternate drug is bithionol, 30 to 50 mg/kg on alternate days for 10 to 15 days.[38]

Pentastomiasis. The *Pentastomida* are blood-sucking, endoparasitic invertebrates that in their adult form live in the lungs of reptiles and birds and in the nasopharynx of mammals, usually carnivores. Most zoologists consider this group to be an aberrant phylum, occupying a position intermediate between the annelids and the arthropods.[154]

Humans become aberrant intermediate hosts by accidental ingestion of food or drink containing ova. In the intestinal tract the viable embryo emerges from the egg and becomes a primary-stage, freely moving larva, which bores through the intestinal wall and migrates for several days until it becomes encysted. The larva molts several times until it becomes a relatively large third-stage form, which reaches a dead end in humans and rarely emerges from its cyst. After 2 years the third-stage larva perishes and undergoes dissolution, leaving a small cyst, or is gradually absorbed and replaced by fibrous tissue. The latter may undergo calcification and thus provide a fairly characteristic diagnostic radiographic appearance. In over 50% of the reported human infections, the liver is the site of involvement (Fig. 35-17).[135]

REFERENCES

1. Acosta–Ferreira W et al: *Fasciola hepatica* human infection: Histopathological study of sixteen cases. Virchow Arch Pathol Anat 383:319, 1979

2. Adams EB, MacLeod IN: Invasive amebiasis: II. Amebic liver abscess and its complications. Medicine 56:325, 1977

3. Aikawa M et al: Freeze fracture study on the erythrocyte membrane during malarial parasite invasion. J Cell Biol 91:55, 1981

4. Alper EI et al: Counterelectrophoresis in the diagnosis of amebiasis. Am J Gastroenterol 65:63, 1976

5. Attah EB et al: Hepatic capillariasis. Am J Clin Pathol 79:127, 1983

6. Badaró R et al: Immunofluorescent antibody test in American visceral leishmaniasis: Sensitivity and specificity of different morphological forms of two *Leishmania* species. Am J Trop Med Hyg 32:480, 1983

7. Barros JL: Hydatid disease of the liver. Am J Surg 135:597, 1978

8. Beaver PC, Jung RC, Cupp EW (eds): Clinical Parasitology, 9th ed. Philadelphia, Lea & Febiger, 1984

9. Bekhti A et al: Treatment of hepatic hydatid disease with mebendazole: Preliminary results in four cases. Br Med J 2:1047, 1977

10. Belli L et al: Resection versus pericystectomy in the treatment of hydatidosis of the liver. Am J Surg 145:239, 1983

11. Benach JL et al: Immunoresponsiveness in acute babesiosis in humans. J Infect Dis 146:369, 1982

12. Bessa SM, Helnry I: Injection sclerotherapy for esophageal varices caused by schistosomal hepatic fibrosis. Surgery 97:164, 1985

13. Bhamarapravati N et al: Liver changes in hamsters infected with liver fluke of man: *Opisthorchis viverrini.* Am J Trop Med Hyg 27:787, 1978

14. Biempica L et al: Liver collagen type characterization in human schistosomiasis: A histological, ultrastructural and immunocytochemical correlation. Am J Trop Med Hyg 32:316, 1983

15. Brasseur PH et al: Impaired cell-mediated immunity in Plasmodium falciparum-infected patients with high parasitemia and cerebral malaria. Clin Immunol Immunopathol 27:38, 1983

16. Bret PM et al: Le traitement de la cholestase par stenose des voies biliaires intrahepatiques au cours de l'echinococcose alveolaire. Gastroenterol Clin Biol 8:308, 1984

17. Bruet A et al: Ileal varices revealed by recurrent hematuria in a patient with portal hypertension and Mekong schistosomiasis. Am J Gastroenterol 78:346, 1983

18. Butterworth AE et al: Damage to schistosomula of *Schistosoma mansoni* induced directly by eosinophil major basic protein. J Immunol 122:221, 1979

19. Bynum TE, Hauser SC: Abnormalities on ERCP in a case of human fascioliasis. Gastrointest Endosc 30:80, 1984

20. Centers for Disease Control: Imported malaria among travelers—United States. MMWR 33:388, 1984

21. Centers for Disease Control: Adverse reactions to Fansidar (R) and updated recommendations for its use in the prevention of malaria. MMWR 33:713, 1985

22. Chadee K, Meerovitch E: The pathogenesis of experimentally induced amebic liver abscess in the gerbil (*Meriones unguiculatus*). Am J Pathol 117:71, 1984

23. Cheever AW: A quantitative post-mortem study of *Schistosomiasis mansoni* in man. Am J Trop Med Hyg 17:38, 1968

24. Chisholm ES et al: *Babesia microti* infection in man: Evaluation of an indirect immunofluorescent antibody test. Am J Trop Med Hyg 27:14, 1978

25. Chulay JD, Bryceson ADM: Quantitation of amastigotes of *Leishmania donovani* in smears of splenic aspirates from patients with visceral leishmaniasis. Am J Trop Med Hyg 32:475, 1983

26. Chulay JD et al: A comparison of three dosage regimens of sodium stibogluconate in the treatment of visceral leishmaniasis in Kenya. J Infect Dis 148:148, 1983

27. Cuarón A, Gordon F: Liver scanning: Analysis of 2,500 cases of amebic hepatic abscesses. J Nucl Med 11:435, 1970

28. D'Alessandro A et al: *Echinococcus vogeli* in man, with a review of polycystic hydatid disease in Colombia and neighboring countries. Am J Trop Med Hyg 28:303, 1979

29. Daly JJ, Baker GF: Pinworm granuloma of the liver. Am J Trop Med Hyg 33:62, 1984

30. Dammin GJ: Babesiosis. In Weinstein L, Fields BN (eds): Seminars in Infectious Disease, vol 1, pp 168–199. New York, Stratton International Medical Book Corp, 1978

31. Davidson RA: Issues in clinical parasitology: The management of hydatid cyst. Am J Gastroenterol 79:397, 1984

32. de Brito PA et al: Host granulomatous response in schistosomiasis mansoni: Antibody and cell-mediated damage of parasite eggs in vitro. J Clin Invest 74:1715, 1984

33. De Cock KM: Human schistosomiasis and its management. J Infection 8:5, 1984

34. de Diego–Choliz J et al: Computed tomography in hepatic echinococcosis. AJR 139:699, 1982

35. de Miguel F et al: CT findings in human fascioliasis. Gastrointest Radiol 9:157, 1984

36. Deroff P et al: Screening blood donors for *Plasmodium falciparum* malariae. Vox Sang 45:392, 1983

37. Dissous C et al: Human antibody response to *Schistosoma mansoni* surface antigens defined by protective monoclonal antibodies. J Infect Dis 149:227, 1984

38. Drugs for parasitic infections. Med Lett 26:27, 1984

39. Dunn MA, Kamel R: Hepatic schistosomiasis. Hepatology 1:653, 1981

40. Eggleston FC: Amebic peritonitis secondary to amebic liver abscess. Surgery 91:46, 1982

41. Facer CA: Erythrocyte sialoglycoproteins and *Plasmodium falciparum* invasion. Trans R Soc Trop Med Hyg 77:724, 1983

42. Files JC et al: Automated erythrocyte exchange in fulminant falciparum malaria. Ann Intern Med 100:396, 1984

43. Flavell DJ: Liver fluke infection as an aetiological factor in bile-duct carcinoma in man. Trans R Soc Trop Med Hyg 75:814, 1981

44. Flavell DJ, Lucas, SB: Potentiation by the human liver fluke, *Opisthorchis viverrini,* of the carcinogenic action of N-nitrosodimethylamine upon the biliary epithelium of the hamster. Br J Cancer 46:985, 1982

45. Foster JR: A study of the initiation of biliary hyperplasia in rats infected with Fasciola hepatica. Parasitology 83:253, 1981

46. Francioli PB et al: Response of babesiosis to pentamidine therapy. Ann Intern Med 94:326, 1981

47. Gadasi H, Kessler E: Correlation of virulence and collagenolytic activity on *Entamoeba histolytica.* Infect Immunol 39:528, 1983

48. Galvao VA: Estudos sobre Capillaria hepatica: Uma avaliacao do seu papel patogenico para o homem. Mem Inst Oswaldo Cruz 76:415, 1981

49. Genta RM: Immunobiology of strongyloidiasis. Trop Geogr Med 30:223, 1984

50. Gil–Grande LA et al: Treatment of liver hydatid disease with mebendazole: A prospective study of thirteen cases. Am J Gastroenterol 78:584, 1983

51. Glickman LT: Toxocariasis. In Warren KS, Mahmoud AAF

(eds): Tropical and Geographical Medicine, pp 431–437. New York, McGraw Hill, 1984

52. Glickman LT, Schantz PM: Epidemiology and pathogenesis of zoonotic toxocariasis. Epidemiol Rev 3:230, 1981
53. Glickman LT et al: Evaluation of serodiagnostic tests for visceral larva migrans. Am J Trop Med Hyg 27:492, 1978
54. González–Robles A, Martínez–Palomo A: Scanning electron microscopy of attached trophozoites of pathogenic *Entamoeba histolytica*. J Protozool 30:692, 1983
55. Grabowski EF et al: Babesiosis transmitted by a transfusion of frozen-thawed blood. Ann Intern Med 96:466, 1982
56. Grimmond TR, Cameron AS: Primaquine-chloroquine prophylaxis against malaria in Southeast-Asian refugees entering South Australia. Med J Aust 140:322, 1984
57. Grove DI, Blair J: Diagnosis of human strongyloidiasis by immunofluorescence, using *Strongyloides ratti* and *S. stercoralis* larvae. Am J Trop Med Hyg 30:344, 1981
58. Guerrero IC et al: Transfusion malaria in the United States, 1972–1981. Ann Intern Med 99:221, 1983
59. Hadidi A: Sonography of hepatic echinococcal cysts. Gastrointest Radiol 7:349, 1982
60. Healy GR, Ruebush TK: Morphology of *Babesia microti* in human blood smears. Am J Clin Pathol 73:107, 1980
61. Hess U et al: Combined chloroquine/Fansidar-resistant falciparum malaria appears in East Africa. Am J Trop Med Hyg 32:217, 1983
62. Hillyer GV: Fascioliasis in Puerto Rico: A review. Bol Asoc Med PR 73:94, 1981
63. Hillyer GV et al: Immunodiagnosis of infection with *Schistosoma haematobium* and *S. mansoni* in man. Am J Trop Med Hyg 29:1254, 1980
64. Hillyer GV et al: The circumoval precipitin test for the serodiagnosis of human schistosomiasis mansoni and haematobia. Am J Trop Med Hyg 30:121, 1981
65. Honma K et al: Hepatic alveolar echinococcosis invading pancreas, vertebrae and spinal cord. Hum Pathol 13:944, 1982
66. Horstmann RD et al: High efficacy of praziquantel in the treatment of 22 patients with Clonorchis/Opisthorchis infections. Tropenmed Parasitol 32:157, 1981
67. Hu X et al: Hepatic damage in experimental and clinical paragonimiasis. Am J Trop Med Hyg 31:1148, 1982
68. Ibarra–Pérez C: Thoracic complications of amebic abscess of the liver. Chest 79:672, 1981
69. Jack RM, Ward PA: *Babesia rhodaini* interactions with complement. Relationship to parasitic entry into red cells. Immunology 124:1566, 1980
70. Jha TK: Evaluation of diamidine compound (pentamidine isoethionate) in the treatment of resistant cases of kala-azar occurring in North Bihar, India. Trans R Soc Trop Med Hyg 77:167, 1983
71. Jones TC: Interactions between murine macrophages and obligate intracellular protozoa. Am J Pathol 102:127, 1981
72. Katzenstein D et al: New concepts of amebic liver abscess derived from hepatic imaging, serodiagnosis, and hepatic enzymes in 67 consecutive cases in San Diego. Medicine 61:237, 1982
73. Kayes SG, Oaks JA: Development of the granulomatous response in murine toxocariasis. Am J Pathol 93:277, 1978
74. Kelton JG et al: Immune-mediated thrombocytopenia of malaria. J Clin Invest 7:832, 1983
75. Khuroo MS, Zargar SA: Biliary ascariasis: A common cause of biliary and pancreatic disease in an endemic area. Gastroenterology 88:418, 1985

76. Knight R: Hepatic amebiasis. Semin Liver Dis 4:277, 1984
77. Kobiler D, Mirelman D: Adhesion of *Entamoeba histolytica* to monolayers of human cells. J Infect Dis 144:539, 1981
78. Krogstad DJ et al: Amebiasis: Epidemiologic studies in the United States 1971–74. Ann Intern Med 88:89, 1978
79. Kune GA et al: Hydatid disease in Australia: Prevention, clinical presentation and treatment. Med J Aust 3:385, 1983
80. Kurathong S et al: Opistorchis viverrini infection and cholangiocarcinoma. Gastroenterology 89:151, 1985
81. Lainson R: The American leishmaniasis: Some observations on their ecology and epidemiology. Trans R Soc Trop Med Hyg 77:569, 1983
82. Laverdant C et al: L'amibiase hépatique: Étude de 152 observations. Gastroenterol Clin Biol 8:838, 1984
83. Levin MH et al: Severe, reversible neutropenia during high-dose mebendazole therapy for echinococcosis. JAMA 249: 2929, 1983
84. Lightner KL et al: Comparison of microscopy and culture in the detection of *Leishmania donovani* from splenic aspirates. Am J Trop Med Hyg 32:296, 1983
85. Long EG et al: Comparison of ELISA, radioimmunoassay and stool examination for *Schistosoma mansoni* infection. Trans Soc Trop Med Hyg 75:365, 1981
86. Lord WD, Bullock WL: Swine ascaris in humans. N Engl J Med 306:1113, 1982
87. Löscher T et al: Praziquantel in clonorchiasis and opistorchiasis. Tropenmed Parasitol 32:234, 1981
88. Lushbaugh WB et al: Isolation of a cytotoxin-enterotoxin from *Entamoeba histolytica*. J Infect Dis 139:9, 1979
89. Lushbaugh WB et al: Proteinase activities of *Entamoeba histolytica* cytotoxin. Gastroenterology 87:17, 1984
90. Lushbaugh WB et al: Relationship of cytotoxins of axenically cultivated *Entamoeba histolytica* to virulence. Gastroenterology 86:1488, 1984
91. Luzzio AJ et al: Quantitative estimation of leishmanial antibody titers by enzyme linked immunosorbent-assay. J Infect Dis 140:370, 1979
92. Lygidakis NJ: Diagnosis and treatment of intrabiliary rupture of hydatid cyst of the liver. Arch Surg 118:1186, 1983
93. Lyra LG et al: Hepatitis B surface antigen carrier state in hepatosplenic schistosomiasis. Gastroenterology 71:641, 1976
94. McBride JS et al: Antigenic diversity in the human malaria parasite *Plasmodium falciparum*. Science 217:254, 1982
95. McGowan K et al: *Entamoeba histolytica* cytotoxin: Purification, characterization, strain virulence and protease activity. J Infect Dis 146:616, 1982
96. McGowan K et al: *Entamoeba histolytica* causes intestinal secretion: Role of serotonin. Science 221:762, 1983
97. McMillan A et al: Amoebiasis in homosexual men. Gut 25:356, 1984
98. Mahmoud AAF: Schistosomiasis: In Warren KS, Mahmoud AAF (eds): Tropical and Geographical Medicine, pp 443–457. New York, McGraw Hill, 1984
99. Maier W: Computed tomographic diagnosis of *Echinococcus alveolaris*. Hepato-gastroenterology 30:83, 1983
100. Marcial-Rojas RA (ed): Pathology of Protozoal and Helminthic Diseases. Baltimore, Williams & Wilkins, 1971
101. Marcial-Rojas RA: Parasitic diseases of the liver. In The Liver. Monographs in Pathology, International Academy of Pathology. Baltimore, Williams & Wilkins, 1973
102. Markell EK et al: Intestinal protozoa in homosexual men of the San Francisco Bay area: Prevalence and correlates of infection. Am J Trop Med Hyg 33:239, 1984

103. Martínez–Maldonado M et al: Liver cell carcinoma (hepatoma) in Puerto Rico: A survey of 26 cases. Am J Dig Dis 10:522, 1965

104. Mathews HM et al: Microvolume, kinetic-dependent enzyme-linked immunosorbent assay for amoeba antibodies. J Clin Microbiol 19:221, 1984

105. Mattern CFT, Keister DB: Experimental amebiasis. II. Hepatic amebiasis in the newborn hamster. Am J Trop Med Hyg 26:402, 1977

106. Meis JFGM et al: An ultrastructural study on the role of Kupffer cells in the process of infection by *Plasmodium berghei* sporozoites in rats. Parasitology 86:231, 1983

107. Milder JE et al: Clinical features of *Strongyloides stercoralis* infection in an endemic area of the United States. Gastroenterology 80:1481, 1981

108. Miller LH et al: Evidence for differences in erythrocyte surface receptors for the malarial parasites, *Plasmodium falciparum* and *Plasmodium knowlesi.* J Exp Med 146:277, 1977

109. Miller LH et al: The Duffy blood group phenotype in American blacks infected with *Plasmodium vivax* in Vietnam. Am J Trop Med Hyg 27:1069, 1978

110. Most H: Treatment of parasitic infections of travelers and immigrants. N Engl J Med 310:298, 1984

111. Muñoz ML et al: *Entamoeba histolytica:* Collagenolytic activity and virulence. J Protozool 31:468, 1984

112. Murray HW: Susceptibility of leishmania to oxygen intermediates and killing by normal macrophages. J Exp Med 153:1302, 1981

113. Murray M, Rushton B: The pathology of fascioliasis, with particular reference to hepatic fibrosis. In Taylor AER, Muller R (eds): Pathogenic Processes in Parasitic Infections, pp 27–41. Oxford, Blackwell Scientific Publications, 1975

114. Nakashima T et al: Primary liver cancer coincident with schistosomiasis japonica: A study of 24 necropsies. Cancer 36:1483, 1975

115. Nakashima T et al: Hepatocellular carcinoma and clonorchiasis. Cancer 39:1306, 1977

116. Nanda R et al: *Entamoeba histolytica* cyst passers: Clinical features and outcome in untreated subjects. Lancet 2:301, 1984

117. Nash TE, Neva FA: Recent advances in the diagnosis and treatment of cerebral cysticercosis. N Engl J Med 311:1492, 1984

118. Nash TE et al: Schistosome infections in humans: Perspectives and recent findings. Ann Intern Med 97:740, 1982

119. Neva FA et al: Comparison of larval antigens in an enzyme-linked immunosorbent assay for strongyloidiasis in humans. J Infect Dis 144:427, 1981

120. Obeid FN et al: Bilharzial portal hypertension. Arch Surg 118:702, 1983

121. Orozco E et al: *Entamoeba histolytica:* Phagocytosis as a virulence factor. J Exp Med 158:1511, 1983

122. Ortega HB et al: Enteric pathogenic protozoa in homosexual men from San Francisco. Sex Transm Dis 11:59, 1984

123. Pachucki CT et al: American paragonimiasis treated with praziquantel. N Engl J Med 311:582, 1984

124. Pandolfo I et al: C. T. findings in hepatic involvement by *Echinococcus granulosus.* J Comput Assist Tomogr 8:839, 1984

125. Patterson M, Schoppe LE: The presentation of amoebiasis. Med Clin North Am 66:689, 1982

126. Patterson M et al: Serologic testing for amoebiasis. Gastroenterology 78:136, 1980

127. Pawlowski FS: Ascariasis: Host-pathogen biology. Rev Infect Dis 4:806, 1982

128. Pearson R, Guerrant R: Praziquantel: A major advance in antihelminthic therapy. Ann Intern Med 99:195, 1983

129. Pearson RD et al: The immunobiology of leishmaniasis. Rev Infect Dis 5:907, 1983

130. Perrin LH et al: The hematology of malaria in man. Semin Hematol 19:70, 1982

131. Phillips SC et al: Sexual transmission of enteric protozoa and helminths in a venereal disease clinic population. N Engl J Med 305:603, 1981

132. Pillai S, Mohimen A: A solid-phase sandwich radioimmunoassay for *Entamoeba histolytica* proteins and the detection of circulating antigens in amoebiasis. Gastroenterology 83:1210, 1982

133. Plorde JJ, Matlock ML: Amebic liver abscess. Med Grand Rounds 2:45, 1983

134. Prata A. Schistosomiasis mansoni. Clin Gastroenterol 7:49, 1978

135. Prathap K et al: Pentastomiasis: A common finding at autopsy among Malaysian aborigines. Am J Trop Med Hyg 18:20, 1969

136. Purtillo DT: Clonorchiasis and hepatic neoplasms. Trop Geogr Med 28:21, 1976

137. Quinn TC et al: Prospective study of infectious agents isolated from the intestines of symptomatic and asymptomatic male homosexuals: The polymicrobial origin of intestinal infections in homosexual men. N Engl J Med 309:576, 1983

138. Raia S et al: Portal hypertension in schistosomiasis. In Benhamou JP, Lebrec D (eds): Portal Hypertension: Clinics in Gastroenterology, pp. 57–82. Philadelphia, WB Saunders, 1985

139. Ralls PW et al: Gray-scale ultrasonography of hepatic amoebic abscesses. Radiology 132:125, 1979

140. Ralls PW et al: Patterns of resolution in successfully treated hepatic amebic abscess: Sonographic evaluation. Radiology 149:541, 1983

141. Ravdin JI, Guerrant RL: Role of adherence in cytopathogenic mechanisms of *Entamoeba histolytica:* Study with mammalian tissue culture cells and human erythrocytes. J Clin Invest 68:1305, 1981

142. Rieckman KH: Falciparum malaria: The urgent need for safe and effective drugs. Annu Rev Med 34:321, 1983

143. Rowin KS et al: Babesiosis in asplenic hosts. Trans R Soc Trop Med Hyg 78:442, 1984

144. Ruebush TK II et al: Human babesiosis on Nantucket Island: Clinical features. Ann Intern Med 86:6, 1977

145. Ruebush TK et al: Experimental *Babesia microti* infections in Macaca mulatta: Recurrent parasitemia before and after splenectomy. Am J Trop Med Hyg 30:304, 1981

146. Sadisgursky M, Andrade ZA: Pulmonary changes in schistosomal cor pulmonale. Am J Trop Med Hyg 31:779, 1982

147. Saimot AG: Traitement médical de l'echinococcose humaine; état actuel. Gastroenterol Clin Biol 8:305, 1984

148. Saimot AG et al: Albendazole as a potential treatment for human hydatidosis. Lancet 2:652, 1983

149. Sargeaunt PG et al: Biochemical homogeneity of *Entamoeba histolytica* isolates, especially those from liver abscess. Lancet 1:1386, 1982

150. Schulman A et al: Sonographic diagnosis of biliary ascariasis. AJR 139:485, 1982

151. Scowden EB et al: Overwhelming strongyloidiasis: An unappreciated opportunistic infection. Medicine 57:527, 1978

152. Seaberg LS et al: Clindamycin activity against chloroquine-resistant *Plasmodium falciparum.* J Infect Dis 150:904, 1984

153. Seah SKK: Digenetic trematodes. Clin Gastroenterol 7:87, 1978

154. Self JT et al: Pentastomiasis in Africans. Trop Geogr Med 27:1, 1975

155. Sepúlveda B: Amebiasis: Host-pathogen biology. Rev Infect Dis 4:836, 1982

156. Sheeby TW et al: Resolution time of an amebic liver abscess. Gastroenterology 55:26, 1969

157. Sher A, Moser G: Schistosomiasis. Immunologic properties of developing schistosomula. Am J Pathol 102:121, 1981

158. Sinniah B, Sinniah D: The antihelminthic effects of pyrantel pamoate, oxantel-pyrantel pamoate, levamisole and mebendazole in the treatment of intestinal nematodes. Ann Trop Med Parasitol 75:315, 1981

159. Sorensen PG et al: Malaria-induced immune thrombocytopenia. Vox Sang 47:68, 1984

160. Soulier JP: Diseases transmissible by blood transfusion: Vox Sang 47:1, 1984

161. Spencer HC et al: The enzyme linked immunosorbent assay (ELISA) for malaria: II. Comparison with the malaria indirect fluorescent antibody test (IFA). Am J Trop Med Hyg 28:933, 1979

162. Spencer HC et al: The enzyme-linked immunosorbent assay (ELISA) for malaria: III. Antibody response in documented *Plasmodium falciparum* infections. Am J Trop Med Hyg 30:747, 1981

163. Strickland GT et al: Clinical characteristics and response to therapy in Egyptian children heavily infected with *Schistosoma mansoni.* J Infect Dis 146:20, 1982

164. Sun T: Pathology and immunology of *Clonorchis sinensis* infection of the liver. Ann Clin Lab Sci 14:208, 1984

165. Sun T et al: Morphologic and clinical observations in human infection with *Babesia microti.* J Infect Dis 148:239, 1983

166. Takahashi S, Simpser E: Granuloma collagenase and EDTA sensitive neutral protease production in hepatic murine schistosomiasis. Hepatology 1:211, 1981

167. Tan EGC, Warren KW: Diseases of the gallbladder and bile ducts. In Schiff L, Schiff ER (eds): Diseases of the Liver, 5th ed, p 1530. Philadelphia, JB Lippincott, 1982

168. Thomas V et al: Assessment of the sensitivity, specificity, and reproducibility of the indirect immunofluorescent technique for the diagnosis of amebiasis. Am J Trop Med Hyg 30:57, 1981

169. Tsutsumi V et al: Cellular basis of experimental amebic liver abscess formation. Am J Pathol 117:81, 1984

170. Uflacker R et al: Parasitic and mycotic causes of biliary obstruction. Gastrointest Radiol 7:173, 1982

171. Upatham ES et al: Morbidity in relation to intensity of infection in *Opisthorchis viverrini:* Study of a community in Khon Kaen, Thailand. Am J Trop Med Hyg 31:1156, 1982

172. van Knapen F et al: Visceral larva migrans: Examination by means of enzyme-linked immunosorbent assay of human sera for antibodies to excretory-secretory antigens of the second-stage larvae of *Toxocara canis.* Z Parasitenkd 69:113, 1983

173. Varela–Díaz VM et al: Evaluation of three immunodiagnostic tests for human hydatid disease. Am J Trop Med Hyg 24:312, 1975

174. Ward PA, Jack RM: The entry process of *Babesia merozoites* into red cells. Am J Pathol 102:109, 1981

175. Warren KS: Schistosomiasis: Host-pathogen biology. Rev Infect Dis 4:771, 1982

176. Warren KS: The kinetics of hepatosplenic schistosomiasis. Semin Liver Dis 4:293, 1984

177. Warren KS, Mahmoud AAF (eds): Tropical and Geographic Medicine. New York, McGraw Hill, 1984

178. Warren KS, Reboucas G: Blood ammonia during bleeding from esophageal varices in patients with hepatosplenic schistosomiasis. N Engl J Med 171:921, 1964

179. Warren KS et al: Morbidity in schistosomiasis japonica in relation to intensity of infection: A study of two rural brigades in Anhui Province, China. N Engl J Med 309:1533, 1983

180. Werner JK, Barreto P: Leishmaniasis in Colombia: A review. Am J Trop Med Hyg 30:751, 1981

181. White NJ et al: Quinine pharmacokinetics and toxicity in cerebral and uncomplicated falciparum malaria. Am J Med 73:564, 1982

182. White NJ et al: Severe hypoglycemia and hyperinsulinemia in falciparum malaria. N Engl J Med 309:61, 1983

183. Wilson JF, Rausch RL: Alveolar hydatid disease: A review of clinical features of 33 indigenous cases of *Echinococcus multilocularis* infection in Alaskan Eskimos. Am J Trop Med Hyg 29:1340, 1980

184. Wilson M et al: Comparison of complement fixation, indirect immunofluorescence and indirect hemagglutination test for malaria. Am J Trop Med Hyg 24:755, 1975

185. Winters C et al: Endoscopic documentation of *Ascaris* induced pancreatitis. Gastrointest Endosc 30:83, 1984

186. Wittner M et al: Successful chemotherapy of transfusion babesiosis. Ann Intern Med 96:601, 1982

187. Wong B: Parasitic diseases in immuno-compromised hosts. Am J Med 76:479, 1984

188. Wyler DJ: Malaria resurgence, resistance and research. N Engl J Med 308:875, 1983

189. Wyler DJ, Suzuki K: In vitro parasite-monocyte interactions in human leishmaniasis: Effect of enzyme treatment on attachment. Infect Immunol 42:356, 1983

190. Wyler DJ et al: Fibroblast stimulation in schistosomiasis: I. Stimulation in vitro of fibroblasts by soluble products of egg granulomas. J Infect Dis 144:254, 1981

chapter 36
Leptospirosis

JAY P. SANFORD

DEFINITION

Leptospirosis is the name applied to disease caused by all leptospires, regardless of specific serotype. Previously, a number of names were used to describe various clinical syndromes, such as Weil's disease for icteric leptospirosis caused by the icterohemorrhagiae serogroup, swineherds' disease for that caused by the pomona serogroup, canicola fever for leptospirosis due to the canicola serogroup, mud fever, autumn fever, field fever, seven-day fever, and Ft. Bragg fever. The recognition of considerable overlap between clinical syndromes and specific serogroups of leptospira has led to the discontinuation of such terminology.

HISTORY

The separation of leptospiral jaundice from other infectious diseases of the liver occurred in two stages, the first, clinical, and the second, nearly 30 years later, bacteriologic.[1] The term "Weil's disease" was first used by Goldschmidt in 1887 to designate the form of infectious jaundice that Professor Weil of Heidelberg had established as a separate entity in 1886 from a study of four patients.[21] Two of the cases had occurred in 1870 and the other two in 1882, but they each presented such similar features that Weil considered them to be the same disease. The four patients were men, and each had a febrile illness with neurologic symptoms, hepatomegaly, splenomegaly, jaundice, and renal involvement. After a relatively short course, the patients recovered. However, three had a recurrence of fever after an afebrile period of 1 to 7 days. Although he could not demonstrate either its anatomic basis or the infective agent, Weil suggested that the cases represented a new entity. Actually, Landouzy had described the disease in 1883 and had associated it with work in sewers.[12] Subsequently, there developed skepticism as to whether Weil's disease was a separate entity. Inada and associates were convinced of the existence of Weil's disease as an illness characterized by conjunctival congestion, muscular pain, fever, jaundice, hemorrhagic diathesis, albuminuria, and a fairly high death rate. They stated that splenic enlargement was uncommon, occurring in about 10% of patients. In November, 1914, in Kyushu,

Inada and co-workers first saw spirochetes in the liver tissue of a guinea pig that had been inoculated with blood from a patient with Weil's disease. They obtained similar results with blood from 13 of 17 other cases of Weil's disease and failed to find spirochetes in guinea pigs inoculated with blood from patients with other infections, including catarrhal jaundice. They named the organism *Spirochaeta icterohaemorrhagiae.* They cultured the organism and showed that it could gain entry into guinea pigs through abraded and even apparently intact skin, that spirochetes could be seen in patient's urine, and that antibodies appeared in patient's serum and persisted for a number of years.[9] Noguchi carefully studied the *Spirochaeta icterohaemorrhagiae* of Inada, strains from British cases in Flanders during World War I, and strains from wild rats in the United States. He considered the morphology to be sufficiently characteristic to justify the creation of a new genus, which he named "leptospira."[14] Stimson described a spirochete in sections of the kidney of a patient in New Orleans who died of presumed yellow fever.[17] He named the organism (?*Spirochaeta*)*interrogans.* His description of the organism and photographs taken in 1940 by Sellards from Stimson's original sections show that the organism was a leptospire.[15]

ETIOLOGY

Leptospires are finely coiled, motile aerobic spirochetes approximately 0.1 μm in width and 6 μm to 20 μm in length. They have bent or hooked ends often resembling question marks; hence the name "interrogans." The cell wall has a three-layered structure similar to that of gram-negative bacteria.[11] Leptospira are resistant to metronidazole.

The genus leptospira contains only one species, *L. interrogans,* so named because of the priority established by Stimson, which is subdivided into two complexes, interrogans and biflexa.[20] The interrogans complex includes the pathogenic strains, whereas the biflexa complex includes saphrophytic strains. Within each complex, the organisms show antigenic variations that are stable and allow them to be classed as serotypes (serovars). Serotypes with common antigens are arranged into serogroups (vars). Despite common usage to the contrary, an example of the correct designation of Leptospira is as follows: "canicola serogroup of *L. interrogans*" or "*L. interrogans*" serovar canicola. The interrogans complex now contains about 170 serotypes of pathogenic leptospires arranged in 18 serogroups (the numbers in the following parentheses refer to the numbers of serotypes within the serogroups): icterohaemorrhagiae (18), hebdomidis (30), autumnalis (17), canicola (12), australis (12), tarassovi (17), pyrogenes (12), bataviae (10), javanica (8), pomona (8), ballum (3), cynoptei (3), celledoni (3), grippotyphosa (5), panama (2), shermani (1), ranarum (2), and bufonis (1). At least 27 serotypes of leptospira occur naturally in the United States.

EPIDEMIOLOGY

Leptospirosis is thought to be the most widespread zoonosis in the world. It occurs throughout the world, except for Antarctica, and is most prevalent in the tropics. In Southeast Asia, the Marquesas Islands, and Trinidad, 15% to 28% of persons are seropositive. Leptospirosis is still endemic in the Po valley of Italy. Although leptospirosis is not common in the United States, it has been reported from all regions including arid areas such as Arizona. Between 1974 and 1984, 40 to 110 cases were reported.[3] Infection in human beings is an incidental occurrence and is not essential in the maintenance of leptospirosis. The disease occurs in a wide range of domestic and wild animal hosts. In many species, such as opossum, skunk, raccoon, and fox, infectivity ratios in the range of 10% to 50% are not unusual. Interspecies spread of specific serotypes of leptospires among animal hosts is frequent; for example, pomona, a serotype principally associated with livestock, has been demonstrated in dogs. Infection in animals may vary from inapparent illness to fatal disease. Asymptomatic host animals may carry high numbers of leptospires in their kidneys ($>10^{10}$ organisms/g). The carrier state, in which the host may shed leptospires in its urine for months or years, develops in many animals. Immunization of dogs may not prevent the carrier or shedder state.[6]

Survival of pathogenic leptospires in nature is governed by factors including pH of the urine of the host, pH of the soil or water into which they are shed, and ambient temperature. Leptospires shed in a carrier's urine have been found in the soil to a depth of 1 cm with a radius 1 cm to 2 cm beyond the "urine spot." Most "spots" retain infective capacity for 6 to 48 hours. Acid urine permits only limited survival; however, if the urine is neutral or alkaline, is shed into a similar moist environment that has low salinity, is not badly polluted with microorganisms or detergents, and has a temperature above 22° C (71.6° F), leptospires may survive for several weeks. Human infection can occur either by direct contact with urine or tissue of an infected animal or indirectly through contaminated water, soil, or vegetation. The usual portals of entry in humans are abraded skin, particularly about the feet, and exposed conjunctival, nasal, and oral mucous membranes. The previously held concept that organisms can penetrate intact skin has been questioned. Although leptospires have been isolated from ticks, these arthropods are unimportant in transmission.

With the ubiquitous infection of animals, leptospirosis in human beings can occur in all age-groups, at all seasons, and in both sexes. However, it is primarily a disease of teenaged children and young adults (about one half of all patients are between the ages of 10 and 39), occurs predominantly in males (80%), and develops most frequently in hot weather (in the United States, one half of infections occur from July to October).[8,23] The wide spectrum of animal hosts results in both urban and rural human disease. Leptospirosis has been considered an occupational disease; however, improved methods of rat control and better standards of hygiene have reduced the incidence among occupational groups such as coal miners and sewer workers. The epidemiologic pattern has changed; in the United States and the United Kingdom water-associated and cattle-associated leptospirosis has become most common. Currently, fewer than 20% of patients have direct contact with animals, and those who have such contact are usually farmers, trappers, or abattoir workers. In the majority of patients, exposure is incidental; two thirds of cases occur in children, students, or housewives. Swimming or partial immersion in contaminated water, such as by riding a motorcycle through contaminated pools of water, has been implicated in one fifth of patients and has accounted for most of the recognized common-source outbreaks. In Hawaii one fourth of cases have been associated with aquaculture industries. In the United Kingdom, fish farm workers show a moderately increased risk. Several soldiers assigned to the British Army on the Rhine have developed leptospirosis after falling into rivers.

PATHOLOGY

Postmortem examinations of patients who died of leptospirosis have been confined almost exclusively to persons with icteric leptospirosis (Weil's disease). Gross examination has revealed bile staining of the tissues. Hemorrhages, petechial or ecchymotic, occur in almost all organs but are most prominent in striated muscle, kidneys, adrenals, liver, stomach, spleen, and lungs.[1] The liver and kidneys are of normal size or slightly enlarged. Lungs are edematous with varying degrees of focal or diffuse hemorrhage.

Histologic alterations in the liver are neither specific nor diagnostic. Proliferation of liver cells as evidenced by mitotic figures and cells with two nuclei, cloudy swelling, dissociation of hepatic cords, enlargement of Kupffer cells, and varying degrees of necrosis (usually slight and focal) occur. Biliary stasis involving the central, but not the peripheral, portion of the lobule is frequent. The degree of functional damage to the liver in fatal cases is often poorly correlated with the degree of histopathologic changes. Leptospires are rarely demonstrated in the liver.

Microscopic changes of the kidneys are often striking. In the acute phase, lesions predominantly involve the tubules and vary from simple dilatation of distal convoluted tubules to degeneration, necrosis, and basement membrane rupture. Interstitial edema and cellular infiltrates consisting of lymphocytes, neutrophilic leukocytes, histiocytes, and plasma cells are uniformly present. Glomerular lesions either are absent or consist of mesangial hyperplasia and focal foot process fusion, which are interpreted as nonspecific changes associated with acute inflammation and protein filtration. Special staining techniques using silver impregnation methods have demonstrated organisms in the lumina of renal tubules but rarely in other organs.

In skeletal muscle, focal necrotic and necrobiotic changes thought to be typical of leptospirosis occur. Biopsies early in the illness demonstrate swelling, vacuolization, and, subsequently, hyalinazation. Leptospiral antigen has been demonstrated in these lesions by the fluorescent antibody technique. Healing ensues with minimum fibrosis through the formation of new myofibrils. Microscopic evidence of myocarditis, including focal hemorrhages, interstitial edema, and focal infiltration with lymphocytes and plasma cells occurs. Pulmonary findings consist of a patchy localized hemorrhagic pneumonitis. Bile staining of leptomeninges and choroid plexus may be seen. Microscopic changes in the brain and meninges are minimal and are not diagnostic.

CLINICAL MANIFESTATIONS

General Features

The incubation period after immersion or accidental laboratory exposure has shown extremes of 2 and 26 days; the usual range is 7 to 13 days and the average is 10 days.[1,6]

Leptospirosis is a typically biphasic illness. During the first, or leptospiremic, phase, leptospires are present in the blood and cerebrospinal fluid.[5] The onset is typically abrupt, and initial symptoms include headache, which is usually frontal, less often retro-orbital, and occasionally bitemporal or occipital.[2] Severe muscle aching occurs in most patients, involving the muscles of the thighs and lumbar areas most prominently, and is often accompanied by severe pain on palpation. The myalgia may be accompanied by extreme cutaneous hyperesthesia (causalgia). Chills followed by a rapidly rising temperature are prominent. Following the abrupt onset, the leptospiremic phase typically lasts 4 to 9 days. Features during this interval include recurrent chills, high spiking temperatures (usually 38.9° C [102° F] or greater), headache, and continued severe myalgia. Anorexia, nausea, and vomiting are encountered in one half or more of the patients. Occasionally, patients have diarrhea. Pulmonary manifestations, usually either a cough or chest pain, have varied in frequency of occurrence from less than 25% to 86%. Hem-

optysis occurs but is rare. Examination during this phase reveals an acutely ill, febrile patient, with a relative bradycardia and normal blood pressure, although European authors comment on early hypotension. Disturbances in sensorium may be encountered in up to 25% of patients. The most characteristic physical sign is conjunctival suffusion, which usually first appears on the third or fourth day. It may be lacking in some patients but more often is overlooked. This may be associated with photophobia, but serous or purulent secretion is unusual. Less common findings include pharyngeal injection, cutaneous hemorrhages, and skin rashes that are usually macular, maculopapular, or urticarial and usually occur on the trunk. Uncommon findings are splenomegaly, hepatomegaly, lymphadenopathy, and jaundice. The first phase terminates after 4 to 9 days, usually with defervescence and improvement in symptoms. This coincides with the disappearance of leptospires from the blood and cerebrospinal fluid.

The second phase, which has been characterized as the immune phase, correlates with the appearance of circulating IgM antibodies.[5] The concentration of C3 in serum remains within normal range. Clinical manifestations show greater variability than those of the first phase. After a relatively asymptomatic period of 1 to 3 days, the fever and earlier symptoms recur, and meningismus may develop. The fever rarely exceeds 38.9° C (102° F) and is usually of 1 to 3 days duration. It is not uncommon for fever to be absent or transient. Even when symptoms or signs of meningeal irritation are absent, routine examination of cerebrospinal fluid after the seventh day has revealed pleocytosis in 50% to 90% of patients.[5] Less common features include iridocyclitis, optic neuritis, and other nervous system manifestations including encephalitis, myelitis, and peripheral neuropathy. Transient ischemic attacks in childhood and adolescence caused by cerebral leptospiral arteritis have been reported by Chinese clinicians.

Some clinicians recognize a third, or convalescent, phase, usually between the second and fourth weeks, when both fever and aching may recur. The pathogenesis of this stage is not understood.

Leptospirosis during pregnancy may be associated with an increased risk of fetal loss.

Specific Features

Weil's syndrome accounts for 1% to 6% of cases of leptospirosis. Serovar *L. icterohaemorrhagiae* accounts for 40% of those with Weil's syndrome and the remainder are caused by multiple serovars. Weil's syndrome is defined as severe leptospirosis with jaundice, usually accompanied by azotemia, hemorrhages, anemia, disturbances in consciousness, and continued fever. There is uncertainty as to the pathogenesis of the syndrome, that is, whether it represents direct toxic damage due to leptospires or whether it is the consequence of immune response to leptospiral antigens. The consensus favors toxic damage.

The onset and first stage are identical with those of the less severe forms of leptospirosis. The distinctive features of Weil's syndrome appear from the third to the sixth days but do not reach their peak until well into the second stage. As in milder forms of leptospirosis, there is a tendency for defervescence on about the seventh day; however, with recurrence, fever is marked and may persist for several weeks. Either renal or hepatic manifestations may predominate. Hepatic disturbances include tenderness in the right upper quadrant and hepatic enlargement, both of which are common when jaundice is present. Serum glutamic-oxaloacetic transaminase (SGOT) values are rarely increased more than fivefold regardless of the degree of hyperbilirubinemia, which is predominantly conjugated (direct); as an example, serum bilirubin is 40 mg/dl, while SGOT is 170 IU. The predominant mechanism appears to be an intracellular block to bilirubin excretion.

Renal manifestations consist primarily of proteinuria, pyuria, hematuria, and azotemia. Dysuria is rare. Serious renal damage usually occurs in the form of acute tubular necrosis associated with oliguria. The peak elevation of blood urea nitrogen is usually seen on the fifth to seventh day. Hemorrhagic manifestations, which are most prevalent in this group of patients, include epistaxis, hemoptysis, gastrointestinal bleeding, hemorrhage into the adrenal glands, hemorrhagic pneumonitis, and subarachnoid hemorrhage. Fatal subarachnoid hemorrhage without thrombocytopenia has been reported. These manifestations have been explained on the basis of diffuse vasculitis with capillary injury. In addition, hypoprothrombinemia and thrombocytopenia have been observed in some patients.

LABORATORY FEATURES

In anicteric patients, leukocyte counts vary from leukopenic levels to mild elevations. In patients with jaundice, leukocytosis as high as 70,000 cells/mm^3 may be present. However, regardless of the total leukocyte count, neutrophilia of greater than 70% is very frequently encountered during the first stage.

Hemolytic substances have been demonstrated in cultures of pathogenic leptospires. In contrast to many hemolysins of bacterial origin that are not hemolytic *in vivo*, leptospiral hemolysins appear to be active *in vivo*. In patients with jaundice, anemia may be severe and most characteristically is due to intravascular hemolysis. Other mechanisms of anemia include that secondary to azotemia and blood loss secondary to hemorrhage. Anemia due to leptospirosis is unusual in anicteric patients.

Thrombocytopenia sufficient to be associated with bleeding may be encountered. Additional hematologic abnormalities include elevation of the erythrocyte sedimentation rate in over one half of patients, although this rate usually remains below 50 mm/hour.

Urinalysis during the leptospiremic phase reveals mild proteinuria, casts, and an increase in cellular elements. In anicteric infections, these abnormalities rapidly disappear after the first week. Proteinuria and abnormalities in the urine sediment usually are not associated with elevations in blood urea nitrogen. Since the anicteric form of the disease has often gone undiagnosed, estimates of the frequency of azotemia and jaundice are probably high. Azotemia has been reported in approximately one fourth of patients. In three fourths of these patients, the blood urea nitrogen is less than 100 mg/dl. Azotemia is usually associated with jaundice. Serum bilirubin levels may reach 65 mg/dl; however, in two thirds of patients, the levels are less than 20 mg/dl. During the first phase, one half of the patients have increased serum creatine phosphokinase (CPK) levels, with mean values of five times normal.[11] Such increases are not seen in viral hepatitis, and a slight increase in transaminase with a definite increase in CPK suggests leptospirosis rather than viral hepatitis.

DIAGNOSIS

Diagnosis is based upon culture of the organism or serologic proof of its existence. The most common initial diagnoses in patients with leptospirosis are meningitis, hepatitis, nephritis, fever of undetermined origin (FUO), and influenza.[2] Leptospires may be isolated quite readily during the first phase from blood and cerebrospinal fluid or during the second phase from the urine. Leptospires may be excreted in the urine for up to 11 months after the onset of illness and may persist despite antimicrobial therapy. Whole blood should be injected immediately into tubes containing semisolid medium such as Fletcher's or EMJH medium. If culture medium is not available, leptospires reportedly will remain viable up to 11 days in blood to which anticoagulants, preferably sodium oxalate, have been added. Citrate should not be used because it inhibits leptospira. Animal inoculation (preferably either suckling hamster or guinea pig) may be used and is of particular value if specimens are contaminated. Direct examination of blood or urine by the dark-field method has been employed; however, this method so frequently results in failure or misdiagnosis that it should not be used.[16] Serologic methods are applicable during the second phase; antibodies appear from the sixth to the twelfth days of illness. Five serologic tests are available: microscopic agglutination (MA), macroscopic agglutination (slide test, ST), hemolytic, indirect hemagglutination (IHA), and complement fixation (CF).[10] The MA test is the standard procedure used for serologic diagnosis, but it is complex, requiring the maintenance of cultures of live leptospira (23 being used). The test is partially serovar specific. Agglutinins elicited by leptospires of a particular serovar often agglutinate leptospires of other serovars in the same serogroup. Absorption studies on serum from an infected person indicate the infecting serovar with a high degree of probability. The ST is commonly used in hospitals to screen sera for infection. Antigens used include ballum, canicola, icterohaemorrhagiae, bataviae, grippotyphosa, pyrogenes, autumnalis, pomona, wolfii, australis, tarasovvi, and georgia. The IHA test uses glutaraldehyde fixation of sheep erythrocytes coated with an alcohol-extracted antigen from a single leptospiral serovar (andaman). Recently an enzyme-linked immunosorbent assay (ELISA) test for leptospirosis has been developed that shows a high degree of specificity and sensitivity compared with the MA test. It is not yet commercially available. Diagnostic criteria are as follows: a case is confirmed by the isolation of leptospires on culture or seroconversion from a titer of <1:50 to ≥1:200 or by a fourfold or greater change in MA titer between acute and convalescent serum specimens studied at the same laboratory; a case is presumed if the finding is an MA titer of ≥1:200 or a positive ST reaction on a single serum specimen obtained after the onset of symptoms.

Differential Diagnosis

Before consideration of specific infections that may be associated with jaundice, it should be noted that, in a patient with underlying liver disease, jaundice may appear or worsen from a variety of causes, including infections. Drugs being used to treat an infected patient may also cause jaundice. Table 36-1 provides a summary of major considerations. In young children, Kawasaki disease (mucocutaneous lymph node syndrome) shares many features with leptospirosis. In older children and young adults, the toxic shock syndrome, which has been associated with an exotoxin produced by some strains of *Staphylococcus aureus* related to phage group I, produces a syndrome that, clinically, is virtually indistinguishable from leptospirosis. Similarly, staphylococcal bacteremia may masquerade as leptospirosis. Through a mechanism that has not been defined, pyelonephritis is sometimes, albeit rarely, associated with jaundice. Consideration of leptospirosis requires a high index of suspicion and a careful epidemiologic history of potential contact with animal urine or water.

TABLE 36-1. Differential Diagnosis of Infectious Causes of Jaundice

MECHANISM OF JAUNDICE	DISEASE ENTITY	CATEGORY OF PATIENT		
		Neonate	Child	Adult
Hemolysis	Infection in patients with abnormal red blood cells	×	×	×
	Malaria	×	×	×
	Babesiosis		×	×
	Bartonellosis		×	×
	Bacteroides bacteremia	×	×	×
	Clostridium perfringens toxemia	×	×	×
Obstruction	Cholangitis with infection	×	×	×
Hepatocellular	Viral hepatitis	×	×	×
	Infectious mononucleosis	×	×	
	TORCH syndrome	×		
	Coxsackievirus	×	×	×
	Yellow fever	×	×	×
	Lassa fever		×	×
	Ebola virus		×	×
	Marburg disease		×	×
	Psittacosis		×	×
	Q fever		×	×
	Gonococcal perihepatitis		×	×
	Kawasaki disease	×	×	
	Toxic shock syndrome (phage group I staphylococci)		×	× (young)
	Granulomatous hepatitis		×	×
	Syphilis			
	Congenital	×		
	Secondary		×	×
	Leptospirosis		×	×
	Bacteremia	×		
	Hepatic abscess	×	×	×
	Pyelonephritis (rare)			×
	Parasites			
	Amebiasis		×	×
	Clonorchiasis			×
	Schistosomiasis			×

TORCH syndrome, toxoplasmosis, rubella, cytomegalovirus, herpes simplex.

PROGNOSIS

The prognosis is dependent upon both the virulence of the organism and the general condition of the patient. Between 1974 and 1981 mortality in reported cases in the United States varied annually between 2.4% and 16.4%, averaging 7.1%.[3] A mortality as high as 48% in 1971 is reported from Barbados.[4] Age is the most significant host factor related to mortality. In a representative series, mortality rose from 10% in men under 50 years of age to 56% in those over 51 years of age. The virulence of the infecting leptospires correlates best with the development of jaundice. In anicteric patients, death is extremely rare, but with the development of jaundice, mortality in various series has ranged from 15% to 40%. The long-term prognosis after the acute renal lesion of leptospirosis is good. Glomerular filtration rates return to normal, usually within 2 months; however, a few patients show residual tubular dysfunction, such as a defect in renal concentrating capacity.

TREATMENT

A variety of antimicrobial drugs, including penicillin, streptomycin, the tetracycline congeners, chloramphenicol, and erythromycin, have been effective *in vitro* and in experimental leptospiral infections. Data concerning the efficacy of antibiotics in human beings have been conflicting. If antimicrobial drugs are to have any beneficial effect, they must be administered within 4 days of the onset of illness. Within 4 to 6 hours after initiation of penicillin G therapy, a Jarisch–Herxheimer type of reaction, which suggests antileptospiral activity, may occur. A recent prospective double-blind study has demonstrated that doxycycline (200 mg taken orally once per week) is highly effective prophylaxis.[18] In a companion prospective double-blind study, doxycycline (100 mg taken orally twice daily for 7 days) reduced duration of illness and favorably affected fever, malaise, headache, and myalgias.[13] Treatment prevented leptospiruria. Both studies were based upon disease acquired in Panama. The epidemiologic conditions and clinical illnesses were typical of leptospirosis generally. It is reasonable to assume that the conclusions are applicable to other areas and would probably apply to other tetracyclines provided appropriate dosage adjustments were made. The efficacy of penicillins is less well proven. Recommendations have included penicillin G (usually 600,000 units intramuscularly every 4 hours) or ampicillin. There is general agreement that antimicrobials administered after the fifth day of illness have no beneficial effect. The clinical impression is that early bedrest may minimize subsequent morbidity. Azotemia and jaundice require meticulous attention to fluid and electrolyte therapy. Since the renal damage is reversible, patients with azotemia should be considered for peritoneal dialysis or hemodialysis.[22] Case reports have suggested that exchange transfusion is beneficial in the management of patients with extreme hyperbilirubinemia.

REFERENCES

1. Alston JM, Broom JC: Leptospirosis in Man and Animals. Edinburgh, E & S Livingstone, 1958
2. Berman SJ et al: Sporadic anicteric leptospirosis in South Vietnam: A study of 150 patients. Ann Intern Med 79:167, 1973
3. Centers for Disease Control: Annual summary 1984: Reported morbidity and mortality in the United States. MMWR 33(54), 1986
4. Damude DF et al: The problem of human leptospirosis in Barbados. Trans R Soc Trop Med Hyg 73:169, 1979
5. Edwards GA, Domm M: Human leptospirosis. Medicine 39:177, 1960
6. Feigin RD, Anderson DC: Human leptospirosis. CRC Crit Rev Clin Lab Sci 5:413, 1975
7. Goldschmidt F: Ein Leintrag zur neuen infections krankheit Weil's. Dtsch Arch Klin Med 40:238, 1877
8. Heath CW Jr, Alexander AD: Leptospirosis in the United States: Analysis of 483 cases in man, 1949–1961. N Engl J Med 273:857, 915, 1965
9. Inada R et al: The etiology, mode of infection, and specific therapy of Weil's disease (spirochaetosis icterohaemorrhagiae). J Exp Med 23:377, 1916
10. Johnson RC: The Biology of Parasite Spirochetes. New York, Academic Press, 1976
11. Johnson WD Jr et al: Serum creatine phosphokinase in leptospirosis. JAMA 233:981, 1975
12. Landouzy LTJ: Fievre bilieuse ou hepatique. Gaz Hop (Paris) 56:809, 1883
13. McClain JB et al: Doxycycline therapy for leptospirosis. Ann Intern Med 100:696, 1984
14. Noguchi H: Spirochaeta icterohaemorrhagiae in American wild rats and its relation to Japanese and European strains. J Exp Med 25:755, 1917
15. Sellards AW: The interpretation of (? Spirochaeta) interrogans of Stimson (1907) in the light of subsequent developments. Trans R Soc Trop Med Hyg 33:545, 1940
16. Smith TF et al: Pseudospirochetes, a cause of erroneous diagnosis of leptospirosis. Am J Clin Pathol 72:459, 1979
17. Stimson AM: Note on an organism found in Yellow Fever tissue. Public Health Rep 22:541, 1907
18. Takafuji ET et al: An efficacy trial of doxycycline chemoprophylaxis against leptospirosis. N Engl J Med 310:497, 1984
19. Turner LH: Leptospirosis. Br Med J 1:537, 1973
20. Turner LH: Classification of spirochetes in general and of the genus *Leptospira* in particular. In Johnson RC (ed): The Biology of Parasitic Spirochetes, pp 95–106. New York, Academic Press, 1976
21. Weil A: Uber eine eigentumliche mit Milztumor, Icterus and Nephirtis einbergehende akute infektions krankheit. Dtsch Arch Klin Med 39:209, 1886
22. Winearls CG et al: Acute renal failure due to leptospirosis: Clinical features and outcome in six cases. Q J Med 53:487 1984
23. Wong ML et al: Leptospirosis: A childhood disease. J Pediatr 90:532, 1977

chapter 37

Surgery of the Liver

MICHAEL E. DeBAKEY and GEORGE L. JORDAN, JR.

TRAUMA TO THE LIVER

Historically, surgeons have relied on reports of experiences with military injuries for information concerning treatment of trauma. One of the largest and most detailed reports of hepatic trauma is based on the World War II experience.[57] Later, however, economic and sociologic changes in the United States made civilian trauma a serious problem in every major city; consequently, the experience reported from civilian hospitals[19,58] now exceeds that reported from World War II. Our own experience also reflects the dramatic increase in hepatic trauma, for before 1950 we treated an average of only 19 patients with hepatic injuries annually. During the next 10 years, this figure had increased 2½ times, and from 1971 to 1974, we were treating 130 patients annually—a sevenfold increase. In a 6-year period prior to 1984, the average number of patients whom we treated for liver injury was approximately 160 per year; there was one year in which we treated 200 hepatic injuries.

Such wounds have increased not only in number, but also in complexity, owing to the change in the type of wounding agent. Two thirds of all patients with hepatic wounds have injuries to one or more additional organs, so that in the treatment of hepatic wounds, the complexity of treating the patient far exceeds the injury to the liver itself. Because serious hepatic injury, however, is usually associated with severe hemorrhage, which is immediately life-endangering, the hepatic wound often must receive the highest priority in treatment.

Mechanism of Injury

The mechanism of injury varies according to the pattern of trauma in different localities. In large cities, assault is so common that penetrating wounds account for most injuries. In rural areas, however, blunt trauma has a higher incidence, owing to automobile accidents. During the past 30 years, the pattern of injuries in our institutions has changed considerably. Whereas penetrating trauma always accounted for most wounds, we noted an equal number of gunshot and stab wounds in our experience of 25 years ago. In many ensuing years, gunshot wounds exceeded

stab wounds by a ratio of 3:1. The development of high-speed expressways has also resulted in an increase in automobile accidents so that the percentage of blunt trauma has increased, whereas the incidence of stab wounds has decreased. Blunt trauma accounted for only 8% of wounds in 1950 and for 19% in 1974, whereas stab wounds decreased in incidence from 45% in 1939 to 19% in recent years (Fig. 37-1.).[19] In more recent years there has been a slight reversal of this trend, with an increasing percentage of patients being injured by knife wounds. The general pattern is that of more severe wounds than were seen 30 years ago. These changes are highly significant in the treatment of patients with hepatic injuries, because gunshot wounds are much more lethal than stab wounds, and blunt trauma to the liver is particularly lethal. Moreover, the weapons causing gunshot wounds are becoming more destructive. In earlier years, the most common were .22 and .32 caliber guns. Now, .357 and .44 magnum handguns are standard weapons for many police, and an increasing number of wounds due to high-velocity hunting rifles are also seen. The most serious injury results from a shotgun blast at close range.[19]

A special type of trauma is iatrogenic, resulting from needle biopsy, percutaneous cholangiography, or percutaneous insertion of catheters into various portions of the hepatic vasculature of the biliary system.

Pathology

A number of authors have tabulated the relative frequency of injury to intra-abdominal structures. In a tabulation of several series of abdominal trauma, Griswold and Collier noted that the liver was fourth in order of frequency among intra-abdominal organs injured, being preceded by the spleen, kidney, and intestine, in that order.[31]

Recent experience at Ben Taub General Hospital in Houston, Texas indicates that the small intestine is the organ most frequently injured, with the liver second; the spleen leads the list in most series of patients sustaining blunt trauma (Tables 37-1 and 37-2).[61]

The hepatic wound varies with the type of wounding agent. Knife wounds, for example, usually make a sharp, relatively superficial incision, whereas pistol or rifle

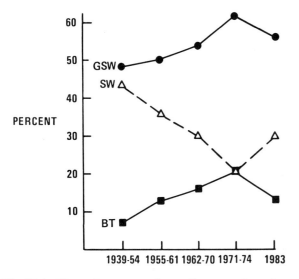

TABLE 37-2. Tabulation of Organs Injured by Blunt Trauma Among 54 Patients

ORGAN INJURED	NUMBER OF PATIENTS TREATED
Spleen	20
Liver	13
Colon	7
Arteries or veins	7
Small intestine	4
Kidney	4
Duodenum	4
Pancreas	3
Urinary bladder	3

Fig. 37-1. Change in patterns of wounding agents in patients treated at the Ben Taub General and Jefferson Davis Hospitals between 1939 and 1974, and in the year 1983. GSW, gunshot wounds; SW, stab wounds; BT, blunt trauma.

wounds produce through-and-through perforations with associated contusion and occasional stellate fracture. The degree of damage by gunshot wounds is proportional to the velocity of the missile. Shotgun wounds at close range may be immediately fatal as a result of severe destruction of the organ, with massive hemorrhage.

Wounds resulting from blunt trauma range from small, subcapsular hematomas to large, stellate fractures that shatter an entire lobe.

The liver is a highly vascular organ, and significant hemorrhage may occur from small wounds, while profuse

hemorrhage should be anticipated from any large wound.[70] Bile leakage occurs uniformly and, if not controlled or drained properly, results in bile peritonitis or intra-abdominal abscess. Rarely does a patient arrive at a hospital alive if his liver has been damaged to such an extent that it cannot support life when hemorrhage is controlled.

In addition to the severe hemorrhage resulting from injury to the liver itself, additional blood may be lost by the development of coagulopathy during the course of treatment. Clagett and Olsen reported the development of coagulopathy in 51% of 33 patients treated for severe hepatic trauma, the highest incidence being in patients undergoing anatomic lobectomy.[13] This problem should therefore be anticipated at the beginning of treatment, and appropriate blood components should be administered during the entire operation as well as in the early postoperative period.

Devitalized segments may give rise to late complications; the most frequent is hemorrhage, which occurs as tissue sloughs. Rarely, an intrahepatic abscess forms, and rare traumatic cysts have been reported. When properly performed, percutaneous needle biopsy usually results in minimal leakage from the liver because the parietal peritoneum rapidly falls against and seals the small opening. In some instances, however, severe hemorrhage may occur. Furthermore, if obstructive jaundice is present, performance of needle biopsy or percutaneous cholangiography may be followed by prolonged leakage of bile, because the bile in the biliary tree is under pressure. The bile peritonitis that results may require an emergency operation. Angiographic studies of patients undergoing percutaneous needle biopsy have shown arteriovenous fistulas in many patients, but these fistulas are not large enough to be of clinical significance and do not require treatment unless complications occur.[72]

Hemobilia probably occurs to some degree in most hepatic wounds of any severity. Rarely, it is serious.[56,90] In such instances, it may represent dissolution of an intrahepatic hematoma with hemorrhage into the biliary tract

TABLE 37-1. Organ Injuries Found at Laparotomy for Trauma at the Ben Taub General Hospital During One 12-Month Period

ORGAN	NUMBER	PERCENT
Small intestine	222	28
Liver	217	27
Colon and rectum	173	22
Diaphragm	122	15
Major vascular structures	117	15
Spleen	102	13
Kidney	97	12
Stomach	87	11
Pancreas	68	8
Urinary bladder	36	4
Mesentery	33	4
Duodenum	24	3
Gallbladder	20	2
Others	19	2

occurring as a late complication, or it may be due to rupture of an arterial aneurysm that formed because of damage to the artery at the time of injury (Chap. 44, Part 4).

Diagnosis

Initial examination of the wounded patient should include a careful history and physical examination. The patient should be totally disrobed and moved sufficiently to examine all areas of the body. This is extremely important because associated wounds are common. Also, lateral and posterior entrance or exit wounds or identification of a subcutaneous missile may be missed if examination is not complete.

Gunshot wounds of the right upper abdominal quadrant almost invariably damage the liver, and in many patients, other abdominal organs as well. Immediate abdominal exploration is indicated in such patients. The management of abdominal stab wounds has undergone considerable change in recent years. In the past, they were explored uniformly, as were gunshot wounds, but today the treatment has become increasingly conservative because many wounds that penetrate the peritoneal cavity do not injure the organ. Even if the liver is injured, the extent may be no greater than that resulting from needle biopsy of the liver, and thus no major operation is required unless severe hemorrhage is evident. Consequently, in many centers, operation is recommended only for those patients with stab wounds of the abdomen who have positive physical findings, changes in hematocrit indicating intra-abdominal hemorrhage, or positive findings on lavage or computed tomography (CT).[16]

Diagnosis of a hepatic wound following blunt trauma may be extremely difficult in the absence of definite signs of hemorrhage or peritonitis. Pain is the most common symptom. Pain may be accentuated with respiration and referred to the shoulder as the result of diaphragmatic irritation. The usual signs of peritonitis are present if the peritoneal cavity has been contaminated and consist of abdominal tenderness, rebound tenderness, muscle spasm, and decreased or absent peristalsis. A fluid wave may be present and is due to free peritoneal fluid. If physical findings are not sufficiently definite to warrant exploration at the time of admission, examination should be repeated at frequent intervals.

Shock is present in most patients with severe wounds, and this finding should suggest hepatic injury in patients with right upper abdominal quadrant pain following blunt trauma.

When clinical observations raise suspicion of injury but the signs are not sufficiently definite to warrant exploration, peritoneal lavage[79] should be performed.

Laboratory studies should include hemoglobin concentration and hematocrit, white blood cell count, and differential count. These are performed repeatedly if necessary. The presence of a high white blood cell count should make one suspicious of visceral injury, and a falling hematocrit should suggest intra-abdominal hemorrhage.

Roentgenograms taken in the supine and upright positions are indicated. Displacement of the stomach or hepatic flexure of the colon or elevation of the right leaf of the diaphragm may be seen with a perihepatic hematoma. Fracture of one of the lower right ribs should always raise suspicion. Diagnosis by angiography has been of interest.[1,44] Freeark and co-workers have suggested total abdominal angiography in patients with suspected abdominal wounds, but this recommendation has not been generally accepted.[26] Angiography is generally believed to offer little diagnostic information about hepatic injury and should therefore be used only for special indications.[44,83] Liver scan with the use of radioactive material and ultrasonography are of value in selected cases. Federle and associates have emphasized the use of the CT scan in the diagnosis of abdominal trauma, and this modality is being used with increasing frequency in many centers in the United States.[22] The value of this test in selected patients is unquestioned, but it is not necessary for appropriate decisions in most patients.

Treatment

Initial therapy should be the same for all patients with severe intra-abdominal trauma regardless of the organ involved. Blood should be drawn immediately for typing and crossmatching as well as for laboratory studies, and intravenous therapy is instituted immediately. An arm or neck vein should be used, or a subclavian catheter inserted, because an associated vena caval wound may preclude proper fluid administration from the lower extremity. Large plastic catheters should be used, for they are less easily dislodged and allow administration of large volumes rapidly. If the patient is in shock, one of the catheters should be passed into the superior vena cava for central venous monitoring during fluid replacement. An airway must be assured, particularly in patients with associated chest trauma, and a thoracostomy tube should be inserted before induction of anesthesia if associated chest trauma exists. A urinary catheter is inserted and fractures are splinted. If the patient is in shock, dextran administration should be instituted until whole blood is available. When hemorrhage is severe, uncrossmatched type-specific blood or low-titer O-negative blood may be used until properly crossmatched blood is available. Excessive time should not be lost trying to "prepare the patient for surgery." In the presence of severe hemorrhage, operative control is perhaps the most important resuscitative measure. Unresponsive shock, therefore, is an urgent indication for operation, and in critical situations the abdomen should be opened in the emergency room without waiting for transport to the operating room.

Adequate exposure is mandatory. A midline incision allows rapid entrance into the abdomen and good exposure for most lesions. When injuries involve the dome, however, it may be necessary to extend the incision into the chest for adequate exposure. This can be accomplished as a classic thoracoabdominal incision, but median sternotomy is used more frequently today. This incision provides good exposure and allows an approach to the inferior vena cava above the liver as well as to the right auricle if special techniques are required. Control of hemorrhage takes priority in treatment. Superficial lacerations are treated by simple suture using large, relatively blunt needles and a suture sufficiently large not to cut through the liver substance (Fig. 37-2). When hemorrhage from deep lacerations is difficult to control, a variety of techniques is advocated.[9] Most surgeons use temporary packing for immediate control. Others advocate the use of special clamps to control bleeding from the liver. A simple method is to place around the liver a tourniquet rapidly constructed from a 1-inch Penrose drain.[69] If these methods are not easily applied or do not control the hemorrhage, temporary occlusion of the hepatic artery and portal vein may be necessary. Fifteen minutes has been believed to be the maximum duration for a single period of total vascular inflow occlusion under normothermic conditions and, as is discussed below, special techniques have been used to maintain hepatic viability while complicated wounds are being treated. The duration of occlusion may be safely increased by local hypothermia, during which the liver is cooled with sterile iced saline solution. Ischemia is safe for as long as 2 hours with hypothermic perfusion. Recently, Huguet and associates presented evidence to indicate that under normothermic conditions, periods of 45 to 65 minutes of occlusion can be tolerated without difficulty[40]; their patients were undergoing elective hepatic resection. Patients with major hepatic injuries have often been in shock before vascular occlusion was accomplished, and we therefore still prefer to keep the duration of vascular occlusion to a minimum.

At times, a through-and-through bullet wound will result in significant blast injury within the substance of the liver although the entrance and exit wounds are small. Also a stellate fracture may result in greater damage deep within the organ than is apparent from inspection of the damage to the several surfaces of the liver. Opening the tract widely for inspection and control of bleeding deep within the liver can be a valuable technique in the treatment of many hepatic injuries but is not justified on a routine basis. The type of wounding as well as the gross findings at the time of surgery will provide information concerning the need for tractotomy.

Necrotic tissue should be debrided and the raw surface repaired with suture (Fig. 37-3). In some patients hemorrhage may be difficult to control even with adequate sutures. The use of hemostatic agents such as Avitene, Gelfoam, or Oxycel gauze should be minimized, for hemostasis is less secure, and these agents may be a focus for infection. Their use, however, may be necessary to obtain good hemostatic control. Plastic adhesives such as methyl 2-cyanoacrylate and other homologues of the cyanoacrylate compounds have been used for hemostasis.[58,102]

The number of recommendations made concerning management of specific problems has led to considerable difference of opinion and controversy in published reports.[16] Each recommendation merits specific discussion.

Packs. Early in our experience, gauze packs were used extensively to control bleeding, and at times a pack was simply left in when bleeding could not be controlled in any other way. As techniques for vascular control improved and the availability of blood transfusions increased, use of packs fell into disrepute. In recent years, however, interest in packs has been revived. In some patients packs have been placed around the liver to control hemorrhage, left in place for 2 or 3 days, and removed at a second operation. At the time of the second operation the packs are removed and the damaged liver examined. A liver that is obviously devitalized should be debrided and any remaining bleeding points controlled with suture. In the occasional patient, repacking will be necessary and a third operation must be performed.[23,51,53,54] Packs can also be

Fig. 37-3. a. Damaged area of right lobe has been débrided. b,c. Repair with mattress sutures.

Fig. 37-2. Simple laceration of the right lobe of the liver and repair by suture.

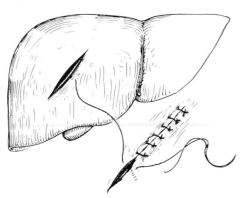

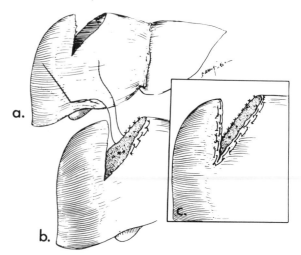

placed in the liver and the ends brought out through a stab wound in the right upper abdominal quadrant so that they can be removed in the ward with the patient under sedation without requiring a second laparotomy. We have removed packs after 4 or 5 days without recurrence of bleeding. Should bleeding recur, however, repacking could be accomplished through the drainage tract without necessarily requiring an additional laparotomy. Stone and Lamb advocated a special type of pack, that is, pedicled omentum, as an autogenous tissue pack for control of hemorrhage. Hemorrhage was controlled in all 37 patients in their report.[92]

Ligation of the Hepatic Artery. Older studies suggested that ligation of the hepatic artery to control hemorrhage was almost uniformly fatal. As experience was gained, however, it was observed that accidental ligation of the right hepatic artery in many persons had no serious consequences, and several years ago, ligation of the hepatic artery was actually recommended for treatment of esophageal varices. The use of hepatic arterial ligation to control massive hemorrhage from hepatic injuries is a relatively recent development. Walt recently reviewed use of this technique.[94] Its primary proponents used it in 59 of 189 patients treated for hepatic injury; 15 of the 59 (24.5%) died. In no other center, however, has hepatic ligation been used as enthusiastically.[59] We have rarely used hepatic arterial ligation and advocate it only after other techniques have failed. If the common hepatic or right hepatic artery is ligated, the gallbladder should be removed, because it may become gangrenous owing to interruption of its blood supply. Interventional radiology has been used to stop hemorrhage by occluding intrahepatic branches of the hepatic artery in selected patients with hepatic trauma.[86]

Major Hepatic Resection. Several years ago, major hepatic resection was enthusiastically advocated to control hemorrhage in the patient with a severely damaged liver. McClelland and associates reported a 20% mortality rate after formal hepatic lobectomy under these circumstances, but most other surgeons were unable to obtain good results, and mortality rates as high as 50% were reported.[61,87] There is general agreement at this writing that conservatism is the preferential approach.[19,49,92,94] Resection of hepatic tissue should, for the most part, be limited to debridement. On rare occasions, a completely shattered lobe may need to be resected, but even under these circumstances, other methods of control of hemorrhage have often been successful (Fig. 37-4).

Management of Hepatic Vein or Retrohepatic Caval Injuries. Because of problems in exposure and because of the need to isolate the liver completely from its vascular supply during the period of repair, hepatic vein and retrohepatic caval injuries have been among the most difficult to treat. A variety of techniques has been advocated, including simple insertion of a Foley catheter into the

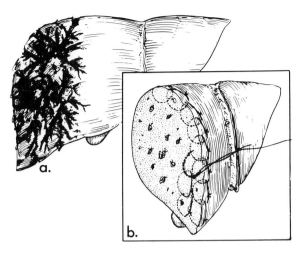

Fig. 37-4. a. Severe contusion and fracture of entire right lobe. **b.** Treatment by right lobectomy. (Redrawn from Shires T: Care of the Trauma Patient. New York, McGraw-Hill, 1966)

vena cava to occlude it, or passage of a catheter into the vena cava through the right atrium and isolation of the liver with tapes around the vena cava above and below the liver to allow return of caval flow to the heart. Coupled with hepatic inflow occlusion, this technique, originally proposed by Schrock, permits complete isolation of the liver.[84] We have used this technique in several additional patients with some success since Bricker and co-workers reported initial success with it in humans (Fig. 37-5).[8] Walt, however, indicated that all nine patients on whom this technique was tried in his institution died, and for that reason, recommended leaving stable, nonexpanding, retroperitoneal, retrohepatic hematomas undisturbed.[94] The technique used in a given patient is dictated by the experience of the surgeon and his assessment of the specific injury.

Drainage. Although many believe that all hepatic wounds should be drained, some think that most patients can be treated without drainage.[25] We advocate drainage of hepatic wounds because secondary hemorrhage or leakage of bile may occur. The drainage allows immediate recognition of bleeding if it occurs and prevents bile peritonitis should a biliary fistula develop (Fig. 37-6).

Drainage of the Common Bile Duct. In 1963, Merendino and associates suggested T-tube drainage of the common bile duct in patients with severe hepatic injuries to maintain minimum pressure in the biliary system and thereby decrease the incidence of biliary fistula.[64] They reported only brief experience, however. Subsequently, Lucas and Walt conducted a controlled study that demonstrated conclusively that the T-tube offered no advantage.[94] In a small duct it might actually impair rather than improve adequate drainage. Biliary fistula is, moreover, rarely a

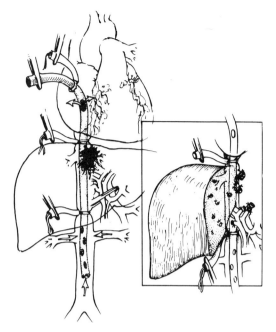

Fig. 37-5. Technique of management of severe wound of left lobe of liver with injury of the left hepatic vein. Total control of hemorrhage is accomplished by placing a vascular clamp across the porta hepatis and passing a shunt through the right atrium into the vena cava to allow occlusion of the hepatic portion of the vena cava without obstructing blood flow from the kidney and lower extremities. The insert demonstrates the completed left hepatic lobectomy. (Bricker DL, et al: Surgical management of injuries to the vena cava: Changing patterns of injury and newer techniques of repair. J Trauma 11:725, 1971)

serious problem, with spontaneous closure the rule; prophylactic insertion of a T-tube is therefore not justified. This method should be reserved for patients with associated injury of the common hepatic or common bile duct.

Although an uncommon complication of hepatic injury, hemobilia may be extremely serious when it does

occur, and surgical control may be difficult. Arteriography provides an accurate diagnosis, and rather than major hepatic resection, as has been required in the past, attempt at treatment with angiographic embolization is justified. Heimbach and associates successfully treated in this manner a patient with false aneurysm that led to hemobilia.[36]

Mortality

The mortality rate for hepatic wounds was extremely high before World War II, exceeding 60% in most series.[4] Madding and Kennedy, however, reported a series of 829 patients treated during World War II with a mortality rate of only 27%,[57] and since that time a progressive decrease has occurred.[1,49,60,98] In the Baylor Affiliated Hospitals, the mortality rate has steadily decreased during the 35 years that we have studied this problem. Despite the fact that, increasingly, more destructive weapons are being used, the mortality rate for gunshot wounds has dropped from 35% in the early years to about 7% in recent years, and for stab wounds the rate has dropped to 1%. Blunt trauma still causes the most lethal injury to the liver. In 1950 the mortality rate for this injury was 70%, but it dropped to 15% in 1983 (Fig. 37-7). This reduction in mortality rates is attributed as much to better overall treatment of the patient with multiple injuries as to the method of treating the hepatic wound.[19] However, these mortality figures represent the result of treatment of those patients who are alive when first seen by a physician. Many patients with hepatic injuries die before reaching the hospital.

Several factors are particularly important in relation to the mortality rate. One is the severity of the injury, for the mortality rate is low in patients who have superficial lacerations. McClelland and associates state that the mortality rate should be 1% or less in patients with small penetrating injuries that involve only the liver,[60] although reports in the literature suggest that this is not achieved by most surgeons. The mortality rate is high for those patients who require resection of large amounts of hepatic tissue. As a corollary, the mortality rate is higher for those patients who are in shock at the time of hospital admission. In the

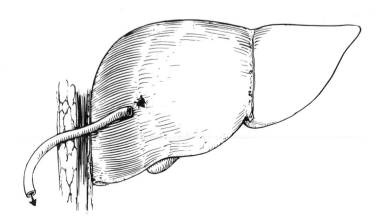

Fig. 37-6. Perforating wound of the liver resulting from passage of a low-velocity bullet. After control of hemorrhage, drainage is instituted.

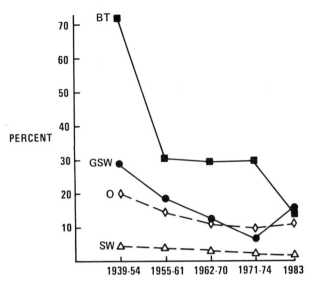

Fig. 37-7. Graph demonstrates changes in mortality rates at the Ben Taub General and Jefferson Davis Hospitals from 1939 to 1974, and the year 1983 according to the wounding agent. BT, blunt trauma; GSW, gunshot wounds; O, overall; SW, stab wounds.

majority of patients, there are injuries to other organs in addition to the wound of the liver. Injuries of the chest occur with greatest frequency, followed by injuries of the stomach. Many patients also sustain fractures and injuries to major vessels (Table 37-3). These injuries are of great importance, for at times the associated injury is more important in prognosis than the injury of the liver (Table 37-4). As the number of associated injuries increases, the complexity of treatment increases. The mortality rate increases with each associated organ or vessel injury (Table 37-5).[19,37,57]

TABLE 37-3. Incidence of Associated Injuries

ASSOCIATED INJURY	INCIDENCE PERCENTAGE
Chest	51
Stomach	31
Small bowel	21
Kidney	20
Colon	19
Major vessel	16
Pancreas	14
Skeletal system	13
Spleen	10
Gallbladder	7
Central nervous system	4
Urinary bladder	1

(Morton JR: Surg Gynecol Obstet 134: 298, 1972)

TABLE 37-4. Mortality Rate with Specific Associated Injuries

ASSOCIATED INJURY	MORTALITY PERCENTAGE
Aorta	73
Inferior vena cava	59
Central nervous system	54
Skeletal	35
Small bowel	27
Colon	23
Kidney	18
Pancreas	18
Esophagus	17

(Morton JR: Surg Gynecol Obstet 134: 298, 1972)

Cause of Death

Hemorrhage with shock is the most common cause of death. In the series of Defore and associates, 71% of deaths were due to this cause, but hemorrhage was more often from another organ or vessel than from the liver itself.[19,20] A variety of factors is responsible for other deaths. Extra-abdominal injuries, such as cerebral trauma, renal insufficiency, pulmonary complications, and infections, are those that occur with greatest frequency. Bile peritonitis is a rare cause of death today and should not exist if proper peritoneal toilet is performed at surgery and adequate drainage instituted.

Complications

A high incidence of nonfatal complications can be anticipated.[50,51] McClelland and associates reported a 20% incidence.[60] The two most common are infection and pulmonary complications. Infections are most often seen in the abdominal wound. Subphrenic abscess, however, is second in frequency, while other intra-abdominal abscesses and intrahepatic infections are uncommon. The

TABLE 37-5. Mortality Rate in Relation to Number of Associated Organs Injured

NUMBER OF ASSOCIATED ORGANS INJURED	MORTALITY RATE	
	Madding and Kennedy[57]	Defore and Associates[19]
0	9.7	4.4
1	26.5	7.7
2	39.7	16.3
3	54.8	25.4
4 (or more—Madding)	84.6	40.7
5 (or more)		72.9

pulmonary complications may be the result of the associated thoracic wounds, whereas others are postoperative atelectasis and pneumonia (Table 37-6). Persistent biliary fistula is unusual and was recorded in only 3% of the Houston series. All biliary fistulas closed spontaneously.[19]

CONGENITAL CYSTS OF THE LIVER

Bristoe is credited with one of the first descriptions of nonparasitic cysts of the liver in a report published in 1856.[52] This author emphasized the association with polycystic renal disease but believed that the association was coincidental. During ensuing years, cystic disease of the liver was recorded relatively infrequently, for as recently as 1955, the report by Melnick indicated that only

two to three cysts were seen per year at the Los Angeles County General Hospital, representing an incidence of one case per 687 autopsies.[62] Recent reports in the literature suggest a possibility that the incidence of congenital hepatic cysts is increasing. Hyde and associates found eight cases during a 10-year period, and Sianesi and associates reported seven cases from the University of Parma in Italy.[41,88] It is entirely possible that more cysts are being found as a result of the more frequent use of ultrasound and CT in the examination of patients with upper gastrointestinal tract complaints.

Primarily Parenchymal

Solitary Cysts

Solitary cysts of the liver may be true cysts with an epithelial lining or false cysts lined by fibrous tissue (Table 37-7).[96] Middleton and Wolper report an experience with a 29-year-old woman with sickle cell disease who developed a fluid-filled cystic mass. They believe that this was a rare complication of sickle cell disease in which hepatic infarct had resulted in the development of a bile cyst.[66] Most true cysts are congenital. Their formation was discussed in detail by Moschcowitz in 1906, and there has been little additional contribution to these concepts in the ensuing years.[68] Moschcowitz presented evidence that cysts arise from aberrant bile ducts or from congenital obstruction caused by inflammatory hyperplasia. This would appear to be adequate explanation for the majority of cysts.

The right lobe is reported to be involved approximately twice as often as the left, although such recordings in most cases are based upon the classic description using the falciform ligament as the line of division of the right and

TABLE 37-6.   Postoperative Complications in 1381 Patients

COMPLICATIONS	PERCENT
Pulmonary	24.4
Atelectasis	9.8
Effusion	5.6
Pneumonia	3.8
Pulmonary insufficiency	2.9
Pneumothorax	1.7
Miscellaneous	0.6
Infection	19.2
Wound	7.8
Subphrenic	5.2
Urinary tract infection	3.1
Sepsis	1.5
Intrahepatic	0.6
Intra-abdominal	0.1
Other	0.9
Fistula	5.7
Biliary	3.0
Pancreatic	1.0
Small bowel	0.7
Colon	0.7
Gastric	0.2
Other	0.1
Hemorrhage	4.2
Liver	1.5
Stress ulceration	1.3
Bleeding diathesis	1.1
Hemobilia	0.2
Intrahepatic hematoma	0.1
Other	6.8
Acute renal failure	2.2
Phlebitis	1.5
Transfusion reactions	1.2
Small-bowel obstruction	1.0
Dehiscence	0.9

(Defore WW Jr et al: Management of 1590 consecutive cases of liver trauma. Arch Surg 111:493, 1976)

TABLE 37-7.   Classification of Hepatic Cysts

I. Congenital
  A. Primarily parenchymal
    1. Solitary
    2. Polycystic disease
  B. Primarily ductal
    1. Localized dilatation of a major intrahepatic duct
    2. Multiple cystic dilatations of intrahepatic ducts ("Caroli's disease")
II. Acquired
  A. Traumatic
  B. Inflammatory
    1. Retention cysts due to inflammatory or calculus obstruction of bile ducts
    2. Hydatid cysts
  C. Neoplastic
    1. Dermoid
    2. Cystadenoma
    3. Degeneration of malignant neoplasms

left lobes, rather than the intrahepatic segmental distribution of bile ducts and vessels (Fig. 37-8). The solitary cyst of congenital origin is unilocular in most instances; in a collection of 189 solitary cysts by Davis in 1937, only 20 were multilocular.[18,30] The cysts are often large, containing 500 ml or more of fluid, and occasionally they become extremely large. One case of a cyst containing 17,000 ml was reported by Burch and Jones.[12]

The contents of the cyst may be thin or thick and vary in color from a clear serous fluid to a bile-colored fluid with a specific gravity of 1.010 to 1.022. Grossly, these cysts are rounded or ovoid, usually well encapsulated and circumscribed. The cyst wall usually comprises an inner layer of cuboidal epithelium surrounded by layers of connective tissue that may contain numerous cellular elements normally found in the liver. There may be large blood vessels in the cyst wall.[33]

Complications that may occur include intracystic hemorrhage, infection, or rupture either into the biliary ductal system or into the free peritoneal cavity. Such complications are rare.

Clinical Features

Solitary cysts are found more frequently in females than in males at a ratio of 4:1. Most occur in the age range of 20 to 50 years, although occasionally cysts are found in the very young or very old. Glanzman and associates, for example, reported a cyst containing 2500 ml of fluid in a 2-year-old child.[29] According to Geist, the oldest patient found in a review of the literature was 82 years old.[28]

Solitary cysts, similar to polycystic lesions, are often asymptomatic and found incidentally at operation or necropsy. A review of the experience at the Mayo Clinic revealed only 38 patients in 47 years, and only 11 of these were operated upon because of symptoms.[38] The rest of the lesions were found incidentally at operation for other conditions. When symptoms do exist, the most common complaint is discomfort due to a large, heavy mass in the right upper abdominal quadrant. Thus, vague abdominal discomfort, nausea and vomiting, and symptoms related to pressure on adjacent viscera are the most common symptoms. The presence of an abdominal mass may also be noted by the patients. Some cysts have appeared so low in the abdomen that the diagnosis of ovarian cyst was entertained preoperatively.[12] The only physical abnormality is a palpable mass in the upper abdomen that moves with respiration. Although the cystic nature of the mass is apparent in some patients, in others is appears to be a hard, solid lesion. In most instances, the mass is located in the right upper abdominal quadrant, although extension to the left upper quadrant may be observed. Torsions with acute pain, strangulation, hemorrhage, and rupture have been reported as complications.

Laboratory Studies. There are no diagnostic laboratory tests. Mild jaundice may occur when pressure on the common bile duct or hepatic ducts occurs, but this is uncommon.[39]

Roentgenographic Findings. Roentgenographic abnormalities depend upon the location of the cyst. The leaf of the diaphragm may be elevated or adjacent organs displaced. Occasionally these cysts develop calcification of the wall, and this may cause confusion in differentiation from echinococcus cyst (Fig. 37-9).

Special radiographic techniques have also been used. An avascular filling defect is visualized by arteriography; this defect suggests the possibility of a cyst but does not permit a definitive diagnosis. Arteriography is indicated in the study of any patient in whom the hepatic lesion may be treated by major hepatic resection. The anatomy of the arterial supply to the liver must be delineated, with special attention to the relation of the lesion to the major hepatic arteries.[65] Recent techniques have proved to be of increasing value. The simplest and least expensive pro-

Fig. 37-8. Large single cyst of right lobe of liver found at necropsy.

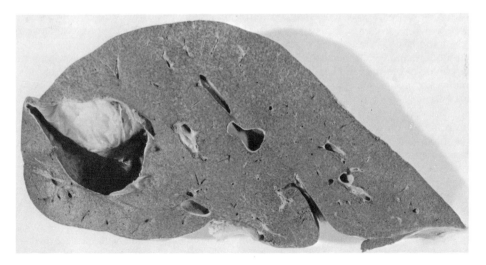

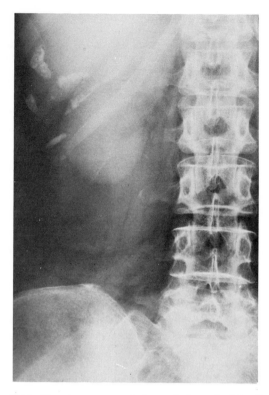

Fig. 37-9. Roentgenogram of a large single cyst arising from the inferior surface of the right lobe of the liver. The overlying renal shadow allows estimation of the large size of this cyst, which measured 5 inches in diameter. On the original film, calcification was visible in the wall, and the possibility of echinococcus cyst was considered.

cedure is ultrasonography.[78,95] Spiegel and co-workers, as well as others, reported use of this technique for diagnosis of primary cysts of the liver.[91] Ultrasonography shows the true cystic nature of a filling defect in the liver. In a study of ten cases by Spiegal and associates, ultrasonography was the most accurate technique for visualizing these lesions and establishing their cystic nature. CT is also accurate in defining intrahepatic cyst and usually will differentiate cystic and solid lesions. Ultrasonography remains the initial study of choice because CT is more expensive.

Liver scanning with use of radioactive materials remains an examination for hepatic lesions. It discloses hepatic pathology but gives no information concerning consistency. Ultrasonography is replacing, or at times complementing, this technique in the evaluation of hepatic cysts.

Treatment. The majority of solitary cysts require no treatment, although if discovered accidentally at time of operation, cysts of less than 8 cm or 10 cm may simply be aspirated. Excision is the treatment of choice for symptomatic superficial cysts, if it can be performed safely. In some patients, the cyst is so large and extends so deeply into the hepatic tissue with proximity to large vessels and bile ducts that excision is hazardous.[18] Longmire and associates have noted that some of the larger cysts have numerous interlacing trabeculae in their walls that may contain sizeable biliary-vascular bundles.[53] Following excision of such a cyst, hemorrhage or the development of biliary fistula may occur as complications. Thus, in some patients, aspiration or unroofing of the cyst and obliteration with suture may be preferable to excision. Furthermore, some of the large cysts may be drained. Simple unroofing of the cyst leaving free communication with the peritoneal cavity has been reported. A preferable approach, however, is internal drainage into a defunctionalized jejunal limb. If the cyst is infected, external drainage is the treatment of choice.

Fernandez and associates have suggested an algorithm for treatment of such cysts. They recommend exploration with simple observation if the cyst is less than 5 cm in diameter.[24] For cysts varying in size from 5 cm to 10 cm, aspiration is performed followed by excision. When the cyst is more than 10 cm in diameter, aspiration also should be performed, but treatment will vary depending upon the contents. When the fluid is clear, partial or total excision is recommended as a treatment of choice. If the cyst contains bile, cholangiography should be performed to determine the exact biliary connection, and treatment is completed with a cystojejunostomy. When blood or pus is aspirated, external drainage should be performed. Roemer and associates have reported patients treated by simple external drainage with a percutaneous catheter placed under radiographic control.[78] Most of these patients, however, refill their cysts with the passage of time, and such treatment cannot be looked upon as definitive.

Few series are large enough to warrant a statement of risk of operative intervention. Beattie and Robertson in 1932 reported a mortality rate of 20% in 62 cases, but Geist, in a review of 122 patients treated from 1924 to 1955, found a mortality rate of only 2.4%.[3,28] In a series reported from the Mayo Clinic there were no deaths.[38] Thus, surgical mortality rates have fallen, and it should be possible to treat such cysts safely.*

Prognosis. Following removal of the cyst the prognosis is excellent. Recurrence is rare.

Polycystic Disease

Polycystic disease of the liver is an embryologic maldevelopment similar to polycystic disease of the kidney. In

---

* The presence of trabeculae on hepatobiliary imagery characterizes hepatobiliary cystadenomas, which are best treated by surgical removal since they may undergo malignant degeneration. (Case Records of the Massachussetts General Hospital. N Engl J Med 313:1275, 1985; Wheeler DA, Edmonson HA: Cystadenoma with mesenchymal stroma (CMS) in the liver and bile ducts. Cancer 56:1434, 1985.)

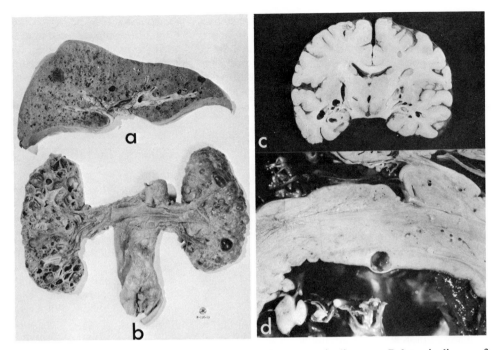

Fig. 37-10. Necropsy specimens from a patient with polycystic disease. **a.** Polycystic disease of the liver with multiple small cysts throughout both lobes. **b.** Bilateral polycystic disease of the kidney. **c.** Cysts of the brain. **d.** Cyst of the myocardium.

fact, when polycystic disease of the liver is found, the possibility of associated cysts of the kidney is high. In collected series, the incidence has been approximately 50%, and other cystic lesions may be found, including cysts of the pancreas, the lung, or the spleen (Fig. 37-10). Furthermore, other congenital abnormalities have been noted.[62] It is of particular significance that cerebrovascular aneurysms have been found in a number of these patients.[11,85] Polycystic liver is diagnosed infrequently during life. Brown reported 8 cases among 11,245 autopsies.[11] The number of cysts varies from two or three to multiple cysts that replace a large portion of hepatic tissue in both lobes (Fig. 37-11). They vary in size from those that are almost microscopic to cysts containing 1000 ml or more of fluid, which usually is brownish in color. Patterson and associates studied the constituents of the cystic fluid in a patient with polycystic disease and compared their findings with information obtained from other reports from the literature on polycystic disease as well as on Caroli's disease and normal human hepatic bile. In their patient the constituents of the fluid resembled the "bile salt–independent" fraction of human bile. It was their belief that their findings supported the hypothesis that such cysts are lined by functioning secretory bile duct epithelium.[74] The hepatic tissue between the cystic lesions is normal in gross appearance and on histologic examination.[15] Rupture, intracystic hemorrhage, and infection represent the pathologic complications, but each of these complications is rare.[62]

Clinical Features. In most reported cases there have been no symptoms, and the cysts were an unsuspected finding at operation or necropsy. In an occasional patient, the large size of the cyst produces abdominal pain due to its weight or due to pressure on surrounding structures. Jaundice due to the pressure of this cyst on bile ducts has been reported, but this complication is rare.[101] When the

Fig. 37-11. Necropsy specimen of polycystic disease of the liver with several cysts in the left lobe only.

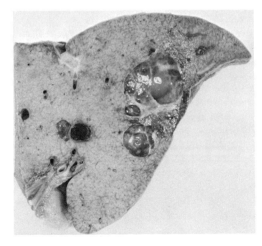

cysts are large, the liver becomes palpable; characteristically it is firm. Although some nodularity may be appreciated, multiple cysts cannot be diagnosed with any degree of certainty on the basis of clinical grounds alone. Temperature is elevated only when infection has occurred or when there has been rupture, and in the latter circumstance there are signs of peritoneal irritation.

Diagnosis. Few patients have symptoms that warrant investigation, and rarely is the diagnosis made preoperatively. Hepatic function tests are usually normal. Roentgenographic studies of the biliary tree and gastrointestinal tract may disclose pressure defects due to an adjacent mass, but there is no characteristic appearance to denote polycystic disease of the liver. Arteriography may suggest cysts by demonstrating filling defects in the liver in the absence of the "tumor stain," but the experience with this test is not sufficient to allow an absolute statement of its reliability. The diagnostic procedures of choice are ultrasonography and CT.

Treatment. No treatment is necessary in most instances. When asymptomatic cysts are found incidentally at operation for other lesions, treatment is not indicated. When symptoms do exist, however, treatment may be directed toward the large cysts that are the cause of symptoms. Occasionally such cysts are present on the surface of the liver and may even be pedunculated such that they can be completely excised. If the cysts cannot be totally excised safely, they may be aspirated and the cyst cavity managed by suture closure, external drainage, or internal drainage through anastomosis to a Roux-en-Y loop of jejunum. Even in symptomatic patients, treatment is limited to the large symptomatic cysts and no effort should be made to eradicate all lesions deeper within the organ.

Other methods of therapy, including the injection of formalin to cause scarring of the cystic cavity, have been suggested, but these can be mentioned only to be condemned. Major hepatic resections have been performed when cysts are limited to one lobe of the liver, but operations of this magnitude are justified only when necessary to relieve life-endangering complications.[7,99]

A rare complication of polycystic disease is the development of portal hypertension. Several cases of esophageal varices have been reported. Ratcliffe and associates reported one patient who died of the complications of her polycystic liver and renal disease, including bleeding from esophageal varices.[77] Laing and associates described bleeding esophageal varices due to portal hypertension in a child treated by percutaneous transhepatic occlusion of the varices and the left gastric vein.[48] During a follow-up period of one year, there was no further hemorrhage. Iannuccilli reported two cases of esophageal varices associated with polycystic disease.[42] In none of these cases was surgical intervention for correction of the esophageal varices undertaken.

Prognosis. Hepatic cysts rarely compromise hepatic function. Surgical treatment of the large cysts relieves symptoms, and the need for a second operation, because of enlargement of the remaining cysts, is uncommon. Prognosis is excellent in contrast to that with cysts of the kidney, which often produce renal insufficiency and death. In fact, the most common cause of death in these patients is renal failure due to polycystic disease of the kidney.

Primarily Ductal

Localized Dilatation of a Major Intrahepatic Duct

Localized dilatation of a major intrahepatic duct is uncommon. Longmire and co-workers reported only three patients in whom there was congenital cystic dilatation of a single duct, all three of which involved the left main duct, although any of the ducts may be involved.[52] Symptoms commonly begin in childhood and consist of recurrent episodes of jaundice, chills, and fever. Diagnosis is made on the basis of cholangiographic findings. The dilatation favors stagnation and incomplete emptying of bile; thus, secondary formation of calculi may develop, and these in turn may cause biliary tract obstruction. The treatment of choice depends upon the site of cystic dilatation and the degree of disease. Those with disease in the peripheral portion of the liver, particularly when excessive stone formation has occurred, are best treated by excision, whereas other patients are best treated by internal drainage with anastomosis to a Roux-en-Y loop.

Multiple Cystic Dilatations of Intrahepatic Ducts ("Caroli's Disease")

Caroli and associates are credited with the first description of general cystic dilatation of the intrahepatic biliary tree. In fact, many authors now refer to it[52] as "Caroli's disease." This lesion is rare, and only a few such cases have been reported. The authors have observed only one such patient (Fig. 37-12). Symptoms consist of abdominal pain, jaundice, and in many instances, weight loss. The liver may be enlarged. Diagnosis is based upon cholangiography, which demonstrates extensive dilatation of all intrahepatic radicals. The treatment of choice is choledochojejunostomy to allow adequate drainage of the ductal system. Following drainage, there may be a decrease in the degree of dilatation, although a decrease to normal size is not anticipated.

ACQUIRED CYSTS OF THE LIVER

Traumatic

Traumatic cysts of the liver appear to be as uncommon as the congenital types, and only a few such cases have

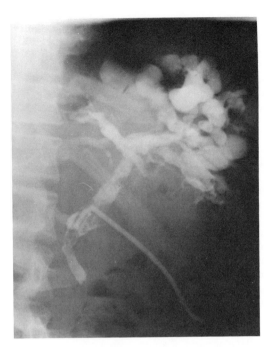

Fig. 37-12. Cystic dilatation of intrahepatic ducts (Caroli's disease).

been reported. Pathologically, they are classified as false cysts, since they are lined by fibrous tissue rather than by epithelial tissue. In our institutions, we have treated more than 2000 patients with liver injuries and to date have not encountered the problem of traumatic hepatic cysts. These cysts have the same potential as other cysts, however. There are no special aspects of treatment.

Inflammatory

Intrahepatic Stones. In the American literature there has often been debate concerning whether or not stones actually form within the liver. Certainly stones may form as a part of congenital cystic disease of the liver. There is considerable evidence, furthermore, that stones do form in the intrahepatic portion of the bile ducts. This, however, appears to be a more common problem in the Oriental population.[2] These patients characteristically have symptoms of right upper abdominal quadrant pain, fever due to secondary infection, and jaundice. Cystic dilatation of the involved ducts may develop. Excision is the treatment of choice, and if there is extensive involvement of an entire lobe, total hepatic lobectomy is justified.[14] In other patients, however, the ductal system may be opened, the stones evacuated, and drainage by Roux-en-Y anastomosis to a loop of jejunum accomplished.

Cystic dilatation of the intrahepatic ducts may occur behind areas of stricture. Symptoms are those of biliary tract obstruction, and treatment consists in elimination of the obstructing lesion.

Hydatid Cysts

Based upon the world experience, the most frequent cyst of the liver is the echinococcus cyst. In fact, in some countries, this probably represents the most common hepatic disease. Even in the United States, hydatid cysts are probably as common as other cysts of the liver, although the majority of cases occur in immigrants from countries in which the disease is endemic. Katz and Pan were able to find only 24 cases in which it appeared that infestation had occurred within the United States.[46] In some other countries of the world, however, particularly where raising of sheep is common and dogs are used as shepherds, the disease is extremely common. Countries with a high incidence include Greece, Uruguay, Argentina, Australia, New Zealand, and South Africa. As recently as 1965, Nicks estimated that 20% to 40% of all dogs in Australia were infected.[71]

Many species of echinococcus have been reported from different parts of the world, but most investigators believe that the same species often has been given a different name when found in a different geographic location. According to D'Alessandro and associates, four species are currently recognized in the genus echinococcus: *Echinococcus granulosus* described by Batsch in 1786, *Echinococcus multilocularis* described by Leuckart in 1863, *Echinococcus oligarthrus* described by Diesing in 1963, and *Echinococcus vogeli* described by Rausch and Bernstein in 1972. D'Alessandro and co-workers consider the status of a fifth species, *Echinococcus cruzi,* to be uncertain.[17]

Echinococcus Granulosus

E. granulosus is the most common form of the disease and has the widest geographic distribution. Two varieties of *E. granulosus* have been described—the pastoral and sylvatic.

Pastoral Form. *Epidemiology.* The dog is the definitive host for this parasitic small tapeworm. The worm is approximately 0.5 cm in length. The characteristic features are a head, commonly termed a scolex, on which are footlets and suckers, a short neck, and three proglottids. The tapeworm grows in the intestine of the dog as the primary host without apparent detriment to the animal. Ova develop in the terminal proglottid, which ruptures and discharges the ova. The ova pass in the feces, thus infecting the intermediate host, the most common of which is the sheep. Pigs, cattle, and humans also serve as intermediate hosts. The intermediate host becomes infected by ingesting material into which ova have passed, and infestation in humans often occurs in childhood because of handling of dogs as pets.

After the intermediate host has ingested the ovum, the outer shell of the ovum is digested by gastric juice and the parasite passes through the portal circulation into the liver, where it may either die or grow into an echinococcus cyst. Infestation may occur in the liver alone, or there may be passage through the liver to involve other organs. At times, other organs are involved in the absence of hepatic disease. Cysts have been reported in virtually all organs of the body; the lungs and brain are two of the most common extrahepatic sites. This cycle is completed when the dogs eat the viscera of infected animals. Thus, this disease can be eliminated if all slaughtered meat is inspected properly and the dog is prevented from ingesting the viscera.

Pathology. The liver is the most common site of echinococcic infestation; approximately 70% of all cysts are found in this organ. The right lobe is most frequently involved, possibly because most of the portal blood from the upper gastrointestinal tract reaches this area. Usually the cysts are single, although multiple cysts may occur. Each cyst consists of an outer layer of adventitia representing a host reaction to the parasite and an inner membrane that contains the growing organism. Typically the cyst fluid is under high pressure and is colorless, although after the passage of time, bile contamination may occur. The cyst grows very slowly and, thus, even with infestation in childhood, symptoms may not occur until adulthood has been reached.

Complications. The most common complication is *rupture* of the cyst as a result of high intracystic pressure (Table 37-8).[55] Harris believed that rupture into the biliary tract is the most common complication.[35] He stated that Deve recorded a 24% incidence of spontaneous cure following such rupture; there was a 30% mortality rate within 6 weeks. In addition to spread of the disease, rupture into the biliary tract may produce obstructive jaundice. The most common site of rupture is into the intrahepatic ducts, although rupture into the common bile duct, cystic duct, and gallbladder has all been reported. Rupture into the peritoneal cavity may occur given that cysts are commonly subserosal. Following rupture into the peritoneum, the cyst may die, and no further difficulty ensues. Hankins

believed that the presence of bile decreases chances of peritoneal implantation.[34] The cysts may implant in the peritoneal cavity, however, and generalized infestation of the peritoneum occurs with slow enlargement of the abdomen. Death may ultimately ensue. The rupture does not usually evacuate the cyst completely; therefore, it may seal with recurrence of the intrahepatic portion of the cyst. It is often stated that rupture of the cyst results in implantation in most instances. Schiller, however, in a long-term follow-up study of 30 patients with documented ruptures of hydatid cysts, found positive evidence of dissemination in only 4.[81] Of the 30 patients, 10 were followed for more than 5 years. All were alive for periods up to 26 years, and 9 were asymptomatic. It thus appears that statistically the chance of dissemination is less than often quoted, but it may constitute a severe problem when it occurs.

Cysts located at the dome of the diaphragm may rupture through the diaphragm into the pleural cavity or into the bronchus. Nicks, in a review of 91 patients with hydatid disease treated in a 5-year period, recorded seven patients with intrapleural rupture from hepatic cysts.[71] This complication may result in a chronic hepatobronchial fistula or the development of an empyema containing both bile and the viable contents of the hepatic cyst. Rupture into other organs may occur because of adherence to the stomach or duodenum. Even rupture into the vena cava has been reported.

The contents of hydatid cysts are usually bacteriologically sterile. Secondary *infection,* however, can occur either from extension to the biliary tract or from septicemia. Active infection of the cyst may result in death of the parasite.

Allergic manifestations to the cyst fluid are common. Urticaria is probably the most common allergic manifestation, but true anaphylactic shock may be observed, particularly in association with rupture of the cyst. Schiller reported a 7% mortality rate from anaphylactic shock after rupture into the peritoneal cavity.[81]

Clinical Features. Many patients with hydatid cysts have no symptoms and remain in good health even though the cyst becomes sufficiently large to be found by palpation on physical examination. In the absence of complications, the only symptoms are vague abdominal distress due to pressure on adjacent organs. With the development of complications, however, significant symptoms develop. Harris described a triad of symptoms typical of rupture into the biliary tract, including (1) biliary colic in an adolescent or young adult; (2) jaundice; and (3) findings of the laminated membrane in the feces.[35] The symptoms are similar to those of cholelithiasis and cholecystitis, and the diagnosis is suspected only if there is other evidence of hydatid disease or if the patient lives in an endemic area. Intraperitoneal rupture, in contrast, is associated with severe symptoms, usually abdominal pain. Shock may occur, as may other signs of sensitivity, and the patient develops the physical findings of an acute abdominal catastrophe. Intrathoracic rupture may be acute or chronic

TABLE 37-8.   Complications of Hydatid Cysts

   I. Rupture
      A. Intrabiliary
      B. Intraperitoneal
      C. Through the diaphragm
         1. Into the pleural space
         2. Into the lung or bronchus
      D. Into other organs
  II. Infection
 III. Allergic manifestations
      A. Urticaria
      B. Anaphylactic shock

and is also characterized by severe pain, as well as dyspnea and coughing when rupture has occurred into the bronchus. When bronchial rupture has occurred, the material expectorated may be bile-stained.

Secondary infection should be suspected if the cyst becomes tender. Chills and fever may follow.

Diagnosis. Several laboratory tests aid in diagnosis. An increase in circulating *eosinophils* (over 7%) is present in one quarter of patients.[76] Eosinophil counts are elevated in a higher percentage of patients with rupture than in those with simple intrahepatic cysts. The standardized *Casoni* test has the widest use and is considered the most reliable immunologic procedure by most investigators. This is performed by injection of 0.2 ml of sterile hydatid fluid intradermally. The positive test is characterized by development of a wheal in 15 minutes and should be compared with a control saline injection. A positive reaction may occur many years after treatment of this disease. In contrast, the *complement fixation test,* which also has a high incidence of positive reaction during the active stage of infection, usually becomes negative within a few months after removal of the cyst. Serologic tests including the indirect hemagglutination, bentonite flocculation, and latex agglutination tests have been reported positive in 82% of patients infected with *E. granulosa.*[45] Recently, immunoelectrophoretic tests have been used with positive results reported in more than 90% of patients. Because no test is uniformly accurate, two tests are often performed. In the past, definite diagnosis of rupture into the common bile duct required surgical intervention, but in recent years, endoscopic retrograde cholangiography has permitted a positive preoperative diagnosis of this complication in some patients.[16] After rupture into the biliary tract, elements of the parasite may be found in the stool, or if there has been rupture into the tracheobronchial tree, the material produced by coughing will contain contents of this cyst.[81]

In endemic areas the roentgenographic finding of a calcific cystic lesion is suggestive of an echinococcic cyst. Uncalcified cysts may also be observed on plain roentgenograms of the abdominal cavity and may displace organs or diaphragm. When gas enters the cyst, the inner membrane falls away from the adventitia and floats on the remaining cyst fluid and produces a picture virtually pathognomonic of the disease. Other roentgenographic techniques include hepatic angiography, tomography, and hepatic scan after the injection of radioactive materials.[47] These tests demonstrate filling defects within the liver but do not allow differentiation from other types of cysts or solid tumors of the same shape.[89] When operation is performed, aspiration of the contents of the cyst will allow identification of the parasite.

Treatment. Treatment of hydatid cysts of the liver was formerly surgical because there was no known drug to which the disease responded favorably. Recently, however, a drug that has some effect on *E. granulosus* has been identified. This drug, mebendazole, has been shown to be effective against the disease in animals. It has also been used in patients with recurrent disease and in those with polycystic disease not amenable to surgical treatment.[5,27] Successful results have been reported, but the reported experience with the drug to date is not large enough to enable definitive evaluation of its efficacy. Present data suggest that it should be used in the treatment of recurrent disease or disease otherwise not amenable to surgical treatment. The treatment of choice for single hepatic cyst today remains surgical, although in the future this drug or other more potent agents conceivably could eliminate the need for surgical treatment in many patients.

Treatment is indicated whenever the diagnosis is made because of the high incidence of complications, many of which terminate fatally. Operation is performed under general anesthesia with an incision made as directly over the cyst as possible. The cyst must be sterilized and removed without contamination of the peritoneal cavity, for spillage of viable parasites may result in development of new cysts in the abdominal cavity. After the liver is well walled off with protective pads and towels, a needle is introduced into the cavity and material aspirated both to relieve pressure within the cyst and to obtain material for microscopic examination. A solution is then injected to kill the parasite before attempts at removal. In the past the most common solution was 2% formalin, which kills the parasite rapidly. Unfortunately, use of this agent has resulted in the deaths of some patients and therefore it is used much less frequently today. A variety of other substances may also kill the parasite. Absolute alcohol (96% alcohol) is as effective as formalin without the same degree of toxicity.[34] Harris advocated the use of 30% saline.[35] After death of the parasite, the lining membrane and all cyst contents are removed. This can be accomplished by surgical resection or aspiration through a large trocar under high negative pressure. The unfortunate consequences of inadvertently spilling viable parasites into the peritoneal cavity with resulting development of intraperitoneal disease have been described by many. This problem is usually avoided by the techniques described above. An ingenious technique for preventing spillage has been reported by Saidi, who devised a funnel to be placed on the dome of the cyst and fused to the cyst cryogenically with use of carbon dioxide to produce a nonleaking connection. The cyst can then be drained through the funnel without danger of spilling into the peritoneal cavity. After evacuation of the cyst, the funnel is removed by thawing and excision of the rim of necrotic tissue around the edge.[80] After the cyst cavity has been evacuated, it may be filled with sterile saline and closed with suture unless it is infected or there is a significant communication with the biliary tree. Most authors advocate external drainage under these circumstances. Harris, however, advocated water-tight closure after filling the cyst with saline even when rupture into the biliary tree has occurred.[35] Other techniques for obliteration of this cyst include filling the cyst with omentum, myoplasty using the rectus muscle,[6] or obliteration around a catheter, producing a method of external drainage.[32]

A variety of other techniques for the treatment of cysts

is advocated in special circumstances. Total excision is recommended for relatively small and easily removed cysts. Some surgeons have used internal drainage by anastomosis to a Roux-en-Y loop or by pericystgastrostomy. Most surgeons reserve pericystgastrostomy for patients who have communication between the biliary tree and the cyst or who have biliary fistulas.[10,21]

When rupture has occurred into the pleural cavity through the diaphragm, a thoracic approach may be necessary. Whether pulmonary lobectomy is required or simple drainage of the pleural cavity suffices depends on the specific complication. In some patients, the intrahepatic portion of the lesion can be treated through the thoracic approach as well, whereas in others, a separate abdominal incision is necessary.

Although most patients can be treated successfully, this disease can be fatal. In a recent report of 212 patients treated surgically, the surgical mortality rate was 3.8% and the recurrence rate was 8.5%.[10]

When complications have occurred, the surgical procedure must be modified to control the problems that result from the complication as well as treatment of the primary cyst. When intrabiliary rupture has occurred, it is important to cleanse the biliary tree and to establish drainage. Following peritoneal rupture, careful cleansing of the peritoneal cavity is important in an attempt to prevent growth of the cyst, although such treatment may not be uniformly successful. Rupture into the pleural cavity may require open drainage and possible decortication, whereas rupture into the bronchus occasionally requires resection of pulmonary tissue for ultimate control.

Sylvatic Form. According to Wilson and associates, a more benign form of *E. granulosus* occurs in North America, particularly in Alaska and Canada.[100] It has a life cycle similar to that of the pastoral form. The dog is the definitive host, and transmittal to humans is almost invariably through contact with dogs. In Alaska and Canada, however, the intermediate hosts are the moose, caribou, and reindeer, rather than cattle and sheep. In the sylvatic form the cystic lesions are reported to be found more commonly in the lungs than in the liver, whereas the reverse is true in the pastoral form. Furthermore, the incidence of serious complications is listed as 0% to 1% for the sylvatic form as compared with 10% to 20% for the pastoral form. Meltzer and co-workers reported cases from West Canada. Wilson and associates reported an additional 101 cases from Alaska with no deaths and few complications in patients with hepatic disease. These writers believe that surgical treatment of hepatic cysts of this type is not justified unless the lesions are symptomatic.[63,100]

Echinococcus Multilocularis

E. multilocularis was originally described by Leukart in 1863. Other authors have identified species that they named *E. alveolaris* and *E. sibiricensis,* as the species were found in different geographic areas of the world. According to Schiller, current opinion supports the concept that these three are all the same species and recommends that the term *E. multilocularis* be used.[82]

Parasitology and Epidemiology. Saidi summarized the comparative parasitology and epidemiology of *E. granulosus* and *E. multilocularis* (Table 37-9).[80] *E. multilocularis* has been found primarily in the Arctic regions, and in North America cases have been reported primarily from Alaskan Eskimos and Canadians. However, cases have been reported in Minnesota.[27] Strains of *E. multilocularis* are very resistant to cold and remain infective even after prolonged exposure to temperatures as low as −50° C (−58° F). The life cycle is similar to that of *E. granulosus.* The dog can serve as the definitive host, although the usual definitive host is the fox, and the usual intermediate hosts are microtine rodents, such as voles, lemmings, and shrews, which form a normal part of the diet for the fox. Some experimental evidence suggests that the domestic cat may also serve as the definitive host in the United States.

Pathology. The pathology differs from that of *E. granulosus* in that the cyst has a minimal laminated membrane. In many instances, there is no true cyst. Saidi described the gross appearance as "a spongy gray gelatinous mass with innumerable small irregular spaces, giving it a Swiss cheese appearance."[80]

Clinical Features. The disease tends to develop slowly over a number of years. Symptoms consist of vague upper gastrointestinal discomfort, anorexia, and loss of weight. Jaundice is often present when the patient is first seen by the physician, in contrast to the findings in *E. granulosus* infection, in which jaundice is not common. The liver is usually palpable and tender.

Diagnosis. The clinical diagnosis of *E. multilocularis* requires a high degree of suspicion. The tests used for *E. granulosus* also yield positive results in alveolar hydatid disease. Little experience with ultrasound has been reported at this writing, but ultrasound or CT might be useful in differential diagnosis.

Treatment. Surgical excision is the recommended treatment.[97] In contrast to the case of *E. granulosus,* however, surgical treatment of *E. multilocularis* requires total excision of all the infected liver for possible cure. In many patients, this requires formal hepatic lobectomy, which some believe is the treatment of choice, because partial lobectomy may be followed by recurrence.[75] In the case reported by Gamble and associates in Minnesota, the patient was asymptomatic 12 months after hepatic lobectomy and the administration of mebendazole.[27] Because hepatic lobectomy may be curative without treatment with mebendazole, the value of this adjuvant therapy remains to be proved.

TABLE 37-9.   Comparative Features of *E. granulosus* and *E. multilocularis*

	E. GRANULOSUS	*E. MULTILOCULARIS*
Geographic distribution	Universal: concentrated in North Africa, South America, Middle East, and Australia	Northern hemisphere: concentrated in the Arctic region, Siberia, and southern Germany
Definitive host	Carnivores, typically dogs, wolves	Carnivores, typically foxes, dogs
Intermediate host	Typically ungulates, exceptionally humans	Typically rodents, exceptionally humans
Adult	4–8 mm in length	2–4 mm in length
No. of testes	Approx. 50	Approx. 25
Distribution of testes	Anterior and posterior to genital pores	From level of genital pores to posterior end of segment
Uterus	Lateral branches	No lateral branches
Larvae		
Rate of development in intermediate host	Slow (years)	Rapid (months), except in humans (years)
Form	Fluid-filled cysts; well encapsulated; well-defined laminated membrane; germinal layer; many scolices	Alveolar, vesicular; interconnected small cysts; poorly differentiated cuticular covering; poorly visible germinal layer and scolices
Growth characteristics	Expanding	Invasive
Host response	Well-defined fibrous adventitial zone	Inflammatory, granulomatous reaction
Organ distribution	Liver 70%, lung 25%, other organs 5%	Liver 90%, lung 5%, brain 5%, other organs?
Immunologic response	Often weak, unless ruptured	Always strong

(Saidi F: Surgery of Hydatid Disease. Philadelphia, WB Saunders, 1976)

Echinococcus Oligarthrus

E. oligarthrus is the only member of the genus known to occur naturally in the strobilar stage in cats. Geographic distribution is limited to Central and South America, including Brazil, Argentina, Panama, and Costa Rica.[17]

Echinococcus Vogeli

D'Alessandro and co-workers reported that *E. vogeli* had been found only in the bush dog, and only recently have human cases been recorded.[17] In 1978 they reported 14 human cases of *E. vogeli* from Colombia, including two polycystic cases involving the liver. The experience in humans with this form of the disease, as well as with *E. oligarthrus,* is limited, and further information will be necessary to define these diseases more specifically.

Neoplastic Cysts

Neuroendocrine Neoplasms. Although cystic neoplasms are rare lesions, a number of types have been reported. Thompson and associates reported one patient in whom there was a cystic neoplasm of neuroendocrine origin that was treated by left hepatic lobectomy.[93] A total of four cysts was found in the specimen.

Cholangiocellular Carcinoma. Imamura and associates performed a right hepatic lobectomy for hepatic tumor.

Four cysts were present in the lobe, one of which was invaded by surrounding cholangiocellular carcinoma, and three of the cysts were epithelialized. They concur with those who believe that cholangiocarcinoma is associated with the development of cysts and is a new entity different from cystadenocarcinoma.[43]

Cystic Hepatoblastoma. Miller notes that cystic hepatoblastoma may resemble simple hepatic cysts on the basis of ultrasonographic characteristics. A distinction can be made by the demonstration of internal septations. This finding is significant because cystic hepatoblastomas have malignant potential and should be treated by removal.[67]

Biliary Cystadenoma. Biliary cystadenomas are rare tumors. Organ and Petrek reviewed this subject in 1984 and stated that fewer than 50 cases have been reported. This tumor is most common in females, with a peak incidence in the fifth decade. Treatment is complete excision, since it is believed that malignant degeneration may occur even though the lesion appears benign.[73]

Hamartoma. Cystic hamartoma is also a rare lesion that has usually been treated by excision.

REFERENCES

1. Baker RJ et al: An assessment of the management of non-penetrating liver injuries. Arch Surg 93:84, 1966

2. Balasegaram M: Hepatic calculi. Ann Surg 175:149, 1972

3. Beattie DA, Robertson HD: A case of simple cyst of the liver, with an analysis of 62 other cases. Lancet 2:674, 1932

4. Beebe GW, De Bakey ME: Battle Casualties. Springfield, IL, Charles C Thomas, 1952

5. Bekhti A et al: Treatment of hepatic hydatid disease with mebandazole: Preliminary results in four cases. Br Med J 2:1047, 1977

6. Bolatzas PC: Myoplasty for the treatment of biliary fistulas due to remaining cavities after surgery for hydatid cysts of the liver. Am J Surg 136:638, 1978

7. Braasch JW: The surgical anatomy of the liver and pancreas. Surg Clin North Am 38:747, 1958

8. Bricker DL et al: Surgical management of injuries to the vena cava: Changing patterns of injury and newer techniques of repair. J Trauma 11:725, 1971

9. Brittain RS: Liver trauma. Surg Clin North Am 43:433, 1963

10. Bros JL: Hydatid disease of the liver. Am J Surg 135:597, 1978

11. Brown RAP: Polycystic disease of the kidneys and intracranial aneurysms. Glasgow Med J 32:333, 1951

12. Burch JC, Jones HE: Large nonparasitic cyst of the liver simulating an ovarian cyst. Am J Obstet Gynecol 63:441, 1952

13. Clagett GP, Olsen WR: Non-mechanical hemorrhage in severe liver injury. Ann Surg 187:369, 1978

14. Clay RC, Finney GG: Lobectomy of the liver for benign conditions. Ann Surg 147:827, 1958

15. Comfort MW et al: Polycystic disease of the liver: Study of 24 cases. Gastroenterology 20:60, 1952

16. Crass RA et al: Selective non-operative management of blunt liver injury using abdominal CT (abstr). J Trauma 24:653, 1984

17. D'Alessandro et al: Echinococcus vogeli in man, with a review of polycystic hydatid disease in Colombia and neighboring countries. Am J Trop Med Hyg 28(2):303, 1979

18. Davis CR: Non-parasitic cysts of the liver. Am J Surg 35:590, 1937

19. Defore WW Jr et al: Management of 1590 consecutive cases of liver trauma. Arch Surg 111:493, 1976

20. Elerding SC et al: Fatal hepatic hemorrhage after trauma. Am J Surg 138:883, 1979

21. Fagarasanu I: Pericystogastrostomy: Internal drainage in the treatment of certain hydatid cysts of the liver. Br J Surg 63:624, 1976

22. Federle MP et al: Computed tomography in blunt abdominal trauma. Arch Surg 117:645, 1982

23. Feliciano DV et al: Intra-abdominal packing for control of hepatic hemorrhage: A reappraisal. J Trauma 21:285, 1981

24. Fernandez M et al: Management of solitary nonparasitic liver cyst. Am Surg 50:205, 1984

25. Fischer RP et al: The value of peritoneal drains in the treatment of liver injuries. J Trauma 18:393, 1978

26. Freeark RJ et al: The role of aortography in the management of blunt abdominal trauma. J Trauma 8:557, 1968

27. Gamble WG et al: Alveolar hydatid disease in Minnesota. JAMA 241:904, 1979

28. Geist DC: Solitary non-parasitic cyst of the liver. Arch Surg 71:867, 1955

29. Glanzman S et al: Treatment of solitary non-parasitic cyst of the liver. NY J Med 60:3684, 1960

30. Gondring WH: Solitary cyst of the falciform ligament of the liver. Am J Surg 109:526, 1965

31. Griswold RA, Collier HS: Blunt abdominal trauma. Surg Gynecol Obstet 112:309, 1961

32. Guedj P et al: Le traitement chirugical actuel du kyste hydatique du foie et de ses principales complications; á propos d'une statistique de 600 kystes opérés. J Chir (Paris) 93:191, 1967

33. Hadad AR et al: Symptomatic nonparasitic liver cysts. Am J Surg 134:739, 1977

34. Hankins JR: Management of complicated hepatic hydatid cysts. Ann Surg 158:1020, 1963

35. Harris JD: Rupture of hydatid cysts of the liver into the biliary tracts. Br J Surg 52:210, 1965

36. Heimbach DM et al: Treatment of traumatic hemobilia with angiographic embolization. J Trauma 18:221, 1978

37. Hellstrom G: Lesions associated with closed liver injury: Clinical study of 192 fatal cases. Acta Chir Scand 131:460, 1966

38. Henson SW Jr et al: Benign tumors of the liver: III. Solitary cysts. Surg Gynecol Obstet 103:607, 1956

39. Hudson EK: Obstructive jaundice from solitary hepatic cyst. Am J Gastroenterol 39:161, 1963

40. Huguet C et al: Tolerance of the human liver to prolonged normothermic ischemia. Arch Surg 113:1448, 1978

41. Hyde GL et al: Solitary nonparasitic hepatic cysts. South Med J 74:1357, 1981

42. Iannuccilli EA, Yu PP: Adult fibropolycystic liver disease and symptomatic portal hypertension. RI Med J 64:551, 1981

43. Imamura M et al: Cholangiocellular carcinoma associated with multiple liver cysts. Am J Gastroenterol 79:790, 1984

44. Judkins MP, Dotter CT: Angiographic diagnosis of intrahepatic rupture secondary to blunt trauma. Northwest Med 64:577, 1965

45. Kagan IG et al: Evaluation of intradermal and serologic tests for the diagnosis of hydatid disease. Am J Trop Med 15:172, 1966

46. Katz AM, Pan CT: Echinococcus disease in the United States. Am J Med 25:759, 1958

47. Kourias B et al: The value of pre- and postoperative scanning in liver echinococcosis. Br J Surg 57:178, 1970

48. Laing IA et al: Percutaneous transhepatic occlusion for bleeding oesophageal varices in polycystic disease. Arch Dis Child 56:954, 1981

49. Levin A et al: Surgical restraint in the management of hepatic injury: A review of Charity Hospital experience. J Trauma 18:399, 1978

50. Lim RC Jr et al: Postoperative treatment of patients after liver resection for trauma. Arch Surg 112:429, 1977

51. Lim RC Jr et al: Prevention of complications after liver trauma. Am J Surg 132:156, 1976

52. Longmire WP et al: Congenital cystic disease of the liver and biliary system. Ann Surg 174:711, 1971

53. Longmire WP Jr: Hepatic surgery: Trauma, tumors, and cysts. Ann Surg 161:1, 1965

54. Lucas CE, Ledgerwood AM: Prospective evaluation of hemostatic techniques for liver injuries. J Trauma 16:442, 1976

55. Macris GJ, Galanis NN: Rupture of echinococcus cysts of the liver into the biliary ducts. Am Surg 32:36, 1966

56. MacVaugh H III et al: Traumatic hemobilia. Surgery 60:547, 1966

57. Madding GF, Kennedy PA: Trauma to the Liver. Philadelphia, WB Saunders, 1965

58. Matsumoto T et al: Higher homologous cyanoacrylate tissue adhesives in surgery of internal organs. Arch Surg 94:861, 1967

59. Mays ET et al: Hepatic artery ligation. Surgery 86:536, 1979

60. McClelland RN et al: Liver trauma. In Shires GT (ed): Care of the Trauma Patient, chap 18, pp 374–383. New York, McGraw-Hill, 1966

61. McClelland RN et al: Hepatic resection for massive trauma. J Trauma 4:282, 1964

62. Melnick PJ: Polycystic liver. Arch Pathol 59:162, 1955

63. Meltzer H et al: Echinococcus in North American Indians and Eskimos. Can Med Assoc J 75:121, 1965

64. Merendino KA et al: The concept of surgical biliary decompression in the management of liver trauma. Surg Gynecol Obstet 117:285, 1963

65. Michels NA: Newer anatomy of the liver and its variant blood supply and collateral circulation. Am J Surg 112:337, 1966

66. Middleton JP, Wolper JC: Hepatic biloma complicating sickle cell disease. Gastroenterology 86:743, 1984

67. Miller JH: The ultrasonographic appearance of cystic hepatoblastoma. Radiology 138:141, 1981

68. Moschcowitz E: Non-parasitic cysts (congenital) of the liver with a study of aberrant bile ducts. Am J Med Sci 131:674, 1906

69. Murray DH Jr et al: Tourniquet control of liver bleeding. J Trauma 18:771, 1978

70. Nelson EW et al: Spontaneous hepatic rupture in pregnancy. Am J Surg 134:817, 1977

71. Nicks R: Intrapleural rupture of hydatid cysts. Med J Aust 1:352, 1965

72. Okuda K et al: Frequency of intrahepatic arteriovenous fistula as a sequela to percutaneous needle puncture of the liver. Gastroenterology 74:1201, 1978

73. Organ B, Petrek J: Biliary cystadenoma. South Med J 77:262, 1984

74. Patterson M et al: Polycystic liver disease, a study of cyst fluid constituents. Hepatology 2:475, 1982

75. Quattlebaum JK, Quattlebaum JK Jr: Technic of hepatic lobectomy. Ann Surg 149:648, 1959

76. Rakower J: Echinococcosis: A survey of 100 cases. Trop Dis Bull 58:344, 1961

77. Ratcliffe PJ et al: Bleeding oesophageal varices and hepatic dysfunction in adult polycystic kidney disease. Br Med J Clin Res 288:1330, 1984

78. Roemer CE et al: Hepatic cysts: Diagnosis and therapy by sonographic needle aspiration. AJR 136:1065, 1981

79. Root HD et al: Diagnostic peritoneal lavage. Surgery 57:633, 1965

80. Saidi F: Surgery of Hydatid Disease. Philadelphia, WB Saunders, 1976

81. Schiller CF: Complications of echinococcus cyst rupture. JAMA 195:220, 1966

82. Schiller EL: Editorial: Echinococcosis in North America. Ann Intern Med 52:464, 1960

83. Schorn L, Coln D: Hepatic angiographic changes after trauma. Am J Surg 134:754, 1977

84. Schrock T et al: Management of blunt trauma to the liver and hepatic veins. Arch Surg 96:698, 1968

85. Schwartz SI: Surgical Diseases of the Liver. New York, McGraw-Hill, 1964

86. Sclafani SJA et al: Interventional radiology in the management of hepatic trauma. J Trauma 24:256, 1984

87. Serge H: Etude sur l'independence anatomique et physiologique des lobes du foie. M Med Bordeaux 32:327, 341, 357, 1902

88. Sianesi M: Symptomatic non-parasitic congenital cysts of the liver. Int Surg 67:453, 1982

89. Sodeman WA Jr, Haynie TP: Hepatic photoscanning in hydatid liver cysts. JAMA 188:318, 1964

90. Sparkman RS: Massive hemobilia following traumatic rupture of the liver. Ann Surg 138:899, 1953

91. Spiegel RM et al: Ultrasonography of primary cysts of the liver. AJR 131:235, 1978

92. Stone HH, Lamb JM: Use of pedicled omentum as an autogenous pack for control of hemorrhage in major injuries of the liver. Surg Gynecol Obstet 141:92, 1975

93. Thompson NW et al: Cystic neuroendocrine neoplasms of the pancreas and liver. Ann Surg 199:158, 1984

94. Walt AJ: The mythology of hepatic trauma—or Babel revisited. Am J Surg 135:12, 1978

95. Weaver RM Jr et al: Gray scale ultrasonographic evaluation of hepatic cystic disease. AJR 130:849, 1978

96. Wellwood JM et al: Large intrahepatic cysts and pseudocysts. Am J Surg 135:57, 1978

97. West JT et al: Alveolar hydatid disease of the liver: Rationale and technics of surgical treatment. Ann Surg 157:548, 1963

98. Williams LF Jr, Byrne JJ: Trauma to the liver at Boston City Hospital from 1955–1965. Am J Surg 112:368, 1966

99. Wilson H, Wolf RY: Hepatic lobectomy: Indications, technique, and results. Surgery 59:472, 1966

100. Wilson JF et al: Cystic hydatid disease in Alaska: A review of 101 autochthonous cases of echinococcus granulosus infection. Am Rev Respir Dis 98:1, 1968

101. Wittig JH et al: Jaundice associated with polycystic liver disease. Am J Surg 136:383, 1978

102. Wojnar VS et al: Liver, spleen, and kidney wounds: Experimental repair with topical adhesive. Arch Surg 89:237 1964

chapter 38
Postoperative Jaundice

FRANK G. MOODY and DAVID A. THOMPSON

A variety of factors during or following an operation may challenge the liver and result in postoperative jaundice. In most cases, however, the jaundice is low grade, of short duration, and of no consequence to the clinical outcome.[20] Progressive jaundice, however, in association with other signs of liver dysfunction, may predict the onset of fulminant hepatic failure, which may result in a devastating illness and death. The purpose of this chapter is to emphasize those features of postoperative jaundice that indicate that careful evaluation be done versus those that are associated with spontaneous resolution. We will discuss strategies in diagnosis and treatment designed to minimize the effects of this potentially disastrous complication. It is important to recognize at the outset that there is no substitute for a well-planned and carefully performed operation in order to minimize disturbances in hepatobiliary function. A thoughtful, logical approach to a problem of postoperative jaundice is far superior to a hasty, ill-conceived reoperation.

PATHOGENESIS

Although postoperative jaundice is usually of multifactorial origin, it can be classified under three basic pathophysiologic headings: (1) overproduction of bilirubin, (2) impaired hepatocellular function, and (3) obstruction to the flow of bile. The major factors leading to postoperative jaundice are listed in Table 38-1.

Overproduction of Bile

When the amount of bilirubin presented to the liver exceeds the metabolic capacity of the organ, then elevation of the serum bilirubin level occurs. Although this bilirubin is predominantly unconjugated, Tisdale and co-workers[64] reported an elevation of the level of conjugated bilirubin in patients who had been infused with unconjugated bilirubin. This outcome suggests that excessive bilirubin may induce an element of cholestatic hepatocellular dysfunction.

The normal turnover of red blood cells results in a production of about 250 mg of bilirubin daily. Acceleration of this turnover is seen in the red blood cells of stored blood. Within 24 hours after transfusion, approximately 10% of 14-day-old blood and 20% of 21-day-old blood undergoes hemolysis. This results in production of 250 mg and 500 mg of bilirubin, respectively.[34,44]

When several units of blood are transfused in a short period of time, the ability of the liver to metabolize and excrete the bilirubin may be exceeded. This is likely to occur when the need for blood transfusion is associated with hypovolemic shock, which impairs the liver's metabolic function.

It has been shown experimentally that infusion of hemoglobin into humans causes a maximal rise in bilirubin 3 to 10 hours after transfusion.[21] Scott and associates,[59] studying battle casualties in Korea, found that hyperbilirubinemia occurred within 48 hours after blood transfusion. Hence, an early rise in the serum bilirubin level may result in cases in which large amounts of stored blood are transfused, especially when it is associated with compromised hepatocellular function.

Extravasated blood sequestered in body tissues or cavities is gradually catabolized to bilirubin. Although the amount of extravasated blood may be difficult to assess accurately, each 500 ml of blood will result in the formation of approximately 2500 mg of bilirubin.[32] A mild to moderate rise in the level of serum bilirubin of from 3 mg to 10 mg/dl may last as long as 7 to 10 days during absorption of large collections of blood.[45]

Hemolytic transfusion reactions due to incompatibility of transfused blood are rare.[73] The intravascular destruction of red blood cells results in the release of free hemoglobin, which may cause renal injury. The intracellular lipid released when the red cells are lysed may precipitate disseminated intravascular coagulation. Although the amount of bilirubin produced from the hemoglobin released may be small, the hepatic parenchyma may be directly injured during the immunologic reaction, thus impairing its ability to metabolize the bilirubin. Also, the renal parenchymal injury may result in a decreased rate of excretion of conjugated bilirubin. These mechanisms may result in significant hyperbilirubinemia. Rudowski[56] reported jaundice in 40% of a large series of cases of hemolytic transfusion reactions.

Patients with congenital or acquired hemolytic anemia may experience an increase in the rate of red cell destruction as a result of an operation. This is probably related to red cell hypoxia, which may occur in cases of systemic hypoxemia and hypotension. Patients with congenital deficiencies of glucose-6-phosphate dehydrogenase (G6PD)

TABLE 38-1. Classification of Postoperative Jaundice

Overproduction of bilirubin
  Hemolysis
  Blood transfusions
  Resorption of hematoma
  Open-heart surgery; prosthetic valves
Impaired hepatocellular function
  Hepatocellular injury
    Drug-related toxicity
    Viral hepatitis
    Ischemic/hypoxia injury
    Hepatic resection
  Cholestatic pattern
    Drugs
    Sepsis
    Benign postoperative cholestasis
Extrahepatic obstruction to bile flow
  Bile duct injury
  Choledocholithiasis
  Pancreatitis

may also experience increases in hemolysis when treated with drugs such as sulfonamides, chloramphenicol, and aspirin.[36] Appropriate preoperative screening should identify most patients with underlying blood dyscrasias of this type. Preoperative screening and appropriate anesthetic management will do much to preclude increased hemolysis in these situations.

Jaundice was observed in 23.4% of patients in a recent prospective study of patients undergoing cardiopulmonary bypass.[10] Of the factors evaluated, hypoxia was found to be the most significant. Other important contributing factors were the preoperative severity of right-sided heart failure and the amount of blood transfused during or shortly after operation. Age, sex, underlying cardiac lesions, operative procedure, and duration of cardiopulmonary bypass were not predictive of postoperative jaundice. Although it is known that cardiopulmonary bypass and prosthetic cardiac valves do shorten the survival of red blood cells, these factors do not contribute significantly to the development of jaundice.[2,39]

Autoimmune hemolytic anemia has been reported following aortic valve replacement.[49] This problem is aggravated by repeated blood transfusions and may require treatment with steroids.

Massive hemolysis resulting in jaundice may occur in association with infection due to *Clostridium welchii*.[31] The problem occurs within 24 to 72 hours after operations on the stomach, biliary tract, or colon. Although fever and leukocytosis may not be dramatic, the diagnosis can be suspected when there is an acute rise in the serum bilirubin level associated with signs of clostridial wound infection. Despite the hemolysis, the majority of the bilirubin may be conjugated in such cases.

Pulmonary embolism, especially when associated with

pulmonary infarction, has been associated with mild degrees of hyperbilirubinemia. The mechanism causing jaundice in this situation appears related to the release of hemoglobin from hemorrhage at the infarct site. Cardiopulmonary dysfunction with its associated hypoperfusion and hypoxia may be implicated in cases with extensive embolization of the pulmonary artery. Also, the resultant increase in pressure in the right side of the heart may cause passive congestion of the liver and result in hepatic dysfunction.[60]

Hepatic Dysfunction

Uncomplicated operations are rarely associated with significant or prolonged hepatic disturbance.[11] The normal liver possesses considerable functional reserve and will tolerate hepatic arterial ligation or major hepatic resection with surprisingly little change in the serum bilirubin value.[1,13,46]

A combination of adverse factors, however, may diminish the functional capacity of the liver sufficiently to cause inadequate bilirubin metabolism, resulting in jaundice. Factors such as shock, hypoxia, sepsis, hepatotoxic drugs, direct liver trauma or resection, and preexisting congenital or acquired hepatic disease may act alone or in combination to produce hepatocellular dysfunction.

This hepatic disturbance can be considered a manifestation of one or the other of two pathologic processes: (1) direct hepatocellular damage (hepatitis-like pattern) and (2) intrahepatic cholestasis (resembling the jaundice caused by obstruction to the biliary tree).

Hepatocellular necrosis is characterized clinically by a marked rise in the serum transaminases, a prolonged prothrombin time, and variable elevations of both unconjugated and conjugated bilirubin. The alkaline phosphatase level is only mildly elevated in most cases.

Intrahepatic cholestasis produces a pattern of enzyme elevation similar to extrahepatic biliary obstruction. The alkaline phosphatase value in such situations may be markedly elevated, and the bilirubin elevation, at least in the initial stages, is predominantly of the conjugated type. The transaminases are usually only mildly elevated initially, but they may increase with longstanding cholestasis.

Ischemia and Hypoxia

Hypoxia results in progressive hepatocellular damage, which may eventually result in centrilobular necrosis.[47] Traditionally, it has been thought that the normal liver would tolerate only 15 to 20 minutes of normothermic total ischemia and that progressively more serious cellular disruption would occur when the period of ischemia was prolonged beyond 30 minutes. This belief resulted from studies in dogs,[16,52] animals which are particularly susceptible to portal sepsis and also have hepatic vein sphincters that may contract in response to ischemia.

Studies in pigs,[27] which are like humans in that they do not have hepatic vein sphincters, have shown that a

90% reduction in blood flow can be tolerated for 90 minutes, but severe disturbances in liver function and some deaths may occur after 180 minutes.

Occlusion of the portal triad at the free edge of the gastrohepatic ligament (Pringle's maneuver) is occasionally necessary for even longer periods of time in the intraoperative management of traumatic liver injuries. Ligation of the main hepatic artery or one of its major branches is also occasionally required to control bleeding in this situation. Unrecognized ligation of the right hepatic artery may sometimes occur during cholecystectomy. The normal liver usually tolerates hepatic arterial ligation without significant sequelae in both of these situations.[1] When significant preoperative liver disease exists, however, or when extensive mobilization of the liver precedes arterial ligation, massive liver necrosis may follow.[18] In the latter case, division of the ligamentum and triangular ligaments of liver may prevent the development of hepatic arterial collateral vessels, which would otherwise occur very rapidly and reduce the extent of the ischemic insult.

In a study by Nunes,[47] only 2% of patients who experience shock following major trauma (excluding liver trauma) developed significant jaundice. Histologic examination of the liver in these cases showed centrilobular congestion and occasionally necrosis with bile stasis. The serum hepatic enzyme changes showed predominantly conjugated hyperbilirubinemia and elevation of the alkaline phosphatase level consistent with intrahepatic cholestasis.

In a study of postoperative massive liver necrosis,[4] it was found that clinical jaundice occurred in only 20% of cases associated with shock. In such cases, shock had usually persisted for several hours and was often associated with severe congestive heart failure.

Kantrowitz[32] reported four cases in which marked hyperbilirubinemia (23 mg to 39 mg/dl) developed following operation for control of massive hemorrhage. The pattern was consistent with intrahepatic cholestasis, and there were only mild abnormalities of hepatic morphology. Rich[53] found that hypoxia leads to decreased hepatic excretory function, but he emphasized that jaundice does not occur unless there is a concomitant increase in bilirubin production. Cooling has a beneficial effect, as has been shown in hepatic transplantation where the donor liver is protected from ischemic injury for up to 12 hours when perfused by a cold salt solution.[8]

Infection

Several types of extrahepatic infections may cause or contribute to the development of postoperative jaundice,[46,75] including pneumonia,[66,74] gram-negative bacteremia (especially in children),[54] intra-abdominal abscess due to a variety of organisms,[42] and pyelonephritis.[3]

The jaundice associated with generalized sepsis usually appears within a few days of the onset of bacteremia.[75] In almost all cases, the infection is but one of several factors that contribute to hyperbilirubinemia. Indeed, in no case

was sepsis the sole cause of the jaundice in a study of a large population of jaundiced hospitalized patients.[30]

Biochemical and histologic parameters indicate that intrahepatic cholestasis occurs in such cases.[43,75] Studies by Utili and co-workers[67] point to the effect of endotoxin on the hepatic sodium potassium ATP-ase as a possible cause of cholestasis.

In a study of 1140 bacteremic patients, Vermillion[68] reported a 0.6% incidence of jaundice. Another study of 30 patients who developed jaundice during the course of severe bacterial infection showed a mortality of 43%[45]; however, a large proportion of the patients in this group had associated renal impairment that would contribute to the hyperbilirubinemia. There was no correlation between the degree or duration of jaundice and prognosis, although all patients who died had persistent jaundice. It seems that hepatic dysfunction associated with sepsis has little effect on the survival compared with the infection itself.[75]

Identification and successful treatment of infection that develops in the postoperative period is usually effective in helping to resolve the associated jaundice.

The viral hepatitides are a well-known cause of postoperative jaundice that adversely affect the operative mortality and morbidity. They have been thoroughly discussed in Chapter 15.

Drugs

Although drugs per se are an infrequent cause of jaundice,[45] many of the drugs used in the postoperative period have been associated with jaundice. Drugs can affect the metabolism of bilirubin at any stage during its production, transportation to and into liver cells, conjugation, and canalicular excretion. Drugs that are hepatotoxic may produce cellular injury directly or indirectly from a metabolite of the drug.[55] Hypersensitivity reactions may also cause hepatocellular dysfunction and on occasion massive liver necrosis and death. In such cases, a clue to the correct diagnosis may be history of allergic manifestations such as urticaria, arthralgia, fever, and eosinophilia.[69]

Hepatic dysfunction may be due primarily to hepatocellular necrosis (Table 38-2) or intrahepatic cholestasis (Table 38-3). An association between the administration of the anesthetic agent halothane and postoperative liver necrosis was reported in 1958.[69] Since then, several similar reports have appeared, but the findings remain inconclusive. A large National Institutes of Health–sponsored study,[7] published in 1969, reported 82 cases of fatal hepatic necrosis following some 850,000 anesthetics. Only seven of those deaths occurred following halothane administration, yielding an overall incidence of fatal halothane-associated hepatic necrosis of approximately 1 in 35,000.

Two prospective studies reported an increased incidence of raised serum transaminase levels in patients receiving halothane.[65,72]

Direct hepatocellular injury seen as centrilobular necrosis is typical in such cases.[51] In an extensive review of

TABLE 38-2.   Hepatotoxic Agents

GENERAL ANESTHETICS
Chloroform
Trichlorethylene
Halothane
Methoxyflurane
Fluroxene
Enflurane

ANTIDEPRESSANTS
Iproniazid and congeners
Amitriptyline

ANTICONVULSANTS
Phenylacetylurea and congeners
Diphenylhydantoin

ANTI-INFLAMMATORY/ANALGESICS
Cinchophen
Zoxazolamine
Ibufenac
Indomethacin
Phenylbutazone
Salicylates
Acetaminophen
Probenecid

DRUGS FOR ENDOCRINE DISEASE
Carbutamide
Propylthiouracil
Methahexamide
Acetohexamide

ANTIMICROBIALS
Tetracycline
Chloramphenicol
Triacetyloleandomycin
Penicillin
Griseofulvin
p-Aminosalicylic acid
Nitrofurantoin
Isoniazid
Ethionamide
Pyrazinamide
Rifampicin
Sulfonamides
Sulfones

DRUGS FOR CARDIOVASCULAR DISEASE
Phenindione
Procainamide
Quinidine
α-Methyldopa
Nicotinic acid
Papaverine

ANTINEOPLASTICS: STEATOSIS
Dactinomycin
4-Aminopyrazolopyrimidine
L-Asparginase
Azacytidine
Azauridine
Bleomycin
Mitomycin
Cycloheximide
Chromomycin
N-Diazocetyglycine hydrade
Puromycin
Methotrexate

ANTINEOPLASTICS: NECROSIS
Calvacin
Mithramycin
Chlorambucil
Urethane
Chlorphosphamide
6-Mercaptopurine

MISCELLANEOUS AGENTS
Tannic acid
Trimethobenzamide
Tripelennamine
Oxyphenisatin
Phenazopyridine
Disulf

INTRINSIC
Iodide ion

the topic, Stock and Stunin[62] concluded that severe liver damage is unlikely to follow a single exposure to halothane in a previously healthy individual, but repeated exposures, especially in obese, middle-aged women, may result in severe liver damage. Administration of repeated halothane anesthesia to children on the other hand seems to be quite safe.[70] The etiology of halothane hepatotoxicity remains unclear.[62]

Prospective studies of hepatic dysfunction after repeated enflurane anesthesia administration have shown very little hepatic dysfunction.[17] As yet, there are no reports of hepatoxicity following isoflurane administration.

Halothane should not be administered subsequently if a patient shows signs of hepatic dysfunction following its administration. In cases of unexplained postoperative jaundice, the patient's record should be reviewed to determine the type of anesthesia used.

The use of cyclosporine as an immunosuppressive agent has been associated with mild elevations of the serum transaminases and alkaline phosphatase values, but clinical jaundice associated with its use has not been reported.

When postoperative jaundice occurs in liver transplant patients, it is often difficult to determine if the jaundice is due to hypoxia, rejection, the toxic effects of many drugs

TABLE 38-3.   Cholestatic Agents

TRANQUILIZERS
Chlorpromazine and related phenothiazines
Ectylurea
Chlordiazepoxide
Diazepam

ANTIDEPRESSANTS
Imipramine

ANALGESICS
Propoxyphene

DRUGS FOR ENDOCRINE DISEASE
Methimazole
Thiouracil
Chlorpropamide
Estradiol
Tolbutamide
C-17 alkylated anabolic
Contraceptive steroids

ANTIMICROBIALS
Erythromycin estolate
Rifampicin
Organic arsenicals
Nitrofurantoin
Idoxuridine
Xenylamine

DRUGS FOR CARDIOVASCULAR DISEASE
Ajmaline

ANTINEOPLASTICS
4,4'-Diaminodiphenylamine
Azathioprine
Busulfan

MISCELLANEOUS
Carbamazepine
Penicillamine

being used, or the amount of blood transfused. Liver biopsy, immunologic testing, and radiologic visualization of the biliary system should be done early in such situations and appropriate treatment begun.[8]

The fasting associated with an operation may contribute to the development of mild hyperbilirubinemia. The unconjugated bilirubin level is increased in such cases and may be clinically apparent in patients with Gilbert's disease.[33] The use of total parenteral nutrition in the perioperative period has also been associated with mild elevation in the serum bilirubin level in 20% to 25% of patients.[26,38] Clinical jaundice is unusual in the absence of shock, infection, or multiple transfusions. Fatty infiltration of the liver has been produced in animals by administering intravenous hypertonic glucose without protein.[9,61] Other evidence suggests that a deficiency of the central fatty acids plays a role in the development of cholestasis.[50] The use of less-concentrated glucose solution and addition of in-

travenous fat preparations may be helpful in patients with postoperative jaundice.

As one might expect, patients with preexisting liver disease, such as congenital metabolic defects, hepatitis, and cirrhosis, are more likely to develop postoperative jaundice, especially following a prolonged or complicated operation.[28,35,37] When possible, the operation should be postponed in such cases. When the operation is mandatory, every effort should be made to prevent hypotension and hypoxia while performing an expeditious operation.

Extrahepatic Obstruction

Mechanical obstruction to the flow of bile in the postoperative period is uncommon.[45] Nevertheless, a technical mishap during the operation in the area of the extrahepatic bile duct may occur with resulting interference to bile flow.[23,41] Injury to the bile duct is most commonly seen following cholecystectomy[24] but may also occur following distal gastrectomy or other operations in the area of the head of the pancreas and blunt and penetrating traumatic injuries.

Theoretically, complete obstruction of the common bile duct results in a daily rise in the level of serum bilirubin of 0.5 mg/dl/day, assuming there is no increase in bilirubin production and normal renal function. As the bilirubin level rises, progressively more is lost in the urine until the rate of renal loss equals the rate of production that occurs at bilirubin levels of 25 mg to 30 mg/dl.[57] When renal failure is present, bilirubin levels of 80 mg/dl may be seen.[45] Complete bile duct obstruction is associated with a marked rise in alkaline phosphatase levels, and the serum glutamic-oxaloacetic transaminase (SGOT) level may temporarily reach very high levels (1000 units).[19]

When choledocholithiasis or common bile duct stricture results in jaundice, it is usually not as severe and often varies in its intensity.[23] Choledocholithiasis may occur after nonbiliary operations or following cholecystectomy or even common bile duct exploration. In the latter case, a T-tube will normally have been placed in the common bile duct. The treatment options in this situation are increased, and, as will be discussed later, the diagnosis can be difficult in a patient who has just undergone laparotomy and is receiving narcotics and sedatives.

On rare occasions, a gallstone impacted in the cystic duct will cause associated obstruction of the hepatic duct. This problem has been termed *Mirizzi's syndrome*.[5] Postoperative acute cholecystitis, however, may be associated with mild jaundice in approximately one third of cases even in the absence of bile duct obstruction.[29] The diagnosis is often difficult in such situations, especially in cases of acalculous cholecystitis, which will be discussed below.

Occasionally blood may collect in the bile duct lumen following cholecystectomy, resulting in obstruction, which may require reoperation for relief.[14]

A biliary fistula may develop proximal to the point of ductal obstruction or following unrecognized ductal injury. In such cases, jaundice may be associated with symptoms and signs of bile peritonitis.

Acute postoperative pancreatitis occasionally occurs after gastric biliary or pancreatic surgery and results in jaundice in approximately 30% of cases.[58] Partial obstruction of the common bile duct occurs as a result of the inflammatory process, which no doubt contributes to the development of hepatocellular dysfunction as well. Jaundice can be expected to clear as the pancreatitis resolves unless a pancreatic pseudocyst or abscess develops.

CLINICAL ASPECTS

Postoperative Assessment

The occurrence of jaundice in the early postoperative period, especially when unexpected, presents a challenge in diagnosis. As discussed extensively previously, a variety of etiologic possibilities exists. The nature of the underlying disease being treated and the nature and details of the surgery are the two most important considerations in the initial phase of evaluating a patient with this problem. Important information can be gleaned from a careful review of the hospital chart. A discussion with the surgeon regarding findings at operation and knowledge of the patient's condition during and immediately after the procedure are essential to the diagnostic process. Attention should be given to the type of anesthetic employed, the drugs administered during the perioperative period, the length of the procedure, and the presence or absence of hypotension, hypoxia, or the need for blood administration. Intra-abdominal operations usually provide information on the status of the liver, gallbladder, biliary tree, and pancreas. One must keep in mind, however, that small gallstones may fail to be detected at the time of exploratory laparotomy and that feeding after an operation may cause the passage of a gallstone into the bile duct.

The immediate postoperative state places serious restraints on the reliability of a history and physical examination. Assisted ventilation, analgesics, and an abdominal incision place formidable barriers to assessment of the status of the liver and adjacent organs. In addition, the patient's general condition may preclude movement to the imaging center for special tests. We will discuss below and present examples as to how some of these challenges can be successfully met in the environment of a tertiary care medical center where the full array of consultants and diagnostic technology exists.

Operations Remote from the Abdomen

Procedures at sites distant from the abdomen usually allow access to a standard diagnostic approach to a jaundiced patient. The abdomen, for example, can be evaluated by auscultation, percussion, and palpation. Distention, absence of bowel sounds, and abdominal tenderness, especially in the right upper quadrant, suggest a primary biliary origin of the jaundice. An infected wound, or signs of pneumonia, on the other hand, would draw attention to the possibility of the jaundice of sepsis.

Initial laboratory evaluation should include a hemogram, white blood cell count, and serum analysis for bilirubin with fractions, transaminase, γ-glutamyl transferase, alkaline phosphatase, albumin, and prothrombin time.

Further tests such as serum amylase, serologic tests for evidence of viral hepatitis, and screening for intravascular hemolysis should be ordered as indicated at this point.

If the enzyme pattern is consistent with hepatocellular damage, careful observation and serial measurements of the hepatic enzymes and discontinuation of hepatotoxic and cholestatic medications are appropriate initial steps (see Tables 38-2 and 38-3). If symptoms and signs of systemic sepsis are present, evaluation should include a chest roentgenogram and blood culture. If intra-abdominal sepsis is suspected, an ultrasound of the abdomen may identify the presence of an abscess. The CT scan is also helpful in evaluating the liver and pancreas, especially in cases in which overlying bowel gas makes an adequate ultrasound examination impossible. In cases in which an intra-abdominal abscess is identified, the CT scan can also be used to guide a percutaneous aspiration catheter, which can be used as a diagnostic and/or therapeutic modality.

If the hepatic enzyme pattern is more consistent with an obstruction pattern, the initial diagnostic imaging procedure should be an abdominal ultrasound examination. It is a simple, safe, relatively precise, and inexpensive procedure that is well tolerated by even a severely ill patient. It may reveal the presence or absence of gallstones, the size of the bile ducts, and the status of the liver parenchyma as to size and consistency. The identification of dilated bile ducts is an indication for contrast visualization of the biliary tree by either percutaneous transhepatic cholangiography (PTC) or endoscopic retrograde cholangiopancreatography (ERCP). We prefer the latter in most situations, since it offers a safer way to identify the point of obstruction and also provides for the possibility of endoscopic sphincterotomy in cases in which a retained bile duct stone is impacted at the ampulla of Vater.

Nuclear imaging studies using technetium-labeled dimethyl acid analogue dimethyliminodiacetic acid (HIDA) and its N-substitute derivative, technetium-labeled para-isopropyliminodiacetic acid (PIPIDA), are also useful in patients suspected of having biliary fistula or in assessing hepatic mass following liver resections or traumatic injury.[71] Biliary scanning is also a useful adjunct in the diagnosis of acute cholecystitis since it allows visualization of the bile duct without filling of the gallbladder even in the clinically jaundiced patient. As discussed below, however, the test may be misleading in patients with acute acalculous cholecystitis, since the thick bile within the gallbladder in this condition may prevent entrance of hepatic bile even when the cystic duct is present.

Abdominal Procedures

The approach to evaluation of the patient who becomes jaundiced after an abdominal operation is not remarkably different from that described previously. Obviously, less reliance can be placed on the examination of the abdomen. This disadvantage, however, is offset by the knowledge gained from the recent inspection of the intra-abdominal viscera.

Operations on the biliary tree and pancreas are often followed by a transient change in hepatic function. Perioperative cholangiography, instrumentation of the biliary tree or the papilla of Vater, and operations in or around the head of the pancreas may provoke a transient rise in the serum bilirubin level. A progressive rise in the bilirubin value after such operations is a cause for concern and requires an aggressive evaluation. Ultrasonography is the favored imaging technique in this situation in our institution. Biliary scanning is preferred by others, with a strong rationale for their points of view.[12] They stress the safety and sensitivity of the procedure in detecting obstruction or disruption of the extrahepatic biliary tree. Furthermore, it is a highly specific test in the presence of acute calculous cholecystitis.

Fig. 38-1. Radiograph of the proximal biliary tree obtained by instilling radiocontrast material through a fine-gauge needle that had been inserted percutaneously through the liver substance into a peripheral bile duct. This technique provides excellent visualization of the anatomy of the intrahepatic ducts and a detailed identification of the point of obstruction in the common hepatic duct.

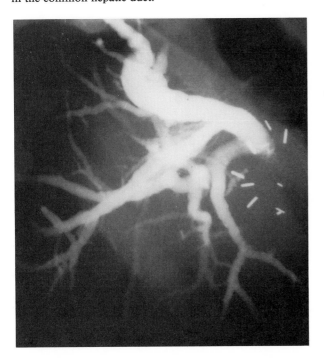

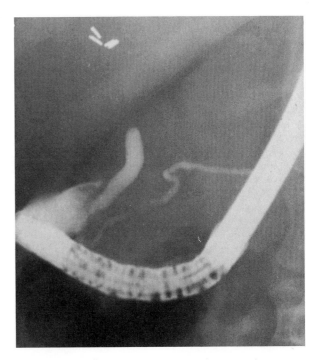

Fig. 38-2. Transendoscopic retrograde cholangiopancreatography as shown here reveals an obstruction in the midaspect of the common bile duct. The pancreatic duct is also well visualized. Lacking, however, is a view of the proximal biliary tree, essential for subsequent repair.

The suspicion of bile duct injury requires visualization of the extrahepatic biliary tree by radiocontrast imaging. We prefer PTC (Fig. 38-1) for this purpose, since it provides a precise localization of the level and extent of injury in contrast to a transendoscopic cholangiogram (Fig. 38-2), which only reveals the anatomy of the normal distal duct. Computed tomography is of little value in the assessment of the jaundiced patient in the early postoperative period. It becomes an important test, however, when ultrasound has failed to reveal an abnormality and an intra-abdominal source of sepsis is suspected.

TREATMENT

In most cases, a thorough evaluation will indicate the type of treatment necessary. Maintenance of adequate ventilatory, cardiovascular, and renal function in this group of patients is especially important. If evaluation has identified any drugs that are potentially hepatotoxic or that may be contributing to hemolysis, these drugs should of course be discontinued. Cases of autoimmune hemolysis may require treatment with corticosteroids.

Postoperative sepsis should be identified and treated quickly and aggressively. A repeat operation must not be delayed because of hepatic dysfunction, if operative drainage of an abscess is indicated. Venous catheters should be changed at least every 2 or 3 days to ensure that they are not the source of sepsis.

A detailed account of the surgical management of extrahepatic biliary obstruction is beyond the scope of this chapter; however, a few general comments are in order. Patients who have retained bile duct stones following cholecystectomy and common duct exploration are best managed with continued T-tube drainage for 4 to 6 weeks. The stones can be extracted safely at this time through the T-tube tract under radiographic control. The treatment of retained stones within the bile duct in the absence of T-tube access is contingent on the patient's overall condition and the nature of the operation. Endoscopic sphincterotomy may provide temporary and, on occasion, definitive management of this situation.

The treatment of retained stones by infusion-dissolution or flushing of the bile duct with bile salts, heparin, or mono-octanoin has not been as successful as mechanical extraction through a T-tube tract or a transendoscopic papillotomy. Infusion of the biliary tree with dissolvants is time consuming and may be associated with septic complications. Possibly, the major application of this

technology will, in the future, relate to the treatment of intrahepatic stones.

Hepatic Ischemia

Ischemia or anoxic insult to the liver will not necessarily be associated with evidence of hepatic dysfunction. Probably the most striking example that we have experienced is the efficiency of the liver in clearing bilirubin after an hepatic transplant. Hepatic transplantation is by necessity associated with a period of several hours of hepatic ischemia. As an example, the ability of a liver to clear bilirubin after 3 hours of cold ischemia is shown in Figure 38-3. There are few experiences more gratifying in a surgeon's work than to see such rapid clearance of bilirubin in a patient who has been deeply jaundiced for several years. Even more amazing is that this can occur after the liver has been without blood flow for such a prolonged period of time.

Contrast this result with that portrayed in Figure 38-4. In this case, a prolonged period of hepatic ischemia was associated with hemoglobin overload from massive transfusion and sequestered blood within the peritoneal cavity. Patience and time allowed gradual return of normal liver

Fig. 38-3. Resolution of jaundice following successful orthotopic liver transplantation in a patient with primary biliary cirrhosis.

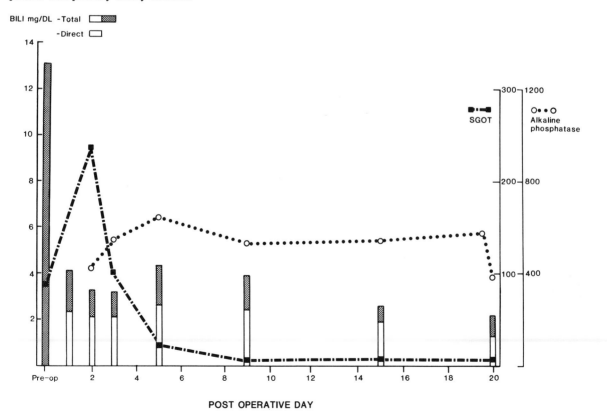

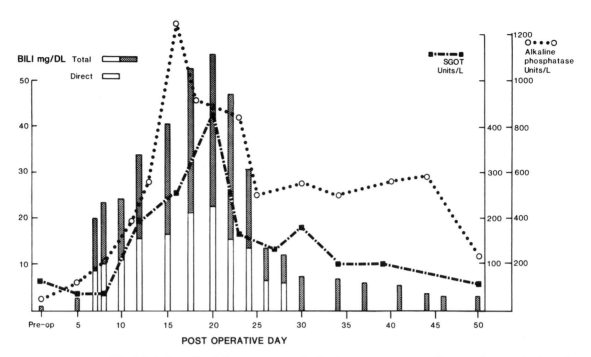

Fig. 38-4. Jaundice following ruptured splenic artery aneurysm. Hypotension required aortic cross-clamping for 45 minutes and transfusion of 70 units of blood. Pneumonia and a urinary tract infection that required antibiotic treatment developed between 7 and 10 days postoperatively. Volatile anesthetics were not used.

function. This case, however, is an exception rather than the rule. Prolonged periods of warm ischemia with multiple blood transfusions and sequestration of blood within the retroperitoneum or free peritoneal cavity are often associated with multiple organ failure and death. The delicate balance between hepatic perfusion and hemoglobin loading has not yet been defined. It is prudent to keep the hepatic ischemia time to a minimum. As a rule of thumb, we attempt to limit total hepatic in-flow occlusion to no longer than 30 minutes, although an hour appears to be well tolerated when the patient (and liver) are hypothermic. Furthermore, we attempt to evacuate all the blood from the peritoneal cavity and to pack it dry when diffuse bleeding cannot be controlled by suture ligature or electrocautery. The problem of massive hemorrhage, such as occurs in pelvic fractures, followed by massive transfusions (greater than 20 units), hypothermia, and generalized bleeding, is unsolved. Patients who survive such a catastrophic event usually have a prolonged period of hepatic dysfunction and jaundice.

Acute Acalculous Cholecystitis

Acute cholecystitis in the postoperative patient is an entity that is difficult to diagnose and is associated with a mortality in excess of 80%. Although the mortality in polytrauma patients may be ascribed to associated injuries, it

is difficult to explain the equally high mortality in patients who have undergone surgical procedures unrelated to the biliary tree.[22] Clearly, the occurrence of jaundice in the injured or postoperative patients presents a quandary in diagnosis and therapy, and delay in surgical intervention is commonplace.[25]

We identified five patients with cases of histologically proven acute acalculous cholecystitis from a total of 4650 cases admitted to the Trauma Service of the University of Texas-Hermann Hospital from 1979 to 1983. The predominant signs were abdominal tenderness, fever, jaundice, and hypoactive bowel sounds. Unfortunately, five patients with sepsis at remote sites during this period had similar signs but recovered without evidence of gallbladder disease. In fact, a positive biliary scan and ultrasound led to the removal of a normal gallbladder in one of these patients.

We have not as yet formed a sure way to diagnose this lethal but, fortunately, rare entity. The algorithm we use to pursue its presence is shown in Table 38-4. A major characteristic of the disease is the presence of thick black bile within the lumen of the gallbladder. This finding suggests that the gallbladder, which is known to become enlarged and empty poorly in the fasting ill patient, develops hyperconcentrated bile within its lumen. This point has been studied experimentally by Bernhoft and his associates,[6] who found that ligation of the cystic duct of the dog

TABLE 38-4.   Management of Acute Acalculous Cholecystitis

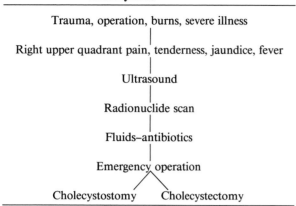

Trauma, operation, burns, severe illness

Right upper quadrant pain, tenderness, jaundice, fever

Ultrasound

Radionuclide scan

Fluids–antibiotics

Emergency operation

Cholecystostomy   Cholecystectomy

will lead to a remarkable accumulation of mucoproteins and solids within the gallbladder lumen. Thomas and his colleagues,[63] in 1952, had shown that ligation of the cystic duct and artery would uniformly lead to acute cholecystitis in the dog. Possibly the combination of a period of ischemia and delayed gallbladder emptying contributes to this rare but lethal lesion, which must always be considered in patients with postsurgical jaundice.

The treatment of acute acalculous cholecystitis is surgical. Cholecystostomy and cholecystectomy appear to be equally effective.[15,40,48] We prefer, however, to remove the gallbladder whenever possible, especially when it appears gangrenous to inspection. Recently, we have treated a patient with presumed acute acalculous cholecystitis by percutaneous cholecystostomy. This offers a safe initial approach but leaves uncertainty as to whether the patient in fact has an inflamed gallbladder. Clearly, seeking ways to prevent this entity would benefit those at risk for its occurrence.

REFERENCES

1. Almersjo O et al: Serum enzyme changes after hepatic dearterialization in man. Ann Surg 167:9, 1966
2. Anderson MN et al: Chronic hemolysis in patients with ball valve prosthesis. J Thorac Cardiovasc Surg 50:501, 1965
3. Arthur AB, Wilson BDR: Urinary infection presenting with jaundice. Br Med J 1:539, 1967
4. Babior BM, Davidson CS: Postoperative massive liver necrosis: A clinical and pathological study. N Engl J Med 276:645, 1967
5. Balthazer EJ: The Mirizzi syndrome, inflammatory stricture of the common hepatic duct. Am J Gastroenterol 64:144, 1975
6. Bernhoft RA et al: Pigment sludge and stone formation in the acutely ligated dog gallbladder. Gastroenterology 85:1166, 1983
7. Bunker JP et al (eds): National Halothane Study: A study of the possible association between halothane anesthesia and postoperative hepatic necrosis. Washington, DC, US Government Printing Office, 1969
8. Calne RY: Preservation of the liver. In Calne RY (ed): Liver Transplantation. New York, Grune & Stratton, 1983
9. Chang S, Silvia SE: Fatty liver produced by hyperalimentation of rats. Am J Gastroenterol 62:410, 1974
10. Chu CM et al: Jaundice after open heart surgery: A prospective study. Thorax 39:52, 1984
11. Clarke RSJ et al: Changes in liver function after different types of surgery. Br J Anaesth 48:1197, 1976
12. Deitch EA, Engel JM: Acute cholecystitis: Ultrasonic diagnosis. Am J Surg 142:290, 1981
13. Donovan AJ et al: Anatomical hepatic lobectomy in trauma to the liver. Surgery 73:833, 1973
14. Dos Reis L, DeAlmeida CC: Post-cholecystectomy jaundice due to intracholedochal blood clots. Br J Surg 68:885, 1981
15. Du Priest RW et al: Acute cholecystitis complicating trauma. Ann Surg 189:84, 1978
16. Farkouh EF et al: Predictive value of liver biochemistry in acute hepatic ischemia. Surg Gynecol Obstet 132:832, 1971
17. Fee JPH et al: A prospective study of liver enzyme and other changes following repeat administration of halothane and influrane. Br J Anaesth 51:1133, 1979
18. Flint LM Jr, Polk HC Jr: Selective hepatic artery ligation: Limitations and failures. J Trauma 19:319, 1979
19. Gardner B: Marked elevation of serum transaminases in obstructive jaundice. Am J Surg 111:576, 1966
20. Geller W, Tagnon HG: Liver dysfunction following abdominal operations: Significance of postoperative hyperbilirubinemia. Arch Intern Med 86:908, 1950
21. Gilligan DR et al: Studies of hemoglobinemia and hemoglobinemia produced in man by intravenous injection of hemoglobin solutions. J Clin Invest 20:177, 1941
22. Glenn F: Acute cholecystitis following the surgical treatment of unrelated disease. Ann Surg 126:411, 1947
23. Glenn F: Complications of biliary tract surgery. Surg Gynecol Obstet 110:141, 1960
24. Glenn F: Postoperative strictures of the extrahepatic bile ducts. Surg Gynecol Obstet 120:560, 1965
25. Glenn F, Becker CG: Acute acalculous cholecystitis. Ann Surg 195:131, 1982
26. Grant JP et al: Serum hepatic enzyme and bilirubin elevations during parenteral nutrition. Surg Gynecol Obstet 145:573, 1977
27. Harris KA et al: Tolerance of the liver to ischemia in the pig. J Surg Res 33:524, 1982
28. Harville DD, Summerskill WHJ: Surgery in acute hepatitis: Causes and effects. JAMA 184:257, 1963
29. Howard RJ, Delaney JP: Postoperative cholecystitis. Am J Dig Dis 17:213, 1972
30. Isbister JP, Soyer A: Incidence and causes of hyperbilirubinemia in a hospital population with particular reference to blood transfusion. Med J Aust 1:261, 1982
31. Isenberg AN: Clostridium welchii infection: A clinical evaluation. Arch Surg 92:727, 1966
32. Kantrowitz RA et al: Severe postoperative hyperbilirubinemia simulating obstructive jaundice. N Engl J Med 276:591, 1967
33. Ketterhagen J, Quadkenbush S: Hyperbilirubinemia of fasting: A case of postoperative jaundice. Arch Surg 118:756, 1983
34. Klatskin G: Bile pigment metabolism. Annu Rev Med 12:211, 1960
35. Koenemann LC, Ceballos R: Massive hepatic necrosis fol-

lowing portacaval shunt: Report of two cases and considerations of liver hemodynamics after shunt. JAMA 198:158, 1966

36. LaMont JT: Postoperative jaundice. Surg Clin North Am 54:637, 1974

37. Lindenmuth WW, Eisenberg MM: The surgical risk in cirrhosis of the liver. Arch Surg 86:235, 1963

38. Lindor KD et al: Liver function values in adults receiving total parenteral nutrition. JAMA 241:2398, 1979

39. Lockey E et al: Early jaundice after open heart surgery. Thorax 22:165, 1967

40. Long TH et al: Acalculous cholecystitis in critically ill patients. Am J Surg 136:31, 1978

41. Longmire WP Jr: Early management of injury to the extrahepatic biliary tract. JAMA 195:623, 1966

42. Miller DF, Irvine RW: Jaundice in acute appendicitis. Lancet 1:321, 1969

43. Miller DJ et al: Jaundice in severe bacterial infection. Gastroenterology 71:94, 1976

44. Mollison PL: Blood Transfusion in Clinical Medicine, 3rd ed. Philadelphia, FA Davis, 1962

45. Morgenstern L: Postoperative jaundice: An approach to a diagnostic dilemma. Am J Surg 128:255, 1974

46. Neale G et al: Effects of intrahepatic and extrahepatic infection on liver function. Br Med J 1:382, 1966

47. Nunes G et al: Mechanism of hepatic dysfunction following shock and trauma. Arch Surg 100:546, 1970

48. Orlando R et al: Acute acalculous cholecystitis in the critically ill patient. Am J Surg 145:472, 1983

49. Pirofsky B et al: Hemolytic anemia complicating aortic-valve surgery: An autoimmune syndrome. N Engl J Med 171:135, 1965

50. Pulito AR et al: Effects of total parenteral nutrition and semistarvation on the liver of beagle puppies. J Pediatr Surg 11:655, 1976

51. Quizilbah AH: Halothane hepatitis. Can Med Assoc J 108:171, 1973

52. Raffuci FL, Wangensteen OH: Tolerance of dogs to occlusion of entire afferent vascular inflow to the liver. Surg Forum 1:191, 1950

53. Rich AR: Pathogenesis of forms of jaundice. Bull Johns Hopkins Hosp 47:338, 1930

54. Rooney JC et al: Jaundice associated with bacterial infection in the newborn. Am J Dis Child 122:39, 1971

55. Rosenoer VM, Tornay AS Jr: Drugs and the liver. Med Clin North Am 63:405, 1979

56. Rudowski WJ: Complications associated with blood transfusion. In Allgower M et al (eds): Progress in Surgery, New York, Karger, 1971

57. Rundle FF et al: Rise in serum bilirubin with biliary obstruction and its decline curve after operative relief. Surgery 43:555, 1958

58. Saidi F, Donaldson GA: Acute pancreatitis following distal gastrectomy for benign ulcer. Am J Surg 105:87, 1963

59. Scott R Jr et al: The systemic response to injury. In Howard JM (ed): Battle Casualties in Korea: Studies of the Surgical Research Team, vol I, pp 149–174. Walter Reed Army Medical Center, Washington DC, 1955

60. Sherlock S: The liver in heart failure: Relation of anatomical, functional and circulatory changes. Br Heart J 13:173, 1951

61. Steiger E et al: Postoperative intravenous nutrition: Effects on body weight, protein regeneration wound healing and liver morphology. Surgery 73:686, 1973

62. Stock JGL, Stunin L: Unexplained hepatitis following halothane. Anesthesiology 63:424, 1985

63. Thomas CG, Womack H: Acute cholecystitis, its pathogenesis and repair. Arch Surg 64:590, 1952

64. Tisdale WA et al: The significance of the direct-reacting fraction of serum bilirubin in hemolytic jaundice. Am J Med 16:214, 1949

65. Trowell J et al: Controlled trial of repeated halothane anesthetics in patients with carcinoma of the uterine cervix treated with radium. Lancet 1:821, 1975

66. Tugswell P, Williams O: Jaundice associated with lobar pneumonia. Q J Med 66:97, 1977

67. Utili R et al: Inhibition of Na^+, K^+–ATPase by endotoxin: A possible mechanism for endotoxin-induced cholestasis. J Infect Dis 136:583, 1977

68. Vermillion SE et al: Jaundice associated with bacteremia. Arch Intern Med 124:611, 1969

69. Virtue RW, Payne K: Postoperative death after fluothane. Anesthesiology 19:562, 1958

70. Wark HJ: Postoperative jaundice in children: the influence of halothane. Anesthesia 38:237, 1983

71. Weissman HS et al: The role of technetium-99m imino diacetic acid (IDA) cholescintigraphy in acute acalculous cholecystitis. Radiology 146:177, 1983

72. Wright R et al: Controlled prospective study of the effect on liver function of multiple exposures to halothane. Lancet 1:814, 1975

73. Young LE: Complications of blood transfusion. Ann Intern Med 61:136, 1964

74. Zimmerman HJ, Thomas LJ: The liver in pneumococcal pneumonia: Observations in 94 cases on liver function and jaundice in pneumonia. J Lab Clin Med 35:556, 1950

75. Zimmerman HJ et al: Jaundice due to bacterial infection. Gastroenterology 77:362, 1979

chapter 39

Amebic and Pyogenic Liver Abscess

KEVIN M. DeCOCK and TELFER B. REYNOLDS

Delay in diagnosis remains a major determinant of the severity of illness and outcome in amebic and pyogenic liver abscess. Lack of familiarity with the clinical features of these conditions on the part of clinicians and failure to consider the diagnosis are among the most important factors contributing to the continued morbidity and mortality.

The management of hepatic abscesses has been greatly influenced by advances in diagnostic imaging and interventional radiology. In amebic liver abscess, medical therapy alone is most often effective. A change has occurred in the therapeutic approach to pyogenic liver abscess, for which surgical drainage had until recently been considered mandatory. In recent times, antibiotic therapy alone, or in combination with percutaneous drainage, has often been shown to be curative, although surgery remains essential in some cases.

Amebic and pyogenic liver abscess share many common features. Clinically, the first diagnostic requirement is demonstration of the presence of an abscess, followed by determination of its nature. We have for these reasons elected to discuss amebic and pyogenic abscess together in the same chapter in an integrated fashion.

AMEBIC LIVER ABSCESS

Historical Aspects

Dysentery and hepatic abscesses were described by British physicians in India in the early 19th century.[79] Ipecacuanha was used for treatment, the active ingredient later being shown to be emetine. Losch,[105] in 1875, was the first author to give a detailed description of amebiasis in his report of a Russian woodcutter who died of the disease. In the same decade, Koch and Gaffky[94] and Kartulis[85] in Egypt reported original observations on amebic dysentery and liver abscess. The first recognized cases of amebic liver abscess in the United States were reported from Johns Hopkins Hospital in 1890 by Osler[136] and Simon.[176] A classic monograph on amebiasis was published from the same institution the following year.[33]

Confusion existed in the early 20th century concerning nomenclature and pathogenicity of different species of amebae. In the Philippines, experimental infections in prisoners made possible the distinction between *Ent-*

amoeba histolytica (pathogenic) and *E. coli* (nonpathogenic), showed that cysts were the infective stage, and demonstrated that not all persons infected with *E. histolytica* became ill.[195]

Important milestones in the history of chemotherapy for amebiasis have been the introduction of emetine for amebic dysentery and liver abscess by Rogers in India in 1912[156]; the demonstration of efficacy of chloroquine in hepatic amebiasis in 1948[29,30]; the introduction in 1959 of dehydroemetine,[22] a synthetic compound closely related to but less toxic than emetine; and the demonstration by Powell and colleagues,[147] in 1966, of cure in all forms of invasive amebiasis using metronidazole. These latter workers form part of a group of medical scientists from Durban, South Africa, whose collective work over more than 20 years has profoundly influenced the modern approach to amebiasis.

Parasitology

The term *amebiasis* signifies infection with the protozoan parasite *E. histolytica* (Fig. 39-1). In the majority of cases infection is noninvasive and parasites are restricted to the intestinal lumen. Trophozoites, the active ameboid forms of the parasite, live in the lower bowel, where they browse on bacteria and other material in the host's feces, dividing by binary fission two or three times daily (Fig. 39-2). Noninvasive trophozoites are 10 μm to 20 μm in diameter and contain a nucleus and a number of vesicles in the granular cytoplasm. Movement is sluggish and involves the formation of blunt pseudopodia limited by the ectoplasmic gel, into which streams the endoplasmic sol. The organisms are actively phagocytic for their food. Although metabolism is essentially anaerobic, the trophozoites can survive under conditions of low oxygen tension.

Under certain circumstances the trophozoites expel their vacuoles and secrete a chitinous wall around themselves to form cysts. Cell division results in each cyst being quadrinucleate when mature. The cysts of *E. histolytica* measure 10 μm to 14 μm in diameter and are distinguishable on the basis of their size and number of nuclei from those of the commensals *E. coli* (14–20 μm; 8 nuclei) and *E. hartmanni* (6–10 μm; 4 nuclei). It is these cysts that are the infective stage; trophozoites die outside the human host and are destroyed by gastric acid when swallowed. Cysts in feces are viable for several days.

1235

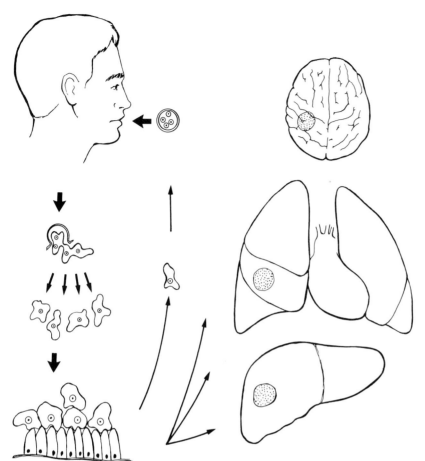

Fig. 39-1. Life cycle of *Entamoeba histolytica.*

When ingested cysts reach the host's small intestine their walls disintegrate and trophozoites are released that mature as they travel down to the large bowel. Any cause of diarrhea or intestinal hurry, including noninfectious conditions, can prevent encystment and result in the passage of active trophozoites in stool.

Undefined factors stimulate trophozoites of *E. histolytica* to become invasive. Invasive organisms are more active and larger than their nonpathogenic predecessors, measuring up to 50 μm in diameter. The hallmark of invasive intestinal amebiasis is the demonstration in stool, or in rectal mucosal scrapings or biopsy specimens, of trophozoites containing ingested red blood cells. It is emphasized that amebic cysts or trophozoites in stool are not diagnostic of invasive disease.

It is unclear what factors render certain strains of *E. histolytica* invasive. Association with bacteria may enhance the pathogenicity of some strains.[198] A number of differences exist in the surface characteristics of trophozoites from different strains when cultured *in vitro*.[170] The injection of amebae from pathogenic human infections into experimental animals resulted in pathology in the new hosts, while noninvasive human infections were of low virulence in the animals.[184] However, invasive strains do not always cause disease, as has been demonstrated in experimental human infections.[195] Resistance to complement-mediated lysis has been demonstrated in some pathogenic strains.[154] Recently, biochemical examination of the isoenzyme characteristics of strains of different geographical origin and of varying pathogenicity associated certain enzyme markers with invasiveness.[166] The association between biochemically distinguishable "zymodenes" of *E. histolytica* and pathogenicity has been the most promising advance in understanding the wide variations in disease.[45]

In contrast to these definable strain differences, no distinguishing features between pathogenic and nonpathogenic organisms are evident on light or electron microscopy, or by examination using immunologic methods.[170]

Host Response

Antigenic determinants capable of eliciting an antibody response have been detected in subcellular fractions of

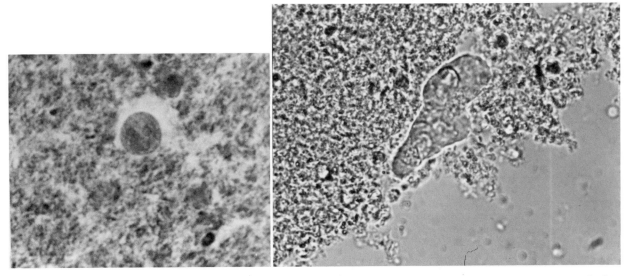

Fig. 39-2. Left. Cyst of *Entamoeba histolytica* in stool. **Right.** Trophozoite of *Entamoeba histolytica* in aspirate from amebic liver abscess.

trophozoites containing ribosomal, lysosomal, and soluble cytoplasmic matter, as well as in material derived from the trophozoite surface.[171] *E. histolytica* antigen has been detected in serum, in feces, and in material from liver abscesses in infected patients.[170]

The complex humoral response to amebic infection results primarily in the production of IgG antibody. IgM class antibody also appears, although IgE is lacking.

Immune serum and antiamebic globulin has been shown experimentally to have a lytic effect on amebae.[170] Complement may be required to mediate this effect; in experimental infections in animals, prior depletion of complement with cobra venom produced more extensive infections.[23]

In general, it seems that cell-mediated immunity, as measured by *in vitro* tests and skin reactivity to amebic antigen, is suppressed early in the course of infection but recovers with successful therapy. The importance of the cellular immune response is uncertain. Immunosuppressive drugs in animals promote the development of experimental amebic liver abscesses,[17] and clinical observations in humans suggest that these drugs enhance invasiveness. *In vitro* studies of the interaction between human white blood cells and virulent amebae suggest that monocyte-derived, activated macrophages may be important effector cells in the immune response against *E. histolytica*.[161]

Alcoholism and malnutrition have frequently been quoted as host factors promoting invasive amebiasis, although definite evidence for this is lacking.[40] The sex of the host is an important factor, with hepatic amebiasis being approximately three to ten times more common in males than females after puberty. Reinfection following successful treatment of invasive amebiasis is possible although relatively uncommon.

Pathogenesis and Pathology

Amebae reach the liver through portal blood. It is unlikely that lymphatic spread can occur since amebae have never been reported in abdominal lymph glands and they do not appear to enter the bloodstream through the thoracic duct.[31,44]

Most amebic abscesses develop in the right lobe of the liver near the dome. The right lobe is probably more often affected than the left lobe because it has a larger volume. In addition, it receives a major part of the venous drainage from the cecum and ascending colon, parts of the bowel frequently affected by amebiasis.[8]

Amebic liver abscesses are well-demarcated lesions (Fig. 39-3) that initially contain yellow-brown fluid that later attains its classic orange-brown "anchovy sauce" appearance (Fig. 39-4). The fluid represents necrotic liver tissue mixed with blood. It is odorless, unless secondarily infected, and usually contains few or no neutrophils. For this reason the term *abscess,* although traditional, is not strictly accurate. The edge of the amebic lesion has a shaggy, fibrinous wall that consists of necrotic material, compressed hepatocytes, and a mixture of inflammatory cells. Amebae are most often found at the periphery of an abscess, although frequently no parasites can be identified in abscess aspirate. Lysis of hepatic cells occurs maximally in periportal regions. The surrounding unaffected liver is hyperemic and edematous, explaining the clinical finding of hepatomegaly that often seems disproportionate to the size of the abscess cavity. A mixed inflammatory cell infiltrate may be seen in adjacent hepatic parenchyma.

Bile is probably lethal to amebae, and infection of the gallbladder and bile ducts does not occur. Healing of

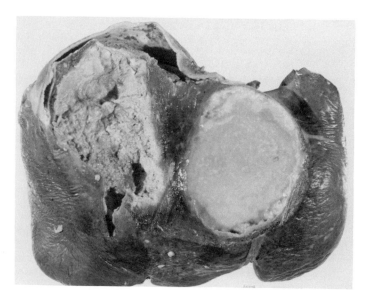

Fig. 39-3. Autopsy specimen of hepatic amebiasis. Two discrete abscesses occupy almost the entire liver.

amebic abscesses progresses without scarring, although the defect in the parenchyma may persist for a long time.

Amebic hepatitis, a term used by some earlier workers,[41] is no longer considered a specific entity. Reports of a diffuse hepatitis with amebae throughout the liver have never been substantiated. There are, however, descriptions by experienced physicians of tender hepatomegaly without overt abscess formation in patients with amebiasis, with improvement following specific chemotherapy.[32,153] Such cases may represent an early stage of hepatic amebiasis, in which microscopic lesions are presumed to coalesce to form a discrete abscess. In addition, in endemic tropical

Fig. 39-4. Amebic liver abscess contents ("anchovy sauce"). The color may vary from light brown (*left*) to orange (*center*) or dark brown (*right*).

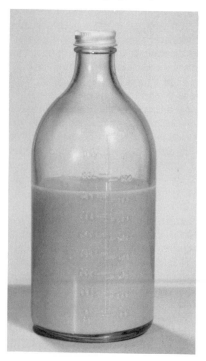
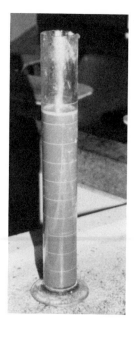
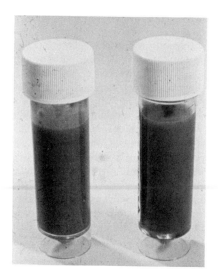

regions nonspecific changes in the liver, including Kupffer cell hyperplasia and portal tract inflammation, are frequent in patients with different intestinal infections.[75]

Epidemiology

Infection with *E. histolytica* affects one tenth of the world's population and is considered responsible for at least 40,000 deaths annually, the majority of infections occurring in the developing countries of the tropics and subtropics.[90,91,110,196] Infection prevalence varies greatly and in some regions exceeds 50%. One study from the Gambia, West Africa, documented infection rates approaching 100% per annum.[20]

The association between amebiasis and warm climates results from the poor sanitation and lack of hygiene that accompany underprivileged living conditions. Infection occurs mainly by the fecal-oral route, with transmission resulting from contamination of food by flies, unhygienic handling of food, and spread within the family. Raw sewage contaminating water supplies occasionally causes infection, as may the use of human feces as fertilizer and of unclean water for freshening food.

Disease incidence is difficult to assess because of the unreliable nature of case reporting. Conclusions from several reviews are that invasive amebiasis, including liver abscess, is especially common in sub-Saharan Africa, Asia, Mexico, and parts of South America.[49,50] Real but ill-defined geographical variations exist in the prevalence of liver abscess among infected individuals. Such regional differences may be partially explained by recent work showing variation in virulence and distribution among parasite strains of differing isoenzyme patterns ("zymodenes").[45]

Transmission of amebiasis can also occur in the developed world.[101] Although amebic liver abscess was recently described in an unfortunate German worker 14 weeks after he fell into a sewage tank,[92] infection is now rarely water-borne.[101] Person-to-person spread, as may occur in institutions or in slum areas with large immigrant populations, accounts for the majority of cases.[173,179,180] An unusual mode of transmission in a recent outbreak was the paramedical practice of colonic irrigation.[24] In occasional patients no source of infection is evident.[149,163]

In recent years an increased incidence of amebiasis has been noted in urban male homosexual populations.[43,88,108,145] Recognition of the association between homosexuality and amebiasis is generally attributed to Most, who, in a lecture entitled "Manhattan: 'A Tropical Isle?'" reported a minor outbreak in New York City.[125] Although amebic liver abscess has been documented in male homosexuals,[119,188,199] no increase in frequency has been reported in the acquired immune deficiency syndrome (AIDS). Homosexual modes of transmission are probably oro-anal or genito-anal with oro-genital contact. Examination of the isoenzyme characteristics of amebae isolated from homosexual subjects has shown a high prevalence of nonpathogenic zymodenes.[117,165] This may help explain the relative rarity of amebic liver abscess in homosexual men compared with the epidemic prevalence of intestinal infection.

Heterosexual venereal transmission with infection of the male and female genitalia has been described, although the reported cases were not associated with liver abscess.[126,186]

Clinical Features[3,6,36,86,103,187,189]

Amebic liver abscess is three to ten times as common in men as in women. Most patients are young adults, although all age-groups can be affected. With care, a relevant epidemiologic history can usually be elicited. Most patients will be emigrants from or residents of endemic areas, and the majority are poor. In the more affluent, a history of international travel by the patient or his close contacts may be relevant. In a patient with compatible symptoms, any history, no matter how remote, of travel to or residence in a developing country should raise the differential diagnosis of amebiasis. Specific questions about homosexual activity should be asked. A history of previous dysentery is infrequent and generally unhelpful unless accompanied by dependable laboratory reports.

Symptoms of amebic liver abscess are slow in onset and usually are present for several days or weeks before medical attention is sought. Initial complaints are vague, and include malaise, fever, anorexia, and abdominal discomfort. In established cases pain is most often the dominant symptom and is maximal in the right hypochondrium. About three fourths of patients complain of fever, often with chills and sweats, particularly at night. Anorexia, nausea, and vomiting are common, and many patients lose weight. Chest symptoms are present in approximately one fourth of patients and include right-sided pleuritic pain and cough. Diaphragmatic irritation may result in right shoulder pain and hiccoughs. Occasional patients recognize abdominal swelling. Concurrent intestinal disease such as dysentery or diarrhea is rare.

Infrequently, the onset of disease is abrupt and the symptoms mimic those of an abdominal surgical emergency.[100] Sometimes patients complain of ill health for many months, with constitutional symptoms such as weight loss and anemia predominating. In a small minority the only manifestation is fever.

On examination, patients are usually ill, sallow, and sweaty, and they may appear anemic and toxic. They tend to remain ambulant until close to hospitalization, by which time movement is clearly painful, and they may seek a certain position on lying down for maximum comfort. Fever and tenderness over the liver are almost invariable, with the tenderness sometimes being most impressive over the right lower intercostal area. Sometimes the liver is visibly enlarged or expands the lower rib cage to give the abdomen an asymmetric appearance. Most often the liver is palpable, and in rare cases it is huge and extends down to the pelvis. The physical signs may be more subtle when the abscess is in the left lobe of the liver.

Epigastric and left hypochondrial tenderness and enlargement of the left lobe could raise this possibility.[8]

Careful examination of the chest reveals abnormalities in up to one half of patients. Movement of the right side may be limited by pain. Dullness to percussion over the right lower lung field is common and implies a raised right hemidiaphragm or pleural effusion. Occasionally there are fine crepitations on auscultation or a pleural or pericardial friction rub.

Jaundice is rare and when present is usually of a minor degree. It generally indicates more severe illness. Deeper jaundice usually results from multiple or large amebic abscesses or from lesions situated near the inferior surface of the liver with compression of the larger intrahepatic ducts.[133,138]

Wherever amebiasis occurs in adults, children also may be infected.[70,112,118,155,168] The majority of reported cases of liver abscess in childhood have been in children under 3 years old, with some affected at only 1 month of life. The sex ratio of cases in children is almost equal. Fever and tender hepatomegaly are the usual physical signs, with the latter sometimes difficult to elicit in a crying child. Associated intestinal amebiasis and multiple hepatic abscesses seem more frequent in children than adults, and malnutrition is an important accompaniment. Amebic liver abscess often seems a more severe disease in childhood.

Treatment with corticosteroids enhances the invasiveness of *E. histolytica*, and cases exist in which administration of such drugs to patients with benign infections apparently resulted in hepatic amebiasis.[11,47,48,81,169,183] Liver abscess sometimes occurs in pregnancy[29,34,39, 122,129,194] and such cases are frequently misdiagnosed. A Nigerian autopsy study demonstrated a higher prevalence and mortality from amebiasis in pregnant compared with nonpregnant women.[2] It has been suggested that the immunologic and hormonal alterations of pregnancy predispose to invasive disease. Finally, there is a widespread clinical impression that amebic liver abscess is rare in patients with cirrhosis, although isolated cases have been documented.[53]

Diagnosis

Conventional Laboratory Tests

Anemia is common in amebic liver abscess, with about one half of patients having hemoglobin values below 12 g/dl. Although usually normochromic and normocytic, a hypochromic blood picture may occur despite adequate iron stores.[111] A neutrophilic leukocytosis is usual, and a high proportion of bands may be seen. Although the white cell count is generally between 10,000 and 20,000/cu mm, isolated cases with leukemoid reactions are described. Eosinophilia is not a feature of amebiasis. The erythrocyte sedimentation rate is generally raised.

Results of liver tests are often abnormal and are of value in focusing attention on the liver, although derangements may be minor and nonspecific. Slight elevation of alkaline phosphatase and reduction of serum albumin levels are the most frequent abnormalities. Normal liver tests do not exclude the diagnosis of hepatic abscess. Significant elevation of the bilirubin level in hepatic amebiasis is unusual.

Diagnostic Imaging

About one half of patients show elevation of the right hemidiaphragm on the chest roentgenogram (Fig. 39-5), the changes in contour being typically most marked anteriorly and medially.[27] Fluoroscopy may demonstrate reduced or absent diaphragmatic movement. Blunting of the right costophrenic angle from a sympathetic pleural effusion is common, as are minor right lower lobe parenchymal abnormalities from atelectasis. Abdominal films may show hepatomegaly but are generally not helpful. Barium studies and infusion tomography are now outdated techniques for diagnosing amebic abscess.[5,150]

Technetium sulfur colloid scanning (Fig. 39-6), the first modality allowing direct assessment of space-occupying liver lesions, is sensitive but lacks specificity.[89,150] Other hepatic masses, such as tumors and cysts, may produce similar "cold" areas. Gallium scans are often used to complement sulfur colloid examinations.[150] Unlike pyogenic abscesses and primary hepatocellular cancers, amebic abscesses generally concentrate gallium only at the periphery of the abscess. The disadvantages of these tests

Fig. 39-5. Chest x-ray film in a young Mexican–American man with amebic liver abscess. Note the elevated right hemidiaphragm.

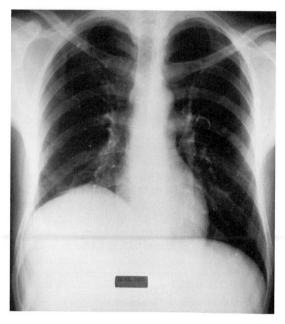

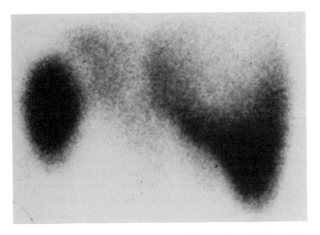

Fig. 39-6. Isotope liver–spleen scan in a patient with amebic liver abscess. Right posterior oblique view. A large defect is seen in the superior aspect of the right lobe of the liver.

include their low specificity, the time required for their completion, and the difficulty of working with isotopes.

Ultrasonography (Fig. 39-7) is quick, safe, economical, and easily repeatable.[4,19,38,150,151,192] Ultrasound scanning readily distinguishes solid from fluid-filled lesions, and if necessary, the apparatus can be brought to the patient's bedside. The technique is applicable even in areas with limited facilities.[38] A disadvantage of ultrasonography is its dependence on the interest and skill of the investigator.

Ultrasonic signs quoted as typical of hepatic amebic abscess are (1) a round or oval shape; (2) a lack of significant wall echoes, so that there is abrupt transition from normal liver to the lesion; (3) a hypoechoic appearance compared with normal liver, with diffuse echoes throughout the abscess; (4) a peripheral location, usually close to the liver capsule; and (5) a distal sonic enhancement.[150,151] Atypical features that have been documented include an irregular shape and a hyperechoic appearance.[35]

Computerized tomography (CT scanning) (Fig. 39-8) shows amebic abscesses as well-defined, round, low-density lesions, which may have a nonhomogeneous internal structure.[150] CT scanning is particularly useful in precise localization and definition of extent of disease, for example, in cases complicated by rupture. Both CT scanning and ultrasound may be used for guidance in cases in which aspiration is indicated. Disadvantages of CT scanning are its cumbersome nature and expense and the ionizing radiation inherent to the investigation.

Parasitology and Serodiagnosis

Concurrent hepatic abscess and amebic dysentery are unusual; stool examinations in large series of patients with amebic abscesses have been negative in three fourths of cases or more. Parasitologic examination of a stool specimen can neither prove nor exclude hepatic amebiasis, although it may be relevant for subsequent management. The quality of practical parasitology in hospital laboratories varies widely. Overdiagnosis is especially common, with stool leukocytes frequently reported as trophozoites of *E. histolytica*.[25,178]

Serodiagnostic tests used include complement fixation, immunodiffusion, indirect fluorescent antibody tests (IFA), indirect hemagglutination (IHA), counterimmunoelectrophoresis (CIE), and enzyme-linked immunosorbent assay (ELISA).[80,92,140,170] Commercially produced di-

Fig. 39-7. Ultrasound of liver in a young Mexican–American with amebic liver abscess. Sagittal view through right lobe of liver.

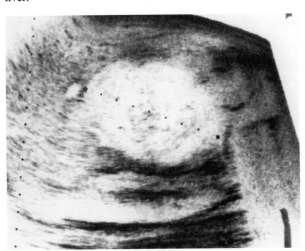

Fig. 39-8. CT scan in a patient with amebic liver abscess. The scan was performed with the patient lying prone. A large right lobe liver abscess is shown. The lesion was subsequently aspirated.

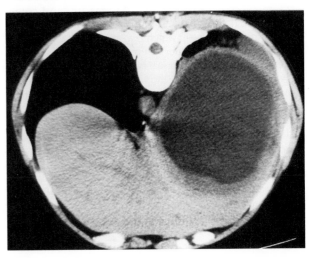

agnostic kits for use at the bedside, such as those using latex agglutination, are also available. Clinicians should familiarize themselves with local facilities and the accepted sensitivity and specificity of the tests in question.

Positive tests are expected in virtually all cases of extraintestinal amebiasis as well as in a majority of cases of amebic dysentery. It is emphasized that serology can only prove that a patient has suffered invasive infection with *E. histolytica*, not that a particular illness is the result of that infection.

The IHA test is highly sensitive and widely available. A serologic titer of 1:512 is usual although not invariable in acute invasive disease. Titers may continue to rise after presentation and on occasion the test is negative when the patient is first seen but positive a few days later. The IHA test may remain positive for months or years after invasive infection.

ELISA is a cheap and sensitive technique that has in recent years been widely applied to the serodiagnosis and seroepidemiologic study of many parasitic diseases.[10] Its use for the diagnosis of amebiasis is likely to increase.

Agreement between the various test systems is not absolute, and it is possible that different antibodies are being detected. Serodiagnostic tests are crucial in diagnosis, but their results must be interpreted in their clinical and epidemiologic context.

Complications

The most frequent complication of amebic liver abscess is rupture, the direction and consequences of which depend on the site of the primary lesion. Rupture can occur into the chest, pericardium, peritoneal cavity, intra-abdominal organs, and through the skin. In one study of fatal amebiasis, 41 of 90 cases with liver abscess had ruptured.[87]

Rupture into the chest may result in hepatobronchial fistula, lung abscess, or amebic empyema, although most pleural effusions in patients with amebic abscess are clear, sterile, "sympathetic" exudates.[7,76,78,191,193] Transdiaphragmatic rupture and pleural effusions are most common on the right side. Symptoms of rupture through the diaphragm include pain (which may be constant, pleuritic, or referred to the shoulder), dyspnea, and shock. Cough is frequent, and when rupture is into the bronchial tree it may be associated with hemoptysis and expectoration of abscess contents. Rare patients suffer silent rupture and present simply with amebic empyema. Reported long-term complications of transdiaphragmatic rupture include pulmonary fibrosis, bronchiectasis, pleural thickening, and chronic empyema.

Left lobe abscesses are especially prone to rupture into the pericardium.[77,106] This very dangerous complication is sometimes preceded by the development of a serous pericardial effusion. Patients present with obscure heart failure, pericarditis, or cardiac tamponade. Constrictive pericarditis may develop later in patients who survive.

Like hepatobronchial fistula, rupture into the bowel may achieve spontaneous drainage.[12] Intraperitoneal rupture is more common and presents as signs of peritonitis, local pain, and tenderness, or simply with ascites.[46,63,123,177] Although such patients may be gravely ill, intraperitoneal rupture of an amebic liver abscess is generally a less serious event than amebic peritonitis from perforation of the large bowel in amebic dysentery. Rare cases have ruptured into kidney or pancreas.

Secondary infection of an amebic liver abscess is unusual and most often iatrogenic, the result of aspiration.[60] Other documented complications, all exceptionally rare, include fulminant hepatic failure,[162] hemobilia,[96,148] reversible portal hypertension,[128] and inferior vena caval obstruction,[74,167] associated in one case with nephrotic syndrome.[74] Amebic cerebral abscess, a very unusual complication, results from hematogenous spread. This must be distinguished from primary amebic meningoencephalitis resulting from infection with certain free-living species of amebae.

PYOGENIC LIVER ABSCESS

Historical Aspects

Liver abscess was recognized by ancient physicians,[65] but modern study of the condition dates back to the late 19th century. In the preantibiotic era, appendicitis was the most frequent underlying cause, accounting for one third of cases reported in the world literature.[135] The first documentation of pyogenic liver abscess secondary to appendicitis is ascribed to Waller in 1846.[135] French physicians referred to the condition as *le foie appendiculaire,* and this complication was observed in up to 4% of patients with appendicitis.[57] The early literature was reviewed by Ochsner and colleagues,[135] who extensively discussed surgical management of pyogenic liver abscess. The first successful use of an antibiotic, sulfanilamide, in conjunction with surgical drainage for multiple hepatic abscesses was reported in 1938.[137] In 1947, anaerobic organisms were cultured from pyogenic liver abscesses and successfully treated with penicillin.[120] Although surgical treatment has remained the most widely accepted form of therapy, McFadzean and colleagues, in 1953, effectively treated pyogenic liver abscesses with antibiotics and closed percutaneous drainage.[116] A report from the University of Southern California in 1979 documented successful treatment of pyogenic liver abscess in selected cases using antibiotics alone.[107]

Epidemiology

Worldwide, pyogenic liver abscess is much less common than amebic abscess, but in Western communities without significant immigrant populations pyogenic abscess is more frequent. Accurate incidence figures are lacking, but 8 to 16 cases/100,000 hospital admissions is an accepted estimate.[65,115,131] The prevalence at autopsy has been quoted as 0.3% to 1.5%.[65,175] Pyogenic liver abscess, therefore, is a rare condition, making prospective controlled studies difficult.

This is generally a disease of middle-aged and older persons, and the sexes are affected approximately equally. Geographic variations in disease frequency are not obvious, and there is no racial susceptibility.

Pathogenesis and Pathology

Pyogenic infection may be carried to the liver in hepatic arterial or portal venous blood and in bile.[13,131,135] Arterial spread results from generalized septicemia or from distant localized infections, whereas portal venous spread more often complicates intra-abdominal sepsis such as diverticulitis or peritonitis from other causes. The classic changes of pylephlebitis, with the portal vein and its branches containing blood clot and pus, are now rarely seen.

A frequent cause of liver abscess is cholangitis, complicating benign or malignant biliary obstruction and endoscopic or operative intervention. Parasitic invasion of the biliary tree by roundworms or flukes also may lead to biliary infection.[32] The important subject of recurrent pyogenic cholangitis (oriental cholangiohepatitis) is outside the scope of the present discussion.

Abscess formation may complicate blunt or penetrating trauma, including liver biopsy and surgery. Foreign bodies have long been recognized as potential sources of infection,[135] and penetration or perforation of bowel by diverse objects such as toothpicks and pins is well described.[18,135] Direct extension of infection to the liver may occur secondary to such conditions as empyema of the gallbladder and subphrenic abscess. Umbilical sepsis is an important cause of liver abscess in infants.

Secondary infection sometimes complicates congenital or acquired hepatic abnormalities such as hydatid or nonparasitic cysts, amebic abscesses, and choledochal cysts. Necrosis and infection of primary or secondary hepatic malignancies is recognized. A significant proportion of cases have no obvious etiology. Spread to the liver via the portal vein is most likely in such instances. Lymphatic spread does not seem to occur.

Abscesses may be multiple or single, with those originating from blood-borne spread of infection usually being multiple. The gross lesions give overlying liver tissue a pale appearance. The abscess cavities are variable in size and frequently coalesce, and advanced cases have a honeycombed appearance. A fibrous capsule may surround the lesions, which contain a polymophonuclear cell infiltrate and necrotic liver tissue. Most abscesses tend to be in the right lobe of the liver.[13,135]

Microbiology

In the preantibiotic era the most common organisms incriminated as causing liver abscess were *Escherichia coli*, streptococci, and staphylococci.[135] About one half of abscesses and all blood cultures were bacteriologically sterile. Today, with awareness of the exacting growth requirements of many organisms, cultures of blood and/or abscess contents will be positive in most cases.

E. coli remains the single bacterium most frequently isolated in the majority of reported series.[13,104,115,121,134,143] Other important aerobic organisms are various gramnegative bacilli, including species of *Klebsiella, Proteus,* and *Pseudomonas,* and gram-positive enteric organisms such as *Streptococcus faecalis* and *Streptococcus faecium.* The latter two agents are referred to as enterococci. Other gram-positive aerobic infections are less common. *Staphylococcus aureus* and *Streptococcus pyogenes* may complicate penetrating trauma, and the former is occasionally associated with unusual immunologic deficiency states such as Job's syndrome[72] or chronic granulomatous disease.[142]

The importance of anaerobic and microaerophilic organisms in liver abscess is a recent recognition.[159,160] Attention to detail concerning the collection of specimens, their transportation to the laboratory, and their subsequent processing increases the recovery of these bacteria. As many as one third to one half of patients may be infected with such organisms. Anaerobic organisms incriminated include *Bacteroides* species, *Fusobacterium* species, anaerobic streptococci (*Peptostreptococcus* and *Peptococcus* species), and, rarely, *Clostridium* species. Microaerophilic streptococci are considered by some authors as the most common of all organisms causing liver abscess.[124] These fastidious organisms require an environment rich in carbon dioxide for successful culture. *Streptococcus milleri* is the most important member of the group. The confusing classification of these organisms has been recently discussed.[21,52] Many lesions are polymicrobial infections.

Unusual organisms documented as causing liver abscess on occasion include species of *Salmonella, Hemophilus,* and *Yersinia.* Actinomycosis, tuberculosis, and melioidosis also may be associated with liver abscess.

Clinical Features[13,14,65,73,82,104,114,115,131,134,135,141,143,157,181]

Clinical presentation is variable with some patients complaining of acute symptoms referable to the right upper quadrant and others having no localizing features. The sex ratio is virtually equal, and most Western patients are middle aged or older. A history of previous abdominal pathology should be carefully sought. Most of the clinical findings in patients with amebic liver abscess may also be associated with pyogenic abscesses. Conditions predisposing to impaired immunity such as diabetes are sometimes present.

Most patients complain of constitutional symptoms such as malaise, anorexia, nausea, vomiting, and weight loss, and many notice fever, rigors, and sweats. Abdominal pain is frequent, most often localized to the right hypochondrium. Some patients present with generalized abdominal pain, mimicking a surgical emergency, while others present simply with fever. The history is most often of short duration but occasionally extends over weeks or months. Very rarely pyogenic liver abscess is virtually asymptomatic[139] or presents as a space-occupying lesion of the liver.

On examination, patients are usually ill and febrile. Anemia and finger clubbing may be present in longstanding cases. Jaundice occurs in about one third of patients. Tachycardia, tender hepatomegaly, and right hypochondrial tenderness are frequent. Respiratory signs indicative of a small right pleural effusion, atelectasis, or raised hemidiaphragm are regularly found.

The complications of pyogenic liver abscess are essentially the same as those of hepatic amebiasis (see above) but, in addition, include the consequences of severe sepsis. Associated diseases such as diverticulitis with peritonitis, Crohn's disease, biliary tract obstruction, or malignancy may all influence the clinical picture. Whether abscesses are solitary or multiple also determines the clinical course, with multiple abscesses carrying a more unfavorable prognosis. Septic complications of pyogenic abscess include septicemia and metastatic abscess, direct extension, hypotension and shock, adult respiratory distress syndrome, mental obtundation, and renal failure.

Diagnosis

Conventional Laboratory Tests

Routine laboratory tests are incapable of distinguishing pyogenic from amebic abscesses. At least one half of patients have hemoglobin levels below 12 g/dl, an elevated white cell count with a left shift is detected in up to three fourths of cases, and the sedimentation rate is invariably raised. Bilirubin and alkaline phosphatase levels are often elevated. Hyperbilirubinemia may result from sepsis but also may reflect biliary tract disease. The latter can also cause alkaline phosphatase elevations, although this may result from the abscess per se or from associated malignancy. Aminotransferase levels are often raised to a minor degree. Albumin levels reflect disease severity, and levels below 2 g/dl carry a poor prognosis.[104] The majority of patients have a prolonged prothrombin time. Although liver tests may be deranged in sepsis of any origin, elevated vitamin B_{12} levels reflect intrahepatic pathology.[130]

Diagnostic Imaging

About one half of patients with pyogenic liver abscess have some abnormality on the chest roentgenogram, and the range of abnormal features is similar to that seen in hepatic amebiasis. If infection is with gas-forming organisms, air–fluid levels may be seen below the diaphragm on chest or abdominal films.

Scintigraphy with technetium sulfur colloid is sensitive for detecting lesions above 2 cm in diameter, although smaller lesions may be missed.[158] Gallium scanning has to be performed in addition if scintigraphy is to be diagnostic. Pyogenic liver abscesses avidly take up gallium, despite occasional false negatives.[62]

Ultrasonography (Fig. 39-9) shows pyogenic abscesses as round, ovoid, or elliptical lesions within the liver parenchyma, most often not contiguous with the liver capsule.[132] The margin of each lesion tends to be irregular and echo poor. Abscesses are mostly hypoechoic compared with normal liver parenchyma, and they contain a variable number of internal echoes. Occasionally a hyperechoic appearance is seen, particularly when gas-forming organisms are present.[102]

Computerized tomography (Fig. 39-10) is highly sensitive for diagnosis of intra-abdominal abscesses.[95,158] The lesions show in the liver as areas of decreased attenuation. An advantage of CT scanning over ultrasound is that the quality of the scan is not affected by bowel gas or foreign objects such as tubes and dressings.

Selective hepatic angiography has been used for diagnosis of hepatic abscesses but is generally no longer a necessary investigation.[13,58]

Microbiology

Multiple blood cultures should be taken prior to the initiation of therapy. Although many authors quote 50% as the expected rate of positive cultures,[115,131] in some recent reports the success rate has been almost 100%.[72] The role of diagnostic aspiration of abscess contents is discussed below. If aspiration is performed, pus, not swabs, should be submitted to the laboratory, and specimens should be dispatched with haste.[51,124] Aspirated pus is creamy yellow and frequently foul smelling. Pus may be transported in a sterile container as well as in blood culture bottles. The clinician should be in close communication with the microbiologist about the handling of specimens. Submitted

Fig. 39-9. Ultrasound of liver in a 38-year-old woman with multiple pyogenic liver abscesses. Transverse view.

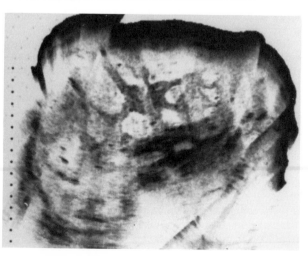

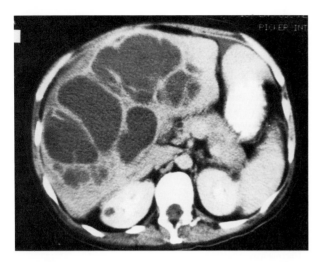

Fig. 39-10. CT scan of liver in the same patient as in Figure 39-9. Aspiration confirmed the lesions to be pyogenic abscesses.

materials must be cultured for aerobic, anaerobic, and microaerophilic organisms.

THE DIAGNOSTIC APPROACH TO LIVER ABSCESS

The presence of a liver abscess may be suggested by the patient's history, physical examination, and results of laboratory tests but is confirmed by imaging techniques. It is unnecessary to subject patients to every type of scan available, and the choice of initial investigation should be governed by local facilities and expertise. Ultrasound is our preferred initial investigation, although it is the most operator dependent of the various imaging modalities. If high quality ultrasound cannot be guaranteed, or if the clinician suspects the presence of an abscess despite negative ultrasound, CT scanning is indicated. We find scintigraphy the least helpful of the scanning modalities.

The features of amebic and pyogenic liver abscess are compared in Table 39-1.[14,64] Diagnosis of the etiology of the abscess should not be made on the results of scans alone. In most cases a confident diagnosis is reached combining epidemiologic, clinical, and radiologic features with the results of blood cultures and amebic serology. If amebic liver abscess is suspected on clinical or epidemiologic grounds, we begin treatment with chloroquine; this treatment is specific for hepatic amebiasis but not for pyogenic abscess. Response to chloroquine, or lack of it, is in itself a useful diagnostic test. Metronidazole may successfully treat anaerobic pyogenic infections, and therapeutic response is therefore not specific for amebiasis.[83] Negative amebic serology virtually excludes the diagnosis of hepatic amebiasis, despite rare cases in which serologic tests become positive after the patient's initial presentation. If

invasive amebiasis seems likely despite an initial negative result, the test should be repeated.

Aspiration of abscesses may be performed for either diagnostic or therapeutic purposes. Diagnostic aspiration is usually performed under ultrasound or CT guidance and involves the removal of a small quantity of abscess material through a fine needle for diagnostic studies. In regions of the world in which sophisticated imaging techniques are not available, aspiration has to be performed blind. In such an event, unless an obvious swelling is present, the needle should be cautiously inserted in the area of maximal hepatic tenderness.

The frequency with which diagnostic aspiration need be undertaken varies with local patterns of disease. Aspiration is rarely indicated in patients with amebic liver abscess, in whom there is usually time to safely await the results of amebic serology and response to therapy with chloroquine. When it is obtained, the aspirate from an amebic abscess is usually orange-brown, odorless, and bacteriologically sterile. In pyogenic abscess, however, diagnostic aspiration may be critically important for microbiologic diagnosis when this has not already been obtained from blood cultures. The detection of malodorous pus and the identification of organisms on Gram stain may provide immediate assistance in the choice of antibiotic therapy.

Diagnostic aspiration is absolutely indicated in the critically ill, in whom there is no time to wait for results of blood cultures and serodiagnostic tests; in patients with negative blood cultures and amebic serology; and in those with either type of abscess not responding to medical therapy. In pyogenic abscess the latter raises the possibility of infection with an organism not covered by administered antibiotics; in hepatic amebiasis bacterial superinfection needs to be excluded.

TREATMENT

Amebic Liver Abscess

The management of amebiasis has been usefully reviewed by Knight.[90,91]

Chemotherapeutic Agents (Table 39-2)

Metronidazole. Metronidazole is currently the treatment of choice for all forms of invasive amebiasis.[55] It is a nitroimidazole that is well absorbed after oral administration, and it is excreted mainly via the kidneys. Reduction of the drug's nitro group by *E. histolytica* produces toxic metabolites that interfere with nucleic acid synthesis. Side-effects include nausea, anorexia, metallic taste, urethral and vaginal burning, dark urine, and a disulfiram-like reaction with alcohol. Central nervous system effects such as vertigo, ataxia, and peripheral neuropathy have also been reported. A transient leukopenia is occasionally ob-

TABLE 39-1.   Comparison of Amebic and Pyogenic Liver Abscess

CRITERIA	AMEBIC	PYOGENIC
Age	Any; mostly younger	Any, mostly older
Sex	Males more than females	Equal
Epidemiologic features	Residence/travel in endemic area; poverty; poor hygiene; homosexuality	None. Occasional association with roundworm or fluke infection
Associated medical conditions	Rare	Common (*e.g.,* surgery; biliary tract disease; diverticulitis; tumors)
Significant jaundice	Rare	Common
Multiple abscesses	Infrequent	Common
Complications	Rupture	Rupture; extension; sepsis
Amebic serology	Positive	Negative (unless previously exposed)
Blood cultures	Negative; if positive, it indicates superinfection	Frequently positive
Response to chloroquine	Yes	No
Response to metronidazole	Yes	Sometimes
Abscess contents	Thick fluid; variable color, yellow-brown, non-odorous	Pus; creamy yellow, mostly foul smelling
Medical therapy effective	Almost always	Often
Percutaneous drainage required	Very rarely	Sometimes
Surgery required	Almost never	Sometimes
Mortality with prompt diagnosis	Very low	Appreciable

served. Reports of possible carcinogenicity, mutagenicity, and teratogenicity under experimental conditions have not been matched by adverse effects in humans, and the advantages of metronidazole for severe disease, including in pregnancy, outweigh its theoretic dangers. In practice, the gastrointestinal side-effects cause the most trouble.

The usual dosage of metronidazole is 750 mg three times daily for 5 to 10 days. In actual fact, a choice of regimens is available, and large single doses (2.4 g) given for shorter periods such as 3 days may be equally effective.[146] The usual pediatric dose is 35 mg to 50 mg/kg/day in three divided doses. In very ill patients some clinicians extend treatment to 15 days or even beyond. As with many infectious diseases, the duration of treatment prescribed is often somewhat arbitrary. Patients unable to take oral metronidazole may be treated with the parenteral preparation.[26,59,98] Metronidazole is effective treatment for invasive intestinal disease but is not completely reliable as a luminal amebicide.

Occasional treatment failures have been reported, in addition to cases of hepatic amebiasis developing after metronidazole therapy for intestinal disease.[1,56,67,68,70,97,144,182,197] Other nitroimidazoles offer no advantage over metronidazole. The best known is tinidazole, which is perhaps associated with less nausea. The usual adult dosage is 2 g/day.

Chloroquine. The antimalarial drug chloroquine, a 4-aminoquinoline, acts by binding to parasite DNA.[90,91] High concentrations in liver tissue are obtained after oral administration. It has a half-life up to a week and is excreted predominantly through the kidneys.

Side-effects are nausea, abdominal discomfort, and pruritus. Retinopathy is only a potential problem in individuals taking long-term chloroquine as for malaria prophylaxis or rheumatoid arthritis. The usual dose is 1 g/day for 2 days followed by 500 mg/day for 20 days. The only controlled trial of chloroquine versus metronidazole for amebic liver abscess showed no difference in efficacy, other than slightly quicker response with metronidazole.[28] Chloroquine has no action against intestinal infection.

Emetine and Dehydroemetine. Emetine is the oldest as well as the most potent amebicidal drug available. It is given by intramuscular or subcutaneous injection and is slowly excreted through the kidneys. The drug acts by interfering with protein synthesis. The usual dosage is 1 mg/kg/day, to a maximum of 60 mg/day for 10 days. Duration of treatment should be kept to a minimum, preferably less than 6 days. Side-effects have rendered this drug obsolete except in the most severe of cases. Adverse effects include vomiting, diarrhea, renal impairment, and pain or necrosis at the site of injection. The most serious

TABLE 39-2.   Drugs in the Treatment of Amebic Liver Abscess

DRUG	CONVENTIONAL DOSAGE	SIDE-EFFECTS
Metronidazole	Adult: 750 mg tid for 5–10 days (alternative schedule 2.4 g once daily for 3–5 days) Pediatric: 35–50 mg/kg/day in three divided doses for 5–10 days Also effective for intestinal amebiasis	Anorexia, nausea, metallic taste, dark urine, disulfiram-like reaction, central nervous system effects, leukopenia. Carcinogenicity in animals; mutagenicity in bacteria.
Chloroquine	Adult: Loading dose 1 g daily for 1–2 days, then 500 mg daily for 20 days Pediatric: 10 mg base/kg Ineffective for intestinal amebiasis	Nausea, vomiting, pruritus; cardiotoxicity in overdose. Retinopathy with long-term ingestion.
Emetine	1 mg/kg by intramuscular or subcutaneous injection (maximum 60 mg/day) for up to 10 days, not to be repeated within 1 month Ineffective as a luminal amebicide	Cardiotoxicity, nausea, vomiting, diarrhea, renal impairment, pain or necrosis at injection site.
Dehydroemetine	1.25 mg/kg intramuscular or subcutaneous injection (maximum 90 mg/day) for up to 10 days. Ineffective as a luminal amebicide.	As for emetine, although less cardiotoxic.
Luminal Amebicides Diloxanide furoate	Adult: 500 mg tid for 10 days Pediatric: 20 mg/kg/day in three divided doses	Very few side-effects: mild gastrointestinal disturbance, flatulence. Available in the United States from Parasitic Diseases Division, Centers for Disease Control, Atlanta, Georgia 30333
Diiodohydroxyquin	Adult: 650 mg tid for 20 days Pediatric: 30–40 mg/kg/day in three divided doses; maximum 2 g daily.	Furunculosis, dermatitis, chills, fever, and abdominal discomfort. Neuropathy, myelopathy, and optic atrophy with longer use. Subacute myelo-optic neuropathy associated particularly with related compound iodochlorhydroxyquin.

side-effect, however, is cardiotoxicity, any sign of which is an absolute indication for stopping the drug. Emetine has no luminal amebicidal activity.

Dehydroemetine is a synthetic preparation with a similar action to emetine but is associated with less cardiotoxicity. It is equally effective therapeutically but is excreted more rapidly. The daily dose is 1.25 mg/kg, given by intramuscular or subcutaneous injection, to a maximum of 90 mg/day. It should be given in preference to emetine, if available. Cardiotoxicity may be more likely with concurrent administration of chloroquine.[172]

Management of the Patient

Therapy with chloroquine is begun while awaiting amebic serology in cases of suspected amebic liver abscess. Metronidazole is substituted once there is firm laboratory support for the diagnosis. Five days of metronidazole is curative in the majority of patients, although in the very ill treatment is continued for 10 to 14 days. Chloroquine is continued as well in such cases. Emetine, or preferably dehydroemetine, is reserved for patients not responding to treatment and is used in conjunction with metronidazole.

Critically ill patients, and those not responding to medical therapy within 48 to 72 hours, should undergo diagnostic aspiration to confirm the diagnosis and exclude bacterial superinfection. Therapeutic percutaneous aspiration is indicated for cases not responding to treatment and for patients in whom rupture seems imminent. Therapeutic aspiration is performed with a large bore needle, preferably under ultrasound or CT guidance, to evacuate as much abscess material as possible. Abscess size should not in itself be a deciding factor about aspiration, although large abscesses are perhaps especially likely to respond slowly to medical treatment. Left lobe lesions must be carefully assessed, in view of their propensity to rupture into the pericardium. Provided diagnosis is not excessively delayed, the great majority of patients can be managed medically without aspiration. Following successful therapy, defects may remain evident on ultrasonography for months or even years (Fig. 39-11).[149,152] Such lesions contain thin, serous fluid.[149] They should not be aspirated and need no specific treatment.

Medical therapy is also the cornerstone of treatment of amebic liver abscess with complications. The role of surgery in such cases is controversial. Amebic empyema should probably be drained, usually by a needle or chest

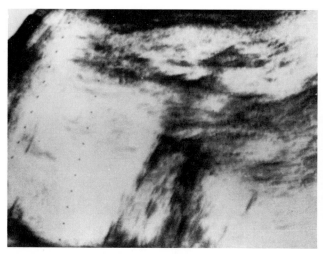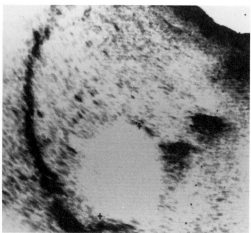

Fig. 39-11. Left. Ultrasound of liver showing a large amebic abscess. Transverse view. **Right.** A cystic residual defect is seen 5 years later and was followed unchanged for another 2 years. Sagittal view.

tube and more rarely by open thoracotomy. Untreated, chronic empyema and pleural thickening may result.[76] Occasionally, amebic empyema is erroneously diagnosed on "thoracentesis" that yields typical amebic pus, when the aspirating needle in such cases has actually traversed the high right diaphragm into the liver abscess cavity. Hepatobronchial fistula may be self-limiting. If secondary lung abscess develops, this can be treated medically, but bacterial contamination must be searched for.

Rupture into the pericardium is an emergency requiring immediate pericardiocentesis. If aspiration through a needle is unsuccessful, then drainage through a pericardial window is indicated. Constrictive pericarditis may develop at a later stage despite appropriate acute management and may require pericardiectomy.[106]

Rupture of an amebic abscess into the peritoneal cavity is frequently only discovered at laparotomy for an undiagnosed acute abdomen. If the diagnosis at operation is clear, the peritoneal cavity should be lavaged, the abscess drained, and medical therapy promptly instituted. Secondary bacterial contamination is a major complication and efforts should be made to avoid it by limiting surgical maneuvers to a minimum. Unless there is failure to respond to therapy, operation is not indicated for peritoneal rupture diagnosed by paracentesis.[63]

It is reasonable to assume that intestinal infection preceded a liver abscess and to treat all patients with a luminal amebicide. Metronidazole is not wholly effective in this regard and does not always eradicate cyst passage. Diloxanide furoate and diiodohydroxyquin are the preferred agents. The respective adult dosages are 500 mg three times daily for 10 days and 650 mg three times daily for 20 days, conventionally given after completion of treatment of hepatic disease.

Prognosis

Amebiasis is an eminently treatable disease, and probably the major factor determining outcome is the rapidity with which the diagnosis is reached. Paradoxically, lack of familiarity with amebic liver abscess in areas well served medically may result in higher mortality than in countries with limited facilities.[42] In uncomplicated disease the case-fatality rate should be less than 1%.[6] The highest death rate is associated with rupture into the pericardium, 32% to 100% in different series.[7,77,106] In general, rupture into the peritoneal cavity or into the chest has a mortality up to 20%. The prognosis of rupture need not be as dire as suggested by autopsy studies,[87] provided diagnosis and treatment are instituted without delay.

Pyogenic Liver Abscess

The traditional treatment for pyogenic liver abscess has been open surgical drainage, combined with broad-spectrum antibiotics.[9] In recent times percutaneous drainage of intra-abdominal abscesses has become widely accepted practice,[54,61,69,84,190] and this technique has also been applied to hepatic abscesses.[15,66,99,109,141,174] This approach is not new; McFadzean and co-workers reported a successful outcome in 13 of 14 patients with pyogenic liver abscess treated by percutaneous needle drainage and antibiotics in 1953.[116] The procedure is now preferably performed under ultrasound or CT guidance, and if aspiration is considered inadequate a pigtailed catheter with side holes may be left *in situ* until drainage stops. The complications of this procedure include bleeding, perforation of intra-abdominal structures, infection, and catheter displacement.

It has now been shown that a significant proportion of patients can be managed medically without aspiration or surgery,[13,16,37,72,107,185] despite some reports to the contrary.[113,121] Although some groups perform diagnostic aspiration in all cases prior to commencing antibiotics, others choose antibiotic therapy on the basis of blood culture results alone. Experience of mixed growths in abscess aspirates with only one organism in the bloodstream and in cases with negative blood cultures suggest that diagnostic aspiration should be routinely performed when pyogenic abscess is suspected. In general, antibiotics effective against gram-negative bacilli as well as against microaerophilic and anaerobic organisms should be prescribed until a microbiologic diagnosis has been established. Duration of treatment is uncertain and should be guided by clinical response. Four to 6 weeks of antibiotic therapy seems appropriate.

Management of the Patient

We consider patients with negative amebic serology who do not respond to chloroquine to be suffering from pyogenic abscess. The results of blood and abscess cultures determine our selection of antibiotics, although we always include an agent effective against anaerobes in the regimen while culture results are pending. *Streptococcus milleri* is sensitive to penicillin-like drugs but not to metronidazole. Frequently used combinations to initiate therapy are ampicillin, an aminoglycoside or third-generation cephalosporin, and clindamycin or metronidazole. Exact microbiologic diagnosis subsequently allows administration of specific antimicrobial therapy. Failure to show some improvement within 48 to 72 hours of beginning appropriate antibiotic therapy leads us to undertake drainage, usually via a catheter. Diagnostic aspiration is performed by the radiologist, under ultrasound or CT guidance, with the internist in attendance to assist in the appropriate handling of specimens. We have used our approach successfully in several dozen patients. In most cases parenteral antibiotics can be replaced by oral medication after 10 to 14 days, with treatment being continued for a further 3 to 4 weeks.

The belief that many patients can be managed medically is tempered by recognition that some patients urgently require drainage. Clinical judgment must be used to carry out swift diagnostic or therapeutic aspiration in those cases in need of it. In addition, surgery remains indicated in a proportion of patients, such as those with biliary tract disease or associated intra-abdominal infection, and cases not responding to the management outlined previously. Surgery will also usually be required for abscesses complicated by rupture or extension. Close supervision of the patient, flexibility in approach, and cooperation between internist, radiologist, microbiologist, and surgeon are essential.

Prognosis

Traditionally, mortality rates approaching 100% have been quoted for undrained liver abscess.[105,121,143] Reports of successful medical management, with or without aspiration, describe case-fatality rates as low as 10%.[72,107] As in amebic abscess, delay in diagnosis and treatment have a major effect on outcome.[164] Prognosis is also related to underlying disease, and an overall mortality of 30% is probably realistic. Mortality seems greater in patients with multiple abscesses. The rarity of pyogenic liver abscess and the wide variation in associated disease make controlled studies of different methods of treatment difficult.

REFERENCES

1. Abioye AA: Drug and immunodiagnostic resistant amoebic liver abscess in Ibadan: An elucidation of a possible mechanism. J Trop Med Hyg 79:252, 1976
2. Abioye AA, Edington GM: Prevalence of amoebiasis at autopsy in Ibadan. Trans R Soc Trop Med Hyg 66:754, 1972
3. Abuabara SF, Barrett JA, Hau T, Jonasson O: Amebic liver abscess. Arch Surg 117:239, 1982
4. Abul-Khair MH, Kenawi MM, Korashy EE, Arafa NM: Ultrasonography and amoebic liver abscesses. Ann Surg 93:221, 1981
5. Adamali N, Wankya BM, Maneno J: Infusion tomography of the liver in the diagnosis of amoebic liver abscess: A preliminary report. East Afr Med J 55:414, 1979
6. Adams EB, MacLeod IN: Invasive amebiasis: II. Amebic liver abscess and its complications. Medicine 56:325, 1977
7. Adeyemo AO, Aderounmu A: Intrathoracic complications of amoebic liver abscess. J R Soc Med 77:17, 1984
8. Alkan WJ, Kalmi B, Kalderon M: The clinical syndrome of amebic abscess of the left lobe of the liver. Ann Intern Med 55:800, 1961
9. Altemeier WA: Pyogenic liver abscess. In Schiff L, Schiff ER (eds): Diseases of the Liver, 5th ed, pp 1221–1238. Philadelphia, JB Lippincott, 1982
10. Ambroise-Thomas P, Desgeorges PT, Monget D: Diagnostic immuno-enzymologique (ELISA) des maladies parasitaires par une micromethode modifiée. Bull WHO 56:797, 1978
11. Amin N: Amoebiasis and corticosteroids. Br Med J 2:1084, 1978
12. Armen RC, Fry M, Heseltine PNR: Spontaneous colonic drainage: A rare complication of an amebic liver abscess. West J Med 142:253, 1985
13. Balasegaram M: Management of hepatic abscess. Curr Probl Surg 18:285, 1981
14. Barbour GL, Juniper K: A clinical comparison of amebic and pyogenic abscess of the liver in sixty-six patients. Am J Med 53:323, 1972
15. Berger LA, Osborne DR: Treatment of pyogenic liver abscesses by percutaneous needle aspiration. Lancet 1:132, 1982
16. Bertoli D, Del Poggio P, Mazzolari M, Randone G: Management of liver abscesses. Lancet 1:743, 1982
17. Biagi FF, Robledo E, Servin H, Marvan G: Influence of some steroids in the experimental production of amebic hepatic abscess. Am J Trop Med Hyg 12:318, 1963
18. Bloch DB: Venturesome toothpick: A continuing source of pyogenic hepatic abscess. JAMA 252:797, 1984
19. Boultbee JE, Simjee AE, Rooknoodeen F, Engelbrecht HE: Experiences with grey scale ultrasonography in hepatic amoebiasis. Clin Radiol 30:683, 1979

20. Bray RS, Harris WG: The epidemiology of infection with *Entamoeba histolytica* in the Gambia, West Africa. Trans R Soc Trop Med Hyg 71:401, 1977

21. Brennan RO, Durack DT: The viridans streptococci in perspective. In Remmington JS, Swartz MN (eds): Current Clinical Topics in Infectious Diseases, vol 5, p 253. New York, McGraw-Hill, 1984

22. Brossi A, Baumann N, Chopard-dit-Jean LH et al: Syntheseversuche in der Emetine-Reihe: 4. Mitteilung Racemisches 2-Dehydroemetine. Helv Chim Acta 42:772, 1959

23. Capin R, Capin NR, Carmona M, Ortiz-Ortiz L: Effect of complement depletion on the induction of amebic liver abscess in the hamster. Arch Invest Med (Mex) 11:173, 1980

24. Centers for Disease Control: Amebiasis associated with colonic irrigation—Colorado. MMWR 30:101, 1981

25. Centers for Disease Control: Pseudo-outbreaks of intestinal amoebiasis—California. MMWR 34:125, 1985

26. Chowcat NL, Wyllie JH: Intravenous metronidazole in amoebic enterocolitis. Lancet 2:1143, 1976

27. Cockshott P, Middlemiss H: Amoebiasis. In Clinical Radiology in the Tropics, pp 130–132. Edinburgh, Churchill-Livingstone, 1979

28. Cohen HG, Reynolds TB: Comparison of metronidazole and chloroquine for the treatment of amoebic liver abscess. Gastroenterology 69:35, 1975

29. Conan NJ: The treatment of amebic hepatitis with chloroquine. Bull NY Acad Med 24:545, 1948

30. Conona NJ: Chloroquine in amebiasis. Am J Trop Med 28:107, 1948

31. Connor DH, Neafie RC, Meyers WM: Amebiasis. In Binford CH, Connor DH (eds): Pathology of Tropical and Extraordinary Diseases, vol 1, pp 308–316. Washington, DC, Armed Forces Institute of Pathology, 1976

32. Cook GC: Tropical Gastroenterology, Oxford, Oxford University Press, 1980

33. Councilman WT, La Fleur HA: Amoebic dysentery. Bull Johns Hopkins Hosp 2:395, 1891

34. Cowan DB, Houlton MCC: Rupture of an amoebic liver abscess in pregnancy. S Afr Med J 53:460, 1978

35. Dalrymple RB, Fataar S, Goodman A et al: Hyperechoic amoebic liver abscesses: An unusual ultrasonic appearance. Clin Radiol 33:541, 1982

36. De Bakey ME, Ochsner A: Hepatic amoebiasis: A 20 year experience and analysis of 263 cases. Int Abstr Surg 92:209, 1951

37. De Cock KM, Bhatt KM, Bhatt SM et al: Management of liver abscesses. Lancet 1:743, 1982

38. De Cock KM, Calder JF: Ultrasonic diagnosis of abdominal disease in Kenya. Trans R Soc Trop Med Hyg 75:632, 1981

39. De Silva K: Intraperitoneal rupture of an amoebic liver abscess in a pregnant woman at term. Ceylon Med J 15:51, 1970

40. Diamond LS: Amebiasis: Nutritional implications. Rev Infect Dis 4:843, 1982

41. Diaz CA: Amebic hepatic abscess. In Padilla y Padilla CA, Padilla GM (eds): Amebiasis in Man. Springfield, IL, Charles C Thomas, 1974

42. Dorrough RL: Amebic liver abscess. South Med J 60:305, 1967

43. Dritz SK, Ainsworth TE, Garrard WF et al: Patterns of sexually transmitted enteric diseases in a city. Lancet 2:3, 1977

44. Edington GM, Gilles HM: Amoebiasis and the liver. In Pathology in the Tropics, 2nd ed, vol 2, pp 71–73. London, Edward Arnold, 1976

45. Editorial: Is that amoeba harmful or not? Lancet 1:732, 1985

46. Eggleston FC, Handa AK, Verghese M: Amebic peritonitis secondary to amebic liver abscess. Surgery 91:46, 1982

47. Eisert J, Hannibal JE, Sanders SL: Fatal amebiasis complicating corticosteroid management of pemphigus vulgaris. N Engl J Med 261:843, 1959

48. El-Hennawy M, Abd-Rabbo H: Hazards of cortisone therapy in hepatic amoebiasis. J Trop Med Hyg 81:71, 1978

49. Elsdon-Dew R: The epidemiology of amoebiasis. In Dawes B (ed): Advances in Parasitology. New York, Academic Press, 1968

50. Elsdon-Dew R: Amebiasis as a world problem. Bull NY Acad Med 47:438, 1971

51. Eykyn S, Phillips I: Pyogenic liver abscess. Br Med J 280:1617, 1980

52. Facklam RR: The major differences in the American and British streptococcus taxonomy schemes with reference to *Streptococcus milleri*. Eur J Clin Microbiol 3:91, 1984

53. Falaiye JM, Okeke GCE, Fregene AO: Amoebic abscess in the cirrhotic liver. Gut 21:161, 1980

54. Ferrucci JT, Van Sonnenberg E: Intra-abdominal abscess: Radiological diagnosis and treatment. JAMA 246:2728, 1981

55. Finegold SM: Metronidazole. Ann Intern Med 93:585, 1980

56. Fisher LS, Chow AW, Lindquist L, Guze LB: Failure of metronidazole in amebic liver abscess. Am J Med Sci 271:65, 1976

57. Fitz RH: Perforating inflammation of the vermiform appendix; with special reference to its early diagnosis and treatment. Am J Med Sci 92:321, 1886

58. Freeny PC: Acute pyogenic hepatitis: Sonographic and angiographic findings. AJR 135:388, 1980

59. Gall SA, Edmisten C, Vernon RP: Intravenous metronidazole in the treatment of ruptured amebic liver abscess. South Med J 73:1274, 1980

60. Gathiram V, Simjee AE, Bhamjee A, et al: Concomitant and secondary bacterial infection of the pus in hepatic amoebiasis. S Afr Med J 65:951, 1984

61. Gerzof SG, Robbins AH, Johnson WC et al: Percutaneous catheter drainage of abdominal abscesses. N Engl J Med 305:653, 1981

62. Gooneratne NS, Imarisio JJ: Decreased uptake of 67 gallium citrate (67 GA) by a bacterial hepatic abscess. Gastroenterology 73:1147, 1977

63. Greaney GC, Reynolds TB, Donnovan AJ: Ruptured amebic liver abscess. Arch Surg 120:555, 1985

64. Greenstein AJ, Barth J, Dicker A et al: Amebic liver abscess: A study of 11 cases compared with a series of 38 patients with pyogenic liver abscess. Am J Gastroenterol 80:472, 1985

65. Greenstein AJ, Lowenthal D, Hammer GS et al: Continuing changing patterns of disease in pyogenic liver abscess: A study of 38 patients. Am J Gastroenterol 79:217, 1984

66. Greenwood LH, Collins TL, Yrizarry JM: Percutaneous management of multiple liver abscesses. AJR 139:390, 1982

67. Gregory PB: A refractory case of hepatic amoebiasis. Gastroenterology 70:585, 1976

68. Griffin FM: Failure of metronidazole to cure hepatic amebic abscess. N Engl J Med 288:1397, 1973

69. Haaga JR, Weinstein AJ: CT-guided percutaneous aspiration and drainage of abscesses. AJR 135:1187, 1980

70. Harrison HR, Crowe CP, Fulginiti VA: Amebic liver abscess in children: Clinical and epidemiologic features. Pediatrics 64:923, 1979

71. Henn RM, Collin DB: Amebic abscess of the liver: Treatment failure with metronidazole. JAMA 224:1394, 1973

72. Herbert DA, Fogel DA, Rothman J et al: Pyogenic liver abscesses: Successful non-surgical therapy. Lancet 1:134, 1982

73. Heymann AD: Clinical aspects of grave pyogenic abscess of the liver. Surg Gynecol Obstet 149:209, 1979

74. Huddle KR: Amoebic liver abscess, inferior vena-caval compression and the nephrotic syndrome. S Afr Med J 61:758, 1982

75. Hutt MSR: Some aspects of liver disease in Ugandan Africans. Trans R Soc Trop Med Hyg 65:273, 1971

76. Ibarra-Perez C: Thoracic complications of amebic abscess of the liver: Report of 501 cases. Chest 79:672, 1981

77. Ibarra-Perez C, Green L, Calvillo-Juarez M, de la Cruz JV: Diagnosis and treatment of rupture of amebic abscess of the liver into the pericardium. J Thorac Cardiovasc Med 64:11, 1972

78. Ibarra-Perez C, Selman-Lama M: Diagnosis and treatment of amebic "empyema". Am J Surg 134:283, 1977

79. Imperato PJ: A historical overview of amebiasis. Bull NY Acad Med 57:175, 1981

80. Juniper KS, Worrell CL, Minshew MC et al: Serologic diagnosis of amebiasis. Am J Trop Med Hyg 21:157, 1972

81. Kanani SR, Knight R: Relapsing amoebic colitis of 12 years' standing exacerbated by corticosteroids. Br Med J 2:613, 1969

82. Kandel G, Marcon NE: Pyogenic liver abscess: New concepts of an old disease. Am J Gastroenterol 79:65, 1984

83. Kane JG, Parker RH: Metronidazole and hepatic abscess: A false-positive response. JAMA 236:2653, 1976

84. Karlson KB, Martin EC, Frankuchen EI et al: Percutaneous abscess drainage. Surg Gynecol Obstet 154:44, 1982

85. Kartulis S: Zur Aetiologie der Dysenterie in Aegypten. Arch Pathol Anat 105:521, 1886

86. Katzenstein D, Rickerson V, Braude A: New concepts of amebic liver abscess derived from hepatic imaging, serodiagnosis, and hepatic enzymes in 67 consecutive cases in San Diego. Medicine 61:237, 1982

87. Kean BH, Gilmore HR, Van Stone WW: Fatal amebiasis: Report of 148 fatal cases from the Armed Forces Institute of Pathology. Ann Intern Med 44:831, 1956

88. Kean BH, William DC, Luminais SK: Epidemic of amoebiasis and giardiasis in a biased population. Br J Vener Dis 55:375, 1979

89. Kew MC, Osler HI, McCann WG et al: Radiocolloid imaging in primary liver cancer and amoebic liver abscess. S Afr Med J 56:127, 1979

90. Knight R: Hepatic amoebiasis. Semin Liver Dis 4:277, 1984

91. Knight R: The chemotherapy of amoebiasis. J Antimicrob Chemother 6:577, 1980

92. Knobloch J, Funke M, Bienzle U: Autochthonous amoebic liver abscess in Germany. Tropenmed Parasitol 31:414, 1980

93. Knobloch J, Mannweiler E: Development and persistence of antibodies to Entamoeba histolytica in patients with amebic liver abscess: Analysis of 216 cases. Am J Trop Med Hyg 32:727, 1983

94. Koch R, Gaffky G: Bericht uber die Thatigkeit der zur Erforschung der cholera in jahre 1883 nach Egypten und Indien Enstandten Kommission. Arb Kaisere Ges 3:1, 1887

95. Koehler PR, Moss AA: Diagnosis of intra-abdominal and pelvic abscesses by computerized tomography. JAMA 244:49, 1980

96. Koshy A, Khuroo MS, Suri S et al: Amebic liver abscess with hemobilia. Am J Surg 138:453, 1979

97. Koutsaimanis KG, Timms PW, Ree GH: Failure of metronidazole in a patient with hepatic amebic abscess. Am J Trop Med Hyg 28:768, 1979

98. Kovaleski T, Malangoni MA, Wheat LJ: Treatment of an amebic liver abscess with intravenous metronidazole. Arch Intern Med 141:132, 1981

99. Kraulis JE, Bird BL, Colapinto ND: Percutaneous catheter drainage of liver abscess: An alternative to open drainage? Br J Surg 67:400, 1980

100. Krettek JE, Goldstein LI, Busuttil RW: The symptoms of an amebic abscess of the liver stimulating an acute surgical abdomen. Surg Gynecol Obstet 148:552, 1979

101. Krogstad DJ, Spencer HC, Healy GR et al: Amebiasis: Epidemiologic studies in the United States, 1971–1974. Ann Intern Med 88:89, 1978

102. Kuligowska E, Connors SK, Shapiro JH: Liver abscess: Sonography in diagnosis and treatment. AJR 138:253, 1982

103. Lamont AC, Wicks ACB: Amoebic liver abscess in Rhodesian Africans. Trans R Soc Trop Med Hyg 70:302, 1976

104. Lazarchick J, de Souza E, Silva NA et al: Pyogenic liver abscess. Mayo Clin Proc 48:349, 1973

105. Losch FA: Massive development of amebas in the large intestine (translated from the original). Am J Trop Med Hyg 24:383, 1975

106. Macleod IN, Wilmot AJ, Powell SJ: Amoebic pericarditis. Q J Med 35:293, 1966

107. Maher JA, Reynolds TB, Yellin AE: Successful medical treatment of pyogenic liver abscess. Gastroenterology 77:618, 1979

108. Marr JS: Amebiasis in New York City: A changing pattern of transmission. Bull NY Acad Med 57:188, 1981

109. Martin EC, Karlson KB, Frankuchen E et al: Percutaneous drainage in the management of hepatic abscesses. Surg Clin North Am 61:157, 1981

110. Martinez-Palomo A, Martinez-Baez M: Selective primary health care: Strategies for control of disease in the developing world: X. Amebiasis. Rev Infect Dis 5:1093, 1983

111. Mayet FGH, Powell SJ: Anemia associated with amebic liver abscess. Am J Trop Med Hyg 13:790, 1964

112. McCarty E, Pathmanand C, Sunakorn P, Scherz RG: Amebic liver abscess in childhood. Am J Dis Child 126:67, 1973

113. McCorkell SJ, Niles NL: Pyogenic liver abscesses: Another look at medical management. Lancet 1:803, 1985

114. McDonald MI: Pyogenic liver abscess: Diagnosis, bacteriology and treatment. Eur J Clin Micro 3:506, 1984

115. McDonald MI, Corey GR, Gallis HA, Durack DT: Single and multiple pyogenic liver abscesses: Natural history, diagnosis and treatment, with emphasis on percutaneous drainage. Medicine 63:291, 1984

116. McFadzean AJS, Chang KPS, Wong CC: Solitary pyogenic abscess of the liver treated by closed aspiration and antibiotics: A report of 14 consecutive cases of recovery. Br J Surg 41:141, 1953

117. McMillan A, Gilmour HM, McNeillage G, Scott GR: Ameobiasis in homosexual men. Gut 25:356, 1984

118. Merritt RJ, Coughlin E, Thomas DW et al: Spectrum of amebiasis in children. Am J Dis Child 136:785, 1982

119. Meyers JD, Kuharic HA, Holmes KK: *Giardia lamblia* infection in homosexual men. Br J Vener Dis 53:54, 1977

120. Michel ML, Wirth RW: Multiple pyogenic abscesses of the liver: Cure by penicillin in case due to anaerobic streptococci. JAMA 133:395, 1947

121. Miedema BW, Dineen P: The diagnosis and treatment of pyogenic liver abscesses. Ann Surg 200:328, 1984

122. Mitchell RW, Teare AJ: Amoebic liver abscess in pregnancy. Br J Obstet Gynaecol 91:393, 1984

123. Monga NK, Wig JD, Sood KC et al: Amebic peritonitis. Int Surg 62:431, 1977

124. Moore-Gillon JC, Eykyn SJ, Phillips I: Microbiology of pyogenic liver abscess. Br Med J 283:819, 1981

125. Most H: Manhattan: "A tropical isle?" Am J Trop Med Hyg 17:333, 1968

126. Mylius RE, Tenseldam REJ: Venereal infection by *Entamoeba histolytica* in a New Guinea native couple. Trop Geogr Med 14:20, 1962

127. Naidoo PM, Keeton G, Stein L et al: Hepatic amoebiasis. S Afr Med J 48:1159, 1974

128. Naik SR, Achar BG, Mehta SK. Reversible portal hypertension in amoebic liver abscess: A case report. J Trop Med Hyg 81:116, 1978

129. Navaratne RA: Postpartum intraperitoneal rupture of an amoebic liver abscess. Ceylon Med J 17:160, 1972

130. Neale G, Caughey DE, Mollin DL, Booth CC: Effects of intrahepatic and extrahepatic infection on liver function. Br Med J 1:382, 1966

131. Neoptolemos JP, Macpherson DS: Pyogenic liver abscess. Br J Hosp Med 26:48, 1981

132. Newlin N, Silver TM, Stuck KJ, Sandler MA: Ultrasonic features of pyogenic liver abscesses. Radiology 139:155, 1981

133. Nigam P, Gupta AK, Kapoor KK et al: Cholestasis in amoebic liver abscess. Gut 26:140, 1985

134. Northover JMA, Jones BJM, Dawson JL, Williams R: Difficulties in the diagnosis and management of pyogenic liver abscess. Br J Surg 69:48, 1982

135. Ochsner A, DeBakey M, Murray S: Pyogenic abscess of the liver: II. An analysis of forty-seven cases with review of the literature. Am J Surg 40:292, 1938

136. Osler W: On the *Amoeba coli* in dysentery and in dysenteric liver abscess. Bull Johns Hopkins Hosp 1:53, 1890

137. Ottenberg R, Berck M: Sulfanilamide therapy for suppurative pylephlebitis and liver abscesses. JAMA 111:1374, 1938

138. Ou Tim L, Segal I, Hodkinson HJ: Amoebic liver abscess in patients presenting with jaundice. S Afr Med J 55:179, 1979

139. Palmer ED: The changing manifestations of pyogenic liver abscess. JAMA 231:192, 1975

140. Patterson M, Healy GR, Shabot JM: Serologic testing for amoebiasis. Gastroenterology 78:136, 1980

141. Perera MR, Kirk A, Noone P: Presentation, diagnosis and management of liver abscess. Lancet 2:629, 1980

142. Perry HB, Boulanger M, Pennoyer D: Chronic granulomatous disease in an adult with recurrent abscesses. Arch Surg 115:200, 1980

143. Pitt HA, Zuidema GD: Factors influencing mortality in the treatment of pyogenic hepatic abscess. Surg Gynecol Obstet 140:228, 1975

144. Pittman FE, Pittman JC: Amebic liver abscess following metronidazole therapy for amebic colitis. Am J Trop Med Hyg 23:146, 1974

145. Pomerantz BM, Marr JS, Goldman WD: Amebiasis in New York City 1958–1978: Identification of the male homosexual high risk population. Bull NY Acad Med 56:232, 1980

146. Powell SJ: Therapy of amebiasis. Bull NY Acad Med 47:469, 1971

147. Powell SJ, MacLeod I, Wilmot AJ, Elsdon-Dew R: Metronidazole in amoebic dysentery and amoebic liver abscess. Lancet 2:1329, 1966

148. Powell SJ, Sutton JB, Lautre G: Haemobilia in amoebic liver abscess. S Afr Med J 47:1555, 1973

149. Price ME: Amoebic liver abscess in a Norfolk factory worker. Br Med J 283:1175, 1981

150. Ralls PW, Colletti PM, Halls JM: Imaging in hepatic amebic abscess. In Ravdin JI (ed): Amebiasis: Human Infection by *Entamoeba histolytica.* New York, John Wiley & Sons, in press

151. Ralls PW, Colletti PM, Quinn MF, Halls J: Sonographic findings in hepatic amebic abscess. Radiology 145:123, 1982

152. Ralls PW, Quinn MF, Boswell WD et al: Patterns of resolution in successfully treated hepatic amebic abscess: Sonographic evaluation. Radiology 149:541, 1983

153. Ramachandran S, De Saram R, Rajapakse CNA, Sivalingam S: Hepatic manifestations during amoebic dysentery. Postgrad Med J 49:261, 1973

154. Reed SL, Sargeaunt PG, Braude AI: Resistance to lysis by human serum of pathogenic *Entamoeba histolytica.* Trans R Soc Trop Med Hyg 77:248, 1983

155. Rode H, Davies MRQ, Cywes S: Amoebic liver abscesses in infancy and childhood. S Afr J Surg 16:131, 1978

156. Rogers L: The rapid cure of amoebic dysentery and hepatitis by hypodermic injections of soluble salts of emetine. Br Med J 1:14, 1912

157. Rubin RH, Swartz MN, Malt R: Hepatic abscess: Changes in clinical, bacteriologic and therapeutic aspects. Am J Med 57:602, 1974

158. Rubinson HA, Isikoff MB, Hill MC: Diagnostic imaging of hepatic abscesses: A retrospective analysis. AJR 135:735, 1980

159. Sabbaj J: Anaerobes in liver abscess. Rev Infect Dis 6:S152, 1984

160. Sabbaj J, Sutter V, Finegold SM: Anaerobic pyogenic liver abscesses. Ann Intern Med 77:629, 1972

161. Salata RA, Pearson RD, Ravdin JI: Interaction of human leukocytes and *Entamoeba histolytica:* Killing of virulent amebae by the activated macrophage. J Clin Invest 76:491, 1985

162. Saltzman DA, Smithline N, Davis JR: Fulminant hepatic failure secondary to amebic abscesses. Dig Dis 23:561, 1978

163. Sanderson IR, Walker-Smith JA: Indigenous amoebiasis: An important differential diagnosis of chronic inflammatory bowel disease. Br Med J 289:823, 1984

164. Sandford NL, Bradbear RA, Powell LW: Pyogenic liver abscess: A neglected diagnosis. Aust NZ J Med 14:597, 1984

165. Sargeaunt PG, Oates JK, MacLennan I et al: *Entamoeba histolytica* in male homosexuals. Br J Vener Dis 59:193, 1983

166. Sargeaunt PG, Williams JE, Grene JD: The differentiation of invasive and non-invasive *Entamoeba histolytica* by isoenzyme electrophoresis. Trans R Soc Trop Med Hyg 72:519, 1978

167. Schmid BD, Lalyre Y, Sigel B et al: Inferior vena cava

obstruction complicating amebic liver abscess. Dig Dis Sci 27:565, 1982

168. Scragg J: Amoebic liver abscess in African children. Arch Dis Child 35:171, 1960

169. Seale JP, Lee JH: An unusual complication of corticosteroid therapy for sarcoidosis. Med J Aust 1:252, 1977

170. Sepulveda B, Martinez-Palomo A: Immunology of amoebiasis by *Entamoeba histolytica.* In Cohen S, Warren KS (eds): Immunology of Parasitic Infections, 2nd ed, pp 170–191. Oxford, Blackwell, 1982

171. Sepulveda B, Martinez-Palomo A: Amebiasis. In Warren KS, Mahmoud AAF (eds): Tropical and Geographical Medicine, pp 305–318. New York, McGraw Hill, 1984

172. Seshadri MS, John L, Varkey K, Koshy TS: Ventricular tachycardia in a patient on dehydroemetine and chloroquine for amoebic liver abscess. Med J Aust 1:406, 1979

173. Sexton DJ, Krogstad DJ, Spencer HC Jr et al: Amebiasis in a mental institution: Serologic and epidemiologic studies. Am J Epidemiol 100:414, 1974

174. Sheinfeld AM, Steiner AE, Rivkin LB et al: Transcutaneous drainage of abscesses of the liver guided by computed tomography scan. Surg Gynecol Obstet 155:662, 1982

175. Sherman JD, Robbins SL: Changing trends in the casuistics of hepatic abscess. Am J Med 28:943, 1960

176. Simon CE: Abscess of the liver: Perforation into the lung; *Amoeba coli* in sputum. Bull Johns Hopkins Hosp 1:97, 1890

177. Singh KP, Sreemannarayana MB, Mehdiratta KS: Intraperitoneal rupture of amebic liver abscess. Int Surg 62:432, 1977

178. Smith JW: Identification of fecal parasites in the Special Parasitology Survey of the College of American Pathologists. Am J Clin Pathol 72:371, 1979

179. Spencer HC, Hermos JA, Healey GR et al: Epidemic amebiasis in an Arkansas community. Am J Epidemiol 104:93, 1976

180. Spencer HC, Muchnick C, Sexton DJ et al: Endemic amebiasis in an extended family. Am J Trop Med Hyg 26:628, 1977

181. Stenson WF, Eckert T, Avioli LA: Pyogenic liver abscess. Arch Intern Med 143:126, 1983

182. Stillman AE, Alvarez V, Grube D: Hepatic amebic abscess: Unresponsiveness to combination of metronidazole and surgical drainage. JAMA 229:71, 1974

183. Stuiver PC, Goud THJLM: Corticosteroids and liver amoebiasis. Br Med J 2:394, 1978

184. Tanimoto-Weki M, Vazquez-Saavedra JA, Calderon P, Aguirre-Garcia J: Resultados de la inoculacion al hamster de trofozoitos obtenidos de portadores asintomaticos de *E. histolytica.* Arch Invest Med 4(suppl 1):105, 1973

185. Thomas CT, Berk SL, Thomas E: Management of liver abscesses. Lancet 1:742, 1982

186. Thomas JA, Antony AJ: Amoebiasis of the penis. Br J Urol 48:269, 1976

187. Thompson JE, Forlenza S, Verma R: Amebic liver abscess: A therapeutic approach. Rev Infect Dis 7:171, 1985

188. Thompson JE, Freischlag J, Thomas DS: Amebic liver abscess in a homosexual man. Sex Transm Dis 10:153, 1983

189. Triger DR: Amoebic liver abscess in Wessex—a retrospective survey of 24 cases. J Trop Med Hyg 81:54, 1978

190. Van Sonnenberg E, Ferruci JT, Mueller PR: Percutaneous radiographically guided catheter drainage of abdominal abscesses. JAMA 247:190, 1982

191. Verghese M, Eggleston FC, Handa AK, Singh CM: Management of thoracic amebiasis. J Thorac Cardiovasc Surg 78:757, 1979

192. Vickary FR, Cusick G, Shirley IM, Blackwell RJ: Ultrasound and amoebic liver abscess. Br J Surg 64:113, 1977

193. Vickers PJ, Bohra RC, Sharma GC: Hepatopulmonary amebiasis—a review of 40 cases. Int Surg 67:427, 1982

194. Wagner VP, Smale LE, Lischke JH: Amebic abscess of the liver and spleen in pregnancy and the puerperium. Obstet Gynecol 45:562, 1975

195. Walker EL, Sellards AW: Experimental entamoebic dysentery. Philippine J Sci 8:253, 1913

196. Walsh JA: Estimating the burden of illness in the tropics. In Warren KS, Mahmoud AAF (eds): Tropical and Geographical Medicine. New York, McGraw-Hill, 1984

197. Weber DM: Amebic abscess of liver following metronidazole therapy. JAMA 216:1339, 1971

198. Wittner M, Rosenbaum RM: Role of bacteria in modifying virulence of *Entamoeba histolytica:* Studies of amebae from axenic cultures. Am J Trop Med Hyg 19:755, 1970

199. Ylvisaker JT, McDonald GB: Sexually acquired amebic colitis and liver abscess. West J Med 132:153, 1980

chapter 40

Transplantation of the Liver

THOMAS E. STARZL, SHUNZABURO IWATSUKI,
ROBERT D. GORDON, and CARLOS O. ESQUIVEL

The ultimate therapeutic step in the treatment of any terminal hepatic disease is the provision of a new liver with or without removal of the afflicted native organ. The first clinical trial of liver transplantation took place in 1963. In the subsequent 22 years, more than 1000 attempts have been made throughout the world, 575 of these by us. The historic aspects of both animal and human liver transplantations have been summarized in a book in which the world literature was brought up to date as of the spring of 1969.[3] The last complete summaries of clinical experience were published in 1982[8] and 1985.[5]

KINDS OF OPERATIONS

Auxiliary Transplantation

Liver transplantation was first performed and recorded by Welch of Albany, New York, in 1955. Welch envisioned treating patients who were dying of cirrhosis or other nonneoplastic diseases for whom the removal of the diseased native liver would not be obligatory. With the Welch operation in dogs, the extra canine liver was placed in the right paravertebral gutter or the right side of the pelvis. Its hepatic arterial supply was derived from the aorta or from the iliac artery. Venous inflow was reconstituted by anastomosis of the distal inferior vena cava or a distal iliac vein to the homograft portal vein. Outflow was into the inferior vena cava.

The use of auxiliary homografts for the treatment of benign hepatic disease initially had a special attractiveness and still does in the minds of a minority of students of liver transplantation. Adherents to auxiliary transplantation argue that sacrifice of the remaining function of the failing recipient liver could be avoided, providing some reserve in the event of poor initial performance by the homograft due to ischemia or to a severe but reversible rejection. This might be a particularly significant advantage in patients with biliary atresia, because the synthesizing functions of the liver are often retained until the terminal stages of this disease. Furthermore, it was initially assumed that the placement of an extra liver would be safer and technically less demanding than the orthotopic

procedure, an assumption that has not been validated by actual experience.

The results in animals with auxiliary transplantation have been inferior to those with liver replacement, partly because coexisting livers have the capacity to damage each other to a variable degree according to which organ is the "dominant" one. Factors favoring dominance include a splanchnic source of the blood for portal venous inflow, perfect biliary drainage, optimal total hepatic blood flow, and unimpeded venous outflow. An auxiliary canine liver graft, which does not enjoy these advantages relative to the host liver, undergoes rapid atrophy. More recently, evidence has been acquired to explain the beneficial effect of perfusing the portal vein with splanchnic venous blood. It has been shown that the "hepatotrophic factors" in this kind of venous blood emanate from the pancreas and that the most important constituent is apparently endogenous insulin.[9] Because insulin is largely removed by a single passage through the liver, the first organ having access to pancreatic blood would deprive the second liver of an adequate supply of this hormone.

Until 1973, clinical auxiliary liver transplantation had never resulted in the significant prolongation of recipient life. The results had been so poor that the number of attempts at the auxiliary operation declined virtually to zero. A contributory factor was that the placement of an extra organ had often proved to be more difficult, rather than technically simpler, than liver replacement.

But early in 1973, Fortner of New York City lightened the pessimism about auxiliary transplantation by revascularizing a homograft, as shown in Figure 40-1, whereby the splanchnic blood was directed through the heterotopically located liver. Fortner's patient suffered from biliary atresia. After operation, the bilirubin level fell to normal, the native liver underwent marked shrinkage, and the splenomegaly and hypersplenism were relieved. The follow-up time in the case is now more than a decade. Another patient treated in Paris with a similar operation also has achieved a long survival.

Our own view is that auxiliary transplantation should be reserved for patients with acute hepatic disease, in which the objective is temporary life support during which recovery of the native liver can be obtained. The feasibility of this approach has been proved in several animal studies but not yet in humans.

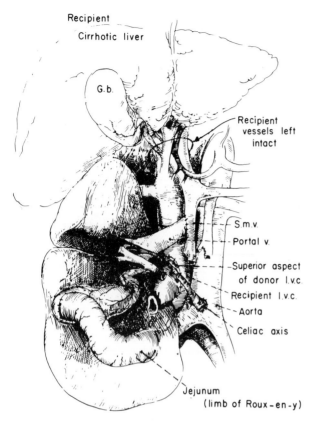

Fig. 40-1. A technique of auxiliary liver transplantation in which the homograft receives through its portal vein venous blood derived from the splanchnic bed. (Starzl TE, Putnam CW: Experience in Hepatic Transplantation, pp 1–553. Philadelphia, WB Saunders, 1969)

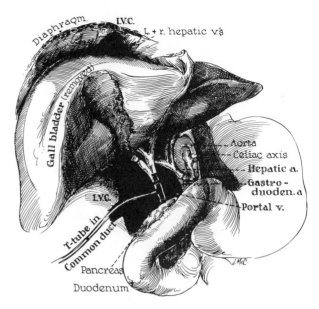

Fig. 40-2. Completed orthotopic liver transplantation. (Starzl TE, Putnam CW: Experience in Hepatic Transplantation, pp 1–553. Philadelphia, WB Saunders, 1969)

Orthotopic Transplantation

The alternative approach to hepatic transplantation is liver replacement (or orthotopic transplantation). With this operation, the diseased host liver is removed, creating a space into which the graft is transplanted with as normal an anatomic reconstruction as possible (Fig. 40-2). Survival exceeding 15 years has been achieved in humans. The remarks in succeeding sections pertain to the more promising orthotopic transplantation as opposed to the auxiliary operation discussed previously.

INDICATIONS

No matter what the underlying disease, certain criteria should be met before patients are accepted for chronic immunosuppression and transplantation. None of the contraindications is absolute, although they may be very strong. For example, preexisting systemic or local infections would create highly unfavorable conditions, as would

diseases of organs other than the liver, such as coexisting severe heart disease, or a history of sociopathic behavior, which would prevent postoperative management. From our experience with renal transplantation, we have learned that persons who are more than 45 or 50 years of age frequently cannot withstand the rigors of intensive immunosuppression. They may develop muscle wasting and other physical incapacities, have steroid-induced pancreatitis more frequently than younger patients, and have a high incidence of a variety of gastrointestinal complications, including gastroduodenal hemorrhage and colonic problems.

The indications for liver replacement in the developmental phase of this field from 1963 through 1979 have been documented elsewere[8] and will not be mentioned here. The perioperative mortality was so high that conclusions were impossible to reach about what diseases were or were not appropriate for consideration of candidacy. This situation has changed drastically since the introduction of cyclosporine-steroid therapy in 1980.

Since the beginning of the cyclosporine era, 244 patients underwent this procedure between March 1980 and July 1984. The principal indications for these operations are shown in Tables 40-1 and 40-2. In about 10% of cases, there were multiple pathologic diagnoses such as the incidental presence of primary hepatic malignancies in livers with a variety of underlying chronic diseases.

The profile of diseases in pediatric patients (under 18 years) has been different than that in adults. In adults, postnecrotic cirrhosis has been the most important reason for proceeding (see Table 40-1). Other common diseases

TABLE 40-1.   Indications for Liver Transplantation in 140 Adults

INDICATION	NUMBER OF PATIENTS	PERCENTAGE
Acute hepatic necrosis	3	2.1
Budd-Chiari syndrome	5	3.6
Cirrhosis	46	32.9
Inborn errors of metabolism	11	7.9
α_1-Antitrypsin deficiency	6	4.3
Wilson's disease	3	2.1
Tyrosinemia	1	0.7
Primary biliary cirrhosis	36	25.7
Primary hepatic tumors	13	9.3
Secondary biliary cirrhosis	5	3.6
Sclerosing cholangitis	19	13.6
Other	2	1.4

in adults have been primary biliary cirrhosis and sclerosing cholangitis. In children, more than half of all the transplantations have been done for biliary atresia, the only other large group being a heterogeneous collection of inborn errors of metabolism (see Table 40-2). The inborn errors if they are hepatic based are cured permanently by liver replacement since the phenotype of the new liver remains that of the original donor.[8] The longest survival of a patient with an inborn error is now 14½ years. The recipient with Wilson's disease has had normal copper metabolism since operation (Fig. 40-3).

The influence of both age and disease on results will be considered later in this chapter.

DONORS

Procurement and Preservation

In most transplantation centers in the United States, the criteria of brain death based on the concept of irreversible brain injury have been accepted for the pronouncement of death. Under these conditions and with an ideal cadaveric donor, the interval of normothermic ischemic injury is reduced essentially to zero, inasmuch as dissection prior to removal of the liver or other organs can be carried out or even completed in the presence of an effective circulation. It is of more than passing interest that public acceptance of these conditions of organ removal has been widespread in America with almost no negative outcries.

The exploitation of liver transplantation has been built on the kidney procurement network in the United States, which was put in place more than a decade ago by federal legislation. At first, renal transplanters were suspicious that removal of the liver and/or the heart would jeopardize the quality of kidney grafts. Fortunately, great advances have been made in multiple organ removal and a relatively standard procedure is being used throughout most of the United States.[4] The operation is done through a complete midline incision from the suprasternal notch to the pubis, including splitting of the sternum. The principle followed is to dissect the aorta for cross-clamping at a level that

TABLE 40-2.   Indications for Liver Transplantation in 104 Children

INDICATION	NUMBER OF PATIENTS	PERCENTAGE
Biliary atresia	56	53.8
Budd-Chiari syndrome	1	1.0
Cirrhosis	10	9.6
Familial cholestasis	7	6.7
Inborn errors of metabolism	23	22.1
α_1-Antitrypsin deficiency	15	14.4
Wilson's disease	4	3.8
Tyrosinemia	3	2.9
Neonatal hepatitis	3	2.9
Secondary biliary cirrhosis	1	1.0
Sclerosing cholangitis	1	1.0
Other	2	1.6

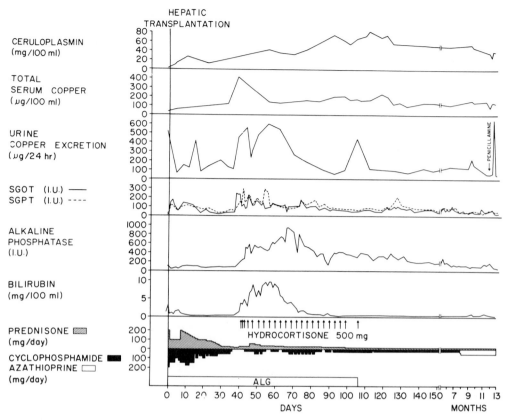

Fig. 40-3. The course of a patient with Wilson's disease who received an orthotopic liver homograft. Note that the ceruloplasmin rose from undetectable to normal levels and that there was a heightened urinary copper excretion for almost a year. In this patient, cyclophosphamide and azathioprine were used interchangeably. The deterioration in liver function, which started just a month after transplantation was caused by serum hepatitis (HBsAg). (Groth CG et al: Transplant Proc 5[1]:829–833, 1973. Reproduced by permission.)

will allow intra-aortic infusion of cold fluids that will pass into the organs to be removed. If the liver is to be one of these organs, dissection of the liver hilum is carried out after which the liver can be infused through both the aorta and portal vein (Fig. 40-4). The kidneys also are cooled by the aortic perfusion. In the example shown in Figure 40-4, the liver and both kidneys are to be removed. With minor modifications, the heart also can be excised.

This procurement technique requires brain death conditions with stable cardiovascular function. An alternative with which we have had recent experience can be done swiftly and in donors who have had cardiac arrest.[5] With this so-called fast method, a cross-clamp is placed on the aorta near the diaphragm and cold solutions (usually the high potassium, high magnesium concentration Collin's solution) are infused rapidly. Blood enters the liver through the normal celiac axis route but also through the portal vein after passing through the splanchnic capillary bed (Fig. 40-5). The portal venous blood quickly becomes almost red cell free.

The cold ischemia limit that is permissible for a human liver graft has been set arbitrarily at 10 hours, but great efforts are made to work within a 5- or 6-hour time frame. One of the most urgent needs in liver transplantation is the development of better methods of preservation. Any technique that would allow safe and easy preservation of livers for the better part of a day would revolutionize the field overnight.

Recipient Matching

With the exception of patients with biliary atresia, most potential recipients of liver homografts have a very brief period of candidacy for transplantation. If an organ cannot be quickly found, death supervenes. Obviously, highly discriminating donor selectivity is not practical under these circumstances, and, for that matter, any selectivity, however supportable on immunologic criteria, may cost the patient his only chance for treatment. It is in the context of such urgency that donor–recipient matching is

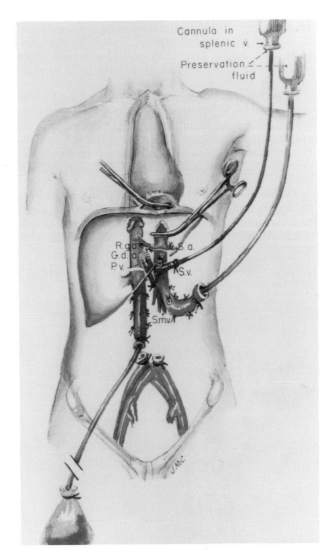

Fig. 40-4. *In situ* infusion technique used when the kidneys and liver are removed from the same donor. R.g.a., right gastric artery; G.d.a., gastroduodenal artery; S.a., splenic artery; S.v., splenic vein; P.v., portal vein; S.m.v., superior mesenteric vein. (Starzl TE et al: Surg Gynecol Obstet 158: 223–230, 1984. By permission of Surgery, Gynecology and Obstetrics.)

conducted. The consequence has been that the HLA antigen matches in our series have been random and consequently uniformly bad.

Because of urgent need, a number of liver transplantations have been performed despite the presence in the recipients of cytotoxic antibodies that were anti-donor-specific. We have carried out several dozen liver transplantations under these circumstances. There were no examples of hyperacute rejection, which almost invariably destroys renal homografts under these conditions; and, in fact, no unequivocal harmful effects were seen later, in comparison to patients without cytotoxic antibodies.[8] We have concluded that the liver is highly privileged in confrontations with preformed cytotoxic antibodies.

Renal homografts are also hyperacutely rejected if there is a breach of blood-group barriers. We proceeded in spite of this adverse factor in a large number of liver recipients who could not wait for blood group–compatible organs. The patients did not behave differently than those given blood group-compatible livers.[8]

With organs other than the liver, preformed antibody states are avoided if at all possible. However, the experience cited with both the ABO red cell and cytotoxic antibodies makes it clear that this kind of positive crossmatch is not a contraindication to liver transplantation.

OPERATIVE PROCEDURES

Preoperative Preparation

Prospective liver recipients are generally poor risks for a major operation. Those with hepatic failure from non-

Fig. 40-5. Method of rapid liver cooling that can be done without any preliminary dissection except for insertion of a distal aortic cannula and cross-clamping of the aorta at the diaphragm. The infusion fluid quickly gets into the portal system by way of the splanchnic capillary bed, providing double inflow cooling. (Starzl TE et al: Transplant Proc 17: 250–258, 1985)

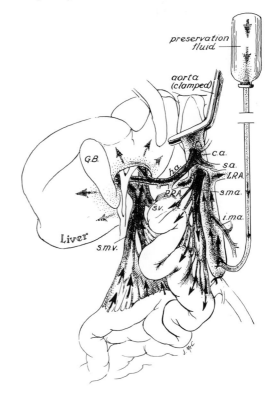

neoplastic disease may even appear at first evaluation to be hopeless. Paracentesis or thoracentesis may be required before anesthesia can be contemplated. Transfusions of blood or albumin may be useful for the correction of blood volume or other fluid space abnormalities. If fresh whole blood, fresh frozen plasma, or platelets are judiciously given, some improvement in coagulation may be possible. Otherwise, there is usually little of real value that can be done to reduce the impending operative hazards.

The surprising ability of these moribund recipients to survive such major surgery may be related partly to the troublesome operative bleeding that is almost invariably encountered. The consequent necessity for major blood replacement frequently results in intraoperative exchange transfusions of at least the magnitude reported to be of benefit in acute liver insufficiency. The coincidental ther-apeutic effect of massive transfusion, as well as the immediate benefits of good hepatic function by the transplant, have usually resulted in patients returning to the ward in better condition than at the time of their departure.

Secondary abnormalities of organs other than the liver can sometimes be effectively ameliorated. For example, the effects of renal failure secondary to the hepatorenal syndrome can be treated with an artificial kidney. Pulmonary manifestations may be improved by simple tracheobronchial toilet, particularly if aspiration has occurred.

The inability to be more specific in preparing patients for surgery means that most prospective recipients cannot be maintained for very long during a search for a suitable donor. At present, only a small fraction of patients with

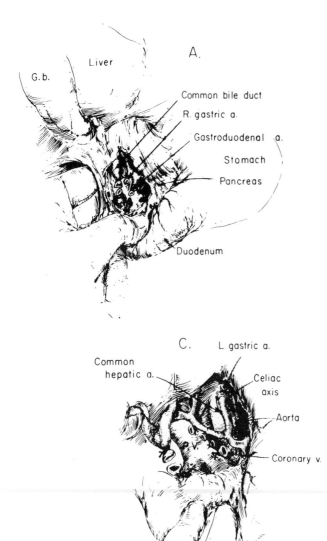

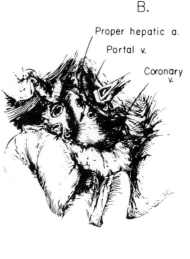

Fig. 40-6. Dissection of the portal triad. **A.** The common duct and the gastroduodenal and right gastric arteries are tied off and divided. Before ligation, it should be determined that the common duct communicates freely with the gallbladder by way of the cystic duct. If anomalies are present, failure to observe these precautions may lead to accidental bile-duct obstruction. **B.** The hepatic artery has been mobilized far enough so that the anterior surface of the portal vein is uncovered. The coronary vein entering the left side of the portal trunk is almost always found; this tributary is ligated and divided. **C.** The portal vein has been freed and the celiac axis mobilized. The splenic artery has not yet been ligated and divided. When the liver is removed, all the celiac axis is usually retained with the specimen; in children, it may be advisable to include a segment of aorta as well. (Starzl TE, Putnam CW: Experience in Hepatic Transplantation, pp 1–553. Philadelphia, WB Saunders, 1969)

truly advanced disease who might be candidates for liver transplantation can actually be treated, because there are no means of providing therapy analogous to that of the artificial kidney to tide over prospective recipients while an organ is being found. Until an artificial liver is developed that provides some of the crucial hepatic functions, liver transplantation will not be able to achieve anything close to its true potential unless the procedure is considered at an earlier time.

Donor Hepatectomy

In removing a liver for eventual transplantation, the essential steps are to incise the restraining ligaments that bind the organ to the diaphragm and body wall and to skeletonize the vessels and duct that must be anastomosed to the companion structures in the recipient (Fig. 40-6). The final steps were described in an earlier section.

Recipient Orthotopic Operation

Reconstruction consists of anastomosing the individual recipient vessels to the vessels of the homograft as quickly as possible. A completed operation is shown in Figure 40-2.

The first anastomosis performed is of the suprahepatic vena cava. As the vena caval anastomoses are constructed, slow infusion of electrolyte solution is continued through the portal vein. Air bubbles can be seen floating out of the graft (Fig. 40-7). If infusion is not provided during this time, the air bubbles in the homograft may be flushed into the circulation after revascularization. They may then pass through abnormal right-to-left venous communications (secondary to liver disease) and on to the brain. A high incidence of cerebral air embolus was encountered in our early experience. This was eliminated with the infusion technique.

Fig. 40-7. Technique to prevent air embolism from orthotopic liver homografts. **A.** Continuous perfusion of solution through the portal vein as vena caval anastomoses are constructed. **B, C.** Escape of air bubbles as the anastomoses are completed. (Starzl TE et al: Ann Surg 187:236–240, 1978)

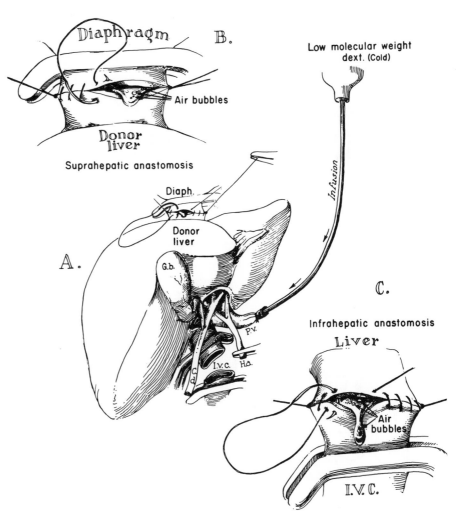

The hilar structures have smaller calibers. Increasingly in infants and young recipients, we have used microvascular techniques, particularly for reconstruction of the hepatic artery and portal vein. If such techniques are not used, pediatric recipients have a high incidence of thrombosis in these vessels.

Biliary tract reconstruction has caused more complications than any other part of the operation.[1,3,8] In our early experience, one of every three recipients subsequently had biliary duct obstruction or biliary fistula. Even without obstruction or fistula, there was a high incidence of bacteremia, probably because of constant contamination of the biliary ducts through the cholecystoduodenostomies (Fig. 40-8A) that were being used in those days.

Since 1974, we have not used cholecystoduodenostomy. We think that duct-to-duct reconstruction (choledochocholedochostomy) is the best method (Figs. 40-2 and 40-8D). If this is not feasible (as, for example, in patients with biliary atresia), we use choledochojejunostomy to a roux-en-Y limb (Fig. 40-8C). Cholecystojejunostomy (Fig. 40-8B) is no longer used.

It is now realized that biliary tract complications (especially obstruction) were frequently the cause of postoperative jaundice that developed after an initial period of bilirubin clearing. When obstruction occurred, it usually was at the narrowed cystic duct after cholecystojejunostomy (Fig. 40-8B). Once the problem was appreciated, it was found safe to secondarily operate, to remove the homograft gallbladder, and to make a conversion to choledochojejunostomy (Fig. 40-8C).

Calne and associates of England have also modified their practices of biliary reconstruction.[1,2] Their presently preferred method is the creation of a cloaca between the homograft gallbladder and common duct, with anastomosis of the common chamber to the recipient common duct. The complexity of this procedure compared with more standard biliary reconstruction militates against its widespread acceptance.

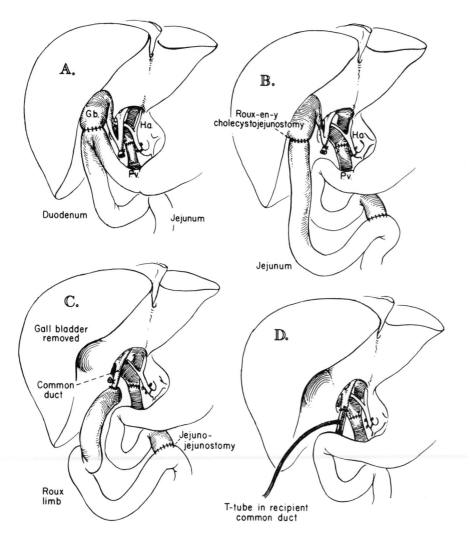

Fig. 40-8. Techniques of biliary-duct reconstruction used for most of the transplantation recipients treated in Colorado. **A.** Cholecystoduodenostomy. This operation is no longer performed. **B.** Cholecystojejunostomy. **C.** Choledochojejunostomy after removal of the gallbladder. **D.** Choledochocholedochostomy. Note that, if possible, the T-tube is placed in the recipient common duct. (Starzl TE et al: Surg Gynecol Obstet 142:487, 1976. By permission of Surgery, Gynecology and Obstetrics.)

The Role of the Veno-Venous Bypass

When liver transplantation was first carried out in dogs, an obligatory condition for success was decompression of the vena caval and portal venous systems that had to be occluded while the native liver was removed and the new organ was sewn in.[3] In the first clinical trials, it was found possible to omit this step and for a number of years bypasses were not used. Without bypasses, the urgency with which the transplantation was performed was comparable to that in the early days of heart surgery when open cardiac operations were performed under inflow occlusion.

In the past 3 years, pump-driven veno-venous bypass techniques without heparin have been developed (Fig. 40-9) that have removed this urgency and that have allowed the avoidance of the venous hypertension that otherwise is inevitable during the anhepatic phase. The advantages of veno-venous bypasses include improved intraoperative cardiovascular stability, preservation of renal function by avoidance of renal-venous hypertension, diminished blood loss, reduced trauma to the gastrointestinal tract by avoidance of the portal venous hypertension, and creation of an operating room ambience compatible with training a new generation of surgeons who in turn will set up numerous new centers in the United States and other countries.

The veno-venous bypass has changed the technical strategy of liver transplantation in important ways. In the past, when time was such a critical factor during the anhepatic phase, it was impossible to obtain meticulous hemostasis in the bare areas opened up by removal of the diseased native liver. Even had there been time, it was often impossible to clean up and make dry the raw surfaces that were exuding blood at a voluminous rate because of venous hypertension. Control of bleeding by mechanical means was frequently impossible until the new liver was in place and until the obstructed venous beds were decompressed by opening the caval and portal venous anastomoses.

If veno-venous bypass is used, techniques can be applied whereby most or all of the bare areas are closed by running sutures.[6] Although these maneuvers may require an hour or longer before the anastomoses are started, the investment pays rich dividends later in ease of hemostasis.

It is curious fact that small pediatric recipients usually did not require veno-venous bypasses. However, the bypasses have revolutionized transplantation in adults.

MANAGEMENT

In view of the enormous difficulty of performing liver transplantation, it is not surprising that the procedure has been followed by a long list of technical complications. Such complications have been responsible for more than half of all deaths within the first year.[2,3,8] Included have been vascular thrombosis, hemorrhage, the unknowing use of ischemically damaged grafts, and biliary tract obstruction or fistulization, to provide a very incomplete accounting. These complications have influenced postoperative immunosuppressive management. For example, better diagnosis and management of biliary complications were made feasible by an increase in the use of cholangiography (percutaneous, retrograde endoscopic, or T-tube).

Another recent change in policy has been the more frequent use of needle biopsy. Evidence of viral hepatitis has thereby been obtained in a surprising number of cases.

Fig. 40-9. Pump-driven bypass. (Griffith et al: Surg Gynecol Obstet 160:270–272, 1985. By permission of Surgery, Gynecology and Obstetrics.)

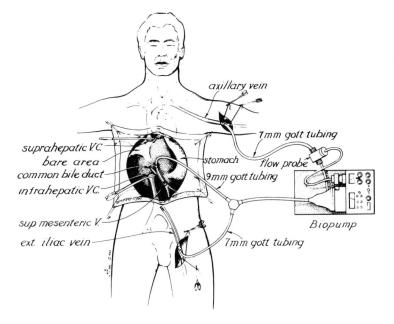

Severe or lethal homograft hepatitis has been caused by HB$_s$Ag virus, herpes, chickenpox, and adenovirus. An example of HB$_s$Ag hepatitis is shown in Figure 40-3. Correct diagnosis helped avoid the lethal error of intensifying immunosuppression at the very moment when the opposite change might have been in order.

The infectious consequences of other major, nonimmunologic complications such as vascular thromboses and enteric fistulas may be difficult to manage under the influence of immunosuppression.

IMMUNOSUPPRESSION AND RESULTS

The unique requirement after transplantation of any organ is immunosuppression. All of our early liver recipients had double drug therapy with a cytotoxic agent, azathioprine (which can be used interchangeably with cyclophosphamide), and prednisone (Fig. 40-3). To the double drug regimen, we often added heterologous antilymphocyte globulin (ALG) (Fig. 40-3). The results were not satisfactory, as summarized elsewhere.[8] None of the therapeutic variations influenced survival (Fig. 40-10). In the first trials from 1963 to 1976, only about one third of the patients lived for as long as 1 year. In a smaller second series of 30 patients treated from 1976 to 1978, the 1-year survival rose to 50%, but this improvement could not be sustained in the next 29 cases (Fig. 40-10).

Fig. 40-10. Results obtained over a 16-year period using the conventional immunosuppression described in the text. Note the failure to improve the results despite the acquisition of considerable experience.

The systematic use of cyclosporine-steroid therapy in liver transplantation was begun in early 1980.[8] Almost immediately, a doubling of 1-year patient survival was noted. Each subsequent year, the case load in our center has increased until in the calendar year of 1984, a total of 166 liver replacements were performed at the University of Pittsburgh. Augmented activity in other centers throughout the world has been documented.[5]

The assessment of whole blood or plasma cyclosporine concentration is possible with radioimmunoassay (RIA) or high-performance liquid chromatography (HLPC). Heavy reliance is now placed on the results of these tests for management decisions. This has been a particularly important development in liver recipients since the intestinal absorption of cyclosporine postoperatively has been unpredictable and to some extent dependent on the quality of graft function. To smooth out the recovery period and to ensure continuity of therapeutic levels of the drug, cyclosporine has been administered both intravenously and orally for several days, weeks, or even months postoperatively.[5] As absorption improves with the oral drug, the intravenous doses are weaned and eventually discontinued.

The chances for living a year after liver replacement under conventional immunosuppression were only about 1 in 3 (Fig. 40-10 and 40-11). Subsequently, 244 liver recipients were provided with cyclosporine-steroid therapy between March 1980 and July 1984 allowing follow-ups of 1 to more than 5 years. The chances of 1-year survival

Fig. 40-11. Marked improvement in results of liver transplantation after the introduction of cyclosporine-steroid therapy in early 1980.

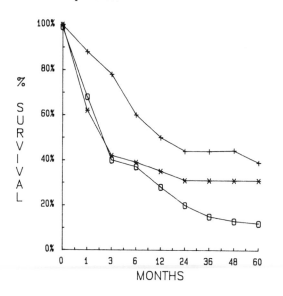

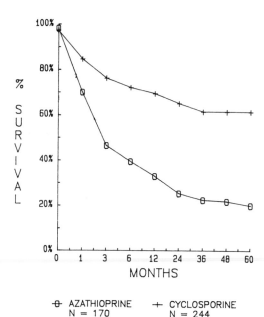

were more than doubled. Actuarial projections beyond 1 year indicate that these gains will be sustained for at least one-half decade (see Fig. 40-11).

Certain risk factors have been carefully looked at for their effect on survival curves. Among the more important has been age. Pediatric recipients throughout the entire history of liver transplantation have fared better by 10 to 25 percentage points than adults, and in the cyclosporine era the age factor has been particularly important (Fig. 40-12).

Somewhat surprisingly, specific diseases that have destroyed the native liver have not for the most part influenced survival. In adults, for example, the outcome has been about the same with such diverse diseases as primary biliary cirrhosis, sclerosing cholangitis, and inborn errors of metabolism. Two high-risk diseases have been identified so far. The results with postnecrotic cirrhosis and with primary hepatic tumors have been inferior. With cirrhosis, the principal explanations have been the technical difficulties of the operation caused by the pathologic process, the generally poor condition of the cirrhotic patient, and the almost universal recapitulation of their original chronic active hepatitis in B-virus carriers.

In patients whose reason for liver replacement was primary hepatic malignancy that could not be removed by conventional subtotal hepatic resection, the early mortality has been quite low, with more than 80% of the recipients being alive at 6 months. A steady decline thereafter has been caused by recurrent tumor, which can be expected in 80% or more of patients who live long enough for me-

tastases to be detected. The only acceptable results thus far have been in patients with the slow-growing and non-aggressive fibrolamellar hepatomas that have been recognized to be a favorable variant within the larger hepatoma category.[6,8]

In children, the results have been about the same in all the main disease categories. It has been interesting that the survival in children with biliary atresia has been competitive with that obtained with other diseases. Transplantation is technically much more difficult in children previously submitted to Kasai operations and re-explorations, but there has not been a demonstrable penalty in terms of either early or late survival (Fig. 40-13).

More complete accounts of underlying disease and other risk factors are being published elsewhere.[7] The improved survival that has been achieved in recent years has been made possible, in part, by an aggressive use of re-transplantation to rescue patients whose first grafts have failed because of rejection or for any other reason. Re-transplantation was not a successful enterprise under conventional immunosuppression,[8] but in the modern times defined by the availability of cyclosporine, the picture has drastically changed.

With the major increases in survival of the past 5 years, liver transplantation has become accepted as a service, as opposed to an experimental procedure. Numerous excellent centers have been or are being set up in all developed countries. The impact of liver transplantation on the practice of hepatology is going to be profound and should be a vitalizing force for this specialty.

Fig. 40-12. Comparison of results in adult and pediatric recipients during the cyclosporine era of 1980–1984.

Fig. 40-13. Lack of influence of underlying disease on the survival of children undergoing liver transplantation.

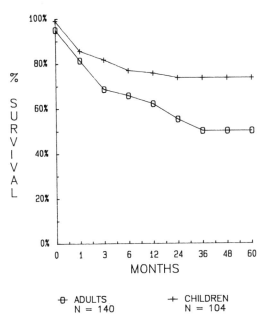

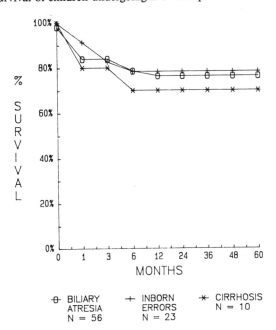

ADDENDUM

The pace of liver transplantation at the University of Pittsburgh program has continued to increase. In 1985, 250 new patients were treated, and in 1986 the total was projected at more than 300. By September 30, 1986, the total number of patients entered into the program was 845, of whom almost 60% were adults. The total of 845 is an understatement of our true experience since more than 1 in 4 patients undergo retransplantation at some time. The greater accrual of experience in data has not changed the slope of the life survival curves and has not altered the opinions expressed more than a year ago when the chapter was written.

REFERENCES

1. Calne RY, Williams R: Liver transplantation. Curr Probl Surg 16:3, 1979
2. Calne RY: Liver Transplantation: The Cambridge-King's College Hospital Experience, pp 3–383. New York, Grune & Stratton, 1983
3. Starzl TE (with the assistance of CW Putnam): Experience in Hepatic Transplantation. Philadelphia, WB Saunders, 1969
4. Starzl TE, Hakala TR, Shaw BW Jr et al: A flexible procedure for multiple cadaveric organ procurement. Surg Gynecol Obstet 158:223, 1984
5. Starzl TE, Iwatsuki S, Shaw BW Jr et al: Orthotopic liver transplantation in 1984. Transplant Proc 17:250, 1985
6. Starzl TE, Iwatsuki S, Shaw BW Jr et al: Factors in the development of liver transplantation. Transplant Proc 17:107–119, 1985
7. Starzl TE, Iwatsuki S, Shaw BW Jr et al: Immunosuppression and other non-surgical factors in the improved results of liver transplantation. Semin Liver Dis (in press)
8. Starzl TE, Iwatsuki S, Van Thiel DH et al: Evolution of liver transplantation. Hepatology 2:614, 1982
9. Starzl TE, Porter KA, Francavilla A: The Eck fistula in animals and humans. Curr Probl Surg 20:687, 1983

chapter **41**

Formation and Treatment of Gallstones

LESLIE J. SCHOENFIELD and JAY W. MARKS

FORMATION OF GALLSTONES

The most prevalent disease of the biliary system is cholelithiasis. In fact, 20 million Americans have gallstones. Moreover, each year about 1 million new cases are discovered and 500,000 cholecystectomies are performed. About 75% of the gallstones in the United States are cholesterol stones, which are subclassified as either pure cholesterol or mixed stones than contain at least 50% cholesterol; virtually all of the remaining stones are pigment stones, which contain mostly calcium bilirubinate.

Gallstones form when the concentration of cholesterol or bilirubin in bile exceeds the limited solubilizing capacity of bile for these substances, which then precipitate from the saturated solution. Research during the past 20 years has clarified substantially our understanding of the pathogenesis of gallstones, especially that of cholesterol gallstones. Furthermore, explanations have been discovered for some of the factors that predispose to the formation of gallstones.

Formation of Cholesterol Gallstones

Stages

The formation of cholesterol gallstones is divided conveniently into three stages: saturation, nucleation, and growth. Because saturation of bile with cholesterol was the first defect that was characterized in the formation of gallstones, saturated bile was referred to as lithogenic bile.[158] However, gallstones form only when crystals of cholesterol nucleate from the saturated bile and then aggregate for growth of the stone. Accordingly, the term *lithogenic bile* more accurately would describe saturated bile that can be shown to be destined to nucleation and growth.

Stage 1: Saturation of Bile with Cholesterol. Saturation of bile with cholesterol is a prerequisite stage for the formation of cholesterol gallstones.[159] Moreover, a direct

correlation has been found between the prevalence of saturated bile and that of cholesterol gallstones in different populations.[122] However, understanding the mechanisms for the saturation of bile requires first an understanding of the mechanisms for the solubilization of cholesterol in bile.[2]

Solubilization of Cholesterol in Bile. The mechanisms for the solubilization of cholesterol in bile are complex, since bile is an aqueous solution and cholesterol is virtually insoluble in water. Most of the cholesterol in bile is solubilized by mixed micelles of bile acids and lecithin. A micelle is a colloidal aggregation of molecules of an amphipathic compound (in this instance, a bile acid) in which the hydrophobic portion of each molecule faces inward and the hydrophilic groups point outward.[45] The cholesterol is solubilized within the hydrophobic center of the micelle.

The formation of simple micelles of bile acids alone depends primarily on the concentration of the bile acids. Thus, micelles form at and not below a critical micellar concentration of bile acids in bile, which is about 2 mM. The formation of micelles also is influenced by the concentrations of biliary solids and counterions, by the type of bile acid (that is, by its degree of hydroxylation and whether it is conjugated with taurine or glycine or not), and by the temperature and *p*H of the bile.

Simple micelles of bile acids are capable of solubilizing and incorporating lecithin. This enables the micelles (then referred to as mixed micelles) to solubilize at least triple the amount of cholesterol solubilized by simple micelles. Solubility of cholesterol in mixed micelles is enhanced when the concentration of total lipids in bile is high. Moreover, maximal solubility occurs when the molar ratio of lecithin to bile acids is between 0.2 and 0.3.

Nevertheless, the solubility of cholesterol in bile is limited.[90] When the maximal effective solubility for cholesterol is reached or exceeded (*i.e.,* when bile becomes saturated or supersaturated), the first requirement for the formation of cholesterol gallstones has been met. The true solubility at equilibrium, which includes metastable solubility, is greater than the maximal effective solubility.[43] These two limits for the solubilization of cholesterol have been determined *in vitro* and can be used to distinguish saturated from unsaturated bile and to estimate the degree of saturation.[18]

The solubilization of cholesterol under standardized conditions of temperature, pH, and concentrations of biliary solids and counterions depends primarily on the relative proportions of cholesterol, bile acids, and lecithin. This can be illustrated graphically by the use of triangular coordinates wherein each of the three axes depicts the percent of the total moles in bile constituted by cholesterol, bile acids, or lecithin (Fig. 41-1). The composition of any bile sample, therefore, can be represented by a single point on such coordinates.

A saturation index for a sample of bile can be estimated directly from the diagram or can be determined by using a formula.[161] The saturation index is the ratio of the actual amount of cholesterol present in a sample to the maximal amount of cholesterol that can be dissolved in it. Bile having a saturation index of one is saturated, that with less than one is unsaturated, and that with greater than one is supersaturated. The degree of saturation also can be expressed as a percent saturation by multiplying the saturation index by 100.

Bile that is not saturated with cholesterol is a single-phase isotropic liquid in which cholesterol is solubilized in micellar solution. When the relative percentage of cholesterol in bile exceeds the maximal effective solubility for cholesterol, the supersaturated solution becomes metastable, that is, liable, albeit reluctantly, to crystallization of cholesterol. In the process of crystallization, the appearance of liquid crystals (*i.e.,* another physical state of cholesterol that is not in a micellar solution or a solid phase) may precede the precipitation of solid crystals of cholesterol.[108]

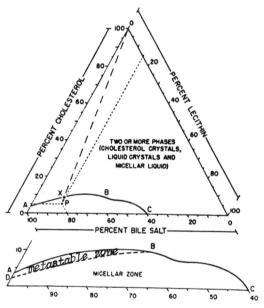

Fig. 41-1. The three major components of bile (bile acids, lecithin, and cholesterol) are plotted on triangular coordinates. Point P represents bile consisting of 80 mol % bile acid, 5% cholesterol, and 15% lecithin (see *dotted lines*). Line ABC represents the maximal effective solubility of cholesterol in varying mixtures of bile acids and lecithin as determined *in vitro*. Point P falls below line ABC and within the zone of a single phase of micellar liquid; therefore, bile that has the composition P is unsaturated with respect to cholesterol. To calculate the percent saturation of this bile, draw a line from P to the cholesterol apex of the triangle (*dashed line*). The intersection of this line with line ABC (*point x*) gives the relative concentration in percentage of cholesterol at 100% effective saturation (*i.e.,* 8% for sample P). Therefore, the percent saturation of bile with a composition at point P = ⅝ (100) = 62.5%. Below is an expanded area of the triangle showing the line (*ABC*) that represents the maximal effective solubility of cholesterol and a line (*DBC*) that represents the true solubility of cholesterol at equilibrium. Bile with a composition above DB but below AB (*i.e.,* in the metastable zone) is supersaturated, but less so than bile with a composition above ABC. The true percent saturation is calculated using the line DBC. Above line DBC, cholesterol exists in micellar, liquid crystalline, and crystalline phases. Bile that falls in the metastable zone maintains cholesterol in solution for prolonged periods, whereas bile that falls above line ABC contains readily precipitable excess cholesterol. (Courtesy of Dr. D. M. Small)

The metastable region for actual bile is larger than that found in artificial systems, reflecting the fact that bile is relatively resistant to crystallization in spite of supersaturation. Thus, normal persons are able to retain cholesterol in metastable solution long enough to discharge the bile from the biliary tree while patients with gallstones precipitate cholesterol from the metastable solution before bile can be evacuated from the gallbladder.

Some patients with gallstones have bile that exhibits an extreme degree of supersaturation. In these patients the true solubility of cholesterol at equilibrium is exceeded and the composition of bile when plotted on the triangular coordinate-diagram is above the metastable zone. In this bile, cholesterol exists in three phases: micellar, liquid crystalline, and solid crystalline.

The triangular coordinate-diagram depicts the physical phases of cholesterol. The diagram suggests that when the quantity of cholesterol in bile exceeds that which can be solubilized by the available bile acids and lecithin, the cholesterol will crystallize out of solution. However, many persons with persistently supersaturated bile do not have crystals or stones of cholesterol. Therefore, other mechanisms besides micellar systems of bile acids must exist for the solubilization of cholesterol in bile.[49] Thus, cholesterol can be solubilized by liposomal vesicles that essentially are micelles containing only lecithin.[150] Also, cholesterol can be solubilized by proteins in bile that have lipid-solubilizing properties similar to the apolipoproteins of plasma lipoproteins.[61] Apolipoproteins, like bile acids, interact with lecithin and provide a hydrophobic core that can solubilize cholesterol. In some samples of bile, more than half of the total biliary cholesterol is solubilized in a lipoprotein-complex that is void of bile acids.[113]

Mechanisms for the Saturation of Bile: Hepatic Secretion. Bile from patients having cholesterol gallstones almost always is saturated with cholesterol. However, many normal persons also secrete saturated bile, at least part of the time.[51] In fact, the biliary saturation of cholesterol normally exhibits a diurnal variation, often reaching supersaturated levels after fasting.[93,97]

Because hepatic bile always is more saturated than cholecystic bile, the liver clearly is the source of the saturated bile.[146] However, the basic abnormality that causes saturation need not be in the liver. Thus, a defect in any intestinal, hepatic, or cholecystic factor that regulates the secretion of bile acids or the composition of biliary lipids could cause the liver to secrete saturated bile.

Hepatic bile theoretically can become saturated with cholesterol through a relative increase in the secretion of cholesterol or through a relative decrease in the secretion of bile acids or lecithin. Actually, in patients with gallstones, usually the secretion of cholesterol has been found to be increased, the secretion of bile acids decreased, and secretion of lecithin normal.[60,104] Other possible mechanisms for saturation (*e.g.,* imbalance in cholecystic absorption of biliary lipids or disorders of the sphincter of Oddi) remain theoretical.

The secretion of bile acids is a major determinant of the secretion of lecithin and cholesterol. Thus a decreased secretion of bile acids results in diminished secretion of both cholesterol and lecithin, but the secretion of lecithin is decreased more than that of cholesterol.[143] Therefore, at low rates of secretion of bile acids, as occurs during fasting or interruption of the enterohepatic circulation, the bile becomes saturated with cholesterol.

Mechanisms for the Saturation of Bile: Alterations in the Metabolism of Bile Acids and Cholesterol. A decreased secretion of bile acids could be caused by a shrunken pool of bile acids. In fact, a small pool has been documented in many patients with cholesterol gallstones.[166] (In one study[13], the size of the pool of chenodeoxycholic acid correlated [inversely] better with the degree of saturation than did the total pool of bile acids.) The diminished pool can result from an increased loss, a decreased synthesis, or an increased frequency of enterohepatic cycling of bile acids.

If bile acids are lost, hepatic synthesis of bile acids would be expected to be increased to compensate for the loss. Therefore, the finding of decreased synthesis when the return of bile acids to the liver is diminished would suggest an inappropriate hepatic response. This abnormality in the regulation of hepatic synthesis of bile acids is best characterized as an oversensitive hepatic response to the feedback of bile acids.

A loss of bile acids because of an increased fecal excretion of bile acids has not been demonstrated in most patients with gallstones. However, patients having Crohn's disease (a condition that predisposes to gallstones) do lose bile acids because of diminished ileal absorption. Other patients with gallstones have been found to have decreased emptying of the gallbladder, a phenomenon that also would decrease the return of bile acids to the liver.

The small pool of bile acids in patients with cholesterol gallstones might be related to appropriately rather than inappropriately decreased synthesis of bile acids. Thus, according to one hypothesis, enhanced emptying of the gallbladder is the basic pathogenic defect that leads to gallstones.[105,165] The resultant increased frequency of recycling of the pool of bile acids appropriately inhibits the synthesis of bile acids, thereby causing a decreased pool of bile acids.

A reduced activity of hepatic cholesterol 7α-hydroxylase, the rate-limiting enzyme for the synthesis of bile acids from cholesterol, has been reported in patients with gallstones.[19,103] This would suggest that the fundamental defect is an inadequate conversion of cholesterol to bile acids, whether or not the low synthesis of bile acids is an appropriate physiologic response. However, the rate of synthesis of bile acids has been found to be normal in other patients with cholesterol gallstones.[21,104]

The hepatic secretion of cholesterol has been found to be greater in patients with cholesterol gallstones than in normal controls,[60,104] especially in those patients who also are obese.[39,40,123] Furthermore, the activity of hepatic HMG-CoA reductase, the rate-limiting enzyme for the synthesis of cholesterol, has been found to be increased in some patients with cholesterol gallstones.[19,103] This might suggest that the excess biliary cholesterol comes from cholesterol that is synthesized in the liver. However, mobilized rather than newly synthesized cholesterol probably is the major source of the excess biliary cholesterol.[91,138] Also, although the rate of intestinal absorption of cholesterol is normal, dietary cholesterol may contribute to biliary cholesterol.[68]

Classification of Defects Leading to Supersaturation. Based on our current understanding of the mechanisms for the saturation of bile with cholesterol, the recognized defects leading to supersaturation can be classified into four types.

Type 1: Excessive Loss of Bile Acids. Excessive loss of bile acids occurs in patients with ileectomy, diseases of the ileum (*e.g.,* Crohn's disease), or surgical bypass of the ileum. This loss results in a decreased return of bile acids to the liver, but the maximal rate of normal hepatic synthesis of bile acids cannot make up for the marked loss. Therefore, the pool and the hepatic secretion of bile acids are decreased, resulting in supersaturated bile despite a normal secretion of cholesterol.

Type 2: Oversensitive Hepatic Response to Feedback of Bile Acids. This defect is found in nonobese whites with gallstones. The findings in these patients can be explained only if relatively low rates of return of bile acids to the liver are adequate to depress the hepatic synthesis of bile acids. During the development of this inappropriate (*i.e.,* oversensitive) hepatic response to the feedback of bile acids, more bile acids are lost from the enterohepatic circulation than are synthesized, although the rate of synthesis is normal or low. This then leads to a decreased pool, hepatic return, and secretion of bile acids, resulting in supersaturated bile. The secretion of cholesterol is normal in these patients. In some of these patients the size of the pool may be normal but the secretion of bile acids still is decreased because of diminished enterohepatic circulations of the pool.

Type 3: Excessive Secretion of Cholesterol. Obese whites with gallstones secrete excessive cholesterol into the bile. This causes supersaturated bile despite normal pools and rates of secretion of bile acids.

Type 4: Mixed Defect. This defect, a combination of types 2 and 3, has been described in both American Indians and whites with gallstones. In these patients, an oversensitive hepatic response to the feedback of bile acids (causing decreased secretion of bile acids) combined with an increased secretion of cholesterol produce supersaturated bile (Fig. 41-2). The decreased synthesis of bile acids (when present) and increased secretion of cholesterol in these patients may be the result of diminished 7α-hydroxylation of cholesterol.

Stage 2: Nucleation of Crystals of Cholesterol. Virtually all patients with cholesterol gallstones have bile that is saturated with cholesterol. However, as already noted, not all persons who have persistently saturated bile will develop gallstones. Therefore, saturation of bile is an essential stage in the evolution of gallstones but is insufficient in itself for the formation of gallstones.

Crystals of cholesterol also can be identified in the saturated bile of most patients with cholesterol gallstones. However, in contrast to saturated bile without crystals, saturated bile with crystals almost invariably contains gallstones.[82,140] Thus, nucleation (*i.e.,* crystallization from a saturated solution) appears to be a sufficient and more immediate precursor of gallstones than saturation.

Saturated bile from the gallbladder of patients having cholesterol gallstones nucleates crystals of cholesterol more rapidly than equally saturated bile from the gallbladder of persons without gallstones.[46] Thus, a rapid nucleation time characterizes lithogenic bile (Fig. 41-3). Moreover, in patients with gallstones, although hepatic bile is consistently more saturated than cholecystic bile, the latter has a more rapid nucleation time than hepatic bile.[15,36] Therefore, the critical defect that induces nucleation is

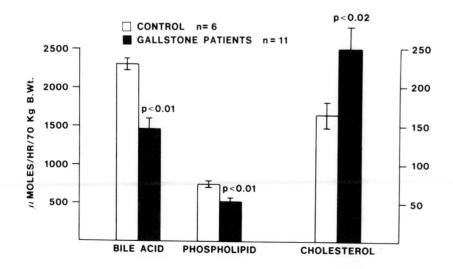

Fig. 41-2. Secretion of biliary lipids in whites with gallstones who were slightly obese ($121 \pm 5\%$ SEM of ideal body weight) compared with matched controls without gallstones. These patients have supersaturated bile because of a type IV defect characterized by [a] decreased secretion of bile acids probably owing to an oversensitive hepatic response to feedback of bile acids and [b] increased secretion of cholesterol that may be due to an inadequate hepatic conversion of cholesterol to bile acids. (Data from Key PH et al: J Lab Clin Med 95: 815, 1980)

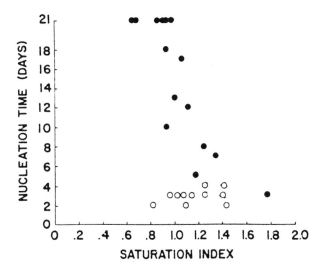

Fig. 41-3. Nucleation time of bile from patients with gall-stones (*open circles*) is more rapid than that from controls without gallstones (*closed circles*), even when the saturation indices are similar. (Reprinted with permission from Holan KR et al: Nucleation time: A key factor in the pathogenesis of cholesterol gallstone disease. Gastroenterology 77:611, 1979. Reprinted with permission of the American Gastroenterological Association)

introduced in the gallbladder. The defect is not a result of the presence of gallstones in the gallbladder because the bile from patients with pigment gallstones, in contrast to that from patients with cholesterol gallstones, does not exhibit accelerated nucleation.

In normal bile, even when the bile is saturated with cholesterol, an equilibrium is maintained between promoters of nucleation and inhibitors of nucleation. In the formation of gallstones, the promoters of nucleation predominate over the inhibitors. This imbalance causes crystals of cholesterol to precipitate from the saturated bile during storage of the bile in the gallbladder.

Efforts in research currently are focused on identifying the promoters and inhibitors of nucleation in bile. Heat-labile proteins[34] and mucous glycoproteins[74] in bile have been shown to promote nucleation. These promoters also may be present in sludge (which is echodense material seen in the gallbladder by ultrasonography and is a possible antecedent of stones). The putative inhibitors of nucleation are other proteins in bile,[50] including apolipoproteins AI and AII,[61] and liposomal vesicles of micellar lecithin.[62,150] These inhibitors have the capacity to solubilize that biliary cholesterol that exceeds the solubilizing capacity of mixed micelles.

The process of nucleation may be homogeneous or heterogeneous.[145] Homogeneous nucleation occurs in the labile zone of supersaturation where crystals of cholesterol form rapidly without the need for nucleating agents. Heterogeneous nucleation occurs in the less supersaturated metastable zone where crystallization of cholesterol occurs more slowly but can be accelerated by nucleating agents. Bile from the gallbladder of most patients with cholesterol gallstones has a composition that falls within the metastable zone and, therefore, is prone to heterogeneous nucleation.

In the process of homogeneous nucleation of crystals of cholesterol from supersaturated bile, initially, liposomal vesicles (*i.e.,* micelles of lecithin that contain cholesterol) separate from the mixed bile acid–lecithin–cholesterol micellar system.[47] This partitioning probably is due to stratification of the particles according to their density in cholecystic bile. Then, these vesicles fuse and aggregate until liquid crystals of cholesterol form. Finally, the liquid crystals fuse and aggregate, culminating in the formation of solid crystals of cholesterol monohydrate. Precipitates of calcium bilirubinate, bile salts, and inorganic salts of calcium, each bound to mucous glycoproteins, have been proposed to provide a nidus for nucleation of crystals of cholesterol.[98]

Stage 3: Growth of Gallstones. The basic units of cholesterol gallstones are crystals of cholesterol monohydrate. The mechanism whereby these crystals assemble to form microscopic stones and eventuate in macroscopic gallstones is not well understood. This process of growth would be encouraged by stasis of bile due to delayed emptying of the gallbladder. When multiple gallstones are in the gallbladder, they often are equal in size, indicating that nucleations for this family of stones occurred simultaneously and that the stones grew at the same rate. Stones of unequal size probably represent different generations.

Crystals of cholesterol in bile (Fig. 41-4) have been observed to aggregate randomly in amorphous groupings as well as to layer radially and concentrically.[110,162] Scanning electron microscopy reveals randomly aggregated crystals of cholesterol in the center of cholesterol gallstones (Fig. 41-5A). The amorphous material in the center of gallstones also contains chemicals (bilirubin, bile acids, mucous glycoproteins, calcium, carbonate, phosphate, copper, and sulfur) that might have provided a nidus for nucleation.[10,135]

In the outer portion of cholesterol gallstones, the crystals are oriented perpendicularly to the surface (Fig. 41-5B). Throughout the gallstones, glycoproteins are thought to provide a matrix for the growth of gallstones. Often, concentric pigmented rings separate layers of crystals of cholesterol that have somewhat different axial orientations. Moreover, the chemical composition of these rings resembles that of the center of gallstones.[81] Therefore, the rings may reflect cyclic deposition of calcium bilirubinate, other calcium salts, and glycoproteins and may have formed when growth of the stones temporarily ceased.

Role of the Gallbladder

The gallbladder must be important in the pathogenesis of cholesterol gallstones because most gallstones form in the

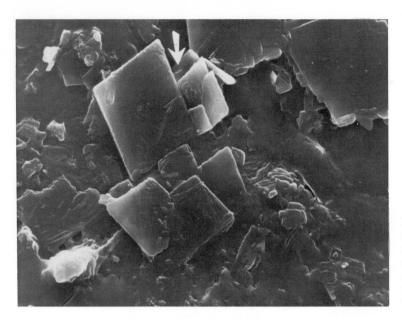

Fig. 41-4. Scanning electron photomicrograph showing typical crystals of cholesterol (*arrow*) in the bile of a patient with cholesterol gallstones. The laminated crystals aggregate radially, concentrically, or randomly. (Original magnification × 200) (Courtesy of Dr. Tashio Osuga)

Fig. 41-5. Left. Scanning electron photomicrograph of the interior of a faceted cholesterol gallstone. Cholesterol crystals are shown: Note their smooth edges, rounded corners, and occasional notches. (Original magnification × 4500) **Right.** Scanning electron photomicrograph of the cortical layer of the same gallstone. The plates of cholesterol are piled one upon another. (Original magnification × 400) (Courtesy of Dr. M. James Phillips).

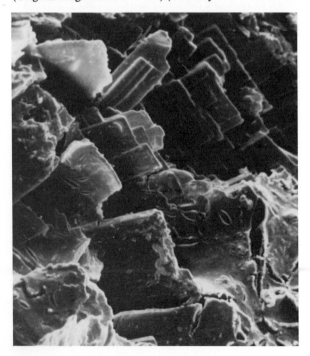

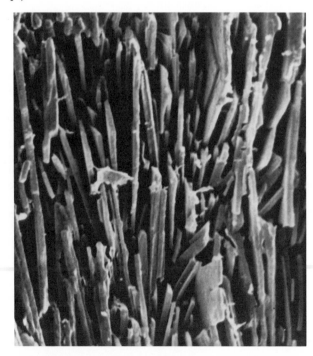

gallbladder and most patients do not have recurrent gall-stones following cholecystectomy. In fact, data suggest that the gallbladder has a role in each of the stages of formation of gallstones: saturation, nucleation, and growth.

If the gallbladder were to have impaired emptying of its bile, whether due to neural, muscular, or hormonal abnormalities, there might result an increased saturation of bile. For example, in patients with gallstones, during fasting (when the gallbladder does not empty), the satu-ration of bile increases due to a decreased secretion of bile acids and an increased ratio of cholesterol to phospho-lipid.[97]

Following cholecystectomy, the rates of secretion of bile salts and lecithin increase and thereby cause a decrease in the saturation of cholesterol in hepatic bile.[141] This does not necessarily mean, however, that the intact, functioning gallbladder serves to increase the saturation index. In fact, the gallbladder, by concentrating the biliary lipids, en-hances the solubilization of cholesterol.[18] This protective role of the normal gallbladder, however, is offset by an-other phenomenon—stasis of bile in the gallbladder.

Between meals the gallbladder stores bile, and during meals the gallbladder discharges its bile incompletely. This stasis of cholecystic bile can provide the time necessary to accommodate nucleation of crystals and growth of gallstones in the gallbladder. Attesting to the importance of stasis in the formation of gallstones is the high incidence of cholelithiasis in patients receiving long-term total par-enteral nutrition (TPN). For example, 49% of patients with Crohn's disease who were receiving TPN had gall-stones.[115] (Crohn's disease alone caused gallstones in 27% of patients.) During TPN, the gallbladder does not empty because the stimulus (ingestion of meals) for the release of cholecystokinin is essentially eliminated.

Although it is unclear whether TPN causes cholesterol or pigment stones, prolonged stasis would promote both nucleation and growth for either type of stone.[126] During TPN, bile stagnates and sludge develops in the gallblad-der.[115] In one study of patients receiving TPN, no patient developed gallstones without first developing sludge.[92] Sludge contains calcium, pigments, bile acids, and gly-coproteins; its contents presumably serve as a nidus for nucleation of crystals.

Prolonged sequestration of bile in the gallbladder causes hepatic bile to become more dilute, a condition that favors the formation of low-density liposomal vesicles in the hepatic bile.[48] These vesicles are rich in lecithin and cho-lesterol and are more buoyant than concentrated biliary micelles. These differing particulate densities probably explain the phenomenon of stratification (*i.e.,* of layering) of biliary lipids in the gallbladder. Stratification has been proposed to favor nucleation of cholesterol.[101]

Several teams of investigators have measured in patients with gallstones and in normal persons the facility of the gallbladder to empty in response to a meal or to admin-istration of cholecystokinin. Unfortunately, the results have been discrepant. Two teams using the technique of cholescintigraphy found slower emptying of the gallblad-der in the patients with gallstones[31] or at least in a subgroup of patients with stones.[119] However, another team using oral cholecystography, found faster emptying in their pa-tients with gallstones.[89] Furthermore, the latter investi-gators, using cholescintigraphy, demonstrated in patients with gallstones an increased sensitivity of the gallbladder to stimulation with cholecystokinin.[106] Nevertheless, the weight of evidence seems to favor slow emptying of the gallbladder in patients with gallstones (Fig. 41-6). More-over, slow emptying and increased volume of the gall-bladder, measured by ultrasonography[27] occur during pregnancy and during administration of oral contracep-tives, two conditions that predispose to the formation of gallstones.

Role of Mucous Glycoproteins

Mucous glycoproteins, collectively referred to as mucin, are an integral part of the structure of both pigment and cholesterol gallstones. The mucin in gallstones extends from the amorphous center to the periphery in either a radial or laminated fashion.[154] Also, mucin is a major component of sludge in the gallbladder, and sludge has been suggested to be a precursor of gallstones.[5,92] Accord-ingly, two roles in the formation of gallstones have been proposed for mucin: (1) as a nucleating agent for the crys-

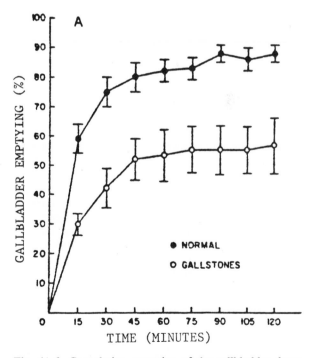

Fig. 41-6. Cumulative emptying of the gallbladder deter-mined by cholescintigraphy after administration of a test meal was slower and less complete in patients with gallstones than in normal subjects. (Reprinted with permission from Fischer RS et al: Dig Dis Sci 27:1019, 1982)

tallization of cholesterol from saturated bile and (2) as a scaffolding for the deposition of crystals during growth of stones.[147]

Mucous glycoproteins have a hydrophobic core of polypeptides linked to hydrophilic, radially arranged side-chains of oligosaccharides. In high concentration, mucin forms polymers of high viscosity. The synthesis of mucous glycoproteins that are secreted by the epithelium of the gallbladder and biliary ducts is thought to be regulated by mucosal prostaglandins. Thus, in prairie dogs that are fed cholesterol blockage of the release of mucous glycoproteins by aspirin, an inhibitor of the synthesis of prostaglandins, prevents the formation of cholesterol crystals and gall-stones.[69]

It has been proposed that in the formation of gallstones the gallbladder hypersecretes mucin, perhaps stimulated by some component of saturated bile. Then, the carbo-hydrate groups of the polymers of mucin avidly bind water to form gels. Meanwhile, the hydrophobic polypeptides in the core of mucous glycoproteins bind the bilirubin and calcium in bile.[64] The resulting water-insoluble com-plex of mucous glycoproteins and calcium bilirubinate provides a surface for nucleation of crystals of cholesterol monohydrate and a framework or matrix for the growth of cholesterol gallstones.[148]

Factors that Predispose to Cholesterol Gallstones

Female Hormones

The incidence of cholelithiasis increases with age in both sexes. However, gallstones are at least two times more prevalent among women than men, probably because of incompletely understood lithogenic effects of female hor-mones.[102] Estrogens increase the saturation of bile by in-creasing the hepatic secretion of cholesterol and perhaps by decreasing the body's pool of bile acids. Moreover, pregnancy further enhances the risk of developing gall-stones, probably because slow emptying of the gallbladder, especially in the last trimester, causes stasis of the saturated bile.[58] More specifically, progesterone (which is increased late in pregnancy) has been shown to retard emptying of the gallbladder. Furthermore, administration of estrogens (to women for contraception or for replacement therapy after menopause or even to men for lowering levels of cholesterol in the serum) approximately doubles the fre-quency of cholesterol gallstones.[59]

Obesity, Fasting, and Diet

Persons who are obese (usually defined as more than 120% of ideal body weight) have a prevalence of cholesterol stones that is almost twice that of people who are not overweight. The reason for this is understood only par-tially. Most overweight persons have an overproduction of cholesterol throughout the body. This leads to an in-creased biliary secretion of cholesterol relative to the se-cretion of bile acids and lecithin.[14] Therefore, most obese persons have bile that is supersaturated with cholesterol, especially during fasting. However, as was discussed pre-viously, not all persons with supersaturated bile, including those who are obese, develop gallstones. The factors that would promote nucleation of crystals of cholesterol spe-cifically in obese persons have not been identified.[168]

During active loss of body weight in obese people (whose bile already is saturated), the cholesterol saturation paradoxically increases even further.[96] This occurs because during diminished caloric intake the synthesis and secre-tion of bile acids are decreased and cholesterol is mobi-lized, probably from adipose tissue, into the bile. Con-ceivably, if the bile becomes sufficiently supersaturated during the loss of weight, homogeneous nucleation of crystals of cholesterol would occur.

After obese persons lose weight, the saturation of bile decreases to less than it was before the loss of weight. Following weight loss, perhaps the mobilizable pool of cholesterol is depleted or inaccessible. It is intriguing to speculate that obese persons form gallstones because of the repeated bouts of loss of weight (and the recidivism) that are so characteristic of these persons.

Fasting itself is potentially lithogenic because it causes decreased hepatic secretion of bile acids and stasis of bile in the gallbladder.[97] Moreover, the cholesterol saturation of bile might be expected to continue to increase during continued fasting. This does occur with fasts up to 18 hours. In fact, in one study, the duration of the overnight fast was found to be greater in young women with gall-stones than in matched controls without gallstones. The formation of gallstones during total parenteral nutrition has been discussed in the section on the role of the gall-bladder.

Although diets that are high in cholesterol or polyun-saturated fatty acids or low in fiber can increase the sat-uration of bile, their role in the formation of cholesterol gallstones in humans is not established.[70] Correlations that have been found between these or other particular char-acteristics of diets and increased frequencies of gallstones in different populations are insufficient to distinguish cause from effect or coincidence.

Race and Heredity

The prevalence of gallstones differs among various racial groups.[17] For example, in one clinical study, among women in the United States, the prevalence was 14.7% in Mexican-Americans, 9% in whites, and 4.5% in blacks.[23] The prevalence reported for Asians generally is even lower than that for the blacks. The percentages for prevalence found in clinical studies are at least doubled in most au-topsy studies because the data in clinical studies usually have been obtained from known cases rather than from screening of populations. Thus, gallstones were found at autopsy in 30% of men and 50% of women above age 20 in Sweden and Czechoslovakia.[169] Contrast this frequency with the virtual absence of cholesterol gallstones in the Masai tribe of East Africa.

The potential for genetic factors to cause cholesterol gallstones is demonstrated best in the American Indians. The extraordinarily high prevalence of stones among Pima women (75% of those over age 30) in itself hints at a genetic etiology.[12] Furthermore, saturated bile develops during puberty in the Pima Indians and precedes nucleation of crystals and detection of gallstones by about 10 years (Fig. 41-7). Most of the Indian women have an inherited decrease in the synthesis of bile acids, which leads to a small pool of bile acids. Also, since many of these women are obese, they have an increased biliary secretion of cholesterol. Therefore, two defects, one genetic (abnormal metabolism of bile acids) and the other environmental (obesity), combine to cause the high prevalence of gallstones in American Indians.[40]

Among whites as well, a predisposition to form gallstones does run in families. Thus, approximately twice as many patients with gallstones than matched controls without gallstones (21% vs 9%) have parents, siblings, or children with gallstones.[35] Also, a significantly higher prevalence of saturated bile was found among the female siblings of patients with gallstones than among the female siblings of matched controls.[22] However, the type of genetic inheritance is not known, and discordance has been found in identical twins.

Diseases and Postoperative States

Patients having diseases of the ileum (particularly, Crohn's disease) or ileal resection are predisposed to form cholesterol gallstones[83] because loss of ileal function causes malabsorption of bile acids. If the malabsorption is severe enough to overcome the compensatory increase in hepatic synthesis of bile acids, the body's pool of bile acids gets depleted. The bile then becomes saturated with cholesterol (Fig. 41-8). The next stage in the formation of gallstones, nucleation, has not been studied in these patients.

A number of other diseases and postoperative states have been claimed to increase the risk for cholesterol gallstones.[57] However, despite the demonstration in these conditions of certain abnormalities that could enhance the formation of gallstones, confounding factors often exist and the actual incidence and type of gallstones have not always been established. For example, in cystic fibrosis, insufficient data are available regarding the purportedly increased incidence of gallstones.[127] Furthermore, the type of gallstone has not been determined, although the bile may be saturated with cholesterol because of abnormal metabolism of bile acids. In addition, aberrant mucin produced by the gallbladder in this disease could enhance nucleation of crystals.

In diabetes mellitus, autonomic dysfunction leads to atony of the gallbladder, which would facilitate nucleation and growth of gallstones.[41] Thus, a diabetic who also is obese would be predisposed to form cholesterol gallstones because the bile in obese persons is saturated with cholesterol and because nucleation is facilitated by stasis of bile in the gallbladder.

Delayed emptying of the gallbladder has been proposed as a mechanism for formation of gallstones in several other conditions, including surgical vagotomy. After vagotomy, however, the gallbladder actually may be supersensitive to cholecystokinin and not all investigators have found the bile to be saturated with cholesterol.[142] After biliopancreatic bypass,[139] an operation done for morbid obesity, and in celiac disease,[88] the gallbladder empties sluggishly because of curtailed release of cholecystokinin from the bypassed or diseased intestinal mucosa. Furthermore, in these two conditions, aberrant metabolism of bile acids could provide saturated bile.

An increased frequency of cholesterol gallstones has been reported in patients having type IIb or type IV hypertriglyceridemic hyperlipoproteinemia.[3] However, these patients often are obese or have diabetes mellitus, and it is not certain whether these hyperlipoproteinemias alone predispose to formation of cholesterol gallstones. Nevertheless, these patients have abnormalities in the metabolism of bile acids and cholesterol that would lead to saturation of bile.

Fig. 41-7. Supersaturated bile preceded the recognition of gallstones by about 10 years in Pima Indian women. (Reprinted with permission from Bennion LJ et al: N Engl J Med 300: 873, 1979)

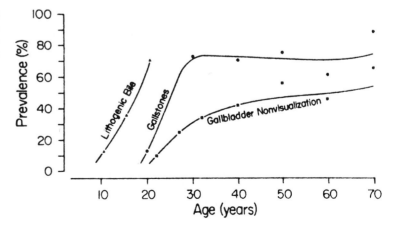

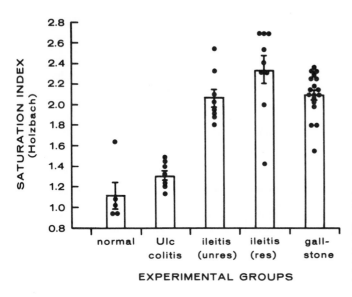

Fig. 41-8. Biliary lipids in inflammatory bowel disease. The biliary cholesterol saturation indices in normal persons and in those with ulcerative colitis were significantly less than those in patients with ileitis (with or without ileal resection) or those with gallstones ($p < 0.01$). (Reprinted with permission from Marks JW et al: Am J Dig Dis 22:1097, 1977)

In other studies, low values of total cholesterol or high values of high density lipoprotein (HDL) cholesterol in serum have been indicated as risk factors because of incriminating statistical correlations between the levels of total or HDL cholesterol in the serum and the presence of gallstones. However, these correlations have not been found consistently.[85]

Drugs

The hypolipidemic agent clofibrate predisposes patients to form cholesterol gallstones.[9] This drug reduces the hepatic synthesis of bile acids and increases the biliary secretion of cholesterol, two effects which result in the formation of supersaturated bile. Gemfibrozil, an analogue of clofibrate, also may cause saturation of bile and produce gallstones. Not all hypolipidemic agents, however, increase the risk for gallstones. For example, probucil, nicotinic acid, and fenofibrate (another analogue of clofibrate) do not increase the saturation of bile.[117] Also, the sequestrants of intestinal bile acids, cholestyramine and cholestipol, might be expected to deplete the body's pool of bile acids and, therefore, cause the formation of gallstones. However, they do neither. Presumably, a compensatory increase in the hepatic synthesis of bile acids offsets the loss of bile acids and thereby prevents the saturation of bile.

A reported association between the use of thiazides and gallstones has been contradicted by a subsequent study.

Formation of Pigment Gallstones

The pathogenesis of pigment gallstones is not as well understood as that of cholesterol gallstones. In fact, only recently has it been recognized that there are two fundamentally different types of pigment stones, descriptively called black pigment stones and brown pigment stones (Fig. 41-9). Although each type probably has a distinctive pathogenesis, they both result from abnormalities in the metabolism of bilirubin.[109]

The bile in patients with both types of pigment gallstones contains an excess of unconjugated bilirubin,[28] analogous to the saturation of bile with cholesterol in patients with cholesterol gallstones. Also, both types of pigment stones are composed primarily of bile pigment and contain a matrix of mucous glycoprotein. However, in black stones the pigment is predominantly an insoluble, highly cross-linked polymer of calcium bilirubinate,[107] whereas in brown stones the main pigment is monomeric calcium bilirubinate. Furthermore, the black and brown stones differ from each other substantially in several additional ways, including their other chemical components, radiodensity, location within the biliary system, geographic distribution, and associations with disease.[80]

Black Pigment Gallstones

Composition. Black pigment gallstones (also known as pure pigment stones because they contain mostly pigment and only minimal cholesterol) are lustrously black, amorphous in form, resistant to manual crushing, and powdery. On microscopic cross-section, their structure is homogeneous and smooth. They contain, in addition to their major component (*i.e.,* the polymer of calcium bilirubinate) lesser amounts of monomeric calcium bilirubinate, calcium carbonate, and calcium phosphate.

Black stones have been subclassified according to the presence or absence of calcium carbonate in the stone. The calcium salts of carbonate and phosphate often render black stones radiopaque. Thus, one half of pigment stones are opaque (the other half are radiolucent) and two thirds

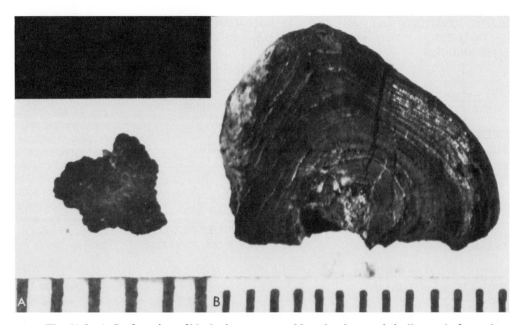

Fig. 41-9. A. Surface view of black pigment stone. Note the characteristically rough, featureless exterior. The cross-section has a similar appearance. **B.** Cross-sectional view of two thirds of a brown pigment stone. Note the characteristically laminated appearance produced by repeated rings of dark and light material of variable width. (Courtesy of Dr. R. D. Soloway)

of opaque stones are pigment stones (the remaining one third are cholesterol stones).

Epidemiology. Black pigment stones are formed primarily in the gallbladder and only occasionally in the biliary ducts. The bile in the gallbladder of these patients is sterile except when acute cholecystitis is present.[155] In most patients with black pigment stones no predisposing condition is recognized. However, black stones are the most common type of stone found in patients having cirrhosis[120] or chronic hemolysis. Thus, up to 60% of patients with sickle cell disease have black stones because of hemolysis.[151] Other conditions in which chronic hemolysis leads to the formation of black stones include thalassemia, hereditary spherocytosis, and cardiovascular prostheses. Whether the gallstones that form during long-term TPN are black stones or cholesterol stones is not yet established.[92,126]

Black stones occur throughout the world in most populations. In the United States, they account for as many as 27% of gallstones.[164] In Japan, the incidence of black stones is increasing (as is that of cholesterol stones) while the incidence of brown stones is decreasing. The frequency of black stones increases with age so that after the seventh decade they are found at cholecystectomy as often as cholesterol stones. In contrast to cholesterol stones, which tend to afflict women and obese persons, black stones occur in men almost as often as in women and without a predilection for the obese.

Pathogenesis. Unconjugated bilirubin is virtually insoluble in bile and normally accounts for less than 3% of total bile pigments in bile. The unconjugated bilirubin that is found in bile either has been secreted as such by the liver or is a hydrolytic product of conjugated bilirubin in bile (Fig. 41-10). The capacity of bile to solubilize unconjugated bilirubin depends primarily on the concentrations of bile acids and hydrogen ions.[99] Thus, bile can become supersaturated with calcium bilirubinate by an increase in the concentration of bilirubinate anions, an increase in the activity of unbound calcium cations, and a decrease in those factors that solubilize unconjugated bilirubin.

In patients having hemolytic disease, the secretion of increased amounts of unconjugated bilirubin into bile leads to the precipitation of calcium bilirubinate. The factors that cause polymerization of the bilirubin are not known. Mucous glycoproteins that are secreted by the epithelium of the gallbladder provide the framework on which microscopic precipitates of calcium bilirubinate, carbonate, and phosphate grow.[65]

Patients with cirrhosis also often have hemolysis; in addition, they may secrete an increased proportion of unconjugated bilirubin into bile (even without hemolysis) and they may have a decreased concentration of biliary bile acids for solubilization of bilirubin. Each of these three abnormalities in patients with cirrhosis can lead to the formation of precipitates of calcium bilirubinate and black pigment stones.

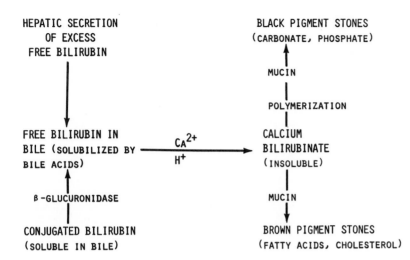

Fig. 41-10. Postulated mechanisms for the pathogenesis of pigment gallstones. In the formation of brown pigment stones, the β-glucuronidase probably is of bacterial origin and the precipitate of calcium bilirubinate is monomeric. Mucous glycoprotein (*mucin*) provides a framework for the growth of both types of pigment stones. The precipitated calcium bilirubinate also could serve as a nidus in the formation of cholesterol gallstones.

Brown Pigment Gallstones

Composition. Brown pigment gallstones (also known as calcium bilirubinate stones because the monomeric form of this compound is their major constituent) are earthy brown to orange, lusterless, laminated, soft, and greasy. On microscopic cross-section, their structure is spongy and porous. They also contain cholesterol (about 15% by dry weight) and calcium soaps of fatty acids (mostly calcium palmitate). Lacking calcium carbonate and phosphate, they are radiolucent.

Epidemiology. Brown pigment stones are formed primarily in the intrahepatic and extrahepatic bile ducts, but also in the gallbladder. The bile is infected in at least 85% of cases, most often with *Escherichia coli*. These stones are found most commonly in patients with chronic infectious cholangitis. This condition occurs virtually only in Asian patients having the biliary parasites, *Ascaris lumbricoides* or *Clonorchis sinensis*. Brown stones are rare in the Western world, where they have been found almost solely in patients having primary sclerosing cholangitis, paravaterian diverticuli, or foreign bodies (sutures or biliary catheters) in the common bile duct.

Pathogenesis. Maki[78] originally proposed that brown pigment gallstones resulted from the hydrolysis of conjugated bilirubin to its unconjugated form. He suggested that this deconjugation was mediated by an increased activity of bacterial β-glucuronidase (an enzyme that hydrolyzes bilirubin diglucuronide and that can be inhibited by glucuronolactone in bile). Calcium bilirubinate then would form and precipitate from bile. Stasis of bile, perhaps due to altered biliary motility or caused by parasite-induced obstruction of the bile ducts, provides the milieu for the development of bacterial infection.[163]

Maki's hypothesis must be expanded to account for the possibility that infection follows rather than precedes the formation of brown pigment stones and to explain the presence of fatty acids and cholesterol in these stones.[149] Thus, hydrolytic enzymes from sources other than bacteria (*e.g.,* from hepatic bile, pancreatic juice, or biliary mucosa) also could generate increased biliary concentrations of unconjugated bilirubin. Furthermore, hydrolysis of biliary lecithin by such enzymes would yield fatty acids and would decrease the amount of lecithin available for the solubilization of cholesterol.[124]

TREATMENT OF GALLSTONES

Gallstones may be eliminated without surgery by either mechanical means or dissolution therapy.

Several different methods are available for removing gallstones mechanically. Instruments that grasp and remove or crush the gallstone may be inserted into the biliary ducts through a T-tube (placed into the common bile duct during prior surgery), through the sphincter of Oddi via a fiberoptic endoscope that is passed orally, or through a cutaneous-biliary duct catheter that is placed radiographically. Mechanical methods are used almost exclusively for gallstones within the biliary ducts and rarely for gallstones within the gallbladder.

Several experimental mechanical methods of eliminating gallstones are being explored, including lithotripsy (shattering of gallstones) by ultrasound, laser, and hydroelectric shock, but none of these methods has been developed to the point of clinical utility.

Dissolution of gallstones can be accomplished by medications that are ingested orally or by solvents that are perfused through the biliary ducts or gallbladder. Dissolution by solvent requires placement of a tube into the biliary tract (*i.e.,* via T-tube, sphincter of Oddi, or the cutaneous-biliary route). Gallstones in either the gallbladder or ducts have been successfully dissolved by medication and solvent.

Oral Medications for Dissolution of Gallstones: Bile Acids

Oral dissolution therapy is the most widely applicable type of dissolution therapy. Estimates of the numbers of patients with gallstones who are candidates for oral therapy vary between 5% and 60%.[56,73] Nevertheless, oral therapy is used infrequently, probably because of the difficulty in predicting efficacy in individual patients and the concern about recurrence of gallstones following their successful dissolution.

Bile acids are the only oral agents available in the United States that have been shown to dissolve gallstones. Chenodeoxycholic acid (chenodiol), a major bile acid of humans, was the first oral agent that was shown to be effective.[136] Ursodeoxycholic acid, the 7B-epimeric metabolite of chenodiol, has also been shown to be effective,[79] and other bile acid metabolites are being studied for efficacy.[144]

Mechanism of Action

Chenodiol. Orally administered chenodiol is absorbed by the small intestine, transported via the portal venous system, and extracted from the portal blood by the liver. The hepatocytes of the liver conjugate the chenodiol, primarily with glycine and taurine, and secrete the conjugated chenodiol into the biliary canaliculi. At clinically useful doses of 10 mg to 15 mg/kg/day, the biliary concentration of conjugated chenodiol increases to 60% to 90% of biliary bile acids,[38] and synthesis of bile acids is inhibited.[60]

Chenodiol unsaturates bile with respect to cholesterol. Bathed in cholesterol-unsaturated bile, cholesterol-rich gallstones lose cholesterol into solution, and, as a result, they dissolve.

The mechanism whereby chenodiol unsaturates bile is not clear. Although it was initially thought that chenodiol unsaturated bile by expanding the bile acid pool and increasing the concentration of biliary bile acids, it was found that doses of chenodiol that did not increase the bile acid pool also reduced biliary cholesterol saturation.[1] Moreover, the bile acid pool could be expanded by either chenodiol or cholic acid (another major bile acid of humans), but only chenodiol desaturated bile.[66] Therefore, expansion of the bile acid pool cannot explain adequately the desaturating effect of chenodiol.

It has been demonstrated by many investigators that desaturation of bile by chenodiol is accompanied by reduced secretion of cholesterol into bile.[60] It is this reduced secretion of cholesterol and not increased secretion of bile acids that primarily is responsible for desaturation of bile.

There are three possible mechanisms whereby chenodiol might decrease cholesterol secretion. It might suppress cholesterol synthesis in the liver (reducing the amount of newly synthesized cholesterol in the liver that is available for biliary secretion), reduce cholesterol absorption from the intestine, or reduce the coupling of cholesterol secretion to bile acid secretion. (A fourth possible mechanism,

decreased mobilization of body stores of cholesterol, seems unlikely.)

Chenodiol has been shown to decrease the activity of HMG-CoA reductase, the rate-limiting enzyme for cholesterol synthesis, in the liver.[19] Nevertheless, the importance of this decreased activity has been questioned since only 20% of biliary cholesterol is newly synthesized in the liver.[138] Moreover, whereas there is a positive correlation between HMG-CoA reductase activity and biliary cholesterol secretion in untreated patients with gallstones, the correlation disappears when patients are treated with chenodiol.[60] Thus, the meaning of reduced HMG-CoA reductase activity in chenodiol-treated patients is unclear.

The effect of chenodiol on absorption of cholesterol by the intestine has been studied by many investigators. Although the data are conflicting, most investigations have shown no effect of chenodiol on cholesterol absorption.[67,72]

Chenodiol may reduce the coupling of cholesterol secretion to bile acid secretion. It has been shown that coupling of cholesterol and bile acid secretion is less with chenodiol than cholic acid.[76] Therefore, replacement of the pool of cholic acid by chenodiol during chenodiol therapy could result in decreased secretion of cholesterol. Decreased secretion of cholestrol may be reflected in the elevated levels of cholesterol in serum that are seen in patients undergoing therapy with chenodiol.[4]

Effects of chenodiol on the secretion of biliary lipids other than cholesterol have been studied. Most studies have shown no effects of chenodiol on bile acid secretion, but both decreased[60] and increased[167] phospholipid secretion have been reported.

Ursodeoxycholic Acid. Ursodeoxycholic acid ("ursodiol") differs from chenodiol only by its steroisomerism at the 7B position. Like chenodiol, ursodiol is absorbed from the intestine, conjugated in the liver, and secreted in bile. Ursodiol also reduces the biliary secretion of cholesterol and unsaturates bile.[152] Despite these similarities between chenodiol and ursodiol, the basic mechanisms whereby ursodiol causes the reduction in biliary cholesterol secretion, the decrease in biliary cholesterol saturation and the dissolution of gallstones are probably different from those of chenodiol.

Several studies have demonstrated a decrease in HMG-CoA reductase activity during ursodiol therapy in a manner similar to chenodiol therapy[86,131]; however, one study found that ursodiol had no effect on HMG-CoA reductase activity.[7]

Ursodiol therapy reduces the intestinal absorption of cholesterol and should, therefore, reduce the availability of cholesterol for biliary secretion. This may be the mechanism of the decrease in secretion of cholesterol associated with ursodiol therapy; however, it has not been shown that decreased intestinal absorption of cholesterol reduces the biliary secretion of cholesterol.[156]

Ursodiol, in contrast to chenodiol, suppresses bile acid synthesis minimally or not at all.[42] (The continued synthesis and secretion of chenodiol and cholic acid explains why biliary ursodiol increases to only 40% to 60% of biliary bile acids during ursodiol therapy.) It has been hypothesized that the continuing (and possibly increased) conversion of cholesterol to bile acids is responsible, in some way, for the decreased availability and secretion of cholesterol. This suggestion is supported by the observation that ursodiol lowers plasma cholesterol,[7] but more studies are needed before this hypothesis can be accepted.

Ursodiol promotes the solubilization of cholesterol in liquid crystals unlike chenodiol, which promotes the solubilization of cholesterol in mixed micelles.[52] Thus, the ability of ursodiol to effect dissolution of gallstones may relate in part to its ability to solubilize cholesterol in a different physical state than chenodiol.

Efficacy

Dissolution. Efficacy may be defined in terms of partial or complete dissolution of gallstones. Since partial dissolution is unlikely to be of benefit to patients, the frequency of complete dissolution is the more clinically relevant measure of efficacy. Reported frequencies for complete dissolution of gallstones in carefully selected patients when optimal doses of chenodiol (approximately 15 mg/kg/day) are used for between 1 and 3 years range from 20% to 40%.[26,125,157] Partial dissolution is seen with comparable frequency. Efficacy with ursodiol is similar to chenodiol[26,125] although dissolution may be faster with ursodiol.

Combination therapy with chenodiol and ursodiol offers two potential advantages. Since these two bile acids solubilize cholesterol through different mechanisms, it is possible that their efficacies for the dissolution of cholesterol gallstones are additive or synergistic. It also may be possible to use smaller doses of each bile acid and thus avoid the side-effects of chenodiol that are dose related. Although combination therapy has been recommended,[116] there are no adequate clinical comparisons of combination therapy and single bile acid therapy.

Most studies have used oral cholecystography to determine the frequency of dissolution. Cholecystography is less sensitive than ultrasonography for detecting small gallstones, and studies have shown an overestimation of complete dissolution varying from 28% to 40% when only cholecystography is used to evaluate dissolution.[29,71] It is important, therefore, to confirm complete dissolution, which is demonstrated by cholecystography with ultrasonography.

Symptoms. Several investigators have claimed efficacy for chenodiol in reducing symptoms of gallstones or dyspepsia, however, carefully conducted placebo-controlled trials have demonstrated no greater decrease in symptoms with chenodiol than with placebo.[29,137] Only patients who experience complete dissolution of their gallstones are likely to be freed of symptoms, and, even then, only those

symptoms caused by their gallstones (i.e., not dyspeptic symptoms).

Need for Surgery. There is no reduction (or increase) in the need for cholecystectomy in patients treated with chenodiol or ursodiol prior to successful dissolution of their gallstones.[29,137]

Recurrence of Gallstones. After discontinuation of dissolution therapy, bile reverts to its cholesterol-saturated state, and, therefore, recurrence of gallstones is possible. The frequency of recurrence has been reported to be from 10% to 50%, 3 to 7½ years after therapy is stopped.[128] A second course of therapy probably will be successful in patients who experience recurrence.

Determinants of Efficacy

Since the efficacy of therapy with bile acids is limited, it is important to select patients for therapy who have a higher likelihood of having dissolution of their gallstones. Several factors are recognized as determinants of efficacy.

Patency of the Cystic Duct. Therapy with bile acids causes hepatic bile to become unsaturated with cholesterol. If the cholesterol-unsaturated hepatic bile is unable to enter the gallbladder due to obstruction of the cystic duct, then therapy will not dissolve the gallstones within the gallbladder.

Permanent obstruction of the cystic duct by gallstones is a common phenomenon, occurring in approximately 7% of patients with gallstones.[100] The simplest means for determining the presence of cystic duct obstruction is oral cholecystography, since nonvisualization of the gallbladder on an oral cholecystogram almost always means obstruction of the cystic duct. Theoretically, radionuclide biliary tract studies would also be able to evaluate cystic duct patency; however, radionuclide studies should not be used for this purpose because of their high cost.

Characteristics of the Gallstones. Bile acid therapy is effective only in those patients whose gallstones are composed entirely or predominantly of cholesterol. Although 85% of gallstones are cholesterol in type, the remaining 15% of gallstones are pigment in type and not responsive to dissolution therapy with bile acids.

There is no simple means of determining which gallstones are pigment and which are cholesterol. Patients with hemolytic diseases or with bile that is cholesterol-unsaturated are much more likely to have gallstones that are pigment in type. On the other hand, patients with cholesterol crystals in their bile or with bile that is saturated with cholesterol are more likely to have gallstones that are cholesterol in type.

Gallstones that appear to float within the gallbladder on the oral cholecystogram (implying that the gallstones have a density that is less than the aqueous mixture of bile and dye) are always cholesterol in type.[24] These gallstones that float respond more frequently to dissolution therapy than gallstones that do not float.[55]

Gallstones that are calcified when they are evaluated radiographically respond poorly to dissolution with bile acid therapy since the calcium-pigment complex that is responsible for the radiographic calcification is resistant to dissolution.[137]

Smaller gallstones are more likely to respond to dissolution therapy than larger gallstones, perhaps because the cholesterol crystals are packed more tightly in the larger gallstones. In one study, 75% of gallstones less than 10 mm in diameter dissolved while only 50% of gallstones between 10 mm and 20 mm dissolved and no gallstone greater than 20 mm dissolved.[53]

Dose of Bile Acid. The optimal dose of chenodiol is in the range of 12 mg to 15 mg/kg/day,[125] although doses as low as 4 mg/kg/day have been reported to be effective.[20] Obese patients may require doses as high as 20 mg/kg/day to unsaturate bile as may occasional nonobese patients who are resistant to the biliary lipid-altering effects of chenodiol.[54,87] In order to identify individuals who are resistant to therapy it is necessary to analyze their bile for the degree of cholesterol saturation during therapy.

Bile acid therapy is as effective for dissolving gallstones in the bile ducts as gallstones in the gallbladder. Thus, 30% of patients with ductal gallstones of the cholesterol type who received ursodiol experienced complete dissolution of their gallstones, as compared with no patients who received placebo.[133] Such patients with cholesterol-type gallstones may be identified by quantitating the cholesterol content of gallstones that have been removed previously at surgery. A high cholesterol content in these gallstones implies that the ductal gallstones are also of the cholesterol type.

One of the difficulties in treating patients with gallstones in the ducts is that complications of ductal obstruction arise frequently and may require surgical intervention before therapy with bile acids can be completed.[153] Therefore, endoscopic sphincterotomy of the papilla of Vater may be a better therapeutic alternative in many patients.[129]

The optimal dose for ursodiol is in the range of 8 mg to 10 mg/kg/day.[125]

Concurrent Drug Therapy, Diet, and Other Factors. Theoretically, drugs that increase the degree of cholesterol saturation of bile, such as contraceptives, estrogens, or clofibrate, should counter the effects of bile acids and impede dissolution of gallstones. Nevertheless, it has been shown that patients may have dissolution of their gallstones while continuing to take oral contraceptives.[26]

Dietary cholesterol is one source of biliary cholesterol, and if dietary cholesterol is reduced, a modest decrease in biliary cholesterol saturation is seen.[68] Therefore, a decrease in dietary cholesterol should enhance the effects of bile acids. Although one study of bile acids combined with a diet low in cholesterol has suggested that reduced dietary cholesterol promotes dissolution of gallstones,[63] another

study has not found a beneficial effect of the low cholesterol diet.[71]

Addition of wheat bran to the diet of patients with gallstones increased the amount of chenodiol in bile and reduced biliary cholesterol saturation; however, the addition of bran to the diets of patients being treated with ursodiol did not have salutary effects on biliary cholesterol saturation or dissolution of gallstones beyond the salutary effects of ursodiol alone.[71,118]

In one very large trial of chenodiol, factors that correlated with greater efficacy were body weight that was less than ideal, female gender, and a pretreatment serum cholesterol level greater than 227 mg/dl.[137] (Serum cholesterol, however, was in the normal range in all patients in this study.)

Side-Effects

Chenodiol. *Hepatic.* Therapy with chenodiol is associated frequently with evidence of hepatotoxicity. In one study 31% of patients receiving 750 mg/day and 19% of patients receiving 375 mg/day of chenodiol developed elevations of serum aminotransferases as compared with 12% of patients receiving placebo.[137] The elevations, however, were usually mild (less than threefold the upper limits of normal) and transient. Therapy was discontinued in only 3% of patients due to aminotransferase elevations that were marked (greater than threefold) or persistent (lasting longer than 8 weeks). In all instances in which therapy was discontinued, the aminotransferase levels reverted to normal.

Serial liver biopsies from 126 patients before and during therapy with chenodiol revealed that approximately two thirds of the patients had minor electron microscopic abnormalities prior to therapy (increased bile pigment, decreased canalicular microvilli, and changes consistent with intrahepatic cholestasis); however, more than three fourths of the patients demonstrated these abnormalities after 9 months of therapy.[30] Abnormalities were not seen more frequently with higher than with lower doses of chenodiol. Because of the lack of biopsies from patients treated with placebo, it was not possible to determine whether the increased prevalence of abnormalities was due to chenodiol or the gallstones.

Despite the high frequency of elevations of serum aminotransferases, no serious or permanent hepatic injury has been reported to result from chenodiol therapy. The elevations, however, may limit therapy in a few patients.

The most likely cause of chenodiol-induced hepatic injury is a metabolite of chenodiol, lithocholic acid, which has been shown to be hepatotoxic in several species of animals.[111,112] Lithocholic acid is formed in the intestine by bacterial dehydroxylation of chenodiol. Like other bile acids, lithocholic acid is absorbed from the intestine, extracted from blood by the liver, conjugated by the hepatocyte and secreted into bile.

Elevated proportions of biliary lithocholic acid have been demonstrated during therapy with chenodiol in several species of animals that are particularly susceptible to chenodiol-induced hepatotoxicity.[112] The hepatotoxicity of chenodiol can be prevented in the rhesus monkey by treatment with lincomycin, an antibiotic that prevents bacterial conversion of chenodiol to lithocholic acid.[130]

Chenodiol is less hepatotoxic in humans than in most species of animals. The lesser hepatotoxicity in humans is probably due to the greater capacity of the liver in humans to sulfate lithocholic acid. Sulfated lithocholic acid is less toxic than nonsulfated lithocholic acid. Moreover, it is less well absorbed and, therefore, is less likely to be recycled through the enterohepatic circulation. In animals such as the rhesus monkey that show serious hepatotoxicity with chenodiol therapy, sulfation of lithocholic acid is poor.[33] In humans, the development of elevations of serum aminotransferases correlates with individuals' abilities to sulfate lithocholic acid. Thus, in one study of therapy with chenodiol, elevations occurred in 75% of patients with a lesser capacity to sulfate lithocholic acid and in only 11% of patients with a greater capacity to sulfate lithocholic acid.[84]

The capacity of an individual to sulfate lithocholic acid does not change during therapy with chenodiol, and, therefore, one would expect the toxic effects of lithocholic acid to persist as long as therapy is continued. Nevertheless, most elevations of aminotransferases are transient. This suggests either that mechanisms other than lithocholic acid production are responsible for the hepatotoxicity of chenodiol in humans or that humans have mechanisms in addition to sulfation that mitigate the toxicity of lithocholic acid. A cause of hepatotoxicity other than lithocholic acid is suggested by the demonstration that chenodiol is directly toxic to isolated human hepatocytes and to the isolated perfused rat liver.[8,95]

Diarrhea. A frequent dose related side-effect of therapy with chenodiol is diarrhea. Persistent or recurrent diarrhea occurred in 50% of patients receiving 750 mg/day compared with 24% of patients receiving placebo.[137] The diarrhea occurred early in the course of therapy and, although usually mild and transient, necessitated a reduction of dose in 11% of patients receiving 750 mg/day. Thus, diarrhea may prevent the use of maximally effective doses of chenodiol.

The most likely cause of the diarrhea is stimulation by chenodiol of the formation of cyclic nucleotides in the intestinal mucosa.[121] The cyclic nucleotides (*e.g.,* cyclic adenosine monophosphate) cause an increase in the net secretion of fluid and electrolytes into the intestine. Mucosal damage may also play a role in the diarrhea caused by chenodiol.[16]

Serum Lipids. Chenodiol has been reported to lower triglyceride levels in serum.[11] The cause of the lower levels may be a decrease in synthesis of triglycerides. Chenodiol therapy has been shown to increase serum levels of total cholesterol.[137] These effects do not appear to be dose related. The increase in the level of total cholesterol is due to an increase in the low density lipoprotein fraction of cholesterol.[4] There is no change in the high density lipoprotein fraction of cholesterol.

The cause of the elevation of low density lipoprotein cholesterol is unknown, but it has been suggested that chenodiol interferes with hepatic uptake and biliary secretion of serum cholesterol.

Although the elevation of cholesterol with chenodiol is small (20 mg/dl as compared with 10 mg/dl with placebo) and the therapy is usually limited to 1 or 2 years, the elevation of low density lipoprotein cholesterol should increase slightly the risk of atherosclerosis, at least theoretically. There has been no evidence of accelerated atherosclerosis when therapy is given, however. The risk would be of more concern if therapy was extended for many years.

Mucosal. Bile acids have been shown to be damaging to gastrointestinal mucosa under experimental conditions and are suspected of being the cause of bile reflux gastritis.[75] Chenodiol has been reported to cause abnormalities in the gastric mucosa of humans when it is ingested.[134] Despite this evidence of mucosal toxicity, therapy with chenodiol is not associated with dyspeptic symptoms on symptomatic ulcer disease.[137]

Carcinogenesis. Bile acids and their metabolites have been implicated in the pathogenesis of intestinal cancer, however, the results of studies that have examined the role of bile acids in carcinogenesis are contradictory, and no conclusions are possible.

Ursodiol. The minor difference between the molecular structure of chenodiol and ursodiol is responsible not only for major differences in the two bile acids' mechanism of action but also for major differences in their side-effects.[26,125] Ursodiol is not associated with clinically evident hepatotoxicity, despite the facts that ursodiol causes a rise in biliary lithocholic acid levels[32] and is capable of causing hepatic damage (although to a lesser degree than chenodiol) in animal models.[94] Ursodiol therapy is not associated with diarrhea (it does not stimulate the formation of intestinal cyclic nucleotides)[121] or elevations of serum cholesterol (perhaps because it allows continued conversion of cholesterol to bile acids). Ursodiol also appears to be less toxic than chenodiol to intestinal mucosa.[75]

Selection of Patients for Dissolution Therapy

The efficacy of dissolution therapy is limited, and alternative methods for the management of gallstones (surgery and observation alone) exist. Therefore, patients who are selected for dissolution therapy should have a high likelihood of having their gallstones dissolve, and dissolution therapy should be the most appropriate form of management.

The characteristics that best identify patients who are likely to have dissolution include a gallbladder that can be visualized on the oral cholecystogram; gallstones that are radiolucent without calcification; gallstones with a diameter of less than 2 cm; and gallstones that float in bile on the oral cholecystogram or bile that is cholesterol-saturated or contains cholesterol crystals.

Dissolution therapy is the most appropriate form of management of gallstones for a subset of patients. The majority of patients with gallstones are asymptomatic from their gallstones, and they remain asymptomatic for many years. In these patients observation may be the best form of management.[37] This is especially true in older patients who are likely to die of natural causes before they become symptomatic from their gallstones.

Patients with frequent or severe symptoms from their gallstones need urgent therapy for relief. Similarly, patients with serious complications of their gallstones such as cholangitis, pancreatitis, or choledocholithiasis, because of the potential for recurrence of these complications, also require urgent therapy. Therefore, frequent symptoms, severe symptoms, or serious complications of gallstones are an indication for surgery.

If asymptomatic patients and patients with frequent symptoms, severe symptoms, or serious complications are eliminated from consideration, then only mildly or moderately symptomatic patients, in particular, those patients with biliary colic or self-limited, acute cholecystitis, remain potential candidates for dissolution therapy. (Needless to say, it is important to be as certain as possible that a patient's symptoms are caused by their gallstones.)

The morbidity and mortality of surgery may alter the choice of management of gallstones. In general, gallbladder surgery is associated with low morbidity and mortality; however, in certain groups of patients, such as those with severe cardiovascular or pulmonary disease, morbidity and mortality is high. Because of the increased risk of surgery, these groups of patients may be more appropriately managed with dissolution therapy.

Patients who refuse surgery despite symptoms that interfere with or threaten their lives are also appropriate candidates for dissolution therapy.

Dissolution therapy does not preclude alternative management. Thus, if dissolution therapy is unsuccessful, management subsequently may be either surgical or observational. Among mildly symptomatic patients, delaying surgery for a trial of dissolution therapy is reasonable since less than 3% per year of such patients will develop symptoms that require urgent surgery during their therapy.[137]

There are several contraindications to the use of dissolution therapy. Severe liver disease, inflammatory bowel disease, and active gastric or duodenal ulcer disease are relative contraindications to the use of chenodiol because of the potential for additive toxicity of chenodiol on the liver and intestinal mucosa. These relative contraindications probably will not apply to ursodiol. Pregnant women should not receive bile acids since the teratogenic potential in humans is unknown and hepatotoxicity has been reported with chenodiol in the fetus of the rhesus monkey.[44] Women who might become pregnant during therapy should use mechanical or spermicidal contraception rather than birth control pills because birth control pills increase the biliary saturation of cholesterol.

Administration and Monitoring of Therapy

At the present time, only chenodiol is available for dissolution of gallstones on a nonresearch basis in the United States.

The dose of chenodiol that has been studied most carefully is 750 mg/day. Although this dose is safe with appropriate monitoring, its efficacy is limited. A dose of 15 mg/kg/day has maximal efficacy. Although the toxicity of this larger dose has not been studied as carefully as the dose of 750 mg/day, there have been no reports of serious or permanent hepatotoxicity with the larger dose.

Chenodiol may be given in divided doses in the morning and evening for the convenience of the patient. The dose should be increased gradually over several weeks until the full therapeutic dose is reached because of the potential for diarrhea.

An oral cholecystogram should be obtained prior to therapy and again after 9 or 12 months of therapy. If the second oral cholecystogram shows that the gallstones have completely dissolved, an ultrasonogram should be done to confirm the dissolution, and therapy should be continued for an additional 3 months. (This allows for the dissolution of remnants of gallstones that are too small to be detected by ultrasonography.) If the ultrasonogram does not confirm dissolution, therapy may be continued for an additional 3 to 6 months and the ultrasonogram repeated. If gallstones still are present, no further therapy is warranted.

If the oral cholecystogram obtained after 9 or 12 months of therapy shows partial dissolution of the gallstones, therapy may be continued for another 9 to 12 months, and then another oral cholecystogram should be obtained. Demonstration of continuing dissolution on the cholecystogram should be followed by further therapy and periodic cholecystograms until the gallstones have dissolved completely. Complete dissolution should be confirmed with ultrasonography as described in the preceding paragraph. If continuing dissolution is not seen, therapy should be stopped.

If the oral cholecystogram obtained after 9 or 12 months of therapy shows no dissolution (partial or complete), continued therapy is unlikely to result in dissolution. Therapy may be discontinued or the dose of chenodiol may be increased, particularly if doses lower than 15 mg/kg/day have been used initially or biliary lipid analysis discloses that bile has not become unsaturated with cholesterol at the dose used initially (i.e., the patient is resistant to therapy).

Patients may develop a gallbladder that cannot be visualized on the oral cholecystogram for the first time during therapy with chenodiol. Therapy does not have to be discontinued since most of these patients will have visualization return on a later cholecystogram.[137] The return of visualization implies that the cystic duct obstruction (which causes the nonvisualization and prevents effective dissolution therapy) is transient.

Calcification within gallstones occurs during dissolution

therapy in a small proportion of patients and probably justifies discontinuing therapy since calcified gallstones respond poorly to therapy.[137]

Patients may develop biliary colic or acute cholecystitis during dissolution therapy. Therapy may be continued in these symptomatic patients if it is warranted clinically since symptoms are not associated with a decrease in the efficacy of therapy.[137]

Serum aminotransferases should be monitored every 2 weeks during the first few months of therapy with chenodiol and every 3 to 4 months thereafter. If elevations of the aminotransferases occur and are either marked (greater than threefold) or prolonged (greater than 8 weeks), therapy should be discontinued. Once the elevations have resolved, therapy may be reinstituted, preferably at a dose lower than the dose that caused the elevation. The dose then may be increased gradually to the desired level. If the elevations recur with reinstitution of therapy, chenodiol should be discontinued permanently.

Should intolerable diarrhea occur during therapy with chenodiol, the dose of chenodiol may be decreased or timing of the doses may be altered (*e.g.,* to three times daily). If the dose is decreased, attempts should be made to reinstitute the full dose for maximal efficacy.

Levels of serum cholesterol should be monitored every 3 to 4 months. If increases in the levels are seen, a diet that is low in cholesterol may be instituted and the levels of cholesterol followed. The risk to the patient depends on the magnitude of the elevation, the duration of therapy, and the extent of preexistent atherosclerotic vascular disease. In general, the risk with minor (less than 20 mg/dl) elevations of cholesterol for periods of 1 to 2 years is small.

Once patients have had complete dissolution of their gallstones, they should have an ultrasonogram of the gallbladder each year to look for recurrence of the gallstones. Recurrences may be managed with reinstitution of dissolution therapy, surgery, or observation.

Ursodiol will be available for use in the United States within the next few years, and it is likely that it will be used more widely than chenodiol because of the lower incidence of side-effects. Administration and monitoring with ursodiol are different than with chenodiol. The optimal dose for ursodiol is 8 mg to 10 mg/kg/day. Dissolution of gallstones with ursodiol may be monitored in the same way as with chenodiol, but serum aminotransferases and cholesterol do not need to be measured since ursodiol does not raise their levels.

Other Oral Medications for Dissolution of Gallstones: Choleretic Agents

No choleretic agents are presently available for use in patients in the United States except in research protocols; however, they are available for general use in Europe and are the only oral medications other than bile acids that are being investigated actively for efficacy in the dissolution of gallstones.

Choleretic agents are absorbed from the intestine, extracted from blood by the liver, and secreted into bile. They stimulate biliary secretion of water and electrolytes and thereby increase the flow of bile.

Choleretic therapy reduces the degree of saturation of bile, but with the doses studied, bile does not become unsaturated.[132] It is unlikely, therefore, that choleretic agents alone will be efficacious for dissolution of gallstones. Nevertheless, it has been suggested on the basis of preliminary studies that the effects of these agents (*e.g.,* the terpene Rowachol) may be additive or synergistic with the effects of bile acids and thus allow smaller doses of bile acids to be used.[25] More experimental work will be necessary to determine whether choleretic agents have a role in dissolution therapy of gallstones.

Perfusion of Solvents for Dissolution of Gallstones

Several agents have been perfused through the biliary tract in an attempt to dissolve gallstones. The agents are perfused by means of catheters that may be placed into the biliary tract through a T-tube, by retrograde cannulation of the common bile duct, or through the liver by percutaneous puncture. Perfusion is considered when nonsurgical mechanical removal of gallstones is not feasible and surgery is undesirable.

The first agents that were perfused, not surprisingly, were bile acids. Perfusion with bile acids was effective, but dissolution required several weeks and the bile acids were associated with toxicity.[77,114]

The next agent to be perfused was mono-octanoin. Mono-octanoin is a monoglyceride that is derived from medium-chain triglycerides. It has an excellent capacity to dissolve cholesterol.[160] Mono-octanoin is effective and safe for dissolving gallstones. Although experience is limited, it has been released for general use in the United States. The problem with mono-octanoin is that it requires 3 to 21 days to effect the dissolution of gallstones.

The agent that has been perfused most recently is methyl tert-butyl ether, a compound that was developed as an octane enhancer for gasoline.[6] Methyl tert-butyl ether, as an aliphatic ether, has prominent cholesterol-solubilizing capabilities and dissolves cholesterol gallstones within hours both *in vitro* and *in vivo*. The use of methyl tert-butyl ether is experimental, and experience is limited. The major concern is its potential toxicity.

REFERENCES

1. Adler RD et al: Effects of low dose chenodeoxycholic acid feeding on biliary lipid metabolism. Gastroenterology 68: 326, 1975
2. Admirand WH, Small DM: The physical basis of cholesterol gallstone formation in man. J Clin Invest 47:1043, 1968
3. Ahlberg J et al: Prevalence of gallbladder disease in hyperlipoproteins. Am J Dig Dis 24:459, 1979
4. Albers JJ et al: The effects of chenodeoxycholic acid on

lipoproteins and apolipoproteins. Gastroenterology 82:638, 1982

5. Allen B et al: Sludge is calcium bilirubinate associated with bile stasis. Am J Surg 141:51, 1981

6. Allen MJ et al: Cholelitholysis using methyl tertiary butyl ether. Gastroenterology 88:122, 1985

7. Angelin B et al: Ursodeoxycholic acid treatment in cholesterol gallstone disease: Effect on hepatic 3-hydroxy-3-methylglutaryl coenzyme A reductase activity, biliary lipid composition, and plasma lipid levels. J Lipid Res 24:461, 1983

8. Barnwell SG et al: Effect of taurochenodeoxycholate or tauroursodeoxycholate on biliary output of phospholipids and plasma-membrane enzymes, and the extent of cell damage, in isolated perfused rat livers. Biochem J 216:107, 1983

9. Bateson MC et al: Clofibrate therapy and gallstone induction. Am J Dig Dis 23:623, 1978

10. Been JM et al: Microstructure of gallstones. Gastroenterology 76:548, 1979

11. Begemann F: Influence of chenodeoxycholic acid on the kinetics of endogenous triglyceride transport in man. Eur J Clin Invest 8:283, 1978

12. Bennion LJ et al: Development of lithogenic bile during puberty in Pima Indians. N Engl J Med 300:873, 1979

13. Bennion LJ et al: Sex differences in the size of bile acid pools. Metabolism 27:961, 1978

14. Bennion LJ, Grundy SM: Effects of obesity and caloric intake on biliary lipid metabolism in man. J Clin Invest 56:996, 1975

15. Burnstein MJ et al: Evidence for a potent nucleating factor in the gallbladder bile of patients with cholesterol gallstones. Gastroenterology 85:801, 1983

16. Camilleri M et al: Pharmacological inhibition of chenodeoxycholate-induced fluid and mucus secretion and mucosal injury in the rabbit colon. Dig Dis Sci 27:865, 1982

17. Capocacchia L et al: Epidemiology and Prevention of Gallstone Disease. Lancaster, MTP Press, 1984

18. Carey MC, Small DM: The physical chemistry of cholesterol solubility in bile: Relationship to gallstone formation and dissolution in man. J Clin Invest 61:998, 1978

19. Coyne MJ et al: Effect of chenodeoxycholic acid and phenobarbital on the rate-limiting enzymes of hepatic cholesterol and bile acid synthesis in patients with gallstones. J Lab Clin Med 87:281, 1976

20. Danzinger RG, Kurtas TK: Very low dose oral chenodeoxycholic acid produced nonlithogenic bile and dissolved gallstones. In Paumgartner G, Steil A, and Gerok W (eds): Biological Effects of Bile Acids, p 103. Lancaster, MTP Press, 1979

21. Danzinger RG et al: Effect of oral chenodeoxycholic acid on bile acid kinetics and biliary lipid composition in women with cholelithiasis. J Clin Invest 52:2809, 1973

22. Danzinger RG et al: Lithogenic bile in siblings of young women with cholelithiasis. Mayo Clin Proc 47:762, 1972

23. Diehl AK et al: Clinical gallbladder disease in Mexican-American, Anglo, and Black women. S Med J 73:438, 1980

24. Dolgin SM et al: Identification of patients with cholesterol or pigment gallstones by discriminant analysis of radiographic features. N Engl J Med 304:808, 1981

25. Ellis WR et al: Pilot study of combination treatment for gallstones with medium dose chenodeoxycholic acid and a terpene preparation. Br Med J 289:153, 1984

26. Erlinger S et al: Franco-Belgian Cooperative Study of ursodeoxycholic acid in the medical dissolution of gallstones: A double-blind randomized, dose-response study, and comparison with chenodeoxycholic acid. Hepatology 4:308, 1984

27. Everson GE et al: Gallbladder function in the human female: Effect of the ovulating cycle, pregnancy, and contraceptive steroids. Gastroenterology 82:711, 1982

28. Fevery J et al: Analysis of bilirubins in biological fluids by extraction and thin layer chromatography of the intact tetrapyrroles: Application to bile of patients with Gilbert's syndrome, hemolysis, or cholelithiasis. Hepatology 3:177, 1983

29. Fisher MM et al: The Sunnybrook Gallstone Study: A double-blind controlled trial of chenodeoxycholic acid for gallstone dissolution. Hepatology 5:102, 1985

30. Fisher RL et al: A prospective morphologic evaluation of hepatic toxicity of chenodeoxycholic acid (CDCA) in patients with cholelithiasis: The National Cooperative Gallstone Study. Hepatology 2:187, 1982

31. Fisher RS et al: Abnormal gallbladder emptying in patients with gallstones. Dig Dis Sci 27:1019, 1982

32. Frenkiel P et al: Effect of ursodeoxycholic acid and diets on biliary lipids. Am J Clin Nutr 43:239, 1986

33. Gadacz TR et al: Impaired lithocholate sulfation in the rhesus monkey: A possible mechanism for chenodeoxycholate toxicity. Gastroenterology 70:1125, 1976

34. Gallinger S et al: Effect of mucous glycoprotein on nucleation time of human bile. Gastroenterology 89:648, 1985

35. Gilat T et al: An increased familial frequency of gallstones. Gastroenterology 84:242, 1983

36. Gollish SH et al: Nucleation of cholesterol monohydrate crystals from hepatic and gallbladder bile of patients with cholesterol gallstones. Gut 24:836, 1983

37. Gracie WA, Ransohoff DF: The natural history of silent gallstones: The innocent gallstone is not a myth. N Engl J Med 307:798, 1982

38. Grundy SM et al: The effects of chenodiol on biliary lipids and their association with gallstone dissolution in the National Cooperative Gallstone Study (NCGS). J Clin Invest 73:1156, 1984

39. Grundy SM et al: Biliary lipid outputs in young women with cholesterol gallstones. Metabolism 23:67, 1974

40. Grundy SM et al: Mechanism of lithogenic bile formation in American Indian women with cholesterol gallstones. J Clin Invest 51:3026, 1972

41. Haber GB, Heaton KW: Lipid composition of bile in diabetics and obesity-matched controls. Gut 20:518, 1979

42. Hardison WG et al: Effect of ursodeoxycholate and its taurine conjugate on bile acid synthesis and cholesterol absorption. Gastroenterology 87:130, 1984

43. Hegardt FG, Dam H: The solubility of cholesterol in aqueous solution of bile salt and lecithin. Z Ernaerungswiss 10:239, 1971

44. Heywood R et al: Pathological changes in fetal rhesus monkey induced by oral chenodeoxycholic acid. Lancet 2:1021, 1973

45. Hofmann AF, Roda A: Physiochemical properties of bile acids and their relationship to biological properties: An overview of the problem. J Lipid Res 25:1477, 1984

46. Holan KR et al: Nucleation time: A key factor in the pathogenesis of cholesterol gallstone disease. Gastroenterology 77:611, 1979

47. Holzbach RT: Factors influencing cholesterol nucleation in bile. Hepatology 4:173S, 1984

48. Holzbach RT: Effects of gallbladder function on human bile: Compositional and structural changes. Hepatology 4: 57S, 1984

49. Holzbach RT, Kibe A: Pathogenesis of cholesterol gallstones. In Cohen S, Soloway RD (eds): Contemporary Issues in Gastroenterology: Gallstones, vol 4, p 73. New York, Churchill Livingstone, 1985

50. Holzbach RT et al: Biliary proteins, unique inhibitors of cholesterol crystal nucleation in human gallbladder bile. J Clin Invest 7:35, 1984

51. Holzbach RT et al: Cholesterol solubility in bile: Evidence that supersaturated bile is frequent in healthy man. J Clin Invest 52:1467, 1973

52. Igimi H, Carey MC: Cholesterol gallstone dissolution in bile: Dissolution kinetics of crystalline (anhydrate and monohydrate) cholesterol with chenodeoxycholate, ursodeoxycholate, and their glycine and taurine conjugates. J Lipid Res 22:254, 1981

53. Iser JH et al: Chenodeoxycholic acid treatment of gallstones: A follow-up report and analysis of factors influencing responses to therapy. N Engl J Med 293:378, 1975

54. Iser JH et al: Resistance to chenodeoxycholic acid (CDCA) treatment in obese patients with gallstones. Br Med J 1: 1509, 1978

55. Jacobus DP et al: The natural history and the therapeutic response to chenodiol in patients with floatable stones in the National Cooperative Gallstone Study (NCGS). Gastroenterology 84:1197, 1983

56. Johansson G: A prospective study of the clinical significance of the treatment of gallstones with chenodeoxycholic acid. Surg Gynecol Obstet 159:127, 1984

57. Kern F: Epidemiology and natural history of gallstones. Semin Liver Dis 3:87, 1983

58. Kern F Jr et al: Biliary lipids, bile acids, and gallbladder function in the human female: Effects of pregnancy and the ovulatory cycle. J Clin Invest 68:1229, 1981

59. Kern F Jr et al: Biliary lipids, bile acids, and gallbladder function in the human female: Effects of contraceptive steroids. J Lab Clin Med 99:798, 1982

60. Key PH et al: Biliary lipid synthesis and secretion in gallstone patients before and during treatment with chenodeoxycholic acid. J Lab Clin Med 95:816, 1980

61. Kibe A et al: Inhibition of cholesterol crystal formation by apolipoproteins in supersaturated model bile. Science 225: 514, 1984

62. Kibe A et al: Factors affecting cholesterol monohydrate crystal nucleation time in model systems of supersaturated bile. J Lipid Res 26:1102, 1985

63. Kuper RM et al: Gallstone dissolution rate during chenic acid therapy: Effects of bedtime administration plus low cholesterol diet. Dig Dis Sci 27:1025, 1982

64. Lamont JT et al: Role of gallbladder mucin in pathophysiology of gallstones. Hepatology 4:51S, 1984

65. Lamont JT et al: Mucin glycoprotein content of human pigment gallstones. Hepatology 3:377, 1983

66. Larusso NF et al: Effect of primary bile acid ingestion on bile acid metabolism and biliary lipid secretion in gallstone patients. Gastroenterology 69:1301, 1975

67. Larusso NF et al: Effect of litholytic bile acids on cholesterol absorption in gallstone patients. Gastroenterology 84:265, 1983

68. Lee DWT et al: Effect of dietary cholesterol on biliary lipids in patients with gallstones and normal subjects. Am J Clin Nutr 42:414, 1985

69. Lee SP et al: Aspirin prevention of cholesterol gallstone formation in prairie dogs. Science 211:1429, 1981

70. Lefkof IR et al: Diet in the formation and treatment of cholesterol gallstones. In Cohen S, Soloway RD (eds): Contemporary Issues in Gastroenterology: Gallstones. New York, Churchill Livingstone, 1985

71. Lefkof IR et al: Effect of diet on dissolution of gallstones by ursodeoxycholic acid, including a comparison between ultrasonography and cholecystography. Mt Sinai J Med 53: 241, 1986

72. Leiss O et al: Effect of three different dihydroxy bile acids on intestinal cholesterol absorption in normal volunteers. Gastroenterology 87:144, 1984

73. Leuschner M: Radiological and ultrasonographic investigations with respect to patient selection and monitoring for chemical gallstone dissolution. Hepatogastroenterology 31: 140, 1984

74. Levy PF et al: Human gallbladder mucin accelerates nucleation of cholesterol in artificial bile. Gastroenterology 87:270, 1984

75. Lillemoe KD et al: Tauroursodeoxycholic acid is less damaging than taurochenodeoxycholic acid to the gastric and esophageal mucosa. Dig Dis Sci 28:359, 1983

76. Linblad L et al: Influence of cholic and chenodeoxycholic acid on biliary cholesterol secretion in man. Eur J Clin Invest 7:383, 1977

77. Mack E et al: Local toxicity of T-tube infused cholate in the rhesus monkey. Surg Forum 28:408, 1977

78. Maki T: Clarification of the nomenclature of pigment gallstones. Am J Surg 144:302, 1982

79. Makino J et al: Dissolution of cholesterol gallstones by ursodeoxycholic acid. Jpn Gastroenterol 72:690, 1974

80. Malet PF et al: Black and brown pigment gallstones differ in microstructure and microcomposition. Hepatology 4: 227, 1984

81. Malet PF et al: Cyclic deposition of calcium salts during growth of cholesterol gallstones. Scan Electron Microsc 2: 775, 1985

82. Marks JW, Bonorris GG: Intermittency of cholesterol crystals in duodenal bile from gallstone patients. Gastroenterology 87:622, 1984

83. Marks JW et al: Gallstone prevalence and biliary lipid composition in inflammatory bowel disease. Dig Dis Sci 22:1097, 1977

84. Marks JW et al: Sulfation of lithocholate as a possible modifier of chenodeoxycholic acid–induced elevations of serum transaminase in patients with gallstones. J Clin Invest 68: 1190, 1981.

85. Marks JW et al: Lack of correlation between lipoproteins and biliary cholesterol saturation in patients with gallstones. Dig Dis Sci 29:1118, 1984

86. Maton PN et al: Hepatic HMG CoA reductase in human cholelithiasis: Effects of chenodeoxycholic and ursodeoxycholic acids. Eur J Clin Invest 10:325, 1980

87. Maton PN et al: Lack of response to chenodeoxycholic acid in obese and non-obese patients. Gut 21:1082, 1980

88. Maton PN et al: Defective gallbladder emptying and cholecystokinin release in celiac disease: Reversal by gluten-free diet. Gastroenterology 88:391, 1985

89. Maudgal DP et al: Postprandial gallbladder emptying in patients with gallstones. Br Med J 1:141, 1980

90. Mazer NA, Carey MC: Quasielastic light scattering studies of aqueous biliary lipid systems: Cholesterol solubilization and precipitation in model bile systems. Biochemistry 22: 426, 1983

91. Mazer NA, Carey MC: Mathematical model of biliary lipid secretion: A quantitative analysis of physiological and biochemical data from man and other species. J Lipid Res 25: 932, 1984

92. Messing B et al: Does total parenteral nutrition induce gallbladder sludge formation and lithiasis? Gastroenterology 84:1012, 1983

93. Metzger AL et al: Diurnal variation in biliary lipid composition: Possible role in cholesterol gallstone formation. N Engl J Med 288:333, 1973

94. Miyai K et al: Hepatoxicity of bile acids in rabbits. Lab Invest 46:428, 1982

95. Miyazaki K et al: Effect of chenodeoxycholic and ursodeoxycholic acids on isolated adult human hepatocytes. Dig Dis Sci 29:1123, 1984

96. Mok HYI et al: Biliary lipid metabolism in obesity: Effects of bile acid feeding before and during weight reduction. Gastroenterology 76:556, 1979

97. Mok HYI et al: Kinetics of the enterohepatic circulation during fasting: Biliary lipid secretion and gallbladder storage. Gastroenterology 78:1023, 1980

98. Moore EW: The role of calcium in the pathogenesis of gallstones: Ca^{++} electrode studies of model bile salt solutions and other biologic systems. Hepatology 4:285, 1984

99. Moore EW: Interactions between ionized calcium and sodium taurocholate: Bile salts are important buffers for prevention of calcium-containing gallstones. Gastroenterology 83:1079, 1982

100. Mujahed Z et al: The nonopacified gallbladder on oral cholecystography. Radiology 112:1, 1974

101. Nakayama F, van der Linden W: Stratification of bile in the gallbladder and gallstone formation. Surg Gynecol Obstet 141:587, 1985

102. Nervi FO et al: Hepatic cholesterologenesis in Chileans with cholesterol gallstone disease: Evidence for sex differences in the regulation of hepatic cholesterol metabolism. Gastroenterology 80:539, 1981

103. Nicolan G et al: Hepatic 3-hydroxy-3-methyl glutaryl CoA (HMG-CoA) reductase and cholesterol 7α-hydroxylase in man. Gastroenterology 64:887, 1973

104. Nilsell K et al: Biliary lipid output and bile acid kinetics in cholesterol gallstone disease: Evidence for an increased hepatic secretion of cholesterol in Swedish patients. Gastroenterology 89:287, 1985

105. Northfield TC, Hofmann AF: Biliary lipid output during three meals and an overnight fast: I. Relationship to bile acid pool size and cholesterol saturation of bile in gallstone and control subjects. Gut 16:1, 1975

106. Northfield TC et al: Gallbladder sensitivity to cholecystokinin in patients with gallstones. Br Med J 1:143, 1980

107. Ohkubo H et al: Polymer networks in pigment and cholesterol gallstones assessed by equilibrium swelling and infrared spectroscopy. Gastroenterology 87:805, 1984

108. Olszewski MF et al: Liquid crystals in human bile. Nature 242:336, 1973

109. Ostrow JD: The etiology of pigment gallstones. Hepatology 4:215S, 1984

110. Osuga T et al: A scanning electron microscope study of gallstone development in man. Lab Invest 31:696, 1975

111. Palmer RH: Toxic effects of lithocholate on the liver and biliary tree. In Taylor W (ed): The Hepatobiliary System: Fundamental and Pathological Mechanisms, pp 227–240. New York, Plenum Press, 1976

112. Palmer RH: Bile acids, liver injury and liver disease. Arch Intern Med 130:606, 1972

113. Pattinson NR: Solubilization of cholesterol in human bile. Febs Lett 181:239, 1985

114. Pitt HA et al: Sodium cholate dissolution of retained biliary stones: Mortality rate following intrahepatic infusion. Surgery 85:457, 1979

115. Pitt HA et al: Increased risk of cholelithiasis with prolonged parenteral nutrition. Am J Surg 145:106, 1983

116. Podda M et al: A combination of chenodeoxycholic acid and ursodeoxycholic acid is more effective than either alone in reducing biliary cholesterol saturation. Hepatology 2: 334, 1982

117. Podda M, Zuin M: Effects of fenofibrate on biliary lipids and bile acid pool size in patients with type IV hyperlipoproteinemia. Atherosclerosis 55:135, 1985

118. Pomare EW et al: The effect of wheat bran upon bile salt metabolism and upon the lipid composition of bile in gallstone patients. Dig Dis Sci 21:521, 1976

119. Pomeranz IS, Shaffer EA: Abnormal gallbladder emptying in a subgroup of patients with gallstones. Gastroenterology 88:787, 1985

120. Raedsch R et al: Hepatic secretion of bilirubin and biliary lipids in patients with alcoholic cirrhosis of the liver. Digestion 26:80, 1983

121. Rahban S et al: The effect of dihydroxy bile acids on intestinal secretion, cyclic nucleotides, and Na^+-K^+-ATPase. Am J Med Sci 279:141, 1980

122. Redinger RM, Small DM: Bile composition, bile salt metabolism, and gallstones. Arch Intern Med 130:618, 1972

123. Reuben A et al: Bile lipid secretion in obese and non-obese individuals with and without gallstones. Clin Sci 69:71, 1985

124. Robins SJ et al: Lipids of pigment gallstones. Biochim Biophys Acta 712:21, 1982

125. Roda E et al: Ursodeoxycholic acid vs. chenodeoxycholic acid as cholesterol gallstone dissolving agents: A comparative randomized study. Hepatology 2:804, 1982

126. Roslyn JJ et al: Gallbladder disease in patients on long-term parenteral nutrition. Gastroenterology 84:148, 1983

127. Roy CC et al: Hepatobiliary disease in cystic fibrosis: A survey of current issues and concepts. J Pediatr Gastroenterol Nutr 1:469, 1982

128. Ruppin DC, Dowling HR: Is recurrence inevitable after gallstone dissolution by bile acid treatment? Lancet 1:181, 1982

129. Safrany L: Duodenoscopic sphincterotomy and gallstone removal. Gastroenterology 72:383, 1977

130. Salen G et al: Prevention of chenodeoxycholic acid toxicity with lincomycin. Lancet 1:1082, 1975

131. Salen G et al: Effect of high and low doses of ursodeoxycholic acid on gallstone dissolution in humans. Gastroenterology 78:1412, 1980

132. Sama C et al: A double-blind comparative trial of dihydroxydibutyl ether in patients with cholesterol gallstones. Int J Clin Pharmacol Ther Toxicol 21:37, 1983

133. Savioli G et al: Medical treatment of biliary duct stones: Effect of ursodeoxycholic acid administration. Gut 24:609, 1983

134. Sawyer WR et al: The morphological effects of chenodeoxycholic acid on human gastric mucosa. Am J Gastroenterol 79:348, 1984

135. Schoenfield LJ et al: Bile acid composition of gallstones from man. J Lab Clin Med 68:186, 1966

136. Schoenfield LJ et al: Dissolution of cholesterol gallstones by chenodeoxycholic acid. N Engl J Med 286:1, 1982

137. Schoenfield LJ et al: Chenodiol (chenodeoxycholic acid) for dissolution of gallstones: The National Cooperative

Gallstone Study: A controlled trial of efficacy and safety. Ann Intern Med 95:256, 1981

138. Schwartz CC et al: Multi-compartmental analysis of cholesterol metabolism in man: Characterization of the hepatic bile acid and biliary cholesterol precursor sites. J Clin Invest 61:408, 1978

139. Scopinaro N et al: Two years of clinical experience with biliopancreatic bypass for obesity. Am J Clin Nutr 33:506, 1980

140. Sedaghat A, Grundy SM: Cholesterol crystals and the formation of cholesterol gallstones. N Engl J Med 302:1274, 1980

141. Shaffer EA et al: Biliary lipid secretion in cholesterol gallstone disease: The effect of cholecystectomy and obesity. J Clin Invest 59:828, 1977

142. Shaffer EA et al: The effect of vagotomy on gallbladder function and bile composition in man. Ann Surg 195:413, 1982

143. Shersten T et al: Relationship between the biliary excretion of bile acids and the excretion of water, lecithin, and cholesterol in man. Eur J Clin Invest 1:242, 1971

144. Singhal AK et al: Prevention of cholesterol-induced gallstones by hyodeoxycholic acid in the prairie dog. J Lipid Res 25:539, 1984

145. Small DM: Cholesterol nucleation and growth in gallstones from man. J Lab Clin Med 68:186, 1966

146. Small DM, Rapo S: Source of abnormal bile in patients with cholesterol gallstones. N Engl J Med 283:53, 1970

147. Smith BF, Lamont JT: Gallbladder mucin and gallstone formation. In Cohen S, Soloway RD (eds): Contemporary Issues in Gastroenterology: Gallstones. New York, Churchill Livingstone, 1985

148. Smith BF, Lamont JT: Identification of gallbladder mucin-bilirubin complex in human cholesterol gallstone matrix: Effects of reducing agents on *in vitro* dissolution of matrix and intact gallstones. J Clin Invest 76:439, 1985

149. Soloway RD, Trotman BW: Bile pigment gallstones. In Ostrow JD (ed): Bile Pigments and Jaundice. Molecular, Metabolic, and Medical Aspects. New York, Marcel Dekker, 1985

150. Somjen GJ, Gilat T: A non-micellar mode of cholesterol transport in human bile. Febs Lett 156:265, 1983

151. Stephens CG, Scott RB: Cholelithiasis in sickle cell anemia: Surgical or medical management. Arch Intern Med 140:648, 1980

152. Stiehl A et al: Effect of ursodeoxycholic acid on biliary bile acid and bile lipid composition in gallstone patients. Hepatology 4:101, 1984

153. Sue SO et al: Treatment of choledocholithiasis with oral chenodeoxycholic acid. Am J Surg 90:32, 1981

154. Sutor DJ, Wooley SE: The organic matrix of gallstones. Gut 15:487, 1974

155. Tabata M, Nakayama F: Bacterial and gallstones: Etiological significance. Dig Dis Sci 26:218, 1984

156. Tangedahl TN et al: Effect of B-sitosterol alone or in combination with chenic acid on cholesterol saturation of bile and cholesterol absorption in gallstone patients. Gastroenterology 76:1341, 1979

157. Tangedahl T et al: Drug and treatment efficacy of chenodeoxycholic acid in 97 patients with cholelithiasis and increased surgical risk. Dig Dis Sci 28:545, 1983

158. Thistle JL, Schoenfield LJ: Induced alterations in composition of bile of persons having cholelithiasis. Gastroenterology 61:488, 1971

159. Thistle JL, Schoenfield LJ: Lithogenic bile among young Indian women: Lithogenic potential decreased with chenodeoxycholic acid. N Engl J Med 284:177, 1971

160. Thistle JL et al: Monooctanoin, a dissolution agent for retained cholesterol bile duct stones: Physical properties and clinical application. Gastroenterology 78:1016, 1980

161. Thomas PJ, Hofmann AF: A simple calculation of lithogenic index of bile: Expressing biliary lipid composition on rectangular coordinates. Gastroenterology 65:698, 1973

162. Toor EW et al: Cholesterol monohydrate growth in model bile solution. Proc Natl Acad Sci USA 75:6230, 1978

163. Trotman BW: Formation of pigment gallstones. In Cohen S, Soloway RD (eds): Contemporary Issues in Gastroenterology: Gallstones. New York, Churchill Livingstone, 1985

164. Trotman BW, Soloway RD: Pigment versus cholesterol cholelithiasis: Clinical and epidemiological aspects. Am J Dig Dis 20:735, 1975

165. Van Berge Henegouwen GP, Hofmann AF: Nocturnal gallbladder storage and emptying in gallstone patients and healthy subjects. Gastroenterology 75:580, 1979

166. Vlahcevic ZR et al: Diminished bile and pool size in patients with gallstones. Gastroenterology 58:165, 1970

167. Von Bergman K et al: Differences in the effects of chenodeoxycholic and ursodeoxycholic acid on biliary lipid secretion and bile acid synthesis in patients with gallstones. Gastroenterology 87:136, 1984

168. Whiting MJ, Watts JMcK: Supersaturated bile from obese patients without gallstones supports cholesterol crystal growth but not nucleation. Gastroenterology 86:243, 1984

169. Zahor et al: Frequency of cholelithiasis in Pregue and Malmo: An autopsy study. Scand J Gastroenterol 9:3, 1974

chapter 42
Diseases of the Gallbladder and Bile Ducts

KENNETH W. WARREN, CAROL I. WILLIAMS, and ERIC G. C. TAN

EMBRYOLOGY

During the fourth week of embryonic life, a diverticulum arises from the ventral floor of the terminal portion of the foregut. The ventral pancreas, the gallbladder, the liver, and their corresponding ductal systems are derived from it. The gallbladder and its cystic duct become evident by the fifth week. About the same time, the proximal portion of the liver primordium arborizes to form the ductal system up to the interlobular level while the distal portion of the primordium proliferates vigorously to form the liver cords, which eventually give rise to the liver cells and the intralobular bile ducts. At this early stage of development, this whole proliferating system, like the duodenum, is solid. Recanalization commences in the sixth week, starting with the common bile duct and progressing slowly distally. The gallbladder gains its lumen in the 12th week. During recanalization, it is not uncommon to find two or three lumina, which usually coalesce to form a single definitive channel.

Aberrations in development can occur at any one of these complicated stages of organogenesis, resulting in agenesis, atresia, duplication, abnormal anatomic arrangement, formation of cysts, and a host of other anomalies that are of clinical importance and therefore are discussed later in greater detail.

While the biliary tract is developing, differential growth of the duodenal wall causes the ventral primordial derivatives to swing to the right and then posteriorly behind the first part of the duodenum, thus enabling the ventral and dorsal pancreas to fuse (Fig. 42-1). This union is sealed with the establishment of an anastomotic channel between the two pancreatic ducts. Eventually, the main pancreatic drainage is by way of the ventral pancreas (duct of Wirsung). Only in about 5% of all patients does the dorsal pancreatic duct (duct of Santorini) persist as the main duct. As part of this differential growth of the duodenal wall, the most proximal portion of the ventral primordial

diverticulum is absorbed to a varying extent into the duodenal wall.

In view of the close association between the development of the biliary tract and that of the pancreas and duodenum, any abnormality in one site indicates the possibility of another abnormality close by.

APPLIED ANATOMY

Gallbladder

The gallbladder is a thin, bluish, pear-shaped organ about 8 cm long lying in a fossa on the visceral surface of the liver along a line separating the right lobe of the liver from the quadrate part of the left lobe. Its capacity is about 50 ml; however, it can undergo great changes in size under various conditions. The distensibility is much impaired when the gallbladder is acutely or chronically inflamed. It is attached to the liver by a reflection of the peritoneum from the liver capsule. In 4% of all persons, a mesentery is present, thus allowing excessive mobility to the organ and predisposing it to torsion.

Anatomically, the gallbladder is divided into a relatively voluminous fundus, a tapering body, an oblique infundibulum, and a tortuous neck that leads into the cystic duct. When it is distended, as in acute cholecystitis, the fundus comes in contact with the anterior abdominal wall in the region of the tip of the right ninth and tenth costal cartilages. This is where Murphy's sign is elicited. Posteroinferiorly, the fundus is closely related to the first and second parts of the duodenum and the hepatic flexure of the colon. The close anatomic relationship between these structures is an important etiologic factor in spontaneous internal biliary fistulas.

The cystic duct is about 3 cm long. Its tortuosity brings the neck of the gallbladder in proximity with the common bile duct. Its redundant mucosa arranges itself in a series

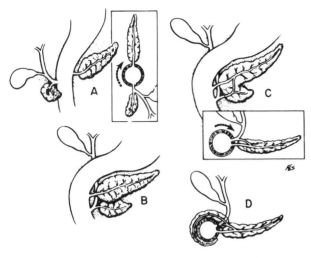

Fig. 42-1. Development around the duodenum. **A.** Rotation of ventral primordial derivatives. **B.** Fusion of the ventral and dorsal pancreas. **C.** Anastomosis between the duct of Wirsung and the duct of Santorini. **D.** Annular pancreas.

of folds, the valves of Heister. Although these folds have no valvular function, they may impede the passage of gallstones and instruments. The cystic duct joins the common hepatic duct as the latter becomes the common bile duct. The mode of union is extremely variable, as indicated in the section on anomalies.

In 80% of instances, a single cystic artery arises from the right hepatic artery in Calot's triangle. This location is marked by a lymph node (the sentinel node). Not infrequently, the parent artery loops dangerously close to the neck of the gallbladder and can be mistakenly ligated as the cystic artery during cholecystectomy. The comparatively large size of the right hepatic artery should alert the surgeon to this peril. In the remaining 20% of cases, the cystic artery has an abnormal origin and therefore an associated abnormal course. Double cystic arteries are also common. The surgeon must appreciate these anatomic variations because the fragile cystic artery is easily avulsed, and, in the attempt to stop the resultant bleeding, bile duct injuries may occur. Most of the venous drainage is through small veins directly into the liver portal system; however, one or more cystic veins frequently accompany the cystic artery to empty into the right branch of the portal vein.

Gallbladder lymphatics drain into the cystic node and then to the nodes alongside the common bile duct, particularly the superior retroduodenal node; eventually, the lymph reaches the celiac nodes. A rich communication exists between the lymphatic vessels of the gallbladder and those of the liver—an important factor in the spread of gallbladder tumors.

A rich plexus of autonomic nerves supplies the gallbladder. The exact role of these fibers is unknown because the primary stimulus for gallbladder contraction is cholecystokinin.

Bile Ducts

The right and left hepatic ducts unite to form the common hepatic duct in the porta hepatis. As the latter descends in the lesser omentum, it is joined by the cystic duct to become the common bile duct. Passing behind the first part of the duodenum, the common bile duct enters a groove in the pancreas to reach its termination in the second part of the duodenum. The simplest topographic arrangement is in the supraduodenal portion of the common bile duct. In this situation, the common bile duct lies along the free edge of the lesser omentum in front of the portal vein and to the right of the common hepatic artery. These structures, in turn, are separated from the inferior vena cava posteriorly by the foramen of Winslow. This is a convenient place for digital control of bleeding (Pringle's maneuver) and for opening of the common bile duct. The anatomy becomes more complex as one proceeds proximally into the porta hepatis and distally into the pancreaticoduodenal area.

The common bile duct is about 8 cm long and 0.5 cm to 1.3 cm in diameter. The supraduodenal segment, which has been described, is about 3 cm to 4 cm long. The remainder of the duct initially lies behind the first part of the duodenum close to the superior pancreaticoduodenal artery. It then enters a groove in the pancreas, running obliquely toward the duodenal papilla. This pancreatic segment of the common bile duct is eventually joined by the pancreatic duct (duct of Wirsung) and empties into the second part of the duodenum. As the two ducts enter the duodenal wall, they become invested with a multilayered fibromuscular structure, the sphincter of Oddi. This results in the marked narrowing of the common bile duct readily seen on cholangiography. Sometimes the narrowing is eccentric, and an infundibulum may be formed where a gallstone can lodge.

Boyden[29] examined the choledochoduodenal junction in humans and stated that the sphincteric mechanism may be divided into two anatomic parts. First is the sphincter choledochus, which ensheathes the submucosal segment of the common bile duct for a distance of 5 mm or more. The tonic contraction of this muscle is responsible for the filling of the gallbladder in the intervals between meals; its relaxation under appropriate stimuli permits discharge of bile into the duodenum. Second, surrounding the tip of the duodenal papilla is another sphincteric component, the sphincter ampullae or sphincter papillae, depending on whether the common bile duct and pancreatic ducts open as a single channel or separately into the duodenum. Contracture of this sphincter impedes drainage of both of these ducts.[29]

The pancreatic duct runs parallel with the common bile duct for 1 cm to 2 cm before opening into its medial wall. Because the common bile duct traverses the duodenal musculature at varying angles of obliquity, the length of the intramural portion of the common bile duct also varies (6 mm–30 mm). This obliquity also accounts for the fact that the pancreatic duct ostium is almost directly behind the opening of the duodenal papilla, whereas the stoma to the common bile duct slopes upward. Thus, in cannulation of the duodenal papilla, it is usually easier to enter the pancreatic duct than the common bile duct (Fig. 42-2).

The blood supply to the common bile duct is essentially arterial; 60% of vessels supplying the common bile duct reach it from below, and the remainder from the hilar region.[158] Because of this pattern of blood supply, longitudinal incisions of the duct are preferred to transverse incisions in surgery of this structure; the latter may severely alter blood supply and affect the viability of tissue with all the attendant complications.

The common hepatic duct is formed by the right and left hepatic ducts in the porta hepatis in 98% of instances. With the cystic duct and the intervening liver tissue, it forms Calot's triangle. Much of the important dissection in cholecystectomy is conducted in this small triangular area.

Porta Hepatis

The porta hepatis is a transverse fissure, 5 cm long, that extends across the visceral surface of the liver, separating the caudate from the quadrate lobes. It is invested by the leaves of the lesser omentum. The ducto-vascular pedicles enter the liver at each end of the liver hilum. The right hepatic duct is short. Within 1 cm of its junction with the left hepatic duct in the porta hepatis, it divides into two or three branches, usually one to the anterosuperior segment, another to the posteroinferior segment, and some-

times one to the caudate lobe. The right hepatic artery crosses behind the common bile duct to lie below and behind the right hepatic duct. Located posteriorly is the portal vein, which divides into the right and left portal veins only high up in the fissure. These three structures—duct, artery, and vein—enter the liver parenchyma through contiguous orifices and not through a common opening.

In 12% of patients, the right hepatic artery arises from the superior mesenteric artery. It may then pursue a course anterolateral to the common bile duct, thus blocking the usual approach to this structure.

The left ductovascular bundle runs a longer extrahepatic course across the whole length of the porta hepatis to enter as its left extremity. The left hepatic duct clings to the anterosuperior aspect of the left portal vein for 3 cm or so before it bifurcates into two major segmental ducts, thereby embracing the left portal vein even more intimately. This point usually forms the limit of dissection in operations on the left hepatic duct. The mode of branching and the interrelationship of the hepatic artery, bile ducts, and the portal vein in the porta hepatis are subject to wide variation.

ANOMALIES

Congenital anomalies in this anatomic area are of importance because they not only influence the safe conduct of biliary operations but they also give rise to serious complications in their own right.[30,91]

Gallbladder

The gallbladder may be congenitally absent[30,92]; obviously, in this case it does not appear on cholecystography or ultrasonography. In the past, patients with congenitally absent gallbladders have erroneously been subjected to operation because of an allegedly "nonfunctioning" gallbladder. Ultrasonography should prevent such mistakes. The incidence of congenitally absent gallbladder is 0.13% of the population.[144] In one fifth of these patients, anomalies are associated with biliary atresia.

Hypoplasia and atresia of the gallbladder represent aborted development of the organ. Varying degrees of duplication occur (Fig. 42-3). Instances of triple gallbladder have also been reported.[180,200]

Fig. 42-2. Obliquity of the common bile duct making the pancreatic duct relatively easier to intubate.

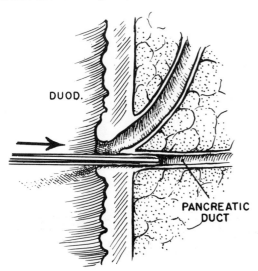

Fig. 42-3. Various degrees of duplication of the gallbladder.

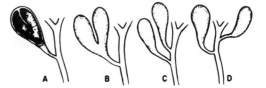

In about 4% of the population, the gallbladder is free from the liver. This resultant increase in mobility predisposes the organ to torsion (Fig. 42-4). Mobile gallbladders are twice as common in women as in men. In contrast, the gallbladder may be intrahepatic in location. Probably the only practical significance of this anomaly is that cholecystectomy is technically more difficult to perform.

The gallbladder is left-sided in situs inversus but may also be in this position without situs inversus.[118] Other unusual locations of the gallbladder include the abdominal wall, the falciform ligament,[154] and even the outside peritoneal cavity.[37]

Finally, deformities of the gallbladder, such as phrygian cap, fish-hook anomaly, hourglass gallbladder, and Hartmann's pouch, are often related to adenomyomatosis and are discussed in that section.

Cystic Duct and Cystic Artery

The most common cystic duct anomaly is a long cystic duct with abnormally low entry into the common bile duct. It occurs in 8.6% of cholecystectomies.[20] This has important implications in the success of cholecystoenteric bypass in malignant diseases involving the distal common bile duct or pancreas. Another important anomaly is the opening of the cystic duct into the right hepatic duct. The cystic duct may be absent, or more than one cystic duct may be present. These are all dangerous anomalies complicating cholecystectomy.

The cystic artery is also important in cholecystectomy because a rash attempt at control of bleeding from this artery is a cause of bile duct injury. The most common vascular anomaly is an accessory cystic artery.[20] Sometimes the right hepatic artery courses close to the gallbladder neck and may mistakenly be divided as the cystic artery.

Congenital Cysts and Cystic Dilatation of the Bile Ducts

Given that the bile ducts form a single system whether they are inside or outside the liver and that congenital cysts may occur in both parts of the system either singularly or in various combinations, an appropriate classification of congenital bile duct cysts and cystic dilatations should include both components of the system.[4,43,79,125,233]

Todani and colleagues[215] have attempted to advance such a classification, bringing together the Alonso-Lej[4] classification and Caroli's disease[43] (Figs. 42-5 and 42-6).

In a review of 955 cases of biliary cysts from the literature, Flanigan[79] found that 81% of the patients were females and that 61% of cases were discovered in children under the age of 10 years. Patients may present from less than one week to more than 40 years after the onset of symptoms. Diagnosis is easier if the patient presents with the classic triad of jaundice, right hypochondrial pain, and a palpable mass. However, 60% of patients lack all three features. Preoperative diagnosis was rare until ultrasonography, computed tomography, percutaneous transhepatic cholangiography, and endoscopic retrograde cholangiopancreatography improved the diagnostic rate.

The most common bile duct cyst is choledochal cyst (86.7%), followed by choledochocele (5.6%), choledochal diverticulum (3.1%), and others (2.6%).[79] In 2% of all cases, biliary atresia is an associated finding.

Fig. 42-5. Anomalies, including congenital cysts, of the bile ducts.

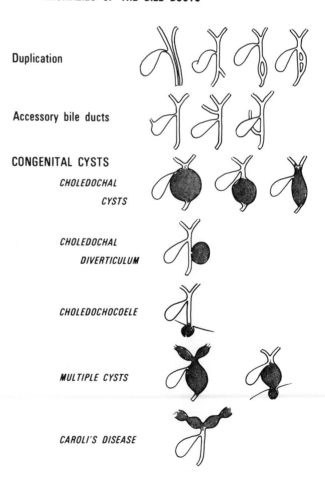

ANOMALIES OF THE BILE DUCTS

Duplication

Accessory bile ducts

CONGENITAL CYSTS

CHOLEDOCHAL CYSTS

CHOLEDOCHAL DIVERTICULUM

CHOLEDOCHOCOELE

MULTIPLE CYSTS

CAROLI'S DISEASE

Fig. 42-4. **A.** Gallbladder with a short mesentery. **B.** Torsion complicating a mobile gallbladder.

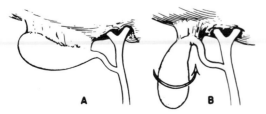

A   B

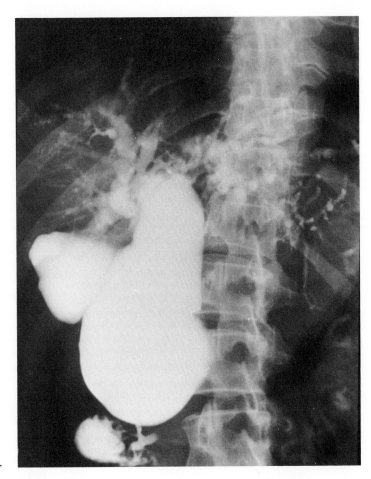

Fig. 42-6. Choledochal cysts.

Biliary cysts and cystic swellings are clinically important because of complications. Biliary obstruction, sludge and stone formation, infection, perforation, bleeding, biliary cirrhosis, and malignant transformation have been reported.[25,221]

Definitive treatment of these conditions is surgical, since the mortality rate of patients managed medically has been reported at 97%. Because of the risk of cancer,[216,245] excision of the cyst is the preferred procedure if it can be performed safely. Failing this, adequate drainage should be provided by a biliary enteric bypass with the understanding that the complexity of this clinical problem may require reoperation and mandate an individualized therapeutic approach.

Deziel and co-workers[66] recently reported on 31 adult patients with bile duct cysts. The median age was 34 years. These patients underwent a total of 86 biliary procedures. Cyst excision was associated with a lower incidence of recurrent cholangitis and the need for reoperative surgery. No increase in mortality was observed for cyst excision. Five of the 31 patients had adenocarcinoma of the bile duct cyst; four of the five died, with a median survival of 6 months.

Other Bile Duct Anomalies

Although the common bile duct normally opens into the second part of the duodenum, in 8% of subjects it opens into the third part. Occasionally, the opening is situated in the first part of the duodenum or even in the pyloric antrum.

Duplication and accessory bile ducts are rare, but failure to appreciate their presence at operation can be disastrous (see Fig. 42-5).

Biliary atresia is discussed in Chapter 36.

APPLIED PHYSIOLOGY OF THE GALLBLADDER

The gallbladder concentrates and stores bile secreted from the liver and discharges its contents in response to a meal.

Concentration of Bile

When hepatic bile enters the gallbladder, it is concentrated by active transport of coupled sodium and anion across the epithelium, which, in turn, is coupled with water in isotonic proportions. This is achieved by a special structural arrangement of the gallbladder epithelium, which consists of long intercellular spaces with tight junctions on their luminal ends and small gaps facing the basal interstitium. These spaces become filled with fluid during reabsorption and collapse when active transport stops. In addition to active transport, there is passive diffusion of calcium and potassium through the tight junctions into the gallbladder lumen. Active secretion of hydrogen ion into the lumen results in acidification of the bile. Conjugated bilirubin and conjugated bile salts are not absorbed to any appreciable extent. The sodium bile salts exist mainly in osmotically inactive micelles. Therefore, although the total concentration of ions in concentrated bile is about twice that of serum, the bile remains isotonic with respect to serum. If bile salts are deconjugated, for example, by bacterial enzymes, their pKa is significantly changed, and absorption by passive nonionic diffusion takes place. Furthermore, the deconjugated bile salts may produce mucosal damage, which further increases bile salt absorption. Thus, the solubility of cholesterol may be reduced and cholelithiasis promoted.

The gallbladder has a resting capacity of about 40 ml. Because of its ability to reabsorb water and electrolytes (90% of water entering the gallbladder is reabsorbed), it is able to handle about ten times that volume of hepatic bile. Even so, only half of secreted hepatic bile enters the gallbladder; the rest is discharged directly into the duodenum. At rest, bile in the gallbladder is stratified into a gradient of density zones. This stratification may play a role in gallstone formation.[117]

Gallbladder Motility

The principal controlling factor in gallbladder emptying is cholecystokinin, which is released from the mucosa of the proximal small bowel in response to amino acids or lipids. The active radical of this peptide hormone is in the C-terminal part of the molecule, which contains a sulfated tyrosine residue. Gastrin and cerulein have a similar molecular configuration and exert the same physiological action, although with different potency.

Cholecystokinin stimulates gallbladder contraction while simultaneously relaxing the sphincter of Oddi. Cholecystokinin acts by stimulating intracellular cyclic 3′,5′-guanosine monophosphate.[7] The mechanism of action on the sphincter of Oddi is unknown.

Bile is delivered to the intestine to aid in fat digestion. The presence of bile salts together with digestive products inhibits cholecystokinin secretion by the intestine, and thus the blood level of cholecystokinin falls. The sphincter of Oddi contracts, the gallbladder relaxes, and hepatic bile again flows into the gallbladder.

The role of the autonomic nervous system on gallbladder contraction is controversial.[6,100,114,188] Some workers have found a loss of tone and power after vagotomy. The organ becomes dilated and flaccid, and this may lead to cholelithiasis. However, a number of other authors disagree with these findings. There is no alteration of gallbladder response to cholecystokinin after vagotomy. It seems that the autonomic nervous system does not play a significant physiologic role in gallbladder contraction. In animal models, stimulation of the sympathetic nervous system causes relaxation of the gallbladder, whereas parasympathetic stimulation causes contraction.

GALLSTONES

Gallstone disease is a major health problem in many parts of the world. About 10% of the population in the United States harbors gallstones; this prevalence is doubled in those over 40 years of age. About 800,000 new cases are discovered each year in the United States.

Types

Gallstones are formed by the precipitation of insoluble bile constituents: cholesterol, bile pigments, calcium salts, and some types of proteins. It is rare to have a chemically pure gallstone. In a given gallstone, the chemical composition often varies from the center to the crust. However, by tradition, gallstones are classified as cholesterol stones, pigment stones, and rare forms, such as calcium carbonate stones. The cholesterol gallstone group includes the large yellowish and round "solitaire" as well as the more common multifaceted "mixed" stone. Mixed stones contain at least 70% cholesterol by weight. Pigment stones, on the other hand, are made largely of calcium bilirubinate. They are usually mulberry-like in shape, homogeneous on section, friable, and very dark in color (Fig. 42-7).

In the United States, 27% to 33% of patients with gallstones have pigment stones.[205] Whereas cholesterol stones are associated with Western countries, pigment stones have been the predominant type in the tropics and the Orient. For example, the proportion of pigment cholelithiasis is nearly 70% in rural Japan. Interestingly, in urban Japan, the composition of gallstones is changing from the pigment to the cholesterol type.

Finally, there is the rare calcium carbonate stone, which is often no more than a mere chalky white paste. It may be bile stained and frequently fills the whole gallbladder. It may coexist with other types of gallstones.

Etiology

Chapter 5 discusses in depth the pathophysiology of gallstone formation. The following discussion is concerned mainly with risk factors for the development of cholelithiasis, with special emphasis on clinical associations. Because the pathogenesis of cholesterol stones is different from that of pigment stones, etiologic factors also differ.

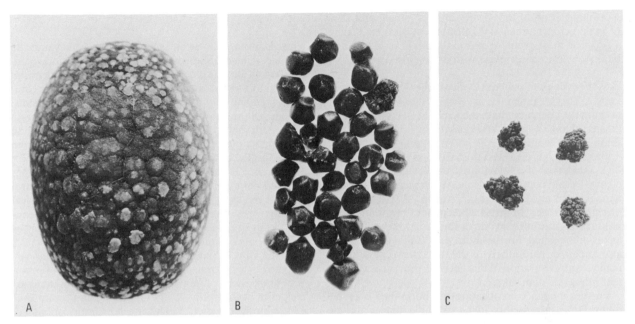

Fig. 42-7. Common types of gallstone. **A.** Solitary cholesterol gallstone. Note that it is made up of a coalescence of multiple small stones. **B.** Faceted gallstones, the main constituent of which is cholesterol (about 70%). **C.** Pigment stones. Typical "mulberry" calcium bilirubinate stones from a patient with hemolytic anemia.

Risk Factors for Cholesterol Stone Formation

Demographic Features. The incidence of cholesterol gallstones varies from country to country.[18] Redinger and Small[177] compared the percentage of cholesterol saturation of gallbladder bile with the respective incidence of gallstones in different populations and found a strong correlation (Fig. 42-8). The Masai, whose bile is only half saturated, have no incidence of cholesterol stones,[24] whereas the Pima Indian women of Arizona, with super-saturated bile, reach an 80% incidence of cholesterol cholelithiasis. Racial tendencies suggest a hereditary mechanism, and this is supported by the finding of Danzinger and co-workers[65] that the younger sisters of young women with cholesterol gallstones have more highly saturated bile than the younger sisters of non–gallstone-bearing control subjects.

Age. Gallstones have been reported in all age-groups, but they are uncommon in the young. The incidence of cho-

Fig. 42-8. Percentage of saturation of control gallbladder bile compared with estimated incidence of gallstones in different populations. Control biles with the lowest percentage of cholesterol saturation appear to come from populations with the lowest incidence of cholesterol gallstones, whereas populations with supersaturated normal biles have a very high incidence of cholesterol gallstones. Several populations with intermediate saturation (*i.e.,* 65–75%) have intermediate incidences of cholesterol stones as estimated from postmortem hospital admission and cholecystographic evidence of gallstones. (Redinger RN, Small DM: Bile composition, bile salt metabolism and gallstones. Arch Intern Med 130:622, 1972)

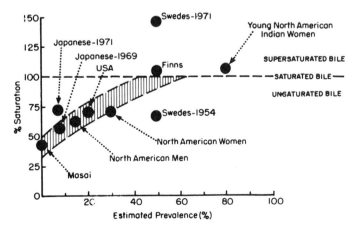

lesterol stones increases with age.[15] Newman and Northup[155] showed that nearly 38% of female and 22% of male octogenarians had gallstones at autopsy (Table 42-1). The most probable reason for this is an increase in biliary cholesterol secretion with advancing years.

Sex. Female preponderance of cholesterol stones is well known. This sex difference in gallstone development starts at puberty. Bennion and associates[19] demonstrated a greater change toward lithogenicity of bile in pubertal Pima Indian women than in corresponding men.

Pregnancy has also been implicated as the cause of the high incidence of cholelithiasis in women. There is a change in bile composition toward lithogenicity in pregnancy. Lynn and co-workers[129] showed that estriol, the principal estrogen in human pregnancy, can induce the production of lithogenic bile in rhesus monkeys. This effect is dose related. Furthermore, gallbladder emptying is also impaired, particularly in the third trimester of pregnancy. Supersaturation of bile coupled with stasis is a potent lithogenic combination.

Further evidence implicating sex hormones may be found in the increased incidence of cholelithiasis among users of exogenous estrogens, such as for postmenopausal replacement and for contraception.[179]

Obesity. Numerous reports have linked obesity with cholelithiasis. The increase in lithogenicity in the bile of obese patients is due to excessive cholesterol secretion secondary to increased cholesterol synthesis. During weight reduction, the bile becomes even more supersaturated before showing an improvement with respect to cholesterol saturation.[196] During caloric restriction and weight loss, the secretion rate of all biliary lipids decreases, and the bile acid pool shrinks. In some, the comparative secretion of bile acids decreases more than that of cholesterol, with a resultant rise in cholesterol saturation. When body weight is stabilized at a reduced level, the bile acid pool expands to normal but cholesterol secretion remains low, and the bile thus becomes less saturated with cholesterol.

Environmental Influences, Including Diet. Nakayama and Miyake[153] have demonstrated a change in gallstone composition in Japan since the world wars. The incidence of cholesterol stones is increasing over that of the more common pigment stones, especially among young patients. This is believed to be due to urbanization and adoption of western dietary habits.[150] Japanese in Hawaii have an even higher incidence of gallstones than their kinsmen in Japan, an incidence that equals that of whites.

In France, Sarles and colleagues[192] have shown a higher caloric intake in subjects with gallstones than in control subjects matched for sex, body size, and level of physical activity. They also have described an increase in the concentration of cholesterol in T-tube bile of postcholecystectomy patients during ingestion of a high-calorie diet.[193]

In the United States, autopsy studies of men who participated in a controlled clinical trial of dietary prevention of complications of atherosclerosis revealed an increased incidence of cholelithiasis in those ingesting a serum cholesterol–lowering diet.[206] The mechanism is unknown. Lack of dietary fiber has been suggested as a cause of cholelithiasis in western societies. Studies of added bran in the diet showed a reduction in the cholesterol saturation of bile in patients with gallstones. However, reports[237] on the effect of bran in normal persons are conflicting. Recently, long-term parenteral nutrition has been implicated in gallstone formation.[183]

Diabetes. A relatively high incidence of gallstones has been found in diabetics of both sexes.[120] The high incidence is thought to be due in part to obesity among diabetics and the associated increase in cholesterol secretion in the bile.

Hyperlipidemia. Hypercholesterolemic patients do not appear to have a propensity to cholesterol cholelithiasis. In contrast, patients with familial hyperlipoproteinemia in general and hypertriglyceridemia (type IV) in particular have a high incidence of cholesterol gallstones. The mechanism is unknown.[73]

Ingestion of Clofibrate (Ethyl Chlorophenoxyisobutrate). Clofibrate is used in the treatment of hyperlipidemia. It inhibits cholesterol synthesis and enhances biliary cholesterol excretion by mobilization of the tissue cholesterol pool, thus lowering the plasma cholesterol level. The increase in biliary cholesterol secretion leads to gallstone formation.[165,209]

Cystic Fibrosis with Pancreatic Insufficiency. Bile acid malabsorption and reduced bile acid pool size in pancreatic insufficiency with cystic fibrosis lead to supersaturation of bile and cholesterol gallstones. Treatment with pancreatic enzyme supplements returns bile composition to normal.

TABLE 42-1.   Age and Sex Incidence of Gallstones at Autopsy

AGE (yr)	WHITE MEN (%)	WHITE WOMEN (%)
0–19	0.1	0.1
20–29	1.0	5.0
30–39	2.0	9.0
40–49	6.0	15.0
50–59	9.0	24.0
60–69	13.0	30.0
70–79	18.0	34.0
80+	22.0	38.0

(Newman HF, Northup UD: The autopsy incidence of gallstones. Surg Gynecol Obstet 109:1, 1959)

Ileal Disease and Extensive Ileal Resection. The rate of bile salt secretion is dependent on bile acid pool size, which is constantly replenished by the enterohepatic circulation. Widespread Crohn's disease of the small bowel or extensive distal small-bowel resection[110] or bypass severely impairs this enterohepatic circulation and thus diminishes the bile acid pool and reduces bile salt secretion. The bile becomes lithogenic. Cohen and associates[56] and Heaton and Read[95,96] have reported gallstones produced by this mechanism.

Risk Factors for Pigment Stone Formation

Age and Sex. Pigment gallstones are more common with increasing age. However, they do not appear to be related to sex or obesity.[18,205]

Infection. Biliary infection, particularly with *Escherichia coli* or *Ascaris,* fosters deconjugation of soluble bilirubin glucuronide by β-glucuronidase to produce free bilirubin, which combines with calcium to form pigment stones. Infection can also promote gallstone formation by providing a nidus of organisms or inflammatory debris around which precipitation occurs by promoting biliary stasis and by altering the *p*H of bile. *E. coli,* for example, is an acid-producing organism. When bile *p*H falls, bile salts become deconjugated. In this form, they compete with cholesterol for sites in the micelle and are readily absorbed by the gallbladder. By these two mechanisms, a drop in the *p*H of bile caused by acid-forming organisms facilitates lithogenesis.

Hemolysis. The association between hemolytic anemias and pigment gallstone formation is well known, particularly in young patients with cholelithiasis. Merendino and Manhas[142] reported gallstones in one third of male patients after prosthetic aortic valve replacement. A mild chronic hemolysis due to mechanical injury of the erythrocytes is considered the cause for a fivefold to tenfold increase in the incidence of gallstones in these patients. This form of hemolysis is now much reduced by improved design of the heart valves.

Cirrhosis. Patients with cirrhosis of the liver have an increased incidence of pigment stones (sixfold to sevenfold) but not cholesterol stones. Although the total bile acid pool size is reduced and secretion of phospholipids is diminished, a corresponding reduction in cholesterol secretion is also seen, with the net result that the bile has a greater cholesterol-holding capacity in patients with cirrhosis than in control subjects. The cause of the production of pigment stones remains unclarified. Although a defect in the conjugation of bilirubin has been postulated, chronic hemolysis secondary to hypersplenism may also contribute to the process.[27,156,227]

Natural History

The natural history of gallstone disease is becoming increasingly important because of two contentious issues: surgery for patients with asymptomatic gallstones and medical therapy for gallstones. Wenckert and Robertson[241] studied a series of 1501 patients in Malmö, Sweden who had either cholelithiasis or nonfunctioning gallbladders on cholecystography. Their radiographic diagnostic accuracy was 98.7%; 781 patients in this large series with a pathologic gallbladder or gallstones had neither cholecystectomy nor complications within the first year of diagnosis. The patients were followed up for 11 years or until cholecystectomy or death intervened. Half of the patients had mild or no symptoms, one third experienced severe symptoms, and serious complications developed in 18%. In the latter two groups of patients, 1 patient had gallstone ileus, 42 had mild acute cholecystitis, 39 had severe acute cholecystitis, and 59 had jaundice, pancreatitis, or both. There were 13 deaths in these groups of patients.

The incidence of severe complications was twice as common for patients with nonvisualization of the gallbladder as for those whose gallbladders continued to function despite the presence of gallstones. Severe complications were also more common in patients over 60 years of age than in the younger age-groups (27% versus 6%). As expected, the complication rate increased steadily with age.

Comfort and co-workers,[59] Kozoll and associates,[113] and Lund[127] reported that symptoms develop in half the patients with silent gallstones with an appreciable complication rate. Both complications and mortality increase with the passage of time, and the first attack may be a serious one, particularly in diabetics. Mortality is also highest in those with complications and in older age-groups.

In contrast, Gracie and Ransohoff[90] studied 123 persons with asymptomatic gallstones. All were white, and the mean age was 54 years (range, 29–87 years). All but 13 were men. No patient died of gallstone disease. The 15-year cumulative probability of the development of biliary pain or complications was only 18%. Nevertheless, 35 persons underwent prophylactic cholecystectomy with no deaths and only one serious complication.

The complications of gallstones are summarized in Figure 42-9. The initial problem is often biliary colic resulting from cystic duct obstruction. This may then lead to acute cholecystitis and its acute and chronic sequelae. The stone may also enter the common bile duct and either cause obstruction or cholangitis or predispose the patient to pancreatitis.

Asymptomatic Gallstones

With the widespread use of organ-imaging techniques, an increasing number of patients with "silent" gallstones are seen.[58,59,69,143] Management of these patients is controversial, since few patients with untreated silent gallstones

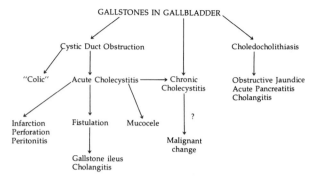

Fig. 42-9. Complications of gallstones.

die of their disease.[90] However, once symptoms supervene, the risk of cholecystectomy in the presence of acute cholecystitis, common duct calculi, or advanced age is increased appreciably.[83]

The risk of elective cholecystectomy is extremely small (less than 0.1% in patients over 50 years of age), and elective cholecystectomy does effectively prevent the serious complications of cholecystitis and choledocholithiasis. Chemical dissolution of gallstones using chenodeoxycholic acid or its analogues is apparently effective in only a minority of patients. When gallstones are or become symptomatic, cholecystectomy is the best treatment.

In the presence of increased operative risk, such as advanced cardiovascular disease or severe pulmonary impairment, silent gallstones are best managed conservatively. Diabetic patients, however, deserve special mention.[147,185,223] The operative mortality for elective cholecystectomy in these patients is 0.7% to 4% but rises to 7.5% to 22% in those operated on emergently with acute cholecystitis. Of diabetics with acute cholecystitis, 20% have gangrene or perforation of the gallbladder on presentation. Elective cholecystectomy is strongly recommended in this high-risk group.

It is reasonable to recommend elective cholecystectomy for silent gallstones because of low operative risk and its effectiveness in the prevention of potentially serious complications. This recommendation should be tempered by any significant increased surgical risk.

A sharp decline in the incidence of gallbladder cancer has accompanied widespread surgery for gallstones. Diehl and Beral[67] have detailed an increase in mortality from gallbladder cancer associated with a decline in cholecystectomy rates in Sweden.

Biliary Dyspepsia and Biliary Colic

Dyspeptic symptoms, such as fat intolerance, flatulence, aerophagia, heartburn, and regurgitation, have variously been attributed to gallbladder disease. Price[171] showed no difference in incidence or character of dyspeptic symptoms between subjects with normal and subjects with abnormal results on cholecystography. This study bears out the clinical impression that cholecystectomy for vague dyspeptic symptoms attributed to cholelithiasis has a considerable failure rate in terms of symptomatic relief.

In biliary colic, the pain arises from a distended obstructed gallbladder. It often starts in the epigastrium and radiates to both hypochondria and to the interscapular region or even the tip of the shoulder. The pain is relatively mild initially but often increases to a level that is almost intolerable. It may make the patient roll around or double up, often with severe nausea and vomiting. Unlike that in intestinal colic, the pain often stays at a high intensity until spontaneous relief occurs or until a potent analgesic is given. The usual duration of each attack is from 1 to 6 hours. Typically, the attacks occur in the early hours of the morning after a heavy meal the night before.

Naturally, this clinical picture varies in terms of intensity, location, radiation, and associated pain. Prolonged obstruction of the gallbladder usually leads to acute cholecystitis and the associated local and systemic manifestations of inflammation. Other causes of severe upper abdominal pain, such as myocardial infarction, perforated peptic ulcer, esophageal spasms, pneumonia and pleurisy, intestinal obstruction, pancreatitis, renal colic, mesenteric infarction, and ruptured aortic aneurysm, must be ruled out.

Treatment involves relief of pain during the acute attack; this usually requires the use of a parenteral narcotic analgesic. Often, an antiemetic is also necessary. Cessation of oral intake and parenteral fluid replacement are needed. Patients with severe biliary colic need no persuasion to undergo surgical treatment, and this is the treatment of choice. The timing of surgical therapy is discussed later in this chapter.

Medical Treatment

When Admirand and Small[2] published their classic paper on cholesterol solubility in bile in 1968, they laid the foundation for medical treatment of gallstones. In 1971, Thistle and Schoenfield[210] showed that it was possible to alter the composition of bile in patients with gallstones with chenodeoxycholic acid.[104] The most common substance used to dissolve gallstones is chenodeoxycholic acid, although ursodeoxycholic acid is attracting some attention as an alternative agent, since it causes no hepatotoxicity or diarrhea and can be used in smaller doses.[11,133,151,152]

Chenodeoxycholic acid improves cholesterol solubility by lowering cholesterol secretion. The exact mode of action is unclear; various theories have been reviewed by Dowling.[70] One theory is that chenodeoxycholic acid inhibits a hepatic enzyme, hydroxymethylglutaryl coenzyme A reductase (HMGCoAR), which controls the production of cholesterol. However, newly formed cholesterol in the liver is not all secreted into bile; some becomes substrate for *de novo* bile acid synthesis, some becomes incorporated into cellular membranes, and some is transported into plasma bound to lipoproteins. Therefore, no consistent relationship exists between HMGCoAR activity, cholesterol synthesis, and biliary cholesterol secretion.

An alternative theory is that chenodeoxycholic acid reduces cholesterol absorption from the intestines and thus affects the equilibrium between various cholesterol pools. One effect may be to reduce biliary cholesterol secretion. This theory is not fully substantiated.

The third possible mechanism of action is based on the "Schersten effect." During passage through the liver, bile acids control the secretion of both phospholipids and cholesterol from liver cells. When cholic acid is substituted for endogenous bile acids in postcholecystectomy patients, some reduction of cholesterol saturation in the T-tube bile occurs, but the bile remains supersaturated. However, when chenodeoxycholic acid is used, the bile becomes unsaturated within 2 hours. This rapidity of action may be accounted for by changes in hepatic HMGCoAR activity.

The usual recommended dose of chenodeoxycholic acid is 13 mg to 15 mg/kg/day. Treatment usually needs to be continued for more than 6 months before appreciable diminution in the size of the gallstone is evident.

Common side-effects include dyspepsia, nausea and vomiting, biliary pain, and diarrhea. The National Cooperative Gallstone Study Group[194] observed that cholesterol levels increased on an average of 20 mg/dl, although low-density lipoproteins accounted for most of the increase in total cholesterol levels. The average serum triglyceride level fell 13% below the mean at enrollment. Minor abnormalities of liver function were manifested in about 7% of patients.

According to Thistle and co-workers,[212] 38% of patients receiving 15 mg/kg/day or less of chenodeoxycholic acid responded, and 83% of patients receiving doses greater than 15 mg/kg/day responded with diminution or disappearance of gallstones based on cholecystographic criteria. The greater sensitivity of ultrasound over cholecystography in demonstrating gallstones, however, as reported in the Canadian Cooperative Gallstone Study, suggests that the United States study may have overestimated the incidence of stone dissolution.

In the United States Cooperative Study,[194] complete dissolution occurred in only 13.5% of patients taking 750 mg/day, 5.2% of patients taking 375 mg/day, and 0.8% of those in the placebo group.

Gallstones recur, and bile reverts to the supersaturated state shortly after treatment stops. The problem of recurrence has not been solved, and long-term maintenance therapy is probably required. Administration of chenodiol has no effect on the incidence of biliary symptoms or on the incidence of cholecystectomy.

That chenodeoxycholic acid is efficacious in improving cholesterol solubility of bile is now established. Nevertheless, chemical dissolution of gallstones is still an experimental treatment. Dissolution of gallstones occurred more frequently in women, thin patients, those with small or floating gallstones, and those whose serum cholesterol level was greater than 2267 mg/dl. The obese patient, the patient with large, multiple, or calcified gallstones, those with underlying liver disease, and those noncompliant with a prolonged medication regimen are probably not good candidates for dissolution therapy.

Thus, it may be said that gallstone dissolution has only a limited place in the management of the patient with cholelithiasis.[219] Only about 10% of patients with gallstones are potential candidates for this approach, and of these only one third will achieve complete resolution after a prolonged period of treatment.

CHOLECYSTITIS

Cholecystitis denotes inflammation of the gallbladder. It is one of the most common clinical problems to confront both physicians and surgeons. Cholecystitis may be acute or chronic. When it is acute, the pathologic process may lead to a multitude of serious complications. In contrast, chronic cholecystitis is associated with chronic ill health.

Acute Calculous Cholecystitis

Inflammation of the gallbladder is associated with gallstones in more than 90% of instances. It is one of the most common causes of the acute abdomen. Although it can occur at any age, cholecystitis is usually seen in patients in the middle years of life. Acalculous cholecystitis, which affects about 3% of patients with cholecystitis, is considered separately.[16,33]

Incidence

The exact incidence of acute cholecystitis is difficult to determine with accuracy. Contributing to this difficulty is the notoriously poor correlation between clinical manifestations and degree of pathologic change. Of 1356 patients operated on at the Lahey Clinic for cholelithiasis or postcholecystectomy symptoms, 5.3% were found to have acute cholecystitis.[33] This low figure probably reflects the nature of the surgery performed at the Lahey Clinic. In acute-care hospitals, 15% to 20% of operations on the biliary tract are performed for acute cholecystitis. This figure is expected to increase in the future because the practice of early operation for acute cholecystitis is gaining in popularity.

Pathogenesis

The crucial step in the pathogenesis of calculous cholecystitis appears to be obstruction of the cystic duct either by a stone impacted in this area or as the result of inflammatory edema secondary to the passage of a stone. The gallbladder becomes distended and its wall edematous. This leads to progressive compression of the capillaries and lymphatics within the wall of the gallbladder and thus causes ischemia and inflammation. An inflamed mucosa allows the reabsorption of bile salts from within the lumen.

The deconjugated bile salts produce mucosal damage and further incite the inflammatory response. In the early stages of acute cholecystitis, the bile is sterile. However, secondary infection with *E. coli* and other enteric organisms occurs in about 40% of all patients. Invasion of an ischemic or necrotic gallbladder wall by gas-forming bacteria may result in emphysematous cholecystitis; this is discussed later in this chapter. There is no good evidence to suggest that bacterial infection has an important initiating role in the development of acute cholecystitis.[10]

Pathology

The inflamed gallbladder is distended, tense, and discolored with edematous thickening of the wall and congestion of overlying serosal vessels. When the inflammation continues unabated, the wall becomes friable, and focal areas of necrosis may develop as a result of thrombosis of the small intramural vessels. Sometimes perforation occurs, the most common sites of which are the fundus of the gallbladder and Hartmann's pouch. With severe acute cholecystitis, surrounding inflammation and inflammatory adhesions to adjacent structures are often seen. When the cholecystitis is mild, there may be only some congestion and edema of the wall of the gallbladder associated with a slight distention of the organ. Histologically, evidence of preexisting chronic inflammation is often found in gallbladders that are acutely inflamed. Edema, extravasated blood, and widespread leukocytic infiltration are present. Areas of necrosis containing young fibroblasts may be seen in disease of some days' duration.

Clinical Features

The manifestations of acute cholecystitis resemble those of acute obstructive appendicitis: an initial period of "colicky" pain is followed by local signs and symptoms of inflammation. Biliary colic often heralds cholecystitis. Right upper quadrant or epigastric in location, the pain may radiate in bandlike fashion around the midtorso to the infrascapular region. Although referred to as "colic," it does not subside completely but persists for several hours with a fluctuating intensity. The patient usually has nausea and vomiting. When cholecystitis is well established, pain is persistent and localized to the right hypochondrium; at times, pain may be felt in the right tip of the shoulder.

Physical findings depend on the stage of disease. Tenderness in the right hypochondrium increases with the severity of inflammation; guarding and rigidity represent peritoneal involvement. In the early phase, tenderness may be elicited at the tip of the right ninth costal cartilage as the patient inspires (Murphy's sign). When the disease has become more established, the gallbladder may be palpable. Systemic manifestations of inflammation, including fever, tachycardia, and tachypnea, are common. Jaundice, which is present in 10% to 30% of patients, suggests an associated mechanical obstruction in the common bile duct. Braasch and associates[33] found that 14.5% of common duct stones were associated with acute cholecystitis, although it is possible to have mild jaundice without choledocholithiasis.

Laboratory Findings

The presence of bile in the urine is supportive evidence of acute cholecystitis, although a negative result does not exclude this condition. A leukocytosis of 10,000 to 15,000/mm^3 is usually present.

The level of serum amylase may be elevated up to 1000 Somogyi units/dl in acute cholecystitis, but this should not be interpreted as indicative of acute pancreatitis without other corresponding clinical evidence.

Diagnosis

Diagnosis can be made in 85% of patients on clinical features alone. At times, it may be difficult to differentiate acute cholecystitis from acute appendicitis, acute pancreatitis, acute peptic ulcer disease, hepatitis, pneumonia, myocardial infarction, early herpes zoster, and acute pyelonephritis.

Some patients, especially the elderly, show remarkably little systemic response to an acutely inflamed gallbladder. In patients with diabetes, control of the blood sugar level may be so severely disturbed by the acute cholecystitis that they may present with ketoacidosis. Finally, the difficulty of diagnosis of any acute intra-abdominal condition during pregnancy is well known, and acute cholecystitis is no exception.

Confirmation of clinical diagnosis is important because early operative intervention is gaining favor as the definitive treatment for this disease. Plain abdominal radiographs are of little confirmatory value because only 10% to 15% of gallstones are radiopaque. Other conditions may be confused with acute cholecystitis, such as perforated peptic ulcer or acute pancreatitis, and radiography should therefore be undertaken.[72]

Real-time ultrasonography and hepatobiliary isotopic scanning have virtually replaced oral and intravenous cholecystography as the investigations of choice in the diagnosis of acute cholecystitis.[174,207,244] Real-time ultrasonography appears to have a greater sensitivity and specificity for chronic cholecystitis, and isotopic scanning has a greater sensitivity for diagnosis of the acute cystic duct obstruction that accompanies acute cholecystitis. Additionally, ultrasonography may be more appropriate and accurate an examination for evaluation of the jaundiced patient with acute right upper quadrant pain.[132]

With these techniques, many of which are complementary, it should be possible to make a firm diagnosis of acute cholecystitis within a short period after hospital admission.

Treatment

The most appropriate definitive treatment for cholecystitis is cholecystectomy. Controversy exists over the timing of operation: early cholecystectomy versus initial medical treatment followed by interval cholecystectomy.[81,116,138,204,226]

The symptomatology may not accurately reflect the pathologic state of the inflamed organ. For example, a patient who has clinically recovered from acute cholecystitis may still harbor an inflamed organ even after 6 to 12 weeks. Therefore, the choice of timing of the operation should not rely on rigid, arbitrary criteria. Rather, it should take into account such factors as age, occupation, associated diseases, clinical picture, duration of attack, past history of biliary disease, and, not least of all, the facilities and technical skill available for the operation.

Cholecystectomy and exploration of the common bile duct may be more difficult in the presence of inflammation and are not recommended as emergency procedures to be performed by one who is not well versed in biliary surgery on an inadequately prepared patient in the middle of the night. However, it has been demonstrated repeatedly that, given the proper facilities and adequate surgical expertise, cholecystectomy with or without exploration of the common bile duct can be performed with safety in the presence of acute cholecystitis. The advantages of early operation are that serious complications of conservative treatment are avoided, that there is no risk of recurrent cholecystitis during the interval preceding cholecystectomy, that all patients receive treatment so that there are no defaulters, and that the hospital stay and period of disability are shortened.

With medical treatment, about 80% of patients with acute gallbladder inflammation achieve a remission. Nasogastric aspiration, intravenous fluid replacement, adequate analgesia, and antibiotics have been the cornerstones of the medical regimen. Patients who do well on this time-honored treatment can be investigated at leisure and submitted to elective cholecystectomy 6 to 12 weeks later. Results of medical treatment are usually good, but patients who do not respond or whose condition deteriorates need prompt surgical intervention.

The laudable results of medical treatment are artificially inflated at the expense of those of surgery by virtue of patient selection. Those who do not respond to medical treatment are likely to be the sickest patients with severe complications and decompensating associated diseases who are forced into the hands of the surgeon. Consequently, the mortality rate is between 5% and 20% in this group of surgical patients.

Van der Linden and Sunzel[226] and McArthur and associates[135] conducted controlled trials of early and delayed operation for acute cholecystitis. No deaths occurred in either group of 70 patients; exploration of the common bile duct was performed whenever indicated. Although low-grade infection was more common in the early operated group, the conservatively treated group had statistically significant prolongation of fever, longer hospital stays, and 50% longer loss of work capacity. In the conservatively treated group, four patients had recurrence during the waiting period before elective cholecystectomy,

and 12 patients refused operation once symptoms disappeared. They were therefore subject to further complications of gallstone disease.[225] These 16 patients (17%) may legitimately be considered failures of medical treatment.

For the patient with acute cholecystitis, given availability of good facilities and sound surgical techniques, early surgery is an attractive alternative to medical treatment. It shortens the period of disability and prevents the situation in which the surgeon is forced to operate in less than ideal circumstances because the patient's condition has deteriorated or severe complications have developed with medical treatment.

Early surgical treatment is always indicated for those patients who present with perforation of the gallbladder and peritonitis, severe toxicity and a markedly distended gallbladder, significant obstructive jaundice, diabetes mellitus that is difficult to control, or pneumocholecystitis. Surgery is also indicated when another abdominal emergency, such as a perforated peptic ulcer or perforated acute appendicitis, cannot be excluded. Elderly patients, especially men with cardiovascular disease, and those immunosuppressed by cancer or corticosteroid therapy in whom the diagnosis of acute cholecystitis may not be readily apparent are also candidates for prompt surgical intervention once the diagnosis has been made.[182]

In some instances, cholecystostomy should be considered as a planned alternative to cholecystectomy,[82] particularly in critically ill patients or in those patients whose biliary anatomy has been obscured by the inflammatory process. All the gallstones in the gallbladder must be removed when cholecystostomy is performed to prevent further complications from the stones. In a patient with jaundice, the ductal system should be examined carefully for calculi. Operative choledochography is helpful in selecting patients for choledochotomy.[30,107]

Pneumocholecystitis

Pneumocholecystitis is acute cholecystitis with secondary infection by gas-forming organisms. It was first described as an operative finding in the English literature by Lobingier in 1908.[121] Because the clinical features are indistinguishable from those of ordinary acute cholecystitis, preoperative diagnosis is possible only with radiographic examination; this was first achieved by Hegner in 1931.[97]

Although the age distribution of patients with pneumocholecystitis is the same as that of patients with acute cholecystitis, male patients predominate.[140] Gallstones are absent in 28% of patients, suggesting that pneumocholecystitis may be different in pathogenesis from the ordinary acute calculous cholecystitis. Of great importance is the strong association with diabetes. Rosoff and Robbins[185] reported that six of ten patients in their series were diabetics; in most series, the incidence of diabetes is about 30%.

Mentzer and associates[140] emphasized that not all patients manifest clinical signs of sepsis. Well-localized tenderness and signs of peritoneal irritation are not typical of this condition.

Organisms most frequently cultured from bile or the gallbladder wall in pneumocholecystitis have been *Clostridium* species, *E. coli, Streptococcus faecalis,* and other enteric bacteria, all probably secondary invaders after establishment of the inflammation. At first, gas is present within the lumen of the gallbladder. As the organisms invade the wall, intramural gas becomes detectable; this process may subsequently spread to pericholecystic tissues. How bacteria reach the gallbladder is still a matter of controversy. The cystic duct is frequently obstructed, and the cystic blood vessels are thrombosed. With this combination of cystic duct obstruction, bacterial destruction, ischemic necrosis of the wall, and gaseous distention of the organ, a relatively high incidence of perforation of the gallbladder is not surprising.[140]

Treatment must be vigorous because of the dangers of perforation and the presence of *Clostridium* species in 46% of patients with positive cultures. Large doses of broad-spectrum antibiotics are given, associated diabetes is controlled, and early operation is recommended as soon as the patient is adequately prepared. Although McCorkle and Fong[137] and Rosoff and Meyers[184] have successfully treated some patients without surgery, it seems judicious to remove an organ that is of doubtful viability and teeming with virulent organisms. Gas gangrene of the abdominal wall is a rare but serious complication after operation for pneumocholecystitis, and steps should be taken to prevent this catastrophe at the time of operation. The reported mortality rate is 15%.

Acalculous Cholecystitis

Less than 5% of cholecystitis is unassociated with stones in the gallbladder. Acalculous cholecystitis is seen as a sequela of torsion, cystic duct obstruction, common bile duct obstruction, multiple transfusions, primary bacterial infections of the gallbladder, direct trauma, and certain arteritides.[84,93] The cause is multifactorial and includes local trauma, blood flow changes, and increased bile pigment load. Removal of the injured gallbladder is recommended when the right or common hepatic artery has been ligated or the organ exhibits signs of injury.

The delineation of the association of acalculous cholecystitis with nonbiliary tract surgery, multiple trauma,[71,87,148] prolonged hyperalimentation, stasis, and multiple organ failure is less clear. Gallbladder stasis secondary to anesthesia, dehydration, fever, narcotics, and parenteral hyperalimentation is thought to be causative.[163,166]

This form of acute cholecystitis is rarely experienced in patients under 50 years of age and affects men twice as often as women. Although the diagnosis is made fairly easily in cholecystitis associated with extra-abdominal surgery, it may be exceedingly difficult when the peritoneal cavity has recently been violated. As in acute cholecystitis complicating trauma, gangrene and perforation can occur.

Early cholecystectomy should be performed.[128] An overall mortality rate of 30% has been reported, reduced to 16% for those treated with prompt cholecystectomy.

Acalculous cystic duct obstruction from fibrosis, anomalous cystic artery, or carcinoma of the cystic and common hepatic ducts has been reported to cause cholecystitis. The mechanism of pathogenesis is similar to that of calculous cystic duct obstruction. Carcinoma of the cystic or the adjacent common hepatic duct must be excluded when acalculous cholecystitis is found at operation.

Because most cases of common bile duct obstruction are not complicated by acute cholecystitis, it is difficult to explain the few cases in which this association exists. Anderson and co-workers[8] stressed the importance of gallstones that pass spontaneously into the common bile duct or the intestine before operation.

Primary infection of the gallbladder causing cholecystitis is exceedingly rare. Although *Salmonella* may be harbored in the gallbladder, it is unusual for it to cause acute inflammation there. Other organisms that have been implicated are *Actinomyces* and *Mycobacteria* species.

Chronic Cholecystitis

Chronic cholecystitis is by far the most common gallbladder disease and is almost invariably accompanied by gallstones. Chronic inflammation may be the aftermath of one or more attacks of acute cholecystitis; more often it is insidious, arising from a combination of mechanical and chemical injury. Scarring results in a contracted, pearly white, thick-walled gallbladder containing bile that is frequently turbid with debris. One or more gallstones are usually present. The mucosa is often ulcerated and scarred. Secondary infection, usually by coliform organisms, is present in 40% to 60% of patients.

Chronic cholecystitis shares many clinical features with other upper abdominal conditions, such as peptic ulcer, hiatus hernia, and chronic pancreatitis. Nonspecific upper abdominal pain, tenderness, fat intolerance, flatulence, nausea, and anorexia are reported. However, in chronic cholecystitis, pain is usually greater in the right hypochondrium than elsewhere; at times typical attacks of biliary "colic" point strongly to the diagnosis. Local tenderness is often present. Diagnosis is made by ultrasonography, which shows stones in a gallbladder that may be thick walled and contracted. Sometimes other investigations, such as barium meal, endoscopy, and radiography of the chest, are needed to exclude or establish the differential diagnosis.

The treatment of choice is cholecystectomy unless pressing contraindications exist. Without cholecystectomy symptoms will persist, and complications may be anticipated in a proportion of patients. These include recurrent attacks of pain, jaundice secondary to calculous obstruction of the common bile duct, cholangitis, pancreatitis, and internal biliary fistula.

The mortality rate from surgery for cholelithiasis is less than 1%. However, in patients over 70 years of age, the mortality rate rises to 2% to 3%. This increase is due largely to associated cardiopulmonary disease.

Postoperative complications occur in about 10% of patients (Table 42-2). The vast majority of these complications are minor and transient.

Mucocele of Gallbladder

Mucocele of the gallbladder occurs as a result of complete cystic duct obstruction either in a normal organ or as a sequela to acute cholecystitis. Bile within the gallbladder is reabsorbed and replaced by a clear watery mucinous fluid secreted by the gallbladder epithelium. The organ is distended and tense. A variable amount of vascular congestion of the serosa is seen. Secondary infection may occur. Symptoms are nonspecific, usually simulating other upper abdominal conditions. The enlarged gallbladder is palpable. Ultrasonography shows the enlarged gallbladder. Removal of the gallbladder is curative. Perforation of a mucocele of the gallbladder may lead to pseudomyxoma peritonei.

CHOLEDOCHOLITHIASIS

Stones in the bile ducts may develop *de novo* (primary) or originate from the gallbladder (secondary). They may reform after operation (recurrent) or may have been overlooked (retained) at cholecystectomy or exploration of the bile ducts. They may be solitary or so numerous as to fill the whole duct (Fig. 42-10).

Primary bile duct stones are seen most commonly in Oriental countries, such as Japan, Korea, China, Hong Kong, and Malaysia, and they are often associated with biliary infections and intrahepatic stones. This condition, recurrent pyogenic cholangitis, is dealt with in the section on cholangitis. A similar disease is encountered in Co-

TABLE 42-2.   Complications in 1356 Cases of Cholelithiasis Treated by Operation

COMPLICATION	NUMBER
PULMONARY	
Atelectasis	18
Pneumonia	6
Pulmonary embolism	6
Pleural effusion	2
Acute pulmonary edema	1
Total	33 (2.5%)
CARDIOVASCULAR	
Venous thrombosis	23
Cerebrovascular accident	3
Myocardial infarction	1
Peripheral arterial embolism	1
Total	28 (2.5%)
WOUND	
Infection	28
Dehiscence	13
Hernia	3
Hematoma	1
Total	45 (3%)
COMMON BILE DUCT	
Retained stone	3
Fibrosis of sphincter of Oddi	1
Sclerosing choledochitis	1
Carcinoma of bile duct	1
Dislodged T tube	1
Total	7 (0.5%)
ABDOMEN	
Subphrenic abscess	7
Pancreatitis	5
Fistula	4
Bowel obstruction	3
Total	19 (1.5%)

(Calcock BP, McManus JE: Experiences with 1,356 cases of cholecystitis and choledocholithiasis. Surg Gynecol Obstet 101:161, 1955)

Fig. 42-10. Faceted stones in the common bile duct.

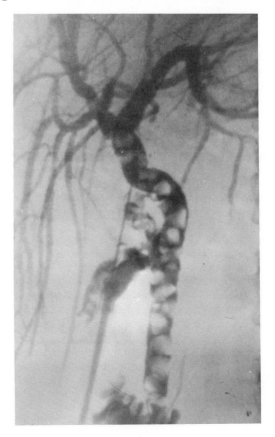

lombia. In western countries in which cholesterol stones predominate and biliary infections and infestations are less common than in the Orient, the incidence of primary common bile duct stones is difficult to determine accurately, although it is a common belief that most stones in the common bile duct have migrated from the gallbladder. Indeed, 10% to 15% of patients with gallbladder stones also have stones in the common bile duct.

When a person presents with a stone in the common bile duct after operation, it is difficult to determine whether the stone has developed anew from the bile constituents or was overlooked at the previous operation. If the interval between operation and the discovery of a common duct stone is short, less than a month, for example, it is likely that the stone was overlooked and therefore should be considered a retained stone.

Unfortunately, no reliable information is available on the rapidity with which a ductal stone may reform. Since both retained and recurrent stones may be asymptomatic for a long time and may present 10 or more years after surgery, it is extremely difficult to distinguish them in this delayed form. The composition of the stone may be of some help in this regard. Recurrent stones are often formed from bile pigments rather than from cholesterol, although this is not an absolute rule. On the other hand, a cholesterol stone that has resided for a long time in the bile duct usually acquires a coat of bile pigments.

Clinical Features

As noted above, stones in the bile duct may be asymptomatic, but symptoms eventually develop in 50% to 80% of patients. The most common complaint is pain. This usually commences at the epigastrium and may radiate to the right or left of the upper abdomen. When severe, it may be associated with nausea and vomiting.

Jaundice secondary to ductal obstruction is also common. Choledocholithiasis features prominently in the differential diagnosis of cholestasis. The jaundice is characteristically fluctuating but may be relentlessly progressive. Dark urine, pale stools, and pruritus develop with the jaundice. The gallbladder is usually not palpable.

Fever and chills are the unwelcome manifestations of cholangitis. They may lead to serious sequelae and should be managed with some urgency and concern (see section on cholangitis). The majority of patients exhibit elevations of serum bilirubin and alkaline phosphatase levels.

Stones in the common bile duct sometimes present with acute pancreatitis. Only rarely is this caused by impaction of a stone in the common channel in the duodenal papilla; rather it is due to the passage of gallstones through the papilla as shown by Acosta and Ledesma.[1]

Rarely, distention or irritation of the biliary ducts by choledocholithiasis may precipitate angina pectoris and induce electrocardiographic changes because of a reflex decrease in coronary blood flow. Equally rare is hemobilia resulting from erosion of the ductal mucosa.

Diagnosis and Management

Choledocholithiasis occurs in many clinical settings, and because the diagnosis and management of this condition may vary in these different conditions, it is advantageous to consider each in turn.

Choledocholithiasis Associated with Cholecystolithiasis

In the preoperative investigation of gallbladder symptoms, choledocholithiasis may be uncovered by ultrasonography. However, few such stones are detected preoperatively. Although ultrasonography shows ductal dilatation well, stones in distal common bile ducts may not be revealed because of technical difficulties with air in the duodenum. Approximately 10% to 15% of patients undergoing gallbladder surgery for gallstones also have stones in the common bile duct.

Most of the former indications for exploration of the common bile duct, such as pancreatitis, small multifaceted stones in the gallbladder, and a past history of jaundice, are now obsolete. The wise surgeon now routinely performs operative cholangiography.[21] When performed properly, this investigation not only reveals unsuspected pathology in the biliary system, including choledocholithiasis, but it also saves many unnecessary duct explorations that would be carried out under the former indications for duct exploration. When a common bile duct stone is shown on operative cholangiography or felt by the surgeon, the common bile duct should be explored. Another indication for duct exploration is dilatation of the common bile duct to more than 15 mm in diameter. In such a dilated duct, operative cholangiography may be technically unsatisfactory because the large volume of contrast material used may obscure the stones within the ducts. Duct exploration should entail obtaining a specimen of bile for microbiologic examination and removing all detectable stones and sludge within the ductal system. Fiberoptic choledochoscopy has been demonstrated[109,122,199] to produce a higher identification rate of ductal stones, particularly those in the hepatic ducts, and is useful in removing stones unreachable by most conventional techniques of extraction. Completion cholangiography is recommended after endoscopic maneuvers.[112]

When the risk of retained or recurrent stones is high or when a second operation on the patient is highly undesirable because of infirmity or old age, consideration should be given to biliary enteric bypass if the common bile ducts are dilated and to transduodenal sphincteroplasty if they are not. In most instances, the recommended practice is to insert a wide-bore T tube into the common bile duct and bring it out through the skin in a direct line so as to facilitate subsequent mechanical extraction of the stone if necessary. T-tube cholangiography is carried out about one week postoperatively, and if results are normal, the T tube is removed 10 to 14 days after operation.

Retained Stones

Despite various preventive measures at the time of surgery, the incidence of retained biliary calculi is still 1% to 5%. The diagnosis is usually made on the basis of postoperative T-tube cholangiography. Should a filling defect be detected and doubt exist as to whether it represents an air bubble or calculus, this investigation should be repeated under fluoroscopy after a few days. If a retained calculus is confirmed, several approaches to the problem are possible, and the approach used will depend mainly on the availability of facilities and expertise. These approaches are chemical dissolution of stones,[3,210,238] surgical reexploration of the common bile duct, endoscopic sphincterotomy and stone extraction,[53,54,178,189,247] and percutaneous nonoperative stone extraction through the T-tube tract.[38,134]

The role of chemical dissolution of retained calculi is in a state of flux. Agents used previously, such as chloroform, ether, and heparin, have not been reliably effective. However, with the advent of bile-salt solutions, such as cholic acid, chenodeoxycholic acid, ursodeoxycholic acid, and recently mono-octanoin,[211] interest in this form of treatment for the dissolution of cholesterol stones has been renewed. Nevertheless, with the advent of mechanical approaches to the problem of retained calculi, chemical dissolution appears to be applicable only to a small group of patients, particularly those in whom other methods have failed. Infusion of any solution into the common bile duct at high pressure may precipitate cholangitis and septicemia if the bile is infected.

Surgical reexploration of the common bile duct carries with it considerable mortality and morbidity and is now reserved for patients in whom other methods have failed or in whom complications have developed during the performance of other procedures. Naturally, the second operation is more difficult technically, and, despite reoperation, a risk of retained stones still exists.

In a large series of patients with choledocholithiasis, Safrany[189] was able to perform endoscopic sphincterotomy in 93%. Most of the patients had retained or recurrent common bile duct stones after cholecystectomy. The procedure was performed to relieve jaundice in 20% of these high-risk patients. Although stones passed spontaneously after sphincterotomy in 188 patients, extraction had to be undertaken with a Dormia basket in 306. Only 29 patients had residual stones after the procedure. Complications, which consisted of bleeding, retroperitoneal perforation, pancreatitis, cholangitis, and stone impaction, occurred in 7%. Complications that necessitated emergency surgery developed in ten patients with five deaths, giving a mortality rate of 1%. Considering that this procedure was performed on a large number of high-risk patients, the morbidity and mortality rates are superior to those for surgical reexploration. In most instances endoscopic sphincterotomy is much less stressful to the patient than a second operation. However, its performance re-

quires a highly skilled team. This procedure has already been used in some instances as primary treatment for all common bile duct stones. However, stone extraction using choledochoscopic control through the T-tube tract has been reported.[51,246]

Mechanical extraction of retained calculi through the T-tube tract was pioneered by Mazzariello[134] with specially designed pliable forceps; later, the use of Dormia stone baskets followed dilatation of the T-tube tract. In 1978, Mazzariello[134] reported nonoperative extraction of residual biliary stones in 1086 patients over a 14-year period with a success rate of 96%. In the same year, Burhenne[39] reported on a series of 661 patients with a similar success rate. This procedure is greatly facilitated if a large T tube has previously been placed in the common bile duct and brought out through the skin in a straight line. In about 30% of patients, multiple sessions are necessary. Failure is due to difficulty with catheterization of a sinus tract too narrow because of the small caliber of the indwelling T-tube, to difficulty recatheterizing a sinus tract after initial removal of a stone or stones, and to inability to engage the stone in a cystic duct remnant, small hepatic ducts, or pockets adjacent to the distal common bile duct. In a survey[38] of 661 patients, the complication rate was remarkably low. Complications consisted mainly of extravasation of bile and infection. Two patients had pancreatitis. No deaths occurred in this series.

Both Burhenne[39] and Mazzariello[134] used fluoroscopic control for this procedure. However, multiple reports[51,64,246] state that successful removal has been accomplished in 90% to 100% of patients with common bile duct stones and in 88% of those with intrahepatic stones. No doubt future developments and refinements will improve both the scope and the results of this form of treatment. Its great attraction is its relative safety compared with the endoscopic retrograde procedure. Obviously, it is possible to use this form of treatment only in patients with a large T-tube tract that has been matured for 4 to 6 weeks.

Spectacular advances have been made in the treatment of choledocholithiasis, particularly with the advent of endoscopic retrograde sphincterotomy with stone extraction and the refinement of percutaneous extraction of retained calculi. By comparison, progress in the prevention of retained calculi has been disappointing despite the widespread use of operative cholangiography and choledochoscopy. The reasons for this must be technical and remediable. The fatalistic acceptance of a minimum irreducible incidence of retained stones after surgery is strongly discouraged.

Choledocholithiasis and Obstructive Jaundice

The current practice in the investigation of patients with clinical and biochemical features of obstructive jaundice is to undertake ultrasonography as the first definitive investigation. If a mechanical obstruction is present, the resultant ductal dilatation is usually detectable by ultrasonography. This investigation can also show concurrent disease in the liver, gallbladder, and pancreas. The level of obstruction, be it at the porta hepatis or in the distal common bile duct, can usually be defined. However, specific demonstration of a common duct stone may be difficult, particularly if the stone is in the retroduodenal portion of the duct. Most surgeons are happy to proceed with operation if a dilated common bile duct together with gallstones in the gallbladder is shown on ultrasonography.

Others prefer further anatomic definition through percutaneous transhepatic cholangiography or endoscopic retrograde cholangiopancreatography (Fig. 42-11). In patients in whom only the intrahepatic bile ducts are shown to be dilated on ultrasonography, preoperative percutaneous transhepatic cholangiography is often requested to define the anatomy and to locate the site of obstruction. In very ill patients, it may be desirable to decompress the biliary tract with an indwelling percutaneous transhepatic tube for a few days before definitive surgery. A recent report,[139] however, suggests an excessive morbidity and mortality associated with lengthy percutaneous drainage of an obstructed biliary tree.

The role of endoscopic retrograde cholangiography in obstructive jaundice is changing.[62] It is used to define the nature of obstruction involving the lower part of the common bile duct with special reference to lesions of the duodenal papilla and head of the pancreas. In some centers,

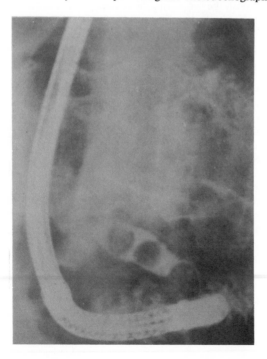

Fig. 42-11. Stones at the lower end of the common bile duct demonstrated by endoscopic retrograde choledochography.

it is the primary treatment for calculous obstruction to the common bile duct, particularly in high-risk patients.

When surgery is undertaken, the usual precautions for operating on jaundiced patients, such as correction of any bleeding tendency, treatment of any infection present, and hydration of the patient to optimize renal function, must be observed carefully. A common bile duct stone causing obstructive jaundice can either be palpated at operation or demonstrated on operative cholangiography.

Gallstone Pancreatitis

The exact relationship between gallstones and pancreatitis remains a contentious issue. Approximately one third of patients with acute pancreatitis are shown to have gallstones either in the gallbladder or in the common bile duct. Therefore, in all patients with acute pancreatitis, investigation of the biliary tract is essential. Ultrasonography is able to show the presence of stones in the gallbladder, but the demonstration of a slightly dilated common bile duct after acute pancreatitis is open to many interpretations and cannot be regarded as an indication of choledocholithiasis.

The trend is toward early, although not emergent, operation for gallstone pancreatitis prompted by the findings that, with early, not immediate, surgery, pancreatic disease is minimized, and recurrent attacks of pancreatitis, which occur during interval periods before elective surgery, are obviated.[1,109,164,218]

Cholangitis

The diagnosis and management of choledocholithiasis associated with cholangitis is discussed elsewhere in this chapter.

Biliary-Type Pain with a History of Cholecystectomy

In patients with a history of cholecystectomy who present with a biliary-type pain, a stone in the common bile duct is suspected. The suspicion is heightened by a raised alkaline phosphatase level. If a common bile duct stone is discovered, it should be treated by surgery, by endoscopic retrograde sphincterotomy with or without stone extraction, or by medical treatment with bile acids. Much depends on the physical condition of the patient, the size and number of stones, the caliber of the common bile duct, and the availability of facilities and expertise. Currently, the most widely practiced approach is surgical exploration, but it can be anticipated that endoscopic sphincterotomy with stone extraction may gain greater favor in the future, particularly in patients who are poor surgical candidates.

CHOLANGITIS

Cholangitis is an inflammatory condition of the bile ducts characterized clinically by a triad of pain, fever, and jaundice. Simple obstructive cholangitis, recurrent pyogenic cholangitis, and sclerosing cholangitis are three distinguishable forms of cholangitis. They differ in their pathology, clinical features, treatment, and prognosis and therefore warrant separate consideration.

Simple Obstructive Cholangitis

Incidence and Etiology

Simple obstructive cholangitis[86,190,214] is the most common type of cholangitis in western countries and is associated with common duct stones, biliary strictures, stenosis of biliary enteric anastomoses, biliary fistulas, choledochal cysts, and, occasionally, malignant obstruction of the biliary tree. Of practical importance is the induction of clinical cholangitis by invasive procedures, such as T-tube choledochography, endoscopic retrograde cholangiography, and percutaneous transhepatic cholangiography.

Pathology

The pathogenesis of obstructive cholangitis is still not well understood. The presence of bacteria in bile does not necessarily result in clinical manifestations or even in histologic evidence of ductal inflammation. The exact route by which enteric organisms enter the bile is still unknown. Dineern[68] has shown in guinea pigs that inoculation of bacteria into regional lymphatics does not cause a high titer of organisms in the bile, the gallbladder wall, or the liver. This is probably because the lymphatic flow is downward toward the celiac nodes rather than to the liver. When bacteria are injected into the portal vein, a significant inoculum can be recovered from both the liver and the extrahepatic biliary tract. Bacterial injection into the systemic circulation does not produce the same result. Therefore, potentially, the portal vein appears to be the significant pathway of biliary bacterial colonization. However, cultures of portal venous blood taken at laparotomy for noninfective diseases are sterile in 98% of all patients. Interestingly, Brooke and associates[36] discovered bacteria in portal blood in 24 of 90 consecutive patients with ulcerative colitis. This is of possible importance in the pathogenesis of sclerosing cholangitis.

Another route of bacterial invasion of the biliary tree is from the small and large intestine either by way of the sphincter of Oddi or by way of various types of direct biliary enteric communications. Heavy colonization of the choledochus by coliform organisms, as in choledochocolostomy in animals, does not necessarily result in overt clinical cholangitis in the absence of obstruction. Biliary obstruction is, therefore, an important prerequisite in the pathogenesis of most patients with cholangitis. Scott and Khan[195] cultured bile obtained during percutaneous cholangiography, and at subsequent operation in four groups of patients they found the incidence of positive cultures to be low in malignant disease and 100% in benign bile duct strictures (Table 42-3). The reason for the rarity of cholangitis in malignant obstruction is not obvious. However, one report[159] showed an increasing proportion of malignant obstruction of the bile ducts giving rise to cholangitis. The common organisms found in the bile in cholangitis are *E. coli, S. faecalis, Clostridium, Klebsiella, Enterobacter, Pseudomonas,* and *Proteus.* Clostridial organisms may constantly be present in any biliary tract infection and should be borne in mind when choosing antibiotics for the treatment of cholangitis.

Biliary infection incites an inflammatory cicatrizing reaction in the bile ducts and produces areas of stricturing and areas of dilatation. The ducts are thickened and often hyperemic. There is frequently much debris in the bile; sometimes calcium bilirubinate stones are formed, especially when *E. coli* is the offending organism. When obstruction is severe and infection unabated, invasion of liver substance by the organism may result in abscesses. With recurrent attacks of cholangitis, biliary cirrhosis and portal hypertension are likely sequelae.

Spillage of bacteria into the bloodstream gives rise to bacteremia and septicemia. The development of septicemia is facilitated by elevated intraluminal pressure of the biliary system, which, in turn, is a reflection of the degree of distal obstruction.[101]

TABLE 42-3.   Percentage of Positive Bile Cultures in Various Conditions

CONDITION	NUMBER OF PATIENTS	POSITIVE CULTURE	PERCENTAGE OF POSITIVE CULTURES
Calculous disease and jaundice	12	10	83
Postoperative stricture and jaundice	13	13	100
Common bile duct tumor and jaundice	10	0	0
Hepatic duct tumor and jaundice	9	0	0

(Scott AJ, Khan GA: Origin of bacteria in bile duct bile. Lancet 2:790, 1967)

Clinical Features

Charcot's triad of intermittent pain, fever, and jaundice is the hallmark of simple obstructive cholangitis. The pain is seldom distressing and is often overshadowed by rigor and fever, which occur one or more times daily for several days. The appearance of dark urine heralds the onset of jaundice, which usually does not become overt until the second or third day of the attack. Nonspecific upper gastrointestinal tract symptoms, such as anorexia and nausea, frequently accompany the other symptoms. With recurrent episodes of cholangitis, weight loss and anemia are common findings. With medical treatment, the attack subsides after 3 or 4 days only to recur at repeated intervals. When cholangitis progresses unabated, the patient's condition deteriorates. Fever and chills become frequent, jaundice deepens, pain worsens, and manifestations of severe sepsis become evident. A fall in urine output is an ominous sign of impending renal failure.

Treatment

The chief danger of cholangitis is bacteremia and septicemia. Therefore, several blood samples should be taken for culture and sensitivity determination. Broad-spectrum antibiotics are then given. Because these patients have a tendency to renal insufficiency, urine output should be well maintained, and blood levels of antibiotics should be measured periodically to ensure effectiveness and to avoid toxicity.

Although antibiotics may abort the symptoms, these agents are not curative unless the associated obstruction is also relieved; this usually requires surgery. Preferably the operation is performed when the acute episode has subsided and the patient has been prepared adequately. Bleeding and clotting profiles should be obtained, and precautionary administration of vitamin K substitute is recommended. Because operative manipulation of the bile ducts is likely to drive bacteria into the bloodstream and to contaminate the operative field, the operation should be performed under an antibiotic cover. The exact procedure depends on the cause of obstruction. Common bile duct stones are removed; strictures and other causes of obstruction are either resected or bypassed. The prime objective is to ensure freedom from obstruction.

In a small number of patients in whom obstruction is complete, cholangitis becomes progressive with frank suppuration within the biliary tree and liver. This condition has been designated acute obstructive suppurative cholangitis.[86] The patient is desperately ill, and anything short of prompt biliary decompression is likely to result in death. Even with decompression, the mortality rate is still about 35% because of associated hepatic and renal failure. In acute suppurative cholangitis, the onset of severe right hypochondrial pain is sudden and tends to be unremitting. Chills, fever, and progressive jaundice follow. The liver becomes enlarged and tender, and the patient is subjected to a fulminating septic course terminating in coma, toxic shock, and death. This patient should be operated on promptly and given vigorous antibiotic treatment and generous intravenous fluid therapy. The operative procedure should be as simple as possible. At times, mere insertion of a T tube in the common bile duct has been lifesaving. After the suppurative process has been brought under control, treatment is that of simple obstructive cholangitis. The use of endoscopic retrograde sphincterotomy has been advocated in the treatment of cholangitis in patients who cannot tolerate surgery and who have an obstruction of the lower common bile duct.[189]

Recurrent Pyogenic Cholangitis (Oriental Cholangiohepatitis)

Incidence

Recurrent pyogenic cholangitis is one of the most common causes of surgical emergency in Hong Kong, Taiwan, Korea, and Malaysia. Because of international travel, it is occasionally encountered in western countries. The incidence is equal in both sexes, and most patients are in the second, third, and fourth decades of life. Most patients are undernourished and in a low socioeconomic class.[240]

Etiology

The cause is unclear. Parasitic infestation can be excluded as a cause except in a few isolated cases because, epidemiologically, clonorchiasis is not known in Taiwan, where the incidence of recurrent pyogenic cholangitis is high. Conversely, *Ascaris* has almost worldwide distribution, but recurrent pyogenic cholangitis is confined mostly to one geographic region. It seems that parasitic infestation in these patients is incidental rather than causative. Distal common duct obstruction has also been implicated as the cause, and Ong's[160] examination of the sphincter of Oddi in patients with recurrent pyogenic cholangitis showed papillitis, stricture, polypoid degeneration of mucosa, and adenoma formation. However, these changes may be secondary to chronic inflammation as a result of stone impaction.

Usually it is not difficult to pass a large dilator through the lower end of the bile duct in these patients.[240] Bile duct colonization by enteric organisms with a colony count rivaling that of the colon is the common finding. In fact, positive cultures can be obtained from the biliary system with macroscopically normal ducts 1 or 2 years before the onset of clinical recurrent pyogenic cholangitis. Most of the positive cultures grow *E. coli*.[243] The level of β-glucuronidase in the common bile duct and gallbladder of these patients is 100 to 1000 times that in normal subjects. It is not known how such a severe degree of biliary infection originates.

Pathology

The most obvious findings at operation are distention of the liver and marked dilatation of the gallbladder, and when previous episodes of inflammation have occurred, the surface of the liver may be scarred. The gallbladder has an edematous wall and is usually free of any binding adhesion. In only one fourth of all patients are stones found within the organ. The common duct is thickened and dilated, in some instances reaching the size of the small intestine. Fibrosis of the duct wall leads to loss of elasticity such that the duct may never return to its normal size. Dilatation usually stops at the sphincter of Oddi, which is characteristically patulous, not offering much resistance to the passage of a large dilator. In contrast to dilatation of the common bile duct, stricturing is a prominent feature of the intrahepatic duct, usually taking place at the confluence of the two ducts. Associated proximal dilatation is sometimes of such proportion that a cystic space is formed with atrophy of overlying liver parenchyma.

Stones, sludge, debris, and pus fill the ducts. Stones are mostly calcium bilirubinate, soft, friable, and often faceted. In the common bile duct, they may pile up like a stack of pancakes. Intrahepatic stones are common in dilated ducts proximal to the strictures. The distribution of stones is about 50% in the common bile duct, 25% in the intrahepatic ducts, and 25% in the gallbladder. These stones lie in an amorphous muddy sludge that is difficult to shift, and this contributes considerably to biliary obstruction.

The complications associated with recurrent pyogenic cholangitis include liver abscesses, which may perforate into the pleural cavity or the bronchial tree, rupture of the gallbladder with resultant bile peritonitis, biliary enteric fistulas, usually between the gallbladder or common bile duct and the duodenum, thrombophlebitis of hepatic veins, and gram-negative septicemia.

Clinical Features

There is usually a history of recurrent attacks of chills, fever, pain, and jaundice similar to that of simple obstructive cholangitis. Each episode lasts for 1 to 2 weeks, and the interval between attacks may range from a week to several months. With progression of the disease, periods of remission shorten. In an acute attack, jaundice with marked upper abdominal tenderness and guarding is present, making adequate examination of the liver, gallbladder, and spleen difficult. Laboratory tests point to infection and obstructive jaundice with an elevated white blood cell count, raised serum bilirubin and alkaline phosphatase levels, and little change in serum transaminase values. Ultrasound examination can be very useful in the diagnosis of this disease. In view of the presence of infection, percutaneous transhepatic cholangiography should be performed only with circumspection. Federle and associates[75] demonstrated the utility of computed tomographic scanning in the diagnosis of these patients. Computed tomography can demonstrate the extent of ductal dilatation and the presence of sludge and soft stones usually undetected by ultrasonography.

Treatment

As in simple obstructive cholangitis, most patients have a remission with medical treatment, thus permitting elective surgery at a later date. The regimen of broad-spectrum antibiotics, parenteral fluid replacement, pain relievers, and vitamin K supplement, together with careful observation of vital signs and general physical condition, is exactly the same as for simple obstructive cholangitis. However, emergency surgery is performed if the patient does not improve rapidly.

The surgical objective is to provide adequate and permanent biliary drainage and the removal of stones and sludge from within the biliary tree. The dilated common bile duct lends itself readily to biliary bypass procedures, such as choledochojejunostomy, which has been found to be the most effective procedure. Strictures are dilated; stones and sludge are removed. At times, when cystic dilatation of an intrahepatic duct develops and the overlying hepatic parenchyma has atrophied, transhepatic lithotomy may be performed with facility. If this is done, the distal obstruction to the cystic space must be relieved or the ectatic bile duct must be bypassed with hepaticojejunostomy. Rarely, hepatic resection is required either to locate an intrahepatic bile duct or to remove a localized diseased or abscessed segment or lobe of the liver. Concomitant cholecystectomy is advocated because of the frequency of associated stones and the risk of perforation.

The prognosis is good when an effective operation is carried out early before serious complications develop. The operative mortality rate ranges from 4% to 20%; most deaths occur because of uncontrolled sepsis and liver failure. The complication rate is about 20%, with wound infection the most common problem.

Retained and recurrent stones and further stricture formation may lead to continuing sepsis. To permit future access to the biliary tree for endoscopic or radiographic manipulation, a part of the biliary enteric bypass is sometimes brought out to the subcutaneous plane. Stone extractions, stricture dilatation, and stenting can be performed repeatedly with ease through this "corridor" without resorting to further operations. Chronic persistent hepatic suppuration or disseminated infection is the usual cause of death in those unsuccessfully treated.[52]

Sclerosing Cholangitis

Much of the mystery and confusion surrounding sclerosing cholangitis[50] can be clarified if it is appreciated that the bile ducts can react only in limited ways to pathologic stimuli. They may become dilated or stenotic, and the dilatation and stenosis may be localized or diffuse. Sclerosing cholangitis merely represents a special pathologic reaction of the biliary tract in which marked narrowing of the lumen is caused by intense subepithelial fibrosis. Usually, the entire extrahepatic biliary tree and almost the whole intrahepatic biliary tree become involved. Not uncommonly, the process is limited to only a section of the biliary system. As a result of progressive sclerosis of the bile ducts, patients with sclerosing cholangitis exhibit progressive biliary obstruction and its sinister sequelae.

Unfortunately, no general agreement exists as to what constitutes primary sclerosing cholangitis. Proposed diagnostic criteria include progressive obstructive jaundice, absence of common duct calculi, no previous biliary surgery, cholangiographic evidence of diffuse multifocal strictures with irregularity and tortuosity of the ductal system, and absence of coexistent bile duct cancer.

The lack of an established cause and effect relationship between inflammatory bowel disease and sclerosing cholangitis has led some authors to designate sclerosing cholangitis as primary regardless of the presence or absence of inflammatory bowel disease. These arbitrary criteria represent attempts to create a single disease entity from a pathologic process that is probably initiated by more than one cause. Indiscriminate addition, alteration, or application of these criteria can only lead to an even more confusing picture of this condition.[12,49,76,124,213,230]

Incidence

Fortunately, sclerosing cholangitis is not a common condition. Almost 70% of the patients are males under the age of 45 years. Despite the well-documented and close association between ulcerative colitis and sclerosing cholangitis, the incidence of sclerosing cholangitis in patients with ulcerative colitis is less than 1%.[119]

Etiology

In most instances of sclerosing cholangitis, no discernible cause can be found. Several theories have been advanced; none has enough good supportive evidence to be outstanding. Bacterial infection is important. Injection of bacteria into the portal vein produces pericholangitis in experimental animals. Patients with ulcerative colitis frequently have organisms in portal venous blood. However, the majority of patients with sclerosing cholangitis have had no demonstrable bacteria in the bile.

The occasional apparently favorable response of this condition to the administration of corticosteroid agents has been cited as evidence that an autoimmune process is the underlying cause of sclerosing cholangitis although results of tests for rheumatoid factor, antimitochondrial antibody, smooth muscle antibody, and antinuclear antibody are negative in the majority of patients.[126,172] The association with ulcerative colitis, Crohn's disease,[12] retroperitoneal fibrosis, Riedel's struma, and lymphoma is suggestive of some genetically determined immunopathy, as are Quigley and co-workers'[172] and Record and co-workers'[176] cases of sclerosing cholangitis associated with a familial immunodeficiency syndrome. A majority of patients with sclerosing cholangitis have been shown to mount a cellular immune response to biliary antigens. Whether this is a cause or effect of ductal injury is unknown.

Results of tests for hepatitis B surface antigen have been negative, virtually excluding hepatitis B virus as an etiologic agent. Reports[14,145] of biliary atresia in rodents and human neonates associated with reovirus infections are suggestive.

Chemical injury of the biliary system by substances excreted from the liver is another possible cause. A lesion similar to that found in sclerosing cholangitis has been produced in rodent bile ducts after injection of 1,4-phenylenediisothiocyanate.[198] However, in humans, the well-recognized relative sparing of ductal mucosa and the patchiness of the involvement in some patients make direct chemical injury a less attractive theory. Some recent data suggest a role for excess hepatic copper.

Gallstones are probably a result rather than a cause of sclerosing cholangitis. Their absence in 70% of patients is proof that they do not play an important, if any, causative role.

Pathology

The entire biliary tree, including the gallbladder, may be sclerosed. Instead of a soft, pliable, and compressible structure, the common bile duct is converted into a thickened cord. When transected, the lumen is often difficult to identify and may admit only the finest of probes. The bile is thick and occasionally so inspissated as to form stones, which are dark and soft. Similar fibrous thickening may affect intrahepatic ducts, which on cholangiography resemble a pruned tree (Fig. 42-12). The gallbladder often has a thick, fibrous wall. Although usually noncalculous,

Fig. 42-12. Sclerosing cholangitis affecting mainly the intrahepatic ducts.

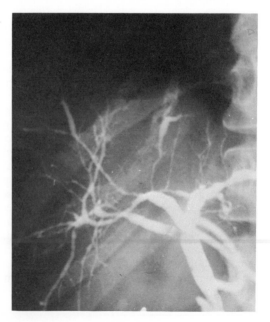

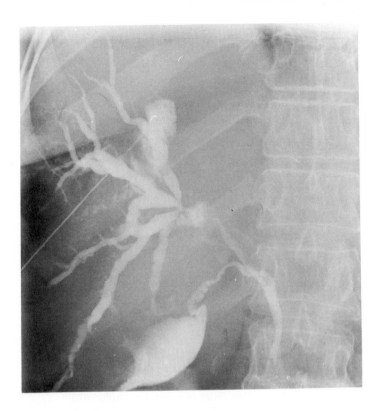

Fig. 42-13. Sclerosing cholangitis affecting the common hepatic and left hepatic duct and simulating ductal carcinoma.

it may contain stones of the same chemical composition as those in the common duct. Enlarged lymph nodes, which exhibit hyperplasia, and vessels may surround extrahepatic strictures. Whether sclerosing cholangitis starts as a diffuse process or begins at one point and later spreads to involve more of the biliary tree is unknown. What is well recognized is that localized sclerosis can occur (Fig. 42-13). The operative findings in our series of 84 patients are of interest in this regard (Table 42-4). Microscopically, the mucosa is essentially normal. The principal changes, in striking similarity to Crohn's disease, are found in the subepithelial and subserosal layers. Fibrosis and chronic

TABLE 42-4.   Operative Findings in 84 Patients with Sclerosing Cholangitis

AREA INVOLVED	NUMBER
Total involvement of biliary tract	45
Involvement of region of ductal bifurcation	22
Diffuse involvement of extrahepatic ducts only	5
Distal common bile duct only	5
Diffuse involvement of intrahepatic ducts only	4
Others	3

inflammation produce thickening of the duct, sometimes to eight times the normal thickness. In the early phase, the liver is relatively spared, but with progression of disease, periportal fibrosis and inflammation lead to biliary cirrhosis. An important but difficult differential diagnosis is sclerosing carcinoma of the bile duct. Both sclerosing cholangitis and sclerosing ductal carcinoma have the same incidence in ulcerative colitis. No data are convincing that sclerosing cholangitis precedes carcinoma.

Clinical Features

The major clinical manifestations of sclerosing cholangitis may be seen in Table 42-5. Jaundice, the dominant clinical feature, was present in the history of 93% of our patients. It is often intermittent but can be expected to become persistent and progressive. The jaundice is accompanied by dark urine, pale stools, and pruritus. Pain is common, affecting two thirds of the patients, and is often situated in the right hypochondrium. Chills and fever are less prominent in sclerosing cholangitis than in other forms of cholangitis, perhaps because only 20% of the patients have positive bile cultures. Weight loss (63%), anorexia and malaise (59%), and nausea and vomiting (45%) are some indications of the poor health associated with sclerosing cholangitis.

About one in three patients had a history of ulcerative colitis. For these patients, the intervals between onset of ulcerative colitis and onset of sclerosing cholangitis may

TABLE 42-5. Clinical Manifestations of 84 Patients with Sclerosing Cholangitis Treated at Lahey Clinic

CLINICAL FEATURE	NUMBER OF PATIENTS	PERCENTAGE OF SERIES
HISTORICAL FEATURES		
Jaundice	78	93
Pain	58	69
Weight loss	53	63
Anorexia and malaise	50	59
Chills and fever	42	50
Pruritus	41	48
Nausea and vomiting	40	45
Colitis	27	32
PHYSICAL FINDINGS		
Jaundice	48	57
Liver enlargement	37	44
Local tenderness	29	34
Ileostomy	5	6

be variable, ranging from less than 1 to more than 20 years. In two patients, sclerosing cholangitis antedated ulcerative colitis by 2 and 4 years, respectively. Colonic and extracolonic manifestations of chronic ulcerative colitis may be superimposed on those of sclerosing cholangitis in these colitic patients. Fortunately, in most instances the colonic disease is quiescent at the time of presentation.

Diagnosis

A history of ulcerative colitis, Crohn's disease, or other associated conditions listed should alert the physician to the possibility of sclerosing cholangitis when a patient with intermittent jaundice, epigastric pain, and fever is being treated. Laboratory tests are nonspecific, usually showing the pattern of obstructive jaundice. More than half of these patients have elevated serum bilirubin levels at the time of hospital admission. Alkaline phosphatase levels are elevated in more than 80% of all patients. Ultrasonography may be misleading in sclerosing cholangitis in not demonstrating a dilated ductal system in the presence of obstructive jaundice. Percutaneous transhepatic cholangiography is technically difficult because of the small caliber of the ducts but will demonstrate areas of stenosis and ductal attenuation. Endoscopic retrograde cholangiopancreatography is helpful in diagnosis provided that sufficient contrast medium is injected to show the peripheries of the ducts.

The characteristic cholangiographic picture includes beaded intrahepatic and extrahepatic ducts; short, band-like areas of stricture; pseudodiverticula; and a "pruned" appearance of the distal biliary radicles.

Liver biopsy specimens may demonstrate a spectrum of histologic changes ranging from cholangitis and portal hepatitis to biliary cirrhosis.

Treatment

Given that no definitive cause of sclerosing cholangitis is known in most instances, treatment[49,149] is empirical and is based mainly on an understanding of the pathology. The primary aim is to relieve biliary obstruction; this may be difficult to achieve because the small caliber of the bile ducts does not lend itself readily to bypass procedures or even to intubation with a T tube for external drainage.

Exploration of the biliary tree is recommended in almost every case. The common bile duct is identified, and operative cholangiography is performed so that the anatomy of the biliary tree may be defined. The common duct is then opened, and any stone found is extracted. A biopsy is then taken of the ductal wall, and mucosal scrapings, particularly at the site of a stricture, are submitted for frozen-section examination in an attempt to exclude cancer. Gentle dilatation of the major ducts is performed with Bakes dilators. After irrigation of the ductal system, a T tube, modified Y tube, or transhepatic U tube of appropriate size is carefully placed in the ductal system. If the distal common bile duct is markedly narrowed and the more proximal biliary tree is dilated, a bypass procedure is performed. Cholecystoduodenostomy, cholecystojejunostomy, choledochojejunostomy, and hepaticojejunostomy have all been used. In these instances, a stent is left in place.

Pitt and associates[168] have reported their experience with a more aggressive surgical approach than has generally been undertaken in the past. They achieved 77% excellent to good results with biliary enteric bypass and (usually) long-term transhepatic stenting after careful dilatation of the major intrahepatic ducts.

Recently a technique of constructing a "corridor" to the biliary tree through a biliary enteric anastomosis and fixation of a Roux-en-Y loop to the parietal peritoneum has allowed repeat access to the biliary tract for various manipulations,[103] including stricture dilatation and replacement of stents without reoperation and their attendant operative risks. This approach is expected to improve the results of treatment of this difficult clinical and mechanical problem.

Sclerosing cholangitis has little bearing on the decision to perform colonic surgery in patients with ulcerative colitis. Sclerosing cholangitis can develop in patients with ulcerative colitis years after they have had colectomy.

Corticosteroid agents produce a temporary beneficial effect in a few patients. Their mechanism of action is not entirely understood, but it is believed to be a combination of choleretic and anti-inflammatory actions. Progressive sclerosing cholangitis can develop in patients with ulcerative colitis who are taking these drugs. Corticosteroids are now seldom given for this condition. The use of immunosuppressants[105] is still experimental, and results so far are not impressive. Both corticosteroids and immunosuppressants are capable of producing serious side-effects and should be used only after careful consideration of all factors. Because 20% of bile cultures are positive for various enteric organisms, the use of antibiotics is recommended for patients who have a history of chills and fever or an elevated white blood cell count.

Liver transplantation has become an important new therapeutic option for patients with sclerosing cholangitis and other advanced liver disease. Special problems in patients with sclerosing cholangitis who undergo liver transplantation include technical details related to difficulties in mucosa-to-mucosa anastomoses, the presence of adhesions, biliary reconstruction, and the presence of portosystemic shunts.

Sclerosing cholangitis is a serious condition. The average duration of survival after onset of biliary symptoms is only 6 years despite one or more attempts at treatment. At the Lahey Clinic, only 13% of patients have no further problems after operation; about 25% continue to have sporadic mild episodes of cholangitis. For more than half the patients, the results of treatment are unsatisfactory; these patients continue to have cholangitis progressing to biliary cirrhosis, liver failure, and portal hypertension. The operative mortality rate is 8%; a further 20% of patients die of the disease during the average follow-up period of 37 months. The early postoperative complications include bacterial cholangitis (12%), biliary fistula (7%), postoperative gastrointestinal tract bleeding (7%), subphrenic abscess (6%), hepatic coma (3%), and septic shock (3%). The problems confronting these patients during the follow-up period are numerous: biliary cirrhosis develops in 34%, 15% have portal hypertension, 9% bleed from esophageal varices, and 21% are troubled by recurrent biliary infections.

BILIARY FISTULA

The incidence of biliary fistula has declined in recent years because of two important developments. First, the pitfalls

of biliary tract operations have been clearly identified, and better operative techniques have been developed, thus contributing to the prevention of operative injuries to bile ducts and to better management of distal biliary obstruction. Second, the increasingly widespread practice of cholecystectomy for calculous disease of the gallbladder even in asymptomatic patients has diminished the number of cholecystoenteric fistulas. The types of biliary fistula, postoperative and spontaneous, are listed in Table 42-6.

Postoperative Biliary Fistulas: Intended External and Internal Biliary Fistulas

The most common type of biliary fistula is one deliberately constructed at operation mainly to relieve or prevent biliary obstruction and sometimes to minimize bile leakage. Cholecystostomy, tubal drainage of the common bile duct, common hepatic duct, and major bile ducts, cholecystoenteric anastomoses, choledochojejunostomy, and hepaticojejunostomy are a few examples of internal and external biliary fistulas used in surgical practice. Usually, external fistulas are intended to be temporary, whereas internal ones are as permanent as possible. To ensure that a temporary artificial external biliary fistula will close, it is absolutely necessary to exclude distal obstruction at the time of operation and again postoperatively by choledochography. To maintain patency of an internal biliary

TABLE 42-6.   Classification of Biliary Fistulas

Postoperative biliary fistulas
  Intended fistulas
    External
      Hepaticostomy
      Choledochostomy
      Cholecystostomy
    Internal
      Hepaticoenterostomy
      Choledochoenterostomy
      Cholecystoenterostomy
  Unintended fistulas
    Cutaneous fistula of major bile ducts
    Cutaneous fistula of minor bile ducts
    Cutaneous fistula of cystic duct
    Persistent cholecystostomy
Spontaneous biliary fistulas
  Gallstone fistulas
    Cholecystoduodenal
    Cholecystogastric
    Cholecystocolic
    Cholecystoduodenocolic
    Cholecystocutaneous
    Others
  Peptic biliary fistulas
  Malignant biliary fistulas
  Bronchobiliary fistulas

bypass, the anastomosis should be mucosa to mucosa and sufficiently wide to compensate for inevitable contracture of the stoma. In many instances, a stent may be used to advantage.

Cutaneous Biliary Fistulas Involving the Major Bile Ducts

Fortunately, unintended postoperative biliary fistulas involving the major bile ducts are uncommon. Three causative mechanisms may be identified: bile duct injury, undetected distal biliary obstruction, and breakdown of a biliary anastomosis.

Ductal injury has been discussed elsewhere in this chapter. It usually occurs during cholecystectomy. Initially, a subhepatic collection of bile develops and becomes localized or spreads to the rest of the peritoneal cavity. This may be followed by copious discharge through the drain tract or the abdominal wound. Major bile duct injury of this type is unlikely to heal spontaneously, and the associated fistula tends to be persistent. Operation is indicated.

Cutaneous fistula of the common bile duct may also occur when the duct has been explored and distal obstruction by a stone, tumor, or fibrous stricture has been overlooked. Drainage through the T tube or its tract persists until the distal obstruction has been relieved.

Breakdown of an anastomosis involving a major bile duct is the third major cause of fistulization. The integrity of the biliary anastomosis is subject to the same factors that govern the integrity of all other types of anastomosis: blood supply, infection, quality of tissues, tension, and surgical technique. This type of fistula is sometimes complicated by escape of intestinal and pancreatic juices, resulting in severe excoriation of the skin and marked metabolic disturbances. Fortunately, most minor breakdowns of anastomosis heal spontaneously, although the risk of subsequent anastomotic stenosis is increased. With a more major breakdown, operative treatment is required. Careful preoperative preparation with respect to sepsis, fluid and electrolyte balance, nutritional state, bleeding and clotting profile, and renal function is required. The surgical procedure to be performed is determined by the operative findings.

Biliary Fistulas Involving the Minor Bile Ducts

Most commonly seen after cholecystectomy, biliary fistulas involving the minor bile ducts also occur in liver injury in which numerous small ducts are torn. Fistulas of the small bile ducts invariably close spontaneously if distal obstruction is not present. The advisability of T-tube drainage of the common bile duct in liver trauma is controversial. If done carefully, insertion of a T tube is attended by few complications; furthermore, it permits choledochography, which may be helpful in the operative and subsequent management of the patient. It also decompresses the biliary tree, thus aiding small torn bile ducts to close spontaneously instead of discharging bile into the peritoneal cavity. On the other hand, the presence of the T tube may introduce infection into a previously sterile system, and this is a serious drawback.

Cutaneous Fistula of the Cystic Duct

Cutaneous fistula of the cystic duct almost invariably follows cholecystectomy. A ligature in the cystic duct may become untied; less frequently, the cystic duct stump may rupture owing to distal obstruction. In the former situation, there is no preceding jaundice, and bile leakage occurs early in the postoperative period. In the latter, jaundice usually precedes the appearance of bile from the fistulous tract. Treatment is operative; the distal obstruction is dealt with appropriately, and the cystic duct is securely ligated.

Cholecystostomy Persisting as a Fistula

When the cholecystostomy tube is removed, the fistulous tract usually closes rapidly, although permanent external biliary fistula followed 30% of all cholecystostomies performed in the late 19th century. Persistent or recurrent bile drainage through the cholecystostomy opening denotes distal obstruction, usually due to a stone in the gallbladder or in the common bile duct. Sometimes a more obscure form of obstruction, such as a malignant or benign stricture of the lower end of the common bile duct, may be responsible. Rarely, after the removal of the cholecystostomy tube, a mucocele of the gallbladder occurs because of cystic duct obstruction. The mucocele discharges intermittently through the cholecystostomy opening as the intraluminal pressure reaches a certain level.

Cholecystography through the fistula readily reveals the underlying cause of obstruction. If it is in the gallbladder or cystic duct, cholecystectomy will be curative. In addition, if distal obstruction is present, such as that from choledocholithiasis, the obstruction should be treated appropriately.

Effects of Prolonged Biliary Drainage

Knochel and associates[111] and Rosato and co-workers[181] reemphasized the potential dangers of prolonged biliary drainage as pointed out by Wangensteen[228] in 1929. Bile contains 97% water and 1% to 3% solids, which consist of bile salts (0.9%–1.8%), mucin and bile pigment (0.5%), cholesterol (0.06%–0.16%), lecithin (0.02%–0.1%), and inorganic salts (0.7%–0.8%). Bile contains more sodium, bicarbonate, and calcium than plasma. The average daily output of an external biliary fistula in humans varies, usually from 300 ml to 500 ml; occasionally, more than 2.5 liters may be produced. When large quantities of bile are lost from the body over a prolonged period, metabolic disturbances often become manifest. As a result of loss of alkaline juice, metabolic acidosis may also develop.[44]

Impairment of fat digestion because of the absence of

bile salts has contributed to steatorrhea in some patients, especially when pancreatic deficiency is a concomitant finding. The fat-soluble vitamins A, D, K, and E are also not well absorbed, but this relatively mild deficiency is usually of no importance clinically.

Spontaneous Biliary Fistulas

Most spontaneous internal biliary fistulas occur in association with gallstones. A much less common cause is a duodenal ulcer penetrating into the common bile duct or the gallbladder. Occasionally, malignant invasion creates a fistula between the biliary tree and the stomach, duodenum, pancreas, or colon. Rarely, a bronchobiliary fistula may result from the transdiaphragmatic rupture of a hepatic or subphrenic abscess.

Gallstone Fistulas

Gallstone fistulas are usually an aftermath of acute cholecystitis. The inflamed gallbladder becomes adherent to various adjacent structures, and subsequently the intervening wall breaks down. Occasionally, after perforation of the gallbladder, a pericholecystic abscess forms that discharges into another organ and, rarely, through the abdominal wall to the exterior. About 70% to 75% of gallstone fistulas are cholecystoduodenal; another 10% to 15% are cholecystocolic, and 3% to 5% are cholecystogastric. Rarer communications, such as those between the gallbladder and renal pelvis, jejunum, abdominal skin, and common bile duct, have also been reported. A stone in the common bile duct may erode through the duodenum, but the most common cause of choledochoduodenal fistula is a penetrating peptic ulcer. Rarely, a compound fistula with more than one enteric opening, such as a cholecystoduodenal fistula, is found.

Cholecystoduodenal Fistula is the most common form of spontaneous internal biliary fistula in the United States, accounting for 70% of fistulas associated with gallstones, and is usually not seen until the sixth or seventh decade of life, with women predominating over men in a ratio of 4:1. Patients usually present with small intestinal obstructions (gallstone ileus). Without obstruction, diagnostic accuracy is only about 20% compared with 63% with gallstone ileus. Nearly half the patients have a previous history of gallbladder symptoms. The fistula permits gas or barium to enter the gallbladder and outline the biliary tree in more than half of the instances (Fig. 42-14); sometimes an opaque stone may be visualized in an abnormal position. In addition to gallstone ileus, other important complications are cholangitis, obstructive jaundice, hemorrhage, and cancer of the gallbladder.

Cholecystocolic Fistula. Although gallstones that have passed through a cholecystocolic fistula may occasionally cause obstruction,[222] especially when they are very large or a stenotic colonic segment is present, the major prob-

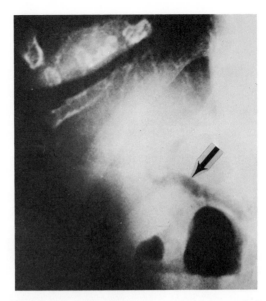

Fig. 42-14. Air in the biliary tree secondary to a cholecystoduodenal fistula.

lems with this type of fistula are diarrhea, recurrent cholangitis, and malabsorption. Diarrhea is a result of bacterial colonization of the small bowel through the bile duct and of the cathartic effect of bile salts. Cholangitis appears when biliary obstruction is associated with infection. These offending enteric organisms may also enter the duodenum and small bowel by way of the common bile duct and cause malabsorption. All of these problems are accentuated in a cholecystoduodenocolic fistula. Preoperative diagnosis is rare but may be made on a plain film of the abdomen or with a barium enema, which shows gas or barium in the biliary tree (Fig. 42-15). Treatment consists of closure of the fistula and cholecystectomy, at which time the common bile duct should be examined carefully.

Cholecystogastric Fistula. The emesis of a large gallstone is a dramatic presentation of cholecystogastric fistula. However, most vomited gallstones originate from a cholecystoduodenal fistula.[77] Cholangitis is a common complication. There has been no report of adverse effects of bile on the stomach mucosa in these patients. Any symptom of alkaline gastritis, if present, is probably attributed to gallbladder disease or to the associated cholangitis. Closure of the fistula and cholecystectomy are curative for gallstone cholecystogastric fistula. Again, the rest of the alimentary tract as well as the common bile duct should be examined carefully for other gallstones.

Gallstone Ileus

Most gallstones entering the small intestine through a spontaneous fistula pass uneventfully, but in 10% of patients the stones are too big to navigate the narrow seg-

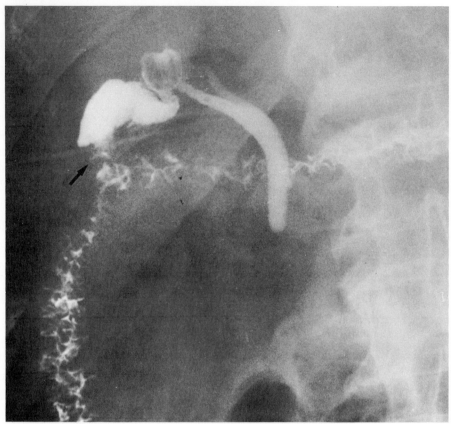

Fig. 42-15. Cholecystocolic fistula (*arrow*) shown on a barium enema study.

ments of the small bowel and thus give rise to mechanical obstruction.[34] It has been suggested that the critical gallstone size is a diameter of 3 cm; however, larger gallstones have traversed without trouble and smaller ones are known to cause intestinal obstruction. When obstruction occurs, the site is usually at the terminal ileum, which is the narrowest portion of the small intestine. In a series of 80 cases of gallstone ileus reported by Raf and Spangen,[173] the duodenum was obstructed in 1 patient, the upper jejunum in 25, the mid–small intestine in 7, the ileum in 46, and the colon in 9.

Gallstone ileus accounts for about 2% of all cases of intestinal obstruction (Fig. 42-16). The age and sex incidence is the same as that for cholecystoduodenal fistula. Because it is a condition affecting the elderly, associated diseases are found in 80% of patients, most commonly cardiovascular and pulmonary diseases and diabetes. The characteristic feature of gallstone ileus is the initial incompleteness of the obstruction. This "tumbling" type of obstruction gives rise to recurrent episodes of intestinal colic, vomiting, and abdominal distention, which may last for several days. Procrastination in seeking proper medical aid because of the intermittency of symptoms may result in severe dehydration and metabolic disturbances. This delayed presentation, together with the as-

sociated disabilities of elderly patients, accounts for a reported mortality rate of about 50%. With earlier and better management of gallstone ileus and associated conditions, it is now possible to reduce the mortality greatly.

Given the associated cardiovascular and metabolic diseases of these relatively fragile patients, treatment consists of fluid and electrolyte replacement. A nasogastric or intestinal tube is used for decompression. When the patient is resuscitated, operation is performed to remove the obstruction. The rest of the bowel and the stomach must be examined carefully so that a second stone (5%–15% occurrence) is not overlooked.[131] The gallbladder and common bile duct should also be examined for stones. Cholecystectomy and closure of the fistula, together with common duct exploration, when indicated, should be performed either concomitantly[22] or as an interval procedure,[88,98] depending on the patient's condition. Recurrent symptoms or serious complications, such as cholangitis, occur in one third of all patients whose gallbladder disease is left untreated.

Peptic Biliary Fistula

Peptic biliary fistula is usually due to the penetration of a posterior duodenal ulcer into the common bile duct.

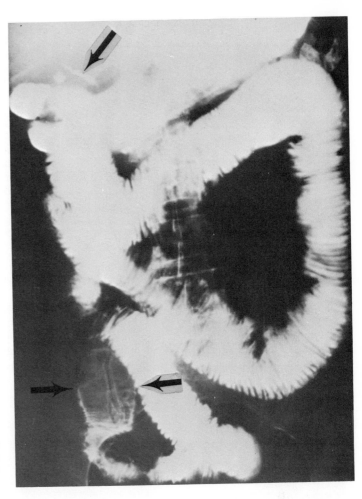

Fig. 42-16. Gallstone ileus. Barium meal study shows small bowel obstruction caused by a large gallstone in the right iliac fossa (*arrows*) and barium in the biliary tree (*arrow*).

Rarely, an anterior duodenal ulcer may perforate the gallbladder. The clinical picture is that of a peptic ulcer. Interestingly, despite the continuous bathing of the ulcer by the alkaline bile, this form of internal biliary fistula is especially prone to bleeding. A Polya gastrectomy is the treatment of choice. When the gallbladder is involved in the fistula, it should also be removed.[102]

Malignant Biliary Fistulas

Carcinoma of the gallbladder, stomach, colon, and, rarely, pancreas may produce a fistula between the biliary tract and these surrounding structures. The most common cause is gallbladder carcinoma, which, like gallstone fistulas, produces cholecystoduodenal, cholecystocolic, and cholecystogastric fistulas. The prognosis is poor, and only palliative procedures can be performed. In view of the possible presence of cancer even when gallstones are present, biopsy and histologic examination should be performed on all biliary fistulas.

Bronchobiliary Fistulas

Persistent expectoration of bile is pathognomonic of bronchobiliary fistula.[28,55,161] As much as 700 ml of bile-stained sputum may be produced each day. If it is not coughed up, a considerable degree of flooding of air passages takes place, causing atelectasis and aspiration pneumonia. Patients with bronchobiliary fistulas are therefore distressingly sick. A classification of bronchobiliary fistulas is offered in Table 42-7. Of interest is congenital bronchobiliary fistula, for which the exact embryologic derivation has not yet been determined.[191] In every reported instance, it has arisen from the proximal portion of the right main bronchus with the distal end usually joining the left hepatic duct system. The proximal segment of the fistula resembles a bronchus in structure, while distally the muscular components become more prominent. The mucosa is lined with squamous epithelium lying on top of the muscularis mucosa. Thus this structure more closely resembles the esophagus than a bile duct. Other associated anomalies of the biliary tract may be present.

TABLE 42-7.   Classification of Bronchobiliary Fistulas

Congenital
Acquired
  Parasitic
    Amebiasis
    Hydatid disease
  Nonparasitic
    Traumatic
    Inflammatory
      Liver abscess
      Subphrenic abscess
      Empyema thoracis
    Neoplastic
      Hodgkin's disease
      Malignancy causing bile obstruction

All infants with congenital bronchobiliary fistula have a severe cough productive of bile-stained sputum starting the first few days of life, with signs of atelectasis and aspiration pneumonia.

Diagnosis is made at bronchoscopy and bronchography. Treatment is ligation of both ends of the fistula and excision of the tract. The biliary system must be free of other congenital anomalies.

Acquired bronchobiliary fistula is usually secondary to an amebic abscess or a hydatid cyst discharging through the diaphragm into the bronchial tree. Occasionally, it is caused by a rupture of a pyogenic liver abscess or subphrenic abscess. The pathology of the various liver diseases that give rise to bronchobiliary fistula has been discussed elsewhere. A particularly difficult clinical problem is bronchobiliary fistula associated with distal biliary obstruction (Fig. 42-17). Patients with this disorder are desperately ill with debilitation, cholangitis, and pneumonia. Often they have several operations with only temporary improvement. To treat the fistula, it is necessary to relieve the distal biliary obstruction. Unfortunately, in some patients distortion of the anatomy and secondary sclerosing cholangitis severely restrict the chances of a satisfactory outcome.

BILE PERITONITIS

Classically, bile peritonitis is an intense inflammatory response of the peritoneum to the presence of infected bile in the peritoneal cavity. In contrast, sterile bile exerts a variable peritoneal reaction, and large volumes may sometimes accumulate with little overt ill effect. Bile peri-

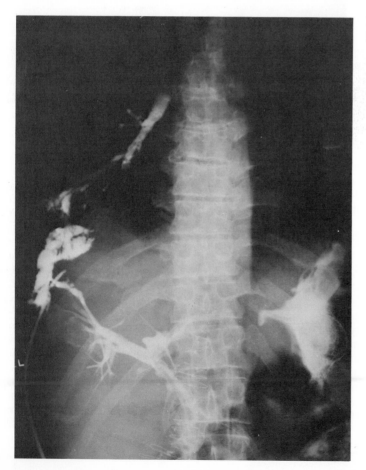

Fig. 42-17. Bronchobiliary fistula caused by subphrenic abscess.

tonitis is a life-threatening condition. It deserves greater mention than the sketchy accounts devoted to it in most texts.[40,60,74,181]

Etiology

Perforation of an acutely inflamed and necrotic gallbladder is the most common cause of bile peritonitis. Depending on the extent of inflammatory adhesions, the bile may discharge freely into the peritoneal cavity or by way of the intermediary of a pericholecystic collection.

Trauma is also a prominent cause of bile peritonitis. The incidence of postoperative bile peritonitis appears to be on the decline because of better surgical techniques. Penetrating and blunt injury to the abdomen may result in immediate or delayed perforation of the gallbladder and peritonitis. Bile peritonitis may develop as a consequence of percutaneous transhepatic cholangiography and liver biopsy, particularly in the presence of obstructive jaundice and cholangitis.

Other rare causes of bile peritonitis include spontaneous rupture of the common bile duct or choledochal cyst, rupture of liver abscesses or liver cysts, and premature removal of T tubes.

Pathophysiology

During operative cholangiography and exploration of the common bile duct, a small amount of bile often escapes into the peritoneal cavity without any consequence. Infants who have spontaneous perforation of the common bile duct may have accumulation of a large quantity of bile in the peritoneal cavity and yet remain afebrile. The only clinical manifestations are often those of increased intra-abdominal pressure. Similarly, in dogs more than 4 liters of bile ascites is tolerated without any difficulty other than intra-abdominal pressure problems. In short, bile may be well tolerated by the peritoneum. What then is the cause of such high fatality in bile peritonitis?

Unconjugated bile salts are cytotoxic and incite an inflammatory response. Most of the bile salt in bile is conjugated; however, bacterial enzymes and alteration in pH may induce deconjugation. The peritoneum, which is affected by the toxic effects of bile salts, becomes much more permeable to fluids, and extensive peritoneal transudation ensues. At the same time, transmigration of enteric organisms occurs. It is the presence of organisms either from the originally infected bile or from transmigration from the colon that is the major cause of death in bile peritonitis. Studies in germ-free animals show that, by control of bacteria in bile peritonitis, death can be prevented. The combined presence of bacteria and bile salts rapidly promotes a profuse outpouring of fluid into the peritoneal cavity. Hypovolemic shock follows. In addition, absorption of toxic products and invasion of the bloodstream by bacteria further compromise the host.

Clinical Features

Like those in other forms of peritonitis, the clinical features in bile peritonitis depend on the extent of involvement.

In diffuse bile peritonitis, the patient has generalized abdominal pain associated with marked tenderness and guarding. Signs of hypovolemic shock and septicemia may be superimposed on the clinical picture. If the condition is untreated, multisystem failure rapidly develops, terminating in death. With the more localized form of bile peritonitis, the patient usually presents with right upper quadrant pain associated with tenderness and guarding, features that are those of acute cholecystitis. Fever and varying degrees of jaundice are present. Pain may be referred to the right tip of the shoulder, and physical signs of right pleural effusion may be found. In postoperative patients receiving strong analgesics, these signs and symptoms may be masked. In children and infants, the clinical manifestations are often different. For example, in spontaneous perforation of the common bile duct, a relatively frequent cause of "bile peritonitis" in young patients, the clinical course tends to be subacute or even protracted, with mild jaundice, nausea, vomiting, pale stools, and ascites.[74]

It is rare to have fever and other signs of peritonitis in these patients in the early phase. This is a picture similar to that of bile ascites seen in older patients.

Treatment

Patients with full-blown bile peritonitis are ill from dehydration and sepsis. Adequate parenteral fluid replacement should be instituted and urine output carefully monitored. After blood cultures, the patient should be given a broad-spectrum antibiotic, such as an aminoglycoside or a cephalosporin. A nasogastric tube is passed to decompress the stomach and to minimize the intestinal distention in the ileus that so frequently accompanies bile peritonitis. It is also essential that the clotting and bleeding profile be checked in these patients.

Laparotomy should be performed early rather than late. The basic principles of treatment are to stop the bile leakage, to evacuate the extravasated bile, and to provide adequate drainage. The definitive procedure depends on operative findings.

Specimens for microbiologic examination should be taken near the area of bile leakage. Copious peritoneal lavage with saline or an antibiotic solution is helpful in reducing the bacterial count in the peritoneal cavity.

Prognosis

The postsurgical course may be complicated by renal failure, pulmonary infection, electrolyte disturbance, ileus, stress ulceration, deep vein thrombosis, pulmonary embolism, pancreatitis, myocardial infarction, and a host of other complications. It is therefore understandable that bile peritonitis carries a mortality rate of about 50%. However, with early diagnosis and operation, careful fluid and electrolyte replacement, appropriate and adequate antibiotic cover, and good surgical techniques, the mortality rate can be reduced substantially.

BILE DUCT INJURIES AND STRICTURES

More than 1000 patients have been treated in more than 1700 operations for benign bile duct strictures at the Lahey Clinic since its inception.[229] Not all strictures are benign, and it behooves the physician to exclude malignant disease in all patients with a ductal stricture.[45] Bile duct carcinoma is discussed elsewhere in this chapter; the rest of this section is confined to benign strictures involving the major bile ducts.[115,231] Although histologically benign, the clinical cause of these strictures may in fact be pernicious and is associated with distressing morbidity and tragic mortality.

Incidence and Etiology

More than 90% of all benign bile duct strictures are iatrogenic, resulting mainly from surgery in the upper abdomen (Table 42-8). The average age of 987 patients seen at the Lahey Clinic between 1940 and 1967 was 42 years.[236] Reflecting the sex ratio of gallstones and cholecystectomy, there were three times more women than men in this series. Maingot[130] estimated that one in 400 to 500 cholecystectomies results in bile duct injury. The skill and experience of the surgeon appear to be important factors in causation. In a random series of 400 postcholecystectomy bile duct strictures reported by Smith,[202] only 16% of the injuries occurred when a consultant surgeon was engaged in the operation, whereas the remaining 84% of the injuries were caused by surgical trainees operating without the help of a consultant surgeon. Other etiologic factors include failure to recognize anatomic anomalies, technical difficulties due to local diseases, and hurried control of bleeding at operation with inadvertent clamping of ductal structures (Table 42-9). In more than two thirds of Lahey Clinic patients, bile duct injury was not recog-

nized at the initial surgical procedure, and most of the operations were described as simple, routine, uncomplicated, uneventful, and so forth. The so-called easy cholecystectomy in the thin visceroptotic patient who has an unduly mobile gallbladder is a trap for the unwary and overconfident surgeon.[130] The sites of injury are summarized in Table 42-10.

Diagnosis

Only 15% of major bile duct injuries are recognized at the time of injury, usually because of excessive pooling of bile in the operative field. In the immediate postoperative period, the onset of deepening obstructive jaundice

TABLE 42-8. Procedures Responsible for Biliary Stricture in 958 Patients, 1940–1965

PROCEDURE	NUMBER OF PATIENTS
Surgical trauma	929 (97%)
Biliary tract surgery	918
Gastric surgery	9
Pancreatic surgery	2
Nonsurgical causes	29 (3%)
Inflammatory obstruction	15
Congenital	5
Erosion by gallstones	3
External blunt trauma	2
Other	4

(Warren KW et al: Management of strictures of the biliary tract. Surg Clin North Am 51:711, 1971)

TABLE 42-9. Recognizable Causes of Biliary Stricture in 310 of 958 Patients, 1940–1965

CAUSE	NUMBER OF PATIENTS
Known duct injury	141
Massive bleeding	58
Difficult cholecystectomy	37
Ligature found on duct at reoperation	35
Difficult gastrectomy	8
Miscellaneous causes, including strictures that were unrelated to surgical trauma (listed in Table 44-8)	31
Total	310

(Warren KW et al: Management of strictures of the biliary tract. Surg Clin North Am 51:711, 1971)

TABLE 42-10. Site of Stricture in 958 Patients, 1940–1965

SITE	NUMBER OF PATIENTS
Common hepatic ducts	379
Common hepatic and common bile duct	265
Common bile duct, including 14 in distal common bile duct	217
Bifurcation of hepatic ducts	59
Individual hepatic ducts only	38
Right	27
Left	11
Total	958

(Warren KW et al: Management of strictures of the biliary tract. Surg Clin North Am 51:711, 1971)

TABLE 42-11.   Clinical Features in 987 Patients with Biliary Stricture, 1940–1967

CLINICAL FEATURE	NUMBER OF PATIENTS	PERCENTAGE
Chills and fever	632	64.0
Abdominal pain	482	48.8
Jaundice and pruritus	433	43.9
Hepatomegaly	369	37.4
External fistula	237	24.0
Portal hypertension	189	19.1
Hepatomegaly and splenomegaly	76	7.7
Splenomegaly	45	4.6
Ascites	24	2.4
None	9	0.9

arouses suspicion that the common bile duct or common hepatic duct has been ligated accidentally. A common presentation of bile duct injury is excessive discharge of bile either through the drain or through the abdominal incision. This biliary discharge may stop temporarily, followed by the onset of jaundice in the patient. The fistula may then reopen with relief of jaundice. This cycle of alternating jaundice and bile discharge may continue. Sometimes the patient may present with a collection of infected bile in the subhepatic space; on drainage of this collection, a biliary fistula develops. Rarely, a spontaneous internal fistula may occur between the bile duct and the duodenum through an abscess cavity. Unfortunately, this does not result in spontaneous cure. Indeed, more often than not, cholangitis supervenes. Associated biliary sludge and calculi are often found within the damaged common bile duct. However, cholangitis may delay its appearance for a considerable time after bile duct injury. Finally, the patient may present with bile ascites.

In a study of traumatic bile duct strictures, Norcross and Dadey[157] found that cholangitis developed in 400 pa-

tients and biliary cirrhosis in one fourth. Sedgwick and Hume[197] noted a 19% incidence of portal hypertension in those with long-standing strictures.

Table 42-11 summarizes the clinical features in 987 patients with biliary strictures. Pain, fever, and jaundice dominate the clinical manifestations. The laboratory findings in these patients are summarized in Table 42-12.

Management

The most important aspect of the management of bile duct injuries is their prevention. Certain principles of safe biliary surgery are worth restating here.

1. Good anesthesia and good illumination of the operative field are vital.
2. Without proper placement of an incision of adequate size, exposure will be compromised.
3. Careful and precise control of bleeding is essential. Blind or hasty clamping of structures in this region to control hemorrhage rapidly only predisposes to bile duct injury.
4. Adequate exposure and clear identification of all important structures in the operative field is essential.
5. No ligation, clamping, or cutting of any tubular structures should be undertaken without first identifying the common bile duct, common hepatic duct, cystic duct, and cystic artery.
6. In circumstances in which the anatomy is distorted and difficult to recognize, cannulation of the bile duct with an appropriate-sized metal dilator permits dissection to proceed while the extrahepatic ducts are guarded (Fig. 42-18).
7. The willingness to perform a simpler, safer procedure, such as cholecystostomy, instead of cholecystectomy in the presence of difficulties is prudent, not cowardly.
8. Removal of every millimeter of a normal cystic duct is unnecessary.
9. The physically or mentally fatigued surgeon and his team are more prone to err than their rested counterparts.

TABLE 42-12.   Laboratory Investigations on Presentation of 987 Patients with Biliary Stricture at the Lahey Clinic, 1940–1967

LABORATORY STUDY	NUMBER OF PATIENTS	PERCENTAGE
Bilirubinemia (>1.5 mg/dl)	551	55.8
Elevated alkaline phosphatase (>7 Bodansky units)	486	49.1
Anemia (hemoglobin, <12 g/dl)	329	33.3
Low serum albumin (<3.5 g/dl)	242	24.5
Leukocytosis (>10,000)	227	23.0
Elevated flocculation tests	113	11.4
Low total serum protein (<5.4 g/dl)	98	9.9
Low prothrombin level (<60%)	75	7.5
Leukopenia (<5000)	66	6.7

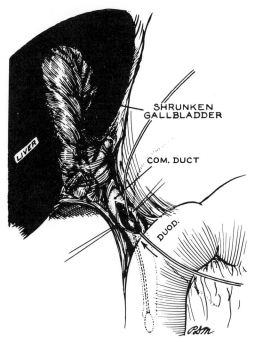

Fig. 42-18. Insertion of a Bakes' dilator in the common bile duct to protect the duct from injury during difficult cholecystectomy.

Appreciation of these principles appears to have resulted in a decline in the incidence of common bile duct injury over the last decade or two. Unfortunately, as long as operations on the gallbladder and bile ducts are carried out, bile duct injuries will continue to remain a risk of the procedure (Fig. 42-19).

A major injury to a bile duct is usually suggested by the onset of jaundice, biliary fistula, or cholangitis; when it is recognized, investigations should be performed to delineate the extent of the injury and to prepare the patient for a possible operation. Depending on the circumstances, good anatomic definition may be obtained by various radiographic procedures. Percutaneous transhepatic cholangiography is probably the single most useful investigation in this situation unless the patient has a T tube or a biliary fistula through which satisfactory cholangiography can be performed.

Careful preoperative preparation of the patient with special attention to control of sepsis, correction of any bleeding dyscrasia, restoration of fluid and electrolyte balance, and support of the nutritional state will help to minimize the appreciable mortality and morbidity associated with the operation for the repair of bile duct injuries. A period of percutaneous transhepatic bile drainage may be helpful in the preoperative preparation of severely jaundiced and debilitated patients.[146,170]

It is now universally accepted that the best chance of successful repair is at the first attempt; the success rate decreases with each subsequent reoperation. Since this is one of the most difficult areas of modern surgery, the operation should be performed by surgeons with specialized knowledge and skill. It is essential for the surgeon to have the ability to assess accurately the nature of injury and complicating factors and the technical expertise to effect a repair with a high chance of success.

A severed bile duct recognized at the time of operation should be reconstructed with fine sutures. A stent should be placed across the anastomosis and left in place for at least 3 months.

In patients with bile duct injury recognized in the postoperative period, the timing of operation depends largely on the effects of the injury. Uncontrolled sepsis needs to be drained and progressive jaundice relieved by early operation. In patients with a biliary fistula, particularly those in whom drainage of bile is adequate, operation may be

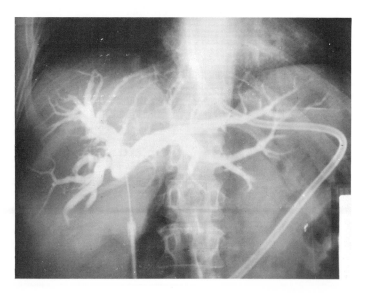

Fig. 42-19. Traumatic stricture of the common hepatic duct.

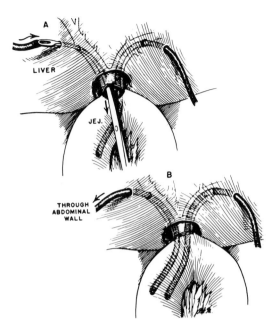

Fig. 42-20. Use of a transhepatic straight rubber tube stent for high hepaticojejunostomy anastomosis.

postponed until the inflammatory reaction has subsided in 6 to 12 weeks.

The types of repair used depend on the nature of the injury; they include choledochal end-to-end anastomosis and plastic repair (unfortunately, seldom possible) and biliary enteric bypass. Roux-en-Y choledochojejunostomy or hepaticojejunostomy[23] has met with success, as has a mucosal graft technique described by Smith,[201,242] particularly appropriate for difficult high strictures. At times, it may be necessary to cut into the liver substance to reach a sizable bile duct. A precise, tension-free anastomosis using unscarred tissue is essential for a successful outcome.[239] As already stated, a period of stenting is helpful in biliary enteric anastomoses (Fig. 42-20); straight, T,

transhepatic U, and modified Cattell Y tubes have been used with success.[32,234]

Both radiologists and endoscopists are attempting to treat bile duct strictures by nonsurgical approaches. Access to the stricture is obtained endoscopically or percutaneously. The strictures are then subjected to dilatation with or without the placement of an endoprosthesis. The role of these new approaches awaits evaluation.

Prognosis

In view of the poor general condition of the patient and the difficulty and magnitude of the operation, repair of biliary strictures is associated with significant operative mortality (13%) and morbidity (25%). The outcome of operative treatment is summarized in Table 42-13. The factors influencing this outcome are the quality of the proximal bile ducts, the presence or absence of inflammation in the area, the number of previous attempts at repair, the presence or absence of liver damage and portal hypertension, and the experience and skill of the surgeon in choosing and performing the most appropriate operation.

The most frequent cause of death is hepatic failure (23.5%) due to associated biliary cirrhosis secondary to prolonged biliary obstruction. Hemorrhage is also an important cause of death (13%); it may occur from the gastrointestinal tract or from the operative site, and it reflects the presence of advanced liver disease with associated abnormality in the coagulation mechanism. The causes of death are summarized in Table 42-14. Nonfatal complications in this series are summarized in Table 42-15. Despite the use of antibiotics, sepsis remains a major problem.

EPITHELIAL TUMORS

Benign Tumors of the Gallbladder

Benign neoplasms of the gallbladder are rare. Kane and co-workers[108] reported eight cases gathered from 42,500

TABLE 42-13. Outcome of Surgical Repair of Biliary Stricture from 1554 Operations in 987 Patients, 1940–1967

RESULT	NUMBER OF PATIENTS	PERCENTAGE	
Excellent	513	52	} 78 Satisfactory
Good	258	26	
Poor	43	4	} 17 Unsatisfactory
Died	132	13	
Lost to follow-up	41	4	

(Warren KW et al: Management of strictures of the biliary tract. Surg Clin North Am 51:711, 1971)

TABLE 42-14. Postoperative Mortality in 987 Patients Treated for Biliary Stricture, 1940–1967

CAUSE	NUMBER OF PATIENTS	PERCENTAGE
Hepatic failure	31	23.5
Hemorrhage	17	12.9
Myocardial infarction	15	11.4
Subphrenic abscess	2 ⎫	
Subhepatic abscess	4 ⎬	9.0
Septicemia	6 ⎭	
Renal failure	12	9.0
Pneumonia	11	8.3
Pancreatitis	9	6.8
Cerebrovascular accident	8	6.0
Other	17	12.9
Total	132	

(Warren KW et al: Management of strictures of the biliary tract. Surg Clin North Am 51:711, 1971)

new patients in whom 2000 cholecystectomies were performed. The only two important forms of benign epithelial tumors are papilloma and adenoma. Papillomas may be single or multiple, sessile or pedunculated, and are usually smaller than 0.5 cm in diameter. Associated gallstones occur in 70% of the patients. Adenomas tend to occur in the infundibulum of the gallbladder where most of the mucous glands are normally situated. These soft reddish sessile tumors usually appear on cholecystography as fixed flat elevations. Gallstones occur in about 50% of the patients. Malignant transformation is extremely rare in both types of tumors. Other exceedingly rare benign gallbladder tumors include leiomyoma, lipoma, myxoma, and fibroma.

TABLE 42-15. Nonfatal Morbidity in 987 Patients Treated for Biliary Stricture in 1553 Operations, 1940–1967

CAUSE	NUMBER OF PATIENTS	PERCENTAGE
Subphrenic abscess	17 ⎫	
Subhepatic abscess	10 ⎬	41.0
Septicemia	55 ⎪	
Wound infection	79 ⎭	
Biliary fistula	45	11.5
Bleeding	41	10.5
Hepatic failure	20	5.1
Pneumonia	19	4.8
Pancreatitis	18	4.6
Urinary tract infection	15	3.8
Wound dehiscence	14	3.6
Myocardial infarction	11	2.8
Renal failure	9	2.3
Thrombophlebitis	9	2.3
Cerebrovascular accident	3	0.8
Other	27	6.9
Total	392	

(Warren KW et al: Management of strictures of the biliary tract. Surg Clin North Am 51:711, 1971)

Primary Carcinoma of the Gallbladder

Carcinoma of the gallbladder is the fifth most common alimentary tract cancer and the most common cancer of the biliary tract, accounting for more than 6500 deaths in the United States each year. About 1% of all surgically removed gallbladders and 4% of all gallbladders in a large random postmortem series have been found to be cancerous. Women outnumber men by a ratio of 3:1 or 4:1. The condition occurs with greatest frequency in the sixth and seventh decades of life; it is uncommon in patients younger than 50 years of age.[42,167,224,232] In countries such as the United States, Canada, and the United Kingdom, with an increased cholecystectomy rate, the mortality associated with gallbladder cancer is falling sharply.

Etiology

The cause of carcinoma of the gallbladder is unknown. Although gallstones are found in 60% to 90% of patients, no good evidence is available to implicate them. Neither is the malignant transformation of benign neoplasms an important factor. Chronic inflammation may have a causative role; the incidence of carcinoma in long-standing cholecystostomy is appreciable, and most cancerous gallbladders show evidence of chronic inflammation. No carcinogen in bile is strongly implicated in gallbladder cancer.

Administration of dimethylnitrosamine to hamsters was found to result in gallbladder carcinoma if the hamsters had previously been implanted with a cholesterol pellet. The hypothesis is that the gallbladder mucosa is damaged by the gallstone, thus making it more susceptible to the carcinogen. Diehl and Beral[67] conducted a case-control study on 81 patients with gallbladder cancer and found that persons with larger gallstones had an increased risk of cancer.

Pathology

Carcinoma of the gallbladder is an infiltrative lesion eventually involving the whole organ. Only in 10% of patients is the tumor limited to the fundus or the neck of the organ. Infiltration is such a feature of this tumor that by the time operation is undertaken, 80% of tumors have invaded the adjacent liver substance, and in half the patients, other structures of the porta hepatis are involved (Fig. 42-21). A massive plaque of malignant tissue is often seen at operation, obliterating the anatomic landmarks. The stomach, duodenum, omentum, hepatic flexure of the colon, right kidney, and even the anterior abdominal wall have all been infiltrated by this tumor. Lymph node metastasis and distant metastasis occur in about one third of patients. Histologically, 85% are adenocarcinomas; the remainder comprise, in order of frequency, undifferentiated carcinomas, squamous cell carcinomas, and adenoacanthomas.

Complications, such as acute cholecystitis, perforation of the gallbladder, malignant fistulous communication with adjacent organs, hemorrhage, obstructive jaundice,

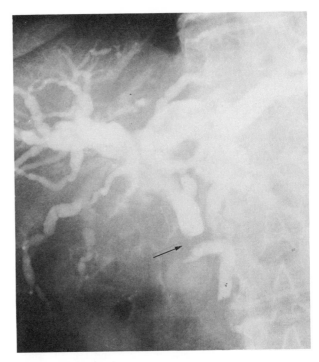

Fig. 42-21. Carcinoma of the gallbladder invading the common bile duct and causing obstructive jaundice.

portal vein compression, and gastric outlet obstruction, are relatively common.

Clinical Features

About one third of all patients have no symptoms referable to the gallbladder. The clinical features of patients with symptomatic disease are almost indistinguishable from those of patients with calculous disease. Pain is by far the most common presenting symptom, is usually intermittent, and is felt in the upper abdomen. Weight loss, anorexia, nausea, and vomiting are common associated complaints. About 50% of the patients present with jaundice, and about the same number have a palpable abdominal mass.

Jaundice denotes a poor prognosis because it signifies involvement of the porta hepatis or massive invasion of the liver. On occasion, carcinoma of the gallbladder presents with one or more of the other complications just listed, most frequently acute cholecystitis.

Radiographic studies are seldom helpful diagnostically; the most frequent finding is nonvisualization of the gallbladder on cholecystography. However, Polk[169] found a high incidence of carcinoma (25%) in the so-called porcelain gallbladder; therefore, a calcified gallbladder detected radiographically is an indication for surgical exploration. Ultrasound examination and percutaneous transhepatic cholangiography have been used, but tumors so diagnosed are usually beyond curative treatment.

Biochemical testing may show only mild nonspecific abnormal liver function. A raised alkaline phosphatase level is the most common finding and may be unassociated with the hyperbilirubinemia, which occurs in one third of patients.

Treatment and Prognosis

Carcinoma of the gallbladder is a highly lethal disease. The 5-year survival rate is 1% to 3%.[9] Surgical resection offers the only hope of cure, and this is possible only in about 23% of patients. Even in this relatively favorable group, the 5-year survival rate is limited to 10.6% of patients. The vast majority of patients die within 6 months of diagnosis. Best results are obtained in the group of patients whose tumors are discovered incidentally on examination of the specimen after cholecystectomy. Almost all the patients who have lived 5 years or more had only cholecystectomy. The decision to perform the sometimes advocated radical procedure of cholecystectomy with contiguous hepatic resection and regional lymphatic clearance must be made only after careful consideration of the high operative risks involved and the uncertain benefit to the patient's survival. It is not routinely recommended.

In the presence of jaundice, palliative biliary bypass or drainage should be attempted to relieve distressing symptoms.[99] Irradiation and chemotherapy have provided some measure of relief to only a few patients.[94,162,203,220]

Benign Tumors of the Bile Ducts

Benign bile duct tumors are exceedingly rare. Papillomas are the most common. They may be firm elevated masses or soft sessile growths or, rarely, pedunculated. They may be either solitary or multicentric and are scattered throughout the biliary tree. Mercadier and co-workers[141] have drawn attention to papillomatosis of bile ducts. In this condition, mucin-secreting papillomas appeared to have arisen in the intrahepatic ducts, and they have progressed relentlessly to involve other parts of the biliary tree. Numerous approaches have been proposed but are not effective for long. The prognosis is bleak. The second most common benign ductal tumor is the adenoma, which can be solid, cystic, or a mixture of both. Other benign neoplasms found are fibroma, lipoma, adenomyofibroma, and leiomyoma. All of these tumors can give rise to pain and produce obstructive jaundice. Malignant transformation is rare, although Cattell and associates[47] reported cases of papillomas of the bile ducts with focal carcinoma that eventually metastasized.

Primary Carcinoma of the Bile Ducts

Carcinoma of the bile duct accounts for 3% of all cancer deaths in the United States.[31,123,235] Men have a slight predominance over women. The highest frequency is in the sixth and seventh decades of life.

Etiology

The cause of bile duct carcinoma is unknown. Although the incidence of associated gallstones is 20% to 50%, no direct evidence exists to establish that gallstones cause ductal carcinoma. A few cases result from malignant transformation of papillomas of the bile duct. An association between ulcerative colitis and bile duct carcinoma has been reported.[175,186] In a series of 103 patients with proximal bile duct carcinoma treated at the Lahey Clinic,[187] 8 patients had associated ulcerative colitis. Interestingly, the age of these patients was 20 to 30 years lower than the median age of patients with ductal cancer.[186] In three patients, carcinoma developed several years after proctocolectomy for colonic disease. Patients with regional enterocolitis have also been found to have bile duct carcinoma. Furthermore, the incidence of malignant transformation in choledochal cysts,[25,221] Caroli's disease, and other cystic conditions of the bile ducts is appreciable. In the majority of patients, however, no etiologic factor is demonstrated. It has been postulated that bile acids are converted into carcinogenic agents, such as methylcholanthrene, which exert their effects on the ductal elements to produce carcinoma. This hypothesis remains unsubstantiated. In a retrospective study of 82 patients with biliary carcinoma, Broden and Bengtsson[35] found a higher than expected prevalence of methyldopa therapy. It is postulated that carcinogenesis is related to electrophil-reactive metabolites of methyldopa.

Pathology

Akin to carcinoma of the gallbladder, bile duct carcinoma has a great tendency to infiltrate extensively in the submucosal plane. Sometimes the tumor is multicentric.[217] Not uncommonly, a localized stricture is formed that is indistinguishable from a benign one. At times, this stricturing may be multifocal or diffuse, mimicking closely sclerosing cholangitis.

Secondary effects of the tumor are important; obstruction of the bile duct gives rise to jaundice, obstruction of the cystic duct may result in a mucocele of the gallbladder or acute cholecystitis, and obstruction of the pancreatic duct may precipitate pancreatitis. It is by its secondary effects that carcinoma of the bile duct frequently manifests itself. By the time operation is performed, one third of all patients have lymph node metastasis, one third have involvement of liver and hilar structures, and one half of patients demonstrate nerve sheath invasion.

The histology is almost invariably adenocarcinoma with varying degrees of differentiation. Only occasionally is a squamous cell carcinoma or an adenoacanthoma found.

Clinical Features

The clinical features of 173 patients with carcinoma of the extrahepatic ducts seen at the Lahey clinic are shown in Table 42-16. The most common presentation is obstructive jaundice, which is usually progressive. Rarely, because of obstruction to the cystic duct, the patient may present with symptoms suggestive of cholecystitis.[31] Occasionally, when the tumor obstructs only a segmental hepatic duct, no jaundice is produced, but the obstruction can lead to proximal ductal infection and liver abscess formation.[31] Finally, bile duct carcinoma has been confused with sclerosing cholangitis.

Diagnosis

The main problems in the diagnosis of bile duct carcinoma are shared by other causes of cholestasis. Jaundice, pruritus, pale stools, and dark urine are often coupled with an obstructive pattern on liver function tests. Various radiographic investigations follow. Ultrasonography can yield useful information regarding the gallbladder, liver, bile ducts, and pancreas. The demonstration of ductal dilatation is particularly useful in separating surgical from nonsurgical causes of obstructive jaundice. Ultrasonography is now favored as the first investigation for the elucidation of obstructive jaundice. For better anatomic definition, it may be necessary to undertake percutaneous transhepatic cholangiography or endoscopic retrograde cholangiography.

Surgical exploration remains the principal method of diagnosis although it may still be impossible at operation to distinguish a benign from a malignant stricture and to distinguish the various forms of periampullary cancers. Even histologic diagnosis of biopsy specimens and intraluminal scrapings can be difficult.

Treatment

Carcinoma of the bile ducts carries a grave prognosis. Operation offers the only hope for cure as well as the best form of palliation. Four features warrant highlighting: (1) Mucosal spread may be extensive without any external signs. Resection should, therefore, be generous. The related problems of biliary reconstruction then ensue; (2) although the affected duct lumen may permit moderate-sized dilators to pass freely, obstructive jaundice may persist after operation. The exact reason for this phenomenon is unknown. It may have to do with the pliability of the ducts; (3) the presence of a collapsed gallbladder usually indicates a tumor above the choledochocystic junction, but a tumor below this junction may also produce collapse of the gallbladder[31]; and (4) histology of these tumors is often difficult to interpret. Intense stromal reaction can obscure malignant cells, resulting in a diagnosis of benign biliary stricture. Tissues for biopsy should be adequate in amount, taken from the most representative sites, and should include the submucosa. Occasionally, several biopsies need to be taken before the correct diagnosis is made. In difficult situations, cytologic examination of mucosal scrapings may reveal the true nature of the condition.

In general, tumors of the distal common bile duct are most amenable to resection by pancreaticoduodenectomy. A new trend is toward preserving the gastric antrum and pylorus to provide better alimentary function.

The main difficulty in this procedure is anastomosis of a soft nondilated pancreatic duct to the jejunum. When these low tumors cannot be resected, palliative biliary enteric bypass is usually possible. For tumors of the middle segment, resection is curative; cholecystectomy is advocated to prevent the complication of cystic duct obstruction. Palliation is usually effected by anastomosis of the jejunum to the hepatic bifurcation. Tumors of the upper segment are not often resectable. Palliation can be difficult, but Cameron and associates[41] described fairly good results with a more aggressive surgical approach than has heretofore been advocated. In their series, tumor resection with stenting was associated with a longer survival than was laparotomy or stenting procedures alone. When biliary enteric anastomosis cannot be achieved, intraductal dilation followed by placement of an indwelling tube can alleviate jaundice and pruritus in some patients (Fig. 42-22).[208] Extensive resection, including partial hepatectomy, has not substantially improved the overall survival of these patients but has contributed to operative mortality and morbidity.

Percutaneous or endoscopically placed tubal drainage of the biliary tract is becoming more common either for relief of obstruction preliminary to definitive surgery or as definitive treatment for unresectable tumors (or benign strictures). In either case, there are hazards as well as benefits. One report[63] suggests that endoscopic placement affords a decreased incidence of septic and hemorrhagic complications.

Thus far, no trial has compared catheter drainage with surgical treatment. Infections introduced by the catheter, hemorrhage, and perforation are serious complications. However, there is a role for these techniques, particularly in patients who are not candidates for surgery.

Conroy and associates[61] and Fletcher[80] described internal radiotherapy of bile duct carcinomas with iridium or radium-bearing percutaneous transhepatic catheters.

TABLE 42-16. Clinical Features of 173 Patients with Extrahepatic Bile Duct Carcinoma

SYMPTOMS AND SIGNS	PERCENTAGE
SYMPTOMS	
Upper abdominal pain	57
Weight loss	46
Pruritus	31
Chills and fever	12
SIGNS	
Jaundice	82
Palpable liver	37
Abdominal mass	10
Palpable spleen	5

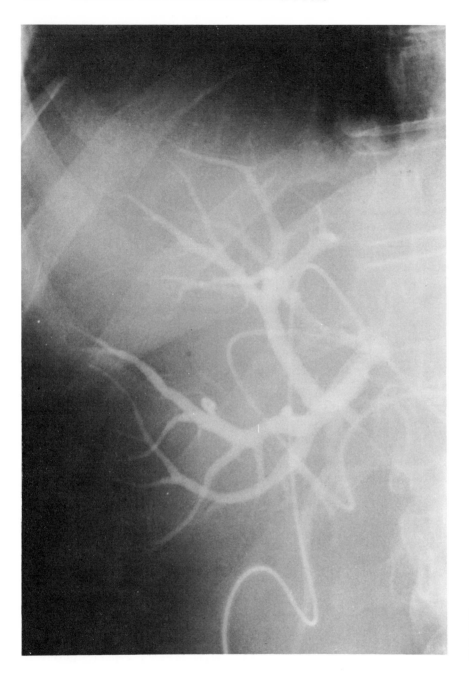

Fig. 42-22. Transhepatic U tubes in palliative treatment for ductal carcinoma of the hepatic bifurcation.

Prognosis

The overall 5-year survival rate is only 5%. In contrast, in tumors of the distal common bile duct, a 25% 5-year survival rate has been achieved with pancreaticoduodenectomy. The operative mortality rate for this procedure is about 10%.

Of all patients with more proximal lesions of the bile duct, 20% died in the postoperative period. Length of survival is determined by the degree of tumor differentiation. With well-differentiated lesions, even when only palliative measures are possible, survival for up to 4 years is not rare. This has been especially true of sclerosing carcinoma of the hepatic ducts as reported by Altemeier and Culbertson.[5]

Death commonly occurs as a result of unrelieved ductal obstruction complicated by sepsis.

MISCELLANEOUS CONDITIONS

Postcholecystectomy Symptoms

Removal of the gallbladder *per se* does not give rise to any specific syndrome in the same sense that gastric resection results in postgastrectomy syndromes. However, about 10% of patients return with symptoms. Most of these are of a trivial nature, but in a small number of patients, they may be sufficiently serious to necessitate a second operation.

When a patient returns with symptoms after cholecystectomy, three groups of conditions should be considered.[26,78] First, the symptoms for which cholecystectomy was performed may not have originated from the gallbladder, even if the organ was found to be diseased. Reflux esophagitis, peptic ulceration, pancreatitis, chronic liver disease, affectations of the right kidney, and some disorders of the small and large intestines have all been treated erroneously by removal of an incidentally diseased gallbladder. It is no wonder, therefore, that such patients return with persistence of preoperative symptoms. The importance of excluding all these lesions by careful clinical, laboratory, radiographic, endoscopic, and operative assessment cannot be overemphasized.

The second group of conditions that may contribute to postcholecystectomy symptoms are the complications of any intra-abdominal operation, such as wound hematoma, infection, occult partial wound dehiscence, adhesions, and intra-abdominal abscesses.

The third group of conditions is much more serious in that operative treatment may be required. In 1960, Cattell and Braasch[46] collected 158 patients who had secondary biliary operations at the Lahey Clinic that year; 87 were for benign biliary strictures, 34 for fibrosis of the sphincter of Oddi with or without common duct stones, 15 for common duct stones without biliary tract obstruction, 6 for removal of retained cystic duct stump or segments of the gallbladder, and 16 for such other conditions as biliary fistula.

Problems relating to bile duct strictures, biliary fistulas, and choledocholithiasis have been discussed in the relevant sections of this chapter.

Fibrosis of the sphincter of Oddi is a chronic inflammatory condition that is usually secondary to a stone in the distal common bile duct or to operative manipulation. Sometimes the cause is not obvious. Such idiopathic cases are thought to be the result of a calculus that has passed through the sphincter, damaging it during transit.

Fibrosis of the sphincter of Oddi is, in many ways, a benign bile duct stricture; the duct is markedly narrowed so that a No. 3 Bakes dilator cannot pass. Histologically, chronic inflammation is present, sometimes with muscular hypertrophy. Obstructive jaundice and cholangitis, as in bile duct strictures, are two serious consequences of fibrosis of the sphincter of Oddi. Fortunately, these complications are rarely florid. Most patients complain of intermittent or constant pain of varying severity. Jaundice and fever are not common.

The diagnosis is suspected on the basis of the history and an obstructive pattern of liver function tests. Endoscopic retrograde cholangiopancreatography is the single most useful study for the investigation of postcholecystectomy pain, especially when sphincteric dysfunction is suspected. It also has the advantage of revealing coincidental pancreatic, gastroduodenal, and biliary disorders as well as effecting treatment by endoscopic sphincterotomy.

Results are more likely to be favorable when stones are found within the bile duct. Of 100 consecutive cases reported by Cattell and co-workers,[48] results were excellent in 83, improved in 9, and poor in 8. Sphincteric tissues should be studied by biopsy in all patients with sphincteric obstruction to rule out the presence of malignant disease.

Cystic Duct and Gallbladder Remnants

In the absence of gallstones, cystic duct and small gallbladder remnants[78] probably do not give rise to any symptoms. In fact, McClenahan and associates[136] found that a cystic duct stump was visible radiographically more often in patients without symptoms than in persons who complained of pain. Therefore, an operation for postcholecystectomy symptoms should not be performed just because such a remnant has been demonstrated. However, gallbladder remnants and large cystic duct stumps are capable of harboring stones. When this occurs, operation is indicated because symptoms and complications can be expected in at least half of such patients. Glenn and McSherry[85] found common duct stones in 22 of 44 patients with cystic duct remnants. Although it is desirable not to leave behind a cystic duct stump or a gallbladder remnant during cholecystectomy, this may be impossible to achieve when dissection is difficult. In these circumstances, it is far better to leave behind a stump than to injure the common bile duct.

Other Conditions

Although cystic duct neuromas have been implicated in postcholecystectomy pain, no good evidence supports this contention. Postoperative biliary dyskinesia is another diagnosis that cannot be advanced with confidence. Even if it is possible to demonstrate abnormalities of biliary dynamics by such means as cinecholecystography, radiomanometry, and operative manometry, it is difficult to relate the abnormality to symptomatology and even more difficult to devise an operation in which the biliary kinetics would not be disturbed further. Perhaps with better understanding of the physiology of biliary motility patterns in the future we will be able to put more meaningful interpretations on abnormal pressure recordings in these patients.

Cholesterolosis

Cholesterolosis is characterized by an accumulation of cholesterol esters in the mucosa and submucosa of the gallbladder. Much of the cholesterol is housed in histiocytes, giving them a foamy appearance. Aggregates of these foamy cells lie on the top of mucosal ridges and are visible to the naked eye as yellowish pinpoint spots. When these spots are diffusely distributed over the mucosa, they simulate the surface of a strawberry, hence the term "strawberry gallbladder." However, the spots may cluster and coalesce into a lobulated polypoid lesion. These cholesterol polyps may break off and become a nidus for gallstone formation or even cause obstructive symptoms. However, many polyps are likely to be missed on radiography.

The therapeutic approach to cholesterolosis is controversial. Asymptomatic patients are best left alone. Those with distressing symptoms suggestive of biliary colic are pressing candidates for cholecystectomy. Preoperative examination of duodenal aspirate for cholesterol crystals is gaining some popularity in suspected cases in which the findings on oral cholecystography are normal. The result of operative treatment is variable. The efficacy of chenodeoxycholic acid and similar substances in the treatment of cholesterolosis awaits further investigation.

Adenomyomatosis (Hyperplastic Gallbladder)

Adenomyomatosis denotes three types of hyperplastic change in the gallbladder: overgrowth of the mucous membrane, thickening of the muscle coat, and intramural diverticular formation known as Rokitansky–Aschoff sinuses.

These changes may involve a small localized area or a segment of the gallbladder or they may affect the whole organ. In the diffuse type of adenomyomatosis, the overgrowth of mucosa gives a thickened rugged pattern to the luminal surface. This is accompanied by an intramural diverticular formation, which on cross-section displays a glandlike structure. This appearance gives rise to the name "cholecystitis glandularis proliferans." Often no inflammatory or neoplastic change is seen. The main features are those of mucosal and muscular hypertrophy; the muscle coat may be five times thicker than normal. Microscopically, some of the diverticula may contain inspissated bile or even intramural calculi, which may erode through the mucosa to become free in the gallbladder cavity or erode through serosa, causing perforation of the gallbladder. The cause of muscular and mucosal hypertrophy is unknown, although increased intraluminal pressure has been implicated.

In the segmental or annular type of adenomyomatosis the gallbladder displays an hourglass deformity surrounded by muscular hypertrophy and intramural diverticula. Sometimes the narrowing may cause a functional obstruction to the distal lobule of the gallbladder and thereby give rise to biliary pain; it may predispose the patient to gallstone formation in the distal lobule. The base of mucosal septa, such as those producing the phrygian cap, fish-hook anomaly of the gallbladder, and the pars spiralis of the cystic duct, are areas that are predisposed to adenomyomatosis. The most common variant of adenomyomatosis is a localized form called adenomyoma. In this condition, hyperplastic changes take the form of a nodular bulge protruding into the gallbladder lumen. Characteristically, adenomyoma occurs in the fundus of the gallbladder. It may be confused with a gallstone on cholecystography, although its fixation to the gallbladder wall despite a postural change is a diagnostic feature.

There is no specific medical treatment for adenomyomatosis of the gallbladder, and no treatment of any type seems necessary when this condition is detected in asymptomatic patients. However, the role of surgery in those patients who have pain suggestive of gallbladder disease but in whom no other pathology is found is controversial. No large reports have been published to give an authoritative answer to this question.

Surgery can be recommended with confidence for patients who have associated gallbladder calculi and for those in whom obstruction of the distal lobule of the gallbladder by a stricture can be demonstrated with cholecystokinin cholecystography. For all other patients, the decision to perform surgery should be based on the merits of each individual case and made with circumspection.

Cystic Duct Syndrome

Cystic duct syndrome is caused by a partial obstruction of the cystic duct, resulting in a biliary type of pain when the gallbladder contracts. The diagnosis is made by cholecystokinin cholecystography, which shows poor emptying of the gallbladder and reproduces the patient's pain.

A variety of structural abnormalities producing partial obstruction of the cystic duct, such as external bands, kinking, and localized stenosis, have been identified. The syndrome may be caused by a small gallstone in the cystic duct. Not uncommonly, the cystic duct syndrome is associated with chronic cholecystitis and adenomyomatosis. These three conditions appear to be related pathogenetically.

The treatment of patients with proved cystic duct syndrome is cholecystectomy. The reported results[89] are good.

REFERENCES

1. Acosta JM, Ledesma CL: Gallstone migration as a cause of acute pancreatitis. N Engl J Med 290:484, 1974
2. Admirand WH, Small DM: The physiochemical basis of cholesterol gallstone formation in man. J Clin Invest 47: 1043, 1968
3. Allen BL et al: Chemical dissolution of bile duct stones. World J Surg 2:429, 1978
4. Alonso–Lej F et al: Congenital choledochal cyst, with a

report of 2, and an analysis of 94, cases (abstr). Surg Gynecol Obstet 108:1, 1959

5. Altemeier WA, Culbertson WR: Sclerosing carcinoma of the hepatic bile ducts. Surg Clin North Am 53:1229, 1973

6. Amdrup BM, Griffith CA: The effects of vagotomy upon biliary function in dogs. J Surg Res 10:209, 1970

7. Amer MS: Cyclic guanosine 3',5'-monophosphate and gallbladder contraction. Gastroenterology 67:333, 1974

8. Anderson A et al: Acalculous cholecystitis. Am J Surg 122:2, 1971

9. Appleman RM et al: Long term survival in carcinoma of the gallbladder. Surg Gynecol Obstet 117:459, 1963

10. Aronsohn HG, Andrews E: Experimental cholecystitis. Surg Gynecol Obstet 66:748, 1938

11. Ashizawa S et al: A clinical study of gallstone dissolution with ursodeoxycholic acid: A controlled double blind trial. Igaku no Ayumi 101:922, 1977

12. Atkinson AJ, Carroll WW: Sclerosing cholangitis: Association with regional enteritis. JAMA 188:183, 1964

13. Banfield WJ: Physiology of the gallbladder. Gastroenterology 69:770, 1975

14. Bangaru B et al: Comparative studies of biliary atresia in the human newborn and reovirus-induced cholangitis in weanling mice. Lab Invest 43:456, 1980

15. Barker DJ et al: Prevalence of gall stones at necropsy in nine British towns: A collaborative study. Br Med J 2:1389, 1979

16. Becker WF et al: A clinical study of 1,060 patients with acute cholecystitis. Surg Gynecol Obstet 104:491, 1957

17. Bell GA, Holubitsky IB: Acute cholecystitis following unrelated surgery. Can Med Assoc J 101:94, 1969

18. Bennion LJ, Grundy SM: Risk factors for the development of cholelithiasis in man (Part II). N Engl J Med 299:1221, 1978

19. Bennion LJ et al: A biochemical basis for the high prevalence of cholesterol gallstones in women. Clin Res 26:496A, 1978

20. Benson EA, Page RE: A practical reappraisal of the anatomy of the extrahepatic bile ducts and arteries. Br J Surg 63:853, 1976

21. Berci G et al: Choledochoscopy and operative fluorocholangiography in the prevention of retained bile duct stones. World J Surg 2:411, 1978

22. Berliner SD, Burson LC: One-stage repair for cholecystduodenal fistula and gallstone ileus. Arch Surg 90:313, 1965

23. Bismuth H et al: Long term results of Roux-en-Y hepaticojejunostomy. Surg Gynecol Obstet 146:161, 1978

24. Biss K et al: Some unique biologic characteristics of the Masai of East Africa. N Engl J Med 284:694, 1971

25. Bloustein PA: Association of carcinoma with congenital cystic conditions of the liver and bile ducts. Am J Gastroenterol 67:40, 1977

26. Blumgart L et al: Diagnosis and management of postcholecystectomy symptoms: The place of endoscopy and retrograde choledochopancreatography. Br J Surg 64:809, 1977

27. Bouchier IA: Postmortem study of the frequency of gallstones in patients with cirrhosis of the liver. Gut 10:705, 1969

28. Boyd DP: Bronchobiliary and bronchopleural fistulas. Ann Thorac Surg 24:481, 1977

29. Boyden EA: The anatomy of the choledochoduodenal junction in man. Surg Gynecol Obstet 104:641, 1957

30. Braasch JW: Congenital anomalies of the gallbladder and bile ducts. Surg Clin North Am 38:627, 1958

31. Braasch JW: Carcinoma of the bile duct. Surg Clin North Am 53:1217, 1973

32. Braasch JW et al: Progress in biliary stricture repair. Am J Surg 129:34, 1975

33. Braasch JW et al: Acute cholecystitis. Surg Clin North Am 44:707, 1964

34. Brockis JG, Gilbert MC: Intestinal obstruction by gallstones: A review of 179 cases. Br J Surg 44:461, 1957

35. Broden G, Bengtsson L: Biliary carcinoma associated with methyldopa therapy. Acta Chir Scand (suppl) 500:7, 1980

36. Brooke BN et al: A study of liver disorder in ulcerative colitis. Postgrad Med J 37:245, 1961

37. Bullard RW Jr: Subcutaneous or extraperitoneal gallbladder (report of unusual case). JAMA 129:949, 1945

38. Burhenne HJ: Nonoperative instrument extraction of retained bile duct stones. World J Surg 2:439, 1978

39. Burhenne HJ: Percutaneous extraction of retained biliary tract stones: 661 patients. AJR 134:888, 1980

40. Cain JL et al: Bile peritonitis in germ-free dogs. Gastroenterology 53:600, 1967

41. Cameron JL et al: Proximal bile duct tumors: Surgical management with Silastic transhepatic biliary stents. Ann Surg 196:412, 1979

42. Carmo MD et al: Natural history study of gallbladder cancer: A review of 36 years experience at M. D. Anderson Hospital and Tumor Institute. Cancer 42:330, 1978

43. Caroli J: Diseases of intrahepatic bile ducts. Israel J Med Sci 4:21, 1968

44. Cass MH et al: Electrolyte losses with biliary fistula: Postcholedochostomy acidotic syndrome. Med J Aust 1:165–169, 1955

45. Cattell RB, Braasch JW: General considerations in the management of benign strictures of the bile duct. N Engl J Med 261:929, 1959

46. Cattell RB, Braasch JW: Management of patients with unsatisfactory results after cholecystectomy. Can Med Assoc J 83:987, 1960

47. Cattell RB et al: Polypoid epithelial tumors of the bile ducts. N Engl J Med 266:57, 1962

48. Cattell RB et al: Stenosis of the sphincter of Oddi. N Engl J Med 256:429, 1957

49. Cello JP: Cholestasis in ulcerative colitis: Long term complications and medical therapy. Gastroenterology 73:372, 1977

50. Chapman RW et al: Primary sclerosing cholangitis: A review of its clinical features, cholangiography, and hepatic histology. Gut 21:870, 1980

51. Chen MF et al: Experience with and complications of postoperative choledochofiberoscopy for retained biliary stones. Acta Chir Scand 148:503, 1982

52. Chou ST, Chan CW: Recurrent pyogenic cholangitis: A necropsy study. Pathology 12:415, 1980

53. Classen M, Demling L: Endoskopische Sphinkterotomie der Papilla Vateri und Steinextraktion aus dem Ductus choledochus. Dtsch Med Wochenschr 99:496, 1974

54. Classen M, Safrany L: Endoscopic papillotomy and removal of gall stones. Br Med J 4:371, 1975

55. Cleve EA, Correa JL: Bronchobiliary fistulas secondary to amebic abscess of liver. Gastroenterology 34:320, 1958

56. Cohen S et al: Liver disease and gallstones in regional enteritis. Gastroenterology 60:237, 1971

57. Colcock BP, McManus JE: Experiences with 1,356 cases

of cholecystitis and choledocholithiasis. Surg Gynecol Obstet 101:161, 1955

58. Colcock BP et al: The asymptomatic patient with gallstones. Am J Surg 113:44, 1967
59. Comfort MW et al: Silent gallstone: 10 to 20 year follow-up study of 112 cases. Ann Surg 128:931, 1948
60. Conn JH et al: Bile peritonitis: An experimental and clinical study. Am Surg 36:219, 1970
61. Conroy RM et al: A new method for treating carcinomatous biliary obstruction with intracatheter radium. Cancer 49:1321, 1982
62. Cotton PB: ERCP. Gut 18:316, 1977
63. Cotton PB: Duodenoscopic placement of biliary prostheses to relieve malignant obstructive jaundice. Br J Surg 69:501, 1982
64. Cotton PB, Vallon AG: British experience with duodenoscopic splenectomy for removal of bile duct stones. Br J Surg 68:373, 1981
65. Danzinger RG et al: Lithogenic bile in siblings of young women with cholelithiasis. Mayo Clin Proc 47:762, 1972
66. Deziel DJ et al: Cystic disease of the bile ducts: Surgical management and reoperation. Probl Gen Surg 2:467, 1985
67. Diehl AK, Beral V: Cholecystectomy and changing mortality from gallbladder cancer. Lancet 2:187, 1981
68. Dineern P: The importance of the route of infection in experimental biliary tract obstruction. Surg Gynecol Obstet 119:1001, 1964
69. Donaldson RM Jr: Editorial: Advice for the patient with "silent" gallstones. N Engl J Med 307:815, 1982
70. Dowling RH: Advances in the medical treatment of gallstones. In Harper PS, Muir JR (eds): Advanced Medicine, p 202, Kent, Sir Isaac Pitman & Sons, 1979
71. DuPriest RW Jr et al: Acute cholecystitis complicating trauma. Ann Surg 189:84, 1979
72. Editorial: Radiography in the diagnosis of acute cholecystitis. Lancet 2:457, 1978
73. Einarsson K et al: Gallbladder disease in hyperlipoproteinaemia. Lancet 1:484, 1975
74. Ericsson NO, Rudhe U: Spontaneous perforation of the bile ducts in infants: Presentation of a case and review of literature. Acta Chir Scand 118:439, 1960
75. Federle MP et al: Recurrent pyogenic cholangitis in Asian immigrants: Use of ultrasonography, computed tomography, and cholangiography. Radiology 143:151, 1982
76. Fee HJ et al: Sclerosing cholangitis and primary biliary cirrhosis: A disease spectrum? Ann Surg 186:589, 1977
77. Feldman M: Choledochoduodenal fistula associated with a large gallstone in the stomach. Am J Gastroenterol 28:466, 1957
78. Feldman M: Postcholecystectomy syndrome, with special reference to cystic duct remnant. Gastroenterology 34:239, 1958
79. Flanigan PD: Biliary cysts. Ann Surg 182:635, 1975
80. Fletcher MS et al: Treatment of high bile duct carcinoma by internal radiotherapy with iridium-192 wire. Lancet 2:173, 1981
81. Gardner B et al: Factors influencing the timing of cholecystectomy in acute cholecystitis. Am J Surg 125:730, 1973
82. Glenn F: Cholecystostomy in the high risk patient with biliary tract disease. Ann Surg 185:185, 1977
83. Glenn F: Editorial: Silent gallstones. Ann Surg 193:251, 1981
84. Glenn F, Mannix H Jr: Acalculous gallbladder. Ann Surg 144:670, 1956

85. Glenn F, McSherry CK: Secondary abdominal operations for symptoms following biliary tract surgery. Surg Gynecol Obstet 121:979, 1965
86. Glenn F, Moody FG: Acute obstructive suppurative cholangitis. Surg Gynecol Obstet 113:265, 1961
87. Glenn F, Wantz GE: Acute cholecystitis following surgical treatment of unrelated diseases. Surg Gynecol Obstet 102:145, 1956
88. Glenn F et al: Biliary enteric fistula. Surg Gynecol Obstet 153:527, 1981
89. Goldstein F et al: Cholecystokinin cholecystography in the differential diagnosis of acalculous gallbladder disease. Am J Dig Dis 19:835, 1974
90. Gracie WA, Ransohoff DF: Editorial: The natural history of silent gallstones: The innocent gallstone is not a myth. N Engl J Med 307:798, 1982
91. Gray SW, Skandalakis JE: Embryology for Surgeons: The Embryological Basis for the Treatment of Congenital Defects. Philadelphia, WB Saunders, 1972
92. Gross RE: Congenital anomalies of gallbladder. Arch Surg 32:121, 1936
93. Gunn A et al: Acalculous gall-bladder disease. Br J Surg 60:213, 1973
94. Hanna SS, Rider WD: Carcinoma of the gallbladder or extrahepatic bile ducts: The role of radiotherapy. Can Med Assoc J 118:59, 1978
95. Heaton KW, Read AE: Association of gallstones with disorders of terminal ileum. Gut 10:414, 1969
96. Heaton KW, Read AE: Gall stones in patients with disorders of the terminal ileum and disturbed bile salt metabolism. Br Med J 3:494, 1969
97. Hegner CF: Gaseous pericholecystitis with cholecystitis and cholelithiasis. Arch Surg 22:993, 1931
98. Hesselfeldt P, Jess P: Gallstone ileus: Review of 39 cases with emphasis on surgical treatment. Acta Chir Scand 148:431, 1982
99. Hoevels J, Lunderquist A, Ihse I: Percutaneous transhepatic intubation of bile ducts for combined internal-external drainage in preoperative and palliative treatment of obstructive jaundice. Gastrointest Radiol 3:23, 1978
100. Hopton DS: The influence of the vagus nerves on the biliary system. Br J Surg 60:216, 1973
101. Huang T et al: The significance of biliary pressure in cholangitis. Arch Surg 98:629, 1969
102. Hutchings VZ et al: Choledochoduodenal fistula complicating duodenal ulcer: Report of 5 cases and review of literature. Arch Surg 73:598, 1956
103. Hutson DG et al: Balloon dilatation of biliary strictures through a choledochojejuno-cutaneous fistula. Ann Surg 199:637, 1984
104. Iser JH et al: Chenodeoxycholic acid treatment of gallstones: A follow-up report and analysis of factors influencing response to therapy. N Engl J Med 293:378, 1975
105. Javett SL: Azathioprine in primary sclerosing cholangitis. Lancet 1:810, 1971
106. Jonsson PE, Andersson A: Postoperative acute acalculous cholecystitis. Arch Surg 111:1097, 1976
107. Kakos GS et al: Operative cholangiography during routine cholecystectomy: A review of 3,012 cases. Arch Surg 104:484, 1972
108. Kane CF et al: Papilloma of gallbladder: Report of 8 cases. Am J Surg 83:161, 1952
109. Kelly TR: Gallstone pancreatitis: Pathophysiology. Surgery 80:488, 1976

110. Kelly TR et al: Alterations in gallstone solubility following distal ileal resection. Arch Surg 105:352, 1972

111. Knochel JP et al: External biliary fistula: Study of electrolyte derangements and secondary cardiovascular and renal abnormalities. Surgery 51:746, 1962

112. Koch H: Operative endoscopy. Gastrointest Endosc 24:65, 1977

113. Kozoll DD et al: Pathologic correlation of gallstones: A review of 1,847 autopsies of patients with gallstones. Arch Surg 79:514, 1959

114. Kramhöft J et al: Vagotomy and function of the gall-bladder. Scand J Gastroenterol 7:109, 1972

115. Lahey FH, Pyrtek JL: Experience with operative management of 280 strictures of bile ducts, with description of new method and complete follow-up study of end results in 229 of the cases. Surg Gynecol Obstet 91:25, 1950

116. Lahtinen J et al: Acute cholecystitis treated by early and delayed surgery: A controlled clinical trial. Scand J Gastroenterol 13:673, 1978

117. LaMorte WW et al: The role of the gallbladder in the pathogenesis of cholesterol gallstones. Gastroenterology 77:580, 1979

118. Large AM: Left-sided gallbladder and liver without situs inversus. Arch Surg 87:982, 1963

119. LaRusso NF et al: Primary sclerosing cholangitis. N Engl J Med 310:899, 1984

120. Lieber MM: The incidence of gallstones and their correlation with other diseases. Ann Surg 135:394, 1952

121. Lobingier AS: Gangrene of the gallbladder. Ann Surg 48:72, 1908

122. Longland CJ: Choledochoscopy in choledocholithiasis. Br J Surg 60:626, 1973

123. Longmire WP. Tumors of the extrahepatic biliary radicals. Curr Probl Cancer 1:1, 1976

124. Longmire WP: When is cholangitis sclerosing? Am J Surg 135:312, 1978

125. Longmire WP Jr et al: Congenital cystic disease of the liver and biliary system. Ann Surg 174:711, 1971

126. Ludwig J et al: Morphologic features of chronic hepatitis associated with primary sclerosing cholangitis or chronic ulcerative colitis. Hepatology 1:632, 1981

127. Lund J: Surgical indications in cholelithiasis: Prophylactic cholelithiasis: Prophylactic cholecystectomy elucidated on the basis of long-term follow-up on 526 nonoperated cases. Ann Surg 151:153, 1960

128. Lygidakis NJ: Surgery for acalculous cholecystitis: An organic and not a functional disease. Am J Gastroenterol 76:27, 1981

129. Lynn J et al: Effects of estrogen upon bile: Implications with respect to gallstone formation. Ann Surg 178:514, 1973

130. Maingot R: Postoperative strictures of the bile ducts: Causes, prevention, repair procedures. Br J Clin Pract 31:117, 1977

131. Malt RA: Experience with recurrent gallstone ileus applied to management of the first attack. Am J Surg 108:92, 1964

132. Matolo NM et al: Comparison of ultrasonography, computerized tomography, and radionuclide imaging in the diagnosis of acute and chronic cholecystitis. Am J Surg 144:676, 1982

133. Maton PN, Murphy GM, Dowling RH: Ursodeoxycholic acid treatment of gallstones: Dose-response study and possible mechanism of action. Lancet 2:1297, 1977

134. Mazzariello RM: A fourteen-year experience with nonoperative instrument extraction of retained bile duct stones. World J Surg 2:447, 1978

135. McArthur P et al: Controlled clinical trial comparing early with interval cholecystectomy for acute cholecystitis. Br J Surg 62:850, 1975

136. McClenahan JL et al: Intravenous cholangiography in postcholecystectomy syndrome. JAMA 159:1353, 1955

137. McCorkle H, Fong EE: Clinical significance of gas in the gallbladder. Surgery 11:851, 1942

138. McCubbrey D, Thieme ET: In defense of the conservative treatment for acute cholecystitis with an evaluation of the risk. Surgery 45:930, 1959

139. McPherson GA et al: Pre-operative percutaneous transhepatic biliary drainage: The results of a controlled trial. Br J Surg 71:371, 1984

140. Mentzer RM Jr et al: A comparative appraisal of emphysematous cholecystitis. Am J Surg 129:10, 1975

141. Mercadier M et al: Papillomatosis of the intrahepatic bile ducts. World J Surg 8:30, 1984

142. Merendino KA, Manhas DR: Man-made gallstones: A new entity following cardiac valve replacement. Ann Surg 177:694, 1973

143. Method HL et al: "Silent" gallstones. Arch Surg 85:338, 1962

144. Monroe SE: Congenital absence of the gallbladder: A statistical study. J Int Coll Surg 32:369, 1959

145. Morecki R et al: Biliary atresia and reovirus type 3 infection. N Engl J Med 307:481, 1982

146. Mori K et al: Percutaneous transhepatic bile drainage. Ann Surg 185:111, 1977

147. Mundth ED: Cholecystitis and diabetes mellitus. N Engl J Med 267:642, 1962

148. Munster AM et al: Acalculous cholecystitis in burned patients. Am J Surg 122:591, 1971

149. Myers RN et al: Primary sclerosing cholangitis: Complete gross and histologic reversal after long-term steroid therapy. Am J Gastroenterol 53:527, 1970

150. Nagase M et al: Present features of gallstones in Japan: A collective review of 2,144 cases. Am J Surg 135:788, 1978

151. Nakagawa S et al: Dissolution of cholesterol gallstones by ursodeoxycholic acid. Lancet 2:367, 1977

152. Nakayama F: Oral cholelitholysis: Cheno versus urso: Japanese experience. Dig Dis Sci 25:129, 1980

153. Nakayama F, Miyake H: Changing state of gallstone disease in Japan: Composition of the stones and treatment of the condition. Am J Surg 120:794, 1970

154. Nelson PA et al: Anomalous position of gall bladder within falciform ligament. Arch Surg 66:679, 1953

155. Newman HF, Northup JD: The autopsy incidence of gallstones. Surg Gynecol Obstet 109:1, 1959

156. Nicholas P et al: Increased incidence of cholelithiasis in Laënnec's cirrhosis: A postmortem evaluation of pathogenesis. Gastroenterology 63:112, 1972

157. Norcross JW, Dadey JL: Medical complications of operative bile-duct injuries. N Engl J Med 257:1216, 1957

158. Northover JM, Terblanche J: A new look at the arterial supply of the bile duct in man and its surgical implications. Br J Surg 66:379, 1979

159. O'Connor MJ et al: Cholangitis due to malignant obstruction of biliary outflow. Ann Surg 193:341, 1981

160. Ong GB: A study of recurrent pyogenic cholangitis. Arch Surg 84:199, 1962

161. Oparah SS, Mandal AK: Traumatic thoracobiliary (pleurobiliary and bronchobiliary) fistulas: Clinical and review study. J Trauma 18:539, 1978

162. Oswalt CE, Cruz AB: Effectiveness of chemotherapy in ad-

dition to surgery in treating carcinoma of the gallbladder. Rev Surg 34:436, 1977

163. Ottinger LW: Acute cholecystitis as a postoperative complication. Ann Surg 184:162, 1976

164. Paloyan D et al: The timing of biliary tract operations in patients with pancreatitis associated with gallstones. Surg Gynecol Obstet 141:737, 1975

165. Pertsemlidis D et al: Effects of clofibrate and of oral contraceptives on biliary lipid composition and bile acid kinetics in man (abstr). Gastroenterology 64:782, 1973

166. Petersen SR, Sheldon GF: Acute acalculous cholecystitis: A complication of hyperalimentation. Am J Surg 138:814, 1979

167. Piehler JM, Crichlow RW: Primary carcinoma of the gallbladder. Surg Gynecol Obstet 147:929, 1978

168. Pitt HA et al: Primary sclerosing cholangitis: Results of an aggressive surgical approach. Ann Surg 196:259, 1982

169. Polk HC Jr: Carcinoma and the calcified gall bladder. Gastroenterology 50:582, 1966

170. Pollock TW et al: Percutaneous decompression of benign and malignant biliary obstruction. Arch Surg 114:148, 1979

171. Price WH: Gall-bladder dyspepsia. Br Med J 2:138, 1963

172. Quigley EMM et al: Familial occurrence of primary sclerosing cholangitis and chronic ulcerative colitis. Gastroenterology 85:1160, 1983

173. Räf L, Spangen L: Gallstone ileus. Acta Chir Scand 137:665, 1971

174. Ralls PW et al: Prospective evaluation of ^{99m}Tc-IDA cholescintigraphy and gray-scale ultrasound in the diagnosis of acute cholecystitis. Radiology 144:369, 1982

175. Rankin JG et al: Liver in ulcerative colitis: Obstructive jaundice due to bile duct carcinoma. Gut 7:433, 1966

176. Record CO et al: Intrahepatic sclerosing cholangitis associated with a familial immunodeficiency syndrome. Lancet 2:18, 1973

177. Redinger RN, Small DM: Bile composition, bile salt metabolism and gallstones. Arch Intern Med 130:618, 1972

178. Reiter JJ et al: Results of endoscopic papillotomy: A collective experience from nine endoscopic centers in West Germany. World J Surg 2:505, 1978

179. Report from Boston Collaborative Drug Surveillance Program: Surgically confirmed gallbladder disease, venous thromboembolism, and breast tumors in relation to postmenopausal estrogen therapy. N Engl J Med 290:15, 1974

180. Roeder WJ et al: Triplication of the gallbladder with cholecystitis, cholelithiasis, and papillary adenocarcinoma. Am J Surg 121:746, 1971

181. Rosato EF et al: Bile ascites. Surg Gynecol Obstet 130:494, 1970

182. Roslyn JJ, Busuttil RW: Perforation of the gallbladder: A frequently mismanaged condition. Am J Surg 137:307, 1979

183. Roslyn JJ et al: Gallbladder disease in patients on long-term parenteral nutrition. Gastroenterology 84:148, 1983

184. Rosoff L, Meyers H: Acute emphysematous cholecystitis: An analysis of ten cases. Am J Surg 111:410, 1966

185. Rosoff L, Robbins FG: Operative treatment of acute cholecystitis. Surg Clin North Am 53:1079, 1973

186. Ross AP, Braasch JW: Ulcerative colitis and carcinoma of the proximal bile ducts. Gut 14:94, 1973

187. Ross AP et al: Carcinoma of the proximal bile ducts: Report of 103 cases. Surg Gynecol Obstet 136:923, 1973

188. Rudick J, Hutchison JS: Effects of vagal-nerve section on the biliary system. Lancet 1:579, 1964

189. Safrany L: Transduodenal endoscopic sphincterotomy and extraction of bile duct stones. World J Surg 2:457, 1978

190. Saharia PC, Cameron JL: Clinical management of acute cholangitis. Surg Gynecol Obstet 142:369, 1976

191. Sane SM et al: Congenital bronchobiliary fistula. Surgery 69:599, 1971

192. Sarles H et al: Diet and cholesterol gallstones: A study of 101 patients with cholelithiasis compared to 101 matched controls. Am J Dig Dis 14:531, 1969

193. Sarles H et al: The influence of caloric intake and of dietary protein on the bile lipids. Scand J Gastroenterol 6:189, 1971

194. Schoenfield LJ, Lachin JM: Chenodiol (chenodeoxycholic acid) for dissolution of gallstones: The National Cooperative Gallstone Study: A controlled trial of efficacy and safety. Ann Intern Med 95:257, 1981

195. Scott AJ, Khan GA: Origin of bacteria in bile duct bile. Lancet 2:790, 1967

196. Screibman PH et al: Lithogenic bile: A consequence of weight reduction. J Clin Invest 53:72, 1974

197. Sedgwick CE, Hume A: Management of bile duct strictures with associated portal hypertension. Surg Gynecol Obstet 108:627, 1959

198. Selye H, Szabo S: Experimental production of cholangitis by 1,4,phenylenediisothiocyanate. Arch Pathol 94:486, 1972

199. Shore JM, Berci G: Operative management of calculi in the hepatic ducts. Am J Surg 119:625, 1970

200. Skielboe B: Anomalies of the gallbladder: Vesica fellea triplex: Report of a case. Am J Clin Pathol 30:252, 1958

201. Smith R: Hepaticojejunostomy with transhepatic intubation: A technique for very high strictures of hepatic ducts. Br J Surg 51:185, 1964

202. Smith R: Obstructions of the bile duct. Br J Surg 66:69, 1979

203. Smoron GL: Radiation therapy of carcinoma of gallbladder and biliary tract. Cancer 40:1422, 1977

204. Sokhi GS, Longland CJ: Early and delayed operation in acute gall-stone disease. Br J Surg 60:937, 1973

205. Soloway RD et al: Pigment gallstones. Gastroenterology 72:167, 1977

206. Sturdevant RA et al: Increased prevalence of cholelithiasis in men ingesting a serum-cholesterol-lowering diet. N Engl J Med 288:24, 1973

207. Suarez CA et al: The role of H.I.D.A./P.I.P.I.D.A. scanning in diagnosing cystic duct obstruction. Ann Surg 191:391, 1980

208. Terblanche J: Is carcinoma of the main hepatic duct junction an indication for liver transplantation or palliative surgery? A plea for the U tube palliative procedure. Surgery 79:127, 1976

209. The Coronary Drug Project Research Group: Clofibrate and niacin in coronary heart disease. JAMA 231:360, 1975

210. Thistle JL, Schoenfield LJ: Induced alteration in composition of bile of persons having cholelithiasis. Gastroenterology 61:488, 1971

211. Thistle JL et al: Effective dissolution of biliary duct stones by intraductal infusion of mono-octanoin (abstr). Gastroenterology 74:1103, 1978

212. Thistle JL et al: Chemotherapy for gallstone dissolution: I. Efficacy and safety. JAMA 239:1041, 1978

213. Thompson BW et al: Sclerosing cholangitis. Arch Surg 104:460, 1972

214. Thompson JE et al: Factors in management of acute cholangitis. Ann Surg 195:137, 1982

215. Todani T et al: Congenital bile duct cysts: Classification, operative procedures, and review of thirty-seven cases including cancer arising from choledochal cyst. Am J Surg 134:263, 1977

216. Todani T et al: Carcinoma arising in the wall of congenital bile duct cysts. Cancer 44:1134, 1979

217. Tompkins RK et al: Operative endoscopy in the management of biliary tract neoplasms. Am J Surg 132:174, 1976

218. Tondelli P et al: Acute gallstone pancreatitis: Best timing for biliary surgery. Br J Surg 69:709, 1982

219. Toouli J et al: Treatment of gallstones by chenodeoxycholic acid. Med J Aust 1:478, 1980

220. Treadwell TA, Hardin WJ: Primary carcinoma of the gallbladder: The role of adjunctive therapy in its treatment. Am J Surg 132:703, 1976

221. Tsuchiya R et al: Malignant tumors in choledochal cysts. Ann Surg 186:22, 1977

222. Turner GG: Giant gall-stone impacted in colon and causing acute obstruction. Br J Surg 20:26, 1932

223. Turrill FL et al: Gallstones and diabetes: An ominous association. Am J Surg 102:184, 1961

224. Vaittinen E: Carcinoma of the gall-bladder: A study of 390 cases diagnosed in Finland 1953–1957. Ann Chir Gynaecol Fenn (suppl) 168:1+, 1970

225. Van der Linden W, Edlund G: Early versus delayed cholecystectomy: The effect of a change in management. Br J Surg 68:753, 1981

226. Van der Linden W, Sunzel H: Early versus delayed operation for acute cholecystitis: A controlled clinical trial. Am J Surg 120:7, 1970

227. Vlahcevic ZR et al: Bile acid metabolism in cirrhosis: III Biliary lipid secretion in patients with cirrhosis and its relevance to gallstone formation. Gastroenterology 64:289, 1973

228. Wangensteen OH: Complete external biliary fistula: Potential serious postoperative complication. JAMA 93:1199, 1929

229. Warren KW, Jefferson MF: Prevention and repair of strictures of the extrahepatic bile ducts. Surg Clin North Am 53:1169, 1973

230. Warren KW et al: Primary sclerosing cholangitis: A study of forty-two cases. Am J Surg 111:23, 1966

231. Warren KW et al: Evaluation and current perspectives of the treatment of benign bile duct strictures: A review. Surg Gastroenterol 1:141, 1982

232. Warren KW et al: Primary neoplasia of the gallbladder. Surg Gynecol Obstet 126:1036, 1968

233. Warren KW et al: Biliary duct cysts. Surg Clin North Am 48:567, 1968

234. Warren KW et al: Use of the modified Y tube splint in the repair of biliary strictures. Surg Gynecol Obstet 134:665, 1972

235. Warren KW et al: Malignant tumours of the bile-ducts. Br J Surg 59:501, 1972

236. Warren KW et al: Management of strictures of the biliary tract. Surg Clin North Am 51:711, 1971

237. Watts JM et al: The effect of added bran to the diet on the saturation of bile in people without gallstones. Am J Surg 135:321, 1978

238. Way LW, Motson RW: Part III. Dissolution of retained common bile duct stones. Adv Surg 10:99, 1976

239. Way LW et al: Biliary stricture. Surg Clin North Am 61:963, 1981

240. Wen CC, Lee HC: Intrahepatic stones: A clinical study. Ann Surg 175:166, 1972

241. Wenckert A, Robertson B: The natural course of gallstone disease: Eleven-year review of 781 nonoperated cases. Gastroenterology 50:376, 1966

242. Wexler MJ, Smith R: Jejunal mucosal graft: A sutureless technic for repair of high bile duct strictures. Am J Surg 129:204, 1975

243. Wong WT et al: The bacteriology of recurrent pyogenic cholangitis and associated diseases. J Hyg 87:407, 1981

244. Worthen NJ et al: Cholecystitis: Prospective evaluation of sonography and ^{99m}TcHIDA cholescintigraphy. AJR 137:973, 1981

245. Yamaguchi M: Congenital choledochal cyst: Analysis of 1,433 patients in the Japanese literature. Am J Surg 140:653, 1980

246. Yamakawa T et al: Experience with routine postoperative choledochoscopy via the T-tube sinus tract. World J Surg 2:379, 1978

247. Zimmon DS et al: Management of biliary calculi by retrograde endoscopic instrumentation (lithocenosis). Gastrointest Endosc 23:82, 1976

chapter **43**
Liver Disease in Infancy and Childhood

WILLIAM F. BALISTRERI and WILLIAM K. SCHUBERT

The liver undergoes major maturational changes in the perinatal period during the transition from an intrauterine existence; the efficiency with which these anatomical and physiological adaptations are established governs the ability to cope with the new environment. Several of the pathophysiological disturbances unique to infants may be a result of faulty or delayed development. Inborn errors of hepatic structure and function will be manifest in this period of life. Infants are subject to complications of severe transplacental and postnatal infection by agents that cause insignificant disease in the adult. The common acquired diseases of the liver seen in adults are rare in the pediatric age-group. Standard methods of investigation of liver disease in adults (percutaneous transhepatic cholangiography and endoscopic cannulation) are seldom of value in children. Use of the Menghini needle for percutaneous liver biopsies has proven to be a safe procedure in both infants and children[312,721]; thus, histologic, biochemical, and ultrastructural definition and management of childhood liver disease have progressed rapidly. There are marked age-related changes in hepatic structure and function[50,53,67,182,384] it is important to keep these varying parameters in mind during clinical evaluation of liver size and liver function, as well as gallbladder structure and function. Differences in drug absorption, distribution, biotransformation, and excretion must be considered when planning therapeutic regimen and monitoring. All of these factors operate to create a fascinating and perplexing field of study.

DEVELOPMENT OF HEPATIC METABOLIC AND EXCRETORY FUNCTION

The fetus is dependent upon the maternal liver; the placenta functions to deliver nutrients, provide a route of elimination of metabolic end products, and expedite biotransformation reactions. After delivery, adaptation to extrauterine existence must be accomplished through differentiation of tissue function (*de novo* enzyme synthesis and enzymatic differentiation). These specific enzymatic processes emerge in certain "clusters" that correlate with dynamic alterations in functional requirements.[272] Fetal liver metabolism is devoted to production of plasma proteins to allow cell proliferation. Near birth the primary needs are production and storage of essential nutrients, excretion of bile, and establishment of processes of elimination. Overall modulation of these developmental processes is presumably through substrate and hormonal input via the placenta and dietary and hormonal input in the postnatal period. There are also intrinsic timing mechanisms.

The fetal liver is very active, metabolically with high blood flow and oxygen consumption rates; gluconeogenesis does not occur. The liver of the newborn, in contrast, has a lower blood flow and oxygen delivery as a result of hemodynamic alterations occurring at birth (closure of ductus venosus and loss of oxygen-rich umbilical venous supply).[68,257] In addition, the carbohydrate-rich placental nutrient flux is discontinued and replaced by a low carbohydrate, high lipid content milk intake. Thereafter, glucose production via gluconeogenesis by the newborn liver is crucial. Fatty acid oxidation, which also provides energy in early life, complements glycogenolysis and gluconeogenesis. There is a restricted capacity for hepatic ketogenesis in the immediate perinatal period, and the newborn tolerates a prolonged period of fasting poorly.

Numerous studies have documented an impairment in hepatic xenobiotic metabolism in the newborn, with a decreased capacity to detoxify certain drugs and age-related differences in pharmacokinetics. The most dramatic example was the "gray baby" syndrome associated with altered chloramphenicol metabolism.[384,439] The major electron transport components of the mono-oxygenase system, such as cytochrome P-450, NADPH, and cytochrome C-reductase, are present in low concentrations in fetal liver microsomal preparations.

There is also evidence of immaturity of hepatic excretory function—"physiologic immaturity of the enterohepatic circulation"—manifest by inefficient lipid digestion, delayed hepatic clearance and metabolism of exogenous (drugs) and endogenous (bile acids and bilirubin) compounds, and a cholestatic phase of liver development. In early fetal life, bile acid pools are localized primarily to an intrahepatic site, a finding that correlates with morphologic and histochemical evidence of perinatal changes in bile canalicular development in the rat.[50,53,181,182,272]

The newborn has a cholestatic propensity that has been attributed to an age-related inefficiency of mechanisms determining the rate of bile flow, which is directly correlated with hepatic bile acid excretion. Hepatic excretory function is subservient to placental excretory function *in utero;* however, following birth there is gradual maturation in this functional capacity. Much experimental data document inefficient metabolism and hepatocyte transport of bile acids (Table 43-1). This was initially suggested by an elevation of serum bile acid concentrations, which is an indirect indicator of impaired hepatic clearance,[50,67,641,672] and confirmed in experimental models in which decreased uptake of bile acids by hepatocytes and membrane vesicles isolated from immature animals was noted.[671,673] A hepatic lobular (periportal to central) gradient for bile acid uptake is noted in the adult rat, suggesting that bile acids are efficiently extracted in the periportal area.[53,675] Inefficient transport, namely decreased uptake and increased efflux, of bile acids by the developing liver results in the absence of a lobular distribution for bile acid uptake.

The intracellular transport and metabolism (binding, translocation, and synthesis) of bile acids may be inefficient in early life. The specific activity of the enzymes involved in bile acid conjugation, sulfation, and glucuronidation is underdeveloped in early life[51,670,674]; the overall capacity to conjugate cholic acid by suckling rat liver was found to be approximately 30% of the adult.[670,674] As a direct reflection of these intracellular events, there is a gradual increase in bile acid pool size in humans and in various animal models.[50,53] In addition to progressive quantitative changes in bile acid synthetic rate, there are qualitative differences, namely, the formation of "atypical" bile acids.[41,50,53,180,279,672] The detection of qualitatively abnormal bile acids suggests the existence of a fetal bio-synthetic pathway as well as a delay in the establishment of a mature synthetic sequence. The physiological importance and pathophysiological effects are unknown. There may be a direct effect on bile flow due to the absence of choleretic/trophic primary bile acids. Certain of the resultant atypical bile acids, such as monohydroxy compounds (3β-hydroxy-5Δ-cholenoic acid) are intrinsically hepatotoxic and may initiate or exacerbate cholestasis. Conversely, polyhydroxylated bile acids (tetrahydroxycholanoic acids), found in the urine of normal infants,[665] are more soluble compounds and may present an efficient alternate route of elimination.

Recent interrelated observations provide a morphologic basis for "physiologic cholestasis" based on cytoskeletal and canalicular immaturity. DeWolf–Peeters and coworkers have documented structural immaturity in developing rat liver bile canaliculi with rapid perinatal differentiation.[180–182] A correlation exists between actin filament distribution, cellular development, and functional maturation of the liver cell. In fetal rat hepatocytes, bile canalicular structure as well as motility characteristics and actin filament distribution differs from that seen in mature liver cells.[471] Spontaneous canalicular contractions, which play a role in canalicular bile flow, are not seen.

Therefore, morphologic and functional differences exist between the neonatal and the mature liver, which create the potential for a decrease in bile flow and the production of abnormal bile acids. Exogenous insults to the unique, vulnerable developing liver, such as *Escherichia coli,* sepsis with endotoxemia, the administration of amino acids during nutritional support, hypoxia, hypoperfusion, and administration of medications, may result in marked cholestasis.

NEONATAL JAUNDICE ASSOCIATED WITH ELEVATION OF UNCONJUGATED BILIRUBIN

Physiologic Jaundice

The most thoroughly studied reflection of immature hepatic function is the phenomenon of "physiologic jaundice." Most normal newborns have a mild elevation of serum bilirubin in cord blood, a gradual rise to a maximum of 8 mg to 9 mg/dl on the third to fifth day, and a fall to normal values in the second week of life. In the premature infant, the peak serum bilirubin levels may be 3 mg to 5 mg/dl higher, occur later, vary inversely with gestational age, and last somewhat longer. This unconjugated hyperbilirubinemia occurs in the absence of hemolytic disease. The neonate is burdened by multiple functional defects, of varying degree, that result in an excess load of unconjugated bilirubin being delivered to an inefficient hepatic excretory system (Table 43-2).

TABLE 43-1.   Evidence That Bile Acid Transport and Metabolism Are Underdeveloped in Early Life[50,53]

↑ Serum bile acid levels[67,641,672]
↓ Hepatic uptake (isolated hepatocytes, membrane vesicles)[671,673]
↑ Efflux[53]
Absence of a lobular gradient[53,675]
↓ Conjugation, ↓ sulfation, ↓ glucuronidation[51,670,674]
Altered synthesis
    Qualitative[41,665]
    Quantitative[50,53]
↓ Pool size
↓ Secretion
↓ Intraluminal concentrations
↓ Ileal active transport

TABLE 43-2. Factors Responsible for Initiation and Perpetuation of "Physiologic Jaundice" in the Normal Neonate

Loss of placental transport and maternal detoxification
Alterations in hepatic blood flow, shunting bilirubin away from the sinusoid[586]
Enhanced bilirubin production due to
    Larger red cell mass
    Shorter red cell life span (~80 days)[531]
    Inefficient erythropoiesis; increased early labeled pigment bilirubin
    Increased heme oxygenase activity
Decreased albumin binding due to
    Lower serum albumin concentration
    Decreased binding capacity
    Stress (*e.g.,* sepsis, acidosis, hypoxia)
Decreased Y protein (↓ uptake and ↓ intracellular binding)[275]
Decreased conjugation (↓ activity of uridine diphosphate [UDP], glucose dehydrogenase, and UDP glucuronyl transferase[220])
Impaired bile secretion[50,53,181,182]
Altered enterohepatic circulation
    ↓ Bacterial flora leading to ↓ formation of urobilinogen
    Hydrolysis of conjugated bilirubin to unconjugated bilirubin by way of intestinal β-glucuronidase with subsequent reabsorption

Mechanism

Upon delivery, the fetus can no longer rely on placental or maternal detoxification of unconjugated bilirubin. Persistent patency of the ductus venosus may divert the portal vein blood flow, which normally provides 80% of hepatic blood flow, away from the sinusoidal bed of the liver.[586] Red cell survival is shortened compared with that in the adult; this effect is even more pronounced in the premature infant. As a result of the normal plethoric state of the infant, an increased red cell mass must be degraded. Shunt bilirubin, from nonhemoglobin sources, is higher (>20%) than that found in adults.[354]

Derangement and immaturity of any or all of the processes involved in the transfer of bilirubin from plasma to bile (uptake into the liver cell, intracellular binding and conjugation, and secretion into the bile canaliculus)[106,598] can exaggerate physiologic hyperbilirubinemia. Of the factors contributing to defective bilirubin kinetics in the newborn and to the pathogenesis of physiologic jaundice in the nonhuman primate, defective bilirubin conjugation is central.[239] Very low levels of glucuronyl transferase activity are detectable in the young of certain animals and in human fetal and newborn liver.[109,198] Variant observations[106,199,235,667] may be related to species or to methodologic differences or to the presence of activators and/or inhibitors of glucuronyl transferase. Progestational steroids, such as pregnanediol present in the sera of normal pregnant women and newborn infants, inhibit conjugation by approximately 50%.[322]

Deficiency of conjugating ability alone is unlikely to account for physiologic jaundice. Impaired hepatic uptake is suggested by studies in fetal and newborn guinea pigs and monkeys of the content of the two hepatic intracellular proteins, (Y and Z), which specifically bind organic anions such as bilirubin, indocyanine green, and sodium sulfobromophthalein (Bromsulphalein).[416,417] In the monkey liver, Z protein content reaches adult levels during fetal development and is normal at birth. Y protein, which has the greatest anion-binding capacity, is absent at birth and reaches adult levels at 10 days of age.[28] Levels of Y protein correlate inversely with the magnitude and duration of "physiologic jaundice" and of impaired anion excretion and delayed plasma clearance found in newborn monkeys. The subsequent return of bilirubin levels and anion excretion to normal is associated with increased binding protein.[416] Similarly, impaired hepatic secretion of bilirubin and organic anions is present in fetal and neonatal animals and humans.[78,384,594,736] Conjugation is essential for secretion under normal (adult) conditions; however, secretion may be the rate-limiting step in the transfer of bilirubin from blood to bile by an immature liver. Impairment in the blood to bile transfer of bilirubin in the human infant seemingly results from a combination of varying degrees of alteration of uptake, conjugation, and secretion.

An enterohepatic circulation of bilirubin may contribute significantly to the genesis of physiologic jaundice.[500] The intestine of the fetus and newborn possesses β-glucuronidase activity and an absence of the bacterial flora that in the adult reduces bilirubin glucuronide to urobilinogen.[105,352] Bilirubin diglucuronide secreted into the intestine in the neonatal period can be hydrolyzed to the unconjugated form, which is more readily absorbed.[245,412,414] *In utero,* if conjugated bilirubin is hydrolyzed to the unconjugated state, it is reabsorbed and excreted via the placenta; after birth the unconjugated bilirubin would be reabsorbed and may elevate the level in serum. Interruption of the enterohepatic circulation, by feeding bilirubin-binding agents such as charcoal, cholestyramine, or agar to infants,[170,413,447,502,538,704] will reduce the maximal level of serum bilirubin attained during the first week in full-term infants. This may be due in part to binding of unconjugated bilirubin transferred across the intestinal mucosa, as in Gunn rats fed cholestyramine.[413]

Delayed feeding of newborn infants, standard practice for many years in pediatrics, is another possible factor in the genesis of physiologic jaundice. Fasted newborn Gunn rats have an exaggerated degree of hyperbilirubinemia and an increased activity of hepatic heme oxygenase. These observations suggest that low caloric intake and/or hypoglycemia is associated with an increased rate of degradation of nonerythroid heme. Early feeding has been shown to lower the maximal bilirubin level in full-term and premature infants as well as in infants of diabetic mothers.[735] The relationship of the increased level of physiologic jaundice in infants in whom feeding is delayed to the hyperbilirubinemia induced by fasting in Gilbert's disease is unclear.[221] Serum bilirubin elevation is associated with fasting in both conditions; however, in the infant the maximal serum bilirubin level can be reduced equally well by water and glucose-water feedings.

Implications: Kernicterus (Bilirubin Encephalopathy)

Kernicterus, classically defined as bilirubin staining of the basal ganglia, pons, or cerebellum, was most often noted in postmortem examination of infants who had severe unconjugated hyperbilirubinemia associated with Rh isoimmune hemolysis.[104,121] The frequency of this postmortem finding has decreased with the decrease in Rh disease and with the introduction of better methods to control serum bilirubin levels in early life. At present the most frequent setting for the detection of kernicterus is in autopsies of critically ill, low-birth-weight infants.[121] Confounding variables noted in these low-birth-weight infants are the frequent presence of respiratory distress, hypoxia, acidosis, intraventricular hemorrhage, sepsis, and extreme prematurity. These insults may open the blood-brain barrier[418] and thereby cause bilirubin encephalopathy to occur at levels of serum unconjugated bilirubin of less than 20 mg/dl.[98,99]

Clinical manifestations of kernicterus vary from lethargy, hypotonia, and poor feeding due to loss of suck reflex, to opisthotonos, spasticity, and death.[711] Survivors may show high-frequency deafness, chorioathetosis, and dental dysplasia. Changes in auditory-evoked brain stem responses (AEBR) may provide a noninvasive monitor of bilirubin encephalopathy.[178,351] In long-term follow-up of apparently normal infants with unconjugated hyperbilirubinemia, subtle neurologic abnormalities, impaired motor performance, hearing loss, and psychological dysfunction have been documented.[356,593]

The brains of jaundiced, clinically affected infants dying acutely show yellow pigmentation of thalamic, hypothalamic, and dentate nuclei and cerebellum. However, visual estimation of color in brain tissue samples is not a reliable criterion for encephalopathy; physiological measures such as AEBR are more reliable. Presumably milder degrees of bilirubin encephalopathy are related to less severe lesions in the same areas.

In plasma, lipid-soluble unconjugated bilirubin is bound to albumin, which provides an efficient biologic buffer; however the binding capacity is limited and can be easily exceeded.[501] Albumin-bound bilirubin is in equilibrium with a small amount of unbound bilirubin (<0.5 mg/dl).[501,503,504] The ratio of available binding sites to true binding capacity may be lowered in the presence of other substances that compete directly with bilirubin or that alter binding sites by attaching to alternate albumin sites.[407] In theory only free bilirubin can diffuse into cells and exert toxic metabolic effects. However, there is the possibility of reversible opening of the blood-brain barrier to albumin as well as to bilirubin in the presence of altered vascular permeability, hypoxia, or acidosis.[98,99,418] Subsequent dissociation of bilirubin from albumin allows passage from serum into the cell. Unbound bilirubin interacts with cell membranes and is toxic to membrane-associated metabolic processes.[595] This is abetted by the fact that bilirubin demonstrates an affinity for cell membrane phospholipids and is relatively insoluble at physiologic pH. Diffusion into mitochondria with subsequent uncoupling of oxidative phosphorylation may be a major mechanism of toxicity. Unconjugated bilirubin inhibits oxidative processes in isolated mitochondria, thereby exerting a cytotoxic effect via a decrease in local adenosine triphosphate (ATP) levels and impairment of energy-dependent cerebral metabolism.[480] Bilirubin toxicity may be initiated by modulation of cerebral-protein phosphorylation. A direct effect on membrane function is suggested by the toxicity of free bilirubin on the non-mitochondria-containing renal papillae of Gunn rats.[501,503] The peculiar vulnerability of the central nervous system to free bilirubin toxicity may be related to the low albumin concentration in brain interstitial fluid, which is one tenth that of plasma.

Any factor that reduces plasma bilirubin binding capacity will predispose to higher tissue bilirubin levels and kernicterus. Factors of clinical importance in the neonate are hypoalbuminemia, acidosis, and the presence of organic anions that bind to albumin such as sulfonamides, salicylates, heparin, caffeine, sodium benzoate, nonesterified fatty acids, and hematin. Plasma free fatty acids (FFA), present in low concentrations, can compete with bilirubin for binding at the primary (high-affinity) site on albumin. This will displace bilirubin and shift the majority to secondary (low-affinity) binding sites, from which it is easily displaced into tissue. If the FFA concentration increases (molar ratio of FFA to albumin $>5:1$), there is competition for the secondary sites as well.[501] Antibiotics such as penicillin and kanamycin, in contrast to sulfonamides, do not alter bilirubin binding capacity. Bilirubin neurotoxicity is exaggerated in the presence of anoxia; the resultant tissue acidosis may further impair mitochondrial oxidation of bilirubin.[103]

These observations suggest that blood levels of bilirubin are not a reliable predictor of toxicity: if drugs displace bilirubin, plasma levels are low while tissue levels are high; conversely, following albumin infusion, blood levels will increase as bilirubin exits from tissue. Therefore monitoring and therapy must be individualized, taking these variables into account.

Nonphysiologic Jaundice

The differential diagnosis of unconjugated hyperbilirubinemia in early life is outlined in Table 43-3.

Increased Bilirubin Production

Increased bilirubin production results from erythrocyte hemolysis, breakdown of blood in enclosed hematomas, and from any condition that further increases red cell mass prior to or at parturition.

Incompatibility. *Rh isoimmunization.* Rh isoimmunization may result in the onset of jaundice in the first 24 hours of life with a rapid increase to pathologic levels that requires treatment. The most severely affected infants are pale, edematous, and suffer circulatory collapse related to the anemia, or are stillborn with hydrops fetalis. The diagnosis is usually anticipated on the basis of prenatal Rh testing. The definitive diagnosis depends on demonstration of maternal antibody coating fetal red cells; 93% of affected mothers have anti-D antibody despite the large number of antigens on the red cell which theoretically could cause isoimmunization. In Rh disease the Coombs' test is strongly positive as opposed to the weakly positive reaction characteristic of ABO incompatibility. Cord blood hemoglobin concentration is reduced, and bilirubin levels are elevated in direct proportion to the severity of the hemolytic process.

Rh disease is rapidly becoming of historical interest only. Prevention of isoimmunization is achieved by the administration of a potent anti-D gamma globulin to the mother after each delivery (or abortion/miscarriage) to destroy fetal Rh^+ red cells that enter the maternal circulation at parturition; intrapartum administration (28th week) has been considered.[139] In women already sensitized, amniocentesis will allow diagnosis prior to 30 weeks by measurement of optical density at 450 μ.[720] Infants may be delivered prematurely by cesarean section if necessary; severely involved infants may be treated with intrauterine transfusion, with reported survival rates of 62% and a low risk of fetal injury.[433]

Affected infants may have elevated levels of conjugated (25%–30% of the total) as well as of unconjugated bilirubin in cord blood; this may be due to *in utero* substrate activation of uptake and conjugation by the large load of bilirubin or a relative failure of excretion.[741] In infants dying within 48 hours of Rh disease, liver histology was

TABLE 43-3.   Differential Diagnosis of Unconjugated Hyperbilirubinemia In Infants

INCREASED BILIRUBIN PRODUCTION	DECREASED BILIRUBIN UPTAKE, STORAGE, METABOLISM	ENTEROHEPATIC RECIRCULATION
Hemolytic disease: isoimmune hemolysis	Crigler–Najjar (I) or Arias (II) syndrome	Breast-milk jaundice
Rh incompatibility	Gilbert's syndrome	Intestinal obstruction
ABO incompatibility	Lucey–Driscoll syndrome	Ileal atresia
Other (Lewis, M, S, Kidd, Kell, Duffy)	Drug inhibition	Hirschprung's disease
Congenital spherocytosis	Hypothyroidism/hypopituitarism	Cystic fibrosis
Hereditary elliptosis	Congestive heart failure	Antibiotic administration
Infantile pyknocytosis	Portacaval shunt	
Erythrocyte enzyme defects	Hypoxia	
Glucose 6-phosphate dehydrogenase	Acidosis	
Pyruvate kinase	Sepsis	
Hexokinase		
Infection		
Enclosed hematoma (cephalohematoma, ecchymoses)		
Polycythemia		
Diabetic mother		
Fetal transfusion (maternal, twin)		
Delayed cord clamping		
Drugs		
Vitamin K		
Maternal oxytocin[113]		
Phenol disinfectants[747]		

the same whether or not conjugated bilirubin levels were elevated.[298] Extramedullary hematopoiesis, hemosiderin deposits, and iron pigment in hepatic and Kupffer cells were present, but there was no hepatic cell necrosis, giant cell change, or cholestasis. Following severe Rh incompatibility, especially prior to widespread use of exchange transfusion, persistent elevation of conjugated bilirubin levels with acholic stools lasting 4 to 8 weeks was not uncommon. "Inspissated bile syndrome" was the term used to designate posterythroblastotic jaundice and originally referred to obstructive jaundice in infancy due to bile plugs in a stenotic or narrowed common duct.[396] The histology (disruption of liver cell cords, hepatocyte necrosis, giant cell transformation, extramedullary hematopoiesis, and portal fibrosis and inflammation of varying degree) was not dissimilar from neonatal hepatitis.[179,321] It is possible that short incubation posttransfusion hepatitis was involved in some cases. Therefore the possibility of mechanical obstruction by bile plugs implied by the term may be incorrect, and the term has largely been discarded. Reports of cirrhosis following documented Rh disease are rare[148] and difficult to interpret.

ABO Incompatibility. In view of the declining incidence of Rh hemolytic disease, the most common cause of newborn hemolytic disease is ABO incompatibility (maternal allo-antibody reacting with fetal red cells).[196] Twenty percent of pregnancies are heterospecific for A, B, and O blood groups. Approximately 5% to 40% are sensitized as shown by the direct Coombs' test; the higher incidence is associated with maternal group O; 50% of sensitized infants have hemolysis, and in about half of these, peak bilirubin exceeds 10 mg/dl. The major problem is the risk of kernicterus; hydrops is rare, anemia is mild. Microspherocytosis on peripheral blood smear is characteristic. Although the direct Coombs' test is not as strongly positive as in Rh disease, the indirect Coombs' test against adult erythrocytes of the infant's type is positive when either infant serum or antibody eluted from the infant's cells is used.[196,754] Amniocentesis is not indicated. First pregnancies may be involved; in subsequent pregnancies, the severity of hemolysis is increased, unchanged, or decreased in about equal proportions.

Others. Less commonly, other hemolytic anemias due to structural and enzymatic red cell defects may produce jaundice and anemia in the first 2 days of life.[647] Congenital spherocytosis may be confused with ABO hemolytic disease, but in at least 60% of cases, one parent is involved and serologic studies are negative.[116] Hereditary elliptocytosis, which has variable clinical manifestations and striking morphologic alterations visible on blood smear, may cause severe neonatal jaundice.[157] Infantile pyknocytosis, limited to premature infants, is associated with peculiar small red cells with spiny projections and produces jaundice in the first few days of life.

At least 14 genetically determined erythrocyte enzyme defects resulting in "nonspherocytic" hemolytic anemia have been described;[709] glucose 6-phosphate dehydrogenase deficiency is capable of causing marked jaundice. In infants of Oriental and Mediterranean descent, the enzyme may be completely absent and hemolysis may occur even in the absence of drugs recognized to cause hemolysis in this condition.[409,706] In the American Negro with glucose 6-phosphate dehydrogenase deficiency, hemolysis in the absence of drug exposure is rare except in prematures. Pyruvate kinase deficiency, second in frequency, may cause jaundice and/or anemia that must be treated.[709] Generally, hemoglobinopathies do not present in the newborn period, presumably because of the normal presence of large amounts of fetal hemoglobin. Homozygous α-chain thalassemia has been associated with hydrops fetalis and stillbirths,[362] γ-β thalassemia with hemolytic disease in the newborn.[363]

Enclosed Hematoma. Blood separated from the circulation (cephalohematoma or extensive bruising of the skin) is degraded promptly and may contribute to the bilirubin load imposed on the neonatal liver.[554] A similar mechanism may occur with subdural hematoma, large vein thrombosis, and ingestion of maternal blood at delivery.[202]

Polycythemia. Senescence of an increased red cell mass, which is physiologic *in utero,* increases the bilirubin load to be excreted after birth. A further increase in the red cell mass occurs in infants of diabetic mothers (increased birth weight, hypoglycemia, and respiratory distress), in fetal transfusion *in utero* from either mother or a twin fetus, from overly aggressive stripping of the umbilical cord at birth, and in congenital adrenal hyperplasia.[465,555] The clinical appearance of excessive plethora may mask the degree of hyperbilirubinemia; treatment is by partial exchange transfusion.

Drugs. Drugs such as water-soluble vitamin K in excessive doses, may produce hemolysis, Heinz bodies, and jaundice in premature infants without erythrocyte enzyme defects.[464] The appropriate dose of 1 mg is harmless. Neonatal hyperbilirubinemia occurred after oxytocin-induced labor as a result of a vasopressin-like effect leading to osmotic swelling, decreased deformability, and rapid destruction of red cells.[113]

Total Parenteral Nutrition. Parenteral infusion of amino acid, carbohydrate, and lipid is frequently used in the support of the low-birth-weight and ill neonate. Amino acids and lipid in solution do not interfere with bilirubin transport; they have no discernible effect on bilirubin kinetics; therefore this mode of nutrition may be used in jaundiced neonates.[693,734] Emulsified fat, given intravenously, may actually serve as a sink to prevent flux of bilirubin into tissue. Further investigation with prospective studies of stressed infants managed in this manner is needed.

Decreased Bilirubin Uptake, Storage, or Conjugation

Crigler–Najjar Syndrome. Seemingly clear examples of deficient hepatic glucuronyl transferase activity in humans, analogous to that found in the Gunn rat,[29,153,598] are associated with extreme jaundice in the neonatal period that persists for life. Two genetic subtypes (I and II) have been described.[29,598] Liver histology is normal in both groups. Type I, originally described by Crigler and Najjar, is recessively inherited.[29,153,598] Serum levels of unconjugated bilirubin are high (20–40 mg/dl), and kernicterus is frequent and may occur at any age.[84] Bile is colorless and contains no bilirubin diglucuronide. Despite the lack of bilirubin in bile in type I, stools are normal color and fecal urobilinogen content is only slightly reduced, presumably because of transfer of unconjugated bilirubin across the intestinal mucosa. Serum bilirubin is maintained at relatively constant (elevated) levels by this mechanism as well as by excretion of water-soluble derivatives.[599] Phenobarbital administration has no effect on serum bilirubin levels.[29,84,264] Type II patients generally have lower serum bilirubin levels (9–17 mg/dl), no neurologic disease, and bile that is slightly pigmented but contains bilirubin glucuronide levels only slightly below the normal range.[26,29,84,152,264,737] Phenobarbital administration results in a prompt fall in serum bilirubin to near normal levels.[29,152,393,598,737,749] In vitro glucuronyl transferase activity does not discriminate between groups.[26,29,73,598] The parents of affected children are anicteric in both groups but may exhibit differences in glucuronide formation. Dominant inheritance of type II with incomplete penetrance is postulated.[29] Kernicterus, reported occasionally in patients otherwise conforming to the type II definition, can be attributed to multiple factors influencing serum bilirubin concentration in the neonatal period, such as hypoxia, acidosis, and drug administration. Very rarely, patients with severe type I disease survive to their teens, emphasizing the importance of alternative excretory pathways and the use of bilirubin-binding agents and phototherapy.[342] In the future, agents such as tin-protoporphyrin, which block heme degradation to bilirubin, may be of great benefit.[195]

Gilbert's Syndrome. A condition characterized by low-grade elevation of unconjugated bilirubin, with mean levels ranging from 2 mg to 3 mg/dl, Gilbert's syndrome is often not diagnosed until puberty.[543] Scleral icterus is the only physical finding. Liver function and histology are normal except for minor alterations noted on electron microscopy. Subjective symptoms such as fatigue, vague abdominal pain, and nausea associated with the disease in the older child may be related primarily to anxiety.

A simple presumptive test is provided by the observation that caloric deprivation (400 cal/day) increases serum bilirubin levels twofold to threefold in adults with Gilbert's disease.[556] Because mild compensated hemolytic states[26,73] and post-hepatitic liver dysfunction[26] may produce similar levels of unconjugated bilirubin, the diagnosis is restricted to patients with normal red cell survival and absence of histologic and functional abnormalities of the liver.[543] Within this definition, Gilbert's disease is probably due to decreased uptake or conjugation of bilirubin. Bilirubin

overproduction (dyserythropoiesis) may be an important coincident factor.[463] Attempts at demonstration of defective conjugation in vitro have yielded conflicting results; in reports in which decreased enzymatic activity was found, the decrease was only partial and insufficient to account for the hyperbilirubinemia.[26,82,462,598] Decreased hepatic uptake of bilirubin is suggested by alterations in bilirubin disappearance curves; organic anion clearance is normal, suggesting that Y and Z proteins are normal.[73,543] A familial incidence has been reported in 15% to 40% of cases[543] and would probably be higher if repeated bilirubin levels and the effect of fasting were determined. Available data suggest an autosomal dominant inheritance (varying penetrance), with males affected more frequently.[543,556]

Transient Familial Neonatal Hyperbilirubinemia. Lucey and Driscoll observed infants with severe hyperbilirubinemia beginning on the first day of life, which if untreated reached levels in excess of 60 mg/dl and caused kernicterus.[31,435] If treated adequately with exchange transfusion, the infants subsequently were normal and had no jaundice or liver disease after the newborn period. Serum and urine from the apparently healthy mothers of such infants inhibited glucuronyl transferase activity in vitro. The inhibitory activity was a threefold to fivefold exaggeration of the inhibitory effect of serum and urine from normal pregnant women.

Drugs. Various compounds, of which novobiocin is a prototype, can result in bilirubin levels that are three times normal in term infants, presumably because of inhibition of glucuronyl transferase.[320,678]

Hypothyroidism. Prolonged elevation of indirect bilirubin may be the first clinical sign of congenital hypothyroidism.[5,130] In an analysis of infants with hypothyroidism, 20% had abnormal and prolonged (up to 7 weeks) jaundice; 33% had hyperbilirubinemia as a presenting sign.[729]

Altered Enterohepatic Circulation

Breast-Milk Jaundice. Breast-fed infants have a higher incidence of elevated serum bilirubin values in the first week of life, which also last longer and reach higher peaks, than do bottle-fed infants.[27,236,383] In a small percentage of infants the unconjugated hyperbilirubinemia is prolonged.[30,661] Typically, the infant is well, and jaundice develops slowly and reaches a peak by the second or third week. Peak bilirubin levels over 20 mg/dl may occur, but the usual range is 10 mg to 20 mg/dl. Despite the jaundice, weight gain continues and neurologic damage does not occur. Interrupting breast feeding for 24 hours may result in a fall in the level of serum bilirubin, confirming the diagnosis and allowing resumption of breast feeding. In the absence of breast-milk restriction, bilirubin levels will fall to normal after 4 to 6 weeks of age. There is no sex predominance, but succeeding infants may be affected.

The mechanism by which certain breast-fed babies exhibit a higher incidence of unconjugated hyperbilirubinemia has been the subject of much study. By studying liver slices, Arias and co-workers[30] demonstrated that breast milk from mothers of these infants had an inhibitory effect on glucuronide formation, and they subsequently isolated from the milk 3 α, 20 β-pregnanediol, which had an inhibitory effect on conjugation. The steroid was fed to four infants, two of whom became jaundiced, and the investigators concluded that it was the cause of jaundice.[30] The inhibitory effect of breast milk on glucuronyl transferase has been confirmed *in vitro* and *in vivo,* but there is not uniform agreement that the inhibitor is 3 α, 20 β-pregnanediol.[137,297] Gartner and co-workers[237] demonstrated an increased enterohepatic circulation of bilirubin in association with ingestion of milk of mothers whose infants developed breast-milk jaundice, suggesting that a constituent of milk affected intestinal bilirubin absorption. Numerous studies have suggested that reabsorption of bilirubin from meconium occurs in neonates and that jaundiced babies had a lower output of bilirubin in the feces. The use of agar feedings to inhibit bilirubin reabsorption has complemented experimental studies that suggest that exaggerated intestinal reabsorption of unconjugated bilirubin is occurring.[170,502] Gourley and associates[266] have detected significant amounts of β-glucuronidase in the breast milk of women whose babies developed jaundice; he has postulated that intraluminal hydrolysis by this enzyme liberates unconjugated bilirubin, which is then efficiently reabsorbed and contributes to the circulating pool.

Bacterial Flora/Transit Time. Alteration of the enterohepatic circulation may cause elevated serum levels of unconjugated bilirubin in other clinical situations. Fifteen percent of infants with pyloric stenosis have significant elevation of unconjugated bilirubin levels, which fall to normal 5 to 10 days after surgery.[87,220] An increase in unconjugated bilirubin may also be present in duodenal stenosis or atresia if the obstruction is above the ampulla of Vater.[70] Late feeding of infants (after 48 hours) results in higher levels of bilirubin whether or not the feeding contains glucose.[323,735] In all three situations, movement of intestinal contents through the gut is decreased, and introduction of bacterial flora to the intestine is delayed. In the relative absence of intestinal bacteria, which function to reduce bilirubin to urobilinogen, reabsorption of unconjugated bilirubin produced in the gut by intestinal β-glucuronidase is possible. Antibiotic administration may similarly exacerbate unconjugated hyperbilirubinemia.

Treatment of Unconjugated Hyperbilirubinemia

The goal of any therapeutic approach to unconjugated hyperbilirubinemia is to lower serum bilirubin levels and prevent toxicity (bilirubin encephalopathy). Current approaches are directed toward removal or degradation of bilirubin: physical removal of unconjugated bilirubin by exchange transfusion or intraluminal binding in the gut; photoconversion of bilirubin (formation of polar derivatives or augmented excretion of unconjugated bilirubin; and stimulation of hepatic excretion of bilirubin (*e.g.,* with phenobarbital). Future therapeutic effort may be directed at blockage of heme conversion to bilirubin.

Exchange Transfusion

Initially used to treat Rh disease, exchange transfusion has been used to treat persistent hyperbilirubinemia in nonsensitized infants since it became obvious that kernicterus can occur in jaundiced infants in the absence of hemolytic disease.[183,318] Exchange transfusion removes bilirubin, corrects hypoalbuminemia, supplies albumin-binding sites, and may remove endogenous metabolites that have saturated potential albumin-binding sites. It can be supplemented with additional albumin to improve the efficiency of bilirubin removal.[503,722] Fortunately, this procedure is rarely indicated.

A serum unconjugated bilirubin level of 20 mg/dl has been widely used as a criterion for exchange or repeat exchange in hemolytic disease and for exchange transfusion in full-term infants with nonhemolytic hyperbilirubinemia.[318] Bilirubin binding-capacity tests may have an improved predictive value over serum bilirubin levels, but their ultimate value in the usual clinical laboratory situation remains to be determined.[121,368,376,406,504] The occurrence of kernicterus at lower serum bilirubin levels in association with drug administration, hypoalbuminemia, hypoxia, acidosis, and in premature infants[98,99,238,377,418,504,656] emphasizes the need to consider other factors in deciding when to treat. The effect of shortened red cell survival in compounding the degree of jaundice has been ameliorated by intramuscular administration of vitamin E (50 mg/kg) on the first day of life.[277] The use of whole blood exchange may be obviated following further development and refinement of techniques such as enzymatic (bilirubin oxidase) removal of bilirubin from blood.[406]

Bilirubin Binding Agents

Oral administration of bilirubin binding agents will decrease absorption and increase fecal excretion of unconjugated bilirubin.[170,502,538,704] Activated charcoal or agar feedings result in significantly lower mean bilirubin levels during the first 5 days of life in healthy infants.[538,704] The potential benefit to jaundiced infants is unknown. Schmid and colleagues found no beneficial effect from cholestyramine feeding begun on the third day of life in premature infants.[601]

Phototherapy

Cremer and co-workers reported the successful treatment of jaundiced infants by exposure to bright light.[151] Photo-enhanced excretion of bilirubin became widely used in

Europe and South America after controlled trials demonstrated efficiency in controlling serum bilirubin levels and in decreasing the need for exchange transfusion in neonatal jaundice. Phototherapy has become the main line of defense against unconjugated hyperbilirubinemia in the United States.[66,436,453]

The mechanism of phototherapy has been extensively studied both in the Gunn rat model, which may not absolutely reflect the *in vivo* human situation, and in jaundiced neonates. Bilirubin is known to be photolabile. In the Gunn rat, phototherapy was noted to cause an accelerated turnover of bilirubin by increased appearance of unconjugated bilirubin in bile and by enhanced excretion of polar derivatives of bilirubin in bile and urine.[519,520]

Bilirubin undergoes several photoreactions *in vivo* and *in vitro* whereby polar photoproducts are formed; these are readily excreted in bile or in urine. In the Z,Z state, intramolecular hydrogen bonds can form, rendering bilirubin insoluble in aqueous solutions. Therefore, a major mechanism of *in vivo* bilirubin photocatabolism is rapid nonoxidative photoisomerization, which occurs in the skin (Fig. 43-1).[133,452,453,454,518,519] This causes the formation of a series of polar photoisomers that will partition into plasma, bind to albumin, and undergo hepatic clearance and secretion into bile. There the less stable photobilirubin will revert spontaneously to the parent compound (bilirubin IX-α) especially in the presence of bile acids. This process accounts for the enhanced excretion of unconjugated bilirubin that is observed.[386,424] Lumirubin formation may be an important route for bilirubin elimination. Bilirubin is activated by a narrow spectrum of blue light; the most effective wavelengths are those near

450 nm, with secondary peaks at 410 nm and 490 nm.[207,208,256] Although blue light is most effective in reducing serum bilirubin levels, daylight fluorescent lamps supplying 200 foot-candles to 400 foot-candles are adequate and may be safer.[207,208]

There are many postulated risks of phototherapy; however, there are very little conclusive data regarding harmful long-term effects. The major concerns are overuse or inappropriate use: failure to recognize instances of cholestasis including sepsis; use in severe hemolysis, thereby delaying definitive management; and use in healthy but mildly jaundiced infants, where the net effect is to prolong the nursery stay.

Potential biological ill effects of phototherapy include indirect effects due to toxicity of photoisomers (*e.g.,* diarrhea, tissue damage, possible neurotoxicity) and direct phototoxic reactions (light-mediated effects on membranes, lipid peroxidation) such as retinal damage, hemolysis, photodecomposition of proteins, and alteration of endocrine function and growth. Exposure of cells to light induces breaks in DNA strands, sister chromatid exchange, and mutations. Bilirubin acts as a photosensitizing agent, thereby enhancing the level of DNA damage in cells exposed to light.[579]

Direct injuries to body tissues, including retinal injury, have been observed in rats and piglets[496,629] but not in human infants.[361] Other postulated hazards are denaturation of albumin with resultant diminished bilirubin binding capacity, platelet or red cell injury with hemolysis, especially in prematures, and a decrease in riboflavin in plasma.[55,390,501,566,584] Concomitant use of riboflavin to improve the efficiency of phototherapy is associated with serious skin reactions.[55] *In vitro* photo-oxidation products may not be cytotoxic;[282,623] *in vivo* products, although rapidly excreted, could have a different toxic potential. A significant portion of these products, which partition into chloroform at neutral *p*H, might diffuse into the brain. Although clinical and laboratory evidence is reassuring, further study of purified, isolated *in vivo* photodegradation products is needed.

Insensible water losses may be significant in low-birth-weight infants. Diarrhea may be suggested by the large green stools occurring during phototreatment.[434,436,490] Overheating may occur from improper light units. The effects on cardiac output and peripheral vascular resistance need to be defined. Eye damage is a potential hazard if eye shields are not properly placed or are dislodged. Jaundice cannot be assessed clinically because the skin is decolorized; therefore serum bilirubin must be measured before and after phototherapy. Clinical experience in over 4800 infants has shown no side-effects on growth or endocrine status.[308,436,490] Phototherapy 10 hours nightly for 3 years in one patient with Crigler–Najjar syndrome has been without ill effect on growth, development, intelligence quotient, or circadian rhythm.[367,447]

The "bronze baby syndrome" may occur in premature infants with jaundice treated with phototherapy.[390,584] Hemolysis and a gray–brown discoloration of the skin,

Fig. 43-1. Photochemical reactions of bilirubin *in vivo*. All these products are less lipophilic than is bilirubin and do *not* require conjugation prior to excretion. Reaction A (geometric isomerization) predominates. Reaction B (intramolecular cyclization to form structural isomer) is less dominant. In experimental models 4E, 15Z, and 4Z, 15E isomers predominate in bile (85%); Z-lumirubin makes up ∼10%. Photo-oxidation photoproducts are excreted in urine. (Modified from Ref. 453)

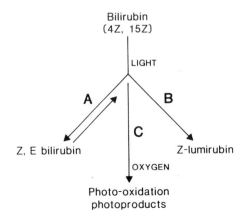

serum, and urine are present, presumably due to retention of photo-oxidation products; this may reflect the effect of light on porphyrins.[584]

Phototherapy has also been used successfully in most of the unconjugated hyperbilirubinemic conditions described above. In hyperbilirubinemia due to hemolytic disease, especially ABO incompatibility, phototherapy will reduce but not eliminate the need for exchange transfusions.[364,630] Perhaps the greatest controversy surrounds the use of prophylactic phototherapy in premature infants. Prophylactic treatment would result in 95% of infants being treated unnecessarily if 15 mg/dl is accepted as a critical level for kernicterus.[66,252] This approach is not recommended until further clinical experience confirms the apparent lack of toxicity. Increase in nursery illumination to 90 foot-candles at the infant's skin, which significantly reduces bilirubin levels in the premature infant and facilitates clinical observation, had been strongly recommended[253]; however, this issue also needs to be clarified in view of the reported deleterious effect of environmental light.

Phenobarbital

Under various circumstances, phenobarbital is capable of inducing microsomal enzymes and hepatic transport, thereby increasing bilirubin uptake, conjugation to glucuronide by the microsomal enzyme cascade, and secretion into bile canaliculus.[29,123,124,134,140,227,501,557,569,749,756] Phenobarbital has also been shown to decrease the efflux of bilirubin as a result of an increase in intracellular binding protein.[744] Prospective controlled studies have shown phenobarbital to be effective in lowering serum bilirubin levels in neonates.[657,699,707,714,752] When barbiturates are administered to infants prophylactically from birth, serum bilirubin levels fall within 48 hours; if administered after jaundice has occurred, serum bilirubin levels require 4 to 5 days to fall. If given to the mother for 14 days prior to delivery, a decrease in cord bilirubin levels can be demonstrated.[448,707] Phenobarbital administration results in a three-fold increase of glucuronyl transferase activity and will decrease peak bilirubin concentration during the first 3 days of life in normal full-term neonates; it is less effective in premature infants.[120,239]

Potential undesirable barbiturate effects include accelerated drug (or vitamin D) metabolism with loss of drug effectiveness[140,141]; altered steroid metabolism,[740] with a consequent potential effect on growth (including brain growth) and development[184]; and depressed vitamin K–dependent clotting factors if administered to the mother.[140] Furthermore, early labeled pigment production may be increased because of increased hepatic heme synthesis.[692] In female rats treated with phenobarbital, diminished litter size and increased neonatal mortality have been reported.[284] In human infants a decreased sucking response and respiratory depression may occur.[740] The availability of phototherapy and exchange transfusion in the United States has obviated routine phenobarbital prophylaxis.

Controlled trials comparing agar feeding, intermittent phototherapy, continuous phototherapy, and phenobarbital administration have shown that continuous phototherapy is the most effective method in lowering serum bilirubin levels in premature infants and that phenobarbital is not additive.[32,447,448,707]

In geographic areas with less access to intensive newborn care facilities and a high incidence of idiopathic hyperbilirubinemia or glucose 6-phosphate dehydrogenase deficiency,[752] prophylaxis both for mother and infant may be of public health value.

Future

The therapeutic modalities used to date are directed at enhancing the metabolic disposition of bilirubin; a more effective approach may be to prevent bilirubin formation. Drummond and Kappas[195] utilized the principle of competitive enzyme inhibition of heme oxygenase to block the degradation of heme; they used a synthetic metalloporphyrin, tin-protoporphyrin, which has a high affinity for the catalytic site on heme oxygenase. A single administration inhibits the enzyme, reduces bilirubin levels, and increases the biliary excretion of unmetabolized heme.[365,624]

PROLONGED CONJUGATED HYPERBILIRUBINEMIA (NEONATAL CHOLESTASIS)

Prolonged conjugated hyperbilirubinemia (neonatal cholestasis) may be the initial manifestation of a heterogeneous group of diseases.[45] This creates a challenge in the evaluation and management of affected infants. Although the list of potential causes of cholestasis in the neonatal period is extensive and diverse (Table 43-4), the relative frequency of "idiopathic neonatal hepatitis" and extrahepatic biliary atresia far exceeds that of any other entity. These two disorders account for 70% to 80% of all cases of neonatal cholestasis.

Neonatal jaundice associated with elevated serum levels of conjugated bilirubin is never physiologic and almost always signifies disease of the liver or biliary tract. Certain rare diseases may represent pure defects in bilirubin excretion, such as Dubin–Johnson or Rotor syndrome.[73]

The neonate presenting with cholestasis (defined as prolonged conjugated hyperbilirubinemia) presents an interesting exercise in differential diagnosis. Neonatal cholestasis can be the result of infectious, genetic, metabolic, or undefined abnormalities that result in either mechanical (anatomic) obstruction to bile flow or a functional impairment in any of the myriad aspects of hepatic excretory function and bile secretion. An example of the former is a stricture or obstruction of the common bile duct; extrahepatic biliary atresia is the prototypic abnormality. Functional impairment in bile secretion can result from generalized damage to liver cells or injury to a specific

TABLE 43-4.   Differential Diagnosis of Conjugated Hyperbilirubinemia (Neonatal Cholestasis)

I. Intrahepatic disorders
- A. Idiopathic
    1. Idiopathic neonatal hepatitis
    2. Intrahepatic cholestasis, persistent
        a. Arteriohepatic dysplasia (Alagille syndrome)
        b. Byler disease (severe intrahepatic cholestasis with progressive hepatocellular disease)
        c. Trihydroxycoprostanic acidemia (defective bile acid metabolism and cholestasis)
        d. Zellweger syndrome (cerebrohepatorenal syndrome)
        e. Nonsyndromic paucity of intrahepatic ducts (apparent absence of bile ductules)
    3. Intrahepatic cholestasis, recurrent (syndromic?)
        a. Familial benign recurrent cholestasis
        b. Hereditary cholestasis with lymphedema (Aagenaes)
- B. Anatomic
    1. Congenital hepatic fibrosis/infantile polycystic disease
    2. Caroli disease (cystic dilatation of intrahepatic ducts)
- C. Metabolic disorders
    1. Disorders of amino acid metabolism: tyrosinemia
    2. Disorders of lipid metabolism
        a. Wolman's disease
        b. Niemann–Pick disease
        c. Gaucher disease
    3. Disorders of carbohydrate metabolism
        a. Galactosemia
        b. Fructosemia
        c. Glycogenosis IV
    4. Metabolic disease in which defect is uncharacterized
        a. α_1-Antitrypsin deficiency
        b. Cystic fibrosis
        c. Idiopathic hypopituitarism
        d. Hypothyroidism
        e. Neonatal iron-storage disease
        f. Infantile copper overload
        g. Multiple acyl-CoA-dehydrogenation deficiency (glutaric acid type II)
        h. Familial erythrophagocytic lymphohistiocytosis

- D. Hepatitis
    1. Infectious
        a. Cytomegalovirus
        b. Hepatitis B virus (? non-A, non-B virus)
        c. Rubella virus
        d. Reovirus type 3
        e. Herpesvirus
        f. Varicella virus
        g. Coxsackievirus
        h. ECHOvirus
        i. Toxoplasmosis
        j. Syphilis
        k. Tuberculosis
        l. Listeriosis
    2. Toxic
        a. Cholestasis associated with parenteral nutrition
        b. Sepsis with possible endotoxemia (urinary tract infection, gastroenteritis)
- E. Genetic/chromosomal
    1. Trisomy E
    2. Down syndrome
    3. Donahue syndrome (leprechaunism)
- F. Miscellaneous
    1. Histiocytosis X
    2. Shock/hypoperfusion
    3. Intestinal obstruction
    4. Polysplenia syndrome

II. Extrahepatic disorders
- A. Biliary atresia
- B. Biliary hypoplasia
- C. Bile duct stenosis
- D. Anomalies of choledochal-pancreatico-ductal junction
- E. Spontaneous perforation of bile duct
- F. Mass (neoplasia, stone)
- G. Bile/mucous plug

(Modified from Balistreri WF: Neonatal cholestasis: Medical progress. J Pediatr 106:171, 1985)

organelle involved in the biliary secretory apparatus. This is clearly a simplistic overview, since there are multiple areas of overlap (clinical, histological, biochemical). Nevertheless, in the absence of more definitive information, our current conceptual approach is to divide neonates presenting with cholestasis into those with primary extrahepatic disease and those with primary intrahepatic disease (Fig. 43-2).

It is critical that prompt diagnosis be attempted so that patients with infectious causes are rapidly managed, those with genetic or metabolic disease are appropriately counseled and treated, and those with surgical lesions are promptly operated. The known causes of cholestasis are reviewed below and an overview of "idiopathic infantile obstructive cholangiopathies" (*i.e.,* biliary atresia and "idiopathic" neonatal hepatitis) presented.

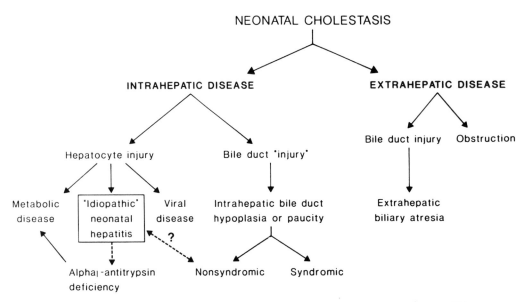

Fig. 43-2. Conceptual scheme of the various forms of neonatal cholestasis. Most cases will be classified as either extrahepatic biliary atresia or "idiopathic neonatal hepatitis." The latter may include early *nonsyndromic* forms of intrahepatic cholestasis. Alpha₁-antitrypsin deficiency, formerly included in the idiopathic category, can now be clearly delineated.

Cholestasis Associated with Infection

Bacterial infection is a frequent cause of an increase in conjugated bilirubin; in one series, 23 of 104 infants had sepsis as the cause of jaundice.[165] *E. coli* has been the most common organism reported. The mechanism of production of cholestasis may be endotoxin-mediated canalicular dysfunction.[89,705] Other gram-negative rods and, less often, staphylococci and streptococci have been etiologic.[75,288] Histologic studies of autopsy material have shown bile stasis and liver cell necrosis as the most striking findings.[75,288] The association of jaundice with bacterial infection in infants not clinically ill is emphasized by a report of 22 infants with positive blood and/or urine cultures, 9 of whom were active and well, with hyperbilirubinemia as the only finding.[574] Urinary tract infection with bacteremia has been emphasized in several series as a cause of neonatal jaundice, especially in infant males.[33,289,495,610,681] There is an absence of associated genitourinary tract anomalies and an occurrence of the disease in clusters or epidemics.[289,495,610] The high incidence in males parallels the increased risk of the male neonate to bacterial infection in general.[169] Thus, urine culture and sediment examination should be obtained in addition to the blood, nasopharyngeal, stool, and cerebrospinal fluid cultures routinely required to evaluate infection as the cause of neonatal jaundice. Appropriate treatment should be initiated immediately after these cultures are obtained in an infant suspected of sepsis.

Syphilis

Conjugated hyperbilirubinemia may be one of the myriad manifestations of congenital syphilis. Syphilitic hepatitis is associated with enlargement of the liver and spleen, rash, anemia, and cutaneous hemorrhage similar to other intrauterine infections such as toxoplasmosis and cytomegalovirus infection. Small granulomatous lesions, diffuse chronic inflammatory cell infiltration, and widespread portal fibrosis may be observed in biopsy samples. Assessment of the cord blood serology, which is obligatory in every infant, usually allows prompt diagnosis; placental morphology may also be abnormal.[17] Nevertheless, every infant with unexplained jaundice should have suitable serologic tests for syphilis repeated regardless of the cord blood result. If positive, prompt treatment with penicillin should be instituted before the classic picture of congenital syphilis develops.

Toxoplasmosis

Forty percent of infants with other clinical manifestations of congenital toxoplasmosis have conjugated hyperbilirubinemia and 60% have hepatomegaly.[119,174] The severe "classic" illness with hydrocephalus, chorioretinitis, and intracranial calcification may not be present; the infant may appear normal at birth and develop hepatosplenomegaly and jaundice later.[146,286,468] Rarely, severe hemolysis is present and produces an erythroblastosis-like illness. Serum aminotransferase levels are elevated, and progressive liver dysfunction with ascites may occur. Parasites are almost never demonstrated in the liver; histologically, extramedullary hematopoiesis, hemosiderosis, canalicular bile stasis, and a scattered periportal mononuclear cell reaction are present.[119,146,468] Multinucleated giant cells resembling "neonatal hepatitis" may be detected.[45,108,223] Diagnosis may be made by demonstration of the organism in Wright-stained smears of spinal fluid sediment.[219] Demonstration of high-titer IgM-specific antibody in the infant may be helpful; occasional transient false-positive test results have been due to placental leak of IgM antibody.[561] The IgM fluorescent antibody (IgM-IFA) test may be useful, although false-negatives have been reported, and an absence of IgM antibody does not rule out the diagnosis.[560] Serologic studies of both mother and child using the Sabin–Feldman dye test will show high titers (1:1024) in the presence of active infection. If positive, the tests should be repeated at 3 to 4 months of age; persistence of elevated titers in both mother and child confirms the infection.[219]

Toxoplasma are present in the placenta of infected infants, and study of this organ may be highly productive and lead to early positive morphologic diagnosis.[16,63] Treatment with a combination of sulfadiazine and pyrimethamine given with leucovorin and fresh bakers' yeast for one month may prevent further progression of tissue damage, although consistent benefit has not been proven. Prevention should be directed toward avoidance of ingestion of infective cysts and contact with sporulated oocysts.

Congenital Viral Infection

Herpesvirus (cytomegalovirus [CMV], herpes simplex [HSV], varicella-zoster) may infect a pregnant woman and be transmitted to the fetus or newborn; the resultant infection may be asymptomatic or may be associated with acute symptoms. The potential for permanent sequelae, such as developmental impairment, is high.[645,646]

Cytomegalovirus. CMV causes a spectrum of liver diseases in infants and in older children.[290,291,451,458,645,646] In view of the ubiquitous nature of CMV, the tendencies of latency, and the ability to be reactivated with stress, it is difficult to implicate this agent in the causation of neonatal cholestasis.

The prevalence of CMV infection is high—50% to 85% depending on socioeconomic background. One in every 50 to 500 live births is infected; 10% are symptomatic at birth.[79,290,649,730] Severely affected infants may present a classic syndrome shortly after birth, with jaundice (conjugated bilirubin elevation), hemolytic anemia, thrombocytopenic purpura, hepatosplenomegaly, and microcephaly uniformly present. This group has a high (20% to 30%) mortality rate, and more than 90% of the survivors have late complications (e.g., hearing loss, mental retar-

dation).[458,731] Chorioretinitis and periventricular calcification are present in about one third of affected infants.[458,731] Of the 90% who are asymptomatic at birth, 5% to 15% are at risk for late sequelae, especially sensorineural hearing loss. This may be related to continuous viral replication.

Affected infants may also present with the "neonatal hepatitis" syndrome of prolonged jaundice and hepatomegaly.[138,291,451,645,646,654,731] Prospective studies have demonstrated hepatomegaly without alteration of liver function tests.[79,645,646] In the jaundiced infant with hepatomegaly and abnormal liver function tests, the liver histology is variable. There may be focal portal inflammatory infiltration with round cells and neutrophils and focal necrosis of hepatocytes with bile stasis and no giant cell formation.[458] In other cases there is extensive giant cell transformation indistinguishable from neonatal hepatitis as described by Landing and Craig.[149,451,731] Extramedullary hematopoiesis is uniformly present. Significant portal or interstitial fibrosis may be present[230,451]; however, these changes are reversible and follow-up studies have demonstrated normal liver size and function or mild residual portal fibrosis.[72,451] Characteristic swollen cells with intranuclear inclusions may be scanty, even in liver specimens from which the virus is cultured. Inclusions are found in bile duct epithelium but rarely in hepatocytes (Fig. 43-3).[41,451,654] Bile ductule obstruction may occur during CMV infection.[205,278] A possible relationship of the biliary epithelial changes to extrahepatic biliary atresia has been suggested by the histologic findings in one case.[516] Obliterative cholangitis due to CMV has been postulated as a precursor of paucity of the intrahepatic bile ducts.[224] Electron microscopy of the liver in CMV infection shows degenerative changes of bile canaliculi with dilatation and loss of microvilli, as well as bile pigment in hepatocytes.[41,739] The frequency of neonatal infection with CMV and the resemblance to "idiopathic" neonatal hepatitis have suggested that CMV is a major cause of idiopathic obstructive cholangiopathy (see below).[290,291,731] However, attempts to isolate the virus from large groups of infants with idiopathic neonatal hepatitis and biliary atresia, without any other manifestation of congenital infection, have not been productive.[415,458,654]

The diagnosis may be made by culture of fresh urine for virus, since viruria persists for many months after birth.[290,451,458,730,731] Examination of the urine sediment for characteristic inclusion-bearing cells is positive in only 20% of the infected cases and is never positive after 7 months of age.[458] Serologic confirmation is possible. The fluorescent antibody test for CMV-specific IgM antibody is rapid and sensitive and is positive in diseased infants and negative in the asymptomatic excretor; high specificity of enzyme-linked immunosorbent assays may enhance detection.

Histologic examination of the placenta may be highly informative in the diagnosis of intrauterine infection; typical inclusions, plasma cell villitis, and focal necrotizing

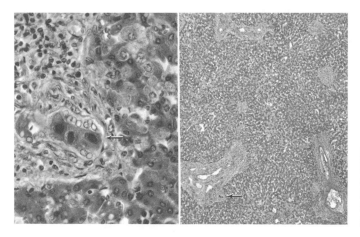

Fig. 43-3. Cytomegalic inclusion disease, autopsy: Extensive inflammatory exudate in all portal areas shown. High power of area (*arrow*) shows three enlarged bile duct epithelial cells with characteristic large intranuclear inclusions. Premature infant weighed 2400 g and died at 5 days of age.

villitis were present in the placenta and the bile duct epithelium[17] in a 19-week fetus.

Antiviral chemotherapeutic agents are of limited value. The brain damage present at birth is probably irreversible. If the infant survives, the liver usually returns to normal.

Herpes Simplex. Herpes infection is a seemingly rare cause of neonatal liver disease and elevation of conjugated bilirubin levels; however, the true incidence remains to be defined as improved detection techniques become available clinically. Neonatal infection with herpesvirus is usually severe, generalized, and characteristically associated with retrograde spread of HSV-2 genital infection in the mother.[299,487,488,550,645,751,758] The overall risk is related to the stage of maternal infection; approximately 10% in women with primary or recurrent HSV-2 and 40% if active infection is present at delivery.[646] Neonatal HSV affects 1 in 2,500 to 10,000 live births; 50% of infected babies are born prematurely. Infection can be limited (neurologic, eye, skin) or disseminated; death occurs in 15% to 50% of the later form, and many of the survivors will have neurologic disability. An affected infant usually appears to be normal at birth and develops a clinical picture indistinguishable from bacterial sepsis on the fourth to seventh day with hepatomegaly, lethargy, jaundice, and hyperthermia or hypothermia progressing to cyanosis, bleeding diathesis, and hypoprothrombinemia, hypoglycemia, and shock.[299,488,550,646,751,758] Jaundice may be minimal and the liver not palpable; the absence of the normally palpable liver in sick infants has been suggested as a clue to the massive hepatic necrosis associated with herpes infection. Vesicles on the skin or mucous membranes of the infant occur in 80% of symptomatic cases and strongly suggest the diagnosis. Keratitis is also suggestive of herpes infection. Direct examination and culture of the mother for genital herpes as well as inquiry as to its presence should be made.

Laboratory studies show evidence of multisystem involvement as in sepsis: elevated bilirubin and serum aminotransferase levels, hypoprothrombinemia, and disseminated intravascular coagulation.[467] Diagnosis is best confirmed by viral culture of throat swabs and vesicle fluid or at autopsy by the finding of intranuclear inclusions in liver, lungs, adrenal glands, and kidney. Monoclonal antibody to HSV antigen may allow for precise diagnosis. The liver grossly shows miliary nodules of necrosis with a hemorrhagic halo about them.[299,549,550,758] Microscopically there are extensive areas of bland necrosis with surrounding hemorrhage but with minimal inflammatory reaction. Intranuclear inclusions typically are located at the junction of normal and necrotic tissue. Central nervous system symptoms may predominate; residual neurologic impairment is frequent. A persistent vesicular rash without liver involvement may be the only manifestation of disease,[315] suggesting that an immune tolerance peculiar to the newborn state may account for the manifestations of herpetic infections in the newborn. Most neonatal infections seem to be acquired during delivery; however, evidence of disease may be present at birth, suggesting intrauterine and possibly transplacental infection.[470,622] Histologic study of the placenta may be of value in confirming the diagnosis. Treatment is not consistently effective; however, adenine arabinoside or other antivirals should be considered in *proven* cases of herpes hepatic or encephalitic infection.[488,646] Prevention of fetal exposure may be possible in mothers with genital herpes diagnosed prepartum by delivery via cesarean section.

Rubella. Intrauterine infection with rubella virus occurred with a frequency of 5 per 1000 live births during the epidemic of 1964[585]; the incidence was 0.7 per 1000 births in a nonepidemic year.[9] Major manifestations include congenital heart disease (80%), hepatomegaly (65%), low birth weight (60%), splenomegaly (59%), purpura (57%), and cataracts (50%). Despite the frequency of hepatomegaly, jaundice is present in only about 15% of cases. The clinical picture may be identical to that of idiopathic "neonatal hepatitis" with elevation of conjugated bilirubin, serum aminotransferase, and alkaline phosphatase levels and acholic stools. Histopathologic findings in the liver in congenital rubella are variable; cholestasis may be the only abnormality.[625] More marked hepatitis with periportal inflammation and cholestasis may be present to a varying degree.[193,211,392,655] Giant cell transformation, with extramedullary hematopoiesis indistinguishable from idiopathic neonatal hepatitis, has been described by several authors.[211,655,666] Hepatocellular disease may be overshadowed by portal tract inflammation, intrahepatic duct obliteration, ductular proliferation and cholestasis, fibrosis, and, in at least one report, changes indistinguishable from biliary atresia.[475,666] Progression to cirrhosis is rare.[724] Diagnosis rests on viral isolation; although virus can be recovered from the liver, the best site is the throat. IgM levels are helpful if elevated, but the frequency of false-negative results is high. Placental histology may be suggestive of congenital rubella.[17] While there is no treatment, mass immunization of prepubertal girls offers the best hope for prevention of the disease.

Coxsackievirus. Rarely, a clinical picture very similar to that produced by herpesvirus is caused by coxsackie B virus infection.[382] The infection may be transplacental or acquired postnatally and is generalized whether or not hepatic manifestations predominate; virus has been isolated from heart, liver, kidney, and central nervous system. Myocarditis is the most common finding in coxsackie infection of infancy (82%); hepatic necrosis and jaundice may occur (15%). The liver may show focal hepatitis or marked central necrosis with little or no inflammation.[218,382] Herpetic intranuclear inclusions are not present. Clinical differentiation from herpes may be difficult and is based on absence of maternal vesicular lesions, the presence of associated myocarditis, and ultimately on viral isolation.

Echovirus. The role of echovirus (types 11, 14, and 19) in the genesis of neonatal hepatic necrosis similar to that produced by herpes simplex has been documented.[247,336,473,536] The illness resembles an overwhelming infection, with bleeding, cholestasis, and progressive liver dysfunction occurring in the first 5 days of life. There is a disparate increase in serum glutamic-oxaloacetic transaminase (SGOT) in many cases, especially in association with echovirus 11. At autopsy the liver shows massive necrosis and varying degrees of extramedullary hematopoiesis; the virus may be recovered from tissues. There is also adrenal necrosis and focal encephalitis. The absence of vesicles is helpful in excluding herpes, but viral isolation is needed for diagnosis. Infection can seemingly be acquired either *in utero* or postnatally; in the series of Modlin and associates,[473] the mothers noted a "viral illness" in the days before delivery. There is no specific therapy available for enteroviral infections.[74,336,536]

Similar cases of neonatal hepatic necrosis without positive viral isolation have been described, suggesting that other, as yet unidentified, viruses may cause liver necrosis in the peculiarly susceptible newborn period.[476]

Metabolic Defects

A wide variety of metabolic diseases may present as cholestasis; this is especially true of inborn errors of carbohydrate metabolism such as galactosemia, which is discussed below. Therefore metabolic screening is a critical facet in the evaluation of the child with cholestasis. However, the detection of reducing substances in urine or of amino acids in urine and serum should be interpreted with caution. For example, an elevation in the serum concentrations of tyrosine and methionine occurs in liver disease of various causes and does not necessarily indicate a specific metabolic disease such as tyrosinemia; the detection of unique metabolites, which reflect an altered pathway of tyrosine degradation, provides much more reliable criteria for the diagnosis of tyrosinemia. There are several other "metabolic" illnesses in which the defect is undefined or poorly characterized (such as alpha$_1$-antitrypsin [α_1-AT] deficiency), which present as cholestasis in early life.

α_1-Antitrypsin Deficiency

Hereditary deficiency of α_1-AT may present in the neonatal period as cholestasis.[616] α_1-AT, the major alpha$_1$ globulin of human plasma, is synthesized in the liver and serves to inhibit several proteolytic enzymes including trypsin.[210,404] Initially deficiency of this protein, inherited as an autosomal recessive trait, was associated with early-onset emphysema in both heterozygotes and homozygotes.[404,684] Sharp and associates next described genetically determined childhood liver disease associated with deficiency of α_1-AT but without lung disease.[613] Subsequently, children with both cirrhosis and lung disease have been described.[255] α_1-AT has been studied extensively by immunoelectrophoresis, and more than 30 variants, designated as Pi (protease inhibitor) phenotypes, have been described. Each is inherited codominantly at a single locus. The normal phenotype of the Pi system is M; these persons have a serum α_1-AT level greater than 2 mg/ml. The Z allele produces a slower moving protein; Pi^{ZZ} persons have α_1-AT levels 10% to 15% of normal and Pi^{MZ} have intermediate levels.[213] To date, children with liver disease have had the Pi^{ZZ} phenotype, but lung disease has been associated with other phenotypes.[213,225,614]

Clinical Features. A perspective on α_1-AT deficiency and liver disease in childhood was provided by the prospective studies of Sveger.[679] He screened (via Pi typing) 200,000 newborn infants, which represented 95% of all births in Sweden during 1972 to 1974, and detected 120 Pi^{ZZ} (incidence = 1 in 2000–4000 live births) and 48 Pi^{SZ} newborn babies. These "at-risk" infants were monitored by periodic clinical evaluation and liver function studies; 12% of the Pi^{ZZ} infants had documented neonatal cholestasis, while an additional 7% had clinical evidence of liver disease in infancy. At 6 months of age, each of these infants appeared to have clinically recovered from liver disease. The remaining Pi^{ZZ} infants were clinically normal; however, 47%

had elevated liver enzymes at 3 months of age, which persisted to at least 4 years of age. Therefore, only 34% of the Pi^{ZZ} infants were found to have had no clinical or laboratory evidence of liver injury. None of the Pi^{SZ} infants had clinical evidence of liver disease. Sveger subsequently noted that of the 120 Pi^{ZZ} children followed prospectively for the first 4 years of life, 2.5% died.[679,680] In the 14 Pi^{ZZ} infants in whom neonatal cholestasis had been documented, two had symptoms of cirrhosis at age 4. The initial observation that of all homozygous deficient persons, fewer than 20% will develop neonatal cholestasis has been confirmed by other series.[548]

When viewed from another perspective, approximately 5% to 10% of all infants presenting with undefined neonatal cholestasis may subsequently be shown to be homozygous α_1-AT deficient.[45,163,165,507,539,616] These patients are clinically indistinguishable from other infants with "idiopathic" neonatal hepatitis (see Fig. 43-2). In a series of 24 patients with α_1-AT deficiency (Pi^{ZZ}) studied by Cutz and Cox,[158] 17 presented with neonatal hepatitis; this group represented 29% of all their infants with "idiopathic" neonatal hepatitis. The biopsies were nonspecific and similar to those seen in other children with idiopathic neonatal hepatitis. Six of the seventeen infants developed cirrhosis and died at 6 to 12 years of age of liver failure or complications of cirrhosis. Postmortem examination revealed a mixed micromacronodular cirrhosis with wide bands of fibrous tissue separating regenerative nodules of varying sizes. Compared with the initial biopsies, inflammatory cell reaction was less and there was a decrease in the number of interlobular bile ductules. In the remaining

11 Pi^{ZZ} infants who presented with a syndrome resembling neonatal hepatitis, there was apparent recovery in that all were clinically asymptomatic; however, at least 5 had elevated aminotransferase levels or hepatomegaly. Follow-up biopsies in 5 of these 11 patients revealed mild to moderate portal fibrosis with few inflammatory cells. Of the original 24 patients, 7 did not manifest neonatal hepatobiliary disease but presented at a later age following an anicteric period.

Hepatic Pathology. The presentation and clinical course of the liver disease are variable. Some have therefore even suggested the possibility of intrauterine hepatic damage in a percentage of cases. The pattern of neonatal liver injury may also be heterogeneous. It may include hepatocellular damage with giant cell transformation, minimal inflammation, and bile stasis, along with varying degrees of portal fibrosis with bile duct proliferation (Fig. 43-4). There may, however, be subsequent complete histologic resolution, persisting liver disease, or the development of cirrhosis.[539,616,683] The jaundice usually clears during the second to fourth month, and the child may appear clinically well. In a similar manner, there may be the presentation of chronic liver disease or undefined cryptogenic cirrhosis in an older child with portal hypertension or another manifestation such as hematemesis.

Diagnosis. The diagnosis of α_1-AT deficiency is best made by determination of the α_1-AT phenotype and confirmed by liver biopsy. The level of α_1-AT measured immunochemically may be deceptive, especially in premature in-

Fig. 43-4. Alpha$_1$-antitrypsin deficiency: Biopsy at age 1 year shows early cirrhosis at low power (*left*). Spherical eosinophilic hyaline bodies resembling erythrocytes, but larger and not biconcave, are visible in periportal hepatocytes at high power (*center,* [*arrow*]). Periodic acid Schiff stain (*right*) shows positive staining diastase-resistant globules adjacent to portal connective tissue.

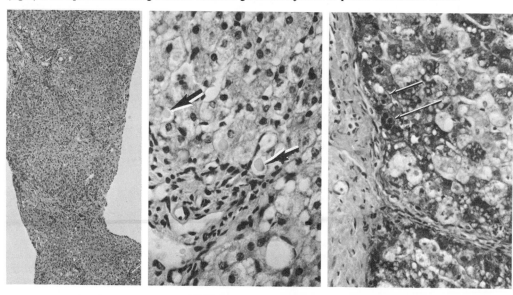

fants in whom low levels may be found despite the normal Pi^{MM} genotype and in heterozygous (Pi^{MZ}) patients in whom a rise of 60% to 80% may occur with inflammation and estrogen therapy or pregnancy. Proper study of a family thus requires quantitation of α_1-AT either by immunodiffusion or chemical measurement of serum trypsin inhibitory capacity and determination of Pi phenotype by acid starch gel electrophoresis.[210,213] The frequency of these conditions (Pi^{MZ}, 3% of the population and Pi^{ZZ}, 0.07%) dictates that all children with liver disease be evaluated for α_1-AT deficiency and that Pi typing be done in those with low levels.[213] Family screening and genetic counseling of affected persons are mandatory.

In patients with α_1-AT deficiency, hepatocyte inclusions can be seen on routine hematoxylin and eosin sections, where they appear as round to oval, slightly eosinophilic hyaline-like globules localized predominantly in periportal hepatocytes (see Fig. 43-4). Periodic acid-Schiff (PAS) stain followed by diastase treatment will highlight the glycoprotein-rich inclusion. Bile duct inclusions may also be noted in α_1-AT–deficient patients with liver disease.[755] Inclusions vary in size with both zygosity and age of the affected person; therefore, they may be difficult to identify in liver tissue from heterozygotes and from infants. The composition of the hepatic inclusions has been demonstrated by immunochemistry to be α_1-AT immunoreactive material. Immunohistochemistry remains a reliable method for identification and confirmation of the deficiency state.

The ultrastructure of the liver inclusions is characteristic, namely, membrane-bound masses of electron-dense material (Fig. 43-5). Electron microscopy has demonstrated the presence of amorphous material in markedly dilated rough endoplasmic reticulum saccules in the liver

Fig. 43-5. Ultrastructural findings in the liver of a patient with homozygous α_1-antitrypsin deficiency include large electron-dense membrane-bound, amorphous inclusions (*i*) along with a mild degree of fat accumulation.

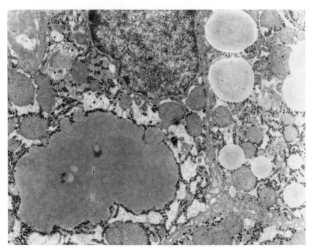

of both homozygous (Pi^{ZZ}) and heterozygous (Pi^{MZ}) deficient persons without liver disease, some of whom were normal and some of whom had emphysema.[423,617]

The presence of the material in the hepatocyte therefore does not seem to be hepatotoxic. The association of low serum levels of α_1-AT with either pulmonary or hepatic disease remains to be explained. Inability to neutralize proteolytic enzymes released by leukocytes or bacteria in response to environmental challenge has been suggested as a mechanism for the pulmonary disease,[210,404] and similar factors may be involved in liver disease.[255,423,539]

Pathogenesis of Hepatic Disease. The cause of the liver disease is uncertain; abnormal biosynthesis of the protein or defective glycosylation may interfere with excretion. The fact that liver involvement is not universal and predominates in early life suggests coexistent factors unique to this age-group. It is well known that uptake of intact proteins from the gut into the systemic circulation occurs frequently in newborns.[702] Udall and co-workers have suggested that in a patient with partial or complete deficiency of protease inhibitors, luminal enzymes (proteases) are absorbed intact from the neonatal gut and enter the systemic circulation. In the absence of protease inhibitors, hepatic inflammation and fibrosis can be initiated.[702] This theoretic postulate may account for the fact that breastfeeding seems to offer some protection against severe liver disease and early death in infants with α_1-AT deficiency. Antiproteases present in breast milk may complex with luminal proteases to neutralize their activity and thereby offer a protective effect. Udall and co-workers subsequently identified infants with α_1-AT deficiency and investigated their early feeding history.[703] Severe liver disease was present in 40% of bottle-fed infants and in 8% of breast-fed infants. This observation needs to be confirmed. An alternative hypothesis suggests that liver fibrosis and cirrhosis may be immunologically mediated.

It is unclear whether patients with partial deficiency states such as Pi^{MZ} and Pi^{SZ} are at a higher risk for hepatic disease. Cox and Smyth reported an increased risk for the development of liver disease in adult men with α_1-AT deficiency, the majority of whom were Pi^{ZZ}.[147] Hodges and associates reported that in a review of more than 1000 biopsies there was an increased prevalence of the MZ phenotype for α_1-AT in subjects with chronic active hepatitis and cryptogenic cirrhosis.[309] However, Roberts and co-workers were unable to conclusively demonstrate an increased occurrence nor an exacerbation of liver disease.[568] Detailed evaluation, including phenotypic analysis and correlation with the liver biopsy, should resolve the issue. However, these studies do indicate that periodic assessment of liver function may be warranted for patients with α_1-AT deficiency who are over 40 years of age.

Treatment and Outcome. There is no specific therapy for the consequences of liver disease associated with α_1-AT deficiency, although replacement therapy looms as a possibility. Danazol, a 17 α-substituted alkyl steroid, is capable of increasing serum α_1-AT levels; however, there is no evidence that this is of clinical value. Rosenberg and associates recently described the synthesis, in yeast, of a functional oxidation-resistant mutant of human α_1-AT.[577] Infusion of a plasma concentrate of α_1-AT or synthetic protease may be a future therapeutic modality. Liver transplantation has been performed and has been curative.[313,757]

The outcome of α_1-AT deficient children with liver disease has been suggested by several studies since the initial observations of Sveger,[679,680] and the results are remarkably uniform.[493,548] There are four equally probable observed patterns: (1) patients may persist in having abnormal liver function tests, develop increasing evidence of cirrhosis, such as portal hypertension and ascites, and die of hepatic complications in the first 10 years of life; (2) patients may have evidence of persistently abnormal liver function but have a slow progression to cirrhosis; (3) patients may have minimal liver dysfunction and less severe fibrosis on liver biopsy and live to adulthood; (4) patients may recover from the initial insult and return to normal liver function and normal liver and spleen size, except for minor evidence of residual fibrosis. Affected persons who develop cirrhosis are often those noted earlier on to have had significant fibrosis. The intrafamilial prognosis is also remarkably similar.

Prenatal diagnosis of α_1-AT deficiency, by direct analysis of the mutation site in the gene using specific oligonucleotide probes, has been suggested.[381] However, there is very little to justify intervention, since no methodology currently available will predict which person with Pi^{ZZ} will have liver disease.

Cystic Fibrosis

As the life expectancy of patients with cystic fibrosis increases, the incidence of hepatobiliary complications increases.[522,547,583] Gallbladder abnormalities are present in 20% of children with cystic fibrosis who are under 5 years of age and in 60% of patients 15 to 20 years of age. Microgallbladder is found in 15% to 20% of all cystic fibrosis patients. Cholesterol gallstones are a frequent finding; most are asymptomatic, but calculous cholecystitis may occur. Cholesterol supersaturation may be related to interruption of the enterohepatic circulation with bile acid loss in feces, an alteration in cholesterol secretion into bile with an uncoupling from bile acid output, or the presence of mucin, which serves as a nucleation factor. Ultrasonography is a useful monitor of biliary tract disease in cystic fibrosis.

A wide variety of hepatic lesions have been described; steatosis is the most common finding. Cholestasis is a relatively rare manifestation of cystic fibrosis.[240,517,619,690,710] In a series of 74 patients with cystic fibrosis, 4 had presented as "neonatal hepatitis."[547] Conjugated bilirubin levels were elevated (up to 15 mg/dl), and jaundice persisted from 20 days to 6 months. Meconium ileus was present in half the infants presenting with cholestasis, approximately five times the incidence expected in patients

with cystic fibrosis. Other series have also emphasized the high rate of neonatal cholestasis in association with meconium ileus and bowel obstruction. Uniformly the liver shows canalicular (inspissated) bile plugs and mucus in intrahepatic bile ducts. In certain cases accumulation of thick, viscid bile was noted at laparotomy and was thought to have caused extrahepatic obstruction[39,710]; "flushing" of the extrahepatic ducts was beneficial in two cases. Drug-induced stimulation of bile flow has not been done.[710]

Aside from steatosis, overall the most common hepatic lesion in cystic fibrosis is focal biliary cirrhosis, which is usually detected later in childhood and found in about 25% of cystic fibrosis autopsies (Fig. 43-6).[150,268,547] A small percent of patients develop severe multilobular biliary cirrhosis eventuating in portal hypertension, esophageal varices requiring shunting, and end-state liver disease (Fig. 43-7).[619,701] Patients with neonatal jaundice may escape severe liver involvement in later life; conversely, most patients with end-stage liver disease gave no neonatal history of jaundice. The role of supplemental taurine in ameliorating gastrointestinal complications of cystic fibrosis is being addressed.[583]

Familial Erythrophagocytic Lymphohistiocytosis

Familial erythrophagocytic lymphohistiocytosis (FEL) is an autosomal recessive disease characterized by anorexia, hepatosplenomegaly, jaundice, thrombocytopenia, liver

Fig. 43-6. Cystic fibrosis, biopsy: Focal biliary cirrhosis in an otherwise normal liver.

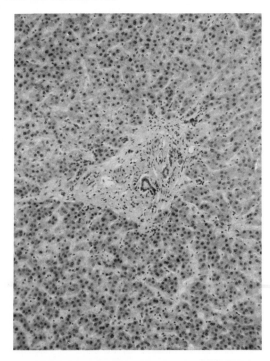

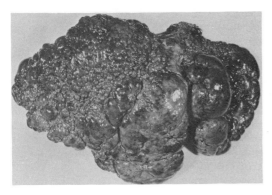

Fig. 43-7. Cystic fibrosis, autopsy: Severe multinodular biliary cirrhosis.

dysfunction, and a rapidly progressive fatal course.[244] Lymphohistiocytic infiltration with marked erythrophagocytosis is noted in multiple organs. Affected patients have a characterized immunodeficiency with altered immunoregulatory activity and hyperlipidemia. A comprehensive analysis of hepatic lipids revealed disproportionate concentrations of most of the major hepatic gangliosides.[746] These findings suggest a role for abnormal lipid metabolism in the causation of the syndrome.

Familial Hepatosteatosis

Unexplained jaundice, hepatomegaly, bleeding diathesis, and death in the neonatal period have been reported in several families.[534,553,592,718] The clinical features are heterogeneous among families, but in a given family the syndrome is stereotyped. The liver is similar histologically in all, showing diffuse large- or small-droplet fat infiltration with displacement of hepatocyte nuclei, no cholesterol crystals, and no inflammation or fibrosis. In one case kernicterus was noted at autopsy.[718] Known causes of fatty infiltration had been ruled out clinically and biochemically in all. There is no associated hypoglycemia, as seen in acyl dehydrogenase deficiencies. The biochemical basis (bases) for the syndrome(s) has not been described.

Endocrine Disorders: Idiopathic Hypopituitarism and Cholestasis

A unique association of congenital hypopituitarism, secondary to hypothalamic hypophysiotropic hormonal deficiency or aplasia of the pituitary, hypoglycemia, microphallus, and neonatal cholestasis has been described.[194,304] Histologically there are changes similar to nonspecific "neonatal hepatitis." Infants may present with cholestasis and symptoms of hypopituitarism such as hypoglycemia or hypothyroidism. Patients with the septo-optic dysplasia syndrome or optic nerve hypoplasia can be discerned clinically. The diagnosis of the latter is often suggested on physical examination by the presence of "wandering nys-

tagmus".[374] Affected patients may have low levels of thyroid hormone, cortisol, and growth hormone. The etiology of the cholestasis in the face of this endocrinopathy is unknown; however, it may be related to a common insult in perinatal life, such as a virus or a toxin. In addition, inadequate development of the hepatobiliary secretory apparatus, in the face of an absence of trophic hormones that modulate or stimulate bile canalicular development or bile acid synthesis, conjugation, or secretion, is also possible. Treatment of the endocrinopathy usually results in resolution of the hepatic dysfunction. It is important to recognize this entity, since hypoglycemia, hypothyroidism, and the attendant endocrine imbalance can be effectively treated.

Liver Disease Associated with Total Parenteral Nutrition

There have been numerous reports of the development of hepatic dysfunction in infants, especially those born prematurely and of low birth weight (<1500 g), who have received intravenous infusion of protein and glucose.[54,541,738] In fact, intrahepatic cholestasis is currently the major complication, other than catheter-related sepsis associated with this modality. Precise delineation and effective management of affected infants are hampered by the context in which the cholestasis occurs; in addition to low birth weight, most have confounding variables such as sepsis, necrotizing enterocolitis, and cardiac failure and are the recipients of blood transfusions and drugs. The incidence of cholestasis in this setting is almost universal with continued duration of therapy. A recent comparison of infants with and without cholestasis who received total parenteral nutrition (TPN) for longer than 2 weeks indicated that both groups were similar in all respects except for the frequency and severity of hyaline membrane disease and shock.[192] Factors such as hypoxia and hypotension may play a role in the development of cholestasis.

The initial description is credited to Peden and coworkers[532] who reported that a premature infant who had received TPN for approximately 10 weeks was found at autopsy to have cholestasis and cirrhosis. There have been numerous subsequent reports. In 62 premature infants studied by Beale and associates, the overall incidence of cholestasis was 23%.[58] In those receiving therapy for more than 60 days, the incidence was 80%, increasing to 90% in those treated for more than 90 days. The incidence was also inversely correlated with birth weight, reflecting the concept of predisposition to cholestasis due to hepatic immaturity.[53,641,672] Recognition of the onset of cholestasis is aided by serial monitoring of all at-risk infants, using standard indices of hepatobiliary dysfunction. We have found the measurement of serum bile acid levels to be a relatively sensitive indicator of disease.[216]

In addition to cholestasis, at-risk low-birth-weight infants receiving parenteral nutrition often have been found to have biliary sludge and gallstones. Gallbladder stasis and ileal dysfunction may be the major predisposing factors. However, sludge and gallstones may also be related to confounding variables such as the administration of diuretics and the attendant alteration of calcium homeostasis. The development of gallbladder sludge has also been demonstrated in both children and adults to be directly related to the duration of therapy[461,581]; the incidence of gallstones was also in direct relationship to duration.[461]

Pathology

As expected, during the administration of parenteral nutrition solutions, fatty change is a universal early finding; however, this does not appear to be related to the subsequent development of cholestasis.[69,77,135] However, subsequent sequential, progressive changes can be noted. After 10 to 14 days, hepatocytic and canalicular cholestasis with accumulation of bile pigment in liver cells and canalicular bile plugs may be noted. Dilated pigment-filled canaliculi are frequently surrounded by pseudorosettes. There is a mild, chronic, inflammatory infiltrate present in more advanced disease (Fig. 43-8). Portal tract expansion with ductular proliferation and portal and lobular fibrosis resembling biliary atresia may be noted after 3 weeks. It appears that these histologic changes are reversible early in the course (<90 days) following discontinuation of intravenous nutrition.[77,135] However, in patients in whom enteral nutrition is unable to be established, persisting cholestasis with moderate to severe portal fibrosis and the development of micronodular biliary cirrhosis have been described.[135,160]

In view of the lack of specificity of histologic changes, the role of liver biopsy may be questioned; however, we feel that TPN-associated cholestasis is a diagnosis made by exclusion. We have noted an alternative, specific cause of cholestasis (e.g., metabolic, endocrine or toxin-based) in 10% of our patients with presumed TPN-related cholestasis.[217] We have recently noted an unusual hepatic lesion, characterized by progressive injury: intralobular cholestasis, inflammation of venules, and extensive sinusoidal veno-occlusion with fibrosis.[95] This vasculocentric hepatotoxicity was directly related to the administration of an intravenous vitamin E supplement to low-birth-weight infants. Affected infants presented with cholestasis, thrombocytopenia, renal failure, and ascites and were often thought to have a severe form of parenteral nutrition–associated cholestasis.

Pathogenesis

An area of intensive study is to define the pathogenesis of parenteral nutrition–related cholestasis. Any postulated theory must account for the epidemiologic features, namely, the high frequency in low birth-weight, ill neonates, and the direct relationship to the duration of therapy. The predisposing role of immaturity of hepatic excretory function and physiologic cholestasis may be a key to the definition of pathogenesis.[50,53,641,672] Much effort has also been devoted to determining whether inherent toxicities or deficiencies are engendered by the infusion of the amino acid and glucose solution. No consistent data have emerged to implicate either the absolute or relative concentrations of glucose or fat; however, there is some indirect evidence to incriminate the protein content or the constituent amino acids.[267,715] Several studies have suggested that the amino acid infusion may directly inhibit hepatic excretory function. Intraperitoneal administration of tryptophan to suckling rats was associated with increased serum bile acid levels.[460] Physiologic concentrations of Na^+-dependent amino acids markedly decrease taurocholate uptake by liver plasma membrane vesicles of suckling rats; this may contribute to the bile secretory failure noted in patients receiving parenteral nutrition.[114] There is decreased bile flow during perfusion of the isolated rat liver with amino acid solutions.[267] Therefore, bile acids, which are the major determinants of bile flow, seemingly undergo a reduced clearance rate in association with the parenteral infusion of amino acids. This might diminish biliary excretion of potentially toxic compounds and increase the risk for development of cholestasis. Conversely, taurine deficiency has frequently been mentioned as a predisposing factor. Taurine has been shown to prevent cholestasis induced by lithocholic acid sulfate in guinea pigs.[191] Recent formulations of parenteral nutrition solutions have incorporated taurine. The simple act of enteral starvation is cholestatic via suppression of trophic and/or secretion-stimulating hormones normally produced by the intestine.[335,432] Affected infants are frequently subjected to prolonged fasting in view of the associated illnesses. Fasting may also be responsible in part for gallbladder stasis and sludge formation.

Fig. 43-8. Cholestasis in an infant receiving prolonged total parenteral nutrition. Biopsy changes include the presence of a low-grade portal inflammation and a mild degree of bile duct proliferation. There is intralobular cholestasis with canalicular plugs and scattered multinucleated hepatocytes.

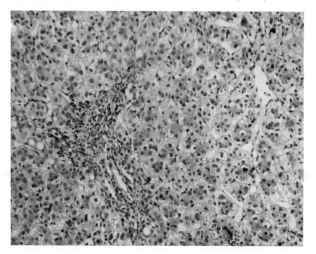

Management

At the present time, there are several approaches to the management of infants with TPN-associated liver and biliary tract disease.[54] Routine serial ultrasonography in a patient receiving TPN for prolonged periods may detect early biliary changes, such as sludge or stones. Modification of the infusate with the inclusion of taurine has been mentioned, although further studies are needed to assess the efficacy in ameliorating cholestasis. Cyclic administration of the infusate has also been suggested. The simplest modality would be to provide some minimal enteral nutrition in hopes of stimulating bile flow. The possible risk of further hepatic injury by continued administration of protein/glucose solutions must be weighed against the known risk of malnutrition in infants who cannot receive adequate oral nutrition.

Choledochal Cyst

Choledochal cyst may be detected at any age, and although cases uncommonly present in the neonatal period, these cysts must be included in the differential diagnosis of neonatal cholestasis. Cysts are present in up to 2% of infants with obstructive jaundice.[108,401] The various types and their relative frequency have been reviewed.[10,56] Infants under one year of age present in a manner simulating biliary atresia and may have progressive disease, with the development of cirrhosis, and a high mortality rate. Older children may have only mild chronic liver disease and a better prognosis. This may reflect variable degrees of common bile duct obstruction. It is also possible that the variability in age and clinical course represents two distinct entities: congenital (infants) versus acquired (older children) disease.

The classic triad of intermittent abdominal pain, jaundice, and right epigastric mass is not present in the infant and indeed is rare in older children, occurring in 21% of cases.[10] Jaundice may be absent, and abdominal pain may be the major symptom. The lesion is three times as common in the female as in the male and may be detected at any age, with 18% appearing before one year. As opposed to biliary atresia, in certain cases the lesion seems to be a true congenital malformation and is associated with other anomalies of the biliary tree such as double common duct, double gallbladder and accessory hepatic ducts, as well as polycystic kidneys and hypoplastic kidneys.[408]

The pathogenesis is undetermined; there are several theories: (1) union of the common bile and the pancreatic ducts proximal to the sphincter of Oddi may permit reflux of pancreatic enzymes into the common bile duct with resultant inflammation, localized weakness, and dilatation of the duct; (2) cysts represent a segmental weakness of the common bile duct wall; (3) cysts are part of the disease spectrum that includes idiopathic neonatal hepatitis and biliary atresia.[398,399]

In infants, the histologic changes in the liver are indistinguishable from biliary atresia.[108] Prolonged obstruction resulting in biliary cirrhosis, portal hypertension resulting from cirrhosis and pressure in the portal vein by the distended cyst, and recurrent pancreatitis are unusual complications of the malformation.[366] Ultrasonography should be the initial procedure in the evaluation of suspected choledochal cyst (Fig. 43-9). Radiographs of the upper gastrointestinal tract may outline the mass as a displacement of the first and second portion of the duodenum (Fig. 43-10). Ultimately the diagnosis requires exploration and operative cholangiography to exclude the presence of a more proximal lesion (Fig. 43-11). Treatment is via complete cyst excision and/or Roux-en-Y cyst choledochojejunostomy proximal to the most distal lesion. This allows direct mucosa to bowel mucosa anastomosis with the lowest risk of stenosis or stricture. The gallbladder is removed in all cases to decrease the risk of cholecystitis with biliary bypass. Cholangitis may occur in up to 15% of patients even with the Roux-en-Y procedure but is much less common than with direct anastomosis to the duodenum; the latter procedure is not advisable.[10,228] Carcinoma has occurred in residual cystic tissue.

Spontaneous Perforation of the Common Bile Duct

Spontaneous perforation of the common bile duct was previously considered to be a rare curiosity; however, over 50 cases have been reported.[316,355,426] The typical onset of

Fig. 43-9. Sonography of the abdomen of a 4-year-old boy with hepatomegaly. Longitudinal scan (4 cm to the right of the midline) demonstrates a large choledochal cyst (*C*) near the hilum anterior to the kidney (*K*). The proximal common hepatic duct (◄) is dilated and branches off the cyst.

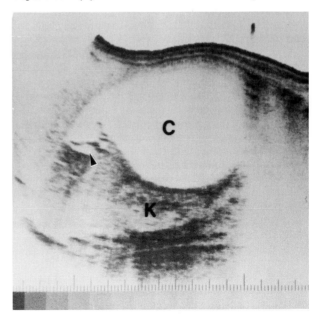

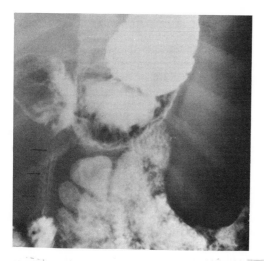

Fig. 43-10. Choledochal cyst, upper gastrointestinal series: Displacement, compression, and elongation of second portion of duodenum (*arrows*) is present. Markedly enlarged spleen, visualized to the left of the midline, resulted from secondary portal hypertension. A 14-year-old girl with upper abdominal enlargement for several years had recent abdominal pain but no jaundice.

symptoms (mild jaundice, ascites, acholic stools, poor weight gain, and vomiting) occurs before 3 months of age. Progressive abdominal distention occurs with bile staining of umbilical and inguinal hernias and the abdominal wall.[316,355,426] The diagnosis is suggested by the relatively mild conjugated hyperbilirubinemia with minimal elevation of aminotransferase levels in association with acholic stools; hepatobiliary scintigraphy may demonstrate evidence of activity outside the biliary tract.[638] Abdominal paracentesis yields clear, bile-stained ascitic fluid. Histologically the liver manifests cholestasis with a normal lobular pattern.

Operative cholangiography will usually demonstrate the presence of the perforation, frequently in association with obstruction at the distal end of the common bile duct, secondary to stenosis, segmental atresia, or "inspissated bile." The rather constant location of the perforation at the junction of the cystic and common bile ducts is highly suggestive of a developmental weakness at this site.[355] Drainage with suture closure of the perforation may be satisfactory treatment. Internal diversion via a Roux-en-Y loop of jejunum may be used for drainage in some infants.

Cholelithiasis

A rare cause of cholestasis in infancy is cholelithiasis. Cholelithiasis in infancy or childhood can be related to anatomic (perforation, malformations) conditions or can be secondary to diseases such as cystic fibrosis, Wilson's disease, ileal dysfunction, hemolysis, metachromatic leu-

kodystrophy, obesity, or the use of TPN. Descos and associates[173] reviewed 32 published reports of cholelithiasis in children under 6 months of age and delineated the following: primary lithiasis, in which the biliary duct exhibited no gross anatomic abnormalities and the stone was usually located in the distal common bile duct; or lithiasis secondary to biliary duct damage, such as perforation, frequently located at the junction of the cystic and common bile duct. For older children with symptomatic lithiasis, cholecystectomy was advocated; however, in infants with lithiasis of the common bile duct, a more conservative operative approach such as flushing with external drainage was curative. In certain of the secondary cases, surgical repair may be required. In most instances, the calculi were found to be pigment stones, often multiple, irregular in shape, with a low percentage of cholesterol composition. It is possible that the genesis of stones in patients without hemolysis or gross anatomic abnormality of the bile duct is similar to that reported for the "inspissated bile syndrome."[76,108]

Bile Plug Syndrome

Rarely, jaundice may be due to obstruction of the common duct by a plug of mucus and bile.[76] This may be different from the "inspissated bile syndrome" occuring after erythroblastosis fetalis, which is often associated with hepatocellular dysfunction and giant cell transformation. In the bile plug syndrome, hemolysis is not present and the liver histology cannot be distinguished from biliary atresia and choledochal cyst. Operative cholangiography

Fig. 43-11. Operative cholangiogram (same patient as in Fig. 43-9) contrast injection into the cystic duct details the cyst with dilated proximal common hepatic duct. (Courtesy of Drs. B. K. Han and D. S. Babcock, Cincinnati)

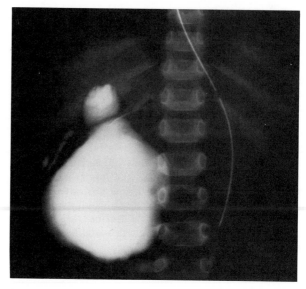

is necessary for diagnosis, and irrigation of the common duct is curative.

Idiopathic Obstructive Cholangiopathies

Once the known causes of conjugated hyperbilirubinemia discussed above (*e.g.,* α_1-AT deficiency, congenital infection) are excluded, the majority of infants with cholestasis will remain unclassified—these infants can be determined to have one of the forms of "idiopathic obstructive cholangiopathy." The spectrum encompassing these neonatal cholestatic syndromes (*i.e.,* idiopathic neonatal hepatitis, extrahepatic biliary atresia, and intrahepatic cholestasis) defies definition, classification, and effective management.[45] The nosology is imprecise, the diagnostic criteria vary, and there is very little information regarding the pathophysiologic basis of specific causes of neonatal cholestasis. Research addressing the development of the hepatocyte excretory pole, the response of the neonatal hepatobiliary tract to injury, and the mechanisms of initiation and perpetuation of impaired bile flow is needed in order to understand more fully this fascinating and challenging group of diseases.

The relative incidence has been defined in a prospective study of Australian infants by Danks and associates.[165] In an 11-year study of 790,000 births, they detected 55 cases of extrahepatic atresia (1 in 14,000 births), 11 cases of intrahepatic cholestasis (1 in 70,000) and 105 cases of idiopathic neonatal hepatitis (1 in 8,000). These relative and absolute estimates have been noted by others.[45,483]

The enigmatic nature of the two most common causes of neonatal cholestasis, namely, biliary atresia and idiopathic neonatal hepatitis, is seemingly related to two features: (1) the neonatal liver is uniquely susceptible to cholestasis; (2) these diseases may actually represent end points of a common initial insult. These features have been stated in the unifying hypothesis of Landing[398,399,489]; however, no consistent congenital or acquired defect has been defined.

Pathogenesis This spectrum of diseases involves either predominant hepatocellular injury or predominant extrahepatic biliary tract injury with intermediate gradations. As mentioned, these entities have been viewed as a continuum with each entity a manifestation of a basic underlying disease process that leads to inflammation at any level of the hepatobiliary tract. The end result represents the sequela of the inflammatory process at the primary site of injury: the hepatocytes or bile ducts. The interrelationship has been further suggested by an apparent postnatal evolution; patients initially shown to have neonatal hepatitis with a patent biliary system were subsequently found to have biliary atresia. Although the initial insult and the sustaining mechanisms remain undefined, there are sufficient provocative characteristics to allow perpetuation and future study of the concept.

Although viral infection is a postulated initial insult, no specific viral agent has been consistently isolated.

Stokes and co-workers suggested that hepatitis B virus transferred across the placenta was causative[662]; however, this could not be substantiated. The presence of hepatitis B or other viruses in tissue or serologic evidence for infection is absent in these patients.[45,49] A similarity exists between the hepatitis with biliary tract inflammation induced by reovirus type 3 infection in weanling mice and the progressive postnatal fibrotic obliteration of the extrahepatic bile ducts and liver cell injury noted in biliary atresia.[478,479] Reovirus type 3 infection may be the "initial insult" in the sequence of events resulting in infantile obstructive cholangiopathy.[45] In our initial study 68% of patients with extrahepatic biliary atresia and over 50% of infants with neonatal hepatitis had serologic evidence of reovirus type 3 infection.[254,478,479] Recently reovirus type 3 has been detected in affected tissue. These findings suggest that this virus may be involved in the pathogenesis of these diseases. Further study of the putative causative role of reovirus type 3 is needed. The observation of immunoglobulin deposits in tissue from a high percentage of patients with extrahepatic biliary atresia may indicate that immunologic injury occurs in conjunction with viral-initiated injury, thereby perpetuating the inflammation and fibrosis.[281]

Despite the postulated common etiopathogenesis and the overlap in clinical features—"obstructive jaundice," acholic stools, hepatomegaly, failure to thrive, pruritus, hemorrhagic disease, and a generally poor prognosis—these diseases may as likely be a diverse group with differing metabolic/anatomic defects.

These concepts present intriguing problems for future investigation. We believe that extrahepatic biliary atresia may be the result of the sporadic occurrence of a virus-induced or initiated progressive obliteration of the extrahepatic bile ducts with some degree of intrahepatic bile duct injury.[45] Viral infection with persisting injury may also account for sporadic (nonfamilial) cases of idiopathic neonatal hepatitis. Conversely, cases of neonatal hepatitis or other forms of intrahepatic cholestasis that demonstrate a familial trend are most likely genetic diseases that represent specific defects in the hepatic excretory process or in the bile secretory apparatus, such as alterations in bile acid metabolism or organellar function.[41,50,223,672] The persistent nature of the presumed enzymatic, metabolic, or structural defects may explain the less favorable prognosis of familial cases. Elucidation of these "inborn errors of liver function" will lead to a better understanding of biliary physiology and to improved therapy.

Differential Diagnosis of the Infant with Cholestasis

On clinical grounds the problem becomes that of separating infants with prolonged conjugated hyperbilirubinemia into those children with idiopathic defects in hepatic excretory function (neonatal hepatitis) from those with possibly remedial defects, namely, galactosemia, sepsis, endocrine disorders and potentially correctable forms of extrahepatic obstruction, such as choledochal cyst or distal biliary atresia.

Evaluation

The workup of an infant with suspected cholestasis is shown in Table 43-5. We recommend the following sequential approach. Prompt differentiation from "physiologic" or breast-milk jaundice is the first goal. Next, early recognition of specific, treatable primary causes of cholestasis is attempted. Neonatal hepatitis must then be differentiated from biliary atresia because the prognosis and management differ significantly.

In infants with neonatal cholestasis, progressive fibrosis rapidly occurs; therefore, significant delay in diagnosis or treatment must be avoided. Jaundice in an infant must not be erroneously attributed to physiologic hyperbilirubinemia or to breast-feeding. Fractionation of the serum bilirubin will usually separate out those conditions that cause a predominant elevation (>80%) of unconjugated bilirubin levels. Matsui suggests that the serum bile acid concentration, obtained from dried blood spots during the first 10 days of life, is significantly higher in cholestatic babies; this finding may allow early discrimination and detection but is impractical at present.[446]

During the evaluation of any infant with cholestasis, certain clinical features need to be addressed. Hypoprothrombinemia may be present regardless of the cause of cholestasis; therefore, administration of vitamin K may prevent spontaneous bleeding, such as intracranial hemorrhage. Expeditious performance of procedures (see Table 43-5) to rule out potentially devastating illnesses such as sepsis, endocrine disorders, and nutritional hepatotoxicity attributable to metabolic disease (galactosemia) can then

TABLE 43-5.   Initial Workup for Infants with Suspected Cholestasis

1. Clinical evaluation
2. Fractionated serum bilirubin/serum bile acid determination
3. Stool color
4. Cultures (blood, urine, spinal fluid)
5. HBsAg, TORCH, and VDRL titers
6. Index of hepatic synthetic function (prothrombin time)
7. Metabolic screen (urine/serum amino acids, urine-reducing substances)
8. Alpha$_1$-antitrypsin phenotype
9. Thyroxine and thyroid-stimulating hormone
10. Sweat chloride
11. Ultrasonography
12. Hepatobiliary scintigraphy or duodenal intubation for bilirubin content
13. Liver biopsy

(Balistreri WF: Neonatal cholestasis: Medical progress. J Pediatr 106:171, 1985)

be accomplished. Definitive detection is usually straightforward, and institution of appropriate treatment may prevent further damage.

No single test is entirely satisfactory in discriminating neonatal hepatitis from biliary atresia; however, historical and clinical features may aid in the differential. Neonatal hepatitis is reported to be more common in males and in premature infants and has a familial incidence of 15% to 20%. The intrafamilial recurrence risk is approximately 1 in 7 for neonatal hepatitis but negligible for biliary atresia.[163,165,166,483] In a study of 137 infants with cholestasis, 80% of the infants with biliary atresia were jaundiced from birth; 63% of infants with neonatal hepatitis had this feature.[483] Acholic stools, an important clue to the presence of biliary atresia, are either intermittent or delayed in onset in 25% of cases and are present in a proportion of cases of neonatal hepatitis. To detect absence of bile pigment in the stool, the center of the specimen must be examined, since bilirubin excreted through the intestinal mucosa and in sloughed cells will coat the outer surface and give a deceptively yellow appearance. The consistent presence of pigmented stools rules out biliary atresia. Duodenal fluid may be obtained to assess the bilirubin content.[45,483] If bile-stained fluid is collected, biliary atresia is excluded. Hepatobiliary scintigraphy, using iminodiacetic acid analogs, has been used by several groups to provide discriminatory data. In biliary atresia, hepatocyte function is intact early in the disease; therefore, uptake of the agent is unimpaired but excretion into the intestine is absent.[242] Conversely, in neonatal hepatitis uptake is sluggish or impaired, but excretion into the bile and intestine eventually occurs. Oral administration of phenobarbital (5 mg/kg/day) for 5 days prior to the study may enhance biliary excretion of the isotope and therefore enhance the sensitivity of the procedure.[45,242] Splenomegaly during the first 3 months of life favors the diagnosis of neonatal hepatitis, as does the presence of Coomb's negative hemolytic anemia. Hypoprothrombinemia is often unresponsive to vitamin K in infants with neonatal hepatitis. Serum 5' nucleotidase activity, which is more hepatobiliary-specific than alkaline phosphatase and has a narrow range of normal values in the infant similar to that in the adult (<15 IU), is a sensitive index of bile flow. An elevated value reflects the degree of bile duct proliferation and is suggestive of biliary obstruction. α-Fetoprotein (AFP), a glycoprotein synthesized and secreted by the fetal liver, is not detectable after birth; therefore reappearance or persistence of values is of diagnostic value; significantly higher mean AFP levels were seen in neonatal hepatitis.[22] Techniques that are used extensively in evaluation of adults with cholestatic disease, such as percutaneous transhepatic cholangiography or endoscopic retrograde cholangiography, have rarely been of value in these children. Ultrasonography may detect dilation of the biliary tract or the presence of a choledochal cyst.

Numerous diagnostic algorithms incorporating clinical and biochemical features have been proposed in an attempt to select those infants who are surgical candidates and to avoid unnecessary surgery. Alagille and associates used discriminative analysis of clinical, biochemical, and histologic data obtained in 288 infants under 3 months of age presenting with neonatal cholestasis and made an accurate differentiation in 85% of the patients studied.[6] In infants with intrahepatic disease the following features occurred significantly more frequently than in infants with extrahepatic biliary atresia: male gender; low birth weight; the presence of other congenital anomalies; later onset of jaundice (mean 23 vs 11 days of age); later onset of acholic stools (mean 30 vs 16 days); and pigmented stools within 10 days after admission (79% vs 26%). Patients with biliary atresia had a greater incidence (87% vs 53%) of liver enlargement, which was usually of a firm or hard consistency.[6] Despite the use of scoring systems such as this, approximately 10% of infants with intrahepatic disease cannot be distinguished from those with biliary atresia.[129,300] Unnecessary explorations are, of course, to be avoided; however, delay in establishing a diagnosis may also be unwarranted since the data suggest that the success rate of portoenterostomy for biliary atresia declines with age.[370,425,511]

In our experience, clinical examination, needle biopsy of the liver, and careful and repeated examination of the stool will correctly identify patients who require surgical diagnosis. In most cases biopsy can be performed using the Menghini technique of percutaneous aspiration with local anesthesia.[45,312] An accurate diagnosis is possible in up to 95% of cases and will avoid unnecessary surgery in patients with intrahepatic disease. The classic histologic features of biliary atresia are bile ductular proliferation, bile plugs, and portal or perilobular fibrosis and edema; the basic hepatic lobular architecture remains intact (Fig. 43-12). This contrasts with neonatal hepatitis, in which severe hepatocellular disease may be accompanied by marked infiltration with inflammatory cells and focal hepatocellular necrosis (Fig. 43-13). Bile ductules show little or no alteration in neonatal hepatitis. In Alagille's series,

bile ductular proliferation was present in only 30% of the patients with intrahepatic disease, compared with 86% of those with extrahepatic biliary atresia.[6] Giant cell transformation is found in a high percentage of infants with either condition and has no diagnostic specificity. When extrahepatic obstruction cannot be ruled out, limited exploration with cholangiography and needle and wedge biopsy of the liver should be performed (Figs. 43-14 and 43-15). If atresia is apparent, the biliary tract can then be further explored (see below). There are reports of the use of laparoscopy with biopsy and cholangiography in differentiation.

Neonatal Hepatitis

Idiopathic neonatal hepatitis is a descriptive term for those cases of prolonged cholestasis in which the characteristic histologic changes described by Craig and Landing are present and in which known infectious agents (such as CMV, HSV, rubella, listeria, syphilis, and toxoplasmosis) and metabolic disease have been excluded (see Fig. 43-2).[45,149,165,223,483] This term has had various connotations and therefore should be subdivided to designate hepatitis in a neonate, that is, infection with a specific virus, such as hepatitis B or CMV; intrahepatic cholestasis, discussed below; and the syndrome of neonatal hepatitis, which implies an idiopathic process associated with inflammatory changes in the liver without evidence of mechanical obstruction. The last entity accounts for the majority of cases, and certain of these patients may prove to have a currently undescribed metabolic or infectious disease. Cholestasis associated with α_1-AT deficiency, formerly included in this idiopathic category, is now clearly separable despite a similar clinical course and hepatic histopathology. Future investigation may permit other discrete diagnoses.[539,613,616] In the absence of one of these specific etiologies, idiopathic neonatal hepatitis is the only diagnosis that can be made in approximately 50% of infants

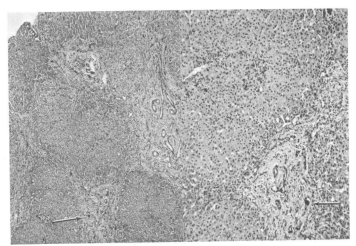

Fig. 43-12. Biliary atresia, biopsy: Well-preserved liver architecture outside the enlarged, fibrotic portal areas that contain proliferated bile ducts. Bile plug (*arrow*) in portal space and adjacent to central vein.

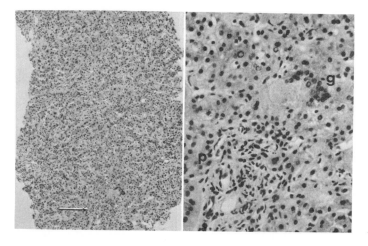

Fig. 43-13. Neonatal hepatitis: Hepatocyte appearance and lobular arrangement diffusely disturbed. Portal area infiltrated with inflammatory cells (*arrow*). Higher power shows multinucleated giant cell (*g*) adjacent to portal area (*p*).

with prolonged neonatal cholestasis. There are familial cases and cases that occur sporadically (nonfamilial). The latter are much more common.

The clinical and pathologic features were first described by Stokes and co-workers, and have been extensively reviewed.[45,149,223,483,662] The presumed heterogeneous nature of the syndrome limits precise definition. Infants with idiopathic neonatal hepatitis present with jaundice in the first week of life in 50% or more of cases and always before 2 months of age.[6,149] Infants with neonatal hepatitis may appear well and gain weight normally; about one third fail to thrive and may have a fulminant course.[6] Hepatosplenomegaly is the major physical finding. Purpura, microcephaly, hydrocephaly, and chorioretinitis do not occur, and if present suggest intrauterine infection with one of the agents described above. The jaundice may be associated with a marked decrease in bile pigment in the stool. Grossly the liver is green to black and smooth in appearance. As noted above, microscopic findings include a variable inflammatory exudate with lymphocytes, eosinophils and neutrophils, swelling of hepatocytes with marked variation in size and degenerative change, individual liver cell necrosis, multinucleated giant cells, up to 400 μm in diameter (see Fig. 43-13) scattered throughout the lobule, and increased extramedullary hematopoiesis.[476] Canalicular bile stasis is present, but ductular bile plugs are absent and bile duct proliferation negligible.[108,150] A similar "hepatitis" can be produced by viral infection during a limited period of susceptibility in the neonatal rat; this has been proposed as an animal model.[440]

Genetic causation has been proposed in view of an increased frequency of neonatal hepatitis in siblings, an in-

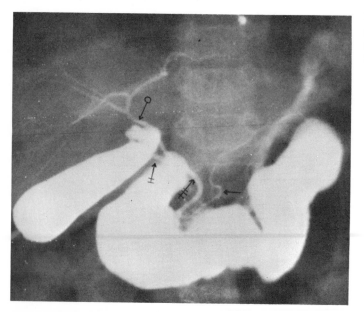

Fig. 43-14. Intrahepatic cholestasis, operative cholangiogram: Common duct of reduced caliber (O→) extends into the liver. Cystic duct (#→), common duct (#→), and pancreatic duct (→) are well visualized.

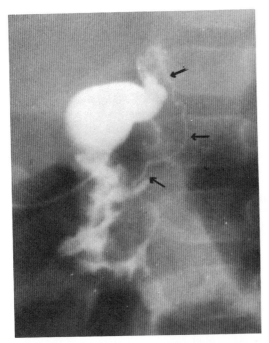 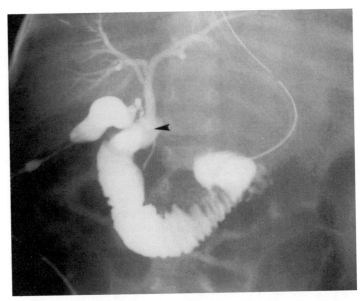

Fig. 43-15. Left. Biliary atresia, operative cholangiogram. Gallbladder is filled, with hypoplastic common duct (←) entering the duodenum, but no duct system is visualized above the gallbladder. Diagnosis proved at autopsy. **Right.** Three-month-old boy presenting with cholestasis. Intraoperative cholangiogram revealed a normal proximal biliary tract and a stricture (◄) near the junction of cystic and hepatic with common bile duct.

crease in consanguinity of parents in one series, and an increased incidence in male infants and in trisomy 21 and trisomy 18.[11,122,163,319]

Once the diagnosis of idiopathic neonatal hepatitis has been made, the goal is to manage the consequences of cholestasis (see below); there is no specific treatment. The outcome in infants with neonatal hepatitis is highly variable. Cumulative data from several series suggest that of patients with sporadic (nonfamilial) neonatal hepatitis, approximately 60% recovered, 10% had persisting fibrosis or inflammation, 2% had cirrhosis, and 30% had died.[166,175,185,506] This outcome differed from that of familial cases, or cases in which consanguinity was present; these patients had a much more severe outcome: 30% recovered, 10% developed chronic liver disease with cirrhosis, and 60% died.

Biliary Atresia

Extrahepatic biliary atresia is responsible for approximately one third of the cases of neonatal cholestasis; the incidence in various series ranges from 1 in 8,000 to 1 in 15,000 live births.[45,165] There is general agreement that the older theory of failure of recanalization of the embryonic duct is not valid and that the lesion is not a true congenital malformation but is acquired in late pregnancy or after birth.[45,165] Theoretic considerations for the etiology of extrahepatic biliary atresia have been based on epidemiologic and clinical features. There are several reports of dizygotic and monozygotic twins discordant for extrahepatic biliary atresia that seemingly exclude genetic causes.[338,668] Documented cases of atresia in premature infants or in stillbirths are rare.[100] Up to 15% to 30% of patients with extrahepatic biliary atresia may have associated anomalies: polysplenia, cardiovascular abnormalities, malrotation. Coexistence with mongolism and duodenal atresia has been reported.[165] Unlike neonatal hepatitis, there is no genetic predisposition or predominance in males and low-birth-weight infants.[163,165,319] Nevertheless, extrahepatic biliary atresia, neonatal hepatitis, and intrahepatic cholestasis may all represent varying morphologic expressions of a continuum of hepatocyte or bile duct injury by a common agent. The concept that an acquired obliterative process underlies infantile obstructive cholangiopathy is attractive and, as discussed above, suggests that a viral-related inflammation may initiate the sequence.[241,281,398,399] Giant cells have been noted in up to 40% of patients with atresia[108]; these decrease in number with advancing age.[476,620] Structural changes suggest a progression of the lesion from acute cholangitis to fibrotic obliteration of the ducts. The dynamic nature of the obliterative process is illustrated by the fact that atresia has been found at autopsy or reexploration in infants previously shown to have patent extrahepatic ducts or neonatal hepatitis.[164,311]

Neither hepatitis A nor hepatitis B virus infection seems to be etiologic.[49] Cytomegalovirus infection characteristically involves the biliary epithelium, and this virus as well as rubella has been suggested as a cause of biliary atresia.[278,516,666] However, there was no apparent increase in incidence of atresia during rubella epidemics, and CMV studies are usually negative in infants with atresia.[415] The role of maternal drug ingestion or exposure has also been fruitlessly explored. Spontaneous extrahepatic biliary atresia has been documented in a nonhuman primate.[576] Jaundice and cholestasis were detected at 6 days in an infant rhesus monkey, and at 6 weeks of age, laparotomy revealed the diagnosis. Histologic examination showed inflammatory and fibrosing lesions, similar to those observed in humans with extrahepatic biliary atresia. Of interest is the fact that sequential serum samples showed persistently high reovirus type 3 titers.[576]

The differential features of biliary atresia and neonatal hepatitis are discussed above. It should be emphasized that infants with extrahepatic biliary atresia may look well, become clinically jaundiced from 3 to 6 weeks of age, have slowly and intermittently progressive elevation of serum bilirubin levels, but seldom have pruritus or skin xanthoma. The liver is enlarged and firm; splenomegaly occurs as cirrhosis develops, and digital clubbing and arterial oxygen desaturation are evident as the disease progresses.[45,47,52,455,511]

Early in the progression of biliary atresia the liver shows preservation of the basic hepatic architecture with bile ductular proliferation, canalicular and cellular bile stasis, and portal or perilobular edema and fibrosis (see Fig. 43-12). Bile plugs in the portal ducts are relatively specific but are present in only 40% of cases. Portal fibrosis with wide swaths of connective tissue extending into the liver substance is common but not directly related to age. Twenty-five percent of infants may have portal inflammatory infiltration and hepatocyte giant cell transformation indistinguishable from neonatal hepatitis.[108,620] When the suspicion of biliary obstruction has been sufficiently established, operative exploration should be performed to document the presence and the site of obstruction and to direct attempts at surgical drainage. Cholangiography and meticulous exploration of the entire biliary tree should be carried out under general anesthesia (see Fig. 43-15). The decision made at the operating table may be aided by observations of the consistency (coarse, fibrotic) and color (green) of the liver usually associated with biliary atresia. The presence of biliary epithelium and the size of residual ducts can be evaluated in frozen sections of the transected porta hepatis.

This approach is not without pitfalls; therefore, caution should be exercised in interpretation of certain studies. In four patients reported by Markowitz and co-workers,[441] scintigraphic evidence of biliary atresia was present and intraoperative cholangiography failed to demonstrate the proximal intrahepatic biliary radicals; therefore, hepatoportoenterostomy was performed. Postoperative results included inadequate drainage with cholangitis, cirrhosis in two, and death from hepatic failure in one infant. Subsequently a histologic and clinical diagnosis of Alagille's syndrome (arteriohepatic dysplasia, see below) was made. The progression of the hepatic disease in these patients demonstrated that portoenterostomy had severely altered the course of this relatively benign disorder. During cholangiography, an absence of retrograde flow into the proximal intrahepatic ducts does not exclude the presence of a patent, albeit hypoplastic (see Fig. 43-14), extrahepatic biliary duct system in a patient with intrahepatic disease. This is not amenable to surgical correction, and no portal dissection should be attempted.

Surgical Management

The anatomy of the abnormal extrahepatic bile ducts is variable. "Correctable" lesions—distal common bile duct atresia along with a patent portion of the extrahepatic duct up to the porta hepatis—allow direct Roux-en-Y drainage. The most commonly (75%–85%) encountered lesion, however, is obliteration of all of the ducts throughout the porta hepatis, presenting an apparently noncorrectable type of atresia. The rates of establishment of bile flow are highly variable despite the rate of potential operability (correctable cases) of approximately 15% to 25%.[300,369,372] Thirty percent of infants thought to have an uncorrectable defect at initial laparotomy have been found at reexploration/autopsy to have a usable dilated hepatic duct.[300,369] Kasai observed that minute bile duct remnants or residual channels are present in the fibrous tissue near the porta hepatis. These channels are often in continuity with the intrahepatic ductal system and therefore should provide drainage.[369,511] If flow is not rapidly established in these ducts, progressive obliteration will ensue. Biliary drainage is attempted by excision of the obliterated extrahepatic ducts and apposition of the resected surface of the porta hepatis to the bowel mucosa (hepatoportoenterostomy).[13,14,372]

Prognosis

A proportion of patients with biliary atresia derive long-term benefit from hepatoportoenterostomy.[13,369,371,372,636] In the majority, however, variable degrees of hepatic dysfunction persist. Even in those patients with transient bile flow whose jaundice does not resolve, some benefit, namely growth to a size sufficient for transplantation, is often achievable. The medical management is similar for all forms of cholestasis (see below).

The variable prognosis after hepatoportoenterostomy is related directly to several factors:

Age at operation. In various series, bile flow has been established in 65% to 90% of infants under 2 months of age.[369,371,636] The success rate drops dramatically, to under 20%, in those older than 90 days at the time of operation. The initial experience of surgeons in the United States was much less successful, probably related to the advanced age of the patients at the time of the operation. Recent reports are more optimistic.[636]

The size of the ducts visualized in tissue from the porta hepatis. Microscopic patency of greater than 150 μm should determine successful postoperative bile flow,[13,14,125] although this concept is not universally recognized. For those patients with smaller or no identifiable epithelial-lined structures in fibrous tissue, the success rate was very low.[13,14,125]

The experience and operative technique of the surgeon is also a determinant.[13,14,371,372,450]

The rate of progression of the liver disease may be the overall limiting factor; a nearly universal finding is the presence of a persistent intrahepatic inflammatory process.[345] This may partially account for the poor results and for the development of portal hypertension. The continuing nature of the disease process may be caused by persistence of an infectious agent, possibly reovirus type 3, immunologically mediated injury, or the presence of an undefined metabolic aberration.

The prevention of secondary postoperative complications, namely bacterial cholangitis, which is a constant threat and can lead to reobstruction.[13,125,387,511] Patients who previously have had good bile excretion may have repeated episodes of fever, increased jaundice, leukocytosis, and evidence of contamination with intestinal flora.

Prognosis following portoenterostomy procedures may also be correlated with the degree of proliferation of the periductular glands. It has been suggested that the hilar biliary plexus may act as a drainage route for bile in these patients.[750]

Several series have emphasized the potential value of reoperation in patients with cessation of bile flow after initial success or with refractory cholangitis. In many cases debridement or revision of the scarred area was associated with the establishment of bile flow.[14,512] Ohi and associates, were successful in obtaining bile drainage after reoperation in 13 of 15 patients in whom flow had initially been established and cessation of bile flow developed.[512] In 12 patients with an initial poor bile flow, reoperation established flow in 4.

Numerous other surgical procedures, including insertion of metal tubes into the liver as artificial bile ducts, drainage of hepatic lymph by anastomosis of lymphatics in the porta hepatis or the thoracic duct to the intestinal tract, and suturing of the raw surface of the liver to the open intestine, have failed.[430,676,677]

Progressive biliary cirrhosis may result in death from hepatic failure, often despite an apparent successful drainage. We have recently seen severe variceal hemorrhage from dilated vessels in the submucosa of the enterostomy loop as a cause of death.

Intrahepatic Cholestasis

A heterogeneous subset of cholestatic diseases, characterized by intrahepatic cholestasis with or without bile duct alterations (hypoplasia or paucity), must be further delineated; these may represent specific syndromes with different prognostic implications. Intrahepatic cholestasis may be the result of hepatocyte or biliary epithelial cell dysfunction induced by a variety of metabolic, genetic, or infectious mechanisms.[45,223,349]

The term bile duct paucity implies that within the portal triad there is an absence or marked reduction in the number of interlobular bile ducts (defined as <0.5 intralobular bile ducts/triad) despite the presence of normal sized branches of the portal venule and hepatic arteriole. The term bile duct hypoplasia is more restrictive pathogenetically and implies a decrease in the size of the bile ducts. These two features may suggest disparate genesis, representing congenital absence, partial failure to form, atrophy secondary to diminished bile flow, or progressive injury with disappearance. Segmental destructive changes or progressive decrease in the number of bile ducts per portal tract on serial sectioning of biopsies has been documented (Fig. 43-16). CMV induced obliterative cholangitis has been suggested as a precursor of liver dysfunction associated with paucity of intrahepatic bile ducts.[224] However, initiating factors and the mechanisms of perpetuation remain to be determined. The histopathological changes may be correlated with presumed physiological alterations; the ductular abnormalities associated with childhood intrahepatic cholestasis may represent a primary functional or enzymatic defect or a change secondary to the toxic effects of retained compounds such as bile acids.

Early descriptions of patients with isolated paucity or hypoplasia of intrahepatic bile ducts, with an intact extrahepatic biliary tree, did not attempt to separate out distinctive syndromes. Recent observations suggest that this is possible. These syndromes are of great theoretic interest—detailed study may enhance our understanding of hepatic excretory function and bile acid metabolism. It is difficult to delineate precisely the ancestral origins of many of the syndromes of intrahepatic cholestasis.[45,53,223,269,349,399] Those associated with bile duct hypoplasia or paucity, often called intrahepatic biliary atresia, may actually represent an end-stage of a neonatal hepatitis-like illness. The genetic basis for these diseases is only partially defined; however, it appears that there are mild forms with varying clinical features.[223]

Clinical Features

The heterogeneous nature of the diseases manifested as intrahepatic cholestasis, with or without bile duct paucity or hypoplasia, precludes an accurate overall statement regarding presentation and prognosis. There are certain progressive, fatal, familial forms such as that seen in Byler's syndrome. However, in patients with syndromic paucity of ducts (the arteriohepatic dysplasia syndrome), the

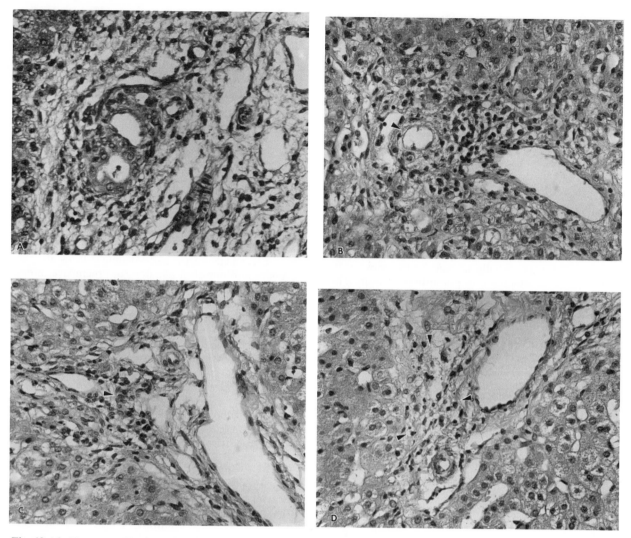

Fig. 43-16. Four portal fields (*A/B/C/D*), observed simultaneously in the same biopsy specimen obtained from a 2½-month-old boy presenting with cholestasis, demonstrate stages of bile duct injury that may result in paucity. **A.** Pericholangitis with bile duct epithelial proliferation. **B.** Damaged bile duct (◄) with patent lumen and pericholangitis. **C.** Inconspicuous bile duct (◄) with minimal surrounding inflammatory process. **D.** Portal area contains no recognizable bile duct; a focal area of cell debris (◄) may represent site of destroyed ductule.

prognosis is much more favorable. Patients with identical syndromic features may show minimal histologic changes of cholestasis, yet a reduction in bile flow is inferred from secondary features such as an elevation of the serum bile acid concentration. A decrease in the number of interlobular ductules may also be observed in some infants with α_1-AT deficiency as part of the wide spectrum of hepatic abnormalities associated with this disorder.[507]

While the diseases in which intrahepatic cholestasis occurs share many clinical features, there are also certain discrete patterns that suggest specific disease entities (see Table 43-4). Hepatomegaly and jaundice are frequently present in the neonatal period; conjugated bilirubin, aminotransferase, cholesterol, and serum bile acid concentrations are variably elevated. Acholic stools may be noted depending on the degree of cholestasis. Jaundice may be transient during the first weeks of life and may be erroneously attributed to "physiologic" unconjugated hyperbilirubinemia of the newborn. In other infants biliary flow may be compromised to such a degree as to indicate the possibility of extrahepatic obstruction.[441] Pruritus and xanthomatous skin eruptions are frequently seen (Fig. 43-17), although jaundice may clear after several months. Affected infants may seem unusually irritable, but obvious

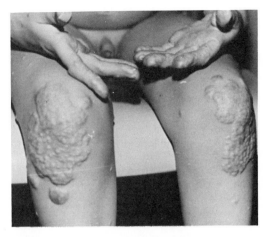

Fig. 43-17. Intrahepatic cholestasis: Characteristic skin xanthomata on hands and knees. Serum cholesterol above 500 mg/100 ml; patient 5 years of age.

pruritus is rare before 3 months of age.[6] Dysmorphoric features and congenital malformations may be evident and suggestive of recognized cholestatic syndromes, such as that described by Alagille and associates.[7]

Intrahepatic cholestasis associated with a paucity of interlobular bile ducts may occur without associated developmental abnormalities and without a benign prognosis; this variant was initially described by Ahrens and associates.[4] The overall prognosis for patients with intrahepatic cholestasis, as noted, appears to be variable based on a compilation of several series.[45] Heathcote and coworkers described a group of 17 patients with intrahepatic cholestasis who were followed for periods of 5 months to 22 years; there were 13 with prolonged survival; however, serial liver biopsies in 11 children showed a decreasing number of small and medium sized bile ducts, increasing portal fibrosis, and eventual cirrhosis.[301] Of the initial 34 cases studied by Alagille, 19 were associated with distinct abnormalities; these "syndromic" patients enjoyed an excellent prognosis. In contrast, no associated malformations were present in the remaining 15; 11 died of cirrhosis in the first 13 years of life.[6,7] Alagille reemphasized the unfavorable course in a group of 18 patients with nonsyndromic intrahepatic cholestasis; 40% of these children died of progressive biliary cirrhosis and hepatic failure.[6] A familial tendency has frequently been noted in this presumably heterogenous form of intrahepatic cholestasis.[45,166,175,185,295]

Evaluation

Initial diagnostic efforts should focus on excluding extrahepatic obstruction and known causes of neonatal liver disease including congenital infection, α_1-AT deficiency, cystic fibrosis, and galactosemia as described above. Histologic findings are nonspecific and common to many liver diseases of early life: variable hepatocellular damage, ballooning of hepatocytes, and giant cell transformation.[223] The ratio of interlobular ducts to the number of portal areas may be reduced in comparison with normal children. However, paucity of intrahepatic ducts may be found in many cholestatic infants and is not pathognomonic of a specific syndrome.[580] Conversely, unless a large enough biopsy, that is, 15 to 20 portal areas, is reviewed, paucity may not be detected. Ultrastructural analysis may be helpful in the diagnosis of specific entities such Zellweger's syndrome and Byler's disease.

Arteriohepatic Dysplasia (Syndromic Paucity of the Intrahepatic Bile Ducts)

The most commonly occurring constellation of findings to incorporate intrahepatic bile duct paucity was described by Alagille.[7] This group of patients is characterized by cholestasis, a decreased number of interlobular ducts, and various congenital malformations.[7,273,723] Jaundice may persist after the neonatal period, and intense pruritus is usually noticed by 4 to 6 months of age. Hepatomegaly is a constant feature. Extrahepatic anomalies are distinctive, but there is considerable variability in phenotypic expression[563,564]: unusual facial characteristics may be recognized in infancy—the forehead is broad, the eyes deeply set and widely spaced, and the chin pointed (these may be nonspecific); vertebral arch defects (butterfly vertebrae, hemivertebrae, and a decrease in the interpedicular distance) are present in the majority of patients; ophthalmologic examination may reveal the presence of posterior embryotoxon (prominent Schwalbe's line); peripheral pulmonic stenosis, the most common cardiovascular defect, is present in over 90% of these cases. Short stature and mental retardation occur and are independent of the severity of cholestasis. Renal abnormalities are frequently associated.

Liver histologic examination demonstrates variable degrees of cholestasis and a paucity of intrahepatic bile ducts. Ballooning of hepatocytes, bile ductular proliferation, portal inflammation, and giant cell transformation may be prominent during the first months of life. The major histopathologic features of arteriohepatic dysplasia are paucity or absence of the intrahepatic interlobular ducts, cholestasis, and an absence of significant fibrosis or cirrhosis. Mild periportal fibrosis may result, but progression to cirrhosis has not been described.[6,563,564] Portal tracts are reduced in size and number.[6,7,161,708] The extrahepatic ductule systems in patients with arteriohepatic dysplasia are patent but are often hypoplastic.[161,441] It has recently been noted that the ultrastructural features suggest distinctive changes.[708] Bile regurgitation into the intercellular space is nearly universal, although the bile canaliculi look normal. Bile pigment retention in the cytoplasm, especially in lysosomes and in vesicles of the outer convex face of the Golgi apparatus, is seen, suggesting a block in the Golgi apparatus or in the pericanalicular cytoplasm. In addition, there is a lack of the ultrastructural pericanalicular changes noted in many forms of cholestasis, such as thickened ectoplasm, an absence of canalicular bile plugs and bile canalicular dilatation; there is no microvillus atrophy.[708] The authors therefore postulate the existence of a bile secretory defect within the hepatocyte that is precanalicular, possibly occurring at the level of the Golgi apparatus.[708]

The histopathologic diagnosis of arteriohepatic dysplasia may not be obvious in infancy. Dahms and colleagues[161] have stressed an evolution of the characteristic pathology of arteriohepatic dysplasia; biopsies were performed on five patients during infancy (i.e., <6 months of age). The histologic features suggested intrahepatic cholestasis and portal inflammation. The infants did not have an absence of intralobular bile ducts (IBD), and only two of the five had paucity (<0.5 IBD/triad). Six biopsies were performed later in life, at 3 to 20 years of age. All had documented paucity or absence of bile ducts, and the cholestasis and inflammation had resolved. If biopsies are evaluated longitudinally, with increasing age portal triads may be noted to contain fewer bile ducts; the progression of the lesion is not associated with inflammation or fibrosis. The mechanism whereby interlobular bile duct deficiency is produced is unknown.

This form of intrahepatic cholestasis carries a relatively good prognosis. Most patients have survived the first decade, and several adults have been reported with this disorder. In most cases, parents are not obviously affected, indicating autosomal recessive transmission; however, typical features have been noted in a father and son.[564] La Brecque and associates have documented the presence of arteriohepatic dysplasia in four successive generations of a single kindred.[395] Of 24 members, 15 had at least some of the characteristics of the arterioehepatic dysplasia syndrome, strongly supporting an autosomal dominant form of transmission.

Hereditary Cholestasis with Lymphedema

Aagenaes and associates have described patients of Norwegian extraction with intrahepatic cholestasis and lymphedema of the legs.[1] Jaundice is consistently present during the neonatal period but occurs episodically in older children. Lymphedema in the lower extremities begins in later childhood and has been attributed to lymphatic vessel hypoplasia. The relationship between the peripheral lymphatic obstruction and liver disease is uncertain. Aagenaes postulates a hepatic lymph-hypoplasia or a functional defect in lymphatic flow leading to cholestasis. Study of reported cases supports an autosomal recessive mode of inheritance of this disorder. Liver histology shows giant cell transformation and cholestasis in infancy. Cirrhosis has been found in several adult patients.[2]

Byler's Disease

A severe form of intrahepatic cholestasis with progressive hepatocellular damage occurs sporadically or on a familial basis[357,509]; paucity of intrahepatic ducts is not a consistent finding. The clinical features and natural progression have been variable in these reports, implying significant heterogeneity among this group of patients. The most completely defined group includes members of several Amish sibships each named Byler.[132] In these children, loose, foul-smelling stools appeared during the first weeks of life. The onset of jaundice was noted later during the first year and was initially episodic but became persistent between 1 and 4 years of age. Mental retardation and growth retardation were usually present; hepatosplenomegaly was a regular feature. Moderate hyperbilirubinemia, elevation of aminotransferase levels, and elevated serum bile acid concentrations were present. A relative increase in the serum concentration of lithocholic acid and hyocholic acid has been reported in the serum of some patients, which probably reflects the severity of cholestasis rather than being specific for this disorder.[427,653]

Liver histology shows severe cholestasis. Slight proliferation of interlobular bile ducts was recorded in the description of Clayton and associates.[132] Progressive intrahepatic cholestasis and cirrhosis are present on subsequent biopsies. Electron microscopy shows dilatation of the canalicular lumen, which is filled with coarse particulate amorphous granular material, reduction in the number of microvilli, and focal interruption of the canalicular membrane.[132] Particularly striking in one report were numerous microfilamentous structures in the pericanalicular ectoplasm and in the hepatocyte cytoplasm. The authors postulate a relationship between the hyperplasia of microfilamentous structures in the liver and a defect in hepatic excretory function.[177]

Death from cirrhosis and liver failure is likely in childhood or early adolescence. Twin brothers with a "Byler-like" illness died during their teenage years of hepatocellular carcinoma.[159] The presence of consanguinity and liver dysfunction in parents of some affected children suggests an autosomal recessive inheritance. Similar inherited syndromes with progressive intrahepatic cholestasis have been reported by others.[357,360,726]

Weber described 14 North American Indian children with a severe form of familial cholestasis.[726] In nine the onset resembled neonatal cholestasis; however, in all, progressive deterioration with the development of portal fibrosis and neoductule proliferation developed. The electron microscopic changes were unique: marked widening of the pericanalicular ectoplasm with abundant pericanalicular microfilaments. Since these contractile proteins make up the hepatocyte cytoskeleton and are involved in bile acid transport and the generation of bile flow, the authors suggest microfilament dysfunction as the underlying disorder.

An unusual form of chronic, slowly progressive intrahepatic cholestasis was recently described in adults. Associated features were dermal hypertrichosis, increased pigmentation, and predisposition to autoimmune conditions, such as chronic thyroiditis with polyneuropathy.[209] High serum levels of α-lipoprotein were found. Prekeratin is an important component of the intermediate filaments in hepatocytes. The authors postulate that a defect in prekeratin-keratin metabolism might be operative, accounting for the hepatic as well as other manifestations.[209]

Benign Recurrent Intrahepatic Cholestasis

Benign recurrent intrahepatic cholestasis most likely represents a variety of defects in hepatic excretory function. This poorly defined group of diseases is mentioned briefly here, since onset is usually noted during childhood.[172] Approximately 20% of patients will experience their first attack by one year of age. The illness may initially be confused with the more common progressive forms of infantile cholestasis and may represent related variants. Complete clinical and biochemical resolution followed by recurrent attacks establishes the diagnosis. Since many of the cases in the literature are inadequately documented, specific criteria have been suggested for this disorder: several episodes of pronounced jaundice with pruritus and biochemical evidence of cholestasis; bile plugs on liver biopsy; apparently normal intrahepatic and extrahepatic bile ducts on cholangiography; absence of factors (e.g., drugs) known to produce cholestasis; and symptom-free intervals of months or years.[172] In infants, other forms of cholestasis, especially the intrahepatic cholestasis syndromes, become prominent considerations in the differential diagnosis. However, in patients affected with intrahepatic cholestasis, while clinical cholestasis may be variable, biochemical abnormalities are persistent. Syndromic features, if present and recognized, may be helpful.

Defective Bile Acid Metabolism

Considerable attention has been directed toward documentation of the existence of possible defects in bile acid metabolism in the pathogenesis of intrahepatic cholestasis.[45,212,292] Hanson and co-workers reported the detection of substantial concentrations of trihydroxycoprostanic acid (THCA) in bile, serum, and urine of two siblings with progressive intrahepatic cholestasis.[292] Both infants developed jaundice in the neonatal period associated with a paucity of intrahepatic bile ducts on liver biopsy. Cirrhosis and death from liver failure occurred at 8 months and 2 years of age. A defect in cholic acid synthesis was considered in light of an elevated total serum bile acid and low serum cholic acid concentration and identification of THCA by gas chromatography/mass spectrometry. THCA is directly converted to cholic acid via mitochondrial oxidative cleavage of the terminal three carbons of the side chain. Infusion of THCA into rats induced hemolysis and hepatic ultrastructural lesions consisting of focal dilation of vesicles within the lumina of the endoplasmic reticulum, decreased matrix density and elongated internal cristae in mitochondria, and filamentous material and vesicles within bile canaliculi.[294] Poulos and Whiting have identified THCA in the plasma of patients with infantile Refsum's disease.[542] It remains to be determined whether this biochemical abnormality reflects specific organelle dysfunction (see below) or is the primary defect in affected children.

Zellweger's Syndrome

Infants with Zellweger's syndrome (cerebrohepatorenal syndrome) have similar defects in bile acid metabolism that have been correlated with altered organellar function and morphology.[293] Clinical manifestations include profound psychomotor retardation, a characteristic facies (narrow cranium, prominent forehead, hypertelorism, and epicanthic folds), cortical cysts of the kidney, and intrahepatic cholestasis.[529,635] Hepatomegaly is usually present at birth, and jaundice appears at 2 to 3 weeks of life. Death from severe hypotonia, sepsis, or intestinal hemorrhage secondary to hypoprothrombinemia occurs in most patients by 6 months of age. The liver reveals variable cholestasis, lobular disarray, focal necrosis, and in some cases paucity of intrahepatic ducts.[246,529,635] A diffuse micronodular cirrhosis is usually present terminally. Ultrastructurally, peroxisomes are absent and mitochondria show disarrangement and twisting of cristae, and angulate lysosomes are visible.[262,477]

The Zellweger syndrome is therefore characterized by the virtual absence of peroxisomes in the liver. These microbodies, which are normally the site of catalases, oxidases, and the like, play an important role in β-oxidation of fatty acids. Several studies have documented increased amounts of C_{27}-bile acid intermediates in serum, urine, and bile of affected infants.[80,168,307] These bile acid precursors, which are characterized by the presence of a partially oxidized side chain, suggest an important role for peroxisomes in bile acid metabolism. This has led to a clear elucidation of a new class of diseases, peroxisomal disorders.[262,263,373,481,482,626,627] Adrenoleukodystrophy, glutaric aciduria type II (multiple acyl-CoA-dehydrogenation defects), and olivocerebellar atrophy share with Zellweger's syndrome altered peroxisomal "chain shortening" function and have distinct patterns of excessive fatty acids. Altered peroxisomal metabolism also accounts for the other biochemical abnormalities that have previously been noted in patients with Zellweger's syndrome, such as the accumulation of pipecolic acid, which is a product of lysine metabolism that accumulates in the presence of deficient peroxisomal oxidase activity; and accumulation of very long chain fatty acids (hexacosanoic C26:0 and hexacosenoic C26:1) in the absence of peroxisomal oxidation.[603,604] Altered organellar function is also suggested by excessive urinary excretion of THCA, dihydroxycoprostanic acid (DHCA), and varanic acid, all precursors of primary bile acids that have undergone incomplete side-chain oxidation.[292]

Since affected infants with Zellweger's syndrome usually die early in life, a precise biochemical diagnosis and differentiation from other causes of hypotonia are important in order to provide genetic counseling. Characteristic dysmorphic, radiologic, biochemical, and pathological findings have been described in four affected fetuses.[544] Prenatal diagnosis of Zellweger's syndrome is possible based on increased levels and impaired degradation of very long chain fatty acids, particularly hexacosanoic acid (C26:0) and hexacosenoic acid (C26:1) in amniotic fluid and in cultured amniocytes.[481,482] The defect in plasmalogen-synthesis in Zellweger's syndrome is restricted to the peroxisome; therefore, microsomal biosynthetic steps are normal. A novel diagnostic assay using fibroblasts and amniocytes is based on the comparison of the ratio of ^{3}H to ^{14}C following incubation with ^{14}C-hexadecanol and ^{3}H-hexadecylglycerol. Quantitative analysis is unnecessary, and the isotopic ratio can be determined within the aldehydes released from plasmalogens by acid hydrolysis.[575] Attempts to induce peroxisomes in two cases of Zellweger's syndrome by treatment with clofibrate have been unsuccessful,[81] suggesting that the protein that is absent is essential for peroxisome formation.

Related Disorders

Idiopathic Neonatal Iron Storage Disease

An entity that resembles, yet is seemingly distinct from, Zellweger syndrome has been noted in infants.[261] Autopsy studies have demonstrated massive amounts of iron in lysosomes (hepatocytes and pancreatic acinar cells).[261] The underlying defect is undefined.

Glutaric Aciduria Type II

Multiple acyl-CoA-dehydrogenation deficiency is characterized by cholestasis with bile duct hypoplasia, siderosis, and fatty degeneration.[88] In addition, congenital polycystic kidneys and symmetric warty dysplasia of the cerebral cortex have been associated. The relationship to peroxisomal dysfunction is suggested by the accumulation of large quantities of carboxylic acids.[88]

Medical Management of Chronic Cholestasis

Following diagnostic evaluation of the infant with neonatal cholestasis or prolonged hyperbilirubinemia, several possibilities exist: specific treatment (*e.g.,* dietary restriction of galactose); surgical attempt at palliation (*e.g.,* hepatoportoenterostomy); and nonspecific management of the consequences of cholestasis (Fig. 43-18). The clinical consequences of prolonged cholestasis attributable directly or indirectly to diminished bile flow must be addressed: retention by the liver of substances normally excreted in

Fig. 43-18. The clinical consequences of prolonged cholestasis result from [1] retention by the liver of substances normally excreted in bile with regurgitation into serum and into tissue, [2] a progressive biliary cirrhosis with complications such as portal hypertension, and [3] a reduction in bile acid delivery to the proximal intestine with inefficient micellar solubilization and malabsorption.

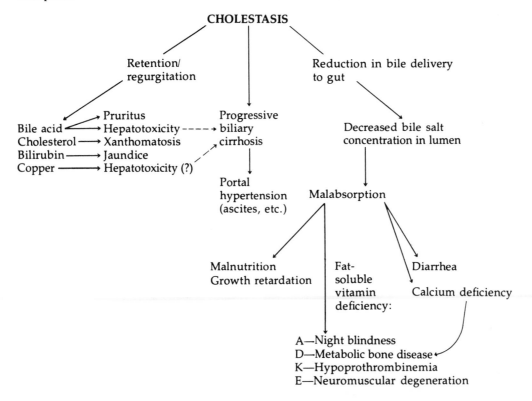

bile, namely bile acids, bilirubin, cholesterol, and trace elements; decreased delivery of bile acids to the proximal intestine, with decreased intraluminal bile acid concentrations resulting in malabsorption of fat and fat-soluble vitamins; and progressive liver damage, with biliary cirrhosis, portal hypertension, and liver failure. Cholestasis, liver damage, and malnutrition interact to alter the metabolism of hormones, somatomedins, or other factors required for growth, and thus result in marked growth failure.[45,47,48,52]

Therefore, for patients with idiopathic neonatal hepatitis, intrahepatic cholestasis, or extrahepatic biliary atresia in whom surgery is unsuccessful, management becomes an effort to minimize growth failure and to reduce discomfort. The limiting factors remain the residual functional capacity of the liver and the rate of progression of the liver disease. Our recommendations for management of cholestasis (Table 43-6) are empiric; therefore, individ-

ualization and careful monitoring serve as the most reliable guide.

Impaired bile secretion can lead to malabsorption and malnutrition due to ineffective intraluminal long-chain triglyceride lipolysis and absorption; therefore medium-chain triglycerides administered in formula or as oil may be beneficial.[136,497] Similarly, fat-soluble vitamin deficiency may occur in patients with chronic cholestasis and may be associated with significant symptoms, most prominently rickets caused by vitamin D deficiency and neuromuscular disease associated with vitamin E deficiency.[48,497,639,640] Malabsorption of these vitamins may be exacerbated by coadministration of cholestyramine. Chronic deficiency of vitamin E (α-tocopherol) results in the development of a progressive disabling degenerative neuromuscular syndrome composed of areflexia, cerebellar ataxia, ophthalmoplegia, posterior column dysfunction, and peripheral neuropathy.[48,578,639,640] The di-

---

TABLE 43-6.   Medical Management of the Effects of Chronic Cholestasis in Children[45,48,497]

A. Malabsorption/malnutrition
   1. Supply medium-chain triglycerides
      a. Formula[136]
      b. Oil[136]
   2. Decrease intake of long-chain triglycerides
   3. Ensure adequate protein intake
B. Vitamin deficiency
   1. Supplement (approximately 2–4 X RDA)
      a. Vitamin A as Aquasol A, up to 25,000 IU/day
      b. Vitamin D
         as D$_2$, 5000 IU/day
         as 25-hydroxycholecalciferol (25 OHCC) oral dose of 3–5 μg/kg/day
      c. Vitamin K as water-soluble derivative of menadione, 2–5 mg/day
      d. Vitamin E as Aquasol E, up to 400 IU/day (? parenteral)
   2. Elemental calcium 50–200 mg/kg/day and elemental phosphorus 25–50 mg/kg/day
C. Pruritus/xanthomata
   a. Phenobarbital, 5–20 mg/kg/day[83,615,660]
   b. Cholestyramine, 8 g (2 packets)/day or more given before and after the first meal of the day
      Complications: Unpalatable; also may lead to obstruction, hyperchloremic acidosis, steatorrhea exacerbation
   c. Other modalities (unproved)
      1. Chlorpromazine
      2. Carbamazepine
      3. Neomycin sulfate (binds bile acids; prevents formation of secondary bile acids)
      4. Cupruretic agents (*e.g.,* penicillamine)
      5. Plasmaperfusion
      6. Phototherapy
D. Ascites/liver failure
   a. Diet, decrease sodium intake (1–2 mEq/kg/day)
   b. Diuretics
      1. Spironolactone, 3–5 mg/kg/day in four doses
      2. Furosemide, 1–2 mg/kg/dose prn
   c. Transplantation

agnosis of vitamin E deficiency in children with chronic cholestasis has been based on low serum levels. However, elevated lipid values allow vitamin E to partition into plasma lipoproteins and falsely raise the serum vitamin E concentration, often into the normal range.[639,640] The neurologic syndrome is partially reversible; therefore, early attempts at repletion should be initiated. The marked impairment of vitamin E absorption may not be compensated by even massive orally administered doses (50–200 IU/kg/day α-tocopherol) of the vitamin.[45,48,639,640] We have used parenterally administered vitamin E in selected patients.[45,48,639,640]

Pruritus and xanthomas, which may cause significant morbidity, are difficult to treat. Compounds such as phenobarbital and cholestyramine will work only if there is an adequate drainage system to allow bile acids to reach the gut lumen.[48,83,497,615,660] Phenobarbital, a known choleretic agent, may also enhance the rate of formation of polar tetrahydroxylated bile acids, which can be readily excreted by the kidney.[45,83,665]

Patients with liver failure associated with chronic cholestasis are candidates for orthotopic liver transplantation. The major indication for liver transplantation in pediatric patients is extrahepatic biliary atresia, which accounts for approximately 50% of all recipients. The high success rates (60%–70%) recently reported for children are the result of excellent preoperative, intraoperative, and postoperative care as well as the use of cyclosporine.[757] These encouraging reports suggest that liver transplantation offers an alternative therapeutic approach that may prolong life in certain patients with severe liver disease.[347,757]

Although the success of biliary–enteric anastomosis in patients with extrahepatic biliary atresia cannot be predicted, we believe it remains the most reasonable initial therapy. Liver transplantation should be delayed as long as possible to permit maximal growth. However, repeated attempts at revision of the hepatoportoenterostomy or portal systemic shunting seem to render eventual transplantation surgery more difficult and more dangerous.[347,757] In that situation, liver transplantation should be seriously considered.

METABOLIC DISEASES OF THE LIVER

Hepatic synthetic, degradative, and regulatory pathways are essential to carbohydrate, lipid, protein, trace element, and vitamin metabolism. Hepatic dysfunction may therefore be primarily or secondarily associated with enzymatic deficiencies or metabolic abnormalities. Hepatic involvement may be manifest as hepatocyte injury with secondary alteration in metabolic function and progression of the injury to cirrhosis; storage of lipid or glycogen; or an absence of true histologic alteration but profound clinical effects of the enzyme deficiency (*e.g.,* in urea cycle defects). In the presence of a metabolic block, a normal nutrient or substrate may become a nonmetabolizable hepatotoxin.

Rapid and precise recognition of inherited enzymopathies will allow treatment by dietary restriction of the offending substrate, replacement of a deficient end product, depletion of a stored substance, administration of metabolic inhibitors, amplification of enzyme activity, or replacement or modification of the mutant protein. The use of amniotic fluid, fibroblasts, and white cells in diagnosis or in screening may have important genetic implications. In addition, organ transplantation offers an alternative modality for many of the diseases to be described.

Inherited metabolic diseases of the liver have protean clinical manifestations often mimicking infections, intoxications, or other systemic diseases; therefore, a high index of suspicion is required. There are clinical features that should suggest the possibility of metabolic disease of the liver: jaundice, hepatomegaly, splenomegaly, hepatic failure, hypoglycemia, organic acidemia, hyperammonemia, hypoprothrombinemia, recurrent vomiting, failure to thrive/short stature, dysmorphic features, developmental delay/psychomotor retardation, hypotonia, progressive neuromuscular deterioration, seizures, unusual odors, rickets, or cataracts. Information obtained from the family or dietary history as well as clinical and laboratory examination can be complemented by analysis of tissue obtained by liver biopsy. This will confirm the suspicion or alert the clinician to new possibilities and allow enzyme assay as well as qualitative and quantitative assay of stored material.[23]

Disorders of Tyrosine Metabolism

There are numerous causes of hypertyrosinemia. For example, transient neonatal tyrosinemia (TNT) has been described in premature infants[35]; this must be differentiated from classic hereditary tyrosinemia. In TNT, immaturity of tyrosine aminotransferase or deficiency of dietary ascorbic acid may be responsible for this mild elevation of serum levels; the liver is normal morphologically. Elevated tyrosine levels in blood may also be an acquired disorder secondary to any form of severe liver injury; therefore, this biochemical finding may be present in infants with galactosemia or neonatal hepatitis. This heterogeneity of symptoms suggests that hypertyrosinemia *per se* does *not* cause neurologic or hepatic damage.

Hereditary tyrosinemia is characterized by hepatic dysfunction, eventuating in liver failure or in cirrhosis, renal tubular dysfunction, and abnormal tyrosine metabolism.[609] There are two apparent forms (acute or chronic), which may occur in the same family. The disease may present in infancy as acute hepatic failure, failure to thrive, ascites, hypoprothrombinemia, bleeding or jaundice, or later in childhood as progressive cirrhosis and rickets.[545,609]

The laboratory features of acute tyrosinemia often indicate disproportionate abnormalities of hepatic synthetic function versus biochemical indices of liver injury. This is evidenced by hypoalbuminemia and a decrease in vitamin K–dependent clotting factors with only a mild to moderate rise in aminotransferase values. There is also a variable rise in total and direct bilirubin; hypophosphatemic rickets; marked elevation of serum tyrosine to levels much higher than those seen in other liver diseases; hypermethioninemia; urinary excretion of phenolic acid byproducts of tyrosine-p-hydroxyphenyl lactic acid, p-hydroxyphenyl pyruvic acid, and p-hydroxyphenyl acetic acid, which can be screened for using Nitrosonaphthol; succinylacetone and succinylacetoacetate in urine; and increased urinary excretion of delta-aminolevulenic acid (ALA). Affected patients are often anemic with evidence of hemolysis, are hypoglycemic, and have renal tubular dysfunction (Fanconi syndrome), which can manifest as hyperphosphaturia, glucosuria, proteinuria, and aminoaciduria. In the acute phase there may be generalized aminoacidemia with a disproportionate elevation of serum levels of tyrosine and methionine; in the older child, aminoacidemia is usually limited to tyrosine, but aminoaciduria is generalized with tyrosine predominating.

The presence of greatly increased amounts of α-fetoprotein in the presence of normal levels of tyrosine in cord blood of affected infants suggests that hypertyrosinemia develops postnatally and that liver disease has a prenatal onset.[314] In the acute form there is fatty infiltration of the liver, iron deposition, varying degrees of liver cell necrosis which may be extreme, and fine diffuse fibrosis with formation of pseudoacini.[545,609] In the older child there is a gross multilobular portal cirrhosis, and bile duct proliferation is often present. In some patients, regenerative nodules resembling a neoplasm may be present, and hepatoma may in fact occur in the older patient.[728]

The primary site of metabolic block in hereditary tyrosinemia has been localized to the level of fumarylacetoacetase (FAH),[428] the final step in the oxidative degradation of phenylalanine and tyrosine. Defective activity of this enzyme accounts for the secondary enzymatic and biochemical defects encountered in tyrosinemia. Accumulated metabolites, such as succinylacetoacetate, fumarylacetoacetate, and maleylacetoacetate, are found in blood and urine.[275] These reactive compounds are capable of binding to sulfhydryl groups and are toxic. Succinylacetone, derived from succinylacetoacetate, is a potent inhibitor of ALA-dehydratase activity and heme formation in humans and may account for the acute porphyria-like symptoms present in these patients.[591] Identification of succinylacetone in the amniotic fluid or assay of fumarylacetoacetase activity in cultured amniotic fluid cells[394] of "at risk" pregnancies will allow for prenatal diagnosis. Autosomal recessive inheritance has been demonstrated, especially in French-Canadians and Scandinavians.[609]

Treatment with dietary restriction of phenylalanine and tyrosine is beneficial in some patients[609] and is especially effective in improving renal tubular dysfunction. The benefit of dietary treatment in patients with the acute infantile disease is unclear; its effect on the ultimate cirrhosis is unknown. Presumably, if a metabolic block occurs at the step mediated by fumarylacetoacetase, therapy in addition to phenylalanine and tyrosine restriction might include the administration of sulfhydryl-containing compounds such as glutathione or penicillamine.[664] Liver replacement in the chronic form, especially in patients with hepatoma, has been successful.[651,727]

Disorders of Carbohydrate Metabolism

Degradation and synthesis of glycogen and the interconversion of glucose, fructose, and galactose are carried out by hepatocytic enzymes of the Embden–Meyerhof–Parnas–Cori pathway (Fig. 43-19). Deficient activity of a specific enzyme results in the hepatic involvement characteristic of galactosemia, fructose intolerance, and the multiple types of glycogen storage disease. In galactosemia and fructosemia, the early course may include cholestasis (see above).

Galactosemia

Classic transferase-deficient galactosemia is a toxicity syndrome characterized by progressive liver and brain injury caused by the ingestion of galactose. The clinical presentation is in the neonatal period, within a short period after starting milk feedings, with vomiting, diarrhea, failure to thrive, hepatomegaly, cholestasis, aminoaciduria, and cataracts.[343] Affected infants have deficient activity of galactose-1-phosphate uridyl transferase (Fig. 43-19).[343] Persistent elevation of conjugated bilirubin levels occurs in over 80% of untreated infants[486]; mental retardation and cirrhosis can occur in untreated patients.

Transferase deficiency results in accumulation of galactose 1-phosphate and galactose in tissue, with resultant toxicity to various organs.[189] Galactose may be reduced to the alcohol galactitol, and the development of cataracts is related to accumulation and toxicity of galactitol in the lens.[251,732] The liver, kidney, ovarian, and brain abnormalities are less well explained but seem related to galactose 1-phosphate or galactosamine accumulation.[375,691] In a related inherited disorder, galactokinase deficiency, accumulation of galactose and galactitol is associated with cataracts; however, there is no liver, brain, or renal disease.[375,691] Hypoglycemia has been related to high tissue levels of galactose 1-phosphate, which will interfere with phosphoglucomutase, the enzyme that catalyzes conversion of glucose 1-phosphate to glucose 6-phosphate; therefore, there is an inability to release glucose from glycogen.

The presence of reducing substance in the urine of cholestatic infants suggests the diagnosis. Testing the urine with both Clinitest (total reducing substance) and Clinistix or glucose oxidase paper (glucose) allows a tentative identification of the sugar at the bedside, which can be confirmed by chromatography. Conversely, routine use of glucose oxidase paper will miss the diagnosis. Vomiting or poor intake of lactose at the time the urine is collected may also result in a false-negative test result. The resemblance of galactosemia to sepsis in the small infant is striking; indeed, gram-negative bacterial sepsis may complicate the disease.[419,486] Specific diagnosis depends on as-

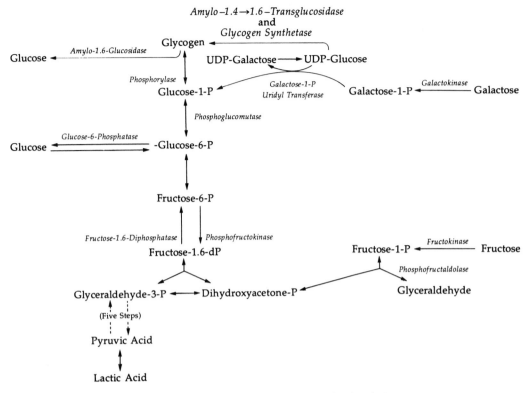

Fig. 43-19. Embden–Meyerhof–Parnas–Cori pathway of anaerobic glycolysis.

say of galactose 1-phosphate uridyl transferase activity in erythrocytes, leukocytes, or liver.[21,249,339] Homozygotes have complete absence of red cell enzymatic-specific activity, and heterozygotes have intermediate values. The galactose tolerance test is unnecessary for diagnosis and may be harmful. Even a remote suspicion of galactosemia is an indication to discontinue dietary lactose feedings until confirmatory tests can be done.

Other laboratory signs of liver injury (serum amino-transferase elevation and prolonged prothrombin time) are present in varying degrees. Hemolytic anemia and erythroid hyperplasia, occasionally severe and resembling erythroblastosis, occur in 40% of patients.[486] Renal tubular dysfunction may be manifest by aminoaciduria and proteinuria as well as galactosuria.

The histopathology of the liver depends on age of the child and duration of galactose ingestion. In the first month of life, the liver is grossly fatty. Hepatocytes contain large droplets of neutral lipid and refractile material viewed with polarized light on frozen section.[633] Bile duct proliferation and very early pseudoglandular proliferation of hepatic cells around bile canaliculi is present, but lobular architecture is preserved.[633] From 1 to 6 months of age, progressive formation of pseudoacini occurs and lipid in hepatocytes decreases (Fig. 43-20). In older infants and children, progressive regenerative pseudolobules replace normal liver parenchyma, and portal cirrhosis ensues.[633] Treatment with dietary elimination of galactose, that is,

with commercial formulas such as Nutramigen or Pregestimil and no milk or milk products, results in remission. Dietary restriction should be continued for several years and possibly for life.[611] Erythrocyte galactose 1-phosphate levels may be monitored to gauge adherence to the diet.[190] Optimally, mothers of homozygous infants should be placed on a galactose-free diet during a subsequent pregnancy. Despite the relative rarity of this autosomal recessive disease (1 in 20,000–50,000 live births), it should be considered in any jaundiced infant because of the disastrous effects of delayed diagnosis.

Hereditary Fructose Intolerance

In the presence of an inherited enzyme deficiency, acute and chronic liver injury and metabolic illness can be caused by the ingestion of fructose. Of the three known defects in fructose metabolism, only fructose 1-phosphate aldolase deficiency leads to significant hepatic injury.

Fructose 1-Phosphate Aldolase Deficiency. A syndrome resembling galactosemia, with vomiting, "colic," hypoglycemia, diarrhea, hepatomegaly, jaundice, failure to thrive, and aminoaciduria, occurs in infants who have deficient activity of fructose 1-phosphate aldolase (phosphofructaldolase, see Fig. 43-19). The onset is later in life, occurring when fructose is added to the diet either as fruit, cane sugar (sucrose, which hydrolyzes to glucose and

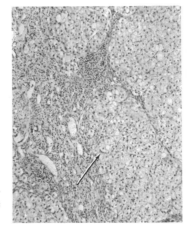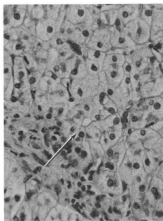

Fig. 43-20. Galactosemia in a 9-week-old infant. Inflammatory portal exudate, fibrosis, and mild bile duct proliferation. Pseudoacinus (*arrow*).

fructose), or as sucrose-containing commercial infant formula.[233] The enzyme deficiency has been demonstrated in liver, kidney and jejunal mucosa. The incidence is approximately 1 in 20,000 newborns[42,510]; the transmission is autosomal recessive. Hypoglycemia and hypophosphatemia occur after fructose ingestion, and fructose appears in the urine. Intravenous fructose, injected rapidly in a single dose, will reproduce these findings, but results may be negative if there is severe liver dysfunction.[233] In homozygotes liver injury occurs within three hours of fructose feeding, as evidenced by elevations in serum aminotransferase levels and changes in the hepatocyte ultrastructure.[537] Fructose and fructose 1-phosphate accumulate in hepatocytes to a considerable degree, with eventual depletion of ATP and inorganic phosphorus.[250] There is an increased rate of purine degradation, with resultant hyperuricemia and increased urate excretion. Phosphorylase is inhibited, impairing glycogenolysis and resulting in hypoglycemia. Hyperchloremic acidosis, hyperlactatemia, and hypokalemia are present. Light microscopy is normal at this time, but peculiar "glycogen-associated membranous arrays" occur in the cytoplasm with rarefaction of a central core of hyaloplasm as evidence of liver cell injury.[537] Prolonged fructose ingestion produces diffuse fatty infiltration, hepatocellular necrosis, and bile duct proliferation (Fig. 43-21). Progressive liver disease and cirrhosis have been described. Deficiency of liver-dependent coagulation factors resembling hemorrhagic disease of the newborn may occur, and bleeding may be a presenting sign.

A version to sugar is present in older children and adults, possibly accounting for an apparent lack of biochemical evidence of liver dysfunction in survivors of the neonatal period.[233,250,537] Hepatic lesions may be reversible, but persistent and variable steatosis is present in some patients, probably due to hidden sources of dietary fructose and sucrose, or possibly the ingestion of sorbitol, which is metabolized to fructose. Isolated reversible growth failure due to disordered adenine nucleotide metabolism may also be associated with chronic low levels of fructose inges-

tion.[472] Treatment is by lifelong exclusion of fruit, vegetables, and sucrose from the diet.

Fructose 1, 6-Diphosphatase. Deficiency of fructose 1, 6-diphosphatase also results in hepatomegaly and hypoglycemia with acidosis precipitated by stress, fasting, or fructose ingestion.[43] Hepatic levels of fructose 1-phosphate aldolase are normal. The liver shows only ballooning of hepatic cells with large fat vacuoles.

Fructokinase. Deficiency of hepatic fructokinase results in a harmless asymptomatic condition, essential fructosuria, in which fructose is present in the urine after ingestion of fructose-containing foods.

Glycogenoses

There are multiple forms of glycogen storage disease (GSD) (Table 43-7); they produce diffuse hepatomegaly

Fig. 43-21. Fructosemia in a 3-month-old infant. All hepatocytes contain large fat droplets that displace the nucleus to one side. Fructose-free diet resulted in normal liver morphology.

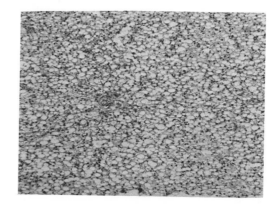

TABLE 43-7. Glycogen Storage Diseases

TYPE	ENZYME DEFICIENCY	TISSUE INVOLVED	CLINICAL SYMPTOMS	SYNONYM
0	Glycogen synthetase[35,326]	Liver, muscle	Fasting hypoglycemia; prolonged hyperglycemia after glucose administration; mental retardation (hypoglycemic). Treatment by frequent protein-rich meals → normal psycho-motor development.	A-glycogenosis; defect convincingly demonstrated in two unrelated families[326]
I	a. Glucose 6-phosphatase[145]	Liver, kidney, intestine	Enlarged liver and kidneys; "doll face," stunted growth, normal mental development; tendency to hypoglycemia, lactic (and pyruvic) acidosis, hyperlipidemia, hyperuricacidemia, gout, bleeding; no rise in blood glucose after IV glucagon.[325] Prognosis fair to good with treatment.[128,270,271]	Von Gierke disease, (hepatorenal glycogenosis).
	b. Translocase (responsible for movement of glucose 6-phosphate across intracellular membranes.	Glucose 6-phosphatase activity is normal in homogenate made of frozen liver but is deficient in isotonic homogenate made of fresh (unfrozen) liver.	Same as in type I; in addition neutropenia may occur.[19,62]	
IIa Infantile[326] IIb Adult[206,326]	Lysosomal acid α-glucosidase (deficient activity of acid α-1,4- and of α-1,6-glucosidase)	In the fatal, infantile, classic form (IIa), glycogen concentration excessive in all organs examined; acid α-glucosidase deficiency may be generalized. Cardiac muscle in IIb normal but deficient in α-glucosidase activity; cardiac glycogen concentration normal.	Clinically normal at birth but with minimal cardiomegaly, abnormal ECG, increased tissue glycogen; abnormal lysosomes in liver and skin, and acid α-glucosidase deficiency demonstrable at birth; within a few months marked hypotonia, severe cardiomegaly, moderate hepatomegaly; normal mental development; death usually in infancy (IIa). Cases with involvement of muscle and liver but without cardiomegaly described in children and adults (IIb). Normal blood glucose response to glucagon.	Pompe's disease (generalized glycogenosis, cardiac glycogenosis). *Note:* Prenatal diagnosis possible: amniocentesis allows electron microscopic demonstration of abnormal lysosomes in uncultured amniotic fluid cells.
III	Amylo-1,6-glucosidase ("debrancher" enzyme)[144] a. Affects liver only	Liver, muscle, heart, etc. in various combinations.	Moderate to marked hepatomegaly; possibly moderate hypotonia or cardiomegaly; no hypoglycemia; no	Limit dextrinosis (debrancher glycogenosis); Cori disease; Forbes disease.

TABLE 43-7.   Glycogen Storage Diseases—*Continued*

TYPE	ENZYME DEFICIENCY	TISSUE INVOLVED	CLINICAL SYMPTOMS	SYNONYM
	b. Generalized		hyperlipemia; glucagon produces a normal rise in blood glucose after a meal but not after fasting[325]; normal mental development. Prognosis fair to good.	
IV	Amylo-1,4→ 1,6-transglucosidase ("brancher enzyme")[110]	Generalized (?); low to normal levels of abnormally structured glycogen (amylopectin-like molecules.	Hepatosplenomegaly, ascites, cirrhosis, liver failure; normal mental development; death in early childhood.	Amylopectinosis (brancher glycogenosis); Andersen disease.
V	Muscle phosphorylase deficiency (congenital absence of skeletal muscle phosphorylase; phosphorylase-activating system intact[600]	Skeletal muscle only.	Temporary weakness and cramping of skeletal muscle after exercise; no rise in blood lactate during ischemic exercise; normal mental development. Fair to good prognosis.	McArdle syndrome (liver and smooth muscle phosphorylase not affected).
VI	Liver phosphorylase deficiency (phosphorylase-activating system intact.[329])	Liver; skeletal muscle normal.	Marked hepatomegaly; no splenomegaly; no hypoglycemia; no acidosis; no hyperlipemia; no rise of blood glucose after IV glucagon; normal mental development. Good prognosis.	Lack of glucagon-induced hyperglycemia distinguishes GSD VI from GSD IX; the latter shows a normal glucagon response.
VII	Phosphofructokinase[687,688]	Skeletal muscle, erythrocytes.	Temporary weakness and cramping of skeletal muscle after exercise; no rise in blood lactate during ischemic exercise. Normal mental development (symptoms identical to those of type-V glycogenosis). Good prognosis.	Reduction of phosphofructokinase activity severe in skeletal muscle, mild in erythrocytes, not established in other tissues.
VIII	No enzymatic deficiency demonstrated (total liver phosphorylase normal, but most in the inactive form; phosphorylase-activating system (intact)[326]	Liver, brain, skeletal muscle normal; cerebral glycogen increased.	Hepatomegaly; truncal ataxia, nystagmus, "dancing eyes" may be present; neurologic deterioration progressing to spasticity, decerebration, and death. Urinary epinephrine increased acutely.	
IX	Liver phosphorylase-kinase deficiency (total liver phosphorylase normal, but most in the inactive form because of deficient endogenous kinase[326,330]	Liver only. Muscle tissue normal biochemically and microscopically.	Marked hepatomegaly, no splenomegaly; no hypoglycemia or acidosis; normal rise in blood glucose after IV glucagon. Prognosis good; treatment may not be necessary.	*Note:* Liver phosphorylase can be activated *in vitro* by addition of exogenous kinase to the homogenate.

(continued)

TABLE 43-7.   Glycogen Storage Diseases—*Continued*

TYPE	ENZYME DEFICIENCY	TISSUE INVOLVED	CLINICAL SYMPTOMS	SYNONYM
IXa	Autosomal recessive			
IXb	X-linked recessive			
IXc	Liver and muscle phosphorylase kinase deficiency			
X	Loss of activity of cyclic 3′,5′-AMP–dependent kinase in muscle and presumably liver (total phosphorylase content of liver and skeletal muscle normal, but the enzyme completely deactivated in both organs; phosphorylase kinase activity 50% of normal, possibly due to loss of cAMP-dependent kinase activity)[331]	Liver and muscle.	Marked hepatomegaly; patient otherwise clinically healthy. No cardiomegaly or hypoglycemia; no rise in blood glucose after IV glucagon or epinephrine.	*Note: In vitro* activation of phosphorylase occurs under assay conditions not requiring cAMP-dependent kinase.
XI	All enzymatic activities measured to date normal (adenyl cyclase, cAMP-dependent kinase, phosphorylase kinase, phosphorylase, debrancher, brancher, glucose 6-phosphatase)	Liver, or liver and kidney.	Tendency for acidosis; markedly stunted growth; vitamin D–resistant rickets (may be cured with high doses of vitamin D and oral supplementation of phosphate); hyperlipidemia, generalized aminoaciduria, galactosuria, glucosuria, phosphaturia; normal renal size; no rise in blood glucose after IV glucagon.	May include patients with varying enzymatic defects.

in all types presently described, except in those that involve skeletal muscle.[326,600] GSD is considered to exist when the concentration (normal = 2% to 6%) or the molecular structure of glycogen is abnormal as the result of an inborn error of metabolism.[326] Classification, as first suggested by Cori, is based on the specific enzymatic deficiency.[144] A recent detailed review, with an approach to evaluation and management of the patient with suspected GSD, is available.[326] Specific diagnosis depends on demonstration of the deficiency of enzyme activity in biopsy specimens of liver and muscle (see Fig. 43-19). If on-site biochemical analysis is available, needle biopsy specimens that can be repeated are ideal. If not, a carefully planned open biopsy should be performed after an overnight fast. After specimens for light and electron microscopy are obtained, the largest part of the biopsy is frozen immediately on dry ice and delivered in the frozen state to the cooperating laboratory.

GSD type O, a deficiency of hepatic glycogen synthetase, has been reported in twins and in an unrelated child.[36,326] There is no response in blood glucose following glucagon administration, since liver glycogen stores are depleted. The presentation is that of idiopathic or ketotic hypoglycemia.

GSD type I in infants produces recurrent severe hypoglycemia, lactic acidosis, hyperlipidemia, and hyperuricemia with massive hepatomegaly, growth failure, asymptomatic renal enlargement, and a potbelly.[326] Hepatic histologic changes are nonspecific. Fat-droplet deposition, marked irregular enlargement of hepatocytes, and prominent nuclear hyperglycogenosis are present (Fig. 43-22).[449] Hepatic tumors have been reported in patients with type-I disease.[644] Autosomal recessive inheritance has been demonstrated.

The severity of the hypoglycemia varies, some infants with GSD type I are severely hypoglycemic but have few

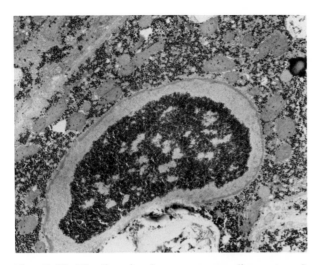

Fig. 43-22. The liver in glycogen storage disease type I. Characteristic changes shown by electron microscopy include [1] marked accumulation of glycogen in the nucleus, [2] abundant glycogen in the cytosol, and [3] the presence of lipid.

symptoms. With increasing age, symptoms moderate, and the liver becomes smaller and abdominal protuberance less evident, although glucose 6-phosphatase activity is still deficient.[145,326] The decrease in blood sugar is due to impaired glucose production.[700] There is, therefore, an overproduction of glucose 6-phosphate due to continuous stimulation of glycogen breakdown; this will increase glycolysis, which in turn results in a net increase in the production of lactate, triglyceride, cholesterol, and uric acid. Avoidance of hypoglycemia and the attendant compensatory hormonal flux is the key to management. Portacaval shunts had been performed; the rationale was delivery of glucose-rich blood from the intestine to peripheral tissue before it reached the liver.[650] Current treatment modalities are based on the rationale that exogenous glucose will inhibit excess glycogenolysis, correct the metabolic abnormalities, and alleviate clinical symptoms.[270,271] This can be accomplished by use of nocturnal intragastric feedings of a high-glucose elemental formula via nasogastric tube to infants, or via an uncooked cornstarch diet for older patients.[128,634] Successful maintenance of blood glucose levels of greater than 70 mg/dl will decrease the hormonal stimulus to the liver to produce glucose. The initiation of continuous nasogastric feedings has been associated with normalization of biochemical parameters and enhanced growth; however, this modality is not without risk, in that it can abolish the tolerance for hypoglycemia. As mentioned, it has been noted by several investigators that prior to the initiation of therapy, children with GSD type I often tolerate hypoglycemia without clinical symptoms. This may be attributable in part to a dependence upon lactate as an alternate cerebral metabolic fuel.[222] Following initiation of therapy, biochemical hypoglycemia may be symptomatic and associated with central nervous system signs; therefore, total suppression of lactate is inadvisable.

A variant of GSD type I, GSD Ib, presents in an identical clinical manner as GSD type I; in addition, there is a tendency toward neutropenia, with infectious and bleeding complications noted.[19,62] This subset is now clearly distinguishable from classic GSD type I. Confusion initially arose due to the fact that glucose 6-phosphatase activity in the liver homogenate was apparently normal. This has subsequently been explained by the observation that when the assay was run in hypotonic homogenate and/or the liver tissue had been frozen prior to the assay, enzyme "latency" was manifest. However, if the homogenate is prepared from fresh liver in isotonic buffer, then the assay for glucose 6-phosphatase will reveal defective activity. It has been suggested that the syndrome is associated with deficiency of a hepatic *translocase* system in GSD Ib patients.[682] This enzyme is thought to transport the substrate glucose 6-phosphate across intracellular membranes, allowing access to the enzyme. Freezing or disruption will abolish intracellular membrane barriers and will increase the amount of measurable activity.

It should also be noted that the clinical picture of GSD type I can be mimicked by carnitine deficiency (see below).

GSD type II is associated with deficient activity of lysosomal acid α-glucosidase.[305] There are two subtypes (IIa and IIb), each associated with very different clinical pictures.[326] The most frequently recognized form is IIa, or Pompe's disease, in which profound hypotonia, cardiomegaly, and death in infancy occur. The liver is only moderately enlarged until congestive heart failure occurs. Type-IIb disease presents as progressive hypotonic muscular dystrophy, and survival until 65 years of age has been observed. The heart is often normal in size, but respiratory failure may eventually occur.[206] The ultrastructural correlates of acid α-glucosidase deficiency are typical large vacuoles filled with monoparticulate glycogen (Fig. 43-23, *left*).[57,327] Although equally severe deficiency of enzyme activity is present in both types, type IIa shows a marked increase in glycogen concentration and many large abnormal lysosomes. Type IIb has normal to slightly elevated glycogen content with fewer and smaller lysosomes.[326] It has been demonstrated in fibroblast culture of a patient with GSD type IIa that the amount of α-glucosidase was normal but that the structure of the enzyme molecule was altered, suggesting that it was catalytically incompetent.[71] In a patient with GSD type IIb, the amount of α-glucosidase was reduced; however, the enzyme molecule was structurally normal.

In type-II disease, hepatocytes are slightly enlarged and pale-staining without disturbance of lobular architecture (Fig. 43-23, *right*). They contain a myriad of 1-μm to 2-μm vacuoles, dispersed evenly throughout the cell, that are PAS-positive and digest with malt diastase.[449] They represent the enlarged lysosomes seen by electron microscopy. Nuclear glycogenosis is not prominent, and fibrosis does not occur. The increased frequency of the disease in males

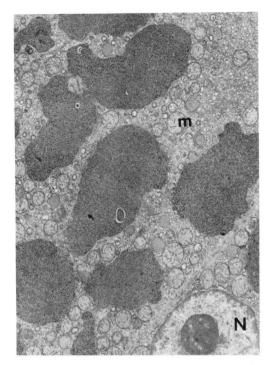
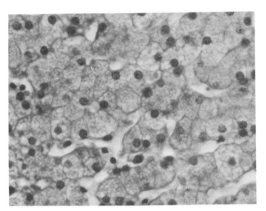

Fig. 43-23. Left. Type II glycogenosis, liver ultrastructure. (Original magnification × 8000) Typical large vacuoles filled with monoparticulate glycogen. Compare size to nucleus (*N*) and mitochondria (*m*). In this necropsy specimen, nonlysosome-bound glycogen is absent, a finding seen also after starvation and prolonged epinephrine administration. **Right.** Type II glycogenosis. (Original magnification × 250) The hepatocytes are slightly enlarged. A myriad of small vacuoles evenly dispersed throughout the cell are visible by light microscopy.

is unexplained, although autosomal recessive inheritance is commonly postulated.[326,621]

Treatment of type IIa patients with multiple agents has been unsuccessful.[326] Infusion of an extract of *Aspergillus niger* containing α-glucosidase for 120 days resulted in return of glycogen concentration, α-glucosidase activity, and ultrastructural appearance of the liver to normal and in a slight clinical improvement, but the enzyme did not enter the cardiac or skeletal muscle, and the patient died.[326,328] Bone marrow transplantation has been unsuccessful in a single case.

Prenatal diagnosis of GSD type IIa by direct electron microscopic examination of amniotic fluid cells for intracellular vacuoles or assay of acid α-glucosidase in cultured amniotic fluid cells is feasible (Fig. 43-24).[326,334]

GSD type III is due to deficiency of amylo-1, 6-glucosidase or debrancher enzyme activity (Fig. 43-25).[144] The liver, muscle, and heart may be involved in various combinations. Hepatomegaly, which may be massive, is the most striking symptom; hypoglycemia, acidosis, and hyperlipemia are not present.[326] Although hypotonia and cardiomegaly may be present, cardiac symptoms are rare. When the patient is in the fed state, administration of glucagon activates hepatic phosphorylase and degrades the outer branches of the glycogen molecule to the 1, 6 branch points with a resultant rise in blood glucose; after a 12-hour fast, the outer branches have been degraded endogenously, and no rise in glucose occurs after glucagon administration.[325] The liver may be indistinguishable from that of type-I disease.[327,449] Liver dysfunction with jaun-

Fig. 43-24. Type II glycogenosis, cultured skin fibroblasts. (Original magnification × 5000) Portion of one fibroblast contains numerous glycogen-filled lysosomes identical to those in the hepatocytes.

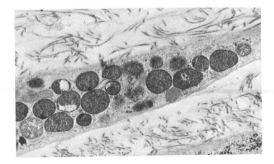

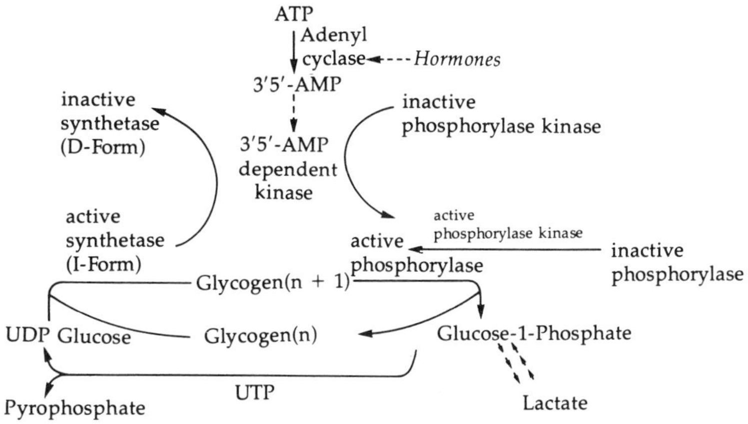

Fig. 43-25. The enzymatic cascade of biologic amplification that results in activation or inactivation of phosphorylase. Inactivation of "active" phosphorylase *kinase* or "active" *phosphorylase* is mediated by the respective phosphatase. GSD type III results from deficiency of "debrancher" (active phosphorylase) activity; GSD type IV results from deficient activity of the "brancher" (active synthetase) enzyme.

dice, aminotransferase elevation, and septal fibrosis may occur.[97,326,652] Family studies suggest autosomal recessive inheritance.[97] Although treatment of one patient with portacaval transposition resulted in improved growth, there seems even less rationale for this procedure in type-III than in type-I disease.[652]

GSD type IV is associated with deficiency of amylo-1,4 → 1,6-transglucosidase or brancher enzyme activity (Fig. 43-25) in liver and leukocytes and storage of an abnormal glycogen with fewer branch points and longer chains than normal.[110] Inheritance appears to be autosomal recessive. The abnormal glycogen is colorless in hematoxylin and eosin, stains positively with PAS, Best carmine, and colloidal iron, and is diastase-resistant.[558] In all cases, onset is in infancy with failure to thrive, gastroenteritis and hepatosplenomegaly, and progressive cirrhosis, with ascites and death usually in the second year, although survival until 7 years of age has been reported.[326] The liver shows a uniform cirrhosis, with broad bands of fibrous tissue extending around and into lobules. Hepatocytes have eccentric nuclei and contain cytoplasmic deposits of the polysaccharide described above.[558] Electron microscopy demonstrates large irregular areas of low-electron density in the cytoplasm. These consist of fibrils and finely granular material and are bordered by normal-appearing alpha particles or glycogen rosettes.[558] Blood-glucose response to glucagon is normal, indicating that at least some glycogen is available for glycolysis.[558] The fact that a branched polysaccharide accumulates in the liver in the absence of branching enzyme is yet to be explained, as is the mechanism by which liver damage occurs, although a toxic effect of the abnormal carbohydrate is postulated.[558] Liver transplantation might be contemplated in the presence of progressive cirrhosis.

GSD types V, VI, VIII, IX, and X have been related to defects occurring in the phosphorylase system.[326,329,330,332,600] Figure 43-25 reviews the complex enzymatic cascade by which inactive phosphorylase is converted to active phosphorylase and glycogen is degraded. Reciprocal inactivation of glycogen production results from inactivation of glycogen synthetase and blood

glucose rises. It is apparent that deficiency of the phosphorylase enzyme, of phosphorylase kinase, of cyclic 3'5'-AMP–dependent kinase, and of adenyl cyclase could all potentially result in deficient phosphorylase activity in either liver or muscle tissue.

GSD type V results from inactivity of muscle phosphorylase activity.[600] Liver phosphorylase is normal, as is the activating system in the muscle.[326]

GSD type VII is due to deficiency of phosphofructokinase (see Fig. 43-19) in muscle; however, symptoms are identical with those of type V. Excess purine degradation occurs in the exercising muscle in both types, suggesting that the ATP pool is deranged because of the defective glycogenolysis or glycolysis.[469] The liver has not been studied.

GSD type VI is due to inactivity of the hepatic phosphorylase enzyme.[329] The activating system is normal as tested against exogenous phosphorylase, and the addition of phosphorylase kinase to the liver homogenate of the patient does not increase the phosphorylase activity of the patient's liver.[329] Glycogen content in the liver is increased, muscle is normal, and the major clinical manifestation is hepatomegaly. Patients with low hepatic phosphorylase activity previously designated as type VI should have activation studies done in order for the enzyme defect to be defined.[329]

GSD type VIII presents as progressive neurologic deterioration and hepatomegaly.[326,332] Hepatic phosphorylase activity is low but can be brought to normal with the addition of ATP and $MgCl_2$. During the active phase of the disease, there is excess urinary excretion of catecholamines, and cerebral biopsy specimens demonstrate excess numbers of α-glycogen particles or rosettes, which are normally present only in liver. *In vivo* glucagon or epinephrine activates the patient's liver phosphorylase. Thus, the disease results from defective control of phosphorylase activation, although phosphorylase and its activating system are intact.

GSD type IX is characterized by asymptomatic hepatomegaly, low hepatic phosphorylase activity, and normal muscle phosphorylase activity.[330] Total liver phosphorylase content is normal but is deactivated because of apparent inactivity of phosphorylase kinase. Addition of exogenous phosphorylase kinase results in normal activation of phosphorylase. Genetic subtypes have been described on the basis of determination of apparent k_m of hepatic phosphorylase kinase.[326] Autosomal recessive inheritance is present in GSD IXa, in which the apparent k_m of the patient's enzyme is close to normal. In GSD IXb, the patient's apparent k_m is significantly higher than normal, and sex-linked recessive inheritance is suggested.[326] The k_m studies suggest that GSD IXa may be a deficiency of regulation, whereas GSD IXb may be due to a structural gene abnormality. This point is of biologic interest because sex-linked deficiency of muscle phosphorylase kinase has been observed in mice, and isoenzymes for phosphorylase exist in liver and muscle that seemingly may be affected independently by genetic defects.[326,437]

GSD type X is represented by a patient with increased glycogen and deactivated phosphorylase in liver and muscle and asymptomatic hepatomegaly.[331] Total phosphorylase was normal, but only 1% was in the active form; phosphorylase kinase activity was present. Type-X disease is apparently due to deficient activity of the cyclic $3'5'$-AMP–dependent kinase.[326,331]

GSD type XI, characterized by increased glycogen concentration in the liver and kidney, is without known enzymatic deficiency. Clinical manifestations include hepatomegaly and the presence of the Fanconi syndrome (with increased urinary excretion of phosphate, amino acids, glucose, and galactose) and growth failure. Florid rickets, resistant to vitamin D, may also be present.

Light microscopy of the liver in GSD types VI, VIII, IX, and X is similar to that of types I and III with irregular enlargement of hepatocytes due to stored glycogen. Nuclear glycogenosis is less prominent than in type I. Similarly, the ultrastructural appearance of all hepatic glycogenoses except type II is similar (Fig. 43-26). There is crowding of endoplasmic reticulum by glycogen particles. Lipid droplets are frequent.[326] Intranuclear glycogen is more prominent in type I, and α-particles have a fractured or splintered appearance in the four types involving the phosphorylase system.[330]

Disorders of Lipid Metabolism

Abetalipoproteinemia

In the familial disorder of lipid transport abetalipoproteinemia, there is absence of β-lipoprotein and an inability to form chylomicrons, the exogenous triglyceride transport particles, and very low density lipoprotein (VLDL), the endogenous triglyceride transport particle.[344,589] This defect in endogenous triglyceride transport results in significant hepatomegaly. The well-known features of this syndrome are steatorrhea, acanthocytosis, retinitis, and an ataxic neuropathy due to vitamin E deficiency. The basic defect seems to be impaired synthesis of an apolipoprotein, which is a major constituent of chylomicrons, low-density lipoprotein, and VLDL.[265]

Grossly, the liver is yellow–white.[527] Microscopically, hepatocytes are distended, with fat droplets ranging from 5 μm to 35 μm in diameter. In frozen sections, the lipid forms one or two large fat droplets in each cell, displacing the nucleus (Fig. 43-27). The lipid is triglyceride chemically and histochemically. Electron microscopy demonstrates a majority of non–membrane-bound fat droplets, an absence from the Golgi apparatus of the budding saccules normally associated with VLDL formation, and de-

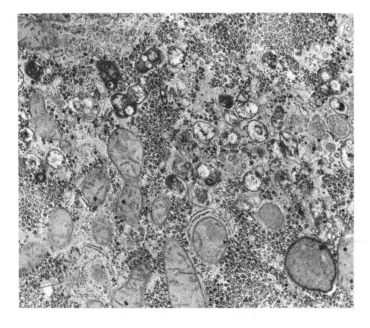

Fig. 43-26. Liver, type IX glycogenosis. (Original magnification $\times$ 20,000) There is crowding of endoplasmic reticulum by numerous glycogen particles that have a "splintered appearance."

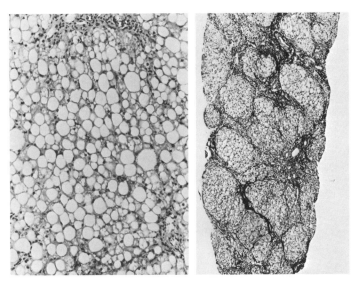

Fig. 43-27. Abetalipoproteinemia, liver biopsy, in a patient at age 10 months (*left*) and at age 30 months (*right*). First biopsy shows mild septal fibrosis with large droplet fat accumulation in each hepatocyte. Second biopsy at lower power shows advanced micronodular cirrhosis and persistence of fat accumulation in hepatocytes.

fective smooth endoplasmic reticulum formation adjacent to the Golgi.[527]

Vitamin E supplementation is imperative, and medium-chain triglycerides (MCT) have been suggested as treatment for the associated malabsorption because they are absorbed and transported to the liver without chylomicron formation.[527] In one patient advanced micronodular cirrhosis was noted to develop during dietary therapy (Fig. 43-27). This may have been unrelated to the MCT. Dietary treatment should be carefully monitored until more information is available.

Lysosomal Storage Disease

Lysosomes, which contain acid hydrolases (hydrolytic enzymes that exhibit a pH optima of 3.5–5.5), are bounded by a single lipoprotein membrane. This organelle can therefore maintain an acidic intralysosomal pH and thereby allow full enzymatic hydrolytic activity. Substrates for acid hydrolases may be endogenous, that is, autophagic as during normal cell turnover where lysosomes degrade material produced by the cell, or exogenous, that is, Kupffer cells mediate phagocytosis of material from blood cells; fusion of lysosomes and phagosomes creates phagolysosomes.

The majority of the hydrolases contained within lysosomes are exolytic and mediate cleavage of sulfates, fatty acids, or sugar moieties from larger molecules. Deficiency of a lysosomal enzyme results in inability to degrade the substrate within the autophagic vacuole, accumulation of the substrate, enlargement of these secondary lysosomes in cells, and organ enlargement. The heterogeneity of this group not unexpectedly accounts for diverse biochemical and clinical manifestations. Many of the lysosomal hydrolases are composed of phosphorylated mannose residues; therefore the possibility of altered mannose–phosphate recognition must be considered in addition to absence of enzyme activity.

Secondary lysosomes often have characteristic ultrastructural appearances; in some conditions, characteristic lysosomes may be present, although liver size and function are normal. Cultured skin fibroblasts usually demonstrate the enzymatic defect, accumulation of the substrate, and the secondary lysosomes by electron microscopy, permitting the option of the intrauterine diagnosis.

Over 40 inherited defects involving the intralysosomal enzymes have been described, many of which affect the liver. These enzymes function to degrade waste macromolecules and enhance elimination; therefore, their failure is associated with the accumulation of the offending compound or abnormal metabolite within the hepatocyte. The net effect is that the hepatocyte is structurally and functionally destroyed by the accumulated waste material. A detailed understanding of the biochemistry and transport mechanisms has brought us closer to treatment of lysosomal diseases by either organ replacement or replacement of the defective gene. Table 43-8 is a partial list of the lysosomal storage disorders of various classes that have been associated with hepatic involvement. There are excellent reviews available in which the biochemical features, clinical manifestations, and diagnostic methods are detailed.[258,391] Only specific aspects of hepatic involvement in lysosomal storage diseases are highlighted below.

Lipidoses. Two distinct clinical syndromes (Wolman's disease and cholesterol ester storage disease [CESD]), which are characterized by the intralysosomal accumulation of lipid, are associated with deficient hydrolytic enzymes. The diagnosis is made by demonstration of deficient lysosomal acid lipase activity in leukocytes or fibroblasts and an elevation of triglycerides and cholesterol ester levels in tissue.

TABLE 43-8.   Lysosomal Storage Disorders Associated with Hepatic Involvement

DISORDER	PRIMARY ENZYME DEFICIENCY	STORAGE PRODUCT
LIPIDOSES		
Wolman's disease	Acid lipase	Triglycerides, cholesteryl esters
Cholesterol ester storage disease	Acid lipase	Triglycerides, cholesteryl esters
SPHINGOLIPIDOSES		
Gaucher's disease		
Type I: adult (nonneuropathic)	β-Glucosidase	Glycosylceramide
Type 2: infantile (neuropathic)	β-Glucosidase	Glucosylceramide
Type 3: juvenile (subacute neuropathic)	β-Glucosidase	Glucosylceramide
Niemann–Pick disease	Sphingomyelinase	Sphingomyelin
GM$_1$ gangliosidosis	β-Galactosidase	Gm$_1$ ganglioside
GM$_2$ gangliosidosis	(Defect in hexosaminidase system)	Gm$_2$ ganglioside
Metachromatic leukodystrophy (3 types)	Arylsulfatase A	Galactocerebroside-3-sulfate
Fabray's disease	α-Galactosidase A	Ceramide trihexoside
Farber's disease	Acid ceramidase	Ceramide
Krabbe's disease	Galactocerebroside: β-galactoside	?
MUCOPOLYSACCHARIDOSES (MPS)		
MPS I	α-L-iduronidase	HS
Hurler (severe)		DS
Scheie (mild)		
Intermediate		
MPS II (Hunter)	Iduronate-2-sulfatase	HS/DS
MPS III (Sanfilippo A-D)	Various[258]	HS and others
MPS IV (Morquio A & B)	Various[258]	KS
MPS VI (Maroteaux–Lamy)	Arylsulfatase B	DS
MPS VII (Sly)	β-glucuronidase	DS/HS
DISORDERS OF GLYCOPROTEIN DEGRADATION		
Mannosidosis	α-Mannosidase	Fragments of glycoproteins (mannose-oligosaccharides)
Sialidosis (mucolipidoses I)	Oligosaccharide neuraminidase (sialidase)	Fragments of glycoproteins (sialyl oligosaccharides)
Fucosidosis	α-L-Fucosidase	Fucoglycoproteins

HS, heparan sulfate; DS, dermatan sulfate; KS, keratan sulfate.

Wolman's Disease. Wolman's syndrome is characterized clinically by steatorrhea, failure to thrive, hepatosplenomegaly, and jaundice; the disease causes death usually within the first year of life.[3,34,745] Stippled calcification of the adrenal glands is uniformly present either early in the course or in association with terminal liver failure.[3,310] Originally described in Jewish infants, the disease has been reported in other ethnic groups including the Japanese, and appears to be inherited as an autosomal recessive trait. Chemically there is diffuse cellular accumulation of triacylglycerol and cholesterol ester in lymph nodes, bone marrow, small intestine, liver, spleen, and adrenal glands. Deficiency of lysosomal acid lipase activity directed toward the hydrolysis of either triglyceride or cholesterol ester was demonstrated by Patrick and Lake and confirmed by others.[115,530,632] Grossly the liver is yellow; frozen sections show large lipid droplets in the parenchymal cells, some of which contain birefringent crystals seen with polarized light. Cholesterol ester crystals are present predominantly in swollen Kupffer cells (Fig. 43-28). Periportal fibrosis may be extensive. Electron microscopy shows liver cell death and dissolution about the portal spaces and crystals

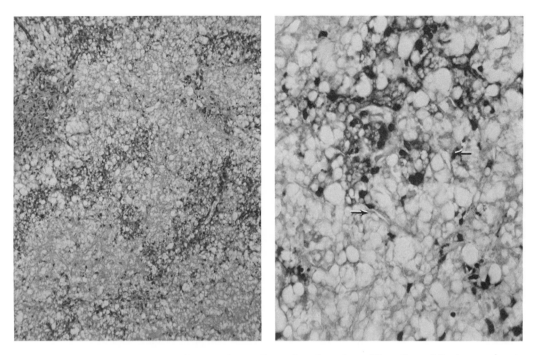

Fig. 43-28. Wolman's disease, biopsy. Extensive alteration of hepatic architecture owing to packing of hepatocytes with lipid vacuoles and pale staining in central lobular area is seen at low power. At high power, normal liver cells are not recognized; angular cholesterol ester crystals (*arrow*) are present.

free in proliferating connective tissue as well as in Kupffer cells.[431] Lipid droplets are surrounded by acid phosphatase–positive single membranes, suggesting that they are within lysosomes.[397] The intestinal mucosa shows neutral lipid in the absorptive epithelium and foam cells containing birefringent lipid packing the lamina propria. Electron microscopy shows lysosomal vacuoles containing crystal-like images.[526] Lymphocytes are vacuolated, and the bone marrow may contain foam cells.

Plasma lipids are generally normal. Diagnosis depends on liver biopsy and study of frozen sections with polarized light in addition to routine staining, analysis of tissue lipid, and demonstration of acid lipase deficiency. Death has occurred in all cases despite therapeutic trials of cholestyramine, adrenal steroids, clofibrate, cyclophosphamide, antibiotics, and thyroxine.[632]

Cholesterol Ester Storage Disease. In CESD, cholesterol ester and triglyceride also accumulate in liver and intestinal mucosa; there is a marked decrease in acid lipase activity against these two substrates.[34,115,524,597,632] Although the same biochemical abnormalities are found in Wolman's disease, patients with CESD have a normal life expectancy and present with only hepatomegaly and hyperbetalipoproteinemia, possibly due to a higher residual enzyme activity. Hepatomegaly is present at birth and increases with increasing age[632]; grossly the liver is a brilliant orange–yellow color. Frozen sections examined un-

stained with polarized light reveal an abundance of needle- or angular-shaped birefringent crystals in every hepatic cell (Fig. 43-29). Lipid stains (oil-red O, Sudan) demonstrate the crystals to be contained in lipid-filled vacuoles in hepatocytes. Paraffin sections show a septal pattern of fibrosis of moderate severity.[597] Hepatocytes are large and polygonal, with fine lacework to the cytoplasm (Fig. 43-30) that does not reflect the high lipid content seen on frozen section.[597] Plastic embedded sections show small droplets clustered about the bile canaliculus that become progressively larger from the canalicular area to the sinusoid of the hepatocyte. By electron microscopy, the larger vacuoles are seen to be surrounded by a single membrane, to contain angular images of cholesterol crystals, and to be secondary lysosomes. The findings are recapitulated in the Kupffer cells. Morphologically, the liver differs from that in Wolman's disease, in which cholesterol crystals are predominantly in Kupffer cells and neutral lipids in hepatocytes and in which disruption of liver architecture is severe.[115] The epithelial cells of the intestinal mucosa are normal, but the lamina propria contains crystals of cholesterol ester and masses of foam cells about the lacteals.[524] Mucosal smooth muscle cells contain crystals of cholesterol ester resembling vascular smooth muscle in atherosclerosis.

Although the genetics are unclear, five of seven children in one large kindred had hepatomegaly, two of whom had

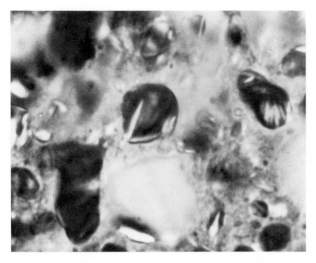

Fig. 43-29. Cholesterol ester storage disease. Unstained frozen section viewed under *polarized* light reveals the presence of anistropic needle-shaped crystals within lipid droplets.

clinical disease.[597] Treatment with cholestyramine had no effect on hepatic lipid content; clofibrate administration (500 mg four times daily for 16 months) resulted in reduction of hepatic lipid content from 22% to 9.5% wet weight, but liver size was unchanged, and cholesterol crystals were still present in large amounts.[596]

Sphingolipidoses. *Gaucher's Disease.* There is accumulation of cerebrosides, specifically glucosylceramide, in lysosomes of reticuloendothelial cells as a result of deficient activity of the β-glucosidase, glucocerebrosidase that catalyzes their breakdown.[94a,95] The reticuloendothelial cells in which glucosylceramide accumulates enlarge and develop the characteristic appearance of the "Gaucher cell." The cells are 20 μ to 100 μ and have an eccentric nucleus and a fibrillar cytoplasm described as "wrinkled tissue paper," in contrast to the foamy appearance of storage cells in other lipidoses. Seen by electron microscopy, the cells contain characteristic secondary lysosomes filled with tubular structures.[716] Symptomatology results from accumulation of these cells in involved organs. Three clinical forms of the disease exist. The most common is type I, also called the adult or chronic nonneuropathic type.[94a,234] Major manifestations are hepatosplenomegaly, thrombocytopenia, bone pain, sometimes with pathologic fractures, pingueculae, and a yellow to brownish skin pigmentation without jaundice. Onset may be at any age, including infancy, but neurologic symptoms do not occur. Infants affected with type II (infantile or acute neuropathic disease) are normal at birth but develop hepatosplenomegaly, cough, and progressive neurologic deterioration associated with strabismus, spasticity, and characteristic persistent retroflexion of the head. Death usually occurs in the first year of life.[94a] Type III (juvenile), a subacute neuropathic form, is less well defined and includes children with Gaucher cells in visceral organs, multiple neurologic

Fig. 43-30. Cholesterol ester storage disease in a 16-year-old: Hepatocytes are large and polygonal, producing a mosaic pattern. The lacy cytoplasm does not reflect the high lipid content. High power shows that the multiple vacuoles contain angular crystals of cholesterol ester (*arrow*).

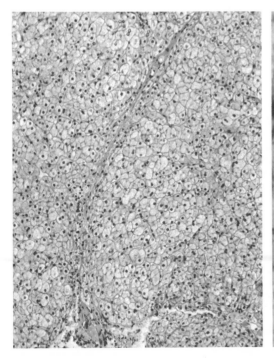
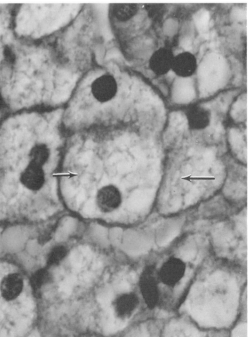

abnormalities, and prolonged survival.[94a] The genetic heterogeneity may reflect differences in processing due to alterations in the active site of the enzyme.

Gaucher cells are usually clearly seen in bone marrow, but in one of our infants, diagnosis was confirmed only after liver biopsy. Definitive diagnosis is by assay of glucocerebrosidase activity. Gaucher's disease is unique among the lysosomal groups in showing elevation of serum acid-phosphatase activity, although tissue levels of this and other acid hydrolases are characteristically increased in lysosomal diseases.

In all three types the liver is similar.[348] Gaucher cells derived from Kupffer cells are scattered throughout the parenchyma in nests about the central vein and encroaching upon and obliterating the sinusoids (Figs. 43-31 and 43-32). Fibrosis varies from strands of fibrous tissue about the Gaucher cells to gross scarring in which clusters of Gaucher cells may be embedded.[234] Portal hypertension and ascites have been reported but are rare, although thrombocytopenia and leukopenia due to splenic sequestration are common. Therapeutic attempts have included administration of purified glucocerebrosidase; future use of encapsulated enzyme may be beneficial.

Niemann–Pick Disease (Sphingomyelin Lipidosis). Multiple clinical variants have been described; all are related to marked or moderate deficiency of sphingomyelinase activity. In acute neuropathic infantile Niemann–Pick disease, marked hepatosplenomegaly occurs

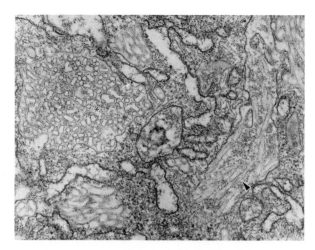

Fig. 43-32. Gaucher's disease. Electron microscopic view of tubules, shown in cross-section (∗) and in longitudinal section (▶), enclosed within lysosomal membranes.

along with neurologic deterioration (hypotonia, difficulty feeding, failure to thrive).

Conjugated hyperbilirubinemia and obstructive jaundice may occur in the neonatal period and resemble neonatal hepatitis.[154,346] More often, asymptomatic hepatosplenomegaly is present, progressing to massive proportions, failure to thrive, and vomiting during the first year of life.[96,346] Neurologic deterioration, both motor and intellectual, begins in the first year and progresses to death usually by the fourth year.[96] The cherry red spot of macular degeneration is present in approximately half of the cases.[96] Accumulation of sphingomyelin in affected organs is characteristic of the disease, but nonesterified cholesterol is also increased.

At least five types have been described, which seem to breed true in affected sibships.[96] Deficiency of sphingomyelinase, a lysosomal enzyme with hydrolytic activity to sphingomyelin, has been found only in type A, the acute infantile form, and to a lesser degree in type B, a chronic disease with early visceral involvement but with no central nervous system dysfunction.[96,346,602] Type C is a subacute disease with visceromegaly but with onset of neurologic symptoms after 2 years of age. Type D resembles type C clinically, is designated the Nova Scotia variant because of its frequency in infants of this ancestry, and often presents with neonatal cholestasis.[96] Type E occurs in adults who have no neurologic disease but visceral storage of sphingomyelin. Sphingomyelin accumulation is greatest in types A and B, presumably secondary to deficient sphingomyelinase activity. In the other types it is unexplained; free cholesterol accumulation in all types is also unexplained.

The liver is pale yellow and fatty and may be brittle.[234] Hepatocytes are vacuolated, and large pale foam cells are scattered among them. Vacuolated lymphocytes may be noted on peripheral smear and may be seen in conjunction with Niemann–Pick foam cells (approximately 15 μm in

Fig. 43-31. Gaucher's disease, biopsy: High-power view of several typical Gaucher cells with eccentric nuclei and typical fibrillar cytoplasm in infantile variety of the disease.

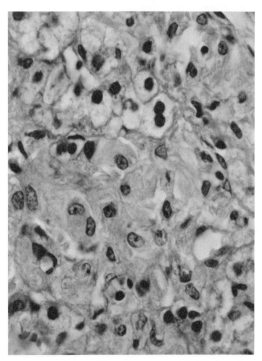

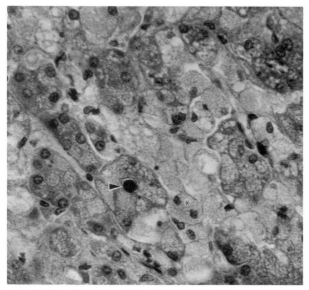

Fig. 43-33. Niemann–Pick disease. Light microscopy shows canalicular bile plug (▶) and fine cytoplasmic vacuoles in liver cells and in the reticuloendothelial cells (Kupffer cells), where they appear as prominent foamy inclusions (∗).

diameter) found in liver biopsy.[733] The foam cells contain peculiar refractile droplets preserved even in paraffin sections but are best studied histochemically in frozen section where they are Sudan and oil red O positive, blue violet with Nile blue sulfate, and have a reticular pattern of acid phosphatase activity.[234,716] In jaundiced infants there is canalicular bile stasis and disruption of lobular architecture[234,346]; giant cell formation and periportal fibrosis may be present (Fig. 43-33). Electron microscopy shows typical inclusions in foam cells (Fig. 43-34), 0.5 μm to 5.0 μm diameter, consisting of swirls of concentric membranes.[716] Hepatocytes contain many membrane-bound inclusions with similar but less dense swirls of membranes.[716] In type A disease, the decreased sphingomyelinase activity, increased sphingomyelin, and lamellated inclusions are present in cultured skin fibroblasts so that intrauterine diagnosis is feasible.[631] There is no treatment.

GM₁ Gangliosidosis. Generalized or type GM_1 gangliosidosis is an autosomal recessive disorder that resembles Gaucher's disease in that three forms have been described: infantile (severe), juvenile, and adult (mild). The infantile form is characterized by severe mental and motor deterioration, hepatosplenomegaly, bony deformities re-

Fig. 43-34. Niemann–Pick disease, electron micrograph: Characteristic swirl-like lipid containing lysosomal inclusion (*arrow*) and normal bile canaliculus (*b*) with adjacent normal mitochondria. (Original magnification × 31,000)

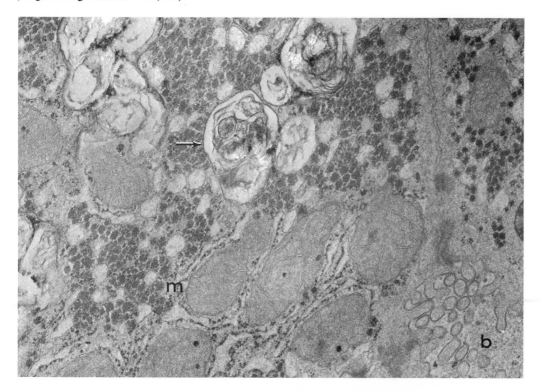

sembling type I mucopolysaccharidosis (Hurler's syndrome), and death by 2 years of age.[400,498] The neurologic deterioration is due to cerebral accumulation of GM$_1$ ganglioside, and there is visceral accumulation of GM$_1$ ganglioside and mucopolysaccharide, all due to deficiency of lysosomal β-galactosidase.[215,400] Affected infants are often retarded, hypoactive, hypotonic, and have facial and peripheral edema. The facies are abnormal, with frontal bossing, a depressed nasal bridge, a wide upper lip, and downy hirsutism of the head and neck. Skeletal deformities include lumbar kyphosis due to one or more hypoplastic vertebrae and midshaft thickening of the long bones.[400,498] The liver is enlarged in all reported cases. Hepatocytes may be vacuolated, but accumulation of stored material is most striking in Kupffer cells, which are foamy in appearance, stain positively with PAS, are diastase-resistant, and are negative with Sudan stain.[400] Inheritance is autosomal recessive. Intrauterine diagnosis with assay of β-galactosidase in cultured amniotic cells is feasible. The juvenile form of GM$_1$ gangliosidosis does not involve the liver.[498]

GM$_2$ Gangliosidosis. In the presence of defects in the hexosaminidase system, GM$_2$ ganglioside accumulates; this is a heterogeneous group of disorders.

Tay–Sachs disease is an excellent example with which to show the value of studying the liver in children with degenerative neurologic disease even though the liver is not enlarged. The disease is due to deficiency of various components (A or B) of hexosaminidase.[514] In the Jewish variety of the disease, component A is deficient; in Sandhoff's disease, the non-Jewish form, both components are deficient.[258,590] The diagnosis can be established by enzyme assay on liver tissue. Both types are characterized clinically by neurologic deterioration beginning at 4 to 6 months of age, followed by dementia, motor loss, and blindness with the cherry-red spot on the retina. The liver is normal by routine light microscopy,[716] but electron microscopy will demonstrate numerous nonlipid vacuoles of variable size; the vacuoles are lysosomes containing tightly laminated concentric inclusions similar to those seen in the less accessible neurons.[716]

Metachromatic Leukodystrophy. There is accumulation of galactocerebroside-3-sulfate due to failure of lysosomal arylsulfatase A to cleave the sulfate group. There are a number of clinical variants described; in multiple sulfatase deficiency, neurologic degeneration progressing to spastic paralysis and dementia begins in the second year of life. Liver biopsy obtained from such patients will demonstrate accumulation of metachromatic granules and macrophages in the portal area of hepatocytes and frozen sections. Similar accumulation may be seen in the gallbladder epithelium.[743] Electron microscopy will reveal residual bodies with laminar organization in liver and skin fibroblasts (Fig. 43-35).[389,540,743] The gallbladder may be small and nonfunctioning with papillomas containing metachromatic material projecting into the lumen.[187,540] Nonopaque gallstones have been reported.[162]

There are a number of other lipidoses in which the

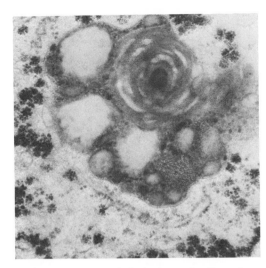

Fig. 43-35. Metachromatic leukodystrophy, liver ultrastructure: Typical abnormal lysosome with concentric lamellar organization. Light microscopy of the liver was normal.

accumulation of undegraded cellular constituents is associated with hepatomegaly.[258,391]

Mucopolysaccharidosis. The generic term *mucopolysaccharidosis* refers to a group of clinically, genetically, and probably biochemically distinct diseases that have in common storage of acid mucopolysaccharides (glycosaminoglycans), heparan sulfate, dermatan sulfate, chondroitin sulfate, and keratan sulfate in tissue, and excretion of one or more of these substances in urine. Multiple clinical types have been described, each the result of a defect in a specific lysosomal hydrolase (see Table 43-8). Comprehensive reviews are available.[258,456] All except X-linked mucopolysaccharidosis II (classic Hunter's disease) are autosomal recessive disorders. All are progressive but of varying severity; there is no effective therapy. The liver is enlarged in all types of mucopolysaccharidoses. Light microscopy in types I, II, and III shows marked vacuolation of hepatocytes and Kupffer cells.[118] There is variation in the size and number of vacuoles in hepatocytes and progressive decrease in vacuole size from peripheral to centrolobular hepatocytes. Electron microscopy demonstrates that the vacuoles are bound by a single membrane and are empty except for remnants of stored material that have not been extracted by tissue preparation (Fig. 43-36).[118] The vacuoles presumably are abnormal lysosomes deficient in the specific degradative enzyme activity. In type-IV disease, similar inclusions are present in large numbers in Kupffer cells and only occasionally in hepatocytes.[695]

Similar abnormal lysosomes are present in cultured skin fibroblasts (Fig. 43-37). Mixing experiments with cells of different genotypes led to the suggestion that specific corrective-factor (or activator) proteins exist that can nor-

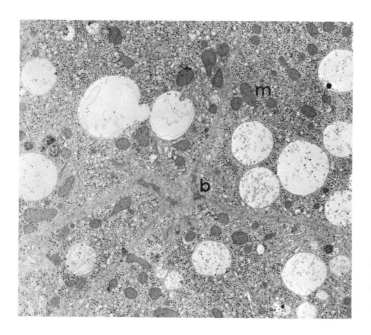

Fig. 43-36. Hurler's disease, liver biopsy ultrastructure: Multiple "abnormal lysosomes" from which most of stored material has been extracted during fixation. b, bile canaliculus; m, mitochondrion. (Original magnification × 5000)

malize mucopolysaccharide metabolism in skin fibroblasts of the respective types.[231,494] The factors have been isolated from cultured fibroblast media and urine and plasma of patients, purified, and in certain subtypes, shown to be the deficient degradative enzyme.[38,258,444,494,499] Treatment of patients with mucopolysaccharidosis types I, II, and III with infusion of fresh frozen plasma in an attempt to restore the deficient enzyme resulted in an increase in degradation products of mucopolysaccharides in urine and in clinical improvement.[186] Subsequent reports did not confirm the clinical benefit. Abnormal lysosomes in hepatocytes were unchanged after plasma infusion. Intrauterine diagnosis is possible through determination of enzyme activity or ^{35}S uptake in cultured amniotic fluid cells.[38,258,444]

Disorders of Urea Cycle

Hyperammonemia

Ammonia is a potent central nervous system toxin if not inactivated via urea formation in the liver. Animal studies have suggested that isolated hyperammonemia is toxic to the immature nervous system, producing sequential depression in the level of consciousness. Neuropathologic changes involve only astrocytes and not neuronal injury, suggesting that the acute neurotoxicity of hyperammonemia is reversible.[717] Repeated and prolonged episodes of hyperammonemic encephalopathy will be associated with permanent impairment of neurologic function.[485]

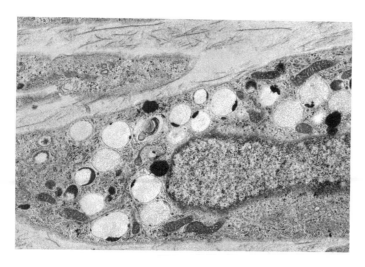

Fig. 43-37. Hurler's disease, cultured fibroblast: Abnormal lysosomes resembling those seen in the patient's liver specimen. (Original magnification × 5000)

The causes of hyperammonemia in infants and children are multiple; the most dramatic examples are inherited defects in the urea cycle enzymes (Table 43-9). The more proximal the enzyme defect is to the point of entry of NH_3 into the cycle, the more severe the disease.[226] Hyperammonemia may also be seen in newborns, especially those born prematurely or with birth asphyxia; it may be seen in older children with Reye's syndrome, in those receiving valproate or other therapeutic agents, or secondary to urinary tract infections.

Rapid clinical deterioration of a full-term newborn, with a clinical picture resembling sepsis, can be the first indication of the presence of one of the hyperammonemic syndromes. Prompt evaluation with measurement of plasma levels of ammonia, pH, amino acids, serum ketones, and bicarbonate can provide a precise diagnosis that will allow the institution of appropriate lifesaving therapy. In most instances, untreated neonatal hyperammonemia due to urea cycle defects is fatal. The incidence of inherited defects in the urea cycle is approximately 1 in 25,000 to 1 in 30,000 newborns. Each represents a specific biochemical defect leading to altered excretion of nitrogenous wastes (Fig. 43-38). In certain subsets molecular dissection of the defect has been attempted. In argininosuccinate synthetase (AS) deficiency, it has been shown that the gene is transcribed and produces a stable m-RNA; however, this is either not translated or the translation product is rapidly degraded or nonreactive, resulting in the clinical state of citrullinemia.[669] Of the known urea cycle defects, carbamyl phosphate synthetase (CPS) deficiency, AS deficiency or citrullinemia, and argininosuccinicaciduria due to arginosuccinate lyase (AL) deficiency are autosomal recessive. Ornithine transcarbamylase (OTC) deficiency is inherited in an X-linked fashion. Therefore, while males with OTC deficiency are severely affected, female patients have inactivation of one X chromosome (Lyon hypothesis) and therefore have heterogeneous symptoms. All of these enzyme defects present in a similar manner, that is, hyperammonemia with the attendant symptoms of lethargy, coma, and episodic vomiting. Marked mental retardation can result in survivors.

It is important to differentiate transient hyperammonemia of the newborn (THN) from inborn errors of metabolism that produce symptomatic neonatal hyperammonemia, namely, the urea cycle defects and the organic acidemias. Differentiation can be made using an algorithm proposed by Hudak and co-workers[324] and based on clinical features and measurement of plasma and urine amino acids, urine ketones and organic acids, and enzyme activities. They reviewed the clinical data of 33 patients with THN and 13 neonates with urea cycle enzyme deficiencies.[324] Neonates with THN were of lower birth weight and younger gestational age and had an earlier onset of profound central nervous system deterioration with coma occurring by the end of the second day. This correlated with a more rapid rise of plasma ammonia levels in THN than in patients with urea cycle defects. In the latter group of patients, coma was seldom noted before the third day of life. The cause of THN is unknown. It is been suggested that decreased hepatic flow, secondary to ductus venosus shunting, contributes to the hyperammonemia.[203] The coincidence with respiratory distress suggests a role for tissue hypoxia.

While the presence of respiratory distress prior to 24 hours of age was highly suggestive of THN, its absence suggested an inborn error of metabolism.[324] The concomitant presence of acidosis or ketosis in an infant with hyperammonemia is suggestive of liver disease or of one of the organic acidemias, that is, an inborn error of methylmalonate, isovalerate, or proprionate metabolism. In the absence of these features, an inborn error of ureagenesis is suggested and plasma citrulline levels serve as an initial screen for urea cycle deects. Plasma citrulline is

TABLE 43-9. **Inherited Urea Cycle Enzyme Defects**

SYNDROME	ENZYME DEFICIENCY	CLINICAL MANIFESTATIONS
CPS deficiency	Carbamyl phosphate synthetase	Lethargy, coma, episodic vomiting, ketoacidosis (provoked by protein ingestion)
OTC deficiency (x-linked dominant) inheritance	Ornithine transcarbamylase	Lethargy, coma, episodic vomiting, ketoacidosis (provoked by protein ingestion)
Citrullinemia	Argininosuccinic acid synthetase	Mental retardation
Argininosuccinic aciduria	Argininosuccinase (lyase)	Mental retardation, seizures, ataxia
Argininemia	Arginase	Spastic diplegia, seizures, mental retardation
N-AGS deficiency	N-acetylglutamate synthetase	Ataxia, mental retardation

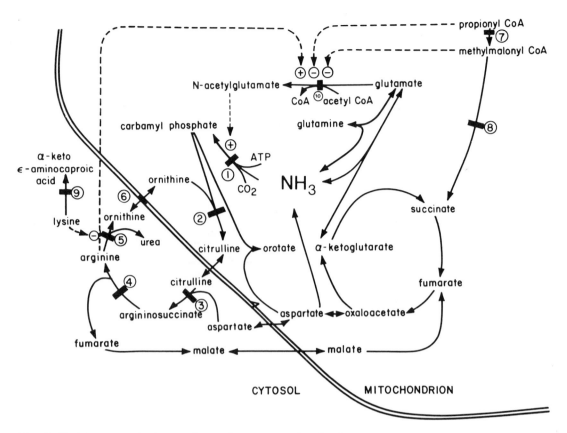

Fig. 43-38. The urea cycle. Excess nitrogen is not stored; therefore it must be excreted by means of this cycle. If a blockage exists (as indicated by numbered bars), accumulation as ammonium ion occurs and toxicity results. (**1**) CPS (carbamylphosphate synthetase): (**2**) OTC (ornithine transcarbamylase); (**3**) ASS (argininosuccinic acid synthetase); (**4**) AL (argininosuccinase); (**5**) arginase; (**6**) mitochondrial ornithine transport; (**7**) propionyl CoA carboxylase; (**8**) methylmalonyl CoA mutase; (**9**) L-lysine dehydrogenase; (**10**) N-AGS (N-acetylglutamate synthetase). Dotted lines indicate site of pathway activation (⊕) or inhibition (⊖). (Reproduced with permission from Flannery DB et al: Current status of hyperammonemic syndromes. Hepatology 2:495, 1982)

greater than 1000 μM in AS deficiency. The plasma citrulline level is in the 100 μM to 300 μM range and argininosuccinate is present in plasma in AL deficiency. If the plasma citrulline levels are low, measurement of urinary orotate levels may help to separate CPS deficiency, which is characterized by low orotate levels, from OTC deficiency, characterized by high urinary orotate levels. Prompt recognition and precise characterization are imperative, since normal plasma ammonia levels can be maintained with therapy; if episodic hyperammonemia is not controlled, coma and death can ensue.

Recent studies suggest a direct relationship between the length of hyperammonemia and the subsequent intellectual performance of the child.[485] There is no apparent relationship between the severity, as measured by serum ammonia levels, and later neurologic development and intelligence. This may be related to the secondary effects of hyperammonemia within the nerve cell, including al-

tered energy metabolism, pH, and changes in electrolyte composition, all of which affect the growth of the neuron.

The treatment of CPS, OTC, AS, and AL deficiencies involves a reduction in nitrogen intake through protein restriction and the provision of essential amino acids. These steps alone are ineffective and must be combined with an attempt to eliminate exogenous ammonia and urea precursors, which has been accomplished in the past by exchange transfusion or dialysis. Recent studies have demonstrated the value of utilization of alternative pathways of nitrogen excretion in the presence of defective ureagenic pathways. Arginine, which is indispensable for affected patients, is partially excreted as urea and will provide substrate for ornithine synthesis and input into the urea cycle.[111] This is effective in the management of AL deficiency. In addition, attempts to bypass the urea cycle by diverting nitrogen from urea synthesis to alternative waste nitrogen products have been successful. For example, administration of sodium benzoate will divert nitrogen from ammonia to glycine and allow excretion as hippurate.[112] Sodium phenylacetate combines with glutamine to form phenylacetylglutamine, leading to excretion of two molecules of ammonia in urine.

Prenatal diagnosis is possible. Two siblings have recently been described with argininosuccinic aciduria in whom the diagnosis was made in the second infant following amniocentesis.[188] As opposed to the first child who had developed severe hyperammonemia and was left with developmental delay, the second child was treated with an arginine infusion beginning at 32 hours of life and never developed hyperammonemia.

Reye's Syndrome

Reye's syndrome (acute encephalopathy and fatty degeneration of the viscera) engendered a great deal of interest in the late 1970s and early 1980s for the following reasons: (1) There was either a marked increase in the incidence or in the ability to recognize all stages of the illness. (2) The pathogenesis is poorly understood; the intriguing enigmatic interaction between the liver and brain that this disease represents has generated substantial research interest. (3) Recently there have been optimistic reports of successful management with early diagnosis and treatment. (4) There is a suggested link to aspirin administration. The resultant media attention has created parental and physician concern.

This disease was initially described almost simultaneously in Australia and in the United States by Reye[562] and Johnson.[353] In the initial report by Reye, 17 of 21 Australian children died; all 16 cases described by Johnson had a fatal outcome. There were sporadic case descriptions[64,91] until the 1974 epidemic in which 379 cases were reported nationwide; the mortality rate was greater than 40%.[142] In recent years, it has become apparent that the incidence varies in direct temporal and geographic relationship to viral epidemics, in particular, those due to influenza B.[142,573] With increased early recognition, the mortality rate has fallen. By January 1985, 190 cases has been reported to the Centers for Disease control (CDC) for 1984; the case fatality rate was 26%. This represents the lowest annual reported incidence of the disease.

Reye's syndrome following type B influenza may be the most common, potentially lethal, virus-associated encephalopathy in the United States, with an incidence of approximately 0.3 cases per 100,000 persons under 18 years of age. Influenza A may also be associated with this syndrome; however, the incidence is less marked.[142] The question remains, is this a new disease or were children with similar symptoms previously classified as having "postviral encephalopathy?" It is possible that milder cases were missed and recovered without event.

Clinical Features. Reye's syndrome is a true, not uncommon, pediatric emergency, capable of rapidly reaching an irreversible state. Clinically, the illness follows a biphasic course.[143,523,605,606] There is a prodromal febrile illness, usually (90%) in the nature of an upper respiratory tract infection, although chickenpox (5%–7%) and other viral illnesses have been associated. The child then seemingly recovers; however, a lucid interval terminates abruptly with the onset of protracted vomiting usually within a week after the onset of the viral illness. Delirium and stupor may occur after the onset of the vomiting and there may be rapid neurologic progression to seizures, coma, and death; there is an absence of focal neurologic signs. There is slight to moderate liver enlargement and biochemical indices to suggest hepatic injury, although the patient remains anicteric. The cerebrospinal fluid is normal except for an elevated pressure.

Diagnostic confusion may arise in view of the frequent prior administration of drugs such as antiemetics and anticonvulsants, which in themselves may cause liver toxicity and central nervous system depression.[86,605] The differential diagnosis includes meningitis, encephalitis, toxic encephalopathy, as well as drug ingestion, such as sodium valproate. Specific metabolic diseases discussed below such as systemic carnitine deficiency, acyl dehydrogenase deficiencies, β-hydroxy-β-methylglutaric acidemia, OTC deficiency, and fructosemia present in a similar manner.

In view of the clinical variability and the rapid progression of the illness, a uniform system of clinical staging has been proposed that divides the clinical illness into five stages, grades I through III representing mild to moderate illness, and grades IV and V representing severe illness (Table 43-10).[605,606]

Laboratory Features. The illness is highlighted by the explosive release of various enzymes such as ALT (liver) and AST (liver or muscle). As a reflection of liver dys-

TABLE 43-10. Clinical Grades of Reye's Syndrome at Time of Admission

CLINICAL GRADE	SYMPTOMS
Mild-moderate	
I	Usually quietness or mild lethargy
II	Deep lethargy, confusion; possibly, brief unconsciousness
III	Extreme lethargy or light coma lasting less than 3 hours; possibly, seizures or agitation.
Severe	
IV	Seizures; possibly, agitation and combativeness; usually protracted deep coma lasting longer than 3 hours; intermittent decerebrate posturing
V	Seizures; deep coma; decerebrate posturing; fixed pupils

function, hypoprothrombinemia unresponsive to vitamin K may occur. The degree of elevation of the serum ammonia level may provide prognostic information. In our institution, of 83 biopsy-proven cases of grade I Reye's syndrome, 78 had no change in coma grade during hospitalization.[306] In the five who progressed to deeper coma grades, the mean level of serum ammonia on admission was significantly higher ($\sim$290 μg/dl) than that in patients whose disease did not progress ($\sim$50 μg/dl). The prothrombin time was also significantly more prolonged (3.9 vs. 1.6 sec) in patients with progressing coma.[306]

As a concomitant of the generalized metabolic injury, there is hyperaminoacidemia (glutamine, alanine, and lysine), as well as an increased concentration of plasma free fatty acids (FFAs), which may in themselves contribute to the central nervous system narcotic effect, and in younger patients there may be hypoglycemia.

Epidemiology. The average age of onset is approximately 6 years, with most children clustering in the 4- to 12-year age range.[605,606,712] Rare reports of adults with Reye's syndrome can be found. There is no difference in the male–female incidence; however, the rural and suburban population appears to be more frequently affected than urban-dwelling children. The significance of this finding is unknown, but a genetic/environmental interaction in causation has been suggested.

The criteria utilized by the CDC for case definition requires the presence of acute noninflammatory encephalopathy—clinical alteration of consciousness with either laboratory (<8 leukocytes per mm^3 in cerebrospinal fluid) or histologic (cerebral edema without inflammation) documentation; fatty metamorphosis of the liver, diagnosed either by biopsy or autopsy or by a threefold or greater rise in aminotransferase or ammonia; and no known other reasonable explanation.[573]

In order to estimate the frequency of Reye's syndrome among children with vomiting and elevated aminotransferase following a prodromal viral illness, all patients presenting to the emergency room at Children's Hospital Medical Center in Cincinnati were carefully evaluated.[420] During this 12-month prospective study, 31 patients met the clinical criteria for diagnosis; 6 were classified on admission as grade II to III and 25 were grade I. Biopsies obtained from 19 of the grade I cases were analyzed using the strict light microscopy, histochemistry, and ultrastructural criteria described below; 14 were determined to have Reye's syndrome. Of the remaining five, two were determined not to have Reye's syndrome, whereas the other three may have had a mild form. None of the 19 patients had evidence of viral or toxic hepatitis or any other recognizable liver disease. During this period, the estimated minimal annual incidence of biopsy-proven Reye's syndrome of all grades was 3.1 per 100,000 persons under 18 years of age. In view of the high frequency and the apparent large number of mildly affected cases, prognostic indicators for severity or progression are needed in order to formulate rational therapeutic decisions. In our

study, ultrastructural changes were most severe in those who progressed; however, biopsies are not indicated for all children. The most practical approach, therefore, may be to utilize as prognostic indicators the serum ammonia level and the correlated prothrombin time as described above.

Pathologic Features. We believe that liver biopsy is essential to define the syndrome precisely and to exclude entities such as metabolic or toxic liver disease. The pathology of Reye's syndrome is striking and characteristic. The liver is grossly yellow to white, reflecting the 20% to 30% triglyceride content. Under light microscopy, there is a uniform foaminess of liver cell cytoplasm with microvesicular fatty accumulation, which may be "concealed" in routine preparations (Figs. 43-39 and 43-40).[93] There is cytoplasmic clarity without inflammation and rare bile stasis; individual cell death is uncommon, and the nuclei are central. The fat stain of a frozen section will strikingly display the histologic abnormality. Triglyceride is distributed throughout the lobule in a monotonous, small droplet pattern in which each cell is affected.[93] Characteristic electron microscopic changes have been described.[526] There is a remarkable alteration in mitochondrial morphology (Fig. 43-41). In mild cases, there is slight rarefaction of the matrix with pleomorphism, swelling, and reduction in the number of mitochondria. In more severely involved cases, glycogen depletion may be noted, matrix expansion is greater, mitochondrial-dense bodies are lost, and mitochondria may assume an ameboid form. Mitochondrial injury is uniformly severe in patients who eventually die and resembles mitochondrial injury with irreversible high-amplitude swelling from uncoupled respiration.[280] During recovery, large mitochondria seem to divide, budding and branching forms appear, and the matrix and mitochondrial-dense bodies return to normal by the third or fourth day (Fig. 43-42). Lysosomes are relatively inconspicuous. The nuclei in nonfatal cases are swollen and spherical; in nonfatal cases, binucleate cells and mitoses are increased, and nucleoli exhibit an open skeinlike structure.

In children who recover, light microscopy of the liver is normal within 2 months except for fat droplets in lipocytes and Kupffer cells.[93] Mitochondria are normal except for an occasional enlarged mitochondrion with a flocculent matrix.[526] Other organs are also involved. There is renal tubular fatty accumulation and infiltration of the cardiac myofibrils; fatty accumulation has also been described in the lungs and pancreatic islet cells as well as in muscle tissue.

Histologic examination of brain tissue obtained during decompressive craniectomy reveals a similar pattern of injury.[525] Grossly there is marked edema, and under light microscopy there is an absence of necrosis or inflammation. Electron microscopic changes include edematous myelin sheaths (blebs), which may account for a substantial portion of the brain swelling. Of interest is the fact that neuronal mitochondria undergo similar structural

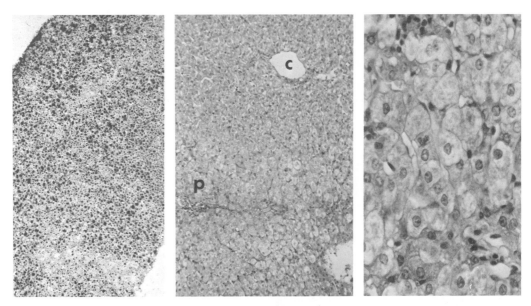

Fig. 43-39. Reye's syndrome: Six-year-old boy, clinical grade IV, who is well after six exchange transfusions. Frozen section (*left*) with oil-red O stain at low power shows universal distribution of small fat droplets in hepatocytes. Routine section (*center*) shows the concealed nature of this fatty infiltration. Large fat droplets are absent and nuclei are not displaced, but hepatocytes are enlarged, compressing sinusoids. p, portal zone; c, central vein. At higher power (*right*), hepatocytes are swollen with lacelike cytoplasm, but no large vacuoles are present.

Fig. 43-40. Nutritional fatty liver in an infant with pancreatic insufficiency: Hepatocytes are distended with one or two large fat vacuoles, and nuclei are displaced to one side. Contrast with "concealed fat" in Reye's syndrome in Figure 43-39.

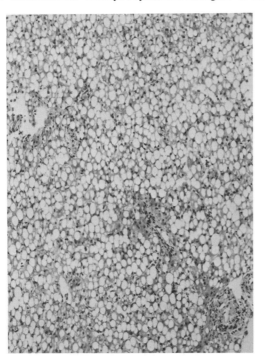

changes as those seen in the liver. These ultrastructural changes appear to be unique to Reye's syndrome. It therefore appears that a generalized mitochondrial dysfunction can account for most findings in Reye's syndrome.

Biochemical Alterations. Abnormal mitochondrial function correlates with the grossly abnormal morphology and results in changes in carbohydrate, amino acid, and fatty acid metabolism, with alterations in serum proteins and coagulation factors, ammonia, and organic acids. Tissue activities of all measured intramitochondrial enzymes including OTC, CPS, pyruvate dehydrogenase, pyruvate carboxylase, succinate dehydrogenase, and cytochrome oxidase are reduced, often to below half normal activity, but are not absent.[605,606] Multiple hepatic cytosolic enzymes including glucokinase, pyruvate kinase, fructose-1,6-diphosphate aldolase, fructose-1,6-diphosphatase, AS, AL, and arginase are normal.

Disturbed mitochondrial function limits oxidation of fatty acids, ketone bodies, and pyruvate, thus increasing glycolysis to meet tissue demands. Increased levels of pyruvate, lactate, and alanine resulting from glycolysis may be inadequately metabolized because of decreased activities of hepatic pyruvate carboxylase and dehydrogenase. The hyperammonemia may result from a decrease in the activity of the two mitochondrial enzymes of the urea cycle, OTC and CPS.

Decreased activity of hepatic enzymes involved in dis-

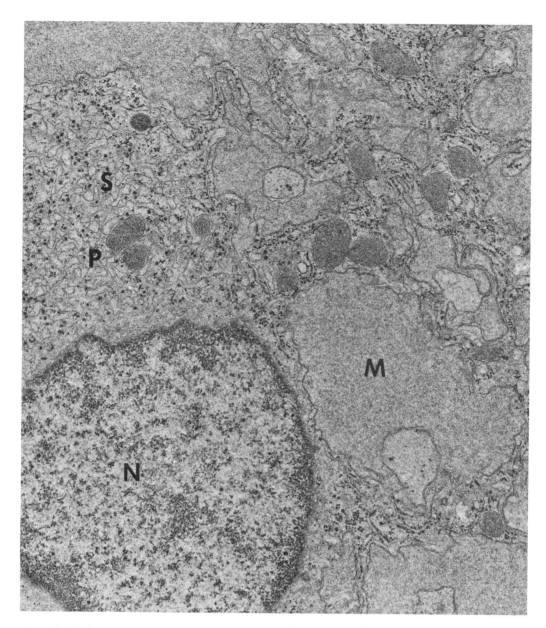

Fig. 43-41. Reye's syndrome, electron micrograph (Original magnification × 23,000) from same specimen as in Figure 43-39. Mitochondria (*M*) are greatly swollen in ameboid configuration. Mitochondrial dense bodies are absent, and matrix density is reduced. Peroxisomes (*P*) are increased in number, and smooth endoplasmic reticulum (*S*) is proliferating. Glycogen particles are small and rare. N, nucleus.

position of FFAs presumably results in elevated FFAs and in esterification of fatty acids in the liver with triglyceride accumulation.

Etiologic Speculations. The specific cause of the generalized mitochondrial dysfunction is unknown; there has been a good deal of etiologic speculation. The most pop-

ular theories implicate virus-related phenomena with or without the concomitant influence of a toxin. Any theory of pathogenesis must account for the known epidemiologic features: the virus-related nature of the illness, the specific and limited age-range affected, the individual susceptibility and the absence of intrafamilial associations, and the absence of a reproducible animal model. Uniformly, there has

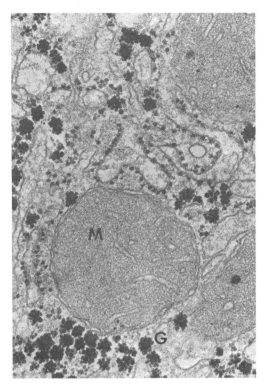

Fig. 43-42. Reye's syndrome in the same patient as in Figure 43-41 4 days after recovery. (Original magnification × 23,000) Mitochondrial morphology (*M*) is nearly normal, glycogen rosettes (*G*) are normal in number and form, and smooth endoplasmic reticulum is distended with lipid particles (*upper left*).

been an association of a prodromal viral illness, and family members frequently have identical uncomplicated viral infections.[562,605,606] The disease has been associated with recognizable viral epidemics, especially influenza B[142,260] and varicella.[259,605,606] Other viral isolates from patients with Reye's syndrome include reovirus 1 and 2, echovirus, coxsackievirus A and B, adenovirus, herpes simplex, Epstein–Barr virus, rubeola, mumps, herpes zoster, as well as influenza A.[200,359,515,552,605,606] There appears to be little doubt that viral infection is part of the illness; however, in view of the multiplicity of viral agents isolated, the presence of identical illnesses without encephalopathy in family members and the limitation of the syndrome to children suggest that a second, as yet unknown, factor is involved in the pathogenesis of the disease. Viral infection may serve to sensitize the host to an ingested toxin or to cause lipolysis and release of fat soluble substances previously ingested and stored in adipose tissue.

Crocker proposed, based on epidemiologic studies in Eastern Canada, that the emulsifying agents or carrier substances used in ubiquitous insecticide sprays could be responsible for Reye's syndrome.[156] Extensive animal work, as well as monolayer cell and organ cultures of human and animal origin, has demonstrated that a benign dose of infective encephalomyocarditis virus (EMV) causes a marked increase in mortality rate if the young animal or tissue is concomitantly treated with the implicated emulsifying agent. To date, examination of tissue from fatal cases of Reye's syndrome has not resulted in identification of hydrocarbons or their derivatives.[588]

Aflatoxin, a toxic metabolite of certain strains of *Aspergillus flavus,* was implicated in the pathogenesis of Reye's syndrome[64,92] based on a seasonal and geographic pattern of contamination that is identical to the incidence of Reye's syndrome. In all species studied, aflatoxin toxicity was greatest in the young. Specific cases of Reye's syndrome had a history of ingestion of food heavily contaminated with the mycotoxin. Thai children had significant amounts of aflatoxin B_1 or B_2 in tissue specimens. Aflatoxin has been sporadically isolated from tissue and body fluids of patients with Reye's syndrome in the United States; however, there is no significant difference between levels found in these patients and those found in a group of control children.[572] Aflatoxin seems to have been effectively ruled out as a cause of this disease.[492]

There is a resemblance of Reye's syndrome to Jamaican vomiting illness, which results from the ingestion of hypoglycin, a toxin found in the unripe fruit of the Ackee tree.[107,562] Hypoglycin ingestion produces vomiting, hypoglycemia, depletion of liver glycogen, fatty infiltration of the liver, coma, and death in up to 80% of the cases. The incidence is higher in young children, especially in those with poor nutritional status. Hypoglycin or α-aminomethylenecycloproprionic acid must be converted to methylenecyclopropylacetic acid (MCPA) to exert toxicity. This may account for the latent period after ingestion before the onset of vomiting. MCPA toxicity results from inhibition of fatty acid oxidation causing increased glucose utilization and a block in gluconeogenesis with resultant hypoglycemia. The inhibition of fatty acid oxidation causes accumulation of an acyl-CoA derivative of MCPA that is slowly metabolized in tissue, with consequent lowering of tissue levels of CoA and carnitine, cofactors needed for fatty acid oxidation.[101] Hypoglycin induces isovaleric and α-methylbutyric acidemia by its interaction with isovaleryl-CoA-dehydrogenase.[685] A possible relation of the neurotoxicity to accumulation of these branched-chain pentanoic acids, both of which are central nervous system depressants, has been suggested. Although hypoglycin ingestion is not the cause of Reye's syndrome, compounds of similar structure possessing a carbon–carbon double bond separated by two carbon atoms from the carboxyl group can have a similar effect.[23] Ingestion of margosa oil, which contains a variety of fatty acids, may produce a Reyelike illness.[628]

Aprille and co-workers suggested that a toxic factor was present in Reye's syndrome serum which was responsible for the mitochondrial dysfunction.[24] In experiments in which rat liver mitochondria were incubated with Reye's syndrome serum, a markedly unusual oxidative activity with stimulation of state 4 respiration and morphologic alterations—mitochondrial swelling and disruption—was seen. The authors postulated that an endogenous factor may be activated by the presence of a virus or an additional toxin and precipitate the cascade responsible for the mitochondrial dysfunction. Serum from patients with hepatic coma due to cirrhosis, chronic active liver disease, or salicylate intoxication did not mediate this effect on respiratory function of isolated rat mitochondria.

The finding of a factor in Reye's syndrome serum that is capable of uncoupling oxidative phosphorylation and impairing the formation of ATP has led to the search for candidate uncouplers. Tonsgard and Getz demonstrated that dicarboxylic acids, which are known uncouplers, are present in the serum and urine of patients with Reye's syndrome; these may be responsible for the generalized impairment of mitochondrial function.[697] The more global implication is the delineation of diseases highlighted by defects of β-oxidation and the accumulation of dicarboxylic acids, especially long-chain dicarboxylic acids, which are clinically similar to Reye's syndrome. These include medium-chain and long-chain acyl-CoA-dehydrogenase deficiencies, systemic carnitine deficiency, and hydroxymethylglutaryl-CoA-lyase deficiency (see below).

Aspirin and Reye's Syndrome. There has been much controversy regarding the association of aspirin and Reye's syndrome. The link was initially established by the finding for case-control studies of a higher frequency of aspirin usage in patients with Reye's syndrome than in controls. For example, in 97 cases of Reye's syndrome in an Ohio study,[287] 97% were reportedly recipients of aspirin; a control group of 156 children had a lower exposure rate (71%).[287] Similar findings were found in case-control studies in Arizona and Michigan. However, in each study, there were several suggested flaws in the epidemiologic design, methods used to identify medication, and the like. The association of salicylates and Reye's syndrome is a reasonable one, since salicylates are mitochondrial toxins, may act as an uncoupler, are known to cause mitochondrial swelling *in vitro,* and may induce aberrations in the immune response. There may be an increased incidence of Reye's syndrome in children with juvenile rheumatoid arthritis who require chronic aspirin therapy. However, classic aspirin toxicity does not seem to be the modality. Not all children with Reye's syndrome are exposed to aspirin, and the number of children exposed to aspirin is extremely high compared with the number of cases of Reye's syndrome. The morphology of aspirin toxicity differs from that of Reye's syndrome.[528] Nevertheless, in 1982, the Surgeon General advised against the use of salicylates and a task force was appointed to carry out a pilot study to address the question of a link between aspirin and Reye's syndrome. The small pilot study demonstrated that of 30 patients with Reye's syndrome, 93% had been exposed to salicylates, whereas in 143 controls selected from emergency room patients, inpatients, and schoolmates chosen at random, the exposure rate to salicylates

ranged from 23% to 59%.[337] The data, therefore, suggested a strong association between Reye's syndrome and the use of aspirin, with an estimated odds ratio of 25:1. Subsequently a request for warning labels on all aspirin products was issued, and there was voluntary compliance by the aspirin industry. The persistent decline in the annual number of cases of Reye's syndrome since 1982 may well reflect the reduction in aspirin use. This remains to be determined as viral cycles continue.

Treatment. Successful management of Reye's syndrome is based upon two key factors. Early diagnosis is essential; therefore the illness should be suspected in any child with unexplained neurologic symptoms with or without vomiting. Also, increased intracranial pressure secondary to cerebral edema appears to be the major factor contributing to the high mortality rate. In the brain there is a loss of the ability to maintain water and electrolyte homeostasis, and marked edema occurs.[176] As intracranial pressure approaches systemic arterial pressure, brain perfusion becomes inadequate with resultant brain damage or death. It is imperative that cell swelling be counteracted and that aerobic metabolism be maintained; vasoconstriction must be induced without further impairment of perfusion. Thus the primary goal of therapy is to decrease intracranial pressure; a secondary goal would be to reverse the metabolic injury. Several methods have been proposed; however, there is no uniform agreement regarding efficacy of specific treatment modalities.

The methods of management vary among institutions and with the severity of the illness; we utilize the following protocol. Patients should initially receive glucose (10%–15%) intravenously, since even with mild illness there may be glycogen depletion. The mitochondrial injury may be associated with initiation of anaerobic metabolism, which in the face of glucose depletion may hasten cellular death.[303] In the presence of cerebral edema, fluid intake should be monitored closely, and the amount administered should be restricted to approximately 1200 ml/m^2/day. Every attempt should be made to prevent fever and to maintain relative hypothermia.

In more severely ill children with coma, endotracheal intubation is indicated. This will allow maintenance of an adequate Po$_2$ (100–120 mm Hg) and hyperventilation to induce hypocarbia (Pco$_2$ of 20–25 mm Hg), which will cause a decrease of cerebral blood flow by causing cerebral vasoconstriction. Patient stimulation should be kept to a minimum, since procedures such as suctioning may generate reactive pressure waves.

Several studies have demonstrated the value of close monitoring of intracranial pressure.[618] This modality will allow for more rational decisions, since clinical signs may not be reliable. Osmotherapy, using mannitol 0.5 g to 1.0 g/kg every 4 to 6 hours, may then be initiated to maintain a serum osmolarity of 310 mOsmol to 320 mOsmol and to induce cerebral dehydration.[618] Pressure monitoring provides an effective guide to therapy with osmotic diuretics and may decrease the rate of renal complications due to hyperosmolarity. Pharmacologically titrated coma, mediated by barbiturates, may have a protective effect on the central nervous system by decreasing cerebral metabolic demands, decreasing cerebral blood flow, and causing cerebral vasoconstriction. Neuromuscular relaxants such as pancuronium bromide have been used in hopes of decreasing cerebral blood volume by decreasing muscular rigidity and causing peripheral pooling.

Whole blood exchange transfusions were initially used in Reye's syndrome in order to normalize blood coagulation factors to allow for safe diagnostic liver biopsy and removal of a postulated, nondialyzable toxin of either endogenous or exogenous origin. Our initial noncontrolled observations of 112 cases managed at Cincinnati Children's Hospital Medical Center (1969–1978) suggested that exchange transfusion was of therapeutic value in more severe grades of Reye's syndrome.[86,607] Following exchange transfusion, 26 of 28 patients in stage III and 25 of 33 patients in stage IV survived. None of the three patients in stage V coma survived.[607] In severely ill patients in whom cerebral edema is not controlled by the above methods, therapeutic bilateral decompressive craniotomy has been performed.[523,525] Success of this procedure will depend on the timing of surgery in this rapidly evolving disease process; however, it should be considered if intracranial pressure is markedly elevated. Controlled trials to establish the merits of various therapeutic methods are needed.

Outcome. There is an association between the severity of the encephalopathy of Reye's syndrome and the behavioral outcome. In the Cincinnati study, the length of the period of disordered central nervous system function during the acute stage of the illness was the best predictor of eventual neuropsychological outcome.[607] In those patients with grade I disease, recovery is rapid and complete. With increasing severity and duration of illness, there may be an apparently normal recovery with subsequent subtle neuropsychological defects noted. The Cincinnati study documented defects in measured intelligence, school achievement, visual–motor integration, and in concept formation.

Diseases That Resemble Reye's Syndrome

There are similarities between Reye's syndrome and diseases associated with specific defects in fatty acid oxidation that involve the liver. In fact, as our understanding of this spectrum of disease increases, a number of patients who might be considered to have Reye's syndrome, especially "recurrent Reye's syndrome," or siblings thought to have Reye's syndrome may be recognized to have a specific inborn error of metabolism. The list of such disorders includes carnitine palmitoyltransferase deficiency, hydroxy-methylglutaryl-CoA-lyase deficiency, type II glutaric aciduria, and the dicarboxylic acidurias.

Carnitine is an essential cofactor in that it allows β-oxidation of long-chain fatty acids by aiding in their transfer across the inner mitochondrial membrane. Recent studies have delineated at least three clinical forms of carnitine deficiency: myopathic, systemic, and mixed.[127] In all states of carnitine deficiency there is accumulation of neutral lipid in liver, skeletal muscle, and heart. There is marked hypoglycemia with an absence of ketonuria. In carnitine deficiency there is extensive fine lipid droplet accumulation in the liver and proliferation of the endoplasmic reticulum; there is an increased number of peroxisomes and lipid vacuoles.[243] Plasma and tissue carnitine levels are very low; replacement therapy has been effective in treatment of the myopathic forms but inconclusively effective in systemic and mixed forms.

Several syndromes in which carnitine deficiency is secondary have been described. Stanley and co-workers studied three children in two families presenting in early childhood with episodes of coma, hypoglycemia, hyperammonemia, and fatty liver associated with fasting.[648] In one case, fatal cerebral edema occurred. These children manifest an absence of ketosis on fasting, despite elevated levels of FFAs, suggesting that hepatic fatty acid oxidation was impaired. Urinary dicarboxylic acid levels were increased during fasting, and a secondary carnitine deficiency was noted. The authors documented that the mid-portion of the intramitochondrial β-oxidation pathway at the medium-chain acyl-CoA-dehydrogenase (MCAD) step was defective.[648]

MCAD and long-chain acyl-CoA-dehydrogenase (LCAD) deficiencies are specific inborn errors of fatty acid oxidation that are now recognized as causes of steatosis, hypoketotic hypoglycemia, and a catastrophic illness distinguishable from Reye's syndrome. Affected patients are young (under 1 year) and present, usually after a prolonged fast, with coma or respiratory arrest, hepatomegaly, vomiting, and hypoglycemia with no ketonuria. Patients with LCAD, the more severe form,[285] are often under 4 months of age and are hypotonic. Liver biopsy will reveal large-droplet fat accumulation.

In MCAD there is isolated excretion of straight-chain C_6-C_{10} dicarboxylic acids due to defective mitochondrial β-oxidation. MCAD is histologically indistinguishable from Reye's syndrome; however, no mitochondrial changes are noticeable by electron microscopy.[20,90] Diagnosis is possible by assessment of acyl-CoA-dehydrogenase activity in liver or fibroblasts or by assessment of the rate of degradation of fatty acid by fibroblasts.[20] Administration of frequent feedings with a carbohydrate-enriched diet, possibly with supplemental carnitine, has been suggested.[571]

HEPATITIS IN CHILDREN

Acute Viral Hepatitis

Recent advances in the diagnosis and management of human infection with the hepatitis viruses have had a major impact on the pediatric patient. Early tracking of hepatitis

A virus (HAV) through day care center clientele and personnel has led to effective measures to prevent further spread throughout the entire community. Perinatal transmission of hepatitis B virus (HBV) remains a major source of spread; early detection and the use of improved methods of immunoprophylaxis are possible. The latter effort may lead to a decrease in the incidence of hepatocellular carcinoma.

Hepatitis A

Non-toilet-trained infants serve as hosts as well as vectors of spread of HAV infection. Several studies have traced outbreaks of HAV infection to day care centers. The high rate of transmission is due to the hygienic condition (overcrowded, understaffed, sharing of fomites such as toys, nonwashed hands, and diaper-changing surfaces) present in implicated centers.[46] Day care center–associated outbreaks of HAV infection have an impact not only on attendees but also on caretakers and parents or siblings of the often asymptomatic yet infected infant. Management consists of identification, suspension of new admissions to the center, exclusion of documented infected infants until fecal viral excretion has ceased, and administration of standard immune globulin to employees and children. The use of immunoglobulin is an effective means of controlling HAV infection both within the day care center and in the community.[283]

Hepatitis B

The epidemiologic and clinical manifestations of HBV infection in children have been reviewed.[46,197] Dupuy and associates studied 80 French children in a 4-year period who had hepatitis B surface antigen (HBsAg) detectable in their serum; 36% were under 1 year of age.[197] The presentations were variable: acute viral hepatitis with recovery was present in 31, yet there was a high rate of fulminant hepatitis (16 cases). Chronic persistent hepatitis (17 cases) and chronic active hepatitis (12 cases) were documented by characteristic biopsy changes; four patients were asymptomatic HBsAg carriers. The peak frequency of HBsAg-related disease in the infants occurred at 2 to 5 months of age, suggesting a perinatal exposure.

Several studies have sought to define the consequences of HBV infection in pregnant women, since transmission of HBV in the perinatal period is responsible for maintenance of a pool of HBsAg carriers. The data suggest that if the mother is a chronic carrier of HBsAg, the antigen is infrequently found in the cord blood or in the infant's serum during the first 6 months of life.[37,637,658] If the mother has HBsAg-positive hepatitis during pregnancy or the immediate postpartum period, HBsAg may be found in the cord blood or in the infant's serum during the first year of life in a high percentage of cases.[608] Several factors, in addition to geographic and ethnic variations, predispose the infant to antigenemia: high maternal HBsAg titer; maternal HBeAg positivity; cord blood HBsAg antige-

nemia; and documented sibling antigenemia.[61,658] Almost all of the offspring of HBeAg-positive mothers were found to be infected with HBV; over 85% became chronic HBsAg carriers. Rarely were the children of anti-HBe–positive mothers found to be infected with HBV, and none developed the carrier state.[513,658] The most common outcome of perinatal infection with HBV is the onset of a mild icteric hepatitis followed by chronic persistent hepatitis and the development of the carrier state. Rare cases of fulminant hepatitis have been described (Fig. 43-43).

Interruption of perinatal transmission is possible by active (vaccination) or passive immunization. High-titer hepatitis B immunoglobulin (HBIG) or standard immune globulin (IG)[696] has been administered to infants of HBsAg-positive mothers in hopes of achieving prophylaxis.[559,659,696,748] Reesink and co-workers gave 0.5 ml/kg HBIG to 21 children born to HBsAg carrier mothers

Fig. 43-43. Fulminant viral hepatitis in 4-year-old patient: Initial biopsy specimen (*above*) at low power shows extensive portal inflammatory infiltrate (*p*) extending into parenchyma of lobule. Higher power (*middle*) shows liver cell necrosis and mitosis (*arrow*). Second biopsy 6 weeks later, shortly before death, shows collapsed reticulum, free of normal hepatocytes, containing proliferating pseudoductules.

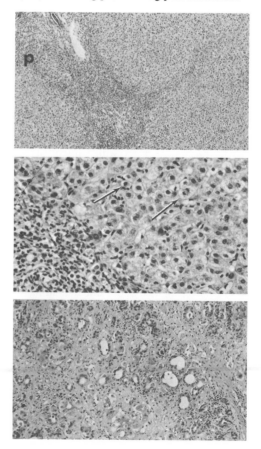

within the first 2 days of life.[559] A follow-up dose (0.16 ml/kg) was given every month for 6 months. Compared with a control group in which 25% became HBsAg positive, none of the treated infants manifested HBV infection and all remained HBsAg negative. Beasley administered 0.5 ml of HBIG at birth and at 3 to 6 months of age to Taiwanese infants and decreased the HBV infection rate from 94% to 75% and decreased the chronic carrier rate from 91% to 22%.[59,60] This data suggest that *early* (within 48 hours of birth) administration of HBIG should be considered for newborns of carrier mothers, especially those HBeAg positive and of those mothers with acute HBV infection in the third trimester.[59,60,696,748] This should be combined with the initiation of a vaccination program beginning at birth.[46,659]

Another group at high risk for acquisition of HBV infection and the development of HBsAg carrier state are residents of institutions for the mentally retarded. The risk of spread of infection to pupils and staff is attributable to improper hygiene, interpersonal contact, and behavioral or medical conditions.[102] Supplemental vaccinations may be necessary in this special group of patients in order to achieve protective levels of anti-HBs.[302] In a recent series of autopsies of all deaths (n = 138) occurring in one such institution, three cases of hepatocellular carcinoma were found; all were carriers of HBsAg without cirrhosis.[530] Serial monitoring of α-fetoprotein levels may allow early detection of carcinoma in this setting.

A unique clinical manifestation of HBV infection in childhood is infantile papular acrodermatitis (Gianotti–Crosti disease), which presents as a diffuse macular or maculopapular rash with arthritis[694]; this is often associated with HBsAg subtype ayw. There is a high incidence of HBsAg in children with membranous glomerulonephropathy; therefore this may represent another immune complex–mediated extrahepatic manifestation of HBV infection.[385,642] Serologic evidence of infection with HBV-associated delta agent has been found in Italian children; the prevalence increased in parallel with the activity of the liver disease and was maximal in the presence of cirrhosis.[214]

Non-A, Non-B Hepatitis

Children at special risk for non-A, non-B hepatitis are hemophiliacs or others who require frequent transfusions or children who receive large volumes of blood.[46] In 18 hemophilic patients, biopsies performed at 2 to 9 years of age revealed chronic persistent hepatitis in 4 children and chronic active hepatitis in 2, one with cirrhosis.[455] Biochemical values were abnormal in 13; none were HBsAg positive. Future development of serologic markers for non-A, non-B viruses and use of techniques to remove, neutralize or inactivate viral particles from blood and blood products will decrease the risk of non-A, non-B hepatitis in children. In an analogy to perinatal HBV transmission, it is possible that mothers infected with non-A, non-B hepatitis may transmit the disease to infants.

This remains to be proven; however, it may be reasonable to give immune globulin as soon as possible after birth, and then to carry out a follow-up study.

Cytomegalovirus Infection in the Older Child

The syndrome of congenital CMV infection is described above; however, acquired CMV infection must also be considered in the differential diagnosis of unexplained hepatomegaly in older children. There will be associated splenomegaly in approximately one third of these patients; mild abnormalities in liver function are common, but serum aminotransferase and total bilirubin levels may be within the normal range.[290] CMV is readily isolated from a fresh urine sample or from liver tissue obtained by biopsy; monoclonal antibodies may be utilized to determine the agent directly.[587] Rare inclusion-bearing cells, characteristic of CMV infection, may be seen in the liver. Other histologic changes vary from minimal hepatocellular unrest to granulomatous hepatitis. A child with hepatomegaly and a positive CMV culture or serology requires complete evaluation, since this agent can be isolated from normal children and may not be related etiologically to the liver disease in the patient. Conversely, definitive diagnosis of CMV infection as causative of liver disease will provide epidemiologic as well as prognostic information.

Herpes Simplex Hepatitis in the Older Child

Hepatitis due to HSV in the nonneonatal age-group is uncommon and is most often observed in patients with postulated defects in cell-mediated immunity, severe malnutrition, in organ transplant patients, and in patients with malignancy, burns, and skin diseases. Herpes simplex hepatitis has been associated with pregnancy and the postmeasles state. HSV infection should be considered in the differential of fulminant hepatic failure.[474] With the introduction of relatively safe and effective antiviral therapy, early diagnosis is important.[645,646] The associated clinical and laboratory features include localized oral or genital herpetic lesions, fever, enlarging hepatomegaly, deteriorating pneumonia, and leukopenia, along with elevations in levels of aminotransferase. Liver biopsy provides a very useful and rapid diagnostic method for evaluation of hepatitis potentially caused by HSV.[551,689] Characteristic intranuclear inclusions can be seen on routine light microscopy, usually in the setting of focal coagulative necrosis surrounded by degenerating liver cells, with hemorrhage. The inflammatory response is minimal. Immunoperoxidase staining to demonstrate viral antigen in affected hepatocytes can be performed rapidly. Electron microscopy and viral cultures can further confirm the diagnosis.

The prognosis for affected adult patients is poor; of 23 patients, 21 sustained a fatal outcome.[689] The outcome of herpes simplex hepatitis has not been well defined in children. In a recent report, five children age 2 to 48 months at risk for disseminated herpes infection were given antiviral agents; one recovered, two survived with cerebral sequelae, and two died.[689]

Chronic Active Hepatitis

It appears that the clinical, biochemical, immunologic, and histologic features of chronic active and chronic persistent hepatitis in children parallel those seen in adults; however, extensive experience has not been accumulated. In this age-group, it is especially important to consider the alternative diagnoses of Wilson's disease, α_1-AT deficiency, and other metabolic liver diseases in the differential of chronic hepatitis. The natural history of the disease spectrum in children is unknown; however, the presentation may be that of acute liver disease, the true nature of which is revealed only by biopsy. Several series have suggested that prednisone (2 mg/kg/day up to 40 mg/day) will be effective in inducing remission in HBsAg-negative chronic active hepatitis.[8,25,421,438,508,713] Alternate-day administration of corticosteroids may lessen the side effects of growth retardation.

Wilson's Disease

In every child with unexplained acute or chronic liver disease, Wilson's disease should be considered because of the potential benefits of early treatment. The disease may present with or without jaundice and without Kayser–Fleischer rings or neurologic involvement. This disease is reviewed elsewhere in this text.

PRIMARY SCLEROSING CHOLANGITIS

Primary sclerosing cholangitis is a rare cause of hepatobiliary disease in childhood.[484,643] Progressive sclerosing cholangitis without apparent associated inflammatory bowel disease was diagnosed by surgical exploration, cholangiography, and biopsy in a 4-year-old child.[643] Secondary causes of biliary obstruction or cholangitis such as gallstones or anomalies were excluded. Cholecystojejunostomy proximal to the area of stenosis did not prevent progression of the inflammatory obliterative process. Mowat reported nine patients (3 males, 6 females; age range 2–7 years) in whom primary sclerosing cholangitis was diagnosed by biopsy and endoscopic retrograde cholangiopancreatography.[484] Seven presented with colitis before clinical or laboratory evidence of liver disease; the two patients without colitis had asymptomatic hepatomegaly.[484] The serum alkaline phosphatase levels were markedly elevated in eight of nine; in contrast to adults all children had very high aminotransferase values, 3 to 20 times greater than normal. In six of eight the IgG level was elevated (>16 g/liter); four were SMA positive. Initial biopsies in three patients suggested chronic active hepatitis with cirrhosis. Despite immunosuppressive therapy, biochemical abnormalities persisted.

CYSTIC DISEASE OF THE LIVER

Multiple hepatic ductal cysts may occur in patients with cystic lesions in other viscera, especially the kidney. In these heritable conditions, the cysts may be diffuse or localized and may or may not communicate directly with the biliary excretory tract. An increase in fibrous tissue and biliary ducts can also be noted in certain subsets. These cystic conditions may resemble other conditions such as Caroli's disease, in which other visceral involvement is not demonstrable. The heterogeneity suggests a variable etiopathogenesis.

The associated renal abnormalities, infectious complications, or hepatic fibrosis may dominate the clinical picture. Affected patients may share common organ involvement and histologic abnormalities yet demonstrate inheritance patterns that suggest a heterogenous etiology.

Morphometric analyses of liver lesions in patients with various forms of cystic diseases of the liver in childhood by Landing and associates[402] have led to our current conceptualization. They demonstrated that various entities previously termed congenital, perinatal, and infantile forms of polycystic disease[85] produce the same liver lesion and recommended that the name infantile polycystic disease (IPCD) of the liver and kidney be used to describe all patients with this autosomal recessive disorder. They associated the entity previously termed the juvenile form of polycystic disease with a liver lesion similar to that classically termed congenital hepatic fibrosis (CHF); these patients present in later childhood with portal hypertension. The authors also suggest that the morphologic features remain constant, and therefore CHF is not IPCD seen at an advanced age.[402] This remains conjectural, however. They have also stressed differences in the pattern of renal lesions between IPCD and CHF.

Infantile Polycystic Disease of the Liver and Kidneys

Massive enlargement of both organs may be present at birth and produce respiratory difficulty in the newborn period. Acidosis, azotemia, and congestive heart failure may be severe and cause death in the first month of life. The kidneys may decrease in size with age in survivors, but the urine specific gravity remains low and progression of renal insufficiency is variable, with survival to 18 years reported.[422] Hepatomegaly is present in all types, but liver function is not impaired. In reported cases serum aminotransferase levels and Bromsulphalein excretion were normal. Grossly the liver is firm, and cysts are not visible; microscopically, the liver shows cystic dilatation of ductules at the periphery of the portal zone, cystic Hering ductules within lobules, and portal fibrosis that increases with age (Fig. 43-44).[401,422] Microdissection studies have shown that the hepatic cysts affect the Hering and interlobular ducts, that is, the terminal duct system, a finding parallel to the cystic dilation in the kidney, which involves the terminal branches of the collecting tubules.[401,402] Portal

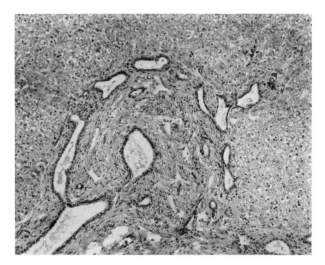

Fig. 43-44. Infantile polycystic disease of the liver and kidneys (IPCD). Characteristic features, shown here, include cystic dilatation of ductules which are located at the periphery of the portal area, and portal fibrosis.

hypertension may occur, but the manifestations of renal insufficiency predominate.[422]

Congenital Hepatic Fibrosis

CHF, a recessive genetic disease, presents in later childhood with hepatomegaly, normal liver function, and portal hypertension with esophageal varices.[167,378-380,422] Functional renal impairment is much less significant or absent (Fig. 43-45).[401,422] There is a relatively characteristic histology: parenchymal lobules separated by broad bands of diffuse periportal or perilobular fibrous tissue. This often is associated with multiple distorted "bile duct–like" structures that do not connect to the biliary tract and portal vein anomalies. Cystic disease of the kidney is reported in approximately half of the cases of CHF.[422] Excretory urograms reveal enlarged kidneys, but excretion of contrast and visualization of the pelvicaliceal system is prompt, as opposed to IPCD, in which the kidneys are massive and visualization is poor. Lesions resembling medullary sponge kidney disease of adults, in which segmental dilatation of the bile ducts also occurs, have been reported in CHF, and the identity of the two diseases is suggested despite the different clinical manifestations.[379]

Treatment of patients with CHF is directed at control of variceal hemorrhage, which may be managed by standard methods, including endoscopic sclerotherapy. These patients have basically normal liver function; therefore, following more severe recurrent hemorrhage, they are candidates for relief of portal hypertension via a portacaval anastomosis. The prognosis is good following a successful shunting procedure; however, survival in some patients may be limited by renal failure.

Progessive renal disease with pathologic features, namely nephrophthisis, which differs from IPCD, has been noted to occur in patients whose hepatic lesion resembles CHF.[742] In these patients the mortality due to renal disease is high.

A diverse group of diseases in which hepatic cystic lesions are encountered is listed below[85,380,401,402,422,742]:

Meckel syndrome, characterized by encephalocele, polydactyly, and distinctive cystic renal disease

Jeune syndrome (asphyxiating thoracic dystrophy), characterized by skeletal dysplasia and late-onset renal disease

Miscellaneous disorders (vaginal atresia, Ellis–Van Creveld syndrome, Ivemark syndrome, and tuberous sclerosis), in which hepatic ductular polycystic disease has been noted

Cystic Dilatation of the Intrahepatic Bile Ducts (Caroli)

Cystic dilatation of the intrahepatic bile ducts is a diverse spectrum of diseases that may include such variants as the Caroli syndrome, in which saccular dilatation of the intrahepatic bile ducts alternating with areas of stenosis is present.[401,402,742] Multiple segments of the biliary tract may be involved. The dilated intrahepatic biliary ducts, which are usually contiguous with the unaffected biliary system, are lined by typical cuboidal epithelium. The major complications include recurrent cholangitis with a predisposition to stone or abscess formation.

CIRRHOSIS

Cirrhosis is the end stage of many of the childhood liver diseases discussed above and summarized in Table 43-11.[296,491] Defining the etiology of cirrhosis is of importance for genetic counseling, even if the severity of the lesion precludes specific treatment. Hepatic fibrosis has been documented to occur in infants born to alcoholic women (the fetal alcohol syndrome); the histologic lesion resembles adult alcoholic liver disease.[410] Management of the complications of cirrhosis is similar in children as in adults. Cases of familial cirrhosis suggest the existence of other undefined infectious or metabolic diseases.[388]

Indian Childhood Cirrhosis

A unique familial form of cirrhosis, Indian childhood cirrhosis (ICC), confined primarily to the Indian subcontinent, affects Hindu children under the age of 3 years. ICC is progressive and results in hepatocellular failure and death.[686] Affected children present with hepatomegaly, abnormal stools, and behavioral changes such as an increased appetite, excessive irritability, and disturbed sleep patterns. Jaundice is uncommon; liver tissue obtained at an early stage reveals only vacuolization of hepatocytes,

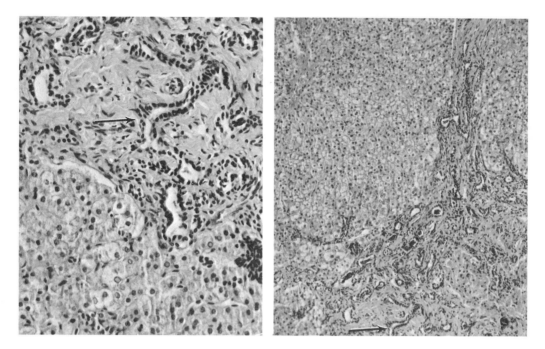

Fig. 43-45. Congenital hepatic fibrosis: liver biopsy in a patient 6 years of age. Liver shows portal fibrosis and dilated cystic bile ductules (*arrow*) at the periphery of the lobule. To the left is a high-power view of the same ductule adjacent to normal liver parenchyma. Intravenous pyelogram was normal.

possibly with focal reticulum condensation. The disease progresses to an intermediate stage in which firm hepatomegaly with splenomegaly and abdominal distention occurs. Liver biopsy at this time will show progressive fibrosis. In the advanced stage, signs of liver failure dominate, with a histopathologic pattern of disorganized liver architecture, widespread necrosis with Mallory's hyaline bodies, and interstitial fibrosis with minimal evidence of regeneration. The suggestion of the proliferative nature of ICC has been complemented by the finding in serum and liver tissue of an oncodevelopmental protein, the Regan isoenzyme, which is a developmental phenotype of alkaline phosphatase isoenzyme.[521] It is possible that the disease has a genesis *in utero*. Tanner has recently suggested that introduction of copper-contaminated milk feeding can explain the epidemiologic features and possibly is etiologic.[686]

Hepatic Copper Overload

Lefkowitch and co-workers described four white American siblings who died in early childhood of an unknown form of cirrhosis.[411] The children presented in the third to fourth year of life with progressive lethargy, abdominal swelling, jaundice, and fever. Hepatic histopathology resembled Indian Childhood Cirrhosis: severe panlobular liver-cell swelling, pericellular fibrosis, cirrhosis, and marked copper deposition. The authors suggest

that this represents a genetically determined disturbance in copper metabolism.[411]

Bacterial Peritonitis

Spontaneous bacterial peritonitis, a well-recognized complication of cirrhosis in adults, has been documented with increasing frequency in children with cirrhosis and ascites. The illness is characterized by increased abdominal distention, fever and abdominal pain often with vomiting, and rapid progression of symptoms. Bowel sounds are reduced and abdominal tenderness is apparent. The episode may precipitate encephalopathy. Leukocyte counts are elevated, and serum bilirubin and aminotransferase levels are also increased. The ascitic fluid contains an increased concentration of leukocytes, with polymorphonuclear leukocytes predominating. In a series of Larcher and co-workers, *Streptococcus pneumoniae* was isolated in 8 of 12 episodes; *Klebsiella pneumoniae* and *Hemophilus influenzae* were noted in other cases.[403] In this series, despite antibiotic therapy, 7 of the 11 patients died. Nevertheless, the importance of early diagnostic paracentesis, with early institution of therapy in hopes of lowering the mortality rate, must be emphasized. In view of the high frequency of pneumococcal infection and the apparent association with complement deficiency, future studies should evaluate prophylactic use of pneumococcal vaccine and plasma infusion.

TABLE 43-11.   Causes of Cirrhosis in Infancy and Childhood

INFECTION
Neonatal viral infection
   Rubella
   Cytomegalovirus
   Coxsackievirus
   ECHOvirus
   Herpes simplex
   "Neonatal hepatitis"
Acute viral hepatitis
Chronic active hepatitis
Syphilis
Cholangitis

METABOLIC
Galactosemia
Fructosemia
Glycogen-storage disease types III, IV
Niemann–Pick disease
Wolman's disease
Cholesterol ester-storage disease
Gaucher's disease
Hurler's disease
Tyrosinemia
Cystinosis
Wilson's disease
α_1-antitrypsin deficiency
Sickle-cell disease
Thalassemia
Hemochromatosis
Cerebrohepatorenal (Zellweger)
Copper overload

OBSTRUCTIVE BILIARY DISEASE
Extrahepatic atresia
Choledochal cyst
Intrahepatic cholestasis
   Familial cholestasis syndromes
   Byler's disease
Congenital hepatic fibrosis
Infantile polycystic disease of liver

VASCULAR DISEASE
Constrictive pericarditis
Pulmonary hypertension
Hepatic vein obstruction
Veno-occlusive disease (Jamaica)
Rendu–Osler–Weber disease
Hemangioendothelioma

MISCELLANEOUS
Cystic fibrosis
Histiocytosis X
Malnutrition
Childhood cirrhosis (India, South Africa, Egypt)
Drugs, toxins
Parenteral nutrition (prolonged)
Inflammatory bowel disease
Obesity
Alcohol

TUMORS

Primary tumors of the liver and tumor-like lesions affecting the liver (Table 43-12) are discussed elsewhere in this text. These are uncommon in infants and children[131,171,232,340,727]; thus, only certain features of hepatic tumors unique to this age-group are discussed below. Approximately 60% to 70% of all hepatic masses found in children are of a malignant nature, especially in the male population. Solitary cysts and hemangioendothelioma are more commonly found in females. The white to black ratio for all tumors is 10:1. The estimated incidence of malignant neoplasms in American white children under 15 years of age is 1.9 cases per million according to the Third National Cancer Survey.[753] The major malignant tumors, hepatoblastoma and hepatocellular carcinoma, have an incidence of approximately 0.2 and 0.7 cases per million, respectively.

Hepatoblastoma usually appears in persons younger than 2 years of age (60% of all cases) but may occur at any age.[341,443] The tumor is usually without symptoms and presents on routine examination as a progressively enlarging nontender nodular abdominal mass.[341,443] Liver function tests are normal, but 80% to 90% of patients have α-fetoprotein detectable in serum.[17] The majority (80%) are single masses, and in a series of 25 patients, 17 tumors were found to involve the right lobe. Associated findings were hemihypertrophy, macroglossia, and sexual precocity presumably due to ectopic gonadotropin production.[65,341,443] Microscopically, there are at least two patterns noted, epithelial and mesenchymal types. The epithelial elements consist of small dark-staining elongated "embryonal" type cells and polyhedral glycogen-containing larger "fetal" type cells that form canalicular and sinusoidal complexes (Fig. 43-46). The mesenchymal element may be represented by fibrous connective tissue, osteoid, and cartilage. Aggressive surgery, with hepatic lobectomy following multidrug chemotherapy to shrink local masses, is the treatment of choice; these tumors are resistant to radiation and chemotherapy.

Hepatocellular carcinoma usually occurs in persons over 3 years of age who often have a cirrhotic liver in the presence of α_1-AT deficiency, tyrosinemia, HBsAg, and the like.[728] It also presents as an abdominal mass (75%), and abdominal pain is frequent (67%). Microscopically,

TABLE 43-12.   Primary Hepatic Tumors and Tumor-like Lesions of Infancy and Childhood

A. *Malignant group*
  1. Tumors of hepatic-cell origin (entodermal)
    a. Hepatoblastoma
      (1) Epithelial ⟵ embryonal
                        fetal
      (2) Mixed
    b. Hepatocellular carcinoma
    c. Cholangiocarcinoma
    d. Adenocarcinoma
  2. Tumors of supporting structure (mesodermal)
    a. Angiosarcoma
    b. Rhabdomyosarcoma
    c. Mesenchymoma
    d. Myxosarcoma
    e. Fibrosarcoma
  3. Secondary tumors
    a. Wilm's tumor
    b. Neuroblastoma
B. *Benign group*
  1. Tumorlike epithelial lesions
    a. Focal nodular hyperplasia
    b. Multiple nodular hyperplasia (with antecedent liver disease)
    c. Accessory lobe
  2. Benign epithelial tumors
    a. Adenoma
    b. Adrenal rest tumor
  3. Cysts and tumor-like mesenchymal lesions
    a. Mesenchymal hamartoma
    b. Nonparasitic cyst
  4. Benign mesenchymal tumors
    a. Cavernous hemangioma
    b. Infantile hemangioendothelioma
    c. Lymphangioma
    d. Fibroma
  5. Teratomas

(Edmondson HA: Differential diagnosis of tumor and tumor-like lesions in infancy and children. Ann Surg 142:214, 1955)

the tumor is identical to the adult type of carcinoma of the liver.[370] Total excision offers the only chance of survival.

Benign tumors include hamartoma, cavernous hemangioma, focal nodular hyperplasia, and infantile hemangioendothelioma.[126,204] Cystic mesenchymal hamartoma typically occurs in males under 2 years of age and presents as a mass on the inferior surface of the liver, often joined by a narrow pedicle. The cut surface may be cystic; the histology is complex. Microscopically there are irregular strands of biliary epithelium in a myxoid stroma. This mass may represent a developmental anomaly rather than a true neoplasm. Cystic lesions can often be drained via Roux-en-Y.

Hemangioma is the most frequent benign tumor of the liver in childhood; the majority are asymptomatic.[126,204]

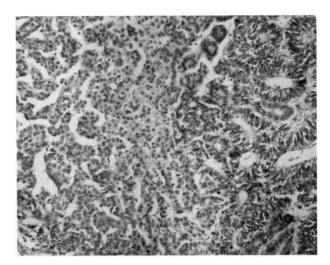

Fig. 43-46. Hepatoblastoma. Tissue present in the *right* half of this biopsy section contains "embryonal-type" cells with rosette formation; the *left* half contains typical "fetal-type" cells.

Hemangioendothelioma is frequently associated with multiple "strawberry" hemangiomata. There is a 2:1 female predominance. The tumor often involves the entire liver and grossly produces solitary or multiple red–purple to gray pulsatile nonencapsulated nodules of various sizes, which have been mistaken for metastatic neuroblastoma.[155,567] Microscopically the lesion has highly cellular endothelial-lined channels (angiosarcoma-like) (Fig. 43-47). While histologically benign, there are possible life-threatening complications. The classic presentation includes the triad of congestive failure in the absence of heart disease, hepatomegaly with a systolic bruit over the liver due to arteriovenous fistulae and cutaneous hemangiomata, often with thrombocytopenia; however, isolated hepatomegaly is the most common presentation. In a series described by McLean,[457] there was a very high (70%) mortality rate, due in most cases to severe high-output cardiac failure. Recent series report much lower mortality rates. Initial evaluation should include sonography of the abdomen; the diagnosis can be confirmed by angiography or computed tomography (Fig. 43-48).[533,698] Localized lesions, if symptomatic, can be resected with care because of a risk of hypotensive complications.[719] In diffuse disease (or if the patient's condition prohibits surgery), treatment with prednisone, diuretics, and digoxin should be used initially. Surgery may then be performed safely in 10 to 14 days. Confirmation of the lesion must first be obtained by open biopsy of nodules.[582] Hepatic artery ligation or embolization of the lesion has replaced radiation therapy. Treatment should be vigorous because complete regression and cure are possible. Cavernous hemangioma is rare and presents as a mass lesion to be distinguished from other tumors only at laparotomy.[201] Surgical resection should

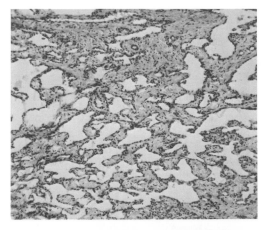

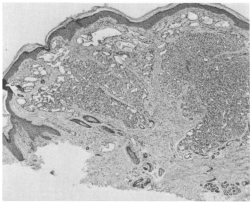

Fig. 43-47. Hemangioendothelioma liver above, "strawberry" skin hemangioma from same patient below. The liver lesion, part of a gray nodule obtained at laparotomy, contains multiple cellular endothelial-lined channels very similar to those of the skin lesion.

be attempted, since rupture with fatal intraperitoneal hemorrhage is frequent.[201,546]

Neuroblastoma may present following widespread metastasis, especially in infancy.[276] All patients with liver tumors, therefore, should have catecholamine studies, ultrasound, computed tomography, and renal imaging performed prior to surgery. There is a high rate of spontaneous regression in infants with stage IV disease. If bone metastasis has not occurred, a high cure rate can be expected with removal of the primary tumor and radiation therapy to the liver.[248,535]

PORTAL HYPERTENSION

Portal hypertension in infants and children can occur as a result of obstruction to flow at several sites, with a disease spectrum similar to that seen in adults. There are, however, several unique features of portal hypertension as it occurs in the pediatric age-group.

Extrahepatic (Presinusoidal) Block

Extrahepatic (presinusoidal) block as is seen in "cavernous transformation of the portal vein" is more commonly seen in children than in adults.[466,612,725] Portal hypertension may be manifest by splenomegaly with or without hypersplenism, hematemesis, or ascites. The natural history of extrahepatic portal venous obstruction has been extensively reviewed.[18,725] A predisposing illness such as intra-abdominal sepsis, omphalitis, or dehydration can be documented in up to 40% of cases. Variceal bleeding has been reported as a late complication of neonatal umbilical vein catheterization; however, the true incidence of this sequela is unknown.[405] The occurrence of congenital anomalies—cardiovascular and biliary malformations—in some cases of "idiopathic" extrahepatic block suggests that a developmental defect underlies the association.[505] Hematemesis is the most common presentation, and ascites occurs in approximately 35% of children, an incidence that is lower than that in adults. Diagnosis is by ultrasound or angiography and by exclusion of liver disease by appropriate function tests, liver biopsy, and screening for known causes of cirrhosis. This is followed by attempts to visualize the portal vein anatomy and the varices. Barium esophagrams are frequently negative in young children, esophagoscopy may require general anesthesia, and wedged hepatic vein pressures are normal in extrahepatic block. Abdominal angiography with selective injection of the splenic artery will visualize the splenic and portal veins and varices if present during the venous filling phase (Fig. 43-49). Direct splenoportography may result in significant hemorrhage and require immediate splenectomy and shunting. In the young child this may produce a suboptimal shunt, less than 1 cm in diameter, which may subsequently thrombose.

In review of 69 patients with extrahepatic portal venous obstruction, Fonkalsrud and co-workers documented 338 episodes of bleeding.[229] However, this and several other series have suggested that portal-system shunting is often avoidable in this condition. Advocates of a conservative approach have emphasized the following: the initial episode is rarely life-threatening, has a low mortality rate, and is usually an opportunity for successful *medical* management; there is a decreased frequency of bleeding with age, and in many patients bleeding has been noted to cease spontaneously; and shunts undertaken at a young age have poor long-term patency rates, often requiring multiple revisions following the initial operative procedure.[229,725] There is a higher long-term mortality rate in those who are subjected to shunt procedures. Despite a concern for the physiological consequences of portal diversion, sequelae are uncommon in patients with normal liver function. Variceal bleeding usually responds to nasogastric lavage and transfusion of fresh blood. Pitressin may be infused intravenously if necessary; sclerotherapy is highly effective.[317] Balloon tamponade is rarely needed. When a definitive shunt procedure is needed following

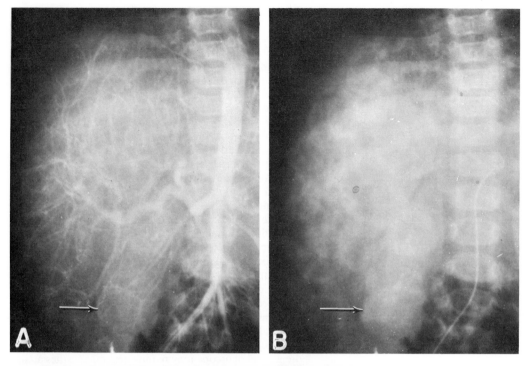

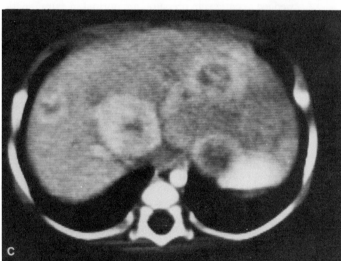

Fig. 43-48. Hemangioendothelioma: aortogram. **A.** Arterial phase shows increased liver vascularity and stretching of small arteries around the hemangiomatous nodules (*arrow*) **B.** Late phase shows similar-sized multiple large nodules retaining contrast material (*arrow*). **C.** Three-month-old girl with hepatomegaly in whom ultrasonography demonstrated multiple intrahepatic echo-free nodules. Computed tomographic examination of the abdomen with rapid bolus injection of contrast material revealed nodular densities with a "donut-like" appearance, subsequently shown to represent hemangioendothelioma. (Courtesy of Dr. Robert A. Kaufman, Cincinnati)

repeated hemorrhagic episodes, it should be delayed until late childhood. There is a high incidence of shunt thrombosis if the patient is under 10 years of age or if the portovenous anastomosis is less than 10 mm in diameter. A standard end-to-side portacaval shunt often cannot be constructed. In these patients the portal vein is often free of thrombosis for a distance of 1.5 cm to 2.0 cm beyond the junction of the superior mesenteric and splenic vein, and it is possible to anastomose this segment end-to-side

to the vena cava or to the central portion of the left renal vein.[442] Because the spleen is not removed, collaterals that have developed about the spleen–diaphragm area are undisturbed.[442] Alvarez and co-workers have advocated a more aggressive approach.[18] They have demonstrated that a portal diversion procedure can be successful in young patients with portal vein thrombosis; adverse sequelae were minimal in their series. Greater than 90% of shunts in their series remained patent.

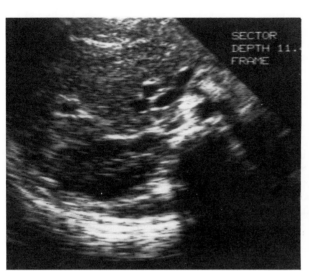

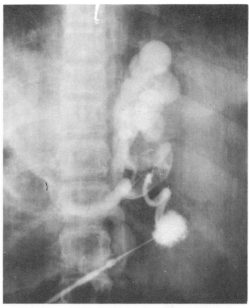

Fig. 43-49. Fifteen-month-old boy presenting with splenomegaly. **Left.** Ultrasound examination (transverse scan) demonstrates round echolucent structures in the hilum of the liver corresponding to collateral vessels. **Right.** Portal hypertension, extrahepatic block. Direct splenoportography demonstrates large gastric varices; splenic vein shadow becomes inapparent in the region of its cavernous transformation to the right of the spine.

Fig. 43-50. Suprahepatic venous obstruction: Infant, aged 6 months, had constrictive pericarditis with protein-losing enteropathy. Liver biopsy (*left*) shows three portal tracts (*arrows*), ectasia of sinusoids and central veins (∗), and fibrosis around other central veins. Biopsy 6 months after pericardiectomy shows resolution of the connective tissue and normal sinusoids.

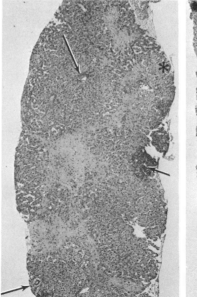
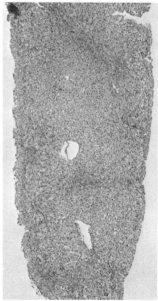

Intrahepatic ("Sinusoidal") Block

Portal hypertension may be associated with congenital hepatic fibrosis or cystic disease of the liver in which liver function is apparently normal despite hepatomegaly and variceal bleeding.[378,380] If, as in adults, cirrhosis underlies the altered flow, the nature of the primary disease should be established (see Table 43-11), since treatment may improve hepatic function in certain metabolic diseases such as Wilson's disease, and genetic counseling can be accomplished. In patients with recurrent bleeding refractory to sclerotherapy, esophageal transection with paraesophagogastric devascularization may be safe and effective. In contrast to patients with extrahepatic block, this group may derive significant benefit from a shunt procedure.[15] The distal splenorenal shunt for selective decompression of the esophageal plexus with maintenance of portal venous flow has been employed successfully in children.[570]

Postsinusoidal Block

Postsinusoidal block (suprahepatic obstruction) is rare in the pediatric group but may occur as a primary or secondary phenomenon and should be ruled out in children with unexplained hepatomegaly and ascites. Hepatic vein occlusion most often is associated with vasculitis, sickle cell anemia, polycythemia, leukemia, or tumor masses obliterating the lumen. The obstruction may occur at any level above the liver up to and including the heart, as in heart failure or constrictive pericarditis (Fig. 43-50). Primary pulmonary hypertension may present as suprahepatic portal hypertension.

Cabrera and co-workers have reemphasized the possible existence of membranous obstruction of the inferior vena cava at the level of the diaphragm as a cause of a Budd–Chiari–like syndrome.[117] This entity is successfully treated by transcardiac membranotomy. Occlusion of central and sublobular hepatic veins by intimal fibrosis or edema or by veno-occlusive disease in association with immuno-deficiency has been well recognized.[459] We have noted occlusive disease of the hepatic venous outflow pathway in patients who are bone marrow transplant recipients, in hypervitaminosis A, and in infants who received an intravenous vitamin E supplement.[94a]

REFERENCES

1. Aagenaes O: Hereditary recurrent cholestasis with lymphoedema: Two new families. Acta Paediatr Scand 63:465, 1974
2. Aagenaes O et al: Hereditary neonatal cholestasis combined with vascular malformations. In Berenberg SR (ed): Liver Diseases in Infancy and Childhood, pp 199–206. Baltimore, Williams & Wilkins, 1976
3. Abramov A et al: Generalized xanthomatosis with calcified adrenals. Am J Dis Child 91:282, 1956
4. Ahrens EH Jr et al: Atresia of the intrahepatic bile ducts. Pediatrics 8:628, 1951
5. Akerren Y: Prolonged jaundice in newborn associated with congenital myxedema. Acta Paediatr 43:411, 1954
6. Alagille D: Cholestasis in the first three months of life. In Popper H, Schaffner F (eds): Progress in Liver Disease, p 471. New York, Grune & Stratton, 1979
7. Alagille D et al: Hepatic ductular hypoplasia associated with characteristic facies, vertebral malformations, retarded physical, mental, and sexual development, and cardiac murmur. J Pediatr 86:63, 1975
8. Alagille D et al: Chronic hepatitis in children. Acta Paediatr Scand 62:566, 1973
9. Alford CA Jr et al: Subclinical central nervous system disease of neonates: A prospective study of infants born with increased levels of IgM. J Pediatr 75:1167, 1969
10. Alonso–Lej et al: Congenital choledochal duct cyst, with a report of 2, and an analysis of 94 cases. Int Abstr Surg 108:1, 1959
11. Alpert LI et al: Neonatal hepatitis associated with trisomy 17-18 syndrome. N Engl J Med 280:16, 1969
12. Alpert ME et al: Alpha-1-fetoglobulin in the diagnosis of human hepatoma. N Engl J Med 278:984, 1968
13. Altman RP: Surgical therapy of cholestasis in the newborn. In Neonatal Cholestasis. Proceedings of the 87th Ross Conference on Pediatric Research, Columbus, Ohio, 1984
14. Altman RP: The portoenterostomy procedure for biliary atresia: A five year experience. Ann Surg 188:351, 1978
15. Altman RP, Potter BM: Portal decompression in infants and children with the interposition mesocaval shunt. Am J Surg 135:65, 1978
16. Altshuler G: Toxoplasmosis as a cause of hydranencephaly: Case report including a description of the placenta. Am J Dis Child 125:251, 1973
17. Altshuler G, McAdams AJ: The role of the placenta in fetal and perinatal pathology. Am J Obstet Gynecol 113:616, 1972
18. Alvarez F et al: Portal obstruction in children: I. Clinical investigation and hemorrhage risk; II. Results of surgical portosystemic shunts. J Pediatr 103:696, 703, 1983
19. Ambruso DR et al: Infectious and bleeding complications in patients with glycogenosis Ib. Am J Dis Child 139:691, 1985
20. Amendt BA, Rhead WJ: Catalytic defect of medium-chain acylco-enzyme A dehydrogenase deficiency: Lack of both cofactor responsiveness and biochemical heterogeneity in eight patients. J Clin Invest 76:963, 1985
21. Anderson EP et al: Defect in the uptake of liver nucleotides in congenital galactosemia. Science 125:113, 1957
22. Andres JM et al: Liver disease in infants: Part I Developmental hepatology and mechanisms of liver function. J Pediatr 90:686, 1977
23. Applegarth DA et al: Laboratory diagnosis of inborn errors of metabolism in children. Pediatr Pathol 1:1071, 1983
24. Aprille JR: Reye's syndrome: Patient serum alters mitochondrial function and morphology in vitro. Science 197:908, 1977
25. Arasu TS et al: Management of chronic aggressive hepatitis in children and adolescents. J Pediatr 95:514, 1979
26. Arias IM: Chronic unconjugated hyperbilirubinemia without overt signs of hemolysis in adolescents and adults. J Clin Invest 41:2233, 1962
27. Arias IM, Gartner LM: Breast-milk jaundice. Br Med J 4:177, 1970
28. Arias IM, Jansen P: Protein binding and conjugation of

bilirubin in the liver cell. In Goresky CA, Fischer MM (eds): Jaundice, pp 175–188. New York, Plenum Press, 1975

29. Arias IM et al: Chronic nonhemolytic unconjugated hyperbilirubinemia with glycuronyl transferase deficiency: Clinical, biochemical, pharmacologic and genetic evidence for heterogeneity. Am J Med 47:395, 1969

30. Arias IM et al: Prolonged neonatal unconjugated hyperbilirubinemia associated with breast feeding and a steroid (pregnane-3 (alpha), 20 (beta) -diol), in maternal milk that inhibits glucuronide formation in vitro. J Clin Invest 43: 2037, 1964

31. Arias IM et al: Transient familial neonatal hyperbilirubinemia. J Clin Invest 44:1442, 1965

32. Arrowsmith WA et al: Comparison of treatments for congenital nonobstructive nonhemolytic hyperbilirubinemia. Arch Dis Child 50:197, 1975

33. Arthur AB, Wilson BDR: Urinary infection presenting with jaundice. Br Med J 1:539, 1967

34. Assmann G et al: Acid lipase deficiency: Wolman's disease and cholesteryl ester storage disease. In Stanbury JB et al (eds): The Metabolic Basis of Inherited Disease, p 803. New York, McGraw Hill, 1983

35. Avery ME et al: Transient tyrosinemia of the newborn. Pediatrics 38:378, 1967

36. Aynsley–Green A et al: Hepatic glycogen synthetase deficiency: Definition of the syndrome from metabolic and enzyme studies on a nine year old girl. Arch Dis Child 52: 573, 1977

37. Aziz MA et al: Transplacental and postnatal transmission of the hepatitis-associate antigen. J Infect Dis 127:110, 1973

38. Bach G et al: The defect in the Hunter syndrome: Deficiency of sulfoiduronate sulfatase. Proc Natl Acad Sci 70:2134, 1973

39. Bachand JP: Un cas inusite de mucoviscidose: Atteinte hepatique neonatale. Laval Med 38:371, 1967

41. Back P, Walter K: Developmental pattern of bile acid metabolism as revealed by bile acid analysis of meconium. Gastroenterology 78:671, 1980

42. Baerlocher K et al: Hereditary fructose intolerance in early childhood: A major diagnostic challenge. Helv Paediatr Acta 33:465, 1978

43. Baker L, Winegrad AI: Fasting hypoglycaemia and metabolic acidosis associated with deficiency of hepatic fructose-1,6-diphosphatase activity. Lancet 2:13, 1970

44. Balazs M: Electron microscopic examination of congenital cytomegalovirus hepatitis. Virchows Arch Pathol Anat 405: 119, 1984

45. Balistreri WF: Neonatal cholestasis: Medical progress. J Pediatr 106:171, 1985

46. Balistreri WF: Viral hepatitis: Implications to pediatric practice. In Barness LA (ed): Advances in Pediatrics, pp 287–320. Chicago, Year Book Medical Publishers, 1985

47. Balistreri WF: The effects of liver disease on nutrition and growth. In Cohen SA (ed): The Underweight Infant, Child, and Adolescent, pp 121–130. Norwalk, Appleton-Century-Crofts, 1986

48. Balistreri WF, Sokol RJ: Nutritional consequences of chronic cholestasis in childhood: Vitamin E deficiency. In Proceedings of Falk Symposium No. 41 on Nutrition, Freiburg, Germany, pp 181–189. MTP Press Limited, 1985

49. Balistreri WF et al: Absence of an association between hepatitis A or B virus and biliary atresia or neonatal hepatitis. Pediatrics 66:269, 1980

50. Balistreri WF et al: Immaturity of the enterohepatic circulation in early life: Factors predisposing to "physiologic" maldigestion and cholestasis. J Pediatr Gastroenterol Nutr 2:346, 1983

51. Balistreri WF et al: Bile salt sulfotransferase: Alterations during maturation and non-inducibility during substrate ingestion. J Lipid Res 25:228, 1984

52. Balistreri WF et al: Elevated cholesterol/phospholipid molar ratio in red cell membranes: An acquired defect in cirrhosis. Pediatrics 67:461, 1981

53. Balistreri WF et al: Immaturity of the enterohepatic circulation of bile acids in early life: Factors responsible for increased peripheral serum bile acid concentrations. In Proceedings of Falk Symposium No. 42, VIII International Bile Acid Meeting, Berne, Switzerland, pp 87–93. MTP Press Limited, 1985

54. Balistreri WF et al: Bile acid metabolism, total parenteral nutrition and cholestasis. In Lebenthal E (ed): Total Parenteral Nutrition: Indications, Complications, and Pathophysiological Considerations in Total Parenteral Nutrition and Home Total Parenteral Nutrition (in press)

55. Ballowitz L et al: Effects of riboflavin on Gunn rats under pathotherapy. Pediatr Res 13:1307, 1979

56. Barlow B et al: Choledochal cyst: A review of 19 cases. J Pediatr 89:934, 1976

57. Barudhuin P et al: An electron microscopic and biochemical study of type II glycogenesis. Lab Invest 13:1139, 1964

58. Beale EF et al: Intrahepatic cholestasis associated with parenteral nutrition in premature infants. Pediatrics 64:342, 1979

59. Beasley RP et al: Efficacy of hepatitis B immune globulin (HBIG) for prevention of perinatal transmission of the hepatitis B virus carrier state: Final report of a randomized double-blind placebo-controlled trial. Hepatology 3:135, 1983

60. Beasley RP et al: Prevention of perinatally transmitted hepatitis B virus infections with hepatitis B immune globulin and hepatitis B vaccine. Lancet 2:1099, 1983

61. Beasley RP et al: The e antigen and vertical transmission of hepatitis B surface antigen. Am J Epidemiol 105:94, 1977

62. Beaudet AL et al: Neutropenia and impaired neutrophil migration in type Ib glycogen storage disease. J Pediatr 97: 906, 1980

63. Beckett RS, Flynn FJ Jr: Toxoplasmosis: Report of two new cases, with classification and with demonstration of organisms in human placenta. N Engl J Med 249:345, 1953

64. Becroft DMO: Syndrome of encephalopathy and fatty degeneration of viscera in New Zealand children. Br Med J 2:135, 1966

65. Behrle FC et al: Virilization accompanying hepatoblastoma. Pediatrics 32:265, 1963

66. Behrman RE: Preliminary report of the committee on phototherapy in the newborn infant. J Pediatr 84:135, 1974

67. Belknap WM et al: Physiologic cholestasis: II. Serum bile acid levels reflect the development of the enterohepatic circulation in rats. Hepatology 1:613, 1981

68. Bendeck JL, Noguchi A: Age-related changes in the adrenergic control of glycogenolysis in rat liver: The significance of changes in receptor density. Pediatr Res 19:862, 1985

69. Benjamin DR: Hepatobiliary dysfunction in infants and children associated with long-term total parenteral nutrition: A clinicopathologic study. Am J Clin Pathol 76:276, 1981

70. Benson CD: Infantile hypertrophic pyloric stenosis. In Mustard WT et al (eds): Pediatric Surgery, vol 2. Chicago: Yearbook Medical Publishers, 1969

71. Beratis NG et al: Characterization of the molecular defect in infantile and adult acid alpha-glucosidase deficiency fibroblasts. J Clin Invest 62:1264, 1978

72. Berenberg W, Nankervis G: Long-term follow up of cytomegalic inclusion disease. Pediatrics 46:403, 1970

73. Berk PD et al: Inborn errors of bilirubin metabolism. Med Clin North Am 59:803, 1975

74. Berkovich S, Smithwick EM: Transplacental infection due to ECHO virus type 22. J Pediatr 72:94, 1968

75. Bernstein J, Brown AK: Sepsis and jaundice in early infancy. Pediatrics 29:873, 1962

76. Bernstein J et al: Bile plug syndrome: Correctable cause of obstructive jaundice in infants. Pediatrics 43:273, 1969

77. Bernstein J et al: Conjugated hyperbilirubinemia in infancy associated with parenteral alimentation. J Pediatr 90:361, 1977

78. Bernstein RB et al: Bilirubin metabolism in the fetus. J Clin Invest 48:1678, 1969

79. Birnbaum G et al: Cytomegalovirus infections in newborn infants. J Pediatr 75:789, 1969

80. Bjorkhem I et al: Urinary excretion of dicarboxylic acids from patients with the Zellweger syndrome: Importance of peroxisomes in beta-oxidation of dicarboxylic acids. Biochim Biophys Acta 795:15, 1984

81. Bjorkhem I et al: Unsuccessful attempts to induce peroxisomes in two cases of Zellweger disease by treatment with Clofibrate. Pediatr Res 19:590, 1985

82. Black M, Billing BH: Hepatic bilirubin UDP-glucuronyl transferase activity in liver disease and Gilbert's syndrome. N Engl J Med 280:1266, 1969

83. Bloomer JR, Boyer JL: Phenobarbital effects in cholestatic liver disease. Ann Intern Med 82:310, 1975

84. Blumenschein SD et al: Familial onset of nonhemolytic jaundice with late onset of neurologic damage. Pediatrics 42:786, 1968

85. Blyth H, Ockenden BG: Polycystic disease of kidneys and liver presenting in childhood. J Med Genet 8:257, 1971

86. Bobo RC et al: Reye syndrome: Treatment by exchange transfusion with special reference to the 1974 epidemic in Cincinnati, Ohio. J Pediatr 87:881, 1975

87. Boggs TR, Bishop H: Neonatal hyperbilirubinemia associated with high obstruction of the small bowel. J Pediatr 66:349, 1965

88. Bohm N et al: Multiple acyl-CoA dehydrogenation deficiency (glutaric aciduria type II), congenital polycystic kidneys and symmetric warty dysplasia of the cerebral cortex in two newborn brothers: II. Morphology and pathogenesis. Eur J Pediatr 139:60, 1982

89. Boler RK, Bibighaus AJ III: Ultrastructural alteration of dog livers during endotoxin shock. Lab Invest 17:537, 1967

90. Bougneres PF et al: Medium-chain acyl-CoA dehydrogenase deficiency in two siblings with a Reye-like syndrome. J Pediatr 106:918, 1985

91. Bourgeois C et al: Encephalopathy and fatty degeneration of the viscera: A clinicopathologic analysis of 40 cases. Am J Clin Pathol 56:558, 1971

92. Bourgeois CH et al: Acute aflatoxin B_1 toxicity in the Macaque and its similarities to Reye's syndrome. Lab Invest 24:206, 1971

93. Bove KE et al: The hepatic lesion in Reye's syndrome. Gastroenterology 69:685, 1975

94. Bove KE et al: Vasculopathic hepatotoxicity associated with E-Ferol syndrome in low-birth-weight infants. JAMA 254:2422, 1985

94a. Brady RO, Barranger JA: Glucosyl ceramide lipidosis (Gaucher's disease). In Stanbury JB et al: (eds): The Metabolic Basis of Inherited Disease, p 842. New York, McGraw-Hill, 1983

95. Brady RO et al: Demonstration of a deficiency of glucocerebrosidase cleaving enzyme in Gaucher's disease. J Clin Invest 45:112, 1966

96. Brady RO et al: The metabolism of sphingomyelin: II. Evidence of an enzymatic block in Niemann–Pick disease. Proc Natl Acad Sci USA 55:366, 1966

97. Brandt IK, DeLuca VA Jr: Type III glycogenosis: A family with an unusual tissue distribution of the enzyme lesion. Am J Med 40:779, 1966

98. Bratlid D et al: Effect of serum hyperosmolality on opening of blood-brain barrier to bilirubin in rat brain. Pediatrics 71:909, 1983

99. Bratlid D et al: Effect of acidosis on bilirubin deposition in rat brain. Pediatrics 73:431, 1984

100. Brent RL: Persistent jaundice in infancy. J Pediatr 61:111, 1962

101. Bressler R et al: Hypoglycin and hypoglycin-like compounds. Pharmacol Rev 21:105, 1969

102. Breuer B et al: Transmission of hepatitis B virus to classroom contacts of mentally retarded carriers. JAMA 254:3190, 1985

103. Brodersen R: Prevention of kernicterus, based on recent progress in bilirubin chemistry. Acta Pediatr Scand 66:625, 1977

104. Brodersen R: Bilirubin transport in the newborn infant, reviewed with relation to kernicterus. J Pediatr 96:349, 1980

105. Brodersen R, Hermann LS: Intestinal reabsorption of unconjugated bilirubin: A possible contributing factor in neonatal jaundice. Lancet 1:1242, 1963

106. Brodersen R et al: Bilirubin conjugation in the human fetus. Scand J Clin Lab Invest 20:41, 1967

107. Brooks SEH, Audretsch JJ: Studies on hypoglycin toxicity in rats: I. Changes in hepatic ultrastructure. Am J Pathol 59:161, 1970

108. Brough AJ, Bernstein J: Conjugated hyperbilirubinemia in early infancy. Hum Pathol 5:507, 1974

109. Brown A, Zuelzer W: Studies on the neonatal development of the glucuronide conjugating systems. J Clin Invest 37:332, 1958

110. Brown BI, Brown DH: Lack of an alpha-1,4-glucan; alpha-1,4-glucan 6-glycosyl transferase in a case of type IV glycogenosis. Proc Natl Acad Sci USA 56:725, 1966

111. Brusilow SW: Arginine, an indispensable amino acid for patients with inborn errors of urea synthesis. J Clin Invest 74:2144, 1984

112. Brusilow SW et al: Treatment of episodic hyperammonemia in children with inborn errors of urea synthesis. N Engl J Med 310:1630, 1984

113. Buchan P: Pathogenesis of neonatal hyperbilirubinaemia after induction of labour with oxytocin. Br Med J 2:1255, 1979

114. Bucuvalas JC et al: Amino acids are potent inhibitors of bile acid uptake by liver plasma membrane vesicles isolated from suckling rats. Pediatr Res 19:1298, 1985

115. Burke JA, Schubert WK: Deficient activity of hepatic acid lipase in cholesterol ester storage disease. Science 176:309, 1972

116. Burman D: Congenital spherocytosis in infancy. Arch Dis Child 33:335, 1958

117. Cabrera J et al: Budd-Chiari syndrome due to a membra-

nous obstruction of the inferior vena cava in a child. J Pediatr 96:435, 1980

118. Callahan WP, Lorincz AE: Hepatic ultrastructure in the Hurler syndrome. Am J Pathol 48:277, 1966

119. Callahan WP Jr et al: Human toxoplasmosis: A clinico-pathologic study with presentation of five cases and review of the literature. Medicine 25:343, 1946

120. Cao A et al: Phenobarbital effect on serum bilirubin levels in underweight infants. Helv Pediatr Acta 28:231, 1973

121. Cashore WJ, Stern L: Neonatal hyperbilirubinemia. Pediatr Clin North Am 29:1191, 1985

122. Cassady G et al: Familial "giant-cell hepatitis" in infancy. Am J Dis Child 107:456, 1964

123. Catz C: Pharmacological modification of bilirubin conjugation in the newborn. Am J Dis Child 104:516, 1962

124. Catz C, Yaffe SJ: Barbiturate enhancement of bilirubin conjugation and excretion in young and adult animals. Pediatr Res 2:361, 1968

125. Chandra RS, Altman RP: Ductal remnants in extrahepatic biliary atresia: A histopathologic study with clinical correlation. J Pediatr 93:196, 1978

126. Chandra RS et al: Benign hepatocellular tumors in the young: A clinicopathologic spectrum. Arch Pathol Lab Med 108:168, 1984

127. Chapoy PR et al: Systemic carnitine deficiency: A treatable inherited lipid-storage disease presenting as Reye's syndrome. N Engl J Med 303:1389, 1980

128. Chen YT et al: Cornstarch therapy in type I glycogen storage disease. N Engl J Med 310:171, 1984

129. Chiba T, Kasai M: Differentiation of biliary atresia from neonatal hepatitis by routine clinical examination. Tohoku J Exp Med 115:327, 1975

130. Christensen JF: Prolonged icterus neonatorum and congenital myxedema. Acta Paediatr 45:367, 1956

131. Clatworthy HW et al: Primary liver tumors in infancy and childhood. Arch Surg 109:143, 1974

132. Clayton RJ et al: Byler disease: Fatal familial intrahepatic cholestasis in an Amish kindred. Am J Dis Child 117:112, 1969

133. Cohen AN, Ostrow JD: New concepts in phototherapy: Photoisomerization of bilirubin IX alpha and potential toxic effects of light. Pediatrics 65:740, 1980

134. Cohen AN et al: Effects of phenobarbital on bilirubin metabolism and its response to phototherapy in the jaundiced Gunn rat. Hepatology 5:310, 1985

135. Cohen C, Olsen MM: Pediatric total parenteral nutrition: Liver histopathology. Arch Pathol Lab Med 105:152, 1981

136. Cohen MI, Gartner LM: The use of medium-chain triglycerides in the management of biliary atresia. J Pediatr 79:379, 1971

137. Cole AP, Hargreaves T: Conjugation inhibitors and early neonatal hyperbilirubinemia. Arch Dis Child 47:415, 1972

138. Collaborative Study: Cytomegalovirus infection in the northwest of England: A report on a two-year study. Arch Dis Child 45:513, 1970

139. Combined Study: Prevention of Rh hemolytic disease: Final results of the "high risk" clinical trial: A combined study from centers in England and Baltimore. Br Med J 2:607, 1971

140. Conney AH: Pharmacological implications of microsomal enzyme induction. Pharmacol Rev 19:317, 1967

141. Conney AH et al: Drug-induced changes in steroid metabolism. Ann NY Acad Sci 123:98, 1965

142. Corey L et al: A nationwide outbreak of Reye's syndrome: Its epidemiologic relationship to influenza B. Am J Med 61:615, 1976

143. Corey L et al: Reye's syndrome: Clinical progression and evaluation. Pediatrics 60:708, 1977

144. Cori GT: Biochemical aspect of glycogen deposition disease. Mod Probl Paediatr 3:344 1958

145. Cori GT, Cori CF: Glucose-6-phosphatase of liver in glycogen storage disease. J Biol Chem 199:661, 1952

146. Couvreu J, Desmonts G: Congenital and maternal toxoplasmosis: Review of 300 congenital cases. Dev Med Child Neurol 4:519, 1962

147. Cox DW, Smyth S: Risk for liver disease in adults with alpha$_1$-antitrypsin deficiency. Am J Med 74:221, 1983

148. Craig JJ: Sequences in the development of cirrhosis of the liver in cases of erythroblastosis fetalis. Arch Pathol 49:665, 1950

149. Craig JM, Landing BH: Form of hepatitis in neonatal period simulating biliary atresia. Arch Pathol 54:321, 1952

150. Craig JM et al: The pathological changes in the liver in cystic fibrosis of the pancreas. Am J Dis Child 93:357, 1957

151. Cremer RJ et al: Influence of light on the hyperbilirubinemia of infants. Lancet 1:1094, 1958

152. Crigler JF, Gold NI: Sodium phenobarbital induced decrease in serum bilirubin in an infant with congenital non-haemolytic jaundice and kernicterus. J Clin Invest 45:998, 1966

153. Crigler JF, Najjar VA: Congenital familial nonhemolytic jaundice with kernicterus. Pediatrics 10:169, 1952

154. Crocker AC, Forbes S: Neimann-Pick disease: A review of 18 patients. Medicine 37:1, 1958

155. Crocker DW, Cleland RS: Infantile hemangioendothelioma of liver: Report of three cases. Pediatrics 19:596, 1957

156. Crocker JFS et al: Lethal interaction of ubiquitous insecticide carrier with virus. Science 192:1351, 1976

157. Cutting HO et al: Autosomal dominant hemolytic anemia characterized by ovalocytosis. A family study of seven involved members. Am J Med 39:21, 1965

158. Cutz E, Cox DW: Alpha-1-antitrypsin deficiency: The spectrum of pathology and pathophysiology. Perspect Pediatr Pathol 5:1, 1979

159. Dahms BB: Hepatoma in familial cholestatic cirrhosis of childhood. Arch Pathol Lab Med 103:30, 1979

160. Dahms BB, Halpin TC: Serial liver biopsies in parenteral nutrition-associated cholestasis of early infancy. Gastroenterology 81:136, 1981

161. Dahms BB et al: Arteriohepatic dysplasia in infancy and childhood: A longitudinal study of six patients. Hepatology 2:350, 1982

162. Dalinka MK et al: Metachromatic leukodystrophy: A cause of cholelithiasis in childhood. Am J Dig Dis 14:603, 1969

163. Danks D, Bodian M: A genetic study of neonatal obstructive jaundice. Arch Dis Child 38:378, 1963

164. Danks DM, Campbell PE: Extrahepatic biliary atresia: Comments on the frequency of potentially operable cases. J Pediatr 69:21, 1966

165. Danks DM et al: Studies of the aetiology of neonatal hepatitis and biliary atresia. Arch Dis Child 52:360, 1977

166. Danks DM et al: Prognosis of babies with neonatal hepatitis. Arch Dis Child 52:368, 1977

167. Darnis F et al: Fibrose hepatique congenitale a precession clinique renale. Presse Med 78:885, 1970

168. Datta NS et al: Deficiency of enzymes catalyzing the biosynthesis of glycerol-ether lipids in Zellweger syndrome. N Engl J Med 311:1080, 1984

169. Davies P: Bacterial infection in the newborn: A review. Arch Dis Child 46:1, 1971

170. Davis DR et al: Activated charcoal decreases plasma bilirubin levels in the hyperbilirubinemic rat. Pediatr Res 17:208, 1983

171. Dehner LP: Hepatic tumors in the pediatric age group: A distinctive clinicopathologic spectrum. Perspect Pediatr Pathol 4:217, 1978

172. De Pagter AGF et al: Familial benign recurrent intrahepatic cholestasis: Interrelation with intrahepatic cholestasis of pregnancy and from oral contraceptives? Gastroenterology 71:202, 1976

173. Descos B et al: Pigment gallstones of the common bile duct in infancy. Hepatology 4:678, 1984

174. Desmonts G, Couvreur J: Congenital toxoplasmosis. N Engl J Med 290:1110, 1974

175. Deutsch J et al: Long term prognosis for babies with neonatal liver disease. Arch Dis Child 60:447, 1985

176. DeVivo DC, Keating JP: Reye's syndrome. Adv Pediatr 22:175, 1976

177. De Vos R et al: Progressive intrahepatic cholestasis (Byler's disease): Case report. Gut 16:943, 1975

178. de Vries LS et al: Relationship of serum bilirubin levels to ototoxicity and deafness in high-risk low-birth-weight infants. Pediatrics 76:351, 1985

179. DeWolf–Peeters C et al: Conjugated bilirubin in foetal liver in erythroblastosis. Lancet 1:471, 1969

180. DeWolf–Peeters C et al: Histochemical evidence of a cholestatic period in neonatal rats. Pediatr Res 5:704, 1971

181. DeWolf–Peeters C et al: Electron microscopy and histochemistry of canalicular differentiation in fetal and neonatal rat liver. Tissue Cell 4:379, 1976

182. DeWolf–Peeters C et al: Electron microscopy and morphometry of canalicular differentiation in fetal and neonatal rat liver. Exp Mol Pathol 21:339, 1974

183. Diamond LK: Replacement transfusion as a treatment for erythroblastosis fetalis. Pediatrics 2:520, 1948

184. Diaz J, Schain RJ: Phenobarbital: Effects of long-term administration on behavior and brain of artificially reared rats. Science 199:90, 1978

185. Dick MC, Mowat AP: Hepatitis syndrome in infancy: An epidemiological survey with 10 year follow up. Arch Dis Child 60:512, 1985

186. Di Ferrante N et al: Induced degradation of glycosaminoglycans in Hurler's and Hunter's syndromes by plasma infusion. Proc Natl Acad Sci 68:303, 1971

187. Dische MR: Metachromatic leukodystrophic polyposis of the gallbladder. J Pathol 97:388, 1969

188. Donn SM, Thoene JG: Prospective prevention of neonatal hyperammonaemia in argininosuccinic aciduria by arginine therapy. J Inherited Metab Dis 8:18, 1985

189. Donnell GN et al: Galactose-1-phosphate in galactosemia. Pediatrics 31:802, 1963

190. Donnell GN et al: Observations on results of management of galactosemic patients. In Hsia D Y-Y (ed): Galactosemia, pp 247–268. Springfield, IL, Charles C Thomas, 1969

191. Dorvil NP et al: Taurine prevents cholestasis induced by lithocholic acid sulfate in guinea pigs. Am J Clin Nutr 37:221, 1983

192. Dosi PC et al: Perinatal factors underlying neonatal cholestasis. J Pediatr 106:471, 1985

193. Driscoll SG: Histopathology of gestational rubella. Am J Dis Child 118:49, 1969

194. Drop SLS et al: Hyperbilirubinemia and idiopathic hypopituitarism in the newborn period. Acta Paediatr Scand 68:227, 1979

195. Drummond GS, Kappas A: An experimental model of postnatal jaundice in the suckling rat: Suppression of induced hyperbilirubinemia by Sn-protoporphyrin. J Clin Invest 74:142, 1984

196. Dufour DR, Monoghan WP: ABO hemolytic disease of the newborn: A retrospective analysis of 254 cases. Am J Clin Pathol 73:369, 1980

197. Dupuy JM et al: Hepatitis B in children: I. Analysis of 80 cases of acute and chronic hepatitis B. J Pediatr 92:17, 1978

198. Dutton GJ: Glucuronide synthesis in foetal liver and other tissues. Biochem J 71:141, 1959

199. Dutton GJ et al: High glucuronide synthesis in newborn liver: Choice of species and substrate. Biochem J 93:4P, 1964

200. Dvorackova I et al: Encephalitic syndrome with fatty degeneration of viscera. Arch Pathol 81:240, 1966

201. Edmondson HA: Differential diagnosis of tumor and tumor-like lesions in infancy and children. Ann Surg 142:214, 1955

202. Egan WA II et al: Neonatal hyperbilirubinemia associated with ingestion of maternal blood. Pediatrics 43:894, 1969

203. Eggermont E et al: Angiographic evidence of low portal liver perfusion in transient neonatal hyperammonemia. Acta Pediatr Belg 33:163, 1980

204. Ehren H et al: Benign liver tumors in infancy and childhood: Report of 48 cases. Am J Surg 145:325, 1983

205. Embil JA et al: Congenital cytomegalovirus infection in two siblings from consecutive pregnancies. J Pediatr 77:417, 1970

206. Engel AG: Acid maltase deficiency in adults: Studies in four cases of a syndrome which may mimic muscular dystrophy or other myopathies. Brain 93:599, 1970

207. Ennever JF et al: Phototherapy for neonatal jaundice: In vivo clearance of bilirubin photoproducts. Pediatr Res 19:205, 1985

208. Ennever JF et al: Phototherapy for neonatal jaundice: In vitro comparison of light sources. Pediatr Res 18:667, 1984

209. Eriksson S, Larsson C: Familial benign chronic intrahepatic cholestasis. Hepatology 3:391, 1983

210. Eriksson SL: Studies in alpha-1-antitrypsin. Acta Med Scand (suppl) 432:177, 1965

211. Esterly JR et al: Hepatic lesions in the congenital rubella syndrome. J Pediatr 71:676, 1976

212. Eyssen H et al: Trihydroxycoprostanic acid in the duodenal bile of two children with intrahepatic bile duct anomalies. Biochim Biophys Acta 273:212, 1972

213. Fagerhol M: Genetics of the Pi system. In Pulmonary Emphysema and Proteolysis, pp 123–133. New York, Academic Press, 1972

214. Farci P et al: Infection with the delta agent in children. Gut 26:4, 1985

215. Farrell DF, MacMartin MP: Gm$_1$ gangliosidosis: Enzymatic variation in a single family. Ann Neurol 9:232, 1981

216. Farrell MK et al: Serum-sulfated lithocholate as an indicator of cholestasis during parenteral nutrition in infants and children. J Parenter Enter Nutr 6:30, 1982

217. Farrell MK et al: All parenteral nutrition associated cholestasis is not due solely to parenteral nutrition. Pediatr Res 20:239A, 1986

218. Fechner RE et al: Coxsackie B virus infection of the newborn. Am J Pathol 42:493, 1963

219. Feldman HA: Toxoplasmosis. N Engl J Med 279:1370, 1431, 1968
220. Felsher BF et al: Hepatic bilirubin glucuronidation in neonates with unconjugated hyperbilirubinemia and congenital gastrointestinal obstruction. J Lab Clin Med 83:90, 1974
221. Felsher BF et al: The reciprocal relation between caloric intake and the degree of hyperbilirubinemia in Gilbert's syndrome. N Engl J Med 283:170, 1970
222. Fernandes J et al: Lactate as a cerebral metabolic fuel for glucose-6-phosphatase deficient children. Pediatr Res 18:335, 1984
223. Finegold MJ: Cholestatic syndromes in infancy. Perspect Pediatr Pathol 3:41, 1976
224. Finegold MJ, Carpenter RJ: Obliterative cholangitis due to cytomegalovirus: A possible precursor of paucity of intrahepatic bile ducts. Human Pathol 13:662, 1982
225. Fisher RL et al: Alpha-1-antitrypsin deficiency in liver disease: The extent of the problem. Gastroenterology 71:646, 1976
226. Flannery DB et al: Current status of hyperammonemic syndromes. Hepatology 2:495, 1982
227. Flodgaard HJ, Brodersen R: Bilirubin glucuronide formation in developing guinea pig liver. Scand J Clin Lab Invest 19:149, 1967
228. Fonkalsrud EW, Boles T: Choledochal cysts in infancy and childhood. Surg Gynecol Obstet 121:733, 1965
229. Fonkalsrud EW et al: Management of extrahepatic portal hypertension in children. Ann Surg 180:487, 1974
230. Frank DJ et al: Fetal ascites and cytomegalic inclusion disease. Am J Dis Child 112:604, 1966
231. Fratantoni JC et al: Hurler and Hunter syndromes: Mutual correction of the defect in cultured fibroblasts. Science 162:570, 1968
232. Fraumeni JF et al: Primary carcinoma of the liver in childhood: An epidemiologic study. J Natl Cancer Inst 40:1087, 1968
233. Froesch ER et al: Hereditary fructose intolerance: An inborn defect of hepatic fructose-1-phosphate splitting aldolase. Am J Med 34:151, 1963
234. Gall EA, Landing BH: Hepatic cirrhosis and hereditary disorders of metabolism. Am J Pathol 26:1398, 1956
235. Gartner LM, Arias IM: The transfer of bilirubin from blood to bile in the neonatal guinea pig. Pediatr Res 3:171, 1969
236. Gartner LM, Arias IM: Studies of prolonged neonatal jaundice in the breast-fed infant. J Pediatr 68:54, 1966
237. Gartner LM et al: Effect of milk feeding on intestinal bilirubin absorption in the rat. J Pediatr 103:464, 1983
238. Gartner LM et al: Kernicterus: High incidence in premature infants with low serum bilirubin concentrations. Pediatrics 45:906, 1970
239. Gartner LM et al: Development of bilirubin transport and metabolism in the newborn rhesus monkey. J Pediatr 90:513, 1977
240. Gatzimos CD, Jowitt RH: Jaundice in mucoviscidosis. (Fibrocystic disease of pancreas.) Am J Dis Child 89:182, 1955
241. Gautier M et al: Morphologic study of 98 biliary remnants. Arch Pathol Lab Med 105:397, 1981
242. Gerhold JP et al: Diagnosis of biliary atresia with radionuclide hepatobiliary imaging. Radiology 146:499, 1983
243. Gilbert EF: Carnitine deficiency. Pathology 17:161, 1985
244. Gilbert EF et al: Familial hemophagocytic lymphohistiocytosis. Pediatr Pathol 3:59, 1985
245. Gilbertson AS et al: Enteropathic circulation of unconjugated bilirubin in man. Nature 196:141, 1962
246. Gilchrist KW et al: Studies of malformation syndromes of man XIB: The cerebro-hepato-renal syndrome of Zellweger: Comparative pathology. Eur J Pediatr 121:99, 1976
247. Gitlin N et al: Fulminant neonatal hepatic necrosis associated with echovirus type 11 infection. Western J Med 138:260, 1983
248. Gitlow SE et al: Diagnosis of neuroblastoma by qualitative and quantitative determinates of catecholamine metabolites in urine. Cancer 25:1377, 1970
249. Gitzelmann R: Hereditary galactokinase deficiency: A newly recognized cause of juvenile cataracts. Pediatr Res 1:14, 1967
250. Gitzelmann R et al: Essential fructosuria, hereditary fructose intolerance, and fructose-1, 6-diphosphatase deficiency. In Stanbury JB et al (eds): The Metabolic Basis of Inherited Disease, p 118. New York, McGraw–Hill, 1983
251. Gitzelmann R et al: Galactitol and galactose-1-phosphate in the lens of a galactosemic infant. Exp Eye Res 6:1, 1967
252. Giunta F: A one year experience with phototherapy for jaundice of prematurity. Pediatrics 47:123, 1971
253. Giunta F, Rath J: Effect of environmental illumination in prevention of hyperbilirubinemia of prematurity. Pediatrics 44:162, 1969
254. Glaser JH et al: The role of Reovirus Type 3 in persistent infantile cholestasis. J Pediatr 105:912–915, 1984
255. Glasgow JT et al: Alpha-1-antitrypsin deficiency in association with both cirrhosis and chronic ostructive lung disease in two sibs. Am J Med 54:181, 1973
256. Glauser SO et al: Action spectrum for the photodestruction of bilirubin. Proc Soc Exp Biol Med 136:518, 1971
257. Gleason CA et al: Hepatic oxygen consumption, lactate uptake, and glucose production in neonatal lambs. Pediatr Res 19:1235, 1985
258. Glew RH et al: Biology of disease: Lysosomal storage diseases. Lab Invest 53:250, 1985
259. Glick TH et al: Acute encephalopathy and hepatic dysfunction associated with chickenpox in siblings. Am J Dis Child 119:68, 1970
260. Glick TH et al: Reye's syndrome: An epidemiologic approach. Pediatrics 46:371, 1970
261. Goldfischer S: Idiopathic neonatal iron storage involving the liver, pancreas, heart and endocrine and exocrine glands. Hepatology 1:58, 1981
262. Goldfischer S et al: Peroxisomal and mitochondrial defects in the cerebro-hepato-renal syndrome. Science 182:62, 1973
263. Goldfischer S et al: Peroxisomal defects in neonatal-onset and X-linked adrenoleukodystrophies. Science 227:67, 1985
264. Gorodischer R et al: Congenital nonobstructive jaundice: Effect of phototherapy. N Engl J Med 282:375, 1970
265. Gotto AM et al: On the protein defect in abetalipoproteinemia. N Engl J Med 284:813, 1971
266. Gourley GR, Arend RA: Neonatal jaundice and breast-milk beta-glucuronidase (abstr). Hepatology 5:959, 1985
267. Graham MF et al: Inhibition of bile flow in the isolated perfused rat liver by a synthetic parenteral amino acid mixture. Hepatology 4:69, 1984
268. Grand RJ: Changing patterns of gastrointestinal manifestations of cystic fibrosis: Survey of recent progress in diagnosis and treatment. Clin Pediatr 9:588, 1970
269. Gray OP, Saunders RA: Familial intrahepatic jaundice in infancy. Arch Dis Child 41:320, 1966
270. Greene HL et al: Continuous nocturnal intragastric feeding for management of type I glycogen-storage disease. New Engl J Med 294:423, 1976

271. Greene HL et al: Type I glycogen storage disease: A metabolic basis for advances in treatment. Adv Pediatr 26:63, 1979

272. Greengard O: Enzymatic differentiation in mammalian liver. Science 163:891, 1969

273. Greenwood RD et al: Syndrome of intrahepatic biliary dysgenesis and cardiovascular malformations. Pediatrics 58:243, 1976

274. Grenier A et al: Detection of succinylacetone and the use of its measurement in mass screening for hereditary tyrosinemia. Clin Chem Acta 123:93, 1982

275. Grodsky GM et al: Effect of age of rat on development of hepatic carriers for bilirubin: A possible explanation for physiologic jaundice and hyperbilirubinemia in the newborn. Metabolism 19:246, 1970

276. Gross RE et al: Neuroblastoma sympatheicum: A study and report of 217 cases. Pediatrics 23:1179, 195

277. Gross SJ: Vitamin E and neonatal bilirubinemia. Pediatrics 64:321, 1979

278. Guburn–Salisachs L: La maladie atresiante des coies biliares extrahepatiques. Arch Fr Pediatr 25:415, 1968

279. Gustafsson J: Bile acid synthesis during development: Mitochondrial 12.-hydroxylation in human fetal liver. J Clin Invest 75:604, 1985

280. Hackenbrock CR: Ultrastructural basis for metabolically linked mechanical activity in mitochondria. J Cell Biol 80:269, 1966

281. Hadchouel M: Immunoglobulin deposits in the biliary remnants of extrahepatic biliary atresia: A study by immunoperoxidase staining in 128 infants. Histopathology 5:217, 1981

282. Haddock JH, Nadler HL: Bilirubin toxicity in human cultivated fibroblasts and its modification by light treatment. Proc Soc Exp Biol Med 134:45, 1970

283. Hadler SC et al: Effect of immunoglobulin on hepatitis A in day-care centers. JAMA 249:48, 1983

284. Halac E Jr, Sicignano C: Re-evaluation of the influence of sex, age, pregnancy and phenobarbital in the activity of UDP-glucuronyl transferase in rat liver. J Lab Clin Med 73:677, 1969

285. Hale DE et al: Long-chain acyl coenzyme A dehydrogenase deficiency: An inherited cause of nonketotic hypoglycemia. Pediatr Res 19:666, 1985

286. Hall EG et al: Congenital toxoplasmosis in the newborn. Arch Dis Child 28:117, 1953

287. Halpin TJ et al: Reye's syndrome and medication use. JAMA 248:687, 1982

288. Hamilton JR, Sass–Kortsak A: Jaundice associated with severe bacterial infection in young infants. J Pediatr 63:121, 1963

289. Handel D, Kitlak W: Jaundice as chief symptom of pyuria during infancy. Dtsch Med Wochenschr 91:1781, 1966

290. Hanshaw JB: Congenital cytomegalovirus infection: A fifteen year perspective. J Infect Dis 123:355, 1971

291. Hanshaw JB et al: Acquired cytomegalovirus infection: Associated with hepatomegaly and abnormal liver function tests. N Engl J Med 272:602, 1965

292. Hanson RF et al: The metabolism of 3 alpha, 7 alpha, 12 alpha, trihydroxy-5 beta-cholestan-26-oic acid in two siblings with cholestasis due to intrahepatic bile duct anomalies. J Clin Invest 56:577, 1975

293. Hanson RF et al: Defects of bile acid synthesis in Zellweger's syndrome. Science 203:1107, 1979

294. Hanson RF et al: Hepatic lesions and hemolysis following administration of 3 alpha, 7 alpha, 12 alpha-trihydroxy-5 beta-cholestan-26 oyl taurine in rats. J Lab Clin Med 90:536, 1977

295. Haratake J et al: Familial intrahepatic cholestatic cirrhosis in young adults. Gastroenterology 89:202, 1985

296. Hardwick DF, Dimmick JE: Metabolic cirrhoses of infancy and early childhood. Perspect Pediatr Pathol 3:103, 1976

297. Hargreaves T, Piper RF: Breast milk jaundice: Effect of inhibitory breast milk and 3 alpha, 20 beta-pregnanediol on glucuronyl transferase. Arch Dis Child 46:195, 1971

298. Harris LE et al: Conjugated serum bilirubin in erythroblastosis fetalis: An analysis of 38 cases. Proc Staff Meet Mayo Clin 37:574, 1962

299. Hass GM: Hepatoadrenal necrosis with intranuclear inclusions: Report of a case. Am J Pathol 11:127, 1935

300. Hays DM et al: Diagnosis of biliary atresia: Relative accuracy of percutaneous liver biopsy, open liver biopsy and operative cholangiography. J Pediatr 71:598, 1967

301. Heathcote J et al: Intrahepatic cholestasis in childhood. N Engl J Med 295:801, 1976

302. Heijtink RA et al: Hepatitis B vaccination in Down's syndrome and other mentally retarded patients. Hepatology 4:611, 1984

303. Herdson PB et al: Fine structural changes produced in rat liver by partial starvation. Am J Pathol 45:157, 1964

304. Herman SP et al: Liver dysfunction and histologic abnormalities in neonatal hypopituitarism. J Pediatr 87:892, 1975

305. Hers HG: Alpha-glucosidase deficiency in generalized glycogen storage disease (Pompe's disease). Biochem J 86:11, 1963

306. Heubi JE et al: Grade I Reye's syndrome: Outcome and predictors of progression to deeper coma grades. N Engl J Med 311:1539, 1984

307. Heymans HSA et al: Severe plasmalogen deficiency in tissues of infants without peroxisomes (Zellweger syndrome). Nature 306:69, 1983

308. Hodgeman JE, Teberg A: Effect of phototherapy on subsequent growth and development of the premature infant. Birth Defects 6, No. 2:75, 1970

309. Hodges JR et al: Heterozygous MZ alpha-1-antitrypsin deficiency in adults with chronic active hepatitis and cryptogenic cirrhosis. N Engl J Med 304:557, 1981

310. Hoeg JM et al: Characterization of neutral and acid ester hydrolase in Wolman's disease. Biochim Biophys Acta 711:59, 1982

311. Holder TM: Atresia of the extrahepatic bile duct. Am J Surg 107:458, 1964

312. Hong R, Schubert WK: Menghini needle biopsy of the liver. Am J Dis Child 100:42, 1960

313. Hood JM et al: Liver transplantation for advanced liver disease with alpha-1-antitrypsin deficiency. N Engl J Med 302:272, 1980

314. Hostetter MK et al: Evidence for liver disease preceding amino acid abnormalities in hereditary tyrosinemia. N Engl J Med 308:1265, 1983

315. Hovig DE et al: Herpes virus hominis infection in the newborn with recurrences during infancy. Am J Dis Child 115:438, 1968

316. Howard ER et al: Spontaneous perforation of common bile duct in infants. Arch Dis Child 51:883, 1976

317. Howard ER et al: Management of esophageal varices in children by injection sclerotherapy. J Pediatr Surg 19:2, 1984

318. Hsia D Y–Y et al: Erythroblastosis fetalis: Studies on serum

bilirubin in relation to kernicterus. N Engl J Med 247:668, 1952

319. Hsia D Y–Y et al: Prolonged obstructive jaundice in infancy: V. The genetic components of neonatal hepatitis. Am J Dis Child 95:485, 1958

320. Hsia D Y–Y et al: Inhibitors of glucuronyl transferase in the newborn. Ann NY Acad Sci 111:326, 1963

321. Hsia D Y–Y et al: Prolonged obstructive jaundice in infancy: General survey of 156 cases. Pediatrics 10:243, 1952

322. Hsia D Y–Y et al: Inhibition of glucuronosyl transferase by steroid hormones. Arch Biochem Biophys 103:181, 1963

323. Hubbell JP et al: "Early" vs. "late" feeding of infants of diabetic mothers. N Engl J Med 265:835, 1961

324. Hudak ML et al: Differentiation of transient hyperammonemia of the newborn and urea cycle enzyme defects by clinical presentation. J Pediatr 107:712, 1985

325. Hug G: Glucagon tolerance test in glycogen storage disease. J Pediatr 60:545, 1962

326. Hug G: Glycogen storage disease. In Kelley VC (ed): Practice of Pediatrics, chap 30. Philadelphia, Harper & Row, 1985

327. Hug G, Schubert WK: Glycogenosis type II: Glycogen distribution in tissues. Arch Pathol 84:141, 1967

328. Hug G et al: Lysosomes in type II glycogenosis: Changes during administration of extract from *Aspergillus niger*. J Cell Biol 35:Cl, 1967

329. Hug G et al: Type VI glycogenosis: Biochemical demonstration of liver phosphorylase deficiency. Biochem Biophys Res Commun 41:1178, 1970

330. Hug G et al: Deficient activity of dephosphorylase kinase and accumulation of glycogen in the liver. J Clin Invest 48:704, 1969

331. Hug G et al: Loss of cyclic 3',5'-AMP dependent kinase and reduction of phosphorylase kinase in skeletal muscle of a girl with deactivated phosphorylase kinase and glycogenosis of liver and muscle. Biochem Biophys Res Commun 40:982, 1970

332. Hug G et al: Liver phosphorylase: Deactivation in a child with progressive brain disease, elevated hepatic glycogen and increased urinary catecholamines. Am J Med 42:139, 1967

333. Hug G et al: Cori's disease (amylo-1, 6-glucosidase deficiency). N Engl J Med 268:113, 1963

334. Hug G et al: Rapid prenatal diagnosis of glycogen storage disease type II by electron microscopy of uncultured amniotic-fluid cells. N Engl J Med 310:1018, 1984

335. Hughes CA et al: Total parenteral nutrition in infancy: Effect on the liver and suggested pathogenesis. Gut 24:241, 1983

336. Hughes JR et al: Echovirus 14 infection associated with fatal neonatal hepatic necrosis. Am J Dis Child 123:61, 1972

337. Hurwitz ES et al: Public health service study on Reye's syndrome and medications: Report of the pilot phase. N Engl J Med 313:849, 1985

338. Hyams JS et al: Discordance for biliary atresia in two sets of monozygotic twins. J Pediatr 107:420, 1985

339. Inouye T et al: Galactose-1-phosphate uridyl transferase in red and white blood cells. Clin Chim Acta 19:169, 1968

340. Ishak KG: Primary hepatic tumors in childhood. In Popper H, Schaffner F (eds): Progress in Liver Diseases V, pp 636–667. New York, Grune & Stratton, 1976

341. Ishak KG, Glunz PR: Hepatoblastoma and hepatocarcinoma in infancy and childhood: Report of 47 cases. Cancer 20:396, 1967

342. Israel JB, Arias IM: Inheritable disorders of bilirubin metabolism. Adv Intern Med 21:77, 1976

343. Isselbacher KJ et al: Congenital galactosemia, a single enzymatic block in galactose metabolism. Science 123:635, 1956

344. Isselbacher KJ et al: Congenital betalipoprotein deficiency: An hereditary disorder involving a defect in the absorption and transport of lipids. Medicine 43:347, 1964

345. Ito T et al: Intrahepatic bile ducts in biliary atresia: A possible factor determining the prognosis. J Pediatr Surg 18:124, 1983

346. Ivemark BI et al: Niemann-Pick disease in infancy: Report of two siblings with clinical, histologic and biochemical studies. Acta Paediatr 52:391, 1963

347. Iwatsuki S et al: Liver transplantation for biliary atresia. World J Surg 8:51, 1984

348. James SP et al: Liver abnormalities in patients with Gaucher's disease. Gstroenterology 80:126, 1981

349. Javitt NB: Cholestasis in infancy. Gastroenterology 70:1172, 1976

350. Jeppesson J–O et al: Properties of isolated human alpha-1-antitrypsins of Pi types M, A and Z. Eur J Biochem 83:143, 1978

351. Jirka JH et al: Effect of bilirubin on brainstem auditory evoked potentials in the asphyxiated rat. Pediatr Res 19:556, 1985

352. Jirsova V et al: Beta-glucuronidase activity in different organs of human fetuses. Biol Neonate 8:23, 1965

353. Johnson G et al: A study of sixteen fatal cases of encephalitis-like disease in North Carolina children. NC Med J 24:464, 1963

354. Johnson JD: Neonatal nonhemolytic jaundice. N Engl J Med 292:197, 1975

355. Johnston JH: Spontaneous perforation of the common bile duct in infancy. Br J Surg 48:532, 1961

356. Johnston WH et al: Erythroblastosis fetalis and hyperbilirubinemia: A five year follow-up with neurological, psychological and audiological evaluation. Pediatrics 39:88, 1967

357. Jones EA et al: Progressive intrahepatic cholestasis of infancy and childhood: A clinicopathological study of a patient surviving to the age of 18 years. Gastroenterology 71:675, 1976

358. Jorgensen MJ: The ductal plate malformation. Acta Pathol Microbiol Scand (A) (Suppl) 257:1, 1977

359. Joske RA et al: Hepatitis-encephalitis in humans with rheovirus infection. Arch Intern Med 113:811, 1964

360. Juberg RC et al: Familial intrahepatic cholestasis with growth retardation. Pediatrics 38:819, 1966

361. Kalina RE, Forrest GL: Ocular hazards of phototherapy for hyperbilirubinemia. J Pediatr Ophthalmol 8:116, 1971

362. Kan YW et al: Hydrops fetalis with alpha thalassemia. N Engl J Med 276:18, 1967

363. Kan YW et al: Gamma-beta thalassemia as a cause of hemolytic disease of the newborn. N Engl J Med 286:129, 1972

364. Kaplan E et al: Phototherapy in ABO hemolytic disease of the newborn infant. J Pediatr 79:911, 1971

365. Kappas A et al: The liver excretes large amounts of heme into bile when heme oxygenase is inhibited competitively by SN-protoporphyrin. Proc Natl Acad Sci 82:896, 1985

366. Karjoo M et al: Choledochal cyst presenting as recurrent pancreatitis. Pediatrics 51:289, 1973

367. Karon M et al: Effective phototherapy in congenital non-

obstructive, nonhemolytic jaundice. N Engl J Med 282: 377, 1970

368. Karp WB: Biochemical alterations in neonatal hyperbilirubinemia and bilirubin encephalopathy: A review. Pediatrics 64:361, 1979

369. Kasai M: Treatment of biliary atresia with special reference to hepatic portoenterostomy and its modification. Progr Pediatr Surg 6:6, 1974

370. Kasai M, Watanabe I: HIstologic classification of liver cell carcinoma in infancy and childhood: Clinical evaluation. Cancer 25:551, 1970

371. Kasai M et al: Follow-up studies of long-term survivors after hepatic portoenterostomy for "noncorrectable" biliary atresia. J Pediatr Surg 10:173, 1975

372. Kasai M et al: Surgical treatment of biliary atresia. J Pediatr Surg 3:665, 1968

373. Kase BF et al: Defective peroxisomal cleavage of the C_{27} steroid side chain in the cerebro-hepato-renal syndrome of Zellweger. J Clin Invest 75:427, 1985

374. Kaufman FR et al: Neonatal cholestasis and hypopituitarism. Arch Dis Child 59:787, 1984

375. Kaufman FR et l: Hypergonadatropic hypogonadism in female patients with galactosemia. N Engl J Med 304:994, 1981

376. Kaufman NA et al: The absorption of bilirubin by Sephadex and its relationship to the criteria for exchange transfusion. Pediatrics 44:543, 1969

377. Keenan WK et al: Kernicterus in small sick premature infants receiving phototherapy. Pediatrics 49:652, 1972

378. Kerr DNS et al: Congenital hepatic fibrosis. Q J Med 30: 91, 1961

379. Kerr DNS et al: A lesion resembling medullary sponge kidney in patients with congenital hepatic fibrosis. Clin Radiol 13:85, 1962

380. Kerr DNS et al: Congenital hepatic fibrosis: The long-term prognosis. Gut 19:514, 1978

381. Kidd VJ et al: Prenatal diagnosis of alpha-1-antitrypsin deficiency by direct analysis of the mutation site in the gene. N Engl J Med 310:639, 1984

382. Kilbrick S, Benirschke K: Severe generalized disease occurring in the newborn period and due to infection with coxsackie virus group B. Pediatrics 22:857, 1958

383. Kivlahan C, James EJP: The natural history of neonatal jaundice. Pediatrics 74:364, 1984

384. Klaassen CD: Development of hepatic excretory function in the newborn rat. In Kitani K (ed): Liver and Aging, p 313. Amsterdam, Elsevier/North-Holland Biomedical Press, 1978

385. Kleinknecht C et al: Membranous glomerulonephritis and hepatitis B surface antigen in children. J Pediatr 95:946, 1979

386. Knox I et al: Urinary excretion of an isomer of bilirubin during phototherapy. Pediatr Res 19:198, 1985

387. Kobayashi A: Ascending cholangitis after successful surgical repair of biliary atresia. Arch Dis Child 48:697, 1973

388. Kocak N, Ozsoylu S: Familial cirrhosis. Am J Dis Child 133:1160, 1979

389. Kolodny EH, Moser HW: Sulfatide lipidosis: Metachromatic leukodystrophy. In Stanbury JB et al (eds): The Metabolic Basis of Inherited Disease, p 881. New York, McGraw-Hill, 1983

390. Kopelman AE et al: The "bronze baby" complication of phototherapy. Pediatr Res 5:642, 1971

391. Kornfeld S, Sly WS: Lysosomal storage defects. Hosp Pract, p 71, August 1985

392. Korones SB et al: Congenital rubella syndrome: Study of 22 infants. Am J Dis Child 110:434, 1965

393. Kreek MJ, Sleisenger M: Reduction of serum-unconjugated bilirubin with phenobarbitone in adult congenital nonhaemolytic unconjugated hyperbilirubinemia. Lancet 1:73, 1968

394. Kvittingen EA et al: Prenatal diagnosis of hereditary tyrosinemia by determination of fumarylacetoacetase in cultured amniotic fluid cells. Pediatr Res 19:334, 1985

395. LaBrecque DR et al: Four generations of arteriohepatic dysplasia. Hepatology 4:467, 1982

396. Ladd WE: Congenital obstruction of bile ducts. Ann Surg 102:242, 1935

397. Lake BD, Patrick AD: Wolman's disease: Deficiency of E 600-resistant acid esterase with storage of lipids in lysosomes. J Pediatr 76:262, 1970

398. Landing BH: Consideration of the pathogenesis of neonatal hepatitis, biliary atresia and choledochal cyst: The concept of infantile obstructive cholangiopathy. Prog Pediatr Surg 6:113, 1974

399. Landing BH: Protracted obstructive jaundice in infancy. In Becker FF (ed): The Liver, Normal and Abnormal Functions, Part B, pp 821–849. New York, Marcel Dekker, 1975

400. Landing BH et al: Familial neurovisceral lipidosis. Am J Dis Child 108:503, 1964

401. Landing BH et al: Diseases of the bile ducts in children. In Gall EA, Mostofi FK (eds): The Liver, vol 13, pp 480–509. Baltimore, Williams & Wilkins, 1973

402. Landing BH et al: Morphometric analysis of liver lesions in cystic diseases of childhood. Hum Pathol 11:549, 1980

403. Larcher VF et al: Spontaneous bacterial peritonitis in children with chronic liver disease: Clinical features and etiologic features. J Pediatr 106:907, 1985

404. Laurell CB, Eriksson S: The electrophoretic alpha-1-globulin pattern of serum in alpha-1-antitrypsin deficiency. Scand J Clin Lab Invest 15:132, 1963

405. Lauridsen UB et al: Oesophageal varices as a late complication to neonatal umbilical vein catheterization. Acta Paediatr Scand 67:663, 1978

406. Lavin A et al: Enzymatic removal of bilirubin from blood: A potential treatment for neonatal jaundice. Science 230: 543, 1985

407. Lee KS, Gartner LM: Bilirubin binding by plasma proteins: A critical evaluation of methods and clinical implications. Rev Perinat Med 2:319, 1978

408. Lee SS et al: Choledochal cyst: A report of nine cases and review of the literature. Arch Surg 99:19, 1969

409. Lee T et al: Increased incidence of severe hyperbilirubinemia among newborn Chinese infants with G-6-PD deficiency. Pediatrics 37:994, 1968

410. Lefkowitch JH et al: Hepatic fibrosis in fetal alcohol syndrome: Pathologic similarities to adult alcoholic liver disease. Gastroenterology 85:951, 1983

411. Lefkowitch JH et al: Hepatic copper overload and features of Indian childhood cirrhosis in an American sibship. N Engl J Med 307:271, 1982

412. Lester R, Schmid R: Intestinal absorption of bile pigments: I. The enterohepatic circulation of bilirubin in the rat. J Clin Invest 42:736, 1963

413. Lester R et al: A new therapeutic approach to unconjugated hyperbilirubinaemia. Lancet 2:1257, 1962

414. Lester R et al: Intestinal absorption of bile pigments: II. Bilirubin absorption in man. N Engl J Med 269:178, 1963

415. Le Tan V et al: Associate de malformation congenitale et de cytomegalie: Etude de 18 observations anatomocliniques. Nouv Presse Med 2:1411, 1973

416. Levi AJ: Two hepatic cytoplasmic protein fractions, Y and Z, and their possible role in the hepatic uptake of bilirubin sulfobromophthalein and other anions. J Clin Invest 48:2156, 1969

417. Levi AJ et al: Deficiency of hepatic organic anion-binding protein, impaired organic anion uptake by liver and "physiologic" jaundice in newborn monkeys. N Engl J Med 283:1136, 1970

418. Levine RL et al: Clearance of bilirubin from rat brain after reversible osmotic opening of the blood-brain barrier. Pediatr Res 19:1040, 1985

419. Levy HL et al: Sepsis due to *Escherichia coli* in neonates with galactosemia. N Engl J Med 297:823, 1977

420. Lichtensten PK et al: Grade I Reye's syndrome: A frequent cause of vomiting and liver dysfunction after varicella and upper-respiratory-tract infections. N Engl J Med 309:133, 1983

421. Lidman K et al: Chronic active hepatitis in children: A clinical and immunological long-term study. Acta Paediatr Scand 66:73, 1977

422. Lieberman E et al: Infantile polycystic disease of the kidneys and liver: Clinical, pathological and radiological correlations and comparison with congenital hepatic fibrosis. Medicine 50:277, 1971

423. Lieberman J et al: Alpha-1-antitrypsin in the livers of patients with emphysema. Science 175:63, 1972

424. Lightner DA et al: Bilirubin photooxidation products in the urine of jaundiced neonates receiving phototherapy. Pediatr Res 18:696, 1984

425. Lilly JR, Altman RP: Hepatic portoenterostomy (the Kasai operation) for biliary atresia. Surgery 78:76, 1975

426. Lilly JR et al: Spontaneous perforation of the extrahepatic bile ducts and bile peritonitis in infancy. Surgery 75:664, 1974

427. Linarelli LG et al: Byler's disease: Fatal intrahepatic cholestasis. J Pediatr 81:484, 1972

428. Lindblad B et al: On the enzymic defects in hereditary tyrosinemia. Proc Natl Acad Sci USA 74:4641, 1977

429. Lohiya G et al: Hepatocellular carcinoma in young, mentally retarded HBsAg carriers without cirrhosis. Hepatology 5:824, 1985

430. Longmire WP, Sanford MC: Intrahepatic cholangiojejunostomy with partial hepatectomy for biliary obstruction. Surgery 24:264, 1949

431. Lough J et al: Wolman's disease: An electron microscopic, histochemical and biochemical study. Arch Pathol 89:103, 1970

432. Lucas A et al: Metabolic and endocrine consequences of depriving preterm infants of enteral nutrition. Acta Pediatr Scand 72:245, 1983

433. Lucey JF: Intrauterine transfusion and erythroblastosis fetalis. In Lucey JF, Butterfield LJ (eds): Ross Fifty-third Conference on Pediatric Research, Columbus, 1966, p 14

434. Lucey JF: Phototherapy of jaundice. Birth Defects 63, 1970

435. Lucey JF, Driscoll JJ: Physiological jaundice re-examined. In Sass-Kortsak A (ed): Kernicterus, p 29, Toronto, University of Toronto Press, 1961

436. Lucey JF et al: Prevention of hyperbilirubinemia of prematurity by phototherapy. Pediatrics 41:1047, 1968

437. Lyon JB Jr, Porter J: The effect of pyridoxine deficiency on muscle and liver phosphorylase of two inbred strains of mice. Biochim Biophys Acta 58:348, 1962

438. Maggiore G et al: Treatment of autoimmune chronic active hepatitis in childhood. J Pediatr 104:839, 1984

439. Mannering GJ: Drug metabolism in the newborn. Fed Proceed 44:2302, 1985

440. Margolis G et al: Rat virus disease, an experimental model of neonatal hepatitis. Exp Mol Pathol 8:1, 1968

441. Markowitz J et al: Arteriohepatic dysplasia: I. Pitfalls in diagnosis and management. Hepatology 3:74, 1983

442. Martin LW: Changing concepts in the management of portal hypertension in childhood. J Pediatr Surg 7:559, 1972

443. Martin LW, Woodman KS: Hepatic lobectomy for hepatoblastoma in infants and children. Arch Surg 98:1, 1969

444. Matalon R, Dorfman A: Hurler's syndrome, an alpha-L-iduronidase deficiency. Biochem Biophys Res Comm 47:959, 1972

445. Mathis RK et al: Liver disease in infants: II: Hepatic disease states. J Pediatr 90:864, 1977

446. Matsui A et al: Serum bile acid levels in patients with extrahepatic biliary atresia and neonatal hepatitis during the first 10 days of life. J Pediatr 107:255, 1985

447. Maurer HM et al: Controlled trial comparing agar, intermittent phototherapy and continuous phototherapy for reducing neonatal hyperbilirubinemia. J Pediatr 82:73, 1973

448. Maurer HM et al: Reduction in concentration of total serum bilirubin in offspring of women treated with phenobarbitone during pregnancy. Lancet 2:122, 1968

449. McAdams AJ, Wilson HE: The liver in generalized glycogen storage disease: Light microscopic observations. Am J Pathol 49:99, 1966

450. McClement JW et al: Results of surgical treatment for extrahepatic biliary atresia in United Kingdom 1980–2. Br Med J 290:345, 1985

451. McCracken GH Jr et al: Congenital cytomegalic inclusion disease: A longitudinal study of 20 patients. Am J Dis Child 117:522, 1969

452. McDonagh AF: Blue light and bilirubin excretion. Science 208:145, 1980

453. McDonagh AF: Molecular mechanisms of phototherapy of neonatal jaundice. In Rubaltelli FF, Jori G (eds): Neonatal Jaundice, p 173. New York, Plenum Press, 1984

454. McDonagh AF, Ramonas LM: Jaundice phototherapy: Micro flow-cell photometry reveals rapid biliary response of Gunn rats to light. Science 201:829, 1978

455. McGrath KM et al: Liver disease complicating severe hemophilia in childhood. Arch Dis Child 55:537, 1980

456. McKusick VA, Neufeld EF: The mucopolysaccharide storage diseases. In Stanbury JB et al (eds): The Metabolic Basis of Inherited Disease, p 751. New York, McGraw–Hill, 1983

457. McLean RH et al: Multinodular hemangiomatosis of the liver in infancy. Pediatrics 49:563, 1972

458. Medearis DN Jr: Observations concerning human cytomegalovirus infection and disease. Bull Johns Hopkins Hosp 114:181, 1964

459. Mellis C et al: Familial hepatic venocclusive disease with probable immune deficiency. J Pediatr 88:236, 1976

460. Merritt RJ et al: Cholestatic effect of intraperitoneal administration of tryptophan to suckling rat pups. Pediatr Res 18:904, 1984

461. Messing B et al: Does total parenteral nutrition induce gallbladder sludge formation and lithiasis? Gastroenterology 84:1012, 1983

462. Metge WR et al: Bilirubin glucuronyl transferase activity in liver disease. J Lab Clin Med 64:89, 1964

463. Metreau JM et al: Role of bilirubin overproduction in revealing Gilbert's syndrome: Is dyserythropoiesis an important factor? Gut 19:838, 1978

464. Meyer TC, Angus J: The effect of large doses of "Synkavit" in the newborn. Arch Dis Child 31:212, 1956

465. Michael AF Jr, Mauer AM: Maternal-fetal transfusion as a cause of plethora in the neonatal period. Pediatrics 28:458, 1961

466. Mikkelsen WP: Extrahepatic portal hypertension in children. Am J Surg 111:333, 1966

467. Miller DR et al: Fatal disseminated herpes simplex virus infection and hemorrhage in the neonate: Coagulation studies in a case and a review. J Pediatr 76:409, 1970

468. Miller MJ et al: Clinical spectrum of congenital toxoplasmosis: Problems in recognition. J Pediatr 70:714, 1967

469. Mineo I et al: Excess purine degradation in exercising muscles of patients with glycogen storage disease types V and VII. J Clin Invest 76:556, 1985

470. Mitchell JE, McCall FC: Transplacental infection by herpes simplex virus. Am J Dis Child 106:207, 1963

471. Miyairi M et al: Cell motility of fetal hepatocytes in short-term culture. Pediatr Res 19:1226, 1985

472. Mock DM et al: Chronic fructose intoxication after infancy in children with hereditary fructose intolerance: A cause of growth retardation. N Engl J Med 309:764, 1983

473. Modlin JF: Fatal echovirus II disease in premature neonates. Pediatrics 66:775, 1980

474. Moedy A et al: Fatal disseminated herpes simplex virus infection in a healthy child. Am J Dis Child 135:45, 1981

475. Moniff GRG et al: Postmortem isolation of rubella virus from three children with rubella syndrome defects. Lancet 1:723, 1965

476. Montgomery CK, Ruebner BH: Neonatal hepatocellular giant cell transformation: A review. Perspec Pediatr Pathol 3:85, 1976 Year Book Medical Publishers

477. Mooi WJ et al: Ultrastructure of the liver in cerebrohepatorenal syndrome of Zellweger. Ultrastruct Pathol 5:135, 1983

478. Morecki R et al: Biliary atresia and reovirus type 3 infection. N Engl J Med 307:481, 1982

479. Morecki R et al: Detection of reovirus type 3 in the porta hepatis of an infant with extrahepatic biliary atresia: Ultrastructural and immunocytochemical study. Hepatology 4:1137, 1984

480. Morphis L et al: Bilirubin-induced modulation of cerebral protein phosphorylation in neonate rabbits in vivo. Science 218:156, 1982

481. Moser AE et al: The cerebrohepatorenal (Zellweger) syndrome: Increased levels and impaired degradation of very-long-chain fatty acids and their use in prenatal diagnosis. N Engl J Med 310:1141, 1984

482. Moser HW et al: Adrenoleukodystrophy: Survey of 303 cases: Biochemistry, diagnosis and therapy. Ann Neurol 16:628, 1984

483. Mowat AP et al: Extrahepatic biliary atresia versus neonatal hepatitis: Review of 137 prospectively investigated infants. Arch Dis Child 51:763, 1976

484. Mowat AP et al: Primary sclerosing cholangitis in childhood. Proceedings 2nd Joint Meeting of the European Society for Pediatric Gastroenterology and Nutrition (ESPGAN) and the North American Society for Pediatric Gastroenterology (NASPG), May 1985

485. Msall M et al: Neurologic outcome in children with inborn errors of urea synthesis. Outcome of urea cycle enzymopathies. N Engl J Med 310:1500, 1984

486. Nadler HL et al: Congenital galactosemia: A study of 55 cases. In Hsia D Y–Y (ed): Galactosemia, pp 127–139. Springfield, IL, Charles C Thomas, 1969

487. Nahmias AJ et al: Newborn infection with herpes virus hominis types 1 and 2. J Pediatr 75:1194, 1969

488. Nahmias AJ et al: Neonatal herpes simplex infection: Role of genital infection in mother as the source of virus in the newborn. JAMA 199:164, 1967

489. Nakai H, Landing BH: Factors in the genesis of bile stasis in infancy. Pediatrics 27:300, 1961

490. National Institute of Child Health and Human Development randomized, controlled trial of phototherapy for neonatal hyperbilirubinemia. Pediatrics 75:385, 1985

491. Nayak NC, Ramalingaswami V: Childhood cirrhosis: In Beck FF, Dekker M (eds): The Liver, Part B, pp 851–882. 1975

492. Nelson DB et al: Aflatoxin and Reye syndrome: A case control study. Pediatrics 66:865, 1980

493. Nemeth A et al: Alpha-1-antitrypsin deficiency and juvenile liver disease: Ultrastructural observations compared with light microscopy and routine liver tests. Virchows Arch Pathol Anat 44:15, 1983

494. Neufeld EF: Replacement of genotype specific proteins in mucopolysaccharidoses: Enzyme therapy in genetic disease. Birth Defects. 9:27, 1972

495. Ng SH, Rawstron JR: Urinary tract infection presenting with jaundice. Arch Dis Child 46:173, 1971

496. Noell WK et al: Retinal damage by light in rats. Invest Ophthalmol 5:450, 1966

497. Novak DA, Balistreri WF: Management of chronic cholestasis. Pediatr Ann 14:488, July, 1985

498. O'Brien JS: Generalized gangliosidosis. J Pediatr 75:167, 1969

499. O'Brien JS et al: Sanfilippo disease type B: Enzyme replacement and metabolic correction in cultured fibroblasts. Science 181:753, 1973

500. Odell GB: "Physiologic" hyperbilirubinemia in the neonatal period. N Engl J Med 277:193, 1967

501. Odell GB et al: The influence of fatty acids on the binding of bilirubin to albumin. J Lab Clin Med 89:295, 1977

502. Odell GB et al: Enteral administration of agar as an effective adjunct to phototherapy of neonatal hyperbilirubinemia. Pediatr Res 17:810, 1983

503. Odell GB et al: Administration of albumin in the management of hyperbilirubinemia by exchange transfusion. Pediatrics 30:613, 1962

504. Odell GB et al: Studies in kernicterus: III. The saturation of serum proteins with bilirubin during neonatal life and its relationship to brain damage at five years. J Pediatr 76:12, 1970

505. Odievre M et al: Congenital abnormalities associated with extrahepatic portal hypertension. Arch Dis Child 52:383, 1977

506. Odievre M et al: Long-term prognosis for infants with intrahepatic cholestasis and patent extrahepatic biliary tract. Arch Dis Child 56:373, 1981

507. Odievre M et al: Alpha-1-antitrypsin deficiency and liver disease in children: Phenotypes, manifestations, and prognosis. Pediatrics 57:226, 1976

508. Odievre M et al: Seroimmunologic classification of chronic hepatitis in 57 children. Hepatology 3:407, 1983

509. Odievre M et al: Severe familial intrahepatic cholestasis. Arch Dis Child 48:806, 1973

510. Odievre M et al: Hereditary fructose intolerance in childhood. Am J Dis Child 132:605, 1978

511. Ohi R et al: Progress in the treatment of biliary atresia. World J Surg 9:285, 1985

512. Ohi R et al: Reoperation in patients with biliary atresia. J Pediatr Surg 20:256, 1985

513. Okada K et al: E antigen and anti-e in the serum of asymptomatic carrier mothers as indicators of positive and negative transmission of hepatitis B virus to their infants. N Engl J Med 294:746, 1976

514. Okada S et al: Ganglioside GM₂ storage diseases: Hexosaminidase deficiencies in cultured fibroblasts. Am J Hum Genet 23:55, 1971

515. Olson LC et al: Encephalopathy and fatty degeneration of the viscera in northwestern Thailand: Clinical syndrome and epidemiology. Pediatrics 47:707, 1971

516. Oppenheimer E, Esterly JR: Cytomegalovirus infection: A possible cause of biliary atresia. Am J Pathol 72:2a, 1973

517. Oppenheimer EH: Hepatic changes in young infants with cystic fibrosis. J Pediatr 86:683, 1975

518. Ostrow JD: Photocatabolism of labeled bilirubin in the congenitally jaundiced (Gunn) rat. J Clin Invest 50:707, 1971

519. Ostrow JD: Effect of phototherapy on hepatic excretory function in normal and Gunn rats. Gastroenterology 62:168, 1972

520. Ostrow JD et al: Effect of phototherapy on bilirubin excretion in man and the rat. In Bergsma E, Blondheim SH (eds): Bilirubin Metabolism in the Newborn, vol 2 New York, American Elsevier, 1976

521. Pakekh SR et al: Detection of Regan variant type of alkaline phosphatase isoenzyme in liver tissue of Indian childhood cirrhosis. Hepatology 3:572, 1983

522. Park RW, Grand RJ: Gastrointestinal manifestations of cystic fibrosis: A review. Gastroenterology 81:1143, 1981

523. Partin JC: Reye's syndrome: Diagnosis and treatment. Gastroenterology 69:511, 1975

524. Partin JC, Schubert WK: Small intestinal mucosa in cholesterol ester storage disease: A light and electron microscopy study. Gastroenterology 57:542, 1969

525. Partin JC et al: Brain ultrastructure in Reye's syndrome (encephalopathy and fatty alteration of the viscera). J Neuropathol Exp Neurol 34:425, 1975

526. Partin JC et al: Mitochondrial ultrastructure in Reye's syndrome (encephalopathy and fatty degeneration of the viscera). N Engl J Med 285:1339, 1971

527. Partin JS et al: Liver ultrastructure in abetalipoproteinemia evolution of micronodular cirrhosis. Gastroenterology 67:107, 1974

528. Partin JS et al: A comparison of liver ultrastructure in salicylate intoxication and Reye's syndrome. Hepatology 4:687, 1984

529. Passarge E, McAdams AJ: Cerebro-hepato-renal syndrome. J Pediatr 71:691, 1967

530. Patrick AD, Lake BD: Deficiency of an acid lipase in Wolman's disease. Nature 222:1067, 1969

531. Pearson HA: Life span of fetal red cells. J Pediatr 70:166, 1967

532. Peden VH et al: Total parenteral nutrition. J Pediatr 78:180, 1971

533. Peremans P et al: Familial metabolic disorder with fatty metamorphosis of the viscera. J Pediatr 69:1108, 1966

534. Pereyra R et al: Management of massive hepatic hemangiomas in infants and children: A review of 13 cases. Pediatrics 70:254, 1982

535. Perez CA et al: Treatment of malignant sympathetic tumors in children: Clinicopathologic correlation. Pediatrics 41:452, 1968

536. Philip AGS, Larson EJ: Overwhelming neonatal infection with ECHO 19 virus. J Pediatr 82:391, 1973

537. Phillips MJ et al: Subcellular pathology of hereditary fructose intolerance. Am J Med 44:910, 1968

538. Poland RL, Odell GB: Physiologic jaundice: The enterohepatic circulation of bilirubin. N Engl J Med 284:1, 1971

539. Porter CA et al: Alpha-1-antitrypsin deficiency and neonatal hepatitis. Br Med J 3:435, 1972

540. Porter MT et al: Metachromatic leukodystrophy: Arylsulfatase-A deficiency in skin fibroblast tissue cultures. Proc Natl Acad Sci USA 62:887, 1969

541. Postuma R, Trevenen CL: Liver disease in infants receiving total parenteral nutrition. Pediatrics 63:110, 1979

542. Poulos A, Whiting MJ: Identification of 3 alpha, 7 alpha, 12 alpha-trihydroxy-5 beta-cholestan-26-oic acid, an intermediate in cholic acid synthesis, in the plasma of patients with infantile Refsum's disease. J Inherited Metab Dis 8:13, 1985

543. Powell LW et al: Idiopathic unconjugated hyperbilirubinemia (Gilbert's syndrome): A study of 42 families. N Engl J Med 277:1108, 1967

544. Powers JM et al: Fetal cerebrohepatorenal (Zellweger) syndrome: Dysmorphic, radiologic, biochemical, and pathologic findings in four affected fetuses. Human Pathol 16:610, 1985

545. Prive L: Pathological findings in patients with tyrosinemia. Can Med Assoc J 97:1054, 1967

546. Pryles CV, Heggestad GE: Large cavernous hemangioma of the liver. Am J Dis Child 88:759, 1954

547. Psacharopoulos HT et al: Hepatic complications of cystic fibrosis. Lancet 2:78, 1981

548. Psacharopoulos HT et al: Outcome of liver disease associated with alpha-1-antitrypsin deficiency (PiZ): Implications for genetic counselling and antenatal diagnosis. Arch Dis Child 58:882, 1983

549. Pugh RCB et al: Hepatic necrosis in disseminated herpes simplex. Arch Dis Child 29:60, 1954

550. Quilligan JJ Jr, Wilson JL: Fatal herpes simplex infection in a newborn infant. J Lab Clin Med 38:742, 1951

551. Raga J et al: Usefulness of clinical features and liver biopsy in diagnosis of disseminated herpes simplex infection. Arch Dis Child 59:820, 1984

552. Rahal JJ, Heule G: Infectious mononucleosis and Reye's syndrome: A fatal case with studies for Epstein-Barr virus. Pediatrics 46:776, 1970

553. Räsänen O et al: Fatal familial steatosis of the liver and kidney in two siblings. Z Kinderheilkd 110:267, 1971

554. Rausen AR, Diamond LK: Enclosed hemorrhage and neonatal jaundice. Am J Dis Child 101:164, 1961

555. Rausen AR et al: Twin transfusion syndrome: A review of 19 cases studied at one institution. J Pediatr 66:613, 1965

556. Redeker AG et al: The reciprocal relationship between caloric intake and degree of hyperbilirubinemia in Gilbert's syndrome. Gastroenterology 58:303, 1970

557. Redinger RN, Small DM: The effect of phenobarbital on bile salt metabolism and cholesterol secretion in the primate. J Clin Invest 50:76a, 1971

558. Reed GB Jr et al: Type IV glycogenosis. Lab Invest 19:546, 1968

559. Reesink HW et al: Prevention of chronic HBsAg carrier state in infants of HBsAg-positive mothers by hepatitis B immunoglobulin. Lancet 2:436, 1979

560. Remington JS, Desmonts G: Congenital toxoplasmosis: Variability in the IgM fluorescent antibody response and some pitfalls in diagnosis. J Pediatr 88:27, 1973

561. Remington JS, Miller MJ: 19S and 7S anti-toxoplasma antibodies in diagnosis of acute congenital and acquired toxoplasmosis. Proc Soc Exper Biol Med 121:357, 1966

562. Reye RDK et al: Encephalopathy and fatty degeneration of the viscera. Lancet 2:749, 1963

563. Riely CA: Familial intrahepatic cholestasis: An update. Yale J Biol Med 52:89, 1979

564. Riely CA et al: Arteriohepatic dysplasia: A benign syndrome of intrahepatic cholestasis with multiple organ involvement. Ann Intern Med 91:520, 1979

565. Riely CA et al: A father and son with cholestasis and peripheral pulmonic stenosis. J Pediatr 92:406, 1978

566. Rivlin RS: Riboflavin metabolism. N Engl J Med 283:463, 1970

567. Robbins BH, Castle RF: Hemangiomas, hepatic involvement, congestive failure. Pediatrics 35:868, 1965

568. Roberts EA et al: Occurrence of alpha-1-antitrypsin deficiency in 155 patients with alcoholic liver disease. Am J Clin Pathol 82:424, 1984

569. Robinson SH et al: Bilirubin excretion in rats with normal and impaired bilirubin conjugation: Effect of phenobarbital. J Clin Invest 50:2606, 1971

570. Rodgers BM, Talbert JL: Distal spleno-renal shunt for portal decompression in childhood. J Pediatr Surg 14:33, 1979

571. Roe CR et al: Diagnostic and therapeutic implications of medium-chain acylcarnitines in the medium-chain acyl-CoA dehydrogenase deficiency. Pediatr Res 19:459, 1985

572. Rogan WJ et al: Aflatoxin and Reye's syndrome: A study of livers from deceased cases. Arch Environ Health 40:91, 1985

573. Rogers MF et al: National Reye syndrome surveillance, 1982. Pediatrics 75:260, 1985

574. Rooney JC et al: Jaundice associated with bacterial infection in the newborn. Am J Dis Child 122:39, 1971

575. Roscher A et al: The cerebrohepatorenal (Zellweger) syndrome: An improved method for the biochemical diagnosis and its potential value for prenatal detection. Pediatr Res 19:930, 1985

576. Rosenberg DP et al: Extrahepatic biliary atresia in a rhesus monkey (Macaca mulatta). Hepatology 3:577, 1983

577. Rosenberg S et al: Synthesis in yeast of a functional oxidation-resistant mutant of human alpha-1-antitrypsin. Nature 312:77, 1984

578. Rosenblum JL et al: A progressive neurologic syndrome in children with chronic liver disease. N Engl J Med 304:503, 1981

579. Rosenstein BS, Ducore JM: Enhancement by bilirubin of DNA damage induced in human cells exposed to phototherapy light. Pediatr Res 18:3, 1984

580. Rosenthal IM et al: Absence of intralobular bile ducts. Am J Dis Child 101:228, 1961

581. Roslyn JJ et al: Gallbladder disease in patients on long-term parenteral nutrition. Gastroenterology 84:148, 1983

582. Rotman M et al: Radiation treatment of pediatric hepatic hemangiomatosis and coexisting cardiac failure. N Engl J Med 302:852, 1980

583. Roy CC et al: Hepatobiliary disease in cystic fibrosis: A survey of current issues and concepts. J Pediatr Gastroenterol Nutr 1:469, 1982

584. Rubaltelli FF et al: Bronze baby syndrome: New insights in bilirubin-photosensitization of copper-porphyrins. In Rubaltelli FF, Jori G (eds): Neonatal Jaundice: New Trends in Phototherapy, p 265. New York, Plenum Press, 1984

585. Rubella Surveillance: National Communicable Disease Center, United States Department of Health, Education and Welfare, June 1969, p 11

586. Rudolph AM: Hepatic and ductus venosus blood flows during fetal life. Hepatology 3:254, 1983

587. Sacks SL, Freeman HJ: Cytomegalovirus hepatitis: Evidence for direct hepatic viral infection using monoclonal antibodies. Gastroenterology 86:346, 1984

588. Safe S et al: The role of chemicals in Reye's syndrome. In Crocker JFS (ed): Reye's Syndrome II, pp 281–308. New York, Grune & Stratton, 1979

589. Salt HB et al: On having no betalipoprotein. Lancet 2:325, 1960

590. Sandhoff K: Variation of beta-N-acetylhexosaminidase pattern in Tay–Sachs disease. Fed Eur Biochem Soc Lett 4:351, 1969

591. Sassa S, Kappas A: Hereditary tyrosinemia and the heme biosynthetic pathway. J Clin Invest 71:625, 1983

592. Satran L et al: Fatal neonatal hepatic steatosis: A new familial disorder. J Pediatr 75:39, 1969

593. Scheidt PC et al: Toxicity to bilirubin in neonates: Infant development during first year in relation to maximum neonatal serum bilirubin concentration. J Pediatr 91:292, 1977

594. Schenker S et al: Bilirubin metabolism in the fetus. J Clin Invest 43:32, 1964

595. Schiff D et al: Bilirubin toxicity in neural cell lines N115 and NBR10A. Pediatr Res 19:908, 1985

596. Schiff L et al: Effects of clofibrate in cholesterol ester storage disease. Gastroenterology 56:414, 1969

597. Schiff L et al: Hepatic cholesterol ester storage disease: A familial disorder: I. Clinical aspects. Am J Med 44:538, 1968

598. Schmid R: Bilirubin metabolism: State of the art. Gastroenterology 74:1307, 1978

599. Schmid R, Hammaker L: Metabolism and distribution of bilirubin in congenital nonhemolytic jaundice. J Clin Invest 42:1720, 1963

600. Schmid R, Mahler R: Chronic progressive myopathy with myoglobinuria: Demonstration of a glycogenolytic defect in the muscle. J Clin Invest 348:2044, 1959

601. Schmid R et al: Lack of effect of cholestyramine resin on the hyperbilirubinemia of premature infants. Lancet 2:938, 1963

602. Schneider PB, Kennedy EB: Sphingomyelinase in normal human spleens and in spleens from subjects with Niemann–Pick disease. J Lipid Res 8:202, 1967

603. Schrakamp G et al: Alkyl dihydroxyacetone phosphate synthase in human fibroblasts and its deficiency in Zellweger syndrome. J Lipid Res 26:867, 1985

604. Schrakamp G et al: The cerebro-hepato-renal (Zellweger) syndrome: Impaired de novo biosynthesis of plasmalogens in cultured skin fibroblasts. Biochim Biophys Acta 833:170, 1985

605. Schubert WK et al: Reye's syndrome. DM 1975

606. Schubert WK et al: Encephalopathy and fatty liver (Reye's syndrome). In Popper H, Schaffner E (eds): Progress in Liver

Diseases, 4th ed, pp 489–510. New York, Grune & Stratton, 1972

607. Schubert WK et al: Management of Reye's syndrome: Cincinnati experience. In Crocker JFS (ed): Reye's Syndrome II, pp 155–176. New York, Grune & Stratton, 1979

608. Schweitzer IL et al: Hepatitis and hepatitis-associated antigen in 56 mother-infant pairs. JAMA 220:1092, 1972

609. Scriver CR et al: Hereditary tyrosinemia and tyrosyluria in a French Canadian geographic isolate. Am J Dis Child 113:41, 1967

610. Seeler RA, Hahn K: Jaundice in urinary tract infection in infancy. Am J Dis Child 118:553, 1969

611. Segal S et al: The metabolism of galactose by patients with congenital galactosemia. Am J Med 38:62, 1965

612. Shaldon S, Sherlock S: Obstruction to the extrahepatic portal system in childhood. Lancet 1:63, 1963

613. Sharp HL: Alpha-1-antitrypsin deficiency. Hosp Pract 6:83, 1971

614. Sharp HL: The current status of alpha-1-antitrypsin, a protease inhibitor, in gastrointestinal disease. Gastroenterology 70:611, 1976

615. Sharp HL, Mirkin BL: Effect of phenobarbital on hyperbilirubinemia, bile acid metabolism and microsomal enzyme activity in chronic intrahepatic cholestasis of childhood. J Pediatr 81:116, 1972

616. Sharp HL et al: Cirrhosis associated with alpha-1-antitrypsin deficiency: A previously unrecognized inherited disorder. J Lab Clin Med 73:934, 1969

617. Sharp HL et al: The liver in noncirrhotic alpha-1-antitrypsin deficiency. J Lab Clin Med 78:1012, 1971

618. Shaywitz B et al: Prolonged continuous monitoring of intracranial pressure in Reye's syndrome. Pediatrics 59:595, 1977

619. Shier KJ, Horn RC Jr: The pathology of liver cirrhosis in patients with cystic fibrosis of the pancreas. Can Med Ass J 89:645, 1963

620. Shirak K: Liver in congenital bile duct atresia: Histological changes in relation to age. Paediatr Univ Tokyo 12:68, 1966

621. Sidbury JB: The genetics of glycogen storage disease. Prog Med Genet 4:3, 1965

622. Sieber OF Jr et al: In utero infection of the fetus by herpes simplex virus. J Pediatr 69:30, 1966

623. Silberberg DH et al: Effects of photodegradation products of bilirubin on myelinating cerebellum cultures. J Pediatr 77:613, 1970

624. Simionatto CS et al: Studies on the mechanism of Sn-protoporphyrin suppression of hyperbilirubinemia: Inhibition of heme oxidation and bilirubin production. J Clin Invest 75:513, 1985

625. Singer DB et al: Pathology of the congenital rubella syndrome. J Pediatr 71:665, 1967

626. Singh I et al: Adrenoleukodystrophy: Impaired oxidation of very long chain fatty acids in white blood cells, cultured skin fibroblasts, and amniocytes. Pediatr Res 18:286, 1984

627. Singh I et al: Lignoceric acid is oxidized in the peroxisome: Implications for the Zellweger cerebro-hepato-renal syndrome and adrenoleukodystrophy. Proc Natl Acad Sci 81:4203, 1984

628. Sinniah D et al: Investigation of an animal model of a Reye-like syndrome caused by margosa oil. Pediatr Res 19:1346, 1985

629. Sisson TRC et al: Retinal changes produced by phototherapy. J Pediatr 77:221, 1970

630. Sisson TRC et al: Phototherapy of jaundice in newborn infants: I. ABO blood group incompatibility. J Pediatr 79:904, 1971

631. Sloan HR et al: Deficiency of sphingomyelin cleaving enzyme activity in tissue cultures derived from patients with Niemann–Pick disease. Biochem Biophys Res Commun 34:582, 1969

632. Sloan HR et al: Enzyme deficiency in cholesterol ester storage disease. J Clin Invest 51:1923, 1972

633. Smetana HF, Olen E: Hereditary galactose disease. Am J Clin Pathol 38:3, 1962

634. Smit GPA et al: The dietary treatment of children with type I glycogen storage disease with slow release carbohydrate. Pediatr Res 18:879, 1984

635. Smith DW et al: A syndrome of multiple developmental defects including polycystic kidneys and intrahepatic biliary dysgenesis in 2 siblings. J Pediatr 67:617, 1965

636. Smith EI et al: Improved results with hepatic portoenterostomy: A reassessment of its value in the treatment of biliary atresia. Ann Surg 195:746, 1982

637. Smithwick EM, Go SC: Hepatitis-associated antigen in cord and maternal sera. Lancet 2:1080, 1970

638. So SKS et al: Bile ascites during infancy: Diagnosis using disofenin Tc 99m sequential scintiphotography. Pediatrics 71:402, 1983

639. Sokol RJ et al: Mechanism causing vitamin E deficiency during chronic childhood cholestasis. Gastroenterology 85:1172, 1983

640. Sokol RJ et al: Vitamin E deficiency with normal serum vitamin E concentrations in children with chronic cholestasis. N Engl J Med 310:1209, 1984

641. Sondheimer JM et al: Cholestatic tendencies in premature infants on and off parenteral nutrition. Pediatrics 62:984, 1978

642. Southwest Pediatric Nephrology Study Group: Hepatitis B surface antigenemia in North American children with membranous glomerulonephropathy. J Pediatr 106:571, 1985

643. Spivak W et al: A case of primary sclerosing cholangitis in childhood. Gastroenterology 82:129, 1982

644. Spycher MS, Gitzelmann R: Glycogenosis type I (glucose-6-phosphatase deficiency): Ultrastructural alterations of hepatocytes in a tumor bearing liver. Virchows Arch Cell Pathol 8:133, 1971

645. Stagno S: Congenital cytomegalovirus infection. N Engl J Med 306:945, 1982

646. Stagno S, Whitley RJ: Herpesvirus infections of pregnancy: Part I. Cytomegalovirus and Epstein-Barr virus infections; Part II. Herpes simplex virus and varicella-zoster virus infections. N Engl J Med 313:1270, 1327, 1985

647. Stamey CC, Diamond LK: Congenital hemolytic anemia in the newborn: Relationship to kernicterus. J Dis Child 94:616, 1957

648. Stanley CA et al: Medium-chain acyl-CoA dehydrogenase deficiency in children with non-ketotic hypoglycemia and low carnitine levels. Pediatr Res 17:877, 1983

649. Starr JG et al: Inapparent cytomegalovirus infection: Clinical and epidemiologic characteristics in early infancy. N Eng J Med 282:1075, 1970

650. Starzl TE et al: Portal diversion in glycogen storage disease. Surgery 65:504, 1969

651. Starzl TE et al: Changing concepts: Liver replacement for hereditary tyrosinemia and hepatoma. J Pediatr 106:604, 1985

652. Starzl TE et al: The effect of portacaval transposition on

carbohydrate metabolism: Experimental and clinical observation. Surgery 57:687, 1965

653. Stellard F et al: Hyocholic acid, an unusual bile acid in Byler's disease. Gastroenterology 77:A42, 1979

654. Stern H: Isolation of cytomegalovirus and clinical manifestations of infection at different ages. Br Med J 1:665, 1968

655. Stern H, Williams BM: Isolation of rubella virus in a case of neonatal giant-cell hepatitis. Lancet 1:293, 1966

656. Stern L, Denton RL: Kernicterus in small premature infants. Pediatrics 35:483, 1965

657. Stern L et al: Effect of phenobarbital on hyperbilirubinemia and glucuronide formation in newborns. Am J Dis Child 120:26, 1970

658. Stevens CE et al: Vertical transmission of hepatitis B antigen in Taiwan. N Engl J Med 292:771, 1975

659. Stevens CE et al: Perinatal hepatitis B virus transmission in the United States: Prevention by passive-active immunization. JAMA 253:1740, 1985

660. Stiehl A et al: The effects of phenobarbital on bile salts and bilirubin in patients with intrahepatic and extrahepatic cholestasis. N Engl J Med 286:858, 1972

661. Stiehm RE, Ryan J: Breast fed jaundice. Am J Dis Child 109:212, 1965

662. Stokes J Jr et al: Viral hepatitis in the newborn: Clinical features, epidemiology and pathology. Am J Dis Child 82:213, 1951

663. Stoll MS et al: Preparation and properties of bilirubin photoisomers. Biochem J 183:139, 1979

664. Stoner E et al: Biochemical studies of a patient with hereditary hepatorenal tyrosinemia: Evidence of glutathione deficiency. Pediatr Res 18:1332, 1984

665. Strandvik B, Wikstrom SA: Tetrahydroxylated bile acids in healthy human newborns. Eur J Clin Invest 12:301, 1982

666. Strauss L, Bernstein J: Neonatal hepatitis in congenital rubella: A histopathological study. Arch Pathol 86:317, 1968

667. Strebel L, Odell GB: U D P glucuronyl transferase in rat liver: Genetic variation and maturation. Pediatr Res 3:351, 1969

668. Strickland AD et al: Biliary atresia in two sets of twins. J Pediatr 107:418, 1985

669. Su T–S et al: Molecular analysis of argininosuccinate synthetase deficiency in human fibroblasts. J Clin Invest 70:1334, 1982

670. Suchy FJ, Balistreri WF: Maturation of bile acid conjugation in hepatocytes from fetal and suckling rats. Gastroenterology 78:1324, 1980

671. Suchy FJ, Balistreri WF: Taurocholate uptake in hepatocytes from developing rats. Pediatr Res 16:282, 1982

672. Suchy FJ et al: Physiologic cholestasis: Elevations of the primary serum bile acid concentrations in normal infants. Gastroenterology 80:1037, 1981

673. Suchy FJ et al: Taurocholate transport by basolateral plasma membrane vesicles isolated from developing rat liver. Am J Physiol 248:G648, 1985

674. Suchy FJ et al: Ontogeny of hepatic bile acid conjugation in the rat. Pediatr Res 19:97, 1985

675. Suchy FJ et al: Absence of a hepatic lobular gradient for bile acid uptake in the suckling rat. Hepatology 3:847, 1983

676. Suruga K et al: A clinical and pathological study of congenital biliary atresia. J Pediatr Surg 71:655, 1972

677. Suruga K et al: The surgery of infantile obstructive jaundice. Arch Dis Child 40:158, 1965

678. Sutherland J, Keller WH: Novobiocin and neonatal hyperbilirubinemia. Am J Dis Child 101:447, 1961

679. Sveger T: Liver disease in alpha-1-antitrypsin deficiency detected by screening of 200,000 infants. N Engl J Med 294:1316, 1976

680. Sveger T: Prospective study of children with alpha-1-antitrypsin deficiency: Eight-year-old follow-up. J Pediatr 104:91, 1984

681. Sweet AY, Wolinsky E: An outbreak of urinary tract and other infections due to E coli. Pediatrics 33:865, 1964

682. Tada K et al: Glycogen storage disease type IB: A new model of genetic disorders involving the transport system of intracellular membrane. Biochem Med 33:215, 1985

683. Talamo RC, Feingold M: Infantile cirrhosis with hereditary alpha-1-antitrypsin deficiency. Am J Dis Child 125:843, 1973

684. Talamo RC et al: Hereditary alpha-1-antitrypsin deficiency. N Engl J Med 278:345, 1968

685. Tanaka K et al: Isovaleric and alpha-methylbutyric acidemias induced by hypoglycin A: Mechanism of Jamaican vomiting sickness. Science 175:69, 1972

686. Tanner MS et al: Early introduction of copper-contaminated animal milk feeds as possible cause of Indian childhood cirrhosis. Lancet 2:992, 1983

687. Tauri S et al: Enzymatic basis for the coexistence of myopathy and hemolytic disease in inherited muscle phosphofructokinase deficiency. Biochem Biophys Res Commun 34:77, 1969

688. Tarui S et al: Phosphofructokinase deficiency in skeletal muscle: A new type of glycogenosis. Biochem Biophys Res Commun 19:517, 1965

689. Taylor RJ et al: Primary disseminated herpes simplex infection with fulminant hepatitis following renal transplantation. Arch Intern Med 141:1519, 1981

690. Taylor WF, Quaquandah BY: Neonatal jaundice associated with cystic fibrosis. Am J Dis Child 123:161, 1972

691. Tedesco TA, Miller KL: Galactosemia: Alterations in sulfate metabolism secondary to galactose-1-phosphate uridyltransferase deficiency. Science 205:1395, 1979

692. Tephly TR et al: Effect of drugs on heme synthesis in the liver. Metabolism 20:200, 1971

693. Thaler MM et al: Influence of intravenous nutrients on bilirubin transport: II. Emulsified lipid solutions; III. Emulsified fat solutions. Pediatr Res. 11:167, 171, 1977

694. Toda G et al: Infantile papular acrodermatitis (Gianotti's disease) and intrafamilial occurrence of acute hepatitis B with jaundice: Age dependency of clinical manifestations of hepatitis B virus infection. J Infect Dis 138:211, 1978

695. Tondeur M, Loeb H: Etude ultrastructurelle du foie dans la maladie de Morquio. Pediatr Res 3:19, 1969

696. Tong MJ et al: Prevention of hepatitis B infection by hepatitis B immune globulin in infants born to mothers with acute hepatitis during pregnancy. Gastroenterology 89:160, 1985

697. Tonsgard JH, Getz GS: Effect of Reye's syndrome serum on isolated chinchilla liver mitochondria. J Clin Invest 76:816, 1985

698. Touloukian RJ: Hepatic hemangioendothelioma during infancy: Pathology, diagnosis and treatment with prednisone. Pediatrics 45:71, 1970

699. Trolle D: Decrease of total serum bilirubin concentration in newborn infants after phenobarbitone treatment. Lancet 2:705, 1968

700. Tsalikian E et al: Glucose production and utilization in children with glycogen storage disease type I. Am J Physiol 247:E513, 1984

701. Tyson KRT et al: Portal hypertension in cystic fibrosis. J Pediatr Surg 3:271, 1968

702. Udall JN et al: The intestinal uptake of trypsin in newborn and weaned rabbits. Am J Physiol 247:G183, 1984

703. Udall JN et al: Liver disease in alpha-1-antitrypsin deficiency: A retrospective analysis of the influence of early breast- vs. bottle-feeding. JAMA 253:2679, 1985

704. Ulstrom RA, Eisenklam E: The enterohepatic shunting of bilirubin in the newborn infants: I. Use of oral activated charcoal to reduce normal serum bilirubin values. J Pediatr 65:27, 1964

705. Utili R et al: Inhibition of Na$^+$,K$^+$-ATPase by endotoxin: A possible mechanism for endotoxin-induced cholestasis. J Infect Dis 136:583, 1977

706. Valaes T et al: Incidence and mechanism of neonatal jaundice related to glucose-6-phosphate dehydrogenase deficiency. Pediatr Res 3:448, 1969

707. Valdes OS et al: Controlled clinical trial of phenobarbital and/or light in reducing neonatal hyperbilirubinemia in a predominantly Negro population. J Pediatr 79:1015, 1971

708. Valencia–Mayoral P et al: Possible defect in the bile secretory apparatus in arteriohepatic dysplasia (Alagille's syndrome): A review with observations on the ultrastructure of liver. Hepatology 4:691, 1984

709. Valentine WN et al: Pyruvate kinase and other enzyme-deficiency disorders of the erythrocyte. In Stanbury JB et al (eds): The Metabolic Basis of Inherited Disease, 5th ed, pp 1606. New York, McGraw-Hill, 1983

710. Valman HB et al: Prolonged neonatal jaundice in cystic fibrosis. Arch Dis Child 46:805, 1971

711. Van Praagh R: Diagnosis of kernicterus in the neonatal period. Pediatrics 28:870, 1961

712. Varma RR et al: Reye's syndrome in nonpediatric age groups. JAMA 242:1373, 1979

713. Vegnente A et al: Duration of chronic active hepatitis and the development of cirrhosis. Arch Dis Child 59:330, 1984

714. Vest M et al: A double blind study of the effect of phenobarbitone on neonatal hyperbilirubinemia and frequency of exchange transfusion. Acta Paediatr Scand 59:681, 1970

715. Vileisis RA et al: Prospective controlled study of parenteral nutrition–associated cholestatic jaundice: Effect of protein intake. J Pediatr 96:893, 1980

716. Volk BJ, Wallace BJ: The liver in lipidosis: An electron microscopic and histochemical study. Am J Pathol 49:203, 1966

717. Voorhies TM et al: Acute hyperammonemia in the young primate: Physiologic and neuropathologic correlates. Pediatr Res 17:970, 1983

718. Wadlington WB, Riley HD: Familial disease characterized by neonatal jaundice, and probable hepatosteatosis and kernicterus: A new syndrome? Paediatrics 51:192, 1973

719. Wagget J et al: Hemangioendothelioma of the liver in an infant: Hypotensive crisis during resection. Surgery 65:352, 1969

720. Walker W: Role of liquor examination. Br Med J 2:220, 1970

721. Walker WA et al: Needle biopsy of the liver in infancy and childhood: A safe diagnostic aid in liver disease. Pediatrics 40:946, 1967

722. Waters WJ, Porter E: Indications for exchange transfusion based upon the role of albumin in the treatment of hemolytic disease of the newborn. Pediatrics 33:749, 1964

723. Watson GH, Miller V: Arteriohepatic dysplasia: Familial pulmonary arterial stenosis with neonatal liver disease. Arch Dis Child 43:459, 1973

724. Watson JRH: Hepatosplenomegaly as a complication of maternal rubella: Report of two cases. Med J Aust 1:516, 1952

725. Webb LJ, Sherlock S: The aetiology, presentation and natural history of extra-hepatic portal venous obstruction. Q J Med 192:627, 1979

726. Weber A et al: Severe familial cholestasis in North American Indian children: A clinical model of microfilament dysfunction? Gastroenterology 81:653, 1981

727. Weinberg AG, Finegold MJ: Primary hepatic tumors of childhood. Hum Pathol 14:512, 1983

728. Weinberg AG et al: The occurrence of hepatoma in the chronic form of hereditary tyrosinemia. J Pediatr 88:434, 1976

729. Weldon AP, Danks DM: Congenital hypothyroidism and neonatal jaundice. Arch Dis Child 47:469, 1972

730. Weller TH: The cytomegalovirus: Ubiquitous agents with protean clinical manifestations. N Engl J Med 285:203, 267, 1971

731. Weller TH, Hanshaw JV: Virological and clinical observations on cytomegalic inclusion disease. N Engl J Med 266:1233, 1962

732. Wells WW et al: The isolation and identification of galactitol from the urine of patients with galactosemia. J Biol Chem 239:3192, 1964

733. Wenger DA et al: Niemann-Pick disease: A genetic model in Siamese cats. Science 208:1471, 1980

734. Wennberg RP, Thaler MM: Influence of intravenous nutrients on bilirubin transport: I. Amino acid solutions. Pediatr Res 11:163, 1977

735. Wennberg RP et al: Early versus delayed feeding of low birth weight infants: Effects on physiologic jaundice. J Pediatr 68:860, 1966

736. Whalen G et al: Impaired biliary excretion of phenol 3,6-dibromophthalein disulfonate in neonatal guinea pigs. Proc Soc Exp Biol Med 137:598, 1971

737. Whelton MJ et al: Reduction in serum bilirubin by phenobarbital in adult nonconjugative hemolytic jaundice. Am J Med 45:160, 1968

738. Whitington PF: Cholestasis associated with total parenteral nutrition in infants. Hepatology 5:693, 1985

739. Wills EJ: Electron microscopy of the liver in infectious mononucleosis, hepatitis and cytomegalovirus hepatitis. Am J Dis Child 123:301, 1972

740. Wilson JT: Phenobarbital in the neonatal period. Pediatrics 43:324, 1969

741. Winsnes A, Bratlid D: Effects of bilirubin loading of pregnant rats on hepatic UDP-glucuronyltransferase activity in the offspring. Biol Neonate 22:367, 1973

742. Witzleben CL, Sharp AR: Nephronophthisis-congenital hepatic fibrosis: An additional hepatorenal disorder. Hum Pathol 13:728, 1982

743. Wolfe HJ, Pictra G: The visceral lesions of metachromatic leukodystrophy. Am J Pathol 44:921, 1964

744. Wolkoff AW et al: Role of ligandin in transfer of bilirubin from plasma into liver. Am J Physiol 236:E638, 1979

745. Wolman M et al: Primary familal xanthomatosis with in-

volvement and calcification of the adrenals. Pediatrics 28: 742, 1961

746. Wong CG et al: Hepatic ganglioside abnormalities in a patient with familial erythrophagocytic lymphohistiocytosis. Pediatr Res 17:413, 1983

747. Wysowski et al: Epidemic neonatal hyperbilirubinemia and use of a phenolic disinfectant detergent. Pediatrics 61:165, 1978

748. Xu ZY et al: Prevention of perinatal acquisition of hepatitis B virus carriage using vaccine: Preliminary report of a randomized, double-blind placebo-controlled and comparative trial. Pediatrics 76:713, 1985

749. Yaffe SJ et al: Enhancement of glucuronide-conjugating capacity in a hyperbilirubinemic infant due to apparent enzyme induction by phenobarbital. N Engl J Med 275: 1461, 1966

750. Yamamoto K et al: Hilar biliary plexus in human liver: A comparative study of the intrahepatic bile ducts in man and animals. Lab Invest 52:103, 1985

751. Yen SSC et al: Herpes simplex infection in female genital tract. Obstet Gynecol 25:479, 1965

752. Yeung CY et al: Phenobarbitone prophylaxis for neonatal hyperbilirubinemia. Pediatrics 48:372, 1971

753. Young JL, Miller RW: Incidence of malignant tumors in U.S. children. J Pediatr 86:254, 1975

754. Yunis E, Bridges R: The serologic diagnosis of ABO hemolytic disease of the newborn. Am J Clin Pathol 41:1964

755. Yunis EJ et al: Fine structural observations of the liver in alpha-1-antitrypsin deficiency. Am J Pathol 82:265, 1976

756. Zaidenberg P et al: Increase in levels of glucuronylating enzymes and associated rise in activities of microsomal oxidative enzymes upon phenobarbital administration in the rat. J Cell Biol 32:528, 1967

757. Zitelli BJ et al: Hepatic homograft survival in pediatric orthotopic liver transplantation with cyclosporine and steroids. Transplant Proc 15 (Suppl 1):2592, 1983

758. Zuelzer WW, Stulberg CS: Herpes simplex virus as the cause of fulminating visceral disease and hepatitis in infancy. Am J Dis Child 83:421, 1952

Original work supported by General Clinical Research Centers Grant RR 123 and Pediatric Liver Research Foundation. The invaluable assistance of Drs. Frederick J. Suchy, George Hug, Janet E. Strife, Kevin E. Bove, A. James McAdams and Veronica Woyshville, Brenda Moore, and Anthony Balistreri of the Children's Hospital Research Foundation is acknowledged.

chapter 44
Miscellaneous Disorders

part 1
Sphincter of Oddi Dysfunction

JOSEPH E. GEENEN and RAMA P. VENU

The existence of a specialized group of muscle fibers at the distal choledochus was established as early as 1681 by Francis Glisson. In 1720, Abraham Vater, the Wittenberg anatomist, described the major duodenal papilla containing the intestinal exodus of the biliary pancreatic ducts. Nearly a century ago, Rugero Oddi pointed out that this strategically located muscle is a dynamic structure with a sphincter-like mechanism that now bears his name, that is, the sphincter of Oddi (SO).[31] Additionally, Oddi first demonstrated that jaundice could be functional in origin owing to spasm of the sphincter. Thirty years later, Meltzer, from his laboratory studies, showed that both jaundice and biliary colic could be caused by SO spasm.[27] Since then, most conclusions regarding the function of SO have been based on indirect evidences of measuring sphincter pressures in experimental animals.

In humans, the majority of pressure measurements have been obtained either at the time of operation or through a T-tube early in the postoperative period. Valuable observation regarding biliary duct emptying was also obtained from cineradiographic observations during T-tube cholangiography. Two new developments in the past decade opened a new era in our understanding of SO motility: (1) The advent of a lateral viewing endoscope with the ability to freely cannulate the papilla of Vater and (2) the miniaturization of a perfusion system. This new perfusion system has minimal compliance, and using a specific flow rate, accurate and reproducible pressure recording of the SO is now possible under acceptable laboratory conditions.

ANATOMY

Our present understanding of the structure of the distal choledochus is largely based on the pioneering anatomical studies of Boyden.[5,6] The terminal ends of the common bile duct and pancreatic duct course obliquely through the duodenal wall as they approach their intestinal exodus. Radiographic anatomy during endoscopic retrograde cholangiopancreatography (ERCP) has shown that the common bile duct and the pancreatic duct form a common channel in 80% of subjects prior to their termination in the duodenum via the papillary orifice.[13] A variable length of this distal segment of common bile duct and pancreatic duct is invested with circular and longitudinal smooth muscle fibers that interdigitate with juxta-ampullary muscle fibers of the duodenal wall to form the SO. Boyden noted a discrete area of muscle thickness situated at the distal choledochus, pancreatic duct, and papilla. These "mini sphincters" have been referred to as sphincter choledochus, sphincter pancreaticus, and sphincter papillae. Manometric studies, however, failed to identify such discrete sphincters at the termination of each duct.

PHYSIOLOGY

Many key observations of the physiology of SO motility came from experimental animals. A brief review of such studies, therefore, seems essential, if not mandatory. The close anatomic relationship between the smooth muscle fibers constituting the sphincter and that of the duodenal wall makes one wonder whether both these groups of muscle fibers function as a single motor unit. Studies in dogs, cats, rabbits, monkeys, and opossum have demonstrated that the sphincter functions independently of duodenal muscle activity.[19,20,25,32] Notable among such studies is the electromyographic studies conducted in the opossum sphincter that revealed distinct electrical spike potential in the sphincter segment that were quite independent of the duodenal spikes. Embryologic studies have also shown that the SO develops from specialized mesenchymal tissue, independent of duodenal musculature, and subsequently migrates into the duodenal wall.[5]

Having realized that the SO is an independent motor unit, let us look at its possible physiologic role. The SO is strategically located at the choledochoduodenal junction to modulate the flow of two important digestive secretions: bile and pancreatic juice. Experimental work in dogs demonstrated that the lower end of the common bile duct exhibited a milking effect on bile, propelling small volumes of bile from the common bile duct into the duodenum.[43]

An excellent animal model developed in American opossums has recently provided valuable information on the sphincter dynamics.[35] In the opossum, the sphincter muscle is located extraduodenally and thus helps to avoid recording interference from the duodenum. Additionally, the opossum SO has forceful phasic wave activity that is similar in amplitude and frequency to that of human sphincter activity. Electromyographic and manometric studies of the opossum SO demonstrate phasic contractions that propagated along the entire length from cephalad to caudad end. At the most distal end of the choledochus, a high pressure zone of 4 mm to 6 mm in length is noted. This so-called SO zone has a basal pressure 5 mm Hg above common bile duct pressure. Superimposed on the resting pressure rhythmically appearing phasic waves are noted at a frequency of 2 to 8 per minute. The common bile duct proximal to this shows no motor activity and appears to be passive conduits for bile.

Simultaneous cineradiography, transsphincteric flow, and electromyographic recordings from the opossum sphincter have demonstrated the influence of phasic wave contractions on bile flow into the duodenum. Antegrade phasic contractions seem to be the predominant mechanism of common bile duct emptying in the opossum. A phasic wave contraction initiated at the junction of the common bile duct and SO milks the bile duct content into the duodenum. During the SO phasic contractions (*i.e.,* sphincter "systole") bile flow ceases from the bile duct into the sphincter segment. Following sphincter systole, relaxation of the sphincter or sphincter "diastole" takes place and passive flow of bile occurs from the common bile duct into the sphincter segment. The next sequence of phasic contractions strips the bile into the duodenum, and the cycle repeats itself, resulting in sequential emptying of the common bile duct.

Based on these observations, the major physiologic role of the sphincter seems to be to keep the SO free of mucus and food, to provide a forceful pump in the event of a partial obstruction, and to clear calculi or debris from the distal bile duct.

Much of the information from the animal studies has been applied to SO motility studies in humans, and glimpses of the physiologic role of human SO are slowly emerging. For years cineradiographic studies of the SO segment have shown spontaneous rhythmic contractions that are comparable to intervals of systolic contractions separated by intervals of diastolic phase.[8]

Manometric studies conducted during biliary tract surgery reveal a zone of resistance at the terminal end of the common bile duct.[12] Both CCK-octapeptide and nitrate cause predictable decrease in the resistance to bile flow. However, direct pressure measurement in the SO was not feasible in humans until the advent of ERCP. Consistent and reproducible manometric studies are now possible in the majority of patients during ERCP under mild sedation.[9,11,18,21]

TECHNIQUE

Two water-perfused infusion (flow rate 0.25 ml/min) side-hole polyethylene catheters are used for manometry. One catheter is inserted through the biopsy channel of the duodenoscope, which can be advanced into the bile duct or pancreatic duct (Fig. 44-1). A second catheter attached

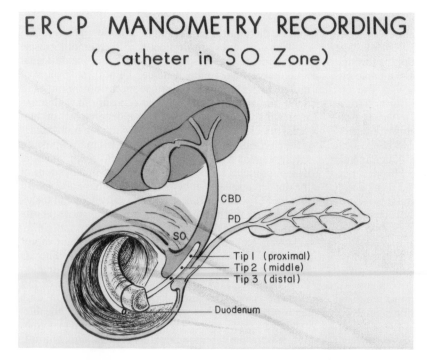

ERCP MANOMETRY RECORDING
(Catheter in SO Zone)

CBD
PD
SO
Tip 1 (proximal)
Tip 2 (middle)
Tip 3 (distal)
Duodenum

Fig. 44-1. Schematic diagram showing the triple lumen catheter position at the sphincter of Oddi zone. Note the manometry catheter advanced through the side-viewing endoscope.

externally to the duodenoscope will record the intraluminal pressures continuously. Initially, the catheter is advanced to at least 2 cm into the bile or pancreatic duct, well beyond the SO zone. The pressure of the common bile duct or pancreatic duct is then recorded. The catheter is then slowly withdrawn and positioned at the SO zone. By station pull-throughs of 2- to 3-mm increments, the SO pressure is determined. For accuracy and reproducibility, the same technique is repeated two or three times in the same patient.

NORMAL SO PRESSURE PROFILE IN HUMANS

The SO demonstrates a basal or resting pressure that averages 8 mm above the common bile duct or pancreatic duct pressure. Superimposed on the basal pressure are high-amplitude phasic wave contractions that occur at a mean frequency of 4 ± 0.5/min (Fig. 44-2). Phasic wave contractions measure 150 ± 16 mm Hg in amplitude and are 4.3 ± 0.5 seconds in duration. Using a triple-lumen pressure catheter with perfused open tips spaced 2 mm apart, these phasic waves are recorded over a 4- to 6-mm

segment of the distal choledochus or SO zone. The direction of the waves recorded between these three recording orifices has been determined during a 3- to 5-minute period. Contraction sequences were antegrade in direction, that is, directed toward the duodenum 61% of the time. Retrograde sequences (*i.e.,* directed away from the duodenum) were noted 30% of the time. In 26%, contraction sequences occurred simultaneously at all three recording orifices.

REGULATORY FACTORS OF SO MOTILITY

Evidence is also accumulating regarding the factors regulating the sphincter motor activity. Histochemical studies of the SO have demonstrated adrenergic as well as cholinergic neurons in the SO segment of cats and dogs. Several hormones and neurotransmitters like CCK, gastrin, secretin, and encephalins have been identified in the sphincter muscle. These observations indicate that the SO muscle might be under a complex neurohumoral control. Vagal transection in dogs results in decreased resistance of transphincteric flow, indicating a cholinergic influence

Fig. 44-2. Manometric tracing of SO showing normal phasic wave. Note the SO shows a basal pressure of 20 mm Hg. Superimposed on the basal pressure are phasic wave contractions of about 100 mm Hg with a frequency of 3/min. Tracing for three recording tips and duodenal pressure is also shown (below).

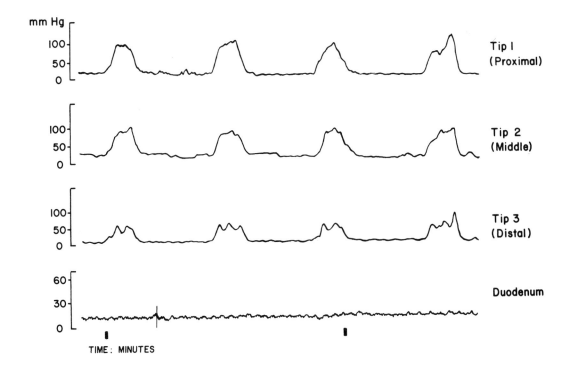

to the basal tone of the sphincter.[4] Similarly, intravenous pulse doses of atropine in humans produced decreased phasic contraction frequency and amplitude.[41] Several enteric hormones have also been known to influence the SO motor activity.[24]

One of the earliest hormones studied is CCK-octapeptide. CCK-octapeptide inhibited phasic wave contractions in humans and certain animals.[36] However, when the animal was pretreated with a neurotoxin (*i.e.*, tetrodotoxin) thus abolishing all the neurons, CCK-octapeptide produced a stimulation of phasic wave contractions.[3] This finding indicated that CCK might have a direct stimulatory effect that is overridden by the indirect inhibitory effect.

The effect of several other enteric hormones on SO motor activity also has been studied during ERCP manometry.[18] Similar to CCK, intravenous pulse doses of glucagon reduce basal SO phasic pressure and markedly inhibit SO phasic wave contractions and frequency rate. Intravenous administration of pentagastrin, on the other hand, causes an increase in the SO phasic waves. Secretin appears to cause an initial increase in SO phasic wave amplitude and frequency, followed within minutes by a profound inhibition of phasic motor activity. Histamine seems to have a dual effect on the sphincter function of the opossum. However, the overall effect seems to be inhibitory. This depressant effect is mediated by actual receptor stimulation of nonadrenergic, noncholinergic inhibitory nerves overriding the H_2 stimulation effect of the sphincter muscle.[37]

Intravenous administration of morphine sulfate in doses of 0.05 μg/kg stimulates the phasic wave contractions.[41] The stimulatory effect of morphine is less pronounced when the subjects are pretreated with naloxone, an opiate antagonist.

In summary, this confusing array of laboratory observations generated during the past decade, although inconclusive, at least suggest to us that the SO is controlled by a multitude of factors. The understanding of the physiologic role of human SO requires further clarification. The sphincter is a superbly adaptive structure that has an ejecting and occluding mechanism. The primary physiologic role of the sphincter seems to be for regulating the pressure within the biliary system. Irrespective of the bile flow rate, pressure within the bile duct is maintained within a narrow range of low pressure that allows the hepatic secretion to proceed. If the pressure inside the bile duct is excessive, sphincter contraction decreases or stops, which then allows transsphincteric passive flow to decrease the pressure. The SO actively participates in regulating the pressure events in the biliary tree by controlling the bile flow.

SO DYSFUNCTION OR BILIARY DYSKINESIA

This poorly understood clinical entity has been defined as a structural or functional disorder involving the SO,

causing a variety of signs and symptoms resulting from an impedance to the flow of biliary and/or pancreatic secretions. A myriad of terminologies have been used to describe SO dysfunction, including dystonia, dyssynergia, spastic and atonic distention, postcholecystectomy syndrome, and sphincterismus. The exact incidence of this entity is unknown, but it may account for 1% to 10% of patients with postcholecystectomy pain syndrome. Ten percent to 20% of patients with idiopathic recurrent pancreatitis may have SO dysfunction. There may be at least two types of SO dysfunction. One is a structural abnormality resulting from chronic inflammation and fibrosis. In this form there is actual stenosis or narrowing of the intraduodenal segment of the distal choledochus. This type is generally designated as papillary stenosis, and it may be etiologically related to chronic irritation from spontaneous migration of gallstones or trauma resulting, for example, from intraoperative manipulation of the distal common bile duct or adenomyosis.[10]

The second variety called SO dyskinesia designates a functional disturbance of the SO. This variety of SO dysfunction may be related to spasm or muscular hypertrophy or denervation; however, little anatomical confirmation exists to support any of these hypotheses. A disturbance in reciprocal dynamics between gallbladder and SO has been postulated for decades and reiterated recently as an explanation for SO dyskinesia.[34] Unfortunately, our knowledge concerning this disintegration mechanism is less than desirable in normal persons, let alone in patients with biliary tract symptoms.

CLINICAL FEATURES

Patients presenting with SO dysfunction have generally been subjected to cholecystectomy with or without any evidence of cholelithiasis. Abdominal pain is the single most common presenting symptom. Typically it is located in the right upper quadrant or epigastrium with radiation to the back or shoulder. It may be intermittent or postprandial and may be "biliary colic." Nausea is the second most common symptom, followed by vomiting. Patients may have intermittent jaundice or fever. Another group of patients may present with recurrent episodes of pancreatitis.[42]

In our clinical attempt to characterize SO dysfunction better, we divided the patients into three groups:

Group I—definitive SO dysfunction (patients must meet all the following criteria): (1) biliary tract pain; (2) elevated serum alkaline phosphatase, bilirubin, or both on two occasions; (3) dilated common bile duct (>12 mm) above a normal-appearing SO segment on ERCP; and (4) delayed drainage of contrast material from the common bile duct (>45 minutes) on ERCP

Group II—presumptive SO dysfunction (patients will meet the following criteria): (1) biliary tract pain; (2) positive findings for one or two of items 2, 3, 4, and 5

Group III—idiopathic recurrent pancreatitis

CLINICAL EVALUATION

Clinical evaluation of patients with SO dysfunction should include history and physical examination, liver function tests, and serum amylase evaluation. Provocative tests using intramuscular injection of morphine sulfate (1 mg) and prostigmine (10 mg) had been advocated as a noninvasive test to select patients with SO dysfunction.[30] These pharmacologic agents cause spasm of the sphincter muscle in patients with SO dysfunction, leading to elevation in amylase, lipase, and/or transaminase. Characteristically, the biliary tract pain is also reproduced.

The early enthusiasm generated by these provocative tests is tempered by the most recent reports indicating that the morphine-prostigmine test (MPT) is not accurate or reliable in selecting patients with SO dysfunction.[26,33]

At present, ERCP seems to be the most valuable investigatory tool for identifying SO dysfunction. ERCP provides us with anatomic information on the diameter of the bile duct, especially to detect dilated biliary ducts as well as biliary drainage time. At the same time, other causes of biliary tract obstruction such as a common bile duct stone may also be ruled out by ERCP. However, the most critical information available through ERCP is SO manometry. At least four distinct manometric abnormalities have been identified in patients with suspected SO dysfunction:

1. *Increased SO basal pressure.* Significant increase in the basal SO pressure has been reported by several investigators.[1,28] A similar increase in the amplitude of phasic contractions also has been noted in some cases. It seems that this increased basal pressure is lowered favorably by intravenous pulse doses of glucagon and inhalation of nitrate by decreasing the pressure. The underlying mechanism of raised basal pressure seems to be spasm or fibrosis involving the intrasphincter muscle. Recent observation made on operative specimens in patients with SO dysfunction lends some credence to this hypothesis.[29]

2. *Paradoxical response to CCK-octapeptide.* The normal response of the SO to intravenous administration of CCK-octapeptide is to abolish phasic wave contractions and significantly decrease the basal pressure. However, a number of patients with clinical findings consistent with SO dysfunction show a paradoxic increase in the basal pressure following intravenous pulse doses of CCK-octapeptide. (Fig. 44-3).[23] This effect is comparable to the paradoxic increase in pressure noted at the lower esophageal sphincter by CCK in patients with achalasia. These findings indicate that perhaps in some patients with SO dysfunction, the sphincter may be denervated by some unknown mechanism and this, in turn, results in a stimulatory effect by CCK-octapeptide.

3. *Retrograde propagation of phasic wave contractions.* The predominant propagation of phasic waves in normal subjects is antegrade (*i.e.,* toward the duodenum).

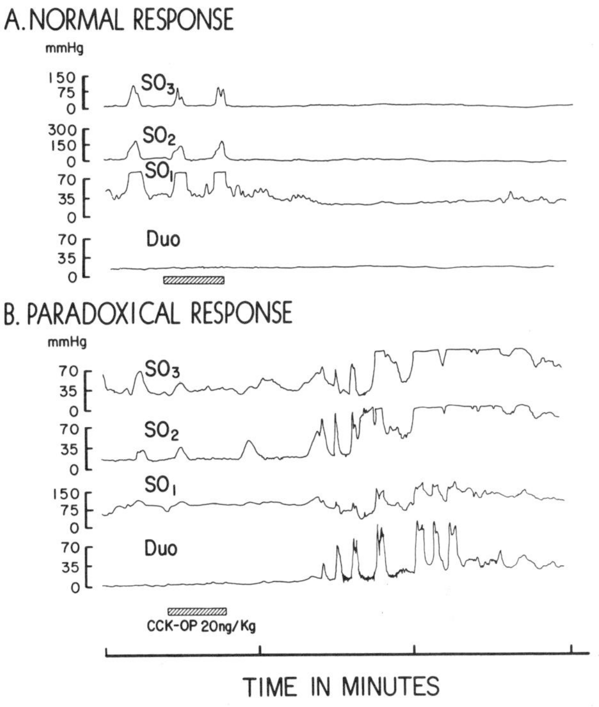

Fig. 44-3. SO manometry showing response to IV CCK-OP. **A.** The normal response. Note the total elimination of phasic wave contractions following CCK administration. **B.** Paradoxical response in a patient with SO dysfunction. Note the increase in basal pressure following CCK.

Retrograde propagation of phasic contraction was initially noted in patients with common duct stones.[39] Soon similar retrograde propagation was reported in patients with SO dysfunction (Fig. 44-4). It is conceivable that such retrograde propagation might be nonperistaltic and might result in impedance to transsphincteric flow.

4. *Increased frequency of phasic wave contractions or "tachyoddia."* Normal SO manometry shows phasic wave contractions at a frequency of 2 to 4/min. Increased frequency of phasic wave contractions has been reported in several patients with suspected SO dysfunction (Fig. 44-5).[22] Such increased frequency of phasic wave activity has been shown to occur following intravenous bolus of morphine sulfate. An impedance to contrast flow into the duodenum resulting from IV bolus of morphine sulfate demonstrated during fluoroscopic monitoring lends support that tachyoddia seen in these patients might cause a functional obstruction to bile flow, causing pain and abnormal results of liver function tests. A similar impedance to biliary flow also has been demonstrated by increasing the phasic wave contraction frequency in American opossums.

These characteristic manometric findings may be seen either alone or in a combination in any single patient with

SO PHASIC WAVE PROPAGATION

A. ANTEGRADE

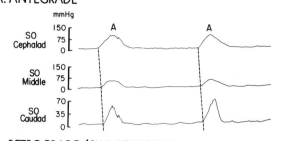

B. RETROGRADE/SIMULTANEOUS

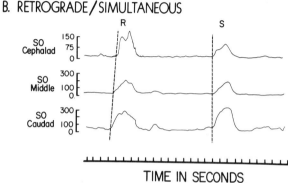

Fig. 44-4. SO manometry recording demonstrating antegrade (*above*) and retrograde progression of phasic waves. In antegrade propagation (*above*), the most proximal recording tip records the phasic contractions followed by the middle tip and then the distal tip. Note the retrograde propagation of phasic waves (*below*), which is exactly opposite of the above.

SO dysfunction.[38] Although these manometric findings may be constant, one must question why is it that the symptoms resulting from SO dysfunction are intermittent. One may be tempted to postulate that high basal pressure, tachyoddia, or other manometric abnormalities may not be responsible for the symptoms and the underlying SO characteristics might make them respond to provocation differently.[7] This hypothesis is partly supported by the paradoxic response to CCK-octapeptide in patients with SO dysfunction.

The validity of any abnormal finding is pertinent only if there is clinical improvement following successful therapeutic intervention directed toward such abnormalities. In this respect, evidence has been accumulated that by operative sphincteroplasty or by endoscopic sphincterotomy, significant clinical improvement may be achieved in patients with SO dysfunction.

In order to categorize patients with suspected SO dysfunction we divided the patients with SO dysfunction into three groups, as indicated earlier. In our series of 18 patients belonging to group I, 17 patients had symptomatic improvement following endoscopic sphincterotomy. All of these 18 patients had increased elevated SO basal pressure. In the presumptive group, 29 of 35 patients who had increased basal pressure showed clinical improvement following endoscopic sphincterotomy. In persons with normal pressures, only 3 were improved, and in 18 there was no change. A similar correlation of clinical improvement and increased basal pressure following endoscopic sphincterotomy was seen in patients with idiopathic recurrent pancreatitis.

To determine whether manometric studies are truly useful in selecting patients who would benefit from en-

Fig. 44-5. Manometry tracing from a patient with tachyoddia. Note that the number of phasic contractions in a minute exceeds 10.

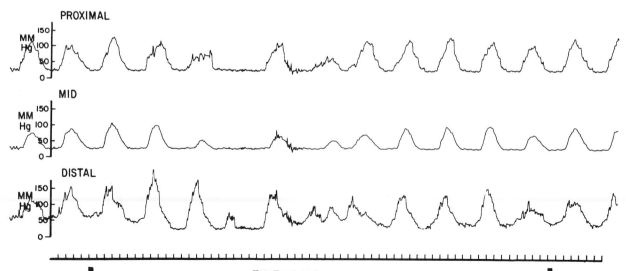

doscopic sphincterotomy, a randomized prospective study also was conducted in patients with presumptive SO dysfunction.[14] Postcholecystectomy patients with recurrent biliary-like pain of greater than 6 months' duration and one or two of the following clinical features were included in the study: (1) dilated bile duct (>12 mm), (2) delayed contrast drainage (>45 minutes) and (3) abnormal results of liver function tests.

Of the 45 patients randomized and followed for 12 months, 22 patients underwent endoscopic sphincterotomy and 23 patients underwent sham sphincterotomy; 68% of patients with sphincterotomy showed clinical improvement, whereas only 30% of patients with sham endoscopic sphincterotomy showed clinical improvement. When the clinical improvement was correlated with SO basal pressure, again a positive correlation was noted, that is, patients who had elevated basal pressures seemed to benefit from endoscopic sphincterotomy while in patients with normal pressures improvement was not that significant.

The next single diagnostic test that helps to select patients with suspected SO dysfunction other than increased pressure is biliary drainage. These carefully conducted studies no doubt support the view that ERCP and SO manometry can certainly identify patients with suspected SO dysfunction, and it can especially select patients for successful endoscopic sphincterotomy. Limited information is also available on the long-term effect of endoscopic sphincterotomy. Endoscopic sphincterotomy virtually eliminates the pressure gradient between the common bile duct and duodenum.[15] Although the resting tone was eliminated for 2 years, the phasic wave contractions returned.[17] Endoscopic sphincterotomy seems to be a reasonable approach to patients with SO dysfunction, however, one should like to keep the options for a less invasive therapeutic approach. This is mainly because endoscopic sphincterotomy is associated with a morbidity rate of 7% and a mortality rate of 0.5%.[40] The incidence of re-stenosis following endoscopic sphincterotomy in patients with SO dysfunction is also higher than in those patients with common bile duct stones.[16] Pharmacologic agents such as nitrates have been reported to be effective in isolated cases of SO dysfunction.[2]

Now that we have made some progress in defining SO dysfunction and characterizing patients with this complex but rare clinical entity, we should look forward to further studies. The day when we can select patients with SO dysfunction with a simple provocative test may not be far off. New pharmacologic agents might appear on the horizon to manage patients with SO dysfunction. Until then, ERCP and SO manometry will remain our only hope to clearly identify patients with SO dysfunction.

REFERENCES

1. Bar-Meir S et al: Biliary and pancreatic duct pressures measured by ERCP manometry in patients with suspected papillary stenosis. Dig Dis Sci 24:209, 1979
2. Bar-Meir S et al: Nitrate therapy in a patient with papillary dysfunction. Am J Gastroenterol 78:94, 1983
3. Behar J, Biancani P: Effect of cholecystokinin and octapeptide of cholecystokinin on the feline sphincter of Oddi and gallbladder. J Clin Invest 66:1231, 1980
4. Benevantano TC et al: The physiological effect of acute vagal resection on canine biliary dynamics. J Surg Res 9:331, 1969
5. Boyden EA: The sphincter of Oddi in man and certain representative mammals. Surgery 1:25, 1937
6. Boyden EA: Anatomy of the choledochoduodenal junction in man. Surg Gynecol Obstet 106:647, 1957
7. Burnett DA: Editorial: Taking the pressure off the sphincter of Oddi. Gastroenterology 87:971, 1984
8. Caroli J et al: Contribution of cineradiography to study of the function of the human biliary tract. Am J Dig Dis 5:677, 1960
9. Carr-Locke DL, Gregg JA: Endoscopic manometry of pancreatic and biliary sphincter zones in man: Basal results in healthy volunteers. Dig Dis Sci 87:971, 1981
10. Classen M et al: Stenosis of the papilla Vateri and common bile duct. Clin Gastroenterol 12:203, 1983
11. Csendes A et al: Pressure measurements in the biliary and pancreatic duct systems in controls and in patients with gallstones, previous cholecystectomy or common bile duct strictures. Gastroenterology 77:1203, 1979
12. Cushieri A et al: Biliary pressure studies during cholecystectomy. Br J Surg 59:267, 1972
13. Geenen JE, Hogan WJ: Endoscopic access to the papilla of Vater. Endoscopy 12:47, 1980
14. Geenen JE et al: A prospective randomized study of the efficacy of endoscopic sphincterotomy in patients with presumptive sphincter of Oddi dysfunction (abstr). Gastroenterology 86:1086, 1984
15. Geenen JE et al: Endoscopic electrosurgical papillotomy and manometry in biliary tract disease. JAMA 237:2075, 1977
16. Geenen JE et al: Resume of a seminar on endoscopic retrograde sphincterotomy (ERS). Gastrointest Endosc 27:31, 1982
17. Geenen JE et al: Endoscopic sphincterotomy: Follow-up evaluation of effects on the sphincter of Oddi. Gastroenterology 87:754, 1984
18. Geenen JE et al: Intraluminal pressure recording from the human sphincter of Oddi. Gastroenterology 78:317, 1980
19. Hauge CW, Mark JBD: Common bile duct motility and sphincter mechanism: Pressure measurements with multilumen catheters in dogs. Ann Surg 162:1028, 1965
20. Hedner P, Rorsman G: On the mechanism of action for the effect of CCK on the choledochoduodenal function in the cat. Acta Physiol Scand 76:248, 1969
21. Hogan WJ et al: Motility and biliary dyskinesia. In Chey WY (ed): Functional Disorders of the GI Tract, pp 267–275. New York, Raven Press, 1983
22. Hogan WJ et al: Abnormally rapid phasic contractions of the human sphincter of Oddi (tachyoddia). Gastroenterology 84:1189, 1983
23. Hogan WJ et al: Paradoxical motor response to the cholecystokinin (CCK-OP) in patients with suspected sphincter of Oddi dyskinesia (abstr). Gastroenterology 82:1085, 1983
24. Honda R et al: Effect of enteric hormones on sphincter of Oddi and gastrointestinal myoelectric activity in fasted conscious opossums. Gastroenterology 84:1, 1983
25. LaMorte WW et al: Choledochal sphincter relaxation in response to histamine in the primate. J Surg Res 28:373, 1980
26. LoGuidice JA et al: Efficacy of the morphine-prostigmine

test for evaluating patients with suspected papillary stenosis. Dig Dis 24:455, 1979

27. Meltzer SJ: Disturbance of law of contrary innervation as a pathogenetic factor in the diseases of the bile ducts and gall-bladder. Am J Med Sci 153:469, 1917

28. Meshkinpour H et al: Bile duct dyskinesia, a clinical and manometric study. Gastroenterology 87:759, 1984

29. Moody FG et al: Transduodenal sphincteroplasty and trans-ampullary septectomy for post-cholecystectomy pain. Ann Surg 197:627, 1983

30. Nardi GL, Acosta JM: Papillitis as a cause of pancreatitis and abdominal pain: Role of evocative test, operative pan-creatography and histological evaluation. Ann Surg 164:611, 1966

31. Oddi R: D'une disposition a sphincter de Pouvesture du canal cholidoque. Arch Ital Biol 8:317, 1887

32. Ono K: The discharge of bile into the duodenum and elec-trical activities of the muscle of Oddi and duodenum. Jap J Smooth Muscle Res 6:123, 1970

33. Steinberg WM et al: The morphine-prostigmine provocative test—is it useful for making clinical decisions? Gastroenter-ology 78:728, 1980

34. Tanaka M et al: Change in bile duct pressure responses after cholecystectomy: Loss of gallbladder as a pressure reservoir. Gastroenterology 87:1154, 1984

35. Toouli J et al: Motor function of the opossum sphincter of Oddi. J Clin Invest 71:208, 1983

36. Toouli J et al: Action of cholecystokinin octapeptide on sphincter of Oddi basal pressure and phasic wave activity in humans. Surgery 92:497, 1982

37. Toouli J et al: Effect of histamine on motor function of opossum sphincter of Oddi. Am J Physiol 241:122, 1981

38. Toouli J et al: Manometric disorders in patients with sus-pected sphincter of Oddi dysfunction. Gastroenterology 88:1243, 1985

39. Toouli J et al: Sphincter of Oddi motor activity—a com-parison between patients with common bile duct stones and cirrhosis. Gastroenterology 82:111, 1982

40. Tedesco FJ, Vennes JA, Dreyer M: In O'Kabe H, Honda T, Oshiba F (eds): Endoscopic Sphincterotomy: The USA Ex-perience in Endoscopic Surgery, pp 41–46. New York, El-sevier, 1984

41. Venu RP et al: Effect of morphine on motor activity of the human sphincter of Oddi (abstr). Gastroenterology 84:1342, 1983

42. Venu RP et al: Idiopathic recurrent pancreatitis (IRP): Di-agnostic role of ERCP and sphincter of Oddi manometry (abstr). Gastrointest Endosc 31:141, 1985

43. Watts JM, Dunphy JE: The role of the common bile duct in biliary dynamics. Surg Gynecol Obstet 122:1277, 1966

part **2**

Intraoperative Biliary Endoscopy: Choledochoscopy

GEORGE BERCI

Since the first common bile duct was explored and stones were removed to cure symptoms of jaundice or cholangitis, the problems of a missed stone perplexes, equally, the operators and patients. One of our greatest surgeons, Hal-stead, died of complications of a retained stone. The in-cidence of retained calculi is not known, and the reports vary from 5% to 28%.[17] The results depend on the accuracy and on the length of the follow up. The incidence can fluctuate from year to year. It is essential, therefore, that all postoperative T-tube cholangiograms should be kept for a minimum period of 5 years to be able to obtain an accurate record of the results. The number of common bile duct explorations is relatively small because only one fifth or one sixth of patients with cholelithiasis coming to surgery need choledochotomies. The increase of endo-scopic papillotomies for retained stones in cholecystec-tomized patients also indicates that more stones are missed than the surgeons are aware of.

Gallstone operations are one of the most frequent types of operations on the surgical schedule. There are 750,000 cholecystectomies performed annually, with approxi-mately 120,000 explorations of the common bile duct in the United States alone. In the case of a 10% incidence of retained stone(s), this would mean that 12,000 patients will require a second procedure.[5,7] The socioeconomic impact of this is significant. If a patient has to accom-modate an indwelling T-tube for a period of 6 weeks, he cannot continue physical activities. The simplest, safest, and most successful second procedure is stone removal through the T-tube tract. This can be performed as an outpatient procedure without mortality and with minimal morbidity.[6] Endoscopic papillotomy requires a short hos-pital stay (1 to 3 days) and has a mortality of 1% to 1.4%, whereby a secondary exploration requires a minimum of 8 to 10 days of institutional care with increased morbidity and mortality.

It became, therefore a logical question to ask how this complication can be decreased in a common, benign, and curable disease. It was also obvious that working in a tu-bular organ semiblindly can result in a missed stone.

In 1923, Bakes was the first surgeon who drew attention to this complication and recommended the use of an ear funnel with a mirror and a little electric globe to look into the distal duct.[1] McIver, in 1941, designed a right-angled cystoscope with a tiny electric globe at the distal end to look into the ducts after the stone extraction attempts were completed.[14] Wildegans was the first in Europe who popularized choledochoscopy.[20] I started my career in bil-iary endoscopy using this instrument, but with less success than the original author.[2] With the introduction of the Hopkins rod-lens system, a smaller instrument could be designed with a better image quality and increased bright-ness.[18] The use of this instrument has become widely ac-cepted. With the advent of the flexible endoscope this technology also became available in the field of biliary endoscopy.[21] The general surgeon is not an endoscopist, and the rigid type of endoscope is easier to manipulate, simpler to use, and more durable for intraoperative performance. I use the flexible endoscope in the postoperative period if a stone retrieval is required through the T-tube tract.

We have to ask the question whether this important intraoperative diagnostic modality really decreased the incidence of a retained stone? Here, too, reports vary. Certain authors praise it and claim that only 0 to 3% of missed stones were confirmed by using the choledochoscope routinely,[10,11,13,16,22] whereby others do not support this claim.[9,15] However, all parties agree that if the choledochoscope is employed properly after standard stone extraction attempts, in 10% to 15% of cases stones that would otherwise have been missed were discovered. This, alone, is an important supporting fact.

A survey was conducted of 184 larger California hospitals, 87% of which had purchased a rigid or flexible choledochoscope. To our greatest surprise the surgeons used it during choledochotomies routinely in only 8% of cases. Another similar study also supports this information, namely, that the instruments are available but that surgeons are reluctant to use them.[19]

In our geographical area, if a surgeon performs 30 to 40 cholecystectomies per year this is regarded as a very good practice. However, this means that the experience of common bile duct exploration is limited to three to five cases during the same time period. We concluded, therefore, that during the past 14 years the concept of intraoperative biliary endoscopy was theoretically accepted but owing to lack of experience the method was not applied in practice on a larger scale.[8]

HOW TO LEARN AND PRACTICE CHOLEDOCHOSCOPY

Animal Model

In hospitals that have an animal laboratory, the vena cava below the renal veins and the lumbar and iliac vessels of a mongrel dog can be ligated, and in an hour or so an isolated vena cava, acting as a "dilated common bile duct," can be created. Choledochoscopy can be practiced with the various stone removal maneuvers. This is a time-consuming dissection, and it is not inexpensive.

Biliary Model

We had previously used plastic models to display the shape or the size of the extrahepatic biliary system with some of the hepatic branches. These models were not suitable because they were rigid and did not simulate the anatomic conditions. We designed a biliary phantom in which the "duodenum" has to be kept on a tension, to keep the distal duct on a stretch, to improve the visualization of the sphincter region.* The Kocher maneuver is essential and overlooked by many surgeons employing choledochoscopy, an important step that should not be omitted. Furthermore, during choledochoscopy, continuous irrigation is required. In this particular model irrigation can be employed because provision is made for it. Another aspect with which a surgeon has to become familiar is working under water.

Team Effort

Choledochoscopy is not a "one-man show" because four hands are required to keep the duodenum on a stretch and to introduce and manipulate the stone basket or grasper. In case a stone comes into vision, accessory instruments are introduced and the stone is withdrawn into the incision. The old concept to introduce the choledochoscope and if a stone is discovered to withdraw the scope and introduce standard instruments semiblindly only extends the operating time and does not provide the visual control. As soon as the surgeon is in a good position to retrieve the stone no further time should be wasted. The assistant should advance the most suitable accessory stone-grasping instrument, and both the surgeon and the assistant together should withdraw the entrapped calculus. During choledochoscopy the first opportunity is the best one, and in an edematous, inflamed duct prolonged manipulations should be avoided. The assistant should be able to follow the movements of the surgeon in a coordinated fashion.

Television Choledochoscopy

Choledochoscopy is greatly improved by television technique. It is made easier by observing the enlarged image of the intraluminal appearance, which can be seen from a convenient distance by the entire surgical team. I learned from orthopedic surgeons that delicate procedures (*e.g.,* meniscectomies, shaving of arthritic surfaces) can be performed with ease from the television screen by the surgeon and his assistant with the use of an arthroscope coupled to a television camera. The television camera can be shared among the orthopedists, general surgeons, and other specialists.[3]

The cost of a biliary phantom or the choledochoscope, with accessories, is minimal compared with the expenses involved if a retained stone is discovered and has to be removed at a later stage.

THE ROLE OF OPERATIVE CHOLANGIOGRAPHY

Choledochoscopy does not exclude cholangiography. These techniques are complementary, and both should

---

* Gaumard Scientific Co., Inc, Miami, FL.

be employed. I routinely use operative cholangiography and have had exceedingly good results.[4] Although this important intraoperative modality has been available for decades, there has been little effort made to improve the technique and to encourage its greater use. Surgeons continue to be skeptical about routine cholangiography because they claim it is too time consuming, its technical failure rate is unacceptably high, as is the false-positive or false-negative rate, and, furthermore, it is not cost effective. When it falls short of expectations, surgeons point to the radiologists, blaming equipment failure, poor exposure techniques, time delay, and interpretative errors, and, therefore, they feel frustrated by the lack of understanding and control of radiologic factors. Radiologists consider the examination as substandard because they lack direct control, blaming the surgeons for not understanding the basic technique, such as the necessity of good scout films, the importance of patient positioning, the careful injection of contrast material, and the removal of foreign bodies from the field. If progress is to be achieved, a cooperative effort must be made by both disciplines to the ultimate benefit of the patient.

An initial cystic duct or initial choledochocholangiogram is preferred because in these conditions there is a closed system without artifacts caused by manipulation. It provides much information to the surgeons early in the course of the operation. The timed display of ductal anatomy aids in subsequent dissection. Attention will be drawn to important anomalies of surgical interest (6%), and the number and location of stones will be displayed. With a well-performed negative cholangiogram, unnecessary exploration of the common bile duct (10% to 20%) accompanied by an increased morbidity can be avoided.[4]

CHOLEDOCHOSCOPY

Despite the frequency of biliary surgery the bile duct was the last hollow viscus for which endoscopy was developed. The biliary tract presents a special challenge for the general surgeon. The technique should be performed under strict sterile conditions. Sometimes the surgeon has to work for an hour or so in an extremely well-illuminated area until he is able to use a scope and then he changes to a small monocular eyepiece. These sudden changes can make perception difficult. These requirements perhaps inhibited successful application until the recent evolution in optical technology. The explosion in electronics with the development of a miniature sterilizable attachable television camera contributes to significant changes in future endoscopic procedures.

There are two types of choledochoscopes available, the rigid one and the flexible one. It does not matter which type of instrument is employed as long as the operator knows how to use it. We prefer the rigid scope because it is simpler to manipulate, easier to learn how to use, and less expensive.[8,12]

The rigid choledochoscope consists of a right-angled telescope with a built-in irrigation channel and a fiberoptic light carrier.* The outside diameter is 5 mm × 3 mm and allows for insertion even into the nondilated duct. The standard 40-mm horizontal limb usually suffices, but on occasion the distal duct can be long (low drainage into the third part of the duodenum) and the 60-mm scope is needed to visualize the sphincter region. Therefore, it is of utmost importance to obtain an initial cholangiogram and to see the drainage site and the configuration of the distal duct, because this will determine which scope will be used and what type of difficulties can be anticipated because of the long and tortuous drainage into the duodenum.

The attachable instrument channel is one of the important accessories. Instead of blind manipulation, a Dormia stone basket or a Fr. No. 4 balloon catheter can be introduced and calculi can be entrapped with precision under visual control. In case of manipulation, the help of the assistant is essential, and, therefore, a teaching attachment or television camera should be used. This provides the possibility of simultaneous observation and coordinated manipulations in extracting a calculus.

Employing the orthodox technique, the physician introduces the biliary balloon catheter inflated and palpated blindly into the duodenum. During withdrawal the balloon has to be deflated to be able to pass the sphincter. During this maneuver the balloon can suddenly jump, and despite immediate reinflation a calculus can be missed in the sphincter area. The same maneuver can be performed now under endoscopic control. The balloon catheter is advanced into the duodenum through the instrument channel. During withdrawal it has to be partially desufflated and reinflated, but this time the position and configuration, in relation to the sphincter, can be well observed. Impacted stones can be removed with an attachable stone forceps. In general, the Dormia basket and the balloon catheter are the major tools for this procedure. To provide adequate irrigation for proper distention and clearing of the ducts, a Fenwal pressure irrigation system, available in every operating room, is used. A cuff pressure of 150 mm Hg, monitored by a manometer, ensures proper visualization. The saline fluid is delivered to the bile ducts under low pressure because of the high resistance of the narrow irrigation channel. A saline drip under hydrostatic pressure only will not suffice. Illumination is provided from an external light source via a flexible optic cable.

Technique

A small standard choledochotomy incision, not exceeding 10 mm, is suitable for the introduction of the scope. The most important step, which is often overlooked and is

---

* Karl Storz Endoscopy Company, Tuttlingen, West Germany; distributed by Karl Storz Endoscopy America, Inc., Culver City, CA.

probably the major factor of an unsuccessful endoscopic procedure of the distal duct (or missed calculus), is the omission or insufficient mobilization of the duodenum. It is not enough to divide the peritoneal reflection of the antimesenteric border of the second part of the duodenum, but it is also important to mobilize it properly with sharp and blunt dissection. Only if the duodenum is widely mobilized can it be kept on a proper stretch to straighten a tortuous distal duct to facilitate proper visualization. During the endoscopic examination one hand should be placed on the mobilized duodenum, whereby the introduced endoscope can be felt as a probe. The wall of the duct in front of the scope is stretched and kept straight to improve vision. It is not necessary to introduce the scope through the sphincter into the duodenum if the sphincter is well observed. By turning the scope 180° the bifurcation, which is similar to the appearance of the carina in the bronchial tree, can be seen and the various orifices of the duct can be well recognized.

Before the procedure is started the surgeon should check that the scope and its accessories are available and that the entire set is in functioning condition. It is advisable to keep the choledochoscope on a separate sterile table and not to mix it with other surgical hand instruments.

The Cystic Stump

In 83% of patients a long parallel or spiral drainage of the cystic duct is present.[4] This will result in a long cystic stump remnant. After prolonged manipulations a small calculus can disappear with ease in this hiding place. In case of multiple stones in a dilated duct, it is advisable to introduce a flexible probe or catheter through the cystic stump into the common bile duct. This will deliver any calculus from this blind pouch into the main duct. On repeated endoscopy this missed stone can be detected and removed.

Complications

I have followed over 500 choledochoscopies and I am not aware of any perforation in the common bile duct or hemobilia from the hepatic ducts after endoscopic procedures.[8] The incidence of wound infections was not increased in cases in which the endoscope was employed intraoperatively.

CONCLUSION

The incidence of retained stones after choledochotomy or choledocholithotomy is far too high. With a little effort the most effective means of recovering a calculus from a difficult position is to use the choledochoscope. This technique should be mastered by the general surgeon. If surgeons would be less reluctant to learn this technique and pay more attention to this intraoperative modality, the realistic incidence of missed stones could be kept below

3%. In addition, if the surgeon could recall the importance to place a larger T-tube without significant curvatures, the patient has a 95% chance in case of a good sinus tract that the missed stones will be removed in the postoperative period. This ancillary procedure (stone removal through the sinus tract) carries no mortality and is therefore the safest and simplest solution. The procedure can be performed in the outpatient setting. Endoscopic sphincterotomy requires hospitalization, and even in the most experienced hands there is a small mortality and morbidity involved.

The surgeon and the assistant performing biliary surgery should be familiar with the intraoperative biliary endoscopic technique. Time should be set aside to practice together in the laboratory or with the biliary phantom. Gallbladder operations are common, but common bile duct explorations are only a small percentage (10%–20%) of the biliary material. These teaching aids can be of great help in becoming familiar with biliary endoscopy.

Our ultimate aim to reduce retained or missed stones can be achieved if choledochoscopy is performed properly.

REFERENCES

1. Bakes J: Die Choledochopapilloskopie. Arch Klin Chir 126: 473, 1923
2. Berci G: Choledochoscopy: The exploration of the extrahepatic biliary system under visual control: Preliminary report. Med J Aust 2:860, 1961
3. Berci G, Cuschieri A, Wood R et al: Television-choledochoscopy. Surg Gynecol Obstet 160:177, 1985
4. Berci G, Hamlin JA: Operative Biliary Endoscopy. Baltimore, Williams & Wilkins, 1981
5. Berci G, Hamlin JA: Operative Biliary Radiology, p 209. Baltimore, William & Wilkins, 1981
6. Berci G, Hamlin JA: Postoperative removal of retained stones. In Cuschieri A, Berci G (eds): Common Bile Duct Exploration, pp 89–97. Boston, Martinus Nijhoff, 1984
7. Cuschieri A, Berci G: Common Bile Duct Exploration, p 3. Boston, Martinus Nijhoff, 1984
8. Cuschieri A, Berci G: Exploration of the CBD. In Cuschieri A, Berci G (eds): Operative Biliary Endoscopy, pp 55–71. Boston, Martinus Nijhoff, 1984
9. Feliciano DV, Mattox KL, Jordan GI: The value of choledochoscopy in the exploration of the CBD. Ann Surg 191: 649, 1980
10. Finnis D, Rowntree T: Choledochoscopy in the exploration of the common bile duct. Br J Surg 64:661, 1977
11. Griffin WT: Choledochoscopy. Am J Surg 132:697, 1976
12. Iseli A, Marshall VC: A comparison of a rigid and a flexible fiberoptic instrument. Med J Aust 1:131, 1978
13. Lennert K: Choledochoskopie. Heidelberg, Springer, 1980
14. McIver MA: An instrument for visualizing the interior of Common Bile Duct at Operation. Surgery 9:112, 1941
15. Rattner DW, Warsaw AL: Impact of choledochoscopy on the management of choledocholithiasis. Ann Surg 194:76, 1981
16. Reitsma BJ: Common duct stones, thesis. University of Maastricht, Holland, 1981

17. Schein CJ, Stern WZ, Jacobson HG: The Common Bile Duct, pp 266–267. Springfield, IL, Charles C Thomas, 1966

18. Shore JM, Morgenstern L, Berci G: An improved rigid choledochoscope. Am J Surg 122:567, 1971

19. Shulman AG, Berci G: Choledochoscopy: A survey of California hospitals. Am J Surg 149:703, 1985

20. Wildegans H: Grenzen der Cholangiographie und Aussichten der Endoskopie der tiefen Gallenwege. Med Klin 48:1270, 1953

21. Yamakawa T: An improved choledocho-fiberscope for removal of retained stones under direct visual control. Gastrointest Endosc 22:160, 1976

22. Yap PC, Atacador M, Yap AG et al: Choledochoscopy as a complementary procedure to operative cholangiography in biliary surgery. Am J Surg 140:648, 1980

part 3
Granulomatous Liver Disease

DAVID J. WYLER and
SHELDON M. WOLFF

Granulomatous inflammation of the liver (granulomatous liver disease) can develop in response to a large number of diverse agents (Tables 44-1 and 44-2). Granulomatous liver disease most frequently represents a manifestation of infectious or noninfectious systemic illness.[7,9] Establishing an etiologic diagnosis may be particularly difficult in the absence of associated systemic manifestations or if no pathogen is isolated, since the histopathologic features of hepatic granulomas are rarely diagnostic. Treatment is directed at the specific inciting agent or systemic process. In roughly one fourth of the cases no etiologic diagnosis can be made. In the latter patients, an empiric trial of antituberculous chemotherapy or corticosteroids may be indicated if systemic manifestations are severe enough to justify a therapeutic trial.

PATHOLOGY AND PATHOGENESIS OF GRANULOMAS

Granulomas in the liver are generally localized near or within the portal tracts and usually do not result in important hepatocellular dysfunction. The morphology and probable pathogenesis of hepatic granulomas are indistinguishable from granulomas in other tissues.[2] Chronic granulomatous inflammation is recognized by a characteristic tightly associated accumulation of predominantly mononuclear cells, including mononuclear phagocytes (macrophages and epithelioid cells) and lymphocytes. Langerhans' or foreign-body giant cells, fibroblasts, eosinophils, and mast cells or basophils may constitute a small subpopulation in granulomas induced by certain agents. Epithelioid cells (so-called because of their resemblance to epithelial cells), the hallmark of granulomas, are modified macrophages with a distinctive morphology (large cytoplasm with expansive endoplasmic reticulum, Golgi apparatus, vesicles, and vacuoles) but uncertain specialized function. The ultrastructural features suggest that these specialized macrophages are probably better adapted for secretion than for phagocytosis.[1] The multinucleated Langerhans' cells form by fusion of macrophages, possibly under the influence of lymphocyte-derived soluble mediators (lymphokines).[12]

Granulomas generally represent either immunologic responses (hypersensitivity granuloma) or apparently nonimmunologic inflammatory responses (foreign body granuloma) to inciting agents.[1] Granulomas can also be classified on the basis of rates of macrophage turnover (recruitment and attrition) as being either high-turnover or low-turnover type.[15] These differences in granulomas have not been shown to be clinically important, however.

The mechanism of granuloma formation has been best defined for hypersensitivity granulomas,[1] largely through studies of schistosomiasis, the most prevalent granulomatous liver disease worldwide. In a process similar to cutaneous delayed hypersensitivity, immobilized or undigestible antigens stimulate specifically sensitized T lymphocytes to secrete lymphokines. These lymphokines act locally to recruit other cellular constituents such as monocytes and fibroblasts and may also promote giant cell formation. It is not certain what prevents cellular egress from these collections; the lymphokine, migration inhibition factor, and the extracellular matrix glycoprotein fibronectin might be involved. Suppressor T cells may subsequently act to reduce ("modulate" or "down-regulate") the magnitude of the granulomatous inflammatory response. In some cases, immune complexes rather than lymphocytes may initiate or down-regulate granuloma formation.

Little is known of the mechanisms whereby granulomas form in response to nonantigenic foreign bodies such as talc and silica particles. Since phagocytosis by both fixed (e.g., Kupffer cells) or circulating mononuclear cells of nondegradable material can stimulate secretion of a variety of biologically active molecules (e.g., monokines), perhaps these mediators directly or indirectly initiate granulomatous inflammation. The possibility that immunologic mechanisms come into play in maintaining and modulating granulomas initiated by foreign bodies has not been excluded.[16] For example, the possibility that autoimmune responses to interstitial matrix proteins such as collagen develop in some patients with foreign body granulomas has not been investigated.

The consequence of granulomatous inflammation appears to depend to some extent on the etiology. In certain infectious diseases such as tuberculosis, activation of granuloma macrophages may serve to restrict replication

TABLE 44-1.   Etiologies of Hepatic Granulomas: Infectious

Bacterial infections	Visceral larva migrans
Mycobacterial diseases	Fascioliasis
Tuberculosis	Capillariosis
BCG	Strongyloidiasis
Atypical mycobacteriosis	Ascariasis
Leprosy	Ancylostomiasis
Brucellosis	Angiostrongyliasis
Typhoid fever	Tongue worm infection
Paratyphoid B	Protozoal diseases
Listeriosis	Amebiasis
Nocardiosis	Toxoplasmosis
Actinomycosis	Malaria
Tularemia	Viral infections
Yersiniosis	Cytomegalovirus
Granuloma inguinale	Infectious mononucleosis
Meliodosis	(Epstein-Barr virus)
Fungal infections	Acute viral hepatitis
Histoplasmosis	Influenza B
Cryptococcosis	Other infections
Coccidiodomycosis	Q fever
Candidiasis	Mediterranean fever (boutonneuse
Torulopsis	fever)
Aspergillosis	Syphilis
Blastomycosis	Lymphogranuloma venereum
Parasitic infections	Psittacosis
Helminthic diseases	
Schistosomiasis	

(Adapted from Harrington PT, Gutierrez JJ, Ramirez-Ronda CH et al: Granulomatous hepatitis. Rev Infect Dis 4:638, 1982)

of the pathogen. In schistosomiasis, establishment of a barrier around helminth eggs deposited in portal venules may protect hepatic parenchymal cells from helminth-derived hepatotoxins. Secretion of interleukin 1 by granuloma macrophages, or by Kupffer cells stimulated by granuloma products, can lead to a variety of host responses including fever.[4] Finally, soluble products secreted by granuloma macrophages and lymphocytes can stimulate fibroblast recruitment, proliferation, and collagen synthesis.[17] The resulting fibrosis and hyalinization are one of the means by which hepatic granulomas heal, although in some situations healing leads to no discernible change in the liver. For unknown reasons, cirrhosis is an infrequent complication of granulomatous liver disease. In the unique case of schistosomiasis, however, extensive periportal fibrosis (Symmer's clay pipe stem fibrosis) can occlude portal venules, resulting in portal hypertension. It has been proposed that this may occur as a result of biologically active factors secreted by granuloma cells.[17]

DIAGNOSIS

Granulomatous liver disease is usually diagnosed as a feature of a systemic disorder, or incidentally on liver biopsy performed for other reasons such as evaluation of patients with fever of undetermined etiology.[14] The frequency with which specific clinical manifestations accompany granulomatous liver disease largely depends on the etiology.[9] Since different etiologies may prevail in different geographic areas, broadly applicable generalizations are difficult to provide. Based on reports from the United States and Europe, fever occurs in about two thirds and hepatomegaly occurs in over one half of patients.[9] Splenomegaly is appreciated less frequently (22%–44%). Massive splenomegaly is more likely to occur in secondary syphilis and schistosomiasis associated with portal hypertension, sarcoidosis, berylliosis, Hodgkin's disease, and chronic granulomatous disease of childhood.[8] Since hepatocellular function is generally preserved, peripheral stigmata of liver disease (spider angiomata, palmar erythema) and severe abnormalities in liver function tests are uncommon. Blood alkaline phosphatase and transaminase levels are mildly or moderately elevated in up to one half to two thirds of patients.[9] Although hyperbilirubinemia occurs in up to one fourth of patients, jaundice is distinctly unusual.[9] Hypoalbuminemia and prolongation of the prothrombin time is rare. In contrast, acceleration of the erythrocyte sedimentation rate and mild hyperglobulinemia are frequently associated abnormalities.

Since granulomas may be randomly scattered throughout the liver, a generous sample of liver tissue should ideally be obtained at laparotomy if a needle biopsy was negative and granulomatous liver disease is strongly suspected. The specimen should be adequate to permit the exami-

TABLE 44-2.   Etiologies and Associations of Hepatic Granulomas: Noninfectious

Sarcoidosis	Clofibrate
Primary liver disease	p-Aminosalicylic acid
Primary biliary cirrhosis	Cromolyn sodium
Laennec's cirrhosis	Diazepam
Postnecrotic cirrhosis	Progesterone-estrogen contraceptives
Nutritional cirrhosis	Copper (vineyard sprayer's lung)
Biliary obstruction	Other (extrinsic allergic alveolitis)
Acute and chronic pericholangitis	Collagen vascular diseases
Fatty infiltration	Wegener's granulomatosis
Toxic or drug-induced hepatitis	Temporal arteritis
Chronic active hepatitis	Polymyalgia rheumatica
Hypersensitivity reactions	Allergic granulomatosis
Erythema nodosum	Immune deficiency diseases
Berylliosis	Chronic granulomatous disease of childhood
Silicone	Malignancies
Drug reactions to	Lymphomas
Sulfonamides	Others
Penicillin	Other diseases
Allopurinol	Crohn's disease
Halothane	Ulcerative colitis
Hydralazine	Whipple's disease
α-Methyldopa	Eosinophilic granuloma of the lung
Procainamide	Starch granuloma of the peritoneum
Quinidine	Post ileal bypass surgery
Hydrochlorothiazide	Lymphomatoid granulomatosis
Phenytoin	Celiac disease
Sulfonylurea derivatives	Foreign bodies (starch, talc, silica)
Phenylbutazone	Idiopathic granulomas
Oxyphenbutazone	

(Adapted from Harrington PT, Gutierrez JJ, Ramirez-Ronda CH et al: Granulomatous hepatitis. Rev Infect Dis 4:638, 1982)

nation of a relatively large area in serial sections and also provide sufficient material for microbiological studies. Granulomas have been identified in 3% to 10% of all needle biopsies performed in large medical centers,[9] indicating that the condition is not rare.

The specific diagnostic tests that should be performed in each case will depend largely on the possible etiologies entertained in the differential diagnosis (see Tables 44-1 and 44-2). Selection of appropriate diagnostic tests will depend on geographic location and historic information regarding travel, diet, and environmental (including animal) and drug exposure history. The nature of associated clinical features should help focus the diagnostic possibilities. Since infectious etiologies (especially tuberculosis) are most common and most readily amenable to specific therapy, these must be most carefully considered. Skin tests, serologic studies, stool examination (for parasites) and special stains (*e.g.*, acid-fast) of biopsy material may be helpful. Even though the successful isolation of organisms may be difficult, liver tissue should be cultured on specialized media for growth of bacteria, mycobacteria, fungi, or viruses.

ETIOLOGIES

Infectious

It is no surprise that blood-borne pathogens should have a propensity to localize in the liver since this is the largest organ of the mononuclear phagocyte (reticuloendothelial) system. Bacteria that can persist within macrophages (*e.g.*, *Mycobacterium, Brucella, Listeria, Salmonella*) are particularly likely to incite granulomatous reactions in the liver, as are fungi and intravascular or migrating parasites.

Tuberculosis is a major reported cause of granulomatous liver disease, accounting for the diagnosis in 10% to 53% of patients.[9] Hepatic granulomas can be found in patients with primary tuberculosis, chronic pulmonary tuberculosis, and miliary dissemination. Clinical features that suggest this etiology include fever with chills, anemia, weight loss, signs of meningeal involvement, and symptoms of less than 6 to 8 months' duration.[8] The diagnostic value of the tuberculin skin test is limited by the fact that some patients with miliary tuberculosis have specific anergy and some individuals with positive skin tests can have hepatic granulomas of nontuberculous origin. Necrosis, destruction of the reticulin framework, irregularity of the granuloma contour with a dense cuff of lymphocytes, and the tendency for granulomas to coalesce are said to be distinctive histopathologic features.[13] Visualization or cultural isolation of acid-free bacilli is exceedingly helpful but achieved in fewer than one third of all tuberculosis cases[9]; identification of the mycobacteria is more common in miliary disease.[3] The favorable response to antituberculous chemotherapy experienced by some patients in whom no etiology was initially established[14] may attest to the limitation of the diagnostic modalities and the importance of tuberculosis as a cause of hepatic granulomas. On the other hand, these patients might have experienced self-limited disease that was not directly influenced by chemotherapy.

Atypical mycobacteria, particularly *M. avium-intracellulare,* can disseminate in immunocompromised patients (including patients with the acquired immune deficiency syndrome) and induce hepatic granulomas. BCG employed in cancer immunotherapy (or for vaccination) can disseminate and incite liver granulomas. Patients with leprosy, especially those with the lepromatous (LL) polar variety, can also develop hepatic granulomas.

Brucellosis occurs worldwide, and in areas where the disease is most prevalent (Rumania, Portugal, Ireland, France, parts of Mexico, and South America, India, South Africa, and Australia) its association with granulomatous liver disease is not unusual. Indeed, in some series, over 50% of patients with brucellosis had some form of liver involvement and 50% of these had documented liver granulomas.[9] *B. abortus* most frequently gives rise to noncaseating hepatic granulomas, whereas *B. mellitensis* is more likely to produce diffuse hepatitis and *B. suis* incites caseating lesions. An appropriate exposure history and positive serology are useful in diagnosis; isolation of *Brucella* is generally more successful from sites other than the liver (*e.g.,* blood, bone marrow).

In the United States, histoplasmosis is by far the most common fungal infection associated with hepatic granulomas,[11] and indeed the liver is second only to the spleen as the organ most commonly infected following dissemination. Microscopic identification and cultural isolation of *Histoplasma* are the only reliable diagnostic tests. The high frequency of positive histoplasmin skin test and serology in certain populations limits their diagnostic value in granulomatous liver disease. Other disseminated fungal infections also can incite granulomatous inflammation in the liver.

Schistosomiasis is unquestionably the most common infection associated with hepatic granulomas, afflicting millions of individuals in developing nations. Eggs of *S. mansoni* and *S. japonicum* are swept into the portal venules after they are released by the adult female worms residing in mesenteric veins. There they incite a granulomatous response.[1] Although extensive perivascular portal fibrosis can result in some patients and give rise to severe portal hypertension, most patients remain asymptomatic or have mild disease. The ease with which helminth eggs can be identified in serial sections of liver biopsy specimens makes this diagnosis relatively simple. Efforts to identify eggs in stool, serologic tests, and rectal biopsies can be useful if eggs are not observed in the biopsy material. Since travelers to endemic areas may be at risk for acquiring schistosomiasis, careful travel history is important when considering this diagnosis.

Migrating helminth larvae (*Toxocara, Strongyloides, Ascaris, Ancylostoma, Angiostrongylis costaricensis*), when they infiltrate the liver, can incite a granulomatous reaction. These granulomas are characteristically rich in eosinophils and may contain the larvae, which is diagnostic. Rarely, hepatic granulomas may occur in association with certain protozoal infections (amebiasis, toxoplasmosis, malaria).

Systemic viral infections may induce focal mononuclear cell infiltrates in the liver but rarely incite genuine granulomatous reactions. Therefore, the occasional reports of the association of hepatic granulomas with certain viral infections are difficult to interpret. In contrast, the rickettsial infection Q fever (due to *Coxiella burnetti*) frequently causes hepatic granulomas that may have the distinctive features of fibrinoid material distributed in a ringlike or broken rod-shaped configuration.[10]

Other infectious causes of hepatic granulomas are rare. Although liver involvement in *syphilis* is common, granulomas are reported rarely in secondary and tertiary cases.[9]

Noninfectious

Sarcoidosis has been identified as the most common cause of granulomatous liver disease in a number of series from the United States and Europe.[9] The liver is involved in over 60% of all sarcoid patients, although symptoms are uncommonly referable to this inflammation. Marked hepatic functional abnormalities with parenchymal destruction and fibrosis can occasionally occur. The liver is palpable in about 20% of sarcoid patients. Hepatic sarcoid granulomas are characteristically located in periportal zones but also can have midcentral and midzonal distribution.[10] They have central eosinophilic necrosis without caseation or destruction of the reticular network. These features are not diagnostic, however. Clinical features that are suggestive of sarcoidosis in patients with hepatic granulomas are symptoms of greater than 16 months' duration; greater occurrence among blacks, especially those 20 to 40 years of age; concomitant cutaneous, ocular, and pulmonary involvement and splenomegaly; and presence of hypergammaglobulinemia, anemia, and leukopenia. Liver biopsy should be used in diagnosis of sarcoid only when biopsy of other sites (*e.g.,* lymph node) are unrevealing.

Primary liver disease, particularly primary biliary cirrhosis and to a lesser extent cirrhosis due to various exogenous causes, may be associated with hepatic granulomas. In primary biliary cirrhosis, granulomas are primarily identified early in disease, at the time of bile duct damage.

Other conditions associated with the presence of hepatic granulomas include erythema nodosum, exposure to beryllium and copper, various rheumatologic disorders, and malignancies. On the other hand, hepatic granulomas have been identified in 5% to 36% of cases of fever of undetermined origin[9,14] in which extensive and thorough evaluation often failed to provide an etiologic diagnosis. Most patients with such "idiopathic granulomatous hepatitis"[14] have responded to corticosteroid therapy, which is usually administered following a course of isoniazid and other antituberculous chemotherapeutic agents. In a few cases, antituberculous chemotherapy alone has been effective, although the possibility that these patients might have healed spontaneously cannot be excluded. When we evaluate patients with prolonged fevers of unknown origin who have had thorough workups,[5,6] we recommend that a liver biopsy be done whether or not the patient has abnormal liver function tests. This recommendation is made since some patients with extensive idiopathic granulomatous hepatitis and fever have had normal results of liver function tests.

REFERENCES

1. Boros DL: Granulomatous inflammation. Prog Allergy 24: 184, 1978
2. Boros DL, Yoshida T (eds): Basic and Clinical Aspects of Granulomatous Diseases. New York, Elsevier/North-Holland, 1980
3. Cucin RL, Coleman M, Eckardt JJ et al: The diagnosis of miliary tuberculosis: Utility of peripheral blood abnormalities, bone marrow and liver biopsy. J Chronic Dis 26:355, 1973
4. Dinarello CA: Interleukinin-1. Rev Infect Dis 6:51, 1984
5. Dinarello CA, Wolff SM: Fever of unknown origin. In Mandell GL, Douglas RG Jr, Bennett JE (eds): Principles and Practice of Infectious Diseases, pp 339–346. New York, Wiley Medical Publishers, 1984
6. Dinarello CA, Wolff SM: Approach to the patient with fever of unknown origin. In Mandell GL, Douglas RG Jr, Bennett JE (eds): Principles and Practice of Infectious Diseases, pp 347–350. New York, Wiley Medical Publishers, 1984
7. Fauci AS, Wolff SM: Granulomatous hepatitis. In Popper H, Schaffner F (eds): Progress in Liver Diseases, vol 5, pp 609–621. New York, Grune & Stratton, 1976
8. Guckian JC, Perry JE: Granulomatous hepatitis: An analysis of 63 cases and review of literature. Ann Intern Med 65: 1081, 1966
9. Harrington PT, Gutierrez JJ, Ramirez-Ronda CH et al: Granulomatous hepatitis. Rev Infect Dis 4:638, 1982
10. Klatskin G: Hepatic granulomata: Problems in interpretation. Ann NY Acad Sci 278:427, 1976
11. Lanza FL, Nelson RS, Somayaji BN: Acute granulomatous hepatitis due to histoplasmosis. Gastroenterology 58:392, 1970
12. Postlethwaite AE, Jackson BK, Beachey EH et al: Formation of multinucleated giant cells from human monocyte precursors: Mediation by a soluble protein from antigen- and mitogen-stimulated lymphocytes. J Exp Med 155:168, 1982
13. Sherlock S: Diseases of the Liver, 6th ed, pp 421–422. Boston, Blackwell Scientific, 1981
14. Simon HB, Wolff SM: Granulomatous hepatitis and prolonged fever of unknown origin: A study of 13 patients. Medicine 52:1, 1973
15. Spector WG: Epithelioid cell, giant cells and sarcoidosis. Ann NY Acad Sci 278:3, 1976
16. Warren KS: A functional classification of granulomatous inflammation. Ann NY Acad Sci 278:7, 1976
17. Wyler DJ: Regulation of fibroblast functions by products of schistosomal egg granulomas: Potential role in the pathogenesis of hepatic fibrosis. In Evered D, Collins GM (eds): Cytopathology of Parasitic Disease, pp 190–204. London, Pitman Books, 1983

part 4

Hemobilia

PHILIP SANDBLOM

Hemobilia, or bleeding into the biliary tract, occurs when disease or trauma produces an abnormal communication between blood vessels and bile ducts. It corresponds to hematuria in urinary tract disease but is probably less common, or at least less often recognized. If the urine becomes bloody, it is noticed immediately; but, if blood enters the intestine through the papilla of Vater, it only comes to light as hematemesis or melena, and its origin may well be mistaken or unidentified. Therefore, hemobilia is a problem of differential diagnosis with regard to other and more common sources of bleeding in the gas-

trointestinal tract, rather than a diagnostic sign of liver or biliary tract disease.

Because of its apparent rarity, hemobilia was late in becoming an acknowledged entity. It was repeatedly discovered only to be forgotten again. As early as 1654, Francis Glisson, in the first detailed description of the anatomy of the liver,[7] discussed the possibility of hemorrhage through the biliary tract in the following words:

I believe that if the liver is injured by a contusion, it may lead to blood leaving the body by way of vomit or the stool for there is no doubt that the biliary duct takes unto itself (to the great good of the patient) some of the blood issuing into the liver and leads it down to the intestines. From there it is either impelled upwards through reverse peristalsis or downwards the usual way.

With better knowledge of the syndrome and with improved diagnostic methods, hemobilia is recognized with increasing frequency. There is, in addition, an absolute increase partly because of the rising number of traffic accidents, which often results in liver injury, and partly because of more invasive diagnostic procedures, which may cause iatrogenic hemobilia.[4,5] The *Index Medicus* did not add the term *hemobilia* until 1980 and now has about 25 references per year, whereas *hematuria* was adopted from the beginning in 1880 and has three times as many references yearly.

Bleeding in hemobilia can be of varying degree, from exsanguinating hemorrhage, leading rapidly to the death of the patient, to occult bleeding, which, if it continues, may result in chronic secondary anemia.

Profuse hemobilia is rare, but, when it occurs, it is not only an essential symptom but also a dangerous, sometimes life-threatening complication of liver or biliary tract disease, which may constitute the main reason for treatment. Minor or occult hemobilia is frequent but generally overlooked or neglected, because it is rarely of clinical significance.[18]

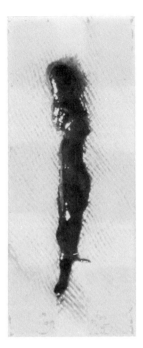

Fig. 44-7. An obstructing blood clot extracted from the common duct in a case of traumatic hemobilia. Note the protuberance, probably a cast of the distal end of the pancreatic duct. (Sandblom P, Mirkovitch V: Ann Surg 190:254, 1979)

Fig. 44-6. Detail of a tubing model of the extrahepatic bile ducts. Blood is injected into bile streaming through the system. **A.** When injected forcefully to imitate major hemobilia, the blood causes turbulence and mixes with the bile. **B.** When injected gently to imitate minor hemobilia, it flows immiscibly to the lower portion and forms a pure coagulum. (Sandblom P: Ann Surg 190:254, 1979)

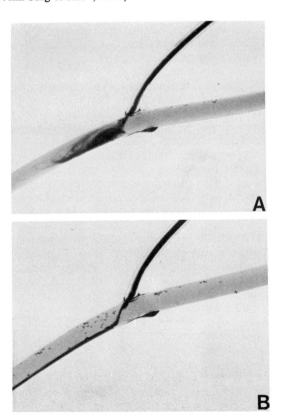

Most hemorrhage of consequence is arterial in origin. When only veins are injured, the bleeding is often slight, but it may be significant if the portal pressure is increased. In minor hemobilia, the blood does not mix with the bile (Fig. 44-6). It either remains fluid and flows unobtrusively into the intestine, or it coagulates to form a cast of the duct when trapped above a closed sphincter of Oddi (Fig. 44-7).[21]

The clot acts like a calculus, causing biliary colic when passed or obstructive jaundice when retained. It generally has a very ephemeral existence, given that it is promptly lysed through the fibrinolytic property of the bile (Fig. 44-8). Through this activity, the bile plays the same role as urine and saliva in clearing fibrin deposits from their respective ducts. When protected from the bile stream, clots may escape this lytic action and remain solid; they are then easily mistaken for gallstones.[17] This can occur when the bile flow is diverted through a T-tube above the clot (Fig. 44-9) or when it is totally obstructed by the clot itself. An excluded gallbladder can offer a hiding place where the clots can remain for long periods and cause cholecystitis[14] or turn into stones. Their role in the formation of so-called primary duct stones is uncertain. With the brown color and brittle consistency they are sometimes misnamed inspissated bile or tissue debris.

The natural history of hemobilia includes gastrointestinal bleeding in 90%, biliary colic in 70%, and jaundice

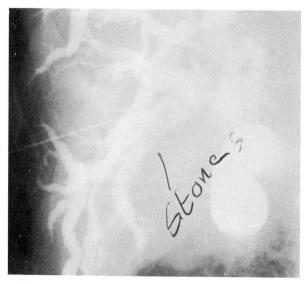

Fig. 44-8. Cholangiogram 30 minutes after liver puncture shows a 4-cm-long defect in a bile duct. This defect was first thought by the radiologist to represent stones but was found to be caused by a coagulum. At operation the next day, it was noted that the coagulum had been nearly dissolved. (Veterans Administration Medical Center, San Diego)

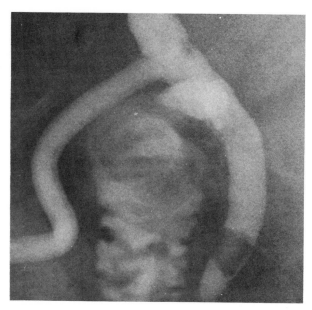

Fig. 44-9. A blood clot in the common duct caused by postoperative hemobilia. Three weeks after the difficult removal of a common duct stone, a cholangiogram showed this defect in the contrast. It was misinterpreted as being due to a retained calculus.

in 60% of the cases. These constitute the pathognomonic symptom triad of hemobilia. The biliary colic caused by passage of coaguli corresponds to the colic in gallstone disease. Such pain may also be produced by an arterial aneurysm bursting into a duct; this event causes violent pain from the sudden increase in intraluminal pressure. The jaundice is usually temporary—it recedes when an obstructive clot is lysed or expelled into the intestine, usually followed by a large gush of blood with hematemesis and melena. Occasionally it has to be removed surgically.

Secondary symptoms are hemorrhagic shock, if the bleeding is substantial, and secondary anemia, if it is prolonged.

Because of the very characteristic and consistent symptom triad, the diagnosis of major hemobilia is easy to establish, provided the physician is aware of the syndrome. It should always be suspected when gastrointestinal hemorrhage is combined with biliary tract symptoms.

Until recently, far too many cases of hemobilia have been diagnosed too late—at autopsy—or with undue delay after one or more inappropriate or inadequate operations such as "blind gastric resection."

The best way of verifying the diagnosis is by selective arteriography, which reveals the source of bleeding in a high percentage of cases (Fig. 44-10). This procedure is of special value in discovering central liver lesions, which may be difficult or impossible to localize even at exploratory laparotomy. Cholangiography, either pre- or postoperatively, may reveal a lesion either by contrast-filling of a cavity or by dislocation of the ducts. Less invasive

methods, such as sonography or computed tomography (CT), run the risk of missing small lesions.[9] Duodenal endoscopy occasionally reveals hemobilia as the cause of upper gastrointestinal bleeding.[2]

The bleeding in hemobilia may originate in the liver parenchyma or in the intrahepatic or extrahepatic biliary tract, including the gallbladder. The pancreas is a rare source.[15]

Common causes of the abnormal communication between blood vessels and the biliary tract that give rise to hemobilia are trauma (due to accident, operation, or liver puncture), inflammation, gallstones, tumors, and vascular disorders. There are many conditions that occasionally give rise to hemobilia, such as echinococci, choledochal cysts, pancreatitis, portal hypertension, and blood coagulation defects. Their relative frequencies are shown in Figure 44-11. The proportion noted in the diagram relates to massive hemobilia. If cases of minor hemobilia had been included, gallstone etiology would have constituted the overwhelming majority, since biliary tract operations and colic from gallstones is nearly always accompanied by minute bleeding from the injured biliary tract mucosa. In the era before cholecystography, the occurrence of microscopic melena was one of the main diagnostic signs of gallstone disease.[12]

The most common cause of hemobilia in the Western world is trauma, accidental or iatrogenic.

The mechanism of penetrating trauma is evident. The first case of hemobilia in the literature, described by Glis-

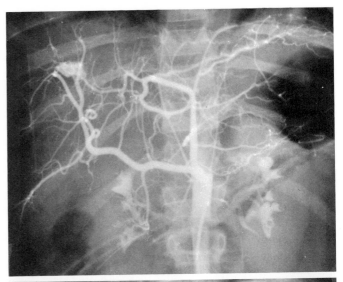

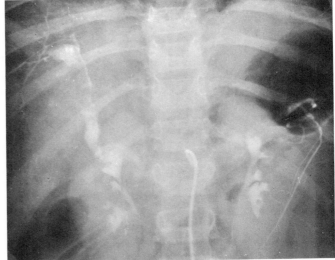

Fig. 44-10. Celiac arteriogram in a case of central liver rupture. **A.** Arterial phase. Pooling of contrast medium in the center of the right lobe. **B.** Early parenchymatous phase. Note filling of the dilated right hepatic duct with contrast medium directly from the lesion. With skill and a measure of good luck, the radiologist has managed to catch the passage of blood and contrast medium from the central lesion down into the common duct. (Enge I et al: Br J Radiol 41:789, 1968)

Fig. 44-11. Distribution of 545 published cases of major hemobilia with respect to cause.

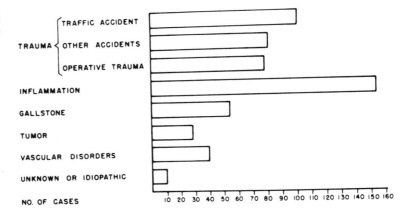

son, was that of a young nobleman who bled to death through the biliary tract after having been pierced by a sword through his liver when fighting a duel. A common "weapon" today in penetrating trauma is the physician's biopsy needle.[25]

The mechanism in blunt trauma is more complicated. If the liver is compressed, the fragile and inelastic parenchyma tears easily (Fig. 44-12). The disrupting force is greatest in the center of the organ, which explains the high frequency of subcapsular liver rupture. This is often combined with smaller superficial rifts caused by the direct force. When the surgeon sees these rifts at emergency exploration, he is apt to be satisfied with repairing them and may miss the central cavity, which is not directly visible. The surgeon may even create a defect if he performs a superficial suture of a deep laceration.[10] One should not expect hemobilia to be a common complication of liver lesions that are open to the peritoneal cavity and in which intra-abdominal bleeding is the predominant and alarming factor. Traumatic hemobilia is rather found in central liver ruptures caused by blunt trauma and has more obscure and less acute symptoms. If a hepatic vein tears there is a risk that bile gets sucked into the circulation, causing bilirubinemia, so-called bilhemia.[3]

Central liver ruptures can be of different sizes, from large cavities extending into both lobes to simple arteriobiliary fistulas. Occasionlly, no or only temporary bleeding occurs, but, most of the time, there is long-standing, often repeated hemobilia. The course of events in these cavities accounts for the typical clinical history in cases of traumatic hemobilia.[16] The rupture tears bile ducts, arteries, and veins, which fill the cavity with bile and blood. If a large artery is torn, exsanguinating gastrointestinal hemorrhage may occur, necessitating emergency surgery to save the patient's life. Usually, the cavity fills slowly, and the escape of bloody bile is delayed by coagulation in the cavity or in the diverting duct assisted by a contracting sphincter of Oddi. Finally, after days or weeks, the pressure in the cavity suddenly forces the clot down the tract into the intestine, followed by a large gush of blood and bile.

During these events, the patient first experiences an increasing, dull pain over the area of the liver. Sometimes, an enlargement of the liver can be detected, and there may be signs of obstructive jaundice. Then, one day, the patient experiences intense biliary colic followed by hematemesis and melena. This classic triad of biliary colic, gastrointestinal hemorrhage, and jaundice should always arouse the suspicion of hemobilia. The patient feels relieved after evacuation of the cavity; the liver size diminishes, and the jaundice subsides. A favorable prognosis may mistakenly be given. Unfortunately, relief is usually only temporary, since the course is repeated over months and years. The syndrome is thus characterized by a distinct

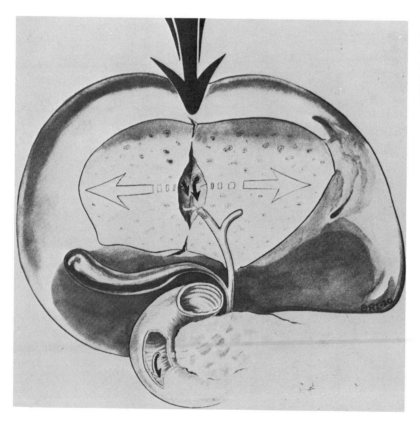

Fig. 44-12. Hemobilia from blunt liver trauma. Compression of the liver (*black arrow*) results in disruptive forces (*white arrows*), thereby producing both superficial rifts and internal rupture. The inflowing blood leaves with the bile through the bile ducts.

periodicity.[16] There is very little hope for spontaneous healing.[8]

The explanation for the curious course of traumatic hemobilia lies in the paradoxic fact that although the liver regenerates quickly local lesions heal slowly. During the first few hours after liver trauma, the parenchymal cells prepare for growth and, in a few days, regeneration is in full swing. In contradistinction, the healing of localized lesions is retarded, even prevented, by a fibrinolytic effect of the bile. There is a striking difference in healing rate between liver wounds open to the peritoneal cavity and liver wounds that heal in the presence of bile. In the latter, there is a very diminished production of fibrinous exudate, granulating tissue, and fibrous scar (Fig. 44-13).[20] As a result, a central cavity is lined by easily damaged parenchymal cells rather than by sturdy granulation tissue. Because spontaneous healing is rare, the only hope for cure is adequate operative treatment. This active surgical approach has considerably lowered mortality.

The surgical treatment may be prophylactic. Adequate handling of a liver lesion at the primary emergency laparotomy can prevent later hemobilia. The operation should include careful exploration of cavities and meticulous hemostasis and suturing of open bile ducts before drainage and closure.[10] If this does not suffice, or if hemobilia occurs in spite of these efforts, a more radical course of action is necessary. The procedure should be preceded by arteriography. The choice is then between hepatic resection and hepatic artery occlusion by ligature or embolization.[24] The decision will depend on the location of injury.

For peripheral and well-localized lesions, resection is preferred. In those close to the hilum, where resection would be difficult or impossible, ligation or embolization of the hepatic artery or one of its branches is the treatment of choice. Excellent results have been reported with obstruction of one of the lobar branches.[11]

Iatrogenic hemobilia from operative trauma is encoun-

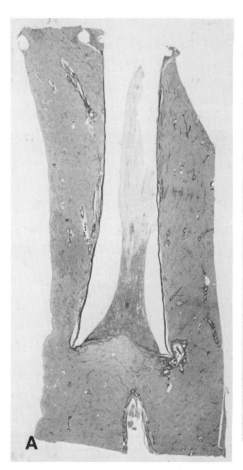

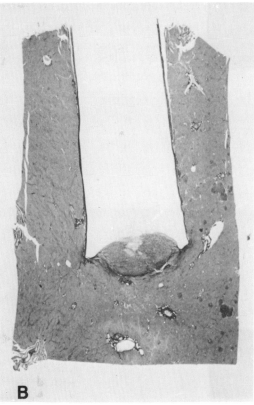

Fig. 44-13. Three months after injury to the liver, there is a marked difference in healing between lesions open to the peritoneal cavity (**A**), where healing is normal, and lesions open to the gallbladder (**B**), where there is striking diminution of fibrinous exudate, granulation tissue, and fibrous scar. (Sandblom P et al: Ann Surg 183:679, 1976)

tered as frequently as hemobilia from traffic accidents. During biliary tract surgery, the hepatic artery may be damaged by a suture or by the dissection, which can result in an arteriobiliary fistula or in a false aneurysm leaking or eroding into the extrahepatic bile ducts. Intrahepatic lesions are caused more commonly by instrumentation of the biliary tree. Not all surgeons are aware of the vulnerability of this region, and efforts to extract intrahepatic calculi may exceed the resistance of the ductal wall. Because the hepatic arteries are in close proximity, there is a potential risk of intrahepatic hematoma due to arterial injury. The result can be profuse hemobilia, often through a T-tube.

Diagnostic liver puncture is a rapidly increasing source of hemobilia. Occult bleeding is reported to occur in between 3%[25] and 10%[1] of patients. Macroscopic hemobilia is very rare, especially if fine-caliber needles are used, but there are still cases reported with exsanguinating hemobilia. Figure 44-14 is taken from a case in which percutaneous transhepatic cholangiography aroused suspicion

of a common duct stone. At operation a blood clot was recovered and postoperative cholangiography demonstrated the source—a lesion caused by the liver puncture. The risk of bleeding increases if a catheter is left in place for biliary drainage.[22]

Hemobilia caused by operations and liver punctures may cease spontaneously, but, generally active intervention, usually obstruction of the damaged artery, is necessary.

The large number of inflammatory cases has a peculiar geographic distribution—all originate in the Orient in China, Vietnam, and Korea. The causative agent in this category is *Ascaris,* a nematode that has a tendency to invade the bile ducts of the patient, where it frequently produces bleeding lesions. This so-called tropic hemobilia is said to be an everyday problem in surgical departments in the Far East.[23]

In gallstone disease, microscopic hemorrhage is frequent and can be proved in every third case. The bleeding occurs when the stones injure the mucosa, especially in connec-

Fig. 44-14. Lesion during transhepatic cholangiography, producing a blood clot in the common duct. **A.** The transhepatic catheter points toward a lesion in the left hepatic duct (*arrow*). A multilobular filling defect in the common duct was caused by a "bile plug," probably a blood clot, which was removed at operation. **B.** A postoperative cholangiogram clearly shows the extravasation from the ductal lesion. The filling defect is gone. (Sandblom P et al: World J Surg 8:41, 1984)

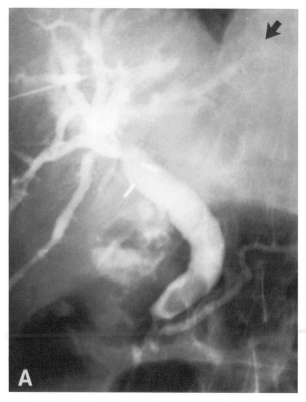
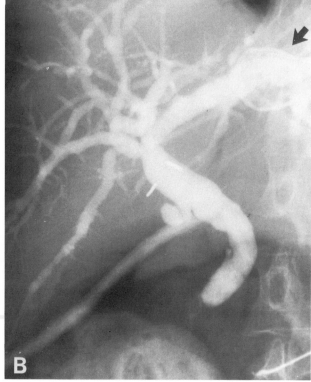

tion with biliary colic. Macroscopic hemobilia is rare, with only 50 cases reported in the literature. It generally occurs when a large stone erodes the cystic artery or penetrates into an adjacent viscus.

As has been mentioned, tumors play an insignificant role as a source of bleeding in the biliary tract. This is especially striking when compared with the urinary tract, where tumors constitute a major cause of hematuria. Tumors are as rare in the gallbladder as they are frequent in the urinary bladder.

The common tumors of the liver are not prone to bleed into the ducts. The hepatomas that cause hemobilia are of the more unusual kind that arise from the ductal epithelium. Benign hemangioma has been the source of bleeding in a few cases. Metastatic tumors in the liver hardly ever bleed, but hemobilia has been described from metastases in such rare locations as the gallbladder wall.

Vascular disease, formerly a common cause, is now responsible for only 10% of gross hemobilia. True aneurysms of the hepatic artery rupturing into the biliary tract are diminishing with the disappearance of the mycotic aneurysm, leaving only those of atherosclerotic origin. Sometimes, vascular lesions associated with arterial hypertension give rise to hemobilia. The structure usually affected is the gallbladder, and the disorder is then designated "apoplexy of the gallbladder" or "hemocholecyst."

In a few cases of portal hypertension, the general congestion in the mucosa of the digestive tract has caused rupture of dilated veins with profuse bleeding into the biliary tract.

Hemobilia has become a generally recognized syndrome. It is not as rare as it was once thought to be. Surgical treatment is often necessary when the hemorrhage is substantial or repeated, and, when an adequate operation is performed with the aid of angiography, the mortality rate is below 20%. Minor hemobilia is frequent, and resulting clots have often been mistaken for gallstones and erroneously treated as such.

Almost 200 years ago, Portal[13] complained that many physicians mistake hemorrhage through the biliary tract for bleeding from other sources and hence prescribe a wrong treatment. With increasing knowledge of the diagnosis and treatment of hemobilia, the number of misinterpreted or mistreated cases should be rare.

REFERENCES

1. Adolph K: Gallengangs- und Pankreasdiagnostik, p. 153. Stuttgart, Enke Verlag, 1968
2. Carr-Locke DL, Westwood CA: Endoscopy and endoscopic retrograde cholangiopancreatography finding in traumatic liver injury and hemobilia. Am J Gastroenterol 73:162, 1980
3. Clemens M, Wittrin G: Bilhämie and Hämobilie nach Reitunfall. Taglich Nordw Dtsch Chirurg. Vortrag 116, 1975
4. Cox EF: Hemobilia following percutaneous needle biopsy of the liver. Arch Surg 95:198, 1967
5. Curet P, Baumer R, Roche A et al: Hepatic hemobilia of traumatic or iatrogenic origin: Recent advances in diagnosis and therapy, review of the literature from 1976 to 1981. World Surg 8:1, 1984
6. Enge I et al: Central rupture of the liver with traumatic haemobilia: A pre- and post-operative angiographic study. Br J Radiol 41:789, 1968
7. Glisson F: Anatomia hepatis, 1654
8. Kelley CJ, Hemingway AP, McPherson GA et al: Non-surgical management of post-cholecystectomy haemobilia. Br J Surg 70:502, 1983
9. Krudy AG, Doppman JL, Bissonette MB et al: Hemobilia: Computed tomographic diagnosis. Radiology 148:785, 1983
10. Madding GF, Kennedy JA: Trauma to the Liver. Philadelphia, WB Saunders, 1971
11. Mays ET: Lobar dearterialization for exsanguinating wounds of the liver. J Trauma 12:397, 1972
12. Naunyn B: Klinik der Cholelithiasis. Leipzig, 1982
13. Portal A: Sur quelques maladies du foie. Hist Acad R 1777: 601, 1790
14. Sandblom P: Hemorrhage into the biliary tract following trauma: "Traumatic hemobilia." Surgery 24:571, 1948
15. Sandblom P: Gastrointestinal hemorrhage through the pancreatic duct. Ann Surg 171:61, 1970
16. Sandblom P: Hemobilia. Springfield, IL, Charles C Thomas, 1972
17. Sandblom P: Clots or stones in the biliary tract. Acta Chir Scand 147:673, 1981
18. Sandblom P, Mirkovitch V: Minor hemobilia. Ann Surg 190:254, 1979
19. Sandblom P, Saegesser F, Mirkovitch V: Hepatic hemobilia: Hemorrhage from the intrahepatic biliary tract, a review. World J Surg 8:41, 1984
20. Sandblom P et al: The healing of liver wounds. Ann Surg 183:679, 1976
21. Sandblom P et al: Formation and fate of fibrin clots in the biliary tract. Ann Surg 185:356, 1977
22. Sarr MG, Kaufmann SL, Zuidema GD et al: Management of hemobilia associated with transhepatic internal biliary drainage catheters. Surgery 95:603, 1984
23. Ton-That-Tung: Les hémobilies tropicales. Chir 98:43, 1972
24. Walter JF, Paaso BT, Cannon WB: Successful transcatheter embolic control of massive hematobilia secondary to liver biopsy. AJR 127:847, 1976
25. Wiechel KL: Percutaneous transhepatic cholangiography. Acta Cir Scand (Suppl) 330:35, 1964

part 5

Hepatobiliary Disorders in Inflammatory Bowel Disease

FRED KERN, JR.

Several types of hepatobiliary disorders may complicate both forms of chronic inflammatory bowel disease, ulcerative colitis and Crohn's disease, especially when the colon is involved. The frequency and severity of some hepatic and biliary tract disorders are related to the extent, duration, and severity of the bowel disease, but others appear to be independent of the activity of the bowel disease.

The reported frequency of hepatic lesions varies widely, depending on the patient population studied, the indications for histologic examination of the liver, and, perhaps, even the type of biopsy performed. Before the introduction of needle liver biopsy, the liver was examined only at operation, which was usually performed late in the illness or at autopsy. The most common hepatic lesion found was fatty infiltration, a frequent complication of any lengthy, severely debilitating illness. It was present in as many as 40% to 50% of such patients, and cirrhosis was found in 2% to 5%. Since then, the incidence of cirrhosis has remained the same, but the incidence of significant fatty infiltration has decreased considerably, especially in groups of patients subjected to nonoperative needle biopsy. Fatty infiltration still occurs, however, in seriously ill patients and in those subjected to prolonged high-dosage adrenal steroid therapy.

The type of biopsy performed may influence the apparent frequency and type of hepatic lesions. For example, when "wedge" biopsies were performed at the time of colectomy, Eade and co-workers found a high incidence of hepatic fibrosis in patients with ulcerative colitis (51%)[17] and Crohn's colitis (35%).[18] Others using needle liver biopsy find hepatic fibrosis much less frequently. Subcapsular fibrosis, a common nonspecific feature of wedge biopsies, may have caused Eade to overestimate the incidence of fibrosis.[19]

The frequency and distribution of hepatic lesions and an understanding of their relationship to the clinical features of inflammatory bowel disease are dependent on the patient population subjected to study. Patients with inflammatory bowel disease have not been studied by needle liver biopsy performed routinely without abnormal biochemical tests suggesting liver disease. Reports from large clinics generally suggest that a biopsy is performed on some, but not all patients with abnormal results of liver function tests. Criteria for liver biopsy are not clearly stated in all reports.[36,42] Some do not clearly separate the findings of needle biopsy from those of wedge biopsy,[16] yielding a mixture that is difficult to interpret. Modern studies, however, have yielded somewhat more consistent results. Wee and Ludwig[62] reported that 160 of 1911 (8.3%) patients with chronic ulcerative colitis had liver biopsies because of clinical and laboratory evidence of hepatobiliary disease. Shepherd and associates[52] reviewed 681 patients with chronic ulcerative colitis and found only 21 (3.0%) with persistently abnormal liver function. Schrumpf and colleagues[50,51] found hepatobiliary disease in 14% of 336 patients with ulcerative colitis. It seems likely, therefore, that minor hepatic abnormalities occur frequently and that 3% to 15% have persistent clinically significant liver disease.

HEPATIC DISORDERS

Fibrosis and Cirrhosis

Cirrhosis is present in 1% to 5% of patients with chronic ulcerative colitis and less commonly in those with Crohn's disease. It is almost always associated with extensive colonic disease and usually begins after inflammatory bowel disease. The cause and pathogenesis of the cirrhosis are obscure, and the anatomic features vary. Macronodular (postnecrotic) cirrhosis is recognized by some authors but not by others. Mistilis attributed macronodular cirrhosis in his patients to progressive pericholangitis,[36,37] but the presumed origin of this type of cirrhosis was not stated in most other series. Dordal and co-workers identified "nutritional" cirrhosis in several patients.[16] They and Eade and associates used the descriptive term *bridging portal hepatofibrosis* for cirrhosis that did not fit the recognized categories. This kind of cirrhosis is characterized by a uniform bridging portal fibrosis, bile duct proliferation, distortion of the lobular architecture, focal collapse, and nodular regeneration. Its appearance suggests biliary cirrhosis, and it was considered to be a possible sequel of pericholangitis. Eade described portal fibrosis without cirrhosis, usually not clinically important, in a large percentage of patients, probably because of the wedge biopsies taken at laparotomy. Edwards and Truelove reported 16 cases of cirrhosis (2.5%) in 624 patients with ulcerative colitis and noted that cirrhosis accounted for 10% of the deaths that occurred during 20 years of observation.[20] In a systematic study involving frequent clinical and biochemical observations for a mean of more than 4 years, Dew and colleagues found portal cirrhosis in 11 (1.5%) of 720 patients with ulcerative colitis and in 3 (0.6%) of 517 with Crohn's disease.[14]

Holdsworth and co-workers described 20 patients with cirrhosis and ulcerative colitis, 5% of their patients with cirrhosis.[23] Given that the prevalence of ulcerative colitis in the general population is about 1 in 1000, this is a 50-fold increase. Of these 20 patients, 19 had macronodular cirrhosis, and one had biliary cirrhosis. Palmer and others found cirrhosis in patients dying with ulcerative colitis to be 12 times more common than in a control series of patients dying with miscellaneous diseases.[41]

The cause of the cirrhosis is usually not clear. The common factors leading to cirrhosis—alcoholism and viral hepatitis—are rarely present. Sequential histologic examinations beginning preferably before cirrhosis and specific indicators of liver injury are needed to help us understand the pathogenesis of cirrhosis occurring in patients with inflammatory bowel disease.

Fatty Infiltration

Fatty infiltration was described commonly in most older series of patients with inflammatory bowel disease.[11,16,19,32,33] In a more recent analysis by Dew and associates of hepatobiliary disorders in 1237 patients with inflammatory bowel disease, fatty infiltration was not seen.[14]

Extensive fatty infiltration is found in seriously ill patients. The fat, which resembles alcohol-induced fat, occurs in large droplets within the parenchymal cells, often pushing the nucleus to the side. There may be small focal collections of inflammatory cells, or inflammation may be completely absent. Minimal to moderate portal fibrosis is also occasionally present, but Mallory bodies are not seen.

The fatty change has been attributed to poor nutrition, anemia, and toxemia. Drugs, except for corticosteroids, are not implicated. Large doses of corticosteroids cause severe fatty infiltration, but the lesion occurs in patients not receiving steroids.

Hepatitis

Acute viral hepatitis, often transmitted by transfusion, occurs in patients with inflammatory bowel disease, but there is no evidence that it is more common in these patients than in other recipients of transfused blood.

Chronic active hepatitis is an uncommon disease in patients with chronic inflammatory bowel disease, but it has been reported in many series of such patients. Although its exact prevalence is not clear, it appears to be increasing. In a series of patients with chronic active hepatitis and cirrhosis, an unexpectedly large number of patients also have chronic ulcerative colitis.[23,26,65] Since both diseases are relatively uncommon, their frequent occurrence in the same patient suggests more than a chance association.

Either inflammatory bowel disease or chronic hepatitis may precede the other. In most patients with these two diseases, a clear history of antecedent acute hepatitis is not elicited. The possibility of a common denominator, perhaps immunologic, has been suggested but has not been supported by direct evidence. The occasional occurrence in the same patient of ulcerative colitis, chronic active hepatitis, and disorders generally regarded as autoimmune, such as Hashimoto's thyroiditis or acquired hemolytic anemia, supports the possibility that autoimmune processes may play a role in all of these diseases.

Miscellaneous Hepatic Disorders

Focal areas of hepatic necrosis associated with inflammatory cell collections are found throughout the hepatic lobule. These nonspecific lesions, which occur in the livers of patients with almost any type of febrile illness or infectious disease, have no known clinical significance.

Granulomatous hepatitis is unusual in patients with inflammatory bowel disease but has been reported by most authors who have studied the liver in a large number of such patients. Slight icterus, hepatomegaly, and fever may be present. Laboratory abnormalities are mild and nonspecific. The hepatic granulomas contain epithelioid cells and giant cells in their centers and lymphocytes at their periphery. Necrosis is not present. These nonspecific granulomas are distributed randomly throughout the liver lobules. In some patients, or perhaps all, they ultimately disappear.

Secondary hepatic amyloidosis is an unusual complication of inflammatory bowel disease. It usually also involves the kidneys, spleen, and other organs.

Pylephlebitis and liver abscesses were frequent complications of fatal cases of ulcerative colitis before the introduction of chemotherapy but today are very uncommon.

BILIARY TRACT DISORDERS

In patients with inflammatory bowel disease, three lesions—pericholangitis, sclerosing cholangitis, and bile duct carcinoma—affect the biliary tract and are probably related to each other. Pericholangitis is common but usually not serious, and the other two, more serious disorders, are generally regarded as less common; however, in recent studies, primary sclerosing cholangitis is identified more frequently than in the past. Wee and Ludwig found primary sclerosing cholangitis in 18 of 160 (11.3%) patients with chronic ulcerative colitis with biopsy evidence of hepatobiliary disease, which was almost 1% of a total of 1911 patients with colitis.[62] An even higher incidence of primary sclerosing cholangitis among patients with chronic ulcerative colitis was reported by Shepherd and associates (2.4%)[52] and Schrumpf and colleagues (5.9%).[50] In each of the latter studies, sclerosing cholangitis accounted for a large portion of ulcerative colitis patients with significant hepatobiliary disease. Cholesterol cholelithiasis, a complication of ileal dysfunction, is usually not related to the other biliary tract disorders.

Pericholangitis

Investigators disagree about the appropriate descriptive term for the most common lesion, pericholangitis. It has also been called *portal triaditis, interlobular hepatitis,* and *intrahepatic cholangitic hepatitis.* The term *pericholangitis* has been declared unacceptable by a conference group concerned with standardizing nomenclature of diseases of the liver and biliary tract. Recently, a new name was introduced, *primary sclerosing cholangitis of the small bile ducts.*[62] This term recognizes the growing understanding of a relationship between the exclusively intrahepatic lesion pericholangitis and primary sclerosing cholangitis,[10,25,33] which almost always involves the extrahepatic bile ducts. However, since "pericholangitis" is not only a generally recognized term but also an appropriate description of most of the usual histologic features, the latter will be employed in this chapter.

In all studies reported since the introduction of percutaneous needle liver biopsy, pericholangitis has been recognized as a common hepatic lesion. However, its exact prevalence is uncertain. It has been found in as many as 20% to 30% of patients with either chronic ulcerative colitis or Crohn's disease who also have clinical or laboratory evidence of liver disease,[11,17,59] but it may be even more common, a view supported by the unexpected discovery of the lesion in liver biopsies of some patients with normal results of tests of liver function.

The lesion is characterized by enlargement of the portal triads by edema and an inflammatory cell infiltrate (Fig. 44-15), usually composed of lymphocytes and plasma cells, and, in some instances, polymorphonuclear leukocytes and eosinophils. The infiltrate is often heaviest around the interlobular bile duct, but it may be evenly distributed throughout the portal spaces. The bile duct epithelium is usually normal, but it may be infiltrated by inflammatory cells. Proliferation of fibroblasts in a loose manner, especially around the interlobular bile ducts, is often present, and dense periductal fibrosis may be quite marked in the later stages. In some patients, it is the only

sign that pericholangitis has existed. Bile duct proliferation may occur with the new ducts enveloped by the inflammatory infiltrate. The degree of involvement of individual portal areas varies even within a single liver biopsy specimen, a feature that makes interpretation and diagnosis difficult. Hepatocytes are usually not affected when the lesion is mild, but, in more severe cases, centrilobular bile stasis, Kupffer cell hyperplasia, and piecemeal necrosis occur (Fig. 44-16). Limited experience with patients with this lesion, which suggests chronic active hepatitis, indicates that the lesion forecasts a progressive course, with cirrhosis being the eventual outcome in some.

Clinical Features and Prognosis

Pericholangitis occurs most commonly in patients with extensive bowel involvement but it may occur when the disease is limited to a small segment, such as the rectum, sigmoid colon, or terminal ileum.

Pericholangitis is often not clinically apparent, requiring laboratory tests for detection. Jaundice, usually slight, is present only in severe cases. The size of the liver is normal or only slightly enlarged, and the spleen is usually not palpable. The most useful laboratory tests for detection of pericholangitis are serum alkaline phosphatase, γ-glutamyl transpeptidase, and 5′-nucleotidase activities.[3,37,58] In more severe cases, the serum transaminase levels are also abnormal. There is no characteristic alteration in serum proteins or lipids.

Pericholangitis is usually a benign disease. Its course often parallels that of the bowel disease. In most patients, inflammation subsides and is replaced by harmless peri-

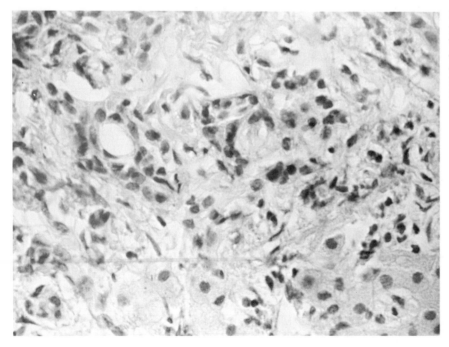

Fig. 44-15. Photomicrograph of a portal area in the liver of a patient with pericholangitis. There is edema and infiltration of lymphocytes and polymorphonuclear leukocytes. (Original magnification × 300; H & E)

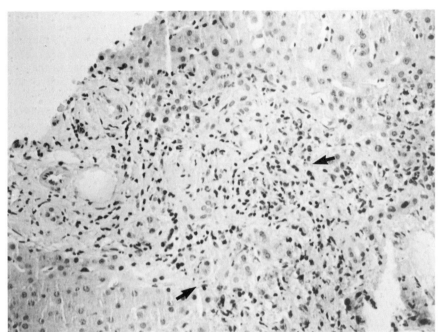

Fig. 44-16. Photomicrograph showing a progressively destructive form of pericholangitis. The expanded portal space is heavily infiltrated by acute and chronic inflammatory cells. The arrows show erosion of the limiting plate by piecemeal necrosis in several areas. Fibrosis is also present. The patient, a young man, had an enlarged liver and spleen, mild jaundice, and elevated serum levels of alkaline phosphatase and transaminases. (Original magnification × 200; H & E)

ductular fibrosis, but, in occasional patients, it appears to progress to chronic liver disease. Such patients may have jaundice and an enlarged, firm liver and spleen. Serum transaminases and γ-globulin levels are usually elevated, and sulfobromophthalein retention may be increased. Tests for antimitochondrial antibodies are uniformly negative. Such patients may ultimately develop all of the complications of hepatic cirrhosis. In some cases, pericholangitis seems to progress to sclerosing cholangitis.

Cause and Pathogenesis

The cause and pathogenesis of pericholangitis are unknown. It has been proposed that harmful substances pass through the wall of the diseased bowel into the portal blood and damage the liver. Three candidate substances have been suggested: bacteria, bile acids, and bacterial antigens.

Portal vein blood is normally sterile, but, in some patients with ulcerative colitis, cultures of portal vein blood at laparotomy are positive for both aerobic and anaerobic fecal organisms.[6,39] Simultaneous cultures of liver tissue may or may not be positive, but blood cultures from the systemic circulation are usually sterile, consistent with the capacity of the liver to remove bacteria from the blood. No direct relationship between portal bacteremia and the presence of pericholangitis or of any other hepatic lesion has been established in reported clinical studies, but positive portal cultures have been generally found in more seriously ill patients. In the only animal experiment reported, a lesion similar to acute pericholangitis was produced by continuous portal vein infusion of *Escherichia coli* in calves.[58]

The secondary bile acid, lithocholic acid, the product of bacterial 7-α-dehydroxylation of chenodeoxycholic acid, has been implicated as a potential hepatic toxin responsible for pericholangitis. Lithocholic acid is normally produced in the distal small intestine and colon, and only a small amount is absorbed. When it is given in large quantities to many types of experimental animals, it is hepatotoxic, and, in several animal species, it produces a lesion very similar to pericholangitis.[40]

Direct supporting evidence implicating lithocholic acid in patients with inflammatory bowel disease is lacking. In such patients, there is no increase of this bile acid in the bile. Furthermore, given that the human liver can sulfate lithocholic acid, converting it into a more polar nontoxic substance, and given that patients with cholesterol gallstones being treated with chenodeoxycholic acid may have a greatly increased amount of lithocholic acid in bile without significant liver damage, it is most unlikely that lithocholic acid is toxic to patients with inflammatory bowel disease. However, the possibility of diminished hepatic sulfating capacity in patients with inflammatory bowel disease and pericholangitis has not been tested.

The third potential mechanism for producing pericholangitis is the increased absorption of immunogenic substances, such as bacterial antigens, that harm the liver either directly or after the formation of antigen–antibody complexes. Again, this hypothesis does not have the support of direct evidence.[6]

Treatment

The treatment of patients with ordinary, nonprogressive pericholangitis is that of the underlying bowel disease. Specific therapy of the liver disease is not warranted. On the other hand, when the hepatic lesion is progressive and the patient is threatened by irreversible liver disease, specific treatment is warranted but not available. Colectomy has been tried, but usually without success.

Primary Sclerosing Cholangitis

Primary sclerosing cholangitis, a disease of obscure cause, is a progressive, sclerosing, obliterative process involving the extrahepatic and, in many patients, the intrahepatic bile ducts. It is an unusual complication of chronic ulcerative colitis and a rare complication of Crohn's disease. It affects men much more often than women. Even though the disease occurs in patients without inflammatory bowel disease, patients with such disease comprise more than 50% of cases.[34,61] In a series of 50 patients seen at the Mayo Clinic over a period of 8 years, 54% had inflammatory bowel disease.[64] In other recently reported studies,[8,29,55] 35% to 70% of patients with sclerosing cholangitis have had inflammatory bowel disease, almost all chronic ulcerative colitis.

The nature of the relationship of sclerosing cholangitis to pericholangitis is uncertain, but the existence of a relationship is suggested by the apparent progression from pericholangitis to sclerosing cholangitis in a few patients and by the appearance of histologic changes resembling pericholangitis in some patients with sclerosing cholangitis.[10,25,33,62] Characteristic bile duct abnormalities primarily involving intrahepatic bile ducts have been reported in patients with the clinical and histologic features of pericholangitis. These observations, made by radiographic visualization of the biliary tree by endoscopic retrograde cholangiography, also suggest that pericholangitis and sclerosing cholangitis may represent the ends of a spectrum.[2,27,47] Cholangiography, performed either endoscopically or percutaneously, in addition to liver biopsy, is essential in the evaluation of patients with inflammatory bowel disease and cholestatic liver disease. Serial studies may further elucidate the relationship between these disorders and lead to a better understanding of their natural history.

Gallstones are usually not present, but the gallbladder is often involved in the same pathologic process.[56] In some patients, stones are found in the biliary tree, possibly secondary to biliary stasis, and may cause further obstruction.

Clinical Features

The principal clinical features of sclerosing cholangitis are fluctuating right upper quadrant and epigastric pain, nausea and vomiting, fever, jaundice, and pruritus—features of bile duct obstruction. However, the disease may be present for years without producing any symptoms. The cholangiogram of a 28-year-old man who had mild ulcerative colitis for 10 years is shown in Figure 44-17A; his sclerosing cholangitis was discovered when investigation (including cholecystectomy and T-tube drainage) was stimulated by the accidental finding of an elevated serum bile acid concentration. Except for a slightly elevated serum alkaline phosphatase level, the patient had no other clinical or laboratory evidence of liver disease. A cholangiogram taken 7 years later, several months after the patient developed fluctuating jaundice, pruritus and laboratory evidence of cholestasis is shown in Figure 44-17B. At this time, his liver and spleen were enlarged and firm and very small esophageal varices were seen at endoscopy. The cholangiogram appears little changed.

Cholangiograms of a man who became jaundiced after 18 years of ulcerative colitis are shown in Figure 44-18A and B. He had a colectomy and an operative cholangiogram that showed mild sclerosing cholangitis. A liver biopsy showed cholestasis, fibrosis, and ductular and periductular changes consistent with the diagnosis. During the next 7 years, he was healthy except for mildly abnormal liver function studies without progression. An episode of biliary colic led to cholecystectomy. He had several 1-mm to 2-mm gallstones and a 5-mm noninvasive papillary carcinoma of the gallbladder. Cholangiography (Fig. 44-18B) showed only modest progression of the large duct disease, and a liver biopsy showed little or no progression of hepatic damage.

In general, the obstructive process eventually progresses to secondary biliary cirrhosis. The liver and spleen become enlarged, signs of portal hypertension develop, and death often occurs from the complications of cirrhosis, bleeding esophageal varices, and hepatic coma.

The characteristic cholangiographic abnormality is diffuse, irregular narrowing of the lumen of the extrahepatic bile ducts. Occasionally, dilated ducts are seen proximal to the sclerotic ducts. Intrahepatic ducts may or may not show irregular narrowing, often without proximal dilatation, but, in some patients, saccular dilatation occurs and may be complicated by bacterial cholangitis.

Microscopic examination of the wall of the large bile ducts shows fibrotic thickening (Fig. 44-19) and often a mononuclear and polymorphonuclear inflammatory infiltrate. Similar changes may be seen in intrahepatic ducts (Fig. 44-20). Sections of the liver may be normal or may reveal inflammatory changes similar to pericholangitis in various stages (acute, subacute, chronic), to cholestasis, and to biliary cirrhosis. In sclerosing cholangitis with an intrahepatic component and in severe pericholangitis alone, one may find dense spherical scars within portal tracts devoid of interlobular bile ducts, presumably representing the sites of destroyed ducts. In other sites, the duct epithelium may be normal, and, in still others, there may be lymphocytic infiltration and destruction of the duct epithelium similar to that seen in primary biliary cirrhosis. Bile duct proliferation and eventual obliteration of ducts may be seen (Fig. 44-21). As the disease progresses, the general architecture of the liver becomes that of sec-

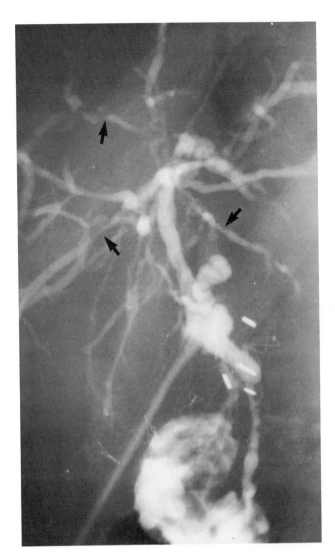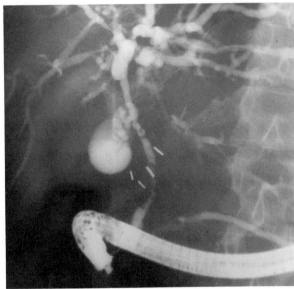

Fig. 44-17. Left. T-tube cholangiogram of a 28-year-old man. The patient had ulcerative colitis for more than 10 years but was clinically well except for an elevated serum bile acid level and a slightly elevated serum alkaline phosphatase level. The common bile duct is narrow and irregular, typical of sclerosing cholangitis. In the intrahepatic bile ducts, there are many areas of narrowing (*arrows*). There is no dilatation of the biliary tract. **Right.** Endoscopic retrograde cholangiogram of the patient shown in *A* 7 years later. Even though the biliary tree has not changed very much, the patient had evidence of chronic cholestatic liver disease at the time this study was done.

ondary biliary cirrhosis. High copper concentrations in hepatic tissue have been described.[4,10,33,64]

Etiology

The cause of the disease is not known. An immunologic hypothesis has been invoked. It has been proposed that immunogenic substances, such as endotoxin, are absorbed in large quantities and combine with antibody to form immune complexes in such a large quantity that they overwhelm the capacity of the liver to remove them, allowing them to enter the systemic circulation.[22,53] The hypothesis is supported by the demonstration of an increase in circulating immune complexes in inflammatory bowel disease, but the immune complexes are no more common in those with than in those without extraintestinal complications. One study identified immune complexes by at least one of two techniques in 16 of 20 patients

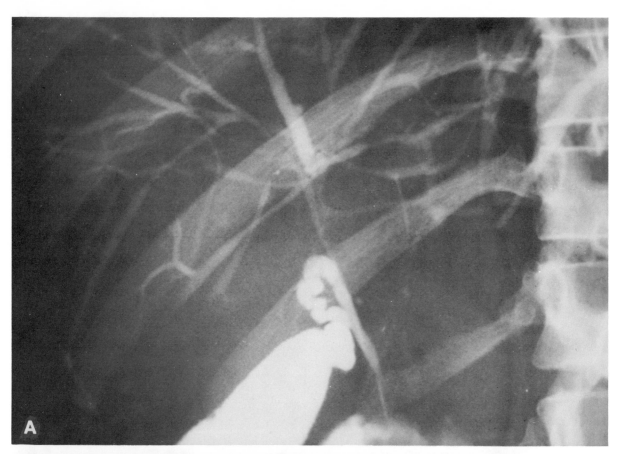

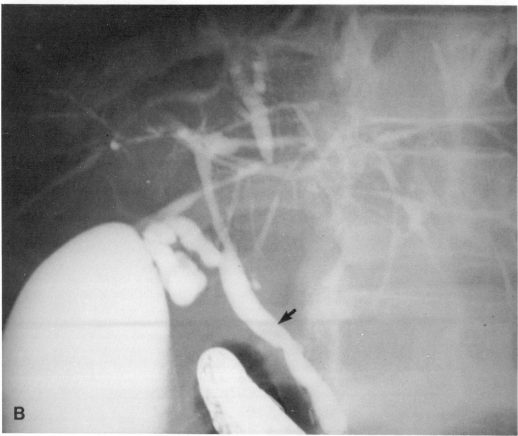

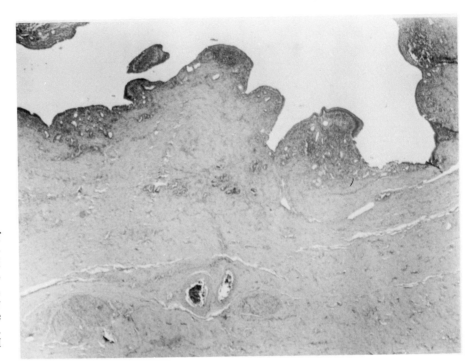

Fig. 44-19. Photomicrograph of a section of the wall of the common bile duct of a 40-year-old man who died from complications of sclerosing cholangitis. The wall consists almost entirely of dense connective tissue. The bile duct epithelium is normal. (Original magnification × 50; H & E)

with primary sclerosing cholangitis.[4] The presence or absence of ulcerative colitis did not appear to affect the results. Minuk and co-workers described delayed plasma clearance of radiolabeled immune complexes in patients with sclerosing cholangitis but not in liver disease control patients.[35] The exact significance of these observations is not clear at this time. Some clinical studies have suggested that immunologic disorders can injure the bile ducts.[45,60] The concurrence of sclerosing cholangitis with lymphocytic thyroiditis, retroperitoneal fibrosis, mediastinal fibrosis, and pernicious anemia is cited as indirect support for an immunologic mechanism. In a mouse model of graft-versus-host disease, bile duct injury resulted in a lesion similar to primary biliary cirrhosis.[49]

Support for a genetic predisposition to an immunologic mechanism comes from studies of HLA antigens. Schrumpf and associates[51] found HLA-B8 in 16 of 20 patients (80%) with chronic ulcerative colitis with hepatobiliary disease (most had primary sclerosing cholangitis) compared with 32% in ulcerative colitis patients without

hepatobiliary disease (34 patients) and 25% in a large number of controls. They found a similar significant increase in HLA-Dr3. Chapman and colleagues[9] studied HLA antigens in 25 patients with primary sclerosing cholangitis, 14 of whom had chronic ulcerative colitis, and found 60% had HLA-B8 compared with 25% in controls. Both HLA-B8 and HLA-Dr3 are associated with diseases involving disordered immunologic function. The genetic hypothesis is further supported by the occurrence of primary sclerosing cholangitis and ulcerative colitis in two siblings in each of three families[5,44] and increase in fractional metabolic rate of C3, a key component of the complement sequence, in patients with hepatobiliary disease associated with ulcerative colitis, suggesting a pathogenetic role for humoral immune factors.

Treatment

The treatment of sclerosing cholangitis is unsatisfactory. Some anecdotal reports suggest that colectomy is bene-

←

Fig. 44-18. **A.** Operative cholangiogram of a young man with ulcerative colitis and evidence of chronic liver disease (see text). Irregular narrowing of the intrahepatic and extrahepatic bile ducts is consistent with primary sclerosing cholangitis. The liver biopsy was also consistent with this diagnosis. **B.** Endoscopic retrograde cholangiogram of the same patient 7 years later, when he had biliary colic. An arrow indicates a gallstone in the common bile duct, which is slightly dilated. The common hepatic duct is narrow. Intrahepatic bile ducts show only slightly more disease than in the earlier cholangiogram (*A*). The liver biopsy also indicated little progression of the disease.

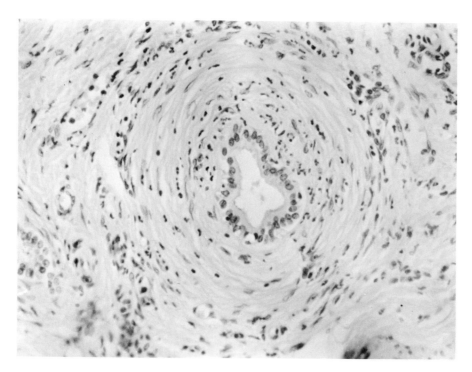

Fig. 44-20. Photomicrograph of an intrahepatic bile duct in the liver of the same patient whose common bile duct is shown in Figure 44-19. There is extensive periductal fibrosis. Inflammatory cells, including polymorphonuclear leukocytes, are apparent in the connective tissue and invading the epithelium itself (shown better in the high-power view in Fig. 44-21B.) (Original magnification × 300)

ficial. No controlled trial of colectomy has been done. Antibiotics and steroids have generally not been helpful. Attempts to relieve the obstruction by surgical drainage are usually disappointing in the long run because of the fibrosis of the duct system, but, when dilated ducts are available for anastomosis to the intestine or for drainage by T-tubes or U-tubes, temporary benefit can be obtained. Anecdotal reports of duct dilatation by balloon, inserted either percutaneously or endoscopically, have appeared, but there are no systematic studies. This approach does not seem likely to provide more than transient palliation.

Bile Duct Carcinoma

Carcinoma of the bile duct is an uncommon complication of ulcerative colitis[12]; however, in a review of cases of concomitant occurrences of the two diseases, it was estimated that such tumors occur 8 to 21 times more frequently in patients with ulcerative colitis than in the general population.[46] In most patients, the entire colon is diseased. Some of the colitis patients who develop this carcinoma do not have evidence of preexisting biliary tract disease, but, in others, sclerosing cholangitis antedates the carcinoma. Cholelithiasis is present in 30% to 50% of noncolitis patients with bile duct carcinoma but not often in colitis patients. Patients with chronic ulcerative colitis who develop bile duct cancer are 20 or more years younger than other patients with bile duct carcinoma. Except for its occurrence in young patients, this adenocarcinoma, which varies in degree of differentiation, has no special biologic features. The tumor may be primary in the extrahepatic or intrahepatic bile ducts or in the gallbladder.

Diagnosis may be difficult, because the symptoms of extrahepatic obstruction are the same as those of sclerosing cholangitis. Cholangiography may reveal a discrete, fairly easily recognized obstructing tumor or a more diffuse, spreading lesion that may be difficult to distinguish from sclerosing cholangitis.

The tumor usually occurs in patients with long standing ulcerative colitis (mean, 15 years), but, in occasional cases, the interval after the onset of colitis may be brief, and, in some, the tumor develops after total colectomy. Ritchie and co-workers described 19 cases of a total of 67 in whom bile duct carcinoma arose 1 to 20 years (mean, 7 to 8 years) after surgery for colitis.[36,37] In these patients, the mean duration of colitis prior to colectomy was 11 years, ranging from 2 to 22.

In summary, the biliary tract seems particularly vulnerable to damage in patients with chronic inflammatory diseases of the bowel. Because pericholangitis, sclerosing cholangitis, and bile duct carcinoma occur in the same patients, it is likely that they are related. It is conceivable that sclerosing cholangitis represents the response of the large bile ducts to the same injury that causes pericholangitis, which involves intralobular ducts, and that bile duct carcinoma is the late sequel of continued injury to the bile duct epithelium. The cause of the presumed bile duct injury remains unknown but a genetic predisposition to an altered immune response may exist. Therapy is not satisfactory.

Cholesterol Cholelithiasis

Cholesterol gallstones occur in 30% to 35% of all patients with ileal resection or with extensive or long standing

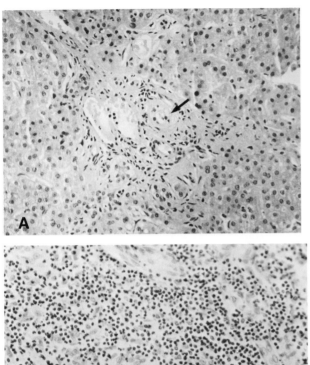

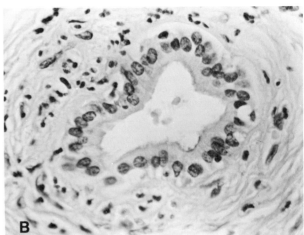

Fig. 44-21. A. Photomicrograph of a liver biopsy specimen from a 21-year-old man who had ulcerative colitis for 9 years. He also had immunoglobulin A deficiency, Hashimoto's thyroiditis and the destructive cholangitic lesion are shown. The arrow indicates a destroyed bile duct. Inflammatory cells, including polymorphonuclear leukocytes, and fibrosis are present. (Original magnification × 200; H & E) **B.** High-power view of the bile duct shown in Figure 44-20. In several areas, the epithelial cells are vacuolated and are being invaded by lymphocytes. Many inflammatory cells surround the epithelium. (Original magnification × 440; H & E) **C.** Photomicrograph of the liver of a patient with primary sclerosing cholangitis showing simultaneous proliferation and destruction of bile ducts. The ductal epithelium is poorly organized and appears to be invaded by acute and chronic inflammatory cells. (Original magnification × 200; H & E)

Crohn's disease of the ileum.[1,11,63] This represents a considerable increase in incidence from that seen in the unaffected population of the same age and sex. The incidence of cholelithiasis is not higher in patients with colitis alone. The increased risk of gallstones in association with ileal dysfunction is consistent with the current understanding of the pathogenesis of cholesterol gallstones. Bile acid malabsorption secondary to ileal disease or resection leads to a decrease in concentration of biliary bile acids and a relative increase in concentration of biliary cholesterol. Under these circumstances, cholesterol crystals precipitate in the gallbladder and gallstones form.

REFERENCES

1. Baker AL et al: Gallstones in inflammatory bowel disease. Am J Dig Dis 19:109, 1974
2. Blackstone MO, Nemchausky BA: Cholangiographic abnormalities in ulcerative colitis associated pericholangitis which resemble sclerosing cholangitis. Am J Dig Dis 23:579, 1978
3. Boden RW et al: The liver in ulcerative colitis: The significance of the raised serum-alkaline-phosphatase levels. Lancet 2:245, 1949
4. Bodenheimer HC et al: Elevated circulating immune complexes in primary sclerosing cholangitis. Hepatology 3:150, 1983
5. Brinch L et al: The *in vivo* metabolism of C_3 in hepatobiliary disease associated with ulcerative colitis. Scand J Gastroenterol 17:523, 1982
6. Brooke BN, Slaney G: Portal bacteremia in ulcerative colitis. Lancet 1:1206, 1958
7. Brooke BN et al: A study of liver disorder in ulcerative colitis. Postgrad Med J 37:245, 1961
8. Cameron JL et al: Sclerosing cholangitis. Ann Surg 200:54, 1984
9. Chapman RW et al: Association of primary sclerosing cholangitis with HLA-B8. Gut 24:38, 1983
10. Chapman RGW et al: Primary sclerosing cholangitis: A review of its clinical features, cholangiography, and hepatic histology. Gut 21:870, 1980
11. Cohen S et al: Liver disease and gallstones in regional enteritis. Gastroenterology 60:237, 1971
12. Converse CF et al: Ulcerative colitis and carcinoma of the bile ducts. Am J Surg 121:39, 1971
13. Dalmark M: Plasma radioactivity after rectal instillation of radioiodine labelled human albumin in normal subjects and in patients with ulcerative colitis. Scand J Gastroenterol 3:490, 1968

14. Dew WF et al: The spectrum of hepatic dysfunction in inflammatory bowel disease. Q J Med 189:113, 1979
15. Doe WF et al: Evidence for complement-binding immune complexes in adult coeliac disease, Crohn's disease, and ulcerative colitis. Lancet 1:402, 1973
16. Dordal E et al: Hepatic lesions in chronic inflammatory bowel disease: Clinical correlations with liver biopsy diagnoses in 103 patients. Gastroenterology 52:239, 1967
17. Eade MN et al: Liver disease in ulcerative colitis: I. Analysis of operative liver biopsy in 138 consecutive patients having colectomy. Ann Intern Med 72:475, 1970
18. Eade MN et al: Liver disease in Crohn's disease: A study of 100 consecutive patients. Scand J Gastroenterol 6:199, 1971
19. Eade MN et al: Liver disease in Crohn's disease: A study of 21 consecutive patients having colectomy. Ann Intern Med 74:518, 1971
20. Edwards FC, Truelove SC: The course and prognosis of ulcerative colitis: III. Complications. Gut 5:1, 1964
21. Greenstein AJ et al: The extra-intestinal complications of Crohn's disease and ulcerative colitis: A study of 700 patients. Medicine 55:401, 1976
22. Hodgson HJF et al: Immune complexes in ulcerative colitis and Crohn's disease. Clin Exp Immunol 29:187, 1977
23. Holdsworth CD et al: Ulcerative colitis in chronic liver disease. Q J Med 34:211, 1965
24. Jewell DP, Maclennan ICM: Circulating immune complexes in inflammatory bowel disease. Clin Exp Immunol 14:219, 1973
25. Kern F Jr, Bloustein PA: The biliary tract in inflammatory bowel disease. In Bianchi L, Gerok W, Sickinger K (eds): Liver and Bile, pp 327–340. London, MTP Press, 1977
26. Kern F Jr et al: The treatment of chronic hepatitis with adrenal cortical hormones. Am J Med 35:310, 1963
27. Kolmannskog F et al: Cholangiographic findings in ulcerative colitis. Acta Radiol Diagn 22:151, 1981
28. Kraft SC: Inflammatory bowel disease (ulcerative colitis and Crohn's disease). In Asquith P (ed): Immunology of the Gastrointestinal Tract, pp 95–128. New York, Churchill Livingstone, 1979
29. La Russo NF et al: Primary sclerosing cholangitis. N Engl J Med 310:899, 1984
30. Leevy CM et al: Diseases of the liver and biliary tract: Standardization of nomenclature, diagnostic criteria, and diagnostic methodology. Fogarty Int Center Proc 22:1, 1976
31. Levitan R, Brudno S: Permeability of the rectosigmoid mucosa to tritiated water in normal subjects and in patients with mild idiopathic ulcerative colitis. Gut 8:15, 1967
32. Ludwig J: Some names hang on like leeches. Dig Dis Sci 24:967, 1979
33. Ludwig J et al: Morphologic features of chronic hepatitis associated with primary sclerosing cholangitis and chronic ulcerative colitis. Hepatology 1:632, 1981
34. Markoff N: Review: Primary sclerosing cholangitis. Acta Hepatogastroenterol 20:77, 1973
35. Minuk GY et al: Abnormal clearance of immune complexes from the circulation of patients with primary sclerosing cholangitis. Gastroenterology 88:166, 1985
36. Mistilis SP et al: Pericholangitis and ulcerative colitis: I. Pathology, etiology and pathogenesis. Ann Intern Med 63:1, 1965
37. Mistilis SP et al: Pericholangitis and ulcerative colitis: II. Clinical aspects. Ann Intern Med 63:17, 1965
38. Morowitz DA et al: Carcinoma of the biliary tract complicating chronic ulcerative colitis. Cancer 27:356, 1971
39. Orloff MJ et al: A bacteriologic study of human portal blood: Implications regarding hepatic ischemia in man. Ann Surg 148:738, 1958
40. Palmer RH: Bile acids, liver injury and liver disease. Arch Intern Med 130:606, 1972
41. Palmer WL et al: Diseases of the liver in chronic ulcerative colitis. Am J Med 36:856, 1964
42. Perrett AD et al: The liver in ulcerative colitis. Q J Med 40:211, 1971
43. Perrett AD et al: The liver in Crohn's disease. Q J Med 40:187, 1971
44. Quigley EMM et al: Familial occurrence of primary sclerosing cholangitis and ulcerative colitis. Gastroenterology 85:1160, 1983
45. Record CO et al: Intrahepatic sclerosing cholangitis associated with a familial immunodeficiency syndrome. Lancet 2:18, 1973
46. Ritchie JK et al: Biliary tract carcinoma associated with ulcerative colitis. Q J Med 170:263, 1974
47. Rohrmann CA et al: Cholangiographic abnormalities in patients with inflammatory bowel disease. Radiol Diagn 127:635, 1978
48. Ross AP, Braasch JW: Ulcerative colitis and carcinoma of the proximal bile ducts. Gut 14:94, 1973
49. Ruderman WB et al: Evolution of hepatic lesions in murine chronic graft-vs-host disease. Gastroenterology 84:1290A, 1983
50. Schrumpf E et al: Sclerosing cholangitis in ulcerative colitis: A follow up study. Scand J Gastroenterol 17:33, 1981
51. Schrumpf E et al: HLA antigens and immunoregulatory T cells in ulcerative colitis associated with hepatobiliary disease. Scand J Gastroenterol 17:187, 1981
52. Shepherd HA et al: Ulcerative colitis and persistent liver dysfunction. Q J Med 208:503, 1983
53. Thomas HC, Vaez-Zadeh F: A homeostatic mechanism for the removal of antigen from the portal circulation. Immunology 26:375, 1974
54. Thomas HC et al: Role of the liver in controlling the immunogenicity of commensal bacteria in the gut. Lancet 1:1288, 1973
55. Thompson HH et al: Primary sclerosing cholangitis: A heterogenous disease. Ann Surg 196:127, 1982
56. Thorpe MEC et al: Primary sclerosing cholangitis, the biliary tree, and ulcerative colitis. Gut 8:435, 1967
57. Vinnik IE et al: Serum 5-nucleotidase and pericholangitis in patients with chronic ulcerative colitis. Gastroenterology 45:492, 1963
58. Vinnik IE et al: Experimental chronic portal vein bacteremia. Proc Soc Exp Biol Med 115:311, 1964
59. Vinnik IE, Kern F Jr: Liver diseases in ulcerative colitis. Arch Intern Med 112:41, 1963
60. Waldram R et al: Chronic pancreatitis, sclerosing cholangitis and sicca complex in two siblings. Lancet 1:550, 1975
61. Warren KW et al: Primary sclerosing cholangitis. Am J Surg 111:23, 1966
62. Wee A, Ludwig J: Pericholangitis in chronic ulcerative colitis: Primary sclerosing cholangitis of the small bile ducts. Ann Intern Med 102:581, 1985
63. Whorwell PJ et al: Ultrasound survey of gallstones and other hepatobiliary disorders in patients with Crohn's disease. Dig Dis Sci 29:930, 1984
64. Weisner RH, La Russo NF: Clinicopathologic features of the syndrome of primary sclerosing cholangitis. Gastroenterology 79:200, 1980
65. Wilcox RG, Isselbacher KJ: Chronic liver disease in young people. Am J Med 30:185, 1961

part **6**

Congenital Hepatic Fibrosis and Caroli's Syndrome

JEAN-PIERRE BENHAMOU

CONGENITAL HEPATIC FIBROSIS

Congenital hepatic fibrosis is an inherited, congenital malformation characterized by large, fibrotic portal spaces, containing multiple bile ductules, the main consequence of which is portal hypertension. The disease was described as fibrocystic disease of the liver by Grumbach and coworkers in 1954.[11] The denomination of congenital hepatic fibrosis was introduced by Kerr and colleagues in 1961.[12]

Pathology and Pathogenesis

The lesion of congenital hepatic fibrosis consists of portal spaces markedly increased in size because of abundant connective tissue and numerous bile ductules, more or less ectatic, communicating with the biliary tree (Fig. 44-22). It must be emphasized that congenital hepatic fibrosis is not simply fibrosis and that bile ductular proliferation is an essential component of the lesion. A few portal spaces remain normal, which explains that congenital hepatic fibrosis may be unrecognized at histologic examination of a small specimen taken by liver biopsy. Some clusters of multiple bile ductule surrounded with fibrosis may be present within the lobules, apart from the portal spaces. Some bile ductules are so markedly dilated that they form microcysts; which communicate with the biliary tree.

Separation between the fibrotic portal spaces and the rest of the liver parenchyma is sharp. Architecture of the liver remains normal. There is no regenerative nodule.

The primary disorder of congenital hepatic fibrosis is likely to be bile ductular proliferation, with fibrosis being secondarily induced by the multiple bile ductules. The initial lesion might be clusters of multiple bile ductules (*i.e.,* von Meyenburgh complexes), resembling the initial lesion of the liver cysts associated with adult polycystic kidney disease. However, in congenital hepatic fibrosis, the abnormal bile ductules maintain their communications with the biliary tree and, as a result, only microcysts are formed; in contrast, in adult polycystic kidney disease, the abnormal bile ductules lose their communication with the biliary tree and, as a result, dilate markedly and form large cysts.

The mechanism for the development of multiple bile ductules in congenital hepatic fibrosis is unknown. It has been suggested that bile ductular proliferation might result from a disproportionate overgrowth of the biliary epithelium.[18] A similar disorder affecting the epithelium of the large bile ducts might account for Caroli's syndrome associated with congenital hepatic fibrosis. A similar mechanism might explain the dilatation of the renal collecting tubules and the dilatation of pancreatic ducts, two extrahepatic malformations that may be associated with congenital hepatic fibrosis.

Etiology and Prevalence

Congenital hepatic fibrosis is an inherited malformation, transmitted as an autosomal recessive trait.[1,12] The parents, presumably heterozygous, are phenotypically normal. Males and females are equally affected. Several siblings may be affected. Consanguinity increases the risk of congenital hepatic fibrosis.

The prevalence of congenital hepatic fibrosis is not established, but it certainly is very low and might be of the

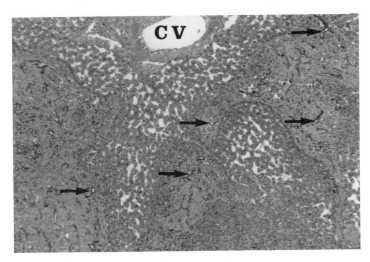

Fig. 44-22. Congenital hepatic fibrosis: liver biopsy. (Original magnification × 70; H & E) The portal spaces are markedly increased in size and contain abundant fibrosis and numerous bile ductules. (Some of them are indicated by arrows.) CV, centrilobular vein.

same order of magnitude than that of another autosomal recessive liver disease, Wilson's disease (*i.e.,* about 1:100,000).[23] There is no ethnic predominance.

Clinical Manifestations and Diagnosis

The main consequence of congenital hepatic fibrosis is portal hypertension, which is likely to have been present since the patient's birth. In most of the patients, the disease is recognized at the first episode of gastrointestinal bleeding due to ruptured esophageal varices, which occurs usually between 5 and 20 years, sometimes later. In a few patients the disease is recognized before any episode of gastrointestinal bleeding because of blood disorders due to hypersplenism, abdominal discomfort due to an enlarged spleen, or the presence of abdominal collateral venous circulation.

At clinical examination, the liver is often, but not constantly, enlarged. Splenomegaly is present in most of the patients. Abdominal collateral circulation (Cruveilhier syndrome in some patients) is often visible. Ascites is absent. There is no symptom or sign indicating liver failure, in particular jaundice or spiders. The results of liver tests are normal, except for moderately increased alkaline phosphatase and gammaglutamyltranspeptidase in a few patients. Endoscopic or radiographic examination demonstrates esophageal varices. Ultrasonography and/or computed tomography show that the liver is often enlarged (often hyperechoic because of fibrosis and ductular proliferation), portal vein is patent (which excludes extrahepatic portal hypertension), spleen is enlarged, and portacaval anastomoses are present; the venous phase of celiac and supramesenteric arteriographies would provide similar information. Histologic examination of a hepatic tissue specimen taken by needle biopsy demonstrates the typical lesion in most of the patients; however, if the specimen is small, the lesion may be missed because, as mentioned above, some of the portal spaces may be normal.

Course and Complications

The course of the disease is dominated by recurrent episodes of gastrointestinal bleeding, the frequency of which widely varies from patient to patient. The episodes of gastrointestinal bleeding are often well tolerated and are usually not followed by hepatic encephalopathy, ascites, or jaundice. The patient's death is due to massive bleeding but not to liver failure. Thus, the course of congenital hepatic fibrosis resembles that of extrahepatic portal hypertension and differs from that of cirrhosis.

Associated Malformations

Congenital hepatic fibrosis is often associated with Caroli's syndrome, either clinically silent (demonstrated by ultrasonography or computed tomography), or determining cholangitis (see below).

Congenital hepatic fibrosis is likewise often associated with a renal malformation consisting of ectatic collecting tubules, resembling sponge kidney.[14] However, dilatation affects the medullary and cortical portions of the collecting tubules in congenital hepatic fibrosis, whereas dilatation is limited to the medullary portion of the collecting tubules in sponge kidney.[5,9] This renal malformation is clinically silent, except for hematuria and/or urinary infection in a few patients. Dilatation of the collecting tubules can be demonstrated by intravenous pyelography showing enlarged kidneys and coarse streaking of the medulla (Fig. 44-23).[14] These radiologic abnormalities are present in about two thirds of the patients[1,14]; their presence is a good evidence for, but their absence is not an argument against, the diagnosis of congenital hepatic fibrosis. In some patients with normal intravenous pyelogram, histologic examination of the kidney may show ectatic collecting tubules.[5]

In most of the patients, dilatation of collecting tubules remains stable. In some of them, the ectatic segments lose their communications with the urinary tree and transform into large renal cysts[7]; the renal malformation then resembles adult polycystic kidney disease. This transformation accounts for the large renal cysts detectable by ultrasonography or intravenous pyelography in a certain number of patients with congenital hepatic fibrosis.[1,5,14]

Fig. 44-23. Congenital hepatic fibrosis: intravenous pyelography. Coarse streaking of the papilla (*arrowheads*) reflects ectatic collecting tubules.

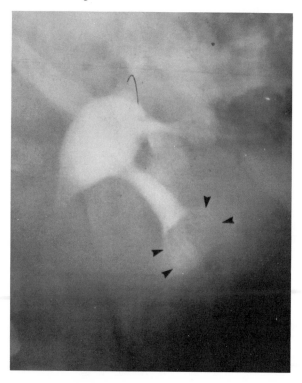

It may be rapid and take place in infancy or, more often, is more progressive, with large renal cysts being formed over 30 or 40 years. In patients with large renal cysts, the renal malformation may cause renal failure and/or arterial hypertension.

Other associated malformations are very uncommon and include duplication of the intrahepatic portal vein branches,[19] cystic dysplasia of the pancreas,[12] intestinal lymphangiectasia,[4] pulmonary emphysema,[30] cerebellar hemangioma,[27] aneurysms of renal and cerebral arteries,[12] and cleft palate.[12]

Treatment

Active bleeding from ruptured esophageal varices requires blood transfusions and esophageal tamponade. Endoscopic sclerotherapy of esophageal varices can be recommended for the prevention of recurrent bleeding, although this procedure has not been specifically evaluated in congenital hepatic fibrosis. However, the efficacy of sclerotherapy has been demonstrated for prevention of variceal bleeding in cirrhosis and can be reasonably expected in congenital hepatic fibrosis.

In patients in whom sclerotherapy is inefficient, poorly tolerated, or not feasible, surgical portacaval shunt can be considered. Hepatic encephalopathy and liver failure after portal-systemic shunt would be less common in patients with congenital hepatic fibrosis than in patients with cirrhosis.[1,13]

Splenectomy, which has been performed in a few patients in whom hypersplenism was not related to congenital hepatic fibrosis, does not prevent occurrence or recurrence of gastrointestinal bleeding and may be followed by portal vein thrombosis, preventing subsequent surgical portacaval shunt. Operations or invasive investigations on the biliary tree, such as cholecystectomy, choledochotomy, T-tube drainage, intraoperative cholangiography, or endoscopic retrograde cholangiography, must be avoided because of the risk of inducing bacterial cholangitis in patients with associated silent Caroli's syndrome.

CAROLI'S SYNDROME

Caroli's syndrome is a congenital malformation characterized by multifocal dilatation of segmental bile ducts, the main consequence of which is recurrent bacterial cholangitis. This malformation was described by Caroli and co-workers in 1958.[3] This malformation is not a single entity and, for this reason, the terms of Caroli's syndrome are more appropriate than those of Caroli's disease.

Pathology, Classification, and Etiology

The lesion of Caroli's syndrome consists of multifocal dilatation of the segmental bile ducts. The ectatic portions form cysts of various size, separated by portions of bile ducts that are normal or regularly dilated. The multifocal dilatation may be diffuse, affecting the whole intrahepatic biliary tree (although it may be more marked in a part of the liver), or it may be confined in a part of the liver, often the left lobe or a segment of the left lobe.[2] The number of cysts is large in the diffuse form and smaller, usually fewer than 10, in the localized form.

Multifocal dilatation of the segmental bile ducts is not a single entity. In the majority of the cases, multifocal dilatation of the segmental bile ducts is associated with congenital hepatic fibrosis.[9] In this type of Caroli's syndrome, the distribution of multifocal dilatation is diffuse; as congenital hepatic fibrosis, the malformation is transmitted as an autosomal recessive trait and may be associated with a renal malformation.

In a few cases, multifocal dilatation of the segmental bile ducts is not associated with congenital hepatic fibrosis. In such cases, multifocal dilatation is often confined to a part of the liver. This type of Caroli's syndrome is not inherited and is usually not associated with a renal malformation, but it may be associated with other malformations of the biliary tree, in particular choledochal cyst.[16]

Manifestations and Diagnosis

Caroli's syndrome, which is likely to be present at birth, remains asymptomatic for the first 5 to 20 years of the patient's life (sometimes longer) and in a few cases during the patient's whole life. Asymptomatic Caroli's syndrome remains unrecognized, except in persons in whom an imaging investigation of the liver is performed for unrelated reasons and in patients in whom congenital hepatic fibrosis has been diagnosed and multifocal dilatation of the segmental bile ducts has been suspected and demonstrated by ultrasonography or computed tomography.

In most of the patients, the first episode of bacterial cholangitis occurs in the absence of any apparent precipitating factor. However, in a few patients, the first episode of bacterial cholangitis is induced by a surgical operation or an invasive investigation on the biliary tree, such as cholecystectomy, choledochotomy, T-tube drainage, intraoperative cholangiography, or endoscopic retrograde cholangiography.[5,8,11]

The main and often the only symptom of bacterial cholangitis due to Caroli's syndrome is fever, in contrast to bacterial cholangitis complicating common bile duct stones in which fever is usually accompanied by pain and/or jaundice. As a consequence, the first episodes of fever may be not attributed to bacterial cholangitis.

At clinical examination, the liver is usually enlarged. There is no sign or symptom indicating liver failure. In patients with Caroli's syndrome associated with congenital hepatic fibrosis, manifestations of portal hypertension are present. Results of liver tests are normal, except for alkaline phosphatase and gammaglutamyl transpeptidase levels, which may be moderately increased.

The best procedures for the diagnosis of Caroli's syndrome are ultrasonography or computed tomography, which show cysts, of various sizes that are distributed throughout the liver or confined to a part of the liver and associated or not associated with tubular dilatation of segmental bile ducts (Figs. 44-24 and 44-25). Computed tomography after intravenous injection of biliary contrast may show opacification of cysts and dilated segmental bile ducts. Cysts may be demonstrated by intraoperative cholangiography, postoperative cholangiography through a T-tube (Fig. 44-26), or endoscopic retrograde cholangiography: these three procedures must not be performed in patients with asymptomatic Caroli's syndrome but can be employed in patients with Caroli's syndrome already complicated by bacterial cholangitis.

The other imaging procedures have less interest for the diagnosis of Caroli's syndrome. Radiocolloid liver scan shows cold areas corresponding to the large cysts. Hepatobiliary scan shows cold areas at the early phase that become hot at the late phase.[24] Intravenous cholangiography, which was used for the diagnosis of Caroli's syn-

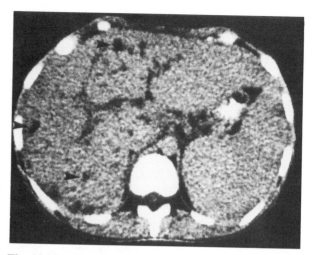

Fig. 44-25. Caroli's syndrome: computed tomography. Numerous water-density formations (*arrowheads*) can be seen in the liver, predominantly in the right lobe.

Fig. 44-24. Caroli's syndrome: static mode of ultrasonography. Transverse view of the right upper quadrant of the abdomen. Multiple, round, or oval fluid-filled formations (*arrowheads*) can be seen, corresponding to multifocal dilatation of the segmental bile ducts. Portal vein branch (*arrows*). D, diaphragm; S, spine; A, aorta.

Fig. 44-26. Caroli's syndrome: T-tube cholangiography. Cystic formation communicating with the biliary tree.

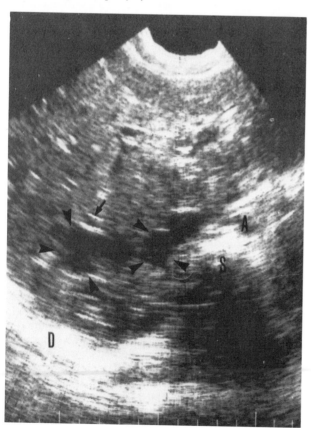

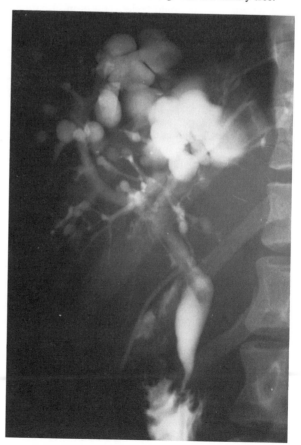

drome before the introduction of ultrasonography and computed tomography, may show cysts opacified by the contrast medium[3]; however, in most cases, opacification is too faint to allow a firm diagnosis.

Course and Complications

The course of Caroli's syndrome is dominated by recurrent episodes of bacterial cholangitis, the frequency of which varies widely: some patients experience 10 to 20, whereas others suffer only 1 or 2 episodes a year. In patients with frequent episodes of bacterial cholangitis, the prognosis is poor, most of such patients died 5 to 10 years after the onset of cholangitis, usually of an uncontrolled biliary bacterial infection. Bacterial cholangitis may be complicated by liver abscesses, septicemia, extrahepatic abscesses, and secondary amyloidosis.[10]

Bacterial cholangitis often induces the formation of intracystic pigment stones,[17] which are easily recognized by ultrasonography or endoscopic retrograde cholangiography but may be missed by computed tomography when not calcified. These stones can migrate from the cysts into the common bile duct and then determine biliary pain and/or cholestasis and/or acute pancreatitis.[22] Cholangiocarcinoma develops in some patients with Caroli's syndrome.[6]

Associated Malformations

In patients with Caroli's syndrome and congenital hepatic fibrosis, the malformations described in association with congenital hepatic fibrosis may be present. In patients afflicted by Caroli's syndrome with or, more often, without congenital hepatic fibrosis, associated choledochal cyst is relatively common.[16] Exceptionally, Caroli's syndrome is associated with Laurence-Moon-Biedl-Bardet syndrome.[25]

Treatment

The treatment of the episodes of bacterial cholangitis is represented by appropriate antibiotics.

The prevention of recurrent bacterial cholangitis is difficult. Periodic administration of antibiotics is efficacious in some patients but completely inefficient in others. T-tube drainage is inefficacious and may be dangerous in patients with associated congenital hepatic fibrosis: large amounts of water and electrolytes secreted by the multiple bile ductules may be lost through the T-tube, which may result in severe dehydration.[26] Administration of chenodesoxycholic acid has been used for the prevention and treatment of intracystic stones; although chenodesoxycholic acid has induced the disappearance of intracystic stones in one patient,[15] this treatment has not been clearly efficacious in others.[17] Transhepatic intubation and drainage of the biliary tree has been used successfully in a small number of patients.[29] Surgical biliointestinal anastomoses or endoscopic papillotomy may facilitate the passage of stones into the intestine; however, this procedure may increase the frequency and severity of the episodes of bacterial cholangitis.[28] In the localized form of Caroli's syndrome, partial hepatectomy is indicated and excellent results can be expected.[20] In the diffuse form, if the cysts predominate in a part of the liver, partial hepatectomy can likewise be envisaged; however, in such patients, partial hepatectomy is difficult because of associated congenital hepatic fibrosis and portal hypertension, and the long-term results may be compromised because multifocal dilatation affecting the remaining liver may be the source of recurrent bacterial cholangitis.[20] In the diffuse form without predominance of the cysts in any part of the liver, complicated by severe recurrent bacterial cholangitis, liver transplantation may be considered.

REFERENCES

1. Alvarez F, Bernard O, Brunelle F et al: Congenital hepatic fibrosis. J Pediatr 99:370, 1981
2. Caroli J, Couinaud C, Soupault R et al: Une affection nouvelle, sans doute congénitale, des voies biliaires: La dilatation kystique unilobaire des canaux hépatiques. Sem Hop Paris 34:136, 1958
3. Caroli J, Soupault R, Kossakowki J et al: La dilatation polykystique congénitale des voies biliaires intra-hépatiques: Essai de classification. Sem Hop Paris 34:488, 1958
4. Chagnon JP, Barge J, Hay JM et al: Fibrose hépatique congénitale, polykystose rénale et lymphangiectasies intestinales primitives. Gastroenterol Clin Biol 6:326, 1982
5. Clermont RJ, Maillard JN, Benhamou JP et al: Fibrose hépatique congénitale. Can Med Assoc J 97:1272, 1967
6. Dayton MT, Longmire WP, Tompkins RK: Caroli's disease: A premalignant condition? Am J. Surg 145:41, 1983
7. Dupond JL, Miguet JP, Carbillet JP et al: Kidney polycystic disease in adult congenital hepatic fibrosis. Ann Intern Med 88:514, 1978
8. Erlinger S, Sakellaridis A, Maillard JN et al: Les formes angiocholitiques de la fibrose hépatique congénitale. Presse Med 77:1189, 1969
9. Fauvert F, Benhamou JP. Congenital hepatic fibrosis. In Schaffner F, Sherlock S, Leevy CM (ed): The Liver and its Diseases, pp 283–288. New York, IMS Co, 1974
10. Fevery J, Tanghe W, Kerremans R et al: Congenital dilatation of the intrahepatic bile ducts associated with the development of amyloidosis. Gut 13:604, 1972
11. Grumbach R, Bourillon J, Auvert JP: Maladie fibrokystique du foie avec hypertension portale chez l'enfant: Deux observations. Arch Anat Pathol 30:74, 1954
12. Kerr DNS, Harrison CV, Sherlock S et al: Congenital hepatic fibrosis. Q J Med 30:91, 1961
13. Kerr DNS, Okonkwo S, Choa RG: Congenital hepatic fibrosis: The long-term prognosis. Gut 19:514, 1978
14. Kerr DNS, Warrick CK, Hart-Mercier J: Lesion resembling medullary sponge kidney in patients with congenital hepatic fibrosis. Clin Radiol 12:85, 1962
15. Kutz K, Mederer SE, Paumgartner G: Chenodesoxycholic acid therapy of intrahepatic radiolucent gallstones in a patient with Caroli's syndrome. Acta Hepatogastroenterol 25:398, 1978
16. Loubeau JM, Steichen FM: Dilatation of intrahepatic bile

ducts in choledochal cyst: Case report with follow-up and review of the literature. Arch Surg 111:1384, 1976

17. Mathias K, Waldmann D, Daikeler G et al: Intrahepatic cystic bile duct dilatations and stone formation: A new case of Caroli's disease. Acta Hepatogastroenterol 25:30, 1978

18. Nakanuma Y, Terada T, Ohta G et al: Caroli's disease in congenital hepatic fibrosis and infantile polycystic disease. Liver 2:346, 1982

19. Odièvre M, Chaumont P, Montagne JP et al: Anomalies of the intrahepatic portal venous system in congenital hepatic fibrosis. Radiology 122:427, 1977

20. Ramond MJ, Huguet C, Danan G et al: Partial hepatectomy in the treatment of Caroli's disease: Report of a case and review of the literature. Dig Dis Sci 29:367, 1984

21. Ratcliffe PJ, Reeders S, Theaker JM: Bleeding oesophageal varices and hepatic dysfunction in adult polycystic kidney disease. Br Med J 288:1330, 1984

22. Sahel J, Bourry J, Sarles H: Maladie de Caroli avec pancréatite aiguë et angiocholite: Intérêt diagnostique et thérapeutique de la cholédoco-wirsungographie endoscopique. Nouvelle Presse Med 5:2067, 1976

23. Scheinberg IH, Sternlieb IM: Wilson's Disease. Philadelphia, WB Saunders, 1984

24. Stillman A, Earnest D, Woolfenden T: Hepatobiliary scanning in diagnosis and management of Caroli's disease (abstr). Gastroenterology 80:1295, 1981

25. Tsuchiya R, Nishimura R, Ito T: Congenital cystic dilatation of the bile ducts associated with Laurence-Moon-Biedl-Bardet syndrome. Arch Surg 112:82, 1977

26. Turnberg LA, Jones EA, Sherlock S: Biliary secretion in a patient with cystic dilatation of the intrahepatic biliary tree. Gastroenterology 54:1155, 1968

27. Wagenvoort CA, Baggenstoss AH, Love JG: Subarachnoid hemorrhage due to cerebellar hemangioma associated with congenital hepatic fibrosis and polycystic kidneys: Report of a case. Proc Mayo Clin 37:301, 1962

28. Watts DR, Lorenzo GA, Beal JM: Congenital dilatation of the intrahepatic bile ducts. Arch Surg 108:592, 1974

29. Witlin LT, Gadacz TR, Zuidema GD et al: Transhepatic decompression of the biliary tree in Caroli's disease. Surgery 91:205, 1982

30. Williams R, Scheuer P, Heard BE: Congenital hepatic fibrosis with an unusual pulmonary lesion. J Clin Pathol 17:135, 1964

part 7
Budd-Chiari Syndrome

TELFER B. REYNOLDS*

The Budd-Chiari syndrome is an uncommon clinical disorder caused by obstruction to hepatic venous outflow. The first published clinical description is attributed to Budd in 1845[6]; Chiari added the first pathologic description of a liver with "obliterating endophlebitis of the hepatic veins" in 1899.[9] Parker summarized the literature in 1959 and was able to find accounts of 164 symptomatic cases with autopsy confirmation, including 18 from his own hospital.[33]

There are a number of known causes of the Budd-Chiari syndrome. Thrombosis of the hepatic veins may complicate the myeloproliferative syndrome or paroxysmal nocturnal hemoglobinuria.[17] Tumors such as hepatocellular carcinoma, hypernephroma,[48] adrenal carcinoma, and leiomyosarcoma[27] may obstruct major hepatic veins directly or in company with a blood clot. The hepatic portion of the inferior vena cava is often occluded with the hepatic veins when the cause is tumor or thrombosis. An hepatic abscess or cyst may cause occlusion of neighboring hepatic veins, although this rarely results in the full clinical expression of the Budd-Chiari syndrome. Radiation can cause obliteration of the smaller hepatic veins. An important cause of the syndrome from the therapeutic standpoint is a fibrous diaphragm or web across the upper

vena cava at or just above the entrance of the left and middle hepatic veins.[3,16] This lesion appears to be more common in South Africa and in the Orient than in the United States,[22,50,52,58] although we have encountered nine cases in Los Angeles in the past 20 years.[41] This lesion has been considered by some to be congenital, related to closure of the ductus venosus.[22] In some cases the membrane is thick and the fibrosis involves one or more of the major hepatic veins. Relationships of hepatic vein thrombosis to pregnancy[21,43] and trauma[8] have been postulated. Three patients have been reported with the lupus anticoagulant,[35,44,49] which has a correlation with venous thrombosis. Very likely this immunoglobulin has not been looked for in many cases of Budd-Chiari syndrome, as is probably the case for deficiencies in protein C and protein S, blood constituents that appear to be protective against thrombosis. A causal relationship with oral contraceptives has been assumed by some on the basis of reports of cases in oral contraceptive users.[19a] However, with the passage of time, it appears that this relationship may be coincidental rather than one of cause and effect. Judging from published reports and my own experience, there has been no obvious increase in the incidence of hepatic vein occlusion since the advent of oral contraceptives. In 1977, Wu and colleagues summarized ten reports of one or two patients in whom hepatic vein thrombosis was attributed to oral contraceptives and added a single case.[57] I found one additional report[7] for a total of 14 cases. But in articles describing larger series of cases published since 1965 and, including my own material, reporting a total of 172 cases,[2,10,11,13,20,25,28,32,36,47,51,53] the frequency of oral contraceptive use in female patients aged 15 to 50 was low (approximately 25%†) and less than some estimates for use in the general population in the United States.[29]

---

* Robert L. Peters, M.D., recently deceased Professor of Pathology at the University of Southern California, contributed importantly to the following material.

† Not all reports listed the ages of the females.

More common than any of the known causes of hepatic vein occlusion is an unexplained partial or complete fibrous obliteration of the major hepatic veins or their ostia. This was found at autopsy in 44% of Parker's series[33] and can be viewed either as a proliferative inflammation or as a result of partial organization of preceding thrombosis. Safouh and colleagues report this type of pathology to be particularly common in Egyptian children with the Budd-Chiari syndrome.[44]

Our experience with the Budd-Chiari syndrome in the Liver Unit at the Los Angeles County-University of Southern California Medical Center includes 39 cases, the causes of which are listed in Table 44-3.

PATHOLOGY

The Budd-Chiari syndrome, produced by any of the processes that impede egress of blood from the liver, is associated in the acute stage with a swollen, blunt-edged, red-purple liver. Cut surface of such a liver reveals the pale, undamaged, periportal tissue regularly demarcating the lobular units and the perivenular, darkened, depressed areas of congestion.

When the obstruction to venous flow is the result of a mechanical process such as a membranous diaphragm or a tumor involving the ostia of hepatic veins, the microscopic pattern during the acute stage is that of severe acute congestion. The sinusoids are engorged with blood, and the centrolobular hepatocytes undergo marked atrophy,

often disappearing with the endothelial processes remaining as a loose stromal network (Fig. 44-27). With continued obstruction, the central veins become obliterated by collapse of the stroma and a small amount of production of new collagen. Fibrin deposition and thrombosis are not prominent features.

The more mysterious "primary" endophlebitis, which represents the disease originally described by Chiari, is characterized by thrombosis or fibrin deposition in the central veins in the earliest stages of the process. The congestion may be so severe as to preclude evaluation of the stromal pattern of the liver. However, in many instances, the striking perivenular pool of blood and fibrin is surrounded by radiating dilated sinusoids devoid of erythrocytes that alternate with thin cords of hepatocytes surrounded by erythrocytes in the space of Disse. On casual inspection, the liver appears congested, but it actually has extravasation of blood into the space of Disse (Figs. 44-28 and 44-29). This may be a fundamental aspect of the pathogenesis of the Budd-Chiari syndrome, in contrast to those conditions that produce only passive congestion of the liver. Leopold and co-workers describe extravasation of blood into the space of Disse in liver biopsies taken from patients who have tumor masses occluding the hepatic veins.[25] Other conditions that produce secondary severe venous stasis may be associated with extravasation of erythrocytes into the trabecula. Confluent necrosis of hepatocytes resulting from an hepatotoxic agent may be associated with a minor degree of dissection of erythrocytes into the trabecular structures.

TABLE 44-3. Causes of Budd-Chiari Syndrome

CAUSE	NUMBER OF CASES	NUMBER OF CASES WITH VENA CAVAL OCCLUSION	CLINICAL COURSE			DEATH	AUTOPSY
			Acute	Subacute	Chronic		
Thrombosis							
Myeloproliferative disease	3	0		3		3	3
Paroxysmal nocturnal hemoglobinuria	1	1			1	1	1
Unknown cause	2*	1		1	1	2	2
Tumor							
Adrenal carcinoma	2	2		2		2	2
Hypernephroma	2	2		2		2	2
Hepatocellular carcinoma	2	1		2		2	2
Choriocarcinoma	1			1		1	1
Fibrous obliteration of unknown cause	3				3	3	3
Venal caval web	9*	9			9	3	1
Radiation	2			2		2	2
Amebic abscess	2		2				
Undetermined cause	10†		2	4	4	1	

* One patient used oral contraceptives.
† Two patients used oral contraceptives.

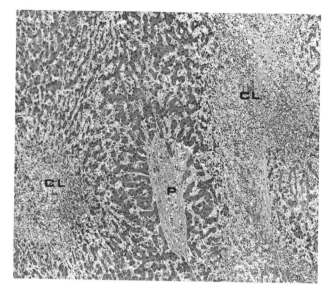

Fig. 44-27. Low-power photomicrograph of the liver of a patient with Budd–Chiari syndrome showing the portal area in the center (*P*) with congested centrolobular areas (*CL*) to either side. Note that the liver cells have disappeared centrally. (Original magnification × 100; H & E)

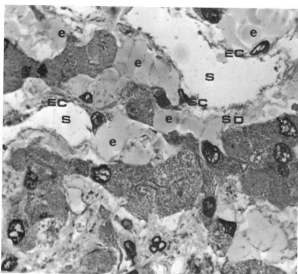

Fig. 44-29. Higher-power photomicrograph showing the shrunken hepatocytes surrounded by erythrocytes (*e*) bloating the space of Disse (*SD*). The space of Disse is separated from the empty sinusoids (*S*) by the endothelial cell processes (*EC*). (Original magnification × 900; H & E)

Fig. 44-28. A portal area surrounded by intact hepatocytes. At the margin between collapsed liver cell stroma and intact hepatocytes, the sinusoids are dilated but not filled with erythrocytes, which are more localized in the space of Disse (see Fig. 44-29). (Original magnification × 165; H & E)

Fig. 44-30. After a prolonged time, the sublobular hepatic veins (*HV*) may be thrombosed and recanalized with extensive loss of hepatocytes. (Original magnification × 160; H & E)

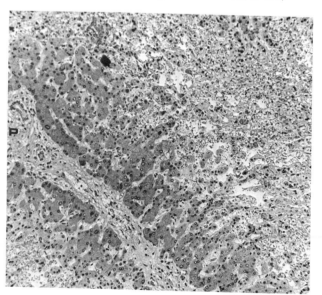

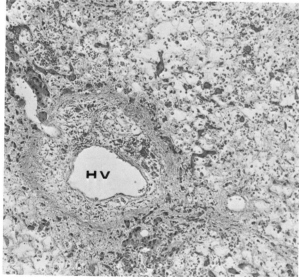

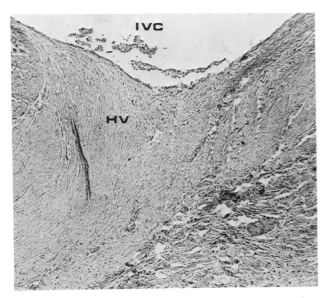

Fig. 44-31. Low-power photomicrograph of an occluded site of entry of the hepatic vein (*HV*) into the inferior vena cava (*IVC*). (Original magnification × 45; H & E)

As the disease moves into chronicity, the fibrin thrombi organize, each producing a fibrous core (Fig. 44-30). Extending in an arachnoid fashion from the central core, thin collagen strands replace the liver cords and the collapsed stroma. The congestion of the sinusoids becomes somewhat less uniform from one area to another. The larger hepatic vein radicles, not usually included in needle biopsy specimens, are sclerotic, usually to the ostia of the hepatic veins into the inferior vena cava (Fig. 44-31). Although it has usually been presumed that the thrombo-sclerotic process had its origin at the outlets of the hepatic veins, thereafter progressing into the liver, there is as much reason to believe that the process may begin in central veins and progress into the large vessels.

After a period of 1 to 3 years, when the liver is studied at autopsy, the ostia of the hepatic veins are filled by sclerotic tissue (Fig. 44-32) that extends to the lobular level. Often, the inferior vena cava has a plastic thickening in its intrahepatic portion. On occasion, the caudate lobe may not be involved in the process and may enlarge as the major functioning unit. In this advanced stage, the liver becomes smaller, irregular, and tough.

Radiation administered to the liver may produce a nearly identical hepatic lesion, but, unless the entire liver or the entire zone of entrance of hepatic veins into the vena cava is irradiated, the veno-occlusive change will involve only a part of the liver and the Budd-Chiari syndrome may not result. Radiation may induce other changes, including sclerotic thickening and even hyalinization of the hepatic arterioles in the portal regions, permitting its identification as the cause of hepatic vein sclerosis. The dissection of erythrocytes into the trabecula of the liver, in contrast to simple congestion of the sinusoids, has been pointed out in Jamaican veno-occlusive disease[5] as well as in experimental monocrotaline poisoning in monkeys.[1] However, only Leopold and colleagues[26] have pointed out this feature in idiopathic Budd-Chiari disease. Budd-Chiari and veno-occlusive diseases may be very similar in etiology and pathogenesis.

A condition pathologically indistinguishable from the Budd-Chiari lesion occasionally occurs in felines housed in zoos in the United States. We have seen examples in a Bengal tiger and two cheetahs. The animals also develop ascites and die in what appears to be hepatic coma.

An interesting association of Budd-Chiari syndrome with hepatocellular carcinoma has been pointed out by Simson[50] in patients with membranous obstruction of the

44-32. Intrahepatic portion of the inferior vena cava (*IVC*) in a fatal case of Budd–Chiari disease. Note the hyalinized thrombotic occlusion of two major hepatic vein radicles (*arrows*).

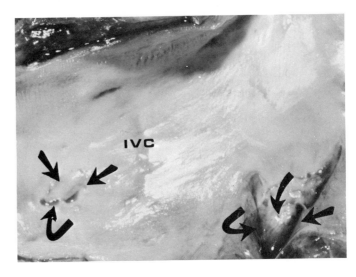

inferior vena cava. Two of our nine patients with the inferior vena cava "web" lesion had hepatocellular cancer.

CLINICAL MANIFESTATIONS

The most important clinical manifestations are abdominal pain, hepatomegaly, and ascites. Seldom is the diagnosis made from the clinical picture alone; clinicians tend to ignore the abdominal pain and to ascribe the ascites and hepatomegaly to cirrhosis.

Astute interpretation of the liver biopsy is often the clue that results in a correct diagnosis. Clinical features in the Budd-Chiari syndrome vary with the extent and rapidity of onset of the venous occlusion and with the manifestations, if any, of the underlying disease. Rarely, there is very acute illness with abdominal pain, hepatomegaly, shock, and a rapid course resulting in death. More commonly, there is a vague illness with abdominal distress weeks or months in duration followed by the appearance of ascites and an enlarged liver. Jaundice may be present but is usually mild. In a few patients there is simply gradual development of hepatomegaly and ascites without prominent abdominal pain; such patients are most likely to receive an erroneous diagnosis of cirrhosis. Portal hypertension develops in all patients with the Budd-Chiari syndrome and may be responsible eventually for hematemesis from esophageal varices.

When there is vena caval occlusion accompanying the Budd-Chiari syndrome and the patient survives long enough, collateral veins often appear on the abdomen or back (Fig. 44-33). Other findings suggesting vena caval involvement include protracted ankle edema, stasis ulceration, or episodes of pulmonary embolization. We described one patient with complete vena caval occlusion and severe hepatic congestion who had no symptoms or findings other than hepatomegaly and episodes of mild abdominal pain.[12]

INVESTIGATIONS

There is nothing distinctive about the biochemical test pattern in patients with the Budd-Chiari syndrome. Hepatic test abnormalities are variable in degree and are similar to those in any chronic liver disease. High ascitic fluid protein content has been said to be characteristic of the Budd-Chiari syndrome,[15,56] but, in my experience, protein levels have more often been in the range usually seen in cirrhosis of the liver. In 15 patients, I found a range of 0.5 g to 4.5 g with a mean of 2.4 g/dl. In three patients, the value was greater than 50% of the serum protein level. Clain and colleagues found values of 0.9 to 2.8 g/dl (mean, 1.8) in six cases.[10] Rarely, the ascitic fluid is blood-stained (in one of our cases and in one of those reported by Clain and associates[10]). Liver scan sometimes shows a marked increase in isotope uptake centrally,[10,53] possibly because of hypertrophy of the caudate lobe related

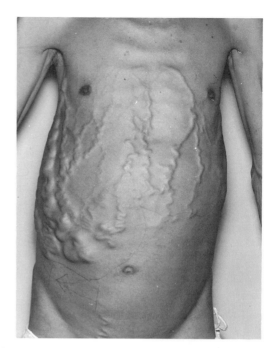

Fig. 44-33. Collateral venous circulation on the abdomen of a patient with the Budd–Chiari syndrome caused by blockage of the inferior vena cava by a "web" lesion cephalad to the hepatic vein orifices.

to its venous drainage directly into the vena cava. This pattern was evident in 6 of the 17 patients in our series who had scans performed (see Fig. 44-34).

Splenoportography and celiac angiography usually show portal collateral flow and failure of opacification of the main portal trunk. Presumably, the portal vein often serves as an outflow vessel when the major hepatic veins are occluded, accounting for the lack of portal visualization with these procedures. Also, portal vein thrombosis sometimes accompanies hepatic vein thrombosis.[10,33]

Hepatic parenchymal contrast injection is useful in the diagnosis and localization of hepatic venous obstruction.[4,10,11,39] Pollard and Nebesar found retrograde portal flow on selective hepatic artery contrast injection in one patient.[34] Celiac and superior mesenteric arteriographies usually show minimal portal opacification with evidence of collateral flow.[13] Rector and Redeker used transhepatic needling of hepatic veins to demonstrate abnormal pressure and abnormal direction of blood flow in three patients.[40] Computed tomography and ultrasonography can be useful adjuncts by showing enlargement of the caudate lobe, absence of major hepatic vein images, and prolonged hepatic opacification after contrast injection.[2]

There are few reports of attempted hepatic vein catheterization in patients with suspected Budd-Chiari syndrome. One would anticipate difficulty with this procedure; however, Clain[10] and Kreel and co-workers[23] were

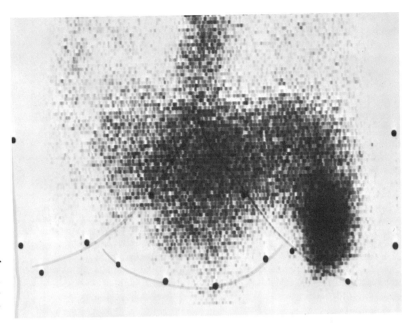

Fig. 44-34. Increased central uptake of isotope in the liver scan of a patient with the Budd–Chiari syndrome caused by hepatic vein thrombosis related to myeloproliferative disease.

Fig. 44-35. An unusual pattern of numerous interlacing vessels is seen after the injection of 7 ml of contrast media through a catheter wedged in the right hepatic vein of a patient with Budd–Chiari syndrome caused by idiopathic hepatic vein occlusion. The catheter could not be passed more than a few centimeters into the hepatic vein.

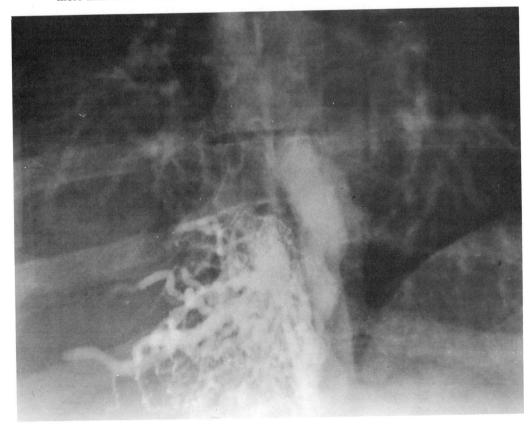

able to place a catheter at least a short distance into one hepatic vein in five of their six patients. The main vessels appeared narrowed and partly occluded, and an unusual pattern of fine interlacing communicating vessels, interpreted as collaterals, was seen on wedged injection of contrast. We found a similar pattern in six of our patients (Fig. 44-35). A technically satisfactory wedged hepatic vein pressure is difficult to obtain in these patients; Clain and colleagues found elevated levels in two of four patients,[10] and we found such levels in three of four.

Vena caval catheterization and angiography are important investigations in patients being evaluated for the Budd-Chiari syndrome. Only if this is done routinely will all cases associated with vena caval occlusion be identified. As emphasized by the case reported from this Liver Unit in 1968, the vena cava may be completely obstructed without the appearance of collateral veins, ankle edema, or stasis ulcers.[12] It is particularly important to catheterize the vena cava in patients with collateral veins visible on the back, because portal hypertension rarely causes collaterals to appear in this area.

TREATMENT

Treatment for hepatic vein occlusion is difficult and limited. Surgery to attempt removal of thrombus from hepatic veins is unlikely to be successful because of the extent of the process and the difficulty of exposure of the hepatic veins. Thrombolytic therapy has been attempted with uncertain results.[54] Decompression of the liver by any of the several existing types of side-to-side portacaval shunt may be very helpful if the inferior vena cava is not occluded.[14,20,25,30,32,37] Liver transplant has been employed in a number of cases, often successfully.[28,38,49]

Surgical treatment may be particularly helpful when the Budd-Chiari syndrome is due to a fibrous diaphragm or web in the vena cava just below the right atrium. The presence and thickness of the web can be assessed when one catheter is placed in the right atrium and another one passed up the inferior vena cava from below. Transcardiac membranotomy has been successfully performed by several groups.[16,18,22,24,46,52,58] Other surgeons have resected the membrane under cardiopulmonary bypass[42,55] or used bypass grafts.[31,58] One of our patients with an incomplete membrane had successful balloon membranotomy,[19] and membrane resection was successful in three of the four patients in whom it was attempted.

Extensive hepatic vein occlusion is usually fatal within weeks or months of the onset of symptoms. Some patients, usually those with gradual onset of the syndrome, survive for extended periods with chronic ascites and portal hypertension and a course resembling that of idiopathic cirrhosis of the liver. It remains to be seen whether more extensive use of side-to-side portacaval shunting procedures will markedly improve the prognosis, both by preventing hemorrhage from esophageal varices and by decreasing hepatic congestion and central necrosis.

REFERENCES

1. Allen JR, Carstens LA: Monocrotaline-induced Budd-Chiari syndrome in monkeys. Dig Dis 16:111, 1971
2. Baert AL et al: Early diagnosis of Budd-Chiari syndrome by computed tomography and ultrasonography: Report of 5 cases. Gastroenterology 84:587, 1983
3. Bennet I: A unique case of obstruction of the inferior vena cava. Bull Johns Hopkins Hosp 87:290, 1950
4. Brink AJ, Botha D: Budd-Chiari syndrome: Diagnosis by hepatic venography. Br J Radiol 28:330, 1955
5. Brooks SEH et al: Acute veno-occlusive disease of the liver. Arch Pathol 89:507, 1970
6. Budd G: On Diseases of the Liver, p 147. London, Churchill, 1845
7. Caroli J, Chevrel B: Syndrome de Budd-Chiari et contraceptifs oraux. Med Chir Dig 5:439, 1976
8. Chamberlain DW, Walter JB: The relationship of Budd-Chiari syndrome to oral contraceptives and trauma. Can Med Assoc J 101:97, 1969
9. Chiari H: Ueber die selbständige Phlebitis obliterans der Hauptstämme der Vanae hepaticae als Todesursache. Beitr Z Pathol Anat 26:1, 1899
10. Clain D et al: Clinical diagnosis of the Budd-Chiari syndrome. Am J Med 43:544, 1967
11. Datta DV et al: Diagnostic value of combined transhepatic venography and inferior vena cavography in chronic Budd-Chiari syndrome. Am J Dig Dis 23:1031, 1978
12. Davis M et al: Budd-Chiari syndrome due to inferior vena cava obstruction. Gastroenterology 54:1142, 1968
13. Deutsch V et al: Budd-Chiari syndrome: Study of angiographic findings and remarks on etiology. AJR 116:430, 1972
14. Erlik D et al: Surgical cure of primary hepatic vein occlusion syndrome by side-to-side portacaval shunt. Surg Gynecol Obstet 114:368, 1962
15. Gibson JB: Chiari's disease and the Budd-Chiari syndrome. J Pathol Bacteriol 79:381, 1960
16. Gips CH et al: Membranous obstruction of the suprahepatic segment of the inferior vena cava. Folia Med Neerl 15:228, 1972
17. Hartmann RC et al: Fulminant hepatic venous thrombosis (Budd-Chiari syndrome) in paroxysmal nocturnal hemoglobinuria: Definition of a medical emergency. Johns Hopkins Med J 146:247, 1980
18. Hirooka M, Kimura C: Membranous obstruction of the hepatic portion of the vena cava. Arch Surg 100:656, 1970
19. Horisawa M et al: Incomplete membranous obstruction of the inferior vena cava: Hemodynamic measurements and correction by balloon membranotomy and surgical resection. Arch Surg 111:599, 1976
19a. Hoyumpa AM et al: Budd-Chiari Syndrome in women taking oral contraceptives. Am J Med 50:137, 1971
20. Huguet C et al: Interposition mesocaval shunt for chronic primary occlusion of the hepatic veins. Surg Gynecol Obstet 148:691, 1979
21. Khuroo MS, Datta DV: Budd-Chiari syndrome following pregnancy. Am J Med 68:113, 1980
22. Kimura C et al: Membranous obliteration of the inferior vena cava in the hepatic portion. J Cardiovasc Surg 4:87, 1963
23. Kreel L et al: Vascular radiology in the Budd-Chiari syndrome. Br J Radiol 40:755, 1967
24. Lam CR et al: Transcardiac membranotomy, for obstruction of the hepatic portion of the inferior vena cava. Circulation 31 and 32(suppl):1, 1965

25. Langer B et al: Clinical spectrum of the Budd-Chiari syndrome and its surgical management. Am J Surg 129:137, 1975

26. Leopold JG et al: A change in the sinusoid-trabecular structure of the liver with hepatic venous outflow block. J Pathol 100:87, 1970

27. McMahon HE, Ball HG: Leiomyosarcoma of hepatic vein and the Budd-Chiari syndrome. Gastroenterology 61:239, 1971

28. Mitchell MC et al: Budd-Chiari syndrome: Etiology, diagnosis and management. Medicine 61:199, 1982

29. National Center for Health Statistics: Contraceptive utilization among currently married women 15–44 years of age: United States, 1973. Monthly Vital Statistics Report 25(suppl):1, 1976

30. Noble JA: Hepatic vein thrombosis complicating polycythemia vera: Successful treatment with a portacaval shunt. Arch Intern Med 120:105, 1967

31. Ohara I: A bypass operation for occlusion of the hepatic inferior vena cava. Surg Gynecol Obstet 117:151, 1963

32. Orloff MJ, Johansen KH: Treatment of Budd-Chiari syndrome by side-to-side portacaval shunt: Experimental and clinical results. Ann Surg 188:494, 1978

33. Parker RGF: Occlusion of the hepatic veins in man. Medicine 38:369, 1959

34. Pollard JJ, Nebesar RA: Altered hemodynamics in the Budd-Chiari syndrome demonstrated by selected hepatic and selective splenic angiography. Radiology 89:236, 1967

35. Pomeroy C et al: Budd-Chiari syndrome in a patient with the lupus anticoagulant. Gastroenterology 86:158, 1984

36. Powell-Jackson PR et al: Budd-Chiari syndrome: Clinical patterns and therapy. Q J Med LI:79, 1982

37. Prandi D et al: Side-to-side portacaval shunt in the treatment of Budd-Chiari syndrome. Gastroenterology 68:127, 1975

38. Putnam CW et al: Liver transplantation for Budd-Chiari syndrome. JAMA 236:1142, 1976

39. Ramsay GC, Britton RC: Intraparenchymal angiography in the diagnosis of hepatic veno-occlusive diseases. Radiology 90:716, 1968

40. Rector WG Jr, Redeker AG: Direct transhepatic assessment of hepatic vein pressure and direction of flow using a thin needle in patients with cirrhosis and the Budd-Chiari syndrome. Gastroenterology 86:1395, 1984

41. Rector WG Jr et al: Membranous obstruction of the inferior vena cava in the United States. Medicine 64:134, 1985

42. Rogers MA et al: Membranous obstruction of the hepatic segment of the inferior vena cava. Br J Surg 54:221, 1967

43. Rosenthal T et al: The Budd-Chiari syndrome after pregnancy: Report of two cases and a review of the literature. Am J Obstet Gynecol 113:789, 1972

44. Roudot-Thoraval F et al: Budd-Chiari syndrome and the lupus anticoagulant. Gastroenterology 88:605, 1985

45. Safouh M et al: Hepatic vein occlusion disease in Egyptian children. Arch Pathol 79:505, 1965

46. Schaffner F et al: Budd-Chiari syndrome caused by a web in the inferior vena cava. Am J Med 42:838, 1967

47. Schramek A et al: New observations in the clinical spectrum of the Budd-Chiari syndrome. Ann Surg 180:368, 1974

48. Schraut WH, Chilcote RR: Metastatic Wilms' tumor causing acute hepatic vein occlusion (Budd-Chiari syndrome). Gastroenterology 88:576, 1985

49. Seltman HJ et al: Budd-Chiari syndrome recurring in a transplanted liver. Gastroenterology 84:640, 1983

50. Simson IW: Membranous obstruction of the inferior vena cava and hepatocellular carcinoma in South Africa. Gastroenterology 82:171, 1982

51. Szoor J et al: The Budd-Chiari syndrome: Report of eight cases. Acta Med Acad Sci Hung 28:127, 1971

52. Takeuchi J et al: Budd-Chiari syndrome associated with obstruction of the inferior vena cava. Am J Med 51:11, 1971

53. Tavill AS et al: The Budd-Chiari syndrome: Correlation between hepatic scintigraphy and the clinical, radiological and pathological findings in nineteen cases of hepatic venous outflow obstruction. Gastroenterology 68:509, 1975

54. Warren RL et al: Treatment of Budd-Chiari syndrome with streptokinase (abstr). Gastroenterology 62:200, 1972

55. Watkins E Jr, Fortin CL: Surgical correction of a congenital coarctation of the inferior vena cava. Ann Surg 159:536, 1964

56. Witte MH et al: Progress in liver disease: Physiological factors involved in the causation of cirrhotic ascites. Gastroenterology 61:742, 1971

57. Wu S-M et al: Budd-Chiari syndrome after taking oral contraceptives. Dig Dis 22:623, 1977

58. Yamamoto S et al: Budd-Chiari syndrome with obstruction of the inferior vena cava. Gastroenterology 54:1070, 1968

part **8**

Idiopathic Benign Recurrent Intrahepatic Cholestasis

LEON SCHIFF

In 1959, Summerskill and Walshe described two patients who had multiple episodes of jaundice accompanied by chemical and histologic evidence of cholestasis, a syndrome they designated as benign recurrent intrahepatic obstructive jaundice.[17]

The age at onset varies from 1 to 27 years. One of the cases reported by Summerskill had its onset at the age of 59.[16] The disease has been reported in siblings.[15] Six cases have been described in which all the patients were natives of a small area of the Apennines and all but one were related. Two cases belonged to the same small community of the Faeroes Islands and were probably related.[17] The clinical features are characterized by recurrent attacks of pruritus, anorexia, and weight loss, followed within 1 to 3 weeks by the development of obstructive jaundice with clay-colored stools and dark urine. A macular eruption has been described preceding attacks of benign recurrent intrahepatic cholestasis, and transient rashes may occur on the shoulders and arms associated with the cholestasis. Abdominal pain, chills, and fever do not occur. Hepa-

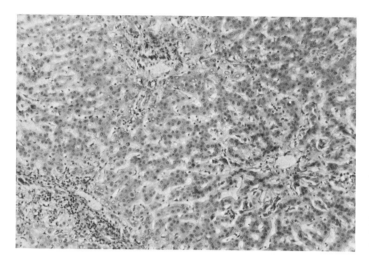

Fig. 44-36. Liver biopsy specimen during exacerbation. Bile plugs are seen in midzone canaliculi, and some pseudoacinar alteration is evident. Small collections of inflammatory cells are seen, usually in portal areas. Nuclear "glycogen" vacuolization, of unknown significance, is prominent. (Original magnification × 150; H & E)

tomegaly is usually absent. Despite numerous episodes of jaundice dating from as early as 1 year of age and extending over a period of 38 years in one case, there may be no persistent impairment of liver function or persistent pathologic changes.[10]

The average duration of an attack is 3 to 4 months, although some have reportedly lasted up to 2 years. An interval of 9 years between attacks has been recorded. The median is four attacks; 25% of the patients have had more than 10 attacks. One patient had only one attack.[16] The exacerbations may be seasonal, and seasonal pruritus may recur for years before the initial appearance of jaundice.

The depth of icterus may vary from one attack to another. In most cases, serum bilirubin is 10 to 20 mg/dl with a major increase in the conjugated fraction. There is a decrease in sulfobromophthalein storage and transport maximum (Tm),[1,22] an increase in serum alkaline phosphatase, serum bile acids, and α-2 and β-globulins, and a slight rise in serum transaminase. During remission, there

is a return to normal in the results of these laboratory tests. A distinctive pattern of serum bile acid and bilirubin concentration has been reported in benign recurrent intrahepatic cholestasis that may prove of diagnostic value.[18] The peak bile acid concentration occurs at the onset of the cholestasis while the bilirubin concentration increases slowly, with the maximum value being reached between 33 and 57 days after the onset of symptoms. On the other hand, the serum bilirubin and serum bile acid concentration change is parallel throughout cholestatic viral hepatitis, chronic active hepatitis, and alcoholic hepatitis. Based on the finding of peak increase of bile acids in the early phase of the cholestatic attack, Van Berge Henegouwen and associates postulated a defective hepatic transport of bile acids as the primary cause of the disease.[21]

Contradictory results have been reported on the rate at which injected unconjugated bilirubin disappears from the plasma. Williams and co-workers[22] found a normal disappearance rate in two cases, in contrast to Brodersen

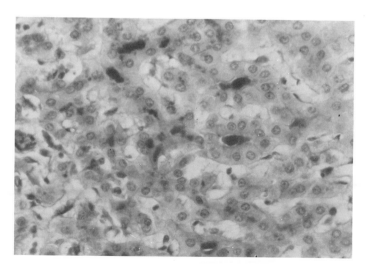

Fig. 44-37. Higher magnification of Figure 44-36. (Original magnification × 500)

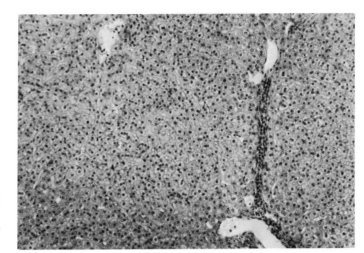

Fig. 44-38. Liver biopsy specimen during remission 90 days later than in Figures 44-36 and 44-37. The liver is essentially normal, except for granules of pigment, histochemically of the lipofuscin type, in a few cells. (Original magnification × 150)

and Tygstrup,[2] who reported an abnormally rapid disappearance in two cases and postulated a hyperactive bilirubin-conjugating mechanism. Summerfield and co-workers reported that the hepatic clearance of unconjugated bilirubin was normal at all times, while during cholestasis conjugated bilirubin refluxed from the liver to the plasma and was then cleared slowly with a half-life of approximately 12 hours.[19] The mechanism of the icterus that occurs in recurrent intrahepatic cholestasis has been assumed to be due to a block in the excretion of bilirubin into the bile with consequent regurgitation of the pigment into the blood, as is also assumed to be true in other forms of cholestasis.

Biopsy specimens of liver obtained during symptomatic periods show marked centrilobular bile stasis and cellular infiltration of the portal areas as viewed under light microscopy (Figs. 44-36 and 44-37). These changes usually disappear during remission (Fig. 44-38). Studies of electron microscopic changes have been carried out by a number of authors.[1,3,11] During periods of exacerbation, bile canalicular changes are similar to those seen in other forms of cholestasis, with distortion and reduction of the microvilli. Other changes include mitochondrial alterations, almost complete cessation of nucleoside phosphatase activity, reduction in the number of acid phosphatase-rich lysosomes, and abundance of lipid spheres, glycogen-rich nuclei, and intracanalicular and intracellular bile pigment (Fig. 44-39).[1] Numerous vesicles, mainly intracellular and of variable size, have been described.[9] During clinical remission, the ultrastructural changes in general return to normal, although small amounts of intracellular and intracanalicular bile pigment, some glycogen-rich nuclei, and crystalloid nucleoids with microbodies may still be present.[1] The round bodies described by Summerskill as

Fig. 44-39. Thin section stained with uranium and lead. A bile canaliculus (*BC*) lies within four continuous cells. A large, clear bleb protrudes into the canalicular lumen with its membrane continuous with the microvilli at the long arrows. The asterisk shows a mass of protruded cytoplasm that may be an enlarged microvillus. Inside the bleb, glycogen aggregates (*GL*) are evident. A dense granular material (*BI*) like the bile pigment described by others is present in the lumen. Glycogen aggregates are seen inside the lumen, possibly a preparative artifact or a result of leakage from the bleb. The canalicular membrane is broken in areas of the bleb (*short arrows*), but junctional complexes (*JC*) are well preserved. (Original magnification × 23,000) (Biempica et al. Gastroenterology 52:521, 1967)

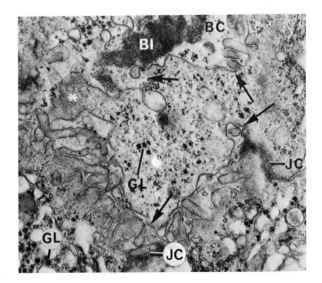

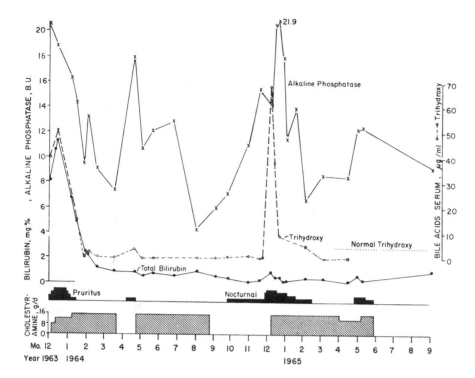

Fig. 44-40. Cholestyramine effect on levels of bile acids, bilirubin, alkaline phosphatase, and pruritus. (This figure appeared, in part, in Spiegel et al. Am J Med 39:682, 1965)

disappearing during remission may still be found in the anicteric phase of the disease.[3]

Extrahepatic biliary obstruction should be excluded by percutaneous or retrograde cholangiography. Failure to determine the cause of the recurrent episodes of jaundice (persisting up to 6 months) may lead to repeated unnecessary laparotomies and peritoneoscopies.

Contradictory results have been recorded on the effects of cholestyramine on the pruritus. This may be explained by inadequate doses in some cases, as exemplified by my own experience, in which it was necessary to increase the dose to 16 g/day in order to obtain relief. Of considerable interest was the simultaneous lowering of levels of serum bilirubin, serum bile acids, and serum alkaline phosphatase that followed the institution of cholestyramine therapy, which in this patient suggested the possibility of a corrective effect on the basic disturbance (Fig. 44-40). The role of bile salts in the experimental production of cholestasis,[4–6] indistinguishable from that which occurs clinically, suggests that bile salts play an etiologic role in the idiopathic recurrent form.

The serum bilirubin level has been reported to drop with the use of steroids (Fig. 44-41), and maintenance of such therapy has been advocated with the hope of reducing the frequency of recurrence.[22]

Stiehl and associates[17] reported treating two children with intrahepatic cholestasis with 10 mg/kg of phenobar-

Fig. 44-41. The effect of prednisolone therapy in case 4 (23rd attack) contrasted with the rate of fall in serum bilirubin level observed during a previous attack (22nd) when the patient was treated with cholestyramine. (Williams et al: Q J Med 33:387, 1964)

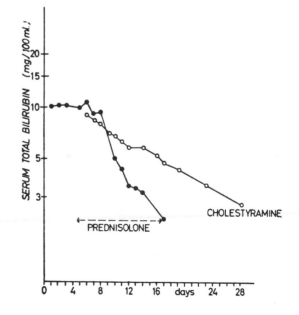

bital for 4 days with a decrease in serum bile salt concentration from 100 mg to 400 mg to 1 mg to 10 mg/liter, a disappearance of pruritus, and a decrease in the serum bilirubin level to 20% to 50% of pretreatment levels. In one case, the ^{131}I-rose bengal fecal excretion increased from 10.1% of the dose before treatment to 71% after phenobarbital was given. In this case, jaundice and pruritus disappeared during the treatment period; however, within 10 days after drug therapy was discontinued, serum bile salt concentrations returned to near pretreatment levels and pruritus returned. In the case reported by Lee and associates,[8] treatment with 60 mg/day of phenobarbital for 30 days and with 8 g/day of cholestyramine for 34 days failed to reduce the jaundice during two respective episodes.

REFERENCES

1. Biempica L et al: Morphological and biochemical studies of benign recurrent cholestasis. Gastroenterology 52:521, 1967
2. Brodersen R, Tygstrup N: Serum bilirubin studies in patients with intermittent intrahepatic cholestasis. Gut 8:46, 1967
3. Da Silva LC, De Brito T: Benign recurrent intrahepatic cholestasis in two brothers: A clinical, light, and electron microscopy study. Ann Intern Med 65:330, 1966
4. Javitt NB: Cholestasis in rats induced by taurolithocholate. Nature 210:1262, 1966
5. Javitt NB, Arias IM: Intrahepatic cholestasis: A functional approach to pathogenesis. Gastroenterology 53:171, 1967
6. King JE, Schoenfield LJ: Lithocholic acid, cholestasis, and liver disease. Mayo Clin Proc 47:725, 1972
7. Kuhn HA: Intrahepatic cholestasis in two brothers. German Med Monthly 8:185, 1963
8. Lee M et al: A case report of benign recurrent intrahepatic cholestasis. Gastroenterol Jpn 19:472, 1984
9. Leibetseder von F et al: Die benigne rezidivierende intrahepatische Cholestase (TYGSTRUP-Syndrom). Wien Klin Wochenschr 83:934, 1971
10. Schapiro RH, Isselbacher KJ: Benign recurrent intrahepatic cholestasis. N Engl J Med 268:708, 1963
11. Schubert WK et al: Idiopathic benign recurrent cholestasis: Biochemical and histologic changes induced by cholestyramine therapy. Clin Res 13:409, 1965
12. Spiegel EL et al: Benign recurrent intrahepatic cholestasis, with response to cholestyramine. Am J Med 39:682, 1965
13. Stathers G et al: Idiopathic recurrent cholestasis. Gastroenterology 52:536, 1967
14. Stiehl A et al: The effects of phenobarbital on bile salts and bilirubin in patients with intrahepatic and extrahepatic cholestasis. N Engl J Med 286:858, 1972
15. Stremmel von W et al: Benigne rekurrierende intrahepatische Cholestase—ein Fallbericht. Z Gastroenterol 22:300, 1984
16. Summerskill WHJ: The syndrome of benign recurrent cholestasis. Am J Med 38:298, 1965
17. Summerskill WHJ, Walshe JM: Benign recurrent intrahepatic "obstructive" jaundice. Lancet 2:686, 1959
18. Summerfield JA et al: A distinctive pattern of serum bile acid and bilirubin concentration in benign recurrent intrahepatic cholestasis. Hepatogastroenterology 28:139, 1981
19. Summerfield JA et al: Benign recurrent intrahepatic cholestasis: Studies of bilirubin, kinetics, bile acids and cholangiography. Gut 21:154, 1980
20. Tygstrup N: Intermittent, possibly familial, intrahepatic cholestatic jaundice. Lancet 1:1171, 1960
21. Van Berge Henegouwen et al: Is an acute disturbance in hepatic transport of bile acids the primary cause of cholestasis in benign recurrent intrahepatic cholestasis? Lancet 1:1249, 1974
22. Williams R et al: Idiopathic recurrent cholestasis: A study of the functional and pathological lesions in four cases. Q J Med 33:387, 1964

Index

Page numbers in italics indicate figures; page numbers followed by *t* indicate tabular material.

1479